The 5-Minute Pediatric Consult Premium

8th EDITION

ASSOCIATE EDITORS

Paul R. Brakeman, MD, PhD
Associate Professor of Pediatrics
Department of Pediatrics
University of California, San Francisco
Medical Director, Pediatric Kidney Transplant Program
UCSF Benioff Children's Hospitals San Francisco and Oakland
San Francisco, California

Megan L. Curran, MD
Assistant Professor of Pediatrics
Department of Pediatrics
University of Colorado School of Medicine
Attending Physician
Section of Rheumatology
Children's Hospital Colorado
Denver, Colorado

Linda A. DiMeglio, MD, MPH
Professor of Pediatrics
Department of Pediatrics, Section of Pediatric Endocrinology and Diabetology
Indiana University School of Medicine
Riley Hospital for Children at Indiana University Health
Indianapolis, Indiana

W. Christopher Golden, MD
Assistant Professor of Pediatrics
Division of Neonatology
Director, Pediatrics Core Clerkship
The Johns Hopkins University School of Medicine
Neonatologist and Medical Director
Newborn Nursery
The Johns Hopkins Hospital
Baltimore, Maryland

Robert E. Goldsby, MD
Professor of Clinical Pediatrics
University of California, San Francisco
Director, Survivors of Childhood Cancer Program
UCSF Benioff Children's Hospital San Francisco
San Francisco, California

Terry Kind, MD, MPH
Associate Professor of Pediatrics
Assistant Dean for Clinical Education
The George Washington University
Children's National Health System
Washington, DC

Carlton K.K. Lee, PharmD, MPH
Associate Professor, Pediatrics
The Johns Hopkins University School of Medicine
Clinical Pharmacy Specialist, Pediatrics
PGY-2 Pediatric Pharmacy Residency Program Director
Department of Pharmacy
The Johns Hopkins Hospital
Baltimore, Maryland

Jenifer R. Lightdale, MD, MPH
Professor of Pediatrics
Department of Pediatrics
University of Massachusetts Medical School
Division Chief, Pediatric Gastroenterology, Hepatology, and Nutrition
Chief Quality Officer
UMass Memorial Children's Medical Center
Worcester, Massachusetts

Camille Sabella, MD
Associate Professor of Pediatrics
Vice-Chair for Education, Pediatric Institute
Director, Center for Pediatric Infectious Diseases
Cleveland Clinic Children's Hospital
Cleveland, Ohio

Ronn E. Tanel, MD
Professor of Clinical Pediatrics
Department of Pediatrics
University of California, San Francisco
Director, Pediatric Arrhythmia Service
Division of Pediatric Cardiology
UCSF Benioff Children's Hospital
San Francisco, California

The 5-Minute Pediatric Consult Premium

8th EDITION

Editor

Michael D. Cabana, MD, MPH
Professor of Pediatrics, Epidemiology & Biostatistics
Director, Division of General Pediatrics
University of California, San Francisco (UCSF)
UCSF Benioff Children's Hospital San Francisco
Zuckerberg San Francisco General Hospital and Trauma Center
Philip R. Lee Institute for Health Policy Studies
San Francisco, California

Wolters Kluwer

Philadelphia • Baltimore • New York • London
Buenos Aires • Hong Kong • Sydney • Tokyo

5MinuteConsult™

Acquisitions Editor: Kate Heaney
Digital Product Development Editor: Leanne Vandetty
Production Project Manager: Bridgett Dougherty
Design Coordinator: Teresa Mallon
Manufacturing Coordinator: Beth Welsh
Marketing Manager: Rachel Mante-Leung
Prepress Vendor: Absolute Service, Inc.

8th Edition

9 8 7 6 5 4 3 2 1

Printed in China

Library of Congress Cataloging-in-Publication Data available from the Publisher upon request.

ISBN-13: 978-1-4963-8177-4

LWW.com

Cover Photograph by Elisabeth Fall

RRS1807

I dedicate this book to my wife Jen and our children. Thanks for being patient with me while I wrote and edited

–PAUL R. BRAKEMAN, MD, PhD

To Cewin, Alex, and Abi

–MICHAEL D. CABANA, MD, MPH

To my parents Donald J. Curran, DO, and Victoria Renz for instilling in me the value of education, to my patients for teaching me on a daily basis, and to Adam for supporting me unconditionally

–MEGAN L. CURRAN, MD

To my patients, colleagues, friends, and family (especially Bob, Richard, Luke, and Max) who infuse my life with purpose and joy

–LINDA A. DIMEGLIO, MD, MPH

To Chinessa and Cadence, how wonderful to have a new sister-in-law and niece and to evidence the love between a new mother and child

–W. CHRISTOPHER GOLDEN, MD

To my family and all of the patients who have allowed me to be part of their lives

–ROBERT E. GOLDSBY, MD

Thanks to my pediatric and medical education colleagues, my patients, and my Kind-Simon family, all of whom inspire me. Let's grow together

–TERRY KIND, MD, MPH

To Joanne, Brendan, Chester, and my parents for all your support

–CARLTON K.K. LEE, PHARMD, MPH

Thank you to my family, as well as to Michael, Leanne, and all of my colleagues in pediatric GI, for their trust, love, support . . . and patience. "Little by little, a little becomes a lot." (African Proverb)

–JENIFER R. LIGHTDALE, MD, MPH

To my family for their love and support and to my father, in memory

–CAMILLE SABELLA, MD

To Sarah, Meghan, and Lauren

–RONN E. TANEL, MD

PREFACE

In a December 30, 1976 cover story interview in *Rolling Stone* magazine, author Maurice Sendak commented, "There's so much more to a book than just the reading. I've seen children touch books, fondle books, smell books, and it's all the reason in the world why books should be beautifully produced."[1] Anyone who has given a book to a 1-year-old child in clinic has probably witnessed a child touch, smell, and even taste a book. For a young child with a new book, every sense is engaged.

My colleagues and I now present a beautifully produced eighth edition of *The 5-Minute Pediatric Consult*. Unlike Mr. Sendak and his young readers, we don't expect you to literally smell or taste this book; however, we have produced a beautiful book that figuratively can be consumed at many different levels.

For those readers who need just a "taste" of each topic, each chapter is designed to give the reader a quick overview. A clinician in a busy office or emergency department can quickly look up a description of each condition, as well as what key questions to ask in a history, what findings to look for during the examination, and what tests are most important to prioritize to confirm a diagnosis. Each chapter also includes a differential of other diagnoses to consider and a concise summary of treatment options. For clinicians who need more than just a brief taste of information, each chapter also includes more information on the etiology, pathophysiology, risk factors, and prognosis of each condition. Finally, for those who want to heavily consume the topic, there are suggestions for additional reading, as well as potential "frequently asked questions" that add even further depth and flavor to each chapter.

There is also a second meaning to Mr. Sendak's comment that "there's so much more to a book than just the reading." Before any reading takes place, there is all the writing and editing that has already been completed. Although each of the chapters is only two pages of reading, each topic represents years of clinical experience as well as countless hours of research, writing, and editing. The authors of these chapters have demonstrated great skill in distilling large amounts of information into an easily accessible 5-minute synopsis or "consult" on a range of clinical topics.

The eighth edition of the book, with over 500 topics, also reflects the continuing achievements and ordeals of the field of pediatrics. With improvements in neonatal care, we now introduce a chapter focused on "Follow-up of the NICU Graduate." With each passing edition, it is also more difficult to find experts on diseases now less common, such as Diphtheria, Measles, Rheumatic Fever, and Reye Syndrome. However, our field also faces new challenges that are represented by new chapters focused on Zika Virus, Chikungunya Virus, Ebola Virus Disease, and even Vaccine Refusal.

To organize this effort, I am fortunate to work with a diverse, distinguished, and talented team of associate editors, who have recruited accomplished authors for each topic. This team of associate editors includes Paul R. Brakeman, MD, PhD; Megan L. Curran, MD; Linda A. DiMeglio, MD, MPH; W. Christopher Golden, MD; Robert E. Goldsby, MD; Terry Kind, MD, MPH; Carlton K.K. Lee, PharmD, MPH; Jenifer R. Lightdale, MD, MPH; Camille Sabella, MD; and Ronn E. Tanel, MD. I have learned from each comment on each draft of each chapter they edited and reviewed. I also give special thanks to Angela Scheuerle, MD who reorganized and updated our Syndromes Glossary for this edition. This updated section includes unique identifiers for dozens of genetic conditions, the associated inheritance pattern, the involved gene(s), mechanism of disease, as well as a description of the associated clinical findings. Finally, I would also like to thank the staff at Wolters Kluwer, especially Leanne Vandetty and Harold Medina, who have helped us present this work so beautifully.

We hope this book will continue to be an indispensable resource for health care professionals who care for children. With these acknowledgments, it is a pleasure to welcome you to this new edition of *The 5-Minute Pediatric Consult*. And in the words of Mr. Maurice Sendak once again, "let the wild rumpus start!"[2]

MICHAEL D. CABANA, MD, MPH
San Francisco, 2018

References

1. Cott J. "Maurice Sendak, King of All Wild Things." *Rolling Stone*. December 30, 1976:48–59.
2. Sendak M. *Where the Wild Things Are*. San Francisco, CA: Harper Collins; 1963.

CONTRIBUTING AUTHORS

Bethlehem Abebe-Wolpaw, MD
Department of Pediatrics
Greater Baltimore Medical Center
Towson, Maryland

Erika L. Abramson, MD, MS[†]
Associate Professor
Pediatrics and Healthcare Policy & Research
Weill Cornell Medical College
New York, New York

Dewesh Agrawal, MD[†]
Associate Professor
Pediatrics and Emergency Medicine
The George Washington University School of Medicine & Health Sciences
Director
Pediatric Residency Program
Children's National Medical Center
Washington, DC

Allison L. Agwu, MD, ScM
Associate Professor
Pediatric and Adult Infectious Diseases
Director, Pediatric and Adolescent HIV/AIDS Program
Medical Director, Accessing Care Early (ACE) Clinic
PI, JHU IMPAACT and ATN
The Johns Hopkins University School of Medicine
Baltimore, Maryland

Jeremy T. Aidlen, MD
Associate Professor of Surgery, Pediatrics, and Urology
University of Massachusetts Medical School
UMass Memorial Children's Medical Center
Worcester, Massachusetts

Akinyemi Ajayi, MBBS, FAAP, FCCP, FAASM
President, Medical Director
Children's Lung, Asthma and Sleep Associates and The Children's Sleep Laboratory
Medical Director, Florida Pediatric Research Institute
Winter Park, Florida

Ibukunoluwa C. Akinboyo, MD
Postdoctoral Fellow
Pediatric Infectious Disease
The Johns Hopkins University School of Medicine
Baltimore, Maryland

Temitope Akinmboni, MBBS
Clinical Assistant Professor, Pediatrics
University of Maryland School of Medicine
Baltimore, Maryland

Noura Al Dhaheri, MBBS
Medical Genetics Resident
McKusick-Nathans Institute of Genetic Medicine
The Johns Hopkins University School of Medicine
Baltimore, Maryland

Stamatia Alexiou, MD
Assistant Professor of Pediatrics
Division of Pulmonary Medicine
The Children's Hospital of Philadelphia
Philadelphia, Pennsylvania

Brittany B. Allen, MD
Clinical Instructor of Pediatrics
Pediatric Hospital Medicine
University of Michigan C.S. Mott Children's Hospital
Ann Arbor, Michigan

Marilee C. Allen, MD
Professor of Pediatrics
The Johns Hopkins University School of Medicine
Co-Director, Infant Developmental Center
Kennedy Krieger Institute
Baltimore, Maryland

Craig A. Alter, MD
Professor of Clinical Pediatrics
Perelman School of Medicine at the University of Pennsylvania
Director, Neuroendocrine Center
The Children's Hospital of Philadelphia
Philadelphia, Pennsylvania

Lusine Ambartsumyan, MD
Assistant Professor of Pediatrics
University of Washington School of Medicine
Director, Gastrointestinal Motility Program
Seattle Children's Hospital
Seattle, Washington

Prina P. Amin, MD
Assistant Professor
Department of Pediatrics
Division of Academic General Pediatrics
Weill Cornell Medical College
New York, New York

Evan J. Anderson, MD
Associate Professor
Departments of Pediatrics and Medicine
Emory University School of Medicine
Atlanta, Georgia

Lauren Andrade, MD
Pediatric Cardiology Fellow
Primary Children's Hospital
Salt Lake City, Utah

John S. Andrews, MD
Associate Dean for Graduate Medical Education
University of Minnesota Medical School
Minneapolis, Minnesota

Ravit Arav-Boger, MD
Professor of Pediatrics
Division of Infectious Disease
Johns Hopkins University School of Medicine
Baltimore, Maryland

Kaveh Ardalan, MD, MS
Instructor
Pediatrics and Medical Social Sciences
Northwestern University Feinberg School of Medicine
Attending Physician
Pediatric Rheumatology
Ann & Robert H. Lurie Children's Hospital of Chicago
Chicago, Illinois

Lisa M. Arkin, MD[†]
Assistant Professor
Department of Dermatology and Pediatrics
University of Wisconsin School of Medicine and Public Health
Director of Pediatric Dermatology
American Family Children's Hospital
Madison, Wisconsin

Stephen S. Arnon, MD, MPH
Chief, Infant Botulism Treatment and Prevention Program
California Department of Public Health
Richmond, California

Allison M. Ast, MD
Pediatric Hematology/Oncology Hospitalist
St. Jude Children's Research Hospital
Memphis, Tennessee

Darlene M. Atkins, PhD
Associate Clinical Professor of Pediatrics
The George Washington University School of Medicine & Health Sciences
Director, Donald Delaney Eating Disorders Clinic
Children's National Health System
Washington, DC

Susan W. Aucott, MD
Associate Professor
Department of Pediatrics
Johns Hopkins University
Program Director
Neonatal-Perinatal Medicine Fellowship
The Charlotte R. Bloomberg Children's Center
Baltimore, Maryland

J. Christopher Austin, MD
Associate Professor of Urology
Oregon Health & Science University
Division Chief, Pediatric Urology
Doernbecher Children's Hospital
Portland, Oregon

Philippe F. Backeljauw, MD
Professor
Department of Clinical Pediatrics
Center for Pediatric and Adult Turner Syndrome Care
Director, Pediatric Endocrinology Fellowship Program
Cincinnati Children's Hospital Medical Center
Cincinnati, Ohio

L. Charles Bailey, MD, PhD
Associate Professor of Clinical Pediatrics
Department of Pediatrics
Perelman School of Medicine
University of Pennsylvania
Divisions of Hematology & Oncology
The Children's Hospital of Philadelphia
Philadelphia, Pennsylvania

Christina B. Bales, MD
Assistant Professor of Clinical Medicine
Perelman School of Medicine at the University of Pennsylvania
Medical Director, Intestinal Rehabilitation Program
Division of Gastroenterology, Hepatology, and Nutrition
The Children's Hospital of Philadelphia
Philadelphia, Pennsylvania

Orkun Baloglu, MD
Clinical Assistant Professor
Department of Pediatrics
Cleveland Clinic Lerner College of Medicine of Case Western Reserve University
Staff Physician
Department of Pediatric Critical Care Medicine
Medical Director, Pediatric Critical Care Transport Team
Cleveland Clinic Children's Hospital
Cleveland, Ohio

Kristin W. Barañano, MD, PhD
Assistant Professor
Department of Neurology
The Johns Hopkins University School of Medicine
Baltimore, Maryland

Jennifer M. Barker, MD
Associate Professor
Pediatric Endocrinology
University of Colorado Anschutz Medical Campus
Program Director
Pediatric Endocrinology Fellowship
Children's Hospital Colorado
Aurora, Colorado

Meagan Barrett, MD
Pediatric Dermatology Fellow
Children's Hospital Los Angeles
Los Angeles, California

Keisha R. Barton, MD
Fellow
Division of Pediatric Gastroenterology, Hepatology, and Nutrition
Baylor College of Medicine
Texas Children's Hospital
Houston, Texas

Laurence S. Baskin, MD
Frank Hinman, Jr., MD Distinguished Professorship in Pediatric Urology
Chief, Pediatric Urology
UCSF Benioff Children's Hospital
University of California, San Francisco
San Francisco, California

Anne S. Bassett, MD, FRCPC
Dalglish Chair in 22q11.2 Deletion Syndrome
Canada Research Chair in Schizophrenia Genetics and Genomic Disorders (Tier 1, 2009 to 2016)
Professor of Psychiatry, University of Toronto
Associate Staff, Division of Cardiology, University Health Network
Associate Member, Canadian College of Medical Geneticists
Director, The Dalglish 22q Clinic for Adults
Director, Clinical Genetics Research Program, Centre for Addiction & Mental Health
Toronto, Ontario, Canada

Hamid Bassiri, MD, PhD
Assistant Professor of Pediatrics
Perelman School of Medicine at the University of Pennsylvania
Attending Physician, Pediatric Infectious Diseases
Faculty Member, Center for Childhood Cancer Research
The Children's Hospital of Philadelphia
Philadelphia, Pennsylvania

Irini D. Batsis, MD
Pediatric Gastroenterology, Hepatology, and Nutrition Fellow
The Charlotte R. Bloomberg Children's Center
Johns Hopkins University
Baltimore, Maryland

Timothy S. Baumgartner, FS, MC, Lt Col, USAF[†]
Pediatric Urology Fellow
Division of Pediatric Urology
The James Buchanan Brady Urological Institute
Department of Urology
The Johns Hopkins Hospital
Baltimore, Maryland

Christopher E. Bayne, MD
Assistant Professor
Department of Urology
Division of Pediatric Urology
University of Florida College of Medicine
Gainesville, Florida

Suzanne E. Beck, MD
Professor of Clinical Pediatrics
Children's Hospital of Philadelphia
University of Pennsylvania School of Medicine
Philadelphia, Pennsylvania

David K. Becker, MD, MPH, MA, LMFT
Clinical Professor of Pediatrics
UCSF Osher Center for Integrative Medicine
Co-Medical Director, Pediatric Pain Management Clinic
UCSF Benioff Children's Hospital San Francisco
San Francisco, California

Shashank P. Behere, MD
Fellow
Nemours Cardiac Center
Nemours Alfred I. duPont Hospital for Children
Wilmington, Delaware
Sidney Kimmel Medical College of Thomas Jefferson University
Philadelphia, Pennsylvania

ElShadey Bekele, MD, MPH
Clinical Instructor
Department of Pediatrics
The George Washington University School of Medicine & Health Sciences
Attending Pediatrician
Children's National Medical Center
Washington, DC

Kelly A. Benedict, MD
Pediatric Nephrologist
Pediatric Kidney Disease and Hypertension Centers
Phoenix, Arizona

Amanda K. Berry, MSN, CRNP, PhD[†]
Pediatric Nurse Practitioner
Division of Urology
The Children's Hospital of Philadelphia
Philadelphia, Pennsylvania

Kate Berz, DO
Assistant Professor of Pediatrics
Divisions of Sports Medicine and Emergency Medicine
University of Cincinnati College of Medicine
Cincinnati Children's Hospital Medical Center
Cincinnati, Ohio

Anita Bhandari, MD
Associate Professor of Pediatrics
University of Pennsylvania
Director, Pulmonary Inpatient Services
The Children's Hospital of Philadelphia
Philadelphia, Pennsylvania

Vineet Bhandari, MD, DM
Professor of Pediatrics, Obstetrics, and Gynecology
Drexel University College of Medicine
Chief, Section of Neonatal-Perinatal Medicine
St. Christopher's Hospital for Children
Philadelphia, Pennsylvania

Sumit Bhargava, MD
Clinical Associate Professor
Department of Pediatrics
Stanford University
Medical Director
Lucile Packard Children's Hospital Pediatric Sleep Laboratory
Palo Alto, California

Diana X. Bharucha-Goebel, MD
Assistant Professor, Neurology
Children's National Health System
Washington, DC

Mihir D. Bhatt, MD, FRCPC
Pediatric Hematologist/Oncologist
McMaster Children's Hospital
McMaster University
Hamilton, Ontario, Canada

Samina S. Bhumbra, MD
Pediatric Infectious Diseases Fellow
Riley Hospital for Children at Indiana University Health
Indianapolis, Indiana

Cara L. Biddle, MD, MPH
Assistant Professor of Pediatrics
The George Washington University School of Medicine & Health Sciences
Associate Division Chief
Division of General Pediatrics and Community Health
Children's National Health System
Washington, DC

Steven Bin, MD
Associate Professor
Department of Emergency Medicine and Pediatrics
University of California, San Francisco
Medical Director
Children's Emergency Department
UCSF Benioff Children's Hospital San Francisco
San Francisco, California

Mercedes M. Blackstone, MD
Associate Professor
Department of Clinical Pediatrics
Perelman School of Medicine at the University of Pennsylvania
Attending Physician
Department of Emergency Medicine
The Children's Hospital of Philadelphia
Philadelphia, Pennsylvania

Seth J. Bokser, MD, MPH
Associate Clinical Professor of Pediatrics
University of California, San Francisco
Pediatric Hospitalist
UCSF Benioff Children's Hospital San Francisco
San Francisco, California

Brett J. Bordini, MD
Assistant Professor
Department of Pediatrics
Section of Hospital Medicine
Nelson Service for Undiagnosed and Rare Diseases
Medical College of Wisconsin
Milwaukee, Wisconsin

Emily C. Borman-Shoap, MD
Assistant Professor of Pediatrics
Director, Pediatric Residency Program
Vice Chair of Education
University of Minnesota
Minneapolis, Minnesota

Renee D. Boss, MD, MHS
Associate Professor
Department of Pediatrics
Division of Neonatology
The Johns Hopkins University School of Medicine
Johns Hopkins Berman Institute of Bioethics
Baltimore, Maryland

John Bower, MD
Associate Professor of Pediatrics
Associate Professor of Microbiology/Immunology/Biochemistry
Northeast Ohio Medical University
Rootstown, Ohio
Division of Pediatric Infectious Diseases
Akron Children's Hospital
Akron, Ohio

Alison Boyce, MD
Endocrinologist
Skeletal Disorders and Mineral Homeostasis Section
National Institute of Dental and Craniofacial Research
National Institutes of Health
Bethesda, Maryland

Paul R. Brakeman, MD, PhD
Associate Professor of Pediatrics
University of California, San Francisco
Medical Director, Pediatric Kidney Transplant Program
UCSF Benioff Children's Hospital San Francisco and Oakland
San Francisco, California

Wendy J. Brickman, MD
Associate Professor
Department of Pediatrics
Division of Endocrinology
Northwestern University Feinberg School of Medicine
Ann & Robert H. Lurie Children's Hospital of Chicago
Chicago, Illinois

Lee J. Brooks, MD
Clinical Professor of Pediatrics
Division of Pediatric Pulmonology and Sleep
Perelman School of Medicine University of Pennsylvania
The Children's Hospital of Philadelphia
Philadelphia, Pennsylvania

Jeffrey P. Brosco, MD, PhD
Professor of Clinical Pediatrics, University of Miami Miller School of Medicine
Associate Director, Mailman Center for Child Development
Faculty Education Development Director, Department of Pediatrics
Director, Population Health Ethics, UM Institute for Bioethics and Health Policy
Chair, Pediatric Bioethics Committee, Holtz Children's Hospital, Jackson Health System
Miami, Florida

Valerie I. Brown, MD, PhD
Associate Professor
Department of Pediatrics
Division of Pediatric Hematology/Oncology
Director, Experimental Therapeutics
Director, Pediatric Hematology/Oncology Fellowship Program
Attending Physician
Hematopoietic Stem Cell Transplant Program
Penn State Hershey Children's Hospital and Penn State College of Medicine
Hershey, Pennsylvania

Terri Brown-Whitehorn, MD
Associate Professor
Department of Clinical Pediatrics
Division of Allergy and Immunology
Perelman School of Medicine at the University of Pennsylvania
The Children's Hospital of Philadelphia
Philadelphia, Pennsylvania

Ann Bruner, MD
Medical Director, Residential Youth Services
Mountain Manor Treatment Center
Baltimore, Maryland

Sara M. Buckelew, MD, MPH
Professor of Pediatrics
University of California, San Francisco
Medical Director, Division of Adolescent and Young Adult Medicine
UCSF Benioff Children's Hospital San Francisco
San Francisco, California

Cynthia Burke, NNP-BC
Clinical Nurse
Neonatal Pediatric Nurse Practice
University of California, San Francisco
San Francisco, California

Vera Joanna Burton, MD, PhD
Assistant Professor of Neurology and Developmental Medicine
Kennedy Krieger Institute
The Johns Hopkins University School of Medicine
Baltimore, Maryland

Melissa A. Buryk, MD, MPH†
LCDR, MC, USN
Assistant Professor
Department of Pediatrics
Uniformed Services University of the Health Sciences
Associate Program Director
Department of Pediatrics
Staff Pediatric Endocrinologist
Portsmouth Naval Medical Center
Portsmouth, Virginia

Amaya L. Bustinduy, MD, MPH, PhD, FRCPCH
Associate Professor in Tropical Pediatrics
Clinical Research Department
London School of Hygiene & Tropical Medicine
London, United Kingdom

Lavjay Butani, MD, MACM
Professor
Department of Pediatrics
Chief of Pediatric Nephrology
University of California, Davis
Sacramento, California

Katherine A. Butler, MD†
Orthopedic Surgery Resident
MedStar Union Memorial Hospital
Baltimore, Maryland

Francesca A. Byrne, MD
Volunteer Clinical Faculty
Department of Pediatrics
Division of Cardiology
University of California, Irvine
Miller Children's & Women's Hospital Long Beach
Long Beach, California

Susanne M. Cabrera, MD†
Assistant Professor
Department of Pediatrics
Medical College of Wisconsin
Children's Hospital of Wisconsin
Max McGee National Research Center for Juvenile Diabetes
Milwaukee, Wisconsin

Mark P. Cain, MD
Robert Garrett Professor of Pediatric Urology
Chief, Division of Pediatric Urology
Indiana University School of Medicine
Riley Hospital for Children at Indiana University Health
Indianapolis, Indiana

Andrew C. Calabria, MD
Assistant Professor of Clinical Pediatrics
Perelman School of Medicine at the University of Pennsylvania
Clinical Director, Division of Endocrinology and Diabetes
The Children's Hospital of Philadelphia
Philadelphia, Pennsylvania

Robert M. Campbell Jr., MD
Professor of Orthopaedic Surgery
University of Pennsylvania
Director, Center of Thoracic Insufficient Syndrome
Division of Orthopaedics
The Children's Hospital of Philadelphia
Philadelphia, Pennsylvania

Ninfa M. Candela, MD
Assistant Professor of Pediatrics, Pediatric Gastroenterology, and Nutrition
University of Massachusetts Medical School
UMASS Memorial Health Care
Worcester, Massachusetts

Joseph B. Cantey, MD
Assistant Professor of Pediatrics
Division of Neonatology
Division of Allergy, Immunology, and Infectious Diseases
University of Texas Health San Antonio
San Antonio, Texas

Katie Carlberg, MD
Pediatric Hematology Oncology Fellow
UCSF Benioff Children's Hospital
Oakland, California

Vanessa S. Carlo, MD
Clinical Assistant Professor
Department of Pediatrics
Sidney Kimmel Medical College
Assistant Residency Director
Jefferson/Nemours Alfred I. duPont Hospital for Children
Philadelphia, Pennsylvania

Michael C. Carr, MD, PhD
Director, Pediatric Urology
KIDZ Multispecialty Group
Naples, Florida

Leslie Castelo-Soccio, MD, PhD
Assistant Professor
Department of Pediatrics and Dermatology
Perelman School of Medicine at the University of Pennsylvania
The Children's Hospital of Philadelphia
Philadelphia, Pennsylvania

Brianna Castillo, MD
University of South Florida Health
Tampa, Florida

Lauren Castner, DO
Pediatric Pulmonary Fellow
University of Michigan C.S. Mott Children's Hospital
Ann Arbor, Michigan

Elizabeth Candell Chalom, MD
Associate Professor, Pediatrics
Robert Wood Johnson Barnabas Health
Director, Pediatric Rheumatology
Saint Barnabas Medical Center
Livingston, New Jersey

Todd P. Chang, MD, MAcM
Associate Professor of Clinical Pediatrics (Educational Scholar)
Keck School of Medicine of USC
Director
Research and Scholarship
Division of Pediatric Emergency Medicine
Associate Fellowship Director
Children's Hospital Los Angeles
Los Angeles, California

Raul Chavez-Valdez, MD
Assistant Professor of Pediatrics
Division of Neonatology
Johns Hopkins University
Baltimore, Maryland

May W. Chen, MD
Postdoctoral Fellow
Division of Neonatology
The Johns Hopkins University School of Medicine
The Charlotte R. Bloomberg Children's Center
Baltimore, Maryland

Pi Chun Cheng, MD, MS
Pediatric Pulmonary Fellow
Division of Pulmonary Medicine and Cystic Fibrosis Center
The Children's Hospital of Philadelphia
Philadelphia, Pennsylvania

David H. Chi, MD
Associate Professor
Department of Otolaryngology
University of Pittsburgh
Clinical Director
Department of Pediatric Otolaryngology
Children's Hospital of Pittsburgh
Pittsburgh, Pennsylvania

Michael F. Chiang, MD
Knowles Professor of Ophthalmology & Medical Informatics and Clinical Epidemiology
Vice-Chair (Research), Department of Ophthalmology
Casey Eye Institute
Oregon Health & Science University
Portland, Oregon

Eric H. Chiou, MD
Assistant Professor of Pediatrics
Division of Pediatric Gastroenterology, Hepatology, and Nutrition
Baylor College of Medicine
Texas Children's Hospital
Houston, Texas

Maribeth Chitkara, MD†
Associate Professor
Department of Clinical Pediatrics
Director, Pediatric Medical Student Education
Stony Brook Long Island Children's Hospital
Stony Brook, New York

Christine S. Cho, MD, MPH, MEd
Associate Professor
Department of Pediatrics
University of Southern California
Fellowship and Education Director
Division of Emergency Medicine
Children's Hospital Los Angeles
Los Angeles, California

Angela Y. Choe, MD
Hospital Medicine Fellow
Cincinnati Children's Hospital Medical Center
Cincinnati, Ohio

Tyler W. Christman, DO, MS
Assistant Professor
Department of Clinical Orthopedic Surgery
Indiana University School of Medicine
Riley Hospital for Children at Indiana University Health
Indianapolis, Indiana

Esther K. Chung, MD, MPH
Professor
Department of Pediatrics
Sidney Kimmel Medical College of Thomas Jefferson University
Jefferson Pediatrics/Nemours-Philadelphia
Philadelphia, Pennsylvania
Director, Department of Newborn Nursery
Director, Advocacy and Community Partnerships
Nemours Alfred I. duPont Hospital for Children
Wilmington, Delaware

Melissa G. Chung, MD
Assistant Professor
Department of Pediatrics
The Ohio State University
Director of Critical Care Neurology
Division of Neurology and Critical Care Medicine
Nationwide Children's Hospital
Columbus, Ohio

Gwynne D. Church, MD
Associate Professor
Department of Pediatric Pulmonology
University of California, San Francisco
Medical Director, Pediatric Sleep Lab
UCSF Benioff Children's Hospital San Francisco
San Francisco, California

Onur Cil, MD, PhD
Clinical Fellow
Department of Pediatrics, Division of Nephrology
University of California, San Francisco
San Francisco, California

Melissa L. Cirillo, MD
Assistant Professor of Pediatrics
Ann & Robert H. Lurie Children's Hospital of Chicago
Chicago, Illinois

Stephanie Clark, MD, MPH
Assistant Professor of Pediatrics
Division of Nephrology
Perelman School of Medicine at the University of Pennsylvania
The Children's Hospital of Philadelphia
Philadelphia, Pennsylvania

Jessica P. Clarke-Pounder, MD
Neonatologist
Atrium Health Levine Children's Hospital
Charlotte, North Carolina

Ronald D. Cohn, MD, FACMG
Associate Professor
Department of Pediatrics and Molecular Genetics
University of Toronto
Chief, Clinical and Metabolic Genetics
Department of Pediatrics
The Hospital for Sick Children
Toronto, Ontario, Canada

Nailah Coleman, MD, FAAP, FACSM
Assistant Professor
Department of Pediatrics
The George Washington University Medical Center
Pediatric Attending
The Goldberg Center for Community Pediatric Health
Children's National Health System
Washington, DC

Ellen Lancon Connor, MD
Professor
Department of Pediatric Endocrinology and Diabetes
University of Wisconsin-Madison
Co-Director, Adolescent PCOS Clinic
American Family Children's Hospital
Madison, Wisconsin

Stephen H. Contompasis, MD
Emeritus Professor
Department of Pediatrics
University of Vermont College of Medicine
Burlington, Vermont

Hillary L. Copp, MD, MS
Assistant Professor
Pediatric Urologist
Department of Urology
University of California, San Francisco
San Francisco, California

Randy Q. Cron, MD, PhD
Arthritis Foundation, Alabama Chapter Endowed Professor of Pediatrics
Director, Pediatric Rheumatology
University of Alabama at Birmingham
Children's of Alabama
Birmingham, Alabama

Megan L. Curran, MD
Associate Professor of Pediatrics
Department of Pediatrics
University of Colorado School of Medicine
Attending Physician
Section of Rheumatology
Children's Hospital Colorado
Aurora, Colorado

Sandra Cuzzi, MD
Assistant Professor
Department of Pediatrics
The George Washington University School of Medicine & Health Sciences
Hospitalist Division
Children's National Medical Center
Washington, DC

Rajesh K. Daftary, MD, MPH
Assistant Professor, Pediatric Emergency Medicine
University of California, San Francisco
Medical Director of Pediatric Emergency Medicine
Zuckerberg San Francisco General Hospital
San Francisco, California

Bertil Damato, MD, PhD, FRCOphth
Director, Ocular Oncology Service
Professor of Ophthalmology and Radiation Oncology
University of California, San Francisco
San Francisco, California

Yalda Serena Dastmalchi, MD
Resident Physician, Emergency Medicine
Maimonides Medical Center
Brooklyn, New York

Diva D. De León, MD, MSCE
Associate Professor of Pediatrics
Perelman School of Medicine at the University of Pennsylvania
Director, Congenital Hyperinsulinism Center
The Children's Hospital of Philadelphia
Philadelphia, Pennsylvania

Jeannine Del Pizzo, MD
Assistant Professor of Clinical Pediatrics
Perelman School of Medicine at the University of Pennsylvania
Attending Physician, Emergency Medicine
The Children's Hospital of Philadelphia
Philadelphia, Pennsylvania

Michelle Denburg, MD, MSCE
Professor of Pediatrics
Department of Pediatrics
Division of Nephrology
The Children's Hospital of Philadelphia
Philadelphia, Pennsylvania

Sanyukta Desai, MD
Clinical Fellow, Division of Hospital Medicine
Cincinnati Children's Hospital Medical Center
Cincinnati, Ohio

Craig C. DeWolfe, MD, MEd
Assistant Professor
Department of Pediatrics
The George Washington University School of Medicine & Health Sciences
Director, Pediatric Medical Student Education
Pediatric Hospitalist
Children's National Health System
Washington, DC

Katherine Deye, MD
Assistant Professor
Department of Pediatrics
The George Washington University School of Medicine & Health Sciences
Child Abuse Pediatrician
Freddie Mac Foundation Child and Adolescent Protection Center
Children's National Medical Center
Washington, DC

Johana Diaz, MD
Assistant Professor, Pediatrics
University of Maryland School of Medicine
Baltimore, Maryland

Francis J. DiMario Jr., MD
Professor
Department of Pediatrics and Neurology
University of Connecticut
Associate Chair Academic Affairs
Department of Pediatrics
Medical Director, Human Research Protection Program
Chief Emeritus, Division of Pediatric Neurology
Connecticut Children's Medical Center
Hartford, Connecticut

Michael DiSandro, MD
Professor of Urology
UCSF Benioff Children's Hospital
San Francisco, California

Danielle G. Dooley, MD, MPhil, FAAP
Assistant Professor of Pediatrics
The George Washington University School of Medicine & Health Sciences
Medical Director
Community Affairs and Population Health
Child Health Advocacy Institute
Children's National Health System
Washington, DC

Rebecca A. Dorner, MD
Postdoctoral Fellow
Division of Neonatology
The Johns Hopkins Hospital
The Charlotte R. Bloomberg Children's Center
Baltimore, Maryland

Morna J. Dorsey, MD, MMSc
Professor of Pediatrics
Section Chief, Allergy & Immunology
Division of Allergy, Immunology, and BMT
University of California, San Francisco (UCSF)
UCSF Benioff Children's Hospital San Francisco
San Francisco, California

Monica Dowling, PhD
Assistant Professor of Clinical Pediatrics
University of Miami Miller School of Medicine
Mailman Center for Child Development
Miami, Florida

Colleen A. Hughes Driscoll, MD
Assistant Professor
Department of Pediatrics
Division of Neonatology
University of Maryland School of Medicine
Baltimore, Maryland

Nancy A. Drucker, MD
Associate Professor of Pediatrics
Robert Larner, MD College of Medicine at the University of Vermont
Pediatric Cardiology
University of Vermont Children's Hospital
Burlington, Vermont

Steven G. DuBois, MD, MS
Associate Professor
Department of Pediatrics
Harvard Medical School
Director, Experimental Therapeutics
Dana-Farber/Boston Children's Cancer and Blood Disorders Center
Boston, Massachusetts

Erin Dunbar, MD, MSc
Pediatric Emergency Medicine Fellow
C.S. Mott Children's Hospital
Michigan Medicine
Ann Arbor, Michigan

Deborah B. Ehrenthal, MD, MPH
Associate Professor of Obstetrics & Gynecology and Population Health Sciences
University of Wisconsin-Madison
Director, Division of Reproductive and Population Health
School of Medicine and Public Health
Madison, Wisconsin

Scott A. Elisofon, MD†
Instructor
Department of Pediatrics
Harvard Medical School
Attending Physician
Division of Gastroenterology, Hepatology, and Nutrition
Medical Director, Liver Transplant Program
Boston Children's Hospital
Boston, Massachusetts

Gary A. Emmett, MD, FAAP
Professor of Pediatrics
Sidney Kimmel Medical College of Thomas Jefferson University
Philadelphia, Pennsylvania

Heidi Engel, PT, DPT
Assistant Clinical Professor
Department of Physical Health and Science
University of California, San Francisco
San Francisco, California

Erica A. Eugster, MD
Professor of Pediatrics
Chief, Division of Pediatric Endocrinology
Riley Hospital for Children at Indiana University Health
Indiana University School of Medicine
Indianapolis, Indiana

Nicholas F. Evageliou, MD
Associate Professor of Clinical Pediatrics
University of Pennsylvania
Division of Oncology
Children's Hospital of Philadelphia
Philadelphia, Pennsylvania

Stephen J. Falchek, MD
Pediatric Neurologist and Clinical Neurophysiologist
Director, Pediatric Neurology Residency and Epilepsy Fellowship Programs
Nemours Alfred I. duPont Hospital for Children
Sidney Kimmel Medical College of Thomas Jefferson University
Wilmington, Delaware

Marni J. Falk, MD
Executive Director, Mitochondrial Medicine Frontier Program
Associate Professor, Division of Human Genetics, Department of Pediatrics
University of Pennsylvania Perelman School of Medicine
Children's Hospital of Philadelphia (CHOP)
Philadelphia, Pennsylvania

Olanrewaju O. Falusi, MD, FAAP
Assistant Professor of Pediatrics
The George Washington University School of Medicine & Health Sciences
Associate Medical Director for Municipal and Regional Affairs
Child Health Advocacy Institute
Children's National Health System
Washington, DC

Azadeh Farzin, MD, MHS
Assistant Professor of Pediatrics and International Health
Johns Hopkins University
International Center for Maternal and Newborn Health
Baltimore, Maryland

Rima Fawaz, MD
Instructor in Pediatrics
Harvard Medical School
Medical Director, Intestinal and Multivisceral Transplant
Division of Gastroenterology, Hepatology, and Nutrition
Boston Children's Hospital
Boston, Massachusetts

Pamela D. Fazzio, MD
Fellow
Pediatric Emergency Medicine
The Children's Hospital of Philadelphia
Philadelphia, Pennsylvania

Jessica L. Fealy, MD
Clinical Instructor, Division of General Pediatrics
Michigan Medicine
C.S. Mott Children's Hospital
Ann Arbor, Michigan

Kristen A. Feemster, MD, MPH, MSHP
Adjunct Associate Professor of Pediatrics, Infectious Diseases
Perelman School of Medicine at the University of Pennsylvania
Director of Research, Vaccine Education Center
The Children's Hospital of Philadelphia
Medical Director, Acute Communicable Diseases and Immunization Programs
Philadelphia Department of Public Health, Division of Disease Control
Philadelphia, Pennsylvania

Daniel E. Felten, MD, MPD
Assistant Professor
Department of Pediatrics
The George Washington University School of Medicine & Health Sciences
Assistant Medical Director
Children's Health Center
Children's National Medical Center
Washington, DC

James H. Feusner, MD
Professor of Pediatrics
Department of Hematology-Oncology
UCSF Benioff Children's Hospital Oakland
Oakland, California

Amy G. Filbrun, MD, MS
Clinical Associate Professor
Department of Pediatrics
Pulmonary Division
University of Michigan C.S. Mott Children's Hospital
Ann Arbor, Michigan

Craig J. Finlayson, MD
Assistant Professor of Orthopaedic Surgery
Northwestern University Feinberg School of Medicine
Ann & Robert H. Lurie Children's Hospital of Chicago
Chicago, Illinois

Anna B. Fishbein, MD, MSc
Assistant Professor of Pediatrics
Division of Allergy & Immunology
Northwestern University
Ann & Robert H. Lurie Children's Hospital of Chicago
Chicago, Illinois

Michael J. Fisher, MD
Associate Professor
Department of Pediatrics
Perelman School of Medicine at the University of Pennsylvania
Chief, Neuro-Oncology Section
Director, Neurofibromatosis Program
Director, Neuro-Oncology Fellowship Program
Center for Childhood Cancer Research and Division of Oncology
The Children's Hospital of Philadelphia
Philadelphia, Pennsylvania

Laurie N. Fishman, MD†
Assistant Professor
Department of Pediatrics
Harvard Medical School
Director, Medical Education for Gastroenterology
Division of Gastroenterology and Nutrition
Boston Children's Hospital
Boston, Massachusetts

Jonathan T. Fleenor, MD, FACC, FAAP
Assistant Professor
Department of Pediatrics
Eastern Virginia Medical School
Medical Director
Department of Pediatric Cardiology
Children's Hospital of the King's Daughters
Norfolk, Virginia

Leah R. Fleming, MD
Genetics and Metabolic Clinic
St. Luke's Children's Hospital
Boise, Idaho

Jay Fong, MD
Assistant Professor of Pediatrics
Division of Pediatric Gastroenterology, Hepatology, and Nutrition
University of Massachusetts Medical School
Worcester, Massachusetts

Michelle Forcier, MD, MPH
Associate Professor
Department of Pediatrics
Division of Adolescent Medicine
Department of Pediatrics
The Warren Alpert Medical School of Brown University
Providence, Rhode Island

Craig M. Forester, MD, PhD†
Assistant Adjunct Professor
Department of Pediatric Hematology/Oncology and HSCT
University of California, San Francisco
UCSF Benioff Children's Hospital
San Francisco, California

Sara F. Forman, MD
Assistant Professor of Pediatrics
Harvard Medical School
Clinical Chief, Division of Adolescent/Young Adult Medicine
Boston Children's Hospital
Boston, Massachusetts

Karen R. Fratantoni, MD, MPH
Assistant Professor
Department of Pediatrics
The George Washington University School of Medicine & Health Sciences
Medical Director
Complex Care Program
Children's National Medical Center
Washington, DC

Melissa B. Freizinger, PhD†
Instructor, Department of Psychiatry
Harvard Medical School
Associate Director
Eating Disorder Program
Adolescent Medicine
Boston Children's Hospital
Boston, Massachusetts

Ilona J. Frieden, MD
Professor of Dermatology and Pediatrics
University of California, San Francisco
UCSF Benioff Children's Hospital San Francisco
San Francisco, California

Linda Y. Fu, MD, MS
Associate Professor of Pediatrics
The George Washington University School of Medicine & Health Sciences
Director, Academic Development
Division of General and Community Pediatrics
Children's National Health System
Washington, DC

Susan Fuchs, MD
Professor
Department of Pediatrics
Northwestern University Feinberg School of Medicine
EMS Medical Director
Division of Emergency Medicine
Ann & Robert H. Lurie Children's Hospital of Chicago
Chicago, Illinois

Ramsay L. Fuleihan, MD
Professor of Pediatrics
Division of Allergy & Immunology
Ann & Robert H. Lurie Children's Hospital of Chicago
Northwestern University Feinberg School of Medicine
Chicago, Illinois

Nora M. Fullington, MD
Assistant Professor of Surgery
Department of Surgery
University of Massachusetts Medical School
UMass Memorial Medical Center
Worchester, Massachusetts

John S. Fuqua, MD
Professor
Department of Clinical Pediatrics
Section of Pediatric Endocrinology
Indiana University School of Medicine
Riley Hospital for Children at Indiana University Health
Indianapolis, Indiana

Steven J. Fusillo, MD
Fellow
Pediatric Gastroenterology
Division of Gastroenterology, Hepatology, and Nutrition
The Children's Hospital of Philadelphia
Philadelphia, Pennsylvania

Payal K. Gala, MD
Assistant Professor of Clinical Pediatrics
Perelman School of Medicine at the University of Pennsylvania
Attending Physician
Pediatric Emergency Medicine
The Children's Hospital of Philadelphia
Philadelphia, Pennsylvania

Theodore J. Ganley, MD
Associate Professor of Orthopedic Surgery
Perelman School of Medicine at the University of Pennsylvania
Director of Sports Medicine
The Children's Hospital of Philadelphia Sports Medicine and Performance Center
Philadelphia, Pennsylvania

George D. Gantsoudes, MD
Assistant Professor of Orthopaedic Surgery
Georgetown University
Pediatric Specialists of Virginia
Fairfax, Virginia

Alejandro V. Garcia, MD
Assistant Professor
Department of Surgery
The Johns Hopkins University School of Medicine
Johns Hopkins Children's Center
Baltimore, Maryland

Ana Catarina Garnecho, MD
Assistant Professor of Pediatrics
Developmental–Behavioral Pediatrics
New England Pediatric Institute of Neurodevelopment
Department of Pediatrics
Women & Infants Hospital
The Warren Alpert Medical School of Brown University
Pawtucket, Rhode Island

Jackie P-D. Garrett, MD
Clinical Assistant Professor
Department of Allergy and Immunology
Department of Pediatrics
Tufts University School of Medicine
Allergy and Immunology Associates of New England
Springfield, Massachusetts

Jordan F. Garris, MD
Child Neurology Resident
Cincinnati Children's Hospital Medical Center
Cincinnati, Ohio

Estelle B. Gauda, MD
Professor of Pediatrics, University of Toronto
Head, Division of Neonatology
Women's Auxiliary Chair in Neonatology at SickKids
Director, Toronto Centre for Neonatal Health
Senior Associate Scientist
The Hospital for Sick Children
Toronto, Ontario, Canada

John P. Gearhart, MD
Professor of Pediatric Urology
The Johns Hopkins University School of Medicine
Chief of Pediatric Urology
The Johns Hopkins Hospital
Baltimore, Maryland

Jeffrey S. Gerber, MD, PhD
Associate Professor of Pediatrics and Epidemiology
Perelman School of Medicine at the University of Pennsylvania
Division of Infectious Diseases
The Children's Hospital of Philadelphia
Philadelphia, Pennsylvania

Donald L. Gilbert, MD, MS, FAAN, FAAP
Professor
Department of Pediatrics and Neurology
Program Director, Child Neurology Residency
Director, Tourette Syndrome and Movement Disorders Clinics
Director, Transcranial Magnetic Stimulation Laboratory
Cincinnati Children's Hospital Medical Center
Cincinnati, Ohio

Maureen M. Gilmore, MD
Assistant Professor
Department of Pediatrics
The Johns Hopkins University School of Medicine
Director of Neonatology
Interim Chair, Pediatrics Department
Johns Hopkins Bayview Medical Center
Baltimore, Maryland

Wendy Robin Glaberson, MD
Pediatric Nephrology Fellow
University of Miami Miller School of Medicine
Holtz Children's Hospital/Jackson Memorial Hospital
Miami, Florida

Nicole S. Glaser, MD
Professor of Pediatrics, Section of Endocrinology
Dean's Endowed Professorship for Pediatric Research
University of California, Davis School of Medicine
Sacramento, California

Jenifer A. Glatz, MD
Clinical Assistant Professor
Department of Pediatrics
Division of Pediatric Cardiology
Children's Hospital at Dartmouth
Manchester, New Hampshire

Jason F. Goldberg, MD, FAAP
Assistant Professor, Pediatric Cardiomyopathy and Heart Transplantation
University of Tennessee Health Sciences Center
Le Bonheur Children's Hospital
St. Jude Children's Research Hospital
Memphis, Tennessee

W. Christopher Golden, MD
Assistant Professor of Pediatrics
Division of Neonatology
Director, Pediatrics Core Clerkship
The Johns Hopkins University School of Medicine
Neonatologist and Medical Director
Newborn Nursery
The Johns Hopkins Hospital
Baltimore, Maryland

Samuel B. Goldfarb, MD
Professor of Clinical Pediatrics
University of Pennsylvania
Medical Director
Pediatric Lung and Heart/Lung Transplant Programs
Division of Pulmonary Medicine
Medical Director, Solid Organ Transplant Center
The Children's Hospital of Philadelphia
Philadelphia, Pennsylvania

Mitchell Goldstein, MD, MBA
Assistant Professor of Pediatrics
Medical Director, Child Protection Team
Johns Hopkins University
Baltimore, Maryland

Stuart L. Goldstein, MD
Clark D. West Endowed Chair
Professor
Department of Pediatrics
University of Cincinnati College of Medicine
Director, Center for Acute Care Nephrology
Co-Director, Heart Institute Research Core
Division of Nephrology and Hypertension
The Heart Institute
Cincinnati Children's Hospital Medical Center
Cincinnati, Ohio

Kandace L. Gollomp, MD
Instructor, Department of Pediatrics
Attending Physician, Division of Hematology
The Children's Hospital of Philadelphia
Philadelphia, Pennsylvania

Michelle Marie Gontasz, MD
Fellow
Department of Neonatology
Johns Hopkins University
Baltimore, Maryland

Blanca E. Gonzalez, MD
Assistant Professor of Pediatrics
Center for Pediatric Infectious Diseases
Cleveland Clinic Lerner College of Medicine of Case Western Reserve University
Pediatric Infectious Diseases
Cleveland Clinic Children's Hospital
Cleveland, Ohio

Zoe M. González-García, MD
Assistant Professor, Pediatric Endocrinology
Children's Hospital and Medical Center
University of Nebraska Medical Center
Creighton University, School of Medicine
Omaha, Nebraska

Eliza M. Gordon-Lipkin, MD
Fellow, Neurodevelopmental Disabilities
Kennedy Krieger Institute
Departments of Pediatrics and Neurology
The Johns Hopkins University School of Medicine
Baltimore, Maryland

Craig H. Gosdin, MD, MSHA
Assistant Professor of Pediatrics
University of Cincinnati
Cincinnati Children's Hospital Medical Center
Cincinnati, Ohio

Kerri Gosselin, MD, MPH
Assistant Professor of Pediatrics
Director, Pediatric Nutrition
University of Massachusetts Medical School
Worcester, Massachusetts

Matthew Grady, MD, CAQSM
Fellowship Director
Primary Care Sports Medicine
Assistant Professor of Clinical Pediatrics
Perelman School of Medicine at the University of Pennsylvania
Pediatric and Adolescent Sports Medicine
Department of Orthopedic Surgery
The Children's Hospital of Philadelphia
Philadelphia, Pennsylvania

Cori Green, MD, MSc
Assistant Professor of Pediatrics
New York-Presbyterian/Weill Cornell Medicine
New York, New York

Benjamin M. Greenberg, MD, MHS
Associate Professor, Department of Neurology and Neurotherapeutics
Associate Professor, Department of Pediatrics
Vice Chair, Translational Research, Department of Neurology and Neurotherapeutics
University of Texas Southwestern
Dallas, Texas

David C. Griffith, MD
Clinical Fellow
Division of Pediatric Infectious Diseases
Johns Hopkins Medical Institutions
Baltimore, Maryland

Jennifer L. Griffith, MD, PhD
Fellow
Pediatric Epilepsy
Washington University in St. Louis School of Medicine
St. Louis Children's Hospital
St. Louis, Missouri

Adda Grimberg, MD
Associate Professor
Department of Pediatrics
Perelman School of Medicine at the University of Pennsylvania
Scientific Director
Diagnostic and Research Growth Center
The Children's Hospital of Philadelphia
Philadelphia, Pennsylvania

Andrew B. Grossman, MD
Assistant Professor of Clinical Pediatrics
Perelman School of Medicine at the University of Pennsylvania
Co-Director, Center for Pediatric Inflammatory Bowel Disease
Division of Gastroenterology, Hepatology, and Nutrition
The Children's Hospital of Philadelphia
Philadelphia, Pennsylvania

Amit S. Grover, MB BCh BAO, MSc
Instructor in Pediatrics
Harvard Medical School
Co-Director, Pancreatic Disorders Program
Division of Gastroenterology, Hepatology, and Nutrition
Boston Children's Hospital
Boston, Massachusetts

Roberto Gugig, MD
Associate Professor
Division of Pediatric Gastroenterology
Director, Endoscopy Unit
Valley Children's Hospital
Lucile Packard Children's Hospital Stanford
Palo Alto, California

Deepti Gupta, MD†
Assistant Professor
Department of Pediatrics
Division of Pediatric Dermatology
University of Washington School of Medicine
Seattle Children's Hospital
Seattle, Washington

Kim Haberer, MD, FRCPC
Fetal and Neonatal Cardiology Fellow
University of Alberta
Edmonton, Alberta, Canada

David J. Hackam, MD, PhD, FACS
Garrett Professor and Chief of Pediatric Surgery
Professor of Surgery, Pediatrics and Cell Biology
Johns Hopkins University School of Medicine
Pediatric Surgeon in Chief and Co-Director, Johns Hopkins Children's Center
The Charlotte R. Bloomberg Children's Center
The Johns Hopkins Hospital
Baltimore, Maryland

Maha N. Haddad, MD†
Associate Professor
Department of Pediatrics
University of California, Davis
Director, Pediatric Dialysis
UC Davis Medical Center
Sacramento, California

Elizabeth J. Hait, MD, MPH
Assistant Professor of Pediatrics
Harvard Medical School
Division of Gastroenterology and Nutrition
Boston Children's Hospital
Boston, Massachusetts

Chad R. Haldeman-Englert, MD
Clinical Geneticist
Fullerton Genetics Center
Asheville, North Carolina

Mark E. Halstead, MD
Associate Professor
Department of Pediatrics and Orthopedics
Washington University
Director, Sports Concussion Clinic
Medical Director, Young Athlete Center
St. Louis Children's Hospital
St. Louis, Missouri

J. Nina Ham, MD
Assistant Professor of Pediatrics
Emory University School of Medicine
Children's Healthcare of Atlanta
Atlanta, Georgia

Ada Hamosh, MD, MPH
Dr. Frank V. Sutland Professor
McKusick-Nathans Institute of Genetic Medicine (IGM)
Clinical Director, IGM
Scientific Director, OMIM
Johns Hopkins University
Baltimore, Maryland

Patrick C. Hanley, MD, FAAP
Pediatric Endocrinology Fellow
The Children's Hospital of Philadelphia
Philadelphia, Pennsylvania

Brian D. Hanna, MD, PhD
Clinical Professor of Pediatrics
University of Pennsylvania School of Medicine
Director, Section of Pulmonary Hypertension
The Children's Hospital of Philadelphia
Philadelphia, Pennsylvania

Cheryl A. Harrow, DNP, FNP-BC, MS, RNC-LRN, IBCLC
Family Nurse Practitioner
Newborn Nursery
Department of Pediatrics
Johns Hopkins Bayview Medical Center
Baltimore, Maryland

Emily A. Hartford, MD, MPH
Assistant Professor, Pediatric Emergency Medicine
University of Washington
Seattle Children's Hospital
Seattle, Washington

Brian P. Hasley, MD
Associate Professor
Department of Orthopedic Surgery
University of Nebraska Medical Center
Children's Hospital & Medical Center
Omaha, Nebraska

Caroline Hastings, MD†
Clinical Professor
Department of Pediatrics
UCSF School of Medicine
Director
Pediatric Hematology/Oncology Fellowship Program
Children's Hospital & Research Center Oakland
Oakland, California

David Hehir, MD, MS
Associate Professor of Pediatrics
Thomas Jefferson University
Philadelphia, Pennsylvania
Chief, Cardiac Critical Care
Nemours Alfred I. duPont Hospital for Children
Wilmington, Delaware

Michelle L. Hermiston, MD, PhD†
Associate Professor
Department of Pediatrics
Division of Pediatric Hematology-Oncology
University of California, San Francisco
UCSF Benioff Children's Hospital San Francisco
San Francisco, California

Christina R. Hermos, MD
Assistant Professor of Pediatrics
Division of Pediatric Immunology and Infectious Diseases
UMass Memorial Children's Medical Center
Associate Program Director, Pediatrics Residency
University of Massachusetts Medical School
Worcester, Massachusetts

Eugene R. Hershorin, MD
Professor
Department of Clinical Pediatrics
Associate Chair, Department of Pediatrics
Chief, Division of General Pediatrics
Director, Developmental and Behavioral Pediatrics
University of Miami Miller School of Medicine
Miami, Florida

Kathryn L. Hillenbrand, MA, CCC-SLP
Master Faculty Specialist
Department of Speech, Language, and Hearing Sciences
Western Michigan University
Kalamazoo, Michigan

Bernadette A. Hillman, MD
Neonatologist
Mt. Washington Pediatric Hospital
Baltimore, Maryland

Tanya Hinds, MD, FAAP
Assistant Professor
Department of Pediatrics
The George Washington University School of Medicine & Health Sciences
Attending Pediatrician
Freddie Mac Foundation Child and Adolescent Protection Center
Children's National Medical Center
Washington, DC

Gurumurthy Hiremath, MD, FACC, FSCAI
Assistant Professor of Pediatrics
Division of Pediatric Cardiology
Director, Pediatric Interventional Cardiology
University of Minnesota Masonic Children's Hospital
Minneapolis, Minnesota

Michael P. Hirsh, MD, FACS, FAAP
Professor
Department of Surgery and Pediatrics
University of Massachusetts Medical School
Surgeon-in-Chief and Chief of Division of Pediatric Surgery
UMass Memorial Children's Medical Center
Worchester, Massachusetts

Adam B. Hittelman, MD, PhD, FACS†
Assistant Professor
Department of Urology
Yale School of Medicine
Pediatric Urology
Department of Urology
Yale–New Haven Hospital
New Haven, Connecticut

Erik R. Hoefgen, MD, MS
Clinical and Research Fellow
Division of Hospital Medicine
Department of Pediatrics
Cincinnati Children's Hospital Medical Center
Cincinnati, Ohio

Robert J. Hoffman, MD, MS
Medical Director, Qatar Poison Center
Department of Emergency Medicine, Sidra Medicine
Doha Qatar
Department of Emergency Medicine
Mount Sinai Beth Israel
New York, New York

Paul L. Hofman, FRACP
Professor Pediatric Endocrinology
University of Auckland
Director of the Paykel CRU
Liggins Institute
Auckland, New Zealand

Kimberlee Honda, RN, MS, FNP
Assistant Clinical Professor, Family Health Care Nursing
University of California, San Francisco
Director, Pediatric Asthma Clinic, Children's Health Center
Zuckerberg San Francisco General Hospital
San Francisco, California

Rachel K. Hopper, MD
Clinical Assistant Professor of Pediatrics (Cardiology)
Stanford University School of Medicine
Associate Director, Pediatric Pulmonary Hypertension Program
Lucile Packard Children's Hospital Stanford
Stanford, California

Biljana N. Horn, MD
Clinical Professor
University of California, San Francisco
Medical Director Pediatric Bone Marrow Transplant
Department of Pediatrics
UCSF Benioff Children's Hospital San Francisco
San Francisco, California

Arvind Hoskoppal, MD, MHS†
Assistant Professor
Department of Pediatrics and Internal Medicine
Director, Utah Adult Congenital Heart Disease Program
University of Utah and Intermountain Healthcare
Salt Lake City, Utah

Renee M. Howard, MD
Professor of Dermatology
University of California, San Francisco
Director, Division of Dermatology
UCSF Benioff Children's Hospital Oakland
Oakland, California

Michael H. Hsieh, MD, PhD
Associate Professor of Urology (Primary) and Pediatrics (Secondary)
The George Washington University
Children's National Health Systems
Washington, DC

Benjamin J. Huang, MD
Assistant Adjunct Professor of Pediatrics
Division of Hematology/Oncology
University of California, San Francisco
UCSF Benioff Children's Hospital San Francisco
San Francisco, California

James N. Huang, MD
Professor of Pediatrics
University of California, San Francisco
Director, Pediatric Hematology
UCSF Benioff Children's Hospital San Francisco
San Francisco, California

Tannie Huang, MD
Kaiser Permanente
Santa Clara, California

Brittany B. Hubbell, MD
Staff Physician, Division of Hospital Medicine
Cincinnati Children's Hospital Medical Center
Cincinnati, Ohio

Jennifer Huffman, MD
Pediatric Neurology
Department of Pediatrics
Randall Children's Hospital
Portland, Oregon

Eva C. Ihle, MD, PhD
Associate Clinical Professor
Department of Health Sciences
University of California, San Francisco
Departments of Psychiatry and Pediatrics
Langley Porter Psychiatric Institute and Weill Institute for Neurosciences
San Francisco, California

Erik A. Imel, MD, MS
Associate Professor
Department of Medicine and Pediatrics
Division of Endocrinology and Metabolism
Indiana University School of Medicine
Department of Internal Medicine and Pediatric Endocrinology/Diabetology Section
Department of Pediatrics
Riley Hospital for Children at Indiana University Health
Indianapolis, Indiana

Rimsha Iqbal, MD
Pediatric Resident
Beaumont Children's Hospital
Royal Oak, Michigan

Allison M. Jackson, MD, MPH
Associate Professor of Pediatrics
The George Washington University School of Medicine & Health Sciences
Division Chief, Child and Adolescent Protection Center
Children's National Health System
Washington Children's Foundation Professor of Child and Adolescent Protection
Washington, DC

Oksana A. Jackson, MD
Assistant Professor, Division of Plastic Surgery
Co-Director, Cleft Lip and Palate Program
Perelman School of Medicine at the University of Pennsylvania
The Children's Hospital of Philadelphia
Philadelphia, Pennsylvania

Shonul A. Jain, MD
Associate Professor
Department of Pediatrics
University of California, San Francisco
Vice-Chief, Department of Pediatrics
Medical Director, Children's Health Center
Zuckerberg San Francisco General Hospital
San Francisco, California

Maria Jacklin Janecek, DO†
General Pediatrician
Downers Grove Pediatrics
Downers Grove, Illinois

Karen E. Jerardi, MD, MEd
Assistant Professor
Division of Hospital Medicine
Cincinnati Children's Hospital Medical Center
Cincinnati, Ohio

Chandy C. John, MD, MS
Ryan White Professor of Pediatrics
Professor of Medicine, Microbiology, and Immunology
Director, Ryan White Center for Pediatric Infectious Diseases and Global Health
Indiana University School of Medicine
Riley Hospital for Children at Indiana University Health
Indianapolis, Indiana

Julia Johnson, MD
Assistant Professor of Pediatrics
Division of Neonatology
Johns Hopkins University
Baltimore, Maryland

Ray J. Jurado, DDS
Division Head, Dentistry
Ann & Robert H. Lurie Children's Hospital of Chicago
Program Director, Pediatric Dentistry
Northwestern University Feinberg School of Medicine
Chicago, Illinois

Dylan C. Kann, MD
Pediatric Infectious Diseases
Department of Pediatric Subspecialties
Kaiser Permanente Santa Clara Medical Center
Santa Clara, California

Chirag R. Kapadia, MD
Associate Professor of Pediatrics
University of Arizona College of Medicine-Phoenix
Fellowship Program Director
Division Chief, Pediatric Endocrinology
Phoenix Children's Hospital
Phoenix, Arizona

Laura E. Kaplan, BA
Medical Student
SUNY Downstate Medical Center College of Medicine
Brooklyn, New York

Wikrom Karnsakul, MD
Associate Professor
Department of Pediatrics
The Johns Hopkins University School of Medicine
Pediatric Liver Center
Baltimore, Maryland

Judith Kelsen, MD
Assistant Professor of Pediatrics
Perelman School of Medicine at the University of Pennsylvania
Director of the Very Early Onset Inflammatory Bowel Disease Program
Division of Gastroenterology, Hepatology, and Nutrition
The Children's Hospital of Philadelphia
Philadelphia, Pennsylvania

Shellie M. Kendall, MD†
Assistant Professor
Department of Pediatrics
Uniformed Services University of the Health Sciences
Bethesda, Maryland
Director, Division of Pediatric Cardiology
Naval Medical Center San Diego
San Diego, California

Sadiqa Kendi, MD, FAAP
Attending Physician, Pediatric Emergency Medicine
Children's National Health System
Washington, DC

Kalpashri Kesavan, MD
Assistant Professor of Pediatrics
University of California, Los Angeles
David Geffen School of Medicine
Los Angeles, California

Seema Khan, MD
Associate Professor of Pediatrics
Division of Gastroenterology, Hepatology & Nutrition
Children's National Medical Centre
George Washington University School of Medicine & Health Sciences
Washington, DC

Amer M. Khojah, MD
Allergy Immunology and Pediatric Rheumatology Fellow
Ann & Robert H. Lurie Children's Hospital of Chicago
Northwestern University
Chicago, Illinois

Jessica M. Khouri, MD
Senior Medical Officer
Infant Botulism Treatment and Prevention Program
California Department of Public Health
Richmond, California

Nadine M. Khouzam, MD
Assistant Professor of Clinical Pediatrics
Keck School of Medicine of USC
Pediatric Nephrologist
Children's Hospital Los Angeles
Los Angeles, California

Harry K.W. Kim, MD
Professor of Orthopedic Surgery
University of Texas Southwestern Medical Center
Director of Research
Director, Center for Excellence in Hip Disorders
Texas Scottish Rite Hospital for Children
Dallas, Texas

Sivan Kinberg, MD, MS, MA
Assistant Professor
Department of Pediatrics
Columbia University Medical Center
Director, Pediatric Intestinal Rehabilitation Clinic
Division of Pediatric Gastroenterology, Hepatology, and Nutrition
New York, New York

Terry Kind, MD, MPH
Associate Professor
Department of Pediatrics
Assistant Dean for Clinical Education
The George Washington University School of Medicine & Health Sciences
Children's National Health System
Washington, DC

Eric S. Kirkendall, MD, MBI, FAAP
Associate Professor of Clinical Pediatrics, Division of Hospital Medicine
University of Cincinnati
Associate Chief Medical Information Officer
Cincinnati Children's Hospital Medical Center
Cincinnati, Ohio

Shyam Kishan, MD
Associate Professor
Indiana University
Pediatric Orthopedics and Scoliosis Surgery
Riley Hospital for Children at Indiana University Health
Indianapolis, Indiana

Eimear Kitt, MB, BCh, BAO (NUI)
Fellow Physician
Division of Infectious Diseases
The Children's Hospital of Philadelphia
Philadelphia, Pennsylvania

Kirsten M. Kloepfer, MD, MS
Assistant Professor
Department of Pediatrics
Section of Pulmonary, Allergy, and Sleep Medicine
Indiana University School of Medicine
Riley Hospital for Children at Indiana University Health
Indianapolis, Indiana

Kelly G. Knupp, MD, MSCS
Associate Professor of Pediatrics and Neurology
University of Colorado Denver, Anschutz Medical Campus
Children's Hospital Colorado
Aurora, Colorado

Aaron E. Kornblith, MD
Assistant Professor
Department of Emergency Medicine and Pediatrics
University of California, San Francisco
UCSF Benioff Children's Hospital San Francisco
San Francisco, California

Sarah A. Korth, MD
Pediatric Rehabilitation Medicine
Co-Director, Keelty Center for Spina Bifida and Related Conditions
Kennedy Krieger Institute
Johns Hopkins University
Baltimore, Maryland

Renee K. Kottenhahn, MD
Clinical Associate Professor of Pediatrics
Department of Pediatrics
Drexel University College of Medicine
Attending Physician
General Pediatrics and Adolescent Medicine
St. Christopher's Hospital for Children
Philadelphia, Pennsylvania

Courtney L. Kraus, MD
Assistant Professor
Department of Ophthalmology
Pediatric Ophthalmology and Adult Strabismus
Krieger Children's Eye Center
Wilmer Eye Institute
Baltimore, Maryland

Richard M. Kravitz, MD
Professor
Department of Pediatrics
Duke University Medical Center
Director, Pediatric Sleep Lab
Co-Director, Duke Children's Neuromuscular Program
Durham, North Carolina

Preetha Krishnan, MD
Clinical Director of Pediatric Neurocritical Care
Attending Physician, Pediatric Critical Care Medicine Randall Children's Hospital at Legacy Emanuel
Portland, Oregon

Matthew P. Kronman, MD, MSCE
Associate Professor
Department of Pediatrics
University of Washington
Director, Pediatric Infectious Diseases Fellowship Training Program
Department of Pediatrics
Division of Infectious Diseases
Seattle Children's Hospital
Seattle, Washington

Elaine Ku, MD, MAS
Assistant Professor
Divisions of Nephrology and Pediatric Nephrology
University of California, San Francisco
San Francisco, California

Johnny I. Kuttab, DDS
Diplomate of the American Board of Pediatric Dentistry
Fellow of the American Academy of Pediatric Dentistry
Ann & Robert H. Lurie Children's Hospital of Chicago
Advocate Lutheran General Hospital
Chicago, Illinois

A. Desiree LaBeaud, MD, MS
Associate Professor
Department of Pediatrics (Infectious Diseases) and Health Research and Policy
Stanford University
Stanford, California

Mitchell R. Ladd, MD, PhD
General Surgery Resident
Department of Surgery
The Johns Hopkins Hospital
Baltimore, Maryland

Meredith C. Laguna, MD, MPH
Clinical Instructor
Department of Pediatrics
Division of General Pediatrics
University of California, San Francisco
UCSF Benioff Children's Hospital San Francisco
San Francisco, California

Michele Puszkarczuk Lambert, MD, MSTR
Associate Professor
Department of Pediatrics
Perelman School of Medicine at the University of Pennsylvania
The Children's Hospital of Philadelphia
Philadelphia, Pennsylvania

Judith Brylinski Larkin, MD, FAAP
Clinical Assistant Professor
Department of Pediatrics
Sidney Kimmel Medical College of Thomas Jefferson University
Nemours duPont Pediatrics, Philadelphia
Philadelphia, Pennsylvania

Javier J. Lasa, MD, FAAP
Assistant Professor
Department of Pediatrics
Divisions of Critical Care Medicine and Cardiology
Baylor College of Medicine
Texas Children's Hospital
Houston, Texas

Phuoc V. Le, MD, MPH, DTM&H
Associate Professor, Internal Medicine and Pediatrics
Co-Founder, HEAL Initiative
University of California, San Francisco
San Francisco, California

Howard M. Lederman, MD, PhD
Professor of Pediatrics, Medicine, and Pathology
The Johns Hopkins University School of Medicine
Director, Immune Deficiency Clinic
Pediatrics
The Johns Hopkins Hospital
Baltimore, Maryland

Christine K. Lee, MD
Instructor
Department of Pediatrics
Harvard Medical School
Attending Physician
Division of Gastroenterology, Hepatology, and Nutrition
Boston Children's Hospital
Boston, Massachusetts

Marsha May Lee, MD
Assistant Clinical Professor of Pediatrics, Pediatric Nephrology
University of California, San Francisco
Medical Director, Pediatric Dialysis Unit
UCSF Benioff Children's Hospital San Francisco
San Francisco, California

Sarah Lee, MD
Clinical Assistant Professor
Department of Neurology and Neurological Sciences
Director, Pediatric Stroke Program at Stanford
Stanford Stroke Center/Stanford Children's Health
Palo Alto, California

Kevin V. Lemley, MD, PhD
Professor
Department of Pediatrics
Keck School of Medicine of USC
Attending Nephrologist
Children's Hospital of Los Angeles
Los Angeles, California

Kieran Leong, DO
Pediatric Cardiology Fellow
Division of Pediatric Cardiology
University of Minnesota
University of Minnesota Masonic Children's Hospital
Minneapolis, Minnesota

Eric B. Levey, MD
Chief Medical Officer
Health Services for Children with Special Needs
Washington, DC
Adjunct Associate Professor
Johns Hopkins University School of Medicine
Baltimore, Maryland

Daniel E. Levin, MD
Pediatric Surgical Fellow
Johns Hopkins Children's Center
Baltimore, Maryland

Leonard J. Levine, MD
Associate Professor of Pediatrics
Assistant Dean for Student Affairs
Drexel University College of Medicine
Attending Physician, Division of Adolescent Medicine
St. Christopher's Hospital for Children
Philadelphia, Pennsylvania

Walter L. Li, MD†
Assistant Clinical Professor
Department of Pediatrics
Division of Cardiology and Electrophysiology
University of California, San Francisco
UCSF Benioff Children's Hospital San Francisco & Modesto Satellite Clinic
San Francisco, California

Cara Lichtenstein, MD, MPH
Assistant Professor
Department of Pediatrics
The George Washington University School of Medicine & Health Sciences
Attending Pediatrician
General and Community Pediatrics
Children's National Medical Center
Washington, DC

Tiffany F. Lin, MD
Adjunct Instructor
Department of Pediatrics, Division of Pediatric Hematology/Oncology
University of California, San Francisco
UCSF Benioff Children's Hospital San Francisco
San Francisco, California

Paul H. Lipkin, MD
Associate Professor of Pediatrics
The Johns Hopkins University School of Medicine
Director, Medical Informatics and the Interactive Autism Network
Kennedy Krieger Institute
Baltimore, Maryland

Richard A. Lirio, MD†
Assistant Professor
Department of Pediatrics
University of Massachusetts Medical School
Director, Pediatric Endoscopy
UMass Memorial Children's Medical Center
Worcester, Massachusetts

Robert Listernick, MD
Professor
Department of Pediatrics
Northwestern University Feinberg School of Medicine
Ann & Robert H. Lurie Children's Hospital of Chicago
Division of Academic General Pediatrics
Chicago, Illinois

Jessica R. Litwin, MD
Assistant Clinical Professor of Child Neurology
UCSF School of Medicine
Pediatric Neurologist
UCSF Benioff Children's Hospital San Francisco
San Francisco, California

Warren D. Lo, MD
Clinical Professor of Pediatrics and Neurology
The Ohio State University
Nationwide Children's Hospital
Columbus, Ohio

Maya B. Lodish, MD, MHSCR
Associate Research Physician
Program Director, Fellowship in Pediatric Endocrinology
National Institute of Child Health and Human Development
Bethesda, Maryland

Kelsey Logan, MD, MPH
Associate Professor of Pediatrics and Internal Medicine
University of Cincinnati College of Medicine
Director, Division of Sports Medicine
Cincinnati Children's Hospital Medical Center
Cincinnati, Ohio

Allison R. Loh, MD
Assistant Professor
Department of Pediatric Ophthalmology and Strabismus
Casey Eye Institute
Oregon Health & Science University
Portland, Oregon

Melissa Long, MD
Assistant Professor
Department of Pediatrics
The George Washington University School of Medicine & Health Sciences
Attending Physician
Children's National Medical Center
Washington, DC

Sahira A. Long, MD, IBCLC, FABM
Assistant Professor
Department of Pediatrics
The George Washington University School of Medicine & Health Sciences
Medical Director, Children's Health Centers-Anacostia
Children's National Health System
Washington, DC

Kathleen M. Loomes, MD
Associate Professor
Department of Pediatrics
Perelman School of Medicine at the University of Pennsylvania
Division of Gastroenterology, Hepatology, and Nutrition
The Children's Hospital of Philadelphia
Philadelphia, Pennsylvania

Katherine Lord, MD
Assistant Professor of Pediatrics
Perelman School of Medicine at the University of Pennsylvania
The Children's Hospital of Philadelphia
Philadelphia, Pennsylvania

Alexander Lowenthal, MD
Pediatric Cardiologist
Department of Pediatric Cardiology
Schneider Children's Medical Center of Israel
Petach Tikvah, Israel

Jeffrey R. Lukish, MD, FACS
Associate Professor
Department of Surgery
The Johns Hopkins University School of Medicine
Baltimore, Maryland

Sarah S. Lusman, MD, PhD
Assistant Professor
Department of Pediatrics
Columbia University Medical Center
Director, Pediatric Gastroenterology Fellowship Training Program
Associate Director, Pediatric Residency Program
Division of Pediatric Gastroenterology, Hepatology, and Nutrition
Morgan Stanley Children's Hospital of New York-Presbyterian
New York, New York

Minnelly Luu, MD
Assistant Professor
Department of Dermatology
Keck School of Medicine of USC
Director, Pediatric Dermatology
Children's Hospital Los Angeles
Los Angeles, California

Ngoc P. Ly, MD, MPH
Professor of Pediatrics
Chief, Division of Pediatric Pulmonology, Cystic Fibrosis and Sleep Medicine
University of California, San Francisco (UCSF)
University of California, San Francisco
UCSF Benioff Children's Hospitals, Oakland and San Francisco
San Francisco, California

Sheela N. Magge, MD, MSCE
Assistant Professor of Pediatrics
Department of Pediatrics
The Children's Hospital of Philadelphia
Philadelphia, Pennsylvania

Melanie M. Makhija, MD, MSc
Assistant Professor
Department of Pediatrics
Northwestern University Feinberg School of Medicine
Attending Physician
Division of Allergy and Immunology
Ann & Robert H. Lurie Children's Hospital of Chicago
Chicago, Illinois

Michael A. Manfredi, MD
Assistant Professor of Pediatrics
Harvard Medical School
Medical Director
Esophageal and Airway Treatment Center
Attending Physician, Gastroenterology and Nutrition
Boston Children's Hospital
Boston, Massachusetts

Courtney W. Mangus, MD
Pediatric Emergency Medicine Fellow
Johns Hopkins Children's Center
Baltimore, Maryland

Melissa L. Mannion, MD, MSPH
Assistant Professor of Pediatrics, Pediatric Rheumatology
The University of Alabama at Birmingham
Birmingham, Alabama

Fiona Marion, MB, BCh, BAO
Primary Pediatric Medical Group
Alameda, California

Andrea Marmor, MD, MSEd
Professor of Pediatrics
University of California, San Francisco
Zuckerberg San Francisco General Hospital
San Francisco, California

Anne M. Marsh, MD
Associate Hematologist/Oncologist
Director, Pediatric Sickle Cell Clinic
UCSF Benioff Children's Hospital Oakland
Oakland, California

Holly H. Martin, MD
Assistant Professor
Department of Pediatrics
University of California, San Francisco
Zuckerberg San Francisco General Hospital
San Francisco, California

Zankhana Master, MD[†]
Assistant Professor
Department of Child Health
Department of Pediatrics
Division of Neonatology
University of Missouri
Columbia, Missouri

Lucy D. Mastrandrea, MD, PhD
Associate Professor
Department of Pediatrics
Jacobs School of Medicine and Biomedical Sciences
University at Buffalo
Associate Division Chief
Pediatric Endocrinology
Women and Children's Hospital of Buffalo
Buffalo, New York

Carol A. Mathews, MD
Brooke Professor of Psychiatry
Director
Center for OCD, Anxiety, & Related Disorders
University of Florida
Gainesville, Florida

Anubhav Mathur, MD, PhD
Assistant Professor of Dermatology, Pediatric Division
University of California, San Francisco
UCSF Benioff Children's Hospital San Francisco
San Francisco, California

Alison T. Matsunaga, MD
Medical Director
General Hematology Program, Hemophilia, and Thrombosis Center
UCSF Benioff Children's Hospital Oakland
Oakland, California

Lindsay J. May, MD, FRCPC
Assistant Professor Pediatrics
University of Utah
Pediatric Cardiology, Heart Failure, and Transplantation
Primary Children's Hospital
Salt Lake City, Utah

Oscar Henry Mayer, MD
Associate Professor of Clinical Pediatrics
Perelman School of Medicine at the University of Pennsylvania
Medical Director, Pulmonary Function Testing Laboratory
Division of Pulmonary Medicine
The Children's Hospital of Philadelphia
Philadelphia, Pennsylvania

Shana E. McCormack, MD, MTR
Attending Physician
Division of Endocrinology and Diabetes
The Children's Hospital of Philadelphia
Assistant Professor of Pediatrics
Perelman School of Medicine at the University of Pennsylvania
Philadelphia, Pennsylvania

Donna M. McDonald-McGinn, MS, LCGC
Clinical Professor of Pediatrics
Perelman School of Medicine at the University of Pennsylvania
Chief, Section of Genetic Counseling
Director, 22q and You Center
Associate Director, Clinical Genetics Center
The Children's Hospital of Philadelphia
Philadelphia, Pennsylvania

Tracey A. McLean, MD
Obstetrics and Gynecology
Kaiser Permanente
Livermore, California

Robert J. McLoughlin, MD
Department of General Surgery
University of Massachusetts Medical School
Worcester, Massachusetts

Maureen C. McMahon, MD
Nemours Pediatrics Villanova
Villanova, Pennsylvania
Assistant Professor of Pediatrics
Sidney Kimmel Medical College of Thomas Jefferson University
Philadelphia, Pennsylvania

Margaret M. McNamara, MD
Professor
Department of Pediatrics
University of California San Francisco
Associate Program Director
Mentoring and Career Development, UCSF Pediatric Residency Program
Co-Director, Foundations of Patient Care and Preceptorships
Site Director, UCSF Bridges Curriculum CMC
Zuckerberg San Francisco General Hospital
San Francisco, California

Maireade E. McSweeney, MD, MPH
Instructor
Department of Pediatrics
Harvard Medical School
Attending Physician
Division of Gastroenterology, Hepatology, and Nutrition
Boston Children's Hospital
Boston, Massachusetts

Jay Mehta, MD, MS
Clinical Director, Pediatric Rheumatology
The Children's Hospital of Philadelphia
Assistant Professor of Pediatrics
Perelman School of Medicine at the University of Pennsylvania
Philadelphia, Pennsylvania

Jondavid Menteer, MD
Associate Professor
Department of Clinical Pediatrics
Keck School of Medicine of USC
Director, Heart Failure Program
Children's Hospital Los Angeles
Los Angeles, California

Laura Mercer-Rosa, MD, MSCE
Assistant Professor of Pediatrics
Director, Echolab Research Unit
Perelman School of Medicine, University of Pennsylvania
Division of Cardiology
Children's Hospital of Philadelphia
Philadelphia, Pennsylvania

Michele Mietus-Snyder, MD
Associate Professor
Department of Pediatrics
The George Washington University
Co-Director Children's National Obesity Institute
Center for Translational Science
Children's National Health System
Washington, DC

Jennifer J. Miller, MD
Neonatology Fellow
Department of Pediatrics
The Charlotte R. Bloomberg Children's Center
The Johns Hopkins Hospital
Baltimore, Maryland

Jane E. Minturn, MD, PhD†
Associate Professor
Department of Clinical Pediatrics
Perelman School of Medicine at the University of Pennsylvania
Division of Oncology
The Children's Hospital of Philadelphia
Philadelphia, Pennsylvania

Hussnain S. Mirza, MD, FAAP
Assistant Professor of Pediatrics
University of Central Florida College of Medicine
Attending Neonatologist
Center for Neonatal Care
Florida Hospital for Children
Orlando, Florida

Nazrat Mirza, MD, ScD
Associate Professor of Pediatrics
George Washington University
Medical Director
I.D.E.A.L Pediatric Weight Management Clinic
Children's National Health System
Washington, DC

Douglas B. Mogul, MD, MPH
Assistant Professor
Pediatric Gastroenterology, Hepatology, and Nutrition
The Johns Hopkins University School of Medicine
Baltimore, Maryland

Angela P. Mojica, MD
Assistant Professor
Department of Pediatrics
State University of New York
Attending Physician
Pediatric Endocrinologist
Upstate University Hospital
Joslin Diabetes Center
Syracuse, New York

Kimberly M. Molina, MD
Assistant Professor of Pediatrics
Medical Director of Heart Transplant
University of Utah
Primary Children's Hospital
Salt Lake City, Utah

Bradley J. Monash, MD
Associate Professor, Internal Medicine & Pediatrics
Associate Chief, Medicine Service
University of California, San Francisco
San Francisco, California

Amaran Moodley, MD
Head
Department of Pediatrics
Division of Infectious Diseases
Blank Children's Hospital
Des Moines, Iowa

Rachel Y. Moon, MD
Professor
Department of Pediatrics
Division Head
General Pediatrics
University of Virginia School of Medicine
Charlottesville, Virginia

Craig Munns, FRACP, MBBS, PhD
Associate Professor
Department of Pediatric Endocrinology
University of Sydney
Director, Division of Diagnostic Services
The Children's Hospital at Westmead
Sydney, Australia

Trish Murphy, RN, MSN
Nurse Coordinator
Survivors Program, Hematology/Oncology/Bone Marrow Transplant
UCSF Benioff Children's Hospital San Francisco/Oakland
San Francisco, California

John R. Mytinger, MD
Assistant Professor
Department of Pediatrics
Division of Pediatric Neurology
Ohio State University
Nationwide Children's Hospital
Columbus, Ohio

Zeina M. Nabhan, MD
Associate Professor of Clinical Pediatrics
Associate Program Director of Pediatric Residency
Indiana University School of Medicine
Riley Hospital for Children
Indianapolis, Indiana

Frances M. Nadel, MD, MSCE
Professor of Clinical Pediatrics
Perelman School of Medicine at the University of Pennsylvania
Attending Physician
Division of Emergency Medicine
The Children's Hospital of Philadelphia
Philadelphia, Pennsylvania

Jessica Rose Nance, MS, MD
Assistant Professor
Division of Pediatric Neurology
The Johns Hopkins Hospital
Baltimore, Maryland

Bhavana Narala, MD
Pediatric Endocrinology Fellow
Medical College of Wisconsin
Children's Hospital of Wisconsin Milwaukee
Milwaukee, Wisconsin

Jessica E. Nash, MD
Assistant Professor
Department of Pediatrics
The George Washington University
General Pediatrician
Children's National Medical Center
Washington, DC

Luz Natal-Hernandez, MD
Pediatric Cardiologist
The Permanente Medical Group
Kaiser Permanente Roseville Medical Center
Roseville, California

Hythem M. Nawaytou, MBBCh, MSc
Assistant Professor of Pediatrics
Division of Cardiology
University of California, San Francisco
UCSF Benioff Children's Hospital San Francisco
San Francisco, California

Pradeep P. Nazarey, MD
Assistant Professor of Pediatrics and Surgery
Division of Pediatric Surgery
University of Massachusetts Medical School
UMass Memorial Healthcare
Boston, Massachusetts

Todd D. Nebesio, MD, FAAP
Associate Professor
Department of Clinical Pediatrics
Section of Pediatric Endocrinology/Diabetology
Indiana University School of Medicine
Riley Hospital for Children at Indiana University Health
Indianapolis, Indiana

Daniel Newman, MD
Assistant Clinical Professor
Department of Pediatrics
Children's Health Centers, Northwest
Children's National Health System
Washington, DC

Jessica R. Newman, DO
Assistant Professor
Department of Internal Medicine
Division of Infectious Diseases
University of Kansas Medical Center
Kansas City, Kansas

Ross Newman, DO, MHPE
Associate Professor of Pediatrics
University of Missouri-Kansas City School of Medicine
Division of General Academic Pediatrics
Children's Mercy, Kansas City
Kansas City, Missouri

Stephanie Nguyen, MD, MAS[†]
Associate Professor
Department of Pediatrics
Division of Nephrology
University of California, Davis
UC Davis Medical Center
Sacramento, California

Graeme A.M. Nimmo, MBBS, MSc
Medical Genetics Resident
The Hospital for Sick Children
University of Toronto
Toronto, Ontario, Canada

Julie M. Nogee, MD
Instructor of Pediatrics
Department of Pediatrics
Division of Newborn Medicine
Washington University School of Medicine
St. Louis, Missouri

Lawrence M. Nogee, MD
Professor of Pediatrics
Department of Pediatrics
Eudowood Neonatal Pulmonary Division
The Johns Hopkins University School of Medicine
Baltimore, Maryland

Frances J. Northington, MD
Professor of Pediatrics
Director, Neurosciences Intensive Care Nursery Program
The Johns Hopkins University School of Medicine
Charlotte Bloomberg Children's Center
Baltimore, Maryland

Adam L. Numis, MD
Assistant Professor of Neurology & Pediatrics
University of California, San Francisco
UCSF Benioff Children's Hospital San Francisco
San Francisco, California

Christopher B. Oakley, MD†
Assistant Professor
Department of Neurology and Nursing
The Johns Hopkins University School of Medicine
Director, Pediatric Headache Center
Director, Headache Medicine Fellowship
Associate Director
Neurology Clerkship
The Johns Hopkins Hospital
Baltimore, Maryland

D. David O'Banion, MD†
Assistant Professor
Department of Pediatrics
Emory University School of Medicine
Atlanta, Georgia

Julie S. O'Brien, MD, MS
Assistant Clinical Professor
Department of Pediatrics
University of California, San Francisco
Medical Director, Pediatric Primary Care
UCSF Benioff Children's Hospital San Francisco
San Francisco, California

Sina Ogholikhan, MD
Pediatric Gastroenterology
Nemours Children's Specialty
Jacksonville, Florida

Kent R. Olson, MD
Clinical Professor
Department of Medicine, Pharmacy, and Pediatrics
University of California, San Francisco
Co-Medical Director
San Francisco Division
California Poison Control System
San Francisco, California

Bruce A. Ong, LTC, MC, MD, MPH, USA†
Deputy Chief of Pediatrics
Department of Pediatrics
Division of Pediatric Pulmonology
Tripler Army Medical Center
Honolulu, Hawaii

Katharine A. Osborn, MD
Pediatric Emergency Medicine Fellow
UCSF Benioff Children's Hospitals Oakland and San Francisco
Oakland, California

Peter T. Osgood, MD
Clinical Fellow in Pediatric Gastroenterology, Hepatology, and Nutrition
Texas Children's Hospital & Baylor College of Medicine
Houston, Texas

Kevin C. Osterhoudt, MD, MS†
Professor
Department of Pediatrics
Perelman School of Medicine at the University of Pennsylvania
Director
Section of Clinical Toxicology
Division of Emergency Medicine
The Children's Hospital of Philadelphia
Philadelphia, Pennsylvania

Mary C. Ottolini, MD, MPH, Med
Professor of Pediatrics
The George Washington University School of Medicine & Health Sciences
Vice-Chair of Education and DIO
Children's National Medical Center
Washington, DC

Vikash S. Oza, MD
Assistant Professor of Dermatology and Pediatrics
Director of Pediatric Dermatology
The Ronald O. Perelman Deparment of Dermatology
New York University School of Medicine
New York, New York

Erica S. Pan, MD, MPH, FAAP
Director, Division of Communicable Disease Control and Prevention (DCDCP)
Deputy Health Officer
Alameda County Public Health Department
Clinical Professor
Pediatric Infectious Diseases
University of California, San Francisco
UCSF Benioff Children's Hospitals San Francisco & Oakland
Oakland, California

Rita Panoscha, MD
Associate Professor
Department of Pediatrics
Institute on Development and Disabilities
Oregon Health & Sciences University
Portland, Oregon

Carolyn A. Paris, MD, MPH
Associate Professor of Pediatrics
University of Washington School of Medicine
Attending Physician
Division of Emergency Medicine
Seattle Children's Hospital
Seattle, Washington

Kristen Park, MD
Associate Professor of Pediatrics and Neurology
Epilepsy Fellowship Program Director
University of Colorado School of Medicine
Aurora, Colorado

Michelle W. Parker, MD
Assistant Professor
Department of Pediatrics
University of Cincinnati
Division of Hospital Medicine
Cincinnati Children's Hospital Medical Center
Cincinnati, Ohio

Akash R. Patel, MD, CEPS, FHRS†
Assistant Professor
Department of Pediatrics
University of California, San Francisco
Electrophysiologist, Pediatric and Congenital Arrhythmia Center
UCSF Benioff Children's Hospital San Francisco
San Francisco, California

Shreena Patel, MD
Department of Pediatric Gastroenterology, Hepatology, and Nutrition
Baylor College of Medicine
Texas Children's Hospital
Houston, Texas

Irina B. Pateva, MD
Assistant Professor
Department of Pediatrics
Case Western Reserve University
Pediatric Hematology/Oncology
Rainbow Babies & Children's Hospital
Angie Fowler AYA Cancer Institute
Cleveland, Ohio

Barry J. Pelz, MD
Assistant Professor
Division of Allergy and Immunology
Medical College of Wisconsin
Children's Hospital of Wisconsin
Milwaukee, Wisconsin

Cheryl A. C. Peretz, MD
Pediatric Hematology/Oncology Fellow
UCSF Benioff Children's Hospital Oakland
Oakland, California

Elena E. Perez, MD, PhD
Allergy Associates of the Palm Beaches
North Palm Beach, Florida

Jessica L. Perniciaro, MD
Clinical Instructor
Department of Pediatrics
Keck School of Medicine of USC
Fellow
Division of Emergency Medicine
Children's Hospital Los Angeles
Los Angeles, California

Farzana Perwad, MD
Assistant Professor of Pediatrics
University of California, San Francisco
Chief, Division of Pediatric Nephrology
UCSF Benioff Children's Hospital San Francisco
San Francisco, California

Shabnam Peyvandi, MD
Assistant Professor of Pediatrics
Division of Pediatric Cardiology
UCSF Benioff Children's Hospital San Francisco
San Francisco, California

Joseph A. Picoraro, MD
Assistant Professor
Department of Pediatrics
Pediatric Gastroenterology, Hepatology, and Nutrition
Columbia University Medical Center
Morgan Stanley Children's Hospital of New York-Presbyterian
New York, New York

Jose A. Pineda, MD, MSCI
Associate Professor
Washington University School of Medicine
Department of Pediatrics and Neurology
Director, Neurocritical Care Program
Division of Critical Care Medicine
St. Louis Children's Hospital
St. Louis, Missouri

Jonathan R. Pletcher, MD
Director, Medical Services
University Health Services
Princeton University
Princeton, New Jersey

Charles A. Pohl, MD
Professor
Department of Pediatrics
Vice Dean of Student Affairs
Sidney Kimmel Medical College of Thomas Jefferson University
Vice Provost of Student Affairs
Thomas Jefferson University
Philadelphia, Pennsylvania

Evelyn Porter, MD, MS
Assistant Professor
Departments of Emergency Medicine and Pediatrics
University of California, San Francisco Medical Center at Parnassus Heights
UCSF Benioff Children's Hospital
San Francisco, California

Anthony F. Porto, MD, MPH†
Assistant Professor
Department of Pediatrics
Yale University
Associate Clinical Chief, Pediatric Gastroenterology
Director, Pediatric Gastroenterology
Greenwich Hospital
New Haven, Connecticut

Amanda Posner, MD
Fellow
Department of Pediatric Gastroenterology
UCSF Benioff Children's Hospital San Francisco
San Francisco, California

Madhura Pradhan, MD
Associate Professor of Clinical Pediatrics
Perelman School of Medicine at the University of Pennsylvania
The Children's Hospital of Philadelphia
Philadelphia, Pennsylvania

Victoria E. Price, MBChB, MSc, FRCPC†
Associate Professor
Department of Pediatrics
Division of Pediatric Hematology/Oncology
IWK Health Centre
Dalhousie University
Halifax, Nova Scotia, Canada

Benjamin T. Prince, MD, MSci†
Assistant Professor
Department of Pediatrics, Allergy & Immunology
The Ohio State University College of Medicine
Nationwide Children's Hospital
Columbus, Ohio

Manisha Punwani, MD
Director, Child and Adolescent Psychiatry Training
Associate Professor
Department of Psychiatry
University of California, San Francisco
San Francisco, California

Kendall Purcell, MD, MPH†
Assistant Professor
Department of Pediatrics
University of Louisville
Louisville, Kentucky

Katherine B. Püttgen, MD
Assistant Professor
Department of Dermatology and Pediatrics
Director, Division of Pediatric Dermatology
The Johns Hopkins University School of Medicine
Baltimore, Maryland

Nashmia Qamar, DO, MSc
Assistant Professor
Department of Pediatrics
Division of Allergy & Immunology
Northwestern University Feinberg School of Medicine
Ann & Robert H. Lurie Children's Hospital of Chicago
Chicago, Illinois

Karen A. Queliza, MD
Clinical Fellow
Pediatric Gastroenterology, Hepatology, and Nutrition
Baylor College of Medicine
Texas Children's Hospital
Houston, Texas

Luis H. Quiroga, MD
Burn & Reconstructive Surgery Fellow
Department of Plastic & Reconstructive Surgery
The Johns Hopkins University School of Medicine
Baltimore, Maryland

Christopher P. Raab, MD
Assistant Professor Pediatrics
Sidney Kimmel College of Medicine
Thomas Jefferson University
Staff Pediatrician
Nemours/A.I. duPont Hospital for Children
Philadelphia, Pennsylvania

Mary Scott Ramnitz, MD
Pediatric Endocrinologist
Section on Skeletal Disorders and Mineral Homeostasis
National Institute of Dental and Craniofacial Research/National Institutes of Health
Bethesda, Maryland

Daniel Ranch, MD
Assistant Professor
Department of Pediatrics
Division of Pediatric Nephrology
University of Texas Health Science Center, San Antonio
San Antonio, Texas

Vamshi K. Rao, MD
Assistant Professor
Northwestern University Feinberg School of Medicine
Attending Physician
Division of Neurology
Ann & Robert H. Lurie Children's Hospital of Chicago
Chicago, Illinois

Robert I. Raphael, MD
Associate Director
Survivors of Childhood Cancer Program
UCSF Benioff Children's Hospital Oakland
Oakland, California

Sergio E. Recuenco, MD, MPH, DrPH†
Professor
Department of Epidemiology
Universidad Nacional Mayor de San Marcos (UNMSM)
Senior Researcher
Department of Preventive Medicine and Public Health
Center for Technological, Biomedical, and Environmental Research
Faculty of Medicine
UNMSM Daniel A. Carrion Tropical Medicine Institute
Lima, Peru

Richard J. Redett, MD
Professor
Plastic and Reconstructive Surgery
The Johns Hopkins University School of Medicine
Director
Pediatric Plastic Surgery
The Charlotte R. Bloomberg Children's Center
Baltimore, Maryland

Rebecca Reindel, MD
Silver Spring, Maryland

Michael X. Repka, MD, MBA
Professor of Pediatrics
The David L. Guyton, MD and Feduniak Family Professor of Ophthalmology
The Johns Hopkins University School of Medicine
Baltimore, Maryland

Leah G. Reznick, MD
Associate Professor
Department of Ophthalmology
Casey Eye Institute
Oregon Health & Sciences University
Portland, Oregon

Hope E. Rhodes, MD, MPH, FAAP
Assistant Professor of Pediatrics
The George Washington University School of Medicine & Health Sciences
Co-Medical Director
Healthy Generations Program
Children's National Medical Center
Washington, DC

Richard C. Rink, MD
Robert A. Garrett Professor of Pediatric Urologic Research
Professor
Department of Urology
Indiana University School of Medicine
Indianapolis, Indiana

Elizabeth Robbins, MD
Clinical Professor
Department of Pediatrics, Hematology/Oncology
University of California, San Francisco
UCSF Benioff Children's Hospital San Francisco
San Francisco, California

Shenandoah Robinson, MD
Professor
Neurosurgery, Neurology, and Pediatrics
Johns Hopkins University
Johns Hopkins Children's Center
Baltimore, Maryland

Rachel G. Robison, MD
Assistant Professor
Department of Pediatrics
Northwestern University Feinberg School of Medicine
Attending Physician
Pediatrics, Division of Allergy & Immunology
Ann & Robert H. Lurie Children's Hospital of Chicago
Chicago, Illinois

Stephen M. Rosenthal, MD
Professor of Pediatrics
Division of Pediatric Endocrinology
University of California, San Francisco
Medical Director, Child and Adolescent Gender Center
Mission Hall: Global Health and Clinical Sciences
San Francisco, California

Tamanna R. Roshan Lal, MBChB
Clinical Genetics Chief Resident
The Johns Hopkins University School of Medicine
Institute of Genetic Medicine
Baltimore, Maryland

Rebecca L. Ruebner, MD, MSCE
Assistant Professor
Department of Pediatrics
Division of Pediatric Nephrology
The Johns Hopkins University School of Medicine
Baltimore, Maryland

Eric T. Rush, MD, FAAP, FACMG
Associate Professor of Pediatrics
University of Missouri - Kansas City
Clinical Geneticist
Children's Mercy Hospital
Kansas City, Missouri

Thomas G. Saba, MD
Assistant Professor
Department of Pediatrics and Communicable Diseases
Pulmonary Division
University of Michigan C.S. Mott Children's Hospital
Ann Arbor, Michigan

Camille Sabella, MD
Associate Professor of Pediatrics
Vice-Chair for Education, Pediatric Institute
Director, Center for Pediatric Infectious Diseases
Cleveland Clinic Children's Hospital
Cleveland, Ohio

Amit J. Sabnis, MD
Assistant Professor, Pediatric Hematology-Oncology
University of California, San Francisco (UCSF)
UCSF Benioff Children's Hospital San Francisco
San Francisco, California

Nina N. Sainath, MD
Pediatric Gastroenterology & Nutrition Fellow
The Children's Hospital of Philadelphia
Philadelphia, Pennsylvania

Amin Salem, MD, MRCPCH, DCH, DPP
Assistant Professor of Clinical Pediatrics
Weill Cornell Medical College Qatar
Senior Attending Physician
Pediatric Emergency Department
Sidra Medicine
Doha, Qatar

Denise A. Salerno, MD
Professor of Clinical Pediatrics
Department of Pediatrics
Temple University School of Medicine
Philadelphia, Pennsylvania

Lauren A. Sanchez, MD
Clinical Fellow, Pediatric Allergy, Immunology, and BMT
University of California, San Francisco
San Francisco, California

Pablo J. Sánchez, MD
Professor of Pediatrics
Divisions of Neonatal-Perinatal Medicine and Pediatric Infectious Diseases
The Ohio State University College of Medicine, Nationwide Children's Hospital
The Research Institute at Nationwide Children's Hospital
Center for Perinatal Research
Columbus, Ohio

Melissa T. Sanford, MD
Resident Physician
Department of Urology
University of California, San Francisco
San Francisco, California

Kara N. Saperston, MD
Staff Pediatric Urologist
St Luke's Children's Hospital
Boise, Idaho

Matthew R. Scheff t, DO, MSHA
Assistant Professor
Department of Pediatrics
Division of Hospital Medicine
Children's Hospital of Richmond at Virginia Commonwealth University
Richmond, Virginia

Adrienne M. Scheich, MD
Attending Physician
Division of Gastroenterology, Hepatology, and Nutrition
Ann & Robert H. Lurie Children's Hospital of Chicago
Northwestern University Feinberg School of Medicine
Chicago, Illinois

Rebecca Schein, MD
Assistant Professor of Pediatrics and Human Development
College of Human Medicine
Michigan State University
East Lansing, Michigan

Angela E. Scheuerle, MD
Professor
Department of Pediatrics
Division of Genetics and Metabolism
University of Texas Southwestern Medical Center
Dallas, Texas

Jocelyn Huang Schiller, MD
Clinical Associate Professor of Pediatrics
University of Michigan Medical School
C.S. Mott Children's Hospital
Ann Arbor, Michigan

Melissa Schoelwer, MD
Assistant Professor
Department of Pediatrics, Endocrinology
University of Virginia Children's Hospital
Charlottesville, Virginia

Amanda C. Schondelmeyer, MD, MSc
Assistant Professor of Pediatrics
University of Cincinnati
Attending Physician
Hospital Medicine
Cincinnati Children's Hospital Medical Center
Cincinnati, Ohio

Alan R. Schroeder, MD
Clinical Professor of Pediatrics (Hospital Medicine and Critical Care)
Stanford University School of Medicine
Associate Chief for Research
Division of Hospital Medicine
Lucile Packard Children's Hospital Stanford
Palo Alto, California

Steven M. Selbst, MD
Professor of Pediatrics
Director, Pediatric Residency Program
Sidney Kimmel Medical College at Thomas Jefferson University
Philadelphia, Pennsylvania
Attending Physician
Division of Emergency Medicine
Nemours/Alfred I. duPont Hospital for Children
Wilmington, Delaware

Mamata V. Senthil, MD
Fellow Physician
Division of Pediatric Emergency Medicine
The Children's Hospital of Philadelphia
Philadelphia, Pennsylvania

Samir S. Shah, MD, MSCE
Professor, Department of Pediatrics
University of Cincinnati College of Medicine
Director, Division of Hospital Medicine
James M. Ewell Endowed Chair
Attending Physician, Infectious Diseases and Hospital Medicine
Cincinnati Children's Hospital Medical Center
Cincinnati, Ohio

Sonal D. Shah, MD
Assistant Clinical Professor
Dermatology & Pediatrics
University of California, San Francisco
UCSF Benioff Children's Hospital San Francisco
San Francisco, California

Pareen Shah Thakral, MD
Attending Physician, General Pediatrics
Ann & Robert H. Lurie Children's Hospital of Chicago
Chicago, Illinois

Hemant P. Sharma, MD, MS, MHS
Assistant Professor
Department of Pediatrics
The George Washington University School of Medicine & Health Sciences
Clinical Chief, Division of Allergy and Immunology
Children's National Medical Center
Washington, DC

Helen M. Sharp, PhD
Professor and Director
School of Communication Sciences and Disorders
Pacific University
Forest Grove, Oregon

Erin E. Shaughnessy, MD, MSHCM
Associate Professor of Child Health
University of Arizona College of Medicine Phoenix
Chief, Division of Hospital Medicine
Phoenix Children's Hospital
Phoenix, Arizona

Jeanne S. Sheffield, MD
Professor of Gynecology and Obstetrics
Division Director, Maternal-Fetal Medicine
The Johns Hopkins University School of Medicine
Baltimore, Maryland

T. Matthew Shields, MD
Assistant Professor of Pediatrics
Division of Pediatric Gastroenterology
UMass Memorial Medical Center
Worcester, Massachusetts

Kristin A. Shimano, MD
HS Associate Clinical Professor
Pediatric Hematology/Oncology and Bone Marrow Transplant
UCSF Benioff Children's Hospital San Francisco
San Francisco, California

Timothy R. Shope, MD, MPH
Associate Professor
Department of Pediatrics
Division of General Academic Pediatrics
Children's Hospital of Pittsburgh
University of Pittsburgh Medical Center
Pittsburgh, Pennsylvania

Stanford T. Shulman, MD
Professor of Pediatrics
Division of Infectious Diseases
Northwestern University Feinberg School of Medicine
Ann & Robert H. Lurie Children's Hospital of Chicago
Chicago, Illinois

Anna Sick-Samuels, MD, MPH
Pediatric Infectious Diseases Clinical and Research Fellow
The Johns Hopkins University School of Medicine
Johns Hopkins Children's Center
Baltimore, Maryland

Melissa A. Simon, MD
Clinical Assistant Professor
Department of Ophthalmology
Brown University
Department of Surgery
Rhode Island Hospital
Providence, Rhode Island

Anne Marie Singh, MD
Assistant Professor
Departments of Pediatrics-Allergy and Immunology, Medicine-Allergy-Immunology
Northwestern University Feinberg School of Medicine
Ann & Robert H. Lurie Children's Hospital of Chicago
Chicago, Illinois

Arunjot Singh, MD, MPH
Assistant Professor
Department of Pediatrics
Perelman School of Medicine at the University of Pennsylvania
The Children's Hospital of Philadelphia
Philadelphia, Pennsylvania

Michael J. Smith, MD, MSCE
Associate Professor of Pediatrics
Division of Pediatric Infectious Diseases
Duke University Medical Center
Durham, North Carolina

Sabrina E. Smith, MD, PhD
Fellow
Academy of Medical Educators
Attending Physician
Pediatric Neurology
Kaiser Permanente Oakland Medical Center
Oakland, California

Lauren G. Solan, MD, MEd
Assistant Professor
Department of Pediatrics
Division of Pediatric Hospital Medicine
University of Rochester
Golisano Children's Hospital
Rochester, New York

Danielle Soranno, MD
Assistant Professor
Pediatrics, Bioengineering & Medicine
Pediatric Nephrology/The Kidney Center
University of Colorado/Anschutz Medical Campus
Children's Hospital Colorado
Aurora, Colorado

Angela M. Statile, MD, MEd
Assistant Professor
Department of Pediatrics
University of Cincinnati College of Medicine
Director, Hospital Medicine Burnet Campus
Division of Hospital Medicine
Cincinnati Children's Hospital Medical Center
Cincinnati, Ohio

Andrew A. Stec, MD[†]
Associate Professor
Department of Urology and Pediatrics
Director of Pediatric Urology
Medical University of South Carolina
Charleston, South Carolina

Andrew P. Steenhoff, MBBCh, DCH
Assistant Professor
Department of Pediatrics
University of Pennsylvania
Medical Director, Global Health Center
Division of Infectious Diseases
The Children's Hospital of Philadelphia
Philadelphia, Pennsylvania

Julie W. Stern, MD
Clinical Professor
Pediatrics, Divisions of Hematology & Oncology
Director, Outreach Services, Division of Oncology
Children's Hospital of Pennsylvania
Philadelphia, Pennsylvania

Christopher C. Stewart, MD
Professor
Department of Pediatrics
University of California, San Francisco
San Francisco, California

C. Matthew Stewart, MD, PhD
Assistant Professor
Otolaryngology, Head and Neck Surgery
The Johns Hopkins University School of Medicine
Baltimore, Maryland

F. Dylan Stewart, MD, FACS
Assistant Professor of Surgery
Johns Hopkins Children's Center
Director, Pediatric Trauma Center
Director, Pediatric Burn Center
Baltimore, Maryland

Rosalyn W. Stewart, MD, MS, MBA
Associate Professor
Departments of Medicine and Pediatrics
The Johns Hopkins University School of Medicine
Medical Director, Care Coordination and Resource Management
Johns Hopkins Hospital
Baltimore, Maryland

Constantine A. Stratakis, MD, D(med)Sci
Scientific Director
Eunice Kennedy Shriver National Institute of Child Health & Human Development (NICHD)
National Institutes of Health (NIH)
Chief, Section on Genetics & Endocrinology (SEGEN), NICHD, NIH
Bethesda, Maryland

Paul K. Sue, MD, CM
Assistant Professor
Department of Pediatrics
Division of Pediatric Infectious Disease
University of Texas Southwestern Medical Center
Children's Medical Center of Dallas
Dallas, Texas

Kathleen E. Sullivan, MD, PhD[†]
Professor
Department of Pediatrics
Perelman School of Medicine at University of Pennsylvania
Chief, Division of Allergy and Immunology
The Children's Hospital of Philadelphia
Philadelphia, Pennsylvania

John I. Takayama, MD, MPH
Professor of Pediatrics
University of California, San Francisco
UCSF Benioff Children's Hospital San Francisco
San Francisco, California

Jie Tang, MD, MS
Pediatric Cardiology Fellow
The Children's Hospital of Philadelphia
Philadelphia, Pennsylvania

Sonny T. Tat, MD, MPH
Assistant Clinical Professor of Pediatric Emergency Medicine
Department of Emergency Medicine
University of California, San Francisco
UCSF Benioff Children's Hospital San Francisco
San Francisco, California

Anupama R. Tate, DMD, MPH
Associate Professor
Department of Pediatrics
The George Washington University School of Medicine & Health Sciences
Director
Oral Health Advocacy & Research
Children's National Health Systems
Washington, DC

Danna Tauber, MD, MPH
Assistant Professor
Department of Pediatrics
Eudowood Division of Pediatric Respiratory Sciences
The Johns Hopkins University School of Medicine
Baltimore, Maryland

Jesse A. Taylor, MD, FACS
Mary Downs Endowed Chair of Pediatric Craniofacial Fellowship
Co-Director, CHOP Cleft Team
Plastic, Reconstructive, and Craniofacial Surgery
The University of Pennsylvania
The Children's Hospital of Philadelphia
Philadelphia, Pennsylvania

David T. Teachey, MD
Associate Professor of Pediatrics
Department of Hematology/Oncology
University of Pennsylvania, Perelman School of Medicine
Children's Hospital of Philadelphia
Philadelphia, Pennsylvania

Peter Tebben, MD
Pediatric Endocrinologist
Departments of Internal Medicine and Pediatrics
Division of Endocrinology
Mayo Clinic College of Medicine and Science
Rochester, Minnesota

Jennifer A. F. Tender, MD, IBCLC
Assistant Professor
Department of Pediatrics
The George Washington University School of Medicine & Health Sciences
Staff Pediatrician
Division of General Pediatrics
The Children's National Health System
Washington, DC

Amit Thakral, MD, MBA[†]
Pediatric Rheumatology Fellow
Ann & Robert H. Lurie Children's Hospital of Chicago
Northwestern University
Chicago, Illinois

Sheila Thampi, MD
Kaiser Permanente
Santa Clara, California

Liu Lin Thio, MD, PhD
Associate Professor
Department of Neurology, Pediatrics, and Neuroscience
Washington University School of Medicine
Director, Pediatric Epilepsy Center
St. Louis Children's Hospital
St. Louis, Missouri

Joanna E. Thomson, MD, MPH[†]
Assistant Professor
Department of Pediatrics
University of Cincinnati College of Medicine
Division of Hospital Medicine
Cincinnati Children's Hospital Medical Center
Cincinnati, Ohio

John E. Tis, MD
Associate Professor of Orthopedic Surgery
Division of Pediatric Orthopedics
Division of Sports Medicine
Johns Hopkins School of Medicine
Baltimore, Maryland

James R. Treat, MD
Associate Professor
Clinical Pediatrics and Dermatology
Perelman School of Medicine at the University of Pennsylvania
Fellowship and Education Directors, Pediatric Dermatology
The Children's Hospital of Philadelphia
Philadelphia, Pennsylvania

Maria Trent, MD, MPH
Professor of Pediatrics
Adolescent/Young Adult Medicine
The Johns Hopkins University School of Medicine
Baltimore, Maryland

Rupal H. Trivedi, MD, MSCR
Associate Professor
Department of Ophthalmology
Storm Eye Institute
Medical University of South Carolina
Charleston, South Carolina

Patrika M. Tsai, MD, MPH[†]
Associate Professor
Department of Pediatrics
Division of Pediatric Gastroenterology, Hepatology, and Nutrition
University of California, San Francisco
UCSF Benioff Children's Hospital San Francisco
San Francisco, California

Nicholas Tsarouhas, MD
Professor of Clinical Pediatrics
Perelman School of Medicine at the University of Pennsylvania
Medical Director, CHOP Emergency Transport Team
Attending Physician, Emergency Department
The Children's Hospital of Philadelphia
Philadelphia, Pennsylvania

Susma Vaidya, MD, MPH
Assistant Professor of Pediatrics
The George Washington University School of Medicine & Health Sciences
Children's National Medical Center
Washington, DC

Pamela L. Valentino, MD, MSc, FRCP(C)
Assistant Professor
Department of Pediatrics
Section of Gastroenterology and Hepatology
Yale University School of Medicine
Yale-New Haven Children's Hospital
New Haven, Connecticut

Kristin L. Van Buren, MD, MEd
Assistant Professor of Pediatrics
Department of Pediatrics
Division of Pediatric Gastroenterology, Hepatology, and Nutrition
Baylor College of Medicine
Texas Children's Hospital
Houston, Texas

Stanley R. Vance Jr., MD
Assistant Professor of Clinical Pediatrics
University of California, San Francisco (UCSF)
UCSF Department of Pediatrics and Division of Adolescent and Young Adult Medicine
UCSF Child and Adolescent Gender Center
San Francisco, California

Hilary Vernon, MD, PhD[†]
Assistant Professor
Department of Pediatrics
The Johns Hopkins University School of Medicine
Director
Medical Biochemical Genetics Fellowship
McKusick-Nathans Institute of Genetic Medicine
Baltimore, Maryland

Elizabeth R. Volkmann, MD, MS
Co-Director, UCLA Connective Tissue Disease-Related Interstitial Lung Disease (CTD-ILD) Program
Department of Medicine
Ronald Reagan UCLA Medical Center
Los Angeles, California

David M. Vu, MD
Instructor
Department of Pediatrics
Division of Infectious Diseases
Stanford University School of Medicine
Stanford, California

Patricia Vuguin, MD, MSc
Associate Professor of Pediatrics
Pediatric Endocrinology
Columbia University College of Physicians and Surgeons
Director, Pediatric Fellowship Program
Division of Pediatric Endocrinology
Morgan Stanley Children's Hospital of New York-Presbyterian
New York, New York

R. Paul Wadwa, MD
Associate Professor
Department of Pediatrics
University of Colorado School of Medicine
Medical Director
Pediatric Division
Barbara Davis Center for Childhood Diabetes
Aurora, Colorado

Lars M. Wagner, MD
Professor of Pediatrics
Chief, Division of Pediatric Hematology/Oncology
University of Kentucky
Kentucky Children's Hospital
Lexington, Kentucky

Justin T. Wahlstrom, MD
Assistant Professor
Department of Pediatrics
University of California, San Francisco
UCSF Benioff Children's Hospital
San Francisco, California

Cynthia X. Wang, MD
Autoimmune Neurology Fellow
Department of Neurology and Neurotherapeutics
University of Texas Southwestern Medical Center
Children's Medical Center of Dallas
Dallas, Texas

Marie E. Wang, MD, MPH†
Clinical Instructor
Division of Pediatric Hospital Medicine
Stanford University School of Medicine
Lucile Packard Children's Hospital Stanford
Palo Alto, California

Ming-Hsien Wang, MD, FAAP†
Associate Professor
Department of Pediatric Urology
Baylor College of Medicine
Texas Children's Hospital
The Woodlands, Texas

Ari Wassner, MD
Assistant Professor
Department of Pediatrics
Harvard Medical School
Director
Thyroid Program
Boston Children's Hospital
Boston, Massachusetts

Ami Waters, MD, MPH
Assistant Professor of Internal Medicine-Pediatrics
University of Texas Southwestern Medical Center
Dallas, Texas
Co-Medical Director, Last Mile Health
Liberia

Andrew J. Wehrman, MD
Fellow Physician
Division of Gastroenterology, Hepatology, and Nutrition
The Children's Hospital of Philadelphia
Philadelphia, Pennsylvania

Dascha C. Weir, MD
Associate Director
The Celiac Disease Program
Boston Children's Hospital
Boston, Massachusetts

Peter Weiser, MD
Associate Professor
Department of Pediatrics
Division of Rheumatology
University of Alabama at Birmingham
Children's of Alabama
Birmingham, Alabama

Dana A. Weiss, MD
Assistant Professor
Department of Surgery in Urology
University of Pennsylvania
Attending Physician
The Children's Hospital of Philadelphia
Philadelphia, Pennsylvania

Benjamin M. Whittam, MD, MS
Assistant Professor of Urology
Riley Hospital for Children at Indiana University Medical Center
Indianapolis, Indiana

Sharon O. Wietstock, MD, MSc†
Child Neurology Resident
University of California, San Francisco
UCSF Benioff Children's Hospital San Francisco
San Francisco, California

Rebekah Williams, MD, MS, FAAP
Assistant Professor
Department of Clinical Pediatrics
Section of Adolescent Medicine
Indiana University School of Medicine
Indianapolis, Indiana

M. Edward Wilson, MD
Professor
Department of Ophthalmology and Pediatrics
Storm Eye Institute
Department of Ophthalmology
Medical University of South Carolina
Charleston, South Carolina

Erica Winnicki, MD
Assistant Professor of Pediatrics
Division of Pediatric Nephrology
University of California, San Francisco
UCSF Benioff Children's Hospital San Francisco
San Francisco, California

Elaine C. Wirrell, MD
Director, Pediatric Epilepsy
Consultant
Professor, Child and Adolescent Neurology and Epilepsy
Mayo Clinic
Rochester, Minnesota

Thomas E. Wiswell, MD
Attending Neonatologist
Kaiser Permanente Moanalua Medical Center
Honolulu, Hawaii

Char M. Witmer, MD, MSCE
Clinical Associate Professor of Pediatrics
Division of Hematology
Perelman School of Medicine, University of Pennsylvania
Assistant Director, Hemostasis and Thrombosis Center
The Children's Hospital of Philadelphia
Philadelphia, Pennsylvania

Margaret S. Wolff, MD
Assistant Professor
Department of Emergency Medicine and Pediatrics
Director, Center for Experiential Learning and Assessment
University of Michigan C.S. Mott Children's Hospital
Ann Arbor, Michigan

Mark L. Wolraich, MD
Shaun Walters Professor of Pediatrics
Chief, Section of Developmental and Behavioral Pediatrics
University of Oklahoma Health Sciences Center (OUHSC)
OU Child Study Center
Oklahoma City, Oklahoma

Lily C. Wong-Kisiel, MD
Assistant Professor
Department of Neurology
Division of Child and Adolescent Neurology
Division of Epilepsy
Department of Neurology
Mayo Clinic
Rochester, Minnesota

George A. (Tony) Woodward, MD, MBA
Professor, Department of Pediatrics
Norcliffe Foundation Endowed Chair Pediatric Emergency Medicine
University of Washington School of Medicine
Medical Director, Emergency and Transport Services
Pediatric Medical Director, Airlift Northwest
Seattle Children's Hospital
Seattle, Washington

Bethany Woomer, MD
Clinical Instructor and Fellow
Division of Pediatric Hospital Medicine
University of California, San Francisco
UCSF Benioff Children's Hospital San Francisco
San Francisco, California

Hsi-Yang Wu, MD
Associate Professor
Department of Urology
Stanford University Medical Center
Director, Pediatric Urology Fellowship Program
Lucile Packard Children's Hospital Stanford
Palo Alto, California

Desale Yacob, MD
Assistant Professor
Department of Clinical Pediatrics
The Ohio State University
Medical Director
Center for Motility and Functional GI disorders
Division of Pediatric Gastroenterology, Hepatology, and Nutrition
Nationwide Children's Hospital
Columbus, Ohio

Jennifer H. Yang, MD[†]
Associate Professor
Department of Urology
Division of Pediatric Urology
University of California, Davis School of Medicine
UC Davis Children's Hospital
Sacramento, California

Michael Yaron, MD
Professor
Department of Emergency Medicine
University of Colorado School of Medicine
Denver, Colorado

Yvette E. Yatchmink, MD, PhD
Associate Professor
Department of Pediatrics
Clinician Educator
Division of Developmental-Behavioral Pediatrics
The Warren Alpert Medical School of Brown University
Hasbro Children's Hospital
Providence, Rhode Island

M. Elizabeth M. Younger, CRND, PhD
Assistant Professor
Department of Pediatrics
The Johns Hopkins University School of Medicine
Baltimore, Maryland

Nazlee Zebardast, MD, MSc
Clinical Fellow
Wilmer Eye Institute, The Johns Hopkins Hospital
Baltimore, Maryland

Ryan W. Zipper, MD[†]
Resident Physician—Urology
Medical University of South Carolina
Charleston, South Carolina

Naamah Levy Zitomersky, MD
Instructor in Pediatrics
Harvard Medical School
Staff Physician, Gastroenterology
Boston Children's Hospital
Boston, Massachusetts

Monica Zlotnicki, MD
Fellow
Pediatric Hematology and Oncology
UCSF Benioff Children's Hospital Oakland
Oakland, California

[†] *The views expressed are those of the authors and do not reflect the official policy of the Department of the Army, Department of the Navy, Department of the Air Force, the Department of Defense, or the United States Government.*

SEVENTH EDITION AUTHOR ACKNOWLEDGMENTS

The editors and authors of the eighth edition gratefully acknowledge the past contributions of the following previous edition authors:

Fizan Abdullah
Garrick A. Applebee
Julia Belkowitz
Anthony Chan
Rohini Coorg
Aarti Dalal
Peter de Blank
Marissa Janel DeFreitas
Sophia D. Delpe
Jennifer DiPace
Mark F. Ditmar
Stacy E. Dodt
Saskia Gex
Rose C. Graham
Daphne M. Hasbani
Mayada A. Helal
Brian M. Inouye
John L. Jefferies
Erin E. Karski
Greggy D. Laroche
Ilse A. Larson
Paul R. Lee
Rebecca K. Lehman
Tobias Loddenkemper
Richard Loffhagen
Kimberly M. Lumpkins
Bradley S. Marino
Renée Marquardt
Heather L. Meluskey
Shina Menon
Caitlin Messner
Avindra Nath
Jason G. Newland
Peter D. Ngo
Heather Olson
Hee-Jung Park
Christopher J. Petit
Laura Robertson
Julia Shaklee Sammons
Gordon E. Schutze
Pirouz Shamszad
David D. Sherry
Stephan Siebel
John Stirling
Waqar Waheed

CONTENTS

ABDOMINAL MASS

Maireade E. McSweeney, MD, MPH

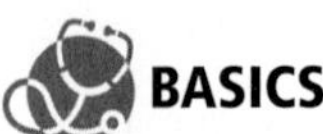

BASICS

DESCRIPTION
A palpable lesion or fullness in the abdominal cavity which may or may not be related to abdominal viscera or a lesion detected on abdominal imaging; the mass may be abdominal or retroperitoneal in origin.

EPIDEMIOLOGY
- Etiologies for abdominal masses are varied, and the differential depends on age and anatomic location.
- Majority are nonsurgical in nature; may be associated with constipation
- Approximately 57% of abdominal masses in children are due to organomegaly (hepatomegaly or splenomegaly).
- Most abdominal masses in infants originate from the kidney and are benign (e.g., hydronephrosis); Wilms tumor is the most common malignant tumor of the kidney seen in childhood.
- Liver masses account for 5–6% of all pediatric intra-abdominal masses; hepatoblastoma is the most common primary liver tumor in children, often presenting at 1 to 3 years of age.

RISK FACTORS
- Certain genetic disorders/syndromes are associated with increased risk of tumor development.
- Patients with Beckwith-Wiedemann syndrome; Wilms tumor, aniridia, genitourinary anomalies, and mental retardation (WAGR); and Denys-Drash syndrome are at increased risk of Wilms tumor and require regular screening.

GENERAL PREVENTION
Dependent on whether or not the mass or lesion is related to a modifiable factor (e.g., a retained foreign body requires parental or patient counseling for prevention)

PATHOPHYSIOLOGY
Varies based on the type of mass seen

ETIOLOGY
- Stomach
  - Gastric distension or gastroparesis
  - Duplication
  - Foreign body or bezoar
  - Gastric torsion
  - Gastric tumor (lymphoma, sarcoma)
- Intestine
  - Feces (constipation)
  - Intestinal distension or toxic megacolon
  - Foreign body
  - Meconium ileus
  - Duplication
  - Volvulus
  - Intussusception
  - Intestinal atresia or stenosis
  - Malrotation
  - Complications of inflammatory bowel disease (abscess, phlegmon)
  - Appendiceal inflammation
  - Meckel diverticulum or abscess
  - Duodenal hematoma (trauma)
  - Lymphoma, adenocarcinoma, GI stromal tumor
  - Carcinoid (appendiceal)
- Liver
  - Hepatomegaly due to intrinsic liver disease
    - Hepatitis (e.g., infectious, autoimmune)
    - Metabolic or storage disorders (e.g., Wilson disease, glycogen storage disease)
    - Infiltration of liver (cyst, tumors)
    - Biliary obstruction
    - Vascular obstruction/impaired venous congestion (Budd-Chiari syndrome, congestive heart failure)
  - Cystic disease (e.g., Caroli disease)
  - Solid tumor (hepatoblastoma; hepatocellular carcinoma; hepatic adenoma; or other diffuse, systemic, neoplastic process)
  - Vascular tumor (hemangioma or hemangioendothelioma)
  - Other: hamartomas, focal nodular hyperplasia
- Gallbladder/biliary tract
  - Choledochal cyst
  - Hydrops of gallbladder
  - Obstruction (stone, stricture, trauma)
- Spleen
  - Congenital cysts
  - Storage disease (e.g., Gaucher, Niemann-Pick)
  - Langerhans cell histiocytosis
  - Leukemia
  - Hematologic (hemolytic disease [e.g., sickle cell] or other RBC disorders [e.g., hereditary spherocytosis])
  - Portal hypertension
  - Wandering spleen
- Pancreas
  - Congenital cysts
  - Pseudocyst (trauma, pancreatitis)
  - Pancreatoblastoma
  - Neuroendocrine tumors (insulinomas, gastrinomas)
  - Solid and papillary epithelial neoplasms
- Kidney
  - Hydronephrosis or ureteropelvic obstruction
  - Multicystic dysplastic kidney
  - Polycystic disease
  - Tumor (mesoblastic nephroma, Wilms tumor, renal cell carcinoma)
  - Renal vein thrombosis
  - Cystic nephroma
- Bladder
  - Bladder distension
  - Neurogenic bladder
- Adrenal
  - Adrenal hemorrhage
  - Adrenal abscess
  - Neuroblastoma
  - Pheochromocytoma
- Uterus
  - Pregnancy
  - Hematocolpos
  - Hydrocolpos or hydrometrocolpos
- Ovary
  - Cysts (dermoid, follicular)
  - Torsion
  - Germ cell tumor
- Peritoneal
  - Ascites
  - Teratoma
- Abdominal wall
  - Umbilical/inguinal/ventral hernia
  - Omphalocele/gastroschisis
  - Urachal cyst
  - Trauma (rectus hematoma)
  - Tumor (fibroma, lipoma, rhabdomyosarcoma)
- Omentum/mesentery
  - Cysts
  - Mesenteric fibromatosis
  - Mesenteric adenitis
- Other
  - Tumors (liposarcoma, leiomyosarcoma, fibrosarcoma, mesothelioma)
  - Intra-abdominal testicle (torsion)
  - Lymphangioma
  - Fetus in fetu
  - Sacrococcygeal teratoma

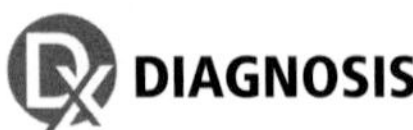

DIAGNOSIS

- Approach to patient
  - When evaluating a pediatric abdominal mass, an organized approach is critical:
    - **Phase 1:** Perform a careful clinical history and abdominal examination in order to help assess clinical symptoms and duration of symptoms and approximate anatomic location of the mass.
    - **Phase 2:** Perform diagnostic tests:
      - Obtain abdominal x-ray to assess for bowel obstruction, fecal load, or mass effect; obtain ultrasound to identify organ of origin and tissue components (e.g., cystic, hemorrhage).
      - Laboratory testing as indicated
  - Tips for screening problems
    - Constipation and fecal impaction can present as a large, hard mass extending from the pubis.
    - In neonates, a palpable liver edge can be normal; assess the total liver span.
    - In infants, a full bladder is often mistaken for an abdominal mass.
    - Gastric distention should be considered in all children who present with a tympanitic epigastric mass.
    - Splenomegaly may be associated with a systemic oncologic or infectious process (e.g., lymphoma or Epstein-Barr virus).

HISTORY
Patients may be asymptomatic or may have some of the symptoms outlined below.
- **Question:** Weight loss?
- *Significance*: malignancy, inflammatory bowel disease
- **Question:** Fever?
- *Significance*: infection, malignancy
- **Question:** Jaundice?
- *Significance*: hepatobiliary or hematologic disease
- **Question:** Hematuria or dysuria?
- *Significance*: renal disease
- **Question:** Vomiting, bilious vomiting, or early satiety?
- *Significance*: intestinal obstruction
- **Question:** Abdominal pain?
- *Significance*: constipation, appendicitis, intussusception, intestinal obstruction
- **Question:** Frequency and quality of bowel movements?
- *Significance*: constipation, intussusception, compression of bowel by mass
- **Question:** Bleeding or bruising?
- *Significance*: liver disease, coagulopathy
- **Question:** Pallor or weakness?
- *Significance*: sign of anemia or blood loss

- **Question:** History of abdominal trauma?
- *Significance*: pancreatic pseudocyst, duodenal hematoma
- **Question:** Sexual activity?
- *Significance*: pregnancy
- **Question:** Age of patient?
- *Significance*:
  - In neonates, the most common origin of abdominal masses are genitourinary (cystic kidney disease, hydronephrosis).
  - In adolescent-aged girls, ovarian disorders, hematocolpos, and pregnancy should be considered.
  - Most common *malignant* abdominal tumors by age: (i) infants: neuroblastoma, Wilms tumor; (ii) children: Wilms tumor, sarcomas, germ cell tumors; (iii) children >10 years of age: sarcomas, germ cell tumors, and abdominal lymphomas

PHYSICAL EXAM

- **Finding:** General appearance?
- *Significance*: ill appearance or cachexia point toward infection or malignancy
- **Finding:** Location of abdominal mass?
- *Significance*:
  - Left lower quadrant: feces, ovarian process, ectopic pregnancy
  - Left upper quadrant: splenomegaly, anomaly of the kidney
  - Right lower quadrant: abscess (inflammatory bowel disease), intestinal phlegmon, appendicitis, intussusception, ovarian process, ectopic pregnancy
  - Right upper quadrant: liver, gallbladder, biliary tree, or intestine
  - Epigastric: abnormality of the stomach (bezoar, torsion), pancreas (pseudocyst), or enlarged liver
  - Suprapubic: pregnancy, hydrometrocolpos, hematocolpos, posterior urethral valves
  - Flank: renal disease (cystic kidney, hydronephrosis, Wilms tumor)
- **Finding:** Characteristics of abdominal mass?
- *Significance*: Mobility, tenderness, firmness, smoothness, and/or irregularity of the surface of the mass can provide clues to its significance.
- **Finding:** Hard and immobile mass?
- *Significance*: tumor
- **Finding:** Extension of mass across midline or into pelvis?
- *Significance*: tumor, hepatomegaly, splenomegaly
- **Finding:** Percussion of mass?
- *Significance*: Dullness indicates a solid mass; tympany indicates a hollow organ.
- **Finding:** Shifting dullness, fluid wave?
- *Significance*: ascites
- **Finding:** Skin exam?
- *Significance*: Bruising and petechiae may occur with coagulopathy related to liver disease and malignant infiltration of bone marrow; café au lait spots are associated with neurofibromas.
- **Finding:** Lymphadenopathy or lymphadenitis?
- *Significance*: systemic process either malignant or infectious
- **Finding:** Peritoneal signs?
- *Significance*: appendicitis, bowel obstruction, or perforation; indication for urgent surgical consultation
- **Finding:** Rectal bleeding?
- *Significance*: intestinal inflammation, polyp, or other bleeding lesion

DIAGNOSTIC TESTS & INTERPRETATION

Initial Tests (screening, lab, imaging)

- **Test:** CBC with differential
- *Significance:* anemia, hemolysis
- **Test:** chemistry panel
- *Significance*:
  - Renal disease: BUN and creatinine levels
  - Liver disease (bilirubin, ALT, AST, alkaline phosphatase, GGT, albumin, PT/PTT)
  - Gallbladder disease (bilirubin, GGT)
  - Pancreatic disease: amylase/lipase levels
  - Intestinal disease: hypoalbuminemia
- **Test:** uric acid and lactate dehydrogenase levels
- *Significance*: elevated in the setting of rapid cell turnover of solid tumors
- **Test:** serum quantitative β-human chorionic gonadotropin (hCG)
- *Significance*: pregnancy, germ cell tumor
- **Test:** elevated α-fetoprotein (AFP) level
- *Significance*: hepatoblastoma
- **Test:** urinalysis
- *Significance*: Blood or protein in the urine may suggest a renal etiology.
- Plain radiographs
  - Evaluate for intestinal obstruction (dilated bowel loops, air-fluid levels), bowel gas pattern, calcifications, or fecal impaction; urinary retention
- Ultrasound
  - Can identify the origin of the mass and differentiate between solid and cystic tissue; Doppler ability can help assess vascularity. Disadvantage is operator variability, and visualization may be limited by overlying bowel gas.
  - May allow for ultrasound guided biopsies of mass lesions
- CT scan
  - Can provide more detail when there is overlying gas or bone; if malignancy is suspected, should also do chest in addition to abdomen and pelvis
- MRI
  - Vascular lesions of liver, major vessels, and tumors
- Nuclear medicine
  - Radioisotope cholescintigraphy (HIDA) scan of liver, gallbladder/biliary tree
  - Meckel scan: can identify gastric mucosa contained within a Meckel diverticulum or intestinal duplication
  - Intravenous urography to assess renal system
- Fluoroscopy
  - Upper GI studies and barium enema studies: may be of benefit when the mass involves the intestine
  - Voiding cystourethrogram (VCUG) to assess renal system

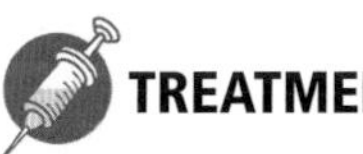

TREATMENT

GENERAL MEASURES

- Immediate hospitalization for patients who present with an abdominal mass and/or signs of dehydration, intestinal obstruction, bleeding, feeding intolerance, or clinical decompensation
- In addition to initial diagnostic and laboratory testing, a pediatric surgical or oncologic consultation should be obtained as indicated.
- The remaining causes of abdominal masses require urgent care and timely evaluation and referral to appropriate specialists depending on location of the lesion.

ISSUES FOR REFERRAL

Except for the diagnosis of constipation, the presence of an abdominal mass in children requires immediate attention, and diagnostic studies should be performed expeditiously at a pediatric health care facility or by pediatric specialists trained in assessment and treatment of these various disorders.

ADMISSION, INPATIENT, AND NURSING CONSIDERATIONS

- Immediate hospitalization for patients who present with an abdominal mass and signs and/or symptoms of intestinal obstruction, distension, or peritoneal symptoms (intussusception, volvulus, gastric torsion, bezoar, foreign body, appendicitis)
  - Toxic megacolon
  - Ovarian torsion
  - Ectopic pregnancy
  - Biliary obstruction (stone, hydrops)
  - Fever
  - Anemia, coagulopathy
  - Pancreatitis (pseudocyst)
- The remaining causes of abdominal masses require urgent care and timely evaluation and referral to appropriate specialists.

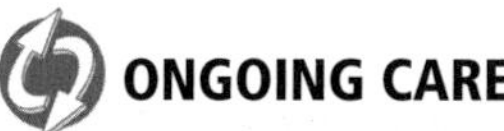

ONGOING CARE

FOLLOW-UP RECOMMENDATIONS

Will be dictated by type of mass or lesion found

ADDITIONAL READING

- Chandler JC, Gauderer MW. The neonate with an abdominal mass. *Pediatr Clin North Am*. 2004;51(4):979–997.
- Golden CB, Feusner JH. Malignant abdominal masses in children: quick guide to evaluation and diagnosis. *Pediatr Clin North Am*. 2002;49(6):1369–1392.
- Ladino-Torres MF, Strouse PJ. Gastrointestinal tumors in children. *Radiol Clin North Am*. 2011;49(4):665–677.
- Potisek NM, Antoon JW. Abdominal masses. *Pediatr Rev*. 2017;38(2):101–103.
- Stevenson RJ. Abdominal masses. *Surg Clin North Am*. 1985;65(6):1481–1504.

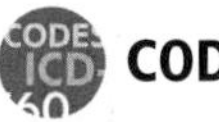

CODES

ICD10

- R19.00 Intra-abd and pelvic swelling, mass and lump, unsp site
- R16.0 Hepatomegaly, not elsewhere classified
- R16.1 Splenomegaly, not elsewhere classified

FAQ

- Q: What congenital anomaly can often serve as a lead point for volvulus or intussusception?
- A: Gastrointestinal duplication cysts
- Q: What type of therapy may result in quick resolution of a benign left lower quadrant fecal mass?
- A: Stool softener or other osmotic laxatives
- Q: What is the most common renal malignancy of childhood?
- A: Wilms tumor

ABDOMINAL MIGRAINE

Desale Yacob, MD

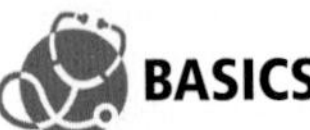

BASICS

DESCRIPTION

Paroxysmal disorder of an acute onset, severe, noncolicky, periumbilical, or diffuse abdominal pain accompanied variably with nausea, vomiting, anorexia, headache, and pallor

EPIDEMIOLOGY

Incidence

- Occurs mostly in children; mean onset at age 7 years (3 to 10 years)
- Peak symptoms 10 to 12 years of age
- More common in girls (3:2)

Prevalence

- May affect as many as 1–4% of children at some point in their lives
- Declining frequency toward adulthood

RISK FACTORS

Genetics

Parents of affected children often have history of migraine headaches and motion sickness.

ETIOLOGY

- May involve neuronal activity originating in the hypothalamus with involvement of the cortex and autonomic nervous system
- Serotonin is implicated and blockade of serotonin receptors may prevent abdominal migraine.
- Recent studies suggest involvement of local intestinal vasomotor factors.
- Abdominal migraine shares pathophysiologic mechanisms and clinical characteristics with cyclic vomiting syndrome and migraine headaches.

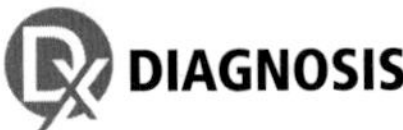

DIAGNOSIS

Rome IV criteria—two episodes fulfilled for at least 6 months meeting all of the following criteria:

- Paroxysmal intense acute periumbilical, midline or diffuse abdominal pain episodes lasting an hour or more
- Episodes are separated by weeks to months.
- Pain that is incapacitating and interferes with normal activity
- Patterns and symptoms are stereotypical in the individual patient.
- Pain associated with ≥2 of the following: anorexia, nausea, vomiting, headache, photophobia, or pallor
- Symptoms cannot be explained by another medical condition based on appropriate evaluation.

HISTORY

- Migraine in the history of patient
- Ask about a family history of migraine headache or unexplained bouts of parental abdominal pain as children.
- Pain typically lasts <6 hours.
- Generalized abdominal pain; can often be localized to the periumbilical or midline areas
- Recurrent abdominal pain that is episodic, intense, stereotypical, and incapacitating
- Intervening periods of baseline health lasting weeks to months between episodes
- Occasionally, other migraine phenomena such as nausea, vomiting, perspiration, body temperature changes, focal paresthesias, radiation of pain to a limb, visual disturbances, or general malaise
- Associated fatigue, lethargy, or impairment of consciousness

PHYSICAL EXAM

- Physical exam, including complete neurologic and abdominal exam, is usually unremarkable.
- Complete eye exam including funduscopic exam should be done to evaluate for papilledema (elevated intracranial pressure), which should be considered inconsistent with diagnosis of abdominal migraine.

DIFFERENTIAL DIAGNOSIS

- Infection
  - Giardia
- Environmental
  - Lead intoxication
- Tumors
- Metabolic
  - Porphyria
  - Lactose intolerance
  - Female carriers of (X-linked) ornithine transcarbamylase (OTC) gene mutation
  - Organic acidemias
- Psychosocial
  - Functional abdominal pain/irritable bowel syndrome
- Surgical
  - Appendicitis
  - Intussusception
  - Biliary colic
- Inflammation
  - Inflammatory bowel disease
  - Peptic ulcer disease
  - Mesenteric adenitis
- GI
  - Irritable bowel syndrome
  - Gastroesophageal reflux
  - Wandering spleen
  - Cyclical vomiting syndrome
  - Functional abdominal pain NOS
  - Constipation
  - Superior mesenteric artery (SMA) syndrome
  - Recurrent pancreatitis
- Anatomic
  - Meckel diverticulum, ureteropelvic junction (UPJ) obstruction
- Neurologic
  - Abdominal epilepsy—but has a shorter duration of pain (minutes), altered consciousness during event, abrupt onset, abnormal discharges in EEG in 80%
  - Temporal lobe epilepsy
  - Intermittent hydrocephalus (possibly secondary to a 3rd-ventricle colloid cyst)

ALERT

When one is able to obtain a detailed history and perform a thorough physical exam, the diagnosis of abdominal migraine should come up on the top of the list of possible diagnosis on the differential. However, it is important to selectively perform a workup to exclude some of the potential serious diagnoses that may present in a similar manner. It is equally important that patients are spared of endless testing including invasive measures such as laparotomy.

DIAGNOSTIC TESTS & INTERPRETATION

- Excluding processes that may cause intense and episodic symptoms is part of the evaluation.
- Exclude increased intracranial pressure and/or other neurologic conditions.
- Exclude intermittent small bowel or urologic obstruction, recurrent pancreatitis, biliary tract disease, familial Mediterranean fever; metabolic disorders such as porphyria and psychiatric disorders should on the differential.

Initial Tests (screening, lab, imaging)

- CBC with differential
- ESR and CRP
- Urinalysis
- Pregnancy test
- Amylase and lipase
- Stool hemoccult
- Lead level
- Evaluation for porphyria or familial Mediterranean fever
- Metabolic evaluation (obtain during symptomatic episode, not during quiescence): urine organic acids, plasma amino acids, ammonia, lactate, blood gas, acylcarnitine profile, imaging

Diagnostic Procedures/Other

- Obstruction series to assess for intermittent or partial bowel obstruction
- Upper GI series to rule out anatomic abnormalities
- US of the abdomen to assess for a mass lesion
- Renal US during episodes to rule out UPJ obstruction
- Air contrast enema (during painful crisis) to rule out intussusception
- Visual evoked response (VER) to red and white flashlight: Children with abdominal migraine may display a specific fast-wave activity response.
- Rarely, brain imaging with CT or MRI may be useful for evaluating causes of intermittent hydrocephalus.

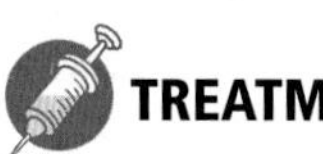

TREATMENT

MEDICATION

- Treatment plan is determined by the severity, frequency, and impact of symptoms on the daily life of the child and family.
- The most important and initial step in addressing the problem is education of the patient and family about the diagnosis.
- Medications can be used to abort acute attacks or be taken as daily prophylaxis.
- For most patients, risks of side effects and complications from the use of these medications may outweigh the relief of pain, especially in children who are experiencing infrequent episodes.
- Limited data exist on abortive agents for abdominal migraines; however, several agents have shown benefit in specialty-based clinical practice, including, intranasal sumatriptan and NSAIDs (although the latter may be avoided if there are clinical concerns for gastritis or peptic ulcer disease). Consider benzodiazepines (i.e., lorazepam) and antiemetics (i.e., ondansetron) for vomiting-predominant symptoms.
- Suggested prophylactic treatments are similar to those for migraine headaches and include tricyclic antidepressants (e.g., amitriptyline), topiramate, propranolol, cyproheptadine, and valproic acid.
- If EEG or other data point to possible epilepsy, empiric treatment with anticonvulsants may be considered.

ADDITIONAL THERAPIES

- Trigger avoidance
  - An event diary should be kept to identify possible migraine triggers.
  - Avoiding triggers is the most optimal strategy for preventing recurrent attacks:
    - Common triggers include caffeine, nitrites, amines, emotional arousal, travel, prolonged fasting, altered sleep, exercise, and/or flickering lights.
- Cognitive therapies
  - Behavioral therapies and lifestyle modification (regular sleep, hydration, and exercise) may also be of benefit. Biofeedback in conjunction with other cognitive therapies and/or relaxation programs may be helpful. Assistance from a trained pediatric mental health professional may be useful.

ONGOING CARE

FOLLOW-UP RECOMMENDATIONS

- Most children outgrow abdominal migraine symptoms (~60%) by early adolescence.
- A substantial percentage of patients (~70%) may develop more typical migraine headaches during adulthood.
- Although nonspecific EEG changes are seen more commonly in this condition, very few children go on to develop epilepsy.
- 10% of children who have a diagnosis of migraine headaches have previously suffered from unexplained recurrent abdominal pain.
- Adult migraine headache sufferers experience abdominal pain more frequently than do tension headache sufferers.

PATIENT EDUCATION

- To help child during bouts of pain, allow the child to do whatever makes him or her comfortable—rest, positioning, being quiet.
- Whether the patient should be excused from school depends on various factors:
  - Frequency, severity, and duration of pain
  - Age, maturity, and coping skills of the child

ADDITIONAL READING

- Catto-Smith AG, Ranuh R. Abdominal migraine and cyclical vomiting. *Semin Pediatr Surg*. 2003;12(4):254–258.
- Cuvellier JC, Lépine A. Childhood periodic syndromes. *Pediatr Neurol*. 2010;42(1):1–11.
- Hyams JS, Di Lorenzo C, Saps M, et al. Functional disorders: children and adolescents [published online ahead of print February 15, 2016]. *Gastroenterology*. doi:10.1053/j.gastro.2016.02.015.
- Lewis DW. Pediatric migraine. *Neurol Clin*. 2009;27(2):481–501.
- Li BU, Balint JP. Cyclic vomiting syndrome: evolution in our understanding of a brain-gut disorder. *Adv Pediatr*. 2000;47:117–160.
- Popovich DM, Schentrup DM, McAlhany AL. Recognizing and diagnosing abdominal migraines. *J Pediatr Health Care*. 2010;24(6):372–377.
- Russell G, Abu-Arafeh I, Symon DN. Abdominal migraine: evidence for existence and treatment options. *Paediatr Drugs*. 2002;4(1):1–8.
- Tan V, Sahami AR, Peebles R, et al. Abdominal migraine and treatment with intravenous valproic acid. *Psychosomatics*. 2006;47(4):353–355.
- Weydert JA, Ball TM, Davis MF. Systematic review of treatments for recurrent abdominal pain. *Pediatrics*. 2003;111(1):e1–e11.

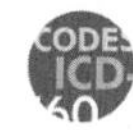

CODES

ICD10

- G43.D0 Abdominal migraine, not intractable
- G43.D1 Abdominal migraine, intractable

FAQ

- Q: Does this diagnosis mean my child will develop migraine headaches?
- A: There is no accurate way to predict whether your child will develop migraine headaches.
- Q: I have two younger children. What chance do they have of developing abdominal migraines?
- A: Although migraine headaches do tend to run in families, there is no known mendelian inheritance pattern.
- Q: What can I do to help my child during bouts of pain?
- A: First, allow the child to do whatever makes him or her comfortable. This approach may mean resting, positioning, or being quiet. Acetaminophen or NSAID-based pain relievers may help to a certain degree. Whether the patient should be excused from school depends on various factors such as the frequency, severity, and duration of the pain as well as the age, maturity, and coping skills of the child.
- Q: My child is having frequent episodes that are affecting his/her quality of life. What can we do?
- A: It may be appropriate to trial him/her on prophylactic daily medications.

ABDOMINAL PAIN

Adrienne M. Scheich, MD

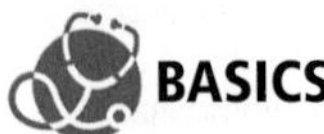

BASICS

DESCRIPTION

- Abdominal pain is a subjective symptom that can originate from any intra-abdominal organ but also be secondary to nonabdominal sources (e.g., peridiaphragmatic conditions [e.g., pneumonia], referred pain, systemic infection [e.g., strep A or viral pharyngitis], depression).
- Acute abdominal pain is often due to benign and self-limited etiologies but may also be due to potentially life-threatening conditions.
- Chronic abdominal pain, defined as present >2 months, can either be of organic origin (anatomic, infectious, inflammatory, or metabolic) or, more frequently, part of a functional gastrointestinal disorder (FGID) based on specific diagnostic criteria (Rome IV).

EPIDEMIOLOGY

- Abdominal pain is one of the most common complaints in pediatric patients.
- Chronic abdominal pain represents 2–4% of general pediatrics office visits and >50% of pediatric gastroenterology visits and can be associated with significant morbidity. Thus, chronic pain also warrants careful consideration and management.

PATHOPHYSIOLOGY

- The nature of abdominal pain is multifactorial and may evolve in nature over time (i.e., in acute appendicitis, pain typically migrates from periumbilical to right lower quadrant).
- Visceral pain (particularly from small intestine) is often poorly localized and is described as dull, diffuse, cramping, or burning. Visceral pain may be associated with autonomic reflex responses (diaphoresis, pallor, nausea, and/ or vomiting).
- More localized, sharp somatoparietal pain typically indicates peritoneal involvement (appendicitis, cholecystitis).
- Referred pain is related to the level of spinal cord entry of visceral afferent nerves (e.g., scapular pain in cholecystitis).

ETIOLOGY

- Right upper quadrant
  - Cholelithiasis/cholecystitis
  - Hepatitis/perihepatitis
  - Nephrolithiasis
  - Ureteropelvic junction obstruction
  - Right lower lobe pneumonia
- Epigastric area
  - Gastroesophageal reflux disease (GERD)
  - Esophagitis (GERD, eosinophilic)
  - Gastritis (NSAID, allergic, *Helicobacter pylori*, Crohn disease)
  - Functional dyspepsia
  - Ulcer disease (NSAID, *H. pylori*)
  - Pancreatitis
  - Cholecystitis
  - Gastric/small intestinal volvulus
- Left upper quadrant
  - Splenic hematoma
  - Renal disease (see above)
  - Left lower lobe pneumonia
  - Constipation
- Right lower quadrant
  - Appendicitis/perforation/psoas abscess
  - Mesenteric adenitis
  - Intussusception
  - Inflammatory bowel disease (IBD)
  - Infection (tuberculosis, *Yersinia*)
  - Ovarian/testicular torsion
  - Ectopic pregnancy
  - Inguinal hernia
- Left lower quadrant
  - Constipation
  - Colitis (inflammatory/infectious)
  - Sigmoid volvulus
  - Genitourinary disease
- Hypogastric area
  - Constipation
  - Colitis
  - Cystitis
  - Dysmenorrhea/uterine disease
  - Pelvic inflammatory disease
- Periumbilical area
  - FGID
  - Constipation
  - Gastroenteritis (infectious/eosinophilic)
  - Pancreatitis
  - Gastric/small bowel volvulus
  - Appendicitis (early)
  - Incarcerated umbilical hernia
- Diffuse
  - Constipation
  - FGID
  - Giardiasis
  - Carbohydrate malabsorption
  - Celiac disease
  - Streptococcal/viral pharyngitis
  - IBD
  - Allergic/eosinophilic gastroenteritis
  - Ischemic necrotizing enterocolitis (NEC)
  - Perforation/peritonitis
  - Malrotation with volvulus
  - Lead/iron poisoning/pica syndrome
  - Cyclic vomiting syndrome
  - Porphyria
  - Sickle cell crisis
  - Familial Mediterranean fever
  - Diabetic ketoacidosis
  - Henoch-Schönlein purpura (HSP)
  - Tumor
  - Trauma
  - Hemolytic uremic syndrome (HUS)

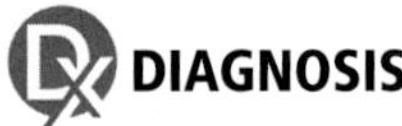

DIAGNOSIS

Initial step is to establish the acuity and severity of symptoms and to rule out a potentially life-threatening emergency (e.g., appendicitis, perforation, bowel obstruction associated with volvulus, adhesions, or intussusception).

HISTORY

- Onset and duration of symptoms
  - Acute versus chronic
- Age of patient may be indicative of certain etiologies particularly in acute presentation.
  - NEC (newborn/prematurity), malrotation/volvulus (80% present in first month of life), intussusception (more frequent in infants/ toddlers), foreign body ingestion in young child
- Localization and radiation of pain
  - May point to specific organ—see etiologies
- Triggering or relieving factors
  - Meals/spices, specific foods (lactose, sucrose)
  - General position with knees bent can be relieving in acute appendicitis.
  - Pain relieved by defecation (constipation) versus pain worsened by defecation (colitis)
- Bowel pattern and stool appearance
  - Stool frequency and consistency: diarrhea versus constipation
  - Urgency or nocturnal diarrhea (colitis)
  - Presence of bloating and excessive flatulence (giardiasis, carbohydrate malabsorption)
  - Presence of mucus (may be normal but can be associated with colitis)
  - Hematochezia (fissure, hemorrhoid, polyp, colitis, HSP); if bright red "currant jelly" appearance, suspect intussusception
  - Melena (upper gastrointestinal bleeding/ulcer)
  - Pale/acholic stools (hepatic or biliary disease)
  - Perirectal disease (IBD)
- Anorexia/nausea/vomiting
  - If postprandial, indicative of upper gastrointestinal condition; nausea may be functional.
  - May indicate extraintestinal disease (urinary tract infection, UPJ obstruction, or pneumonia)
  - Hematemesis suggests esophagitis/gastritis; more significant blood volume suggests ulcer disease, Mallory-Weiss tear (lower esophagus).
  - Bilious emesis indicates intestinal obstruction (volvulus, intussusception, NEC in newborns).
- Dysphagia/food impaction
  - In older children, suspect eosinophilic esophagitis
  - GERD
- Fever
  - Acute infection, acute appendicitis, chronic inflammatory process
- Weight loss/growth failure/delayed puberty
  - Chronic inflammatory process, celiac disease
- Extraintestinal symptoms
  - Dysuria
  - Skin rash (atopy may point to eosinophilic process; purpura: abdominal pain may be first symptom of HSP)
  - Respiratory symptoms (pneumonia)
  - Arthralgias (IBD, HSP)
- Preexisting conditions (infectious diarrhea preceding HUS; hemoglobinopathy or cystic fibrosis risk factors for cholecystitis)
- Exposures
  - Lead/iron in young children
  - Travel/well water/pets (giardiasis)
  - Insect bite (HSP)
  - NSAID use (gastritis)
  - Tetracycline (pill esophagitis)
- Dietary history to assess fiber and fluid intake; excessive use of sugar-free gum (sorbitol malabsorption); intake of sucrose-, fructose-, or lactose-containing foods (disaccharidase deficiencies, most commonly lactose intolerance)
- Prior abdominal surgical history (adhesions)
- Family history of IBD, *H. pylori*, celiac disease, atopy, migraine
- Social history and identification of stressors, school attendance, signs of mood disorder

PHYSICAL EXAM

- In an acute setting, an abdominal exam may need to be serially performed, as location of pain may change over time.
- Signs of acute appendicitis:
  - Exquisite pain at McBurney point on percussion or palpation
  - Involuntary guarding
  - Rovsing sign (palpation LLQ), psoas sign, obturator sign
  - Rebound tenderness (peritoneal inflammation)
  - Pain on movement (walking, jumping)
  - Pain may be relieved temporarily if the appendix ruptures followed by signs of peritonitis.
  - Right upper quadrant pain on inspiration (cholecystitis)
  - Flank tenderness (renal pathology)
  - Perianal examination may reveal skin tags/fissures (constipation, IBD), perianal abscess (IBD), hemorrhoids.
- Rectal examination done carefully can be indicative of
  - Peritoneal irritation (appendicitis/peritonitis)
  - Hematochezia (IBD, HSP), perianal disease
  - Fecal retention/abnormal sphincter tone (anal stricture, absent relaxation of IAS suggesting anal achalasia)
- Skin rashes (eczema, purpura)
- Other signs of chronic disease include pallor, clubbing, edema.

DIAGNOSTIC TESTS & INTERPRETATION

- Laboratory testing, if any, should be carefully guided by the history and clinical picture.
  - If a benign acute condition such as acute viral gastroenteritis is suspected, any further testing can be delayed with close follow-up (in absence of clinical evidence of dehydration).
  - In the presence of "red flags" (see "Issues for Referral"), blood and stool testing should be performed.
- CBC/differential
  - Leukocytosis (appendicitis/abscess, acute infectious process); normal white blood cell count may indicate low risk for acute appendicitis.
  - Anemia (gastrointestinal blood loss)
  - Microcytosis (chronic inflammation, IBD, celiac disease)
- Elevated ESR or CRP (acute infection, chronic inflammation)
- Hypoalbuminemia and low ferritin (IBD, celiac disease); diarrhea may be absent.
- Pancreatic enzymes, hepatic enzymes
- Fecal cultures in the presence of bloody diarrhea (colitis); ova and parasites (giardiasis)
- Fecal calprotectin and lactoferrin (inflammation or infection)
- Urinalysis to rule out urinary tract infection (leukocyturia may be present in acute appendicitis)
- Celiac screening (anti-tissue transglutaminase IgA or anti-endomysial IgA in presence of normal total IgA levels) should be considered if abdominal pain and/or constipation do not respond to bowel regimen or if unexplained diarrhea, weight loss/growth failure; also at-risk groups: type 1 diabetes, autoimmune thyroiditis, Down/Turner syndrome
- Thyroid screen if abdominal pain/chronic constipation unresponsive to therapy

ALERT
H. pylori testing is not indicated in the evaluation of chronic/functional abdominal pain, nonulcer dyspepsia, or newly diagnosed GERD unless the patient has endoscopically documented peptic ulcer disease, a family history of gastric cancer, documented mucosa-associated lymphoid tissue (MALT) lymphoma, or unexplained iron deficiency anemia.

- Radiologic evaluation (abdominal decubitus and upright films)
  - Dilatation or air–fluid levels: acute obstruction
  - "Double bubble" sign and airless abdomen: midgut volvulus/malrotation
  - Air–fluid level or fecalith in right lower quadrant: acute appendicitis if suspected
  - Radiopaque renal stones or dilated ureters
- Upper gastrointestinal contrast study to document anatomic anomalies (i.e., malrotation)
- Ultrasound/CT scan in the evaluation of trauma, acute appendicitis, intussusception, suspected abscess in IBD, tumors, pancreatitis/pseudocyst, cholecystitis
- Use of CT scan in suspected acute appendicitis should be carefully considered, as it can both lead to unnecessary appendectomies or be falsely negative. In patients identified as "low risk" for appendicitis (absent leukocytosis with left shift), ultrasound and/or close observation should be considered as alternative to CT scan.

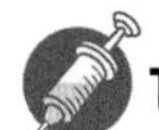

TREATMENT

GENERAL MEASURES

- In the acute setting of abdominal pain suggesting a potential life-threatening condition (acute appendicitis, acute obstruction, volvulus), the patient should be stabilized and referred appropriately for further management including surgery if indicated.
- In the setting of extraintestinal conditions (i.e., pneumonia, pharyngitis, or urinary tract infection), antibiotic therapy should be initiated if indicated.
- In the setting of chronic pain and in the absence of red flags (see "Issues for Referral"), diagnosis most likely falls into abdominal pain—related FGIDs. These include functional dyspepsia, IBS, abdominal migraine, and functional abdominal pain not otherwise specified. The diagnosis of these entities is based on specific symptom-based criteria (Rome IV).
- Functional dyspepsia: trial of proton pump inhibitor (PPI) therapy for 4 weeks to rule out postviral dyspepsia. Avoid use of NSAIDs, spicy and fatty foods, and caffeine. If no response or unable to tolerate progressive taper of PPIs, refer to a gastroenterologist for endoscopic evaluation.
- Irritable bowel syndrome: Address bowel pattern: diarrhea (antidiarrheals); constipation (nonstimulating laxatives); peppermint oil or antispasmodics may alleviate pain
- Functional abdominal pain: Use biopsychosocial approach; behavioral treatment with or without trial of tricyclic antidepressants or SSRIs (particularly in presence of anxiety)

ALERT
Psychological comorbidities should be addressed in all FGIDs.

ISSUES FOR REFERRAL

The presence of clinical red flags, in the setting of acute or chronic abdominal pain, may indicate an underlying mucosal pathology of the gastrointestinal tract (other than infectious), warranting referral to a gastroenterologist for further endoscopic evaluation and management. These include the following:

- Nocturnal pain: pain that wakes from sleep
- Persistent vomiting and/or dysphagia
- GERD nonresponsive to PPI trial
- Hematemesis
- Nocturnal diarrhea
- Hematochezia
- Perianal disease
- Weight loss/delayed growth and/or puberty
- Family history of PUD or IBD

ADDITIONAL READING

- Chitkara DK, Rawat DJ, Talley NJ. The epidemiology of childhood recurrent abdominal pain in Western countries: a systematic review. *Am J Gastroenterol*. 2005;100(8):1868–1875.
- Hyams JS, Di Lorenzo C, Saps M, et al. Functional disorders: children and adolescents [published online ahead of print February 15, 2016]. *Gastroenterology*. doi:10.1053/j.gastro.2016.02.015.
- Jones NL, Koletzko S, Goodman KJ, et al. Joint ESPGHAN/NASPGHAN guidelines for the management of *Helicobacter pylori* in children and adolescents (Update 2016). *J Pediatr Gastroenterol Nutr*. 2017;64(6):991–1003.
- Kharbanda AB, Dudley NC, Bajaj L, et al; for Pediatric Emergency Medicine Collaborative Research Committee of the American Academy of Pediatrics. Validation and refinement of a prediction rule to identify children at low risk for acute appendicitis. *Arch Pediatr Adolesc Med*. 2012;166(8):738–744.
- Koppen IJ, Nurko S, Saps M, et al. The pediatric Rome IV criteria: what's new? *Expert Rev Gastroenterology Hepatol*. 2017;11(3):193–201.
- Korterink JJ, Ockeloen L, Benninga MA, et al. Probiotics for childhood functional gastrointestinal disorders: a systematic review and meta-analysis. *Acta Paediatr*. 2014;103(4):365–372.
- Newlove-Delgado TV, Martin AE, Abbott RA, et al. Dietary interventions for recurrent abdominal pain in childhood. *Cochrane Database Syst Rev*. 2017;(3):CD010972.
- Ross A, LeLeiko NS. Acute abdominal pain. *Pediatr Rev*. 2010;31(4):135–144.
- Saps M, Youssef N, Miranda A, et al. Multicenter, randomized, placebo-controlled trial of amitriptyline in children with functional abdominal gastrointestinal disorders. *Gastroenterology*. 2009;137(4):1261–1269.

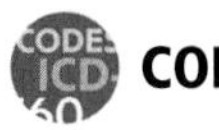

CODES

ICD10

- R10.9 Unspecified abdominal pain
- R10.0 Acute abdomen
- R10.31 Right lower quadrant pain

ABNORMAL BLEEDING

Char M. Witmer, MD, MSCE

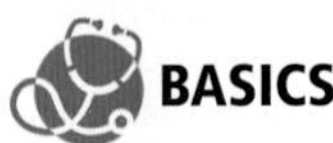

BASICS

DESCRIPTION

Abnormal bleeding may present as

- Frequent or significant mucocutaneous bleeding (epistaxis, bruising, gum bleeding, or menorrhagia)
- Bleeding in unusual sites such as muscles, joints, or internal organs
- Excessive postsurgical bleeding

ETIOLOGY

Abnormal bleeding can be the result of a coagulation factor deficiency, an acquired or congenital disorder of platelet number or function, or inherited or acquired collagen vascular disorders.

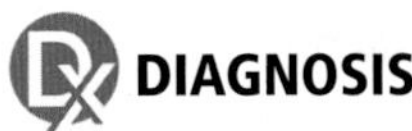

DIAGNOSIS

Approach to patient

- Phase 1
  - Includes a thorough history and physical exam
  - Familial history specifically of bleeding or consanguinity
  - Standard screening laboratory tests include PT, aPTT, and platelet count.
- Phase 2
  - If a bleeding disorder is suspected but the initial screening tests are negative, testing for von Willebrand disease, qualitative platelet disorders, dysfibrinogenemia, or factor XIII deficiency is warranted.
- Phase 3
  - Any abnormal screening tests need further evaluation with additional testing to define the specific disorder (e.g., factor assays).

HISTORY

By taking into account the patient's age, sex, clinical presentation, past medical history, and family history, the most likely cause of bleeding can be usually determined.

- Hemophilia is X-linked, most common in males.
- A family history of bleeding suggests an inherited bleeding disorder.
- Bleeding in unusual places without significant trauma (intracranial, joints) indicates a significant bleeding disorder.
- Persistent palpable bruising is highly suggestive of a bleeding disorder.
- Several surgeries without bleeding makes an inherited bleeding disorder less likely.
- Mucocutaneous bleeding (gum bleeding, bruises, epistaxis, recurrent petechiae, menorrhagia) may indicate thrombocytopenia, a platelet disorder, or von Willebrand disease.
- The use of aspirin and NSAIDs (e.g., ibuprofen) negatively affect platelet function and result in an acquired bleeding disorder.
- Some congenital syndromes may have accompanying bleeding diathesis, which may be unrecognized until they face a hemostatic challenge.

PHYSICAL EXAM

- Children with bleeding disorders are more likely to have large bruises (>5 cm), palpable bruises, and bruises on more than one body part.
- Uncommon sites for bruising for all ages include the back, buttocks, arms, and abdomen.
- **Finding:** Petechiae in skin and mucous membranes?
- *Significance*: disorder of platelet number or function, von Willebrand disease, or vasculitis
- **Finding:** Bruises in unusual places?
- *Significance*: possible platelet disorder, von Willebrand disease, or coagulation deficiency
- **Finding:** Large bruises or palpable bruises?
- *Significance*: coagulation deficiencies, severe platelet disorders, or von Willebrand disease
- **Finding:** Delayed wound healing?
- *Significance*: factor XIII deficiency or dysfibrinogenemia
- **Finding:** Purpura localized to lower body (buttocks, legs, ankles)?
- *Significance*: Henoch-Schönlein purpura

DIFFERENTIAL DIAGNOSIS

Platelet disorders may be quantitative or qualitative, collagen vascular disorders can be acquired or inherited, and disorders of coagulation factors can be congenital or acquired.

- Thrombocytopenia: defective production
  - Congenital/genetic
    - Thrombocytopenia with absent radii syndrome
    - Amegakaryocytic thrombocytopenia
    - Fanconi anemia
    - Metabolic disorders
    - Wiskott-Aldrich syndrome
    - Bernard-Soulier syndrome
    - Other rare familial syndromes (e.g., MYH9-related disorders, *RUNX1* mutations)
  - Acquired
    - Aplastic anemia
    - Drug-associated marrow suppression
    - Virus-associated marrow suppression
    - Chemotherapy
    - Radiation injury
    - Nutritional deficiencies (e.g., vitamin B_{12} and folate)
  - Marrow infiltration
    - Neoplasia (e.g., leukemia, solid tumor)
    - Histiocytosis
    - Osteopetrosis
    - Myelofibrosis
    - Hemophagocytic syndromes
    - Storage diseases
- Thrombocytopenia: increased destruction
  - Idiopathic thrombocytopenia
  - Neonatal alloimmune thrombocytopenia
  - Maternal autoimmune thrombocytopenia
  - Drug-induced (heparin, sulfonamides, digoxin, chloroquine)
  - Disseminated intravascular coagulation
  - Infection: viral, bacterial, fungal, rickettsial
  - Microangiopathic process (e.g., thrombotic thrombocytopenic purpura or hemolytic uremic syndrome)
  - Kasabach-Merritt syndrome
- Thrombocytopenia: sequestration
  - Hypersplenism
  - Hypothermia
- Platelet function disorders
  - Storage pool disorders (e.g., dense granule deficiency, Hermansky-Pudlak or Chédiak-Higashi syndrome)
  - Platelet receptor abnormalities (e.g., Glanzmann thrombasthenia, adenosine 5′-diphosphate receptor defect)
  - Drugs (e.g., aspirin, NSAIDs, guaifenesin, antihistamines, phenothiazines, anticonvulsants)
  - Uremia
  - Paraproteinemia
- Coagulation disorders
  - Prolongation of activated partial thromboplastin time (aPTT)
    - Deficiency of factors VIII, IX, XI, or XII; prekallikrein; or high-molecular-weight kininogen
    - Acquired inhibitor or lupus anticoagulant
  - Prolongation of prothrombin time (PT)
    - Deficiency of factor VII
    - Mild vitamin K deficiency
    - Liver disease, mild to moderate
  - Prolongation of PT and aPTT
    - Deficiency of factors II, V, or X or fibrinogen
    - Liver disease, severe
    - Disseminated intravascular coagulation
    - Severe vitamin K deficiency
    - Hemorrhagic disease of the newborn
    - Dysfibrinogenemia
    - Hypoprothrombinemia associated with a lupus anticoagulant
  - Normal screening (PT, aPTT) laboratory tests
    - Von Willebrand disease
    - Factor XIII deficiency
    - α_2-Antiplasmin deficiency
    - Plasminogen activator inhibitor-1 deficiency

- Vessel wall disorders
  - Congenital
    - Hereditary hemorrhagic telangiectasia
    - Ehlers-Danlos syndrome
    - Marfan syndrome
  - Acquired
    - Vasculitis (systemic lupus erythematosus, Henoch-Schönlein purpura, and others)
    - Scurvy (vitamin C deficiency)

ALERT

Always consider nonaccidental injury as a cause of increased bruising.

DIAGNOSTIC TESTS & INTERPRETATION

- Phase 1: initial laboratory screening
  - Platelet count
  - PT and aPTT
- Phase 2: test for von Willebrand disease
  - Factor VIII:C
  - Von Willebrand factor antigen (VIIIR:Ag)
  - Von Willebrand factor activity (ristocetin cofactor)
  - Von Willebrand factor multimeric analysis—only send after the diagnosis of von Willebrand disease has been established
  - Thrombin time and fibrinogen assay to screen for afibrinogenemia and dysfibrinogenemia
  - Definitive platelet testing includes platelet aggregation and secretion studies with specific agonists.
  - Factor XIII deficiency suspected: factor XIII assay (Urea clot lysis study is a screening test.)
- Phase 3: discriminating laboratory studies for abnormal phase 1 or 2 tests
- The aPTT may be extremely prolonged in patients with deficiencies of the contact factors (prekallikrein, high-molecular-weight kininogen, factor XII). These deficiencies do *not* result in bleeding.
- Improper specimen collection including heparin contamination or underfilling of the specimen tube can result in artificially prolonged clotting times.
- When thrombocytopenia is present:
  - Inspection of blood smear
  - Mean platelet volume (may be normal or elevated in destructive causes, elevated in congenital macrothrombocytopenias, low in Wiskott-Aldrich syndrome)
  - Bone marrow aspiration (rarely necessary)
- Prolonged aPTT
  - Inhibitor screen (50:50 mixing study of patient's and normal plasma)
  - If aPTT fully corrects with mixing, this is consistent with a factor deficiency:
    - Assess for specific factor deficiencies: factors VIII, IX, XI, or XII; prekallikrein; and high-molecular-weight kininogen
  - If partial or no correction after mixing study:
    - Inhibitor is present.
    - Confirmatory test for the presence of a lupus anticoagulant with a platelet-neutralizing procedure or dilute Russell viper venom time (DRVVT)
- Prolonged PT
  - Inhibitor screen should also be considered for prolonged PT.
  - Specific factor level (VII)
- Prolonged PT and aPTT
  - Factor assays: II (prothrombin), V, X, and fibrinogen
  - Potential other causes: disseminated intravascular coagulation, liver disease, and fibrinogen disorders, as described previously
  - Vitamin K deficiency, moderate to severe

ALERT

Pitfalls of testing:

- Platelet Function Assay (PFA)-100
  - Low specificity and sensitivity
  - Affected by medications (NSAIDs)
  - *Not* recommended as a screening test
- Bleeding time
  - Prolonged when platelets $<100{,}000/\text{mm}^3$
  - Affected by medications such as aspirin, NSAIDs, antihistamines
  - Does not correlate with bleeding risk
  - Highly operator dependent
  - *Not* recommended as a screening test
- PT and aPTT
  - Normal ranges are age-dependent.
  - Polycythemia (hematocrit 65%) or underfilling of the specimen tube may result in a spuriously prolonged result.
  - Heparin contamination results in a spuriously prolonged result.
- Von Willebrand disease studies
  - Values fluctuate over time and may be periodically normal in affected individuals.
  - May require repeated testing to make diagnosis
- Emergency care
  - Pressure, elevation, and ice are generally helpful for most bleeding disorders when active bleeding is present.
  - More definitive care is dictated by the nature of the underlying hemostatic defect:
  - Platelet transfusions are useful in disorders of thrombocytopenia owing to decreased production and for intrinsic qualitative platelet disorders but not for immune platelet disorders.
  - Frozen plasma should be used only in severe cases when the exact diagnosis is not readily available but a defect in coagulation is suspected.
  - Head injuries in patients with thrombocytopenia or hemophilia require immediate medical attention.

TREATMENT

GENERAL MEASURES

- Pressure on wound
- Elevation
- Topical application of thrombin
- Topical application of clot-activating polymers

ADDITIONAL READING

- Buchanan GR. Bleeding signs in children with idiopathic thrombocytopenic purpura. *J Pediatr Hematol Oncol*. 2003;25(Suppl 1):S42–S46.
- Khair K, Liesner R. Bruising and bleeding in infants and children—a practical approach. *Br J Haematol*. 2006;133(3):221–231.
- Koreth R, Weinert C, Weisdorf DJ, et al. Measurement of bleeding severity: a critical review. *Transfusion*. 2004;44(4):605–617.
- Lillicrap D, Nair SC, Srivastava A, et al. Laboratory issues in bleeding disorders. *Haemophilia*. 2006; 12(Suppl 3):68–75.
- Sarangi SN, Acharya SS. Bleeding disorders in congenital syndromes. *Pediatrics*. 2017;139(2).
- Sarnaik A, Kamat D, Kannikeswaran N. Diagnosis and management of bleeding disorder in a child. *Clin Pediatr (Phila)*. 2010;49(5):422–431.

CODES

ICD10

- D68.9 Coagulation defect, unspecified
- R04.0 Epistaxis
- T14.8 Other injury of unspecified body region

FAQ

- Q: What are the proper preoperative screening tests for bleeding disorders prior to elective surgery such as tonsillectomy?
- A: A thorough personal history, familial history, and physical exam are by far the most important screening tests. A bleeding time or PFA-100 is not recommended. A CBC, PT, and aPTT are often requested by the surgeon, but normal results do not ensure that a bleeding complication will not occur. Overall, the sensitivity and specificity of these screening tests is poor.
- Q: Bruising is a normal part of childhood. How does one know when bruising is "too much"?
- A: Small bruises on bony prominences on the front of the body are common in children and probably reflect trauma rather than a bleeding disorder. Children with bleeding disorders are more likely to have large bruises (>5 cm), palpable (raised) bruises, and bruises on more than one body part. Uncommon sites for bruising for all ages include the back, buttocks, arms, and abdomen.

ACETAMINOPHEN (PARACETAMOL) POISONING

Kevin C. Osterhoudt, MD, MS

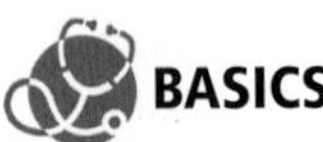

BASICS

DESCRIPTION

- Acetaminophen poisoning may occur after acute or chronic overdose.
- Acetaminophen is sold under many brand names and is often an ingredient in combination pain reliever preparations.
- Acetaminophen poisoning may be clinically occult until frank hepatic or renal injury becomes evident.
- After acute overdose, a serum acetaminophen level above the treatment line of the Rumack-Matthew acetaminophen poisoning nomogram should be considered possibly hepatotoxic.
- Serious hepatotoxicity after a single acute exploratory ingestion by young children is rare compared with that from intentional overdose by adolescents.
- Most toddlers with acetaminophen hepatotoxicity suffer from repeated supratherapeutic dosing.

EPIDEMIOLOGY

- Analgesics are the most common drugs implicated in poisoning exposures reported to United States poison control centers.
- Acetaminophen preparations make up ~45% of all analgesic poisoning exposures reported to poison control centers.
- Acetaminophen poisoning is the most common cause of acute liver failure in the United States.

RISK FACTORS

- Depression
- Pain syndromes
- Glutathione depletion: prolonged vomiting, alcoholism, etc.
- CYP2E1 induction (e.g., alcoholism, isoniazid therapy)

GENERAL PREVENTION

- Acetaminophen should be stored with child-resistant caps, out of sight of young children.
- Proper use of acetaminophen products should be taught to patients with pain or fever.

PATHOPHYSIOLOGY

- Most absorbed acetaminophen is metabolized through formation of hepatic glucuronide and sulfate conjugates.
- Some acetaminophen is metabolized by the CYP450 mixed-function oxidase system, leading to the formation of the toxic *N*-acetyl-p-benzoquinoneimine (NAPQI).
- NAPQI is quickly detoxified by glutathione under usual circumstances.
- After overdose, metabolic detoxification can become saturated:
  - Drug elimination half-life becomes prolonged.
  - More NAPQI is produced.
  - Glutathione supply cannot meet detoxification demand.
  - Hepatic or renal toxicity may ensue.

ETIOLOGY

- Single acute overdose of >200 mg/kg or 10 g
- Repeated overdose of >150 mg/kg/24 h or 6 g/24 h, for >2 days (or >100 mg/kg/24 h or 4 g/24 h if "susceptible")

COMMONLY ASSOCIATED CONDITIONS

- Acetaminophen is often marketed in combination with other pharmaceuticals, which may complicate a drug overdose situation.
- Adolescents frequently overdose on >1 drug preparation.

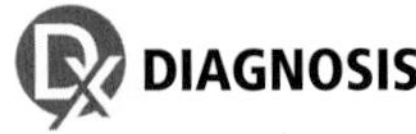

DIAGNOSIS

HISTORY

- Medical history of pain or fever
  - Acetaminophen ingestion should be explored in any patient being treated for pain or fever.
- Amount of acetaminophen ingested
  - A single, acute ingestion of <200 mg/kg (≤10 g in adolescents) is unlikely to cause significant toxicity among otherwise healthy individuals.
- Timing of ingestion
  - Allows application of the Rumack-Matthew nomogram
- Sustained-release preparation
  - Acetaminophen is now available in sustained-release form.
- Medication list
  - Use of isoniazid or other CYP2E1 hepatic enzyme inducers may increase risk for toxicity.
- Signs and symptoms
  - Initially may be clinically silent
  - Vomiting
  - Anorexia

PHYSICAL EXAM

Right upper quadrant tenderness may suggest acetaminophen-induced hepatitis.

DIFFERENTIAL DIAGNOSIS

- Infectious hepatitis
- Other drug-induced hepatitis

DIAGNOSTIC TESTS & INTERPRETATION

Initial Tests (screening, lab, imaging)

- Serum acetaminophen level
  - Allows application of the Rumack-Matthew nomogram after acute overdose
  - Rumack-Matthew nomogram applies only to single, acute acetaminophen overdose scenarios.
- Hepatic transaminases
  - Aspartate aminotransferase (AST) is the most sensitive of the widely available measures to assess acetaminophen hepatotoxicity and begins to rise 12 to 24 hours after significant overdose.
- Liver and kidney function tests
  - As the AST rises, it is important to follow liver and kidney function with tests such as serum glucose, prothrombin (PT) and partial thromboplastin (PTT) times, serum creatinine, plasma pH, and serum albumin.
  - The PT and PTT may be slightly elevated owing to direct effect of elevated blood acetaminophen concentrations or *N*-acetylcysteine therapy, without signifying liver injury.
  - The decline of an elevated serum AST may indicate either liver recovery or profound liver failure and must be interpreted in context.
- Salicylate level
  - May be a coingestant in the setting of analgesic drug overdose
- Pathologic findings
  - Hepatic zone III (centrilobular) necrosis

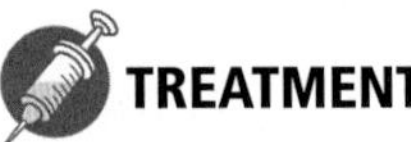

TREATMENT

GENERAL MEASURES

Evaluate for possible polypharmacy overdose.

MEDICATION

First Line

- Single acute overdose
  - Activated charcoal, 1 to 2 g/kg (maximum 75 g), may be administered if acetaminophen is judged to be present in the stomach or proximal intestine (usually within 1 hour of ingestion).
  - *N*-Acetylcysteine should be administered if a serum acetaminophen level obtained >4 hours after overdose falls above the treatment line of the Rumack-Matthew nomogram (see Appendix, Figure 4).

- Patients presenting to medical care >7 hours after overdose should be given a loading dose of *N*-acetylcysteine while waiting for the serum acetaminophen level result.
- IV *N*-acetylcysteine dose: 150 mg/kg (maximum 15 g) loading dose over 1 hour, then 12.5 mg/kg/h for 4 hours (maximum 5 g over 4 h), and then 6.25 mg/kg/h for 16 hours (maximum 10 g over 16 h) (see "FAQ")

ALERT

Some toxicologists suggest higher *N*-acetylcysteine dosing for very large acetaminophen overdoses. Please contact an expert for a serum acetaminophen concentration >400 mcg/mL or for evidence of mitochondrial failure.

- Oral *N*-acetylcysteine dose: 140 mg/kg (maximum 15 g) loading dose, followed by 70 mg/kg (maximum 7.5 g) maintenance doses q4h (see "FAQ")

- Repeated supratherapeutic ingestion
  - Consider *N*-acetylcysteine therapy if
    - Ingestion of >150 mg/kg or 6 g/24 h for consecutive days
    - Patient is symptomatic.
    - Serum AST concentration is elevated.
    - Acetaminophen level is higher than would be expected given dosing, and AST level is normal.
- Once started, *N*-acetylcysteine therapy should be continued until
  - The serum acetaminophen level is nondetectable
  - A simultaneous serum AST has not risen or, if elevated, liver enzymes and liver function are clearly improving
- Precautions
  - IV *N*-acetylcysteine has been associated with anaphylactoid reactions, which may require cessation or slowing of infusion, antihistamines, corticosteroids, and/or epinephrine.
  - Acetaminophen poisoning and oral *N*-acetylcysteine are emetogenic: Chill and cover the *N*-acetylcysteine. Consider antiemetic therapy or slow nasogastric administration if necessary.

ISSUES FOR REFERRAL

- Patients with AST approaching 1,000 IU/L should be considered for transfer to a liver transplant center.
- Mental health services should be provided to victims of intentional overdose.

SURGERY/OTHER PROCEDURES

Liver transplant should be considered per transplant center protocols. The King's College Hospital Criteria include the following:

- pH <7.30 after resuscitation, or
- PT >1.8 times control, plus
- Serum creatinine >3.3 mg/dL, plus
- Encephalopathy

ADMISSION, INPATIENT, AND NURSING CONSIDERATIONS

- Admission criteria
  - *N*-acetylcysteine therapy
  - Psychiatric evaluation warranted
- Discharge criteria
  - *N*-acetylcysteine therapy concluded
  - No concern for developing liver injury

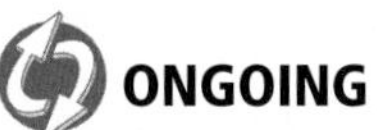

ONGOING CARE

FOLLOW-UP RECOMMENDATIONS

Patient Monitoring

- Cardiorespiratory monitoring is warranted during IV *N*-acetylcysteine therapy.
- Intensive care monitoring is warranted during fulminant hepatic failure.

PATIENT EDUCATION

- Drug administration education should be offered to victims of chronic overdose.
- Home safety education should be provided after pediatric exploratory ingestions.

PROGNOSIS

- Among previously healthy children, hepatotoxicity is rare with single doses <150 to 200 mg/kg.
- After single acute acetaminophen overdose, likelihood of hepatotoxicity may be determined by using the Rumack-Matthew nomogram.
- *N*-Acetylcysteine therapy prevents fulminant hepatic failure in >99% of acetaminophen-poisoned patients if administered within 8 hours of overdose.
- *N*-Acetylcysteine therapy is less efficacious when administered >8 hours after overdose but should still be offered.
- Repetitive dosing of acetaminophen >75 mg/kg/24 h should be evaluated cautiously, especially in the presence of the following:
  - Febrile illness
  - Vomiting or malnourishment
  - Anticonvulsant or isoniazid therapy

COMPLICATIONS

- Hepatic failure
- Renal insufficiency
- Anaphylactoid shock may complicate IV *N*-acetylcysteine therapy.

ADDITIONAL READING

- American College of Medical Toxicology. ACMT position statement: duration of intravenous acetylcysteine therapy following acetaminophen overdose. *J Med Toxicol*. 2017;13(1):126–127.
- Chun LJ, Tong MJ, Busuttil RW, et al. Acetaminophen hepatotoxicity and acute liver failure. *J Clin Gastroenterol*. 2009;43(4):342–349.
- Dart RC, Erdman AR, Olson KR, et al; for American Association of Poison Control Centers. Acetaminophen poisoning: an evidence-based consensus guideline for out-of-hospital management. *Clin Toxicol (Phila)*. 2006;44(1):1–18.
- Heard KJ. Acetylcysteine for acetaminophen poisoning. *New Engl J Med*. 2008;359(3):285–292.
- Rumack BH, Bateman DN. Acetaminophen and acetylcysteine dose and duration: past, present and future. *Clin Toxicol*. 2012;50(2):91–98.

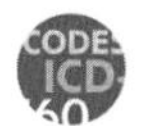

CODES

ICD10

- T39.1X4A Poisoning by 4-Aminophenol derivatives, undetermined, init
- K71.9 Toxic liver disease, unspecified
- T39.1X1A Poisoning by 4-Aminophenol derivatives, accidental, init

FAQ

- Q: What is "patient-tailored" *N*-acetylcysteine therapy?
- A: The duration of *N*-acetylcysteine therapy used to depend on the pharmaceutical form administered but is now tailored to the patient based on serum acetaminophen level and liver function.
- Q: Should *N*-acetylcysteine be given PO or IV?
- A: Both seem to be similarly efficacious. Oral administration of *N*-acetylcysteine is complicated by taste aversion and vomiting. IV *N*-acetylcysteine may lead to anaphylactoid shock. Few cost–benefit studies are available for direct comparison of patient-tailored courses of oral *N*-acetylcysteine and IV *N*-acetylcysteine.

ACNE

Deepti Gupta, MD • Renee M. Howard, MD

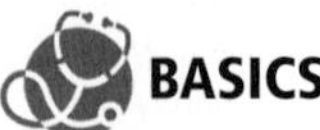

BASICS

DESCRIPTION

Acne vulgaris is one of the most common skin conditions in children and adolescents. It is a disorder of pilosebaceous units (PSUs). PSUs are found predominantly on the face, chest, back, and upper arms. Acne presents as comedonal or inflammatory lesions and can cause depressed scars and hyperpigmentation. Presentation, treatment, and associated systemic manifestations differ by age of presentation, pubertal status, and severity of disease.

- Classification of acne by age:
  - Neonatal (birth to 6 weeks): affects up to 20% of neonates. Also known as neonatal cephalic pustulosis. Presents with a papulopustular eruption predominantly on face. Thought to be due to *Malassezia* colonization. No treatment necessary; for severe cases can use ketoconazole cream 2%
  - Infantile acne (6 weeks to 1 year): presents with comedonal and inflammatory lesions on face. Some evidence that it may predispose to severe adolescent acne. Often, no underlying endocrine abnormality; self-limited but in severe cases can use topical acne treatments
  - Midchildhood acne (1 to 6 years): uncommon. Presents with comedonal and inflammatory lesions on face. Suspect an underlying endocrinopathy.
  - Preadolescent (7 to 11 years): presents with predominantly comedonal lesions in "T-zone," central face; can be first sign of onset of puberty
  - Adolescent (12 to 19 years): very common presentation, affects 85% of adolescents

RISK FACTORS

Genetics

Familial patterns exist, but no inheritance pattern has been demonstrated.

GENERAL PREVENTION

- Effective and early treatment limits scarring, postinflammatory pigment alteration, and minimizes psychosocial impact.
- Use of oil-free and noncomedogenic moisturizers, sunscreens, and make-up

PATHOPHYSIOLOGY

Pathogenesis of acne is multifactorial and involves four different components:

- Increased sebum production: stimulated by an increase in androgen levels. The adrenal gland is active during the 1st year of life and then reawakens in preadolescent time period. Production peaks in teens and decreases in 20s.
- Alteration in follicular growth and differentiation leading to the creation of a microcomedone, a precursor of inflammatory and comedonal acne lesions
- Follicular colonization with *Propionibacterium acnes*, an anaerobic, gram-positive diphtheroid bacteria. *P. acnes* produces free fatty acids (FFAs) leading to inflammation.
- Inflammation and immune response through the innate immune system

ETIOLOGY

- Androgen excess (physiologic vs. pathologic)
- Medication-induced (corticosteroids, anticonvulsants, lithium, etc.)
- Occlusion (from topical- or oil-based products)
- Frictions from clothing or athletic gear such as helmets, shoulder pads, chin straps, or bra straps may worsen acne.

COMMONLY ASSOCIATED CONDITIONS

- Polycystic ovarian syndrome (PCOS)
- SAPHO syndrome: synovitis, acne, pustulosis, hyperostosis, and osteitis
- Adrenal or gonadal/ovarian tumors
- Late-onset congenital adrenal hyperplasia

DIAGNOSIS

HISTORY

- Age of onset: Early or late onset of acne may indicate androgen excess.
- Medications and supplement use: Hormonal (including some oral contraceptive products (OCPs), progestin implants, depot medroxyprogesterone), steroids (topical, inhaled, or oral), anticonvulsants (lithium, isoniazid, nicotine products) may worsen acne.
- Menstrual history: Premenstrual flares may occur due to androgenic effects of progesterone.
- Androgen excess (history of or current):
  - Prepubertal: early-onset acne or body odor, increased linear growth, axillary or pubic hair, genital maturation, or clitoromegaly
  - Postpubertal: alopecia, hirsutism, truncal obesity, acanthosis nigricans, irregular menses, increased muscle mass
- Previous acne treatments tried, effect of previous treatments, and reason treatment failed (cost, adherence, tolerability, ease of use)

ALERT

Psychological impact: Ask patients about self-esteem, depression, and suicidal ideations.

PHYSICAL EXAM

- Skin
  - Distribution of lesions
  - Type of acne lesions: comedonal (open: blackhead, due to oxidation of lipids and not dirt; closed: whitehead), inflammatory (erythematous papule, pustule, nodule, pseudocyst)
  - Scarring and hyperpigmentation
- Global assessment of acne severity (number, size, extent, and scarring)
- Note signs of androgen excess (see "History").
- Height, weight, growth curve
- Blood pressure

DIFFERENTIAL DIAGNOSIS

- Adenoma sebaceum (facial angiofibromas)
- Keratosis pilaris
- Flat warts
- Molluscum contagiosum
- Periorificial dermatitis
- Milia
- Miliaria
- Syringomas
- Demodex folliculitis
- *Malassezia* (*Pityrosporum*) folliculitis
- Gram-negative folliculitis
- Staphylococcal folliculitis
- Chloracne (exposure to chlorinated aromatic hydrocarbons)
- Papular sarcoidosis

DIAGNOSTIC TESTS & INTERPRETATION

Initial Tests (screening, lab, imaging)

- Consider for patients with signs of androgen excess, midchildhood acne, or acne unresponsive to traditional therapy.
  - Serologic testing (LH, FSH, testosterone total and free, dehydroepiandrosterone sulfate (DHEA-S), androstenedione prolactin, 17-hydroxyprogesterone)
  - Bone age
  - Referral to pediatric endocrinology
  - Imaging for adrenal or gonadal tumor
- Lab monitoring while using isotretinoin should include baseline complete blood count (CBC), fasting lipid panel (triglycerides and cholesterol), transaminases, and pregnancy test for females and monthly fasting lipid panel (triglycerides and cholesterol), transaminases, and pregnancy test for females. Prior to starting, females need two negative pregnancy tests 30 or more days apart.

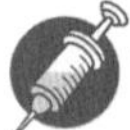

TREATMENT

- Choose regimen based on previous therapies used and effect, cost, vehicle selection, regimen complexity, active scarring, and psychosocial impact.
- Vehicle selection:
  - Creams and lotions less drying than gels and solutions
  - Creams better for sensitive skin/eczema
  - Gels and solutions may be better for oily skin or for use with make-up.
- Manage patient expectations.
- Treatment may take 2 to 3 months to be effective.
- Acne may initially flare prior to improving.
- Counsel about medication side effects.

- General approach: categorized by acne severity and age of patient
  - Mild acne: comedonal, inflammatory, or mixed
    - Initial:
      - Topical monotherapy:
        - Benzoyl peroxide (BP)
        - Topical retinoid
      - Topical combination therapy:
        - BP + antibiotic
        - Retinoid + BP
        - Retinoid + BP + antibiotic
    - Inadequate response:
      - Assess adherence.
      - Add BP or retinoid if not already prescribed.
      - Change:
        - Topical retinoid concentration, type, or formulation
        - Change topical combination therapy.
  - Moderate acne: comedonal, inflammatory, or mixed
    - Initial:
      - Topical combination therapy:
        - Retinoid + BP
        - Retinoid + BP + antibiotic
      - Oral antibiotic + topical retinoid + BP
    - Inadequate response:
      - Assess adherence.
      - Change topical retinoid concentration, type, or formulation.
      - Add or change oral antibiotic.
      - Females: Consider hormonal therapy.
      - Consider oral isotretinoin.
      - Consider dermatology referral.
  - Severe acne: inflammatory, mixed, and/or nodular lesions; extensive involvement often with significant scarring
    - Initial:
      - Oral antibiotic + topical retinoid + BP ± topical antibiotic
      - Consider oral isotretinoin.
      - Consider dermatology referral.
    - Inadequate response:
      - Assess adherence.
      - Change topical retinoid concentration, type, or formulation.
      - Change oral antibiotic.
      - Females: Consider hormonal therapy.
      - Consider oral isotretinoin.
      - Scars warrant aggressive treatment targeting inflammation.

MEDICATION

- Topical agents/over the counter
  - Gentle cleansers:
    - Using gentle soap-free, pH-balanced cleansers is recommended for everyday washing.
    - BP:
      - Bactericidal, mild comedolytic, and anti-inflammatory properties
      - Limits antibiotic resistance and provides increased efficacy in combination with retinoids
      - Available as lotion, cream, wash, and gel in 2.5–10%
      - Increased concentration does not increase efficacy but can cause more irritation.
      - 5% concentration generally effective; can start with lower concentration or decrease number of days of use if too irritating
      - Side effects: drying, erythema, burning, peeling, stinging, and rarely contact dermatitis
      - Cautions: can cause bleaching of hair, clothing, and linen; increased risk of photosensitivity; rare but serious and potentially life-threatening allergic reactions or severe irritation have been reported.
    - Salicylic acid (SA):
      - Promotes comedolysis with drying and peeling
      - Not as effective as BP
    - Sulfur/sulfacetamide:
      - Mild antibacterial and keratolytic properties
      - Very well-tolerated
      - Distinctive odor

ALERT
Avoid vigorous cleansing of the skin or harsh facial astringents and toners that may irritate the skin.

- Prescription topical medications
  - Topical antibiotics (erythromycin, clindamycin):
    - Reduce *P. acnes* concentration and inflammatory mediators
    - Available in combination products to increase compliance, but these products are often more expensive
    - Combine with BP to decrease antibiotic resistance
    - Combine with retinoids to help yield faster results
    - Side effects: well-tolerated but may include drying or irritation
  - Topical retinoids:
    - Prevent formation of microcomedones, clear existing microcomedones, anti-inflammatory
    - Available in three forms
    - Adapalene
      - Available as cream or gel and as a combination product with BP
      - Pregnancy class C (see Appendix IV; Table 10)
      - Photostable
      - Better tolerability than tretinoin but weaker in strength
    - Tretinoin
      - Available as cream, gel, microsphere gel of various strengths
      - Pregnancy class C (see Appendix IV; Table 10)
      - Apply to dry skin.
      - Apply pea-sized amount to entire face.
      - Can be very irritating and drying
      - Start with low concentration (0.025%) and decreased frequency (few times a week) of application and titrate up as tolerated.
      - Inactivated by sunlight; use at nighttime.

ALERT
BP inactivates tretinoin when used together. Apply BP in the morning and tretinoin at night.

    - Tazarotene
      - Available in cream and gel
      - Pregnancy class X; contraindicated in pregnancy
      - Apply to dry skin.
      - More irritating than other retinoids
      - Inactivated by sunlight; use at nighttime.
      - Not 1st-line therapy for most patients
      - Side effects: erythema, dryness, irritation, initially acne flares, and photosensitivity (Advise use of daily noncomedogenic sunscreen with sun protection factor (SPF) 30+ and facial moisturizer tazarotene.)
      - Apply pea-sized amount to entire face.
      - Start with lowest strength 3 times a week and increase frequency slowly to every night as tolerated. Some patients may not tolerate medication every night.
      - Increase concentration of medication if patient still with oily skin or getting new acne lesions.
  - Azelaic acid:
    - Comedolytic and antibacterial; decreases hyperpigmentation
    - 15% gel or 20% cream, applied twice daily
    - Pregnancy class B (see Appendix IV; Table 10)
    - Side effects include itching, burning, stinging, and erythema.
    - Consider for patients with comedonal acne who cannot use retinoids.

- Topical dapsone:
  - Synthetic sulfone has antimicrobial and anti-inflammatory effects.
  - Available in 5% gel, twice-daily application recommended
  - Most effective against inflammatory acne lesions
  - Safe in patients with G6PD deficiency
  - Enhanced efficacy when combined with retinoids
  - Side effects: erythema and dryness
  - Caution: When used with BP, a temporary orange staining of skin can occur.

ALERT

Do not use antibiotics as monotherapy due to slow onset of action and development of antibiotic resistance. Use with BP.

- Oral antibiotics: reduce *P. acnes* concentration and inflammatory mediators
  - Tetracyclines (doxycycline, minocycline, tetracycline): pregnancy class D; must be >8 years of age due to staining of tooth enamel
    - Doxycycline and minocycline are preferred due to 1 to 2×/24 h dosing and greater follicular penetration.
      - Dosing: 50 to 100 mg daily or b.i.d.
    - Tetracycline is cheap but has least efficacy.
    - Increasing antibiotic resistance. Limit treatment length and do not use as monotherapy. Use with BP or topical retinoid.
    - Taper or switch to topical retinoid monotherapy after 12 weeks and when patient is no longer getting new acne lesions.
    - Systemic side effects and cautions:
      - Doxycycline: GI upset, vaginal candidiasis, pill esophagitis, photosensitivity (phototoxicity), benign intracranial hypertension; take with food and large glass of water, stay upright 1 hour after taking medication, photoprotection, can use enteric-coated form
      - Minocycline: acute vestibular reaction (vertigo, dizziness), vaginal candidiasis, hyperpigmentation, drug-induced hypersensitivity reaction 2 to 8 weeks after starting medication, lupus-like syndrome, autoimmune hepatitis, Stevens-Johnson syndrome (SJS), benign intracranial hypertension
  - Sulfa (trimethoprim-sulfamethoxazole):
    - Dosing: 160 to 800 mg PO b.i.d.
    - Used judiciously, refractory cases
    - Systemic side effects: severe cutaneous reactions (SJS, toxic epidermal necrolysis, drug-induced hypersensitivity reaction, fixed drug eruption), bone marrow suppression
    - Check baseline CBC and periodically thereafter.
  - Cephalosporins (cephalexin, cefadroxil):
    - Dosing: 500 mg PO b.i.d.
    - Well-tolerated
    - Systemic side effects: GI upset
  - Penicillins (amoxicillin):
    - Well-tolerated
    - Systemic side effects: GI upset
  - Macrolides (erythromycin, azithromycin)
    - High prevalence of *P. acnes* resistance to erythromycin
    - Systemic side effects: erythromycin GI upset, drug–drug interactions
- Oral retinoids (isotretinoin): decreases sebum production, anti-inflammatory, and reduces *P. acnes*
  - Used as monotherapy
  - Used for recalcitrant acne and/or with significant scarring
  - Dosing:
    - Start with 0.5 mg/kg/24 h for first 4 weeks and then advance to 1 mg/kg/24 h.
    - Goal cumulative treatment course is generally 120 to 150 mg/kg. Higher courses up to 220 mg/kg have been reported.
    - For patients with severe inflammatory and nodulocystic acne, start at lower dose and consider starting oral corticosteroids to prevent acne fulminans.
  - Need baseline and monthly labs (see "Initial Tests (screening, lab, imaging)")
  - Side effects:
    - Common: dry skin, dry eyes, cheilitis, photosensitivity, myalgias
    - Teratogen
      - Two forms of birth control need to be used while on medication or abstinence.
      - FDA-mandated registry (iPledge: see https://www.ipledgeprogram.com/); prescribed only by registered users
    - Depression and suicide have been reported in patients on isotretinoin; counsel about this risk and assess if patient a candidate for medication.
    - Inflammatory bowel disease: conflicting data. Association may exist but rare, and there are many confounding factors.
    - Bone effects: conflicting data regarding increased risk of fractures and demineralization. Hyperostoses and premature epiphyseal closure are rare and uncommon side effects.
    - Rare, sporadic reports of serious skin infections including erythema multiforme, SJS, and toxic epidermal necrolysis

ALERT

Do not use tetracycline antibiotics with oral retinoids due to risk of pseudotumor cerebri.

- Hormonal therapy: 2nd-line therapy for women; usually used in combination with other acne treatments
  - OCPs (for women): suppress ovarian androgen production
  - Can be used as an adjunct for females with moderate to severe acne not responding to topical retinoids
  - Three OCPs are FDA-approved for acne:
    - Ethinyl estradiol (35 mcg) and norgestimate (≥15 years of age)
    - Ethinyl estradiol (20–30–35 mcg) and norethindrone (≥15 years of age)
    - Ethinyl estradiol (30 mcg) and drospirenone (3 mg) (≥14 years of age)
  - Screen for personal tobacco use and family history of thromboembolic event.
    - Use caution in girls who smoke tobacco.
  - May need 3 to 6 months to see improvement
  - Side effects include nausea, breast tenderness, headache, weight gain, breakthrough menstrual bleeding, myocardial infarction, ischemic stroke, and deep venous thrombses.
  - Controversial effect on bone density and growth; recommendation to start at least 1 year after onset of menstruation

- Spironolactone (for women): a potassium-sparing diuretic; blocks androgen receptor in sebaceous glands reducing sebocyte proliferation
  - Dose 25 to 150 mg daily start low and titrate to minimum effective dose.
  - Off-label use
  - Can be used in combination with OCP
  - Side effects: hyperkalemia (lab monitoring may be indicated in some cases), teratogen (controversial/limited studies in animal models; the American College of Obstetricians and Gynecologists [ACOG] recommends not using during pregnancy especially during the first trimester due to antiandrogenic effects), hypotension, dizziness, dry mouth

COMPLEMENTARY & ALTERNATIVE THERAPIES

- Limited empiric studies on CAM and acne
- Randomized controlled trials of the following showed that they were not as effective as 5% BP but resulted in less skin irritation:
  - Tea tree oil: a mixture of terpenes and alcohols with antibiotic and antifungal properties; 5% solution may be effective in treating comedonal and inflammatory acne; may be associated with male gynecomastia
  - Gluconolactone 14% solution may be effective on comedonal and inflammatory acne.

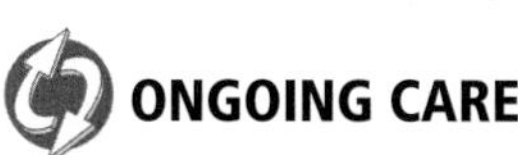

ONGOING CARE

PATIENT EDUCATION

- http://www.aad.org/dermatology-a-to-z/diseases-and-treatments/a–d/acne
- http://www.nlm.nih.gov/medlineplus/acne.html (handout in Spanish also available)
- https://pedsderm.net/for-patients-families/patient-handouts/#Anchor-Acne (handout and patient education video)

COMPLICATIONS

- Scarring may be permanent.
- Hyperpigmentation: occurs more in dark-skinned individuals; self-resolves but may take months to years
- Self-esteem: acne severity correlated to social variables including embarrassment and lack of enjoyment in social activities among teenagers
- Patients with mild to moderate acne showed clinical depression and >5% suicidal ideation. Depression scores improve in correlation with response to acne treatment.

ADDITIONAL READING

- Eichenfield LF, Krakowski AC, Piggott C, et al; for American Acne and Rosacea Society. Evidence-based recommendations for the diagnosis and treatment of pediatric acne. *Pediatrics*. 2013;131(Suppl 3):163–186.
- Friedlander SF, Eichenfield LF, Fowler JF Jr, et al. Acne epidemiology and pathophysiology. *Semin Cutan Med Surg*. 2010;29(2)(Suppl 1):2–4.
- Lam C, Zaenglein A. Contraceptive use in acne. *Clin Dermatol*. 2014;32(4):502–515.
- Yan AC, Baldwin HE, Eichenfield LF, et al. Approach to pediatric acne treatment: an update. *Semin Cutan Med Surg*. 2011;30(Suppl 3):S16–S21.

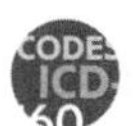

CODES

ICD10

- L70.9 Acne, unspecified
- L70.4 Infantile acne
- L70.0 Acne vulgaris

FAQ

- Q: Can I modify my diet to improve my acne?
- A: Limited and variable data is available. There is suggestion that high glycemic diets and skim milk consumption (not full-fat milk) may be associated with increased acne via activation of insulin and insulin-like growth factor 1 (IGF-1), which activates sebocyte production. Limited data is also available on the use of zinc and Nicomide supplementation and their potential to improve acne.
- Q: Does poor hygiene cause acne?
- A: No. Use of harsh astringents, exfoliating scrubs, and vigorous scrubbing can worsen acne by causing more inflammation and scarring. They also can be more irritating and drying, decreasing tolerability of acne treatments. Recommend use of a gentle, soap-free, pH-balanced cleanser for daily use in addition to noncomedogenic moisturizers and sunscreen in conjunction with acne treatments.
- Q: Do cosmetics worsen acne?
- A: Recommend use of oil-free, noncomedogenic make-up, which have been proven not to delay treatment response or worsen acne severity.
- Q: Any other factors that I should know about that can affect acne?
- A: Yes. Smoking also has shown to worsen acne through a mechanism of nicotinic acid binding to acetylcholine receptors and increasing follicular plugging and epithelial hyperplasia.

ACUTE DRUG WITHDRAWAL

Robert J. Hoffman, MD, MS

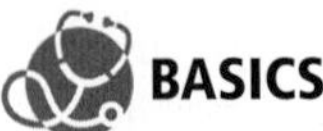

BASICS

DESCRIPTION

- Drug withdrawal is a physiologic response to an effectively lowered drug concentration in a patient with tolerance to that drug.
- Withdrawal results in a predictable pattern of symptoms that are reversible if the drug in question or another appropriate substitute is reintroduced.
- Sedative-hypnotic withdrawal is the most common life-threatening withdrawal syndrome in children. This includes withdrawal from barbiturates, benzodiazepines, baclofen, as well as γ-hydroxybutyrate and similar substances.
- Other substances that are associated with withdrawal syndromes include nicotine, opioids, selective serotonin reuptake inhibitors (SSRIs), and caffeine.

EPIDEMIOLOGY

- The most common life-threatening withdrawal syndrome, alcohol withdrawal, rarely occurs in children.
- Neonates born to alcohol-dependent mothers are at risk.

RISK FACTORS

- Patients receiving sedatives or analgesics capable of causing tolerance are at risk.
- Any inpatient use of sedative or opioids >5 days is a risk factor for withdrawal.
- This risk is particularly important to consider with infusions or high doses of such substances in previously naive patients.

GENERAL PREVENTION

- Clinician familiarity with tolerance and withdrawal associated with prescribed medications allows appropriate drug tapering.
- Drug abuse prevention is appropriate for all children.

PATHOPHYSIOLOGY

- Altered CNS neurochemistry is the most important and clinically relevant aspect of withdrawal pathophysiology.
- Under normal conditions, the CNS maintains a balance between excitation and inhibition. Although there are several ways to achieve this balance, excitation is constant and actions occur through removal of inhibitory tone.
- Relative to adults and younger children, adolescents are more prone to develop dependence and withdrawal syndrome due to immaturity of their prefrontal cortex.

ETIOLOGY

- Neonates
  - Maternal alcohol, caffeine, opioid, sedative-hypnotic, or SSRI use may result in a neonatal abstinence syndrome.
  - Treatment with caffeine, opioids, or sedative-hypnotics and subsequent discontinuation may result in subsequent development of an abstinence syndrome.
- Older children
  - Subsequent to treatment with opioids, or sedative-hypnotics, an abstinence syndrome may result.
  - Substance abuse, particularly opioids, γ-hydroxybutyrate, or other sedative-hypnotics, may result in an abstinence syndrome.
  - Frequent caffeine or nicotine use may lead to an abstinence syndrome.
- Use of opioid antagonists such as naloxone, naltrexone, and nalmefene is associated with development of opioid withdrawal.

DIAGNOSIS

- Drug withdrawal is a clinical diagnosis.
- Patients should be evaluated for associated diagnoses (e.g., traumatic injury, pneumonia).

HISTORY

- Typically, a history of substance exposure, either direct exposure or maternal use, will be elicited.
  - Exposure may be to prescribed medication or abusable substances.
  - Substance use by the mother or child might intentionally be concealed.
- The timing of withdrawal varies depending on the half-life of the substance involved.
  - Shorter half-life causes quicker onset of withdrawal with greater severity.
- Alcohol or sedative-hypnotics
  - Causes tremor, diaphoresis, agitation, insomnia, altered mental status, or withdrawal seizures
  - Baclofen withdrawal is more frequently severe or life-threatening relative to benzodiazepine withdrawal. History of pump manipulation or malfunction should be sought.
- Caffeine
  - Withdrawal may result in dysphoria, headache, behavioral changes, or agitation.
- Opioids
  - Nausea, vomiting, diarrhea, irritability, yawning, sleeplessness, diaphoresis, lacrimation, tremor, and hypertonicity may result.
  - Neonates can also have seizures, a high-pitched cry, skin mottling, and excoriation. These latter signs and symptoms are more typical of opioid withdrawal and rarely occur with neonatal alcohol withdrawal.
- Nicotine
  - Dysphoria, agitation, behavioral changes, and increased appetite may all occur.
- SSRIs
  - Neonatal withdrawal from SSRIs may result in jitteriness, agitation, crying, shivering, increased muscle tone, breathing and sucking problems, as well as seizure.
  - Children withdrawing from SSRIs may have jitteriness, agitation, dysphoria, behavioral changes, shivering, increased muscle tone, and seizure.

PHYSICAL EXAM

- A clinically appropriate, validated scoring tool (e.g., Withdrawal Assessment Tool, Version 1 [WAT-1] for children or adolescents or the Finnegan Neonatal Abstinence Syndrome Scale for newborns) should be completed with the physical exam to obtain objective, valid assessment of severity of withdrawal.
- Vital signs including temperature should be evaluated regularly. Vital sign changes such as tachycardia and hypertension may occur concomitantly with acute drug withdrawal.
- Technology-dependent patients, such as children with an intrathecal baclofen pump, should have evaluation of the machine to determine if it is working properly.
- Most cases of substance withdrawal only result in behavioral changes. Opioid withdrawal may be accompanied by diaphoresis, mydriasis, yawning, and lacrimation.
- Sedative-hypnotic withdrawal may result in hypertension, tachycardia, hyperthermia, agitation, hallucinations, and seizure.

DIFFERENTIAL DIAGNOSIS

- Hypoglycemia
- Intoxication with sympathomimetics, anticholinergics, theophylline, caffeine, aspirin, or lithium
- Thyroid storm
- Serotonin syndrome
- Neuroleptic malignant syndrome
- Encephalitis
- Meningitis
- Sepsis

DIAGNOSTIC TESTS & INTERPRETATION

Initial Tests (screening, lab, imaging)

Neuroimaging to rule out intracranial pathology may rarely be indicated.

Diagnostic Procedures/Other

- No routine lab tests are indicated for patients with substance withdrawal.
- Tests necessary to rule out differential diagnoses should be obtained when appropriate.

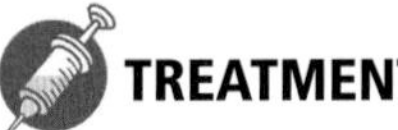

TREATMENT

GENERAL MEASURES

- Initial stabilization
  - Initial management is aimed at evaluating and supporting airway, breathing, circulation, serum glucose, and ECG ("A, B, C, D, E").
- Supportive care is the most important general principle.
- The illness is managed with intent of close monitoring and addressing issues as they arise.

MEDICATION

- In adolescents and probably most children, symptom-triggered treatment is superior to fixed-regimen treatment in terms of patient outcome and length of stay.
- For neonates, a standardized regimen of drug tapering appears to be superior with regard to shorter length of stay.

- Patients with benzodiazepines or barbiturate withdrawal may be treated by reinstituting the drug and then tapering.
- Iatrogenic withdrawal induced by use of opioid antagonists should not be treated by opioid administration.
  - Withdrawal induced by naloxone should abate rapidly due to the brief half-life of naloxone.
  - Withdrawal induced by naltrexone or nalmefene will be much longer lasting. Symptomatic treatment may be indicated.
- There is no fixed quantity of drug to use for any withdrawal syndrome. Each patient requires a unique quantity of drug, and use of 80% of the previous dosing is a useful rough estimate.
  - Repeated dosing should continue until the symptoms are controlled, at which point maintenance and then tapering can occur.
- Sedative-hypnotic withdrawal
  - Ideally, withdrawal is treated with the same class of substance, such as benzodiazepine or barbiturate, if not the precise same drug.
  - Benzodiazepines are particularly useful due to the rapid onset of effect.
  - Diazepam has active metabolites that may assist in tapering the drug in older children and neonates.
  - In neonates, diazepam efficacy is poor.
  - Lorazepam 0.1 mg/kg IV (maximum initial dose 4 mg) may be repeated q30min until symptoms have improved.
  - Propofol is an outstanding medication for treatment of severe alcohol or sedative-hypnotic withdrawal in adults.
    - Propofol may be used in pediatric cases refractory to benzodiazepines and barbiturates.
    - Use is associated with respiratory depression.
    - Clinicians must be capable of airway management and expect airway support to be necessary when propofol is used.
    - Propofol use is safe in children, but rare cases of metabolic acidemia have occurred when prolonged infusions are used. Prolonged use of propofol infusion should be accompanied by close observation for acidemia.
- Opioid withdrawal
  - Heroin (as well as other opioids) withdrawal is best treated with an opioid of similar potency and equal or longer duration of action.
  - Buprenorphine, which has been introduced to pediatric and neonatal practice recently, is extremely promising as therapy for opioid withdrawal.
  - Buprenorphine is a partial opioid agonist, does not cause respiratory depression, and does not result in the pleasurable or euphoric sensation associated with morphine or methadone.
  - Buprenorphine is currently only prescribable by specific clinicians with a special Drug Enforcement Agency (DEA) approval to give this therapy.
  - Methadone is currently a preferred treatment for withdrawal in adolescents and adults.
  - 5 to 10 mg of methadone empirically is an appropriate initial dose to treat adolescents and adults.
  - For neonates, 0.05 mg/kg/dose PO or IV q6h with increase in dose by 0.05 mg/kg until symptoms are controlled, then the dosing interval can be increased to q12–24h
  - Patients who experience opioid withdrawal in the setting of chronic or intensive care may be treated by reinstituting infusion or dosing of the drug they were on before withdrawal symptoms and then tapering this, typically by 10% daily.
- Caffeine withdrawal
  - Caffeine as soft drink or tea taken to treat headache or agitation
  - Neonatal caffeine abstinence symptoms may be treated by reinstituting 75–100% of the caffeine dosage that was discontinued. This amount is then tapered, typically by 10% daily.
- Nicotine withdrawal is not typically treated in children.
- Use of nicotine patch, gum, or other delivery methods is used to increase success rate of abstinence rather than for medical management of the withdrawal syndrome.
- SSRI withdrawal in neonates may be treated with phenobarbital or a benzodiazepine such as diazepam or lorazepam.
  - Lorazepam dosing for SSRI withdrawal is 0.05 mg/kg IV q6h.
  - Phenobarbital dosing for SSRI withdrawal is 2.5 mg/kg/dose q12h. An optional loading dose either IV or PO may be used.
  - The quantity of SSRI excreted in breast milk varies between these medications, but generally, they are in breast milk in low quantities.
  - It is reasonable to permit or recommend breastfeeding for neonates experiencing SSRI withdrawal syndrome, despite medication instruction warnings to avoid breastfeeding.

ISSUES FOR REFERRAL

- Any patient with substance abuse issues should be referred for appropriate psychiatric or drug counseling.
- Most cases of substance withdrawal are best handled by an addiction specialist, medical toxicologist, intensivist, or other clinician experienced with management of withdrawal.

ADMISSION, INPATIENT, AND NURSING CONSIDERATIONS

- Inpatient treatment for alcohol or sedative-hypnotic withdrawal is mandatory.
- Although withdrawal from opioids and SSRIs is not life-threatening, admission with initial management as an inpatient may be preferable.
- Maintenance IV fluid may be required in patients who are unable to take PO.
- Dehydration was once a leading cause of death among patients with alcohol withdrawal.
- Inpatients who have been converted from parenteral to oral medications and are controlled with oral medications may be discharged for home tapering.
- Patients who never require parenteral therapy may be discharged with oral replacement medication after consultation with the appropriate specialist.

ONGOING CARE

FOLLOW-UP RECOMMENDATIONS

- If disposition will be discharge, it is crucial to ensure that the patient's condition is stable before discharge.
- If there is any question regarding whether the patient can be appropriately managed as an outpatient, initial inpatient management is preferable.

Patient Monitoring

- Sedative-hypnotic withdrawal or any other withdrawal syndrome with severe symptoms is best cared for with initial cardiopulmonary monitoring until vital sign abnormalities are controlled with appropriate replacement therapy.
- Patients should be closely monitored until vital signs are within acceptable limits.
- Vigilance for agitation or delirium with sedative-hypnotic withdrawal is necessary.
- Vigilance to detect oversedation and respiratory depression is necessary.

PATIENT EDUCATION

Patients or parents should be aware of withdrawal symptoms to be vigilant for detecting future events.

PROGNOSIS

- With appropriate therapy, withdrawal is well tolerated.
- Poor prognostic factors are primarily related to comorbidities.

COMPLICATIONS

Complications of hypertension, tachycardia, hyperthermia, and CNS agitation or seizure may occur with sedative-hypnotic withdrawal.

ADDITIONAL READING

- Franck LS, Scoppettuolo LA, Wypij D, et al. Validity and generalizability of the Withdrawal Assessment Tool-1 (WAT-1) for monitoring iatrogenic withdrawal syndrome in pediatric patients. *Pain*. 2012;153(1):142–148.
- Galinkin J, Koh JL; for Committee on Drugs, Section on Anesthesiology and Pain Medicine, American Academy of Pediatrics. Recognition of and management of iatrogenically induced opioid dependence and withdrawal in children. *Pediatrics*. 2014;133(1):152–155.
- Hall ES, Isemann BT, Wexelblatt SL, et al. A cohort comparison of buprenorphine versus methadone treatment for neonatal abstinence syndrome. *J Pediatr*. 2016;170:39–44.e1.
- McQueen K, Murphy-Oikonen J. Neonatal abstinence syndrome. *N Engl J Med*. 2016;375(25):2468–2479.
- Nordeng H, Lindeman R, Perminov KV, et al. Neonatal withdrawal syndrome after in utero exposure to selective serotonin reuptake inhibitors. *Acta Paediatr*. 2001;90(3):288–291.

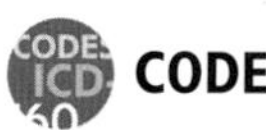

CODES

ICD10

- P96.1 Neonatal w/drawal symp from matern use of drugs of addiction
- P96.2 Withdrawal symptoms from therapeutic use of drugs in newborn
- F13.939 Sedatv/hyp/anxiolytc use, unsp w withdrawal, unsp

ACUTE KIDNEY INJURY

Stuart L. Goldstein, MD

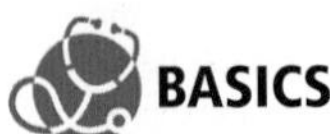

BASICS

DESCRIPTION

- Acute kidney injury (AKI) is defined as an abrupt (within 48 hours) reduction in kidney function with an absolute increase in serum creatinine of more than or equal to 0.3 mg/dL, or a 1.5-fold increase from baseline or a reduction in urine output (documented oliguria of <0.5 mL/kg/h for >6 hours).
- In AKI, the urine output is variable: anuria, oliguria and, in some cases, polyuria can all be observed at presentation.

EPIDEMIOLOGY

- The epidemiology of AKI has changed over the recent years from primary kidney disease to a syndrome secondary to other systemic illness.
- AKI may be seen in up to 10% of all hospitalized children. The incidence is higher in intensive care unit (ICU) admissions and with increasing multiorgan disease severity.
- AKI is seen in 27% of children admitted to an ICU.

PATHOPHYSIOLOGY

The pathogenesis of AKI is multifactorial. It may be initiated by ischemia or toxins, and the subsequent injury involves a complex interplay between vasoconstriction, leukostasis, vascular congestion, cell death, and abnormal immune modulators.

ETIOLOGY

Previously, AKI was subcategorized into three groups: prerenal, renal, and postrenal. The differentiation between "prerenal" and "intrinsic" causes can be difficult because renal hypoperfusion may coexist with any stage of AKI. For that reason "functional" has replaced prerenal and "structural" has replaced intrinsic in the terminology.

- Functional
  - Decreased glomerular filtration rate (GFR) resulting from renal hypoperfusion in a structurally intact kidney
  - Often rapidly reversible when the underlying cause is corrected
- Structural
  - Disorders that directly affect the kidney
  - Acute tubular necrosis (ATN) was used in the past to describe a form of intrinsic AKI from severe and persistent hypoperfusion of the kidneys. However, the histologic diagnosis of tubular necrosis is rarely confirmed by biopsy.
  - Glomerular disorders include the various forms of acute glomerulonephritis (AGN) (e.g., postinfectious, rapidly progressive [crescentic]).
  - Vascular lesions compromise glomerular blood flow. Hemolytic uremic syndrome (HUS) is the most common vascular disorder that causes intrinsic AKI in children.
  - Acute interstitial nephritis (AIN) most often occurs as a result of exposure to medications such as NSAIDs. It may also be associated with infections (e.g., pyelonephritis), systemic diseases, or tumor infiltrates.
- Postrenal
  - Obstructive process (either structural or functional)
  - Obstruction can be in the lower tract or bilaterally in the upper tracts (unless the patient has a single kidney).
  - More common in newborns

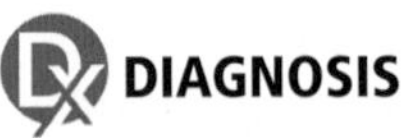

DIAGNOSIS

HISTORY

- Previous infection, neurogenic bladder, single kidney
- Exposure to nonsteroidal anti-inflammatory agents, β-lactam antibiotics, acyclovir, aminoglycosides, amphotericin B, cisplatin
- Gross hematuria: AGN (tea colored), renal calculi (bright red blood)
- Trauma: crush injury
- Signs and symptoms: fever, rash bloody diarrhea, pallor, severe vomiting or diarrhea, abdominal pain hemorrhage, shock, anuria, polyuria

PHYSICAL EXAM

- General: weight and hydration status; shock, edema (calculation of percent fluid overload based on body weight), jaundice
- Lungs: rales
- Heart: gallop
- Abdomen/pelvis: mass
- Skin: rash, petechiae
- Joints: arthritis

DIFFERENTIAL DIAGNOSIS

- Chronic kidney disease: insidious, associated with poor growth, normocytic anemia, hyperparathyroidism
- Azotemia (elevated BUN): hypercatabolic states including corticosteroid therapy or upper GI bleeding
- Elevated creatinine: caused by rhabdomyolysis, drugs (trimethoprim-sulfamethoxazole, cimetidine)

DIAGNOSTIC TESTS & INTERPRETATION

Initial Tests (screening, lab, imaging)

- All patients with AKI should have a urinalysis with microscopic exam, serum chemistries, and a CBC:
  - Urinalysis: specific gravity (>1.020 suggests prerenal AKI), proteinuria (>3+ structural, glomerular AKI), eosinophiluria (AIN), pyuria (pyelonephritis), granular casts (functional, ATN), pigmenturia (ATN), erythrocyte casts (glomerulonephritis, AIN, ATN)
  - Serum chemistries: hyponatremia, acidosis, hyperkalemia, hypocalcemia, hyperphosphatemia
  - CBC: microangiopathic hemolytic anemia, thrombocytopenia (i.e., HUS), eosinophilia (i.e., AIN)
  - Selected patients require further studies, including serologies, urine electrolytes, imaging, and renal biopsy:
    - Serologies: hypocomplementemia, antineutrophil cytoplasmic antibodies, antinuclear antibodies (AGN)
- Fractional excretion of sodium (FE_{Na})
  - Can be useful to assess tubular function; $FE_{Na} = [(U_{Na} / P_{Na}) / (U_{creat} / P_{creat})] \times 100$
  - The FE_{Na} should not be obtained after diuretics are administered; $FE_{Na} > 2$: ATN; $FE_{Na} < 1$: AGN, prerenal
  - FE_{Na} can be <1% despite ATN in case of radiocontrast nephropathy or pigment nephropathy.
- Fractional excretion of urea (FE_{Urea})
  - Less affected by diuretics
  - $FE_{Urea} = [(U_{Urea} / P_{Urea}) / (U_{creat} / P_{creat})] \times 100$
  - $FE_{Urea} < 35$: prerenal AKI; $FE_{Urea} > 50$: ATN
- Chest radiograph: cardiomegaly or pulmonary edema (fluid overload)
- Renal US: hydronephrosis, trabeculated bladder (i.e., obstruction), increased echogenicity (i.e., ATN, AIN, AGN, HUS), abnormal Doppler study (renal venous thrombosis)

Diagnostic Procedures/Other

Renal biopsy: indicated in patients with prolonged, unexplained AKI or suspicion for crescentic glomerulonephritis

TREATMENT

MEDICATION

- Clearance of many medications is impaired in AKI. Careful monitoring of drug dosing and levels can minimize toxicity.
- Low-dose (renal dose) dopamine is ineffective in improving kidney function in AKI. Loop diuretics (furosemide) and osmotic diuretics (mannitol) do not affect the progression or outcome of AKI and may be harmful.
- Bicarbonate may be useful to treat AKI in rhabdomyolysis.
- *N*-Acetylcysteine and bicarbonate, used prophylactically, may prevent contrast nephropathy.

ADDITIONAL THERAPIES

- Supportive
  - Avoid nephrotoxic medications when possible.
  - Monitor electrolytes closely. Avoid drugs, fluids, or foods containing potassium in patients with oliguria or anuria.
  - Hyponatremia is usually due to free water excess and should be managed with fluid restriction. Hypertonic saline should be used only if CNS symptoms are present.
- Fluid management
  - Can be divided into three phases based on the clinical status
  - Fluid resuscitation/repletion: The goal is to restore end-organ perfusion.
  - Fluid balance maintenance: After initial resuscitation, the patient's ongoing fluid needs (blood products, medications, nutrition) should be balanced with the output (urine and insensible losses). Fluid restriction may be needed to avoid worsening fluid overload. Increasing degrees of fluid overload (%FO) at initiation of renal replacement therapy (RRT) are independently associated with mortality.
  - Fluid overload may be calculated as:
    - $\%FO = (\text{Fluid Input [L]} - \text{Fluid Output [L]}) / \text{Patient ICU admission weight (kg)} \times 100$
  - Fluid removal/recovery: If the fluid conservative strategy does not work, RRT may be needed to remove the volumes associated with patient needs.
- RRT is indicated for fluid overload, refractory acidosis, severe hyperkalemia, and uremic symptoms (e.g., pericarditis, lethargy, bleeding diathesis). The modality of RRT (hemodialysis or continuous RRT) depends on the hemodynamic status of the patient.
- Provision of adequate nutrition is essential due to the high prevalence of malnutrition in this group and the associated morbidity and mortality. Protein restriction with the aim of delaying RRT is not recommended.
- Specific treatment based on etiology: Each cause of AKI may necessitate specific treatment, such as fluid resuscitation (i.e., renal hypoperfusion), urologic intervention (i.e., obstruction), and corticosteroids (i.e., AIN, some forms of AGN).

ADMISSION, INPATIENT, AND NURSING CONSIDERATIONS

- If hypovolemic, rapidly establish euvolemia with 0.9% NS or balanced solution boluses.
- If urine output remains low after euvolemia is established, begin fluid restriction (insensible losses and urine output).
- In severe hyperkalemia (>6.5 mEq/L), consider the following:
  - Calcium gluconate (100 mg Ca gluconate salt/kg IV) over 5 to 10 minutes if symptomatic
  - Glucose (0.5 g/kg) and insulin (0.1 U/kg) IV over 30 minutes
  - Sodium bicarbonate (1 to 2 mEq/kg) IV over 10 to 30 minutes if acidotic
  - When administering sodium bicarbonate, monitor serum calcium carefully because the hypocalcemia may worsen.
  - Sodium polystyrene sulfonate (Kayexalate) (1 g/kg) PO or PR in sorbitol; avoid use of sorbitol-containing products in the presence of risk for colonic necrosis, GI bleeding, ischemic colitis, and GI perforation.
  - Furosemide (1 to 2 mg/kg) if renal function is adequate
  - RRT

ONGOING CARE

FOLLOW-UP RECOMMENDATIONS

- The likelihood of recovery from AKI depends on the underlying cause.
- AKI may result in full recovery or incomplete recovery leading to chronic kidney disease. In severe cases, nonrecovery may lead to end-stage renal disease.
- Long-term follow-up to monitor renal function is recommended.

PROGNOSIS

The mortality rate increases in patients with multisystem organ failure despite good supportive care. AKI is independently associated with increased mortality in ICU patients.

COMPLICATIONS

- A significant postobstructive diuresis can be seen after treatment for obstructive AKI.
- Fluid overload, resulting in congestive heart failure, hypertension, or hyponatremia
- Hyperkalemia, affecting cardiac function by causing arrhythmias
- Uremia, manifest by mental status changes, increased risk of bleeding, and infection
- Metabolic acidosis
- Hypocalcemia, causing tetany

ADDITIONAL READING

- Fortenberry JD, Paden ML, Goldstein SL. Acute kidney injury in children: an update on diagnosis and treatment. *Pediatr Clin North Am*. 2013;60(3):669–688.
- Kaddourah A, Basu RK, Baghsaw SM, et al; for AWARE Investigators. Epidemiology of acute kidney injury in ill children and young adults. *N Eng J Med*. 2017;376:11–20.
- Kidney Disease: Improving Global Outcomes. KDIGO clinical practice guideline for acute kidney injury. *Kidney Int Suppl*. 2012;2(1):1–138.
- Singri N, Ahya SN, Levin ML. Acute renal failure. *JAMA*. 2003;289(6):747–751.
- Zappitelli M. Epidemiology and diagnosis of acute kidney injury. *Semin Nephrol*. 2008;28(5):436–446.

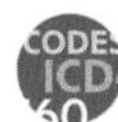

CODES

ICD10

- N17.9 Acute kidney failure, unspecified
- N17.0 Acute kidney failure with tubular necrosis
- N00.9 Acute nephritic syndrome with unsp morphologic changes

FAQ

- Q: What is the expected recovery time in patients with AKI who present with anuria?
- A: Recovery time depends on the etiology of the AKI. Children with HUS may recover in days to weeks. In severe HUS or AKI requiring RRT, ongoing recovery to new, baseline renal function occurs over several months. Those with ATN recover days after treatment for the cause. Children with AKI secondary to an obstructive process usually recover as soon as the obstruction is removed.
- Q: When should renal function return to normal?
- A: Renal function may never return to normal in patients with long-standing anuria. In other cases, after recovery occurs, serum creatinine levels return to normal within weeks.
- Q: Which indices should be observed after a patient recovers from AKI?
- A: Patients recovering from AKI should have renal function (serum creatinine and cystatin C), BP, and urinalysis for proteinuria monitored regularly.

ACUTE LIVER FAILURE

Shreena Patel, MD • K. Lynette Van Buren, MD, MEd • Eric H. Chiou, MD

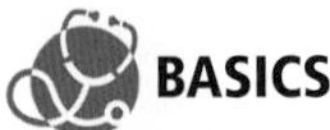

BASICS

DESCRIPTION

- A set of criteria has been proposed to diagnose pediatric acute liver failure (ALF).
  - Biochemical evidence of liver injury due to rapid loss of hepatocyte function
  - No previous history of chronic liver disease
  - Coagulopathy not responsive to vitamin K administration
  - International normalized ratio (INR) >1.5 in presence of encephalopathy or INR >2 without encephalopathy
- In older children, in whom hepatic encephalopathy can be more easily assessed, ALF may more simply be defined as follows:
  - Onset of encephalopathy <8 weeks after the onset of symptoms referable to liver dysfunction in a patient without preexisting liver disease

EPIDEMIOLOGY

- Exact frequency of ALF in children is unknown but accounts for 10–15% of pediatric liver transplants in the United States annually.
- In infants and children <3 years of age, indeterminate and metabolic etiologies predominate.
- In older children, drug-induced toxicity (especially acetaminophen), autoimmune hepatitis become more common.
- Infectious etiologies (e.g., viral hepatitis) vary in prevalence based on geographic region.

PATHOPHYSIOLOGY

- Hepatocellular necrosis leads to release of growth factors that promote hepatic regeneration.
- Hepatic failure may become irreversible if:
  - The initial insult overcomes the liver's regenerative capacity.
  - The offending agent or derangement is not eliminated or corrected.
  - Secondary complications, such as shock or disseminated intravascular coagulation, lead to further injury.

ETIOLOGY

The major causes of ALF can be grouped into the following broad categories:

- Indeterminate
- Drug-induced/toxin
- Metabolic/genetic
- Infectious
- Vascular/ischemic
- Malignancy
- Immune dysregulation

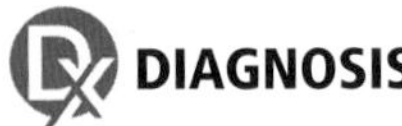

DIAGNOSIS

HISTORY

- Age: may suggest possible etiologic subgroup
- Toxin exposure: prescription, over-the-counter, herbal, or supplemental medications
- Symptoms of viral prodrome (fever)
- Travel history, exposure history
- Length of symptoms, acuity of onset
- History of developmental delay or seizures may suggest metabolic defect.
- Associated symptoms/ROS:
  - Jaundice, bleeding, bruising
  - Weakness, fatigue
  - Abdominal distension, pain, diarrhea
  - Pruritus secondary to cholestasis
  - Change in mental status

PHYSICAL EXAM

- Skin: jaundice, bruising
- Eyes: scleral icterus
- Abdomen: hepatomegaly, ascites with dullness to percussion or fluid wave, splenomegaly
- Neurologic
  - Sequential mental status exams are paramount to monitor for change and should include age-appropriate questions.
  - Assess for presence of encephalopathy:
    - Grade I: confused, altered sleep; reflexes normal, may have tremor or apraxia
    - Grade II: drowsy, inappropriate behavior; hyperreflexic or asterixis; dysarthria or ataxia
    - Grade III: stupor but may obey simple commands, sleepy; hyperreflexic, asterixis, Babinski-positive; increased general tone
    - Grade IV: comatose; reflexes absent; decerebrate or decorticate posturing

DIFFERENTIAL DIAGNOSIS

The cause of ALF can be indeterminate in up to 50% of cases across all age groups. Etiologic subgroups include the following:

- Intrinsic hepatotoxins and idiosyncratic hepatotoxic effects:
  - Acetaminophen: most common in older children and adolescents
  - Salicylates, iron compounds, anticonvulsants, antibiotics
  - Recreational drugs (cocaine, MDMA)
  - *Amanita* species (mushrooms)
- Metabolic/genetic/misc: early infancy
  - Galactosemia, tyrosinemia
  - Gestational alloimmune liver disease (neonatal hemochromatosis)
  - Storage diseases
  - Mitochondrial disorders
  - Fatty acid oxidation disorders
  - Hereditary fructose intolerance
  - α_1-antitrypsin deficiency
- Metabolic/genetic/misc: older children
  - Autoimmune hepatitis
  - Wilson disease
  - Pregnancy (HELLP syndrome, AFL)
  - Reye syndrome
- Infectious
  - Hepatitis virus: A, B, E; less commonly C
  - Herpes virus: HSV, EBV, CMV, VZV, HHV6
  - Echovirus, especially in neonates
  - Parvovirus, adenovirus
- Vascular/ischemic
  - Congestive heart failure
  - Hypotensive shock
  - Budd-Chiari syndrome: hepatic venous outflow obstruction
  - Venoocclusive disease: Nonthrombotic occlusion of hepatic venules typically occurs following stem cell transplantation.
- Malignancy
  - Primary: hepatoblastoma, hepatocellular carcinoma
  - Other: leukemia, lymphoma, hemophagocytic lymphohistiocytosis
- Heatstroke, hyperthermia, rhabdomyolysis

DIAGNOSTIC TESTS & INTERPRETATION

Initial Tests (screening, lab, imaging)

- Abdominal ultrasound with Doppler: visualization of both hepatic parenchyma and vasculature (direction of portal flow, presence of thrombosis)
- Head CT scan without IV contrast in presence of encephalopathy or neurologic signs to rule out intracranial hemorrhage or cerebral edema

Diagnostic Procedures/Other

- Initial laboratory testing
  - Hepatocellular injury: aminotransferases (AST, ALT) often markedly elevated; degree of elevation may depend on mechanism and time frame of injury.
  - Biliary injury/obstruction: elevated alkaline phosphatase, γ-glutamyl transpeptidase (GGT), total/conjugated bilirubin
  - General labs: CBC with differential, electrolytes, glucose, blood urea nitrogen and creatinine, amylase/lipase
- Assessment of synthetic function
  - Prolonged PT/INR (with adequate supply of vitamin K)
  - Depressed factors V, VII levels
  - Hypoalbuminemia
  - Hypoglycemia: Frequent glucose measurements should be followed during initial evaluation and with any mental status or neurologic change.
- Encephalopathy: ammonia level (has not been proven to correlate directly to presence or grade of encephalopathy)
- Tests to determine etiology
  - Testing priority should be guided by the age group and population and for conditions amenable to specific therapies.
  - Toxin: urine or serum drug screen, serum acetaminophen and aspirin levels
  - Infectious: hepatitis virus serologic testing, comprehensive viral cultures; PCR testing for EBV, CMV, HSV, and other viruses; antibody tests
  - Autoimmune hepatitis: antinuclear, anti–smooth muscle/F-actin, anti-LKM antibodies, total IgG
  - Wilson disease: decreased serum ceruloplasmin (may not be reliable in setting of ALF), increased serum or urinary copper, Coombs-negative hemolytic anemia
  - Pregnancy test in adolescent females
  - Metabolic: urine succinylacetone, reducing substances, and organic acids; plasma amino acids, acylcarnitine profile, lactate/pyruvate, creatinine kinase; newborn screen
  - α_1-antitrypsin deficiency: Pi type
  - Hemophagocytic lymphohistiocytosis: ≥2 cytopenias, elevated ferritin, elevated triglycerides, and low fibrinogen
  - Gestational alloimmune liver disease (neonatal hemochromatosis): severe hypoglycemia and coagulopathy, elevated ferritin with near-normal aminotransferase; evidence of iron deposition on buccal biopsy or abdominal MRI
- Liver biopsy: generally, not considered critical for management or diagnosis due to substantial risks of hemorrhage. Transjugular approach may reduce risks. May be appropriate to attempt to identify a specific etiology that may influence treatment strategy (e.g., Wilson disease). Severity of necrosis may not predict potential liver recovery.

TREATMENT

GENERAL MEASURES

- Close monitoring, preferably in an ICU setting with a liver transplant program
- General supportive care:
  - Fluid restriction: 75–95% of maintenance requirements to prevent worsening of portal hypertension, ascites, and pulmonary edema
  - Sodium restriction: Patients should typically not receive >0.25 NS as maintenance fluids. A total sodium intake of 1 mEq/kg/24 h is usually adequate. Hyponatremia should not be corrected with hypertonic saline, as this can worsen fluid overload and encephalopathy.
  - Glucose infusion: Maintenance fluid typically should include 10% dextrose; glucose infusion may need to be increased to maintain serum glucose between 90 and 110 mg/dL.
  - Nutrition: Adequate nutrition should be maintained either via enteral route or TPN.
  - Blood products should be given slowly to avoid rapid expansion of intravascular space.
  - Minimize invasive catheterization when possible due to infection risk.

MEDICATION

- Hematologic
  - Vitamin K: Administer IV or SQ/IM for prolonged PT/INR, and monitor response with repeat PT/INR 4 to 6 hours afterward.
  - PT and INR however are not good markers for risk of bleeding in ALF due to decreased production of both procoagulant and anticoagulant proteins.
  - FFP and cryoprecipitate should be reserved for acute severe bleeding or prior to invasive procedure; their use prohibits subsequent monitoring of PT/INR or specific factor levels.
  - Recombinant factor VIIa can be used in cases of acute severe bleeding.
- Neurologic/hepatic encephalopathy
  - Sedatives, especially benzodiazepines, should be avoided, as they may worsen encephalopathy.
  - Lactulose (oral, enema forms) should be used if encephalopathy present; goal is to acidify stool (pH <6) and increase frequency of stool but not cause diarrhea.
  - Oral or rectal administration of antibiotics (neomycin, rifaximin) may be effective by reducing ammonia production in the gut.
  - Restriction of protein intake to no more than 1 g/kg/24 h may help reduce ammonia production.
  - Elevated arterial ammonia levels may help predict development of encephalopathy and intracranial hypertension.
- Infectious disease
  - Prophylactic antibiotics and antifungal medications if febrile, after obtaining cultures from any central venous access or catheterization
- Renal
  - Nephrotoxic drugs should be avoided when possible. Diuretics should be used with caution; renally dose medications if renal compromise present
  - Renal replacement therapy as indicated
- Other:
  - *N*-acetylcysteine is the treatment for acetaminophen-induced hepatic toxicity.
  - Plasma exchange may be helpful for removal of copper in Wilson disease.
  - IV acid suppression should be considered.
  - Removal of offending agent when identified

SURGERY/OTHER PROCEDURES

- Those more likely to require liver transplantation include children with ALF secondary to indeterminate cause, idiosyncratic drug toxicity, hepatic vein thrombosis, or Wilson disease.
- Transplant-free survival >50% for ALF due to acetaminophen, hepatitis A, shock liver or pregnancy-related disease, whereas all other etiologies have <25% transplant-free survival.
- Currently, artificial liver support systems, such as molecular adsorbent recirculating system (MARS) are not recommended outside of clinical trials.

ADMISSION, INPATIENT, AND NURSING CONSIDERATIONS

- Initial evaluation should include assessment of neurologic status.
- Elective intubation as well as ICP monitoring should be considered in grade III or IV encephalopathy with somnolence.
- Aggressive initial fluid resuscitation should be avoided unless there is evidence of hemodynamic compromise.
- Central venous access should be considered to allow for higher glucose infusion rates and for central nutrition.

ONGOING CARE

PROGNOSIS

- Etiology of ALF provides good indicator of prognosis and also dictates management.
- One half of pediatric ALF patients will die or receive liver transplant.
- Existing liver failure scoring systems based on biochemical markers (e.g., INR) and/or clinical features, including the King's College Hospital Criteria, have not been shown to be useful for predicting survival or death in pediatric ALF.
- Decisions for liver transplantation in pediatric ALF are often challenging due to uncertainty of diagnosis and possibility of spontaneous recovery, potential morbidity/mortality of the transplant procedure itself, and the limited number of organs available.
- Overall 1-year survival following liver transplant is lower in patients transplanted for ALF compared to chronic liver failure; however, after the 1st year, this trend is reversed and ALF patients have better long-term survival.

COMPLICATIONS

- Complications are a direct consequence of loss of hepatic metabolic function:
  - Hepatic encephalopathy: decreased elimination of neurotoxins or depressants
  - Cerebral edema: pathogenesis incompletely understood
  - Coagulopathy: failure of hepatic synthesis of clotting and fibrinolytic factors
  - Hypoglycemia: impaired glucose synthesis and release, decreased degradation of insulin
  - Acidosis: failure to eliminate lactic acid or free fatty acids
  - Hepatorenal syndrome: typically, low urine sodium and no improvement with volume expansion; continuous venovenous hemofiltration or dialysis may be necessary.
- In cases of suspected hepatic encephalopathy, consider other etiologies of neurologic change including hypoglycemia, intracranial hemorrhage, acute infection, or sepsis.
- There is often rapid progression through the stages of encephalopathy. Increased intracranial pressure can develop quickly and can lead to irreversible neurologic sequelae.

ADDITIONAL READING

- Bass NM, Mullen KD, Sanyal A, et al. Rifaximin treatment in hepatic encephalopathy. *N Engl J Med*. 2010;362(12):1071–1081.
- Bucuvalas J, Yazigi N, Squires RH Jr. Acute liver failure in children. *Clin Liver Dis*. 2006;10(1):149–168.
- Kortsalioudaki C, Taylor RM, Cheeseman P, et al. Safety and efficacy of N-acetylcysteine in children with non-acetaminophen-induced acute liver failure. *Liver Transpl*. 2008;14(1):25–30.
- Lee WM, Stravitz RT, Larson AM. Introduction to the revised American Association for the Study of Liver Diseases Position Paper on acute liver failure 2011. *Hepatology*. 2012;55(3):965–967.
- Li R, Belle SH, Horslen S, et al; for Pediatric Acute Liver Failure Study Group. Clinical course among cases of acute liver failure of indeterminate diagnosis. *J Pediatr*. 2016;171:163–170.e3.
- Miyake Y, Sakaguchi K, Iwasaki Y, et al. New prognostic scoring model for liver transplantation in patients with non-acetaminophen-related fulminant hepatic failure. *Transplantation*. 2005;80(7):930–936.
- Squires RH Jr, Shneider BL, Bucuvalas J, et al. Acute liver failure in children: the first 348 patients in the pediatric acute liver failure study group. *J Pediatr*. 2006;148(5):652–658.
- Sundaram SS, Alonso EM, Narkewicz MR, et al; and Pediatric Acute Liver Failure Study Group. Characterization and outcomes of young infants with acute liver failure. *J Pediatr*. 2011;159(5):813–818.

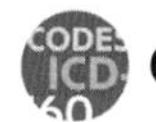

CODES

ICD10

- K72.00 Acute and subacute hepatic failure without coma
- K71.10 Toxic liver disease with hepatic necrosis, without coma

FAQ

- Q: What are the most common causes of ALF in infants?
- A: Up to 40–50% of cases are indeterminate, followed by neonatal hemochromatosis, viral infection, and metabolic disorders.
- Q: What is the risk of bleeding in ALF-associated coagulopathy?
- A: Spontaneous, clinically significant bleeding in ALF is generally rare, despite abnormal INR. Thromboelastography (TEG), which assesses overall hemostasis including the cumulative effects of procoagulant and anticoagulant proteins, fibrinogen, platelets, and red blood cells, may be a better guide for administration of blood products in ALF than INR.
- Q: Is the initial level of elevation of transaminases directly correlated to the prognosis of patient?
- A: No. In viral hepatitis and acetaminophen toxicity, initial transaminases can be in 1,000s, but patients can have complete recovery.

ACUTE LYMPHOBLASTIC LEUKEMIA

Monica Zlotnicki, MD • Caroline Hastings, MD

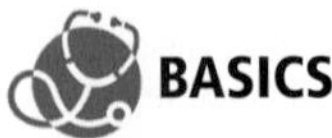

BASICS

DESCRIPTION

- Acute lymphoblastic leukemia (ALL) is a hematopoietic malignancy that results from malignant proliferation of immature WBC (B cells and T cells).
- Risk group classification:
  - Infant ALL: age <1 year
  - Standard risk ALL: age 1 to <10 years; initial WBC count <50,000/μL
  - High-risk ALL: age ≥10 years; WBC ≥50,000/μL
- Further risk stratification done based on multiple factors including National Cancer Institute (NCI) criteria (age and WBC count), biologic, cytogenetic characteristics, and response to initial therapy. This classification determines the intensity of therapy and prognosis.
  - Low-risk ALL: NCI standard risk group
    - Favorable cytogenetic changes (hyperdiploidy, double trisomies of 4, 10, *ETV6/RUNX1* fusion)
    - Pre–B lymphoblasts and negative minimal residual disease (MRD = number of leukemic cells detected by flow cytometry in bone marrow) at end of induction
  - Average-risk ALL: NCI standard risk group
    - Noncontributory cytogenetics
    - Negative MRD at end of induction (<0.01%)
    - No extramedullary (CNS or testicular) involvement, CNS 1
    - Negative MRD at end of induction
  - High-risk ALL: NCI high-risk group
    - Age >10 years regardless of WBC count, extramedullary (CNS 2, 3, or testicular) involvement
    - T-cell phenotype
    - No or very low MRD at end of induction
  - Very high-risk ALL
    - Unfavorable cytogenetics (t[9;22] Philadelphia-positive ALL)
    - Hypodiploidy
    - *MLL* gene rearrangement, iAMP21
    - Induction failure (>25% lymphoblasts in bone marrow at end of induction)
    - Positive MRD at the end of induction (>0.01%)
  - Other prognostic factors
    - Steroid pretreatment (poor)
    - Down syndrome (poor)
    - Evidence of CNS or testicular disease (poor)

EPIDEMIOLOGY

- ALL is the most common childhood malignancy.
- Accounts for approximately 35% of cancer in children
- More common in Caucasians and males
- ALL incidence: 3 to 4 cases per 100,000 per year
- Peak incidence is between ages 2 and 5 years.

RISK FACTORS

- Prior cancer therapy (chemotherapy or radiation)
- Twin with ALL
- Genetic syndrome listed in the following sections

Genetics

- Increased risk of leukemia, higher with monozygotic twin
- Associated genetic syndromes
  - Trisomy 21 (Down syndrome)
  - Fanconi anemia
  - Bloom syndrome
  - Shwachman-Diamond syndrome
  - Ataxia telangiectasia
  - Diamond-Blackfan anemia
- Neurofibromatosis type 1
- Li-Fraumeni syndrome (a familial cancer syndrome due to *P53* gene mutation)
- Congenital immunodeficiencies (Wiskott-Aldrich syndrome)

PATHOPHYSIOLOGY

- Leukemia arises from lymphoid progenitor cells that have sustained multiple specific genetic damages that lead to malignant transformation and proliferation, lack of cell maturation, and resistance to normal cell death processes (apoptosis).
- This lymphoblastic proliferation replaces the normal bone marrow precursor cells, causing ineffective hematopoiesis and infiltration of lymphatic tissue and end organs.

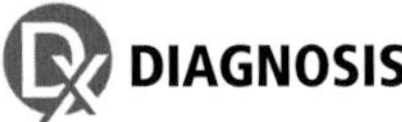

DIAGNOSIS

- Clinical features due to direct invasion of the bone marrow:
  - Pancytopenia: anemia, thrombocytopenia, leukopenia, and/or neutropenia
  - Anemia: irritability, fatigue, anorexia, headache, pallor
  - Thrombocytopenia: Bleeding is usually mild and manifests as petechiae, bruising, gingival oozing, epistaxis.
- Fever: may be a sign of presumed cytokine release or underlying infection due to neutropenia and immunosuppression
- Bone pain
  - Typically long bones
  - Could be due to direct leukemic infiltration of the periosteum or expansion of marrow cavity by leukemic cells
  - Pathologic fractures, leukemic lines on plain radiographs, or T2-weighted changes on MRI
- Testicular involvement (2–5% of the boys, more in T-cell ALL), unilateral or bilateral painless testicular enlargement
- CNS involvement (2–5% of patients on presentation for B-cell ALL, 10–15% for T-cell ALL)
  - Increased intracranial pressure (morning headache, vomiting, lethargy, visual changes, seizures, CN VI palsy, diplopia, and esotropia)
- Superior vena cava (SVC) syndrome (due to a mediastinal mass)
  - Swelling of the face, neck, chest, and, rarely, upper arms with or without visual venous distension, cough, dyspnea, dysphagia
- Leukostasis (large number of deformable blasts plugging the microcirculation)
  - Respiratory symptoms: dyspnea, hypoxia
  - Neurologic symptoms: visual changes, headache, dizziness, tinnitus, lethargy
  - Rare symptoms including renal insufficiency, priapism, acute limb ischemia
- Spinal cord compression (due to a chloroma, an extramedullary collection of lymphoblasts): extremity weakness, numbness, and tingling

PHYSICAL EXAM

- Pallor (anemia)
- Tachycardia/murmurs (anemia)
- Lymphadenopathy (leukemic infiltration)
- Hepatosplenomegaly (leukemic infiltration)
- Testicular enlargement (leukemic infiltration)
- Bone: tenderness, fracture (marrow infiltration)
- Skin: bruises, petechiae, rash in form of subcutaneous nodules (leukemia cutis, most commonly seen in infants)
- Mouth sores (related to neutropenia)
- Papilledema (CNS involvement)
- Focal neurologic signs (CNS involvement, chloroma)

DIFFERENTIAL DIAGNOSIS

- Infectious: infectious mononucleosis, Epstein-Barr virus (EBV), pertussis, parapertussis, parvovirus; cytomegalovirus (CMV), acute infectious lymphocytosis
- Juvenile idiopathic arthritis
- Hematologic: immune thrombocytopenic purpura (ITP), aplastic anemia, Evans syndrome (ITP and autoimmune hemolytic anemia)
- Malignant disorders: round blue cell tumors with bone marrow involvement (neuroblastoma, rhabdomyosarcoma, Langerhans cell histiocytosis, lymphoma, retinoblastoma), myelodysplastic syndrome (MDS), acute myeloid leukemia (AML), chronic myeloid leukemia (CML)

DIAGNOSTIC TESTS & INTERPRETATION

Initial Tests (screening, lab, imaging)

- CBC
  - Increased or decreased WBC (50% present with WBC <10,000/μL and 20% present with WBC ≥50,000/μL)
  - Anemia: Hgb <10 g/dL (80% of cases)
  - Thrombocytopenia (platelets <100,000/μL in 75% at presentation)
  - Peripheral smear: may see circulating lymphoblasts, especially with high WBC (>10,000/μL)
- Serum chemistry
  - Signs of tumor lysis: elevated uric acid, hyperkalemia, hyperphosphatemia (with secondary hypocalcemia), elevated lactate dehydrogenase (LDH)
  - Elevated liver enzymes (leukemic infiltrate)
  - Elevated creatinine (due to uric acid/calcium phosphate crystal deposition in renal tubules or leukemic infiltrates)
- CXR: mediastinal mass (5–10% of cases)
- Plain films of long bones in case of bone pain/tenderness may show leukemic lines.

Diagnostic Procedures/Other

- Bone marrow aspirate and biopsy (presence of ≥25% blasts consistent with diagnosis of leukemia). Immunophenotyping and cytochemistry is then used to differentiate ALL from AML and identify T-cell or B-cell phenotype.
- Lumbar puncture is also performed for CSF analysis for lymphoblasts.
- Immunophenotyping
  - B cell: CD 10+, 19+, 20+, 22+, TdT+
  - Pre–T cell: CD 3+, 5+, 7+, TdT+
  - Myeloid markers: CD 13+, 33+, 34+ (in minority)
  - CNS 1: no detectable blasts
  - CNS 2: <5 WBC/μL, blasts present (higher risk)
  - CNS 3: ≥5 WBC/μL and blasts or symptoms of CNS leukemia (higher risk)

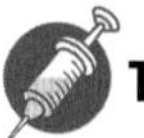

TREATMENT

- Patient suspected with ALL must be referred to a pediatric oncologist as soon as possible for further evaluation and management.
- Initial emergent stabilization may be required in case of
  - Hyperleukocytosis, defined as a WBC $\geq$100,000/μL
  - Tumor lysis syndrome with renal insufficiency
  - Spinal cord compression
- Mediastinal mass causing SVC syndrome
- Therapy is aimed at inducing permanent biologic and clinical remission and is divided into various phases. Many children and adolescents are enrolled on.
- Clinical trials through the Children's Oncology Group or local institution. Treatment is standardized by prognostic indicators and provided by highly specialized teams with expertise in childhood cancer.
  - Induction (first 28 to 35 days); typically includes the following drugs:
    - A glucocorticoid (prednisone or dexamethasone)
    - Vincristine
    - PEG L-asparaginase
    - Anthracycline (in high-risk patients only)
    - Intrathecal chemotherapy (initial dose of cytarabine; subsequent treatment with methotrexate) with two additional IT doses if CNS 2
  - Consolidation (28 days): focuses on CNS prophylaxis; weekly intrathecal chemotherapy with
    - Low/average-risk patients: weekly vincristine, oral 6-mercaptopurine (6-MP), PEG L-asparaginase, intensified with cyclophosphamide and cytarabine in certain subsets of patients
    - High-risk patients: more intensive systemic therapy with cyclophosphamide, cytarabine, methotrexate, vincristine, and PEG L-asparaginase
    - Patients with initial involvement of the CNS or testes may receive radiation during this phase.
  - Interim maintenance (56 days): similar to maintenance therapy but more intensified
    - Vincristine, methotrexate, PEG L-asparaginase
    - Intrathecal methotrexate
  - Delayed intensification (56 days): (reintensification and reconsolidation)
    - Combination of intensive therapy similar to induction and consolidation
  - Maintenance: continuation of therapy (lasts for 2 to 3 years)
    - Daily 6-MP, weekly oral methotrexate, pulse glucocorticoids, and vincristine with periodic intrathecal chemotherapy
    - The course of maintenance is longer for boys than girls.
- Length of treatment from 2 to 3.5 years, depending on protocol and gender
- Ph+ patients t(9;21) receive continuous tyrosine kinase inhibitors (imatinib or dasatinib).
- Patients with CNS and/or testicular involvement receive radiation therapy. Those with CNS disease also receive additional intrathecal chemotherapy in addition to radiation. Although this is still standard of care with CNS 3 disease, studies are being performed to include more CNS-directed therapy to replace radiation therapy.
- T-cell ALL with high WBC count are at high risk for relapse and receive radiation.
- Patients with Down syndrome and ALL have increased treatment-related morbidity and mortality and require some treatment modifications.
- Very high-risk or relapsed patients may be treated with bone marrow transplant (BMT), following remission induction.
- Therapies in clinical trial
  - Blinatumomab—anti-CD19 monoclonal antibody being studied in relapsed ALL
  - Rituximab—anti-CD20 monoclonal antibody being studied in relapsed ALL
  - Nelarabine—purine analog being studied relapsed ALL
  - Immunotherapy: studies have shown that engineered T cells (chimeric antigen receptor [CAR] modified T cells) can be used to treat leukemia.

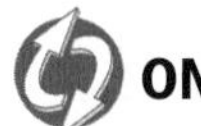

ONGOING CARE

FOLLOW-UP RECOMMENDATIONS

Early intensification has led to an increase in relapse-free survival.

Patient Monitoring

After completion of therapy:

- CBC, complete metabolic panel with LDH, liver and renal function tests every month for the 1st year, every 2 months for the 2nd year, every 3 months for the 3rd year, every 6 months for the 4th year, and yearly thereafter
- Cardiac evaluation every year, dependent on cumulative dose of anthracycline and possible radiation scatter
- Endocrine evaluation close to puberty, especially in children who have received cranial or testicular radiation
- Monitor for late effects in cancer survivor's clinic.

PROGNOSIS

Long-term event free survival

- Overall: approaches 90%
- Low-risk patients: 90–95%
- Standard risk group: 85%
- High-risk group: 60–75%
- Very high-risk group: ~20–50%
- Infant group: 50%
- B-cell ALL: ~85%
- T-cell ALL: ~75%

COMPLICATIONS

- Bone marrow suppression (anemia and thrombocytopenia requiring transfusion support)
- Possible transfusion-related infection or iron overload
- Neutropenia leading to increased risk of infection
- L-asparaginase: anaphylaxis, pancreatitis, thrombosis, stroke
- Anthracyclines (daunorubicin and doxorubicin): cardiac toxicity, secondary AML
- Intrathecal methotrexate: neurotoxicity (frequently reversible)
- Steroids: avascular necrosis of bone, decreased bone density, mood instability
- Radiation: growth retardation, learning difficulties and/or cognitive impairment, increased risk of secondary malignancies
- Testicular radiation: lack of pubertal development, sterility
- Relapse
  - Approximately 15–20% of children and adolescents with ALL will relapse, usually within 5 years of diagnosis.
  - If relapse occurs while the patient is receiving therapy and in bone marrow, outcomes are poor (<20%) even with systemic retreatment and possible BMT.
  - If relapse occurs >36 months from diagnosis or is isolated to an extramedullary site such as the CNS or testis, survival is improved to 40–70% with systemic chemotherapy and possible focal radiation therapy.

ADDITIONAL READING

- Cooper SL, Brown PA. Treatment of pediatric acute lymphoblastic leukemia. *Pediatr Clin North Am*. 2015;62(1):61–73.
- Hunger SP, Loh ML, Whitlock JA, et al. Children's Oncology Group's 2013 blueprint for research: acute lymphoblastic leukemia. *Pediatr Blood Cancer*. 2013;60(6):957–963.
- Hunger SP, Mullighan CG. Acute lymphoblastic leukemia in children. *N Engl J Med*. 2015;373(16): 1541–1552.

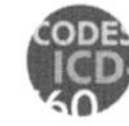

CODES

ICD10

- C91.00 Acute lymphoblastic leukemia not having achieved remission
- C91.01 Acute lymphoblastic leukemia, in remission
- C91.02 Acute lymphoblastic leukemia, in relapse

FAQ

- Q: Can a child on treatment for ALL go to school or leave the house?
- A: Yes. Most centers encourage the child to live a normal life, including school, activities, and travel.
- Q: Will hair fall out and will the child be sick for ALL 3 years on chemotherapy?
- A: The hair usually falls out within a few weeks of initiating therapy and grows back when maintenance therapy begins (6 to 8 months). Most children feel relatively well during therapy, especially maintenance chemotherapy, and can resume a lot of normal activities.
- Q: Does the child need to be isolated from other children?
- A: The most serious infections a child on chemotherapy gets come from bacteria that the child is already colonized with, not community-acquired viruses. That being said, the child should be isolated from any child who has varicella or other known symptomatic infection.
- Q: What should I tell the family if they develop a fever at home during therapy?
- A: This is an oncologic emergency. Direct them to present to the nearest emergency room, where a CBC with differential should be assessed. Blood culture should be drawn and antibiotics started. Alert their primary oncology team at their treatment center for further management recommendations.
- Q: What else should I be monitoring when I am seeing a survivor of ALL in my clinic?
- A: There is a high prevalence of issues with concentration and school performance. Many kids require evaluation for 504 and individualized education program (IEP) plans. Thus, monitoring for school performance status at visits is warranted.
  - Due to steroid exposure: Weight and height should be monitored. Evaluate for orthopedic issues as well as avascular necrosis, decreased bone density.
  - These children are at risk for secondary malignancies possibly related to therapy (including radiation) including hematologic (AML, MDS, CML, Hodgkin), CNS tumors, and other tumors (bone, melanoma, germ cell, thyroid).

ACUTE MYELOID LEUKEMIA

Allison M. Ast, MD

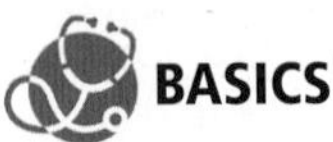

BASICS

DESCRIPTION

- Acute myeloid leukemia (AML) results from a block in differentiation and unregulated proliferation of myeloid progenitor cells.
- AML is classified according to the World Health Organization (WHO) classification (2008).
- Formerly classified by French-American-British (FAB) classification
- WHO classification is based on genetic alterations, whereas FAB is based on morphology.

EPIDEMIOLOGY

- AML is the seventh most common pediatric malignancy.
- Leukemia that occurs in first 4 weeks of life is usually AML.
- Ratio of AML to acute lymphoblastic leukemia (ALL) throughout childhood is 1:5.
- Boys and girls are equally affected.
- Rates are highest in Asian and Pacific Islanders followed by Hispanics, Caucasians, and African Americans.
- AML incidence peaks in infants <1 year of age and again in children 10 to 14 years of age.
- Around 500 children per year in the United States

RISK FACTORS

Genetics

- 20–30% of pediatric blast cells have normal karyotype versus 40–50% in adults.
- 60% of abnormal karyotypes fall into known subgroups.
- Translocations or duplications of the *MLL* gene at 11q23 or monosomy 7 carry a poor prognosis.
- These genetic abnormalities are found in many cases of therapy-induced AML.
- FLT3-ITD with high allelic ratio, a drug targetable lesion, has also been shown to carry a poor prognosis.
- Translocations t(8;21), t(15;17), and inv(16), as well as *NPM* and *CEPBα* mutations carry a good prognosis.
- AML associated with Down syndrome has an excellent prognosis.
- Certain congenital syndromes that carry an increased risk of AML:
  - Fanconi anemia
  - Bloom syndrome
  - Neurofibromatosis type 1
  - Down syndrome
  - Severe congenital anemia (i.e., Kostmann disease treated with granulocyte colony-stimulating factor)
  - Diamond-Blackfan anemia
  - Paroxysmal nocturnal hemoglobinemia
  - Li-Fraumeni syndrome
  - Shwachman-Diamond syndrome
  - Dyskeratosis congenita
  - Noonan syndrome (RASopathies)

PATHOPHYSIOLOGY

- Principal defect is a block in the differentiation of primitive myeloid precursor cells.
- Two mechanisms predominate:
  - Defect at the level of transcriptional activation
  - Defects in the signaling pathway of hematopoietic growth factors. For example, the proto-oncogene *Ras* is mutated in up to 1/3 of patients with AML.

ETIOLOGY

- Exact cause unknown in most cases
- Acquired risk factors include the following:
  - Exposure to benzene
  - Exposure to ionizing radiation
  - Therapy induced, from chemotherapy for a prior malignancy
  - Alkylating agents such as cyclophosphamide, nitrogen mustard, chlorambucil, and melphalan (typically presents several years after therapy)
  - Epipodophyllotoxins such as VP16, VM26 (typically occurs within 2 years after therapy and is characterized by rearrangements involving 11q23)

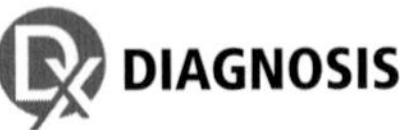

DIAGNOSIS

HISTORY

Children with AML can present with very few symptoms or with life-threatening sepsis or hemorrhage. Common symptoms include the following:

- Fever: 30–40%
- Pallor: 25%
- Weight loss/anorexia: 22%
- Fatigue: 19%
- Bleeding (i.e., cutaneous, mucosal, menorrhagia): 33%
- Bone or joint pain: 18%

PHYSICAL EXAM

- Signs of anemia:
  - Pallor
  - Fatigue
  - Headache
  - Dyspnea
  - Systolic flow murmur
- Signs of thrombocytopenia:
  - Petechiae
  - Bruising
  - Epistaxis
  - Gingival bleeding
- Signs of infection:
  - Fever
  - Bacterial infections of lung, sinuses, gingiva, perirectal area, skin
- Other exam findings:
  - Hepatomegaly
  - Splenomegaly
  - Lymphadenopathy
  - Gingival hyperplasia
  - Papilledema, cranial nerve palsies (rare)
  - Colorless or slightly purple subcutaneous nodules: "blueberry muffin" lesions of leukemia cutis (more commonly seen in neonates)
  - Chloroma is an extramedullary collection of leukemic cells that can present as a mass.

DIFFERENTIAL DIAGNOSIS

- Myeloid blast crisis of chronic myeloid leukemia (Philadelphia chromosome positive)
- Transient myeloproliferative disorder of the newborn (in Down syndrome)
- ALL
- Leukemoid reaction
- Exaggerated leukocytosis
- Myelodysplastic syndrome

DIAGNOSTIC TESTS & INTERPRETATION

Techniques such as fluorescence in situ hybridization, flow cytometry, Southern blotting, and reverse transcriptase-polymerase chain reaction are used to diagnose and classify AML.

Initial Tests (screening, lab, imaging)

- CBC
  - Anemia, thrombocytopenia, elevated or low total WBC peripheral smear
  - Circulating myeloblasts may be seen.
- Prothrombin time (PT)/partial thromboplastin time (PTT), fibrin spit products
  - Elevated in some cases, especially with acute promyelocytic leukemia (M3)
  - Can have severe, life-threatening disseminated intravascular coagulation (DIC)
- Electrolytes (abnormalities associated with tumor lysis syndrome)
  - Hyperkalemia
  - Hypocalcemia
  - Hyperphosphatemia
  - Hyperuricemia
- CSF analysis for cell count and cytology:
  - >5 WBC/μL is suggestive of CNS disease.
  - 5–15% of cases have CNS involvement at diagnosis.

Diagnostic Procedures/Other

Bone marrow aspirate:

- >20% myeloblasts are typically seen.
- To differentiate between AML with low blast count and myelodysplastic syndrome, serial bone marrow aspirates and biopsies are required as well as detailed cytogenetic analysis.
- At diagnosis, morphology, cytochemistry, immunophenotyping, and molecular and cytogenetics of the bone marrow aspirate are required.

- Pathologic findings
  - Immunophenotyping
    - Precursor stage: CD34, CD117
    - Myelomonocytic markers: CD11b, CD11c, CD13, CD14, CD15, CD33, CD64, CD65, i-lysozyme
    - Lymphoid markers: T- and B-cell markers may be present on 30–60% of pediatric blasts.
    - CD41, CD42, and CD61 (megakaryocytic): particularly prevalent in patients with Down syndrome
  - Morphology
    - Large blasts with low nuclear/cytoplasmic ratio
    - Multiple nucleoli and cytoplasmic granules (Auer rods are clumps of azurophilic granular material that form elongated needles and seen in the cytoplasm of certain AML blasts.)
  - Cytochemistry
    - Blasts are positive for myeloperoxidase and Sudan Black and usually negative for periodic acid–Schiff (PAS) and terminal deoxynucleotidyl transferase (TdT).

TREATMENT

MEDICATION

- Patients are treated with 6 to 9 months of intensive chemotherapy given in cycles.
- The most effective drugs for remission induction in AML combine anthracyclines (e.g., doxorubicin, daunorubicin, and mitoxantrone), actinomycin, and cytarabine (Ara-C)
- Other agents sometimes used in combination chemotherapy include etoposide (VP-16), gemtuzumab (anti-CD33 monoclonal antibody), fludarabine, dexamethasone, L-asparaginase, and 6-thioguanine.
- Patients with acute promyelocytic leukemia can be cured with all-*trans*-retinoic acid and arsenic.
- Intrathecal Ara-C for CNS prophylaxis
- FLT3 inhibitors including sorafenib are being used in some patients with FLT3-ITD.
- Hematopoietic stem cell transplant is recommended for patients with high-risk cytogenetics (monosomy 7, monosomy 5, 5q-, FLT3-ITD) or those whom not in remission following two courses of induction therapy.

ADDITIONAL THERAPIES

- Hydration and allopurinol during induction; hydration particularly important to try and prevent leukostasis
- Consider rasburicase in patients with marked elevations in uric acid and renal compromise (contraindicated in patients with G6PD deficiency).
- Blood product support
  - Avoid products from family members as sensitization can lead to poor engraftment after allogeneic bone marrow transplant.
- Broad-spectrum antibiotics and antifungal therapy for fever and neutropenia
- Prophylactic trimethoprim-sulfamethoxazole for *Pneumocystis* infection
- Allogeneic bone marrow transplant is recommended for high-risk AML in first remission.

ADMISSION, INPATIENT, AND NURSING CONSIDERATIONS

Children with suspected AML should have immediate evaluation with physical exam, history, and laboratory data including CBC, PT/PTT, electrolytes, calcium, phosphorus, uric acid, and creatinine.

ONGOING CARE

FOLLOW-UP RECOMMENDATIONS

Patient Monitoring

- Blood counts monthly for 1st year, every 4 months for the 2nd year, and every 6 months thereafter
- Liver and kidney function tests every 3 to 6 months
- Cardiac function every 12 months
- Endocrine function should be tested in pubertal children.

PROGNOSIS

- 85% achieve remission with intensive chemotherapy.
- ~60–70% achieve long-term survival (>5 years after diagnosis).
- Factors associated with poor prognosis:
  - WBC count >100,000/μL
  - Monosomy 7, monosomy 5, or del(5q)
  - Secondary AML or prior myelodysplastic syndrome
  - FLT3-ITD
  - Presence of multiple other genetic translocation events or mutations
  - Poor initial response to therapy (induction failure or presence of >0.1% minimal residual disease [MRD] in the bone marrow at the end of induction)
  - MRD testing measures quantities of residual leukemia not seen on morphologic exam using flow cytometry or standard cytogenetics.

COMPLICATIONS

- Bleeding (usually secondary to thrombocytopenia)
- DIC occurs in some types of AML, including acute promyelocytic leukemia (M3).
- Treat bleeding aggressively with fresh frozen plasma and platelets.
- Other cytopenias require blood product support.
- Infection
  - 40% of patients are febrile at diagnosis.
  - Empiric antibiotic therapy must be started after blood cultures are obtained.
- Leukostasis
  - Intravascular clumping of blasts causing hypoxia, infarction, and hemorrhage
  - Usually occurs when WBC >200,000/μL
  - Brain and lung are commonly affected.
  - Leukapheresis or exchange transfusion may be indicated for patients who are symptomatic with extremely high blast counts.
- Tumor lysis syndrome
  - Refers to the metabolic consequences from the release of cellular contents of dying leukemic cells
  - Hyperuricemia can lead to renal failure.
  - Hyperkalemia, hyperphosphatemia, and secondary hypocalcemia can be life-threatening.
  - Patients should be hydrated with fluid-containing bicarbonate and given allopurinol.

ADDITIONAL READING

- Creutzig U, van den Heuvel-Eibrink M, Gibson B, et al; for AML Committee of the International BFM Study Group. Diagnosis and management of acute myeloid leukemia in children and adolescents: recommendations from an international expert panel. *Blood*. 2012;120(16):3187–3205.
- Kersey JH. Fifty years of studies of the biology and therapy of childhood leukemia. *Blood*. 1997;90(11):4243–4251.
- Pui CH, Carroll WL, Meshinchi S, et al. Biology, risk stratification, and therapy of pediatric acute leukemias: an update. *J Clin Oncol*. 2011;29(5):551–565.
- Puumala S, Ross J, Aplenc R, et al. Epidemiology of childhood acute myeloid leukemia. *Pediatr Blood Cancer*. 2013;60(5):728–733.
- Rubnitz JE, Gibson B, Smith FO. Acute myeloid leukemia. *Hematol Oncol Clin North Am*. 2010;24(1):35–63.
- Vardiman JW, Thiele J, Arber DA, et al. The 2008 revision of the World Health Organization (WHO) classification of myeloid neoplasms and acute leukemia: rationale and important changes. *Blood*. 2009;114(5):937–951.

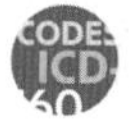

CODES

ICD10

- C92.00 Acute myeloblastic leukemia, not having achieved remission
- C92.01 Acute myeloblastic leukemia, in remission
- C92.02 Acute myeloblastic leukemia, in relapse

FAQ

- Q: Is an indwelling line required for therapy?
- A: The majority of time. There may be exception in patients with acute promyelocytic leukemia and coagulopathy.
- Q: Are repeated hospitalizations likely?
- A: Repeated hospitalizations are needed for chemotherapy and infectious complications.

ADENOVIRUS INFECTION

Jessica R. Newman, DO

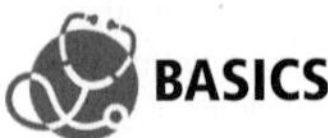

BASICS

DESCRIPTION
Adenoviruses are ubiquitous, nonenveloped, double-stranded DNA viruses capable of causing respiratory tract disease, ocular disease, and gastroenteritis.

EPIDEMIOLOGY
- Primary infection usually occurs early in life (by age 5 years) and is, most often, characterized by upper respiratory symptoms.
- Peaks in the first 2 years of life
- Military trainees are especially susceptible to infection, probably due to crowded living conditions.
- Respiratory and enteric infections may occur at any time of year. In temperate climates, peaks tend to occur in winter months.
- Cause approximately 5% of all pediatric respiratory tract infections and 5–10% of pneumonias
- Transmission of respiratory disease occurs via infected droplets.
  - Transmission of enteric adenoviruses is via the fecal–oral route.
  - Transmission can less commonly occur via contact with infected conjunctiva.
- Outbreaks of pharyngoconjunctival fever have been associated with inadequately chlorinated swimming pools and shared towels.
- One of the most common causes of viral myocarditis in children and adults

RISK FACTORS
Exposure to adenovirus

GENERAL PREVENTION
- A live oral vaccine for prevention of acute respiratory tract disease is used in military personnel.
- For hospitalized patients:
  - Respiratory symptoms: contact/droplet precautions
  - Gastrointestinal symptoms: contact precautions
  - Conjunctivitis: contact precautions

PATHOPHYSIOLOGY
- Adenoviruses may cause a lytic infection or a chronic/latent infection.
- In addition, they are capable of inducing oncogenic transformation of cells, although the clinical significance of this observation remains unclear.

ETIOLOGY
There are at least 67 identified human serotypes classified into seven species (species A to G).

COMMONLY ASSOCIATED CONDITIONS
- Respiratory infections
  - Upper respiratory tract infections: otitis media, common cold, pharyngitis
  - Lower respiratory tract infection: pneumonia, pertussis-like syndrome, croup, necrotizing bronchitis, bronchiolitis (serotypes 3, 7, and 21 predominant in pneumonia epidemics)
- Pharyngoconjunctival fever
  - Low-grade fever associated with conjunctivitis, pharyngitis, rhinitis, and cervical adenitis
  - 15% of patients may have meningismus.
  - Increased incidence in summer months
  - Common source outbreaks most often associated with type 3
- Epidemic keratoconjunctivitis
  - Bilateral conjunctivitis with preauricular adenopathy
  - May persist for up to 3 to 4 weeks
  - Corneal opacities may persist for several months.
  - Most commonly associated with types 8, 19, and 37
- Myocarditis preceding viral illness
  - Presents with cardiovascular collapse, congestive heart failure, respiratory distress, or ventricular tachycardia
  - Prognosis is poor.
  - High mortality; a large number require transplant, and a portion develop dilated cardiomyopathy.
- Hemorrhagic cystitis may cause microscopic or gross hematuria.
  - If present, gross hematuria persists on average for 3 days.
  - Often associated with dysuria and urinary frequency
  - More common in males than females
  - Associated with types 11 and 21
  - Can occur in both immunocompetent and immunocompromised hosts
- Infantile diarrhea
  - Watery diarrhea associated with fever
  - Symptoms may persist for 1 to 2 weeks.
  - Associated with types 40, 41, and less often 31
- CNS infection epidemics (associated with outbreaks of respiratory disease) and sporadic cases of encephalitis and meningitis have been observed; often associated with pneumonia
- Immunocompromised hosts
  - Can cause disseminated disease including pneumonia, hepatitis, and gastroenteritis
  - Frequently observed in transplanted patients; up to 40% of pediatric human stem cell transplant recipients and in 5–10% of solid organ transplant recipients
  - Fatality rates much higher, up to 30–75% in hematopoietic stem cell transplant patients
- Miscellaneous: associated with intussusception (isolated in up to 40% of cases) and fatal congenital infection

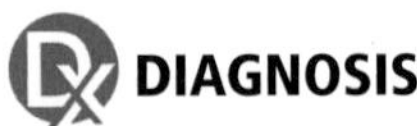

DIAGNOSIS

HISTORY
- Fever
  - Nonspecific
- Rhinitis
  - Upper respiratory infection (URI)
- Laryngitis, sore throat
  - URI
- Nonproductive or croupy cough
  - Respiratory infection
- Headache, myalgias
  - CNS infection
- Hematuria (gross or microscopic), dysuria, urinary frequency
  - Hemorrhagic cystitis
- Watery diarrhea
  - Enteric adenovirus
- Conjunctivitis, rhinitis, exudative pharyngitis, and meningismus
  - Typical findings of adenovirus

PHYSICAL EXAM
- Pulmonary tachypnea, wheezing, rales
  - Pneumonia
- Tachycardia, tachypnea, gallop rhythm, hepatomegaly
  - Myocarditis
- Abdominal tenderness, distention
  - Gastroenteritis

DIFFERENTIAL DIAGNOSIS
- Respiratory infection
  - Influenza
  - Parainfluenza
  - Human metapneumovirus
  - Pertussis
  - Mycoplasma pneumonia
  - Bacterial pneumonia
  - Bocavirus

- Pharyngoconjunctival fever
  - *Group A Streptococcus*
  - Epstein-Barr virus
  - Parainfluenza
  - Enterovirus
  - Measles
  - Kawasaki disease
- Epidemic keratoconjunctivitis
  - Herpes simplex
  - *Chlamydia*
  - Enterovirus
- Myocarditis
  - Enteroviruses
  - Herpes simplex
  - Epstein-Barr virus
  - Influenza
  - Bacterial myocarditis
- Hemorrhagic cystitis
  - Glomerulonephritis
  - Vasculitis
  - Renal tuberculosis
- Infantile diarrhea
  - *Rotavirus*
  - *Calicivirus* (including norovirus)
  - *Astrovirus*
  - *Salmonella*
  - *Shigella*
  - *Campylobacter*
- CNS infection
  - Enterovirus
  - Herpes simplex virus
  - *Mycoplasma*
  - Bacterial meningitis

DIAGNOSTIC TESTS & INTERPRETATION

Initial Tests (screening, lab, imaging)

- CBC
  - Leukocytosis or leukopenia, often with left shift in the differential counts
- Erythrocyte sedimentation rate (ESR)
  - Often elevated
- Viral isolation
  - From nasopharyngeal secretions, urine, conjunctivae, or stool
- Viral identification
  - Observe viral antigen in infected cells by immunofluorescence; amplify genome by polymerase chain reaction (PCR).
  - Stool antigen enzyme immunoassay (EIA) test
  - Highest yield from nasopharyngeal swab or stool
  - Adenovirus PCR is helpful in narrowing differential diagnosis, especially in the immunocompromised host, and can be used for prognostic purposes.
- ECG
  - Low-voltage QRS
  - Low-amplitude or inverted T waves
  - Small or absent Q wave in V_5 and V_6
- Echocardiogram (ECHO) or cardiac magnetic resonance imaging (MRI) for suspected myocarditis
  - Left ventricular hypertrophy, wall motion abnormalities (ECHO)
  - Increase in T1 and T2 signal intensity, increased early myocardial contrast enhancement, and presence of late gadolinium enhancement (MRI)
- Chest radiograph
  - Bilateral patchy interstitial infiltrates (lower lobes) or enlarged heart

TREATMENT

GENERAL MEASURES

- Supportive care
- Monitor for secondary bacterial infections.
- Avoid steroid-containing ophthalmic ointments.

MEDICATION

First Line

- Cidofovir
  - Has been shown to have benefit in immunocompromised patients with disseminated disease, specifically in hematopoietic stem cell transplant (HSCT) patients, where a reduction in adenovirus-related mortality compared with historical controls has been reported
  - However, a risk of developing a dose-limiting nephrotoxicity exists, and optimal dosing is not known. Prehydration with IV NS and probenecid is used to reduce risk for nephrotoxicity.
  - Reducing immunosuppression in transplanted patients should be considered for those with adenovirus disease.
- Infusion of adenovirus-specific cytotoxic T cells or intravenous immunoglobulin (IVIG) may have some benefit in immunocompromised patients, particularly HSCT patients.
- Brincidofovir (an orally bioavailable lipid conjugate of cidofovir) has shown promise in immunocompromised patients, and clinical trials are ongoing.

ONGOING CARE

PROGNOSIS

Most syndromes are self-limited in the immunocompetent host.

COMPLICATIONS

- Bronchiolitis obliterans (rare)
- Corneal opacities with visual disturbance (usually resolves spontaneously)
- Congestive heart failure
- Dilated cardiomyopathy

ADDITIONAL READING

- Hammond S, Chenever E, Durbin JE. Respiratory virus infection in infants and children. *Pediatr Dev Pathol*. 2007;10(3):172–180.
- Leruez-Ville M, Minard V, Lacaille F, et al. Real-time blood plasma polymerase chain reaction for management of disseminated adenovirus infection. *Clin Infect Dis*. 2004;38(1):45–52.
- Lion T. Adenovirus infections in immunocompetent and immunocompromised patients. *Clin Microbiol Rev*. 2014;27(3):441–462.
- Matthes-Martin S, Feuchtinger T, Shaw PJ, et al; for Fourth European Conference on Infections in Leukemia. European guidelines for diagnosis and treatment of adenovirus infection in leukemia and stem cell transplantation: summary of ECIL-4 (2011). *Transpl Infect Dis*. 2012;14(6):555–563.
- Tebruegge M, Curtis N. Adenovirus: an overview for pediatric infectious diseases specialists. *Pediatr Infect Dis J*. 2012;31(6):626–627.

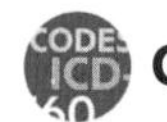

CODES

ICD10

- B34.0 Adenovirus infection, unspecified
- A08.2 Adenoviral enteritis
- B97.0 Adenovirus as the cause of diseases classified elsewhere

FAQ

- Q: Is there anything one can do to prevent these infections?
- A: Washing hands and avoiding contact with ill persons will help slow the spread of these infections.
- Q: Is there any role of antiviral medications in immunocompetent hosts?
- A: No. Generally, disease is self-limited in immunocompetent hosts, and antiviral therapy can be associated with significant toxicities.
- Q: Given mortality risk, is there a role for prophylactic antiviral therapy for adenovirus in immunosuppressed individuals?
- A: No. Prophylactic antiviral therapy with currently available antiviral drugs is not recommended; however, preemptive therapy (treating at-risk patients who have viremia) may be helpful and is recommended in certain patient populations.

ALCOHOL (ETHANOL) INTOXICATION

Ann Bruner, MD

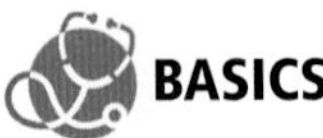

BASICS

DESCRIPTION

- Acute ingestion (accidental or intended) of alcohol, resulting in loss of inhibition, often associated with unruly/violent behavior, impaired judgment and/or coordination, diminished alertness/responsiveness, and sedation or coma
- Accidental ingestion is more common in toddlers and younger children.
- Frequency of intentional alcohol use increases with age.
- Alcohol–drug interactions are common because acute intoxication reduces hepatic clearance for other drugs, thereby increasing their serum concentrations.
- Signs and symptoms of intoxication vary depending on the type and quantity of alcohol, the rate of consumption, and the patient's pattern of prior use of alcohol.

EPIDEMIOLOGY

Alcohol is the most used drug by young people: 30% of 8th graders, 69% of 12th graders, and 81% of college students have consumed alcohol.

Prevalence

- 71% of high school students have consumed alcohol in their lifetime.
  - 21% had their first drink before age 13 years.
  - 39% had one drink in past 30 days.
  - 54% of 12th graders and 13% of 8th graders have been drunk at least once.
- Underage (12 to 20 years old) drinkers are 3 times more likely than adults to use illicit drugs with alcohol.
- >90% of alcohol is consumed through binge drinking (>5 drinks for males or >4 drinks for females); prevalence of binge alcohol use in past 2 weeks in 2012 was 5% of 8th graders, 16% of 10th graders, 24% of 12th graders, 37% of college students, and 36% of young adults.
- Among college students, 20% of males and 8% of females report having consumed double the binge threshold (>10 drinks for males and >8 for females).
- 24% of high school students have ridden in a car driven by someone who had been drinking alcohol; 8% had driven a car when they had been drinking.
- 56% of college students mixed energy drinks with alcohol in the past month.
- Household products (medicinal, cosmetic, cleaning, hygiene) can contain up to 100% ethanol; rates of accidental exposure to and intentional intoxication from hand sanitizers are increasing.

RISK FACTORS

Patients with psychiatric conditions are at an increased risk for abuse of alcohol and other drugs.

GENERAL PREVENTION

- Promote family discussions about alcohol use and abuse.
- Provide safety recommendations to prevent accidental ingestions.

PATHOPHYSIOLOGY

- Effects of alcohol ingestion are related to dose, the time in which alcohol was consumed and then absorbed, and the patient's history of alcohol exposure; peak serum concentrations occur 30 to 60 minutes after ingestion.
- Alcohol absorption, decreased by the presence of food in the stomach and increased if liquid is carbonated, occurs rapidly and largely in the small intestine.
  - Minimal quantities of alcohol are excreted in urine, sweat, and breath.
  - >90% of alcohol oxidized in liver follow zero-order kinetics, primarily by alcohol dehydrogenase (ADH) and then acetaldehyde dehydrogenase (ALDH).
  - Rate of metabolism is fixed (not related to dose or time) and is proportional to body weight.
  - Ethnic/racial and gender variabilities exist on quantity and efficacy of ADH.
  - Ethanol is metabolized by ADH to acetaldehyde, then to acetate, and finally to ketones, fatty acids, or acetone; ketosis and, infrequently, metabolic acidosis can occur.
- Respiratory acidosis can occur secondary to carbon dioxide retention from respiratory depression due to ethanol intoxication.
- Hypoglycemia occurs during acute ethanol intoxication due to impaired gluconeogenesis resulting from changes in the NADH/NAD+ ratio associated with ethanol metabolism.
- Alcohol affects the CNS primarily through the γ-aminobutyric acid (GABA) and glutamate neurotransmitter systems.

ETIOLOGY

- Alcohol is produced from fermentation/distillation of sugar from grapes (wine), grains/corn (beer/whiskey), potatoes (vodka), or sugar cane (rum) and then mixed into solution to make specific beverages.
  - Products are marketed according to alcohol content or proof (twice the percent).
  - Alcohol content ranges from 3–6% (6 to 12 proof) in beer to 40–75% (80 to 150 proof) in vodka/rum/whiskey.
- Alcohol is often consumed concurrently with other substances (licit and illicit), presenting a mixed clinical picture of intoxication.

COMMONLY ASSOCIATED CONDITIONS

- Alcohol is involved in 30% of all drug overdoses.
- A significant percentage of adolescent trauma patients, especially victims of gunshot wounds, have positive toxicology screens for alcohol and other drugs. Ethanol use increases trauma risk by 3- to 7-fold.
- A blood alcohol concentration (BAC) of 50 mg/dL doubles the risk of involvement in a motor vehicle crash.
- Among college students, alcohol use is highly associated with intimate partner violence and sexual assault.

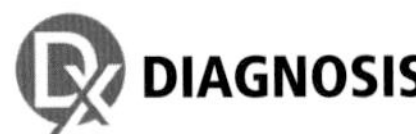

DIAGNOSIS

HISTORY

- Medical: Baseline health will affect patient's response to alcohol; diabetics, for example, may have worse hypoglycemia.
- Type and dose of other drugs ingested:
  - Clinical effects and treatment for other ingestions can vary depending on substance.
  - Polysubstance ingestion is very common.
- Psychiatric history: Evaluate for possible suicidal ideation.
- Gathering details regarding the alcohol consumed (type, amount, and over what time period) may help predict clinical course. For example, BAC may continue rising if ingestion occurred recently.
- Intoxication presents clinically with signs ranging from lack of coordination, slurred speech, and confusion (BAC of 20 to 200 mg/dL) to ataxia and nausea/vomiting (BAC 200 to 300 mg/dL) to amnesia, seizures, or coma (BAC >300 mg/dL).

PHYSICAL EXAM

- Bruises, lacerations, and fractures may suggest trauma and raise concern about CNS injury.
- Neurologic exam, including mental status, will assess degree of intoxication and consciousness, including patient's ability to protect his or her airway, and risk for aspiration.
- Tachycardia and hypotension may indicate dehydration.
- Fever may suggest infection.
- Mental status
  - Average time for normalization of mental status in intoxicated adults is 3 to 3.5 hours.
  - Patients without clinical improvement in 3 hours should be evaluated for other causes of altered mental status.

DIFFERENTIAL DIAGNOSIS

- Environmental
  - Other ingestions (overdose of sedatives or illicit drugs, such as benzodiazepines, marijuana, narcotics, lysergic acid diethylamide [LSD], and phencyclidine [PCP])
  - Toxic exposures (ethylene glycol, methanol, carbon monoxide)
  - Head trauma
- Infection
  - Meningitis
  - Encephalitis
  - Sepsis

- Tumor: brain tumor
- Metabolic
  - Hypoglycemia
  - Ketoacidosis
  - Hyperammonemia
  - Electrolyte imbalances (hyponatremia, hypernatremia)
- Miscellaneous
  - Increased intracranial pressure from hydrocephalus, mass, other
  - Stroke

DIAGNOSTIC TESTS & INTERPRETATION

Initial Tests (screening, lab, imaging)

- BAC
  - Generally correlates with clinical picture
  - In children, signs of intoxication may be present at levels of 50 mg/dL.
  - Serum levels of 600 to 800 mg/dL can be fatal.
- Blood and/or urine toxicology screen
  - Most urine toxicology screens do not test for alcohol.
  - Concurrent ingestions are common.
- Acetaminophen level
  - Usually not part of the general serum toxicology screen
  - Consider if polysubstance ingestion suspected and/or if patient has suicidal ideation.
- Serum electrolytes
  - Alcohol is a diuretic. The associated nausea and vomiting seen with intoxication may result in severe dehydration.
  - Ketosis and, infrequently, metabolic acidosis can occur.
- Serum glucose level: Ethanol inhibits gluconeogenesis and can be associated with hypoglycemia.
- Blood gas can show both respiratory and metabolic acidosis.

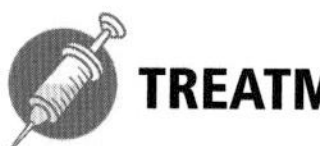

TREATMENT

GENERAL MEASURES

- Assess airway, breathing, and circulation (ABC).
- Protect airway: The patient may require intubation and mechanical ventilation.
- Mainstay is supportive therapy as no specific ethanol antidote exists.
- Appropriate trauma management as needed
- Because alcohol is absorbed rapidly, gastric lavage is indicated only if the patient is seen immediately after ingestion (within minutes).

MEDICATION

IV dextrose as needed for hypoglycemia

ISSUES FOR REFERRAL

- Refer to substance abuse specialist (addiction medicine, psychiatrist, or certified addictions counselor) for detailed evaluation and treatment.
- Refer for psychiatric evaluation if depression, anxiety, suicidal ideation, or any other mental health condition is suspected.
- Assess for other risk-taking behaviors—including other substance use, sexual activity, use of motor vehicles while intoxicated, weapon carrying, and delinquency—and their sequelae, including pregnancy, sexually transmitted infections, and violence.

ADMISSION, INPATIENT, AND NURSING CONSIDERATIONS

- Keep patient awake; watch for vomiting as patients are at risk for choking owing to depressed gag reflex.
- Admission criteria
  - Unstable vital signs (hypotension)
  - Persistent CNS depression/impaired mental status
  - Potential severity of comorbid psychiatric conditions (depression/suicidality)
  - Inability to contact a parent/guardian
- IV fluids for dehydration and hypotension
- Observe and monitor vital signs and neurologic status.
- Discharge criteria
  - Stable vital signs
  - Patient awake, alert, responsive, and oriented
  - Decreasing BAC
  - Parent/guardian fully informed about patient's alcohol use

DIET

NPO secondary to depressed gag reflex

PROGNOSIS

BAC serum levels of 600 to 800 mg/dL can be fatal.

COMPLICATIONS

- Diuresis and dehydration
- Vasodilation, hypotension, and tachycardia
- Vomiting, aspiration, potential respiratory arrest
- Hypoglycemia
- Metabolic acidosis
- Impaired mental status
- Engagement in risk-taking behaviors (e.g., other drug use, unprotected intercourse) while intoxicated
- CNS depression
- Gastritis
- GI bleeding
- Acute pancreatitis
- Motor vehicle collisions associated with driving while intoxicated
- Alcoholism
- Alcohol withdrawal following a period of intoxication in chronic users (symptoms include tachycardia, elevated blood pressure, irritability, nausea, vomiting, and tremor)

ADDITIONAL READING

- Centers for Disease Control and Prevention. 2011 Youth Risk Behavior Survey. http://www.cdc.gov/yrbs. Accessed September 1, 2013.
- Howland J, Rohsenow DJ. Risks of energy drinks mixed with alcohol. *JAMA*. 2013;309(3):245–246.
- Johnston LD, O'Malley PM, Bachman JG, et al. *Monitoring the Future National Results on Drug Use: 2012 Overview, Key Findings on Adolescent Drug Use*. Ann Arbor, MI: Institute for Social Research, The University of Michigan; 2013.
- Merrill JE, Carey KB. Drinking over the lifespan: focus on college ages. *Alcohol Res*. 2016;38(1):103–114.
- Rayar P, Ratnapalan S. Pediatric ingestions of house hold products containing ethanol: a review. *Clin Pediatr (Phila)*. 2013;52(3):203–209.
- The Center on Alcohol Marketing and Youth. Prevalence of underage drinking. http://www.camy.org/factsheets/sheets/Prevalence_of_Underage_Drinking.html. Accessed March 15, 2018.

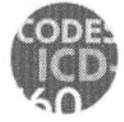

CODES

ICD10

- F10.920 Alcohol use, unspecified with intoxication, uncomplicated
- F10.929 Alcohol use, unspecified with intoxication, unspecified
- T51.0X4A Toxic effect of ethanol, undetermined, initial encounter

FAQ

- Q: How quickly is alcohol metabolized?
- A: The liver metabolizes approximately 10 g of ethanol per hour, which corresponds to a decline in BAC of 18 to 20 mg/dL/h; clearance rates are related to prior exposure to alcohol, ranging from 15 to 20 mg/dL in inexperienced drinkers to 25 to 35 mg/dL in patients with chronic alcohol abuse.
- Q: What is binge drinking in youth?
- A: For children 9 to 13 years old and girls 14 to 17 years old, 3 or more drinks; for boys 14 to 15 years old, 4 or more drinks
- Q: Are younger children at any increased risk from alcohol poisoning?
- A: Ethanol inhibits gluconeogenesis; younger children have an increased risk of hypoglycemia because they have relatively smaller hepatic glycogen stores; however, children tend to have more rapid clearance rates (up to 30 mg/dL/h).
- Q: How is alcohol smoked?
- A: Alcohol can be vaporized and inhaled using dry ice or by using purchased or homemade vaporizers. The inhaled vapor bypasses the stomach and liver and thus reaches the brain much faster. Vaporizing or smoking alcohol has a higher risk for alcohol poisoning.

ALLERGIC CHILD

Barry J. Pelz, MD • Anne Marie Singh, MD

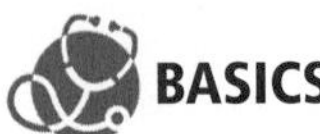

BASICS

Allergic diseases include atopic dermatitis, food allergy, asthma, and allergic rhinitis. Atopic or allergic diseases are becoming more and more prevalent in the population.

- Food allergy in its most severe form may manifest as anaphylaxis.
- These conditions may present in a variety of ways as described below.

DESCRIPTION

- Atopic dermatitis
  - Atopic dermatitis (or eczema) is characterized by chronic, relapsing, pruritic inflamed skin, which is often erythematous, xerotic, and/or excoriated.
  - Atopic dermatitis may occur in isolation without other atopic diseases or it may be the beginning of the "atopic march" preceding the onset of other atopic conditions, which may include food allergy, asthma, and/or allergic rhinitis.
- Urticaria
  - Refers to hives or the erythematous wheals that occur when histamine is released from mast cells
  - May be caused by a number of triggers
  - Viral infection is the most common cause of urticaria in children.
  - The allergic child may develop urticaria when an antigen such as a food causes IgE-mediated release of mast cell mediators.
- Food allergy
  - Presents with an IgE-mediated reaction after exposure to a food to which the child is sensitized
  - Reactions may involve any number of allergic symptoms, including urticaria, lip or tongue swelling, closing of the throat, wheezing, shortness of breath, hypotension, lethargy, repeated vomiting after allergen ingestion, diarrhea, or any combination of the above.
  - The most common food allergens include cow's milk, egg, peanut, tree nuts, wheat, soy, fish, and shellfish.
  - Food allergy should be distinguished from food intolerance, which does *not* have an IgE basis and does not carry a risk of anaphylaxis.
- Asthma
  - An obstructive airway disease characterized by recurrent wheezing, bronchoconstriction, increased mucous production, and airway inflammation
  - Asthma is one of many potential causes of wheezing in children.
  - Wheezing with RSV and human rhinovirus infection are associated with the development of asthma.
- Allergic rhinitis and conjunctivitis
  - A condition in which children are sensitized to perennial allergens, seasonal allergens, or both
  - Perennial allergens include dust mite, cockroach, animal dander, and some molds.
  - Seasonal allergens include tree pollens, grass pollens, weed pollen, ragweed pollen, and other molds.
  - Symptoms may include watery eyes, itchy eyes, rhinorrhea, nasal discharge, itchy nose, sneezing, postnasal drip, throat clearing, headache, sinus pressure, nasal obstruction, mouth breathing, or snoring.
  - Symptoms may be seasonal, year-round, or triggered by exposure to specific allergens (such as cats or dogs).

RISK FACTORS

Genetics

- Children who do not have a family history of atopy have approximately a 25% chance of being atopic.
- For children with at least one parent who is atopic, the risk of atopy approximately doubles compared to the general population.

PATHOPHYSIOLOGY

Most of these allergic conditions are IgE mediated, and all result from a complex interaction between multiple genetic and environmental factors.

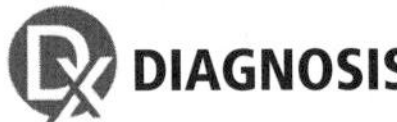

DIAGNOSIS

A thorough history and physical examination are the keys to diagnosing the allergic child. Confirmatory tests should be used when indicated.

HISTORY

- History should elicit signs and symptoms of allergic diseases while at the same time exploring other potential etiologies for the child's symptoms.
- The allergic child should have symptoms of atopic dermatitis, urticaria, wheezing, reactions to foods, or symptoms of allergic rhinitis and conjunctivitis such as sneezing, itchy eyes, watery eyes, itchy nose, runny nose, or itchy throat.
- The practitioner should also review the family history because atopic disease often runs in families.

PHYSICAL EXAM

A complete physical exam is essential to rule out systemic diseases that can mimic allergic disease.

- Ocular signs may include the following:
  - Dark circles under the eyes or the "allergic shiners" which result from venous stasis secondary to passive congestion in the nose, impeding venous return from the vessels under the eyes
  - Cobblestoning of the conjunctiva
  - Erythematous injection of the conjunctiva
  - Dennie-Morgan lines or infraorbital folds associated with suborbital edema secondary to chronic inflammation from atopic dermatitis
  - Clear stringy ocular discharge
- Nasal allergic signs may include the following:
  - Pale edematous nasal mucosa
  - Clear nasal discharge with or without occlusion
  - Nasal crease across the bridge of nose secondary to repeated upward rubbing of the nose from "the allergic salute"
  - Nasal polyps may be present, although they are much more common in adults and should prompt consideration of diseases such as cystic fibrosis when seen in children.
- Ear allergic signs may include the following:
  - Fluid in the middle ear or retracted tympanic membranes
  - Eustachian tube dysfunction associated with allergic inflammation
- Throat allergic signs may include the following:
  - Cobblestoning of the posterior pharynx secondary to submucosal lymphoid hyperplasia
- Lung allergic signs may include the following:
  - Wheezes, rhonchi, decreased air entry, prolonged expiration, and chronic obstruction secondary to allergic responses
- Skin allergic signs may include the following:
  - Eczema, hives, angioedema, and/or dermatographism

DIFFERENTIAL DIAGNOSIS

The differential for allergic diseases is extensive and should focus on considering other etiologies for the symptoms.

- Ear/nose symptoms
  - Eye findings may be caused by physical or chemical irritants or by viral or bacterial infection.
  - Allergic rhinitis symptoms may resemble upper respiratory infections, sinusitis, nasal foreign bodies, or nonallergic rhinitis.
  - A number of medications can lead to rhinitis medicamentosa or symptoms of nasal congestion due to medication use.
  - Systemic diseases such as cystic fibrosis, immotile cilia syndrome, Kartagener syndrome, or immunodeficiencies may present with recurrent nasal or lung symptoms, or sinopulmonary infections.
  - Lung symptoms may be caused by physical or chemical irritants including tobacco smoke, environmental pollution, and inhalants.
- Chest symptoms
  - Lung symptoms may also result from gastroesophageal reflux leading to cough (often nocturnal) or cough with recumbency.
  - Foreign body aspiration may produce lung symptoms and auscultatory signs, although typically, foreign bodies create more focal lung findings.
  - Anatomic defects in the airway may also result in symptoms that are similar to allergic symptoms.
- Skin symptoms
  - Skin findings may be caused by a number of etiologies including irritant dermatitis; viral exanthems; autoimmune disorders; bacterial, fungal, or parasitic infections.
- Multisystem findings
  - Anaphylaxis may sometimes be confused with angioedema, vocal cord dysfunction, globus sensation, or with other causes of shock (sepsis, hypovolemia, cardiogenic).
  - Food allergy may sometimes be confused with food intolerance, but food intolerances typically present with abdominal discomfort, bloating, flatulence, or nonspecific malaise, whereas food allergy presents with true IgE-mediated reactions.

DIAGNOSTIC TESTS & INTERPRETATION

The diagnosis of allergic diseases can be strongly suggested based on history and physical alone. Specific tests can be done by a specialist in allergy and immunology in order to be properly interpreted. Often, initial therapy can be initiated without definitive tests.

Once the allergic child is referred to the allergist, testing may include the following:

- Immediate hypersensitivity testing
  - Skin prick tests (percutaneous testing) to suspected allergens based on history may demonstrate IgE sensitization if positive.
  - Intradermal skin tests for patients who have a negative skin prick test and a suspicious history pose a greater risk of systemic reactions but can be done for environmental allergens, not for foods.
- Blood-specific IgE testing
  - ImmunoCAP® tests measure free serum IgE to a specific antigen to which a particular patient may be sensitized.
  - Although panels are available, these tests are best done for targeted potential allergens that are suggested by the history. These should be interpreted by an allergist with experience in interpreting and guiding therapy.
  - Incorrect use or interpretation of ImmunoCAP® testing may result in inappropriate dietary restrictions, nutritional deficits, and undue anxiety.
  - ImmunoCAP® levels may be trended over time to help monitor for the development of tolerance.
- Eosinophilia
  - Eosinophils in peripheral blood, respiratory secretions, or nasal samples may be indicative of an allergic diathesis.
- Pulmonary function tests (PFTs)
  - PFTs or spirometry should be obtained on asthmatic children or in children with respiratory allergic histories to evaluate for obstructive diseases.

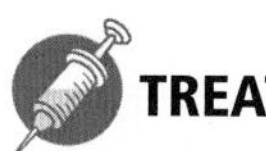

TREATMENT

GENERAL MEASURES

- The main principle of therapy for allergic diseases is avoidance of allergic triggers.
- For atopic dermatitis, general treatment methods include measures to help lock moisture into skin, treat inflammation when present, control pruritus, minimize skin irritants, and treat infection when present.
- For food allergy, the most important therapeutic measure is strict avoidance of the food that causes the allergy in order to prevent an allergic reaction.
  - Children at risk for a reaction to a food allergen should be prescribed an epinephrine autoinjector to use in the event of systemic symptoms or anaphylaxis.
  - An emergency action plan should be provided, reviewing the signs and symptoms of a reaction and the doses and medications that should be used in the event that an accidental ingestion occurs.
  - Infants with food allergy or moderate to severe atopic dermatitis should be evaluated by an allergist who will screen for the possible early introduction of peanut to prevent development of peanut allergy.
- For allergic rhinitis, systemic antihistamines may be helpful in controlling symptoms. Many patients also benefit from intranasal corticosteroids when indicated.
  - Specific environmental control measures may be indicated based on specific skin testing results.
  - Pets should be kept out of the bedroom if a child has allergic stigmata due to animal dander.
  - To minimize exposure to dust mite allergen, bedding should be placed in dust mite encasements and washed in hot water at least once every 2 weeks.
  - Immunotherapy may be indicated for patients with allergic rhinitis or venom allergy.
- For patients with asthma, treatment should follow the latest National Heart, Lung, and Blood Institute (NHLBI) of the National Institutes of Health (NIH) asthma guidelines with consideration to the child's symptomatology, impairment, and risk. Therapies may include use of rescue inhalers, controller medications such as inhaled corticosteroids, leukotriene antagonists, and others (see Appendix). Control of comorbidities such as allergic rhinitis and gastroesophageal reflux disorder (GERD) are also important therapeutic steps.

ISSUES FOR REFERRAL

- Any child with allergic symptoms may benefit from referral to an allergist-immunologist.
- A patient failing medical management of upper respiratory or ocular allergies with routine antihistamine/decongestant medications may be referred to an allergist who can help identify triggers contributing to the problem.
- Poorly controlled asthma not responding to intermittent inhaled β-agonists or an asthmatic child who is symptomatic between exacerbations or has an atypical pattern of exacerbations should be referred.
- Asthma patients with frequent hospitalizations or steroid courses should be referred.
- Patients who are absent from school frequently because of allergic or asthmatic symptoms should be referred.
- Patients with food allergy, drug allergy, latex allergy, or difficult-to-manage atopic dermatitis should also be referred to an allergist.
- Infants with moderate to severe atopic dermatitis or other food allergy should be referred to an allergist.

ONGOING CARE

PROGNOSIS

- In general, environmental allergies that cause rhinitis and asthma persist into adulthood.
- About 50% of milk-allergic children may outgrow their allergy by school age and about 80% by age 16 years. Those who tolerate baked milk have a higher likelihood of outgrowing the allergy.
- About 70% of egg-allergic children may outgrow their egg allergy by age 16 years. Children who tolerate baked egg seem more likely to outgrow the allergy.
- Children may occasionally outgrow peanut (~20% obtain natural tolerance), tree nut (~10%), or shellfish allergy.
- Allergic diseases may have a significant impact on the patient and family's quality of life and may lead to issues with anxiety and mental health.
- Early introduction of peanut in high-risk children significantly lowers the risk of peanut allergy.

ADDITIONAL READING

- Adkinson NF, Bochner BS, Busse WW, et al. *Middleton's Allergy Principles and Practice*. 7th ed. Philadelphia, PA: Mosby; 2009.
- Du Toit G, Roberts G, Sayre PH, et al; for LEAP Study Team. Randomized trial of peanut consumption in infants at risk for peanut allergy. *N Engl J Med*. 2015;372(9):803–813.
- Hatzler L, Hofmaier S, Papadopoulos NG. Allergic airway diseases in childhood—marching from epidemiology to novel concepts of prevention. *Pediatr Allergy Immunol*. 2012;23(7):616–622.
- Langley EW, Gigante J. Anaphylaxis, urticaria, and angioedema. *Pediatr Rev*. 2013;34(6):247–257.
- Papadopoulos NG, Arakawa H, Carlsen KH, et al. International consensus on (ICON) pediatric asthma. *Allergy*. 2012;67(8):976–997.
- Wood RA, Sicherer SH, Vickery BP, et al. The natural history of milk allergy in an observational cohort. *J Allergy Clin Immunol*. 2013;131(3):805–812.

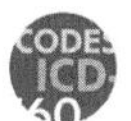

CODES

ICD10

- L20.9 Atopic dermatitis, unspecified
- L27.2 Dermatitis due to ingested food
- J45.909 Unspecified asthma, uncomplicated

FAQ

- Q: Do children outgrow allergies?
- A: In general, environmental allergies that cause rhinitis and asthma persist into adulthood. However, most children outgrow food allergies to milk, egg, soy, and wheat. Children may occasionally outgrow peanut, tree nut, or shellfish allergies.
- Q: If a parent is allergic to a specific allergen, can the child inherit this allergy?
- A: Children inherit the tendency to be allergic, but they do not inherit specific allergies.
- Q: How can allergies be prevented?
- A: In general, allergy prevention is currently not possible, but research in this field is ongoing. Early introduction of peanut in the 1st year of life may prevent the development of peanut allergy in high-risk infants.

ALOPECIA (HAIR LOSS)

Hope E. Rhodes, MD, MPH, FAAP • Terry Kind, MD, MPH

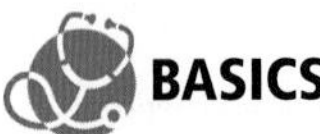

BASICS

DESCRIPTION

- Absence of hair where it normally grows
- Categorized as acquired or congenital
  - Most cases are acquired: Tinea capitis is most common, followed by traumatic alopecia and alopecia areata.
- Also categorized as diffuse or localized
  - Most cases of alopecia are localized and, of these, tinea capitis is the most common.
- Many normal healthy newborns lose their hair in the first few months of life.
  - Hair loss may be exacerbated by friction from bedding/sleep surface, especially in atopic infants.
- Normally, about 50 to 100 hairs are shed and simultaneously replaced every day.
- 90% of alopecia cases are due to the following disorders:
  - Tinea capitis
  - Alopecia areata
  - Traction alopecia
  - Telogen effluvium
    - Alopecia is preceded by a psychologically or physically stressful event 6 to 16 weeks prior to the onset of hair loss.
    - Growing hairs convert rapidly to resting hairs.

RISK FACTORS

Genetics

- Alopecia areata
  - Polygenic with variety of triggering factors
  - Family history in 10–42% of cases
  - Males and females equally affected
  - Onset usually before age 30 years
- Monilethrix (also called beaded hair)
  - A rare autosomal dominant disorder

COMMONLY ASSOCIATED CONDITIONS

Trichotillomania is frequently associated with a finger-sucking habit.

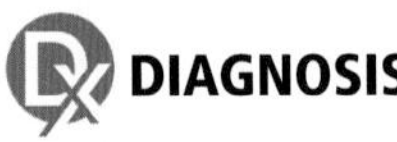

DIAGNOSIS

HISTORY

Attempt to classify the alopecia. This will guide the diagnosis and treatment plan.

- **Question:** Is the loss acquired or congenital? Is the alopecia treatable? Is it likely to be self-limited?
- *Significance*: Consider most likely diagnoses, including tinea capitis, traumatic alopecia, and alopecia areata.
- **Question:** Associated abnormalities?
- *Significance*: may be part of a syndrome
- **Question:** Is there an endocrine abnormality or a toxin/medication effect?
- *Significance*: Some of these would require prompt attention.
- **Question:** Assess extent of hair loss.
- *Significance*:
  - Increased amount of hair in the brush or in the shower/tub drain?
  - Does hair appear or feel thinner?
  - Patches of hair loss or broken hairs noted?
- **Question:** Considering trichotillomania?
- *Significance*: Note that patients often deny hair-pulling. Direct confrontation is rarely helpful.

PHYSICAL EXAM

Assess localized versus diffuse hair loss.

- **Finding:** appearance of the scalp
- *Significance*:
  - Alopecia areata: Except for well-demarcated hair loss, scalp appears normal with smooth surface.
  - Tinea capitis: Scalp is often scaly and may be erythematous; areas of hair loss with broken hair stubs, referred to as *black-dot* alopecia
- **Finding:** bizarre configuration and irregular border; hairs of varying lengths
- *Significance*: distinguishes traction/traumatic alopecia from alopecia areata
- **Finding:** short broken hairs but not black dots
- *Significance*: Short hairs are usually associated with trichotillomania, whereas black-dot alopecia is seen with tinea capitis.
- **Finding:** frontal, vertex, or bitemporal decreased hair density in adolescents
- *Significance*: may be adolescent-onset, androgenetic alopecia
- **Finding:** Hair shaft varies in thickness, with small node-like deformities (like beads), increased breakage, and partial alopecia.
- *Significance*:
  - Monilethrix
  - Other hair-shaft abnormalities with increased fragility include pseudomonilethrix, trichorrhexis, pili torti, pili bifurcati, Menkes kinky hair syndrome, and trichothiodystrophy.
- **Finding:** cervical or occipital lymphadenopathy
- *Significance*:
  - Often associated with infectious etiology (e.g., tinea capitis)
- **Finding:** associated systemic signs or any nonscalp findings
- *Significance*: may signify a genetic syndrome or endocrine abnormality
- **Finding:** nail defects such as dystrophic changes and fine stippling
- *Significance*:
  - Nail defects are seen in 10–20% of cases of alopecia areata.
  - Nail defects accompanying localized alopecia along with syndactyly, strabismus, and dermal hypoplasia may be found in Goltz syndrome.
  - In ectodermal dysplasias, nails, hair, teeth, or glands may be affected.
- **Finding:** pubic hair and eyebrow hair loss
- *Significance*:
  - Found in a form of alopecia areata called *alopecia universalis*, where nearly all body hair is lost (alopecia totalis involves the loss of all scalp hair)
  - Body hair loss such as pubic hair or eyebrow hair may also occur in trichotillomania.

DIFFERENTIAL DIAGNOSIS

Consider the most likely diagnoses first.

- Infectious
  - Tinea capitis
  - Varicella
  - Syphilis
- Congenital
  - Aplasia cutis congenita
  - Incontinentia pigmenti
  - Oculomandibulofacial syndrome (sparse hair, hypoplastic teeth, cataracts, short stature)
  - Goltz syndrome (alopecia, focal dermal hypoplasia, strabismus, nail dystrophy)
  - Triangular alopecia of the frontal scalp
  - Focal dermal hypoplasia
  - Hair-shaft defects (trichodystrophies)
  - Ectodermal dysplasias
  - Nevi
  - Progeria
- Nutritional
  - Zinc deficiency
  - Marasmus
  - Kwashiorkor
  - Anorexia or bulimia
  - Hypervitaminosis A
  - Celiac disease
- Endocrinologic
  - Androgenetic alopecia
  - Hypothyroidism
  - Hyperthyroidism
  - Hypoparathyroidism
  - Hypopituitarism
  - Diabetes mellitus
- Autoimmune
  - Alopecia areata
  - Systemic lupus erythematosus
  - Scleroderma
- Trauma
  - Traction alopecia
  - Trichotillomania
  - Scalp electrode scar from in utero monitoring
- Toxic exposures
  - Antimetabolites
  - Anticoagulants
  - Antithyroid medications
  - Heavy metals (e.g., arsenic, lead)
  - Radiation
- Stress
  - Trichotillomania
- Miscellaneous:
  - Telogen effluvium
  - Darier disease (keratotic crusted papules, keratosis follicularis)
  - Lichen planus
  - Burn
  - Stress

DIAGNOSTIC TESTS & INTERPRETATION

- **Test:** fungal culture
- *Significance*:
  - Recommended when assessing for tinea capitis as a cause of alopecia
  - Definitive results may take up to several weeks; may treat while awaiting results
  - Using a cotton-tipped applicator, culturette, toothbrush, or direct plating on Sabouraud dextrose agar, culture will be positive for *Trichophyton tonsurans* in >90% of cases in North America. This species is often involved in human to human transmission.
  - Less common are *Microsporum canis*, *Microsporum audouinii*, *Trichophyton mentagrophytes*, and *Trichophyton schoenleinii*.
- **Test:** dermatophyte test medium (DTM)
- *Significance*:
  - Assessing for tinea capitis
  - Definitive results may take from days to weeks. If dermatophyte colonies grow on the medium, the phenol red indicator in the agar will turn from yellow to red.
- **Test:** Wood light (lamp) examination
- *Significance*:
  - *M. canis*, *M. audouinii*, or *T. schoenleinii* fluoresces green.
  - *T. tonsurans* does not fluoresce.
- **Test:** potassium hydroxide (KOH) exam
- *Significance*:
  - The KOH exam is another way to assess for tinea capitis.
  - Hyphae and spores within hair shaft indicate tinea capitis.
  - With *Microsporum*, spores surround the hair shaft.
- **Test**: endocrine testing
- *Significance*:
  - Alopecia areata or diffuse alopecia is associated with several endocrine disorders (e.g., hyperthyroidism, diabetes).
  - Based on history of physical exam, consider relevant screening tests or referral to an endocrinologist or dermatologist for further evaluation.
  - Routine screening for autoimmune disorders is generally not indicated.
- **Test:** hair-pluck test
- *Significance*:
  - Used to determine the ratio of telogen (resting) to anagen (growing) hairs
  - ~50 hairs are plucked (with one firm tug using a hemostat clamped around the hair ~1 cm from the scalp) and examined under the low-power lens of a microscope to determine the percentage of hairs that are telogen and anagen hairs.
  - >25% telogen hairs are indicative of telogen effluvium.
- **Test:** scalp biopsy
- *Significance*:
  - Can help to distinguish alopecia areata and trichotillomania
  - In alopecia areata, hair follicles become small but continue to produce fine hairs; there is mitotic activity in the matrix and often inflammation is present.
  - In trichotillomania, follicles are not small. They are usually in a transitional (catagen) phase and no longer produce normal hair shafts. Keratinous debris, fibrosis, and clumps of dark melanin pigment are present. Significant inflammation is absent.
  - In telogen effluvium, follicles remain intact without inflammation.

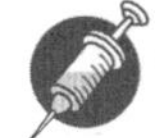

TREATMENT

GENERAL MEASURES

- Treatment of alopecia is guided by the underlying cause.
- Most patients with alopecia areata do not need treatment, as regrowth will occur spontaneously. Other than reassurance and waiting, there is no proven effective long-term therapy. Topical steroids may show short-term benefit. There are no randomized clinical trials on the use of topical immunotherapy or intralesional steroids.
- Systemic treatment is needed for tinea capitis; topical antifungals alone are not adequate. Topicals are recommended to decrease fungal shedding and risk of spread to others.
- Infectious causes of alopecia (such as with tinea capitis) should be treated promptly.
- If alopecia signifies a toxic exposure or an endocrine abnormality, the underlying condition may require prompt diagnosis and treatment.
- Caution regarding side effects of all potential treatments.

MEDICATION

First Line

- For tinea capitis: microsize griseofulvin 20 to 25 mg/kg/24 h (maximum 1 g) or ultramicrosize griseofulvin 10 to 15 mg/kg/24 h (maximum 750 mg) orally once per day for 4 to 6 weeks; approved for children >2 years of age
- Most alopecia areata does not require treatment.

Second Line

- For tinea capitis: Terbinafine may be equally as effective in treating tinea caused by *T. tonsurans* but is still considered 2nd-line therapy. Itraconazole or fluconazole may be effective. Only terbinafine is FDA-approved for this condition.
- For alopecia areata: There is limited evidence for long-term effectiveness of any treatment. For trial of other therapies (intralesional steroid, topical immunotherapy), seek consultation with a dermatologist.

COMPLEMENTARY & ALTERNATIVE THERAPIES

- Hypnotherapy, massage, acupuncture, and onion juice are among the complementary therapies that have been tried for conditions like alopecia areata and trichotillomania.
- Of note, although many patients try CAM for alopecia, more research is needed.

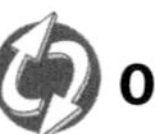

ONGOING CARE

PROGNOSIS

- Tinea capitis, alopecia areata, and traction alopecia
  - Hair will regrow, may take months
  - There is a poorer prognosis with alopecia universalis. <10% have full recovery.
- Telogen effluvium
  - Spontaneous regrowth is expected unless the stressful event continues/recurs.
- Alopecia areata may spontaneously remit and then recur.

ADDITIONAL READING

- Alkhalifah A, Alsantali A, Wang E, et al. Alopecia areata update: part II. Treatment. *J Am Acad Dermatol*. 2010;62(2):191–202.
- Castelo-Soccio L. Diagnosis and management of alopecia in children. *Pediatr Clin North Am*. 2014;61(2):427–442.
- Chen X, Jiang X, Yang M, et al. Systemic antifungal therapy for tinea capitis in children: an abridged Cochrane Review. *J Am Acad Dermatol*. 2017;76(2):368–374.
- Haynes JW, Persons R, Jamieson B. Clinical inquiries: childhood alopecia areata: what treatment works best? *J Fam Pract*. 2011;60(1):45–52.
- Hunt N, McHale S. The psychological impact of alopecia. *BMJ*. 2005;331(7522):951–953.
- National Alopecia Areata Foundation: http://www.naaf.org
- Sardesai V, Prasad S, Agarwal T. A study to evaluate the efficacy of various topical treatment modalities for alopecia areata. *Int J Trichology*. 2012;4(4):265–270.
- van den Biggelaar FJ, Smolders J, Jansen JF. Complementary and alternative medicine in alopecia areata. *Am J Clin Dermatol*. 2010;11(1):11–20.

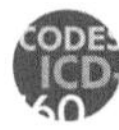

CODES

ICD10

- L65.9 Nonscarring hair loss, unspecified
- B35.0 Tinea barbae and tinea capitis
- L63.9 Alopecia areata, unspecified

FAQ

- Q: When can children with tinea capitis return to school?
- A: Once treatment with a systemic antifungal has begun, the child may return to school. A topical shampoo such as selenium sulfide or ketoconazole is recommended to decrease fungal shedding and the risk of spread.
- Q: Will the hair grow back?
- A: For the three most common causes of childhood alopecia—accounting for 90% of cases; tinea capitis, alopecia areata, and traction alopecia—hair will regrow but may take months to do so.

ALPHA-1 ANTITRYPSIN DEFICIENCY

Christine K. Lee, MD

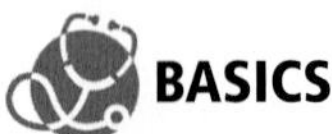

BASICS

DESCRIPTION

- α_1-antitrypsin (AAT) deficiency is an autosomal codominant genetic disorder that causes lung, liver, and skin disease.
- Lung disease in AAT deficiency can develop after the 3rd decade of life and progress to emphysema.
- Liver disease may present as jaundice in infants or as elevated liver enzymes, portal hypertension, or cirrhosis in older patients.
- Skin disease is more rare and presents as necrotizing panniculitis in adults (mean age of onset is 40 years).
- AAT deficiency is caused by a deficiency of AAT, which is a serine protease inhibitor (Pi), comprised of a 55-kDa glycoprotein that is primarily synthesized in the liver and released into the circulation.
- AAT is the main inhibitor of neutrophil proteases.
- Classic PiZZ AAT deficiency is caused by homozygosity for Z mutant allele of AAT.

EPIDEMIOLOGY

Most common genetic cause of liver disease in children and of emphysema in adults

Incidence

- Incidence of the PiZZ genotype is highest in Caucasians in North America, Australia, and Europe, particularly in Scandinavia, British Isles, Northern France, and the Tyrol region of Italy.
- In the United States, the PiZ allele is found in ~14.5 per 1,000 people, with higher frequency in Caucasians and lower frequency in Asians, blacks, and Hispanics.
- The incidence of classic AAT deficiency (PiZZ) is 1 in 1,800 to 2,000 live births.

Prevalence

- It has been estimated that approximately 70,000 to 100,000 individuals are affected in the United States.
- Of these genetically affected individuals, fewer than 10% are estimated to have been diagnosed with AAT deficiency.
- Approximately 25 million people in the United States are thought to be carriers of a mutant allele.

RISK FACTORS

Genetics

- AAT is a serine Pi encoded by the *SERPINA1* gene, which is located on the long arm of chromosome 14.
- The normal allele is M, with >100 variant alleles identified.
- The classic PiZZ genotype is the result of a point mutation at position 342 in the AAT gene, which encodes a substitution of lysine for glutamate.
- The S allele (second most common mutation) occurs from a substitution of valine for glutamate at position 246.
- Patients with PiZZ alleles have serum AAT levels, which are <15% of normal.
- Heterozygous carriers of the Z allele are found in 1.5–3% of the population. In and of itself, this genetic mutation is not a cause of liver disease, but it may contribute to pathophysiology of other liver diseases.
- PiMS, PiMZ, and PiSS are also not directly associated with liver disease, although referral center data reports patients with chronic liver disease having a higher frequency of PiMZ than would be predicted by chance.
- The mutant S protein, when coexpressed with Z-protein, can form abnormal polymers leading to liver disease, which is identical to PiZZ patients.
- Because ~10% of affected PiZZ or PiSZ individuals have clinically significant liver disease, there may be other genetic or environmental factors that are important modifiers of AAT.

PATHOPHYSIOLOGY

- Lung disease in patients with PiZZ results from inadequate levels of AAT to protect the lungs from destructive enzymes, such as elastase, leading to early emphysema.
  - This process is further worsened by exposure to cigarette smoke and environmental pollutants.
- Liver disease occurs from accumulation of the abnormal Z mutant protein within liver cells.
  - The mutant Z gene is transcribed, translated, and then translocated into the endoplasmic reticulum (ER).
  - Some molecules undergo proteolytic degradation, others aggregate to form large protein polymers, and few are secreted, leading to intrahepatocyte accumulation and thereby resulting in low AAT serum levels.
  - ER-associated degradation of mutant Z-protein is less efficient, leading to a great burden of protein in the liver and increased liver injury.
  - Autophagy degradation has also been proposed as an important route for degradation of the AAT mutant Z polymers.
- Panniculitis involves inflammation of the fat underneath the skin, causing hardening in lumps and patches, likely due to the unrestrained, destructive action of neutrophil elastase.

ETIOLOGY

Mutations in the *SERPINA1* gene result in lung disease through unopposed protease activity and in liver disease by intracellular retention of mutant AAT.

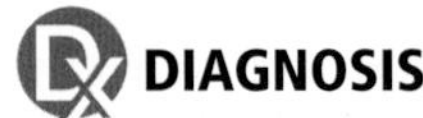

DIAGNOSIS

HISTORY

- Highly variable presentation in neonates and young children
- Most infants develop cholestatic jaundice, hepatosplenomegaly, poor feeding, and poor weight gain.
- Jaundice typically improves around 1 year of age and can then lead to either a continuation of liver disease, progression to cirrhosis, or normal liver function.
- Older children can present as asymptomatic chronic hepatitis, poor feeding, failure to thrive, hepatosplenomegaly, or complications of portal hypertension and cirrhosis.
- Risk of hepatocellular carcinoma in AAT may be independent of cirrhosis.
- Fulminant hepatic failure is rare but has been reported.

PHYSICAL EXAM

There may be signs of jaundice, hepatosplenomegaly, abdominal distention, and other stigmata of chronic liver disease.

DIFFERENTIAL DIAGNOSIS

- The differential diagnosis varies with age at presentation.
- Infants generally present with jaundice; the differential diagnosis in infants should include biliary atresia, anatomic biliary abnormalities, congenital infections, galactosemia, and tyrosinemia (see "Neonatal Cholestasis" and "Jaundice" for complete listing).
- In older children, viral (hepatitis viruses, EBV, and CMV), toxic (ethanol, acetaminophen), metabolic (Wilson disease), and obstructive causes should be considered.

DIAGNOSTIC TESTS & INTERPRETATION

Initial Tests (screening, lab, imaging)

- Elevated total and conjugated bilirubin, elevated serum transaminases, hypoalbuminemia, or coagulopathy
- Gold standard assessment is protein electrophoresis to determine the Pi phenotype.
- Serum levels of AAT can be helpful to guide workup before phenotype results are available.

- Quantitative serum AAT levels
  - PiMM: 80 to 200 mg/dL
  - PiZZ: ≤20 to 45 mg/dL
  - Pi null/null phenotype: 0 mg/dL
  - As an acute-phase reactant, AAT levels can be falsely negative, as they may rise into the normal range in an ill patient.
- Abdominal ultrasound with Doppler can be useful to assess for portal hypertension and/or for pretransplantation evaluation in the setting of end-stage liver disease.

Diagnostic Procedures/Other

- Diagnosis is determined by identification of the AAT phenotype by serum protein electrophoresis.
- Liver biopsy is not required for diagnosis but can help to support it.
- Pathologic findings
  - Liver biopsy findings can be variable in infants and may include giant cell transformation, lobular hepatitis, steatosis, fibrosis, hepatocellular necrosis, bile duct paucity, or bile duct proliferation.
  - Globular eosinophilic inclusions in some hepatocytes can be seen under H&E stain, which represent dilated ER membranes with polymerized mutant protein.
  - Staining with periodic acid–Schiff (PAS) followed by digestion with diastase to stain glycoproteins can be performed to highlight these globules.
  - These findings are sometimes seen in other liver diseases, are not visible in all hepatocytes, and may even be absent in neonates.

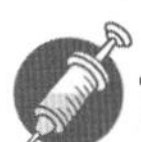

TREATMENT

- There is no specific treatment for the liver disease associated with AAT deficiency.
- Management involves supportive care to try to prevent complications of chronic liver disease.
- Patients with advanced liver disease should avoid alcohol and other hepatotoxins.
- Liver transplantation can be considered for end-stage liver disease. When transplanted, the graft will secrete normal AAT and stop further progression of lung disease.
- Due to increased risk of hepatocellular carcinoma, surveillance imaging and/or α-fetoprotein levels should be considered.
- Patients should be cautioned to avoid smoking, secondhand smoking, and other inhalation injury.
- Although enzyme replacement therapy can be used in adults to prevent progression of lung disease, it has no effect on liver disease.
- Vaccination against hepatitis A and B

MEDICATION

- Ursodeoxycholic acid, a choleretic agent, can be used to manage cholestasis and pruritus in patients with liver disease.
- Augmentation therapy
  - Pooled human plasma–derived AAT (alpha-1 antiprotease) is the most efficient way to increase the circulating levels of AAT in the plasma and lung.
  - Therapy has been reported to decrease the rate of decline in 1-second forced expiratory volume (FEV_1) and mortality rate during the period of study.

SURGERY/OTHER PROCEDURES

- There is no primary therapeutic surgical intervention for AAT deficiency aside from liver transplantation.
- Surgery in patients with native livers can be used to treat complications of portal hypertension.
- Orthotopic liver transplantation should be considered in patients with end-stage liver disease.
- Following transplantation, serum phenotype, and AAT level return to donor levels. Lung damage will not progress but is unlikely to be reversed after liver transplantation.
- For lung disease, volume reduction surgery or lung transplantation may be considered.

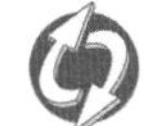

ONGOING CARE

FOLLOW-UP RECOMMENDATIONS

Patient Monitoring

- Annual liver and pulmonary function testing
- Surveillance for hepatocellular carcinoma in PiZZ patients is suggested, but consensus on frequency and methodology is lacking.

PROGNOSIS

Approximately 10% of PiZZ and PiSZ individuals will have clinically significant liver disease during childhood; ~50% of the remaining individuals will have mildly elevated aminotransferases. Further significant liver disease may develop later in life.

COMPLICATIONS

- Patients with liver disease may develop complications of chronic liver disease including portal hypertension, cirrhosis, and/or hepatocellular carcinoma.
- Lung disease may progress to early-onset lower lobe emphysema.

ADDITIONAL READING

- Miranda E, Pérez J, Ekeowa UI, et al. A novel monoclonal antibody to characterize pathogenic polymers in liver disease associated with alpha1-antitrypsin deficiency. *Hepatology*. 2010;52(3):1078–1088.
- Perlmutter DH. Alpha-1-antitrypsin deficiency: diagnosis and treatment. *Clin Liver Dis*. 2004;8(4):839–859.
- Perlmutter DH. Pathogenesis of chronic liver injury and hepatocellular carcinoma in alpha-1-antitrypsin deficiency. *Pediatr Res*. 2006;60(2):233–238.
- Steiner SJ, Gupta SK, Croffie JM, et al. Serum levels of alpha1-antitrypsin predict phenotypic expression of the alpha1-antitrypsin gene. *Dig Dis Sci*. 2003;48(9):1793–1796.
- Stoller JK, Brantly M. The challenge of detecting alpha-1 antitrypsin deficiency. *COPD*. 2013;(10 Suppl 1):26–34.
- Teckman J. Alpha1-antitrypsin deficiency in childhood. *Semin Liver Dis*. 2007;27(3):274–281.
- Teckman J. Liver disease in alpha-1 antitrypsin deficiency: current understanding and future therapy. *COPD*. 2013;(10 Suppl 1):35–43.
- Teckman J, Jain A. Advances in alpha-1-antitrypsin deficiency liver disease. *Curr Gastroenterol Rep*. 2014;16(1):367.

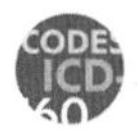

CODES

ICD10

E88.01 Alpha-1-antitrypsin deficiency

FAQ

- Q: Do all patients with presumed AAT require liver biopsy for diagnosis?
- A: No. A liver biopsy is not required for diagnosis but may help be performed to support it.
- Q: Are PAS-positive, diastase-resistant globules on liver biopsy diagnostic for AAT deficiency?
- A: No. Diagnosis is made by identification of the AAT phenotype by serum protein electrophoresis. Evidence of these globules on liver biopsy can support the diagnosis but may be absent in PiZZ neonates.
- Q: Will liver transplantation for AAT deficiency have any effect on the lungs?
- A: Yes. When a patient with AAT deficiency gets an orthotopic liver transplant, serum levels of AAT usually return to normal. This halts further progression of lung disease but does not reverse lung damage, which has already occurred.

ALTITUDE ILLNESS

Michael Yaron, MD

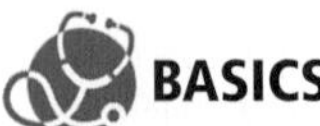

BASICS

DESCRIPTION

High-altitude illness represents a spectrum of clinical entities with neurologic and pulmonary manifestations that overlap presentations and share elements of pathophysiology. Acute mountain sickness (AMS) is the relatively benign and self-limited presentation, whereas high-altitude pulmonary edema (HAPE) and high-altitude cerebral edema (HACE) represent the potentially life-threatening manifestations.

EPIDEMIOLOGY

- Altitude illness common with rapid ascent to *moderate altitude* (8,000 to 11,500 feet); most serious cases occur at *very high altitude* (11,500 to 18,000 feet).
- Children risk developing altitude illness when travelling to high locations with their families.

Incidence

- Children have the same or lower incidence of altitude illness as adults.
- The rapid ascent profile associated with air travel to high-altitude locations results in higher AMS rates. Among skiers who fly or drive to resorts in the western United States, AMS frequency is approximately 25%.
- HACE is extremely rare in children primarily occurring after prolonged stays at very high altitudes; a place most children should not be
- HAPE frequency in children is <1% with primary ascent, but reentry HAPE may occur in 6–17% of children who are permanent altitude residents. A concurrent viral illness increases risk.
- In most cases, altitude illness can be prevented by employing proper precautions and/or instituting early treatment before any serious illness occurs.

RISK FACTORS

- Incidence depends on rate of ascent, sleeping altitude, degree of physical exertion, cold weather, and previous altitude exposure.
- Individual (genetic) susceptibility plays a key role in risk assessment. Children with a previous history of AMS and HAPE can experience similar symptoms with similar ascent profiles.
- Underlying medical conditions resulting in hypoxia sensitivity or pulmonary hypertension are significant risk factors: acute respiratory infection or otitis, incomplete postnatal circulatory transition (term infants <6 weeks of age or premies <46 weeks postconceptual age), atrial or ventricular septal defects, PFO, PDA, pulmonary vein stenosis, congenital absence of pulmonary artery, pulmonary hypertension, obstructive sleep apnea, cystic fibrosis, hypoplastic lung, Down syndrome, sickle cell disease, and children <1 year of age with a history of oxygen requirement or pulmonary hypertension
- Reentry HAPE risk in residents from >9,000 feet that travel to low altitude for short period and return home

GENERAL PREVENTION

- Assess risk factors and plan rate of ascent:
  - Slow ascent is the best prevention strategy; sleeping altitude: ideally first night no higher than 9,200 feet and then 2 to 3 nights at 8,200 to 9,800 feet, with subsequent increases limited to 1,500 feet each night and 1 extra day without ascent for every 3,000 feet gained
- Formulation of emergency communication and evacuation plan
  - Difficult descent situations (i.e., additional ascent needed before descent possible) should be avoided.
  - Cell or satellite communication may fail.
- Prompt recognition of symptoms
  - Train parents in symptom recognition and treatment principles.

PATHOPHYSIOLOGY

- Severe AMS/HACE: rising intracranial volume and pressure from vasogenic edema (HACE). Mechanism for mild AMS remains unclear. A "tight-fitting" CNS within the skull and spine has less ability to buffer early edema. Activation of the trigeminovascular system may play a role.
- HAPE: elevated pulmonary artery pressure, uneven vasoconstriction, pulmonary overperfusion injury and leakage, inflammation, and impaired alveolar fluid clearance
- Among children who reside at high altitude, reentry HAPE decreases with increasing age suggesting a role in pulmonary vasculature remodeling.

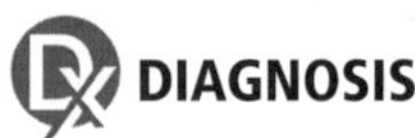

DIAGNOSIS

HISTORY

- AMS:
  - All symptoms may range from mild to severe and incapacitating. AMS occurs in the setting of recent altitude gain, a headache, and at least one of the following: anorexia, nausea or vomiting, general weakness or fatigue, dizziness or light-headedness, or difficulty sleeping. These are the adult criteria for AMS and may be used in older children and adolescents who are able to verbally express headache or hunger. Headache can be assessed by asking if the "head hurts" and GI symptoms by asking the child if they are "hungry" rather than evaluating appetite. Sleep disturbance is common in all visitors to high altitudes but is exacerbated in the setting of AMS.
  - Among infants and older preverbal children (up to 3 years of age), signs of AMS are less specific and diagnosed using nonverbal criteria. AMS is manifested by increased fussiness (headache equivalent), decreased playfulness, decreased appetite, and sleep disturbance. In most cases, all of these symptoms are present. Fussiness is a state of irritability that is not easily explained by a cause, such as tiredness, wet diaper, hunger, teething, or pain from an injury. Fussy behavior includes crying, restlessness, or muscular tension. Decreased playfulness may be profound, vomiting may occur, and sleep disturbance is most often manifest as decreased sleep and the inability to nap.
  - Parents can learn to recognize AMS in preverbal children using the Children's Lake Louise Score (LLS).
    - To calculate score, combine the fussiness score with the symptom score.
    - Children's LLS ≥7 with fussiness score ≥4 + symptom score ≥3 is considered diagnostic of AMS.

Fussiness Score	0	1	2	3	4	5	6
Amount	None			Intermittent			Constant
Intensity	Not fussy			Moderately fussy			Extremely fussy

Symptom Score	0	1	2	3
Eating	Norm	Slightly less	Much less	Not eating; vomiting
Playing	Norm	Slightly less	Much less	Not playing
Sleeping	Norm	Slightly less or more	Much less or more	Not able to sleep

  - Symptoms generally develop 6 to 12 hours after ascent but may be seen 1 to 2 hours after ascent and reach maximum severity by 24 hours, followed by resolution over the next day without any further ascent. Symptoms developing 2 or more days after ascent to a given altitude should prompt consideration of alternative diagnoses (see "Differential Diagnosis"). AMS may reappear upon additional ascent. Rarely symptoms persist for several days requiring descent if treatment fails.

ALERT

The vague nature of AMS presentation has resulted misdiagnoses and morbidity. These symptoms warrant a presumptive diagnosis of AMS and limitation of further ascent, until proven otherwise.

- HACE:
  - Extremely rare in children but rapidly fatal if unrecognized; develops 2 to 3 days after ascent
  - Differentiated from AMS by the presence of neurologic signs
  - Most common are ataxia and altered mental status including confusion, progressive unresponsiveness, and coma.
  - Less common are focal cranial nerve palsies, motor and sensory deficits, and seizures.
- HAPE:
  - Generally, develops gradually over 24 to 72 hours and may be associated with concurrent viral illness; may also occur suddenly
  - Although all children have dyspnea on exertion at altitude, dyspnea out of proportion to effort or dyspnea at rest is an early indicator of HAPE. AMS precedes HAPE development in approximately 1/2 of cases. General malaise progresses to the more specific sign of dyspnea at rest, then cardiopulmonary distress.
  - Young children may show agitation and general debility. Older children may complain of headache, and all ages frequently experience nausea and vomiting. Cough is common in all ages.
  - Dyspnea at rest, orthopnea, cyanosis, chest pain, and tachycardia, herald worsening compromise leading to production of pink-tinged sputum, increasing hypoxia with eventual coma, and death.

PHYSICAL EXAM

- There are no diagnostic physical signs in cases of mild AMS. Any evidence of CNS dysfunction, such as mild ataxia or altered mentation is early evidence of HACE.
- Similarly, although dyspnea on exertion is universal at high altitudes, dyspnea at rest or out of proportion to effort is an early indicator of HAPE.

- HAPE exam findings are often less severe than a patient's chest radiograph and the hypoxemia on pulse oximetry would predict. Children appear pale, with or without visible cyanosis. Auscultation reveals rales, usually greater in the right lung. Fever (<38.5°C) and tachypnea are common. Higher fevers are unusual from HAPE alone and should prompt consideration of infection or other diagnoses. Respiratory infection may precede HAPE development (see "Risk Factors") thus coexist with HAPE.

DIFFERENTIAL DIAGNOSIS

- If AMS symptoms develop without a headache or begin several days after ascent, an alternative diagnosis should be considered. AMS symptoms resolve quickly with oxygen administration (2 to 4 L/min for 20 minutes) and may be used to support the diagnosis.
- If AMS is not clear, viral or bacterial illness, sepsis, metabolic/toxic abnormalities, hypothermia, occult trauma including corneal abrasion, and dehydration should be considered.
- Differential of HAPE includes pneumonia, bronchitis/bronchiolitis, asthma, heart failure, other noncardiogenic pulmonary edema, and pulmonary embolism. HAPE is most frequently misdiagnosed as pneumonia.

DIAGNOSTIC TESTS & INTERPRETATION

Initial Tests (screening, lab, imaging)

- EKG: HAPE: may reveal RV strain
- Pulse oximetry: HAPE: Arterial oxygen desaturation is a consistent finding, with saturations frequently <75%.
- No lab studies needed for AMS. Labs may be needed for evaluation of differential diagnoses when altitude illness is complicated or unclear.
- Chest x-ray
  - HAPE—pulmonary edema pattern variable, from patchy/peripheral to homogeneous in severe cases. Right lung shows more radiographic changes of edema than left. Peribronchial and perivascular cuffing and enlargement of pulmonary artery are common.
- Brain CT/MR imaging
  - HACE—CT imaging consistent with edema and increased intracranial pressure. MRI: high T2 signal in the white matter, specifically in the splenium of the corpus callosum, with diffusion-weighted technique

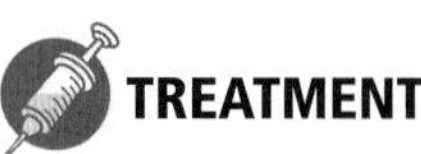

TREATMENT

GENERAL MEASURES

- After development of altitude illness, further ascent is contraindicated until resolution occurs.
- Descent (of 1,600 to 3,300 feet) from altitude of illness onset is effective treatment for all forms of altitude illness.
- Mild AMS
  - Usually self-limited not requiring treatment. Stop ascent and rest until symptoms improve.
  - May be treated without descent if monitoring by reliable caregiver available
- Moderate to severe AMS
  - Symptomatic treatment with analgesics and antiemetics: ibuprofen, acetaminophen, ondansetron; oxygen if available; may use acetazolamide if above measures inadequate; descend if persistent or severe.
- HACE
  - Descend immediately.
  - Supplemental oxygen to keep Spo_2 >90%, bed rest, dexamethasone, portable hyperbaric chamber while awaiting descent
- HAPE
  - Without medical expertise, descend immediately. Otherwise, if mild may treat by stopping ascent, rest, and oxygen to keep Spo_2 >90%. Use nifedipine in severe cases if descent is delayed or oxygen unavailable.

MEDICATION

- Oxygen relieves AMS symptoms (1 to 4 L/min), easily available in most resorts, reserved for severe cases in remote settings; hyperbaric therapy also effective, as it simulates descent
- Acetazolamide (carbonic anhydrase inhibitor)
  - AMS prevention: 2.5 mg/kg PO q12h, max 125 mg/dose; not routinely used in children; indicated with unavoidable rapid ascent profile or previous significant/recurrent history with similar ascent planned
  - AMS treatment: 2.5 mg/kg PO q8–12h, max 250 mg/dose;
  - Caution if patient has a sulfa allergy
  - Paresthesia and taste alteration with carbonated beverages common
  - Liquid solution can be made by crushing 250 mg tablet and suspend in sweet solution to hide bitter taste.
- Dexamethasone (steroid)
  - Prevention of AMS: risk of adverse effects; use not warranted; use slow ascent or acetazolamide.
  - AMS treatment: Oxygen/descent is treatment of choice for severe AMS; acetazolamide preferred, if patient has a sulfa allergy; dexamethasone may be used.
  - HACE treatment: immediate descent plus oxygen and dexamethasone, 0.15 mg/kg PO/IM/IV q6h, max 4 mg/dose
- Nifedipine (calcium channel blocker)
  - Prevention and treatment of HAPE: small children: immediate-release 0.5 mg/kg/dose q8h, max 20 mg/dose. If >60 kg, 30 mg sustained-release (SR) PO q12h. Indicated for treatment in emergency setting where oxygen and descent are not an option (oxygen alone provides maximal treatment, no advantage adding nifedipine); may cause hypotension
- Sildenafil (phosphodiesterase inhibitor)
  - Prevention/treatment of HAPE: 0.5 mg/kg/dose PO q8h, max 50 mg/dose q8h
  - For treatment, only indicated in emergency setting where oxygen and descent are not an option, alternative if nifedipine not well-tolerated

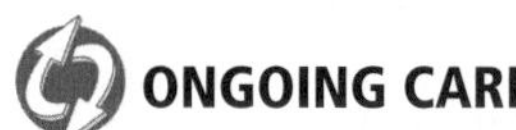

ONGOING CARE

FOLLOW-UP RECOMMENDATIONS

Refer to primary care physician for education of prevention strategies and consideration of prophylaxis with future ascent. History of HAPE or severe hypoxemia warrants cardiopulmonary evaluation for pulmonary hypertension or structural cardiac abnormality.

PROGNOSIS

- Excellent if recognized quickly, ascent stopped, and descent and/or therapy initiated
- Prognosis can be poor if symptoms go unrecognized or noted without appropriate descent and therapy.

ADDITIONAL READING

- Joy E, Van Baak K, Dec KL, et al. Wilderness preparticipation evaluation and considerations for special populations. *Wilderness Environ Med*. 2015;26(Suppl 4): S76–S91.
- Luks AM, McIntosh SE, Grissom CK, et al. Wilderness Medical Society consensus guidelines for the prevention and treatment of acute altitude illness. *Wilderness Environ Med*. 2010;21(2):146–155.
- Niermeyer S. Going to high altitude with a newborn infant. *High Alt Med Biol*. 2007;8(2):117–123.
- Pollard AJ, Niermeyer S, Barry P, et al. Children at high altitude: an international consensus statement by an ad hoc committee of the International Society for Mountain Medicine. *High Alt Med Biol*. 2001;2(3):389–403.
- Yaron M, Niermeyer S. Travel to high altitude with young children: an approach for clinicians. *High Alt Med Biol*. 2008;9(4):265–269.

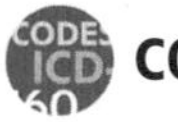

CODES

ICD10

- T70.20XA Unspecified effects of high altitude, initial encounter
- T70.29XA Other effects of high altitude, initial encounter
- R09.02 Hypoxemia

FAQ

- Q: Can one develop AMS at moderate altitudes, such as during a ski vacation?
- A: Yes. 25% of visitors from sea level will get AMS symptoms, although the altitudes encountered rarely lead to the development of severe symptoms.
- Q: When can we bring our newborn term baby to our mountain house at 9,000 feet?
- A: The postnatal cardiopulmonary transition is nearly complete by 6 weeks and then most babies can safely ascend to moderate altitudes.
- Q: Should I give prophylactic medication to my child to prevent high altitude illness?
- A: Not usually. Gradual ascent is the primary method of preventing illness. Only children with a significant risk/history or unavoidable rapid ascent should be given prophylaxis.
- Q: Is it safe to take my child on a 3-week trek crossing several mountain passes in Nepal?
- A: Not necessarily. Balance the benefits against the risks of being in a remote environment with exposure to environmental dangers (altitude, weather, infectious disease), without easy medical care, evacuation, or communication.
- Q: Should I treat my child with acetazolamide if she develops AMS.
- A: Usually not needed. Rest, stopping further ascent and symptomatic treatment are generally adequate (see "General Measures" section)

AMBIGUOUS GENITALIA (DISORDERS OF SEXUAL DEVELOPMENT)

J. Nina Ham, MD

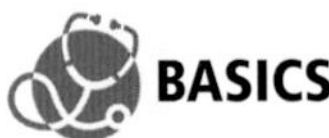

BASICS

DESCRIPTION

- Genital ambiguity occurs when it is not possible to categorize the gender of the child based on outward genital appearance.
- Can result from various disorders of sexual development (DSD), a generic term defined as a congenital condition in which development of chromosomal, gonadal, or phenotypic sex is atypical
  - General DSD categories are sex chromosome DSD; 46,XX DSD; 46,XY DSD; ovotesticular DSD; 46,XX testicular DSD; and 46,XY complete gonadal dysgenesis. Specific diagnoses (when available) are preferable to these broad categories.
  - Previous terms such as "intersex," "pseudohermaphroditism," or "sex reversal" should be avoided.
- Criteria that suggest that a child may have a DSD include the following:
  - Bilateral nonpalpable testes
  - Micropenis (stretched length <2.5 cm at full term)
  - Severe hypospadias or mild hypospadias with a unilateral undescended testis
  - Clitoromegaly (width >6 mm or length >9 mm), posterior labial fusion
  - An inguinal/labial mass
  - Family history of a DSD
  - Discordance between genital appearance and prenatal karyotype
- Note: The term "DSD" also comprises sex chromosome disorders including Turner (45,X) and Klinefelter syndromes (47,XXY). However, these usually do not present as ambiguous genitalia.

EPIDEMIOLOGY

- Genital anomalies at birth have a prevalence as high as 1 in 300.
- Genital ambiguity has a prevalence of approximately 1 in 5,000 births.
- Congenital adrenal hyperplasia (CAH) is the most common cause of DSD. CAH is discussed in detail in a separate chapter.
- Partial androgen insensitivity syndrome (PAIS) is the next most common cause of DSD (classified as a 46,XY DSD).
- Disorders causing genital ambiguity are congenital and usually present in the newborn period.
- Later presentations can occur in older children and young adults. Examples:
  - 46,XY individuals with complete 17α-hydroxylase/17,20-lyase deficiency may present in adolescence with hypertension and delayed puberty.
  - Women with complete androgen insensitivity syndrome (CAIS) may present during adolescence with primary amenorrhea.
  - Children with 5α-reductase deficiency may become virilized during puberty.

RISK FACTORS

Genetics

- Several single-gene disorders causing gonadal dysgenesis have been described. However, only 15–20% of patients with DSDs are diagnosed at the molecular level.
- 46,XY DSD may be associated with mutations in the following genes:
  - Genes involved in testicular development: sex-determining region on Y (*SRY*), *SOX9*, steroidogenic factor 1 (*SF-1*), Wilms tumor suppressor (*WT1*) gene, *WNT4* duplication, and *DAX1* duplication
  - Genes involved in steroid hormone action or synthesis (autosomal recessive, except for the androgen receptor [AR])
    - LH/choriogonadotropin receptor (*LHCGR*) gene, leading to Leydig cell hypoplasia and decreased testosterone (T) production
    - Genes encoding adrenal steroidogenic enzymes, causing undervirilization: 17α-hydroxylase (*CYP17A1*), 3β-hydroxysteroid dehydrogenase (*HSD3B2*), P450 oxidoreductase, and StAR protein (lipoid hyperplasia)
    - 5α-reductase gene (*SRD5A2*), leading to defective conversion of T to dihydrotestosterone (DHT). DHT is necessary for the development of male external genitalia in utero.
    - AR gene located on the X chromosome (X-linked recessive), leading to impaired androgen action
- 46,XX DSD may be associated with mutations in the following genes:
  - Genes involved in ovarian development and leading to gonadal dysgenesis: FSH receptor (*FSHR*), *SF-1*
  - Genes involved in testicular development: presence of *SRY*, *SOX9* duplication
  - Genes encoding adrenal steroidogenic enzymes, leading to virilizing CAH: 21-hydroxylase (*CYP21A*), the most common form; 11β-hydroxylase (*CYP11B1*); 3β-hydroxysteroid dehydrogenase (*HSD3B2*)
  - Aromatase gene (*CYP19A1*), leading to impaired placental conversion of fetal adrenal androgens to estrogens
- Sex chromosome DSDs (45,X; 47,XXY; 45,X/46,XY; and 46,XX/46,XY) are caused by meiotic or mitotic nondisjunction.

PATHOPHYSIOLOGY

- 46,XY DSD
  - Incomplete masculinization of the male fetus can be caused by disorders of T synthesis (e.g., CAH, 5α-reductase deficiency), unresponsiveness to T action (androgen insensitivity syndromes), or defects in testicular development (complete or partial gonadal dysgenesis).
- 46,XX DSD
  - Masculinization of the female fetus is caused by exposure to androgens, either endogenous or exogenous. The most common cause is CAH in which the fetal adrenal glands overproduce androgens in an attempt to produce cortisol.
  - The ovaries and müllerian derivatives are normal, and the sexual ambiguity is limited to masculinization of the external genitalia.
- Ovotesticular DSD
  - Presence of both ovarian and testicular elements. Combinations may include one ovary and one testis, two ovotestes, or one ovotestis with either an ovary or a testis. Differentiation of internal and external genitalia often coincides with the gonad on the ipsilateral side.
  - Karyotypes are 46,XX most commonly; the molecular basis of this disorder may not be known; 46,XX/46,XY and 46,XX/47,XXY reported.
- Gonadal dysgenesis
  - Mixed gonadal dysgenesis (MGD) (classically 45,X/46,XY) involves a streak gonad on one side and a testis, often dysgenetic, on the other side. Phenotype is highly variable and ranges from female external genitalia through all stages of ambiguous genitalia to a normal male.
  - Pure (complete) gonadal dysgenesis (46,XX, 46,XY, or a Turner syndrome karyotype) involves replacement of gonads by streak gonads. Neonates have female external genitalia and often present later in life with delayed puberty and primary amenorrhea.

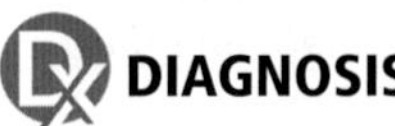

DIAGNOSIS

- Genital ambiguity in the neonate should be treated as an emergency, and diagnostic evaluation undertaken as soon as possible.
- CAH, the most common cause of DSD, can be life-threatening when accompanied by salt wasting.
- A diagnosis of DSD is difficult and may be disturbing for families and calls for immediate investigation, counseling, and support.

HISTORY

Obtain a careful gestational and family history addressing the following:

- Drug ingestions or exposure to teratogens
- Infections during the pregnancy
- Androgenic changes in the mother
- Family history of DSDs may not be known or disclosed, but hypospadias, amenorrhea, or infertility in the family may be more commonly known.
- History of consanguinity

PHYSICAL EXAM

Notable features include phallic structure size, labial fusion, symmetry of external genitalia, presence and location of palpable gonads, and presence of additional anomalies.

- Gonads: Palpable gonads are nearly always testes and the presence of Y-chromosome material, whereas bilateral undescended testes may indicate 46, XX DSD.
- Labial fusion: measurement of the anogenital ratio (distance from anus to posterior fourchette divided by distance from anus to base of phallus). If >0.5, this suggests virilization with posterior labial fusion.
- Position of the urethra
- Length and breadth of penis/clitoris: In term newborns, stretched penile length is usually ≥2.5 cm; clitoral size is usually <1 cm in length and <6 mm breadth.
- Presence of a vagina
- Development of the scrotum: Bifid scrotum suggests undervirilization.

- Inguinal hernia in the presence of female external genitalia: may indicate testes
- Asymmetry of external genitalia: suggests ovotesticular or 45,X/46,XY DSDs
- Hypertension is seen with CAH due to 17α-hydroxylase and 11-hydroxylase deficiencies.
- Other dysmorphic features

DIFFERENTIAL DIAGNOSIS

- Gonadal dysgenesis
- 46,XY DSD
  - CAH causing undervirilization of boys
  - 5α-Reductase deficiency prevents in utero formation of male external genitalia.
  - Syndromes of androgen resistance due to abnormalities in AR or postreceptor defects
- 46,XX DSD
  - CAH causing virilization in female
  - Maternal androgen exposure
  - Exogenous androgens or endogenous production (e.g., maternal virilizing tumor)
- Ovotesticular DSD
- Multiple congenital anomalies: Ambiguous genitalia can be a part of a spectrum of congenital anomalies involving the rectum and urologic system.
- Idiopathic

DIAGNOSTIC TESTS & INTERPRETATION

Initial Tests (screening, lab, imaging)

- Initial evaluation should be targeted to help with sex assignment and assessment of gonadal and adrenal steroids. First-line investigation includes the following:
  - Karyotype, or fluorescence in situ hybridization (FISH) (X- and Y-specific probes)
  - Measurement of 17α-hydroxyprogesterone (17-OHP), T, anti–müllerian hormone (AMH) (reliable indicator of testicular tissue), and serum electrolytes
- Second-line investigations depend on the karyotype, the presence of palpable gonads, and the 17-OHP levels. These can be ordered simultaneously or after initial tests, depending on the clinical situation.
  - Karyotype is 47,XY: Labs include tests to determine if testes are present and functional:
    - LH, FSH, müllerian-inhibiting substance (MIS), T, and DHT
    - hCG stimulation test will help differentiate disorders of abnormal response to androgen from disorders of androgen synthesis.
  - Karyotype is 46,XX and nonpalpable gonads:
    - Most commonly due to CAH
- Ultrasonography (US) of the abdomen and pelvis
  - Part of the first-line investigation
  - Can help determine the presence of gonads, uterus, and/or vagina
  - Lack of US visualization of gonads not definitive; only 50% accurate in identifying intra-abdominal testes
- Retrograde urethrogram can help evaluate the urogenital sinus.
- MRI can further delineate the internal anatomy.

Diagnostic Procedures/Other

- Cystoscopy/vaginoscopy is gold standard method to assess the urethral and vaginal anatomy.
- Laparoscopy +/− gonadal biopsy may be required for definitive evaluation of the reproductive structures.

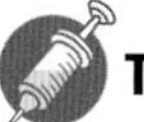

TREATMENT

GENERAL MEASURES

- Emphasis is on patient-centered care.
- Medical staff should use terms such as "your child" or "your baby" rather than "he," "she," or "it."
- Counsel family to not make announcements describing gender until gender assignment is determined.
- Parents should be counseled that the diagnostic information, surgical factors, prediction of hormone function, and potential for fertility will be taken together as a whole.
- Gender assignment should be made through a family-centered and multidisciplinary team approach with consultations from endocrinology, urology, neonatology, genetics, psychiatry/psychology, and social work. If these services are not available, the family may benefit from transfer to a pediatric tertiary care facility that can provide this multidisciplinary approach.
- Surgical management
  - If the gender assignment is female, feminizing genitoplasty should be considered in severe virilization. Given the potential risk for disturbance of sensation, clitoroplasty should not be performed for cosmetic purposes alone. Vaginoplasty may be acceptable in infancy given the potential for improved functional outcome.
  - If gender assignment is male, phallic reconstruction can be done when the team and parents are comfortable with the timing. Urethral reconstruction for hypospadias is usually scheduled between 6 and 24 months of age.
  - Reconstructive surgery timing is an area of controversy in recent years. Some advocate for delay in surgery until individual gender identity is established, and the child is fully able to consent. There is no clear consensus as to timing of surgery except for need to engage in fully informed discussion with the family.
  - Gonadectomy or repositioning may be recommended in patients at risk of gonadal malignancy (gonads bearing the Y chromosome). Tumor risk is heterogeneous among DSDs (e.g., high in MGD and low in AR), and the optimal age and type of surgery can vary substantially.

MEDICATION

- With the exception of CAH, most DSD conditions do not require specific medical treatment until puberty.
- At the time of expected puberty, hormonal therapy is usually started in patients with hypogonadism: between 10.5 and 12 years for females and 12.5 and 14 years for males.

ADDITIONAL THERAPIES

Psychosocial management

- Long-term counseling for the child and parents by mental health staff with expertise in DSDs is critical to promote psychological adaption at all stages of cognitive and psychosocial development.
- The team can facilitate decision-making processes involving gender assignment/reassignment, timing of surgery, and hormonal replacement.

ONGOING CARE

FOLLOW-UP RECOMMENDATIONS

- Long-term follow-up may involve monitoring hormone levels, linear growth, and sexual and psychological development.
- Follow-up also involves monitoring for gonadal malignancy. Surveillance imaging and testicular palpation should be performed in all DSD patients with abdominal or scrotal testes respectively.

PROGNOSIS

- Approach to surgical management has changed over time. Cosmetic and functional outcomes vary; there continues to be, however, a need for further data on long-term outcomes.
- Potential for reproductive function depends on the specific diagnosis.
- Long-term studies of psychological adjustment are underway.

ADDITIONAL READING

- Barbaro M, Wedell A, Nordenström A. Disorders of sex development. *Semin Fetal Neonatal Med.* 2011;16(2):119–127.
- Lambert SM, Vilain EJ, Kolon TF. A practical approach to ambiguous genitalia in the newborn. *Urol Clin North Am.* 2010;37(2):195–205.
- Lee PA, Houk CP, Ahmed SF, et al; and International Consensus Conference on Intersex organized by the Lawson Wilkins Pediatric Endocrine Society and the European Society for Paediatric Endocrinology. Consensus statement on management of intersex disorders. *Pediatrics.* 2006;118(2):e488–e500.
- MacLaughlin DT, Donahoe PK. Sex determination and differentiation. *N Engl J Med.* 2004;350(4):367–378.
- Mouriquand PD, Gorduza DB, Gay CL, et al. Surgery in disorders of sex development (DSD) with a gender issue: if (why), when, and how? *J Pediatr Urol.* 2016;12(3):139–149.
- Nokoff NJ, Palmer B, Mullins AJ, et al. Prospective assessment of cosmesis before and after genital surgery. *J Pediatr Urol.* 2017;13(1):28.e1–28.e6.
- Wherrett DK. Approach to the infant with a suspected disorder of sex development. *Pediatr Clin N Am.* 2015;62:983–999.

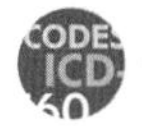

CODES

ICD10

- Q56.4 Indeterminate sex, unspecified
- E25.0 Congenital adrenogenital disorders assoc w enzyme deficiency
- Q56.3 Pseudohermaphroditism, unspecified

FAQ

- Q: Should a child's sex assignment be consistent with the karyotype?
- A: This is a major decision that should involve the family and the treatment team. Future potential for sexual, hormonal, and reproductive function, in addition to genetics, are all important factors.
- Q: What clues can the physical exam give to the timing of in utero events causing sexual ambiguity?
- A: In the virilized female, labioscrotal fusion results from androgen exposure prior to 12 weeks of gestation. After 12 weeks, androgen exposure only can result in clitoromegaly.

AMBLYOPIA

Melissa A. Simon, MD • Michael F. Chiang, MD

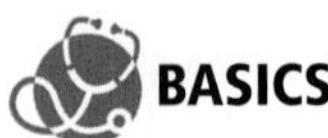

BASICS

DESCRIPTION

Amblyopia is a decrease in best corrected visual acuity, usually in an otherwise anatomically normal eye. It is generally classified by cause, with three primary types:

- Refractive amblyopia: resulting from uncorrected refractive error (improper focusing of light by the eye which generally requires correction by eyeglasses or contact lenses), with the following subtypes:
  - Anisometropic amblyopia: resulting from asymmetric refractive error and resultant unilateral blurring. This condition is the most common cause of refractive amblyopia.
  - Ametropic amblyopia: resulting from significant refractive error in both eyes
  - Meridional amblyopia: resulting from large uncorrected astigmatism in one or both eyes
- Strabismic amblyopia: resulting from strabismus (misalignment of the eyes) and subsequent lack of an image that can be "fused" or integrated into a single image in the brain. This condition is most likely with early onset, constant strabismus. Approximately 50% of patients with strabismus will also have amblyopia.
- Deprivation amblyopia: resulting from optical or anatomic pathology (e.g., cataract, ptosis, corneal opacity, prolonged patching), which prevents the formation of a clear image in one or both eyes. Deprivation, especially if it begins early in life, is associated with the most severe amblyopia.

EPIDEMIOLOGY

Amblyopia is the most common cause of unilateral vision loss in children and young adults.

Prevalence

Large population-based studies indicate that 0.8–3.3% of the adult population has amblyopia.

PATHOPHYSIOLOGY

- Visual acuity in amblyopic eyes varies from minimal impairment (20/25) to legal blindness (<20/200) or worse. Other significant impairments in amblyopic eyes may include reduced contrast sensitivity, reduced or absent binocularity and depth perception, and impaired or distorted spatial perception. Peripheral visual fields are preserved, and vision is never completely lost (no light perception) from amblyopia alone.
- Asymmetric input between the two eyes (e.g., unilateral cataract, anisometropia, etc.) is more likely to cause amblyopia than symmetrically poor images due to competitive influences between the two eyes. As a result, amblyopia is usually unilateral.
- Bilateral amblyopia may result from severe, symmetric bilateral image degradation such as bilateral cataract, bilateral high ametropia (high refractive error), etc.

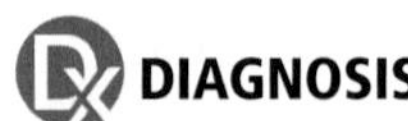

DIAGNOSIS

Signs and symptoms: poor vision

HISTORY

- Age when poor vision was first noted
- Eye trauma, injury, or surgery
- Refractive error or glasses
- Ptosis or ocular occlusion (Because amblyopia related to ptosis is often due to resultant astigmatism, this can occur even if the affected eye is not completely occluded.)
- Family history of strabismus, anisometropia, or amblyopia
- History of prematurity or developmental delay

PHYSICAL EXAM

- Because the outcome of amblyopia depends entirely on early detection and treatment within the first few years of life, all children should be screened by monocular recognition visual acuity as early as possible, and testing has traditionally been recommended to be repeated annually until 8 years of age (although evidence now suggests potential benefits of screening through adolescence).
- The United States Preventive Services Task Force recommends screening beginning at age 3 years. Ongoing research is investigating potential benefits of screening children as early as age 1 year. In general, children who are not capable of accurate visual acuity testing by 4 years of age should be referred for complete evaluation.
- Visual acuity is the single most significant sign in detection of amblyopia. Vision must be tested in each eye separately with reliable occlusion (ideally an adhesive patch). Because most amblyopia is monocular, testing vision with both eyes open is inadequate as a screening tool.
- Children must be tested with each eye separately.
- Binocularity tests such as Titmus stereopsis (3D fly) will detect suppression, which is frequently associated with amblyopia.

DIFFERENTIAL DIAGNOSIS

- Amblyopia is diagnosed by exclusion: Conditions that cause vision loss without easily recognized pathology might be mistaken for amblyopia.
- In children, the differential diagnosis of vision loss in eyes that appear normal by penlight includes the following:
  - Uncorrected refractive error (hyperopia, myopia, astigmatism)
  - Optic nerve hypoplasia
  - Optic atrophy
  - Compressive, toxic, or hereditary optic neuropathies
  - Retinopathies, including retinopathy of prematurity, Leber congenital amaurosis, Stargardt disease, retinitis pigmentosa, and others
  - Central visual impairment (cortical blindness)
  - Glaucoma
  - Nonorganic or functional causes

DIAGNOSTIC TESTS & INTERPRETATION

- Vision testing in young children is difficult and, sometimes, unreliable. Repeating the tests and adjunctive tests including the Titmus test, cover testing, photoscreening, and Brückner red reflex test will increase the sensitivity of screening.
- Photoscreening has become a sensitive, specific, and recommended way to screen preverbal and nonverbal children for the risk factors that lead to amblyopia, but these devices do not yet identify amblyopia itself. Only visual acuity testing can identify amblyopia directly.
- The American Association for Pediatric Ophthalmology and Strabismus published online "Vision Screening Recommendations" and referral criteria by age. For every cohort, multiple exam techniques and data collection approaches are recommended.
- Imaging studies of the optic nerves and posterior visual pathways may be useful in selected cases to exclude other causes of vision loss.

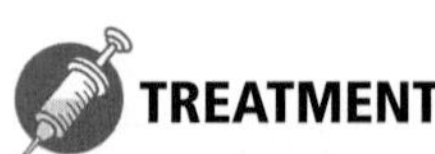

TREATMENT

GENERAL MEASURES

- Refractive correction, when needed, is critical and can improve amblyopia before additional treatment.
- Unilateral amblyopia
  - Treat underlying cause of vision loss (strabismus, anisometropia, optical opacity) and force preferential use of the amblyopic eye.
  - The classic and most common treatment is occlusion with an adhesive patch worn over the opposite (unaffected) eye for hours daily.

- The amount of time of occlusion necessary to reverse amblyopia depends on variables including the severity of amblyopia, cause of amblyopia, age, and other associated ocular conditions.
- Typical duration of treatment is 6 months but can be longer in some cases.
- Infants and very young children require closer observation to prevent reversing the amblyopia to the previously preferred eye (occlusion amblyopia) from excessive patching.
- Optical penalization of the opposite (unaffected) eye using topical cycloplegic eye drops, such as atropine 1%. Studies by the Pediatric Eye Disease Investigator Group have shown that atropine penalization is as effective as patching to treat mild or moderate amblyopia.

- Successful outcomes are far more likely when treatment is initiated early. However, treatment can still be effective after age of 8 years (the classically considered sensitive period) in teenagers, especially those who have not been previously treated. In strabismic amblyopia, initiation of treatment for amblyopia need not wait for correction of the strabismus. Moreover, the stability of the surgical strabismus correction is improved if amblyopia therapy is initiated before surgery.
- Novel therapies using binocular viewing to complete tablet or computer games have shown success, but studies show varied results in comparison to patching.
- Treatment is usually continued until visual acuity in both eyes is equal or until vision in the amblyopic eye shows no further improvement after several examinations over a period of time.
- The primary risk of treatment is overcorrection, with iatrogenic amblyopia in the occluded opposite eye.

ISSUES FOR REFERRAL

Prompt referral of failures and children suspected of poor vision for complete ophthalmic examination is essential for successful amblyopia screening programs.

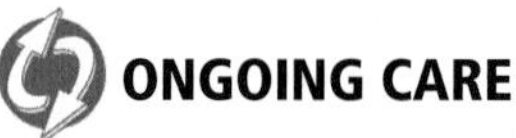

ONGOING CARE

FOLLOW-UP RECOMMENDATIONS

- Patients will be followed on a schedule of weeks to months depending on age and severity of amblyopia.
- In younger children, amblyopia may regress after successful treatment.

Patient Monitoring

- Children should be retested frequently and retreated if vision drops after finishing successful initial treatment.
- Approximately 1/4 of children treated for amblyopia experience a regression in the 1st year after treatment.
- Testing should continue at least annually until the child is at least 8 years old, and recent trials suggest there may be benefit to monitoring through adolescence.

PATIENT EDUCATION

- For all treatment options, compliance is a challenge that has been studied. Patient education may improve compliance.
- Children are generally motivated to avoid the temporary vision impairment from patching and will peek or remove patches frequently.

PROGNOSIS

- Vision loss from amblyopia will persist even after the condition that originally caused the amblyopia has resolved. In some cases, when there is no obvious cause, a history of episodes of anisometropia, occlusion, or strabismus must be considered.
- Despite successful amblyopia treatment, the dominant eye usually maintains better vision compared to the fellow (other) eye, and binocular vision and stereopsis may not improve.
- Patients with an amblyopic eye are at increased risk for injury to the fellow (other) eye. Polycarbonate lenses are often recommended for this reason.

COMPLICATIONS

- Left untreated, amblyopia results in irreversible, uncorrectable vision loss after visual maturity.
- Usually, the vision loss is unilateral, and the functional effects may be minimal if vision in the remaining eye is normal.
- In bilateral cases, or if other diseases or injury affects the remaining eye, the outcome can be significant functional impairment, including legal blindness.

ADDITIONAL READING

- American Academy of Ophthalmology Pediatric Ophthalmology/Strabismus Panel. *Preferred Practice Pattern Guidelines. Amblyopia*. San Francisco, CA: American Academy of Ophthalmology; 2012.
- American Association for Pediatric Ophthalmology and Strabismus. Vision screening recommendations. https://aapos.org//client_data/files/2014/1076_aapos_visscreen.pdf. Accessed June 8, 2018.
- Gunton KB. Advances in amblyopia: what have we learned from PEDIG trials? *Pediatrics*. 2013;131(3):540–547.
- Longmuir SQ, Boese EA, Pfeifer W, et al. Practical community photoscreening in very young children. *Pediatrics*. 2013;131(3):e764–e769.
- Sloper J. New treatments for amblyopia—to patch or play? *JAMA Ophthalmol*. 2016;134(12):1408–1410.

CODES

ICD10

- H53.009 Unspecified amblyopia, unspecified eye
- H53.029 Refractive amblyopia, unspecified eye
- H53.039 Strabismic amblyopia, unspecified eye

FAQ

- Q: My child refuses to wear a patch. Are there alternatives to patching?
- A: Yes. Optical penalization with glasses, atropine cycloplegic penalization, and even contact lens occlusion can be effective. Research shows that patching and atropine can be similarly effective depending on severity of amblyopia and refractive error. Parental support, encouragement, and reward are essential for treatment compliance.
- Q: How long will patching or atropine be necessary?
- A: It is not possible to predict exactly how long treatment will be necessary to restore vision. In general, the younger the patient, the milder the impairment, and the more intensive the patching, the more quickly vision is restored. In general, patching is usually continued for 1 to 6 months in most cases of anisometropic or strabismic amblyopia. Normalization of vision or lack of further improvement is usually the treatment end point.
- Q: Will vision be normal after treatment?
- A: The degree of recovery with amblyopia therapy depends on the density of the amblyopia, the cause, and the age at which treatment is initiated. In almost all children <6 to 8 years of age, some visual improvement can be expected with amblyopia treatment, although not all patients will improve to 20/20 vision.
- Q: Will patching eliminate the need for glasses?
- A: No. Patching does not influence the outcome of refractive errors (power of glasses, refractive error). Glasses may still be needed after patching or atropine is completed. In fact, glasses can improve amblyopia before additional treatment is introduced.
- Q: Will treatment for amblyopia improve the strabismus?
- A: No. In most cases, patching for amblyopia will not eliminate strabismus or the need for strabismus surgery. However, in most cases, it is best to begin amblyopia treatment before surgery to improve the surgical outcome.
- Q: Is "vision therapy" without patching an effective treatment for strabismus?
- A: Although eye exercises, pleoptics, and other vision therapies have been used to treat amblyopia, none is as effective as patching or other occlusive therapy. Current vision therapy techniques have not been proven to improve amblyopia.

AMEBIASIS

John Bower, MD

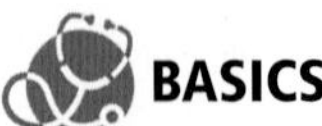

BASICS

DESCRIPTION

Amebic intestinal infection is generally noninvasive and most often due to infection with *Entamoeba histolytica*. Extraintestinal spread can occur and usually involves the liver.

EPIDEMIOLOGY

- Fecal–oral transmission
- Transmission also via contaminated water and food
- The incubation period is typically 1 to 3 weeks but can range from a few days to months or years.

Incidence

- Amebiasis accounts for 40 to 50 million cases of colitis worldwide.
- 40,000 to 110,000 deaths annually

Prevalence

- The estimated prevalence in the United States is 4%, although there have been no recent serosurvey in developed countries.
- Many asymptomatic individuals with *Entamoeba* identified in their stool likely have *Entamoeba dispar* which is nonpathogenic but morphologically indistinguishable from *E. histolytica*.
- Worldwide distribution involving an estimated 10% or more of the world's population
  - Most common in tropical areas, with infection rates as high as 20–50%
  - Highest morbidity and mortality are seen in developing countries in Central America, South America, Africa, and Asia.

RISK FACTORS

- The very young, the elderly, and patients with underlying immunosuppression or malnutrition are at highest risk for severe disease.
- Patients in whom the diagnosis should be considered include the following:
  - Immigrants from or travelers to endemic areas
  - Children with bloody stools or mucus in stools
  - Children with hepatic abscess
  - The febrile child with right upper quadrant pain and tenderness, abdominal pain, or discomfort
  - The child with hepatomegaly, typically without jaundice

GENERAL PREVENTION

- Treatment of drinking water
- Hand washing
- Appropriate disposal of human fecal waste
- Use of condoms
- Infection-control measures: Standard precautions are recommended for the hospitalized patient.

PATHOPHYSIOLOGY

- *E. histolytica* is excreted as cysts or trophozoites in the stool of infected patients.
- Ingested cysts are unaffected by gastric acid and become trophozoites that colonize and invade the colon.
  - Amebae attach to epithelial cells via a galactose/*N*-acetylgalactosamine (Gal/GalNac)–binding lectin
  - The parasite has the ability to lyse human epithelial cells or kill by inducing apoptosis.
  - Then cytokines and chemokines released attract neutrophils, macrophages, and lymphocytes. The host immune response contributes significantly to the reduction of epithelial integrity.
  - Amebae then use cysteine protease to cleave extracellular matrix proteins to invade the submucosal layers.
  - The EhCPDH112 complex interacts with mucosal tight junction proteins to produce mucosal damage.
- Amebae can then disseminate directly from the intestine to the liver in up to 10% of patients. Dissemination from the liver to the lung, heart, brain, and spleen has been described.

ETIOLOGY

- *E. histolytica* is a nonflagellated protozoan parasite.
- Other species of the *Entamoeba* family are nonpathogenic, including the morphologically identical *E. dispar*.

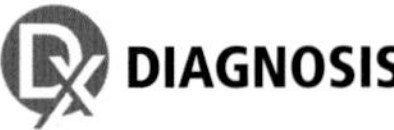

DIAGNOSIS

HISTORY

- Intestinal disease may be asymptomatic or have mild symptoms such as abdominal discomfort, flatulence, constipation, and occasionally diarrhea.
- Nondysenteric colitis is characterized by intermittent diarrhea and abdominal pain.
- Acute amebic colitis (dysenteric) is associated with grossly bloody stools with mucus, abdominal pain, and tenesmus.

PHYSICAL EXAM

- Fever may be present.
- Abdominal tenderness, abdominal rigidity, and rebound are variably present.
- Right upper quadrant tenderness and jaundice may be present in cases of liver abscess.

DIFFERENTIAL DIAGNOSIS

ALERT

The diagnosis is often missed in children because the diagnosis is not considered in the differential. Because it is not common in the United States, amebiasis may initially be misdiagnosed as bacterial dysentery.

Differential diagnosis includes the following:

- Infection
  - *Salmonella* species
  - *Shigella* species
  - *Campylobacter* species
  - *Yersinia* species
  - *Clostridium difficile*
  - *Escherichia coli* (enteroinvasive and enterohemorrhagic)
- Pyogenic abscess
- Echinococcal cyst
- Inflammatory bowel disease
  - Crohn disease
  - Ulcerative colitis
- Ischemic colitis
- Diverticulitis
- Arteriovenous malformations
- Hepatoma

DIAGNOSTIC TESTS & INTERPRETATION

The diagnosis of amebiasis depends on the recognition of typical symptoms and routine laboratory tests.

- CBC typically reveals a leukocytosis.
- Hepatic enzymes are often not elevated.
- Occult blood is detected in stool.
- Stool samples
  - Isolation and visualization
    - Serial stool samples, usually three, are recommended.
    - Samples obtained within 1 to 2 hours of passage should be examined by wet mount and fixed in formalin and polyvinyl alcohol.
    - Serial stool samples are necessary because cysts may be shed intermittently. Three serial stool samples will detect up to 70% of patients with amebic colitis and 50% of patients with hepatic abscess.
    - Stool samples should not be contaminated by urine, water, barium, enema substances, laxatives, or antibiotics because these substances may destroy or interfere with identification of the trophozoites.

- ○ Microscopy has a sensitivity of <60% and specificity of 10–50% on a single sample.
- ○ Nonpathogenic *Entamoeba*, such as *E. dispar* and *Entamoeba moshkovskii*, cannot be distinguished microscopically from *E. histolytica*
- – Stool antigen testing for *E. histolytica* has demonstrated excellent sensitivity and specificity and is preferable to microscopic examination of the stool.
- – Rapid multiplex PCR GI panels appear to have excellent sensitivity and specificity for *E. histolytica* and allow for screening of other common parasitic, viral, and bacterial agents of gastroenteritis.
- Serology
  - Serologic testing for *E. histolytica* is commercially available and is particularly valuable for diagnosing extraintestinal amebic infection.
  - ~85% of patients with amebic dysentery and 99% of patients with liver amebiasis will have positive serology. However, up to a third of those living in endemic areas may be seropositive.
  - Serology is most useful for travelers returning from endemic regions who are unlikely to have been previously exposed.
- Imaging
  - US, CT, or MRI of the liver may reveal liver abscess.
  - In patients with hepatic amebiasis, chest x-ray may reveal elevation of the right hemidiaphragm.

Diagnostic Procedures/Other

- Amebae are difficult to visualize in abscess aspirates, and substantial risk is associated with CT- or US-guided procedures, including bleeding, peritonitis secondary to spillage of amebae, or rupture of echinococcal cysts.
- Colonoscopy

Test Interpretation

- Identification of trophozoites or cysts in the stool
- Colonic or rectal mucosa visualized by colonoscopy reveals ulcerations, and amebae can often be found around these lesions.

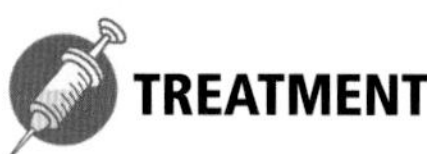

TREATMENT

GENERAL MEASURES

- The goal of treatment is the elimination of tissue-invading trophozoites and intestinal cysts.
- The choice of treatment regimens depends on the clinical presentation.
- Agents that are active against *E. histolytica* are divided into two categories: drugs with activity against intraluminal amebae and drugs with activity against extraintestinal and invasive amebiasis.

MEDICATION

First Line

- Asymptomatic intestinal amebiasis: intraluminal agents
  - Iodoquinol is the drug of choice. The recommended dosage is 30 to 40 mg/kg/24 h (max, 1,950 mg) PO in 3 divided doses for 20 days.
- Acute amebic colitis or extraintestinal amebiasis
  - Metronidazole (a tissue-active agent) 35 to 50 mg/kg/24 h PO in 3 divided doses for 10 days (max, 2,250 mg/24 h) plus a course of treatment with an intraluminal-active agent (as the preceding)
  - ~1/3 of patients treated with metronidazole alone will relapse.

Second Line

- Asymptomatic intestinal amebiasis
  - Paromomycin, 25 to 35 mg/kg/24 h PO in 3 divided doses for 7 days
- Acute amebic colitis or extraintestinal amebiasis
  - One study has reported good efficacy using nitazoxanide in children; however, the sample size was small and the analyses combined *E. histolytica* and *E. dispar* into one stratum.
  - Nitazoxanide is not FDA-approved for treatment of *Entamoeba* infection.

SURGERY/OTHER PROCEDURES

Patients with large liver abscesses or who have failed medical therapy should be considered candidates for surgical or percutaneous drainage.

ONGOING CARE

FOLLOW-UP RECOMMENDATIONS

Patient Monitoring

- Follow-up stool examination is always necessary to ensure eradication of intestinal amebae.
- For amebic abscesses, drainage should be considered if response to medical therapy has not occurred in 4 to 5 days.

PROGNOSIS

Clinical improvement is expected within 72 hours of initiation of therapy.

COMPLICATIONS

- Amebic liver abscess
  - Second most common presentation of amebiasis, often not associated with amebic dysentery
- Ameboma
  - Abdominal mass representing granulation tissue in the colon
- Progressive infection of the colon can uncommonly result in toxic megacolon, mucosal ulceration, and perforation.
- Extraintestinal manifestations of amebiasis are presumed to be a result of direct extension from liver abscesses. These include the following:
  - Pericarditis
  - Pleuropulmonary abscess or empyema
  - Bronchohepatic fistula
  - Genitourinary tract abscess
  - Cerebral abscess
  - Cutaneous amebiasis
    - ○ This is a rare finding in children, with ~6,510 cases reported in the literature.
    - ○ Shallow painful cutaneous ulcers in the diaper area, usually found in association with amebic colitis or dysentery
  - Epidemiologic studies from countries with high prevalence of amebiasis show an association between amebic diarrhea and poor growth. The negative effect on growth was significantly more deleterious than diarrhea caused either by *Giardia* or *Cryptosporidium*.

ADDITIONAL READING

- Haque R, Huston CD, Hughes M, et al. Amebiasis. *N Engl J Med*. 2003;348(16):1565–1573.
- Magaña ML, Fernández-Díez J, Magaña M. Cutaneous amebiasis in pediatrics. *Arch Dermatol*. 2008;144(10):1369–1372.
- Marie C, Petri WA Jr. Regulation of virulence of *Entamoeba histolytica*. *Annu Rev Microbiol*. 2014;68:493–520.
- Mondal D, Petri WA Jr, Sack RB, et al. *Entamoeba histolytica*-associated diarrheal illness is negatively associated with the growth of preschool children: evidence from a prospective study. *Trans R Soc Trop Med Hyg*. 2006;100(11):1032–1038.
- Ravdin JI, Stauffer WM. *Entamoeba histolytica* (amebiasis). In: Mandell GL, Bennett JE, Dolin R, eds. *Principles and Practice of Infectious Diseases*, Vol 2. 6th ed. Philadelphia, PA: Churchill Livingstone; 2005:3097–3111.
- Stauffer W, Ravdin JI. *Entamoeba histolytica*: an update. *Curr Opin Infect Dis*. 2003;16(5):479–485.
- Tanyuksel M, Petri WA Jr. Laboratory diagnosis of amebiasis. *Clin Microbiol Rev*. 2003;16(4):713–729.

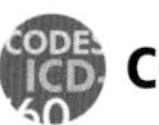

CODES

ICD10

- A06.9 Amebiasis, unspecified
- A06.0 Acute amebic dysentery
- A06.4 Amebic liver abscess

FAQ

- Q: How often does a liver abscess complicate intestinal amebiasis?
- A: About 10% of children with intestinal amebiasis will develop a liver abscess.
- Q: What is the best diagnostic study for a suspected amebic liver abscess?
- A: Serology is the best way to diagnose amebiasis as the cause of a liver abscess. Stool studies are usually negative at the time that a liver abscess has complicated intestinal amebiasis; thus, the yield of stool studies is low.

AMENORRHEA

Renee K. Kottenhahn, MD • Deborah B. Ehrenthal, MD, MPH

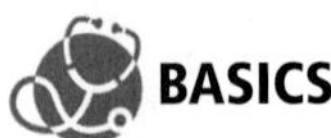

BASICS

DESCRIPTION

Amenorrhea is the absence of menstruation. It is divided into two categories:

- Primary amenorrhea
  - The failure to begin menstruation by 15 years of age in girls with otherwise appropriate pubertal development or by age 13 years in the absence of secondary sexual characteristics
  - This diagnosis should also be considered if a girl has not menstruated within 3 years of thelarche (after breast development begins) regardless of her age.
- Secondary amenorrhea
  - The cessation of menstruation for 3 cycles or 6 months in girls and women with previously established regular cycles
  - Should not be used when referring to girls who are within 2 years of menarche because regular ovulatory cycles have not yet been established; their periods are unpredictable.

EPIDEMIOLOGY

There is insufficient information about the incidence of amenorrhea in contemporary pediatric populations.

RISK FACTORS

Common preventable risk factors for amenorrhea include:

- Pregnancy
- Extremes in weight (including that related to obesity, eating disorders and energy imbalance from athleticism)
- Psychosocial stress

GENERAL PREVENTION

- Healthy lifestyle, maintaining a healthy weight
- Avoidance of excessive athletic activity or training
- Management of emotional stress
- Adherence with chronic disease management

PATHOPHYSIOLOGY

- Amenorrhea related to estrogen deficiency is associated with poor bone health. These patients may fail to reach peak bone mass and have increased risk of fractures.
- Depending on the underlying etiology, future fertility may be impacted.
- Patients with polycystic ovary syndrome (PCOS) may experience long periods of unopposed estrogens and therefore have an elevated risk of endometrial hyperplasia and an increased risk for endometrial cancer.

ETIOLOGY

Menstruation requires the presence of functional female internal genitalia with an intact and patent outflow tract and appropriate stimulation and regulation of the endometrial lining by the hypothalamic–pituitary–ovarian axis. Disruption at any level of the hormonal axis can lead to amenorrhea.

COMMONLY ASSOCIATED CONDITIONS

- The most common chromosomal abnormality associated with primary amenorrhea is Turner syndrome.
- Amenorrhea associated with obesity or PCOS is becoming a common cause of both primary and secondary amenorrhea among adolescents in developing countries.

DIAGNOSIS

A stepwise approach to the evaluation, guided by the history and physical exam, is recommended.

- Phase 1: Exclude pregnancy by urine or serum β-hCG testing.
- Phase 2: Obtain a complete menstrual history to differentiate between primary and secondary amenorrhea to help identify the underlying cause.
- Phase 3: Perform a directed physical exam.
- Phase 4: Initiate stepwise diagnostic testing to assess for causes of amenorrhea.

HISTORY

- Age of patient
  - Genetic abnormalities should be considered in younger patients with primary amenorrhea.
  - Premature ovarian failure becomes more likely with increasing patient age.
- Past and current medical history
  - Prior/current/chronic illness including autoimmune, renal, thyroid, or liver disease; diabetes; or cancer (radiation or chemotherapy) may be the underlying cause of amenorrhea.
- Stressful life events
  - Stress can lead to amenorrhea but should be considered a diagnosis of exclusion.
- Growth and weight changes
  - Consider endocrinopathy, genetic disease, PCOS, rapid weight gain, eating disorder, or other chronic disease.
- Behavioral
  - Eating disorder and/or excessive exercise
- Headaches
  - Assess for visual field defects, dizziness (suggesting pituitary tumor or other intracranial process).
- Reproductive and sexual history
  - Age at menarche
  - Menstrual cycle history: regularity, flow, duration; characteristics of last menstrual period
  - A history of symptoms of pre/perimenstrual molimina (breast tenderness, fluid retention, cramping) suggests prior ovulatory cycles.
  - Risk factors for uterine scarring, such as prior gynecologic surgery
  - Sexual history, including sexual activity and prior pregnancy
  - Current or prior contraceptive use:
    - It is important to recognize current or recent use of hormonal contraception that may not be readily disclosed by the patient.
    - Amenorrhea can be seen with "extended cycling"/continuous use of either oral contraceptives, vaginal ring, or transdermal patch and unpredictably with various progestin delivery systems including oral progestins, implants (Nexplanon), intrauterine systems (various IUDs).
- Depo-Provera can cause amenorrhea for up to 18 months.
- Galactorrhea
  - Spontaneous milky breast discharge suggests elevated prolactin or, more rarely, thyroid abnormality.
  - Also can be due to manual nipple stimulation, medications, illicit drugs (cannabis, opiates, and amphetamines), or herbal supplement use
- Abdominal or pelvic pain
  - Cyclic or intermittent severe abdominal/pelvic pain suggests a uterine anomaly or obstruction.
- Skin and hair
  - Excess hair growth (inquire about shaving, plucking, or waxing), acne, balding, and acanthosis nigricans are symptoms of androgen excess and suggest PCOS, congenital adrenal hyperplasia (rare), or a tumor (rare).
  - Easy bruising or violaceous striae suggest Cushing syndrome.
- Medications
  - Hormonal medications (e.g., Depo-Provera or hormonal contraceptives), cytotoxic medications, illicit drugs, antidepressant drugs, antipsychotic drugs (e.g., risperidone), and other medications including opiates

PHYSICAL EXAM

- General appearance, height, and weight with calculation of body mass index (BMI, in kg/m^2):
  - Obesity raises suspicion of PCOS or possible Cushing syndrome.
  - Athleticism or underweight suggests female athlete triad or eating disorder, respectively.
  - Stigmata of Turner syndrome (short stature, webbed neck, etc.) or other genetic syndromes
  - Abnormal growth pattern suggests endocrinopathy, dietary restriction, chronic disease, or genetic disorder.
- Skin exam
  - Acne, hirsutism (increased facial hair, midline hair over sternum and lower abdomen), acanthosis nigricans, and balding are suggestive of virilization or PCOS.
  - Bruises or pigmented striae suggest Cushing syndrome.
- Tanner staging and breast exam
  - Abnormal Tanner stage for chronologic age suggests an endocrine, metabolic, or genetic abnormality.
  - Galactorrhea suggests abnormalities in prolactin or thyroid.
- Thyroid nodule or enlargement
  - Evaluate for hyperthyroidism or hypothyroidism.
- Abdominal mass
  - Evaluate for uterine obstruction, tumor.
- Genitourinary exam
  - Abnormal external genitalia suggest outflow tract abnormalities.
  - Clitoral enlargement is a sign of virilization and raises suspicion for an androgen-secreting tumor or congenital adrenal hyperplasia.
  - The decision to do a digital or speculum pelvic exam should be based on the patient's age/maturity/gynecologic history/and ability to tolerate the exam.

DIFFERENTIAL DIAGNOSIS

- Pregnancy
- Anatomical abnormalities
  - Imperforate hymen, transverse vaginal septum, müllerian agenesis, androgen insensitivity syndrome
- Ovarian failure
  - Chromosomal abnormalities (e.g.,Turner syndrome), androgen insensitivity syndrome, and other inherited defects
  - Radiation- or chemotherapy-induced ovarian failure, autoimmune premature ovarian failure, idiopathic premature ovarian failure
- Chronic anovulation
  - Androgen excess: PCOS (common), congenital adrenal hyperplasia, ovarian or adrenal tumor
  - Elevated prolactin: prolactinoma, medications, hypothyroidism, others. Remember that stress can cause mild elevations in serum prolactin that are not pathologic.
  - Chronic or systemic illness, eating disorders, extreme obesity, excessive exercise (female athlete triad), psychological stress, hypopituitarism
  - Thyroid disease
  - Cortisol excess: Cushing syndrome
- Medications (including, but not limited to the following)
  - Hormonal contraception
  - Gonadotropin-releasing hormone (GnRH) analogs
  - Cytotoxic medications
  - Opiates
  - Psychiatric medications

DIAGNOSTIC TESTS & INTERPRETATION

Initial Tests (screening, lab, imaging)

Standard initial testing: pregnancy test, FSH/LH, estradiol, TSH, free T_4, prolactin (8 a.m.)

Follow-up Tests & Special Considerations

- For primary amenorrhea (elevated FSH/LH and low estradiol), include genetic testing by checking a karyotype for sex chromosome abnormalities.
- If PCOS is suspected or virilization is identified, also include total and free testosterone, dehydroepiandrosterone-sulfate (DHEA-S), and 17-hydroxyprogesterone.
- If Cushing syndrome is suspected, consider an overnight dexamethasone suppression test or measurement of 24-hour urinary free cortisol excretion.
- Imaging should be used selectively:
  - Transvaginal or pelvic ultrasound to confirm presence of normal müllerian structures (uterus and ovaries) and exclude vaginal or cervical outlet obstruction for patients with primary amenorrhea and those with an abnormal karyotype
  - Exclude renal malformations with an abdominal ultrasound if there are abnormalities of müllerian structures identified by pelvic ultrasound.
  - MRI of the pituitary gland if indicated based on neurologic symptoms, galactorrhea, and/or laboratory results (elevated prolactin)
  - The role of bone densitometry is complex in this age group but should be considered for patients with anorexia or female athlete triad.

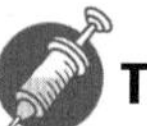

TREATMENT

GENERAL MEASURES

Identification and management depends on the underlying disorder. Premature use of hormonal therapy may alter subsequent testing and should be discouraged.

MEDICATION

- Medical management will be guided by the underlying cause of amenorrhea.
- Estrogen/progestin hormonal therapy may have a role but should not be initiated prior to completing a full evaluation.
- Contraindications to hormone therapy must be considered (refer to Centers for Disease Control and Prevention *Medical Eligibility Criteria* at https://www.cdc.gov/reproductivehealth/contraception/mmwr/mec/summary.html).

ISSUES FOR REFERRAL

- Pregnant patients should be referred.
- Appropriate specialty consultation may be needed based on suspected etiology (e.g., endocrine, genetics). In addition, patients with eating disorders require tailored management by a skilled multidisciplinary team.

ADDITIONAL THERAPIES

An interdisciplinary team may be required to effectively manage eating disorders, complex behavior problems, or emotional symptoms.

SURGERY/OTHER PROCEDURES

Teens with outflow tract obstruction or anomalies should be evaluated by a qualified surgeon.

ADMISSION, INPATIENT, AND NURSING CONSIDERATIONS

Patients with severe recalcitrant eating disorders may require hospitalization.

ONGOING CARE

FOLLOW-UP RECOMMENDATIONS

Most patients with amenorrhea can be managed in an outpatient setting.

DIET

Address underlying nutritional disorders and bone health. Multidisciplinary support may be needed for the care of eating disorders or extreme obesity.

PATIENT EDUCATION

- Patients and their families should be counseled that normal menstruation is a sign of good health. Education needs will be guided by the underlying etiology. Long-term consequences of amenorrhea on bone and reproductive health should be emphasized. Appropriate time should be allocated to interview the adolescent patient alone, both to obtain an accurate history and to provide effective counseling.
- Adolescents should not feel falsely reassured that amenorrhea eliminates the risk of pregnancy, in many circumstances, ovulation can occur unpredictably and may precede menarche/resumption of menses. Additionally, precaution for sexually transmitted disease should be included in the care of sexually active teens.

PROGNOSIS

Long-term prognosis is related to the underlying etiology, the duration of amenorrhea, and the effectiveness of interventions. A tailored approach is needed to guide counseling given the breadth of underlying causes for both primary and secondary amenorrhea.

ADDITIONAL READING

- ACOG Committee Opinion No. 651: menstruation in girls and adolescents: using the menstrual cycle as a vital sign. *Obstet Gynecol*. 2015;126(6):e143–e146.
- Azurah AG, Zainuddin AA, Jayasinghe Y. Diagnostic pitfalls in the evaluation and management of amenorrhea in adolescents. *J Reprod Med*. 2013;58(7–8):324–336.
- Dominé F, Dadoumont C, Bourguignon JP. Eating disorders throughout female adolescence. *Endocr Dev*. 2012;22:271–286.
- Gray SH. Menstrual disorders. *Pediatr Rev*. 2013;34(1):6–17.
- Klein DA, Poth MA. Amenorrhea: an approach to diagnosis and management. *Am Fam Physician*. 2013;87(11):781–788.
- Roupas ND, Georgopoulos NA. Menstrual function in sports. *Hormones (Athens)*. 2011;10(2):104–116.
- Santoro N. Update in hyper- and hypogonadotropic amenorrhea. *J Clin Endocrinol Metab*. 2011;96(11):3281–3288.
- Viswanathan V, Eugster EA. Etiology and treatment of hypogonadism in adolescents. *Pediatr Clin North Am*. 2011;58(5):1181–1200.

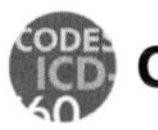

CODES

ICD10

- N91.2 Amenorrhea, unspecified
- N91.0 Primary amenorrhea
- N91.1 Secondary amenorrhea

FAQ

- Q: Does a patient who says she has never had sexual intercourse still need a pregnancy test?
- A: Yes.
- Q: What menstrual patterns should patients expect after stopping hormonal contraception?
- A: Normal menstruation is anticipated within 1 to 3 months of stopping combined oral contraceptive pills. If this does not occur, evaluation for secondary amenorrhea is appropriate. Depo-Provera is associated with menstrual disturbance that can persist; return of normal menstrual cycles is anticipated within 6 to 18 months after the last injection. Amenorrhea should not be attributed to prior IUD or Nexplanon (etonogestrel implant) use as return to fertility after removal is rapid.

ANAEROBIC INFECTIONS

Eimear Kitt, MB, BCh, BAO (NUI) • Hamid Bassiri, MD, PhD

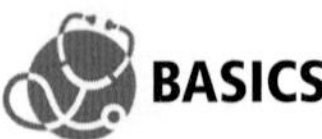

BASICS

DESCRIPTION

- Anaerobic bacteria are organisms capable of growing in a reduced oxygen environment, either exclusively (obligate anaerobes) or in addition to growing in air (facultative anaerobes).
- Anaerobic bacteria can cause invasive and serious infections.
- Anaerobic bacteria tend to participate with other anaerobic and aerobic flora in causing polymicrobial infections.

EPIDEMIOLOGY

- Although anaerobic bacteremia is less frequent in children than in adults, other anaerobic infections such as chronic sinusitis or chronic otitis media are common in children.
- Because of their fastidious nature, the ability of microbiology laboratories to identify anaerobic bacteria is highly dependent on proper collection and transport of culture specimens; hence, anaerobic bacteria are often missed and likely underreported.

RISK FACTORS

- Impaired host immunity
  - Malignancy
  - Splenic dysfunction
  - Hypogammaglobulinemia
- Presence of devitalized tissue
- Surgery, trauma
- Vascular insufficiency
- Poorly controlled diabetes
- Presence of foreign bodies
- Colitis

PATHOPHYSIOLOGY

- Anaerobic infections commonly derive from the normal flora of the oropharynx, skin, intestines, or the female genital tract; thus, anaerobic infections occur when there is a loss of integrity of anatomic or epithelial barriers at these sites.
- Virulence factors include production of exotoxins (e.g., *Clostridia* spp.), endotoxins (e.g., *Fusobacterium* spp.), and presence of phagocyte-inhibiting capsules (e.g., *Bacteroides* spp.).

ETIOLOGY

The most common clinically-relevant anaerobes include the following:

- Gram-negative rods (*Bacteroides*, *Prevotella*, *Porphyromonas*, *Fusobacterium*)
- Gram-positive cocci (*Peptostreptococcus*, *Peptococcus*)
- Spore-forming gram-positive bacilli (*Clostridia*)
- Non–spore-forming gram-positive bacilli (*Eubacterium*, *Bifidobacterium*, *Propionibacterium*, *Actinomyces*, *Lactobacillus*)
- Gram-negative cocci (*Veillonella*, *Acidaminococcus*)
- Spirochetes (many of which are anaerobic)

COMMONLY ASSOCIATED CONDITIONS

- CNS infections:
  - Brain abscess due to bacteremia
  - Subdural empyema
  - Epidural abscess (most commonly due to complications from sinusitis)
- Head and neck infections:
  - Sinusitis (generally polymicrobial)
  - Chronic otitis media
  - Ludwig angina (infection of the submandibular space)
  - Cervical adenitis
  - Peritonsillar abscess
  - Dental abscess
  - Gingivitis
  - Actinomycosis of jaw
  - Lemierre disease
    - Septic thrombophlebitis of the internal jugular vein owing to anaerobic bacteremia
    - Most commonly with *Fusobacterium* spp., often resulting in pulmonary abscess formation and metastatic infection
- Pleuropulmonary infections:
  - Aspiration of infected amniotic or vaginal secretions in neonates
  - Aspiration of oral or gastrointestinal fluids in children (severe gingival or periodontal may be a risk factor)
  - Pneumonia, abscess formation due to aspirated foreign bodies
  - Actinomycosis
- Peritonitis/peritoneal abscess:
  - Appendiceal abscess
  - Perforated viscus
  - Postoperative complication
  - Trauma-related
  - Actinomycosis
- Cholangitis
  - Ascending infection may occur following biliary tract surgery (e.g., Kasai procedure).
- Soft tissue infections:
  - Paronychia
  - Pilonidal cyst
  - Hidradenitis suppurativa
  - Crepitant cellulitis
  - Necrotizing fasciitis
  - Gas gangrene (*Clostridium* spp.)
  - Infected decubitus ulcers (may result in contiguous osteomyelitis)
  - Penetrating wounds (may lead to tetanus)
- Infections of the female genital tract:
  - Endometritis
  - Salpingitis
  - Tubo-ovarian or adnexal abscess
  - Pelvic inflammatory diseases
  - Pelvic abscess
  - Bartholin gland, vulvar, or perineal abscess
  - Bacterial vaginosis
- Infected bite wounds
  - Anaerobes isolated from 50% of human or animal bites
- Bacteremia
  - Often associated with focal primary site of involvement (gastrointestinal disease, abscess)
- Neonatal infections:
  - Cellulitis at fetal monitoring sites
  - Aspiration pneumonia
  - Omphalitis
  - Conjunctivitis
  - Infant botulism

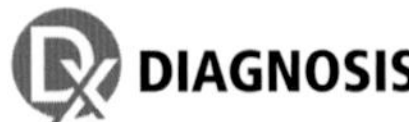

DIAGNOSIS

Involvement of anaerobic bacteria should be suspected in infections with suppuration or foul smell, abscess formation, tissue necrosis, or in hosts with systemic disease or defective immunity.

HISTORY

- Impaired mental status
  - Increased risk of aspiration
- History of sore throat or neck pain in an adolescent
- History of thumb sucking
  - Anaerobes frequently isolated from paronychia
- History of animal or human bites
- History of unprotected sexual intercourse
- Recent surgery or trauma
  - Poor drainage or devitalized tissue associated with anaerobic infection
- Underlying immunodeficiency or chronic illness
  - Impaired phagocytic function
- History of pus that is "sterile" (no growth on routine cultures)

PHYSICAL EXAM

- Location of infection
  - See "Commonly Associated Conditions."
- Poor dentition
  - Increased colonization of oropharynx with anaerobic organisms
- Necrotic tissue
- Crepitus with gas gangrene
- "Dishwater" pus or discharge with foul odor
  - Characteristic of anaerobic infections
- Lower abdominal pain with adnexal tenderness
- Lateral neck pain in association with respiratory distress:
  - Lemierre disease results in septic thrombophlebitis of the internal jugular vein and formation of lung abscesses; untreated or undiagnosed Lemierre disease carries a significant mortality rate.

DIAGNOSTIC TESTS & INTERPRETATION

Initial Tests (screening, lab, imaging)

- Certain anaerobic bacteria have unique morphology on Gram stains:
  - *Bacteroides* spp.: small, pleomorphic gram-negative bacilli
  - *Clostridium* spp.: large gram-positive organisms with "boxcar" morphology
- Anaerobic cultures
  - Should be performed on tissue or aspirated fluid obtained directly from the infected sites in a sterile fashion
  - Anaerobically collected specimens should be transported to the laboratory promptly.
  - Swabs should not be sent for anaerobic cultures.
- Radiographs may show the following:
  - Air–fluid levels
  - Cavity formation
  - Gas in tissue
- CT and/or MRI scans
  - Often important to define anatomic location and extent of disease and to determine surgical approaches to drainage or debridement

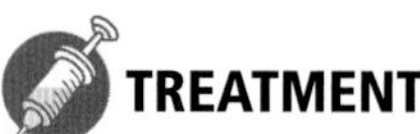

TREATMENT

MEDICATION

- Empiric antibiotics for anaerobic infections include the following:
  - Metronidazole
  - Carbapenems (e.g., meropenem or imipenem)
  - Chloramphenicol (Supplies in the United States may be limited.)
  - β-Lactam/β-lactamase inhibitor combinations (e.g., amoxicillin-clavulanate, ampicillin-sulbactam, ticarcillin-clavulanate, or piperacillin-tazobactam)
  - Clindamycin
  - Cephamycins (e.g., cefoxitin or cefotetan)
  - Vancomycin has activity against gram-positive but not gram-negative anaerobes.
  - Penicillins, cephalosporins, tetracyclines, macrolides, aminoglycosides, trimethoprim-sulfamethoxazole, and monobactams have either variable or poor activity against anaerobes and should not be used empirically.
  - Most fluoroquinolones also have variable activity, but exceptions exist (e.g., moxifloxacin).
  - Antibiotic resistance is increasing in certain anaerobes, especially *Bacteroides* spp.; not all microbiology laboratories routinely test anaerobes for antibiotic susceptibility.
    - If a patient with a documented anaerobic infection does not appear to be responding to empiric therapy, it is advisable to consult with an infectious diseases specialist for further recommendations.
- Empiric drug therapy reflects the polymicrobial nature of infections in which anaerobic bacteria are predominantly found:
  - CNS infections
    - Vancomycin + 3rd- or 4th-generation cephalosporin (e.g., ceftriaxone) + metronidazole
    - Avoid using β-lactam/β-lactamase inhibitor combinations for brain abscesses, as β-lactamase inhibitor penetration across blood–brain barrier may be suboptimal.
  - Head and neck infections
    - Ampicillin-sulbactam, amoxicillin-clavulanate, or clindamycin alone if gram-negative aerobic bacteria are of little concern
  - Pleuropulmonary infections due to aspiration
    - Ampicillin-sulbactam, amoxicillin-clavulanate, or clindamycin
  - Peritonitis/peritoneal abscess
    - Ampicillin-sulbactam, piperacillin-tazobactam, cefoxitin, meropenem, or imipenem
  - Cholangitis
    - Piperacillin-tazobactam, meropenem, or imipenem
  - Soft tissue infection
    - Clindamycin, ampicillin-clavulanate
  - Infections of the female genital tract
    - Ampicillin-sulbactam, ticarcillin-clavulanate, piperacillin-tazobactam, cefoxitin, meropenem, or imipenem
  - Infected bite wounds
    - Ampicillin-sulbactam, piperacillin-tazobactam, amoxicillin-clavulanate
  - Bacteremia
    - Isolate-dependent, but it may be reasonable to start with vancomycin + 3rd- or 4th-generation cephalosporin (e.g., ceftriaxone) + metronidazole until isolate speciated and bacteremia confirmed to be due to anaerobic bacteria.

ADDITIONAL THERAPIES

- Neutralization of toxins, especially in the case of botulism or tetanus, is critical.
- Hyperbaric oxygen, although still sometimes used (especially in clostridial infections), has not been shown to be of proven benefit, although it may help define and demarcate the borders of devitalized tissues.

SURGERY/OTHER PROCEDURES

- Effective drainage of abscesses and debridement of devitalized tissue is essential to obtain source control.
- Cultures should be obtained by aspirating fluids into sterile syringes, capping them, and transporting these to the laboratory promptly.
- Cultures can also be obtained from intact tissues that are transported to the laboratory promptly.
- Swabs should not be sent for anaerobic cultures.

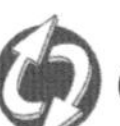

ONGOING CARE

PROGNOSIS

- Determined by speed with which infection is appropriately treated with antibiotics and/or drainage
- High rates of morbidity and mortality associated with untreated anaerobic bacteremia
- Specific prognosis depends on the bacterial species involved and the status of the patient's immune system.
- Soft tissue infections, necrotizing fasciitis, or gas gangrene caused by *Clostridium* spp. may cause up to 20% mortality despite aggressive therapy.

COMPLICATIONS

- Vary with nature of infection but can include extension of infection to adjacent structures
- Development of bacteremia

ADDITIONAL READING

- Brook I. Anaerobic infections in children. *Adv Exp Med Biol*. 2011;697:117–152.
- Brook I. Clinical review: bacteremia caused by anaerobic bacteria in children. *Crit Care*. 2002;6(3):205–211.
- Japanese Society of Chemotherapy Committee on Guidelines for Treatment of Anaerobic Infections; Japanese Association for Anaerobic Infections Research. Chapter 1-1. Anaerobic infections (General): epidemiology of anaerobic infections. *J Infect Chemother*. 2011;17(Suppl 1):4–12.
- Nagy E. Anaerobic infections: update on treatment considerations. *Drugs*. 2010;70(7):841–858.

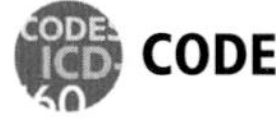

CODES

ICD10

- A49.9 Bacterial infection, unspecified
- A49.8 Other bacterial infections of unspecified site
- J32.9 Chronic sinusitis, unspecified

FAQ

- Q: My patient has a suspected brain abscess. What is the appropriate antibiotic regimen to initiate pending further tests?
- A: Like many anaerobic infections, a brain abscess must be assumed to be polymicrobial in etiology. An appropriate regimen would be triple therapy with ceftriaxone, vancomycin, and metronidazole. β-Lactam/β-lactamase inhibitors such as ampicillin-sulbactam must be avoided in this setting given the suboptimal CNS penetration associated with these agents.

ANAPHYLAXIS

Benjamin T. Prince, MD, MSci • Rachel G. Robison, MD

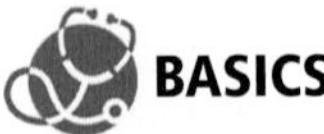

BASICS

DESCRIPTION

- Anaphylaxis is a serious, life-threatening, systemic allergic reaction that is rapid in onset and is a result of mast cell and basophil activation and degranulation.
- Skin and mucosal symptoms such as flushing, itching, urticaria, or angioedema are present in 80–90% of patients with anaphylaxis. However, absence of skin findings does not exclude anaphylaxis.
- In fatal anaphylaxis, initial signs and symptoms may include respiratory distress without urticaria resulting in delayed diagnosis and treatment.

EPIDEMIOLOGY

- Rate of occurrence appears to be increasing.
- Estimated to be fatal in 0.7–2% of cases

RISK FACTORS

Genetics

There are few studies of genetic factors in human anaphylaxis; however, individuals with a previous history of anaphylaxis or a history of atopy are at increased risk for future anaphylaxis episodes.

PATHOPHYSIOLOGY

- In anaphylaxis, mast cells and basophils are activated via an IgE-mediated (most common) or non–IgE-mediated mechanism releasing preformed and newly generated mediators of inflammation.
  - Mediators include histamine, tryptase, proteoglycans, leukotrienes, prostaglandins, platelet-activating factor, and cytokines.
  - Local or systemic effects can include increased vascular permeability, vasodilation, smooth muscle contraction, complement activation, and coagulation.
- IgE-mediated anaphylaxis occurs when IgE is synthesized in response to allergen exposure (sensitization) and becomes fixed to high-affinity IgE receptors located on the surface of mast cells and basophils. Subsequent allergen exposure results in receptor-bound IgE aggregation and cell activation.
- Non–IgE-mediated anaphylaxis generally results from nonimmune stimulation of mast cells or basophils. Rarely, IgG and complement can be implicated.

ETIOLOGY

- IgE-mediated:
  - Foods (peanut, tree nuts, fish, shellfish, milk, egg, wheat, soy)
  - Medications (antibiotics especially β-lactams, NSAIDs, biologic products)
  - Venoms (usually from stinging insects including fire ants)
  - Latex (direct exposure to natural rubber or ingestion of cross-reacting foods)
  - Other (vaccines, occupational allergens, and rarely inhaled allergens)
- Non–IgE-mediated:
  - Radiocontrast media (can also trigger IgE-dependent anaphylaxis)
  - Medications (opiates, NSAIDs, dextrans, vancomycin, polymyxin B)
  - Physical stimuli (exercise, cold, heat, sunlight/UV radiation)
  - Ethanol
- If no identifiable trigger is found, anaphylaxis may be idiopathic in origin.

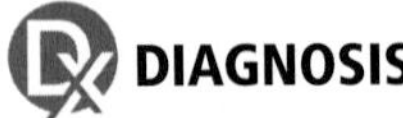

DIAGNOSIS

Anaphylaxis is a clinical diagnosis that is considered highly likely when any one of the following three criteria is met:

- Acute onset of illness (minutes to hours) with involvement of skin, mucosa, or both and at least one of the following: (i) respiratory compromise or (ii) reduced blood pressure or associated symptoms of organ dysfunction.
- Two or more of the following occurring acutely (minutes to hours) after exposure to a likely allergen: (i) involvement of skin-mucosal tissue, (ii) respiratory compromise (dyspnea, wheezing, stridor, hypoxemia), (iii) reduced blood pressure or associated symptoms of organ dysfunction, (iv) persistent gastrointestinal symptoms (abdominal cramping, vomiting)
- Reduced systolic blood pressure acutely (minutes to hours) after exposure to known allergen for that patient; defined by age-specific normals or >30% decrease from patient's baseline

HISTORY

- A detailed history of exposures and events in minutes to hours prior to onset should be obtained after treatment is initiated.
- Any previous history of anaphylaxis?
  - Can help direct history and patient education, especially if epinephrine was indicated but not given or if a known allergen was not recognized
- Food triggers
  - Most common: peanut, tree nuts, fish, shellfish, milk, egg, wheat, soy, sesame, additives (spices, contaminants)
  - Foods need to be ingested for a reaction to occur, but rarely anaphylaxis can be caused by inhalation of aerosolized vapors from cooking or processing (including fish and shellfish).
  - Gastrointestinal symptoms tend to be more prominent than in other etiologies.
- Medication triggers
  - Specifically inquire about NSAIDs, supplements, and herbal treatments.
  - β-blockers and ACE inhibitors can increase severity and/or make treatment of anaphylaxis more difficult.

ALERT

For patients with anaphylaxis who are taking β-blockers or ACE inhibitors and have persistent hypotension and bradycardia despite epinephrine, consider giving glucagon.

- Insect stings
  - If possible, attempt to identify the insect. Honeybees leave stinger at sting site.
  - All patients should be referred to an allergist, as immunotherapy is effective in preventing up to 98% of future anaphylactic reactions.
- Natural rubber latex
  - Latex-allergic patients can develop anaphylaxis after ingestion of cross-reactive foods including banana, kiwi, papaya, avocado, potato, and tomato.

PHYSICAL EXAM

- Skin and mucosa
  - Flushing, itching, conjunctival erythema, urticaria, angioedema
- Respiratory
  - Upper airway: nasal itching, congestion, rhinorrhea, sneezing, dysphonia, hoarseness, stridor, drooling (can be a sign of angioedema or obstruction)
  - Lower airway: tachypnea, cough, wheezing/bronchospasm, decreased peak expiratory flow
  - Cyanosis, respiratory arrest
- Cardiovascular system
  - Tachycardia or bradycardia (less common), hypotension, arrhythmias, shock, urinary or fecal incontinence, cardiac arrest
- Gastrointestinal
  - Abdominal pain/cramping, vomiting, diarrhea, dysphagia
- Central nervous system
  - Patients may appear uneasy or describe a sense of impending doom.
  - Altered mental status, confusion, tunnel vision

DIFFERENTIAL DIAGNOSIS

- Allergic/immunologic
  - Acute urticaria
  - Acute asthma
  - Pollen-food syndrome
  - Mast cell activation syndrome
- Cardiovascular
  - Myocardial infarction
  - Pulmonary embolus
- Genetic/metabolic
  - Hereditary or acquired angioedema
- Infectious
  - Septic shock
- Neoplastic
  - Mastocytosis/clonal mast cell disorders
  - Carcinoid
  - Basophilic leukemia
  - Pheochromocytoma
- Neurologic
  - Syncope
  - Seizure
- Nonorganic disease
  - Panic attack
  - Vocal cord dysfunction
  - Munchausen syndrome

- Other:
  - Foreign body aspiration
  - Scombroidosis (ingestion of fish containing high levels of histamine)
  - Red man syndrome

DIAGNOSTIC TESTS & INTERPRETATION

Anaphylaxis is a clinical diagnosis; however, certain tests can aid in confirming the diagnosis. Treatment of anaphylaxis should be initiated immediately if a patient presents with a clinical picture that is consistent with anaphylaxis.

Initial Tests (screening, lab, imaging)

- Serum total tryptase
  - Elevated 15 minutes to 3 hours after onset of anaphylaxis
  - Elevated in patients with anaphylaxis due to injected medications, insect stings, and when hypotension is present
  - Can be normal in anaphylaxis due to foods or in those who are normotensive
  - Normal serum tryptase does not rule out anaphylaxis.
  - Laboratory test that is routinely used in practice
- Plasma histamine
  - Elevated if measured 15 to 60 minutes after onset of anaphylaxis due to its short half-life
  - Blood sample requires special handling.
  - Normal level does not rule out anaphylaxis.
- Urine histamine and *N*-methylhistamine
  - 24-hour urine histamine and *N*-methylhistamine (a metabolite) can be elevated in the context of anaphylaxis.
- Chest radiograph: may be useful to rule out foreign body aspiration or congenital malformations of the respiratory or gastrointestinal tract

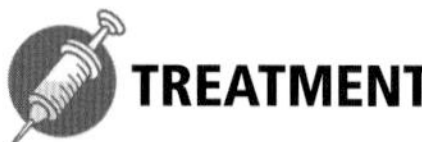

TREATMENT

MEDICATION

First Line

IM epinephrine 1:1,000 (1 mg/mL) solution

- 0.01 mg/kg, maximum of 0.3 mg (child) or 0.5 mg (adult), repeated q5–15min as needed (most respond to 1 or 2 doses)
- Delayed administration of epinephrine is associated with higher rates of hospitalization and is an independent risk factor for mortality.

Second Line

- Diphenhydramine IV or PO (or equivalent H_1-antihistamine)
  - 1 mg/kg, maximum of 50 mg, q4–6h
- Albuterol 2.5 mg/3 mL solution
  - Nebulized and inhaled via face mask
- Ranitidine IV
  - 1 mg/kg, maximum 50 mg
- Methylprednisolone IV (or equivalent glucocorticoid)
  - 1 to 2 mg/kg, maximum of 60 mg (may be continued PO once daily for 1- to 3-day course)
  - Steroids have no role in the acute management of anaphylaxis and have not been shown to decrease prolonged or biphasic reactions. Consider in patients with other comorbidities such as uncontrolled asthma.

ADDITIONAL THERAPIES

- Maintain airway:
  - Supplemental oxygen
  - Bag mask or intubation if necessary
- Maintain circulation:
  - Place patient supine and elevate lower extremities if possible.
  - Volume resuscitation with 0.9% saline
  - IV vasopressors may be necessary in patients with refractory hypotension or shock.

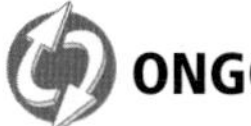

ONGOING CARE

FOLLOW-UP RECOMMENDATIONS

Most patients who are diagnosed with anaphylaxis will benefit from a referral to an allergist/immunologist for further evaluation, recommendations, and management.

Patient Monitoring

Biphasic anaphylaxis, in which symptoms recur within 1 to 72 hours (usually 8 to 10 hours) after resolution of initial symptoms, occurs in up to 23% of adults and up to 11% of children with anaphylaxis.

- A prescription for autoinjectable epinephrine should be provided on discharge in any patient diagnosed with anaphylaxis.
- Medical monitoring after return to baseline should be individualized and depends on degree of symptoms and other risk factors.
  - Patients presenting with moderate respiratory compromise, hypotension, or requiring >1 dose of epinephrine should be monitored for a minimum of 4 hours or longer if indicated (especially young patients or patients with comorbidities).

PATIENT EDUCATION

All patients should be instructed on allergen avoidance measures and provided with a written personalized emergency plan detailing appropriate management of future anaphylactic episodes.

PROGNOSIS

Good with trigger identification and avoidance

COMPLICATIONS

- Laryngeal edema and airway obstruction
- Pulmonary edema, pulmonary hemorrhage, and pneumothorax
- Myocardial ischemia and infarction
- End-organ ischemia and damage
- Death secondary to airway obstruction (asphyxiation) and/or shock

ADDITIONAL READING

- Greenberger PA, Rotskoff BD, Lifschultz B. Fatal anaphylaxis: postmortem findings and associated comorbid diseases. *Ann Allergy Asthma Immunol*. 2007;98(3):252–257.
- Lieberman P, Nicklas RA, Randolph C, et al. Anaphylaxis—a practice parameter update 2015. *Ann Allergy Asthma Immunol*. 2015;115(5): 341–384.
- Simons FE. Anaphylaxis. *J Allergy Clin Immunol*. 2010;125(2 Suppl 2):S161–S181.
- Simons FE, Ardusso LR, Bilò MB, et al. World Allergy Organization guidelines for the assessment and management of anaphylaxis. *World Allergy Organ J*. 2011;4(2):13–37.

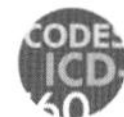

CODES

ICD10

- T78.2XXA Anaphylactic shock, unspecified, initial encounter
- T78.00XA Anaphylactic reaction due to unspecified food, init encntr
- T63.891A Toxic effect of contact with other venomous animals, accidental (unintentional), initial encounter

FAQ

- Q: Can a patient have an anaphylactic reaction on first exposure to an allergen?
- A: In IgE-mediated anaphylaxis, a patient must have been previously exposed to the offending allergen for sensitization to occur with a subsequent exposure potentially resulting in anaphylaxis. Remember, however, that the absence of a previous exposure on history does *not* exclude an allergen as causal because sensitization may have previously occurred unknowingly (through skin contact, in breast milk, in utero). Non–IgE-mediated anaphylaxis can occur on first exposure to the offending allergen.
- Q: Should patients with a history of anaphylaxis carry more than one autoinjectable epinephrine device?
- A: Yes, up to 30% of patients with anaphylaxis are reported to require a second dose of epinephrine either because of ongoing symptoms or because of biphasic anaphylaxis.
- Q: Can a patient develop anaphylaxis to an allergen that they have tolerated previously?
- A: Yes, this often occurs with medications or foods (particularly peanut, tree nuts, fish, and shellfish) especially if there is a long period of time between exposures.

ANEMIA OF CHRONIC DISEASE (ANEMIA OF INFLAMMATION)

Kandace L. Gollomp, MD • Michele Puszkarczuk Lambert, MD, MSTR

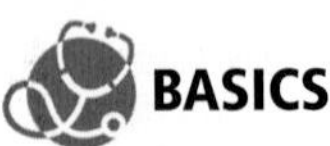

BASICS

DESCRIPTION

- Anemia that accompanies a variety of systemic diseases, with the common features of chronicity and inflammation
- Anemia of chronic disease is more properly called anemia of inflammation (AI) and is the combined result of mildly increased destruction of RBCs, relative erythropoietin resistance, and iron-restricted erythropoiesis.

PATHOPHYSIOLOGY

Typically mild to moderate anemia (Hgb 7 to 12 g/dL); develops in the setting of infection, inflammatory disorders, and some malignancies

- Deficient cellular iron in the setting of hepcidin excess (functionally inaccessible iron)
- Typically normochromic, normocytic but, if long-standing, can be hypochromic, microcytic (especially in children)
- Main mechanism appears to be
  - Hepcidin is increased by interleukin-6 (IL-6), causing depletion of ferroportin, the only known membrane iron transporter.
  - Elevated hepcidin results in macrophage inability to release iron recycled from senescent RBCs, hepatocyte inability to release stored iron, and enterocyte inability to absorb dietary iron.
  - These changes lead to iron restriction with decreased iron available for erythropoiesis.
- Other factors contributing to anemia in various degrees include the following:
  - Increased red cell destruction
  - Diagnostic phlebotomy or other blood loss
  - Inflammatory cytokines suppress erythropoiesis
  - Cytokine-mediated suppression of erythropoiesis
  - Cytokines such as interleukin-1 (IL-1) and IL-6 can activate ferritin synthesis, leading to sequestration of iron, which eventually is converted into hemosiderin.

ETIOLOGY

Underlying disease process

COMMONLY ASSOCIATED CONDITIONS

- Underlying disease process
  - Infections, both acute and chronic
  - Inflammatory disease
  - Collagen vascular diseases
  - Malignancies
  - Renal failure
- Anemia of chronic disease often coexists with other causes of anemia, including:
  - Occult blood loss
  - Hemolysis
  - Dietary iron deficiency
  - Drug-related marrow suppression

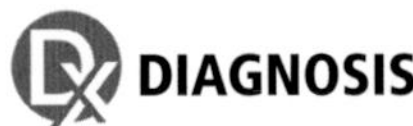

DIAGNOSIS

Signs and symptoms

- Various abnormal physical findings may be present, depending on the underlying chronic disease process.
- May have mild pallor but will not have signs of circulatory collapse
- Similar disease can be seen more acutely in the setting of anemia of critical illness (also part of AI).

HISTORY

Anemia develops over the 1st month of the underlying disease process and then remains fairly stable over time.

PHYSICAL EXAM

- Mild pallor
- Mild tachycardia, may be inapparent at rest
- Very rarely more overt signs of anemia such as:
  - Flow murmur
  - Gallop
  - Hepatomegaly
- Physical findings of the underlying disease

DIFFERENTIAL DIAGNOSIS

Anemia of chronic disease is often confused with iron deficiency anemia.

- In anemia of chronic disease:
  - Mild to moderate anemia (rarely <8 g/dL)
  - Mild anisocytosis
  - Usually normochromic, normocytic but can be hypochromic with microcytosis
  - Decreased plasma iron
  - Decreased iron-binding capacity
  - Normal or slightly low transferrin saturation
  - Decreased marrow sideroblasts
  - Normal or elevated reticuloendothelial iron
  - Elevated free erythrocyte protoporphyrin
  - Normal or elevated ferritin
  - Increased hepcidin
- In iron deficiency:
  - Decreased plasma iron
  - Increased iron-binding capacity
  - Decreased transferrin saturation
  - Decreased marrow sideroblasts
  - Decreased reticuloendothelial iron
  - Increased free erythrocyte protoporphyrin
  - Decreased serum ferritin
  - Decreased hepcidin
- In both iron deficiency and anemia of chronic disease:
  - Decreased plasma iron
  - Decreased transferrin saturation
  - Decreased marrow sideroblasts
  - Elevated free erythrocyte protoporphyrin
  - Decreased reticulocyte count
- Tests that help differentiate iron deficiency from anemia of chronic disease:
  - Iron-binding capacity
  - Serum ferritin
  - Reticuloendothelial iron stain in marrow
  - Hepcidin level (although not available everywhere)

DIAGNOSTIC TESTS & INTERPRETATION

If only the serum iron is obtained, without other iron studies, the child may be inappropriately diagnosed with iron deficiency.

Initial Tests (screening, lab, imaging)

- CBC with indices
  - Normocytic, normochromic (can be microcytic, hypochromic when very long-standing) anemia with hematocrit rarely <20%
  - Reticulocyte count usually in the normal range but low for the level of anemia
- Iron studies
  - Low plasma iron, with low total iron-binding capacity
  - Low iron transferrin saturation
  - Normal or high ferritin level
- Elevated free erythrocyte protoporphyrin
- If bone marrow biopsy performed, can visualize increased hemosiderin in bone marrow macrophages with an iron stain
- Albumin and transferrin are both low.
- Acute-phase reactants such as C-reactive protein may be elevated.
- Hepcidin levels will be elevated.

Diagnostic Procedures/Other

Bone marrow aspiration is generally not indicated.

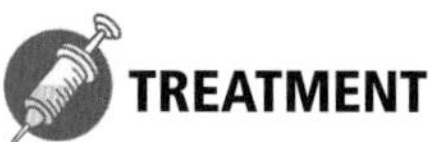

TREATMENT

GENERAL MEASURES

- Iron
  - Generally, no role for iron therapy unless there is coexisting iron deficiency anemia.
  - However, recent studies in patients with renal disease have shown improved response to erythropoietin with coadministration of IV iron and it may have similar activity in AI.
- Recombinant human erythropoietin
  - Effective, but indications for use are still not universally accepted
  - Often used in chronic renal failure
  - Has been used in inflammatory bowel disease, with good results
  - Should be used for more severe and symptomatic anemia in which the underlying disease is likely to be prolonged and difficult to treat
- Treatment should be directed at the underlying disease process.
- Experimental therapeutics include IL-6 inhibitors and hepcidin blockers.

ADDITIONAL THERAPIES

Transfusion of packed RBCs is sometimes indicated intermittently in severe anemia with hemodynamic compromise.

ONGOING CARE

FOLLOW-UP RECOMMENDATIONS

Patient Monitoring

Treatment of underlying disease process may promote slow resolution of associated anemia. Hematocrit increases ~6 to 8 weeks after start of recombinant human erythropoietin therapy; continues to rise over 6 months

COMPLICATIONS

If severe, patients may be transfusion dependent and, thus, be at risk for complications associated with packed RBC transfusions.

ADDITIONAL READING

- Cullis J. Anaemia of chronic disease. *Clin Med (Lond)*. 2013;13(2):193–196.
- Fraenkel PG. Anemia of Inflammation: a review. *Med Clin North Am*. 2017;101(2):285–296.
- Ganz T. Molecular pathogenesis of anemia of chronic disease. *Pediatr Blood Cancer*. 2006;46(5):554–557.
- Goodnough LT, Skikne B, Brugnara C. Erythropoietin, iron, and erythropoiesis. *Blood*. 2000;96(3):823–833.
- Nemeth E, Ganz T. Anemia of inflammation. *Hematol Oncol Clin North Am*. 2014;28(4):671–681.

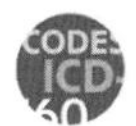

CODES

ICD10

- D63.8 Anemia in other chronic diseases classified elsewhere
- D63.1 Anemia in chronic kidney disease
- D63.0 Anemia in neoplastic disease

FAQ

- Q: Does anemia that is associated with a chronic disease require further evaluation?
- A: If the anemia fits within the usual expectations for the patient's diagnosis, there is no need to pursue further investigation, except in specific cases. If there is an associated malignancy for which marrow metastasis is possible, a bone marrow aspirate and biopsy should be done. In conditions with malabsorption, nutritional deficiencies and blood loss should be ruled out.

ANKYLOGLOSSIA

Timothy R. Shope, MD, MPH • David H. Chi, MD • Melissa A. Buryk, MD, MPH

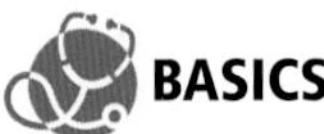

BASICS

DESCRIPTION

Anatomic variation of the tongue in which the lingual frenulum is unusually tight and short. Also known as tongue-tie. This condition may result in impaired tongue mobility with early breastfeeding problems, maternal nipple pain, and, later speech problems.

EPIDEMIOLOGY

- Prevalence ranges from 2 to 10% in various studies.
- About half of breastfeeding infants with ankyloglossia will have difficulty feeding or will cause maternal nipple pain during feeds.
- Incidence of speech articulation disorders due to ankyloglossia is unknown.
- Male-to-female ratio of 3:1

RISK FACTORS

No known environmental risk factors

PATHOPHYSIOLOGY

- Pedigree analysis suggests significant hereditary component, possibly X-linked.
- Studies show 40–50% of patients with ankyloglossia had a relative with the same condition and an inheritance rate of about 21%.
- Mutations in the T-box transcription factor TBX22 have been associated with heritable ankyloglossia with or without cleft lip, cleft palate, or hypodontia.
- Newborns with ankyloglossia
  - Are often asymptomatic but problems can occur with breastfeeding
  - May have poor or ineffective latch or may cause maternal nipple pain due to poor tongue mobility and prolonged feeding times
- Later in childhood, the effect of ankyloglossia is controversial.
  - May cause problems with articulation of certain sounds that require tongue to reach teeth, palate, and lips (e.g., "t," "d," "z," "s," "th," "n," "l")
  - Not a cause of speech delay
  - May also result in mechanical problems including difficulty with oral hygiene (inability to lick lips), inability to lick ice cream cone, play wind instruments, or French kiss (cataglottism)

COMMONLY ASSOCIATED CONDITIONS

- Smith-Lemli-Opitz syndrome
- Simpson-Golabi-Behmel syndrome
- Oral-facial-digital syndrome
- Beckwith-Wiedemann syndrome

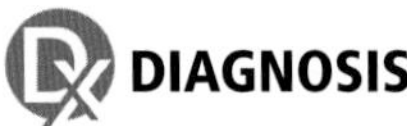

DIAGNOSIS

Diagnosis based on physical appearance and functional impairment of breastfeeding or speech

HISTORY

- Maternal report of difficulty with infant latch or nipple pain while breastfeeding
- Report of inability of infant/child to extrude tongue beyond alveolus/teeth
- Ankyloglossia varies in severity. Some children can protrude tongue past alveolus/teeth but not past lower lip and still have difficulties.

PHYSICAL EXAM

- Commonly missed finding on newborn exam because the mouth is usually not open
- Examiner should pass the small finger, pad-side down, under the infant's tongue to feel for resistance at the site of the lingual frenulum.
- Examiner should also visualize the floor of mouth and lingual frenulum when the infant cries or by using tongue depressors, Q-tips, or fingers to open the mouth.
- Visualization of the tongue will show
  - Abnormally short frenulum, inserting at or near the tip of the tongue
  - Difficulty lifting tongue to upper alveolus/palate
  - Inability to protrude tongue beyond lower alveolus/teeth
  - Notching or "heart shape" of tip of tongue when protruded
  - Note: Some children can protrude tongue past alveolus/teeth but not past lower lip and still have difficulties.

DIFFERENTIAL DIAGNOSIS

- Consider other causes of poor breastfeeding including inexperience, poor positioning, poor suck, or an undetected partial cleft palate.
- Consider other causes of speech articulation difficulties including incoordination and neuromuscular disease.

DIAGNOSTIC TESTS & INTERPRETATION

Initial Tests (screening, lab, imaging)

- No imaging indicated
- Functional ultrasound of tongue movement during breastfeeding has been used experimentally to quantify milk transfer.

Diagnostic Procedures/Other

- Mothers of infants with ankyloglossia and difficulty breastfeeding should meet with lactation consultant to rule out other potential causative factors.
- Children with speech articulation difficulty should meet with speech therapist for therapy and to assess for other causes.

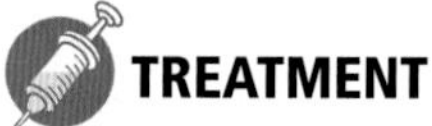

TREATMENT

GENERAL MEASURES

- Observation if there is no functional impairment of breastfeeding or speech
- Surgical treatment if functional impairment is present
- Treatment is frenotomy—incision of lingual frenulum.
  - For most healthy newborns, this may be performed in an outpatient setting.
  - The newborn is swaddled. An assistant keeps the head in midline and opens the mouth with gentle pressure on the chin. The tongue is retracted superiorly with a grooved guide or two-gloved fingers or cotton tip applicators on both sides of the frenulum. Sterile scissors are then used to divide the frenulum with care not to cut into the tongue or floor of mouth. Topical lidocaine and oxymetazoline on a cotton ball may be applied before and after the frenotomy.
  - For older children unlikely to cooperate and any patient with medical comorbidities or coagulopathy, the procedure should be performed in the operating room under general anesthesia.

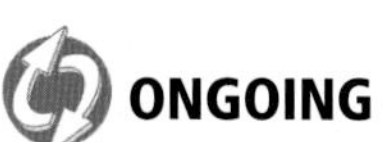

ONGOING CARE

FOLLOW-UP RECOMMENDATIONS

- Infants should be seen about 1 week after frenotomy to assess feeding and weight gain.
- Older children should be seen about 6 weeks after surgery to assess function and to determine whether a revision procedure for scar formation is needed.

PROGNOSIS

- Infants treated for tongue-tie have an excellent prognosis.
- <1% require repeat frenotomy or local flaps.
- Frenotomy has been shown to be effective for improving infant breastfeeding problems such as infant weight gain and maternal nipple pain. There are five randomized controlled trials with similar positive results.
- Breastfeeding rates in infants treated with frenotomy for ankyloglossia appear similar to healthy infants (approximately 40–45% at 6 months and 25% at 12 months).
- Studies evaluating frenotomy for speech articulation problems are inconclusive, of low quality, with lack of randomization, and small sample sizes. Further studies are needed.
- Complications have rarely been reported including severe infection or severe bleeding. Severe bleeding was associated with untrained individuals performing the procedure.

ADDITIONAL READING

- Buryk M, Bloom D, Shope T. Efficacy of neonatal release of ankyloglossia: a randomized trial. *Pediatrics*. 2011;128(2):280–288.
- Chinnadurai S, Francis D, Epstein R, et al. Treatment of ankyloglossia for reasons other than breastfeeding: a systematic review. *Pediatrics*. 2015;135(6):e1467–e1474.
- Francis D, Krishnaswami S, McPheeters M. Treatment of ankyloglossia and breastfeeding outcomes: a systematic review. *Pediatrics*. 2015;135(6): e1458–e1466.
- Han SH, Kim MC, Choi YS, et al. A study on the genetic inheritance of ankyloglossia based on pedigree analysis. *Arch Plast Surg*. 2012;39(4):329–332.
- Opara PI, Gabriel-Job N, Opara KO. Neonates presenting with severe complications of frenotomy: a case series. *J Med Case Rep*. 2012;6:77.

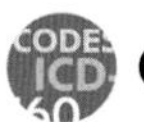

CODES

ICD10

- Q38.1 Ankyloglossia
- P92.8 Other feeding problems of newborn

FAQ

- Q: What is the appropriate time to perform frenotomy in breastfeeding newborns with ankyloglossia?
- A: Optimal timing is not known. A reasonable approach is to allow enough time to establish that there is a problem with breastfeeding caused by ankyloglossia. Some infants with ankyloglossia will not have problems. Usually, this issue is evident in the first 2 days of life. Newborns with identified breastfeeding difficulty should have frenotomy performed quickly to allow for continued breastfeeding. Delay may cause some mothers to abandon breastfeeding due to pain or difficulty. Optimal timing is probably between 2 and 7 days of life.
- Q: In infants with ankyloglossia who are either bottlefeeding or breastfeeding with no difficulty, should frenotomy be performed to help "prevent" future problems with speech or functional difficulties?
- A: Data regarding speech/functional outcome in these children are not known at present.
- Q: Who does frenotomies?
- A: ENT or oral surgeons most commonly perform the procedure. In areas where access to these specialists is difficult, general pediatricians, family practitioners, neonatologists, or newbornists may perform the procedure after sufficient training. The procedure is not difficult. It can be done in the inpatient or outpatient setting. It is billed under the Common Procedural Terminology (CPT) Code 41010 (frenotomy).
- Q: What are the postoperative instructions after frenotomy?
- A: For all patients after frenotomy: acetaminophen for pain. Although complications are rare, patients should go to an emergency department if bleeding, infection, or swelling occurs. For older children, avoid citrus; spicy; or hard, scratchy foods for 1 week after the procedure.
- Q: What is a posterior tongue-tie?
- A: A frenulum that originates more posteriorly and may not be visually apparent as those that extend to the tip of the tongue. Palpation and superior retraction of the tongue reveals a tight band that may still be symptomatic during nursing.

ANOMALOUS LEFT CORONARY ARTERY FROM THE PULMONARY ARTERY (ALCAPA)

Shellie M. Kendall, MD

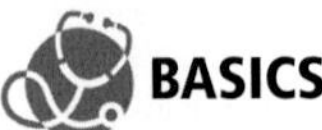

BASICS

DESCRIPTION

The anomalous coronary artery arises from the pulmonary artery rather than from its usual origin, the aorta. Most commonly, the anomalous left coronary artery arises from the pulmonary artery in a condition known as ALCAPA or Bland-White-Garland syndrome.

EPIDEMIOLOGY

- The majority of patients present in infancy at approximately 2 months of age when pulmonary vascular resistance falls.
- There are case reports of patients presenting as late as the 4th to 8th decades of life.

Incidence

Very rare anomaly affecting 1 in 300,000 live births and occurring in 0.2–0.5% of cases of congenital heart disease

PATHOPHYSIOLOGY

- In the fetal and neonatal period, pulmonary vascular resistance is increased relative to systemic vascular resistance providing the driving force for antegrade flow from the pulmonary artery through the anomalous coronary artery to supply the ventricle.
- As pulmonary vascular resistance drops, pulmonary arterial pressure drops. When the diastolic blood pressure in the pulmonary artery decreases below myocardial perfusion pressure (or diastolic aortic pressure), pulmonary run-off "steals" blood from the myocardium, resulting in myocardial ischemia. In ALCAPA, ischemia of the anterolateral left ventricular wall occurs leading to left ventricular and mitral valve papillary muscle dysfunction.
- The fact that the ventricle is perfused with desaturated blood plays a less important role than the overall perfusion-related imbalance between myocardial oxygen demand and supply.

ETIOLOGY

- Abnormal septation of the conotruncus into the aorta and pulmonary artery
- Persistence of the pulmonary buds and involution of the aortic buds that usually form the coronary arteries
- As-yet-unspecified genetic predisposition

DIAGNOSIS

HISTORY

- Typically presents with paroxysms of poor feeding, pallor, cough, tachypnea, respiratory distress, and diaphoresis
- Irritability, crying, appearance of being in pain (especially after meals)
- Can be asymptomatic
- Can be symptomatic in infancy and then gradually improve if adequate coronary collateralization develops
- Older children may have exercise intolerance, dyspnea, syncope, chest pain, palpitations.
- Sudden death, especially with exertion

PHYSICAL EXAM

- Signs of congestive heart failure (CHF) such as cachexia, tachycardia, tachypnea, increased work of breathing, lethargy, diaphoresis
- Signs of low cardiac output such as pallor, diminished peripheral pulses, and perfusion
- Gallop rhythm
- Narrowly split S2 with a loud P2 component (if left ventricular heart failure raises pulmonary arterial pressure)
- Murmur of mitral regurgitation or a continuous murmur reminiscent of a coronary arteriovenous fistula
- Diagnosis should be entertained in any infant presenting with cardiomegaly or perplexing cardiorespiratory symptoms.

DIFFERENTIAL DIAGNOSIS

- Dilated cardiomyopathy
- Myocarditis
- Coronary artery fistula
- Left ventricular failure from other causes
- Mitral valve regurgitation from other causes
- Respiratory distress from other causes
- Colic

DIAGNOSTIC TESTS & INTERPRETATION

Initial Tests (screening, lab, imaging)

- Chest radiograph: cardiomegaly, pulmonary edema
- Electrocardiography: anterolateral infarct pattern in an infant (Q in I, aVL, V4–V6), abnormal R-wave progression in precordial leads
- Echocardiogram: attachment of coronary artery to pulmonary artery by two-dimensional imaging. Doppler interrogation shows flow passing from coronary artery to great artery rather than vice versa (if pulmonary vascular resistance has fallen). False negative studies can occur. If the echocardiogram demonstrates normal appearing coronary arteries but clinical suspicion persists, perform cardiac magnetic resonance imaging (MRI), coronary computed tomography (CT) angiography, or cardiac catheterization with angiography.
  - Dilation of the right coronary artery
  - Left ventricular function impairment, wall motion abnormalities, and dilation
  - Mitral regurgitation
  - Highly echogenic papillary muscles and myocardium
- Cardiac MRI: excellent diagnostic modality for patients of all ages; provides assessment of anatomy, left ventricular function, and myocardial fibrosis
- Coronary CT angiography: excellent diagnostic modality for patients of all ages. Rapidly advancing technology permits minimizing radiation exposure.
- Cardiac catheterization: Angiographic and hemodynamic parameters may correlate with degree of cardiovascular dysfunction.
  - Low cardiac output
  - High left atrial filling pressures
  - Pulmonary arterial hypertension
  - Aortic root angiography shows passage of contrast medium from normally connected right coronary artery to the left coronary arterial system to the pulmonary artery.
  - Pulmonary artery angiogram shows reflux of contrast medium into the left coronary artery or a "negative wash-in" of unopacified blood flowing from left coronary to pulmonary artery.

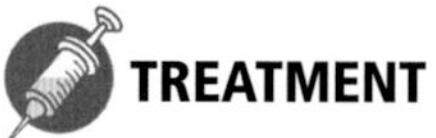

TREATMENT

GENERAL MEASURES

The first priority is to safely institute supportive care measures while expeditiously planning for surgical intervention.

SURGERY/OTHER PROCEDURES

- Direct reimplantation of the left coronary artery into the aorta using a button of pulmonary arterial tissue and/or an extension-tube graft of anterior and posterior pulmonary arterial wall tissue sewn into a narrow cylinder to avoid tension, distortion, and stenosis of the coronary artery
- Creation of an aortopulmonary window and tunnel that directs blood from aorta to the left coronary ostium (Takeuchi procedure)
- Ligation of the origin of the left coronary artery and reconstitution with a coronary artery bypass graft; performed with or without the use of cardiopulmonary bypass
- Ligation of the origin of the left coronary artery (to prevent flow runoff into the pulmonary artery or "steal") is rarely ever performed in the current era.

ADMISSION, INPATIENT, AND NURSING CONSIDERATIONS

- Attention to basic life support measures (airway, breathing, and circulation) and prompt referral to a pediatric cardiac center are indicated immediately on presentation.
- As myocardial ischemia can be worsened with traditional heart failure treatments such as oxygen administration, afterload reduction, and inotropic support, these therapies should be administered in consultation with a pediatric cardiac care center.
- An excess of procedures, interventions, and manipulation is poorly tolerated by this group of critically ill patients.

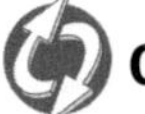

ONGOING CARE

PROGNOSIS

- Untreated, 90% of those who present in infancy will die before the age of 1 year, usually at 1 to 2 months of age (when pulmonary vascular resistance falls).
- Late results after surgery are excellent in many centers. Hospital mortality in larger selected series is ≤5%, with very little subsequent attrition.
- Mitral regurgitation commonly resolves completely after surgery establishes a patent dual-coronary system, but this may take 6 to 12 months to be fully realized. Follow-up evaluation is warranted, as mitral regurgitation may progress despite surgery and valve repair may be required later.
- Complete normalization of global left ventricular systolic function is common. However, evidence of chronic regional left ventricular function impairment is apparent with echocardiographic myocardial strain evaluation. Cardiac MRI commonly reveals wall motion abnormalities, perfusion deficits, and myocardial fibrosis.
- Residual coronary artery lesions, such as coronary artery stenosis or aneurysms can occur.
- At least moderate pulmonary valve insufficiency typically develops after the Takeuchi procedure.

ADDITIONAL READING

- Azakie A, Russell JL, McCrindle BW, et al. Anatomic repair of anomalous left coronary artery from the pulmonary artery by aortic reimplantation: early survival, patterns of ventricular recovery and late outcome. *Ann Thorac Surg.* 2003;75(5):1535–1541.
- Bland E, White P, Garland J. Congenital anomalies of the coronary arteries: report of an unusual case associated with cardiac hypertrophy. *Am Heart J.* 1933;8:787–801.
- Cabrera A, Chen D, Pignatelli R, et al. Outcomes of anomalous left coronary artery from pulmonary artery repair: beyond normal function. *Ann Thorac Surg.* 2015;99(4):1342–1347.
- Castaldi B, Vida V, Reffo E, et al. Speckle tracking in ALCAPA patients after surgical repair as predictor of residual coronary disease. *Pediatr Cardiol.* 2017;38(4):794–800.
- Ginde S, Earing M, Bartz P, et al. Late complications after Takeuchi repair of anomalous left coronary artery from the pulmonary artery: case series and review of literature. *Pediatr Cardiol.* 2012;33(7):1115–1123.
- Lange R, Vogt M, Hörer J, et al. Long-term results of repair of anomalous origin of the left coronary artery from the pulmonary artery. *Ann Thorac Surg.* 2007;83(4):1463–1471.
- Michielon G, Di Carlo D, Brancaccio G, et al. Anomalous coronary artery origin from the pulmonary artery: correlation between surgical timing and left ventricular function recovery. *Ann Thorac Surg.* 2003;76(2):581–588.
- Schmitt B, Bauer S, Kutty S, et al. Myocardial perfusion, scarring, and function in anomalous left coronary artery from the pulmonary artery syndrome: a long-term analysis using magnetic resonance imaging. *Ann Thorac Surg.* 2014;98(4):1425–1436.

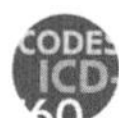

CODES

ICD10

Q24.5 Malformation of coronary vessels

FAQ

- Q: How do you differentiate crying from the symptoms of myocardial ischemia from crying from colic?
- A: This is not easy, but clinical assessment should manifest the signs of CHF, shock, and low cardiac output, which are decidedly atypical for the usual patient with colic. If the patient is still feeding, the crying in patients with this lesion classically occurs after meals, when blood is shunted to the liver and intestines. This is not a highly sensitive finding, and concern should lead to further objective evaluation.

ANOREXIA NERVOSA

Darlene M. Atkins, PhD • Sara M. Buckelew, MD, MPH

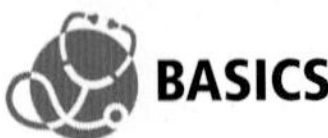

BASICS

DESCRIPTION

Anorexia nervosa (AN) is a complex biopsychosocial illness.

- *Diagnostic and Statistical Manual of Mental Disorders 5th edition* (*DSM-5*) criteria:
  - Restriction of energy intake relative to requirements, leading to a significantly low body weight in the context of age, sex, developmental trajectory, and physical health. Significantly low weight is defined as weight that is less than minimally normal or, for children and adolescents, less than minimally expected.
  - Intense fear of gaining weight or becoming fat, or persistent behavior that interferes with weight gain, even though at a significantly low weight
  - Disturbance in the way in which one's body weight or shape is experienced, undue influence of body weight or shape on self-evaluation, or persistent lack of recognition of the seriousness of current low body weight
- Types: restricting (no binge eating or purging) or binge eating/purging (purging includes vomiting, laxatives, and/or diuretic use)
- Reprinted with permission from the American Psychiatric Association. *Diagnostic and Statistical Manual of Mental Disorders*. 5th ed. Arlington, VA: American Psychiatric Association; 2013:171.

EPIDEMIOLOGY

- Approximately 0.5% of adolescent girls in the United States have AN.
- 10% of all patients with eating disorders are males.
- In younger patients, approximately equal numbers of females and males
- Increasing prevalence of eating disorders is seen in preadolescents, in males, and in minority populations within the United States.

RISK FACTORS

- Early physical/pubertal development
- Personality traits such as perfectionism and eagerness to please
- Family history of eating disorders, alcoholism, or mood disorders
- Involvement in sports or activities that emphasize shape/weight
- "Dieting" itself is a risk factor for developing an eating disorder.

Genetics

- Family studies demonstrate that 1st-degree relatives have a 10-fold increased lifetime risk of developing AN.
- Twin studies also support role of genetics and familial concordance of AN.

GENERAL PREVENTION

- Assess height, weight, and BMI at every preventive visit at a minimum; evaluate for deviations.
- Discourage "dieting" behavior. Instead, focus on promoting healthy eating behaviors and lifestyle change.
- Strongly encourage regular family meals. Research suggests that regular family meals are a protective factor for all types of eating disorders and obesity.

PATHOPHYSIOLOGY

- Physical manifestations are primarily the result of caloric restriction and consequences of malnutrition, which can affect all organ symptoms. The degree of symptoms seen may be due in part to the duration and severity of caloric restriction.
- Associated changes may also be due to purging, including vomiting, laxative use, or diet pill use.
- Bradycardia and hypothermia may result from significantly decreased metabolic rate due to malnutrition and caloric restriction.
- Hormonal changes due to starvation include resumption of prepubertal gonadotropin secretion.

ETIOLOGY

Evidence for specific etiology is not definitive; most likely multifactorial, including genetic risk factors, environmental triggers, and individual and family life experiences

COMMONLY ASSOCIATED CONDITIONS

- Amenorrhea
- Osteopenia/osteoporosis
- Female athlete triad (disordered eating, amenorrhea, osteoporosis)
- Depression
- Anxiety disorders including obsessive-compulsive disorder
- Substance abuse

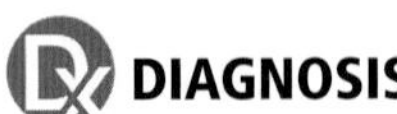

DIAGNOSIS

Diagnosis is made using *DSM-5* criteria. However, many patients exhibit marked symptoms but do not meet the full criteria for AN; for example, despite drastic weight loss, the patient's weight remains in the normal range. These patients may be diagnosed with other specified feeding or eating disorder, also called subclinical or atypical AN. These patients likely still require close monitoring and potential intervention.

HISTORY

- Weight history:
  - Highest and lowest weight in last year; patient's "target weight" they were attempting to reach with restriction
  - Ask, "How often do you weigh yourself? What is the most you have weighed in past year? The least? What do you think of as your own ideal weight?"
- Psychological assessment:
  - Interviews with patient and parents, detailed history of body image concerns, obsession with weight and/or shape, developmental and family history, social and academic history, cognitive and personality traits, and premorbid and current level of functioning
  - Critical in establishing a diagnosis and developing a treatment plan
- Other psychological symptoms: Assess mood and anxiety symptoms, suicidal ideation, substance use, and other risky or self-injurious behaviors.
- Diet and nutrition history: 24-hour dietary recall, history of binge eating, purging (including use of diuretics, laxatives, diet pills, or emetics), food restrictions, or calorie counting
- Exercise history: type, how much and intensity
- Menstrual history: last menstrual period (LMP), weight at LMP, history of skipped periods

PHYSICAL EXAM

- Vital signs, specifically orthostatic heart rates (HR) and blood pressures (to evaluate for vital sign instability that may be an indicator of severity and need for inpatient management), and temperature
- Weight, height, and BMI plotted in comparison to historical growth curve
- HEENT: Evaluate for signs of dehydration, dental exam for erosion due to purging.
- CV: cardiac status
- GI: Evaluate for pain, tenderness, organomegaly.
- Derm: lanugo, Russell sign (callousing of the finger from self-induced purging), evidence of self-injurious behavior
- GU: Tanner staging for pubertal development
- Neurologic: complete exam including funduscopic exam to rule out brain tumor

DIFFERENTIAL DIAGNOSIS

- Medical conditions such as
  - Pregnancy
  - Oncologic: brain tumor, other cancers
  - GI: inflammatory bowel disease (including Crohn and ulcerative colitis), celiac disease
  - Endocrinologic: diabetes mellitus, thyroid disease, hypopituitarism, Addison disease
  - HIV or other chronic infections
- Psychiatric or psychological conditions such as
  - Psychiatric: depression, obsessive-compulsive disorder, substance abuse, psychotic symptoms
- *DSM-5* avoidant/restrictive food intake disorder: food aversions/hypersensitivity, extreme picky eating, decreased intake due to fears of swallowing/choking

DIAGNOSTIC TESTS & INTERPRETATION

Initial Tests (screening, lab, imaging)

- Serum electrolytes, BUN/creatinine, glucose: typically normal if patient is not purging
- Serum calcium, magnesium, phosphorous: may all be low. If hospitalized, follow phosphorous daily to assess for refeeding syndrome.
- TSH; if indicated, free T_4, T_3: to rule out thyroid disease; if abnormal, may be due solely to starvation
- CBC with differential: Anemia may be present due to iron deficiency or chronic disease but may be falsely normal if patient is dehydrated; low WBC count is seen with malnutrition.
- ESR: generally low due to malnutrition
- AST, ALT: occasionally abnormal due to fatty liver
- β-hCG: Rule out pregnancy if amenorrheic.
- Urinalysis: Evaluate specific gravity to assess for dehydration or may have diluted urine if patients water load to falsely increase their weight.
- Consider EKG: may demonstrate bradycardia, prolonged QTc
- Patients amenorrheic for >6 months:
  - Dual-energy x-ray absorptiometry (DEXA) scan: Evaluate bone density, risk of compression fracture, and bone loss; may be helpful motivator for treatment as may not be reversible
  - Serum LH, FSH, prolactin, if persistent amenorrhea with normal weight: LH and FSH will generally be low.

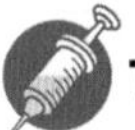

TREATMENT

- Multidisciplinary team approach is considered the state of the art standard of care and includes medical monitoring, nutritional counseling, and psychological treatments.
- Family-based treatment (FBT) is the only evidence-based psychological treatment for pediatric and adolescent AN. Parents/caregivers are viewed as an integral part of the treatment team.
- Initially, all meals and snacks are prepared by and supervised by the parents. Gradually, age-appropriate autonomy regarding eating is returned to the child/adolescent as physical and psychological progress is made.

MEDICATION

- Medications are not the primary mechanism for treating AN but may be helpful in the treatment of co-occurring illnesses such as depression and anxiety.
- Medications to treat constipation may be necessary but should be used with caution.
- Supplements such as multivitamin, calcium, and vitamin D should be considered.
- Refeeding is the treatment of choice for amenorrhea rather than starting oral contraceptive pills (OCPs).

ISSUES FOR REFERRAL

Depending on severity and availability, refer to an adolescent medicine specialist or other eating disorder specialist.

ADMISSION, INPATIENT, AND NURSING CONSIDERATIONS

- Criteria for inpatient hospitalization:
  - Severe malnutrition with weight <75% ideal body weight or weight loss despite treatment
  - Bradycardia including daytime HR <50 bpm and/or nighttime HR<45 bpm
  - Systolic blood pressure <90 mm Hg
  - Orthostatic hypotension or significant orthostatic changes in pulse
  - Severe hypothermia
  - Arrhythmia
  - Acute food refusal
  - Severe electrolyte abnormalities
- Suicidality may require psychiatric hospitalization.
- Once a patient is medically stable and no longer meets admission criteria, insurance companies may limit lengths of hospital stays. Most patients are treated solely as outpatients.

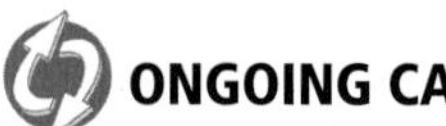

ONGOING CARE

- Ongoing medical monitoring with emphasis placed on overall vital signs and not on weight alone
- Goals are set for nutritional rehabilitation. Meal plans are established and reassessed at each subsequent visit.
- Physical activity is also monitored with appropriate goals set in collaboration with patient, physician, and therapist.
- Referral to a family therapist with this expertise is advised. Individual psychotherapy may also be useful for many patients.
- Group psychotherapy can be a useful adjunct particularly for some older adolescent and young adult patients.
- More intensive services include intensive outpatient, day, or residential treatment.
- Other adjunctive therapies include mindfulness training, expressive arts, etc.

PROGNOSIS

- Most adolescent patients recover fully but generally not without a long course of treatment. Overall, children and adolescents have better outcomes than adults.
- Better outcomes are associated with shorter duration of symptoms, earlier diagnosis, absence of purging behaviors, and less severity of psychiatric comorbidity. However, outcome findings vary depending on factors such as length of follow-up and definitions of recovery.
- Mortality rates for adolescents with AN are reported to be 1.8%, primarily from effects of starvation (especially cardiac) or from suicide.

COMPLICATIONS

- Majority of complications may be reversed with improved nutrition.
- Refeeding syndrome:
  - As the patient is refed, the body may shift from a catabolic state to an anabolic state.
  - This change may result in a release of insulin which may drive phosphorous and potassium intercellularly and drop extracellular levels resulting in delirium, coma, arrhythmias, cardiac failure, and death.
- CV: arrhythmias, pericardial effusions
- GI: delayed gastric emptying, slowed intestinal motility and constipation, pancreatitis; elevated cholesterol
- Endocrine: amenorrhea, osteoporosis, sick euthyroid syndrome, growth delay
- Complications related to purging include Mallory-Weiss tears, esophagitis, electrolyte and fluid imbalances (particularly hypokalemia).
- Neuropsychological: anxiety, poor concentration, depressed mood, cognitive impairment, cortical atrophy

ADDITIONAL READING

- Academy for Eating Disorders. *Critical Points for Early Recognition and Medical Risk Management in the Care of Individuals with Eating Disorders*. 3rd ed. http://www.aedweb.org/images/MCG_06.02.16.pdf. Accessed February 14, 2017.
- American Academy of Child and Adolescent Psychiatry. Practice parameter for the assessment and treatment of children and adolescents with eating disorders. http://www.jaacap.com/article/S0890-8567%2815%2900070-2/fulltext. Accessed February 14, 2017.
- Bulik CM, Kleiman SC, Yilmaz Z. Genetic epidemiology of eating disorders. *Curr Opin Psychiatry*. 2016;29(6):383–388.
- Golden NH, Katzman DK, Sawyer SM, et al. Position paper of the Society for Adolescent Health and Medicine: medical management of restrictive eating disorders in adolescents and young adults. *J Adolesc Health*. 2015;56(1):121–125.
- Golden NH, Schneider M, Wood C; for Committee on Nutrition, Committee on Adolescence, Section on Obesity. Preventing obesity and eating disorders in adolescents. *Pediatrics*. 2016;138(3):e20161649.
- Rosen DS; for American Academy of Pediatrics Committee on Adolescence. Identification and management of eating disorders in children and adolescents. *Pediatrics*. 2010;126(6):1240–1253.

SEE ALSO

- National Eating Disorders Association (www.nationaleatingdisorders.org)
- www.maudsleyparents.org
- www.feast-ed.org
- Bulimia chapter

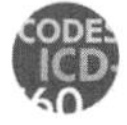

CODES

ICD10

- F50.00 Anorexia nervosa, unspecified
- F50.01 Anorexia nervosa, restricting type
- F50.02 Anorexia nervosa, binge eating/purging type

FAQ

- Q: If the patient presents with severe low mood, why not start them on an antidepressant right away?
- A: Many of their depressive symptoms may be secondary to the effects of their malnourished state. It's best to begin nutritional rehabilitation and reassess as intake improves.
- Q: Can patients have AN if they do not report feeling fat or intentionally dieting?
- A: Yes. Denial is very often associated with AN. Rely on behavioral signs and parental report.
- Q: Can AN be diagnosed in preadolescents?
- A: Yes. The age of onset of AN has continued to decrease. If they present with weight preoccupation, pursuit of thinness, and other diagnostic criteria, their diagnosis is AN.

ANTHRAX

Eimear Kitt, MB, BCh, BAO (NUI) • Andrew P. Steenhoff, MBBCh, DCH

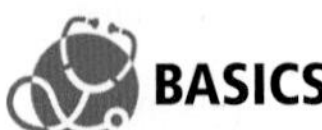

BASICS

DESCRIPTION

Bacillus anthracis is a spore-forming, aerobic gram-positive rod that can cause acute infection (anthrax) in humans and animals and has the potential to be used as a biologic weapon due to its rapid systemic progression and high mortality in those who are exposed and untreated.

EPIDEMIOLOGY

- Anthrax is primarily a zoonotic disease. Most naturally acquired anthrax infections are cutaneous (95%). Inhalational (5%) and gastrointestinal (GI) (<1%) forms are particularly rare.
  - In recent times, injection anthrax has been described in Europe and is associated with injecting drug users.
  - This form has not yet been reported in the United States nor in the pediatric population.
- Incidence is extremely low, averaging 1 to 2 cases of cutaneous anthrax per year in the United States.
- Prior to October 2001, only 18 cases of inhalational anthrax were reported in the United States during the 20th century.
- No human-to-human spread of inhalational anthrax has been reported.
- Rare cases of human-to-human transmission of cutaneous anthrax have been reported after direct contact with infected skin lesions.
- Anthrax has been used as an agent of bioterrorism.

GENERAL PREVENTION

- Antibiotics are effective against germinating *B. anthracis* but not against the spores. Therefore, if prophylactic antibiotics are stopped prematurely, remaining spores can cause disease when they germinate. This phenomenon of delayed-onset disease occurs with inhalational anthrax and not with cutaneous or GI exposures.
- Where the threat of transmission of *B. anthracis* spores is deemed credible, decontamination of skin and potential fomites (e.g., clothing) may be considered to reduce the risk for cutaneous and GI forms of the disease.
- Anthrax vaccine absorbed (AVA) is the only licensed human anthrax vaccine in the United States.
  - Primary vaccination consists of subcutaneous injections at 0, 2, and 4 weeks and three booster vaccinations at 6, 12, and 18 months.
  - Annual booster injections are required to maintain immunity.
  - The most common adverse event is injection-site discomfort (e.g., edema, pain, local hypersensitivity).
- Infection control
  - Immediately notify the hospital epidemiologist, infection control department, or local health department of suspected cases.
  - No data suggest that patient-to-patient transmission of inhalational anthrax occurs.
  - Standard barrier isolation precautions are recommended for all hospitalized patients with all forms of anthrax infection.
  - High-efficiency particulate air-filter masks or other measures for airborne precautions are not indicated.
  - There is no need to immunize or provide prophylaxis to patient contacts unless they, like the patient, were exposed to the aerosol.
  - If anthrax is used as a bioweapon, spores may be detected on environmental surfaces. The risk of inhalation anthrax from secondary aerosolization of these spores is uncertain.

ALERT

Pulmonary disease caused by anthrax is a hemorrhagic mediastinitis with pleural effusions and *not* a bronchopneumonia.

PATHOPHYSIOLOGY

- After inhalation, wound inoculation, or ingestion, *B. anthracis* spores infect macrophages, germinate, and proliferate.
  - Proliferation occurs at the site of infection and in regional lymph nodes.
  - Replicating bacteria release toxins, leading to edema, hemorrhage, and necrosis.
- Incubation period depends on the route of transmission.
  - Inhalational anthrax: Infection requires inhalation of >8,000 spores; incubation period is 2 to 60 days.
  - Cutaneous anthrax: Spores enter a cut or abrasion in the skin; incubation period is 1 to 12 days.
  - GI anthrax: Spores are ingested in undercooked, infected meat; incubation period is 1 to 7 days; infection occurs in the upper (oropharyngeal lesions) or lower (intestinal lesions) GI tract.
  - Injection anthrax: Spores enter injection site in injection drug users.
- Hematogenous spread of the bacteria causes infection at other sites, including the CNS, liver, spleen, and kidney.

COMMONLY ASSOCIATED CONDITIONS

If anthrax is intentionally released, physicians must be alert for diseases caused by other potential biologic warfare agents (e.g., plague, tularemia, Q fever, smallpox, and botulism).

DIAGNOSIS

HISTORY

- Inhalational anthrax
  - Clinical presentation is a two-stage illness.
  - Initial symptoms are nonspecific and last 1 to 3 days. They include low-grade fever, dry cough, headache, vomiting, chills, weakness, abdominal pain, and substernal discomfort. This stage may be followed by a brief period of apparent recovery.
  - Second-stage symptoms develop abruptly 2 to 5 days later: fever, hemoptysis, dyspnea, chest pain, and profuse diaphoresis. Death may occur within 1 to 2 days.
- Cutaneous anthrax
  - Painless lesions develop on affected areas soon after exposure.
  - Systemic symptoms of fever, malaise, and headache may occur.
- GI anthrax
  - Oropharyngeal form causes sore throat, dysphagia, and fever.
  - Intestinal form also causes nausea, vomiting, anorexia, severe abdominal pain, and bloody diarrhea.
- Injection anthrax
  - Similar presentation to cutaneous anthrax but with suspected history of injection drug use
  - Systemic illness results from hematogenous and lymphatic dissemination.

PHYSICAL EXAM

- Clinical presentation of anthrax in children is varied; rapid diagnosis and effective treatment require recognition of the broad spectrum of clinical presentations.
- Inhalational anthrax
  - Tachypnea, hypoxia, cyanosis
  - Stridor, rales, signs of pleural effusion
  - Hemoptysis, hematemesis, melena
- Cutaneous anthrax
  - Initial painless, pruritic macule or papule enlarges into a 1- to 3-cm round ulcer by the 2nd day.
  - 1- to 3-mm vesicles with clear or serosanguineous fluid surround the ulcer.
  - A painless, depressed, black eschar follows, often with extensive local edema.
  - Over 1 to 2 weeks, the eschar dries, loosens, and falls off, occasionally with scarring.
  - Painful, regional lymphadenopathy may occur.
- GI anthrax
  - Unilateral oral or esophageal ulcers, cervical lymphadenopathy
  - Cecal or terminal ileal ulcers (Intestinal anthrax progresses to massive ascites and acute abdomen.)
- Injection anthrax
  - Painless blisters or sores surrounding where the drug was injected
  - Can disseminate faster than cutaneous anthrax
- Disseminated anthrax (potential complication of any of the above forms of anthrax):
  - Sepsis syndrome: tachycardia, hypotension, septic shock
  - Meningitis: meningismus, delirium, obtundation

DIFFERENTIAL DIAGNOSIS

- The prodromal illness of inhalational anthrax may resemble a lower respiratory tract infection, although upper respiratory infection symptoms are characteristically absent.
- Patients with inhalational anthrax may have a widened mediastinum on chest radiograph, which may resemble an aortic aneurysm or bacterial mediastinitis.
- Necrotic skin lesions may resemble plague, tularemia, ecthyma gangrenosum, and brown recluse spider bite.
- The combination of necrotic skin lesions with respiratory findings may be mistaken for a vasculitis.
- GI anthrax may be confused with other infectious enteritides (e.g., *Shigella*, *Salmonella*, *Yersinia*, *Campylobacter*, enterohemorrhagic *Escherichia coli*, *Clostridium difficile*, colitis), intussusception, Meckel diverticulum, and inflammatory bowel disease.

DIAGNOSTIC TESTS & INTERPRETATION

Initial Tests (screening, lab, imaging)

- Gram stain smear and culture from vesicular fluid
  - Diagnose cutaneous anthrax
  - Gram stain reveals large, gram-positive, boxcar-shaped bacilli.
  - Capsule is visualized in red on polychrome methylene blue stain smears.
  - *B. anthracis* grows readily on blood agar.

- Anthraxin skin test
  - Measures anthrax cell-mediated immunity
  - It is positive in 80% of patients within 72 hours of infection and in >95% of cases within 3 weeks.
  - The test was positive in 72% of patients >16 years after recovery.
- Serologic enzyme-linked immunosorbent assay (ELISA)
  - Measures antibodies to the lethal and edema toxins of *B. anthracis*
  - Positive if a single acute-phase titer is >1:32 or if there is a 4-fold or greater rise between acute and convalescent titers collected 4 weeks apart
- Polymerase chain reaction assay or immunohistochemistry
  - Bacterial DNA detection in blood, CSF, or exudates by polymerase chain reaction assay, tissue immunohistochemistry, or matrix-assisted laser desorption ionization time-of-flight (MALDI-TOF) mass spectrometry assay may be available through state health departments.
- Nasopharyngeal swab or induced respiratory secretion culture
  - Used for epidemiologic investigation
  - The sensitivity, specificity, and predictive value of nasal swab testing are unknown; therefore, this test should not be used to guide the use of postexposure prophylactic antibiotics.
- Blood culture
  - Patients with cutaneous anthrax may have bacteremia with *B. anthracis* even without significant signs of systemic disease.
- CBC
  - Often normal initially
  - May later develop anemia, leukocytosis, and thrombocytopenia
- Serum electrolytes, glucose, and calcium
  - Hypokalemia, acidosis, hypoglycemia, and hypocalcemia occurred during experimental anthrax infection in animals.
- Chest radiograph (or chest CT scan)
  - Inhalational anthrax causes a hemorrhagic mediastinitis.
  - May show a widened mediastinum and pleural effusions
  - No infiltrates are present.

TREATMENT

GENERAL MEASURES

Direct physical contact with a substance alleged to be anthrax:

- Wash exposed skin and articles of clothing with soap and water.
- Administer postexposure prophylaxis until the substance is proved not to be anthrax.
- Contact the public health department or the Centers for Disease Control and Prevention (CDC).
- For severe anthrax, anthrax-specific hyperimmune globulin 5% should be considered in consultation with CDC.

MEDICATION

Postexposure prophylaxis (PEP)

- Ciprofloxacin 15 mg/kg (up to 500 mg) *or* doxycycline 2.2 mg/kg (up to 100 mg) or levofloxacin 8 mg/kg (up to 250 mg) PO b.i.d. for 60 days
- Pediatric: Use ciprofloxacin for initial prophylaxis. Switch to amoxicillin or penicillin if susceptibility testing permits.
- The 3-dose anthrax vaccine series may be given in addition to PEP to those deemed to have significant anthrax exposure.
- For all forms of anthrax, begin with IV therapy and switch to oral therapy when clinically appropriate. Duration of therapy: Treat for 60 days (IV and PO combined) for biologic weapon–related events; for naturally acquired infection: 7 to 10 days
- Inhalational or GI anthrax: ciprofloxacin 10 mg/kg (up to 400 mg) *or* doxycycline 2.2 mg/kg (up to 100 mg) IV q12h *plus* clindamycin or rifampin
- Cutaneous anthrax: ciprofloxacin or doxycycline IV. (Pediatric: Begin therapy with ciprofloxacin [plus clindamycin or rifampin for inhalational/GI anthrax] and convert to penicillin G IV if susceptibility testing permits and when clinical improvement is documented.)
- If meningeal involvement is suspected, regimen should include agents with CNS penetration: ciprofloxacin plus meropenem plus linezolid IV.

ONGOING CARE

PROGNOSIS

- Inhalational anthrax
  - Case fatality rates were previously estimated to be >85% after symptoms develop. However, early use of appropriate antibiotic therapy appears to improve survival to approximately 55%.
  - Survival rate is higher if symptoms develop >30 days after exposure.
- Cutaneous anthrax
  - Case fatality rate is 20% without antibiotic treatment and <1% with antibiotic treatment.
- GI anthrax: Case fatality rate is 25–60%.

COMPLICATIONS

- Antibiotic therapy of cutaneous anthrax limits the likelihood of developing systemic symptoms but does not change the course of the eschar formation.
- Systemic dissemination of inhalational, cutaneous, or GI anthrax may lead to sepsis, meningitis, and death.

ADDITIONAL READING

- Advisory Committee on Immunization Practices. Use of anthrax vaccine in the United States. *MMWR Recomm Rep*. 2000;49(RR-15):1–20.
- Akbayram S, Doğan M, Akgün C, et al. Clinical findings in children with cutaneous anthrax in eastern Turkey. *Pediatr Dermatol*. 2010;27(6):600–606.
- Alexander JJ, Colangelo PM, Cooper CK, et al. Amoxicillin for postexposure inhalational anthrax in pediatrics: rationale for dosing recommendations. *Pediatr Infect Dis J*. 2008;27(11):955–957.
- Bradley JS, Peacock G, Krug SE, et al; and American Academy of Pediatrics Committee on Infectious Diseases and Disaster Preparedness Advisory Council. Pediatric anthrax clinical management. *Pediatrics*. 2014;133(5):e1411–e1436.
- Bravata DM, Holty JE, Wang E, et al. Inhalational, gastrointestinal, and cutaneous anthrax in children: a systematic review of cases: 1900 to 2005. *Arch Pediatr Adolesc Med*. 2007;161(9):896–905.
- Centers for Disease Control and Prevention. Update: investigation of bioterrorism-related anthrax and interim guidelines for exposure management and antimicrobial therapy, October 2001. *MMWR Morb Mortal Wkly Rep*. 2001;50(42):909–919.
- Hendricks KA, Wright ME, Shadomy SV, et al. Centers for Disease Control and Prevention expert panel meetings on prevention and treatment of anthrax in adults. *Emerg Infect Dis*. 2014;20(2):e130687.
- Kyriacou DN, Adamski A, Khardori N. Anthrax: from antiquity and obscurity to a front-runner in bioterrorism. *Infect Dis Clin North Am*. 2006;20(2):227–251.
- Li F, Nandy P, Chien S, et al. Pharmacometrics-based dose selection of levofloxacin as a treatment for post-exposure inhalational anthrax in children. *Antimicrob Agents Chemother*. 2010;54(1):375–379.
- Scorpio A, Blank TE, Day WA, et al. Anthrax vaccines: pasteur to the present. *Cell Mol Life Sci*. 2006;63(19–20):2237–2248.
- Stocker JT. Clinical and pathological differential diagnosis of selected potential bioterrorism agents of interest to pediatric health care providers. *Clin Lab Med*. 2006;26(2):329–344.

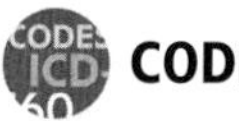

CODES

ICD10

- A22.9 Anthrax, unspecified
- A22.0 Cutaneous anthrax
- A22.1 Pulmonary anthrax

FAQ

- Q: Does the United States federal government have a plan in place if there were mass exposure to anthrax?
- A: Yes. Under emergency plans, the federal government would ship appropriate antibiotics from its stockpile to wherever they are needed. The government also has two antitoxin products—anthrax immune globulin (AIG—a polyclonal human immunoglobulin) and raxibacumab (a humanized monoclonal antibody approved by the FDA for use in children for the prevention and treatment of anthrax).
- Q: Should individuals ask their physicians to write a prescription for ciprofloxacin (or other antibiotic) so they have prophylaxis available?
- A: No. Ciprofloxacin and other antibiotics should not be prescribed unless there is a clearly indicated need. In addition, indiscriminate prescribing and widespread use of ciprofloxacin could hasten the development of drug-resistant organisms.
- Q: Can a person get screened or tested for anthrax?
- A: No screening test is available to determine whether anthrax exposure has occurred. The only way exposure can be determined is through a public health investigation.
- Q: Is a vaccine universally available for protection against anthrax?
- A: There is an anthrax vaccine, but it is not approved for universal use. It may be administered to people who are at high risk of exposure, such as military personnel, or to patients who have been deemed to have a significant exposure to anthrax.
- Q: What are the clues to differentiate pulmonary or inhalational anthrax from RSV in children?
- A: Children with pulmonary anthrax must have had direct exposure to the spores. They may display a high WBC count with left shift compared to the relatively normal WBC of those with RSV. Blood O_2 levels may be severely depressed in inhalational anthrax.

APLASTIC ANEMIA

Craig M. Forester, MD, PhD • James N. Huang, MD

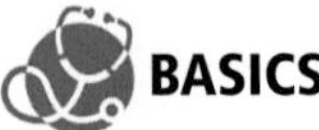

BASICS

DESCRIPTION

Aplastic anemia represents a heterogenous group of disorders characterized by peripheral pancytopenia and bone marrow hypocellularity.

EPIDEMIOLOGY

Incidence

- Estimated incidence of 2:1,000,000 per year in Western Hemisphere and Europe with increased incidence of 5 to 7:1,000,000 per year in Far East and those of Asian descent
- In the pediatric population, most commonly presents between ages 15 and 25 years

RISK FACTORS

Genetics

Patients with a number of inherited bone marrow failure syndromes are at increased risk of developing aplastic anemia. Recent evidence implicates somatic clonal mutations of genes involved in immune regulation and cellular proliferation in acquired aplastic anemia.

GENERAL PREVENTION

Aside from avoidance of environmental toxins (as described below), there are no practical preventive measures for acquired aplastic anemia.

PATHOPHYSIOLOGY

- Most instances of acquired aplastic anemia are thought to occur through a T-cell dependent autoimmune process leading to apoptosis of hematopoietic stem or progenitor cells.
- Additionally, exposure to certain toxins, chemicals, medications (classically chloramphenicol), and high doses of radiation can also lead to marrow aplasia.

ETIOLOGY

Acquired

- Idiopathic (70% of cases)
- Toxin: exposure to arsenic, benzene, radiation, organophosphates, organochlorines
- Drugs: chloramphenicol, numerous chemotherapeutic agents
- Radiation
- Paroxysmal nocturnal hemoglobinuria (PNH)
- Seronegative hepatitis (non-A, non-B, and non-C)
- HIV-1, Epstein-Barr virus (EBV), human herpes virus 6 (HHV-6), cytomegalovirus (CMV)
- Malnutrition
- Pregnancy

COMMONLY ASSOCIATED CONDITIONS

- Congenital or inherited bone marrow failure syndromes
  - Fanconi anemia, Shwachman-Diamond syndrome, Diamond-Blackfan anemia, dyskeratosis congenita, congenital amegakaryocytic thrombocytopenia, germline GATA2 mutations, Pearson syndrome
- Acquired
  - Differentiating aplastic anemia from refractory cytopenia of childhood (RCC) is crucial as RCC is considered a form of myelodysplastic syndrome (MDS) and should be considered for hematopoietic stem cell transplantation (HSCT).

DIAGNOSIS

HISTORY

- Detailed history including birth history, growth trajectory, antecedent illnesses, infections, environmental exposures
- Comprehensive review of systems with emphasis on neurologic (including developmental delay and learning disabilities), dermatologic, cardiac, pulmonary, endocrine (hypogonadism, growth delay), and hematologic systems
- Family history of cancer predisposition, excessive toxicity to chemotherapy, unexplained fetal loss, anemia/cytopenias, or congenital anomalies

PHYSICAL EXAM

- Thorough physical exam combined with plotting of growth curves
- Head: Evaluate for eye, epicanthal folds, jaw, palate abnormalities, oral mucosal lesions/bleeding, thrush.
- Cardiopulmonary: auscultation for cardiac anomalies, dyspnea, diminished aeration, asymmetry
- GI: hepatosplenomegaly, palpation for masses
- GU: renal/urinary/ureter abnormalities, gonadal abnormalities, or undescended testes
- Skeletal: dysmorphisms, forearms, thumbs, vertebral anomalies, osteopenia
- Skin: pigmentation changes, eczematous rash, nail abnormalities, bruising, petechiae, pallor
- Lymphadenopathy

DIFFERENTIAL DIAGNOSIS

- Myelosuppression secondary to ongoing infection (viral, tuberculosis)
- MDS (including RCC)
- Hematologic malignancy
- Nutritional deficiency: vitamin, mineral, or starvation/anorexia
- Autoimmune disease: systemic lupus erythematosus (SLE), thyroid disease, rheumatoid arthritis
- PNH
- Metastatic disease
- Hemophagocytic histiocytosis

DIAGNOSTIC TESTS & INTERPRETATION

Initial Tests (screening, lab, imaging)

- To confirm the diagnosis:
  - Diagnosis requires exclusion of other disease processes associated with pancytopenia (see "Etiology" and "Differential Diagnosis" sections) as well as the following:
    - Empty or hypoplastic bone marrow
    - Two out of three of the following:
      - Absolute neutrophil count (ANC) $<1{,}500/\mu L$
      - Platelets $<50{,}000/\mu L$
      - Hemoglobin (Hgb) <10 g/dL
  - Severe aplastic anemia (sAA)
    - Bone marrow cellularity <25%
    - Two out of three of the following:
      - ANC $<500/\mu L$
      - Platelets $<20{,}000/\mu L$
      - Absolute reticulocyte count <20,000/mL
  - Very severe aplastic anemia: The criteria are the same as for sAA, except for ANC $<200/\mu L$.
- To exclude other causes:
  - Complete blood count, + reticulocyte count
  - Peripheral blood smear
  - Hgb F %
  - Liver function tests, lactate dehydrogenase (LDH), uric acid
  - Direct and indirect Coombs assay
  - Baseline serum iron, ferritin, total iron-binding capacity (TIBC)
  - Flow cytometry for glycosylphosphatidylinositol (GPI)-anchored proteins CD55/CD59
  - Vitamin B_{12}, folate, copper levels
  - Viral studies: hepatitis A, B, and C; EBV, CMV, HIV, HHV-6, varicella-zoster virus (VZV), parvovirus
  - Antinuclear antibody (ANA), anti-double stranded DNA (dsDNA)
  - Acid-fast bacillus (AFB) staining of bone marrow aspirate
  - Human leukocyte antigen (HLA) typing of patient and family members
  - Ruling out inherited bone marrow failure syndromes:
    - Chromosomal breakage (mitomycin C or diepoxybutane): Fanconi anemia
    - Telomere length: dyskeratosis congenita
    - Exocrine pancreatic testing: serum trypsinogen and pancreatic isoamylase: Shwachman-Diamond syndrome
    - Erythrocyte adenosine deaminase: Diamond-Blackfan anemia
    - c-MPL mutation: congenital amegakaryocytic thrombocytopenia
- Imaging
  - Chest x-ray
  - Abdominal ultrasound (US)
  - Echocardiogram

Diagnostic Procedures/Other

- Bone marrow aspirate and biopsy
- Cytogenetics of bone marrow with fluorescence in situ hybridization (FISH) for monosomy 5, 7, 8
  - Bone marrow fragments are hypocellular with prominent fat spaces and reduced erythropoiesis, megakaryocytes, and granulocytes. Lymphocytes, macrophages, plasma cells, or mast cells may be prominent. Appearance of dysplasia in megakaryocyte or granulocytic lineage, blasts, hypercellularity, or increased reticulin staining is not consistent with aplastic anemia.

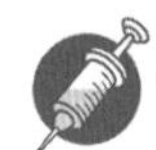

TREATMENT

Treatment for aplastic anemia that does not meet the severe or very severe criteria is individualized and controversial as some patients do spontaneously improve. However, patients with severe or very severe aplastic anemia should be promptly treated because of their high risk of infection.

MEDICATION

First Line

In all patients with sAA who are <40 years and without significant comorbidities, the treatment of choice is HSCT with a matched sibling donor (MSD). Superior and durable outcomes for MSD transplants conditioned with cyclophosphamide/antithymocyte globulin (ATG) as 1st-line therapy stresses importance of timely workup and HLA typing.

Second Line

For patients without an MSD or with significant comorbidities:

- Immunosuppressive therapy (IST) with combination horse ATG (hATG) and cyclosporine (antithymocyte globulin/CsA) followed by prolonged taper of cyclosporine
- If patients do not show clinical improvement within 3 to 6 months, consider an alternative donor HSCT such as with a matched unrelated donor (MUD) HSCT, if available, or repeat trial of IST.

ISSUES FOR REFERRAL

Pediatric hematology/oncology/bone marrow transplant (BMT): As a rare disorder, patients are typically managed by centers with hematologic experience and transplant capabilities.

ADDITIONAL THERAPIES

- Patients should be transfused when symptomatic with leukocyte-reduced, irradiated PRBCs, and platelets. Transfusions are weighed against the risk of alloimmunization and graft rejection with allogeneic BMT, but most institutions will transfuse to keep Hgb >7 to 8 g/dL and platelets above 10,000/μL. Transfusions should be with CMV-negative blood (if patient is CMV seronegative), if patient is likely to undergo transplant.
- Use of *Pneumocystis carinii* (*jiroveci*) pneumonia (PCP) prophylaxis prior to BMT is institution-dependent, but some recommend use of pentamidine (with atovaquone or dapsone as second line), avoiding sulfamethoxazole/trimethoprim due to its myelosuppressive properties.
- Antifungal prophylaxis is also used by many institutions.
- Granulocyte colony-stimulating factor (G-CSF) support may be used in setting of acute infection but has not been shown to improve overall survival or remission rates.
- Supportive care, androgens, cyclosporine, or growth factors alone are not definitive therapies. Corticosteroids alone are also not proven to be effective and lead to increased susceptibility to fungal infections.

ADMISSION, INPATIENT, AND NURSING CONSIDERATIONS

- Patients should be transfused slowly initially with PRBC 5 cc/kg over 4 hours to avoid pulmonary overcirculation.
- Platelet transfusions for symptomatic bleeding
- Cultures of blood and urine should be obtained with all fevers, and empiric broad-spectrum antibiotics coverage should be started while awaiting culture results.
- Symptomatic anemia, fever, severe thrombocytopenia, or any evidence of clinical bleeding must be admitted for supportive care and monitoring.
- Unless the patient has had a recent history of inadequate intake or losses, IV fluids are not usually necessary at the outset. Bear in mind that the patient will likely be receiving additional volume due to transfusions.
- Patients should be roomed in isolation if possible.

ONGOING CARE

FOLLOW-UP RECOMMENDATIONS

Regardless of whether IST or BMT is chosen for treatment modality, follow-up should be lifelong given risk of recurrence of aplastic anemia or transformation to MDS or malignancy. Long-term retrospective studies have demonstrated rates of relapse of up to 38%, with incidence of clonal transformation in 10–25% of patients who undergo IST.

Patient Monitoring

- Those who undergo HSCT are expected to have hematopoietic reconstitution as they engraft. Hematologic recovery in those who undergo IST may take several months: 90% of patients who respond will do so by 3 months, but some patients may take up to 6 months from antithymocyte globulin to recover marrow function.
- Parameters of recovery
  - Improve overall hematopoiesis to reduce transfusion dependency and no longer fulfill criteria for sAA by 6 months. Neutrophil recovery may be the first cytopenia to improve.
  - Relapse or clonal evolution commonly occurs at 2 to 4 years from time of IST. Some centers recommend monitoring bone marrow aspirates with biopsy at 6-month intervals for 1st year after IST and then annually.

DIET

Recommend low bacterial content diet.

PATIENT EDUCATION

- NIH site: http://www.nhlbi.nih.gov/health/health-topics/topics/aplastic/
- Aplastic Anemia & MDS International Foundation: http://www.aamds.org/about/aplastic-anemia
- North American Pediatric Aplastic Anemia Consortium: http://www.napaac.org/

PROGNOSIS

- Aplastic anemia has a high rate of mortality if left untreated. Death is predominantly from infection and hemorrhage. If patients are treated with antibiotics and transfusions alone, mortality is 80% in 2 years.
- First line
  - MSD: HSCT with MSD from bone marrow source has a predicted 6-year outcome of 80–91% in children <20 years of age.
- Second line
  - IST: Response rate of IST in children is 75%.
- Relapse/salvage: Aplastic anemia refractory to IST at 6 months should be considered for salvage therapy: MUD-HSCT for younger patients; repeat IST for older patients and those with significant comorbidities.
- MUD: Recent trials have shown improved survival of >60% and as high as 94% in children who have undergone MUD-HSCT for sAA.
- Repeat IST: Patients refractory to the initial course of IST had a response rate of 30–40% at 6 months to antithymocyte globulin/CsA.

COMPLICATIONS

- Infection
- Hemorrhage
- Iron overload requiring phlebotomy or chelation therapy
- Allosensitization to transfusion products

ADDITIONAL READING

- Bacigalupo A, Passweg J. Diagnosis and treatment of acquired aplastic anemia. *Hematol Oncol Clin North Am*. 2009;23(2):159–170.
- Marsh JC, Ball SE, Cavenagh J, et al; for British Committee for Standards in Haematology. Guidelines for the diagnosis and management of aplastic anemia. *Br J Haematol*. 2009;147(1):43–70.
- Miano M, Dufour C. The diagnosis and treatment of aplastic anemia: a review. *Int J Hematol*. 2015;101(6):527–535.
- Niemeyer CM, Baumann I. Classification of childhood aplastic anemia and myelodysplastic syndrome. *Hematology Am Soc Hematol Educ Program*. 2011;2011:84–89.
- Scheinberg P, Nunez O, Weinstein B, et al. Horse versus rabbit antithymocyte globulin in acquired aplastic anemia. *N Engl J Med*. 2011;365(5):430–438.
- Scheinberg P, Young NS. How I treat acquired aplastic anemia. *Blood*. 2012;120(6):1185–1196.
- Shimamura A. Clinical approach to marrow failure. *Hematology Am Soc Hematol Educ Program*. 2009;1:329–337.
- Young NS, Scheinberg P, Calado RT. Aplastic anemia. *Curr Opin Hematol*. 2008;15(3):162–168.

CODES

ICD10

- D61.9 Aplastic anemia, unspecified
- D61.89 Oth aplastic anemias and other bone marrow failure syndromes
- D61.3 Idiopathic aplastic anemia

FAQ

- Q: When starting IST, should I choose hATG or rabbit ATG (rATG) as part of the antithymocyte globulin/cyclosporine/prednisone regimen?
- A: A head-to-head comparison of hATG versus rATG in immunosuppressive regimens showed inferiority of rATG in 1st-time treatment for sAA.
- Q: When should patient and family members be HLA typed when considering aplastic anemia?
- A: HLA typing should be performed on patient and family members once peripheral pancytopenia and bone marrow hypocellularity is confirmed.
- Q: What are common side effects of the IST regimen?
- A: Antithymocyte globulin may cause hypersensitivity reactions, whereas cyclosporine A may cause hypertension, electrolyte abnormalities, nephropathy, and hirsutism.

APPENDICITIS

Robert J. McLoughlin, MD • Michael P. Hirsh, MD, FACS, FAAP

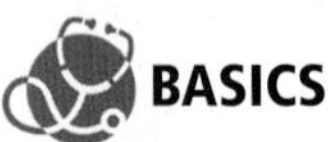

BASICS

DESCRIPTION

Acute inflammation or infection of the vermiform appendix

EPIDEMIOLOGY

- Most common surgical emergency of childhood
- Incidence rate (per 10,000 person-years):
  - 2 in 0- to 4-year olds
  - 10 in 5- to 9-year olds
  - 15 in 10- to 14-year olds
- 293,000 admissions in the United States in 2010
- 80,000 pediatric appendectomies per year in United States
- Most commonly seen in 2nd decade of life; <5% are aged 0 to 4 years old.
- Affects boys more commonly than girls

PATHOPHYSIOLOGY

- Acute inflammation of the appendiceal lumen is caused by obstruction (i.e., by a fecalith, calculi, parasites, hyperplastic lymphoid tissue, or tumor).
- Appendix is innervated by somatic afferent nerves of the 10th dermatome overlying the epigastrium and periumbilical areas.
- In the first phase of pain, occlusion causing increasing wall tension results in vague pain poorly referred to this area.
- Increasing wall tension and full-thickness serositis results in inflammation of surrounding tissues, and the second phase of pain is localized to the area in which the appendix is lying.
- In 85% of patients, this tenderness is located at McBurney point; however, pelvic, retrocecal, retroperitoneal, inguinoscrotal, or other orientations will result in variance of location and intensity of this pain.

COMMONLY ASSOCIATED CONDITIONS

Neonatal appendicitis is associated most commonly with prematurity, inguinal hernia, and Hirschsprung disease.

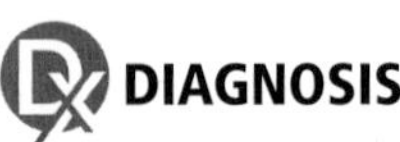

DIAGNOSIS

Classic signs and symptoms include right lower quadrant pain, anorexia, nausea and vomiting, and fever.

HISTORY

- Abdominal pain is most common symptom.
- Pain usually begins in the periumbilical or epigastric regions prior to migrating to the right lower quadrant. Pain is followed by nausea and vomiting with fever.
- Leukocytosis occurs later.
- Timing of pain preceding nausea and vomiting and absence of diarrhea in most cases are distinguishing factors from gastroenteritis.
- Anorexia is present in the majority of cases but may not be a prominent symptom if the appendix is retrocecal or retroperitoneal.
- Perforation of the inflamed appendix may result in temporary relief of pain. These patients can proceed to develop distension, dehydration, diarrhea from perirectal irritation, and dysuria from perivesicular irritation.
- Delayed diagnosis and perforation occur more frequently in young children, presumably because they are less able to articulate their symptoms.

PHYSICAL EXAM

- Low-grade fever is common unless perforation has already occurred.
- Perforation can result in worsened fever, tachypnea, and tachycardia.
- Pain and tenderness at McBurney point (1/3 the distance from the anterior superior iliac spine [ASIS] in a line from the umbilicus to the ASIS)
- Findings may include abdominal rebound tenderness, guarding, and focal tenderness on rectal exam.
- Other signs:
  - Rovsing sign: pain in the right lower quadrant with palpation in the left lower quadrant
  - Psoas sign: pain in the right lower quadrant with passive right hip extension and may be associated with a retrocecal appendix
  - Obturator sign: pain in right lower quadrant with right hip and knee flexion followed by internal rotation and may be associated with a pelvic appendix

DIFFERENTIAL DIAGNOSIS

- Infection
  - Gastroenteritis (e.g., *Yersinia*, *Campylobacter*)
  - Right lower lobe pneumonia
  - Mesenteric adenitis
  - Typhlitis
  - Urinary tract infection
  - Pelvic inflammatory disease, tubo-ovarian abscess, or ectopic pregnancy
  - Parasitic infection (*Trichuris trichiura*, *Ascaris lumbricoides*)
- Inflammatory processes
  - Inflammatory bowel disease
  - Anaphylactic purpura
  - Cholecystitis
  - Pancreatitis
  - Diverticulitis
- Genetic/metabolic
  - Diabetes
  - Sickle cell disease
  - Hypernatremia
- Miscellaneous
  - Constipation
  - Functional abdominal pain
  - Small bowel obstruction
  - Renal stones
  - Torsion of testes or ovaries
  - Ovarian cyst
  - Endometriosis
  - Mittelschmerz

DIAGNOSTIC TESTS & INTERPRETATION

Initial Tests (screening, lab, imaging)

- CBC, expect elevated WBC count (10,000 to 17,000 cells per μL range) with left shift
- Erythrocyte sedimentation rate is usually normal.
- C-reactive protein can be elevated but is nonspecific.
- Diagnosis can often be made with history, physical exam, and laboratory studies without imaging with a diagnostic accuracy of 80–90% in some studies.
- Abdominal radiograph
  - Often normal
  - May show fecalith, indistinct psoas margins, cecal wall thickening
  - Free air or pneumoperitoneum may indicate a perforation.
- Ultrasound
  - Currently considered the initial imaging study of choice for the diagnosis of appendicitis
  - Findings include edema, inflammation, or abscess formation.
  - Most specific finding is an appendiceal maximum outer diameter (MOD) of ≥7 mm (associated with a sensitivity of 98.7% and a specificity of 95.4% for the diagnosis).

- CT scan
  - Has a high diagnostic accuracy for appendicitis and may have a higher sensitivity than ultrasound; however, requires exposure to ionizing radiation and may be avoidable with careful history and physical exam, use of labs, and less invasive imaging
  - Findings include fat stranding, abscess or phlegmon, appendicolith when present, and focal cecal thickening.

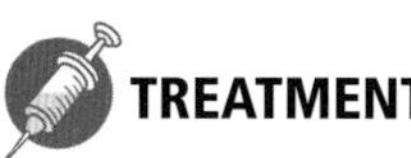

TREATMENT

GENERAL MEASURES

- IV fluids to correct hypovolemia, electrolyte abnormalities
- Broad-spectrum antibiotics (e.g., cefoxitin, piperacillin and tazobactam, or ceftriaxone and metronidazole)
- Pain medications

SURGERY/OTHER PROCEDURES

- Emergency appendectomy
  - Laparoscopic technique is now practiced by most surgeons in the United States.
  - It shows comparable results to open technique, allows wider exploration, and is associated with faster recovery in adults to daily activity.
  - Laparoscopic approaches now include single-port technology that limit the incision to the umbilical location.
- Given the relative risk and delay of care with CT prep, there is some evidence that immediate surgery may be preferential to radiologic investigation.
- Perforated appendicitis
  - Can also be treated via a laparoscopic approach and use of suction/irrigation devices to cleanse the abdomen of collections
  - In many patients with perforated appendicitis, nonoperative management with percutaneous abscess drainage and broad-spectrum antibiotics followed by interval appendectomy may be preferable.
  - Typical interval appendectomy performed 6 to 8 weeks after initial appendicitis
  - Does not appear to be different in initial laparoscopic appendectomy versus nonoperative management and interval appendectomy in terms of total hospitalization, recurrent abscess rate, or total cost
- Nonoperative management
  - Managed with broad-spectrum IV antibiotics, percutaneous drainage if perforated, and admission
  - Studies have suggested immediate and 30-day success rates of nonoperative management were 93% and 90%.
  - Presence of appendicolith associated with a 72% rate of recurrent appendicitis compared with a recurrence rate of 26% in those with no appendicolith
  - Associated with increased length of stay versus surgical management but with quicker return to school, less disability days

ONGOING CARE

PROGNOSIS

- Recovery is rapid.
- Prognosis is excellent.
- Overall current survival rate in United States is 98%.
- It is estimated that 35,000 people die yearly from appendicitis worldwide.

COMPLICATIONS

- Rate of wound complication postlaparoscopic appendectomy is 3.1%.
- Rate of abscess formation postappendectomy is 0–4% for nonperforated appendicitis and 14–20% for perforated appendicitis.
- Perforated appendicitis may result in greater risk of postoperative ileus and small bowel obstruction or fertility issues longer term.
- Complications associated with perforated appendicitis most profound in those aged <4 years

ADDITIONAL READING

- Amyand C. Of an inguinal rupture, with a pin in the appendix caeci, incrusted with stone, and some observations on wounds in the guts. *Phil Trans Royal Soc London*. 1735;39:329–342.
- Bansal S, Banever GT, Karrer FM, et al. Appendicitis in children less than 5 years old: influence of age on presentation and outcome. *Am J Surg*. 2012;204(6):1031–1035.
- Fitz RH. Perforating inflammation of the vermiform appendix: with special reference to its early diagnosis and treatment. *Trans Assoc Am Physicians*. 1886;1:107–144.
- Gasior AC, St Peter SD, Knott EM, et al. National trends in approach and outcomes with appendicitis in children. *J Pediatr Surg*. 2012;47(12):2264–2267.
- Lee SL, Islam S, Cassidy LD, et al. Antibiotics and appendicitis in the pediatric population: an American Pediatric Surgical Association Outcomes and Clinical Trials Committee Systematic Review. *J Pediatr Surg*. 2010;45(11):2181–2185.
- McBurney C. Experience with early operative interference in cases of disease of the vermiform appendix. *NY Med J*. 1889;50:676–684.
- Semm K. Die endoskopische appendektomie. *Gynakol Prax*. 1983;7:131–140.
- Trout AT, Sanchez R, Ladino-Torres MF, et al. A critical evaluation of US for the diagnosis of pediatric acute appendicitis in a real-life setting: how can we improve the diagnostic value of sonography? *Pediatr Radiol*. 2012;42(7):813–823.

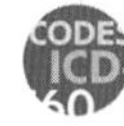

CODES

ICD10

- K37 Unspecified appendicitis
- K35.80 Unspecified acute appendicitis
- K35.89 Other acute appendicitis

FAQ

- Q: What were historical milestones in the treatment of appendicitis?
- A: Milestones include:
  - 1735: Dr. Claudius Amyand performed an appendectomy in a situation of an appendicitis within a right inguinal hernia. This condition is now referred to as Amyand hernia. The patient was an 11 year-old boy named Hanvil Anderson.
  - 1886: Dr. Reginald Heber Fitz first described what we recognize as appendicitis in his treatise "Perforating Inflammation of the Vermiform Appendix: With Special Reference to Its Early Diagnosis and Treatment."
  - 1887: Dr. Thomas Morton performed the first successful appendectomy under ether anesthesia.
  - 1889: Dr. Charles McBurney described the localization of pain from appendicitis.
  - 1980: Dr. Kurt Semm performed the first laparoscopic appendectomy.

ARTHRITIS, JUVENILE IDIOPATHIC (RHEUMATOID)

Elizabeth Candell Chalom, MD

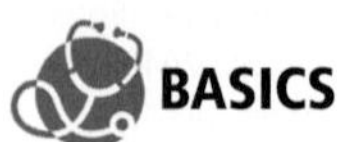

BASICS

DESCRIPTION

Juvenile idiopathic arthritis (JIA) is defined as chronic synovial inflammation of unknown etiology in at least one joint, for at least 6 weeks. Age of onset must be <16 years old. It is classified as one of seven subtypes:

- Oligoarticular arthritis affects <5 joints during the first 6 months of the disease. Tends to involve large joints, especially the knee. Peak age of onset is 1 to 6 years. Up to 80% are antinuclear antibody (ANA)-positive.
  - Persistent oligoarticular JIA remains in <5 joints after the 6th month of disease.
  - Extended oligoarticular JIA spreads to involve five or more joints (cumulatively) after the 6th month of disease; has worse prognosis than persistent oligoarthritis
- Polyarticular JIA affects ≥5 joints. Can occur at any age; peak ages of onset are 1 to 4 years and 7 to 10 years; divided into two subtypes
  - Rheumatoid factor–positive (RF+) polyarticular JIA is like adult-onset rheumatoid arthritis (RA) that occurs in a child; often quite aggressive
  - Rheumatoid factor–negative (RF−) polyarticular JIA is usually less aggressive and easier to control.
- Systemic-onset idiopathic juvenile arthritis
  - Characterized by high spiking, quotidian or diquotidian fevers and an evanescent pink/salmon-colored macular rash
  - Affected children may also have lymphadenopathy, hepatosplenomegaly, pericarditis, or pleuritis.
  - Arthritis may not appear until weeks to months after the onset of the systemic symptoms.
  - Can occur at any age
- Enthesitis-related arthritis (ERA)
  - Entheses (e.g., osteotendinous junctions, osteoligamentous junctions) are sites where tendons or ligaments attach to bone.
  - ERA generally affects boys in late childhood or adolescence.
  - Many are human leukocyte antigen-B27–positive.
- Psoriatic arthritis is associated with psoriasis. It often begins in a few joints and then becomes polyarticular. It often involves small joints of hands and feet, as well as knees. Dactylitis (inflammation of an entire digit with joint and tendon involvement) is seen in nearly 50% of patients.
- Undifferentiated arthritis is arthritis that does not fall into any of the other categories or falls into more than one of the above categories.

EPIDEMIOLOGY

Incidence

Incidence ranges from 1 to 23/100,000 per year.

Prevalence

- Prevalence ranges from 3.8 to 400/100,000; varies but is thought to be ~1/1,000
- Affects >100,000 children in the United States
- Girls are affected twice as often as boys, but boys are affected more frequently with ERA.
- ~50% of children with JIA have the oligoarticular type.
- 30% have the polyarticular type.
- 10% have systemic-onset JIA.

RISK FACTORS

Genetics

- Rare in siblings, but many studies have demonstrated increased frequencies of various human leukocyte antigen markers in JIA
- Each marker may be associated with a different subtype of JIA:
  - Human leukocyte antigen-DR4: RF+ polyarticular JIA
  - Human leukocyte antigen-DR1: oligoarticular disease without uveitis
  - Human leukocyte antigen-DR5: oligoarticular JIA with uveitis
  - Human leukocyte antigen-B27: ERA
  - Human leukocyte antigen-A2: early-onset oligoarticular JIA
- Etiology is multifactorial and likely differs between onset types. Other susceptibility loci in immune response genes, both adaptive and innate, have been reported. Environmental (including infectious) and hormonal factors can also play a role in pathogenesis.
- Activated T cells and macrophages produce synovitis.

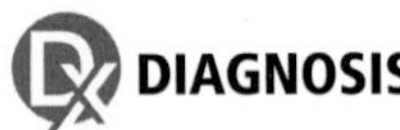

DIAGNOSIS

HISTORY

- Morning stiffness that improves after a warm shower/bath or with stretching and mild exercise is common in JIA. Many young children do not complain of pain but walk with a limp or refuse to walk down stairs in the morning.
- Joints often become sore/painful again in the late afternoon or evening.
- Patients with JIA generally do not complain of severe pain, but rather, they avoid using joints that are particularly affected.
  - If a child has severe pain in a joint, especially pain that seems out of proportion to the physical findings, diagnoses other than JIA should be entertained.
- In systemic JIA, the fever curve is important to document.
  - Between fever spikes, the child is often completely afebrile.
  - The rash is evanescent, and patients often have a history of fatigue, malaise, and weight loss.

PHYSICAL EXAM

- Arthritis must be present, not just arthralgias:
  - In addition to swelling, warmth, and tenderness, there may be restricted range of motion in the affected joints and soft tissue contractures.
- Enthesitis and sacroiliac tenderness are often seen in ERA.
- In systemic JIA, the rash, if present, is very suggestive of this disease.
- Lymphadenopathy and hepatosplenomegaly may be seen in systemic JIA.
- A careful cardiac and pulmonary examination must be done to assess for pericarditis and pleuritis.

ALERT

Arthritis must be present for at least 6 weeks before a patient can be diagnosed with JIA. Many viral illnesses can produce joint pain and swelling that mimics JIA but resolves within 4 to 6 weeks.

DIFFERENTIAL DIAGNOSIS

- Monoarticular JIA
  - Septic joint
  - Toxic synovitis
  - Trauma
  - Hemarthrosis
  - Villonodular synovitis
- Monoarticular or oligoarticular JIA
  - Lyme disease
  - Acute rheumatic fever or poststreptococcal arthritis
  - Viral/postviral arthritis
  - Malignancies
  - Sarcoidosis
  - Inflammatory bowel disease
- Polyarticular JIA
  - Viral or postviral illness (especially parvovirus)
  - Lyme disease
  - Lupus
- Systemic-onset JIA
  - Infection
  - Oncologic process (leukemia, lymphoma)
  - Inflammatory bowel disease
  - Lupus

DIAGNOSTIC TESTS & INTERPRETATION

Initial Tests (screening, lab, imaging)

- No laboratory finding is diagnostic for JIA.
- Many patients with JIA, especially the polyarticular and systemic types, have elevated sedimentation rates and anemia.
- ANA is a useful test in classifying patients with JIA and determining the risk of uveitis; positive in the following:
  - 80% of oligoarticular
  - 40–60% of polyarticular
  - 15–20% of normal population
- RF will be positive in 15–20% of patients with polyarticular arthritis and usually indicates a more aggressive form of arthritis.
- Radiography is often normal early in JIA.
- Later, if arthritis persists, bone demineralization, loss of articular cartilage, erosions, and joint fusion may be seen.

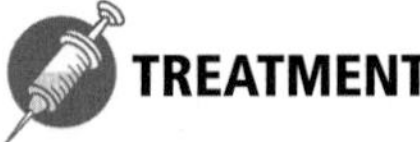

TREATMENT

GENERAL MEASURES

- Responses to treatments for JIA vary tremendously:
  - Some patients may respond to NSAIDs within 1 to 2 weeks. Others take 4 to 6 weeks to improve, and some may not respond at all.
  - Steroids usually start to relieve symptoms within a few days.
  - Methotrexate usually takes 4 to 8 weeks until a benefit is noted.
  - Biologic therapy can start decreasing symptoms in as little as a few days to 2 weeks or may take up to a few months to see the full benefit.
- The waxing and waning nature of JIA adds to the variability of response to treatment.

MEDICATION

First Line

- Steroids (glucocorticoids)
  - Intra-articular steroids are often used when patients have only one or two active joints.
  - Systemic steroids
    - Systemic steroids are often needed to control flares or with the initial presentation of polyarticular or systemic JIA. Because of the many side effects, patients should be weaned off steroids as soon as possible.
    - Glucocorticoids can be given orally (daily or every other day) or as IV pulses (every 1 to 8 weeks).
- NSAIDs
  - 1st-line therapy for mild JIA
  - If there is an inadequate response to the initial NSAID after 4 to 6 weeks, consider changing to another NSAID or adding a 2nd-line agent. Patients may respond differently to the various NSAIDs.
  - If arthritis remains active after 2 to 3 months, a 2nd-line treatment should be added.
- Disease-modifying antirheumatic drugs (DMARDs)
  - If NSAIDs are ineffective in controlling the disease, or the patient has moderate to severe arthritis, a DMARD, such as methotrexate or leflunomide, is often added.
  - Methotrexate
    - Methotrexate is the most common 2nd-line agent for active arthritis. It can be given orally or subcutaneously, once weekly.
    - Laboratory values must be monitored closely, looking for bone marrow suppression or elevation of transaminase levels. Nausea/vomiting are common adverse effects.
  - Leflunomide is often used when methotrexate is ineffective or patients cannot tolerate the nausea associated with methotrexate. It is a daily tablet and can also cause liver toxicity.
  - Both methotrexate and leflunomide cause mild immune suppression.
- Biologic agents
  - Biologic agents are often added when patients do not respond adequately to methotrexate, cannot tolerate its side effects, or have moderate to severe arthritis. All biologic agents suppress the immune system, and infections are the most common adverse effects.
    - Antitumor necrosis factor (anti-TNF) therapy is frequently used for moderate to severe polyarticular JIA.
      - Etanercept is a receptor for TNF, given SC once or twice a week.
      - Infliximab is a chimeric antibody to TNF, given IV every 4 to 8 weeks.
      - Adalimumab is a fully humanized antibody to TNF, given SC every other week.
    - Anti–IL-6 therapy (tocilizumab)
      - An IV medication given every 2 to 4 weeks
      - Approved for children with systemic-onset and polyarticular JIA
    - IL-1 inhibition is often used as a 1st-line agent, along with corticosteroids, in severe systemic JIA. It can also be used in patients with polyarticular JIA who do not respond to TNF inhibition.
      - Anakinra is a recombinant IL-1 receptor antagonist, given as a daily SC injection.
      - Canakinumab is a human monoclonal antibody against IL-1 β. It is given monthly as an SC injection.
    - Costimulation blocker: Abatacept blocks the interaction of CD28 on T cells with CD80 and CD86 receptors on antigen presenting cells.
      - IV is given at 2 and 4 weeks after first infusion and then every 4 weeks thereafter.
      - SC is given once weekly.
      - Approved as an SC or IV injection in children and adults
- Rituximab
  - An antibody to CD20, which is present on certain B cells
  - Approved for use in adult RA but not JIA
- Medications such as cyclophosphamide or thalidomide are sometimes necessary to control severe systemic-onset JIA when biologic treatments are ineffective.

ADDITIONAL THERAPIES

- Physical and occupational therapy are important in the management of JIA.
- The goal is to maintain range of motion, muscle strength, and function.

ONGOING CARE

PROGNOSIS

- Varies considerably
- Children with oligoarticular JIA usually fare well and often go into remission within a few years of starting treatment. They may have flares, however, even up to 10 years after being symptom-free and off all medications.
- Patients with polyarticular JIA who are RF+ often develop a severe arthritis that may persist into adulthood.
- RF− polyarticular patients generally fare better and may outgrow their disease.
- 50% of patients with systemic-onset JIA will develop severe chronic polyarticular arthritis.

COMPLICATIONS

- Joint degeneration with loss of articular cartilage
- Soft tissue contractures
- Leg length discrepancy
- Micrognathia
- Cervical spine dislocation
- Rheumatoid nodules
- Growth retardation
- Uveitis
  - Oligoarticular JIA, especially with a positive ANA test, is associated with chronic uveitis, which can lead to loss of vision if not detected early with routine slit-lamp eye examinations.
  - May be seen in polyarticular JIA but is less common
- Pericarditis, pleuritis, and severe anemia may develop in patients with systemic-onset JIA.
- Macrophage activation syndrome or hemophagocytic syndrome
  - Rare, but potentially lethal complication of systemic-onset JIA, resulting from an overproduction of inflammatory cytokines
  - May present as an acute febrile illness with pancytopenia and hepatosplenomegaly
  - Bone marrow aspiration can be diagnostic.
  - Treatment is often high-dose steroids and high-dose IL-1 inhibitors, or cyclosporine.

ADDITIONAL READING

- Andersson Gäre B. Juvenile arthritis—who gets it, where and when? A review of current data on incidence and prevalence. *Clin Exp Rheumatol*. 1999;17(3):367–374.
- Beukelman T, Patkar NM, Saag KG, et al. 2011 American College of Rheumatology Recommendations for the Treatment of Juvenile Idiopathic Arthritis: initiation and safety monitoring of therapeutic agents for the treatment of arthritis and systemic features. *Arthritis Care Res (Hoboken)*. 2011;63(4):465–482.
- Patel H, Goldstein D. Pediatric uveitis. *Pediatr Clin North Am*. 2003;50(1):125–136.
- Prakken B, Albani S, Martini A. Juvenile idiopathic arthritis. *Lancet*. 2011;377(9783):2138–2149.
- Ravelli A, Martini A. Juvenile idiopathic arthritis. *Lancet*. 2007;369(9563):767–778.
- Ringold S, Weiss PF, Beukelman T, et al. 2013 Update of the 2011 American College of Rheumatology recommendations for the treatment of juvenile idiopathic arthritis: recommendations for the medical therapy of children with systemic juvenile idiopathic arthritis and tuberculosis screening among children receiving biologic medications. *Arthritis Rheum*. 2013;65(10):2499–2512.
- Weiss J, Ilowite N. Juvenile idiopathic arthritis. *Pediatr Clin North Am*. 2005;52(2):413–442.

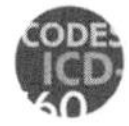

CODES

ICD10

- M08.80 Other juvenile arthritis, unspecified site
- M08.849 Other juvenile arthritis, unspecified hand
- M08.879 Other juvenile arthritis, unspecified ankle and foot

FAQ

- Q: Will the patient outgrow JIA?
- A: Prognosis depends on the type of JIA. In some studies, up to 50% of patients with JIA still had active disease 10 years after diagnosis, but only 15% had loss of function.
- Q: Will siblings of patients with JIA develop the disease?
- A: Rarely, but it can occur.

ASCARIS LUMBRICOIDES (ASCARIASIS)

Amaya L. Bustinduy, MD, MPH, PhD, FRCPCH

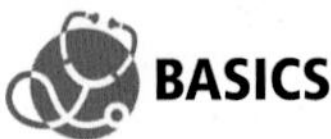

BASICS

DESCRIPTION

Ascaris lumbricoides is a large parasitic nematode (roundworm), 15 to 40 cm in length, which infects humans via eggs found in soil.

EPIDEMIOLOGY

- Geographic distribution: South America, sub-Saharan Africa, China, and East Asia
- All ages may be affected; however, children are more frequent hosts owing to oral behavior and tend to have a higher worm burden.
- Ascariasis is more common where sanitation is poor and population is dense.
- Eggs are viable in the soil for >6 years in temperate climates.
- It is the most prevalent helminth infection in the world.
- 800 million cases worldwide and estimated 400 million children infected
  - Around 51 million children suffer severe morbidity, mostly from moderate and heavy worm loads.

GENERAL PREVENTION

Infection control

- Sanitary disposal of human excrement, not using human feces as fertilizer, and hand washing has the potential to eliminate this infection.
- In communities with high transmission of *Ascaris*, community-wide mass drug delivery of anthelmintics is effective in controlling morbidity.

PATHOPHYSIOLOGY

- Fertilized eggs are ingested from soil contaminated with human feces.
- Larvae hatch in the small intestine and migrate to cecum and colon.
- Larvae invade the mucosa into the venous system and travel to the portal circulation, inferior vena cava, and finally, pulmonary capillaries.
- During migration through the pulmonary vessels, an eosinophilic response is evoked.
- Larvae penetrate the alveoli, are expelled by coughing, and swallowed back (days 10 to 14).
- Larvae become adult worms in the small intestine (day 24).
- Female worms excrete up to 200,000 eggs per day.
- Ingestion to excretion takes 2 to 3 months.
- Once in soil, fertilized eggs require 2 to 3 weeks of incubation in soil to become infectious and restart cycle.

ETIOLOGY

Children commonly acquire this infection from playing in dirt contaminated with *Ascaris* eggs.

COMMONLY ASSOCIATED CONDITIONS

This infection may be associated with other soil-transmitted helminths:

- Hookworm (*Necator americanus*, *Ancylostoma duodenale*)
- *Trichuris trichiura*
- *Strongyloides stercoralis*
- *Toxocara canis*

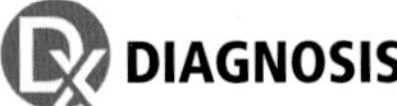

DIAGNOSIS

HISTORY

- Gastrointestinal symptoms include the following:
  - Abdominal distention
  - Pain
  - Nausea
  - Diarrhea
  - Decreased appetite
- In the chronic phase, ascariasis is associated with the following:
  - Growth stunting
  - Cognitive delays
- Severe respiratory symptoms during the pulmonary migratory stage, when larvae cause an inflammatory response (Löeffler syndrome), characterized by the following:
  - Dyspnea
  - Cough
  - Fever
  - Shifting pulmonary infiltrates
  - Eosinophilia
- Severe presentation during the intestinal phase, when symptoms are due to the presence of worms:
  - Pain
  - Obstruction (2 per 1,000)
  - Peritonitis from perforation
  - Biliary colic, hepatitis, or pancreatitis from blockages due to worms
- History of passage of large worms in the stool or vomitus is suggestive of ascariasis.
- History of wheezing may precede passage of worms by 2 to 3 months.

PHYSICAL EXAM

- Chest: may have rales or wheezing if *Ascaris* larvae are in the lungs
- Abdomen
  - Distended
  - Auscultate and palpate for signs of obstruction or perforation.

DIFFERENTIAL DIAGNOSIS

Ascariasis should be considered in the differential diagnosis when a patient presents with pneumonia, peripheral eosinophilia, and/or intestinal obstruction in returned traveler or resident from an endemic area.

DIAGNOSTIC TESTS & INTERPRETATION

Initial Tests (screening, lab, imaging)

- Microscopic examination of stool specimens will demonstrate the characteristic *Ascaris* eggs (round with thick shell).
- During the pulmonary phase, may have peripheral eosinophilia and larvae in sputum but negative stool examinations
- Serologic tests are unnecessary and are poorly specific to the diagnosis.
- Molecular diagnostics (PCR) are becoming more widely available and are more sensitive test particularly in low-prevalence areas.
- Chest radiograph, if cough is present, may demonstrate shifting pulmonary infiltrates.
- Abdominal imaging, if abdominal signs or symptoms of obstruction or perforation

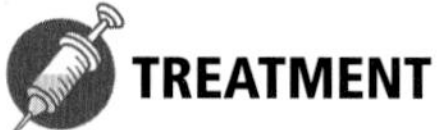

TREATMENT

MEDICATION

First Line

- Oral
  - Albendazole
    - 400 mg, single dose
    - The World Health Organization (WHO) recommends 200 mg single dose for children <1 year old.
  - Mebendazole
    - 100 mg, b.i.d. for 3 days or 500 mg once
  - Ivermectin
    - 150 to 200 mcg/kg, single dose
  - Nitazoxanide
    - 100 mg b.i.d. for 3 days (12 to 47 months of age)
    - 200 mg b.i.d. for 3 days (4 to 11 years of age)
    - 500 mg b.i.d. for 3 days (12 years and above)
- Alternatives (oral):
  - Pyrantel pamoate
    - 11 mg/kg to max 1 g per day for 3 days
  - Piperazine citrate
    - 75 mg/kg/24 h for 2 days; maximum, 3.5 g
    - Has been used historically for cases of intestinal obstruction (causes worm paralysis), but it is no longer available in the United States

SURGERY/OTHER PROCEDURES

Surgery or endoscopic retrograde cholangiopancreatography may be required for severe intestinal or biliary tract obstruction.

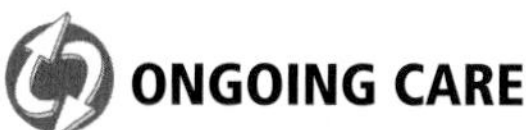

ONGOING CARE

FOLLOW-UP RECOMMENDATIONS

- Treatment is highly effective.
- Reexamination of stool specimens 2 weeks after therapy can be considered but is not essential.
- Reinfection is common in endemic areas and has led to mass drug administration programs.

Patient Monitoring

Warn parents about passage of worms in stool with treatment.

PROGNOSIS

- Once intestinal infection is detected and treated, the prognosis is excellent.
- If obstructive or respiratory complications have occurred, the prognosis is less favorable.
- The case fatality rate in cases with complications is up to 5%, most from obstruction.

COMPLICATIONS

- Bronchopneumonia may be seen during the pulmonary migrational stage, producing fever, cough, dyspnea, wheeze, eosinophilia, and pulmonary infiltrates (Löeffler syndrome).
- Heavy infestations may cause abdominal pain, malabsorption, and growth failure.
- Children may experience obstruction (ileocecal), malabsorption, or intussusception.
- Perforation or migration into the appendix, biliary, or pancreatic ducts may rarely occur.
- Hepatitis, acute cholecystitis, or pancreatitis can occur. Liver abscess can occur if intrahepatic ducts are obstructed.

ADDITIONAL READING

- American Academy of Pediatrics. *Ascaris lumbricoides* infections. In: Kimberlin DW, Brady MT, Jackson MA, et al, eds. *Red Book: 2015 Report of the Committee on Infectious Diseases*. Elk Grove Village, IL: American Academy of Pediatrics; 2015:247–248.
- Capello M, Hotez PJ. Intestinal nematodes. In: Long S, Pickering L, Prober C, eds. *Principles and Practice of Pediatric Infectious Diseases*. 4th ed. Churchill Livingstone/Elsevier; 2012:1326–1334.
- Centers for Disease Control and Prevention. Parasites—ascariasis. http://www.cdc.gov/parasites/ascariasis/. Accessed January 27, 2017.
- Dold C, Holland CV. *Ascaris* and ascariasis. *Microbes Infect*. 2011;13(7):632–637.
- Hall A, Hewitt G, Tuffrey V, et al. A review and meta-analysis of the impact of intestinal worms on child growth and nutrition. *Matern Child Nutr*. 2008;4(Suppl 1):118–236.
- Lamberton PH, Jourdan PM. Human ascariasis: diagnostics update. *Curr Trop Med Rep*. 2015;2(4):189–200.
- Mitchell PD, Yeh HY, Appleby J, et al. The intestinal parasites of King Richard III. *Lancet*. 2013;382(9895):888.
- O'Lorcain P, Holland CV. The public health importance of *Ascaris lumbricoides*. *Parasitology*. 2000;121(Suppl):S51–S71.
- World Health Organization. Intestinal worms. http://www.who.int/intestinal_worms/disease/en/. Accessed January 27, 2017.

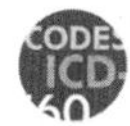

CODES

ICD10

- B77.9 Ascariasis, unspecified
- B77.0 Ascariasis with intestinal complications
- B77.81 Ascariasis pneumonia

FAQ

- Q: What are the long-term effects of untreated *Ascaris* infection in children?
- A: Growth stunting and cognitive delays are the most common long-term effects of untreated infections. Given the prevalence of this infection in the world, this is a major cause of morbidity in the world.
- Q: Which King of England, who was also the subject of a play by William Shakespeare, was infected with *A. lumbricoides*?
- A: In 2012, the remains of Richard III were excavated and identified in Leicester, England. Further analysis of sediment samples from the sacral area suggested evidence of roundworm eggs (*A. lumbricoides*) and intestinal roundworm infection.

ASCITES

Rima Fawaz, MD

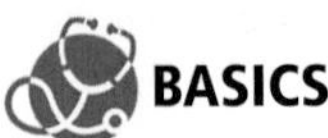

BASICS

DESCRIPTION

- Ascites is defined as a pathologic accumulation of intraperitoneal fluid.
- Peritoneal fluid formation is a dynamic process of production and absorption.
- In children, ascites is usually the result of liver or renal disease.
- In adults, ascites is most often due to portal hypertension from cirrhosis.
- Ascites is the most common of the three major complications of cirrhosis; the other two complications of cirrhosis are hepatic encephalopathy and variceal hemorrhage.

PATHOPHYSIOLOGY

- Normal circulation
  - Blood enters the liver from the hepatic artery and portal vein, perfuses the hepatic sinusoids, and exits the liver via the hepatic veins.
  - Hepatic lymph, formed by the filtration of sinusoidal plasma into the space of Disse, drains from the liver via the transdiaphragmatic lymphatic vessels to the thoracic duct.
  - Hepatic lymph is isosmotic to plasma, as the sinusoidal endothelium is highly permeable to albumin.
  - In the intestine, the mesenteric capillary membrane is impermeable to albumin. The osmotic gradient favors the return of interstitial fluid/lymph into the capillary.
  - Intestinal lymph from regional lymphatics combines with hepatic lymph in the thoracic duct.
- Portal hypertension
  - Ascitic fluid production is due to a net transfer of fluid that exceeds the drainage capacity of the lymphatics.
- Cirrhotic ascites results from three pathophysiologic process:
  - Portal hypertension
  - Vasodilation: mediated predominantly by nitric oxide
  - Hyperaldosteronism: Decreased effective volume sensed by the kidneys stimulates the renin-angiotensin-aldosterone system, leading to increased sympathetic activity and antidiuretic hormone secretion.
- Noncirrhotic ascites can be the result of the following:
  - Proteinaceous material produced by malignant cells or by inflammation of visceral and/or parietal peritoneum: peritoneal carcinomatosis, tuberculous ascites
  - Obstruction of lymphatic flow by mass, tumor, or external pressure
  - Impaired portal flow: right-sided heart failure, Budd-Chiari syndrome, portal venous malformations
  - Decreased effective arterial blood volume: heart failure
  - Decreased oncotic pressure/hypoalbuminemia: nephrotic syndrome, protein-losing enteropathy, severe malnutrition
  - Primary (congenital) abnormalities of the lymphatics, metabolic disorders (lysosomal storage diseases including sialidosis, Wolman disease, GM1 gangliosidosis, Gaucher disease, and Niemann-Pick type C)
  - Rupture of intra-abdominal viscus or peritoneal/mesenteric cyst, bowel perforation, ureteral rupture

ETIOLOGY

Accumulation of fluid occurs with the following:

- Inflammatory conditions (e.g., mesenteric adenitis, tuberculosis, pancreatitis, secondary to inflammation of visceral, and/or parietal peritoneum)
- Portal hypertension or obstruction of portal vein flow and/or lymphatic flow by mass, tumor, or external pressure; tumors of abdominal viscera, retroperitoneum, thorax, or mediastinum (often characterized by chylous ascites)
- Infectious processes: abscess, tuberculosis, *Chlamydia* infection, schistosomiasis
- Gastrointestinal: infarcted bowel/perforation, pancreatitis, ruptured pancreatic duct, parenchymal liver disease
- Gynecologic: ovarian tumors, torsion, or rupture
- Renal: nephrotic syndrome, obstructive uropathy, perforated urinary tract, peritoneal dialysis
- Cardiac: congestive heart failure (CHF), constrictive pericarditis, inferior vena cava web
- Neoplastic: lymphoma, neuroblastoma
- Miscellaneous: systemic lupus erythematous, eosinophilic ascites, chylous ascites, hypothyroidism, ventriculoperitoneal shunt

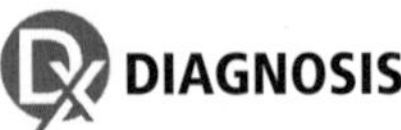

DIAGNOSIS

HISTORY

- Duration of symptoms
- Weight gain
- Respiratory distress
- Change in bowel habits or urinary color (evidence of GI bleeding)
- Use of umbilical catheters in newborn period (increased risk of portal vein thrombosis)
- History of chronic liver disease
- Exposure to hepatotoxins
- Concurrent illnesses (acute decompensation in hepatocellular function (e.g., massive bleeding, sepsis, superimposed infections)
- Developmental delay or growth failure suggestive of metabolic disease

PHYSICAL EXAM

- Vital signs:
  - Fever
  - Increased heart rate (reflecting increased cardiac output)
  - Lower blood pressure seen in cirrhotics
- General appearance: cachexia, icterus
- Auscultation of the pericardium: pericardial friction rub (pericarditis), cor pulmonale
- Abdominal exam
  - Protuberant abdomen
  - Bulging flanks
  - Fluid wave
  - Caput medusae
  - Umbilical hernia
  - Dullness to percussion
  - Shifting dullness
  - Peritoneal signs
  - Abdominal tenderness
  - Splenomegaly
- Neurologic exam: Signs of hepatic encephalopathy include irritability, somnolence, mood and behavior changes.
- Skin
  - Jaundice
  - Spider angioma
  - Palmar erythema
  - Scratch marks
  - Striae
  - Xanthomas
- Extremities
  - Clubbing
  - Edema

DIFFERENTIAL DIAGNOSIS

- Organomegaly: enlarged liver or spleen
- Mesenteric cyst or ovarian cyst: does not have shifting dullness when position is changed
- Bowel obstruction
- Cancer
- Heart failure
- Nephrotic syndrome

DIAGNOSTIC TESTS & INTERPRETATION

- Complete blood count
- Electrolytes
- Liver tests: transaminases, prothrombin time/international normalized ratio, total protein, albumin, total and fractionated bilirubin
- Amylase and lipase (to exclude pancreatitis)
- Creatinine and blood urea nitrogen
- Fluid cultures: blood, urine, ascitic fluid
- Urinalysis
- Specific testing for etiologies of ascites from chronic liver disease and other causes as deemed appropriate
- Ultrasound of the abdomen with Doppler study
  - Best study for differentiating between free and loculated fluid collection and the presence of intra-abdominal masses
  - Can be used to evaluate patency of hepatic and portal vasculature and directionality of flow
- Plain radiography (centralized bowel loops)
- Abdominal computed axial tomography
- Abdominal magnetic resonance imaging
- Abdominal paracentesis
  - Ascitic fluid analysis is essential and should include:
    - Cell count and differential
    - Albumin, total protein
    - Culture, Gram stain
    - Glucose (will be low in infection)
    - Lactate dehydrogenase concentration (will be high in infection, bowel perforation, or tumor)
    - Other optional tests include amylase (high in perforated viscus or pancreatitis), triglycerides (high in chylous ascites), and cytology (peritoneal carcinomatosis).
  - Serum to ascites albumin gradient (SAAG)
    - (Serum albumin) – (ascites albumin)
    - Blood and ascitic fluid analysis should be obtained on same day.
    - SAAG $\geq$1.1 g/dL suggests presence of portal hypertension.
    - If SAAG $<$1.1 g/dL, suspect other causes.

ALERT
- Ultrasonography should be the initial diagnostic imaging of choice for evaluation of ascites.
- With congenital ascites, evaluate for lysosomal storage diseases.
- Diagnostic paracentesis is crucial in the evaluation of new-onset ascites.
- Calculate SAAG to differentiate between portal hypertension and other causes.
- In patients with liver disease and new-onset ascites, evaluate for etiologies to explain acute decompensation.

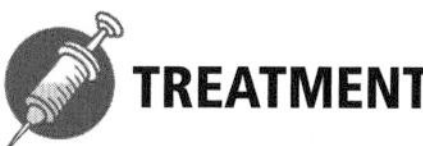

TREATMENT

GENERAL MEASURES
- The management of the ascites should be directed toward the underlying etiology.
- Benefits of treatment of ascites should always be weighed against risks and complications of treatment.
- Mobilization of cirrhotic ascitic fluid is best accomplished by creating a negative sodium balance and then maintaining the balance.
- In patients with cirrhosis, causes of decompensation should be sought, such as sodium and fluid overload, infection, esophageal hemorrhage, spontaneous bacterial peritonitis (SBP).
- In adults, dietary sodium intake is restricted to 44 to 88 mEq (1 to 2 g/24 h) or approximately 17 to 35 mEq (0.4 to 0.8 g) per thousand calories.
- In pediatrics, restricting dietary sodium intake should be balanced against palatability of food and nutritional needs: diet with no extra salt to a maximum 2 mEq/kg/24 h. Water is only restricted in patients with profound hyponatremia (<125 mEq/L): 50–75% of maintenance requirements.
- Attention to unintentional sodium intake from IV fluids in hospitalized patients

MEDICATIONS
- Goal of diuretic therapy is negative fluid balance limited to 10 mL/kg daily until ascites is resolved.
- Spironolactone (PO)
  - Most effective single diuretic; counteracts the hyperaldosteronism present in cirrhotic ascites
  - Acts on the distal collecting system; inhibits reabsorption of 2% of filtered sodium
  - Bioactive metabolites have long half-lives, hence, need >5 days to achieve steady state.
  - Start at 2 to 3 mg/kg/24 h as a single morning dose (max 100 mg initial dose). In adults, typical starting dose is up to 100 mg/24 h and can be increased to max 400 mg/24 h; in pediatrics, max dose 6 mg/kg/24 h
  - Most effective in combination with furosemide given at same time
  - Adverse effects: azotemia, hyperkalemia, and volume contraction
- Adequacy of spironolactone therapy can be monitored with urinary sodium excretion (desired >50 mEq/L). If no response, furosemide is added.
- Furosemide (PO)
  - Loop diuretic: can increase sodium excretion by 30%
  - Start at 1 mg/kg/24 h (max initial dose 40 mg), may increase every few days if needed.
  - Adults maintain ratio of 100 mg of spironolactone to 40 mg of furosemide to maintain eukalemia (max 400 mg spironolactone to 160 mg of furosemide daily).
  - Adverse effects: hypokalemia, ototoxicity, nephrocalcinosis
- When diuretics are used, urine output and serum electrolytes should be closely monitored to prevent prerenal azotemia and decreased effective blood flow to the kidneys.
- Albumin: Supplementation may aid fluid mobilization if albumin is <2.5 g/dL (use 1 g/kg of 25% albumin until level >2.5 g/dL).

SURGERY/OTHER PROCEDURES
Diuretic-refractory ascites derives from a lack of response to dietary sodium restriction and maximal diuretic therapy. Treatment options are the following:
- Therapeutic paracentesis
  - Therapeutic abdominal paracentesis (large-volume paracentesis); used in adults with refractory ascites
  - In children, therapeutic abdominal paracentesis is used to relieve respiratory distress or other sequelae of rapidly increasing intra-abdominal pressure.
  - Paracentesis of volumes >1 L should be accompanied by IV infusion of 25% albumin during the procedure.
- Transjugular intrahepatic portosystemic shunting (TIPS) may be valuable in cases where portal hypertension is felt to be the underlying etiology of ascitic accumulation.
- Orthotopic liver transplantation is the only curative therapy for refractory ascites from liver disease and the only definitive treatment that has been shown to improve survival.

ONGOING CARE

PROGNOSIS
- Development of ascites in the setting of cirrhosis is a landmark in the natural history of cirrhosis: 15% of adult patients succumb in 1 year and 44% in 5 years.
- Liver transplantation dramatically improves survival.
- Prognosis depends on etiology of ascites: nephrotic syndrome (ascites will regress as proteinuria clears), infection, hepatic decompensation (prognosis improves if able to reverse cause of liver injury).

COMPLICATIONS
- SBP
  - Spontaneous ascitic fluid infection: Infection of the peritoneal fluid may occur in the absence of secondary cause (e.g., bowel perforation or intra-abdominal abscess).
  - Fever, irritability, abdominal tenderness, and distention are common signs; vomiting and diarrhea may occur.
  - Abdominal paracentesis must be performed and ascitic fluid must be analyzed before a confident diagnosis of ascitic fluid infection can be made. The blood culture bottle should be injected with peritoneal fluid at the bedside in order to increase the culture yield.
  - Diagnosis: ascitic fluid absolute polymorphonuclear leukocytes ≥250 cells/mm^3 without evidence of an intra-abdominal process
  - Bacterial organisms commonly identified are the following: *Streptococcus pneumoniae*, *Escherichia coli*, *Klebsiella pneumoniae*, enterococci, and *Haemophilus influenzae*.
  - Broad-spectrum antibiotics with gram-negative coverage such as 3rd-generation cephalosporin can be used until identification of bacterial pathogen allows narrower coverage.
  - Prophylaxis for recurrent SBP has been recommended in certain situations.
- Other complications:
  - Respiratory distress from decreased lung volume and diaphragmatic limitation
  - Hepatic hydrothorax (large symptomatic pleural effusion that occurs in a cirrhotic patient in the absence of primary cardiopulmonary disease)
  - Abdominal wall hernias with rupture
  - Tense ascites with leakage (especially after paracentesis)
  - Conservative management consists of appropriate initial therapy for most of these except hernia rupture, which requires surgical reduction.

ADDITIONAL READING

- European Association for the Study of the Liver. EASL clinical practice guideline on the management of ascites, spontaneous bacterial peritonitis, and hepatorenal syndrome in cirrhosis. *J Hepatol*. 2010;53(3):397–417.
- Giefer MJ, Murray KF, Colleti RB. Pathophysiology, diagnosis, and management of pediatric ascites. *J Pediatr Gastroenterol Nutr*. 2011;52(5):503–513.
- Hou W, Sanyal AJ. Ascites: diagnosis and management. *Med Clin North Am*. 2009;93(4):801–817.
- Lane ER, Hsu EK, Murray KF. Management of ascites in children. *Expert Rev Gastroenterol Hepatol*. 2015;9(10):1281–1292.
- Runyon BA; for American Association for the Study of Liver Diseases Practice Guidelines Committee. Management of adult patients with ascites due to cirrhosis: an update. *Hepatology*. 2009;49(6):2087–2107.

CODES

ICD10
- R18.8 Other ascites
- R18.0 Malignant ascites
- A18.31 Tuberculous peritonitis

FAQ
- Q: What etiologies are likely in cases of congenital ascites?
- A: Lysosomal storage disorders and/or other metabolic diseases should be excluded. If hepatic function is impaired, causes of neonatal liver failure should also be investigated.
- Q: What is the best test to discriminate the type of ascites?
- A: Analysis of the peritoneal fluid collected by abdominal paracentesis is required for this purpose. The SAAG is helpful to discriminate ascites due to portal hypertension from other etiologies.
- Q: Where does the word "ascites" come from?
- A: It is thought that the word ascites is derived from the Greek word "askos" which refers to a container of wine or a wineskin.

ASPERGILLOSIS

Rebecca Schein, MD

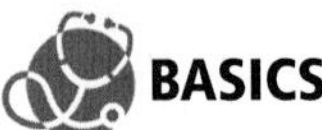

BASICS

DESCRIPTION

Aspergillosis is an infection caused by species of the mold *Aspergillus*. Invasive, allergic or chronic (saprophytic) disease occurs based on the immune status of the host.

- Invasive disease is seen mainly in immunocompromised patients and primarily involves the lungs, sinuses, central nervous system (CNS), or skin; rarely, endocarditis, osteomyelitis, eye/orbital disease, esophagitis, or peritonitis occurs.
- Children with asthma or cystic fibrosis may develop allergic bronchopulmonary aspergillosis (ABPA) due to a hypersensitivity reaction.
- Aspergillomas are fungal balls that grow primarily in the bronchi or lungs causing a chronic, noninvasive disease.

EPIDEMIOLOGY

- *Aspergillus* species are common, ubiquitous molds that grow on decaying vegetation and can be found in soil, plants, household dust, building material, animal droppings, and water.
- The primary route of transmission is the inhalation of aerosolized conidia or spores.
- Spores are aerosolized when soil is disturbed due to construction or gardening. Aerosolization can occur via water or ventilation systems and may result in nosocomial infections.
- Person-to-person spread does not occur.
- The incubation period is unknown.
- Risk of aspergillosis varies by the population studied.
  - ABPA occurs in 1–15% of patients with cystic fibrosis and 2.5% of adults with asthma.
  - Invasive disease is fairly rare and primarily occurs in stem cell and solid organ transplant patients.

RISK FACTORS

- Invasive aspergillosis occurs primarily in immunocompromised patients with prolonged neutropenia due to chemotherapy, chronic steroids or impaired phagocyte function (i.e., chronic granulomatous disease), hematologic malignancies, stem cell or solid organ transplant.
- ABPA is seen in patients with cystic fibrosis or asthma. Allergic sinusitis may be seen in children with nasal polyps or after sinus surgery.
- Aspergillomas occur in children with underlying lung disease like cystic fibrosis or tuberculosis.

GENERAL PREVENTION

- Hospitalized allogenic hematopoietic stem cell transplant (HSCT) patients and other high-risk immunocompromised patients like those undergoing induction chemotherapy should be placed in a protective environment.
- A protective environment should minimally be a private room isolated from construction and fresh plants. High-efficiency particulate air filtration, positive pressure, and frequent air exchanges are recommended.
- High-risk persons should avoid gardening, composting, and exposure to construction or renovation.
- As nosocomial outbreaks occur, hospitals should perform surveillance with environmental cultures as needed.

PATHOPHYSIOLOGY

Invasive aspergillosis usually occurs when airborne spores are inhaled but not effectively cleared by alveolar macrophages and occasionally by direct invasion through damaged skin.

- Invasion of blood vessels by *Aspergillus* leads to infarction, necrosis, and hematogenous dissemination.
- Progression to disease depends largely on its ability to evade host defenses.
- Macrophages and neutrophils can typically eliminate *Aspergillus* without difficulty, explaining its rarity in normal hosts.

ETIOLOGY

Most human disease is caused by *Aspergillus fumigatus*. Several other species including *Aspergillus flavus*, *Aspergillus terreus*, *Aspergillus versicolor*, *Aspergillus niger*, and *Aspergillus nidulan* are capable of causing disease.

- Invasive aspergillosis is typically a bilateral pulmonary infection and can disseminate to the sinuses, brain, or skin. Rarer presentations include endocarditis, meningitis, osteomyelitis, esophagitis, hepatitis, peritonitis, renal or eye infections.
- Sinusitis may be acute invasive disease characterized fungal balls in the maxillary sinuses or a hypersensitivity reaction resulting in allergic fungal rhinosinusitis (AFRS).
- Cutaneous infection typically follows trauma.
- Chronic pulmonary aspergillosis may be cavitary with fungal balls or fibrotic.
- Aspergilloma are saprophytic fungus balls that grow in preexisting lung cavities due to chronic lung disease.
- ABPA is an IgE-mediated hypersensitivity response to inhaled spores.

COMMONLY ASSOCIATED CONDITIONS

- Hematologic malignancy
- HSCT and solid organ transplant
- Chronic granulomatous disease
- Asthma
- Cystic fibrosis

DIAGNOSIS

HISTORY

- Pulmonary and invasive disease typically presents with a high fever, dry cough, and chest pain. Shortness of breath and hemoptysis can occur.
- Sinusitis causes facial pain or swelling, ear pain, and drainage. Nasal polyps are common with allergic disease.
- CNS disease presents with headache, nausea and vomiting. Altered mentation, hemiparesis, and cranial nerve palsies are rare.
- Cutaneous disease is seen in burn victims, neonates, and after skin injury in patients with solid organ transplantation.
- Chronic aspergillosis presents with >3 months of respiratory symptoms, fatigue, and weight loss.
- Aspergillomas are often asymptomatic but many cause a persistent productive cough, hemoptysis, and weight loss.
- ABPA presents as asthma symptoms including wheezing and a productive cough with brown sputum.
- Otomycosis is a chronic otitis externa that causes ear pain, drainage, pruritus, and hearing loss.

PHYSICAL EXAM

- Lung disease is often indistinguishable from other causes of pneumonia on physical examination. Fever, tachypnea, rales, hypoxemia, and hemoptysis. Patients with severe immune compromise may appear progressively sicker without focal findings.
- Sinusitis disease causes pallor of the nasal mucosa, nasal obstruction, polyps, mucosal crusting or ulceration, or blackened areas of necrosis.
- CNS disease is typically a brain abscess and may have findings of increased intracranial pressure.
- Cutaneous disease begins as red raised lesions that progress to purple, then black, and then ulcerates. Progressive necrosis may be present.
- ABPA findings include wheezing, pulmonary infiltrates, bronchiectasis, and fibrosis.

DIFFERENTIAL DIAGNOSIS

- Bacterial infections: *Nocardia*, *Streptococcus pneumoniae*, and *Staphylococcus aureus* with abscess or cavitary lesions; tuberculosis and atypical mycobacterial infections
- Sinus: *Mucor* or *Rhizopus*
- Cutaneous lesions: *Pseudomonas* or *Candida*

DIAGNOSTIC TESTS & INTERPRETATION

Initial tests (screening, lab, imaging)

- Proven invasive *Aspergillus* is diagnosed by histopathologic or cytologic staining of tissue or growth in culture. *Aspergillus* may be isolated from blood, cerebrospinal fluid, sputum, urine, bronchoalveolar lavage (BAL) fluid, and tissue biopsy specimens.
- A CT scan should be performed when there is a clinical suspicion of invasive pulmonary disease regardless of chest x-ray findings.
  - Pulmonary disease: Classic CT findings of "halo sign" (an area of low attenuation surrounding a nodule) initially and later the "crescent sign" (an air crescent near the periphery of a lung nodule, caused by contraction of infarcted tissue) are seen infrequently in children but may be present in adolescents.
- BAL is recommended in all patients with concern for invasive pulmonary aspergillosis.
- Diagnosis is often difficult especially in patients with severe immune dysfunction.

ALERT

Evaluation for *Aspergillus* should be performed in immunocompromised patients with persistent fever.

- Galactomannan is an *Aspergillus* cell wall polysaccharide that can be detected from serum or BAL fluid and used to diagnose infection in high-risk patients.
  - Recommended to assist in diagnosis in patients with hematologic malignancies or HSCT
  - BAL specimens (not serum) may be used for screening in patients on antifungal prophylaxis.
  - Not useful in patients with chronic granulomatous disease or solid organ transplant
  - False-positive tests do occur most notably in patients on piperacillin-tazobactam.
- β-D glucan detected in the serum of patients with hematologic malignancies or HSCT is suggestive of disseminated fungal infection but not specific for aspergillosis.

- *Aspergillus* nucleic acid testing is available; however, there is currently no consensus recommendation on how this test should be used or interpreted.
- Chronic cavitary pulmonary aspergillosis:
  - >3 months of pulmonary symptoms, chronic illness, or progressive radiographic abnormalities
  - Positive *Aspergillus* IgG antibody
  - No evidence of immune compromise
- ABPA:
  - Elevated *Aspergillus* specific IgE
  - Supported by elevated total IgE >1,000 ng/mL, *Aspergillus* IgG, total eosinophil count >500 cells/microliter, and positive skin testing for *Aspergillus*

Follow-up Tests & Special Considerations

- Serial monitoring of serum galactomannan may be used to monitor therapeutic response in patients with hematologic malignancies or HSCT.
- Susceptibility testing should be performed only if there is failure to respond to initial therapy or recent treatment that would suggest the development of resistance.
- *Aspergillus* species are very common in the environment and growth from sputum and nasal specimens may represent colonization in the immunocompetent host. The entire clinical picture should be considered when interpreting culture results.

Test Interpretation

- *Aspergillus* species are septate hyphae that branch at 45-degree angles detected with potassium hydroxide or silver staining of biopsy specimens.
- In high-risk patients, 50–65% of with positive cultures have invasive disease, whereas only 8–28% of low-risk patients have invasive aspergillosis.

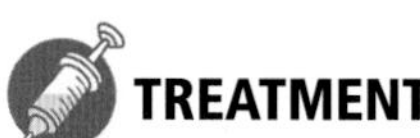

TREATMENT

GENERAL MEASURES

- Pediatric patients with prolonged neutropenia at risk for invasive aspergillosis should receive prophylaxis with voriconazole or micafungin. Posaconazole, which is approved for use in children >13 years of age, is the 1st-line drug for prophylaxis in adults.
- Patients with graft versus host disease and those who recently underwent lung transplant should also receive prophylaxis.
- Other solid organ transplant patients should be assessed on an individual basis regarding the need for prophylaxis.
- Aspergillosis in a normal host often does not require antifungal therapy.

MEDICATION

First Line

Voriconazole is primary therapy for invasive and chronic pulmonary aspergillosis.

- Voriconazole dosing is based on weight.
  - Children <50 kg
    - 9 mg/kg IV every 12 hours for 2 loading doses
    - 8 mg/kg IV or 9 mg/kg orally every 12 hours for maintenance
  - Children >50 kg dose as adults
    - 6 mg/kg IV every 12 hours for 2 loading doses
    - 4 mg/kg IV or 200 mg orally every 12 hours for maintenance
- Therapeutic drug monitoring should be performed because of variability between patients with a goal trough level of 1.5 to 6 mcg/mL.
- Voriconazole while generally well tolerated can cause nausea, vomiting, visual changes, skin rash, fever, and chills as well as drug–drug interactions. Patients should be monitored while on therapy.
- Treatment is typically 6 to 12 weeks and may be longer depending on the clinical presentation.
- Patients with ongoing immune compromise are often continued on prophylaxis.

Second Line

- For invasive aspergillosis is liposomal amphotericin B.
- Salvage therapy for invasive aspergillosis includes the lipid-based amphotericin B, micafungin, caspofungin, and posaconazole.
- Isavuconazole is used for salvage therapy in adults but is not approved for use in children.

ADDITIONAL THERAPIES

ABPA is treated primarily with corticosteroids. Itraconazole is often used in combination therapy.

SURGERY/OTHER PROCEDURES

Surgical excision or localized debridement, in addition to antifungal medication, may be required for invasive disease. Mortality may be improved with surgical excision of lung lesions, but the procedure itself is often risky.

- Aspergilloma is treated with surgical excision and antifungals may be used as 2nd-line therapy.
- AFRS is treated with polypectomy and sinus washout.

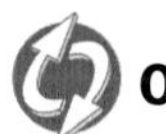

ONGOING CARE

FOLLOW-UP RECOMMENDATIONS

Patient Monitoring

- Pulmonary aspergillosis should have a repeat chest CT scan 2 weeks into therapy to assess the response to treatment.
- Other follow-up imaging should be based on clinical presentation and the response to treatment.
- Antifungal therapy typically requires monitoring.

PROGNOSIS

- Noninvasive disease in the normal host usually resolves but may take several weeks.
- ABPA has variable outcomes. Resolution, steroid dependence, and ongoing lung destruction due to inflammatory dysregulation are all possible.
- Immunosuppressed or neutropenic patients may have rapid extension or dissemination of disease; prognosis is often very poor. Early recognition and aggressive treatment and debridement are necessary.

COMPLICATIONS

- Progression to invasive disseminated disease can occur as the initial manifestation if host factors are altered. Involvement of CNS, heart, or bones worsen prognosis.
- Otitis and sinusitis can erode through cranial bones to involve the orbits or CNS.
- Pulmonary disease can progress to pulmonary hemorrhage, respiratory failure, or pneumothorax.

ADDITIONAL READING

- Burgos A, Zaoutis TE, Dvorak CC, et al. Pediatric invasive aspergillosis: a multicenter retrospective analysis of 139 contemporary cases. *Pediatrics*. 2008;121(5):e1286–e1294.
- Choi SH, Kang ES, Eo H, et al. *Aspergillus* galactomannan antigen assay and invasive aspergillosis in pediatric cancer patients and hematopoietic stem cell transplant recipients. *Pediatr Blood Cancer*. 2013;60(2):316–322.
- Pascual A, Calandra T, Bolay S, et al. Voriconazole therapeutic drug monitoring in patients with invasive mycoses improves efficacy and safety outcomes. *Clin Infect Dis*. 2008;46(2):201–211.
- Patterson TF, Thompson GR III, Denning DW, et al. Practice guidelines for the diagnosis and management of aspergillosis: 2016 update by the Infectious Diseases Society of America. *Clin Infect Dis*. 2016;63(4):e1–e60.
- Schubert MS. Allergic fungal sinusitis: pathophysiology, diagnosis and management. *Med Mycol*. 2009;47(Suppl 1):S324–S330.
- Segal BH. Aspergillosis. *N Engl J Med*. 2009;360(18):1870–1874.
- Stevens DA, Melikian GL. Aspergillosis in the "nonimmunocompromised" host. *Immunol Invest*. 2011;40(7–8):751–766.

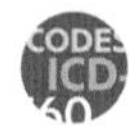

CODES

ICD10

- B44.9 Aspergillosis, unspecified
- B44.1 Other pulmonary aspergillosis
- B44.81 Allergic bronchopulmonary aspergillosis

FAQ

- Q: Does *Aspergillus* grown a respiratory culture from a healthy child require treatment?
- A: No. *Aspergillus* is common in the environment and colonization may occur. Healthy, asymptomatic children do not require treatment.
- Q: Who is at risk for ABPA and when should I consider this diagnosis?
- A: ABPA is primarily seen in children with asthma or cystic fibrosis. Children with cystic fibrosis are screened regularly for *Aspergillus*. A child with asthma that is not responding to treatment and has worsening pulmonary function testing should be evaluated for ABPA.
- Q: Who requires prophylaxis for invasive aspergillosis?
- A: Children with prolonged neutropenia, lung transplant within the last 4 months, and chronic granulomatous disease. Other high-risk children may require prophylaxis on a case by case basis.

ASPLENIA/HYPOSPLENIA

Joseph A. Picoraro, MD • Sarah S. Lusman, MD, PhD

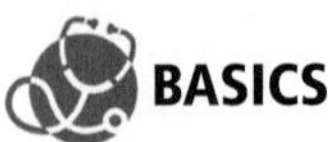

BASICS

DESCRIPTION

- Asplenia is the absence of the spleen due to either a congenital anomaly or a surgical procedure.
- Hyposplenia is the reduced or absent function of the spleen, impairing the capacity to prevent bacterial infections.

EPIDEMIOLOGY

- The exact incidence is not known.
- Asplenia is present in about 3% of neonates with structural heart disease.
- Isolated asplenia is most often recognized at autopsy.

PATHOPHYSIOLOGY

- The spleen is a major component of the reticuloendothelial system; it is important both for antibody synthesis and for clearance of opsonized organisms by phagocytosis.
- Antibody-mediated phagocytosis is the primary mechanism to destroy encapsulated microbes, such as pneumococcus, meningococcus, and *Haemophilus*.
- In the absence of the spleen's phagocytic pathway, the polysaccharide-rich capsules of these bacteria protect them from destruction and permit them to effect systemic bacterial infection that may lead to overwhelming sepsis.
- For patients $<$4 years of age in whom few alternate routes of bacterial clearance exist, significant pathology can result from impaired splenic function.

ETIOLOGY

- Surgical splenectomy
- Congenital asplenia
- In association with certain diseases or conditions (see "Differential Diagnosis")

COMMONLY ASSOCIATED CONDITIONS

- Besides splenectomy, when asplenia is known, patients with certain diseases are at risk of asplenia or hyposplenia (see "Differential Diagnosis").
- Asplenia or hyposplenia should be suspected in any patient with overwhelming infection with an encapsulated organism.

DIAGNOSIS

HISTORY

- Any patient with a condition known to be associated with asplenia/hyposplenia (see "Differential Diagnosis") deserves evaluation for splenic function.
- In the apparently healthy child with no identified risk factors who presents with an overwhelming infection with an encapsulated organism, a blood smear should be examined for signs of hyposplenism (see "Initial Tests (screening, lab, imaging)").

PHYSICAL EXAM

- The spleen may be normal, large, or nonpalpable. Therefore, the size of the spleen cannot be used as an indicator of splenic function.
- The size is most closely linked to the underlying etiology.
  - Portal hypertension or complete splenic replacement by cysts, neoplasm, or amyloid can lead to splenomegaly.
  - Sequestration crises such as those associated with sickle cell disease and malaria clog the spleen with cellular debris, which may also result in increased spleen size.
  - Patients with sickle cell disease typically have splenomegaly early in life, as the spleen tends to sequester the abnormal red cells. With time, the spleen slowly autoinfarcts and eventually becomes nonpalpable.

DIFFERENTIAL DIAGNOSIS

Diminished splenic function is associated with the following:

- Congenital
  - Isolated congenital asplenia
  - Heterotaxy syndrome
- Hematologic
  - Sequestration crises (e.g., sickle hemoglobinopathies, essential thrombocytosis, malaria)
  - Sickle cell disease
  - Hereditary hemoglobinopathies
- Autoimmune
  - Glomerulonephritis
  - Systemic lupus erythematosus
  - Rheumatoid arthritis
  - Sarcoidosis
  - Sjögren syndrome
  - Graves disease
  - Graft-versus-host disease
- GI/hepatic
  - Celiac disease
  - Inflammatory bowel disease
  - Chronic liver disease/portal hypertension
- Space-occupying lesions
  - Tumors, such as lymphoma
  - Amyloidosis
  - Cysts
- Postsplenectomy
  - Trauma
  - β-Thalassemia
  - Hereditary spherocytosis
- Vascular
  - Splenic artery occlusion
  - Splenic vein thrombosis
- Miscellaneous
  - Normal infants
  - Elderly
  - Bone marrow transplant
  - HIV infection
- Splenic irradiation

DIAGNOSTIC TESTS & INTERPRETATION

Initial Tests (screening, lab, imaging)

- The reduction or absence of splenic function can be determined by specific hematologic changes detectable on a blood smear.
  - The spleen normally removes intercellular debris such as Howell-Jolly bodies (nuclear remnants), Heinz bodies (denatured hemoglobin), and Pappenheimer bodies (iron granules).
  - Findings of target cells (red cells with a bull's eye center due to excessive membrane relative to the amount of iron and hemoglobin), Howell-Jolly bodies, Heinz bodies, Pappenheimer bodies, and pitted (or pocked) erythrocytes are indicative of hyposplenia or asplenia.
- Surface indentations, pits or "pocks," of the red cell surface when seen in $>$12% of red blood cells are the most sensitive indicator of hyposplenia. These are submembranous vacuoles that can be seen only in wet preparations of red cells fixed in 1% glutaraldehyde and viewed using direct interference-contrast microscopy.
- US with Doppler: to assess spleen size and direction of flow in splenic vein and portal vessels
- CT/MRI: to detect spleen shape, location, number (i.e., polysplenia), size, and characterization of parenchymal disease
- Radionucleotide (technetium-99m) liver/spleen scan: to detect functional reticuloendothelial cells

TREATMENT

GENERAL MEASURES

- Immunization with pneumococcal, meningococcal, and *Haemophilus* vaccines should be carried out in all patients with asplenia/hyposplenia.
- In those patients who will be undergoing a scheduled splenectomy, the pneumococcal, meningococcal, and *Haemophilus* vaccines should be given at least 14 days prior to the operation.
- All children between 6 weeks and 59 months of age should receive the 4-dose series of the 13-valent pneumococcal conjugate vaccine (PCV13).
  - In children 2 to 5 years of age with asplenia/hyposplenia, the 23-valent pneumococcal polysaccharide vaccine (PPSV23) should be administered following the 4-dose series of PCV13.
  - A repeat of the PPSV23 should be administered 5 years after the initial dose.
- Infants between 2 and 23 months of age with asplenia/hyposplenia should receive a 4-dose series of the meningococcal groups C and Y, *Haemophilus influenzae* b, and tetanus toxoid conjugate vaccine (Hib-MenCY-TT) or the meningococcal groups A, C, W, and Y and diphtheria protein CRM (MenACWY-CRM).
  - Children >19 months should wait until 2 years of age and then receive the 2-dose series of the quadrivalent meningococcal conjugate vaccine with diphtheria toxoid (MenACWY-D).
  - Children should receive first booster of either MenACWY-CRM or MenACWY-D 3 years after completion of primary series.
  - Revaccination is recommended every 5 years (MenACWY-CRM or MenACWY-D).
  - Vaccination against serogroup B for adolescents and young adults is recommended by the Centers for Disease Control and Prevention (CDC).
- Children should also receive the *H. influenzae* type b vaccine if not completed as above.
- Antimicrobial prophylaxis should be strongly considered in all children with asplenia/hyposplenia.
  - Penicillin or amoxicillin is most commonly used; however, with increasing penicillin resistance, it may be replaced by amoxicillin-clavulanic acid, fluoroquinolones, or cefuroxime.
- Patients with sickle cell disease have impaired splenic function at all stages and should receive antimicrobial prophylaxis.

ADMISSION, INPATIENT, AND NURSING CONSIDERATIONS

Any patient with asplenia/hyposplenia with a febrile illness should be evaluated for systemic bacterial illness. Blood culture with broad-spectrum antibiotic coverage should be strongly considered.

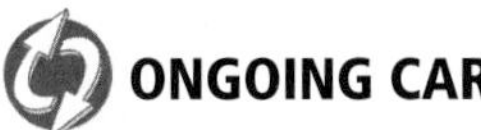

ONGOING CARE

PATIENT EDUCATION

- Patients should be counseled regarding the risk of bacterial infection and considerations in setting of febrile illness.
- MedicAlert bracelets/necklaces can be used to indicate splenic function and risk of sepsis.

COMPLICATIONS

Bacteremia

- For asplenic or hyposplenic patients, risk of bacteremia is highest in younger children and in the years immediately following splenectomy.
- The most common pathogens causing bacteremia are the encapsulated organisms, *Streptococcus pneumoniae*, *H. influenzae*, and *Neisseria meningitidis*.
- There is also an increased risk of infection with *Babesia microti* and *Plasmodium falciparum* (intraerythrocytic parasites) and *Capnocytophaga canimorsus* (via dog bites).

ALERT

Generally, for patients <4 years, splenectomy is contraindicated because of the risk of developing bacterial infection.

ADDITIONAL READING

- Centers for Disease Control and Prevention. Use of 13-valent pneumococcal conjugate vaccine and 23-valent pneumococcal polysaccharide vaccine among children aged 6–18 years with immunocompromising conditions: recommendations of the Advisory Committee on Immunization Practices (ACIP). *MMWR Morb Mortal Wkly Rep.* 2013;62(25):521–524.
- Di Sabatino A, Carsetti R, Corazza GR. Post-splenectomy and hyposplenic states. *Lancet.* 2011;378(9785):86–97.
- MacNeil JR, Rubin L, McNamara L, et al; for Centers for Disease Control and Prevention. Use of MenACWY-CRM vaccine in children aged 2 through 23 months at increased risk for meningococcal disease: recommendations of the Advisory Committee on Immunization Practices, 2013. *MMWR Morb Mortal Wkly Rep.* 2014;63(24):527–530.
- Rubin LG, Schaffner W. Clinical practice. Care of the asplenic patient. *N Engl J Med.* 2014;371(4):349–356.
- Yawn BP, Buchanan GR, Afenyi-Annan AN, et al. Management of sickle cell disease: summary of the 2014 evidence-based report by expert panel members. *JAMA.* 2014;312(10):1033–1048.

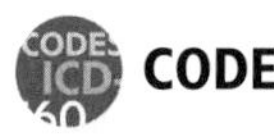

CODES

ICD10

- Q89.01 Asplenia (congenital)
- Z90.81 Acquired absence of spleen
- D73.89 Other diseases of spleen

FAQ

- Q: What should I do if my child has a fever?
- A: All patients with asplenia/hyposplenia should be evaluated for a serious bacterial infection and treated appropriately.
- Q: Are there any special times I need to worry about infections?
- A: Patients with asplenia/hyposplenia receiving dental work or GI endoscopy should be considered on a case-by-case basis. Antibiotic prophylaxis should be strongly considered in patients undergoing high-risk endoscopic procedures (i.e., sclerotherapy or stricture dilation).

ASTHMA

Kimberlee Honda, RN, MS, FNP • Andrea Marmor, MD, MSEd

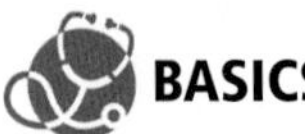

BASICS

DESCRIPTION

- Characterized by three components:
  - Reversible airway obstruction
  - Airway inflammation
  - Airway hyperresponsiveness to a variety of stimuli
- Diagnosis (the three "R"s)
  - Recurrence: Symptoms are recurrent.
  - Reactivity: Symptoms are brought on by a specific occurrence or exposure (trigger).
  - Responsiveness: Symptoms diminish in response to bronchodilator or anti-inflammatory agent.

EPIDEMIOLOGY

- 1 out of 10 school-aged children in the United States has asthma, making it one of the common chronic illnesses in children.
- Current asthma prevalence among children in the United States is 8.6% and has been rising since the early 1980s across all age, sex, and ethnic groups.
- Incidence is >5 times higher in younger children (age 0 to 4 years) than older children (age 5 to 17 years).
- Incidence and prevalence vary widely based on geographic, ethnic, and socioeconomic factors.
  - Prevalence and rate of exacerbations is highest in Puerto Ricans compared to all ethnic groups.
- Up to 75% of adolescents who wheeze will have asthma which persists in to adulthood, especially if comorbidities are present.
- Impact
  - Asthma accounts for 25% of all emergency room visits annually and is the third ranking cause of hospitalization in children <15 years.
  - Asthma is leading cause of school absenteeism in children ages 5 to 17 years, accounting for nearly 14 million missed school days per year.
- Disparities
  - Morbidity and mortality are disproportionately higher among low-income, minority, and inner-city children likely due to limited access to culturally sensitive care.
  - African American children are >3 times more likely to be hospitalized or die from asthma compared to Caucasian children.
  - Minority children are less likely to use controller medications, which may be due in part to underprescribing, limited access to care, and poor adherence.
- Mortality
  - Overall, death from asthma in children has decreased by 26% since 1999, perhaps owing to better recognition and increased use of anti-inflammatory medications.
  - Death from asthma may occur in any asthma of any severity but is more likely when asthma is poorly recognized and under controlled.

RISK FACTORS

- Family history of asthma
  - Parental history of asthma increases a child's risk of asthma 3 to 6 fold, with slightly higher risk thought to be conferred in maternal asthma.
- Prematurity
- Allergic rhinitis and atopic dermatitis
- Obesity/overweight
- History of viral infections in early childhood
- Tobacco smoke exposure
- Exposure to inhaled allergens (such as dust mite, mold) or chemical irritants

Genetics

- Asthma is a heterogenous condition; identification of phenotype can help stratify asthma subgroups and better predict individual clinical response to therapy.
- In addition to previously identified allergic and nonallergic phenotypes, other features such as age at onset, degree of airway obstruction, and endotype have been included in the refinement of asthma phenotypes.
- Several studies have suggested that epigenetics may have a role in the pathogenesis of asthma via mechanisms such as DNA methylation (reversible DNA modification in response to environmental influence).
- Emerging methods such as genome-wide association studies (GWASs) have identified genetic polymorphisms that help explain certain ethnic disparities as well as variations in atopic pathogenesis, severity, and response to medications.

GENERAL PREVENTION

- Currently, no known methods for primary prevention of asthma
- Once asthma is diagnosed, strategies focus on preventing of severe exacerbations and lost work/school days as well as comorbidities such as obesity, depression.
- All children with asthma should receive the inactivated influenza vaccine annually, starting at age 6 months.
- Effective measures (see "Patient Education") include:
  - Good adherence with environmental, behavioral, and medical treatment plan
  - Written asthma action plan: shown to reduce emergency department visits and lost school/work days
  - Education about and avoidance of triggers

PATHOPHYSIOLOGY

- Immune and inflammatory responses in the airways are triggered by an array of environmental antigens, irritants, or infectious organisms.
- Airway is stimulated and primary inflammatory mediators released
- Airway is invaded by inflammatory cells (mast cells, basophils, eosinophils, macrophages, neutrophils, B and T lymphocytes).
- Inflammatory cells respond to and produce various mediators (cytokines, leukotrienes, lymphokines), augmenting the inflammatory response.
- Airway epithelium is inflamed and becomes disrupted, and basal membrane is thickened.
- Airway smooth muscle is hyperresponsive, and bronchoconstriction ensues.
- Eosinophilia and the ability to make excess IgE in response to antigen are associated with increased airway reactivity.
- Viral infections, particularly respiratory syncytial virus (RSV) during infancy, may play a role in the development of asthma or may modify the severity of asthma.
- Airway smooth muscle hypertrophy and airway epithelial hyperplasia are characteristic chronic changes resulting from poorly controlled asthma.

DIAGNOSIS

- Asthma is primarily a clinical diagnosis, based on evidence of recurrent, reversible bronchoconstriction and/or inflammation.
- Initial diagnosis focuses on establishing asthma as the cause of the patient's symptoms.
- Once the diagnosis of asthma is confirmed, focus should be on classifying *either* severity or control.
  - *Severity* in patients not currently taking a controller medication
  - *Control* in patients currently taking a controller

ALERT

- Asthma can manifest with cough alone (wheezing may not be evident).
- Reluctance to "label" child with having asthma (using terms such as reactive airway disease or bronchitis) may result in underrecognition of chronicity and/or severity of condition.
- Children may underreport symptoms (e.g., a child who "doesn't like to play sports" may have learned that exercise causes dyspnea).
- Exam may be normal between exacerbations or even during mild exacerbations.

HISTORY

- Inquire about coughing, wheezing, shortness of breath, chest tightness:
  - Consider alternate causes (allergy, postnasal drip, deconditioning, GERD).
  - Document responsiveness of symptoms to bronchodilators.
- Document impairment: frequency, severity, pattern, and triggers.
  - Frequency: Consider occurrence of daytime and nighttime symptoms during a typical 2-week period (when child is not ill); frequency of use of rescue medications
  - Severity: degree of impairment during usual activities, missed school/work
  - Pattern: perennial versus seasonal, diurnal versus nocturnal, continuous versus episodic
  - Triggers: infections, allergens, weather, temperature, exercise/play, medications, emotions (stress/laughter), environmental irritants (smoke, odors), hormonal factors (menses)
- Document risk for severe exacerbations:
  - Use of systemic steroids in the last year
  - Emergency room visits in the last year
  - Hospitalizations (lifetime and in the last year)
  - History of ICU/intubation
- Past medical history
  - History of atopy, important comorbidities (prematurity, lung disease), breastfeeding
- Family/social/environmental history
  - Family history of asthma or atopy
  - Type and location of home (urban, suburban, rural)
  - Exposure to cigarette smoke
  - Pets
  - Presence of molds, cockroaches, rodents
  - Heating system/air conditioning
  - Carpeting, stuffed animals, drapes

- Review of systems:
  - Symptoms of complicating factors/alternate diagnoses (gastroesophageal reflux, sinusitis, allergies)
  - Dyspepsia, sour taste (gastroesophageal reflux); throat clearing, purulent nasal discharge, facial pain (sinusitis); nasal itching ("allergic salute"), eye rubbing, sneezing, watery nasal discharge (allergies)

PHYSICAL EXAM

- General exam (vital signs):
  - Blood pressure (pulsus paradoxus)
  - Respiratory rate (tachypnea)
  - Hypoxia (Note: Hypoxia may be absent in severe asthma exacerbation.)
- Pulmonary exam/auscultation
  - Physical exam pearl: forced-exhalation maneuver to observe for wheezes or for precipitating coughing
  - Work of breathing/level of distress
    - Intercostal/supraclavicular muscle retractions
    - Abdominal breathing, head-bobbing, grunting, nasal flaring
  - Auscultation
    - Wheezing (inspiratory, expiratory, or both)
    - Air entry and symmetry (Poor air entry in severe obstructions may result in lack of wheeze.)
    - End-expiratory involuntary cough
    - Prolonged expiratory phase
    - Adventitious sounds (crackles, rhonchi)
    - Stridor (indicates extrathoracic airway obstruction)
  - Chest shape (i.e., normal vs. barrel-shaped)
- Cardiac: Murmur may suggest alternative diagnosis.
- HEENT: signs of allergies or sinusitis:
  - Injected eyes, swollen palpebral conjunctivae
  - Allergic shiners
  - Dennie-Morgan lines
  - Thin, watery nasal secretions
  - Boggy, pale, or blue-gray nasal turbinates
  - Nasal polyps
  - Septal deviation
  - Nasal crease
  - Cobblestoning of posterior oropharynx
  - Tonsillar hypertrophy
- Malocclusion skin: evidence of atopic dermatitis
- Extremities: digital clubbing (very rare in asthma; suggests alternative diagnosis)

DIFFERENTIAL DIAGNOSIS

- Infectious
  - Pneumonia
  - Bronchiolitis
  - Laryngotracheobronchitis
  - Sinusitis
  - Immune deficiency
- Mechanical
  - Extrinsic airway compression
  - Vascular ring
  - Foreign body
  - Vocal cord dysfunction
  - Tracheobronchomalacia
- Miscellaneous:
  - Cystic fibrosis
  - Bronchopulmonary dysplasia
  - Pulmonary edema
  - Gastroesophageal reflux
  - Recurrent aspiration
  - Bronchiolitis obliterans

DIAGNOSTIC TESTS & INTERPRETATION

Initial Tests (screening, lab, imaging)

ALERT

- Overuse of chest radiograph may result in misdiagnosis of pneumonia (subsegmental atelectasis misdiagnosed as an infiltrate).
- Spirometry is not necessary to establish the diagnosis of asthma.

- Spirometry
  - Recommended, if available, for confirmation of initial asthma diagnosis and during ongoing assessment
  - Children as young as 4 to 5 years old can usually perform spirometry with practice and proper coaching.
  - Improper technique or poor effort will produce unreliable results.
  - Assesses lung volume, type of obstruction (intrathoracic vs. extrathoracic), airflow and airway reactivity
  - Decreased FEV1/FVC (<80% of predicted) is indicative of large airway obstruction.
  - Decreased midexpiratory flow (FEF 25–75%) is most sensitive finding for small airway obstruction in children and can occur even when the physical exam is normal.
  - A bronchodilator challenge with pre- or post-spirometry testing can demonstrate reversibility (>8–12% change in FEV1 following bronchodilator is supportive of asthma).
- Serial values can follow progress of disease and response to long-term treatment; provocational testing
  - Exercise challenge: determines effect of exercise on triggering airway obstruction
  - Methacholine challenge (indicated only in cases for which history is equivocal and pulmonary function test is normal): measures the degree of airway hyperreactivity; a positive test supports the diagnosis of asthma.
- Exhaled nitric oxide: may help assess bronchial reactivity and glucocorticoid responsiveness
  - Identifies Th2-mediated airway inflammation or other asthma phenotype
  - May identify/exclude steroid responsive airway inflammation but is not recommended for routine use to guide asthma treatment
- Allergy evaluation:
  - Skin prick testing is the preferred test for assessing sensitivity to environmental agents or foods.
    - Strong negative predictive value and is both rapid and cost-effective
    - Contraindicated for patients with high risk for anaphylaxis
    - Use of antihistamine within previous 5 days will impair results.
  - Immunoassay (or "RAST") testing is less sensitive than skin prick testing but may be considered when skin prick testing is contraindicated.
  - In select cases, may consider additional serum tests such as eosinophil count or total IgE.
- Chest radiograph
  - Should not be routinely obtained
  - Consider if the diagnosis is uncertain, if patient fails to respond to treatment, or to rule out congenital lung malformations or obvious vascular malformations
  - Findings most often normal
  - In severe chronic disease or during acute exacerbation, may show peribronchial thickening, subsegmental atelectasis, and hyperinflation
- Chest CT should only be performed if bronchiectasis or anatomic abnormality is strongly suspected.

Diagnostic Procedures/Other

Bronchoscopy: in select cases only, can rule out anatomic malformations, foreign bodies, mucous plugging, vocal cord dysfunction, and aspiration (lipid-laden macrophages)

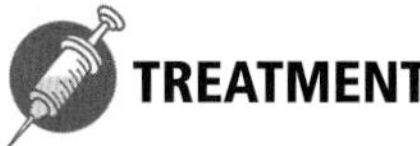

TREATMENT

ALERT

- High risk of poor adherence with therapy when symptoms are controlled
- Proper technique must be used to ensure efficacy of inhaled medications.

GENERAL MEASURES

- Goals of acute therapy are to reduce acute symptoms and prevent hospitalization.
- Goals of long-term therapy are to reduce impairment (ongoing symptoms, interference with activity) and risk (likelihood of serious exacerbation).
- Long-term treatment should be based on classification of severity or control.
  - Those with persistent asthma should be started on a daily controller.
  - Those whose asthma is not well-controlled should have treatment increased to the next step.
- A quick rule of thumb: if patient has:
  - ≥2 days per week with symptoms OR
  - ≥2 nights per month with symptoms OR
  - ≥2 steroid bursts per year (inpatient or outpatient) and then they have persistent or not well-controlled asthma
- See Figure 5 in Appendix for Stepwise Approach for Managing Asthma Long Term.

MEDICATION

- Acute asthma symptoms/exacerbation
  - Short-acting β_2-agonists (SABAs) (bronchodilators):
    - Indicated for relief of acute bronchospasm (quick-relief medicine)
    - Use as needed for breakthrough symptoms; use prior to exercise in exercise-induced bronchospasm.
    - Regular use or overuse associated with worsened control of asthma
    - Routes include metered-dose inhaler (MDI) with valved holding chamber (VHC; preferred) or nebulizer (less efficient, not portable).
    - Recommended for use every 4 hours at home, but during acute exacerbation or in hospital/clinic setting, may be given as frequently as needed to relieve bronchospasm
    - Side effects generally mild (tachycardia, flushing, hyperactivity)
    - Preparations include
      - Albuterol (Ventolin®, Proventil®, ProAir®): MDI or ampule for nebulization
      - Levalbuterol (Xopenex®): a single-isomer preparation of albuterol; MDI or ampule for nebulization, covered by some insurance plans but has not been shown superior
      - Terbutaline (Brethine®): injectable

- Anticholinergic agents (bronchodilators):
  - Adjunctive bronchodilators, used in conjunction with SABA in acute severe asthma exacerbation
  - Preparations include
    - Ipratropium bromide MDI or ampule for nebulization (Atrovent®); no clear recommendations for outpatient use in pediatrics
    - Tiotropium (Spiriva®), MDI, or DPI approved for children >6 years old
- Short-course systemic corticosteroids: for acute asthma exacerbations that do not respond to intermittent SABA alone or for patients at risk for severe exacerbation
  - Shown to both reduce and shorten hospitalization; most effective when given early in exacerbation
  - 2 doses of dexamethasone (0.3 to 0.6 mg/kg/dose) 24 to 36 hours apart may cause hyperglycemia due to stronger glucocorticoid effect.
  - Prednisone or prednisolone 1 to 2 mg/kg/24 h for 3 to 7 days or longer; usually tapered if >7 days of therapy required or if systemic steroids are used frequently
  - IV: methylprednisolone (Solu-Medrol®) 1 to 2 mg/kg/24 h IV divided q6–12h until improved and able to take oral medication—not shown to be more effective than oral corticosteroids
- Miscellaneous drugs used in severe cases
  - Magnesium sulfate ($MgSO_4$): used intravenously as a bronchodilator in severe acute asthma exacerbation
  - IV theophylline or IV terbutaline (systemic bronchodilators)
    - 2nd line after $MgSO_4$ for status asthmaticus
    - For theophylline, serum levels must be routinely monitored (therapeutic levels are 10 to 20 mg/mL).
    - Many factors affect theophylline levels. Increased levels are seen with erythromycin, ciprofloxacin, cimetidine, viral illnesses, fever. Decreased levels are seen with phenobarbital, phenytoin, rifampin.
  - Heliox (helium/O_2 mixture)
    - May improve airflow in severe asthma
    - Limits FiO_2 to 40%—contraindicated in severely hypoxic patients

• Control of persistent asthma
- Inhaled corticosteroids (ICS)
  - When used daily, the safest and most effective controller medications for asthma
    - Select patients with infrequent exacerbations may be well-controlled on a moderate dose ICS only during exacerbations.
  - Control symptoms, prevent exacerbations, reduce airway inflammation and hyperresponsiveness more than any other inhaled agents.
  - Inhibit production and release of cytokines and arachidonic acid–associated metabolites; enhance β-adrenoreceptor responsiveness.
  - Side effects: oral thrush; may minimally affect growth velocity (~1 cm) during 1st year of use at moderate or high doses
  - Dosage individualized to each patient (see Figure 5 in Appendix for Stepwise Approach for Managing Asthma Long Term)
  - Agents vary in topical potency and systemic bioavailability (see Table 14 in Appendix for Comparative Doses).
  - Available as MDIs, dry-powder inhalers (DPIs), or nebulized
  - Fluticasone propionate (Flovent®) 44, 110, 220 mcg/puff MDI and 50, 100, 250 mcg DPI for b.i.d. administration
  - Fluticasone furoate (Arnuity Ellipta®) 100, 200 mcg/puff breath activated inhalation for once daily administration, currently approved for children ≥12 years old
  - Budesonide (Pulmicort®) 90, 180 mcg/puff DPI and 250, 500, and 1,000-mcg vials for nebulizer
  - Beclomethasone (Qvar®) 40, 80 mcg/puff
  - Flunisolide (AeroBid®) 80 mcg/puff
  - Ciclesonide (Alvesco®) 80, 160 mcg/puff
  - Mometasone (Asmanex®) 100 mcg/puff MDI and 110, 220 mcg DPI
- Long-acting β_2-agonists (LABAs)
  - Preparations include salmeterol (Serevent®) and formoterol (Foradil®).
  - Indicated for patients not well-controlled on ICS alone
  - Only available in fixed combination products with ICS
  - Fluticasone/salmeterol (Advair®): DPI = 100/50, 250/50, 500/50 mcg/puff; MDI = 45/21, 115/21, 230/21 mcg/puff MDI; also available as fluticasone/salmeterol (AirDuo RespiClick®) DPI = 55/14, 113/14, 232/14 mcg/puff
  - Mometasone/formoterol (Dulera®) MDI: 100/5, 200/5 mcg/puff
  - Budesonide/formoterol (Symbicort®) MDI: 80/4.5, 160/4.5 mcg puff
  - Black box warning: Some studies have shown an increased risk of asthma-related deaths in patients using salmeterol, and it is suggested that LABAs be prescribed only for patients not adequately controlled on other asthma-controller medications or whose disease severity warrants initiation of treatment with two maintenance therapies.
- Leukotriene modifiers (anti-inflammatory agents)
  - Block the synthesis and/or action of leukotrienes
  - Indicated as a 2nd-line step up from low-dose ICS (not as effective as medium-dose ICS or ICS/LABA combo)
  - Rarely as monotherapy for very mild persistent or exercise-induced asthma
  - Leukotriene receptor antagonists: zafirlukast (10, 20 mg; Accolate®) and montelukast (4, 5, and 10 mg; Singulair®)
  - 5-lipoxygenase inhibitors, zileuton: may cause hepatic dysfunction
- Mast-cell stabilizers
  - Weak anti-inflammatory agents, not routinely used as less effective than other options
  - Inhaled: nebulizer; MDI
  - Preparations: cromolyn sodium (nebulizer only); nedocromil sodium (Tilade®, available in Canada)
  - Omalizumab (Xolair®): monoclonal antibodies against IgE; can be given as a monthly SC injection in severe asthma patients with moderately high IgE levels
  - Immunotherapy
    - Efficacy in asthma is controversial.
    - Most effective if a single antigen can be identified
    - Used only in select cases if medical management and environmental control measures are ineffective
- Steroid-sparing agents:
  - Troleandomycin (TAO): Macrolide antibiotic decreases clearance of corticosteroids, thus prolonging the effects of corticosteroids on the lung; lower corticosteroid dosing required
  - Methotrexate: Potent immunosuppressive drug needs further investigation in children.
  - Cyclosporine: shown to have steroid-sparing effect in adult population with asthma; side effects are significant and may limit use.

ISSUES FOR REFERRAL

- A patient who requires hospitalization more than once a year or who has required intensive care or intubation
- A patient who requires frequent bursts of systemic corticosteroids
- A patient whose airway obstruction is not easily reversible
- A patient who has clinical features suggesting another pulmonary process

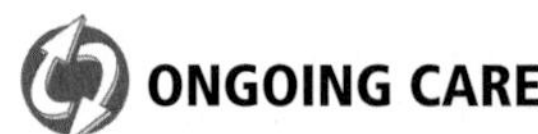

ONGOING CARE

FOLLOW-UP RECOMMENDATIONS

- Asthma is highly variable over time, and regular, long-term follow-up is essential to maintain normal activity and pulmonary function.
- Assess medication adherence, proper medication use technique, and access to medications.
- Patients who are well-controlled may be evaluated every 3 to 4 months.
- Patients for whom therapy is initiated or undergo a change in regimen should have follow-up at 4- to 6-week intervals.
- For those patients at high risk for exacerbation or who demonstrate minimal response to medication, close follow-up (i.e., 2 to 4 weeks) is recommended.

Patient Monitoring

- At each visit: Monitor lung function and reported symptoms, adjust medication using a stepwise approach, and provide individualized patient education on trigger avoidance.
- For patients requiring a daily controller medication, regularly assess level of asthma control.
  - Increase in daytime symptoms, increased use of bronchodilator medication, and/or nighttime awakenings due to asthma represent a loss of asthma control and indication for step up in treatment.
  - In certain populations, use of a validated screening tool may help quantify symptoms (e.g., the childhood asthma control test [C-ACT®] or Asthma Therapy Assessment Questionnaire for children and adolescents [pediatric ATAQ®]).
- Peak flow meter may be recommended for certain patients but is not shown to be superior to symptom monitoring at home.
  - May be helpful in patients who have poor symptom recognition or labile asthma but not a sensitive test for airflow limitation
  - Effort-dependent, measures peak expiratory flow rate (PEFR)
  - Technique and adherence are highly variable.
  - Peak flow rate values are divided into three zones:
    - Green: ≥80% of baseline
    - Yellow: 50–80% of baseline
    - Red: 50% of baseline
  - Specific peak flow rate guidelines should be individualized for each patient based on the best measurement obtained during a 14-day period when the child is well.

DIET

- Encourage healthy eating habits to prevent or manage obesity.
- Food-induced asthma is *not* common; however, cold foods or strong smells may trigger asthma symptoms.
- Vitamin D: potential role in the development of asthma and severity of exacerbations, no clear recommendations

- Breastfeeding: in some studies, associated with reduced atopy in early childhood
- Prenatal: correlation shown between maternal intake of Omega 3/maternal vitamin D levels and wheezing/atopic disease in offspring; however, RCTs have failed to show causality.

PATIENT EDUCATION

- Goals: Establish provider/caregiver partnership, improve adherence to treatment plan, improve quality of life, decrease frequency/severity of exacerbations.
- An individualized approach encourages self-management and, when possible, involves the child and family in treatment planning and decision making.
- Consider literacy level when providing written material.
  - General education: Every patient/caregiver should be taught that asthma is a chronic, inflammatory condition that can be controlled with proper therapy.
  - Other important teaching points for families:
    - Basic asthma pathophysiology
    - Prevention of asthma attacks/trigger avoidance
    - Role of controller versus quick-relief medication in managing symptoms
  - Action plan: Provide with any medication change, should include specific instructions for:
    - Use of daily controller medication
    - Symptom recognition and escalation of rescue medication
    - When to seek emergency care
- Medications
  - Explore patient/family goals of treatment, and address barriers to medication adherence.
  - Purpose and indication for all medications should be explained, and potential risks, side effects, and benefits reviewed.
  - Regardless of patient age, a VHC, "spacer" device should always be used with a MDI.
    - Use a VHC with appropriately sized pediatric mask for infants and young children.
    - A VHC with mouthpiece may be used for children >7 years old who can demonstrate correct breath coordination.
  - Proper device technique for MDI with VHC, DPI, or nebulizer or should be taught by demonstration and reviewed at subsequent visits
    - MDIs should be refilled based on the number of doses used, not by estimating contents by shaking or spraying (MDIs with a built-in dose counter are preferred).
- Environmental counseling
  - Avoid airborne irritants (tobacco smoke, wood stoves, noxious fumes, scented cleaning products, or air fresheners).
  - Offer a home visit evaluation if feasible.
  - Identify and reduce exposure to the most common airborne triggers such as dust, mold, animal dander, and pollens.
    - Carpet removal or frequent vacuuming is recommended for children with dust mite allergy.
    - Use dust mite–proof mattress and pillow encasings.
    - Wash pillows, blankets, and sheets in hot water weekly.
    - Minimize stuffed animals, quilts, books, and clutter.
    - Avoid molds by decreasing relative humidity to 50%.
    - Remove pets from child's bedroom and from house if patient is allergic to the animal.
    - Eliminate indoor pests (cockroaches, rats, fleas, bedbugs).
- Activity/school
  - Encourage physical activity.
    - With close follow-up, most patients with asthma can participate fully in sports, even at a high level.
    - Patients with exercise-induced bronchospasm may require use of quick-relief medication 20 minutes prior to activity.
    - All athletes should have their quick-relief medications on hand at all times.
  - School and daycare facilities must be notified of the child's asthma.
    - Written medication forms to permit use of quick-relief medication while at school
    - Include instructions for emergency care as well as medication use during exercise.
    - Establish good communication between school, family, and provider regarding frequency of symptoms and medication use.

PROGNOSIS

With proper therapy, individualized education and good adherence to treatment regimen: excellent

COMPLICATIONS

- Frequent hospitalizations/need for systemic corticosteroids
- Absence from school or poor school performance
- Obesity/poor cardiovascular health from poor physical conditioning
- Parental loss of wages/work, decreased productivity
- Psychological impact of having a chronic illness
- Decline in lung function over time

ADDITIONAL READING

- Chauhan BF, Chartrand C, Ducharme FM. Intermittent versus daily inhaled corticosteroids for persistent asthma in children and adults. *Cochrane Database Syst Rev*. 2013;(2):CD009611.
- Chauhan BF, Ducharme FM. Addition to inhaled corticosteroids of long-acting beta2-agonists versus anti-leukotrienes for chronic asthma. *Cochrane Database Syst Rev*. 2014;(1):CD003137.
- Chong J, Haran C, Chauhan BF, et al. Intermittent inhaled corticosteroid therapy versus placebo for persistent asthma in children and adults. *Cochrane Database Syst Rev*. 2015;(7):CD011032.
- Compalati E, Braido F, Canonica GW. An update on allergen immunotherapy and asthma. *Curr Opin Pulm Med*. 2014;20(1):109–117.
- Corren J. Asthma phenotypes and endotypes: an evolving paradigm for classification. *Discov Med*. 2013;15(83):243–249.
- D'Amato G, Vitale C, Molino A, et al. Asthma-related deaths. *Multidiscip Respir Med*. 2016;11:37.
- DeVries A, Vercelli D. Epigenetic mechanisms in asthma. *Ann Am Thorac Soc*. 2016;13(Suppl 1):S48–S50.
- Gunaratne AW, Makrides M, Collins CT. Maternal prenatal and/or postnatal n-3 long chain polyunsaturated fatty acids (LCPUFA) supplementation for preventing allergies in early childhood. *Cochrane Database Syst Rev*. 2015;(7):CD010085.
- Kaiser SV, Huynh T, Bacharier LB, et al. Preventing exacerbations in preschoolers with recurrent wheeze: a meta-analysis. *Pediatrics*. 2016;137(6):e20154496.
- Kew KM, Quinn M, Quon BS, et al. Increased versus stable doses of inhaled corticosteroids for exacerbations of chronic asthma in adults and children. *Cochrane Database Syst Rev*. 2016;(6):CD007524.
- Litonjua AA, Carey VJ, Laranjo N, et al. Effect of prenatal supplementation with vitamin D on asthma or recurrent wheezing in offspring by age 3 years: the VDAART randomized clinical trial. *JAMA*. 2016;315(4):362–370.
- National Institutes of Health, National Heart, Lung, and Blood Institute. *NHLBI Third Expert Panel Report (EPR3): Guidelines for the Diagnosis and Management of Asthma*. Bethesda, MD: National Institutes of Health, National Heart, Lung, and Blood Institute; 2007. NIH Publication 08-405.
- Ober C, Yao TC. The genetics of asthma and allergic disease: a 21st century perspective. *Immunol Rev*. 2011;242(1):10–30.
- Pruteanu AI, Chauhan BF, Zhang L, et al. Inhaled corticosteroids in children with persistent asthma: dose-response effects on growth. *Cochrane Database Syst Rev*. 2014;(7):CD009878.
- Reddel HK, Bateman ED, Becker A, et al. A summary of the new GINA strategy: a roadmap to asthma control. *Eur Respir J*. 2015;46(3):622–639.
- Reddel HK, Foster JM. Inconclusive evidence about the efficacy of diverse strategies for intermittent versus daily inhaled corticosteroids for persistent asthma in adults and children. *Evid Based Med*. 2014;19(1):e2.
- Sullivan P, Ghushchyan VG, Navaratnam P, et al. School absence and productivity outcomes associated with childhood asthma in the USA. *J Asthma*. 2018;55(2):161–168.
- Zhang L, Prietsch SO, Ducharme FM. Inhaled corticosteroids in children with persistent asthma: effects on growth. *Cochrane Database Syst Rev*. 2014;(7):CD009471.

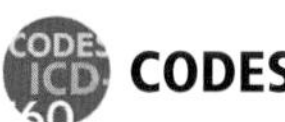

CODES

ICD10

- J45.909 Unspecified asthma, uncomplicated
- J45.901 Unspecified asthma with (acute) exacerbation
- J45.990 Exercise induced bronchospasm

FAQ

- Q: Will my child outgrow his or her asthma?
- A: Family history is the biggest predictor of ultimate outcome. Wheezing during the first 3 years of life is extremely common. Many of these children do not develop asthma and "outgrow" their wheezing by school age. Some patients develop asthma again as young adults. If others in your family have asthma as an adult, there's a good chance your child will too.
- Q: Can my child become dependent on asthma medications?
- A: When asthma medications are used correctly, children will not become "dependent" on these medications as they would with narcotic agents. If daily medication is recommended for your child, its goal is to decrease the need for stronger medications by keeping airways open and reducing inflammation. If medications are not used correctly, or are overused, they may become less effective over time.
- Q: Will my child be on medications for the rest of his or her life?
- A: This depends on the severity of their asthma. Most children need less daily medication over time, but most will always need to keep their short-acting rescue medication handy. The types, doses, and frequency of asthma medications will likely change over your child's lifetime. Unfortunately we are not very good at predicting which children will continue to need medications for a long time and which will need less medication over time.

ATAXIA

Kristin W. Barañano, MD, PhD

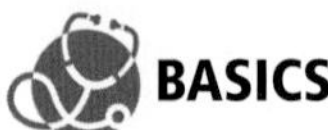

BASICS

DESCRIPTION

- Ataxia refers to incoordination of movement out of proportion to weakness.
- Can be caused by dysfunction of cerebellum, proprioception, or vestibular system
- Careful history of timing of onset and antecedent events key in framing differential: acute, subacute, chronic/progressive, episodic

EPIDEMIOLOGY

- Acute cerebellar ataxia (ACA) was previously seen in 1 per 5,000 cases of varicella, accounting for 25% of total cases. The risk following varicella-zoster virus (VZV) vaccination is 1.5 per 1,000,000 doses.
- Most cases of ACA are still postviral, followed by ingestions, then Guillain-Barré syndrome (GBS) (combined account for 80% of total).
- Dominantly inherited spinocerebellar ataxias (SCAs) are 1 to 5 per 100,000 but tend to have a later age of onset.
- More likely to see autosomal recessive (AR) ataxias in childhood; most common is Friedreich ataxia (FRDA) at 1 in 30,000 to 50,000.

PATHOPHYSIOLOGY

- The cerebellum does not generate motor commands; instead, it modifies them to make them accurate and adaptive.
- The cerebellum receives input from the vestibular apparatus, spinal cord, and the cerebral cortex (via the pons).
- Both input and output is ipsilateral (i.e., right-sided cerebellar lesions cause right-sided ataxia).
- Midline cerebellum (vermis) controls gait, head and trunk stability, eye movements; lesions of vermis result in wide-based ("drunken sailor") gait, truncal sway, and head titubation (bobbling movements).
- Cerebellar hemispheres control limb tone and coordination, motor learning, speech, eye movements; lesions of the cerebellar hemispheres cause limb dysmetria (trouble with finger-nose-finger testing).
- Function can be impaired by chemicals, autoimmune processes, genetic mutations; typical pathologic finding is loss of Purkinje cells and injury to their elaborate dendritic arbor.

ETIOLOGY

- Acute onset
  - Ingestions/intoxications: alcohol, anticonvulsants including phenytoin, benzodiazepines, antihistamines, heavy metals, carbon monoxide
  - Infections (e.g., *Bartonella*, *Mycoplasma*, Epstein-Barr virus)
  - Postinfectious
  - Postvaccination
  - Demyelinating events: multiple sclerosis, acute disseminated encephalomyelitis (ADEM) (can be associated with altered mental status and seizure), Miller Fisher variant of GBS (triad of ataxia, ophthalmoplegia, areflexia; look for eye movement abnormalities and areflexia)
  - Initial presentation of recurrent ataxia
- Subacute onset
  - Cerebellar hemorrhage
  - Ischemic stroke
  - Encephalitis or cerebellitis
  - Acute labyrinthitis/vestibular neuronitis (often prominent nausea/vomiting, hearing affected)
  - Posterior fossa tumors (e.g., medulloblastoma)
  - Paraneoplastic syndromes (opsoclonus-myoclonus syndrome, with multidirectional chaotic eye movements; evaluate for neuroblastoma)
- Chronic or progressive
  - Developmental defects: Dandy-Walker syndrome, cerebellar agenesis, rhombencephalosynapsis, Chiari I malformation
  - Ataxic cerebral palsy
  - Tumors
  - Paraneoplastic
  - Metabolic/degenerative
    - With pathologic accumulation: hexosaminidase deficiency, Niemann-Pick type C, metachromatic leukodystrophy, Wilson disease
    - Hypomyelinating leukodystrophies (e.g., Pelizaeus-Merzbacher disease)
    - SCAs
    - AR ataxias including FRDA (associated pes cavus, cardiomyopathy, diabetes, polyneuropathy), ataxia telangiectasia (frequent infections, increased susceptibility to leukemia/lymphoma; telangiectasias are a late finding)
- Recurrent
  - Migraine (Vestibular migraine can present with ataxia and vertigo without headache.)
  - Episodic ataxia (EA1 and EA2 best characterized, at least six loci identified)
  - Metabolic disorders: mitochondrial disorders, Hartnup disease, urea cycle defects, intermittent forms of maple syrup urine disease

DIAGNOSIS

HISTORY

- Focus on the time course of onset.
- Elicit possible ingestions, access to medications at homes of friends, family
- Antecedent infections or vaccinations (fever, especially upper respiratory infection [URI] and GI symptoms)
- Recent trauma (concussion, possible vertebral artery dissection)
- Past medical history: similar episodes, migraines, congenital heart defect, multiple organ system involvement suggestive of metabolic/mitochondrial disease, unusual susceptibility to infection
- Family history: recurrent or progressive ataxias, migraines
- Symptoms to elicit: altered mental status, headache, diplopia, vertigo (illusion of movement or dizziness), history of seizure, nausea/vomiting, diminished hearing, or tinnitus

PHYSICAL EXAM

- Vital signs: presence of fever
- General exam: presence of meningismus; otoscopic examination for otitis; assess for pharyngitis, lymphadenopathy, splenomegaly, rash, skin and eyes for telangiectasias
- Neurologic exam
  - Mental status: altered with ingestions, CNS infections, ADEM
  - Cranial nerves: funduscopic exam for papilledema, eye movement abnormalities, presence of nystagmus, head impulse (thrust) test for vestibular function, hearing with tuning fork (Weber and Rinne tests), dysarthria or scanning speech
  - Motor: presence of hypotonia or tremor, exclude weakness as cause of incoordination
  - Reflexes: absence suggestive of GBS
  - Sensory: Assess for sensory ataxia due to lack of proprioceptive input.
  - Coordination: presence of head titubation, truncal ataxia, intention tremor; limb dysmetria with finger-nose-finger, overshoot with finger chase; dysdiadochokinesia with rapid alternating movements, and heel to shin test
  - Gait: ability to tandem walk, sway with Romberg test (either cerebellar or proprioceptive defect)

DIFFERENTIAL DIAGNOSIS

- Movement disorders: Tremor, chorea, athetosis may be mistaken for ataxia.
- Weakness: incoordination in proportion to weakness (myasthenia gravis, GBS)
- Conversion disorder: variability, distractibility, lack of associated cerebellar signs, astasia-abasia (exaggerated factitious inability to walk or stand)
- Epileptic ataxia (pseudoataxia): episodic, associated alteration of awareness
- Optic ataxia: difficulty reaching for target due to lesions in posterior parietal lobe resulting in impaired visual input to cerebellum

DIAGNOSTIC TESTS & INTERPRETATION

Initial Tests (screening, lab, imaging)

- Initial ER screening labs for acute presentation:
  - CBC, comprehensive metabolic panel (CMP)
  - Lactate, ammonia
  - Toxicology screen and drug levels for specific intoxications
- Additional investigations for chronic/progressive ataxias:
  - Rule out reversible/potentially treatable causes:
    - Exposures: heavy metals, zinc (chelated copper)
    - Autoimmune: celiac, anti-glutamic acid decarboxylase (GAD), paraneoplastic panel, urine homovanillic acid/vanillylmandelic acid (HVA/VMA) for neuroblastoma
    - Metabolic: TSH, vitamin E, coenzyme Q, vitamin B_{12} and B_1 levels, copper, ceruloplasmin, lactate, ammonia, plasma amino acids, urine organic acids, urine amino acids (for Hartnup disease), very-long-chain fatty acid (VLCFA) with phytanic acid (Refsum), paired CSF and serum glucose levels or *SLC2A1* sequencing for GLUT1 deficiency, cholestanol (cerebrotendinous xanthomatosis), lysosomal enzymes
  - Other potential screening laboratories: lipid panel, IgA levels
  - Serum α-fetoprotein (AFP) level is sensitive screening lab after 1 year of age for AT
  - Ataxia panels for inherited cerebellar ataxias (e.g., SCAs); most not clinically distinguishable in early stages
- Head CT in the acute setting for altered mental status or concern for hemorrhage
- MRI of brain more sensitive in assessing posterior fossa pathology; consider administration of contrast if concern for infection/demyelination; MRA of brain and neck if concern for stroke/dissection

Diagnostic Procedures/Other

- Lumbar puncture
  - For infection or ADEM: cell counts, protein, glucose, bacterial culture and viral polymerase chain reactions (PCRs), IgG index, oligoclonal bands
  - For suspected metabolic disorders: glucose, protein, cell counts, lactate, pyruvate, 5-methyltetrahydrofolate (5-MTHF), amino acids; pair with serum glucose and amino acids
- Metaiodobenzylguanidine (MIBG) scan and body CT for potential neuroblastoma
- Nerve conduction studies: suspected GBS
- Electronystagmography (ENG) for potential vestibular involvement
- EEG for consideration of epileptic ataxia

TREATMENT

- Treatment of many of the acute ataxias (ingestions, postviral) is supportive.
- Specific therapies
  - ADEM: corticosteroids
  - GBS: intravenous immunoglobulin (IVIG), plasmapheresis
  - Paraneoplastic: treatment of malignancy, immunosuppression
  - Migraine: avoidance of food triggers, preventive medications (e.g., calcium channel blockers, tricyclic antidepressants [TCAs])
  - Episodic ataxias: acetazolamide
  - Inherited ataxias: some evidence for use of medications such as amantadine, riluzole, varenicline
  - Possible role for treatment with specific vitamins and cofactors (carnitine, coenzyme Q, vitamin E, riboflavin, folinic acid) for mitochondrial disorders

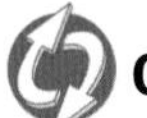

ONGOING CARE

PROGNOSIS

- Most acute ataxias are ingestions and postviral and have a good prognosis. If recovery from a presumed postviral ataxia is delayed (>2 weeks), evaluation for neuroblastoma should be undertaken.
- Recovery from GBS is generally good but can be incomplete.
- Specific diagnosis of an inherited cerebellar ataxia is helpful in predicting clinical course (time to wheelchair, potential for cognitive decline, death).

COMPLICATIONS

- Risk of injury due to falls
- Risk of aspiration due to swallow dysfunction
- Autonomic instability can be associated with GBS.
- With inherited cerebellar ataxias: Some patients also develop neuropathy, spasticity, and cognitive decline.
- Risk of depression and cognitive impairment given increasingly recognized role of cerebellum in cognition and emotion

ADDITIONAL READING

- Blaser SI, Steinlin M, Al-Maawali A, et al. The pediatric cerebellum in inherited neurodegenerative disorders: a pattern-recognition approach. *Neuroimaging Clin N Am*. 2016;26(3):373–416.
- Caffarelli M, Kimia AA, Torres AR. Acute ataxia in children: a review of the differential diagnosis and evaluation in the emergency department. *Pediatr Neurol*. 2016;65:14–30.
- National Ataxia Foundation: www.ataxia.org
- Neuromuscular Disease Center of Washington University: http://neuromuscular.wustl.edu/ataxia/aindex.html
- Paulson HL, Shakkottai VG, Clark HB, et al. Polyglutamine spinocerebellar ataxias—from genes to potential treatments. *Nat Rev Neurosci*. 2017;18(10):613–626.

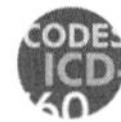

CODES

ICD10

- R27.0 Ataxia, unspecified
- G11.9 Hereditary ataxia, unspecified
- G11.1 Early-onset cerebellar ataxia

FAQ

- Q: Which ingestions are most likely to cause ataxia?
- A: Alcohol, anticonvulsants, antihistamines, benzodiazepines, TCAs
- Q: What is the typical time course of postinfectious ataxia?
- A: Typically, it will be maximal in onset in the first day or two, then improve within 2 weeks. Ataxia persisting beyond 2 weeks should prompt evaluation for neuroblastoma.
- Q: What is the role of physical therapy for cerebellar ataxia?
- A: Studies have demonstrated that intensive coordination training improves motor performance in progressive cerebellar disorders and translates into improved activities of daily living.
- Q: What is the risk of transmitting a hereditary cerebellar ataxia?
- A: It depends on the mode of inheritance: AR (25%), autosomal dominant (50%, with risk of anticipation for disorders with polyglutamine expansion), maternal (mitochondrial and X-linked disorders).

ATELECTASIS

Richard M. Kravitz, MD

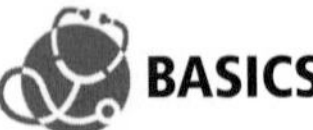

BASICS

DESCRIPTION
- State of collapsed and airless alveoli
- May be subsegmental, segmental, or lobar or may involve the entire lung
- A radiographic sign of an underlying disease and not a diagnosis unto itself

EPIDEMIOLOGY
- Depends on the underlying disease causing atelectasis
- Resorption atelectasis is the most common form.

RISK FACTORS
Genetics
Depends on the underlying disease causing atelectasis (i.e., cystic fibrosis, primary ciliary dyskinesia)

GENERAL PREVENTION
- Maintaining adequate cough
- Good airway clearance techniques in patients at risk for atelectasis

PATHOPHYSIOLOGY
- Reduced lung compliance
- Loss of alveoli (if extensive) may lead to hypoxia.
- Intrapulmonary shunting develops from hypoxia-induced pulmonary arterial vasoconstriction, which may lead to areas of ventilation–perfusion (V/Q) mismatch and further hypoxia.
- If atelectasis is extensive and long-term, pulmonary hypertension may develop.
- Atelectatic areas are prone to bacterial overgrowth and possible secondary infection.

ETIOLOGY
- Airway obstruction (resorption atelectasis)
  - Most common cause of atelectasis in children
  - Obstructed communication between alveoli and trachea
- Large airway obstruction
  - Intrinsic
    - Foreign body aspiration
    - Mucous plug
    - Tumor
    - Plastic bronchitis
  - Extrinsic
    - Hilar adenopathy
    - Mediastinal mass
    - Congenital lung malformations
- Small airway obstruction
  - Acute infection
    - Bronchiolitis
    - Pneumonia
    - Respiratory infections are the most common cause of acute atelectasis.
  - Altered mucociliary clearance:
    - CNS depression
    - Smoke inhalation
    - Pain
- Mechanical compression of the pulmonary parenchyma or pleural space (compressive atelectasis)
  - Intrathoracic compression
    - Pneumothorax
    - Pleural effusion
    - Lobar emphysema
    - Intrathoracic tumors
    - Cardiomegaly
    - Diaphragmatic hernias
  - Abdominal distention
    - Large intra-abdominal tumors
    - Hepatosplenomegaly
    - Massive ascites
    - Morbid obesity
- Decreased surface tension in the small airways and alveoli (adhesive atelectasis)
  - Stems from surfactant deficiency
  - Diffuse surfactant deficiency
    - Hyaline membrane disease
    - Acute respiratory distress syndrome
    - Smoke inhalation
  - Localized surfactant deficiency
    - Acute radiation pneumonitis
    - Pulmonary embolism
- Neuromuscular weakness (hypoventilation)
  - Inherent weakness
    - Duchenne muscular dystrophy
    - Spinal muscular atrophy
    - Paralysis
  - Acquired weakness (e.g., postanesthesia hypoventilation)

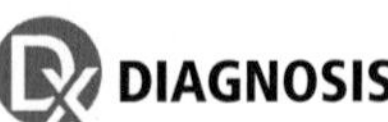

DIAGNOSIS

HISTORY
- Depends on the underlying disease process
- May be asymptomatic
- Cough and/or wheeze can be present.
- Dyspnea
- Chest pain
- Special questions:
  - Is the atelectasis acute, recurrent, or chronic in terms of its duration?
  - Is there a history of asthma, chronic lung disease, or exposure to smoke or toxic fumes that would increase the risk for atelectasis?

PHYSICAL EXAM
- May be normal
- Tachypnea
- Rales or rhonchi
- The most specific sign is localized decrease or loss of breath sounds.
- Dullness to percussion if large area involved
- Tracheal deviation and shift of heart sounds toward atelectatic side
- Localized wheezes in cases of partial obstruction
- Cyanosis (seen when extensive atelectasis is present, causing impairment of oxygenation and areas of ventilation/perfusion mismatch)

DIFFERENTIAL DIAGNOSIS
- Pneumonia
  - Viral pneumonia versus subsegmental atelectasis
  - Bacterial pneumonia versus segmental or lobar atelectasis
- Thymus (may often be mistaken for atelectasis in an upper lobe)
- Congenital malformations (e.g., sequestration, bronchogenic cyst)
- Pleural effusion
- Asthma (acute exacerbation or poorly controlled)

DIAGNOSTIC TESTS & INTERPRETATION
Initial Tests (screening, lab, imaging)
- Appropriate test depends on the underlying etiology:
  - Asthma
    - Spirometry
  - Cystic fibrosis
    - Sweat test
  - Infection
    - Cultures (sputum, blood, bronchoalveolar lavage fluid)
    - Nasal washing (especially for viruses)
    - PPD (when tuberculosis is suspected)
  - Foreign body aspiration
    - Bronchoscopy (to remove the obstructing agent. Rigid bronchoscopy is indicated if the obstructing agent is a foreign body; flexible: can be used for mucous plugs, plastic bronchitis, or infectious etiology)

- Immunodeficiency
  - CBC with differential
  - Immunoglobulins (IgG, IgA, IgM)
  - HIV testing
- Congenital malformations
  - CT scan of the chest (for lung malformation)
  - Bronchoscopy (for H-type tracheoesophageal fistula [TEF] or bronchial stenosis)
- Chest radiograph
  - Most important diagnostic tool
  - Radiographic signs of atelectasis:
    - Loss of lung volume from the affected lobe
    - Compensatory hyperexpansion of the remaining lobes on the affected side
    - Shift of interlobar fissures
    - Elevation of diaphragm
    - Mediastinal shift toward the affected side
    - Approximation of ribs on the affected side
- CT of chest
  - Confluence of bronchi and blood vessels converge toward the affected side.
  - Provides information regarding precise location and extent of any obstructing process

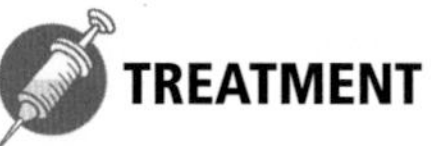

TREATMENT

GENERAL MEASURES

- Treat underlying disease (i.e., removal of aspirated foreign body, clearance of mucous plugs, treatment of any underlying infection).
- Chest physical therapy +/− bronchodilators (duration is dependent of the extent of the atelectasis)
- If no improvement with conservative therapy, a bronchoscopy with lavage to remove possible mucous plug(s) is indicated (lavage may be with saline or, in select cases, with recombinant human DNase, *N*-acetylcysteine, or hypertonic saline).
- Consider surgery to remove the affected region:
  - Chronic or recurrent atelectasis
  - Unresponsive to therapy
  - Focal bronchiectasis has developed.
  - Significant morbidity documented
- Prevention of recurrent or future atelectasis: directed toward underlying cause, when applicable
- Airway clearance is important in clearing areas of atelectasis.
- Various techniques are available including the following:
  - Manuel chest physiotherapy
  - Mechanical chest physiotherapy (high-frequency chest wall oscillation—the Vest)
  - Incentive spirometry
  - Acapella or Flutter devices
  - Intermittent positive pressure breathing (IPPB) or intrapulmonary percussive ventilator (IPV)
  - Mechanical insufflator–exsufflator (Cough Assist):
    - For patients with weakened cough (i.e., neuromuscular weakness)

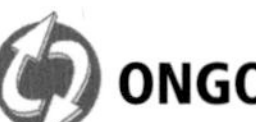

ONGOING CARE

FOLLOW-UP RECOMMENDATIONS

Patient Monitoring

Expect improvement: 1 to 3 months in typical, uncomplicated cases.

PROGNOSIS

- Depends on the underlying disease process
- In otherwise healthy individuals: excellent

COMPLICATIONS

- Recurrent infections
- Bronchiectasis
- Hemoptysis
- Abscess formation
- Fibrosis of the pulmonary parenchyma

ADDITIONAL READING

- Altunhan H, Annagür A, Pekcan S, et al. Comparing the efficacy of nebulizer recombinant human DNase and hypertonic saline as monotherapy and combined treatment in the treatment of persistent atelectasis in mechanically ventilated newborns. *Pediatr Int*. 2012;54(1):131–136.
- Birnkrant DJ, Pope JF, Eiben RM. Management of the respiratory complications of neuromuscular diseases in the pediatric intensive care unit. *J Child Neurol*. 1999;14(3):139–143.
- Hough JL, Flenady V, Johnston L, et al. Chest physiotherapy for reducing respiratory morbidity in infants requiring ventilatory support. *Cochrane Database Syst Rev*. 2008;(3):CD006445.
- McCool FD, Rosen MJ. Nonpharmacologic airway clearance therapies: ACCP evidence-based clinical practical guidelines. *Chest*. 2006;129(Suppl 1):250S–259S.
- Oermann CM, Moore RH. Foolers: things that look like pneumonia in children. *Semin Respir Infect*. 1996;11(3):204–213.
- Redding GJ. Atelectasis in childhood. *Pediatr Clin North Am*. 1984;31(4):891–905.
- Riethmueller J, Kumpf M, Borth-Bruhns T, et al. Clinical and in vitro effect of dornase alfa in mechanically ventilated pediatric non-cystic fibrosis patients with atelectases. *Cell Physiol Biochem*. 2009;23(1–3):205–210.
- Slattery DM, Waltz DA, Denham B, et al. Bronchoscopically administered recombinant human DNase for lobar atelectasis in cystic fibrosis. *Pediatr Pulmonol*. 2001;31(5):383–388.

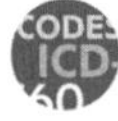

CODES

ICD10

- J98.11 Atelectasis
- P28.10 Unspecified atelectasis of newborn
- P28.0 Primary atelectasis of newborn

FAQ

- Q: What should be considered if atelectasis is recurrent in nature but in different segments?
- A: Asthma should always be considered if atelectasis is recurrent and in varying segments.
- Q: When is the optimal time for bronchoscopy?
- A: There are no established criteria for when a bronchoscopy should be performed. A bronchoscopy should be done early in the course of illness when:
  - There is a high suspicion of a foreign body.
  - Significant respiratory distress is present.
  - Cases of acute chest syndrome in patients with sickle cell disease
  - The atelectasis is extensive and conservative treatment is ineffective.
  - Bronchoscopy is infrequently performed in patients with cystic fibrosis secondary to its recurrent nature.

ATOPIC DERMATITIS

ElShadey Bekele, MD, MPH

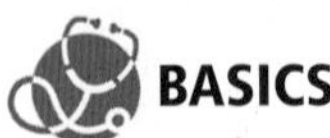

BASICS

DESCRIPTION

Atopic dermatitis (AD) is a chronic inflammatory state of the skin characterized by pruritus, erythema, induration, and scale of the skin. It is the result of chronic inflammation resulting from abnormalities of skin barrier structures, an immunologic response to environmental allergens, defects in innate immunity, and an altered microbiome.

EPIDEMIOLOGY

- 45% of those with AD have symptoms in the first 6 months of life; 60% during the 1st year and 85% before the age of 5 years old
- There is higher prevalence in urban versus rural populations.
- Prevalence of AD is 20% in the United States. Internationally, estimates range widely between 0.3% and 20.5%.
- 13.4% have AD by the age of 1 year and 21.5% have AD by 2 years of age.

RISK FACTORS

Genetics

- Genetic predisposition in affected patients with 30–70% of family members having atopy (allergies, asthma, eczema)
- Mode of inheritance is not well-defined and is likely multifactorial.
- Exact causes of AD are unknown, but defects in the filaggrin genes are known to increase the risk of AD and conditions such as ichthyosis vulgaris by impairing keratinization and causing defects in the epidermal barrier.

GENERAL PREVENTION

- One key factor in preventing AD flares is through using emollients to retain moisture of the skin.
- Another useful tactic is the avoidance of exacerbating factors. These include heat, low humidity, sweat, excess saliva, nonbreathable clothing fabrics, infections, bathing without moisturizing immediately afterwards, harsh solvents, and detergents.

PATHOPHYSIOLOGY

- AD is due to a combination of impairment of skin barrier and an abnormal immune response.
- Defects in skin barrier integrity result in increased water loss in both skin marked with lesions as well as unaffected skin. Irritants and allergens impair the skin's barrier functions leading to cytokine production, inflammation, and development of eczematous lesions. Defects in the skin barrier lead to allergen penetration leading to sensitization.
- Abnormalities of the immunologic reaction such as a strong type 2 T-helper cell (TH2) response to environmental allergens and defects in innate immunity lead to an increased inflammatory state.
- On histology typical findings of AD include spongiosis (edema of the epidermis), acanthosis, hyperkeratosis, and lymphohistiocytic infiltrate of the dermis. Spongiosis leads to stretching and rupture of intercellular attachments with vesicle formation.
- AD is a disorder of immune dysregulation with increased T-cell activation and increased cytokine production of interleukin (IL)-4, IL-5, and IL-13, which lead to increased IgE production.

ETIOLOGY

- The exact cause of AD is still under debate but it is the result of dysfunction of the innate skin barrier, genetic predisposition, environmental exposures, and immune dysregulation. Increased viral (warts and molluscum) and dermatophyte infections seen in atopic patients appear to be related to cytokine-induced suppression of endogenous antimicrobial peptides.
- Patients often have elevated IgE levels and decreased chemotaxis of neutrophils.

DIAGNOSIS

HISTORY

- Diagnosis is based on history of symptoms, family history, and physical exam.
- Important elements of the history include sleep impairment, age of onset, pruritus, soap and detergent use, family history of atopy, asthma, or allergic rhinitis.
- Assessment of sleep disturbance, itching, impact on daily activities, area of body covered by lesions, skin thickening, bleeding, alteration of pigmentation, oozing or cracking of skin

PHYSICAL EXAM

- Skin findings include erythema, xerosis, diaper area spared, lichenification, dyspigmentation.
- Infants have red, scaly pruritic, crusted lesions on extensor surfaces, trunk, extensor surfaces, cheeks, or scalp with sparing of diaper area.
- Children: flexor surfaces (wrists, ankles, antecubital, or popliteal fossae)
- Older children and adolescents often have lichenified plaques with distribution in flexural surfaces especially antecubital and popliteal fossae, volar aspect of wrists, ankles, and neck; also may have reticulate pigmentation of the neck
- Adults have more localized and lichenified lesions in skin flexures also involving the face, neck, or hands.
- Acute flares reveal erythematous and scaly maculopapular exudative patches.
- Chronic disease is characterized by hyperpigmentation or hypopigmentation, lichenification, and scaling.
- Severe AD can present as exfoliative erythroderma with diffuse scaling and erythema.
- Other associated findings include Dennie-Morgan folds (infraorbital folds), pityriasis alba (dry white patches), hyperlinear palms, facial pallor, infraorbital darkening, follicular accentuation, keratosis pilaris (dry, rough hair follicles on extensor surfaces of upper arms and thighs), and ichthyosis.

DIFFERENTIAL DIAGNOSIS

- Tinea corporis
- Severe seborrheic dermatitis
- Contact dermatitis
- Allergic or irritant psoriasis
- Wiskott-Aldrich syndrome
- Langerhans cell histiocytosis
- Acrodermatitis enteropathica
- Secondary syphilis
- HIV/AIDS related skin changes
- Netherton syndrome
- Viral exanthema
- Ichthyosis vulgaris
- Food allergy
- Drug eruptions
- Phenylketonuria
- Nutritional deficiencies
- Scabies
- Xerosis
- Hyper-IgE syndrome
- Metabolic deficiencies (carboxylase or prolidase)

DIAGNOSTIC TESTS & INTERPRETATION

- AD is a clinical diagnosis without a diagnostic test. Laboratory testing may be used to distinguish from other conditions or to diagnose complications such as infections.
- Biopsy can be helpful to rule out other skin disorders, such as psoriasis.
- IgE levels can be elevated but need not be checked.
- Bacterial cultures of skin can be obtained to rule out superinfections.
- Rapid fluorescent antibody studies, polymerase chain reaction studies, or viral cultures, and Tzanck smear can identify the presence of eczema herpeticum (EH).

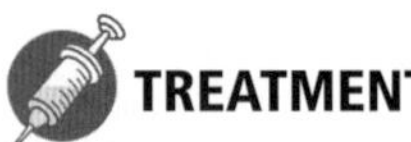

TREATMENT

GENERAL MEASURES

- Treatment approaches address restoration of skin barrier, removal of allergens, and hydration of the skin.
- Avoid factors such as heat and low humidity.
- Frequent use of emollients to promote moisture retention; creams with low water and high oil content or ointments at least twice a day and immediately after bathing
- Treat skin infections.
- Antihistamines to control itching
- Avoidance of irritants and allergens that could trigger a flare. Common agents are soaps, lotions, and detergents with fragrances.
- Dilute bleach bath: Apply topical steroids to the affected areas and moisturizer to the rest of the skin. Moist gauze or cotton clothing dampened by warm water is then applied with a layer of dry cotton clothing on top. The dressings can be left on for 3 to 8 hours. They can also be used for 24 to 72 hours or overnight for up to 1 week.

MEDICATION

First Line

- Topical corticosteroids starting with low potency and progressively increasing potency based on severity of disease. The face, neck, and skin folds are sensitive to local side effects so lower potency steroids should be used in these areas. (see Appendix: Table 15).
- Adverse effects include skin atrophy, telangiectasias, folliculitis, intraocular hypertension, cataracts, periorificial dermatitis, and contact dermatitis.

Second Line

- Topical calcineurin inhibitors have been approved for children >2 years of age and include tacrolimus and pimecrolimus. They are used in moderate to severe AD.
- Due to case reports, animal studies and known risks of systemic calcineurin inhibitors, in 2006 the FDA issued a black box warning for cancer for topical calcineurin inhibitors although a direct causal relationship has not been established.

- The most common adverse effects are localized burning and stinging sensation at the site of application.
- These topical agents act to suppress T-cell function.
- Sun damage can be potentiated, so children who receive these medications should receive instructions for diligent sun protection and sunscreen use.
- Systemic steroids are generally not used because of the chronicity of AD. They are reserved for refractory AD, and if used, it should only be for a short duration.
- Phototherapy with UVB can be used in patients with extensive disease resistant to other therapies. Not used for infants or young children. Side effects include erythema, herpes simplex reactivation, and polymorphic light eruption. Carcinogenic risk is unknown.
- Crisaborole is a topical phosphodiesterase-4 inhibitor approved by FDA in December 2016 for patients >2 years old with mild to moderate AD. Applied topically twice a day. The most frequently reported adverse effect is application site pain and paresthesias. Data on long-term safety and efficacy are still needed.
- Oral antibiotics are indicated when there is superinfection of lesions.
- Oral antivirals are indicated in cases of EH.
- Oral antihistamines such as diphenhydramine or hydroxyzine can be effective in reducing the itching sensation but may cause sedation. Other antihistamines such as cetirizine or loratadine do not have sedating effects but are less effective although may be useful for those who have environmental triggers. Topical antihistamines are not effective and may have irritants that can worsen AD.
- Topical barrier repair agents including N-palmitoylethanolamine cream, MAS063DP cream, and various ceramide formulations may be useful adjuncts to therapy.

ISSUES FOR REFERRAL

Referral should be considered in the following circumstances:

- If the diagnosis of AD is in question
- The patient does not respond to treatment.
- If high potency steroids are being considered for sensitive areas such as face or skin folds
- If the child may need immunosuppressive therapy

ADMISSION, INPATIENT, AND NURSING CONSIDERATIONS

- Admission for AD alone is uncommon but may be necessary for severe AD flares unresponsive to outpatient therapy.
- Superinfections with bacteria or herpes herpticum requiring IV treatment
- Persistent AD requiring further workup for alternative diagnosis

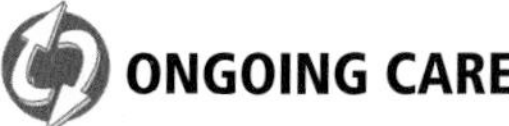

ONGOING CARE

FOLLOW-UP RECOMMENDATIONS

Patient Monitoring

- AD is a chronic disease which has multiple relapses. The chronicity of the disease should be highlighted for families as prevention of flares through daily use of emollients is crucial.
- It should be emphasized to parents that AD is a chronic disease and that good skin care is necessary to control disease activity and enhance quality of life.
- To improve compliance with treatment, providers should use therapeutic patient education techniques so parents and patients can manage this chronic disease.
- Address parental concerns about the safety of topical steroids in order to reduce steroid phobia.

PROGNOSIS

The majority of children with AD have resolution of symptoms by adulthood. Studies have shown that by 8 years after diagnosis, 80% did not have persistence of symptoms and 20 years after <5% had persistence of symptoms. About 40–70% of children with AD no longer have symptoms by age 6 to 7 years. Children with later onset and severe AD are more likely to have persistent disease into adolescence and adulthood.

COMPLICATIONS

- The major complications are viral and bacterial infections.
- Decreased cell-mediated immunity, decreased chemotaxis, and decreased production of endogenous antimicrobial peptides can result in increased infection. In addition, given the fissures and open excoriations, there is a risk of superinfection. The decreased integrity of the skin can result in widely spread cutaneous infections.
- The most common bacterial infection is with *Staphylococcus aureus*. AD is a risk factor for MRSA colonization. Colonization rates of MRSA are higher in those with AD (11–34%) than the general population (1–3%). The virulence of this bacteria in patients with AD is partially due to the production of staphylococcal enterotoxins which act as superantigens. MRSA is associated with increased skin infections. Those colonized are less responsive to topical corticosteroids.
- *S. aureus* infections can be superficial or invasive leading to bacteremia, endocarditis, septic arthritis, or osteomyelitis.
- The most commonly associated fungal infection is *Malassezia* species and can induce inflammation by cell-mediated immunity and IgE production.
- EH is caused by the herpes simplex virus (HSV). Those with EH usually have more severe or earlier onset of AD as well as increased risk of food allergies and asthma compared to AD patients without EH. EH can cause disseminated vesicles with skin breakdown, viremia, lymphadenopathy, or more severe infections such as meningitis or keratoconjunctivitis. Can be life-threatening. Infections are treated with acyclovir.
- Similar problems can also be seen with coxsackievirus or molluscum contagiosum and used to occur with the smallpox vaccine.
- Early growth delay is not uncommon among children with AD, although later catch-up growth is generally seen. This may be related to impaired growth hormone release. Growth delay can occur independent of topical steroid exposure.
- Increased prevalence of emotional, behavioral, and psychological issues secondary to sleep disturbance

ADDITIONAL READING

- Kim JP, Chao LX, Simpson EL, et al. Persistence of atopic dermatitis (AD): a systematic review and meta-analysis. *J Am Acad Dermatol*. 2016;75(4):681–687.e11.
- Montes-Torres A, Llamas-Velasco M, Pérez-Plaza A, et al. Biological treatments in atopic dermatitis. *J Clin Med*. 2015;4(4):593–613.
- Paller AS, Tom WL, Lebwohl MG, et al. Efficacy and safety of crisaborole ointment, a novel, nonsteroidal phosphodiesterase 4 (PDE4) inhibitor for the topical treatment of atopic dermatitis (AD) in children and adults. *J Am Acad Dermatol*. 2016;75(3):494–503.e6.
- Pyun BY. Natural history and risk factors of atopic dermatitis in children. *Allergy Asthma Immunol Res*. 2015;7(2):101–105.
- Siegfried E, Hebert A. Diagnosis of atopic dermatitis: mimics, overlaps, and complications. *J Clin Med*. 2015;4(5):884–917.
- Tollefson MM, Bruckner AL; for Section On Dermatology. Atopic dermatitis: skin-directed management. *Pediatrics*. 2014;134(6):e1735–e1744.

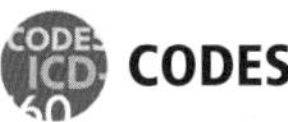

CODES

ICD10

- L20.9 Atopic dermatitis, unspecified
- L20.83 Infantile (acute) (chronic) eczema
- L20.89 Other atopic dermatitis

FAQ

- Q: If my child has AD will he/she develop food allergies or asthma?
- A: Children with AD are more likely to develop allergic rhinitis and asthma than the general population, referred to as the atopic march. These children also produce higher levels of IgE and have a higher incidence of sensitization to allergens with a higher likelihood of developing food allergies. One theory for this progression is introduction of allergens through an impaired skin barrier leading to food sensitization.
- Q: What can I do to prevent my child from having eczema flares?
- A: With AD that is responsive to topical therapies one approach to preventing flares is a proactive method. Topical corticosteroids can be used intermittently, twice a day, 2 days per week for 16 weeks. For infants and children, low potency topical steroids can be used and for adolescents and adults moderate to high potency.
- Q: What new treatments are being developed for AD?
- A: Currently under investigation is a monoclonal antibody, dupilumab, which targets IL-4 and inhibits IL-4 and IL-13.
- Q: What are the systemic adverse effects with topical steroid use?
- A: Systemic absorption of topical steroids can result in suppression of the hypothalamic pituitary adrenal axis, iatrogenic Cushing syndrome, impaired growth in infants and children, glaucoma, vision loss, avascular necrosis of femoral head, and severe disseminate CMV. Several factors increase the risk of such side effects including young age, impaired skin barrier, penetration through mucous membranes and scrotal skin, high potency steroids, frequency and duration and occlusion of application, and/or simultaneous use of drugs classified as CYP3A4 inhibitors.

ATRIAL SEPTAL DEFECT

Jonathan T. Fleenor, MD, FACC, FAAP

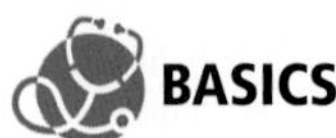

BASICS

DESCRIPTION

- An opening in the atrial septum, other than a patent foramen ovale (PFO)
- Four major types of atrial septal defects (ASDs)
  - Secundum ASD
  - Primum ASD
  - Sinus venosus ASD
  - Coronary sinus ASD
- PFO
  - Usually does not cause a significant intracardiac shunt
  - A probe-patent PFO can be found in up to 15–25% of normal hearts at pathologic exam.
- Secundum defects
  - Make up 60–70% of all ASDs
  - Usually, there is a shunt from the left atrium to the right atrium.
- Primum defects
  - Occur in ~30% of all ASDs
  - They are usually associated with a cleft mitral valve. This defect is the result of an abnormality of the endocardial cushions and therefore is also referred to as an incomplete atrioventricular (AV) canal defect.
- Sinus venosus defects
  - Can be of the superior or inferior vena caval type and occur in ~5–10% of all ASDs
  - In ASDs of the superior vena caval type, the right pulmonary veins (usually right upper lobe) may drain anomalously to the superior vena cava or right atrium.
- Coronary sinus ASDs
  - Rare and occur in <1% of all ASDs
  - They are often associated with absence of the coronary sinus and a persistent left superior vena cava that joins the roof of the left atrium (also known as an "unroofed coronary sinus").

EPIDEMIOLOGY

Females > males (2:1)

Incidence

- Difficult to determine
- Represents 6–10% of all cardiac anomalies encountered

PATHOPHYSIOLOGY

- A left-to-right shunt occurs through the ASD. For large defects, this results in right atrial and right ventricular volume overload.
- There is usually increased pulmonary blood flow.
- The left-to-right shunt generally increases with time as pulmonary resistance drops and right ventricular compliance normalizes.
- Moderate and large defects are associated with a Qp/Qs ratio of >2:1.
- The direction of atrial shunting is determined by the relative compliance of the right and left ventricles.

ETIOLOGY

- ASDs may be associated with partial or total anomalous pulmonary venous drainage, mitral valve anomalies, transposition of the great arteries, or tricuspid atresia.
- Although usually isolated, ASDs may occur as part of a syndrome (Holt-Oram [autosomal dominant]).

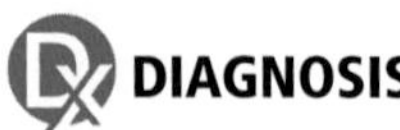

DIAGNOSIS

HISTORY

- Most infants are asymptomatic.
- Older children with moderate left-to-right shunts are often asymptomatic but may have mild fatigue or dyspnea, especially with exercise.
- Children with large left-to-right shunts may complain of fatigue and dyspnea, which may become noticeable as the child gets older.
- Growth failure is uncommon.
- Older patients with large atrial shunts may develop atrial arrhythmias.

PHYSICAL EXAM

- Inspection and palpation of the precordium are usually normal, although older children with a large ASD may have a hyperdynamic precordium, right ventricular heave, or precordial bulge.
- Auscultation reveals three important features:
  - Wide and "fixed" splitting of S2. Splitting of S2 (A2 and P2 components) is caused by a delay in emptying of a volume-loaded right ventricle.
  - A systolic ejection murmur at the upper left sternal border. This murmur is caused by an increase in blood flow across a normal pulmonary valve. It may be differentiated from the murmur of pulmonary stenosis because there is no click.
  - A diastolic murmur at the lower sternal border, indicating a Qp/Qs ratio of at least 2:1. This murmur is caused by increased flow across the tricuspid valve.

DIFFERENTIAL DIAGNOSIS

- Ventricular septal defect
- Patent ductus arteriosus
- AV canal defect
- Valvar pulmonary stenosis

DIAGNOSTIC TESTS & INTERPRETATION

Initial Tests (screening, lab, imaging)

- ECG
  - Usually normal sinus rhythm with an rSR′ (incomplete right bundle branch block pattern) in leads V1, V3R, and V4R, indicating right ventricular volume overload
  - For larger shunts, ECG may show evidence of right atrial enlargement as well as 1st-degree AV block. A late finding suggestive of pulmonary hypertension is right ventricular hypertrophy.
- Chest radiograph
  - Cardiomegaly (right atrium and right ventricle), increased pulmonary vascular markings, and a dilated pulmonary trunk are seen in patients with significant left-to-right shunts.

- Echocardiogram
  - A 2D echo study is diagnostic; it reveals the location, size, and associated defects, if any.
  - It may demonstrate dilated right heart structures. Color Doppler generally permits visualization of the direction of shunt flow.
  - Older children and adolescents may require transesophageal echo to best define the ASD.
- Cardiac catheterization
  - Generally unnecessary
  - It is indicated when pulmonary vascular disease is suspected (determination of pulmonary vascular resistance) or for associated cardiac defects.

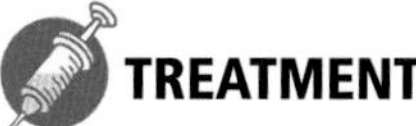

TREATMENT

GENERAL MEASURES

- Infants with congestive heart failure should be treated with diuretics.
- Elective closure is indicated for ASDs associated with large left-to-right shunts, cardiomegaly, or symptoms.
  - The timing of closure is usually deferred until 3 to 5 years of age.
  - For most secundum-type ASDs, device closure of the defect can be performed in the cardiac catheterization laboratory, thus avoiding surgery.
- Prevention of paradoxical emboli and cerebrovascular accidents is an uncommon but possible indication for closure of ASDs or PFO.
- Irreversible pulmonary hypertension from a long-term left-to-right shunt usually does not occur until adolescence or young adulthood.
- Sinus venosus, primum, and coronary sinus–type ASDs require surgical closure. The mortality of surgical repair for an uncomplicated ASD approaches 0%.
- There is some anecdotal evidence suggesting that PFOs are a cause of migraine headaches in certain populations. Prospective adult studies are currently ongoing to further investigate this question, but to date, no study has found an indication for PFO closure in migraine patients.

ONGOING CARE

FOLLOW-UP RECOMMENDATIONS

Patient Monitoring

- Children with typical auscultation, chest radiograph, and ECG findings should undergo an echocardiographic evaluation to determine the location and size of the ASD.
- Children with ASDs should have regular follow-up to assess for signs of congestive heart failure or right ventricular volume overload. Restriction of activity is unnecessary. Subacute bacterial endocarditis (SBE) prophylaxis is not indicated for an isolated secundum ASD. Residual ASD after surgery is rare.
- SBE prophylaxis is indicated for the first 6 months (assuming no residual defect) after closure of a secundum defect.
- Complications related to surgery include the following:
  - Sinus node dysfunction
  - Venous obstruction (facial or pulmonary edema) may occur after a sinus venosus ASD repair.
  - Postpericardiotomy syndrome, which manifests with nausea, vomiting, chest pain, abdominal pain, or fever, may occur a few weeks after surgical repair. Although a friction rub may not be present, the chest radiograph may show cardiomegaly and the echocardiogram may reveal a pericardial effusion.

PROGNOSIS

- The prognosis for small ASDs seems excellent without specific therapy.
- Spontaneous closure of small secundum ASDs can occur in up to 80% of infants in the 1st year of life. Isolated secundum ASDs of moderate and large size do not typically cause symptoms in most infants and children.
- Pulmonary hypertension is rare in childhood.
- Atrial flutter and fibrillation occur in up to 13% of unoperated patients >40 years of age.
- Bacterial endocarditis is rare in children with isolated ASD.
- Paradoxical emboli may occur and should be considered in patients with cerebral or systemic emboli.

ADDITIONAL READING

- Horton SC, Bunch TJ. Patent foramen ovale and stroke. *Mayo Clin Proc.* 2004;79(1):79–88.
- Kharouf R, Luxenberg DM, Khalid O, et al. Atrial septal defect: spectrum of care. *Pediatr Cardiol.* 2008;29(2):271–280.
- Meijboom F, Roos-Hesselink J, Sievert H. The role of the atria in congenital heart disease. *Cardiol Clin.* 2002;20(3):351–366.
- Ohye RG, Bove EL. Advances in congenital heart surgery. *Curr Opin Pediatr.* 2001;13(5):473–481.
- Radzik D, Davignon A, van Doesburg N, et al. Predictive factors for spontaneous closure of atrial septal defects diagnosed in the first 3 months of life. *J Am Coll Cardiol.* 1993;22(3):851–853.
- Rocchini AP. Pediatric cardiac catheterization. *Curr Opin Cardiol.* 2002;17(3):283–288.
- Zanchetta M, Rigatelli G, Pedon L, et al. Role of intracardiac echocardiography in atrial septal abnormalities. *J Interv Cardiol.* 2003;16(1):63–77.

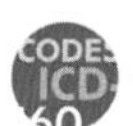

CODES

ICD10

- Q21.1 Atrial septal defect
- Q21.2 Atrioventricular septal defect

FAQ

- Q: When should a moderate secundum ASD be closed?
- A: This can generally be electively performed in children prior to their starting grade school.
- Q: What is the significance of a patient having gastrointestinal complaints (nausea and vomiting) 2 to 3 weeks after surgical closure of an ASD?
- A: This may represent a pericardial effusion (postpericardiotomy syndrome).

ATTENTION-DEFICIT/HYPERACTIVITY DISORDER

D. David O'Banion, MD • Mark Wolraich, MD

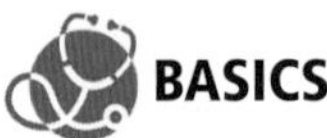

BASICS

DESCRIPTION

- Attention-deficit/hyperactivity disorder (ADHD) is a chronic condition that is characterized by a persistent pattern of developmentally inappropriate inattention and/or hyperactivity/impulsivity interfering with function or development.
- *DSM-5* criteria for diagnosis lists 18 core symptoms:
  - At least 6 of 9 symptoms of inattention and/or 6 of 9 hyperactivity/impulsivity symptoms (5 of 9 in individuals >17 years of age)
  - These maladaptive symptoms have been persisting for at least 6 months.
  - Clear impairment, interference, or reduction in quality of academic, social, occupational function
  - Several symptoms existed before age 12 years, several symptoms present in two or more settings (e.g., home, school, day care, after-school activities, church, and community activities).
- Classified into three subtypes:
  - Hyperactive/impulsive
  - Inattentive
  - Combined type (most frequently comes to clinical attention)
- Symptoms not solely due to opposition and cannot be better explained by another mental health disorder. Autism spectrum disorder is no longer an exclusion criterion.

EPIDEMIOLOGY

- 2:1 male-to-female ratio
- 3–10% prevalence of school-age children
- Females more likely to have inattentive type

RISK FACTORS

Studies using MRI and other imaging demonstrate differences in brain anatomy, function and connectivity between executive functioning networks and reward networks, implicating dopamine and noradrenergic transmission in ADHD.

Genetics

- Risk of ADHD in 1st-degree relatives is ~25%.
- Concordance in monozygotic twins: 59–81%; dizygotic twins: 33%

COMMONLY ASSOCIATED CONDITIONS

- Learning disorders
- Language disorders
- Anxiety and mood disorders
- Sleep disorders
- Tic disorder (may affect treatment decisions)
- Oppositional defiant disorder and conduct disorder
- Poor social skills

DIAGNOSIS

- Primary care clinicians should consider an extended visit to evaluate any child, age 4 to 18 years, presenting with behavioral and/or academic problems related to ADHD symptoms.
- To make the diagnosis, the clinician should ensure *DSM-5* criteria are met, document impairments in at least one major setting (e.g., home, school, day care). Information should be gathered from more than one reporter, ideally (e.g., caregivers and teachers).

ALERT

Avoid the common mistake of delaying diagnosis indefinitely due to inability to obtain Teacher Rating Scale. Informal teacher report (letter) or parent report of school symptoms may suffice.

- In general, the diagnosis does not require any specific psychological test, laboratory test, or referral.
- Watchful waiting is not recommended, as evidence-based treatments can make significant improvements even at a young age.

HISTORY

- A detailed history of the child's behavior at home, school, and with peers
- Onset and duration of noted behaviors: Sudden onset should prompt consideration of other conditions (mood disorder, trauma, abuse, substance use, etc.).
- Timing of behaviors with respect to developmentally appropriate expectations placed on the child
- Frequent or excessive need of supervision and redirection in age-appropriate common tasks and routines
- Not following rules/requests—oppositional and/or "forgetful" (getting lost or side-tracked)
- Academic progress with particular attention to problems with specific subjects and behaviors during specific subjects
- Disruption of peer relationships
- Developmental history (developmental delay is *not* characteristic of ADHD)
- Sleep history—adequate length, hygiene
- Participation in age-appropriate organized activities (e.g., scouts, camp, team sports)
- History of trauma
- Family history of dropping out of school, ADHD, or learning disorders
- Family history of early cardiac disease including arrhythmias, hypertrophic cardiomyopathy, sudden cardiac death or unexpected death in children or young adults
- Social history: those who live with patient, recent family discord, separation, recent death in the family, recent change in schools
- Past medical history and medication history
- Adverse pregnancy or birth history

ALERT

Concentrating for hours on video games is *not* evidence *against* the diagnosis. This requires sustained attention of mere seconds before the game's next action.

PHYSICAL EXAM

- Comprehensive physical and neurologic examination with attention to specific systems based on the history
- Vital signs: weight, height, pulse, BP, visual and hearing acuity
- Note any dysmorphology.
- Assess motor coordination.

DIFFERENTIAL DIAGNOSIS

- Developmental
  - Learning disabilities (common comorbidity)
  - Intellectual disability (not mutually exclusive)
  - Autism spectrum disorder (not mutually exclusive)
  - Language or speech disorder (pragmatic language disorder)
- Psychiatric
  - Depression and anxiety disorders (determine whether ADHD is primary or secondary)
  - Obsessive-compulsive disorder
  - Oppositional defiant disorder
  - Conduct disorder
  - Adjustment disorder
  - Posttraumatic stress disorder or victim of bullying
- Medical
  - Genetic disorder
  - Sleep disorder
  - Sensory impairment (vision, hearing)
  - Medication side effects
  - Toxins (lead)
  - Iron deficiency anemia
  - Postconcussion syndrome
- Educational
  - Inappropriate school environment
  - Developmentally inappropriate expectations
- Social
  - Disorganized/chaotic family environment
  - Child abuse and neglect or sexual abuse
  - Psychosocial stressors

DIAGNOSTIC TESTS & INTERPRETATION

- Validated rating scales of behavior help the clinician review *DSM-5* criteria. These can be distributed, collected, and reviewed prior to a scheduled evaluation.
  - Vanderbilt ADHD Diagnostic Rating Scale, Conners Rating Scales-Revised, SNAP, ADHD RS
  - Most clinicians choose a single tool and gain familiarity with it. Most scales are useful for measuring change over time with treatment. Ideally, collect rating scales from parents and teachers. *DSM-5* highly recommends, but doesn't require both teacher and parent scales.
  - Some assess only for ADHD; others include assessment of comorbidities such as anxiety, oppositional defiant disorder, and depression (Vanderbilt).
  - Some are proprietary (Conners), and some are freely distributed (Vanderbilt).
- IQ, cognitive, and achievement testing are not required but should be guided by specific concerns for learning and intellectual disabilities.
  - Evaluation for an Individualized Educational Program (IEP) or 504 plan may be obtained following parental written request to the child's school.
  - No neuropsychological "testing" for ADHD has been found to be necessary in children. These tests may differentiate true cases from false in older adolescents and young adults.

Initial Tests (screening, lab, imaging)

Not required except as guided by history and physical. Screening ECGs are not recommended or considered cost-effective.

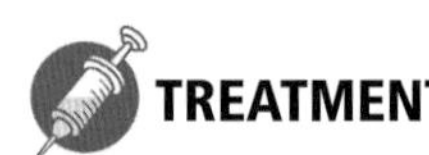

TREATMENT

GENERAL MEASURES

- Treat ADHD as a chronic disease and use the medical home model. Partner and discuss treatment options with families (both parents and patients). Include the school when possible.
- The family and patient choose target goals and actively participate in measuring/monitoring achievement of these goals.
- Three treatment modalities:
  - Behavior therapy (evidence-based programs exist)
  - Educational support and accommodations
  - Medication (strongest evidence for effect)

- Nonpharmacologic
  - Behavior therapy and parent training
    - Reduces core symptoms of ADHD in multiple settings
    - Parent education, parent training programs, and behavior therapies usually have a planned number of weeks (10 to 16 weeks). Their focus is increasing positive behavior through rewards and extinguishing negative behavior with effective discipline.

ALERT

Common "counseling" and talk/play therapy have *not* been found efficacious.

- Psychological support may be helpful for:
  - Poor peer relations, such as peer groups or social training groups
  - Patient with a comorbidity
  - Commonly, families have difficulty with parenting a child with ADHD.
- Cognitive behavioral therapy (CBT) may be helpful for older children and adults.
- Educational support options:
  - 504 plans benefit many children with ADHD. Request through patient's school an evaluation for accommodations (different than an IEP).
  - Small teacher-to-student ratio is ideal.
  - Suggest ways to improve communication between school and home (i.e., school-home daily report). Card relieves forgetful child of responsibility for turning in homework dutifully completed at home.

MEDICATION

Consider treatment goal, family preferences, other family member's reaction to specific medications, duration of coverage (shorter school day in younger child), ability to swallow pills, and concern for divergence (or abuse).

First Line

CNS stimulants: FDA-approved. All are either methylphenidate or amphetamine-class derivatives. Both classes increase synaptic dopamine and norepinephrine by inhibiting reuptake, thereby improving signal transmission of "planning" networks.

- Efficacy: extensive evidence supporting efficacy and safety. 80% of children with ADHD show significant improvement if titrated appropriately.
- Pharmacokinetics: Individual response is highly variable. Effectiveness and side effects can be seen within hours of starting medication. Duration varies by preparation. Younger children may metabolize stimulants more slowly, giving a longer duration than expected for immediate-release preparations. Does not "build up" in the system, so no known permanent effects; daily dosing required for symptom relief and weekend med breaks do not impede weekday efficacy.
- Dose: Weight-based dosing is not appropriate due to differences in metabolism and idiosyncratic responses. Start with smallest dose and titrate up in single-dose increments weekly as needed. Base titrations on changes in rating scales and achievement toward target goals, weighing improvements against side effects. Start with short-acting medication in children <7 years. For some younger children, this may provide a sufficient duration of therapy for school. Consider long-acting/extended-release in older children. Start medication when the parents are available to watch for side effects and duration of action (typically over a weekend). Follow closely with the parents; ask them to get feedback from school on a weekly basis until dose is properly adjusted. This process may take 1 to 2 months to be completed with frequent communication with caregivers. If at highest dose and still not having good effect, or having significant side effects at a lower dose, switch to the lowest dose of the other class of stimulants and repeat the titration process.
- Side effects: Side effects last <24 hours. Families should know that any unacceptable side effects will abate if the medication is stopped. Medication is safe to stop "cold turkey." Most side effects can be managed expectantly.
  - Decreased appetite is common, although sustained weight loss is not.
  - Abdominal pain, tics, headache, difficulty falling asleep, and jitteriness
  - Difficulty shifting attention, overfocus (the "zombie effect"), indicates too high dose for that patient.
  - Severe movement disorders, obsessive-compulsive thoughts, or psychotic symptoms are rare and cease when medication is stopped.
  - Growth velocity may slow. Final adult height is small to minimally decreased.
- Contraindications: glaucoma, symptomatic cardiovascular disease (except with guidance by cardiology), hyperthyroidism, hypertension

Second Line

- Atomoxetine: selective norepinephrine uptake inhibitor. Once-a-day or b.i.d. dosing. Must be taken daily during treatment. 6 weeks before effects are at maximum. Side effect profile similar to stimulants but with slightly increased chance of suicidal thinking. Less evidence for use, less efficacious than stimulants. Start with 0.5 mg/kg/24 h for 1 week, if no side effects (often GI upset); increase to 1.2 mg/kg/24 h, max 1.4 mg/kg/24 h or 100 mg/24 h if >70 kg.
- Adjuvants: extended-release α-adrenergic agonists (clonidine, guanfacine). Must take daily; commonly causes sedation that may improve with time

ISSUES FOR REFERRAL

- Young children not responding to effective behavior therapy or therapy not available (i.e., considering meds)
- When comorbidities are suspected or when contraindications for treatment are present
- If patient is not responding to titration attempts of both stimulant classes
- If the patient is having difficulty tolerating different stimulants or having unexpected or severe side effects

COMPLEMENTARY & ALTERNATIVE THERAPIES

- Most complementary and alternative medicine (CAM) treatments have not been found to be efficacious. Polyunsaturated fatty acid supplementation may be of variable benefit. No dietary changes have proven efficacy.
- Studies of EEG neurofeedback do not support its use as a stand-alone treatment.

ONGOING CARE

FOLLOW-UP RECOMMENDATIONS

- Initially, follow-up by phone/email may be every 1 to 2 weeks until proper dosing is achieved. First follow-up in clinic in 1 month. After successful titration, patients should be seen every 3 to 6 months specifically for ADHD visits.
- Consider mailing refills once titrated to prevent burden on families who'd otherwise pick up the paper prescription monthly; monthly clinic visits usually not medically necessary
- Monitor weight, height, BP, and heart rate.
- Weight loss is not usually sustained.
- Encourage meals when patient is hungry, perhaps later than family's usual dinner or large breakfast.
- Assess for change in growth velocity.
- Assess family and peer relationship.
- Assess school performance.
- Assess for ongoing need for medication. Be prepared for most adolescents to desire stopping their medication.
- Transition planning to adult care—identify a capable adult medical provider.

ADDITIONAL READING

- Graham J, Banaschewski T, Buitelaar J, et al; for European Guidelines Group. European guidelines on managing adverse effects of medication for ADHD. *Eur Child Adolesc Psychiatry*. 2011;20(1):17–37.
- Weber W, Newmark S. Complementary and alternative medical therapies for attention-deficit/hyperactivity disorder and autism. *Pediatr Clin North Am*. 2007;54(6):983–1006.
- Wolraich M, Brown L, Brown RT, et al; for Subcommittee on Attention-Deficit/Hyperactivity Disorder; Steering Committee on Quality Improvement and Management. ADHD: Clinical practice guideline for the diagnosis, evaluation, and treatment of attention-deficit/hyperactivity disorder in children and adolescents. *Pediatrics*. 2011;128(5):1007–1022.

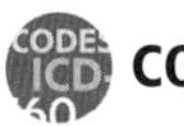

CODES

ICD10

- F90.9 Attention-deficit hyperactivity disorder, unspecified type
- F90.1 Attn-defct hyperactivity disorder, predom hyperactive type
- F90.0 Attn-defct hyperactivity disorder, predom inattentive type

FAQ

- Q: Is medication needed every day?
- A: Not exactly, but stimulants only help on days when taken. Some patients need medication daily in order to function successfully with peers or in structured environments. Others need help mainly with focus and do well with medication only on school days.
- Q: How long will my patient be on medication?
- A: A large percentage of children with ADHD will continue to have symptoms as adults. Some patients may need to continue medication through formal learning (high school and college). During this time, they should be able to learn coping strategies to minimize the effects of their symptoms. If treatment goals are being met, it is reasonable to have a trial of medications to see if performance of medications can be sustained (sometimes called a drug holiday).
- Q: Are there support groups available?
- A: A widely recognized advocacy and support organization for families is Children and Adults with Attention Deficit/Hyperactivity Disorder (www.chadd.org). Use discretion when using online resources; there are many websites sponsored by pharmaceutical companies and others that actively discourage use of currently recommended treatments.

AUTISM SPECTRUM DISORDER

Eliza Gordon-Lipkin, MD • Paul H. Lipkin, MD

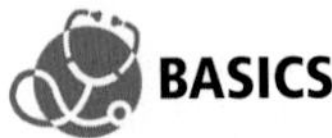

BASICS

DESCRIPTION

- Neurodevelopmental disorder characterized by:
  - Delays/impairments in development of social communication and social interaction
  - Restricted, repetitive patterns of behavior, interests, or activities
  - Symptoms present in early childhood
  - Significant impairment in functioning
- Diagnostic criteria changes since 2013:
  - *DSM-IV* previously included autistic disorder, Asperger disorder, Rett disorder, childhood disintegrative disorder, and pervasive developmental disorder, not otherwise specified within overall category
  - *DSM-5* has eliminated these separate diagnoses due to insufficient evidence.
  - *DSM-5* added severity levels (1 to 3) based on the level of support required.
- Associated with specific known genetic disorder (e.g., fragile X) in a minority (15%) of cases
- Behaviors exist along continuum with unclear boundaries between trait and disorder.

EPIDEMIOLOGY

Prevalence

- Approximately 1 in 68 (14.6 per 1,000) of 8 year-old children, according to the Centers for Disease Control and Prevention (CDC) 2016 report
- Rate rising over past decades
- 4 times more common in males than females
  - Females are more frequently severely impaired with intellectual disability.

RISK FACTORS

- Strong genetic influence: risk in 1st-degree relatives 2–18%; identical twins 35–95%
- Multiple genes implicated (>100), suggesting polygenic risk. Approximately 15% of children with autism have identifiable genetic anomaly.
- Other risk factors: closer spacing of pregnancies, advanced maternal or paternal age, extreme premature birth (<26 weeks), possible maternal inflammation in utero
- Link to vaccinations not supported by scientific evidence
- Pathophysiology unknown but may be associated with abnormalities in cortical laminar architecture during prenatal brain development

COMMONLY ASSOCIATED CONDITIONS

- Intellectual disability
- Gastrointestinal (GI) problems
- Epilepsy
- Sleep disorders
- ADHD
- Anxiety, depression, mood disturbances
- Aggression and self-injury

DIAGNOSIS

ALERT

Typically, primary care providers are the first point of contact. Developmental screening in all preschool-age children is aimed at identifying early signs that lead to diagnosis rather than waiting for a child to present with symptoms. Therefore, children with autism may present by (i) a positive developmental screen in a previously asymptomatic child or (ii) a parental or educational concern for autism.

HISTORY

- A detailed prenatal, developmental, medical, family (three generation), and social history are essential.
- Delays/impairments in social communication and social interaction:
  - Delayed language development
  - Impairment in eye contact, facial expression, nonverbal social behaviors (pulling parents by hand but not looking at them)
  - Lack of social smile, pointing, or joint attention
  - Impaired social interactions and relationships
  - Lack of imaginary play appropriate to developmental level
  - Doesn't include others in play
- Stereotyped behaviors and restricted interests:
  - Stereotypies (e.g., rocking, hand flapping)
  - Echolalia
  - Restricted range of interests/activities
  - Attachment to unusual objects, fascination with parts of objects
  - Behavioral rigidity, distress with changes in routine
  - Hyper- or hyporeactivity to sensory input or unusual sensory interests in objects or persons (smelling, touching, sensitivity to clothing)

PHYSICAL EXAM

- Growth: Failure to thrive, short stature, or overgrowth may point to genetic etiologies.
- Head circumference: 20–30% have macrocephaly, >4 SD above mean associated with *PTEN* mutations; microcephaly may be associated with TORCH infection, Angelman syndrome, Rett disorder.
- Dysmorphic features: long, thin face, prominent ears in fragile X (Macroorchidism may not be present until after puberty.)
- Skin exam: signs of self-injurious behavior; neurocutaneous syndromes, hypopigmented macules on Wood lamp exam/fibromas suggest tuberous sclerosis.
- Motor exam: stereotypical movements, motor coordination abnormalities, mirror/overflow movements; spasticity or ataxia may suggest leukodystrophy.

DIFFERENTIAL DIAGNOSIS

- Deafness: delayed/absent oral language acquisition; behavioral/social difficulties may relate to language delays.
- Intellectual disability: common comorbidity
- Social (pragmatic) communication disorder: lack of restricted, repetitive patterns of behavior or interests
- Language disorder: no deficits in social interactions or restricted range of interests
- Selective mutism: Early development is not disturbed.
- Anxiety, ADHD, obsessive-compulsive disorder, or schizophrenia: common comorbidity but have overlapping features that may lead to diagnostic overshadowing
- If regression, consider alternative diagnoses like inborn errors of metabolism or autoimmune encephalitis.

ALERT

Intellectual disability is a common comorbidity (~50%). The patient *may not* have autistic spectrum disorder if communication, behavior, play, and social skills are appropriate to developmental age.

DIAGNOSTIC TESTS & INTERPRETATION

Initial Tests (screening, lab, imaging)

- Modified Checklist for Autism in Toddlers, Revised with Follow-Up (M-CHAT-R/F) version downloadable free online (with translations in >30 languages) at mchatscreen.com
- Social Communication Questionnaire (SCQ)
- Autism spectrum disorder (ASD) is a clinical diagnosis. There is no diagnostic biomarker. To assess for comorbidities:
  - CBC: evaluation of growth delay or pica
  - Blood lead level: R/O lead intoxication
  - Thyroid function tests: R/O hyper-/hypothyroidism
- To evaluate etiology of ASD:
  - Chromosomal microarray (SNP)
  - Fragile X
  - *MECP2* (if girl with regression)
  - *PTEN* (if HC >2.5 SD)
  - Consider whole exome sequencing or karyotype if SNP/fragile X negative.
  - Consider workup for inborn errors of metabolism if above negative or plateau or loss of developmental skills.
  - Consider TORCH (toxoplasmosis, syphilis, varicella-zoster, parvovirus B19, rubella, cytomegalovirus, HIV, and herpes) infection workup if microcephaly present.

Diagnostic Procedures/Other

- Audiology (audiogram or brainstem auditory evoked response): to R/O hearing deficits
- Ophthalmologic exam to R/O visual deficits
- Electroencephalogram if epilepsy is suspected (~25%)
- Head MRI/CT: if focal neurologic deficit is present or if suspected neurocutaneous disease
- Autism Diagnostic Observation Schedule (ADOS) and Autism Diagnostic Interview-Revised (ADI-R)—structured interviews and assessments usually performed by a trained professional: provides diagnostic confirmation in children with concerns on surveillance or screening
- Social Responsiveness Scale (SRS)—quantifies severity of ASD symptoms

TREATMENT

GENERAL MEASURES

- Early intervention: referral to state/local programs beginning on first diagnosis to institute therapies, preferably before age 3 years
- Applied behavior analysis (ABA) and related techniques highly beneficial in many children
- Psychoeducational assessment:
  - Cognitive ability and adaptive skills
  - Speech language assessment for receptive and expressive language measures
  - OT may be beneficial for sensory or motor difficulties.
- Special education eligibility until age 21 years; some go on to "postsecondary education" and/or job training.
- Social skills training, especially for higher functioning patients, may be helpful.
- Cognitive behavioral therapy for related comorbidities such as anxiety or ADHD; not indicated to address core features of autism

MEDICATION

- Pharmacotherapy treats associated behavior symptoms but does not treat the primary disorder.
- Symptoms/medications to consider:
  - Hyperactivity/attention difficulties: Psychostimulants (amphetamine/methylphenidate), atomoxetine, clonidine, guanfacine
  - Anxiety: SSRIs, venlafaxine, benzodiazepines (may increase disorganization and agitation)
  - Aggression: atypical antipsychotics, SSRIs, anticonvulsants, guanfacine
  - Self-injurious behavior: atypical/typical antipsychotics, guanfacine, clonidine
  - Sleep disturbances: melatonin, clonidine, trazodone
  - Seizures: newer anticonvulsants, carbamazepine, phenytoin, valproate, barbiturates (may worsen hyperactivity/irritability)
  - Tic disorders: guanfacine, clonidine, atypical/typical antipsychotics
  - Depression: SSRIs, venlafaxine
- FDA-approved medications include aripiprazole for ages 6 to 17 years and risperidone for ages 5 to 16 years.
  - Important to monitor baseline glucose and lipids as atypical antipsychotics are associated with metabolic syndrome
  - Used for associated aggression and irritability

ALERT

- ASDs vary greatly in symptom presentation. Discordancy among clinicians' diagnoses and under- and over-diagnosis of these disorders are common.
- Intellectual disability, anxiety, and ADHD are common comorbidities, which may change management.
- Medication often not helpful for core autistic features but may treat comorbidities
- Wandering, elopement, and suicidal ideation/action are major causes of morbidity and mortality.
- Genetic workup is recommended upon diagnosis. 1st-line testing includes chromosomal microarray (SNP), fragile X.

COMPLEMENTARY & ALTERNATIVE THERAPIES

- Almost 1/3 of children with ASD receive some form of complementary and alternative medicine (CAM). Clinicians should counsel families on evidence for/against efficacy and potential side effects (resources include nccih.nih.gov and clinicaltrials.gov).
- For those patients using CAM, quantitative assessments by therapists or neuropsychologists may be helpful to determine baseline and response to therapy or lack thereof.
- Children with ASD often require lifelong treatment and support related to the associated medical (e.g., GI, sleep), developmental, and psychiatric comorbidities.
- Primary care clinician should remain active in long-term treatment planning and individual and family treatment and support, offering medical home services.
- "First 100 Days Kit" available online for families with newly diagnosed child with ASD along with other resources at autismspeaks.org
- Information regarding safety for children with ASD may be found at nationalautismassociation.org.
- Prognosis linked to cognitive ability, acquisition of social/communication skills, and psychiatric comorbidities

ONGOING CARE

DIET

No systematic evidence to support specific diets

PROGNOSIS

Early intervention and provision of services can improve prognosis.

ADDITIONAL READING

- Johnson CP, Myers SM; for American Academy of Pediatrics Council on Children with Disabilities. Identification and evaluation of children with autism spectrum disorders. *Pediatrics*. 2007;120(5):1183–1215.
- Levy SE, Hyman SL. Complementary and alternative medicine treatments for children with autism spectrum disorders. *Child Adolesc Psychiatr Clin N Am*. 2015;24(1):117–143.
- McGuire K, Fung LK, Hagopian L, et al. Irritability and problem behavior in autism spectrum disorder: a practice pathway for pediatric primary care. *Pediatrics*. 2016;137(Suppl 2);S136–S148.
- Moeschler JB, Shevell M; and Committee on Genetics. Comprehensive evaluation of the child with intellectual disability or global developmental delays. *Pediatrics*. 2014;134(3):e903–e918.
- Myers SM, Johnson CP; for American Academy of Pediatrics Council on Children with Disabilities. Clinical report: Management of children with autism spectrum disorders. *Pediatrics*. 2007;120(5):1162–1182.
- Schaefer GB, Mendelsohn NJ; for Professional Practice and Guidelines Committee. Clinical genetics evaluation in identifying the etiology of autism spectrum disorders: 2013 guideline revisions. *Genet Med*. 2013;15(5):399–407.
- Simms MD, Jin XM. Autism, language disorder, and social (pragmatic) communication disorder: DSM-V and differential diagnoses. *Pediatr Rev*. 2015;36(8):355–362.
- Stoner R, Chow ML, Boyle MP, et al. Patches of disorganization in the neocortex of children with autism. *N Engl J Med*. 2014;370(13):1209–1219.
- Volkmar F, Siegel M, Woodbury-Smith M, et al; and American Academy of Child and Adolescent Psychiatry Committee on Quality Issues. Practice parameter for the assessment and treatment of children and adolescents with autism spectrum disorder. *J Am Acad Child Adolesc Psychiatry*. 2014;53(2):237–257. www.aacap.org

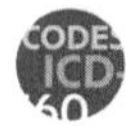

CODES

ICD10

- F84.0 Autistic disorder
- F84.2 Rett's syndrome
- F84.5 Asperger's syndrome

FAQ

- Q: What are the chances of having a second child with autism?
- A: In families with one child with autism, the recurrence risk for subsequent children is 3–18%. This is in contrast to the risk in the general population of 0.1–0.2%.
- Q: What is the value of brain imaging in autism?
- A: MRI may help diagnose a heritable syndrome with genetic counseling implications (e.g., tuberous sclerosis) but is usually unhelpful in high-functioning cases without severe intellectual impairment and focal neurologic findings. Benefits versus risks should be weighed if anesthesia is needed.
- Q: Do vaccines cause autism?
- A: There is no causal association between the MMR or other vaccines and autism.

AUTOIMMUNE HEMOLYTIC ANEMIA

Kandace L. Gollomp, MD • Michele Puszkarczuk Lambert, MD, MSTR

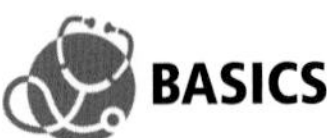

BASICS

DESCRIPTION

- Autoimmune hemolytic anemia (AIHA) is characterized by shortened red cell survival caused by autoantibodies directed against RBC surface antigens, with or without the participation of complement on the red cell membrane.
- Natural history
  - Acute disease
    - Onset with rapid fall in hemoglobin level over hours to days
    - Usual course: complete resolution of disease within 3 to 6 months
    - Resolution more likely in children who present between 2 and 12 years of age
  - Chronic disease
    - Slower onset of anemia over weeks to months, with some having persistence of hemolysis or intermittent relapses
    - More likely to be associated with underlying chronic illness
    - More common in adults and children <2 years or >12 years of age

EPIDEMIOLOGY

- Less common in children and adolescents than in adults
- No apparent racial or sexual predisposition (in childhood)

Incidence

- ~1 to 3:100,000 persons/year
- Peak incidence in childhood is in first 4 years of life with most cases due to warm AIHA.

PATHOPHYSIOLOGY

- Warm autoantibodies (~80% cases)
  - Maximal activity of in vitro antibody RBC binding at 37°C
  - IgG-class antibody usually
  - IgG-coated RBCs cleared, predominantly extravascularly in the spleen, by macrophages
- Cold autoantibodies (cold agglutinins) (7–25%)
  - Maximal activity of in vitro RBC binding at temperatures between 0°C and 30°C
  - Almost always caused by IgM antibody with specificity for antigens of the i/I system on RBCs
  - Anti-I antibodies characteristic of *Mycoplasma pneumoniae*—associated hemolysis and can be associated with infectious mononucleosis
  - Hemolysis is complement-dependent.
- Paroxysmal cold hemoglobinuria
  - IgG autoantibody binds RBC at cooler areas of the body (i.e., extremities), causing irreversible binding of complement components (C3 and C4). When coated RBCs enter warmer areas of the body, IgG falls off and complement causes hemolysis (Donath–Landsteiner biphasic hemolysin).
  - Unusual IgG antibody with anti-P specificity
  - Most frequently found in children with viral infections (30%)

ETIOLOGY

- Idiopathic
- Passive transfer of maternal antibodies
- Secondary to an underlying disorder
  - Infection: viral (e.g., Epstein-Barr virus, cytomegalovirus, hepatitis, HIV) or bacterial (e.g., *Mycoplasma, Streptococcus*, typhoid fever, *Escherichia coli* septicemia)
  - Drugs: antimalarials, antipyretics, sulfonamides, penicillin, ceftriaxone, rifampin
  - Hematologic disorders: leukemia, lymphoma
  - Autoimmune disorders: lupus, mixed connective tissue disorders, Wiskott-Aldrich syndrome, ulcerative colitis, rheumatoid arthritis, common variable immunodeficiency, scleroderma, Evans syndrome, autoimmune lymphoproliferative syndrome (ALPS), 22q11.2 deletion syndrome
  - Tumors: ovarian, carcinomas, thymomas, dermoid cysts
  - Following hematopoietic stem cell transplant due to alloimmunity and immunosuppression or after solid organ transplants where there is ABO incompatibility between donor and recipient

DIAGNOSIS

HISTORY

- Pallor
- Jaundice
- Dark urine
- Fever
- Weakness
- Dizziness
- Syncope
- Exercise intolerance

PHYSICAL EXAM

- Pallor
- Jaundice
- Splenomegaly
- Hepatomegaly
- Tachycardia, systolic flow murmur, S_3 gallop
- Orthostasis in acute onset

DIFFERENTIAL DIAGNOSIS

- Defects intrinsic to RBC:
  - Membrane defects such as hereditary spherocytosis
  - Enzyme defects including hemolytic episode due to G6PD deficiency
  - Hemoglobin defects
  - Congenital dyserythropoietic anemias
  - Paroxysmal nocturnal hemoglobinuria
- Defects extrinsic to RBC:
  - Immune-mediated
    - Isoimmune: hemolytic disease of the newborn, blood group incompatibility
    - Autoimmune (see "Etiology")
    - Drug-dependent RBC antibodies
    - Hemolytic transfusion reaction
- Non–immune-mediated
  - Idiopathic
  - Secondary to an underlying disorder (i.e., hemolytic uremic syndrome, thrombotic thrombocytopenic purpura)
  - Mechanical: march hemoglobinuria, heart valves

DIAGNOSTIC TESTS & INTERPRETATION

Initial Tests (screening, lab, imaging)

- CBC
  - Hemoglobin level decreased (Other cell lines may be decreased in Evans syndrome or ALPS.)
  - Mean corpuscular volume may be normal or increased due to RBC agglutination.
  - Mean corpuscular hemoglobin concentration may be increased due to spherocytosis.
- Reticulocyte count
  - Usually increased
  - May also be decreased if reticulocytes bear the target antigen
- Peripheral smear:
  - Spherocytes
  - Polychromasia
  - Macrocytes
  - Agglutination
- Direct antiglobulin test (Coombs)—positive in ~95% of cases
  - Single most important test
  - Warm AIHA will have IgG ± C3-positive.
  - Cold AIHA and paroxysmal cold hemoglobinuria will have C3-positive.
- Haptoglobin level decreased
- Indirect hyperbilirubinemia
- Elevated lactate dehydrogenase
- Urinalysis:
  - Hemoglobinuria
  - Increased urobilinogen
- Bone marrow aspiration: erythroid hyperplasia (to rule out leukemia or lymphoma associated with AIHA)
- Cold agglutinin titer: positive (usually >1:64)
- Donath–Landsteiner test should be performed in cases of suspected paroxysmal cold hemoglobinuria.

ALERT

- A negative Coombs test can occur when small numbers of IgG or C3 molecules are present on the red cell membrane or if most of the coated red blood cells are cleared from circulation (i.e., in cases of less severe hemolysis, low-affinity antibodies, or in cases of very severe, rapid clearance).
- Radiolabeled Coombs test or enzyme immunoassays are more sensitive diagnostic tests in these circumstances.
- Reticulocytopenia may occur in some cases where the antibody coats and removes reticulocytes.

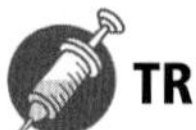

TREATMENT

MEDICATION

First Line

- Corticosteroids
  - Indication:
    - In IgG-mediated disease, steroids have been shown to interfere with macrophage Fc and C3b receptors responsible for RBC destruction. In addition, they have been shown to elute IgG Ab from the RBC surface (improving survival); induces remission in 80–85% of cases
    - In chronic, warm, AIHA, pulsed high-dose dexamethasone has been shown to be effective in some cases.
  - Complications:
    - Both short- and long-term side effects
    - Generally not effective in cold agglutinin disease
  - Dose:
    - Start prednisone PO/methylprednisolone IV at 2 mg/kg/24 h in divided doses.
    - Tapering of steroids should begin after a therapeutic response is achieved (may take several days to weeks).
  - Goal:
    - Initially, to return to normal hemoglobin level with tolerable doses of steroid or off steroids entirely
    - In some patients, goal may be achieving decreased hemolysis and a clinically asymptomatic state with minimal steroid side effects.
    - Alternative treatments should be considered for patients unresponsive to steroids or who require high doses for maintenance of hemoglobin level.

Second Line

- IV immunoglobulin
  - Indication:
    - May be useful in selected cases of immune hemolytic anemia unresponsive to steroids
  - Mechanism of action is not entirely clear.
  - Effect is usually temporary; retreatment may be required every 3 to 4 weeks.
  - Complications:
    - Aseptic meningitis
    - Theoretical risk of transfusion-transmitted viral infection
    - Large doses of IVIG have been associated with hemolytic anemia.
  - Expensive
  - Dose: Up to 1 g/kg/24 h for 5 days has been required to achieve a beneficial effect.
- Plasmapheresis/exchange transfusion
  - Indication:
    - Will slow the rate of hemolysis in severe disease, especially if IgM-mediated
  - Indicated if thrombotic thrombocytopenic purpura cannot be excluded
  - Complications:
    - Only of short-term benefit
  - Expensive
- Rituximab: Monoclonal anti-CD20 antibody likely works through depletion of B cells.
  - Indicated in refractory AIHA (375 mg/m^2 weekly for 2 to 4 weeks)
  - Response 40–100%
  - Particularly useful in warm AIHA
  - Adverse effects: infusion associated: fever, chills, rigors, hypertension, bronchospasm; Late onset: rare risk of viral infections, hypogammaglobulinemia
- Immunosuppressive agents (antimetabolites and alkylating agents)
  - Indication:
    - When there is a clinically unacceptable degree of hemolysis that is refractory to 1st-line agents
    - May be used in conjunction with steroids
    - Some have been effective in cold agglutinin disease.
  - Complications:
    - There are varying side effects dependent on the agent used. Therefore, clinical indications must be strong and exposure to drug should be limited.
  - Dose:
    - Adjusted to maintain WBC >2,000, absolute neutrophil count (ANC) >1,000, and platelet count at 50,000 to 100,000 cells/mm^3
- Alemtuzumab (anti-CD52): may be effective very refractory AIHA particularly secondary to B-cell chronic lymphocytic leukemia (B-CLL)

ADDITIONAL THERAPIES

Blood transfusion:

- Should only be used with great caution in this setting in patients with very low hemoglobin/brisk hemolysis because of difficulty with appropriate cross-matching
- Indication: physiologic compromise from the anemia (usually only in severe acute onset)
- Considerations:
  - The blood bank may be unable to find compatible blood. In IgG-mediated disease, autoantibody is usually pan-reactive; therefore, you must use the least incompatible unit of blood.
  - In cold agglutinin disease, use a blood warmer for all infusions to decrease IgM binding, and monitor for acute hemolysis during transfusion.

SURGERY/OTHER PROCEDURES

Splenectomy

- Indication: Patients unresponsive to medical management, who require moderate- to high-maintenance doses of steroids or who develop steroid intolerance may be candidates.
- Not effective in cold agglutinin disease
- Response rate is 50–70%, with many partial remissions.

ONGOING CARE

FOLLOW-UP RECOMMENDATIONS

Patient Monitoring

- Hemoglobin level q4h–q12h (depending on severity) until stable
- Reticulocyte count: daily
- Spleen size: daily
- Hemoglobinuria: daily
- Coombs: weekly

PROGNOSIS

- Dependent on age, underlying disorder (if any), and response to therapy. See also "Description" section (natural history).
- Mortality in pediatric series ranged from 9% to 19%.

COMPLICATIONS

- May be increased risk of venous thrombosis in patients with AIHA
- May be associated with a predisposition to lymphoproliferative disorders
- Gallstones related to chronic hemolysis

ADDITIONAL READING

- Barros MMO, Blajchman MA, Bordin JO. Warm autoimmune hemolytic anemia: recent progress in understanding the immunobiology and treatment. *Transfus Med Rev*. 2010;24(3):195–210.
- Hoffman PC. Immune hemolytic anemia—selected topics. *Hematology Am Soc Hematol Educ Program*. 2009:80–86.
- Miano M. How I manage Evans syndrome and AIHA cases in children. *Br J Haematol*. 2016;172(4):524–534.
- Petz LD. Cold antibody autoimmune hemolytic anemias. *Blood Rev*. 2008;22(1):1–15.
- Teachey DT, Lambert MP. Diagnosis and management of autoimmune cytopenias in childhood. *Pediatr Clin North Am*. 2013;60(6):1489–1511.
- Vagace JM, Bajo R, Gervasini G. Diagnostic and therapeutic challenges of primary autoimmune haemolytic anaemia in children. *Arch Dis Child*. 2014;99(7):668–673.

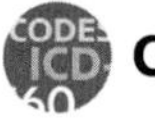

CODES

ICD10

- D59.1 Other autoimmune hemolytic anemias
- D59.0 Drug-induced autoimmune hemolytic anemia

FAQ

- Q: Will the anemia go away?
- A: Children with cold autoantibodies tend to have short-lived illness, whereas children with warm antibodies often have a chronic clinical course characterized by periods of remissions and relapses.
- Q: Is this contagious?
- A: No. Another child may acquire the same viral illness; however, the body's response to produce an autoantibody is dependent on the individual patient.

AVASCULAR (ASEPTIC) NECROSIS OF THE FEMORAL HEAD (HIP)

Craig Munns, FRACP, MBBS, PhD

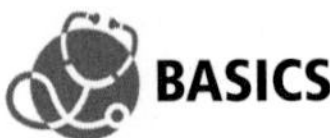

BASICS

DESCRIPTION

- Avascular (aseptic) necrosis results from the interruption of the blood supply to bone (either traumatic or nontraumatic occlusion).
- The femoral head is the most common site.
- A self-limiting idiopathic avascular necrosis of the hip that occurs in children is known as Perthes disease (see "Perthes Disease" chapter).

RISK FACTORS

Genetics

- Variable, depending on cause
- Steroid-induced avascular necrosis may have an underlying genetic predisposition.

PATHOPHYSIOLOGY

- Death and necrosis of bone with gradual return of blood supply
- Necrotic bone gradually resorbed and replaced by new bone
- During bone resorption, structural integrity of femoral head may be reduced, leading to collapse.

ETIOLOGY

- Traumatic
  - Slipped capital femoral epiphysis
  - Hip fracture
  - Hip dislocation
  - Complication of casting, bracing, surgery
- Nontraumatic
  - Steroids or chemotherapy
  - Malignancy (leukemia)
  - Idiopathic (older, after physeal closure); similar to adult avascular necrosis
  - Idiopathic (younger, before physeal closure, Perthes disease)
  - Caisson disease
  - Sickle cell disease
  - Septic arthritis
  - Gaucher disease
  - Viral infection (HIV, CMV)
  - Radiation therapy
  - Hypercoagulable states

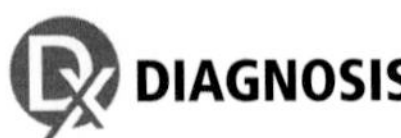

DIAGNOSIS

HISTORY

- Onset (gradual or after traumatic event)
- Association with the following:
  - Trauma
  - Medications (steroids or chemotherapy)
  - Casting, splinting, surgery (iatrogenic)
  - Pain, limping
  - Stiffness (decreased range of motion)
  - Perthes disease may occasionally be bilateral or occur in contralateral hip at a later time point.

PHYSICAL EXAM

- Gait
  - Limping
  - Antalgic ("against pain") gait (shortened stance phase relative to swing phase)
  - Trendelenburg gait (tilting of pelvis during the stance phase of gait; pelvis rises on the side not taking weight)
- Test and note range of motion:
  - Flexion and extension
  - Abduction and adduction
  - Internal and external rotation
- Hip joint irritability (short arc rotation)
- Signs of other disease processes associated with avascular necrosis (e.g., sickle cell disease)
- Physical examination pearl
  - Loss of internal rotation usually first and most affected loss of motion

DIFFERENTIAL DIAGNOSIS

- Trauma
  - Osteochondral fracture
  - Impaction fracture
  - Epiphyseal/physeal fracture
- Infection
  - Osteomyelitis
  - Septic arthritis
- Neoplastic process: epiphyseal tumors (chondroblastoma, Trevor disease, etc.)
- Rheumatologic processes
- Skeletal dysplasia, particular if bilateral hip involvement

DIAGNOSTIC TESTS & INTERPRETATION

- Laboratory examinations should be normal in most forms of avascular necrosis of the femoral head.
- Exceptions:
  - Sickle cell disease
  - Septic arthritis
  - Chemotherapy
- Radiographic findings:
  - Sclerosis
  - Subchondral fracture
  - Collapse
  - Reossification
  - Repair
- Magnetic resonance imaging (MRI)
  - Bone edema
  - If contrast medium used, area of reduce blood flow evident
- Bone scan
  - Reduced signal in affected hip
- Other potential findings:
  - Cysts
  - Physeal growth arrest (young)
  - Early osteoarthritis
  - Subluxation

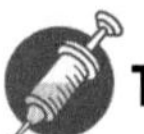

TREATMENT

MEDICATION

- NSAIDs may reduce pain by decreasing associated inflammation but may also reduce new bone formation.
- If associated with corticosteroid use, discontinuation or elimination of steroids may be helpful.
- Antiresorptive therapy (bisphosphonate/receptor activator of nuclear factor-κB (RANK) ligand inhibitor) may reduce pain and preserve joint shape; research studies using this approach are ongoing.

GENERAL MEASURES

- Maintain range of motion (physical therapy, traction, continuous passive motion).
- Contain the femoral head in the acetabulum (see treatment principles listed in "Perthes Disease" chapter).
- Duration of therapy variable, depending on cause
- Reduced weight bearing on affected hip may help prevent collapse.

SURGERY/OTHER PROCEDURES

Redirectional osteotomy

- Femoral or acetabular reorientation
- Core decompression to stimulate new blood supply

ONGOING CARE

DIET

- Thought not to alter disease process
- Recommend general balanced diet.
- During immobilization, excessive weight gain may occur.

PROGNOSIS

- Depends on extent of femoral head collapse
- Good if mild involvement and patient is young
- Timing of improvement is variable, dependent on etiology.
- Moderate to severe cases often have significant collapse and end up requiring a total hip replacement.

COMPLICATIONS

- Joint collapse with decreased range of motion, pain, limping
- Osteoarthritis
- Physeal arrest with growth disturbance

ALERT

Signs to watch for:

- Subluxation
- Early osteoarthritis
- Growth arrest

ADDITIONAL READING

- Lahdes-Vasama T, Lamminen A, Merikanto J, et al. The value of MRI in early Perthes' disease: an MRI study with a 2-year follow-up. *Pediatr Radiol*. 1997;27(6):517–522.
- Mont MA, Cherian JJ, Sierra RJ, et al. Nontraumatic osteonecrosis of the femoral head: where do we stand today? A ten-year update. *J Bone Joint Surg Am*. 2015;97(19):1604–1027.
- Padhye B, Dalla-Pozza L, Little DG, et al. Use of zoledronic acid for treatment of chemotherapy related osteonecrosis in children and adolescents: a retrospective analysis. *Pediatr Blood Cancer*. 2013;60(9):1539–1545.
- Roposch A, Mayr J, Linhart WE. Age at onset, extent of necrosis, and containment in Perthes disease. Results at maturity. *Arch Orthop Trauma Surg*. 2003;123(2–3):68–73.
- Sharma S, Leung WH, Deqing P, et al. Osteonecrosis in children after allogeneic hematopoietic cell transplantation: study of prevalence, risk factors and longitudinal changes using MR imaging. *Bone Marrow Transplant*. 2012;47(8):1067–1074.
- Shipman SA, Helfand M, Moyer VA, et al. Screening for developmental dysplasia of the hip: a systematic literature review for the US Preventive Services Task Force. *Pediatrics*. 2006;117(3):e557–e576.
- Tokmakova KP, Stanton RP, Mason DE. Factors influencing the development of osteonecrosis in patients treated for slipped capital femoral epiphysis. *J Bone Joint Surg Am*. 2003;85-A(5):798–801.

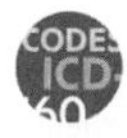

CODES

ICD10

- M87.059 Idiopathic aseptic necrosis of unspecified femur
- M91.10 Juvenile osteochondrosis of head of femur, unspecified leg
- M87.052 Idiopathic aseptic necrosis of left femur

FAQ

- Q: What type of medication is most often associated with avascular necrosis of the hip?
- A: Corticosteroids
- Q: For avascular necrosis in children (Perthes disease of the hip, for example), is younger or older age associated with a better prognosis?
- A: Younger age (<8 years)

BABESIOSIS

Frances M. Nadel, MD, MSCE

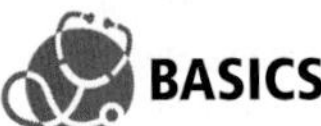

BASICS

DESCRIPTION

- Human babesiosis is a tick-borne, malaria-like illness characterized by fever, malaise, and hemolytic anemia.
- Most infected individuals are asymptomatic.

EPIDEMIOLOGY

- Human babesiosis is a protozoal illness caused by the intraerythrocytic parasite of the *Babesia* genus.
  - *Babesia microti* is responsible for most cases of babesiosis in the United States.
  - *Babesia duncani* has been the causative agent in older men on the Pacific coast of the United States.
  - *Babesia divergens* is responsible for most European cases.
  - *Babesia venatorum* has been the causative agent in China.
- Most cases in the United States occur in the Northeast and Upper Midwest.
  - 94% of reported cases in 2014 occurred in Connecticut, Massachusetts, New Jersey, New York, Rhode Island, Minnesota, and Wisconsin.
- Human infection most commonly occur in the warm months—late spring to early fall.

Incidence

- In 2011, babesiosis became a nationally notifiable disease monitored by the Centers for Disease Control and Prevention (CDC).
- According to the CDC, 1,744 cases were reported in the United States in 2014. Six of the cases were transfusion related.

Prevalence

Prevalence is difficult to ascertain, as asymptomatic infection appears to be common in endemic areas. For instance, seroprevalence is as high as 9% in some endemic areas of Rhode Island.

RISK FACTORS

- Asplenia (functional or anatomic)
- Extremes of age, especially age >50 years
- HIV/AIDS
- Immunosuppressive medications
- Malignancy
- Primary immunodeficiency syndrome

Genetics

There is no known genetic predisposition.

GENERAL PREVENTION

- Prevention begins with avoidance of tick bites.
- Simple measures include wearing long-sleeved shirts and long pants, with pants tucked into the socks in tick-infested areas.
- Avoid endemic regions during the peak months of May to September.
- Light clothing will make ticks easier to see.
- Use N,N-Diethyl-meta-toluamide (DEET)-containing insect repellents during outdoor activities.
- Spraying one's clothing with a permethrin tick repellent may be helpful.
- Children and dogs should be inspected daily for ticks after being outside.
- Prophylaxis is not recommended after a tick bite.
- No vaccine is currently available.
- There is currently no universal laboratory screening of blood products.

PATHOPHYSIOLOGY

- Babesial infection of the erythrocyte causes membrane damage and lysis, which promotes adherence to the endothelium and microvascular stasis.
- This process results in a hemolytic anemia.
- The spleen plays an important role in decreasing the protozoal load through antibody production and filtering of abnormally shaped infected red blood cells.

ETIOLOGY

- The protozoa is transmitted by a bite from the tick *Ixodes scapularis* (deer tick), the same vector responsible for transmission of *Borrelia burgdorferi* (the causative agent in Lyme disease).
- The white-footed mouse (*Peromyscus leucopus*) is the primary reservoir host of *Babesia*.
- Incubation period
  - Usually 1 to 4 weeks for tick-transmitted disease
  - 1 to 9 weeks for transfusion-associated disease
- Human-to-human transmission is limited to infection through contaminated blood.
  - Babesiosis is currently the most common transfusion-transmitted infection in the United States.
  - Rare cases of transplacental and perinatal infection have been reported.

COMMONLY ASSOCIATED CONDITIONS

- Two thirds of patients have concurrent Lyme disease.
  - Coinfections with *Borrelia* account for 80% of tick-borne coinfections.
- One third may have concurrent human granulocytic anaplasmosis (HGA).
- Less common coinfection may occur with other tick-borne agents.

DIAGNOSIS

HISTORY

- Few patients recall a tick bite.
- Patients live in or have recently traveled to an endemic region.
- Initial symptoms begin 1 to 4 weeks after the tick bite and are vague. They may include progressive fatigue, malaise, headaches, and anorexia, accompanied by intermittent fevers as high as 40°C.
- Chills, myalgias, and arthralgias may follow these symptoms.
- Less common complaints include cough, sore throat, neck stiffness, abdominal pain, and emotional lability.

PHYSICAL EXAM

- Fever and tachycardia are often the only findings.
- Mild conjunctival injection and pharyngeal erythema occasionally occur.
- Mild hepatomegaly and/or splenomegaly may be present.
- Jaundice or hematuria may also be observed.
- Petechiae and ecchymosis occur in rare cases, most often in the presence of severe illness with associated shock and/or DIC.

DIFFERENTIAL DIAGNOSIS

- HGA
- Malaria
- Leptospirosis
- Sepsis associated with hemolytic anemia
- Noninfectious causes of hemolytic anemia
- Influenza
- Nonspecific viral syndrome

DIAGNOSTIC TESTS & INTERPRETATION

- Giemsa or Wright thin blood smears may demonstrate the intraerythrocytic ring form:
  - This is often confused with the ring form of *Plasmodium falciparum*, the etiologic agent of malaria.
  - Rarely, the pathognomonic "Maltese cross" forms of the *Babesia* parasite may be seen on the blood smear.
  - Multiple smears should be performed as initial smears may be falsely negative early in the disease.
- Polymerase chain reaction (PCR) is highly sensitive and specific when available.
- Indirect immunofluorescent serology may help support or confirm the diagnosis.
  - Antigen-specific for *B. microti*
  - In endemic areas, the test has a sensitivity of 91% and a specificity of 99%.
  - Can be used when blood smears are negative
  - In general, a titer = 1:64 indicates exposure.
  - A 4-fold rise in antibody titer in acute and convalescent sera confirms the diagnosis.
  - Immunoglobulin levels decline rapidly within months of recovery.
- Other tests: Most of the abnormal routine test results are the result of hemolysis.
- Urinalysis
  - Proteinuria
  - Hemoglobinuria
- CBC
  - Normal leukocyte count/leukopenia
  - Normocytic/normochromic anemia
  - Thrombocytopenia
  - Atypical lymphocytosis
  - Reticulocytosis

- Possible positive Coombs test
- Elevated ESR
- Liver function tests: elevated bilirubin, lactate dehydrogenase, and liver transaminases
- Elevated BUN and creatinine
- In asymptomatic patients, these tests are often normal.

ALERT

False negatives:
- Blood smears may not demonstrate the protozoa at low levels of parasitemia.
- Serologic false positives for *B. microti* include cross-reactivity with other *Babesia* sp. or malarial organisms.
- Serology titers may be low in the 1st week of symptoms.

TREATMENT

GENERAL MEASURES

Those with mild clinical disease usually recover without treatment.

MEDICATION

- For asymptomatic patients who are otherwise healthy, treatment is only recommended if their babesial PCR or blood smear remains positive for more than 3 months.
- For symptomatic patients, treatment is generally for 7 to 10 days regardless of regimen; more severely ill patients may require a longer duration of therapy.

First Line

- Atovaquone in combination with azithromycin
  - Has similar treatment effectiveness with fewer side effects (such as vertigo, tinnitus, and GI upset) than clindamycin and quinine
- Pediatric dosing:
  - Atovaquone 40 mg/kg/24 h PO every 12 hours (max 750 mg/dose)
  - Azithromycin 10 mg/kg/24 h (max 500 mg) PO on day 1 and 5 mg/kg/24 h (max 250 mg) PO once daily thereafter
- Adult dosing:
  - Atovaquone 750 mg PO every 12 hours
  - Azithromycin 500 to 1,000 mg PO on day 1 and 250 to 1,000 mg PO once daily thereafter

Second Line

- Clindamycin in combination with quinine
  - Standard therapy for asplenic, immunodeficient, or severely ill patients
  - IV route for clindamycin is recommended for the severely ill patient.
- Pediatric dosing:
  - Clindamycin: 20 to 40 mg/kg/24 h IV/PO divided every 6 to 8 hours (max 600 mg/dose)
  - Quinine: 24 mg/kg/24 h PO every 8 hours (max dose 650 mg/dose)
- Adult dosing:
  - Clindamycin: 600 mg PO every 8 hours or 300 to 600 mg IV every 6 hours
  - Quinine: 650 mg PO every 6 to 8 hours
- In areas endemic for Lyme disease and ehrlichiosis, consider adding doxycycline to either regimen until lab confirmation of absence of either disease in the patient with babesiosis.

ADDITIONAL THERAPIES

- For life-threatening infections, exchange transfusion has been successful. Consider in patients with severe parasitemia ($\geq$10%), severe hemolysis, or renal/hepatic/pulmonary compromise.
- Progressive respiratory distress may require mechanical ventilation.

ALERT

- Signs to watch for:
  - Respiratory distress, especially after treatment has begun
  - Pancytopenia and lymphadenopathy: may indicate the development of hemophagocytic syndrome
- Pitfalls
  - Children who are from endemic areas and have an acute febrile illness may be misdiagnosed with a nonspecific viral illness.
  - One should be suspicious for a coinfection with Lyme disease or HGA in those who are not responding to standard therapy.
  - Delayed recognition of this uncommon disease may be life-threatening in the immunocompromised patient.
  - In endemic areas, babesiosis should be considered in a posttransfusion febrile illness in at-risk populations.

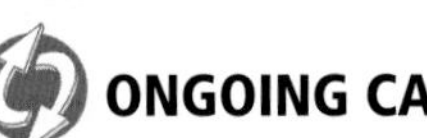

ONGOING CARE

FOLLOW-UP RECOMMENDATIONS

When to expect improvement:
- Some improvement of symptoms should be noted within 24 to 48 hours of onset of therapy.
- Those who are only mildly affected usually have resolution of their symptoms over a few weeks.
- For severely affected and immunodeficient patients, the convalescent period may be as long as 18 months.
- In untreated asymptomatic individuals, parasitemia may persist for months to years.
- Long-term complications are rare.
- Recrudescence has been reported.

COMPLICATIONS

- Rarely fatal in the United States
- Pancytopenia and overwhelming secondary bacterial sepsis may occur.
- Serious and fulminant complications have been described:
  - Pulmonary edema and adult respiratory distress syndrome often happening after treatment has begun.
  - CHF
  - Renal failure
  - Hemophagocytic syndrome/DIC
  - Seizures/coma
- Those coinfected with Lyme disease are susceptible to more severe disease and complications.

ADDITIONAL READING

- American Academy of Pediatrics. Babesiosis. In: Kimberlin DW, Brady MT, Jackson MA, et al, eds. *Red Book: 2015 Report of the Committee on Infectious Diseases*. 30th ed. Elk Grove Village, IL: American Academy of Pediatrics; 2015:253–254.
- Centers for Disease Control and Prevention. *Surveillance for Babesiosis—United States, 2014 Annual Summary*. Atlanta, GA: U.S. Department of Health and Human Services, CDC; 2016.
- Diuk-Wasser MA, Vannier E, Krause PJ. Coinfection by ixodes tick-borne pathogens: ecological, epidemiological, and clinical consequences. *Trends Parasitol*. 2016;32(1):30–42.
- Mukkada S, Buckingham SC. Recognition of and prompt treatment for tick-borne infections in children. *Infect Dis Clin North Am*. 2015;29(3): 539–555.
- Sanchez E, Vannier E, Wormser GP, et al. Diagnosis, treatment, and prevention of Lyme disease, human granulocytic anaplasmosis, and babesiosis: a review. *JAMA*. 2016;315(16):1767–1777.
- Vannier E, Krause PJ. Human babesiosis. *N Engl J Med*. 2012;366(25):2397–2407.

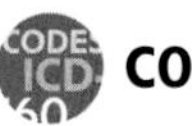

CODES

ICD10

B60.0 Babesiosis

FAQ

- Q: How long does a tick have to be attached for infection to occur?
- A: In general, successful transmission requires at least 24 hours of attachment.
- Q: How should a tick be removed?
- A: The tick should be grasped with forceps as close to its head as possible and pulled straight up. If possible, it should be saved for identification. Wash the area with soap and water after removal.
- Q: Does infection confer lifetime immunity?
- A: No. Reinfection is possible.

BACK PAIN

Kate Berz, DO • Kelsey Logan, MD, MPH

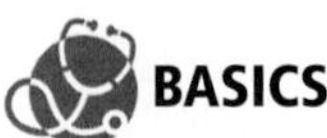

BASICS

DESCRIPTION

Any condition causing pain of the thoracic, lumbar, or sacral spine

EPIDEMIOLOGY

- 12-month period prevalence: 10–20% of children
- Lifetime prevalence: 12–50%

PATHOPHYSIOLOGY

- Dependent on underlying cause
- Until skeletal maturity, partially ossified posterior column and vertebral body are weak points.
- Hyperextension with rotational spinal loading in the case of pars defects (e.g., spondylolysis or spondylolisthesis)
- Autoimmune or autoinflammatory processes as with juvenile idiopathic arthritis (JIA) or juvenile ankylosing spondylitis

ETIOLOGY

- Unidentified in 50% of cases
- 30% of chronic cases (back pain >3 years) without clear etiology despite workup

RISK FACTORS

- Poor conditioning or high athletic performance
- Joint hypermobility
- Role of backpack weight and style of wear undetermined
- Role of overweight or obesity yet to be determined

GENERAL PREVENTION

- Back muscle strengthening and hamstring stretching exercises may be helpful.
- Maximum backpack load: 10–15% body weight
- Weight loss and increased physical activity in overweight or obese children
- 3 months off from sport per year, 1 day off from scheduled activity per week

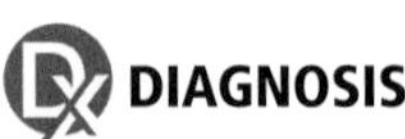

DIAGNOSIS

HISTORY

- History to elucidate most likely cause
- Musculoskeletal/trauma
  - Direct trauma
  - Worsening pain after activity
  - Repetitive movements causing microtrauma
- Inflammatory
  - Morning stiffness (variable pain)
  - Pain/stiffness improves with movement.
  - Family history of rheumatic disease
- Infectious
  - Fever
  - Recent exposure to infection or tuberculosis (TB)
  - Recent illness
- Malignancy
  - Night sweats, fever, weight loss, malaise, pain waking at night
  - Previous history of malignancy
  - Severe, unrelenting pain despite supine position or adequate analagesia
- Neurologic
  - Radiating pain or foot drop
  - Loss of bowel or bladder function
- Endocrine/metabolic
  - Long-term steroid use
  - Vitamin D deficiency
- Psychosocial stressors (e.g., family coping mechanisms and response to pain and stress)
- Age differentiation
  - <10 years: diskitis, tumor
  - >10 years: pars defects, inflammatory disorders

PHYSICAL EXAM

- Observe from behind patient: sacral dimple, vascular anomalies, posture, spinal curvature, anterior superior iliac spine (ASIS) height, limb length discrepancy, foot arch, lower limb alignment, rib rotation
  - Consider occult problem; mechanical or musculoskeletal problem
  - Scoliosis is rarely painful.
  - Increased fixed kyphosis of 40 degrees is indicative of Scheuermann disease.
- Palpate for point or focal tenderness along spine; sacroiliac (SI) joint tenderness
  - If bony tenderness present, consider fracture, vertebral osteomyelitis.
  - If paraspinal tenderness present, consider muscle strain; if SI tenderness, consider spondylitis or overuse.
- Assess range of motion: pain with spinal extension (causing strain of posterior elements of spine)
  - Consider spondylolisthesis (forward vertebral displacement), spondylolysis (pars interarticularis defect), fracture, vertebral osteomyelitis, or tumor.
- Assess range of motion: forward spinal flexion limitation
  - If painful, consider diskitis, vertebral osteomyelitis, vertebral body tumor, and herniated disk if pain radiates.
  - If limited as noted by flattening of lumbosacral region with movement, consider spondylitis.
- Assess range of motion: restriction of spine with pain (especially with neck extension) and other associated joint abnormalities (swelling or pain/tenderness with limitation). If positive, consider JIA.
- Special tests:
  - Assess for pain with straight-leg raise: Consider tight hamstrings, psoas strain, or disk herniation if pain goes past the knees.
  - Assess for back pain with FABER (hip **f**lexion, **ab**duction, **e**xternal **r**otation with foot on opposite knee) testing or direct palpation of SI joint: SI joint irritation or inflammation or hip etiology if hip pain
  - Assess for symmetric Achilles and patellar reflexes, sensation, Babinski (upper motor neuron), pain, and proprioception; deficits may indicate neuronal involvement; nerve testing: gastrocsoleus, L5 extensor hallucis longus, L4 to L5 tibialis anterior, L3 to L4 quadriceps, L2 to L3 hip flexors
- Abdominal or pelvic exam may be helpful.

DIFFERENTIAL DIAGNOSIS

- Mechanical/trauma
  - Overuse injury
  - Disk herniation
- Direct trauma, contusion
  - Musculoskeletal strain in children with closed growth plates
  - Apophyseal ring fracture
- Structural
  - Pars defects: children usually >10 years of age
  - Spondylolysis/spondylolisthesis (anterior displacement/"slip" of vertebral body, evolution of bilateral spondylolysis)
  - Scheuermann kyphosis: deformity of thoracic spine associated with vertebral body wedging
  - Scoliosis: not usually associated with significant back pain
  - Backpack weight not clearly shown to correlate with back pain
- Inflammatory
  - JIA
  - Juvenile ankylosing spondylitis
  - Chronic recurrent multifocal osteomyelitis
- Neoplastic
  - Ewing sarcoma
  - Lymphoma, leukemia
- Infectious
  - Osteomyelitis
  - Epidural abscess
  - Pyelonephritis
  - Diskitis
- Endocrine/metabolic
  - Osteoporosis
  - Vitamin D deficiency
- Other
  - Pain amplification syndrome (fibromyalgia, myofascial pain)
  - Sickle cell crises, abdominal disease (pancreatitis, pyelonephritis)

DIAGNOSTIC TESTS & INTERPRETATION

Initial Tests (screening, lab, imaging)

- **Tests:** CBC with differential, sedimentation rate, C-reactive protein (CRP), and comprehensive metabolic panel with uric acid and LDH
  - *Significance*: malignancy, infection, inflammatory
- Antinuclear antibody, rheumatoid factor, anticyclic citrullinated antibody, and HLA-B27 only if obvious other associated joint abnormalities found
  - *Significance*: inflammatory/autoimmune disorders
- Cultures, PPD, or other TB study
  - *Significance*: infection
- 25(OH)D, PTH, calcium, phosphorus, alkaline phosphatase
  - *Significance*: vitamin D deficiency or rickets
- Abnormal exam/history or focal symptoms warrant imaging.
- Plain radiographs if trauma, bony tenderness, 3 to 4 weeks of pain
  - AP and lateral; oblique (if warranted) of the spine, standing full AP spine for curve
  - Assess for fracture, osteomyelitis, and masses.
  - Intra-articular pars defect commonly in L4/L5 indicates spondylolysis.
  - Bilateral pars defect with anterior vertebral body displacement indicates spondylolisthesis.
- Bone scan with single photon emission CT (SPECT)
  - Occult/subtle bony lesions, stress fractures, spondylolysis, and spondylolisthesis
- Plain CT spine: rarely used
  - Osteoid osteoma, unstable fracture
- MRI
  - Tumor, infection, diskitis, disk injuries, synovitis (including effusions or erosions—with contrast), and neurologic findings
  - Becoming test of choice for spondylolysis requires specific protocol.

B

ALERT

Warning signs of potentially serious causes of back pain in children include the following:

- Young age: <7 years old
- Duration of pain: >4 weeks
- Acute trauma
- Night pain, fever, weight loss, or malaise
- Abdominal mass
- Early morning stiffness
- History of tumor
- Exposure to TB
- Limp
- Chronic interference with normal activity (e.g., school, sports, play)
- Postural changes causing scoliosis or kyphosis
- Other associated joint abnormalities (swelling OR pain/tenderness with joint limitation)

TREATMENT

GENERAL MEASURES

- If no warning signs, conservative management with nonsteroidal anti-inflammatory drugs (NSAIDs) and relative rest (avoiding activities that cause or increase pain)
- Supervised exercise programs through home exercises or physical therapy have moderate evidence of effectiveness for low back pain without apparent anatomic cause.
- Close follow-up is appropriate.
- Spondylolysis: Compliance with relative rest from offending activities is variable and should be addressed to improve adherence; there is evidence that more relative rest, up to 3 months, improves outcome.
- Diskitis: antistaphylococcal coverage
- Bed rest/activity limitation: Adult data do not support this strategy.

MEDICATION

- NSAIDs for overuse, sprains, or strains in adolescents and for patients with arthritis
- Additional medication may be necessary depending on underlying condition such as antibiotics for infection, chemotherapy for malignancy, immunosuppression for inflammatory/autoimmune, or vitamin D and calcium supplementation for vitamin D deficiency or osteoporosis.
- Oral steroids are not considered effective treatment for acute or chronic back pain.

ISSUES FOR REFERRAL

- Sports medicine or orthopedics appropriate with Scheuermann disease, spondylolysis, or spondylolisthesis
- Concern for malignancy or long-standing inflammatory process such as JIA or juvenile ankylosing spondylitis warrants referral to hematology/oncology or rheumatology, respectively.
- Endocrinology referral for suspected osteoporosis

ADDITIONAL THERAPIES

- Physical therapy or a home exercise program with focus on core strength and flexibility is helpful in most cases.
- For overuse injuries, removal from activity with slow gradual return
- Structural problems such as spondylolysis, spondylolisthesis, and Scheuermann disease often respond to rest, ice, and NSAIDs.
- Thoracolumbar bracing has not been shown to improve healing or time back to full activity but may be used for pain control if needed.
- Biopsychosocial approach is needed for patients with pain amplification syndromes in conjunction with physical and cognitive behavioral therapies and emphasis on functionality.

COMPLEMENTARY & ALTERNATIVE THERAPIES

- Yoga and Pilates emphasizing core strength and flexibility may be useful in the adolescent.
- Cochrane systematic review determined massage may be useful in the setting of acute or subacute back pain in adults.
- Acupuncture has been shown to be safe and may be effective for low back pain.

SURGERY/OTHER PROCEDURES

- May be indicated in patients with spondylolisthesis of >50%
- Epidural steroid injection for lumbar disk herniation is safe in children and adolescents; efficacy is variable.

ONGOING CARE

FOLLOW-UP RECOMMENDATIONS

- Patients managed conservatively should be reevaluated within 2 weeks and then visits spaced further out as their pain improves.
- If symptoms not improving with conservative measures, then consider workup as outlined and appropriate referral depending on results.

Patient Monitoring

No specific lab tests need to be routinely followed.

PATIENT EDUCATION

- Patients and families need to be aware that musculoskeletal and structural causes may take several weeks or months to heal.
- Bony healing in spondylolysis is not correlated with clinical outcome in many cases.
- Patients should be told to report changes in symptoms, especially any red flags.
- Higher body mass index (BMI) has been associated with low back pain; weight counseling in overweight or obese patients may be of benefit.

PROGNOSIS

- Dependent on the underlying cause
- With proper diagnosis and treatment, the majority do well, without significant sequelae.
- Muscular or functional back pain often abates as biomechanical issues are corrected through rehab.
- Bony fractures and stress fractures: Expect to take normal bony healing course with appropriate treatment.

COMPLICATIONS

- Weakness in core and hip muscles
- Paralysis, other permanent neuromuscular injury
- Chronic back pain or development of pain amplification syndrome

ADDITIONAL READING

- Agabegi SS, Kazemi N, Sturm PF, et al. Natural history of adolescent idiopathic scoliosis in skeletally mature patients: a critical review. *J Am Acad Orthop Surg*. 2015;23(12):714–723.
- Brenner JS; for American Academy of Pediatrics Council on Sports Medicine and Fitness. Overuse injuries, overtraining, and burnout in child and adolescent athletes. *Pediatrics*. 2007;119(6):1242–1245.
- Furlan AD, Imamura M, Dryden T, et al. Massage for low back pain: an updated systematic review within the framework of the Cochrane Back Review Group. *Spine (Phila Pa 1976)*. 2009;34(16):1669–1684.
- Hershkovich O, Friedlander A, Gordon B, et al. Associations of body mass index and body height with low back pain in 829,791 adolescents. *Am J Epidemiol*. 2013;178(4):603–609.
- Jackson C, McLaughlin K, Teti B. Back pain in children: a holistic approach to diagnosis and management. *J Pediatr Health Care*. 2011;25(5):284–293.
- Michaleff ZA, Kamper SJ, Maher CG, et al. Low back pain in children and adolescents: a systematic review and meta-analysis evaluating the effectiveness of conservative interventions. *Eur Spine J*. 2014;23(10):2046–2058.
- Shah SA, Saller J. Evaluation and diagnosis of back pain in children and adolescents. *J Am Acad Orthop Surg*. 2016;24(1):37–45.
- Taxter AJ, Chauvin NA, Weiss PF. Diagnosis and treatment of low back pain in the pediatric population. *Phys Sportsmed*. 2014;42(1):94–104.
- Tsirikos AI, Garrido EG. Spondylolysis and spondylolisthesis in children and adolescents. *J Bone Joint Surg Br*. 2010;92(6):751–759.

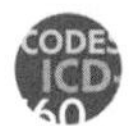

CODES

ICD10

- M54.9 Dorsalgia, unspecified
- M54.6 Pain in thoracic spine
- M54.5 Low back pain

FAQ

- Q: Which children with back pain should have activity restriction?
- A: Activities should be able to be performed with normal mechanics (no limping or adjustment of skills due to pain). Resting is indicated if this is not possible. Workup and ultimate diagnosis will determine further activity restriction.
- Q: When can/should the child resume activities after an acute back injury?
- A: Children with a normal neurologic exam, normal range of motion, and normal strength may resume tolerable activities if diagnostic studies are normal.
- Q: Should a trial of steroids be used to rule out inflammatory back pain?
- A: Pain improvement with glucocorticoids may suggest an inflammatory condition but is not diagnostic. It is not recommended in children. It can often complicate the clinical picture, as noninflammatory back pain will sometimes respond to treatment as well.

BAROTITIS

Judith Brylinski Larkin, MD, FAAP

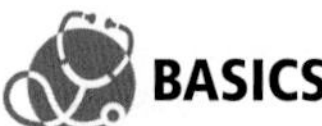

BASICS

DESCRIPTION
- Barotrauma of the middle or inner ear, most commonly caused by flying in an airplane or scuba diving but also caused by travel in elevators and travel to high altitudes
- May also be seen in those who have used a hyperbaric oxygen chamber and in people involved in explosions—blast injuries
- Referred to as "middle ear squeeze" by scuba divers

EPIDEMIOLOGY
- Severe disease is uncommon in commercial aircraft because of pressurization.
- Significant disease is more common in scuba divers, in those who fly military aircraft, and during use of hyperbaric oxygen chambers.
- There is wide variation, with studies reporting an incidence of 8–55% for children after a single flight.
- Most studies agree that the incidence is ~20% in adults after a single flight.
- 40% frequency in scuba diving

RISK FACTORS
- Age: Infants or toddlers are at higher risk because of small eustachian tubes.
- Disease states that impede normal eustachian tube function: otitis media, upper respiratory tract infection (URI), allergic rhinitis
- Smoking
- Vigorous use of Valsalva maneuver

GENERAL PREVENTION
- Gradual descent during scuba diving—never rapid
- When ascending, divers should avoid rising more quickly than their air bubbles.
- Yawning, swallowing, chewing, or doing Valsalva maneuver during takeoff and landing in planes and during ascent and descent when scuba diving
- Gentle Valsalva—never vigorous
- Avoid flying or diving when you have a URI or allergic rhinitis.
- Avoid sleeping on plane during takeoff and landing.
- Break seal of wet suit hood to allow water to fill external canal before descent.
- Avoid use of earplugs.

PATHOPHYSIOLOGY
- Boyle's law states that as pressure of a gas decreases, volume increases, and as pressure of a gas increases, volume decreases.
- Ambient pressure decreases during airplane/scuba diving ascent and increases during descent.
- During ascent, the tympanic membrane (TM) bulges outward and the eustachian tube vents the excess middle ear pressure. Pressure is easily equalized.
- During descent, the TM bulges inward and the eustachian tube resists inward flow of air. Pressure equalization is difficult.
- At a pressure differential of 60 mm Hg (greater ambient to middle ear pressure), subjective discomfort is reported.
- At a pressure differential of 90 mm Hg, the eustachian tube collapses and becomes obstructed. Autoinflation is unsuccessful.
- TM can rupture at pressure differentials >100 to 400 mm Hg.
- Barotitis is sometimes classified using Teed classification of disease severity (see "Physical Exam").

ETIOLOGY
Differences in the atmospheric pressure between the inner ear, middle ear, and environment result in injury to the middle and/or inner ear.

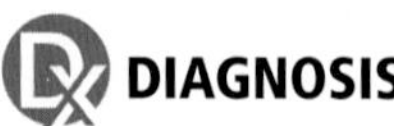

DIAGNOSIS

HISTORY
- Ear pain, pressure sensation, diminished hearing
- Symptoms of inner ear damage may include vestibular and/or auditory complaints including tinnitus, vertigo, nausea, and vomiting.
- History of recent airplane flying, scuba diving, or hyperbaric oxygen chamber use

PHYSICAL EXAM
- Nystagmus
- Hearing loss
- Teed classification to describe appearance of the TM:
  - Grade 0: symptoms without physical signs
  - Grade 1: diffuse redness and retraction of TM
  - Grade 2: grade 1 plus slight hemorrhage into TM
  - Grade 3: grade 1 plus gross hemorrhage into TM
  - Grade 4: bulging TM with air–fluid level, blood in TM
  - Grade 5: free hemorrhage into TM and ear canal with perforation of TM

DIFFERENTIAL DIAGNOSIS
- Otitis media with effusion
- Acute otitis media
- Otitis externa
- Blunt trauma to the TM
- Exposure to extremely loud noise

DIAGNOSTIC TESTS & INTERPRETATION

Initial Tests (screening, lab, imaging)
CT of the inner ear may be indicated in patients with vestibular symptoms or hearing loss to rule out inner ear damage.

Diagnostic Procedures/Other
Hearing tests should be performed on all patients who have signs of barotrauma and on patients with normal physical exams but who are symptomatic.

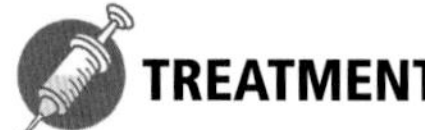

TREATMENT

GENERAL MEASURES
- Valsalva maneuver (blowing the nose while pinching the nostrils closed) may be helpful when diving or descending and will force air into the middle ear via the eustachian tube, thereby equalizing the pressure between the middle ear and the environment. This should be done gently.
- Swallowing, yawning, and chewing can help to release pressure through the eustachian tube when descending in an airplane or when returning to the water surface while scuba diving.
- Politzer bag: instrument used for clearing pressure disequilibrium that has not improved with Valsalva maneuvers and a trial of decongestants
- Otovent: Another instrument that may be used for treatment or prevention; usage can be taught to children as young as 2 to 6 years of age.
- Myringotomy with or without tubes may be required to relieve pressure in severe disease. It may also be used as a preventive measure in those with a history of barotitis.
- Myringotomy is effective for the patient with excruciating pain or unrelenting eustachian tube dysfunction; this is best performed by an otolaryngologist.

MEDICATION

- Nasal decongestant sprays (oxymetazoline [Afrin®])
  - Have been reported by some to be helpful, but a randomized clinical trial showed no advantage over placebo
  - Theory: By constricting mucosal arterioles, eustachian tube function is enhanced.
  - Topical decongestants are used 1 hour prior to plane travel/diving and 1/2 hour prior to plane descent.
  - 2 drops/sprays per nostril
  - Use in children >6 years of age.
- Oral decongestants
  - Two randomized controlled trials suggest that oral decongestants may be effective, although a trial in children did not show a beneficial effect.
  - May be helpful through the same physiologic pathway as topical agents
  - Should be initiated 1 to 2 days prior to the expected pressure change
- Antihistamines
  - May also be helpful by reducing mucosal edema and enhancing the eustachian tube orifice
  - Can be used on the day of the expected pressure change
- Nasal surfactants may be useful, but ongoing studies are needed.
- Pain relievers such as acetaminophen, ibuprofen, and naproxen may be useful for severe pain.

SURGERY/OTHER PROCEDURES

Rarely, myringotomy with or without tube insertion is required to relieve pressure and pain as well as prevent complications. Myringotomy is a surgical procedure where a small incision is made in the TM. This opens the middle ear space and equalizes the pressure on both sides of the TM. Myringotomy without tube insertion will relieve pressure, but the opening may close very quickly and may not allow time for the barotrauma to heal; on occasion, myringotomy with tube insertion is necessary. Tympanostomy tubes are not appropriate for scuba divers.

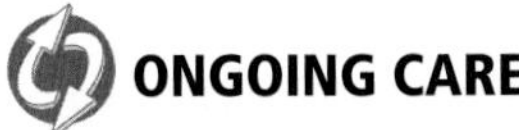

ONGOING CARE

FOLLOW-UP RECOMMENDATIONS

Patient Monitoring

Most patients with barotitis can be managed conservatively. Those with complications noted earlier require specialist referral.

PROGNOSIS

- Complete spontaneous resolution in mild cases
- Middle ear barotrauma is usually self-limited and correctable with the techniques described in the "General Measures" section. In rare instances, where there is severe pain or eustachian tube dysfunction, myringotomy with or without tube insertion will relieve the pressure differential.
- Pressure differential without damage to the middle or inner ear usually resolves within a few days of returning to normal atmospheric pressure.
- Barotitis that results in injury to the middle or inner ear has a variable rate of improvement; some damage may be permanent (e.g., that to the organ of Corti), whereas other injury is reversible (e.g., that involving the TM).
- Variable outcome for auditory and vestibular symptoms and injuries to the inner ear

COMPLICATIONS

- Vertigo
- Tinnitus
- Hearing loss
- TM rupture
- Oval or round window rupture
- Hemorrhage

ADDITIONAL READING

- Buchanan BJ, Hoagland J, Fischer PR. Pseudoephedrine and air travel-associated ear pain in children. *Arch Pediatr Adolesc Med*. 1999;153(5):466–468.
- Janvrin S. Middle ear pain and trauma during air travel. *Clin Evid*. 2002;7:466–468.
- Jones JS, Sheffield W, White L, et al. A double-blind comparison between oral pseudoephedrine and topical oxymetazoline in the prevention of barotrauma during air travel. *Am J Emerg Med*. 1998;16(3):262–264.
- Mirza S, Richardson H. Otic barotrauma from air travel. *J Laryngol Otol*. 2005;119(5):366–370.
- Rosenkvist L, Klokker M, Katholm M. Upper respiratory infections and barotraumas in commercial pilots: a retrospective survey. *Aviat Space Environ Med*. 2008;79(10):960–963.
- Stangerup SE, Klokker M, Vesterhauge S, et al. Point prevalence of barotitis and its prevention and treatment with nasal balloon inflation: a prospective, controlled study. *Otol Neurotol*. 2004;25(2):89–94.
- Weiss MH, Frost JO. May children with otitis media with effusion safely fly? *Clin Pediatr (Phila)*. 1987;26(11):567–568.

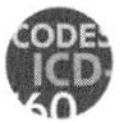

CODES

ICD10

- T70.0XXA Otitic barotrauma, initial encounter
- H92.09 Otalgia, unspecified ear
- H93.19 Tinnitus, unspecified ear

FAQ

- Q: Is the Valsalva maneuver also effective on plane ascent?
- A: Yes. Creating even greater pressure in the middle ear by performing the Valsalva maneuver can overcome a resistant eustachian tube and result in sudden venting of increased middle ear pressure.
- Q: Can children with otitis media travel in airplanes?
- A: Yes. Weiss and Frost (1987) have shown that commercial air travel did not result in worsening of symptoms and, in fact, the presence of otitis media with effusion seemed to be protective against barotitis.
- Q: How can I minimize my child's ear pain when traveling in an airplane?
- A: For infants: Have them nurse, take a bottle, or suck on a pacifier during ascent and descent. Older children may eat or chew gum or suck on hard candies. This will result in pharyngeal movements that will repeatedly open the eustachian tube and equalize middle ear pressure to environmental pressure. Children can also be taught the Valsalva maneuver. If the child is currently experiencing a URI, use of decongestants prior to flight may be helpful.

BELL PALSY

Stephen J. Falchek, MD

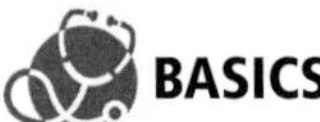

BASICS

DESCRIPTION

- This paralysis may involve all of the modalities affected by the 7th cranial nerve:
  - Mimetic facial movement
  - Taste
  - Cutaneous sensation
  - Hearing acuity
  - Lacrimation
  - Salivation
- The most important feature in diagnosis and management of Bell palsy is the distinction between a peripheral and a central 7th nerve palsy.

EPIDEMIOLOGY

Incidence

- Annually, incidence ranges from 3/100,000 in patients <10 years to 25/100,000 in adults.
- Only 1% of cases have bilateral involvement.

PATHOPHYSIOLOGY

Nearly all cases of true Bell palsy are believed to arise from a viral infection of the facial nerve and, in particular, the geniculate ganglion.

ETIOLOGY

- Idiopathic: pregnancy-related
- Infectious
  - Herpes simplex virus 1
  - Human herpesvirus 6
  - Herpes zoster (without Ramsay Hunt syndrome)

COMMONLY ASSOCIATED CONDITIONS

- Associated illnesses can cause or predispose to an isolated facial nerve palsy but are important to distinguish from a classic Bell palsy.
- Rubella
- Lyme disease (*Borrelia burgdorferi*)
- Epstein-Barr virus (EBV)
- Cytomegalovirus (CMV)
- Mumps
- HIV
- *Mycoplasma pneumoniae*
- Sarcoidosis

DIAGNOSIS

HISTORY

- Mastoid or retroauricular pain ipsilateral to the side of developing symptoms (40–50% of patients)
- 50% of patients will have no clear sensory prodrome.
- Bell palsy often follows some identifiable infectious illness, such as viral upper respiratory tract infection (URI) symptoms, *M. pneumoniae* infection, Lyme disease, or infectious mononucleosis. However, an identified antecedent illness is not requisite for the diagnosis.
- The onset is almost always rapid, with progression to a fairly constant state of unilateral paresis or paralysis within hours to 2 to 3 days.
- As the weakness progresses, the patient (and family members) may note the following:
  - Difficulty with oral motor tasks (e.g., eating and drinking) due to inability to maintain mouth closure
  - Inability to completely close the eye on the affected side (sometimes leading untrained observers to note an eyelid "droop" on the normal side due to the contrast with normal eyelid closure and movements)
  - Decreased lacrimation and eye itching and burning
  - Hyperacusis
  - Ipsilateral facial numbness (less commonly)
  - Distortion of the taste of foods (dysgeusia)
- Bilateral symptoms (<1%) are distinctly rare and suggest an alternative diagnosis, such as Guillain-Barré syndrome or other infectious, inflammatory, or metabolic disease.

PHYSICAL EXAM

- Weakness of all muscles of mimetic facial movement is noted on the affected side.
- A classic feature of peripheral facial nerve palsies is symmetric weakness or paralysis of the upper (frontalis), middle (orbicularis oculi), and lower (orbicularis oris) muscles on voluntary and involuntary mimetic movements. Having the patient wrinkle his or her forehead, raise his or her eyebrows, close his or her eyes tightly, and bare his or her teeth or smile, respectively, test these muscles.
- Occasionally, slow or absent spontaneous blinking on the affected side
- The corneal reflex should be decreased or absent on the affected side, but the consensual response on the unaffected side should be preserved.
- The sensory division of the 7th cranial nerve is tested by examining taste perception on the anterior tongue:
  - This is done by applying, ipsilaterally, swabs soaked in a sugar solution and a salt solution to the anterolateral aspect of the tongue, without allowing for mouth closure and dispersion of the substances to the other side. Taste sensation should be ipsilaterally decreased.
  - Despite complaints of retroauricular pain and unilateral facial "numbness," abnormalities of cutaneous sensation typically are not verifiable by sensory testing in pure 7th nerve palsies. The presence of true diminution of sensation should raise the question of other cranial nerve involvement (e.g., 5th cranial nerve).
- Examination of the external auditory canal on both sides is crucial.
  - Vesicular lesions of the tympanic membrane indicate a zoster-associated palsy (i.e., Ramsay Hunt syndrome).
  - Purulent acute otitis media or evidence of trauma mandates aggressive antibiotic treatment and possibly urgent surgical subspecialty evaluation and imaging of the temporal bone.

DIFFERENTIAL DIAGNOSIS

- Trauma
  - Birth (especially forceps pressure to lateral face)
  - Congenital facial palsies should not be regarded as Bell palsy but rather symptomatic of some other cause.
  - Temporal bone/petrous bone fractures
  - Deep lacerations or trauma to parotid region
- Infection
  - Purulent acute otitis media/mastoiditis
  - Basilar meningitis
  - Petrous apicitis (Gradenigo syndrome)
  - Varicella-zoster virus (VZV; Ramsay Hunt syndrome)
  - Syphilis
  - Trichinosis
  - Tuberculosis
  - Leprosy
- Inflammatory
  - Sarcoidosis
  - Behçet disease
  - Giant cell arteritis
  - Polyarteritis nodosa
  - Guillain-Barré syndrome
  - Melkersson-Rosenthal syndrome: rare neurologic disorder characterized by recurring facial paralysis, swelling of the face and lips (usually the upper lip), and the development of folds and furrows in the tongue
- Tumors
  - Cerebellopontine angle tumors, osteosarcomas, cholesteatomas, neurofibromas, lymphoma
  - Hyperostosis cranialis interna, osteopetrosis
- Metabolic
  - Diabetes (nerve ischemia)
  - Hyperparathyroidism
  - Hypothyroidism
  - Porphyria
- Congenital/genetic
  - Congenital absence or hypoplasia of depressor anguli oris muscle
  - Möbius syndrome
  - Chiari malformation
  - Syringobulbia

DIAGNOSTIC TESTS & INTERPRETATION

Initial Tests (screening, lab, imaging)

- The decision to defer medical imaging in the evaluation of a typical Bell palsy should be based on a sound clinical history and physical examination. Unusual features should provoke thoughtful review and broader investigation where indicated.
- MRI of the head with gadolinium enhancement: recommended in cases of unusual presentation or progression (e.g., bilateral involvement, slow progression [>1 week], or other cranial nerve findings). Several small series have proposed that gadolinium enhancement of the involved 7th nerve predicts a slower or less optimal recovery.

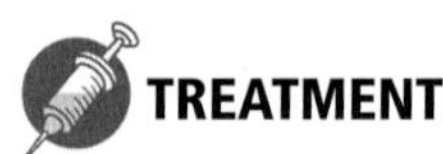

TREATMENT

Identifying treatable causes of 7th nerve palsy (e.g., Lyme borreliosis and Ramsay Hunt syndrome) is crucial for optimizing outcome and preventing comorbidities of these illnesses.

GENERAL MEASURES

- Eye protection and lubrication: A significant risk for corneal injury is best managed by applying artificial tear solutions at least 3 to 4 times daily and lubricating gels (e.g., Lacri-Lube) at night. Patching and protective eyewear, during active play and sleep, are usually prescribed based on the degree of remaining eyelid closure.
- Corticosteroids: prednisone, considered only within the first 72 hours of symptoms. Recommended dose: 1 mg/kg/24 h PO (maximum 80 mg) once daily for 5 days, with a taper over the following 5 days. Recent evidence suggests that corticosteroids may worsen long-term outcomes in cases of facial palsy associated with Lyme disease. Therefore, careful consideration of this etiology prior to prescribing steroids, and prompt follow-up of laboratory results/Lyme serologies, ought to be priority. Consider adjustment of treatment strategy if Lyme serologies are positive for acute infection.
- Famciclovir: most clearly indicated for the treatment of Ramsay Hunt syndrome. It is also used empirically by some practitioners in standard Bell palsy management, although evidence for its supplementary use to

corticosteroids is still relatively weak; see discussion in the following text. Recommended dose for children ≥45 kg and adolescents: 250 mg t.i.d. PO for 5 to 7 days. Valacyclovir 20 mg/kg/dose (max dose: 1,000 mg/dose) t.i.d. PO for 7 days may be used as an alternative agent for children <45 kg. Generally, any evidence of vesicular eruption in the ear canal or face should be treated promptly with antiherpetic agents (famciclovir or valacyclovir preferred over acyclovir), as outcomes from VZV-associated palsies are reported to be worse in general.

MEDICATION

- Corticosteroids: Recent large series and meta-analyses indicate that treatment with corticosteroids is effective in reducing the risk of incomplete recovery; however, this treatment seems to be only effective if initiated within the first 48 hours of symptoms. The occurrence of synkinesias is less likely in patients treated with steroids within 48 hours across all age groups.
- Antivirals: There is little or no benefit to therapy with antivirals alone. Recent meta-analyses suggest that antivirals may provide benefit when used in combination with corticosteroids, both in functional recovery and reduction of long-term sequelae. However, the quality of evidence remains low to moderate. Famciclovir, when used in combination with corticosteroids, provides superior benefit compared to acyclovir, and so famciclovir seems to be the antiviral drug of choice for idiopathic facial palsy. The best evidence for added efficacy of antivirals in combination with corticosteroids still seems to be in cases with particularly severe degrees of paralysis or in cases with suspected herpes zoster infection.
- Antibiotics: In areas where Lyme disease is endemic, many practitioners will begin treatment with oral antibiotics presumptively, while awaiting serologies (recall that the IgM titer is the most useful in the acute setting). (See "Lyme Disease" chapter.)

First Line

- Prednisone, 1 mg/kg/dose (max 80 mg/24 h) PO once daily for 5 days, with a subsequent taper over 5 days; total treatment course 10 days; must be initiated in the first 48 hours for significant results
- Amoxicillin, 50 mg/kg/24 h PO divided in 3 doses for 21 to 28 days, when Lyme disease suspected

Second Line

For presumed Lyme disease:

- Patients >8 years: doxycycline, 100 mg PO b.i.d. for 21 to 28 days
- Patients of all ages: cefuroxime, 30 mg/kg/24 h PO in 2 divided doses for 21 to 28 days
- In cases where zoster infection is suspected or with particularly severe paralysis at onset: famciclovir 250 mg t.i.d. for 5 to 7 days, as adjunct to corticosteroids; treatment guidelines are not well-established.
- Valacyclovir, 20 mg/kg/dose (max 1 g/dose) divided t.i.d. for 5 days as adjunct to corticosteroids; treatment guidelines are not well-established.

SURGERY/OTHER PROCEDURES

Surgical decompression: Previously, surgical decompression of the 7th nerve had been proposed as a possible treatment in cases where recovery was delayed or the clinical course more severe. No clinical evidence to support the benefit of this strategy has emerged. Surgical decompression is best reserved for "other" cases of facial nerve palsy in which there is a definable syndrome of nerve compression due to extrinsic factors, such as exostoses, tumor, etc.

ISSUES FOR REFERRAL

Subspecialty consultation: In general, patients are referred if their recovery time is prolonged or if there is a relapsing pattern or other deviations from the expected course. However, the presence of other questionable cranial nerve involvement, recent trauma, meningeal symptoms, or neurologic findings (e.g., eye movement abnormalities, acute hemiparesis, etc.) should be viewed with great concern and evaluated in an urgent care setting.

ADDITIONAL THERAPIES

The decision to pursue physical therapy after Bell palsy is a matter of personal preference for the practitioner and family.

- A recent study of a large number of patients, comparing oral corticosteroids versus corticosteroids plus Kabat physical rehabilitation, showed a significant degree of improvement in the latter group in functional facial movement outcomes, at a much faster rate. There was no statistically significant difference in the incidence of synkinesias (abnormal involuntary movements that accompany a normally executed voluntary movement).
- However, the application of physical therapy in Bell palsy recovery remains controversial, and the latest clinical practice guidelines from the American Academy of Otolaryngology—Head and Neck Surgery include no recommendation for facial physical therapy. There is no evidence that facial physiotherapy is harmful.

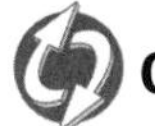

ONGOING CARE

DIET

There are no dietary restrictions that affect the outcome of Bell palsy.

PATIENT EDUCATION

Minimizing risk for injury to the cornea ipsilateral to the facial palsy may require either restricting some activities where debris or contusions to the eye are likely or wearing protective eyewear during such activities (e.g., beach activities and competitive sports). These restrictions only need to be in effect so long as there is inadequate closure of the eyelid on the affected side.

PROGNOSIS

- 60–70% full-recovery rate from isolated 7th nerve palsy
- Signs of recovering function (generally improving control of mimetic movement) are typically apparent by the 3rd week after onset.
- Prognosis for recovery seems to be worse with either a secondary deterioration in function after 2 to 4 days, no signs of recovery after 3 weeks, or demonstrated gadolinium enhancement of the affected facial nerve on MRI.
- Of patients with less than total recovery, many will experience at least partial return to normal function; cosmetic results vary in this group.
- Outcome of idiopathic facial palsy as a pregnancy complication seems to be less favorable (~55% full recovery).
- Up to 7% of patients may experience a second occurrence at some point in the future.

COMPLICATIONS

- Corneal injury, due to decreased lacrimation and poor eye closure
- Several sequelae, generally related to aberrant reinnervation of affected end organs, are observed after an episode of Bell palsy.
  - Various synkinesias including the Marin-Amat phenomenon (spontaneous eye closure with mouth opening or its converse)
  - Blepharospasm, hemifacial spasm, facial contractures
  - The "crocodile tears" phenomenon (eating provokes ipsilateral tearing) results from crossed reinnervation between lacrimal and salivary parasympathetic fibers.

ADDITIONAL READING

- Baugh RF, Basura GJ, Ishii LE, et al. Clinical practice guideline: Bell's palsy. *Otolaryngol Head Neck Surg*. 2013;149(Suppl 3):S1–S27.
- Gronseth GS, Paduga R; for American Academy of Neurology. Evidence-based guideline update: steroids and antivirals for Bell palsy: report of the Guideline Development Subcommittee of the American Academy of Neurology. *Neurology*. 2012;79(22):2209–2213.
- Hernandez JM, Sherbino J. Do antiviral medications improve symptoms in the treatment of Bell's palsy? *Ann Emerg Med*. 2017;69(3):364–365.
- Jowett N, Gaudin R, Banks C, et al. Steroid use in Lyme disease-associated facial palsy is associated with worse long-term outcomes. *Laryngoscope*. 2017;127(6):1451–1458.
- Kim HJ, Kim SH, Jung J, et al. Comparison of acyclovir and famciclovir for the treatment of Bell's palsy. *Eur Arch Otorhinolaryngol*. 2016;273(10): 3083–3090.
- Lee HY, Byun JY, Park MS, et al. Steroid-antiviral treatment improves the recovery rate in patients with severe Bell's palsy. *Am J Med*. 2013;126(4): 336–341.
- Madhok VB, Gagyor I, Daly F, et al. Corticosteroids for Bell's palsy (idiopathic facial paralysis). *Cochrane Database Syst Rev*. 2016;(7):CD001942.
- Monini S, Iacolucci CM, Di Traglia M, et al. Role of Kabat rehabilitation in facial nerve palsy: a randomised study on severe cases of Bell's palsy. *Acta Otorhinolaryngol Ital*. 2016;36(4):282–288.
- Pereira LM, Obara K, Dias JM, et al. Facial exercise therapy for facial palsy: systematic review and meta-analysis. *Clin Rehabil*. 2011;25(7):649–658.
- Teixeira LJ, Soares BG, Vieira VP, et al. Physical therapy for Bell's palsy (idiopathic facial paralysis). *Cochrane Database Syst Rev*. 2008;(3):CD006283.

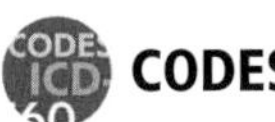

CODES

ICD10

G51.0 Bell's palsy

FAQ

- Q: How does one differentiate between peripheral facial nerve palsy and a CNS lesion?
- A: A critical step in diagnosis is the differentiation of peripheral from central (upper motor neuron) lesions. With upper motor neuron lesions (above the level of the 7th nerve nucleus), there is preferential weakness of lower facial musculature and, sometimes, differential paresis of voluntary versus spontaneous emotional mimetic movements. Brainstem lesions, on the other hand, may produce a peripheral-appearing lesion but almost always have involvement of other pathways and cranial nerve nuclei, for example, ipsilateral lateral rectus palsy and contralateral somatic hemiplegia (Millard-Gubler syndrome).

BEZOARS

Andrew B. Grossman, MD

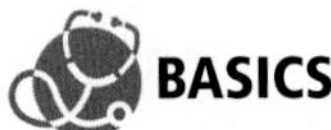

BASICS

DESCRIPTION

- Accumulation of foreign material in the gastrointestinal (GI) tract
- Commonly divided into three categories based on the substances from which the bezoar is derived:
  - Phytobezoar (from vegetables/fruits)
  - Trichobezoar (hair)
  - Lactobezoar (milk/formula)
- Documented to occur in humans for >2 millennia, suggesting formation of bezoars may have been/still be culturally important for certain societies

EPIDEMIOLOGY

- Phytobezoars occur almost exclusively in adults.
- 90% of trichobezoars occur in female patients <20 years of age.
- Lactobezoars occur mostly in premature, low-birth-weight infants.

PATHOPHYSIOLOGY

- Trichobezoars
  - Associated with developmental delay, pica, trichotillomania, and trichophagia; may ingest own hair but also rugs and animal or doll hair
  - Most cases of trichophagia do not result in bezoar formation (~1%).
  - History of trichophagia is obtained in only 50% of cases.
  - Retention and accumulation of hair strands in the gastric folds
  - Trichobezoars may become large and form a cast in the stomach leading to abdominal mass.
  - Bezoar may extend through the pylorus into the small bowel. This phenomenon is commonly referred to as Rapunzel syndrome. The "tail" may obstruct the ampulla of Vater, leading to jaundice and pancreatitis.
- Phytobezoars
  - Most common form among adults, rare in children
  - Associated with gastric dysmotility and poor gastric emptying (either primary or following gastric surgery) and hypochlorhydria
  - Composed primarily of cellulose, hemicellulose, lignins, and tannins
- Lactobezoars (milk)
  - Most often reported in premature, low-birth-weight infants being fed high-calorie premature formula (although there are reports in full-term infants and exclusively breastfed infants)
  - Factors contributing to lactobezoar formation include the following:
    - Formulas with high casein content
    - Early and rapid feeding advancement in small infants
    - High-caloric-density formulas
    - Formulas with high calcium/phosphate content
    - Continuous tube feedings
    - Altered gastric motility in low-birth-weight infants

ETIOLOGY

Classification of bezoars is dependent on the most prominent substance from which they are formed, including:

- Trichobezoars: hair, carpet
- Phytobezoars: indigestible fruit and vegetable matter
- Lactobezoars: milk
- Less common materials include the following:
  - Foreign bodies
  - Gallstones
  - Medications, including vitamins, antacids, psyllium, sucralfate, cimetidine, and nifedipine
- Can occur in cystic fibrosis (CF) patients after lung transplantation
- Colonic and rectal bezoars
  - Due to indigestible sunflower seeds, popcorn, and chewing gum have been reported in children and adults
  - These usually present with obstruction, although encopresis and colitis-type symptoms have been described.

COMMONLY ASSOCIATED CONDITIONS

- Iron deficiency anemia
- Steatorrhea
- Protein-losing enteropathy

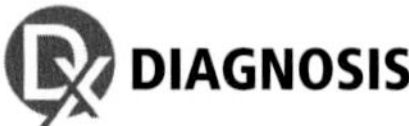

DIAGNOSIS

HISTORY

- Signs and symptoms of bezoar formation include the following:
  - Pain
  - Halitosis
  - Nausea
  - Vomiting
  - Diarrhea
  - Gastric ulceration
  - Upper GI bleeding and perforation
  - Left upper quadrant mass
- Lactobezoars
  - Diarrhea
  - Emesis
  - Increased gastric residuals

PHYSICAL EXAM
- Trichobezoars
  - Unusual patterns of balding
  - Palpable left upper quadrant mass in the abdomen is often detected.
  - Hair found in the stool
- Phytobezoars
  - Abdominal mass is palpable in <50% of patients.
- Lactobezoars
  - Abdominal distention

DIFFERENTIAL DIAGNOSIS
Any gastric foreign body can mimic a gastric mass and may be present on palpation.

DIAGNOSTIC TESTS & INTERPRETATION
Initial Tests (screening, lab, imaging)
- Assess for iron deficiency anemia.
- Assess for presence of steatorrhea or protein-losing enteropathy.
- Plain abdominal x-ray
  - Heterogeneous intragastric mass that could be mistaken for food-filled stomach
- Upper GI barium studies
  - May identify and outline the mass
- Ultrasound and CT can also be helpful.

Diagnostic Procedures/Other
Endoscopy allows for direct visualization and elucidation of composition of bezoar.

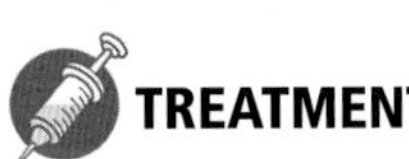

TREATMENT

GENERAL MEASURES
- Trichobezoars
  - Difficult to remove endoscopically; attempts to fragment may result in migration and small bowel obstruction.
  - Treatment is usually surgical removal: Trichobezoars are normally large and hair is not dissolvable.
- Phytobezoars
  - Medications such as prokinetic agents to stimulate gastric motility
  - Enzyme therapy to help dissolve the material
  - *N*-acetylcysteine treatment via nasogastric tube has been documented in one case report.
  - Endoscopic fragmentation or extraction
  - Coca-Cola administration with or without endoscopic extraction has been reported to be effective.
  - Surgical extraction
  - Diet alteration
- Lactobezoars
  - Withholding feedings for 48 hours while the patient is sustained on IV fluids will resolve most lactobezoars.
  - Gentle gastric lavage may be helpful.

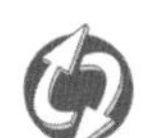

ONGOING CARE

FOLLOW-UP RECOMMENDATIONS
Based on the type of bezoar removed, dietary counseling, medications regimen modification, behavioral modification therapy, and/or correction of underlying motility problems may help prevent future recurrence.

PROGNOSIS
Dependent on type, size, and location of bezoar

COMPLICATIONS
- Protein-losing enteropathy
- Steatorrhea
- Vitamin deficiencies
- Pancreatitis
- Gastric ulcer or gastritis
- GI bleeding
- Intestinal obstruction
- Perforation

ADDITIONAL READING

- Chogle A, Bonilla S, Browne M, et al. Rapunzel syndrome: a rare cause of biliary obstruction. *J Pediatr Gastroenterol Nutr*. 2010;51(4):522–523.
- DuBose TM V, Southgate WM, Hill JG. Lactobezoars: a patient series and literature review. *Clin Pediatr (Phila)*. 2001;40(11):603–606.
- Ladas SD, Kamberoglou D, Karamanolis G, et al. Systematic review: Coca-Cola can effectively dissolve gastric phytobezoars as a first-line treatment. *Aliment Pharmacol Ther*. 2013;37(2):169–173.
- Lynch KA, Feola PG, Guenther E. Gastric trichobezoar: an important cause of abdominal pain presenting to the pediatric emergency department. *Pediatr Emerg Care*. 2003;19(5):343–347.
- Taylor JR, Streetman DS, Castle SS. Medication bezoars: a literature review and report of a case. *Ann Pharmacother*. 1998;32(9):940–946.

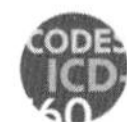

CODES

ICD10
- T18.9XXA Foreign body of alimentary tract, part unspecified, initial encounter
- T18.2XXA Foreign body in stomach, initial encounter
- T18.3XXA Foreign body in small intestine, initial encounter

FAQ
- Q: What are some commonly used medications that can lead to bezoar formation?
- A: Vitamins, antacids, psyllium, sucralfate, cimetidine, and nifedipine
- Q: What may place an infant at risk for formation of a bezoar?
- A: The literature suggests that formulas with high casein content may be linked with lactobezoar formation. Other possible contributing factors include early and rapid feeding advancement in small infants, high-density formulas, formulas with a high calcium/phosphate content, continuous tube feedings, and altered gastric motility in low-birth-weight infants.

BILIARY ATRESIA

Sina Ogholikhan, MD • Douglas B. Mogul, MD, MPH

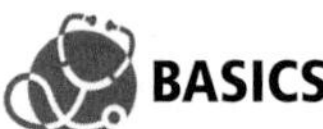

BASICS

DESCRIPTION

Biliary atresia (BA) is a congenital disease characterized by fibrosis, obstruction, and obliteration of the biliary system that is universally fatal without intervention.

EPIDEMIOLOGY

- BA accounts for approximately 30% of cases of neonatal cholestasis.
- BA is the most common cause of persistent cholestasis in infants and children and the most frequent indication for pediatric liver transplantation.
- The disease affects 1:8,000 to 1:18,000 live births.

RISK FACTORS

Genetics

- No single genetic mutation has been identified as the sole cause of BA, and there is no clear pattern of inheritance.
- Genes influencing morphogenesis may contribute to pathophysiology.

PATHOPHYSIOLOGY

- Biliary obstruction begins at, or near, the time of birth and progresses throughout early infancy, leading to damage and ultimately scarring of liver parenchyma.
- Approximately 20% of biliary patients have at least one other major congenital anomaly (i.e., embryonal form) including splenic malformation, interrupted inferior vena cava, midline liver, situs inversus, preduodenal portal vein, and intestinal malrotation.
- More common form is the perinatal form that is not associated with malformations.

ETIOLOGY

Etiology is not completely defined, but many different pathogenic mechanisms have been proposed, including the following:

- Perinatal infection of the liver and biliary tract with potential organisms including cytomegalovirus, rotavirus, and reovirus
- Immune dysregulation
- Defective morphogenesis
- Environmental toxin exposure
- Vascular insufficiency

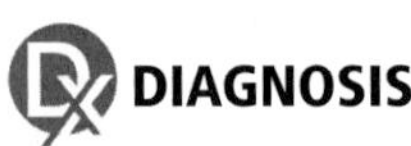

DIAGNOSIS

HISTORY

- Newborns appear healthy at birth with good growth and development. However, jaundice of the skin and eyes persists beyond the 2-week interval of physiologic jaundice.
- Acholic stools and dark urine may be noted.
- In addition, infants with BA may present with poor weight gain, bleeding (due to vitamin K deficiency), and/or increased stool frequency.

PHYSICAL EXAM

- Jaundice can be seen in the eyes, skin, or buccal mucosa.
- Infants may have hepatomegaly and splenomegaly.
- Rectal exam, including digital exam, may reveal acholic stools.

ALERT

- One of the most important factors determining outcomes in BA, including survival and need for transplantation, is the age at which a patient is referred for workup.
- The 10-year survival rate of patients diagnosed and treated prior to 60 days versus after 90 days is 73% and 11%, respectively.

DIFFERENTIAL DIAGNOSIS

- Intrahepatic
  - Infection: sepsis, UTI, gastroenteritis, toxoplasmosis, other viruses, rubella, cytomegalovirus, herpes virus (TORCH) infections, HIV, viral hepatitis (A, B, C, D, E), Epstein-Barr virus, adenovirus, coxsackie B virus, echovirus, enterovirus
  - Systemic disease: panhypopituitarism, congestive heart failure, ischemic hepatopathy, trauma
  - Metabolic: galactosemia, tyrosinemia, α_1-antitrypsin, cystic fibrosis, citrin deficiency, respiratory chain disorders, hereditary fructose intolerance, disorders of bile acid synthesis, storage disorders, neonatal iron storage disease
  - Genetic: Alagille syndrome, Zellweger syndrome, Down syndrome, Turner syndrome
  - Progressive familial intrahepatic cholestasis (i.e., PFIC 1, 2, and 3)
  - Toxins and drugs: total parenteral nutrition, antibiotics, and other medications
  - Miscellaneous: neonatal hepatitis, neonatal lupus, congenital hepatic fibrosis, Caroli syndrome, inspissated bile syndrome, histiocytosis X
- Extrahepatic
  - Choledochal cyst
  - Choledocholithiasis
  - Neonatal sclerosing cholangitis
  - Tumor/mass compression
  - Spontaneous perforation of common bile duct

DIAGNOSTIC TESTS & INTERPRETATION

Initial Tests (screening, lab, imaging)

- An infant stool color card that identifies acholic and normal stool has been used in Taiwan, where it was shown to decrease the time to diagnosis in BA and improve outcomes for children with BA.
- Infants with BA have elevated direct bilirubin at 24 hours of life, suggesting a potential role for screening with this blood test.
- Conjugated hyperbilirubinemia (defined as a conjugated fraction >2 mg/dL or a conjugated bilirubin >20% of the total bilirubin) may be elevated *as early as the first 24 hours of life*.
- Additional laboratory findings may include mild to moderate elevations in AST, ALT, and alkaline phosphatase as well as significant elevations in γ-glutamyltransferase (GGT)
- Additional diagnostic testing should be done as clinically indicated.
- Bacterial cultures (blood, urine, stool), viral studies (hepatitis B, hepatitis C, Epstein-Barr virus, TORCH infections, HIV, adenovirus, enterovirus)
- Metabolic profiles (plasma amino acids, urine organic acids and urine succinylacetone, lactate/pyruvate ratio)
- Serum α_1-antitrypsin level and phenotype
- Thyroid function tests (TSH, free T_4)
- Urine-reducing substances to evaluate for galactosemia (if infant has taken breast milk or lactose-containing formula)
- CBC, coagulation studies (prothrombin time/international normalized ratio/partial thromboplastin time [PT/INR/PTT]), total protein, albumin, and fat-soluble vitamins
- Abdominal ultrasound
  - Should be obtained to rule out choledochal cyst but has poor sensitivity and specificity for BA unless "triangular chord" sign seen (80% sensitive, 98% specific)
  - May also assist in defining embryonal versus perinatal form
- Hepatobiliary iminodiacetic acid (HIDA) scan/hepatobiliary scintigraphy can be obtained to evaluate biliary excretion.

Follow-up Tests & Special Considerations

- Discussion with pediatric gastroenterologist should be obtained following evidence of persistent cholestasis.
- Liver biopsy: In BA, findings may include:
  - Bile duct proliferation
  - Bile stasis
  - Periportal inflammation
  - Periportal fibrosis
- Sweat chloride test (cystic fibrosis)
- Ophthalmology exam to assess for Alagille syndrome (posterior embryotoxon) and congenital infections
- Spine film to evaluate butterfly vertebrae of Alagille syndrome
- Echocardiogram to evaluate cardiac anomalies in Alagille syndrome
- Urine bile acid analysis
- Intraoperative cholangiogram
  - Gold standard for diagnosis of BA but is an invasive test
  - Reserved for individuals with high suspicion of BA

TREATMENT

SURGERY/OTHER PROCEDURES

- A hepatoportoenterostomy (Kasai procedure)
  - The Kasai procedure is the only effective therapy for BA other than a liver transplant.
  - The goal of the Kasai procedure is to restore bile flow from the liver to the intestine.
- Despite the Kasai procedure, 70–80% of patients with BA ultimately require liver transplantation.
  - At 3 months after Kasai procedure, a total serum bilirubin <2 mg/dL is associated with low likelihood of requiring hepatic transplant within 2 years.
  - A total serum bilirubin ≥6 mg/dL is associated with failure of adequate bile flow and higher likelihood of need for liver transplantation.
- Indications for transplantation include the following:
  - Synthetic dysfunction of the liver
  - Complications of portal hypertension (PHTN) such as life-threatening hemorrhage, ascites, and spontaneous bacterial peritonitis
  - Persistent cholestasis with impaired quality of life such as intractable pruritus
  - Recurrent cholangitis

ALERT

- Without surgical intervention, 50–80% of patients with BA will die from biliary cirrhosis by 1 year of age and 90–100% by 3 years of age.
- If diagnosed within the first 3 months of life, surgical therapy can successfully restore bile flow from liver into the intestinal tract in 30–80% of patients.

MEDICATIONS

- After the Kasai operation, patients receive
  - Ursodeoxycholic acid to promote bile flow
  - Supplemental fat-soluble vitamins
  - Oral prophylactic antibiotics to prevent ascending cholangitis
- Corticosteroids have not been shown to improve outcomes in patients with BA.

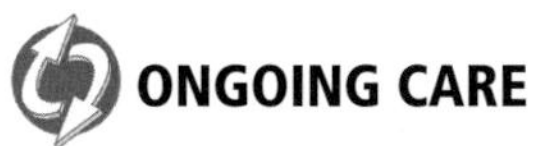

ONGOING CARE

FOLLOW-UP RECOMMENDATIONS

- In conjunction with a GI specialist, obtain routine serum biomarkers including CBC, liver function tests, and GGT to determine progression of disease.
- Physicians should also monitor closely fat-soluble vitamins as well as coagulation studies to evaluate liver function including production of clotting factors and absorption of vitamin K.

DIET

- Anthropometrics should be performed consistently and frequently to evaluate growth as patients tend to have decreased fat stores and decreased lean body mass.
- For individuals with poor weight gain on breast milk or receiving standard formula supplementation, patients should use formulas enriched with medium-chain triglycerides because these fats do not require bile for absorption.
- If patients exhibit poor weight gain on oral feedings, an enteric feeding tube for supplemental nutrition should be strongly considered.
- Due to decrease bile acid excretion, patients with BA malabsorb fat-soluble vitamins (A, D, E, and K) and likely need supplementation.

COMPLICATIONS

- Ascending bacterial cholangitis:
  - Patients are predisposed to this infection after the portoenterostomy procedure given the absence of the ampulla of Vater and present with fever, elevated liver function tests, hypopigmented stools, increased pruritus, and/or increased GGT.
  - Recurrent ascending cholangitis can lead to sclerosis and loss of remaining intrahepatic bile ducts.
  - Antibiotic prophylaxis is helpful in preventing recurrent infections.
- Pruritus:
  - Occurs frequently and is due to elevated circulating bile acid
  - Ursodeoxycholic acid, antihistamines, rifampin, naloxone, and cholestyramine may be used to alleviate itching.
- Ascites:
  - Spironolactone, chlorothiazide, and furosemide are commonly used diuretics; however, their use should be monitored closely in order to avoid the development of hepatorenal syndrome.
- PHTN:
  - Monitoring liver firmness, texture, and span along with splenomegaly will be helpful.
  - Progressive thrombocytopenia suggests further splenomegaly.
  - PHTN can also manifest as ascites, spontaneous bacterial peritonitis, portosystemic encephalopathy, portopulmonary syndrome, or GI hemorrhage from esophageal or gastric varices.
- Very young children with BA display a characteristic profile of early developmental deficits before transplantation, with significant delays in gross motor and language skills.

ADDITIONAL READING

- Caudle SE, Katzenstein JM, Karpen SJ, et al. Language and motor skills are impaired in infants with biliary atresia before transplantation. *J Pediatr*. 2010;156(6):936–940.e1.
- Chen SM, Chang MH, Du JC, et al; for Taiwan Infant Stool Color Card Study Group. Screening for biliary atresia by infant stool color card in Taiwan. *Pediatrics*. 2006;117(4):1147–1154.
- Cowles RA, Lobritto SJ, Ventura KA, et al. Timing of liver transplantation in biliary atresia—results in 71 children managed by a multidisciplinary team. *J Pediatr Surg*. 2008;43(9):1605–1609.
- Davenport M, Tizzard SA, Underhill J, et al. The biliary atresia splenic malformation syndrome: a 28-year single-center retrospective study. *J Pediatr*. 2006;149(3):393–400.
- Garcia A, Cowles R, Kato T, et al. Morio Kasai: a remarkable impact beyond the Kasai Procedure. *J Pediatr Surg*. 2012;47(5):1023–1027.
- Hartley JL, Davenport M, Kelly DA. Biliary atresia. *Lancet*. 2009;374(9702):1704–1713.
- Karrer FM, Bensard DD. Neonatal cholestasis. *Semin Pediatr Surg*. 2000;9(4):166–169.
- Mack CL. The pathogenesis of biliary atresia: evidence for a virus-induced autoimmune disease. *Semin Liver Dis*. 2007;27(3):233–242.
- Shneider BL, Brown MB, Haber B, et al. A multicenter study of the outcome of biliary atresia in the United States, 1997 to 2000. *J Pediatr*. 2006;148(4):467–474.
- Sokol RJ, Mack C, Narkewicz MR, et al. Pathogenesis and outcome of biliary atresia: current concepts. *J Pediatr Gastroenterol Nutr*. 2003;37(1):4–21.

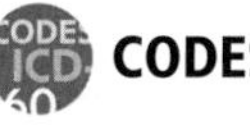

CODES

ICD10

- K83.1 Obstruction of bile duct
- Q44.2 Atresia of bile ducts
- R16.0 Hepatomegaly, not elsewhere classified

FAQ

- Q: How soon should parents contact their primary care provider when they see pale-colored stools?
- A: The first time they notice these stools are acholic.
- Q: What should a physician do if he or she is concerned about persistent jaundice?
- A: Obtain a thorough history, perform a thorough physical exam, and measure both total and direct bilirubin. If there is significant conjugated bilirubinemia, contact your local pediatric gastroenterologist and begin neonatal cholestasis diagnostic workup, ruling out the most immediately dangerous etiologies (including potentially fatal metabolic diseases and infections) as well as common etiologies such as BA.
- Q: Who developed the Kasai procedure?
- A: Morio Kasai, MD (1922–2008) is credited with helping develop the field of pediatric surgery in Japan. He was a 1947 graduate of National Tohoku University School of Medicine (Sendai, Japan). He completed a research fellowship in 1959 with C. Everett Koop, MD at the Children's Hospital of Philadelphia. He served as Chair of the Department of Surgery at Tohoku University. He performed the first Kasai procedure in 1955 on a 72 day-old infant and published the description of the procedure in 1959. The description of the procedure was published in English in the 1960s and gained popularity thereafter.

BLADDER AND BOWEL DYSFUNCTION

Kara N. Saperston, MD • Laurence S. Baskin, MD

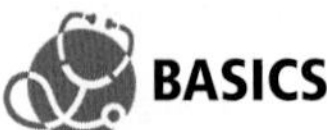

BASICS

DESCRIPTION

- Bladder and bowel dysfunction (BBD) is the appropriate term that the International Children's Continence Society has agreed upon to define combined bowel and bladder disturbance.
- Children's symptoms can then be subcategorized as either lower urinary tract dysfunction and/or bowel dysfunction.
- 5 years is the minimum age for a child to be defined as having lower urinary tract symptoms (LUTS).
- 4 years is the minimum age for a child to have functional bowel dysfunction.
- Incontinence is the leakage of urine that is continuous or intermittent.
- Intermittent incontinence can occur during the day (daytime incontinence) or exclusively at night (enuresis).
- Dysfunctional voiding is defined as tightening of the pelvic floor muscles before completely emptying the bladder, which may leave a large amount of urine in the bladder.
- BBD also encompasses the underactive ("flaccid") bladder, which is seen in children who postpone voiding and only empty a few times a day.
- Constipation has a major role to play in affecting the bladder's ability to store urine and also affects the bladder's ability to empty completely and in a timely fashion.
- Patients with BBD may experience daytime and/or nighttime incontinence.

EPIDEMIOLOGY

- 15% of 6-year-olds have abnormal voiding patterns. Children with BBD can have
  - Abnormal renal ultrasound (US)
  - Higher rates of urinary tract infections (UTIs)
  - A decreased ability to resolve vesicoureteral reflux (VUR)
- 89% of children who are treated for their constipation completely resolve their daytime urinary incontinence, and 63% resolve their nighttime incontinence.
- 50% of children with BBD may have had adverse childhood experiences.
- 16% of 5-year-olds complain of LUTS, whereas only 5% of children >14 years old complain of LUTS.

RISK FACTORS

- Recurrent UTIs
- Constipation

GENERAL PREVENTION

- Daily soft, formed bowel movements
- Timed voiding—goal between 5 to 7 times a day

PATHOPHYSIOLOGY

- A child who is holding his or her stool and not having regular daily bowel movements has increased stool in the rectal vault.
- As stool builds up in the rectal vault (constipation), it begins to push on the bladder. This process causes decreased bladder filling.
- In addition, the rectal vault shares sensory input with the bladder in the same spot of the sacral spinal cord, and the full rectal vault can be confused at this level and trigger bladder spasms, leakage, and/or incomplete emptying of the bladder.
- As a child struggles to stay dry in the face of bladder spasms, he or she overcontracts the external sphincter of the bladder, has a hard time relaxing the external sphincter during voiding, and develops increased pressure during voiding. This increased pressure can be transmitted to the kidneys.

ETIOLOGY

The etiology of BBD is broad and can have multiple causes. Increased rectal volume will mechanically compress the bladder and decrease bladder capacity and cause urgency and frequency. This can also change the neural stimuli in the bladder and the pelvic floor muscles leading to decreased urge to evacuate, poor coordination of the sphincter and the bladder muscles, increased residuals, and decreased awareness of evacuation leading to stool and bladder accidents.

COMMONLY ASSOCIATED CONDITIONS

- ADHD
- Autism spectrum disorder

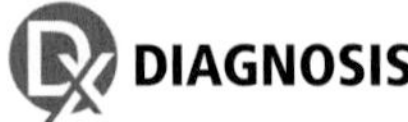

DIAGNOSIS

HISTORY

- A child will present after toilet training with symptoms of daytime and/or nighttime incontinence.
- In addition, he or she may have a history of recurrent UTIs or VUR.
- Bowel dysfunction may present as encopresis, constipation, or as fecal impaction.
- It is important to know frequency of voiding, maximum and average bladder volumes, fluid intake.
- Symptoms of urgency, holding maneuvers, dribbling or straining to urinate
- Change in gross motor coordination in the lower extremities; that is, new clumsiness or falling (tethered cord)
- Birth history or trauma during birth, neurodevelopmental delay
- Family conflict or social stressors
- History of urologic or renal disorders
- Define constipation using the Rome III criteria

PHYSICAL EXAM

- Most commonly, the exam will be normal.
- Abdomen: palpable bladder or stool in the colon
- Evaluate the spine for skin discoloration, dimples, or hair patches to rule out occult spinal dysraphism.
- Evaluate female genitalia and rule out labial adhesions that can trap urine and cause incontinence.
- Consider possible ectopic ureter if there is vaginal pooling of urine.
- Evaluate male genitalia and rule out prior hypospadias repair or severe phimosis in which urine trapping can occur as a result of urethral strictures.
- Rectal exam can reveal fecal impaction.

DIFFERENTIAL DIAGNOSIS

- Ectopic ureter to the vagina
- Spinal cord abnormalities (tethered cord)
- Brain tumors
- Urethral strictures

DIAGNOSTIC TESTS & INTERPRETATION

Initial Tests (screening, lab, imaging)

- Voiding drinking diary over 3 days has a lower false negative rate for frequency compared to a 2-day diary.
- Dysfunctional Voiding Symptom Score helps guide response to treatment.
- Short Screening Instrument for Psychological Problems in Enuresis
- Urinalysis to rule out bacteriuria or glucosuria
- First morning urine osmolality to assess renal concentrating ability in nocturnal enuresis

Follow-Up Tests & Special Considerations

- Radiograph of kidneys, ureters, and bladder (KUB): constipation, normal spine
- Renal US: pre- and postvoid images to evaluate the bladder and kidneys
- Pelvic US to measure the transverse radius of the rectum if >3 cm is indicative of rectal fecal impaction.

Diagnostic Procedures/Other

- Uroflow with EMG and PVR is noninvasive and can be helpful in more recalcitrant cases to better define synergy of the sphincter during voiding
- Voiding cystourethrogram (VCUG)
  - Used to evaluate for VUR and to look at the urethra and bladder neck during voiding
  - Only to be done in cases with multiple febrile UTIs
- Urodynamic studies
  - Tools used to define bladder function if there is a poor response to initial management
  - Uroflow is used to evaluate bladder outflow.
  - Cystometry and perineal EMG studies give information about bladder function during filling and voiding.

Test Interpretation

Children with severe BBD may need to go on for MRI testing of the spine to rule out tethered cord, in these scenarios the children will have abnormal urodynamic studies and potential VCUG/RBUS with thickened bladder wall, trabeculations +/− hydronephrosis, and/or VUR.

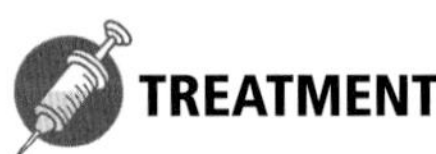

TREATMENT

GENERAL MEASURES

Behavior modification

- Educate proper voiding mechanics.
- Timed voiding every 2 hours; may use a watch with a repeating alarm
- Correct sitting and standing positions during voiding
- Modify drinking and voiding habits based on diaries to attain frequent voiding and regular stooling.

- Encourage plenty of water intake; fiber for management of constipation
- Time set aside to attempt regular morning bowel movements
- When a provider is treating a child with BBD, it is imperative that the focus begins with daytime management first, specifically focusing on soft daily bowel movements and timed voiding.
- The nighttime wetting will not improve until the daytime wetting and the constipation have been properly managed.

MEDICATION

- First line: bowel management
  - Goal: full clean out
    - Clean out usually lasts 3 days.
    - Use polyethylene glycol 3350 (MiraLax®)/lactulose and enemas and/or mineral oil.
  - If severe, can use KUB to confirm clean out is complete
- Daily management
  - Goal: 1 to 2 soft bowel movements daily
  - Polyethylene glycol 3350 (MiraLax®)/lactulose daily dosing and/or mineral oil help for daily maintenance.
- Consider a referral at this point if no progress.
- Second line: antimuscarinics
  - Are used for overactive bladders
  - Work by reducing the frequency and intensity of the bladder contraction
  - Can be supplied in short-acting and long-acting formulas or transdermally
  - Constipation is a potential side effect.
- Third line: mirabegron
  - Targets smooth muscle in the bladder to help with relaxation
  - Promotes bladder storage
  - Hypertension is a possible side effect.

ALERT

Make sure the patient has truly had a good bowel clean out and is focusing first on one to two daily soft bowel movements before adding medications to treat the bladder symptoms.

ISSUES FOR REFERRAL

- If a child's symptoms do not respond to a bowel clean out and daily maintenance then consider referral to pediatric urology.
- If a child has had multiple febrile UTIs then consider referral to pediatric urology.

ADDITIONAL THERAPIES

- Biofeedback
- Physical therapy
- Acupuncture
- Botox
- Neuromodulation

SURGERY/OTHER PROCEDURES

- A pediatric urologist will be crucial in deciding whether or not a child should move forward with more invasive testing such as urodynamics and whether or not a child should have an MRI to rule out tethered cord.
- Sacral neuromodulation and botulinum A are also used as an intervention for children with refractory urge incontinence after failure of more standard therapies.

COMPLEMENTARY & ALTERNATIVE THERAPIES

Transcutaneous posterior tibial nerve stimulation and parasacral transcutaneous neuromodulation have shown improvement in bladder volumes, overactivity, and dysfunctional voiding scores. However, it is still unknown how many treatments and for how long a child may require the therapy.

ADMISSION, INPATIENT, AND NURSING CONSIDERATIONS

Nursing education regarding bowel clean outs and daily bowel management are crucial. A nurse can make all the difference between a child staying cleaned out and on a good maintenance course to one who does not stay cleaned out.

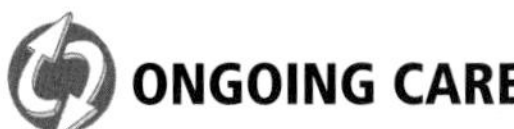

ONGOING CARE

FOLLOW-UP RECOMMENDATIONS

Patient Monitoring

Patients need follow-up around 1 month after commencing treatment of the constipation, at that point, improvement in the LUTS becomes evident. They need reminding that a good bowel cleanout and maintenance of the bowel function needs to go on consistently for 3 to 6 months before there is persistent change. They also need reminding of a good timed voiding schedule.

DIET

Optimal hydration is key to good bladder cycling and avoiding constipation. Increased fiber intake and physical activity also help with preventing constipation.

PATIENT EDUCATION

Mobile apps for tracking voiding and drinking diaries may be helpful.

PROGNOSIS

- 80% of children are able to resolve their symptoms, with attention given to their bowel function and timed voiding.
- Because this treatment predominantly involves making behavioral changes, this process does not occur quickly. Time and patience are required by both the parents and the children.

COMPLICATIONS

- Children with recurrent febrile UTIs should be referred to pediatric urology.
- Children with abnormal renal US should be referred to pediatric urology.
- Children who don't resolve their incontinence after initial management of the bowel dysfunction should be referred to pediatric urology.

ADDITIONAL READING

- Austin P, Bauer S, Bower W, et al. The standardization of terminology of lower urinary tract function in children and adolescents: update report from the Standardization Committee of the International Children's Continence Society. *Neurourol Urodyn*. 2016;35(4):471–481.
- Dohil R, Roberts E, Jones KV, et al. Constipation and reversible urinary tract abnormalities. *Arch Dis Child*. 1994;70(1):56–57.
- Issenman RM, Filmer RB, Gorski PA. A review of bowel and bladder control development in children: how gastrointestinal and urologic conditions relate to problems in toilet training. *Pediatrics*. 1999;103(6, Pt 2):1346–1352.
- Koff SA, Wagner TT, Jayanthi VR. The relationship among dysfunctional elimination syndromes, primary vesicoureteral reflux and urinary tract infections in children. *J Urol*. 1998;160(3, Pt 2):1019–1022.
- Loening-Baucke V. Urinary incontinence and urinary tract infection and their resolution with treatment of chronic constipation of childhood. *Pediatrics*. 1997;100(2, Pt 1):228–232.
- Santos JD, Lopes RI, Koyle MA. Bladder and bowel dysfunction in children: an update on the diagnosis and treatment of a common, but underdiagnosed pediatric problem. *Can Urol Assoc J*. 2017;11(1–2 Suppl 1):S64–S72.
- Van Hoecke E, Baeyens D, Vanden Bossche H, et al. Early detection of psychological problems in a population of children with enuresis: construction and validation of the Short Screening Instrument for Psychological Problems in Enuresis. *J Urol*. 2007;178(6):2611–2615.

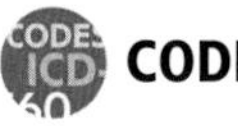

CODES

ICD10

- R32 Unspecified urinary incontinence
- K59.00 Constipation, unspecified
- R15.9 Full incontinence of feces

FAQ

- Q: Should children with BBD have urodynamic evaluation?
- A: Rarely. A patient should undergo standard therapy with timed voiding and treatment of constipation as the 1st-line therapy. If that fails, then a referral to pediatric urology is appropriate and the need for further testing will be assessed.
- Q: Will the child outgrow this?
- A: 66% of children had improvement of the daytime and nighttime symptoms with management of the bowel function alone and up to 89% of all children will respond well to education also known as urotherapy and bowel management.
- Q: How many children with BBD have psychological comorbidities?
- A: In a recent study it was found that 51% of children with BBD had an adverse childhood encounter compared to only 25% of children with a neuropsychiatric disorder. One should consider screening and possible referral of these children for psychological counseling to aid with treatment. The "Short Screening Instrument for Psychological Problems in Enuresis" is one screening questionnaire that can be helpful.

BLASTOMYCOSIS

Evan J. Anderson, MD

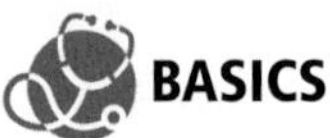

BASICS

DESCRIPTION

- Systemic infection caused by the dimorphic soil fungus *Blastomyces dermatitidis*
- Dimorphism is characterized by a mold phase (mycelial form) that grows at room temperature and a yeast form that grows at body temperature.
- Incubation period estimated at 30 to 45 days

EPIDEMIOLOGY

- Similar to other dimorphic fungi, *B. dermatitidis* is a soil saprophyte (mycelial form).
- Congenital infections occur rarely.
- Infection is endemic in the Upper Midwest and Southern United States, particularly in the wooded Mississippi and Ohio River valleys and the Great Lakes. The highest incidence in the United States is in Wisconsin, Mississippi, and Tennessee followed by Minnesota, Illinois, North Dakota, Alabama, and Louisiana.
- Substantial disease occurs in the Canadian provinces of Manitoba and northwestern Ontario. Other reported areas of infection include Africa, India, and South America.
- Children account for 3–11% of all cases of blastomycosis.
- Blastomycosis is a very uncommon diagnosis even in endemic regions.

RISK FACTORS

- Blastomycosis is more common in males. This is thought to be due to occupational or recreational activities that increase risk of exposure.
- Underlying immunodeficiency is rarely observed among children with blastomycosis.

GENERAL PREVENTION

- No special precautions for hospitalized patients are indicated.
- The natural reservoir is undetermined.

PATHOPHYSIOLOGY

- Inhalation of the fungus into the lung is followed by an inflammatory response with neutrophils and macrophages.
- Blastomycosis most commonly presents as subacute pulmonary disease, but the clinical spectrum of the disease extends from asymptomatic to disseminated disease that can involve lung, skin, bone, and central nervous system (CNS).
- As many as 50% of infections are asymptomatic.

ETIOLOGY

- Infection is almost always caused by inhalation of spores from *B. dermatitidis*.
- Rarely, blastomycosis has occurred through accidental inoculation, dog bites, conjugal transmission, and intrauterine transmission.
- Point-source outbreaks have occurred with occupational and recreational activities that occur in areas with moist soil and decaying vegetation, such as along streams and rivers.
- Natural infection occurs in humans and dogs.

COMMONLY ASSOCIATED CONDITIONS

- Pulmonary blastomycosis
  - Most common form of infection by *Blastomyces* in children
  - Can be acute, subacute, or chronic
  - Illness severity can vary greatly, from asymptomatic to upper respiratory tract infection, bronchitis, pleuritis, pneumonia, or severe respiratory distress.
- Cutaneous blastomycosis
  - Skin manifestations are variable and include nodules, verrucous lesions, subcutaneous abscesses, or ulcerations.
  - Cutaneous disease usually occurs after pulmonary infection with dissemination to the skin, rarely by direction inoculation.
- Bone blastomycosis
  - Bone disease usually occurs after pulmonary infection with dissemination to the bone resulting in osteomyelitis and bone destruction.
- Disseminated blastomycosis
  - Recent series suggest that this occurs in $<1/2$ of children.
  - Usually begins as pulmonary infection, with subsequent spread to involve skin, bone, genitourinary tract, and/or CNS
  - Can disseminate to virtually any organ
  - The classic triad of lung, bone, and skin disease occurs in $\leq 15\%$ of children.

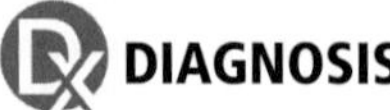

DIAGNOSIS

HISTORY

- History of residence or travel to an endemic area is very important.
- For children with acute pulmonary blastomycosis, the most common presenting symptoms are the following:
  - Cough (may be productive)
  - Fever
  - Chest pain
  - Malaise
- Children with chronic pulmonary disease present with the following:
  - Chronic (>2 weeks) nonproductive cough
  - Pleuritic chest pain
  - Poor appetite
  - May also be a history of fever, chills, weight loss, fatigue, night sweats, or, rarely, hemoptysis

PHYSICAL EXAM

- Initial pulmonary infection may present with physical exam findings similar to those of bacterial pneumonia.
- Respiratory signs and symptoms often have resolved by the time cutaneous manifestations are apparent.
- Skin involvement appears as nodules, nodules with ulceration, or granulomatous lesions.
- Bone involvement usually presents with progressive focal pain and point tenderness.

DIFFERENTIAL DIAGNOSIS

- Acute bacterial infection
- Neoplasm
- Tuberculosis
- Sarcoidosis
- Other fungal infections causing pneumonia (e.g., histoplasmosis)

DIAGNOSTIC TESTS & INTERPRETATION

Diagnostic Procedures/Other

- Definitive diagnosis requires the growth of *B. dermatitidis* from a clinical specimen. In the cooler temperature at which fungal culture is performed in the laboratory, *B. dermatitidis* usually switches back to the mold form.
- Direct visualization of the yeast form may be performed on samples of sputum, urine, cerebrospinal fluid (CSF), bronchoalveolar lavage sample, or tissue biopsy.
- Although the most accurate serologic test is the enzyme immunoassay, all serologic tests have poor sensitivity and specificity.
- An assay to detect *Blastomyces* antigen in urine is available and is about 93% sensitive. The sensitivity of the urinary antigen is lower in extrapulmonary disease. Cross-reactivity occurs in patients with histoplasmosis, paracoccidioidomycosis, and *Penicillium marneffei* infections.
- Blastomycosis can also cause a false positive *Histoplasma* urinary antigen.
- Chest radiography commonly reveals lobar consolidation. Cavitation, fibronodular patterns, mass, and mass effect may also be seen.

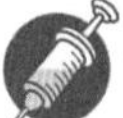

TREATMENT

MEDICATION

First Line

- Although acute pulmonary infections may resolve without treatment, the high rate of progression to extrapulmonary disease leads many experts to recommend treatment for all cases of blastomycosis.
- Mild or moderate pulmonary or extrapulmonary disease
  - Oral itraconazole
  - Alternative agents include fluconazole or voriconazole.
- Severe pulmonary disease, other severe infection, or immunosuppression
  - IV amphotericin B: Many experts prefer a lipid formulation of amphotericin B over amphotericin B deoxycholate.
  - Therapy may be switched to oral itraconazole after clinical stabilization with amphotericin B.
- CNS blastomycosis
  - Lipid formulation of amphotericin B at 5 mg/kg/24 h over 4 to 6 weeks, followed by an oral azole
- During pregnancy
  - IV amphotericin B
  - Azoles should be avoided owing to potential teratogenicity.
- Length of therapy is site dependent:
  - ≥6 months or longer for pulmonary disease
  - ≥12 months or longer for bone or CNS disease
- Lifelong suppressive therapy with oral itraconazole may be required for immunosuppressed patients and in patients who experience relapse despite appropriate therapy.

Second Line

Voriconazole, a newer azole, has in vitro activity against *B. dermatitidis* and penetrates the CSF better than itraconazole. Anecdotal reports support its use as an option for step-down therapy for CNS infection.

ISSUES FOR REFERRAL

Follow-up should occur with an infectious disease specialist until therapy is completed.

SURGERY/OTHER PROCEDURES

Occasionally, drainage of abscesses and debridement of bone are necessary.

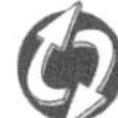

ONGOING CARE

FOLLOW-UP RECOMMENDATIONS

Patient Monitoring

- All azoles can cause hepatitis. Thus, hepatic enzymes should be measured before starting therapy, 2 to 4 weeks after therapy has begun, and every 3 months during therapy.
- All azoles interact with P450 enzymes. Consider drug–drug interactions when the patient is taking other medications.
- Itraconazole capsules are poorly absorbed; the oral solution is poorly tolerated due to taste.
- Monitoring adherence to therapy is important and many recommend following itraconazole levels.
- Amphotericin B commonly causes acute kidney injury and electrolyte wasting (particularly potassium and magnesium). Infusion-related toxicity is also common. Lipid formulations are typically better tolerated than the deoxycholate.
- The *Blastomyces* urinary antigen has been used to monitor response to therapy.

PROGNOSIS

- Before antifungal medications were available, the mortality associated with blastomycosis was up to 90%.
- Appropriate treatment with antifungal medications results in excellent cure rates and mortality rates of <10%.
- Worse outcomes tend to occur in association with a delay between onset of symptoms and establishment of a diagnosis.

COMPLICATIONS

- Dissemination is the main complication of the infection, occurring in <50% of children with blastomycosis.
- Residual orthopedic issues can persist in children with bone involvement.
- Systemic infection may be well advanced before symptoms are noted, requiring long-term therapy and follow-up.

ADDITIONAL READING

- Anderson EJ, Ahn PB, Yogev R, et al. Blastomycosis in children: a study of 14 cases. *J Pediatric Infect Dis Soc.* 2013;2(4):386–390.
- Baddley JW, Winthrop KL, Patkar NM, et al. Geographic distribution of endemic fungal infections among older persons, United States. *Emerg Infect Dis.* 2011;17(9):1664–1669.
- Chapman SW, Dismukes WE, Proia LA, et al. Clinical practice guidelines for the management of blastomycosis: 2008 update by the Infectious Diseases Society of America. *Clin Infect Dis.* 2008;46(12):1801–1812.
- Chu JH, Feudtner C, Heydon KH, et al. Hospitalizations for endemic mycoses: a population-based national study. *Clin Infect Dis.* 2006;42(6):822–825.
- Fanella S, Skinner S, Trepman E, et al. Blastomycosis in children and adolescents: a 30-year experience from Manitoba. *Med Mycol.* 2011;49(6):627–632.
- Montenegro BL, Arnold JC. North American dimorphic fungal infections in children. *Pediatr Rev.* 2010;31(6):e40–e48.

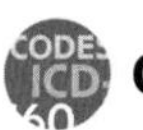

CODES

ICD10

- B40.9 Blastomycosis, unspecified
- B40.2 Pulmonary blastomycosis, unspecified
- B40.7 Disseminated blastomycosis

FAQ

- Q: When should I suspect blastomycosis?
- A: Consider blastomycosis in a child with exposure to an endemic blastomycosis area that is presenting with subacute to chronic pneumonia. Oftentimes, these children will have been treated with multiple prior antibiotics and have ongoing or progressive pneumonia or develop skin or bone lesions.
- Q: Blastomycosis is on my differential; how can I best test for it?
- A: The urine antigen test is the most sensitive test for the detection of blastomycosis but can be falsely positive. Usually, a clinical specimen is ultimately needed to establish a diagnosis.
- Q: I have a child hospitalized with blastomycosis; should I start with itraconazole or amphotericin B?
- A: If the child is not in the ICU, is not acutely worsening, and is able to take itraconazole by mouth, then it is reasonable to start with itraconazole. Itraconazole is generally much better tolerated than are amphotericin B formulations.

BLEPHARITIS

Prina P. Amin, MD • Erika L. Abramson, MD, MS

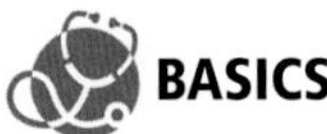

BASICS

DESCRIPTION

- Inflammatory or infectious process of the eyelid margin, typically involving skin, lashes, and meibomian glands
  - Associated with itchiness, redness, flaking, and crusting of the eyelids
  - Usually chronic, intermittent with exacerbations and remissions
  - Typically bilateral
  - No universal classification system
- Historically classified according to location, anterior versus posterior
  - Anterior blepharitis: affects the base of the eyelashes and eyelash follicles
  - Posterior blepharitis: affects the meibomian glands
- Can also be classified by etiology
  - Inflammatory: seborrheic, meibomian gland dysfunction, allergic, associated with rosacea
  - Infectious: bacterial (most commonly *Staphylococcus aureus* or *Staphylococcus epidermidis*), viral, fungal, or parasitic

EPIDEMIOLOGY

One of the most common ocular disorders (37–47% of patients seen by ophthalmologists and optometrists)

- Presents in patients of all ages
- Mean age of presentation is age 50 years.
- No gender differences seen

RISK FACTORS

- Presence of atopic, allergic, or seborrheic dermatitis
- Rosacea
- Tear deficiency and dysfunction
- Contact lens use
- Isotretinoin used to treat severe cystic acne
- Less common risk factors include underlying immunologic disorders such as lupus, eyelid tumors, trauma, and other dermatoses.

PATHOPHYSIOLOGY

- Multifactorial:
  - Results from the complex interplay between abnormal lid margin secretions, lid margin organisms, and dysfunction of the tear film
- Infectious blepharitis:
  - Bacteria such as *Staphylococcus* may cause direct infection of the eyelids, evoke reaction to the exotoxin, or provoke an allergic reaction to the staphylococcal antigens.
- Inflammatory blepharitis:
  - Inflammation of the meibomian glands leads to impaired gland secretions and instability of the tear film.
- This condition can have a direct toxic effect and promote bacterial overgrowth.

ETIOLOGY

- Complex and poorly understood
- Likely multifactorial
  - Infectious conditions
  - Systemic diseases
  - Environmental factors
- Posterior blepharitis more commonly associated with seborrhea or rosacea

COMMONLY ASSOCIATED CONDITIONS

- Seborrheic dermatitis
- Allergic or contact dermatitis
- Down syndrome (trisomy 21)
- Ocular rosacea
- Dry eye (keratoconjunctivitis sicca)
- Hordeolum
- Chalazion

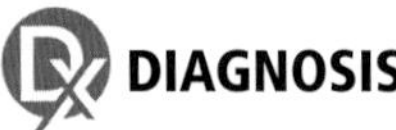

DIAGNOSIS

Signs and symptoms

- Redness of eyelid margin
- Irritation
- Burning
- Tearing
- Gritty sensation
- Dry or watery eyes
- Increased blinking
- Loss of eyelashes
- Photophobia
- Contact lens intolerance
- Eye discharge or crust, particularly along lashes
- Eyelid sticking, especially in the morning

HISTORY

- Duration of symptoms: Blepharitis is often chronic, with periods of exacerbation and remission.
- Symptoms and signs of systemic disease
- Current and previous systemic and topical medications (in particular: antihistamines, drugs with anticholinergic effects, and isotretinoin)
- Contact lens use
- Exacerbating conditions such as eye makeup use, smoke, allergens
- Previous intraocular or eyelid surgery
- Trauma
- Past medical and family histories of atopy
- Recent exposure to lice

PHYSICAL EXAM

- Use a focused direct light source to carefully evaluate the eyelids for abnormal eyelid position, eyelash loss, hyperemia of the eyelid margins, abnormal deposits at the base of the eyelids, ulceration, vesicles, scaling, chalazion/hordeolums, and scarring.
- Examine the conjunctiva and sclera to look for signs of inflammation, which warrants a slit-lamp examination.
- Assess visual acuity.
- Perform a general exam looking for signs of systemic disease such as seborrhea, atopic dermatitis, rosacea, and lupus.

DIFFERENTIAL DIAGNOSIS

- Acute conjunctivitis (bacteria, viral, or allergic)
- Atopic or contact dermatitis
- Keratitis
- Iritis
- Glaucoma
- Chemical burn
- Corneal abrasion
- Foreign body
- Hordeolum

- Chalazion
- Lice
- Trichotillomania

DIAGNOSTIC TESTS & INTERPRETATION

Initial Tests (screening, lab, imaging)

- Diagnosis is made clinically. There are no specific diagnostic tests to confirm the diagnosis of blepharitis.
- In refractory cases or cases of recurrent anterior blepharitis with severe inflammation, cultures of the eyelid margins may be useful.

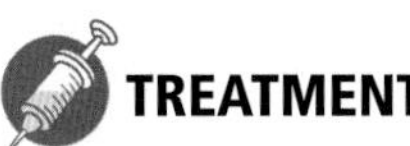

TREATMENT

GENERAL MEASURES

- Several treatments may be helpful and are generally used in combination.
- Treatments may provide symptomatic relief but usually do not result in cure for chronic cases.
- Treatments include the following:
  - Warm compresses
  - Eyelid hygiene
  - Antibiotics (topical and/or systemic)
  - Topical short course anti-inflammatory agents
- Warm compresses should be applied for 15 minutes at least twice daily to loosen crusts.
- Eyelid hygiene
  - Consists of massaging the eyelid margins daily and carefully removing the crusts using cotton swabs, cotton balls, commercial eyelid scrubs, and/or diluted baby shampoo
  - Children should be instructed to avoid rubbing their eyes if possible and to wash hands frequently.
- Wearing contact lens or eye makeup should be avoided during exacerbations.
- Activities that result in decreased blinking can dry out the eye and worsen exacerbations. Such activities may include television watching and use of computers or video games.

MEDICATION

- Warm compresses and eyelid hygiene are the traditional mainstay of therapy.
- Medications can be added in conjunction with conservative measures.
- A topical antibiotic ophthalmic ointment (such as bacitracin or erythromycin) may be applied 1 to 4 times daily until inflammation resolves.
- A brief course of topical corticosteroids are generally reserved for severe inflammation and in cases of severe conjunctival injection or marginal keratitis.
- The minimal effective dose of corticosteroid should be used and for as short a time as possible.
- Long-term use of oral antibiotics (such as erythromycin or tetracycline) may be useful in severe cases.
- Calcineurin inhibitors may be useful in severe cases as alternatives to topical corticosteroids.

SURGERY/OTHER PROCEDURES

Novel interventional procedures are in development

- Mechanical opening and dilation of obstructed meibomian gland orifices
- Thermal pulsation
- Intense pulsated light

ISSUES FOR REFERRAL

- Moderate or severe pain
- Vision loss
- Severe or chronic redness
- Corneal involvement
- Traumatic eye injury
- Recent ocular surgery
- Distorted pupil
- Recurrent episodes
- More severe eyelid inflammation with nodular mass, ulceration, or extensive scarring
- Lack of improvement with conservative measures and topical antibiotics

COMPLIMENTARY & ALTERNATIVE THERAPIES

Dietary supplementation with omega-3 fatty acids for 12 months has been shown to improve subjective and objective symptoms.

ONGOING CARE

- No additional care is needed if symptoms resolve completely.
- Patients should be educated about the potential for recurrence and chronicity with blepharitis.
- Warm compresses and eyelid hygiene treatment may be required long term.

PROGNOSIS

- Disease usually mild and benign
- Lack of uniformally successful therapies makes it a chronic condition with exacerbations and remissions for most patients.

COMPLICATIONS

Severe disease can result in:

- Eyelid deformity
- Vision loss from keratopathy

ADDITIONAL READING

- American Academy of Ophthalmology Cornea/External Disease Panel. *Preferred Practice Pattern® Guidelines. Blepharitis: Limited Revision*. San Francisco, CA: American Academy of Ophthalmology; 2011. https://www.aao.org/preferred-practice-pattern/blepharitis-ppp--2013. Accessed February 17, 2017.
- Duncan K, Jeng B. Medical management of blepharitis. *Curr Opin Ophthalmol*. 2015;26(4):289–294.
- Jackson WB. Blepharitis: current strategies for diagnosis and management. *Can J Ophthalmol*. 2008;43(2):170–179.
- Lindsley K, Matsumura S, Hatef E, et al. Interventions for chronic blepharitis. *Cochrane Database Syst Rev*. 2012;(5):CD005556. doi:10.1002/14651858.CD005556.pub2.

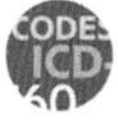

CODES

ICD10

- H01.009 Unspecified blepharitis unspecified eye, unspecified eyelid
- H01.019 Ulcerative blepharitis unspecified eye, unspecified eyelid
- L21.8 Other seborrheic dermatitis

FAQ

- Q: Is blepharitis contagious?
- A: Blepharitis is not contagious. However, if blepharitis is due in part to bacterial infection, the bacteria can be transmitted to other family members and result in conjunctivitis. Thus, good hand hygiene is important.
- Q: Will the child outgrow this?
- A: Although some children may be cured, for many, blepharitis is a chronic condition in which symptomatic control is the goal.
- Q: Is blepharitis common in children?
- A: Although blepharitis can occur in patients of all ages, it tends to be seen much more frequently in adults.

BONE MARROW AND STEM CELL TRANSPLANT

Justin T. Wahlstrom, MD • Biljana N. Horn, MD

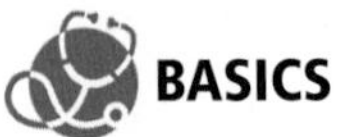

BASICS

DESCRIPTION

- Hematopoietic stem cell transplantation (HSCT) is the infusion of progenitor stem cells with the intention of restoring hematopoiesis and immunity. HSCT can be classified by
  - Donor type: syngeneic (derived from an identical twin), allogeneic (derived from a related or unrelated donor), or autologous (derived from the patient prior to stem cell-toxic therapy)
  - Product type
    - Bone marrow transplantation (BMT): Stem cells are obtained by harvesting bone marrow under anesthesia.
    - Peripheral blood stem cell transplantation (PBSCT): Stem cells are mobilized to the periphery with cytokines (GCSF) and collected by apheresis.
    - Umbilical cord blood transplantation (UCBT): Stem cells are collected from the umbilical cord and placenta immediately after birth.
- Stem cells are infused in the peripheral blood of the recipient using a central venous catheter, similar to a blood transfusion. They then home to the bone marrow niche and over the next 2 to 4 weeks differentiate into mature blood components.

EPIDEMIOLOGY

- In 2013, >1,900 pediatric allogeneic HSCTs were performed worldwide. Approximately 40% of allogeneic transplants are from matched related donors.
- The use of unrelated PBSCT and unrelated UCBT has been gradually increasing since the late 1990s, whereas the use of related BMT has remained stable.

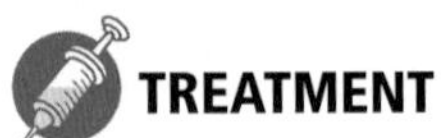

TREATMENT

- Indications
  - HSCT is typically used to provide stem cell rescue following myeloablative therapy (cancers), to provide new stem cells to correct an intrinsic cellular defect (inborn errors of metabolism, other stem cell defects), or to alter the immune system to improve or correct an immunologic defect (e.g., autoimmune disease).
  - Examples of diseases for which HSCT can be beneficial include the following:
    - Leukemia (acute lymphoblastic leukemia [ALL], acute myeloid leukemia [AML], juvenile myelomonocytic leukemia [JMML], and chronic myeloid leukemia [CML])
      - High-risk ALL (indications for transplant include lack of response to chemotherapy or early relapse)
      - High-risk AML (indication based on cytogenetic markers, response to therapy, or early relapse)
      - All JMML patients require HSCT for cure.
      - CML only if not well-controlled on tyrosine-kinase inhibitor therapy (imatinib, dasatinib)
    - Solid tumors (lymphoma, neuroblastoma, brain tumors, some sarcomas)—often autologous source
    - Severe primary immunodeficiencies (severe combined immunodeficiency [SCID], Wiskott-Aldrich syndrome [WAS], chronic granulomatous disease [CLD], hyper IgM, X-linked lymphoproliferative [XLP] syndrome,Chédiak-Higashi syndrome, Griscelli syndrome)
    - Stem cell defects (aplastic anemia, myelofibrosis, Fanconi anemia, thalassemia major, sickle cell disease)
    - Inborn errors of metabolism (Hurler syndrome, Hunter syndrome, adrenoleukodystrophy)
    - Autoimmune disease (lemophagocytic lymphohistiocytosis [HLH], severe systemic lupus erythematosus [SLE])
- Donor selection
  - Optimal major histocompatibility antigen (HLA) matching of the donor to the recipient minimizes the risks of rejection and graft-versus-host disease (GVHD).
  - HLA matching is important at the A, B, C, and DRB1 loci (8/8 match is recommended in most cases).
  - Additional HLA matching at the DQ and DP loci (12/12) may be important in some cases.
  - For nonmalignant disease, donor preference is syngeneic > matched familial > unrelated.
  - Matched unrelated donor: >18 million potential donors registered worldwide. Disadvantages include long search time (2 to 3 months), lower chance of finding an 8/8 match for minorities, increased risk of graft failure and GVHD, and slower immune reconstitution.
  - Alternative donors include mismatched unrelated donor (match at ≥7/8 HLA Ag), umbilical cord blood (match at ≥4/6 HLA Ag), or haploidentical (related) donor (<7/8 matching requires ex vivo manipulation of the graft to deplete T cells in order to prevent fatal GVHD, resulting in prolonged T-cell reconstitution).
  - Other donor characteristics to consider include age, gender, and CMV status.
  - CMV reactivation risk is based on donor/recipient serologies:
    - D−/R−: very low risk
    - D+/R−: intermediate risk
    - R+: high risk; CMV+ donor is preferred.
- Conditioning and toxicity
  - Three goals of conditioning (depending on disease):
    - Myeloablation (M): Clear marrow space to allow stem cell engraftment.
    - Immunosuppression (I): Prevent rejection and GVHD.
    - Antineoplastic effect (N): Eradicate any remaining leukemia/tumor cells.
  - Agents used during conditioning differ by their M/I/N effects and are used in combination to produce the desired outcome; side effects of conditioning agents:
    - Total body irradiation (M/I/N): cognitive delay, poor growth, cataracts, abnormal dental development, pulmonary and cardiac dysfunction, pituitary dysfunction, infertility, second malignancy
    - Busulfan (M/N): restrictive lung disease, seizures and possibly neurocognitive deficits, skin rash and hyperpigmentation, second malignancy
    - Thiotepa (M/I/N): skin rash, hemorrhagic cystitis, second malignancy
    - Melphalan (M/N): mucositis, cardiac dysfunction, second malignancy
    - Cyclophosphamide (I/N): cardiac dysfunction, SIADH, hemorrhagic cystitis, second malignancy
    - Etoposide (M/N): allergic reaction, hypotension, second malignancy
    - Fludarabine (I/N): cerebellar syndrome, peripheral neuropathy
    - Carmustine (M/N): pulmonary toxicity, second malignancy
    - Alemtuzumab (Campath®) (I): anaphylaxis, fever, hypotension, hives, viral and fungal infection
    - Antithymocyte globulin (ATG) (I): anaphylaxis, fever, hypotension, hives, serum sickness, viral and fungal infection
  - Nonmyeloablative or reduced toxicity regimens
    - Goal of reduced toxicity regimens is to allow partial donor stem cell engraftment, while limiting toxic effects of conditioning agents.
    - Indications include preexisting organ toxicity precluding full-dose chemotherapy; low performance status, often in the elderly; and primary DNA repair defects resulting in sensitivity to ionizing radiation and alkylating agents (Fanconi anemia, dyskeratosis congenita).
    - Uses immunoablative agents and lower doses of myeloablative agents or radiation
    - Relies more heavily on the GVL effect of alloreactive donor T cells to control or eradicate any remaining neoplastic disease

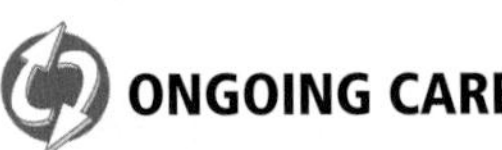

ONGOING CARE

FOLLOW-UP RECOMMENDATIONS

Long-term follow-up should include evaluations of disease, immune status and response to immunizations, cardiopulmonary function, growth, metabolic and endocrine function reproductive function, hepatic function, renal function, bone health, ophthalmologic exam, dental exam, audiology, educational and vocational progress, and surveillance for second cancers.

PROGNOSIS

- Immune reconstitution
  - Innate immunity recovers within 2 to 4 weeks posttransplant and includes monocytes, followed by granulocytes and NK cells.
  - Adaptive immunity recovers over months to years, with peripheral expansion of donor memory T cells (first wave) followed by thymic development of donor stem cells (second wave). Measurements of adaptive immune reconstitution include ALC, donor chimerism, lymphocyte phenotyping, T-cell function (proliferation to mitogen and antigen), B-cell function (serum IgA/IgM and isohemagglutinin titers), and vaccine titers before and after revaccination.
  - Revaccination: Effects of conditioning require revaccination with killed vaccines when adaptive immunity has recovered (approximately 1 year posttransplant). If titers demonstrate an immunologic response, live-attenuated vaccines are administered (approximately 2 years posttransplant).
- Overall outcomes:
  - 10–20% transplant-related mortality from rejection (<1–8%); toxicity (including infection, 5–20%); and GVHD (5–15%)
  - Additional risk of relapse ranges from 15% to 40%.

- Risks are modified by several factors:
  - Rejection risks: disease, donor match, cell dose
  - Toxicity risks: infectious risks, conditioning, performance status/organ function
  - GVHD risks: HLA match, number of donor T cells infused, GVHD prophylaxis
  - Relapse risks: disease, disease status, conditioning regimen, donor type
- Long-term effects
  - Risk is based on doses of chemotherapy and/or TBI received and presence/severity of GVHD.
  - Incidence at 10 years (and etiologies):
    - Pulmonary: 20% (TBI, busulfan, GVHD/bronchiolitis obliterans)
    - Ophthalmologic: 44% (TBI, steroids, GVHD)
    - Hypothyroidism: 36% (TBI, busulfan)
    - Osteoarticular: 29% (steroids, GVHD)
    - Cardiac: 11% (TBI, Cytoxan, prior anthracyclines)
    - Hepatic: 16% (iron overload, GVHD)
    - Dental: 15% (TBI, GVHD)
    - Secondary malignancy: 5–10% (TBI, alkylators, VP16, immunodeficiency)
    - Infertility: 50% to >90% (TBI, alkylators)
    - Other effects include GH deficiency, hearing loss, hypogonadism, chronic renal insufficiency, neurocognitive defects.

COMPLICATIONS

Treatment-related mortality (TRM) has been declining over time (40% in 1987 to 1995 to 15% in 2003 to 2006) and is attributable to the following complications:

- Infection
  - Correlates with immunologic defect; divided into early and late infections (<100 days vs. >100 days from transplant)
  - Bacterial
    - Early bacterial infections are due to neutropenia, mucositis, or central line (*Staphylococcus* spp, gram-negative rods, *Clostridium difficile*, VRE, atypicals). Later, prolonged adaptive immunity defect and chronic GVHD are risks for mycobacteria and encapsulated bacteria.
    - Treat neutropenic fever empirically with broad-spectrum antibiotics.
  - Viral
    - Early viral infections are due to lymphopenia, T-cell depletion, cord blood source, and previous viral exposures. Common infections include RSV, rhinovirus, adenovirus, influenza, and herpes virus reactivation (HSV, CMV, HHV-6). Persistent defect in adaptive immunity contributes to later infections such as CMV, VZV, and EBV/PTLD.
    - Acyclovir prophylaxis to prevent HSV reactivation
    - At detection of CMV viremia, rule out CMV retinitis with funduscopic exam and begin preemptive therapy for CMV viremia with foscarnet or ganciclovir. For CMV organ involvement, consider Cytogam, IVIG, or intravitreal foscarnet for CMV retinitis. Continue maintenance therapy with ganciclovir or valganciclovir once viremia is cleared.
  - Fungal
    - Combined innate and adaptive immunity defects (early) and persistent T-cell dysfunction (late) confer risk for *Candida*, *Aspergillus*, *Pneumocystis*, and other fungal infection (*Fusarium*, *Zygomycetes/Mucor*, *Cryptococcus*, *Histoplasma*, *Coccidioides*).
    - Fungal prophylaxis is risk-based and may include yeast prophylaxis with azoles (fluconazole or voriconazole) or echinocandins (caspofungin); *Pneumocystis* prophylaxis is with cotrimoxazole before conditioning and after engraftment. Voriconazole, posaconazole, or isavuconazole are used empirically for sustained fever without source (strong mold/*Aspergillus* coverage).
    - Decrease calcineurin inhibitor (tacrolimus or cyclosporine) or sirolimus dose when starting azoles due to moderate or strong CYP3A inhibition.
    - Document infection (BAL) whenever possible.
- Mucositis
  - Grades 1 to 4 based on WHO classification (mild to severe)
  - Prevention: reduced intensity protocols, glutamine, palifermin; consider holding posttransplant methotrexate if severe mucositis.
  - Treatment: IV pain control, TPN, suction
- Veno-occlusive disease (VOD)/sinusoidal obstruction syndrome (SOS)
  - Due to hepatic accumulation of toxic metabolites leading to reduced hepatic venous outflow and postsinusoidal intrahepatic portal hypertension
  - Overall risk of VOD is 10–25%. Risk factors include mismatched or unrelated donor, previous hepatic tumor involvement or abdominal RT, pretransplant elevation of AST, and medications such as busulfan.
  - Diagnosis
    - Modified Seattle criteria: Any two of the following present by day +20: jaundice (bilirubin >2 mg/dL); painful hepatomegaly; or ascites ± weight gain of >2% from baseline
    - Baltimore criteria: bilirubin >2 mg/dL before day +21 and any two of the following: hepatomegaly, ascites, or weight gain (>5% from baseline)
    - Reversal of portal venous flow on ultrasound (US) is characteristic but not part of diagnostic criteria.
  - Prophylaxis may include ursodiol and/or defibrotide.
  - Treatment
    - Defibrotide: porcine intestinal mucosal oligonucleotide; anticoagulant with effects on endothelial cells, platelets, and fibrinolysis
    - Supportive care: restriction of sodium and fluid intake; diuresis to keep fluid balance even (spironolactone if able to take PO)
  - Complications of VOD include renal insufficiency, altered mental status, cardiac failure, and bleeding.
- Thrombotic microangiopathy
  - Generalized endothelial dysfunction with microangiopathy
  - Calcineurin GVHD prophylaxis is a risk factor (CSA > tacrolimus). Combination with sirolimus triples the risk from 4.2% to 10.8%.
  - Common symptoms: RBC fragmentation, thrombocytopenia with increased need for frequent platelet transfusions, elevated LDH, proteinuria, hypertension, elevation in creatinine, neurologic dysfunction
  - Treatment: Discontinue calcineurin inhibitors; supportive care; limited data for plasmapheresis, eculizumab (anti-C5 monoclonal antibody), and defibrotide
- Engraftment syndrome
  - Cytokine-mediated inflammation due to increasing neutrophil activity
  - Usually occurs by day +28 (earlier for autos, later for cord blood transplants)
  - Characterized by rash, fever, and pulmonary edema at the time of engraftment or before neutrophil recovery
  - Treatment: Rule out infection and then methylprednisolone for 3 to 7 days.
- Acute lung injury
  - Complication of TBI, chemotherapy (busulfan, cyclophosphamide), or infection (fungal, CMV); idiopathic pneumonia syndrome (IPS) if no etiology is found
  - Diagnosis:
    - Cough, dyspnea, hypoxemia, fever
    - CXR/CT: diffuse versus focal consolidations, nodules or cavitary lesions suggestive of fungus
    - BAL: sensitive for CMV, RSV, PCP, other respiratory viruses; less sensitive for fungus
  - Treatment: early empiric broad-spectrum antibiotics and antifungals, respiratory support. Consider corticosteroids or TNF blockade for IPS.
- GVHD
  - See GVHD chapter

ADDITIONAL READING

- Chow E, Anderson L, Baker KS, et al. Late effects surveillance recommendations among survivors of childhood hematopoietic cell transplantation: a children's oncology group report. *Biol Blood Marrow Transplant*. 2016;22(5):782–795.
- Fisher BT, Alexander S, Dvorak CC, et al. Epidemiology and potential preventative measures for viral infections in children with malignancy and those undergoing hematopoietic cell transplantation. *Pediatr Blood Cancer*. 2012;59(1):11–15.
- Pai SY, Logan BR, Griffith LM, et al. Transplantation outcomes for severe combined immunodeficiency, 2000–2009. *N Engl J Med*. 2014;371(5):434–446.
- Spellman SR, Eapen M, Logan BR, et al; for National Marrow Donor Program; Center for International Blood and Marrow Transplant Research. A perspective on the selection of unrelated donors and cord blood units for transplantation. *Blood*. 2012;120(2):259–265.

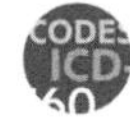

CODES

ICD10

- Z94.81 Bone marrow transplant status
- Z94.84 Stem cells transplant status
- Z52.3 Bone marrow donor

FAQ

- Q: Should friends and family of a patient needing a transplant be tested as a potential match?
- A: If family contacts are willing to donate for an unrelated patient in need of a stem cell transplant, they should join the National Marrow Donor Program (NMDP) registry. However, extended family members are not likely to be a match for a related patient.
- Q: Can transplant recipients meet their donors?
- A: The NMDP has guidelines for donor/recipient contact. If both parties agree, contact is allowed 1 to 2 years after the transplant.

BOTULISM AND INFANT BOTULISM

Jessica M. Khouri, MD • Stephen S. Arnon, MD, MPH

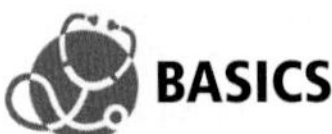

BASICS

DESCRIPTION

- An acute illness caused by neurotoxins produced by *Clostridium botulinum* or related neurotoxigenic species, which results in cranial nerve palsies and a symmetric, descending, flaccid paralysis
- The neurotoxin may be elaborated either in the large intestine of individuals temporarily colonized with the bacterium, or ingested, or absorbed from infected wounds.
- There are three main forms of the disease:
  - Infant botulism (IB) is the intestinal toxemia form in which swallowed spores germinate and colonize the infant's colon and elaborate toxin in situ.
  - Foodborne botulism in children and adults occurs when preformed toxin is ingested with improperly prepared or stored foods.
  - Wound botulism occurs when spores of the bacterium contaminate the wound, germinate, and produce toxin that is then absorbed.

EPIDEMIOLOGY

- IB is the most common form of human botulism in the United States.
- IB occurs in the 1st year of life, with ~90% of cases reported in the first 6 months of life.
- IB affects infants of all racial backgrounds and socioeconomic groups.
- Male to female ratio is 1:1.
- Toxin types A and B represent 98.5% of cases in United States (1976 to 2015), with dual toxin types (e.g., Ba, Bf) and more rare type E and type F comprising the remaining 1.5%.
- IB has been recognized in all 50 states, with a greater proportion of toxin type B cases east of the Mississippi River and toxin type A cases west of the Mississippi.
- Recognized on five of the six inhabited continents, Africa being the exception.
- Often, a history of a recent change in feeding practice is found.
- Honey is an identified food reservoir of *C. botulinum* spores. Honey consumption in U.S. IB patients from 1976 to 2015 was only approximately 4.8%.
- For the majority of IB cases, spore acquisition likely occurs from the natural environment, that is, infants inhale and then swallow spores attached to airborne microscopic dust particles. Nearby soil disruption may play a role.
- Breastfed infants who acquire IB tend to be older at onset than are formula-fed infants.
- Foodborne cases are usually associated with home-processed, low acid foods—especially vegetables, fruits, and condiments. Restaurant-associated outbreaks have occurred. Recent outbreaks in U.S. prisons have been associated with fermented alcoholic beverage commonly referred to as *pruno*.
- Wound botulism has been associated with "black tar" heroin injection drug use and traumatic injuries in teenagers.

Incidence

- U.S. IB incidence: 2.2 cases per 100,000 live births (1976 to 2014). The states with the highest incidence in descending order include Delaware, Utah, Hawaii, Pennsylvania, and California.
- Approximately 100 to 150 IB cases annually in United States
- Since the disease was first recognized >40 years ago, >4,400 cases of IB have been reported worldwide, of which >3500 are U.S. cases (~80%).
- Foodborne cases occur sporadically yet may result from a common exposure.
- Wound botulism is very rare.

RISK FACTORS

- Infants who have <1 bowel movement per day may be at increased risk of developing IB.
- Honey is an identified, avoidable food source of *C. botulinum* spores.
- Ingestion of improperly canned or preserved low-acid foods may result in foodborne botulism.

GENERAL PREVENTION

- Do not feed honey or raw honey–containing products to infants.
- Botulinum toxin is heat-labile; 5 minutes of boiling will destroy the toxin.
- Spores are heat-resistant.
- Proper food preservation, storage, and preparation will prevent foodborne botulism.

PATHOPHYSIOLOGY

- Neurotoxin is endocytosed at peripheral cholinergic nerve endings; it blocks release of acetylcholine at the neuromuscular junction.
- Cranial nerves are usually affected first and most severely, leading to ptosis, ophthalmoplegia, decreased facial expression, difficulty swallowing, and loss of airway-protective reflexes. Respiratory failure may ensue.
- Sensation and sensorium remain intact.
- Recovery occurs through regeneration of motor neuron axon terminals and the formation of new motor end plates.
- Infants are particularly prone to temporary colonic colonization by *C. botulinum*. When foods other than breast milk are introduced to breastfed infants, perturbation of the intestinal microbiome may predispose to illness.

ETIOLOGY

C. botulinum, the etiologic agent, is a gram-positive, spore-forming, obligate anaerobic bacterium that is found in dust, soil, and marine sediments worldwide. Rarely, neurotoxigenic *Clostridium butyricum* and *Clostridium baratii* may cause disease due to toxin type E and type F, respectively.

DIAGNOSIS

HISTORY

- IB
  - Symptoms include constipation, poor feeding/poor latch, diminished facial expression, droopy eyelids, difficulty swallowing, and generalized weakness.
  - Fever is typically absent (barring concomitant infections).
  - Infants may appear lethargic (from ptosis and decreased facial expression).
  - Occasionally, rapid progression of symptoms may result in respiratory arrest or an apparent life-threatening event (ALTE).
- Foodborne botulism
  - ~50% of patients report emesis.
  - There may initially be complaints of diarrhea followed by constipation.
  - The incubation period from ingestion to the onset of symptoms is usually 18 to 36 hours (range, a few hours to several days).
  - Patients complain of weakness and dry mouth.
  - Visual complaints include blurry vision, loss of accommodation, and diplopia.
  - Patients may complain of difficulty swallowing or slurred speech.
  - Patients may have urinary retention.
  - Occasionally, progression may be quite rapid, and the abrupt onset of lethargy and weakness may suggest bacterial sepsis or meningitis.
- Wound botulism
  - Often history of IV drug use
  - Incubation period ranges from 4 to 14 days.
  - Fever may be present from wound infection not botulism.
  - Patients often report constipation but rarely nausea or vomiting.
  - Patients may complain of purulent discharge from the wound.

PHYSICAL EXAM

- IB
  - Patients are typically afebrile and appear lethargic.
  - Cranial nerve findings include ptosis, diminished facial expression, weak cry, poor latch/suck, drooling/dysphagia, weak gag, and poor head control.
  - Pupils
    - Often midposition initially; may be normal to sluggishly reactive but fatigue with repetitive stimulation
    - In some cases, pupils appear fixed and dilated for a period.
  - Frog-leg positioning due to weakness of hip girdle musculature
  - Generalized weakness and loss of motor milestones
  - Flaccid, descending paralysis, and hyporeflexia
  - The remainder of the physical examination is normal.
  - In infants, early in the course of the disease, pupillary and corneal reflexes may fatigue easily (refer to physical examination tools under "For Physicians—Clinical Diagnosis" tab at www.infantbotulism.org)
- Older children and adults
  - May appear alert and are afebrile
  - Ptosis, extraocular palsies, and dilated, sluggishly reactive pupils are often the first signs of descending paralysis.
  - Dysphagia, dysarthria, and hypoglossal weakness indicate lower cranial nerve involvement.
  - Respiratory failure may rapidly ensue from upper airway obstruction resulting from loss of pharyngeal tone, loss of airway-protective reflexes, and respiratory muscle weakness.
  - The triad of bulbar palsies, clear sensorium, and absence of fever should prompt immediate consideration of botulism.
  - Signs of autonomic instability may include unexpected fluctuations in skin color, BP and heart rate, and urinary retention.

DIFFERENTIAL DIAGNOSIS

- Top 2 clinical mimics of IB are spinal muscular atrophy (SMA) type I and metabolic disorders.
- Infections
  - In infants, sepsis, meningitis and polio-like enteroviruses may present in a similar way.
  - In older children and adults, bacterial sepsis, meningitis, poliomyelitis, tick paralysis, and diphtheric polyneuritis are considerations.

- Postinfectious demyelinating processes may mimic botulism but generally have asymmetric findings.
- Absence of fever and a clear sensorium make sepsis and meningitis less likely.
- Neurologic
  - Myasthenia gravis spares the pupillary constrictor response, which in botulism is either fatigable, sluggish, or absent.
  - In SMA type I (Werdnig-Hoffmann disease), extraocular and sphincter muscles are spared.
- Metabolic/genetic
  - Certain metabolic or genetic conditions may closely mimic IB.
- Toxins: Drug ingestions may lead to weakness and lethargy.

DIAGNOSTIC TESTS & INTERPRETATION

Initial Tests (screening, lab, imaging)

- For IB, stool or enema is submitted for diagnostic testing to a state health department or the Centers for Disease Control and Prevention (CDC). Diagnosis is established by identification of toxin by mouse neutralization assay and/or isolation of a toxigenic organism. Serum testing is not routinely performed. Clinicians should request specific instructions on specimen submission from their state health departments.
- In foodborne and wound botulism, tests for the presence of toxin or organisms can be conducted on patient samples (serum, gastric aspirates, feces, or wound exudate) or suspected foodstuffs.
- Anaerobic cultures of wound material may yield the organism.
- In infant and foodborne botulism, excretion of toxin and organisms in feces may persist for weeks to months after symptom onset.
- EEG, MRI, and CT are nonspecific and usually normal in the absence of complications.

Diagnostic Procedures/Other

- Most tests for toxin and organism are done by state health departments or the CDC.
- The most common test performed is an assay for botulinum toxin in stool.
- Specimens must be shipped in sealed, break-proof, and leak-proof containers. Even minute amounts of toxin, if inhaled or ingested, can lead to disease.
- Suspect foods should be shipped refrigerated and in their original containers if possible.
- Electromyography (EMG) may demonstrate a characteristic pattern of brief, small, overly abundant motor unit action potentials (BSAPs). EMG results may be normal or inconclusive in botulism patients. Nerve conduction velocities are normal.

TREATMENT

GENERAL MEASURES

- Patients with suspected botulism should be hospitalized and have continuous monitoring of heart rate, respiratory rate, and oxygenation, as well as frequent assessment of respiratory effort and airway-protective reflexes.
- The mainstay of therapy is meticulous supportive care.
  - Particular attention should be paid to respiratory and nutritional needs.
- Cases of suspected toxin ingestion should be treated early with induced emesis and/or gastric lavage in an attempt to decrease toxin exposure.
- All suspect cases should be immediately reported to the state health department and the CDC.

MEDICATION

- Prompt recognition of IB and early treatment with intravenous human botulism immune globulin (BIG-IV; BabyBIG) significantly shortens hospital stay, time in intensive care, and duration of respiratory and nutritional support. BIG-IV is available through the California Department of Public Health's Infant Botulism Treatment and Prevention Program (IBTPP).
- Treatment with BIG-IV should be *promptly* initiated based on clinical findings and *not* delayed for laboratory diagnostic studies.
- Antibiotics are not helpful in IB:
  - In suspected IB, avoid aminoglycoside antibiotics (e.g., gentamicin); an abrupt worsening of weakness and respiratory failure may result from potentiating effects at the neuromuscular junction.
- Equine-derived antitoxin is not recommended for the treatment of IB but has been used to treat type-F IB cases.
- Antibiotics are indicated only for documented complications such as pneumonia or urinary tract infections.
- Cathartics are not beneficial.
- Foodborne or wound botulism
  - Should be treated with the licensed, equine-derived heptavalent botulinum antitoxin (BAT), available from the CDC
  - Antitoxin should not be administered to asymptomatic individuals who have only eaten suspect foods.
- Wound botulism should be treated with IV penicillin G 250,000 U/kg/24 h or equivalent and BAT antitoxin.

ADMISSION, INPATIENT, AND NURSING CONSIDERATIONS

- Meticulous supportive care with particular emphasis on respiratory and nutritional needs is the most important consideration.
- Endotracheal intubation is necessary for patients with respiratory failure or loss of airway-protective reflexes.
- Wounds should be explored and debrided and anaerobic cultures obtained.

ONGOING CARE

PROGNOSIS

- IB has an estimated mortality rate of <1% in hospitalized patients. Complete recovery can be expected when the disease is recognized early and treated appropriately.
- The mortality rate of adult foodborne botulism is 20–25%. In patients <20 years old it is 10%.
- Foodborne botulism patients with a shorter incubation period usually have more severe involvement and a worse prognosis, probably related to an increased amount of toxin ingested.
  - Recovery can generally be expected, but fatigability may persist for up to 1 year.

COMPLICATIONS

- Fatal respiratory failure from paralysis of respiratory muscles is the most serious complication.
- Bulbar dysfunction in IB may lead to dehydration and starvation ketosis before presentation.
- Loss of airway-protective reflexes can lead to aspiration and pneumonia.
- Constipation and urinary retention may precede the onset of paralysis and may complicate later management. Cases of severe *Clostridium difficile* enterocolitis with hypovolemia, hypotension, and prolonged ICU stays have occurred in IB patients.
- Recurrent urinary tract infections and syndrome of inappropriate antidiuretic hormone secretion (SIADH) are rare complications of IB.

ADDITIONAL READING

- Arnon SS, Schechter R, Maslanka SE, et al. Human botulism immune globulin for the treatment of infant botulism. *N Engl J Med*. 2006;354(5):462–471.
- Francisco AM, Arnon SS. Clinical mimics of infant botulism. *Pediatrics*. 2007;119(4):826–828.
- Koepke R, Sobel J, Arnon SS. Global occurrence of infant botulism, 1976–2006. *Pediatrics*. 2008;122(1):e73–e82.
- Mitchell WG, Tseng-Ong L. Catastrophic presentation of infant botulism may obscure or delay diagnosis. *Pediatrics*. 2005;116(3):e436–e438.
- Passaro DJ, Werner SB, McGee J, et al. Wound botulism associated with black tar heroin among injecting drug users. *JAMA*. 1998;279(11):859–863.
- McCarty CL, Angelo K, Beer KD, et al. Large outbreak of botulism associated with a church potluck meal—Ohio, 2015. *MMWR Morb Mortal Wkly Rep*. 2015;64(29):802–803.

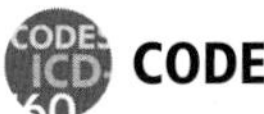

CODES

ICD10

- A05.1 Botulism food poisoning
- A48.51 Infant botulism
- A48.52 Wound botulism

FAQ

- Q: Can IB recur?
- A: True recurrence of IB has not been documented.
- Q: Should antitoxin be given to persons who have ingested food that they think might be contaminated with botulinum toxin (foodborne botulism)?
- A: Because the equine-derived antitoxin carries a risk of serum sickness, it should be given only to persons exhibiting symptoms consistent with foodborne or wound botulism.
- Q: Where is antitoxin obtained?
- A: For suspected IB cases human-derived antitoxin, BIG-IV (BabyBIG), may be obtained from the IBTPP, California Department of Public Health at 510-231-7600; www.infantbotulism.org. The call center is open 24 hours per day for 365 days per year. For non-IB patients, the licensed heptavalent (A to G) equine-derived antitoxin, BAT, may be obtained from the CDC, Atlanta, Georgia; 24/7/365 Ph: 770-488-7100.
- Q: How is the human-derived antitoxin BabyBIG produced?
- A: BIG-IV, BabyBIG, is produced from pooled human plasma from screened adult volunteers immunized against botulinum toxin for occupational protection.

BRACHIAL PLEXUS PALSY (PERINATAL)

Luis H. Quiroga, MD • Richard J. Redett, MD

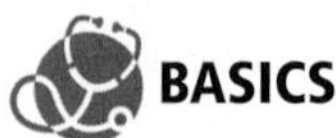

BASICS

DESCRIPTION

- The brachial plexus contains sensory and motor nerves to the upper extremities, stemming from the cervical and thoracic spine (commonly C5–T1 roots).
- The brachial plexus contains a consistent pattern of nerves that innervate predictable muscles and skin regions.
- Brachial birth palsy is a flaccid upper extremity paralysis caused by traction injury of the brachial plexus during birth.
- It can produce a proximal stretch, avulsion, or rupture type injury. Classifications are as follows:

Common Terminology	Affected Nerve Roots	Paralysis
Erb palsy (type I)	C5–C6	Bicep and deltoid
Extended Erb (type II)	C5–C7	Same + triceps and wrist extensor (wrist flexion = waiter's tip)
Pan plexus (type III)	C5–T1	Entire limb (flail arm)
Pan plexus with Horner syndrome (type IV)	C5–T1 and sympathetic chain	Flail arm + Horner syndrome (ptosis, miosis, and anhidrosis)
Klumpke	C8–T1	Paralyzed hand

EPIDEMIOLOGY

- There is no predominance of gender, but variations in clinical care, preventive measures, and birth weight may explain estimates of incidence to range from 0.4 to 4 per 1,000 live births.
- Incidence drops from 0.2% with vaginal delivery to 0.02% after cesarean section as there is a probable mechanical basis for the plexopathy.
- Erb palsy is the most commonly encountered plexus injury.

RISK FACTORS

- Large size for gestational age, multiparity, prolonged labor, breech position, difficult delivery—especially when forceps- or vacuum-assisted
- Diabetic mothers and/or neonatal birth weight >4.5 kg
- Although there is no genetic basis *per se*, previous delivery leading to obstetric palsy is a risk factor.

GENERAL PREVENTION

- Careful positioning of the upper extremity during childbirth and conversion to cesarean section when necessary
- Prevention of long-term disability and contracture can be minimized with exercise of the child's joints and functioning muscles every day beginning at 3 weeks of age.

PATHOPHYSIOLOGY

- Seddon and Sunderland have described classification systems to describe degree of injury.
  - Neuropraxia
    - Mildest form, interruption of conduction
    - The myelin sheath is disrupted, but the axons and surrounding connective tissue remain intact.
    - Good recovery
  - Axonotmesis
    - The myelin sheath and the axon are both interrupted and the surrounding connective tissue remain undamaged.
  - Neurotmesis
    - Most severe
    - There is a complete disruption of the myelin sheath, axon, and surrounding connective tissue (epineurium and perineurium).
    - Nerve may be grossly intact; recovery difficult to predict
- Lesions also can be classified according to their relation to the dorsal root ganglion (preganglionic or postganglionic).
  - Preganglionic lesions occur proximal to the dorsal root ganglion and involve avulsion from the spinal cord. Implementation of nerve transfer is usually a better strategy for these lesions.

ETIOLOGY

- Downward mechanical force on the shoulder during delivery can lead to stepwise stretch injury, resulting in either transient or permanent damage or total avulsion of nerve roots.
- Upward mechanical force (i.e., after face delivery) is less frequent and leads to isolated lower plexus palsy (C8–T1 injury = Klumpke).
- Avulsion injury carries the worst prognosis, particularly if proximal to the cell body of the motor nerve (preganglionic), as these injuries cannot spontaneously recover.

COMMONLY ASSOCIATED CONDITIONS

Horner syndrome, phrenic nerve injury, and long thoracic nerve injury (winged scapula) may be observed and are associated with preganglionic injury and a poor prognosis.

DIAGNOSIS

HISTORY

- In neonates: obstetric history including birth weight, use of assistive devices, multiparity, perinatal difficulties, previous difficult deliveries, and so forth
- Despite a prominent association between shoulder dystocia and neonatal brachial plexus palsy injury, some of these injuries occur without any shoulder dystocia.
- In older children: Consider recent infectious processes (viruses), tetanus shots, trauma, and tumor.

PHYSICAL EXAM

- Serial examination is key for predicting recovery.
- Active and passive ROM testing, bulk, deep tendon reflexes (DTRs), autonomic function, and evaluation for phrenic nerve injury and paravertebral muscle weakness are important adjunctive exams.
- Sensory testing may be more challenging because of age and overlap of dermatomes.
- Because of invariability of brachial plexus anatomy, injury patterns yield predictable disabilities.
- Erb palsy
  - Associated with downward force on the head and neck during delivery, leading to upper plexus injuries
  - Shoulder limp, adducted, internally rotated
  - Elbow extended, forearm pronated, wrist and fingers flexed ("waiter's tip" posture)
  - Hand grip and intrinsic function generally preserved. Shoulder and elbow flexion is weak.
  - DTRs: biceps and brachioradialis absent, Moro asymmetric
- Klumpke palsy
  - Risk of injury to the lower brachial plexus results from traction on an abducted arm, as with an infant being pulled from the birth canal by an extended arm above the head.
  - Shoulder intact, elbow flexed, forearm supinated, wrists and fingers extended
  - Hand grip is weak, whereas shoulder and elbow function may be normal. Horner syndrome can be present.
  - DTRs: triceps absent; Horner sign suggests ipsilateral T1 injury.
- Complete plexus injury ("flail"):
  - Entire extremity and shoulder girdle is flaccid, anesthetic, and areflexic.

DIFFERENTIAL DIAGNOSIS

- Important to rule out clavicular, shoulder, elbow, and humeral injury as primary cause of limb paresis or weakness
- Central lesions resulting from tumors and strokes, as well as spinal cord lesions, should be considered.
- Congenital contractures and limb deformities can resemble brachial plexus injuries.
- Central paralysis is generally spastic and peripheral (i.e., brachial plexus or lower motor neuron) is flaccid.
- Horner syndrome may be associated with proximal injury.
- Parsonage-Turner syndrome may cause plexus inflammation and symptoms without obvious injury.

DIAGNOSTIC TESTS & INTERPRETATION

- Plain radiographs may demonstrate clavicle injury and shoulder and elbow subluxation and dislocation.
- Routine imaging is not recommended. It is reserved for preoperative evaluation of refractory brachial plexus injury.
- MRI neurography is generally favored over CT myelography and electromyography (EMG) and is less invasive. MRI provides high-quality images to evaluate nerve avulsion (preganglionic injuries) and preoperative planning.
- Ultrasound is helpful in assessing postganglionic injuries and it can detect infantile shoulder dislocation.
- Previous cases using EMG data to determine whether an injury occurred *in utero* has been investigated; interpretation of all these modalities may lead to false positives and negatives. EMG results may overestimate clinical recovery.
- Somatosensory and motor evoked potentials are less useful as they generally corroborate physical exam findings.

Follow-up Tests & Special Considerations

- Following the diagnosis of brachial plexus palsy, neonates should be followed closely to determine if the injury will resolve spontaneously or will require further treatment.
- Patients should be followed by an experienced multidisciplinary brachial plexus team of therapists, pediatricians, and pediatric surgery subspecialists.

TREATMENT

- Therapy is paramount in managing symptoms of plexopathy.
- Goals include comfort, optimizing recovery, and assessing improvement.
- Stretching exercises, splints to prevent contracture, joint taping to stabilize shoulder, and sensory awareness activities are commonly used.

GENERAL MEASURES

- Palsies must be observed during the first weeks to months of life.
  - Immobilization of a flaccid limb encouraged very early for pain control
  - After 3 weeks of immobilization and fractures/dislocation have been ruled-out, ROM exercises should commence to prevent deformity and contracture.
- Majority of neonates with obstetric brachial plexus injury will resolve spontaneously.

Type of Injury	Paralysis	Likelihood of Spontaneous Recovery
Erb palsy (type I)	Bicep and deltoid	~90 %
Extended Erb (type II)	Same + triceps and wrist extensor	~65 %
Pan plexus (type III)	Entire limb (flail arm)	<50%
Pan plexus with Horner syndrome (type IV)	Flail arm + Horner syndrome (ptosis, miosis, and anhidrosis)	~0%
Klumpke	Paralyzed hand	~0%

- Classic Erb palsy has the best prognosis.
- The majority of upper brachial plexus birth injuries are transient.
- Global palsies have a poor prognosis with nonoperative treatment.
- Failure to recover antigravity biceps function by 3 to 6 months of age is a poor prognostic sign.
- Infants with C5–C6 or C5–C7 injuries may continue to demonstrate spontaneous improvement up to 9 months of age, thus precluding the need for early surgery.

SURGERY/OTHER PROCEDURES

- Indications for early surgical intervention
  - Pan-plexus ("flail") lesions (generally warrant early intervention as soon as 3 months if no improvement)
  - All brachial plexus injuries should be evaluated by a multidisciplinary team at 3, 6, and 9 months of age.
  - Failure to improve at each examination is usually an indication for surgery. There are several different grading systems, which can be used to assess an infant's healing progress.
- Nonsurgical measures
  - Neuromuscular electrical stimulation can be used as part of an infant's comprehensive therapy to help improve blood flow, preserve muscle bulk, and minimize atrophy.
  - Botulinum toxin A therapy to impair preserved muscle groups allow weaker muscle groups to strengthen.
- Primary surgery
  - Surgical outcome is best if performed by 6 to 12 months and probably not useful if done after 24 months; ongoing care
  - Exploration generally confirms clinical and radiographic findings.
  - Injured nerves generally present as neuromas.
    - Neurolysis to free uninjured nerve from scar versus
    - Excision of neuroma en bloc with interpositional nerve grafting
    - Excision is favored when nerve transmission across the injured site is significantly diminished (<50%) or absent; immobilization of a flaccid limb encouraged very early for pain control
- Autologous sural nerve is an excellent donor and it is reversed when interposed to maximize signaling to the CNS.
- When there is insufficient nerve graft, neurotization—attachment of functional motor nerves to distal recipient nerves—is a useful adjunct.
- Common donor nerves include the spinal accessory, contralateral C7 nerve root, and intercostal nerves.
- Use of nerve conduits and adjunctive neurotrophic factors is under investigation.
- Secondary surgery
  - Tendon transfers (generally wait 2 to 4 years to assess long-term nerve recovery) improve flexibility and functional mobility of affected joints.
    - Shoulder: transfer of preserved internal rotators to impaired abductors and external rotators
    - Elbow: triceps to biceps repair, pectoralis to biceps repair, latissimus to biceps repair
    - Forearm: Biceps rerouting and pronator lengthening can relieve pronation and supination contractures.
    - Scapula: contralateral rhomboid, trapezius, and latissimus transfer to anchor and support a winged scapula
    - Osteotomies (late presentation)
      - External rotational osteotomy of humerus to improve upper extremity function with fixed, internally rotated shoulder
      - Radius rotational osteotomy to address pronation and supination deformities
  - Soft tissue (late presentation)
    - Capsulotomies and joint manipulation under anesthesia can facilitate movement in a contracted joint.
    - Local flaps and tissue transfer can augment a contracted flexor or extensor zone.

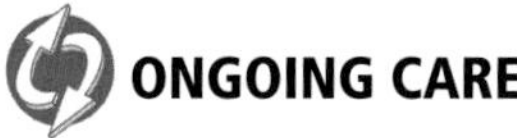

ONGOING CARE

PROGNOSIS

~75–85% of all patients regain very good to full strength and function, with 1/2 doing so rapidly (the mild group) and 1/2 more slowly (the moderate group).

ADDITIONAL READING

- Borschel GH, Clarke HM. Obstetrical brachial plexus palsy. *Plast Reconstr Surg*. 2009;124(Suppl 1):144e–155e.
- Chuang DC, Ma HS, Wei FC. A new evaluation system to predict the sequelae of late obstetric brachial plexus palsy. *Plast Reconstr Surg*. 1998;101(3):673–685.
- Chuang DC, Ma HS, Wei FC. A new strategy of muscle transposition for treatment of shoulder deformity caused by obstetric brachial plexus palsy. *Plast Reconstr Surg*. 1998;101(3):686–694.
- Hale HB, Bae DS, Waters PM. Current concepts in the management of brachial plexus birth palsy. *J Hand Surg Am*. 2010;35(2):322–331.
- Somashekar D, Yang LJ, Ibrahim M, et al. High-resolution MRI evaluation of neonatal brachial plexus palsy: a promising alternative to traditional CT myelography. *AJNR Am J Neuroradiol*. 2014;35(6):1209–1213.
- Tse R, Kozin SH, Malessy MJ, et al. International Federation of Societies for Surgery of the Hand Committee report: the role of nerve transfers in the treatment of neonatal brachial plexus palsy. *J Hand Surg Am*. 2015;40(6):1246–1259.
- Wolfe SW, Strauss HL, Garg R, et al. Use of bioabsorbable nerve conduits as an adjunct to brachial plexus neurorrhaphy. *J Hand Surg Am*. 2012;37(10):1980–1985.

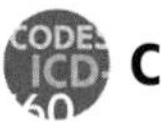

CODES

ICD10

P14.3 Other brachial plexus birth injuries

FAQ

- Q: My baby was diagnosed with a brachial plexus injury. What are the odds she will recover completely?
- A: Most (roughly 80%) children recover completely. Stretched and inflamed nerves should recover. However, babies with more significant injuries causing axonotmesis and neurotmesis may not recover completely or at all.
- Q: My last baby suffered a brachial plexus injury at birth but since got better. What are the odds my next child will have the same problem?
- A: Your next child has a 14-fold increase in risk for brachial plexus injury compared to the general population.
- Q: My baby is 3 months old and cannot move his left arm? Whom should I call?
- A: A center for brachial plexus injury is ideal. A well-organized team includes physical and occupational therapists, neurologists, and surgeons (neurosurgeon, plastic surgeon, orthopedic surgeon, or combination thereof).
- Q: Could my obstetrician have prevented this injury?
- A: Likely, not. Although there may be increased risk for shoulder dystocia in some women, it is not a diagnosable problem. Preemptive cesarean section in at-risk women may be unnecessarily risky to mother and fetus.
- Q: My child had a brachial plexus injury that hasn't improved and our surgeon is recommending surgery. Will my baby have a normal arm after surgery?
- A: The goals of nerve reconstruction in children with brachial plexus injuries is to improve the arm enough to make it functional. The amount of improvement your child's arm has after surgery is greatly dependent on the extent of the initial nerve injury.

BRAIN ABSCESS

Karen E. Jerardi, MD, MEd • Samir S. Shah, MD, MSCE

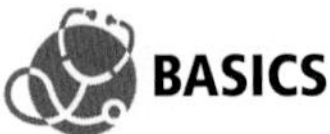

BASICS

DESCRIPTION

- Suppurative infection involving the brain parenchyma
- May be a single or multiple lesions

EPIDEMIOLOGY

- Males more commonly affected (2:1 male-to-female predominance)
- Typical age of presentation is 4 to 7 years but varies according to predisposing factor.
- 85% of cases have a predisposing risk factor.

Incidence

~1,500 to 2,500 cases (adults and pediatric combined) occur per year with up to 25% being children.

RISK FACTORS

- Cyanotic congenital heart disease (tetralogy of Fallot is most common)
- Otorhinolaryngologic infections such as sinusitis, mastoiditis, and chronic otitis media
- Meningitis (especially in neonates)
- Penetrating head trauma
- Surgical manipulation of the brain (ventriculoperitoneal shunts, tumor removal)
- Congenital lesions of the head and neck
- Cystic fibrosis
- Dental infections
- Lung infections
- Patients who have traveled to endemic areas where neurocysticercosis (Latin America, parts of Africa, Asia, and the Indian subcontinent) is endemic
- Immunocompromised patients (congenital or acquired)

GENERAL PREVENTION

- During recreational activities, wearing helmets may prevent penetrating head trauma.
- Appropriate management of acute otitis media and acute sinusitis as well as timely recognition of treatment failure

PATHOPHYSIOLOGY

- Microorganisms enter the brain parenchyma by contiguous or hematogenous extension.
- Location of brain abscesses:
  - Cyanotic congenital heart disease patients tend to have abscesses within the middle meningeal artery distribution: frontal, parietal, and temporal lobes.
  - Frontal abscesses are commonly seen with sinus and dental infections.
  - Temporal, parietal, or cerebellar abscesses tend to occur with mastoiditis or otitis media.
  - Brain abscesses can occur anywhere in the brain parenchyma, regardless of a predisposing risk factor, secondary to hematogenous metastasis.

ETIOLOGY

- Bacteria are the most common causes.
- *Streptococcus milleri* (*anginosus*) group and *Staphylococcus* spp. are the most commonly cultured microorganisms.
- Neonates may develop brain abscesses as a complication of gram-negative meningitis (*Proteus*, *Citrobacter*, *Enterobacter*, and *Cronobacter* species).
- Polymicrobial infections occur in 30–50% of cases.
- Anaerobic organisms are found with increasing incidence with improved laboratory and culture techniques. Common pathogens include *Bacteroides*, *Peptostreptococcus*, *Fusobacterium*, *Propionibacterium*, *Actinomyces*, *Veillonella*, and *Prevotella*.
- Neurocysticercosis is caused by the parasite, *Taenia solium*. Fungi and protozoa can cause brain abscess in immunocompromised patients.

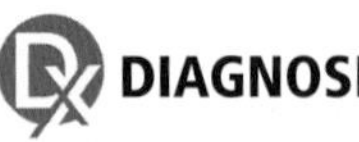

DIAGNOSIS

HISTORY

The location of the brain abscess or abscesses will influence the clinical presentation.

- Classic triad of fever, headache, and focal neurologic findings occurs in <30% of cases.
- Fever, headache, and vomiting each occur in ~60–70% of cases.
- Headache is the most common complaint.
- Vomiting and mental status changes can be the presenting chief complaints.
- Neonates will often have a history of meningitis before developing a brain abscess.
- Questions should focus on acute or chronic otolaryngologic infections.
- A history of cyanotic congenital heart disease should be obtained, as well as partially repaired cyanotic congenital heart disease.

PHYSICAL EXAM

- Neonates may present with a full fontanel, increasing head circumference, seizures, or vomiting.
- Older children may have signs of a focal neurologic deficit, hemiparesis, or even papilledema.
- Meningeal symptoms occur in ~30% of patients.
- Location of abscess also affects presenting signs.
  - Frontal lobe: behavioral changes, emotional lability
  - Temporal lobe: cranial nerve dysfunction, motor abnormalities, aphasia
  - Parietal lobe: visual abnormalities, dysphagia, perceptive abnormalities
  - Cerebellum: ipsilateral ataxia, tremor, 6th cranial nerve palsy

DIFFERENTIAL DIAGNOSIS

- Infectious
  - Meningitis
  - Encephalitis
  - Subdural empyema
  - Epidural abscess
- Vascular
  - Venous sinus thrombosis
  - Migraine
  - Cerebral infarct
  - Cerebral hemorrhage
- Miscellaneous
  - Primary or secondary tumor
  - Pseudotumor cerebri
  - Hydrocephalus

DIAGNOSTIC TESTS & INTERPRETATION

Initial Tests (screening, lab, imaging)

- Routine lab tests are not helpful and cannot rule out the diagnosis.
- <10% of blood cultures are positive.
- Peripheral WBC may be mildly elevated, but <10% will show band forms.
- Erythrocyte sedimentation rate (ESR) is a poor indicator of brain abscesses.
- Electrolytes may show low sodium, indicating syndrome of inappropriate secretion of antidiuretic hormone (SIADH).
- A lumbar puncture is contraindicated if any intracranial mass lesion is suspected, but if CSF is obtained:
  - It may show a mild to moderate pleocytosis (20% of patients may have normal values).
  - Opening pressure may be elevated.
  - Glucose is decreased in 30% of patients.
  - Protein is elevated in 70% of cases.
  - CSF Gram stain and cultures are often negative.
- CT with contrast and MRI scans are the studies of choice in diagnosing brain abscesses and identifying potential sources (e.g., sinus, orbit).

- Although CT can provide more rapid results, occult intracranial infections can be missed in up to 50% of cases.
- Cranial ultrasound may be useful in premature neonatal cases.

ALERT

- Not all patients with brain abscesses have fever.
- Pitfalls
  - Failure to consider a brain abscess in a child with altered mental status, fevers, and meningismus or in a child with nonspecific symptoms but risk factors, such as cyanotic congenital heart disease
  - Failure to recognize symptoms not typically seen in sinusitis, such as vomiting

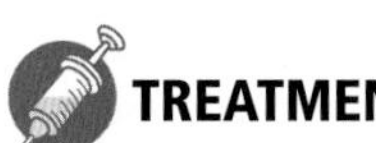

TREATMENT

MEDICATION

- Broad-spectrum antibiotics that penetrate the central nervous system (CNS) should be given at the time of diagnosis directed at most likely pathogens. The combination of a 3rd-generation cephalosporin (e.g., ceftriaxone), vancomycin, and metronidazole provides good empiric coverage.
  - Add gentamicin if concomitant endocarditis is present.
  - Consider antipseudomonal antibiotics (e.g., cefepime) in lieu of ceftriaxone in immunocompromised patients.
- Culture-directed antimicrobial therapy is recommended whenever possible. Typical antibiotic courses are 4 to 6 weeks.
- Systemic corticosteroids, although not routinely recommended, should be considered if there is severe or progressive elevation in intracranial pressure.
- Some patients are managed successfully with antibiotics alone, especially if there is a single, small (<2 cm) abscess.
- Antiparasitic medications (albendazole) with or without corticosteroids should be considered for treatment of neurocysticercosis.
- Antifungals should be considered for immunocompromised patients.

SURGERY/OTHER PROCEDURES

- Consider neurosurgical and/or otolaryngology consultation.
- MRI or CT-guided stereotactic aspiration is encouraged to obtain cultures and identify the causative organism(s).

ADMISSION, INPATIENT, AND NURSING CONSIDERATIONS

- All patients with concern for brain abscess should be admitted for clinical monitoring, diagnostic evaluation, and treatment.
- Evaluation by cardiology, dental, otorhinolaryngology, and/or immunology may help identify predisposing factors.
- If a patient is manifesting signs and symptoms of increased intracranial pressure (Cushing triad: bradycardia, hypertension, and abnormal respirations) or if the patient is unable to protect his or her airway, endotracheal intubation is indicated. Hyperventilation and mannitol should be considered.
- Electrolyte abnormalities such as SIADH may occur. Frequent monitoring of electrolytes is warranted.
- Seizures and focal neurologic deficits can occur early in presentation. They typically resolve with drainage of the lesion. Careful and frequent neurologic exams should be part of the hospital care.
- Generally, patients may be discharged home once their symptoms have resolved and antibiotic therapy is complete or can be completed at home.

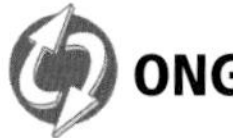

ONGOING CARE

FOLLOW-UP RECOMMENDATIONS

- Follow-up with neurosurgical, rehabilitation, and neurology clinics is usually required.
- Repeat imaging prior to cessation of antibiotic therapy should be done to document resolution of the abscess.

PROGNOSIS

- Overall mortality is <5%.
- Improved outcomes come with early diagnosis and treatment, compliance with completing the complete prescribed antibiotic course, and adhering to rehabilitation/therapy recommendations when appropriate.

COMPLICATIONS

- Long-term complications arise from the location, size, and number of intracranial abscesses.
- Multiple abscesses, coma on presentation, age <2 years, and rupture of abscess into the ventricle carry a higher mortality rate.
- 30–40% of patients have some morbidity associated with brain abscess; seizures, hydrocephalus, focal neurologic deficits (motor and sensory dysfunction), and behavioral or personality changes are potential complications. Mortality rates have decreased because of advances in imaging to assist in rapid diagnosis and surgical management.

ADDITIONAL READING

- Bonfield CM, Sharma J, Dobson S. Pediatric intracranial abscesses. *J Infect*. 2015;71(Suppl 1):S42–S46.
- Goodkin HP, Harper MB, Pomeroy SL. Intracerebral abscess in children: historical trends at Children's Hospital Boston. *Pediatrics*. 2004;113(6):1765–1770.
- Herrmann BW, Chung JC, Eisenbeis JF, et al. Intracranial complications of pediatric frontal rhinosinusitis. *Am J Rhinol*. 2006;20(3):320–324.
- Sáez-Llorens X. Brain abscess in children. *Semin Pediatr Infect Dis*. 2003;14(2):108–114.
- Yogev R, Bar-Meir M. Management of brain abscesses in children. *Pediatr Infect Dis J*. 2004;23(2):157–159.

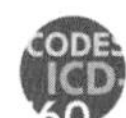

CODES

ICD10

G06.0 Intracranial abscess and granuloma

FAQ

- Q: Do all brain abscesses require surgery?
- A: No. Often times, brain abscesses will respond to intravenous antibiotics and will not require drainage. Close clinical and radiographic follow-up is imperative in these cases. Stereotactic aspiration of a brain abscess can be very helpful in identifying the microbiology of a brain abscess and help direct specific treatment.
- Q: What is the best imaging study to definitively diagnose a brain abscess?
- A: MRI can detect smaller abscesses than CT. MRI also has the advantage over CT in being able to identify potential sources of infection such as the frontal sinuses and the orbits.

BRAIN INJURY, TRAUMATIC

Mark E. Halstead, MD • Jose A. Pineda, MD, MSCI

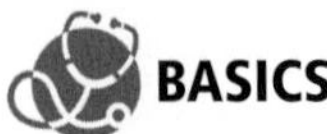

BASICS

DESCRIPTION

Traumatic brain injury (TBI): damage to the brain from accidental or nonaccidental trauma

- Children >1 year: Glasgow Coma Scale (GCS) <14, amnesia >15 minutes for event, penetrating head injury (see Appendix, Table 5)
- Children <1 year: any loss of consciousness (LOC), protracted emesis, suspected abuse (see Appendix, Table 6)
- Mild brain injury: GCS >14
- Severe brain injury: usually initial GCS <9

EPIDEMIOLOGY

- Trauma, number 1 cause of death of children >1 year; head injury most common contributor to morbidity and mortality
- Almost 500,000 emergency department visits each year for TBI for those aged 0 to 14 years; males age 0 to 4 years highest rate of TBI emergency department visits
- 75% of TBIs each year are mild.
- <2 years old: Nonaccidental trauma is principal cause of TBI.
- >2 years old: Falls (~37%) are most common cause of trauma.
- For severe TBI, nonaccidental trauma remains principal cause in young children.
- Motor vehicle accidents in older children, although penetrating injuries becoming more common

PATHOPHYSIOLOGY

- Primary
  - Focally applied forces: lacerations, penetration injuries, skull fractures
  - Contusions, intracerebral hematomas uncommon; epidurals, classic subdurals <10% in children
  - Acceleration–deceleration/shearing forces: cervical spine injuries, diffuse axonal injury (DAI), nonaneurysmal subarachnoid hemorrhage, subdural hematoma (SDH) from shear forces
- Secondary
  - Extension of injury to viable tissue/entire brain
  - Dysautoregulation of cerebral blood flow, neuroexcitotoxicity, and inflammatory mediators. In severe TBI, CT or MRI signs of edema may progress over 3 to 5 days (see "Treatment").
- Age-specific pathophysiology:
  - Infants/toddler
    - Shear forces on the brain due to acceleration/deceleration avulse axons from their cell bodies causing DAI; often compounded by tearing and bleeding of dural veins
    - Unmyelinated infant brain absorbs rather than transfers impact. Immature, distensible skull renders brain less likely to contuse or herniated but more likely to sustain diffuse secondary injuries, with swelling.
    - Subgaleal hematoma, cephalohematoma (below the periosteum), and caput succedaneum (confined to the superficial scalp) at birth do not predict brain injury.
    - More severe birth trauma can result in SDH.
    - Bilateral interhemispheric SDH suggests nonaccidental trauma.
    - Diffuse injuries secondary to shaken impact syndrome can lead to cerebral swelling with secondary infarction and/or decreased central respiratory control, leading to apnea, hypoxia, seizures, and cerebral edema.
    - Suspect nonaccidental trauma with growing skull fracture, if >1 cranial bone involved or if other injuries are present.
  - Older children/adolescents
    - Mild TBI likely due to neuronal disruption, potassium efflux with release of glutamate; increases demand of ATP and glucose
    - Still more subject to DAI than adults due to incomplete myelination
    - Projectile injuries in adolescent population may cause prolonged brain swelling (particularly close-range gunshot wounds).

DIAGNOSIS

HISTORY

- Eyewitness accounts are invaluable.
- Details of who was caring for the child
- Falls: Did LOC precede fall? Height of fall, surface of impact
- History of epilepsy, cardiac problems
- History of previous concussions (consider "second impact syndrome") or trauma
- Intoxication (of child, caregiver, others in the environment)
- Prior physical abuse/neglect?
- Restrained motor vehicle passenger? Angle of impact
- How did patient act or change over time? Unresponsive? Confused? Headache? Visual changes? Vomiting? Seizure?
- Consider use of published concussion symptom checklists.

PHYSICAL EXAM

Rapid neurologic exam in trauma

- Can derive some of these by observation. Note presence of neuromuscular blockers/sedation:
  - Level of arousal: awake, lethargic, stuporous, unresponsive
  - Resting posture: spontaneous, restless, still normal, flexor, extensor
  - Respiration: in context of arousal and posture, hyperpnea, or Cheyne-Stokes respiration
  - Response to stimulation: voice, pain (of supraorbital nerve or earlobe to avoid spinal withdrawal response); note localization, withdrawal, posturing.
  - Pupils: equal, anisocoria >1 mm, unequal/sluggish pupil, unequal/wide/fixed pupil. Consider funduscopic exam if suspected nonaccidental trauma.
  - Extraocular movements: disconjugate gaze nonlocalizing with drugs/trauma, 3rd nerve palsy uncal herniation sign, 4th nerve palsy common in head injuries, 6th nerve palsy from trauma or increased ICP
  - Brainstem reflexes: corneals (V and VII), oculocephalic if patient unable to cooperate with eye exam and cervical spine cleared. Avoid gag—raises ICP.
  - Muscle reflexes/motor exam: Lateralizing signs may indicate contralateral hemispheric lesion, with ipsilateral dilated pupil may indicate uncal herniation.
  - Sensory: brief for four limbs/spinal level if indicated
  - Bruising behind the ear (Battle sign) or around the eyes (raccoon-eyes) may indicate presence of a skull fracture.
  - In patients with severe TBI abnormal flexion or extension on exam may indicate presence of intracranial hypertension.
- This exam should be repeated often according to the patient's level of acuity. A more detailed exam tailored to degree of arousal can be done as the patient is stabilized.
- Mild TBI can be assessed with standard neurologic exam as outlined earlier. Balanced assessment and neurocognitive assessment (short-term memory, months of the year in reverse, digits in reverse) may be useful. Use of SCAT5 in sport concussion assessment may be beneficial on sideline or emergency department.

DIFFERENTIAL DIAGNOSIS

- Neurologic presentation varies in severity from a normal examination through coma similar to hypoxic-ischemic brain injuries (e.g., near-drowning), other causes of stupor/coma, seizure activity (postictal encephalopathy).
- Distinction between simple concussion, DAI, and hypoxic-ischemic injury may be difficult at initial presentation, becoming clear as clinical picture/neuroimaging evolves.

DIAGNOSTIC TESTS & INTERPRETATION

Initial Tests (screening, lab, imaging)

In all patients with suspected TBI, consider:

- CBC (Infants can have a large amount of intracranial blood loss.)
- PT/PTT (to evaluate a possible bleeding disorder as a possible preoperative laboratory test)
- Electrolytes
- LFTs if suspected nonaccidental trauma
- Toxin screen
- Laboratory studies likely not necessary in mild TBI unless laboratory abnormality suspected as contributor to TBI
- In mild TBI, imaging most likely not needed. High risk for lesion includes GCS <15 at 2 hours postinjury, suspicion of open skull fracture, worsening headache, and irritability. Medium risk for lesion includes large, boggy hematoma, signs of basal skull fracture, and dangerous mechanism of injury.
- Unenhanced CT scan of the brain is the imaging study of choice for initial evaluation of a patient with suspected TBI.
- Abnormal CT: lesion density, midline shift, compression of cisterns, bone fragments
- MRI: useful for DAI (with a negative head CT) as well as showing small lesions (e.g., punctate contusions)
- In suspected cervical spine injury where patient is unresponsive, CT scan initially with consideration for MRI of the spine to rule out noncontiguous unstable ligamentous injury.
- Long bone films if degree of injury is not consistent with history or history of fall from unclear height
- Consider EEG and lumbar puncture if a non-traumatic etiology for altered mental status is suspected, if CT normal.

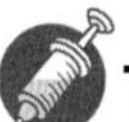

TREATMENT

- Airway, breathing, circulation
- Cervical spine stabilization in unconscious patient
- Prehospital stabilization: Avoid hypoxemia, hyperventilation, and hypotension (strong, possibly modifiable, independent predictors of outcome in TBI).

GENERAL MEASURES

- For acute mild TBI, initially recommend reducing cognitive stress in school and rest from full sports participation while symptomatic. Allowing some light cardiovascular activity may be acceptable if it does not worsen symptoms until fully recovered.
- AAP guidelines set conditions for return to play depending on symptoms:
  - An AAP concussion statement outlines graduated return to activity if no return of symptoms and suggests (i) no same-day return (ii) and medical clearance needed before initiating return to activity progression
- A rapid neurologic exam repeated over time is instrumental in directing the patient's care.
- For more severe trauma or in infants, emergent referral to a trauma center with pediatric neurosurgical capabilities is indicated.
- Secondary survey: external evidence of head injury/deformities, ecchymoses (periorbital-orbital roof fracture; mastoid-petrous temporal fracture), lacerations, penetrations; CSF leak nasal/otic
- Seizures: lorazepam 0.05 to 0.1 mg/kg IV at 2 mg/min or rectal Diastat 0.3 to 0.5 mg/kg if no IV access. Then load fosphenytoin 15 to 20 mg/kg IV; important to treat to avoid increased ICP, neurotoxicity, brain metabolic crisis
- No evidence that seizure prophylaxis >1 week posttrauma prevents late seizures
- No evidence that steroids improve outcome
- Hypothermia may decrease ICP in severe TBI; no difference in long-term outcome
- No evidence for prophylactic use of mannitol, although it is effective for control of increased ICP. Bolus doses 0.25 g/kg of body weight to 1 g/kg of body weight to goal ICP <20 mm Hg. Avoid dehydration and hypotension.
- Hypertonic 3% saline IV for increased ICP as above; may also be used as initial fluid resuscitation (central venous access ideal but not required under emergent situations)
- Rapid sequence intubation by experienced airway provider in patients with severe TBI
- Reserve hyperventilation (P_{CO_2} 30 to 25 mm Hg) for patients with signs of brain herniation (abnormal pupils, hypertension, bradycardia, and abnormal respiration).
- The postresuscitation GCS score should be recorded in all trauma patients.
- Involvement of neurosurgery with moderate GCS <13 injury, even if patient initially stable
- Survival for children with severe TBI is greater when treated in pediatric ICU. Management based Brain Trauma Foundation guidelines may result in better outcomes.
- Decompressive craniectomy may be considered given the following conditions:
  - Diffuse cerebral swelling or midline shift on CT imaging
  - Secondary clinical deterioration
  - Persistent intracranial hypertension (ICP >20 mm Hg) despite maximal medical treatment
  - Evolving cerebral herniation syndrome

ADMISSION, INPATIENT, AND NURSING CONSIDERATIONS

- Cervical spine stabilization and clearance; in severe TBI, entire spine is stabilized:
  - If necessary, orotracheal intubation with rapid sequence induction; avoid hypotension and hypoxia.
  - Hyperventilation may induce regional cerebral ischemia in children, especially in first 24 hours; transient hyperventilation with 100% oxygen indicated in patients with cerebral herniation while other therapies are being administered
  - Increased ICP managed by bed elevation of 30 degrees, hypertonic fluids, sedation, and blood pressure (BP) support to maintain cerebral perfusion pressure
- Hemodynamic stabilization (normal high systolic BP ~135) predictor of better outcome in TBI (median systolic BP = 90 mm Hg + [2 × age in years])
  - Hemodynamic instability indicative of systemic hemorrhage (abdomen, long bone fractures), pericardial tamponade (narrow pulse pressure), or cardiac contusion. Consider presence of neurogenic shock.
  - Hypotension late sign; early: ↑HR, ↓capillary refill, ↓urine output
  - Fluid resuscitation: Consider hypertonic saline. Mounting evidence of improved outcomes especially with hemorrhagic shock and TBI (initial dose 5 to 10 mL/kg bolus; titrate continuous 3% saline infusion 0.1 to 1 mL/kg/h to maintain serum sodium between 150 to 160 mmol/L).
  - Fluid overload may worsen intracranial hypertension (ICP).
  - Consider use of short-acting sedatives and analgesics (i.e., fentanyl and propofol) to facilitate serial neurologic exam during initial stabilization. Avoid hypotension.
  - Consider monitoring ICP to maintain <20 mm Hg for abnormal admission CT scan, and GCS 3 to 8 after CPR, or normal CT and GCS 3 to 8, and posturing, asymmetric pupils or hypotension, or if serial neurologic exams precluded by sedation.

ONGOING CARE

PROGNOSIS

- Majority of mild TBI patients recovery without significant sequelae
- Presence of both hypoxemia and hypotension or traumatic cardiac arrest on arrival to ER bode poorly
- 24-hour GCS better predictor of outcome than postresuscitation; PRISM score also helpful
- GCS <3 with abnormal pupils poor prognosis unless secondary to epidural hematoma; rapid evacuation can minimize permanent deficits.
- Diffuse white matter, subcortical gray, or brainstem lesions on MRI portend long periods of coma and poorer outcome.
- Somatosensory-evoked potentials (VEPS or BAEPs) are less sensitive but have high specificity in predicting neurologic outcome.
- Degree of injury on head CT can be predictive.
- Patients who have sustained moderate to severe head injury (GCS = 13) often have academic difficulties, memory abnormalities, and disinhibition.
- Monitoring for cognitive difficulties (executive function in particular), hyperactivity, seizures, hydrocephalus, movement disorders, paralysis, visual/hearing disturbance, headache; psychologists, neurologists, neurosurgeons, ophthalmologists, audiologists, and physical therapists may be helpful.
- Refer any patient with known skull fracture who manifests a new swelling in area of old fracture to neurosurgeon for 3D CT imaging of the head.
- Patients with severe head injury may require inpatient rehabilitation and significant support when returning to school. Long-term prognosis usually evaluated 1 year postinjury. ~10% will develop epilepsy.

ADDITIONAL READING

- Badjatia N, Carney N, Crocco TJ, et al. Guidelines for prehospital management of traumatic brain injury 2nd edition. *Prehosp Emerg Care*. 2008;12(Suppl 1):S1–S52.
- Centers for Disease Control and Prevention: www.cdc.gov/concussion/HeadsUp/high_school.html
- Halstead ME, Walter KD; for Council on Sports Medicine and Fitness. American Academy of Pediatrics. Clinical report—sport-related concussion in children and adolescents. *Pediatrics*. 2010;126(3):597–615.
- Hymel KP, Makoroff KL, Laskey AL, et al. Mechanisms, clinical presentations, injuries, and outcomes from inflicted versus noninflicted head trauma during infancy: results of a prospective, multicentered, comparative study. *Pediatrics*. 2007;119(5):922–929.
- Jagannathan J, Okonkwo DO, Dumont AS, et al. Outcome following decompressive craniectomy in children with severe traumatic brain injury: a 10-year single-center experience with long-term follow up. *J Neurosurg*. 2007;106(Suppl 4):268–275.
- Kochanek PM, Carney N, Adelson PD, et al. Guidelines for the acute medical management of severe traumatic brain injury in infants, children, and adolescents—second edition. *Pediatr Crit Care Med*. 2012;13(Suppl 1):S1–S82.
- McCrory P, Meeuwisse W, Dvořák J, et al. Consensus statement on concussion in sport-the 5th international conference on concussion in sport held in Berlin, October 2016. *Br J Sports Med*. 2017;51(11):838–847.
- Osmond MH, Klassen TP, Wells GA, et al; for Pediatric Emergency Research Canada Head Injury Study Group. CATCH: a clinical decision rule for the use of computed tomography in children with minor head injury. *CMAJ*. 2010;182(4):341–348.
- Pineda JA, Leonard JR, Mazotas IG, et al. Effect of implementation of a paediatric neurocritical care programme on outcomes after severe traumatic brain injury: a retrospective cohort study. *Lancet Neurol*. 2013;12(1):45–52.
- White JR, Farukhi Z, Bull C, et al. Predictors of outcome in severely head-injured children. *Crit Care Med*. 2001;29(3):534–540.

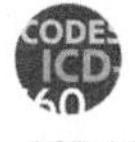

CODES

ICD10

- S06.9X0A Unsp intracranial injury w/o loss of consciousness, init
- S06.9X9A Unsp intracranial injury w LOC of unsp duration, init
- S06.9X1A Unspecified intracranial injury with loss of consciousness of 30 minutes or less, initial encounter

BRAIN TUMOR

Jane E. Minturn, MD, PhD • Michael J. Fisher, MD

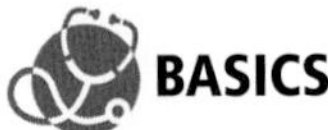

BASICS

DESCRIPTION

A primary neoplasm arising in the central nervous system (CNS)

EPIDEMIOLOGY

- Most common solid neoplasm of childhood (second to leukemia in overall incidence)
- Most common cause of cancer death in children 0 to 14 years
- Slight male predominance
- Majority arise infratentorially (within cerebellum or brainstem) in children 1 to 14 years of age.
- Majority arise supratentorially in children <1 year of age.

Incidence

- Incidence >3,000 new cases/year
- 5.4 cases/100,000 children/year (age-adjusted incidence rate, ages 0 to 19 years, between 2007 and 2011)
- Peak incidence in children ≤7 years of age
- Approximately 1 in 2,000 children born 2009 to 2011 will be diagnosed with a primary malignant CNS tumor by age 14 years.

RISK FACTORS

Genetics

- Brain tumors are not inherited.
- About 5% of primary brain tumors may be linked to hereditary genetic syndromes:
  - Neurofibromatosis with optic pathway gliomas (NF1) and meningiomas, vestibular schwannomas (NF2)
  - Tuberous sclerosis with gliomas and rarely ependymomas
  - Li-Fraumeni syndrome with astrocytomas
  - von Hippel-Lindau with cerebellar hemangioblastoma
  - Turcot syndrome with medulloblastoma

PATHOPHYSIOLOGY

Tumors are now classified based on histology and molecular genetic features. The most common are the following:

- Diffuse gliomas/other astrocytic tumors
  - Arises from glial cells (e.g., astrocytes most common in children)
  - ~50% of childhood CNS tumors
  - Ranges from low-grade (grade I to II; often in the cerebellum or optic pathway) to high-grade (grade III to IV; in the cerebrum or brainstem)
  - Locally recurrent and invasive when high grade
  - Molecular alterations distinguish pediatric from adult gliomas.
- Embryonal tumors
  - Heterogenous group of tumors that arise from malignant embryonic cells
  - Comprises ~15% of childhood CNS tumors
  - Most common malignant brain tumor in children
  - Most common embryonal tumor (60%) is medulloblastoma (cerebellum).
  - Predisposition for leptomeningeal dissemination
- Ependymoma
  - Arises from ependymal cells that line the ventricular system
  - 5–8% of childhood CNS tumors
  - Most commonly occurs in the 4th ventricle; may arise in the spinal cord
  - Locally recurrent and invasive; spinal metastases rare at initial diagnosis
- Germ cell tumors
  - Derived from totipotent germ cells
  - 3–5% of childhood CNS tumors
  - Majority are located in the pineal or suprasellar region.
- Atypical teratoid/rhabdoid tumor
  - Now classified under embryonal tumors
  - <3% of childhood CNS tumors
  - Majority arise in children <5 years of age.
  - Propensity to arise in the posterior fossa with frequent leptomeningeal dissemination; reported in association with malignant rhabdoid tumors of the kidney
- Neuronal and mixed neuronal-glial tumors: 6% of childhood CNS tumors
- Craniopharyngioma: 3–5% of childhood CNS tumors
- Choroid plexus tumors (papilloma and carcinoma)
- Meningioma and hemangioblastoma, rare in children

ETIOLOGY

- No specific causative agents are known, but there is an association with exposure to ionizing radiation, other malignancies, familial/heritable diseases, immunosuppression/immunodeficiency (CNS lymphoma).
- Molecular markers and variants of individual tumor types are being identified.

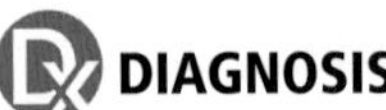

DIAGNOSIS

Tumor location dictates symptoms and signs.

HISTORY

- Headache and vomiting (particularly in the morning), irritability, and lethargy are associated with increased intracranial pressure.
- Difficulty swallowing, slurred speech and diplopia may indicate brainstem tumor.
- Visual field deficits (bumps into things) could indicate optic pathway lesion.
- Focal weakness hints at pyramidal tract lesion.
- Ataxia may be a sign of cerebellar lesion.
- Changes in behavior or school performance, new-onset seizures, and weakness could be signs of supratentorial lesion.
- Polyuria/polydipsia may indicate hypothalamic/pituitary lesion.
- Failure to thrive, emaciation, euphoria, and increased appetite in an infant may indicate hypothalamic lesion (diencephalic syndrome).
- Back pain, extremity weakness, and bowel/bladder dysfunction could signify spinal cord metastases (often seen with medulloblastoma and germ cell tumors).

PHYSICAL EXAM

- Papilledema, impaired upgaze and/or lateral gaze, macrocephaly (infants), and bulging fontanelle are signs of increased intracranial pressure.
- Focal deficit on neurologic exam helps localize the mass lesion:
  - Isolated cranial nerve VI and VII palsies may indicate brainstem tumor.
  - Ataxia and dysmetria could indicate cerebellar mass.
  - Decreased visual acuity, visual field deficit, absent pupillary light response, and strabismus may all be signs of optic pathway tumor.
  - Changes in cognitive function, mood, and affect could indicate supratentorial lesion.
  - Impaired upgaze, convergence nystagmus, and pupils responding to accommodation but poorly to light are signs of pineal lesion (Parinaud or dorsal midbrain syndrome).
- Signs of neurocutaneous disease (e.g., café au lait spots, axillary freckling, Lisch nodules) may indicate a syndrome such as NF1.

DIFFERENTIAL DIAGNOSIS

- Infection: cerebral abscess
- Demyelination:
  - Inflammatory demyelinating or white matter lesions
  - Usually differentiated on imaging
- Tumors:
  - Metastatic tumor to brain
  - Uncommon with childhood cancers
- Trauma: hemorrhage unlikely to be confused with tumor
- Congenital
  - Arteriovenous malformation
  - Hamartoma
  - Dysplastic brain
- Psychosocial: Some patients with nausea, vomiting, or behavior changes are first diagnosed with psychiatric disorders, gastrointestinal disorders, failure to thrive, or anorexia nervosa prior to discovery of a brain tumor.

ALERT

New onset of psychoses should prompt imaging to rule out tumor.

DIAGNOSTIC TESTS & INTERPRETATION

Initial Tests (screening, labs, imaging)

- MRI
  - With and without gadolinium enhancement
  - The "gold standard" for identification, localization, and characterization of tumors
- CT
  - Can be used as an initial study; but if negative and a high index of suspicion, follow with MRI.
  - Useful to evaluate for hydrocephalus and hemorrhage

Diagnostic Procedures/Other

Staging of tumor

- Postoperative brain MRI within 24 to 48 hours to determine residual disease before postoperative inflammatory changes are prominent
- Spine MRI and cerebrospinal fluid (CSF) cytology required for neuraxis staging of tumors with high risk of leptomeningeal dissemination
- Elevated α-fetoprotein and quantitative β-human chorionic gonadotropin in CSF and serum are markers for germ cell tumors.

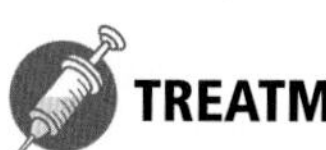

TREATMENT

SURGERY/OTHER PROCEDURES

- Both for histology/molecular characterization and to attempt maximal tumor debulking; should be performed by experienced pediatric neurosurgeon
- Rarely indicated in diffuse midline glioma; although biopsy for molecular profiling increasingly in use
- Ventriculoperitoneal shunt or endoscopic third ventriculostomy when needed for obstructive hydrocephalus (risk of peritoneal seeding minimal)

ALERT
Patient should be referred to a pediatric brain tumor/oncology center at diagnosis (preoperatively).

- Radiotherapy
  - Volume and dose vary depending on histology.
  - Radiation therapy to the tumor bed is used for most patients with brain tumors.
  - Medulloblastoma patients need craniospinal radiation therapy. The one exception is infants and young children (<3 years of age) in whom cognitive deficits from radiation therapy are devastating.
  - Duration of radiation therapy: usually 6 weeks
  - Newer approaches to limit exposure of normal brain include proton radiotherapy.

MEDICATION

- Dexamethasone to control increased intracranial pressure
- Chemotherapy
  - Drugs are most often used in combination:
    - Carboplatin, vincristine, or 6-thioguanine, procarbazine, lomustine, vincristine for low-grade glioma
    - Cisplatin, lomustine, vincristine, etoposide, and cyclophosphamide are active agents for medulloblastoma and other embryonal tumors.
    - Temozolomide for glioma
  - New protocols currently being evaluated:
    - High-dose chemotherapy with autologous stem cell rescue for high-risk medulloblastoma
    - Molecularly targeted therapies, angiogenesis inhibitors, vaccine and immunotherapies
  - Duration of chemotherapy: 6 months to 2 years

ALERT
Possible drug interactions with other treatments: Chemotherapy can alter anticonvulsant levels.

ONGOING CARE

- Neurologic deficits can take months to improve or stabilize with permanent deficit.
- Any worsening or relapse of symptoms must be evaluated for tumor recurrence.
- MRI every 3 months the 1st year, every 6 months for the next 2 years, and annually thereafter. Benefit of routine surveillance imaging is controversial.

PROGNOSIS

- Dependent on histology of tumor, location, and extent of initial resection
- Glioma
  - Low-grade: ≥90% 5-year progression-free survival (PFS) following gross total resection; 45–65% for subtotal resection
  - High-grade: median survival 8 to 31 months; depends on grade and extent of resection
  - Diffuse midline (location in pons): median overall survival of 9 to 13 months from diagnosis
- Medulloblastoma
  - 79–83% PFS at 5 years if localized, gross total resection achieved, and >3 years old at diagnosis
  - <50% PFS if disseminated
- Ependymoma
  - 50–70% survival at 5 years with total resection
  - <30% survival with subtotal resection
- Infants overall have a worse prognoses, possibly due to the limitations of therapy and/or the aggressiveness of the tumor.

ALERT
Even benign tumors may be life threatening if their location precludes resection.

COMPLICATIONS

- Secondary to disease
  - Increased intracranial pressure
    - Obstruction of CSF flow
    - Requires immediate neurosurgical evaluation
- Secondary to radiotherapy
  - Neurocognitive sequelae (age- and dose-related)
  - Endocrinopathy (growth hormone deficiency, hypothyroidism, gonadal dysfunction)
  - Risk of second malignancies (meningioma, glioma, sarcoma)
  - Increased risk of stroke
- Secondary to chemotherapy
  - Risks associated with bone marrow suppression (infection, bleeding, anemia)
  - Hearing loss
  - Risk of secondary leukemia

ADDITIONAL READING

- Fleming AJ, Chi SN. Brain tumors in children. *Curr Probl Pediatr Adolesc Health Care*. 2012;42(4):80–103.
- Liu KW, Pajtler KW, Worst BC, et al. Molecular mechanisms and therapeutic targets in pediatric brain tumors. *Sci Signal*. 2017;10(470):eaaf7593.
- Louis DN, Perry A, Reifenberger G. et al. The 2016 World Health Organization classification of tumors of the central nervous system: a summary. *Acta Neuropathol*. 2016;131(6):803–820.
- Ostrom QT, de Blank PM, Kruchko C, et al. Alex's Lemonade Stand Foundation infant and childhood primary brain and central nervous system tumors diagnosed in the United States in 2007–2011. *Neuro Oncol*. 2015;16(Suppl 10):x1–x36.
- Parsons DW, Pollack IF, Haas-Kogan DA, et al. Gliomas, ependymomas, and other nonembryonal tumors of the central nervous system. In: Pizzo PA, Poplack DG, eds. *Principles and Practice of Pediatric Oncology*. 7th ed. Philadelphia, PA: Lippincott Williams & Wilkins; 2015:628–662.

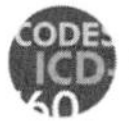

CODES

ICD10

- D49.6 Neoplasm of unspecified behavior of brain
- C71.9 Malignant neoplasm of brain, unspecified
- D33.2 Benign neoplasm of brain, unspecified

FAQ

- Q: Are my other children at risk for getting a brain tumor?
- A: No (except in rare cases of certain familial syndromes).
- Q: Did something I do cause this?
- A: No. In addition, the claims made about high-power lines and cellular phones causing brain tumors or cancer are unproven.

BRANCHIAL CLEFT MALFORMATIONS

Pi Chun Cheng, MD, MS • Anita Bhandari, MD

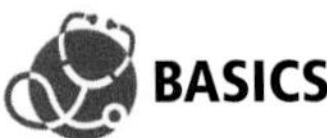

BASICS

DESCRIPTION

- Phylogenetically, the branchial apparatus represents the "gills" seen in fish and amphibians.
- The fetal branchial apparatus is a foregut derivative and develops in the 2nd fetal week.
- Five paired pharyngeal arches are separated by four endodermal pouches internally and four ectodermal clefts externally.
- Overgrowth of the second through fourth cleft creates the cervical sinus and occurs during weeks 4 and 5.
- Persistence of the cervical sinus produces a spectrum of cysts, sinus tracts, and fistulae.
- Classification
  - First branchial cleft anomalies
    - Site: anywhere from external auditory canal to angle of mandible, usually superior to or within parotid
    - Fistula tract: external auditory canal
  - Second branchial cleft anomalies
    - Site: ventral to anterior border of sternocleidomastoid muscle, lateral to carotid sheath, and dorsal to submandibular gland
    - Fistula tract: palatine tonsil
  - Third branchial cleft anomalies
    - Site: posterior triangle in middle to lower left side of the neck near level of upper thyroid lobe
    - Fistula: upper lateral piriform sinus wall to lower lateral neck posterior to sternocleidomastoid muscle
  - Fourth branchial cleft anomalies
    - Site: close association to thyroid gland associated with clinical thyroiditis if cyst infected
    - Fistula: apex of piriform sinus to base of neck anterior to sternocleidomastoid muscle

EPIDEMIOLOGY

- Overwhelming majority of cysts in newborns and infants are developmental, whereas in children and adults, they are inflammatory or neoplastic.
- Branchial cleft cysts are the most common congenital neck lesion. Although congenital, usually present in older children and adults.
- Branchial fistula and sinuses are common in children, but cysts are more commonly seen in adults.
- Midline malformations are most often thyroglossal duct cysts or dermoids.
- Cysts occurring in the laterocervical region are usually branchial cleft malformations; the most common of these are derivatives of the second cleft, followed by those of the first cleft, of the fourth pouch and thymic cysts.
- Third and fourth branchial cleft anomalies are rare, with most presenting as sinus tracts rather than cysts.
- Suspect congenital anomaly in the clinical setting of recurrent infection.

RISK FACTORS

Genetics

Familial history of branchial defects occasionally noted

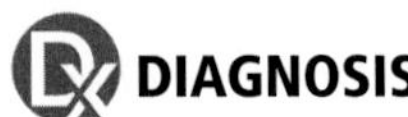

DIAGNOSIS

HISTORY

- Present since birth
- Recurrent neck infections
- Intermittent discharge from neck
- Fever
- Tenderness

PHYSICAL EXAM

- Mass usually mobile
- Usually a single lesion
- Nonpulsatile
- Lesion usually nontender (unless actively infected)
- Assess for sites of drainage:
  - At the anterior or posterior border of the sternocleidomastoid muscle
  - In the posterior pharynx at the tonsillar fossa or piriform sinus

DIFFERENTIAL DIAGNOSIS

- Congenital
  - Anterior triangle of neck
    - Thymic cyst
  - Midline and anterior triangle of neck
    - Ranula
    - Laryngocele
    - Sialocele
    - Thyroglossal cyst
    - Dermoid/teratomatous cyst
    - Bronchogenic cyst
  - Posterior triangle of neck
    - Lymphangioma
    - Hemangioma
- Inflammatory
  - Adenitis
  - Granulomatous disease (sarcoidosis, tuberculosis)
  - Lymphoepithelial cysts (HIV)
  - Otorrhea
  - Parotiditis
  - Retropharyngeal abscess
  - Thyroiditis
- Tumors
  - Lymphoma
  - Rhabdomyosarcoma
  - Cystic schwannoma (anterior triangle of neck)
  - Pilomatrixoma

DIAGNOSTIC TESTS & INTERPRETATION

Initial Tests (screening, lab, imaging)

- Complete blood count with differential: increased white blood cell count with left shift seen with infection
- Tuberculin test and interferon-γ release assays: to rule out mycobacterial infection, including atypical mycobacteria
- Microbiology: Oral cavity flora in neck abscess is suspicious for a branchial pouch anomaly.
- Chest radiography to assess for hilar adenopathy, suggesting a systemic process (such as tuberculosis or malignancy)
- Lateral neck radiography to assess for airway compromise (not usually seen)
- Ultrasound to help differentiate solid masses from cystic masses
- Fistulogram to inject contrast into the fistula to delineate its course
- Computed tomography (CT) scan of neck for superior spatial delineation and definition of anatomic compartment of the lesion
- Magnetic resonance imaging (MRI) for more detailed soft tissue characterization and recognition of solid components within cystic masses. It can also aid in determining the presence and path of sinus formation.
- CT scans and MRI may be used for preoperative planning in patients with recurrent neck masses or clinically complex cases.

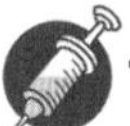

TREATMENT

MEDICATION

Antibiotics are indicated if the lesion is infected.

SURGERY/OTHER PROCEDURES

- Excision of the entire lesion is the standard approach.
- Novel endoscopic and marsupialization approaches have been reported.
- Surgery should be delayed if infection is present.

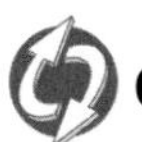

ONGOING CARE

FOLLOW-UP RECOMMENDATIONS

- Postoperative follow-up as outpatient for wound inspection
- Observation for recurrence or reinfection

ALERT

- Lesion may recur if not completely excised.
- High incidence of reinfection if not properly treated

PROGNOSIS

If lesion completely excised: excellent. Many patients require multiple procedures.

COMPLICATIONS

- Cysts, sinus tracts, and fistulas can become recurrently infected (especially with abscess formation).
- Surgery is more difficult if there has been previous infections or previous surgery.
- Damage to facial, hypoglossal, glossopharyngeal, and recurrent laryngeal nerves, internal jugular vein, or carotid artery can occur during surgical repair.
- Cyst, fistula, or sinus recurrence
- Thyroiditis
- Parotiditis (more common in first branchial arch malformation)

ADDITIONAL READING

- Acierno SP, Waldhausen JH. Congenital cervical cysts, sinuses and fistulae. *Otolaryngol Clin North Am*. 2007;40(1):161–176.
- Adams A, Mankad K, Offiah C, et al. Branchial cleft anomalies: a pictorial review of embryological development and spectrum of imaging findings. *Insights Imaging*. 2016;7(1):69–76.
- Brown RE, Harave S. Diagnostic imaging of benign and malignant neck masses in children—a pictorial review. *Quant Imaging Med Surg*. 2016;6(5):591–604.
- Geddes G, Butterly MM, Patel SM, et al. Pediatric neck masses. *Pediatr Rev*. 2013;34(3):115–125.
- Goins MR, Beasley MS. Pediatric neck masses. *Oral Maxillofac Surg Clin North Am*. 2012;24(3):457–468.
- Graham A. Development of the pharyngeal arches. *Am J Mes Genet A*. 2003;119A(3):251–256.
- Mandell DL. Head and neck anomalies related to the branchial apparatus. *Otolaryngol Clin North Am*. 2000;33(6):1309–1332.
- Nicollas R, Guelfucci B, Roman S, et al. Congenital cysts and fistulas of the neck. *Int J Pediatr Otorhinolaryngol*. 2000;55(2):117–124.
- Nicoucar K, Giger R, Jaecklin T, et al. Management of congenital third branchial arch anomalies: a systematic review. *Otolaryngol Head Neck Surg*. 2010;142(1):21–28.e2.
- Nicoucar K, Giger R, Pope HG Jr, et al. Management of congenital fourth branchial arch anomalies: a review and analysis of published cases. *J Pediatr Surg*. 2009;44(7):1432–1439.
- Pahlavan S, Haque W, Pereira K, et al. Microbiology of third and fourth branchial pouch cysts. *Laryngoscope*. 2010;120(3):458–462.
- Prabhu V, Ingrams D. First branchial arch fistula: diagnostic dilemma and improvised surgical management. *Am J Otolaryngol*. 2011;32(6):617–619.

CODES

ICD10

- Q18.2 Other branchial cleft malformations
- Q18.0 Sinus, fistula and cyst of branchial cleft

FAQ

- Q: Can the cyst, fistula, or sinus recur?
- A: Only a 3% recurrence rate is seen if the lesion is completely excised. A higher rate of recurrence is seen in cases of incomplete excision or with previous surgeries.
- Q: Should the lesion be removed as soon as it is discovered?
- A: The lesion should not be removed if there is an active infection present; treat the infection first and then schedule elective surgery.
- Q: What is the likelihood that a pediatric neck mass is malignant?
- A: Most neck masses in childhood are either developmental or inflammatory but up to 15% may be neoplastic.
- Q: What is branchio-oto-renal syndrome (BOR syndrome)?
- A: It is an association of branchial cleft malformations, auricular malformations, deafness, and hypoplastic renal anomalies. BOR syndrome is found in approximately 2–3% of children with profound deafness (prevalence 1/40,000).

BREAST ABSCESS

Charles A. Pohl, MD

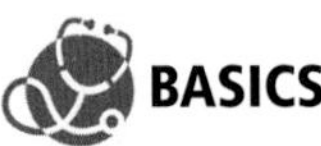

BASICS

DESCRIPTION
- Breast abscess: infection of the breast bud or tissue associated with localized pus and inflammation
- Mastitis: infection of the breast tissue observed primarily during lactation

EPIDEMIOLOGY
- 3–11% of women with breastfeeding mastitis develop a breast abscess.
- Affects primarily infants (peak age 1 to 6 weeks) and adolescents
- Bilateral abscesses, seen among neonates, are rare.
- Male-to-female ratio is 1:2 in neonates.

RISK FACTORS
- In lactating teens, primiparity
- Gestational age >40 weeks
- Mastitis
- Obesity, black race, tobacco use

GENERAL PREVENTION
- Avoid breast manipulation (including piercing).
- In lactating teens, establish good breastfeeding techniques.
- Recognize and treat mastitis early.

PATHOPHYSIOLOGY
- Newborns
  - Trauma, breast hypertrophy from maternal estrogen, or compromised host defenses enable spread of bacteria that often colonize the nasopharynx and umbilicus.
  - The bacteria and/or its toxin, in turn, cause(s) subcutaneous destruction and loculated pus formation.
- Adolescents/adults: Trauma (e.g., sexual manipulation, nipple rings, tight-fitting bras, incorrect latching during breastfeeding), contiguous spread of a local infection (e.g., mastitis, acne), or underlying structural abnormalities (e.g., mammary duct ectasia, epidermal cysts) cause breast tissue edema and destruction by bacteria and/or its toxin.
- When mastitis is associated with breastfeeding, the inflammation inhibits milk release. The stasis of milk, in turn, may allow for bacterial proliferation.

ETIOLOGY
- Newborn infection: *Staphylococcus aureus* (most common), group A or B *Streptococcus*, *Bacteroides* species, and gram-negative enteric bacteria, including *Escherichia coli*, *Pseudomonas aeruginosa*, *Proteus mirabilis*, *Salmonella* species
- Adolescent/adult infection: *S. aureus* (most common) with up to 19% being methicillin-resistant, *E. coli*, *P. aeruginosa*, *Mycobacterium tuberculosis*, *Neisseria gonorrhoeae*, and *Treponema pallidum* are infrequent pathogens.

DIAGNOSIS

HISTORY
- Ask about history of breast trauma or manipulation, concomitant illness or infections, and patient's immunologic status.
- Constitutional symptoms including irritability and lethargy usually are absent unless the infection involves deeper tissue or the bloodstream (1/3 of cases).
- Low-grade fever
- *Salmonella* infections generally present with GI symptoms.

PHYSICAL EXAM
- Firm, tender breast mass with overlying erythema and warmth. Fluctuant mass may be present.
- Regional adenopathy
- Purulent nipple discharge (rare)
- Necrotizing fasciitis is distinguished from breast abscess by pain out of proportion to the cutaneous signs, crepitus, or presence of straw-colored bullae.

DIFFERENTIAL DIAGNOSIS
- Physiologic conditions:
  - Breast engorgement (usually bilateral; absence of fever, erythema, and tenderness)
  - Mastodynia (painful breast engorgement; associated with ovulatory cycles; cyclic pattern)
- Infectious: cellulitis including mastitis (absence of a loculated breast mass)
- Tumors (rare):
  - Fibroadenomas
  - Rhabdomyosarcoma
  - Non-Hodgkin lymphoma
  - Fibrocystic disease
  - Intraductal papilloma
  - Cystosarcoma phyllodes
  - Hemangioma
- Trauma:
  - Contusion (firm, tender, poorly defined mass)
  - Hematoma (sharply defined mass with ecchymosis)
  - Fat necrosis (firm, nontender, circumscribed, mobile mass)
- Miscellaneous: Mondor disease (thrombophlebitis of the subcutaneous veins in the breast)
  - Typically seen in adults
  - Presents with tenderness and pain
  - Associated with trauma
  - Spontaneously resolves
- Vascular malformation

DIAGNOSTIC TESTS & INTERPRETATION

Initial Tests (screening, lab, imaging)
- Gram stain and culture of nipple discharge, needle aspirate, and/or surgical incision and drainage help(s) guide therapeutic decisions if a fluctuant mass or discharge is present.
- Blood culture
  - Useful in neonates
  - Consider full sepsis workup if patient is febrile and toxic appearing or <28 days old.
- CBC: Leukocytosis (>15,000 cells/mm^3) is present in 1/2 to 2/3 of patients.
- CSF: Consider LP in 2 month olds who are ill-appearing, febrile ≥38°C, or abnormal WBC (>15,000 cells/mm^3 or <5,000 cells/mm^3). Surveillance cultures of nasopharynx and umbilicus should be considered in neonates to rule out colonization with *S. aureus*.
- Ultrasound may be useful if fluctuant mass is suspected or if poor response to antimicrobial therapy.

Diagnostic Procedures/Other
If fluctuant, needle biopsy may be diagnostic and therapeutic.

ALERT
- Neonatal infections require prompt recognition, intervention, and identification of other involved sites to avoid widespread infection and poor outcome.
- Unrecognized fluctuant mass and its subsequent drainage will delay therapeutic response.
- Incidence of community-acquired methicillin-resistant *S. aureus* (CA-MRSA) is increasing in many regions of the country.

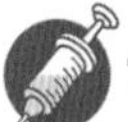

TREATMENT

GENERAL MEASURES

- Warm compresses
- Nonsteroidal anti-inflammatory agents (NSAIDs) help control the inflammation and pain in older children.
- Continuation of breast milk expression helps prevent engorgement and further milk stasis.

MEDICATION

- Neonatal infection (specific dosage interval based on degree of prematurity)
  - Parenteral β-lactamase–resistant antistaphylococcal antibiotics (e.g., nafcillin 75 to 100 mg/kg/24 h)
  - Aminoglycosides (e.g., gentamicin) or 3rd-generation cephalosporin should be included if the infant appears ill or if the Gram stain reveals gram-negative bacilli.
  - Consider vancomycin (40 mg/kg/24 h) if MRSA suspected in neonate >1 month of age.
- Adolescent infection
  - Parenteral antistaphylococcal antibiotics (e.g., nafcillin 50 to 100 mg/kg/24 h; maximum 12 g/24 h)
  - Consider amoxicillin-clavulanic acid orally (45 mg/kg/24 h or 875 mg b.i.d.) or clindamycin (450 to 1,800 mg/24 h orally with max dose 1.8 g/24 h; 1,200 to 1,800 mg/24 h parenterally with max dose 4.8 g/24 h) in patients with penicillin allergies and those who are well-appearing and without systemic symptoms.
  - Consider adding aminoglycosides in situations as described earlier.
  - Consider vancomycin, clindamycin, or trimethoprim-sulfamethoxazole if MRSA suspected. Avoid latter if mother nursing newborn because of risk of hyperbilirubinemia.
- Duration
  - Usually for 10 to 14 days
  - Length of parenteral treatment is based on isolate and the clinical response. Oral agents may be used after a few days if a good clinical response occurs.

ISSUES FOR REFERRAL

Consider referral to an infectious disease specialist if recurrent.

SURGERY/OTHER PROCEDURES

- Incision and drainage if a fluctuant mass is present
- Surgical exploration is necessary if necrotizing fasciitis is suspected.

COMPLEMENTARY & ALTERNATIVE THERAPIES

A specific probiotic strain of *Lactobacillus salivarius* PS2 when given to women during late pregnancy may prevent lactational mastitis.

ADMISSION, INPATIENT, AND NURSING CONSIDERATIONS

Admission criteria

- Ill appearance
- Neonates
- Inability to tolerate oral medications
- Concern for medication nonadherence

ONGOING CARE

FOLLOW-UP RECOMMENDATIONS

Clinical improvement should be evident after 48 hours of parenteral antibiotics.

ALERT

Signs to watch for are the following:

- A poor or delayed clinical response to antibiotic therapy suggests a resistant organism, an unusual pathogen, or a different diagnosis.
- An evolving fluctuant mass warrants surgical intervention.
- Reaccumulation of fluctuant mass
- Toxic appearance, prolonged fever, purulent discharge, or progressive erythema postoperatively
- Crepitus associated with excessive pain and/or straw-colored bullae suggests necrotizing fasciitis.

PATIENT EDUCATION

- Continue breastfeeding.
- Establish good breastfeeding techniques.

PROGNOSIS

- Most children recover without any sequelae.
- Neonates are more likely to have bilateral abscesses (<5% cases).
- Neonates have higher morbidity and complications.

COMPLICATIONS

- Cellulitis (most common; 5–10%)
- Abscess rupture with disseminated infection (e.g., bacteremia, pneumonia)
- Septicemia
- Toxin syndromes (e.g., toxic shock syndrome)
- Necrotizing fasciitis
- Scar formation from mammary gland destruction (associated with a reduced breast size after puberty)
- Mammary duct fistula

ADDITIONAL READING

- Al Ruwaili N, Scolnik D. Neonatal mastitis: controversies in management. *J Clin Neonatol*. 2012;1(4):207–210.
- Barbosa-Cesnik C, Schwartz K, Foxman B. Lactation mastitis. *JAMA*. 2003;289(13):1609–1612.
- Bharat A, Gao F, Aft RL, et al. Predictors of primary breast abscesses and recurrence. *World J Surg*. 2009;33(12):2582–2586.
- Fernández L, Cárdenas N, Arroyo R, et al. Prevention of infectious mastitis by oral administration of *Lactobacillus salivarius* PS2 during late pregnancy. *Clin Infect Dis*. 2016;62(5):568–573.
- Fortunov RM, Hulten KG, Hammerman WA, et al. Community-acquired *Staphylococcus aureus* infections in term and near-term previously healthy neonates. *Pediatrics*. 2006;118(3):874–881.
- Moazzez A, Kelso RL, Towfigh S, et al. Breast abscess bacteriologic features in the era of community-acquired methicillin-resistant *Staphylococcus aureus* epidemics. *Arch Surg*. 2007;142(9):881–884.
- Stricker T, Navratil F, Forster I, et al. Nonpuerperal mastitis in adolescents. *J Pediatr*. 2006;148(2):278–281.

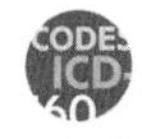

CODES

ICD10

- N61 Inflammatory disorders of breast
- P39.0 Neonatal infective mastitis
- O91.219 Nonpurulent mastitis associated w pregnancy, unsp trimester

FAQ

- Q: How can you differentiate a breast abscess from mastitis?
- A: Although both illnesses involve signs of inflammation (i.e., warmth, erythema, swelling, tenderness), a breast abscess is distinguished from mastitis in that the former presents as a firm, well-defined mass (with or without fluctuant material).
- Q: Should a mother discontinue breastfeeding if she has a breast abscess?
- A: To avoid milk stasis, breastfeeding should be continued unless impeded by a surgical incision site or the overall clinical condition of the mother.
- Q: What is the role of homeopathic remedies (e.g., belladonna, *Phytolacca*) in the treatment of mastitis and breast abscess?
- A: Currently, there is insufficient scientific evidence to support their routine use. A specific probiotic strain of *Lactobacillus salivarius* PS2 when given to women during late pregnancy may prevent lactational mastitis.
- Q: Are anaerobic organisms common pathogens for breast abscesses?
- A: No. Although anaerobic pathogens are isolated in up to 40% of infections, their role is controversial, and therapy directed at them is unnecessary.

BREASTFEEDING

Jennifer A. F. Tender, MD, IBCLC • Sahira A. Long, MD, IBCLC, FABM

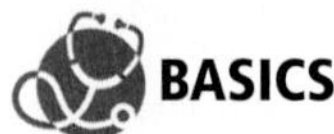

BASICS

DESCRIPTION

- Human milk is recognized as the optimal nutrition for infants by the American Academy of Pediatrics (AAP), the World Health Organization (WHO), the Surgeon General, and all major medical groups.
- Physiology
  - Breast milk production
    - Lactogenesis I: Milk production begins around 16 weeks prenatally.
    - Lactogenesis II: onset of copious milk secretion around 2 to 3 days after vaginal delivery; under hormonal control initiated by the expulsion of placenta and decrease in progesterone levels
    - Lactogenesis III: Mature milk production (maintenance) depends on autocrine (local) control. The amount of milk removed influences milk volume. If milk is not removed, a protein (feedback inhibitor of lactation) accumulates and inhibits prolactin release.
    - Prolactin is released from the anterior pituitary in response to nipple stimulation and triggers milk secretion into the lumen of breast alveoli.
    - Oxytocin is released from the posterior pituitary gland, causing ejection of milk into the breast ducts (milk ejection reflex).
    - Let-down can be triggered by physical stimulation of the breast or by mental stimulation such as hearing a baby cry.
  - Composition
    - Largely independent of maternal diet, except for fatty acids and water-soluble vitamins
    - Colostrum contains high levels of secretory immunoglobulin A for immune protection. Lactoferrin stimulates meconium passage and promotes colonization with protective lactobacillus bifidus.
    - High whey-to-casein ratio
    - Milk changes within a feed and throughout the day. Hindmilk and milk at night contains higher fat and calories.

EPIDEMIOLOGY

Prevalence

- 81% of infants born in the United States in 2013 initiated breastfeeding, according to the Centers for Disease Control and Prevention.
- At 3 months, 44% breastfed exclusively.
- At 6 months, 52% breastfed, 22% exclusively
- At 12 months, 31% breastfed.
- Racial and economic disparities in breastfeeding exist; lower rates in the SE United States among African American women and women living in poverty

RISK FACTORS

- Contraindications to breastfeeding:
  - Infant with classic galactosemia
  - Maternal conditions:
    - HIV (in industrialized countries)
    - Illicit drug use
    - Active, untreated tuberculosis
    - Herpes simplex virus lesions on breast
    - HTLV-I– or HTLV-II–positive
    - Exposure to radioactive material, while there is radioactivity in the milk
    - Use of some medications, such as cytotoxic drugs
- Infant conditions that may interfere with breastfeeding:
  - Prematurity
  - Low birth weight
  - Hypotonia
  - Cleft lip or palate
  - Ankyloglossia (tongue-tie)
- Maternal conditions that may interfere with breastfeeding:
  - History of breast surgery
  - Abnormal breast shape (glandular insufficiency)
  - Inverted nipples
  - Medications that inhibit lactation
  - Endocrine: infertility, hypothyroidism, polycystic ovary, retained placenta, Sheehan syndrome, obesity
- Common reasons cited for early termination of breastfeeding:
  - Perceived insufficient milk supply
  - Poor latch
  - Sore nipples
  - Returning to work or school

DIAGNOSIS

HISTORY

- Experience breastfeeding previous children
- Prior breast surgery
- Breast enlargement during pregnancy
- Frequency and duration of feedings
  - Feed >8 to 12 times a day in the 1st few weeks of life, with no more than 4 hours between feedings.
  - Newborns typically need >8 to 10 minutes of active suckling.
- Signs of adequate milk intake:
  - Adequate hydration: 1 wet diaper for each day of life until more copious milk production around day 4 of life
  - Adequate nutrition: Stool changes from meconium to transitional to yellow seedy by 4th day of life. Infant typically has >3 to 4 yellow stools/24 h in the 1st month. Stool pattern often changes at 1 month, and infant may only stool every 3 to 7 days.
- Infant may lose up to 8% of birth weight until onset of more copious milk production around day 4 or 5.
- Infant should gain 15 to 30 g/24 h and be back to birth weight by 10 to 14 days.
- The WHO growth charts better represent typical growth of breastfed infants.
- Breast/nipple pain: Women may experience discomfort at first, but breastfeeding should not hurt. The most common cause of pain is poor latch. Other causes include candidal infection of the nipple or mastitis.

PHYSICAL EXAM

- Direct observation of a feeding is crucial:
  - Examine the infant's oropharynx for thrush, ankyloglossia, or anatomic abnormalities.
  - Examine the mother's breasts for scars (prior surgery), nipple inversion, erythema (possible candida, mastitis), or cracking (poor latch).
  - Infant feeding cues: Rooting, lip smacking, and sucking are early signs of hunger; crying is a late sign.
  - The mother should be positioned comfortably and not have to bend down.
- Two types of infant positioning:
  - Infant-led: The mother is semireclined in bed with the infant's head at breast height. The infant initiates the latch.
  - Mother-led:
    - Cross-cradle: easy visualization of latch. Mother holds her baby with the arm opposite the breast she is using, holds the back of the baby's neck, and brings the baby to breast height. Her other hand supports and compresses her breast. The infant should be in a straight line with ear, shoulder, and hip aligned.
    - Other positions include cradle, football, and sidelying.
- For an effective latch, the mother touches the infant's nose or upper lip to her nipple and waits until the infant opens wide. She brings the infant to her breast. She may compress her breast with her thumb by the infant's nose parallel to upper lip.
- Evaluating the latch: Lips should be everted and mouth wide open approaching a 180 degrees angle. As much as possible of the areola is in the infant's mouth. More of the areola shows above the infant's mouth than below. The mother's nipple should not be distorted after the infant suckles.
- Signs of good milk transfer: Infant relaxed and breasts less full after nursing, infant has deep movement of the jaw and sucks/swallows/breathes rhythmically, milk visible in infant's mouth

DIAGNOSTIC TESTS & INTERPRETATION

Initial Tests (screening, lab, imaging)

- Total/direct bilirubin level, if clinically indicated
- Electrolytes (especially sodium) in infant, if there is concern for dehydration

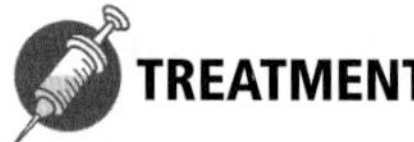

TREATMENT

GENERAL MEASURES

- Cracked nipples should be treated by correcting the latch. Women can apply breast milk or purified lanolin. Keep nipples dry.
- Engorgement can be relieved by frequent and effective feeding or pumping, therapeutic breast massaging, and applying cool compresses.
- Clogged milk ducts may be treated with warm compresses, frequent emptying of the breast, massaging the area, and varying feeding positions.

B

- Pumping may help with inverted nipples. A nipple shield can be tried if inverted nipples cause trouble latching. Prolonged nipple shield use is controversial, as concerns exist regarding their impact on milk supply; thus, their use should be limited to a short period of time (~1 month).
- Mastitis can be treated with antibiotics, frequent and effective feeding, and maternal rest.
- Infants with ankyloglossia that affects latch or impedes milk transfer should be referred for frenotomy.

MEDICATION

- Vitamin D, 400 IU/24 h orally for all infants starting at the first visit if not given at hospital discharge, even if supplementing with formula
- The AAP Section on Breastfeeding recommends starting iron-rich complementary foods at 6 months. Elemental iron at 2 mg/kg/24 h starting by age 1 month is recommended for preterm infants.
- Symptomatic candidal infection of the nipples requires simultaneous treatment of both mother and infant with a topical antifungal agent and thorough washing of all artificial nipples. Treatment options include nystatin or oral fluconazole for resistant cases.
- Most maternal medications are compatible with breastfeeding. Mothers should not breastfeed if using illicit or cytotoxic drugs or radioactive compounds until cleared from the mother's milk. Choose medications with short half-lives, high protein binding, low oral bioavailability, high molecular weight, and low lipid solubility. Refer to databases such as the National Library of Medicine's LactMed.

COMPLEMENTARY & ALTERNATIVE THERAPIES

Herbs traditionally used to try to increase milk supply (galactagogues) include the following:

- Fenugreek (*Trigonella foenum-graecum*): taken as tea or capsules; may be effective; probably safe in moderate doses
- Milk thistle (*Silybum marianum*): usually taken as a tea; no scientifically valid clinical trials support this use.

ADMISSION, INPATIENT, AND NURSING CONSIDERATIONS

If a breastfed infant is hospitalized, encourage continued breastfeeding if possible. If the infant is not able to breastfeed, provide a hospital-grade double electric pump and encourage pumping at least 8 times per day.

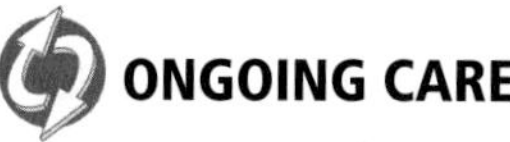

ONGOING CARE

FOLLOW-UP RECOMMENDATIONS

Patient Monitoring

- In general, 2 to 3 days after hospital discharge; weight check, physical exam, and observation of feeding
- Close follow-up 1 to 2 days later if concern about milk intake or jaundice and then as needed
- At age 2 to 3 weeks: weight check and breastfeeding support
- Patient education: Mother should be assisted with latch and positioning and should know signs/symptoms of adequate milk intake (urine output, stooling), dehydration, and illness.

DIET

- For the infant:
  - Except for vitamin D, no food or fluid other than breast milk is needed for the first 6 months of life.
  - After 6 months, iron-rich foods and other complementary foods may be introduced.
- For the mother:
  - ~500 kcal/24 h are used for breastfeeding.
  - Women should avoid breastfeeding for at least 2 hours after alcohol consumption.
  - If infant has G6PD deficiency, mother should avoid fava beans and certain medications.

COMPLICATIONS

- Infant
  - Hyperbilirubinemia
  - Dehydration/hypernatremia
  - Poor weight gain
- Mother
  - Engorgement
  - Clogged milk duct
  - Mastitis
  - Candidal nipple infection
  - Cracked nipples

ADDITIONAL READING

- Academy of Breastfeeding Medicine. The Academy of Breastfeeding Medicine protocols. http://www.bfmed.org/Resources/Protocols.aspx. Accessed March 29, 2018.
- Bartick MC, Schwarz EB, Green BD, et al. Suboptimal breastfeeding in the United States: maternal and pediatric health outcomes and costs. *Matern Child Nutr*. 2017;13(1).
- Centers for Disease Control and Prevention. CDC breastfeeding report card. https://www.cdc.gov/breastfeeding/pdf/2016breastfeedingreportcard.pdf. Accessed March 29, 2018.
- Kramer MS, Kakuma R. Optimal duration of exclusive breastfeeding. *Cochrane Database Syst Rev*. 2009;(1):CD003517.
- LactMed, National Institutes of Health: https://toxnet.nlm.nih.gov/newtoxnet/lactmed.htm
- La Leche League International: www.lalecheleague.org
- Office on Women's Health, U.S. Department of Health and Human Services: www.womenshealth.gov/breastfeeding
- U.S. Department of Health and Human Services. *The Surgeon General's Call to Action to Support Breastfeeding*. Washington, DC: U.S. Department of Health and Human Services, Office of the Surgeon General; 2011. http://www.surgeongeneral.gov/library/calls/breastfeeding/calltoactiontosupportbreastfeeding.pdf. Accessed February 18, 2017.

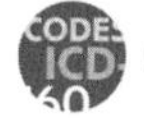

CODES

ICD10

- P92.5 Neonatal difficulty in feeding at breast
- Q38.1 Ankyloglossia
- P92.6 Failure to thrive in newborn

FAQ

- Q: How do I know if my baby is getting enough milk?
- A: Look for signs of effective feeding as described earlier. Your baby should suck deeply and rhythmically during a feeding, seem satisfied after a feeding, and gain approximately 15 to 30 g/24 h. A baby's elimination pattern may be variable, but, in general, most adequately breastfed infants will have 3 or more stools a day by 4 days of life.
- Q: How do I alleviate nipple pain associated with nursing?
- A: Most pain is due to poor latch. Ensure deep latch. Compress the breast and make sure the baby takes as much of the areola as possible. If stinging occurs throughout nursing, consider candidal infection. Seek advice from a lactation expert if pain does not improve.
- Q: How can I increase my milk supply?
- A: Increase frequency and effectiveness of feeding or pumping. Place infant skin to skin. Pump after nursing sessions. If pumping often, use a hospital-grade double pump. Get plenty of sleep and try to reduce stress.
- Q: How long can expressed breast milk be stored safely (applies to term infants only)?
- A: At room temperature (up to 77°F) for 3 to 6 hours. In the back of a refrigerator for 3 (ideal) to 8 days if very clean container. For 6 to 12 months if in the freezer. Thawed breast milk should be refrigerated and used within 24 hours of thawing.
- Q: How long should breastfeeding be continued?
- A: The AAP recommends breastfeeding at least until 12 months of age and as long afterward as is mutually desired. The WHO recommends breastfeeding for at least 2 years. Exclusive breastfeeding is nutritionally adequate for the first 6 months.
- Q: Can adoptive mothers breastfeed?
- A: Induced lactation is possible. Lactation experts should be consulted.
- Q: What are the risks of *not* breastfeeding?
- A: There are potential risks and consequences associated with a lack of breastfeeding at several levels.
  - For child: increases risk of postneonatal death; gastroenteritis, necrotizing enterocolitis, lower respiratory infections requiring hospitalization, acute otitis media, bacterial meningitis, obesity, sudden infant death syndrome (SIDS), acute lymphoblastic leukemia, and inflammatory bowel disease
  - For mother: increases risk of ovarian and premenopausal breast cancer, diabetes, hypertension, myocardial infarction, and postpartum hemorrhage. Loss of benefit of lactational amenorrhea and child spacing
  - For family: increased expenditures, more workdays lost to care for ill child
  - For society: increases environmental impact and costs $18.5 billion annually (in 2014 dollars) for medical, nonmedical, and premature deaths due to an increase in childhood and maternal diseases

BREATH-HOLDING SPELLS

Nailah Coleman, MD, FAAP, FACSM

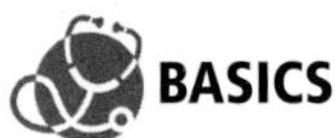

BASICS

DESCRIPTION

- Breath-holding spells are the general term for emotionally provoked attacks that occur in young children. These attacks can progress from a strong emotion to "breath holding" to decreased sensorium and either limpness or stiffness, which can appear as seizure-like activity.
- Disease essentials
  - Provoked by anger, pain, or frustration
  - Association with altered respiratory effort
  - Results in decreased muscle tone
  - Can be classified as simple (brief, no loss of consciousness) or severe (prolonged, associated loss of consciousness)
- Subtypes
  - Cyanotic (80%)
    - Classic breath-holding spells
    - Typically associated with anger
    - Progress from crying to exhalation to apnea and syncope to decreased muscle tone and falling
    - May also note generalized clonic jerks, opisthotonos, and bradycardia
    - Ages: 6 months to a peak at 2 years, with resolution by 5 years
  - Pallid (20%)
    - Typically associated with pain, frustration, or surprise
    - Progress from quieting to apnea (at the end of expiration) to syncope to decreased muscle tone and falling
    - May also note clenched hands and clonic jerks and bradycardia

EPIDEMIOLOGY

- Incidence: not reported
- Prevalence: 4.6% (severe), up to 27% (simple)
- No gender difference
- 20–35% have a positive family history
- Age/frequency
  - Median age of onset 6 to 12 months of age
  - Typically ages 1 to 5 years but can occur up to 7 years of age
  - Usually resolve by school age
  - Frequency
    - Can occur several times per day to only once a year
    - Age of peak frequency of spells is from 1 to 2 years of age.

RISK FACTORS

- Underlying autonomic regulatory dysfunction
- Inheritance
  - 20–35% of patients with breath-holding spells have a positive family history.
  - 11% of patients with epilepsy or other chronic, but nonneurologic disorder have a positive family history of breath-holding spells.
  - For 80% of patients with severe spells and a positive family history, the affected family members are mainly on the maternal side.
  - An autosomal dominant trait with reduced penetrance has been noted in some.

GENERAL PREVENTION

- There are no known methods, medications, or treatments for preventing breath-holding spells.
- Although the term breath-holding spells implies volition, these attacks are involuntary and reflexive.
- For a variety of reasons, emotional outbursts are common in this age group; however, appeasing a child to prevent a spell is not recommended as it may lead the child to develop other, similar-appearing behaviors encouraging parental concession.

PATHOPHYSIOLOGY

- Cyanotic breath-holding spells
  - Syncope due to a Valsalva maneuver increasing the intrathoracic pressure, decreasing cardiac blood return and eventually cardiac output, which causes cerebral hypoperfusion and unconsciousness
- Pallid breath-holding spells
  - Abnormal vagal response to emotional stimulation causing bradycardia and/or asystole, leading to decreased cardiac output and cerebral ischemia and unconsciousness

ETIOLOGY

Always provoked by anger, pain, or frustration

COMMONLY ASSOCIATED CONDITIONS

- No definitive associated conditions
- There have been reports of some children with breath-holding spells going on to have syncope and/or seizures.
- Anemia:
  - Some studies have noted an increased prevalence of anemia in children with breath-holding spells; the anemia and spells improved over time with iron treatment.
  - Although these findings also coincide with the expected timing for resolution of breath-holding spells, anemia might complicate an individual child's picture.
  - The suggested mechanisms for iron deficiency associated with breath-holding spells include lowered oxygen levels in the central nervous system, catecholamine disruption, and increased crying/fussiness (known trigger) with iron deficiency.
- New research has found an association between the frequency of breath-holding spells and the frequency of respiratory sinus arrhythmia.
- There is an increased risk of vasovagal syncope in adolescents and adults, who had pallid breath-holding spells as children.

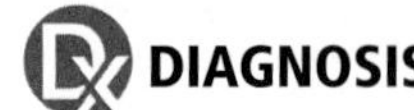

DIAGNOSIS

HISTORY

Important to elicit history of

- Provocation by anger, pain, or frustration
- Altered respiratory effort, decreased responsiveness, and altered muscle tone (either limpness or stiffness)
- Lack of trauma
- Not volitional

PHYSICAL EXAM

- Vital signs: normal on exam; perform orthostatic blood pressures.
- Focal findings: none, normal cardiac, and neurologic exams

DIFFERENTIAL DIAGNOSIS

- Syncope: not usually preceded by crying; altered muscle tone typically accompanied by efforts to prevent falling
  - Neurocardiogenic (vasovagal syncope, fainting)
    - Associated with bradycardia, vasodepression, and/or hypotension leading to decreased cerebral perfusion
    - More common in adolescents
  - Cardiac
    - Dysrhythmias
      - Prolonged QT syndrome
      - Wolff-Parkinson-White syndrome
      - Complete heart block
    - Structural
      - Hypertrophic cardiomyopathy
      - Severe pulmonary or aortic stenosis
      - Coronary artery aneurysm
      - Anomalous origin of the left coronary artery
      - Pulmonary hypertension
      - Myxoma
  - Orthostatic
  - Neuropsychiatric
    - Panic attacks or hyperventilation syndrome
    - Benign paroxysmal vertigo
    - Cataplexy
    - Hysterical syncope
  - Cough
    - Most common in asthmatics
    - Increased intrapleural pressure from coughing leads to decreased venous return and eventually decreased cardiac output and cerebral perfusion
  - Metabolic: hypoglycemia
- Epilepsy or epilepsy equivalent: altered muscle tone precedes color change; abnormal EEG
- Central or obstructive apnea: not typically associated with crying; abnormal sleep study
- Brainstem pathology such as tumor or malformation: other abnormal findings on history and exam
- Familial dysautonomia: other abnormal findings on history and exam
- Rett syndrome: other abnormal findings on history and exam

DIAGNOSTIC TESTS & INTERPRETATION

Initial Tests (screening, lab, imaging)

- If anemia is of concern, CBC should be obtained.
- If hypoglycemia is high on differential acutely, plasma glucose should be obtained.
- No specific imaging is necessary to diagnosis breath-holding spells. However, if trauma, brain pathology, or abnormal cardiac morphology is suspected, the following imaging could be obtained:
  - Head CT
  - Brain MRI
  - Cardiac echocardiogram (EKG)
  - Cardiac MRI
  - Chest x-ray: Evaluate lung hyperinflation in asthmatics (not needed for diagnosis).

Diagnostic Procedures/Other

- For evaluation of potential dysrhythmias, consider the following:
  - EKG
  - Holter monitor
  - Electrophysiology study
  - Stress test
- For evaluation of epilepsy or other neuroelectric disorder, consider an EEG.
- For evaluation of apnea, consider a sleep study.

TREATMENT

GENERAL MEASURES

Reassurance is the primary treatment.

MEDICATION

- No medication has been found to be definitively useful in preventing or treating breath-holding spells.
- It is important to note that breath-holding spells can occur in the presence of other conditions that can present with syncope and seizure-like activity. Should those conditions be present or suspected, additional treatments may be necessary.
- Multiple studies have evaluated the use of various medications to prevent and/or treat breath-holding spells. However, they are limited by inadequate sample size, power, and/or statistical significance.
  - Iron therapy may be useful in breath-holding spells, particularly in children found to be anemic and/or iron deficient; however, benefits have been seen in children without anemia.
  - Atropine and pacemakers have been used for those with severe bradycardia to good effect.
  - Fluoxetine was noted to improve pallid breath-holding spells in another small study.
  - Piracetam has been shown to decrease breath-holding spell severity; however, it still lacks approval from the United States Food and Drug Administration (FDA) for this indication.

ISSUES FOR REFERRAL

Referral is not necessary unless diagnoses on the differential could not be excluded or if the spells do not conform to the normal pattern and/or the normal age range.

ADDITIONAL THERAPIES

- Should loss of consciousness occur with a breath-holding spell, it is important to place the child on his or her side and ensure a clear airway.
- With the potential for altered muscle tone and additional injury, parents should ensure the environment around the child is safe.

ADMISSION, INPATIENT, AND NURSING CONSIDERATIONS

- Inpatient hospital admission for breath-holding spells is not necessary as they are a benign condition. However, if other diagnoses are being considered, if the patient required resuscitation, or if the patient requires ongoing support, an inpatient hospital admission and medical evaluation is warranted.
- Should an inpatient admission be warranted, other diagnoses should be considered and evaluated.

ONGOING CARE

PATIENT EDUCATION

The primary goal for ongoing care is parental education as to the natural history of breath-holding spells.

PROGNOSIS

- As they are a benign condition, isolated breath-holding spells have an excellent prognosis without sequelae.
- Breath-holding spells typically resolve by school age.
- Should breath-holding spells not follow the typical course or time frame, additional diagnoses should be considered (could impact the prognosis).

COMPLICATIONS

Although some have postulated the potential for the development of syncope, epilepsy, and neurodevelopmental disorders, no definitive associations have been found.

ADDITIONAL READING

- Azab SF, Siam AG, Saleh SH, et al. Novel findings in breath-holding spells: a cross-sectional study. *Medicine (Baltimore)*. 2015;94(28):e1150.
- DiMario FJ Jr. Prospective study of children with cyanotic and pallid breath-holding spells. *Pediatrics*. 2001;107(2):265–269.
- Lombroso CT, Lerman P. Breathholding spells (cyanotic and pallid infantile syncope). *Pediatrics*. 1967;39(4):563–581.
- Mocan H, Yildiran A, Orhan F, et al. Breath holding spells in 91 children and response to treatment with iron. *Arch Dis Child*. 1999;81(3):261–262.
- Narchi H. The child who passes out. *Pediatr Rev*. 2000;21(11):384–388.
- Singh P, Seth A. Breath holding spells—a tale of 50 years. *Indian Pediatr*. 2015;52(8):695–696.
- Walsh M, Knilans TK, Anderson JB, et al. Successful treatment of pallid breath-holding spells with fluoxetine. *Pediatrics*. 2012;130(3):e685–e689.
- Yilmaz U, Doksoz O, Celik T, et al. The value of neurologic and cardiologic assessment in breath holding spells. *Pak J Med Sci*. 2014;30(1):59–64.

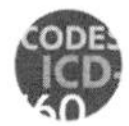

CODES

ICD10

R06.89 Other abnormalities of breathing

FAQ

- Q: What is the age range of the typical child with breath-holding spells?
- A: The typical age range of the child with breath-holding spells is 1 to 5 years of age.
- Q: What is the typical provocation and pathophysiology of the most common type of breath-holding spells?
- A: The most common breath-holding spells are cyanotic (80%). These are typically provoked by anger, which leads to crying, a Valsalva maneuver, decreased cardiac return, decreased cardiac output, decreased cerebral perfusion, and syncope.
- Q: Is there a genetic basis for breath-holding spells?
- A: An autosomal dominant trait has been found in some patients with breath-holding spells.
- Q: What are the common diagnostic tools used to diagnose breath-holding spells?
- A: Breath-holding spells are diagnosed primarily by obtaining a good history and performing a physical exam, the latter of which should be normal. Additional diagnostic tools should only be used if a separate diagnosis is being considered due to unusual history or abnormal physical exam findings.
- Q: How are breath-holding spells managed and prevented?
- A: Breath-holding spells require reassurance provided to the family about acute management and their natural history. At this time, there is no way to prevent breath-holding spells.

BRIEF RESOLVED UNEXPLAINED EVENT (APPARENT LIFE-THREATENING EVENT)

Craig C. DeWolfe, MD, MEd

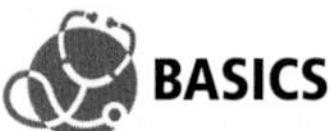

BASICS

DESCRIPTION

- Brief resolved unexplained event (BRUE) is a term suggested by the American Academy of Pediatrics (AAP) to replace the term apparent life-threatening event (ALTE).
- BRUE is a resolved episode in an infant <1 year of age that was sudden, brief, and characterized by any of the following:
  - Absent, decreased, or irregular breathing
  - Cyanosis or pallor
  - Marked change in muscle tone (hyper- or hypotonia)
  - Altered responsiveness
- ALTE was originally described in 1986.
  - It disassociated apnea, color change, change in tone, choking or gagging with sudden infant death syndrome (SIDS), and triggered a research agenda for managing these patients.
  - It was faulted for including diagnoses such as choking or gagging, including actively symptomatic patients, and labeling an event as "life-threatening" without clear justification.
- BRUE, by contrast, is used to describe a well-appearing patient with an event and symptoms that have resolved by the time of presentation to a medical practitioner.
  - Identifies low risk for recurrence or a serious underlying disorder based on:
    - Age >60 days
    - Born ≥32 weeks' gestation and have corrected age ≥45 weeks
    - No CPR performed by trained medical provider
    - Event lasting <1 minute
    - First event
  - Offers management recommendations for lower risk patients

EPIDEMIOLOGY

- 43% of healthy term infants have at least one 20-second apneic episode over a 3-month period.
- 5.3% of parents recall seeing apnea.
- 0.2–0.9% of infants have an episode of apnea that results in an admission to the hospital.

RISK FACTORS

A greater risk for a future adverse event and/or serious underlying diagnosis is conferred by:

- Prematurity and <45 weeks postconceptual age
- Age ≤60 days
- Multiple events
- Events lasting >1 minute
- CPR by trained medical provider
- Suspected child maltreatment

PATHOPHYSIOLOGY

No unifying pathophysiology because of the numerous potential presentations and underlying diagnoses

- Central apnea: disrupted propagation of respiratory signals from the brainstem along the descending neuromuscular pathways. Example diagnoses with similar presentations include:
  - Apnea of prematurity
  - Congenital central hypoventilation syndrome
- Obstructive apnea: neuromuscular respiratory effort disrupted by an occluded airway. Example diagnoses with similar presentations include:
  - Obstructive sleep apnea
  - Pierre Robin
- Mixed apnea: combination of central and obstructive apnea. Example diagnoses with similar presentations include:
  - Laryngomalacia with a sedating ingestion
  - Prematurity with superimposed upper respiratory viral infection
- Color change from decreased oxygenation or differential blood flow. Example diagnoses with similar presentations include:
  - Cyanotic heart disease
  - Acrocyanosis
- Altered muscle tone from central or autonomic nervous system disruption. Examples include:
  - Seizure
  - Breath-holding spell
- Altered responsiveness from effects on the cerebral hemispheres and/or reticular activating system. Example diagnoses with similar presentations include:
  - Toxic ingestion
  - Traumatic brain injury

ETIOLOGY

By definition, a BRUE is unexplained. ALTE could have had multiple different etiologies or be labeled as idiopathic.

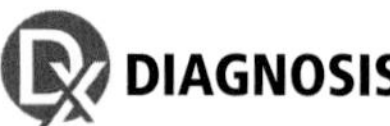

DIAGNOSIS

ALERT

The practitioner should attempt to identify key symptoms and persisting physical exam findings to focus the workup and pursue an underlying diagnosis.

HISTORY

A description of the event by a witness should explore the following features:

- Presence of apnea
  - Type suggests different causes.
    - Obstructive symptoms
    - Central symptoms
  - Duration may suggest severity: <20-second central apnea is physiologic if not associated with other symptoms such as cyanosis.
- Presence of color change and distribution
  - Perioral and peripheral cyanosis alone are not suggestive of hypoxia.
  - Central cyanosis is indicated by blue/purple discoloration of face, lips, or core body and suggests hypoxia.
- Change in tone, rhythmic shaking, and/or eye deviation may suggest a seizure.
- Ability to see the witness or respond to voice may suggest loss of consciousness.
- Relationship to feeds and/or milk in the mouth may suggest aspiration.
- Fatigue or diaphoresis with feeds may suggest a cardiac condition.
- Coryza may suggest an upper or lower respiratory infection.
- Fever may suggest an infectious etiology.
- History of trauma may suggest an intracranial bleed.
- State of alertness prior to ALTE may suggest sleep apnea.
- Changing versions of the history, discrepancies among witnesses, bleeding, and/or features inconsistent with the infant's developmental stage may suggest nonaccidental trauma.
- Type of resuscitation needed may provide a sense of severity or an opportunity for anticipatory guidance.
- Current condition of child and/or time required to reach baseline: may suggest an ongoing, evolving condition and/or postictal period
- Location of event, position of child (i.e., supine/prone), and objects nearby could suggest suffocation or choking.
- Medications dosed or taken by a breastfeeding mother
- Prematurity
- Prior history of ALTE/BRUE
- Family history of ALTE/BRUE, SIDS, arrhythmia, or sudden unexpected death in family members <35 years
- Social history including exposure to smoke, drugs, or previous involvement with Child Protective Services

PHYSICAL EXAM

- Ongoing abnormal symptoms may suggest an evolving and/or underlying condition and should not be labeled a BRUE.
  - Arousal
  - Vital signs
  - Signs of trauma
    - Irritability
    - Full fontanelle
    - Pupil reactivity, conjunctival/retinal hemorrhage
    - Bruising or bleeding
  - Craniofacial abnormalities
  - Persisting signs of disordered breathing
  - Heart rhythm/murmurs
  - Neurologic exam
- Consider observing a feeding.

ALERT

Recurrent ALTEs; historical discrepancies; a family history of ALTE, SIDS, or unexplained death; parents calling emergency services; unexplained facial bruising or bleeding; and the presence or irritability at the time of presentation would warrant a thorough assessment for possible child maltreatment.

DIFFERENTIAL DIAGNOSIS

Estimated frequency of the involved system given as a percentage of patients presenting with ALTE

- Gastrointestinal: 34%
  - Colic
  - Dysphagia
  - Esophageal dysfunction
  - Gastroenteritis
  - Gastroesophageal reflux (GER)
  - Surgical abdomen
- Neurologic: 17%
  - Apnea of prematurity
  - Brain tumor
  - Central hypoventilation syndrome (Ondine curse)
  - Congenital malformation of the brainstem

- Head injury (intraventricular hemorrhage, subarachnoid hemorrhage)
- Hydrocephalus
- Meningitis/encephalitis
- Neuromuscular disorders
- Seizure
- Vasovagal reaction

- Respiratory: 11%
  - Aspiration pneumonia
  - Foreign body
  - Other lower or upper respiratory tract infection
  - Reactive airway disease
  - Respiratory syncytial virus
  - Pertussis
- Otolaryngologic: 4%
  - Laryngomalacia or tracheomalacia
  - Anatomic airway stenosis or obstruction
  - Obstructive sleep apnea
- Child maltreatment syndrome: 1–2%
  - Intentional suffocation
  - Munchausen syndrome by proxy
  - Shaken baby syndrome
  - Head injury
  - Ingestion
- Cardiovascular: 1%
  - Cardiac arrhythmia/prolonged QTc
  - Cardiomyopathy
  - Congenital heart disease
  - Myocarditis
- Metabolic/endocrine: 1%
  - Electrolyte disturbance
  - Hypoglycemia
  - Inborn error of metabolism
- Other infections: 2%
  - Sepsis
  - Urinary tract infections
- Other: 6%
  - Anemia
  - Breath-holding spell
  - Choking
  - Drug or toxin reaction
  - Hypothermia
  - Physiologic event (periodic breathing, acrocyanosis)
  - Unintentional smothering
- Idiopathic/apnea of infancy: 23%

DIAGNOSTIC TESTS & INTERPRETATION

- Routine testing is unlikely to be helpful in patients who are well-appearing and have no other findings suggestive of a particular diagnosis.
- In addition to discomfort, inconvenience, risk, and costs of various tests, an indiscriminate number of screening tests may affect the reliability of the results and initiate an inappropriate and unnecessary testing cascade.

Initial Tests (screening, lab, imaging)

In patients meeting criteria for a "lower risk" BRUE, the following diagnostic recommendations have been offered.

- May obtain:
  - Pertussis testing
- Need not obtain:
  - Bicarbonate
  - CBC
  - Glucose
  - Lactate
  - Urinalysis
  - Viral respiratory studies
  - Neuroimaging
- Should not obtain:
  - Ammonia
  - Blood culture
  - Blood gas
  - CSF studies nor culture
  - Electrolytes
  - Inborn error of metabolism testing
  - Chest x-ray
  - GER testing

Follow-Up Tests & Special Considerations

In patients meeting criteria for a "lower risk" BRUE, the following diagnostic recommendations have been offered.

- May obtain:
  - 12-lead electrocardiography
- Should not obtain:
  - Echocardiogram
  - Electroencephalogram
  - Overnight polysomnogram

TREATMENT

ADMISSION, INPATIENT, AND NURSING CONSIDERATIONS

Hospital admission is not necessary in the patient with a "lower risk" BRUE. In patients with a "higher risk" BRUE, a period of observation on a cardiorespiratory monitor with pulse oximetry is typically warranted. Patients presenting with continued signs and symptoms should be managed according to the working differential diagnosis and risk.

ONGOING CARE

- All patients should be offered the following anticipatory guidance: safe sleep practices and other SIDS prevention techniques
- CPR overview and resources

FOLLOW-UP RECOMMENDATIONS

Return to medical attention for routine follow-up within 24 hours or sooner for recurrence.

PROGNOSIS

Studies on morbidity and mortality are generally incomplete and often contradictory. Differences in reported prognoses from such studies may reflect differences in study design (e.g., patient inclusion criteria, definitions, and follow-up periods, etc.).

- Studies report mortality between 0% and 6%.
- Insufficient data to quantify risk of subsequent event or underlying diagnosis in the higher risk BRUE
- No developmental repercussions among patients who are discharged without a serious underlying diagnosis and have no subsequent events

ADDITIONAL READING

- DeWolfe CC. Apparent life-threatening event: a review. *Pediatr Clin North Am*. 2005;52(4):1127–1146.
- National Institutes of Health Consensus Development Conference on Infantile Apnea and Home Monitoring, Sept 29 to Oct 1, 1986. *Pediatrics*. 1987;79(2):292–299.
- Ramanathan R, Corwin MJ, Hunt CE, et al; for The Collaborative Home Infant Monitoring Evaluation. Cardiorespiratory events recorded on home monitors: comparison of healthy infants with those at increased risk for SIDS. *JAMA*. 2001;285(17):2199–2207.
- Tieder JS, Altman RL, Bonkowsky JL, et al. Management of apparent life-threatening events in infants: a systematic review. *J Pediatr*. 2013;163(1):94–99.e6.
- Tieder JS, Bonkowsky JL, Etzel RA, et al. Brief resolved unexplained events (formerly apparent life-threatening events) and evaluation of lower-risk infants: executive summary. *Pediatrics*. 2016;137(5):e20160591.

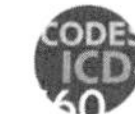

CODES

ICD10

- R68.13 Apparent life threatening event in infant (ALTE)
- P28.4 Other apnea of newborn
- R23.0 Cyanosis

FAQ

- Q: How should patients with "higher risk" BRUE be managed?
- A: No testing recommendations are offered, although indiscriminate testing is discouraged. Admission for a brief period of cardiorespiratory monitoring with pulse oximetry (typically for at least 24 hours after the last event) is recommended to monitor for evolving symptomatology, clustering, and a targeted workup.
- Q: Why aren't there established guidelines with respect to the evaluation and management of patients presenting with higher risk BRUE?
- A: No study has compared diagnostic or treatment strategies among first presenters with a sample size large enough to detect rare events in a prospective fashion.
- Q: What is the relationship between ALTE and SIDS?
- A: There is no established relationship between ALTE and SIDS. The use of the terms "near-miss SIDS" and "aborted crib death" are discouraged. 4–13% of patients diagnosed with SIDS had a preceding history of apnea, a percentage only slightly higher than healthy controls. The "Back to Sleep" campaign, which has dramatically decreased the SIDS rate, has had no effect on ALTE presentations.
- Q: What is the role of home monitoring in ALTE?
- A: Home monitors are not efficacious in preventing mortality among patients with ALTE. In fact, there is evidence that caregivers may have increased anxiety, depression, and hostility, whereas patients may have worse developmental consequences. The AAP suggests that home monitors may have a role in certain situations such as a known unstable airway, abnormal respiratory control, or symptomatic and technologically dependent chronic lung disease.

BRONCHIOLITIS (SEE ALSO: RESPIRATORY SYNCYTIAL VIRUS)

Matthew R. Schefft, DO, MSHA • Alan R. Schroeder, MD

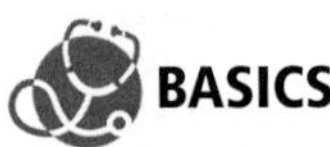

BASICS

DESCRIPTION

Acute infection of the lower respiratory tract in infants and young children leading to mononuclear infiltration of the bronchiolar epithelium, causing edema and mucus plugging of the small airways

EPIDEMIOLOGY

- Peak season is November through April, with some variation by state in the United States (begins earlier in the Southeast).
- Most common cause of infant hospitalization
  - ~150,000 hospitalizations per year in the United States
  - Hospitalization rates tripled from 1980 to 1997 with the advent of pulse oximetry but have decreased slightly over the last decade.
- Most recent estimate ~15 hospitalizations per 1,000 person-years for children <2 years of age
- Approximately 1/3 of all children will get bronchiolitis in the first 2 years of life.

GENERAL PREVENTION

- Hand hygiene is the only preventative measure for otherwise healthy infants and children.
- Palivizumab can be given to high-risk infants and young children (see "Respiratory Syncytial Virus" [RSV] section for discussion of RSV immunoprophylaxis).

ETIOLOGY

- RSV is the most common causative organism, but other organisms include the following:
  - Human rhinovirus
  - Adenovirus
  - Human metapneumovirus
  - Enterovirus
  - Coronaviruses
  - Influenza viruses
  - Parainfluenza viruses
  - *Mycoplasma pneumoniae*
  - *Human bocavirus*
- Majority of bronchiolitis cases are caused by one virus, but viral coinfections (two or more viruses) may occur in ~1/4 of cases.

RISK FACTORS

- Patients at high risk of severe bronchiolitis:
  - Premature infants (<36 weeks' gestation)
  - Young infants (<2 to 3 months of age)
  - Congenital heart disease
  - Chronic lung disease (including bronchopulmonary dysplasia [BPD])
  - Low birth weight
  - Cystic fibrosis
  - Immunodeficiency
  - Neuromuscular diseases
  - Trisomy 21
- Exposure to cigarette smoke is a risk factor for more severe disease.

DIAGNOSIS

HISTORY

- Generally begins as an upper respiratory infection with rhinorrhea but spreads to lower respiratory tract within 2 to 3 days
- Often multiple sick contacts in household
- Variable timing of symptoms. The unpredictability of the time course of the disease may be partly explained by viral coinfections.
- Poor feeding and increased insensible water loss may lead to dehydration and decreased urine output.
- Fever in approximately 50% of patients
- Restlessness or lethargy may indicate impending respiratory failure (hypoxemia and/or CO_2 retention).
- Apnea can be sole presenting sign in younger infants. Apnea is more common in infants who are younger (particularly <2 weeks), lower birth weight, and born prematurely.

PHYSICAL EXAM

- General appearance
  - Interactive versus ill-appearing
  - Paroxysmal cough common
- HEENT exam
  - Nasal congestion with copious secretions
  - Otitis media is common.
- Pulmonary exam
  - Pattern of breathing: apnea or periodic breathing
  - Tachypnea: >70 breaths/minute is associated with severe illness.
  - Grunting, nasal flaring, and accessory muscle use (supracostal, intercostal, subcostal retractions) are signs of more severe disease.
  - Thoracoabdominal asynchrony ("abdominal breathing")
  - Hyperresonance to percussion
  - On auscultation: diffuse, high-pitched heterophonic wheezing; prolonged expiratory phase; inspiratory crackles; diffuse rhonchi
  - Lung exam can change rapidly.
- Other findings:
  - Signs of dehydration (sunken fontanelle, dry mucus membranes, poor skin turgor)
  - Poor peripheral perfusion (delayed capillary refill time, cool extremities, weak peripheral pulses, mottling of skin) is a concerning sign.
  - Liver and spleen often caudally displaced by hyperinflated lungs.

DIFFERENTIAL DIAGNOSIS

- Pneumonia (viral or bacterial)
- Foreign body aspiration
- Asthma
- Gastroesophageal reflux disease (GERD)
- Pulmonary edema (e.g., congestive heart failure)
- Cystic fibrosis
- Airway abnormalities (tracheomalacia, bronchomalacia, vascular ring)

DIAGNOSTIC TESTS & INTERPRETATION

- The majority of bronchiolitis cases do not warrant any laboratory investigation.
- Blood gas
  - In severe cases, can help determine acid–base status and effectiveness of ventilation; however, decisions to escalate support can generally be based on clinical assessment.
  - Arterial Po_2 generally does not add much information beyond that provided by a pulse oximeter.
- CBC +/− differential:
  - low yield; bandemia common
- Serum electrolytes:
  - Also low yield, but on occasion, may assist with assessment of hydration (BUN, creatinine), and hyponatremia rarely occurs due to antidiuretic hormone release.
- Viral testing
  - Rarely changes management
  - Some hospitals require it for cohorting but can be misleading given the broad number of potentially causative viruses and the high frequency of viral coinfections.
  - Best obtained by nasopharyngeal aspirate; can also be obtained by nasal swab
  - Viral cultures are accurate but may take up to 14 days for results.
- Chest radiography is of little value in the majority of bronchiolitis cases, and multiple recent efforts have attempted to limit unnecessary radiographic testing.
- When obtained, findings may include the following:
  - Hyperinflation, flattened diaphragms
  - Peribronchial thickening
  - Patchy or more extensive atelectasis
  - Possible collapse of a segment or a lobe
  - Diffusely increased interstitial markings are common.

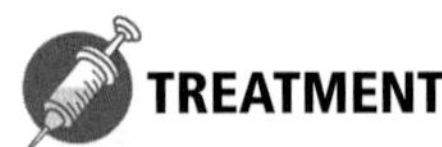

TREATMENT

GENERAL MEASURES

- There is substantial variation in the use of diagnostic testing, hospitalization, and treatments, but bronchiolitis is a self-limited condition that generally improves without intervention.
- Most cases are mild and may be managed at home.
  - Ensure adequate fluid intake.
  - Antipyretics may be used for comfort.
  - For rhinorrhea, nasal suction with bulb syringe may be of use particularly prior to feeding.
  - Home oxygen use is an alternative and has been shown to successfully and safely reduce hospital admission rates from the emergency department (ED) and to shorten length of stay in hospitalized patients.
- The following medications/therapies are of *no* proven benefit in bronchiolitis and should be avoided:
  - Corticosteroids (systemic or inhaled)
  - Ipratropium bromide
  - Leukotriene modifiers
  - Magnesium sulfate

B

ADMISSION, INPATIENT, AND NURSING CONSIDERATIONS

- Common indications for hospitalization include the following:
  - Need for nonoral hydration
  - Need for frequent suctioning
  - Moderate to severe distress (respiratory rate >60 to 70 breaths/minute, accessory muscle use, agitation, cyanosis, poor perfusion)
  - Apnea
- Monitoring
  - Intermittent measurement of vital signs is generally safe for patients.
  - Pulse oximetry
    - Intermittent pulse oximetry is preferred in infants who are not requiring oxygen.
    - Continuous pulse oximetry can be useful as a monitoring device in order to titrate oxygen therapy, but it may also prolong length of stay by contributing to overdiagnosis of hypoxemia (i.e., transient desaturations in otherwise comfortable infants).
    - Additionally, overreliance on pulse oximetry in the ED setting may drive hospital admission rates.
- Supplemental oxygen
  - Although hypoxemia is often used as an indication for hospitalization, exact oxygen saturation thresholds are uncertain. The American Academy of Pediatrics (AAP) suggests using supplemental oxygen for saturations <90%, and this threshold has been associated with a shorter length of stay and duration of oxygen use than a threshold of 94%, with equivalent safety profiles for both thresholds.
  - Can be given humidified via nasal cannula, high-flow nasal cannula, face mask cannula, noninvasive positive pressure ventilation, or via endotracheal tube
  - Should be titrated based on oxygen saturations, and choice of oxygen delivery modality should be based on respiratory distress
- Hydration
  - IV crystalloid boluses of 10 to 20 mL/kg should be given to infants with signs of poor perfusion.
  - For infants who are unable to maintain adequate PO intake, hydration can be maintained with nasogastric feeds or maintenance IV fluids. Because of the risk of hyponatremia, hypotonic fluids should be avoided.
- Suctioning
  - Nasal suctioning may improve work of breathing and facilitate feeding. Noninvasive suctioning (i.e., a nasal aspirator placed over the naris) is preferable to deep suctioning, which may cause trauma to the nasopharynx and worsen edema.
- Aerosols
  - β-Adrenergic agonists have no clear benefit in bronchiolitis. Although some trials have suggested transient improvements in respiratory scores, none has demonstrated any impact on clinically meaningful outcomes such as hospitalization rates or hospital length of stay. β-Agonists increase heart rate and overall metabolic demand.
  - Racemic epinephrine, with its α-adrenergic properties is not recommended and has demonstrated no benefit compared to hypertonic saline (HTS).
  - Neither β- or α-adrenergic agonists are recommended by the AAP for routine use.
  - Recent studies of nebulized HTS did not demonstrate improvement in length of stay, respiratory score, or readmission rate compared to nebulized normal saline.
  - If aerosols are to be used in bronchiolitis, careful attention should be paid to the clinical exam before and after administration (preferably with the use of a respiratory score) in order to support their ongoing use. Administering treatments on an as needed basis, rather than scheduled, may reduce length of stay.
- Antimicrobials
  - Antibiotics are overused in bronchiolitis and should be avoided in most cases.
  - Special considerations include the following:
    - In severe cases of respiratory distress, with clinical findings suggestive of pneumonia, the risk–benefit profile of antibiotics may favor treatment.
    - Urinary tract infection
    - Otitis media
  - See RSV chapter for discussion of ribavirin and RSV immunoprophylaxis.
- The following inpatient medications/therapies are of *no* proven benefit in bronchiolitis and should be avoided:
  - Corticosteroids (systemic or inhaled)
  - Ipratropium bromide
  - Leukotriene modifiers
  - Methylxanthines (theophylline, aminophylline)
  - Recombinant human DNAse
  - *N*-Acetylcysteine
  - Chest physiotherapy

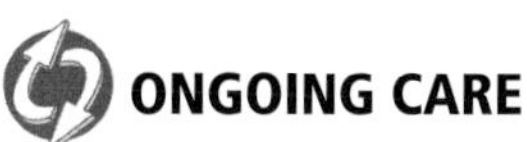

ONGOING CARE

FOLLOW-UP RECOMMENDATIONS

Patient Monitoring

- Most infants with no underlying disease improve within 1 week.
- A fraction of infants (~20%) will have symptoms for 3 weeks or more.
- Clinical course is prolonged in younger infants (<6 months) and those with comorbid conditions.

PROGNOSIS

- For most previously healthy infants, the prognosis is good.
- A small fraction of infants, especially young or chronically ill ones, need support in the ICU with positive pressure ventilation.
- Mortality rates are very low (<0.1%).
- Infants with chronic underlying disease may have a protracted course and are at risk for repeated hospitalizations.
- Although up to 50% of infants with bronchiolitis develop subsequent episodes of wheezing, the direction of causality between bronchiolitis and asthma is unclear.
- Elevated eosinophil count may be suggestive of more severe disease and greater likelihood of future asthma with atopy.

COMPLICATIONS

- Complications are rare in otherwise healthy children.
- Harm associated with medical interventions may occur including antibiotic side effects, IV infiltration, hyponatremia related to hypotonic fluids. Additionally, direct harms may occur secondary to oxygen exposure (e.g., resorption atelectasis or toxicity from reactive oxygen intermediates).

ALERT

- Almost all infants with bronchiolitis get better and do not need testing or therapies.
- Be aware of viral coinfections—1/4 or more of hospitalized patients with bronchiolitis have evidence of infection with at least two viruses.

ADDITIONAL READING

- Brooks CG, Harrison WN, Ralston SL. Association between hypertonic saline and hospital length of stay in acute viral bronchiolitis: a reanalysis of 2 meta-analyses. *JAMA Pediatr*. 2016;170(6):577–584.
- Cunningham S, Rodriguez A, Adams T, et al; for Bronchiolitis of Infancy Discharge Study Group. Oxygen saturation targets in infants with bronchiolitis (BIDS): a double-blind, randomised, equivalence trial. *Lancet*. 2015;386(9998):1041–1048.
- Florin TA, Plint AC, Zorc JJ. Viral bronchiolitis. *Lancet*. 2017;389(10065):211–224.
- Mansbach JM, Piedra PA, Teach SJ, et al. Prospective multicenter study of viral etiology and hospital length of stay in children with severe bronchiolitis. *Arch Pediatr Adolesc Med*. 2012;166(8):700–706.
- Ralston S, Garber M, Narang S, et al. Decreasing unnecessary utilization in acute bronchiolitis care: results from the value in inpatient pediatrics network. *J Hosp Med*. 2013;8(1):25–30.
- Ralston SL, Lieberthal AS, Meissner HC, et al. Clinical practice guideline: the diagnosis, management, and prevention of bronchiolitis. *Pediatrics*. 2014;134(5):e1474–e1502. *Pediatrics*. 2015;136(4):782.

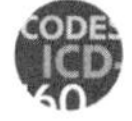

CODES

ICD10

- J21.9 Acute bronchiolitis, unspecified
- J21.0 Acute bronchiolitis due to respiratory syncytial virus
- J21.8 Acute bronchiolitis due to other specified organisms

FAQ

- Q: How did my child get bronchiolitis?
- A: Viral bronchiolitis is a common, seasonal, respiratory tract infection that is easily transmissible. It is acquired in much the same way as the common cold.
- Q: Can my child become reinfected?
- A: Children can become reinfected with RSV bronchiolitis, and infection can occur more than once during the same respiratory season. Furthermore, some patients can get two viral infections at the same time.
- Q: Do patients with bronchiolitis need to be isolated?
- A: Ideally, all patients with bronchiolitis are kept in isolation from other patients with and without bronchiolitis. If cohorting is necessary, patients with the same virus can be roomed together, although contact precautions should still be taken.
- Q: Will my child develop asthma?
- A: There is an ~50% chance that a patient with bronchiolitis will wheeze again. However, it is not clear whether the virus causes asthma or if infants who are predisposed to asthma are more likely to get bronchiolitis.

BRONCHOPULMONARY DYSPLASIA (BPD)

Vineet Bhandari, MD, DM • Anita Bhandari, MD

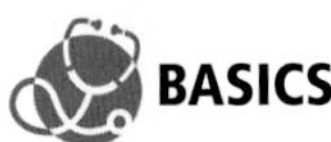

BASICS

DESCRIPTION

- A chronic lung disease (CLD) of premature infants defined as the need for supplemental oxygen for 28 days and a need for supplemental oxygen +/− positive pressure at 36 weeks postmenstrual age (PMA)
- It is categorized as mild, moderate, and severe based on the following at 36 weeks PMA or discharge (whichever comes first).
  - Mild: breathing room air
  - Moderate: need for <30% oxygen
  - Severe: need for >30% oxygen, with or without positive pressure ventilation or continuous positive pressure

EPIDEMIOLOGY

- BPD is the most common CLD in infants.
- Infants with birth weight (BW) <1,250 g account for 97% of all patients with BPD.
- Prevalence based on BW:
  - 501 to 750 g: 42%
  - 751 to 1,000 g: 25%
  - 1,001 to 1,250 g: 11%
  - 1,251 to 1,500 g: 5%

RISK FACTORS

- Infants with gestational age (GA) <28 weeks and BW <1,000 g
- Invasive ventilation
- Exposure to hyperoxia
- Sepsis (*in utero* and postnatal (PN); local/systemic)
- Genetic predisposition

GENERAL PREVENTION

- Prevention of premature birth
- Noninvasive ventilation approaches
- Avoidance of hyperoxia
- Decreasing perinatal infections

PATHOPHYSIOLOGY

- Multifactorial with gene–environmental interactions
- Antenatal (AN)—chorioamnionitis
- PN—ventilator injury, hyperoxia, and sepsis
- AN and PN factors act on a genetically predisposed immature lung, causing release of multiple molecular mediators of inflammation, resulting in activation of cellular death pathways, followed by resolution or repair.
- Repair of the injured developing lung results in decreased alveolarization and dysregulated pulmonary vasculature, the pathologic hallmarks of BPD.

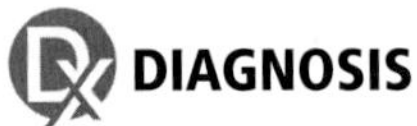

DIAGNOSIS

HISTORY

- AN: pregnancy-induced hypertension, preterm/prolonged rupture of membranes, chorioamnionitis, steroids
- Perinatal: resuscitation at birth
- PN: GA, BW, small for GA (SGA), respiratory distress syndrome (RDS), surfactant use, duration of invasive/noninvasive ventilation, supplemental oxygen
- Family: premature birth, asthma

PHYSICAL EXAM

- Early phase (up to 1 PN week): normal to severe RDS (i.e., tachypnea, dyspnea)
- Evolving phase (>1 PN week to 36 weeks PMA): increasing respiratory distress and FiO_2
- Established phase (>36 weeks PMA): tachypnea, dyspnea, crackles, stridor (subglottic stenosis), wheezing, "BPD spells" (tracheobronchomalacia), evidence of pulmonary hypertension (PHTN), gastroesophageal reflux (GER), poor growth parameters

DIFFERENTIAL DIAGNOSIS

- Pneumonia
- Aspiration
- Congenital heart disease
- Wilson-Mikity syndrome
- Interstitial lung disease
  - Surfactant protein deficiency
  - Pulmonary lymphangiectasia

DIAGNOSTIC TESTS & INTERPRETATION

Initial Tests (screening, lab, imaging)

- Blood gases: monitoring of acid–base status, hypo/hyperoxia, hypo/hypercapnia
- Chest radiography:
  - Early—reticular-granular pattern with air bronchograms (RDS)
  - Evolving—pulmonary edema, atelectasis
  - Established—hyperinflation, increased interstitial markings, cysts

Follow-Up Tests & Special Considerations

- Echocardiogram:
  - Evidence of PHTN-tricuspid regurgitant jet, flattening of the interventricular septum, accelerated pulmonary regurgitation velocity, right atrial enlargement, right ventricular hypertrophy and dilation
  - It is recommended that all patients with BPD undergo echocardiography to rule out PHTN.
- Cardiac catheterization in selective infants to confirm PHTN
- Pulmonary function testing:
  - Majority have abnormal spirometry with decreased forced expiratory volume at 1 second (FEV_1) and decreased small airway forced expiratory flows (FEF, 25–75%) and impaired diffusion capacity.
  - Majority of studies reveal no decrease in exercise capacity in former premature babies, although response to exercise differs.
- CT scan: persistent findings which include linear densities, subpleural triangular densities, and emphysema

Diagnostic Procedures/Other

- Bronchoscopy for subglottic stenosis, tracheo-/bronchomalacia
- Sleep studies for persistent hypoxia and suspected central or obstructive apnea
- pH probe for GER

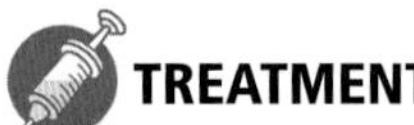

TREATMENT

GENERAL MEASURES

Fluids/nutrition

- Early phase: Restricting fluids to ~140 cc/kg/day may decrease BPD.
- Early/evolving/established phase: Aim to achieve 120 to 140 kcal/kg/day.

MEDICATION

- Oxygen supplementation
  - Prevention of hypoxia and as a pulmonary vasodilator
  - Early/evolving phases: Titrate FiO_2 by pulse oximeter 88–92%, generally, >85–<95%.
  - Established phase: generally ~95%, for prevention of PHTN
- Methylxanthines
  - Acts as a respiratory stimulant, increase diaphragmatic contractility, weak bronchodilator and diuretic action
  - Caffeine use has been associated with decreased BPD and improved neurodevelopmental outcomes.
  - Early/evolving phases: caffeine citrate (IV/PO) 20 mg/kg loading dose, 5 mg/kg/24 h maintenance dose
  - Side effects include feeding intolerance, tachycardia.
  - Therapeutic levels of 5 to 25 mg/L
  - Cardiovascular, neurologic, or GI toxicity reported at serum levels >50 mg/L
- Vitamin A
  - Helpful in maintaining epithelial cell integrity of the respiratory tract
  - Early/evolving phases: 5,000 IU IM 3 times per week for 4 weeks
- Steroids
  - Decreases inflammation, pulmonary edema
  - Evolving phase: dexamethasone (IV/PO, 0.5 mg/kg/24 h × 2 days, then 0.25 mg/kg/24 h × 2 days and then 0.15 mg/kg/24 h × 1 day) may be used to assist with extubation attempts after 3 to 4 PN weeks.
  - Established phase: Prednisolone (PO, 2 mg/kg/24 h × 5 days, then 1 mg/kg/24 h × 3 days and then 1 mg/kg/24 h every other day for 3 doses) may be helpful in weaning oxygen.
  - Side effects include hyperglycemia and hypertension in the short term.

- Diuretics
  - Evolving/established phases: furosemide (PO/IV, 1 to 2 mg/kg/24 h or every other day); chlorothiazide (PO/IV, 20 to 40 mg/kg/24 h) alone or with spironolactone (PO, 2 to 4 mg/kg/24 h) for transient improvement of lung function
  - Side effects include electrolyte abnormalities, nephrocalcinosis, and osteopenia of prematurity.
- Bronchodilators
  - Evolving/established phases: Inhaled β-agonists (e.g., albuterol 1.25 to 2.5 mg given via nebulizer or 2 puffs [180 mcg] given via MDI with spacer device, every 3 to 4 hours as needed) are effective treatment for reversible bronchospasm, although safety and efficacy of long-term use has yet to be established.
  - Muscarinic antagonists (e.g., ipratropium bromide 250 to 500 mcg via nebulizer or 18 mcg/puff via MDI with spacer device, every 6 to 8 hours as needed) may be useful adjuncts, especially in patients who are not significantly responsive to albuterol. It may be better tolerated than albuterol in patients with significant tracheomalacia.
  - Cromolyn has been used for its anti-inflammatory effects and has a low side-effect profile. It has no role in prevention of BPD.

ALERT

- Many patients have oral aversion and feeding difficulties; close monitoring of growth and nutrition is recommended.
- Patients <2 years of age are candidates for respiratory syncytial virus (RSV) immune globulin injections (palivizumab; Synagis®), and those >6 months of age should be offered influenza immunization.
- Childhood immunizations are based on chronologic age rather than corrected age.
- There are no evidence-based guidelines regarding diuretic use or weaning of supplemental oxygen therapy in patients with established BPD.

ADDITIONAL THERAPIES

Ventilator strategy

- Early phase: Avoid intubation; if intubated, give early surfactant (<2 hours of PN life), use short inspiratory times (0.24 to 0.4 second), rapid rates (40 to 60/min), low peak inspiratory pressure (14 to 20 cm H_2O), moderate positive end-expiratory pressure (4 to 6 cm H_2O), and tidal volumes (3 to 6 mL/kg), with blood gas targets pH 7.25 to 7.35, Pa_{O_2} 40 to 60 mm Hg, Pa_{CO_2} 45 to 55 mm Hg; "rescue" high-frequency ventilation; attempt extubation to nasal intermittent positive pressure ventilation (NIPPV) or nasal continuous positive airways pressure (NCPAP) in the first PN week.
- Evolving phase: Use noninvasive ventilation with blood gas targets pH 7.25 to 7.35, Pa_{O_2} 50 to 70 mm Hg, Pa_{CO_2} 50 to 65 mm Hg.
- Established phase: Use noninvasive ventilation with blood gas targets pH 7.35 to 7.45, Pa_{O_2} 60 to 80 mm Hg, Pa_{CO_2} 45 to 60 mm Hg.

ONGOING CARE

FOLLOW-UP RECOMMENDATIONS

- Multidisciplinary approach with primary care physician; pediatric pulmonologist; pediatric cardiologist; nutritionist; and speech, respiratory, occupational, and physical therapists as well as social worker is recommended.
- Monitor linear growth and nutritional status.
- Immunization: prophylaxis against RSV (palivizumab monthly during respiratory season) and influenza
- Neurodevelopmental follow-up

PROGNOSIS

- Infants with BPD have high rates of rehospitalization in the 1st year of life (up to 50%).
- Long-term pulmonary sequelae that may persist into adulthood include airway obstruction, airway hyperreactivity, and concern regarding development of chronic obstructive pulmonary disease (COPD) with aging.
- Long-term neurodevelopmental sequelae associated with BPD is not a specific neuropsychological impairment but more of a global deficit.
- Noninvasive ventilation approaches (NIPPV and NCPAP) hold promise in decreasing BPD.

COMPLICATIONS

- Prolonged intubation may lead to subglottic stenosis, tracheobronchomalacia.
- Undiagnosed PHTN may result in a prolonged oxygen requirement or need for ventilation, poor growth, and cor pulmonale.

ADDITIONAL READING

- Bhandari A, Bhandari V. "New" bronchopulmonary dysplasia: a clinical review. *Clin Pulm Med*. 2011;18:137–143.
- Bhandari A, Bhandari V. Pitfalls, problems, and progress in bronchopulmonary dysplasia. *Pediatrics*. 2009;123(6):1562–1573.
- Bhandari A, McGrath-Morrow S. Long-term pulmonary outcomes of patients with bronchopulmonary dysplasia. *Semin Perinatol*. 2013;37(2):132–137.
- Bhandari V. Hyperoxia-derived lung damage in preterm infants. *Semin Fetal Neonatal Med*. 2010;15(4):223–229.
- Bhandari V. The potential of non-invasive ventilation to decrease BPD. *Semin Perinatol*. 2013;37(2):108–114.

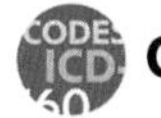

CODES

ICD10

P27.1 Bronchopulmonary dysplasia origin in the perinatal period

FAQ

- Q: Can my patient with BPD receive influenza vaccine?
- A: Yes. Influenza vaccination should be considered for babies >6 months of age and their contacts.
- Q: The American Academy of Pediatrics (AAP) Committee on Infectious Diseases recommends monthly immunoprophylaxis for infants with BPD who are <2 years old and have been on medical therapy for 6 months prior to onset of second RSV season. What should I do if my patient turns 2 years old, 2 months after the respiratory season started?
- A: Once initiated, immunoprophylaxis should be completed even if the child turns 2 years old before the respiratory season has ended.
- Q: If my patient gets RSV infection while on immunoprophylaxis (palivizumab), should the monthly injections be stopped?
- A: Monthly prophylaxis with palivizumab should be discontinued because of extremely low likelihood of a second RSV hospitalization in the same season based on the revised AAP 2014 policy statement.
- Q: Will my patient with BPD continue to have respiratory problems?
- A: Survivors of BPD are more likely to be rehospitalized with respiratory illnesses in the first 2 years of their life, but the rate of hospitalization decreases after 2 years of age and is rare after 14 years of age. They are more likely to develop asthma, have abnormal pulmonary function tests, and require respiratory medications as compared to their peers. There is also some concern that survivors may develop a COPD phenotype as they age.
- Q: If my patient with BPD has recurrent croup, should I refer the patient to a pediatric pulmonologist for evaluation of asthma?
- A: Survivors of BPD are more likely to develop asthma as compared to peers born full term. However, upper and large airway problems such as subglottic stenosis and tracheomalacia are common in this population. Recurrent croup may result from a narrowing of the upper airway and hence, referral to a pediatric otolaryngologist should be considered to rule out causes such as subglottic stenosis.
- Q: Will my patient with BPD likely to have neurodevelopmental issues as well?
- A: Yes. Children with BPD are more likely to have delayed speech and language development, visual-motor integration impairments, and behavior problems. They may also have low average IQ, memory and learning deficits, and attention problems.
- Q: My patient with BPD has not been growing well and has not been able to come off supplemental oxygen. What else should I consider?
- A: PHTN has been shown to occur in 1/4 to 1/3 of patients with BPD; it is worthwhile to refer for a cardiac evaluation to rule out PHTN.

BRUISING

Julie W. Stern, MD

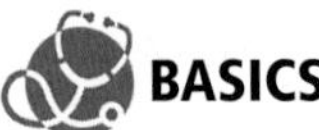

BASICS

DESCRIPTION

Bruises are the result of extravasation of blood into the skin. Conventional usage often groups petechiae and bruises (or ecchymoses) together as purpura and defines them as follows:

- Petechiae: flat, red, or reddish purple; 1 to 3 mm; nonblanching
- Ecchymoses: larger than petechiae, local extravasation, nonpulsatile, sometimes palpable, color depends on age of lesion

EPIDEMIOLOGY

Prevalence

- <1% nonmobile babies
- 17% cruising and crawling infants
- 53% walkers
- Majority of school age children

RISK FACTORS

Underlying bleeding disorders (e.g., von Willebrand disease, platelet disfunction, thrombocytopenia), child abuse/trauma, medications, infections, etc. may all be risk factors leading to bruising in childhood.

Genetics

- Hemophilia is an X-linked disorder affecting males.
- von Willebrand disease may be autosomal dominant.
- Other platelet disorders have a variety of inheritance patterns.

PATHOPHYSIOLOGY

Extravasation of blood from blood vessels leading to a collection of blood below the surface of the skin

ETIOLOGY

- Disorders of blood vessels and surrounding tissue
- Platelet abnormalities (function, number)
- Coagulation disorders

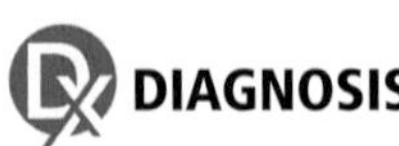

DIAGNOSIS

General goal is to determine if the cause of the bruising is thrombocytopenia, a coagulation disorder, or an extrinsic factor (such as trauma, infection).

- **Phase 1:** Determine if the history of bruising and/or petechiae is acute or chronic in onset and if there is known trauma versus spontaneous lesions
  - General estimates
    - New (purple, dark red)
    - ~ 1 to 4 days (dark blue to brown)
    - ~ 5 to 7 days (greenish to yellow)
    - ~ >7 days (yellow)
  - Acute onset of diffuse subcutaneous bleeding with bruises of different ages may indicate severe thrombocytopenia.
  - Generally, children will not bruise or develop petechiae spontaneously until the platelet count is $<20{,}000/\text{mm}^3$.
  - Idiopathic thrombocytopenic purpura, leukemia, aplastic anemia, and so forth, can cause this bleeding.
  - A hematologist should be consulted because of the risk of potentially life-threatening bleeding.
  - Chronic history of recurrent bleeding may indicate an inherited coagulation defect such as von Willebrand disease or hemophilia. Familial history may be positive, although von Willebrand disease often goes undiagnosed into adulthood if there has been no challenge such as surgery.
  - Various bleeding scores available but not fully validated in pediatrics; may be helpful to direct history taking
- **Phase 2:** Perform screening tests for bleeding disorders to categorize the abnormality.
  - Platelet count to assess level of thrombocytopenia
  - PT/PTT: Prolongation of either one or both of these may aid in diagnosis of von Willebrand disease, coagulation factor deficiencies, liver disease, and vitamin K deficiency.
  - Testing for von Willebrand disease and platelet aggregation disorders generally need to be done by a hematologist for accuracy and interpretation.

HISTORY

- **Question:** Significant bruising in the neonatal period?
- *Significance*: may indicate neonatal thrombocytopenia, congenital infections, and sepsis with disseminated intravascular coagulation
- **Question:** Bleeding in the neonatal period?
- *Significance*: Hemophilia. Other inherited disorders of coagulation may not be diagnosed until a child is older; tend to be mild; may be uncovered with preoperative testing or postoperative bleeding complications. Idiopathic thrombocytopenic purpura may occur at any age.
- **Question:** Pattern of bruising?
- *Significance*: in a younger child, may indicate normal toddler activity, child abuse, or religious practices such as coining
- **Question:** Use of aspirin, ibuprofen, cough syrups with guaifenesin, and/or antihistamines?
- *Significance*: platelet dysfunction; use of these drugs may also unmask an otherwise mild inherited bleeding disorder.
- **Question:** Ecchymosis or petechiae?
- *Significance*: Infections such as meningococcemia or viruses and collagen vascular diseases may present with these.
- **Question:** Familial history?
- *Significance*: Positive familial history of inherited disorders of coagulation factors or platelet aggregation may aid in directing the workup. Negative familial history does not rule out any of these disorders.

PHYSICAL EXAM

- **Finding:** Good appearance, with a history of an antecedent viral illness?
- *Significance*: Those with idiopathic thrombocytopenic purpura often appear well, although often with a history of an antecedent viral illness.
- **Finding:** Ill appearance?
- *Significance*: It should raise concerns about malignancy, infection (especially meningococcemia), or other acquired coagulation factor deficiencies such as those seen with liver failure.
- **Finding:** Bruising in unusual locations (back, genitalia, thorax)?
- *Significance*: should raise suspicions of child abuse, especially if lesions are in different stages of healing or suggest the pattern of a hand or belt
- **Finding:** Purpura confined mostly to the legs?
- *Significance:* typical of Henoch-Schönlein purpura

ALERT

The amount of bruising may not correlate with the amount of internal bleeding that has occurred.

- Hemophiliacs can significantly drop their hemoglobin during a thigh or psoas bleed without having much in the way of ecchymosis.
- A child presenting with idiopathic thrombocytopenic purpura may have bruises and petechiae from head to toe without changing the hemoglobin much at all.

- **Finding:** Multiple ecchymoses in the pretibial regions?
- *Significance*: This is typical of normal toddler activity.
- **Finding:** Petechiae entirely above the nipple line?
- *Significance*: consistent with Valsalva maneuver, severe cough, and viral infections
- **Finding:** Deeper bleeding in muscles and joints?
- *Significance*: hemophilia
- **Finding:** Bleeding in mucous membranes?
- *Significance*: Severe thrombocytopenia, streptococcal pharyngitis, varicella, measles, and other viral infections can cause this.
- **Finding:** Gingival and/or mucous membrane bleeding?
- *Significance*: von Willebrand disease can present with this. Severe thrombocytopenia and ITP may also present with oral bleeding.
- **Finding:** Involvement of the reticuloendothelial system?
- *Significance*: can be found with malignancies such as leukemia or with viral or bacterial infections, indicated by hepatosplenomegaly or lymphadenopathy
- **Finding:** Upper extremity limb malformations and bruising?
- *Significance*: may present with syndromes such as Fanconi anemia and thrombocytopenia absent radii (TAR)

DIFFERENTIAL DIAGNOSIS

- Congenital/anatomic
  - Coagulation factor abnormality: hemophilia, von Willebrand disease
  - Platelet defect: Bernard-Soulier syndrome, Glanzmann thrombasthenia, and storage pool defects
  - Congenital alloimmune or isoimmune thrombocytopenia
  - Neonatal extramedullary hematopoiesis
  - Hereditary hemorrhagic telangiectasia
- Infectious
  - Meningococcemia
  - Viral infections (coxsackievirus, echovirus)
  - Rocky Mountain spotted fever
  - Syphilis
  - Pertussis—secondary to severe cough
  - Septic or fat emboli
  - Disseminated intravascular coagulation—acquired factor deficiency
- Toxic, environmental, drugs
  - Warfarin—acquired factor deficiency
  - Corticosteroids—striae caused by increased capillary fragility
  - Aspirin and ibuprofen—cause a qualitative platelet abnormality
  - Sulfonamides
  - Bismuth
  - Chloramphenicol

B

- Trauma
  - Normal activity
  - Child abuse
  - Valsalva, crying, forceful coughing
  - Cupping or coin rubbing
  - Tight garments
- Tumor (quantitative platelet abnormality)
  - Bone marrow replacement—leukemia, myelofibrosis, or (rarely) metastatic solid tumors
- Genetic/metabolic
  - Uremia
  - Vitamin C deficiency
  - Vitamin K deficiency—owing to antibiotics, biliary atresia, malabsorption (acquired factor deficiency)
- Allergic/inflammatory/vasculitic
  - Henoch-Schönlein purpura
  - Bone marrow failure: aplastic anemia (including Fanconi, paroxysmal nocturnal hemoglobinuria)
  - Increased destruction: idiopathic thrombocytopenic purpura, Evans syndrome, lupus
  - Nephrotic syndrome
  - Collagen vascular disease
  - Ehlers-Danlos syndrome, other joint hypermobility syndromes
  - Snake bite (copperhead)
- Miscellaneous (disorders that simulate bruises)
  - Ataxia telangiectasia
  - Cherry angiomas
  - Kaposi sarcoma

DIAGNOSTIC TESTS & INTERPRETATION

Initial Tests (screening, lab, imaging)

- **Test:** CBC
- *Significance*: Platelet count is the most important; abnormalities of WBC or Hgb may aid in diagnosis of bone marrow infiltration or failure.
- **Test:** PT
- *Significance*: Elevation may indicate warfarin ingestion or factor VII and/or vitamin K deficiencies.
- **Test:** aPTT
- *Significance*: Prolongation is seen with hemophilia and may be seen in von Willebrand disease.
- **Test:** both PT and aPTT
- *Significance*: Both are prolonged in disseminated intravascular coagulation, liver failure, and severe vitamin K deficiency.

Follow-up Tests & Special Considerations

- **Test:** bleeding time (rarely performed in children any longer)
- *Significance*: lengthened in platelet aggregation disorders and with drug effects
- **Test:** fibrinogen
- *Significance*: decreased in liver failure, disseminated intravascular coagulation
- **Test:** urinalysis
- *Significance*: Hematuria and/or proteinuria may indicate Henoch-Schönlein purpura, nephrotic syndrome, or other vasculitis.

Diagnostic Procedures/Other

- **Test:** bone marrow aspirate
- *Significance:* for suspected malignancy, bone marrow failure syndromes, aplastic anemia
- **Test:** platelet function, specific coagulation studies
- *Significance*: indicated for patients with personal or family histories suggestive of a new onset or inherited coagulopathy

ALERT

Factors that make this condition an emergency include the following:

- Severe thrombocytopenia below 10,000 to 20,000/mm^3 carries a higher risk of spontaneous internal bleeding including intracranial bleeding.
- Bleeding or bruising accompanied by evidence of leukemia or other malignancy
- Evidence of sepsis (disseminated intravascular coagulation) or meningococcemia

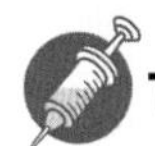

TREATMENT

GENERAL MEASURES

Thrombocytopenia precautions for platelets <20,000 to 50,000—toddlers may need a helmet until platelet count recovers; patients with hemophilia may need restricted activity, generally not needed for patients with mild Type 1 von Willebrand disease; depends on underlying cause

MEDICATION

- Factor replacement for hemophilia
- DDAVP, Humate P®, amicar, tranexamic acid for von Willebrand disease
- DDAVP and/or platelet transfusions for mild platelet function abnormalities
- Platelet transfusion for thrombocytopenia due to decreased production
- IVIG, steroids, thrombopoietin (TPO) mimetics, splenectomy for ITP, (Rh immune globulin rarely used any longer)

ISSUES FOR REFERRAL

- Persistent, multiple bruises >1 cm without significant thrombocytopenia
- Family history of bleeding disorder
- Additional personal bleeding sites (menorrhagia, epistaxis, gingival, etc.)
- Suspected child abuse
- Abnormal bleeding laboratory studies

ADMISSION, INPATIENT, AND NURSING CONSIDERATIONS

- Severe thrombocytopenia, suspected child abuse, significant bleeding, significant head trauma
- Level of care (floor vs. ICU) depends on clinical situation

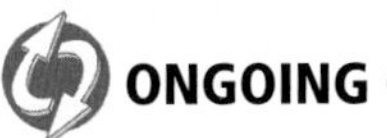

ONGOING CARE

FOLLOW-UP RECOMMENDATIONS

Patient Monitoring

Recurrent and chronic ITP possible

- Rapidity of platelet recovery in ITP difficult to predict
- Most will recover within 6 to 12 months

DIET

Rarely an issue

PATIENT EDUCATION

Avoid contact activities for platelet count <20,000/mm^3, some bleeding disorders (i.e., hemophilia).

COMPLICATIONS

Significant bleeding with a bleeding disorder, thrombocytopenia

ADDITIONAL READING

- Berntorp E. Progress in haemophilic care: ethical issues. *Haemophilia*. 2002;8(3):435–438.
- Buchanan GR. Bleeding signs in children with idiopathic thrombocytopenic purpura. *J Pediatr Hematol Oncol*. 2003;25(Suppl 1):S42–S46.
- Geddis AE, Balduini CL. Diagnosis of immune thrombocytopenic purpura in children. *Curr Opin Hematol*. 2007;14(5):520–525.
- Horton TM, Stone JD, Yee D, et al. Case series of thrombotic thrombocytopenic purpura in children and adolescents. *J Pediatr Hematol Oncol*. 2003;25(4):336–339.
- Khair K, Liesner R. Bruising and bleeding in infants and children—a practical approach. *Br J Haematol*. 2006;133(3):221–231.
- Kos L, Shwayder T. Cutaneous manifestations of child abuse. *Pediatr Dermatol*. 2006;23(4):311–320.
- Maguire S, Mann MK, Sibert J, et al. Are there patterns of bruising in childhood which are diagnostic or suggestive of abuse? A systematic review. *Arch Dis Child*. 2005;90(2):182–186.
- O'Brien SH. An update on pediatric bleeding disorders: bleeding scores, benign joint hypermobility, and platelet function testing in the evaluation of the child with bleeding symptoms. *Am J Hematol*. 2012;87(Suppl 1):S40–S44.
- Wight J, Paisley S. The epidemiology of inhibitors in haemophilia A: a systematic review. *Haemophilia*. 2003;9(4):418–435.

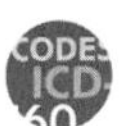

CODES

ICD10

- T14.8 Other injury of unspecified body region
- R23.3 Spontaneous ecchymoses
- D68.9 Coagulation defect, unspecified

FAQ

- Q: Is hemophilia always diagnosed in the newborn period?
- A: No. A familial history may provide clues, but a significant number of patients represent a spontaneous mutation. Additionally, not all boys with hemophilia will bleed with circumcision, and the diagnosis may not be made until the infants become more active.
- Q: What is a common cause of bruising among girls?
- A: Girls may first come to attention at menarche and be diagnosed at that time with von Willebrand disease. Rarely, girls whose fathers have hemophilia may be unfavorably lyonized and, therefore, have decreased factor levels consistent with mild hemophilia.
- Q: Can boys with a family history of von Willebrand disease be circumcised?
- A: Yes, but only within the first few days of life, and testing does not need to be completed prior to procedure. If procedure is not completed in the neonatal period, testing may need to be delayed until 6 months of life or later.

BRUXISM

Anupama R. Tate, DMD, MPH • Karen R. Fratantoni, MD, MPH

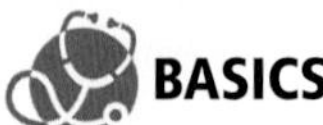

BASICS

DESCRIPTION

- Bruxism is defined as habitual nonfunctional forceful contact of teeth, which is involuntary. These movements can include excessive grinding, clenching, or rubbing of teeth.
- Other nonfunctional (or "parafunctional") oral habits include movements not involved with normal chewing, swallowing, or speaking, such as chewing pencils, nails, cheek, or lip.
- Sleep bruxism should be distinguished from daytime awake bruxism. Sleep bruxism has been classified as a sleep-related movement disorder.
- Awake bruxism is rare with little or no audible sound during clenching, compared to the loud grinding sound commonly occurring in sleep bruxism.

EPIDEMIOLOGY

- Age/onset
  - In children, prevalence in the literature is highly variable with a range of 4–40%. Prevalence decreases with increasing age.
  - May occur throughout life but frequently tends to peak in early childhood, then decreases with age
  - Sleep bruxism progressively diminishes around 9 to 10 years of age.
  - Infants have been known to grind their teeth during the eruption of primary teeth.
  - May be temporarily or intermittently present, which makes diagnosis difficult
- Gender
  - Recent systematic review of literature reported no gender differences in prevalence.
  - Previous studies suggested girls may be more affected than boys.
- Some studies support higher incidence in children with developmental disabilities, Down syndrome, sleep disorders, and autism.

RISK FACTORS

Genetics

- No genetic mechanism has been explained.
- Based on self-reports, 20–50% of children with sleep bruxism have an immediate family member who experienced bruxism as a child.

ETIOLOGY

- The exact cause is not known. It is likely to be a multifactorial process including oral motor activities, regulation of sleep–wake cycle, autonomic, catecholaminergic, hereditary, and psychosocial influences.
- Awake bruxism is more commonly associated with psychosocial factors and psychopathologic symptoms.
- Dental factors (current evidence suggests that they play a small role, only ~10% of cases)
  - Occlusal interferences, including malocclusions, in which teeth do not interdigitate smoothly
  - High dental restorations (e.g., fillings or crowns)
  - Intraoral irritation (e.g., sharp tooth cusp)
  - Teething
- Psychological factors
  - Nervous tension (related to stress, anger, and aggression)
  - Personality disorders
  - Posttraumatic stress disorder
- Common systemic factors
  - Moving between levels of sleep
  - Sleep-disordered breathing
  - Snoring and obstructive sleep apnea
  - Tonsil/adenoid hypertrophy
  - Mouth breathing
  - Neurodevelopmental disorders (e.g., cerebral palsy)
  - Brain injury
  - ADHD
- Other possible factors
  - Asthma
  - Allergies
  - Nasal obstruction
  - Exposure to secondhand smoke
  - Medications (amphetamines, barbiturates, antidepressants—particularly serotonin reuptake inhibitors)

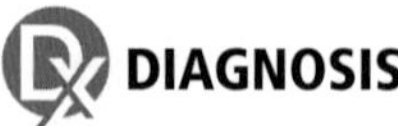

DIAGNOSIS

HISTORY

- Teeth
  - Wearing of facets, abraded areas
  - Extreme wear of primary teeth is occasionally observed; however, pulp or nerve damage is rare.
  - Broken dental restorations
  - Loose teeth
  - Progression of periodontal disease (gingival inflammation, recession, and alveolar bone loss)
  - Pain or sensitivity
- Muscular symptoms of the head and neck muscles, most often seen in the lateral pterygoids followed by the medial pterygoids and masseters
  - Pain
  - Trismus
  - Spasm
- Frequent headache or migraines
- Parasomnias
- Temporomandibular joint (TMJ) disorders
  - Symptoms (pain, clicking, popping when opening or closing)
  - Limited mandibular range of motion

DIFFERENTIAL DIAGNOSIS

- Dental erosion
- Drug reaction
- Gastroesophageal reflux
- Seizures
- Sleep disorder
- Stress

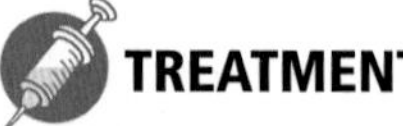

TREATMENT

GENERAL MEASURES

- Often, children outgrow bruxism and no treatment is indicated.
- When palliative management is not adequate and treatment is needed, it is best managed in a multiprofessional team approach including a dentist.
- Patient and family education: Ensure that the bruxism itself does not become an issue, generating increased stress for the child.
- Plastic or vinyl bite guard (must not interfere with normal dental growth and development)
- Stress counseling
  - Identify and address sources of stress.
  - Meditation
  - Music therapy
  - Biofeedback exercises
  - Acupressure and/or acupuncture
- Counseling/psychotherapy
  - Hypnosis

B

MEDICATION
- Analgesics or anti-inflammatory medications (e.g., ibuprofen) for management of symptoms
- Rarely used
  - Muscle relaxants for symptoms
  - Mild anxiolytics if anxiety plays an etiologic role

ADDITIONAL THERAPIES
Rarely used
- Occlusal adjustment (selective tooth grinding to balance the bite): There is no evidence-based support. Because of inadequate data regarding their usefulness, irreversible therapies should be avoided.
- Tonsillectomy and adenoidectomy

COMPLEMENTARY & ALTERNATIVE THERAPIES
- Warm compresses for muscle or TMJ symptoms
- Limiting affected muscle activity (e.g., "do not open wide," "take small bites," "avoid chewing gum") may help reduce TMJ symptoms.

ADMISSION, INPATIENT, AND NURSING CONSIDERATIONS
- Treatment for bruxism is rarely indicated for children in the inpatient setting.
- Therapy is justified if damage to the permanent dentition or periodontal structures is observed.
- For neurologically impaired patients with acute self-injurious issues, bite blocks, or mouth props can be used with caution to avoid oral injury. Patients who exhibit chronic chewing may require the fabrication of custom-fitted mouth guards, which may require the use of deep sedation or general anesthetic procedures to construct the appliance. The risk of these procedures would need to be weighed against the benefit of the bite guard.

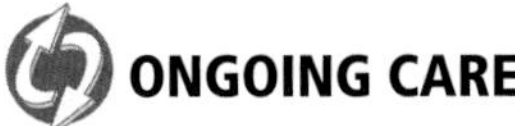

ONGOING CARE

FOLLOW-UP RECOMMENDATIONS

Patient Monitoring
The large majority of bruxism in children stops without any therapy. Monitor for significant associated problems; recommend treatment if damage to permanent dentition and/or periodontal structures occurs.

PROGNOSIS
- There are no data to indicate a cause-and-effect relationship exists for bruxism in childhood continuing into adulthood.
- Preschool- and school-age children
  - Ensure that all children establish a dental home by 1 year of age.
  - Typically ceases without therapeutic intervention
  - Associated problems are rare.
  - Monitor for associated conditions.
- Adolescents
  - More commonly benefit from therapeutic intervention
  - Associated problems (e.g., attrition of teeth; muscular, TMJ symptoms) may also require therapy.
- Special-needs children
  - Long-term prognosis is poor.
  - Children who are comatose or those who have suffered traumatic brain injuries or neurologically impaired may be managed using prefabricated bite blocks or, in rare cases, by the fabrication of custom-fitted mouth guards to minimize risk of damage to lips or tongue. Intraoral botulinum-A injections have relieved the spasticity.

ADDITIONAL READING

- American Academy of Sleep Medicine. Sleep related bruxism. In: *International Classification of Sleep Disorders: Diagnostic and Coding Manual*. 3rd ed. Westchester, IL: American Academy of Sleep Medicine; 2014:182–185.
- Cheifetz AT, Osganian SK, Allred EN, et al. Prevalence of bruxism and associated correlates in children as reported by parents. *J Dent Child (Chic)*. 2005;72(2):67–73.
- Dahshan A, Patel H, Delaney J, et al. Gastroesophageal reflux disease and dental erosion in children. *J Pediatr*. 2002;140(4):474–478.
- Ferreira NM, Dos Santos JF, dos Santos MB, et al. Sleep bruxism associated with obstructive sleep apnea syndrome in children. *Cranio*. 2015;33(4):251–255.
- Guideline on acquired temporomandibular disorders in infants, children, and adolescents. *Pediatr Dent*. 2016;38(6):308–314.
- Lavigne GJ, Khoury S, Abe S, et al. Bruxism physiology and pathology: an overview for clinicians. *J Oral Rehabil*. 2008;35(7):476–494.
- Manfredini D, Lobbezoo F. Role of psychosocial factors in the etiology of bruxism. *J Orofac Pain*. 2009;23(2):153–166.
- Manfredini D, Restrepo C, Diaz-Serrano K, et al. Prevalence of sleep bruxism in children: a systematic review of the literature. *J Oral Rehabil*. 2013;40(8):631–642.
- Motta LJ, Martins MD, Fernandes KP, et al. Craniocervical posture and bruxism in children. *Physiother Res Int*. 2011;16(1):57–61.
- Norwood KW Jr, Slayton RL; for Council on Children with Disabilities, Section on Oral Health. Oral health care for children with developmental disabilities. *Pediatrics*. 2013;131(3):614–619.
- Ortega AO, Dos Santos MT, Mendes FM, et al. Association between anticonvulsant drugs and teeth-grinding in children and adolescents with cerebral palsy. *J Oral Rehabil*. 2014;41(9):653–658.

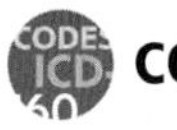

CODES

ICD10
- F45.8 Other somatoform disorders
- G47.63 Sleep related bruxism

FAQ
- Q: What is the recommendation for nighttime bruxism management in a preschool child?
- A: The majority of bruxism in children stops without any therapy. Considering the controversial nature of treatment modalities, it is prudent to advise no treatment for childhood bruxism and to advise the parents that the condition is common and the child will outgrow the condition.
- Q: Does bruxism in a child result in problems with the permanent teeth or with the TMJ?
- A: There is no evidence that bruxism in children leads to problems during adolescence or later.
- Q: What is the recommendation for bruxism management in a child with snoring or tonsil/adenoid hypertrophy?
- A: Studies have shown a higher incidence of bruxism among children with tonsil hypertrophy and sleep apnea and a decrease in bruxism after adenotonsillectomy. Bruxism alone, without evidence of upper airway obstruction, would not currently be an indication for adenotonsillectomy. Physicians should assess children with bruxism for upper airway obstruction and refer when indicated.
- Q: When should patient be referred to multiprofessional team including a dentist?
- A: Monitor for significant associated problems; recommend referral if damage to permanent dentition and/or periodontal structures occurs or pain persist.

BULIMIA

Sara F. Forman, MD • Melissa B. Freizinger, PhD

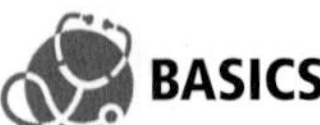

BASICS

DESCRIPTION

Bulimia nervosa is an eating disorder (ED) characterized by the following:

- Recurrent binge eating episodes with rapid consumption of large amounts of food in discrete periods of time (approximately 2 hours)
- Feeling of lack of control over eating behavior during eating binges
- Compensatory behaviors such as self-induced vomiting, laxative or diuretic use, strict dieting, or vigorous exercise
- Minimum average of one binge eating/compensatory behavior episode per week for at least 3 months
- Associated feelings of guilt, shame, low self-esteem, and depression
- Persistent overconcern with body shape and weight
- Symptoms and psychopathology may overlap with anorexia nervosa, but bulimia does not occur exclusively during episodes of anorexia nervosa.

EPIDEMIOLOGY

- Onset in adolescence to young adulthood
- Approximately 10:1 female-to-male ratio
- 70% of the adolescents who meet criteria for full and partial syndrome eating disorders also meet criteria for an Axis I disorder.

Prevalence

- Adolescents have a 1–1.5% 12-month prevalence of bulimia according to the *Diagnostic and Statistical Manual of Mental Disorders* 5th edition (*DSM-5*).
- Up to 25% of college-aged women use bingeing and purging as a weight management technique.
- Bulimia nervosa prevalence rates in Western countries for females range from 0.3% to 7.3%.

RISK FACTORS

Genetics

Recent studies, including twin studies, suggest that bulimia nervosa and binge eating may have a genetic vulnerability and familial transmission.

GENERAL PREVENTION

- Emphasize healthy self-esteem/body image with preadolescents and adolescents.
- Regular family dinners may have some protective effect against eating disorders.

ETIOLOGY

- Personality traits of low self-esteem, self-regulatory difficulties, frustration, intolerance, and impaired ability to recognize and express feelings directly described in bulimia nervosa
- Small positive association between childhood sexual abuse and eating disorders but size and nature of this association not known
- Neuroendocrine abnormalities may also play a role: Abnormalities in serotonergic and vagal function have been demonstrated in patients with bulimia nervosa.
- Cholecystokinin response to a meal is decreased in bulimia nervosa, which may also indicate abnormal satiety signaling.
- May be abnormalities in other hormones or neurotransmitters such as leptin, dopamine, and endorphins; unclear if cause or effect

COMMONLY ASSOCIATED CONDITIONS

- Mood lability, impulsivity, and emotional dysregulation are common in patients with bulimia or subthreshold bulimia.
- Lifetime rates of major depressive disorder in individuals with eating disorders 50–75%
- In adolescents, bulimia is associated with persistent depressive disorder, (formerly known as *dysthymia*), more than major depression.
- 63.5% of bulimic patients have lifetime history of an anxiety disorder.

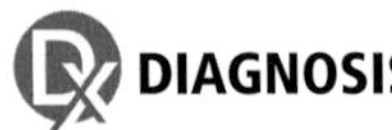

DIAGNOSIS

HISTORY

- ED specific
  - Eating habits
  - Presence of binge or purge behavior
  - Food rituals
  - Body image
  - Exercise history
  - Actual and desired weights, minimum and maximum weights
  - Use of laxatives, diuretics, diet pills, emetics, ipecac, or weight loss supplements
  - Menstrual history—amenorrhea or oligomenorrhea
  - Unease with others watching them eat
  - Preoccupation with food/eating
  - Preoccupation with body weight/shape concerns
  - Fear of loss of control over one's body
- General
  - Weakness or fatigue or hyperactivity
  - Facial fullness
  - Headaches
  - Dizziness
  - Abdominal pain, fullness, or bloating; nausea
  - Constipation or diarrhea
  - Dental caries
  - Irregular menses
- Psychiatric
  - Mood disorder
  - Substance abuse
  - Anxiety
  - Personality disorders
  - Suicidal thoughts
  - Low self-esteem
  - Impulsivity
- Family
  - Medical and psychiatric histories
- Specific questions
  - Do you have a weight goal?
  - How do you control your weight?
  - How do you feel about yourself?
  - Do you ever vomit, use diuretics, laxatives, or other substances to control your weight? If so, how often?
  - Do you exercise? How much?

PHYSICAL EXAM

- Vital signs: Check for hypotension, orthostasis, and hypothermia.
- Weight: may be normal, overweight, or underweight
- Erosion of dental enamel: exposure to gastric acid secondary to frequent vomiting
- Parotid gland enlargement due to vomiting
- Calluses on knuckle or hands: Russell sign secondary to inducing vomiting
- Muscle weakness or cramps: electrolyte disturbance

DIFFERENTIAL DIAGNOSIS

- Psychogenic vomiting
- Drug abuse
- GI obstruction
- Hiatal hernia
- Achalasia, gastroesophageal reflux
- Brain tumor

DIAGNOSTIC TESTS & INTERPRETATION

Initial Tests (screening, lab, imaging)

- Part of the diagnostic workup. Most useful for assessing complications; no diagnostic or confirmatory laboratory test for bulimia nervosa. Many patients have normal labs.
- CBC: iron deficiency anemia
- Erythrocyte sedimentation rate (ESR): almost invariably normal; if elevated, consider occult organic process.
- Electrolytes, including calcium, magnesium, and phosphate: Abnormalities may occur as a result of prolonged vomiting or laxative use. Most common pattern for vomiting is hypokalemic-hypochloremic alkalosis.
- Bicarbonate level: metabolic alkalosis from vomiting or metabolic acidosis if using laxatives or dehydrated
- Glucose: Patient may be hypoglycemic.
- BUN and creatinine: renal function usually normal, but BUN may be elevated secondary to dehydration or altered intake
- Cholesterol, lipids: may be elevated in starvation state
- Amylase: increased secondary to vomiting
- Lipase: increases may indicate severe complications such as pancreatitis
- Total protein, albumin, prealbumin: usually normal, but may be low if with malnutrition
- Liver function tests: Transaminases may be mildly elevated from starvation.
- Urine toxicology screen (optional): may be positive as this disorder often is associated with substance abuse
- Electrocardiogram with rhythm strip: may see U waves with hypokalemia, check QTc
- Consider upper GI series with small bowel follow-through if unclear etiology of vomiting.
- Consider dual-energy x-ray absorptiometry (DXA) study if prolonged amenorrhea to evaluate bone mineral density.

Diagnostic Procedures/Other

Eating Disorder Examination Questionnaire (EDE-Q): Questionnaire assessments may be helpful and augment the diagnostic interview in diagnosing bulimia nervosa.

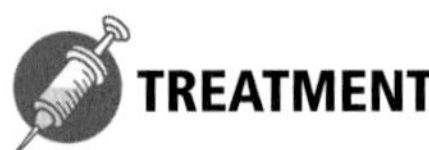

TREATMENT

MEDICATIONS

- Antidepressants
  - Decrease the binge–purge behavior
  - Improve attitudes about eating
  - Lessen preoccupation with food and weight
  - Fluoxetine (Prozac®), sertraline (Zoloft®), desipramine (Norpramin®), citalopram (Celexa®), and fluvoxamine (Luvox®) used with good results
  - Antidepressant effect may diminish over time; may relapse when drug stopped
  - Psychotherapy and cognitive behavioral therapy (CBT) combined with antidepressant therapy appears to yield the best outcome.

- Low response rate to alternative treatments after CBT and 1st-line antidepressant therapy
- Few studies either of medication or psychotherapy in those <18 years of age; however, CBT and family-based therapy appear promising.
- Stool softeners: often of little use for constipation; consider nonstimulating osmotic laxatives if severe.
- Ondansetron: shown in one study to decrease vomiting frequency; may help normalize the physiologic mechanism controlling satiation

ADDITIONAL THERAPIES

- CBT adapted for adolescents (CBT-A) has shown promise. CBT with family involvement may also be effective. Enhanced CBT (CBT-E) has been shown to reduce ED pathology on the EDE-Q. In general, CBT:
  - Can be done in group or individual formats
  - Is more effective than interpersonal psychotherapy or behavioral therapy alone
  - Helps patients determine other ways to cope with the feelings that precipitate purging and to try to correct maladaptive thoughts and beliefs about body image
  - EDE-Q may also be effective in a self-help format, including self-help manual format (CBT-guided self-care).
- Family-based treatment for bulimia nervosa (FBT-BN): Therapist empowers parents to disrupt behaviors such as binge eating, purging, restrictive eating, and other compensatory behaviors. The treatment has shown positive research outcomes. FBT-BN shown to be more effective than CBT-A in reducing binge/purge behaviors at the end of treatment and 6-month follow-up. There were no differences between the two therapies at the year follow-up.
- Dialectical behavioral therapy (DBT): skill-based treatment helpful for adult patients with binge ED and less severe symptoms of bulimia nervosa
- Integrated FBT and DBT for adolescents with bulimia nervosa: This new treatment shows promise: a reduction in binge/purge episodes but not emotional regulation
- Individual interpersonal psychotherapy (IPT) is helpful but takes longer to have an effect.
- Family therapy
- Group therapy
- Outpatient supportive psychotherapy
- Multifamily therapy for bulimia nervosa (MFT-BN) is a new family therapy conducted in a closed group with multiple families >20 weeks. Preliminary findings show reduced ED behaviors.
- Physical activity shown in one study to reduce pursuit of thinness and decrease bingeing/purging behavior. Both physical activity and yoga have shown promise as adjunct treatments.

ADMISSION, INPATIENT, AND NURSING CONSIDERATIONS

Hospitalize in cases of the following:

- Dehydration
- Severe electrolyte disturbances
- Intractable vomiting
- Acute psychiatric emergencies (e.g., suicidal ideation, acute psychosis)
- Medical complication of malnutrition (e.g., aspiration pneumonia, cardiac failure, pancreatitis, Mallory-Weiss syndrome)
- Comorbid diagnosis that interferes with the treatment of the ED (e.g., severe depression, obsessive-compulsive disorder, severe family dysfunction)
- Failure of outpatient therapy

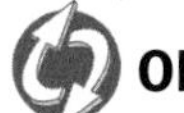

ONGOING CARE

FOLLOW-UP RECOMMENDATIONS

- Encourage routine meals and snacks.
- Reduction in binge and purge episodes may take time.
- Behavioral and thought disorders associated with bulimia nervosa may be of long duration.

Patient Monitoring

Signs to watch for:

- Weight loss or major weight fluctuations
- Electrolyte abnormalities
- Muscle cramps
- Fatigue
- Depression or mood disturbance
- Mood swings/irritability
- Increasing emotional lability
- Menstrual function/irregular menses
- Suicidality

PROGNOSIS

Eating disorders have the highest mortality rate of any mental disorder. Reported mortality rates vary between studies. Part of the variance is because those with an ED may ultimately die of heart failure, organ failure, malnutrition, or suicide. Anorexia nervosa has the highest mortality rate compared with bulimia nervosa and ED not otherwise specified (NOS).

- Most patients have episodic course with trend toward improvement.
- No studies of long-term prognosis in adolescents
- Adult studies at 22 years follow-up
  - 68% of patients achieve recovery from bulimia nervosa.
- Poor prognostic indicators: concomitant depression, personality disorder, substance abuse, frequent vomiting
- Good prognostic indicators
  - High motivation for treatment
  - No concurrent disruptive psychopathology
  - Good self-esteem

COMPLICATIONS

- Pulmonary
  - Aspiration pneumonia
  - Pneumomediastinum
- GI
  - Parotid or salivary gland enlargement
  - Gastric and esophageal irritation and gastroesophageal reflux
  - Mallory-Weiss tears
  - Paralytic ileus (from laxative abuse/hypokalemia)
  - Severe constipation (due to laxative abuse and subsequent dependence)
  - Pancreatitis
- Metabolic
  - Electrolyte imbalances, including hypomagnesemia; acid–base disturbances
  - Hypokalemia (due to laxative abuse/emesis)
  - Secondary cardiac dysrhythmias, myopathy
  - Fluid imbalances
  - Hyperamylasemia
  - Edema (secondary to hypoproteinemia or renal sodium and water retention secondary to hypovolemia and secondary hyperaldosteronism)
  - Bone loss (if amenorrhea; significantly more common in anorexia nervosa)
- Dental
  - Enamel erosion
  - Caries and periodontal disease
- Hormonal
  - Irregular menstrual bleeding

ADDITIONAL READING

- American Psychiatric Association. *Diagnostic and Statistical Manual of Mental Disorders*. 5th ed. Arlington, VA: American Psychiatric Association; 2013.
- Crow SJ, Peterson CB, Swanson SA, et al. Increased mortality in bulimia nervosa and other eating disorders. *Am J Psychiatry*. 2009;166(12):1342–1346.
- Eddy KT, Tabri N, Thomas JJ, et al. Recovery from anorexia nervosa and bulimia nervosa at 22-year follow-up. *J Clin Psychiatry*. 2017;78(2):184–189.
- Kreipe RE, Birndorf SA. Eating disorders in adolescent and young adults. *Med Clin North Am*. 2000;84(4):1027–1049.
- Le Grange D, Lock J, Agras SW, et al. Randomized clinical trial of family-based treatment and cognitive-behavioral therapy for adolescent bulimia nervosa. *J Am Acad Child Adolesc Psychiatry*. 2015;54(11):886–894.e2.
- Lock J. An update on evidence-based psychosocial treatments for eating disorders in children and adolescents. *J Clin Child Adolesc Psychol*. 2015;44(5):707–721.
- Mairs R, Nicholls D. Assessment and treatment of eating disorders in children and adolescents. *Arch Dis Child*. 2016;101(12):1168–1175.
- Smink FR, van Hoeken D, Hoek HW. Epidemiology of eating disorders: incidence, prevalence, and mortality rates. *Curr Psychiatry Rep*. 2012;14(4):406–414.

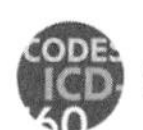

CODES

ICD10

- F50.2 Bulimia nervosa
- F50.9 Eating disorder, unspecified

FAQ

- Q: How do I determine if a patient has anorexia with vomiting or bulimia?
- A: The key feature of anorexia nervosa that distinguishes it from bulimia nervosa is the degree of malnutrition and presence of bingeing. There is a definite crossover between patients with anorexia nervosa and bulimia nervosa. If bingeing and purging is seen in the setting of significant malnutrition with restriction and low weight, the patient is diagnosed with anorexia nervosa.
- Q: What laboratory abnormalities should I look for in my patients with bulimia?
- A: Clinicians should look for electrolyte abnormalities, particularly hypokalemia and bicarbonate elevation. Patients may develop a hypochloremic metabolic alkalosis. If electrolytes are significantly abnormal, hospitalize until normalized.

CAMPYLOBACTER INFECTIONS

Matthew P. Kronman, MD, MSCE

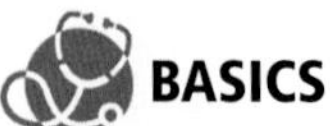

BASICS

DESCRIPTION

Campylobacter species are motile, curved, gram-negative bacilli that are commensal flora of birds, pigs, and cattle and commonly cause bacterial gastroenteritis in humans.

EPIDEMIOLOGY

- *Campylobacter* infections are among the most common causes of enteritis worldwide, with the highest attack rates in children <4 years of age.
- Asymptomatic infection occurs in 30–100% of chickens, turkeys, and water fowl. Other reservoirs of infection include swine, cattle, sheep, horses, rodents, and household pets (especially young pets).
- Contaminated water and unpasteurized milk and milk products are other sources of infection.
- Infections typically occur sporadically, without outbreaks.

Incidence

- Estimated rates of *Campylobacter* infection vary widely worldwide. In the United States, the estimated annual incidence in 2014 was 13.45/100,000 overall, 13% higher than in 2006 to 2008.
- The highest U.S. incidence is for those <5 years of age, at approximately 24/100,000 population.
- Among speciated U.S. infections, historically 90% have been *Campylobacter jejuni* and 8% *Campylobacter coli*. Of all U.S. infections in 2014, 17% resulted in hospitalization and 0.2% in death.
- The incidence is seasonal and generally peaks in summer worldwide.

Prevalence

- Although surveillance data are limited, the highest prevalence of *Campylobacter* infections occur in resource-poor settings.
- *Campylobacter* is the most common cause of travelers' diarrhea in Southeast Asia, accounting for a third of all infections.

RISK FACTORS

- Approximately 40% of *Campylobacter* enteritis is estimated to be attributable to undercooked chicken consumption.
- Other risk factors for *Campylobacter* enteritis include international travel, direct contact with farm animals, chronic disease, poor food preparation hygiene, consumption of chicken prepared outside the home, and use of acid-suppressive medications.
- Children are at higher risk relative to adults.
- In low resource settings, breastfeeding and routine treatment of drinking water are protective among children <2 years of age.
- Frequent exposure to *Campylobacter* (e.g., among food handlers and abattoir workers) may protect against disease.
- Person-to-person transmission of *C. jejuni* has been reported when index cases were young children incontinent of feces or as vertical transmission from mother to neonate.
- Asymptomatic hospital personnel or food handlers have not been implicated as sources.

GENERAL PREVENTION

- Hand washing after contact with animals or animal products, cleaning cooking utensils and cutting boards after contact with raw poultry, proper cooling and storage of foods, pasteurization of milk, and chlorination of water supplies decrease the risk for infection.
- Diapered infants with symptomatic infection should be excluded from child care until resolution of diarrhea.
- No licensed vaccines currently exist, but *C. jejuni* strains with decreased risk of secondary Guillain-Barré syndrome (GBS) are being developed as candidates for capsular polysaccharide conjugate vaccines.

PATHOPHYSIOLOGY

- Transmission of disease is by the fecal–oral route from contaminated food and water or by direct contact with fecal material from animals or persons infected with the organism.
- As few as 500 organisms may be required to produce infection.
- *Campylobacter* spp. possess one or two flagella that provide the organism's motility and facilitate intestinal colonization.
- *C. jejuni* adheres to epithelial cells and mucus, secretes cytotoxins (which play a role in the development of watery diarrhea), can invade intestinal epithelial cells using a microtubule entry system, and induces an inflammatory ileocolitis.
- *Campylobacter* can cause a range of clinical manifestations, including enteritis and rare localized extraintestinal infections.
- Bacteremia, although uncommon, can occur, especially in the neonate and immunocompromised host; *Campylobacter fetus* is the species most likely to be isolated. *C. fetus* can also cause neonatal meningitis.
- *Campylobacter upsaliensis*, *Campylobacter lari*, and *Campylobacter hyointestinalis* have been identified in immunocompromised individuals and are usually associated with a self-limiting enteritis but can occasionally cause systemic illness.

ETIOLOGY

- *Campylobacter* is a motile, curved, microaerophilic, non–lactose-fermenting, oxidase-positive, gram-negative rod that requires oxygen and carbon dioxide for optimal growth.
- Three main *Campylobacter* species involved in human infections include *C. jejuni*, *C. coli* (which cause enteritis), and *C. fetus* (implicated in systemic illness in neonates and compromised hosts). Rarer human pathogens include *Campylobacter concisus*, *Campylobacter curvus*, *C. hyointestinalis*, *C. lari*, *Campylobacter rectus*, *Campylobacter sputorum*, and *C. upsaliensis*.

COMMONLY ASSOCIATED CONDITIONS

Campylobacteriosis occurs in both healthy and immunocompromised individuals.

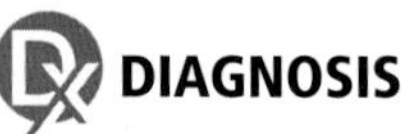

DIAGNOSIS

HISTORY

- Enteritis is characterized by fever, abdominal pain, and bloody diarrhea.
- Symptoms can last for 24 hours and be indistinguishable from viral gastroenteritis or appendicitis, or can be relapsing, thus mimicking inflammatory bowel disease.
- In some patients, illness can be severe, resembling dysentery.
- Incubation period is usually 2 to 5 days, and symptoms are usually self-limited and resolve within 5 to 7 days.

PHYSICAL EXAM

- Abdominal tenderness, diarrhea, malaise, and fever are common signs and symptoms of infection.
- Stools can contain occult or visible blood.
- Inflammatory ileocolitis is the most common manifestation in children.
- If the infection establishes a chronic phase (20% of infected patients), symptoms may mimic inflammatory bowel disease and other immunoreactive complications may occur.

ALERT

Not all bacterial colitis presents with blood or mucus in the stool. Therefore, increased suspicion for bacterial colitis should exist if the diarrhea is prolonged or the patient has appropriate exposures.

DIFFERENTIAL DIAGNOSIS

- *Campylobacter* infection should be considered in all patients with a diarrheal illness, especially those with blood or mucus in their stool, recurrent gastritis, or in immunocompromised hosts.
- Symptoms can overlap with those of appendicitis or inflammatory bowel disease.
- Additional intestinal bacterial pathogens include *Aeromonas*, *Campylobacter*, *Clostridium difficile*, *Escherichia coli*, *Listeria*, *Plesiomonas*, *Salmonella*, *Shigella*, *Vibrio* species, and *Yersinia*.
- Other viral and parasitic pathogens include amebiasis, adenovirus types 40 and 41, *Cryptosporidium*, *Cyclospora*, *Cystoisospora*, *Giardia*, norovirus, rotavirus, and astrovirus.

DIAGNOSTIC TESTS & INTERPRETATION

Initial Tests (screening, lab, imaging)

- Stool culture requires selective media (Skirrow, Butzler, or campy-BAP), microaerophilic conditions, and an incubation temperature of 42°C to isolate important *Campylobacter* species.
- *C. fetus*, *C. hyointestinalis*, and *C. upsaliensis* may not be detected on *Campylobacter*-selective media due to their sensitivity to antimicrobial agents in the media.

Diagnostic Procedures/Other

Rapid multiplex assays using quantitative real-time PCR to detect and differentiate *Campylobacter* spp. from other enteropathogens have been developed and a number have excellent sensitivity (>97%) and specificity (>98%) compared to stool culture. These methods may identify *Campylobacter* spp. twice as often as routine culture methods.

Test Interpretation

Examination of fecal specimens for darting motility of *C. jejuni* by darkfield or phase-contrast microscopy within 2 hours of passage can permit presumptive diagnosis.

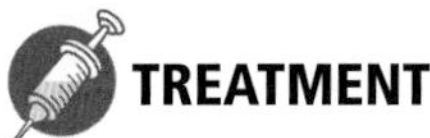

TREATMENT

GENERAL MEASURES

Immunocompetent children with diarrhea usually improve with rehydration alone.

MEDICATION

First Line

- Most patients have self-limited infection.
- Selected patient populations (HIV and other immunocompromised individuals, pregnant women) may benefit from early therapy.
- If treated in the first 3 days of enteritis, the macrolides erythromycin (40 mg/kg/24 h orally in 4 divided doses for 5 days) or azithromycin (10 mg/kg/24 h orally once daily for 3 days) appear effective in eradicating the organism from the stool within 2 to 3 days and shortening the course of diarrhea.
- Ampicillin (50 to 100 mg/kg/dose IV every 6 hours), ciprofloxacin (10 mg/kg/dose IV every 12 hours), tetracycline (25 to 50 mg/kg/24 h orally divided every 6 hours), gentamicin (2.5 mg/kg/dose IV every 8 hours), and imipenem (60 to 100 mg/kg/day IV divided every 6 hours) are alternatives if resistant or bacteremic strains are present, although fluoroquinolone resistance is increasingly common and thought to be related to human and agricultural antibiotic use.
- Macrolide resistance is approximately 5%.
- Treatment duration for enteritis is 3 to 5 days.
- Appropriate bacteremia treatment should be based on antimicrobial susceptibility testing.

ISSUES FOR REFERRAL

Specific follow-up is unnecessary.

ADDITIONAL THERAPIES

Antimotility agents can prolong symptoms and should be avoided.

ADMISSION, INPATIENT, AND NURSING CONSIDERATIONS

- Correct initial dehydration.
- Admit those requiring IV fluids.
- Use normal saline to correct dehydration. IV fluids should contain dextrose if being used for maintenance fluid requirements.
- Contact precautions are recommended for admitted infected infants and children incontinent of stool and should be maintained until they receive 48 hours of antibiotics or have remained asymptomatic for 48 hours.
- Discharge rehydrated patients able to maintain hydration orally.

ONGOING CARE

FOLLOW-UP RECOMMENDATIONS

Patient Monitoring

- In untreated patients, the median organism excretion is 2 to 3 weeks but can be up to 3 months.
- Asymptomatic carriage is uncommon.

DIET

Avoid undercooked poultry and unpasteurized milk and milk products. Resume a normal diet when tolerated.

PATIENT EDUCATION

Symptoms resolve in 1 week for most people.

PROGNOSIS

For patients with enteritis, the prognosis is very good, regardless of whether antibiotic treatment is given.

COMPLICATIONS

- Postinfectious immunologic complications include reactive arthritis, GBS, Miller-Fisher syndrome (a GBS variant predominantly affecting eye movement), reactive arthritis, and erythema nodosum.
- GBS is estimated to affect 1 in 1,000 patients with *Campylobacter* infection.
- *C. jejuni* (serotypes O:19 and O:41) is the most frequently identified GBS cause and is responsible for up to 40% of U.S. GBS cases.
- HLA-B27 antigen is associated with reactive arthropathy. The estimated incidence of reactive arthritis after *Campylobacter* infection ranges from 0% to 7%, but a systematic review identified the incidence as approximately 2.9%.
- Children with high fever may develop seizures.
- Some studies have demonstrated associations between *Campylobacter* infection and both irritable bowel syndrome and inflammatory bowel disease.
- Spontaneous abortion and hemolytic uremic syndrome are described with *C. upsaliensis*.

ADDITIONAL READING

- Amour C, Gratz J, Mduma E, et al; for Etiology, Risk Factors, and Interactions of Enteric Infections and Malnutrition and the Consequences for Child Health and Development Project Network Investigators. Epidemiology and impact of *Campylobacter* infection in children in 8 low-resource settings: results from the MAL-ED study. *Clin Infect Dis*. 2016;63(9):1171–1179.
- Buss SN, Leber A, Chapin K, et al. Multicenter evaluation of the BioFire FilmArray gastrointestinal panel for etiologic diagnosis of infectious gastroenteritis. *J Clin Microbiol*. 2015;53(3):915–925.
- Crim SM, Griffin PM, Tauxe R, et al. Preliminary incidence and trends of infection with pathogens transmitted commonly through food—Foodborne Diseases Active Surveillance Network, 10 U.S. sites, 2006–2014. *MMWR Morb Mortal Wkly Rep*. 2015;64(18):495–499.
- Domingues AR, Pires SM, Halasa T, et al. Source attribution of human campylobacteriosis using a meta-analysis of case-control studies of sporadic infections. *Epidemiol Infect*. 2012;140(6):970–981.
- Keithlin J, Sargeant J, Thomas MK, et al. Systematic review and meta-analysis of the proportion of *Campylobacter* cases that develop chronic sequelae. *BMC Public Health*. 2014;14:1203.
- Kirkpatrick BD, Tribble DR. Update on human *Campylobacter jejuni* infections. *Curr Opin Gastroenterol*. 2011;27(1):1–7.
- Lal A, Hales S, French N, et al. Seasonality in human zoonotic enteric diseases: a systematic review. *PLoS One*. 2012;7(4):e31883.
- Liu J, Platts-Mills JA, Juma J, et al. Use of quantitative molecular diagnostic methods to identify causes of diarrhoea in children: a reanalysis of the GEMS case-control study. *Lancet*. 2016;388(10051):1291–1301.
- Ross AG, Olds GR, Cripps AW, et al. Enteropathogens and chronic illness in returning travelers. *N Engl J Med*. 2013;368(19):1817–1825.

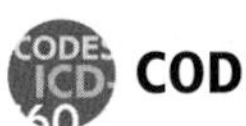

CODES

ICD10

A04.5 Campylobacter enteritis

FAQ

- Q: Is treatment necessary for asymptomatic children when *Campylobacter* is isolated as the pathogen causing the enteritis?
- A: No treatment is needed in this situation.
- Q: Can one develop immunity to *Campylobacter* infections?
- A: Immunity to *C. jejuni* is acquired after one or more infections. For children living in endemic areas, effective natural immunity is a result of significant repeated early exposure.
- Q: How are *C. jejuni* infection and GBS related?
- A: Many strains of *C. jejuni* have surface glycolipids that are similar to gangliosides, which are abundant in the central and peripheral nervous systems. Anti-*Campylobacter* antibodies bind to the gangliosides through molecular mimicry, causing the demyelinating process characteristic of GBS.

CANCER THERAPY LATE EFFECTS

Trish Murphy, RN, MSN • Robert I. Raphael, MD

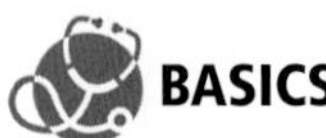

BASICS

DESCRIPTION

The majority of children diagnosed with cancer will reach adulthood. Childhood cancer survivors require unique medical follow-up. Risks of late effects depend on the treatments received as well as the type and site of cancer. The Children's Oncology Group's long-term follow-up guidelines serve as the basis for many of the recommendations in this chapter.

EPIDEMIOLOGY

- Long-term survival into adulthood for a child diagnosed with cancer is nearly 80%.
- Among adults treated for childhood cancer:
  - Nearly 2/3 of survivors will develop one or more chronic health condition.
  - Nearly 1/3 of survivors will experience severe or life-threatening complications during adulthood.
- Approximately 450,000 childhood cancer survivors live in the United States.
- These numbers will continue to grow as new cancer therapies become available and more children survive.

RISK FACTORS

Late effects of cancer therapy are influenced by tumor-related, treatment-related and host factors.

PATHOPHYSIOLOGY

Risk of organ dysfunction is related to primary cancer location and treatment used. See detailed systems-based evaluations in the following sections.

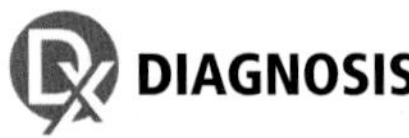

DIAGNOSIS

HISTORY

It is essential for the primary care physician to obtain a thorough cancer treatment summary, including the following:

- Date of diagnosis/age at diagnosis
- Type of cancer, stage, histology
- Site of primary tumor and metastatic sites
- Relapse(s) and date(s)
- Treatment modalities
  - Significant surgical procedures
  - Treatment protocol(s)
  - Chemotherapy
    - Drugs and cumulative dosages
    - Age of first anthracycline therapy
  - Radiation therapy (XRT)
    - Type
    - Site/dose
    - Total/boost doses
  - Hematopoietic stem cell transplant (HSCT)
    - Type and date of transplant
    - Source: bone marrow, cord blood, or peripheral blood stem cells
    - Conditioning regimen
  - Immunotherapy: types/cumulative doses

PHYSICAL EXAM

Annual physical exam of the entire body with particular attention to organ systems as listed in the following sections

TREATMENT

Treatment depends on specific long-term effects; see discussion for organ system-specific ongoing care and screening.

ONGOING CARE

The following section reviews organ systems at risk (alphabetically), risk factors to consider and recommending screening

- General issues
  - Regular visits with primary care provider and oncologist or long-term follow-up program
  - Dental exams and cleanings every 6 months
  - Promptly assess signs or symptoms of subsequent neoplasms (SNs).
  - Assess psychosocial functioning at each visit.
  - Maintain health insurance coverage.
  - Immunizations may require updates.

ALERT

- Reimmunize after chemotherapy per oncologist and using Centers for Disease Control and Prevention (CDC) guidelines.
- Psychosocial assessment of the patient should be performed at each clinic visit.

- Bladder toxicity
  - Chronic infections
    - Risk factors: cystectomy
  - Hemorrhagic cystitis, fibrosis, dysfunctional voiding
    - Risk factors: ≥30 Gy XRT to spine, flank, abdomen, pelvis, bladder, or total body irradiation (TBI), cyclophosphamide, ifosfamide
  - Urinary incontinence or tract obstruction
    - Risk factors: pelvic surgery, hysterectomy
  - Screening: annual detailed voiding history; bladder ultrasound and urinalysis as needed
- Bone toxicity
  - Decreased bone mineral density, osteopenia, osteonecrosis, increased risk of fractures
    - Risk factors: corticosteroids, high-dose methotrexate, ≥40 Gy XRT to any field, or HSCT
    - Screening: Consider bone density evaluation with DEXA scan at entry to long-term follow-up, ensure adequate vitamin D intake.
  - Scoliosis or kyphosis
    - Risk factors: spine or thoracic surgery, XRT to spine, chest, lungs, or abdomen
    - Spine exam annually until growth is complete
  - Bone growth failure
    - Risk factors: XRT to any field, especially cranium, spine, trunk, or TBI
    - Screening: Measure height, weight, sitting height yearly.
- Cardiovascular toxicity
  - Cardiomyopathy, left ventricular dysfunction, and arrhythmias
    - Risk factors: anthracyclines (daunorubicin, doxorubicin/adriamycin, epirubicin, idarubicin, mitoxantrone) and/or XRT to the thorax or abdomen
    - Screening: echocardiogram (ECHO)/multigated acquisition (MUGA) every 1 to 5 years, depending on cumulative dose of anthracyclines, age at first dose, and field of XRT (involving heart).
    - Consider close monitoring during pregnancy.

ALERT

Anthracycline and XRT to the heart/chest/lungs/neck increases risk of cardiovascular disease; at-risk patients require detailed history, exam, and frequent ECHO/MUGA screening.

  - Carotid artery or subclavian artery disease
    - Risk factors: ≥40 Gy XRT to head, neck, chest, lungs, or TBI
    - Examine for carotid bruits or diminished carotid/brachial/radial pulses.
  - Thrombosis at prior central venous catheter site
    - Inspect site for pain/swelling.
  - Dyslipidemia
    - Risk factors: TBI
    - Screening: fasting lipid panel every 2 years
  - Vasospastic attacks (Raynaud phenomenon)
    - Risk factors: vincristine or vinblastine
- Dermatologic toxicity
  - Skin cancer, dysplastic nevi, fibrosis, alopecia, telangiectasias, nail/pigmentation changes
    - Risk factors: any XRT, HSCT with chronic graft-versus-host disease (cGVHD)
    - Encourage monthly self-skin exams.
- Endocrine toxicity
  - Thyroid dysfunction, nodules, and cancer
    - Risk factors: XRT to neck, head, spine, mediastinum, TBI, or therapeutic systemic metaiodobenzylguanidine (MIBG)
    - Screening: thyroid exam and TSH/free T_4 annually
  - Growth hormone deficiency
    - Risk factors: XRT to cranium or TBI, brain neurosurgery
    - Height, weight, BMI, Tanner stage every 6 months until mature and then annually
    - If at risk: insulin-like growth factor (IGF)-1, IGF-2, and IGFBP-3
  - Central adrenal insufficiency
    - Risk factors: ≥30 Gy XRT to cranium, TBI, brain neurosurgery
    - Screening: annual endocrinology visit
  - Hyperprolactinemia
    - Risk factors: ≥40 Gy XRT to cranium, TBI
    - If symptomatic, screen with prolactin level
  - Hypopituitarism
    - Risk factors: brain neurosurgery, ≥30 Gy XRT to cranium, TBI
    - Screening labs: cortisol, prolactin, testosterone/estradiol, IGF-1, TSH, FSH, LH
  - Diabetes mellitus/impaired glucose metabolism
    - Risk factors: abdominal radiation, TBI, prolonged corticosteroid use, family history
    - Screening labs: fasting blood glucose or HgbA1c at least every 2 years
  - Obesity
    - Risk factors: XRT to cranium, brain neurosurgery, prolonged corticosteroid use
    - Height, weight, BMI, BP annually
- Gastrointestinal toxicity
  - Esophageal stricture
    - Risk factors: ≥30 Gy XRT to spine, neck, chest, lung, mediastinum, mantle, abdomen, TBI or HSCT with cGVHD
  - Cholelithiasis
    - Risk factors: ≥30 Gy XRT to abdomen, flank, liver, kidneys, TBI
  - Strictures, fistula, chronic enterocolitis
    - Risk factors: ≥30 Gy XRT to neck, chest, spine, abdomen, liver, kidneys, pelvis, TBI

- Bowel obstruction/adhesions
  - Risk factors: laparotomy or ≥30 Gy XRT to abdomen, pelvis, or spine
- Fecal incontinence
  - Risk factors: pelvic or spinal cord surgery, cystectomy
- Hepatic toxicity
  - Chronic hepatitis C
    - Risk factor: blood products prior to 1993
    - Screening: hepatitis C antibody, PCR if positive
  - Hepatic dysfunction
    - Risk factors: methotrexate, mercaptopurine (6-MP), thioguanine (6-TG), HSCT
  - Veno-occlusive disease
    - Risk factors: mercaptopurine or thioguanine
    - Obtain baseline: ALT/AST/bilirubin; ferritin after HSCT
- Musculoskeletal toxicity
  - Orthopedic complications
    - Risk factors: amputation, limb-sparing surgery
    - Screening evaluation of affected limb or prosthesis every 6 months until skeletally mature and then annually; annual radiographs after limb-sparing procedure
- Neurologic toxicity
  - Peripheral neuropathy
    - Risk factors: cisplatin, carboplatin, vincristine, or vinblastine
  - Cerebrovascular complications
    - Risk factors: ≥18 Gy XRT to cranium or TBI
  - Neurocognitive difficulties
    - Risk factors: brain neurosurgery, methotrexate (intrathecal or high-dose), high-dose IV cytarabine, XRT to cranium, TBI
  - Seizures, motor/sensory deficits, or hydrocephalus following brain neurosurgery
  - Clinical leukoencephalopathy following methotrexate, high-dose IV cytarabine, or XRT to cranium or TBI
  - Neuropathic pain risk following amputation
  - Neurogenic bowel/bladder, incontinence, sexual dysfunction risk after spinal cord neurosurgery
- Ophthalmologic toxicity
  - Cataracts/ocular issues
    - Risk factors: corticosteroids, busulfan, XRT to orbit/eye, cranium, or TBI
    - Annual funduscopic and visual acuity exams
    - Annual ophthalmologist exam as indicated
- Ototoxicity
  - Hearing loss, vertigo, or tinnitus
    - Risk factors: cisplatin, carboplatin: myeloablative or any does <1 year; XRT >30 Gy to ear, cranium, or TBI
    - Baseline audiogram (annually if loss detected)
    - Otoscopic exam annually
- Oral toxicity
  - Tooth enamel dysplasia and root/tooth agenesis or root thinning/shortening
    - Risk factors: any chemotherapy (particularly at a young age), XRT to head/neck
  - Xerostomia or salivary gland dysfunction
    - Risk factors: head/neck XRT or cGVHD
  - Osteoradionecrosis
    - Risk factors: ≥40 Gy XRT to head, neck, TBI
  - Screening: oral exam annually; dental cleaning and exam every 6 months
- Pulmonary toxicity
  - Fibrosis, dyspnea, decreased lung function
    - Risk factors: bleomycin, busulfan, carmustine, lomustine, XRT to chest or lungs, or TBI
    - If at risk, obtain baseline pulmonary function testing, and as clinically indicated.
- Psychosocial disorders
  - Neurocognitive, educational, or vocational difficulties
    - Risk factors: any treatment, especially high-dose/intrathecal methotrexate, high-dose cytarabine, brain neurosurgery or XRT to head or TBI
    - Educational/vocational assessment annually
    - Formal neuropsychological evaluation as indicated
  - Posttraumatic stress, depression, anxiety, risky behaviors, body image disturbance
    - Risk factors: any cancer treatment
    - Assess mental health at each clinic visit.
- Renal toxicity
  - Hypertension or renal dysfunction
    - Risk factors: nephrectomy or carboplatin, cisplatin, ifosfamide, high-dose methotrexate, or XRT to liver, kidneys, flank, abdomen, TBI, or HSCT
  - Hydronephrosis, dysfunctional voiding, vesicoureteral reflux
    - Risk factors: cyclophosphamide, ifosfamide, ≥30 Gy XRT to abdomen, flank, or pelvis
  - Urinary incontinence or tract obstruction
    - Risk factor: pelvic surgery
  - Baseline: BUN/Cr, Na/K/Cl/CO_2, Mg, phosphorus, Ca
  - Screening: annual UA and BP if at risk or after nephrectomy
- Reproductive toxicity
  - Gonadal dysfunction: infertility, azoospermia, oligospermia, hypogonadism, delayed or arrested puberty, sexual dysfunction, early menopause, testosterone deficiency
    - Risk factors: spinal neurosurgery, orchiectomy, alkylating agents (busulfan, carmustine, chlorambucil, cyclophosphamide, ifosfamide, lomustine, mechlorethamine, melphalan, procarbazine, thiotepa), carboplatin, cisplatin, dacarbazine, temozolomide, XRT to gonads, pelvis, abdomen, cranium, or TBI
    - Assess Tanner stage yearly until mature.
    - Males: Screen with FSH/LH/testosterone at 14 years or if symptomatic and semen analysis as requested.
    - Females: Screen with FSH/LH/estradiol at 13 years or with delayed puberty/amenorrhea/irregular menses/estrogen deficiency symptoms.
- Subsequent neoplasms (SNs)
  - Increased risk varies by host factors, primary cancer therapy, and environmental exposures.
  - The Childhood Cancer Survivor Study reported a 30-year cumulative incidence of 20.5%.
  - The risk of SNs remains elevated for >30 years following primary cancer diagnosis.
  - Patients with genetic cancer predisposition syndromes are at increased risk of SNs.
  - 80% of SNs are solid tumors and demonstrate a strong relationship with ionizing radiation.
  - Blood cancer: acute lymphoblastic leukemia (ALL), acute myeloid leukemia (AML), and therapy-related myelodysplastic syndrome (t-MDS)
    - Risk factors: alkylating agents, anthracyclines, carboplatin, cisplatin, dacarbazine, temozolomide
    - Topoisomerase II inhibitor–associated AML occurs 6 months to 3 years after exposure.
    - Alkylating agent–associated t-MDS/AML occurs 3 to 5 years after exposure.
    - Screen with annual complete blood count with differential for 10 years following treatment.
    - Perform dermatologic exam for petechiae, purpura, and pallor at each visit.
  - Bladder cancer
    - Risk factors: cyclophosphamide, XRT to bladder, prostate, abdomen, pelvis, vagina, flank, inguinal region, or sacral/whole spine
    - Obtain annual detailed voiding history.
  - Bone cancer in any XRT field
    - Perform annual inspection/palpation of the bones/soft tissues/skin in XRT field.
  - Brain tumors
    - Risk factors: XRT to cranium or TBI
    - Perform annual neurologic exam.
  - Breast cancer
    - Risk factors: XRT to chest, lungs, mediastinum, axilla, mantle, or TBI
    - Annual breast exam from puberty to age 25 years; after age 25 years, perform every 6 months.
    - ≥20 Gy XRT: annual mammogram and breast MRI beginning at age 25 or 8 years post-XRT (whichever is last); 10 to 19 Gy XRT: Consider testing.
  - Colorectal cancer
    - Risk factors: ≥30 Gy XRT to spine, liver, kidneys, flank, abdomen, pelvis, or TBI
    - Perform colonoscopy at age 35 years or 10 years after XRT (whichever is last), every 5 years.
    - Familial adenomatous polyposis (FAP), start colonoscopy at 21 years; hereditary nonpolysis colorectal cancer (HNPCC), start at puberty
  - Skin cancer
    - Risk factors: any XRT
    - Perform annual dermatologic exam in XRT field.
    - Encourage monthly self-skin exams.
  - Thyroid cancer
    - Risk factors: XRT to cranium, neck, spine, supraclavicular, mediastinum, mantle, chest, lungs, or TBI
    - Perform annual thyroid exam.

ADDITIONAL READING

- Armstrong GT, Liu Q, Yasui Y, et al. Late mortality among 5-year survivors of childhood cancer: a summary from the Childhood Cancer Survivor Study. *J Clin Oncol*. 2009;27(14):2328–2338.
- Centers for Disease Control and Prevention. Immunization schedules. http://www.cdc.gov/vaccines/schedules/. Accessed February 5, 2015.
- Children's Oncology Group. Long-term follow-up guidelines for survivors of childhood, adolescent, and young adult cancers. http://wwwsurvivorshipguidelines.org/. Accessed February 5, 2015
- Oeffinger KC, Mertens AC, Sklar CA, et al; for Childhood Cancer Survivor Study. Chronic health conditions in adult survivors of childhood cancer. *N Engl J Med*. 2006;355(15):1572–1582.

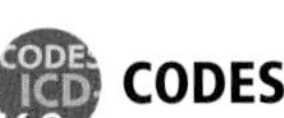

CODES

ICD10

- T88.7XXS Unspecified adverse effect of drug or medicament, sequela
- Z85 Personal history of malignant neoplasm
- Z92.21 Personal history of antineoplastic chemotherapy

FAQ

- Q: Who is considered a cancer "survivor"?
- A: Anyone from time of cancer diagnosis until end of life. Many long-term follow-up clinics specialize in patients who are 2 years post-cancer therapy.
- Q: Where can I find the latest long-term follow-up guidelines for childhood cancer survivors?
- A: http://www.survivorshipguidelines.org/

CANDIDIASIS

Rebecca Schein, MD

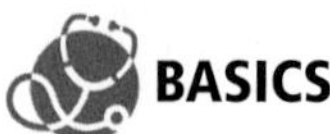

BASICS

DESCRIPTION

Candidiasis is an infection caused by species of the yeast *Candida* resulting in a wide spectrum of disease.

- Mucocutaneous infections include oral thrush, vaginitis, and infections of skin folds as well as esophagitis or laryngitis.
- Invasive disease includes bloodstream infection or candidemia, disseminated candidiasis, endocarditis, central nervous system (CNS) infection, osteomyelitis, and catheter-associated peritonitis and urinary tract infections.

EPIDEMIOLOGY

- *Candida* species are common, ubiquitous yeast. *Candida albicans* is part of the normal human microbiome and lives on the skin, in the mouth, intestinal tract, and vaginal mucosa.
- Vulvovaginitis is associated with pregnancy and can be transmitted to the newborn infant in utero, during delivery or after birth.
  - Neonatal thrush and vaginal candidiasis occur mainly in healthy hosts.
- Candidiasis is an opportunistic infection.
  - Invasive disease and chronic or recurrent mucocutaneous disease are associated with AIDS, primary immunodeficiency, and cancer treatment.
- Person-to-person transmission is rare.
- The incubation period is unknown.
- Oral candidiasis occurs in 5–7% of normal newborns and about 20% of persons with AIDS or cancer.
- Genital or vulvovaginal candidiasis is very common with nearly 75% of women reporting at vaginal yeast infection.
- Invasive candidiasis is a common health care associated infection with ~46,000 U.S. cases a year.

RISK FACTORS

- General risk factors:
  - Corticosteroid use
  - Broad-spectrum antibiotic use
  - Diabetes mellitus
  - AIDS
  - Cancer chemotherapy
  - Neutrophil defects
  - Organ transplantation
- Oral thrush
  - Occurs mainly in babies in the 1st month of life, the elderly, and persons with immune compromise
  - *Candida* may live on oral devices like bottle nipples, pacifiers, and dentures causing recurrent or prolonged infection.
- Intertriginous candidiasis is associated with obesity.
- Genital candidiasis is more common in pregnancy.
- Invasive candidiasis is often a health care–associated infection and is associated with central venous catheters, intensive care unit (ICU) stay, dialysis, renal failure, and gastrointestinal surgery.

GENERAL PREVENTION

- Clean bottles, nipples, and pacifiers in hot water.
- Avoid unnecessary antibiotic use and limit antibiotic duration.
- Remove indwelling catheters as soon as possible.
- Hospitals should use bundles to prevent catheter infections. Consider daily chlorhexidine baths.
- Ensure proper hygiene with urine catheters and peritoneal dialysis catheters.

PATHOPHYSIOLOGY

- *Candida* species are yeast that reproduce via budding.
- Mucocutaneous disease is typically caused by the hosts own organisms.
  - Changes in vaginal pH or hormonal changes may predispose to genital disease.
  - Oral and skin infections occur when diseases like cancer or diabetes or medications like antibiotics or steroids cause imbalance in the normal environment.
- Invasive disease occurs when *Candida* species enter the bloodstream and spread through the body. Invasive infection is typically health care–associated and related to catheter use including blood stream central venous lines, urinary and peritoneal catheters.

ETIOLOGY

- >15 species of *Candida* cause human disease with 95% of infections caused by *C. albicans*, *Candida glabrata*, *Candida tropicalis*, *Candida parapsilosis*, and *Candida krusei*. *Candida* spp. may cause disease at any site.
- Superficial infections include thrush or oropharyngeal candidiasis and diaper dermatitis both of which are most common in infancy and intertriginous candidiasis which occurs in skinfolds generally in healthy patients with chronic moisture, recent antibiotic use, or obesity.
- Esophagitis results in mucosal irregularities and swallowing difficulty and is seen with primary immune deficiencies and is an AIDS defining illness.
- Chronic mucocutaneous candidiasis is caused by a T-cell defect resulting in decreased production of *Candida*-specific antibody resulting in a superficial infection of the skin, hair, mucous membranes, and nails.
- Congenital cutaneous candidiasis is a rare ascending infection into the uterus prior to birth that causes a diffuse red rash.
- Invasive candidiasis may be isolated to the blood stream; that is, candidemia or disseminated candidiasis with fungal invasion of the liver, spleen, bone, kidneys, and/or brain. Fungal sepsis may occur.

COMMONLY ASSOCIATED CONDITIONS

- Diabetes mellitus
- Cancer
- Organ transplant
- Primary neutropenia
- AIDS
- Obesity

DIAGNOSIS

HISTORY

- Thrush causes pain with eating or swallowing.
- Esophageal symptoms are dysphagia, odynophagia, and retrosternal pain.
- Diaper dermatitis is a bright red rash that may be painful when the diaper is soiled.
- Vulvovaginitis symptoms include pruritus, vaginal discharge, and dysuria.
- Candidemia and invasive disease signs and symptoms are nonspecific and include persistent fever and eventually signs of sepsis.
- In neonates, disseminated disease causes temperature instability, lethargy, hypothermia, hypotension, respiratory distress, abdominal distension, hyperglycemia, and feeding intolerance.
- Chronic mucocutaneous candidiasis manifests as severe, recurrent thrush, onychomycosis, vaginitis, and chronic skin lesions.
- Endophthalmitis causes decreased visual acuity.
- CNS disease is a meningoencephalitis with fever, stiff neck, altered mentation, and headache and may be asymptomatic in infants.
- Renal disease manifests as pyelonephritis, flank mass, or urinary obstruction.

PHYSICAL EXAM

- Thrush
  - White cottage cheese–like adherent plaques on the tongue, buccal mucosa, pharynx, and gingiva
  - The lesions are difficult to scrape away and the underlying mucosa may be ulcerated.
- Diaper dermatitis
  - An erythematous rash with pustules and papules and superficial scale that become confluent over time
  - Satellite lesions are classic.
- Vulvovaginitis results in a white or watery vaginal discharge and erythematous vaginal mucosa with adherent white plaques.
- Candidiasis typically has minimal clinical findings but can present with a macular or pustular rash.
- Endophthalmitis causes focal, white, infiltrative, mound-like lesions on the retina and sometimes a vitreal haze.
- CNS infection, endocarditis, osteomyelitis, and peritonitis are clinically indistinguishable from bacterial infections and diagnosed via culture.

DIFFERENTIAL DIAGNOSIS

- Invasive: acute bacterial infections including *Pseudomonas* and fungal disease like *Aspergillus* and *Cryptococcus*
- Genital: bacterial vaginitis and *Trichomonas*
- Oral: aphthous ulcers, herpes simplex

DIAGNOSTIC TESTS & INTERPRETATION

Initial Tests (screening, lab, imaging)

- Mucocutaneous candidiasis is primarily a clinical diagnosis.
  - In difficult cases, yeast may be identified microscopically from a skin scraping.
  - The rash or lesion should be gently scraped with a scalpel to obtain a few cells on a slide. The slide is then stained with potassium hydroxide and fungal elements are visualized under the microscope.
- Bloodstream and invasive disease are diagnosed by growth of *Candida* from sterile body fluid or tissue. *Candida* will grow from blood, urine, CSF, bone marrow, or biopsy specimens.
- *Candida* will grow rapidly on standard blood culture media.

ALERT
Candida from a blood culture should never be considered a contaminant.

- β-D glucan is a cell wall constituent of various fungi and can be detected in the serum of patients with disseminated candidiasis. Although not specific for candidiasis, an elevated β-D glucan is suggestive of an invasive fungal infection.
- *Candida* nucleic acid testing is available and may be used on blood specimens for earlier detection of candidemia.
- *Candida* antibody-antigen testing is widely available in Europe but limited in the United States and role in diagnosis and management remains unclear.

Diagnostic Procedures/Other
- Blood cultures may miss deep-seated infections. Tissue biopsy may be required to make the diagnosis.
- As 16% of patients with candidemia have eye involvement, a dilated funduscopic exam by an ophthalmologist is recommended.
- A lumbar puncture and retinal exam should be performed on infants with *Candida* in blood or urine.
- A CT scan or ultrasound or the liver, spleen, and genitourinary (GU) tract looking for fungal mass should be performed if candidiasis persists.

Test Interpretation
- *Candida* species appear as budding yeast. *C. albicans* is pleomorphic and forms branching pseudohyphae.
- *Candida* species grown from respiratory specimens are rarely pathogenic.

ALERT
Maintain a high index of suspicion for invasive candidiasis in an immunocompromised patient. Persistent fevers despite antibiotic therapy, a diffuse rash, and visual complaints are important clues.

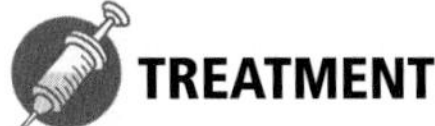

TREATMENT

GENERAL MEASURES
- Critically ill patients at risk for invasive candidiasis should receive empiric therapy with micafungin, caspofungin, or alternatively high-dose fluconazole.
- Central venous lines should be removed from nonneutropenic patients with candidiasis and from neutropenic patients with line-related infections.
- Infected hardware including CNS drains and cardiac devices should be removed or replaced.
- Nurseries with high rates (>10%) of invasive candidiasis should place low-birth-weight infants on fluconazole (3 to 6 mg/kg twice a week) prophylaxis.
- Adult ICUs with >5% invasive candidiasis can consider prophylaxis fluconazole.

MEDICATION
First Line
- Oral and esophageal candidiasis:
  - Nystatin suspension is 1st-line therapy for thrush in infants, whereas clotrimazole lozenges may be used in older patients.
  - Fluconazole (3 to 6 mg/kg) is the treatment for moderate to severe oral thrush (10 to 14 days) and esophageal infection (14 to 21 days).
- Cutaneous
  - Topical agents like clotrimazole, miconazole, and nystatin
- Vaginal candidiasis
  - Topical agents like clotrimazole, miconazole, butoconazole, and terconazole are highly effective and 1st-line therapy.
  - Fluconazole (10 mg/kg up to 150 mg as a single dose) is an alternative.
- Urinary infections—cystitis or pyelonephritis
  - Only treat high-risk patients.
  - Fluconazole (10 mg/kg or 200 mg daily) for 14 days is primary therapy.
  - Amphotericin B deoxycholate for 1 to 7 days is the alternative.
- Systemic or disseminated candidiasis
  - Echinocandins like micafungin (2 mg/kg daily dose) and caspofungin (70 mg/m^2 loading dose, then 50 mg/m^2 daily dose) are 1st-line therapy.
  - Lipid-based amphotericin B (3 to 6 mg/kg daily) is an alternative.
  - Fluconazole (12 mg/kg single loading dose followed by a 6 mg/kg daily dose) may be used in patients not severely ill and not on fluconazole prophylaxis.
  - Voriconazole may be used empirically in febrile neutropenic patients when dual coverage for *Aspergillus* is required.
  - Treatment is a minimum of 2 weeks from culture sterility and may be longer depending on organ involvement.
- Neonatal candidiasis
  - Traditional amphotericin B deoxycholate (1 mg/kg daily dose) is 1st-line therapy.
  - Fluconazole (25 mg/kg single loading dose followed by a 12 mg/kg daily dose) is an alternative. As resistance can occur fluconazole should be avoided in infants who received fluconazole prophylaxis.

Second Line
- Oral and esophageal candidiasis
  - Itraconazole and posaconazole are alternatives for fluconazole-resistant disease. An echinocandin may be used in patients unable to tolerate oral therapy.
- Vaginal candidiasis severe or recurrent
  - Fluconazole (10 mg/kg up to 150 mg daily) for 3 days for severe acute infection
  - Fluconazole (10 mg/kg up to 150 mg) daily for 10 to 14 days then weekly for 6 months for recurrent infection
  - *C. glabrata* is resistant to azoles and can be treated with intravaginal boric acid or nystatin.
- Neonatal candidiasis
  - Lipid-based amphotericin B (3 to 6 mg/kg daily) should be used with caution as penetration to the CNS and kidney is limited.
  - Echinocandins should be used with caution and limited to salvage therapy.
  - Flucytosine (25 mg/kg 4 times a day) may be added to salvage therapy for CNS disease.

SURGERY/OTHER PROCEDURES
Septic joints require surgical debridement, and infected hardware requires surgical removal.

ADMISSION, INPATIENT, AND NURSING CONSIDERATIONS
- Patients with invasive infection should be admitted initially and treated with IV therapy.
- Step down to oral therapy may occur once candidemia is resolved, patient is clinically improved, and susceptibility to oral therapy is verified.

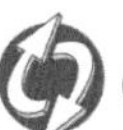

ONGOING CARE

FOLLOW-UP RECOMMENDATIONS
Patient Monitoring
- Multiple subsequent daily blood cultures are required to ensure candidemia is resolved.
- Itraconazole, voriconazole, posaconazole, and flucytosine require therapeutic drug monitoring.

PROGNOSIS
- Mucocutaneous disease typically responds well to therapy.
- Invasive candidiasis has 30% overall mortality.
- Drug resistance especially in *C. glabrata* and *C. krusei* may lead to a delayed response and require alternate therapy.
- *Candida auris* is an emerging strain associated with severe systemic illness and high mortality.

ADDITIONAL READING

- Benjamin DK Jr, Stoll BJ, Gantz MG, et al; for Eunice Kennedy Shriver National Institute of Child Health and Human Development Neonatal Research Network. Neonatal candidiasis: epidemiology, risk factors, and clinical judgment. *Pediatrics*. 2010;126(4):e865–e873.
- Hacimustafaoglu M, Celebi S. Candida infections in non-neutropenic children after the neonatal period. *Expert Rev Anti Infect Ther*. 2011;9(10):923–940.
- Pappas PG, Kauffman CA, Andes DR, et al. Clinical practice guideline for the management of candidiasis: 2016 update by the Infectious Diseases Society of America. *Clin Infect Dis*. 2016;62(4):e1–e50.
- Steinbach WJ, Roilides E, Berman D, et al. Results from a prospective, international, epidemiologic study of invasive candidiasis in children and neonates. *Pediatr Infect Dis J*. 2012;31(12):1252–1257.

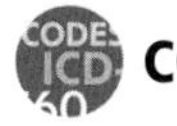

CODES

ICD10
- B37.9 Candidiasis, unspecified
- B37.0 Candidal stomatitis
- B37.81 Candidal esophagitis

FAQ
- Q: When should an older child with thrush be evaluated for possible immunodeficiency?
- A: Thrush in the older child is usually caused by recent antibiotic or steroid treatment or diabetes. If no explanatory cause is identified, further evaluation that includes HIV testing should be considered.
- Q: Does *Candida* isolated from respiratory or urine cultures or healthy children require treatment?
- A: No. *Candida* is a commensal organism, part of the normal flora and therefore can be cultured from healthy persons while not causing disease. In general, respiratory cultures do not require treatment and urine infections only occur when urinary catheters are used.
- Q: When should invasive candidiasis be considered?
- A: Consider and empirically treat for candidiasis in children with neutropenia or critical illness and persistent fevers.

CARBON MONOXIDE POISONING

Kevin C. Osterhoudt, MD, MS

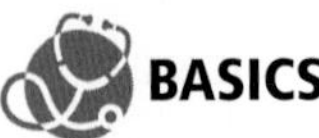

BASICS

DESCRIPTION

- Carbon monoxide (CO) is an odorless gas produced via incomplete combustion of carbonaceous fuels.
- CO poisoning occurs when carboxyhemoglobin and CO accumulation leads to impaired physiologic function.

EPIDEMIOLOGY

CO poisoning is a leading cause of death by poisoning within the United States.

Incidence

- >14,000 CO exposures were reported to the American Association of Poison Control Centers in 2015, with ~1/3 of such exposures occurring in children.
- There are >400 deaths per year in the United States.
- Seasonal cold weather and other natural disaster events lead to increases in incidence of exposure.

GENERAL PREVENTION

- Furnaces should receive regular maintenance by skilled technicians.
- Automobiles, gas-powered machinery, and nonelectrical space heaters should only be used with proper ventilation.
- CO detectors should be installed within living spaces.

PATHOPHYSIOLOGY

- On inhalation, some CO binds to hemoglobin to form carboxyhemoglobin.
- Carboxyhemoglobin does not carry oxygen.
- Carboxyhemoglobin produces an allosteric leftward shift of the oxyhemoglobin dissociation curve.
- Carboxyhemoglobin elimination half-life
  - ~4 hours in room air
  - 1 to 2 hours in 100% oxygen
  - 20 minutes in 100% oxygen at 3 atmospheres
- CO interacts with cellular proteins, leading to impaired mitochondrial function.
- CO is a source of oxidative stress and poisoning may begin a cascade of inflammatory vasculitis within the CNS and heart.

ETIOLOGY

- Common sources of CO exposure include the following:
  - Automobile or boat exhaust
  - Smoke inhalation from house fires
  - Oil, gas, or kerosene space heaters or cooking stoves
  - Portable electricity generators and construction equipment
  - Faulty home furnaces
- The solvent methylene chloride is metabolized to CO by the liver after ingestion, inhalation, or dermal absorption.
- CO is a component of cigarette smoke and environmental air pollution.
- CO is a naturally occurring by-product of the heme biosynthesis pathway.

COMMONLY ASSOCIATED CONDITIONS

Victims of house fires may suffer from thermal injury and/or cyanide poisoning.

DIAGNOSIS

Many emergency medical services crews carry CO detectors.

HISTORY

- Health of family members?
  - CO is an environmental gas that often sickens multiple household members.
- Use of furnace or space heaters?
  - May suggest source of exposure
- Time of exposure?
  - Carboxyhemoglobin levels must be interpreted with consideration to their timing.
- Duration of exposure?
  - Toxicity is related to both magnitude and duration of exposure.
- Loss of consciousness?
  - Syncope appears to be the best clinical predictor of delayed neurologic sequelae.
- Signs and symptoms
  - Mild CO intoxication
    - Malaise
    - Nausea
    - Light-headedness
    - Headache
    - Vomiting
  - Moderate to severe CO intoxication
    - Confusion
    - Syncope
    - Weakness
    - Angina

PHYSICAL EXAM

- Soot on nasal mucosa: suggests possibility of thermal pulmonary injury
- Hypotension: suggests severe CO poisoning
- Cherry red skin: This classic sign is mostly a postmortem finding.

DIFFERENTIAL DIAGNOSIS

- Influenza
- Gastroenteritis
- Vasomotor syncope
- Asphyxia
- Stroke

DIAGNOSTIC TESTS & INTERPRETATION

Initial Tests (screening, lab, imaging)

- CO-oximetry: allows quantitation of carboxyhemoglobin
- Arterial blood gas: allows accurate assessment of oxygenation
- Hemoglobin quantitation: The percentage of carboxyhemoglobin concentration must be considered in relation to the total hemoglobin.
- Serum bicarbonate: A wide anion gap metabolic acidosis suggests the accumulation of lactate, which may result from severe CO poisoning or concomitant cyanide poisoning.
- Creatine kinase: CO poisoning victims are susceptible to rhabdomyolysis.
- Troponin: CO poisoning may lead to myocardial injury.
- ECG: Hypoxemia and metabolic poisoning may lead to cardiac ischemia.
- Transcutaneous carboxyhemoglobin measurement devices are now marketed.
- Neuroimaging
  - Not routinely helpful in acute management
  - Globus pallidus and subcortical white matter changes may be seen after severe or chronic CO poisoning.

ALERT

Pitfalls

- Pulse oximetry frequently overestimates the percentage of oxyhemoglobin.
- Smokers may have carboxyhemoglobin levels up to 10%.
- Hemolysis, or the presence of fetal hemoglobin, may lead to mild elevation of carboxyhemoglobin.
- In-hospital carboxyhemoglobin levels are not good at predicting risk of delayed neurologic sequelae.

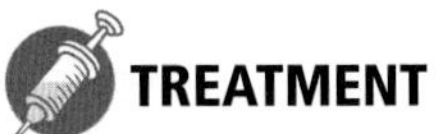

TREATMENT

GENERAL MEASURES

- Recognize CO exposure.
- Remove patient from source of CO.
- Initial stabilization
  - Administer 100% oxygen at least until patient is asymptomatic and carboxyhemoglobin level is <5–10%.

ADDITIONAL THERAPIES

- Use local care standards to consider hyperbaric oxygen treatment referral to prevent delayed neurologic sequelae.
- Relative indications
  - Loss of consciousness
  - Seizures
  - Pregnancy
  - Persistent neurologic symptoms
  - CO concentration >25%
- Contraindications
  - Concurrent illness or injury requiring ongoing acute care
  - Unvented pneumothorax
  - Lack of accessible hyperbaric oxygen chamber
- Complications
  - Barotitis media
  - Tympanic membrane rupture
  - Claustrophobic anxiety
  - Seizure
  - Pneumothorax

ALERT

Pitfalls

- Failure to differentiate CO poisoning from winter viral illness
- Syncope may be hard to discern in young infants.
- Undue delay in hyperbaric oxygen therapy, which is most effective in first 6 hours after exposure

ISSUES FOR REFERRAL

- Neuropsychological testing may benefit individuals with perceived neurocognitive deficits.
- Cardiac evaluation for those with myocardial ischemia

ADMISSION, INPATIENT, AND NURSING CONSIDERATIONS

- Admission criteria
  - Perceived merit of hyperbaric oxygen therapy
  - Persistent neurologic symptoms
  - Evidence of myocardial ischemia
  - Associated injuries that merit hospitalization
- Discharge criteria
  - Conclusion of hyperbaric therapy
  - Stable cardiovascular and neurologic systems after elimination of excess carboxyhemoglobin

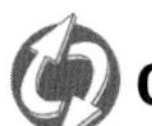

ONGOING CARE

FOLLOW-UP RECOMMENDATIONS

Delayed neurologic sequelae may develop 2 to 40 days after exposure.

PROGNOSIS

- Acute mortality appears to be caused by carboxymyoglobin formation and ischemic ventricular dysrhythmia.
- Patients stable on presentation to medical care have a good prognosis for recovery.
- Delayed neurologic sequelae may manifest in as many as 10–40% of patients after a CO-mediated syncopal episode.

COMPLICATIONS

- Death
- Delayed neurologic sequelae, for example
  - Neurocognitive deficits
  - Personality changes
  - Parkinsonism

ADDITIONAL READING

- Baum CR. What's new in pediatric carbon monoxide poisoning? *Clin Pediatr Emerg Med*. 2008;9:43–46.
- Macnow TE, Waltzman ML. Carbon monoxide poisoning in children: diagnosis and management in the emergency department. *Pediatr Emerg Med Pract*. 2016;13(9):1–24.
- Sircar K, Clower J, Shin MK, et al. Carbon monoxide poisoning deaths in the United States, 1999 to 2012. *Am J Emerg Med*. 2015;33(9):1140–1145.
- Teksam O, Gumus P, Bayrakci B, et al. Acute cardiac effects of carbon monoxide poisoning in children. *Eur J Emerg Med*. 2010;17(4):192–196.
- Weaver LK. Clinical practice. Carbon monoxide poisoning. *N Engl J Med*. 2009;360(12):1217–1225.

CODES

ICD10

- T58.91XA Toxic effect of carb monx from unsp source, acc, init
- T58.8X1A Toxic effect of carb monx from oth source, accidental, init
- T58.01XA Toxic effect of carb monx from mtr veh exhaust, acc, init

FAQ

- Q: At what carboxyhemoglobin level should hyperbaric oxygen therapy be recommended?
- A: In practice, most dissociation of carboxyhemoglobin occurs with administration of normal pressure oxygen before hyperbaric therapy can be administered.
  - The advocated value of hyperbaric oxygen is to limit cerebral ischemic reperfusion injury in an effort to ameliorate delayed neurologic sequelae.
  - Carboxyhemoglobin levels may not directly correlate in this risk stratification, and the occurrence of syncope or seizure may be used as a surrogate marker.
  - Currently, patients with CO concentrations >25% may be considered as potential candidates for hyperbaric oxygen.
- Q: In a household, which family member is at greatest risk of CO poisoning?
- A: Smaller and younger children have greater minute ventilation rates and may attain higher carboxyhemoglobin concentrations at a given exposure level.
  - It is possible that developing brain tissue is more susceptible to the deleterious effects of CO poisoning.

CARDIOMYOPATHY

Kimberly M. Molina, MD • Lindsay J. May, MD, FRCPC

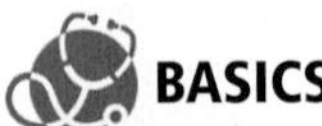

BASICS

DESCRIPTION

Cardiomyopathy (CM) is a disease of the heart muscle, which impairs function (systolic, diastolic, or both). It is classified based on structural and functional abnormalities:

- Dilated cardiomyopathy (DCM): impairment of systolic function with ventricular dilation; predominantly involves the left ventricle (LV) and 70% of children with DCM will present in congestive heart failure (CHF)
- Hypertrophic cardiomyopathy (HCM): excessive thickening of the LV that is not secondary to load conditions, such as aortic stenosis or hypertension. Up to 20–25% of patients exhibit LV outflow tract obstruction.
- Restrictive cardiomyopathy (RCM): a rare disease characterized by normal or decreased volume of both ventricles associated with biatrial enlargement, normal LV wall thickness, impaired ventricular filling with restrictive physiology, and normal systolic function

EPIDEMIOLOGY

Incidence

Overall incidence of CM is 1 to 2 cases per 100,000 children per year. There is a peak incidence during the 1st year of life and a second peak in adolescence.

- DCM: 0.3 to 2.6 cases/100,000 children/year
- HCM: 0.3 to 0.5 cases/100,000 children/year
- RCM: 0.03 to 0.04 cases/100,000 children/year

Prevalence

- DCM: 36 cases per 100,000 people
- HCM: ~10–20 cases per 100,000 people
- RCM: least common form of CM (<5%)

RISK FACTORS

Genetics

- DCM: familial DCM ~20% of cases
  - Autosomal dominant most common pattern. >20 genes have been identified in DCM.
  - Can be associated with diseases of X-linked inheritance: Duchenne and Becker muscular dystrophy and Barth syndrome
  - May also be inherited via mitochondrial DNA, with variable penetrance
- HCM: ~60% of cases are thought to be inherited; traditionally inherited in an autosomal dominant pattern with incomplete penetrance
- RCM: Idiopathic cases may have a familial occurrence and may be associated with a skeletal myopathy. An autosomal dominant form with variable penetrance has been associated with Noonan syndrome.

GENERAL PREVENTION

There are no relevant factors in prevention, although for patients undergoing chemotherapy, there are cardioprotective strategies that can be used.

PATHOPHYSIOLOGY

- DCM: inadequate systolic function with a low cardiac index (hypoperfusion) and a high central venous pressure (systemic congestion). There can be left atrial (LA) hypertension and pulmonary hypertension (PH) from left heart dysfunction.
- HCM: Diastolic dysfunction and LV outflow tract obstruction are the most problematic and lead to LA hypertension.
- RCM: Diastolic dysfunction over time leads to LA hypertension and PH. There can also be RV dysfunction and hepatic venous congestion as a result.

ETIOLOGY

- DCM: A clear etiology identified in only 30% of cases
  - Of known causes, the most common is myocarditis (coxsackievirus B, adenovirus). DCM can also occur from toxin exposure (anthracyclines), ischemic coronary artery disease (anomalous left coronary artery from the pulmonary artery [ALCAPA], coronary aneurysms), and chronic tachyarrhythmias.
  - Can be associated with X-linked muscular dystrophies, inborn errors of fatty acid oxidation, disorders of mitochondrial oxidative phosphorylation, nutritional deficiencies, and carnitine deficiency
  - It may be familial and genetically inherited.
  - Most commonly idiopathic. Many of these "idiopathic" cases have unidentified familial DCM.
- HCM: genetic etiology in up to 70% of cases; caused by myocyte hypertrophy with fibrillin disarray
- RCM: most commonly idiopathic, although known causes include the following:
  - Systemic disease such as lupus erythematosus, sarcoidosis, amyloidosis, infiltrative diseases (Gaucher disease, Hurler syndrome), storage diseases (Fabry disease), carcinoid syndrome, and radiation-induced fibrosis
  - Familial/inherited forms

COMMONLY ASSOCIATED CONDITIONS

CM is most commonly identified in otherwise healthy children but can be associated with:

- DCM: neuromuscular disorders (9%), inborn errors of metabolism (4%), or rarely with malformation syndromes (1%)
- HCM: neuromuscular disorders (8%), inborn errors of metabolism (9%), or malformation syndromes (9%)
- RCM: In some tropical regions, endomyocardial fibrosis associated with RCM is common.

DIAGNOSIS

In the early stages of all three forms of CM symptoms are nonspecific and can mimic other disease processes. The cardiac examination can be completely normal.

HISTORY

DCM:

- Irritability, failure to thrive
- Respiratory distress, dyspnea with exertion
- Anorexia, abdominal pain, nausea
- Exercise intolerance
- Syncope, palpitations

> **ALERT**
> In older children and adolescents gastrointestinal complaints (abdominal pain, nausea, vomiting, decreased appetite, weight loss) can be the first symptoms of CHF.

- HCM: often referred for evaluation based on family history or for murmur evaluation. Symptoms can include:
  - Chest pain with exertion
  - Dizziness, syncope, palpitations
- RCM: Symptoms are usually evident late in the disease process:
  - Dyspnea with exertion
  - Abdominal or chest pain, palpitations

PHYSICAL EXAM

- Cardiac
  - DCM: tachycardia, cardiomegaly, hepatomegaly, S_3 or S_4; evidence of CHF and low cardiac output
  - HCM: may have systolic murmur (mitral regurgitation and/or LV outflow tract obstruction). The presence of outflow tract obstruction produces a systolic ejection murmur of variable intensity related to the degree of obstruction; the murmur increases in intensity with Valsalva and decreases in magnitude with squatting. A parasternal or carotid thrill or S_4 may be present.
  - RCM: Jugular venous pulse either fails to fall or rises during inspiration (Kussmaul sign): the presence of S_3 or S_4. Advanced cases may exhibit weak peripheral pulses as evidence of low cardiac output.
- Respiratory (DCM, RCM): tachypnea, rales, wheezing
- Abdominal (DCM, RCM): hepatomegaly, ascites

DIFFERENTIAL DIAGNOSIS

- DCM: Presentation may mimic other diseases:
  - Right upper quadrant pain, nausea, anorexia indicate right heart failure but could be mistaken for hepatic or gallbladder disease.
  - Wheezing, tachypnea, and dyspnea on exertion may be diagnosed as asthma.
  - Cardiomegaly on x-ray may be mistaken for a large pericardial effusion.
  - There is often diagnostic uncertainty as to whether a patient presenting with LV failure has acute myocarditis or DCM.
- HCM: Must be differentiated from LV hypertrophy seen in a well-trained athlete.
- RCM: Should be distinguished from constrictive pericarditis. A history of tuberculosis, trauma, or cardiac surgery may suggest constrictive pericarditis.

DIAGNOSTIC TESTS & INTERPRETATION

Initial Tests (screening, lab, imaging)

DCM: Inflammatory markers as well as:

- Metabolic: acylcarnitine profile, serum organic acids, and urine organic and amino acids, pyruvate, lactate, thyroid function tests, creatine kinase, ammonia, lactate
- Genetic: directed chromosomal analysis if appropriate
- Infectious: enterovirus, coxsackievirus A/B, hepatitis, cytomegalovirus, Epstein-Barr virus, adenovirus, parvovirus, herpes simplex virus, and human immunodeficiency virus
- Brain natriuretic peptide (BNP)
- Chest radiograph: cardiomegaly, pulmonary venous congestion, pulmonary edema, and pleural effusions; segmental atelectasis from bronchiole compression
- Echocardiogram: assessment of systolic and diastolic function, ventricular dimensions, basic anatomy
  - DCM: significant dilation of left (and right) ventricle with decreased systolic function
  - HCM: LV hypertrophy and systolic anterior motion of the mitral valve. LV function is hyperdynamic until late in the disease process.
  - RCM: disproportionately dilated atria with impaired diastolic filling by Doppler. LV function is normal until late stages.

> **ALERT**
> It is essential in an infant with newly diagnosed DCM to rule out structural abnormalities (coarctation or ALCAPA)

- Cardiac magnetic resonance imaging (MRI)
  - DCM: MRI can provide diagnostic information when there is a question of possible myocarditis.
  - HCM: MRI can be used to look for myocardial fibrosis as a risk factor for sudden death.

Follow-Up Tests & Special Considerations

- Developmental and nutritional services are essential.
- In arranging investigations, be aware that sedation for many patients with CM can lead to life-threatening complications and should be performed at an experienced center only.

Diagnostic Procedures/Other

- Electrocardiogram: Supraventricular or ventricular arrhythmia may be seen.
  - DCM: sinus tachycardia, nonspecific ST segment, and T-wave changes
  - HCM: hypertrophy, deep Q waves
  - RCM: atrial enlargement, nonspecific ST and T-wave changes
- Holter monitoring
  - DCM: Rule out arrhythmia secondary to CM but also helps rule out arrhythmia as the primary etiology.
  - HCM: surveillance for VT or atrial fibrillation
- Cardiac catheterization
  - DCM: rarely used as the primary diagnostic tool; enables biopsy and identifies coronary anatomy
  - HCM: evaluates diastolic function and pulmonary vascular resistance (PVR), classic spike, and dome arterial pulse tracing; Brockenbrough phenomenon (a beat following a premature ventricular contraction exhibits an arterial pulse pressure less than that of a control beat)
  - RCM: Atrial pressures are elevated from increased LV and right ventricle (RV) end diastolic pressures. Ventricular pressures exhibit a rapid and deep early decline at the onset of diastole followed by a rapid rise to a plateau in early diastole (dip and plateau or square root sign). Evaluate PVR.

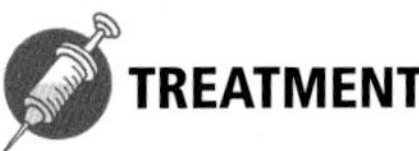

TREATMENT

GENERAL MEASURES

The initial assessment evaluates their degree of compensation in heart failure and whether they are congested/dry, warm/cold. This will guide initial treatment and should be done with the assistance of cardiology. An assessment of end organ function (including neurologic) in patients with newly diagnosed heart failure is essential.

MEDICATION

Dosing is tailored to the status of the patient.

First Line

- DCM
  - At diagnosis, a trial of IV immunoglobulin (IVIG) and/or other immunomodulators (prednisone) to treat possible myocarditis, although impact on outcomes is unclear
  - Inotropes (milrinone, dobutamine) may be first line depending on the status of the patient.
  - Diuretics
  - Afterload reduction (enalapril, captopril)
  - β-Adrenergic blockers (metoprolol, carvedilol)
  - Aldactone, digoxin
  - Anticoagulation to avoid embolic complications
  - Antiarrhythmics as needed
- HCM: β-Adrenergic blockers remain first line.
- RCM: Diuretics can be used with caution to treat venous congestion without reducing ventricular preload.

Second Line

- DCM: inotropic agents
  - Milrinone, dobutamine
- HCM: calcium channel blockers or disopyramide
  - Diuretics are seldom used because of preload-dependence. Antiarrhythmics may be used.
- RCM: antiarrhythmics
  - Anticoagulation due to high risk of thrombus formation and embolic complications from hemostasis in the dilated atrium

ISSUES FOR REFERRAL

- Patients with CM will have lifelong follow-up with a cardiologist, ideally a specialist in heart failure and transplantation. The interval of follow-up depends on the status of the patients.
- Genetic specialists should be involved to guide specific gene testing and family screening, to consider underlying genetic disorders associated with CM.

SURGERY/OTHER PROCEDURES

- If a patient deteriorates despite inotropic support, extracorporeal membrane oxygenation (ECMO) may be needed.
- Ventricular assist devices have been used for end-stage heart failure as a bridge to transplantation.
- DCM: Cardiac resynchronization with a pacemaker may be helpful in only selected pediatric patients.
- HCM: If medical therapy is not effective, other options may include septal myectomy (for severe outflow obstruction). Placement of an implantable cardioverter-defibrillator (ICD) may be indicated depending on the patient's risk profile.
- DCM, HCM: Heart or heart–lung (if the PVR is elevated) transplantation may be necessary.
- RCM: Transplantation is typically indicated due to the prognosis associated with RCM.

ADMISSION, INPATIENT, AND NURSING CONSIDERATIONS

Many patients with CM will present in compensated heart failure and are likely to require admission for work-up and treatment. If patients with CM present with acute hemodynamic compromise, stabilization should be done in an ICU. In addition, noninvasive positive pressure can support the LV.

ALERT

Intubation and sedation pose significant risk of causing hemodynamic collapse, as does aggressive fluid resuscitation.

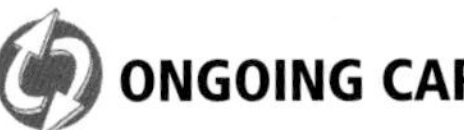

ONGOING CARE

PATIENT EDUCATION

The Children's Cardiomyopathy Foundation includes helpful resources for families of those affected by CM.

PROGNOSIS

- DCM: The rate of death or transplant is ~30% at 1-year and 40% at 5-year follow-up. Age (<1 month and >6 years), ventricular function, and symptoms of CHF at diagnosis are risk factors for a worse outcome. Myocarditis is associated with improved outcome.
- HCM: Between the ages of 12 and 35 years and in young athletes, HCM is the most common cause of sudden death. Heart failure symptoms usually do not occur until adulthood. Survival is poorer for those diagnosed at <1 year of age.
- RCM: The reported median survival in RCM is 1.4 years in children with <20% freedom from death or transplant at 5 years.
- LV noncompaction CM: 5-year survival free of death or transplantation is 75%.

COMPLICATIONS

- CHF can occur in all forms of CM.
- Arrhythmias are not uncommon in CM.
- There is no consensus as to prophylactic anticoagulation in children with heart failure.

ADDITIONAL READING

- Alvarez JA, Orav EJ, Wilkinson JD, et al. Competing risks for death and cardiac transplantation in children with dilated cardiomyopathy: results from the pediatric cardiomyopathy registry. *Circulation*. 2011;124(7):814–823.
- Ammash NM, Seward JB, Bailey KR, et al. Clinical profile and outcome of idiopathic restrictive cardiomyopathy. *Circulation*. 2000;101(21):2490–2496.
- Gersh BJ, Maron BJ, Bonow RO, et al. 2011 ACCF/AHA guideline for the diagnosis and treatment of hypertrophic cardiomyopathy: executive summary: a report of the American College of Cardiology Foundation/American Heart Association Task Force on Practice Guidelines. *Circulation*. 2011;124:2761–2796.
- Kantor PF, Lougheed J, Dancea A, et al. Presentation, diagnosis, and medical management of heart failure in children: Canadian Cardiovascular Society guidelines. *Can J Cardiol*. 2013;29(12):1535–1552.
- Kirk R, Dipchand AI, Rosenthal DN, et al. *International Society for Heart and Lung Transplantation Monograph Series, Volume 8. ISHLT Guidelines for the Management of Pediatric Heart Failure*. Birmingham, United Kingdom: UAB Printing; 2014.
- Towbin JA. Hypertrophic cardiomyopathy. *Pacing Clin Electrophysiol*. 2009;32(Suppl 2):S23–S31.
- Towbin JA, Lowe AM, Colan SD, et al. Incidence, causes, and outcomes of dilated cardiomyopathy in children. *JAMA*. 2006;296(15):1867–1876.
- Wilkinson JD, Landy DC, Colan SD, et al. The pediatric cardiomyopathy registry and heart failure: key results from the first 15 years. *Heart Fail Clin*. 2010;6(4):401–413.

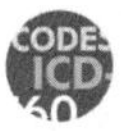

CODES

ICD10

- I42.9 Cardiomyopathy, unspecified
- I42.0 Dilated cardiomyopathy
- I42.5 Other restrictive cardiomyopathy

FAQ

- Q: Should family members be evaluated once CM is diagnosed in a 1st-degree relative?
- A: Yes. In some forms of CM, there is a strong genetic component, and family members should be evaluated. If the CM is known to be acquired, evaluation of relatives is not required.
- Q: What are the differentiating features of HCM and the benign physiologic hypertrophy of an athlete's heart?
- A: A familial history of HCM raises the suspicion of this entity. Specific echocardiographic LV dimensions may differentiate benign hypertrophy and HCM (i.e., wall thickness of ≥15 mm or LV cavity dimension <45 mm are more consistent with HCM). Also, evidence of abnormal mitral valve inflow is suggestive of HCM.

CATARACT

M. Edward Wilson, MD • Courtney L. Kraus, MD • Rupal H. Trivedi, MD, MSCR

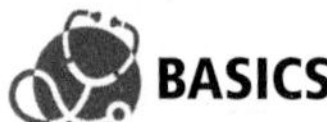

BASICS

DESCRIPTION
Cataract is the term used for any opacification of the crystalline lens of the eye.

EPIDEMIOLOGY
- Prevalence of childhood cataracts is 1 to 15:10,000, with the range being attributable to reporting, definition, age, and variance in populations.
- Approximately four children per million total population will be born with bilateral congenital cataracts in developed countries.
- Adjusted cumulative incidence is 2.49 per 10,000 in the 1st year of life, increasing to 3.46 by age 15 years.

GENERAL PREVENTION
- There is currently no known way to prevent congenital cataracts. Timely prenatal diagnosis and treatment of intrauterine infections can prevent associated infant morbidities, including secondary cataracts. Correcting an underlying metabolic abnormality and minimizing exposure to inciting agents also reduces risk.
- It is essential that all newborns (and all children) receive screening eye examinations by health care providers. In much of the world, early diagnosis and referral is still the limiting factor for a child's ultimate visual prognosis.

PATHOPHYSIOLOGY
- Derangement of the normal developmental growth of the crystalline fibers of the central lens nucleus or peripheral lens cortex. The location of the opacity often suggests the congenital or early acquired onset.
- Frequently classified according to morphology or etiology
- Dense central opacities of ≥3 mm are visually significant and may produce visual disability.

ETIOLOGY
- Congenital or developmental: About 2/3 are idiopathic, the remainder being inherited or associated with systemic disorders.
- Hereditary: Autosomal dominant transmission is responsible for 75% of bilateral hereditary cataracts. Most affected individuals are otherwise healthy.
  - Phenotypically identical cataracts can occur with mutations at different genetic loci, and phenotypically variable cataracts can be found within a single family.
  - Multiple contributing genetic loci have been identified.
  - Rare hereditary syndromes combine cataracts with systemic disease. These are listed in the following discussion.
- Acquired
  - Toxic: may result from chronic steroid use or radiation exposure
  - Traumatic: may result from either blunt or penetrating ocular trauma
  - Inflammatory: from chronic uveitis
- Ocular abnormalities: Cataracts may be associated with primary ocular abnormalities such as aniridia, Peters anomaly, coloboma, and microcornea.

COMMONLY ASSOCIATED CONDITIONS
- Prenatal factors: intrauterine infection, fetal alcohol syndrome
- Metabolic and endocrine:
  - Galactosemia
  - Neonatal hypoglycemia
  - Hypoparathyroidism
  - Diabetes mellitus
  - Homocystinuria
  - Fabry disease
  - Wilson disease
  - Mannosidosis
- Chromosomal:
  - Trisomy 21 (Down syndrome), 18, 13, or 15
  - Turner syndrome
- Dermatologic:
  - Congenital ichthyosis
  - Hereditary ectodermal dysplasia
  - Infantile poikiloderma
  - Gorlin syndrome
- Renal:
  - Lowe syndrome
  - Alport syndromes
- Musculoskeletal:
  - Marfan syndrome
  - Conradi syndrome
  - Albright syndrome
  - Myotonic dystrophy
- Rheumatologic:
  - Juvenile idiopathic arthritis
  - Other uveitis (psoriatic, HLA-B27, etc.)
- Other:
  - Craniofacial and mandibulofacial syndromes
  - Neurofibromatosis

DIAGNOSIS

HISTORY
- Decreased visual fixation and tracking? Cataracts may decrease vision.
- Sun sensitivity or squinting in bright light? Cataracts may cause glare and light scatter.
- Strabismus (ocular misalignment)? May indicate loss of vision in one eye
- White pupil? Cataracts may appear as a white spot in or under the pupil.
- Asymmetric or abnormal pupillary reflections (red eyes) with flash photography? Cataract may block the normal red reflex.
- Nystagmus (rhythmic oscillations)? May be a sign of severe, usually bilateral, vision loss
- Ocular trauma? Cataract can occur from blunt or penetrating trauma.
- Delayed development? Especially with significant bilateral congenital cataracts
- Careful family and prenatal history? Congenital cataracts can be inherited as an isolated condition. Intrauterine infection or alcohol exposure can cause cataracts.
- Positive family history, known history of an associated systemic condition or history of trauma?

PHYSICAL EXAM
- Decreased visual acuity:
  - In preverbal child, assess and compare ability to fixate and follow with each eye.
  - In verbal child, assess with pictures, "HOTV" chart matching, or alphabet (Snellen) eye chart.
- Leukocoria: white pupil
- Red reflex:
  - Absent, asymmetric, or irregular
  - How much of the pupil is obscured?
  - Use direct ophthalmoscope held at an arm's length to illuminate both eyes and compare the red reflex from each eye.
- Strabismus: often an indication; cataract is long-standing and amblyopia likely.
- Nystagmus:
  - Will first appear at 2 to 3 months of age if vision deprivation from cataract is present at birth
  - Very poor prognostic sign for full vision recovery unless treatment is prompt
- Laterality of disease: Bilateral cataracts may be due to systemic disease.
- Globe (eyeball) size: Microphthalmia (small eye) suggests congenital cataracts.
- Complete physical exam: to assess for associated conditions

DIFFERENTIAL DIAGNOSIS
- Childhood cataracts can be readily identified as such. However, they represent one of the many etiologies on the differential diagnosis for leukocoria.
- Cataracts may also be an expression of an underlying systemic disease, which must be diagnosed for the child's overall benefit.
- Leukocoria or poor red reflex differential diagnosis:
  - Retinoblastoma
  - Retinopathy of prematurity
  - Persistent fetal vasculature
  - Uveitis
  - Retinal detachment
  - Coats disease
  - Toxocariasis

DIAGNOSTIC TESTS & INTERPRETATION

Initial Tests (screening, labs, imaging)
For cases with a definitive etiology, laboratory evaluation is typically not necessary. For bilateral cataracts without a clear cause, a selective workup to rule out associated conditions may be indicated.
- Serologies: titers to rule out toxoplasmosis, syphilis, HIV, rubella, cytomegalovirus, herpes simplex infections
- Blood glucose, calcium, and phosphate to exclude metabolic disorders such as diabetes and hypoparathyroidism
- Urine tests: reducing substances to rule out galactosemia; protein, amino acids, and pH to rule out Lowe syndrome
- Red blood cell enzyme levels: galactokinase and galactose-1-phosphate uridyltransferase as part of galactosemia workup
- Karyotype: in conjunction with genetic consultation and ocular examination of parents and siblings
- Ophthalmologist may perform ocular ultrasonography if unable to visualize structures posterior to the opacity.

Diagnostic Procedures/Other

- Complete, timely ophthalmic evaluation by a pediatric ophthalmologist, including slit-lamp biomicroscopy and dilated fundus examination
- Examination under anesthesia may be required if office-based exam is inadequate; coupled with intent to remove cataract when necessary

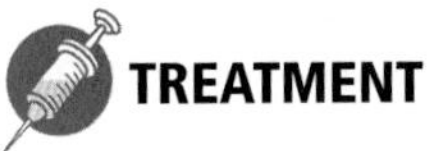

TREATMENT

GENERAL MEASURES

- Importance of timely referral:
  - Congenital cataracts may require surgical removal by 4 to 6 weeks of age to prevent irreversible deprivation amblyopia, so timely identification and quick referral is critical.
  - Acquired pediatric cataracts may also cause amblyopia, typically prior to 7 years of age.
- Conservative management:
  - Partial cataracts that do not block the visual axis may be managed with observation, pharmacologic pupillary dilatation, and/or amblyopia treatment as needed (occlusion of the contralateral eye). Glasses may or may not be of additional help.
  - A small or partial cataract may progress, so close follow-up is required.

SURGERY/OTHER PROCEDURES

- Visually significant cataracts must be removed surgically. In addition to the size of cataract, blackening of the retinoscopic reflex is the most important factor determining need for a surgery. In an older child, any opacity causing a decrease in quality of life should be considered for surgery.
- An intraocular lens (IOL) may be inserted at the time of cataract surgery or later when the child is older.
- Successful intervention must occur very early in life in the case of visually significant congenital cataracts or as soon as possible after progression of later onset or partial cataracts.
- To prevent deprivation amblyopia in bilateral cases, both cataracts are typically removed within 1 or 2 weeks of each other. Rarely, the eyes are operated simultaneously if anesthesia risks are high.
- Postoperative care
  - Overview: Removing the lens leaves the child aphakic (without a lens). Postoperative optical correction with contact lens, glasses, and/or IOL and amblyopia treatment are essential for optimal visual prognosis.
  - Contact lens/glasses: In children <1 year of age, initial optical correction of aphakia is frequently accomplished with contact lenses or glasses. Silicone contact lenses are often chosen for infants and are designed for long-term wear, with removal and cleaning once a week. An IOL is then implanted after eye growth (often in the preschool years or later) as a secondary procedure.
  - IOL: In children >1 year of age, IOLs are frequently placed at the time of cataract surgery. Glasses are needed as well, even when an IOL is placed. The glasses power is changed as the eyes grow. A bifocal is usually added at age 3 years.
  - Amblyopia therapy: In unilateral cataract cases, successful visual rehabilitation usually requires aggressive occlusion therapy to the normal eye, possibly for years.

ONGOING CARE

FOLLOW-UP RECOMMENDATIONS

- Without treatment, visually significant cataracts result in progressive visual loss. When an opacity that is present at birth or very early in life is not promptly addressed, the visual loss quickly becomes irreversible.
- Once surgical removal is performed and optical correction is started, the child, the parents, and the ophthalmologist enter into an intensive and long rehabilitation period, lasting until visual maturity is reached (usually 7 to 10 years of age). Afterward, yearly eye examinations remain a minimum requirement.
- Parental and educational support services as well as special local, state, and federal services for the visually handicapped and blind may be required as not all children with successful surgical results will have good vision.

ALERT

Pitfalls include (i) lack of early diagnosis, referral, and treatment; (ii) lack of understanding of irreversible deprivation amblyopia; (iii) lack of adherence with postoperative optical correction and occlusion therapy; and (iv) lack of continued long-term follow-up to detect and treat late glaucoma or shift in refractive errors with continued eye growth.

PROGNOSIS

- Early surgery and rapid postsurgical optical correction result in best-corrected visual acuities of 20/40 to 20/200 for monocular cataracts and 20/40 or better for bilateral cataracts. 20/20 is obtained in some patients.
- With dense unilateral cataracts, good vision is more likely if the surgery is completed between 30 days and the end of the 6th week of life for a baby born at term. After this time, visual restoration becomes progressively more difficult because of deprivation amblyopia.
- The prognosis for visual rehabilitation in children with bilateral congenital cataracts is better than for unilateral, as long as treatment is before vision deprivation nystagmus develops. For best outcomes, surgery is most often completed in both eyes between 4 and 8 weeks of life.
- Later onset and partial, slowly progressing cataracts have the best prognosis.
- Family adherence with both postsurgical optical correction and amblyopia treatment is critical and directly affects the child's ultimate visual outcome later in life.

COMPLICATIONS

- Lack of removal of a visually significant cataract at the appropriate time leads to irreversible deprivation amblyopia.
- Cataract removal in children leaves the eye without the natural crystalline lens—a structure that normally changes to offset the effects of eye growth. Even when an IOL is placed, glasses are often needed, and the prescription changes frequently as the eyes grow. Unless appropriate optical correction is maintained, irreversible amblyopia may still occur after the cataract is removed, particularly if the cataract is unilateral.
- Congenital cataract eyes often have immature outflow (trabecular meshwork) and 30% or more will eventually develop glaucoma (often years after surgery), requiring drops or surgery to control eye pressure.
- Short- and long-term postoperative complications also include visual axis opacification, retinal detachment, and, very rarely, endophthalmitis (intraocular infection). These complications may lead to vision loss or loss of the eye, and long-term ophthalmology follow-up is required.

ADDITIONAL READING

- Amaya L, Taylor D, Russell-Eggitt I, et al. The morphology and natural history of childhood cataracts. *Surv Ophthalmol*. 2003;48(2):125–144.
- Infant Aphakia Treatment Study Group. A randomized clinical trial comparing contact lens with intraocular lens correction of monocular aphakia during infancy: grating acuity and adverse events at age 1 year. *Arch Ophthalmol*. 2010;128(7):810–818.
- Infant Aphakia Treatment Study Group. Comparison of contact lens and intraocular lens correction of monocular aphakia during infancy: a randomized clinical trial of HOTV optotype acuity at age 4.5 years and clinical findings at age 5 years. *JAMA Ophthalmol*. 2014;132(6):676–682.
- Lambert SR, Drack AV. Infantile cataracts. *Surv Ophthalmol*. 1996;40(6):427–458.
- Serafino M, Trivedi RH, Levin AV, et al. Use of the Delphi process in paediatric cataract management. *Br J Ophthalmol*. 2016;100(5):611–615.

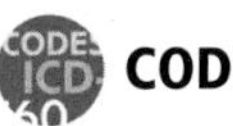

CODES

ICD10

- H26.9 Unspecified cataract
- Q12.0 Congenital cataract
- H26.40 Unspecified secondary cataract

FAQ

- Q: Is surgical removal of the cataract a visual cure?
- A: No. Surgery is only the beginning of treatment, which also includes optical correction and amblyopia therapy.
- Q: Once the cataract is removed, will intensive, extensive follow-up be needed?
- A: Yes. The visual prognosis is directly related to postsurgical treatment compliance.
- Q: Is the cataract easier to treat when the child is older?
- A: No. Irreversible deprivation amblyopia develops as the child grows, precluding any chance for normal vision. In newborns, cataracts must typically be removed at 4 to 6 weeks of age.
- Q: In congenital bilateral cataracts, are both eyes ever operated at the same time?
- A: Yes. Although it is customary to operate one eye at a time, with the second eye operated one week later, a growing trend for infants is to operate both eyes under the same anesthesia. Precautions, like using a different set of instruments on each eye, are needed to reduce the chances of a bilateral infection.

CAT-SCRATCH DISEASE

Camille Sabella, MD

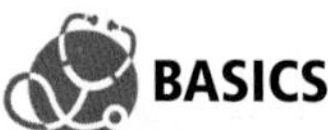

BASICS

DESCRIPTION

Cat-scratch disease (CSD) is a zoonotic infection caused by *Bartonella henselae*, which most commonly causes a subacute, regional lymphadenitis syndrome but is also more rarely associated with visceral organ, neurologic, and ocular manifestations.

EPIDEMIOLOGY

- Cats are the primary reservoir for *B. henselae* and the major vector for transmission to humans.
- CSD most commonly results from a cat scratch or bite; flea bites are also implicated in transmission.
- Kittens are more likely to transmit the organism than adult cats.
- 90% of patients with CSD have history of recent cat contact, most commonly with an apparently healthy kitten.
- Person-to-person transmission is not thought to occur.
- More common in males
- Most cases of CSD occur in the autumn and winter.
- Incubation period is 7 to 12 days (from time of the scratch to appearance of primary skin lesion).

Incidence

- There are an estimated 12,000 cases annually in the United States each year.
- Incidence highest among those living in the southeastern United States (6.4/100,000 persons) and in children aged 5 to 9 years (9.4/100,000 persons).
- Most common cause of subacute/chronic regional lymphadenitis in U.S. children

GENERAL PREVENTION

- Avoiding cats is an effective but unpractical method of preventing CSD.
- Cat bites and scratches should be immediately and thoroughly cleaned.
- Immunocompromised individuals should avoid contact with cats that scratch or bite; avoid kittens as new pets and stray cats.
- Care of cats should involve effective flea control.

PATHOPHYSIOLOGY

- Infection can result in local invasion, causing lymphadenopathy or disseminated infection, leading to visceral organ spread.
- Involved nodes initially develop generalized lymphoid hyperplasia, followed by the development of stellate granulomas; the centers are acellular and necrotic and may be surrounded by histiocytes and peripheral lymphocytes.
- Progression leads to microabscesses, which may become confluent and lead to pus-filled pockets within the infected nodes.

ETIOLOGY

The etiologic agent is *B. henselae*, a fastidious, small, curved, pleomorphic gram-negative bacillus.

DIAGNOSIS

HISTORY

- Cat contact
  - 90% of patients have an antecedent cat contact.
- A cutaneous lesion
  - A red papule generally appears on the skin at the site of inoculation 7 to 12 days after the initial cat scratch.
  - This papule persists for 1 to 4 weeks, often progresses through a vesicular and crusty stage, and then regresses spontaneously.
- Appearance of large lymph nodes
  - Within 1 to 4 weeks after appearance of a skin lesion, lymphadenopathy in the region of drainage (generally immediately proximal to the skin lesion) is often noted.
- Other symptoms
  - Most persons with CSD do not have fever or other constitutional symptoms; fever and mild systemic symptoms (such as generalized achiness, malaise, and anorexia) are present in up to 30% of patients.

PHYSICAL EXAM

- An erythematous papule at the inoculation site may be detectable. Rarely, the lesion may be pustular or nodular.
- Chronic or subacute regional lymphadenitis proximal to the inoculation site is present in approximately 90% of cases:
  - The groups affected, in decreasing order of frequency, are the axillary, cervical, submandibular, periauricular, epitrochlear, femoral, and inguinal lymph nodes.
  - Affected nodes are usually tender, with overlying erythema, warmth, and induration.
  - ~10–30% spontaneously suppurate or form a sinus tract to the skin.
- The finding of conjunctivitis/conjunctival granuloma along with ipsilateral preauricular lymphadenitis is a unique presentation of CSD (Parinaud oculoglandular syndrome), in which the conjunctiva or eyelid is the site of inoculation.

DIFFERENTIAL DIAGNOSIS

- Includes infectious and noninfectious causes of lymphadenopathy
- Infectious:
  - *Mycobacterium tuberculosis*
  - Nontuberculous mycobacterial infection
  - Acute bacterial lymphadenitis caused by *Staphylococcus aureus* and *Streptococcus pyogenes*)
  - Tularemia
  - Viral causes: EBV, CMV, HIV
  - Toxoplasmosis
- Noninfectious
  - Malignancy, especially lymphoma
  - Congenital cysts
  - Kawasaki disease
  - Kikuchi disease
  - Sarcoidosis

DIAGNOSTIC TESTS & INTERPRETATION

- Indirect fluorescent antibody (IFA) testing
  - For detection of serum antibodies to *B. henselae*
  - Available at many commercial laboratories and the Centers for Disease Control and Prevention (CDC)
  - Can be used to confirm CSD
  - A single IgG titer of >1:256, a 4-fold rise in titer, or seroconversion is necessary for serologic diagnosis of CSD.
  - IgM titers are less sensitive than IgG titers, even in acute disease.
  - Overall sensitivity and specificity of IFA IgG testing is 88% and 98%, respectively.
- Enzyme immunoassay (EIA) testing
  - Also for detection of serum antibodies to *B. henselae*
  - Not clear whether these are more sensitive or specific than IFA
- Blood cultures
  - Because this is a fastidious, slow-growing organism, it requires specific culture techniques to optimize isolation.
  - Using lysed or centrifuged blood may, at times, yield *B. henselae* growth from infected individuals in whom bacteremia is suspected.
  - Growth typically is obtained on blood agar after 12 to 15 days but may require incubation period of up to 45 days.
- Polymerase chain reaction (PCR)
  - Available in some commercial and research laboratories
  - Sensitive and specific method for diagnosis of *Bartonella* infection in tissue specimens (e.g., needle aspiration of lymph node)
  - PCR testing of blood can be used for atypical manifestations, such as endocarditis, although the sensitivity appears to be low.
- Histologic findings of lymph nodes are characteristic of CSD but not pathognomonic.
  - Early findings include lymphocytic infiltration with epithelioid granulomas.
  - Later findings include neutrophilic infiltration with necrotic granulomas (stellate microabscesses).
- Warthin-Starry silver stain
  - May demonstrate *B. henselae* bacilli in chains, clumps, or filaments within necrosed areas of lymph node or within primary inoculation site of the skin
  - Not specific for *B. henselae* and not definitively diagnostic of CSD but is strongly suggestive in conjunction with compatible clinical findings

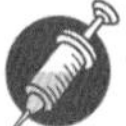

TREATMENT

GENERAL MEASURES

- The management of typical CSD is supportive.
- Severe, systemic disease or infection in immunocompromised patients generally warrant antimicrobial therapy.

MEDICATION

- Antimicrobial therapy may hasten recovery in acutely or severely ill patients with systemic symptoms and is recommended for all immunocompromised people.
  - Macrolides, doxycycline, ciprofloxacin, and trimethoprim-sulfamethoxazole appear to be effective.
  - Rifampin may be effective but is often used in combination with a macrolide or doxycycline.
  - Azithromycin or doxycycline is recommended for patients with bacillary angiomatosis and bacillary peliosis.
- The optimal duration of therapy for complicated infections is not clear but may be prolonged for systemic disease.
- Azithromycin (500 mg initially then 250 mg daily for a total of 5 days in patients >45.5 kg and 10 mg/kg on the 1st day and 5 mg/kg for the subsequent 4 days in patients ≤45.5 kg) has been shown to be of modest clinical benefit in children with uncomplicated CSD.

ISSUES FOR REFERRAL

- Consider infectious disease consult to aid in evaluation, diagnosis, and management, especially in complicated disease or in immunocompromised hosts.
- Consider general surgery consult for needle aspiration if needed.

SURGERY/OTHER PROCEDURES

- Percutaneous needle aspiration of painful, fluctuant nodes can be performed for relief of pain.
- Incision and drainage should be avoided to reduce the risk of sinus tract formation, and surgical excision is generally not necessary.

ADMISSION, INPATIENT, AND NURSING CONSIDERATIONS

Admission is warranted for:

- Severe pain refractory to oral analgesics
- Workup to rule out serious other causes of lymphadenopathy or symptomatology
- Severe or unusual complications of CSD

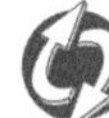

ONGOING CARE

PROGNOSIS

- Typical CSD is self-limited. Slow resolution of enlarged or painful lymph nodes will occur over 2 to 4 months.
- ~10–30% of affected lymph nodes will spontaneously suppurate.
- Most immunocompetent patients have a benign course with complete recovery.
- Patients with significant complications, such as encephalopathy, thrombocytopenic purpura, or bone lesions, usually have a more prolonged course but generally have a good long-term prognosis.

COMPLICATIONS

- Systemic CSD
  - Usually characterized by fever, arthralgia, malaise, myalgia, and hepatosplenic involvement
  - Cause of fever of unknown origin (FUO) in children
  - Hepatosplenic involvement may manifest with abdominal pain; microabscesses or granulomas may be visualized on ultrasound or CT of the liver and spleen.
- Encephalopathy/encephalitis
  - May occur 1 to 3 weeks after the initial symptoms of CSD
  - Seizures, lethargy, combative behavior, and coma may occur.
  - Cerebrospinal fluid (CSF) analysis typically normal or slight lymphocytic pleocytosis and elevated protein
  - Recovery is generally complete.
- Optic neuritis or neuroretinitis
  - Acute (usually unilateral) painless vision loss
  - Associated with stellate macular exudates
- Erythema nodosum
  - Likely represents a delayed hypersensitivity reaction to the infection
  - Most often involves the subcutaneous fat of the legs and, at times, dorsum of arms, hands, and feet
- Osteolytic bone lesions
- Endocarditis
- Other, rare complications
  - Thrombotic thrombocytopenic purpura
  - Henoch-Schönlein purpura
  - Mesenteric lymphadenitis
  - Pneumonia
  - Osteomyelitis
  - Hypercalcemia
  - Guillain-Barré syndrome
  - Transverse myelitis
- Bacillary angiomatosis and bacillary peliosis can occur in the immunocompromised host.

ADDITIONAL READING

- American Academy of Pediatrics. Cat-scratch disease. In: Kimberlin DW, Brady MT, Jackson MA, Long SS, eds. *Red Book: 2015 Report of the Committee on Infectious Diseases*. American Academy of Pediatrics; 2015;280–283.
- Bass JW, Freitas BC, Freitas AD, et al. Prospective randomized double blind placebo-controlled evaluation of azithromycin for treatment of cat-scratch disease. *Pediatr Infect Dis J*. 1998;17(6):447–452.
- Ciervo A, Mastroianni CM, Ajassa C, et al. Rapid identification of *Bartonella henselae* by real-time polymerase chain reaction in a patient with cat scratch disease. *Diagn Microbiol Infect Dis*. 2005;53(1):75–77.
- English R. Cat-scratch disease. *Pediatr Rev*. 2006;27(4):123–128.
- Florin TA, Zaoutis TE, Zaoutis LB. Beyond cat scratch disease: widening spectrum of *Bartonella henselae* infection. *Pediatrics*. 2008;121(5):e1413–e1425.
- Nelson CA, Saha S, Mead PS. Cat-scratch disease in the United States, 2005–2013. *Emerg Infect Dis*. 2016;22(10):1741–1746.
- Schutze GE. Diagnosis and treatment of *Bartonella henselae* infections. *Pediatr Infect Dis J*. 2000;19(12):1185–1187.

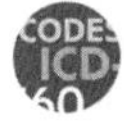

CODES

ICD10

A28.1 Cat-scratch disease

FAQ

- Q: Can a sibling develop CSD from an infected patient?
- A: No. There is no evidence of person-to-person transmission; however, asymptomatic household contacts of the index case are more likely to be seropositive than the general population. This situation is likely related to exposure to the same animal.
- Q: Should the parents of a child with CSD get rid of the cat?
- A: In general, this is not recommended. These animals are not ill; the capacity to transmit disease appears to be transient, and recurrent disease is rare.
- Q: What is the benefit of azithromycin in the treatment of uncomplicated CSD lymphadenitis?
- A: In a prospective, randomized, double-blind study, azithromycin given for 5 days was shown to result in significantly greater decrease in lymph node volume during the 1st month of treatment as compared to placebo. However, there was no difference in outcome between the two groups after 30 days.

CAVERNOUS SINUS SYNDROME

Sabrina E. Smith, MD, PhD

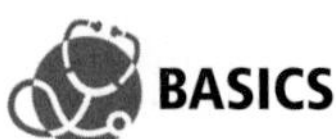

BASICS

DESCRIPTION

- Cavernous sinus syndrome comprises disease processes that localize to the cavernous sinus—a venous plexus that drains the face, mouth, tonsils, pharynx, nasal cavity, paranasal sinuses, orbit, middle ear, and parts of the cerebral cortex.
- Small lesions in this region may produce dramatic neurologic signs.

EPIDEMIOLOGY

Cavernous sinus syndrome is a rare but serious condition.

PATHOPHYSIOLOGY

- The cavernous sinus is located lateral to the pituitary gland and sella turcica, superior to the sphenoid sinus, and inferior to the optic chiasm.
- Within the cavernous sinus are the carotid artery, the pericarotid sympathetic fibers, and the abducens nerve (VI); within its lateral wall are the oculomotor nerve (III), the trochlear nerve (IV), and the ophthalmic and maxillary divisions of the trigeminal nerve (V_1, V_2).
- Cavernous sinus syndrome is typically caused by septic or aseptic sinus thrombosis, neoplasm, or trauma. Acute obstruction by mass or thrombosis may progress rapidly if not diagnosed and treated quickly.

ETIOLOGY

- Infectious agents include *Staphylococcus aureus*, *Streptococcus pneumoniae*, gram-negative rods, and anaerobes; mucormycosis and *Aspergillus* in immunocompromised patients
- Aseptic venous thrombosis has been associated with sickle cell anemia, trauma, dehydration, vasculitis, pregnancy, oral contraceptive use, congenital heart disease, inflammatory bowel disease, and hypercoagulable states.
- Neoplasms involving the cavernous sinus include pituitary adenomas, meningiomas, trigeminal schwannomas, craniopharyngiomas, lymphomas, neuromas, chordomas, chondrosarcomas, rhabdomyosarcomas, nasopharyngeal carcinomas, and very rarely, teratomas. Neoplasms may present with diplopia, visual field deficits, headache, or isolated cranial nerve deficits.
- The lateral extension of pituitary neoplasms into the cavernous sinus usually affects the 3rd cranial nerve, with the 4th and 6th nerves less commonly involved. Rupture of a cystic craniopharyngioma may present as acute cavernous sinus syndrome.
- Carotid-cavernous fistulas, often with a more chronic course, are direct high-flow shunts between the internal carotid artery and the cavernous sinus. Most often sequelae of trauma, they may present with a history of ocular motility deficits, arterialization of conjunctival vessels, and a bruit usually heard best over the orbit. Less commonly, rupture of a carotid cavernous aneurysm may lead to fistula formation.
- Nonspecific and idiopathic inflammation of the cavernous sinus, also called idiopathic cavernous sinusitis or Tolosa-Hunt syndrome, has been reported in patients as young as 3 1/2 years. This is a diagnosis of exclusion. However, MRI may show enlargement of the affected cavernous sinus with an adjacent soft tissue mass that resolves after treatment with steroids.

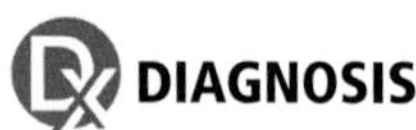

DIAGNOSIS

HISTORY

- Recent facial furuncle or cellulitis, sinusitis, dental infection, otitis, or orbital cellulitis may predispose to cavernous sinus syndrome.
- Fever, headache, eye pain, diplopia, and facial paresthesias may be present.

PHYSICAL EXAM

- Conjunctival injection with lid swelling and proptosis indicates cavernous sinus venous congestion.
- Ptosis, anisocoria, ophthalmoparesis, and facial sensory changes are signs of cranial nerve involvement.
- Horner syndrome: Sympathetic nerve fibers traveling with V_1 may be affected; usually occurs in conjunction with an abducens nerve (CN VI) palsy with an inability to abduct the eye
- Signs and symptoms begin unilaterally but may rapidly spread bilaterally.
- The optic nerve and visual acuity are spared early in cavernous sinus syndrome but can be affected as it progresses.
- Funduscopic findings include venous dilatation and hemorrhages.
- Ocular bruit may be heard in any acute cavernous sinus syndrome but especially in carotid-cavernous fistula.
- Signs of meningitis and systemic toxicity rapidly evolve if infections are untreated.

DIFFERENTIAL DIAGNOSIS

Other disorders that may resemble cavernous sinus syndrome include the following:

- Orbital cellulitis
- Sphenoid sinusitis
- Thyroid eye disease
- Cavernous carotid aneurysm
- Orbital apex tumor
- Orbital pseudotumor
- Ocular migraine
- Ocular trauma
- Burkitt lymphoma

ALERT

- Ophthalmoplegic migraine or cluster headache must be distinguished from cavernous sinus syndrome by neuroimaging studies and history.
  - Proptosis does not occur in migraine or cluster headache.
  - Ophthalmoplegic migraine is a diagnosis of exclusion, especially on first presentation.
- Acute infection and hemorrhage of the pituitary gland—pituitary apoplexy—may present with acute bilateral ophthalmoplegia and signs of acute pituitary insufficiency; most commonly occurs with pituitary neoplasms but may also occur in pregnant women at the time of delivery
- Chronic granulomatous disorders such as sarcoid and tuberculosis may underlie cavernous sinus syndrome.

DIAGNOSTIC TESTS & INTERPRETATION

Initial Tests (screening, lab, imaging)

- CBC, ESR, PT/PTT, blood culture: Basic studies in any child with suspected acute cavernous sinus syndrome. Blood cultures are positive in 70% of cases of septic venous sinus thrombosis.
  - Lumbar puncture should be performed if there is no contraindication and infection is suspected.
  - ~35% of patients with septic cavernous sinus thrombosis have CSF findings consistent with bacterial meningitis—excess neutrophils, increased protein, and/or decreased glucose.

- Evaluation for a prothrombotic state should be considered in patients with cavernous sinus thrombosis, especially in the absence of infection or trauma. Specific labs include protein C activity, protein S activity, antithrombin III activity, factor V Leiden gene mutation, prothrombin gene mutation, anticardiolipin antibodies, β-2-glycoprotein antibodies, dilute Russell viper venom time, homocysteine, lipoprotein(a), and factor VIII activity.
- Antinuclear antibody panel, angiotensin-converting enzyme level, and HIV test should be obtained before diagnosis of Tolosa-Hunt syndrome (diagnosis of exclusion).
- Any child with proptosis, cranial nerve findings, or an ocular bruit should have an urgent MRI or CT.
  - MRI, with and without gadolinium, with special attention to the cavernous sinus and parasellar region, is the imaging study of choice.
  - Magnetic resonance venography may be helpful.
  - CT angiography may be the preferred study to evaluate for carotid-cavernous fistula.

Diagnostic Procedures/Other

- Diagnosis of carotid-cavernous fistulas requires angiography.
- Nasopharyngeal biopsy and culture if mucormycosis or *Aspergillus* is suspected

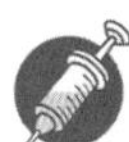

TREATMENT

First priority is to rule out septic cavernous sinus thrombosis, life-threatening infections of the face, sinuses, middle ear, teeth, and orbit.

MEDICATION

First Line

- For septic cavernous sinus thrombosis, broad-spectrum antibiotics (including coverage of penicillinase-resistant staphylococci and anaerobes) are begun immediately. Duration of therapy is usually 2 to 4 weeks beyond the resolution of symptoms.
- Amphotericin B if mucormycosis or *Aspergillus* is suspected
- Idiopathic cavernous sinusitis, a diagnosis of exclusion, responds to corticosteroids. Treatment should not be started until neoplasm and infection have been ruled out.

Second Line

Anticoagulation is controversial, but recent studies in children found that heparin is safe and may be beneficial in treatment of septic cavernous sinus thrombosis.

SURGERY/OTHER PROCEDURES

- Surgical drainage of the primary infection (i.e., sinusitis) may be indicated (avoiding surgical manipulation of the cavernous sinus itself).
- Posttraumatic carotid-cavernous fistulas rarely close spontaneously and have been treated with endoarterial balloon embolization.

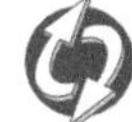

ONGOING CARE

- Septic cavernous sinus thrombosis may relapse, or embolic abscesses may develop 2 to 6 weeks after therapy has been stopped.
- Repeat MRI with gadolinium should be considered, especially if symptoms recur or new symptoms develop.
- Mortality is 8%, and 25% of patients with cavernous sinus thrombosis have persistent neurologic deficits.
- Patients with carotid-cavernous fistulas frequently have persistent cranial nerve deficits even after embolization.
- Idiopathic cavernous sinusitis responds to steroids, but relapses can be problematic. Clinical follow-up and serial MRI scans are indicated to rule out a low-grade neoplasm or fungal infection.
- Consultation with a neurooncologist and a neurosurgeon is important for suspected neoplasms or surgical lesions.

PROGNOSIS

- Prognosis depends on the underlying cause.
- Bacterial infections usually respond if diagnosed and treated promptly.

COMPLICATIONS

- Vary with the cause of cavernous sinus syndrome. Septic cavernous sinus thrombosis and fungal infections may rapidly evolve to bilateral thrombosis, life-threatening sepsis, and meningitis.
- Visual impairment and cranial nerve palsies may persist.
- Mucormycosis, usually seen in patients with diabetic ketoacidosis, is especially dangerous.
- Carotid arteritis with resulting stenosis, occlusion, or embolism may occur, resulting in focal neurologic deficits.
- Aseptic cavernous sinus thrombosis may evolve to more extensive intracranial venous sinus thrombosis.
- Local spread of neoplasms will continue if not treated appropriately.

ADDITIONAL READING

- Chen CC, Chang PC, Shy CG, et al. CT angiography and MR angiography in the evaluation of carotid cavernous sinus fistula prior to embolization: a comparison of techniques. *AJNR Am J Neuroradiol*. 2005;26(9):2349–2356.
- Lee AG, Quick SJ, Liu GT, et al. A childhood cavernous conundrum. *Surv Ophthalmol*. 2004;49(2):231–236.
- Leiba H, Jaqqi GP, Boltshauser E, et al. Prediction of the clinical outcome of cavernous sinus lesions in children. *Neuropediatrics*. 2013;44(4):191–198.
- Press CA, Lindsay A, Stence NV, et al. Cavernous sinus thrombosis in children: imaging characteristics and clinical outcomes. *Stroke*. 2015;46(9): 2657–2660.
- Smith DM, Vossough A, Vorona GA, et al. Pediatric cavernous sinus thrombosis: a case review and review of the literature. *Neurology*. 2015;85(9):763–769.

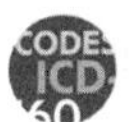

CODES

ICD10

- I67.6 Nonpyogenic thrombosis of intracranial venous system
- G08 Intracranial and intraspinal phlebitis and thrombophlebitis
- H49.889 Other paralytic strabismus, unspecified eye

FAQ

- Q: Will my child's eye movements return to normal?
- A: In most cases, oculomotor nerves regain function as other signs improve, although they may take the longest to recover.
- Q: Can more pain medicine be given?
- A: There is often an attempt to balance side effects of sedation and hypoventilation against the need for pain control, especially when intracranial pressure is a concern.

CAVERNOUS TRANSFORMATION AND PORTAL VEIN OBSTRUCTION

Richard A. Lirio, MD

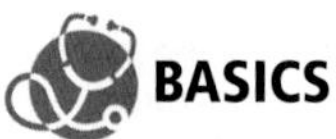

BASICS

DESCRIPTION

- Cavernous transformation
  - Is a term used to describe the collection of collaterals that develop around an obstructed vessel
  - Often develops with obstruction of the portal vein
- Portal vein obstruction
  - Can occur anywhere along the course of the main portal vein or splenic vein, between the hilum of the spleen and the porta hepatis
  - In pediatrics, obstruction is most typically of the portal vein.
  - Major cause of prehepatic or noncirrhotic portal hypertension

EPIDEMIOLOGY

- Most children with portal vein thrombosis present between birth and 15 years of age.
- Acute presentation is rare.
- Chronic cases present with complications of portal hypertension.
- Gastrointestinal (GI) bleeding is more typical in patients presenting <7 years of age.
- Splenomegaly in the absence of symptoms is more typical for patients aged 5 to 15 years.

RISK FACTORS

Genetics

A genetic basis of this problem has not been identified, although congenital abnormalities of the heart, major blood vessels, biliary tree, and renal system are often found.

PATHOPHYSIOLOGY

- In cirrhosis and hepatic malignancies, the thrombus usually begins intrahepatically and spreads to the extrahepatic portal vein.
- In most other etiologies, the thrombus usually starts at the site of origin along the portal vein.
- Occasionally, thrombosis of the splenic vein propagates to the portal vein, most often resulting from an adjacent inflammatory process (e.g., severe pancreatitis).
- Asymptomatic splenomegaly or upper GI hemorrhage results from extrahepatic portal hypertension.
- Less commonly, ascites or failure to thrive can occur, as well as portopulmonary hypertension

ETIOLOGY

50% of portal vein obstructions are idiopathic. Identified causes include the following:

- Congenital vascular anomaly
  - Portal vein malformation
  - Webs or diaphragms within the portal vein
- Clot resulting from a hypercoagulable state
- Clot from other causes:
  - Omphalitis
  - Umbilical vein catheterization
  - Portal pyelophlebitis
  - Intra-abdominal sepsis
  - Surgery near the porta hepatis
  - Sepsis
  - Cholangitis
  - Dehydration
  - Trauma
- Other causes for portal vein obstruction in older children:
  - Ascending pyelophlebitis from perforated appendicitis
  - Primary peritonitis, cholangitis, and pancreatitis causing a splenic vein thrombosis
  - Inflammatory bowel disease

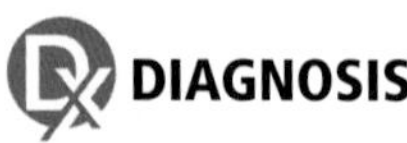

DIAGNOSIS

HISTORY

- Often asymptomatic
- Acutely, can present as sudden onset hematemesis from bleeding varices
- Clinical history and examination should concentrate on identifying possible causes predisposing to portal vein obstruction.
- May present with history of splenomegaly presumed due other causes (see "Splenomegaly" chapter for complete differential diagnosis)
  - Exposure to infectious mononucleosis
  - Metabolic storage disease (e.g., Gaucher disease)
  - Malignancy (e.g., chronic myelogenous leukemia)
- History of prematurity and admission to NICU
  - May be associated with umbilical vein catheterization and increased risk of portal vein thrombosis

PHYSICAL EXAM

- Splenomegaly
  - Spleen is measured from the left anterior axillary line at the costal margin diagonally toward the umbilicus and inferiorly toward the iliac crest.
- Hemorrhoids

DIFFERENTIAL DIAGNOSIS

The differential diagnosis must exclude other causes of splenomegaly and portal hypertension.

DIAGNOSTIC TESTS & INTERPRETATION

Initial Tests (screening, lab, imaging)

- General comments
  - There may be no elevation of liver enzymes, as portal vein obstruction does not affect liver function unless the patient has an underlying liver disease (e.g., cirrhosis).
  - This situation is partially due to a compensatory increased flow of the hepatic artery maintaining the total hepatic blood flow.
  - There may be mild coagulation profile abnormalities.
- CBC:
  - Leukopenia and thrombocytopenia will be present if there is hypersplenism.
  - Anemia, if presents acutely with hematemesis/variceal bleeding
- Aspartate aminotransferase/alanine aminotransferase/γ-glutamyl transferase: should be normal
- PT/PTT: may be abnormal if malabsorption is present but commonly normal
- Additional testing associated with hypercoagulable states (as clinically indicated)
  - Protein C
  - Protein S
  - Antithrombin III levels
  - Factor V Leiden mutation
  - Activated protein C resistance
  - Lupus anticoagulation evaluation
  - Anticardiolipin antibodies (IgA, IgG, IgM)
  - Antinuclear antibody
  - Blood homocysteine
  - Prothrombin 20-21-0 mutation
  - Methylene tetrahydrofolate reductase mutation evaluation
  - Factor VIII coagulant
  - Reptilase time
  - Heparin cofactor II
  - Tissue plasminogen activator
  - Plasminogen activator inhibitor-1
  - Sticky platelet evaluation
  - Paroxysmal nocturnal hemoglobinuria (genetics or flow cytometry evaluation)
- Ultrasound with Doppler
  - To examine portal vein flow and to identify collateral veins that develop with cavernous transformation of the portal vein
  - Liver may be slightly small but is generally normal in texture.
  - Remains the most useful imaging study
- CT angiography or MRV can give additional information if needed, especially prior to planning a surgical portosystemic shunt procedure.

Diagnostic Procedures/Other

- Upper endoscopy and sigmoidoscopy: to define extent of varices
- Liver biopsy
  - Not required for diagnosis nor performed routinely unless to exclude other etiologies
- Pathologic findings
  - Portal hypertension: spider nevi, prominence of abdominal veins, splenomegaly
  - Bruising: may be prominent when coexistent consumption of clotting factors
  - Normal liver palpation and percussion
  - Ascites rarely present

TREATMENT

- General goals of therapy are (1) to manage variceal hemorrhage and (2) to identify an underlying cause and/or determine if the patient is at risk for additional venous thrombosis or malignancy.
- Therapy for GI variceal hemorrhage:
  - Octreotide infusion: 1 mcg/kg/h maximum 50 mcg/h
  - Prophylactic endoscopic variceal banding for large esophageal varices
  - β-Blocker therapy
  - Rex shunt (mesenterico–left intrahepatic portal vein shunt):
    - Involves surgically connecting the internal jugular vein, internal iliac vein, or dilated coronary vein with the superior mesenteric vein and the umbilical portion of the left portal vein (in the liver)
    - Restores the physiologic intrahepatic portal vein perfusion
    - Avoids the consequences of long-term portosystemic shunting, especially hepatic encephalopathy
- Portosystemic shunts: divert portal blood into the low-pressure systemic venous circulation. Classified into
  - Nonselective shunts: These communicate the entire portal venous system to a systemic venous circulation such as the mesocaval shunt, proximal splenorenal shunt, and portacaval shunts. Nonselective shunts divert more blood into the systemic venous system, and patients are more likely to have encephalopathy.
  - Selective shunts: These divert the gastrosplenic portion of the portal venous flow into the left renal vein or the inferior vena cava. The most common selective shunt is the distal splenorenal shunt (also known as the Warren shunt).

ONGOING CARE

FOLLOW-UP RECOMMENDATIONS

Focus on growth parameters, early detection of malabsorption, presence of GI hemorrhage, and indications for nutritional intervention

- Aggressive contact sports should be actively discouraged in children with hepatosplenomegaly.
- All patients should be advised to restrict activities that could injure their already enlarged spleen. Spleen guards may be recommended.
- Patients should be told to avoid medicines that interfere with platelet function, unless recommended by hematology for hypercoagulable states.
- In addition, patients should avoid medications that increase BP, including many over-the-counter cold medications (e.g., phenylephrine), as this can increase splanchnic pressures and may provoke variceal bleeds.

PROGNOSIS

- Long-term prognosis overall is considered good.
- Upper GI hemorrhage becomes less problematic as children become older.
- Most patients receive β-blockers or undergo repeated prophylactic banding. If the liver function remains normal, as in most cases, it is rare for encephalopathy to develop unless a large portosystemic shunt is created.
- Rex shunt restores normal physiology and decreases portal pressure.

COMPLICATIONS

- Variceal hemorrhage from the upper tract or from the perianal varices
- Splenomegaly with hypersplenism:
  - Thrombocytopenia
  - Consumption coagulopathy
  - Leukopenia
- Steatorrhea and protein-losing enteropathy occur secondary to venous congestion of the intestinal mucosa.
- Degree of portal hypertension is variable and depends on the formation of spontaneous shunts or collaterals that may decompress the portal hypertension. These autoshunts may predispose to the development of complications such as hepatic encephalopathy or hepatopulmonary syndrome.
- Spleen can undergo autoinfarction, resulting in intermittent episodes of pain.
- A large spleen is susceptible to traumatic rupture.
- Spontaneous splenic rupture may also occur (classically associated with infectious mononucleosis).

ADDITIONAL READING

- Fuchs J, Warmann S, Kardorff R, et al. Mesenterico—left portal vein bypass in children with congenital extrahepatic portal vein thrombosis: a unique curative approach. *J Pediatr Gastroenterol Nutr*. 2003;36(2):213–216.
- Mileti E, Rosenthal P. Management of portal hypertension in children. *Curr Gastroenterol Rep*. 2011;13(1):10–16.
- Ryckman FC, Alonso MH. Causes and management of portal hypertension in the pediatric population. *Clin Liver Dis*. 2001;5(3):789–818.
- Superina RA, Alonso EM. Medical and surgical management of portal hypertension in children. *Curr Treat Options Gastroenterol*. 2006;9(5):432–443.
- Superina R, Shneider B, Emre S, et al. Surgical guidelines for the management of extra-hepatic portal vein obstruction. *Pediatr Transplant*. 2006;10(8):908–913.
- Wang RY, Wang JF, Sun XG, et al. Evaluation of rex shunt on cavernous transformation of the portal vein in children. *World J Surg*. 2017;41(4):1134–1142.

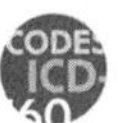

CODES

ICD10

- I81 Portal vein thrombosis
- K76.6 Portal hypertension
- Q26.9 Congenital malformation of great vein, unspecified

FAQ

- Q: In a patient with cavernous transformation of the portal vein, should I recommend restriction of activities and avoidance of certain medications?
- A: Contact sports should be limited or a spleen guard should be used. NSAIDs, including aspirin, should be avoided because of the risk of hemorrhage. Medications that increase blood pressure, including many nonprescription cold preparations, should also be avoided.

CELIAC DISEASE

Dascha C. Weir, MD

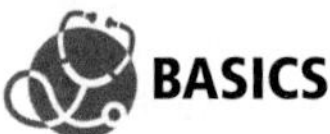

BASICS

DESCRIPTION

- Celiac disease (CD) is a systemic immune-mediated disorder caused by a permanent sensitivity to gluten in genetically susceptible individuals.
- "Gluten"
  - The collective term for specific alcohol-soluble proteins (called prolamines) that are found in wheat, rye, and barley
- "Classic CD"
  - Refers to children who present predominately with malabsorptive symptoms including diarrhea, abdominal pain, vomiting, and abdominal distention in the setting of suboptimal growth and irritability
  - The majority of children presenting with CD do not have classic symptoms. For example, the majority have constipation rather than diarrhea.
- "Silent CD"
  - Defines a minority of people with CD who have no identifiable symptoms but have consistent intestinal mucosal lesions and elevated serum antibodies
- "Celiac crisis"
  - A rare but serious manifestation of CD
  - Consists of severe watery diarrhea, electrolyte disturbances, dehydration, hypotension, and lethargy
- "Potential CD"
  - Patients with positive serologic testing but normal intestinal histology
  - Some, but not all, of these "potential CD" patients develop CD over time on a gluten-containing diet

EPIDEMIOLOGY

- CD is present in approximately 1% of the U.S. population, but only a small proportion have been diagnosed.
- Average age at diagnosis of pediatric CD in the United States is approximately 9 years old.
- Females are more affected than males.

RISK FACTORS

Genetics

- There is increased prevalence in patients with 1st-degree relatives with CD (10–15%).
- HLA-DQ2 and HLA-DQ8 haplotypes are "necessary but not sufficient" for CD.
  - >90% of CD patients carry HLA-DQ2, 5% carry HLA-DQ8.
  - High negative predictive value for negative DQ2/DQ8 testing
  - Low positive predictive value (30% of general population in North America is HLA-DQ2 positive.)
- Numerous other genes have been identified as increasing CD susceptibility.
- A family or personal history of autoimmune disease is also associated with CD.

PATHOPHYSIOLOGY

- In people with CD, ingestion of gluten leads to an enteropathy of the small intestine characterized by mucosal inflammation and villous atrophy.
- Generation of unique serologic autoantibodies and development of a diverse spectrum of signs and symptoms also occur.
- Elimination of gluten, via implementation of a strict gluten-free diet (GFD), leads to intestinal healing, normalization of elevated antibody levels, and resolution of related symptoms.

COMMONLY ASSOCIATED CONDITIONS

- Autoimmune thyroiditis
- Type 1 diabetes mellitus
- Sjögren syndrome
- Selective IgA deficiency
- Williams syndrome
- Down syndrome
- Turner syndrome

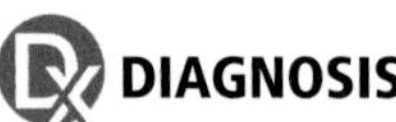

DIAGNOSIS

- The range of signs and symptoms secondary to CD is broad. Malabsorptive symptoms such as diarrhea and weight loss are more commonly seen in early childhood. Other more subtle gastrointestinal (GI) symptoms in pediatric CD can be recurrent intermittent abdominal pain, intermittent diarrhea, constipation, and nausea.
- Extraintestinal manifestations of CD may be more prominent, especially in the older child. "Atypical" or "nonclassic" symptoms can include the following:
  - Aphthous stomatitis
  - Arthritis/arthralgias
  - Delayed puberty
  - Dental enamel hypoplasia
  - Dermatitis herpetiformis (a pruritic blistering symmetric rash)
  - Elevated transaminases
  - Elevated pancreatic enzymes
  - Fatigue
  - Iron deficiency anemia
  - Neuropsychiatric symptoms (including headaches, cognitive impairment, neuropathy, epilepsy, and ataxia)
  - Osteopenia
  - Short stature
  - Thyroiditis
  - Vitamin deficiencies
- Awareness of the wide range of clinical presentation and the high prevalence of CD coupled with a careful history and physical exam is essential to making the diagnosis of CD.
- Obtaining celiac-specific serologic markers is also integral to making the diagnosis.
- Currently, small bowel biopsies remain the gold standard and are required for confirmation of CD.
- Treatment with a GFD should not be initiated before confirmation of disease.

HISTORY

- Review the patient's stooling pattern as well as symptoms of abdominal pain, nausea/ vomiting, low appetite, and bloating/distension.
- Investigate extraintestinal manifestations of CD including fatigue, arthralgias, recurrent oral sores, unusual rashes, and headaches.
- Attention to family history of CD, long-standing undiagnosed GI symptoms, and autoimmune diseases

PHYSICAL EXAM

- Focus on growth patterns:
  - Some patients may have short stature or suboptimal weight gain as the only manifestation of CD.
  - Many children with CD have normal growth or even overweight status.
- Assess pubertal development.
- Although patients with classic CD often have a distended abdomen with wasted buttocks, most patients do not have clear physical signs of CD.
- Observe for dental enamel defects, oral sores, or dermatitis herpetiformis.

DIFFERENTIAL DIAGNOSIS

- Presumed infectious causes:
  - Giardiasis
  - Rotavirus, parasites
  - Chronic gastroenteritis
  - Postenteritis enteropathy
  - Intractable diarrhea of infancy
  - Tropical sprue
  - Intestinal bacterial overgrowth
  - Immunodeficiency syndromes (HIV)
- Presumed noninfectious:
  - Milk or soy protein intolerance
  - Protein-calorie malnutrition
  - Eosinophilic gastroenteritis
  - Autoimmune enteropathy
  - Graft-versus-host disease
  - Collagenous sprue
  - Peptic duodenitis
  - Immunodeficiency syndromes
  - Crohn disease
  - Congenital enteropathies (microvillus inclusion disease, tufting enteropathy)
  - Bowel ischemia
  - Radiation
  - Chemotherapy

DIAGNOSTIC TESTS & INTERPRETATION

All evaluation for CD should be done while a patient is consuming gluten regularly. Testing for the disease while on a GFD can lead to false-negative results. Both serologic testing and histopathologic changes can normalize with gluten removal.

Initial Tests (screening, lab, imaging)

- Total IgA quantification is essential. IgA deficiency is associated with CD and can contribute to false-negative results.
- Celiac serologic markers with high specificity and sensitivity
  - Tissue transglutaminase antibody IgA (tTG IgA): best general screening test
  - Endomysial antibody IgA (EMA IgA): more subjective and expensive than tTG IgA
- Celiac serologic markers with low specificity and sensitivity
  - Antigliadin IgA and IgG (AGA IgA, AGA IgG) are NOT recommended for screening.
- Deamidated gliadin peptide antibody IgG is a newer test with high sensitivity and specificity that should be used in cases of IgA deficiency.
- Nonspecific testing to screen for associated nutritional deficiencies
  - Vitamin levels
  - CBC
  - Iron panel
  - Bone densitometry
  - Tests of absorption (fecal fat, D-xylose uptake)
- Endoscopic evaluation
  - Small bowel biopsies obtained by esophagogastroduodenoscopy (EGD) is required in most cases to confirm CD.
    - It is recommended to obtain multiple small bowel biopsies during endoscopy due to the patchy distribution of lesions.
    - The duodenal bulb, in addition to the duodenum, should be biopsied.
    - The current recommendation is to obtain six small bowel biopsies on a gluten-containing diet.
    - European guidelines outline a "no biopsy" approach to diagnosis in a specific subset of children. However, the "no biopsy" approach should only be utilized with the guidance and monitoring of a pediatric gastroenterologist.
- Pathologic findings
  - CD has a number of cardinal histopathologic findings on small bowel biopsy:
    - Increased intraepithelial lymphocytosis
    - Villous atrophy (partial, subtotal, or total)
    - Crypt hyperplasia
    - Infiltration of lamina propria with excess lymphocytes (CD4 T cells mainly) and plasma cells

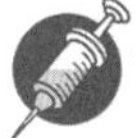

TREATMENT

- Current treatment of CD consists of a strict, lifelong GFD.
  - Elimination of all wheat, rye, and barley is essential, with close care to avoid cross-contamination during the preparation and serving of food.
  - Oats, unless specifically certified as gluten free, should also be avoided, as they are standardly contaminated with wheat.
- Consultation with a specialized dietitian with expertise in the GFD is recommended for all cases.

MEDICATION

- There are no medications currently available to treat CD. However, people on a GFD should take a multivitamin. It is imperative to confirm that all vitamins and medications are also GF.
- It may be appropriate to consider recommending the following:
  - Calcium and vitamin D
  - Iron for iron deficiency anemia
  - In patients with symptoms of lactose intolerance, lactase enzyme replacement

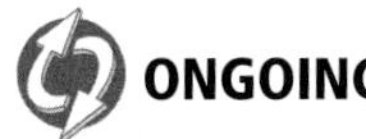

ONGOING CARE

FOLLOW-UP RECOMMENDATIONS

Patient Monitoring

- Close clinical monitoring of patients with newly diagnosed CD is important. Patients should be seen several times within the 1st year of diagnosis to monitor symptom response to the GFD, adherence to the GFD, and patient/family coping with the lifestyle changes associated with the GFD. After the 1st year, yearly follow-up is recommended.
- Special attention should be paid to growth at each visit. Catch-up growth is typically noted within the 1st year on the GFD.
- Monitor for other autoimmune disease, especially thyroiditis and diabetes mellitus, with targeted history and exam.
- Assessing for adequate calcium intake and vitamin D deficiency is also recommended to optimize bone health. Bone density in children with CD typically normalizes on a GFD. Bone densitometry can be considered but, in most cases, is recommended after a year on a GFD.
- tTG levels typically normalize within a year on the GFD and, coupled with clinical status, can be helpful in assessing response to the GFD. Obtaining a tTG IgA is recommended after 6 months on a GFD and then on a yearly basis.
- Repeat endoscopic evaluation is not currently recommended in patients who respond clinically to a GFD and who have normalization of tTG IgA. However, repeat endoscopic evaluation in cases of clinical nonresponse to the GFD or persistent serologic elevation should be considered.

PROGNOSIS

In patients with CD, it is strongly recommended to remain on a GFD for life. In patients on a strict GFD, there is lower risk for malignancies and other complications associated with CD. However, increased risk of other autoimmune diseases seems to persist.

COMPLICATIONS

- Adults with CD have increased risk of intestinal lymphoma and other GI malignancies. This risk is magnified in suboptimally treated CD.
- Other complications include the following:
  - Osteopenia/osteoporosis
  - Infertility
  - Development of other autoimmune disorders
  - Nutritional deficiencies
- Refractory CD is a diagnosis of exclusion that is defined by persistent symptoms and villous atrophy on a strict GFD.
  - Refractory CD is rare in children but affects up to 5% of adults with CD, most of whom harbor an abnormal clonal intraepithelial T-lymphocyte population.
  - Complications of refractory CD: "Cryptogenic enteropathy-associated T-cell lymphoma," ulcerative jejunoileitis, and collagenous sprue
  - Treatment: immunosuppressives including corticosteroids, azathioprine, cyclosporine, and total parenteral nutrition, in addition to GFD

C

ADDITIONAL READING

- Fasano A, Catassi C. Clinical practice. Celiac disease. *N Engl J Med*. 2012;367(25):2419–2426.
- Hill ID, Dirks M, Liptak G, et al. Guideline for the diagnosis and treatment of celiac disease in children: recommendations of the North American Society for Pediatric Gastroenterology, Hepatology and Nutrition. *J Pediatr Gastroenterol Nutr*. 2005;40(1):1–19.
- Husby S, Koletzko S, Korponay-Szabó IR, et al. European Society for Pediatric Gastroenterology, Hepatology, and Nutrition guidelines for the diagnosis of coeliac disease. *J Pediatr Gastroenterol Nutr*. 2012;54(1):136–160.
- Leffler DA, Schuppan D. Update on serologic testing in celiac disease. *Am J Gastroenterol*. 2010;105(12):2520–2524.
- Olsson C, Hernell O, Hörnell A, et al. Difference in celiac disease risk between Swedish birth cohorts suggests an opportunity for primary prevention. *Pediatrics*. 2008;122(3):528–534.

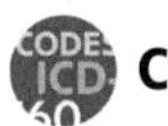

CODES

ICD10

K90.0 Celiac disease

FAQ

- Q: Is biopsy confirmation necessary if my patient is already doing better on a GFD?
- A: Yes. Referral to a pediatric gastroenterologist who can obtain small bowel biopsy is recommended in almost all cases of suspected pediatric CD.
- Q: Are oats included in the gluten-containing cereal group?
- A: Strictly speaking, wheat, rye, and barley are more closely related in their development from the primitive grains than are oat, rice, corn, sorghum, and millets, which do not activate CD. Gluten-free means a diet devoid of all wheat, rye, and barley. Several studies have shown that ingestion of pure oats did not cause histologic or clinical deterioration. However, it is important to use a brand of oats that has been tested and demonstrated to not be contaminated with gluten.

CELLULITIS

Nicholas Tsarouhas, MD

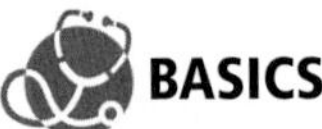

BASICS

DESCRIPTION

- Cellulitis is an acute, spreading pyogenic inflammation of the dermis and subcutaneous tissue, often complicating a wound or other skin condition.
- Cellulitis may be further classified by the unique area of the body it affects (e.g., periorbital or orbital cellulitis, peritonsillar cellulitis).

EPIDEMIOLOGY

- The most common cause of cellulitis in children is *Staphylococcus aureus* or *Streptococcus pyogenes* infection, which develop secondary to local trauma of the integument.
- In purulent cellulitis (presence of a pustule, abscess, or purulent drainage), *S. aureus* infection is more likely.
- Community-acquired methicillin-resistant *S. aureus* (CA-MRSA) infections continue to increase in incidence but more commonly cause purulent abscesses rather than cellulitis.
- The prevalence of CA-MRSA among purulent skin and soft tissue infections is >60% in some communities.
- Bacteremic disease is rare, owing to the tremendous efficacy of vaccines against both *Haemophilus influenzae* type b (Hib) and *Streptococcus pneumoniae*.

GENERAL PREVENTION

- Good wound care is paramount.
- All wounds should be cleaned with soap and water and then covered with a clean, dry cloth.
- Topical antibiotic ointment is optional with minor wounds.

PATHOPHYSIOLOGY

- Cellulitis usually occurs after local trauma that breaches in the integument (abrasions, lacerations, bite wounds, excoriated dermatitis, varicella, etc.).
- Cellulitis may result from local invasion or infection (e.g., sinusitis leading to orbital cellulitis).
- Hematogenous dissemination is rare.

ETIOLOGY

- *S. aureus:* methicillin-susceptible *S. aureus* (MSSA) and MRSA.
- Group A β-hemolytic streptococci (GABHS, or *S. pyogenes*).
- *S. aureus* and *S. pyogenes* are by far the most common causes of uncompleted cellulitis.
- *S. pyogenes* is also the usual cause of erysipelas, a superficial cellulitis.
- *S. pneumoniae* (uncommon)
- Group B streptococci (GBS) and gram-negative rods (GNRs): neonates
- Hib (rare)
- *Pseudomonas aeruginosa* and anaerobic bacteria: immunocompromised children
- *Pasteurella* species: cat and dog bites
- *Eikenella corrodens*: human bites

COMMONLY ASSOCIATED CONDITIONS

- Periorbital
  - Usually from local trauma (scratch, impetigo, eczema, excoriated varicella)
  - Hematogenous spread is very uncommon.
  - Rarely associated with infectious conjunctivitis
- Orbital
  - Commonly associated with severe sinusitis
  - Less commonly: dental abscess, trauma, hematogenous spread
- Buccal: usually from local trauma; hematogenous seeding also very rare
- Peritonsillar
  - Commonly due to GABHS pharyngitis
  - Cellulitis may progress to a peritonsillar abscess.
- Extremity: usually secondary to local trauma
- Breast: usually with mastitis (neonates)
- Perianal
  - Seen in infants and young children
  - Etiology: GABHS
  - Perianal pain, pruritus, and erythema; sometimes associated with bloody stools
- Cellulitis–adenitis syndrome
  - Neonates and infants
  - Etiology: GBS most common; *S. aureus*, GNRs
  - Bacteremia/meningitis commonly associated

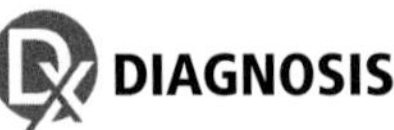

DIAGNOSIS

HISTORY

- An expanding, red, painful area of swelling is the most common presentation.
- Mild constitutional symptoms (with or without fever) are commonly associated with cellulitis.
- A history of local trauma to the integument is the clue to the portal of bacterial entry.
- Visual changes, proptosis, and painful or limited eye movements are classic findings in orbital cellulitis.
- Painful swallowing, pain with opening the mouth (trismus), and muffled ("hot potato") voice are classic presenting symptoms of peritonsillar cellulitis/abscess.

PHYSICAL EXAM

- Erythema, edema, tenderness, and warmth: usual clinical findings of cellulitis
- Spreading, irregular margins of erythema are classic, and distinguish cellulitis from erysipelas, which has well-demarcated margins.
- A red streak extending proximally from the extremity: lymphangitis, which usually implies more serious involvement
- Regional adenopathy: commonly associated with minor cellulitis; occasionally complicated by lymphadenitis

DIFFERENTIAL DIAGNOSIS

- Allergic angioedema can be excluded by its lack of tenderness and the absence of fever.
- Allergic reactions to insect stings are usually pruritic and may present with mild to severe local erythema; a bite history confirmatory
- Red giant urticarial lesions, similarly, may masquerade as cellulitis.
- Contact dermatitis is distinguished by its painlessness, pruritus, and the Koebner phenomenon (appearance of isomorphic lesions in the lines of scratching).
- Nummular eczema is a pruritic dermatitis consisting of one or more circular lesions with papules, scales, and/or crusting, typically distributed on the trunk or extremities.
- The erythema migrans rash of Lyme disease starts as a red macule at the tick bite site, then expands to a large, annular, erythematous lesion; the classic "bull's eye" lesion with central clearing is not always seen.
- A traumatic contusion may be mistaken for cellulitis; the history confirms the diagnosis.
- Severe conjunctivitis presents with conjunctival injection, chemosis, and discharge.
- "Popsicle panniculitis," a cold-induced fat injury to the cheeks of infants; mimics buccal cellulitis; a history of cold weather exposure, eating ice, or popsicle sucking are classic.
- Erythema nodosum, a panniculitis with raised, tender lesions that are frequently over the shins; this may present as a single erythematous lesion; associated with systemic disorders, including inflammatory bowel disease
- Superficial thrombophlebitis is distinguished by a tender cord palpable along the course of the affected superficial vein.
- An eye malignancy (retinoblastoma), invasive tumor (rhabdomyosarcoma), or metastatic disease (neuroblastoma, leukemia, lymphoma) may simulate periorbital or orbital cellulitis.
- Necrotizing fasciitis is a serious skin and soft tissue infection of the subcutaneous tissue and fascia that is rapidly progressive and has a high mortality rate; it may resemble cellulitis, with spreading skin erythema; however, the skin may initially be spared.

DIAGNOSTIC TESTS & INTERPRETATION

- WBC, C-reactive protein (CRP), and erythrocyte sedimentation rate (ESR): normal or elevated
- Bacterial cultures
  - Via needle aspiration or biopsy at the leading edge or point of maximal inflammation
  - Usually not helpful, often yielding negative results
- Blood culture:
  - Rarely positive
  - Children who are ill-appearing, immunocompromised, or have extensive areas of cellulitis may warrant a blood culture.
- Open wound and abscess culture: As resistance continues to rise (especially MRSA), open wound and abscess content cultures are quite useful.
- Plain radiographs:
  - Sometimes helpful to rule out complications such as osteomyelitis
  - Also useful in cases of suspected foreign bodies
- Ultrasound: often useful to distinguish cellulitis from abscess, which might need incision and drainage (I&D).
- Head/sinus/orbital CT scan:
  - Important in cases when clinical distinction between periorbital and orbital cellulitis is difficult.
  - Useful in orbital cellulitis to delineate extent of disease

Diagnostic Procedures/Other

In some cases, a cutaneous biopsy, examined by an experienced pathologist, may be needed to identify the correct diagnosis.

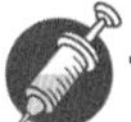

TREATMENT

GENERAL MEASURES

Local care of cellulitis involves elevation and immobilization of the limb to reduce swelling, and cool sterile saline dressings to remove purulence from open lesions.

MEDICATION

- Most cases of uncomplicated, superficial "nonpurulent" cellulitis (cellulitis with no purulent drainage or exudate, and no associated abscess) may be treated with β-lactam oral antibiotics active against β-hemolytic streptococci and MSSA (e.g., cephalexin or amoxicillin-clavulanate).
- Coverage for MRSA is indicated in patients who do not respond to initial therapy, patients with signs of systemic illness, patients with recurrent infection in the setting of underlying predisposing conditions, and patients with a previous episode of MRSA infection.
- Additionally, MRSA coverage should be considered in patients with MRSA risk factors, and in areas where the prevalence of MRSA is >30%.
- Patients with purulent cellulitis (cellulitis associated with purulent drainage or exudate, in the absence of a drainable abscess) should be treated with antibiotics active against MRSA.
- Clindamycin is a good initial choice due to its activity against β-hemolytic streptococci and both MSSA and MRSA; however, clindamycin resistance for both MSSA and MRSA is increasingly being recognized. Susceptibility patterns are geographically dependent.
- Trimethoprim-sulfamethoxazole covers both MSSA and MRSA but not β-hemolytic streptococci; consequently, some combine it with amoxicillin to add the streptococcal coverage.
- Some feel that initial coverage against β-hemolytic streptococci is not always mandatory in patients with purulent cellulitis; thus, monotherapy with trimethoprim-sulfamethoxazole is also occasionally employed.
- Doxycycline and minocycline are additional alternatives with good MRSA coverage, especially for penicillin-allergic patients.
- Erythromycin is also sometimes used in patients allergic to penicillin; isolates resistant to erythromycin exist, however, and may be cross-resistant to clindamycin as well.
- Ill-appearing children or those with extensive cellulitic lesions require IV antibiotics.
- The presence of fever may predict failure of empirical outpatient antibiotic therapy.
- Younger age children are also more likely to require hospitalization, although a specific age cutoff is not clear.
- As MRSA infections continue to rise, most experts now recommend clindamycin as initial parenteral therapy; however, resistance of MSSA to clindamycin is increasing.
- Oxacillin, nafcillin, cefazolin, and ampicillin-sulbactam are reasonable alternatives when MRSA is not strongly suspected.
- Vancomycin is used as empiric therapy in ill-appearing children or in cases of severe or rapidly progressive infections.
- Linezolid, a newer antibiotic that can be given IV or PO, is very effective against MRSA, but it is expensive and should mostly be reserved for multiresistant organisms.
- If hematogenous dissemination is a strong possibility, an agent active against Hib also should be added (e.g., ceftriaxone, cefotaxime).
- The duration of antibiotics (IV and PO) should generally be 7 to 10 days.
- Patients can be switched from IV to oral antimicrobial therapy when they are afebrile for 24 hours or longer, improving clinically, and able to take oral medications.
- Bite wounds should have tetanus and rabies prophylaxis issues addressed.

ALERT

- Remember to consider the possibility of MRSA in all deep, invasive, or persistent infections (i.e., consider adding clindamycin in these cases).
- Increasing rates of resistance of MSSA to clindamycin are being reported, which may limit the use of clindamycin monotherapy for cellulitis caused by MSSA.
- Penicillin and amoxicillin are never good empiric choices for cellulitis because they have poor *S. aureus* coverage.

SURGERY/OTHER PROCEDURES

- Abscesses should always be drained.
- Antibiotics are often unnecessary for management of uncomplicated skin abscesses, if I&D are properly performed.

ONGOING CARE

FOLLOW-UP RECOMMENDATIONS

- Steady improvement should be expected.
- If daily improvement is not noted, consider the following:
  - Inappropriate antimicrobial coverage
  - A deeper infection or abscess that needs drainage
  - Immunocompetency issues
  - Foreign body

PROGNOSIS

The prognosis for complete recovery is good as long as appropriate antimicrobials are administered in a timely fashion.

COMPLICATIONS

- Local or distant spread of infection is possible.
- Suppuration and abscess formation may occur (e.g., peritonsillar abscess).
- Extremity cellulitis may extend into the deep tissues to produce an arthritis or osteomyelitis, or it may extend proximally as a lymphangitis.
- Orbital cellulitis may be complicated by visual loss and/or cavernous sinus thrombosis.
- Prior to widespread immunization against Hib, the bacteremia associated with facial cellulitis was associated with pneumonia, meningitis, pericarditis, epiglottitis, arthritis, and osteomyelitis.

ADDITIONAL READING

- Amin AN, Cerceo EA, Deitelzweig SB, et al. Hospitalist perspective on the treatment of skin and soft tissue infections. *Mayo Clin Proc.* 2014;89(10):1436–1451.
- Elliott DJ, Zaoutis TE, Troxel AB, et al. Empiric antimicrobial therapy for pediatric skin and soft-tissue infections in the era of methicillin-resistant *Staphylococcus aureus*. *Pediatrics.* 2009;123(6):e959–e966.
- Hyun DY, Mason EO, Forbes A, et al. Trimethoprim-sulfamethoxazole or clindamycin for treatment of community-acquired methicillin-resistant *Staphylococcus aureus* skin and soft tissue infections. *Pediatr Infect Dis J.* 2009;28(1):57–59.
- Larru B, Gerber JS. Cutaneous bacterial infections caused by *Staphylococcus aureus* and *Streptococcus pyogenes* in infants and children. *Pediatr Clin North Am.* 2014;61(2):457–478.
- Liu C, Bayer A, Cosgrove SE, et al; for Infectious Diseases Society of America. Clinical practice guidelines by the Infectious Diseases Society of America for the treatment of methicillin-resistant *Staphylococcus aureus* infections in adults and children. *Clin Infect Dis.* 2011;52(3):e18–e55.
- Mistry RD. Skin and soft tissue infections. *Pediatr Clin North Am.* 2013;60(5):1063–1082.
- Odell CA. Community-associated methicillin-resistant *Staphylococcus aureus* (CA-MRSA) skin infections. *Curr Opin Pediatr.* 2010;22(3):273–277.
- Pallin DJ, Binder WD, Allen MB, et al. Clinical trial: comparative effectiveness of cephalexin plus trimethoprim-sulfamethoxazole versus cephalexin alone for treatment of uncomplicated cellulitis: a randomized controlled trial. *Clin Infect Dis.* 2013;56(12):1754–1762.
- Raff AB, Kroshinsky D. Cellulitis: a review. *JAMA.* 2016;316(3):325–337.

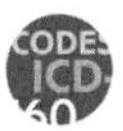

CODES

ICD10

- L03.90 Cellulitis, unspecified
- H05.019 Cellulitis of unspecified orbit
- J36 Peritonsillar abscess

FAQ

- Q: Is IV ampicillin-sulbactam adequate initial parenteral therapy for cellulitis with abscess?
- A: No. MRSA should be covered in these patients. IV clindamycin is a better choice when MRSA is most likely. Ampicillin-sulbactam may be adequate for the child with cellulitis without abscess who does not have risk factors for MRSA.
- Q: When should IV vancomycin be used?
- A: IV vancomycin should be reserved for ill-appearing children or those with severe or rapidly progressive infections. These are cases when any treatment delay waiting for definitive culture and sensitivity results could be life-threatening.

CEREBRAL PALSY

Stephen H. Contompasis, MD

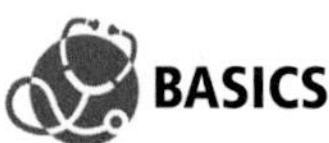

BASICS

DESCRIPTION

Cerebral palsy (CP) describes a group of disorders of movement and posture, limiting activity, attributed to nonprogressive underlying brain pathology. The motor disorders of CP are often accompanied by disturbances of sensation, cognition, communication, perception, and/or behavior or by a seizure disorder:

- Spastic (pyramidal; 75%): increased deep tendon reflexes, sustained clonus, hypertonia, and the clasp-knife response:
  - Spastic diplegia: lower extremity involvement
  - Spastic hemiplegia: one side of the body involved
  - Spastic quadriplegia: total body involvement; usually associated with dystonia, dysphagia, and dysarthria
- Dyskinetic (10%): fluctuating tone, rigid total body involvement by definition; persistent primitive reflex patterns (asymmetric tonic neck reflex, labyrinthine)
  - Athetoid: slow writhing movements (or chorea; rapid, random, jerky movements)
  - Dystonic: posturing of the head, trunk, and extremities
- Ataxic (<10%): characterized by cerebellar signs (ataxia, dysmetria, past pointing, tremor, nystagmus) and abnormalities of voluntary movement
- Mixed (10%): two or more types codominant, most often spastic and dyskinetic
- Other (10%): criteria for CP met, but specific subtype cannot be defined
- Extrapyramidal: sometimes applied to nonspastic types of CP as a group

EPIDEMIOLOGY

- ~50% of cases are associated with prematurity.
- Increased concordance among monozygotic versus dizygotic twins in some studies (not in others)
- Intrauterine growth retardation (IUGR) more common in CP than controls, especially for full-term infants in whom CP develops
- Male > female (1.3:1)
- Inconsistent relationship to maternal age, socioeconomic status, and parity
- Prenatal factors are more strongly associated with subsequent CP than are perinatal or postnatal factors; however, individual risk factors are poorly predictive of subsequent CP in the individual child.
- Perinatal asphyxia accounts for only ~9% of CP; diagnosis requires evidence of hypoxic-ischemic insult, severe encephalopathy (e.g., neonatal seizures, severe hypotonia), and consistent laboratory/radiologic findings.
- Increased with multiple gestation (10% were twins in one study)
- Prevalence ~2–3/1,000

ETIOLOGY

- Not apparent in most cases. Some studies suggest that the presence of chorioamnionitis; mild or even subclinical infection may have increased association with CP.
- Epidemiologic studies indicate two types of associated vulnerability to CP:
  - Prematurity: Vulnerability of the periventricular white matter between 28 and 32 weeks of gestation results in periventricular leukomalacia.
  - IUGR: fetal growth retardation associated with CNS dysgenesis, non-CNS malformation, teratogens, growth retardation, evidence of hypoxic-ischemic encephalopathy

COMMONLY ASSOCIATED CONDITIONS

- Sensory
  - Sensorineural and conductive hearing loss
  - Impaired visual acuity
  - Oculomotor dysfunction
  - Strabismus
  - Cortical visual impairment
  - Somatosensory impairments
- Cognitive/developmental
  - Intellectual disability in ~50%, especially in spastic quadriparesis
  - Autism, ADHD
  - Language and learning disabilities
  - Dysarthria
  - Sleep and behavioral disturbances
- Neurologic
  - Seizures
  - Hydrocephalus
- Musculoskeletal
  - Contractures
  - Hip subluxation/dislocation
  - Scoliosis
  - Osteoporosis
- Cardiorespiratory
  - Upper airway obstruction
  - Aspiration pneumonitis
  - Restrictive lung disease/thoracic deformity
  - Reactive airway disease
- GI/nutritional
  - Poor growth
  - Gastroesophageal reflux
  - Constipation
  - Oral motor dysfunction/dysphagia
- Urinary: neurogenic bladder
- Skin: decubitus ulcers
- Dental
  - Malocclusions
  - Caries
  - Gingival hyperplasia
  - Abnormalities of enamel (congenital)

DIAGNOSIS

HISTORY

- Prenatal
  - Exposure to toxins/drugs
  - Infections or fever
  - HIV/STD risk
  - Vaginal bleeding
  - Abnormal fetal movement
  - Preeclampsia (especially proteinuria)
  - Breech position
  - Poor maternal weight gain
  - Premature labor
  - Fetal distress
  - IUGR
  - Prenatal testing
  - Placental disorders
- Perinatal
  - Premature delivery
  - Neonatal resuscitation
  - Low Apgar scores (<5 at 5 minutes)
  - Birth trauma
  - Evidence of neonatal encephalopathy (seizures, lethargy, hypotonia)
  - Complicated neonatal course (intraventricular hemorrhage, prolonged respiratory support, meningitis, sepsis, hyperbilirubinemia)
- Postnatal
  - Hospitalization for severe infection or trauma
  - Periodic or persistent deterioration in function (suggests neurodegenerative/metabolic disease)
- Development
  - Significant delay in motor milestones/motor quotient (age of typical skill attainment/age of attainment <0.5) (e.g., not rolling at 10 months, not sitting at 12 months, not walking at 24 months)
  - Associated with persistent primitive reflexes (e.g., prominent tonic neck and labyrinthine responses at 1 year of age) and delayed or absent development of protective reactions (e.g., lateral prop at 7 months, parachute at 13 months)
  - Associated delays in language, play, social, and adaptive behavior

PHYSICAL EXAM

- General observation:
  - Evidence of dysmorphism
  - Pigmentary skin changes
  - Growth abnormalities
- Head circumference:
  - Evaluate for microcephaly, macrocephaly, and hydrocephaly.
  - Growth velocity points to timing of brain pathology
- Eye exam:
  - Assess for strabismus, cataracts, iris or retinal abnormalities.
  - May suggest cranial nerve damage, muscle imbalance, metabolic disease, or congenital infection

- Musculoskeletal
  - Decreased range with contractures
  - Leg length discrepancy: hip dislocation
  - Spinal curvature/scoliosis
- Neurologic
  - Documentation of best level of visual motor/manipulative skills (transfer, hold a cup): to follow course of motor impairment
  - Cranial nerves: strabismus, speech and swallowing, vision and hearing
  - Tone: spasticity versus rigidity versus hypotonia
  - Strength: typically decreased
  - Hyperactive deep tendon reflexes and clonus in spasticity; Babinski reflex (extensor response to plantar stimulation)
  - Persistent primitive reflexes
  - Protective reactions: head and trunk righting, prop reactions, parachute; cerebellar signs
  - Balance, stability

ALERT

Pitfalls

- Overdiagnosis of CP in premature infants with spastic hypertonia; normalization of tone/function may take up to 2 years.
- False or premature assumption of cognitive deficit in children with severe dysarthria; may take years of augmentative communication supports to determine true potential
- Slowly progressive neurodegenerative diseases and pediatric neurotransmitter disorders may masquerade as CP.
- Cervical cord lesions may masquerade as diparetic or quadriparetic spastic CP.
- Determination of ideal body weight/caloric requirements may be complex in CP; skinfold measuring <10th percentile is the best indicator of poor nutrition.
- Pain is a common problem, with more than half of adults and children with CP reporting pain as an ongoing health concern.

DIFFERENTIAL DIAGNOSIS

- Motor syndromes related to spinal cord, lower motor neuron, peripheral nerve, primary muscular disease, or progressive disorders of the basal ganglia (dopa-responsive dystonia)
- Connective tissue disorders (primary and secondary) resulting in musculoskeletal abnormalities (e.g., arthrogryposis multiplex, skeletal dysplasias)
- Inborn errors of metabolism and CP: protean manifestations, dyskinesia, ataxia, postnatal growth failure, neurologic deterioration, recurrent vomiting

DIAGNOSTIC TESTS & INTERPRETATION

Initial Tests (screening, lab, imaging)

- Genetic and metabolic studies: if history or physical suggests a progressive or hereditary disorder
- Blood chemistries, liver function studies, cell counts: Evaluate nutritional/metabolic status, anticonvulsant levels.
- Brain imaging: Perform when hydrocephalus is suspected; can help determine etiology
- Radiography: should be done routinely in spastic diparesis for hip dislocation; consider scoliosis films.
- GI studies to evaluate gastroesophageal reflux, slow gastric emptying, aspiration risk

Diagnostic Procedures/Other

- Hearing and vision: all in 1st year, with regular follow-up exams
- Audiologic evaluation required per guidelines
- Urodynamic studies: spastic bladder in those with recurrent UTIs or voiding dysfunction
- Sleep study: may disclose treatable obstructive sleep apnea in those with somnolence or abnormal sleep–wake cycles
- Pulmonary function studies: document progressive restrictive pulmonary dysfunction (e.g., in severe scoliosis)
- Consider bone density: liability to fracture
- Brain wave (EEG): if seizure suspected

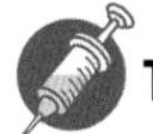

TREATMENT

- Family-centered care and coordination in a medical home directed toward optimizing health, activity, and participation
- Interdisciplinary clinics: services (medical, surgical, therapy) coordinated with primary physician and medical home
- More frequent health maintenance visits and coordination meetings from a medical home practice may assist in managing multiple chronic associated health conditions.
- Spasticity reduction with IM injections of botulinum toxin is well-supported; oral or intrathecal baclofen used increasingly, although consensus on functional improvement long term is variable
- Orthopedic management with directed procedures to reduce contractures and improve posture has more evidence on improving functional outcomes long term.
- Education services: emphasis on inclusion/mainstreaming and mandated special education services and accommodations
- Augmentative communication supports especially for nonverbal/dysarthric children.
- Physical, occupational, speech/language therapy, other interdisciplinary health professionals: therapy provided in home, school, and hospital settings; directed primarily at improved mobility, self-care, and communication; orthodontists for dental malocclusion
- Counseling support for children coping with chronic disability
- Social services: provided in a variety of contexts to aid in the coordination of care
- Vocational counseling and employment options, assistance with transition to adulthood, self-advocacy, self-determination
- Transition to adult health care system and medical home

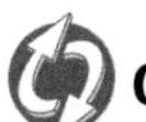

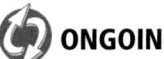

ONGOING CARE

FOLLOW-UP RECOMMENDATIONS

- Requirements for specialty care vary greatly with the degree of disability and impairment. An interdisciplinary clinic setting may be more appropriate for a child with severe CP.
- Early referral to a pediatric orthopedist or physiatrist is indicated, especially for monitoring of the hip.
- Early referral for developmental assessment: need for early intervention to optimize development and promote family coping

DIET

Nutritional assessment and support for those with dysphagia or poor growth (especially calcium, vitamin D intake)

ADDITIONAL READING

- Delgado MR, Hirtz D, Aisen M, et al; for Quality Standards Subcommittee of the American Academy of Neurology and the Practice Committee of the Child Neurology Society. Practice parameter: pharmacologic treatment of spasticity in children and adolescents with cerebral palsy (an evidence-based review): report of the Quality Standards Subcommittee of the American Academy of Neurology and the Practice Committee of the Child Neurology Society. *Neurology*. 2010;74(4):336–343.
- Liptak GS, Murphy NA; for Council on Children with Disabilities. Providing a primary care medical home for children and youth with cerebral palsy. *Pediatrics*. 2011;128(5):e1321–e1329.
- Novak I. Evidence-based diagnosis, health care, and rehabilitation for children with cerebral palsy. *J Child Neurol*. 2014;29(8):1141–1156.
- Pakula AT, Van Naarden Braun K, Yeargin-Allsopp M. Cerebral palsy: classification and epidemiology. *Phys Med Rehabil Clin N Am*. 2009;20(3):425–452.
- Rosenbaum P, Paneth N, Leviton A, et al. A report: the definition and classification of cerebral palsy April 2006. *Dev Med Child Neurol Suppl*. 2007;109:8–14.

CODES

ICD10

- G80.9 Cerebral palsy, unspecified
- G80.1 Spastic diplegic cerebral palsy
- G80.2 Spastic hemiplegic cerebral palsy

FAQ

- Q: Is severe clumsiness a form of CP?
- A: Mild spastic diplegia or hemiplegia may present this way, but tone abnormalities and significant functional impairments distinguish CP from the milder specific developmental disorder of motor function (ICD-F82).
- Q: Do all children with CP also have intellectual disability?
- A: Only ~50% have intellectual disability.

CERVICITIS

Camille Sabella, MD

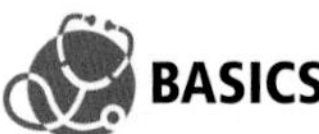

BASICS

DESCRIPTION

Infection of the endocervix resulting in inflammation, leading to mucopurulent cervical discharge, edema, erythema, bleeding, and friability of the cervix and endocervical canal

EPIDEMIOLOGY

- The true incidence of cervicitis is unknown; however, the primary causes (gonorrhea/chlamydia) are more common in adolescents and young adults than any other age group.
- Because many patients are asymptomatic and the interpretation and presence of the clinical signs are quite variable, many cases are undiagnosed.

RISK FACTORS

- Early age of coitarche
- Multiple sexual partners
- Absent or inconsistent condom use

ETIOLOGY

In most cases of cervicitis, no pathogen is isolated. Common causes include the following:

- *Chlamydia trachomatis*
- *Neisseria gonorrhoeae*
- *Herpesvirus hominis*
- *Trichomonas vaginalis*
- *Mycoplasma genitalium*

COMMONLY ASSOCIATED CONDITIONS

The presence of other sexually transmitted infections (STIs) must be considered, including the following:

- Syphilis
- Hepatitis B
- HIV
- Bacterial vaginosis

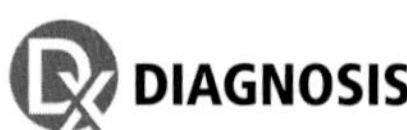

DIAGNOSIS

HISTORY

- Often asymptomatic
- If symptomatic: The following symptoms are consistent with but not diagnostic of cervicitis:
  - Abnormal vaginal bleeding and/or discharge? Inflamed cervix may bleed spontaneously or following sexual intercourse.
  - Dysuria? May indicate urethritis or bladder infection
  - Vulvar itching? May be associated discharge from cervical inflammation or a coexisting vaginal infection
  - Dyspareunia? Common complaint owing to the sensitive cervix
- Past medical history—important to evaluate risk factors related to sexual health but not diagnostic of cervicitis
  - Previous STI? Identifies patients at increased risk for reinfection
  - Last menstrual period? Symptomatic infection often occurs within 7 days of the last menstrual period because of loss of the protective endocervical mucous plug.
  - Birth control method? Condoms are protective.
  - Exposure to infected partner? Identifies patient at increased risk
  - Gravity?
  - Parity?

PHYSICAL EXAM

- Abdominal exam
  - No tenderness on palpation of the abdomen suggests that infection is limited to the cervix.
- Vaginal exam
  - Assess for signs of vaginal/external lesions consistent with herpes simplex virus (HSV).
- Pelvic exam
  - Mucopurulent discharge from the cervical os or yellow exudative discharge present on a cotton-tipped swab from the endocervical canal: clinical evidence of cervical infection
  - No cervical motion or adnexal tenderness or masses: Pathology has not extended beyond the cervix to the upper genital tract.
  - Friability of the exocervix: easily induced bleeding from the cervical canal not to be confused with normal cervical ectopy (area of columnar epithelium around the cervical os presenting as a discrete, nonfriable, reddish circle)

ALERT

Pitfalls:

- Failure to recognize the importance of evaluating the internal pelvic organs by physical examination with the presenting symptoms of dysuria, vaginal discharge, or abnormal menstrual bleeding in the postpubertal female
- Imperative not to confuse normal cervical ectropion (i.e., cervical eversion) in an adolescent with cervicitis

DIFFERENTIAL DIAGNOSIS

- It is helpful to consider cervicitis/vaginitis as a single disease in the evaluation process because the symptoms of these two entities are the same.
- Inflammation of the vulva, urethra, and/or bladder, and vagina
- In patients presenting with abnormal menstrual bleeding, these infectious causes are common.
- Pregnancy is a frequent cause of abnormal vaginal bleeding.
- Foreign body can be associated with both discharge and bleeding.
- Polycystic ovary syndrome (PCOS), thyroid dysfunction, and hyperprolactinemia can all present with abnormal vaginal bleeding.
- Noninfectious cervicitis occurs and is primarily caused by mechanical or chemical irritation (foreign objects, latex, vaginal douches, contraceptive creams).

DIAGNOSTIC TESTS & INTERPRETATION

Initial Tests (screening, lab, imaging)

- Nucleic acid amplification tests done on the patient's urine offers the least invasive method to detect *Chlamydia*, gonococcal, and *Trichomonas* infections. Cervical or vaginal swabs may also be used for nucleic acid amplification tests, provided that there is no bleeding:
  - Cervical swabs, vaginal swabs obtained by the health care provider, and urine have similar sensitivity and specificity.
  - Cervical cultures for chlamydia and gonorrhea will also identify the pathogen but require a speculum examination.
  - Identifies the pathogen, which is important for patient and partner treatment and disease surveillance
- HSV culture if vesicular rash or ulcers are present: important to identify the cause of the ulcers for treatment and patient counseling
- Wet preparation and vaginal pH may be helpful in diagnosing bacterial vaginosis.

TREATMENT

MEDICATION

- Gonorrhea
  - Ceftriaxone ≤45 kg: 50 mg/kg (max 125 mg) IM × 1, >45 kg: 250 mg IM × 1, PLUS azithromycin 20 mg/kg (max 1 g) PO, single dose or doxycycline 100 mg PO b.i.d. for 7 days. Oral cefixime is no longer recommended as first line due to resistance. If cefixime is used because ceftriaxone is not available, a test of cure is necessary.
  - Recently, noticed patterns of resistance to fluoroquinolones have caused the Centers of Disease Control and Prevention (CDC) to no longer recommend this class as first line of treatment of gonococcal cervicitis in the United States.
  - If fluoroquinolones are used, a test of cure is necessary.
- *C. trachomatis*
  - Azithromycin ≥45 kg: 1 g PO, single dose, OR
  - Doxycycline 100 mg PO b.i.d. for 7 days, OR
  - Erythromycin <45 kg: 50 mg/kg/24 h (base or ethylsuccinate) PO divided q6h for 7 days; ≥45 kg: 500 mg (base) or 800 mg (ethylsuccinate) PO q.i.d. for 7 days
- *T. vaginalis*
  - Metronidazole <45 kg: 45 mg/kg/24 h (max 2,000 mg/24 h) PO divided TID for 7 days; ≥45 kg: 2 g PO, single dose, OR 500 mg PO b.i.d. for 7 days OR
  - Tinidazole >3 years old: 50 mg/kg (max 2 g) PO as a single dose
- *H. hominis*
  - Acyclovir 400 mg PO t.i.d. for 7 to 10 days or until resolution, OR
  - Acyclovir 200 mg PO 5 times daily for 7 to 10 days or until resolution, OR
  - Famciclovir 250 mg PO t.i.d. for 7 to 10 days or until resolution, OR
  - Valacyclovir 1 g PO b.i.d. for 7 to 10 days or until resolution

ADMISSION, INPATIENT, AND NURSING CONSIDERATIONS

- Patients meeting the criteria for the clinical diagnosis of cervicitis or those who have a high likelihood of infection should receive presumptive therapy for *N. gonorrhoeae* and *C. trachomatis*.
- Treat other pathogens if clinically indicated or if documented by laboratory studies.

ONGOING CARE

FOLLOW-UP RECOMMENDATIONS

- The recommended treatment regimens have excellent cure rates.
- The patient should have resolution of symptoms 3 to 5 days after starting therapy.
- Patients should abstain from intercourse until 7 days after both partners have been treated to prevent reinfection.
- Routine follow-up cultures are not necessary unless the patient remains symptomatic or in the case of pregnancy.
- Nucleic acid amplification tests done <6 weeks following treatment may yield false-positive results because of persistence of dead organisms.
- Detection of an STI at follow-up is most likely the result of reexposure and reinfection.

Patient Monitoring

- Partners should be referred for evaluation and treatment if laboratory diagnosis of gonorrhea/chlamydia or *Trichomonas* is made.
- Gonorrhea/chlamydia are reportable STIs.

PROGNOSIS

If treated appropriately, patients are cured and have no sequelae from the infection.

COMPLICATIONS

The patient with endocervical infection is at risk for the following:

- Reinfection
- Other STIs
- Pregnancy
- Symptomatic or asymptomatic upper genital tract disease (pelvic inflammatory disease), with all its sequelae:
  - Tuboovarian abscess
  - Infertility
  - Ectopic pregnancy
  - Chronic pelvic pain

ADDITIONAL READING

- American Academy of Pediatrics. Sexually transmitted infections in adolescents and children. In: Kimberlin DW, Brady MT, Jackson MA, et al, eds. *Red Book: 2015 Report of the Committee on Infectious Diseases*. 30th edition. Elk Grove, IL: American Academy of Pediatrics; 2015:177.
- Centers for Disease Control and Prevention. Sexually transmitted diseases treatment guidelines, 2015. *MMWR Recomm Rep*. 2015;64(RR-3):1–137.
- Centers for Disease Control and Prevention. Update to CDC's sexually transmitted diseases treatment guidelines, 2006: fluoroquinolones no longer recommended for treatment of gonococcal infections. *MMWR Morb Mortal Wkly Rep*. 2007;56(14):332–336.
- Centers for Disease Control and Prevention. Update to CDC's sexually transmitted diseases treatment guidelines, 2010: oral cephalosporins no longer a recommended treatment of gonococcal infections. *MMWR Morb Mortal Wkly Rep*. 2012;61(31):590–594.
- Committee on Adolescence and Society for Adolescent Health and Medicine. Screening for nonviral sexually transmitted infections in adolescents and young adults. *Pediatrics*. 2014;134(1):e302–e311.

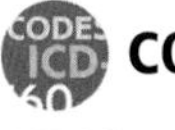

CODES

ICD10

- N72 Inflammatory disease of cervix uteri
- A54.03 Gonococcal cervicitis, unspecified
- A56.09 Other chlamydial infection of lower genitourinary tract

FAQ

- Q: How much cervical motion tenderness is present in patients with cervicitis?
- A: None. Patients with cervicitis have inflammation and infection of the cervix only. They do not have any evidence of peritoneal inflammation on physical examination; therefore, patients with tenderness should be treated with the protocols recommended by the CDC for pelvic inflammatory disease. This does not include the use of a single dose of azithromycin.
- Q: Which partners should be referred for treatment?
- A: Sex partners from the preceding 60 days should be referred for evaluation and treatment. Treatment is based on documented or presumptive etiologies.
- Q: What is the appropriate treatment for *M. genitalium*?
- A: *M. genitalium* has clearly been implicated in the development of urethritis in males and is thought to play some role in the development of cervicitis in females (although that role is not entirely clear). Data suggests that azithromycin may be the best treatment for this infection.
- Q: How often should asymptomatic sexually active adolescents be screened for STIs?
- A: Sexually active men and women <25 years of age should be screened annually for STIs.

CHANCROID

Evelyn Porter, MD, MS • Christine S. Cho, MD, MPH, MEd

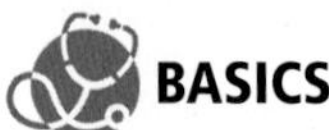

BASICS

DESCRIPTION
Sexually transmitted infection caused by *Haemophilus ducreyi* that manifests as painful genital skin ulcerations and inguinal lymphadenopathy

EPIDEMIOLOGY
- Low incidence in the United States with sporadic outbreaks
- In underdeveloped countries, a major cause of genital ulcer syndrome
- Probably underreported due to difficulty with definitive diagnosis via culture in developing areas
- Increases the risk of HIV transmission
- Seen more commonly in males; females are more likely to be asymptomatic.
- Sexual contact is the only known route of transmission.
- If diagnosed in children, sexual abuse should be considered.
- The United States has seen a 99% decline in cases between 1990 and 2010; since then, the incidence has fluctuated.
- In 2016, there were seven reported cases.

RISK FACTORS
Increased association with sex workers and individuals involved in drug use

GENERAL PREVENTION
Condom use

PATHOPHYSIOLOGY
- Transmission suspected via microabrasions sustained during sexual intercourse, allowing the organism to penetrate the epidermis
- 3 to 10 days later, an erythematous, tender papule develops and progresses to a pustule.
- The pustule ruptures after 2 to 3 days, leaving a shallow ulcer with a painful, necrotic base with undermined edges.
- Single or multiple ulcers may be present.

ETIOLOGY
H. ducreyi, a gram-negative coccobacillus

COMMONLY ASSOCIATED CONDITIONS
- Associated with HIV transmission and infection
- Coinfection with syphilis and human herpesvirus may occur (10%).

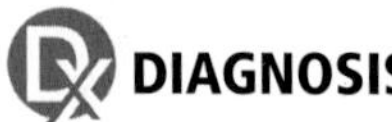

DIAGNOSIS

- Diagnosis of chancroid is routinely based on clinical findings after the exclusion of other causes of genital ulcer disease.
- Males usually present with symptoms referable to an acute, painful genital ulcer.
- Females may be asymptomatic or present with nonspecific symptoms (dysuria, vaginal discharge, pain with stooling or sexual intercourse, rectal pain, or bleeding).

PHYSICAL EXAM
Classic findings:
- Extremely painful ulcer with an irregular, undermined border and a gray, necrotic center
  - In males: found on prepuce or coronal sulcus
  - In females: found on the vulva, cervix, or perianal area
- Painful, unilateral, inguinal lymphadenopathy (bubo) in 50% which may spontaneously drain
- Extragenital sites are rare and include the inner thigh area, breasts, fingers, and mouth.

DIFFERENTIAL DIAGNOSIS
- Chancroid must be distinguished from the other causes of genital ulcers, including:
  - Syphilis
  - Herpes simplex virus (HSV)
  - Lymphogranuloma venereum
  - Granuloma inguinale
  - More than one of these pathogens may be present in individual cases.
- Uncommon etiologies include:
  - Trauma
  - Fixed drug eruptions
  - Inflammatory bowel disease
  - Behçet syndrome

DIAGNOSTIC TESTS & INTERPRETATION
Diagnosis is made by clinical findings and exclusion of other causes of genital ulcers.

Initial Tests (screening, lab, imaging)
- Gram stain from the base of the ulcer: may show short gram-negative coccobacilli in parallel "school of fish" arrangement. Not reliable as a screening test as ulcers may contain multiple organisms; routine use is not helpful.
- Cultures from the ulcer
  - *H. ducreyi* is a fastidious organism and requires specialized media and technique for successful isolation.
  - Compared with newer amplification techniques, it has been proven to be 75% sensitive.
  - Currently the only method routinely available for the definite diagnosis of chancroid
- DNA amplification
  - A genital ulcer multiplex (GUM) polymerase chain reaction test has been developed for simultaneous amplification of DNA targets from *H. ducreyi*, *Treponema pallidum*, and HSV types 1 and 2; offers improved sensitivity when compared with culture
  - This technology is not routinely available.
- Monoclonal antibody
  - Monoclonal antibody against the outer membrane protein of *H. ducreyi* using immunofluorescent antibody has also proven to be more sensitive than culture.
  - Could provide easy, rapid, inexpensive, sensitive testing but not available currently
- Additional testing
  - Evaluation for the common causes of genital ulcer syndrome should be done routinely: culture and PCR for HSV 1 and 2 and dark field examination of ulcer or serologic testing for syphilis performed 7 days after ulcer onset
  - HIV test

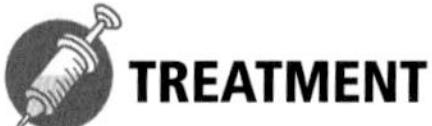

TREATMENT

GENERAL MEASURES

Condom use if consenting teen and sexually active

MEDICATION

- Azithromycin 20 mg/kg (max 1 g) PO, once
- Ceftriaxone 50 mg/kg (max 250 mg) IM, once
- Ciprofloxacin 500 mg b.i.d. for 3 days (patients >18 years)
- Erythromycin base 500 mg PO q.i.d. for 7 days (≥18 years)
- One-time directly observed dosing with azithromycin or ceftriaxone is recommended.

ISSUES FOR REFERRAL

Patients should follow up 1 week after diagnosis for monitoring symptom resolution.

SURGERY/OTHER PROCEDURES

Persistent inguinal fluctuant adenitis may be treated with either needle aspiration or incision and drainage.

ADMISSION, INPATIENT, AND NURSING CONSIDERATIONS

Patients should be admitted to the hospital if they are systemically ill and unwell appearing or for concerns of ongoing sexual abuse and safety.

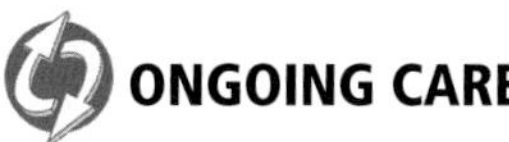

ONGOING CARE

FOLLOW-UP RECOMMENDATIONS

- Patients should be followed weekly until symptoms resolve.
- Recent sexual partners (within the preceding 10 days) should be treated.
- If initial HIV and syphilis test results are negative, they should be repeated in 3 months following diagnosis of chancroid.

PATIENT EDUCATION

Prevention: condom use with all sexual activity

PROGNOSIS

- Symptoms improve within 3 to 7 days.
- Ulcers heal between 1 and 4 weeks.
- Lymphadenopathy may take longer to regress; may become fluctuant despite adequate therapy
- For patients who do not follow the typical course, consider other causes of genital ulcers; noncompliance; presence of a coexisting sexually transmitted disease, especially HIV; and, rarely, presence of a resistant organism.

COMPLICATIONS

- Draining bubo
- Coinfection with syphilis and HSV
- HIV infection

ADDITIONAL READING

- American Academy of Pediatrics. Chancroid. In: Pickering LK, Baker CJ, Kimberlin DW, et al, eds. *Red Book: 2012 Report of the Committee on Infectious Diseases*. 29th ed. Elk Grove Village, IL: American Academy of Pediatrics; 2012:271–272.
- Centers for Disease Control and Prevention. 2016 Sexually transmitted diseases surveillance. https://www.cdc.gov/std/stats16/other.htm. Accessed October 30, 2017.
- Kaliaperumal K. Recent advances in management of genital ulcer disease and anogenital warts. *Dermatol Ther*. 2008;21(3):196–204.
- Lewis DA. Chancroid: clinical manifestations, diagnosis, and management. *Sex Transm Infect*. 2003;79(1):68–71.
- Mackay IM, Harnett G, Jeoffreys N, et al. Detection and discrimination of herpes simplex viruses, *Haemophilus ducreyi*, *Treponema pallidum*, and *Calymmatobacterium* (*Klebsiella*) *granulomatis* from genital ulcers. *Clin Infect Dis*. 2006;42(10):1431–1438.
- Trager JD. Sexually transmitted diseases causing genital lesions in adolescents. *Adolesc Med Clin*. 2004;15(2):323–352.
- World Health Organization; Communicable Disease Surveillance and Response; Epidemiology, Distribution, Surveillance and Control. Guidelines for sexually transmitted infections surveillance. UNAIDS/WHO Working Group on Global HIV/AIDS/STI surveillance. http://apps.who.int/iris/bitstream/10665/66421/1/WHO_CDS_CSR_EDC_99.3.pdf. Accessed October 30, 2017.

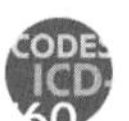

CODES

ICD10

A57 Chancroid

FAQ

- Q: If the culture is negative should I still consider chancroid?
- A: Yes. Sensitivity for cultures of genital ulcers caused by chancroid are only 75% sensitive.
- Q: Can a diagnosis of chancroid be made by clinical findings alone?
- A: In the United States, it is recommended that a combination of both clinical features as well as negative testing for HSV and syphilis be used for the diagnosis of chancroid.
- Q: Will the inguinal bubo heal with the recommended treatment?
- A: Inguinal lymphadenopathy and associated fluctuance may require incision and drainage.

CHEST PAIN

Steven M. Selbst, MD

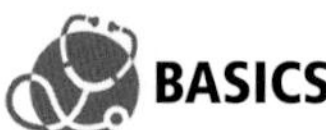

BASICS

DESCRIPTION

Chest pain is a common pain syndrome in childhood. It is less common than abdominal pain and headache. Cardiac disease is an uncommon etiology. Musculoskeletal cause is most common. Boys and girls are equally affected. Etiology is often unclear (idiopathic).

COMMONLY ASSOCIATED CONDITIONS

- Asthma
- Cystic fibrosis
- Diabetes mellitus (long-standing)
- Hypertrophic cardiomyopathy
- Kawasaki disease
- Marfan syndrome
- Sickle cell disease
- Systemic lupus erythematosus

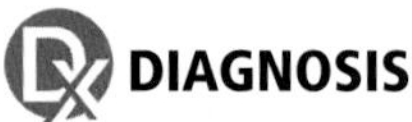

DIAGNOSIS

- Approach to patient
  - Identify the rare child with a serious cause for chest pain (see discussion in "Physical Exam"—important physical findings on general examination of child with chest pain)
    - **Phase 1:** Is the patient in acute distress? If so, begin emergency management and proceed rapidly to find the cause of pain.
    - **Phase 2:** For most stable children with chest pain, determine whether laboratory tests are needed to help identify the cause.
    - **Phase 3:** Treat specific conditions as appropriate. Begin analgesics, reassure the family, and arrange for follow-up care.
- Hints for screening problems
  - Take a thorough history and perform a careful physical exam. Examine the chest last—do not focus only on this area. Use laboratory tests sparingly, only to confirm clinical suspicions.

HISTORY

- **Question:** How severe, how often is the pain?
- *Significance*: Constant, frequent severe pain is more likely to be distressing and interruptive of daily activity. Serious etiology is not well correlated with frequency and severity of pain.
- **Question:** What is the type of pain? Where is its location?
- *Significance*: Burning pain is associated with esophagitis. Sharp, stabbing pain relieved by sitting up or leaning forward is typical of pericarditis. Young children do not describe or localize chest pain well.
- **Question:** When was the onset of pain?
- *Significance*: Acute pain (<48 hours) is more likely to have an organic cause. Chronic pain (>6 months) is more likely to be psychogenic or idiopathic. In an older child with sudden onset of pain, consider an arrhythmia, pneumothorax, or musculoskeletal injury. In a young child with sudden onset of pain, consider a foreign body (coin) in the esophagus or injury.
- **Question:** Is the pain induced by exercise?
- *Significance*: Exercise-induced chest pain may be related to serious cardiac disease or asthma.
- **Question:** Recent trauma, rough play, or muscle overuse?
- *Significance*: musculoskeletal (chest wall) pain
- **Question:** Eaten spicy foods? Taken tetracycline or other pills?
- *Significance*: Esophagitis. Teens often take pills with little water and then lie down. The undissolved pill may lodge in the esophagus and cause pain.
- **Question:** Recent use of "street drugs" such as cocaine?
- *Significance*: hypertension, tachycardia, myocardial ischemia, or pneumothorax
- **Question:** Use of oral contraceptives, clotting disorder, or recent leg trauma?
- *Significance*: pulmonary embolism. This is rare in the pediatric age group.
- **Question:** Recent significant stress (e.g., move, death of loved one, serious illness)?
- *Significance*: psychogenic pain. Children may have headaches and abdominal pain related to stress. Chest pain may also relate to unusual stress.
- **Question:** Associated complaints?
- *Significance*: Fever may imply pneumonia (common), myocarditis, or pericarditis (less common but serious). Syncope and palpitations may imply cardiac arrhythmias or severe anemia. Joint pain or rash may relate chest pain to collagen vascular disease. Pain that resolves with parental attention may indicate an emotional cause.
- **Question:** Positive familial history?
- *Significance*: Hypertrophic cardiomyopathy is often familial. Those with this disorder may have familial history positive for sudden death. When there is a positive familial history of heart disease or chest pain, the parents may be unusually concerned about the symptom in a child. Such a child often has a nonorganic cause.
- **Question:** Past medical history?
- *Significance*: Previous Kawasaki disease, long-standing insulin-dependent diabetes mellitus, and sickle cell disease may have serious cardiac or pulmonary complications leading to chest pain. Marfan syndrome has increased risk for aortic dissection and pneumothorax. Asthma has increased risk for pneumonia and pneumothorax. Collagen vascular disease has increased risk for pleural effusion and pericarditis. Most underlying structural cardiac lesions rarely produce chest pain. Hypertrophic cardiomyopathy is a high-risk situation.

PHYSICAL EXAM

- Important physical findings on general examination of child with chest pain
  - Severe distress
  - Chronically ill appearance
  - Fever
  - Skin rash or bruising
  - Abdominal pathology
  - Arthritis present
  - Anxiety apparent
  - Obesity (BMI >25)
- **Finding:** Child is in significant distress?
- *Significance*: requires emergency care; stabilization. Consider pneumothorax, arrhythmia, or ischemia.
- **Finding:** Child appears chronically ill?
- *Significance*: Chest pain may be found in serious illnesses such as malignancy (Hodgkin lymphoma) or systemic lupus erythematosus.
- **Finding:** Fever?
- *Significance*: Consider pneumonia, myocarditis, or pericarditis.
- **Finding:** Skin bruising present?
- *Significance*: Chest pain may be related to unrecognized trauma. Osteomyelitis of the rib is a rare cause.
- **Finding:** Abdominal pathology?
- *Significance*: Pain may be referred to the chest.
- **Finding:** Arthritis present?
- *Significance*: Collagen vascular disease may manifest as pleural effusion or chest pain.
- **Finding:** Unusually anxious child?
- *Significance*: Underlying stress may lead to pain.
- **Finding:** Obesity?
- *Significance*: higher risk for pulmonary embolism
- Important physical findings on chest examination of child with chest pain
  - Breast abnormality
  - Subcutaneous emphysema
  - Heart murmur, rub, arrhythmia
  - Chest wall tenderness
- **Finding:** Breast enlargement, asymmetry, tenderness?
- *Significance*: Physiologic breast changes in young teens may be painful. Consider pregnancy in teenage girls.
- **Finding:** Decreased breath sounds, wheezing?
- *Significance*: may suggest pneumonia, asthma with overuse of chest wall muscles
- **Finding:** Subcutaneous emphysema palpable on chest or neck?
- *Significance*: pneumothorax, pneumomediastinum
- **Finding:** Heart murmur, rub, arrhythmia?
- *Significance*: congenital heart disease, hypertrophic cardiomyopathy, cardiac infections such as myocarditis, pericarditis, supraventricular tachycardia, ventricular tachycardia
- **Finding:** Tenderness of chest wall, costochondral junctions?
- *Significance*: musculoskeletal pain, costochondritis

ALERT

Factors that make this an emergency include the following:

- Pneumothorax: may present with severe sudden chest pain, respiratory distress, cyanosis, hypotension
- Cardiac arrhythmia: Ventricular tachycardia or supraventricular tachycardia in an older child may progress to heart failure or a lethal rhythm.
- Cocaine intoxication: may present with pneumothorax, cardiac arrhythmia, hypertension
- Direct chest trauma: may lead to cardiac contusion and arrhythmia
- Caustic ingestions or esophageal foreign bodies require prompt attention.

DIFFERENTIAL DIAGNOSIS
- Musculoskeletal disorders
  - Chest wall strain
  - Costochondritis
  - Direct chest trauma
  - Slipping rib syndrome
- Cardiac pathology
  - Arrhythmia (supraventricular tachycardia, premature ventricular contractions)
  - Coronary artery anomalies
  - Coronary artery aneurysms (Kawasaki disease)
  - Infections (myocarditis, pericarditis)
  - Myocardial infarction/ischemia
  - Structural abnormalities: hypertrophic cardiomyopathy
- GI disorders
  - Caustic ingestions
  - Esophageal foreign bodies
  - Esophagitis (sometimes tetracycline or "pill" induced)
- Psychogenic causes
  - Anxiety/stress
  - Hyperventilation
- Respiratory disorders
  - Asthma
  - Cough (prolonged)
  - Pleural effusion
  - Pneumonia
  - Pneumothorax: spontaneous, trauma related, drug related (cocaine)
  - Pneumomediastinum
  - Pulmonary embolism
- Miscellaneous
  - Breast mass
  - Cigarette smoke
  - Pleurodynia
  - Precordial catch syndrome ("Texidor twinge")
  - Shingles
  - Sickle cell crisis—acute chest syndrome
  - Thoracic tumor

DIAGNOSTIC TESTS & INTERPRETATION
- **Test:** EKG
- *Significance*
  - Obtain if history suggests cardiac pathology (e.g., acute onset of pain, pain on exertion, pain associated with syncope, dizziness, palpitations, history of congenital heart disease, serious associated medical problems [Kawasaki disease, diabetes mellitus], use of cocaine).
  - Obtain also if physical exam is abnormal; for instance, respiratory distress, cardiac abnormality, fever, significant trauma
- **Test:** Holter monitor
- *Significance*: Arrange for this study if cardiac arrhythmia is suspected. EKG may fail to detect intermittent arrhythmia.
- **Test:** exercise stress test
- *Significance*: Obtain if pain is induced by exertion. Usefulness is debated but may identify cardiac disease or asthma.
- **Test:** drug screen
- *Significance*: Obtain if cocaine use is suspected.
- **Test:** troponins
- *Significance*: Obtain in older child with concerns for ischemia.
- **Test:** D-dimer
- *Significance*: Consider with suspected pulmonary embolism, although sensitivity varies in children.
- Chest radiograph
  - Obtain also if history suggests cardiac or pulmonary pathology, tumor, Marfan syndrome, or foreign body (coin ingestion).
  - Obtain also if physical exam suggests decreased breath sounds or palpation of subcutaneous air.
- Chest CT scan
  - Obtain if strong suspicion for pulmonary embolism.

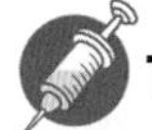

TREATMENT

GENERAL MEASURES
Chest pain in children is rarely related to cardiac pathology. However, not all children with chest pain have a benign etiology; pain associated with exertion, syncope, dizziness is concerning for heart disease; if the child is febrile, consider pneumonia or viral myocarditis. Treat specific cause when found. OTC analgesics (acetaminophen 15 mg/kg/dose, ibuprofen 10 mg/kg/dose) suffice for most pain. Antacids may be diagnostic and therapeutic for esophagitis pain. Rest, heat, and relaxation techniques may be useful. Avoid expensive, invasive laboratory studies with chronic pain and normal physical exam or benign history.

ISSUES FOR REFERRAL
- Acute distress
- Significant trauma
- History of heart disease or related serious medical problem
- Pain with exercise, syncope, palpitations, dizziness
- Serious emotional disturbance
- Esophageal foreign body, caustic ingestion
- Pneumothorax, pleural effusion
- Abnormal heart (or sometimes lung) exam
- Abnormal EKG

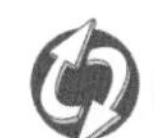

ONGOING CARE

PROGNOSIS
40% will have continued chest pain for 6 to 24 months. Follow-up care is important. Serious pathology is unlikely to be found if not diagnosed initially. However, watch for signs of exercise-induced asthma or for emotional problems that were not obvious initially. Encourage return to normal activity if evaluation is negative. Most have an excellent prognosis.

ADDITIONAL READING

- Agha BS, Sturm JJ, Simon HK, et al. Pulmonary embolism in the pediatric emergency department. *Pediatrics*. 2013;132(4):663–667.
- Blake JM. A teen with chest pain. *Pediatr Clin North Am*. 2014;61(1):17–28.
- Friedman KG, Alexander ME. Chest pain and syncope in children: a practical approach to the diagnosis of cardiac disease. *J Pediatr*. 2013;163(3):896–901.e3.
- Miller AJ, Texidor TA. Precordial catch, a neglected syndrome of precordial pain. *J Am Med Assoc*. 1955;159(14):1364–1365.
- Smith N, DelGrippo E, Selbst SM. Approach to the adolescent with chest pain. In: Goyal MK, Rowlett JD, eds. *AM:STARs: Acute Emergencies in Adolescents. Vol. 26, No. 3*. Itasca, IL: American Academy of Pediatrics; 2016:528–551.
- Yeh TK, Yeh J. Chest pain in pediatrics. *Pediatr Ann*. 2015;44(12):e274–e278.

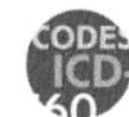

CODES

ICD10
- R07.9 Chest pain, unspecified
- R07.89 Other chest pain
- J45.909 Unspecified asthma, uncomplicated

FAQ
- Q: How common is chest pain in children?
- A: Chest pain is a common pain syndrome reported in 6/1,000 children who present to an urban emergency department. The complaint is less common than abdominal pain or headache. Although children of all ages may complain of chest pain, the mean age is about 12 years.
- Q: Which features in the history are worrisome?
- A: Acute onset of pain, it occurs with exercise, associated syncope, dizziness or palpitations, heart disease or chronic conditions that can affect the heart, trauma, fever, drug use (e.g., cocaine).
- Q: Which findings on physical exam are most worrisome?
- A: Respiratory distress, decreased/abnormal breath sounds, cardiac abnormality, fever, trauma, subcutaneous air, Marfan features
- Q: Which children with chest pain do not need extensive evaluation with laboratory studies?
- A: Those with chronic pain (>6 months) and none of the worrisome features mentioned earlier. Individualized management—analgesics, reassurance, and follow-up usually suffice.
- Q: Why should clinicians be concerned about chest pain in children?
- A: Heart disease is an uncommon cause, but serious pathology is found in some cases. Parental fears must be addressed.

CHICKENPOX (VARICELLA, HERPES ZOSTER)

Camille Sabella, MD

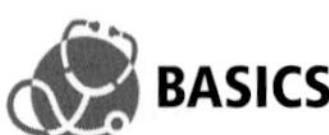

BASICS

DESCRIPTION

Varicella-zoster virus (VZV) is a highly contagious herpesvirus. Primary infection with the virus results in varicella (chickenpox), whereas reactivation from latency results in herpes zoster (shingles).

EPIDEMIOLOGY

- Transmission occurs by droplet and airborne transmission of infectious respiratory secretions or direct contact with vesicles and respiratory secretions.
- Incubation 10 to 21 days (usually 14 to 16 days) after exposure; cases most contagious 12 days before the rash appears until skin lesions have fully crusted
  - Immunocompromised patients may have longer or shorter incubation.
  - Post–intravenous immunoglobulin (IVIG), incubation may be up to 28 days.
- The attack rate for susceptible household contacts exposed to varicella is 90%.
- Disease is more severe in immunocompromised persons, infants >3 months of age, adolescents, adults, persons with pulmonary disorders (asthma), persons with chronic skin disorders (eczema), and persons on oral and/or IV steroids or long-term aspirin therapy.
- Congenital varicella embryopathy: Risk is 1–2% when maternal primary VZV infection occurs before the 20th week of gestation.
- The incidence of chickenpox has declined by 90% since the introduction of universal varicella vaccination.
- The rate of complications from varicella has declined dramatically since the licensure of the varicella vaccine.

GENERAL PREVENTION

- Varicella vaccine
  - Live attenuated vaccine (Oka strain)
  - 2-dose series for routine immunization of all healthy, susceptible children, adolescents, and adults
- Immunogenicity: 76–85% of immunized children developed protective levels of humoral and cellular immunity after 1 dose, ~100% with 2 doses.
- Effectiveness
  - Effectiveness after 1 dose of vaccine: 86%
  - Effectiveness after 2 doses of vaccine: 98%
  - >97% effective in preventing severe varicella
  - 3.3 times less likely to have breakthrough disease when 2 doses of vaccine (as compared to 1 dose) were administered
- Herpes zoster can occur following varicella vaccination, but clinical severity of the zoster is milder and the risk of acquiring zoster following immunization is lower than following wild-type chickenpox.
- Contraindications
  - Anaphylaxis to vaccine components (e.g., neomycin, gelatin)
  - Pregnant, immunocompromised, or <12 months of age
  - HIV is an exception: Vaccine is recommended for HIV-positive children if CD4+ T-cell counts are ≥15%. Give doses 3 months apart.
  - High-dose corticosteroid doses of ≥2 mg/kg/day or ≥20 mg/day of prednisone, or its equivalent, for ≥14 days are considered immunosuppressive doses: VZV vaccine should not be given until systemic corticosteroid therapy has been discontinued for at least 1 month.
- Postexposure prophylaxis
  - If no contraindication to VZV vaccine: Administer VZV vaccine to susceptible hosts (first or second dose) within 3 days (possibly up to 5 days) of exposure.
  - If contraindications to VZV vaccine exist: Consider passive immunization (see below).
- Give passive immunization if
  - (i) No evidence of immunity in exposed person, (ii) probability that exposure will result in infection, and (iii) likelihood of complications of VZV in the exposed person due to risk factors
  - Susceptible immunocompromised people, pregnant women, and neonates whose mothers develop varicella infection 5 days prior to 2 days after delivery should be especially considered for passive immunization upon exposure.
  - Administer varicella zoster immune globulin (VariZIG®) or IVIG as per protocol within 10 days of exposure.
  - If VariZIG® or IVIG is unavailable, some experts recommend postexposure prophylaxis with oral acyclovir (20 mg/kg q6h; max dose: 3,200 mg/24 h) or valacyclovir (20 mg/kg/dose q8h; max dose: 3,000 mg/24 h), beginning 7 to 10 days after exposure and continuing for 7 days.

PATHOPHYSIOLOGY

- After primary infection, the virus establishes latency in dorsal root ganglia cells.
- Immunity from natural disease is usually lifelong, but symptomatic and asymptomatic reinfections do occur, boosting antibody levels.

DIAGNOSIS

HISTORY

- Chickenpox
  - Fever, malaise; decreased appetite common prior to onset of rash
  - Fever low grade to moderate and persists after rash appears
  - Pruritic rash begins on scalp, face, or trunk.
  - New lesions appear as some begin to crust; multiple stages (macules, vesicles, crusted lesions) apparent at one time.
  - Vesicles may appear in the mouth, conjunctiva, vagina, and urethra.
- Zoster
  - Prodrome of pain, pruritus, hyperesthesias
  - Vesicular lesions are clustered unilaterally in a dermatomal distribution of one or more adjacent sensory nerves.
  - Mildly painful in children

PHYSICAL EXAM

- Chickenpox
  - Evolution of rash from macules to vesicles, which appears as "dewdrop on a rose petal," then crust
  - Lesions in multiple stages of formation is pathognomonic.
  - Most children have <300 lesions; higher numbers are found among children who develop varicella after household contact.
  - New lesions appear for up to 7 days in otherwise healthy children.
  - Assess for complications: interstitial pneumonia, encephalitis, secondary bacterial infection (especially group A *Streptococcus*).
- Zoster
  - Discrete vesicles appear first, then enlarge and coalesce.
  - New lesions cease to form after 3 to 7 days and crusting occurs within 2 weeks.
  - Severe local dermatomal infection, cutaneous dissemination, and visceral dissemination may occur in immunocompromised children.

DIFFERENTIAL DIAGNOSIS

The differential diagnosis includes other causes of vesicular rash:

- Coxsackievirus infection (hand, foot, mouth)
- Eczema herpeticum
- Herpes zoster with dissemination
- Impetigo
- Insect bites
- Monkeypox
- *Mycoplasma* (erythema multiforme)
- *Pseudomonas* (ecthyma gangrenosum)
- Rickettsialpox
- Scabies
- Toxic epidermal necrosis
- Stevens-Johnson syndrome

DIAGNOSTIC TESTS & INTERPRETATION

- Studies generally not needed for typical cases in healthy children
- VZV is difficult to isolate in cell culture.
- Polymerase chain reaction (PCR) testing of vesicular fluid is the diagnostic method of choice.
- Direct fluorescent antibody assay from scrapings of a vesicle base can provide rapid diagnosis but is less sensitive than PCR.
- Serology
  - Utilized to determine susceptibility to infection
  - Acute and convalescent sera can determine acute infection.
  - IgM assays not reliable for diagnosing acute infection

TREATMENT

GENERAL MEASURES

- Isolation of hospitalized patients with chickenpox:
  - Contact and airborne precautions of the index case for the duration of vesicular eruption and all vesicles crusted (usually 5 days, longer in immunocompromised patients)
  - Use negative-pressure rooms, if possible.
  - Exposed susceptible persons should be in contact and airborne precautions from day 8 to 21 after the onset of rash in the index patient.
  - Neonates born to mother with VZV: contact and airborne precautions until day 28
  - Embryopathy does not require precautions if there are no active lesions.
  - Persons who received VariZIG® or IVIG should be kept in contact and airborne precautions for 28 days after exposure.
- Isolation of hospitalized patients with zoster:
  - Immunocompromised patients who have zoster (localized or generalized) and immunocompetent patients with disseminated zoster should remain in contact and airborne precautions for the duration of the illness, as above.
  - Immunocompetent patients with localized zoster: contact precautions until all lesions crusted
- Isolation of outpatients with chickenpox:
  - Child should remain at home, away from susceptible and high-risk persons, until no new eruptions and all vesicles have crusted.
- Isolation of outpatients with zoster:
  - For immunocompetent patients with localized zoster, contact precautions are recommended until all lesions are crusted.
  - If lesions can remain completely covered, child may return to school; however, active lesions are infectious.

MEDICATION

- Acyclovir is the drug of choice for varicella or zoster in children.
- IV acyclovir is indicated for infected immunocompromised hosts and neonates and those with associated pneumonia or encephalitis:
  - <1 year old: 10 to 20 mg/kg q8h
  - ≥ 1 year old: 500 mg/m^2 q8h or 10 to 20 mg/kg q8h
  - ≥ 12 years old: 10 mg/kg q8h
- Treat for 7 to 10 days or until no new lesions for 48 hours.
- Oral acyclovir may be considered for those with increased risk of severe infection, including those with cutaneous disorders, chronic diseases that may be exacerbated by acute varicella infection, adolescents, and those who acquire infection after household contact.
  - Acyclovir (PO): 20 mg/kg q6h to max of 800 mg q6h, for 5 days
  - Valacyclovir (PO): (≥ 2 years old) 20 mg/kg (max 1,000 mg) q8h for 5 days; better bioavailability
- Children with VZV should not receive salicylates because of the risk of Reye syndrome. Use acetaminophen to control fever.

ONGOING CARE

FOLLOW-UP RECOMMENDATIONS

Patient Monitoring

For normal healthy individuals, follow-up is not necessary.

PROGNOSIS

- For most children, this childhood exanthema is a benign disease that lasts 6 to 8 days.
- Postherpetic neuralgia can cause significant morbidity following zoster in adults but is very rare in children.

COMPLICATIONS

Complications are associated with significant morbidity and may occur regardless of the use of acyclovir:

- Secondary bacterial infection—especially group A streptococcal infections and *Staphylococcus aureus*
- CNS (1 in 4,000): transverse myelitis, myelopathy, encephalitis (60 cases/year prevaccine), meningoencephalitis, acute cerebellar ataxia, necrotizing retinitis
- Varicella interstitial pneumonitis (more common in adults and infants)
- GI: pancreatitis, appendicitis, and hepatitis
- Heme: idiopathic thrombocytopenia, disseminated intravascular coagulation (hemorrhagic VZV)
- Nephritis
- Vasculopathy of small and large cerebral vessels, causing strokes
- Zoster sine herpete: radicular pain without rash but virologic confirmation of reactivation; can be dermatomal or CNS; very rare in the pediatric population
- Individuals with AIDS may have chronic VZV, including progressive myelopathy.
- Congenital varicella syndrome: characterized by limb atrophy and scarring of the extremity (cicatrices), CNS and eye manifestations
- Postherpetic neuralgia: Neuropathic pain is more common in zoster patients >60 years.
- Death: Varicella-related deaths continue to occur despite the recommended vaccine. Secondary bacterial infections and pneumonia are most frequent causes of death.

ADDITIONAL READING

- American Academy of Pediatrics. Varicella-zoster virus infections. In: Kimberlin DW, Brady MT, Jackson MA, et al, eds. *Red Book®: 2015 Report of the Committee on Infectious Diseases*. 30th ed. American Academy of Pediatrics; 2015:846–860.
- American Academy of Pediatrics, Committee on Infectious Diseases. Policy statement—prevention of varicella: update of recommendations for use of quadrivalent and monovalent varicella vaccines in children. *Pediatrics*. 2011;128(3):630–632.
- Baxter R, Ray P, Tran TN, et al. Long-term effectiveness of varicella vaccine: a 14-year, prospective cohort study. *Pediatrics*. 2013;131(5):e1389–e1396.
- Centers for Disease Control and Prevention. Updated recommendations for use of VariZIG—United States, 2013. *MMWR Morb Mortal Wkly Rep*. 2013;62(28):574–576.
- Marin M, Güris D, Chaves SS, et al; for Advisory Committee on Immunization Practices, Centers for Disease Control and Prevention. Prevention of varicella: recommendations of the Advisory Committee on Immunization Practices (ACIP). *MMWR Recomm Rep*. 2007;56(RR-4):1–40.
- Rubin LG, Levin MJ, Ljungman P, et al. 2013 IDSA clinical practice guideline for vaccination of the immunocompromised host. *Clin Infect Dis*. 2014;58(3):e44–e100.

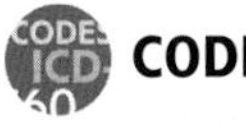

CODES

ICD10

- B01.9 Varicella without complication
- B02.9 Zoster without complications
- B01.89 Other varicella complications

FAQ

- Q: What do you do for a patient on corticosteroids who has not had VZV and is exposed to VZV?
- A: Patients receiving ≥ 2 mg/kg/24 h or ≥ 20 mg/24 h of prednisone or its equivalent cannot be immunized with VZV vaccine. If the child is susceptible, has had sufficient exposure, and deemed at risk for serious infection, passive immunization with VariZIG® or IVIG can be given.
- Q: Can children receiving inhaled steroids for asthma be immunized safely with VZV vaccine?
- A: Yes. Asthmatics on inhaled steroids can be safely immunized because the dose of inhaled steroid is not immunosuppressive.
- Q: For whom is VZV vaccine contraindicated?
- A: Immunosuppressed individuals, pregnant patients, infants <1 year old, and anyone who has a history of an allergic reaction to a vaccine component such as neomycin should not receive the VZV vaccine. Additionally, any child with a moderate to severe acute illness should have his or her VZV vaccination deferred until his or her illness has resolved. Patients with HIV infection can be vaccinated if their CD4+ T-cell percentages are $\geq 15\%$.
- Q: Can a child get shingles after vaccination with VZV vaccine?
- A: Yes. Zoster can occur following VZV vaccination. However, cases of shingles following vaccination tend to be milder and less frequent than after wild-type varicella.
- Q: What are the most common adverse effects of VZV vaccination?
- A: Mild local reactions are most common, occurring in 20–25% of vaccine recipients. 1–3% of children will develop a localized rash after vaccination, whereas 3–5% will develop a more generalized varicella-like rash. These rashes typically consist of 2 to 5 maculopapular or vesicular lesions and occur 5 to 26 days after vaccination.
- Q: What are the characteristics of breakthrough infection in a child who has been immunized with VZV vaccine?
- A: Breakthrough varicella can occur in children who have been appropriately immunized with VZV vaccine. Breakthrough infection is usually milder than that occurring in unimmunized children, often with fewer than 50 lesions, lower fever, and faster recovery. Although these children are less contagious than those with wild virus infection, they can transmit the virus to susceptible individuals.

CHIKUNGUNYA VIRUS

David M. Vu, MD • A. Desiree LaBeaud, MD, MS

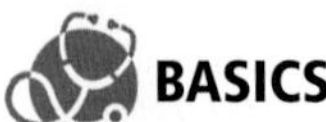

BASICS

DESCRIPTION

- Chikungunya virus (CHIKV) is an arthropod-borne virus (arbovirus) that causes a febrile illness (chikungunya fever) characterized by rash and arthralgia and arthritis of one or more joints.
- Arthralgia from CHIKV infection can last months to years and can be debilitating.

EPIDEMIOLOGY

- In the past decade, there have been explosive outbreaks of CHIKV infection occurring in Sub-Saharan Africa and Asia, followed by epidemics in South and Central America.
- During outbreaks, attack rates are high (80–90%).

RISK FACTORS

- Travel to or residing in an area with an active CHIKV outbreak
- Exposure to *Aedes* spp. mosquitoes
- Elderly (>65 years) individuals with underlying conditions have higher risks for more severe disease.
- Neonates born to CHIKV viremic women have high risk of infection and neuroinvasive disease.

GENERAL PREVENTION

- Mosquito avoidance
  - Wear clothing that maximizes skin coverage.
  - Use insect repellants such as N,N-Diethyl-meta-toluamide (DEET).
  - Cover crib, stroller, and baby carrier with mosquito netting.
- Empty open containers of standing water.
  - Stagnant water is a breeding ground for mosquitoes.
  - The Centers for Disease Control and Prevention (CDC) recommend emptying and scrubbing, turning over, covering or throwing out items that hold stagnant water, such as tires, buckets, planters, toys, pools, birdbaths, flowerpots, or trash containers on a weekly basis.
- As of publication of this book in 2018, no vaccine exists to prevent CHIKV infection or disease.

PATHOPHYSIOLOGY

Pathogenic mechanisms contributing to persistent arthritis/arthralgia remain poorly understood.

ETIOLOGY

- CHIKV is transmitted by *Aedes aegypti* and *Aedes albopictus* mosquitoes. *Aedes* mosquitoes are:
  - Endemic in many tropical and subtropical areas of the world
  - Highly adapted to thrive in peri-urban settings, often entering homes and laying eggs in man-made containers
  - Able to lay eggs in as little as a tablespoon of water
  - Expanding their habitat range due to global warming
- CHIKV is a member of the *Alphaviridae* family of arthritogenic viruses, including O'nyong nyong, Ross River, and Mayaro viruses.
  - Single-stranded RNA virus
  - First reported in 1952 to 1953 during an epidemic of fever, rash, and arthralgia in a region in present day Tanzania

COMMONLY ASSOCIATED CONDITIONS

Unknown

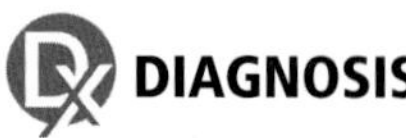

DIAGNOSIS

Most patients infected with CHIKV develop symptoms of fever and arthralgia.

HISTORY

- Travel to or residence in an area known to be experiencing an outbreak of CHIKV infection
- Self-reported history of mosquito bites is not a sensitive predictor of mosquito exposure.
- Sudden onset of high fevers
- Nausea and vomiting
- History of rash
  - Maculopapular rash affecting much of the body, with desquamation at resolution
  - There have been some reports of bullous lesions in infants.
- Debilitating polyarthralgia interfering with performing activities of daily living.
- Retro-orbital headaches associated with dengue virus infection are *absent*.

PHYSICAL EXAM

- Skin: maculopapular rash that affects most of the body and can be coalescent in areas
- Joints: arthralgia out of proportion to arthritis
- Extremities: swelling of hands due to symmetric polyarthritis of metacarpophalangeal and interphalangeal joints
- Eye exam: Conjunctivitis may be present.

DIFFERENTIAL DIAGNOSIS

- Septic arthritis
- Dengue virus infection
- Rheumatic fever

DIAGNOSTIC TESTS & INTERPRETATION

Initial Tests (screening, lab, imaging)

- Reverse-transcriptase PCR (RT-PCR) of blood samples can detect CHIKV RNA during initial 5 to 7 days of febrile illness.
- Serum IgM to CHIKV may be detectable by ELISA within the first several days of illness.

Follow-Up Tests & Special Considerations

CHIKV IgG seroconversion between acute and 1-month convalescent blood samples as measured by ELISA

Test Interpretation

Positive RT-PCR confirms CHIKV infection.

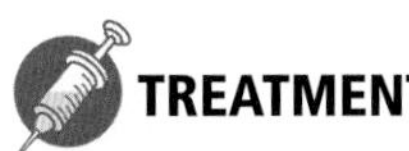

TREATMENT

GENERAL MEASURES

- Treatments specifically for CHIKV infection are not available.
- Therapy is generally supportive.
  - Anti-inflammatory agents
  - Rehydration

MEDICATION

First Line

Nonsteroidal anti-inflammatory agents such as ibuprofen

ISSUES FOR REFERRAL

- Occupational and physical therapy in cases of persistent debilitating arthralgia
- Since 2015, CHIKV disease is a nationally notifiable condition. Cases should be reported to local health departments based on standard case definitions.

COMPLEMENTARY & ALTERNATIVE THERAPIES

Unknown

ADMISSION, INPATIENT, AND NURSING CONSIDERATIONS

Primarily for pain management

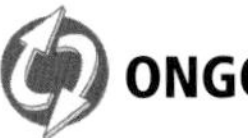

ONGOING CARE

FOLLOW-UP RECOMMENDATIONS

- Follow-up symptomatic treatment of arthralgia, which can last for months to years
- Closely follow neonates born to mothers who are viremic at delivery.

DIET

No special dietary considerations

PATIENT EDUCATION

- Mosquito avoidance
  - Wear clothing that maximizes skin coverage.
  - Use mosquito repellants such as DEET.
  - Empty containers of standing water.
  - Cover crib, stroller, and baby carrier with mosquito netting.
- Travel guidance
  - The CDC issues travel notices to inform travelers about the status of current health issues related to specific travel destinations in the world.
  - See: https://www.nc.cdc.gov/travel/notices

PROGNOSIS

In general, children recover more quickly and completely from CHIKV infection than adults.

COMPLICATIONS

- Death is rare but occurs.
- Rare complications:
  - Encephalitis/encephalopathy
  - Myocarditis
  - Hepatitis
  - Multiorgan failure
- Disability due to persistent arthralgia

ADDITIONAL READING

- Burt FJ, Chen W, Miner JJ, et al. Chikungunya virus: an update on the biology and pathogenesis of this emerging pathogen. *Lancet Infect Dis*. 2017;17(4):e107–e117.
- Ritz N, Hufnagel M, Gérardin P. Chikungunya in children. *Pediatr Infect Dis J*. 2015;34(7):789–791.
- Robinson MC. An epidemic of virus disease in Southern Province, Tanganyika Territory, in 1952-53. I. Clinical features. *Trans R Soc Trop Med Hyg*.1955;49(1);28–32.
- Vu DM, Jungkind D, LaBeaud AD. Chikungunya virus. *Clin Lab Med*. 2017;37(2):371–382.

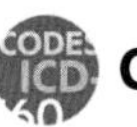

CODES

ICD10

A92.0 Chikungunya virus disease

FAQ

- Q: What can I do to prevent chikungunya infection?
- A: Wear clothing that protects arms and legs, and use insect repellant.
- Q: In what areas of the world do I have to worry about chikungunya infection?
- A: The most up-to-date information and guidance on chikungunya outbreaks is at www.cdc.gov.
- Q: What is the origination of the name "chikungunya"?
- A: CHIKV was first reported in the Makonde Plateau of Tanganyika (present day Tanzania). The symptoms of arthralgia were so severe that patients contorted their bodies and were unable to change position without assistance. "Chikungunya" is the Makonde (Bantu) term that means "that which bends up."

CHILD ABUSE, PHYSICAL

Allison M. Jackson, MD, MPH

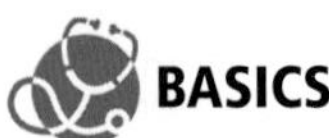

BASICS

DESCRIPTION

Physical abuse is an act inflicted on a child or youth by a parent or caregiver resulting in mucocutaneous, musculoskeletal, visceral, or intracranial injury and/or death. Although a medical diagnosis, physical abuse is also defined legally in state statutes.

EPIDEMIOLOGY

Incidence

- Of those cases reported to child protective service agencies in the United States in 2014, 702,000 children were victims of abuse and neglect.
  - Child abuse rate was 9.4 per 1,000 children per year.
  - 17% of abused children were found to be victims of physical abuse.
  - >1,500 child deaths were attributed to maltreatment in 2014, of which nearly 42% resulted from physical abuse.
  - Nearly 70% of all child maltreatment fatalities occurred in children age of <3 years.
- Abuse can happen in any family regardless of race, ethnicity, or socioeconomic class.

Prevalence

Not all child maltreatment is reported. In a nationally representative sample of >4,000 children, >18% reported experiencing maltreatment in their lifetime.

GENERAL PREVENTION

- Assessing risk (parental history of mental illness or childhood victimization, parental substance abuse, economic stressors, difficult child temperament, unreasonable developmental expectations, children living with single mothers and an unrelated male)
- Screening for family violence (intimate partner violence)
- Providing anticipatory guidance regarding infant crying/toddler tantrums, toileting, and discipline techniques
- Nurse home visitation for at-risk families
- Parenting classes for all parents, although classes usually only target at-risk parents of young children

ETIOLOGY

- Although child abuse occurs in families regardless of race, ethnicity, or socioeconomic status, there are individual, family, community, and societal factors that place children at increased risk for maltreatment.
- Examples of risk factors include the following:
  - Difficult temperament
  - Parental history of childhood victimization
  - Parental substance abuse
  - Parental mental illness
  - Poverty and unemployment
  - Family violence
  - Unrelated male caregiver in the home

COMMONLY ASSOCIATED CONDITIONS

- Emotional abuse
- Neglect
- Sexual abuse
- Domestic violence exposure
- Chronic runaway status
- Domestic sex trafficking
- Posttraumatic stress disorder
- Depression
- Anxiety disorder

ALERT

Pitfalls

- Failing to consider abuse in the differential diagnosis of all pediatric trauma
- Failing to consider abuse in the differential diagnosis of all infants and toddlers with mental status changes (especially brief resolved unexplained events [BRUEs]), even without bruising
- Failing to recognize the significance of subconjunctival hemorrhages and bruises in locations on the body atypical for accidental trauma
- Failing to consider trauma as a cause for bloody CSF
- Failing to consider alternative medical diagnoses in children for whom you suspect abuse
- Failing to document the history, physical findings, and assessment clearly

DIAGNOSIS

HISTORY

- As in all of medicine, the history is paramount to diagnosing child physical abuse. The history yields information useful in creating a timeline, determining plausibility of the injury event, and in formulating a differential diagnosis. Tips for gathering history when abuse is suspected:
  - Be curious but nonjudgmental.
  - Use open-ended, nonleading questions.
  - Speak with the verbal child and parent separately when abuse is suspected.
- Eliciting a narrative history about the injury event and the evolution of symptoms helps to establish a timeline and determine plausibility of the explanation. Asking, "Tell me what happened," is the best place to begin. Eliciting achieved developmental milestones also aids in determining plausibility.
- In cases in which no injury event is reported, it is important to gather information of when the child was last well, how signs and symptoms evolved, and what prompted the caregiver(s) to seek medical attention.
- It is also important to elicit who was caring for the child at the time of the injury event or when the child became acutely and persistently ill. When children are verbal, ask them "what happened?" or "how did you get that?" regarding identified injuries.
- Past medical history, review of systems, and family history can also be helpful in formulating a differential diagnosis.

PHYSICAL EXAM

A comprehensive physical exam should be performed on any child for whom maltreatment is suspected. Tips include the following:

- Plot growth parameters.
- Conduct a head-to-toe physical exam, including an anogenital exam.
- Suspicion for physical abuse is raised with injuries in the mouth (such as frenula injuries), subconjunctival hemorrhages, bruises in infants, bruises in locations atypical for accidental trauma (ears, neck, abdomen, buttocks, thighs), or cutaneous injuries with a pattern (e.g., loop marks, human bites).
- When head trauma is suspected, a dilated funduscopic exam should be completed by an ophthalmologist. Retinal hemorrhages that are in multiple layers of the retina and that extend to the ora serrata have a high specificity for inflicted head trauma.
- Not all injuries can be detected on physical exam; therefore, it is important to use other modalities to screen for other injuries.

DIFFERENTIAL DIAGNOSIS

Should be based on the physical exam, patient history, and family history

- Bruises
  - Trauma: accidental or inflicted
  - Dermatologic: congenital intradermal nevi, hemangiomas, phytophotodermatitis
  - Hematologic: hemophilia, platelet disorders, idiopathic thrombocytopenic purpura, leukemia
  - Infectious: meningococcemia
  - Genetic: Ehlers-Danlos syndrome
  - Congenital indifference to pain
  - Cultural healing practices: coining (*Cao gio*), cupping, spooning (*Quat sha*)
  - Vasculitis: Henoch-Schönlein purpura, hypersensitivity vasculitis
- Burns
  - Trauma: accidental or inflicted
  - Dermatologic: contact dermatitis, fixed drug reaction
  - Infectious: impetigo, staphylococcal scalded skin
  - Genetic: congenital indifference to pain
  - Cultural practices: moxibustion (burning moxa herb at therapeutic points on skin), *maquas* (small deep burns at therapeutic points), garlic (used topically for infections)
  - Other: brown recluse spider bite
- Fractures
  - Trauma: birth, accidental, or inflicted
  - Metabolic: rickets, scurvy, copper deficiency, osteogenesis imperfecta, hypervitaminosis A, prostaglandin E toxicity
  - Neoplastic: leukemia, Langerhans cell histiocytosis, metastatic
  - Infectious: congenital syphilis, osteomyelitis
  - Other: infantile cortical hyperostosis
- Head injury
  - Trauma: accidental or inflicted
  - Hematologic disorder: late hemorrhagic disease of the newborn (vitamin K), clotting factor deficiencies, thrombocytopenia, platelet function disorder, von Willebrand disease
  - Infectious: bacterial meningitis
  - Metabolic: glutaric aciduria type I

DIAGNOSTIC TESTS & INTERPRETATION

Initial Tests (screening, lab, imaging)

- In patients with bruising or intracranial hemorrhage and/or a history or exam in which a bleeding disorder should be considered:
  - Urinalysis (UA) for myoglobinuria
  - Creatine kinase for muscle injury
  - Prothrombin time (PT)/partial thromboplastin time (PTT) for prolonged bleeding
  - CBC with platelets for anemia and thrombocytopenia
  - von Willebrand antigen and activity
  - Factors VIII and IX levels for hemophilia
  - Disseminated intravascular coagulation (DIC) panel
- In patients with multiple fractures, screen for metabolic bone disease:
  - Alkaline phosphatase
  - Calcium and phosphorus
  - 25-hydroxy vitamin D
  - Intact parathyroid hormone (PTH)
- To screen for abdominal trauma (bruising not usually present):
  - AST and ALT for liver injury
  - Amylase, lipase for pancreatic injury
  - UA for genitourinary injury
- In patients with altered mental status or concerns for poisoning:
  - Toxicology screen
- To evaluate for skeletal trauma:
  - Skeletal survey for all children <2 years old with suspected abuse (occasionally useful in children 2 to 5 years old)
    - Fractures with high specificity for abuse include posterior rib fractures, classic metaphyseal lesions (i.e., bucket handle or corner fractures), scapular fractures, sternal fractures, and vertebral fractures.
    - A reported injury event that fails to mechanistically or developmentally provide a plausible mechanism should raise suspicions for abuse.
  - Radionuclide bone scans can augment the assessment for skeletal injury.
- To evaluate for head trauma:
  - CT of the brain and MRI of the brain and spine in children <1 year old or with signs or symptoms suggestive of head injury
    - Subdural hemorrhages are associated with abusive head trauma.
    - MRI may be helpful in assessing hemorrhages of different ages and detecting brain injury and soft tissue neck trauma.
  - To evaluate for thoracic, abdominal, and/or pelvic trauma:
    - CT chest, abdomen, and/or pelvis
- Pathologic findings
  - An autopsy by a qualified medical examiner should be completed when maltreatment is in the differential diagnosis.

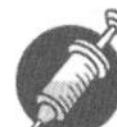

TREATMENT

GENERAL MEASURES

- Medical treatment according to injuries
- Report suspicions for physical abuse to the Child Protective Services agency in the jurisdiction of occurrence.
- Incorporate other disciplines into the treatment plan, in particular, social work and trauma-informed mental health care providers.

ADMISSION, INPATIENT, AND NURSING CONSIDERATIONS

- Admission criteria
  - Primarily based on medical needs of patient
  - For patient safety to allow for initial investigation to assess for a safe caregiver
- Discharge criteria
  - When medically prepared for discharge and a safe caregiver has been established by child welfare

ONGOING CARE

FOLLOW-UP RECOMMENDATIONS

Patient Monitoring

- Reports will be investigated by the appropriate child welfare and/or law enforcement agency.
- The child may or may not be placed into foster care. In either case, if a child welfare case is opened, measures to monitor and strengthen the family and parents would be implemented. These measures are not always successful.
- Because toxic stressors like maltreatment effect the developing brain and the traumatic brain injury in some cases, developmental assessment and monitoring should be established.
- Primary care and ongoing providers should monitor patients for physical and mental health sequelae of the abuse as well as ongoing abuse or neglect.

PROGNOSIS

Depends on nature and extent of injuries, the response of the child welfare and criminal justice system, and the timely implementation of medical and mental health services

COMPLICATIONS

- Death
- Intellectual disability
- Cerebral palsy
- Seizure disorder
- Learning disabilities
- Psychiatric disorders (depression, anxiety, posttraumatic stress disorder)

ADDITIONAL READING

- Anderst JD, Carpenter SL, Abshire TC; for Section on Hematology/Oncology and Committee on Child Abuse and Neglect of the American Academy of Pediatrics. Evaluation for bleeding disorders in suspected child abuse. *Pediatrics*. 2013;131(4):e1314–e1322.
- Christian CW; for Committee on Child Abuse and Neglect, American Academy of Pediatrics. The evaluation of suspected child physical abuse. *Pediatrics*. 2015;135(5):e1337–e1354.
- Finkelhor D, Turner H, Ormrod R, et al. Violence, abuse, and crime exposure in a national sample of children and youth. *Pediatrics*. 2009;124(5):1411–1423.
- Flaherty EG, Perez-Rossello JM, Levine MA, et al; for American Academy of Pediatrics Committee on Child Abuse and Neglect, Section on Radiology, Section on Endocrinology and Section on Orthopaedics, and the Society for Pediatric Radiology. Evaluating infants and young children with fractures for child physical abuse. *Pediatrics*. 2014;133(2):e477–e489.
- Flaherty EG, Stirling J Jr; for American Academy of Pediatrics Committee on Child Abuse and Neglect. Clinical report—the pediatrician's role in child maltreatment prevention. *Pediatrics*. 2010;126(4):833–841.
- Hinds T, Shalaby-Rana E, Jackson AM, et al. Aspects of abuse: abusive head trauma. *Curr Probl Pediatr Adolesc Health Care*. 2015;45(3):71–79.

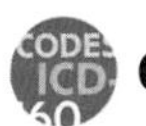

CODES

ICD10

- T74.12XA Child physical abuse, confirmed, initial encounter
- T74.4XXA Shaken infant syndrome, initial encounter
- Z69.010 Encounter for mental health services for victim of parental child abuse

FAQ

- Q: When do I need to report child abuse?
- A: Whenever there is suspicion that your patient has experienced maltreatment based on your clinical evaluation. You do not have to prove abuse; you just need to suspect it.
- Q: What happens when a report is taken?
- A: Many jurisdictions proceed with a multidisciplinary investigation. Investigators and attorneys may need to speak with you to clarify your findings and assessment.

CHLAMYDIA TRACHOMATIS INFECTION

Sumit Bhargava, MD

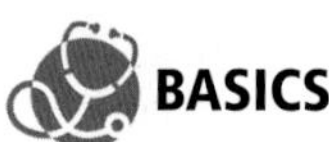

BASICS

DESCRIPTION

Chlamydiae are obligate intracellular bacteria responsible for pulmonary infections, ocular trachoma, sexually transmitted diseases, and infections of the genital tract in the pediatric and adult population.

- The genus *Chlamydophila* has three species known to affect humans:
  - *Chlamydia trachomatis*
  - *Chlamydophila psittaci*
  - *Chlamydophila pneumoniae*
- All three species can produce the clinical picture of the so-called atypical or interstitial pneumonia.
- *C. trachomatis* can cause afebrile pneumonia in 10–20% of infants born to infected mothers. Infected infants usually present prior to 2 months of age. Up to 50% of patients have a history of inclusion conjunctivitis.
- *C. psittaci* is mainly pathogenic for birds and occasionally affects humans, typically causing interstitial pneumonitis with associated fever, headache, malaise, and nausea.
- *C. pneumoniae* causes pneumonia, pharyngitis, sinusitis, and bronchitis in humans.

GENERAL PREVENTION

- Adequate surveillance and treatment of *C. trachomatis* colonizing the genital tract of pregnant women is the best way of preventing disease in the infant.
- Annual chlamydia screening for all sexually active women <25 years and for all pregnant women in the first trimester of pregnancy is recommended.

ALERT

Ocular prophylaxis at birth does not reliably prevent *C. trachomatis* conjunctivitis or extraocular infection, even if erythromycin ointment is used. Topical treatment alone is not recommended because it does not eradicate the nasopharyngeal colonization.

EPIDEMIOLOGY

C. trachomatis

- There are at least 18 serologically distinct variants with different associations:
  - A–C: trachoma
  - D–K: genital, oculogenital, and perinatal infection
  - L1–L3: lymphogranuloma venereum (LGV)
- *C. trachomatis* is the most frequent cause of epididymitis in sexually active young men.
- Incubation period: 5 to 14 days after delivery for conjunctivitis and 3 to 19 weeks for neonatal pneumonia
- The possibility of sexual abuse should be considered in older infants and children with vaginal, urethral, or rectal *C. trachomatis*.

Incidence

- This is the most common reportable sexually transmitted infection in the United States. The number of new infections exceeds 1.3 million annually.
- Most infections occur in 15- to 19-year and 20- to -24-year age groups.
- *C. trachomatis* is responsible for neonatal conjunctivitis, trachoma, pneumonia in young infants, genital tract infection, and LGV.
- Rates of infection in adolescent girls are 15–20%.
- 23–55% of all cases of nongonococcal urethritis in men are caused by *C. trachomatis*. Up to 50% of men with gonorrhea may be coinfected with *C. trachomatis*.
- *C. trachomatis* pneumonia usually develops in infected infants <2 months of age (2 weeks to 5 months). The contagiousness of pulmonary disease is unknown but is considered low.
- 50–75% of the neonates born to infected mothers via vaginal delivery will acquire *C. trachomatis*. Conjunctivitis may develop in 30–50%.

ALERT

C. trachomatis infection can occur in infants delivered by cesarean section, even without rupture of amniotic membranes.

- Pneumonia may develop in up to 30% of infants with nasopharyngeal infection.
- Ocular trachoma caused by serovars A, B, Ba, and C is the most common cause of preventable blindness in the world but is rare in the United States.
- Rates among African Americans are 8 times that of Caucasians, followed by American Indians/Alaska natives (4.3 times) and Hispanics (2.7 times).

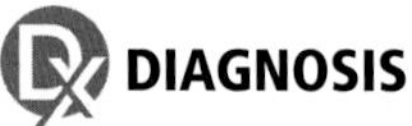

DIAGNOSIS

HISTORY

- Presents between 4 and 12 weeks of age
- Insidious onset
- Afebrile illness
- Rhinorrhea
- Repetitive cough
  - Staccato type in >50% of infants
  - Sometimes, pertussis-like coughing spells
- Conjunctivitis in up to 50% of infants
- Mild to moderate respiratory distress

PHYSICAL EXAM

- Afebrile
- 50% of patients will have conjunctivitis with discharge (can be seen up to several weeks after birth).
- Rhinitis with mucoid discharge or nasal stuffiness, sometimes causing significant airway obstruction
- Hypoxia is frequently present.
- Apneic episodes may be seen in preterm infants.
- Moderate tachypnea (50 to 60 breaths/minute)
- Staccato cough
- Scattered rales on chest auscultation
- Wheezing is an uncommon finding.

DIFFERENTIAL DIAGNOSIS

- Viral respiratory pathogens:
  - Respiratory syncytial virus (RSV)
  - Adenovirus
  - Influenza A
  - Influenza B
  - Parainfluenza
- Other agents that can cause pneumonitis:
  - Cytomegalovirus
  - *Pneumocystis carinii*
  - *Ureaplasma urealyticum*
  - *Bordetella pertussis*

DIAGNOSTIC TESTS & INTERPRETATION

Initial Tests (screening, lab, imaging)

- Cell culture
  - Definitive diagnosis is by isolation of the organism in tissue culture.
  - Confirmation is by microscopy of the characteristic inclusions by fluorescent antibody staining.
  - Specimens are obtained from the nasopharynx, conjunctiva, vagina, or rectum.
  - Dacron, rayon, and cotton-tipped swabs on plastic/aluminum should be used for collection.
- Nucleic acid amplification methods (NAAT):
  - U.S. Food and Drug Administration (FDA)-approved nucleic acid amplification methods such as polymerase chain reaction (PCR), strand displacement amplification (SDA), and transcription-mediated amplification (TMA) are more sensitive (98%) than cell culture and more specific and sensitive than DNA probe, direct fluorescent antibody (DFA), or enzyme immunoassay (EIA).
  - In addition, these have been approved for urine studies in both men and women, making them useful noninvasive tests for adolescents.
- Direct antigen tests:
  - DNA probe, DFA, and EIA are the most common nonculture direct antigen-detection tests approved by the FDA.
  - These are most sensitive (90%) and specific (95%) in conjunctival specimens.
  - These methods can have false-positive results when used for vaginal or rectal specimens.
- Serum antibody detection
  - Difficult to perform
  - Tests are not widely available.
- Eosinophilia of 300 to 400/mm^3, hyperinflation, bilateral diffuse infiltrates on chest radiograph, and elevation of IgM (>110 mg/dL) and IgG (>500 mg/dL) are indirect evidence that indicate *C. trachomatis* pneumonia.
- Only culture should be used for sexual abuse or other forensic purposes. NAAT have been sanctioned for screening in girls only, but positive results must be reconfirmed.
- Chest radiography
  - Hyperinflation with bilateral diffuse infiltrates

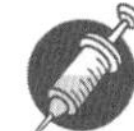

TREATMENT

MEDICATION

- Erythromycin, 50 mg/kg/24 h divided q.i.d. for 14 days (therapy is effective in 80–90% of cases). Additional topical therapy is unnecessary. An association between oral erythromycin and infantile hypertrophic pyloric stenosis (IHPS) has been reported in infants <6 weeks of age. Parents should be informed of the possible risk of IHPS and its signs.
- If the patient does not tolerate erythromycin, oral sulfonamides may be used after the immediate neonatal period. Children >8 years can be treated with tetracycline, 25 to 50 mg/kg/24 h divided q.i.d. for 7 days.
- A single 1-g oral dose of azithromycin may be used in children ≥45 kg or ≥8 years of age.
- In adults and adolescents, a single 1-g dose of azithromycin or doxycycline 100 mg b.i.d. orally for 7 days is 1st-line treatment.

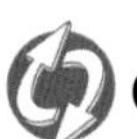

ONGOING CARE

PROGNOSIS

- In general, good
- Infection with *C. trachomatis* has been associated with long-term respiratory sequelae, such as an increased incidence of reactive airway disease and abnormal pulmonary function tests.
- Slow recovery
- Cough and malaise may persist for several weeks.

COMPLICATIONS

- 40% of women whose chlamydial infection is untreated develop pelvic inflammatory disease. 20% of these women may become infertile.
- Role of chlamydia in pathogenesis of asthma and atherosclerosis is under investigation.

ADDITIONAL READING

- Centers for Disease Control and Prevention. Sexually transmitted disease guidelines 2002. *MMWR Recomm Rep*. 2002;51(RR-6):1–78.
- Geisler WM. Management of uncomplicated *Chlamydia trachomatis* infections in adolescents and adults: evidence reviewed for the 2006 Centers for Disease Control and Prevention sexually transmitted diseases treatment guidelines. *Clin Infect Dis*. 2007;44(Suppl 3):S77–S83.
- Harris JA, Kolokathis A, Campbell M, et al. Safety and efficacy of azithromycin in the treatment of community-acquired pneumonia in children. *Pediatr Infect Dis J*. 1998;17(10):865–871.
- Siqueira LM. Chlamydial infections in children and adolescents. *Pediatrics Rev*. 2014;35(4):145–154.
- U.S. Preventative Services Task Force. Screening for chlamydial infection: U.S. Preventative Services Task Force recommendation statement. *Ann Intern Med*. 2007;147(2):128–133.

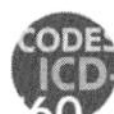

CODES

ICD10

- A74.9 Chlamydial infection, unspecified
- P23.1 Congenital pneumonia due to Chlamydia
- A71.1 Active stage of trachoma

FAQ

- Q: If the mother has an untreated genital infection, should we treat the asymptomatic newborn?
- A: Yes. The child should receive oral erythromycin for 14 days.
- Q: Do we need to pursue the diagnosis of other sexually transmitted diseases?
- A: Yes. Gonorrhea, syphilis, hepatitis B, and human immunodeficiency virus infection need to be ruled out. If conjunctivitis is present, an ocular swab to exclude *Neisseria gonorrhoeae* infection must be included.
- Q: When do we need to suspect *C. trachomatis* pneumonia?
- A: In any infant <4 months of age who presents with cough, tachypnea, and rales on examination, when the chest radiograph shows bilateral infiltrates with hyperinflation

CHLAMYDOPHILA (FORMERLY *CHLAMYDIA*) *PNEUMONIAE* INFECTION

Amanda C. Schondelmeyer, MD, MSc • Angela M. Statile, MD, MEd

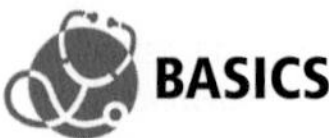

BASICS

DESCRIPTION

Chlamydiae are obligate intracellular organisms classified as bacteria but which possess qualities of both bacteria and viruses. They cause a variety of infections from the respiratory to the urogenital tract. The genus has been divided into *Chlamydia* (*Chlamydia trachomatis*, others) and *Chlamydophila* (*Chlamydophila pneumoniae*, *Chlamydophila psittaci*, others). Three species are known to affect humans:

- *C. trachomatis*: a leading cause of sexually transmitted infections in the United States, which can be vertically transmitted during childbirth
- *C. psittaci*: a rare zoonosis
- *C. pneumoniae*: an important cause of respiratory infections in the school-aged child; will be the focus of this chapter

EPIDEMIOLOGY

- Spread person to person by respiratory droplets; no seasonal trend
- Asymptomatic carriage and prolonged nasopharyngeal shedding occurs.
- Peak ages of infection are 5 to 15 years.
- Coinfection with other respiratory pathogens is common.
- Serum antibodies are positive in about 50% of adults by age 20 years, and reinfection commonly occurs in adults.

RISK FACTORS

School-aged children are at highest risk.

GENERAL PREVENTION

Cough etiquette (coughing into elbow or tissue) and proper hand hygiene are important control measures.

PATHOPHYSIOLOGY

- Chlamydiae exist in two forms:
  - Elementary body (EB): infectious form
  - Reticulate body (RB): reproductive form
- Life cycle:
  - EB is taken into cell by endocytosis and reorganizes into an RB to replicate.
  - After replication, RB transformed to EB and are released by exocytosis or cytolysis.
  - Cycle between endocytosis and release is 2 to 3 days.

DIAGNOSIS

HISTORY

- *C. pneumoniae* incubation period is approximately 21 days.
- Most commonly presents with prolonged cough (2 to 6 weeks), developing into atypical pneumonia
- Sore throat may precede onset of cough.
- Infection may be asymptomatic; symptomatic patients are often mild to moderately ill.
- Immunocompromised hosts at risk for severe illness

PHYSICAL EXAM

- Nasal discharge
- Nonexudative pharyngitis
- Laryngitis, otitis media, and sinusitis may be present.
- Lung exam may be notable for wheezing and rales.

DIFFERENTIAL DIAGNOSIS

- Atypical pneumonia due to *Mycoplasma pneumoniae*
- Pneumonia due to typical pathogens such as *Streptococcus pneumoniae*
- Viral pneumonia
  - Influenza
  - Parainfluenza
  - Adenovirus
  - Respiratory syncytial virus (RSV)
- Less frequently
  - *Coxiella burnetii*
  - *Legionella pneumophila*

DIAGNOSTIC TESTS & INTERPRETATION

Initial Tests (screening, lab, imaging)

Treatment should be initiated empirically if atypical pneumonia is suspected. Confirmatory laboratory tests include:

- United States Food and Drug Administration (FDA)-approved polymerase chain reaction (PCR) test now available
- Serologic testing and culture are also available.
- Chest radiography
  - May have focal or diffuse infiltrates
  - May demonstrate pleural effusion

TREATMENT

MEDICATION

1st-line therapy is recommended based on national guidelines, as antimicrobial therapy is usually initiated empirically when suspicion is high for atypical pathogens. Alternative therapies are targeted at *C. pneumoniae*.

- First line
  - Azithromycin 10 mg/kg (max 500 mg) for 1 day followed by 5 mg/kg (max 250 mg) for 4 days
  - In hospitalized patients, if clinical picture may also be consistent with typical pathogens, add ampicillin IV 150 to 200 mg/kg/24 h divided every 6 hours (300 to 400 mg/kg/24 h may be used for suspected *S. pneumoniae* with penicillin MICs ≥4 mcg/mL; max 4,000 mg/24 h) or amoxicillin 90 mg/kg/24 h divided every 8 or 12 hours (max 4,000 mg/24 h) if tolerating oral medications.
- Alternatives:
  - If >8 years, doxycycline
  - Levofloxacin if unable to tolerate macrolides
- Appropriate length of antimicrobial therapy in *C. pneumoniae* infections is unclear.

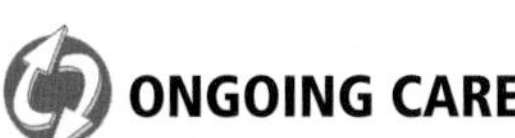

ONGOING CARE

PROGNOSIS

For *C. pneumoniae*, full recovery is expected in general.

COMPLICATIONS

- Immunocompromised individuals, such as those with cystic fibrosis and sickle cell disease, can experience a fulminant course, including pulmonary exacerbations and acute chest syndrome.
- Rarely, immunocompetent patients may also experience complications such as pulmonary abscess or respiratory distress syndrome.

ADDITIONAL READING

- Bradley JS, Byington CL, Shah SS, et al. Executive summary: the management of community-acquired pneumonia in infants and children older than 3 months of age: clinical practice guidelines by the Pediatric Infectious Diseases Society and the Infectious Diseases Society of America. *Clin Infect Dis*. 2011;53(7):617–630.
- Burillo A, Bouza E. *Chlamydophila pneumoniae*. *Infect Dis Clin North Am*. 2010;24(1):61–71.
- Kicinski P, Wisniewska-Ligier M, Wozniakowska-Gesicka T. Pneumonia caused by *Mycoplasma pneumoniae* and *Chlamydophila pneumoniae* in children—comparative analysis of clinical picture. *Adv Med Sci*. 2011;56(1):56–63.

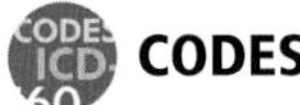

CODES

ICD10

A70 Chlamydia psittaci infections

FAQ

- Q: What is the best way to diagnose *C. pneumoniae* in a patient with suspected atypical pneumonia?
- A: Empiric treatment is recommended in patients with suspected atypical pneumonia. Confirmatory laboratory tests may be indicated in patients with severe disease and include PCR, serologies, or culture.
- Q: What counseling should be provided to patients with *C. pneumoniae* infection?
- A: Cough may be prolonged, lasting 2 to 6 weeks. If difficulty breathing, prolonged fever, or other concerning symptoms develop, patients should seek immediate care to assess for complications.
- Q: How can *C. pneumoniae* infectious be prevented?
- A: Common infection control methods, such as appropriate hand washing, are appropriate. Outbreaks can occur in crowded living conditions, such as among college students or armed services members. This is a consideration for hosts at risk, for high for severe infection, but there is currently no vaccine available and asymptomatic infection is common, making prevention of transmission a challenge.

CHOLELITHIASIS (GALLSTONES)

Karen A. Queliza, MD • Eric H. Chiou, MD • Kristin L. Van Buren, MD, MEd

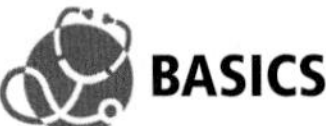

BASICS

DESCRIPTION

Cholelithiasis is defined by the presence of cholesterol or pigmented stones in the gallbladder. Risk factors in children include obesity, hemolytic disease, cystic fibrosis (CF), Crohn disease, and long-term total parenteral nutrition (TPN). Gallstone disease can affect the pancreaticobiliary system, liver, and small bowel.

EPIDEMIOLOGY

- Cholelithiasis is relatively uncommon in childhood and adolescence. However, the incidence is increasing secondary to improved diagnostic modalities and the rise in pediatric obesity.
- Gallstones occurring in utero and in infancy have been described.
- Canadian Eskimos and Native Africans have the lowest risk of cholelithiasis.
- Native Americans (Pima Indians), Hispanics, Swedes, Scandinavians, and Czechs have the highest risk.

Incidence

- Ascertaining the incidence of gallstones in otherwise healthy children is difficult because the majority of cases are asymptomatic.
- The incidence of cholecystectomy for gallstones in children appears to be rising, especially in association with nonhemolytic or cholesterol gallstones
- Incidence is believed to be equal in males and females before puberty. After puberty, the incidence increases in females.

Prevalence

- The prevalence of cholelithiasis in children and adolescents reported in the literature is ~1.9–4.0%.
- In children with sickle cell disease (SCD), the prevalence of gallstones has been reported to be anywhere between 15% and 36%.
- Pigment stones are more prevalent in prepubertal children, whereas cholesterol stones are predominant in adolescence and adulthood.

RISK FACTORS

- Acute renal failure
- Age
- Anatomic abnormalities (biliary stricture, duodenal diverticulum)
- CF
- Chronic hemolysis (SCD, thalassemia, hereditary spherocytosis, pyruvate kinase deficiency, malaria)
- Dehydration
- Diabetes mellitus
- Down syndrome
- Dyslipidemia
- Ethnic background (e.g., Hispanic)
- Family history
- Female gender
- Genetic predilection
- Hepatobiliary disease/cirrhosis
- Ineffective erythropoiesis (vitamin B_{12} and folate deficiencies)
- Lack of physical activity
- Medications (estrogens, octreotide, clofibrate, furosemide, cyclosporine, ceftriaxone, oral contraceptives)
- Necrotizing enterocolitis
- Obesity/metabolic syndrome: Pediatric obesity is estimated to increase the risk of gallstones by over 5-fold.
- Pregnancy/parity
- Prematurity
- Prolonged fasting/low-calorie diets/rapid weight loss
- Severe Crohn disease of ileum and/or ileal resection
- TPN
- Trauma, surgery (i.e., abdominal, bariatric, cardiac)

Genetics

- Mutations have been identified in genes encoding the ABC transporters for phosphatidylcholine (adenosine triphosphate–binding cassette, subfamily B), bile salts (*ABCB11*), and cholesterol 7α-hydroxylase (*CYP7A1*).
- CCK-A receptor (*CCKAR*) and CF gene (*CFTR*) mutations have been reported as well.
- *ABCB4* is also known as multidrug-resistant 3 glycoprotein (*MDR3*). *MDR3* codes for a phospholipid translocator in the hepatocyte membrane involved in biliary phosphatidylcholine excretion. MDR3 deficiency can cause severe neonatal liver disease, but mutations in *MDR3* have also been associated with cholelithiasis, cholestasis of pregnancy, and biliary cirrhosis.
- Variants of *ABCG8* and *UGT1A1* associated with bile acid metabolism and Gilbert syndrome are risk factors for cholelithiasis.
- Other gene polymorphisms are currently under investigation in humans.

GENERAL PREVENTION

- Exercise and dietary modifications can decrease gallstone formation. This includes high-fiber intake, diet low in saturated fatty acids and refined carbohydrates, and moderate physical activity.
- Prevention of gallstone formation involves treating underlying risk factors (small enteral feedings in addition to TPN, early pancreatic enzyme supplements in CF patients, alternative forms of contraception in high-risk patients, and weight control in obese patients with known hemolytic disease).

PATHOPHYSIOLOGY

- Bile is an aqueous solution of bile salts, bilirubin, phospholipids, and cholesterol. Changes in the proportion of bile constituents (e.g., cholesterol supersaturation), nucleation (aggregation of cholesterol crystals), gallbladder hypomotility, or infection can lead to stone formation.
- Biliary sludge may progress to stone formation.
- Stone types are classified depending on constituents: pigment (black and brown), cholesterol, and mixed.

ETIOLOGY

- Black pigment stones are associated with:
  - Increased unconjugated bilirubin
    - Congenital or acquired hemolytic anemias
    - Abnormal erythropoiesis
    - Enterohepatic circulation of unconjugated bilirubin
  - TPN
  - Cirrhosis
- Brown pigment stones are associated with common bile duct infection. Parasitic etiologies are public health concerns in developing countries.
- Cholesterol stones are the most common and are associated with the following:
  - A decrease in bile salt pool
  - Decreased bile acid synthesis
  - Gallbladder stasis (weight loss, pregnancy, long-term TPN)
  - Hypersecretion of cholesterol into bile
  - Increased biliary mucus secretion
  - Medications: furosemide, ceftriaxone, cyclosporine
  - Obesity
- Cholesterol or pigment stones have been reported with ileal resection, ileal Crohn disease, and CF.

COMMONLY ASSOCIATED CONDITIONS

- Hemolytic disease
- CF
- Crohn disease (terminal ileal disease) or ileal resection
- TPN dependence

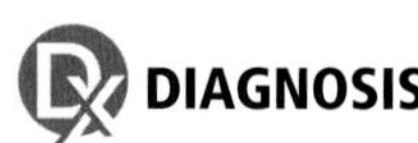

DIAGNOSIS

HISTORY

- Gallstones in children are most commonly asymptomatic ("silent," up to 50%). Silent gallstones present coincidentally on abdominal ultrasounds of infants and young children.
- When symptomatic, young children present with nonspecific symptoms including obstructive jaundice and mild elevation in transaminases
- Right upper quadrant (RUQ) abdominal pain is the most common complaint.
  - Classically involves sharp, intermittent, cramping pain radiating to the right shoulder, along with nausea and vomiting
  - These symptoms are more common in older children and adolescents.
- Fatty food intolerance rarely exists in young children.
- Fever is unusual in all age groups and often indicates the development of cholecystitis. The history should always include questions concerning
  - Previous episodes of RUQ abdominal pain
  - Family history of cholelithiasis
  - Nutritional history
  - Medication use
  - Surgical history
  - Associated medical conditions (e.g., short bowel syndrome, ileal disease)
  - See "Risk Factors" section.

PHYSICAL EXAM

- The physical exam may be completely normal or may uncover the acute abdomen of pancreatitis.
- Murphy sign (tenderness on palpation of RUQ of abdomen associated with inspiration) may be elicited in adolescents.

DIFFERENTIAL DIAGNOSIS

- Acalculous gallbladder disease
- Acute hepatitis
- Biliary dyskinesia
- Cholecystitis (inflammation of the gallbladder)
- Choledocholithiasis (common bile duct stones)
- Congenital biliary anomalies
- Gastritis
- Hydrops of the gallbladder (may be associated with Kawasaki disease)
- Peptic ulcer disease
- Pneumonia

DIAGNOSTIC TESTS & INTERPRETATION

Initial Tests (screening, lab, imaging)

- Laboratory tests should include a complete blood count, urinalysis, amylase, lipase, fractionated bilirubin, alkaline phosphatase, γ-glutamyltransferase, and transaminase levels.
  - Results should typically be within normal ranges.
  - Abnormal results may suggest infection, obstruction, or another disease process.
- Ultrasound
  - Diagnostic procedure of choice
  - Noninvasive with high sensitivity and specificity (>95%)

- Plain radiography
  - The high concentration of calcium salts causes black pigment stones to be radiopaque.
  - Brown and cholesterol stones are radiolucent. However, calcified cholesterol stones may appear on abdominal radiographs.
  - May not be useful as most gallstones in children are not radiopaque
- Magnetic resonance cholangiopancreatography is useful to define anatomy in hepatobiliary disease and identify choledocholithiasis.

Follow-Up Tests & Special Considerations

- Consider sending a blood culture if workup is concerning for cholangitis.
- In obese patients with gallstones, a lipid panel may be helpful to diagnose dyslipidemia and the potential need for medical therapy.

Diagnostic Procedures/Other

- Endoscopic retrograde cholangiopancreatography
  - Diagnostic for choledocholithiasis
  - Therapeutic for removal of stones, stenting, or decompression of the biliary tree
- Cholecystectomy should be considered for symptomatic patients.

Test Interpretation

- Black pigment stones can be black to dark brown in color. They are associated with hemolysis.
- Brown pigment stones can be brown to orange and are associated with biliary tract infections. They are not found in the gallbladder.
- Cholesterol stones are yellow-green and develop from genetic and environmental influences.

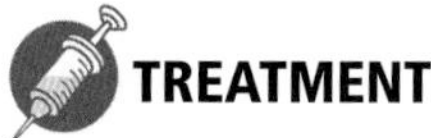

TREATMENT

GENERAL MEASURES

- Asymptomatic gallstones should only be observed.
- Gallstones should be removed in children who are dependent on TPN and in patients with short bowel syndrome, pseudo-obstruction, inflammatory bowel disease, or a hemoglobinopathy.
- Stone formation increases with age.
  - Sickle cell patients should therefore undergo cholecystectomy when stones are identified.
  - This will decrease the risk of cholecystitis and other complications and also help to differentiate between biliary colic and sickle cell crisis.
- Patients with a history of cholecystitis are at increased risk for further episodes (69% will have biliary colic within 2 years and 6% will require cholecystectomy).

MEDICATION

- There is no approved medical therapy for pediatric cholelithiasis.
- Ursodeoxycholic acid (UDCA) has been described for cholesterol gallstone dissolution in select patients. It suppresses hepatic cholesterol synthesis and secretion and can improve gallbladder muscle contractility by decreasing muscle cell cholesterol content in the plasma membranes.

ISSUES FOR REFERRAL

- Bile duct obstruction and gallstone pancreatitis are reasons for GI referral.
- A patient with symptomatic cholelithiasis should also be seen by general surgery.

ADDITIONAL THERAPIES

Consultation with a dietitian can be helpful for patients requiring weight management.

SURGERY/OTHER PROCEDURES

- Laparoscopic cholecystectomy is the procedure of choice in symptomatic children.
- Lithotripsy using shock waves has not been approved for use in children.

ADMISSION, INPATIENT, AND NURSING CONSIDERATIONS

Admission is indicated for patients with symptomatic cholelithiasis and related complications requiring pain medications and rehydration.

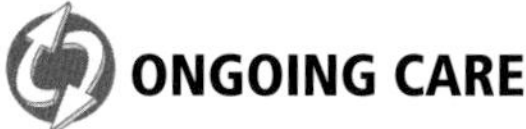

ONGOING CARE

FOLLOW-UP RECOMMENDATIONS

Patient Monitoring

- Asymptomatic patients: Monitor for onset of symptoms; no use for repeat imaging or labs unless symptomatic
- Symptomatic patients: Consider cholecystectomy.

DIET

- Patients with cholelithiasis should continue to eat a healthy diet, including high fiber and low saturated/trans fats.
- There is no specific diet recommended after a cholecystectomy. However, a healthy well-balanced diet is still encouraged.

PATIENT EDUCATION

- If a child with cholelithiasis does not have symptoms, observation is appropriate.
- Surgical treatment is warranted if symptoms develop.
- If a patient requires gallbladder removal, there are typically no significant detrimental effects as the bile directly flows from the liver into the intestine.

PROGNOSIS

- Resolution of gallstones is well documented in infants.
- Spontaneous resolution of gallstones in older children is infrequent.
- Spontaneous resolution of TPN-induced stones has been reported among patients who are not chronically dependent on TPN.

COMPLICATIONS

- Complications of cholelithiasis are rare in children.
- Acute pancreatitis develops in 8% of patients with gallstones and is the most common complication. It is more common in obese adolescents who have undergone rapid weight reduction.
- Cholecystitis
- Choledocholithiasis
- Cholangitis (infection of the bile duct)
- Gallbladder perforation
- Gallstone ileus (mechanical obstruction of small bowel by impacted gallstone)
- Mirizzi syndrome (impacted gallstone in cystic duct or gallbladder neck resulting in common hepatic duct obstruction)

ADDITIONAL READING

- Bogue CO, Murphy AJ, Gerstle JT, et al. Risk factors, complications, and outcomes of gallstones in children: a single-center review. *J Pediatr Gastroenterol Nutr*. 2010;50(3):303–308.
- Buch S, Schafmayer C, Völzke H, et al. Loci from a genome-wide analysis of bilirubin levels are associated with gallstone risk and composition. *Gastroenterology*. 2010;139(6):1942–1951.
- Guarino MP, Cong P, Cicala M, et al. Ursodeoxycholic acid improves muscle contractility and inflammation in symptomatic gallbladders with cholesterol gallstones. *Gut*. 2007;56(6):815–820.
- Koebnick C, Smith N, Black MH, et al. Pediatric obesity and gallstone disease. *J Pediatr Gastroenterol Nutr*. 2012;55(3):328–333.
- Lucena JF, Herrero JI, Quiroga J, et al. A multidrug resistance 3 gene mutation causing cholelithiasis, cholestasis of pregnancy, and adulthood biliary cirrhosis. *Gastroenterology*. 2003;124(4):1037–1042.
- Mehta S, Lopez ME, Chumpitazi BP, et al. Clinical characteristics and risk factors for symptomatic pediatric gallbladder disease. *Pediatrics*. 2012;129(1):e82–e88.
- Murphy PB, Vogt KN, Winick-Ng J, et al. The increasing incidence of gallbladder disease in children: a 20 year perspective. *J Pediatr Surg*. 2016;51(5):748–752.
- Portincasa P, Moschetta A, Palasciano G. Cholesterol gallstone disease. *Lancet*. 2006;368(9531):230–239.
- Rosmorduc O, Hermelin B, Boelle PY, et al. ABCB4 gene mutation-associated cholelithiasis in adults. *Gastroenterology*. 2003;125(2):452–459.
- Rothstein DH, Harmon CM. Gallbladder disease in children. *Semin Pediatr Surg*. 2016;25(4):225–231.
- Suell MN, Horton TM, Dishop MK, et al. Outcomes for children with gallbladder abnormalities and sickle cell disease. *J Pediatr*. 2004;145(5):617–621.

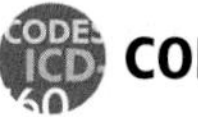

CODES

ICD10

- K80.20 Calculus of gallbladder w/o cholecystitis w/o obstruction
- K80.21 Calculus of gallbladder w/o cholecystitis with obstruction
- K80.01 Calculus of gallbladder w acute cholecystitis w obstruction

FAQ

- Q: Does my child with CF have a greater risk for gallstones?
- A: Yes. Children with CF may have more frequent development of gallstones than children without CF. Reports of gallstones while on UDCA therapy have also been noted.
- Q: Why does my child with SCD have gallstones?
- A: Because the hemolytic process involves breakdown of hemoglobin, which produces bilirubin. This process may accelerate the formation of pigmented gallstones.
- Q: If my child has repeated attacks of RUQ abdominal pain and there are gallstones in the gallbladder, should he have surgery? What kind?
- A: Yes. Laparoscopic cholecystectomy is typically recommended.
- Q: Does obesity increase my child's risk of gallstones?
- A: Yes. Obesity is associated with up to 40% of gallstones observed in all children.

CHOLERA

Matthew P. Kronman, MD, MSCE

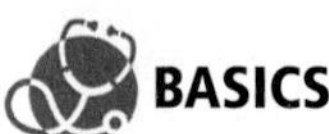

BASICS

DESCRIPTION

Cholera is an acute-onset infection producing profuse secretory diarrhea with the potential for epidemic spread.

EPIDEMIOLOGY

- Diarrheal disease, including cholera, is the second leading cause of mortality in children <5 years old worldwide.
- The first 6 recorded cholera pandemics occurred prior to 1923, but the current seventh pandemic began in 1961 and has continued through several waves of global transmission.
- Most cholera occurs in Asia and Africa, but *Vibrio cholerae* is now endemic in many countries. Regions previously free of cholera have become susceptible to severe outbreaks, as occurred in Haiti since 2010.
- In the United States, most cases result from travel. Cases have been reported in the Gulf Coast of Louisiana and Texas related to undercooked shellfish consumption.
- Case fatality rates are ~1% with timely treatment but can rise to 35–50% in severe cases in extremely resource-limited settings.

Incidence

- Although underreported, approximately 2.8 million cholera cases occur in endemic countries annually, with an additional 87,000 cases annually in nonendemic countries.
- An estimated 91,000 deaths occur in endemic countries annually.

Prevalence

Given the relatively short duration of illness and lack of chronic carrier state, cholera prevalence generally matches its incidence.

RISK FACTORS

- Inadequate drinking water and sanitation increase transmission; peri-urban slums, refugee camps, disaster areas, etc., are high risk for cholera epidemics.
- Floods and surface water temperature changes lead to increased cholera density.
- Low gastric acidity (which decreases killing of ingested organisms), blood group O, and retinol deficiency are risk factors.
- Young children are at risk for severe cholera.

Genetics

Because cholera pathophysiology involves chloride loss at the cystic fibrosis transmembrane conductance regulator (CFTR) chloride channel, it is hypothesized that those heterozygous or homozygous for mutations in CFTR have less severe cholera disease.

GENERAL PREVENTION

- Transmission
  - Hand washing after defecation and before food preparation is essential. Boiling or disinfection of water also prevents infection.
  - Thorough cooking of shellfish (which can be naturally contaminated) prevents infection.
  - During travel to endemic areas, avoid swimming or bathing in fresh water.
  - Report confirmed cholera cases to the local department of health.
  - Antibiotic prophylaxis of cholera contacts is debated but was shown in a meta-analysis to prevent disease among the contacts, although the analysis noted a risk of bias.
- Vaccines
  - No vaccines are available in the United States.
  - Whole cell killed oral cholera vaccines have 52% efficacy in preventing cholera over the subsequent year, but protective efficacy is lower in children <5 years of age at 38%. In some studies, vaccine efficacy remains this high up to 5 years after vaccination.
  - Single-dose oral vaccines with a vaccine efficacy ranging from 40–80% are also being studied.
  - Herd immunity occurs among unvaccinated people living near vaccinees.

PATHOPHYSIOLOGY

- Infection follows ingestion of large numbers of organisms from contaminated water or food (raw or undercooked shellfish and fish, or room temperature damp vegetables).
- The infectious dose for severe cholera is $\sim 10^8$ organisms but can be as little as 10^3 organisms in young children or those with decreased gastric acidity (such as persons on acid suppression medication or after certain meals).
- The typical incubation period is usually 2 to 3 days but ranges from ~12 hours to 5 days.
- 75% are infected asymptomatically; symptomatic illness ranges from moderate to severe.
- Cholera toxin is the key virulence factor responsible for the profuse watery diarrhea.
- Cholera toxin has 1A and 5B subunits.
  - The B subunits facilitate toxin attachment to intestinal cells.
  - The A subunit activates adenylate cyclase, increasing intracellular levels of cyclic adenosine monophosphate (cAMP), which causes chloride and sodium to be secreted into the gut lumen.
  - Water follows via osmosis.
- Severely ill patients can progress rapidly to dehydration, circulatory collapse, and death.
- Symptomatic patients may shed as many as 10^{10} to 10^{12} organisms per liter of stool and will shed organisms for 2 days to 2 weeks.

ETIOLOGY

- *V. cholerae* is a curved, motile gram-negative rod. >200 serogroups exist, but only serogroups O1 and O139 cause epidemics.
- *V. cholerae* serogroup O1
  - Divided into two biotypes: classical and El Tor
  - The classical biotype was formerly predominant, but the El Tor biotype is causing the seventh pandemic.
- *V. cholerae* serogroup O139
  - First identified in 1992
  - Resembles the O1 El Tor biotype but possesses a distinct lipopolysaccharide and capsule.
- Humans are the only known host, but organisms can also exist freely in water, potentially contaminating fish and shellfish.

COMMONLY ASSOCIATED CONDITIONS

Cholera occurs in healthy individuals.

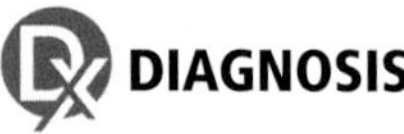

DIAGNOSIS

HISTORY

- Vomiting and profuse watery diarrhea:
  - Severe illness is characterized by voluminous watery diarrhea (up to 1 L per hour) flecked with mucus ("rice-water stools").
- Sick contacts with similar symptoms: Cholera epidemics can spread rapidly.
- Exposures
  - Return from travel within the last 5 days: Cholera is endemic in much of the world; the incubation period is typically 2 to 3 days.
  - Patient's water source: Contaminated water serves as a reservoir.
  - History of inadequately cooked shellfish: Shellfish (e.g., oysters, crabs) can harbor the organism.

PHYSICAL EXAM

- Patients with cholera display signs of dehydration (tachycardia, dry mucous membranes, sunken fontanelle or eyes, loss of skin turgor, lethargy) varying with severity.
- Arm and leg cramps occur due to secondary hypokalemia and hypocalcemia.
- Fever and obtundation secondary to hypoglycemia are more common in children.

DIFFERENTIAL DIAGNOSIS

- Other *Vibrio* species can cause gastroenteritis (commonly caused by *Vibrio parahaemolyticus* but also by *Vibrio fluvialis, Vibrio hollisae,* and *Vibrio mimicus*) or wound infections and sepsis (*Vibrio vulnificus*). Of these, only *V. parahaemolyticus* and *V. vulnificus* cause outbreaks.
- Additional intestinal bacterial pathogens include *Aeromonas, Campylobacter, Clostridium difficile, Escherichia coli, Listeria, Plesiomonas, Salmonella, Shigella, Vibrio* species, and *Yersinia*.
- Other viral and parasitic pathogens include amebiasis, adenovirus types 40 and 41, *Cryptosporidium, Cyclospora, Giardia,* norovirus, astrovirus, and rotavirus.

DIAGNOSTIC TESTS & INTERPRETATION

Initial Tests (screening, lab, imaging)

- Cholera is generally a clinical diagnosis.
- The World Health Organization (WHO) has a clinical case definition of cholera: In an area where the disease is not known to be present, a patient >5 years develops severe dehydration or dies from acute watery diarrhea (sensitivity, 91.3%), or in an area known to have cholera, a patient >5 years develops acute watery diarrhea with or without vomiting (sensitivity, 63.1%).
- Electrolytes, BUN, creatinine, serum calcium, and glucose can be useful if available. Acidosis can occur from stool bicarbonate losses and lactic acidosis from poor perfusion.

Diagnostic Procedures/Other

- Use selective media (thiosulfate citrate bile salts sucrose agar) to isolate *V. cholerae*. Alert the microbiology laboratory if culture testing for *V. cholerae* is desired.
- Serologic testing on acute and convalescent sera is also available through the Centers for Disease Control and Prevention (CDC).
- Stool culture may not always be positive in suspected cases of cholera, and rapid dipstick methods to identify cholera toxin and lipopolysaccharide, direct fluorescent antibody assays, and polymerase chain reaction (PCR)–based rapid diagnostic methods also exist and are being studied.
- Rapid molecular tests for other stool pathogens have been developed and can be used to exclude other agents in the differential diagnosis in some settings.

Test Interpretation

Diagnosis can also be made with the identification of darting, curved bacilli in 400× darkfield microscopy of stool.

TREATMENT

GENERAL MEASURES

- The mainstay of cholera treatment is rapid rehydration, accounting for both initial and ongoing fluid losses.
- Patients with moderate disease may require only oral rehydration solutions (ORS).
- Administer ORS in frequent small sips to those with vomiting. These solutions should contain at minimum 75 mEq/L of sodium to replete the significant sodium losses associated with cholera.
- ORS with total osmolality ≤270 mOsm/L is associated with increased risk of biochemical hyponatremia but not with other symptomatic outcomes compared to ORS ≥310 mOsm/L in a meta-analysis of a few existing trials.
- Those with more severe disease (volume loss >10%) require IV fluids.

MEDICATION

- Overall, it is estimated that antibiotics can reduce duration of diarrhea by 36 hours, stool volume by 50%, and amount of rehydration fluids by 40%.
- Give antibiotics as an adjunct to fluid replacement for those with moderate to severe cholera.
  - Single-dose doxycycline (4 to 6 mg/kg, up to 300 mg maximum) in those >8 years of age
  - Alternately, single-dose azithromycin (20 mg/kg up to 1,000 mg maximum) in children <8 years of age and pregnant women
  - Ciprofloxacin (15 mg/kg, up to 500 mg maximum, twice daily for 3 days) is another alternative.
- Single-dose azithromycin can reduce symptom duration by 50% and may reduce excretion of the organism to 1 to 2 days.
- *V. cholerae* isolates resistant to sulfonamides and tetracyclines are common. Resistance to fluoroquinolones, macrolides, and β-lactams is increasingly reported.
- Administer zinc for 10 to 14 days: 10 mg/24 h for those <6 months of age and 20 mg/24 h for those 6 months to 5 years of age.
- Consider vitamin A supplementation for children in developing countries.
- Avoid antiemetics and antimotility agents.

ADDITIONAL THERAPIES

During outbreaks, rapid institution of improved sanitation and safe water availability are critical to decrease the extent of the outbreak.

ADMISSION, INPATIENT, AND NURSING CONSIDERATIONS

- Rapid correction of severe (>10%) dehydration is critical.
- Admit those requiring IV fluids.
- Dhaka solution is an optimal IV fluid containing dextrose and more bicarbonate and potassium than lactated Ringer (LR).
- LR is an acceptable, more available alternative; D5LR contains 5% dextrose.
- Normal saline lacks potassium and bicarbonate and is second line.
- Measure ongoing fluid losses carefully.
- Use contact precautions for infected infants and children who are incontinent of stool.
- Discharge rehydrated patients able to maintain hydration orally.

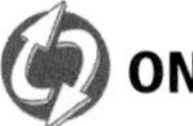

ONGOING CARE

FOLLOW-UP RECOMMENDATIONS

Patient Monitoring

In the untreated patient, the typical period of *V. cholerae* shedding is 1 to 2 weeks. Asymptomatic carriage is uncommon.

DIET

Resume a high-energy diet immediately after the initial fluid deficit is replaced. Infants should be encouraged to breastfeed.

PATIENT EDUCATION

- Improved sanitation and safe drinking water can help prevent future episodes.
- Secondary transmission can occur in households with affected members if strict hand washing and hygiene is not followed.

PROGNOSIS

For patients with prompt rehydration, the prognosis is very good regardless of whether antibiotic treatment is given.

COMPLICATIONS

- The main complications are those of severe dehydration: renal failure, thrombosis, stroke, and cardiovascular collapse.
- Cholera itself causes no complications.

ADDITIONAL READING

- Bhattacharya SK, Sur D, Ali M, et al. 5 year efficacy of a bivalent killed whole-cell oral cholera vaccine in Kolkata, India: a cluster-randomised, double-blind, placebo-controlled trial. *Lancet Infect Dis*. 2013;13(12):1050–1056.
- Chen WH, Cohen MB, Kirkpatrick BD, et al. Single-dose live oral cholera vaccine CVD 103-HgR protects against human experimental infection with *Vibrio cholerae* O1 El Tor. *Clin Infect Dis*. 2016;62(11):1329–1335.
- Leibovici-Weissman Y, Neuberger A, Bitterman R, et al. Antimicrobial drugs for treating cholera. *Cochrane Database Syst Rev*. 2014;(16):CD008625.
- Lucien MA, Schaad N, Steenland MW, et al. Identifying the most sensitive and specific sign and symptom combinations for cholera: results from an analysis of laboratory-based surveillance data from Haiti, 2012–2013. *Am J Trop Med Hyg*. 2015;92(4):758–764.
- Musekiwa A, Volmink J. Oral rehydration salt solution for treating cholera: ≤270 mOsm/L solutions vs ≥310 mOsm/L solutions. *Cochrane Database Syst Rev*. 2011;(12):CD003754.
- Qadri F, Wierzba TF, Ali M, et al. Efficacy of a single-dose, inactivated oral cholera vaccine in Bangladesh. *N Engl J Med*. 2016;374(18):1723–1732.
- Reveiz L, Chapman E, Ramon-Pardo P, et al. Chemoprophylaxis in contacts of patients with cholera: systematic review and meta-analysis. *PLoS One*. 2011;6(11):e27060.
- Sinclair D, Abba K, Zaman K, et al. Oral vaccines for preventing cholera. *Cochrane Database Syst Rev*. 2011;(3):CD008603.

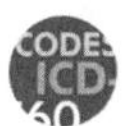

CODES

ICD10

- A00.9 Cholera, unspecified
- A00.0 Cholera due to Vibrio cholerae 01, biovar cholerae
- A00.1 Cholera due to Vibrio cholerae 01, biovar eltor

FAQ

- Q: What foods should I avoid while traveling?
- A: Foods associated with cholera include untreated or unboiled water and ice, undercooked fish and shellfish, raw vegetables, food from street vendors, and cooked food stored at ambient temperature.
- Q: Does cholera pose a risk to pregnant patients?
- A: Given the severe fluid losses, cholera can be life-threatening to the fetus; fetal loss occurs in up to 50% of women in their third trimester despite aggressive fluid resuscitation.
- Q: What is the risk of developing cholera among household contacts of those with disease?
- A: Up to 50% of household contacts may develop diarrheal symptoms, typically within 2 days of exposure to the index case.

CHRONIC DIARRHEA

Kerri Gosselin, MD, MPH

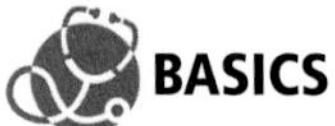

BASICS

DESCRIPTION

- Chronic diarrhea is defined as stool output >200 g/24 h in children and adults, or 10 g/kg/24 h in infants, that has occurred for >30 days.
- Should be differentiated from acute diarrhea, which is generally caused by enteric pathogens, is self-limiting, and has a duration of symptoms <14 days; as well as persistent diarrhea, which lasts 14 to 29 days

EPIDEMIOLOGY

- Gender and genetic factors do not play a significant role in most cases of chronic diarrhea.
- Infectious chronic diarrhea is seen most commonly in low-resource settings.

PATHOPHYSIOLOGY

The two major categories of chronic diarrhea are osmotic and secretory. Inflammatory and motility disorders are important subcategories to consider.

- Osmotic diarrhea occurs when unabsorbable solute accumulates in the lumen of the small intestine and colon, increasing intraluminal osmotic pressure and resulting in excessive fluid and electrolyte losses in stool.
  - Osmotic diarrhea will improve with fasting.
  - Osmotic diarrhea is usually related to malabsorption of dietary products or to the presence of congenital or acquired disaccharidase deficiency or glucose–galactose defects.
- Secretory diarrhea occurs when the net secretion of fluid and electrolyte is in excess of absorption in the intestine:
  - Secretory diarrhea occurs independently of the osmotic load in the intestinal lumen
  - Will not improve with fasting
  - The mechanisms for secretory diarrhea include the activation of intracellular mediators such as cAMP, cGMP, and calcium-dependent channels.
  - These mediators stimulate active chloride secretion from the crypt cells and inhibit the neutral coupled sodium chloride absorption.
- Inflammation in the intestine can cause an alteration in mucosal integrity resulting in exudative loss of mucus, blood, and/or protein. Increased permeability and altered mucosal surface area may affect absorption and result in diarrhea due to malabsorption.
- Motility disorders affect intestinal transit time. Hypomotility can allow stasis from bacterial overgrowth and can lead to diarrhea.

DIAGNOSIS

HISTORY

- Evaluation of the stool pattern, including consistency, frequency, and appearance
  - The characteristics of the onset of diarrhea should be noted as precisely as possible (e.g., congenital, abrupt, or gradual).
  - Overall duration of the diarrhea and pattern of intermittent versus continuous may also help in determining the underlying process.
  - Stool characteristics should be investigated including:
    - A history of blood and mucus in stool is strongly suggestive of inflammation.
    - Large-volume stools (>750 mL/24 h) imply small bowel disease and/or a secretory process.
    - Watery stools tend to be more associated with carbohydrate malabsorption, small bowel processes, medications, and functional processes.
    - Steatorrhea (fatty stools) can be greasy, oily, foul-smelling, and bulky and may be indicative of pancreatic insufficiency, bacterial overgrowth, and short bowel syndrome.
- Epidemiologic factors (e.g., travel before onset of illness, antibiotic exposure, and illness in other family members) should be elicited.
- Dietary intake including the types of food and the occurrence of diarrhea in close relationship to specific foods (e.g., dairy products) may be diagnostic. The quantity and type of liquid ingested may also be helpful in diagnosis.
- Nutritional status and growth parameters should be assessed. The presence of growth failure or malnutrition in the setting of chronic diarrhea warrants further investigation.
- Exposure to medications (antibiotics, laxatives, chemotherapeutic agents) or herbal therapies
- Iatrogenic causes of diarrhea should be investigated by obtaining a detailed medication history and history of radiation therapy and surgery.
- Other symptoms associated with the diarrhea are important to assess and include abdominal pain, fever, bloating, tenesmus, soiling, rashes, and joint complaints.
- The presence or absence of abdominal pain should be evaluated. Pain is often present in patients with inflammatory bowel disease, irritable bowel syndrome, and mesenteric ischemia.
- Family history (e.g., celiac disease, inflammatory bowel disease, cystic fibrosis, and other pancreatic processes)

PHYSICAL EXAM

- Nutritional and anthropometric measurements including height-for-weight and weight-for-age Z-scores.
- Anthropometric measurements are important in assessing loss of body fat and muscle mass.
- Peripheral edema, ascites, rash, dystrophic nails, alopecia, chronic chest findings, and pallor may all be indicative of nutritional deficiencies secondary to chronic diarrhea.
- A rectal exam may reveal stool impaction with overflow diarrhea.
- A perirectal examination may reveal signs of perianal inflammatory bowel disease (perianal fistula, skin tag, abscess)
- Aphthous lesions, arthritis, and clubbing
- Other features of diagnostic significance include rashes on the skin, mouth ulcers, thyroid masses, wheezing, arthritis, heart murmurs, hepatomegaly or abdominal masses.

DIFFERENTIAL DIAGNOSIS

- Infants (<1 year of age)
  - Cow's milk and/or soy protein intolerance
  - Intractable diarrhea of infancy is associated with diffuse mucosal injury beginning at <6 months of age, resulting in malabsorption and malnutrition (sucrose and lactase deficiency).
  - Infectious/protracted postinfectious diarrhea
  - Microvillus inclusions disease
  - Tufting enteropathy
  - Autoimmune enteropathy
  - IPEX (immune dysregulation, polyendocrinopathy, enteropathy, X-linked)
  - Congenital glucose–galactose malabsorption
  - Transport defects (e.g., congenital chloridorrhea)
  - Nutrient malabsorption (e.g., congenital glucose–galactose malabsorption and congenital lactase deficiency, sucrase-isomaltase deficiency)
  - Cystic fibrosis
  - AIDS enteropathy
  - Primary immune defects
  - Munchausen syndrome by proxy (factitious)
  - Drug-, toxin-induced
  - Short bowel syndrome
- Children (1 to 5 years of age)
  - Chronic nonspecific diarrhea of infancy (toddler's diarrhea)
  - Infectious/postinfectious enteritis
  - Giardiasis
  - Eosinophilic gastroenteritis
  - Sucrase-isomaltase deficiency
  - Tumors (neuroblastoma, VIPoma with secretory diarrhea)
  - Inflammatory bowel disease
  - Celiac disease
  - Cystic fibrosis
  - Small bowel bacterial overgrowth
  - AIDS enteropathy
  - Constipation with (overflow) encopresis
  - Acquired short bowel syndrome
  - Shwachman syndrome
  - Factitious
- Children (>5 years of age)
  - Similar to above
  - Acquired lactose deficiency (early adolescent)
  - Inflammatory bowel disease
  - Celiac disease
  - Constipation with (overflow) encopresis
  - Irritable bowel syndrome (adolescent)
  - Laxative abuse (adolescents)
  - Infection
- Bacterial (*Aeromonas*, *Plesiomonas*, *Campylobacter*, *Salmonella*, *Mycobacterium tuberculosis*, *Yersinia*, recurrent *Clostridium difficile*)
- Viral (rotavirus, adenovirus, Norwalk virus, norovirus)
- Parasites (*Amoeba*, *Trichuris*, *Cryptosporidium*, *Giardia*, *Schistosoma*, *Cyclospora*)
- Small bowel bacterial overgrowth
- Tumors (neuroblastoma, VIPoma with secretory diarrhea)
- Primary bowel tumors (rare, adolescent)
- Complex congenital heart disease with protein-losing enteropathy
- Pancreatic insufficiency/chronic pancreatitis
- Hyperthyroidism
- Diabetes

DIAGNOSTIC TESTS & INTERPRETATION

Initial Tests (screening, lab, imaging)

- Stool samples
  - Stool should be cultured for bacteria, ova and parasites, and viral organisms.
  - *C. difficile* can be investigated with PCR testing.
  - Stool samples can be analyzed for a number of characteristics and contents, including stool pH, reducing substances, electrolytes, occult blood and for the presence of fecal leukocytes.
    - If stool is positive for reducing substances and/or the pH is <5.5, carbohydrate malabsorption with or without proximal small bowel injury is likely.
      - Note: Sucrose is *not* a reducing substance. If sucrose malabsorption is suspected, stool sample has to be hydrolyzed with hydrochloric acid and heat before analysis.
    - Stool may be collected for electrolyte and osmolality measurements. Osmotic gap >100 mOsm/kg is indicative of an osmotic diarrhea.
    - A positive Sudan stain of the stool is indicative of fat malabsorption. However, a 72-hour fecal fat collection remains the gold standard to diagnose fat malabsorption.
    - Stool for fecal elastase can also be used to assess fat malabsorption.
    - Spot or 24-hour collection for fecal α_1-antitrypsin can help assess protein loss.
    - Stool collection for fecal calprotectin or lactoferrin (proteins contained in neutrophils) are reliable noninvasive screening tests for intestinal inflammation.
- CBC
  - Serum hemoglobin levels and measurements of mean corpuscular volume (MCV) may provide evidence and characteristics of anemia (i.e., microcytotic, macrocytotic, normochromic).
  - Leukocytosis suggests the presence of inflammation.
  - Eosinophilia can be seen with neoplasm, allergy, collagen vascular disease, parasitic infection, and eosinophilic gastroenteritis, or colitis.
- Other blood tests:
  - Prealbumin and albumin can provide parameters of protein and overall nutritional status.
  - Erythrocyte sedimentation rate (ESR) and C-reactive protein (CRP) can serve as markers for inflammatory conditions.
  - Hormonal studies to assess for secretory tumors (vasoactive intestinal peptide [VIP], gastrin, secretin, urine assay for serotonin [5-HT])
  - Serologic screening for celiac disease should be performed by obtaining serum antitissue transglutaminase antibody and antiendomysial antibodies (presuming a normal level of total serum IgA)
  - Hepatic panel, coagulation profile, and fat-soluble vitamin levels (25-OH vitamin D; vitamins E, A, K) may be helpful to assess fat malabsorption.
  - Viral serologies such as HIV and cytomegalovirus need to be considered in the immunocompromised host with diarrhea.
  - Thyroid studies in patients with large-volume watery diarrhea
- Specialized studies:
  - A D-xylose absorption test is helpful in screening for small bowel injury. Timed serum D-xylose following oral ingestion is significantly lower in diseases causing diffuse mucosal damage to the small bowel (i.e., postviral enteropathy, celiac disease).
  - A hydrogen breath test may be helpful in evaluating for the possibility of small bowel bacterial overgrowth.
- Sweat chloride if cystic fibrosis is suspected
- Plain radiograph studies are usually not helpful; may demonstrate presence or absence of formed stool and/or fecal impaction which may present paradoxically with a complaint of "chronic diarrhea"
- Upper GI series with small bowel follow-through may show partial small bowel obstruction, strictures, or evidence of inflammatory bowel disease.
- Abdominal CT scan may help in assessing the pancreas for calcifications and inflammation.

Diagnostic Procedures/Other

- Endoscopy with small bowel biopsy and small bowel aspirate for culture may be required to diagnose certain congenital, immunologic, or infectious causes of diarrhea
  - Small bowel disaccharidase studies can be used to identify carbohydrate malabsorption.
- Colonoscopy will diagnose colitis related to inflammatory bowel disease or infection.
- Video capsule endoscopy may also be used to further evaluate the small bowel for evidence of inflammation.

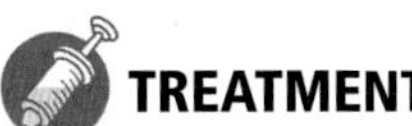

TREATMENT

MEDICATION

- Pancreatic enzymes may be used in patients with pancreatic insufficiency.
- Luminal (nonabsorbed) antibiotics for small bowel bacterial overgrowth

ALERT

- In certain cases in which the diet is altered as a therapeutic intervention, the physician must ensure that the patient is still absorbing adequate calories and micronutrients, so that the nutritional status of the patient is not further compromised.
- The use of antimotility and antisecretory agents should be judicious and as an adjunct to other therapy but not as the mainstay in the treatment regimen.
- In patients with cow's milk and/or soy allergy, rechallenge after 12 months of age in a controlled environment in case anaphylaxis occurs.
- Children with the following symptoms should see a health care provider:
  - Signs of dehydration
  - Failure to thrive
  - A fever of 102°F or higher
  - Stools containing blood or pus
  - Stools that are black and tarry

ADDITIONAL THERAPIES

- The first goal is to ensure adequate hydration status, nutritional intake, and to permit normal growth and development.
- Many causes of congenital diarrhea do not have specific therapy available, and treatment is supportive.
- Diet: If infection is severe or protracted, an elemental formula may be necessary early in the recovery phase. If oral nutrition appears inadequate, the formula can be given in a slow, continuous fashion via a nasogastric/jejunal tube. Remove offending agent (e.g., cow's milk protein, soy protein, lactose, or gluten).
- In cases in which there is increased motility and thus rapid transit time, such as in chronic nonspecific diarrhea, alterations in the diet can be very helpful.
- Elimination of sorbitol-containing juices, which increases the osmotic load, and low-carbohydrate diet will help to lower the osmotic load delivered to the intestine. Furthermore, a high-fat diet will slow the intestinal transit time and increase the time available to absorb fluid, electrolytes, and nutrients from the intestinal tract.

ADDITIONAL READING

- Berni Canani R, Terrin G, Cardillo G, et al. Congenital diarrheal disorders: improved understanding of gene defects is leading to advances in intestinal physiology and clinical management. *J Pediatr Gastroenterol Nutr*. 2010;50(4):360–366.
- Bhutta ZA, Nelson EA, Lee WS, et al. Recent advances and evidence gaps in persistent diarrhea. *J Pediatr Gastroenterol Nutr*. 2008;47(2):260–265.
- Lee SD, Surawicz CM. Infectious causes of chronic diarrhea. *Gastroenterol Clin North Am*. 2001;30(3):679–692.
- Pawlowski SW, Warren CA, Guerrant R. Diagnosis and treatment of acute or persistent diarrhea. *Gastroenterology*. 2009;136(6):1874–1886.
- Savilahti E. Food-induced malabsorption syndromes. *J Pediatr Gastroenterol Nutr*. 2000;30:S61–S66.

CODES

ICD10

K52.9 Noninfective gastroenteritis and colitis, unspecified

FAQ

- Q: If my infant has cow's milk allergy, when can he have cow's milk?
- A: In patients with cow's milk and/or soy allergy, rechallenge should be around 12 months of age and should be in a controlled environment in case anaphylaxis occurs.

CHRONIC GRANULOMATOUS DISEASE

Benjamin T. Prince, MD, MSci • Ramsay L. Fuleihan, MD

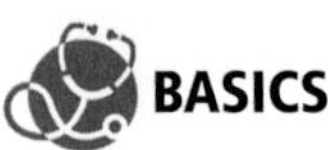

BASICS

DESCRIPTION

Chronic granulomatous disease (CGD) is a rare, primary immunodeficiency caused by a genetic defect that results in an inability of phagocytes to generate superoxide, which is important in microbial killing. Affected individuals are susceptible to recurrent, life-threatening bacterial and fungal infections.

EPIDEMIOLOGY

Incidence

1:200,000 to 1:250,000 live births in the United States and Europe. Rates in other countries vary depending on ethnic practices and degree of intermarriage.

RISK FACTORS

Genetics

- Mutations in any of the five genes that code for the five subunits of the phagocyte NADPH oxidase complex (phox) can result in CGD.
- Mutations in the gp91phox subunit (CYBB) are responsible for 65% of cases and are inherited in an X-linked manner (1/3 of these cases are the result of a de novo mutation).
- Mutations in p47phox, p22phox, p67phox, and p40phox subunits account for the remaining cases and have an autosomal recessive inheritance.
- Mutations in the p47phox subunit are the most common cause of autosomal recessive CGD (25% of all cases).

PATHOPHYSIOLOGY

- Phagocytes (neutrophils, monocytes, and macrophages) require NADPH oxidase to generate reactive oxygen species (ROS) in a process called the respiratory burst.
- During this process, the NADPH oxidase complex transfers an electron to molecular oxygen forming superoxide, which is eventually converted to hydrogen peroxide.
- Superoxide plays a significant role in killing bacterial and fungal pathogens both directly and through the activation of more important intraphagosomal proteases.
- The clinical phenotype of CGD is related to the level of residual superoxide production; patients who have higher levels of superoxide production have better long-term survival rates.
- Only the X-linked subunit gp91phox is phagocyte specific, and patients with defects in the autosomal subunits may also have other abnormalities such as vascular disease, diabetes, and inflammatory bowel disease.

ETIOLOGY

CGD is the result of a spontaneous or inherited genetic mutation that is present at birth.

DIAGNOSIS

The diagnosis of CGD should be considered in patients with

- Recurrent lymphadenitis
- Staphylococcal hepatic abscess
- Infections with *Burkholderia cepacia*, *Serratia marcescens*, *Nocardia*, or *Aspergillus*
- *Salmonella* sepsis
- Perirectal or deep tissue abscesses
- Colitis in infancy
- Granulomatous lesions of the gastrointestinal or genitourinary systems

HISTORY

- Patients most commonly present in early childhood with recurrent or severe bacterial or fungal infections of the lung, ski, lymph nodes, liver, bones, and blood.
- Patients may also have a history of failure to thrive, diarrhea, anemia, abnormal wound healing, or granulomatous inflammation.
- Infecting organisms are typically catalase producing; however, catalase alone does not appear to be a significant virulence factor in animal models.
- Most common organisms include *Staphylococcus aureus*, *B. (Pseudomonas) cepacia*, *S. marcescens*, *Nocardia*, *Aspergillus*, *Salmonella*, Bacillus Calmette-Guérin (BCG), *Mycobacterium*, *Klebsiella pneumoniae*, *Candida*, *Actinomyces, and Granulibacter bethesdensis*.
- Obtain a good maternal family history, given that most common inheritance is X-linked. There may also be family history of lupus, especially maternal.

PHYSICAL EXAM

- Skin and mucosa
  - Dermatitis, cellulitis, impetigo, abscesses, stomatitis, gingivitis
- HEENT
  - Conjunctivitis, chorioretinitis, sinusitis
- Lymphatic
  - Lymphadenopathy, suppurative lymphadenitis
- Respiratory
  - Pneumonia, pneumonitis
- Gastrointestinal
  - Gastric outlet obstruction hepatomegaly, splenomegaly, colitis, diarrhea, malabsorption, perirectal abscess, fistulae
- Genitourinary
  - Urethral strictures, urinary tract infections

DIFFERENTIAL DIAGNOSIS

- Genetic/metabolic
  - Sarcoidosis
  - Glucose-6-phosphate dehydrogenase (G6PD) deficiency
  - Glutathione synthetase (GS) deficiency
  - Cystic fibrosis
- Immunology
  - Myeloperoxidase deficiency
  - Hyper IgE syndrome
  - Humoral immunodeficiencies
  - IRAK4 deficiency
  - MyD88 deficiency
- Gastrointestinal
  - Inflammatory bowel disease

DIAGNOSTIC TESTS & INTERPRETATION

Initial Tests (screening, lab, imaging)

- Dihydrorhodamine 123 (DHR) test
  - Uses flow cytometry to directly measure NADPH oxidase function in phagocytes
  - Phagocytes take up nonfluorescent DHR. Oxidation by a normal functioning NADPH oxidase complex causes DHR to fluoresce, which is identified by flow cytometry.
  - More sensitive and quantitative than older nitroblue tetrazolium (NBT) test
  - Can identify NADPH positive and negative subpopulations of phagocytes, easily identifying a carrier of CGD
  - May be falsely positive in patients with myeloperoxidase deficiency and SAPHO (synovitis, acne, pustulosis, hyperostosis, osteitis) syndrome
- NBT test
  - Historical test for CGD that is no longer widely used by immunologists
  - Neutrophils with a normal NADPH complex can reduce the dye, resulting in a color change from yellow to dark blue. Neutrophils from patients with CGD cannot reduce the dye, and it remains colorless.
  - Color change is assessed with microscopy, and results may be inaccurate if not performed by experienced technician.
- Genetic testing
  - A diagnosis of CGD should be confirmed with genetic testing to identify the specific genetic defect.
  - Identification of specific mutation can better predict the patient's clinical course.
  - Identification of specific mutation is necessary for a future prenatal diagnosis.
- Obtain chest radiograph, ultrasound, CT scan, or MRI as appropriate to aid in the diagnosis and evaluation of acute infections.

TREATMENT

MEDICATION
- Prophylaxis
  - Trimethoprim-sulfamethoxazole (TMP-SMX)
    - First line for antibacterial prophylaxis; also can be used for the treatment of acute bacterial infections
    - Prophylaxis dosing: 5 mg/kg/24 h TMP PO divided b.i.d., maximum 320 mg b.i.d.
    - Has been shown to significantly decrease frequency and severity of infections in CGD patients
  - Itraconazole
    - First line for antifungal prophylaxis
    - Prophylaxis dosing: 5 mg/kg PO daily, maximum 200 mg daily
  - Interferon γ-1b
    - Effective in reducing the frequency and severity of infections when used prophylactically; however, it is unclear how much additional benefit is gained when used in conjunction with TMP-SMX and itraconazole prophylaxis
    - Prophylaxis dosing: 50 mcg/m^2 subcutaneously 3 times weekly
  - Ciprofloxacin
    - Should be started prophylactically before any invasive procedure and continued for at least 24 hours afterward
    - Prophylaxis dosing: 7.5 mg/kg PO q12h, maximum 500 mg q12h
- Acute infections
  - Broad-spectrum IV antimicrobials: Severe infections should be treated empirically until a specific organism is identified. Treatment should cover both gram-negative and gram-positive bacteria along with fungi.
  - First line: TMP-SMX, fluoroquinolones, and voriconazole
  - Carbapenems, vancomycin, and amphotericin B may be considered depending on site or severity of infection.

ISSUES FOR REFERRAL
Factors that may help alert you to make a referral:
- New diagnosis of CGD
  - Immunologists can assist with antibiotic prophylaxis and with parameters for when to seek medical attention.
  - Can help establish the specific molecular diagnosis of the patient and offer genetic counseling for the future
  - Can discuss treatment options, including the possibility of hematopoietic stem cell transplant (HSCT)
- Fever or suspected infection
  - Patients with CGD tend to develop infections in unusual sites with unusual organisms.
  - Both an infectious disease specialist and an immunologist can help with the evaluation and appropriate treatment of infections.
- Gastrointestinal symptoms or malabsorption
  - Gastroenterologists can help identify and treat strictures, obstruction, and colitis.

ADDITIONAL THERAPIES
- HSCT
  - HSCT can be a definitive cure for CGD.
  - Younger patients with absence of preexisting overt infection, and HLA matched donors have the best prognosis.
- Gene therapy
  - Alternative treatment of CGD with newer vectors showing a higher rate of success
  - Should be considered in patients with more severe phenotypes that don't have a viable HSCT option

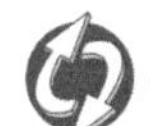

ONGOING CARE

FOLLOW-UP RECOMMENDATIONS

Patient Monitoring
- Regular screening blood tests
  - CBC with differential and LFTs should be performed every 6 months to monitor for any adverse effects of prophylactic medications.
  - CRP and ESR should be performed regularly and at times of acute infection.
- Pulmonary function testing should be followed annually to screen for chronic lung disease.
- Patients should be screened regularly by ophthalmology for chorioretinal lesions.
- Closely monitor CGD patients and carriers for signs of systemic lupus erythematosus and other autoimmune disorders.

PROGNOSIS
- CGD is a lifelong disease.
- Survival beyond the 4th decade is now common with antimicrobial prophylaxis and early and aggressive treatment of infections.
- Successful HSCT is curative.

COMPLICATIONS
CGD patients have an increased susceptibility to bacterial and fungal infections that usually are not pathogenic in normal hosts:
- Recurrent infections (see previous sections)
- Sepsis
- Chronic lung disease (secondary to recurrent infections)
- Chronic liver disease (secondary to recurrent infections)
- Chronic osteomyelitis of large and small bones
- Malabsorption
- Systemic and discoid lupus erythematosus
  - Increased incidence in female carriers

ADDITIONAL READING

- Cole T, Pearce MS, Cant AJ, et al. Clinical outcome in children with chronic granulomatous disease managed conservatively or with hematopoietic stem cell transplantation. *J Allergy Clin Immunol*. 2013;132(5):1150–1155.
- Damen GM, van Krieken JH, Hoppenreijs E, et al. Overlap, common features, and essential differences in pediatric granulomatous inflammatory bowel disease. *J Pediatr Gastroenterol Nutr*. 2010;51(6):690–697.
- Kuhns DB, Alvord WG, Heller T, et al. Residual NADPH oxidase and survival in chronic granulomatous disease. *N Engl J Med*. 2010;363(27):2600–2610.
- Song E, Jaishankar GB, Saleh H, et al. Chronic granulomatous disease: a review of the infectious and inflammatory complications. *Clin Mol Allergy*. 2011;9(1):10.
- Thomsen IP, Smith MA, Holland SM, et al. A comprehensive approach to the management of children and adults with chronic granulomatous disease. *J Allergy Clin Immunol Pract*. 2016;4(6):1082–1088.

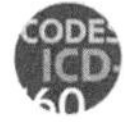

CODES

ICD10
D71 Functional disorders of polymorphonuclear neutrophils

FAQ
- Q: Should patients with CGD receive dental prophylaxis?
- A: Yes. Antibiotic prophylaxis should be started before and continued for 24 hours after any dental treatment likely to cause bleeding.
- Q: Can patients with CGD receive live viral vaccines?
- A: Yes. The only routine immunization that adults and children with CGD should NOT receive is BCG as it has been associated with disseminated infection.
- Q: Are all CGD patients with fever automatically admitted to the hospital?
- A: No. Although CGD patients are more prone to invasive and systemic infections, they are not necessarily admitted with every febrile episode. If there is evidence of a minor bacterial or viral infection without any concern for a more serious infection, patients may be treated as an outpatient with close monitoring. Subtle signs of an invasive infection must be taken very seriously.
- Q: Can CGD be diagnosed prenatally?
- A: Yes. Testing involves chorionic villus sampling; however, it can only be done on families with a history of CGD in which the specific mutation is known.

C

CHRONIC HEPATITIS

Pamela L. Valentino, MD, MSc, FRCP(C)

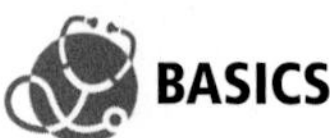

BASICS

DESCRIPTION

- Chronic hepatitis is a continuous inflammation of the liver that can lead to cirrhosis.
- Features of chronic inflammation include raised transaminases for >6 months and histologic evidence of hepatocellular injury, cholestasis, or presence of inflammatory infiltration.

EPIDEMIOLOGY

Depends on the cause of the underlying disease

- Nonalcoholic steatohepatitis (NASH) is a leading cause of elevated alanine aminotransferase (ALT)/ aspartate aminotransferase (AST).
- Hepatitis B: common in immigrant children from Asia and Eastern Europe
- Hepatitis C: common in those who had blood products before screening became available, history of IV drug use, tattoos, or in immigrant children with shared vaccination needles
- Hepatitis E: can cause chronic hepatitis in pregnant women
- Wilson disease presents mainly in older children (>2 years of age) and adolescents.
- Autoimmune hepatitis (AIH) is more common in females and patients >6 months of age. AIH may be associated with other autoimmune conditions such as primary sclerosing cholangitis (PSC), type I diabetes, inflammatory bowel disease, autoimmune thyroiditis, and celiac disease.
- Cystic fibrosis (CF) may present with cholestasis of the newborn; 5–10% of patients with CF develop advanced liver disease in childhood.
- α_1-antitrypsin (AAT) deficiency phenotype (Pi) Pi*MM is wild type; Pi*ZZ or Pi*SZ cause liver disease.

PATHOPHYSIOLOGY

Chronic hepatitis involves a continuous process of liver injury and regeneration.

- Pattern of liver injury and histopathology varies depending on the clinical diagnosis.
- The response to chronic liver injury is the same across most liver diseases: development of fibrosis.
- The liver is in a constant equilibrium between the production and breakdown of extracellular matrix (ECM) proteins, which includes collagen and others.
- Hepatitis causes increased cellular activation and transformation (e.g., activated stellate cells differentiate to myofibroblasts), which leads to the accumulation of ECM.
- Over time, as the connective tissue bands thicken they can extend from portal triad to portal triad (bridging fibrosis) or to central veins with eventual formation of nodules (cirrhosis).

ETIOLOGY

- Autoimmune liver disease: AIH or PSC
- Celiac disease associated with hepatitis
- Viral hepatitis
- Nonalcoholic fatty liver disease (NAFLD), or specifically NASH
- Congenital hepatic fibrosis
- Genetic disease
  - AAT deficiency
  - Alagille syndrome
  - CF
  - Progressive familial intrahepatic cholestasis (PFIC) syndromes
  - Wilson disease
- Metabolic disease
  - Mitochondrial disease
  - Lysosomal acid lipase deficiency (LAL-D)
  - Lysosomal storage disorders
  - Peroxisomal disease
  - Lipid storage disease
  - Glycogen storage disease (GSD)
  - Wilson disease and others
- Drug-induced liver injury (DILI)
  - Parenteral nutrition–associated liver disease
  - Chemotherapy: methotrexate, 6-mercaptopurine, thioguanine
  - Isoniazid
  - Valproate
- Liver disease associated with other chronic diseases
  - Hypothyroidism, hyperthyroidism
  - Growth hormone deficiency/panhypopituitarism
  - Diabetes mellitus (uncontrolled hyperglycemia)
  - Congestive hepatopathy (cardiac: right-sided heart failure or hypertension, such as post-Fontan procedure; pulmonary hypertension)
  - Autosomal recessive polycystic kidney disease
  - Langerhans cell histiocytosis
  - Immunodeficiency

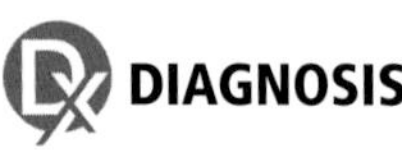

DIAGNOSIS

HISTORY

- Complete medical history including the following clinical signs and symptoms:
  - Use of medications, complementary or alternative medications, supplements, or IV drugs
  - Foreign travel
  - History of blood transfusions
  - Social circumstances that predispose to liver diseases including multiple sexual partners
  - Jaundice in infancy
  - Vaccination history
  - Family history of liver or autoimmune disease, consanguinity
- Symptoms of chronic illness can be nonspecific:
  - Poor growth
  - Intermittent jaundice
  - Pruritus (especially without a preceding rash)
  - Easy bruising or bleeding
  - Abdominal pain
  - Fever
  - Amenorrhea
  - Poor school performance
- Variceal bleeding may be a presenting symptom in patients with portal hypertension.
- Mental status changes with memory loss, irregular hand writing, poor academic performance (hepatic encephalopathy)

PHYSICAL EXAM

Stigmata of chronic liver disease are as follows:

- Poor weight gain/FTT, weight loss
- Oxygen desaturation (hepatopulmonary syndrome)
- Jaundice
- Pruritus/scratch marks
- Spider nevi, palmar erythema
- Dilated veins on abdomen/cutaneous shunts
- Palmar erythema
- Clubbing
- Acanthosis nigricans (NAFLD)
- Hypercholesterolemic xanthomas
- Enlarged liver or hard, shrunken liver
- Splenomegaly, bruising (hypersplenism)
- Ascites; males may develop scrotal edema.
- Rickets
- Fetor hepaticus associated with high ammonia or dimethyl sulfide

DIFFERENTIAL DIAGNOSIS

Nonhepatic etiologies

- Hepatomegaly: respiratory diseases with lung hyperexpansion
- Splenomegaly
  - Blood malignancies
  - Storage diseases
  - Hematologic disease with hemolysis
  - Infection
  - Vascular
- Jaundice: often confused with hypercarotenemia
- Elevated transaminases: Consider nonhepatic sources such as skeletal muscles in myopathies.
- Alkaline phosphatase: may be elevated in growing children, bone fractures, and in rickets; may not indicate biliary obstruction
- γ-Glutamyl transferase
  - Produced in renal tubules, pancreatic and biliary ducts as well as hepatocytes
  - Can be elevated due to enzymatic induction from anticonvulsants, without any liver injury
- Abnormal coagulation: anticoagulant medications, bacterial overgrowth with malabsorption, inherited disorders of coagulation, sepsis

DIAGNOSTIC TESTS & INTERPRETATION

Initial Tests (screening, lab, imaging)

- General liver testing: ALT (normal <25 in boys and <22 in girls), AST, γ-glutamyl transferase, albumin, direct or conjugated bilirubin, PT/INR, CBC, creatinine
- Viral serologies: hepatitis B surface antigen, hepatitis C antibody
- Autoantibodies: AIH: type 1: smooth muscle (also called F-actin), antinuclear, antisoluble liver antigen; type 2: liver kidney microsomal; PSC: perinuclear antineutrophil cytoplasmic antibody (p-ANCA) with elevated GGT; celiac: tissue transglutaminase (tTG-IgA)
- Immunoglobulins: IgG elevated in autoimmune liver disease, immunoglobulin A deficiency associated with celiac disease
- AAT level and phenotype
- Serum ceruloplasmin, 24-hour urine copper (+/− penicillamine challenge) (Wilson disease)
- Fasting glucose, insulin levels, lipid profile, hemoglobin A1c (NAFLD)
- Cholesterol, triglycerides elevated in cholestatic syndromes, glycogen storage, Alagille syndrome, certain lysosomal disease, steatohepatitis
- TSH, free T_4
- CPK level to rule out muscle source of elevated ALT/AST

- Serum bile acids, total and fractionated (to confirm cholestasis with symptoms of pruritus)
- Ultrasound with Doppler flow studies: should focus on liver and spleen

Follow-Up Tests & Special Considerations

Other testing as indicated by the specific clinical presentation

- Hepatitis E IgM in pregnant patients
- Ophthalmologic exam for Kayser-Fleischer rings (Wilson disease) or for posterior embryotoxon (Alagille syndrome)
- Metabolic workup as indicated
- Urinary succinylacetone: tyrosinemia
- Urinary bile acids: bile acid synthetic defects
- Sweat test and CF genotyping
- α-Fetoprotein (AFP) level
- Fibrosis markers (FibroSURE; FibroTest; ActiTest) are not validated for children but may be useful in older patients.

Diagnostic Procedures/Other

Other testing as indicated by specific clinical presentation

- Liver biopsy
- Quantitative liver copper (Wilson disease)
- MRI: Evaluate masses or vascular abnormalities.
- Endoscopic retrograde cholangiopancreatography (ERCP) or magnetic resonance cholangiopancreatography (MRCP) for PSC
- Colonoscopy: PSC-inflammatory bowel disease
- FibroScan can measure liver stiffness/fibrosis.
- Bone marrow aspirate to exclude Niemann-Pick type C or other storage disorders
- Enzyme analysis to evaluate for lysosomal storage disease, GSD
- Angiography: congenital or acquired venous or arterial malformations, assessment of portosystemic shunt
- Echocardiogram and cardiac catheterization to assess cardiac function and pulmonary hypertension
- Bubble echocardiogram to assess for hepatopulmonary syndrome in the setting of portal hypertension and oxygen desaturation
- Muscle biopsy to assay respiratory chain enzymes in mitochondrial disorders
- Genotyping: CF, PFIC, and others

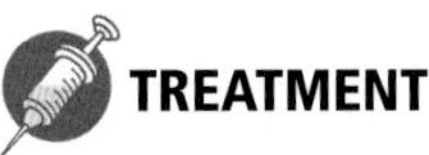

TREATMENT

GENERAL MEASURES

The management of patients is dictated by the underlying diagnosis.

- General management
  - Maintaining growth and development is paramount.
  - Anthropometric parameters must be recorded: skinfold thickness, mid arm circumference, body mass index.
  - Proactive involvement of clinical psychologist and play therapist can help alleviate problems such as depression and fear.
  - Aggressive weight management in patients with obesity/metabolic syndrome with steatohepatitis; dietary changes including portion size control, curbing passive activities such as television, computer games
  - Timely and accurate diagnosis of spontaneous bacterial peritonitis with paracentesis in febrile patients with ascites—treat with antibiotics
  - Complete immunization schedule including hepatitis A, hepatitis B, and annual flu shots.
  - Early referral to a liver transplant center
  - Specific management depends on the underlying liver disease.

MEDICATION

- Management of cholestasis
  - Fat-soluble vitamins (A, D, E, K) given orally are poorly absorbed in cholestasis; levels must be monitored and supplementation provided. Phytonadione (Vitamin K) can be administered IM.
  - Preference for medium-chain triglyceride (MCT)–rich formulas can reduce fat malabsorption.
  - Ursodeoxycholic acid (UDCA): choleretic
  - Encourage bolus feedings; minimizing continuous feeding and total parenteral nutrition may reduce gallbladder sludge.

ALERT

Phytonadione (vitamin K) can be given IM; anaphylaxis can occur with the IV formulation.

- Management of chronic debilitating pruritus may include:
  - Keeping nails short and skin well-hydrated
  - UDCA—maximum 20 mg/kg/24 h
  - Antihistamines (diphenhydramine, hydroxyzine)
  - Rifampicin
  - Naltrexone
  - Ondansetron
  - Cholestyramine
  - Ultraviolet light
- Liver transplantation may be indicated with failure of medical therapy.

SURGERY/OTHER PROCEDURES

Early referral to a liver transplant center

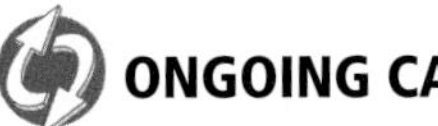

ONGOING CARE

FOLLOW-UP RECOMMENDATIONS

Patient Monitoring

- Provide hepatocellular carcinoma surveillance with cirrhosis or diseases at high risk (tyrosinemia, GSD, etc.).
- Obtaining an ultrasound scan of liver and AFP every 6 to 12 months is considered a reasonable schedule.
- Advise patients with splenomegaly to wear a spleen guard and avoid activities (e.g., contact sports) that can cause splenic rupture.
- Surveillance for esophageal varices with development of splenomegaly and thrombocytopenia

PROGNOSIS

Some cases of chronic hepatitis are associated with diseases that are treatable. Others are progressive and not amenable to treatment. A subset of patients will progress to end-stage liver disease and require liver transplantation.

ADDITIONAL READING

- Mieli-Vergani G, Vergani D. Autoimmune hepatitis in children: what is different from adult AIH? *Semin Liver Dis*. 2009;29(3):297–306.
- Murray KF, Shah U, Mohan N, et al; for Chronic Hepatitis Working Group. Chronic hepatitis. *J Pediatr Gastroenterol Nutr*. 2008;47(2):225–233.
- Nel E, Sokol R, Comparcola D, et al. Viral hepatitis in children. *J Pediatr Gastroenterol Nutr*. 2012;55(5):500–505.
- Schwimmer JB, Dunn W, Norman GJ, et al. SAFETY study: alanine aminotransferase cutoff values are set too high for reliable detection of pediatric chronic liver disease. *Gastroenterology*. 2010;138(4): 1357–1364.
- Sheiko MA, Sundaram SS, Capocelli KE, et al. Outcomes in pediatric autoimmune hepatitis and significance of azathioprine metabolites. *J Pediatr Gastroenterol Nutr*. 2017;65(1):80–85.
- Tangerman A, Meuwese-Arends MT, Jansen JB. Cause and composition of foetor hepaticus. *Lancet*. 1994;343(8895):483.
- Vos MB, Abrams SH, Barlow SE, et al. NASPGHAN Clinical Practice Guideline for the diagnosis and treatment of nonalcoholic fatty liver disease in children: recommendations from the Expert Committee on NAFLD (ECON) and the North American Society of Pediatric Gastroenterology, Hepatology and Nutrition (NASPGHAN). *J Pediatr Gastroenterol Nutr*. 2017;64(2):319–334.
- Woodruff SA, Sontag MK, Accurso FJ, et al. Prevalence of elevated liver enzymes in children with cystic fibrosis diagnosed by newborn screen. *J Cyst Fibros*. 2017;16(1):139–145.

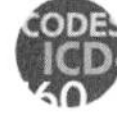

CODES

ICD10

- K73.9 Chronic hepatitis, unspecified
- K73.0 Chronic persistent hepatitis, not elsewhere classified
- B18.9 Chronic viral hepatitis, unspecified

FAQ

- Q: What are the risks of providing very young patients with a liver transplant?
- A: Lifetime risks of immunosuppression and rejection. Although transplant in the very young is more difficult, with the increased use of split liver techniques and improved use of immunosuppressives, outcomes of orthotopic liver transplantation in infants have improved.
- Q: Why should we be aggressive with vitamin supplementation?
- A: Chronic hepatitis is associated with significant malabsorption of vitamins A, D, E, and K. Vitamins D and E deficiencies in particular can cause rickets and neuropathy.
- Q: How can I optimally administer oral supplements of vitamins in the very young?
- A: It is common practice in some centers to give vitamins K as an intramuscular injection on a monthly basis, with levels done in between.
- Q: What stigmata of chronic liver disease can be seen in children?
- A: Jaundice, spider nevi, liver palms (palmar erythema), splenomegaly, cutaneous shunts, and clubbing are very common.

CHRONIC KIDNEY DISEASE

Rebecca L. Ruebner, MD, MSCE • Madhura Pradhan, MD

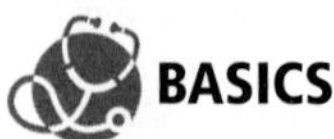

BASICS

DESCRIPTION

- The Kidney Disease: Improving Global Outcomes (KDIGO) 2012 clinical practice guideline defines pediatric chronic kidney disease (CKD) based on a child meeting one of the following criteria for >3 months:
  - Glomerular filtration rate (GFR) <60 mL/min/1.73 m^2 with implications for health, regardless of whether other CKD markers are present.
  - GFR >60 accompanied by markers of kidney damage including structural abnormalities, proteinuria, renal tubular disorders, or histologic abnormalities
- The criteria for >3 months duration does not apply to infants <3 months of age.
- The criteria for GFR does not apply to children <2 years of age.
- CKD is classified based on cause, GFR category, and albuminuria category.
- GFR categories
  - G1: GFR ≥90
  - G2: GFR 60 to 89
  - G3a: GFR 45 to 59
  - G3b: GFR 30 to 44
  - G4: GFR 15 to 29
  - G5: GFR <15
- Albuminuria categories—albumin to creatinine ratio in mg/g
  - A1 <30
  - A2 30 to 300
  - A3 >300

EPIDEMIOLOGY

Incidence

~5 to 12 cases per year per million of age-related population

Prevalence

- Prevalence of CKD has been reported to be between 21 and 74 cases per million of age-related population from various studies in Europe and Latin America.
- Incidence and prevalence of CKD are higher among males, due to higher incidence of congenital anomalies of the kidney and urinary tract (CAKUT).

RISK FACTORS

- Risk factors for CAKUT include genetic and environmental factors (maternal diabetes, exposure to medications such as ACE inhibitor/NSAIDs).
- Low birth weight, prematurity, and rapid weight gain in early childhood increase risk of CKD.
- Hypertension and proteinuria increase risk of CKD progression.

PATHOPHYSIOLOGY

- Cardiovascular: Hypertension secondary to activation of renin-angiotensin system, fluid overload, and anemia from erythropoietin deficiency contribute to cardiovascular morbidity.
- Bone and mineral bone disorder of CKD: Decreased excretion of phosphorous and decreased synthesis of 1,25-dihydroxy vitamin D leads to hyperparathyroidism and bone disease.
- Growth: Metabolic acidosis, anemia, and perturbations in the growth hormone insulin-like growth factor-1 (GH-IGF-1) axis lead to poor growth.

ETIOLOGY

- CAKUT constitute ~60% of cases of childhood CKD and include the following:
  - Renal dysplasia/hypoplasia
  - Obstructive uropathy (posterior urethral valves [PUV], prune belly syndrome)
- Cystic disorders
  - Autosomal recessive and dominant polycystic kidney disease
  - Juvenile nephronophthisis
- Hereditary metabolic disorders
  - Cystinosis
  - Oxalosis
- Glomerular diseases
  - Focal segmental glomerulosclerosis (FSGS)
  - Hemolytic uremic syndrome (HUS)
  - Systemic lupus erythematosus (SLE)
  - IgA nephropathy
  - Alport syndrome
  - Others—membranoproliferative glomerulonephritis (MPGN), membranous nephropathy, pauci-immune glomerulonephritis, congenital nephrotic syndrome

COMMONLY ASSOCIATED CONDITIONS

- Many genetic syndromes are associated with CAKUT including Alagille, Bardet-Biedl, Beckwith-Wiedemann, branchio-oto-renal, and Townes-Brocks syndromes.
- CAKUT also occurs with congenital malformation syndromes such as VACTERL association (vertebral defects, anal atresia, cardiac defects, tracheo-esophageal fistula, renal anomalies, and limb abnormalities), CHARGE syndrome (coloboma, heart defects, atresia choanae, retardation of growth, genital abnormalities, and ear abnormalities), and in patients with conditions causing neurogenic bladder such as spina bifida.

DIAGNOSIS

HISTORY

- Past history
  - Birth history for oligohydramnios, perinatal events
  - Recurrent urinary tract infections (UTIs)
  - Enuresis
  - Abnormal urinary stream (PUV)
- Family history
  - CKD, dialysis, kidney transplant
  - Kidney stones
  - Hearing impairment (Alport syndrome)
  - Kidney cysts
- Signs and symptoms
  - Poor growth
  - Poor appetite
  - Fatigue, malaise
  - Headache (if hypertensive)
  - Polyuria (in patients with CAKUT or tubular disorders)
  - Gross hematuria, edema, oliguria (in patients with glomerulonephritis)

PHYSICAL EXAM

- General
  - Short stature
  - Decreased weight for age
  - Pallor
  - Fetid breath
  - Elevated blood pressure (BP)
- Head, ears, eyes, nose, and throat
  - Retinal changes
  - Presence of preauricular pits/tags, branchial cysts (associated with CAKUT)
  - Hearing deficit (associated with CAKUT or Alport syndrome)
- Chest
  - Rales (if fluid overloaded)
- Heart
  - Flow murmur (if anemic)
  - Gallop
  - Pericardial rub
- Abdomen
  - Palpable kidneys (cystic kidney disease or obstruction)
  - Suprapubic mass (lower urinary tract obstruction)
- Extremities
  - Rachitic changes
  - Edema
- Neurologic system
  - Developmental delay
  - Altered mental status
  - Hypotonia
  - Irritability

DIFFERENTIAL DIAGNOSIS

Differentiate acute kidney injury from CKD

DIAGNOSTIC TESTS & INTERPRETATION

Initial Tests (screening, lab, imaging)

- Serum chemistries: azotemia, hyperkalemia, acidemia, hypocalcemia, hyperphosphatemia, elevated alkaline phosphatase
- CBC: normocytic anemia with low reticulocyte count (CKD stage 3, GFR <60)
- Urinalysis: isosthenuria in CAKUT or tubular disorders; proteinuria, hematuria with glomerular disease
- Intact parathyroid hormone: elevated
- 25-vitamin D: often low
- GFR measurement
  - Inulin clearance is the gold standard for GFR measurement but is not practical. A simple and commonly used method to estimate GFR in children >1 year of age with CKD is the CKiD bedside equation, an update to the traditional Schwartz formula.
  - The calculation is already corrected for surface area and does not require a urine collection: height (cm) × 0.413 correction factor/serum creatinine in mg/dL.
  - Cystatin C is another marker of kidney function which can be used to estimate GFR when creatinine may not be a reliable marker of kidney function (i.e., in patients with decreased muscle mass).
- Chest radiograph: pulmonary edema, cardiomegaly
- Bone radiographs: delayed bone age, rickets, osteomalacia, osteitis fibrosa
- Renal ultrasound: small echogenic kidneys, cystic kidneys, hydronephrosis, thickened bladder wall (PUV)
- VCUG: PUV, vesicoureteral reflux

Diagnostic Procedures/Other

A renal biopsy is indicated for diagnosis of acquired or glomerular kidney diseases such as FSGS. It is not necessary when there is radiologic evidence of CAKUT such as small or echogenic kidneys or urologic abnormalities.

TREATMENT

GENERAL MEASURES

- Avoid nephrotoxic medications including NSAIDs.
- Fluid restriction may be necessary in patients with glomerular disease.
- Monitor BP closely and initiate therapy for patients with hypertension.
- Evaluate nutritional status and provide supplemental nutrition if necessary.
- Dietary restriction of sodium, potassium, and phosphate may be necessary in progressive CKD.

MEDICATION

- Disease-specific therapies:
  - Some acquired causes of CKD such as FSGS and SLE may be treated with immunosuppressive medications.
  - ACE inhibitors may be used for renoprotection and reduction of proteinuria.
- Hypertension:
  - Anti-hypertensives including calcium channel blockers, ACE inhibitors, β-blockers, and others
  - Strict BP control is important as hypertension can contribute to CKD progression.
- Anemia:
  - Iron
  - Erythropoietin-stimulating agents
- Metabolic bone disease:
  - Phosphate binders (e.g., calcium carbonate, calcium acetate, sevelamer; avoid aluminum)
  - 25-hydroxy vitamin D and/or 1,25-dihydroxy vitamin D
- Acidosis: sodium bicarbonate/citrate
- Growth delay: recombinant human growth hormone
- Hyperlipidemia: statins

ISSUES FOR REFERRAL

Pediatric primary care physicians should observe patients with CKD in consultation and with assistance from a pediatric nephrologist.

ADDITIONAL THERAPIES

Renal replacement therapy (dialysis/kidney transplantation) is indicated when GFR is <10 mL/min/1.73 m^2 or when medical management fails to control signs/symptoms of CKD.

SURGERY/OTHER PROCEDURES

- Urologic: Patients with obstructive uropathies may require surgical interventions such as ablation of PUV, ureteral reimplantation, vesicostomy, and bladder augmentation.
- Nephrectomy may be indicated in patients on dialysis with severe hypertension.
- Transplantation: In some cases, a preemptive transplant may be offered instead of dialysis.
- Consider arteriovenous fistula or graft placement for patients who will require long-term hemodialysis.

COMPLEMENTARY & ALTERNATIVE THERAPIES

Treatment of hypertension, proteinuria (with ACE inhibitor/angiotensin receptor blockers), and dyslipidemia delays progression of CKD.

ADMISSION, INPATIENT, AND NURSING CONSIDERATIONS

- Patients with CKD may need to be admitted to the hospital in the setting of acute illnesses such as gastroenteritis in order to provide IV hydration and UTIs to provide IV antibiotics.
- As patients progress toward end-stage kidney disease, they may be admitted to the hospital for medical management of comorbidities and to initiate dialysis.
- Weights should be obtained daily, and all intake and output should be documented.
- BPs should be obtained with an appropriately sized cuff in the upper extremity.
- Avoid placing IV and checking BP in the nondominant arm of any patient with CKD when admitted to the hospital in order to preserve future vascular access for dialysis.
- When admitted to the hospital, patients with CKD may be on a restricted diet including sodium, potassium, and phosphate.
- When admitted to the hospital, avoid all nephrotoxic medications including NSAIDs, CT contrast, etc.

ALERT

During episodes of gastroenteritis, infants with CKD may be prone to dehydration because they have obligatory polyuria due to a concentrating defect. Do not use urine output level or specific gravity of urine as indices for hydration. If hospitalized, fluid levels considered "maintenance" may be insufficient due to polyuria.

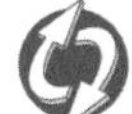

ONGOING CARE

FOLLOW-UP RECOMMENDATIONS

Patient Monitoring

Children with CKD need close outpatient follow-up every 1 to 3 months, depending on the level of GFR to monitor BP, growth, and lab tests.

DIET

Restrictions depend on the underlying condition but may include limitation of

- Phosphate
- Potassium
- Sodium (indicated if patient has edema/hypertension)
- Fluid (indicated in conditions related to oliguria)
- Infants with CKD may require a gastrostomy tube to provide adequate nutrition.

PROGNOSIS

Prognosis of CKD depends on the underlying cause. Patients with glomerular disease tend to progress faster than patients with nonglomerular diseases. Ultimately, CKD progression may lead to need for renal replacement therapy. Prognosis of children with renal transplantation is excellent with 5-year survival of >85%.

COMPLICATIONS

- Growth retardation is particularly severe when CKD develops in the first year of life. Growth failure may be secondary to poor nutrition, bone disease, acidosis, or a direct effect on the GH-IGF-1 axis.
- Mineral and bone disorders may be seen early in association with CKD, manifesting with growth failure, bowing of the lower extremities, and slipped epiphysis. Vitamin D deficiency and secondary hyperparathyroidism are the major factors leading to bone disease.
- Anemia develops secondary to decreased erythropoietin secretion and decreased erythrocyte survival. The anemia is a normocytic variant associated with a low reticulocyte count.
- Cardiovascular disease including left ventricular hypertrophy and coronary artery disease often develops in early adulthood. Uncontrolled hypertension, anemia, hyperlipidemia, and hyperparathyroidism all contribute to this leading cause of death in adults with CKD.
- Neurodevelopmental delay increases in children with CKD. This dely is probably due to uremic effects on the development of the brain.
- Hypertension may be seen in some patients with CKD due either to hyperreninemia or hypervolemia.
- Platelet abnormalities, protein-calorie malnutrition, and immunologic disturbances are also seen in patients with uremia.

ADDITIONAL READING

- Friedman AL. Etiology, pathophysiology, diagnosis, and management of chronic renal failure in children. *Curr Opin Pediatr*. 1996;8(2):148–151.
- Kidney Disease: Improving Global Outcomes CKD Work Group. KDIGO 2012 clinical practice guideline for the evaluation and management of chronic kidney disease. *Kidney Inter Suppl*. 2013;3:1–150.
- Schwartz GJ, Muñoz A, Schneider MF, et al. New equations to estimate GFR in children with CKD. *J Am Soc Nephrol*. 2009;20(3):629–637.
- Staples A, Wong C. Risk factors for progression of chronic kidney disease. *Curr Opin Pediatr*. 2010;22(2):161–169.
- Wong CJ, Moxey-Mims M, Jerry-Fluker J, et al. CKiD (CKD in children) prospective cohort study: a review of current findings. *Am J Kidney Dis*. 2012;60(6):1002–1011.

CODES

ICD10

- N18.9 Chronic kidney disease, unspecified
- Q63.9 Congenital malformation of kidney, unspecified
- N18.3 Chronic kidney disease, stage 3 (moderate)

FAQ

- Q: Which OTC medications should be avoided in children with CKD?
- A: NSAIDs, pseudoephedrine (if patient is hypertensive), enemas containing phosphate, and antacids containing magnesium or aluminum should not be taken.
- Q: Can children with CKD receive immunizations?
- A: Children with CKD should especially receive all necessary immunizations because some vaccines are contraindicated after transplantation. In some cases, booster immunizations are necessary because of an inadequate response to the initial series (e.g., hepatitis B virus, measles, mumps, rubella; varicella). Additionally, children with CKD should receive the polyvalent pneumococcal vaccine after age 2 years.
- Q: When is recombinant human erythropoietin indicated?
- A: Generally, this medication should be considered when the hematocrit level is <33% (Hgb <11.0 g/dL).
- Q: Can patients with CKD undergo MRI with gadolinium?
- A: There is a risk of nephrogenic systemic fibrosis, a condition characterized by diffuse hardening and thickening of the skin, when gadolinium is administered to patients with severe CKD. Consultation with a pediatric nephrologist is recommended before gadolinium is administered to a patient with CKD.

CIRRHOSIS

Rima Fawaz, MD

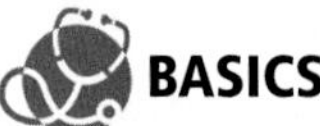

BASICS

DESCRIPTION

- Cirrhosis is the end stage of progressive hepatic necrosis, fibrosis, and regenerative nodule formation that may occur as a result of many different liver diseases.
- Results in distortion of liver architecture and compression of hepatic vascular and biliary structures
- Cirrhosis is clinically defined by outcomes as either compensated or decompensated:
  - Compensated cirrhosis: typically asymptomatic with normal synthetic function
  - Decompensated cirrhosis: defined as loss of normal synthetic function, development of jaundice, and/or the clinical complications of portal hypertension such as ascites, variceal hemorrhage, spontaneous bacterial peritonitis, hepatic encephalopathy, hepatorenal syndrome, hepatopulmonary syndrome, and portopulmonary hypertension
- In its decompensated form/advanced form, cirrhosis is irreversible and often requires liver transplantation for survival of the patient.

EPIDEMIOLOGY

- There are varying causes of cirrhosis; accordingly, no specific epidemiologic pattern can be identified.
- Cirrhosis due to chronic hepatitis C virus (HCV) infection, alcoholic liver disease, and nonalcoholic fatty liver disease (NAFLD) are the most common indications for liver transplantation in adults.
- Biliary cirrhosis due to biliary atresia is the most common indication for liver transplantation in children.

RISK FACTORS

Genetics

- Many distinct genetic disorders can cause cirrhosis, such as Wilson disease and hereditary hemochromatosis.
- Human leukocyte antigen (HLA) associations have been identified in several autoimmune disorders, including sclerosing cholangitis and autoimmune hepatitis.

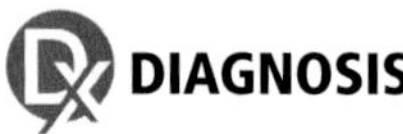

DIAGNOSIS

HISTORY

Based on the varying etiologies, one should elicit pertinent historical features characteristic of specific problems:

- Exposure to infectious hepatitis, antecedent viral illnesses
- Exposure to drugs/hepatotoxins
- Family or personal history of genetic, metabolic, or autoimmune diseases
- Neurologic problems, deteriorating school performance, sleep disturbances, depression (Wilson disease)

PHYSICAL EXAM

- General:
  - Poor growth, malnutrition, cachexia
  - Obesity (NAFLD)
  - Cyanosis
  - Fever
- Eyes:
  - Scleral icterus
  - Kayser-Fleischer rings (Wilson disease)
- Skin:
  - Jaundice, flushing, pallor, cyanosis
  - Palmar erythema
  - Spider angiomata, fine telangiectasia (face and upper back)
  - Easy bruising
- Abdomen:
  - Ascites (distention, fluid wave, shifting dullness); see "Ascites" chapter.
  - Caput medusa (prominent periumbilical veins)
  - Splenomegaly
  - Hepatomegaly or a shrunken liver
- Extremities:
  - Digital clubbing
  - White nails due to decreased vascularity of the nail bed (Terry nails)
  - Hypertrophic osteoarthropathy
  - Muscle wasting
  - Peripheral edema
- Endocrine:
  - Gynecomastia
  - Testicular atrophy
  - Delayed puberty/maturation
- Central nervous system:
  - Asterixis
  - Positive Babinski sign
  - Mental status changes
  - Hyperreflexia

DIFFERENTIAL DIAGNOSIS

- Biliary
  - Extrahepatic biliary atresia
  - Choledochal cyst
  - Tumors
  - Common bile duct and biliary lithiasis
  - Alagille syndrome
  - Biliary hypoplasia
  - Sclerosing cholangitis
  - Graft-versus-host disease
  - Vanishing bile duct syndrome due to drugs (e.g., trimethoprim–sulfamethoxazole)
  - Langerhans cell histiocytosis
- Hepatic
  - Infectious hepatitis, including viral hepatitis B, C, D, other viruses
  - Autoimmune hepatitis
  - Nonalcoholic steatohepatitis (NASH)
  - Drugs/toxins and alcohol
- Genetic/metabolic (examples for each category, not a complete list)
  - Cystic fibrosis
  - α_1-Antitrypsin deficiency
  - Congenital hepatic fibrosis
  - Progressive familial intrahepatic cholestasis (PFIC)
  - Wilson disease
  - Hereditary hemochromatosis
  - Carbohydrate defects: galactosemia, hereditary fructose intolerance, glycogen storage III and IV
  - Amino acid defects: tyrosinemia
  - Lipid storage diseases: Gaucher disease, Niemann-Pick type C
  - Mitochondrial disorders: fatty acid oxidation defects, respiratory chain defects
  - Peroxisomal disorders: Zellweger syndrome
  - Porphyrias: erythropoietic protoporphyria
- Vascular
  - Budd-Chiari syndrome
  - Venoocclusive disease
  - Congestive heart failure

DIAGNOSTIC TESTS & INTERPRETATION

Initial Tests (screening, lab, imaging)

Can be useful in determining the etiology and the severity of liver disease prior to a liver biopsy

- Tests of liver cell injury:
  - Alanine aminotransferase (ALT) more liver specific
  - Aspartate aminotransferase (AST)
- Tests of synthetic function:
  - Albumin
  - Prothrombin time (PT), international normalized ratio (INR)
  - Clotting factors (VII shortest half-life)
  - Ammonia
- Tests of cholestasis:
  - Fractionated bilirubin
  - Alkaline phosphatase
  - γ-Glutamyltransferase
  - Cholesterol
  - Serum bile acids
- Tests of fibrosis: serum markers to evaluate hepatic fibrosis (not used routinely in clinical practice)
- α-Fetoprotein (AFP)
- Miscellaneous disease-specific serum tests:
  - Viral serologies: hepatitis B, hepatitis C, other viruses
  - Wilson disease: serum ceruloplasmin, 24-hour urine copper, and slit-lamp exam for Kayser-Fleischer rings
  - α_1-Antitrypsin deficiency: α_1-antitrypsin serum level and protease inhibitor (Pi) phenotype
  - Autoimmune hepatitis: autoantibodies (antinuclear, anti–smooth muscle, anti-liver/kidney microsomal, anti–F-actin), serum immunoglobulins
  - Hemochromatosis: serum iron, total iron binding capacity, ferritin
  - Metabolic/genetic: fasting blood sugar, lactate, pyruvate, ammonia, uric acid, sweat test, carnitine, creatine phosphokinase (CPK), porphyrins, serum amino acids, urine organic acids, urine reducing substances, urine succinylacetone, fatty acid degeneration products
- Ultrasound with Doppler images:
  - Evaluate for anatomy of the liver and biliary tree and vessels, presence of ascites, signs of portal hypertension such as splenomegaly, varices, flow in portal vein, hepatic artery, and hepatic veins.

- Hepatobiliary radioisotope scanning:
  - Assess biliary patency in neonatal cholestasis.
- Cholangiography (magnetic resonance cholangiopancreatography [MRCP]):
  - Assess for intra- and extrahepatic biliary disease (stones, choledochal cyst, sclerosing cholangitis).
- Angiography:
  - CT or magnetic resonance angiography to evaluate for vascular anatomy and portosystemic shunts
- Noninvasive assessment of liver fibrosis: CT, MRI, elastography (by ultrasound or MRI)

Diagnostic Procedures/Other

- Liver biopsy
  - Percutaneous needle biopsy, intraoperative wedge biopsy, transjugular liver biopsy
  - Confirms the presence (stage), activity (grade), and type of cirrhosis
  - Various hepatic diseases that progress to cirrhosis have characteristic histologic findings. However, the process of cirrhosis may obscure the nature of the original insult, rendering morphologic and histologic classifications unhelpful.
- Hepatic venous pressure gradient (HVPG)
  - Rarely used in children but the most accurate prognostic indicator of outcome in adults with cirrhosis
  - HVPG >10 mm Hg is classified as clinically significant portal hypertension beyond which complications of portal hypertension are found.
- Cholangiography
  - Intraoperative cholangiography: assesses for extrahepatic biliary atresia in neonates
  - Endoscopic retrograde cholangiopancreatography (ERCP): assesses for extrahepatic biliary disease in older patients where MRCP is not helpful or therapeutic interventions possible (i.e., stent placement)

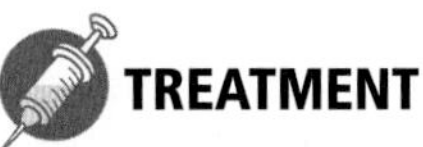

TREATMENT

GENERAL MEASURES

If significant splenomegaly, prescribe spleen guard and avoidance of contact sports/activities, which could increase risk abdominal trauma.

MEDICATION

First Line

- Fat-soluble vitamin supplementation (vitamins A, D, E, and K) in patients with cholestasis (direct bilirubin >1 mg/dL)
- Diuretic therapy (furosemide, spironolactone) for patients with ascites
- Albumin infusions for patients with refractory ascites and albumin <2.5 g/dL
- β-Blockers have been shown in adults to reduce the risk of variceal bleeding in patients with small varices and decompensated cirrhosis, or with medium to large esophageal varices.
- Antibiotics should be used in patients with suspected variceal bleeding, cholangitis, and/or spontaneous bacterial peritonitis; may improve mortality
- Avoid use of nephrotoxic agents, including nephrotoxic antibiotics.
- Lactulose and rifaximin may be helpful for patients with hepatic encephalopathy.

SURGERY/OTHER PROCEDURES

- Endoscopic variceal band ligation or sclerotherapy for variceal GI bleeding
- Paracentesis for diagnosis of spontaneous bacterial peritonitis, refractory ascites, and ascites compromising respiratory status
- Portosystemic shunt placement (surgical or radiologic transjugular intrahepatic portosystemic shunt [TIPS] procedure) for complications of uncontrolled portal hypertension
- Liver transplantation

ONGOING CARE

DIET

- Malnutrition is common in chronic liver diseases because of several metabolic derangements, as well as fat malabsorption, anorexia, and increased energy requirements.
- Adequate caloric intake is critical and, often, will require supplemental nasogastric tube feedings.
- Some dietary fat should be provided as medium-chain triglycerides, which do not require bile for absorption.
- Fat-soluble vitamin levels should be monitored and supplemented, if necessary.
- Careful attention must also be paid to fluid and electrolyte balance; sodium restriction (<2 mEq/kg/24 h) may be necessary in the presence of ascites.

PROGNOSIS

- The prognosis for cirrhosis leading to decompensation depends on the underlying cause.
- The underlying condition should be treated when possible (e.g., Wilson disease, autoimmune hepatitis, hepatitis C).
- Poor prognostic features in children include prolonged INR unresponsive to vitamin K, ascites, malnutrition, hyponatremia <130 mEq/L, low plasma cholesterol, elevated bilirubin level, and presence of hepatorenal syndrome.

COMPLICATIONS

- Malnutrition and growth failure
- Malabsorption (diarrhea, steatorrhea, fat-soluble vitamin deficiencies)
- Portal hypertension and variceal bleeding
- Chronic gastritis, peptic ulcer disease, gastroesophageal reflux
- Ascites
- Encephalopathy
- Hypersplenism (associated with anemia, thrombocytopenia, and neutropenia)
- Anemia
- Coagulopathy
- Hepatopulmonary syndrome (hypoxemia, cyanosis, dyspnea, digital clubbing)
- Hepatorenal syndrome (rapidly progressive renal failure in patients with cirrhosis)
- Bacterial infections, spontaneous bacterial peritonitis
- Hepatocellular carcinoma

ADDITIONAL READING

- Albillos A, Garcia-Tsao G. Classification of cirrhosis: the clinical use of HVPG measurements. *Dis Markers*. 2011;31(3):121–128.
- Feldstein AE, Charatcharoenwitthaya P, Treeprasertsuk S, et al. The natural history of non-alcoholic fatty liver disease in children: a follow-up study for up to 20 years. *Gut*. 2009;58(11): 1538–1544.
- Goyal NP, Schwimmer JB. The progression and natural history of pediatric nonalcoholic fatty liver disease. *Clin Liver Dis*. 2016;20(2):325–338.
- Kohli R, Cortes M, Heaton ND, et al. Liver transplantation in children: state of the art and future perspectives. *Arch Dis Child*. 2018;103(2):192–198.
- Leonis MA, Balistreri WF. Evaluation and management of end-stage liver disease in children. *Gastroenterology*. 2008;134(6):1741–1751.
- Mouzaki M, Ng V, Kamath BM, et al. Enteral energy and macronutrients in end-stage liver disease. *JPEN J Parenter Enteral Nutr*. 2014;38(6):673–681.
- Pinto RB, Schneider AC, da Silveira TR. Cirrhosis in children and adolescents: an overview. *World J Hepatol*. 2015;7(3):392–405.

CODES

ICD10

- K74.60 Unspecified cirrhosis of liver
- K74.5 Biliary cirrhosis, unspecified
- Q44.2 Atresia of bile ducts

FAQ

- Q: Will my child with cystic fibrosis develop cirrhosis?
- A: The medical literature suggests a 5–10% incidence of cirrhosis in children with cystic fibrosis. Children with cystic fibrosis liver disease who develop cirrhosis are at risk for complications of portal hypertension.
- Q: Will every child with cirrhosis need a liver transplant?
- A: If cause of cirrhosis cannot be treated, most children who develop cirrhosis will ultimately require a liver transplant.

CLEFT LIP AND PALATE

Oksana A. Jackson, MD • Jesse A. Taylor, MD, FACS

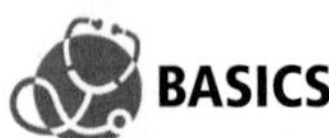

BASICS

DESCRIPTION
- Cleft lip
  - Deformity of the upper lip that may include a discontinuity of vermilion, skin, muscle, and mucosa as well as the underlying gingiva and bone
  - May be unilateral or bilateral
  - A complete cleft extends into the nose. An incomplete cleft has a bridge of intact tissue between the oral and nasal cavities.
- Cleft palate
  - May involve the gingiva, hard palate, and/or soft palate
  - Represents a visible separation between the two halves of the roof of the mouth, involving mucosa, muscle, and often the bones of the hard palate
  - A submucous cleft palate has intact mucosa, but the underlying muscle and bone are at least partially divided.

EPIDEMIOLOGY
- Incidence of cleft lip with or without cleft palate is approximately 1 in 700 births.
- Isolated cleft palate is present in 1 in 2,000 births across races.
- Racial heterogeneity noted in cleft lip and palate (Asians, 2.1 in 1,000 births; Caucasians, 1 in 1,000; African-Americans, 0.41 in 1,000)
- Gender heterogeneity noted in Caucasians (male-to-female ratio: cleft lip with or without cleft palate, 1.5 to 2:1; cleft palate only, 0.7:1)

RISK FACTORS
- Incidence of cleft lip with or without cleft palate increases with parental (especially paternal) age >30 years. Some association with low socioeconomic class may be nutrition-related.
- Some recognized patterns of malformation that include cleft lip and/or cleft palate may be caused by exposure to teratogens, but there is little evidence linking isolated clefts to exposure to any single teratogenic agent.
  - Exceptions include phenytoin (use during pregnancy has been associated with a 10-fold increase in the incidence of cleft lip) and isotretinoin (~26 relative risk of congenital malformations including cleft palate).
- Incidence of cleft lip in infants born to mothers who smoke during pregnancy is twice that in those born to nonsmoking mothers.

Genetics
- 1/3 of patients with cleft lip and/or cleft palate have a positive family history; positive family history is noted twice as often in cleft lip with or without cleft palate compared to cleft palate alone.
- The recurrence risk for cleft lip with or without cleft palate is 4% if one 1st-degree relative is affected and 9% if two are affected.

PATHOPHYSIOLOGY
- Muscle fibers are atrophic and disorganized in the region of the cleft.
- Mitochondrial abnormalities are noted at the cleft margins by histochemical and electromyographic studies.

ETIOLOGY
- Cleft lip may result from failure of the medial nasal and maxillary processes to join in utero or possibly from lack of adequate mesenchymal reinforcement, leading to subsequent breakdown and separation.
- Cleft palate results from failure of the palatal shelves to fuse.
- Prenatal dietary supplementation with folic acid and vitamin B_6 has led to lower-than-expected incidence of cleft lip and cleft palate and to a decreased incidence of neural tube defects.
- Bilateral cleft lip is associated with cleft palate in 86% of cases. Unilateral cleft lip is associated with cleft palate in 68% of cases.
- Cleft lip/cleft palate is more common on the left, particularly in boys.

COMMONLY ASSOCIATED CONDITIONS
- Most clefts are nonsyndromic and may be either multifactorial in origin or the result of changes at a major single-gene locus.
- >400 genetic syndromes are associated with facial clefts.
- Among patients with clefts of the secondary palate alone, syndromes associated with microdeletions of chromosome 22q11.2 are currently the most common syndromic diagnoses.
  - Collectively known as 22q11.2 deletion syndrome, includes velocardiofacial syndrome, DiGeorge syndrome, and conotruncal anomaly face syndrome
  - Inheritance is autosomal dominant with considerable variability in phenotypic expression, which may include facial dysmorphism, developmental delay, cardiovascular anomalies, immunologic abnormalities, cleft palate, and velopharyngeal dysfunction.
- Next most common syndrome associated with palatal clefts is Stickler syndrome:
  - Characterized by autosomal dominance, cleft palate, epicanthal folds, flat facies, joint hyperflexibility, severe myopia, retinal detachment, and glaucoma
  - Caused by a mutation of the gene for type 2 collagen (chromosome 12q)
- Most common syndrome associated with clefts of the lip and/or palate is van der Woude syndrome (autosomal dominant, lower lip pits, IRF6 mutations, 1q32).
- Other genetic syndromes associated with cleft lip and/or palate:
  - CHARGE (coloboma of the eye, heart defects, atresia of the choanae, retardation of growth and/or development, genital and/or urinary abnormalities, and ear abnormalities and deafness) syndrome has an autosomal dominant pattern of malformation with majority of patients having CHD7 microdeletion or mutation.
  - Ectrodactyly–ectodermal dysplasia–cleft (EEC) syndrome is associated with p63 gene mutations.
  - Smith-Lemli-Opitz (defect in cholesterol synthesis, *DHCR7* gene mutation, 7q34)
  - Pierre Robin sequence is a condition usually associated with a wide U-shaped cleft palate.
    - Characterized by a small mandible, retropositioned tongue, and subsequent upper airway obstruction
    - May occur in infants with or without genetic syndromes (Stickler most common)

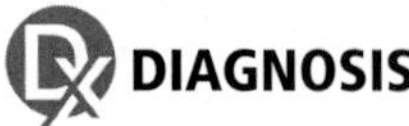

DIAGNOSIS

HISTORY
- Prenatal exposure to alcohol, cigarettes, phenytoin, and isotretinoin
- Family history of cleft lip or cleft palate
- Speech problems in 1st-degree relative

PHYSICAL EXAM
- Incomplete or complete cleft of lip, alveolus, hard and soft palate, or uvula. Soft palate and uvula clefts are always midline, whereas lip, alveolar, and hard palatal clefts can be unilateral or bilateral.
- A bifid uvula or a notch in the bone at the posterior hard palate may indicate a submucous cleft.
- A small mandible and retropositioned tongue may indicate a risk for airway obstruction (Pierre Robin sequence).
- Look for associated anomalies of the face, heart, and extremities that may indicate a clefting syndrome.
- Examination tips
  - Examine the palate from the top of the patient, with the head in your lap, using a tongue depressor and flashlight.
  - Palpate the posterior hard palate for a possible notch in the bone.
  - Palpate the gums and maxilla for a possible notch in the floor of the nose.

DIAGNOSTIC TESTS & INTERPRETATION
- Hearing evaluation
- Complete ophthalmologic examination to check for myopia, glaucoma, and retinal detachment and rule out Stickler syndrome
- Pulse oximetry to check for desaturation while feeding or while supine
- Polysomnography to distinguish central from obstructive apnea; increased serum 7-dehydrocholesterol and decreased serum cholesterol to rule out Smith-Lemli-Opitz syndrome
- Karyotype to rule out specific genetic abnormalities
- Fluorescence in situ hybridization to rule out a chromosome 22q11.2 deletion
- Echocardiography, renal ultrasound, and endocrine laboratory studies if indicated
- Prenatal diagnosis of cleft lip is reliable by ultrasound; prenatal diagnosis of cleft palate remains unreliable by ultrasound. 3D ultrasound has improved the reliability of prenatal diagnosis.
- Fetal MRI provides excellent soft tissue definition and can be used when the diagnosis is uncertain on ultrasound or to better delineate the severity of the cleft.
- After birth, no additional radiologic imaging is indicated in patients with isolated cleft lip and/or palate.

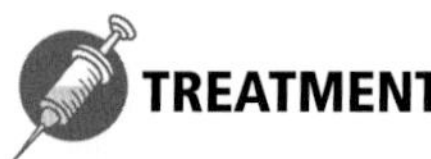

TREATMENT

GENERAL MEASURES
- Airway management
  - Prone positioning if the tongue is causing airway obstruction
  - Plastic surgery and ENT consultation if airway obstruction persists

- Orthodontics
  - Preoperative orthodontics may include obturators to facilitate feeding and speech; nasoalveolar molding and lip taping to narrow the cleft and reshape the nose before lip repair; palatal expansion prior to bone grafting; conventional orthodontics including braces, maxillary appliances, prosthetic teeth, bridgework; and maxillary and/or mandibular distraction to advance the mid- or lower face.

SURGERY/OTHER PROCEDURES

- Significant airway obstruction and desaturation in the neonatal period refractory to prone positioning may indicate the need for a tongue–lip adhesion, release of the floor of the mouth musculature, mandibular distraction, or tracheostomy.
- Wide clefts of the lip may benefit from either nasoalveolar molding or preliminary lip adhesion at 2 to 3 months of age. Timing of definitive lip repair varies from 2 to 6 months of age.
- Palate repair is generally done at <1 year of age to decrease speech and language difficulties.
- Otitis media is more common with cleft palate, and bilateral myringotomy tubes can be inserted at the time of cleft repair.
- Correction of secondary deformities may include the following:
  - Lip scar revision
  - Cleft nasal deformity correction (infancy to adulthood)
  - Alveolar bone grafts (usually when permanent canines are erupting, age 6 to 10 years)
  - Pharyngoplasty for soft palate–velopharyngeal incompetence (childhood to adolescence)
  - Closure of palatal fistulas
  - Orthognathic surgery for severe jaw deformities (after facial growth is complete)

ADMISSION, INPATIENT, AND NURSING CONSIDERATIONS

- Admission criteria
  - Airway obstruction or severe feeding difficulties in the neonate
- Discharge criteria
  - Stable airway
  - Tolerating feedings
  - Pain controlled on an oral regimen

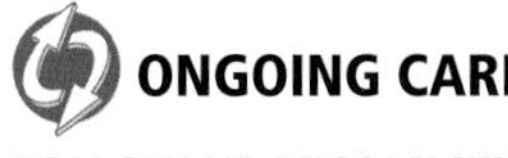

ONGOING CARE

FOLLOW-UP RECOMMENDATIONS

Multidisciplinary team for routine visits from infancy to adolescence:

- Pediatrician
- Plastic surgeon
- Speech pathologist
- Orthodontist
- Pediatric dentist
- Otolaryngologist
- Oral surgeon
- Psychologist
- Social worker
- Anthropologist (facial growth specialist)
- Geneticist
- Support groups

DIET

- Cleft patients may have significant feeding problems because of an inability to generate negative intraoral pressure necessary to feed efficiently.
- Preemie nipples with enlarged or cross-cut openings, or soft plastic squeezable bottles, can facilitate milk flow.
- Specially designed cleft bottles are commercially available.
- Poor weight gain may necessitate nasogastric tube feedings.

PROGNOSIS

Very good. Most patients undergo normal growth and development. Long-term follow-up by a multidisciplinary team and parental support are critical for optimal outcomes.

COMPLICATIONS

- Airway obstruction and feeding disorders, particularly with Pierre Robin sequence
- Chronic otitis media
- Speech problems, including hypernasality and articulation errors
- Associated malformations
  - ~1/3 of patients with cleft palate has associated anomalies, with isolated cleft palates having the highest. CNS, cardiac and urinary tract malformations, and clubfoot are commonly associated with clefting.
- Potential problems
  - Hypernasal resonance and nasal air emission during speech may indicate velopharyngeal incompetence or palatal fistula. 8–30% of patients may require additional palatal or pharyngeal surgery following initial palate repair.
  - Multiple ear infections may require prolonged use of myringotomy tubes to prevent hearing impairment. Audiograms should be obtained regularly.
  - Delays in speech and language development may require detailed evaluation, early intervention programs, and speech therapy.
  - Poor dentition, occlusal problems (crossbite), gingivitis, and crowding
  - Learning disabilities are increased in children with clefts.
  - Behavior disorders and psychosocial adjustment disorders
  - ~25% of affected individuals will manifest maxillary hypoplasia that requires jaw surgery to correct occlusal abnormalities.

ALERT

- Failure to diagnose airway obstruction in infants with Pierre Robin sequence may lead to failure to thrive or, in severe cases, death.
- Failure to diagnose associated anomalies may lead to missed syndromes and inaccurate genetic counseling.
- A submucous cleft palate can be easily missed until hypernasal speech is noted later in life.

ADDITIONAL READING

- Fisher DM, Sommerlad BC. Cleft lip, cleft palate, and velopharyngeal insufficiency. *Plast Reconstr Surg.* 2011;128(4):342e–360e.
- Heinrich A, Proff P, Michel T, et al. Prenatal diagnostics of cleft deformities and its significance for parent and infant care. *J Craniomaxillofac Surg.* 2006;34 (Suppl 2):14–16.
- Mulliken JB, Wu JK, Padwa BL. Repair of bilateral cleft lip: review, revisions, and reflections. *J Craniofac Surg.* 2003;14(5):609–620.
- Murray JC. Gene/environment causes of cleft lip and/or palate. *Clin Genet.* 2002;61(4):248–256.
- Nasser M, Fedorowicz Z, Newton JT, et al. Interventions for the management of submucous cleft palate. *Cochrane Database Syst Rev.* 2008;(1):CD006703.
- Redford-Badwal DA, Mabry K, Frassinelli JD. Impact of cleft lip and/or palate on nutritional health and oral-motor development. *Dent Clin North Am.* 2003;47(2):305–317.
- Strong EB, Buckmiller LM. Management of the cleft palate. *Facial Plast Surg Clin North Am.* 2001;9(1):15–25.

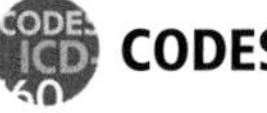

CODES

ICD10

- Q37.9 Unspecified cleft palate with unilateral cleft lip
- Q36.9 Cleft lip, unilateral
- Q35.9 Cleft palate, unspecified

FAQ

- Q: Will there be a scar?
- A: All cleft lip repairs will leave some type of permanent scar, with potential asymmetry that may benefit from later additional lip scar revision or additional nasal surgery.
- Q: What is the goal of surgery?
- A: Goal is to create a lip that does not attract undue attention.
- Q: What is the most difficult part of surgery?
- A: The nose is often the most difficult to correct because of asymmetry in cartilage and skin contour.
- Q: Will my child be able to speak clearly?
- A: Most children will achieve velopharyngeal competence and normal speech but may require additional speech therapy to achieve this goal.
- Q: Is cleft palate inherited?
- A: Cleft palate is inherited in two ways:
  - For nonsyndromic cleft lip with or without cleft palate:
    - Risk of having a second child with a cleft, if neither parent has a cleft: 4%
    - Child's risk of later having a child with a cleft: 4%
    - Risk of having a third child with a cleft, if parents have two affected children but neither parent is affected: 9%
    - Risk of having a second child with a cleft, if one parent also has a cleft: 17%
  - For nonsyndromic isolated cleft palate:
    - Risk of having a second child with a cleft, if neither parent has a cleft: 2%
    - Child's risk of later having a child with a cleft: 3%
    - Risk of having a third child with a cleft, if parents have two affected children but neither parent is affected: 1%
    - Risk of having a second child with a cleft, if one parent also has a cleft: 15%

C

CLUBFOOT

Tyler W. Christman, DO, MS • Shyam Kishan, MD

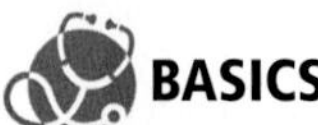

BASICS

DESCRIPTION

- Clubfoot (talipes equinovarus) is a complex foot deformity consisting of four components:
  - Equinus (plantar flexion)
  - Hindfoot varus (toward the midline)
  - Forefoot adductus
  - Midfoot cavus (high arch with overextension)
- Untreated clubfoot can prevent the development of normal gait and result in secondary bone changes leading to lifetime disability.

EPIDEMIOLOGY

- Familial occurrence in 25%
- Male > female (2.5:1)
- 50% of cases are bilateral.
- Clubfoot is the most common congenital deformity of the lower extremity.
- 1 to 2:1,000 births in United States
- Lowest prevalence in Chinese, 0.39:1,000
- Highest prevalence in Polynesians, 7:1,000

PATHOPHYSIOLOGY

- Both intrinsic and extrinsic causes have been associated with the development of clubfoot.
- Intrinsic causes:
  - Neurogenic (spina bifida)
  - Muscular (anomalous or atrophic musculature)
  - Vascular (hypoplastic anterior tibial artery)
  - Connective tissue diseases (arthrogryposis, Loeys-Dietz syndrome)
  - Abnormal primary bone formation
  - Interruption of the transcriptional pathway PITX1-TBX4 which is critical to early limb development has been linked to development of clubfoot and similar deformities.
- Extrinsic causes:
  - Intrauterine immobility (multiple gestations, malpresentation, uterine abnormalities, oligohydramnios)
  - Maternal cigarette smoke exposure

ETIOLOGY

- Most cases (80%) are idiopathic (multifactorial with genetic and environmental influences).
- Remaining cases likely associated with associated structural, genetic, and/or chromosomal anomalies
- Rapid recurrence of deformity should prompt a thorough examination for possible underlying neuromuscular etiologies.

DIAGNOSIS

Prenatal diagnosis

- Obstetric ultrasound improvements have led to a significant increase in the prenatal diagnosis of clubfoot.
- The 16- to 20-week ultrasound often shows the classical features (plantar surface of fetal foot in same sagittal plane as both lower extremity bones) of a clubfoot, allowing for early prenatal counseling which can be helpful for easing parental anxiety.
- False positive for bilateral clubfoot is 7% and up to 40% in unilateral clubfoot.
- Deformity severity is difficult to predict prenatally.

HISTORY

- Family history of clubfoot
- Birth history and environmental factors
- Onset of deformity (congenital or developmental)

PHYSICAL EXAM

- Careful examination of
  - The neuromuscular system for spasticity, asymmetry, muscle imbalance/atrophy, lumbosacral sinuses/dimples, and lipomas
  - The hips for hip dysplasia
  - The neck for torticollis
- Physical exam of foot
  - Passively, move the foot into corrected position. Is the deformity ridged? Fully correctable? Over correctable?
  - Ridged clubfeet or "complex idiopathic clubfoot" demonstrates rigid equinus (limited upward bending), midfoot (metatarsal) plantarflexion, a deep heel crease at the posterior ankle, a transverse midsole or midfoot crease, and a short hyperextended hallux.
  - Complex idiopathic clubfoot accounts for approximately 1 in 15 cases and is more difficult to treat.

DIFFERENTIAL DIAGNOSIS

Distinguish other deformities of the foot:

- Metatarsus adductus (medial deviation of forefoot, heel remains in normal position)
- Calcaneovalgus (excessively dorsiflexed hindfoot, hindfoot valgus)
- Vertical talus (hindfoot equinovalgus, midfoot dorsiflexion, forefoot abduction and dorsiflexion)
- Many children with clubfoot also have tibial torsion, which is a normal variant that rarely requires treatment.

DIAGNOSTIC TESTS & INTERPRETATION

Initial Tests (screening, lab, imaging)

- The diagnosis is established clinically.
- Radiographs may confirm bone position but are typically not needed for initial diagnosis.
- Anteroposterior and dorsiflexion lateral (Turco view) radiograph films (after 3 months of age) may help in defining residual deformity.
- Decreased talocalcaneal angle on the anteroposterior (<20 degrees) and dorsiflexion lateral views (<35 degrees)
- Medial displacement of the navicular and cuboid on the calcaneus and persistent plantar flexion of the forefoot on the hindfoot (negative talus-1st metatarsal angle) indicate more complex deformities.

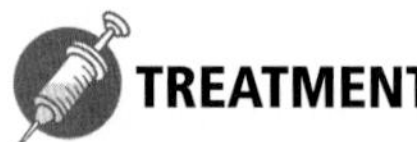

TREATMENT

The goal of treatment is to have a pain-free, plantigrade foot, without calluses, that demonstrates good mobility and functions well without the need for modified shoes.

GENERAL MEASURES

- The Ponseti method (casting and bracing) as and its variations have become the standard of initial treatment.
- Initial treatment:
  - Care may begin in the 1st week after birth, although new studies suggest initiating treatment after the 1st month may be preferred as the foot is larger and more easily manipulated, with less risk for cast slippage.
  - Treatment begins with weekly serial manipulation of the foot and casting with long leg casts (short leg casts poorly control rotation and result in higher failure rates [37.5%] with significantly longer treatment times).

- Serial casting systematically corrects deformity; first, correcting the cavus deformity, then gradually, with subsequent cast applications correcting forefoot adductus and hindfoot varus
- During casting, the talar head is stabilized with the physician's thumb while the contralateral hand slightly supinates and abducts the foot in a plantigrade fashion.
- Lateral pressure on the calcaneus should be avoided. The foot should never be placed in a pronated position.
- Percutaneous Achilles tenotomy is recommended to correct residual equinus contracture in approximately 80% of cases.
- Following tenotomy, the operated foot is stabilized for 3 to 4 weeks in a Ponseti-type cast to allow for tendon healing.
- Bracing is an integral part of the Ponseti method with recommendation for Denis Browne (DB) bar and shoes bracing to be worn full time for 3 months following final casting and continued nightly and during naps until the child is age 3 to 4 years.

• With the Ponseti method, 11–48% of patients may have various forms of recurrence requiring repeated casting and/or surgical release (3–29%).
• Treatment of complex idiopathic clubfoot may require up to five additional casts to abduct the forefoot at the midfoot. Recurrence of deformity is more common in this type.

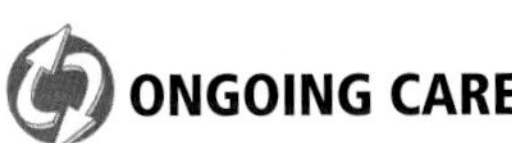

ONGOING CARE

FOLLOW-UP RECOMMENDATIONS

Patient Monitoring

• Deformity recurrence is more common during periods of rapid growth and can be significantly reduced through strict adherence to bracing with DB bar and shoes.
• Initial treatments for recurrence are heel cord stretching and repeat casting.
• Persistent deformity in children >2.5 years of age may show improvement with anterior tibial tendon transfer (ATTT) to the lateral cuneiform or require posterior medial release and tendon lengthening.
• The risk of relapse following ATTT is 15.2%
• Refractory clubfoot may require triple arthrodesis (joint fusion) during early adolescence.
• Further careful evaluation is warranted in patients with refractory clubfoot to identify neuromuscular or syndromic causes that might have been undiagnosed as an infant.
• Infants with clubfoot will likely begin walking later than typically expected; however, walking will likely occur by 15 to 18 months.
• Depending on the severity of the deformity, all corrected clubfeet can be expected to demonstrate various amounts of generalized hypoplasia of the affected limb, weakness, ankle and subtalar stiffness, shoe size discrepancy, and leg length discrepancy, usually <2 cm.
• Athletic performance of school-age children is not significantly impaired following satisfactory treatment of clubfoot.

ADDITIONAL READING

• Dobbs M, Rudzki JR, Purcell D, et al. Factors predictive of outcome after use of the Ponseti method for the treatment of idiopathic clubfeet. *J Bone Joint Surg Am*. 2004;86-A(1):22–27.
• Changulani M, Garg NK, Rajagopal TS, et al. Treatment of idiopathic club foot using the Ponseti method. Initial experience. *J Bone Joint Surg Br*. 2006;88(10):1385–1387.
• Hamel J, Becker W. Sonographic assessment of clubfoot deformity in young children. *J Pediatr Orthop B*. 1996;5(4):279–286.
• Kenmoku T, Kamegaya M, Saisu T, et al. Athletic ability of school-age children after satisfactory treatment of congenital clubfoot. *J Pediatr Orthop*. 2013;33(3):321–325.
• Ponseti IV, Zhivkov M, Davis N, et al. Treatment of the complex idiopathic clubfoot. *Clin Orthop Relat Res*. 2006;451:171–176.

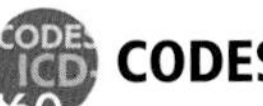

CODES

ICD10

• Q66.89 Other specified congenital deformities of feet
• Q66.7 Congenital pes cavus
• Q66.0 Congenital talipes equinovarus

FAQ

• Q: What percentage of clubfoot is successfully treated by casting?
• A: At least 94% of patients with idiopathic clubfoot treated with serial casting and manipulation achieve good initial correction. Rigid or complex clubfeet are more difficult to treat and less likely to be fully corrected by casting and heel cord tenotomy alone.
• Q: What will be the permanent disability of a congenital clubfoot deformity?
• A: Although casting and surgical correction of a congenital clubfoot can realign the foot, this does not address underlying neuromuscular problems. As a result, all children with clubfeet are likely to have a leg length discrepancy (usually <1.5 inches), a smaller foot (mean 1.3 cm shorter and 0.4 cm narrower than normal foot), calf circumference narrowing (mean 2.3 cm) that cannot be significantly improved with exercise, and some degree of joint stiffness (ankle, subtalar, and midfoot). Recent studies report no significant impairment in the athletic performance of school-age children who have undergone satisfactory treatment of congenital clubfoot.
• Q: How soon should an infant with congenital clubfoot be referred to an orthopedic surgeon?
• A: Casting typically begins within the 1st to 2nd week of life. Studies have shown that excellent results can be obtained from the Ponseti method even when initiated after the 1st year of life. Medical and life-threatening conditions should take precedence over the treatment of the clubfoot. An orthopedic surgery referral should be done as soon as is practical.

COARCTATION OF AORTA

Luz Natal-Hernandez, MD

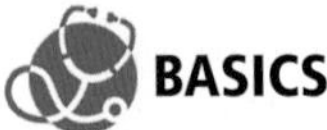

BASICS

DESCRIPTION

- Discrete stenosis of the upper thoracic aorta, usually just opposite the site of insertion of the ductus arteriosus (juxtaductal). A segment of tubular hypoplasia and/or a remnant of ductal tissue give rise to a prominent posterior infolding ("the posterior shelf").
- The hemodynamic lesion is most often discrete but may be a long segment or tortuous in nature. It is usually juxtaductal but may occur in other sites (i.e., the abdominal aorta).
- The prevalence of other associations (bicuspid aortic valve) and long-term complications (hypertension) indicate that this lesion may be part of a broader spectrum arteriopathy and/or endothelial disorder.

EPIDEMIOLOGY

Prevalence

- ~6–8% of patients with congenital heart disease have coarctation.
- More common in males

RISK FACTORS

Genetics

- Occurs in 35% of patients with Turner syndrome (XO)
- Has been described in cases of monozygotic twins
- Mutations of several genes, including *NOTCH1* and *MCTP2*, have been identified in some patients.
- Many studies document the prevalence of a microdeletion at 22q11 in patients with arch anomalies and ventricular septal defects.

PATHOPHYSIOLOGY

- Decreased systemic blood flow to lower body after ductal closure
- Increased afterload to left ventricle (LV) causes LV hypertrophy. Relative underperfusion of the renal vessels, baroreceptors, and multiple other mechanisms combine to induce compensatory hypertension.
- If the coarctation is severe, LV dysfunction and congestive heart failure (CHF) result, with low cardiac output and increased LV end-diastolic pressure.
- Decreased myocardial perfusion may be present in cases of very low output.

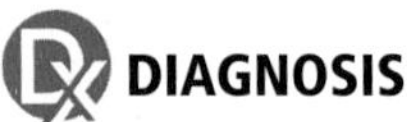

DIAGNOSIS

HISTORY

There are two typical patterns for the clinical presentation of coarctation:

- An infant with CHF or shock: typically precipitated by ductal closure
  - Respiratory distress (dyspnea/tachypnea)
  - Poor feeding
  - Pallor
  - Diaphoresis
  - Poor weight gain
  - Oliguria
- A child or adolescent with systolic hypertension and/or a heart murmur
  - Lower extremity claudication
  - Headaches
  - May be asymptomatic

PHYSICAL EXAM

- Tachypnea and tachycardia
- Discrepant arterial pulses and systolic blood pressure (BP) in the upper and lower extremities
- Gallop rhythm in an infant with CHF
- Ejection click of a bicuspid aortic valve
- Heart murmur:
  - Several types of murmurs may be present (depending of the presence of other abnormalities) but it is commonly a grade 2/6 to 3/6 systolic ejection murmur.
  - Murmur best heard at the upper left sternal border and radiating to the left interscapular area posteriorly
- An infant with severe coarctation and a patent ductus arteriosus (PDA) may have "differential cyanosis." The lower part of the body appears cyanotic because the descending aortic flow is provided by the right ventricle (RV) through the PDA (check postductal saturation).

ALERT

- The most reliable clinical findings to diagnose native, residual, or recurrent coarctation are the presence of pressure differences in the upper and lower extremities and decreased or absent femoral pulses. Palpable pulses alone do not exclude coarctation.
- Four-extremity BP measurement is very important in assessing infants and children with possible congenital heart disease. Proper cuff size must be used.
- Bowel ischemia can be present in the ill patient, and emesis or poor feeding are hallmark signs.

DIFFERENTIAL DIAGNOSIS

- Other left-sided heart obstructive lesions
- Hypoplastic left heart syndrome
- Cardiomyopathy and/or myocarditis
- Critical aortic stenosis (aortic obstruction to a degree that adequate systemic perfusion depends on patency of the ductus arteriosus)
- Sustained tachyarrhythmia
- Shock from sepsis, metabolic disease, or other entities

DIAGNOSTIC TESTS & INTERPRETATION

Initial Tests (screening, lab, imaging)

- Electrocardiogram:
  - In infants, the electrocardiogram may be normal, may show RV hypertrophy, or may show LV hypertrophy with strain pattern if aortic stenosis or myocardial disease is present.
  - The electrocardiogram is often normal in children.
  - LV hypertrophy is apparent with more severe coarctation or longer standing coarctation, particularly in older children.
- Blood tests:
  - In the patient presenting in extremis, management, initial therapy, and timing of surgery can be guided by arterial blood gas analyses and markers of end organ dysfunction.
- Chest x-ray:
  - In infant, moderate to severe cardiomegaly with increased pulmonary vascular markings (PVMs) is seen.
  - In an asymptomatic child, the heart size is often normal, with normal PVMs.
  - Rib notching may be seen in older children secondary to dilated intercostal collateral vessels.
- Echocardiography:
  - Localization, degree of coarctation, and associated findings (PDA, arch hypoplasia, other defects)
  - Assessment of associated left-sided obstruction: mitral valve abnormality, LV outflow obstruction, and aortic stenosis (bicuspid aortic valve)
- Magnetic resonance imaging:
  - Clearly defines the location and severity of coarctation
  - Useful for serial postoperative follow-up (especially aortic aneurysms)

Diagnostic Procedures/Other

Cardiac catheterization and angiography: usually not indicated unless there are further questions to be answered and/or a planned intervention

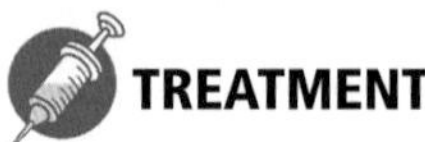

TREATMENT

GENERAL MEASURES

- For the sick neonate who presents with severe CHF or shock (ductal-dependent systemic blood flow):
  - Alprostadil (PGE1) prostaglandin infusion: 0.05 to 0.1 mcg/kg/min (anticipating adverse effects, including apnea and need for intubation)
  - Inotropic support: Dopamine 3 to 5 mcg/kg/min
  - Diuretics for pulmonary venous hypertension or pulmonary edema
  - Correction of metabolic disturbances (acidosis, hypothermia, hypoglycemia, anemia)
  - Surgical intervention should follow as soon as possible.
- For the asymptomatic child, elective repair, and assessment for systemic hypertension are appropriate; however, aggressive antihypertensive pharmacotherapy is not indicated prior to surgical intervention.

SURGERY/OTHER PROCEDURES

- Types of surgical repair: end-to-end anastomosis, subclavian flap aortoplasty, prosthetic patch aortoplasty, bypass graft.
  - Infancy
    - Surgical repair of severe coarctation and coarctation associated with intracardiac anomalies
    - The surgical mortality rate for infants with isolated coarctation approaches 0%. In those with coarctation and a large ventricular septal defect, mortality ranges from 2% to 10% and is higher for children with more complex intracardiac anomalies.
  - Childhood
    - Elective coarctation repair between ages 18 months and 3 years in asymptomatic children without severe upper extremity hypertension.
    - Later repair is associated with an increased risk of sustained hypertension and other late complications.
- Other: interventional cardiology
  - Percutaneous balloon angioplasty of native coarctation in infants and children is pursued in some centers. Others have concern about rates of recurrent stenosis, hypertension, aneurysm formation, and iliofemoral arterial injury.
  - Use of vascular stents to relieve the area of stenosis, particularly in older children and adolescents, has provided an alternative to surgical intervention.

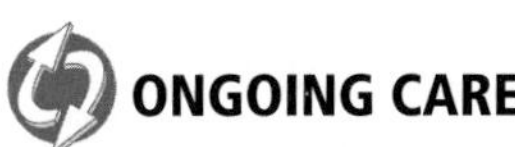

ONGOING CARE

FOLLOW-UP RECOMMENDATIONS

Patient Monitoring

- Reexamine every 12 months with four-extremity pulse and BP assessment.
- Residual or recurrent coarctation
  - Occurs most commonly in those patients requiring repair in early infancy and can depend on the method of intervention (e.g., higher incidence with patch aortoplasty and coarctation ridge resection)
  - Most centers delay percutaneous balloon angioplasty of residual or recurrent lesions until 2 months postoperatively.
- Persistent systemic hypertension: most common in patients whose coarctation repair is delayed beyond early childhood
- Aortic aneurysm formation
- Intracranial aneurysms and/or cerebrovascular accidents
- May have hypertension with exercise, even if normotensive at rest
- Exercise-induced hypertension without anatomic stenosis may respond to β-blocker therapy.

PROGNOSIS

- Untreated coarctation has a poor natural history with the onset of CHF, especially in those patients with other intracardiac malformations. Claudication is common in older children with previously undiscovered coarctation.
- Generally, the short-term prognosis following successful intervention for isolated coarctation in infancy or childhood is excellent. Procedure-related mortality in every modern series is very near zero.
- Clinical conditions that may affect long-term prognosis after repair of coarctation include the following:
  - Residual or recurrent coarctation
  - Hypertension (rest and exercise)
  - Aortic aneurysm (associated with repair technique)
  - Associated intracardiac lesions
  - Intracranial aneurysms
  - Occurrence or progression of aortic valve disease
  - Premature coronary arterial and cerebrovascular disease
- Associated lesions
  - Bicuspid aortic valve
  - Ventricular septal defect
  - Valvar or subvalvar aortic stenosis
  - Mitral stenosis: often associated with structural mitral valve abnormalities (i.e., supravalvar mitral ring, thickening of mitral leaflet, single papillary muscle with parachute deformity, or short dysplastic chordae tendineae)
  - Shone syndrome: multiple left-sided obstructive lesions, including supravalvar mitral ring, parachute mitral valve, subaortic obstruction, and coarctation
  - Berry aneurysm of the circle of Willis
  - Renal artery stenosis associated with abdominal coarctation
  - Congenital diaphragmatic hernia

COMPLICATIONS

- Shock, if severe untreated obstruction
- CHF, if severe untreated obstruction
- Systemic hypertension, before and after intervention
- Intracranial aneurysms
- Mesenteric ischemia
- Paraplegia
- Postoperative complications
  - Bleeding
  - Postcoarctectomy syndrome/mesenteric ischemia
  - Paradoxical hypertension
  - Spinal cord ischemia (0.4%)
  - Residual coarctation
  - Chylothorax
  - Stridor
  - Diaphragm paralysis
  - Aortic aneurysm or dissection
  - Paralysis

ADDITIONAL READING

- Carr JA. The results of catheter-based therapy compared with surgical repair of adult aortic coarctation. *J Am Coll Cardiol*. 2006;47(6):1101–1107.
- Celermajer DS, Greaves K. Survivors of coarctation repair: fixed but not cured. *Heart*. 2002;88(2):113–114.
- Cowley CG, Orsmond GS, Feola P, et al. Long-term randomized comparison of balloon angioplasty and surgery for native coarctation of the aorta in childhood. *Circulation*. 2005;111(25):3453–3456.
- Rosenthal E. Coarctation of the aorta from fetus to adult: curable condition or life long disease process? *Heart*. 2005;91(11):1495–1502.
- Shah L, Hijazi Z, Sandhu S, et al. Use of endovascular stents for the treatment of coarctation of the aorta in children and adults: immediate and midterm results. *J Invasive Cardiol*. 2005;17(11):614–618.
- Toro-Salazar OH, Steinberger J, Thomas W, et al. Long-term follow-up of patients after coarctation of the aorta repair. *Am J Cardiol*. 2002;89(5):541–547.

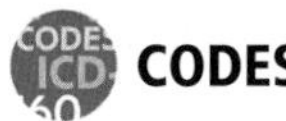

CODES

ICD10

Q25.1 Coarctation of aorta

FAQ

- Q: When is the most appropriate time to perform surgical repair of simple coarctation?
- A: Recommendations vary regarding the age at which asymptomatic children (without severe upper extremity hypertension) should undergo intervention. Advances in technique no longer require patients to be "grown" to a threshold size or weight, and there is increasing evidence that severity and incidence of late complications correlate directly with older age at repair. Although some authors mention 3 to 5 years of age, others recommend repair as early as 18 months to 2 years of age.
- Q: What is the incidence of systemic hypertension after surgical repair of coarctation?
- A: Greatly depends on age at repair, surgical method or technique, length of follow-up interval, and how one defines or measures hypertension. In no situation is the answer zero, and this important complication is one of several reasons patients require lifelong detailed follow-up. 1 year after a technically perfect repair via resection with end-to-end anastomosis, the patient operated on in early childhood is unlikely to have hypertension at rest. However, 20 years further along, a patient of older age at repair is quite likely to have significant hypertension on exercise stress testing.

COCCIDIOIDOMYCOSIS

Camille Sabella, MD

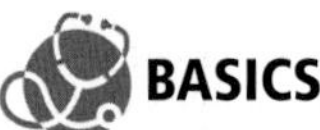

BASICS

DESCRIPTION

Coccidioidomycosis is an endemic systemic mycosis resulting in both asymptomatic and life-threatening disseminated infections.

EPIDEMIOLOGY

- *Coccidioides* spp. are dimorphic fungi that live in the soil.
- Endemic to the southwestern United States (southern California, Arizona, western and southern Texas, New Mexico), northern Mexico, and parts of South and Central America
- Infection is acquired from exposure to aerosolized spores (arthroconidia) usually during recreational or occupational activities; clusters of cases may involve dust storms and earthquakes.
- The average incubation period is 10 to 16 days (range 1 to 4 weeks) for primary infection.
- There is no person-to-person spread except in rare instances of draining lesions or donor derived transmission through organ donation.
- 60% of acute infections are subclinical (asymptomatic).

Incidence

- Rising incidence reported in the United States over the past 2 decades
- Annual incidence in 2011 was 42.6 per 100,000 population.
- Highest rate of infection in the summer and early fall

Prevalence

Seropositivity rates in children living in endemic area for 1 year approach 20%, whereas rates in children living in endemic area for 10 or more years approach 80%.

RISK FACTORS

- The course of illness is highly variable and depend on host immune response and amount of exposure.
- Risk factors for disseminated infection:
  - Immunosuppression (especially organ transplant recipients, those receiving immunosuppressive therapies and immunomodulators, and those with HIV infection)
  - Male gender (adult)
  - Neonates, infants, and the elderly
  - Filipino, African American, Native American, Hispanic ethnicity
  - Pregnancy
- Risk of dissemination is less in children than in adults.

GENERAL PREVENTION

- No special isolation or precautions for the hospitalized patient
- Contaminated dressings from skin lesions should be handled and discarded with care.
- Inhalation of aerosolized spores from culture can be hazardous to laboratory personnel.
- Preventive efforts are aimed at dust control and trials to eliminate organisms from soil.
- Immunocompromised people should be counseled to avoid activities that may expose them to aerosolized spores in endemic areas.

PATHOPHYSIOLOGY

- Spores (arthroconidia) are the infectious forms of *Coccidioides* organisms; they are released from the mold and propagate the mold in the soil.
- Inhalation of arthroconidia from disturbed, arid soil is the major route of infection.
- In tissues, arthroconidia enlarge to form spherules. Mature spherules release endospores that propagate in the host and continue the tissue cycle.
- Primary infection occurs in the lungs.
- Most patients have infection limited to a localized area of lung and hilar lymph nodes after mounting an intense inflammatory response with granuloma formation.
- Extrapulmonary dissemination occurs via lymphatic or hematologic spread and usually involves the skin, bones and joints, and central nervous system but can spread to virtually any organ system.

ETIOLOGY

- *Coccidioides immitis* and *Coccidioides posadasii* are the etiologic agents of coccidioidomycosis.
- Asymptomatic infection is the most common outcome, occurring in 60% of infected individuals.
- Primary pulmonary infection accounts for most symptomatic cases; nonspecific illness most common feature (cough, malaise, chest pain, fever); self-limited in most cases; may be accompanied by reactive rashes such as erythema multiforme or erythema nodosum
- Disseminated disease occurs in <1% of infected individuals and may manifest with
  - Osteomyelitis:
    - Subacute or chronic and frequently involves more than one bone (40%)
    - Common sites are the hands, feet, ribs, skull, and vertebrae.
  - Meningitis:
    - Develops within 6 months of initial infection
    - Hydrocephalus is a common complication.
    - Central nervous system vasculitis and intracerebral abscesses are rare.
  - Cutaneous disease:
    - Papules or pustular lesions that ulcerate are most common.
    - Most commonly seen on the face but can occur anywhere
    - Regional adenitis is common.

DIAGNOSIS

HISTORY

- Travel or residence in an endemic area is typical. Risk factors for disseminated infection should be sought.
- Acute pneumonia
  - Fever, dry or productive cough, and pleuritic chest pain; hemoptysis is rare in children.
  - Systemic symptoms include headache, malaise, arthralgias, sore throat, and fatigue; rash may be reported.
  - Also known as "valley fever"
- Myalgias, arthralgias, chills, night sweats, and anorexia suggest systemic dissemination.
- Headache, vomiting, and altered mental status suggest meningitis.
- Most infections (60%) are asymptomatic.

PHYSICAL EXAM

- Signs of pneumonia and pleural effusions are often present with symptomatic pulmonary infection.
- Reactive rashes
  - Contain no live organisms
  - Erythematous maculopapular rash and erythema multiforme are seen in 50% of symptomatic children.
  - Erythema nodosum and fever may occur following the onset of symptoms and correlate with the development of cell-mediated immunity (hypersensitivity reactions).
  - Hypersensitivity reactions may occur in the absence of pulmonary symptoms.
- Hematogenous dissemination to the skin
  - Lesions may consist of papules, nodules, abscesses, pustules, sinus tracts, and verrucous ulcers.
  - May be single or multiple
  - Can occur anywhere but are most common on the nasolabial folds
- Stridor is present with infection of the subglottic tissues.
- Signs of increased intracranial pressure are often seen with central nervous system infection. Classic signs of meningeal irritation and fever may be absent.

ALERT

- Clinicians in endemic areas should maintain a high level of clinical suspicion of primary as well as disseminated infection.
- Diagnosis in nonendemic areas may be missed owing to low clinical suspicion or missed travel history.
- False-negative serologic results may occur during the initial weeks of infection or in an immunocompromised host.

DIFFERENTIAL DIAGNOSIS

- Other pulmonary mycoses (e.g., *Histoplasma capsulatum*, *Aspergillus fumigatus*, and *Blastomyces dermatitidis*)
- *Mycobacterium tuberculosis* (lung or CSF)
- *Mycoplasma pneumoniae*
- Influenza and other viral infections that present as bronchopneumonia
- Skin lesions may mimic other endemic mycoses, tuberculosis, actinomycetes, or syphilis.

DIAGNOSTIC TESTS & INTERPRETATION

- Direct examination and culture
  - Cytologic examination of bronchoalveolar fluid is diagnostic in only about 1/3 of persons and is less sensitive than culture. Visualization of large spherules is possible in stained specimens of sputum, tracheal aspirates, urine, or tissue biopsy. They are rarely seen in CSF.
  - The organisms can be detected by culture in experienced laboratories. The yield is highest from purulent material. The yield from other sources, such as pleural fluid, blood, and gastric aspirates, is lower.
  - A DNA probe can identify *Coccidioides* species in cultures.
- Coccidioidin or spherulin skin intradermal testing has been used as an epidemiologic tool in the past but is no longer commercially available.

- Serologic studies
  - Serve as valuable diagnostic and prognostic tools but may be hampered by false-negative results early in the course of infection and in immunocompromised hosts; false-positive reactions occur as a result of cross-reactivity with other endemic mycoses.
  - *C. immitis*–specific IgM antibody is detectable in 90% of patients 3 weeks after symptom onset and usually is absent after 6 months. False-positive results are seen in 15% of patients with cystic fibrosis.
  - IgG is detected by the complement fixation (CF) assay from serum or CSF. It is positive in 50% of patients at 4 weeks and 83% at 3 months following symptomatic primary infection. In general, higher titers reflect more extensive infection, and rising CF antibody concentrations are associated with worsening disease.
  - Enzyme immunoassay (EIA) for qualitative detection of IgM and IgG is sensitive but can yield false-positive results. It can be useful for screening, but a positive EIA should be confirmed with another test.
  - Hematologic findings include elevated erythrocyte sedimentation rate, leukocytosis, and eosinophilia (in 10%).
- Other studies
  - CSF findings in meningitis include hypoglycorrhachia and pleocytosis with mononuclear cell predominance.
- Radiologic studies
  - Chest radiograph may reveal well-circumscribed nodules, lobar or patchy pulmonary infiltrates, pleural effusions, cavitary lesions, and hilar adenopathy.
  - Radiographs of involved bones may reveal lytic lesions. Scintigraphy or MRI of bone is more sensitive for the diagnosis of osteomyelitis.

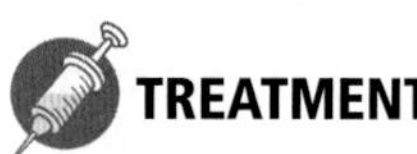

TREATMENT

MEDICATION

- Uncomplicated or minor disease is self-limited and usually resolves without specific antifungal therapy.
  - Controversial whether treatment reduces illness severity or risk of severe complications
- Treatment of uncomplicated respiratory infection is recommended for infants, pregnant women, and patients with continuous fever for >1 month, >10% weight loss, extensive or progressive pulmonary disease, or immunodeficiency (either from HIV or as a result of immunosuppressive medications). Use either oral fluconazole or itraconazole for 3 to 6 months.
- Diffuse pneumonia: amphotericin B or high-dose fluconazole. The total length of therapy should be at least 1 year, and for patients with severe immunodeficiency, oral azole therapy should be continued as secondary prophylaxis.
- Disseminated infection, nonmeningeal: Treat with oral fluconazole or itraconazole. Amphotericin B may be used as an alternative. The duration of therapy may be longer than for those with pneumonia only.
- Meningitis: Oral fluconazole is preferred (12 mg/kg/24 h once daily or divided b.i.d., max 800 to 1,000 mg/24 h). Therapy should be continued indefinitely. Intrathecal amphotericin B may be useful in central nervous system infections for those who fail to respond to azole therapy.

SURGERY/OTHER PROCEDURES

Surgical debridement is used for localized and persistent lesions in bone and lung.

ONGOING CARE

FOLLOW-UP RECOMMENDATIONS

Patient Monitoring

- Patients with mild primary respiratory tract infections who are not treated with antifungal therapy should be assessed at 3 to 6 months intervals for up to 2 years to ensure that their clinical and radiographic findings have resolved.
- Periodic assessment should be done for all patients treated with antifungal therapy throughout their treatment and after cessation of antifungal therapy.
- Patients who are being treated for meningeal infections should undergo CSF assessment every 3 months for life.
- Rising or unchanging CF titers while the patient is receiving treatment may indicate treatment failure, most often due to noncompliance or an occult focus that may require surgical drainage.
- All azoles inhibit P450 enzymes. Consider drug–drug interactions when the patient is taking other medications.

PROGNOSIS

- Most infections are asymptomatic (60%) or mild (35%) and self-limited.
- Primary infection of the lungs is usually self-limited, with a course of illness lasting 1 to 3 weeks; complications (see below) may prolong the course.
- Fatigue can last for several months.
- Dissemination is infrequent (see earlier section for risk factors). Morbidity and mortality have improved with use of antifungal therapy, but immunocompromised patients still have a poor prognosis after the development of disseminated infection. The mortality rate is 70% in HIV-infected patients with diffuse pulmonary coccidioidomycosis.
- Meningitis, untreated, is nearly always fatal within 2 years of diagnosis.

COMPLICATIONS

- Localized complications of primary pulmonary infection are infrequent and include pleural effusions and pericarditis.
- ~5% of lung infections result in residual pulmonary sequelae, usually nodules or abscess cavities. 1/3 of these cavities spontaneously resolve within 2 years. Hemoptysis and rupture of the abscess, with formation of an empyema, are potential complications in patients with unresolved cavities.
- Extrapulmonary dissemination usually develops within a year after the initial infection but may appear much later if immunity is impaired (e.g., HIV infection, malignancy, immunosuppressive or immunomodulatory therapy).
- Hospital admission seems to be more common in patients with comorbid conditions and frequently necessitates surgical intervention.
- Hydrocephalus may occur with central nervous system involvement.

ADDITIONAL READING

- Ampel NM. New perspectives on coccidioidomycosis. *Proc Am Thorac Soc*. 2010;7(3):181–185.
- Centers for Disease Control and Prevention. Increase in reported coccidioidomycosis—United States, 1998–2011. *MMWR Morb Mortal Wkly Rep*. 2013;62(12):217–221.
- Dimitrova D, Ross L. Coccidioidomycosis: experience from a children's hospital in an area of endemicity. *J Pediatric Infect Dis Soc*. 2016;5(1):89–92.
- Fisher BT, Chiller TM, Prasad PA, et al. Hospitalizations for coccidioidomycosis at forty-one children's hospitals in the United States. *Pediatr Infect Dis J*. 2010;29(3):243–247.
- Galgiani JN, Ampel NM, Blair JE, et al; for Infectious Diseases Society of America. Coccidioidomycosis. *Clin Infect Dis*. 2005;41(9):1217–1223.
- Montenegro BL, Arnold JC. North American dimorphic fungal infections in children. *Pediatr Rev*. 2010;31(6):e40–e48.
- Nguyen C, Barker BM, Hoover S, et al. Recent advances in our understanding of the environmental, epidemiological, immunological, and clinical dimensions of coccidioidomycosis. *Clin Microbiol Rev*. 2013;26(3):505–525.
- Shehab ZM. Coccidioidomycosis. *Adv Pediatr*. 2010;57(1):269–286.

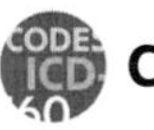

CODES

ICD10

- B38.9 Coccidioidomycosis, unspecified
- B38.2 Pulmonary coccidioidomycosis, unspecified
- B38.3 Cutaneous coccidioidomycosis

FAQ

- Q: Do all patients with symptomatic primary respiratory infection due to *C. immitis* require treatment?
- A: No. Because >95% of initial pulmonary infections are self-limited, treatment is not always required. Patients with concurrent risk factors (e.g., HIV, organ transplant, or high doses of corticosteroids) or evidence of unusually severe infections should always be treated. Factors suggesting increased severity of infection include weight loss of >10%, symptoms for 3 or more weeks, infiltrates involving more than half of one lung or portions of both lungs, and CF antibody to *C. immitis* >1:16.
- Q: What is the best option for treatment of the child with coccidioidal meningitis?
- A: Fluconazole has become the treatment of choice because of its ease of administration, excellent central nervous system penetration, and safety profile. Intravenously and intrathecally administered amphotericin B is considered a 2nd-line agent because of its inconvenience and adverse effect profile.

COLIC

Cori Green, MD, MSc

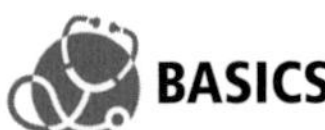

BASICS

DESCRIPTION

- Crying is considered a normal part of human behavior and is a baby's most effective form of communication. However, when crying is perceived to be in excess than what is expected, it can cause a family a great deal of distress.
- Colic is a syndrome of excessive crying for which no organic cause can be identified. It is described as unexplained end-of-the-day crying that begins at age 2 to 3 weeks, peaks at 8 weeks, and tapers at 12 weeks.
- No standard definition of colic exists. Dr. Brazelton defined it as any excessive crying that worried parents. However, the consensus definition is from 1954 (Wessel) and referred to as the rule of 3's. He defined colic by the amount of crying:
  - >3 hours a day
  - >3 days a week
  - And lasting at least 3 weeks
- Colic episodes usually begin suddenly, with no clear reason, and at the end of the day or evening. The crying is intense and high pitched. Infants may have a flushed face, furrowed brow, and postural changes such as bending or drawing up of the knees, clenched fists, and tensed abdominal muscles. Episodes may end with a bowel movement or passing of gas.

EPIDEMIOLOGY

- Crying is one of the most common reasons families present to a health care professional during the 1st months of life.
- One in six families who have children with colic seek care from a health care professional.
- Estimates are difficult to make due to lack of standard definition; literature suggests a prevalence of 3–40%.
- Incidence is similar in male and females and in breastfed and bottle-fed infants.

RISK FACTORS

- Possible risk factors include maternal smoking, increased maternal age, and being the first-born child.
- In addition, colic has been associated with higher levels of maternal stress, anxiety, and depression.

GENERAL PREVENTION

Although no study has shown any certain way to prevent colic, educating parents about infant crying can be helpful. Remind parents that crying is an infant's way to communicate, inform them of the expected average hours a day and infant may cry, and teach them soothing techniques.

ETIOLOGY

- The term colic is now considered a misnomer because it derives from the Greek word for colon. Studies in the early 1900s suggested colic was a result of gastrointestinal (GI) dysfunction, whereas today, there are many theories.
- Causes of colic are multifactorial, and it is typically considered to result from an interaction between infant, maternal, and paternal factors and the environment at a unique time of biologic vulnerability. No single cause has been identified. Several hypotheses for the etiology exist.
  - GI disturbances are often implicated in colic. Abnormal motility has been hypothesized and is somewhat supported by the fact that anticholinergics may improve symptoms. Other studies have shown infants with colic have decreased amounts of lactobacilli and increased amounts of coliform bacteria. Although another theory is that increased gas production can cause colic, this theory is not supported based on radiographs taken during crying spells. Recent studies have suggested an association with *Helicobacter pylori* and infantile colic. Others theorized that colic is a form of milk protein allergy. However, these studies are limited, and no causality has been established.
  - Psychosocial issues have been implicated including family tension, parental anxiety, or inadequate parent–infant interactions. However, in studies where infants are cared for by trained occupational therapists, symptoms did not improve.
  - A neurodevelopmental etiology is supported by the fact that infants with colic have similar patterns of crying to infants without colic and that colic is outgrown. Excessive crying has also been considered a manifestation of normal emotional development where colic is on the end of a spectrum of crying.

DIAGNOSIS

HISTORY

- Obtain a detailed history about the crying including the frequency, intensity, time of day, duration, the infant's behavior around the crying episode, and whether there is a common trigger for the crying.
- Include a detailed psychosocial history and what the parents have tried so far to soothe the baby during crying episodes.
- Prenatal history and history of fever in the infant is important to assess infant's risk of infection.
- Elicit history about stooling and vomiting to eliminate organic etiologies of crying such as gastroesophageal reflux, malabsorption, or pyloric stenosis.
- History of color changes, apnea, or respiratory distress should help assess for a cardiac or respiratory etiology for crying.

PHYSICAL EXAM

- For the diagnoses of colic, vital signs, growth, and physical exam should be normal.
- Observation of the infant's behavior, reactions, and parent–infant interactions are useful.
- Look for signs of trauma or evidence of nonaccidental injuries. Look for bruises and palpate bones to look for fractures. A thorough GI and neurologic exam should also be performed.

DIFFERENTIAL DIAGNOSIS

- Normal crying
  - As studied by Brazelton in 1962, at 2 weeks, normal infants cried for a median of 1 3/4 hour a day, just under 3 hours at 6 weeks, and ~1 hour by 12 weeks. Normal crying, like colic, tends to occur predominantly in the evening and can vary from day to day.
- Organic causes of excessive crying:
  - Cardiac: congenital heart disease, supraventricular tachycardia
  - Respiratory: upper respiratory infection, pneumonia, foreign body aspiration, pneumothorax
  - GI: constipation, cow's milk protein allergy, gastroesophageal reflux, lactose intolerance, intussusception, rectal fissures, and strangulated inguinal hernias, failure to thrive
  - Neurologic: hydrocephalus, subdural hematoma, infantile migraine, neonatal drug withdrawal
  - Metabolic: hypoglycemia, electrolyte abnormalities, ingestions, inborn errors of metabolism
  - Infectious: meningitis, otitis media, urinary tract infections, and viral illnesses
  - Trauma: child abuse, corneal abrasions, foreign bodies in the eye, fractures, and hair tourniquets

DIAGNOSTIC TESTS & INTERPRETATION

No tests are indicated if there are no concerning signs on history or physical exam.

ALERT

Although organic causes are found in <5% of infants who present with crying, it is important to look for red flags in the history and physical such as the following:

- Symptoms elicited in history:
  - Vomiting that is frequent, large quantity (>1 oz), bilious, or projectile
  - Bloody stools
  - Poor weight gain
  - Respiratory difficulties including apneic or cyanotic episodes
  - Fever, lethargy, poor feeding
- Signs observed on physical exam:
  - Irritability, tachycardia, pallor, mottling, poor perfusion
  - Abnormal neurologic findings including hypotonia, a full fontanelle, or a head circumference >95%
  - Petechiae, bruising, tachypnea, cyanosis, nasal flaring
  - Weight decreasing

TREATMENT

GENERAL MEASURES

The most important and effective treatment is for health care providers to acknowledge the difficulty of the situation and to provide reassurance. Parents of a colicky infant often feel tired and inadequate and need their concerns to be substantiated by a provider who acknowledges how difficult of a time this must be. Main points to reassure and guide parents include the following:

- The crying of colic can be persistent, but there is no evidence of disease, a physical problem, or proof that the infant is in pain. Periods of wellness each day followed by periods of crying is reassuring.
- Nothing bad will happen to the baby despite the crying and perceived pain.
- Colic is benign and self-limited; the majority of infants improve by age 3 to 4 months.
- During crying spells, the infant is probably overaroused and tired.
- On average, a healthy infant will cry 2 to 3 hours per day.
- Strategies for soothing their infant such as swaddling, making "shh" sounds, swinging the baby (no more than 1 inch back and forth), pacifier use, repetitive sounds, and decreasing environmental stimulation
- Anticipatory guidance on child abuse prevention (e.g., encouraging parents to take a break when their infant's crying is causing them excessive distress or to turn to each other or others for support)

MEDICATION

The literature does not support the use of pharmacologic interventions in colic. Although some studies have shown certain pharmacologic agents to be effective, these studies lack methodologic rigor or involve medications with serious adverse effects.

- Meta-analyses and systematic reviews have shown that specific probiotic strains, such as *Lactobacillus reuteri* DSM 17938, can decrease the amount of time infants cry each day. The evidence is strongest for breastfed infants, but there is some data to suggest it works for mixed- and formula-fed infants as well. However, some of these studies show that the impact occurs only after 3 weeks which may just represent the normal course of crying. Further studies are needed before probiotics should be routinely recommended.
- Anticholinergic medications such as dicyclomine hydrochloride and cimetropium are contraindicated in infants <6 months in the United States due to side effects such as apnea and drowsiness.
- Simethicone is an over-the-counter medication that decreases intraluminal gas. Studies of its efficacy have been mixed, and any reduction of symptoms has been attributed to a placebo effect.

ADDITIONAL THERAPIES

- Diet modification
  - Breastfeeding mothers are encouraged to continue to breastfeed. There is conflicting evidence about whether mothers should eliminate allergenic foods from their diet. There is some evidence that mothers who take probiotics while breastfeeding could prevent colic or reduce symptoms.
  - Although hydrolyzed formulas have been shown to reduce symptoms of colic, most of these studies lack methodologic rigor. In addition, if symptoms do improve, milk protein allergy must be considered. Switching formulas is not recommended for infants with colic and no signs of milk protein allergy or failure to thrive.
  - Although soy milk formula has been shown to reduce crying, it is not recommended in the treatment of colic due to the prevalence of allergy to soy.
  - High-fiber formulas and lactase drops have not been shown to be effective.
- Behavioral modifications
  - Car-ride simulators, crib vibrators, and increased carrying have not been shown to be effective.
  - Other interventions such as modified parent and infant interactions involving decreased stimulation, "contingent music," and assisting parents in acquiring effective coping and consoling methods have shown some benefit. However, none of these studies involve randomization and blinding, and most are of small sample size.

COMPLEMENTARY & ALTERNATIVE THERAPIES

- Although teas containing chamomile, vervain, licorice, fennel, and lemon balm have been shown to be effective if used 3 times a day with 150 mL per dose, they are not recommended. Adverse events have been reported. The dose is a large volume. In addition, there is no standard dosing or formulations of these products.
- Sucrose solutions have been found to improve symptoms compared to placebo, yet evidence is limited, and there are concerns about nutritional effects and lack of standardization for formulation of preparations.
- Chiropractic care and infant massage have also been studied, but due to mixed results and lack of methodologic rigor, they are not recommended in treating colic. There is increasing evidence that acupuncture may reduce crying; however, safety has been an issue in some studies.

ONGOING CARE

FOLLOW-UP RECOMMENDATIONS

Patient Monitoring

- It is important to keep in close touch with parents of an excessively fussy baby. Telephone contact every 2 to 3 days is essential until improvement.
- Although reexamination may not be needed, consistent follow-up from a supportive physician may help reassure parents.

DIET

Breast milk and formula changes are not recommended unless milk protein allergy is suspected.

PATIENT EDUCATION

Educate parents regarding the average number of hours an infant is expected to cry and provide soothing techniques. Reassure that colic is benign and self-limited.

PROGNOSIS

- Without intervention, this prolonged crying usually diminishes around 3 to 4 months of age.
- Some studies suggest infants with colic can have difficulties later in life in family communication; dissatisfaction; and sleeping, psychological, or GI disorders; however, other research has shown no long-term consequences.
- There is no association between colic and later diagnosed asthma or allergic disease.

COMPLICATIONS

Most complications are related to the fatigue, anxiety, and distress that colic can cause in families. The most serious outcome is if parental exasperation leads to the physical abuse of the infant.

ADDITIONAL READING

- Brazelton TB. Crying in infancy. *Pediatrics*. 1962;29(4):579–588.
- Harb T, Matsuyama M, David M, et al. Infant colic—what works: a systematic review of interventions for breast-fed infants. *J Pediatr Gastroenterol Nutr*. 2016;62(5):668–686.
- Radesky JS, Zuckerman B, Silverstein M, et al. Inconsolable infant crying and maternal postpartum depressive symptoms. *Pediatrics*. 2013;131(6):e1857–e1864.
- Schreck Bird A, Gregory PJ, Jalloh MA, et al. Probiotics for the treatment of infantile colic: a systematic review. *J Pharm Pract*. 2017;30(3):366–374.
- Wessel MA, Cobb JC, Jackson EB, et al. Paroxysmal fussing in infancy, sometimes called colic. *Pediatrics*. 1954;14(5):421–435.

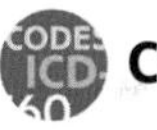

CODES

ICD10

- R10.83 Colic
- R68.11 Excessive crying of infant (baby)

FAQ

- Q: What is colic?
- A: Excessive crying in an infant for which no organic etiology is identified. Crying usually is for at least 3 hours a day, for 3 days a week, for a minimum of 3 weeks.
- Q: Why do certain infants get colic?
- A: The etiology of colic is poorly understood. Although there is evidence that GI dysfunction can cause colic, most believe colic is a neurodevelopmental syndrome.
- Q: How is colic treated?
- A: Pharmacologic, nutritional, and behavioral interventions are not recommended. The most important treatment a health care provider can provide is to substantiate a parent's concern, provide reassurance, educate, and provide anticipatory guidance about colic.

COMA

Jennifer Huffman, MD • Preetha Krishnan, MD

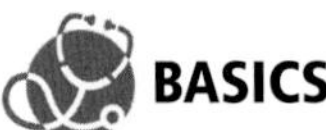

BASICS

DESCRIPTION

Coma is defined as a state in which the patient appears to be asleep, shows no awareness of his or her surroundings, and cannot be aroused. Coma frequently is only a transient state, whereby patients recover, die, or progress to a permanent state of impairment. Often a medical emergency, immediate intervention may be required to preserve life and brain function.

- Coma is at the far end of a spectrum of acute impaired consciousness, which also includes the following:
  - Lethargy or stupor: patient arousable but does not stay awake; impaired responses to commands
  - Delirium: a confused, agitated or hypoactive patient with fragmented attention, concentration, and memory
- Coma may progress to
  - Persistent vegetative state: chronic state of unconsciousness with no awareness or cognition, no voluntary responses, and no language abilities; preserved autonomic functions and sleep–wake cycles
  - Brain death: lack of cortical and brainstem responses

EPIDEMIOLOGY

Incidence varies by age, season (infection), and ethnicity (inborn errors of metabolism [IEM]).

PATHOPHYSIOLOGY

Dysfunction of the reticular activating system in the brainstem or bilateral cerebral dysfunction causes impaired arousal and consciousness.

ETIOLOGY

Coma etiology can be traumatic or nontraumatic. Infection is a common cause of nontraumatic coma.

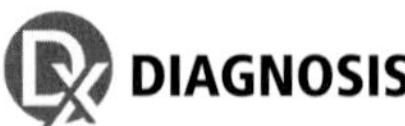

DIAGNOSIS

HISTORY

- **Question:** Evidence or history of head trauma, drowning, or other trauma?
- *Significance*: Are there concerns for nonaccidental trauma?
- **Question:** What medications are in the home? Has the patient been depressed or displayed suicidal behaviors? Is there a history of illicit drug use?
- *Significance*: ingestion/drugs/toxins
- **Question:** Recent fevers, viral or bacterial illnesses, mental status changes, sick contacts, immunosuppression, infectious risk factors?
- *Significance*: infection
- **Question:** Past medical history risk factors?
- *Significance*: epilepsy, diabetes, heart disease, neurologic disease including previous episodes of coma, history of failure to thrive (IEM)
- **Question:** Recent nausea, vomiting, mental status change?
- *Significance*: increased intracranial pressure (ICP)

PHYSICAL EXAM

Vital sign changes: Hyperthermia suggests infection, intoxication, and neuroleptic malignant syndrome. Tachycardia suggests fever, pain, hypovolemia, arrhythmia, and heart failure.

ALERT

Hypertension, bradycardia, and irregular respirations (Cushing triad) herald impending brain herniation.

- Skin changes: Look for rashes suggesting infection, bruising, and other evidence of trauma; neurocutaneous stigmata may be associated with seizures; feel anterior fontanelle in infants for evidence of ICP.
- Neurologic exam: Focus on general level of awareness, eye movements, and motor responses to accurately define coma versus lethargy or delirium. Findings can be used in various coma scales.
- Eye movements: Persistent eye deviation is associated with contralateral seizure activity or ipsilateral brain lesions. Impaired upward gaze may indicate high ICP. Nystagmus can be seen in intoxications.
- Pupillary reaction: Small reactive or large reactive pupils suggest intoxication. Anisocoria suggests unilateral brainstem compression. Fixed, dilated pupils can indicate brain herniation/death.
- Motor exam: Assess tone, reflexes, and motor responses to stimuli. Flaccid tone and areflexia are serious signs if not related to medications or lower motor neuron disease. Pressure on the supraorbital notch beneath medial eyebrow will avoid reflex pain responses. Localizing pain entails purposeful movements to remove the stimulus. Withdrawal from pain is less purposeful. Decorticate (adduction with elbow and wrist flexion) and decerebrate (extension, internal rotation of arms) may be provoked by stimulation. They can be asymmetric and intermittent and should not be mistaken for seizures.
- Glasgow Coma Scale/Pediatric Glasgow Coma Scale (see Appendix, Tables 5 and 6)
  - Eye opening (score range 1 to 4)
  - Verbal response (score range 1 to 5)
  - Motor response (score range 1 to 6)

DIFFERENTIAL DIAGNOSIS

- Trauma
  - Epidural/subdural or intracerebral bleeding, cerebral swelling, and/or diffuse axonal injury
- Intoxication
  - Household drug ingestion including barbiturates, opiates, psychotropics, and salicylates; street drugs; alcohol; smoke or carbon monoxide inhalation; ethylene glycol; lead; and others
- Hypoxia/diffuse ischemia
  - Drowning, suffocation/strangulation, cardiac disease
- Infection
  - Bacterial or viral meningitis, encephalitis, postinfectious encephalomyelitis, toxic or systemic shock, subdural empyema. Pathogens leading to coma include HSV, *Mycoplasma pneumoniae*, influenza, and *Neisseria meningitidis*.
- Postinfectious/autoimmune mediated
  - Anti-NMDA receptor encephalitis, acute disseminated encephalitis (ADEM), acute necrotizing encephalitis (ANE), febrile infection–related epilepsy syndrome (FIRES), CNS lupus
- Metabolic disorders
  - Hypoglycemia (salicylate or ethanol intoxication, insulin overdose/hyperinsulinemia), diabetic ketoacidosis (DKA), hyperglycemic nonketotic coma, Reye syndrome, electrolyte abnormalities (Na, K, Ca, Mg), hepatic/uremic encephalopathy, IEM, endocrine abnormalities (hypothyroidism, Addisonian crisis), hypothermia/hyperthermia
- Tumor
  - Can cause ICP and herniation
- Seizure
  - Nonconvulsive status
- Vascular
  - Infarction, hemorrhage from arteriovenous malformation (AVM), aneurysm, cerebral venous thrombosis, hypertensive encephalopathy, basilar-type migraine
- Hydrocephalus
  - Ventriculoperitoneal (VP) shunt obstruction, mass/bleed obstructing ventricular outflow
- Disorders mimicking coma include the following:
  - Psychogenic coma
    - Patient may resist passive eye opening, regard self in a mirror, and avoid passive arm fall over face and other noxious stimuli.
  - Catatonia
    - A form of psychogenic coma; patients may hold a posture, sit, or stand.

- Locked-in state/complete paralysis
  - Patient is paralyzed with intact cerebral function; may occur in severe neuromuscular disorders or in ventral pontine lesions
- Botulism toxicity
  - Botulism toxicity presents as a descending flaccid paralysis which may include dilated or fixed pupils.

DIAGNOSTIC TESTS & INTERPRETATION

- Recommended initial studies:
  - Glucose, electrolytes, blood urea nitrogen/creatinine, calcium, magnesium, phosphorous
  - CBC and blood culture
  - Arterial blood gas
  - Urine toxicology screen (Consider EKG)
  - Urine analysis and culture
  - Ammonia, liver transaminases, CK
- Other helpful studies based on the clinical picture may include the following:
  - Metabolic labs (urine organic acids, serum amino acids, lactate), thyroid function tests, cortisol, coagulation studies, carboxyhemoglobin (CO poisoning), ANA, anti-NMDA receptor antibodies
  - LP (opening pressure, glucose, cell count, protein, Gram stain, culture) to rule out infection or bleed; defer until after CT if focal exam or signs of increased ICP. Simultaneous fingerstick blood glucose is ideal. If concerned about traumatic tap, evaluate CSF for xanthochromia (see "FAQ").
  - EEG can be helpful to rule out nonconvulsive status epilepticus, especially in patients with a history of seizures or clinically suspected seizures. Continuous EEG may be needed to make this diagnosis.
  - Electrophysiologic studies including somatosensory evoked potential (SEP), brainstem auditory evoked, and visual evoked potentials may be helpful for diagnosis and prognosis.
  - Head CT: Quick noncontrast scan can detect hemorrhage, hydrocephalus, herniation, and masses; should be done prior to LP to rule out a mass (risk for herniation from LP)
  - Cervical spine imaging if indicated based on history and physical exam.
  - Brain MRI: can help with diagnosis and prognosis if prior workup is unrevealing. Consider MRA to evaluate arteries and MRV to rule out venous thrombosis. MRS can help clarify hypoxic and metabolic etiologies.

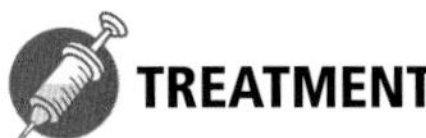

TREATMENT

SURGERY/OTHER PROCEDURES

Neurosurgical intervention may be required in cases of head trauma, hemorrhage, mass lesion, or hydrocephalus. Neurology consultation is usually indicated.

ADMISSION, INPATIENT, AND NURSING CONSIDERATIONS

- First priority is airway, breathing, and circulation management.
- If head trauma is suspected, stabilize the cervical spine with a collar while securing the airway.
- Endotracheal intubation: often required for airway protection and adequate oxygenation
- Place large-bore IV lines for isotonic fluids to maintain intravascular volume and blood pressure as needed.
- Evidence of increased ICP
  - Maintain normocarbia.
  - Consider 3% hypertonic saline (HS) as bolus or continuous infusion.
  - Consider mannitol (0.5 to 1 g/kg IV).
  - Prevent hyperthermia with antipyretics and environmental cooling methods.
  - Elevate head to 30 degrees above horizontal; avoid head-turned posture to maximize cerebral venous drainage.
  - Hospitalization in the intensive care unit for close monitoring of changes in respiratory status or signs of increased ICP
  - Neurosurgical consultation; consider role for decompression craniectomy.
- If fingerstick glucose is low, give 2 to 4 mL/kg of 25% dextrose (D25) IV.
- If opiate ingestion is suspected, administer naloxone.
- Correct electrolyte and acid–base abnormalities.
- Empiric treatment with IV antibiotics and acyclovir should be started if bacterial or viral meningitis is suspected.
- Consider benzodiazepine (lorazepam 0.05 to 0.1 mg/kg IV) for suspected seizure activity, although this may compromise neurologic examination.

ONGOING CARE

PROGNOSIS

- Prognosis depends on underlying etiology and patient's clinical course. It is not advised to prognosticate too early.
- Serial exams combined with diagnostic tests (electrophysiology, imaging) will provide more complete information.
- The following portend poor prognosis: absent motor responses to painful stimuli on day 3, no spontaneous eye opening after 1 week, bilaterally absent SEP, and isoelectric baseline or burst suppression on EEG at 1 week
- Conversely, a reactive EEG is associated with improved outcomes. Some of these findings are more firmly established in adults but, in the right clinical context, may be applicable to pediatric patients.

COMPLICATIONS

- Acute coma
  - Brain injury
  - Respiratory failure/aspiration
  - Seizures
  - Infection
- Chronic sequelae
  - Epilepsy
  - New cognitive and/or motor baseline

ADDITIONAL READING

- Abend NS, Licht DJ. Predicting outcome in children with hypoxic ischemic encephalopathy. *Pediatr Crit Care Med*. 2008;9(1):32–39.
- Kochanek PM, Carney N, Adelson PD, et al. Guidelines for the acute medical management of severe traumatic brain injury in infants, children, and adolescents—second edition. *Pediatr Crit Care Med*. 2012;13(Suppl 1):S1–S2.
- McCoy B, Sharma R, Ochi A, et al. Predictors of nonconvulsive seizures among critically ill children. *Epilepsia*. 2011;52(11):1973–1978.
- Seshia SS, Bingham WT, Kirkham FJ. Nontraumatic coma in children and adolescents: diagnosis and management. *Neurol Clin*. 2011;29(4):1007–1043.

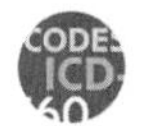

CODES

ICD10

- R40.20 Unspecified coma
- R40.1 Stupor
- R40.3 Persistent vegetative state

FAQ

- Q: When a bacterial infection is suspected as a potential etiology of coma, should antibiotic therapy be delayed until CSF has been obtained for testing?
- A: Antibiotics should not be delayed if patient is unstable or there is difficulty obtaining CSF. The administration of antibiotics does not change leukocyte number or composition in the CSF cell count within the first 48 hours.
- Q: When should we obtain an EEG?
- A: Approximately 1/3 of critically ill children will have seizures detected in 24 hours of continuous EEG monitoring. High-risk comatose patients include those with nonaccidental trauma, meningitis, and TBI
- Q: What is the significance of CSF xanthochromia?
- A: If blood has been present in CSF for 12 or more hours, RBC breakdown creates a visible pigment. This xanthochromia will be absent if RBCs are the result of a traumatic tap.

COMMON VARIABLE IMMUNODEFICIENCY

Elena E. Perez, MD, PhD

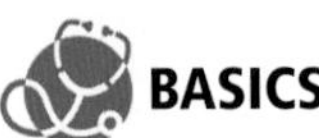

BASICS

DESCRIPTION

- Common variable immunodeficiency is the most common clinically important primary immunodeficiency syndrome, characterized by
  - Low IgG, IgA, and/or IgM
  - Recurrent infections
  - A wide spectrum of immunologic abnormalities, including autoimmune disease, inflammatory conditions, and the development of lymphomas
- Diagnosis of exclusion, requiring low IgG and variable reduction in IgA and/or IgM, impaired specific antibody responses

EPIDEMIOLOGY

- Prevalence has been estimated at between 1:100,000 and 1:10,000 of the population.
- Prevalence can vary across different populations.
- Can present at any age
  - Most diagnosed between 20 and 40 years old
  - Diagnosis is usually made several years after the onset of recurrent infections (pneumonia, sinusitis, otitis).
- A subgroup of children has been described in which the onset of disease was most often <5 years of age. This group was characterized by a relapsing and remitting course in which autoimmune disease predominated.
- About 20–25% of patients with common variable immunodeficiency have one or more autoimmune conditions at time of diagnosis.
- Affects males and females equally

RISK FACTORS

Genetics

- Complex genetics
- Rare recessive mutations described in
  - T-cell inducible costimulatory (ICOS) in one kindred, <1% of patients
  - CD19 in a few unrelated families
  - B-cell activating factor (BAFF)
  - CD20 and CD81
  - Transmembrane activator and calcium-modulating cyclophilin ligand interactor (TACI, TNFRSF13B) in 8% of patients, associated with autoimmunity and lymphoid hyperplasia; heterozygous mutation more common than homozygous; significance not clear due to similar mutation found in healthy family members
- IgA deficiency more likely in offspring of parents with common variable immunodeficiency
- Incidence of IgA deficiency, autoimmune disease, and malignancies is increased in family members of patients with common variable immunodeficiency.

PATHOPHYSIOLOGY

- Main characteristic is hypogammaglobulinemia.
- Impaired immunoglobulin and specific antibody production despite normal B cell numbers
- Often increased proportion of immature B cells
- Deficiency of class-switched memory B cells associated with more complex disease (autoimmunity, granulomatous disease, hypersplenism, and lymphoid hyperplasia)
- Functional defects of both B and T lymphocytes are described.

ETIOLOGY

- The primary immunologic defect(s) leading to this syndrome is unknown.
- Multiple defects have been associated with common variable immunodeficiency, including the following:
  - Lack of somatic mutation within variable region genes
  - Lack of memory B cells
  - Impaired maturation, IL-12 secretion, and upregulation of costimulatory molecules by antigen-presenting cells may impair T cells, which are important for providing help to B cells for antibody production.
  - Toll-like receptor 9 (TLR9) response and expression by B cells may also be impaired. TLR signaling pathways are being investigated for their potential role in pathogenesis of common variable immunodeficiency.
- Some genetic defects have been described but do not account for the majority of cases.

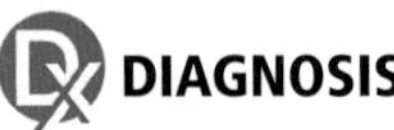

DIAGNOSIS

HISTORY

- Recurrent sinopulmonary infections, especially sinusitis and pneumonia, with encapsulated bacteria
- Autoimmune diseases such as autoimmune hemolytic anemia (AIHA), idiopathic thrombocytopenic purpura (ITP), thyroid disease, and chronic active hepatitis
- Localized or systemic granulomatous disease that can be diagnosed years before low IgG is discovered. Lungs, spleen, and lymph nodes are most commonly affected; can be misdiagnosed as sarcoidosis
- Persistent diarrhea of infectious (e.g., *Giardia lamblia*) or noninfectious causes
- Inflammatory bowel disease–like disorder in 6–10% of patients
- A subset of patients may have a severe norovirus-associated enteropathy leading to intestinal villous atrophy and malabsorption.
- Noninfectious, diffuse pulmonary complications described as granulomatous-lymphocytic interstitial lung disease (GLILD) exhibit granulomatous and lymphoproliferative histologic patterns (lymphocytic interstitial pneumonia [LIP], follicular bronchiolitis, and lymphoid hyperplasia).
- Patients at high risk for GLILD may also have splenomegaly, ITP, AIHA, low IgA, and expansion of CD21 low B cells.
- Severe or unusual viral infections with herpes simplex, cytomegalovirus, and varicella, such as pneumonitis, hepatitis, or encephalitis. Chronic meningoencephalitis can be seen with enteroviral infection.

PHYSICAL EXAM

- Evaluation should focus on the presence of infection.
- 30% of patients will have lymphadenopathy and/or splenomegaly.

DIFFERENTIAL DIAGNOSIS

- Other primary antibody deficiency disorders: X-linked agammaglobulinemia, transient hypogammaglobulinemia of infancy, and selective antibody deficiency
- Severe malabsorption with protein-losing enteropathy
- HIV infection
- Chronic lung disease: cystic fibrosis, immotile cilia syndrome, and α_1-antitrypsin deficiency
- Primary autoimmune diseases: immune ITP, AIHA, systemic lupus erythematosus, thyroiditis

DIAGNOSTIC TESTS & INTERPRETATION

Initial Tests (screening, lab, imaging)

- IgG, IgA, IgM below age-appropriate norms
- CBC with differential: Examine smear for evidence of hemolysis in AIHA.
- Autoimmune antibody screen: antinuclear antibody, autoantibody panel
- Stool culture for bacteria and ova/parasites to evaluate chronic diarrhea
- Isohemagglutinins as well as functional antibody titers to bacterial antigens such as tetanus, diphtheria, and pneumococcus are usually low to absent.
- Spirometry may be helpful in following chronic lung disease.
- Mitogen/antigen stimulation studies will help assess lymphocyte function.
- T- and B-lymphocyte enumeration by flow cytometry
- B-cell phenotyping becoming more available
- Absent B lymphocytes in males suggest X-linked agammaglobulinemia rather than common variable immunodeficiency.
- Appropriate cultures based on site of infection
- Chest and sinus x-ray studies/CT scans may be warranted for evaluation of bronchiectasis and chronic disease.

Diagnostic Procedures/Other

- GI endoscopy with biopsies for cases of idiopathic persistent diarrhea
- Lymph node biopsy in suspected malignancy

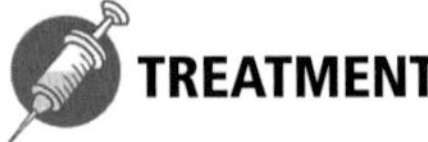

TREATMENT

MEDICATION

First Line

Immunoglobulin replacement (lifetime) therapy

Second Line

Antibiotics as needed for infection may also be used as adjunct to immunoglobulin replacement as prophylaxis.

ADDITIONAL THERAPIES
- Monthly IV immunoglobulin replacement
  - Starting dose is usually 400 to 600 mg/kg/month IV to maintain a trough IgG level of at least 500 mg/dL or FDA-approved formulation(s) for SC administration, given weekly or biweekly following the establishment of intravenous immunoglobulin (IVIG) dosage.
- Appropriate antibiotics for acute infections
- Prophylactic antibiotics may be helpful in chronic/recurrent infections.
- Cautious use of corticosteroids may be necessary in the treatment of GI and autoimmune manifestations.

ISSUES FOR REFERRAL
- Autoimmune manifestations
- GI: chronic abdominal pain or signs of possible lymphoid hyperplasia
- Suspicion for underlying monogenic immunodeficiency

ADMISSION, INPATIENT, AND NURSING CONSIDERATIONS
- Supervision during IVIG administration
- Monitor for side effects of therapy.
- Have anaphylaxis medications available.

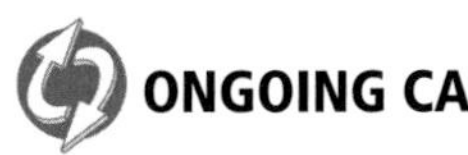

ONGOING CARE

FOLLOW-UP RECOMMENDATIONS
- Close and frequent follow-up is warranted for patients with severe, recurrent symptoms. It may be as frequent as monthly, depending on symptoms.
- Signs and symptoms suggesting malignancy (e.g., persistent adenopathy in absence of infection, significant weight loss, or abdominal mass) should be evaluated expeditiously.
- Abdominal pain may indicate infection or lymphoid hyperplasia.

Patient Monitoring
CBC with differential, LFT, creatinine, IgG level

PATIENT EDUCATION
Several Web sites available to patients and families:
- Immune Deficiency Foundation: http://primaryimmune.org
- International Patient Organisation for Primary Immunodeficiencies: www.ipopi.org
- The Jeffrey Modell Foundation: www.jmfworld.org
- National Institute of Allergy and Infectious Diseases: www.niaid.nih.gov

PROGNOSIS
- Immunoglobulin replacement therapy, prophylactic antibiotics when necessary, and close follow-up by immunology have greatly improved the overall prognosis.
- The newer challenge with this disease is detection and management of autoimmune and other disease-associated complications.
- Phenotypic classifications based on memory B cell numbers divide patients into two major categories: those that do well with IgG replacement alone and others with more likely autoimmune and granulomatous complications.
- A new study notes that low IgA at diagnosis may be a poor prognostic indicator.

COMPLICATIONS
- Autoimmune disease in 20% of common variable immunodeficiency patients; most common are AIHA and ITP.
- GI complications include chronic diarrhea, malabsorption, and weight loss. Inflammatory bowel disease and *Helicobacter pylori* infection have also been observed.
- Granulomatous infiltrations may mimic sarcoidosis.
- Lymphoproliferative disease: Overall risk is 8–10%. The most common are lymphomas, usually non-Hodgkin lymphoma, well differentiated, mostly Epstein-Barr virus negative.
- Chronic sinusitis and lung disease with abnormal pulmonary function tests
- Progressive decline in T-lymphocyte function

ADDITIONAL READING

- Azizi G, Abolhassani H, Asgardoon MH, et al. Autoimmunity in common variable immunodeficiency: epidemiology, pathophysiology and management. *Expert Rev Clin Immunol*. 2017;13(2):101–115.
- Ballow M. Primary immunodeficiency disorders: antibody deficiency. *J Allergy Clin Immunol*. 2002;109(4):581–591.
- Bonilla FA, Barlan I, Chapel H, et al. International Consensus Document (ICON): common variable immunodeficiency disorders. *J Allergy Clin Immunol Pract*. 2016;4(1):38–59.
- Castigli E, Geha R. Molecular basis of common variable immunodeficiency. *J Allergy Clin Immunol*. 2006;117(4):740–746.
- Chapel H. Common variable immunodeficiency disorders (CVID)—diagnoses of exclusion, especially combined immune defects. *J Allergy Clin Immunol Pract*. 2016;4(6):1158–1159.
- Cunningham-Rundles C. How I treat common variable immune deficiency. *Blood*. 2010;116(1):7–15.
- Graziano V, Pecoraro A, Mormile I, et al. Delay in diagnosis affects the clinical outcome in a cohort of CVID patients with marked reduction of iga serum levels. *Clin Immunol*. 2017;180:1–4.
- Hartono S, Motosue MS, Khan S, et al. Predictors of granulomatous lymphocytic interstitial lung disease in common variable immunodeficiency. *Ann Allergy Asthma Immunol*. 2017;118(5):614–620.
- Jolles S, Chapel H, Litzman J. When to initiate immunoglobulin replacement therapy (IGRT) in antibody deficiency: a practical approach. *Clin Exp Immunol*. 2017;188(3):333–341.
- Jørgensen SF, Reims HM, Aukrust P, et al. CVID and celiac disease. *Am J Gastroenterol*. 2017;112(2):393.
- Kienzler AK, Hargreaves CE, Patel SY. The role of genomics in common variable immunodeficiency disorders. *Clin Exp Immunol*. 2017;188(3):326–332.
- Mooney D, Edgar D, Einarsson G, et al. Chronic lung disease in common variable immune deficiency (CVID): a pathophysiological role for microbial and non-B cell immune factors. *Crit Rev Microbiol*. 2017;43(4):508–519.
- Orange JS, Glessner JT, Resnick E, et al. Genome-wide association identifies diverse causes of common variable immunodeficiency. *J Allergy Clin Immunol*. 2011;127(6):1360–1367.e6.
- Seppänen M, Aghamohammadi A, Rezaei N. Is there a need to redefine the diagnostic criteria for common variable immunodeficiency? *Expert Rev Clin Immunol*. 2014;10(1):1–5.
- Woodward J, Gkrania-Klotsas E, Kumararatne D. Chronic norovirus infection and common variable immunodeficiency. *Clin Exp Immunol*. 2017;188(3):363–370.

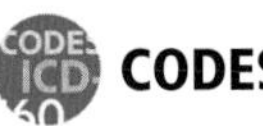

CODES

ICD10
- D83.0 Common variable immunodeficiency with predominant abnormalities of B-cell numbers and function
- D83.2 Common variable immunodeficiency with autoantibodies to B- or T-cells
- D83.9 Common variable immunodeficiency, unspecified

FAQ

- Q: What is the life expectancy of patients with the diagnosis of common variable immunodeficiency?
- A: Because the clinical presentations and symptoms are variable, it is difficult to predict the life expectancy in individual patients. IVIG replacement, in addition to antibiotic therapy, has greatly improved the outlook for these patients. However, despite adequate therapy, a large percentage of patients with common variable immunodeficiency have a progressive decline in immune function. Major morbidity and mortality usually result from the associated complications of malignancy, chronic lung disease, and severe autoimmune disease. In one study, the mortality is estimated at 23–27% over a median follow-up of 7 years (0 to 25 years). The 20-year survival after diagnosis for males is 64% and for females 67% versus 92% and 94%, respectively, for the general population. Main causes of death include respiratory complications, granulomatous disease of organs, liver disease, malnutrition due to GI pathology, uncontrolled autoimmune manifestations, and lymphoma.
- Q: Should patients with common variable immunodeficiency receive live viral vaccines?
- A: In general, patients receiving IVIG replacement therapy do not require any vaccinations. Live viral vaccines should be avoided in these patients, especially if they have deteriorating immune function.
- Q: Can common variable immunodeficiency be diagnosed prenatally?
- A: Because there are no clear genetic inheritance patterns, prenatal diagnosis is unavailable.

C

COMPLEMENT DEFICIENCY

Melanie M. Makhija, MD, MSc

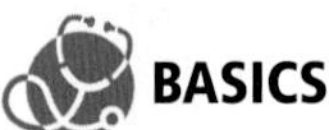

BASICS

DESCRIPTION

- Complement is a major component of the innate immune system.
  - Consists of plasma and membrane proteins which mediate three pathways of cascading enzyme reactions (classical, alternative, and lectin pathways)
  - Pathway activation leads to inflammatory and immune responses.
- Deficiencies can arise in any of the proteins, leading to loss of activity of the deficient protein as well as loss of function of proteins that follow in the cascade.
- Inherited deficiencies of the complement components may predispose individuals to bacterial infections and autoimmunity.
- Secondary/acquired deficiencies are much more common than inherited deficiencies and are most often caused by increased consumption by immune complexes.

EPIDEMIOLOGY

- Complement deficiency accounts for 1–6% of all primary immune deficiencies (PIDs); up to 10% in some registries.
- Homozygous C2 deficiency 1 in 20,000
- Partial C4 deficiency in 1–3% of Caucasian population
- C9 deficiency almost always found in people of Japanese descent
- C6 deficiency more common in African Americans
- Alternative pathway deficiencies (properdin, factor D) are rare.

RISK FACTORS

Genetics

- Properdin deficiency is X-linked.
- Most other complement deficiencies are autosomal recessive.
- C1 inhibitor deficiency is autosomal dominant.
- Heterozygotes are usually phenotypically normal.

Clinical Manifestations of Complement Deficiencies

Deficiency	Clinical Manifestations
C1q,r,s, C2	Systemic lupus erythematosus (SLE)-like, bacterial infections, invasive pneumococcal infections
C4	SLE-like, autoimmune disorders, infections
C3	Severe infections with encapsulated bacteria (i.e., *Haemophilus influenzae*), glomerulonephritis, immune complex diseases (i.e., atypical hemolytic uremic syndrome [aHUS])
Factor H, I	Secondary C3 deficiency, aHUS, age-related macular degeneration (AMD), hemolysis, elevated liver enzymes, and low platelet count (HELLP) syndrome
Properdin	Males with neisserial and sinopulmonary infections
Factor B	Neisserial infections, aHUS, AMD
Factor D	Neisserial infections
MBL, MASP	Infections with encapsulated bacteria, respiratory infections
Ficolin-3	Respiratory infections, necrotizing enterocolitis
C5, 6, 7, 8, 9	Disseminated neisserial infections, SLE
DAF, CD59	Paroxysmal nocturnal hemoglobinuria
C1 inhibitor	Hereditary angioedema (HAE)

PATHOPHYSIOLOGY

- Classic complement pathway is activated when IgM or IgG antibodies bind to antigen.
- Lectin pathway is activated when a serum lectin such as mannose-binding lectin (MBL) binds to antigen.
- Alternative pathway does not need antibody or lectins to be activated.
- Main goal of all three pathways is to deposit C3b fragments on the target antigen to mark the target for immune response.

ETIOLOGY

- Primary complement deficiencies are hereditary.
- Acquired deficiencies: accelerated consumption by immune complexes (most common), decreased hepatic production (less common), or loss through the urine (rare)

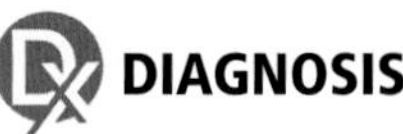

DIAGNOSIS

HISTORY

Indications for evaluating complement system:

- Recurrent pyogenic infections in patients with normal white blood cell count and immunoglobulin levels
- Recurrent neisserial infections (meningitis, sepsis, gonococcal arthritis) at any age
- Meningococcal meningitis >5 years of age
- Multiple family members who have had neisserial infections
- Autoimmune manifestations including SLE, especially familial lupus
- Renal and ophthalmic inflammatory disorders
- Recurrent angioedema without urticaria: Evaluate for C1 inhibitor deficiency (HAE).

PHYSICAL EXAM

- Depends on which component is deficient
- Assess for signs and symptoms of autoimmunity (i.e., SLE) and also of bacterial infections and sequelae.
- Failure to thrive
- Recurrent angioedema without urticaria for HAE

DIFFERENTIAL DIAGNOSIS

- Antibody (humoral) deficiency syndromes
- Secondary complement deficiencies

DIAGNOSTIC TESTS & INTERPRETATION

Initial Tests (screening, lab, imaging)

- Total hemolytic complement (CH50):
  - Screens for homozygous deficiencies in the classical pathway; all nine components (C1 to C9) required for normal CH50
  - Complement activity is thermolabile and reduced quickly at room temperature; low levels often due to improper specimen handling
  - Complete deficiency of any component gives undetectable CH50 level.
  - Heterozygotes may have normal CH50.
- AH50
  - To assess integrity of alternate pathway
  - Most commonly used to evaluate some renal diseases of childhood
- Individual component testing
  - C3, C4 levels most commonly measured
  - Based on clinical history
- HAE testing
  - Based on clinical history
  - C4, C1 esterase inhibitor level and function may be used to evaluate for HAE.

ALERT

- Most common cause of low complement levels is improper specimen handling. It is essential that blood samples are processed as quickly as possible to serum tubes and frozen if not running tests immediately.
- Secondary deficiency may be caused by consumption of complement components.

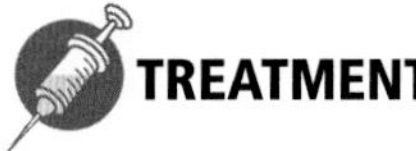

TREATMENT

GENERAL MEASURES

- Consider prophylactic antibiotics to prevent recurrent infections.
- Vaccination with *Streptococcus pneumoniae* and *Neisseria meningitidis* conjugate vaccines as well as *Haemophilus influenzae* for patients and household contacts
- Immunization against *Neisseria* decreases recurrence due to activation of adaptive immunity.
- Can receive other routine vaccines (including live viral vaccines) safely
- Wear medical identification tag identifying condition.
- Plasma infusions impractical over lifetime and risk of development of antibody against missing component

MEDICATION

- There are no specific treatments for most complement deficiencies.
- Aggressive diagnosis and treatment of infections with antibiotics is imperative.
- HAE prophylaxis and treatment for C1 inhibitor deficiency

ISSUES FOR REFERRAL

- Should be followed by immunologist
- Monitor for autoimmune disease and refer to rheumatologist for autoimmunity management.
- Genetic counseling for family members

ONGOING CARE

COMPLICATIONS

- Severe infections and sequelae including death
- Immune complex disease
- Autoimmunity

ADDITIONAL READING

- Bonilla FA, Geha RS. 12. Primary immunodeficiency diseases. *J Allergy Clin Immunol*. 2003;111(Suppl 2):S571–S581.
- Frank MM. Complement deficiencies. *Pediatr Clin North Am*. 2000;47(6):1339–1354.
- Frank MM. Complement disorders and hereditary angioedema. *J Allergy Clin Immunol*. 2010;125(2 Suppl 2):S262–S271.
- Grumach AS, Kirschfink M. Are complement deficiencies really rare? Overview on prevalence, clinical importance and modern diagnostic approach. *Mol Immunol*. 2014;61(2):110–117.
- Ingels H, Schejbel L, Lundstedt AC, et al. Immunodeficiency among children with recurrent invasive pneumococcal disease. *Pediatr Infect Dis J*. 2015;34(6):644–651.
- Merle NS, Chruch SE, Femaux-bacchi V, et al. Complement system part I—molecular mechanisms of activation and regulation. *Front Immunol*. 2015;6:262.
- Merle NS, Noe R, Halbwachs-Mecarelli L, et al. Complement system part II: role in immunity. *Front Immunol*. 2015;6:257.
- Walport MJ. Complement. First of two parts. *N Engl J Med*. 2001;344(14):1058–1066.
- Walport MJ. Complement. Second of two parts. *N Engl J Med*. 2001;344(15):1140–1144.

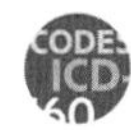

CODES

ICD10

D84.1 Defects in the complement system

FAQ

- Q: When should I evaluate for a complement deficiency?
- A: Any child with recurrent sinopulmonary infections/invasive pneumococcal infections or >1 episode of a neisserial infection.

C

CONCUSSION

Andrea Marmor, MD, MSEd

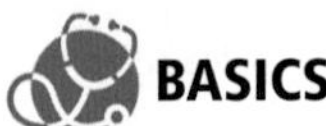

BASICS

DESCRIPTION

- Concussion is defined by short-term clinical symptoms and/or impairment of neurologic function after head/brain trauma, with or without loss of consciousness, and without abnormality on standard neuroimaging studies.
- Concussion may be caused either by a direct blow to the head or a blow to the face, neck, or elsewhere on the body with an "impulsive" force transmitted to the head.
- Concussion may result in pathologic changes, but the acute clinical symptoms largely reflect a functional rather than structural injury, and by definition, there is no evidence of intracranial injury (ICI) in imaging.
- The symptoms of concussion typically resolve spontaneously over hours to days; however, postconcussive symptoms may be prolonged.

EPIDEMIOLOGY

- Concussion can occur after any type of head trauma, but sports-related concussions are of particular interest.
- Since 2000, there has been an increase in diagnosis of sports-related concussions, which account for 25–50% of those reported to the emergency department (ED).
- The Centers for Disease Control and Prevention (CDC) estimates that approximately 3.8 million recreation- and sport-related concussions occur annually in the United States.
- Concussion may be underreported by athletes, trainers, and coaches.
- Although concussion is overall more common in boys, girls have higher rates of concussion than boys in similar sports (e.g., soccer).

RISK FACTORS

- Risk of sports concussion depends on sex, sport, position, and history of prior concussion.
- For boys, concussions are most likely in rugby football, ice hockey, and lacrosse.
- For girls, concussions are most likely in soccer, lacrosse, and field hockey.

GENERAL PREVENTION

- Helmet use is the single most important preventive measure for serious traumatic brain injury. However, helmets have not been consistently shown to prevent concussion.
  - Helmets are not effective at preventing movement of the brain within the skull.
- At preparticipation medical visits, providers should emphasize that reporting concussion immediately is essential and that loss of consciousness is not the only manifestation of concussion.
- Children with more than one concussion should be cleared by a physician before returning to activity.
- Baseline neuropsychological testing (prior to concussion) is being performed by many school athletic departments via widely available computerized testing modules.
  - Research is still needed regarding the optimum timing of this testing and whether baseline testing improves outcome.

ALERT

Retirement should be considered when any athlete who has sustained three concussions in an individual season, when an athlete has had postconcussive symptoms for >3 months, when recovery requires an increasing amount of time, or when concussions occur with less forceful injury.

PATHOPHYSIOLOGY

- Concussion occurs with rapid rotational acceleration of the brain.
- With acceleration–deceleration, the brain experiences continued momentum after impact and strikes against bone. The temporal and frontal lobes are particularly prone to injury because of their location adjacent to irregular parts of the skull.
- Depressed level of consciousness is thought to be the result of rotational stretch injury to the reticular activating system in the dorsal aspect of the brainstem.
- Pathologic changes after concussion include alterations in neuronal depolarization and neurotransmitter release, impaired axonal function, lactic acid accumulation, and decreased cerebral blood flow/autoregulation and glucose metabolism.
- Children may respond to brain trauma differently than adults due to developmental factors such as brain size, brain water content, myelination level, skull and suture geometry and elasticity, and differential skull to body proportions.

DIAGNOSIS

- Concussion is primarily a clinical diagnosis based on a history of trauma and typical acute signs and symptoms including headache, nausea, dizziness, confusion, imbalance, impaired memory, slow speech, inattentiveness and emotional lability.
- Consider referral to ED or trauma center for: Glasgow Coma Scale (GCS) score <15, repeated vomiting, severe or worsening headache, seizure, unsteady gait, slurred speech, weakness, or numbness in the extremities, unusual behavior or signs of basilar skull fracture.
- Neurosurgical evaluation should be obtained if any abnormalities on neuroimaging.
- Postconcussive symptoms may develop later and may be prolonged. These include:
  - Somatic: headaches, fatigue, decreased energy, nausea, vision change, tinnitus, dizziness, incoordination, and balance difficulty
  - Emotional/behavioral: irritability, increased emotionality, personality change, depression, or anxiety
  - Cognitive: slowed thinking and response time; impaired concentration, learning, and/or memory; and reduced problem-solving ability
  - Sleep disturbances

ALERT

Symptoms of serious head injury may be delayed and may occur with or without skull fracture and without an initial loss of consciousness.

HISTORY

- Detailed history of traumatic event, including possible LOC and/or preceding event such as a seizure
- Detailed symptom evaluation
- History of prior concussions, including surrounding circumstances
- History of preexisting cognitive or attention problems to help guide interpretation of postinjury testing

PHYSICAL EXAM

- Onsite and acute evaluation should include the usual ABCs and evaluation for potential associated injuries such as cervical spinal injury.
- A detailed mental status and neurologic examination should be performed to detect focal signs suggestive of serious neurologic impairment and to allow accurate observation over time.
- Consider exertion provocative tests: 5 push-ups, 5 sit-ups, 5 knee bends, 40-yard sprint; look for change in symptoms/exam.

DIAGNOSTIC TESTS & INTERPRETATION

Initial Tests (screening, lab, imaging)

- Standardized, validated instruments for sport concussion are available and can be administered quickly on the sideline (e.g., Sport Concussion Assessment Tool-5th edition [SCAT-5]).
- Imaging is not indicated for diagnosis, and structural lesions are absent on standard CT and MRI in concussion.
- Evidence-based decision rules should be used to identify children at low risk of ICI who do not need neuroimaging.
- Imaging should be performed in children with increased suspicion of ICI, such as those with abnormal mental status, non-frontal scalp hematoma, prolonged loss of consciousness, severe injury mechanism, palpable skull fracture, vomiting, or severe headache.
- Head CT is the test of choice in the acute evaluation of suspected ICI or skull fracture in head trauma. Low radiation protocols should be used when available.

Follow-Up Tests and Special Considerations

- MRI is the imaging modality of choice in the subacute or chronic evaluation of concussion.
- MRI may be used in the acute setting in centers where experience and technique deem it sufficiently accurate for identifying ICI.
- Neuropsychological evaluation should be considered in children with multiple concussions or when recovery is not progressing as expected (e.g., not improving or still symptomatic after 14 days).

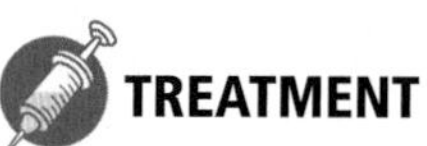

TREATMENT

GENERAL MEASURES

- Remove the child from the activity with no return to play if concussion is suspected.
- Provider or caregiver should monitor the child for several hours after the injury to evaluate for any deterioration.
- Complete rest from physical and cognitive activity is recommended only for the acute phase (24 to 48 hours) after concussion. After the acute phase, the exact duration and amount of rest is not known.
  - Recent evidence suggests that early return to nonimpact aerobic activity and light cognitive activity may be associated with earlier and more complete recovery.
- Most consensus guidelines recommend a gradual and progressive return to normal activity with reassessment at each step (activity should not reactivate or worsen symptoms).
- Before considering return to play, athletes must be symptom-free off medications and free of physical, cognitive, or behavioral symptoms, at rest or during exertion.

MEDICATION

- Occasional use of over-the-counter pain medications such as NSAIDs or acetaminophen may be recommended for headache or discomfort.
  - Caution against frequent or prolonged use as rebound headaches may occur
- Ondansetron may be used for occasional nausea.
- Benzodiazepines should be avoided due to interference with accurate assessment of recovery

ISSUES FOR REFERRAL

- Neuropsychological evaluation
  - Referral for should be considered in children with prolonged symptoms or multiple concussions.
  - Neuropsychological evaluation can document impairment, identify factors contributing to persisting difficulties, and guide school accommodations or formal intervention.
- Some centers have a concussion program that brings together providers from medicine, surgery, physical therapy, psychology, and neurology.

ADMISSION, INPATIENT, AND NURSING CONSIDERATIONS

- Most children with concussion can be managed as outpatients.
- Consider admission if the child continues to have altered level of consciousness, if focal neurologic signs are present, or if patient remains severely symptomatic.
- Nursing staff must be able to perform neurologic assessments at regular intervals.
- Consults by speech therapy, physical therapy, neuropsychology, and neurology should be considered to evaluate for subtle sequelae.
- Discharge planning must be individualized depending on severity of symptoms, family support, and presence of associated injuries.

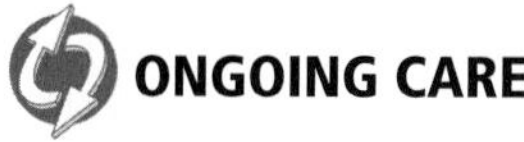

ONGOING CARE

FOLLOW-UP RECOMMENDATIONS

Patient Monitoring

If patient is being monitored at home, the guardian should have detailed instruction regarding reasons to return to the ED.

- These include difficulty awakening or staying awake, worsening headache or dizziness, emesis, seizures, blood or clear fluid from the ears or nose, major changes in behavior, or any focal weakness/sensory/vision changes.

PATIENT EDUCATION

- Complete physical and cognitive rest is recommended for the first 24 to 48 hours.
- Families should be educated on activities with a high cognitive demand, including television, computer, videogames, and texting.
  - School accommodations may be needed.
- Instruct families on instituting a graduated return to normal activity if asymptomatic for 24 hours, reducing activity if symptoms return.
  - Student athletes should receive specific return to play guidelines.
  - Consider in sequence:
    - Light aerobic activity
    - Noncontact sport–related activity
    - Full practice, and then
    - Game play
- Review symptomatic care, emphasizing rest and recovery over pharmacotherapy.

PROGNOSIS

- In general, the prognosis is excellent.
- Severity of acute symptoms is the best predictor of prolonged or incomplete recovery. Loss of consciousness and location of impact do not predict severity.
- Children usually recover by 48 hours. However, children with previous head injury, learning difficulties, or neurologic, psychiatric, or family problems may continue to show significant ongoing problems at 3 months.

COMPLICATIONS

- Postconcussion symptoms may take several months to resolve.
- Concussions have a cumulative effect and result in increased vulnerability to future injuries.
- With repeated concussions, patients may experience sequelae such as chronic headaches, persistent difficulty with short- and long-term memory, and episodic confusion.

ALERT

"Second-impact syndrome" is a controversial and rare but potentially fatal condition involving diffuse cerebral swelling from a second head injury sustained while still recovering from a concussion.

ADDITIONAL READING

- CDC HEADS UP for Health Care Providers: https://www.cdc.gov/headsup/providers/index.html
- Centers for Disease Control and Prevention. Nonfatal traumatic brain injuries related to sports and recreation activities among persons aged ≤19 years—United States, 2001–2009. *MMWR Morb Mortal Wkly Rep*. 2011;60(39):1337–1342.
- Davis GA, Purcell L, Schneider KJ, et al. The Child Sport Concussion Assessment Tool 5th Edition (Child SCAT5). *Br J Sports Med*. 2017;51(11):859–861.
- Giza CC, Kutcher JS, Ashwal S, et al. Summary of evidence-based guideline update: evaluation and management of concussion in sports: report of the Guideline Development Subcommittee of the American Academy of Neurology. *Neurology*. 2013;80(24):2250–2257.
- Grool AM, Aglipay M, Momoli F, et al; for Pediatric Emergency Research Canada Concussion Team. Association between early participation in physical activity following acute concussion and persistent postconcussive symptoms in children and adolescents. *JAMA*. 2016;316(23):2504–2514.
- Halstead ME, Walter KD; for Council on Sports Medicine and Fitness. American Academy of Pediatrics. Clinical report—sport-related concussion in children and adolescents. *Pediatrics*. 2010;126(3):597–615.
- Kuppermann N, Holmes JF, Dayan PS, et al; for Pediatric Emergency Care Applied Research Network. Identification of children at very low risk of clinically-important brain injuries after head trauma: a prospective cohort study. *Lancet*. 2009;374(9696):1160–1170.
- McCrory P, Meeuwisse W, Dvořák J, et al. Consensus statement on concussion in sport—the 5th international conference on concussion in sport held in Berlin, October 2016. *Br J Sports Med*. 2017;51(11):838–847.
- Sport Concussion Assessment Tool-5th edition available at BMJ.com: http://dx.doi.org/10.1136/bjsports-2017-097506SCAT5
- Thomas DG, Apps JN, Hoffmann RG, et al. Benefits of strict rest after acute concussion: a randomized controlled trial. *Pediatrics*. 2015;135(2):213–223.

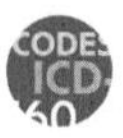

CODES

ICD10

- S06.0X0A Concussion without loss of consciousness, initial encounter
- F07.81 Postconcussional syndrome
- R41.3 Other amnesia

CONGENITAL ADRENAL HYPERPLASIA

Erica A. Eugster, MD

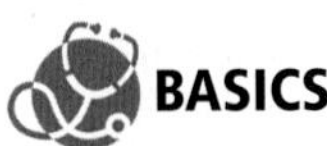

BASICS

DESCRIPTION

Congenital adrenal hyperplasia (CAH) refers to a group of autosomal recessive disorders that have in common deficiency of an enzyme needed for cortisol biosynthesis. The disease exists along a spectrum of severity and is typically subdivided into "classic" (severe) and "nonclassic" (milder) forms.

- There are five specific causes of CAH:
  - 21-hydroxylase deficiency (21OHase)
  - 11-hydroxylase deficiency
  - 3β-hydroxysteroid dehydrogenase deficiency
  - 17α-hydroxylase deficiency
  - Congenital lipoid hyperplasia (stAR mutation)
- The vast majority of cases of CAH (~95%) are due to 21OHase deficiency, which will therefore be the focus of this chapter. The 21OHase enzyme is in the glucocorticoid and mineralocorticoid biosynthetic pathways.

EPIDEMIOLOGY

- The incidence of classic CAH is 1:10,000 to 1:20,000 live births.
  - More common in certain ethnic groups and in remote areas
  - Approximately 75% of cases are characterized by overt salt wasting due to mineralocorticoid deficiency, whereas the remaining cases are described as simply virilizing.
- The prevalence of nonclassic CAH (also called late onset) is approximately 1:1,000.
  - More common in some ethnicities such as Ashkenazi, Italian, and persons from the former Yugoslav Republic and may be as common as 1:50 individuals in these groups

RISK FACTORS

Genetics

- CAH is caused by mutations in the *CYP21A2* gene, which is located on chromosome 6p21.3 and encodes for the 21OHase enzyme. This locus is characterized by many overlapping transcripts and a high rate of recombination.
- Most mutations involve large deletions or arise from the transfer of small sequences of the nearby pseudogene *CYP21A1P* during meiosis. >100 different *CYP21A2* mutations have been reported. Most patients are compound heterozygotes, with the phenotype reflecting the milder mutation.
- Approximately 1% of mutations are estimated to arise de novo and uniparental disomy has been reported. Although genotype–phenotype correlations are generally high, the genetic complexity of CAH renders them sometimes problematic.

PATHOPHYSIOLOGY

- The enzymatic block in cortisol biosynthesis results in diminished negative feedback at the level of the hypothalamus and pituitary gland with a subsequent increase in corticotropin-releasing hormone (CRH) and adrenocorticotropic hormone (ACTH). Precursor buildup proximal to the block results in increased adrenal androgen production (Appendix, Table 13).
- Variable degrees of mineralocorticoid deficiency cause salt wasting and contribute to the risk of adrenal crisis. The clinical consequences of this process vary according to gender and to the severity of the CAH.
- Classic CAH; genetic females
  - Androgen excess during early prenatal life (first trimester) results in ambiguous genitalia. Typical features include elongation of the urethra, development of a urogenital sinus, and enlargement of the clitoris.
  - Internal reproductive structure development is unaffected.
  - If not diagnosed and treated early, progressive virilization occurs postnatally. Girls with salt-wasting CAH are also at risk for an adrenal crisis.
- Classis CAH; genetic males
  - Prenatal androgen exposure has no clinical consequence in infant boys with CAH. However, infant boys with salt-wasting CAH are at risk for an adrenal crisis.
  - As with girls, if not diagnosed and treated early, progressive virilization occurs postnatally.
- Nonclassic CAH; females
  - The far milder degree of androgen excess in nonclassic CAH has no effect during embryologic development but can result in symptoms of hyperandrogenism during childhood, adolescence, or adulthood.
- Nonclassic CAH; males
  - Symptoms of androgen excess can occur during childhood, adolescence, or adulthood.

DIAGNOSIS

HISTORY

- Any family history of CAH should be sought as well as any history of exposures and/or maternal virilization during pregnancy.
- In infants, poor feeding, lethargy, and vomiting are important potential clues to an impending adrenal crisis.
- Children with previously undiagnosed CAH typically present with precocious puberty due to androgen excess. Typical symptoms in classic CAH in young children include adult body odor, acne, pubic and axillary hair, penile enlargement in boys, clitoromegaly in girls, and linear growth acceleration. Symptoms of nonclassic CAH during childhood are usually limited to adult body odor and early pubic/axillary hair.
- Symptoms of CAH in adolescent girls include irregular periods, hirsutism, and acne.

PHYSICAL EXAM

- Classic CAH; genetic females
  - Ambiguous genitalia in infant girls with classic CAH exists along a continuum known as the Prader scale. Prader 1 is a typical female, whereas Prader 5 denotes the most extreme degree of masculinization in which the urethral opening is at the tip of the clitoris and complete labial fusion has occurred. Thus, a male sex assignment is sometimes mistakenly made. This scenario is the rationale for the admonition "Never circumcise a male infant with bilaterally nonpalpable testes!"
  - Most girls with classic CAH are Prader 3 or 4. Significant clitoromegaly will be present along with increased rugation and pigmentation of the labioscrotal structures but no palpable gonads. Posterior labial fusion and a single perineal opening is usually found.
  - Physical findings in the setting of salt wasting are nonspecific but would include low weight percentile, poor skin turgor, dry mucous membranes, and vital signs suggesting dehydration.
  - Although the vast majority of infant girls with classic CAH are diagnosed in the newborn period, occasional cases are missed. If this occurs, the external genitalia will exhibit the same features as in infancy. Other signs of hyperandrogenism will be present such as pubic hair and extreme tall stature from linear growth acceleration. The presence of a urogenital sinus and posterior labial fusion indicate 1st-trimester androgen excess, whereas androgen exposure after this critical period results in clitoromegaly only.
- Classic CAH; genetic males
  - Although average penile size in newborn boys with classic CAH is increased, the external genitalia appear normal, and thus there is nothing on physical exam to alert providers to the presence of CAH. As is the case in girls, physical exam findings associated with salt wasting include low weight percentile, poor skin turgor, dry mucous membranes, and vital signs indicating dehydration.
  - Boys with classic CAH who are missed in infancy come to medical attention due to early secondary sexual development. On physical exam, tall stature, adult body odor, acne, pubic and axillary hair, and penile enlargement are seen. A hallmark of CAH and other forms of peripheral precocious puberty in boys is a prepubertal testicular volume, indicating a source of sex steroids other than the hypothalamic-pituitary-gonadal axis.
- Nonclassic CAH; females
  - Girls with nonclassic CAH have pubic and/or axillary hair, adult body odor, and ± acne. Adolescent girls typically have hirsutism. Mild clitoromegaly may also be seen.
- Nonclassic CAH; males
  - Boys with nonclassic CAH will also have signs of mild androgen excess on physical exam including pubic and axillary hair, adult body odor, and acne.

DIFFERENTIAL DIAGNOSIS

- CAH is the most common 46,XX disorder of sex development. Other causes for ambiguous genitalia are outlined in other chapters.
- The differential diagnosis of classic CAH presenting during childhood includes etiologies of androgen excess such as an androgen-secreting tumor or exogenous exposures. In boys, a β-hCG–producing tumor, McCune-Albright syndrome, and familial male precocious puberty should be considered.
- Nonclassic CAH presenting during childhood is often indistinguishable from premature adrenarche. In adolescent girls, the differential diagnosis includes polycystic ovary syndrome (PCOS), which also shares many clinical features with nonclassic CAH.

DIAGNOSTIC TESTS & INTERPRETATION

Initial Tests (screening, lab, imaging)

- CAH is included on the newborn screen in all 50 states. The biochemical hallmark is an elevated 17-hydroxyprogesterone (17OHP). Depending on the 17OHP concentration, a repeat newborn screen or a serum concentration is obtained. In any presumptive positive case, serum electrolytes need to be monitored closely for early detection of an adrenal crisis. False positives are extremely common in preterm and sick neonates. An elevated plasma renin will confirm overt salt wasting.
- Any report of an abnormal newborn screen for CAH, particularly in a term infant male, should be considered an emergency.
- Serum 17OHP is also the diagnostic test for classic CAH that was missed in the newborn period and for nonclassic CAH. Testosterone, dehydroepiandrosterone-sulfate (DHEAS), and androstenedione should also be measured.
- In infants with ambiguous genitalia, a pelvic ultrasound and genitogram are often performed. In girls with CAH, a normal uterus is seen on ultrasound, whereas a urogenital sinus, "male-type" urethra, and cervical impression are typical findings on genitogram. No routine imaging is performed in infant boys with CAH. However, periodic testicular ultrasound to detect adrenal rest tumors is recommended starting in adolescence, particularly in boys whose CAH is poorly controlled as evidenced by chronic elevations in 17OHP concentrations.
- A bone age radiograph is an important part of the evaluation in children with precocious puberty. In the setting of undiagnosed classic CAH, skeletal maturation will be markedly advanced.

Diagnostic Procedures/Other

- In equivocal cases, a full ACTH stimulation test can distinguish between classic and nonclassic CAH, affected individuals and heterozygous carriers, and between 21OHase deficiency and other forms of CAH.
- Genotyping can also confirm the diagnosis and is helpful for genetic counseling. However, complete sequencing (rather than targeted mutation analysis) of the *CYP21A2* gene may be necessary to accurately determine genotype because complex genetic variations are often present.
- CAH may also be diagnosed prenatally through chorionic villus sampling, amniocentesis, or cell-free fetal DNA in maternal plasma.

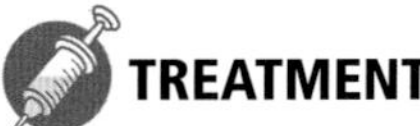

TREATMENT

GENERAL MEASURES

ALERT
Stress-dose glucocorticoid coverage during illness or injury is essential in patients with CAH.

MEDICATION

- Medical treatment of CAH consists of glucocorticoid therapy in doses sufficient to suppress adrenal androgen overproduction, which are generally considered to be 10 to 15 mg/m^2/24 h hydrocortisone equivalent.
- Striking variability in individual sensitivity to different glucocorticoids has been observed, and the use of pharmacogenetics may someday lead to targeted therapy in children with CAH.
- A sustained-release form of hydrocortisone and a CRH receptor antagonist are under investigation as alternative therapeutic approaches in patients with CAH.
- Regardless of salt-wasting status, current recommendations also endorse mineralocorticoid therapy in all patients with classic CAH in the form of Florinef 0.05 to 0.2 mg/24 h.
- Salt supplementation (NaCl 3 to 5 mEq/kg/24 h) is also needed during infancy and until children can control their own salt intake which is generally considered to be around age 2 years.

ADDITIONAL THERAPIES

Girls with CAH usually undergo genital surgery in the form of a feminizing genitoplasty. However, whether and when such surgery should be performed is controversial.

ONGOING CARE

- Ongoing clinic visits and monitoring of growth, puberty, and hormonal studies (including serial measurements of 17OHP) are standard of care.
- Psychological support and educational materials should be provided on a regular basis.

PROGNOSIS

- Adult height is normal when CAH is well controlled but is compromised in poorly controlled or late-diagnosed cases.
- Girls with classic CAH may exhibit boy-typical behaviors but typically have female gender identity.
- Fertility is decreased in women with classic CAH compared to the general population.
- Fertility may be impaired in men with CAH if testicular adrenal rest tumors are present.
- Transition to adulthood ideally takes place in the context of a multidisciplinary team.

ADDITIONAL READING

- Auchus RJ, Witchel SF, Leight KR, et al. Guidelines for the development of comprehensive care centers for congenital adrenal hyperplasia: guidance from the CARES Foundation initiative. *Int J Pediatr Endocrinol*. 2010;2010:275213.
- Finkielstain GP, Chen W, Mehta SP, et al. Comprehensive genetic analysis of 182 unrelated families with congenital adrenal hyperplasia due to 21-hydroxylase deficiency. *J Clin Endocrinol Metab*. 2011;96(1):E161–E172.
- Nebesio TD, Eugster EA. Growth and reproductive outcomes in congenital adrenal hyperplasia. *Int J Pediatr Endocrinol*. 2010;2010:298937.
- Nebesio TD, Renbarger JL, Nabhan ZM, et al. Differential effects of hydrocortisone, prednisone, and dexamethasone on hormonal and pharmacokinetic profiles: a pilot study in children with congenital adrenal hyperplasia. *Int J Pediatr Endocrinol*. 2016;2016:17.
- Speiser PW, Azziz R, Baskin LS, et al. Congenital adrenal hyperplasia due to steroid 21-hydroxylase deficiency: an Endocrine Society clinical practice guideline. *J Clin Endocrinol Metab*. 2010;95(9):4133–4160.

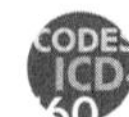

CODES

ICD10

E25.0 Congenital adrenogenital disorders assoc w enzyme deficiency

FAQ

- Q: When does a salt-wasting crisis usually occur in newborns with CAH?
- A: The most common time is between days 5 and 10 of life. However, it may occur as early as on day 1 of life or not until many weeks or months later.
- Q: When should children with CAH be given a "stress dose" and what does this consist of?
- A: Double or triple the usual glucocorticoid dose is considered a stress dose. This should be given at times of illness or psychological stress. However, if a child is vomiting, an emergency Solu-Cortef® injection should be given. Hydrocortisone 100 mg/m^2 IV is given prior to any surgery.
- Q: What is the best form of glucocorticoid treatment in children with CAH?
- A: Hydrocortisone has long been considered the optimal glucocorticoid in CAH. However, this is controversial, and some patients do well on prednisone or dexamethasone.
- Q: Should extremely virilized girls with CAH be sex-assigned male?
- A: Because fertility and gender identity are normal in girls with CAH, the current consensus is to raise these girls female regardless of the extent of virilization.

CONGENITAL HEPATIC FIBROSIS

Peter T. Osgood, MD • Eric H. Chiou, MD • Kristin L. Van Buren, MD, MEd

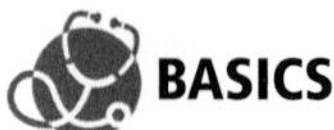

BASICS

DESCRIPTION

- Congenital hepatic fibrosis (CHF) is an inherited, noncirrhotic liver disease.
- Prominent clinical features include the following:
  - Portal hypertension (portal HTN)
  - Increased risk of ascending cholangitis
  - Very likely to have associated renal disease
- Liver biopsy is the gold standard for diagnosis and shows the classic lesion of ductal plate malformation.
- Majority of patients with CHF have associated autosomal recessive polycystic kidney disease (ARPKD). However, CHF has a number of potential genetic associations.

EPIDEMIOLOGY

The incidence of ARPKD is 1/20,000 live births, and all individuals with ARPKD have some degree of hepatic involvement, although the spectrum of disease phenotype is broad (asymptomatic to severe fibrosis and portal HTN).

RISK FACTORS

Genetics

- Inheritance is autosomal recessive in most families, but X-linked and autosomal dominant patterns are also seen.
- Penetrance is 100%, but marked intrafamilial variation in severity is observed.
- *PKHD1*, the ARPKD disease gene, is located on chromosome 6p12.
- >300 mutations of the *PKHD1* gene have been reported, yet even those with the same *PKHD1* mutation may have variable rates of hepatic/renal disease progression indicating the presence of modifier genes or epigenetic factors.
- The presence of two truncating mutations leads to the most severe phenotype, associated with death in the neonatal period.
- The *PKHD1* gene product is a transmembrane protein called fibrocystin (or polyductin).
- Located mostly on the primary cilia and apical surface of renal tubular cells and cholangiocytes
- It complexes with polycystin 1 (PC1) and polycystin 2 (PC2), the mutated proteins in autosomal dominant polycystic kidney disease (ADPKD).Together, the complex is thought to function as a mechanotransducer, detecting the shear force from urine and bile flow and transducing signals via a phosphorylation cascade.

PATHOPHYSIOLOGY

- Ductal plate malformation is a characteristic histologic lesion of the liver, implying a disturbance of the normal development of the bile ducts.
- The primary defect in ARPKD may be linked to ciliary dysfunction.
- Defects lead to impaired calcium signaling with imbalanced proliferation and apoptosis of the ductal plate starting around the 6th to 7th week of gestation.
- Hallmarks include the following:
  - Irregularly shaped, dilated, proliferating bile ducts, often described as staghorn shaped or saccular
  - Noninflammatory periportal fibrosis characterized by a dense extracellular matrix
  - Normal appearance of hepatocytes and lobular architecture
  - The ciliary structure is abnormal in ARPKD renal tubule cells and cholangiocytes.
- Developmental abnormalities involve the liver and kidneys and, less commonly, the vasculature and the heart.
  - In concurrent cases of CHF and ARPKD, renal and liver disease progress at independent rates.
- Portal HTN is thought to result from the fibrosis in the portal tracts as well as, in some patients, from portal vein abnormalities.

COMMONLY ASSOCIATED CONDITIONS

- Portal HTN leading to varices, hypersplenism, and some reports of hepatopulmonary syndrome (HPS)
- Hepatomegaly
- Systemic HTN
- Renal dysfunction
- Cholangitis
- Urinary tract infections (UTIs)
- Growth impairment
- Neurocognitive delays
- Conditions associated with the finding of ductal plate malformation/CHF:
  - ARPKD; most frequent association
  - ADPKD; rare
  - Caroli syndrome (CHF and intrahepatic bile duct dilation, seen especially with the neonatal phenotype)
  - Juvenile nephronophthisis
  - Congenital malformation syndromes
    - Meckel-Gruber syndrome
    - Joubert syndrome
    - Jeune syndrome
    - Bardet-Biedl syndrome
    - Oral-facial-digital syndrome

DIAGNOSIS

HISTORY

- Severely affected patients are usually diagnosed in utero or shortly after birth due to massively enlarged cystic kidneys.
- Prenatal renal enlargement and dysfunction may result in oligohydramnios, pulmonary hypoplasia, and limitations to enteral feeding.
- Older patients may present with systemic HTN or signs of portal HTN and esophageal variceal bleeding.
- Patients may present with symptoms of cholangitis such as fever, jaundice, right upper quadrant tenderness or, rarely, with signs of liver failure.

PHYSICAL EXAM

- Firm, enlarged liver with a prominent left lobe
- Splenomegaly in cases of portal HTN
- Kidneys may be palpable on abdominal exam.

DIFFERENTIAL DIAGNOSIS

Varies with presentation. Usually, differential diagnosis is that of early cirrhosis or idiopathic portal HTN.

DIAGNOSTIC TESTS & INTERPRETATION

Initial Tests (screening, lab, imaging)

- Thrombocytopenia and leukopenia are associated with hypersplenism.
- Liver enzymes and bilirubin are typically normal but may be elevated in some patients.
- Usually, hepatic synthetic function (albumin, prothrombin time) is normal.
- Urinalysis and urine culture should be obtained to assess for UTI in a febrile child with known urinary anomalies, especially females.
- May see elevated blood urea nitrogen and creatinine with renal involvement
- Genetic testing is available but, given the wide variation in phenotypes, prognostic information is limited.
- Complete abdominal ultrasound with Doppler:
  - Increased hepatic echogenicity
  - Splenomegaly
  - Evidence of portal HTN, portal vein patency, and decreased flow variability
  - Cystic kidneys likely (all patients found to have CHF should be screened for renal cystic disease)
- Magnetic resonance cholangiopancreatography (MRCP) can further characterize the biliary system in Caroli syndrome.

Diagnostic Procedures/Other

- Liver biopsy (recommended in the presence of signs and symptoms):
  - Characteristic histology of ductal plate malformation
  - If cholangitis is suspected clinically, send specimen for bacterial culture (although biopsy is not routinely done for this diagnosis alone).
- May need upper gastrointestinal (GI) endoscopy to screen for varices

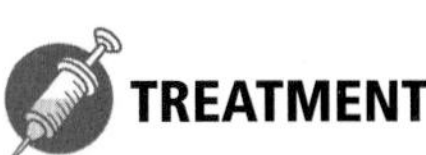

TREATMENT

GENERAL MEASURES

- Monitor growth, weight gain, nutritional status, and for vitamin A, D, E, K malabsorption, with supplementation as needed.
- Vaccinate against encapsulated bacteria as patients may have splenic dysfunction
- Symptoms of cholangitis such as jaundice, rise in serum bilirubin and/or gamma-glutamyl transferase (GGT) levels, right upper quadrant pain, and fever should prompt immediate evaluation (serum liver markers, blood counts, blood culture, possible liver biopsy) and empiric antibiotics to cover gram-negative rods and anaerobes.
- Endoscopic variceal banding and/or sclerotherapy provide prevention and treatment of esophageal variceal hemorrhage in many cases.
- Activity
  - No contact sports if splenomegaly is present
  - Spleen guard may be used to protect against injury from abdominal trauma.

MEDICATION

- Choleretic agents, including ursodeoxycholic acid, are used in cases of bile stasis.
- Some patients with chronic cholangitis *may* require antibiotic prophylaxis.
- Currently no clear safety profile or dosing recommendations for β-blockers in children with portal HTN

ISSUES FOR REFERRAL

- Patients with diseases on the spectrum of CHF or its associated renal diseases should be referred, respectively, to a pediatric hepatologist and/or nephrologist.
- Depending on gene(s) affected, patients and families may also benefit from referral to a geneticist or genetic counselor.

SURGERY/OTHER PROCEDURES

- Portosystemic shunting may be needed if endoscopic therapy cannot sufficiently prevent GI bleeding but should be considered in the context of kidney function because ammonia disposal occurs renally.
- Liver transplant may be indicated for chronic cholangitis, recurrent bleeding related to portal HTN, decompensated cirrhosis, or HPS.
- Children who require transplantation should be considered for combined liver and renal transplantation.

ONGOING CARE

FOLLOW-UP RECOMMENDATIONS

Patient Monitoring

- Acute upper GI tract bleeding or melena requires urgent esophagogastroduodenoscopy (EGD) for bleeding control, frequent Hgb/Hct checks, blood cultures, IV proton pump inhibitor, antibiotics, and possible need for octreotide drip in the ICU setting.
- Morbidity and mortality occurs mainly from variceal bleeding and cholangitis.
- Systemic HTN and kidney function must be monitored.
- Early referral to a hepatologist, nephrologist, and transplant center is indicated in neonatal disease.

DIET

No restrictions are needed unless secondary to renal disease.

PROGNOSIS

- Substantial variability in severity and progression of clinical manifestation exists.
- Those presenting during childhood have better prognosis compared to those presenting within the neonatal period.
- Bleeding from varices is a major cause of morbidity and mortality.
- Ascending cholangitis with resultant sepsis is a major cause of morbidity and mortality. Need for eventual liver +/− kidney transplantation needs to be considered.

COMPLICATIONS

- Portal HTN with hypersplenism and variceal bleeding (chronic, common)
- Cholangitis (acute and recurrent, common [especially with Caroli syndrome])
- Renal and/or hepatic failure
- Associated vascular anomalies in the liver and brain
- Increased risk of hepatocellular or cholangiocarcinoma in adulthood; screening in pediatric population is not warranted.
- Systemic HTN owing to renal involvement

ADDITIONAL READING

- Chandar J, Garcia J, Jorge L, et al. Transplantation in autosomal recessive polycystic kidney disease: liver and/or kidney? *Pediatr Nephrol*. 2015;30(8):1233–1242.
- Ebner K, Schaefer F, Liebau MC, et al. Recent progress of the ARegPKD registry study on autosomal recessive polycystic kidney disease. *Front Pediatr*. 2017;5:18.
- Gunay-Aygun M, Avner ED, Bacallao RL, et al. Autosomal recessive polycystic kidney disease and congenital hepatic fibrosis: summary statement of a first National Institutes of Health/Office of Rare Diseases conference. *J Pediatr*. 2006;149(2):159–164.
- Hartung EA, Guay-Woodford LM. Autosomal recessive polycystic kidney disease: a hepatorenal fibrocystic disorder with pleiotropic effects. *Pediatrics*. 2014;134(3):e833–e845.
- Rawat D, Kelly DA, Milford DV, et al. Phenotypic variation and long-term outcome in children with congenital hepatic fibrosis. *J Pediatr Gastroenterol Nutr*. 2013;57(2):161–166.
- Rock N, McLin V. Liver involvement in children with ciliopathies. *Clin Res Hepatol Gastroenterol*. 2014;38(4):407–414.

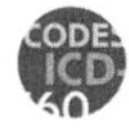

CODES

ICD10

- P78.89 Other specified perinatal digestive system disorders
- K76.6 Portal hypertension
- K83.0 Cholangitis

FAQ

- Q: Will other children of mine be affected?
- A: Maybe. If the inheritance pattern is autosomal recessive, the possibility of having an affected sibling is 1:4.
- Q: Is my child at increased risk if he contracts viral hepatitis?
- A: Yes. The underlying liver disease places these patients at increased risk. They should be immunized against hepatitis A and B.
- Q: If my child has a fever, does she need to be seen by her doctor?
- A: Yes. Patients with CHF who have fever without an obvious source should be evaluated for possible cholangitis and/or UTI, at least by obtaining a blood culture, urine culture, and liver enzymes.

CONGESTIVE HEART FAILURE

Jondavid Menteer, MD

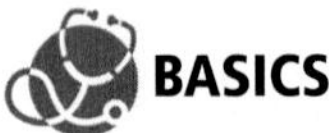

BASICS

DESCRIPTION

- Heart failure (HF) is the pathophysiologic state in which the heart is unable to pump sufficient blood to meet the metabolic demands of the body.
- HF can manifest without cardiac dysfunction (e.g., severe anemia, large arteriovenous malformation [AVM]), but this chapter will concentrate on cardiac causes.
- The most common cardiac causes of HF in pediatric patients include:
  - Congenital heart disease (CHD) with left-to-right shunting, where cardiac performance is normal, but flow is wastefully circular.
  - Congenital causes of LV failure include coarctation of the aorta, aortic stenosis, anomalous coronary origins.
  - Primary cardiomyopathies with inborn issues of structure or function of the myocardium
  - Acute myocarditis
  - Secondary cardiomyopathies due to neuromuscular disease, arrhythmias, history of cardiotoxic chemotherapy, or longstanding renal failure.
- The management of HF in pediatrics is highly specialty-dependent. Immediate pediatric cardiology consultation is important whenever a cardiac cause of HF is suspected.

EPIDEMIOLOGY

- Although minor CHD may occur in up to 5% of live births, CHD manifesting as HF is much rarer, <0.1% of the population.
- Cardiomyopathy (CM) can be divided into:
  - Dilated CM (DCM) (40%)
  - Hypertrophic CM (HCM) (50%) (obstructive or nonobstructive)
  - Restrictive CM (RCM) (<5%)
  - RV cardiomyopathies (<1%) (arrhythmogenic right ventricular dysplasia and Uhl anomaly)
  - Other (5%)

RISK FACTORS

- In utero
  - Arrhythmias: chronic supraventricular or ventricular tachycardia, complete heart block (CHB)
  - Volume overload: atrioventricular (AV) valve regurgitation (e.g., Ebstein anomaly)
  - AVM
  - Primary myocardial disease: CM (dilated, hypertrophic), myocarditis
  - Anemia: Rh isoimmune disease, thalassemia, twin-twin transfusion
  - Premature closure of ductus arteriosus with isolated right ventricular failure
- In neonates
  - Myocardial dysfunction: asphyxia, acidosis, myocarditis, hypoglycemia, CM, ischemia (anomalous left coronary artery from the pulmonary artery), metabolic defects, or pressure overload imposed by aortic stenosis, pulmonary hypertension, or coarctation of the aorta
  - Volume overload: ventricular septal defect (VSD) (large), patent ductus arteriosus (PDA) (large), truncus arteriosus, aortopulmonary window, anomalous pulmonary venous return, AVM in any location
  - Arrhythmias: supraventricular or ventricular tachycardia, CHB
  - Left heart inlet obstruction: mitral stenosis, cor triatriatum, pulmonary venous obstruction
  - Note: Certain cyanotic heart diseases such as hypoplastic left heart syndrome may present with elevated pulmonary blood flow, depressed systemic blood flow, and minimal desaturation. These patients may have HF in the 1st day of life.
- In infants
  - Myocardial dysfunction: CM (any type), metabolic/mitochondrial diseases, myocarditis, Kawasaki disease, anomalous left coronary artery from pulmonary artery, or chronic pressure overload due to coarctation of the aorta or aortic stenosis
  - Volume overload: large atrial septal defect (ASD), VSD, or PDA; common AV canal defect, partial anomalous pulmonary venous connections.
  - Secondary causes: renal disease (volume overload), severe hypertension, hypothyroidism
  - Arrhythmias: supraventricular or ventricular tachycardia, CHB
  - Pericardial effusion/tamponade due to inflammatory diseases, or following heart surgery
- In childhood and adolescence:
  - Repaired heart defects with volume and/or pressure overload (e.g., repaired TOF)
  - Acquired: pericarditis, myocarditis, endocarditis, acute rheumatic fever
  - Cor pulmonale (primary pulmonary hypertension, Eisenmenger syndrome, chronic lung disease)
  - CM due to primary or secondary myocardial disease (dilated, hypertrophic, restrictive, ventricular noncompaction), cancer therapies, neuromuscular disease (e.g., Duchenne or Becker muscular dystrophy)

Genetics

- For about 2/3 of primary cardiomyopathies (not due to metabolic defect or other medical condition), a genetic cause can be identified; higher odds for HCM than DCM
- Examples:
  - HCM: α-tropomysin, troponin T, β-myosin, etc.; Noonan spectrum (RASopathies)
  - DCM: myosin heavy chain, laminin, RYR2, troponin C, more
  - CM with arrhythmia: lamin A/C, desmin
  - Arrhythmogenic right ventricular dysplasia: desmosomal genes and regulators

GENERAL PREVENTION

- Limited use of anthracycline drugs in cancer therapy
- Prompt treatment (within 10 days) of streptococcal pharyngitis to prevent rheumatic fever
- Angiotensin converting enzyme (ACE) inhibitors slow the progression of CM in muscular dystrophy.
- Appropriate endocarditis prophylaxis

ETIOLOGY

- Low cardiac output HF (e.g., all CM, severe AV valve regurgitation)
- High cardiac output HF (left-to-right shunts [e.g., ASD, VSD, PDA], AVM, severe anemia, hyperthyroidism)

DIAGNOSIS

The keys to successful triage of HF are recognition appreciation of its severity, and appropriate referral to appropriate level of care.

- Assessment of degree of illness
- If perfusion is compromised (decreased mentation, somnolence, acidosis, hypotension, abdominal pain, or angina), ICU care is indicated.
- Hospitalization may be necessary to initiate treatment or prepare for surgery (e.g., coronary abnormalities, aortic coarctation).
- Many patients diagnosed as outpatients with CHD or CM, but not in symptomatic HF, may not require inpatient treatment. Immediate consultation with a pediatric cardiologist should be arranged.

HISTORY

- Infants and neonates
  - Prolonged feedings
  - Tachypnea, retractions, or diaphoresis
  - Emesis, inadequate caloric intake, poor growth
  - Orthopnea: "Spoiled baby" becomes distressed when supine.
  - Sweating, especially when supine/sleeping
- Childhood and adolescence
  - Exercise intolerance with exertional dyspnea
  - Palpitations or chest pain, especially during exercise
  - Chronic cough, wheezing, orthopnea, fatigue, weakness, anorexia, nausea, and edema
  - Gradual weight loss (anorexia, nausea, and increased metabolic demands)
  - Sudden weight gain (fluid retention)
  - Family history of HF or sudden unexpected deaths

PHYSICAL EXAM

- General
  - Tachycardia
  - Gallop rhythm
  - Hyperactive precordium, displaced point of maximal impulse; poor pulses (Check all four extremities.)
  - Abdominal or cranial bruit (AVMs)
  - Murmur of outflow obstruction, increased flow, AV valve regurgitation, VSD, or semilunar valve incompetence
  - Manifestations of Kawasaki disease, rheumatic fever, or endocarditis on mucous membranes, skin, and extremities
- Right HF:
  - Hepatomegaly, abdominal distension
  - Jugular venous distension
  - Abnormal second heart sound (fixed split, loud P2 component)
  - Edema (eyes in infants, peripheral for older children)
- Left HF:
  - Tachypnea, wheezing, crackles, rales, nasal flaring, grunting, retractions
  - Pulsus alternans
  - Cool and/or mottled extremities, poor capillary refill
- Tamponade:
  - Dull heart sounds
  - Pulsus paradoxus

DIFFERENTIAL DIAGNOSIS

- Tachycardia
  - Fever
  - Dehydration
  - Anxiety
  - Anemia
  - Supraventricular tachycardia or ventricular tachycardia without HF
  - Hyperthyroidism
  - Pericardial effusion
- Tachypnea
  - Respiratory disease or infection
  - Acidosis (metabolic disease, poisoning)
  - Pneumothorax, pleural effusion
  - Carbon monoxide poisoning

- Edema
  - Hypoalbuminemia
  - Systemic inflammatory conditions/allergies
  - Hypothyroidism
- Sepsis
- Hepatomegaly
  - Liver disease
  - Storage disease
  - Extramedullary hematopoiesis

DIAGNOSTIC TESTS & INTERPRETATION

Diagnostic Procedures/Other

- Chest radiograph
  - Cardiomegaly, pulmonary vascular markings, hyperinflation, effusions
- Electrocardiography
  - Abnormal P waves
  - ST-T wave changes (ischemia, strain, inflammation/myocarditis)
  - Heart block (1st-, 2nd-, 3rd-degree) or tachyarrhythmia
  - Left or right ventricular hypertrophy
  - Disease-specific findings: anomalous left coronary artery from the pulmonary artery (Q waves and inverted T waves in leads I and aVL with ischemic changes), RCM (global strain and biatrial enlargement), pericarditis pattern (diffuse ST segment changes, low voltages), Pompe disease (massive hypertrophy)
- Blood testing: chemistries, blood gas, B-type natriuretic peptide (BNP), creatine kinase level (muscular dystrophies), troponin I (ischemia/infarct), thyroid function, erythrocyte sedimentation rate, C-reactive protein, blood counts.
- Depending on the etiology and degree of HF, echocardiography, Holter monitoring, cardiac magnetic resonance imaging (MRI), metabolic evaluation, cardiac catheterization and/or stress testing may be suggested.
- Echocardiography: Assess anatomy and function.
- Cardiac catheterization (in select cases)
  - Assessment of hemodynamics
  - Endomyocardial biopsy may be helpful in the diagnosis of myocarditis, storage disease, or CM.
- Cardiac MRI or computed tomography (CT) (in select cases)
  - Delineation of complex anatomic relationships
  - Right ventricular performance
  - HCM prognosis markers—perfusion, septal thickness
- Further screening labs:
  - Urine: urinalysis, urine organic acids
  - Metabolic screening—lactate, pyruvate, amino acid quantification, urine organic acids, carnitine, selenium, acylcarnitine profile, liver function tests
  - Suspected myocarditis viral evaluation (adenovirus, coxsackievirus, Epstein-Barr virus, cytomegalovirus, parvovirus, echovirus)

ALERT

Beware the patient with very high BNP level may be extremely unstable. A patient with extremely high BNP should be assessed by a cardiologist immediately, even if HF is chronic.

TREATMENT

GENERAL MEASURES

- Treatment of underlying cause
  - Surgical palliation or correction of CHD
  - Interventional cardiac catheterization (e.g., balloon dilation of aortic or pulmonary stenosis, coil embolization of PDA, device closure of ASD, dilation, or stenting of coarctation of the aorta)
  - Targeted medical treatment of endocarditis, myocarditis, anemia, rheumatic fever, Kawasaki disease, or hypertension
  - Radiofrequency ablation of tachyarrhythmia
  - Medical therapy for patients or mothers of fetuses with tachyarrhythmia
  - Carnitine, coenzyme Q10, riboflavin, per geneticist recommendations for metabolic myopathies
  - Pacing for bradyarrhythmias (e.g., heart block)
  - Control of chronic inflammatory conditions, such as systemic lupus erythematosus or juvenile rheumatoid arthritis
  - Intravenous immunoglobulin (IVIG) for myocarditis or Kawasaki disease
- Immediate/acute management
  - Activity restriction
  - Oxygen to maintain saturation >95%
  - Loop diuretics (e.g., furosemide)
- Emergency department of intensive care unit care:
  - Drainage of pericardial effusion, if needed
  - Inotropic agents (digoxin, milrinone, dobutamine in refractory cases)
  - Nesiritide (synthetic BNP) for refractory fluid overload
  - Mechanical respiratory support
  - Mechanical circulatory support (extracorporeal membrane oxygenation, ventricular assist device)

ALERT

Care must be used in the administration of oxygen to the undiagnosed infant with heart disease. A patient with single-ventricle physiology (e.g., hypoplastic left heart syndrome) can have manifestations of HF and mild desaturation (92–98%). Providing oxygen in this situation can result in shock due to excessive pulmonary blood flow and inadequate systemic blood flow.

- Chronic therapy
  - Antagonism of activated neurohormonal systems: ACE inhibitor or angiotensin receptor blocker, spironolactone, β-blocker
  - Sacubitril/valsartan can replace ACE inhibitor.
  - Loop diuretics (e.g., furosemide) for fluid overload/edema or orthopnea
  - Afterload reduction: ACE inhibitors, or angiotensin receptor blocker; anticoagulation or antiplatelet therapy (especially in restrictive and severe DCM)
  - Digoxin for contractility
  - Biventricular or multisite pacing/resynchronization in some cases
  - HCM: β-blockers, verapamil, disopyramide, surgically treated with septal myectomy for obstruction, or implantable cardioverter-defibrillator for arrhythmia risk.
  - Assess nutrition in chronic cases.
  - Heart transplantation in select cases

ONGOING CARE

FOLLOW-UP RECOMMENDATIONS

- For the patient with new onset HF, immediate cardiology consultation is needed.
- Dependent on the etiology and degree of HF. Generally, initial follow-up of a patient with HF should be intensive, focused on assessing response to therapy. Initial follow-up will be frequent, perhaps even weekly, spreading to monthly or quarterly over time, under the supervision of a pediatric cardiologist.

PATIENT EDUCATION

- Patients with newly recognized HF should be restricted from physical education class and intense physical activity until cleared by a cardiologist. Toddlers and young children are difficult to activity restrict but usually self-limit their activity.
- Warning signs of worsening HF: chronic cough, orthopnea, morning nausea/vomiting, abdominal pain with eating, dyspnea with activity, decreased activity level, chest pain, palpitations, syncope, swelling. These symptoms should prompt an evaluation.

ADDITIONAL READING

- Auerbach SR, Richmond ME, Lamour JM, et al. BNP levels predict outcome in pediatric heart failure patients: post hoc analysis of the Pediatric Carvedilol Trial. *Circ Heart Fail*. 2010;3(5):606–611.
- Kay JD, Colan SD, Graham TP Jr. Congestive heart failure in pediatric patients. *Am Heart J*. 2001;142(5):923–928.
- Kindel SJ, Miller EM, Gupta R, et al. Pediatric cardiomyopathy: importance of genetic and metabolic evaluation. *J Card Fail*. 2012;18(5): 396–403.
- Rosenthal DN. Cardiomyopathy in infants: a brief overview. *Neoreviews*. 2000;1(8):e139–e145.
- Shaddy RE. Optimizing treatment for chronic congestive heart failure in children. *Crit Care Med*. 2001;29(Suppl 10):S237–S240.
- Towbin JA, Bowles JA. The failing heart. *Nature*. 2002;415(10):227–233.

CODES

ICD10

- I50.9 Heart failure, unspecified
- P29.0 Neonatal cardiac failure
- Q23.4 Hypoplastic left heart syndrome

FAQ

- Q: My child has HF. Should I take salt out of his diet?
- A: No. Excessive salt restriction is seldom enforceable and is not necessary. A no-added-salt diet is generally sufficient.
- Q: β-blockers slow the heart rate. Isn't that bad if you already have HF?
- A: True, severe bradycardia may be poorly tolerated in patients with HF and a relatively fixed stroke volume. But chronic sympathetic activation causes progression of HF and β-blockers slow this process.
- Q: What are the major causes of death to HF patients?
- A: Patients may die of progressive HF or arrhythmia. Ventricular arrhythmias are the most common cause of sudden death in older children and adults with cardiomyopathies. Other causes of mortality include infection (causing HF exacerbation) and stroke.
- Q: My patient has a normal blood pressure, but the cardiologist says more ACE inhibition is necessary. Why?
- A: Blood pressure is the weight that the myocardial muscle must "lift" with every beat. Decreasing the blood pressure reduces the work done by the heart and myocardial oxygen consumption. Reduction of the systemic blood pressure also potentially reduces the amount of left-to-right shunting through VSD or PDA.

CONJUNCTIVITIS

Shonul A. Jain, MD

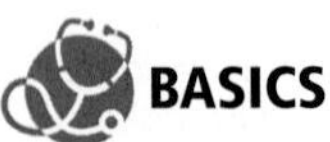

BASICS

DESCRIPTION

An inflammatory process of the conjunctiva, the membrane covering the eye and inside of the eyelids, manifested by erythema and edema, frequently with tearing and discharge. Also known as "pink eye." There is a wide range in severity and many potential causes. It is critical to rule out gonococcus and herpes simplex virus (HSV) infection because of the destructive nature of the eye disease and potential for vision loss.

EPIDEMIOLOGY

- Children: Viral infection is the most common cause and is highly contagious.
- Neonates: Ophthalmia neonatorum, conjunctivitis in the 1st month of life, is the most common infection in neonates. Remains a significant cause of blindness in children worldwide. *Chlamydia trachomatis* is the most common infectious cause.

PATHOPHYSIOLOGY

- Results from bacterial, viral, allergic, or toxic activation of the inflammatory response that causes dilation and exudation from conjunctival blood vessels
- Pathology involves dilated conjunctival capillaries with leukocytic infiltration and edema of conjunctiva and substantia propria.

ETIOLOGY

- Ophthalmia neonatorum
  - If present in the first 24 hours of life, most likely due to chemical irritation from silver nitrate or povidone-iodine (e.g., Wokadine, Betadine) eye drops
  - Gonococcal conjunctivitis is treatable if recognized early but devastating if diagnosis is delayed or missed.
  - Chronic *Chlamydia* infection can lead to scarring and corneal opacity. Chlamydial pneumonia develops in 20% of patients with chlamydial conjunctivitis.
- Bacterial
  - Agents include staphylococci, streptococci, *Haemophilus*, *Moraxella*, and *Pseudomonas*.
  - Serious complications of these are rare.
- Viral
  - Adenovirus is the most common agent.
  - Recurrent HSV infection can lead to significant visual loss from corneal scarring, even with proper therapy.
  - Other viral etiologies usually follow a benign course but rarely can lead to conjunctival scarring.
- Allergic
  - IgE-mediated hypersensitivity response

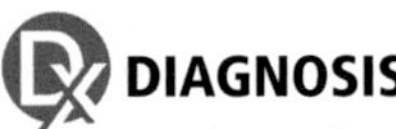

DIAGNOSIS

HISTORY

- Ophthalmia neonatorum
  - Gonococcus: typically presents 2 to 4 days after birth with mucopurulent discharge
  - *Chlamydia*: typically presents 4 to 14 days after birth with mucopurulent discharge
- Bacterial
  - Eye redness, mucopurulent discharge, eye edema. Patient complain of sticky eyelids upon waking with discharge that continues throughout the day. Mild photophobia and discomfort may be present but are typically not painful; often unilateral but can be bilateral
- Viral
  - HSV ocular infection may present as conjunctivitis; often associated with corneal anesthesia, so can be painless. In neonates, it occurs 1 to 2 weeks after birth as unilateral serous discharge and conjunctival injection.
  - Other viral causes often present similar to bacterial infection with eye redness, tearing, serous discharge, eyelid edema. Eyes may be sticky upon waking but discharge tends to be more serous during the day. Typically begins in one eye but spreads to the other within a few days. History of URI symptoms or similar infection in siblings or contacts is common.
- Allergic
  - Bilateral itching and tearing; classically, a complaint of itching or foreign body sensation in an older child with red eyes

PHYSICAL EXAM

- General
  - Cornea is clear.
  - Vision, pupils, and ocular motility are normal.
  - Red flags (refer to an ophthalmologist): reduction in visual acuity, vesicular rash on eyelids, limbic injection, or corneal changes, as the condition may be caused by HSV and can be vision threatening
- Bacterial
  - Wide range of clinical presentation, from mild hyperemia to significant injection and mucopurulent discharge (opaque and thick)
  - Injected conjunctiva, episcleral vessels, palpebral conjunctival papillae
  - Preauricular lymphadenopathy less common
- Viral
  - HSV ocular infection may involve corneal ulceration or dendritic or disciform keratitis.
  - Serous discharge (clear and watery)
  - May involve pseudomembrane formation, pinpoint subconjunctival hemorrhages, and palpable preauricular lymph nodes
- Allergic
  - Bilateral conjunctival edema and chemosis

ALERT

- Failure to diagnose gonococcal conjunctivitis may lead to corneal perforation or visual loss.
- HSV ocular infection is associated with a significant risk of blindness; have high suspicion for HSV with any recurrent unilateral eye redness, decrease in visual acuity, corneal changes, or vesicular rash on eyelids
- Corticosteroids can activate or accelerate unrecognized HSV infection, and chronic use can lead to raised intraocular pressure or cataract formation.
- Chronic use of empiric broad-spectrum antibiotics for self-limited conjunctivitis can promote bacterial resistance, although less so than for systemic antibiotic administration.

DIFFERENTIAL DIAGNOSIS

- Ophthalmia neonatorum
  - Chemical conjunctivitis: noninfectious, mild, self-limited; result of silver nitrate or povidone-iodine administration
  - Birth trauma: often unilateral subconjunctival hemorrhage, may have associated eyelid contusion, history of forceps use or difficult delivery
  - Congenital glaucoma: mild redness, minimal discharge. Look for enlarged eye, cloudy cornea, tearing, and photophobia.
  - Nasolacrimal duct obstruction: unilateral or bilateral discharge, may be clear to mucopurulent with reflux from nasolacrimal sac. Conjunctiva is usually noninjected.
- All conjunctivitis
  - Preseptal cellulitis: early eyelid edema/erythema; looks like conjunctivitis, especially in young children with a difficult exam. Motility deficit, proptosis, decreased vision, and afferent pupillary defect are consistent with orbital cellulitis.
  - Foreign body
  - Blepharitis: inflammation of eyelids, history of gritty/burning sensation, excessive tearing, significant eyelid swelling
  - Corneal abrasion: history of pain, associated trauma; significant tearing, photophobia, erythema. Diagnose with fluorescein and blue light.
  - Keratitis: signifies corneal infection; may have associated conjunctivitis. Primary herpes keratitis is associated with vesicular eyelid rash and pain. Consult an ophthalmologist. Bacterial keratitis may be caused by staphylococci, streptococci, and *Pseudomonas*; Lyme spirochete; or vitamin A deficiency.
  - Episcleritis: inflammation of the thick loose connective tissue between the clear conjunctiva and the white-appearing stroma of the sclera; rare disease in childhood; can be associated with rheumatologic disease
  - Scleritis: presents as red eye; severe disease involving inflammation of the sclera; rare in childhood; associated with systemic disease; requires oral or IV steroids
  - Iritis/uveitis: frequently unilateral, with or without a history of trauma; photophobia, decreased vision, and constant pain (except if associated with juvenile rheumatoid arthritis). Contagious history is rare. Consult an ophthalmologist for full evaluation, including pupillary dilation.
- Systemic diseases with red eye
  - Varicella: ocular involvement in rare cases. Treat with antiviral medications.
  - Stevens-Johnson syndrome: secondary to viruses, mycoplasma, or adverse drug reaction. Mucous membrane involvement may lead to conjunctival bullae with risk of rupture and subsequent scarring.
  - Kawasaki disease: acute vasculitis. Classic symptoms include fever $\times$ 5 days, plus four out of five of the following: bilateral, limbic-sparing nonexudative conjunctivitis; oropharyngeal changes (including strawberry tongue); cervical adenopathy; polymorphous rash; and extremity changes/swelling of palms and soles with peeling around nail beds.
  - Measles: presents with fever, rash, cough coryza, and conjunctivitis
  - Cat-scratch disease: Parinaud syndrome includes granulomatous conjunctivitis and adenopathy.
  - Reactive arthritis triad: large joint inflammatory arthritis, conjunctivitis or uveitis, and urethritis in men or cervicitis in women

DIAGNOSTIC TESTS & INTERPRETATION

Initial Tests (screening, lab, imaging)

- Diagnosis tends to be clinical; cultures are not generally used even by ophthalmology except in cases of ophthalmia neonatorum.
- Gram stain
  - Gonococcus: gram-negative intracellular diplococcus
  - *Chlamydia*: intracytoplasmic, paranuclear inclusion bodies on Gram stain and conjunctival scraping with Giemsa stain for basophilic intracytoplasmic inclusion bodies
  - Viral or chemical: polymorphonuclear leukocytes without bacteria
- Culture
  - Viral: Cultures for HSV and adenovirus are not clinically useful.
  - Bacterial: blood agar and chocolate agar
  - Gonococcus: Thayer-Martin media
  - *Chlamydia*: Culture techniques are not widely available. However, they remain the gold standard for diagnosis. Specimens should be obtained using an aluminum-shafted Dacron-tipped swab and processed within 24 hours. A positive test is confirmed when the organism is identified using fluorescein-conjugated monoclonal antibody. Other equally effective methods involve polymerase chain reaction or direct fluorescent antibody.
- Conjunctival scrapings
  - Allergic: mast cells and eosinophils
- Serum tests
  - Allergic: IgE may be elevated.
  - *Chlamydia*: The diagnosis of chlamydial pneumonia can be made with a serum test but is not reliable for chlamydial conjunctivitis.

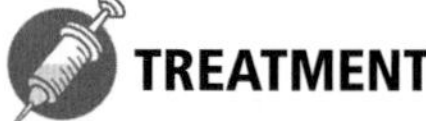

TREATMENT

GENERAL MEASURES

- Ophthalmia neonatorum
  - Hospitalization for suspected gonococcal conjunctivitis for workup for sepsis
  - For suspected chlamydial infection, topical and oral therapy is usually appropriate.
- Bacterial
  - Usually self-limited, but treatment may help shorten course and prevent spread of infection. Contact lens users should remove lenses until infection clears and consider use of fluoroquinolone.
- Viral
  - Suspected HSV warrants hospitalization for IV antiviral therapy.
  - For suspected adenovirus, children should stay home from school until discharge is minimal and discomfort has subsided; cool compresses for comfort
- Allergic
  - Remove/avoid offending allergen if possible.
  - Mild symptoms can be treated with preservative-free artificial tears. Consider topical or systemic antiallergy medicine if symptoms persist.
  - Consider treating other atopic conditions which are often present.
- Chemical
  - Close observation only. Remove offending agent; self-limited

MEDICATION

- Ophthalmia neonatorum
  - Gonococcus: ceftriaxone, 25 to 50 mg/kg/dose (max 125 mg) IV or IM as a single dose and ocular irrigation followed by topical 0.5% erythromycin ophthalmic ointment q.i.d. for 14 days. Also treat for *Chlamydia*.
  - *Chlamydia*: oral erythromycin suspension, 12.5 mg/kg/dose q6h for 14 days. Topical 0.5% erythromycin ophthalmic ointment q.i.d. both eyes for 14 days as above. (Povidone-iodine 1.25% ophthalmic drops q.i.d. can be used if other antibiotics are not readily available.)
  - Important to treat both of these conditions systemically as well as topically
- Bacterial
  - Often self-limited; however, studies have shown empiric antibiotic treatment can shorten duration of symptoms and reduce transmission.
  - Treatment includes erythromycin ointment or polymyxin-trimethoprim drops. Alternatives include bacitracin or sulfacetamide 10% ointment, fluoroquinolone drops, or azithromycin drops.
- Viral
  - Herpes simplex: topical trifluorothymidine (Viroptic solution), 1 drop q2h while awake (max 9 drops/24 h) until reepithelialization of ulcer and then 1 drop q4h for 7 days (do not exceed 21 days of treatment) with or without systemic acyclovir
  - Topical glucocorticoid therapy is contraindicated.
  - Other viral: over-the-counter antihistamine or decongestant drops for symptom relief; may also use nonantibiotics eye lubricating drops for comfort
- Allergic
  - Topical antihistamine/mast cell stabilizers such as olopatadine (0.1% strength dosed at 1 drop to affected eye[s] b.i.d., and 0.2% and 0.7% strengths dosed at 1 drop once daily) are effective for acute symptoms in more involved cases. Side effects include increased ocular dryness.
  - Consider systemic antiallergic therapies such as oral antihistamines.

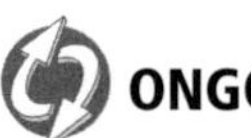

ONGOING CARE

FOLLOW-UP RECOMMENDATIONS

Patient Monitoring

- Daily follow-up is necessary for gonococcus, *Chlamydia*, and HSV.
- No office follow-up is recommended for routine conjunctivitis as long as symptoms resolve.
- Follow atypical conjunctivitis closely until a more serious disease can be excluded.
- A nonresponsive or worsening condition needs ophthalmic consultation.

COMPLICATIONS

- Significant complications are extremely rare for common bacterial, viral, or allergic conjunctivitis.
- Blindness may result from untreated neonatal conjunctivitis or from HSV ocular infection.

ADDITIONAL READING

- American Academy of Ophthalmology. *Conjunctivitis. Preferred Practice Pattern*. San Francisco, CA: American Academy of Ophthalmology; 2013.
- Azari AA, Barney NP. Conjunctivitis: a systematic review of diagnosis and treatment. *JAMA*. 2013;310(16):1721–1729.
- Bielory L, Mongia A. Current opinion of immunotherapy for ocular allergy. *Curr Opin Allergy Clin Immunol*. 2002;2(5):447–452.
- Brook I. Ocular infections due to anaerobic bacteria in children. *J Pediatr Ophthalmol Strabismus*. 2008;45(2):78–84.
- Credé CSF. Reports from the obstetrical clinic in Leipzig. Prevention of eye inflammation in the newborn. *Am J Dis Child*. 1971;121(1):3–4.
- Greenberg MF, Pollard ZF. The red eye in childhood. *Pediatr Clin North Am*. 2003;50(1):105–124.
- Hillenkamp J, Reinhard T, Ross RS, et al. The effects of cidofovir 1% with and without cyclosporin a 1% as a topical treatment of acute adenoviral keratoconjunctivitis: a controlled clinical pilot study. *Ophthalmology*. 2002;109(5):845–850.
- Rietveld RP, van Weert HC, ter Riet G, et al. Diagnostic impact of signs and symptoms in acute infectious conjunctivitis: systematic literature search. *BMJ*. 2003;327(7418):789.
- Sethuraman U, Kamat D. The red eye: evaluation and management. *Clin Pediatr (Phila)*. 2009;48(6):588–600.
- Sheikh A, Hurwitz B, van Schayck CP, et al. Antibiotics versus placebo for acute bacterial conjunctivitis. *Cochrane Database Syst Rev*. 2012:(9):CD001211.
- Strauss EC, Foster CS. Atopic ocular disease. *Ophthalmol Clin North Am*. 2002;15(1):1–5.
- Trocme SD, Sra KK. Spectrum of ocular allergy. *Curr Opin Allergy Clin Immunol*. 2002;2(5):423–427.

CODES

ICD10

- H10.9 Unspecified conjunctivitis
- B30.9 Viral conjunctivitis, unspecified
- P39.1 Neonatal conjunctivitis and dacryocystitis

FAQ

- Q: Is conjunctivitis contagious?
- A: All infectious conjunctivitis is contagious but to varying degrees. Viral or epidemic keratoconjunctivitis (EKC) is the most contagious. Careful handling of secretions, tissues, towels, and bed linens and strict hand washing usually prevent spread. Wipe surfaces with isopropyl alcohol or dilute bleach to prevent recontamination. Gonococcus, *Chlamydia*, and HSV can be transmitted through infected discharge or secretions, but this is less common. The most common source is the infected birth canal.
- Q: Should the patient with "pink eye" (non-gonococcus, non-*Chlamydia*, non-HSV conjunctivitis) be treated with empiric antibiotics?
- A: There is some benefit to empiric antibiotic treatment in bacterial conjunctivitis but not in viral or allergic etiologies. Practically, it is often difficult to distinguish viral and bacterial conjunctivitis based on symptoms alone, and return to school is often contingent on initiation of antibiotic therapy. Providers should be aware that empiric treatment with topical antibiotics can cause harm in the case of sulfa-containing compounds. Antibiotic toxicity, including Stevens-Johnson reactions, can occur from sulfa antibiotics, and use of antibiotics long term promotes selection of resistant strains of bacteria. Empiric treatment also increases manipulation of the infected eye and thus increases the risk of spread.
- Q: How long is the patient with pink eye (non-gonococcus, non-*Chlamydia*, non-HSV conjunctivitis) contagious, and when can the patient return to school?
- A: The organism can be recovered from the eye for up 2 weeks after onset of symptoms, demonstrating that patients are infectious during this time. Practically, children should probably be kept out of school at least 24 hours after onset of therapy, if indicated, ideally until discharge is minimal and discomfort has subsided.

CONSTIPATION

Jay Fong, MD

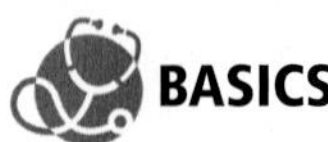

BASICS

DESCRIPTION

Delay or difficulty in defecation; infrequent (<2) stools per week; defecation resulting in pain and/or rectal bleeding, and/or fecal soiling; may also refer to a decrease in frequency of bowel movements compared with the patient's usual bowel pattern

GENERAL PREVENTION

- Maintain adequate fluid intake.
- Consume a high-fiber diet with fruits and vegetables.
- Avoid excessive caffeine and milk (calcium) intake.
- Engage in regular physical activity.

PATHOPHYSIOLOGY

- Delay in colonic passage and/or retention of stool allows fluids mixed in stool to be resorbed across cellular membranes, increasing stool caliber and leading it to be harder in consistency.
- Decreased motility leads to a buildup of desiccated stool causing painful defecation, which is a risk factor for ongoing stool retention.
- As the rectosigmoid enlarges over time with retained stool, a child's ability to sense rectal fullness diminishes, and he or she may not appreciate the need to defecate.
- Often, there is a family history of motility disturbances or constipation.

ETIOLOGY

- Most patients have idiopathic or functional constipation with no identifiable cause.
- Personal history of constipation may be traceable to an acute event (i.e., passage of large, painful stool) followed by chronicity.
- Intentional or unintentional withholding of stool may result in hard stools, anal pain, and fissures that perpetuate and lead to constipation. Rectal dilatation, decreased sensation of the urge to defecate, shortening of the anal canal, decreased tone of the external anal sphincter, and encopresis can result.
- Precipitating events may include the following:
  - Transition from breast milk to cow's milk
  - Excessive cow's milk intake
  - Insufficient water intake
  - Refusal to use toilets outside the home
  - Premature toilet training
  - Perianal streptococcal infection
  - Food allergies
  - Transient viral illness (diarrhea followed by constipation)
- Constipation also can be caused by anatomic anomalies in the lower GI tract, decreased propulsion, increased rectal sensitivity threshold, a functional outlet obstruction (muscular spastic levator ani or impaired relaxation of the puborectalis).
- Neurologic causes:
  - Abnormalities of the myenteric plexus
  - Intestinal pseudoobstruction
  - Congenital aganglionosis (Hirschsprung disease)
  - Nonrelaxing internal anal sphincter
  - Visceral neuropathies
  - Visceral myopathies
  - Familial dysautonomia
- Lesions of the spinal cord can result in loss of rectal tone and sensation and reduced anal closure, affecting the sacral reflex center (e.g., meningocele, myelomeningocele, tethered cord, schwannoma).
- Anatomic disorders of anus and rectum (stricture, stenosis, mass, ectopic anus, imperforate anus, fistula)
- Endocrine abnormalities (hypothyroidism), drugs, and electrolyte abnormalities

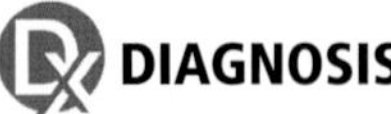

DIAGNOSIS

HISTORY

- **Question:** What was the timing after birth of passage of meconium?
- *Significance*: If it is delayed for >48 hours, consider Hirschsprung disease.
- **Question:** Is the child able to pass a bowel movement unaided by a suppository or enema?
- *Significance*: If rectal stimulation is required for passage of a bowel movement, consider Hirschsprung disease or habituation to rectal stimulation.
- **Question:** What are the size, frequency, and consistency of bowel movements?
- *Significance*: 1 to 3 normal (in size and consistency), painless bowel movements may be passed every 1 to 3 days. The size of bowel movements reflects the caliber of the colon.
- **Question:** Does the child experience frequent urination, bed-wetting, or urinary tract infections?
- *Significance*: Chronic UTIs are frequently linked to chronic constipation.
- **Question:** Does fecal soiling occur?
- *Significance*: Soiling occurs with stool impaction or with nerve damage involving the anus.
- **Question:** Is there the presence of rectal sensation?
- *Significance*: Patients with long-standing constipation or stool withholding may develop a dilated rectum and lose the sensation of rectal distention.
- **Question:** Is there a history of painful bowel movements or rectal fissure?
- *Significance*: Pain with defecation and/or fissuring can further lead to withholding secondary to fear of painful bowel movements.
- **Question:** Is the child experiencing any stressful events (i.e., new sibling, family death)?
- *Significance*: Stress can precipitate stool withholding.
- **Question:** Is there an unsteady gait?
- *Significance*: This may suggest neuromuscular problems.
- **Question:** Did the child experience difficult toilet training?
- *Significance*: May be associated with encopresis

PHYSICAL EXAM

- General: Look for evidence of systemic illness and alarm signals: weight loss, anorexia, delayed growth, delayed passage of meconium, urinary incontinence, passage of bloody stools (in the absence of anal fissure), fever, vomiting, and diarrhea.
- Abdomen: abdominal distention (indicative of the presence of stool or gas), presence of stool masses (size, location), distended bladder, and bowel sounds (may be decreased in intestinal pseudoobstruction)
- Rectal examination
  - Perianal soiling
  - Size and position of anus (Evaluate for signs of imperforate, stenosed, or ectopic anus.)
  - Presence of skin tags and fissures (can contribute to pain with defecation; may indicate Crohn disease)
  - Perianal or anal erythema (streptococcal proctitis)
- Evidence of child abuse
- Digital examination is not routinely recommended and should not be used to diagnose functional constipation. If suspicious for other etiologies, a digital exam can be used to assess anal tone (long and tight anal canal in Hirschsprung), amount and consistency of stool, size of rectum (dilated rectum with chronic constipation, tight and empty anus with Hirschsprung disease), presence of blood.
- Absence of anal wink or cremasteric reflex suggests neurologic abnormalities.
- Neurologic examination: decreased reflexes in the lower extremities
- Back: Check for sacral dimple, tuft of hair (underlying sacral abnormality), flat buttocks, and patulous anus.

ALERT

- Grunting baby syndrome: Infants cry, scream, and draw up their legs during a bowel movement. They respond to rectal distention by contracting their pelvic floor. This is not constipation.
- Always rule out an organic cause.
- Always consider medications as a cause.

DIFFERENTIAL DIAGNOSIS

- Celiac disease (more likely in younger children)
- Hypothyroidism, hypercalcemia, hypokalemia
- Diabetes mellitus
- Dietary protein allergy
- Drugs, toxics:
  - Opiates, anticholinergics, antidepressants, chemotherapy, and heavy metal ingestion (lead)
- Vitamin D intoxication
- Botulism
- Cystic fibrosis
- Hirschsprung disease
- Anal achalasia
- Colonic inertia
- Anatomic malformations (imperforate anus, anal stenosis)
- Pelvic mass (sacrococcygeal teratoma)
- Spinal cord anomalies, trauma, tethered cord
- Abnormal abdominal musculature (prune belly, gastroschisis, Down syndrome)
- Pseudoobstruction
- Multiple endocrine neoplasia type 2B

DIAGNOSTIC TESTS & INTERPRETATION

Initial Tests (screening, lab, imaging)

- Testing for possible underlying thyroid disease and/or celiac disease may be recommended in patients with likely functional constipation with alarm symptoms. Patients with a personal or family history of atopy may be screened for suspected and/or common food allergies (i.e., milk, soy, egg, wheat). Other lab testing is not routinely recommended.
- Abdominal radiography:
  - May demonstrate presence or absence of fecal impaction
  - Should not be used routinely for the evaluation and diagnosis of functional constipation

- Water-soluble contrast enema:
  - An unprepped study is useful to diagnose Hirschsprung disease.
  - A prepped study is useful to diagnose a stricture.
  - Most patients with constipation will not require this test, especially those with functional constipation.

Diagnostic Procedures/Other

- Measurement of abdominal transit time with radio-opaque markers may help discriminate between children with and without clinical constipation, but evidence does not support its routine use in diagnosis.
- Anorectal manometry: analyzes rectal sensation, resting and squeezing pressures, and pelvic floor dyssynergia (anismus)

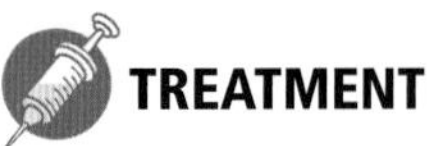

TREATMENT

GENERAL MEASURES

- Treatment of functional constipation:
  - Disimpaction
    - The use of polyethylene glycol (PEG) (e.g., MiraLAX® or other generics) with or without electrolytes orally at 1 to 1.5 g/kg/24 h for 3 to 6 days is recommended as first line for children presenting with impaction.
    - If the patient is not tolerating PO, or PEG unavailable, enemas may be needed for initial disimpaction.

ALERT

Multiple phosphate enemas can cause severe electrolyte imbalances (hyponatremia, hypokalemia, hypocalcemia, hypomagnesemia).

- Children >2 to 3 years of age require adult-size enemas, whereas younger children require pediatric-size enemas. Enemas can be given once per day for 3 to 6 days.
  - Evacuation
    - Following rectal disimpaction, further evacuation can be achieved by using PEG solution (GoLytely®), orally or via nasogastric tube over 6 to 8 hours until the effluent is clear.
  - Maintenance stool softeners
    - Infants ≤6 months of age may be given sorbitol- or pectin-containing juices (i.e., prune, pear) (1/2 to 1 oz 1 to 2 times per day dilute 1:1 with breast milk, formula, or water), lactulose (0.7 to 2 g/kg/24 h [1 to 3 mL/kg/24 h], max 40 g/24 h [60 mL/24 h]), or Karo syrup (>1 month old: 5 to 10 mL once daily; dark Karo syrup may not be effective).
    - Children >6 months of age may be given lactulose (0.7 to 2 g/kg/24 h [1 to 3 mL/kg/24 h], max 40 g/24 h [60 mL/24 h]) or MiraLAX (0.5 to 1 g/kg, max 17 g/24 h).
    - Mineral oil or Kondremul (>15 months of age 1 to 3 mL/24 h, >6 years 10 to 25 mL/24 h) is added as an adjunctive lubricant to aid in the passage of stool but contraindicated in children <15 months as well as in children at risk for aspiration.
    - Maintenance treatment should continue for at least 2 months with all symptoms of constipation resolved at least 1 month before discontinuation of treatment, which should be decreased gradually.
- Rescue stimulant laxatives:
  - Bisacodyl or senna may be used as a stimulant laxative for short period of time. Long-term use has been associated with colonic nerve damage in adults.
- Diet: A balanced diet of whole grains, fruits, and vegetables is recommended. A normal-fiber diet is recommended (toddler 14 g/24 h; school-aged 17 to 25 g/24 h; adolescent 25 to 31 g/24 h). Fiber should be increased gradually to minimize side effects of flatulence. Caffeine and excessive milk-product intake (>16 oz/24 h of milk) may be constipating.
- Fluid intake: Normal fluid intake is important.
- Toilet sitting: Regular toilet sitting (1 min/year of age to a maximum of 10 minutes) 1 to 2 times per day (ideally after a meal, tailored to the age of the child). Calendar: It is important to keep a record of stools, accidents, toilet sitting, and medications in order to identify causes of failure.
- Biofeedback has not been shown to be helpful in patients who fail conventional therapy and who have abnormalities on anorectal manometry.
- There may be some benefit in referring a patient with constipation and behavioral abnormalities to a cognitive behavioral psychologist or other mental health professional with expertise in childhood constipation.

ONGOING CARE

FOLLOW-UP RECOMMENDATIONS

- Schedule regular visits to make certain therapy is maintained, decreasing the frequency of visits when patient is doing well.
- Parents should be encouraged to call when problems develop.
- Compliance and good follow-up are key to successful management of constipation.

PROGNOSIS

For functional constipation, the success rate is variable (45–90%). Presence of abdominal pain at the time of presentation, close follow-up, and maintenance use of stool softeners are good prognostic factors. Presence of soiling, use of stimulant laxatives, and lack of follow-up were associated with failure.

COMPLICATIONS

- Anal fissures: Infrequent hard stools can cause a tear of the anal mucosa, causing pain and withholding.
- Encopresis: Chronic constipation leads to progressive rectal dilatation and decreased rectal sensation. Fecal impaction results in secondary soiling or encopresis (see "Encopresis").
- Intestinal obstruction: manifests as vomiting, abdominal pain, and constipation. Abdominal radiograph films show intestinal obstruction and presence of large amounts of stool.
- Sigmoid volvulus: A chronically constipated child may present with symptoms of acute abdomen, fever, tender abdomen, and palpable mass. Abdominal radiograph shows obstruction in the colon. Barium enema may be both diagnostic and therapeutic by achieving reduction.
- Treatment of complications:
  - Encopresis (soiling or diarrhea): Disimpaction and clean out as necessary, followed by treatment of constipation, is recommended (see previous discussion).
  - Intestinal obstruction from fecal mass: Presents with vomiting, abdominal pain, and constipation. Abdominal radiograph film shows intestinal obstruction. Make NPO, provide IV fluids, and rule out an acute abdomen. Then give enemas and clear out stool from below. Avoid oral laxatives or a PEG solution in a case of obstruction.
  - Sigmoid volvulus: Chronically constipated child with symptoms of acute abdomen, fever, tender abdomen, and palpable mass. Abdominal radiograph shows obstruction in the colon. Contrast enema may reveal and possibly reduce a volvulus.

ADDITIONAL READING

- Bekkali NLH, van den Berg MM, Dijkgraaf MGW, et al. Rectal fecal impaction treatment in childhood constipation: enemas versus high doses oral PEG. *Pediatrics*. 2009;124(6):e1108–e1115.
- Croffie JM, Fitzgerald J. Idiopathic constipation. In: Walker WA, Kleinman RE, Sherman PM, et al, eds. *Pediatric Gastrointestinal Disease*. 4th ed. Philadelphia, PA: BC Decker; 2004:1000–1055.
- Hyman PE, Milla PJ, Benninga MA, et al. Childhood functional gastrointestinal disorder: neonate/toddler. *Gastroenterology*. 2006;130(5):1519–1526.
- Rasquin A, Di Lorenzo C, Forbes D, et al. Childhood functional gastrointestinal disorders: child/adolescent. *Gastroenterology*. 2006;130(5):1527–1537.
- Tabbers MM, DiLorenzo C, Berger MY, et al. Evaluation and treatment of functional constipation in infants and children: evidenced-based recommendations from ESPGHAN and NASPGHAN. *J Pediatr Gastroenterol Nutr*. 2014;58(2):265–281.
- U.S. Department of Health and Human Services. Dietary guidelines for Americans, 2010. http://www.health.gov/dietaryguidelines/2010.asp. Accessed March 1, 2015.

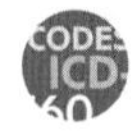

CODES

ICD10

- K59.00 Constipation, unspecified
- K59.09 Other constipation
- K59.02 Outlet dysfunction constipation

FAQ

- Q: When is constipation an emergency?
- A: When intestinal obstruction, sigmoid volvulus, or Hirschsprung enterocolitis occurs.
- Q: Does polyethylene glycol-3350 taste bad?
- A: Advantages of polyethylene glycol-3350 include its lack of taste, smell, or odor and that it can be mixed in any liquid.
- Q: What is the overall prognosis of functional constipation in children?
- A: 50% of patients referred to pediatric gastroenterologists will recover and be without laxatives after 6 to 12 months. Approximately 10% do well taking laxatives and 40% will still be symptomatic despite being on treatment. 80% of children with functional constipation are generally recovered at 10 years.

CONTACT DERMATITIS

Jocelyn Huang Schiller, MD • Brittany B. Allen, MD

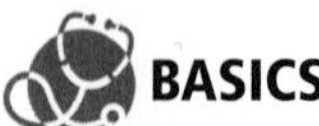

BASICS

DESCRIPTION

An acute or chronic inflammation of the dermis and epidermis as result of either direct irritation to the skin (irritant contact dermatitis) or delayed-type (type IV) hypersensitivity reaction to a contact allergen (allergic contact dermatitis)

EPIDEMIOLOGY

Incidence

Incidence in children is not known.

Prevalence

- Irritant contact dermatitis: Most cases of contact dermatitis (>80%) are due to irritants.
  - Skin reactivity is highest in infants and tends to decrease with age.
- Allergic contact dermatitis
  - Because children have less time to develop sensitivities, it is less common in infants and children than in adults.
  - Prevalence increases with age.
  - Overall prevalence is ~13–23% and has been increasing in children, perhaps due to more frequent exposure to allergens at a younger age or improved diagnosis.
  - Contact sensitization may complicate the course in >40% of patients with atopic dermatitis.

RISK FACTORS

- Irritant contact dermatitis
  - Frequent hand washing or water immersion
  - Atopic dermatitis: Chronically impaired barrier function increases susceptibility to irritants.
  - Genetic factors
  - Environmental factors such as cold/hot temperatures or high/low humidity disrupt the skin barrier.
- Allergic contact dermatitis
  - Atopic dermatitis
  - Skin barrier disruption from injuries or wounds
  - Genetic factors
  - Increased exposure to allergens

GENERAL PREVENTION

Minimize contact exposure to known or potential irritants and allergens and maintain the barrier function of the skin.

PATHOPHYSIOLOGY

- Irritant contact dermatitis does not involve an immune response and thus can occur with the first exposure to the irritant. Multiple mechanisms are involved, including:
  - Direct damage to keratinocytes by chemicals (soaps, detergents) or physical irritants (moisture, friction) with resulting disruption of the epidermal barrier and localized release of proinflammatory cytokines
  - Chronic exposure may stimulate cell proliferation, resulting in acanthosis and hyperkeratosis with postinflammatory hypo- or hyperpigmentation.
- Allergic contact dermatitis requires initial exposure and sensitization to an allergen and only occurs in susceptible individuals. Repeated exposure leads to the development of a type IV hypersensitivity reaction resulting in proliferation of sensitized T lymphocytes.
  - Strong antigens may require only one exposure, whereas weaker antigens may require multiple.
  - Exposure can occur transepidermally or systemically.
- Both processes result in nonspecific findings of dermal and epidermal edema and inflammation and may be indistinguishable from other forms of inflammatory dermatitis.

ETIOLOGY

- Irritant contact dermatitis
  - Frequent hand washing or water immersion
  - Soaps and detergents
  - Saliva (lip licking or thumb sucking)
  - Urine and feces (see "Diaper Rash")
  - High concentrations of most chemicals can induce irritant contact dermatitis, whereas mild irritants may induce inflammation only in susceptible individuals.
- Allergic contact dermatitis
  - Nickel and other metals (gold, cobalt)
  - Hair products (ammonium, 5-diamine)
  - Solvents (toluene-2)
  - Cleansers, shampoos (cocamidopropyl betaine)
  - Additives to medications, cosmetics (thimerosal, mercuric chloride)
  - Rubber
  - Fragrances (balsam of Peru [BOP])
  - Dyes (cobalt, potassium dichromate, black henna)
  - Formaldehydes
  - Topical antibiotics (neomycin, bacitracin)
  - Topical corticosteroids
  - Emollient components (lanolin alcohol)
  - Plants (*Toxicodendron* species; e.g., poison ivy, poison oak, and poison sumac, which contain the allergen urushiol)

COMMONLY ASSOCIATED CONDITIONS

Atopic dermatitis or other chronic dermatoses

DIAGNOSIS

HISTORY

- Patients may present with either acute or chronic localized, pruritic dermatitis.
- Patients should be asked about all chemicals, potential irritants, or allergens to which they are intermittently or frequently exposed.
- Many patients are unable to associate a specific allergen with symptom development.
- Timing of symptoms
  - Irritant contact dermatitis: immediate inflammation
  - Allergic contact dermatitis: inflammation 48 to 72 hours, but occasionally longer, after exposure. Two or more exposures may be required to trigger reaction.
- Location of skin changes may provide clues, as reactions are typically localized to the areas that come in contact with the allergen.

PHYSICAL EXAM

- Irritant contact dermatitis
  - Acute: ranges from mild skin dryness and mild erythema to erythematous papules and patches, edema, vesicles, and oozing; in severe cases, may result in a chemical burn (skin necrosis)
  - Chronic: erythema, dryness, lichenification, hyperkeratosis, and cracking
  - A perioral rash often signifies an irritant contact dermatitis from lip licking.
- Allergic contact dermatitis
  - Acute: pruritus, erythema, and edema with vesicles or bullae that often rupture, leaving a crust
  - Chronic: lichenification, erythema, scaling
- Often an unusual pattern or distribution that correlates with pattern of exposure (e.g., a linear pattern as patient brushes against poison ivy, round lesion on abdomen where skin contacts nickel button on jeans)
- Can have activation of dermatitis at distant, prior sites of exposure
- Autoeczematization or "id" reaction: A more generalized dermatitis may develop distal to the original site of contact one or more weeks after the initial localized dermatitis.

DIFFERENTIAL DIAGNOSIS

- Infection
  - Impetigo and cellulitis: Bacterial infections of the skin (*Staphylococcus aureus* or group A *Streptococcus*) may manifest as erythematous, edematous, crusted patches and plaques. Pustules and/or deep-seated inflammatory nodules may be present. Infection is usually associated more with pain and tenderness than with pruritus.
  - Fungal infection: KOH examination can clarify the diagnosis.
  - Scabies: intensely pruritic papules and nodules with a predilection for the hands and feet (especially the web spaces), the axillae, and the groin. Close contacts are often affected.
  - Herpes simplex virus may present with vesicles but is less erythematous and pruritic and more painful.
- Metabolic
  - Acrodermatitis enteropathica: a genetic or acquired zinc deficiency with characteristic bullae and erosions involving hands, feet, and periorificial areas (perioral, periocular, and perineal); associated with failure to thrive, diarrhea, and alopecia
- Immunologic
  - Atopic dermatitis: may favor the face and extremities or occur more diffusely with truncal involvement; usually spares diaper, perinasal, and periocular areas; usually symmetric; associated with erythematous, excoriated, and crusted papules, patches, and plaques and with chronic pruritus, often worse at night; often accompanied by a personal or family history of atopy. Skin breakdown from atopic dermatitis may predispose to contact dermatitis, and contact dermatitis may trigger an atopic dermatitis flare.
  - Fixed drug reaction: cutaneous drug reaction that recurs in the same locations with reexposure. Well-demarcated round red-brown macules, usually solitary lesions; frequently seen with NSAIDs, sulfas, penicillins, tetracyclines, acetaminophen, and barbiturates
  - Seborrheic dermatitis: usually affects infants <1 year of age or adolescents; erythema and greasy scaling patches that favor scalp, face, ears, and intertriginous areas; usually asymptomatic
  - Nummular eczema: a chronic, often intensely inflammatory and pruritic dermatitis with multiple round, crusted, edematous, erythematous patches and plaques, often on extremities
  - Psoriasis vulgaris: a chronic dermatitis with recurrent well-defined erythematous plaques with silvery scale; commonly affects scalp, elbows, and knees; nail changes may be present.

- Other
  - Ichthyoses: diffuse, severely dry, scaly, and hyperkeratotic skin; acquired or inherited
  - Pityriasis rosea: may begin with a single round, sharply demarcated, pink "herald" patch on the torso which becomes scaly and develops central clearing, followed by crops of oval lesions on the trunk and proximal extremities
  - Child abuse: inflicted trauma or burns

DIAGNOSTIC TESTS & INTERPRETATION

Initial Tests (screening, lab, imaging)

- Removal of suspected allergens identified on history should be the first diagnostic step; look for improvement/resolution of symptoms, usually within 2 to 4 weeks.
- Formal epicutaneous patch testing may be considered in the setting of uncontrollable or worsening chronic dermatitis or failure to improve with standard treatment.
  - Distinguishes irritant and allergic contact dermatitis and identifies inciting allergens
  - Involves the controlled exposure of multiple allergens to the skin. Positive reactions manifest with the development of erythema, edema, and vesicles at the site of exposure, usually within 48 to 96 hours. It may be performed using a standard panel of allergens or by the application of selected allergens at the discretion of the specialist. Patch testing for poison ivy or oak is not recommended because reactions may be severe. Oral and topical steroids should be held prior to patch testing to avoid suppression of reactions.

Diagnostic Procedures/Other

- Skin biopsy is rarely necessary but may help differentiate between contact dermatitis and psoriasis or other inflammatory dermatoses.
- Skin biopsy findings may not be specific, and histopathologic features may not differentiate irritant from allergic contact dermatitis.

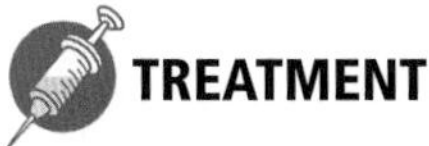

TREATMENT

GENERAL MEASURES

- The most effective treatment involves identification and avoidance of the offending allergens or exposures. This often requires extensive education of the patient and family regarding potential sources of exposure.
- Emollients restore epidermal barrier function. Petrolatum-based products are preferred to emollients containing lanolin or fragrances to reduce the risk of contact sensitization. Frequent application is recommended.
- Prompt bathing with soap and water immediately after exposure to poison ivy, oak, or sumac may help reduce exposure to the allergen in susceptible individuals.
- Chemical inactivators of urushiol may decrease dermatitis, but oil-removing compounds and soap also decrease dermatitis when used promptly after exposure.
- Acute allergic contact dermatitis: Application of cool compresses and shake lotions with drying properties (e.g., calamine lotion) can be helpful. Products containing colloidal oatmeal may also be helpful in soothing inflamed skin.

MEDICATION

First Line

- Topical corticosteroids: may help with the pruritus and inflammation associated with both acute and chronic contact dermatitis
  - In irritant contact dermatitis, topical corticosteroids are controversial, as efficacy has not been evaluated in randomized controlled studies. Potential benefits must be weighed against the adverse effects.
  - Milder forms not involving the face or flexural areas can be treated with class 3 to 5 topical corticosteroids for a short duration.
  - For severe or chronic contact dermatitis with lichenification not involving the face of flexural areas, a medium- to high-potency topical corticosteroid (class 2 to 4) should be used for a short duration (≤2 weeks).
  - If involving the face or flexural areas, medium- to high-potency topical corticosteroids should be avoided; instead, use a low-potency topical corticosteroid (class 6 or 7).
  - Remember that topical corticosteroids can induce an allergic contact dermatitis.
- Systemic antihistamines (diphenhydramine or hydroxyzine) are generally not necessary but can be considered if pruritus is extreme. There is no evidence that topical antihistamines are useful in treatment of pruritus.
- In severe cases involving a large body surface area or associated with significant facial, genital, or extremity edema, a short course (7 to 10 days) of systemic corticosteroids (prednisone 1 to 2 mg/kg/24 h) may be appropriate, with tapering over 1 to 2 weeks to avoid a rebound of the dermatitis.

Second Line

- The intermittent use of a topical calcineurin inhibitor such as tacrolimus or pimecrolimus, which have anti-inflammatory and steroid-sparing properties, may be considered as adjunctive therapy in patients with chronic contact dermatitis. They are beneficial in that they do not cause the skin atrophy that topical steroids may. These agents are less effective than midpotency corticosteroids. The U.S. Food and Drug Administration (FDA) issued an advisory about the possible link between their use and malignancy. They should not be used in children <2 years of age.
- Use of oral immunomodulators such as cyclosporine, methotrexate, azathioprine, and mycophenolate mofetil may be considered in recurrent disease under the supervision of a specialist.

ONGOING CARE

FOLLOW-UP RECOMMENDATIONS

Patient Monitoring

Patients who do not improve after 1 to 2 weeks of therapy should be reevaluated.

DIET

Patients with allergy to nickel or BOP may experience continued dermatitis from ingestion of foods containing these products.

- Nickel can be found in canned foods, cocoa, chocolate, soy beans, oatmeal, almonds, cashews, legumes, tuna, herring, shellfish, salmon, and mackerel.
- BOP can be found in citrus, spices (cinnamon, cloves, vanilla), pickles, chocolate, colas, and tomato products.

PATIENT EDUCATION

Prevention

- Patients should be instructed on allergen avoidance, including the use of protective gloves and clothing as well as dietary avoidance where appropriate.
- Barrier creams containing quaternium-18 bentonite (bentoquatam 5%) may prevent exposure to the allergen in poison ivy if applied prior to anticipated exposure. Protective clothing may be helpful but can harbor the allergenic resin for many days.

PROGNOSIS

Complete resolution can be expected after appropriate treatment and elimination of further exposure to the allergen.

COMPLICATIONS

Generally, there are no long-term complications, although secondary bacterial infections may occur.

ADDITIONAL READING

- Admani S, Jacob SE. Allergic contact dermatitis in children: review of the past decade. *Curr Allergy Asthma Rep*. 2014;14(4):421.
- De Waard-van der Spek FB, Andersen KE, Darsow U, et al. Allergic contact dermatitis in children: which factors are relevant? (review of the literature). *Pediatr Allergy Immunol*. 2013;24(4):321–329.
- Goldenberg A, Silverberg N, Silverberg JI, et al. Pediatric allergic contact dermatitis: lessons for better care. *J Allergy Clin Immunol Pract*. 2015;3(5):661–667.
- Pelletier JL, Perez C, Jacob SE. Contact dermatitis in pediatrics. *Pediatr Ann*. 2016;45(8):e287–e292.

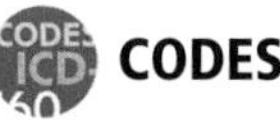

CODES

ICD10

- L25.9 Unspecified contact dermatitis, unspecified cause
- L24.9 Irritant contact dermatitis, unspecified cause
- L23.9 Allergic contact dermatitis, unspecified cause

FAQ

- Q: Can the fluid from blisters caused by poison ivy spread the rash to other parts of the body?
- A: The contents of blisters from rhus dermatitis are not contagious. After exposure is eliminated, new lesions may appear because of the variable sensitivity of various areas of the body to the allergen.
- Q: How does saliva cause a perioral rash in some kids?
- A: "Lip-licker dermatitis" is an irritant dermatitis that results from chronic and/or excessive exposure to moisture. It is not caused by any specific substances in the saliva.
- Q: Can someone have a contact dermatitis at a site that was not exposed to the trigger?
- A: Autoeczematization can occur, in which a generalized dermatitis develops following a localized flare at sites distant from the original exposure. This is felt to be an autoimmune reaction. Additionally, some patients with allergic contact dermatitis can experience dermatitis after ingestion of allergens, such a nickel and BOP.

CONTRACEPTION

Michelle Forcier, MD, MPH

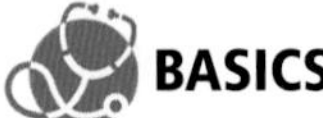

BASICS

DESCRIPTION

- Prevention of conception or pregnancy. Ideal contraceptive is 100% effective, has no side effects, is easily reversed, and is readily used by adolescents.
- Efficacy issues:
  - In practice, contraceptive efficacy is based on two core concepts:
    - Adherence or ability to adequately "do" the method
    - Continuation or length of time over which patient uses method
  - Adherence and continuation improved by superior effectiveness of long-acting reversible contraceptives (LARCs), such as intrauterine devices (IUDs) or subdermal implants. LARCs have failure rates of <1% and approximately 80% continuation rates.
  - The most effective methods should be offered as 1st-line contraceptive options for sexually active persons of all ages.
- Methods of contraception:
  - LARCs:
    - Etonogestrel implant
      - Single-rod subdermal implant containing 68 mg of progestin etonogestrel. Implant provides contraception for 3 years.
      - Benefits: easy to insert and remove device, insertion site easy to access (nondominant upper arm)
      - Can be placed in not yet sexually active patients considering future sexual activity or for heavy or painful menses
    - Levonorgestrel-releasing IUDs
      - T-shaped polyethylene IUDs containing progestin hormones
      - Ovulation may be suppressed in some women. However, not main mechanism of action. Between 45% and 75% of women ovulate on the 52-mg device, and almost all women ovulate on the lower dose levonorgestrel IUDs.
      - Ovulation on lower dose levonorgestrel IUDs may result in less amenorrhea and more regular menses which can be a desired effect for some women.
      - Mirena®, Liletta® contain 52 mg of levonorgestrel and a release rate of 20 mcg/24 h. Mirena is approved by the U.S. Food and Drug Administration (FDA) for use for 5 years but is effective up to 7 years. Liletta is approved for 4 years, may be similar to Mirena; significantly reduces menstrual bleeding and dysmenorrhea
      - Skylar® IUD is minimally smaller, 28 mm × 30 mm, contains 13.5 mg levonorgestrel, releasing 5 to 14 mcg/24 h, with decline to 5 mcg/24 h after 3 years.
      - Phase II and III trials are being conducted with 8, 12, 16 mcg/24 h products.
    - Copper T380 IUD
      - Contraceptive effect related to in utero oxidation with release of copper ions
      - FDA-approved for use up to 10 years but may be effective for up to 12 years
      - May also be placed as very effective emergency contraceptive and then retained for ongoing pregnancy prevention
  - Moderate-duration contraceptives:
    - Depot-medroxyprogesterone acetate (DMPA or Depo-Provera®)
      - IM injection administered every 13 weeks. Failure rates in real-world settings estimated as low as 6%, likely much higher for adolescents
      - 1-year continuation: 56% for users of all ages, likely lower for adolescents
      - Effective up to 14 weeks, so patients within the dosing window do not need additional pregnancy testing before readministration
  - Short-acting estrogen-progestin contraceptives:
    - General issues:
      - Typically use both estrogen (to minimize breakthrough bleeding) and progestin (to block ovulation) in variety of delivery systems
      - Typical use failure rates at 9% but higher in adolescent populations. Continuation rates are 67%, likely lower in adolescents; 99.9% effective with perfect use but real-life use, difficulties with adherence, and continuation significantly reduce effectiveness
      - Some estrogen-progestin agents such as combined oral contraceptive pills (COCs) and vaginal rings may be used almost continuously for extended cycling. Such extended cycling may be useful for patients with dysmenorrhea, heavy periods, anemia, or times (life events) when delaying a period desired.
    - COCs:
      - Monophasic COCs contain fixed doses of estrogens (ethinyl estradiol) and progestins. Phasic COCs vary doses of estrogens, progestins, or both; no practical difference between monophasic and phasic COCs
      - Benefits: reduce incidence of endometrial and ovarian cancers after as little as 3 months of use, protect against salpingitis (pelvic inflammatory disease [PID]) and subsequent ectopic pregnancies, and decrease incidence of benign breast disease and dysmenorrhea
      - Effective treatment for abnormal or heavy uterine bleeding (AUB), perimenstrual mood and physiologic symptoms, hygiene and behavior changes around menses for some developmentally delayed individuals, and sequelae of hyperandrogenism or polycystic ovary syndrome (AUB, hirsutism, acne)
    - Transdermal patch
      - Contains ethinyl estradiol and norelgestromin. Each patch left in place for 7 days, changed weekly, allowing 1 patch-free week per month for menses; convenient due to once-weekly change
      - Typically not recommended for extended cycling, as studies demonstrate 60% more circulating estrogen than with other estrogen-progestin methods
      - Unclear if this increases vascular thrombotic event (VTE) risk
    - Vaginal ring
      - Soft, flexible, polymer ring containing ethinyl estradiol and etonogestrel
      - FDA-approved for vaginal insertion for 3 weeks and then removed for 1 week for menses
      - May be effective over a 4-week insertion and for extended cycling
      - Benefits: avoids 1st-pass liver effects and lower hormone doses
  - Emergency contraceptives: postcoital contraceptives, "morning-after" pills
    - General issues:
      - Safe but less effective (estimated 75%) than other hormonal/inserted contraceptives
      - Not abortifacient but blocks ovulation, as do other hormonal methods of contraceptives
      - Advance provision improves patient use but does not decrease overall pregnancy rates over time.
      - May be offered to all women using short- or moderate-acting contraceptives
    - Ulipristal acetate (UPA) 30 mcg
      - Should be 1st-line option as efficacy seems less effected by timing and patient weight
      - Administered in a single oral dose up to 5 days post unprotected sex with equal effectiveness across time
      - Is more effective in overweight or obese women than progestin methods
      - Not carried by all pharmacies, both community and hospital-based as of 2015
      - Often requires insurance preauthorization (unlike progestin only methods) which may delay administration
    - Progesterone-only methods:
      - Most effective when used within 72 hours of intercourse; treatment less likely to be effective up to 5 days
      - Levonorgestrel administered one time at a dose of 1.5 mg available by prescription and over the counter in the United States
      - Male patients should be educated about the use of emergency contraceptives and may purchase this method over the counter as well.
    - Yuzpe method of emergency contraception with COCs
      - Consists of 100 mcg ethinyl estradiol + 0.5 mg levonorgestrel given with repeated second dose 12 hours later
      - This method has higher rates of nausea and vomiting.
      - Generally used as a matter of urgent timing, convenience and expense if a woman has a COC pack of pills at home and prefers to use these for her emergency contraception method because other methods are more effective and have fewer side effects

- Additional contraceptive methods:
  - General issues:
    - Well-known but with significantly lower efficacy
    - Include barrier methods to sperm entry (male and female condoms, diaphragms)
  - Male condoms
    - 88% effective with typical use; likely higher failure rates in adolescents
    - Female condom and diaphragm are 79% and 88% effective, respectively.
    - Proper condom use can prevent transmission of sexually transmitted infections such as HIV, HPV, HSV, syphilis, *Neisseria gonorrhoeae*, and *Chlamydia trachomatis*.
    - Important to inform adolescents that condoms are superior for sexually transmitted infection (STI) prevention but inferior to other methods as a sole agent of contraception
  - Spermicidal agents
    - Include: foam, film, vaginal inserts, as well as nonoxynal-9 as the active agent most widely used
    - Only 72% effective in preventing pregnancy with typical use. May reduce transmission of *C. trachomatis* and *N. gonorrhoeae*; when used with condoms, overall efficacy 93% with typical use
    - Irritant effect linked in some high-risk populations with increased risk of HIV transmission
    - Spermicides must be inserted with each intercourse, near the time of intercourse; some formulations require 10 to 15 minutes for activation. Most have an unpleasant taste.
  - Progestin-only pills (POPs) ("mini-pill")
    - Much less effective than most other hormonal methods, as effectiveness is highly dependent on perfect use
    - May offer some measure of benefit for women who are immediately postpartum (up to 6 months) and breastfeeding on demand
    - Typically not a good method for most women
  - Abstinence
    - Sexual activity is a normal part of adolescent and adult human development.
    - Abstinence or refraining from vaginal-penile sexual intercourse is the most effective way to prevent unintended or unwanted pregnancy as well as transmission of STIs. Provider counseling and recommendations should promote a 4-pronged approach to sexual decision making: personal maturity and readiness, thoughtful partner selection and communication, family planning and pregnancy prevention, as well as prevention of STIs.

ALERT

- Advising women to abstain from all forms of physical intimacy may be both unrealistic and counterproductive in the context of their psychosocial development.
- Providers should emphasize at every visit that only 100% use of condoms (or abstinence) protects against sexually transmitted diseases but is not the most effective form of birth control available.
- All forms of birth control are not "equal"—long-acting reversible contraceptives are significantly more effective contraceptives than all other methods, even sterilization.
- Long-acting reversible contraceptive implants are both highly desirable and well tolerated in all patients and should be offered as 1st-line contraceptives to all women at risk for unintended pregnancy.
- Include male patients in discussions about both condom use as well as contraceptive use.

GENERAL PREVENTION

- Encourage consistent use of latex condoms.
- Patients using oral contraceptive pills may be strongly encouraged to cease tobacco use, but tobacco use does not preclude estrogen-progestin methods in women <35 years.

PATHOPHYSIOLOGY

- Combined estrogen-progestin hormonal therapy suppresses ovulation by directly decreasing release of hypothalamic gonadotropin-releasing hormone (GnRH) and pituitary follicle-stimulating hormone (FSH) and luteinizing hormone (LH).
- Progesterone thickens cervical mucus, thins the endometrium, and decreases tubal motility. Higher dose systemic progestins inhibit the hypothalamic-ovarian axis and halt ovulation.
- Copper: Copper ions inhibit transtubal sperm migration and act in both an ovicidal and spermicidal way to prevent zygote formation.
- Emergency contraception: Mechanisms of action include ovulation disruption, endometrial impairment to prevent implantation, and possibly sperm or ova transport alteration.
- Spermicides (nonoxynol-9 and octoxynol-9) destroy sperm cell membranes. Most spermicidal preparations contain an inert base (foam, cream, or jelly) to support the spermicidal agent and provide a barrier to sperm entry.

DIAGNOSIS

HISTORY

General considerations in family planning interviews and methods counseling:

- Open queries about family planning intentions should be included in all reproductive age anticipatory guidance or reproductive health visits.
- One Key Question: "Do you want to be pregnant in the next 6 months or year?" opens the conversation to all potential family planning intentions: intention to become pregnant, ambivalence about pregnancy, and desire for contraception and no immediate pregnancy plan.
- Method selection should consider and include the following:
  - Past use
  - Failures
  - Side effects (both real and perceived) of contraceptives
  - Priorities and goals for family planning
- Does the patient want a pregnancy and parenting? Does his or her partner? Is this patient ambivalent about pregnancy and parenting?
- What is the patient's sexual history? Ask about sexual debut, recent partners, lifetime number of partners, gender and risk behaviors of partners, types of sexual behaviors (may be receptive or giving/insertive, penile-vaginal, penile-anal, oral, digital, devices and other objects).
- Is sexual activity spontaneous or planned? Coerced or desired? Is the adolescent happy and confident about his or her sexual activity? Does sex give pleasure, feel uncomfortable, any other sexual concerns?
- What methods has the youth tried in the past? What worked, what did not work and why? Does the patient feel that she or he can be compliant with a daily pill or barrier methods? Can the adolescent demonstrate this ability with other medications or regimens?
- Does the patient require privacy and confidentiality? Does an adolescent have a parent or guardian's support regarding contraception and safer sex?
- Is the patient comfortable applying a condom or asking their partner to put on a condom?
- Does the patient have open communication with his or her partner? Does the partner respect the patient's decisions? Does the patient feel safe and respected by his or her partner?
- Are there any other barriers to adherence and continuation with the chosen contraceptive method? Is the patient comfortable with the level of efficacy and potential side effects with the current plan?

PHYSICAL EXAM

- Is not essential for some patients who need to start contraception on an urgent or emergency basis. A thorough medical history that excludes current pregnancy, medical conditions that would be a contraindication to particular methods, and a plan for follow-up can allow some providers to begin a method without a physical exam at that time.
- Exams may be helpful in obtaining baseline weight, blood pressure (BP), and other physical stigmata (hirsutism, acne) that may benefit from hormones.
- It is not necessary to perform a pelvic exam on asymptomatic young women initiating hormonal contraception. It is not recommended to perform a pelvic exam (bimanual and speculum) for an adolescent who has never been sexually active but requests contraception.
- A pelvic exam to assess and diagnose an STI or to evaluate for pregnancy in a patient with amenorrhea may be indicated.
  - The Centers for Disease Control and Prevention (CDC) recommends screening for STIs after sexual debut and at least annually until age 25 years.
  - Papanicolaou (Pap) cancer screening begins after sexual debut and by 21 years of age. Pap guidelines have been evolving and changing over recent years.

DIAGNOSTIC TESTS & INTERPRETATION

- Pregnancy test prior to initiating hormonal contraceptives:
  - Urine pregnancy tests are typically adequate for diagnosing most pregnancies.
  - Serum human choriogonadotropin hormone (B-hCG) is useful when trying to differentiate between normal and abnormal (miscarriage, ectopic) pregnancies.
- It is helpful to ask patients "when was your last sexual activity without a condom and without birth control?" to determine the accuracy of your current pregnancy test, not exclude very early pregnancy, potentially offer emergency contraception, and create a follow-up plan for possible future pregnancy testing in 2 to 4 weeks.

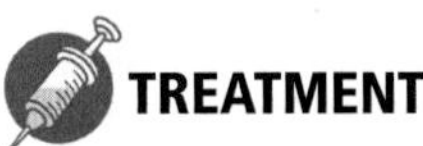

TREATMENT

GENERAL MEASURES

- Barrier methods: Trained personnel can teach the proper technique for application of condoms and spermicidal agents.
- Fertility (and ovulatory cycles) should return within 6 months of the last DMPA injection.
- Etonogestrel implant is a simple procedure easily done in outpatient settings but requires training and certification by the manufacturer.
- IUDs are also simple outpatient procedures for primary care providers with pelvic and uterine exam skills. Insertion of an IUD should be scheduled when one can be as certain as possible that the adolescent is not pregnant. DMPA may be offered as a bridging medicine prior to placement to avoid insertion delays that place patient at risk for unintended pregnancy.
- All methods offer contraceptive protection immediately if inserted days 0 to 5 of their menstrual cycle. Most methods require 7 days to reach effectiveness. Most patients return to ovulation soon after discontinuation of most contraceptives.

ALERT

- Drugs that activate the cytochrome P450 enzyme will diminish the efficacy of hormonal contraceptives and may include the following: phenobarbital, carbamazepine, primidone, rifampin, griseofulvin, HIV protease inhibitors, and tetracyclines (including doxycycline).
- Hormonal contraceptives can increase concentrations of phenytoin, benzodiazepines, antidepressants, corticosteroids, β-blockers, theophylline, and alcohol.
- Hormonal contraceptives can decrease the efficacy of acetaminophen, oral anticoagulants, hypoglycemics, and methyldopa.
- Always check for potential drug interactions as many other medications metabolized by and can alter the cytochrome P450 enzyme system.

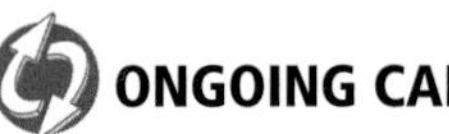

ONGOING CARE

FOLLOW-UP RECOMMENDATIONS

Patient Monitoring

- Patients using hormonal contraceptives may be seen within 6 weeks to 3 months of initiation, to evaluate effectiveness and determine what methods are most optimal for patient adherence, continuation, and side effects.
- BP, weight, and STIs may continue to be monitored.

PROGNOSIS

- There is an estimated 80% risk of pregnancy for pregnancy over the course of 1 year of unprotected sex.
- Use of COCs declines over time:
  - 45% in 3 months
  - 33% at 1 year

COMPLICATIONS

- Barrier methods
  - Latex allergy:
    - Patients may use polyurethane rather than latex condoms.
    - Animal skin condoms are permeable to viral pathogens.
  - Breakage or permeability:
    - Oil-based lubricants and most intravaginal medications used with latex condoms will increase the risk of these complications.
- Spermicides
  - Local irritation or allergic reaction
  - May increase risk of HIV infection in adolescents with high-risk sexual partners
- Hormonal estrogen-progestin contraceptives
  - Contraindications to COC pills are uncommon in most women and include the following: pregnancy, history of thromboembolic event, structural heart disease, breast cancer, active liver disease, migraine headaches with an aura, prolonged immobilization, or severe hypertension.
  - Caution should be taken with women <6 weeks postpartum, with gallbladder disease, and those who use medications that affect liver enzymes.
  - Minor, and usually self-limited, side effects of COCs may include intermenstrual spotting, nausea, breast changes, fluid retention, leukorrhea, minor headache, and depression.
  - Thromboembolic events and liver disease are extremely rare in nonsmoking adolescents using estrogen-containing oral contraceptive pills. Placing risk in perspective is essential for adequate consent. Estimates of VTE may be communicated as follows:
    - Baseline risk: 10 in 100,000 women-years
    - COC user risk: 15 in 100,000 women-years
    - 3rd-generation COC (desogestrel) or patch risk: 30 in 100,000 women-years
    - Pregnancy risk: 60 in 100,000 women-years
  - Mortality from estradiol-containing methods estimated at 1 in 1.5 million per year.
    - Mortality from bike riding, motor vehicle crashes, and other causes is much higher.
    - Death from gynecologic and related causes was 7/100,000 in 15- to 19-year-old adolescents per year.
    - If no fertility control measures were used, the mortality is 0.3/100,000 per year in nonsmoking oral contraceptive pill users and 2.2/100,000 per year in smoking oral contraceptive pill users.
- Progestin-only methods
  - POPs side effects include weight gain, rapid hair turnover, and menstrual irregularities.
  - DMPA can reduce bone mineral density (BMD), which typically rebounds to normal after DMPA discontinuation.
    - Because adolescence is the period of peak bone mass accretion, there is concern that DMPA use during adolescence may increase the risk for osteopenia or osteoporosis later in life.
    - This risk has not been proven or validated at present.
    - For adolescents with anorexia nervosa, chronic steroid use, chronic renal failure, there may be better LARCs available that have no BMD impact.

- Most common side effect reported with etonogestrel implant is abnormal bleeding.
  - A wide range of bleeding patterns may be experienced, and it is not possible to predict the bleeding pattern for any one individual.
  - Overall, in the 90-day reference periods of clinical trial experience, 33.3% had infrequent bleeding, 21.4% had amenorrhea, 6.1% had frequent bleeding, and 16.9% had prolonged bleeding.
- The lower androgenic effect of etonogestrel may make side effects of acne and weight gain less frequent than with other progestins.

- IUDs
  - Contraindications to IUD placement are those who are pregnant or suspected to be pregnant, have active PID or puerperal or post abortion sepsis, malignancy of the genital tract, uterine abnormalities that distort the uterine cavity, an allergy to any component of IUDs, or Wilson disease (for the copper T IUD only).
  - PID risk
    - IUDs have been associated with a slightly higher risk of PID within the first 21 days after insertion, especially if cervical infection is present.
    - IUDs do not increase risk of PID above baseline after this time.
  - Younger age may confer a 5% risk of IUD failure from expulsion because of smaller uterus and higher incidence of nulliparity.
  - The copper T IUD has been associated with increased menstrual bleeding and spotting, especially in first 3 to 6 months after insertion. In addition, some women may experience menstrual pain and heavy bleeding throughout use.
- Emergency contraception
  - Ulipristal is a well-tolerated 1st-line emergency contraceptive yet may not be covered by insurances.

ADDITIONAL READING

- Bellanca HK, Hunter MS. ONE KEY QUESTION®: preventive reproductive health is part of high quality primary care. *Contraception*. 2013;88(1):3–6.
- Curtis KM, Tepper NK, Jatlaoui TC, et al. U.S. medical eligibility criteria for contraceptive use, 2016. *MMWR Recomm Rep*. 2016;65(3):1–103.
- Dean G, Schwarz EB. Intrauterine contraceptives (IUCs). In: Hatcher RA, Trussell J, Nelson AL, et al, eds. *Contraceptive Technology*. 20th ed. New York, NY: Ardent Media; 2011:147–191.
- Fok WK, Blumenthal PD. Update on emergency contraception. *Curr Opin Obstet Gynecol*. 2016;28(6):522–529.
- Mestad R, Secura G, Allsworth JE, et al. Acceptance of long-acting reversible contraceptive methods by adolescent participants in the Contraceptive CHOICE Project. *Contraception*. 2011;84(5): 493–498.
- Sitruk-Ware R, Nath A, Mishell DR Jr. Contraception technology: past, present and future. *Contraception*. 2013;87(3):319–330.
- Tepper NK, Curtis KM, Jatlaoui TC, et al. Updated guidance for safe and effective use of contraception. *J Womens Health (Larchmt)*. 2016;25(11): 1097–1101.
- Winner B, Peipert JF, Zhao Q, et al. Effectiveness of long-acting reversible contraception. *N Engl J Med*. 2012;366(21):1998–2007.
- Yuzpe AA, Thurlow HJ, Ramzy I, et al. Post coital contraception—a pilot study. *J Reprod Med*. 1974;13(2):53–58.

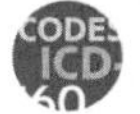

CODES

ICD10

- Z30.9 Encounter for contraceptive management, unspecified
- Z30.09 Encounter for oth general cnsl and advice on contraception
- Z30.8 Encounter for other contraceptive management

FAQ

- Q: My adolescent, minor patient asks for confidentiality regarding contraception. Can I comply?
- A: Yes. Adolescents benefit from private and confidential contraceptive services. Adolescents should have right to confidentiality regarding contraception and treatment of STIs, even though some states do not have specific laws protecting these rights. The benchmark of care supported by all professional medical societies supports private and confidential contraceptive care for adolescents. Do not assume, however, that an adolescent may not have or benefit from parental support in her efforts to prevent pregnancy. It may be in the patient's best interest to have a caring adult involved. Which adult and how he or she is involved should be negotiated with the adolescent.
- Q: My patient has been on and off short-acting birth control methods? I am worried about her risk of pregnancy? How might I better help her?
- A: There are several parts to managing this issue.
  - First, in an open and supportive manner, ask her whether she wants to become pregnant and parent or would she like to delay pregnancy?
  - Second, if she wishes to delay pregnancy over the next 6 to 12 months, offer her a LARC. Educate her on the superior efficacy and ease of use. Insert a LARC that day or facilitate an urgent referral to an adolescent-friendly provider if she continues to express an interest.
  - While she waits for that appointment, offer to help her protect from unintended pregnancy with a single dose of DMPA providing coverage for the next 12 weeks. Offer her emergency contraceptives as well.
  - Applaud efforts to be smart and safely sexually active.
  - Engage her partner, if present and supportive, in contraceptive discussions and discussions about safe, satisfying, and responsible sexuality.
- Q: One of my patients has asked me to prescribe emergency contraception in advance for her. Is this something that I should do?
- A: Yes. Emergency contraception is now over the counter, but if a patient is more likely to access using insurance coverage, this may increase use. Studies done clearly show that use of emergency contraceptives is safe. In fact, there are no absolute contraindications to using progestin-only emergency contraceptives. Because unprotected sexual encounters often take place at a time when adolescents do not have access to their health care providers (e.g., evenings or weekends), advanced prescription may be of benefit for many adolescents.
- Q: What should I tell my patient if she misses or is late for her birth control?
- A: Missed doses or delays in reapplying/reinjecting contraceptives put women at risk for pregnancy. Women who have trouble with adherence and continuation should be counseled on the value of inserted long-acting reversible methods which offer superior effectiveness for contraception, are completely reversible, and easy to use over time.
- Q: Who is Yuzpe?
- A: Abraham Albert Yuzpe, MD, MSc is a Canadian obstetrician-gynecologist. He received his MD and MSc at the University of Western Ontario (London, Ontario). In 1974, he published an emergency contraception method that uses a combination of ethinyl estradiol and levonorgestrel.

COR PULMONALE

Brian D. Hanna, MD, PhD • Rachel K. Hopper, MD

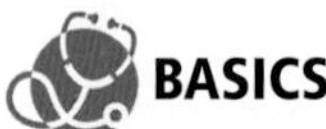

BASICS

DESCRIPTION

- Cor pulmonale refers to right ventricular (RV) failure secondary to a pulmonary process that results in a loss of functional capillary vascular bed and in increased pulmonary artery pressure and pulmonary vascular resistance (PVR).
- Cor pulmonale is not used to describe right heart failure associated with congenital heart defects or primary pulmonary vascular disease. It results from pulmonary hypertension (PH) associated with diseases of the lung, termed "Group 3 PH" in recent World Health Organization (WHO) classifications.

ALERT

- RV failure from PH occurs but is rare in newborns. At birth, RV muscle mass is normally comparable to that of the left ventricle.
- RV failure in newborns is usually a consequence of hypoxemia, ischemia, metabolic acidosis (e.g., persistent fetal circulation), and/or premature restriction/closure of the intrauterine ductus arteriosus.

EPIDEMIOLOGY

- Cor pulmonale may be found at any age but is the result of acute or long-standing pulmonary processes.
- Severe bronchopulmonary dysplasia is an increasingly common cause of neonatal PH and cor pulmonale.

Incidence

The incidence of cor pulmonale is unknown and is disease-specific.

Prevalence

- Upwards of 2 per 1,000 neonatal intensive care unit patients will develop significant cor pulmonale.
- At least 20% of infants with severe bronchopulmonary dysplasia will develop PH and are at risk for cor pulmonale.

RISK FACTORS

Genetics

- Pediatric patients with trisomy syndromes are at high risk for PH and cor pulmonale, often related to airway obstruction.
- To date, seven genes have been associated with heritable pulmonary arterial hypertension, most notably bone morphogenetic protein type 2 (*BMPR2*). Genetic etiologies are less frequently found in patients with secondary etiologies of PH, including those related to lung disease.
- Genetic causes have been identified for various developmental lung diseases, including alveolar capillary dysplasia (ACD) and surfactant protein abnormalities.

PATHOPHYSIOLOGY

- Chronic hypoxia is a principal factor, resulting in a cascade of endothelial dysfunction with pulmonary vasoconstriction, followed by the development of PH.
- A variety of vasoactive mediators may be responsible for the effect on vasomotor tone.
- Alveolar hypercarbia and/or acidemia worsen the increased RV afterload and decreased RV systolic function.

ETIOLOGY

- Parenchymal lung disease (most common)
- Chronic obstructive pulmonary disease
  - Cystic fibrosis
  - Asthma
- Restrictive lung disease
  - Infectious
  - Pulmonary toxins
  - Pulmonary fibrosis
  - Bronchopulmonary dysplasia (combined)
- Upper airway diseases causing obstructive sleep apnea (OSA): tonsillar/adenoidal hypertrophy
- Syndromes (Down, Treacher Collins)
- Neuromuscular disorders: Duchenne muscular dystrophy
- Chest wall and thoracic insufficiency syndromes
- Acute causes include pulmonary embolism and acute respiratory distress syndrome (ARDS).

COMMONLY ASSOCIATED CONDITIONS

- Genetic syndromes
- Pulmonary vascular abnormalities
- Pulmonary arterial hypertension
- Collagen vascular diseases
- Pulmonary veno-occlusive disease
- Pulmonary thromboembolism

DIAGNOSIS

HISTORY

- Fatigue
- Failure to thrive/weight loss
- Dizziness
- Syncope
- Dyspnea on exertion
- Exercise intolerance
- Chest pain (secondary to RV ischemia)
- Palpitations
- Hemoptysis

ALERT

- Hemoptysis is a life-threatening emergency and heralds a poor prognosis for any patient with PH.
- Cyanosis may not be from the lung parenchymal disease but from intracardiac shunt.

PHYSICAL EXAM

- Tachycardia
- Parasternal RV impulse
- Cyanosis may be evident.
- Hepatomegaly, jugular venous distention, peripheral edema
- A loud, narrowly split or single second heart sound (P_2); RV gallop; holosystolic murmur right of the sternum (tricuspid regurgitation); and/or diastolic murmur at the left upper sternal border (pulmonary insufficiency)

ALERT

In the newborn period to puberty, an abnormally increased RV impulse is best felt under the xiphoid.

DIFFERENTIAL DIAGNOSIS

- Congenital heart disease with PH and right-to-left shunt (Eisenmenger syndrome)
- Pulmonary arterial hypertension (previously termed primary PH) or pulmonary veno-occlusive disease
- Obstruction of pulmonary venous returns, either anatomic obstruction or left ventricular failure

DIAGNOSTIC TESTS & INTERPRETATION

Initial Tests (screening, lab, imaging)

- Brain-type natriuretic peptide can be a useful biomarker of RV dysfunction and is elevated with worsening cor pulmonale.
- Decreased Pa_{O_2}, increased Pa_{CO_2}, and a compensatory metabolic alkalosis
- Polycythemia may be consistent with chronic hypoxemia.
- Chest radiograph: cardiomegaly from RV dilation and main pulmonary artery enlargement
- Echocardiography: RV dilation, tricuspid annular plane systolic excursion (TAPSE) as a marker of RV function, RV hypertrophy, pulmonary valve insufficiency, elevated RV pressure estimate from tricuspid regurgitation and/or intraventricular septal position, RV systolic and diastolic dysfunction
- Ventricular/perfusion (V/Q) scan is beneficial to rule out thromboembolic disease.
- Chest computed tomography scan with contrast and lung volumes to assess lung hypoplasia, interstitial lung disease, thromboembolic disease, and large pulmonary vein disease

Diagnostic Procedures/Other
- Electrocardiogram: may show right axis deviation, right atrial enlargement, RV hypertrophy, and T-wave inversion
- Polysomnogram if OSA suspected
- 6-minute walk: measures functional capacity and limitations and may be useful for serial assessments
- Cardiac catheterization, although invasive, remains the gold standard for PH diagnosis and to guide therapy.
- Lung biopsy is diagnostic in certain scenarios (e.g., ACD) but may be contraindicated in the face of severe PH and significant lung disease due to procedural risk.
- Pathologic findings
  - Pulmonary vascular lesions, including arterial hypertrophy in longstanding PH
  - Parenchymal fibrotic lesions
  - RV dilation and hypertrophy

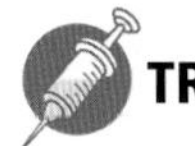

TREATMENT

GENERAL MEASURES
- The primary goal is reduction of the abnormally elevated pulmonary artery pressure and the RV workload.
- If at all possible, address the primary pulmonary etiology (i.e., tonsillectomy/adenoidectomy in a patient with obstructive upper airway disease).
- Fluid boluses are poorly tolerated by the right ventricle and rarely augment systemic blood pressure.

MEDICATION
First Line
- Oxygen to keep saturations >90%
- Diuretics, especially with pulmonary congestion

Second Line
- Bronchodilators (theophylline)
- Digoxin (may improve RV contractility)
- Inotropes
- Anticoagulation (if thromboembolic event)
- Pulmonary vasodilator therapy may be helpful, although there is risk of worsening intrapulmonary shunt and V/Q mismatch with systemic administration.
- Pulmonary vasodilators:
  - Inhaled nitric oxide
  - Calcium channel blockers rarely are indicated or helpful and definitely not recommended in patients <1 year of age and/or with compromised cardiac output.
  - Phosphodiesterase-5 inhibitors
  - Endothelin receptor antagonists
  - Prostacyclin agonists

ISSUES FOR REFERRAL
Guideline recommendations suggest early consultation with expert pediatric PH specialists for any symptomatic patient with PH.

ADDITIONAL THERAPIES
- Atrial septostomy (in select cases, may improve cardiac output but at the expense of worsening hypoxemia)
- Lung, or rarely, heart–lung transplantation
- Usually self-limited activity
- No competitive sports

SURGERY/OTHER PROCEDURES
Consider tracheostomy for chronic ventilation, Nissen fundoplication, and gastrostomy tube (G-tube) if chronic aspiration is contributing to parenchymal lung injury.

ONGOING CARE

FOLLOW-UP RECOMMENDATIONS
Patient Monitoring
Home oxygen saturation monitoring may be indicated when night oxygen is necessary to keep saturations >90%.

PROGNOSIS
- Patients with reversible lung disease usually have a better prognosis.
- Patients with cor pulmonale are at risk for sudden death because of the inability to augment cardiac output with exercise, growth, or febrile illnesses.
- Numerous medical therapies and lung transplantation may improve long-term survival.
- Long-term survival is variable and depends on the age at onset of pulmonary changes and the underlying conditions (e.g., Down syndrome) that may adversely affect survival.

COMPLICATIONS
- As a result of the underlying lung process, the chronic hypoxia leads to polycythemia and the risk for thrombotic complications
- RV failure secondary to the inability of the RV to handle the excessive afterload can lead to poor cardiac output.

ADDITIONAL READING

- Abman SH, Hansmann G, Archer SL, et al; for American Heart Association Council on Cardiopulmonary, Critical Care, Perioperative and Resuscitation, Council on Clinical Cardiology, Council on Cardiovascular Disease in the Young, Council on Cardiovascular Radiology and Intervention, Council on Cardiovascular Surgery and Anesthesia, American Thoracic Society. Pediatric pulmonary hypertension: guidelines from the American Heart Association and American Thoracic Society. *Circulation*. 2015;132(21):2037–2099.
- Cerro MJ, Abman S, Diaz G, et al. A consensus approach to the classification of pediatric pulmonary hypertensive vascular disease: report from the PVRI Pediatric Taskforce, Panama 2011. *Pulm Circ*. 2011;1(2):286–298.
- Koestenberger M, Ravekes W, Everett AD, et al. Right ventricular function in infants, children and adolescents: reference values of the tricuspid annular plane systolic excursion (TAPSE) in 640 healthy patients and calculation of z score values. *J Am Soc Echocardiogr*. 2009;22(6):715–719.
- Lammers AE, Adatia I, Cerro MJ, et al. Functional classification of pulmonary hypertension in children: report from the PVRI Pediatric Taskforce, Panama 2011. *Pulm Circ*. 2011;1(2):280–285.

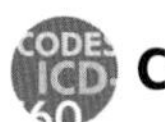

CODES

ICD10
- I27.81 Cor pulmonale (chronic)
- I26.09 Other pulmonary embolism with acute cor pulmonale

FAQ
- Q: Is cardiac catheterization indicated in all patients with cor pulmonale?
- A: Yes. Although a great deal of information can be learned from echocardiogram and other diagnostic tests, direct pulmonary artery pressure/resistance measurements require an invasive procedure. In addition, assessment of the reactivity of the pulmonary vascular bed to various agents (oxygen, prostacyclin, and nitric oxide) is best performed in the catheterization laboratory. Catheterization may be delayed in acutely unstable patients.
- Q: Is nocturnal oxygen therapy beneficial?
- A: Nocturnal oxygen has been speculated to delay the progression of cor pulmonale in some select patients with obstructive sleep hypoxemia.

COSTOCHONDRITIS

Richard M. Kravitz, MD

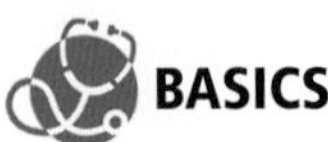

BASICS

DESCRIPTION

Costochondritis is chest pain that emanates from a costal cartilage and is reproducible on compression of that cartilage.

EPIDEMIOLOGY

- Frequency of sternal wound infections following median sternotomy is 0.1–1.6%.
- Costochondritis accounts for 10–31% of all pediatric chest pain.
- Peak age for chest pain in children is 12 to 14 years.

PATHOPHYSIOLOGY

- Inflammation of unknown etiology (Histologic examination is usually normal.)
- Infection
  - Can present months to years after surgery (The costal cartilage is avascular, making it vulnerable to infection if it has been exposed, injured, or denuded of perichondrium.)
  - Complication of median sternotomy
  - Occurs by spread from adjacent osteomyelitis or may arise de novo during surgery

ETIOLOGY

- Infectious
  - Bacterial
    - *Staphylococcus aureus* (especially after thoracic surgery)
    - *Salmonella* (in sickle cell disease)
    - *Escherichia coli*
    - *Pseudomonas* sp.
    - *Klebsiella* sp.
  - Fungal
    - *Aspergillus flavus*
    - *Candida albicans*
- Posttraumatic injury

DIAGNOSIS

HISTORY

- Inflammatory costochondritis
  - Pain usually preceded by exercise or an upper respiratory tract infection
  - Description of pain
    - Usually sharp
    - Affects the anterior chest wall
    - Localized or radiates to the back or abdomen
    - Usually unilateral (left side greater than right side)
  - The 4th to 6th costochondral junction is the usual site of pain.
  - Motion of the arm and shoulder on the affected side elicits the pain.
  - Girls are affected more often than are boys.
- Tietze syndrome
  - Onset is usually abrupt but can be gradual.
  - Believed to be caused by a minor trauma, although etiology is unknown
  - Description of pain
    - Radiates to arms or shoulder
    - May last up to several weeks
    - Swelling at the sternochondral junction may persist for several months to years.
  - Usually affects the 2nd or 3rd costochondral joint
  - Pain is aggravated by sneezing, coughing, deep inspiration, or twisting motions of the chest.
  - No differences in frequency between sexes
- Infectious costochondritis
  - Slow, insidious course
  - Usually unimpressive clinical symptomatology

PHYSICAL EXAM

- Usually normal
- Inspect for evidence of trauma, scars, bruising, and swelling.
- Palpation and percussion of the costochondral and costosternal junctions should reproduce and localize the pain.
- In Tietze syndrome, spindle-shaped swelling is visible at the sternochondral junction.

DIFFERENTIAL DIAGNOSIS

- Cardiovascular
  - Myocardial infarction
  - Pericarditis
  - Pericardial effusion
  - Myocarditis
  - Endocarditis
  - Cardiomyopathy
  - Premature ventricular contractions
  - Supraventricular tachycardia
  - Dissecting aneurysm
- Pulmonary
  - Asthma
  - Exercise-induced bronchospasm
  - Pneumonia
  - Pleural effusion
  - Pneumothorax
  - Pulmonary embolism
- GI
  - Gastroesophageal reflux
  - Esophagitis
  - Gastritis
  - Achalasia
- Mechanical
  - Muscle strain
  - Stress fractures
  - Precordial catch syndrome
  - Trauma
- Rheumatologic
  - Rheumatoid arthritis
  - Ankylosing spondylitis
- Oncologic
  - Rhabdomyosarcoma
  - Leukemia
  - Ewing sarcoma
- Miscellaneous
  - Tietze syndrome
  - Psychogenic chest pain
  - Breast tissue pain (both sexes)

DIAGNOSTIC TESTS & INTERPRETATION

Initial Tests (screening, lab, imaging)

- WBC count not helpful (even when infection present)
- EKG (may be helpful if cardiac etiology is being considered)
- Radiologic studies (chest x-ray, CT) usually not helpful
- Gallium scan
  - May be useful in some cases of infectious origin
  - Not highly specific
  - May show increased radionuclide uptake
  - No evidence of osteomyelitis of the sternum in most cases
- Technetium bone scan
  - Not highly specific

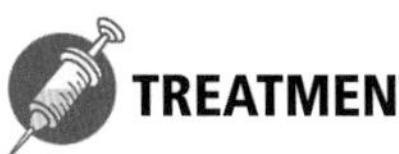

TREATMENT

GENERAL MEASURES

- Inflammatory costochondritis
  - Anti-inflammatory and analgesic agents
  - Reassurance
  - If pain disturbs normal activities and sports, infiltration with local anesthetic may prove useful.

ALERT

Inflammatory costochondritis

- Important cause of school absence
- Adolescents tend to limit physical activity unnecessarily for long periods.
- Restriction of activities is usually not required.
- Most adolescents still worry about cardiac problems, even after the diagnosis has been made.

- Infectious costochondritis
  - Prolonged course of IV antibiotics
  - Prompt surgical resection of all involved cartilage
  - Reconstructive surgery with muscular flaps should be done.

ALERT

Infectious costochondritis

- Long-term IV antibiotics alone do not resolve the problem; surgical resection and repair also are required.
- There is a tendency for the infection to spread to adjacent costal cartilages and across the sternum to the contralateral chest wall.
- In general, avoid costochondral junctions when performing surgical procedures in the chest (e.g., chest tube placement).

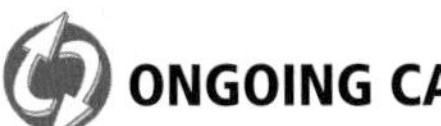

ONGOING CARE

FOLLOW-UP RECOMMENDATIONS

Patient Monitoring

- Inflammatory costochondritis
  - Long-lasting condition
  - Follow-up once a year is recommended.
- Infectious costochondritis
  - Long-term follow-up after surgery is mandatory.

PROGNOSIS

- Inflammatory costochondritis: excellent
- Infectious costochondritis: prognosis relates to
  - Underlying clinical condition of the patient (i.e., immunocompromised, postradiation therapy for cancer, postcardiac surgery)
  - Extent of surgery required to reconstruct the area damaged by the infection

ADDITIONAL READING

- Brown RT, Jamil K. Costochondritis in adolescents. A follow-up study. *Clin Pediatr (Phila)*. 1993;32(8): 499–500.
- Kocis KC. Chest pain in pediatrics. *Pediatr Clin North Am*. 1999;46(2):189–203.
- Mendelson G, Mendelson H, Horowitz SF, et al. Can (99m)technetium methylene diphosphonate bone scans objectively document costochondritis? *Chest*. 1997;111(6):1600–1602.
- Selbst SM. Consultation with the specialist. Chest pain in children. *Pediatr Rev*. 1997;18(5):169–173.
- Son MB, Sundel RP. Musculoskeletal causes of pediatric chest pain. *Pediatr Clin North Am*. 2010;57(6):1385–1395.
- Talner NS, Carboni MP. Chest pain in the adolescent and young adult. *Cardiol Rev*. 2000;8(1):49–56.

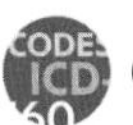

CODES

ICD10

M94.0 Chondrocostal junction syndrome [Tietze]

FAQ

- Q: Am I having or will I have a heart attack?
- A: Chest pain does not imply a heart problem. This pain arises from the chest wall; there is no risk of a myocardial infarction. A cardiac etiology to chest pain in an adolescent is usually uncommon.
- Q: Is costochondritis related to arthritis?
- A: There is no relation to any form of arthritis.
- Q: Where does the name Tietze syndrome come from?
- A: The syndrome is named after German surgeon Alexander Tietze (1864 to 1927), who first described the syndrome in 1921.

COUGH

Margaret M. McNamara, MD • Gwynne D. Church, MD

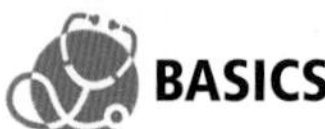

BASICS

DESCRIPTION

A high-velocity expulsion of gas from the airways that serves to clear them of mucus, cellular and microbial debris, or foreign bodies. An absence or inability to cough can lead to recurrent pneumonia. Cough can be acute (<2 weeks), subacute/protracted (2 to 4 weeks), or chronic (>4 weeks).

EPIDEMIOLOGY

- Cough is the most common symptom presenting to primary care physicians in the United States and worldwide.
- Chronic cough accounts for up to 38% of pulmonary outpatient visits.
- Healthy children can have a nonpathologic cough.
- School-age children typically experience up to 10 instances of cough per day.

PATHOPHYSIOLOGY

- Cough results from a complex reflex phenomenon initiated by cough receptors that is mediated through the brainstem.
- The receptors are located in the respiratory tract from the larynx to the segmental bronchi, paranasal sinuses, external auditory canal, and stomach and are triggered by thermal, chemical, mechanical, or inflammatory stimuli.
- Cough is generally reflexive but may sometimes be voluntarily initiated or suppressed.

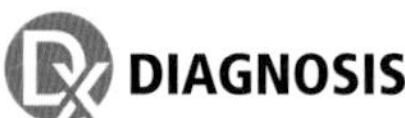

DIAGNOSIS

DIFFERENTIAL DIAGNOSIS

- Infection and asthma are the most common causes of cough in all pediatric age groups and should always be considered.
- Children have an average of 6 to 8 upper respiratory infections (URIs) per year, with each lasting up to 2 to 3 weeks. Roughly 1/3 of preschool-aged children cough >10 days after a cold, and 10% of preschool children cough >25 days after a cold.
- In children with wheezing, the term reactive airway disease (RAD) is used for children <3 years old, and asthma is used in children >3 years of age.
- Causes of *acute* (<2 weeks) or *subacute/protracted* (2 to 4 weeks) cough
  - Infection—URI
  - Lower respiratory infection
  - RAD or asthma
  - Irritants
  - Allergy
  - Foreign body
- Causes of *chronic* (>4 weeks) cough
  - Bronchitis
  - Postinfectious
  - Sinusitis
  - Asthma
  - Irritants (cigarette smoke exposure, air pollution)
  - Allergic rhinitis
  - Foreign body
  - Gastroesophageal reflux disease (GERD)
  - Habit or psychogenic
  - Bronchiectasis
  - Cystic fibrosis (CF)
  - Ciliary dyskinesia
  - Immunodeficiency states that result in recurrent respiratory infections: HIV, immunoglobulin deficiencies (IgA, IgG), phagocytic defects, complement deficiency
  - Interstitial lung disease
  - Angiotensin-converting enzyme inhibitors
  - Stimulation of external auditory canal cough receptors (Arnold reflex cough)
  - Anatomic abnormalities: tracheoesophageal fistula (TEF), tracheobronchomalacia, laryngeal cleft, polyps, adductor vocal cord paralysis, pulmonary sequestration, bronchogenic cyst, cystic hygroma, vascular ring, tumor
- Approach to patient
  - Given the common nature of cough and the large differential diagnosis it generates, an extremely thorough history and physical exam (H&P) should direct a rational, stepwise approach.

HISTORY

- **Question:** How long has the child coughed?
- *Significance*: Most acute and subacute coughs are associated with viral URIs. Pediatric chronic cough is defined as daily cough that lasts for >4 weeks.
- **Question:** Is there a recent history of URI?
- *Significance*: Serial URIs, the most common cause of chronic cough in children, can be diagnosed by a careful history of waxing and waning symptoms and will avoid unnecessary tests. Also consider postinfectious cough (due to heightened cough receptor sensitivity) or sinusitis. Overall, 8–12% of children with URIs develop complications.
- **Question:** What are the associated symptoms?
- *Significance*:
  - Fever and nasal discharge suggest infection.
  - Fever with chills or night sweats suggests TB in children with chronic cough.
  - With rhinorrhea, halitosis, headache, or facial edema, consider sinusitis.
  - With respiratory distress, suspect RAD, infection, or foreign body.
- **Question:** What is the quality of the cough?
- *Significance*:
  - Acute wet cough suggests upper or lower airway respiratory infection or asthma.
  - Subacute wet cough suggests sinusitis, bronchitis, or asthma.
  - Chronic wet cough is always abnormal and can be associated with sinusitis, bronchitis, asthma, bronchiectasis, CF, ciliary dyskinesia, or anatomic lower airway abnormality such as tracheomalacia.
  - Dry cough can suggest asthma.
  - Acute barking cough is usually associated with croup.
  - Chronic barking cough is associated with tracheomalacia or vascular ring.
  - A honking or barking chronic cough that increases during times of stress and is absent during sleep is typical for habit cough.
  - Staccato cough suggests chlamydial pneumonia in infants.
  - Paroxysmal cough, with or without whoop, suggests pertussis or parapertussis.
- **Question:** What is the pattern of the cough?
- *Significance*:
  - Chronic nighttime cough suggests RAD/asthma, postnasal drip from allergic rhinitis, or GERD.
  - With nighttime/early morning cough, consider sinusitis or allergic rhinitis.
  - Seasonal cough suggests allergy.
- **Question:** Are there any known triggers of cough (e.g., smoke, cold air, dust, URI)?
- *Significance*: Consider irritant, allergy, or RAD/asthma.
- **Question:** Is there any personal or familial history of atopy?
- *Significance*: Consider RAD/asthma.
- **Question:** Are there recurrent infections?
- *Significance*: Consider immunodeficiency, CF. Consider anatomic abnormality if patient has recurrent pneumonias in same location.
- **Question:** Is there any relation of cough to feedings?
- *Significance*: Consider aspiration, GERD, laryngeal cleft, and TEF.
- **Question:** Is there a history of a choking episode?
- *Significance*: Consider retained foreign body.
- **Question:** Is there exercise intolerance?
- *Significance*: Consider asthma, interstitial lung disease.
- **Question:** What is the parental level of concern?
- *Significance*: Children's cough generates significant parental stress and concerns, and appreciation of parental worries is valuable when addressing this problem.

PHYSICAL EXAM

Assess patient's general appearance.

- **Finding:** Evidence of failure to thrive?
- *Significance*: Consider TB, CF, immunodeficiency, aspiration.
- **Finding:** Cyanosis or pallor?
- *Significance*: Consider pneumonia, asthma, apnea, or nonpulmonary disease.
- **Finding:** Signs of respiratory distress such as tachypnea, accessory muscle use?
- *Significance*: Consider pneumonia, asthma, congenital anatomic abnormalities.
- **Finding:** Barrel chest?
- *Significance*: suggests air trapping due to chronic disease
- **Finding:** Clubbing?
- *Significance*: Consider CF, ciliary dyskinesia, interstitial lung disease, chronic aspiration.
- **Finding:** Nasal polyp?
- *Significance*: must rule out CF; also seen with allergic rhinitis
- **Finding:** Tracheal deviation?
- *Significance*: suggests mediastinal mass or foreign body aspiration
- **Finding:** Signs of atopic disease such as eczema, allergic shiners, transverse nasal crease, rhinitis, mucosal cobblestoning, injected conjunctivae?
- *Significance*: allergic rhinitis
- **Finding:** Rhinorrhea/purulent posterior pharyngeal drainage, sniffling, halitosis, periorbital edema, sinus tenderness?
- *Significance*: suggest sinusitis
- **Finding:** Crackles (rales)?
- *Significance*: Coarse crackles suggest bronchiectasis; fine crackles suggest pneumonia, atelectasis, pulmonary edema, and interstitial lung disease.
- **Finding:** Rhonchi?
- *Significance*: bronchitis, protracted bacterial bronchitis, impaired cough (from weakness, tracheostomy)
- **Finding:** Decreased breath sounds?
- *Significance*: suggests pneumonia, pleural effusion, chest mass

- **Finding:** Wheezing?
- *Significance*:
  - Polyphonic inspiratory or expiratory wheezes suggest RAD.
  - Monophonic or fixed wheezes should make one consider foreign body or mass/congenital lesion.

DIAGNOSTIC TESTS & INTERPRETATION

- Laboratory investigation should reflect a rational, stepwise approach based on likely etiologies after a thorough H&P.
- Evidence-based clinical practice guidelines for evaluating chronic cough in pediatrics were published in 2006. In general, children with chronic cough should have a chest radiograph, and spirometry should be considered for children >4 years of age.
- **Test:** chest radiograph posteroanterior/lateral
- *Significance*: detect infection, foreign body, chronic aspiration, interstitial lung disease, pulmonary edema, diaphragmatic hernia, signs typical for asthma, CF
- **Test:** spirometry
- *Significance*: detect airway obstruction or lung restriction. Pre- and postbronchodilator response is useful to diagnose asthma.
- **Test:** microbiology workup as indicated (e.g., polymerase chain reaction [PCR] for pertussis, direct fluorescent antibody [DFA] for viral panel, culture for *Chlamydia*)
- *Significance*: aids in precise diagnosis and treatment as needed
- **Test:** paranasal sinus CT scan
- *Significance*: should be used judiciously to evaluate sinus disease, that is, for complications of sinusitis, recurrent sinusitis
- **Test:** CBC
- *Significance*: Eosinophilia suggests atopic disease or, rarely, parasitic infection; anemia should prompt one to consider chronic disease or, rarely, pulmonary hemosiderosis; leukocytosis suggests infection.
- **Test:** bronchoscopy
- *Significance*: diagnose presence of foreign body and airway anomalies (laryngeal cleft, tracheobronchomalacia, TEF, vascular ring) and perform alveolar lavage for cultures, cytology, hemosiderin-laden macrophages (suggest alveolar bleeding), lipid-laden macrophages (suggest aspiration)
- **Test:** barium swallow
- *Significance*: aspiration
- **Test:** upper GI series
- *Significance*: vascular ring
- **Test:** Mantoux test: purified protein derivative (PPD) skin test or Quantiferon level
- *Significance*: to diagnose TB
- **Test:** serum IgE
- *Significance*: Significant elevation indicates allergy or, rarely, allergic bronchopulmonary aspergillosis.
- **Test:** sweat test
- *Significance*: to diagnose CF, but need to be sure that laboratory has experience with this test
- **Test:** immune workup
- *Significance*: HIV, immunodeficiency
- **Test:** pH probe
- *Significance*: GERD
- **Test:** high-resolution CT scan of the thorax, video fluoroscopy, echocardiogram, or nuclear medicine scans
- *Significance*: may be judiciously used; generally reserved until after referral to a specialist
- **Test:** genetic testing (in consultation with specialist)
- *Significance*: CF, ciliary dyskinesia, surfactant deficiency
- Chest radiograph
  - Infiltrates may suggest pneumonia, bronchiolitis, pneumonitis, TB, CF, bronchiectasis, or foreign body.
  - Volume loss may be seen with foreign body aspiration; sometimes need to obtain lateral decubitus views in young children who cannot cooperate with inspiratory/expiratory views
  - Hyperinflation suggests RAD/asthma or CF; may represent foreign body
  - Peribronchial cuffing suggests asthma/RAD or lower airway inflammation/infection; chronic aspiration
  - Mediastinal nodes may indicate infection (especially TB or fungal) or malignancy.

TREATMENT

GENERAL MEASURES

- Cough should be treated based on etiology.
- Over-the-counter (OTC) cough medicines are widely prescribed, overused, and may have negative consequences.
- The U.S. Food and Drug Administration (FDA) and Consumer Healthcare Products Association recommend avoiding OTC cough and cold medicines in children <4 years of age. An American Academy Pediatrics position statement questions the efficacy and safety of these medications in children <6 years of age.
- To avoid overuse of antibiotics, parents should be informed that viral URI can cause cough that commonly lasts up to 2 to 3 weeks.
- Educate parents about the beneficial function of cough to remove irritants and about the potential harm of suppressing a productive cough or cough secondary to RAD.
- Honey may be used in children >1 year of age. Acute cough from URI or chronic nonspecific cough (i.e., dry cough in the absence of asthma or other identifiable disease) may be safely, effectively, and inexpensively treated with honey.
- Specific pharmacologic interventions:
  - RAD/asthma: bronchodilators ± inhaled anti-inflammatory agents, oral or inhaled steroids, removal of irritants
  - Infection: appropriate antibiotics as indicated; should be considered in cases of chronic productive cough (e.g., protracted bacterial bronchitis, pneumonia, infant/toddler adenoiditis)
  - Antihistamines (nonsedating) should be used only when cough coexists with rhinitis in order to treat postnasal drip.
- Self-hypnosis is a safe, effective treatment for children with habit cough.
- Children with "nonspecific cough" (i.e., without specific indicators by H&P as noted earlier) generally do not derive much benefit from medications and may undergo a period of "watchful waiting." If medications are used, patients need to be reassessed in 2 to 3 weeks.

ISSUES FOR REFERRAL

- The vast majority of cases of cough, even when chronic, can be diagnosed and managed by the primary care physician.
- Factors in making a referral:
  - The cough is unresponsive to treatment.
  - The cause is likely to be an anatomic malformation or foreign body aspiration.
  - There appears to be involvement of other organ systems (e.g., failure to thrive, CF, congestive heart failure, immunodeficiency, unusual infection).
- Hemoptysis

ADMISSION, INPATIENT, AND NURSING CONSIDERATIONS

- Cough should be considered an emergency if there are associated signs or symptoms of respiratory distress.
- Routine emergency airway assessment should be undertaken on presentation and appropriate supportive measures started in cases in which there is concern.

ADDITIONAL READING

- Anbar RD, Hall HR. Childhood habit cough treated with self-hypnosis. *J Pediatr*. 2004;144(2):213–217.
- Chang AB, Robertson CF, van Asperen PP, et al. A cough algorithm for chronic cough in children: a multicenter, randomized controlled study. *Pediatrics*. 2013;131(5):e1576–e1583.
- Chang AB, van Asperen PP, Glasgow N, et al. Children with chronic cough: when is watchful waiting appropriate? Development of likelihood ratios for assessing children with chronic cough. *Chest*. 2015;147(3):745–753.
- Goldsobel AB, Chipps BE. Cough in the pediatric population. *J Pediatr*. 2010;156(3):352–358.
- Gupta D, Verma S, Vishwakarma SK. Anatomic basis of Arnold's ear-cough reflex. *Surg Radiol Anat*. 1986;8(4):217–220.
- Lowry JA, Leeder JS. Over-the-counter medications: update on cough and cold preparations. *Pediatr Rev*. 2015;36(7):286–297.
- Marchant JM, Morris P, Gaffney J, et al. Antibiotics for prolonged moist cough in children. *Cochrane Database Syst Rev*. 2005;(4): CD004822.
- Mulholland S, Chang AB. Honey and lozenges for children with non-specific cough. *Cochrane Database Syst Rev*. 2009;(2):CD007523.

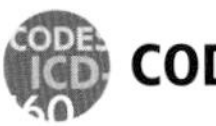

CODES

ICD10

- R05 Cough
- J00 Acute nasopharyngitis [common cold]
- J45.909 Unspecified asthma, uncomplicated

FAQ

- Q: Is whooping cough still a problem despite routine childhood immunization?
- A: Yes. Pertussis often goes unrecognized as a cause of acute and chronic cough, particularly in infants who have not completed their immunization series and in older children, adolescents, and adults. Immunity from vaccination or natural infection may wane within 5 years, thus providing a reservoir of pertussis in the community. Tdap vaccination is recommended for all 11 years of age and older.
- Q: How can an ear examination help explain the cause of chronic cough?
- A: For some patients, the presence of cerumen, a foreign body, or irritation of the external auditory ear canal can stimulate the auricular branch of the vagus nerve ("Arnold nerve") and trigger a cough. This is also known as the oto-respiratory reflex. One study conducted in India suggests a 4% prevalence of this phenomenon.

CROHN DISEASE

Steven J. Fusillo, MD • Andrew B. Grossman, MD

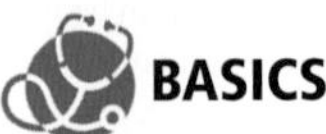

BASICS

DESCRIPTION

Crohn disease (CD) is a chronic inflammatory bowel disease (IBD) that may affect any part of the gastrointestinal (GI) tract from the mouth to the anus. CD is generally characterized by transmural skip lesions as well as periods of exacerbations and quiescence.

EPIDEMIOLOGY

- ~20–25% of patients with CD are diagnosed in childhood or adolescence.
- Family history of CD is present in 30% of patients <30 years old.
- In adulthood, male = female; in childhood, male > female (1.6:1)
- Higher prevalence in the developed world; increasingly more common in developing countries
- Although the prevalence is highest in Ashkenazi Jews, CD may occur in individuals of all racial and ethnic backgrounds.

RISK FACTORS

Genetics

- 1st-degree relatives have a 5–25% higher risk of developing CD.
- Children of one parent with CD have a 7–16% risk of developing either CD or ulcerative colitis (UC); if both parents affected, risk of child developing the disease is 33%.
- Sibling relative risk for developing CD is 13–26%.
- CD concordance in monozygotic twins is 30% and in dizygotic twins, 4%.
- CD is complex genetic disease:
  - >300 gene loci have been associated with CD.
  - >30 known amino acid polymorphisms
  - Most associated susceptibility genes are involved in host defense.
  - *NOD2/CARD15*: first gene associated with increased CD susceptibility
  - A *NOD2* risk allele confers a 2- to 3-fold relative risk of developing CD; risk increases 17-fold if two alleles present.
  - Several causative gene defects have been identified in very early-onset IBD (children diagnosed <6 years).
  - 8–15% of the healthy population possess at least one of these mutations, and 1% of healthy individuals are homozygous or compound heterozygous; suggests phenotypic expression of disease is subject to polygenic factors, variable penetrance, and other environmental mediators

PATHOPHYSIOLOGY

- Interaction and combination of environmental and genetic factors, intestinal microbiota, and likely one or more undetermined triggers (such as bacterial metabolic products) lead to a dysregulated immune response and chronic intestinal inflammation.
- CD pathogenesis is now attributed to dysfunction of both innate and adaptive immunity.
  - Innate immunity: Defects have been identified in epithelial barrier, microbial sensing, and autophagy in CD, for example, patients with the *CARD15/NOD2* mutation have dysregulated response to bacterial products.
  - Adaptive immunity: abnormal activation of T-helper-1 and Th17 lymphocytes leads to overproduction of inflammatory cytokines such as IL-2, IFNγ, IL-6, TNF-α, and IL-17 which cause invasive intestinal inflammation in CD.
- IL-23 is a significant cytokine in CD. Polymorphisms in the IL-23R gene have been associated with aberrant responses of both the innate and adaptive immune systems.

DIAGNOSIS

HISTORY

- Abdominal pain (85%)
- Weight loss (85%)
- Diarrhea (80%)
- Rectal bleeding (50%)
- Fever (40%)
- Growth failure (35%)
- Perianal disease (25%)
- Nausea and vomiting (25%)
- Delayed puberty
- Menstrual irregularity
- Extraintestinal disease (25%)
  - Arthritis
  - Erythema nodosum
  - Pyoderma gangrenosum
  - Mouth ulcers
  - Episcleritis
  - Uveitis
  - Thromboembolic disease
  - Vasculitis
  - Renal stones
  - Amyloidosis
  - Sclerosing cholangitis
  - Pancreatitis
- May present as acute intestinal obstruction or with abdominal abscess

PHYSICAL EXAM

- Fever, tachycardia, dehydration, pallor
- Growth delay and weight loss, delayed puberty
- Abdominal examination:
  - Right lower quadrant mass
  - Abdominal tenderness
- Rectal and perianal examination: skin tag, fissure, fistula, or abscess
- Evaluation for extraintestinal manifestations, such as arthritis, oral ulcers, and dermatologic involvement

DIFFERENTIAL DIAGNOSIS

- Ulcerative colitis
- Appendicitis
- Celiac disease
- Infection:
  - *Mycobacterium tuberculosis*
  - *Salmonella*, *Shigella dysenteriae*
  - *Campylobacter jejuni*, *Aeromonas* spp.
  - *Yersinia enterocolitica*, *Clostridium difficile*
  - *Escherichia coli*, *Giardia lamblia*, *Cryptosporidium*, *Strongyloides*
- Hemolytic uremic syndrome
- Henoch-Schönlein purpura
- Irritable bowel syndrome
- Peptic ulcer disease
- Autoimmune enteropathy, immunodeficiency
- Cow's milk protein allergy
- Small intestinal lymphoma
- Functional disorders

DIAGNOSTIC TESTS & INTERPRETATION

Initial Tests (screening, lab, imaging)

- CBC—microcytic anemia common (due to iron deficiency); may also have normocytic anemia due to chronic disease or a macrocytosis from nutritional deficiency (such as vitamin B_{12} or folate)
- ESR, CRP, stool calprotectin, stool lactoferrin—markers of inflammation/disease activity
- Comprehensive metabolic panel—hypoalbuminemia (sign of protein losing enteropathy), elevated transaminases (concomitant liver disease)
- Stool for occult blood and infectious studies, including stool bacterial cultures, *C. difficile* toxin assay, ova and parasites, and *Cryptosporidium*
- Serologic profiles, including perinuclear antineutrophil cytoplasmic antibody (pANCA) and anti–*Saccharomyces cerevisiae* antibody (ASCA), may be helpful in differentiating among types of IBD.
- Genetic screening among healthy, asymptomatic patients is not recommended.
- Consider plain abdominal radiograph in acute presentation to rule out obstruction, perforation, or toxic megacolon.
- In CD, the terminal ileum is the most commonly affected site in the GI tract. Other sites, in order of decreasing frequency, include right colon, isolated colon, proximal small bowel, and upper GI tract (stomach, duodenum, or esophagus).
- MRI enterography to assess disease extent and activity: preferred modality of imaging as it, spares radiation and provides information about small bowel and colonic disease, including abscesses and fistulae
- Barium upper GI and small bowel follow-through may also be used to evaluate extent of disease in small bowel but involve exposure to radiation.
- CT scan or ultrasound may be necessary to evaluate complications (abscess, phlegmon).
- Macroscopic findings:
  - Ulcerations
  - "Creeping fat" (increased mesenteric fat surrounding inflamed small intestinal loops)
  - Sinus tracts (extension of deep ulcerations beyond the intestinal wall)
  - Fistulae (communications between intestine and skin, other intestinal loops, or other organs)
  - Strictures
- Colonoscopy and upper endoscopy with multiple biopsies are the gold standard tests for initial evaluation and diagnosis of CD.
- Microscopic findings:
  - Transmural inflammation
  - Cryptitis and crypt abscesses
  - Granulomas (hallmark of CD)—present in 20–40% of biopsies
- Video capsule endoscopy can be used to assess small bowel not visualized with endoscopy.

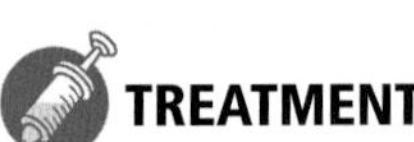

TREATMENT

MEDICATION

- The goal of therapy is resolution of all symptoms in the acute phase and microscopic healing of the intestinal mucosa, steroid-free long-term remission, appropriate growth, and good quality of life.
- 5-aminosalicylic acid (5-ASA)
  - Works locally to decrease inflammation in the bowel. These medications may be used for both

induction and maintenance of remission in mild to moderate disease but have modest efficacy. Various oral and topical preparations are available:
  - Oral mesalamine can be used to target terminal ileum and colon (Asacol®, Lialda®, Apriso®, Delzicol®: 50 to 100 mg/kg/24 h [max 4.8 g/24 h for active disease and 3.2 g/24 h to maintain remission]) or to target duodenum, jejunum, ileum, colon (Pentasa®: 50 to 100 mg/kg/24 h [max 4 g/24 h for active disease and 3 g/24 h to maintain remission])
  - Sulfasalazine (Azulfidine®): 40 to 60 mg/kg/24 h (max 4 g/24 h) for active disease and 30 mg/kg/24 h (max 2 g/24 h) for maintenance of remission (liquid preparation available)
  - Balsalazide (Colazal®; 6.75 g/24 h; 110 to 170 mg/kg/24 h)
  - Rectal mesalamine (Rowasa®/Canasa®): 4-g enemas and 500-mg suppositories daily to b.i.d. PR
- Corticosteroids
  - May be used to control intestinal inflammation in the acute setting and to induce remission of disease
  - Long-term use should be avoided given the unfavorable side-effect profile. Effective dosing for CD is 1 to 2 mg/kg/24 h IV methylprednisolone or oral prednisone (max 60 mg/24 h). Initial treatment course of ~10 to 14 days, with dosing taper initiated as soon as clinically indicated.
  - Topical hydrocortisone is useful in localized left-sided colonic disease and is available in liquid or foam enemas.
  - Corticosteroid with controlled ileal release, budesonide (9 mg/24 h) is also available.
- Enteral nutrition therapy
  - With exclusive enteral nutrition (EEN), all calories are given via an elemental or polymeric diet. EEN may be administered orally or via NG tube feeds (typically given overnight). This option is frequently used in Europe and Canada as a 1st-line therapy to induce remission in lieu of steroids.
  - Enteral nutrition therapy providing at least 80–90% of daily calories has been shown to be effective in inducing remission, especially in active small bowel disease and may also help to correct growth failure.
  - Enteral nutrition has the appeal of being drug-free but does involve a large commitment from the patient and may be difficult to maintain long-term.
- Immunomodulators
  - Azathioprine, 2 to 3 mg/kg/24 h PO, and its metabolite 6-mercaptopurine (6-MP) 1 to 1.5 mg/kg/24 h PO, may be used as maintenance therapy in patients who have achieved remission. Adverse events include liver toxicity, leukopenia, pancreatitis, and slightly increased risk of malignancy, specifically lymphoma.
  - Methotrexate is also used for the maintenance of remission, at 10 to 25 mg IM or PO once weekly. Adverse effects are similar to azathioprine and 6-MP, with the addition of nausea and vomiting and pulmonary fibrosis.
  - Frequent laboratory follow-up is necessary when immunomodulators are used. WBC and platelet count should be monitored carefully. In the case of azathioprine and 6-MP, thiopurine methyltransferase (TPMT)—an enzyme catabolizing these drugs—activity or genotype should be determined prior to drug initiation. If TPMT activity is absent (homozygous), these immunomodulators should not be used due to severe risk of myelosuppression. If TPMT activity is intermediate (heterozygous), they should be used in adjusted decreased doses with close monitoring of WBC count.
  - Other immunomodulatory therapy used infrequently: cyclosporine, tacrolimus (FK-506), thalidomide, etc.
- Biologics
  - Infliximab, a biologic, chimeric anti–TNF-α antibody (5 mg/kg IV infusion; induction doses given at 0, 2, and 6 weeks), followed by maintenance infusions, typically every 8 weeks, for treatment of moderate to severe CD
  - Adalimumab, a humanized anti–TNF-α antibody (80 to 160 mg SC at week 0, 40 to 80 mg at week 2, and 20 to 40 mg at week 4, and bimonthly thereafter) also approved for use in children with moderate to severe CD
  - Both infliximab and adalimumab can be used for both induction and maintenance of remission. Serum drug levels and antidrug antibodies can be monitored to help guide medication dosing. Dose escalation is often required. Side effects include serious infections, anaphylactic reactions, rash and possibly slightly increased risk of malignancy (lymphoma).
  - Vedolizumab, a monoclonal antibody that blocks the $\alpha_4\beta_7$ integrin resulting in gut-specific anti-inflammatory activity, is approved for adults with moderate to severe CD and is currently being studied in pediatric IBD.
  - Ustekinumab is a monoclonal antibody directed against IL-12 and IL-23 that was recently approved for use in adult CD and is currently being studied in pediatrics as well.
- Antibiotics
  - Antibiotics can be used for induction of remission, fistulizing disease, or postoperative maintenance of remission; however, their efficacy is modest, and side effects frequently preclude their long-term use.
  - Metronidazole: 15 mg/kg/24 h
  - Ciprofloxacin: 20 mg/kg/24 h
  - Rifaximin: 200 mg t.i.d. to 800 mg b.i.d.
- Complementary therapy (probiotics, prebiotics)

SURGERY/OTHER PROCEDURES

- Surgery may be considered for localized CD that is unresponsive to other therapies or that is causing intractable bleeding.
- Surgery may be necessary in stricturing and/or penetrating disease, especially in cases of proximal intestinal dilatation, obstruction, or perforation.
- Several types of procedures are available: stricture-plasty, abscess drainage, seton placement (for perianal fistulae), and intestinal resection (side-to-side anastomosis is widely accepted).
- Surgery for CD is not curative, and postoperative recurrence at the site of anastomosis is common. Postoperative surveillance at the anastomosis is recommended.

ONGOING CARE

FOLLOW-UP RECOMMENDATIONS

Patient Monitoring

- The morbidity of CD is high. The majority of patients experience recurring disease.
- Most patients have good general health in between episodes and go on to lead productive lives.
- Carcinoma surveillance is necessary on a regular basis.
- Routine health maintenance should include bone density scan, 25-OH Vitamin D monitoring, yearly influenza vaccination, and ophthalmologic evaluation.

COMPLICATIONS

- Intestinal obstruction due to strictures or adhesions
- Abscess or phlegmon formation
- Enteroenteric, enterovesical, enterovaginal, or enterocutaneous fistulae
- Perforation
- Gallstones, kidney stones
- Intestinal lymphoma, colon cancer
- Malabsorption resulting in nutritional deficiencies (e.g., vitamin B_{12} or iron deficiency)
- Short bowel syndrome due to repeated bowel resections
- Massive hemorrhage is rare (1%).
- Growth failure is frequent; final height is reduced, and puberty is delayed in CD affecting prepubertal children.
- Future infertility due to inflammation involving the fallopian tubes and ovaries
- Osteopenia and osteoporosis secondary to inflammation, nutritional deficiency, and/or therapeutic side effects (corticosteroids)
- Toxic megacolon is a rare but serious complication.

C

ADDITIONAL READING

- Benchimol EI, Fortinsky KJ, Gozdyra P, et al. Epidemiology of pediatric inflammatory bowel disease: a systematic review of international trends. *Inflamm Bowel Dis*. 2011;17(1):423–439.
- Cabré E, Gassull MA. Nutritional and metabolic issues in inflammatory bowel disease. *Curr Opin Clin Nutr Metab Care*. 2003;6(5):569–576.
- Day AS, Ledder O, Leach ST, et al. Crohn's and colitis in children and adolescents. *World J Gastroenterol*. 2012;18(41):5862–5869.
- Henderson P, van Limbergen JE, Wilson DC, et al. Genetics of childhood-onset disease. *Inflamm Bowel Dis*. 2011;17(1):346–361.
- Hildebrand H, Karlberg J, Kristiansson B. Longitudinal growth in children and adolescents with inflammatory bowel disease. *J Pediatr Gastroenterol Nutr*. 1994;18(2):165–173.
- Kugathasan S, Baldassano RN, Bradfield JP, et al. Loci on 20q13 and 21q22 are associated with pediatric-onset inflammatory bowel disease. *Nat Genet*. 2008;40(10):1211–1215.
- Maltz R, Podberesky DJ, Saeed SA. Imaging modalities in pediatric inflammatory bowel disease. *Curr Opin Pediatr*. 2014;26(5):590–596.
- Rufo PA, Denson LA, Sylvester FA, et al. Health supervision in the management of children and adolescents with IBD: NASPGHAN recommendations. *J Pediatr Gastroenterol Nutr*. 2012;55(1):93–108.

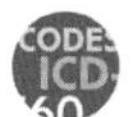

CODES

ICD10

- K50.90 Crohn's disease, unspecified, without complications
- K50.913 Crohn's disease, unspecified, with fistula
- K50.911 Crohn's disease, unspecified, with rectal bleeding

FAQ

- Q: Should the diet of patients with CD be restricted?
- A: One approach to inducing remission in active disease can be to use EEN. However, this approach can be difficult to maintain long-term and should be reserved for those patients who are committed to excluding all other foods. In general, a careful, balanced approach to nutrition in children with CD is required to assure appropriate growth and development. The only foods not recommended are poorly digestible, high-residue vegetables, nuts, and popcorn, which can cause obstruction in the narrowed, inflamed intestine. Patients with secondary lactose intolerance should use lactase supplements or avoid milk products while ensuring adequate calories and calcium intake.

CROUP (LARYNGOTRACHEOBRONCHITIS)

Lauren Castner, DO • Steven Bin, MD • Amy G. Filbrun, MD, MS

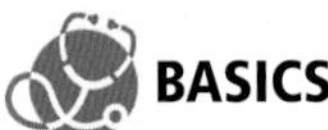

BASICS

DESCRIPTION

- Croup (laryngotracheobronchitis) is a common respiratory illness in children that presents with hoarseness, a characteristic barking cough, rhinorrhea, and fever.
- Spasmodic croup (subglottic allergic edema) refers to an illness characterized by sudden inspiratory stridor at night followed by sudden resolution. Mild cold symptoms may be present but are often absent. The child can have frequent attacks on the same night or for multiple, successive nights.

EPIDEMIOLOGY

- Accounts for 3–5% of total visits to the emergency department (ED)
- Most commonly occurs in children between 6 and 36 months of age
  - Although cases can be seen up to 6 years of age, it is uncommon in children >6 years.
  - Mean age at presentation is 18 months.
- Timing
  - Most prevalent in the fall to early winter
  - Major peak in October with parainfluenza type 1, with minor peaks later during respiratory syncytial virus (RSV) and influenza season
  - ED visits for croup are most frequent between the hours of 10 p.m. and 4 a.m.
- More common in males (ratio 1.4:1)

RISK FACTORS

- Anatomic narrowing of the airway such as in subglottic stenosis or laryngeal cysts or hemangiomas
- Prior history of croup
- Hyperactive airway triggered by atopy or reflux seen in recurrent croup
- Preexisting airway swelling

ETIOLOGY

- In children, the cricoid ring of the trachea, located in the immediate subglottic area, is the narrowest part of their upper airway. A small amount of edema in this region can lead to significant airway obstruction, which is what makes children especially susceptible to this illness.
- Caused mainly by respiratory viruses including the following:
  - Parainfluenza virus types 1 to 3, most commonly; accounting for 65% of cases
  - Adenovirus
  - RSV—in some cases, patients may also have wheezing present
  - Influenza virus A, B
  - Rhinoviruses
  - Enteroviruses
  - Metapneumovirus
  - Enteric cytopathogenic human orphan virus (echovirus)
  - Human coronavirus NL63
  - Measles—in areas where measles is prevalent
  - *Mycoplasma pneumoniae*—associated with mild cases of croup
  - Bacterial infection may occur secondarily by *Staphylococcus aureus*, *Streptococcus pyogenes*, and *Streptococcus pneumoniae*.

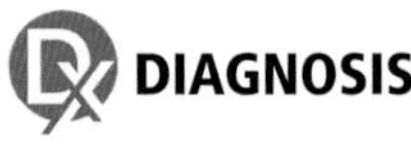

DIAGNOSIS

HISTORY

- Croup typically starts with an upper respiratory infection (URI)—rhinorrhea, cough, and congestion.
- Fever is often present.
- Within 12 to 48 hours, upper airway obstruction occurs abruptly resulting in hoarseness, "barky cough," and inspiratory stridor. Symptoms persist for 3 to 7 days.
- Usually presents as hoarseness in children >6 years of age or adults

ALERT

The sudden development of inspiratory stridor without URI symptoms or fever should prompt the clinician to maintain a high index of suspicion for a foreign body aspiration or upper airway mass.

- Foreign body aspiration is usually preceded by a history of choking or sudden onset cough.
- Recurrent episodes of stridor should lead to the consideration of spasmodic croup, an anatomic abnormality, or an underlying condition such as atopy.
- In a child with truncal or multiple strawberry hemangiomas, a sudden episode of stridor without fever or URI symptoms should raise the concern for a hemangioma in the child's airway.
- Bacterial tracheitis should be suspected in a child who presents with high fever and toxic appearance, or develops marked worsening of symptoms after having mild croup symptoms.

PHYSICAL EXAM

- Examine the child in a comfortable position and make every effort to not agitate the child, as this can often worsen their symptoms.
- Observe for stridor at rest, irritability, and fatigue. Assess respiratory status and level of consciousness.
- Vital signs:
  - Fever and tachypnea may be present.
  - A child with croup is usually not hypoxic because croup affects the upper airway.
  - Hypoxia is a sign of an impending complete airway obstruction.
- A child with croup will likely have a hoarse voice, inflamed pharynx, and varying degrees of respiratory distress.
- The degree of respiratory distress should be observed by assessing for tachypnea, nasal flaring, retractions, grunting, and use of accessory muscles.
- Children with significant upper airway obstruction may sit in a "sniffing" position with their neck mildly flexed and head mildly extended.
  - This position contrasts with the "tripod" position noted in epiglottitis where the child is in a sitting position with the chin pushed forward and refusing to lie down.
- The presence of inspiratory stridor should be determined.
  - Stridor may be present at rest or only with agitation, and this difference will affect the patient's management.
  - Stridor at rest is a sign of significant upper airway obstruction and needs urgent treatment with racemic epinephrine.
- The hydration status of the child should be assessed.
  - Drooling should not be present with croup.
  - Drooling may indicate a different diagnosis such as epiglottitis or peritonsillar abscess.
- The severity of croup can be determined by a clinical scoring system known as the modified Westley Croup Score (see "Table 1").
  - Score <3: mild disease
  - Score of 3 to 6: moderate disease
  - Score >6: severe disease

DIFFERENTIAL DIAGNOSIS

ALERT

Cases of epiglottitis still occur in unimmunized and underimmunized children; therefore, it is important to check the child's immunization status.

Other important diseases to consider in the differential include the following:

- Infectious
  - Acute epiglottitis
  - Bacterial tracheitis
  - Retropharyngeal abscess
  - Adenotonsillitis
  - Diphtheria
  - Pneumonia
  - Ulcerative laryngitis
- Allergic/inflammatory
  - Asthma
  - Anaphylaxis
  - Angioedema
  - Microaspiration secondary to gastroesophageal reflux or hypotonia
- Environmental
  - Foreign body aspiration
  - Caustic ingestion or burn
  - Smoke inhalation
  - Paraquat poisoning
- Traumatic
  - Subglottic edema/stenosis postintubation
  - Laryngeal or subglottic hematoma
  - Laryngeal fracture
- Obstruction/masses
  - Papillomatosis
  - Hemangioma
  - Cystic hygroma
  - Lymphoma
  - Rhabdomyosarcoma
  - Thymoma
  - Teratoma
  - Thyroglossal duct cyst
  - Branchial cleft cyst
- Congenital anomalies of the upper airway
  - Tracheomalacia/laryngomalacia
  - Vascular ring
  - Laryngeal web
- Genetic/metabolic
  - Hypocalcemia

DIAGNOSTIC TESTS & INTERPRETATION

Initial Tests (screening, lab, imaging)

- Croup is a clinical diagnosis.
- The anxiety associated with invasive laboratory and imaging studies may worsen the child's condition and are often not needed.
- Obtaining rapid antigen tests and cultures are not recommended. If intubation is attempted, trachea cultures should be obtained to evaluate for the presence of bacterial tracheitis.
- Radiographs may be helpful to rule out other causes of stridor; they should be considered in children with atypical courses, recurrent episodes, failure to respond to treatment, or if a foreign body is suspected (although of note, most foreign bodies are not radio-opaque).
- Classically, an anteroposterior view demonstrates the "steeple" sign, which is a narrowed air column in the subglottic area.

Table 1. Croup (Laryngotracheobronchitis)—Severity Score for Croup Patients (Westley Croup Score)

Indicator of Severity of Illness	Score
Inspiratory stridor	
None	0
At rest, with stethoscope	1
At rest, w/o stethoscope	2
Retractions	
None	0
Mild	1
Moderate	2
Severe	3
Air entry	
Normal	0
Decreased	1
Severely decreased	2
Cyanosis	
None	0
With agitation	4
At rest	5
Level of consciousness	
Normal	0
Altered mental status	5

Diagnosis Procedures/Other
- Pulse oximetry
- Visual inspection of the airway via bronchoscopy and direct or fiberoptic laryngoscopy may be helpful in cases of recurrent croup to rule out an anatomic abnormality. In spasmodic croup, noninflammatory edema may be seen of the airway suggesting atopy.
- Pathologic findings
  - Gross pathology: edema and erythema of the subglottic trachea; occasionally, pseudomembranes or exudate are noted.
  - Microscopic: edema of airway lining with infiltration of neutrophils, histiocytes, plasma cells, and lymphocytes

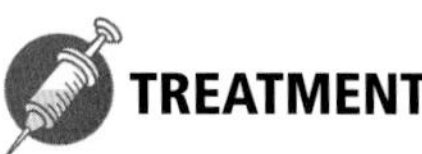

TREATMENT

Initial stabilization
- Racemic epinephrine
- Corticosteroids
- Oxygen (if needed)
- Endotracheal intubation is very rarely required, noted to occur about 1% of the time in studies.

GENERAL MEASURES
- Children with mild symptoms can be treated with humidity, antipyretics, and oral hydration at home. However, randomized controlled trials (RCTs) have not demonstrated a benefit for the use of humidity.
- Short, acute episodes of stridor can be treated with cool mist, a bathroom filled with steam from a shower or cold night air. If the stridor persists, worsens, or occurs at rest, the child should be seen in the ER.
- It is important to try to keep the child calm, as agitation or anxiety can worsen symptoms and increase work of breathing.

ALERT

In the child with impending respiratory failure, prompt intubation and direct visualization of the airway in the operating room is imperative. Do not wait for x-rays to confirm a diagnosis.

MEDICATION
- Corticosteroids and nebulized racemic epinephrine, which are the main treatments for croup, have resulted in a dramatic reduction in the number of admissions and length of hospital stays in patients with croup.
- Dexamethasone (PO or IM; half-life 36 to 54 hours) 0.6 mg/kg single dose (max 10 mg) has been shown to reduce symptoms in patients with moderate to severe croup.
  - Oral dexamethasone is the most cost-effective steroid treatment available.
  - Comparable efficacy between oral and IM
  - Reduces risk of returning to the ED 7 to 10 days after initial visit
  - It has been shown to start having an effect within 30 minutes.
- Alternatively, prednisolone 1 to 2 mg/kg for 1 to 3 daily doses can be used to treat a patient with mild to moderate croup. Efficacy does not differ from dexamethasone, but there may be more return ED visits; can be used if dexamethasone is not readily available
- Budesonide given via nebulizer at a dose of 2 mg administered q12h—shown to be as effective as dexamethasone in reducing symptoms; less systemic absorption compared with dexamethasone, with maximum deposition of drug in the upper airway. Can reduce symptoms for up to 24 hours. Onset of action is between 1 and 2 hours. Consider if the patient is vomiting or is unable to take oral medications.
- Racemic epinephrine: A nebulized racemic epinephrine treatment offers immediate reduction in swelling of the laryngeal airway in children who present with at least moderate croup; dose: 0.5 mL of 2.25% solution (D- and L-isomers) in 2.5 mL normal saline delivered via nebulizer as needed
- Helium-oxygen can be used in 70:30 or 80:20 concentrations for severe respiratory distress. When used in combination with corticosteroids, heliox may provide improvement in croup scores 60 to 90 minutes into treatment but does not have a long-term benefit.

ADMISSION, INPATIENT, AND NURSING CONSIDERATIONS
- Admission criteria
  - Persistent stridor at rest and/or respiratory distress (chest wall retractions) despite treatment with steroids and racemic epinephrine
  - Requirement of treatment of racemic epinephrine more than once over a 3- to 4-hour period
  - Dehydration or risk for dehydration
  - Admission should be strongly considered for children who present symptomatically to an ER more than once and have significant stridor on day 1 of illness as croup is usually worse on days 2 to 3.
- Discharge criteria
  - Croup score of ≤3 over a 1- to 3-hour period of observation
  - Received 1 dose of corticosteroid and observed for at least 2 hours
  - Does not require racemic epinephrine in the 3 to 4 hours prior to discharge
  - Able to take adequate PO fluids

ISSUES FOR REFERRAL
- The vast majority of children with croup do well. However, transfer to a facility where trained individuals can address pediatric airway problems should be considered if the patient is inadequately responding to treatment or has increasing respiratory distress.
- A recent study showed heliox during transport for children with severe croup provided added benefit to their prognosis.

PROGNOSIS
- The vast majority of patients do not require hospitalization.
- Almost all patients go on to complete recovery.

COMPLICATIONS
- Poor oral intake/dehydration
- Hypoxia
- Upper airway obstruction
- Respiratory failure (rare)

C

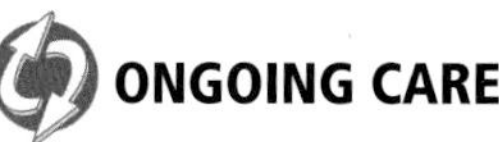

ONGOING CARE

FOLLOW-UP RECOMMENDATIONS

Patient Monitoring
- In most cases, the illness is self-limited, lasting 3 to 5 days.
- A "rebound phenomenon" with worsening of stridor and respiratory distress after initial relief with the racemic epinephrine treatment may be seen up to 2 hours posttreatment in some patients.
- Dexamethasone has a half-life of 36 to 54 hours so parents should be warned that some children may have worsening in 2 days after treatment with this medication.
- Several studies have shown that children can be safely discharged 3 to 4 hours after racemic epinephrine treatment.

ALERT

Recurrent croup may signal an underlying anatomic problem and needs evaluation for other causes.

ADDITIONAL READING

- Bjornson CL, Johnson DW. Croup in Children. *CMAJ*. 2013;185(15):1317–1323.
- Bjornson CL, Russell KF, Vandermeer B, et al. Nebulized epinephrine for croup in children. *Cochrane Database Syst Rev*. 2011;(2):CD006619.
- Donaldson D, Poleski D, Knipple E, et al. Intramuscular versus oral dexamethasone for the treatment of moderate-to-severe croup: a randomized, double-blind trial. *Acad Emerg Med*. 2003;10(1):16–21.
- Kline-Krammes S, Reed C, Giuliano JS Jr, et al. Heliox in children with croup: a strategy to hasten improvement. *Air Med J*. 2012;31(3):131–137.
- Miller EK, Gebretsadik T, Carroll KN, et al. Viral etiologies of infant bronchiolitis, croup and upper respiratory illness during 4 consecutive years. *Pediatr Infect Dis J*. 2013;32(9):950–955.
- Moraa I, Sturman N, McGuire T, et al. Heliox for croup in children. *Cochrane Database Syst Rev*. 2013;(12):CD006822.
- Petrocheilou A, Tanou K, Kalampouka E, et al. Viral croup: diagnosis and a treatment algorithm. *Pediatr Pulmonol*. 2014;49(5):421–429.
- Toward Optimized Practice (TOP) Working Group for Croup. *Diagnosis and Management of Croup: Clinical Practice Guideline*. Edmonton, Canada: Toward Optimized Practice; 2008.

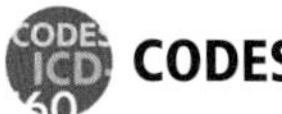

CODES

ICD10
- J05.0 Acute obstructive laryngitis [croup]
- J40 Bronchitis, not specified as acute or chronic

CRYING

Maria Jacklin Janecek, DO

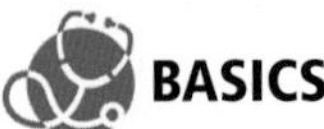

BASICS

DESCRIPTION

- Crying is usually a normal physiologic response to stress, discomfort, unfulfilled needs such as hunger, pain, over- or understimulation, or temperature change.
- Crying is felt to be potentially pathologic if it is interpreted by caregivers as differing in quality and duration without apparent explanation and/or persists without consolability beyond a reasonable time (generally 1 to 2 hours).

EPIDEMIOLOGY

Excessive crying in the 1st months of life, per parental reports, occurs in about 1 in 5 infants.

ETIOLOGY

- The most likely cause of inconsolable crying in the first few months of life is infantile colic.
  - However, colic is a diagnosis of exclusion.
  - Practitioners must be familiar with the clinical pattern of infantile colic so that deviations are readily recognized.
- Organic problems are identified in 5% or less of afebrile excessively crying infants.

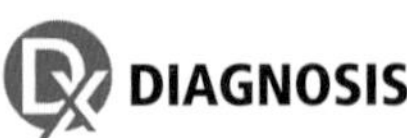

DIAGNOSIS

A thorough history and physical exam with removal of all clothing is the key to diagnosis and can provide clues to the etiology in the majority of cases.

HISTORY

- **Question:** Colic?
- *Significance*:
  - Colic less likely as a cause if onset after 1 month of age or persistent in infants >4 months of age
  - Recurrent episodes, particularly with a diurnal or late afternoon/evening pattern, are more likely due to colic.
- **Question:** Feeding?
- *Significance*:
  - Crying shortly after feeding suggests aerophagia or gastroesophageal reflux; 1 hour after feeding suggests formula intolerance. A rare cause of postprandial crying is anomalous coronary arteries.
  - Overfeeding or underfeeding, excessive air swallowing, inadequate burping, and improper formula preparation may contribute to excessive crying.
- **Question:** Fever?
- *Significance*: indicates potential need for evaluation of sepsis, meningitis, other infections
- **Question:** Paradoxically increased crying (attempts at consolation make the crying worse, especially with lifting, rocking)?
- *Significance*: can be seen in meningitis, peritonitis, long bone fractures, arthritis
- **Question:** Stridor?
- *Significance*: implies possible upper airway obstruction (mechanical, functional)
- **Question:** Expiratory grunting?
- *Significance*: indicates higher likelihood of a significant pathologic cause of crying (especially cardiac, respiratory, and/or infectious disease)
- **Question:** Cold symptoms and/or day care attendance?
- *Significance*: increases likelihood of otitis media
- **Question:** Vomiting?
- *Significance*: increases likelihood of pathologic GI cause (e.g., pyloric stenosis, obstruction, gastroesophageal reflux with possible esophagitis), particularly in infant <3 months of age, or CNS disease
- **Question:** Recent fall or trauma?
- *Significance*: may indicate possible fracture, increased intracranial pressure, abuse
- **Question:** Documented weight loss outside of the 2-week neonatal period?
- *Significance*: suggests an organic cause if insufficient caloric intake is excluded, especially in the breastfed newborn

PHYSICAL EXAM

- **Finding:** Infant appears ill (e.g., pallor, grunting, poor arousability, poor response to social overtures)?
- *Significance*: implies much higher likelihood of an organic cause
- **Finding:** Tenderness on palpation of extremities, clavicle, scalp, or painful or decreased range of motion of joints?
- *Significance*: suggests fracture, subluxation, osteomyelitis, septic arthritis
- **Finding:** Conjunctival redness, eye tearing, scratches near the eye?
- *Significance*: suggest corneal abrasion (fluorescein testing of eye warranted) or foreign body in eye (eversion of lid recommended). Cessation of crying with ophthalmic anesthetic drops while doing fluorescein staining suggests corneal injury as a cause.
- **Finding:** Impacted or bloody stool on rectal exam, abdominal mass?
- *Significance*: suggest constipation or intussusception
- **Finding:** Geographic scars, frenulum tears, retinal hemorrhages, suspicious bruises, burns (e.g., palatal), decreased weight/height ratio?
- *Significance*: suggest neglect/abuse (physical, emotional). Bruises are rare in preambulatory children (particularly <6 months of age); if found, particularly in patterns, consider inflicted injuries.
- **Finding:** Bulging or full fontanel (especially in upright, quiet infant)?
- *Significance*: indicates possible increased intracranial pressure (e.g., meningitis, subdural hematoma, hydrocephalus, vitamin A toxicity)
- **Finding:** Edema of individual toes, fingers, or penis?
- *Significance*: suggests hair tourniquet syndrome
- **Finding:** Tender swelling in inguinal or scrotal area?
- *Significance*: may indicate incarcerated hernia, testicular torsion
- **Finding:** Heart rate >200 bpm with minimal variability?
- *Significance*: indicates possible supraventricular tachycardia
- **Finding:** Hypothermia?
- *Significance*: suggests infections or hypothyroidism

DIFFERENTIAL DIAGNOSIS

- Congenital/anatomic
  - Intussusception
  - Gastroesophageal reflux/esophagitis
  - Malrotation/volvulus
  - Gaseous distention (secondary to improper feeding or burping)
  - Incarcerated inguinal hernia
  - Peritonitis (acute abdomen)
  - Pneumothorax
  - Testicular/ovarian torsion
  - Constipation
  - Anal fissure
  - Meatal ulceration
  - Glaucoma
  - Nephrolithiasis
  - Urinary retention (secondary to posterior urethral valves)
  - Cardiac—anomalous coronary artery, hypoxia, congestive heart failure (CHF)
  - Increased intracranial pressure (hydrocephalus, tumor, pseudotumor cerebri)
- Infectious
  - Otitis media/externa
  - UTI/pyelonephritis
  - Stomatitis/gingivitis
  - Meningitis/encephalitis
  - Endocarditis/myocarditis/pericarditis
  - Diskitis
  - Gastroenteritis
  - Appendicitis
  - Mastitis
  - Arthritis, septic
  - Osteomyelitis
  - Perianal cellulitis
  - Balanitis
  - Dermatitis (especially pruritic as in scabies or painful as in staphylococcal scalded skin syndrome)
- Toxic, environmental, drugs
  - Neonatal drug withdrawal
  - Prenatal/perinatal cocaine exposure
  - Immunization reactions (especially DTP)
  - Isolated fructose intolerance
  - Drug reactions (especially antihistamines, pseudoephedrine, phenylpropanolamine), including maternal medications in breast milk
  - Vitamin A toxicity
  - Carbon monoxide exposure
  - Emotional/physical neglect
  - Foreign body ingestion (coin, pin)
  - Ear foreign body (cockroach)
- Trauma
  - Corneal abrasion
  - Foreign body (hypopharynx, eye, ear, nose)
  - Skull fracture/subdural hematoma
  - Intracranial hemorrhage
  - Retinal hemorrhage (shaken baby syndrome)
  - Other fractures (especially extremities)
  - Subluxation
  - Hair tourniquet syndrome (encircling finger, toe, penis, clitoris)
  - Open diaper pin
  - Bite (human, animal, insect)
  - Burns

- Genetic/metabolic
  - Sickle cell crisis
  - Phenylketonuria
  - Hypothyroidism
  - Electrolyte abnormalities (especially sodium)
  - Hypoglycemia
  - Hypocalcemia
  - Hypercalcemia
  - Inborn error of metabolism
- Allergic/inflammatory
  - Cow milk allergy/allergic colitis
  - Celiac disease (gluten enteropathy)
  - Hemolytic uremic syndrome
  - Henoch-Schönlein purpura
  - Kawasaki disease
  - Pancreatitis
- Functional
  - Parental expectations/responses
- Miscellaneous
  - Overstimulation
  - Persistent night awakening
  - Night terrors
  - Caffey disease (infantile cortical hyperostosis)
  - Dysrhythmia (especially supraventricular tachycardia)
  - IV infiltration
  - Autism
  - Teething
  - Headache/migraine
  - Temperament
  - Colic
  - Discomfort (cold, heat, itching, hunger)

DIAGNOSTIC TESTS & INTERPRETATION

Diagnostic testing should be based on history and physical exam findings. In <1% of children, will testing contribute to a diagnosis in the absence of a suggestive clinical picture.

- **Test:** stool for occult blood
- *Significance*: possible intussusception, anal fissure
- **Test:** fluorescein testing of eye
- *Significance*: corneal abrasion (may occur without significant conjunctival redness)
- **Test:** urinalysis/urine culture
- *Significance*: UTI
- **Test:** urine toxicology screen
- *Significance*: drug withdrawal (neonatal), ingestions, passive exposures (e.g., cocaine)
- **Test:** pulse oximetry
- *Significance*: Hypoxia (from cardiac causes) may cause increased irritability.
- **Test:** electrolyte panel/blood glucose
- *Significance*: endocrine or metabolic disturbance, especially if abnormal sodium, hypoglycemia, significant acidosis, or elevated anion gap
- **Test:** skeletal survey
- *Significance*: suspected abuse; also consider MRI or head CT scan for infants <6 months with evidence of abuse and children <1 year of age with high-risk injuries (rib fractures, multiple fractures, or facial injury).

ALERT

Factors that make this an emergency include the following:

- Suspicion of meningitis: stiff neck, bulging fontanel, fever (especially infants <2 to 3 months of age)
- Suspicion of intestinal obstruction: vomiting (especially bilious or projectile), mass on abdominal palpation, and/or bloody stools
- Suspicion of incarcerated hernia or testicular/ovarian torsion
- Evidence of cardiac compromise (CHF, supraventricular tachycardia): tachycardia, poor perfusion (capillary refill >3 seconds, poor distal pulses), rales
- Evidence of acute dehydration: weight loss, decreased urine output, orthostatic changes, poor perfusion
- Evidence of child abuse or neglect

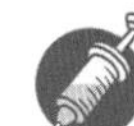

TREATMENT

- General goal is to decide if the crying represents a normal physiologic response, a protracted multifactorial physiologic/developmental response (colic), or a potentially pathologic problem.
- Triage: How urgent is the need for evaluation? A classic and difficult triage issue. One must identify the periodicity of the problem, associated symptoms, impression of wellness, and parental anxiety/reliability. If colic seems unlikely, see the patient as soon as possible.
- Management is then based on the most likely diagnosis following evaluation.
  - Crying that has resolved prior to the arrival or early in the assessment is less likely to be caused by serious illness but still warrants follow-up by phone or in the office, in order not to miss conditions characterized by intermittent symptoms or paroxysms (e.g., intussusception).
  - If crying is persistent or recurrent during the initial exam then observation is recommended.
  - If after a period of observation the child appears well or is easily consoled and parental anxiety is alleviated then 24-hour follow-up is recommended.
- In those patients in whom the history, physical exam, and initial workup are not diagnostic and who continue to show signs of excessive crying, continued observation and serial exams with possible admission is recommended. Be wary of the infant who, despite a period of observation, is not noted at any time to be calm when awake.

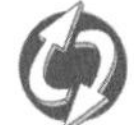

ONGOING CARE

FOLLOW-UP RECOMMENDATIONS

24-hour-follow up is recommended to be assured the crying has improved/resolved and the correct diagnosis and appropriate treatment was given. If the crying is persistent then reevaluation may be necessary.

ADDITIONAL READING

- Bolte R. The crying child: what are they trying to tell you? Parts I and II. *Contemp Pediatr*. 2007;24:74–81, 90–95.
- Chau K, Lau E, Greenberg S, et al. Probiotics for infantile colic: a randomized, double-blind, placebo-controlled trial investigating *Lactobacillus reuteri* DSM 17938. *J Pediatr*. 2015;166(1):74–78.
- Douglas P, Hill P. Managing infants who cry excessively in the first few months of life. *BMJ*. 2011;343:d7772.
- Douglas P, Hill P. The crying baby: what approach? *Curr Opin Pediatr*. 2011;23(5):523–529.
- Freedman SB, Al-Harthy N, Thull-Freedman J. The crying infant: diagnostic testing and frequency of serious underlying disease. *Pediatrics*. 2009;123(3):841–848.
- Herman M, Le A. The crying infant. *Emerg Med Clin North Am*. 2007;25(4):1137–1159.
- McKenzie SA. Fifteen-minute consultation: troublesome crying in infancy. *Arch Dis Child Educ Pract Ed*. 2013;98(6):209–211.
- Poole SR. The infant with acute, unexplained, excessive crying. *Pediatrics*. 1991;88(3):450–455.
- Rubin DM, Christian CW, Bilaniuk LT, et al. Occult head injury in high-risk abused children. *Pediatrics*. 2003;111(6, Pt 1):1382–1386.

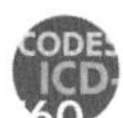

CODES

ICD10

- R68.11 Excessive crying of infant (baby)
- R10.83 Colic
- K21.9 Gastro-esophageal reflux disease without esophagitis

FAQ

- Q: How might the quality of cry be helpful in the diagnosis?
- A: Subjective interpretation can be helpful.
  - High-pitched (shrill, piercing) crying in short bursts: associated with CNS pathology, especially with increased intracranial pressure
  - High-pitched crying in longer bursts: seen in small-for-gestational age infants, neonatal drug withdrawal
  - Hoarse crying: seen in hypothyroidism, laryngeal diseases, hypocalcemic tetany
  - Weak crying: may be seen in neuromuscular disorders, infant botulism, and/or the very ill infant
  - Catlike cry: can be associated with cri du chat syndrome (5p-syndrome or absence of short arm of chromosome 5)
- Q: How common is teething as a cause of excessive crying?
- A: Patients' families often suggest teething as a cause of excessive crying (as well as fever, diarrhea, rashes, etc.). Objective data do not support a strong association. Be careful in ascribing symptoms and signs to teething.
- Q: What role does over-the-counter supplements take in helping to reduce crying attributable to colic?
- A: A specific probiotic strain, *Lactobacillus reuteri* DSM 17938 given for 21 days or longer to infants with colic was shown to reduce crying time in breastfed infants by >50% compared to placebo. This is the only over-the-counter supplement that has been consistently proven beneficial for breastfed infants with colic in clinical trials.
- Q: Are there any other measures such as changing formulas or antireflux medications that may be helpful for colic?
- A: Changing of formulas or the prescription of antireflux medications is not recommended in the absence of other symptoms suggestive of milk protein intolerance/allergic colitis or without any other symptoms of reflux pathology causing gastroesophageal reflux disease.

CRYPTOCOCCAL INFECTIONS

Eric S. Kirkendall, MD, MBI, FAAP • Samir S. Shah, MD, MSCE

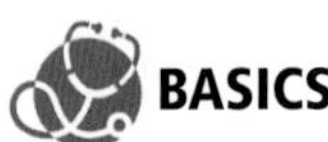

BASICS

DESCRIPTION

Cryptococcosis is an opportunistic fungal infection caused by *Cryptococcus neoformans* that may involve several organ systems, including the CNS, lungs, bones, visceral organs, and skin. *Cryptococcus gattii* is a less common human pathogen.

EPIDEMIOLOGY

- Most pediatric infections occur in immunocompromised hosts, including those with malignancy, HIV, and solid organ or bone marrow transplantation.
- 20% of infections requiring hospitalization occur in normal hosts.
- Occurs in 5–15% of HIV-infected adults, usually with CD4+ lymphocyte counts <50 cells/mm^3; occurs in 0.8–2.3% of HIV-infected children. The lower infection rate in children reflects lower exposure to sources of *C. neoformans*. Seroprevalence varies by age: neonates, 0%; school-aged children, 4.1%; and adults, 69%.
- 1–3% of solid organ transplant recipients develop *C. neoformans* infections, typically >1 year after transplantation. It is the third most common invasive fungal infection in these patients.

GENERAL PREVENTION

- Use of highly active antiretroviral therapy (HAART) prevents most cases of cryptococcosis in HIV-infected patients. Incidence remains high in developing countries.
- Primary prophylaxis with fluconazole prevents new-onset cryptococcal disease in HIV-infected patients but is not routinely recommended except for those with limited access to HAART and with high levels of antiretroviral drug resistance.
- Maintenance (suppressive) therapy after completion of therapy for cryptococcal infection is recommended for HIV-infected patients. In those with low CD4+ lymphocyte counts, relapse is 100% without maintenance antifungal therapy, 18–25% with amphotericin B or itraconazole, and 2–3% with fluconazole.
  - Prophylaxis may be discontinued in asymptomatic children 6 years or older receiving HAART with CD4+ lymphocytes >100/mm^3 and undetectable viral loads for at least 3 months.
- There is no consensus on the duration of fluconazole suppressive therapy after treatment of cryptococcosis in HIV-negative immunocompromised patients. Most experts provide maintenance (suppressive) antifungal therapy with fluconazole PO (6 mg/kg/24 hr) for at least 1 year after the completion of acute treatment and then reassess ongoing use based on the level of immunosuppression.

PATHOPHYSIOLOGY

- Primary infection occurs through the inhalation of aerosolized soil particles containing the yeast forms. The skin and GI tract are also portals of entry.
- Protective immune response requires specific T cell–mediated immunity.
- CNS infection with *C. neoformans* results from hematogenous dissemination.

COMMONLY ASSOCIATED CONDITIONS

- *C. neoformans* is the most common cause of fungal meningitis in the United States.
- Dissemination is rare in immunocompetent patients.
- Concurrent *Pneumocystis jiroveci* pneumonia was detected in 13% of adults with cryptococcal meningitis.
- Pulmonary involvement is asymptomatic in up to 50% of cases, and disease may be either focal or widespread.
- Bone involvement occurs in 10% of cases of disseminated cryptococcal infection.
- Cutaneous involvement mimics acne-type eruptions that ulcerate and results from hematogenous spread of the organism or from direct extension of bone infection.

DIAGNOSIS

HISTORY

- Cryptococcal meningitis may present as either an indolent infection or acute illness.
- Symptoms of cryptococcal meningitis include headache, malaise, and low-grade fever. Nausea, vomiting, altered mentation (including behavioral changes), and photophobia are less common. Stiff neck, focal neurologic symptoms (e.g., decreased hearing, facial nerve palsy, or diplopia), and seizures are rare.
- Primary pulmonary cryptococcal disease is not well described in children because most cases are disseminated at the time of diagnosis. 50% of adults have cough or chest pain, and fewer have sputum production, weight loss, fever, and hemoptysis.
- In immunocompromised hosts, the onset of infection is more rapid and the course more severe. Pulmonary involvement is minimal when dissemination occurs quickly.

PHYSICAL EXAM

- None of the presenting signs of cryptococcal infection are sufficiently characteristic to distinguish it from other infections, particularly in immunocompromised patients.
- CNS involvement: nuchal rigidity, photophobia, and focal neurologic deficits
- Respiratory tract involvement: cough, tachypnea, grunting, and subcostal or intercostal retractions. May present as acute respiratory distress syndrome. Decreased breath sounds or dullness to percussion may be present, or the lung exam may be normal.
- Cutaneous manifestations: erythematous or verrucous papules, nodules, pustules, acneiform lesions, ulcers, abscesses, or granulomas. Lesions can occur anywhere but are found most often on the face and neck.
  - Mucocutaneous findings are present in 10–15% of cases of disseminated disease.

DIFFERENTIAL DIAGNOSIS

- Although cryptococcosis occurs most commonly in HIV-infected patients with low CD4+ lymphocyte counts, the diagnosis warrants consideration in all febrile immunocompromised children (e.g., solid organ transplant, leukemia).
- Meningitis: viruses, *Mycobacterium tuberculosis*, and other fungal causes
- Pneumonia: other pulmonary mycoses, including aspergillosis, histoplasmosis, and blastomycosis; also consider *Mycoplasma pneumoniae* and *M. tuberculosis*.
- Bone: osteogenic sarcoma
- Cutaneous: molluscum contagiosum, herpes simplex virus infection, pyoderma gangrenosum, and cellulitis

DIAGNOSTIC TESTS & INTERPRETATION

Initial Tests (screening, lab, imaging)

- There are many excellent rapid diagnostic tests for suspected cryptococcal meningitis available, although a large quantity of CSF may be needed as specimens may contain only a few organisms.
- Lumbar puncture: to diagnose cryptococcal meningitis
  - Opening pressures should be obtained if possible, to assess for increased intracranial pressure. Patients with signs and symptoms consistent with increased pressures may require repeat therapeutic lumbar punctures.
  - CSF should be sent for cell count and differential; protein; glucose; bacterial and fungal cultures; and cryptococcal antigen. Consider herpes simplex virus (HSV) or other viral PCR tests.
  - Examination of the CSF reveals <500 WBC/mm^3 (usually <100 WBC/mm^3), mostly mononuclear leukocytes, with minimal changes in protein. CSF glucose is <50 mg/dL in ~65% of patients.
  - India ink stain (less commonly performed) shows budding yeast in 50% of cases.
  - CSF cultures are positive in ~90% of cases.
  - The latex agglutination test for cryptococcal polysaccharide antigen is specific, sensitive, and rapid. Titers ≥1:4 suggest the diagnosis of cryptococcal infection if appropriate controls are negative.
  - HIV-infected patients with pneumonia and CD4+ T-lymphocyte counts <200 cells/mm^3 should be evaluated with sputum fungal culture, blood fungal culture, and a serum cryptococcal antigen test. A lumbar puncture to exclude the possibility of occult meningitis should be considered. If any test is positive for *C. neoformans*, then a lumbar puncture should be performed to exclude cryptococcal meningitis.
- Blood culture and serum cryptococcal antigen titers: diagnose disseminated cryptococcal infection. Serum cryptococcal antigen tests are positive in >90% of patients with cryptococcal meningitis.
- Sputum culture: diagnose cryptococcal pneumonia
- Skin or bone biopsy: diagnose cutaneous or osteoarticular cryptococcal infection
- HIV testing: Evaluation for immunodeficiencies, including HIV, is warranted in any patient with cryptococcosis.

- CBC with differential: may reveal hypereosinophilia (absolute eosinophil count >1,500/mm^3)
- Serum electrolytes: detect hyponatremia, a complication of cryptococcal meningitis
- Chest radiographs: Focal or solitary nodules, diffuse infiltrates, and pleural effusions may be seen in cryptococcal pneumonia.
- Head CT or MRI: may demonstrate granulomatous lesions (cryptococcomas; ~15% of patients with meningitis) or elevated intracranial pressure. MRI reveals dilation of perivascular spaces in almost half the cases.

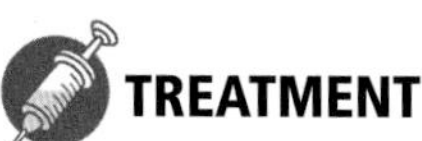

TREATMENT

- Clinical management depends on extent of disease and immune status of the host.
- Pulmonary and extrapulmonary disease (*HIV-negative, nontransplant*)
  - Normal hosts with isolated pulmonary nodules may not need treatment if the serum cryptococcal antigen is negative and the patient is asymptomatic.
  - Patients with symptoms, extensive pulmonary disease, or evidence of extrapulmonary disease require treatment.
  - Fluconazole 6 to 12 mg/kg/24 h PO (max 400 mg) for 6 to 12 months for mild/moderate disease; alternate regimen: itraconazole 5 to 10 mg/kg/24 h PO (max 400 mg) for 6 to 12 months (steady-state trough level >1 mcg/mL and ≤10 mcg/mL) or amphotericin B 0.7–1 mg/kg/24 h IV for 3 to 6 months
  - Severe disease: same as CNS (see below)
  - Maintenance therapy with fluconazole should be considered for immunocompromised patients (see "General Prevention").
- Pulmonary and extrapulmonary disease (*HIV-infected or transplant*)
  - Fluconazole (PO) 6 to 12 months for mild/moderate disease; same as CNS infection for severe disease
  - Consider surgical debridement for patients with persistent or refractory pulmonary or bone lesions.
- CNS disease (*HIV-negative, nontransplant*)
  - Induction/consolidation: amphotericin B (1 mg/kg/24 h) plus flucytosine (100 mg/kg/24 h PO, divided q6h; therapeutic levels: 30 to 80 mcg/mL) for 2 weeks and then fluconazole PO (10 to 12 mg/kg/day, max 800 mg daily dose) for a minimum of 8 weeks or until CSF is sterile. Alternate induction/consolidation regimen: amphotericin B plus flucytosine for 6 to 10 weeks. Additional regimens are available for children with renal impairment, less severe disease, or in children who do not tolerate flucytosine.
- CNS disease (*HIV-infected or transplant*)
  - Recommendations for treatment of cryptococcal infections in HIV-positive children are largely extrapolated from adult studies.
  - Induction/consolidation: amphotericin B (IV) plus flucytosine (PO) for at least 2 weeks, followed by fluconazole PO (10 to 12 mg/kg/day) for at least 8 weeks; consider subsequent long-term suppressive therapy with fluconazole PO (6 mg/kg/24 h).
  - Intrathecal amphotericin B is very toxic but may be used in refractory cases.
  - HIV-infected patients require continuation of antifungal drugs indefinitely because of the high recurrence rate of cryptococcosis.
  - Liposomal amphotericin (5 mg/kg/24 h) or amphotericin B lipid complex (5 mg/kg/24 h) IV may be substituted for amphotericin B, especially in patients with renal dysfunction and those receiving calcineurin inhibitors.
  - Flucytosine is used only in combination with amphotericin B and not as a single agent because of the rapid emergence of drug resistance.
- Voriconazole, a triazole antifungal agent, demonstrates excellent in vitro activity against *C. neoformans* but requires clinical study.
- Caspofungin, an echinocandin antifungal agent, is *not active* against *C. neoformans*.

ONGOING CARE

FOLLOW-UP RECOMMENDATIONS

Patient Monitoring

- Because of the risk of relapse, patients should be seen at 3-month intervals for 12 to 18 months following treatment. Immunocompromised patients should be evaluated every 2 to 3 months, even while on suppressive therapy, to monitor clinically for relapse.
- Repeat lumbar punctures documenting a decrease in CSF cryptococcal antigen and sterility of culture are useful in evaluating response to treatment. During therapy for acute meningitis, an unchanged or increased titer of CSF antigen correlates with clinical and microbiologic failure to respond to treatment. Serum antigen titers are not helpful for this purpose.
- Evaluate patients with cryptococcal meningitis for neurologic sequelae.
- HIV-infected patients require suppressive antifungal therapy (see "General Prevention").

PROGNOSIS

- Mortality is rare in patients with isolated pulmonary or cutaneous disease.
- In-hospital, mortality is ~20% for cryptococcal meningitis and ~8% for non-CNS cryptococcal infections.
  - In normal hosts with meningitis, poor prognostic factors include serum or CSF cryptococcal titers >1:32 or CSF WBC <20/mm^3.
  - In HIV-infected patients with meningitis, poor prognostic factors include hyponatremia, concomitant growth of *C. neoformans* from another site, increased intracranial pressure, and any alteration of mental status.
- Up to 40% of patients with cryptococcal meningitis have residual neurologic deficits.
- Relapse rates are high in HIV-infected patients (see "General Prevention").

COMPLICATIONS

- Elevated intracranial pressure with meningitis
- Pulmonary, cutaneous, and bone involvement may occur (see "Commonly Associated Conditions").
- In solid organ transplant patients, tacrolimus recipients are less likely to have CNS involvement and more likely to have skin, soft tissue, or osteoarticular involvement.
- Cryptococcal immune reconstitution inflammatory syndrome (C-IRIS) may lead to a new presentation of the disease and/or a clinical deterioration after reversal of a host immune deficiency state, often weeks to months after initiating therapy. Cases have been described in children, but most information comes from the adult literature. The most common presentation is mediastinal lymphadenitis.

ADDITIONAL READING

- Joshi NS, Fisher BT, Prasad PA, et al. Epidemiology of cryptococcal infection in hospitalized children. *Pediatr Infect Dis J*. 2010;29(12):e91–e95.
- Pappas PG, Perfect JR, Cloud GA, et al. Cryptococcosis in human immunodeficiency virus-negative patients in the era of effective azole therapy. *Clin Infect Dis*. 2001;33(5):690–699.
- Perfect JR, Dismukes WE, Dromer F, et al. Clinical practice guidelines for the management of cryptococcal disease: 2010 update by the Infectious Diseases Society of America. *Clin Infect Dis*. 2010;50(3):291–322.
- U.S. Department of Health and Human Services. *Panel on Opportunistic Infections in HIV-Exposed and HIV-Infected Children*. Guidelines for the Prevention and Treatment of Opportunistic Infections in HIV-Exposed and HIV-Infected Children. Rockville, MD: U.S. Department of Health and Human Services; 2013. http://aidsinfo.nih.gov/contentfiles/lvguidelines/oi_guidelines_pediatrics.pdf. Accessed February 27,2018.

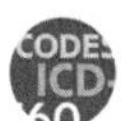

CODES

ICD10

- B45.9 Cryptococcosis, unspecified
- B45.0 Pulmonary cryptococcosis
- B45.8 Other forms of cryptococcosis

FAQ

- Q: What are the sources of *Cryptococcus* in nature?
- A: Pigeon droppings and soil. Naturally acquired infections occur in lower mammals, especially cats. However, neither animal-to-human nor human-to-human infections have been reported.
- Q: Should all children with *Cryptococcus* infection be evaluated for immunodeficiency?
- A: Yes, most cases of symptomatic cryptococcal infections are related to a defect in T cell–mediated immunity.
- Q: Are repeat assessments of CSF necessary in cryptococcal meningoencephalitis?
- A: Yes, to prove achievement of sterility and guide length of treatment.

CRYPTORCHIDISM

Hsi-Yang Wu, MD

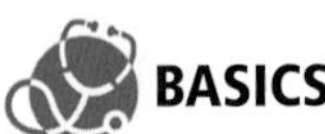

BASICS

DESCRIPTION

Cryptorchidism is a condition characterized by one or both testes being undescended. An undescended testis does not remain at the bottom of the scrotum after the cremaster muscle has been fatigued by overstretching. Cryptorchidism is commonly confused with a retractile testis. A retractile testis may not always lie in the scrotum but will stay at the bottom of the scrotum after overstretching the cremaster.

EPIDEMIOLOGY

- 3% of full-term newborn boys have cryptorchidism.
- This percentage falls to 1% by 3 months of age.
- There are two peaks for detection of undescended testes: at birth and at 5 to 7 years of age. The latter group probably represents those patients with low undescended testes that become apparent with linear growth.
- Bilateral undescended testes occur in 10% of patients with undescended testicles.
- Unilateral anorchia is found in 5% of patients with cryptorchidism.

RISK FACTORS

Genetics

- Of boys with undescended testes, 4% of their fathers and 6–10% of their brothers also had undescended testes. There is a 23% prevalence of cryptorchidism in family members of cases compared to 7.5% in relatives of controls.
- Abnormalities in *HOXA10*, *HOXA11*, *HOXD13*, *ESR1*, *INSL3*, and the *LGR8/GREAT* receptor genes account for only 2–3% of patients with nonsyndromic cryptorchidism. Androgen receptor gene mutations are not linked to isolated cryptorchidism. A genome-wide association study failed to identify significant genetic markers.

PATHOPHYSIOLOGY

- Normal testicular descent occurs during the 7th month of gestation.
- The majority of testes that are undescended at birth but descend spontaneously will do so by 3 months of age, possibly due to the gonadotropin surge that is responsible for germ cell maturation.
- The undescended testis fails to show normal maturation at both 3 months and 5 years of age.
  - At 3 months of age, the fetal gonocytes are transformed into adult dark spermatogonia.
  - At 5 years of age, the adult dark spermatogonia become primary spermatocytes.
  - Both of these steps are abnormal in the undescended testis and, to a lesser extent, the contralateral descended testis.
  - It was previously believed that the undescended testis was normal between birth and 1 year of age. However, this is incorrect because these data were derived from counts of all germ cells without taking into account whether maturation was occurring.
  - After 5 years of age, thermal effects on the testis left out of position are seen independent of the endocrinologic effects.

ETIOLOGY

- Multifactorial mechanisms involving two theories have been postulated:
  - Hypogonadotropic hypogonadism
  - Abnormal mechanical factors (gubernaculum, epididymis, genitofemoral nerve innervation, intra-abdominal pressure)
- Although boys with undescended testes do have abnormal attachment of the gubernaculum, the mechanical theories do not consistently explain the testis histology found in cryptorchidism.
- Many boys with cryptorchidism have lower morning urinary luteinizing hormone and a decreased luteinizing hormone/follicle-stimulating hormone response to gonadotropin-releasing hormone, corresponding to the abnormal germ cell development in both the undescended and contralateral descended testis.
- The normal initial postnatal gonadotropin surge at 60 to 90 days of age is absent or blunted in some boys with cryptorchidism. Without this surge, Leydig cells do not proliferate, testosterone does not increase, germ cells do not mature, and infertility may develop. This indicates that a mild endocrinopathy is responsible, and cryptorchidism may be a variant of hypogonadotropic hypogonadism.
- Exposure to the environmental antiandrogen polybrominated diphenyl ether is linked to an increased cryptorchidism risk, with an odds ratio of 1.5 to 1.9.
- Secondary undescended testes can occur after inguinal surgery, either due to scar tissue or difficulty in diagnosing an undescended testis in a young boy with a hernia.

COMMONLY ASSOCIATED CONDITIONS

- Patients with prune belly, Klinefelter, Noonan, and Prader-Willi syndromes have a higher likelihood of undescended testes.
- Cryptorchidism associated with hypospadias should also raise the possibility of a disorder of sex development (DSD), which occurs in 30–40% of patients, mainly due to defects in gonadotropin or testosterone synthesis.

DIAGNOSIS

HISTORY

- Exogenous maternal hormones (e.g., those used in infertility treatment)
- Maternal oral contraceptive use
- Consanguinity
- Family history of urologic abnormalities or neonatal deaths
- Prematurity
- CNS lesions
- Previous inguinal surgery
- Precocious puberty
- Infertility

PHYSICAL EXAM

- An undescended testis may be found at the upper scrotum, in the superficial inguinal pouch, or in the inguinal canal. For treatment purposes, the main distinction that needs to be made is whether or not the testis is palpable.
- The patient should be examined sitting in the frog-leg position.
  - With warmed hands, check the size, location, and texture of the contralateral descended testis.
  - Begin the examination of the undescended testis at the anterior superior iliac spine.
  - Sweep the groin from lateral to medial with the nondominant hand.
  - Once the testis is palpated, grasp it with the dominant hand and continue to sweep the testis toward the scrotum with the other hand.
  - With a combination of sweeping and pulling, it is sometimes possible to bring the testis to the scrotum.
  - Maintain the position of the testis in the scrotum for a minute so that the cremaster muscle is fatigued.
  - Release the testis, and if it remains in place, it is a retractile testis.
  - If it immediately pops back, it is an undescended testis.
- For difficult-to-examine patients (e.g., chubby 6-month-olds or obese youth), having them sit with heels together and knees abducted can help relax the cremaster. Wetting the fingers of the nondominant hand with lubricating jelly or soap can increase the sensitivity of the fingers in palpating the small, mobile testis.

DIFFERENTIAL DIAGNOSIS

- Retractile testes are commonly confused with undescended testes. The key to distinguishing them from undescended testes is the physical exam.
  - All retractile and many undescended testes can be delivered into the scrotum.
  - The retractile testis will stay in the scrotum after the cremaster muscle has been overstretched.
  - The low undescended testis will immediately pop back to its undescended position after being released.
- Atrophic or "vanishing" testes are found anywhere along the normal path to the scrotum.
  - They are believed to be due to neonatal vascular ischemia.
  - The contralateral testis can be hypertrophied in these boys, but this is not a reliable diagnostic sign.
- Anorchia or DSD
  - On evaluation, 80% of nonpalpable testes are present in either the abdomen or in the inguinal canal.
  - All child with bilateral nonpalpable testes should have an endocrine evaluation to rule out anorchia or DSD.
  - Any newborn with bilaterally undescended testicles should be considered a female with virilizing congenital adrenal hyperplasia until evaluation proves otherwise.

DIAGNOSTIC TESTS & INTERPRETATION

Initial Tests (screening, lab, imaging)

- For the typical patient with a unilateral palpable or nonpalpable undescended testis, no further laboratory evaluation is necessary.
- For the patient with bilateral undescended testes, with one testis palpable, no further workup is necessary.
- The patient with bilateral nonpalpable testes should have a chromosomal and endocrinologic evaluation, as should the patient with one or two undescended testes and hypospadias. For newborns with bilaterally nonpalpable testes, this evaluation is emergent and needs to rule out the possibility that the baby is a female with virilizing congenital adrenal hyperplasia.
- If the patient has bilateral nonpalpable testes and is <3 months of age, serum luteinizing hormone, follicle-stimulating hormone, testosterone, and anti-müllerian hormone levels will determine whether testes are present.
- After that age, human chorionic gonadotropin stimulation will result in a measurable serum testosterone if testes are present. A failure to respond to human chorionic gonadotropin stimulation in combination with elevated luteinizing hormone/follicle-stimulating hormone levels is consistent with anorchia.
- Ultrasound, CT, and MRI can detect testes in the inguinal region, but this is also the region where they are most easily palpable. They are only 50% accurate in showing intra-abdominal testes. Imaging is not necessary preoperatively because for nonpalpable testes; surgical planning is based on the exam performed in the clinic and under anesthesia.

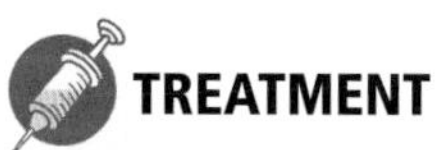

TREATMENT

GENERAL MEASURES

- Patients with undescended testes should be referred for surgical evaluation no later than 3 months of age.
- Hormonal therapy
  - For many years hormonal therapy was widely used in Europe for inducing descent of undescended testes. Both gonadotropin-releasing hormone and human chorionic gonadotropin were used, with long-term success rates of 20%.
    - Treatment is most successful for low undescended testes, but there is a 25% relapse rate.
    - More recent recommendations from European pediatric endocrinologists indicate that surgery is the preferred therapy.
  - For these reasons, as well as that gonadotropin-releasing hormone and human chorionic gonadotropin are not approved for this indication in the United States, most therapy in the United States to bring the testis down to the scrotum is surgical (orchiopexy).
  - The use of hormonal therapy after orchiopexy to improve semen analyses in high-risk patients remains investigational.

SURGERY/OTHER PROCEDURES

Goals in bringing testes into the scrotum:

- Prevent ongoing thermal damage to the testis.
- Treat the associated hernia sac.
- Prevent testis torsion/injury against the pubic bone.
- Achieve a good cosmetic result/avoid psychological effects of empty scrotum.
- Allow the older child to perform testicular self-exam for cancer.

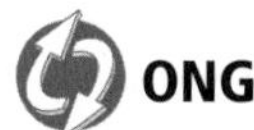

ONGOING CARE

FOLLOW-UP RECOMMENDATIONS

Patient Monitoring

After successful orchiopexy, patients are examined at 6 to 12 months to check on testicular size and position. They are rechecked at puberty to explain the technique and need for monthly testis self-exam concerning early recognition of testis cancer. Patients with retractile testes should be examined annually until age 7 years because ~5% will be found to have a testis out of the scrotum.

PROGNOSIS

- Surgery cannot reverse the maturational failure of the undescended testis, but it can prevent ongoing thermal injury.
- Parents are often concerned about future fertility:
  - In patients who have undergone orchiopexy at an early age, it appears that 90% of boys with unilateral cryptorchidism and 65% with bilateral cryptorchidism will achieve paternity.
  - Patients who are interested in their risk for infertility may have a semen analysis performed at age 18 years.
- Surgery decreases the relative risk of testicular cancer if the surgery is performed before 13 years of age.
  - All patients should be taught proper monthly testicular self-exam at the time of puberty. Some patients with cryptorchidism are at a higher risk of cancer (prune belly syndrome, ambiguous genitalia, karyotypic abnormalities, or the postpubertal boy).

ADDITIONAL READING

- Barthold JS, Wang Y, Kolon TF, et al. Pathway analysis supports association of nonsyndromic cryptorchidism with genetic loci linked to cytoskeleton-dependent functions. *Hum Reprod*. 2015;30(10):2439–2451.
- Callaghan P. Undescended testis. *Pediatr Rev*. 2000;21(11):395.
- Hauser R, Skakkebaek NE, Hass U, et al. Male reproductive disorders, diseases, and costs of exposure to endocrine-disrupting chemicals in the European Union. *J Clin Endocrinol Metab*. 2015;100(4):1267–1277.
- Lee PA. Fertility after cryptorchidism: epidemiology and other outcome studies. *Urology*. 2005;66(2): 427–431.
- Pettersson A, Richiardi L, Nordenskjold A, et al. Age at surgery for undescended testis and risk of testicular cancer. *N Engl J Med*. 2007;356(18):1835–1841.
- Pyörälä S, Huttunen NP, Uhari M. A review and meta-analysis of hormonal treatment of cryptorchidism. *J Clin Endocrinol Metab*. 1995;80(9): 2795–2799.
- Ritzén EM. Undescended testes: a consensus on management. *Eur J Endocrinol*. 2008;159(Suppl 1): S87–S90.
- Tasian GE, Yiee JH, Copp HL. Imaging use and cryptorchidism: determinants of practice patterns. *J Urol*. 2011;185(5):1882–1887.
- Virtanen HE, Bjerknes R, Cortes D, et al. Cryptorchidism: classification, prevalence and long-term consequences. *Acta Paediatr*. 2007;96(5):611–616.
- Virtanen HE, Cortes D, Rajpert-De Meyts E, et al. Development and descent of the testis in relation to cryptorchidism. *Acta Paediatr*. 2007;96(5):622–627.

CODES

ICD10

- Q53.9 Undescended testicle, unspecified
- Q53.10 Unspecified undescended testicle, unilateral
- Q53.20 Undescended testicle, unspecified, bilateral

FAQ

- Q: If there is only one testicle in the scrotum, will fertility be affected?
- A: In general, the outlook for paternity is good in a patient with only one descended testicle. Paternity is more significantly affected with a history of two undescended testicles.
- Q: Why do patients with retractile testes require follow-up?
- A: The ability to distinguish between retractile and undescended testes can be difficult in some patients. Some of the patients will be found to have true undescended testes as they grow. Boys should be taught how to perform a monthly testicular self-exam at puberty.

CRYPTOSPORIDIOSIS

Michelle W. Parker, MD

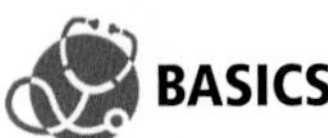

BASICS

DESCRIPTION

Cryptosporidiosis is protozoal infection causing a self-limited acute gastroenteritis characterized by nonbloody watery diarrhea.

- Symptoms, when present, can also include abdominal pain, fever, fatigue, weight loss, vomiting, headache, and joint pain and typically last 1 to 2 weeks.
- In an immunocompromised patient, gastrointestinal symptoms can be chronic, relapsing, and severe, causing profound and life-threatening wasting and malabsorption.
- Extraintestinal: Pulmonary, biliary tract (sclerosing cholangitis, acalculous cholecystitis, pancreatitis), or disseminated infection rarely occurs among immunocompromised individuals.

EPIDEMIOLOGY

- Oocysts of *Cryptosporidium* are shed in the stool of infected hosts (humans, cattle, and other mammals) and are transmitted by fecal–oral contamination.
- Disease is most commonly associated with contamination of water sources, both drinking and recreational, and transmission is also seen in association with child care centers or livestock.
- *Cryptosporidium* has been found in all parts of the world and is a cause of traveler's diarrhea.
- Because of summer recreational water use, the incidence of cryptosporidiosis is highest in children and typically peaks in summer through early fall.

Incidence

In the United States, an estimated 748,000 cases of cryptosporidiosis occur annually.

RISK FACTORS

- Those most at risk for infection are children who attend child care centers, people who take care of others with cryptosporidiosis (including child care workers, parents of infected children, and health care workers), those who swim in or drink from contaminated water sources such as streams or unprotected wells, and people who handle livestock including those visiting petting zoos.
- Because *Cryptosporidium* are chlorine tolerant, swimming in chlorinated pools does not decrease the risk of infection.

GENERAL PREVENTION

- Drinking water should be adequately filtered to a particle size of 1 μm or smaller in order to ensure oocyst removal.
- If a recreational water supply becomes contaminated, it should be closed, and proper decontamination measures should be implemented.
- Those diagnosed with cryptosporidiosis should not swim for at least 2 weeks after diarrhea stops to help protect others.
- Good hand hygiene, washing with soap and water vigorously for at least 20 seconds, is key after contact with animals or stool.
- Children with diarrhea should not attend day care settings until diarrhea is resolved.
- In day care settings, disinfection of diapering areas after each use and frequent disinfection of toys, tabletops, and highchairs during outbreaks is recommended.
- Oocysts can survive for long periods and are resistant to many disinfectants including chlorine, iodine, and dilute bleach. Boiling water or full-strength bleach disinfectant is most effective.
- Contact precautions are recommended for the length of the hospital stay for hospitalized patients.
- Immunocompromised persons should avoid contact with any person or animal with cryptosporidiosis.

PATHOPHYSIOLOGY

- Transmission occurs via fecal–oral passage of oocysts from food, water, or poor hand hygiene.
- The incubation period is typically 3 to 14 days with a median of 7 days, and oocyst shedding may occur for weeks to months after symptoms resolve. In the majority of people, shedding stops after 2 weeks. Immunocompromised patients can shed for several months.
- Invasion of intestinal epithelial cells in the small intestine and proximal colon leads to a secretory diarrhea.
- Intestinal destruction occurs with villous atrophy and subsequent malabsorption and increased intestinal permeability.

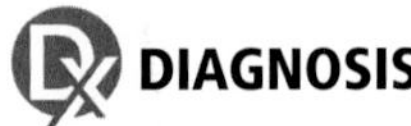

DIAGNOSIS

HISTORY

- Acute onset of symptoms combined with exposure to any of the transmission sources discussed above should prompt consideration. Fever and vomiting are symptoms more commonly found in children and can lead to the misdiagnosis of viral gastroenteritis.
- Immunocompromised patients such as those with AIDS may have chronic severe symptoms with significant wasting.

PHYSICAL EXAM

- Acute weight loss
- Fever
- Tenderness to palpation of abdomen
- Dehydration
- Immunocompromised patients may rarely exhibit respiratory symptoms (dyspnea) or biliary tract symptoms (colicky right upper quadrant pain).

DIFFERENTIAL DIAGNOSIS

- Other infectious etiology of diarrheal illness:
  - Viral gastroenteritis including rotavirus, adenovirus, astrovirus; caliciviruses including norovirus, cytomegalovirus
  - Bacterial gastroenteritis including *Salmonella*, *Shigella*, *Yersinia*, *Campylobacter*, enterotoxigenic *Escherichia coli*, *Vibrio cholerae*
  - *Clostridium difficile* enterocolitis
  - Parasitic gastroenteritis including *Giardia*, *Entamoeba*, *Cyclospora*, *Isospora*, *Microsporidia*
- Noninfectious etiology of diarrheal illness:
  - Allergic colitis, inflammatory bowel disease, irritable bowel syndrome, appendicitis, intussusception, malrotation/volvulus, celiac disease, or other malabsorption

DIAGNOSTIC TESTS & INTERPRETATION

Initial Tests (screening, lab, imaging)

- Detection of organisms in stool specimens is diagnostic. Oocysts are small and may be missed on routine light microscopic examination of stool; modified acid-fast staining may aid in diagnosis.
  - Fluorescent stains such as auramine O are rapid but have high false-positive rates.
  - Immunofluorescent assays and enzyme-linked immunosorbent assays for antigen detection are also available.
  - The direct immunofluorescent stain is the diagnostic test of choice.
- Tests for *Cryptosporidium* are not routinely performed and should be specifically requested.

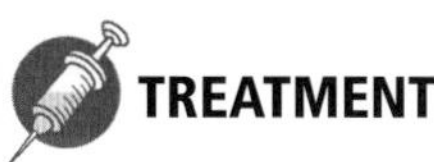

TREATMENT

GENERAL MEASURES

Fluids and electrolytes should be replaced by either oral or intravenous routes.

MEDICATION

- In immunocompetent patients, disease is typically self-limited, and no treatment is necessary.
- For those who are malnourished where treatment is preferred, oral nitazoxanide may be given for 3 days.
- Dosage for children 1 to 3 years of age is 100 mg b.i.d.; for children 4 to 11 years of age, 200 mg b.i.d.; and for children ≥12 years of age and adults, 500 mg b.i.d.
- For immunosuppressed patients, antiretroviral therapy to improve CD4+ count has been associated with decreasing duration of illness. Nitazoxanide, paromomycin, and bovine immunoglobulin have also been tried without strong data to support efficacy.

ONGOING CARE

PATIENT EDUCATION

- Because the oocysts can be shed in the stool for weeks after clinical resolution, it is important to realize that asymptomatic patients can still transmit the infection to household and day care contacts.
- Requiring patients whose diarrhea has resolved to have a negative stool test for *Cryptosporidium* before reentry to day care has not been evaluated as an outbreak control measure. Repeated testing is expensive.

PROGNOSIS

- For immunocompetent hosts, gastrointestinal disease is self-limited, usually lasting approximately 10 days. Supportive therapy is usually all that is necessary.
- For immunocompromised patients, diarrhea can be severe, debilitating, and often life-threatening. Aggressive supportive therapy is usually required, along with antimicrobial therapy and immune reconstitution.

ADDITIONAL READING

- American Academy of Pediatrics. Cryptosporidiosis. In: Kimberlin DW, Brady MT, Jackson MA, et al, eds. *Red Book: 2015 Report of the Committee on Infectious Diseases*. 30th ed. Elk Grove Village, IL: American Academy of Pediatrics; 2015:312–315.
- Centers for Disease Control and Prevention. Parasites—*Cryptosporidium* (also known as "Crypto"). http://www.cdc.gov/parasites/crypto/. Accessed February 14, 2017.
- Painter JE, Hlavsa MC, Kreiner PW, et al; for Centers for Disease Control and Prevention. Cryptosporidiosis surveillance—United States, 2011–2012. *MMWR Surveill Summ*. 2015;64(3):1–14.

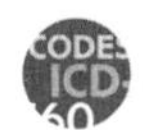

CODES

ICD10

A07.2 Cryptosporidiosis

FAQ

- Q: For whom should cryptosporidiosis be considered as a differential diagnosis?
- A: For anyone with acute onset of watery diarrhea with any of the mentioned risk factors
- Q: When is it safe for a child with cryptosporidiosis to return to day care?
- A: When the diarrhea has resolved
- Q: For how long is an immunocompetent patient with cryptosporidiosis contagious?
- A: A healthy person may continue to shed for weeks to months after diarrhea has resolved.

CUSHING SYNDROME

Maya B. Lodish, MD, MHSCR • Constantine A. Stratakis, MD, D(med)Sci

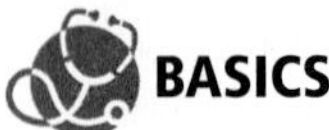

BASICS

DESCRIPTION

Cushing syndrome is a multisystem disorder resulting from prolonged exposure to excess glucocorticoid.

- Characterized by growth deceleration, truncal obesity, characteristic skin changes, muscle weakness, and hypertension
- Most common cause in childhood is exogenous glucocorticoid administration.
- Endogenous Cushing syndrome may be caused by adrenocorticotropic hormone (ACTH)-secreting tumor of the pituitary gland (Cushing disease), ectopic secretion of ACTH, or ACTH-independent secretion of glucocorticoids by the adrenal glands.
- Accurate diagnosis and classification of Cushing syndrome in children is crucial to guide appropriate therapeutic intervention.
- In endogenous Cushing syndrome, the hypothalamic-pituitary-adrenal axis has lost its ability to self-regulate due to excessive secretion of either ACTH or cortisol and loss of the negative feedback function.
- Diagnostic tests help to distinguish the cause of this disorder.
- Key differences exist between children and adults in the diagnosis and management of Cushing syndrome.

EPIDEMIOLOGY

- The overall incidence of Cushing syndrome is approximately 2 to 5 new cases per million people per year. Only approximately 10% of the new cases each year occur in children.
- In older children with Cushing syndrome, there is a female-to-male predominance, whereas in younger children, there may be a male predominance.
- Exogenous Cushing syndrome caused by chronic administration of glucocorticoids (by any route) or, more rarely, by administration of ACTH (e.g., for infantile seizures) is the most common cause of this syndrome in children.
- The pituitary-dependent form (Cushing disease) accounts for >80% of all cases of Cushing syndrome in children >7 years of age.

ETIOLOGY

- Cushing disease:
  - In most cases, the genetic etiology of pituitary corticotropinomas remains unknown. In rare cases, a germline mutation in Menin (multiple endocrine neoplasia type 1 [MEN1]) or aryl hydrocarbon receptor interaction protein (*AIP*) gene is found.
  - Recently, somatic mutations in ubiquitin-specific protease 8 (*USP8*) gene, resulting in increased activity of the epidermal growth factor receptor (EGFR) signaling pathway have been found to be associated with 30% of cases of Cushing disease in pediatrics.
- Adrenal sources of Cushing syndrome:
  - In very young children, Cushing syndrome is usually caused by adrenal sources.
  - 10–15% of all cases of Cushing syndrome in childhood are due to ACTH-independent Cushing syndrome from unregulated secretion of cortisol from the adrenal glands.
  - Adrenocortical neoplasms
    - Often malignant in young children
  - Primary pigmented nodular adrenocortical disease (PPNAD)
    - PPNAD is a genetic disorder often associated with Carney complex and related to mutations of the *PRKAR1A* gene.
    - Cushing syndrome in PPNAD may be cyclical and difficult to diagnose.
  - Isolated micronodular adrenocortical disease (iMAD)
    - If no *PRKAR1A* mutations are found or if the patient does not have Carney complex, and Cushing syndrome is due to bilateral adrenal hyperplasia without massive enlargement of the adrenal glands on imaging, then the most likely diagnosis is iMAD.
    - Like in PPNAD, Cushing syndrome in iMAD can be difficult to diagnose due to an often atypical and/or cyclical clinical course.
  - Massive macronodular adrenocortical disease (MMAD)
    - Another form of ACTH-independent bilateral adrenal disease seen (rarely) in children
    - Easier to diagnose due to massive enlargement of the adrenal glands on imaging studies
  - Adrenal hyperplasia and/or adenomas can also be seen in the McCune-Albright and Beckwith-Wiedemann syndromes, usually in the infantile period.
- Ectopic ACTH production accounts for <1% of the cases of Cushing syndrome in children and may be due to a variety of neuroendocrine (NE) tumors.
  - NE tumors include carcinoid tumors in the lungs, pancreas (and other locations in the gastrointestinal tract), or thymus; medullary carcinomas of the thyroid; and pheochromocytomas, as well as small cell carcinoma of the lungs that may be seen rarely in adolescents.
  - Other causes of ectopic ACTH secretion include infantile neuroblastomas (and related tumors) and paraneoplastic syndromes in all ages.
- Corticotropin-releasing hormone (CRH) secretion by an ectopic CRH-producing source, typically an NE tumor such as the ones producing ectopical ACTH, is an extremely rare cause of Cushing syndrome in children.
- Exogenous steroids: Iatrogenic Cushing syndrome is the most common cause in pediatrics. Cushing syndrome can be caused by chronic systemic, topical, or intranasal steroid use, or ACTH use.

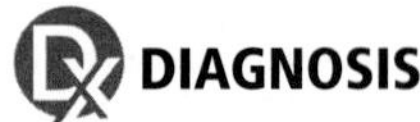

DIAGNOSIS

HISTORY

- The most common presenting symptom of the syndrome in childhood is weight gain accompanied by poor linear growth.
- Additional pertinent features in the history of presenting illness often include headaches, hypertension, weakness, hirsutism, irregular menses, and delayed puberty.
- Dermatologic features include facial flushing, striae (in older children and adolescents only), acne, bruising, and acanthosis nigricans.
- Fractures and/or kidney stones related to Cushing syndrome are also relatively frequent.
- Cushing syndrome is a hypercoagulable state; patients are at higher risk of thrombosis especially in the setting of a family history of blood clots.

PHYSICAL EXAMINATION

- Check growth chart and document height velocity and weight change.
- Note fat distribution (characteristic central obesity, dorsocervical, subclavicular, and bitemporal fat pads).
- Skin examination
  - Document striae (usually wide, violaceous) and acanthosis.
  - Look for characteristic dermatologic features that may be associated with genetic forms of Cushing (café au lait spots for McCune-Albright syndrome, lentigines for Carney complex).
- Neurologic examination
  - Check for proximal muscular weakness by having patient rise from a squatting position. (Note: typically not present in younger children)
  - Check visual fields and perform funduscopic examination.
- Document Tanner staging and note any discrepancy between pubic hair and gonadal or breast size (which may point to ACTH-dependent or independent causes of Cushing syndrome).

DIAGNOSTIC TESTS & INTERPRETATION

Diagnostic tests: The first step in the diagnosis of Cushing syndrome is to document hypercortisolism.

Initial Tests (screening, lab, imaging)

- Screening
  - 24-hour urine-free cortisol excretion
  - Low-dose dexamethasone test
    - 1 mg dexamethasone (adjust for pediatric patients 15 mcg × weight [kg]; maximum dose 1 mg) PO at 11 p.m. Measure plasma cortisol at 8 a.m. next day.
  - Circadian cortisol profile
    - Measure serum or salivary cortisol at 8 a.m. and midnight.

- Confirmation: The following results are suspicious for Cushing syndrome:
  - 24-hour urine-free cortisol excretion above normal limits for assay (corrected for body surface area)
  - Post–low-dose dexamethasone 8 a.m. plasma cortisol >1.8 mcg/dL
  - Blunted circadian rhythm: a single midnight cortisol value of >4.4 mcg/dL highly sensitive and specific for Cushing syndrome
- Differentiate causes:
  - Measure plasma ACTH.
  - If low ACTH (<29 pg/mL) = likely ACTH-independent but need to confirm with dexamethasone testing; only completely undetectable ACTH levels indicate undoubtedly an adrenal source of Cushing syndrome.
  - Proceed with high-dose dexamethasone suppression test (adjust dexamethasone dose for weight 120 mcg × kg; max dose 8 mg).
  - Lack of suppression in response to high-dose dexamethasone indicates that an adrenal tumor is the likely diagnosis.
  - If high ACTH (>29 pg/mL) = likely ACTH-independent
    - Proceed with CRH testing (generally done by an endocrine specialist).
    - 1 mcg/kg CRH is given, and serial cortisol and ACTH levels are measured. The criterion for the diagnosis of the pituitary-dependent Cushing disease is a mean increase of 20% above baseline for cortisol values at 30 to 45 minutes and an increase in the mean corticotropin concentrations of at least 35% over basal value at 15 to 30 minutes after CRH administration.
    - If CRH testing is negative: Likely diagnosis is ectopic ACTH production.
    - If CRH testing is positive: consistent with Cushing disease
- When Cushing disease (ACTH-secreting pituitary tumor) is suspected, pituitary magnetic resonance imaging (MRI) should be done in thin sections with high resolution with gadolinium.
- Computed tomography (CT) of the adrenal glands useful in the distinction between pituitary Cushing disease and adrenal causes of Cushing syndrome. MRI of the adrenal glands is less useful for the detection of PPNAD or iMAD but may be used for the detection of MMAD, single large tumors, and cancer.
- Bilateral inferior petrosal sinus sampling (IPSS) is a catheterization study used to confirm the source of ACTH secretion in ACTH-dependent Cushing syndrome. IPSS needed only when the pituitary MRI is negative or tests are contradictory but may be performed only if ACTH-dependent disease is confirmed and cortisol levels are consistently high.

TREATMENT

- The treatment of choice for Cushing disease is transsphenoidal surgery (TSS).
- In most specialized centers with experienced neurosurgeons, the success rate of the first TSS is close to, or even higher than, 85%.
- The treatment of choice for adrenal tumors is surgical resection, and if metastatic carcinoma, chemotherapy and radiation may be employed.
- Bilateral total adrenalectomy is usually the treatment of choice in PPNAD, iMAD, and MMAD.
- Adrenalectomy may also be used in patients with refractory Cushing disease or with difficult-to-treat ectopic ACTH-dependent Cushing syndrome.

COMPLICATIONS

- After TSS, patients may have persistent disease or recurrence.
- Postoperative complications may include transient diabetes insipidus and syndrome of inappropriate antidiuretic hormone secretion, central hypothyroidism, growth hormone deficiency, hypogonadism, bleeding, infection (meningitis), and pituitary apoplexy.
- Children and adolescents may be at higher risk of developing depression, anxiety, and poor school performance following cure of Cushing syndrome.
- Patients who undergo bilateral adrenalectomy with Cushing disease must be aware of the potential of Nelson syndrome, characterized by increased pigmentation, elevated ACTH levels, and a growing pituitary ACTH-producing pituitary tumor.

ADDITIONAL THERAPIES

- Pituitary irradiation following a failed TSS will lead to remission in approximately 80% of patients, although commonly results in hypopituitarism. Newer forms of stereotactic radiotherapy are now available as options for the treatment of Cushing syndrome, including proton beam and gamma knife.
- A number of medications are available to inhibit corticosteroid biosynthesis, although none of these agents are specifically approved for use in children. These pharmacotherapies include metyrapone and ketoconazole, which may be employed in cases of refractory Cushing or when bridging the patient to definitive therapy. In addition, dopamine receptor agonists such as pasireotide and cortisol receptor antagonists, such as mifepristone, are also under clinical investigation for use in children.

ONGOING CARE

- Following TSS in Cushing disease, patients will be transiently adrenally insufficient while the hypothalamic-pituitary-adrenal axis is recovering.
- Stress doses of cortisol are necessary in the perioperative period.
- These should be weaned relatively rapidly to a physiologic replacement dose.
- The patient should be followed every few months, and adrenocortical function should be periodically assessed with a 1-hour 250 mcg ACTH test. Most patients recover hypothalamic-pituitary-adrenal function within 1 year after TSS.
- Following bilateral adrenalectomy, lifetime replacement with glucocorticoids and mineralocorticoids (fludrocortisone 0.1 to 0.3 mg daily) is required.
- All patients who are status postcure of Cushing need to be taught precautions for adrenal insufficiency, including emergency injection of hydrocortisone and carrying/wearing medical alert identification.

ALERT

- Falsely high urine-free cortisol may be obtained with stress, obesity, pregnancy, chronic exercise, depression, poor diabetes control, alcoholism, anorexia, narcotic withdrawal, anxiety, malnutrition, and high water intake. A combined dexamethasone–CRH test may help to differentiate pseudo-Cushing syndrome from true Cushing syndrome.
- Falsely low urine-free cortisol may be present if inadequate collection or intermittent cortisol hypersecretion.

ADDITIONAL READING

- Batista DL, Riar J, Keil M, et al. Diagnostic tests for children who are referred for the investigation of Cushing syndrome. *Pediatrics*. 2007;120(3):e575–e586.
- Lodish M. Cushing's syndrome in childhood: update on genetics, treatment, and outcomes. *Curr Opin Endocrinol Diabetes Obes*. 2015;22(1):48–54.
- Lodish M, Stratakis CA. A genetic and molecular update on adrenocortical causes of Cushing syndrome. *Nat Rev Endocrinol*. 2016;12(5):255–262.
- Stratakis CA. Cushing syndrome in pediatrics. *Endocrinol Metab Clin North Am*. 2012;41(4):793–803.

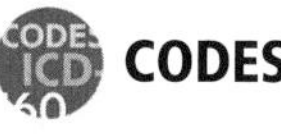

CODES

ICD10

- E24.9 Cushing's syndrome, unspecified
- E24.0 Pituitary-dependent Cushing's disease
- E24.2 Drug-induced Cushing's syndrome

FAQ

- Q: What clinical clue is most useful to determine which children have obesity alone versus those with Cushing syndrome?
- A: Cushing syndrome is associated with growth failure, whereas obesity is associated with adequate linear growth.
- Q: Are most patients on lifetime glucocorticoid replacement after surgery for Cushing disease?
- A: No. The majority of patients recover their hypothalamic-pituitary-adrenal axis within 1 year of their TSS and can be weaned off glucocorticoids.

CUTANEOUS LARVA MIGRANS

Ross Newman, DO, MHPE

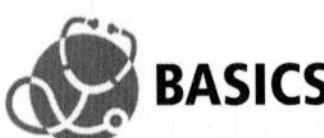

BASICS

DESCRIPTION

Infestation of the epidermis by the infectious larvae of certain nematodes, classically manifesting with an intensely pruritic, serpiginous skin lesion

EPIDEMIOLOGY

Worldwide distribution but most frequent in warmer climates, including the Caribbean, Africa, South America, Southeast Asia, and southeastern United States

RISK FACTORS

- Contracted from soil contaminated with dog and cat feces
- Occupational exposures occur from crawling under buildings, such as among plumbers and pipefitters.

PATHOPHYSIOLOGY

- Route of spread
  - Primary host (dog or cat) passes eggs to ground through feces.
  - Warm, sandy soil acts as an incubator.
  - Eggs mature into *rhabditiform larvae* (noninfectious), which molt in 5 days to *filariform larvae* (infectious).
- Humans are accidental hosts.
- *Filariform larvae* penetrate the epidermis either through hair follicles, skin fissures, or through intact skin with the use of proteases.
- Larvae are unable to penetrate the basement membrane of the dermis; therefore, the infection remains limited to the epidermis.
- Larvae cannot complete their life cycle in the human host and die within weeks to months.
- Symptoms are due to hypersensitivity to the organism or its excreta.

ETIOLOGY

- Most common organism is the dog or cat hookworm, *Ancylostoma braziliense*.
- Other species include *Ancylostoma caninum*, *Uncinaria stenocephala*, and *Bunostomum phlebotomum*.

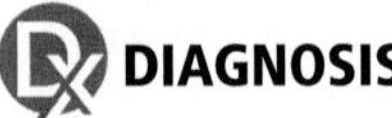

DIAGNOSIS

Diagnosis is clinical. Organisms are rarely recovered from biopsy, and antibody titers are unreliable.

HISTORY

- Incubation period
  - Usual time from infectious exposure to symptoms is 7 to 10 days but may last for up to several months.
- Rash
  - Intensely pruritic, raised, serpiginous, and linear
  - Most commonly located on feet, buttocks, and abdomen; also found on face, extremities, and genitalia
- Pruritus
  - Symptoms typically begin with some tingling in the affected area with the development of the typical rash with intense pruritus.
- Speed at which rash spreads
  - Rash typically lengthens by a few millimeters to 2 to 3 cm daily.
- Source of infection
  - History of contract with beaches in tropical countries where dogs are frequently found
  - In the United States: most frequently contracted from moist soil in southeastern United States contaminated with animal feces

PHYSICAL EXAM

The classic rash is described as an erythematous, raised, serpiginous rash. In addition, it may begin as vesicular and/or form bullae along the track. Tracks under the skin reflect the course of the larvae. The active end is not part of the track.

DIFFERENTIAL DIAGNOSIS

- Cutaneous larva migrans should be considered in anyone with an intensely pruritic, raised, serpiginous, linear, cutaneous eruption.
- Hookworm infections
  - *Strongyloides stercoralis*
  - *U. stenocephala*
  - *B. phlebotomum*
  - *Gnathostoma spinigerum*
- Free-living nematodes (*Pelodera strongyloides*) and insect larvae
- Other cutaneous eruptions that may mimic cutaneous larva migrans include the following:
  - Scabies
  - Tinea pedis
  - Erythema migrans of Lyme disease
  - Jelly fish stings
  - Contact dermatitis
  - Photosensitivity

DIAGNOSTIC TESTS & INTERPRETATION

- Biopsy: not indicated because it rarely yields organisms
- Serologic testing: not helpful and unreliable, as immunity does not usually develop
- Diagnosis is based on clinical presentation.

TREATMENT

MEDICATION

- Albendazole
  - 1st-line recommendation by the Centers for Disease Control and Prevention (CDC)
  - Used by the World Health Organization (WHO) in children 1 year and older at reduced dosing
  - Contraindicated in children <2 years
  - Administered as 400 mg PO once a day for 3 to 7 days
- Ivermectin
  - Preferred treatment by multiple sources
  - Oral ivermectin is contraindicated in children who weigh <15 kg or are <5 years old.
  - 200 mcg/kg once a day for 1 to 2 days
- Topical treatments:
  - Used in mild disease cases and in young children
  - Topical thiabendazole 10–15% applied 3 times a day for 5 to 7 days; not readily available for prescription
  - Topical albendazole 10% applied 3 times a day for 10 days; not readily available for prescription

ONGOING CARE

FOLLOW-UP RECOMMENDATIONS

Patient Monitoring

- Symptoms persist for 8 weeks but up to 1 year in untreated patients.
- Those with extensive involvement should be seen after treatment to be certain of improvement in symptoms.

PROGNOSIS

- This is a self-limited disease and will resolve without treatment when the larvae die.
- Cure rates with oral ivermectin range from 77% to 100% after 1 dose, with a second dose usually providing complete resolution. Oral albendazole for 5 to 7 days has cure rates of 92–100%.

COMPLICATIONS

- Most common complication is secondary bacterial infection of the involved skin.
- Self-limited disease: If untreated, larvae die within 2 to 8 weeks but may persist for up to 1 year.
- Rarely, the larvae can invade the dermis and, subsequently, the bloodstream, leading to a peripheral eosinophilia and pulmonary infiltrates (Löffler syndrome).

ADDITIONAL READING

- American Academy of Pediatrics. Cutaneous larva migrans. In: Kimberlin DW, Brady MT, Jackson MA, et al, eds. *Red Book: 2015 Report of the Committee on Infectious Diseases*. 30th ed. Elk Grove Village, IL: American Academy of Pediatrics; 2015:315–316.
- Blackwell V, Vega-Lopez F. Cutaneous larva migrans: clinical features and management of 44 cases presenting in the returning traveler. *Br J Dermatol*. 2001;145(3):434–437.
- Bouchaud O, Houzé S, Schiemann R, et al. Cutaneous larva migrans in travelers: a prospective study, with assessment of therapy with ivermectin. *Clin Infect Dis*. 2000;31(2):493–498.
- Brenner MA, Patel MB. Cutaneous larva migrans: the creeping eruption. *Cutis*. 2003;72(2):111–115.
- Caumes E. Treatment of cutaneous larva migrans. *Clin Infect Dis*. 2000;30(5):811–814.
- Heukelbach J, Feldmeier H. Epidemiological and clinical characteristics of hookworm-related cutaneous larva migrans. *Lancet Infect Dis*. 2008;8(5):302–309.
- Tan SK, Liu TT. Cutaneous larva migrans complicated by Löffler syndrome. *Arch Dermatol*. 2010;146(2):210–212.

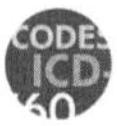

CODES

ICD10

- B76.9 Hookworm disease, unspecified
- B76.8 Other hookworm diseases

FAQ

- Q: Can children spread the infection to each other?
- A: The usual spread of infection is from direct contact with the larvae. Person-to-person spread does not occur.
- Q: What is the role of treatment in cutaneous larva migrans?
- A: Although the infestation is self-limited, as the larvae die with time, antiparasitic therapy helps to control the symptoms and prevent complications such as secondary bacterial infection.
- Q: What are preventive strategies for avoiding cutaneous larva migrans when visiting tropical beaches?
- A: When on tropical beaches frequented by dogs, wear shoes, avoid lying directly on dry sand, and only lie in sand that has been washed by the tide.
- Q: What are other names for cutaneous larva migrans?
- A: Creeping eruption, sandworms, and plumber's itch

CYCLIC VOMITING SYNDROME

Desale Yacob, MD

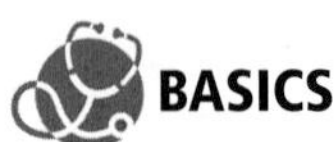

BASICS

DESCRIPTION

- Cyclic vomiting syndrome (CVS) is characterized by recurrent and stereotypical episodes of vomiting with intervening periods of normal health.
- Essential clinical features of CVS are two or more periods of intense nausea and paroxysmal vomiting lasting hours to days within a 6-month period, return to baseline health between episodes, stereotypical episodes with regard to timing of symptoms and duration as well as the absence of an identifiable organic cause for vomiting.

EPIDEMIOLOGY

- CVS commonly starts in early childhood with approximately 46% of children developing symptoms at ≤3 years of age.
- Prevalence of 0.2–1% has been reported.
- The syndrome is more common in Caucasians.

COMMONLY ASSOCIATED CONDITIONS

- 2/3 of CVS patients have symptoms of irritable bowel syndrome (IBS).
- 11% of CVS patients have migraine headaches and a third of patients later develop migraine headaches.

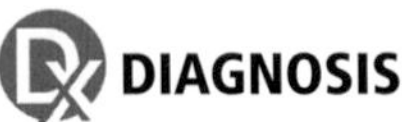

DIAGNOSIS

- A consensus statement by the North American Society for Pediatric Gastroenterology, Hepatology and Nutrition (NASPGHAN) expert task force suggests the diagnosis can be made if the following criteria are met:
  - A minimum of two attacks during a 6-month period or at least five attacks in any interval
  - Episodic attacks of intense nausea and vomiting lasting 1 hour to 10 days and occurring at least 1 week apart
  - Stereotypical pattern and symptoms in the individual patient
  - Vomiting during attacks occurs at least 4 times per hour for at least 1 hour.
  - Return to baseline health between episodes
  - Not attributed to another disorder
- If the above criteria is met, the diagnosis should be considered most likely to be CVS and the workup should consist of the following tests only:
  - Electrolytes, glucose, BUN, and creatinine
  - An upper GI (UGI) series to evaluate for malrotation
- Red flags that CVS is not the correct diagnosis include the following:
  - Episode of vomiting is characterized by the presence of the following:
    - Bilious emesis
    - Severe localized abdominal pain or tenderness
    - Hematemesis
- If episodes are triggered by intercurrent illness, fasting, or high-protein meal, the following labs should be obtained at the beginning of the attack prior to IV fluid:
  - Glucose, electrolytes for anion gap, urine ketones serum lactate, ammonia and amino acids, urine organic acids. Optional metabolic labs include plasma carnitine and acylcarnitine.
- If episodes occur in the context of an abnormal neurologic exam, including severe altered mental status, papilledema, abnormal eye movements, motor asymmetry, and gait abnormality, consultation with a neurologist is indicated and a brain MRI should be obtained.
  - Consider at any given time:
    - US of abdomen and pelvis
    - UGI series
    - Amylase and lipase
    - Esophagogastroduodenoscopy
  - During an attack, obtain LFTs, lipase ± amylase to rule out hepatitis and pancreatitis.
  - During an attack, consider US of kidneys to evaluate for ureteropelvic junction (UPJ) obstruction.
  - During an attack, consider metabolic workup, especially in young children.

HISTORY

- Children with CVS experience a stereotypical pattern of vomiting characterized by a consistent time of onset, duration, and associated symptoms.
- Vomiting frequency is high, with median of six bouts of emesis per hour, often bilious and associated with severe nausea.
- The intense vomiting results in dehydration and need for IV hydration.
- Accompanying symptoms include nausea, retching, headache, abdominal pain, pallor, listlessness, anorexia, and photophobia.
- Physical and psychological stresses are common triggers.
- CVS episodes are most likely to start in the early morning hours.

PHYSICAL EXAM

Physical exam is often consistent with dehydration, and young children may appear listless.

DIFFERENTIAL DIAGNOSIS

- Cannabinoid hyperemesis syndrome
- Malrotation
- Ureteropelvic junction (UPJ) obstruction
- Rumination syndrome
- Gastroparesis
- Pseudo-obstruction
- CNS lesion
- Increased intracranial pressure
- Infectious illness
- Pancreatitis
- Mitochondrial disorder

DIAGNOSTIC TESTS & INTERPRETATION

The consideration of established criteria is important when diagnosing CVS, as is a thorough workup to rule out other etiologies that may explain the symptoms. These tests may include blood, urine, and imaging studies depending on the history and physical exam of the individual child.

Initial Tests (screening, lab, imaging)

- Basic metabolic panel: Na^+, K^+, Cl^-, HCO_3, glucose, BUN, and creatinine
- Liver and pancreas: ALT, GGT, lipase ± amylase
- Other: urine ketones, lactate, ammonia, serum amino acids, urine organic acids, plasma carnitine, and acylcarnitine
- UGI series
  - A UGI should be performed in all patients who present with bilious emesis and who are suspected to have CVS.
- Abdominal US
  - Helpful in evaluation of the hepatobiliary and urinary systems
  - Helpful during attack to identify UPJ obstruction
- Brain MRI
  - Should be obtained when episodes of emesis are associated with progressive or acute as well as diffuse or focal, neurologic symptoms or signs
  - MRI, rather than CT or skull x-ray is the preferred modality for visualization of the posterior fossa.

DIAGNOSTIC PROCEDURES/SURGERY

Esophagogastroduodenoscopy

- May be indicated if hematemesis occurs following multiple episodes of emesis in a patient with CVS
- Most likely etiologies of hematemesis in a child with CVS are mild esophagitis, Mallory-Weiss tear, or prolapse gastropathy.
- Endoscopy may also be indicated if patients have persistent symptoms between episodes suggestive of peptic/bacterial, allergic, inflammatory or celiac disease, or hematemesis of large quantity that may require endoscopic hemostasis.

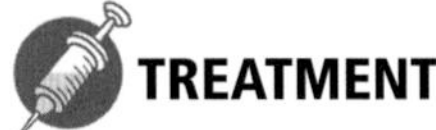

TREATMENT

- The treatment strategy should be tailored to an individual taking into account the following:
  - The frequency and severity of attacks as well as how badly it impacts the patient
  - Potential side effects of the treatment have to also be taken into consideration.
- Treatment of children with CVS can be as follows:
  - Prophylactic or preventive measures
  - Abortive and supportive interventions

GENERAL MEASURES

There are a number of lifestyle changes that can be implemented that may prevent recurrence of CVS attacks without resorting to daily medications. Targeted lifestyle changes that can be effective are best found by reviewing a detailed vomiting diary to identify triggers for episodes. Generally speaking, the following are effective measures:

- Reassurance and education of patients and their families about CVS to decrease stress
- Avoidance of triggers and precipitating factors, including prolonged fasting, poor sleep hygiene, chocolate, cheese, monosodium glutamate, antigenic foods, and excessive exercise

- If episodes are induced by fasting, the child should have supplemental carbohydrate by having snacks between meals, before exertion, or at bedtime.
- Considering CVS to be in the migraine spectrum, migraine headache lifestyle interventions by doing regular aerobic exercise, regular meal times, and regulated consumption of caffeine

MEDICATION

- Children >5 years of age
  - Amitriptyline, a tricyclic antidepressant (TCA), has been shown to be very effective.
    - It is recommended to initially prescribe a dose of 0.25 to 0.5 mg/kg PO at bed time.
    - Doses should be increased by 5 to 10 mg weekly to a maximum dose of 1 to 1.5 mg/kg if symptoms continue to occur.
    - Patients should be evaluated prior to starting amitriptyline with an EKG for QT_c abnormality and 10 days after achieving peak dose.
    - Side effects of this drug consist of arrhythmia (prolongation of the QT interval), sedation, behavioral changes, and constipation.
    - Nortriptyline is another TCA that can be used as an alternative.
  - Propranolol, a β-blocker, is considered a 2nd-line therapy.
    - This should be dosed at 0.25 to 1 mg/kg/24 h PO, with a typical maximum dose of 10 mg b.i.d. or t.i.d.
    - Heart rate should be monitored and maintained ≥60 bpm.
    - Side effects include lethargy and reduced exercise intolerance.
    - Propranolol is contraindicated in children with asthma, diabetes, heart disease, and depression. Propranolol must be tapered for 1 to 2 weeks when it is discontinued.
- Children ≤5 years of age can be treated by the following:
  - Cyproheptadine, which is an antihistamine, is first choice.
  - Dosed at 0.25 to 0.5 mg/kg/24 h PO divided b.i.d. or t.i.d., the β-blocker propranolol can be used as a second choice as discussed above.
  - Nutritional supplements including the following:
    - L-carnitine 50 to 100 mg/kg/24 h PO divided b.i.d. or t.i.d. (side effects reported include diarrhea and fishy body odor)
    - Coenzyme Q_{10} 10 mg/kg/24 h PO divided b.i.d. or t.i.d. (max 100 mg t.i.d.)
  - Other medications and supplements that have been used in treating CVS in a prophylactic measure include the following and are generally only prescribed by neurologists: phenobarbital or alternative anticonvulsants; topiramate, valproic acid, gabapentin, levetiracetam.
- A plan that combines lifestyle changes and medications with careful attention to dosing, side effects, and specialist referrals should be put in place and clearly communicated with the patients and parents.

ADDITIONAL THERAPIES

When children with CVS have an acute episode, they will require both supportive and abortive interventions.

- Decreasing stimulation by situating the patient in a quiet and dark area
- Providing fluid replacements with electrolytes and calories along with antiemetics and analgesics
- Identifying possible metabolic decompensation by paying attention to the following:
  - Anion gap, lactic acidosis, and hyperglycemia
  - Using fluids with higher dextrose concentration such as 10% may also be very helpful.
- Abortive intervention
  - Sumatriptan, an antimigraine drug, can be given at the time of onset at a dose of 20 mg intranasally.
    - Possible side effects: neck pain or burning and coronary vasospasm
    - A contraindication for its use is comorbidity with basilar artery migraines.
- Supportive care
  - Fluids: D10 1/2 NS with or without KCl at 1 1/2 times maintenance
    - Peripheral parenteral nutrition may be necessary if the patient had no enteral intake for 3 to 5 days.
  - Antiemetic
    - Ondansetron at a dose of 0.15 mg/kg/dose (max dose: 16 mg) IV given every 4 to 6 hours
  - Sedatives
    - Diphenhydramine 1 to 1.25 mg/kg/dose (max dose: 50 mg) IV every 6 hours
    - Lorazepam 0.05 to 0.1 mg/kg/dose (max dose: 2 mg) IV every 6 hours
  - Analgesics
    - Ketorolac 0.4 to 1 mg/kg IV every 6 hours with a max dose of 30 mg and total daily max of 120 mg. Do not exceed 3 to 5 days of continuous use.
  - It is also important to treat any abdominal pain, diarrhea, hypertension, and complications that may result from the persistent emesis such as dehydration, weight loss, hematemesis, metabolic acidosis, and syndrome of inappropriate antidiuretic hormone secretion (SIADH).
  - Once the episode of emesis is over, the child can be fed ad libitum.

ONGOING CARE

FOLLOW-UP RECOMMENDATIONS

Referral to either pediatric gastroenterologists or neurologists with special interest in CVS should be made.

PATIENT EDUCATION

Patients and parents should be directed to visit the following:

- The Cyclic Vomiting Syndrome Association Web site: http://www.cvsaonline.org
- International Foundation for Functional Gastrointestinal Disorders Web site: http://www.aboutkidsgi.org/site/about-gi-health-in-kids/functional-gi-and-motility-disorders/cyclic-vomiting-syndrome
- The Rome Foundation Web site: http://www.theromefoundation.org

ADDITIONAL READING

- Boles RG. High degree of efficacy in the treatment of cyclic vomiting syndrome with combined co-enzyme Q10, L-carnitine and amitriptyline, a case series. *BMC Neurol*. 2011;11:102.
- Fleisher DR, Matar M. The cyclic vomiting syndrome: a report of 71 cases and literature review. *J Pediatr Gastroenterol Nutr*. 1993;17(4):361–369.
- Hyams JS, Di Lorenzo C, Saps M, et al. Functional disorders: children and adolescents [published online ahead of print February 15, 2016]. *Gastroenterology*. doi:10.1053/j.gastro.2016.02.015.
- Li BU, Lefevre F, Chelimsky GG, et al. North American Society for Pediatric Gastroenterology, Hepatology, and Nutrition consensus statement on the diagnosis and management of cyclic vomiting syndrome. *J Pediatr Gastroenterol Nutr*. 2008;47(3):379–393.
- Li BU, Murray RD, Heitlinger LA, et al. Heterogeneity of diagnoses presenting as cyclic vomiting. *Pediatrics*. 1998;102(3, Pt 1):583–587.
- Robinson TL, Cheng FK, Domingo CA, et al. Spicing up the differential for cyclical vomiting. *Am J Gastroenterol*. 2013;108(8):1371.

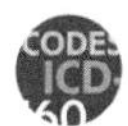

CODES

ICD10

- G43.A0 Cyclical vomiting, not intractable
- G43.A1 Cyclical vomiting, intractable

FAQ

- Q: How should I evaluate a child with presumed CVS who presents with progressive or focal neurologic findings?
- A: The child should be evaluated for increased intracranial pressure as well as a metabolic disorder.
- Q: How can one distinguish true encephalopathy from CVS-associated listlessness in child presenting to the ED?
- A: The child with CVS will respond to commands appropriately and is oriented despite the desire to remain low key due to the severe nausea. In contrast, a child with metabolic encephalopathy is most likely to be confused, disoriented, and difficult to arouse.

CYCLOSPORA

Jessica R. Newman, DO

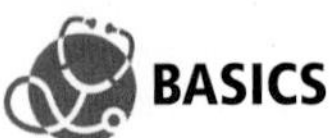

BASICS

DESCRIPTION

Cyclospora cayetanensis, a coccidian protozoan, causes a diarrheal illness first described in humans in 1979.

EPIDEMIOLOGY

- Worldwide distribution, with areas of endemic infection (Nepal, Peru, Haiti, Guatemala, Indonesia)
- People living in endemic areas have a shorter illness or may be asymptomatic carriers.
- *Cyclospora* can be an opportunistic infection in human immunodeficiency virus patients.
- In the United States, infection occurs primarily in spring and summer.
- In the United States and Canada, cases are associated with consumption of imported fresh produce.

GENERAL PREVENTION

- Fresh produce, especially raspberries, cilantro, and salad mixes, should be washed thoroughly before being eaten, although this still may not entirely eliminate the risk of transmission.
- Avoid consumption of waste water and, in endemic areas, avoid consumption of tap water.

PATHOPHYSIOLOGY

- Infected patients excrete noninfectious unsporulated oocysts in their stool.
- Sporulation then occurs days to weeks after release into the environment.
- Ingestion of sporulated oocysts occurs and sporozoites are released that invade the intestinal epithelial cells.
- Sporozoites develop into trophozoites, which undergo schizogony and form merozoites.
- Merozoites may develop into macro- or microgametes, which become fertilized, resulting in oocysts.
- Entire life cycle is completed in the host.
- Incubation period is between 2 and 14 days, with an average of 7 days.

ETIOLOGY

- Outbreaks have been associated with the consumption of raspberries, mesclun (young salad greens), salad mixes, cilantro, and basil.
- Infection occurs through the consumption of contaminated food and water.
- Transmission does not occur through person-to-person spread.

DIAGNOSIS

HISTORY

- Fever
  - Low-grade fever is common.
- Clinical prodrome
  - Acute onset of diarrhea is typical, but a flulike prodrome may occur.
- Nature of the diarrhea
  - Profuse, nonbloody, watery diarrhea that may be foul smelling
  - Can alternate with constipation
- Other symptoms experienced:
  - Abdominal cramping
  - Fatigue
  - Anorexia
  - Flatulence
  - Vomiting
- Foods that have been consumed in the past 2 weeks
  - Illness has been attributed to contaminated raspberries, water, mesclun, salad mix, cilantro, and basil.

PHYSICAL EXAM

Dehydration

- Due to profuse diarrhea
- Signs of dehydration (tachycardia, dry mucous membranes, sunken eyes, poor skin turgor, and weight loss) may be present.

DIFFERENTIAL DIAGNOSIS

- *Cryptosporidium*
  - Outbreaks are associated with contaminated water sources (municipal pools).
  - Person-to-person transmission may occur.
  - Clinically indistinguishable from *Cyclospora*
- *Cystoisospora belli*
  - Outbreaks are associated with food and water.
  - Clinically indistinguishable from *Cyclospora*, although fever may be more common
- *Microsporidia*
  - Outbreaks are associated with contaminated water sources.
  - Chronic diarrhea occurs in immunocompromised patients, especially HIV patients.
  - Fever is uncommon.
- *Giardia lamblia*
  - Community epidemics are associated primarily with contaminated water sources.
  - Person-to-person transmission may occur and has led to outbreaks in day care centers.
  - Clinical presentation may vary from occasional acute watery diarrhea to a severe, protracted diarrheal illness.
- Viral gastroenteritis
  - *Rotavirus*
  - Adenovirus
- Bacterial gastroenteritis
  - *Clostridium difficile*
  - *Vibrio cholerae* and non-*cholerae Vibrio* species
  - *Escherichia coli* (especially toxin-producing strains)
  - *Shigella* species
  - *Salmonella* species
  - *Yersinia enterocolitica*
  - *Campylobacter* species

C

DIAGNOSTIC TESTS & INTERPRETATION

Initial Tests (screening, lab, imaging)

- Ova and parasites with modified acid-fast staining
  - Identification of *Cyclospora*, *Cystoisospora*, and *Cryptosporidium*
  - Three samples are preferable due to intermittent shedding.
- Ova and parasites: identify common protozoans including *Giardia*
- *Cryptosporidium* and *Giardia* antigen test: immunoassay with high sensitivity and specificity
- Electron microscopy of stool: gold standard for diagnosing microsporidia
- Bacterial stool cultures: identify common bacterial pathogens
- Stool for *C. difficile* PCR: identify a common cause of diarrhea
- Gastrointestinal multiplex nucleic acid testing: simultaneous qualitative detection and identification of multiple viral, parasitic, and bacterial nucleic acids in stool specimens from individuals with gastroenteritis (some panels include *Cyclospora*)
- Electrolytes, blood urea nitrogen, creatinine: may be helpful in some cases to determine extent of dehydration

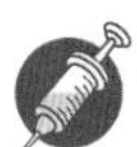

TREATMENT

MEDICATION

- Immunocompetent patient: trimethoprim-sulfamethoxazole (5 mg/kg) IV/PO twice a day for 7 to 10 days
- HIV patient: trimethoprim-sulfamethoxazole 3 times a day for 10 days and then prophylactic dosing 3 times per week to prevent relapse
- Ciprofloxacin or nitazoxanide for 7 days may be alternatives in patients with sulfa allergy.
- Based on severity of dehydration, treatment with IV fluids may be indicated.

ADMISSION, INPATIENT, AND NURSING CONSIDERATIONS

Moderate to severe dehydration should warrant admission.

ONGOING CARE

FOLLOW-UP RECOMMENDATIONS

Patient Monitoring

- Infected patients need to be observed closely for dehydration.
- Relapse may occur in HIV patients, so close follow-up is essential.

PROGNOSIS

- Most cases are self-limited.
- Diarrhea may last up to 3 months in untreated patients who acquired the parasite in a foreign country where *Cyclospora* is endemic.
- In U.S. outbreaks, the average duration of diarrhea ranged from 10 to 24 days.
- Relapses may occur in untreated patients.
- Patients with HIV have more severe and prolonged diarrhea, which may recur.

COMPLICATIONS

- Dehydration and weight loss are the most common complications.
  - Severe, prolonged diarrhea may lead to dehydration.
  - Malabsorption of D-xylose and excretion of fecal fat occurs, leading to weight loss.
- May cause ascending biliary tract disease in AIDS patients
- Rare associated complications
  - Guillain-Barré syndrome
  - Reactive arthritis

ADDITIONAL READING

- Centers for Disease Control and Prevention. Outbreaks of cyclosporiasis—United States, June–August 2013. *MMWR Morb Mortal Wkly Rep*. 2013;62(43):862.
- Herwaldt BL. *Cyclospora cayetanensis*: a review, focusing on the outbreaks of cyclosporiasis in the 1990s. *Clin Infect Dis*. 2000;31(4):1040–1057.
- Legua P, Seas C. *Cystoisospora* and *Cyclospora*. *Curr Opin Infect Dis*. 2013;26(5):479–483.
- Ortega YR, Sanchez R. Update on *Cyclospora cayetanensis*, a food-borne and waterborne parasite. *Clin Microbiol Rev*. 2010;23(1):218–234.

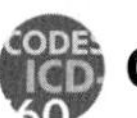

CODES

ICD10

A07.4 Cyclosporiasis

FAQ

- Q: Does routine ova and parasites testing detect *Cyclospora*?
- A: Rarely. Therefore, modified acid-fast staining must be done to improve the laboratory's ability to detect the oocysts.
- Q: Can person-to-person transmission occur in *Cyclospora* illness?
- A: No. It takes days to weeks for oocysts to sporulate and become infectious.
- Q: Can animals/pets be affected by this same pathogen?
- A: Humans are the only natural hosts of *Cyclospora* infection.

CYSTIC FIBROSIS

Samuel B. Goldfarb, MD • Bruce A. Ong, LTC, MC, MD, MPH, USA

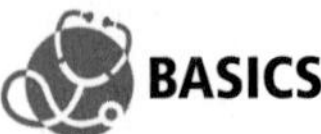

BASICS

DESCRIPTION

Cystic fibrosis (CF) is an inherited autosomal recessive disorder, characterized by chronic obstructive lung disease, pancreatic exocrine insufficiency, and elevated sweat chloride concentration.

ALERT

- Due to variability in presentation, the most common pitfalls are failure to diagnose and initiate therapies in a timely manner.
- Diagnosis may be delayed in patients with mild or atypical symptoms.

EPIDEMIOLOGY

- Most common lethal inherited disease in the Caucasian population
- Carrier frequency of mutations in the CF transmembrane conductance regulator (CFTR) gene:
  - 1:29 in Caucasians
  - 1:49 in Hispanics
  - 1:53 in Native Americans
  - 1:62 in African Americans
  - 1:90 in Asians

Prevalence

- 1:3,300 in Caucasians
- 1:9,500 in Hispanics
- 1:11,200 in Native Americans
- 1:15,300 in African Americans
- 1:32,100 in Asians

RISK FACTORS

Genetics

CFTR gene

- Located on the long arm of chromosome 7
- Most common mutation results in deletion of phenylalanine at position 508 in the CFTR glycoprotein.
- The Δ508 mutation occurs in ~70% of CF patients.
- >1,700 mutations have been reported in the CFTR gene.
- Presence of gene modifiers may cause incomplete phenotypic presentations.

GENERAL PREVENTION

Prepregnancy carrier detection

PATHOPHYSIOLOGY

- CFTR
  - Membrane glycoprotein, which functions as a cyclic AMP–activated chloride channel at the apical surface of epithelial cells
  - An abnormality in CFTR results in defective chloride conductance.
  - May have other roles in the regulation of membrane channels and the pH of intracellular organelles; may affect cell apical sodium channel regulation
  - CFTR abnormalities may act as binding sites for *Pseudomonas aeruginosa*, promoting proinflammatory responses in the lung.
- In the respiratory system
  - Increased mucus viscosity
  - Early bacterial colonization despite a robust neutrophilic inflammatory response
  - Mucous plugging and atelectasis
  - Bronchiectasis and emphysema develop.
  - Abnormal nasal sinus development
- In the gastrointestinal (GI) tract
  - Progressive pancreatic damage leads to exocrine pancreatic insufficiency.
  - Endocrine pancreatic dysfunction
  - Focal biliary cirrhosis of the liver
  - Hypoplasia of the gallbladder and impaired bile flow

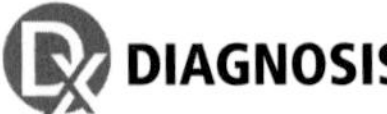

DIAGNOSIS

HISTORY

- Most common presenting respiratory symptoms: chronic cough, recurrent pneumonia, nasal polyps, chronic pansinusitis
- Most common presenting GI symptoms:
  - Meconium ileus (15–20% of patients present with this symptom); pancreatic insufficiency occurs in 85% of patients.
  - In infants, fat malabsorption may lead to chronic diarrhea and failure to thrive.
  - In older patients, pancreatitis, rectal prolapse (occurs in 2% of the patients; must consider CF until proven otherwise)
  - Distal obstruction of the small intestine (meconium ileus equivalent, seen in older children and adults)
- Evidence of heat intolerance: In summer, increased sweating may lead to dehydration with hyponatremia or hypochloremic metabolic alkalosis.

PHYSICAL EXAM

- Respiratory findings:
  - Frequent cough, often productive of mucopurulent sputum
  - Rhonchi, crackles, wheezing, hyperresonance to percussion
  - Nasal polyposis
- Other common findings:
  - Digital clubbing
  - Hepatosplenomegaly in patients with cirrhosis
  - Growth retardation
  - Delayed puberty
  - Osteoporosis

DIFFERENTIAL DIAGNOSIS

- Pulmonary:
  - Recurrent pneumonia or bronchitis
  - Asthma
  - Aspiration pneumonia
  - Ciliary dyskinesia
  - Airway anomalies
  - Chronic sinusitis
  - Chronic aspiration
  - Non-CF bronchiectasis
  - Allergic bronchopulmonary aspergillosis
  - α_1-Antitrypsin disease
- GI:
  - Celiac disease
  - Protein-losing enteropathy
  - Gastroesophageal reflux
  - Chronic pancreatitis
- Other:
  - Metabolic alkalosis
  - Immune deficiency
  - Shwachman-Diamond syndrome

DIAGNOSTIC TESTS & INTERPRETATION

Initial Tests (screening, lab, imaging)

- Immunoreactive trypsinogen test (IRT): used by all 50 states in the United States as part of newborn screening for CF. Blood drawn 2 to 3 days after birth is analyzed for elevated trypsinogen levels.
- Positive IRT testing must be followed by sweat and/or genetic testing to confirm diagnosis.

ALERT

Reflexive DNA testing for positive newborn screening IRT tests may vary from state to state.

- Sweat chloride test: measures CFTR functionality and is keystone for the diagnosis of CF
  - Sweat chloride ≥60 mmol/L consistent with CF
  - Sweat chloride 30 to 59 mmol/L: CFTR dysfunction possible; CFTR gene and functionality testing required to establish or rule out CF/cystic fibrosis metabolic disorder (CRMS)
- Diagnostic criteria include the following:
  - In infants: positive newborn screen and sweat test and clinical features consistent with CF or a positive family history of CF
  - All populations: positive sweat test and two disease causing mutations in *trans* in CFTR genetic analysis and clinical features consistent with CF
  - Individuals with clinical symptoms consistent with CF and intermediate test results should be referred to an accredited CF center for further evaluation.
- Other causes of elevated sweat chloride:
  - Malnutrition
  - Adrenal insufficiency
  - Nephrogenic diabetes insipidus
  - Ectodermal dysplasia
  - Fucosidosis
  - Hypogammaglobulinemia
  - False negatives seen in CF patients with edema
- Mutation analysis:
  - Can detect >90% of CF patients
  - Failure to identify two mutations reduces but does not eliminate CF diagnosis.
- Basic metabolic panel may be required to evaluate for hyponatremia, hypokalemia, and hypochloremia.
- Frequently recovered organisms in sputum cultures:
  - *Haemophilus influenzae*
  - *Staphylococcus aureus*
  - Methicillin-resistant *S. aureus* (MRSA)
  - *P. aeruginosa* (nonmucoid and mucoid)
  - *Burkholderia cepacia*
  - *Stenotrophomonas maltophilia*
  - *Aspergillus* and other fungal species
  - Nontuberculous mycobacterial species
- Pulmonary function test: usually reveals obstructive lung disease, although some patients may have a restrictive pattern
- Analysis of stimulated pancreatic secretions: degree of pancreatic exocrine deficiency
- Fecal elastase measurements can detect pancreatic insufficiency.
- Functional CFTR testing to include nasal potential difference (NPD) or intestinal current measurement (ICM) may be used in specialized centers to make diagnosis of CF.
- Chest radiography
  - Typical features include hyperinflation, peribronchial thickening, atelectasis, and bronchiectasis.
- Computed tomography
  - Bronchiectasis
  - Cystic and interstitial changes
  - Focal consolidation or scarring

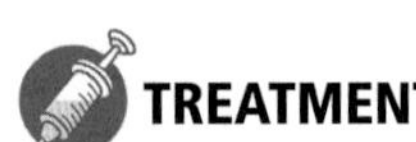

TREATMENT

MEDICATION

First Line

- Antibiotic therapy based on sputum culture results and clinical improvement:
  - Oral antibiotics:
    - Cephalexin
    - Linezolid
    - Trimethoprim-sulfamethoxazole

- Doxycycline
- Ciprofloxacin
- Inhaled antibiotics:
  - Tobramycin, colistin, or aztreonam in selected patients
- IV antibiotics:
  - To treat *S. aureus*, consider oxacillin, trimethoprim-sulfamethoxazole, linezolid, or vancomycin.
  - To treat *P. aeruginosa* and *B. cepacia*, consider aminoglycoside plus ceftazidime or piperacillin with tazobactam.
- Severe cases with resistant strains may benefit from aztreonam, imipenem, or meropenem.
- Two or more antibiotics may be used during treatment of pulmonary exacerbations.
- The use of regular azithromycin is as effective as an anti-inflammatory agent. If used, monitoring for atypical *Mycobacterium* should be performed due to concerns for emerging mycobacterial resistance. Recent concerns of potential antagonism when used in combination with inhaled tobramycin.
- Indwelling catheters may be needed for frequent antibiotic therapy.

- Clearance of pulmonary secretions
  - Chest physical therapy or with high-frequency oscillatory vest device. Adjunct therapy such as positive expiratory pressure (PEP) mask may also be used.
  - Bronchodilator: aerosol or metered-dose inhaler (β_2 agonist)
  - Mucolytics: RhDNase
  - Anti-inflammatory: short-term oral steroid course. Inhaled corticosteroids may benefit patients with asthma and/or those demonstrating an oral steroid response.
  - Hypertonic saline
- GI disease
  - Pancreatic enzyme replacement therapy: used in CF patients who are pancreatic insufficient; dosage adjusted for frequency and character of the stools and for growth pattern; generic substitutes are not bioequivalent to name brands. The maximum recommended dose is 2,500 U of lipase/kg per meal and 10,000 U of lipase/kg/24 h.
  - Adjunctive H_2 antagonist or PPI use can enhance pancreatic enzyme replacement therapy.
  - Vitamin supplements: multivitamin, fat-soluble vitamins A, D, E, and K
  - Salt supplementation
  - Patients with cholestasis may benefit from therapy with ursodeoxycholic acid.
- Other medications
  - CFTR potentiators and correctors
    - Ivacaftor (potentiator) and ivacaftor-lumacaftor (potentiator/corrector) both improve CFTR function in CF patients with specific class mutations, resulting in improved lung function and decreased exacerbations.
    - Management of these medications requires knowledge of genetic mutations eligible for therapy and close monitoring for side effects.

ONGOING CARE

FOLLOW-UP RECOMMENDATIONS

Patient Monitoring

- Newborns should be seen in a CF center within 48 to 72 hours after a diagnosis has been established.

ALERT

In infants with positive newborn screen and poor growth, it is appropriate to make a presumptive diagnosis of CF and treat empirically with pancreatic enzyme replacement therapy and salt until diagnosis can be confirmed or ruled out. If clinically indicated, evaluation and intervention of electrolyte derangements may be required.

- Specialized care should be at a CF center.
- Frequency of visits depends on age and severity of illness:
  - Infants should be seen at least monthly for the first 12 months and then every 2 to 3 months.
- Respiratory
  - Sputum cultures for fungi, acid-fast bacteria, and aerobic organisms are used to direct antimicrobial therapy.
  - Duration of antibiotic therapy is generally 14 to 21 days; more frequent use is required as pulmonary function deteriorates.

DIET

- High-calorie diet with added salt
- Lifelong nutritional support usually required
- Gastrostomy tube placement may be necessary to increase caloric intake and maintain growth.

PROGNOSIS

- Current median survival is ~38 years.
- Variable course of the disease
- The median survival has been increasing for the past 4 decades, although the rate of increase in age has slowed in the past decade.

COMPLICATIONS

- Respiratory complications:
  - Recurrent bronchitis and pneumonia
  - Atelectasis
  - Bronchiectasis
  - Pneumothorax
  - Hemoptysis
  - Chronic sinusitis and nasal polyps
- Cardiovascular complications:
  - Pulmonary hypertension in patients with severe obstructive lung disease
- GI complications:
  - Pancreatic insufficiency in 85–90% of CF patients
  - Patients usually have steatorrhea and poor growth and nutritional status.
  - Decreased levels of vitamins A, E, D, and K
  - Rectal prolapse
  - 10–15% of patients have meconium ileus.
  - Distal intestinal obstruction syndrome
  - Clinically significant focal biliary cirrhosis; hepatobiliary disease in 5% of CF patients
  - Esophageal varices
  - Splenomegaly
  - Hypersplenism
  - Cholestasis
- Reproductive complications:
  - Sterility in 98% of males due to absence or atresia of the vas deferens
  - Slight decrease in fertility for females secondary to abnormalities of cervical mucus
- Endocrine complications:
  - Glucose intolerance
  - CF-related diabetes occurs with increasing frequency in adolescent and adult patients.
- Skeletal complications:
  - Osteoporosis
  - Joint pain
- Psychosocial complications:
  - Anxiety or depressive disorders

ADDITIONAL READING

- Baumer JH. Evidence based guidelines for the performance of the sweat test for the investigation of cystic fibrosis in the UK. *Arch Dis Child*. 2003;88(12):1126–1127.
- Farrell PM, White TB, Howenstine MS, et al. Diagnosis of cystic fibrosis in screened populations. *J Pediatr*. 2017;181(Suppl):S33–S44.e2.
- Farrell PM, White TB, Ren CL, et al. Diagnosis of cystic fibrosis: consensus guidelines from the Cystic Fibrosis Foundation. *J Pediatr*. 2017;181(Suppl):S4–S15.e1.
- Flume PA, O'Sullivan BP, Robinson KA, et al; for Cystic Fibrosis Foundation, Pulmonary Therapies Committee. Cystic fibrosis pulmonary guidelines: chronic medications for maintenance of lung health. *Am J Respir Crit Care Med*. 2007;176(10):957–969.
- Pier GB. CFTR mutations and host susceptibility to *Pseudomonas aeruginosa* lung infection. *Curr Opin Microbiol*. 2002;5(1):81–86.
- Ryan G, Mukhopadhyay S, Singh M. Nebulised anti-pseudomonal antibiotics for cystic fibrosis. *Cochrane Database Syst Rev*. 2003;(3):CD001021.
- Smyth A, Walters S. Prophylactic antibiotics for cystic fibrosis. *Cochrane Database Syst Rev*. 2000;(2):CD001912.
- Southern KW, Barker PM. Azithromycin for cystic fibrosis. *Eur Respir J*. 2004;24(5):834–838.
- Stallings VA, Stark LJ, Robinson KA, et al; for Clinical Practice Guidelines on Growth and Nutrition Subcommittee, Ad Hoc Working Group. Evidence-based practice recommendations for nutrition-related management of children and adults with cystic fibrosis and pancreatic insufficiency: results of a systematic review. *J Am Diet Assoc*. 2008;108(5):832–839.
- Wainwright CE, Elborn JS, Ramsey BW, et al; for the TRAFFIC and TRANSPORT Study Groups. Lumacaftor-Ivacaftor in patients with cystic fibrosis homozygous for Phe508del *CFTR*. *N Engl J Med*. 2015;373(3):220–231.
- Yankaskas JR, Marshall BC, Sufian B, et al. Cystic fibrosis adult care: consensus conference report. *Chest*. 2004;125(Suppl 1):1S–39S.

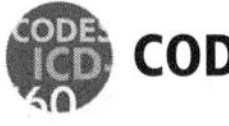

CODES

ICD10

- E84.9 Cystic fibrosis, unspecified
- E84.0 Cystic fibrosis with pulmonary manifestations
- E84.11 Meconium ileus in cystic fibrosis

FAQ

- Q: Should relatives be tested?
- A: All siblings should have a sweat test.
- Q: How well will a child with CF do?
- A: The course of the illness is variable. It is difficult to predict the course of disease in an individual.
- Q: How should a borderline sweat test be interpreted?
- A: Borderline sweat tests should always be correlated with other findings such as physical exam, sputum cultures, pulmonary function, radiographic findings, nutritional evaluation, and/or mutation analysis. Referral to a CF center for further evaluation is indicated.
- Q: Can an infant with a positive newborn screen and only one CF mutation found on reflex CFTR genetic testing have CF if mother was the carrier of the mutation and the father was negative for CF mutations on the prenatal 23 mutation panel?
- A: Yes. Although the infant is at least a carrier of a CF mutation, the negative screening panel for the father only rules out common mutations, and he could be a carrier for an untested CF mutation. The infant requires further testing to confirm or rule out CF.

CYTOMEGALOVIRUS INFECTIONS

Michelle Marie Gontasz, MD • Ravit Arav-Boger, MD

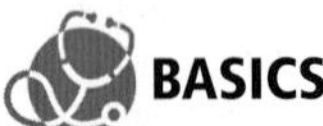

BASICS

DESCRIPTION

Cytomegalovirus (CMV) is a ubiquitous double-stranded DNA virus that is a member of the herpesvirus family. It establishes latency in peripheral blood mononuclear cells and endothelial cells.

EPIDEMIOLOGY

- Primary infection occurs from early childhood into adolescence and childbearing years.
- Transmission occurs by contact with infected body fluids such as saliva, urine, blood, or breast milk through sexual contact or solid organ transplantation. Intrauterine transmission is the most common route of acquiring congenital infection.

Prevalence

Seroprevalence increases with age and varies with socioeconomic status; 50% of middle- and 80% of lower socioeconomic status adults are seropositive.

GENERAL PREVENTION

- Pregnant women should receive education about CMV transmission. Precautions should be instituted for hospitalized patients known to be shedding CMV.
- Seriously ill neonates should receive blood products from CMV-negative donors.
- CMV-seronegative solid organ transplantation recipients should receive organs (and all blood products) from CMV-negative donors whenever possible.
- Hyperimmunoglobulin has been used in high-risk CMV-negative recipients of CMV-positive donors to prevent severe CMV disease.

PATHOPHYSIOLOGY

Infection leads to intranuclear inclusions with massive enlargement of cells. Almost any organ may become infected with CMV in severe disseminated infection.

COMMONLY ASSOCIATED CONDITIONS

- Congenital infection
  - Occurs in about 1% of newborns in United States
  - Intrauterine transmission is more common in pregnant women mothers with primary infection during pregnancy (40–50%) compared to recurrent infection (<1%).
  - Postnatal acquisition of CMV via breast milk: Controversy exists over whether this precludes breastfeeding in premature infants (has a lower risk for neurologic sequelae than congenital infection).
  - 10% of infected infants are symptomatic at birth, with severe disease characterized by growth retardation, hepatosplenomegaly, thrombocytopenia, and central nervous system (CNS) involvement.
  - 10–20% of infants who are asymptomatically infected at birth may develop sensorineural hearing loss.
  - Of symptomatically infected infants, 90% will have some neurologic sequelae. Degree of impairments may be predicted by CT findings and microcephaly at birth.
- Mononucleosis syndrome
  - Syndrome similar to that caused by Epstein-Barr virus (EBV) infection in immunocompetent patients
  - The most common symptoms are malaise (67%) and fever (50%). ~70% of patients have abnormal liver enzymes.
  - Pharyngitis and splenomegaly less common and severe than observed with EBV-induced mononucleosis
- Interstitial pneumonitis
  - Seen primarily in severely immunosuppressed children and adults
  - Begins with fever and nonproductive cough but may progress to dyspnea and severe hypoxia over 1 to 2 weeks
  - Mild, self-limited pneumonitis may occur in immunocompetent patients.
- Retinitis
  - Observed in infants with symptomatic congenital infection and in patients with advanced AIDS
  - Immunosuppressed children should have regular eye exams.
- Hepatitis
  - Occurs in healthy individuals with primary infections and in immunosuppressed patients with either primary or reactivated disease
  - Fever, mild elevation of liver enzymes, and hepatomegaly are typical. Jaundice and severe hepatitis are uncommon.
- Gastrointestinal (GI) disease
  - Severely immunosuppressed patients may experience esophagitis, gastritis, colitis, or pancreatitis.
  - Diagnosis requires endoscopy with biopsy.
- CNS disease
  - Commonly seen in infants with symptomatic congenital infection
  - Characterized by microcephaly, periventricular calcifications, seizures, developmental delay, and sensorineural hearing loss
  - Encephalitis or meningoencephalitis may occur in immunocompromised patients and very rarely reported in literature in immunocompetent hosts.
- Hearing loss
  - Congenital CMV is the most common infectious cause of deafness.
  - Onset of deafness often seen after 1st month of life and is progressive; may be missed by newborn hearing screen (if only done in first 2 weeks of life)

DIAGNOSIS

HISTORY

- Relevant exposures include
  - Day care attendance; increased risk of infection
  - Recent blood transfusion; risk of transfusion-associated CMV
  - Use of immunosuppressive medications; associated with increased cause of serious infection
- Prolonged fever
  - Mononucleosis-like syndrome
- Blurred vision
  - CMV retinitis
- Cough, dyspnea, wheezing
  - CMV pneumonitis
- Vomiting, abdominal pain, diarrhea (watery or bloody)
  - CMV colitis
- Hearing loss (may require audiogram, brainstem evoked auditory responses) or failed hearing screening test
  - Congenital infection

PHYSICAL EXAM

- Microcephaly
  - Congenital infection
- White, perivascular retinal infiltrates and hemorrhage
  - Retinitis
- Photophobia, headache, nuchal rigidity
  - Meningitis/encephalitis
- Tachypnea, rales
  - Pneumonitis
  - Hepatomegaly and/or splenomegaly
  - Mononucleosis-like syndrome
- Rash
  - Petechiae, purpura, "blueberry muffin" lesions, rubelliform rash
- Adenopathy
  - Mononucleosis-like syndrome

DIFFERENTIAL DIAGNOSIS

- Congenital infection
  - Congenital rubella syndrome
  - Toxoplasmosis
  - Syphilis
  - Neonatal herpes simplex virus
  - HIV
  - Enteroviral infection
- Mononucleosis syndrome
  - EBV infection
  - Toxoplasmosis
  - Hepatitis A or B infection
- Interstitial pneumonitis
  - Respiratory syncytial virus
  - Adenovirus
  - Measles
  - Varicella
  - *Pneumocystis jiroveci* (previously *carinii*)
  - *Chlamydia*
  - *Mycoplasma*
  - Fungal
  - Drug/toxin-induced pneumonitis
- Retinitis
  - Ocular toxoplasmosis
  - Candidal retinitis
  - Syphilis
  - Herpes simplex virus
- Hepatitis
  - EBV infection
  - Hepatitis A, B, or C infection
  - Enterovirus
  - Adenovirus
  - Herpes simplex virus
  - Drug/toxin-induced
- GI disease
  - Herpes simplex virus
  - Adenovirus
  - *Salmonella*
  - *Shigella*
  - *Campylobacter*
  - *Yersinia*
  - *Clostridium difficile*
  - *Giardia*
  - *Cryptosporidium*
- CNS disease
  - Congenital disease (see congenital infection earlier)
  - Meningoencephalitis in immunocompetent host: herpes simplex virus, EBV, varicella-zoster virus, enterovirus, arbovirus. Meningoencephalitis in immunocompromised host: in addition to organisms listed previously, should include HIV encephalitis, fungal meningitis, toxoplasmosis

DIAGNOSTIC TESTS & INTERPRETATION

Initial Tests (screening, lab, imaging)

- Shell-vial assay:
  - Staining for immediate early antigen production
  - Allows detection of virus 24 to 48 hours after inoculation
- Viral culture:
  - Virus may be isolated from nasopharyngeal/oropharyngeal secretions, urine, stool, and WBC.
  - Isolation may take up to 4 weeks.
  - Urine or saliva samples are most common way to diagnose congenital disease.
- Highly sensitive CMV quantitative polymerase chain reaction (PCR) assay:
  - Measures viral DNA in plasma, whole blood, urine, and CSF
  - Real-time PCR has replaced most diagnostic tests in monitoring response to therapy or identifying viral quantitation; recently standardized to be reported as IU/mL
- Quantitative antigenemia assay:
  - Detection of circulating CMV-infected polymorphonuclear cells by indirect immunofluorescence
  - In an immunocompromised patient, may monitor response to therapy or identify viral reactivation.
- Serology:
  - Enzyme-linked immunosorbent assay or indirect fluorescent antibody assay to detect the presence of CMV IgM or IgG has a limited role.
  - IgG avidity test can be used in certain circumstances, particularly in pregnant women, to diagnose a recent infection.

ALERT

- Due to frequency of asymptomatic shedding, mere isolation of virus does not necessarily establish an etiologic association.
- Severely immunocompromised patients who are actively infected with CMV may be seronegative. 4-fold rise in CMV IgG is not diagnostic of primary infection. Increased antibody titers may occur with reactivation. DNA quantification by real-time PCR is useful in these circumstances to make a timely diagnosis.

- Noncontrast head CT
  - Periventricular calcifications, cystic abnormalities, ventriculomegaly, periventricular leukomalacia
- Brain MRI
  - Has higher sensitivity than ultrasound for brain abnormalities and greater predictor of symptomatic infection

TREATMENT

Majority of transplant experts prefer prophylaxis over preemptive therapy in high-risk patients (donor CMV positive, recipient negative).

MEDICATION

First Line

- Ganciclovir: suppresses viral replication by inhibiting the viral DNA polymerase
  - Indications: symptomatic congenital CMV in a neonate meeting clinical criteria; CMV chorioretinitis in immunocompromised patients; tissue diagnosis (hepatitis, enteritis, pneumonitis) of CMV infection; and in immunocompromised patients with CMV disease (viremia + symptoms)
  - Dosing: 6 mg/kg/dose given IV every 12 hours
  - Side effects: neutropenia (60%), thrombocytopenia (~5%)
- Valganciclovir: an oral prodrug that is rapidly converted to ganciclovir
  - Indications: same as ganciclovir
  - Dosing: 16 mg/kg/dose given orally twice daily
  - Side effects: neutropenia (>20%), headache (6–22%), GI upset (10–20%)

Second Line

Foscarnet: suppresses viral replication by inhibiting viral DNA polymerase

- Indications: same as earlier, but in patients who have failed to improve on ganciclovir therapy or who have experienced significant bone marrow toxicity related to ganciclovir use or with resistance to ganciclovir
- Dosing: 60 mg/kg/dose IV every 8 hours in combination with ganciclovir; continue until symptom improvement, followed by chronic maintenance therapy 90 to 120 mg/kg/dose daily.
- Side effects: renal impairment (12–33%), headache (26%), seizures (10%)

ONGOING CARE

PROGNOSIS

Varies with nature of infection (see "Commonly Associated Conditions")

COMPLICATIONS

Varies with nature of infection (see "Commonly Associated Conditions")

ADDITIONAL READING

- Alexander BT, Hladnik LM, Augustin KM, et al. Use of cytomegalovirus intravenous immune globulin for the adjunctive treatment of cytomegalovirus in hematopoietic stem cell transplant recipients. *Pharmacotherapy*. 2010;30(6):554–561.
- Boeckh M, Ljungman P. How we treat cytomegalovirus in hematopoietic cell transplant recipients. *Blood*. 2009;113(23):5711–5719.
- Cannon MJ, Schmid DS, Hyde TB. Review of cytomegalovirus seroprevalence and demographic characteristics associated with infection. *Rev Med Virol*. 2010;20(4):202–213.
- Dollard SC, Schleiss MR, Grosse SD. Public health and laboratory considerations regarding newborn screening for congenital cytomegalovirus. *J Inherit Metab Dis*. 2010;33(Suppl 2):S249–S254.
- Foulon I, Naessens A, Foulon W, et al. Hearing loss in children with congenital cytomegalovirus infection in relation to the maternal trimester in which the maternal primary infection occurred. *Pediatrics*. 2008;122(6):e1123–e1127.
- Grangeot-Keros L, Mayaux MJ, Lebon P, et al. Value of cytomegalovirus (CMV) IgG avidity index for the diagnosis of primary CMV infection in pregnant women. *J Infect Dis*. 1997;175(4):944–946.
- Istas AS, Demmler GJ, Dobbins JG, et al. Surveillance for congenital cytomegalovirus disease: a report from the National Congenital Cytomegalovirus Disease Registry. *Clin Infect Dis*. 1995;20(3):665–670.
- James SH, Kimberlin DW. Advances in the prevention and treatment of congenital cytomegalovirus infection. *Curr Opin Pediatr*. 2016;28(1):81–85.
- Kimberlin DW, Jester PM, Sánchez PJ, et al; for National Institute of Allergy and Infectious Diseases Collaborative Antiviral Study Group. Valganciclovir for symptomatic congenital cytomegalovirus disease. *N Engl J Med*. 2015;372(10):933–943.
- Kimberlin DW, Lin CY, Sánchez PJ, et al; for National Institute of Allergy and Infectious Diseases Collaborative Antiviral Study Group. Effect of ganciclovir therapy on hearing in symptomatic congenital cytomegalovirus disease involving the central nervous system: a randomized, controlled trial. *J Pediatr*. 2003;143(1):16–25.
- Noyola DE, Demmler GJ, Nelson CT, et al. Early predictors of neurodevelopmental outcome in symptomatic congenital cytomegalovirus infection. *J Pediatr*. 2001;138(3):325–331.
- Revello MG, Zavattoni M, Sarasini A, et al. Human cytomegalovirus in blood of immunocompetent persons during primary infection: prognostic implications for pregnancy. *J Infect Dis*. 1998;177(5):1170–1175.
- Wreghitt TG, Teare EL, Sule O, et al. Cytomegalovirus infection in immunocompetent patients. *Clin Infect Dis*. 2003;37(12):1603–1606.

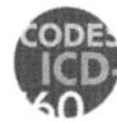

CODES

ICD10

- B25.9 Cytomegaloviral disease, unspecified
- P35.1 Congenital cytomegalovirus infection
- B25.0 Cytomegaloviral pneumonitis

FAQ

- Q: Should children with congenital CMV infection be excluded from day care settings?
- A: No. Due to the high frequency of shedding of CMV in the urine and saliva of asymptomatic children, especially those <2 years of age, exclusion from out-of-home care is not justified for any child known to be infected with CMV. Careful attention to hygienic practices, especially hand washing, is important.
- Q: Up to what age can congenital CMV infection be diagnosed?
- A: The diagnosis of congenital CMV infection can be made up to 21 days of life. After this time, it is unclear if the infection was acquired congenitally or postnatally.
- Q: Do children with CMV infection who are hospitalized require isolation?
- A: No, standard precautions should be sufficient to interrupt transmission of CMV.

DAYTIME INCONTINENCE

Amanda K. Berry, MSN, CRNP, PhD • Dana A. Weiss, MD

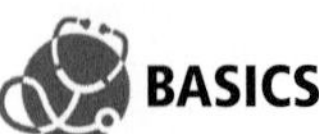

BASICS

DESCRIPTION

- Daytime wetting in a child ≥5 years of age warrants evaluation.
- Causes of functional incontinence include an array of bladder storage and voiding disorders.
- Voiding dysfunction is abnormal behavior of the lower urinary tract without a recognized organic cause, generally in the form of pelvic floor hyperactivity or bladder–sphincter discoordination.
- Bowel bladder dysfunction (BBD) describes the association between abnormal bladder and bowel behavior.

EPIDEMIOLOGY

Prevalence

- Studies in children 6 to 7 years of age have shown that 3.1% of girls and 2.1% of boys had an episode of wetting at least once per week.
- Daytime incontinence is 2 to 5 times more common in girls than boys from age 7 years to adolescence.
- Spontaneous cure rate of 14% per year without treatment
- Of all children who wet, 10% have only daytime wetting, 75% wet only at night, and 15% wet during the day and at night.

RISK FACTORS

- Constipation
- Recurrent urinary tract infections (UTIs)
- Diabetes mellitus/diabetes insipidus
- Attention deficit disorder (ADD)/attention deficit hyperactivity disorder (ADHD)
- Neurodevelopmental conditions
- Developmental delay
- Obesity
- History of abuse

Genetics

- Only anecdotal relationships have been seen in functional daytime incontinence, unlike studies showing genetic tendencies in nocturnal enuresis.
- Increased rates of daytime wetting have been reported in:
  - Urofacial (Ochoa) syndrome, an autosomal recessive condition
  - Williams syndrome, which is the result of a deletion involving the elastin gene in chromosome 7

PATHOPHYSIOLOGY

- Detrusor instability or over active bladder (OAB), which results from involuntary and uninhibited detrusor contractions during bladder filling
- Dysfunctional voiding, or detrusor sphincter discoordination, caused by incomplete relaxation of the pelvic floor muscles during urination and often resulting in incomplete bladder emptying
- Detrusor underactivity characterized by a large capacity, hypotonic bladder. This condition may be the result of longstanding dysfunctional voiding or voiding postponement.
- Neurogenic bladder

ETIOLOGY

- Bladder irritability caused by UTI
- Constipation
- Increased urinary output—polyuria
- Infrequent or deferred voiding
- Overactive bladder
- Low functional bladder capacity, with detrusor instability during filling
- Vaginal reflux
- Giggle incontinence
- Temperamental factors (e.g., short attention span, inattentiveness to body signals) in children who ignore the urge to void
- Developmental differences in age at which toilet training is achieved
- Obstructive uropathy (e.g., posterior urethral valves)
- Neurogenic bladder (e.g., myelomeningocele)
- Anatomic anomalies (e.g., ectopic ureter)

COMMONLY ASSOCIATED CONDITIONS

- Constipation (common)
- Nocturnal enuresis (common)
- UTIs (common)
- Vesicoureteral reflux is more common in children with voiding dysfunction due to elevated detrusor pressures that overcome a marginal vesicoureteral junction.

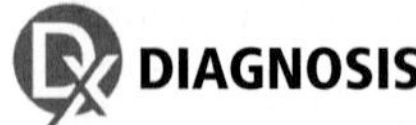

DIAGNOSIS

HISTORY

- Onset (primary vs. secondary)
- Frequency and degree of wetting
- Presence or absence of any dry interval
- Frequency of voiding
- Signs of urgency, use of hold maneuvers, waiting until the last minute to void
- Description of stream (i.e., strong/weak, continuous/interrupted)
- Straining or pushing during voiding
- Nocturnal enuresis or nocturia
- Frequency and description of bowel movements
- Presence or history of fecal soiling
- Quality and quantity of fluid intake
- History of UTIs, vesicoureteral reflux
- ADD/ADHD, learning disabilities, or developmental delays
- Level of concern on part of child/family
- History or concern for abuse
- Medications

PHYSICAL EXAM

- Abdomen: signs of constipation, distended bladder
- Rectal: if constipation is suspected
- Spine: sacral abnormalities
- Genitalia: labial adhesions, labial erythema, phimosis, urethral stenosis, evidence of leakage
- Neurologic: sensation, reflexes, and gait

DIFFERENTIAL DIAGNOSIS

- UTI
- Constipation
- Developmental variations in toilet training
- Neurogenic bladder
- Spinal cord abnormality
- Giggle incontinence
- Stress incontinence
- Genitourinary tract abnormality (posterior urethral valve, ectopic ureter)
- Vaginal reflux
- Benign increased urinary frequency (pollakiuria)
- Sexual abuse

DIAGNOSTIC TESTS & INTERPRETATION

Initial Tests (screening, lab, imaging)

- First morning urinalysis to check concentrating ability, rule out occult renal disease
- Urine culture to rule out infection
- Renal and bladder ultrasound (RBUS) in children who wet with a history of UTIs and in children with persistent wetting despite regular voiding
- Kidneys, ureter, and bladder (KUB) radiograph to assess for constipation
- MRI of lumbosacral spine if sacral abnormality or refractory to treatment
- MR urogram if any abnormality on RBUS concerning for ectopic ureter

Diagnostic Procedures/Other

- Uroflowmetry and assessment of postvoid residual urine
- Invasive urodynamic testing is not indicated in neurologically normal children unless refractory to treatment.

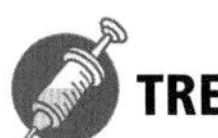

TREATMENT

GENERAL MEASURES

- Aggressive management of bowels so that child is passing at least one soft bowel movement daily (see "Constipation") ≥5 years old
- Adequate hydration
- Bolus water drinking
- Elimination schedule, with voids every 2 to 3 hours and time to defecate at least once a day. A reminder watch may be helpful.
- Voiding diary provides concrete data and focus for child.
- Positive reinforcement for regular voiding
- Avoid acidic/diuretic beverages (caffeine, carbonation, chocolate, citrus).
- Local management of perineal irritation/vulvovaginitis to ensure comfort during voiding
- Girls with postvoid dribbling due to vaginal reflux should void with their legs wide apart, sitting backward on the toilet when possible, to minimize backflow of urine into the vagina. Wipe after standing up.

ALERT

- Failure to recognize and manage constipation before attempting to manage wetting will lead to poorer outcomes.
- Use of anticholinergic medications in children with benign frequency of childhood is generally ineffective.
- Increased risk of UTIs when child is placed on anticholinergic medication due to infrequent voiding/incomplete emptying

MEDICATION

- A trial of an anticholinergic may be indicated if the child wets despite conservative medical/behavioral management.
- Extended-release formulations are available.
- Common side effects include constipation, dry mouth, and decreased diaphoresis with flushing. Blurred vision and dizziness are less common.

First Line

≥5 years old

- Oxybutynin (Ditropan®/Ditropan XL®): 5 to 15 mg/24 h
- Tolterodine (Detrol®/Detrol LA®): 2 to 4 mg/24 h (adult dose; pediatric dose not established)
- Solifenacin (Vesicare®): 5 to 10 mg/24 h (adult dose; pediatric dose not established)

ISSUES FOR REFERRAL

Referral to pediatric urologist

- When wetting is accompanied by recurrent UTIs
- When wetting is refractory to behavioral management, child may benefit from a noninvasive urodynamic evaluation to assess flow pattern, voiding mechanics, and ability to empty the bladder.

ADDITIONAL THERAPIES

Pelvic floor muscle retraining through biofeedback can help children learn to identify and relax the pelvic floor muscles to empty the bladder smoothly and completely.

ONGOING CARE

PROGNOSIS

- Spontaneous cure rate of 14% per year without treatment
- 72% of patients sustained improvement 1 year after simple behavioral therapy.

COMPLICATIONS

- Local irritation and inflammation of the perineum
- Recurrent UTIs and vesicoureteral reflux
- Reduced self esteem and potential for impaired interactions with peers
- Persistence of symptoms into adulthood

ADDITIONAL READING

- Deshpande AV, Craig JC, Smith GH, et al. Management of daytime urinary incontinence and lower urinary tract symptoms in children. *J Paediatr Child Health*. 2012;48(2):E44–E52.
- Franco, I. Functional bladder problems in children: pathophysiology, diagnosis and treatment. *Pediatr Clin North* Am. 2012;59(4):783–817.
- Loening-Baucke V. Urinary incontinence and urinary tract infection and their resolution with treatment of chronic constipation of childhood. *Pediatrics*. 1997;100(2, Pt 1):228–232.
- Thibodeau BA, Metcalfe P, Koop P, et al. Urinary incontinence and quality of life in children. *J Pediatr Urol*. 2013;9(1):78–83.
- Wiener JS, Scales MT, Hampton J, et al. Long-term efficacy of simple behavioral therapy for daytime wetting in children. *J Urol*. 2000;164(3, Pt 1): 786–790.

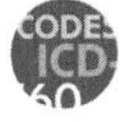

CODES

ICD10

- R32 Unspecified urinary incontinence
- N39.498 Other specified urinary incontinence

FAQ

- Q: What is normal voiding frequency for a child?
- A: Children between 5 and 12 years of age should void 6 to 7 times per day, or about every 2 to 3 hours. This pattern sometimes doesn't fit into the daily school schedule and so communication with school teachers and nurses is essential in creating a care plan.
- Q: What is a normal bladder capacity for a child?
- A: Normal bladder capacity (in ounces) can be estimated as the child's age plus 1 oz. A child's bladder capacity can be determined by measuring voided volumes for 2 consecutive days when the child is well-hydrated. The largest voided volume (not including the first morning void) is considered the child's functional capacity.
- Q: How much water should a child drink each day to cycle the bladder well?
- Adequate water drinking is important to keep the urine more dilute and less irritating to the bladder and to help cycle the bladder. In addition to other fluids, children 5 to 7 years old should drink at least 20 to 28 oz of water per day, children 8 to 12 years old should drink at least 28 to 32 oz of water per day, and teens should drink at least 36 to 48 oz of water per day.

DEHYDRATION

Sonny T. Tat, MD, MPH • Katharine A. Osborn, MD

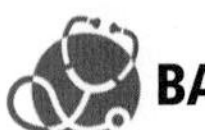

BASICS

DESCRIPTION

- Dehydration is a pathologic state of negative fluid balance in the body. Severity is generally expressed as a percentage of body weight. Mild, moderate, and severe dehydration correspond to volume loss of <5%, 5–10%, and >10%, respectively.
- Dehydration can also be classified as isotonic (Sodium [Na] 130 to 150 mmol/L), hypotonic (Na <130 mmol/L), or hypertonic (Na >150 mmol/L).
- Dehydration can be the result of a wide range of illnesses.
- Accurate clinical recognition and classification of dehydration determines rehydration treatment options.

EPIDEMIOLOGY

- Globally, dehydration from diarrheal illness is one of the leading causes of mortality in children <5 years old.
- Incidence of moderate to severe dehydration in the United States has declined since the introduction of routine rotavirus immunization.
- Despite a reduction in morbidity attributed to routine rotavirus vaccination, >100,000 children per year are hospitalized in the United States for dehydration from diarrheal illness.

PATHOPHYSIOLOGY

Dehydration is caused by either excessive fluid and salt losses or inadequate intake of fluids.

ETIOLOGY

- Common sources of fluid loss include
  - GI losses: vomiting, diarrhea (most common cause of dehydration in pediatric patients)
  - Renal losses: diabetes mellitus, diabetes insipidus, diuretics
  - Insensible losses: sweating, fever, tachypnea, increased ambient temperature, large burns
- Common causes of inadequate fluid intake include
  - Pain from stomatitis, pharyngitis, herpangina, oral trauma
  - Anorexia or malaise
  - Altered mental status
  - Inadequate access to fluids or neglect

DIAGNOSIS

- Accurate diagnosis of dehydration determines therapy options. Over diagnosis may lead to unnecessary interventions while under diagnosis can result in significant complications and morbidity.
- The gold standard for dehydration is weight loss from preillness baseline. Each gram of weight loss can be estimated as 1 mL of fluid loss.
- Reliable preillness weights are often not available.
- Diagnosis of dehydration and its severity should focus on important features of the history and physical exam.

HISTORY

- Frequency and duration of emesis and/or diarrhea gives an estimate of risk of dehydration.
- Parental report of decreased urine output may be helpful but nonspecific.
- Estimating frequency of urination is difficult when diarrhea is also present.
- Fever increases insensible water loss.
- Exertion or heat exposure increases insensible water loss.

PHYSICAL EXAM

- Acute change in weight is the best indicator of fluid deficit.
- Vital signs:
  - Tachycardia
  - Orthostatic increase in heart rate or hypotension
  - Hyperpnea
- Skin:
  - Capillary refill at fingertip >2 seconds
  - Mottling
  - Poor turgor
- Eyes: decreased or absent tears, sunken eyes
- Mucous membranes: dry or parched
- Anterior fontanelle: sunken

ALERT

Diagnostic pitfalls

- A combination of clinical features is a better predictor of dehydration than any one finding. The number and severity of physical signs increase with the degree of dehydration.
- Capillary refill time may be falsely prolonged by cool ambient temperature and is not affected by fever.
- Deep, rapid breathing with clear lung sounds may be a sign of acidosis.
- In diabetic ketoacidosis (DKA), decreased urine output is not a reliable indicator of dehydration because of the associated inappropriate polyuria.
- From a practical standpoint, patients should be classified into one of three levels of dehydration severity based on history and physical exam.
  - No dehydration
  - Mild to moderate dehydration
  - Severe dehydration

DIAGNOSTIC TESTS & INTERPRETATION

- Diagnostic testing is not typically useful in mild to moderate dehydration.
- Consider diagnostic testing in severe dehydration requiring IV fluid hydration, young patients (<6 months), altered mental status, or suspicious presentations.
- Serum Na
  - Classifies type of dehydration
  - Consider if there is a history of excessive free water intake, especially in young infants.
- Serum glucose
  - Consider rapid glucose testing in lethargic patient.
- Urine specific gravity
  - This may be elevated early in dehydration but is an unreliable marker of dehydration.
- Serum bicarbonate
  - Can be low with diarrhea due to bicarbonate loss in stool
  - Low bicarbonate can identify acidosis in severe dehydration.
- Blood urea nitrogen (BUN)
  - May rise late in dehydration but is nonspecific in children
- Ultrasound measurement of inferior vena cava (IVC) diameter has been studied in the assessment of intravascular volume but has not proved accurate in children and is not currently recommended.

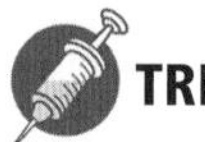

TREATMENT

GENERAL MEASURES

- Most patients can be treated safely and effectively with oral rehydration therapy (ORT). A smaller number of patients need IV rehydration.
- Treatment strategy depends on level of dehydration.
  - No dehydration: Patients can be safely sent home with ORT to maintain fluid balance.
  - Mild to moderate dehydration: ORT is the preferred therapy for rehydration.
  - Severe dehydration: requires IV hydration with isotonic fluids
- ORT:
  - Give a low osmotic solution that contains equimolar concentrations of Na and glucose, such as World Health Organization (WHO) solution, Pedialyte®, or Infalyte®.
  - In mild dehydration, ORT with apple juice diluted 1:1 with water, followed by the patient's preferred fluids may improve compliance and be more affordable.

- For mild to moderate dehydration, aim to give 50 mL/kg observed ORT.
- Replace entire deficit in 4 hours: Reassess hydration status and tolerance of ORT frequently.
- Give additional ORT to replace ongoing losses (vomiting, diarrhea).
- Start with small amounts (5 to 15 ml every 5 minutes). For infants and children who refuse to drink, use a syringe rather than bottle or cup to administer ORT. After 30 minutes, increase the volume and rate if tolerated.
- Oral intake can be improved with the use of ondansetron when nausea and vomiting are a primary cause of dehydration.
- Have the child's caregiver give the fluids and provide education on fluid replacement and signs of dehydration.
- Failure of ORT includes intractable vomiting, refusal to drink ORT, clinical deterioration, or lack of improvement after 4 hours.
- Contraindications to ORT include severe dehydration, altered mental status, persistent vomiting, excessive stool losses, and severe electrolyte abnormalities.

- IV fluids
  - IV fluids are required when ORT is contraindicated or fails.
  - Administer IV bolus of normal saline 20 mL/kg. Dehydration resulting in clinical instability or shock may require more rapid fluid administration. Repeat 20 ml/kg boluses as needed until signs of severe dehydration resolve.
  - Boluses of dextrose-containing solutions do not improve outcomes and are not typically used. Dextrose may be needed to correct documented hypoglycemia.
  - Initiate ORT as soon as tolerated.
  - If the patient does not tolerate ORT or has ongoing losses after the initial fluid deficit has been replaced, maintenance IV fluids can be used.
  - The 4-2-1 rule is a practical estimate of hourly maintenance fluid requires in most cases.
    - 4 mL/kg/h for the first 10 kg, plus 2 mL/kg/h for the next 10 kg, plus 1 mL/kg/h for the remaining weight
  - Use isotonic fluids (normal saline) for maintenance fluids. Hypotonic solutions (1/2 or 1/4 normal saline) are associated with increased risk of hyponatremia. Dextrose may be included in maintenance fluids.
- Alternative routes of fluid administration
  - Enteral fluids may safely be given via nasogastric (NG) tube when oral fluids are refused.
  - In severe dehydration and shock and when multiple IV attempts have been unsuccessful, intraosseous administration of fluids is safe and effective.
  - Subcutaneous fluid administration using recombinant hyaluronidase to facilitate fluid delivery may be an alternative rehydration therapy in patients who have mild to moderate dehydration but cannot tolerate ORT.

MEDICATION

- Most children with dehydration do not require specific medication therapy.
- In children with significant vomiting, ondansetron 0.15 mg/kg PO decreases vomiting and facilitates oral rehydration. Ondansetron may be repeated as needed q8h until symptoms resolve. However, if symptoms persist, consider reevaluation.
- Children with either fever or pain contributing to decreased oral intake may benefit from ibuprofen 10 mg/kg PO or acetaminophen 15 mg/kg PO.

ADMISSION, INPATIENT, AND NURSING CONSIDERATIONS

- Admission criteria
  - Failure of oral or IV rehydration within 4 hours
  - Severe electrolyte abnormalities
  - Substantial ongoing losses indicating a high likelihood of recurrence of dehydration
- Discharge criteria
  - After initiating ORT, children who are tolerating oral fluids at an acceptable rate to replace their deficit over 4 to 6 hours and whose dehydration is not caused by an illness that will likely complicate the clinical course may be discharged with a willing and reliable caregiver to complete the ORT at home.

ONGOING CARE

FOLLOW-UP RECOMMENDATIONS

Patient Monitoring

- After rehydration, children with ongoing losses, as in gastroenteritis, should receive a maintenance solution in addition to regular feedings to maintain a positive fluid balance.
- Avoid liquids with excessive glucose, such as fruit juices, punches, and soft drinks, as these can promote osmotic fluid losses in the stool.
- In infants <6 months old, do not give large amounts of free water, which can lead to hyponatremia.

PROGNOSIS

Excellent with appropriate rehydration therapy

COMPLICATIONS

- Severe dehydration may lead to hypovolemic shock and acute renal failure.
- Hyponatremia is associated with hypotonia, hypothermia, and seizures.
- Overly rapid correction of chronic (>36 to 48 hours) severe hypernatremia or hyponatremia can produce cerebral edema.

ADDITIONAL READING

- Desai R, Curns AT, Steiner CA, et al. All-cause gastroenteritis and rotavirus-coded hospitalizations among US children, 2000–2009. *Clin Infect Dis*. 2012;55(4):e28–e34.
- Freedman SB, Vandermeer B, Milne A, et al. Diagnosing clinically significant dehydration in children with acute gastroenteritis using noninvasive methods: a meta-analysis. *J Pediatr*. 2015;166(4):908–916.e6.
- Freedman SB, Willan AR, Boutis K, et al. Effect of dilute apple juice and preferred fluids vs electrolyte maintenance solution on treatment failure among children with mild gastroenteritis: a randomized clinical trial. *JAMA*. 2016;315(18):1966–1974.
- Liu L, Johnson HL, Cousens S, et al; for Child Health Epidemiology Reference Group of World Health Organization and United Nation Children's Fund. Global, regional, and national causes of child mortality: an updated systematic analysis for 2010 with time trends since 2000. *Lancet*. 2012;379(9832):2151–2161.
- Niescierenko M, Bachur R. Advances in pediatric dehydration therapy. *Curr Opin Pediatr*. 2013;25(3):304–309.
- Wang J, Xu E, Xiao Y. Isotonic versus hypotonic maintenance IV fluids in hospitalized children: a meta-analysis. *Pediatrics*. 2014;133(1):105–113.

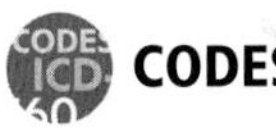

CODES

ICD10

- E86.0 Dehydration
- E87.1 Hypo-osmolality and hyponatremia

22Q11.2 DELETION SYNDROME (DIGEORGE SYNDROME, VELOCARDIOFACIAL SYNDROME)

Anne S. Bassett, MD, FRCPC • Donna M. McDonald-McGinn, MS, LCGC

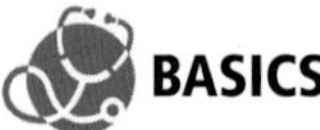

BASICS

DESCRIPTION

22q11.2 deletion syndrome, formerly known as DiGeorge or velocardiofacial syndrome, is a multisystem disorder with variable severity and number of associated features, classically including developmental delay, learning difficulties, congenital cardiac anomalies, palatal abnormalities, especially velopharyngeal insufficiency, hypocalcemia, and subtle facial dysmorphism.

- Intellectual disabilities are usually borderline to mild; rarely severe
- Treatable psychiatric illness is common.
- Rarely (≤1%), neonates have a severe T-cell immunodeficiency.

EPIDEMIOLOGY

Prevalence is estimated at up to 1 in 2,000 live births.

RISK FACTORS

Genetics

- Associated hemizygous microdeletion of 22q11.2
- Up to 10% of newly diagnosed cases are inherited.
- 50% recurrence risk at each pregnancy for affected individuals

PATHOPHYSIOLOGY

A developmental defect of the 3rd and 4th pharyngeal arches may be part of the mechanism; molecular disturbances of neurodevelopment are yet to be identified.

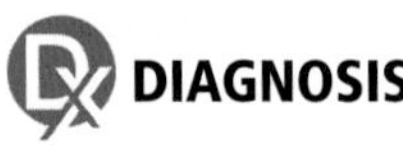

DIAGNOSIS

HISTORY

- This syndrome is underrecognized at all ages; thus, an index of suspicion is needed for any child with multisystem features.
- Neonatal and more commonly later onset hypocalcemia may be present secondary to hypoparathyroidism in up to 60% of cases.
- Congenital anomalies of any organ system
- Cardiac defects include interrupted aortic arch type B, septal defects, tetralogy of Fallot ± pulmonary atresia, truncus arteriosus, and vascular ring.
- Failure to thrive/dysphagia/gastroesophageal reflux disease (GERD), occasional growth hormone deficiency
- Recurrent infections/autoimmune disease
- Developmental delays, any, including speech
- Seizures
- Anxiety, attention-deficit disorder, OCD, autism spectrum, and schizophrenia

PHYSICAL EXAM

Subtle facial dysmorphism (e.g., malar flatness, hooded eyelids, auricular anomalies, small mouth, micrognathia; tubular nose, bulbous nasal tip with hypoplastic alae nasi), not as recognizable in non-Caucasians

- Developmental/cognitive/behavioral disorders
- Hypernasal speech; disarticulation
- Heart murmur
- Hypothyroidism; hyperthyroidism
- Renal/urogenital abnormalities
- Scoliosis; other skeletal abnormalities, for example, polydactyly and butterfly vertebrae
- Recurrent otitis media; hearing deficits
- Thrombocytopenia; splenomegaly
- Juvenile rheumatoid arthritis
- Enamel hypoplasia; chronic caries

DIAGNOSTIC TESTS & INTERPRETATION

Initial Tests (screening, lab, imaging)

- Genome-wide microarray, multiplex ligation-dependent probe amplification (MLPA), or fluorescence in situ hybridization (FISH) using specific probe (may miss smaller deletions)
  - Most common microdeletion in humans
  - Parents also require testing for the deletion.
- CBC with differential
- Calcium and parathyroid hormone (PTH)
- TSH
- Newborns
  - Flow cytometry
- Age 9 to 12 months (before live vaccines)
  - Flow cytometry
  - Immunoglobulins
  - T-cell function
- Echocardiogram
- Renal ultrasound
- Cervical spine radiographs
- Other, as indicated by history and signs
- Audiology assessment
- Ophthalmology assessment

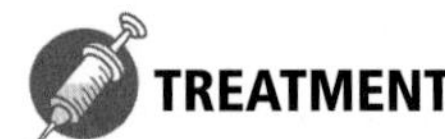

TREATMENT

GENERAL MEASURES

- Standard treatments are generally effective for each associated feature.
- Vitamin D supplements (those with hypocalcemia may need 1,25-D calcitriol supplementation and calcium supplements)
- Special consideration for infants:
  - Initially withhold live vaccines.
  - Irradiated blood products
  - Influenza vaccinations
  - Respiratory syncytial virus prophylaxis
  - If severe T-cell dysfunction: Avoid live viral vaccines; consider immunoglobulin replacement therapy.
  - Consider varicella zoster immune globulin in a patient with either unknown humoral immunity status or definitive humoral abnormalities and a history of exposure. IV acyclovir may be necessary if varicella develops with severe T-cell defect.
  - Most patients with CD4+ cell counts >500 cells/mm^3 can be safely and effectively vaccinated with live viral vaccines.

ISSUES FOR REFERRAL

- Depending on the features the child manifests, issues may need consultation and/or follow-up:
  - Infant stimulation; educational consultant
  - Speech and cognitive intervention for speech and language delays
  - Palate team, otolaryngology
  - Developmental pediatrics
  - Child psychiatry
  - Neurology
  - Endocrinology
  - Cardiology to define aortic arch anatomy (side and branching pattern); monitoring for aortic root dilation
  - Gastroenterology/feeding team
  - Dentistry

- Immunology to monitor T-cell disorder, recurrent infections, allergy, autoimmune disease
- Severe immunodeficiency may require bone marrow transplant or thymic transplant.

- Special consideration with surgery/obstetrics/acute injury
  - Risk of hypocalcemia with biologic stress
  - Increased risk of any complication

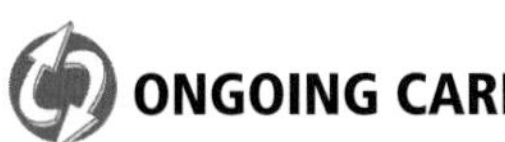

ONGOING CARE

FOLLOW-UP RECOMMENDATIONS

Patient Monitoring

- Monitor growth and development.
- Monitor hearing.
- Monitor for emerging endocrine, psychiatric, autoimmune, skeletal, obesity, and other disorders.
- Cardiac monitoring for aortic root dilation
- Genetic and reproductive counseling for adolescents and at transition to adult care

PROGNOSIS

- Most patients survive childhood. Exceptions include those with severe congenital cardiac anomalies, severe immunodeficiency, other major anomalies.
- Associated conditions that arise through development and into adulthood include an increased risk for treatable psychiatric illness (anxiety disorders and psychotic disorders; ~1 in 4 develop schizophrenia).
- Other later onset conditions include autoimmune diseases and neurologic sequelae, including seizure disorder, movement disorders, early-onset Parkinson disease.
- Functioning in adults is correlated most highly with the degree of intellectual deficit and to a lesser degree with severe psychiatric illness.
- Age at death of adults is on average several decades younger than population expectations.

COMPLICATIONS

- In the newborn period, patients may present with hypocalcemic tetany/seizures, manifestation of cardiac abnormality, nasal regurgitation, GERD, dysphagia, and/or recurrent infections.
- In childhood and adolescence, patients present more commonly with speech, neurologic, developmental and/or behavioral issues, endocrine disorders, and/or psychiatric illness.
- Patients are at increased risk for developing multiple later onset conditions, including autoimmune disease, obesity, and psychiatric illness.

ADDITIONAL READING

- Al-Sukaiti N, Reid B, Lavi S, et al. Safety and efficacy of measles, mumps, and rubella vaccine in patients with DiGeorge syndrome. *J Allergy Clin Immunol*. 2010;126(4):868–869.
- Bassett AS, Chow EW, Husted J, et al. Premature death in adults with 22q11.2 deletion syndrome. *J Med Genet*. 2009;46(5):324–330.
- Bassett AS, McDonald-McGinn DM, Devriendt K, et al; and International 22q11.2 Deletion Syndrome Consortium. Practical guidelines for managing patients with 22q11.2 deletion syndrome. *J Pediatr*. 2011;159(2):332–339.e1.
- Butcher NJ, Chow EW, Costain G, et al. Functional outcomes of adults with 22q11.2 deletion syndrome. *Genet Med*. 2012;14(10):836–843.
- Carotti A, Digilio MC, Piacentini G, et al. Cardiac defects and results of cardiac surgery in 22q11.2 deletion syndrome. *Dev Disabil Res Rev*. 2008;14(1):35–42.
- Fung W, Butcher N, Costain G, et al. Practical guidelines for managing adults with 22q11.2 deletion syndrome. *Genet Med*. 2015:17(8):599–609.
- Habel A, McGinn MJ II, Zackai EH, et al. Syndrome-specific growth charts for 22q11.2 deletion syndrome in Caucasian children. *Am J Med Genet A*. 2012;158A(11):2665–2671.
- McDonald R, Dodgen A, Goyal S, et al. Impact of 22q11.2 deletion on the postoperative course of children after cardiac surgery. *Pediatr Cardiol*. 2013;34(2):341–347.
- McDonald-McGinn DM, Sullivan KE. Chromosome 22q11.2 deletion syndrome (DiGeorge syndrome/velocardiofacial syndrome). *Medicine (Baltimore)*. 2011;90(1):1–18.
- McDonald-McGinn DM, Sullivan KE, Marino B, et al. 22q11.2 deletion syndrome. *Nat Rev Dis Primers*. 2015;1:15071.
- McLean-Tooke A, Barge D, Spickett GP, et al. Immunologic defects in 22q11.2 deletion syndrome. *J Allergy Clin Immunol*. 2008;122(2):362–367.
- Repetto GM, Guzmán ML, Delgado I, et al. Case fatality rate and associated factors in patients with 22q11 microdeletion syndrome: a retrospective cohort study. *BMJ Open*. 2014;4(11):e005041.
- Repetto GM, Guzmán ML, Puga A, et al. Clinical features of chromosome 22q11.2 microdeletion syndrome in 208 Chilean patients. *Clin Genet*. 2009;76(5):465–470.
- Voll S, Boot E, Butcher NJ, et al. Obesity in adults with 22q11.2 deletion syndrome. *Genet Med*. 2017;19(2):204–208.
- Vorstman JA, Breetvelt EJ, Duijff SN, et al; and International Consortium on Brain and Behavior in 22q11.2 Deletion Syndrome. Cognitive decline preceding the onset of psychosis in patients with 22q11.2 deletion syndrome. *JAMA Psychiatry*. 2015;72(4):377–385.

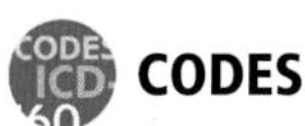

CODES

ICD10

- Q93.81 Velo-cardio-facial syndrome
- D82.1 Di George's syndrome

FAQ

- Q: Can patients have severe intellectual impairments?
- A: They can but relatively rarely. Most patients with 22q11.2 deletion syndrome have IQs in the borderline range, about 30% fall in the mild intellectual deficit range; a minority are in the average range. A minority fall in the moderate to severe intellectual deficit range. Some children have a >10 point split between their verbal and performance IQ, and thus, the full-scale IQ may not reflect the true functional potential. Over development in childhood, the IQ tends to decline. Most patients have particular difficulties in the areas of arithmetic, auditory working memory, and executive functioning such as social judgment. Cognitive remediation should be tailored to the individual's relative strengths and weaknesses.
- Q: How often are 22q11.2 deletions found in the general (unaffected) population?
- A: The penetrance of any individual associated clinical feature, when considering the multisystem nature of 22q11.2DS, is very high, approaching 100%. The typical 22q11.2 deletion is almost never found in control populations.

D

DENGUE VIRUS

David M. Vu, MD • A. Desiree LaBeaud, MD, MS

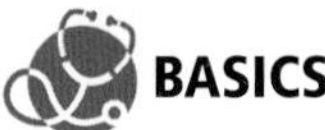

BASICS

DESCRIPTION

- Dengue virus (DENV) is an arthropod-borne virus (arbovirus) that causes a febrile illness characterized by intense headache (classically retro-orbital), rash, abdominal pain, nausea, and joint pain.
- The majority of DENV infections is subclinical or asymptomatic, but some people with DENV infection develop severe dengue disease, which:
  - Manifests when the fever from the initial illness subsides
  - Is characterized by plasma leak leading to hypovolemic shock and death
  - Can be anticipated based on the presence of warning signs
- Identification of severe dengue-associated warning signs is important for determining need for additional monitoring and hydration.

EPIDEMIOLOGY

DENV has been reemerging over the last 50 years as a significant cause of febrile illness in tropical and subtropical areas of the world.

- Approximately 50 to 60 million symptomatic infections per year worldwide
- Estimated 300 million infections per year worldwide, including subclinical or asymptomatic infections

RISK FACTORS

- Travel to or residing in an area that is experiencing an outbreak of or is endemic for DENV.
- Exposure to *Aedes* spp. mosquitoes
- Previous DENV infection of a serotype that is different than the circulating serotype

GENERAL PREVENTION

- Mosquito avoidance
  - Wear clothing that maximizes skin coverage.
  - Use insect repellants such as N,N-diethyl-meta-toluamide (DEET).
- Empty open containers of standing water.

PATHOPHYSIOLOGY

- DENV has a tropism for monocytes, macrophages, and dendritic cells.
- After invading a cell, it hijacks the cellular machinery to produce more infectious virus.
- Massive activation of the host inflammatory response is thought to lead to severe dengue disease.
- DENV nonstructural protein 1 (NS1) also directly affects vascular endothelium leading to plasma leakage.

ETIOLOGY

- DENV is transmitted by *Aedes aegypti* and *Aedes albopictus* mosquitoes.
- *Aedes* mosquitoes are
  - Endemic in many tropical and subtropical areas of the world
  - Highly adapted to thrive in peri-urban settings, often entering homes and laying eggs in man-made containers
  - Able to lay eggs in as little as a tablespoon of water
  - Expanding their habitat range due to global warming
- DENV is endemic in many parts of South and Southeast Asia, Central and South America, and Australia.
- Humans are only known reservoir for DENV.
- DENV can be categorized into four serotypes.
  - One or more serotypes may be circulating in an area.
  - Infection from one serotype is thought to protect against reinfection from the same (homologous) serotype but does not provide durable protection against the other (heterologous) serotypes.
  - Antibodies produced against one serotype (during primary infection) can cross-react with a heterologous serotype (during secondary infection) and increase the risk for developing severe dengue disease via a mechanism called antibody-dependent enhancement of infection.
- Single-stranded RNA virus
- DENV is a member of the *Flaviviridae* family of viruses that includes yellow fever virus, Japanese encephalitis virus, Zika virus, hepatitis C virus.

COMMONLY ASSOCIATED CONDITIONS

Other tropical and subtropical infections, including other mosquito-borne infections such as malaria or other arboviruses

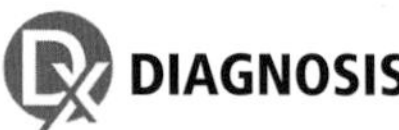

DIAGNOSIS

HISTORY

- Travel to or residence in an area known to be endemic for DENV
- Febrile phase lasting 3 to 7 days with:
  - Headache, classically severe retro-orbital pain
  - Myalgias and arthralgias
  - Maculopapular to petechial rash
  - Mucosal bleeding from gums and nose (observed more frequently in adults)
- Critical phase lasting 2 to 3 days that:
  - Starts when fever subsides
  - Consists of a vascular leak syndrome resulting in hypoproteinemia, ascites, pleural effusions or hypovolemic shock
  - Is characterized by leukopenia and thrombocytopenia
- Recovery phase during which hemodynamic status stabilizes followed by diuresis of fluids administered during the critical phase.

PHYSICAL EXAM

- Mucosal bleeding from the nose or gums (more frequent in adults than children)
- Maculopetechial rash
- Abdominal tenderness
- Hepatosplenomegaly
- Tourniquet sign
  1. Take the patient's blood pressure (BP) and record it, for example, 100/70.
  2. Inflate the cuff to a point midway between SBP and DBP and maintain for 5 minutes. $(100 + 70) \div 2 = 85$ mm Hg
  3. Release pressure and wait 2 minutes.
  4. Count petechiae below antecubital fossa. A positive test is 10 or more petechiae per 1 square inch.

ALERT

- Risk for developing severe dengue disease is associated with the following warning signs:
  - Abdominal pain or tenderness
  - Persistent emesis
  - Volume overload (edema)
  - Mucosal bleeding
  - Lethargy or restlessness
  - Hepatomegaly
  - Hemoconcentration
- Children with dengue with warning signs require hospital admission for:
  - IV fluids
  - Possible transfusions
  - Monitoring of hematocrit, peripheral perfusion, urine output, blood glucose

DIFFERENTIAL DIAGNOSIS

- Sepsis
- Meningitis
- Acute gastroenteritis
- Chikungunya infection
- Malaria infection
- Zika virus infection

DIAGNOSTIC TESTS & INTERPRETATION

Initial Tests (screening, lab, imaging)

- Rapid diagnostic point-of-care test to detect DENV NS1 and/or serum IgM antibodies against DENV (not available in the United States)
- Reverse-transcriptase PCR (RT-PCR) to detect DENV RNA in blood
- Serum antibodies against DENV can be measured by enzyme-linked immunosorbant assay (ELISA).

Follow-Up Tests & Special Considerations

Plaque reduction neutralization test (PRNT) is a more virus-specific test for antibody.

Test Interpretation
- A blood sample positive by DENV RT-PCR is diagnostic of acute DENV infection.
- Positive anti-DENV IgM suggests acute primary infection.
  - Because antibodies to other flaviviruses may cross-react in this assay, a DENV IgM-positive sample is confirmed by PRNT.
- Positive anti-DENV IgG during the febrile phase raises the concern for secondary DENV infection, which is associated with higher risk for developing severe DENV disease.

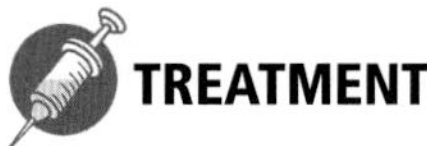

TREATMENT

GENERAL MEASURES
- Identify any dengue warning signs:
  - Abdominal pain or tenderness
  - Persistent vomiting
  - Edema
  - Mucosal bleeding
  - Lethargy or restlessness
  - Hepatomegaly
  - Hemoconcentration
- Management is based on the World Health Organization (WHO) dengue classification
- Probable dengue
  - Criteria
    - Live in or travel to a dengue endemic area
    - Fever and at least two of the following: nausea, vomiting, rash, leukopenia, arthralgia, myalgia, and a positive tourniquet test
  - Management
    - Outpatient management with daily monitoring
    - Oral rehydration solution
    - Acetaminophen for treatment of fever
    - Do not use nonsteroidal anti-inflammatory agents
- Dengue without warning signs (dengue fever)
  - Criteria
    - Laboratory-confirmed dengue
    - Fever and at least two of the following: nausea, vomiting, rash, leukopenia, arthralgia, myalgia, and a positive tourniquet test
  - Management
    - Hospital admission of infants, consider outpatient management with daily monitoring in children >1 year
    - Oral rehydration solution if tolerated
    - Closely monitor temperature pattern, fluid balance, urine output, warning signs, hematocrit, white blood cell and platelet counts
- Dengue with warning signs (dengue hemorrhagic fever)
  - Criteria
    - Laboratory-confirmed dengue
    - Fever and at least two of the following: nausea, vomiting, rash, leukopenia, arthralgia, myalgia, and a positive tourniquet test
    - Any of the following warning signs: abdominal pain or tenderness, persistent emesis, volume overload (edema), mucosal bleeding, lethargy or restlessness, hepatomegaly, hemoconcentration
  - Management
    - Intravenous crystalloid solutions
    - Blood transfusions if necessary
    - Monitor hematocrit, vital signs, peripheral perfusion, urine output, blood glucose and other organ functions.
- Severe dengue (dengue shock syndrome)
  - Criteria
    - Laboratory-confirmed dengue
    - One of the following: shock, significant volume overload with respiratory distress, severe clinical bleeding, organ failure
  - Management
    - Intensive care treatment
    - Intravenous crystalloid or colloid solutions
    - Blood transfusion with fresh-packed red cells or fresh whole blood
    - Platelet concentrates in case of massive bleeding

MEDICATION

First Line
Maintain hydration.
- Oral rehydration for dengue without warning signs
- IV hydration for dengue with warning signs or for infants <1 year

Second Line
- Acetaminophen
- Avoid nonsteroidal anti-inflammatory agents such as ibuprofen.

ADMISSION, INPATIENT, AND NURSING CONSIDERATIONS
- For dengue with warning signs or severe dengue, monitor:
  - Hematocrit
  - Peripheral perfusion
  - Urine output
  - Blood glucose
- Blood or platelet transfusions may be needed.

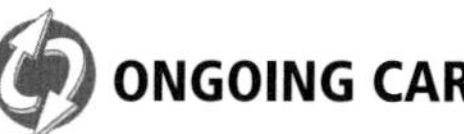

ONGOING CARE

FOLLOW-UP RECOMMENDATIONS
Monitor for warning signs as fever subsides (usually day 4 to 5 of illness).

PATIENT EDUCATION
Encourage mosquito avoidance.
- Wear clothing that covers the arms and legs.
- Protect infants in strollers by covering strollers with netting. Do not place netting directly on infant's face.
- Use insect repellants such as DEET.

PROGNOSIS
- Most patients with dengue fever without warning signs recover fully.
- Severe dengue disease has high mortality.

COMPLICATIONS
Multisystem organ failure and death

ADDITIONAL READING

- Guzman MG, Gubler DJ, Izquierdo A, et al. Dengue infection. *Nat Rev Dis Primers*. 2016;2:16055.
- Verhagen LM, de Groot R. Dengue in children. *J Infect*. 2014;69(Suppl 1):S77–S86.
- World Health Organization. *Dengue: Guidelines for Diagnosis, Treatment, Prevention, and Control—New Edition*. Geneva, Switzerland: World Health Organization; 2009.

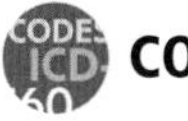

CODES

ICD10
- A90 Dengue fever [classical dengue]
- A91 Dengue hemorrhagic fever

FAQ
- Q: What can I do to prevent dengue infection?
- A: Wear clothing that protects arms and legs, and use insect repellant.
- Q: In what areas of the world do I have to worry about dengue infection?
- A: Up-to-date information and guidance on areas with endemic dengue or areas experiencing dengue outbreaks is at www.cdc.gov.

D

DENTAL CARIES

Ray J. Jurado, DDS

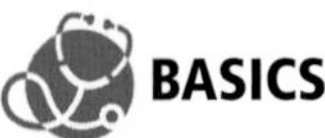

BASICS

DESCRIPTION

Dental caries is the process of tooth structure demineralization, ultimately leading to cavitation (cavities). Over time, bacterial metabolism of carbohydrates produces acid, leading to tooth demineralization. The presence of one or more decayed, missing, or filled primary tooth surfaces in children <6 years old constitutes "early childhood caries" (ECC).

EPIDEMIOLOGY

- 28% of 2- to 5-year-olds suffer from ECC, which is most prevalent in disadvantaged populations, with those <3 years old largely untreated.
- Although the prevalence of ECC has not changed in the last few years, filled teeth have increased, indicating more treatment is being provided.
- ECC may lead to increased emergency department visits and hospital admissions, higher treatment costs, loss of school days, delayed growth and development, and diminished ability to learn.

RISK FACTORS

- Dental caries is multifactorial
  - Factors increasing duration of sugar on teeth: frequent consumption of sugars (including prolonged bottlefeeding), sugary beverages, sticky sugars, medications sweetened with sucrose, inconsistent brushing/flossing after meals, pouching of food, tightly spaced teeth that are difficult to clean
  - Factors leading to dry mouth (less saliva, less acid buffering): mouth breathing, albuterol inhalers, psychiatric medications
  - Factors leading to weaker tooth enamel: lack of systemic or topical fluoride, developmental enamel defects
  - Epidemiologic factors: low socioeconomic status, previous caries experience
  - Microbial risk markers: mutans streptococci (MS) and *Lactobacillus* species
- Health-related risk factors
  - Developmental delay—oral hygiene difficult
  - Cerebral palsy—crowded dentition, difficult to brush
  - Conditions requiring frequent, high nutrient oral feedings
  - Conditions treated with medications that dry the mouth—psychiatric conditions

PATHOPHYSIOLOGY

Dental caries develops when oral bacteria, primarily MS, ferment carbohydrates into organic acids, over time demineralizing tooth enamel. Continuous demineralization of tooth enamel leads to enamel cavitation.

ALERT

MS has been shown to be vertically transmitted from caregiver to child, leading to the concept of ECC as an infectious disease. Horizontal transmission between family members and caregivers also can occur.

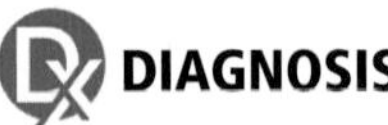

DIAGNOSIS

HISTORY

- Frequent carbohydrate challenge (bottle, juice, snacks, sweets, meds, etc.)
- Inconsistent brushing and flossing after meals
- Sensitivity or pain to cold or hot foods, sweets, or biting
- Past medical history may reveal caries risk factors discussed earlier.

ALERT

Spontaneous or nocturnal pain (waking up at night) may be a sign of advanced caries and dental infection. See chapter on "Dental Infections."

PHYSICAL EXAM

- Tooth discoloration: chalky white (initial caries demineralization), yellow, or brown (advanced cavitation)
- Locations on teeth: in-between (interproximal) front incisors, biting surfaces (occlusal) of molars, at gum line (cervical)
- Soft tissue swelling (advanced caries with infection)
- Dental instrument exploration of affected areas helps confirm diagnosis and severity.
- To document and communicate the location of the lesion, a Universal Numbering System is used to identify the specific tooth/teeth involved (Appendix; Figure 2). Each tooth has a unique letter or number.
  - Primary teeth are identified by uppercase letters (A to T).
  - Permanent teeth are identified by numbers (1 to 32).

DIFFERENTIAL DIAGNOSIS

- Developmental tooth hard tissue defects—hypoplastic or hypomineralized enamel; dental fluorosis
- Dark staining—iron supplements, tea
- Dental calculus (tartar) formation

DIAGNOSTIC TESTS & INTERPRETATION

Initial Tests (screening, lab, imaging)

- Intraoral radiographs (bitewing and periapical views) help to identify radiolucent/carious tooth structure.
- Tooth percussion testing and hot and cold testing (inconsistent diagnostic potential) help to identify extent of caries and/or infection.

TREATMENT

MEDICATION

Acetaminophen or ibuprofen for symptomatic pain management. See antibiotic therapy in the chapter "Dental Infections."

ADDITIONAL THERAPIES

- Timely restorative care (fillings, crowns) by a pediatric dentist
- Supplemental topical fluoride (high concentration, prescription only, dentifrice, mouthwash, gel, varnish) with the goal of temporarily arresting caries
- Silver diamine fluoride application by pediatric dentist to arrest decay (arrested areas stain black) when conventional restorative treatment is not feasible
- Treatment of infected teeth with tooth extraction (primary teeth) or root canal (permanent teeth)

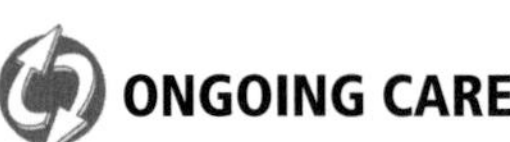

ONGOING CARE

FOLLOW-UP RECOMMENDATIONS

- Dental caries essentially results from sugar exposure over the course of time. Prevention of dental caries should focus on minimizing frequency of sugary beverages/snacks and brushing (with fluoridated toothpaste) and flossing after as many meals/medication administrations as possible.
- Children should have their first dental visit 6 months after the eruption of their first tooth or around 1 year of age. This first visit is to assess for dental caries risk factors and give appropriate anticipatory guidance to the parent with the goal of preventing ECC.
- Dental caries can advance quickly, therefore periodic preventive visits (at least every 6 months) are recommended throughout childhood.

PROGNOSIS

- Timely caries risk assessment as well as restoration of tooth structure and function will minimize the child's caries experience and its consequences.
- Initial signs of caries (chalky white demineralization) may be remineralized with excellent oral hygiene and fluoride supplementation. Untreated advanced dental caries leads to irreversible pulpitis, dental infection, and tooth extraction.

ADDITIONAL READING

- American Academy of Pediatric Dentistry. 2014 Guideline on fluoride therapy. http://www.aapd.org/media/Policies_Guidelines/G_FluorideTherapy1.pdf. Accessed May 31, 2017.
- American Academy of Pediatric Dentistry. 2016 Policy on early childhood caries (ECC): classifications, consequences, and preventive strategies. http://www.aapd.org/media/Policies_Guidelines/P_ECCClassifications1.pdf. Accessed May 31, 2017.
- American Academy of Pediatric Dentistry. 2016 Policy on early childhood caries (ECC): unique challenges and treatment options. http://www.aapd.org/media/Policies_Guidelines/P_ECCUniqueChallenges1.pdf. Accessed May 31, 2017.
- Kawashita Y, Kitamura M, Saito T. Early childhood caries. *Int J Dent*. 2011;2011:725320.
- Meyer-Lueckel H, Paris S, Elkstrand KR. *Caries Management—Science and Clinical Practice*. New York, NY: Thieme Medical Publishers; 2013.
- U.S. Department of Health and Human Services, U.S. Public Health Service. Oral health in America: a report of the surgeon general (Executive Summary). http://www.nidcr.nih.gov/datastatistics/surgeongeneral/report/executivesummary.htm. Accessed May 31, 2017.

CODES

ICD10

- K02.9 Dental caries, unspecified
- K04.0 Pulpitis
- K04.7 Periapical abscess without sinus

FAQ

- Q: When should I refer my patient for his/her first dental visit?
- A: Children should have their first dental visit 6 months after the eruption of their first tooth or around 1 year of age. This first visit is to assess for dental caries risk factors and give appropriate anticipatory guidance to the parent, with the goal of preventing ECC.
- Q: Why do baby teeth need to be treated if they are just going to fall out?
- A: Dental pain can affect a child's daily activities, leading to delayed growth and development and diminished ability to learn. Premature primary tooth loss due to infection and extraction can lead to eruption and crowding issues in the permanent dentition.
- Q: Does breastfeeding result in caries?
- A: ECC may not result from breast milk alone; however, in combination with other dietary carbohydrates, caries can arise.

DENTAL HEALTH AND PREVENTION

Johnny I. Kuttab, DDS

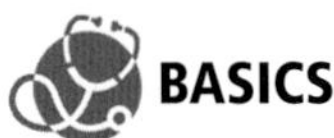

BASICS

DESCRIPTION

- Dental health and prevention is the practice of maintaining proper oral health to prevent the initiation or progression of oral disease. It is composed of effective oral hygiene, appropriate dietary practices, fluoride exposure, and the establishment of a dental home.
- Dental caries is a disease that is generally preventable. Early risk assessment allows for identification of parent–infant groups who are at risk for early childhood caries (ECC) and would benefit from early preventive intervention.
- The ultimate goal of early assessment is the timely delivery of educational information to populations at high risk for developing caries in order to prevent the need for later surgical intervention.

EPIDEMIOLOGY

- 42% of children 2 to 11 years old have had dental caries in their primary teeth.
- 23% of children 2 to 11 years old have untreated dental caries.
- Children 2 to 11 years old have an average of 1.6 decayed primary teeth and 3.6 decayed primary surfaces.
- 21% of children 6 to 11 years old have had dental caries in their permanent teeth.
- Tooth decay is 5 times more common than asthma and 7 times more common than hay fever.
- >51 million school hours are lost due to dental-related illness each year.

RISK FACTORS

- Poor oral hygiene
- Poor dietary practices
  - Frequent nighttime bottlefeeding with milk or juice
  - Breastfeeding >7 times daily after 12 months of age
  - Ad libitum breastfeeding after introduction of other dietary carbohydrates
  - A diet high in natural or added sugars
  - Frequent sugar-containing snacking between meals
- Delayed establishment of dental home
- Previous caries
- Lack of exposure to fluoride
- Low socioeconomic status
- Immigrant status
- Poor salivary flow
- Special health care needs or chronic conditions

GENERAL PREVENTION

- Caries risk assessment is the determination of the likelihood of the incidence of caries (i.e., the number of new cavitated or incipient lesions) during a certain time period or the likelihood that there will be a change in the size or activity of lesions already present.
- Establishment of a dental home no later than the child's first birthday allows the dental practitioner to educate and promote the use of caries-preventing strategies such as dietary recommendations and appropriate oral hygiene.
- Anticipatory guidance is the process of providing practical, developmentally-appropriate information about children's health to prepare parents for the significant physical, emotional, and psychological milestones.
- Dietary guidelines include the following:
  - Eating a variety of nutrient-dense foods and beverages
  - Balancing foods eaten with physical activity to maintain a healthy body mass index
  - Maintaining a caloric intake adequate to support normal growth and development
  - Choosing a diet with plenty of vegetables, fruits, and whole grains and low in fat
  - Using sugars and salt (sodium) in moderation
  - The American Academy of Pediatrics (AAP) recommends children 1 to 6 years of age consume no more than 4 to 6 oz of fruit juice per day from a cup (i.e., not a bottle or covered cup) and as part of a meal or snack.
- Oral hygiene measures should be implemented no later than the time of eruption of the first primary tooth.
  - Brushing the infant's teeth after eruption with a toothbrush will help reduce bacterial concentrations.
  - Brushing should be performed for children by a parent twice daily.
  - Flossing should be initiated when adjacent tooth surfaces touch.
  - Parents and caregivers should help or watch over their kids' tooth brushing abilities until they're at least 8 years old.
- Optimal exposure to fluoride is an important preventive measure for children. The use of fluoride for the prevention and control of caries is documented to be both safe and effective.
  - When determining the risk–benefit ratio of fluoride, the key issue is mild fluorosis versus preventing devastating dental disease.
  - In children considered at moderate or high caries risk of age <2 years, a "smear" of fluoridated toothpaste should be used.
  - In all children ages 2 to 5 years, a "pea-size" amount should be used.
  - Professionally applied topical fluoride, such as fluoride varnish, should be considered for children at risk for caries.
  - Systemically administered fluoride should be considered for all children at caries risk who drink fluoride-deficient water (<0.6 ppm) after determining all other dietary sources of fluoride exposure.

ALERT

54% of U.S. preschool children were given some form of over-the-counter medications, most commonly as analgesics, antipyretics, and cough and cold medications. Numerous oral liquid medications contain a high sugar content to increase palatability and acceptance by children. Frequent ingestion of sugar-sweetened medications has demonstrated a higher incidence of caries in chronically ill children.

- To motivate children to consume vitamins, numerous companies have made "gummy" vitamin supplements.
  - Cases of vitamin A toxicity have been reported as a result of excessive consumption.
  - The AAP recommends that the optimal way to obtain adequate amounts of vitamins is to consume a healthy and well-balanced diet.

PATHOPHYSIOLOGY

- The oral cavity contains a diverse microbiota that is essential for maintaining normal physiology in the oral cavity.
  - Oral bacteria metabolize sugar and produce lactic acid. Lactic acid is responsible for the demineralization of tooth structure and may lead to cavitation and the advancement of caries through the various dental structures.
  - Furthermore, lactic acid alters the oral environment to a more acidic one and thus disrupts the balance of the oral microbiota, causing the appearance of more pathogenic organisms, thereby enhancing the process.
- Dental caries is a common chronic infectious and transmissible disease resulting from primarily mutans streptococci (MS) that metabolize sugars to produce acid which, over time, demineralizes and cavitates tooth structure (enamel).
  - MS colonization of an infant may occur from the time of birth by "vertical transmission" from mother to infant. The higher the levels of maternal salivary MS, the greater the risk of the infant being colonized, the greater risk for caries.
  - Along with salivary levels of MS, mother's oral hygiene, periodontal disease, snack frequency, and socioeconomic status also are associated with infant colonization.
- The initial acquisition of MS occurs at the median age of 26 months during the "window of infectivity."
  - Mothers are recommended to minimize or eliminate saliva-sharing habits such as sharing spoons.

DIAGNOSIS

HISTORY
- Poor oral hygiene
- Poor dietary practices
  - Frequent nighttime bottlefeeding with milk or juice
  - Breastfeeding >7 times daily after 12 months of age
  - Ad libitum breastfeeding after introduction of other dietary carbohydrates
  - A diet high in natural or added sugars
  - Frequent sugar-containing snacking between meals
- Delayed establishment of dental home
- Previous caries
- Lack of exposure to fluoride
- Low socioeconomic status
- Immigrant status
- Poor salivary flow
- Special health care needs or chronic conditions
- Maternal caries
- Dental pain

PHYSICAL EXAM
- Visible plaque buildup
- "Chalky" teeth
- Cavitated teeth
- Gingivitis
  - Red, swollen gingival
  - Spontaneous bleeding
- Abscessed teeth
- Lymphadenopathy
- Pain

DIFFERENTIAL DIAGNOSIS
- Viral infections such as primary herpetic gingivostomatitis, hand-foot-and-mouth disease, herpangina
- Gingivitis
- Periodontal disease

DIAGNOSTIC TESTS & INTERPRETATION
- Oral swabbing to assess MS bacterial load
- Plaque index
  - Use of disclosing tablets to highlight plaque and score teeth
- Caries risk assessment

Initial Tests (screening, lab, imaging)
Dental radiographs as needed at discretion of the pediatric dentist

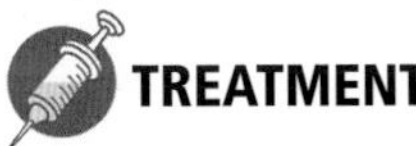

TREATMENT

MEDICATION
Treatment of dental caries does not involve medication but rather the restoration of decayed teeth along with the establishment of a dental home. Proper oral hygiene and dietary measures need to be introduced to the patient and the parent.

ADDITIONAL THERAPIES
- Probiotics
  - Probiotics are living microbes that beneficially influence the health of the host when used in adequate numbers.
  - Specific probiotic strains (e.g., *Lactobacillus rhamnosus* LB21, *Lactobacillus rhamnosus* GG) have been shown in some studies to act as antagonists toward pathogenic bacteria by a variety of different mechanism.
  - Restoring the oral health to a more balanced one creates a more suitable environment for the prevention of dental caries and proper oral health.
- Increased fluoride exposure
  - When used appropriately, fluoride is both safe and effective in preventing and controlling dental caries.
  - Topically, low levels of fluoride in plaque and saliva inhibit the demineralization of sound enamel and enhance the remineralization of demineralized enamel.
- Sealant application
  - Sealants reduce the risk of pit and fissure caries in susceptible teeth and are cost-effective when maintained.
  - They are indicated for primary and permanent teeth with pits and fissures that are predisposed to plaque retention.
  - At-risk pits and fissures should be sealed as soon as possible.
- Xylitol chewing gum
  - Xylitol is a five-carbon sugar alcohol derived primarily from forest and agricultural materials.
  - Xylitol reduces plaque formation and bacterial adherence (i.e., is antimicrobial), inhibits enamel demineralization (i.e., reduces acid production), and has a direct inhibitory effect on MS.

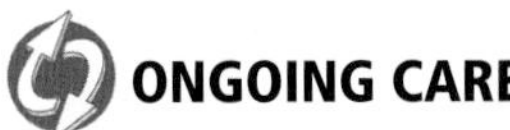

ONGOING CARE

FOLLOW-UP RECOMMENDATIONS
The most common interval of examination is 6 months; however, some patients may require examination and preventive services at more or less frequent intervals based on historical, clinical, and radiographic findings.

PROGNOSIS
The practice of pediatric dentistry is based on prevention. If a dental home is established early, a pediatric dentist can guide the parent and the child on proper oral hygiene and diet, minimizing the risk for the development of caries.

ADDITIONAL READING

- American Academy of Pediatric Dentistry. 2015-16 Definitions, oral health policies, and clinical guidelines. http://www.aapd.org/policies/. Accessed September 2013.
- American Academy of Pediatric Dentistry. Symposium on the prevention of oral disease in children and adolescents. Chicago, Ill; November 11–12, 2005: conference papers. *Pediatr Dent*. 2006;28(2):96–198.
- Dye BA, Shenkin JD, Ogden CL, et al. The relationship between healthful eating practices and dental caries in children aged 2–5 years in the United States, 1988–1994. *J Am Dent Assoc*. 2004;135(1):55–66.
- Näse L, Hatakka K, Savilahti E, et al. Effect of long-term consumption of a probiotic bacterium, *Lactobacillus rhamnosus* GG, in milk on dental caries and caries risk in children. *Caries Res*. 2001;35(6):412–420.
- Stecksén-Blicks C, Sjöström I, Twetman S. Effect of long-term consumption of milk supplemented with probiotic lactobacilli and fluoride on dental caries and general health in preschool children: a cluster-randomized study. *Caries Res*. 2009;43(5):374–381.
- U.S. Department of Health and Human Services, Office of the Surgeon General. *A National Call to Action to Promote Oral Health*. Rockville, MD: U.S. Department of Health and Human Services, Public Health Service, National Institutes of Health, National Institute of Dental and Craniofacial Research; 2003.

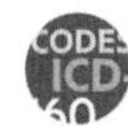

CODES

ICD10
- K02.9 Dental caries, unspecified
- K05.10 Chronic gingivitis, plaque induced
- K05.6 Periodontal disease, unspecified

FAQ
- Q: It's just a baby tooth. Isn't it going to fall out?
- A: Untreated dental caries in children can lead to pain and infection and affect speech and communication, eating and dietary nutrition, sleeping, learning, playing, and quality of life, even into adulthood.
- Q: My child cannot spit yet and swallows the toothpaste. Can I use a fluoride-free "safe-to-swallow" toothpaste?
- A: Latest research has strongly and unequivocally supported the safety and efficacy of fluoride toothpaste in children. The benefit of fluoride far outweighs any potential risks of toxicity. However, use of fluoride should be based on individual risk factors. In children considered at moderate or high caries risk of age <2 years, a smear of fluoridated toothpaste should be used. In all children ages 2 to 5 years, a pea-size amount should be used.

DENTAL INFECTIONS

Johnny I. Kuttab, DDS

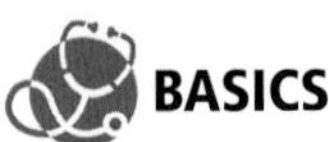

BASICS

DESCRIPTION

A dental infection is an acute or chronic inflammatory response of the dental pulp (pulpitis) tissue caused by the invasion of bacteria secondary to caries or trauma. Pulpal infection can lead to necrosis of the pulp tissue and cause an abscess (localized collection of pus) to form.

- Reversible pulpitis is a condition when pulpitis can be reversed such as the placement of a filling in a tooth.
- Irreversible pulpitis is a condition that cannot be reversed and rather leads to necrosis of the nerve and eventual abscess deposition.

EPIDEMIOLOGY

Periapical abscesses account for 47% of all dental-related attendances at pediatric emergency rooms in the United States.

RISK FACTORS

- Poor diet (high in sugar)
- Poor hygiene (visible plaque on teeth)
- Dental caries
- Low socioeconomic status
- Lack of dental home due to access to care

PATHOPHYSIOLOGY

- Most dental infections are a result of the advancement of dental caries from the enamel, into the dentin, and finally, into the pulp tissue of the tooth.
  - Advancement occurs due to the production of acid by a group of bacteria that metabolize sugar from diet.
  - As more acid is created, the pH of the oral cavity is lowered, which further enhances the cycle.
  - Demineralization of the tooth layers occurs. As the caries process progresses, the bacteria then invade the pulp where an inflammatory response is initiated.
  - Necrosis of the pulp tissue occurs and forms an abscess at the apex of the root, resulting in bone destruction.
- Depending on host factors, infection may remain localized and drain through a sinus tract or may spread into the marrow, perforate the cortical plate, and invade surrounding tissues and facial planes.
- Typically, once full necrosis of the nerve has occurred, the pain subsides, and abscess formation is present.
  - This situation is particularly dangerous because the abscess can remain localized at the apex of the tooth or proceed between muscles, arteries, and veins into fascial spaces and cause significant and potentially life-threatening problems.
  - However, most are self-limiting and establish intraoral localized drainage.

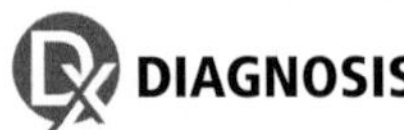

DIAGNOSIS

HISTORY

- Nocturnal pain
  - Waking up due to pain
- Inability to eat due to pain
- Sensitivity to cold
- Fever
- Swelling
- Pain secondary to reversible pulpitis
  - Typically, symptoms of reversible pulpitis include sensitivity to hot/cold/sugary foods or sensitivity to air/brushing.
  - Pain is acute in nature.
  - When the stimulus is removed, the spontaneous pain subsides. When the tooth is restored, the pain disappears.
- Pain secondary to irreversible pulpitis
  - Irreversible pulpitis symptoms include a dull achy pain that is constant, whether a stimulus is present or not.
  - Most patients present to the dentist or the emergency room with irreversible pulpitis or abscess/infection.

PHYSICAL EXAM

- Lymphadenopathy
- Extraoral asymmetry due to swelling
- Intraoral swelling
  - Sublingual, submandibular, vestibular, palatal swelling adjacent to tooth
- Sinus tract or fistula adjacent tooth
- Limited oral opening
- Tenderness to palpation
- Low-grade fever
- Dehydration

DIFFERENTIAL DIAGNOSIS

- Reversible pulpitis
- Gingival abscess due to foreign body
- Ulceration (herpetic or aphthous)
- Eruption of permanent tooth

DIAGNOSTIC TESTS & INTERPRETATION

Initial Tests (screening, lab, imaging)

- Periapical or panoramic radiograph
  - Localized bone destruction or widened periodontal ligament (PDL) space
- CT scan in cases of serious extraoral swelling

Diagnostic Procedures/Other

Dentists perform pulp vitality tests to assess the health of the nerve, which can dictate treatment. Depending on the response of the nerve to cold, electricity, or percussion, a proper diagnosis can be reached.

- Percussion test (tapping on tooth elicits pain)
- Vitality test
  - Cold test
  - Electric pulp test (EPT)
- Mobility of tooth

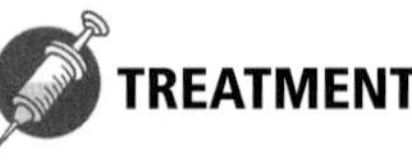

TREATMENT

GENERAL MEASURES

Space maintenance

- Space maintenance is important to allow proper growth and development of the permanent teeth.
- The primary tooth is the best space maintainer.
- Without opposing or adjacent primary teeth, others may drift or tip into the space left by the extracted tooth, causing the development of malocclusions.
- Spacers are used for space maintenance.

MEDICATION

Antibiotic use should be considered when symptoms include nocturnal pain, fever, lymphadenopathy, and extraoral swelling.

First Line

- Amoxicillin 20 to 40 mg/kg/24 h PO in 2 divided doses
- Amoxicillin/clavulanate 25–45 mg/kg/24 h PO in 2 divided doses
- Acetaminophen 10 to 15 mg/kg/dose PO every 4 to 6 hours as needed
- Ibuprofen 5 to 10 mg/kg/dose PO every 6 to 8 hours as needed

Second Line

- Clindamycin 10 to 30 mg/kg/24 h PO in 3 divided doses
- Azithromycin 10 mg/kg/dose PO × 1 on day 1, followed by 5 mg/kg/dose PO once daily on days 2 to 5

ADDITIONAL THERAPIES

- Treatment of irreversible pulpitis or dental infection in primary teeth includes extraction of offending primary tooth or pulpectomy (primary tooth root canal).
  - Extraction is preferred, as the goal is to create the most ideal environment for the permanent tooth to continue to develop.
  - It is not uncommon for the permanent tooth to undergo damage in the presence of a long-term chronic infection.
- Treatment of irreversible pulpitis in permanent teeth includes root canal therapy (removal of the nerve and replacing the nerve with a synthetic filling material) followed by crown.

ADMISSION, INPATIENT, AND NURSING CONSIDERATIONS

- Significant extra- or intraoral swelling due to abscess
- Unusual drowsiness, headache, or a stiff neck; weakness or fainting
- Difficulty swallowing or breathing
- Significant eyelid swelling (e.g., eye swollen shut)
- A rising fever, dehydration, and inability to eat
- Although rare, a dental infection or abscess may spread to fascial planes and cause facial cellulitis.
  - An infection in the buccal space can cause extraoral swelling in the infraorbital, zygomatic, and buccal regions. This most often involves maxillary molars.
  - An infection in the submental space can cause extraoral swelling secondary to infection the mandibular incisors.
  - An infection in the submandibular space can cause extraoral swelling unilaterally in the submandibular region secondary to infection in the mandibular molars.
  - The spread of dental infection through the fascial planes can end at the parapharyngeal or retropharyngeal spaces.
- Dental infections can also spread via lymphatics, veins, and arteries.
  - The cavernous sinus is involved in most fatal spread of dental infection due to the lack of retrograde valves in the veins leading into the sinus.
  - The result may be a cavernous sinus thrombosis.

ALERT

An infection in the submental, sublingual, and bilateral submandibular spaces is referred to as Ludwig angina. Infection may spread down the anterior cervical triangle to the clavicles. Speaking, swallowing, and breathing are severely compromised. This is a medical emergency and requires establishment of a safe airway (intubation).

ONGOING CARE

FOLLOW-UP RECOMMENDATIONS

- Referral to pediatric dentist for treatment
  - Extraction, root canal therapy, restorative treatment
- Thorough dental workup for other caries
- Resolution of abscess/swelling
- Management of space issues caused by extraction
- Establish proper dental home with proper dietary and hygiene intervention and guidance.

PROGNOSIS

The prognosis for a dental infection or abscess is good with timely proper medical and dental treatment.

ADDITIONAL READING

- American Academy of Pediatric Dentistry. 2015-16 definitions, oral health policies, and clinical guidelines. http://www.aapd.org/policies/. Accessed September 2013.
- American Academy of Pediatrics, American Society for Microbiology. *Your Child and Antibiotics: Unnecessary Antibiotics Can Be Harmful*. Atlanta, GA: Centers for Disease Control and Prevention; 1997.
- American Association of Oral and Maxillofacial Surgeons. Parameters of care: clinical practice guidelines for oral and maxillofacial surgery (AAOMS ParCare 07 Ver 4.0). *J Oral Maxillofac Surg*. 2007;32(Suppl):238–245.
- Centers for Disease Control and Prevention, U.S. Food and Drug Administration, National Institutes of Health. A public health action plan to combat antimicrobial resistance; 1999. http://www.cdc.gov/drugresistance/actionplan/aractionplan.pdf. Accessed September 2013.
- Dodson T, Perrott D, Kaban L. Pediatric maxillofacial infections: a retrospective study of 113 patients. *J Oral Maxillofac Surg*. 1989;47(4):327–330.
- Graham DB, Webb MD, Seale NS. Pediatric emergency room visits for nontraumatic dental disease. *Pediatr Dent*. 2000;22(2):134–140.
- Kaban L, Troulis M. Infections of the maxillofacial region. In: Kaban L, Troulis M, eds. *Pediatric Oral and Maxillofacial Surgery*. Philadelphia, PA: Saunders; 2004:171–186.
- Seow W. Diagnosis and management of unusual dental abscesses in children. *Aust Dent J*. 2003;48(3):156–168.

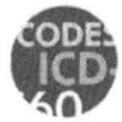

CODES

ICD10

- K04.0 Pulpitis
- K04.1 Necrosis of pulp
- K04.7 Periapical abscess without sinus

FAQ

- Q: It's just a baby tooth. Isn't it going to fall out?
- A: Dental pain can affect a child's daily activities, leading to delayed growth and development and diminished ability to learn. Delayed treatment for a dental infection may cause damage to the permanent teeth or may proceed to a facial cellulitis. Premature primary tooth loss due to infection and extraction can lead to eruption and crowding issues in the permanent dentition.
- Q: I had horrible teeth growing up. Is this genetic?
- A: Genetic variation of the host factors may contribute to increased risks for dental caries; however, research suggests that other risk factors contribute greater such as diet and hygiene.
- Q: I see a pimple on my child's gums, but he does not complain of pain and is sleeping fine. Does this require treatment?
- A: All dental infections involving primary or permanent teeth require some form of treatment. If the body's host factors have localized the infection, drainage may occur with the absence of pain; however, the source of the infection remains. This may lead to damage to succedaneous (permanent) teeth or spread of the infection into a cellulitis.
- Q: I started the course of antibiotics and my child is feeling better. Is it necessary to complete the antibiotic?
- A: It is necessary to complete the entire course of the antibiotic unless an allergic reaction is occurring. Resolution of pain or swelling does not ensure the infection has fully responded to the antibiotic. Follow-up studies suggest that antibiotic use should continue at least 5 days beyond the point of improvement of symptoms.

DENTAL TRAUMA

Ray J. Jurado, DDS

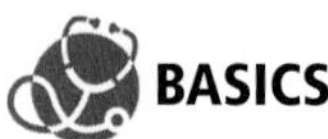

BASICS

DESCRIPTION

Dental trauma is defined as fractured, displaced, or lost primary or permanent teeth.

EPIDEMIOLOGY

- 30% of children suffer from traumatic dental injuries to the primary dentition, with the highest incidence at 2 to 3 years of age.
- 22% of children suffer from traumatic dental injuries to the permanent dentition occurring secondary to falls, traffic accidents or bicycles, violence, sports, and physical abuse
- 70% of cases involve maxillary incisors.
- Displacement injuries are most common in the primary dentition. Crown fractures are more common in the permanent dentition.

RISK FACTORS

- Sex:
  - In the primary dentition, the prevalence of injuries ranges from 31% to 40% in boys and from 16% to 30% in girls.
  - In the permanent dentition, the prevalence of dental trauma in boys ranges from 12% to 33% as opposed to 4–19% in girls.
- Age:
  - The most common age for trauma in the primary dentition is from 1.5 to 2.5 years of age when the child is learning to walk.
  - In the permanent dentition, the peak age ranges from 8 to 10 years of age.
- Season:
  - Injuries occur more in summer months than in winter, depending on the population and demographics being studied.
- Occlusion:
  - Increased "overjet" (protrusion of upper incisors) and insufficient lip closure are predisposing factors to traumatic injuries.

GENERAL PREVENTION

- Most sports injuries can be prevented with appropriate use of mouth guards.
- The American Academy for Sports Dentistry lists 40 sports for which it recommend the use of mouth guards, including: acrobatics, baseball, basketball, cycling, discus, shot put, horseback riding, gymnastics, handball, racquetball, squash, judo, karate, rollerblading, rugby, motor cross, parachuting, skiing, soccer, surfing, skateboarding, ice skating, trampoline, tennis, volleyball, wrestling, weight lifting, and water polo.

PATHOPHYSIOLOGY

- Basic tooth structures: enamel (white outer layer), dentin (yellow inner layer), pulp (nerves, blood vessels, connective tissue), cementum (layer covering roots), periodontal ligament (PDL; supports tooth in socket)
- Types of injuries (Figure 3)
  - Infraction: fracture of the enamel without loss of tooth structure; a "crack" in the enamel
  - Uncomplicated crown fracture: fracture with loss of tooth substance confined to enamel or dentin and not involving the pulp
  - Complicated crown fracture: fracture involving enamel and dentin with a pulp exposure
  - Crown/root fracture: fracture involving enamel, dentin, and cementum
  - Root fracture: dentin and cementum fracture involving the pulp
  - Concussion: injury to tooth-supporting structures, no abnormal loosening or displacement
  - Subluxation: injury to tooth-supporting structures with abnormal loosening, no displacement
  - Lateral luxation: lateral displacement of the tooth in its socket with fracture of alveolar bone plate
  - Intrusion: tooth forced into the socket and locked into position in the bone
  - Extrusion: tooth displacement partially out of the socket
  - Avulsion: complete displacement totally out of the socket
  - Alveolar process fracture: fracture of alveolar bone containing tooth

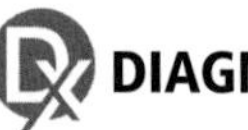

DIAGNOSIS

HISTORY

- Medical history
  - Family history of bleeding disorders
  - History of drug allergies
- Where did the injury occur?
  - Possible contamination
  - Assess need for tetanus prophylaxis.
- How did the injury occur?
  - Mechanism of impact should be consistent with injury.
- When did the injury occur?
  - Time elapsed affects treatment and prognosis (e.g., avulsions).
- Loss of consciousness
  - May indicate need to assess for other injuries
- Bite discrepancy
  - May indicate luxation injury or jaw fracture
- Sensitivity to cold or hot
  - May indicate crown fracture

ALERT

- Missing teeth should be located. If not, consider aspiration, swallowing, or even displacement to a sinus.
- The history of injury should correlate with the trauma to rule out physical abuse.

PHYSICAL EXAM

- Pediatric advanced life support if life-threatening emergency (ABCD, cervical assessment, etc.)
- Clean face and oral cavity with water or saline.
- Extraoral exam:
  - Assess face and lips for soft tissue injuries and palpate mandible and maxilla for possible fractures.
- Intraoral exam:
  - Assess for intraoral soft tissue injuries, tooth fractures, abnormal tooth position, and tooth mobility.

ALERT

To help determine whether the tooth is primary or permanent, classify the dentition according to age: primary dentition (<6 years of age), mixed dentition (6 to 12 years of age), permanent dentition (12 years of age and older). Upper primary incisors begin to loosen and exfoliate around 6 years of age.

DIFFERENTIAL DIAGNOSIS

Soft tissue lesions must correlate with history and mechanism of trauma to rule out physical abuse.

DIAGNOSTIC TESTS & INTERPRETATION

Initial Tests (screening, lab, imaging)

- A soft tissue radiograph helps to identify foreign bodies. A dental film is placed in the vestibule between the lips and a radiograph is taken at 25% normal exposure time.
- Intraoral radiographs (periapical and occlusal views) help to identify root fractures and/or extent of displacements.
- Panoramic radiograph helps to identify jaw fractures.
- CT helps to identify tooth fractures in relation to surrounding bone as well as accurately determine alveolar fracture location and morphology.
- Tooth percussion testing helps to identify severity of tooth concussions.
- Hot and cold testing assess tooth vitality.

Diagnostic Procedures/Other

None

TREATMENT

MEDICATION

- Acetaminophen for pain management
- Consider antibiotic therapy for severe injuries in cases of infection risk (subacute bacterial endocarditis [SBE] risk, immunosuppression, etc.).

ADDITIONAL THERAPIES

- Primary dentition
  - Infraction: no treatment necessary
  - Crown fracture: restoration of tooth structure (tooth colored filling); pulp therapy if indicated
  - Root fracture: extraction of crown and root
  - Luxation: soft diet × 1 week if minor; if severe or interfering with bite, extraction is recommended
  - Intrusion: allow to reerupt if not impinging on permanent tooth bud (determined by intraoral radiograph); extract if impinging
  - Extrusion: if minor: allow for spontaneous realignment; if severe: extraction
  - Avulsion: leave out, do not reimplant, to protect permanent tooth bud
  - Alveolar fracture: reposition alveolar segment and tooth-bonded splint
- Permanent dentition
  - Infraction: tooth sealant
  - Crown fracture: restoration of tooth structure (tooth colored filling); pulp therapy if indicated
  - Root fracture: reposition, tooth-bonded splint
  - Luxation: reposition, tooth-bonded splint
  - Intrusion: immediate repositioning or spontaneous reeruption
  - Extrusion: reposition, tooth-bonded splint
  - Alveolar fracture: reposition alveolar segment and tooth-bonded splint
- Permanent avulsion
  - Rinse tooth in cold water if dirty and reimplant into socket immediately and stabilize with finger. Refer to dentist immediately for assessment and splint stabilization.
  - If reimplantation is not possible, place tooth in physiologic media—milk, saline, or Hanks balanced storage medium (avoid touching root).
  - Refer to dentist *immediately* for reimplantation, tooth-bonded splint, and eventual root canal therapy.
  - Treatment options and prognosis depend on stage of tooth development, time out of socket, and storage medium.
- Mandibular fracture
  - Immediate referral to an emergency department or oral surgeon who will be able to determine management options.

ALERT

Every minute counts! Permanent tooth avulsions require immediate reimplantation. Prognosis worsens the longer the tooth is out of the socket.

ONGOING CARE

FOLLOW-UP RECOMMENDATIONS

- For most dental traumas, the child should be seen by a pediatric dentist as soon as possible for immediate assessment and treatment to optimize prognosis. Regular follow-up is necessary to reassess site of trauma.
- It is very difficult to prevent the majority of trauma. It is recommended that mouth/tongue piercings be avoided.
- Recommend use of mouth guards for appropriate sport activities.
- The social impact of dental trauma can be emotional (e.g., school, pictures, social) and financial. The total costs for replacing a single knocked-out tooth can be >20 times the preventive cost of a professionally, custom-made mouth guard.

PROGNOSIS

- Prognosis depends on severity of trauma. Minor traumas have relatively good outcomes with timely treatment. Severe traumas highly depend on timely, skilled management and the child's healing abilities.
- In the case of any primary tooth trauma, informing parents about possible pulpal complications, appearance of a vestibular sinus tract, or color change of the crown associated with a sinus tract can help assure timely management.
- Primary tooth displacement may also result in complications involving the developing permanent tooth, including enamel hypoplasia, hypocalcification, crown/root dilacerations, or disruptions in eruption patterns or sequence.

ADDITIONAL READING

- American Academy of Pediatric Dentistry. Guideline of management of acute dental trauma. http://www.aapd.org/media/Policies_Guidelines/G_Trauma.pdf. Accessed February 18, 2018.
- The Dental Trauma Guide: http://www.dentaltraumaguide.org/

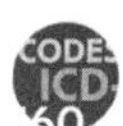

CODES

ICD10

- S02.5XXA Fracture of tooth (traumatic), init for clos fx
- S02.5XXB Fracture of tooth (traumatic), init encntr for open fracture
- K08.119 Complete loss of teeth due to trauma, unspecified class

FAQ

- Q: Why not reposition or reimplant primary teeth?
- A: The treatment strategy in primary teeth trauma is dictated by the concern for the safety of the permanent tooth bud. If the displaced primary tooth has invaded the developing permanent tooth bud, extraction is indicated to minimize damage. Reimplantation may encroach on the permanent tooth bud as well.

DEPRESSION

John I. Takayama, MD, MPH • Eva C. Ihle, MD, PhD

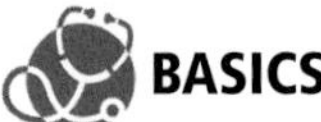

BASICS

DESCRIPTION

- General term that includes major depressive disorder (MDD), persistent depressive disorder (dysthymic disorder), depression associated with bipolar disorder, disruptive mood dysregulation disorder and adjustment disorder with depressed mood
- Syndrome of persistent sadness or irritability associated with a variety of symptoms, resulting in functional impairment in the following:
  - Interpersonal (family, friends) relationships
  - Health (somatic complaints, unhealthy habits)
  - Work or school (task completion, grades)
  - Safety (high-risk behaviors including suicide)

EPIDEMIOLOGY

- 12-month prevalence of MDD: 7.5% of adolescents (age 13 to 18 years), 3–4% in younger children
- Lifetime prevalence: 11% will have diagnosable depression by adolescence.
- Ratio of females to males: 1:1 in school-aged children, 2:1 in adolescents
- Often chronic with high rate of recurrence and comorbidity with other psychiatric disorders
- <45% of affected individuals receive disorder-specific care.

RISK FACTORS

- Family history of depression, bipolar disorder, suicidal behavior in 1st-degree relative
- Personal history of anxiety disorders, ADHD, learning disabilities, and conduct problems
- Prior depressive episodes
- Family dysfunction or caregiver–child conflict
- Negative style of interpreting events and coping with stress
- Substance abuse
- Exposure to adversity (e.g., victim of abuse, bullying)
- Chronic illness (including obesity)
- Not everyone with exposure to adversity or chronic illness will go on to have MDD (some moderators are resilience and response to treatment).

COMMONLY ASSOCIATED CONDITIONS

40–70% of children and adolescents with depression have comorbid psychiatric disorders:

- Anxiety disorders
- Somatization disorders
- Disruptive behavioral disorders (e.g., oppositional defiant and conduct disorders)
- Eating disorders
- ADHD
- Substance abuse
- Physical or sexual abuse

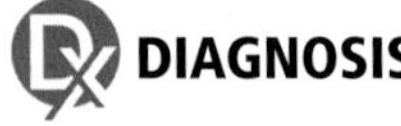

DIAGNOSIS

- U.S. Preventive Services Task Force recommends routine screening of adolescents for depression in clinical settings that can ensure accurate diagnosis and appropriate management and follow-up and universal surveillance for younger children.
- If screening identifies depression, diagnosis should be established through formal assessment, and risk for suicidal behavior assessed.
- Screening tools include Patient Health Questionnaire for Adolescents (PHQ-A; sensitivity 73%, specificity 94%), Beck Depression Inventory for Primary Care (BDI-PC, sensitivity 91%, and specificity 91%), and Strengths and Difficulties Questionnaire (SDQ, sensitivity 33–63%) for identifying depression in adolescents.
- Additional tools: Kutcher Adolescent Depression Scale, Reynolds Adolescent Depression Screen, Mood and Feelings Questionnaire

HISTORY

- Obtain detailed history of child's mood and functioning at home, at school, and with parents, siblings, teachers, and peers.
- Determine onset and duration of depressive symptoms, associated stressors, and personal impact (distress or impairment).
- Diagnosis of MDD according to the *DSM-5* requires at least 2 weeks of symptoms one or two, and four or more of the remaining symptoms:
  - Depressed or irritable mood: feeling down, sad, or blue most of the time or being "annoyed" or "bothered" by everything and everyone
  - Diminished interest or pleasure in previously enjoyable activities (events, hobbies, interests)
  - Change in appetite or weight
  - Sleep disturbance: not feeling well rested, difficulty in waking up in the morning or in falling asleep at night, waking up in the middle of the night or too early in the morning, daytime napping or sleeping, and nighttime arousal
  - Psychomotor retardation or agitation: talk or move more slowly than typical, exhibit less speech, and have longer response latencies; difficulty sitting still, pacing, hand wringing, tantrums, yelling, shouting, and nonstop talking
  - Fatigue or loss of energy: feeling chronically tired, exhausted, listless, and without energy or motivation (Parents may interpret as laziness.)
  - Feelings of worthlessness or guilt leading to reluctance to do things, excessive self-criticism, difficulty identifying positive self-attributes, "I don't care" attitude, envy or preoccupation with success of others, marked self-reproach or guilt for events that are not their fault
  - Impaired concentration or indecisiveness: problems with attention and concentration, slowed thinking and processing of information, indecisiveness and procrastination, helplessness or paralysis in taking action
  - Running or recurrent thoughts of death or suicide or attempts suicide
- Diagnosis should also include assessment of distress and impairment of functioning.
- Patient should not have manic or hypomanic behavior, and symptoms should not be attributable to substance use or another medical condition.
  - Manic/hypomanic symptoms
    - Ask about episodes of elevated or irritated mood associated with increased energy and activity, decreased need for sleep, grandiose thinking, and impulsive behavior.
    - History of manic symptoms suggests bipolar disorder.
  - If depressive symptoms occur only in the context of substance use or another medical condition, then the symptoms are considered secondary and not an MDD proper.
- If symptoms do not fulfill criteria of MDD, consider persistent depressive disorder or unspecified depressive disorder (*DSM-5*).
- Persistent depressive disorder (previously dysthymic disorder): symptoms less intense but more persistent; depressed or irritable for at least 1 year with two of the following: appetite disturbance, sleep disturbance, fatigue, low self-esteem, poor concentration, difficulty making decisions, or feelings of hopelessness
- Disruptive mood dysregulation disorder: clinically significant chronic, persistent irritability present between frequent verbal or behavioral outbursts
- Adjustment disorder with depressed mood is diagnosed when depressive symptoms occur only in the context of a specific stressor.
- Important to assess for the following symptoms:
  - Premenstrual timing of symptoms
    - If depressed mood is primarily in the days prior to menses, diagnosis may be premenstrual dysphoric disorder.
  - Psychotic symptoms
    - Ask about auditory or visual hallucination, paranoid ideation, and odd beliefs, which suggest either a more serious depression or a separate psychotic diagnosis.
    - If family reports patient as withdrawn and less motivated, with no clear evidence for sad or irritable mood, this may also suggest a psychotic disorder.

PHYSICAL EXAM

Weight loss or gain may be associated with depression. Somatic complaints (i.e., headaches, abdominal pain) are common in depression. Physical exam should focus on identifying other medical conditions that cause depressive symptoms (hypothyroidism, neurologic conditions, and underlying chronic illness) and evaluating for signs of comorbid psychiatric conditions such as eating disorders.

- Vital signs: weight loss or weight gain
- Goiter (hypothyroidism)
- Lymphadenopathy (chronic illness, infection)
- Sexual development (Delayed puberty may be related to hypothyroidism, anorexia nervosa.)
- Extremities: arthritis (rheumatologic disease)
- Neurologic exam (postconcussive symptoms)
- Skin: pale, cool, dry (hypothyroidism); evidence of self-injurious behavior (i.e., scars from repetitive cutting)
- Mental status exam
  - Appearance, alertness, speech, behavior
  - Awareness of environment (orientation)
  - Assessment of mood (patient's own words)
  - Assessment of affect (outward manifestation of emotional state)
  - Memory, judgment, reasoning
  - Motoric slowing indicates severe depression.
  - Abnormal thought content, such as current suicidal ideation or psychotic thoughts, should prompt immediate referral to a psychiatrist.

DIFFERENTIAL DIAGNOSIS

- Other medical
  - Mood disorder related to a medical condition
  - Endocrine: hypothyroidism, Addison disease
  - Neurologic: postconcussion syndrome
  - Metabolic: vitamin B_{12} deficiency
  - Autoimmune: systemic lupus erythematosus
  - Infectious: mononucleosis, HIV/AIDS
- Behavioral
  - Substance-induced mood disorder
- Psychiatric
  - Adjustment disorder with depressed mood
  - Bipolar disorder

DIAGNOSTIC TESTS & INTERPRETATION

Initial Tests (screening, lab, imaging)

- Vitamin B_{12}, free T4, TSH, or other labs based on history and exam to identify contributing or associated medical condition
- Screening for substance abuse as indicated

TREATMENT

- Assessment of severity of depression
  - Determine severity by considering number of symptoms, thought content and process, risk for suicidal behavior, and impact on functioning.
  - Mild depression: five or six symptoms with mild impairment in functioning
  - Moderate depression: six to eight symptoms with mild to moderate impairment in functioning
  - Severe depression: all nine symptoms or five or more symptoms and reports specific suicide plan, clear intent, or recent attempt; psychotic symptoms; severe impairment in functioning (i.e., inability to leave home)
- Safety assessment and planning
  - Instruct family to restrict access to lethal means and monitor risk factors for suicidal behavior.
  - Provide patient and family with emergency contacts if risks for suicidal behavior increase.
  - Establish clear follow-up plan.
- Initial management of mild depression
  - Supportive management including education of patient and family about depression and stress reduction, clinical and community support, and management of identified stressors
  - Schedule visits with primary care clinician weekly or biweekly for 6 to 8 weeks for monitoring.
  - If depression worsens or does not improve in 4 to 6 weeks, additional intervention is needed.
- Management of moderate or persistent (lasting >6 to 8 weeks) depression
  - Education, support, stress reduction
  - Psychosocial interventions (counseling, therapy), antidepressant medication, or combination of both
  - Among adolescents, psychosocial and medical interventions are equally effective, with slightly increased benefit with combination. Choice of intervention depends on resources, patient/family preference, and individual clinical factors (i.e., age, severity of depression, family history of treatment response).
  - Among adolescents, 1st-line antidepressant medication is selective serotonin reuptake inhibitors (SSRIs).
  - Among preadolescent children, there is little evidence for effectiveness of antidepressant medication with elevated risk of serious side effects; refer to child psychiatrist if antidepressants are being considered.
  - Antidepressant use in adolescents and young adults may be associated with a slight increase in risk of suicidal thoughts and behaviors. These medications, however, have a favorable risk benefit ratio and can be used safely with appropriate patient education and monitoring.
  - Omega-3 fatty acids (1,000 mg/day) may be effective in both children and adolescents.
  - If patient is referred for therapy, continue frequent monitoring until depression is resolved.
  - Several types of therapy can be used for depression. For adolescents, there is evidence for effectiveness of cognitive behavioral therapy (CBT) and interpersonal psychotherapy (IPT).
- Special diagnostic considerations
  - Premenstrual dysphoric disorder: SSRIs can be used as the 1st-line treatment.
  - Adjustment disorder: When depressed mood is only in context of a specific stressor, psychosocial interventions, rather than medications, are recommended.

ISSUES FOR REFERRAL

Patients with depression can be successfully managed by primary care clinicians. Referral to a mental health provider is recommended for the following:

- Risk for acute suicidal behavior: Refer to emergency services.
- History of suicide attempts
- Presence of substance abuse
- Presence of manic or psychotic symptoms
- No improvement after 6 to 8 weeks of treatment
- Recurrent or chronic depression
- Severe functional impairment
- Psychiatric comorbidities
- Complicated psychosocial factors, such as dysfunctional family dynamics
- After initiating referral to a mental health provider, primary care clinician should continue to follow patient while he or she waits for first appointment and throughout treatment course.

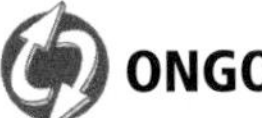

ONGOING CARE

FOLLOW-UP RECOMMENDATIONS

- In the initial phase (6 to 9 months or longer), the primary care clinician must identify medical conditions associated with depression, provide support and resources, assess patient safety and review safety plan, and monitor response to psychosocial and medical treatments.
- In the continuation phase (6 to 12 months), patients continue psychosocial or pharmacologic treatments used to achieve remission in the acute phase for at least 6 months, 12 months if difficulties in achieving remission, history of recurrent depression, or presence of ongoing risk factors; patients are typically seen biweekly or monthly by mental health providers depending on clinical status, functioning, support systems, stressors, motivation for treatment, and comorbid psychiatric or medical disorders.
- When asymptomatic for 6 to 12 months, patients may be recommended for either maintenance phase or discontinuation of treatment.

PROGNOSIS

- Up to 30–40% of patients with MDD can be expected to recover by 6 months and 70–80% by 12 months; 5–10% have protracted episodes lasting longer than 2 years.
- Time to recovery is influenced by age at onset of illness, severity, presence of comorbid disorders, and parental history of depression.
- Shorter duration of symptoms at the time of diagnosis is associated with better outcomes; thus, early identification and treatment are recommended.
- Probability of recurrence following recovery of a major depressive episode is approximately 40% by 2 years and 70% by 5 years.

ADDITIONAL READING

- Avenevoli S, Swendsen J, He JP, et al. Major depression in the National Comorbidity Survey—Adolescent Supplement: prevalence, correlates, and treatment. *J Am Acad Child Adolesc Psychiatry*. 2015;54(1):37–44.e2.
- Cheung AH, Zuckerbrot RA, Jensen PS, et al; for GLAD-PC Steering Group. Guidelines for adolescent depression in primary care (GLAD-PC): II. Treatment and ongoing management. *Pediatrics*. 2007;120(5):e1313–e1326.
- Deacon G, Kettle C, Hayes D, et al. Omega 3 polyunsaturated fatty acids and the treatment of depression. *Crit Rev Food Sci Nutr*. 2017;57(1):212–223.
- Greydanus DE, Calles JL, Patel DR. *Pediatric and Adolescent Psychopharmacology: A Practical Manual for Pediatricians*. Cambridge, United Kingdom: University Press; 2008.
- Klein DN, Kotov R. Course of depression in a 10-year prospective study: evidence for qualitatively distinct subgroups. *J Abnorm Psychol*. 2016;125(3):337–348.
- Lewandowski RE, Acri MC, Hoagwood KE, et al. Evidence for the management of adolescent depression. *Pediatrics*. 2013;132(4):e996–e1009.
- March J, Silva S, Petrycki S, et al; for Treatment for Adolescents with Depression Study Team. Fluoxetine, cognitive-behavioral therapy, and their combination for adolescents with depression: Treatment for Adolescents with Depression Study (TADS) randomized controlled trial. *JAMA*. 2004;292(7):807–820.
- Rao U, Chen LA. Characteristics, correlates, and outcomes of childhood and adolescent depressive disorders. *Dialogues Clin Neurosci*. 2009;11(1):45–62.
- Williams SB, O'Connor EA, Eder M, et al. Screening for child and adolescent depression in primary care settings: a systematic evidence review for the US Preventive Services Task Force. *Pediatrics*. 2009;123(4):e716–e735.
- Zuckerbrot RA, Cheung AH, Jensen PS, et al; for GLAD-PC Steering Group. Guidelines for adolescent depression in primary care (GLAD-PC): I. Identification, assessment, and initial management. *Pediatrics*. 2007;120(5):e1299–e1312.

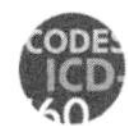

CODES

ICD10

- F32.9 Major depressive disorder, single episode, unspecified
- F33.9 Major depressive disorder, recurrent, unspecified
- F34.1 Dysthymic disorder

FAQ

- Q: What is the PHQ-9?
- A: The PHQ-9 is a self-completed screening survey composed of nine questions that ask about the frequency of symptoms of depression. If a patient reports five or more symptoms more than half the days during the past 2 weeks, the clinician must consider MDD as a diagnosis.
- Q: How should clinicians interpret the "black box warning" about SSRIs?
- A: In 2004, the Food and Drug Administration issued the black box warning about increased risk of suicidal thoughts or behavior in children and adolescents treated with SSRI. The meta-analyses that led to this warning are now considered flawed. Given evidence for improvement of depression with SSRIs and increased rates of suicide in the years following the black box warning, clinicians should weigh the risks and benefits with the patient and family in deciding treatment; adolescents treated with SSRIs must be closely monitored for any worsening in depression, emergence of suicidal thinking or behavior, or unusual changes in behavior, such as sleeplessness, agitation, or withdrawal from normal social situations.
- Q: What is CBT?
- A: In CBT, the therapist guides and helps a patient to understand and modify dysfunctional thoughts, feelings, and behaviors. If a patient believes that he is worthless, the therapist may encourage him to challenge the negative and irrational belief by understanding patterns in his thinking that relate to such a belief.

DERMATOMYOSITIS/POLYMYOSITIS

Megan L. Curran, MD

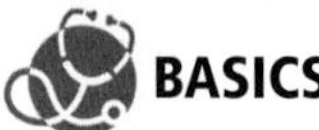

BASICS

DESCRIPTION

Juvenile dermatomyositis (JDM) and juvenile polymyositis (JPM) are inflammatory myopathies in which inflammation within tissues and capillary endothelium of muscle, skin, and other organs causes vascular and tissue damage. JDM patients present with characteristic rashes and muscle weakness. JPM patients have inflammatory myopathy but lack skin findings. Both disorders have a wide range of severity and presenting findings.

EPIDEMIOLOGY

- The average age of onset is 7 years, but 25% of cases are diagnosed by 4 years of age.
- Male-to-female ratio in the United States is 1:2.3.
- JDM incidence is 3.2 new cases per 1 million children per year; JPM is extremely rare.

RISK FACTORS

- Underlying genetic susceptibility
- Environmental triggers
  - Ultraviolet light exposure
  - Infectious triggers are inconsistently reported, including group A β-hemolytic streptococci, coxsackievirus B, toxoplasma, enterovirus, and parvovirus.
  - Reports of drug exposure, vaccination, and psychological stress prior to diagnosis, but no causation has been found

Genetics

- Genetic factors, including the following:
  - HLA alleles: B8, DRB1*0301, DQA1*0501, DQA1*0301
  - Cytokine polymorphisms: TNFα-308A promoter, various IL-1 genes, interferon regulatory factor 5, and others, all resulting in upregulated inflammation
  - Polymorphisms of immunoglobulin constant regions
- Epigenetic factors likely exist: Monozygotic twin studies show low concordance.

PATHOPHYSIOLOGY

- Vasculopathy in patients with underlying inflammatory genetic susceptibility, triggered by environmental factors
- JDM: immune attack on muscle capillary endothelium with infiltration of plasmacytoid dendritic cells causing a type I interferon response and upregulation of myofiber MHC class I expression
  - Immune complex deposition and complement activation drive vasculopathy
  - Upregulation of ICAM-1 and von Willebrand factor antigen indicates endothelial injury.
  - After vasculopathy and MHC class I upregulation, plasmacytoid dendritic and other immune cells infiltrate perivascular and perimysial tissue, resulting in upregulated type I interferon response which perpetuates inflammatory processes including increased production of proinflammatory cytokines
- JPM: CD8 T cell and myeloid dendritic cell-mediated attack on myofibers causing myonecrosis; no increased interferon response
- Myositis-specific and associated autoantibodies directed against vascular and muscle antigens implicated in pathogenesis of JDM and JPM
- Maternal cell chimerism reported in peripheral blood T cells and muscle tissue of JDM patients may be autoreactive toward host cells.

COMMONLY ASSOCIATED CONDITIONS

- Dermatomyositis in children is not associated with presence of malignancy as seen in adults.
- Celiac disease is rarely associated with JDM.

DIAGNOSIS

Bohan and Peter criteria (1975): not validated in children and becoming outdated, but nonetheless used. Definite JDM requires rash plus three other criteria; probable JDM requires rash plus two other criteria:

- Characteristic rashes: heliotrope discoloration of eyelids and/or erythematous papules over extensor surfaces of joints (Gottron papules)
- Symmetric proximal muscle weakness
- Elevated serum skeletal muscle enzymes
- Electromyography (EMG) findings of myopathy and denervation; characteristic MRI findings are often substituted to fulfill EMG criteria in children, although are not specific.
- Muscle biopsy with characteristic abnormalities

HISTORY

- Onset is often insidious but can be rapid.
- Constitutional
  - Fever and adenopathy in some children
  - Anorexia, weight loss
  - Fatigue is a sign of muscle weakness and immune activation.
- Skin: characteristic rashes, skin ulceration, sun sensitivity; Raynaud phenomenon and erythema around fingernails due to vasculopathy
- Weakness such as difficulty rising, climbing stairs, getting out of bed or chair, combing hair
- Gastrointestinal (GI)
  - Dysphonia, dysphagia, choking, and regurgitation of liquids through nose indicate pharyngeal muscle weakness.
  - Constipation, early satiety from muscle weakness
  - Abdominal pain and hematochezia from gut vasculopathy
- Musculoskeletal: myalgia, arthralgia, arthritis, joint contractures
- Often strong family history of various autoimmune diseases

PHYSICAL EXAM

ALERT

Findings requiring immediate evaluation: tachycardia, dyspnea, dysphagia, hematochezia, severe abdominal pain, and inability to stand up from the floor or walk

- Classic rashes in JDM:
  - Heliotrope rash: violaceous discoloration of upper eyelids; can be accompanied by lid swelling, capillary telangiectasia, discoloration below eyes
  - Gottron papules: scaly, erythematous, symmetric, usually hypertrophic but sometimes atrophic papules over extensor surfaces of joints, especially fingers, elbows, knees, and ankles
- Other cutaneous findings in JDM:
  - Malar rash
  - V-sign: erythema of upper chest; shawl-sign includes erythema of shoulders.
  - Nailfold capillary telangiectasia
  - Overgrown, ragged cuticles
  - Edema of skin overlying inflamed muscles
  - Erythema, dilated vessels, ulcerations of hard palate and buccal mucosa
  - Dermatitis of scalp
  - Ulcerations of skin especially of inner canthi, elbows, or at sites of calcinosis
  - Calcinosis cutis is a late finding:
    - Tumorlike calcium deposits at pressure points: elbows, scapulae, ischia
    - Sheetlike or nodular calcification around joints, axillae
- Musculoskeletal findings in JDM and JPM
  - Core weakness: neck, abdominal muscles
  - Proximal weakness: symmetric weakness of shoulder abductors, hip flexors
  - Distal muscle weakness in severe cases
  - Muscle tenderness
  - Waddling (Trendelenburg), wide-based or marching gait due to weak hip flexors
  - Arthritis and joint contractures

ALERT

Some JDM patients have little to no muscle weakness (amyopathic/hypomyopathic JDM). Patients seemingly without weakness with facial, hand, and/or other vasculopathic rashes can be misdiagnosed with eczema or psoriasis.

- Rarely, patients may have myositis and vasculopathic skin findings but lack heliotrope changes and Gottron papules.
- GI: diffuse abdominal tenderness, distension, palpable stool
- CV: tachycardia, murmurs, tachypnea
- Physical exam tips
  - Gower sign: inability to rise from floor without using hands
  - Lying supine on flat exam table without a pillow, patients with neck and abdominal weakness will have difficulty lifting head (chin to chest) or shoulders off bed.
  - Objective measure of strength: duration of straight-leg raise (normal = 20 seconds)
  - Use ophthalmoscope or otoscope to examine nailfolds for telangiectasia.
  - Evaluate for dysphonia by asking child to say "Nancy" or "jug"—listen for a nasal quality.

DIFFERENTIAL DIAGNOSIS

- Infectious/postinfectious: influenza A and B, coxsackievirus B, schistosomiasis, trypanosomiasis; bacterial/pyomyositis if focal
- Trauma (physical, toxic, or drug-induced)
- Myositis with other connective tissue diseases
  - Systemic lupus erythematosus
  - Systemic sclerosis
  - Overlap syndromes including mixed or undifferentiated connective tissue disease
  - Other forms of idiopathic inflammatory myopathy (extremely rare in children): inclusion body myositis, cancer-associated myositis, eosinophilic myositis/fasciitis
- Childhood neuromuscular diseases
  - Muscular dystrophies
  - Congenital myopathies (nemaline rod)
  - Myotonic disorders
  - Metabolic myopathies (glycogen metabolism disorders, mitochondrial myopathies, familial periodic paralysis, lipid myopathies [carnitine deficiencies], myoadenylate deaminase deficiency, myopathy secondary to endocrinopathy)
  - Neurogenic atrophies (spinal muscular atrophy and anterior horn cell dysfunction, peripheral nerve dysfunction, neuromuscular transmission disorders)
- The differential diagnosis for JPM is broader than JDM due to lack of skin findings.

DIAGNOSTIC TESTS & INTERPRETATION

Initial Tests (screening, lab, imaging)

- Muscle enzymes: creatine kinase, aldolase, lactate dehydrogenase, aspartate aminotransferase, alanine aminotransferase
  - One or more is elevated in most cases.

ALERT

Creatine kinase and/or other muscle enzymes can be normal or low in patients with hypomyopathic JDM or long duration of untreated disease.

- Markers of immune activation
  - ESR and C-reactive protein often normal
  - Inflammatory findings in complete blood count often not present
  - Elevated neopterin: secreted by activated macrophages and dendritic cells
  - Elevated von Willebrand factor antigen: marker of endothelial activation
  - Complement generally normal; if low, consider overlap syndrome.
- Autoantibodies
  - Antinuclear antibodies with various antigen specificities may be present.
  - ~63% of JDM/JPM patients have a myositis-specific antibody (MSA). Anti-p-155 and MJ antibodies most common; antisynthetase antibodies (i.e., Jo-1), anti-Mi-2, and antisignal recognition particle are rare in childhood-onset disease.
  - Myositis-associated antibodies (MAAs) are seen in ~16% of JDM/JPM patients, including anti-Ro, anti-U1RNP, and anti-PM-Scl.
  - MSAs and MAAs should be tested by immunoprecipitation using validated assays.
  - Rheumatoid factor and double-stranded DNA antibodies are usually negative; if positive, consider overlap syndrome.
  - Consider celiac disease testing if with GI symptoms, anemia, and weight loss.
- Occult blood in stool; anemia if blood loss
- MRI: Inflamed muscles are identified by signal enhancement on short T1 inversion recovery (STIR) or fat-suppressed T2 sequences; useful to locate site for biopsy
- Video swallow study to identify palatal or proximal esophageal weakness, aspiration
- PFTs to evaluate for respiratory musculature weakness and interstitial lung disease
- EKG and possibly ECHO to evaluate for myocarditis, myocardial dysfunction

Diagnostic Procedures/Other

- Muscle biopsy
- Skin biopsy
- EMG is rarely used in children but can help support diagnosis.
- Pathologic findings
  - Skeletal muscle: perifascicular atrophy; variation in fiber size due to degeneration and regeneration; focal necrosis; lymphocytic and mononuclear infiltrates in the perimysium and perivascular spaces; overexpression of MHC class I
  - Skin: epidermal atrophy, dermal and perivascular lymphocytic infiltrates

TREATMENT

MEDICATION

- Early aggressive therapy improves overall outcome and reduces frequency of calcinosis.
- Prednisone 1 to 2 mg/kg/24 h PO (maximum 60 mg) for 1 month, taper over months to years
- IV methylprednisolone 30 mg/kg/24 h (maximum 1,000 mg) for three infusions at treatment onset; may also be given weekly if concerns for poor oral absorption
- Methotrexate, usually 15 mg/m^2 (maximum generally 25 mg) weekly; SC or IV preferred—PO absorption is poor due to gut vasculopathy.
- IV gammaglobulin, especially helpful for rash
- Hydroxychloroquine, especially useful for rash
- 2nd-line immunosuppressants: cyclosporine, mycophenolate mofetil
- Biologic agents for refractory disease including rituximab and abatacept under investigation
- Topical calcineurin inhibitors for rash
- Aggressive broad-spectrum photoprotection with physical blockers (i.e., titanium dioxide) and chemical blockers (i.e., avobenzone)
- Calcium and vitamin D supplementation
- Treatment of calcinosis may include sodium thiosulfate, diltiazem, and bisphosphonates.

ISSUES FOR REFERRAL

- Pediatric rheumatologist for diagnosis and management
- Speech therapist for dysphagia and dysphonia
- Gastroenterology, cardiology, or pulmonary referral depending on involved organ system
- Plastic surgery referral may be indicated for excision of severe calcifications, but there is risk of recurrence and infection.

ADDITIONAL THERAPIES

Physical and occupational therapy

- Initially to maintain range of movement
- Strengthening after acute inflammation resolves
- Depending on disease severity, patients may require extensive, long-term therapy.

ADMISSION, INPATIENT, AND NURSING CONSIDERATIONS

Respiratory compromise occasionally requires mechanical ventilation.

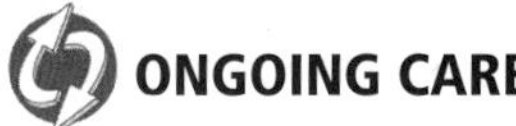

ONGOING CARE

FOLLOW-UP RECOMMENDATIONS

Patient Monitoring

- Serial evaluation of muscle strength and function using validated measures such as the Childhood Myositis Assessment Scale or Manual Muscle Testing
- Muscle enzyme levels to monitor treatment efficacy and flare of inflammation
- Joint range of motion
- Skin exams to check for ulceration, calcinosis
- Steroid-induced myopathy is possible: Consider if weakness worsens or does not improve during treatment.

PATIENT EDUCATION

- Lifelong sun avoidance and sun protection
- Steroid side effects and warnings about physiologic dependence

PROGNOSIS

- Presence of myositis-specific or associated antibodies can predict disease course.
- Normal to good functional outcome: 65–80%
- Muscle atrophy or joint contractures: 25–30%
- Calcinosis cutis: 12–47%
- Wheelchair dependent: 5%
- Death: 1–2% (sepsis, GI bleeding or perforation, respiratory failure, myocarditis)

COMPLICATIONS

- Infections, sepsis due to immunosuppression
- Ulcerative rash and scarring
- Calcinosis cutis
- Skin infections at sites of ulceration, calcinosis
- Lipoatrophy, lipodystrophy
- Muscle fibrosis or arthritis causing joint contractures
- Restrictive, interstitial lung disease
- Aspiration pneumonia due to respiratory weakness and swallowing dysfunction
- Myocarditis (rare)
- GI tract vasculitis causing ulcerations, perforation
- Osteoporosis due to inflammation and glucocorticoids

ADDITIONAL READING

- Feldman BM, Rider LG, Reed AM, et al. Juvenile dermatomyositis and other idiopathic inflammatory myopathies of childhood. *Lancet*. 2008;371(9631):2201–2212.
- Pagnini I, Vitale A, Selmi C, et al. Idiopathic inflammatory myopathies: an update on classification and treatment with special focus on juvenile forms. *Clin Rev Allergy Immunol*. 2017;52(1):34–44.
- Ravelli A, Trail L, Ferrari C, et al. Long-term outcome and prognostic factors of juvenile dermatomyositis: a multinational, multicenter study of 490 patients. *Arthritis Care Res (Hoboken)*. 2010;62(1):63–72.
- Rider LG, Katz JD, Jones OY. Developments in the classification and treatment of the juvenile idiopathic inflammatory myopathies. *Rheum Dis Clin North Am*. 2013;39(4):877–904.
- Rider LG, Pachman LM, Miller FW, et al, eds. *Myositis and You: A Guide to Juvenile Dermatomyositis for Patients, Families, and Healthcare Providers*. Washington, DC: The Myositis Association; 2007.
- Rider LG, Shah M, Mamyrova G, et al; for Childhood Myositis Heterogeneity Collaborative Study Group. The myositis autoantibody phenotypes of the juvenile idiopathic inflammatory myopathies. *Medicine (Baltimore)*. 2013;92(4):223–243.
- Sanner H, Sjaastad I, Flatø B. Disease activity and prognostic factors in juvenile dermatomyositis: a long-term follow-up study applying the Paediatric Rheumatology International Trials Organization criteria for inactive disease and the myositis disease activity assessment tool. *Rheumatology (Oxford)*. 2014;53(9):1578–1585.

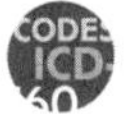

CODES

ICD10

- M33.00 Juvenile dermatopolymyositis, organ involvement unspecified
- M33.02 Juvenile dermatopolymyositis with myopathy

FAQ

- Q: Is it mandatory to perform a muscle biopsy to confirm the diagnosis?
- A: Biopsy is indicated if diagnosis is in any way uncertain. In patients with classic rash, weakness, and elevated muscle enzymes, MRI may suffice. However, biopsy results potentially provide prognostic information so the risks and benefits should be discussed in detail with patients/families.

DEVELOPMENTAL DELAY

Rita Panoscha, MD

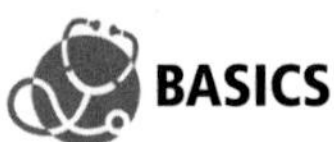

BASICS

DESCRIPTION

- Developmental delay is a descriptive term, not a specific diagnosis, comprising many disorders and encompassing a broad category of etiologies.
- The term describes any situation where a child is not meeting age-appropriate milestones as expected in one or more streams of development. These streams of development include gross motor, fine motor, receptive and expressive language, adaptive, and social (Appendix, Table 1).
- The key feature is that the rate of progress has been slow over time in the area(s) of delay.

ALERT

- Children with behavioral problems may also be masking developmental delays.
- Children with delays in one stream of development may also have delays in other areas of development. For example, language delay may be an indication of general cognitive delays.
- Hearing impairment may present as a delay in development.

EPIDEMIOLOGY

Found in both sexes and all racial and socioeconomic groups

Prevalence

This is a heterogeneous group of disorders with different prevalence rates.

GENERAL PREVENTION

There is no known prevention of developmental delays, although prevention of some of the underlying causes is possible.

PATHOPHYSIOLOGY

- This is highly variable depending on etiology, which can include genetic, familial, metabolic, infectious, endocrinologic, traumatic, anatomic brain malformations, environmental toxins, and degenerative disorders as causes. These disorders often result in some neurologic or neuromuscular injury causing the delay. In many cases, the etiology is never determined.
- Prevalence of this group of disorders may vary depending on the inclusiveness of the definition. The milder delays are quite common and can be found in any pediatric practice. Some disorders in this grouping are more prevalent in boys. The long-term outcome depends on the severity and type of delay, with the more involved children usually having lifelong disability.

ETIOLOGY

Specific etiologies are too numerous to list completely, but a partial list of the more common causes includes the following:

- Genetic/familial
  - Fragile X syndrome
  - Trisomy 21 (Down syndrome)
  - Other chromosomal abnormalities
  - Tuberous sclerosis
  - Neurofibromatosis
  - Phenylketonuria
  - Muscular dystrophy
- Nervous system anomalies
  - Hydrocephalus
  - Lissencephaly
  - Spina bifida
  - Seizures
- Infections
  - Prenatal cytomegalovirus
  - Rubella
  - Toxoplasmosis
  - HIV
  - Postnatal bacterial meningitis
  - Neonatal herpes simplex
- Endocrinologic
  - Congenital hypothyroidism
- Environment
  - Heavy metal poisoning such as lead
  - In utero drug or alcohol exposure
- Trauma/injury
  - Closed head trauma
  - Asphyxia
  - Stroke
  - Perinatal cerebral hemorrhages

COMMONLY ASSOCIATED CONDITIONS

- There are numerous associated findings including seizures, sensory impairments, feeding disorders, psychiatric disorders (especially depression), and behavioral disorders.
- Having a child with significant developmental delays can also add stress to the family in terms of time, finances, and emotions.

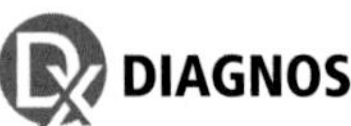

DIAGNOSIS

HISTORY

A complete and detailed history is needed, including the following:

- Pregnancy history
  - Maternal age and parity
  - Maternal complications (including infections and exposures)
  - Medications/drugs used
  - Tobacco or alcohol used, along with quantities
  - Fetal activity
- Birth history
  - Gestational age
  - Birth weight
  - Route of delivery
  - Maternal or fetal complications/distress
  - Apgar scores
- General health
  - Significant illnesses, hospitalizations, or surgeries
  - Accidents or injuries
  - Hearing and vision status
  - Medications used
  - Known exposures to toxins
  - Any new or unusual symptoms
- Developmental history
  - Current developmental achievement in each stream of development
  - Age when developmental milestones were achieved
  - Any loss of skills
  - Where parents think their child is functioning developmentally
- Educational history
  - Type of schooling and services received, if any
  - Any previous educational/developmental testing
- Behavioral history
  - Any perseverative or stereotypical behaviors
  - Interaction skills
  - Attention and activity level
- Family history
  - Anyone with developmental delays, neurologic disorders, syndromes, consanguinity

PHYSICAL EXAM

- A complete physical exam including growth parameters is needed looking for etiology.
- Key features to include:
  - Observation of interactions and behavior: any atypical behaviors and general impression
  - Head circumference: Assess for macrocephaly or microcephaly.
  - Skin: Examine for neurocutaneous lesions.
  - Major or minor dysmorphic features: any indication of a syndrome or anatomic malformation
  - Neurologic examination: Assess for cranial nerve deficits, neuromuscular status, reflexes, balance and coordination, and any soft signs.
  - Developmental testing: Although considerable information will already be available on history and observation, a more formal developmental screening or testing should be done. Possible office tests include the Ages & Stages Questionnaires, the Parents' Evaluation of Developmental Status, or the Capute Scales (formerly called the CAT/CLAMS). Referral to a specialist or a multidisciplinary team for more detailed testing is indicated when delay is suspected.

DIFFERENTIAL DIAGNOSIS

- The differential can be extensive and may become more evident with further workup.
- Broad diagnoses include the following:
  - Intellectual disability
  - Developmental language disorder
  - Autism spectrum disorder
  - Learning disability
  - Cerebral palsy
  - Attention-deficit/hyperactivity disorder
  - Significant visual or hearing impairment
  - Degenerative disorders

DIAGNOSTIC TESTS & INTERPRETATION

Initial Tests (screening, lab, imaging)

- There is no specific laboratory test battery for general developmental delays. The testing needs to be tailored to the individual situation based on the history and physical exam. A high index of suspicion should be maintained for any associated findings and delays in the other streams of development.
- Some of the more common studies ordered for developmental delay workup:
  - Genetic testing: warranted for any dysmorphic features, a family history of delays, or genetic disorder. A karyotype and fragile X DNA testing should be considered, particularly for significant cognitive delays. The comparative genomic hybridization (CGH) microarray is now increasingly recommended as a 1st-line test for developmental delays.
  - Metabolic tests: Tests such as quantitative plasma amino acids, quantitative urine organic acids, lactate, pyruvate, or ammonia should be considered if there is any loss of skills, indication of a metabolic disorder, or newborn metabolic screen has not been done.
  - Thyroid function tests: Most infants will have had screening for hypothyroidism shortly after birth. This should be rechecked if symptoms indicate.
- Head MRI: Consider a head MRI for head abnormalities, significant neurologic findings, loss of skills, or for workup of a specific disorder such as trauma or leukodystrophy.

Diagnostic Procedures/Other

- Audiologic: Hearing should be checked in any child with speech and language and/or cognitive delays.
- EEG: An EEG should be considered if there is any concern about seizures.
- Subspecialists: Referral to other medical specialists may also be indicated. These specialists may include developmental pediatrics, neurology, genetics, orthopedics, or ophthalmology.

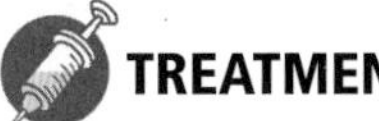

TREATMENT

GENERAL MEASURES

- Therapy should include appropriately treating any medical conditions and associated findings, for example, anticonvulsants for seizures or hearing aids when appropriate for hearing impairment. In addition, traditional therapy has included early intervention or special education services specifically addressing the areas of delay.
- Therapy could include physical therapists, occupational therapists, speech/language therapists, special educators, psychologists, and audiologists, depending on the needs of the child.

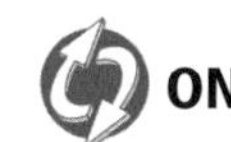

ONGOING CARE

FOLLOW-UP RECOMMENDATIONS

Patient Monitoring

- General pediatric care for well-child visits and to monitor any underlying medical conditions is indicated.
- These children need ongoing monitoring of their therapy and educational programs to ensure that it is still meeting their individual needs as these needs change over time.
- The families will also need ongoing counseling and support in dealing with a child having special needs.

PROGNOSIS

Variable depending on the type and severity of delay and the etiology

ADDITIONAL READING

- Battaglia A, Carey JC. Diagnostic evaluation of developmental delay/mental retardation: an overview. *Am J Med Genet C Semin Med Genet*. 2003;117C(1):3–14.
- Council on Children With Disabilities, Section on Developmental Behavioral Pediatrics, Bright Futures Steering Committee, et al. Identifying infants and young children with developmental disorders in the medical home: an algorithm for developmental surveillance and screening. *Pediatrics*. 2006;118(1):405–420.
- Gerber RJ, Wilks T, Erdie-Lalena C. Developmental milestones: motor development. *Pediatr Rev*. 2010;31(7):267–277.
- Gropman AL, Batshaw ML. Epigenetics, copy number variation, and other molecular mechanisms underlying neurodevelopmental disabilities: new insights and diagnostic approaches. *J Dev Behav Pediatr*. 2010;31(7):582–591.
- Liptak GS. The pediatrician's role in caring for the developmentally disabled child. *Pediatr Rev*. 1996;17(6):203–211.
- Marks KP, LaRosa AC. Understanding developmental-behavioral screening measures. *Pediatr Rev*. 2012;33(10):448–458.
- McQuiston S, Kloczko N. Speech and language development: monitoring process and problems. *Pediatr Rev*. 2011;32(6):230–239.
- Moeschler JB, Shevell M; for American Academy of Pediatrics Committee on Genetics. Clinical genetic evaluation of the child with mental retardation or developmental delays. *Pediatrics*. 2006;117(6):2304–2316.
- Scharf RJ, Scharf GJ, Stroustrup A. Developmental milestones. *Pediatr Rev*. 2016;37(1):25–37, quiz 38, 47.
- Shevell M. Global developmental delay and mental retardation or intellectual disability: conceptualization, evaluation, and etiology. *Pediatr Clin North Am*. 2008;55(5):1071–1084.

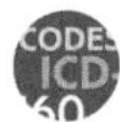

CODES

ICD10

- F89 Unspecified disorder of psychological development
- F82 Specific developmental disorder of motor function
- F80.9 Developmental disorder of speech and language, unspecified

FAQ

- Q: When do you test a child for delays?
- A: A child can have developmental assessments at any age, including infancy. Making a specific diagnosis, for example, for level of intellectual disability, may need to wait until the child is older.
- Q: When can a child start receiving services?
- A: Children who qualify can receive therapy services starting at birth and in some cases extending up to age 21 years.
- Q: The parents are raising a concern about delays, but the general impression in the office is that the child is doing okay. What should be done next?
- A: Parents or grandparents may be the first to express concerns, especially in a child with milder delays. A more detailed developmental history and more formal developmental screening or testing may be indicated as an initial step.

DEVELOPMENTAL DYSPLASIA OF THE HIP

Katherine A. Butler, MD • John E. Tis, MD

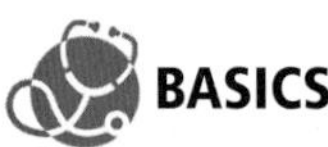

BASICS

DESCRIPTION

Developmental dysplasia of the hip (DDH) is a range of hip pathology including dysplasia (shallow acetabulum), subluxation (partial femoral head–acetabulum contact), and dislocation (no hip joint contact). Abnormalities can be present at birth or develop over time. A teratologic dislocation is a different condition that occurs during fetal development usually from genetic/syndromic causes. Discussion of teratologic dislocation is beyond the scope of this chapter.

EPIDEMIOLOGY

- Female-to-male ratio is 4:1.
- Clinical hip instability occurs in approximately 1 to 2 in 100 newborns.
- Dislocation incidence is about 1 in 1,000 births.
- Bilateral hip dysplasia in approximately 20%

RISK FACTORS

- Compressive factors:
  - Breech position (newborn DDH risk: male 2.6%, female 12%)
  - Oligohydramnios
  - Firstborn child
  - High birth weight
- Demographic factors:
  - Female gender (newborn DDH risk 1.9%)
  - Family history (newborn DDH risk: male 0.9%, female 4.4%)
  - Ethnicity: Native American, Laplander

Genetics

No defined mode of inheritance; family history, gender, and ethnicity association

GENERAL PREVENTION

- Although DDH cannot be prevented, treatment is directed at preventing early arthritis.
- Screening programs have reduced the newborn dislocation rate to 1 in 5,000 children by the age of 18 months.

PATHOPHYSIOLOGY

- The acetabular depth (growth) is determined by healthy cartilage and development around a concentrically reduced/stable femoral head. Cartilage damage occurs from continued instability.
- Untreated subluxation/dislocation can result in an everted labrum, hypertrophic cartilage/labrum complex (neolimbus), and false acetabulum (pseudoacetabulum).
- In early adulthood, this condition can lead to abnormal wear of the joint, limb length differences, and arthritic pain. Compensatory problems may include spinal malalignment (scoliosis/lordosis) and gait abnormalities.

ETIOLOGY

- Scientific understanding is still evolving, but both genetic and environmental factors play a role.
- Mechanical factors: attributed to a smaller in utero environment from oligohydramnios, breech position, increased birth weight, or an unstretched uterus (first pregnancy)
- Female predominance: unclear etiology but has been attributed to estrogen-induced ligamentous laxity
- Left side predominance: attributed to fetal positioning of left hip adduction against the mother's lumbosacral spine
- Native American predominance: attributed to the hip extension/adduction position of swaddling

COMMONLY ASSOCIATED CONDITIONS

- Neurologic conditions (e.g., myelomeningocele)
- Connective tissue disorders (e.g., Ehlers-Danlos)
- Syndromic conditions (e.g., Larsen syndrome)
- Myopathic disorders (e.g., arthrogryposis)

DIAGNOSIS

HISTORY

Gestational age, gender, birth weight, order, delivery method/position (breech), and family history (DDH or associated conditions)

PHYSICAL EXAM

- Ensure that the child is relaxed and calm.
- Screening should be done at all well-child visits until normal ambulatory development.
- Newborn exam
  - Hard signs (<3 months old):
    - Ortolani test: The contralateral hip is flexed, abducted, and held with one hand to stabilize the pelvis. The other hip is held with the thumb in the groin crease and the index/middle finger over the trochanter. With the hip flexed (90 degrees), the trochanter is lifted (anteriorly) as the hip is abducted. An unstable hip will "clunk" as it reduces.
    - Barlow test: similar hand position as the Ortolani test. The hip is flexed (90 degrees), and as the hip is adducted, a posterior stress is applied. An unstable hip will palpably slip out of socket.
    - Galeazzi sign: With bilateral hip and knee flexion, an asymmetry in knee height occurs from apparent femoral shortening on the dislocated side.
  - Soft signs:
    - "Packaging" abnormalities: torticollis, limb deformity (metatarsus adductus), joint contractures, or dislocation of other joints
    - Asymmetric skinfolds (low sensitivity)
    - Sacral dimple
- Ambulatory child exam:
  - Stiffness: limited or asymmetric abduction (normally abduction >75 degrees, adduction >30 degrees)
  - Limb length difference: unilateral toe walking, abnormal Galeazzi sign, scoliosis
  - Gait: lurching to one side (Trendelenburg gait)
  - Bilateral dislocation: may have waddling gait and hyperlordosis. Galeazzi sign will be normal; may be difficult to recognize

ALERT

- Early diagnosis and referral are paramount.
- Main instability indicators are the Barlow and Ortolani exams. Perform these gently.
- Soft tissue clicks superficial in sound and most asymmetric thigh folds are normal.
- An unreducible hip may have a falsely normal Ortolani/Barlow exam but will be Galeazzi positive.
- Hip exam should be performed before referral for further imaging.

DIFFERENTIAL DIAGNOSIS

- Septic hip
- Congenital coxa vara
- Proximal femoral focal deficiency

DIAGNOSTIC TESTS & INTERPRETATION

Initial Tests (screening, lab, imaging)

- If the clinical exam findings are clearly abnormal, orthopedic referral is indicated. No further imaging is needed for referral.
- Imaging is used to clarify an equivocal examination and to monitor treatment progress.
- Ultrasound
  - Optimal age: 3 weeks to 5 months
  - Static examination: Superior acetabular coverage (α-angle) and femoral head position (β-angle) are assessed.
  - Dynamic examination: assesses stability
  - Can be used to monitor improvement in bony acetabular development over time
  - Used to ensure reduction of previously dislocated hips after treatment initiation
- Plain radiographs (AP pelvis ± frog lateral)
  - Optimal age: after 3 to 6 months
- CT scan/MRI
  - May be used to assess concentric hip reduction after closed reduction and cast application or open hip reduction

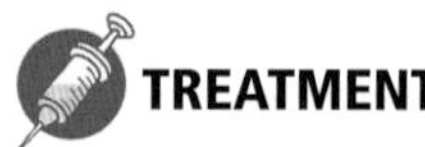

TREATMENT

GENERAL MEASURES

Treatment principle: Acetabular remodeling potential rarely exists after 4 years of age. When remodeling potential exists, treatment goals are to redirect the femoral head into the acetabulum with minimal force while avoiding complications of avascular necrosis and cartilage damage.

ISSUES FOR REFERRAL

Primary care providers (PCPs) algorithm of care:

- Initial (newborn) exam
  - Abnormal (Ortolani or Barlow positive, asymmetric hip abduction after 4 weeks, positive Galeazzi sign): orthopedic referral
  - Inconclusive (soft exam findings only): Send for ultrasound after 2 to 3 weeks of age. If abnormal, refer.

- Normal exam
  - If no risk factors: Reexamine at every well-child visit until normal ambulatory development.
  - If one or more risk factors (breech, breech position, family history, or history of improper swaddling): Consider imaging be performed at 6 weeks to 6 months of age (ultrasound 6 weeks to 4 months or AP pelvis after 4 months).
  - If patient has imaging with abnormalities, referral is indicated. Immediate bracing was previously indicated, although there is emerging evidence that close clinical and radiographic follow-up may be adequate in some cases.
- Follow-up (postnewborn) exam: if abnormalities exist after the initial newborn period, then referral with ultrasound (if <5 months of age) or radiographs (if >4 to 6 months of age)

ADDITIONAL THERAPIES

Pavlik harness

- Indications: if earlier criteria is met for referral, but referral is not possible and child is <6 months of age or the PCP is trained in Pavlik harness use
- Abduction brace (more rigid) can be used if treatment extends past 6 months of age.
- For a reducible hip:
  - Place harness full time with joint reduced (may confirm with ultrasound).
  - Reexamine hips and readjust harness every 3 weeks.
  - Monitor patient for femoral nerve palsy at each follow-up visit. If palsy develops, decrease hip flexion in harness.
  - Repeat ultrasound ~6 to 12 weeks.
  - Once hip exam is normal, continue full-time Pavlik harness use for additional 6 to 12 weeks.
  - Radiograph at 6, 12 months
- For hip dislocation (nonteratologic):
  - Follow the earlier protocol except
    - Initial ultrasound and radiographs for documentation of dislocation
    - Clinically reassess every 7 to 10 days until hip reduces.
    - If hip reduces, document with ultrasound.
    - Radiographs at 3 months
    - Refer patient and abandon harness treatment if not reduced by 3 weeks.
- Pavlik harness application:
  - Chest strap: nipple level, snug but should be able to comfortable fit examiner's index finger underneath strap
  - Shoulder strap: should cross posteriorly, snug
  - Stirrup: should start distal to the popliteal fossa
  - Anterior strap: midaxillary line strap adjusted so hip is flexed at 90 to 100 degrees
  - Posterior strap: attaches over the scapula, adjusted so hips do not adduct (do not force abduction)

ALERT

- Pavlik harness use is safe when properly placed.
- Never force the hip into position.
- If a Pavlik harness is placed on a dislocated hip, patient should be followed closely to reduction after harness placement. If no reduction after 3 weeks, discontinue brace and refer.
- Improper use can lead to cartilage damage, femoral nerve palsy, and avascular necrosis.

SURGERY/OTHER PROCEDURES

- Closed reduction:
  - Used when Pavlik harness treatment fails
  - Spica cast is applied for 2 to 6 months.
- Open reduction:
  - Used when closed reduction fails usually due to soft tissue interposition and/or muscle contracture
  - Common after 6 months of age
  - Adductor tenotomy is usually done.
  - Spica cast is applied after hip is reduced.
- Osteotomy:
  - After about age 2 years, excessive force is needed for a closed/open reduction.
  - Femoral osteotomy reduces this risk along with an open reduction.
  - For residual dysplasia, acetabular osteotomies are performed.

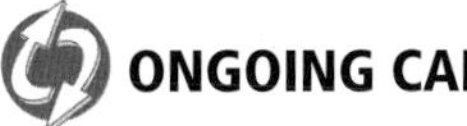

ONGOING CARE

FOLLOW-UP RECOMMENDATIONS

Patient Monitoring

See "Issues for Referral" section.

PROGNOSIS

- 95% successful resolution of an abnormal Ortolani exam when Pavlik harness treatment is initiated in a newborn
- 85% success when the same treatment is started after 1 month of age

COMPLICATIONS

- Pavlik harness
  - Tight shoulder strap: brachial plexopathy, skin breakdown
  - Hip hyperflexion: femoral nerve palsy, inferior dislocation
  - Forced abduction. Compression of vascular structures may lead to avascular necrosis and growth arrest.
  - Poor hygiene: skin breakdown (groin crease and popliteal fossa)
- Failure or lack of treatment: residual dysplasia, instability/growth arrest resulting in limb length difference, scoliosis/lordosis, decreased hip arc of motion, premature osteoarthritis, gait disturbance

ADDITIONAL READING

- American Academy of Orthopaedic Surgeons. Detection and nonoperative management of pediatric development dysplasia of the hip in infants up to six months of age: evidence based clinical practice guideline. http://www.aaos.org/research/guidelines/DDHGuidelineFINAL.pdf. Accessed April 19, 2018.
- American Academy of Pediatrics. Clinical practice guideline: early detection of developmental dysplasia of the hip. *Pediatrics*. 2000;105(4 Pt 1):896–905.
- American Institute of Ultrasound in Medicine. AIUM practice guideline for the performance of an ultrasound examination for detection and assessment of developmental dysplasia of the hip. *J Ultrasound Med*. 2013;32(7):1307–1317.
- Guille JT, Pizzutillo PD, MacEwen GD. Development dysplasia of the hip from birth to six months. *J Am Acad Orthop Surg*. 2000;8(4):232–242.
- Mahan ST, Katz JN, Kim YJ. To screen or not to screen? A decision analysis of the utility of screening for developmental dysplasia of the hip. *J Bone Joint Surg Am*. 2009;91(7):1705–1719.
- Nemeth BA, Narotam V. Developmental dysplasia of the hip. *Pediatr Rev*. 2012;33(12):553–561.
- Shaw BA, Segal LS; for AAP Section on Orthopaedics. Evaluation and referral for developmental dysplasia of the hip in infants. *Pediatrics*. 2016;138(6):e20163107.
- Storer SK, Skaggs DL. Developmental dysplasia of the hip. *Am Fam Physician*. 2006;74(8):1310–1316.
- Vitale MG, Skaggs DL. Developmental dysplasia of the hip from six months to four years of age. *J Am Acad Orthop Surg*. 2001;9(6):401–411.
- Weinstein SL, Mubarak SJ, Wenger DR. Developmental hip dysplasia and dislocation: part I. *Instr Course Lect*. 2004;53:523–530.
- Weinstein SL, Mubarak SJ, Wenger DR. Developmental hip dysplasia and dislocation: part II. *Instr Course Lect*. 2004;53:531–542.
- Westacott D, Pattison G, Cooke S. Developmental dysplasia of the hip. *Community Pract*. 2012;85(11):42–44.

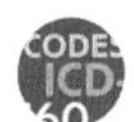

CODES

ICD10

Q65.89 Other specified congenital deformities of hip

FAQ

- Q: Is emergent or urgent orthopedic referral required if hip instability in the newborn is diagnosed?
- A: No. Although referral should not be delayed for months, it can be obtained 2 to 3 weeks after diagnosis.
- Q: Why are ultrasound and radiographs used at different age ranges?
- A: After about 3 months of age, radiographs become easier to assess, as radiographs require ossification, and ultrasound waves cannot penetrate ossified bone. The hip is not fully ossified at birth, rendering early radiographic examination difficult.
- Q: Why are the Barlow/Ortolani exams used before 3 months of age but not as useful later?
- A: These exams become less useful as the hip naturally stiffens after 3 months, as stiffness results in asymmetric motion and may mask instability.

D

DIABETES INSIPIDUS

Todd D. Nebesio, MD, FAAP

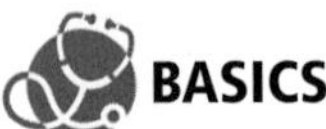

BASICS

DESCRIPTION

Polyuria and polydipsia caused by the inability to produce or respond to antidiuretic hormone; also called arginine vasopressin

EPIDEMIOLOGY

Because most cases are secondary to another disease, the incidence depends on the primary cause.

RISK FACTORS

Genetics

- Rare genetic causes of central diabetes insipidus (DI) are usually autosomal dominant mutations (neuronal degeneration) and rarely recessive (biologically inactive hormone).
- Nephrogenic DI is usually familial (autosomal recessive or dominant and X-linked).

PATHOPHYSIOLOGY

- Antidiuretic hormone stimulates the formation of cyclic adenosine monophosphate (cAMP) in the renal collecting ducts, thereby increasing water permeability and increasing reabsorption of free water.
- Lack of antidiuretic hormone effect results in urinary loss of free water.
- Patients with an intact thirst mechanism drink copiously (polydipsia) to compensate for free water loss.
- If the thirst mechanism is not present or if access to free water is limited (e.g., infants, developmentally delayed child, or vomiting), severe dehydration can occur.

ETIOLOGY

- Insufficient antidiuretic hormone secretion
  - Traumatic or postsurgical
  - Nonaccidental injury
  - Related to tumor invasion of posterior pituitary
  - Extension from anterior pituitary/suprasellar region: optic glioma, rarely adenomas
  - Hypothalamic: germinoma, craniopharyngioma, meningioma
  - Lymphoma
  - Granulomas: histiocytosis, sarcoidosis
  - Metastatic carcinoma
  - Post–severe ischemic or hypoxic injury to the brain
  - Familial (autosomal dominant)
  - Congenital malformation of CNS
  - Infection: viral encephalitis, meningitis, tuberculosis
  - Increased metabolic clearance of antidiuretic hormone (gestational DI)
  - Drug or toxin related: snake venom, tetrodotoxin
  - Autoimmune disorders: hypophysitis (inflammation of the pituitary gland)
  - Psychogenic: excessive water drinking
  - Idiopathic: must observe for many years to exclude slow-growing tumors
- Unresponsive to antidiuretic hormone
  - Familial or nephrogenic (X-linked dominant and autosomal recessive forms)
  - Tumor related
  - Urinary tract obstruction, especially in utero
  - Renal medullary cystic disease
  - Electrolyte disturbances: hypokalemia, hypercalcemia (hypercalciuria)
  - Drugs: usually reversible (diuretics, diphenylhydantoin, reserpine, cisplatin, rifampin, lithium [may become permanent], demeclocycline, ethanol, chlorpromazine, volatile anesthetics, foscarnet, amphotericin B)
  - Loss of the medullary concentrating gradient due to excessive free water intake relative to solute intake

ALERT

Pitfalls

- Management of patients without an intact thirst mechanism and of newborns is difficult.
- Patients with psychogenic polydipsia may fail a water deprivation test because prolonged excessive water intake can wash out the renal medullary gradient required for concentrating the urine.
- Surreptitious water intake during water deprivation test
- Idiopathic, acquired DI can be caused by slowly growing brain tumors not visible on the initial magnetic resonance image.

DIAGNOSIS

HISTORY

- Abnormal growth can be a sign of DI.
- Waking up during the night to drink or void:
  - True DI is associated with polyuria throughout the day and night. Enuresis may be the first sign in a child who previously acquired bladder control. Patients, including infants, prefer ice-cold water to other liquids.
- Number of hours the patient goes without drinking:
  - Patients with complete DI do not voluntarily stop drinking for >1 to 2 hours unless the thirst mechanism is also abnormal.
  - Patients with DI have such overwhelming thirst that they will drink anything, including bath and toilet water.
- Volume of urine output in a day (not just frequency of urination):
  - The daily volume of urine can be as high as 4 to 10 L.
  - Younger or dehydrated children with DI tend to make less urine daily than older or hydrated children with DI.
- Familial history of DI:
  - Nephrogenic DI will typically affect maternal uncles during infancy, and mothers may have a mild form.
- Frequent episodes of dehydration requiring medical attention:
  - Families may disregard the polydipsia as normal behavior.
  - Repeated episodes of severe dehydration can lead to brain damage.
- Treatment of adrenal insufficiency in a patient with panhypopituitarism can unmask DI (i.e., one needs cortisol to excrete free water).

PHYSICAL EXAM

- Signs of dehydration:
  - DI is typically associated with dry, pale skin and mucous membranes. Because this is hyperosmolar dehydration, the patient may not look as severely dehydrated as she or he is.
- Complete neurologic exam:
  - Check for impaired visual fields, which can be the first sign of brain tumor.

DIFFERENTIAL DIAGNOSIS

- Psychogenic polydipsia
- Abnormal thirst mechanism (dipsogenic DI)
- Hypernatremic dehydration
- Diabetes mellitus
- Polyuric renal failure (e.g., renal tubulopathy)
- Hypercalcemia
- Cerebral salt wasting
- Hyperthyroidism
- Hypokalemia

DIAGNOSTIC TESTS & INTERPRETATION

- Morning urinary osmolality with simultaneous serum sodium and serum osmolality
  - If urine osmolality is at least 2 times higher than serum osmolality, patient does not have complete DI but may still have partial DI.
- Water deprivation test
  - Although definitive, it requires admission to the hospital for controlled testing under the close supervision of a pediatric endocrinologist. Patient fails test if urinary osmolality cannot concentrate to more than twice serum osmolality at the same time that serum osmolality exceeds 305 mOsm/kg; serum osmolality exceeds 305 mOsm/kg at any time; or patient loses >5% of body weight and becomes symptomatic from hypovolemia.
  - Once patient fails the water deprivation test, a dose of aqueous vasopressin should be given followed by close monitoring of urinary osmolality to document responsiveness to antidiuretic hormone.
  - Never attempt a water deprivation trial at home. Tell parents to allow free access to water at home in any suspected cases.

- Urinary specific gravity (nonspecific)
  - Insufficient by itself and nondiagnostic during a water deprivation test
- 24-hour urine collection (home testing)
  - To obtain accurate urinary volume while patient has free access to water
- MRI of the brain with and without contrast, with special cuts of the pituitary and hypothalamus: to confirm the bright spot normally seen in the posterior pituitary and to search for tumors. Its absence is not pathognomonic of central DI.

ALERT
Do not restrict water intake unless the patient is in the hospital under close surveillance. Pitfall: Checking random (nonfasting) labs are often normal in those with an intact thirst mechanism and may be misleading and falsely reassuring.

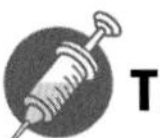

TREATMENT

MEDICATION

- Desmopressin (DDAVP®): intranasal spray or oral tablets
- Aqueous vasopressin: SC
  - Comes as 4 mcg/mL solution and doses range from 0.05 mcg up to 1 mcg SC b.i.d. daily. Titrate dose as you would with DDAVP®.
- Duration of action of DDAVP® is variable from patient to patient. Titration and frequency of dosing should be made under supervision of a pediatric endocrinologist.
- Control of DI in infants is more difficult.
  - These patients may increase fluid intake because of hunger or increase caloric intake because of thirst, thereby causing an imbalance between free water intake and output.
  - Infants can be treated with diluted formula—the volume and frequency of feedings will be increased, but intake of free water will better match urine output.
  - DDAVP® should not be used in infants.
  - In some cases, low renal solute load formula (e.g., Similac PM 60/40®) and/or thiazide diuretics have been used in infancy.
  - Strict record keeping of intake/output and accurate daily weighing are usually necessary for infants or patients without an intact thirst mechanism.
  - All infants with DI must be treated by experienced providers.
- Nephrogenic DI may be treated with diuretics and solute restriction as these patients are resistant to DDAVP®.
- Side effects:
  - Facial flushing
  - Increased blood pressure
  - Headache
  - Nasal congestion
  - Hyponatremia: caused by water overdose (intoxication), not by overdose of drug. Taking a higher dose of DDAVP® will generally extend the period of antidiuresis but will not cause hyponatremia. Drinking too much water in the setting of antidiuresis causes hyponatremia. Water intoxication most often occurs in antidiuresed patients who also are on IV fluids, lack an intact thirst mechanism, or have psychogenic polydipsia.
- Treatment duration is generally lifelong; some tumors regress with radiation, allowing recovery of antidiuretic hormone secretion.
- Possible conflicts with other treatments:
  - Nasal congestion or gastrointestinal illness can affect the absorption of DDAVP® administered.

ONGOING CARE

FOLLOW-UP RECOMMENDATIONS

Patient Monitoring

- Depends on the patient and underlying disease causing the DI
- When to expect improvement:
  - Effects of DDAVP® are immediate.
  - Most cases of DI are lifelong; one exception is DI that occurs during the 7 to 10 days immediately after neurosurgery because this postsurgical DI may resolve spontaneously within 1 to 2 weeks after surgery (part of the triple-phase response).
- Signs to watch for:
  - Lethargy
  - Somnolence
  - Irritability
  - Hyperpyrexia
  - Any sign of dehydration
  - Seizures

DIET

- Patients with an intact thirst mechanism should drink only when thirsty.
- Patients without an intact thirst mechanism should drink only a carefully calculated fluid volume.

PROGNOSIS

- Generally good but depends on the primary cause
- May cause developmental delay if the hypernatremia is prolonged

COMPLICATIONS

- Without treatment and without access to water:
  - Hypernatremia
  - Dehydration
  - Coma
- When overdosed with water:
  - Hyponatremia
  - Seizures
  - Cerebral edema

ADDITIONAL READING

- Al Nofal A, Lteif A. Thiazide diuretics in the management of young children with central diabetes insipidus. *J Pediatr*. 2015;167(3):658–661.
- Dabrowski E, Kadakia R, Zimmerman D. Diabetes insipidus in infants and children. *Best Pract Res Clin Endocrinol Metab*. 2016;30(2):317–328.
- Di Iorgi N, Napoli F, Allegri AE, et al. Diabetes insipidus—diagnosis and management. *Horm Res Paediatr*. 2012;77(2):69–84.
- Ghirardello S, Garrè ML, Rossi A, et al. The diagnosis of children with central diabetes insipidus. *J Pediatr Endocrinol Metab*. 2007;20(3):359–375.
- Linshaw MA. Back to basics: congenital nephrogenic diabetes insipidus. *Pediatr Rev*. 2007;28(10):372–380.
- Maghnie M, Cosi G, Genovese E, et al. Central diabetes insipidus in children and young adults. *N Engl J Med*. 2000;343(14):998–1007.

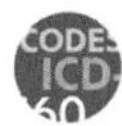

CODES

ICD10

- E23.2 Diabetes insipidus
- N25.1 Nephrogenic diabetes insipidus

FAQ

- Q: In a patient with an intact thirst mechanism and partial DI, is the use of DDAVP® necessary?
- A: No, as long as the patient has constant access to free water.
- Q: How does therapy of DI affect daily life? Is it easily integrated into normal activity and eating patterns?
- A: DDAVP® is used in a patient with an intact thirst mechanism to facilitate the daily routine as well as to allow patients to sleep without the need to void frequently during the night.
- Q: Is there a longer acting preparation or an implantable pump for dosing?
- A: The longest acting form of antidiuretic hormone is an injected medication and can have effects for 3 days, increasing the risks of hyponatremia. Home use of the nasal spray or tablets, therefore, is easier and safer than the use of injections.
- Q: In cases of central DI, is it necessary to screen for anterior pituitary hormone deficiencies?
- A: Yes—at diagnosis of DI and during follow-up as other pituitary hormone deficiencies can occur over time.

D

DIABETES MELLITUS, TYPE I

R. Paul Wadwa, MD

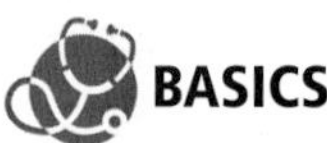

BASICS

DESCRIPTION

Type 1 diabetes is an autoimmune disorder that causes pancreatic β-cell destruction. This destruction leads to insulin deficiency that results in hyperglycemia and disrupts energy storage and metabolism. Severe insulin deficiency can lead to ketosis, acidosis, dehydration, shock, and death.

EPIDEMIOLOGY

- Most common endocrine disorder of childhood
- More common in whites of Northern European descent

Incidence

- Annual U.S. incidence is <19/100,000 in children 10 to 19 years old.
- Incidence of type 1 diabetes is rising by 3% per year overall and faster in young children.

Prevalence

- Prevalence of type 1 diabetes in youth 0 to 19 years in United States is <2/1,000.
- Note: At least 2% of diabetes in children may be due to maturity-onset diabetes of youth (MODY) or other genetic forms.

RISK FACTORS

Genetics

- Increased susceptibility to type 1 diabetes associated with HLA region of chromosome 6, 5-fold greater risk with MHC antigen types DR3 and DR4
- MODY is a group of autosomal dominant syndromes of partial insulin deficiency due to monogenic defects of pancreatic development or insulin secretion; they comprise a small fraction of childhood diabetes.

PATHOPHYSIOLOGY

- Loss of pancreatic β cells results in insulin deficiency, leading to hyperglycemia and predominance of catabolic processes.
- Hyperglycemia causes hyperosmolality, polyuria, and damage to small blood vessels.
- Catabolic processes produce ketosis, weight loss, and metabolic acidosis.

ETIOLOGY

- An environmental trigger (likely viral) induces expression of antigens on β-cell surface.
- Recruitment of cytotoxic lymphocytes
- Production of anti-insulin and anti-islet cell antibodies (including GAD65, ICA512, ZnT8)
- Progressive inflammatory, autoimmune loss of β-cell mass results in insulin deficiency.
- Autoimmunity precedes hyperglycemia; development of two or more antibodies will inevitably lead to dysglycemia due to type 1 diabetes.
- The autoimmune destruction of β cells is more likely in genetically susceptible persons.

COMMONLY ASSOCIATED CONDITIONS

- Autoimmune thyroid disease
  - Hashimoto (hypothyroidism) more common than Graves (hyperthyroidism)
- Celiac disease
- More rarely other autoimmune diseases, such as alopecia areata, rheumatoid arthritis
- Depression
- After prolonged hyperglycemia: vascular complications:
  - Microvascular
    - Nephropathy
    - Retinopathy
    - Neuropathy
    - (See "Patient Monitoring" for screening recommendations.)
  - Macrovascular
    - Peripheral vascular disease
    - Cardiovascular disease

DIAGNOSIS

HISTORY

- Duration of symptoms prior to diagnosis varies by age: may be days in toddlers, months in adolescents.
- Polyuria, nocturia, and enuresis are related to hyperglycemia >180 mg/dL.
- Polydipsia: due to polyuria, hyperosmolality
- Polyphagia: appetite amplified by loss of calories from glycosuria; this is often absent.
- Weight loss: dehydration, loss of calories
- Malaise, nausea, vomiting, abdominal pain, hyperventilation, lethargy due to ketosis, acidosis, electrolyte depletion, hyperosmolality
- MODY is usually asymptomatic.

PHYSICAL EXAM

- Weight loss common at presentation of type 1 diabetes
- Candidal vaginitis and balanitis common in young children with type 1 diabetes
- In ketoacidosis: dehydration, hyperventilation

DIFFERENTIAL DIAGNOSIS

- MODY
- Type 2 diabetes (in obese pubertal youth)
- Urinary tract infection (polyuria)
- Renal glycosuria
- Stress-related hyperglycemia
- Drug-induced hyperglycemia (steroids)
- Psychogenic polydipsia
- Pneumonia (in diabetic ketoacidosis [DKA])
- Sepsis (in DKA)
- Acute surgical abdomen (in ketoacidosis)

DIAGNOSTIC TESTS & INTERPRETATION

- Diagnosis based on blood glucose (BG) concentration:
  - Fasting BG ≥126 mg/dL, random BG ≥200 mg/dL, or 2-hour BG ≥200 mg/dL on oral glucose tolerance test (OGTT), and exclusion of stress hyperglycemia
  - Asymptomatic hyperglycemia requires repeat confirmation.
- HgbA1c reflects BG levels of previous 2 to 3 months and is nearly always elevated at diagnosis.
- Glycosuria may be intermittent.
- Ketonuria may occur with both type 1 and type 2 diabetes.
- With presence of ketonuria or ketosis, DKA should be ruled out by checking serum bicarbonate.
- GAD, islet cell, ZnT8, and/or insulin autoantibodies are positive in most persons with type 1 diabetes at onset (85–90%).
- In some patients presenting with hyperglycemia and ketosis, not possible to distinguish type 1 from type 2 until the course over several months has been followed

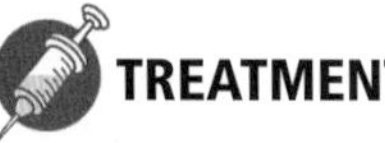

TREATMENT

GENERAL MEASURES

- Insulin is administered as a fixed or flexible regimen.
- Total daily dose (TDD)—calculated by adding up all short- and long-acting insulin given over 24 hours—usually ~0.7 to 1.2 U/kg/24 h; choose higher range for ketoacidosis presentation, obesity, and puberty.
- Doses may decline during "honeymoon period."
- Fixed insulin regimens require fewer shots but consistent schedule and eating; generally providing suboptimal glycemic control
- Historically, common fixed regimen is split-mixed: 2/3 of TDD in morning (1/3 as short-acting and 2/3 long-acting) and 1/3 of TDD in evening (with 1/2 as short-acting and 1/2 as long-acting), either at dinner or split between dinner and bedtime.
- Flexible insulin regimens consist of basal insulin plus a short-acting bolus for every carbohydrate meal and for high blood sugar.
- Basal dosing
  - 40–50% of TDD is given as one injection of a long-acting insulin such as glargine (Lantus, Basaglar) or detemir (Levemir).
  - Sometimes, these long-acting insulins are split into twice daily doses given ~12 hours apart.
- Boluses of short-acting insulin (lispro, aspart, faster acting insulin aspart, or glulisine) are given for meals and snacks based on carbohydrate content and BGs.
  - Carbohydrate coverage (grams of carbohydrate covered by 1 unit) can be estimated by dividing the TDD by 500.
  - Hyperglycemia coverage ("corrective dose") can be estimated by dividing the TDD to 1,800 to find how much 1 unit of insulin may lower blood sugar.
- Another flexible method uses SC insulin infusion by pump that administers a continuous basal infusion.
  - Patient gives manually administered bolus doses of rapid-acting analog insulin at mealtimes and corrective doses.
  - Dosing guidelines are similar.
  - Insulin pump use has increased within the past few years.
  - Recently, a "hybrid closed loop" systems that adjusts infusion rates based on glucoses from a continuous glucose monitor has become available.
- Blood sugars are generally monitored using fingerstick blood sugars and a glucose meter before meals and snacks, at bedtime, and as needed for symptoms of hypo- and hyperglycemia for a total of 6 to 10 times per day.
  - Continuous glucose monitoring (CGM) provides glucose monitoring in addition to standard fingerstick blood sugars using a sensor placed subcutaneously, a transmitter and receiver.
  - CGM use provides sensor glucose values every 5 minutes and alarms may be set for high and low glucose thresholds.
  - Some CGM is able to be used "nonadjunctively" to replace fingerstick glucose testing, although it requires calibration with fingerstick blood sugars.
  - "Flash" glucose monitors are also now available that do not need calibration and provide an "intermittently viewed" glucose reading without fingerstick.

MEDICATION

(See insulin regimens under "General Measures.") Insulin is required to treat type 1 diabetes.

- Insulins:
  - Rapid-acting analogs:
    - Aspart (NovoLog®), lispro (Humalog®), glulisine (Apidra®), faster acting insulin aspart (Fiasp®)
    - Onset of action 5 to 15 minutes, peak action 60 to 90 minutes, and duration 2 to 5 hours

- Short-acting
  - Regular insulin—used for IV delivery, can be used for SC injection
  - Onset of action when given SC—30 to 60 minutes, peak 2 to 3 hours, duration 6 to 9 hours
- Intermediate-acting
  - NPH (Humulin N®, Novolin N®)
    - Onset 1 to 2 hours, peak action 3 to 8 hours, duration 12 to 15 hours
    - Use is less common when long-acting analogs available.
- Long-acting analogs
  - Detemir (Levemir®), glargine (Lantus®, Basaglar®, Toujeo®), degludec (Tresiba®)
  - Onset—3 to 4 hours, no significant peak, duration 20 to 24 hours (glargine, detemir), up to 42 hours (degludec)
  - Different concentrations (U200, U300) available but rarely used in pediatrics

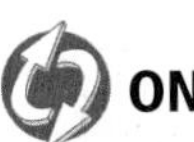

ONGOING CARE

FOLLOW-UP RECOMMENDATIONS

Patient Monitoring

- Regular appointments with diabetes specialist every 3 months to assess management:
  - HgbA1c assessment at each visit (with generally recommended goal of <7.5% for children)
  - Is diabetes interfering with emotional health, family relationships, school attendance, athletic activities, or social development?
  - Is family minimizing hospitalization risks from hypoglycemia or DKA with appropriate adjustment of insulin, recognition of lows, glucagon availability, ketone testing, and telephone contact?
  - Is family reducing long-term complication risk by keeping HgbA1c lower and by avoiding or treating other risk factors?
  - Exam: growth, weight, blood pressure, thyromegaly, liver size, pubertal status, injection/infusion sites, feet, skin lesions
- Meet with nutritionist periodically/as needed to reassess meal plan.
- Meet with psychologist or social worker as needed to address psychosocial issues.
- Regular screening for long-term complications:
  - Annual urine for microalbumin after 12 years of age, 3 to 5 years diabetes duration
  - Periodic lipid profile, thyroid screening (T_4, TSH or TSH and thyroid antibodies), celiac screen
  - Annual eye exam to detect early retinopathy after 10 years of age, 3 to 5 years diabetes duration

DIET

- Dietary education for type 1 diabetes is directed toward healthy distribution and matching of carbohydrate intake with insulin action:
  - Recommended distribution of calories: 55% from carbohydrates (mostly complex), 30% from fats, 15% from protein
  - Fixed insulin regimens require snacks spaced between meals and before bedtime.
  - Carbohydrate counting is essential for flexible insulin regimens and helpful for maintaining consistency for fixed regimens.
- Reduction of saturated and trans fats, rapidly digested carbohydrates, and salt may be beneficial in both types of diabetes.

PATIENT EDUCATION

- Insulin injection/infusion and site rotation
- Home BG monitoring at least 6 to 10 times per day. Many patients will need to test more frequently: before meals, when feeling hypoglycemic, or ill.
- In 2016, the U.S. Food and Drug Administration (FDA) approved "nonadjunctive" CGM use permits using certain CGM values in place of fingerstick blood sugars for some diabetes treatment decisions (see "General Measures" section under "Treatment" above for CGM information).
- Diet: carbohydrate counting
- Oral carbohydrate for mild hypoglycemia; glucagon 0.5 to 1 mg IM for severe hypoglycemia (lower dose given in children <20 kg)
- Activity:
  - Frequent exercise reduces BG and insulin requirements in both types of diabetes.
  - Exercise may require extra carbohydrate intake or reduced insulin doses to prevent hypoglycemia in type 1 diabetes.
  - Detecting or preventing hypoglycemia during or after physical exercise
- Prevention: checking urine for ketones when blood sugar is high or child feels ill; extra insulin for ketones

COMPLICATIONS

DKA: most common cause of hospitalization and death in type 1 diabetes in childhood. See "Diabetic Ketoacidosis."

ALERT

DKA should be treated in the emergency department or inpatient setting. The risk for morbidity and mortality due to cerebral edema or other complications of DKA is high.

- Hypoglycemia
  - This most common acute complication; limits achievable glycemic control
  - If severe, may cause seizure, unconsciousness
- Long-term harm may be reduced by better glycemic control:
  - Nephropathy: Microalbuminuria and hypertension are first manifestations before adulthood.
  - Retinopathy: Blood vessel changes may occur in childhood but not vision loss.
  - Neuropathy: diminished nerve conduction velocity common; paresthesias are earliest symptoms.
  - Vasculopathy: Large vessel disease begins in childhood, but clinical effects occur in adults.
  - Prenatal harm to infants of diabetic mothers: Birth defects occur early, large size late.
  - Growth failure (Mauriac syndrome) and delayed sexual maturation
- Depression, family stress, higher divorce rate

ADDITIONAL READING

- American Diabetes Association. 2. Classification and diagnosis of diabetes: *Standards of Medical Care in Diabetes-2018*. *Diabetes Care*. 2018;41(Suppl 1):S13–S27.
- Atkinson MA, Eisenbarth GS, Michels AW. Type 1 diabetes. *Lancet*. 2014;383(9911):69–82.
- Chiang JL, Kirkman MS, Laffel LM, et al; for Type 1 Diabetes Sourcebook Authors. Type 1 diabetes through the life span: a position statement of the American Diabetes Association. *Diabetes Care*. 2014;37(7):2034–2054.
- Insel RA, Dunne JL, Atkinson MA, et al. Staging presymptomatic type 1 diabetes: a scientific statement of JDRF, the Endocrine Society, and the American Diabetes Association. *Diabetes Care*. 2015;38(10):1964–1974.
- Kovatchev B, Tamborlane WV, Cefalu WT, et al. The artificial pancreas in 2016: a digital treatment ecosystem for diabetes. *Diabetes Care*. 2016;39(7):1123–1126.
- Nguyen TM, Mason KJ, Sanders CG, et al. Targeting blood glucose management in school improves glycemic control in children with poorly controlled type 1 diabetes mellitus. *J Pediatr*. 2008;153(4):575–578.
- Skyler JS, Bakris GL, Bonifacio E, et al. Differentiation of diabetes by pathophysiology, natural history, and prognosis. *Diabetes*. 2017;66(2):241–255.
- Steinke JM, Mauer M; for International Diabetic Nephropathy Study Group. Lessons learned from studies of the natural history of diabetic nephropathy in young type 1 diabetic patients. *Pediatr Endocrinol Rev*. 2008;5(Suppl 4):958–963.
- Tamborlane WV, Beck RW, Bode BW, et al; and Juvenile Diabetes Research Foundation Continuous Glucose Monitoring Study Group. Continuous glucose monitoring and intensive treatment of type 1 diabetes. *N Engl J Med*. 2008;359(14):1464–1476.

D

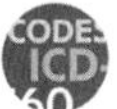

CODES

ICD10

- E10.9 Type 1 diabetes mellitus without complications
- E10.8 Type 1 diabetes mellitus with unspecified complications
- E10.21 Type 1 diabetes mellitus with diabetic nephropathy

FAQ

- Q: What is the risk of diabetes in a sibling or child of a person with type 1 diabetes?
- A: It is 5–10% in 1st-degree relatives (siblings, offspring) and 40–50% in identical twins.
- Q: Should children be screened for type 1 diabetes?
- A: Screening for asymptomatic youth with antibody screening tests are not currently recommended; however, the American Diabetes Association recommends at-risk relatives of persons with type 1 diabetes be informed of the opportunity to have screening through clinical research through Type 1 Diabetes TrialNet at www.trialnet.org (ages 1 to 45 years with a 1st-degree relative with type 1 diabetes and for young people, ages 1 to 20 years with a 2nd-degree relative with type 1 diabetes). Other studies are beginning to offer screenings in the general population in a small number of communities. Evaluation of a *symptomatic* child is clinically important and, if abnormal, should be treated as an urgent situation.
- Q: What are the newest management tools?
- A: Continuous glucose monitors allow patients to avoid symptomatic high and low glucoses by detecting trends, to see the outcome of management decisions, and to reduce the risk of severe nocturnal hypoglycemia. Insulin pumps using data from sensors are in development ("artificial pancreas" systems). A pump with a feature to suspend insulin delivery for low glucose detected by sensor is now available. Additionally, in 2016, the FDA approved the first "hybrid closed loop" insulin pump/CGM system for persons with type 1 diabetes age >14 years. Clinical use of the system (outside of clinical trials) began in 2017. Other systems for clinical use will likely become available for patients within the next few years.

DIABETES MELLITUS, TYPE 2

Wendy J. Brickman, MD

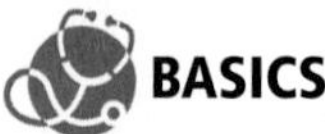

BASICS

DESCRIPTION

Type 2 diabetes mellitus (T2DM) refers to abnormalities in glucose homeostasis characterized by insulin resistance and relative defects in insulin secretion. T2DM is often associated with microvascular and macrovascular complications.

EPIDEMIOLOGY

- Increased prevalence over past 3 decades
- Estimated 5,000 new cases per year in the United States
- T2DM accounts for 15–86% of newly diagnosed cases of diabetes in youth (10 to 19 years); wide variation depending on population
- Prevalence (per 1,000 youth <20 years)
  - American Indian/Alaskan Native 0.63
  - Non-Hispanic black 0.56
  - Hispanic 0.40
  - Asian/Pacific Islander 0.19
  - Non-Hispanic white 0.09

RISK FACTORS

- Female gender
- Adiposity
- Ethnic minorities
- Adolescence (10 to 19 years)
- Offspring of mothers with gestational diabetes
- Family history of type 2 diabetes
- History of the following:
  - Large for gestational age at birth
  - Intrauterine growth retardation
- Impaired fasting glucose
  - Fasting glucose 100 mg/dL (5.6 mmol/L) to 125 mg/dL (6.9 mmol/L)
- Impaired glucose tolerance
  - Based on 2-hour glucose from oral glucose tolerance test (OGTT; see the following) of 140 mg/dL (7.8 mmol/L) to 199 mg/dL (11 mmol/L)

PATHOPHYSIOLOGY

- Insulin resistance
  - Major abnormality in youth with T2DM
  - Tissues (muscle, hepatic, adipose) have a decreased response to insulin, mediated by abnormal phosphorylation of insulin receptor.
- Ideally, a compensatory hyperinsulinemia develops to maintain euglycemia.
- In the presence of β-cell dysfunction, inadequate amounts of insulin are secreted to meet demands from insulin resistance.
- This relative deficiency of insulin secretion leads to hyperglycemia and diabetes.

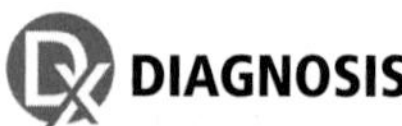

DIAGNOSIS

T2DM usually presents in setting of the following:

- Family history of T2DM
- Overweight or obesity
- Other abnormalities associated with insulin resistance (i.e., acanthosis nigricans, polycystic ovary syndrome [females], hypertension)
- Residual (yet abnormal/insufficient) β-cell function
- Absence of diabetes autoimmunity

HISTORY

- Asymptomatic (most common)
- Polyuria
- Polydipsia
- Weight loss
- Blurry vision
- Increase in nocturia
- Family history of type 2 diabetes
- Maternal gestational diabetes
- Medications such as atypical antipsychotics

PHYSICAL EXAM

- Overweight (BMI ≥85th percentile but <95th percentile) or obese (BMI ≥95th percentile)
- Hypertension
- Acanthosis nigricans
- Vaginal candidiasis

DIFFERENTIAL DIAGNOSIS

- Type 1 diabetes
- Atypical diabetes
- Medication-induced diabetes
- Maturity-onset diabetes of youth (MODY)
  - Monogenic disorders of glucose regulation
  - Abnormalities of β-cell function common
  - BMI range: normal, overweight, or obese
  - Genetic testing for MODY available
- Renal glycosuria
- Stress-induced hyperglycemia

ALERT

When differentiation of type 1 and type 2 diabetes unclear, treat youth with possible type 2 diabetes and significant hyperglycemia with insulin, as if they have type 1 diabetes, until clinical course and laboratory findings prove otherwise.

DIAGNOSTIC TESTS & INTERPRETATION

- Diagnosis of diabetes mellitus:
  - HgbA1c ≥6.5%
    - Using NGSP-certified method
    - False negatives when increased blood cell turnover is present
  - Fasting glucose ≥126 mg/dL (7 mmol/L)
  - 2-hour OGTT glucose ≥200 mg/dL (11.1 mmol/L)
    - At time 0, give oral glucose 1.75 g/kg (maximum dose 75 g) over 5 minutes.
    - At time 120 minutes, measure glucose.
    - If asymptomatic, do second OGTT on a subsequent day to confirm.
  - Random glucose >200 mg/dL with symptoms of hyperglycemia
- Distinguish type 1 from type 2 diabetes.
  - Serum c-peptide or insulin in setting of hyperglycemia
    - Usually normal or elevated in type 2 diabetes
    - Can be low
  - Diabetes autoimmunity
    - Usually absent in type 2 diabetes
- Evaluate for acute complications.
  - Diabetic ketoacidosis (DKA)
    - Ketones present
    - Venous gas: pH <7.30
    - Metabolic panel: HCO_3—<15 mEq/L
  - Hyperglycemic hyperosmolar state (HHS)
    - Ketones absent or minimal
    - Serum glucose: >600 mg/dL (33 mmol/L)
    - Serum osmolality: >330 mOsm/kg
    - Metabolic panel: HCO_3—≥15 mEq/L

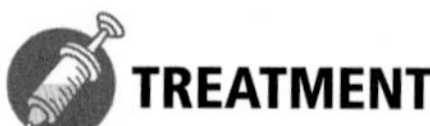

TREATMENT

- See also "Diabetic Ketoacidosis" chapter for treatment of DKA.
- Goals of treatment:
  - HgbA1c in target range per American Diabetes Association (ADA) and International Society for Pediatric and Adolescent Diabetes (ISPAD)
    - <7.5% for youth
    - <7% for adults
  - Limit hypoglycemia and hyperglycemia.
  - Minimize likelihood and delay onset of microvascular and macrovascular disease.
- Treatment is multifaceted and includes lifestyle changes, pharmacotherapy, psychosocial support as needed and, in rare occasions, bariatric surgery.

ALERT

A portion of youth with T2DM can have rapid deterioration in β-cell function requiring escalating intervention.

MEDICATION

- Only two medications are approved for treatment of T2DM in adolescents: insulin and metformin.
- New diagnosis:
  - Random glucose <250 mg/dL and HgbA1c <9%
    - Start metformin.
  - Random glucose is >250 mg/dL or HgbA1c ≥9% and no acidosis.
    - Start metformin.
    - Start basal insulin (can consider adding bolus insulin as well to regimen).
    - Once good glucose management is achieved, wean insulin down by 30–50% (and eventually off) each time metformin is increased.
    - If acidosis reoccurs, reconsider type of diabetes.
  - Acidosis at presentation or possible type 1 diabetes
    - Start multiple dose or basal-bolus insulin regimen.
    - When acidosis resolves and type 2 diabetes diagnosis confirmed, start metformin and attempt to wean insulin.
- Established diagnosis
  - If not reaching goal HgbA1c—escalate therapy (in addition to refocus of lifestyle changes).
    - Add basal insulin (long acting) to metformin regimen.
    - Add bolus insulin (short acting) to metformin and basal insulin regimen.
- Metformin
  - First line of therapy for youth with type 2 diabetes with random glucose <250 mg/dL and HgbA1c <9%
  - Begin at 500 mg once a day. Increase by 500 mg every 1 to 2 weeks as tolerated to reach goal of 1,000 b.i.d. or 2,000 mg daily extended release.
  - Take with food to minimize gastrointestinal side effects.
  - Counsel females as metformin can lead to increased pregnancy risk in teens with ovulatory abnormalities.
  - Stop during gastrointestinal illness.
  - Stop 48 hours prior to elective surgery or contrast study with dye.
  - Do not use with renal failure, pulmonary or cardiac insufficiency, possibly liver disease.
  - For long-term use, consider supplement with vitamin B_{12}.

- Side effects:
  - Short-term: anorexia, flatus, abdominal pain
  - Long-term: lactic acidosis and vitamin B_{12} deficiency
- Insulin—basal
  - Begin at 0.25 to 0.5 U/kg.
  - Increase (up to 1.2 U/kg) as indicated for poor glucose control.
    - If needed to optimize glucose control
    - As tolerated without hypoglycemia
- Insulin—basal bolus
  - Initiate basal-bolus insulin regimen (may need to individualize).
    - Total daily dose (TDD) often 0.5 to 1 U/kg/24 h
    - 40% in long acting usually given at bedtime
    - For meals and snacks, calculate number of carbohydrates to be eaten and cover with short-acting insulin (lispro, aspart, glulisine).
      - Calculate carbohydrate coverage: 1 unit of insulin for every X grams of carbohydrates, often start with X = 500/TDD.
    - For hyperglycemia prior to mealtimes, give short-acting insulin corrective dose by using the sensitivity factor to lower glucose to goal range.
      - Insulin sensitivity factor: 1 unit of insulin will drop glucose by X, often start with X = 1,800/TDD.
      - Correct until goal blood glucose is reached: Begin with goal 120 to 150 mg/dL.
- Insulin—alternative regimens
  - Psychosocial factors may make a regimen with fewer injections, but more rigid eating schedules a more favorable choice.
  - Two examples with TDD starting at 0.7 to 1 U/kg/24 h
    - Two injections per day: premixed insulin of short and intermediate analogs
      - 2/3 of TDD with breakfast
      - 1/3 of TDD with dinner
    - Three injections per day: split-mixed
      - 2/3 of TDD with breakfast (2/3 NPH, 1/3 short acting)
      - 1/9 of TDD with dinner (short acting)
      - 2/9 of TDD at bedtime (NPH)
- Side effect of all insulin regimens is hypoglycemia, especially with increased activity, decreased oral intake, and/or addition of oral antihyperglycemic agent. Adjust dose to prevent.

ADDITIONAL THERAPIES

- Frequently, youth with T2DM come from families with multiple stressors (i.e., other family members with T2DM, low socioeconomic status).
  - Consider resources and team members to help address these complex dynamics.
- Account for these realities in prescribed treatment plans.
- Lifestyle changes—tailor to individual's and family's cultural and personal beliefs, and resources
- Physical activity
  - 60 minutes moderate to vigorous activity a day
  - Can be split throughout the day
  - Start with shorter periods of daily activity and gradually increase to 60-minute goal.
  - Treat orthopedic, respiratory issues.
- Sedentary activity
  - Decrease sedentary activity.
  - Limit screen time to <2 hours a day.
  - Remove televisions/screens from bedrooms.
  - Choose walking or biking over driving, stairs over elevator.
- Nutrition
  - Replace sugar-containing drinks with water or noncaloric options.
  - Limit simple sugars and high-fructose corn syrup.
  - Increase fruits and vegetables.
  - Decrease portion sizes.
  - Increase fiber.
  - Increase intake of low (rather than high) glycemic index foods.
- Smoking
  - In adults, tobacco is associated with increased risk of type 2 diabetes and worsening complications.
  - Counsel patients and parents on risks of tobacco exposure.
  - Assist with referrals for smoking cessation.

ONGOING CARE

FOLLOW-UP RECOMMENDATIONS

- Blood glucose monitoring
  - Metformin monotherapy:
    - Consider fasting and bedtime.
    - Increase when ill, changing dose, concern for low or high glucose.
    - Decrease when stable, in good control.
  - Insulin pharmacotherapy
    - Preprandial and bedtime (Consider less often if only on basal insulin.)
    - Testing to uncover asymptomatic hypoglycemia, calculate corrective doses, and dose efficacy
    - Increase when ill, changing dose, concern for low or high glucose.
- Clinic visits
  - Every 3 months
  - Consider less frequent if goals are reached on metformin only.
  - Check HgbA1c and glucose logs at each visit.
  - Recommend medication, lifestyle changes to reach HgbA1c goals.
  - Assess for comorbidities and complications.
- Challenges of persistently elevated HgbA1c
  - Reassess approach to lifestyle changes.
  - Research protocols underway in pediatrics for some of the many other medications available for adults which have not been approved in youth
  - Bariatric surgery:
    - Remission of diabetes reported after surgery
    - Surgical intervention is still uncommon, and follow-up is continuing to better understand long-term course and complications.
    - Refer to multidisciplinary, experienced bariatric surgery program focused on weight loss and metabolic surgery in adolescents.
- Minor complications can be detected at presentation, and major complications may develop rapidly.
  - Renal and neurologic complications have been reported within 5 years of diagnosis.
  - Major complications such as dialysis, blindness have been reported within 10 years of diagnosis.
- Assessment of microvascular and macrovascular complications
  - Retinopathy
    - Examination at diagnosis, then annually
    - Treatment includes laser photocoagulation.
  - Nephropathy
    - Measure at diagnosis, then annually.
    - Microalbuminuria: 30 to 299 mg/g
    - Macroalbuminuria: ≥300 mg/g
    - If random urine is abnormal, repeat with overnight sample collected in the morning immediately after waking. Abnormalities in two of three consecutive samples are considered abnormal.
    - Treat with angiotensin converting enzyme (ACE) inhibitor.
    - Monitor urine in 3- to 6-month intervals.
    - Goal is to normalize excretion of protein.
    - If macroalbuminuria is present, consider consultation and evaluation of other causes.
  - Peripheral neuropathy
    - Comprehensive foot exam at time of diagnosis
      - Repeat annually.
    - Foot exam includes inspection; palpation of lower pulses; assessment of patellar and Achilles reflexes; proprioception, vibration, and monofilament sensation.
  - Autonomic neuropathy
    - Assess at diagnosis, then annually.
    - Examples include resting tachycardia, orthostasis, gastroparesis, urologic dysfunction, and abnormal sweat patterns.
  - Cardiovascular disease
    - Screen and optimize therapy for hypertension, dyslipidemia, smoking cessation.

ALERT

Complications can be present at time of diagnosis, and deterioration may be accelerated in adolescents with T2DM.

ISSUES FOR REFERRAL

- Comorbidities are often associated with type 2 diabetes and may need referral to specialists for full evaluation and therapeutic implementation.
- Some comorbidities, such as depression, have the potential to worsen glucose control.
- Examples include (but not limited to):
  - Depression and mental health issues
  - Hypertension
  - Dyslipidemia
  - Obstructive sleep apnea
  - Nonalcoholic fatty liver disease
  - Orthopedic abnormalities (e.g., slipped capital femoral epiphysis)
  - Polycystic ovary syndrome
  - Dental abnormalities

ADDITIONAL READING

- American Diabetes Association. Standards of medical care in diabetes—2014. *Diabetes Care*. 2014;37(Suppl 1):S14–S80. doi:10.2337/dc14-S014.
- Copeland KC, Silverstein J, Moore KR, et al; for American Academy of Pediatrics. Management of newly diagnosed type 2 diabetes mellitus (T2DM) in children and adolescents. *Pediatrics*. 2013;131(2):364–382.
- Pettitt DJ, Talton J, Dabelea D, et al; for SEARCH for Diabetes in Youth Study Group. Prevalence of diabetes in U.S. youth in 2009: the SEARCH for Diabetes in Youth study. *Diabetes Care*. 2014;37(2):402–408.
- Springer SC, Silverstein J, Copeland K, et al; for American Academy of Pediatrics. Management of type 2 diabetes mellitus in children and adolescents. *Pediatrics*. 2013;131(2):e648–e664. doi:10.1542/peds.2012-3496.
- Zeitler P, Fu J, Tandon N, et al; for International Society for Pediatric and Adolescent Diabetes. ISPAD Clinical Practice Consensus Guidelines 2014. Type 2 diabetes in the child and adolescent. *Pediatr Diabetes*. 2014;15(Suppl 20):26–46.
- Zeitler P, Hirst K, Pyle L, et al; and TODAY Study Group. A clinical trial to maintain glycemic control in youth with type 2 diabetes. *N Engl J Med*. 2012;366(24):2247–2256.

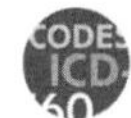

CODES

ICD10

- E11.9 Type 2 diabetes mellitus without complications
- Z83.3 Family history of diabetes mellitus
- E11.51 Type 2 diabetes w diabetic peripheral angiopath w/o gangrene

DIABETIC KETOACIDOSIS

Nicole S. Glaser, MD

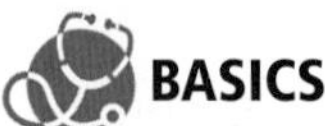

BASICS

DESCRIPTION

- Severe metabolic derangement in patients with diabetes mellitus secondary to insulin deficiency and/or stress hormone excess
- Clinical features include hyperglycemia, ketosis, metabolic acidosis, dehydration, and electrolyte deficits.

EPIDEMIOLOGY

- Diabetes ketoacidosis (DKA) occurs more commonly in type 1 diabetes (T1D) but can also occur in type 2 diabetes (T2D).
- 20–40% of children with new-onset T1D present in DKA
- Risk of DKA in established T1D is 1–10% per patient per year (most episodes caused by insulin omission/diabetes mismanagement).
- DKA accounts for majority of diabetes-related deaths in childhood (most secondary to cerebral edema/brain injury).

RISK FACTORS

- For T1D presenting as DKA:
  - Very young children (<5 years)
  - Ethnic minority
  - Inadequate health insurance
  - A missed diagnosis of diabetes in preceding clinic visits is frequent in DKA patients (~35%).
- For DKA in established diabetes:
  - Adolescence
  - Lack of health insurance
  - Poor glycemic control
  - Ethnic minority
  - Low socioeconomic status (SES)

GENERAL PREVENTION

- Prompt diagnosis of new-onset diabetes (e.g., urinalysis in patients with poor weight gain, polyuria, influenza-like symptoms, vomiting)
- Patient/parental education regarding ketone testing (with any symptoms of illness or unexplained high blood glucose level)
- Strict supervision of long-acting (glargine, detemir) insulin injections by parents
- Detection and avoidance of insulin pump interruptions by frequent blood glucose testing and strict protocols for changing infusion sets

PATHOPHYSIOLOGY

- Excess of counterregulatory "stress" hormone concentrations (glucagon, cortisol, and epinephrine) in relation to insulin concentrations occurs, either as a result of insulin absence (new-onset diabetes or insulin omission) or illness (raising stress hormone levels).
- Imbalance between counterregulatory hormones and insulin results in increased glycogenolysis and gluconeogenesis and decreased peripheral glucose uptake (causing hyperglycemia) as well as lipolysis and ketogenesis (causing ketosis).
- Hyperglycemia causes osmotic diuresis resulting in dehydration and electrolyte losses.
- Ketogenesis results in metabolic acidosis, causing vomiting and tachypnea.
- Dehydration causes poor tissue perfusion, raising lactate levels and is contributing to metabolic acidosis.

ETIOLOGY

- Insulin deficiency
  - New diagnosis of diabetes
  - Insulin omission (diabetes mismanagement or insulin pump malfunction)
- Acute illness (leading to rise in counterregulatory hormone levels)

COMMONLY ASSOCIATED CONDITIONS

- Acute illness as a precipitating factor
- Autoimmune disorders (especially hypothyroidism) for persons with T1D

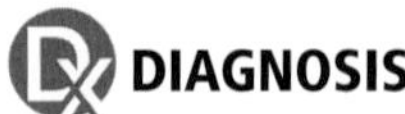

DIAGNOSIS

HISTORY

- Symptoms of new-onset diabetes (polyuria, polydipsia, weight loss)
- Nausea, vomiting, abdominal pain, weakness, lethargy

PHYSICAL EXAM

- Vital signs: tachycardia, tachypnea (deep, "Kussmaul" respirations), occasional hypothermia
- Dehydration: dry mucous membranes, sunken eyes, poor distal perfusion
- Fruity breath odor
- Abdominal tenderness and decreased bowel sounds (intestinal ileus)
- Altered mental status, lethargy, obtundation

DIFFERENTIAL DIAGNOSIS

- Gastroenteritis
- Acute abdomen (pancreatitis, appendicitis, bowel ischemia)
- Urinary tract infection
- Pneumonia, bronchiolitis
- Stress hyperglycemia (particularly during gastroenteritis in young children—ketosis may also be present due to lack of oral intake and may be difficult to differentiate from DKA)
- Salicylate ingestion
- Rare inborn errors of ketolysis (succinyl-CoA: 3-ketoacid CoA transferase deficiency)

DIAGNOSTIC TESTS & INTERPRETATION

- Glucose: >200 mg/dL (usual range 200 to 1,200 mg/dL)
- Urinalysis: glucosuria and ketonuria
- Electrolytes: total body depletion of sodium, chloride, potassium, phosphate, calcium, magnesium (depletion generally not reflected in serum electrolyte concentrations which may be low, normal, or high at presentation)
- Sodium: initial Na usually normal or low
  - Hyperglycemia depresses serum Na by about 1.6 mEq/L for every 100 mg/dL—elevation in glucose >100 mg/dL.
  - Elevated Na at presentation implies extreme dehydration.
- Potassium: Initial serum levels typically normal or elevated may fall rapidly with therapy.
- Serum bicarbonate (total CO_2) is low, consistent with metabolic acidosis.
  - Bicarbonate <18 mEq/L suggests pH <7.3.
  - Bicarbonate <10 mEq/L suggests pH <7.1.
- Phosphate: typically normal or slightly elevated at presentation
- Blood pH low (<7.3) due to metabolic acidosis; low P_{CO_2} secondary to respiratory compensation for metabolic acidosis
- CBC:
  - White blood cell counts frequently elevated and may be left shifted (even in the absence of infection)
  - Hematocrit may be elevated due to hemoconcentration.
- Serum ketones (β-hydroxybutyrate) are elevated (typically >5 mmol/L).
- Liver enzymes (ALT, AST) may be mildly elevated.
- Amylase and lipase are often mildly elevated.

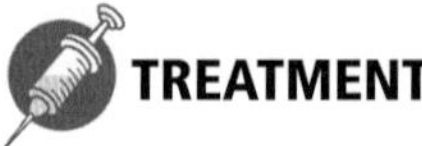

TREATMENT

GENERAL MEASURES

Initial emergency treatment consists of fluid resuscitation to insure hemodynamic stability. Most DKA patients require admission to a pediatric critical care unit or other unit with similar capabilities.

ISSUES FOR REFERRAL

The pediatric endocrinology service should be advised of all DKA admissions. New-onset diabetes patients will require diabetes education. Patients with recurrent DKA may require reeducation or other counseling.

ADMISSION, INPATIENT, AND NURSING CONSIDERATIONS

- IV fluids
  - Initial isotonic IV fluid bolus (0.9% saline) of 10 to 20 cc/kg—may be repeated as necessary to restore perfusion and hemodynamic stability
  - IV fluid rate after initial bolus(es)
    - Average fluid deficit is ~7% of body weight.
    - Replace deficit evenly over 24 to 48 hours.
    - Add maintenance fluids to deficit replacement (minus initial boluses) to calculate total rate.
    - Replacement of ongoing urinary fluid losses is generally unnecessary, but urine output should be monitored.
    - Urine output and specific gravity do not reflect state of hydration.
    - Adjust fluid infusion rate based on fluid intake and output balance, clinical measures of perfusion, and laboratory indicators of hydration.
  - Composition of IV fluids:
    - After initial isotonic fluid bolus(es), IV fluids should consist of 0.45–0.9% saline.
    - Potassium replacement is essential and should be added to IV fluids as soon as renal failure or extreme hyperkalemia is ruled out.
    - Typical initial K replacement is 40 mEq/L, using 1/2 KCl and 1/2 K phosphate.
    - Dextrose should be added to IV fluids when serum glucose level is below ~250 mg/dL. The "2 bag method" (which involves customizing the glucose infusion rate by titrating two bags of IV fluids with the same electrolyte concentrations but glucoses of 0% and 10%) is ideal.
    - Dextrose concentrations in IV fluids should be adjusted to maintain serum glucose in the range of 100 to 200 mg/dL. Rates of insulin infusion generally should not be decreased until acidosis resolves.
- Insulin
  - Insulin treatment should begin after initial isotonic fluid bolus(es).
  - Insulin should be administered via continuous IV infusion at a rate of 0.1 units/kg/h.
  - An initial insulin "bolus" or "loading dose" is not necessary.
- Other
  - Treatment with bicarbonate is generally unnecessary and has been associated with increased risk of cerebral edema.

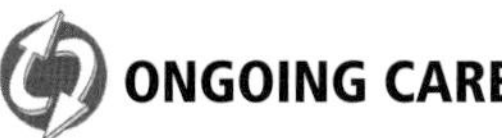

ONGOING CARE

FOLLOW-UP RECOMMENDATIONS

Patient Monitoring

Recommended monitoring:

- Frequent (at least hourly) assessment of mental status and perfusion
- Hourly vital signs
- Cardiac monitor and pulse oximeter
- Hourly intake and output
- Hourly fingerstick or serum glucose
- Electrolytes and venous blood gas every 2 to 4 hours
- Ca, Mg, phosphate every 4 to 6 hours

PROGNOSIS

Mortality of DKA in children is ~0.2–0.3%, (most frequently caused by cerebral edema/cerebral injury).

COMPLICATIONS

- Cerebral injury is the most frequent DKA-related cause of death (57–87% of DKA deaths).
  - Patients at highest risk for cerebral injury are those with the most severe dehydration and acidosis (often younger children).
  - The cause of brain injury in DKA is unclear but may be related to reduced cerebral perfusion during untreated DKA, followed by injury related to reperfusion.
  - Commonly occurs 2 to 12 hours after starting treatment with insulin and saline
    - Symptoms may include mental status changes in association with severe headache, recurrence of vomiting, inappropriate slowing of heart rate or hypertension.
    - Loss of consciousness, seizures, apnea, or signs of increased intracranial pressure may also occur.
  - Treatment of suspected cerebral edema includes mannitol (0.5 to 1 g/kg by IV infusion over 15 minutes) or hypertonic saline.
  - Cerebral imaging studies should be done to evaluate edema or other signs of cerebral injury, but treatment should not be delayed to obtain imaging studies.
- Cardiovascular collapse from shock is rare and usually due to delayed or inadequate IV fluids.
- Other complications:
  - Hypokalemia is frequent and can be avoided with frequent serum K reassessments and adjustment of potassium content of IV fluids.
  - Hypoglycemia may occur but can be avoided with frequent glucose checks and adjustment of dextrose concentration of IV fluids.
  - Mild hypophosphatemia is common, but severe hypophosphatemia is rare. Severe hypophosphatemia has been associated with rhabdomyolysis and hemolytic anemia.
  - Hyperchloremic acidosis may occur, particularly with higher NaCl concentrations in IV fluids.
  - Other rare complications include the following:
    - Pulmonary edema or acute respiratory distress syndrome (ARDS)
    - Pneumomediastinum from hyperventilation
    - Arrhythmias due to electrolyte disturbances
    - Thrombosis, especially at central line site
    - Disseminated intravascular coagulation (DIC)
    - Rhinocerebral mucormycosis
    - Pancreatitis

ADDITIONAL READING

- Glaser N. Cerebral injury and cerebral edema in children with diabetic ketoacidosis: could cerebral ischemia and reperfusion injury be involved? *Pediatr Diabetes*. 2009;10(8):534–541.
- Glaser NS, Ghetti S, Casper TC, et al; for Pediatric Emergency Care Applied Research Network DKA FLUID Study Group. Pediatric diabetic ketoacidosis, fluid therapy and cerebral injury: the design of a factorial randomized controlled trial. *Pediatr Diabetes*. 2013;14(6):435–446.
- Orlowski JP, Cramer CL, Fiallos MR. Diabetic ketoacidosis in the pediatric ICU. *Pediatr Clin North Am*. 2008;55(3):577–587.
- Wolfsdorf JI, Allgrove J, Craig ME, et al; for International Society for Pediatric and Adolescent Diabetes. ISPAD Clinical Practice Consensus Guidelines 2014. Diabetic ketoacidosis and hyperglycemic hyperosmolar state. *Pediatr Diabetes*. 2014;(15 Suppl 20):154–179.

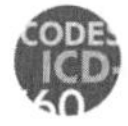

CODES

ICD10

- E10.10 Type 1 diabetes mellitus with ketoacidosis without coma
- E13.10 Oth diabetes mellitus with ketoacidosis without coma

FAQ

- Q: Is DKA in children with known diabetes usually caused by infection or other illness?
- A: Diabetes mismanagement resulting in inappropriate insulin omission is a far more frequent cause of DKA in children than infection. It is generally unnecessary to evaluate children with DKA for infection unless fever or other symptoms of infection are present.
- Q: Does rapid infusion of IV fluids or excessive administration of insulin cause cerebral edema in DKA?
- A: At present, neither the IV fluid administration rate nor the rate of insulin administration has been convincingly shown to increase the risk of DKA-related cerebral edema. Recent data suggest that cerebral edema may be related to alterations in cerebral perfusion occurring in the setting of elevated levels of inflammatory mediators stimulated by DKA. The impact of IV fluid protocols on risk of DKA-related cerebral injury is currently under investigation in a multicenter randomized clinical trial.
- Q: How can DKA episodes in children with diabetes be prevented?
- A: Greater supervision of diabetes care by parents or guardians can decrease the likelihood of insulin omission. Parents should also be instructed to test for ketones at the first sign of any illness or with unexplained high glucose levels and to contact the diabetes care team immediately if ketones are positive.

DIAPER RASH

Jocelyn Huang Schiller, MD • Jessica L. Fealy, MD

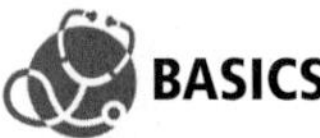

BASICS

DESCRIPTION

Diaper dermatitis is a general term used to describe any inflammatory skin rash that develops in the perineal region. Also known as diaper or napkin rash, there are several causes of diaper dermatitis. Most often, diaper rash is caused by an acute irritant contact dermatitis, which is the focus of this chapter.

ALERT

- Severe cases of diaper dermatitis may be complicated by bacterial or fungal infection, which may require treatment with topical or systemic antibiotics and/or antifungals.
- If severe cases fail to respond to conventional therapies, consider other diagnoses such as Langerhans cell histiocytosis, acrodermatitis enteropathica, or seborrheic dermatitis.

EPIDEMIOLOGY

Incidence

- The reported incidence varies worldwide due to differences in diaper use, toilet training, hygiene, and child-rearing practices.
- Can develop in the 1st week of life but unlikely once the child is no longer in diapers

Prevalence

Estimated prevalence ranges from 7% to 35%.

RISK FACTORS

- Diarrhea increases the risk of irritant diaper rash.
- The presence of oral thrush or recent antibiotic use increases the risk of secondary *Candida albicans* infection.
- Formula-fed infants may have higher risk of diaper dermatitis due to higher stool pH.

GENERAL PREVENTION

- Frequent diaper changes and proper skin care help prevent diaper rash.
- Diapers should be changed as often as every 2 hours or sooner if diaper is wet and/or soiled.
- Superabsorbent diapers (disposable diapers containing gelling materials) keep moisture away from skin and may prevent diaper dermatitis compared to cloth diapers.
- Some experts recommend soft cloths and water for cleansing due to preservatives in baby wipes. As manufacturers have decreased the number of additives, contact dermatitis due to wipes has become less common.
- Petrolatum and/or zinc oxide provide effective barriers against potential perineal skin irritants and moisture. Several authors advise caregivers to refrain from rubbing barrier products off completely during diaper changes to prevent further skin damage.

ETIOLOGY

The pathophysiology is multifactorial, including moisture, friction, warmth, urine, and feces.

- Friction: Rubbing of wet diapers against exposed skin can result in chafing, maceration, and irritation.
- Moisture trapped against skin causes increased permeability and susceptibility to damage from friction.
- Irritation: Urine raises the pH, which activates fecal enzymes resulting in skin damage.
- As the skin barrier breaks down, microbes are more likely to cause a secondary infection.
  - Common causes of secondary infections include *C. albicans*, group A β-hemolytic *Streptococcus*, and *Staphylococcus aureus*.

DIAGNOSIS

HISTORY

- Associated symptoms: Acute or chronic diarrhea suggests a primary irritant dermatitis.
- The presence of oral thrush or recent antibiotic use increases the risk of secondary *C. albicans* infection. Presence of the rash for >3 days also increases likelihood of candidal infection.
- Treatment with topical corticosteroid, antifungal, or antibacterial products can change the appearance of the rash.
- Chemicals, dyes, and fragrances in lotions, wipes, diapers, and detergents can cause irritant or allergic contact dermatitis.
- Infrequent or poor hygiene can result in diaper rash, whereas excessive bathing may result in increased friction on the skin and worsening of a preexisting rash.
- Moderate to severe rashes and rashes infected with group A β-hemolytic *Streptococcus* or *S. aureus* cause discomfort for the child.

PHYSICAL EXAM

- Ranges from asymptomatic, generalized erythema to skin breakdown leading to an open wound
- Irritant and allergic dermatitis occurs on skin surfaces in direct contact with the diaper, urine, and feces. Skinfolds are typically spared.
  - Affected intertriginous areas suggest seborrheic dermatitis, candidal infection, or group A β-hemolytic *Streptococcus* infection.
  - Perianal rashes suggest group A β-hemolytic *Streptococcus* (more common) or *S. aureus* (less common) infection.
- The morphology of the dermatitis is important:
  - Well-demarcated, shiny, erosive, erythematous perianal patches suggest group A β-hemolytic *Streptococcus*.
  - Scattered inflammatory papules or pustules suggest *S. aureus*.
  - Erythematous patches with peripheral erythematous papules (satellite lesions) suggest candidal infection.
  - Greasy erythema and scaling suggest seborrheic dermatitis.
- Infants with diaper dermatitis may have palpable inguinal lymphadenopathy.
- A complete physical exam may reveal other features of the underlying diagnosis:
  - Scalp seborrhea (cradle cap) suggests seborrheic dermatitis.
  - Thrush (oral candidiasis) raises the possibility of a candidal infection.
  - Hepatosplenomegaly suggests Langerhans cell histiocytosis.

DIFFERENTIAL DIAGNOSIS

- Candidal dermatitis:
  - Irritant dermatitis may become secondarily infected with *C. albicans*.
  - Results in beefy red plaques with satellite lesions and superficial pustules
  - Common during or after antibiotic use
- Allergic contact dermatitis:
  - Can result from allergens in the diaper, wipes, or topical creams including dyes, detergents, fragrances, or elastic
  - Only in areas in contact with trigger
  - May result in erythema, edema, and superficial erosions
- Impetigo:
  - Due to group A β-hemolytic *Streptococcus* (common) or *S. aureus* (less common)
  - 1- to 2-mm pustules and honey-colored, crusted erosions
  - Bullous impetigo appears as large, fluid-filled bullae.
- Perianal group A β-hemolytic *Streptococcus*:
  - Presents as bright red, sharply demarcated perianal rash with pain or pruritus
  - May also have streptococcal pharyngitis
- Coxsackievirus (particularly the A6 strain):
  - Becoming more common in North America since 2012
  - Often accompanied by viral prodrome and concurrent palmar or plantar and oral lesions
  - May have vesicles, bullae, erosions, or scabbed lesions; may extend down posterior thighs
- Seborrheic dermatitis:
  - Associated with scalp, face, and skinfold involvement
  - In the diaper region, it is characterized by well-circumscribed erythematous papules and plagues.
- Atopic dermatitis:
  - Usually spares the diaper region due to the moist environment
  - If affected, characterized by increased skin lines and excoriations due to scratching
- Psoriasis:
  - May involve the diaper area either exclusively or may occur in the setting of more diffuse presentation, including other intertriginous areas and the face and scalp
  - Presents with sharply demarcated erythematous and silvery scaly papules and plaques

- Scabies:
  - Pruritic, erythematous papules and nodules may involve the genitalia, abdomen, web spaces of extremities, and axilla.
  - Often, there is a history of multiple affected family members and more widespread involvement.
- Herpes simplex virus:
  - May manifest as grouped vesicular, papular, or pustular lesions
  - May be transmitted through sexual contact or herpetic whitlow
- Child abuse:
  - An unusual history or morphology suggests the possibility of abuse.
  - Especially consider in cases if the lesions appear geometric or resemble scalds, burns, or bruises or if sexually transmitted disease diagnosed.
- Langerhans cell histiocytosis:
  - Usually presents with multiple reddish-brown crusted papules and/or vesicles and petechiae in conjunction with hepatosplenomegaly and anemia
- Acrodermatitis enteropathica:
  - Caused by impaired zinc metabolism (either inherited or acquired)
  - Leads to an erosive acrodermatitis involving the face in a perioral and periocular distribution, the diaper area, and the hands and feet
- Jacquet erosive diaper dermatitis:
  - Rare and likely represents severe irritant diaper dermatitis
  - Characterized by well-demarcated papules, nodules, and punched out ulcerations
- Granuloma gluteale infantum:
  - Rare, benign inflammatory dermatosis associated with the use of high-potency topical corticosteroids
  - Characterized by reddish-purplish nodules

DIAGNOSTIC TESTS & INTERPRETATION

Initial Tests (screening, lab, imaging)

- Rarely helpful
- Candidal infections can be verified by a potassium hydroxide preparation or fungal culture of skin scraping if diagnosis is unclear.
- Group A β-hemolytic *Streptococcus* and *S. aureus* infection can be confirmed by swabbing affected area for bacterial culture.
- Pathologic findings
  - Skin biopsy is rarely required unless the rash is atypical and unresponsive to therapy.
  - Skin biopsy may be helpful in diagnosing psoriasis, Langerhans cell histiocytosis, or granuloma gluteale infantum.

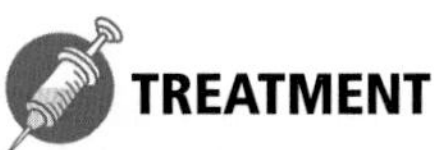

TREATMENT

GENERAL MEASURES

- Similar to primary prevention, frequent diaper changes and proper skin care are the primary treatments for diaper dermatitis.
- Skin should be gently washed with a mild cleanser and/or infant wipe and patted dry or air-dried. Vigorous rubbing of the skin or use of washcloths may cause further irritation and skin breakdown.
- Rinsing the bottom in a sink with warm water or with a squeezable bottle and then patting dry may also be helpful if skin is open and sensitive.
- Frequent diaper changes are helpful in minimizing exposure to irritants.
- If feasible, remove diaper and expose skin to air to avoid friction and trapped moisture.
- If unable to leave open to air, cool and low setting on a blow dryer for 30 to 60 seconds may help achieve the same effect; may also use a clean diaper to fan the bottom before rediapering
- Baking soda baths may help soothe the skin and neutralize any acid on the skin from stool, especially in infants eating solid/acidic foods.
- Routine use of a barrier ointment and pastes such as zinc oxide with each diaper change is recommended. Barriers should be applied thickly and can be covered with petroleum jelly to prevent sticking to the diaper.

MEDICATION

- Candidal infections should be treated with topical antifungal cream such as nystatin, miconazole, ketoconazole, or clotrimazole cream.
- If secondary bacterial infection is present, topical antibiotics such as mupirocin or oral antibiotics are necessary. Neomycin and bacitracin can incite an allergic contact dermatitis, so they should be avoided.
- Low-potency topical steroids, such as hydrocortisone and hydrocortisone acetate, may be used sparingly in moderate to severe cases.
- Topical application of sucralfate suspension can be useful in recalcitrant cases. It acts as a physical barrier and has antibacterial activity.

ALERT

- Mid- to high-potency topical corticosteroids should not be used because absorption is increased in areas of thin skin and under occlusion. Skin atrophy or systemic effects may result.
- Similarly, prolonged use of any potency topical steroids (>7 days) in the diaper area should be avoided.
- Combination topical corticosteroids and antifungal creams should not be used because these contain mid- to high-potency corticosteroids. Separate corticosteroid and antifungal creams allow the discontinuation of corticosteroid earlier (when the rash starts to improve) while continuing antifungal until rash resolves.
- Products containing boric acid, camphor, phenol, benzocaine, and salicylates should be avoided because of the potential for systemic toxicity.
- Use of powders such as talcum and corn starch is controversial. Powders can reduce moisture and friction but pose the risk of accidental aspiration and should not be used on open wounds.

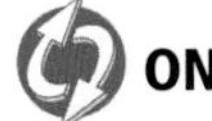

ONGOING CARE

FOLLOW-UP RECOMMENDATIONS

Patient Monitoring

With proper care, the rash should improve within 4 to 7 days. If it does not resolve with appropriate treatment, other causes must be sought.

PROGNOSIS

- Diaper dermatitis usually resolves with the institution of appropriate skin care and the treatment of any underlying cause.
- Irritant diaper dermatitis resolves once the child is potty trained.

COMPLICATIONS

- Generally no long-term complications although secondary bacterial or fungal infections may lead to ulceration
- Chronic topical corticosteroid use in diaper area may lead to skin atrophy or systemic effects.
- Some experience postinflammatory hypo- or hyperpigmentation that is typically self-limited.

ADDITIONAL READING

- Adam R. Skin care of the diaper area. *Pediatr Dermatol*. 2008;25(4):427–433.
- Coughlin C, Eichenfield L, Frieden I. Diaper dermatitis: clinical characteristics and differential diagnosis. *Pediatr Dermatol*. 2014;31(Suppl 1):19–24.
- Ravanfar P, Wallace JS, Pace NC. Diaper dermatitis: a review and update. *Curr Opin Pediatr*. 2012;24(4):472–479.

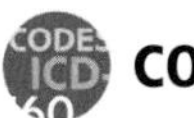

CODES

ICD10

- L22 Diaper dermatitis
- B37.2 Candidiasis of skin and nail

FAQ

- Q: Should I switch from cloth to disposable diapers?
- A: There is no definitive answer; however, some studies indicate that the superabsorbent disposable diapers may be better for preventing diaper rashes. Cloth diapers used with plastic outer layer probably irritate the skin more because they trap moisture against the skin. Frequent changing of diapers and the use of a barrier paste are very helpful in preventing diaper rash.
- Q: Is the diaper rash due to not keeping the skin clean enough?
- A: Although stool and urine may release enzymes that help break down skin integrity, vigorous and frequent scrubbing with relatively abrasive materials on the damaged skin can be more harmful. This rough cleaning allows introduction of bacteria and yeast into the skin and results in a diaper rash. Gentle cleaning materials should be used. It is not usually necessary to clean the skin of barrier ointments every time; rather, patting the infant dry with a soft cloth or baby wipe, gently reapplying barrier products, and then replacing the diaper is all that is generally required.

DIAPHRAGMATIC HERNIA (CONGENITAL)

Ngoc P. Ly, MD, MPH • Fiona Marion, MB, BCh, BAO

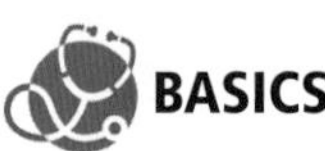

BASICS

DESCRIPTION
- Defect in the diaphragm allowing herniation of abdominal contents into the thoracic cavity, causing varying degrees of pulmonary hypoplasia
- There are four types of congenital diaphragmatic hernia (CDH):
  - Bochdalek hernia (posterolateral location)
  - Morgagni hernia (lateral retrosternal location)
  - Pars sternalis (medial retrosternal)
  - Anterolateral

EPIDEMIOLOGY
- 1:2,000 to 5,000 live births
- Left sided in 85–90%
- Right-sided and bilateral defects less common
- Familial recurrence 2%

RISK FACTORS
Pregestational diabetes and alcohol use associated with increased risk

PATHOPHYSIOLOGY
- Diaphragm arises from four elements and is complete by 8 weeks' gestation.
  - Septum transversum, which becomes the central tendon of the diaphragm
  - Pleuroperitoneal membranes, which extend from the lateral body wall and fuse with the septum transversum and esophageal mesentery
  - Mesentery of the esophagus, which becomes the crura of the diaphragm
  - Lateral body wall from which myocytes migrate to muscularize the diaphragm
- Posterolateral (Bochdalek defect) in 70%, anterior (Morgagni) in 25–30%, central in 2–5%
- Main problem concerns pulmonary hypoplasia, which results in pulmonary hypertension.
  - Smaller lungs with fewer airway branches, fewer alveoli per terminal lung unit, and decreased surfactant production
  - Decreased pulmonary vascular surface area and smaller muscular arterioles with abnormal vasoreactivity results in pulmonary hypertension.
- Both ipsilateral and contralateral lungs are hypoplastic, worse on ipsilateral side.
- Degree of pulmonary hypoplasia and pulmonary hypertension determines illness severity both in acute and chronic settings.

ETIOLOGY
- Unknown
- Most cases occur sporadically.
- Experimental rat models suggest role of vitamin A deficiency in pathogenesis.

COMMONLY ASSOCIATED CONDITIONS
40–50% of cases associated with another type of congenital malformation
- Cardiac: 10–35%
- Genitourinary: 23%
- Gastrointestinal malformations: 14%
- Central nervous system abnormalities: 10%
  - Approximately 10% of cases with associated congenital anomalies have a syndrome.
  - Associated syndromes include Beckwith-Wiedemann and trisomies 13, 18, and 21.

DIAGNOSIS

HISTORY
- Prenatal history:
  - CDH is detected by prenatal ultrasound in >70% cases.
  - Mean gestational age at diagnosis is 24 weeks.
- Poor prognostic factors:
  - Severe associated anomalies
  - Liver herniation
  - Right-sided defect
  - Low fetal lung volume
    - Observed/expected lung-to-head ratio as determined by ultrasound
    - Observed/expected fetal lung volume ratio by fetal magnetic resonance imaging (MRI)
- Postnatal history:
  - Large defects present at birth with respiratory distress
  - May be easily identified on chest radiograph (CXR); however, computed tomography (CT) scan may be required to confirm the diagnosis.
  - Smaller defects may be undetected until late childhood/adolescence or even adulthood.
  - Symptoms may include the following:
    - Recurrent cough
    - Recurrent chest infections
    - Intestinal obstruction
    - Feeding intolerance
- Important to evaluate for associated congenital abnormalities to guide management

PHYSICAL EXAM
- Scaphoid abdomen (abdominal contents in thoracic cavity) and asymmetry of chest wall
- Decreased breath sounds with dullness to percussion on the affected side
- Bowel sounds heard in the chest
- Heart sounds shifted to the contralateral chest

DIFFERENTIAL DIAGNOSIS
- Pulmonary
  - Pulmonary sequestration
  - Congenital pulmonary airway malformation (CCAM)
  - Pneumatocele
  - Pulmonary cyst
  - Diaphragmatic eventration
  - Hiatal hernia
  - Congenital lobar emphysema
  - Pneumonia
  - Atelectasis
  - Pleural effusion
  - Pneumothorax
  - Pulmonary agenesis
  - Anterior mediastinal mass
- Cardiac
  - Dextrocardia
  - Congenital heart disease

DIAGNOSTIC TESTS & INTERPRETATION

Initial Tests (screening, lab, imaging)
- Ultrafast fetal MRI to confirm the diagnosis and to estimate lung volumes
- Amniocentesis and genetic consultation recommended to screen for chromosomal anomalies
- Arterial blood gas
  - Po_2 low: reflects significant hypoxemia
  - Pco_2 high: reflects inadequate ventilation
  - pH, bicarbonate, lactate: acid–base balance
- Karyotype: to assess for associated syndromes and chromosomal abnormalities
- CXR
  - Opacified hemithorax with contralateral shift of mediastinum
  - Decreased lung volumes
  - Esophageal portion of nasogastric tube deviated toward opposite side
  - May see loops of bowel in the thoracic cavity
  - Bowel remaining in the abdomen usually gasless
- Chest CT/MRI to confirm diagnosis of CDH

ALERT
- CXR findings in the newborn period may be subtle.
- Small CDH defects may present outside of newborn period.

- Echocardiogram
  - Right ventricular function is an important determinant of disease severity.
  - Can estimate degree of pulmonary hypertension
  - Determine presence of associated congenital cardiac defects

Follow-Up Tests & Special Considerations
- Pulmonary function testing
- Audiology to detect hearing loss
- Serial echocardiogram to monitor pulmonary hypertension
- Endoscopy may be required in the setting of severe reflux.
- If recurrence is suspected, CT may be required to make the diagnosis.

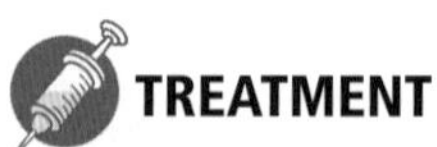

TREATMENT

GENERAL MEASURES
- Intubation and ventilation
  - Intubate in delivery room.
  - Avoid bag and mask ventilation.
- Nasogastric tube insertion and continuous suction to decompress herniated contents and reduce lung compression
- Cardiovascular support

ALERT
- It is important to assess and treat pulmonary hypertension.
- Avoid aggressive ventilation. It is important to minimize barotrauma.

ISSUES FOR REFERRAL
Long-term multidisciplinary follow-up required to monitor for complications and recurrence of hernia

SURGERY/OTHER PROCEDURES
- Delaying surgery until infant is stabilized has been associated with better outcome.
- Primary repair versus prosthetic patch
- Minimally invasive thoracoscopic approach now possible, although is associated with an increased recurrence rate compared with the open approach
- Up to 50% will require patch repair of diaphragmatic defect.

- Recurrence of hernia occurs in up to 50% of patch closures.
- Patch closure of abdomen or creation of surgical silo may be required with very large defects.
- Prenatal: Fetal endoscopic tracheal occlusion (FETO) is an investigational procedure for treatment of isolated severe CDH: trial ongoing at limited centers

ADMISSION, INPATIENT, AND NURSING CONSIDERATIONS

- Goal is to limit barotrauma, maintain peak pressures ≤25 mm Hg and positive end-expiratory pressure (PEEP) at physiologic levels (3 to 5 mm Hg).
- Permissive hypercapnia: Tolerate $Paco_2$ up to 60 mm Hg.
- Aim for preductal oxygen saturation >85%.
- Consider high-frequency oscillatory ventilation and extracorporeal membrane oxygenation (ECMO) when earlier measures are not effective (e.g., pH <7.25, $Paco_2$ >60 mm Hg, preductal saturation <85% on FiO_2 0.6).
- Pulmonary hypertension
  - Severity predicts outcome.
  - 50% of patients are responsive to inspired nitric oxide (iNO), but the effect may be temporary. iNO has no influence on overall outcome.
  - Sildenafil: Phosphodiesterase 5 inhibitor may be used as an adjunct to iNO to prevent rebound hypertension when weaning iNO or in management of chronic pulmonary hypertension.
  - In setting of left ventricular dysfunction with a right ventricle–dependent systemic circulation, milrinone and prostaglandin may be used to decrease afterload and maintain ductal patency.
  - In setting of pulmonary hypertension, aim for higher mean arterial blood pressure.

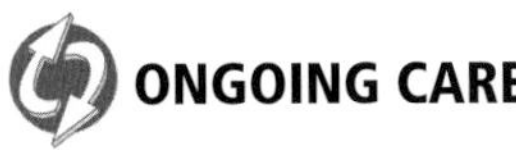

ONGOING CARE

PATIENT EDUCATION

- Many babies with CDH have long-term problems including:
  - Breathing or other lung problems
  - Not gaining weight
  - Digestive problems
  - Learning problems or hearing loss
- Routine vaccinations and yearly influenza vaccine are recommended.

PROGNOSIS

- Depends on the size of the defect and in turn, the degree of pulmonary hypoplasia and pulmonary hypertension
- 70% postnatal survival, with up to 90% survival described by some centers
- 50% survival in those requiring ECMO
- Prematurity associated with worse prognosis

COMPLICATIONS

- Up to 75% with pulmonary, neurologic, or gastrointestinal morbidities at discharge
- Pulmonary
  - Chronic lung disease: Up to 50% require supplemental oxygen at 28 days and 16% at the time of discharge from hospital.
  - Prevalence of long-term pulmonary morbidity unclear: Some series report chronic pulmonary symptoms in up to 50% of survivors.
  - Spirometry shows obstructive pattern of lung disease.
  - Scoliosis and chest wall defects may cause restrictive lung disease.
- Gastrointestinal/nutrition
  - Growth failure secondary to chronic lung disease, increased work of breathing, gastroesophageal reflux, and oral aversion
  - Failure to thrive is common. Up to 1/3 require gastrostomy tube.
  - Gastroesophageal reflux (45–90%): may lead to recurrent bronchitis, worsening bronchopulmonary dysplasia, aspiration pneumonia. Persists into adulthood. Consider an H_2 blocker in all patients.
- Cardiac
  - Pulmonary hypertension may persist in up to 30%.
- Neurodevelopmental
  - Behavioral, cognitive, and motor problems are common.
  - High risk of speech and language delay
  - Greatest risk in those with large defects or those requiring ECMO
- Sensorineural hearing loss
  - Incidence varies: up to 40% described by some
  - Underlying cause unknown
  - Deficit is progressive.
- Musculoskeletal
  - Chest wall deformities and scoliosis are common, occurring in up to 30% of patients.
- Surgical
  - Orthopedic: pectus deformity and scoliosis
  - Recurrence of hernia (in up to 50%): risk greater in those who required patch closure
    - May present with vomiting, bowel obstruction, pulmonary symptoms, or may be asymptomatic
    - Serial CXR recommended for screening

ALERT

- Recurrence of CDH is common and typically presents with vague gastrointestinal symptoms (in contrast to a dramatic presentation of the newborn period).
- Hearing impairment may be progressive. Therefore, serial screening through childhood is essential.

ADDITIONAL READING

- Bohn D. Congenital diaphragmatic hernia. *Am J Respir Crit Care Med*. 2002;166(7):911–915.
- Danzer E, Gerdes M, D'Agostino JA, et al. Longitudinal neurodevelopmental and neuromotor outcome in congenital diaphragmatic hernia patients in the first 3 years of life. *J Perinatol*. 2013;33(11):893–898.
- Kotecha S, Barbato A, Bush A, et al. Congenital diaphragmatic hernia. *Eur Respir J*. 2012;39(4):820–829.
- Lally KP, Engle W; and American Academy of Pediatrics Section on Surgery, American Academy of Pediatrics Committee on Fetus and Newborn. Postdischarge follow-up of infants with congenital diaphragmatic hernia. *Pediatrics*. 2008;121(3):627–632.
- van den Hout L, Sluiter I, Gischler S, et al. Can we improve outcome of congenital diaphragmatic hernia? *Pediatr Surg Int*. 2009;25(9):733–743.

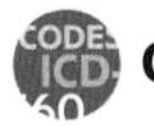

CODES

ICD10

- Q79.0 Congenital diaphragmatic hernia
- Q33.6 Congenital hypoplasia and dysplasia of lung

FAQ

- Q: What is the recurrence rate?
- A: Reported rates of recurrence vary from 10% to 50%. Serial screening with CXR and a high index of suspicion is necessary. The typical presentation includes emesis, gastrointestinal obstruction, or respiratory symptoms.
- Q: Is pulmonary impairment lifelong?
- A: Although pulmonary function improves with growth, studies (spirometry, plethysmography, ventilation–perfusion [V/Q] scan) show persisting deficits. Most patients report decreased pulmonary morbidity/symptoms with increasing age.
- Q: What follow-up is necessary?
- A: Long-term multidisciplinary follow-up is essential. Complications involving multiple organ systems are common.
- Q: Why is long-term gastrointestinal follow-up necessary?
- A: Although complications such as failure to thrive and oral aversion are less common with increasing age, the risk of reflux is lifelong. Treatment into adulthood may be required to control reflux and prevent Barrett esophagus.

DIARRHEA

Kerri Gosselin, MD, MPH

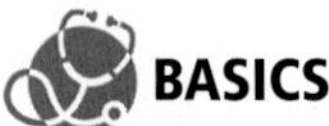

BASICS

DESCRIPTION

- Diarrhea is an increase in frequency, volume, or fluidity of a patient's stool as compared to the normal bowel movement pattern.
- On the basis of its duration, diarrhea can be classified as acute (<14 days), persistent (14 to 29 days), or chronic (>30 days).
- Acute diarrhea typically presents abruptly with increased fluid content of the stool >10 mL/kg/24 h and lasts <14 days; usually involves the passage of >250 g/24 h of unformed stool
- Persistent diarrhea can also begin acutely but last for ≥14 days.
- Diarrhea is caused whenever there is disruption of the normal absorptive and secretory functions of intestinal mucosa.
- Malabsorption, maldigestion, cellular electrolyte pump dysfunction, and intestinal colonization or invasion by microorganisms can cause diarrhea.
- Tenesmus, perianal irritation or discomfort, and fecal incontinence may occur with all forms of diarrhea.

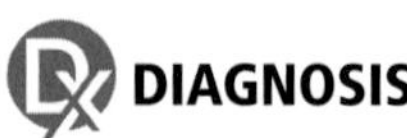

DIAGNOSIS

Approach to patient

- The first step in the clinical appraisal of the patient with diarrhea is to identify what the patient "means" by diarrhea; exclude the possibility of fecal impaction with overflow diarrhea and/or incontinence; rule out drug-induced diarrhea; distinguish acute from chronic; categorize as inflammatory, fatty, or watery; and consider the possibility of factitious diarrhea.
- It is important to determine the type of diarrhea (osmotic vs. secretory), as this will alter your diagnostic and therapeutic plan.
  - Secretory diarrhea
    - Absorption of intestinal fluid and electrolytes is accomplished through multiple cellular pumps transporting sodium (Na), glucose, and amino acids.
    - Factors that interrupt these pumps (e.g., cholera toxin, prostaglandin E, vasoactive intestinal peptide, secretin, acetylcholine) can cause a severe active isotonic secretory state manifested by profuse diarrhea, dehydration, and acidosis. Other causes include bile acid malabsorption, inflammatory bowel disease, disordered regulation (postvagotomy, diabetic neuropathy), peptide-secreting endocrine tumors, and neoplasia (colon carcinoma, lymphoma, villous adenoma).
  - Osmotic diarrhea
    - In general, the solute composition of intestinal fluid is similar to that of plasma.
    - Osmotic diarrhea occurs when poorly absorbed or nonabsorbable solute is present in the intestinal lumen (this may result in low stool pH <6).
    - This can occur with the ingestion of nonabsorbable sugars (e.g., sorbitol), cathartics (e.g., magnesium citrate); carbohydrate malabsorption secondary to mucosal damage (e.g., lactose); maldigestion (e.g., pancreatic dysfunction), rapid transit of intestinal fluid; or with a rare congenital transport defect.

HISTORY

- **Question:** Duration? (<14 days, >30 days)
- *Significance*: A distinction should be made between acute and chronic diarrhea. The cause of acute diarrhea is almost always related to an infection, a medication, or the addition of a new food.
- **Question:** Travel history?
- *Significance*: Questions should be asked regarding travel to areas where drinking water is contaminated (e.g., *Entamoeba* in Mexico) or food handling/preparation is prolonged or unsanitary (e.g., *Campylobacter*, *Bacillus cereus*, or *E. coli*); exposure to freshwater streams or ponds (e.g., *Cryptosporidium*, *Giardia*)
- **Question:** Recent use of antibiotics?
- *Significance*: A variety of antibiotics can be associated with *C. difficile* colitis or antibiotic-related diarrhea.
- **Question:** Adolescents?
- *Significance*: Questions should be asked regarding body image and weight. Laxative abuse causing an osmotic diarrhea is common among adolescents who have an eating disorder or athletes attempting to lose weight rapidly.
- **Question:** Family history?
- *Significance*: conditions with genetic susceptibility (e.g., inflammatory bowel disease, celiac disease)
- **Question:** Systemic symptoms?
- *Significance*: It is important to ask about concomitant fever, GI bleeding, rashes, or vomiting. Certain GI infections and inflammatory bowel disease have specific associated systemic symptoms.
- **Question:** Hematochezia?
- *Significance*: The occurrence of acute, bloody stools and fever generally indicates a bacterial infection. However, these same symptoms coupled with fatigue, poor urine output, and history of easy bruising may suggest hemolytic uremic syndrome. Bloody stools in combination with a history of crampy abdominal pain, arthritis, and purpuric rash can indicate HSP, a completely different entity. Chronic bloody diarrhea, abdominal pain, and weight loss are characteristic of inflammatory bowel disease.
- **Question:** Steatorrhea? (greasy or bulky stools)
- *Significance*: indicates fat malabsorption (e.g., cystic fibrosis)
- **Question:** Age? (congenital vs. acquired)
- *Significance*: The age of the child is important because a number of diseases present between birth and 3 months of life including cystic fibrosis, milk or soy protein intolerance, and congenital enteropathies (e.g., microvillus inclusion disease, tufting enteropathy).
- **Question:** Previously well infant with recent viral illness and subsequent protracted diarrhea?
- *Significance*: Postviral enteritis should be suspected. This disorder is characterized by severe mucosal injury resulting in transient disaccharidase deficiency and potentially prolonged malabsorption.
- **Question:** Normal preschool-aged children who have 2 to 10 watery stools per day with normal growth?
- *Significance*: Chronic nonspecific diarrhea of childhood (a.k.a. functional diarrhea) should be considered. Assess juice and dietary sugar intake.
- **Question:** Lactose intolerance?
- *Significance*: commonly occurs in many older children and adults, with >95% occurrence rate in some ethnic groups
- **Question:** Chronic diarrhea with weight loss?
- *Significance*: Inflammatory or immunologic disorders such as ulcerative colitis, Crohn disease, and celiac disease must be ruled out. Celiac disease is an immune-mediated enteropathy caused by dietary gluten intake in genetically susceptible individuals; occurs in ~1:130 of the U.S. population with a genetic predisposition and should be considered in any child with chronic diarrhea and poor weight gain

PHYSICAL EXAM

- **Finding:** Stool in left lower quadrant and/or a history of encopresis?
- *Significance*: Chronic loose stools are common in children with functional constipation and large fecal impaction due to overflow incontinence and can be easily mistaken for diarrhea.
- **Finding:** Child's growth parameters?
- *Significance*: Previous measurements and growth curves are necessary to make an accurate evaluation. Findings of a chronically malnourished child with years of weight loss or poor growth velocity would indicate a divergent differential diagnosis from that of a healthy-appearing child with a history of normal growth.
- **Finding:** Arthritis and rash?
- *Significance*: Diarrhea accompanied by these signs can occur in diseases such as inflammatory bowel disease, celiac disease, HSP, and specific bacterial infections.
- **Finding:** Oral ulcers?
- *Significance*: occur in inflammatory bowel disease and celiac disease
- **Finding:** Dehydration?
- *Significance*: Capillary refill >3 seconds, tachycardia without pain or fever, and dry mucous membranes provide clues to dehydration.
- **Finding:** Nail bed clubbing?
- *Significance*: This finding may direct questioning to rule out cystic fibrosis or chronic inflammatory bowel disease.
- **Finding:** Masses?
- *Significance*: A right lower quadrant mass could suggest an abscess (e.g., terminal ileitis in Crohn disease or appendiceal abscess) or intussusception (e.g., irritable child with currant jelly-like stools).

DIFFERENTIAL DIAGNOSIS

- Acute diarrhea
  - Dietary causes
    - Sorbitol, fructose, lactose, and intolerance to specific foods (beans, fruit, peppers, etc.)
  - Infectious causes:
    - Bacterial (e.g., *Escherichia coli*, *Clostridium difficile*, *Salmonella*, *Shigella*, *Campylobacter*, *Yersinia*)
    - Viral (e.g., rotavirus, norovirus, adenovirus)
    - Parasites (e.g., *Giardia*, *Cryptosporidium*, *Entamoeba histolytica*)
  - Medications
    - Antibiotics, laxatives
- Chronic diarrhea
  - Allergic/autoimmune
    - Milk/soy protein allergy, eosinophilic enteritis, Henoch-Schönlein purpura (HSP), celiac disease, autoimmune enteropathy, or microscopic colitis
  - Immunodeficiency
    - HIV/AIDS, chronic granulomatous disease, hyper IgM, severe combined immunodeficiency

- Anatomic abnormalities
  - Short bowel syndrome (e.g., history of necrotizing enterocolitis, Hirschsprung, malrotation, inflammatory bowel disease)
- Bile acid malabsorption
- Congenital
  - Cystic fibrosis, microvillus inclusion disease, tufting enteropathy, or IPEX syndrome
- Encopresis
- Endocrine disorders
  - Hyperthyroidism, diabetes, congenital adrenal hyperplasia
- Bacterial overgrowth (e.g., blind loop, ostomy)
- Inflammatory bowel disease
  - Ulcerative colitis, Crohn disease
- Intestinal lymphangiectasia
  - Primary and secondary
- Irritable bowel syndrome
- Lactose intolerance
  - Primary, secondary, and congenital
- Pancreatic exocrine dysfunction
  - Shwachman-Diamond syndrome, cationic trypsinogen deficiency, Jeune syndrome, Pearson syndrome, and Johanson-Blizzard syndrome
- Postinfectious enteropathy
- Secretory tumors
  - VIPoma, somatostatinoma, gastrinoma, carcinoid, glucagonoma

DIAGNOSTIC TESTS & INTERPRETATION

- **Test:** stool culture
- *Significance*: Stool examination for blood, mucus, inflammatory cells, and microorganisms is an important first step in determining the cause of the diarrhea. Stool cultures for parasites (e.g., *Giardia*, *Cryptosporidium*, *Entamoeba*), bacterial pathogens (e.g., *Salmonella*, *Campylobacter*, *Shigella*, *Yersinia*, *Aeromonas*, *Plesiomonas*), viral particles, and *C. difficile* toxin should be appropriately obtained in all children with unexplained diarrhea.
- **Test:** stool pH and reducing substances
- *Significance*: These tests are useful in identifying carbohydrate malabsorption. A stool pH <5 to 6 and stool-reducing substances >0.5–1% is suggestive of malabsorption.
- **Test:** stool osmolality and electrolytes
- *Significance*: Stool osmolality, stool Na, and stool K can be used to calculate an ion gap and differentiate between secretory and osmotic diarrhea.
  - Stool osmotic gap = measured stool osmolality − estimated stool osmolality
  - Estimated stool osmolality = 2 (Na stool + K stool)
  - An increased stool osmotic gap is >50 mOsm/kg.
- **Test:** stool guaiac test (Hemoccult®)
- *Significance*: Sensitive and specific test is helpful in distinguishing truly heme-positive stools from ingested foods/drinks with artificial or natural red coloring. Stool positive for blood is suggestive of bacterial or inflammatory causes.
- **Test:** 72-hour quantitative fecal fat evaluation
- *Significance*: This is a sensitive test for steatorrhea. Patients need to be placed on a high-fat diet (2 to 4 g/kg) for a minimum of 1 day prior to testing.
  - Over 3 days, all stool is collected, refrigerated, and tested. A diet record needs to be performed for the 3 days that correspond to the stool collection period.
  - The coefficient of fat absorption is calculated: grams of fat ingested − grams of fat excreted/grams of fat ingested × 100.
  - Normal values are as follows:
    - Premature infants: 60–75%
    - Newborns: 80–85%
    - Children 10 months to 3 years: 85–95%
    - Children >3 years: 93%
  - When fat malabsorption is present, disorders of pancreatic function (e.g., cystic fibrosis, Shwachman-Diamond syndrome) or severe intestinal disease should be suspected.
- **Test:** lactose breath test
- *Significance*: This noninvasive test measures hydrogen levels and or methane. It is based on the principle that hydrogen gas is produced by colonic bacterial fermentation of malabsorbed carbohydrates. When abnormal in older healthy-appearing children, primary lactase deficiency is likely. However, in young children, a secondary lactase deficiency should be considered and small-bowel disease should be ruled out.
- **Test:** D-xylose test
- *Significance*: This serum test is an indirect measure of functional small bowel surface area. D-xylose absorption in the blood occurs independent of bile salts, pancreatic enzymes, and intestinal disaccharidases. A specific dose of D-xylose (1 g/kg, maximum 25 g) is given orally after an 8-hour fast, and the serum level of D-xylose is determined after 1 hour. Levels <15 to 20 mg/dL in children is abnormal and suggestive of disorders that alter or disrupt intestinal mucosa absorption.
- **Test:** fecal calprotectin
- *Significance*: Calprotectin is a neutrophilic protein detected in stools in inflammatory conditions.
- **Test:** endoscopy and colonoscopy
- *Significance*: Direct visualization of the intestinal mucosa as well as intestinal culture, disaccharidase collection, and biopsies can provide clues to diagnosis.
- **Test:** celiac panel
- *Significance*: This includes a tissue transglutaminase IgA, quantitative IgA level, and endomysial antibody.

TREATMENT

GENERAL MEASURES

- The key elements in treatment of diarrhea are as follows: (i) correction of hydration, (ii) correction of electrolytes, and (iii) specific treatment of underlying cause when indicated.
- Rehydration is the cornerstone of treatment.
- Oral rehydration therapy with glucose concentrations of 111 mmol/L and 90 mmol/L Na is recommended.
- IV rehydration is indicated for patients who are severely dehydrated and unable to tolerate oral feedings.

ISSUES FOR REFERRAL

Children who present with growth failure, noninfectious heme-positive diarrhea, or unexplained chronic diarrhea should be considered for referral to a pediatric gastroenterologist.

ADMISSION, INPATIENT, AND NURSING CONSIDERATIONS

Diarrhea can lead to significant dehydration and electrolyte imbalance. Any child suspected of clinical dehydration should be closely observed. Only if oral rehydration is ineffective is IV therapy indicated. Culture-negative GI bleeding associated with severe abdominal pain and diarrhea should always be treated urgently.

- Antibiotics
  - *Vibrio cholerae*, *Shigella*, and *Giardia lamblia* require antimicrobial therapy (i.e., trimethoprim/sulfisoxazole, azithromycin, tetracycline, ciprofloxacin, metronidazole).
  - Prolonged courses of enteropathogenic *E. coli*, *Yersinia* in patients with sickle cell disease, and *Salmonella* species infections in the very young febrile or bacteremic infant require antimicrobial therapy.

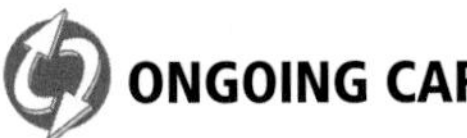

ONGOING CARE

DIET

- Breastfeeding should continue during episodes of gastroenteritis, as it promotes mucosal healing.
- A regular diet should be resumed as soon as possible. Dietary limitations are not indicated and can delay nutritional recovery.
- Micronutrient supplementation
  - Zinc supplementation at a dose of 20 mg/24 h for children >6 months and 10 mg/24 h in those <6 months for 10 to 14 days during episodes of acute diarrhea has been shown to decrease severity and duration as well as preventing future episodes in malnourished children.
- Probiotics and Prebiotics
  - Have been used for both prevention and treatment of diarrhea
  - *Lactobacillus rhamnosus GG* has been shown to shorten the duration of diarrheal illness and viral shedding (e.g., rotavirus).
  - Best evidence for effectiveness in antibiotic-associated diarrheas, rotavirus, and recurrent *C. difficile*

ADDITIONAL READING

- Aomatsu T, Yoden A, Matsumoto K, et al. Fecal calprotectin is a useful marker for disease activity in pediatric patients with inflammatory bowel disease. *Dig Dis Sci*. 2011;56(8):2372–2377.
- Castelli F, Saleri N, Tomasoni LR, et al. Prevention and treatment of traveler's diarrhea. Focus on antimicrobial agents. *Digestion*. 2006;73(Suppl 1):109–118.
- Gore JI, Surawicz C. Severe acute diarrhea. *Gastroenterol Clin North Am*. 2003;32(4):1249–1267.
- Guandalini S. Probiotics for prevention and treatment of diarrhea. *J Clin Gastroenterol*. 2011;(Suppl 45):S149–S153.
- Hartling L, Bellemare S, Wiebe N, et al. Oral versus intravenous rehydration for treating dehydration due to gastroenteritis in children. *Cochrane Database Syst Rev*. 2006;(3):CD004390.
- Patel K, Thillainayagam AV. Diarrhea. *Medicine*. 2009;37(1):23–27.
- Scharf RJ, Deboer MD, Guerrant RL. Recent advances in understanding the long-term sequelae of childhood infectious diarrhea. *Curr Infect Dis Rep*. 2014;16(6):408.
- Surawicz CM. Mechanisms of diarrhea. *Curr Gastroenterol Rep*. 2010;12(4):236–241.
- Thielman NM, Guerrant RL. Clinical practice. Acute infectious diarrhea. *N Engl J Med*. 2004;350(1):38–47.

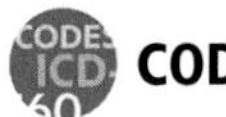

CODES

ICD10

- R19.7 Diarrhea, unspecified
- K52.9 Noninfective gastroenteritis and colitis, unspecified
- A09 Infectious gastroenteritis and colitis, unspecified

DIPHTHERIA

Michael J. Smith, MD, MSCE

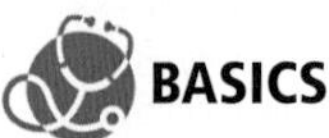

BASICS

DESCRIPTION

Acute infectious disease caused by *Corynebacterium diphtheriae*; affects primarily the membranes of the upper respiratory tract with the formation of a gray-white pseudomembrane

EPIDEMIOLOGY

- The only known reservoir for *C. diphtheriae* is humans; disease is acquired by contact with either a carrier or a diseased person.
- Most cases occur during the cooler autumn and winter months in individuals <15 years of age who are unimmunized.
- Recent outbreaks have occurred, most notably in the countries of the former Soviet Union, and supply additional evidence that disease occurs among the socioeconomically disadvantaged living in crowded conditions.

Incidence

- Although the disease is distributed throughout the world, it is endemic primarily in developing regions of Africa, Asia, and South America.
- In the Western world, the incidence of diphtheria has changed dramatically in the past 50 to 75 years as a result of the widespread use of diphtheria toxoid after World War II.
- The incidence has declined steadily and is now a rare occurrence.

GENERAL PREVENTION

Active immunization with diphtheria toxoid is the cornerstone of population-based diphtheria prevention. Current recommendations from the Advisory Committee on Immunization Practices (ACIP) of the Centers for Disease Control and Prevention (CDC) are as follows:

- Ages 2 months to 7 years: 5 doses of diphtheria vaccine (with tetanus toxoid and acellular pertussis)
  - First three given as DTaP vaccine 0.5 mL IM at 2-month intervals beginning at 2 months of age
  - Fourth dose of DTaP should be given at 15 to 18 months of age.
  - Fifth dose of DTaP at 4 to 6 years of age
- In 2005, 2 tetanus toxoid, reduced diphtheria toxoid, and acellular pertussis (Tdap) vaccines were licensed for use in adolescents 11 to 18 years of age.
- 1 booster dose of Tdap should be given to all adolescents at the 11- to 12-year-old visit, provided they have completed the childhood series. Subsequent tetanus and diphtheria (Td) boosters should be administered every 10 years.
- Tdap should replace the first dose of Td in children 7 to 10 years of age who are undergoing primary immunization.
- Isolation of patients with diphtheria is required until culture from the site of infection is negative on two consecutive specimens.

PATHOPHYSIOLOGY

- The initial entry site for *C. diphtheriae* is via airborne respiratory droplets, typically the nose or mouth but occasionally the ocular surface, genital mucous membranes, or preexisting skin lesions.
- Following 2 to 4 days of incubation at one of these sites, the bacterium elaborates toxin.
- Locally, the toxin induces formation of a necrotic coagulation of the mucous membranes (pseudomembrane) with underlying tissue edema; respiratory compromise may ensue.
- Elaborated exotoxin may also have profound effects on the heart, nerves, and kidneys in the form of myocarditis, demyelination, and tubular necrosis, respectively.

ETIOLOGY

C. diphtheriae, a gram-positive pleomorphic bacillus

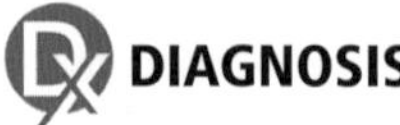

DIAGNOSIS

- Respiratory tract diphtheria
  - Nasal diphtheria starts with mild rhinorrhea that gradually becomes serosanguineous, then mucopurulent, and often malodorous; it occurs most often in infants.
  - Tonsillar and pharyngeal diphtheria begin with anorexia, malaise, low-grade fever, and pharyngitis.
    - A membrane appears within 1 to 2 days.
    - Cervical lymphadenitis and edema of the cervical soft tissues may be severe.
    - Disease course varies with extent of toxin elaboration and membrane production.
    - Respiratory and cardiovascular collapse may occur.
  - Laryngeal diphtheria most often represents extension of a pharyngeal infection.
    - Clinically presents as typical croup
    - Acute airway obstruction may occur.
    - In severe cases, the membrane may invade the entire tracheobronchial tree.
  - Cutaneous diphtheria occurs in warmer tropical regions.
    - It is characterized by chronic nonhealing ulcers with gray membrane.
    - May serve as a reservoir in endemic and epidemic areas of respiratory diphtheria
- Other sites: Rarely, vulvovaginal, conjunctival, or aural forms occur.

HISTORY

- Exposure to an individual with diphtheria is not necessarily elicited because contact with an asymptomatic carrier may be the only source of infection.
- Incubation period
  - Incubation period is 1 to 6 days.
  - Respiratory diphtheria, depending on the site of infection, may begin with nasal discharge alone or with pharyngitis accompanied by mild systemic symptoms.
  - Progression of symptoms thereafter occurs as outlined earlier (see "Diagnosis").
- Previous diphtheria immunization history, diphtheria exposure

PHYSICAL EXAM

- Classic findings
  - Nasal discharge
  - Nasal or pharyngeal membrane
  - Heart rate out of proportion to body temperature
  - Respiratory distress
  - Stridor
  - Cough
  - Hoarseness
  - Palatal paralysis
  - Neck swelling
  - Cervical lymphadenitis
  - Attempt to remove any membrane present results in bleeding.
- Conjunctival diphtheria: palpebral conjunctival involvement with a red, edematous, membranous appearance
- Aural diphtheria: otitis externa with a purulent, malodorous discharge
- Cutaneous diphtheria: See "Diagnosis."

DIFFERENTIAL DIAGNOSIS

- Nasal diphtheria
  - Common cold
  - Nasal foreign body
  - Sinusitis
  - Adenoiditis
  - Snuffles (congenital syphilis)

- Tonsillar or pharyngeal diphtheria
  - Streptococcal pharyngitis
  - Infectious mononucleosis
  - Primary herpetic tonsillitis
  - Thrush
  - Vincent angina
  - Posttonsillectomy faucial membranes
  - Oropharyngeal involvement caused by toxoplasmosis, cytomegalovirus, tularemia, and salmonellosis
- Laryngeal diphtheria
  - Croup
  - Acute epiglottitis
  - Aspirated foreign body
  - Peripharyngeal and retropharyngeal abscess
  - Laryngeal papillomas
  - Other masses

DIAGNOSTIC TESTS & INTERPRETATION

Diagnosis should be on clinical grounds: Delay in treatment increases morbidity and mortality.

- Culture of material from the membrane or beneath the membrane. Because special growth media are required, the lab should be notified of suspicion of diphtheria.
- If a strain of *C. diphtheriae* is isolated, additional testing for presence or absence of toxin production should be done by a laboratory prepared to conduct an animal neutralization test or, alternatively, neutralization (with antitoxin) in tissue culture.

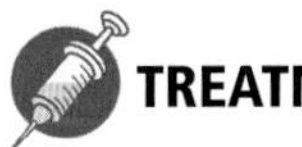

TREATMENT

MEDICATION

Antibiotic therapy: Use in addition to, not in place of, diphtheria antitoxin (DAT).

- Respiratory diphtheria
  - Penicillin G
    - Aqueous crystalline 150,000 to 250,000 U/kg/24 h IV in 4 divided doses for 14 days or
    - Procaine (IM route): ≤10 kg: 300,000 U once daily; >10 kg: 600,000 U once daily for 14 days or
  - Erythromycin 40 to 50 mg/kg (maximum 2 g/24 h) PO or parenterally for 14 days
- DAT antiserum, produced in horses, must be administered as soon as possible. DAT is available from the CDC. (Note: For patients with known horse serum sensitivity, a test dose should be administered first; if positive, the patient should be desensitized.)
  - Pharyngeal or laryngeal disease of <48 hours duration: 20,000 to 40,000 U IV
  - Nasopharyngeal lesions: 40,000 to 60,000 U IV
  - Extensive disease of ≥3 days duration or diffuse neck swelling: 80,000 to 120,000 U IV

ADDITIONAL THERAPIES

Cutaneous diphtheria: requires local care of the lesion with soap and water and administration of antimicrobials for 10 days

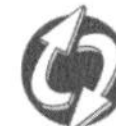

ONGOING CARE

FOLLOW-UP RECOMMENDATIONS

Patient Monitoring

- Mild cases: After membrane sloughs off in 7 to 10 days, recovery is usually uneventful.
- More severe cases: Recovery may be slower; serious complications may occur.

PROGNOSIS

- Most strongly dependent on the immunization status of the host. Those without prior adequate immunization have significantly higher morbidity and mortality.
- Delay in onset of treatment also increases mortality.
  - When appropriate treatment has been administered on day 1 of illness, mortality may be as low as 1%.
  - When treatment has been delayed until day 4, the mortality rate is ≤20-fold higher.
- Organism virulence: Toxigenic strains are associated with more severe disease and a poorer prognosis.
- Location of membrane: Laryngeal diphtheria has a higher mortality due to airway obstruction.
- A megakaryocytic thrombocytopenia and WBC count <25,000/mm^3 are associated with poor outcome.

COMPLICATIONS

- Cardiac toxicity: Myocarditis may develop secondary to elaborated toxin anytime between the 1st and 6th week of illness. Although cardiac failure may occur, most cases are transient.
- Neurologic toxicity occurs secondary to toxin elaboration and mainly reflects bilateral motor involvement.
- Paralysis of the soft palate is most common, but ocular paralysis, diaphragm paralysis, peripheral neuropathy of the extremities, and loss of deep tendon reflexes also occur.
- The frequency of all complications, including those listed above, increases with increasing time between symptom onset and antitoxin administration and also with extent of membrane formation.

ADDITIONAL READING

- American Academy of Pediatrics. Diphtheria. In: Kimberlin DW, Brady MT, Jackson MA, et al, eds. *Red Book: 2015 Report of the Committee on Infectious Diseases*. 29th ed. Elk Grove Village, IL: American Academy of Pediatrics; 2015:325–329.
- Broder KR, Cortese MM, Iskander JK, et al. Preventing tetanus, diphtheria, and pertussis among adolescents: use of tetanus toxoid, reduced diphtheria toxoid and acellular pertussis vaccines recommendations of the Advisory Committee on Immunization Practices (ACIP). *MMWR Recomm Rep*. 2006;55(RR-3):1–34.
- Centers for Disease Control and Prevention. Updated recommendations for use of tetanus toxoid, reduced diphtheria toxoid and acellular pertussis (Tdap) vaccine from the Advisory Committee on Immunization Practices, 2010. *MMWR Morb Mortal Wkly Rep*. 2011;60(1):13–15.
- Enhanced surveillance of non-toxigenic *Corynebacterium diphtheriae* infections. *Commun Dis Rep CDR Wkly*. 1996;6(4):29–32.
- Galazka A. The changing epidemiology of diphtheria in the vaccine era. *J Infect Dis*. 2000;181(Suppl 1):S2–S9.

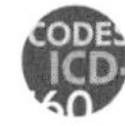

CODES

ICD10

- A36.9 Diphtheria, unspecified
- A36.1 Nasopharyngeal diphtheria
- A36.3 Cutaneous diphtheria

FAQ

- Q: What is the incidence of diphtheria in the United States?
- A: One probable case of diphtheria was reported in the United States in 2012, the first since 2003. Cutaneous diphtheria still occurs but is not a reportable disease.
- Q: Are there currently places in the world where diphtheria is a problem?
- A: Yes. An epidemic began in 1990 in Russia, spread in 1991 to Ukraine, and during 1993 and 1994, spread to the remaining countries of the former Soviet Union where it remains endemic. Other endemic regions include the Middle East and Asia and some countries in Africa and Central and South America. Travelers to these regions should check the CDC Web site for the latest information.
- Q: What precautions should be taken by travelers to areas of the world with diphtheria outbreaks?
- A: The Advisory Committee on Immunization Practices (ACIP) recommends that travelers to such areas be up to date with diphtheria immunization. Infants traveling to areas where diphtheria is endemic or epidemic should ideally receive 3 doses of DTaP before travel.

DISKITIS

Melissa L. Mannion, MD, MSPH • Randy Q. Cron, MD, PhD

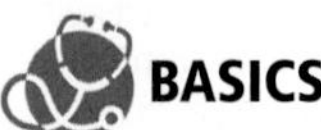

BASICS

DESCRIPTION
Often benign, self-limited inflammatory process of an intervertebral disk

EPIDEMIOLOGY
>50% of the cases occur in children <4 years of age.

Incidence
- Peak incidence is between 0 and 2 years of age.
- Second peak: >10 years

Prevalence
Rare

PATHOPHYSIOLOGY
- Probably of infectious etiology by an indolent organism
- Usually none identified; occasionally, *Staphylococcus aureus*, *Moraxella*, or the Enterobacteriaceae are cultured.
- *Kingella kingae* has been implicated in ages 6 months to 4 years old.
- Can be a late complication after ingested button battery is removed

ETIOLOGY
Idiopathic, infectious, or traumatic

DIAGNOSIS

HISTORY
- Uncomfortable, irritable child
- Refusal to walk
- Fever
- Back or abdominal pain
- Symptoms of short duration prior to presentation

PHYSICAL EXAM
- Usually, rigid posture and pain elicited on movement (sits in tripod position)
- Loss of lumbar lordosis
- Pain exacerbated by flexion
- Focal tenderness to palpation
- Most common locations: L4–L5 and L3–L4

DIFFERENTIAL DIAGNOSIS
- Infection
  - Vertebral osteomyelitis (e.g., *Staphylococcus*, *Salmonella*)
  - Pott disease (tuberculous spondylitis)
  - Pyelonephritis
  - Retrocecal appendicitis
  - Pelvic inflammatory disease
  - Psoas or epidural abscess
- Trauma
  - Fracture
  - Disk herniation
- Tumors
  - Osteoid osteoma
  - Langerhans cell granulomatosis of the spine
- Vascular: avascular necrosis of vertebral body
- Congenital: spondylolisthesis
- Immunologic
  - Spondyloarthropathy or ankylosing spondylitis
  - Nonbacterial osteitis
- Miscellaneous:
  - Scheuermann disease (osteochondritis of the vertebral bodies)
  - Disk calcification

ALERT
There is difficulty distinguishing early vertebral body osteomyelitis from diskitis.

DIAGNOSTIC TESTS & INTERPRETATION

Initial Tests (screening, lab, imaging)
- Purified protein derivative (PPD) or interferon-γ release assay (IGRA)
- WBC count
- Erythrocyte sedimentation rate (ESR)
- C-reactive protein (CRP)
- Blood cultures
- Procalcitonin has been used in adults.
- Plain radiographic studies
  - Usually normal, although may demonstrate disk narrowing as illness progresses

- MRI
  - Useful to confirm diagnosis and location of pathology
  - Demonstrates disk edema
- Bone scan
  - Demonstrates increased uptake at affected area
  - May be used to screen for other sites of infection

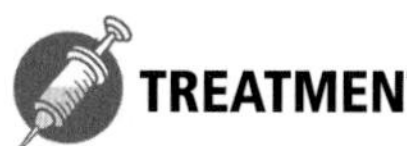

TREATMENT

MEDICATION

- Usually quite responsive to NSAIDs
- Toddlers are usually treated with antibiotics for *S. aureus* and *Kingella*.

SURGERY/OTHER PROCEDURES

Surgery indicated for compression of neural elements, instability, severe bone destruction, and intractable pain

COMPLEMENTARY & ALTERNATIVE THERAPIES

Physical therapy

- Patient should be immobilized during acute period.
- Casting may be required.

ADMISSION, INPATIENT, AND NURSING CONSIDERATIONS

Duration

- Follow CBC, CRP, and ESR.
- Continue treatment until child is asymptomatic.

ALERT

Neonates are at risk for sepsis and multifocal infections.

ONGOING CARE

FOLLOW-UP RECOMMENDATIONS

Patient Monitoring

- When to expect improvement: Most patients are asymptomatic in 6 to 8 weeks.
- Signs to watch for:
  - Recurrence of symptoms due to reactivation of the disease
  - Progressive loss of disk height
  - Destruction of adjacent vertebral bodies
  - Development of neurologic symptoms

PROGNOSIS

- Usually excellent
- Scoliosis may occur.
- Radiologic disk space narrowing almost always occurs.

COMPLICATIONS

- Occasionally, scoliosis or kyphosis
- Ankylosis of adjacent vertebrae may occur.
- Osteomyelitis of vertebral body most common in adolescents
- Neurologic deficits possible

ADDITIONAL READING

- Arthurs OJ, Gomez AC, Heinz P, et al. The toddler refusing to weight-bear: a revised imaging guide from a case series. *Emerg Med J*. 2009;26(11):797–801.
- Chandrasenan J, Klezl Z, Bommireddy R, et al. Spondylodiscitis in children: a retrospective series. *J Bone Joint Surg Br*. 2011;93(8):1122–1125.
- Fernandez M, Carrol CL, Baker CJ. Discitis and vertebral osteomyelitis in children: an 18-year review. *Pediatrics*. 2000;105(6):1299–1304.
- Kang HM, Choi EH, Lee HJ, et al. The etiology, clinical presentation and long-term outcome of spondylodiscitis in children. *Pediatr Infect Dis J*. 2016;35(4):e102–e106.
- Kayser R, Mahlfeld K, Greulich M, et al. Spondylodiscitis in childhood: results of a long-term study. *Spine (Phila Pa 1976)*. 2005;30(3):318–323.
- Marin C, Sanchez-Alegre ML, Gallego C, et al. Magnetic resonance imaging of osteoarticular infections in children. *Curr Probl Diagn Radiol*. 2004;33(2):43–59.
- Mitha A, Boutry N, Nectoux E, et al. Community-acquired bone and joint infections in children: a 1-year prospective epidemiological study. *Arch Dis Child*. 2015;100(2):126–129.
- Principi N, Esposito S. Infectious discitis and spondylodiscitis in children. *Int J Mol Sci*. 2016;17(4):539.
- Spencer SJ, Wilson NI. Childhood discitis in a regional children's hospital. *J Pediatr Orthop B*. 2012;21(3):264–268.

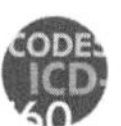

CODES

ICD10

- M46.40 Discitis, unspecified, site unspecified
- M46.46 Discitis, unspecified, lumbar region
- M46.42 Discitis, unspecified, cervical region

FAQ

- Q: When are a biopsy and tissue culture indicated?
- A: If there is bony destruction of adjacent vertebral bodies, if clinical course is prolonged or recurrent, or if the lesion mimics a tumor
- Q: When are antibiotics indicated?
- A: In situations with positive cultures or clear infective focus, or if course is atypical or prolonged
- Q: What organism should be considered as a cause of diskitis in not only developing or emerging countries but also is reported in industrialized nations?
- A: *Mycobacterium tuberculosis*

D

DISSEMINATED INTRAVASCULAR COAGULATION

Char M. Witmer, MD, MSCE

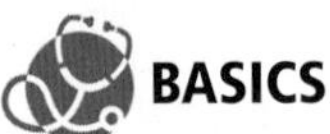

BASICS

DESCRIPTION

- Disseminated intravascular coagulation (DIC) is an acquired syndrome that is always secondary to an underlying etiology.
- It is a systemic life-threatening process characterized by an uncontrolled activation of the coagulation and fibrinolytic systems with excessive thrombin generation and the consumption of coagulation factors and platelets.
- Widespread deposition of microthrombi can compromise perfusion and lead to organ failure.
- Ongoing activation and consumption of coagulant factors and platelets can result in diffuse and profuse bleeding.

EPIDEMIOLOGY

- Most commonly secondary to infections
- Overall incidence is difficult to determine secondary to the many conditions that cause DIC.

PATHOPHYSIOLOGY

- Not a disorder in itself; occurs as a result of various initiating events
- Characterized by microvascular thrombosis and hemorrhage
- May be acute (e.g., meningococcemia) or chronic (e.g., malignancy/leukemia)
- There is a systemic intravascular deposition of fibrin as a result of increased thrombin generation, suppression of anticoagulant pathways, impaired fibrinolysis, and activation of inflammatory pathways.
- The initiation of coagulation activation leading to thrombin formation in DIC is mediated via the tissue factor/factor VIIa pathway.
- The tissue factor/factor VIIa pathway is activated via tissue factor expression from damaged endothelial cells.
- Anticoagulant pathways are diminished because of a decrease in the plasma levels of antithrombin and the protein C system through impaired production and increased destruction.
- The increase in fibrinolytic activity is likely secondary to the release of plasminogen activators from damaged endothelial cells.

ETIOLOGY

Most common causes are sepsis (particularly gram-negative), hypotensive shock, and trauma.

- Sepsis/severe infection
  - Bacterial: gram-negative and gram-positive
  - Malaria: *Plasmodium falciparum*
  - Fungal: *Aspergillus*
  - Rickettsial: Rocky Mountain spotted fever
  - Viral
- Trauma
  - Multiple fractures with fat emboli
  - Massive soft tissue injury
  - Severe head trauma
  - Multiple gunshot wounds
- Malignancies
  - Acute promyelocytic leukemia
  - Widespread solid tumors (e.g., neuroblastoma, adenocarcinoma)
- Obstetric
  - Retained intrauterine fetal demise
  - Preeclampsia/eclampsia
  - Amniotic fluid embolism
  - Abruptio placentae
  - Posthemorrhagic shock
- Neonatal
  - Necrotizing enterocolitis
  - Perinatal asphyxia
  - Amniotic fluid aspiration
  - Obstetric complications (see above)
  - Sepsis (bacterial and viral)
  - Erythroblastosis fetalis
  - Respiratory distress syndrome
- Vascular malformations
  - Kasabach-Merritt syndrome
  - Large vascular aneurysms
- Miscellaneous
  - Acute hemolytic transfusion reaction
  - Snake bite
  - Homozygous protein C/S deficiency (purpura fulminans)
  - Transplant rejection
  - Severe collagen vascular disease
  - Recreational drugs
  - Profound shock or asphyxia
  - Hypothermia or hyperthermia
  - Extensive burn injuries
  - Fulminant hepatitis/hepatic failure
  - Severe pancreatitis

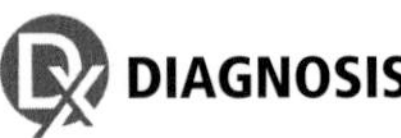

DIAGNOSIS

HISTORY

- Presence of one of the underlying conditions (see "Etiology")
- Abrupt onset of bleeding
- Prolonged bleeding from venipuncture sites
- Bleeding from multiple sites, especially venipunctures, cutdown sites, mucous membranes, skin, GI tract, and genitourinary tract
- Pulmonary or intracranial hemorrhage
- Major organ dysfunction: pulmonary, renal, hepatic

PHYSICAL EXAM

- Signs of underlying disease
- Generally, a very toxic-appearing patient
- Ecchymosis and petechiae
- Bleeding from previously intact venipuncture sites or surgical wounds
- Skin infarctions (purpura fulminans) secondary to thrombosis of dermal vessels

DIFFERENTIAL DIAGNOSIS
- Coagulopathy of liver disease
- Vitamin K deficiency
- Pathologic fibrinolysis
- Other microangiopathic diseases, for example, thrombotic thrombocytopenic purpura or hemolytic uremic syndrome

DIAGNOSTIC TESTS & INTERPRETATION

Initial Tests (screening, lab, imaging)
- There is no single test that can reliably diagnose DIC.
- Laboratory testing for DIC should be followed closely because results can change rapidly.
- CBC: Decreased platelet count is often the earliest abnormality, but this finding is nonspecific.
- Peripheral smear: schistocytes, microspherocytes (50% of cases)
- Prothrombin time (PT) and activated partial thromboplastin time (aPTT): normal to prolonged
  - Prolonged PT in 50–75% of cases
  - Prolonged aPTT in 50–60% of cases
- Fibrinogen: in the initial phase is increased as an acute-phase reactant and then decrease with consumption
  - Sensitivity is only 28%.
- Fibrin degradation products or fibrin split products: increased
  - Sensitivity 90–100% but low specificity
- Soluble fibrin monomer complexes (D-dimers): increased
  - Elevated D-dimer in 93–100% of patients with DIC but low specificity
  - A normal D-dimer rules out DIC.
- Antithrombin, protein C or S levels: decreased
  - Not routinely sent to assess for DIC
- Factor VIII: in the initial phase could be increased as an acute-phase reactant and then decrease with consumption
  - Factor VIII is normal in coagulopathy associated with liver disease.
- Multiple scoring systems using common laboratory results have been developed to help determine if a patient is in DIC. These scoring systems have not been validated in pediatric patients.

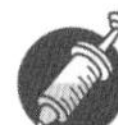

TREATMENT

GENERAL MEASURES
- The most important therapy for DIC is to treat the underlying disorder.
- Supportive therapy may be required to treat symptomatic coagulation abnormalities.
- Hemostatic therapy should not be used to treat isolated laboratory abnormalities.
- Correction of the coagulopathy should only occur to treat bleeding or prior to an invasive procedure.
- Replacement therapy
  - Cryoprecipitate: for fibrinogen replacement
  - Platelets
  - Fresh frozen plasma: contains all pro and anticoagulant proteins
- The role of heparin for DIC is controversial. It has been used in chronic DIC, arterial thromboses, or large vessel venous thromboses.
- Antithrombin at supraphysiologic dosing has been studied with mixed results.
  - Antithrombin is currently not recommended for the treatment of DIC in pediatric patients.
- In pediatric DIC, recombinant activated protein C has not been shown to be beneficial and was associated with an increased risk of bleeding.
- Off-label use of recombinant activated factor VII has been reported for patients with severe bleeding that is refractory to replacement therapy. There are significant concerns about the prothrombotic potential of this medication.
- Antifibrinolytic agents (aminocaproic acid or tranexamic acid) have been used for patients with intense fibrinolysis (e.g., Kasabach-Merritt syndrome, acute promyelocytic leukemia, or trauma). These medications are not routinely recommended for the treatment of DIC.
- Supportive care: Manage other organ system failure.

ONGOING CARE

PROGNOSIS
- Poor unless underlying disease is treated
- The intensity and duration of DIC depend on the degree of activation of the coagulation system, liver function, blood flow, and ability to reverse underlying etiology that has led to DIC.

COMPLICATIONS
- Hemorrhage
  - Pulmonary
  - Intracranial
- Thrombosis
- Multiorgan system failure

D

ADDITIONAL READING

- Levi M. Disseminated intravascular coagulation. *Crit Care Med*. 2007;35(9):2191–2195.
- Levi M, Meijers JC. DIC: which laboratory tests are most useful. *Blood Rev*. 2011;25(1):33–37.
- Montagnana M, Franchi M, Danese E, et al. Disseminated intravascular coagulation in obstetric and gynecologic disorders. *Semin Thromb Hemost*. 2010;36(4):404–418.
- Rajagopal R, Thachil J, Monagle P. Disseminated intravascular coagulation in paediatrics. *Arch Dis Child*. 2017;102(2):187–193.
- Veldman A, Fischer D, Nold MF, et al. Disseminated intravascular coagulation in term and preterm neonates. *Semin Thromb Hemost*. 2010;36(4):419–428.

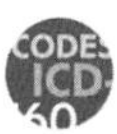

CODES

ICD10
- D65 Disseminated intravascular coagulation
- P60 Disseminated intravascular coagulation of newborn

DOWN SYNDROME (TRISOMY 21)

Esther K. Chung, MD, MPH

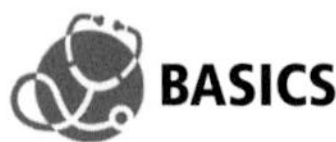

BASICS

DESCRIPTION

Syndrome first described by John Langdon Down in 1866 consisting of multiple abnormalities, including hypotonia, flat facies, upslanting palpebral fissures, and small ears; also called "trisomy 21"; other abnormalities include the following:

- Congenital heart disease (40–50%; most not symptomatic as a newborn)
  - Atrioventricular (AV) canal (60% of those with congenital heart disease)
  - Ventricular septal defect (VSD)
  - Patent ductus arteriosus (PDA)
  - Atrial septal defect (ASD)
  - Aberrant subclavian artery
  - Tetralogy of Fallot
- Hearing loss (66–75%): sensorineural and conductive
- Strabismus (33–45%)
- Nystagmus (15–35%)
- Fine lens opacities (by slit-lamp examination 59%), cataracts (1–15%)
- Refractive errors (50%)
- Nasolacrimal duct stenosis
- Delayed tooth eruption
- Tracheoesophageal fistula
- Airway anomalies, including tracheo- and laryngomalacia
- Obstructive sleep apnea (30–60%)
- Gastrointestinal atresia (12%)
- Celiac disease
- Meckel diverticulum
- Hirschsprung disease (<1%)
- Imperforate anus
- Renal malformations
- Hypospadias (5%)
- Cryptorchidism (5–50%)
- Testicular microlithiasis
- Thyroid disease (15–33%): hypothyroidism, hyperthyroidism
- Transient myeloproliferative disorder (3–10%), neonatal (leukemoid reaction)
- Transient neonatal polycythemia, neutrophilia, thrombocytopenia
- Leukemia (<1%; 10 to 20 times greater risk than in general population, acute lymphoblastic and myeloid leukemias)
- Decreased T and B lymphocytes
- Testicular germ cell tumors
- Infertility, especially in males
- Obesity
- Alopecia areata (10–15%)
- Seizures (5–10%), usually myoclonic
- Alzheimer disease (Nearly all age >40 years show neuropathologic signs.)
- Mild to moderate mental retardation (IQ range 25 to 70)
- Dry, hyperkeratotic skin (75%)

EPIDEMIOLOGY

- Population prevalence: 8.3/10,000 population
- 14/10,000 live births
- Male > female (1.3:1)
- Best recognized and most frequent chromosomal syndrome of humans
- One of the three most common autosomal trisomies in humans (Others are trisomies 18 and 13.)
- Most common autosomal chromosomal abnormality causing mental retardation
- >50% of trisomy 21 fetuses are spontaneously aborted in early pregnancy.

Incidence

1/600 to 1/800 live births, although incidence varies with maternal age:

- 1/1,500 for maternal ages 15 to 29 years
- 1/800 for maternal ages 30 to 34 years
- 1/270 for maternal ages 35 to 39 years
- 1/100 for maternal ages 40 to 49 years

RISK FACTORS

Genetics

- Approximately 90% of cases are the result of chromosomal nondisjunction (failure to segregate during meiosis) in the maternal DNA.
- <5% of cases are the result of paternal nondisjunction.
- 3–4% of cases are the result of translocations; mostly chromosomes 21 and 14 [t(14q21q)]; rarely between chromosome 21 and 13 or 15; 75% of translocations are sporadic de novo events; the others result from balanced translocations in one parent.
- Of live births, 1–2% are mosaic (nondisjunction occurs after conception; two cell lines are present); generally less severely affected

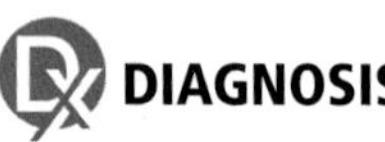

DIAGNOSIS

HISTORY

- Check for previous history of infant with Down syndrome in the family.
- Growth and developmental status
- Feeding problems
- Snoring, signs of sleep apnea (e.g., restless sleep)
- Stool habits
- Hearing concerns

PHYSICAL EXAM

The phenotype is variable from person to person.

- General
  - Short stature
  - Hypotonia (80–100%), with an open mouth and a protruding tongue
  - Midface hypoplasia
- Head
  - Brachycephaly with a flattened occiput
  - Microcephaly
  - False fontanelle (95%)
  - Late closure of fontanelles
- Eyes
  - Upslanting palpebral fissures (98%)
  - Inner epicanthal folds
  - Brushfield spots (speckling of the iris)
  - Fine lens opacities on slit-lamp examination
  - Cataracts, refractive error, strabismus, and nystagmus
- Ears
  - Small, prominent, low set; overfolding of upper helix and small canals
- Nose: small (85%); flat nasal bridge
- Tongue
  - Relative but not true macroglossia (Tongue mass is normal.)
  - Fissuring of tongue
- Mouth: high-arched or abnormal palate
- Teeth
  - Missing (50%), small, hypoplastic
  - Irregular placement
- Neck
  - In infancy, excess skin at the nape
  - Short appearance
  - Occasionally webbed
- Heart: murmur, arrhythmia, cyanosis
- Abdomen
  - In neonate, distention may be present owing to obstruction or atresia.
  - Diastasis recti
- Genitals
  - In adolescents, straight pubic hair
  - In males, small penis, cryptorchidism
- Extremities
  - Broad hands, with short metacarpals and phalanges
  - 5th finger with hypoplasia of the midphalanx (60%) and clinodactyly (50%)
  - Simian crease (single transverse palmar crease) in ~50%. A newborn with a simian crease has a 1 in 60 chance of having Down syndrome.
  - Wide gap between the 1st and 2nd toes (96%)
  - Syndactyly of 2nd and 3rd toes
  - Hyperflexibility of joints
- Skin
  - Cutis marmorata (43%)
  - In older children, hyperkeratotic dry skin (75%)
  - Fine, soft, sparse hair

DIAGNOSTIC TESTS & INTERPRETATION

Initial Tests (screening, lab, imaging)

- Prenatal
  - 2nd-trimester prenatal quad screen test (α-fetoprotein [AFP], unconjugated estriol, human chorionic gonadotropin [hCG], and inhibin A):
    - Performed at 15 to 18 weeks
    - These serum markers together can detect 67–76% of pregnancies affected by trisomy 21, with a false-positive rate of ~5%.
    - A positive test is an indication for karyotyping with amniocentesis.
  - 1st-trimester maternal serum screening (pregnancy-associated plasma protein A and free β-hCG)
  - When 1st- and 2nd-trimester tests are combined, there is a detection rate of 95%.
  - 2nd-trimester noninvasive prenatal screening (NIPS) tests are available to assess fetal DNA in the maternal circulation as a supplement to other tests.
- Postnatal
  - Chromosomal karyotype on cultured lymphocytes from peripheral blood: may be performed postnatally for confirmation if there is a clinical suspicion of Down syndrome
  - Complete blood count (CBC)
    - In the newborn period to check for polycythemia and transient myeloproliferative disorder; repeat test in adolescence.
  - Down syndrome patients may have an increased mean corpuscular volume (MCV), making the diagnosis of iron deficiency anemia difficult.
  - Thyroid function tests: to rule out hypothyroidism or hyperthyroidism
- 1st-trimester ultrasound measurement of nuchal translucency: performed in the first trimester along with maternal serum screening

- Fetal ultrasound
  - May show polyhydramnios if bowel obstruction is present
  - A thickened nuchal fold, an absent nasal bone in the first trimester, and echogenic intracardiac foci have been associated with an increased risk for Down syndrome.
- Echocardiography and chest radiography: done in the 1st month of life to rule out cardiac disease
- When symptoms suggestive of atlantoaxial instability (e.g., neck and/or radicular pain, weakness, change in tone, difficulties walking, or changes in bowel and bladder function) are present, lateral cervical spine radiographs in flexion, neutral, and extension: to rule out atlantoaxial instability, defined as >5-mm space between atlas and odontoid process of the axis. Important measures include the following:
  - Atlantodens interval (ADI; normal <4.5 mm): the distance between the posterior surface of the anterior arch of C1 and the anterior surface of the dens
  - Neural canal width (NCW; normal ≥14 mm): the distance between the posterior surface of the dens and the anterior surface of the posterior arch of C1
  - Distance of subluxation at the occipitoatlantal joint: normally ≥7 mm

Diagnostic Procedures/Other

- Prenatal karyotyping via amniocentesis (16 to 18 weeks' gestation) or chorionic villus sampling (9 to 11 weeks' gestation)
  - Performed for any woman who presents with a positive triple or quad screen
  - May be offered if prenatal ultrasound reveals a finding associated with Down syndrome
  - Because this test fails to detect 10–15% of Down syndrome in older women, amniocentesis is typically offered to all women >35 years of age.
- Tissue sample other than blood (usually skin): to check for mosaicism

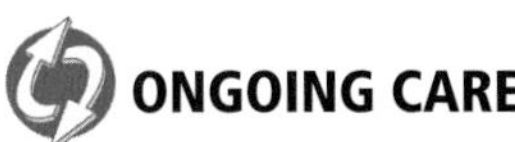

ONGOING CARE

FOLLOW-UP RECOMMENDATIONS

- Genetic counseling and evaluation is recommended.
- Referral to organizations (e.g., Down Syndrome International), parent-to-parent support groups, and other community supports available to families of children with Down syndrome

Patient Monitoring

- Annually: growth and development:
  - Current recommendations by the American Academy of Pediatrics (AAP) are to use standard growth charts for all children, including those with Down syndrome, because the previously used Down syndrome growth charts are no longer felt to represent the current body proportion.
  - Average age for acquiring developmental milestones differs from normal population.
  - Early intervention services for hypotonia and developmental delay are recommended.
  - Review need for physical, occupational, and speech therapy at each health maintenance visit.
  - Discuss psychosocial and behavioral progress and concerns, and screen for mental health disorders (e.g., autism, ADHD).
- Assessment of nutrition and activity for obesity prevention/counseling
- Evaluation/referrals for available family support including medical, financial, and social services, and school transitions
- Injury and abuse prevention
- Cardiac:
  - Early evaluation in newborn period, with follow-up until the presence or absence of disease is evident
  - Subacute bacterial endocarditis prophylaxis for patients with certain types of cardiac disease
- Ophthalmologic
  - Early evaluation for cataracts and glaucoma
  - Visit to ophthalmologist by 6 months, annually until age 5 years, and then every 2 to 3 years
- Ear, nose, and throat (ENT)/audiologic
  - Audiologic evaluation; if newborn evaluation was normal, repeat at 6 months of age in the first 3 years of life, and then every other year.
- Obstructive sleep apnea
  - Review symptoms with family in first 6 months and screen for symptoms at each well-child visit.
  - Refer all children for sleep study or polysomnography by 4 years of age and at any age if symptomatic.
- Orthopedic: Routine screening by x-ray for atlantoaxial instability in asymptomatic children is no longer recommended by the AAP.
- Endocrine: thyroid function tests in newborn period, ages 6 months and 12 months, and then yearly
- Gastrointestinal: Screen for symptoms of celiac disease (i.e., diarrhea, poor growth, failure to thrive), and if symptomatic, obtain tissue transglutaminase immunoglobulin A (IgA) level and quantitative IgA.
- For adolescents, discuss personal hygiene and issues related to reproductive health.

PATIENT EDUCATION

- Information, medical forms and resources for Special Olympics Athletes: http://resources.specialolympics.org/Topics/General_Rules/Article_02.aspx
- Down syndrome. See: http://kidshealth.org/parent/medical/genetic/down_syndrome.html

PROGNOSIS

- Life expectancy is mildly decreased, with many living into the 6th decade; median age of death is 49 years.
- Clinical signs of Alzheimer disease occur later in life, with reports as high as 51% in the 4th decade.
- As adults, most patients with Down syndrome can work in supported positions.

COMPLICATIONS

- Otitis media with effusion (50–70%)
- Sinusitis
- Tonsillar and adenoidal hypertrophy
- Obstructive airway disease with associated sleep apnea (50–79%), cor pulmonale
- Obstructive bowel disease (12%, newborn period)
- Constipation (owing to low tone and decreased gross motor mobility)
- Subluxation of the hips (secondary to ligamentous laxity)
- Atlantoaxial instability (10–30%; secondary to ligamentous laxity, which is most severe prior to age 10 years)

ALERT

- Use caution with endotracheal intubation if absence or presence of atlantoaxial instability is unknown in order to avoid spinal cord injury, which may be seen in rare cases.
- Hearing loss may be misinterpreted as a behavioral problem.
- Use care with atropine and pilocarpine for ophthalmologic evaluation because of possible cholinergic hypersensitivity.

ADDITIONAL READING

- Bruwier A, Chantrain CF. Hematological disorders and leukemia in children with Down syndrome. *Eur J Pediatr*. 2012;171(9):1301–1307.
- Bull MJ; and Committee on Genetics. Health supervision for children with Down syndrome. *Pediatrics*. 2011;128(2):393–406.
- Bunt CW, Bunt SK. Role of the family physician in the care of children with Down syndrome. *Am Fam Physician*. 2014;90(12):851–858.
- Dykens EM. Psychiatric and behavioral disorders in persons with Down syndrome. *Ment Retard Dev Disabil Res Rev*. 2007;13(3):272–278.
- Gregg AR, Gross SJ, Best RG, et al. ACMG statement on noninvasive prenatal screening for fetal aneuploidy. *Genet Med*. 2013;15(5):395–398.
- Maris M, Verhulst S, Wojciechowski M, et al. Prevalence of obstructive sleep apnea in children with Down syndrome. *Sleep*. 2016;39(3):699–704.
- Presson AP, Partyka G, Jensen KM, et al. Current estimate of Down syndrome population prevalence in the United States. *J Pediatr*. 2013;163(4):1163–1168.
- Purdy IB, Singh N, Brown WL, et al. Revisiting early hypothyroidism screening in infants with Down syndrome. *J Perinatol*. 2014;34(12):936–940.

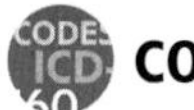

CODES

ICD10

- Q90.9 Down syndrome, unspecified
- Q90.2 Trisomy 21, translocation
- Q90.1 Trisomy 21, mosaicism (mitotic nondisjunction)

FAQ

- Q: Why was Down syndrome referred to as mongolism in the past?
- A: There was a mistaken notion about a racial cause for this syndrome because of the facial appearance, which was thought to be similar to that of those of Mongoloid origin.
- Q: Do all children with Down syndrome have mental retardation?
- A: No. Although all persons with nonmosaic Down syndrome have some degree of cognitive disability, some have IQs >70 and are not considered to have mental retardation.
- Q: Can a normal cardiac examination rule out the presence of a cardiac anomaly?
- A: No. The AAP recommends that all patients with Down syndrome have a cardiology consultation within the 1st month of life. Timely surgery may be necessary to prevent serious complications.
- Q: Are patients with atlantoaxial instability symptomatic?
- A: No. Most are asymptomatic, but symptoms of cord compression may be seen in 1–2% of patients. Patients with neck and/or radicular pain, weakness, change in tone, difficulties walking, or changes in bowel and bladder function should undergo radiologic evaluation for atlantoaxial instability.

DROWNING

Mercedes M. Blackstone, MD

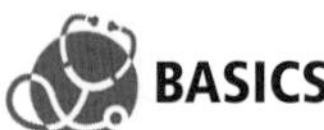

BASICS

DESCRIPTION

- Drowning is defined as respiratory impairment from submersion in a liquid medium.
- The term "drowning" does not imply outcome; drowning can be fatal or nonfatal.
- Historically "near drowning," or submersion injury, was defined as survival, at least temporarily, after suffocation by submersion in water.
  - The World Congress on Drowning and the World Health Organization advocate abandoning confusing terms such as "near drowning," "wet drowning," "dry drowning," and "secondary drowning"; they suggest that the literature should only use the term "drowning."

EPIDEMIOLOGY

- Drowning is second only to motor vehicle collisions as the most common cause of death from unintentional injury in childhood.
- For every drowning death, another five children present to emergency departments for nonfatal submersion events.
- Bimodal age distribution, with peak in children <5 years of age and again among adolescents 15 to 19 years of age
- Bathtub drowning is common in babies; child neglect or abuse should be considered.
- Adolescent submersion injuries usually involve substance abuse or risk-taking behavior.

RISK FACTORS

- Males, children <5 years of age, African Americans, and children of low socioeconomic status are at greatest risk.
- Other significant risk factors include the following:
  - Direct access to swimming pools (There are more drowning in southern states.)
  - Poor swimming ability or overestimation of ability
  - Use of alcohol and illicit drugs
  - Inadequate adult supervision
  - Underlying medical conditions such as seizure disorders or primary cardiac arrhythmias like long QT syndrome

GENERAL PREVENTION

- Most drownings are preventable.
- Quality prevention efforts include:
  - Legislation to require adequate four-sided isolation fencing and rescue equipment for public and residential pools
  - Restriction of sale and consumption of alcohol in boating areas, pools, and beaches
  - Life vests for children of all ages near bodies of water
  - Parental education regarding adequate supervision during bathing and around bodies of water
  - Cardiopulmonary resuscitation (CPR) courses for pool owners, parents, and older children
  - Parental education about dangers of bathtubs, buckets, and inflatable pools for babies and toddlers
  - Swimming lessons and lifeguard supervision

PATHOPHYSIOLOGY

- Drowning begins with a loss of the normal breathing pattern as panic ensues and subsequent apnea, laryngospasm, or aspiration occurs.
- Water aspirated into the trachea and lungs washes out surfactant and leads to atelectasis, intrapulmonary shunting, poor lung compliance, increased capillary permeability, and hypoxemia, ultimately resulting in acute respiratory distress syndrome (ARDS).
- Severe hypoxemia is the final common pathway and results in multisystem organ failure.
- Cerebral hypoxia results in cerebral edema and increased intracranial pressure (ICP) and causes the majority of morbidity and mortality associated with drowning.

COMMONLY ASSOCIATED CONDITIONS

- Cervical spine injuries should be considered in older children who have experienced diving accidents but are otherwise relatively rare in drowning events.
- Signs of child abuse or neglect should be sought in young children.
- Adolescents may have associated toxic ingestions.
- Hypothermia (see management below)

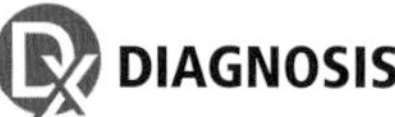

DIAGNOSIS

HISTORY

- Mechanism
  - History of diving or other high-impact injury
  - Intoxication
  - Seizure disorder
  - Cardiac arrhythmia
  - Child abuse
- Prognostic indicators; the following have been correlated with a poor prognosis and may be helpful to ask about:
  - Age >14 years
  - Length of submersion >5 minutes
  - Time to effective CPR >10 minutes
  - Lack of vital signs at the scene
  - Length of resuscitation >25 minutes
  - Warmer water: Submersion in cold water (<5°C [41°F]) may have a good prognosis despite submersion time >5 minutes.

PHYSICAL EXAM

- Vital signs with core temperature
- Drowning victims with unclear histories must be treated as trauma victims.
- Neurologic
  - Pupillary response, cranial nerve findings, Glasgow Coma Scale (GCS) score, gag reflex
  - Serial neurologic exams should be performed to assess neurologic outcome. Children with a GCS score <5 after resuscitation usually have a poor neurologic outcome.
- Respiratory
  - Lower airway findings (rales, tachypnea, wheezing, retractions, nasal flaring)
  - Drowning victims may have deteriorating pulmonary involvement despite an initially normal exam. Watch closely for signs of lower airway involvement.
- Circulation
  - Perfusion, strength of distal pulses, capillary refill, urine output, cardiac rhythm
- GI tract
  - Abdominal distention from swallowed water or ventilation
- Musculoskeletal
  - Neck injuries in high-impact drownings

DIAGNOSTIC TESTS & INTERPRETATION

Initial Tests (screening, lab, imaging)

- Blood gases
  - To detect and facilitate treatment of respiratory/metabolic acidosis in the child with respiratory distress or apnea
- Electrolytes
  - Not indicated in the seemingly well child; aspiration of huge amounts of water is required to generate electrolyte shifts.
- Blood glucose
  - An elevated level correlates with poor outcome for comatose submersion victims.
- Anticonvulsant levels for victims with seizure disorders
- Toxicology screening when ingestion suspected
- Children with severe submersion injuries are at risk of multiorgan system failure, and in these patients, end organ labs should be checked including coagulation studies.
- A chest radiograph is indicated for children with signs of pulmonary involvement and after intubation.
  - Caution: Initial chest radiographs may be normal in the drowning victim.
- Cervical spine films are indicated for victims of high-impact events.
- Neuroimaging for cerebral anoxic injury

Diagnostic Procedures/Other

- ECG to document normal rhythm and evaluate for prolonged QT_C if indicated by history
- Serial pulse oximetry to detect early signs of pulmonary involvement

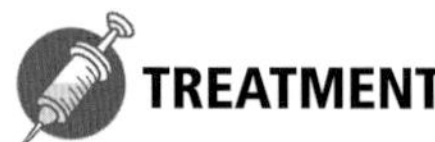

TREATMENT

GENERAL MEASURES

- Good prehospital care and effective bystander CPR dramatically improve chances of neurologically intact survival.
- Attempts to remove water from the lungs such as abdominal thrusts or Heimlich maneuver delay care are not recommended.
- Cervical spine immobilization can interfere with airway management and should *only* be performed when injury is suspected based on mechanism of drowning or exam findings.
- Patients who are breathing spontaneously should be placed in the right lateral decubitus position to prevent aspiration.
- CPR in drowning victims should follow the traditional ABC approach rather than compression-only CPR because prompt rescue breathing increases the chance of survival.
- Even patients who respond well to bystander resuscitation need to be transported to an emergency department for further monitoring.
- Pulses may be difficult to appreciate as they can be weak and slow due to hypothermia; some common arrhythmias such as sinus bradycardia and atrial fibrillation need no immediate treatment.
- The hypothermic patient who is a warm water (>20°C [86°F]) drowning victim does not have a good prognosis or need vigorous rewarming.

MEDICATION

- Patients may experience bronchospasm and typically respond to conventional management with inhaled β-agonists.
- Prophylactic antibiotics or steroids are not indicated.
- For patients who develop pneumonia, antimicrobial therapy should cover waterborne pathogens (e.g., *Pseudomonas*, *Aeromonas*).
- Seizures should be aggressively controlled with antiepileptics because they increase oxygen consumption.
- A trial of naloxone should be considered if concomitant opioid ingestion is suspected.

ADMISSION, INPATIENT, AND NURSING CONSIDERATIONS

- Airway
  - Protect the cervical spine if indicated by history.
  - Ensure a patent airway in the comatose victim or patient in cardiac arrest.
- Breathing
  - Supplemental oxygen via facemask with any respiratory compromise or desaturation
  - Treatment of bronchospasm
  - Noninvasive ventilation with CPAP or BiPAP can often be used for respiratory compromise.
  - Intubate for apnea, airway protection, or inadequate oxygenation or ventilation on noninvasive modalities. A nasal/orogastric tube should be placed for gastric decompression as well.
- May need escalating ventilator support as in other types of acute lung injury
- Circulation
  - Because capillary leak may occur after an ischemic/anoxic episode, isotonic fluids (e.g., normal saline solution or Ringer lactate, 10 mL/kg aliquots) should be given for signs of intravascular volume depletion until normalized.
  - Patients can also develop hypotension from a "cold diuresis."
  - ECG monitoring should be provided with appropriate response to dysrhythmias, especially for the hypothermic, cold-water drowning victim.
  - For severely hypothermic patients with a core temperature <28°C (82.4°F), aggressive rewarming is indicated. Electrical defibrillation and pharmacotherapy may not be successful until rewarmed.
- Disability: focused on prevention of secondary injury
  - Maintenance of eucapnia and adequate oxygenation to prevent further hypoxemia
  - Elevate the head of the bed once cervical spine is cleared.
  - Other measures for reducing ICP have not proven effective, likely because the brain injury and swelling is secondary to hypoxic cell injury rather than a traumatic lesion.
- Exposure
  - The drowning victim should be dried and warmed.
  - Most thermometers do not register temperatures below 34°C (93.2°F) so a hypothermia thermometer may be necessary:
    - For core temperatures 32°C (89.6°F) to 35°C (95.0°F), active external rewarming with heating blankets or radiant warmers
    - For <32°C (89.6°F), active internal rewarming added (heated aerosolized oxygen and IV fluids, gastric and bladder lavage with warm saline)
    - For severe hypothermia (<28°C [82.4°F]) and where available, peritoneal dialysis or hemodialysis, mediastinal irrigation, and cardiac bypass
    - The cold water drowning victim with hypothermia should be rewarmed to a temperature >34°C (93.2°F) before CPR is terminated.
- Remember: The saying, "The patient is not dead until he or she is warm and dead" only applies to drownings in very cold water.
- Severely ill children require admission to the intensive care unit.
- Children who were apneic, cyanotic, or pulseless at the scene should be admitted for close observation even if they appear well.
- Patients who are at all symptomatic should be admitted to a monitored setting.
- A subset of asymptomatic children may be discharged from the emergency department after being monitored for 6 to 8 hours.

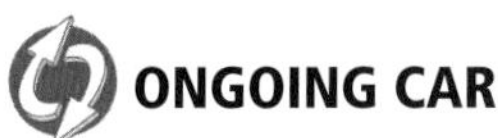

ONGOING CARE

FOLLOW-UP RECOMMENDATIONS

- Long-term follow-up of apparently neurologically intact survivors has shown mild coordination or gross motor deficiencies.
- Potential increased risk for chronic lung disease, depending on pulmonary involvement

Patient Monitoring

- Victims who appear well and had a relatively minor event:
  - Monitor with pulse oximetry for progressive respiratory distress.
  - If asymptomatic at 6 to 8 hours postimmersion, can be discharged
- Victims with significant neurologic injury: Key is to prevent secondary injury.
  - Maintain euvolemia, euglycemia.
  - Aggressively treat fevers or seizures.

PROGNOSIS

- Most children (about 75%) recover with intact neurologic survival.
- ~5–10% of survivors have severe neurologic impairment.
- Duration and severity of initial hypoxic insult are most important determinants of brain injury and death.
- See prognostic factors in "History" section. Additional indicators of poor prognosis:
  - Coma on arrival
  - Needing CPR in the emergency department
  - Initial arterial blood pH <7.1
- Children with warm water submersion time >4 minutes who do not receive CPR at the scene and who have absent vital signs or a GCS score <5 in the emergency department usually have a poor prognosis.
- Victims who have prolonged submersions in very cold water (<5°C [41°F]) may have a good prognosis because of core cooling with a concomitant decrease in metabolic rate while the brain is still being perfused.
- A good prognostic indicator is continuing improvement in the neurologic examination over the first several hours.

COMPLICATIONS

- Pneumonia
- Pneumomediastinum or pneumothorax in the patient undergoing ventilation therapy
- Brain injury secondary to hypoxia
- Pulmonary injury with intrapulmonary shunting secondary to damage of the alveoli
- ARDS
- Metabolic acidosis secondary to hypoxemia
- Ischemic injury to organs such as liver, kidneys, and intestines
- Disseminated intravascular coagulation
- Hypothermia in cold water drowning

ADDITIONAL READING

- American Academy of Pediatrics Committee on Injury, Violence, and Poison Prevention. Prevention of drowning. *Pediatrics*. 2010;126(1):178–185.
- Brenner RA. Prevention of drowning in infants, children, and adolescents. *Pediatrics*. 2003;112(2):440–445.
- Centers for Disease Control and Prevention. Web-based Injury Statistics Query and Reporting System (WISQARS) [online]. http://www.cdc.gov/injury/wisqars. Accessed November 30, 2014.
- Hwang V, Shofer FS, Durbin DR, et al. Prevalence of traumatic injuries in drowning and near drowning in children and adolescents. *Arch Pediatr Adolesc Med*. 2003;157(1):50–53.
- Noonan L, Howrey R, Ginsburg CM. Freshwater submersion injuries in children: a retrospective review of seventy-five hospitalized patients. *Pediatrics*. 1996;98(3, Pt 1):368–371.
- Papa L, Hoelle R, Idris A. Systematic review of definitions for drowning incidents. *Resuscitation*. 2005;65(3):255–264.
- Szpilman D, Bierens JJ, Handley AJ, et al. Drowning. *N Engl J Med*. 2012;366(22):2102–2110.
- Thompson DC, Rivara FP. Pool fencing for preventing drowning in children. *Cochrane Database Syst Rev*. 2000;(2):CD001047.
- Tobin JM, Ramos WD, Pu Y, et al. Bystander CPR is associated with improved neurologically favourable survival in cardiac arrest following drowning. *Resuscitation*. 2017;115:39–43.
- Vanden Hoek TL, Morrison LJ, Shuster M, et al. Part 12: cardiac arrest in special situations: 2010 American Heart Association Guidelines for Cardiopulmonary Resuscitation and Emergency Cardiovascular Care. *Circulation*. 2010;122(18 Suppl 3):S829–S861.

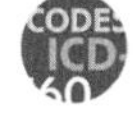

CODES

ICD10

T75.1XXA Unsp effects of drowning and nonfatal submersion, init

FAQ

- Q: Should the drowning victim who arrives at the hospital with cardiopulmonary arrest be resuscitated?
- A: Yes. A brief (10 to 15 minutes) attempt at resuscitation is indicated until circumstances of the drowning and core temperature are known. Warm water drowning victims who require CPR in the emergency department may rarely (0–25%) have good neurologic recovery, but these patients usually respond quickly (<15 minutes) to therapy.
- Q: Is artificial surfactant useful in drowning victims?
- A: Surfactant has not been found to be beneficial for acute lung injury secondary to drowning. Further investigation is needed before it can be recommended for clinical use.
- Q: Is there a significant difference in management of fresh water versus salt water drownings?
- A: No, because victims seldom aspirate the large volumes of water required to create fluid shifts, electrolyte derangements are quite rare. If the victim develops pneumonia, the location of the drowning may be relevant when considering causative organisms.

DYSFUNCTIONAL (ABNORMAL) UTERINE BLEEDING

Leonard J. Levine, MD • Jonathan R. Pletcher, MD

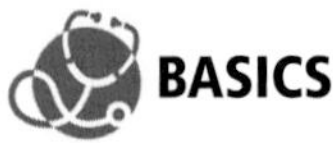

BASICS

DESCRIPTION

- Bleeding that is excessive in flow, outside of regular menstrual cycles, or occurs daily for >8 days
- Adolescents typically do not establish regular ovulatory cycles until their mid to late teens, therefore "normal" periods can last 2 to 7 days, can occur every 21 to 45 days, and blood loss can vary from 20 to 80 mL per cycle.
- Abnormal uterine bleeding (AUB) can vary in presentation from menses that lasts for weeks and varies in flow followed by long periods of amenorrhea to shorter but heavy flow menses, occurring more frequently.
- In teens, AUB most commonly results from an immature hypothalamic–pituitary–ovarian (HPO) axis and consequent anovulatory cycles.

EPIDEMIOLOGY

- AUB commonly occurs within 5 to 7 years after menarche, most often in the first 2 years when >50% of cycles are anovulatory.
- Later age at menarche is associated with longer duration of anovulatory cycles.
- Most females who experience anovulatory cycles do not develop AUB.

RISK FACTORS

Genetics

Patients with disorders, such as blood dyscrasias and polycystic ovary syndrome (PCOS), usually have familial histories of similar disorders.

PATHOPHYSIOLOGY

- In anovulatory cycles, failure to ovulate results in a lack of progesterone production due to corpus luteum absence.
- Without the secretory effect of progesterone from the corpus luteum, endometrial proliferation continues because of unopposed estrogen.
- The thickened endometrium eventually outgrows support from the basal endometrium, resulting in sloughing of the highest endometrial levels. Alternatively, cyclic estrogen withdrawal may occur, which will lead to sloughing of the endometrium in the absence of progesterone.
- As subsequent levels of endometrium are shed, bleeding increases. Profuse bleeding may result when the basal endometrium is exposed.
- Anovulatory cycles occur as a result of maturity, PCOS, pregnancy, thyroid dysfunction, or hypothalamic dysfunction as a result of weight loss, obesity, autoimmune or other chronic disease, or exercise.
- AUB can also result or be exacerbated by underlying blood dyscrasia or infection.

DIAGNOSIS

HISTORY

- A complete history should be obtained both with and without the presence of adolescent's caregiver.
- A complete menstrual history includes:
  - Assessment of the amount of bleeding and confirmation that it is vaginal bleeding
  - Timing, including when the bleeding began, and any variations in flow can be helpful in estimating amount of blood loss.
  - Having the patient keep a menstrual record using a smartphone app or a calendar can be very useful in determining the pattern of bleeding.
- The pattern of AUB can help guide the diagnostic workup.
  - Normal cyclic intervals with increased bleeding during each cycle may suggest a bleeding disorder.
  - Normal intervals with bleeding between cycles may suggest infection or foreign body.
  - Abnormal intervals with no cycle regularity may suggest anovulatory cycles or be a side effect of inconsistent use of hormonal contraception.
- Irregular periods and the absence or inconsistent menstrual symptoms such as cramps or breast tenderness are consistent with anovulatory cycles.
- Assessing the amount of blood loss is nearly impossible outside of an inpatient setting.
- Easy bruisability, epistaxis, and/or bleeding gums may be suggestive of a bleeding disorder.
- A family history of thyroid disease, bleeding disorder, PCOS, or AUB will help guide the laboratory workup.
- Personal and immediate family history of thromboembolism or known familial risk factors
- A complete review of systems and medication history may indicate a pattern of underlying illness or medication use that could interfere with menstrual function such as hormonal contraception or corticosteroid use.
- A confidential social history is essential in identifying underlying potential causes such as a sexually transmitted infection (STI) or other consequence of sexual activity, trauma, or substance use, such as marijuana, that can interfere with hypothalamic function.

PHYSICAL EXAM

- Often normal in patients with AUB
- Assess vital signs, including orthostatic blood pressure (BP), for signs of cardiac instability resulting from severe blood loss.
- Pallor of skin or mucous membranes, elevated heart rate, or flow murmur may be indicative of anemic state.
- Look for signs of androgen excess (e.g., hirsutism, acne), which may be reflective of disrupted ovulatory function.
- Check skin for acanthosis nigricans, bruising, or petechiae.
- Bitemporal hemianopsia is suggestive of a pituitary adenoma leading to hyperprolactinemia.
  - Hyperprolactinemia can result in anovulation.
  - Only 1/3 of adolescents with hyperprolactinemia will experience galactorrhea.
- Assess for evidence of thyroid disease (goiter) or systemic disease (e.g., poor nutritional status).
- Assess sexual maturity rating (SMR, or Tanner stage). Menarche usually does not occur before SMR 3, so bleeding before this stage suggests a nonmenstrual source of bleeding.
- External genital exam for clitoromegaly, signs of trauma, and hymenal integrity
- Speculum-assisted pelvic examination may help determine source of bleeding. Bimanual examination is helpful in assessing ovarian or uterine masses, cervical motion or adnexal tenderness, and uterine sizing.

DIFFERENTIAL DIAGNOSIS

- Most cases of AUB in adolescents can be attributed to anovulatory cycles resulting from immaturity of the HPO axis. Because there is no confirmatory laboratory or imaging test for HPO axis immaturity, it is important to rule out underlying and alternate causes of irregular or heavy bleeding.
- Pregnancy testing should be considered in every patient, regardless of patient's reported sexual history. If positive, possible causes of AUB include:
  - Ectopic pregnancy
  - Threatened abortion, incomplete abortion
  - Placenta previa
  - Hydatidiform mole
- Infection
  - Vaginitis (e.g., trichomoniasis)
  - Cervicitis or endometritis (e.g., gonorrhea or chlamydia)
  - Pelvic inflammatory disease
- Hematologic conditions
  - Thrombocytopenia (e.g., immune thrombocytopenic purpura [ITP], leukemia)
  - Platelet dysfunction
  - Coagulation defect (e.g., von Willebrand disease)
- Endocrinologic disorders
  - Hyper- or hypothyroidism
  - Hyperprolactinemia
  - PCOS
  - Adrenal disorders
- Trauma: laceration to vagina or cervix
- Foreign body: usually associated with strong, foul odor
- Medications
  - Direct effect on hemostasis (e.g., Coumadin, chemotherapeutic agents)
  - Hormonal effects (e.g., oral contraceptives, Depo-Provera, other exogenous steroid hormones)
- Systemic disease
  - Disruption of HPO axis
  - Other examples include systemic lupus erythematosus and chronic renal failure.
- Primary gynecologic disorders
  - Endometriosis
  - Uterine polyps, submucosal myomas
  - Hemangioma, arteriovenous malformation

DIAGNOSTIC TESTS & INTERPRETATION

Initial Tests (screening, lab, imaging)

- Obtain urine or serum human chorionic gonadotropin (β-hCG), regardless of sexual history. Urine hCG testing can reliably detect pregnancy as early as 2 weeks postconception; however, it may be positive for up to 2 weeks following a miscarriage or abortion.
- CBC: Degree of anemia guides treatment plan. Assess for thrombocytopenia. In the setting of acute blood loss, a normal hemoglobin may be falsely reassuring. It is wise to recheck hemoglobin after IV hydration as decreases may be dramatic.
- For *Chlamydia trachomatis* and *Neisseria gonorrhoeae*, obtain nucleic acid amplification tests (NAATs) (e.g., PCR or LCR) on urine, vaginal, or cervical swabs. Obtain cervical cultures if abuse is suspected or reported.
- Consider prolactin level and thyroid function tests (TSH, T_4): Hyperprolactinemia may have several causes, including pituitary microadenoma, and result in amenorrhea or AUB.
- Follicle-stimulating hormone (FSH) level obtained in the 1st week of the menstrual cycle can be helpful in identifying ovarian insufficiency if elevated.
- Prothrombin and partial thromboplastin time, von Willebrand factor: to assess for hematologic causes of bleeding

- Androgen levels, including testosterone (total and free), dehydroepiandrosterone sulfate (DHEAS), androstenedione: Abnormal levels are supportive of PCOS or other hyperandrogenic state.
- Pelvic ultrasound
  - Indicated when pregnancy is suspected (ectopic or intrauterine)
  - Consider when a pelvic mass is felt, uterine anomaly is being considered, or bimanual examination cannot be completed.
  - May reveal contributing cause of AUB including vaginal outlet obstruction, uterine leiomyoma, polycystic ovaries, or ovarian mass
  - May also identify adrenal mass if indicated based on signs of hyperandrogenism
- MRI of the pelvis: indicated for patients with a suspected pelvic or adrenal mass when ultrasonography does not clearly define the anatomy

ALERT
Pitfalls
- Neglecting to assess hemodynamic stability by obtaining orthostatic BP and heart rate
- Neglecting to perform pregnancy testing in an adolescent who denies sexual activity
- Neglecting to reassess hemoglobin concentration after volume expansion

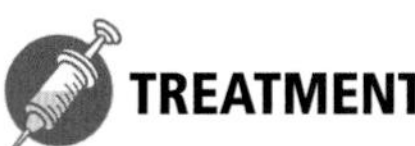

TREATMENT

GENERAL MEASURES

- The initial step in evaluating AUB is to determine pregnancy status and assess hemodynamic stability.
- Any adolescent who exhibits signs or symptoms of hemodynamic instability or who has AUB in the setting of pregnancy should be stabilized and transported to an emergency department for further care.
- Adolescents who are assessed to be nonpregnant and are hemodynamically stable can be triaged to three categories: mild, moderate, and severe AUB.
- For mild AUB (inconvenient, unpredictable bleeding, normal hemoglobin in setting of hemodynamic stability)
  - Reassurance until ovulatory cycles resume, encourage menstrual calendar maintenance, with follow-up in 3 to 6 months
  - Iron supplementation
  - If the problem persists, consider hormonal therapy with a daily combined oral contraceptive pill (OCP), 1 tablet daily to regulate menstrual cycle. If estrogen is contraindicated, may use progesterone-only pill, medroxyprogesterone acetate 5 to 10 mg/24 h PO for 5 to 10 days every month starting on day 16 or 21 of menstrual cycle.
  - For mild to moderate AUB, a progestin-containing intrauterine device may be indicated.
- For moderate AUB (irregular, prolonged, heavy bleeding with a hemoglobin >10 g/dL)
  - Hormonal therapy, as described previously; may start combination OCP containing 35 mcg of ethinyl estradiol twice a day until bleeding stops, then taper to once a day
  - Menstrual calendar with follow-up every 1 to 3 months
- For severe AUB (i.e., heavy, prolonged bleeding with a hemoglobin <10 g/dL), treatment depends on the presence of active bleeding.
  - If no active bleeding, hemodynamically stable patients can be started on daily OCPs and iron supplementation, with follow-up in 1 to 2 months.
  - In the presence of active bleeding: hormonal therapy using combined OCP containing higher dose of estrogen (50 mcg ethinyl estradiol)—1 pill every 6 hours until bleeding stops, followed by pill taper (e.g., 4 times a day for 4 days, 3 times a day for 3 days, twice a day for 2 weeks, then 1 pill daily); switch to lower dose pill (30 to 35 mcg) after taper is complete.
  - Hospitalization of patient during treatment if with severe anemia (hemoglobin <7 g/dL), if hemodynamically unstable, or with compliance concerns; blood transfusion as necessary
  - If patient is hemodynamically unstable or unable to tolerate oral pill regimen, can give IV conjugated estrogen up to every 4 hours for 24 hours to stop bleeding. Add PO or IM progesterone as soon as possible to prevent rebound or severe breakthrough bleeding.
  - Iron replacement when tolerated
  - Dilation and curettage rarely necessary; may be needed if hormonal therapy fails
- Possible side effects
  - Estrogen, given in high doses, will cause nausea and/or vomiting. An appropriate antiemetic should be used for prophylaxis against these symptoms.
  - High-dose estrogen may have vascular side effects and should be used with caution in patients particularly at risk for vascular events (e.g., patients with a history of lupus, stroke, or thrombotic phenomena and those who smoke cigarettes). In these cases, consult a gynecologist or adolescent medicine specialist for an alternative progesterone-only therapy.

ALERT
Pitfalls
- Neglecting to provide both estrogen and progesterone in a timely fashion
- Neglecting to adequately assess or mediate risk for thromboembolic event related to estrogen therapy
- Neglecting to consider a retained foreign body (e.g., tampon)

ADMISSION, INPATIENT, AND NURSING CONSIDERATIONS

If AUB is attributed to anovulatory cycles, or if a complete workup fails to yield a diagnosis, treatment is guided by the severity of AUB, associated signs or symptoms that may develop over time, and the presence of active bleeding.

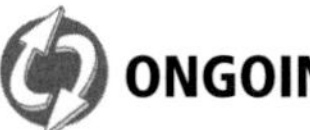

ONGOING CARE

FOLLOW-UP RECOMMENDATIONS

Patient Monitoring

When to expect improvement
- Bleeding usually tapers after the first few doses of hormone therapy.
- After 6 to 12 months, if patient does not wish to remain on OCPs, a trial off medication might reveal normal ovulatory cycles.
- Ongoing follow-up with an adolescent medicine or adolescent gynecologist may be warranted.

PROGNOSIS

AUB persists for 2 years in 60% of patients, 4 years in 50%, and up to 10 years in 30%.

COMPLICATIONS

- Mild to severe anemia resulting from blood loss
- Thromboembolic event from procoagulant effects of estrogen therapy

ADDITIONAL READING

- ACOG Committee Opinion No. 651: menstruation in girls and adolescents: using the menstrual cycle as a vital sign. *Obstet Gynecol*. 2015;126(6):e143–e146.
- Bradley LD, Gueye NA. The medical management of abnormal uterine bleeding in reproductive-aged women. *Am J Obstet Gynecol*. 2016;214(1):31–44.
- Hickey M, Higham JM, Fraser I. Progestogens with or without oestrogen for irregular uterine bleeding associated with anovulation. *Cochrane Database Syst Rev*. 2012;(9):CD001895.
- LaCour DE, Long DN, Perlman SE. Dysfunctional uterine bleeding in adolescent females associated with endocrine causes and medical conditions. *J Pediatr Adolesc Gynecol*. 2010;23(2):62–70.

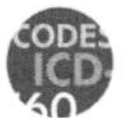

CODES

ICD10

- N93.8 Other specified abnormal uterine and vaginal bleeding
- N92.3 Ovulation bleeding
- N93.9 Abnormal uterine and vaginal bleeding, unspecified

FAQ

- Q: If most girls have anovulatory cycles, why do only some present with AUB?
- A: Most girls do have irregular menstrual cycles during the first 2 years after menarche. However, in most, the negative-feedback system of estrogen leads to cyclic endometrial shedding in an anovulatory pattern.
- Q: If AUB from anovulatory cycles is caused by lack of progesterone, why does the initial treatment of severe AUB with active bleeding involve large doses of estrogen?
- A: Estrogen has procoagulation effects that promote hemostasis (e.g., effects on platelet aggregation and levels of fibrinogen and clotting factors). In addition, severe AUB may lead to an exposed endometrial base that bleeds profusely; for progesterone to exhibit its secretory effects, the endometrium in that area must be restored by estrogen.
- Q: When hormonal therapy fails, and the basal endometrium continues to bleed, how does a dilation and curettage act as the final treatment?
- A: The curettage removes any remaining bleeding vessels and stimulates local prostaglandins to create a uterine contracture that inhibits bleeding. This procedure is rarely needed in adolescent patients, as they usually respond to hormonal therapy.
- Q: Are there other causes of vaginal bleeding in adolescents in addition to AUB?
- A: The differential diagnosis for vaginal bleeding in an adolescent includes ovarian hemorrhage, cervical friability, or urinary or gastrointestinal source. Bleeding can also occur from the vaginal wall or vulva, typically from trauma or infection.

D

DYSMENORRHEA

Rebekah Williams, MD, MS, FAAP

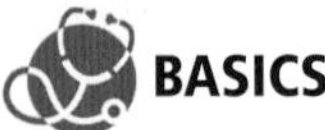

BASICS

DESCRIPTION

Menses-associated pain in the pelvis, lower abdomen, or lower back

- Primary dysmenorrhea: functional menses-associated pain due to amplification of normal menstrual physiologic processes
- Secondary dysmenorrhea: menses-associated pain due to other pelvic pathology, such as endometriosis or Müllerian anomaly

EPIDEMIOLOGY

- Primary dysmenorrhea
  - Typically begins 6 to 24 months post-menarche
  - More likely as more cycles become ovulatory
- Secondary dysmenorrhea
  - More common later in adolescence and in young adults

Prevalence

- Most common gynecologic condition among women of reproductive age, affecting 45–95% of menstruating women
- Up to 62% of adolescents with dysmenorrhea have endometriosis.

RISK FACTORS

- Early menarche
- Increased duration or amount of menstrual flow
- Nulliparity
- Cigarette smoking
- Alcohol consumption
- Family history of dysmenorrhea
- Higher body mass index

Genetics

- Dysmenorrhea more common in patients with a positive family history
- Hereditary predisposition to endometriosis; polygenic mode of inheritance, multifactorial, with expression varying with interaction with environmental factors
- Even when not in pain, women with primary dysmenorrhea have upregulation of proinflammatory cytokine genes and downregulation of anti-inflammatory response genes.

PATHOPHYSIOLOGY

- Ovulation is followed by increased progesterone release by the corpus luteum in the second half of the menstrual cycle. With the drop in progesterone late in the menstrual cycle, arachidonic acid and other omega-6 fatty acids are released, triggering an inflammatory response cascade involving prostaglandins (PGs) and leukotrienes (LTs).
- Uterine PGs and LTs cause myometrial contractions and endometrial artery vasoconstriction, resulting in uterine ischemia with ensuing pain.
  - PGF_{2alpha} is thought to stimulate the myometrium and cause vasoconstriction.
  - Dysmenorrhea severity is directly proportional to endometrial PGF_{2alpha} concentrations.
- Vasopressin, also elevated among women with dysmenorrhea, may play a secondary role by potentiating uterine contractions and ischemic pain.
- PGs and LTs can affect other body systems/organs, leading to dysmenorrhea-associated symptoms such as nausea/vomiting, diarrhea, and headache.
- Inappropriate local aromatase activity in endometriosis lesions leads to a local rise in estrogen, which induces cyclooxygenase (COX)-2 transcription and PGE_2 synthesis. Aberrant cytokine expression also mediates inflammation/pain.
- Secondary dysmenorrhea may be caused by a Müllerian abnormality.

DIAGNOSIS

HISTORY

- Primary dysmenorrhea
  - Painful, often spasmodic cramps of varying severity in the pelvis, lower abdomen or back, starting hours to a few days prior to menses and lasting up to 2 to 3 days after the start of menses
  - Pain is most severe initially and wanes by the end of menses. Referred pain to thighs may occur.
- Secondary dysmenorrhea
  - More likely to present with both menstrual and intermenstrual pain (chronic pelvic pain), menstrual irregularity, menorrhagia, and/or dyspareunia
- Menstrual pain
  - Ask about quality and intensity of pain (use pain scales); constant or intermittent occurrence; location; onset, timing, and duration; aggravating or alleviating factors; extent to which the pain limits activities (school, work, sports, social).
- Menstrual history
  - Age at menarche: Dysmenorrhea is more common in girls with earlier menarche.
  - Last menstrual period
  - Cycle regularity and length
  - Menstrual flow: dysmenorrhea more common in women with heavy/long menstrual flow
- Menstruation-associated symptoms: nausea, vomiting, diarrhea, headache, irritability, fatigue, insomnia, breast tenderness, dizziness, bloating, and acne
- Confidential sexual history
  - Parity, current sexual activity, contraception, and history of sexually transmitted infections (STIs) or pelvic inflammatory disease (PID)
- History of sexual, physical, or emotional abuse
- Family history
  - Gynecologic diseases, including endometriosis, infertility, breast or gynecologic cancer
  - Complications with estrogen-containing contraceptives including deep vein thrombosis (DVT), stroke, or myocardial infarction
- Medications: current medications, response to analgesic medications including name, dose, and perceived effectiveness

ALERT

- The adolescent health care provider should screen for menstrual symptoms at every encounter with an adolescent female.
- Confidential history taking is essential to assess for possible pregnancy or STI, trauma or abuse, comorbid mental health conditions that can cause or exacerbate chronic pain, and substance use.
- Severe menstrual pain that started at menarche or immediately after menarche is unlikely to be primary dysmenorrhea, as most girls are still having anovulatory cycles.

PHYSICAL EXAM

- Abdominal exam
  - Lower abdomen/suprapubic tenderness
  - With outflow tract obstructions, may palpate an enlarged uterus
- Inspection of external genitalia: for sexual maturity rating (Tanner staging), evaluation of normal anatomy, presence of patent vaginal opening. A cotton-tipped swab can be inserted into the vagina to evaluate for a transverse vaginal septum or vaginal agenesis.
- Internal pelvic exam
  - Defer in patients with classic symptoms and normal external genitalia.
  - Perform bimanual exam in patients with history suggesting secondary dysmenorrhea, or those who have failed 1st- or 2nd-line treatments.

DIFFERENTIAL DIAGNOSIS

- Primary dysmenorrhea is a diagnosis of exclusion.
- Secondary dysmenorrhea should be ruled out based on history, physical exam, response to initial treatment, and imaging if warranted.
- Causes of secondary dysmenorrhea
  - Endometriosis, congenital vaginal or uterine anomalies, adenomyosis, ectopic pregnancy, ovarian cysts or tumors, pelvic adhesions, pelvic inflammatory disease, fibroids, or polyps
- Other diagnoses to rule out:
  - Pregnancy, ectopic
  - Gastrointestinal: constipation, diverticulitis, inflammatory bowel disease, irritable bowel syndrome
  - Urologic: interstitial cystitis, nephrolithiasis, urinary tract infection
  - Neurologic: fibromyalgia, herniated disk, lower back pain

DIAGNOSTIC TESTS & INTERPRETATION

Lab studies generally not warranted unless needed to rule out other potential abdominal or pelvic pathology as indicated by history and physical examination

Initial Tests (screening, lab, imaging)

Consider pregnancy and STI testing as indicated by history.

Follow-Up Tests and Special Considerations

- Consider pelvic ultrasound (US) for patients who fail a trial of NSAIDs.
  - US can rule out genital tract abnormalities and ovarian pathologies.
  - Pelvic magnetic resonance imaging (MRI) may be indicated if US does not provide sufficient anatomic detail.
- Although US and MRI can detect ovarian, vaginal, and bladder endometriosis and deeply infiltrative lesions, there are no good imaging modalities to detect intraperitoneal endometriosis lesions.

Diagnostic Procedures/Other

Consider a diagnostic laparoscopy with resection/ablation of lesions if indicated in patients with dysmenorrhea refractory to treatments with NSAIDs and oral contraceptive products (OCPs), particularly if they have a 1st-degree relative with endometriosis.

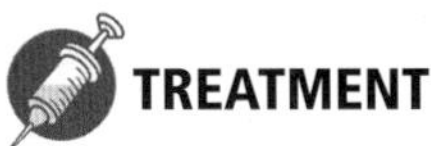

TREATMENT

GENERAL MEASURES

Only 6% of adolescents with dysmenorrhea are treated by a medical professional, but 70% self-manage with over-the-counter or complementary and alternative therapies.

ALERT

A number of over-the-counter medicines and supplements are marketed for treating cramps in women. Only those formulations that contain NSAIDs are effective in treating dysmenorrhea.

MEDICATION

First Line

- NSAIDs
  - Conventional PG synthetase (COX) inhibitors
  - If a patient fails to respond to the first choice at a therapeutic level, try a different NSAID.
  - There is no evidence that any given NSAID is more effective than another for dysmenorrhea.
- A COX-2 inhibitor should be considered in patients with prior history of peptic ulcer or gastrointestinal bleeding.
- 90% of patients have relief with proper dosing.
- Most effective when used on a regular basis for the first 2 to 3 days of menses
- If possible, start 1 day prior or at the onset of menses.
- Choices include:
  - Ibuprofen: 800 mg initially, followed by 400 to 800 mg PO q8h as needed
  - Naproxen sodium: 440 to 550 mg initially, followed by 220 to 550 mg PO q12h as needed
  - Mefenamic acid: 500 mg PO initially, followed by 250 mg PO q6h as needed
- Side effects of conventional NSAIDs
  - Black box warnings: increased risk of adverse cardiovascular events, including myocardial infarction, stroke, and new-onset or worsening of preexisting hypertension; increased risk of gastrointestinal irritation, ulceration, bleeding, and perforation

Second Line

- Hormonal contraceptives may be first line based on patient preference or if there is another indication (e.g., contraception, menorrhagia, irregular menses, acne, premenstrual syndrome/premenstrual dysphoric disorder).
- Significant improvement may not be seen until 3 months of therapy.
- Long-acting and progestin-only contraceptives
  - Levonorgestrel intrauterine devices: The 52 mg 5-year intrauterine device (IUD) suppresses ovulation in approximately 15% of cycles, decreases menstrual blood loss by 90%, and is U.S. Food and Drug Administration (FDA)–approved for the treatment of dysmenorrhea.
  - Etonogestrel subdermal implant: The 3-year subdermal implant is the most effective method for suppression of ovulation. Menstrual patterns are variable, and breakthrough bleeding is the main reason for discontinuation.
  - Depot medroxyprogesterone acetate (DMPA) injection: 150 mg intramuscular or 104 mg subcutaneous formulations given every 12 weeks suppress ovulation, thin the endometrium, and decrease menstrual blood loss and cramping.
  - Side effects: breakthrough menstrual bleeding, weight gain (DMPA only), reversible bone mineral density loss (DMPA only)
- Combined hormonal contraceptives
  - Suppress ovulation and decrease uterine PG secretion following reduction in progesterone levels
  - Can be given via (i) monthly intravaginal ring, (ii) weekly transdermal patch, or (iii) daily oral pill
  - Monthly cycling is achieved with 21 to 24 days of hormone administration, followed by 3 to 7 days hormone-free interval.
  - Shorter hormone-free intervals (≤4 days) and lengthened hormone intervals (extended or continuous cycling, 42 days or longer) are more effective for treatment of dysmenorrhea.
  - Side effects: nausea, vomiting, breast tenderness, breakthrough menstrual bleeding, headaches; rare: DVT, stroke, myocardial infarction
- Secondary dysmenorrhea is treated by addressing the underlying cause. An extended OCP regimen is the first line of treatment for endometriosis. Medical management in patients refractory to extended OCP may proceed to treatment with a gonadotropin-releasing hormone (GnRH) agonist.

ALERT

Starting hormonal contraception other than intrauterine devices does not require a pelvic exam.

ISSUES FOR REFERRAL

Consider referral to adolescent gynecology specialist for patients who do not respond to 1st- or 2nd- line therapies. These patients may require additional evaluation or laparoscopy to identify other pathology, or multidisciplinary teams to address chronic pain management and functional limitations.

SURGERY/OTHER PROCEDURES

Laparoscopic techniques for interruption of the uterosacral nerves have been used as treatment for primary dysmenorrhea when other modalities have failed.

- Laparoscopic uterine nerve ablation (LUNA) is effective for long-term (≥12 months) pain relief in primary dysmenorrhea.
- Laparoscopic presacral neurectomy is more effective than LUNA for pain relief at ≥6 months follow-up but has significant side effects especially constipation; it should only be performed by pelvic laparoscopic surgeons with special training.
- Cochrane review shows insufficient evidence to support routine use of these interventions.

COMPLEMENTARY & ALTERNATIVE THERAPIES

- Transcutaneous electrical nerve stimulation (TENS): Electrodes on the skin stimulate nerves at different current frequencies and intensities. Better results are reported with high frequency than with low frequency.
- Exercise may help to reduce dysmenorrhea due to release of endorphins.
- Behavioral interventions, Chinese herbal medicine, yoga, and heat therapy may reduce dysmenorrhea.
- Some evidence suggests that supplementation with vitamin B_1, fenugreek, ginger, valerian, zataria, zinc sulphate, and/or fish oil may alleviate dysmenorrhea symptoms.
- Cochrane reviews show insufficient evidence for acupuncture, heat therapy, dietary supplements, or spinal manipulation.

ONGOING CARE

FOLLOW-UP RECOMMENDATIONS

Patient Monitoring

- Patients should be followed up at least every 3 months until dysmenorrhea is controlled and not limiting functioning. Visits that are more frequent may be necessary for more severe cases.
- 3 months is considered a sufficient trial to see some benefit from most 1st- and 2nd-line therapies.

DIET

Most clinicians encourage healthy nutrition, consistent exercise, and sufficient sleep to help with dysmenorrhea. Data supporting these recommendations are lacking.

PATIENT EDUCATION

- Patients should track days of menses, pain ratings (0 to 10 scale), limited activities (school or work) due to pain, and associated symptoms in a calendar or diary.
- Multiple tablet and smart phone applications are available for menstrual symptom tracking.
- Websites for patient education materials
  - The Center for Young Women's Health. Menstrual Cramps. http://youngwomenshealth.org/2010/04/21/menstrual-cramps/
  - American College of Obstetricians and Gynecologists. Dysmenorrhea. http://www.acog.org/~/media/For%20Patients/faq046.pdf?dmc=1&ts=20121119T1244369567

PROGNOSIS

Improvement in dysmenorrhea symptoms may occur with increasing age or after pregnancy.

COMPLICATIONS

- 30–50% miss school or work at least 1 day each cycle.
- Many have decreased academic performance, sports participation, and peer socialization.

ADDITIONAL READING

- De Sanctis V, Soliman A, Bernasconi S, et al. Primary dysmenorrhea in adolescents: prevalence, impact and recent knowledge. *Pediatr Endocrinol Rev*. 2015;13(2):512–520.
- Iacovides S, Avidon I, Baker FC. What we know about primary dysmenorrhea today: a critical review. *Hum Reprod Update*. 2015;21(6):762–778.

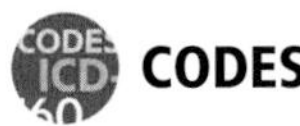

CODES

ICD10

- N94.6 Dysmenorrhea, unspecified
- N94.4 Primary dysmenorrhea
- N94.5 Secondary dysmenorrhea

FAQ

- Q: My period app has an "advice" group—can I go there for good information?
- A: Information quality and medical oversight of online and in-app message boards and question and answer features are highly variable. Patients should be encouraged to go to reputable electronic resources (such as those above) for online medical information or to contact their health care provider's office.
- Q: Will starting birth control for dysmenorrhea cause patients to have sex at earlier ages?
- A: Treatment of dysmenorrhea and other menstrual disorders with contraceptives does not affect age at first sex, or frequency of sex among adolescents.
- Q: For patients with chronic illnesses, is it safe to use contraceptives for dysmenorrhea?
- A: For guidance on contraindications to use of various contraceptives including drug interactions, see the Centers for Disease Control and Prevention 2016 Medical Eligibility Criteria for Contraceptive Use. https://www.cdc.gov/reproductivehealth/contraception/mmwr/mec/summary.html. Accessed May 8, 2018.

DYSPNEA

Thomas G. Saba, MD • Amy G. Filbrun, MD, MS

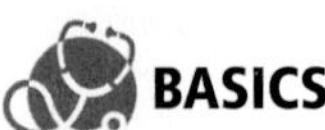

BASICS

DESCRIPTION

A subjective experience of breathing discomfort that consists of qualitatively distinct sensations that varies in intensity

PATHOPHYSIOLOGY

Abnormality in one of the following elements:

- Respiratory controller (breathing rate, depth)
- Ventilatory pump (chest wall, pleura, airways)
- Gas exchanger (alveoli, capillaries)
- Cardiovascular derangements (cardiac output)

ETIOLOGY

- Respiratory
  - Upper airway
    - Infection (croup, tracheitis, peritonsillar abscess, epiglottitis)
    - Foreign body
    - Anaphylaxis
    - Anatomic abnormalities
    - Vocal cord dysfunction (VCD)/paradoxical vocal fold movement (PVFM)
  - Lower airway
    - Asthma
    - Aspiration
    - Airway malacia
    - Hemorrhage
    - Internal/external fixed compression (tumor, cyst, vascular)
  - Parenchymal lung disease
    - Infection (viral, bacterial, fungal)
    - Interstitial lung disease (ILD)
    - Atelectasis
    - Chronic lung disease (chronic obstructive pulmonary disease [COPD], cystic fibrosis)
  - Chest wall disorder
    - Neuromuscular weakness (Duchenne muscular dystrophy [DMD], spinal muscular atrophy [SMA])
    - Scoliosis
    - Pectus excavatum
  - Pleural
    - Pleural effusion
    - Pneumothorax
- Cardiovascular
  - Cardiac
    - Elevated pulmonary venous pressure
    - Congestive heart failure (CHF)
  - Vascular
    - Pulmonary hypertension (PH)
    - Pulmonary embolism (PE)
- Toxic/metabolic
  - Metabolic acidosis (diabetic ketoacidosis [DKA], salicylate intoxication, renal tubular acidosis [RTA])
  - Renal failure causing fluid overload
- Other
  - Anemia
  - Deconditioning
  - Obesity
  - Panic attack
  - Pregnancy
  - Trauma
  - Gastroesophageal reflux disease (GERD)

DIAGNOSIS

- Secure the airway and address life-threatening emergencies.
- Identify those who will need intensive/emergency care and those who can be worked up in the office.
- Distinguish new-onset dyspnea from deterioration of chronic disease.
- Detailed history is key to diagnosis.

HISTORY

- Onset
  - Recurrent, discrete episodes associated with anxiety
    - Panic attacks
  - Sudden
    - Foreign body
    - Pneumothorax
- Associated signs and symptoms
  - "Tightness"
    - Bronchoconstriction (asthma)
  - Stridor
    - Upper airway obstruction
  - Wheezing
    - Lower airway obstruction
  - Chest pain
    - Pneumothorax
    - PE
    - Pleural effusion
  - Hemoptysis
    - Hemorrhage
  - Worse when supine
    - Pulmonary edema
- Temporal association
  - Exercise-induced
    - PVFM
    - Asthma
    - Deconditioning
    - GERD
  - Nocturnal
    - Asthma
    - GERD
  - Persistent and progressive
    - Neuromuscular disease
    - ILD
- Infectious signs and symptoms
  - Fever, cough, rhinorrhea
    - Pneumonia
    - Bronchiolitis
  - Stridor, cough, rapid onset
    - Croup
    - Tracheitis
    - Abscess
    - Epiglottitis
- Gastrointestinal signs and symptoms
  - Choking, gagging with feeds
    - Aspiration
  - Epigastric pain, discomfort
    - GERD
- Exposures
  - Salicylates, allergens
- PE risk factors include immobilization, surgery, smoking, pregnancy, central catheter, history of deep vein thrombosis
- History of cardiac disease
  - PH, CHF
- Diabetes history
  - Polyuria, polydipsia, polyphagia

PHYSICAL EXAM

- Vital signs, oxygen saturation, temperature
  - Fever
    - Infection
  - Hypoxia suggestive of pulmonary and cardiac causes
- Weight, BMI
  - Chronic disease, obesity
- Breath sounds
  - Generalized decreased air entry
    - Bronchoconstriction, atelectasis
  - Localized decreased intensity
    - Pneumothorax, pleural effusion, local obstruction, elevated hemidiaphragm, foreign body, pneumonia
  - Egophony, bronchial breath sounds
    - Consolidation/pneumonia
  - Wheezing
    - Bronchoconstriction, foreign body, bronchiolitis
  - Crackles
    - Infection, ILD (especially if crackles don't clear with coughing)
  - Barking quality of cough
    - Croup
  - Stridor
    - Upper airway obstruction
- Cardiac exam
  - Crackles, peripheral edema, hepatomegaly, gallop
    - CHF
  - Loud P_2
    - PH
- Extremities
  - Clubbing
    - Chronic pulmonary/cardiac disease
  - Cyanosis
    - Shunting
  - Calf tenderness
    - DVT
- Musculoskeletal
  - Generalized muscle weakness
    - DMD, SMA, other neuromuscular diseases
- Head and neck
  - Pharyngeal cobblestoning
    - GERD, allergic rhinitis
  - Allergic shiners, nasal crease, swollen nasal turbinates
    - Allergic rhinitis
  - Rhinorrhea
    - Allergic rhinitis, infection
  - Pharyngeal erythema, uvular deviation
    - Peritonsillar abscess

DIAGNOSTIC TESTS & INTERPRETATION

Initial Tests (screening, lab, imaging)

- Arterial blood gas
  - Hypercarbia suggests impending respiratory failure; distinguishes metabolic from respiratory acidosis
- Complete blood count with differential
  - Anemia; leukocytosis with left shift is a sign of infection.
- Glucose
  - Hyperglycemia can lead to DKA.
- Viral testing (polymerase chain reaction [PCR], direct fluorescent antibody [DFA], culture)
  - Diagnose viral infection; consider influenza in winter months.
- B-type natriuretic peptide (BNP)
  - Diagnostic marker to help recognize heart disease when access to echocardiography not readily available
- Chest radiograph
  - Identify pleural effusion, pneumothorax, consolidation, cardiomegaly, hyperinflation
- CT
  - High-resolution CT to diagnose ILD; multidetector CT to diagnose PE
- Echocardiography
  - Signs of PH; heart failure; structural abnormalities

Diagnostic Procedures/Other

- Pulmonary function tests
  - Spirometry
    - Obstructive lung disease (asthma); distinguish upper from lower airways obstruction
  - Lung volumes
    - Restrictive lung disease (ILD, neuromuscular and chest wall diseases)
  - Diffusion capacity
    - ILD
  - Mean inspiratory and expiratory pressure
    - Neuromuscular disease/weakness
- Bronchoscopy with bronchoalveolar lavage (BAL)
  - Dynamic visualization of airways to diagnose fixed (vascular) or dynamic (bronchomalacia) airway compression; bacterial, viral, and fungal cultures; lipid-laden macrophages (aspiration); hemosiderin-laden macrophages (hemorrhage)
- Electrocardiogram
  - Readily available test to rapidly diagnose heart disease
- Cardiopulmonary exercise testing
  - Indicated when initial evaluation fails to yield diagnosis; distinguish cardiac and respiratory causes and deconditioning

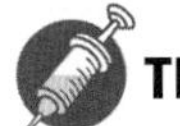

TREATMENT

- Secure airway and stabilize the patient.
- Treatment should be directed at the underlying cause of dyspnea.
- Consider palliative/symptomatic treatment once underlying or reversible cause has been addressed.

MEDICATION

- Opioids (parenteral/oral/inhaled)
- Anxiolytics

ISSUES FOR REFERRAL

- Unstable vital signs, unsecure airway, inability to oxygenate, and need for critical care services
- Surgical consultation for foreign body removal with rigid bronchoscopy
- Pulmonary referral for severe asthma, hemorrhage, ILD, CF, DMD, SMA, flexible bronchoscopy, chronic mechanical ventilation
- Cardiac referral for cardiac disease, PH
- Endocrinology referral for diabetes
- Nephrology referral for RTA and renal failure

ADDITIONAL THERAPIES

- Oxygen
- Pulmonary rehabilitation/speech therapy for PVFM
- Movement of cool air (face fan)

ALERT

In patients with hypercapnic chronic respiratory failure, hypoxemia might be the primary drive to breathe; supplemental oxygen will remove the hypoxic respiratory drive and cause apnea.

SURGERY/OTHER PROCEDURES

- Evacuation of tension pneumothorax with chest tube
- Pleural drainage/video-assisted thoracic surgery for loculated empyema
- Rigid bronchoscopy for foreign body retrieval
- Flexible bronchoscopy and laryngoscopy for visual diagnosis and BAL

ADDITIONAL READING

- Kurland G, Deterding RR, Hagood JS, et al; for American Thoracic Society Committee on Childhood Interstitial Lung Disease and the Childhood Interstitial Lung Disease Research Network. An official American Thoracic Society clinical practice guideline: classification, evaluation, and management of childhood interstitial lung disease in infancy. *Am J Respir Crit Care Med*. 2013;188(3):376–394.
- Lands LC. Dyspnea in children: what is driving it and how to approach it. *Paediatr Respir Rev*. 2017;24:29–31.
- Maher KO, Reed H, Cuadrado A, et al. B-type natriuretic peptide in the emergency diagnosis of critical heart disease in children. *Pediatrics*. 2008;121(6):e1484–e1488.
- Morris MJ, Christopher KL. Diagnostic criteria for the classification of vocal cord dysfunction. *Chest*. 2010;138(5):1213–1223.
- National Asthma Education and Prevention Program. *Expert Panel Report 3: Guidelines for the Diagnosis and Management of Asthma*. Bethesda, MD: National Asthma Education and Prevention Program; 2007. NIH Publication No. 07-4051.
- Parshall MD, Schwartzstein RM, Adams L, et al; for American Thoracic Society Committee on Dyspnea. An official American Thoracic Society statement: update on the mechanisms, assessment, and management of dyspnea. *Am J Respir Crit Care Med*. 2012;185(4):435–452.
- Ullrich CK, Mayer OH. Assessment and management of fatigue and dyspnea in pediatric palliative care. *Pediatr Clin North Am*. 2007;54(5):735–756.

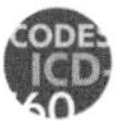

CODES

ICD10

- R06.00 Dyspnea, unspecified
- R06.1 Stridor
- R06.2 Wheezing

FAQ

- Q: In most pediatric cases, is dyspnea pulmonary in nature?
- A: In most cases, yes. Nonetheless, a systematic approach looking at all organ systems should be employed when addressing a patient with dyspnea.
- Q: How does the etiology of dyspnea differ in adults?
- A: In adults, the most common causes of dyspnea are asthma, COPD, ILD, myocardial dysfunction, and obesity/deconditioning. Whereas asthma and obesity are common in children, COPD, ILD, and myocardial disease are much more common in adults.

DYSURIA

Stephanie Clark, MD, MPH • Rebecca L. Ruebner, MD, MSCE

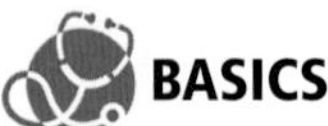

BASICS

DESCRIPTION

Symptoms of pain and/or burning on urination

ETIOLOGY

- Infectious
  - Cystitis
    - Bacterial
    - Viral
    - Interstitial
  - Pyelonephritis
  - Urethritis
    - Viral infection
    - Herpes simplex
    - *Neisseria gonorrhoeae*
    - *Chlamydia trachomatis*
  - Balanitis/balanoposthitis
  - Vaginitis
    - *Candida albicans*
    - Group A *Streptococcus*
    - *Shigella* species
  - Cervicitis
  - Pelvic inflammatory disease (PID)
  - Varicella
  - Tuberculosis
  - Pin worms
    - Pruritus rather than true dysuria
- Congenital/anatomic
  - Urethral stricture
  - Meatal stenosis
  - Labial adhesions
  - Lichen sclerosis
  - Posterior urethral diverticula
  - Vesicovaginal fistula
  - Virginal vaginal ulcers
  - Passage of gross hematuria
- Trauma
  - Masturbation
  - Sexual abuse
  - Foreign body
  - Diaper dermatitis
  - Bicycle injury
  - Irritation (e.g., sand, tight pants)
- Toxic/environmental/drugs
  - Bubble baths
  - Detergents
  - Fabric softeners
  - Perfumed soaps
  - Spermicides/douches
  - Cyclophosphamide
- Urolithiasis
  - Hypercalciuria
  - Hyperoxaluria
  - Hyperuricosuria
  - Cystinuria (autosomal recessive)
- Systemic illnesses
  - Stevens-Johnson syndrome
  - Behçet syndrome
  - Reactive arthritis
  - Food allergy
  - Contact dermatitis
- Functional
  - Dysfunctional voiding
  - Psychogenic
- Tumor
  - Sarcoma botryoides

PATHOPHYSIOLOGY

- Muscular contraction of the bladder and peristaltic activity of the urethra
  - Stimulates pain fibers in inflamed mucosa
- Pain when urine contacts inflamed mucosa

COMMONLY ASSOCIATED CONDITIONS

- Congenital anomalies of the kidney and urinary tract (CAKUT)
- Kidney stones

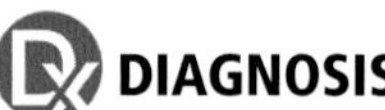

DIAGNOSIS

HISTORY

- Are there associated symptoms?
  - Fever, urinary frequency, urinary urgency, and urinary incontinence can indicate a urinary tract infection (UTI).
  - The addition of flank pain, vomiting, and abdominal pain may indicate pyelonephritis.
  - Abdominal pain, flank pain, and intermittent symptoms may indicate urolithiasis.
  - Conjunctival injection, oral ulcers, joint pain/swelling, or rash may suggest a systemic disease.
- Is there associated gross hematuria?
  - May suggest UTI, bladder abnormalities (tumor/cystitis), hypercalciuria, or urolithiasis
- What is the frequency and quality of bowel movements?
  - Constipation can cause dysfunctional voiding and dysuria. Constipation can also be a risk factor for UTI.
- Has the patient suffered any recent trauma?
  - Ask specifically about falls, playground accidents, and foreign bodies.
- Does the patient take bubble baths?
  - Bubble baths may deplete the protective lipids in the urethra causing irritation.
- In male patients, what is the quality and strength of the urinary stream?
  - Patients with posterior valves may have urinary dribbling, poor urinary stream, difficulty with potty training, or diurnal enuresis.
- Do the symptoms occur at a particular time or day of the week?
  - If symptoms only occur on weekends or before school, may be psychogenic
- Has the patient been exposed to any new foods or do they have known food allergies?
  - Milk allergy may cause dysuria. Citrus fruits may increase the acidity of the urine and cause dysuria in some patients.
- What medications does the patient take?
  - Some medications such as cyclophosphamide can cause urethral irritation and dysuria.
- Has the patient ever had imaging such as a renal and bladder ultrasound or past urologic surgery?
  - This will elicit a history of CAKUT or kidney stones.
- Is the patient sexually active?
  - If so, consider sexually transmitted infection (STI) testing.
- Is there associated vaginal discharge?
  - Suggestive of an STI or yeast infection

PHYSICAL EXAM
- Vital signs: Assess for fever, tachycardia.
- Abdominal exam: Evaluate for suprapubic tenderness, mass, or palpable stool.
- Back exam: Evaluate for costovertebral angle (CVA) tenderness, which is suggestive of pyelonephritis.
- Genital exam: Evaluate for signs of trauma (erythema, tears, ecchymoses), bleeding, foreign body, discharge, anatomic abnormalities (adhesions).
- Skin exam: Thorough skin exam may reveal systemic infections such as varicella, HSV, allergies.
- Genital exam may reveal a prolapsed urethra.
- A grapelike structure in the vagina suggests sarcoma botryoides.
- Visualize a urine specimen to assess for gross hematuria.

DIFFERENTIAL DIAGNOSIS
- See "Etiology"
- Sexual abuse
- Appendicitis
- Pinworms

DIAGNOSTIC TESTS & INTERPRETATION
Initial Tests (screening, lab, imaging)
- Urinalysis
  - Dipstick may show microscopic hematuria, proteinuria, positive leukocyte esterase, and positive nitrites which is concerning for a UTI.
  - Formal urinalysis may show pyuria.
- Urine culture
  - Gold standard for diagnosis of a UTI
- Urine calcium
  - If persistent dysuria with microscopic hematuria, evaluate for hypercalciuria.
- Basic metabolic panel, magnesium, phosphorus, uric acid
  - If known history of kidney stones, a metabolic workup is indicated.
- STI testing
  - If patient is sexually active and there is associated vaginal discharge
  - DNA amplification by polymerase or ligase chain reaction on freshly voided urine has 95% sensitivity and 100% specificity.

Follow-Up Tests & Special Considerations
- Consider renal and bladder ultrasound if there is concern for kidney stones, CAKUT, or pyelonephritis.
- A 24-hour urine collection to assess stone risk may be indicated if a diagnosis of kidney stones is suspected.

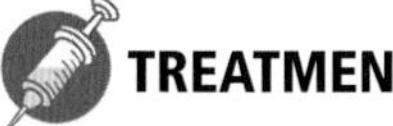

TREATMENT

GENERAL MEASURES
- See treatment of UTI, vaginitis, urethritis.
- Increase fluid intake if concern for hypercalciuria and/or kidney stones.
- Warm water sitz baths may be helpful for symptomatic treatment.

MEDICATION
Phenazopyridine (Pyridium®) may be used for symptomatic relief while documenting cause of dysuria.

ISSUES FOR REFERRAL
- Evidence of congenital anomaly—pediatric urologist
- Recurrent febrile UTIs—pediatric urologist
- Kidney stones and/or hypercalciuria—pediatric nephrologist
- Persistent microscopic hematuria—pediatric nephrologist

ADDITIONAL READING

- Claudius H. Dysuria in adolescents. *West J Med*. 2000;172(3):201–205.
- Hellerstein S, Linebarger JS. Voiding dysfunction in pediatric patients. *Clin Pediatr (Phila)*. 2003;42(1):43–49.
- Lee HJ, Pyo JW, Choi EH, et al. Isolation of adenovirus type 7 from the urine of children with acute hemorrhagic cystitis. *Pediatr Infect Dis J*. 1996;15(7):633–634.
- Rushton HG. Urinary tract infections in children. Epidemiology, evaluation, and management. *Pediatr Clin North Am*. 1997;44(5):1133–1169.

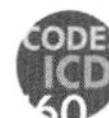

CODES

ICD10
- R30.0 Dysuria
- N39.0 Urinary tract infection, site not specified
- N34.2 Other urethritis

FAQ
- Q: How does bubble bath cause dysuria?
- A: The bubble bath depletes lipids that protect the urethra, causing the tissue to swell and become inflamed.
- Q: Can allergies cause dysuria?
- A: It is difficult to directly prove allergies as a cause of dysuria; however, in some cases, elimination of certain foods such as spices, citrus fruits, or known skin allergens has improved symptoms.
- Q: How do children get infected with gonorrhea or chlamydia?
- A: This is a red flag for sexual abuse, which must be investigated.
- Q: Which viruses cause dysuria?
- A: Adenovirus has been associated with cystitis and dysuria.

EARACHE

Vanessa S. Carlo, MD

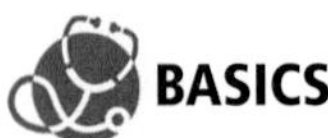

BASICS

DESCRIPTION

- *Otalgia*, classified as primary or secondary, means ear pain or an earache.
- Primary (or otogenic) otalgia is ear pain that originates inside the ear, either from the external auditory canal or from the middle ear structures.
- Secondary (or referred) otalgia is ear pain that originates from outside of the ear. Any anatomic area that shares innervation with the ear can be the primary source of perceived ear pain.

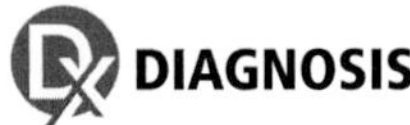

DIAGNOSIS

The first decision that must be made is whether the patient's symptoms require emergent, urgent, or nonurgent intervention. Emergency treatment is rarely required for pediatric patients with otalgia.

- **Phase 1:** thorough history—must include a full assessment of ear symptoms, followed by questions to determine possible involvement of other head and neck structures
- **Phase 2:** physical exam—thorough examination of external and internal ear, followed by inspection of the head, neck, and inside of the mouth
- **Phase 3:** treatment of identifiable conditions
- **Phase 4:** referral to otolaryngologist (ENT physician), dentist, or other specialist as needed

HISTORY

- **Question:** Duration of symptoms?
- *Significance*: acute (more likely infection or trauma) versus chronic
- **Question:** Quality of the pain?
- *Significance*:
  - Constant (more likely otogenic) versus intermittent (more likely referred)
  - Dull (more likely due to inflammation) versus sharp (more likely due to trauma or neuralgia)
- **Question:** Severity of pain?
- *Significance*:
  - Severe—usually otogenic
  - Mild to moderate—more likely to be referred
- Worsening factors
  - **Question:** Movement of auricle or pressure on tragus?
  - *Significance*: characteristic of otitis externa; can also be associated with furunculosis
  - **Question:** Movement of the jaw (biting, chewing)?
  - *Significance*: Temporomandibular joint (TMJ) dysfunction; furunculosis
- Associated symptoms
  - **Question**: Fever?
  - *Significance*: infection
  - **Question**: Upper respiratory infection (URI) symptoms?
  - *Significance*: acute otitis media (AOM) or otitis media with effusion (OME)
  - **Question**: Sore throat?
  - *Significance*: referred otalgia
  - **Question**: Ear discharge, tinnitus, or vertigo?
  - *Significance*: otogenic causes
  - **Question**: Mouth pain?
  - *Significance*: dental issues or stomatitis
  - **Question**: Hoarseness?
  - *Significance*: gastroesophageal reflux
  - **Question**: Multiple somatic complaints?
  - *Significance*: psychogenic
  - **Question:** Recent swimming?
  - *Significance*: otitis externa
  - **Question:** Recent travel? Hobbies?
  - *Significance*:
    - Barotrauma from scuba diving or air travel
    - Wrestling—auricular trauma
  - **Question:** History of recurrent AOM or OME?
  - *Significance*: cholesteatoma
  - Note: Serous otitis media or OME is common in pediatrics but is usually painless. Children usually complain of fullness or hearing loss.

PHYSICAL EXAM

- **Finding:** Erythematous, dull, bulging tympanic membrane, with decreased mobility?
- *Significance*: suggestive of AOM
- **Finding:** Retracted, immobile tympanic membrane?
- *Significance*: suggestive of OME or eustachian tube dysfunction
- **Finding:** Pain with pressure on the tragus or traction on the pinna?
- *Significance*: suggestive of otitis externa or furunculosis
- **Finding:** Erythema and edema of the external auditory canal?
- *Significance*: suggestive of otitis externa
- **Finding:** Purulent discharge in external auditory canal?
- *Significance*: suggestive of otitis externa or AOM with a ruptured tympanic membrane
- **Finding:** Redness, swelling, and/or tenderness of the auricle?
- *Significance*:
  - With earlobe involvement—cellulitis
  - Without earlobe involvement—perichondritis
- **Finding:** Swelling behind the pinna with its lateral displacement?
- *Significance:* suggestive of mastoiditis
- **Finding:** Normal ear exam?
- *Significance*: suggestive of secondary otalgia, thus other possible sources must be carefully examined
- **Finding:** Multiple dental caries?
- *Significance*: may be the source of pain; can indicate the presence of a dental abscess
- **Finding:** Foreign body within the ear or in the oropharynx?
- *Significance*: may be the source of pain from direct pressure or secondary to inflammation
- **Finding:** Enlarged, asymmetric tonsils or uvular deviation from midline?
- *Significance*: suggestive of tonsillitis or peritonsillar abscess
  - Look for signs of trauma inside or outside of the ear.

DIFFERENTIAL DIAGNOSIS

- Primary otalgia
  - Infectious
    - AOM—most common cause of otalgia in children
    - Otitis externa—inflammation of external auditory canal, usually associated with swimming and/or localized trauma; second most common cause of otalgia in children
    - Cellulitis of the auricle—usually caused by *Streptococcus pyogenes*; typically involves the earlobe
    - Perichondritis—inflammation of the auricle without earlobe involvement
    - Furunculosis—infection of the cartilaginous portion of the external auditory canal. Most commonly caused by *Staphylococcus aureus*. Pain is usually made worse by chewing.
    - Mastoiditis—now a rare complication of AOM, characterized by the auricle being pushed out and forward, away from the head
    - Myringitis (bullous myringitis)—inflammation of the tympanic membrane, usually with painful blisters on the eardrum
    - Varicella and herpes zoster infection within the ear
    - Herpes simplex virus infection within the ear
  - Trauma
    - Blunt trauma
    - Laceration or abrasion—if inside the ear canal, usually due to cleaning with cotton swabs
    - Thermal injury—frostbite of the ear or burn from a heat source
    - Barotrauma—associated with pressure changes on airplanes and scuba diving
    - Traumatic perforation of the tympanic membrane—frequently presents with tinnitus
  - Tumors—rare; usually associated with weight loss, voice changes, dysphagia, and persistent cervical lymphadenopathy
  - Allergic/inflammatory
    - Otitis media with effusion
    - Eczema
    - Psoriasis
    - Allergic reaction to topical antibiotics and cerumenolytic agents
  - Functional
    - Eustachian tube dysfunction—symptoms are due to pressure differences between the middle ear and the Eustachian tube.
  - Miscellaneous
    - Foreign body—can lead to pain, fullness, and minor hearing loss
    - Impacted cerumen—may cause pain if the cerumen presses against the tympanic membrane

- Secondary otalgia
  - Infectious
    - Dental infections—cavities, abscesses, gingivitis
    - Pharyngitis
    - Parotitis
    - Tonsillitis
    - Peritonsillar abscess
    - Retropharyngeal abscess
    - Sinusitis
    - Cervical lymphadenitis
    - Neck abscess
    - Stomatitis
    - Sialadenitis
    - Ramsay Hunt syndrome—viral neuritis of the facial nerve secondary to herpes zoster infection
  - Trauma
    - Dental trauma
    - Postsurgical—tonsillectomy, adenoidectomy
    - Oropharyngeal trauma—penetrating injuries, burns
    - Neck and cervical spine injuries
  - Allergic/inflammatory
    - Allergic rhinitis
    - Cervical spine arthritis
    - Subacute thyroiditis
    - Esophagitis—secondary to gastroesophageal reflux
    - Bell palsy
  - Functional
    - TMJ dysfunction—less common in children. Pain is usually unilateral and aggravated by chewing and biting.
  - Miscellaneous
    - Foreign body—in oropharynx or esophagus
    - Aphthous ulcers
    - Esophagitis
    - TMJ disease
    - Migraine
    - Aural neuralgia
    - Pillow otalgia (otalgia from sleep position)
    - Psychogenic pain

DIAGNOSTIC TESTS & INTERPRETATION

Labs, imaging studies, and other diagnostic tests are usually unnecessary as a thorough history and physical exam can lead to a diagnosis in the majority of cases.

- **Test:** culture of ear discharge
- *Significance*: indicated when otitis externa or AOM with perforation of the tympanic membrane does not resolve as expected with routine antibiotic treatment
- **Test:** audiometry
- *Significance*: Evaluate for hearing loss, which would suggest primary otalgia.
- **Test:** tympanometry
- *Significance*: Evaluate for OME, eustachian tube dysfunction, or tympanostomy tube obstruction.

Initial Tests (screening, lab, imaging)

- CT scan: rarely needed
  - CT of neck—evaluates for retropharyngeal abscess, mass, or hematoma
  - CT of sinuses—evaluates for sinusitis
  - CT of temporal bone—evaluates for AOM, mastoiditis, and other bony pathology
- MRI: rarely needed unless intracranial lesion is suspected

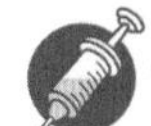

TREATMENT

GENERAL MEASURES

- Therapy is directed at the identified underlying cause.
- Pain medications such as acetaminophen and ibuprofen are important because many of the infectious causes are exquisitely painful.
- Topical benzocaine and other otic drops for pain control are no longer recommended as they have not been evaluated by the FDA for safety, quality, or effectiveness.
- Observation without antibiotic therapy ("watchful waiting") is indicated in certain groups of children with AOM.

MEDICATION

- Treat the underlying cause, which may or may not warrant medications.
- Manage the pain, which may or may not warrant medications.

ISSUES FOR REFERRAL

Referral to ENT when otalgia is primary in origin and any of the following:

- Pain with unexplained hearing loss, vertigo, or tinnitus
- Unexplained or persistent otorrhea
- Suspected neoplasm
- History suggestive of severe barotrauma
- AOM with complications
- Foreign bodies that cannot be removed easily from the ear
- Potential for auricle destruction (e.g., perichondritis may lead to permanent deformation, cauliflower ear)
- Persistent ear pain without an identifiable source should prompt a referral.

ADMISSION, INPATIENT, AND NURSING CONSIDERATIONS

- Emergency care rarely needed with most causes of otalgia but may be required if
  - Potential airway compromise from foreign body, mass, or abscess
  - Significant trauma—possible basilar skull fracture
  - Infection with a toxic-appearing child
- For all of the above situations, first establish "ABCs" as needed, hospitalize, and consult ENT promptly.

ADDITIONAL READING

- Conover K. Earache. *Emerg Med Clin North Am*. 2013;31(2):413–442.
- Leung AK, Fong JH, Leong AG. Otalgia in children. *J Natl Med Assoc*. 2000;92(5):254–260.
- Licameli GR. Diagnosis and management of otalgia in the pediatric patient. *Pediatr Ann*. 1999;28(6):364–368.
- Lieberthal AS, Carroll AS, Chonmaitree T, et al. The diagnosis and management of acute otitis media. *Pediatrics*. 2013;131(3):e964–e999.
- Majumdar S, Wu K, Bateman N, et al. Diagnosis and management of otalgia in children. *Arch Dis Child Educ Pract Ed*. 2009;94(2):33–36.
- Neilan RE, Roland PS. Otalgia. *Med Clin North Am*. 2010;94(5):961–971.

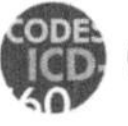

CODES

ICD10

- H92.09 Otalgia, unspecified ear
- H66.90 Otitis media, unspecified, unspecified ear
- H60.90 Unspecified otitis externa, unspecified ear

FAQ

- Q: What are the most common organisms that cause AOM?
- A:
  - *Streptococcus pneumoniae*
  - *Haemophilus influenzae*
  - *Moraxella catarrhalis*
  - Viruses
- Q: What are the most common organisms that cause otitis externa?
- A:
  - *Pseudomonas aeruginosa*
  - *S. aureus*
  - *Staphylococcus epidermidis*
  - Gram-negative rods
  - Fungal (*Aspergillus*) or yeast (*Candida*)—rare
- Q: What is the most common cause of referred ear pain?
- A: Dental disease

E

EBOLA VIRUS DISEASE

Ami Waters, MD, MPH • Phuoc V. Le, MD, MPH, DTM&H

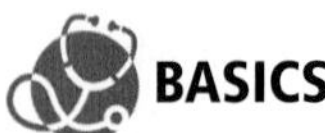

BASICS

DESCRIPTION

- Ebola virus disease (EVD) is a zoonotic illness that affects multiple organ systems and has high mortality.
- Previously called Ebola hemorrhagic fever (EHF) but renamed due to the inconsistent hemorrhage presentation.
- Prior to 2014, EVD was known for causing localized but deadly outbreaks, usually in remote areas in Central Africa. From 2014 to 2016, there was an EVD outbreak in West Africa caused by the Zaire strain that infected >29,000 people and led to 11,315 deaths. Although the outbreak predominantly affected the West African countries of Guinea, Liberia, and Sierra Leone, cases were identified and treated in 12 other countries, including the United States.
- Increased globalization, with increasing numbers of people traveling across country borders, supports the importance of continued vigilance

EPIDEMIOLOGY

- Endemic in Central, Western, and Eastern Africa
- Although it can infect animals and be further transmitted to humans, most transmission in outbreaks is human-to-human through contact with bodily fluids including blood, saliva, sperm, vomit, feces, vaginal secretions, and breast milk.
- Neonates are at high risk for vertical transmission in-utero and peripartum.
- Incubation period of 2 to 21 days, average of 8 to 10 days from exposure to first symptoms
- Infectivity increases as illness progresses.
- Subclinical infection indicated by seroprevalence studies, although uncommon
- Ebola virus is known to remain in certain sanctuary sites including CSF, intraocular fluid, breast milk, vaginal secretions, and semen.
- No significant difference between incidence in males and female overall

RISK FACTORS

- Contact with a person with EVD or their bodily fluids in last 21 days
- Risk is often stratified by
  - Duration of contact
  - Type of contact
  - Point of illness at which contact occurs
- Highest risk are those who have direct contact with symptomatic patient or their bodily fluids while not wearing personal protective equipment (PPE).
- Risk increases as illness progresses and is high for those who have direct contact with a dead body.
- Risk of transmission is less for those who only have close contact (within 3 feet) but not direct contact with a person or bodily fluids of a person with EVD while not wearing PPE.
- Wearing appropriate PPE with adherence to donning and doffing practices decreases risk considerably.

GENERAL PREVENTION

ALERT

If EVD is suspected, the patient should be isolated in a separate room with private bathroom. Notify local or state public health officials to ensure appropriate protocols are followed to minimize transmission.

- Standard, droplet and contact precautions to be employed along with the following PPE:
  - Two sets of gloves
  - N95 mask with face shield or goggles
  - Hood with neck and shoulder coverage
  - Boot covers
- Safe burial practices, including not touching corpses
- Not handling or eating animals that have been sick
- Vaccine (rVSV-ZEBOV) has shown promising results in safety and immunogenicity efficacy.

PATHOPHYSIOLOGY

- Ebola virus enters the body through direct inoculation with needles, through mucous membranes, or through areas in the skin with a loss of integrity.
- Ebola virus affects multiple systems by infecting monocytes, macrophages, and dendritic cells.
- Inhibition of type 1 interferon response and induction of inflammatory mediators and cytokines (which can vary between children and adults) triggering systemic inflammatory response and immune dysregulation

ETIOLOGY

- Ebola is a zoonotic disease with an unknown reservoir.
- The Ebola virus is of the *Filoviridae* family and has five different strains including *Zaire ebolavirus*, *Sudan ebolavirus*, *Bundibugyo ebolavirus*, *Tai Forest ebolavirus*, and *Reston ebolavirus* (which have not caused disease in humans to date).
- The Zaire strain was the first identified in 1976 and has the highest mortality.

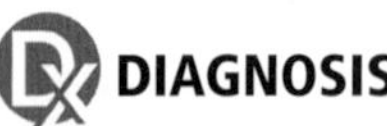

DIAGNOSIS

HISTORY

ALERT

When an EVD diagnosis is suspected, ask about travel history and a history of exposure to sick patient with suspected or confirmed EVD.

The disease often starts with nonspecific signs and symptoms and then progresses:

- Fever >38°C (up to 100% of confirmed pediatric cases in some outbreaks)
- "Dry symptoms"
  - Headache, fatigue, myalgia, abdominal pain, anorexia, and cough
  - Older children may complain of chest pain, back pain, sore throat.
- "Wet symptoms"
  - Nausea and vomiting, diarrhea
  - Can become the dominant symptoms
- Unexplained bleeding
  - As infrequent as 18%, as reported in the West African outbreak
  - More frequent in other outbreaks; however, <50% of cases
  - Usually occurs around day 5 to 7 of illness
  - Hematochezia most common type of bleeding
- As disease progresses further, can present with hiccups, somnolence, dizziness, seizures, and coma

PHYSICAL EXAM

- Vital signs: fever, potential hypotension, relative bradycardia, tachypnea
- HEENT: conjunctival injection and dark red discoloration of soft palate
- Skin: petechiae, bruising, diffuse maculopapular rash (day 5 to 7 of illness)
- Neurologic: gait imbalance, delirium, encephalopathy
- Anuria

DIFFERENTIAL DIAGNOSIS

- The differential will be greatly influenced by the other epidemiologically common infectious diseases.
  - Malaria
  - Typhoid
  - Measles
  - Influenza
  - Meningitis
  - Pneumonia
  - Cholera
  - Traveler diarrhea
  - Viral gastroenteritis
- Hemorrhagic symptoms
  - Lassa fever: West Africa, usually milder but 20% with severe disease
  - Yellow fever: fever, jaundice
  - Crimean-Congo hemorrhagic fever
  - Marburg hemorrhagic fever: Central Africa

DIAGNOSTIC TESTS & INTERPRETATION

Initial Tests (screening, lab, imaging)

ALERT

State or local health departments must be notified if a diagnosis of EVD is being considered and/or testing is pursued. Diagnostic testing should be done at selected state public health laboratories in the United States. The Centers for Disease Control and Prevention (CDC) will perform confirmatory testing.

- Testing
  - PPE should be worn by all lab personnel and health workers drawing blood, having direct contact with patient, or handling any body fluids.
  - 4 mL of whole blood is to be collected in plastic tubes (not glass) preserved ideally with ethylenediaminetetraacetic acid (EDTA) and stored at 2–8°C (or frozen and kept on cold packs).
- Reverse transcription-polymerase chain reaction (RT-PCR) testing Ebola antigen
  - Gold standard for diagnosis
  - Sensitivity 94–98%, specificity 100%
- ELISA for IgM and IgG antibodies
  - Quick turnaround, lower cost
- Other tests for appropriate settings
  - EBOV-RPA:
    - Point of care (POC) rapid testing in 15 minutes
    - Sensitivity 97%, specificity 97%
  - Urine dipstick
    - POC use with little training needed
    - 100% PPV, but sensitivity varies with cycling times of tests

Follow-Up Tests & Special Considerations

- Daily monitoring of electrolytes and kidney function
- Liver function tests, fibrinogen and coagulation studies, blood culture, complete blood count help influence treatment; however, be aware of context and risk of venipuncture to both patient and to health staff.

Diagnostic Procedures/Other

All children with appropriate travel history should have thick blood smear done to rule out malaria.

Test Interpretation

- RT-PCR usually positive 3 days after symptoms begin; repeat RT-PCR if done prior to day 3 with negative result.
- Seroconversion typically occurs around day 8 to 12, may be negative prior to day 12.

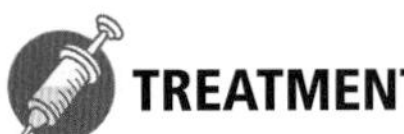

TREATMENT

GENERAL MEASURES

- Supportive care is the mainstay of treatment.
- Fluid and electrolyte management of hydration
  - Should be instituted early with close attention to hemodynamic status
  - Oral or IV; however, IV preferred for those who already have significant losses through diarrhea and vomiting
- Symptomatic treatment of fever, pain, vomiting
  - Treatment of fever/pain with acetaminophen
  - Avoid NSAIDs due to bleeding risk and renal complications.

MEDICATION

First Line

Transfusions as necessary for replacement of coagulation factors and platelets in DIC

ALERT

There is a lack of data for children regarding specific therapies targeting EVD. This situation requires careful consideration of ethical issues as well as the potential risk/benefit of investigational treatment.

Second Line

- ZMapp®
  - Investigational drug
  - Three monoclonal antibodies directed against Ebola surface glycoprotein
  - Promising decrease in mortality in preliminary results
- Favipiravir
  - Investigational drug
  - A nucleoside analog
  - Conflicting results in recent trials
  - Pediatric dosing is available.

ISSUES FOR REFERRAL

ALERT

If clinically stable, institution should seek assistance of local and state public health officials to transfer suspected patients to identified hospitals with Biosafety Level 4 capabilities and staff who have been trained in EVD Infection and Prevention Control.

- Avoid transfer if patient is deteriorating, as transferring patient could place staff at higher risk and lead to poor outcome for patient.

ADDITIONAL THERAPIES

Convalescent serum was used as therapy in the West African outbreak, but the benefit was not significant.

SURGERY/OTHER PROCEDURES

ALERT

Consider risk/benefit ratio for any proposed procedure, as any procedure requires high vigilance to avoid complications and environmental decontamination.

- Consider central line to minimize blood draws and to give opportunity for therapeutics.
- Surgery and invasive procedures are generally avoided in the period of active illness to avoid further complications, increased risk of bleeding, and increased risk of transmission to health providers.
- Elective tracheal intubation or intubation may be safer for patient and health providers than noninvasive positive pressure ventilation due to droplet dissemination.
- Continuous renal replacement therapy (CRRT) has been utilized in intensive care settings for those with renal failure who are treated in hospitals with advanced technology.

ADMISSION, INPATIENT, AND NURSING CONSIDERATIONS

- While awaiting transfer, patient should be placed in single bed isolation room with private bathroom and dedicated medical equipment.
- Consider pediatric intensive care unit admission independent of patient's current clinical status.
- Limit care to essential staff and only to those who have been trained in appropriate infection prevention and control procedures and PPE.
- Parental presence for pediatric patient with EVD should be considered in consultation with state and/or local public health authorities.

ONGOING CARE

FOLLOW-UP RECOMMENDATIONS

Postdischarge, patients will need close follow-up to mobilize services, to prevent further complications, and to ensure recovery. Specific services needed include:

- Nutrition services
- Depression screening and counseling
- Opthalmology: baseline exam and subsequent regular exams for uveitis and cataracts
- Physical therapy

Patient Monitoring

- RT-PCR should be conducted twice (48 hours apart) on breast milk prior to mother breastfeeding.
- Barrier methods should be used during sexual intercourse for 12 months or for males until semen has tested negative by RT-PCR 2 times with tests separated by a week.
- Monitoring of contacts of patient will be determined by public health officials based on risk of contact. Monitoring period is 21 days.
- Testing of neonates born to mothers with suspected EVD should be undertaken proactively prior to symptom development to initiate early treatment as necessary.
- Newborn infants of infected mothers should be monitored for 21 days prior to discharge.

DIET

- Infants: formula feeding by mouth as tolerated or through NG tube (if safe to place NG tube without inducing bleeding)
- Older children: as tolerated diet if patient is alert and not vomiting. NG tube feeds are alternative.
- Consider total parenteral nutrition for those who are critically ill if appropriate monitoring can be performed.
- No restrictions on discharge

PATIENT EDUCATION

- https://www.cdc.gov/vhf/ebola/pdf/is-it-flu-or-ebola.pdf
- https://www.cdc.gov/vhf/ebola/index.html

PROGNOSIS

- Recovery timing
  - Nonfatal cases usually improve 6 to 11 days after onset of illness.
  - Risk for mortality peaks at day 9 of illness in fatal cases but can range from day 6 to 11.
- Factors associated with mortality
  - Strain:
    - Mortality varies across strains from 25% to 90%.
    - For Zaire strain, mortality rates range from 40% to 90%.
  - Age: Mortality varies for different age groups.
    - In the West African outbreak, children <1 year of age had approximately 90% mortality.
    - Those <5 years of age had 80% mortality.
    - In other outbreaks, older adults have experienced higher mortality compared to children and adolescents.
  - Sex: Females had lower case fatality rates in West African outbreak (63% vs. 67%).
  - Location: For those treated in the United States and Europe, mortality was <20%.
- For survivors, the recovery period is prolonged with many patients developing post-Ebola syndrome, a constellation of symptoms including neurologic problems (68%), eye problems (60%), musculoskeletal problems (53%), fatigue, somnolence, inability to regain weight. Sloughing of skin and hair loss can also occur.

COMPLICATIONS

- Electrolyte disturbances
- Myocarditis or pericarditis with heart failure
- DIC, bleeding
- Sepsis, especially at risk for gram-negative bacteremia due to loss of gut integrity
- Acute renal failure: usually resulting from prerenal causes
- Liver failure
- Acute uveitis, cataracts, and blindness
- Post-Ebola syndrome

ADDITIONAL READING

- Centers for Disease Control and Prevention. Ebola virus disease (EVD) information for clinicians in U.S. healthcare settings. https://www.cdc.gov/vhf/ebola/healthcare-us/preparing/clinicians.html. Accessed June 7, 2018.
- Eriksson CO, Uyeki TM, Christian MD, et al. Care of the child with Ebola virus disease. *Pediatr Crit Care Med*. 2015;16(2):97–103.
- Kourtis AP, Appelgren K, Chevalier MS, et al. Ebola virus disease: focus on children. *Pediatr Infect Dis J*. 2015;34(8):893–897.
- Olupot-Olupot P. Ebola in children: epidemiology, clinical features, diagnosis and outcomes. *Pediatr Infect Dis J*. 2015;34(3):314–316.
- Shorten RJ, Brown CS, Jacobs M, et al. Diagnostics in Ebola virus disease in resource-rich and resource-limited settings. *PLoS Negl Trop Dis*. 2016;10(10):e0004948. doi:10.1371/journal.pntd.0004948.

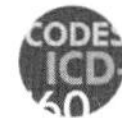

CODES

ICD10

A98.4 Ebola virus disease

FAQ

- Q: Can EVD spread through the air?
- A: There are no documented cases of airborne transmission. EVD is spread via respiratory droplets and direct contact with infected person or their bodily fluids.

EDEMA

Stephanie Clark, MD, MPH • Rebecca L. Ruebner, MD, MSCE

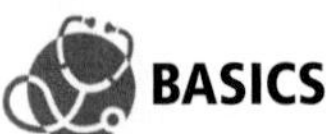

BASICS

DESCRIPTION

Presence of abnormal amount of fluid in the interstitial spaces of the body; usually secondary to low albumin, obstruction of venous or lymphatic channels, or trauma

PATHOPHYSIOLOGY

- Altered capillary hemodynamics
  - Increased capillary hydrostatic pressure
  - Decreased capillary oncotic pressure
  - Increased capillary permeability
- Lymphatic obstruction or dysfunction

ETIOLOGY

- Increased capillary hydrostatic pressure
  - Congestive heart failure
  - Pericardial effusion
  - Kidney disease (due to retention of salt and water)
    - Acute glomerulonephritis
    - Acute kidney injury
    - Chronic kidney disease
  - Cirrhosis
  - Venous obstruction
    - Superior vena cava syndrome
    - Deep vein thrombosis
- Decreased capillary oncotic pressure
  - Inadequate intake/production of protein
    - Protein malnutrition
    - Liver disease
  - Excessive losses of protein
    - Nephrotic syndrome
    - Protein-losing enteropathy
- Increased capillary permeability
  - Sepsis
- Lymphatic obstruction
  - Congenital lymphatic malformations
  - Obstruction from tumor
  - Filariasis
  - Radiation therapy
- Medications (calcium channel blockers, vasodilators)

COMMONLY ASSOCIATED CONDITIONS

- Nephrotic syndrome
- Congestive heart failure
- Liver disease

DIAGNOSIS

HISTORY

- Is the edema localized or generalized?
  - Localized edema more suggestive of trauma, infection, allergy, or lymphatic obstruction
  - Generalized edema more suggestive of congestive heart failure, nephrotic syndrome, protein-losing enteropathy, cirrhosis
- Has the patient experienced difficulty fitting into clothes or shoes?
  - Indicates degree of fluid overload
- It may be helpful to see a picture of the patient before symptoms started and/or determine previous baseline weight prior to onset of edema.
- Does the edema affect different parts of the body at different times of the day?
  - Generalized edema tends to be dependent, so periorbital edema may be more pronounced after being recumbent overnight and more significant in the lower extremities at the end of the day.
- Does the patient take any medications that can cause edema?
- Does the patient have a history of cardiac, renal, or liver disease?
- Does the patient have a history of chronic diarrhea suggestive of protein-losing enteropathy?
- Does the patient have shortness of breath?
  - Could be a result of pleural effusions, pulmonary edema, or ascites causing compression on the diaphragm
- Does the patient have difficulty walking, respiratory distress, or painful scrotal edema?
  - Symptomatic edema leading to distress may indicate a more urgent need for medical treatment.
- Does the patient have fever and severe abdominal pain?
  - These can be signs of spontaneous bacterial peritonitis, which can occur in the setting of ascites.

PHYSICAL EXAM

- Location of edema—edema is typically dependent and may change in location depending on patient position.
  - Periorbital
  - Pedal
  - Lumbosacral
  - Ascites
  - Scrotum/labia
- Pitting edema:
  - Assess by applying pressure to edematous area for 5 seconds.
  - Pitting edema is seen in most etiologies listed here.
  - Nonpitting edema is more suggestive of lymphatic obstruction or myxedema seen in thyroid disease.
- Pulmonary exam: Evaluate for pleural effusions, pulmonary edema.
- Cardiac exam: Evaluate for signs of congestive heart failure.
- Abdominal exam:
  - Determine degree of ascites by assessing shifting dullness and fluid wave.
  - Assess for hepatosplenomegaly.
  - Severe abdominal tenderness can be a sign of spontaneous bacterial peritonitis.
- Soft ear cartilage is a common finding in nephrotic syndrome.
- Skin exam: thorough skin exam to evaluate for cellulitis, which can develop in cases of severe edema

DIFFERENTIAL DIAGNOSIS

- Trauma
- Bee stings or insect bites
- Allergic reaction
- Angioedema: medications (angiotensin-converting enzyme inhibitors), acquired or inherited deficiency of C1 esterase inhibitor
- Myxedema—seen in thyroid disease
- Sickle cell dactylitis

DIAGNOSTIC TESTS & INTERPRETATION

Initial Tests (screening, lab, imaging)

- Urinalysis
  - High-grade proteinuria is suggestive of nephrotic syndrome.
  - Gross hematuria with or without proteinuria is suggestive of glomerulonephritis.
- Urine protein to creatinine ratio: to confirm the presence of nephrotic-range proteinuria if protein is seen on urinalysis
- Serum albumin
  - Hypoalbuminemia in the setting of generalized edema and proteinuria supports a diagnosis of nephrotic syndrome.
  - Hypoalbuminemia in the setting of generalized edema with no proteinuria is suggestive of liver disease, protein-losing enteropathy.
  - Generalized edema with normal serum albumin should prompt evaluation for other causes of edema including cardiac, lymphatic obstruction, and others.
- Comprehensive metabolic panel to evaluate electrolytes, creatinine, and liver enzymes
- Total cholesterol: will be elevated in nephrotic syndrome
- Complete blood count
  - Anemia can be seen in conditions including protein-losing enteropathy.
  - Patients with nephrotic syndrome often have elevated hemoglobin, due to hemoconcentration and thrombocytosis.

Follow-Up Tests & Special Considerations

- Consider chest radiograph if there are clinical signs of pulmonary edema or pleural effusions.
- Consider echocardiogram if there are clinical signs of heart failure.
- Consider abdominal imaging if there are clinical signs of liver disease.
- Consider additional evaluation of lymphatic system if there are clinical signs of lymphatic obstruction.
- α_1-Antitrypsin level in stool: will be elevated in protein-losing enteropathy

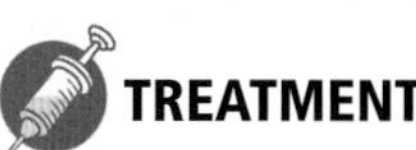

TREATMENT

GENERAL MEASURES

- Moisturize skin.
- Avoid pressure sores.
- Decrease sodium intake: Amount is age-dependent, but typical goal is <2,000 mg of sodium intake per day for older children.
- Active or passive leg exercise to avoid venous thromboses
- Elevate head of the bed to prevent periorbital edema upon awakening.
- If there is scrotal edema, compression shorts will help support the scrotum and protect the skin from breaking down. Scrotal elevation while recumbent can also be helpful.

MEDICATION

For severe edema with respiratory distress, severe abdominal discomfort, or severe scrotal edema, consider treatment with diuretics such as furosemide with or without IV albumin.

ISSUES FOR REFERRAL

- Nephrotic syndrome—pediatric nephrologist
- Protein-losing enteropathy or hepatobiliary disease—pediatric gastroenterologist
- Congestive heart failure, pericardial effusion—pediatric cardiologist
- Myxedema due to thyroid disease—pediatric endocrinologist
- Lymphatic or other mechanical obstructions—vascular surgeon or pediatric surgeon
- Angioedema—pediatric allergist/immunologist
- The duration and frequency of follow-up depends on the underlying etiology of edema.

ADMISSION, INPATIENT, AND NURSING CONSIDERATIONS

- Patients with edema that compromises either cardiorespiratory function or the vascular integrity of a peripheral organ or limb should be referred immediately to an appropriate specialist for emergency care.
- Patients with significant edema leading to respiratory distress, inability to walk, or severe scrotal edema may need inpatient admission for medical management of edema.

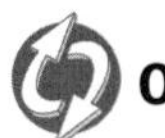

ONGOING CARE

FOLLOW-UP RECOMMENDATIONS

Patient Monitoring

Determined based on the underlying cause of edema

DIET

- Patients with edema due to salt and water retention may benefit from a sodium-restricted diet and a total fluid limit based on their age and size.
- Patients with edema due to malnutrition or protein-losing enteropathy should be followed closely by a dietitian.

PROGNOSIS

Depends on the underlying cause of edema

COMPLICATIONS

- Patients with ascites can develop spontaneous bacterial peritonitis. This usually presents with fever, severe abdominal pain, vomiting, and/or diarrhea. Diagnosis is made by paracentesis with measurement of peritoneal cell count and bacterial culture. Immediate diagnosis and treatment with IV antibiotics is necessary.
- Skin breakdown due to edema can lead to cellulitis. Close monitoring of skin for early signs of infection is important.

ADDITIONAL READING

- Braamskamp MJ, Dolman KM, Tabbers MM. Clinical practice. Protein-losing enteropathy in children. *Eur J Pediatr*. 2010;169(10):1179–1185.
- Hisano S, Hahn S, Kuemmerle NB, et al. Edema in childhood. *Kidney Int Suppl*. 1997;59:S100–S104.
- Rosen FS. Urticaria, angioedema, and anaphylaxis. *Pediatr Rev*. 1992;13(10):387–390.
- Vande Walle JG, Donckerwolcke RA. Pathogenesis of edema formation in the nephrotic syndrome. *Pediatr Nephrol*. 2001;16(3):283–293.

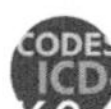

CODES

ICD10

- R60.9 Edema, unspecified
- R60.0 Localized edema
- R60.1 Generalized edema

FAQ

- Q: At what level of serum albumin does edema occur?
- A: Edema is generally associated with serum albumin <2.5 g/dL.
- Q: How does angioedema present differently from other forms of edema?
- A: Angioedema typically has a rapid onset (within minutes to hours), has an asymmetric distribution, and can involve the lips, upper airway, and bowel. Angioedema due to hereditary deficiency in C1 esterase inhibitor typically presents with recurrent episodes of edema.
- Q: How can allergies be differentiated from nephrotic syndrome or other causes of edema?
- A: Edema due to nephrotic syndrome will not respond to antihistamines or epinephrine. If edema is suspected to be due to allergies but does not improve after these therapies, workup for nephrotic syndrome and other causes of edema should be initiated.
- Q: What bacteria typically cause spontaneous bacterial peritonitis?
- A: The most commonly isolated bacteria include gut bacteria such as *Escherichia coli* and *Klebsiella pneumoniae*. Patients with ascites due to nephrotic syndrome are particularly at risk for infection with *Streptococcus pneumoniae*. Additional organisms can include *Staphylococcus* and other *Streptococcus* species.

EHRLICHIOSIS AND ANAPLASMOSIS

Camille Sabella, MD

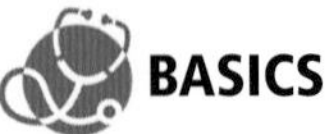

BASICS

DESCRIPTION

Two clinically described, tick-borne infections are human monocytic ehrlichiosis (HME), most commonly caused by *Ehrlichia chaffeensis*, and human granulocytic anaplasmosis (HGA), caused by *Anaplasma phagocytophilum*. HME can also be caused by two other *Ehrlichia* species in the United States: *ewingii* and *emuris*-like agent.

EPIDEMIOLOGY

- HME typically occurs in the midwest, south central, and southeastern United States, mirroring the pattern of Rocky Mountain spotted fever (RMSF). In addition, it has been found in Europe, South America, Asia, and Africa.
- HGA typically occurs in the north central, northeastern United States, and northern California, similar to Lyme disease. Most patients are infected during April through September, the months of greatest tick and human outdoor activity.
- A second peak of HGA occurs from late October to December.

GENERAL PREVENTION

- Avoid tick-infested areas.
- Clothes should cover arms and legs.
- Use tick repellents, but with caution in young children.
- A thorough body search should always be done after returning from a tick-infested area:
  - If a tick is found, the area should be cleaned with a disinfectant, and the tick should be removed immediately.
  - To remove the tick, grasp the tick at the point of origin with forceps, staying as close to the skin as possible.
  - Applying steady, even pressure, slowly pull the tick off the skin. After the tick has been removed, clean the skin with a disinfectant.
- Instruct parents to seek medical attention only if symptoms develop.
- No vaccine is available.

PATHOPHYSIOLOGY

- Obligate intracellular, pleomorphic, gram-negative bacteria.
- Transmission to humans by a tick vector
- Incubation period from 5 to 14 days for HME and 5 to 21 days for HGA
- HME infects monocytes and macrophages, whereas HGA infects neutrophils.
- The bacteria reside and divide within cytoplasmic vacuoles of circulating leukocytes, called morulae.
- There is overinduction of the inflammatory and immune response, resulting in clinical manifestations of disease, including multiorgan system involvement.

ETIOLOGY

- HME is transmitted by *Amblyomma americanum*, the lone star tick. The white-tailed deer is the major reservoir.
- HGA is transmitted by *Ixodes scapularis*, the black-legged or deer tick, or the Western black-legged tick (*Ixodes pacificus*). Small mammals such as the white-footed mouse are the major reservoirs.
- Congenital infection is very rare but has been described in case reports.

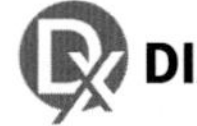

DIAGNOSIS

Classic presentation: fever, headache, and myalgias, followed by the development of a progressive leukopenia, thrombocytopenia, and anemia

HISTORY

- History of tick bite or exposure to wooded areas that are endemic for tick-borne diseases is helpful but is not always present.
- Fever, severe headache, chills, and myalgias
- Complaints of abdominal pain, vomiting, anorexia, and diarrhea may be present.
- Cough and sore throat are often described.

PHYSICAL EXAM

- Fever is described in all children.
- A pleomorphic rash occurs in ~60% of pediatric patients with HME and less commonly with HGA:
  - Rash is described as macular, maculopapular, petechial, erythematous, vesicular, or a combination of these.
  - Usually distributed on the trunk and extremities; spares palms, soles, and face
- Mental status change due to meningoencephalitis
- Cardiac murmur (II/VI systolic ejection murmur at the left lower sternal border)
- Hepatosplenomegaly
- Conjunctival or throat injection

DIFFERENTIAL DIAGNOSIS

- Tick-borne infection
  - RMSF
  - Tularemia
  - Relapsing fever
  - Lyme disease
  - Colorado tick fever
  - Babesiosis
- Other infections
  - Toxic shock syndrome
  - Kawasaki disease
  - Meningococcemia
  - Pyelonephritis
  - Gastroenteritis
  - Hepatitis
  - Leptospirosis
  - Epstein-Barr virus
  - Influenza
  - Cytomegalovirus
  - Enterovirus
  - *Streptococcus* pharyngitis
- Miscellaneous
  - Leukemia
  - Idiopathic thrombocytopenia purpura
  - Hemolytic uremic syndrome

DIAGNOSTIC TESTS & INTERPRETATION

Initial Tests (screening, lab, imaging)

- CBC with differential (with smear)
  - Thrombocytopenia, $<150,000/mm^3$ (77–92% incidence)
  - Lymphopenia, $<1,500/mm^3$ (75%) with HME
  - Neutropenia, $<4,000/mm^3$ (58–68%) with HGA
  - Anemia, hematocrit <30% (38–42%)
  - Intracytoplasmic morulae within leukocytes (20–60%); more common with HGA
- Electrolytes with BUN and creatinine: hyponatremia (33–65%)
- Liver function tests: elevated alanine aminotransferase, >55 U/L (90%)
- Coagulation labs, type and cross, as indicated
- CSF
  - Leukocytosis, with an average cell count of $100/mm^3$
  - Lymphocytic predominance
  - Elevated protein and borderline low glucose (less common in children, more common in adults)
  - Microbiology cultures are negative.
  - Intraleukocytoplasmic *Ehrlichia* microorganisms (morulae) have been described on CSF smears.

- Serum studies
  - Acute and convalescent antibody titers of *Ehrlichia* (a 4-fold rise or fall is considered positive) or *Anaplasma* obtained 2 to 4 weeks apart
  - An acute antibody titer of ≥1:128 is considered diagnostic.
  - Polymerase chain reaction assays are available for both HME and HGA. These are sensitive and offer a means for early diagnosis.
  - The detection of intraleukocytoplasmic *Ehrlichia* or *Anaplasma* microcolonies (morulae) on blood or bone marrow monocytes or granulocytes is diagnostic but is not present in all patients.

Diagnostic Procedures/Other
- Bone marrow biopsy is not necessary to diagnose the ehrlichiosis but may be carried out amid concern for other hematologic diseases.
- Bone marrow is usually hypercellular, but normocellularity and hypocellularity have also been found.

ALERT
- Failing to consider the diagnosis of ehrlichiosis or a delay in treatment pending confirmatory serum titers increases morbidity and mortality.
- Thus, treatment should be started if infection is suspected based on history, physical, and initial laboratory data.
- Alternative diagnoses should be considered in children who do not rapidly improve with doxycycline.
- Simultaneous infections have been documented with HGA and Lyme disease.

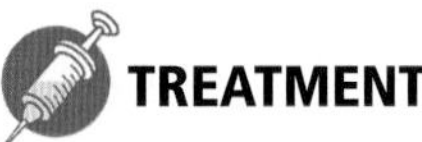

TREATMENT

GENERAL MEASURES
- Volume and blood pressure medications as needed
- Intubation for respiratory failure
- Dialysis for renal failure
- Platelets for thrombocytopenia
- Packed red blood cells for anemia
- Fresh frozen plasma, cryoprecipitate, and vitamin K for disseminated intravascular coagulation (DIC)
- Antifungal or antibiotics for secondary infections

MEDICATION
First Line
- Doxycycline, either PO or IV
- Drug of choice regardless of age of child
- Dose: 4.4 mg/kg/24 h divided q12h (max dose 100 per dose)
- Treatment duration: standard course is 5 to 10 days. Continue for 3 to 5 days after defervescence, longer if there is CNS involvement.

Second Line
- Rifampin has been reported to be an effective antibiotic for children <8 years of age who have HGA infection, but data regarding this option are limited.
- Children treated with rifampin must be carefully monitored to assure clinical resolution of illness.
- Rifampin has been used effectively to treat a small number of pregnant women who have HGA.
- Unlike Lyme disease, neither amoxicillin nor ceftriaxone has been shown to be effective for the treatment of ehrlichiosis.

ONGOING CARE

PROGNOSIS
- >60% of patients are hospitalized.
- Case fatality rate for HME is 1–3%; for HGA, <1%
- Elevated BUN and creatinine have been associated with a more severe course.
- Children appear to have an excellent outcome: Blood, renal, and liver abnormalities resolve in 1 to 2 weeks after initiating antibiotics.
- Cognitive and behavioral problems have been reported.
- Neuropathy has been described.

COMPLICATIONS
- Neurologic
  - Headache, described as severe
  - Mental status changes
  - Seizures
  - Coma
  - Focal neurologic findings
  - Cognitive learning deficits
- Hematologic
  - DIC
  - Thrombocytopenia
  - Leukopenia
  - Lymphopenia
  - Anemia
- GI
  - Hemorrhage
  - Elevated liver enzymes
  - Hepatosplenomegaly
- Respiratory
  - Pulmonary hemorrhage
  - Interstitial pneumonia
  - Pleural effusions
  - Noncardiogenic pulmonary edema
- Infectious
  - Fungal superinfection
  - Nosocomial infections
  - Opportunistic infections
- Renal
  - Renal failure
  - Proteinuria
  - Hematuria
- Cardiac
  - Cardiomegaly
  - Murmurs

ADDITIONAL READING

- Dhand A, Nadelman RB, Aguero-Rosenfeld M, et al. Human granulocytic anaplasmosis during pregnancy: case series and literature review. *Clin Infect Dis*. 2007;45(5):589–593.
- Dumler JS, Madigan JE, Pusterla N, et al. Ehrlichioses in humans: epidemiology, clinical presentation, diagnosis, and treatment. *Clin Infect Dis*. 2007;45(Suppl 1):S45–S51.
- Havens NS, Kinnear BR, Mató S. Fatal ehrlichial myocarditis in a healthy adolescent: a case report and review of the literature. *Clin Infect Dis*. 2012;54(8):e113–e114.
- Nichols Heitman K, Dahlgren FS, Drexler NA, et al. Increasing incidence of ehrlichiosis in the United States: a summary of National Surveillance of *Ehrlichia chaffeensis* and *Ehrlichia ewingii* infections in the United States, 2008–2012. *Am J Trop Med Hyg*. 2016;94(1):52–60.
- Schutze GE, Buckingham SC, Marshall GS, et al. Human monocytic ehrlichiosis in children. *Pediatr Infect Dis J*. 2007;26(6):475–479.

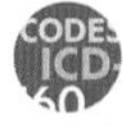

CODES

ICD10
- A77.40 Ehrlichiosis, unspecified
- A77.41 Ehrlichiosis chafeensis [E. chafeensis]
- A77.49 Other ehrlichiosis

FAQ
- Q: If a tick is removed from my child, should antibiotics be started?
- A: No. Antibiotics should be started if a child becomes symptomatic. Prophylactic use of antimicrobial agents does not prevent the development of disease.
- Q: What is the most common chief complaint in children with ehrlichiosis?
- A: Intense, unremitting headache and fever are the most common features.

ENCEPHALITIS

Lily C. Wong-Kisiel, MD • Elaine C. Wirrell, MD

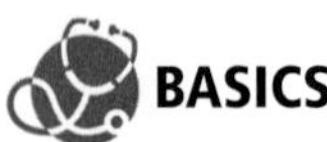

BASICS

DESCRIPTION

Encephalitis is inflammation of the brain parenchyma, which results in alterations in mental status, motor or sensory symptoms, speech problems, or seizures. This inflammation may be due to direct brain invasion by an infectious pathogen or immune-mediated from an inflammatory process due to acute or chronic illnesses.

EPIDEMIOLOGY

- Exact incidence is unknown, but infants and children are predominantly affected.
- Encephalitis due to enterovirus or arbovirus has a peak incidence between summer and early autumn. Many cases of viral encephalitis occur in epidemics.

RISK FACTORS

- Unimmunized state (measles, mumps, rubella, influenza)
- Travel or residence in an endemic region

GENERAL PREVENTION

- Routine immunization for measles, mumps, rubella, and influenza, and if travelling to endemic area (e.g., Southeast Asia), consideration of immunization for Japanese encephalitis
- Careful hand washing, avoid tick and mosquito exposure (DEET [*N,N*-diethyl-meta-toluamide] repellant, mosquito netting, appropriate dress), and insect control (drainage of stagnant water, insecticides)

PATHOPHYSIOLOGY

- Transmission of infectious pathogens can be by the blood-borne route, by retrograde spread through peripheral nerves (such as HSV or rabies), or rarely by direct inoculation of the brain.
- Encephalitis may also result indirectly, by immune-mediated injury due to parainfectious (i.e., acute disseminated encephalomyelitis [ADEM] or mycoplasma) or inflammatory/paraneoplastic causes (i.e., anti-NMDA receptor encephalitis). Such immune-mediated mechanisms involve cytokine effects and cytotoxic antibodies on neurons.

ETIOLOGY

- In most cases, the underlying cause remains unknown. Of those with known etiology, the majority are due to viral agents, followed by bacterial, autoimmune, parasitic, and fungal causes.
- The most common viral causes include HSV-1 and HSV-2, enteroviruses, arboviruses (West Nile virus [WNV]), and other herpesviruses (CMV, EBV, HHV-6, VZV).
  - HSV-1 typically presents with focal seizures, often of temporal lobe origin and encephalopathy.
  - HSV-2 is the predominant cause of neonatal HSV infection.
  - Enteroviruses and arboviruses typically cause disease in the summer and fall.
  - WNV presents as an acute flaccid paralysis, extrapyramidal symptoms, and cranial nerve palsies.
  - Zika virus may rarely result in meningoencephalitis but is more commonly associated with low-grade fever and rash and with congenital microcephaly.
  - Other viruses may be considered given specific historical features (rabies with animal bite or bat exposure or with prominent hydrophobia) or history of travel (Japanese encephalitis virus).
- Bacterial causes include *Listeria, Francisella tularensis, Bartonella, Mycobacterium, Rickettsia, Mycoplasma, Borrelia*, and *Chlamydia*.
- Fungal and parasitic causes include *Cryptococcus, Blastomyces, Histoplasma, Paracoccidioides, Naegleria, Toxoplasma, Plasmodium*, and *Toxocara*.
- Parainfectious etiologies include ADEM, acute hemorrhagic leukoencephalitis, postinfectious cerebellitis, and *Mycoplasma* encephalopathy. ADEM typically presents with encephalopathy and focal neurologic symptoms, with an MRI showing multifocal white matter lesions.
- Other inflammatory or paraneoplastic etiologies include anti-NMDA receptor encephalitis, voltage-gated potassium channel complex antibody, aquaporin-4 autoimmunity, SREAT (steroid-responsive encephalopathy associated with thyroid disease), systemic lupus erythematosus, and other vasculitis. Anti-NMDA receptor encephalitis typically presents subacutely with encephalopathy, sleep disturbance, seizures, perioral dyskinesias, and autonomic disturbances.

COMMONLY ASSOCIATED CONDITIONS

Children with autoimmune encephalitis have higher rates of other autoimmune disorders such as diabetes mellitus or juvenile rheumatoid arthritis.

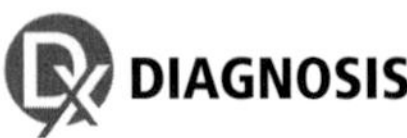

DIAGNOSIS

HISTORY

- Symptoms include fever, headache, photophobia, altered mental status, irritability, gait disturbance, and seizures.
- Ask about focal neurologic symptoms.
- A recent viral illness, recent travel, animal exposures, tick or mosquito bites, immunizations, and immune status may provide clues to etiology.
- A history of maternal herpes infection or prolonged rupture of membranes should be queried in neonates.

PHYSICAL EXAM

- Hypertension, bradycardia, or apnea may suggest impending herniation due to brain swelling.
- Altered mental status is the hallmark of encephalitis and ranges from mild confusion to stupor and coma. Distinguishing infectious from postinfectious encephalitis usually cannot be done reliably on clinical grounds.
- Specific neurologic findings suggestive of a specific etiology include focal seizures and focal neurologic findings (HSV); hydrophobia, pharyngeal spasms, and mood disturbance (rabies); facial nerve palsy (Lyme disease); flaccid paralysis or polio-like syndrome (WNV); and ataxia (VZV).
- Nonneurologic findings suggesting a specific etiology include respiratory symptoms (*Mycoplasma*), adenopathy and splenomegaly (EBV), petechial skin rash (*Rickettsia*), morbilliform rash (measles), erythematous maculopapular rash (enterovirus), and parotitis (mumps).

DIFFERENTIAL DIAGNOSIS

- Several conditions or disorders can resemble encephalitis.
  - Metabolic (acute electrolyte disturbance, inborn errors of metabolism)
  - Toxic (ingestions)
  - Structural (acute obstructive hydrocephalus or shunt obstruction)
  - Vascular (cerebral vasculitis, ischemic or hemorrhagic stroke, septic embolization, sinus thrombosis)
  - Endocrine (hypothyroid crisis, pituitary infarction)
  - Infectious (bacterial meningitis, brain abscess, subdural empyema, viral meningitis)
  - Epileptic disorders (status epilepticus)
- Febrile infection-related epilepsy syndrome (FIRES) is a rare, devastating disorder that presents in school-aged children, following a nonspecific febrile illness with refractory status epilepticus. This condition is likely related to a fever-induced, proinflammatory, proexcitatory process, and an underlying infectious or immune etiology has not been found.

DIAGNOSTIC TESTS & INTERPRETATION

Initial Tests (screening, lab, imaging)

- Routine labs such as electrolytes, glucose, renal and liver function, and CBC are usually nonspecific.
- Selected serologic testing depending on the suspected agent (e.g., WNV and *Mycoplasma*) can provide confirmatory diagnosis of underlying etiology.
- Toxicology screen should be done to rule out overdose or toxin exposure as the cause for altered mental status.
- Lumbar puncture is performed urgently, once the patient is stabilized and signs and symptoms of intracranial pressure are excluded (broad-spectrum treatment should commence if these conditions are not met).
- In addition to measuring opening pressure (frequently elevated), other studies should include:
  - CSF cell count and differential (lymphocytic predominance suggests a viral process, whereas neutrophilic predominance suggests bacterial or early viral processes)
  - Red blood cells (in the absence of a traumatic tap, red blood cells are suggestive of necrotizing encephalitis associated with HSV)
  - Protein (often elevated)
  - Glucose (usually normal)
  - Gram stain and bacterial culture (20% of patients with suspected encephalitis are diagnosed with bacterial meningitis.)
  - HSV polymerase chain reaction (PCR)
  - Initial studies may be normal, which does not rule out the diagnosis of encephalitis if clinical suspicion is high.
- Other PCR-based tests on CSF including enterovirus, *Borrelia burgdorferi*, and WNV may be considered depending on the situation.
- In immunocompromised hosts, CSF should be sent for fungal stains and culture (and serum for cryptococcal serum antigen).

- In those patients suspected of paraneoplastic etiology, an extended panel of autoimmune antibodies should be investigated in the serum and CSF. Voltage-gated potassium channel antibodies in children are a nonspecific marker of inflammatory neurologic disease, especially associated with encephalopathy. These are usually nonspecific and rarely test positive for a known protein (LGI1 or CASPR2).
- Imaging is performed urgently to rule out surgically remediable conditions (e.g., abscess or hematoma). MRI (or if not available, CT) of the brain with and without contrast medium is preferred. Neuroimaging can be normal or demonstrate focal or diffuse parenchymal enhancement (HSV-2 has a preference for the medial temporal lobe).

Diagnostic Procedures/Other
- An EEG usually shows diffuse generalized slowing. Findings of periodic lateralized discharges are suggestive but not diagnostic of HSV.
- Brain biopsy: rarely performed

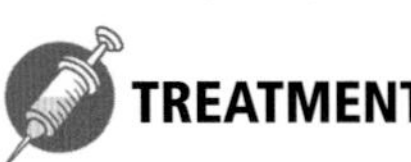

TREATMENT

GENERAL MEASURES
Children suspected of encephalitis should be admitted for empiric antibacterial and antiviral treatments with expedited diagnostic workup.

MEDICATION
Initial treatment should target bacterial and viral agents until culture results are confirmed or negative.
- Bacterial meningitis: vancomycin (15 to 20 mg/kg IV q6–8h, monitor levels) plus either cefotaxime (225 to 300 mg/kg/24 h IV q6–8h) or ceftriaxone (100 mg/kg/24 h IV divided q12–24h; use for ≥1 month old). Treat until cultures are negative at 48 hours.
- HSV encephalitis: acyclovir (>28 days–<12 years: 20 mg/kg/dose IV q8h; ≥12 years: 10 mg/kg/dose IV q8h). Acyclovir is continued for a minimum of 21 days if HSV is confirmed. PCR may be falsely negative in 5–10% of cases—contact an infectious diseases consultant if there is a high clinical suspicion. Monitor renal function while on acyclovir.
- Rickettsial infection (characteristic rash with exposure to ticks in an endemic region) or ehrlichiosis (headache, rash, leukopenia, thrombocytopenia, typical blood smear, transaminase elevation, with exposure to ticks in an endemic region): Consider empiric doxycycline.
- There is no evidence from controlled clinical trials that corticosteroids, IVIG, and therapeutic hypothermia are useful in cases of infectious encephalitis.
- *Mycoplasma* encephalopathy: erythromycin (Benefit sustained from this medication is controversial given probable parainfectious mechanism.)
- ADEM: high-dose IV methylprednisolone 20 to 30 mg/kg/24 h for 3 days followed by prednisolone taper. In refractory cases, either IVIG or plasmapheresis can be considered.
- Anti-NMDA receptor encephalitis: high-dose IV corticosteroids, IVIG, or plasmapheresis. Rituximab has been used in combination with 1st-line agents.
- Immunotherapy is also recommended for other inflammatory or paraneoplastic causes of encephalitis.

ISSUES FOR REFERRAL
Subspecialty consultations should include pediatric infectious disease and neurology. Transfer to intensive care unit may be needed should there be concerns with cardiorespiratory status, status epilepticus, and cerebral edema.

ADMISSION, INPATIENT, AND NURSING CONSIDERATIONS
- Careful attention to cardiorespiratory status is essential as is ruling out potential cerebral herniation. Children with severe encephalitis require intensive care with careful cardiorespiratory monitoring.
- Isolation precautions are based on type of suspected organism.
- Seizures:
  - IV benzodiazepines (lorazepam, midazolam, or diazepam) are used acutely. Status epilepticus should be aggressively managed with a loading dose of fosphenytoin or levetiracetam.
  - Barbiturate coma or midazolam infusion may be needed in refractory cases.
  - In children with reduced level of consciousness, or those treated for refractory status epilepticus, EEG monitoring should be considered.
- Cerebral edema:
  - Cerebral perfusion pressure should be kept at 70 mm Hg or higher for children >2 years of age. Conservative measures including fluid restriction, elevation of the head of the bed, and hyperventilation are most commonly used. With impending herniation, mannitol should be considered.
  - Rarely, in malignant cases of cerebral edema, craniectomy can be considered for decompression.
- Occult tumors
  - Investigation for occult tumors should be done with anti-NMDA receptor or other autoantibody-mediated encephalitis. Among girls with anti-NMDA receptor encephalitis, 9% age <14 years and 30% age <18 years were found to have an ovarian teratoma. Tumor resection is required to improve symptoms. Testicular teratoma has been rarely reported.
- Closely monitor electrolytes, anticipating possible syndrome of inappropriate antidiuretic hormone or diabetes insipidus.

ONGOING CARE

FOLLOW-UP RECOMMENDATIONS
- Physical and occupational therapists should be consulted early in the course and will be helpful during the convalescence.
- Neuropsychological testing is helpful to identify cognitive deficits and direct appropriate services.
- Follow-up with speech pathologists and developmental pediatricians may be indicated.

PROGNOSIS
- Outcome varies greatly and depends on age, etiologic agent, and disease severity at the time of presentation (e.g., patients presenting in coma do worse).
- Outcomes range from complete recovery to focal neurologic deficits, persistent vegetative state, and death.
- Potential complications include aphasia, ataxia, developmental delay, learning disabilities, quadriparesis/hemiparesis, and epilepsy.

ADDITIONAL READING

- DuBray K, Anglemyer A, LaBeaud AD, et al. Epidemiology, outcomes and predictors of recovery in childhood encephalitis: a hospital-based study. *Pediatr Infect Dis J*. 2013;32(8):839–844.
- Gable MS, Sheriff H, Dalmau J, et al. The frequency of autoimmuine *N*-methyl-D-aspartate receptor encephalitis surpasses that of individual viral etiologies in young individuals enrolled in the California Encephalitis Project. *Clin Infect Dis*. 2012;54(7):899–904.
- Rosenfeld MR, Dalmau J. Anti-NMDA-receptor encephalitis and other synaptic autoimmune disorders. *Curr Treat Options Neurol*. 2011;13(3):324–332.
- Sonneville R, Klein IF, Wolff M. Update on investigation and management of postinfectious encephalitis. *Curr Opin Neurol*. 2010;23(3):300–304.
- Tunkel AR, Glaser CA, Bloch KC, et al; for Infectious Diseases Society of America. The management of encephalitis: clinical practice guidelines by the Infectious Diseases Society of America. *Clin Infect Dis*. 2008;47(3):303–327.

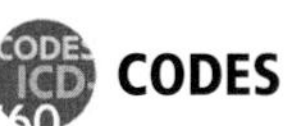

CODES

ICD10
- G04.90 Encephalitis and encephalomyelitis, unspecified
- A85.8 Other specified viral encephalitis
- B00.4 Herpesviral encephalitis

FAQ
- Q: Will the child suffer permanent brain injury from encephalitis?
- A: The complications following encephalitis vary greatly from severe mental retardation and cerebral palsy to full recovery. There is a correlation between degree of brain destruction and outcome; however, children frequently recover better than adults with a similar degree of illness. Outcomes depend on the neurologic status of the patient at presentation and the causative organism. Although many children will make a full recovery, some have persisting neurologic problems including cognitive or motor difficulties, vision or hearing deficits, epilepsy, or personality change. Children with focal deficits or markedly impaired level of consciousness in the acute stage or those with HSV encephalitis are at highest risk of sequelae.
- Q: Is encephalitis highly contagious?
- A: Most cases of encephalitis are not highly contagious, although precautions should be followed with blood or body fluid exposure.
- Q: When should autoimmune encephalitis be considered?
- A: Subacute presentations, movement disorders, insomnia, focal and generalized seizures, developmental regression, and status epilepticus are diverse neurologic presentations of autoimmune encephalitis. Clinical triad of acute or subacute onset of CNS dysfunction, serologic detection of the pertinent antibody, and a response to immunotherapy increase the suspicion of autoimmune etiology. Because of the potential associations with occult neoplasm, early recognition through clinical and serologic diagnosis is important because this may lead to an early diagnosis of cancer, expedited implementation of immunotherapy, and improved neurologic long-term outcome.

ENCOPRESIS

Jay Fong, MD

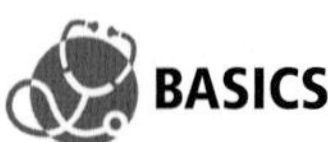

BASICS

DESCRIPTION

- Repeated unintentional soiling of underwear
- Most commonly associated with functional constipation with stool retention and subsequent overflow incontinence:
  - 80–90% cases of encopresis fall into this category.
- Another less common type of functional encopresis is nonretentive fecal incontinence; refers to the entity of repeated passage of feces into inappropriate places (usually clothing or floor) after the age of 4 years in the absence of constipation and structural or inflammatory diseases

EPIDEMIOLOGY

- The reported ratio of boys to girls with encopresis ranges from 2:1 to 6:1.
- Boys are more likely to experience nonretentive fecal incontinence than girls at a ratio of 9:1.
- Encopresis is reported in 1.5–2.8% of children >4 years of age.
- Between 10% and 30% of children with encopresis have nonretentive fecal incontinence.

RISK FACTORS

There is no association with family size, ordinal position in the family, age of parents, or socioeconomic status.

Genetics

Monozygotic twins have a 4-fold higher incidence than do dizygotic twins.

ALERT

- Constipation with a rectal fecal mass is most common risk for encopresis.
- Children with nonretentive fecal incontinence have more behavioral problems, poor self-esteem, and higher prevalence of attention deficit disorder.

PATHOPHYSIOLOGY

Chronic constipation with fecal impaction results in overflow incontinence and reduced sensation secondary to rectal distention. The pattern of holding fecal matter, leading to chronic constipation and overflow incontinence, may result from a variety of causes, such as a painful experience from a fissure, difficult toilet training, or reluctance to use school bathrooms. However, eliciting a medical history often does not reveal a triggering event.

ETIOLOGY

- Chronic constipation leads to a dilated rectum, decreased rectal sensation, shortening of the anal canal, and decreased anal sphincter tone in some patients.
- Findings on anorectal manometry include increased rectal sensory threshold and paradoxic contraction of the external anal sphincter during attempts at defecation (known as *anismus*).
- Nonretentive fecal incontinence occurs in children without constipation. The soiling may be a manifestation of an emotional disturbance. In some children, it can be associated with specific triggers (person or place) or may represent a voluntary impulsive action. Laboratory, imaging, and motility studies in these patients are normal, including normal anorectal manometry and normal colonic transit times.

COMMONLY ASSOCIATED CONDITIONS

- Urinary tract infections (UTIs)
- Enuresis
  - More frequently seen in patients with nonretentive fecal incontinence (45% have daytime urinary incontinence and 40% have nighttime enuresis) compared to constipated children

DIAGNOSIS

HISTORY

- Toileting habits:
  - Constipation: frequency and size of bowel movements (Large-diameter bowel movements are common in children with encopresis associated with functional constipation.)
  - Bowel movements that obstruct the toilet and/or chronic abdominal pain relieved by enemas or laxatives
  - Retentive posturing: avoiding defecation by contraction of pelvic floor, squeezing the buttocks together (leg scissoring, crossing the legs, standing on tiptoes)
- Irritability, abdominal cramps, decreased appetite (Symptoms improve after passage of large stool.)
- Onset: Elicit history of triggering events (perianal infection, diet changes, toilet training, avoidance of school bathrooms, sexual abuse, or other stressful events).
- Urinary incontinence (may occur in patients with megarectum compressing the bladder)
- Timing in the neonatal period of meconium passage, as well as past surgeries, medical history, and medications, are relevant.
- Unsteady or clumsy gait may suggest a neuromuscular disorder.
- Children with nonretentive fecal incontinence do not have any history of constipation and have daily bowel movements. The incontinence is diurnal, usually in the afternoon.

PHYSICAL EXAM

- Encopresis with functional constipation
  - Fecal mass palpable in 40% of patients; fecal soiling in the perianal region
  - Dilated rectum with a normally positioned anus
- Digital rectal exam is not recommended to routinely diagnose fecal impaction functional encopresis or nonretentive fecal incontinence.
  - Anal sphincter tone may be normal or slightly decreased; the anal canal is usually shorter than normal.
  - Hard stool or a large amount of "mushy" stool present in rectal vault
- Nonretentive fecal incontinence
  - No palpable fecal mass
  - Normal-size rectum
  - Normal sphincter length
- Examine deep tendon reflexes, anal wink, rectal exam, lumbosacral spine exam to look for sacral dimpling, and documentation of normal growth.
- In patients with extreme fear of anal exam, attempt a perianal inspection and obtain a plain radiograph of the abdomen to establish a fecal impaction.

DIFFERENTIAL DIAGNOSIS

Determine whether stool leakage is caused by functional constipation or an underlying anatomic, metabolic, or neurologic abnormality. Fecal incontinence may be secondary to diarrheal diseases or defective neuromuscular control, such as in children with spinal defects.

- Neuromuscular
  - Spinal cord tumor
  - Tethered spinal cord
  - Meningomyelocele
- Anal abnormalities
  - Anteriorly displaced anus
  - Ectopic anus
- Inflammatory
  - Proctitis (infectious or ulcerative)
  - Fistula secondary to Crohn disease
  - Celiac disease
- Stricture (after necrotizing enterocolitis or inflammatory bowel disease)
- Abdominal pelvic mass (sacral teratoma, meningomyelocele)
- Hypotonia (cerebral palsy, amyotonia congenita, familial visceral myopathy)
- Hirschsprung disease (constipation common, fecal incontinence rarely seen) or ultra-short-segment Hirschsprung disease
- Postsurgical repair of imperforate anus or Hirschsprung disease
- Endocrine
  - Hypothyroidism
  - Panhypopituitarism
  - Diabetes mellitus
- Constipating medications
  - Opiates
  - Calcium supplements
  - Psychotropics

DIAGNOSTIC TESTS & INTERPRETATION

Referral to a pediatric gastroenterologist for further evaluation, including anorectal manometry, may be useful for patients who are not responding to standard management.

Initial Tests (screening, lab, imaging)

- No tests are needed if both the history and physical exam are consistent with functional constipation and associated encopresis. If the patient's history or physical exam is atypical and a systemic disorder is suspected, appropriate diagnostic tests should be done.
- Abdominal radiography is often necessary for patients who refuse a rectal exam or when a rectal impaction is not palpable on abdominal exam (e.g., in obese patients).
- Enema with water-soluble contrast material can be both helpful diagnostically to look for areas of narrowing and therapeutically as a clean out procedure.
- MRI of the spine can be done for children with suspected spinal abnormalities. This is rarely necessary if the neurologic exam is normal.
- Colonic transit study with radio-opaque markers to confirm the patients' complaints or assess for slow transit constipation

Diagnostic Procedures/Other

- Rectal suction biopsy can be performed to evaluate for ganglion cells within the colonic mucosa and definitively evaluate for Hirschsprung disease.
- Anorectal manometry can be done in selected cases to evaluate anorectal function. The main indication is to demonstrate the rectoanal inhibitory reflex to exclude Hirschsprung disease and ultra-short-segment Hirschsprung disease. It may also show an increased threshold to rectal sensation, providing important information to the patient and the parents.
- Patients with spinal cord abnormalities may show changes in anorectal manometry.

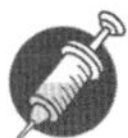

TREATMENT

MEDICATION

- Evidence suggests fecal disimpaction can be equally achieved with either oral polyethylene glycol (PEG) (with or without electrolytes at 1 to 1.5 g/kg/24 h) for 3 to 6 days of enemas or enema therapies.
  - Severe cases may require PEG ingestion by NG tube after disimpaction in a hospital setting.
  - Sedated manual disimpaction is rarely required.
- Stimulant laxatives:
  - Magnesium citrate
  - Bisacodyl
  - Senna
- Oral stool softeners:
  - PEG-3350 (0.75 mg/kg/24 h) is the preferred agent because of its palatability and ease of administration.
  - Lactulose (2.5 to 10 mL/24 h for infants and 40 to 90 mL/day in older children) is recommended as the 1st-line treatment if PEG-3350 is not available.
  - Milk of magnesia (0.5 to 1 mL/kg/24 h) is a good option.
  - Mineral oil (5 to 20 mL in divided doses) may also be used in older children who have no risk of aspiration.

ISSUES FOR REFERRAL

Patients with nonretentive fecal incontinence usually require referral to a mental health professional for more intensive behavioral intervention.

COMPLEMENTARY & ALTERNATIVE THERAPIES

- Behavior modification therapy: Decrease family stress. Have the child sit on toilet for defined amount of time (1 min/year of age to a maximum of 10 minutes) 1 to 2 times per day (ideally after a meal, tailored to the age of the child) and try to perform a Valsalva maneuver. Have young children blow into a pinwheel or a balloon to try to make them bear down.
- Use a sticker incentive chart if age-appropriate.
- Delay toilet training if the child is in diapers (to reduce stress).
- Motivate using positive reinforcement strategies. Biofeedback can be successful in some cases.

ADMISSION, INPATIENT, AND NURSING CONSIDERATIONS

Management combines pharmacology, behavioral modification, and dietary alterations.

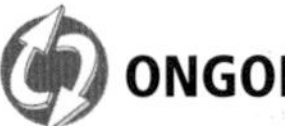

ONGOING CARE

FOLLOW-UP RECOMMENDATIONS

Patient Monitoring

- First follow-up visit is at 2 weeks to ensure compliance and success with the initial management.
- If the fecal impaction has been successfully removed, a reward system is started.
- The patient is followed at monthly intervals to ensure motivation and to be supportive.
- Treatment with stool softeners is needed until behavior and diet have improved and until rectal dilation has resolved.
- Medication is often needed for 2 to 6 months or longer.

ALERT

- Parents may misconstrue stool-withholding behavior as an attempt to defecate.
- Parents may think that the soiling represents diarrheal illness, causing a delay in diagnosis and treatment.
- Parents may think their child's soiling is deliberate. They may not understand that the child can neither feel the passage of stool nor prevent it. The usual urge to defecate, which comes from stretching of the ampulla and internal anal sphincter, is not felt because the rectal ampulla is massively distended.
- Patients or their parents often stop stool softeners as soon as a normal stool pattern starts. If therapy has been ended prematurely, the patient's constipation and encopresis returns immediately because rectal tone is still poor and no other behavior or dietary modifications have been made.

DIET

- Normal fiber intake
- Adequate fluid intake

COMPLICATIONS

- Social problems
- UTIs, especially in girls
- Abdominal discomfort
- Decreased appetite and weight loss

ADDITIONAL READING

- Burgers RB, Benninga MA. Functional nonretentive fecal incontinence in children: a frustrating and long-lasting clinical entity. *J Pediatr Gastroenterol Nutr*. 2009;48(Suppl 2):S98–S100.
- Desantis DJ, Leonard MP, Preston MA, et al. Effectiveness of biofeedback for dysfunctional elimination syndrome in pediatrics: a systematic review. *J Pediatr Urol*. 2011;7(3):342–348.
- Di Lorenzo C, Benninga MA. Pathophysiology of pediatric fecal incontinence. *Gastroenterology*. 2004;126(1 Suppl 1):S33–S40.
- Griffiths DM. The physiology of continence: idiopathic fecal constipation and soiling. *Semin Pediatr Surg*. 2002;11(2):67–74.
- Har AF, Croffie JM. Encopresis. *Pediatr Rev*. 2010;31(9):368–374.
- Koppen IJ, von Gontard A, Chase J, et al. Management of functional nonretentive fecal incontinence in children: recommendations from the International Children's Continence Society. *J Pediatr Urol*. 2016;12(1):56–64.
- Siddiqui A, Rosen R, Nurko S. Anorectal manometry may identify children with spinal cord lesions. *J Pediatr Gastroenterol Nutr*. 2011;53(5):507–511.
- Tabbers MM, DiLorenzo C, Berger MY, et al. Evaluation and treatment of functional constipation in infants and children: evidence-based recommendations from ESPGHAN and NASPGHAN. *J Pediatr Gastroenterol Nutr*. 2014;58(2):258–274.

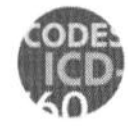

CODES

ICD10

- R15.9 Full incontinence of feces
- F98.1 Encopresis not due to a substance or known physiol condition

FAQ

- Q: Is it possible to become "addicted" to laxative medicines?
- A: Stool softeners, rather than cathartic laxatives or per rectal therapies, are chosen for long-term therapy because the colon does not become dependent on stool softeners.
- Q: Will my child become sick if this problem is not resolved?
- A: Most children with chronic constipation and encopresis grow well and do not develop other health problems. The major problems are social and should be taken seriously. Social continence is crucial for the school-aged child.

ENDOCARDITIS

Jenifer A. Glatz, MD

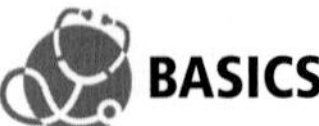

BASICS

DESCRIPTION

Infective endocarditis (IE) is a microbial infection of the endocardium of the heart, especially of the heart valves.

EPIDEMIOLOGY

Incidence

- IE is relatively uncommon in children, accounting for 0.05 to 0.12 cases per 1,000 pediatric admissions.
- Recent increase in frequency has been associated with improved survival of patients with congenital heart disease and the more widespread and often prolonged use of central vascular catheters, especially in premature infants.
- No gender or race predisposition in children

RISK FACTORS

- Preexisting heart disease (congenital or acquired such as rheumatic heart disease)
- Prior history of endocarditis
- Cardiac surgery/intervention (Risk increases 5-fold with a procedure within the last 6 months.)
- Intracardiac pacemakers and implantable cardioverter-defibrillators
- Prosthetic valves or conduits
- Indwelling catheters
- IV drug use
- IE occurs in 8–10% of children without known risk factors.

GENERAL PREVENTION

- The degree to which antibiotics decrease the incidence, duration, or extent of bacteremia with at-risk procedures is controversial. In 2007, the guidelines for subacute bacterial endocarditis (SBE) prophylaxis from the American Heart Association (AHA) were changed due to the lack of evidence that prophylactic antibiotic administration prevents IE.
- SBE prophylaxis is recommended by the AHA only for the following cardiac conditions:
  - Prosthetic cardiac valve or prosthetic material used for cardiac valve repair
  - Prior history of IE
  - Unrepaired cyanotic congenital heart disease, including palliative shunts and conduits
  - Congenital heart defect repaired with prosthetic material or device for the first 6 months after the procedure
  - Repaired congenital heart disease with residual defect near the site of prosthetic patch or device
  - Cardiac transplantation recipients with cardiac valvulopathy
- SBE prophylaxis is recommended only for the following procedures:
  - Dental procedures involving manipulation of the gingival or periapical region of teeth or perforation of the oral mucosa
  - Surgery involving prosthetic intravascular or intracardiac material, including heart valves
  - Invasive respiratory tract procedures involving incision or biopsy, such as tonsillectomy/adenoidectomy or abscess drainage
- Prevention should focus on education regarding rationale behind current guidelines, discussion of potential risk, signs and symptoms of IE, and maintaining optimal oral hygiene.
- Risk can be further decreased by correction of the cardiovascular anomaly by surgery or interventional catheterization techniques if indicated and by minimizing or decreasing the use of central lines.

PATHOPHYSIOLOGY

- IE is primarily seen in patients with preexisting heart disease (congenital or acquired) who develop bacteremia with organisms that are likely to cause infection.
- IV drug abusers and patients with indwelling central venous catheters may develop endocarditis even in the absence of prior heart disease.
- Local turbulence secondary to the cardiovascular abnormality is thought to result in damage of the endocardial surface. The development of a fibrin and platelet network occurs in which bacteria may then become entrapped, leading to formation of a vegetation.
- Bacteremia may be a complication of focal infection (e.g., pneumonia, cellulitis, or urinary tract infection) or may be associated with various dental and surgical procedures. Bacteremia, however, occurs most commonly with daily activities, such as chewing, flossing, and brushing teeth.
- Peripheral manifestations in chronic endocarditis are mediated by embolic or immune complex reactions.

ETIOLOGY

- Gram-positive cocci account for 90% of culture-positive endocarditis.
  - *Streptococcus viridans and Staphylococcus aureus* are the most common agents.
  - Other organisms that can cause endocarditis are enterococci sp., coagulase-negative staphylococci, β-hemolytic streptococci, and the HACEK group (*Haemophilus aphrophilus*, *Haemophilus paraphrophilus*, *Haemophilus parainfluenzae*, *Actinobacillus actinomycetemcomitans*, *Cardiobacterium hominis*, *Eikenella corrodens*, *Kingella* species). IE can also be caused by *Candida*, *Aspergillus*, *Abiotrophia*, and *Granulicatella* species.
- Approximately 5% of endocarditis cases in children are reported as culture negative.

DIAGNOSIS

HISTORY

- Signs and symptoms of IE in children are typically nonspecific, so a meticulous history is essential.
- General symptoms include:
  - Fever, chills, rigors, diaphoresis
  - Malaise, fatigue
  - Anorexia, weight loss
  - Symptoms of heart failure
  - Arthralgia/myalgia
  - Neurologic symptoms
- Occasionally, a recent infection, surgical procedure, or dental visit can be identified.
- Acute endocarditis is associated with a more rapidly progressive, fulminant course.

PHYSICAL EXAM

- General
  - Fever (usually low grade with α-hemolytic streptococci and high grade with *S. aureus*)
  - Petechiae
- Embolic or immunologic phenomena
  - Renal: glomerulonephritis, infarct
  - Pulmonary embolus
  - Splinter hemorrhages
  - Retinal hemorrhages (Roth spots)
  - Osler nodes (painful, red lesions found on hands/feet)
  - Janeway lesions (painless macular/nodular lesions on palms/soles)
  - Splenomegaly
  - Arthritis, osteomyelitis
  - Neurologic signs secondary to cerebral infarction, meningitis, or hemorrhage
- Cardiac/valvulitis
  - New or change in heart murmur
  - Signs of congestive heart failure (CHF)
  - Cyanosis
- Newborns with IE may present with feeding difficulty, respiratory distress, tachycardia, hypotension, seizures, apnea, and evidence of septic emboli.
- Splinter hemorrhages, Roth spots, Osler nodes, and Janeway lesions are rare in children.

DIFFERENTIAL DIAGNOSIS

- Other infections
- Acute rheumatic fever
- Malignancy
- Connective tissue disorders

DIAGNOSTIC TESTS & INTERPRETATION

Initial Tests (screening, lab, imaging)

- Blood cultures
  - Most important diagnostic test for endocarditis
  - Positive in 85–95% of reported cases
  - Obtain in any child with fever of unknown origin with a history of heart disease, central venous catheter, a new murmur, or prior endocarditis.
  - Obtain three blood cultures from different sites during the 1st day of suspected endocarditis. If no growth by day 2 of incubation, draw 2 to 3 more cultures.
  - The bacteremia of endocarditis is continuous; therefore, it is not necessary to wait to obtain the blood cultures during a fever spike.
  - Culture of arterial blood is not more beneficial than a venous sample.
- Nonspecific data
  - Anemia
  - Leukocytosis
  - Thrombocytopenia
  - Elevated erythrocyte sedimentation rate (ESR) and C-reactive protein
  - Hematuria and red cell casts
  - Positive rheumatoid factor
  - Hypocomplementemia
- Echocardiography, transthoracic
  - Valuable noninvasive technique in the identification of vegetations
  - Specificity is 98%, but sensitivity is approximately 60–70%, so a negative echocardiogram does not rule out endocarditis. Sensitivity in children depends on image quality and improves with weight <60 kg.

- IE should be suspected with presence of a vegetation, abscess, pseudoaneurysm, or new dehiscence of a prosthetic valve.
  - Also invaluable for follow-up, including evaluation for potential cardiac complications
- Echocardiography, transesophageal
  - Especially helpful for smaller vegetations, obese patients, paravalvular leakage, root abscess, prosthetic valve involvement, or when image quality is limited as is often seen in patients following recent open heart surgery
  - Recommended in patients with an inconclusive transthoracic study but a high index of suspicion for endocarditis
- Echocardiography, intracardiac
  - Helpful with pacemaker lead infections or prosthetic valves
- The modified Duke criteria define diagnostic categories (definite endocarditis, possible endocarditis, and rejected cases) based on combinations of major and minor criteria.
  - Criteria:
    - Major: organism specific for IE demonstrated by positive blood culture and evidence of endocardial involvement
    - Minor: predisposing heart disease, fever, vascular/immunologic phenomena, or microbiologic evidence not within major criteria
  - Definitive endocarditis requires two major, or one major plus three minor, or five minor criteria.
  - Several studies have confirmed the high sensitivity of these criteria, although specificity is controversial.

ALERT

- The absence of vegetation(s) by echocardiography does not rule out endocarditis.
- In patients with a prosthetic valve, echocardiography is not always helpful as there is frequently artifact from the prosthetic valve. Abnormal movements of the valve leaflets may suggest a vegetation.
- The ESR may remain elevated for some time, even after cessation of bacteremia.

Diagnostic Procedures/Other

Electrocardiogram: New-onset abnormalities such as atrioventricular block (even 1st-degree) or a rhythm disorder may represent conduction system and myocardial involvement from invasive disease.

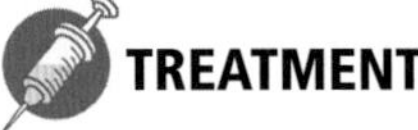

TREATMENT

GENERAL MEASURES

- Rest
- Optimal nutrition and hydration
- Careful dental hygiene

MEDICATION

Antibiotics

- Prolonged IV therapy (at least 4 weeks and often 6 to 8 weeks) is needed.
- Choice of antibiotic(s) and duration of treatment depend on the infecting organism, sensitivity pattern, and patient risk factors. Often combination therapy is used.
- If the blood cultures are initially negative and the patient is not acutely ill, consider withholding antibiotics to determine the definitive etiology.
- If the patient is acutely ill or septic, obtain three blood cultures over 1 to 2 hours and empirical antibiotics should be initiated.
- Bactericidal rather than bacteriostatic antibiotics should be chosen.

ISSUES FOR REFERRAL

Consider microbiology lab consultation, especially if there is a high index of suspicion for IE and cultures are negative.

SURGERY/OTHER PROCEDURES

Consider surgical intervention for:

- Severe/worsening CHF
- Valvular disease with unstable hemodynamics
- Failing medical therapy
- Large (>10 mm), mobile vegetations
- ≥2 major embolic events
- Fungal endocarditis
- Abscess formation/periannular extension
- Prosthetic valve endocarditis

ADMISSION, INPATIENT, AND NURSING CONSIDERATIONS

- Antipyretics
- Monitor for conduction or rhythm disturbances.
- Blood pressure support if needed
- Consider removal of central venous catheter if present.

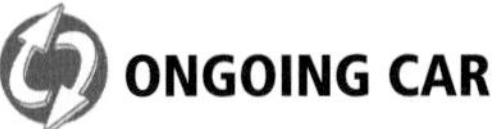

ONGOING CARE

FOLLOW-UP RECOMMENDATIONS

Patient Monitoring

- Obtain repeat blood cultures after a few days of antibiotic or antifungal therapy to ensure organism eradication.
- Repeat blood cultures after completion of a full course of antibiotic therapy could be considered, although may result in identification of a contaminant.
- Can consider outpatient IV therapy in select patients after stabilization in the hospital once the patient is afebrile, blood cultures are negative, and risk for complications is minimized
- Frequent monitoring with home nursing should be considered to monitor for complications and ensure adherence to the medical plan.
- Patients should be educated regarding risk of future recurrence and the importance of maintaining good oral hygiene. SBE prophylaxis is currently recommended by the AHA for patients with a prior history of IE.
- Cardiology follow-up is essential as residual valvular regurgitation can lead to heart failure even following clearance of the infecting organism.

PROGNOSIS

If diagnosed in a timely fashion and appropriate therapy is instituted, prognosis is relatively good for bacterial endocarditis. *S. aureus* and fungal endocarditis are associated with higher morbidity and mortality. Patients with underlying congenital heart disease are at higher risk for morbidity and mortality. In-hospital mortality for children with IE is approximately 5–10%.

COMPLICATIONS

Despite improvements in diagnosis and treatment, IE continues to be a disease with significant morbidity. Approximately 30% of patients have complications including:

- Cardiac: valve destruction and perforation leading to incompetence, abscess and fistula formation, ruptured sinus of Valsalva, heart failure, myocardial dysfunction, shunt or conduit obstruction, pericardial effusion, or conduction abnormalities
- Embolic events may occur to multiple organ systems (central nervous system, bowel, coronary arteries, kidneys, spleen, skin, lungs).
- Vascular: mycotic aneurysms
- Increased risk of complications seen in patients with prosthetic valves, *S. aureus* or fungal IE, prior episode of IE, cyanotic heart disease, and the presence of a systemic to pulmonary shunt

ADDITIONAL READING

- Baltimore RS, Gewitz M, Baddour LM, et al. Infective endocarditis in childhood: 2015 update: a scientific statement from the American Heart Association. *Circulation*. 2015;132(15):1487–1515.
- Ferrieri P, Gewitz MH, Gerber MA, et al. Unique features of infective endocarditis in childhood. *Circulation*. 2002;105(17):2115–2126.
- Johnson JA. Boyce TG, Cetta F, et al. Infective endocarditis in the pediatric patient: a 60-year single-institution review. *Mayo Clin Proc*. 2012;87(7):629–635.
- Wilson W, Taubert KA, Gewitz M, et al. Prevention of infective endocarditis: guidelines from the American Heart Association: a guideline from the American Heart Association Rheumatic Fever, Endocarditis, and Kawasaki Disease Committee, Council on Cardiovascular Disease in the Young, and the Council on Clinical Cardiology, Council on Cardiovascular Surgery and Anesthesia, and the Quality of Care and Outcomes Research Interdisciplinary Working Group. *Circulation*. 2007;116(15):1736–1754.

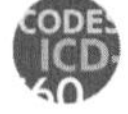

CODES

ICD10

- I38 Endocarditis, valve unspecified
- I33.0 Acute and subacute infective endocarditis

FAQ

- Q: I forgot to give my child antibiotics prior to the procedure. Should I give him a dose afterward?
- A: The dosage may be administered up to 2 hours after the procedure.
- Q: SBE prophylaxis is recommended for my child, but she already is on long-term antibiotic therapy with that recommended antibiotic. Should she use an additional antibiotic or increase her current dose for the procedure?
- A: An antibiotic from a different class should be selected.
- Q: My child has a congenital heart defect. Does he/she require SBE prophylaxis?
- A: The answer depends on the type of the congenital heart defect and the status of any needed intervention. The child's physician should be contacted regarding the need for prophylaxis.

ENURESIS

Eugene R. Hershorin, MD • Wendy Robin Glaberson, MD

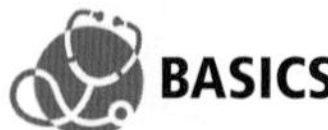

BASICS

DESCRIPTION

- Involuntary, urinary incontinence after age of expected bladder control; term generally reserved for children ≥5 years of age; may be
  - Primary: has never been "dry" for 6 months (80%)
  - Secondary: patient previously "dry" for 6 months or longer
- Classified as
  - Monosymptomatic nocturnal enuresis (MNE)
  - Non-monosymptomatic nocturnal enuresis (NMNE) if there is evidence of lower urinary tract malfunction (e.g., delayed voiding, frequency, urgency, holding maneuvers)

EPIDEMIOLOGY

- Male > female, although some recent reports state that nocturnal enuresis is more common in girls than in boys
- Prevalence
  - 10–15% of children at age 5 years
  - 7–15% of children at 7 years
  - 5% of children at 10 years
  - 0.5–1% in teenagers and adults

RISK FACTORS

- Constipation
- Lower urinary tract dysfunction
- Sleep disorders (e.g., obstructive sleep apnea [OSA])
- Neuropsychiatric disorders

Genetics

- 60–70% have a positive family history of enuresis.
- Risk of severe enuresis is greater with maternal enuresis history compared with paternal history (odds ratio 3.6 vs. 1.8).
- Autosomal dominant pattern seen in 50%, whereas 30% of cases are sporadic
- Risk is twice as high in monozygotic twin of a child with enuresis compared with a dizygotic twin.
- Several loci on chromosomes 8q, 12q, 13q, and 22q associated with a nocturnal enuresis phenotype; candidate genes include *ENUR1* and *ENUR2*.

ETIOLOGY

- Primary nocturnal enuresis: results from interplay of one or more of the following:
  - Nocturnal polyuria
  - Decreased functional bladder volume
  - Increased detrusor activity
  - Increased arousal threshold when asleep
  - Inadequate secretion of antidiuretic hormone
- Daytime incontinence and enuresis, day and night
  - As above
  - More concerning for underlying urologic and neurologic disorder
  - Urinary reflux into vagina with seepage after conclusion of voiding
  - Insertion of ureter into urethra or vagina
  - Stress incontinence with increased abdominal pressure (laughing, coughing, increased intravesicular pressure)
- Secondary enuresis can result from:
  - Any condition causing polyuria (including diabetes, hypercalcemia)
  - Urinary tract infection (UTI)
  - Encopresis
  - Emotional stress or trauma including physical and sexual abuse, parental divorce, depression, new sibling, household moving, new school

COMMONLY ASSOCIATED CONDITIONS

Neuropsychiatric comorbidities: ADHD, anxiety, and oppositional behavior are more commonly associated with secondary nocturnal enuresis.

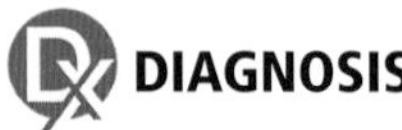

DIAGNOSIS

HISTORY

- Onset
  - Nocturnal versus diurnal
  - Dry period (even if only weeks)
    - Concomitant recent onset of polydipsia (sometimes accompanied by candidal infections, weight loss) suggests new-onset diabetes.
  - Frequency
    - A frequency–volume chart provides information on daily fluid intake and volumes and timing of voids; identifies subtle lower urinary tract symptoms and can aid in treatment approach
  - Pattern of urination
    - Constantly wet pants (dribbling)
    - Frequent small amounts of urine
    - Presence of weak urinary stream
    - Dysuria
    - Frequency
    - Hesitancy
    - Urine holding maneuvers (e.g., pressing the heel into perineum)
    - Nocturia
- Past medical history
  - Obstipation/constipation/fecal incontinence (encopresis)
  - History of UTI
  - Behavioral/developmental history
  - Toilet training history
  - Medications
  - Neurologic symptoms
  - Other medical problems
- Family history
  - One parent or both parents
- Social history
  - For whom does this pose problem—parent or child?
  - Effect on child
    - Ability to sleep away from home without embarrassment
    - Teasing at school
    - Emotional effects
- Social changes
  - Divorce
  - New significant other for parent
  - New sibling
  - Household move
  - New school

PHYSICAL EXAM

- Vital signs
- Growth parameters and pattern
- Neurologic exam
  - Gait, tone, sensory, motor, deep tendon reflexes, cremasteric reflex
- Funduscopy: to rule out raised intracranial pressure
- Abdominal exam: to rule out masses, especially renal mass, fecal impaction, bladder distention
- Genitalia: Rule out adhesions, vulvovaginitis, balanitis, stenosis, foreign bodies.
- Urinary stream
- Rectal exam: tone, perianal sensation, anal wink
- Spine: bony defects, cutaneous signs of underlying spinal defects

DIFFERENTIAL DIAGNOSIS

- UTI/urethritis
- Obstipation/constipation
- Water intoxication
- Type 1 or type 2 diabetes
- Diabetes insipidus
- Hypercalcemia
- Sickle cell disease or trait
- Nephritis/nephrosis
- Anatomic abnormalities of the urinary tract
- Sleep disorders
- Depression
- Anxiety
- Behavioral disorders
- Medications (sedatives, soporifics, antihistamines, diuretics, caffeine, methylxanthines)
- Spinal cord disease
  - Cognitive disorders
  - Seizure disorders
- Legitimate safety issues in going to bathroom alone
- Substandard living conditions (cold bathrooms, poor facilities)

DIAGNOSTIC TESTS & INTERPRETATION

Initial Tests (screening, lab, imaging)

- Urinalysis
  - Specific gravity (first morning void)
  - Glucose
  - Protein
  - Blood
- Urine culture: usually not necessary if no symptoms are present
- Rarely necessary in primary enuresis
- Perform if suggestion of anatomic or functional abnormality of genitourinary tract
- Ultrasound least invasive modality
- Renal/bladder ultrasound with pre-/postvoid bladder images to assess residual urine volume and look at bladder contour
- Noninvasive uroflow with pelvic floor electromyography—done by pediatric urologists

ALERT

Laboratory evaluation rarely yields a specific diagnosis. Balance risks and costs with unlikelihood of yield. Evaluation should generally not involve more than urinalysis.

TREATMENT

GENERAL MEASURES

- If the problem is affecting only the parents and child is not affected, the treatment should be education and support for the parents.
- Avoid all negative interventions.
- Minimize fluid intake during evening.
  - Success rate: low
- Encourage child to void regularly during the day and immediately prior to retiring to bed.
- Alarm therapy
  - Most effective in motivated patient and family
  - Improves arousal and nocturnal bladder function as a reservoir through conditioning
  - Use nightly for at least 2 to 3 months until 14 consecutive dry nights are achieved.
  - "Overlearning" (after dryness is achieved, have child drink modest amount of water 1 hour before bedtime) reduces risk of relapse if dryness is maintained for 1 month on this regimen.
  - High relapse rate; second remission very frequent with reintroduction of alarm system; second relapse rare
  - May not be appropriate for those with developmental disabilities

MEDICATION

- Avoid medication use before age 6 to 8 years.
- Desmopressin (DDAVP®)
  - Dose not based on age or weight
    - Standard dose 0.2 to 0.4 mg PO given 1 hour before bedtime
    - Use oral formulation only (nasal formulation is associated with increased risk of hyponatremia and seizures).
  - Caution against excessive fluid intake
  - Can be used intermittently or continuously
  - Sudden discontinuation results in high likelihood of relapse
  - Planned drug holidays are advised to assess for resolution of symptoms.
- Anticholinergics (e.g., oxybutynin)
  - Often used in combination with DDAVP
  - Usual dose: 5 mg given at bedtime
  - Exclude postvoid residual bladder volume.
  - Adverse effects: constipation, decreases saliva (hence, stress proper dental hygiene), hallucinations/agitation
  - Can be discontinued 6 months after resolution of symptoms
- Imipramine
  - Tricyclic antidepressant
  - 80% effective
  - No longer 1st- or 2nd-line choice for benign condition because of risk of QTc prolongation and controversial risk of sudden cardiac death and risk of ingestion by siblings
  - Usual dose: 25 mg for children <6 years old (20 to 25 kg), 50 mg for children 6 to 11 years old, and 50 to 75 mg for those <11 years old; given 1 hour before sleep

ADDITIONAL THERAPIES

- Urotherapy: aims toward normalizing bladder emptying and storage by teaching relaxed voiding techniques (e.g., biofeedback programs)
- Cognitive behavioral interventions
  - Formal programs developed and used by pediatric psychologists: high rate of success; involve "overcorrection techniques"—frequent practice and rewards for voiding procedures along with enuresis alarm
  - Positive reinforcement for dry nights
  - Use of praise, stickers, token economies
- Hypnotism
  - Appears to work by increasing subconscious awareness of bladder pressure during sleep, allowing increased awareness during sleep of intravesicular pressure
- Parasacral transcutaneous electrical nerve stimulation (PTENS)
  - Used when 1st-line alarm therapy and medications fail
  - Effective treatment of overactive bladder and MNE
  - Requires weekly office visits for treatment

ADMISSION, INPATIENT, AND NURSING CONSIDERATIONS

- Specific therapy to address specific anatomic, infectious, or functional genitourinary problems
- Address constipation and lower urinary tract dysfunction, as both may lead to treatment failure, whereas addressing these problems may result in spontaneous enuresis resolution.

ALERT

Decision to treat is a balance of the effect on the child of nontreatment (social, emotional) with the potential side effects of medication.

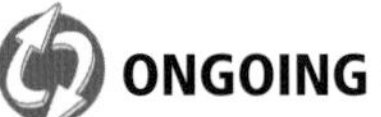

ONGOING CARE

PROGNOSIS

- 99% of cases resolve without treatment.
- Spontaneous resolution is ~15% per year after age 5 years.

COMPLICATIONS

- Physical
  - Vulvovaginitis
  - Diaper dermatitis
- Emotional
  - Embarrassment
  - Poor self-esteem
  - Reluctance to sleep out with peers or nonimmediate family
  - Depression
  - Poor school learning

ADDITIONAL READING

- Arda E, Cakiroglu B, Thomas DT. Primary nocturnal enuresis: a review. *Nephrourol Mon*. 2016;8(4):e35809.
- Fagundes SN, Lebl AS, Azevedo Soster L, et al. Monosymptomatic nocturnal enuresis in pediatric patients: multidisciplinary assessment and effects of therapeutic intervention. *Pediatr Nephrol*. 2017;32(5):843–851.
- Franco I, von Gontard A, De Gennaro M; for International Children's Continence Society. Evaluation and treatment of nonmonosymptomatic nocturnal enuresis: a standardization document from the International Children's Continence Society. *J Pediatr Urol*. 2013;9(2):234–243.
- International Children's Continence Society: www.i-c-c-s.org. Accessed May 19, 2018.
- Maternik M, Krzeminska K, Zurowska A. The management of childhood urinary incontinence. *Pediatr Nephrol*. 2015;30(1):41–50.
- Neveus T, Eggert P, Evans J, et al; for International Children's Continence Society. Evaluation of and treatment for monosymptomatic enuresis: a standardization document from the International Children's Continence Society. *J Urol*. 2010;183(2):441–447.
- von Gontard A, Heron J, Joinson C. Family history of nocturnal enuresis and urinary incontinence: results from a large epidemiological study. *J Urol*. 2011;185(6):2303–2306.

CODES

ICD10

- R32 Unspecified urinary incontinence
- N39.44 Nocturnal enuresis

FAQ

- Q: Do the medications cure the enuresis?
- A: None of the medications cure the problem. DDAVP works as an anti-diuretic, reducing the amount of water that is released as urine, resulting in decreased bladder volumes. Tricyclic antidepressants cause urinary retention by the noradrenergic effects on bladder contraction and detrusor relaxation. Oxybutynin decreases detrusor irritability, resulting in larger bladder capacity before emptying. The medications result in nonemptying of the bladder during sleep but do not affect the underlying cause. Any resolution that occurs after cessation of medication treatment is probably from the natural resolution of the problem with age.
- Q: Isn't it important to treat the enuresis when the parents bring it up as a problem?
- A: Developmental resolution of nocturnal enuresis occurs at a range of ages, and in almost all cases, the enuresis resolves spontaneously. It is important to elicit for whom the enuresis is a problem. If the child is not affected by the enuresis, and it is only the parents who desire a cure, the important intervention is to educate them on the natural history of the problem and to let them know about the available interventions and their success rates for when the child desires a cure.
- Q: Are there any other interventions available for use only on sleep-out nights?
- A: One helpful tip is to allow the child to take a sleeping bag with him or her on sleep-outs. Place a pull-up inside the sleeping bag. When the child gets into the sleeping bag, he or she can change into the pull-up without anyone knowing. In the morning, the child puts his or her underwear back on, leaving the damp pull-up in the sleeping bag; the parent can take it out when the child gets home.

EOSINOPHILIC ESOPHAGITIS

Seema Khan, MD • Hemant P. Sharma, MD, MS, MHS

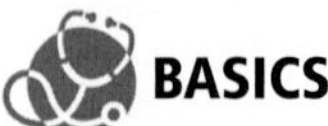

BASICS

DESCRIPTION

- Eosinophilic esophagitis (EoE) is a chronic immune-mediated esophageal disease characterized clinically by variable symptoms of esophageal dysfunction and pathologically by localized eosinophilic inflammation.
- The diagnosis is established in symptomatic patients who have the following:
  - At least 15 eosinophils/high powered field (HPF) confined to the esophagus on endoscopic biopsies
  - Reliable exclusion of other potential causes of esophageal eosinophilia
  - Persistent eosinophilic infiltrate in esophageal biopsies after a trial of high-dose proton pump inhibitor (PPI) therapy

EPIDEMIOLOGY

- Incidence rates are 5.1 and 7 per 100,000 person-years in children and adults, respectively.
- Prevalence in children is 29.5, lower than 43.4 per 100,000 in adults, and higher in United States compared to Europe.
- 3:1 male-to-female ratio
- Peaks of onset in childhood and 3rd to 4th decade

PATHOPHYSIOLOGY

- The exact pathophysiology of EoE is unknown but likely involves an immune response to environmental antigens in genetically predisposed individuals.
- Environmental factors (food and possibly aeroallergens) trigger inflammatory response mediated by T-helper type 2 (Th2) cells.
- Genetic polymorphisms which predispose to EoE include eotaxin-3, thymic stromal lymphopoietin, and calpain-14.

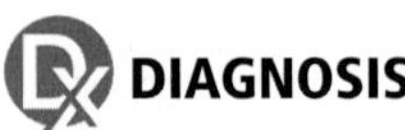

DIAGNOSIS

ALERT

Any patient who presents with esophageal food impaction should be evaluated for EoE. More than half of patients with food impaction are ultimately diagnosed with EoE.

HISTORY

- Although majority of children and adults are symptomatic, a small proportion of children are diagnosed when esophageal biopsies are obtained due to an esophageal foreign body impaction (e.g., coin) or ENT/respiratory symptom-based presentations (e.g., chronic cough).
- Symptoms of EoE vary with age:
  - In younger children, symptoms may include feeding difficulty or refusal (median age 2 years), vomiting (median age 8 years), and abdominal pain (median age 12 years).
    - Assess for:
      - Failure to thrive (poor weight gain, weight loss)
      - Feeding difficulties (not advancing past liquids, refusal of previously tolerated solids)
      - Gastroesophageal reflux disease (GERD) (arching, irritability/fussiness)
      - Vomiting
  - In adolescents and adults, symptoms include dysphagia, food impaction, refractory heartburn, epigastric abdominal pain, chest pain.
  - Questions to assess dysphagia:
    - Sensation of difficulty swallowing or food getting stuck?
    - Is the child a slow eater? Does the child overchew or overcut food? Does the child avoid specific foods?
    - Personal history of esophageal food impaction?
  - EoE is often associated with atopic disease (asthma, allergic rhinitis, atopic dermatitis, food allergy). Ask about the following:
    - Personal or family history of atopic disease?
    - Family history of EoE, dysphagia, refractory GERD, esophageal food impactions, or esophageal dilations?
  - No relief of symptoms after acid-blocking medication (minimum 8 weeks)

PHYSICAL EXAM

- Typically normal
- Poor nutritional status (rare but may occur if feeding dysfunction or significantly decreased appetite)
- Signs of comorbid atopic disease: allergic shiners, wheezing, eczematous skin lesions

DIFFERENTIAL DIAGNOSIS

- GERD
- Eosinophilic gastrointestinal disorder
- Crohn disease
- Celiac disease
- Graft versus host disease
- Parasitic infection
- Connective tissue disease
- Vasculitis
- Drug allergy
- Hypereosinophilic syndrome
- Candida esophagitis
- Viral esophagitis (HSV, CMV)
- Achalasia
- Peptic stricture

DIAGNOSTIC TESTS & INTERPRETATION

Initial Tests (screening, lab, imaging)

- Blood tests
  - No diagnostic serum markers for EoE
  - Peripheral eosinophilia observed in <50% of patients
  - Elevated serum IgE present in 50–60%.
- Food allergy testing
  - Performed after biopsies confirm EoE
  - In vitro–specific IgE testing: serum testing for food-specific IgE antibodies; no studies of predictive value, limited or no role
  - Skin prick testing (SPT): assesses for IgE-mediated reactions; good specificity (>82%) for identifying EoE triggers but poor sensitivity
  - Atopy patch testing (APT): assesses for non–IgE-mediated reactions; application of fresh or rehydrated food in occlusive chambers for 48 hours on back; similar specificity as SPT but better sensitivity
  - Combination of SPT and APT identified causative food antigens in 70% of patients at one center. More studies, especially prospective randomized controlled studies are needed.
- Aeroallergen testing
  - SPT may identify aeroallergen triggers of EoE and inform timing of follow-up endoscopies relative to pollen seasons.
- Upper GI series fluoroscopy
  - Provides complementary information to an upper endoscopy
  - Evaluates esophageal anatomy for strictures, hiatal hernia, Schatzki ring (lower esophageal ring), and achalasia
  - Is not recommended to make a diagnosis of EoE but useful in evaluation of sequelae of EoE (stenosis, stricture) in anticipation of dilation
- Endoscopic ultrasound
  - Findings include thickened mucosal and muscular layer.

Diagnostic Procedures/Other

- Esophagogastroduodenoscopy (EGD)
  - Required for diagnosis of EoE
  - Used to evaluate appearance of esophagus and obtain biopsies for pathology
  - As some forms of EoE are responsive to high doses of PPI, the diagnostic endoscopy is usually performed after an 8-week trial of a twice-daily PPI.
  - 4 to 6 esophageal biopsies are obtained by cold forceps, usually two to three biopsies sampled separately from the distal and mid/proximal esophagus. A pathologist experienced with the diagnosis of EoE should examine the biopsies for the presence of ≥15 eosinophils/HPF. Corroborating features include surface layering of eosinophils, eosinophilic microabscesses, degranulating eosinophils, basal zone hyperplasia, papillary elongation, other inflammatory cells, dilated intercellular spaces, and lamina propria fibrosis.
  - Gastric and duodenal biopsies should also be obtained to rule out other causes of esophageal eosinophilia. In EoE, there is no associated gastric or duodenal eosinophilic infiltrate.
- Esophageal pH-impedance probe
  - Use in diagnosis and management of EoE is unclear.
  - Some patients clearly suffer from both pathologic reflux and EoE.
- Esophageal manometry
  - Limited usefulness in routine clinical evaluation and best applied to those with dysphagia
  - Allows insight into extent of esophageal dysmotility
- Functional lumen imaging probe (FLIP)
  - Currently regarded as an investigational test; used to assess luminal compliance and stiffness in the context of esophageal remodeling

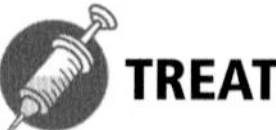

TREATMENT

Dietary therapy
- Elemental diet
  - Use amino acid–based formula for 100% of caloric requirements.
  - Highest efficacy with a histologic response in nearly 91%
  - Reintroduction of foods into diet should be stepwise and guided by allergist.
- Empiric food elimination diet
  - Generally entails avoidance of the four to six most common food allergens: (i) milk, (ii) soy, (iii) wheat, (iv) egg, (v) peanuts and tree nuts, (vi) fish and shellfish.
  - Histologic response in 72%, although not as high as with elemental diet but comparable to topical swallowed steroids
  - Limited data has demonstrated complete or partial histologic response to removal of cow's milk in 65% children.
- Targeted elimination diet
  - Use results from multimodal allergy testing to guide food eliminations from diet.
  - Efficacy comparable to empiric elimination diet
- When reintroducing foods into the diet following one of the above dietary therapies, caution should be taken to do so stepwise with reevaluation of esophageal biopsies after each food reintroduction to determine the actual dietary trigger that should continue to be avoided.

MEDICATION

- PPIs
  - Part of the diagnostic criteria for EoE is that the esophageal eosinophilia persists after treatment with high-dose PPI (e.g., omeprazole, pantoprazole, esomeprazole, lansoprazole, dexlansoprazole, or rabeprazole). If the eosinophilia persists after an 8-week course of PPI, then the diagnosis of EoE is applied.
  - Useful as adjunctive therapy to treat associated reflux symptoms
  - Insufficient to treat EoE
- Nonsystemic corticosteroids
  - Description
    - Swallowed topical steroids (fluticasone propionate and budesonide) are an alternative to dietary therapy.
    - Discontinuation is associated with recurrence of disease. They are safe for short-term administration.
    - Oropharyngeal and esophageal fungal infections, adrenal insufficiency, and bone demineralization are known potential complications.
    - Data on long-term safety are lacking.
  - Fluticasone propionate
    - Use metered-dose inhaler without a spacer.
    - Dose is sprayed into mouth and swallowed.
    - Initial doses:
      - Adults: 440 to 880 mcg twice daily
      - Children: 88 to 440 mcg 2 to 4 times daily
    - Avoid eating or drinking for 30 minutes after each dose.
  - Budesonide (viscous suspension)
    - Liquid budesonide inhaled solution ampules are mixed with sucralose/maltodextrin (e.g., Splenda®, 5 packets per ampule) or other sweetener to form thick slurry that coats the esophagus when ingested (see Liacouras CA, Furuta GT, Hirano I, et al, 2011 in "Additional Reading").
    - Initial doses:
      - Older children and adults: 2 mg daily
      - Children (<10 years): 1 mg daily
    - Avoid eating or drinking for a minimum of 30 minutes after dose.
    - Bedtime dosing is optimal.
- Systemic corticosteroids
  - Are effective but should only be used in cases of severe dysphagia and weight loss affecting growth
  - Long-term use should be avoided.
  - Prednisone (PO) or methylprednisolone (IV)
    - 1 to 2 mg/kg/24 h (max 60 mg daily)

ADDITIONAL THERAPIES

Endoscopic therapy
- Dilation of esophageal strictures
  - Useful in alleviating dysphagia
  - Does not address underlying problem
  - A trial of medical or dietary therapy is advisable prior to dilation unless a high-grade stricture is present.
  - Complications include chest pain (5%) and esophageal rupture (<1–5%).
- Removal of esophageal food impaction
  - Should be performed within 24 hours of food impaction to decrease risk of esophageal rupture

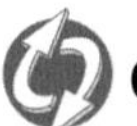

ONGOING CARE

COMPLICATIONS

- Feeding difficulties
- Esophageal strictures
- Small-caliber esophagus
- Esophageal perforation
- Esophageal fungal or viral superinfection

ADDITIONAL READING

- Arias A, González-Cervera J, Tenias JM, et al. Efficacy of dietary interventions for inducing histologic remission in patients with eosinophilic esophagitis: a systematic review and meta-analysis. *Gastroenterology*. 2014;146(7):1639–1648.
- Arias Á, Pérez-Martínez I, Tenías JM, et al. Systematic review with meta-analysis: the incidence and prevalence of eosinophilic oesophagitis in children and adults in population-based studies. *Aliment Pharmacol Ther*. 2016;43(1):3–15.
- Dellon ES, Liacouras CA. Advances in clinical management of eosinophilic esophagitis. *Gastroenterology*. 2014;147(6):1238–1254.
- Furuta GT, Katzka DA. Eosinophilic esophagitis. *N Engl J Med*. 2015;373(17):1640–1648.
- Greenhawt M, Aceves SS, Spergel JM, et al. The management of eosinophilic esophagitis. *J Allergy Clin Immunol Pract*. 2013;1(4):332–342.
- Liacouras CA, Furuta GT, Hirano I, et al. Eosinophilic esophagitis: updated consensus recommendations for children and adults. *J Allergy Clin Immunol*. 2011;128(1):3–20.e6, quiz 21–22.
- Soon IS, Butzner JD, Kaplan GG, et al. Incidence and prevalence of eosinophilic esophagitis in children. *J Pediatr Gastroenterol Nutr*. 2013;57(1):72–80.

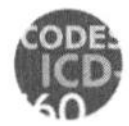

CODES

ICD10

K20.0 Eosinophilic esophagitis

FAQ

- Q: What are the goals of EoE treatment?
- A: There is no agreed on definition of EoE remission. Treatment goals include symptom reduction, decrease in esophageal eosinophilia to <15 eosinophils/HPF, and improvement in histologic and visual endoscopic changes. However, several studies show discordance between symptoms and histologic findings.
- Q: Do patients who have symptom response but persistent esophageal eosinophilia require further treatment?
- A: There is insufficient natural history data to answer this question. The concern is that untreated esophageal eosinophilia may progress to dysphagia, strictures, and esophageal fibrosis, but predictors of this progression are not well-defined.
- Q: Why might the empiric and targeted elimination diet have similar efficacy?
- A: The targeted elimination diet is guided by allergy testing (SPT and APT) results, but data on their diagnostic use are poorly reproducible. For certain foods (milk, wheat), they have poor reliability. Also, the APT process is not standardized, and interpretation may be subjective and variable. More prospective controlled trials are needed to evaluate the diagnostic use of these tests.
- Q: What is the best 1st-line therapy for EoE?
- A: The approach to each patient is individualized, as there is no agreement on the single best 1st-line therapy for EoE. Younger children may be more amenable to dietary restrictions. Children with failure to thrive benefit from elemental formula either as monotherapy or as a nutritional supplement in conjunction with either an elimination diet or topical corticosteroids. Dietary compliance in teenagers makes topical corticosteroids a popular option.

EPIDIDYMITIS

Melissa T. Sanford, MD • Hillary L. Copp, MD, MS

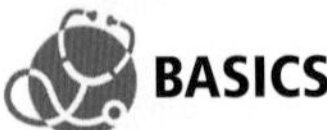

BASICS

DESCRIPTION

Epididymitis is an acute inflammation of the epididymis which can cause severe scrotal pain. It is important to differentiate epididymitis from testicular torsion or testicular appendage torsion.

EPIDEMIOLOGY

- Epididymitis is the most common cause of acute scrotum, approximately 37–65% of cases. The incidence ranges between 0.8 and 1.2 cases per 1,000 persons per year.
- There is a bimodal distribution with a peak in incidence in infants <1 year of age and peripubertal boys.

RISK FACTORS

Urologic manipulation (cystoscopy, intermittent self-catheterization, surgery of the urethra)

PATHOPHYSIOLOGY

- The majority of epididymitis is idiopathic (73%).
- Viral epididymitis: second most common cause
  - Urinalysis and culture are negative.
  - Often elevated titers of enterovirus, *Mycoplasma pneumoniae*, and adenoviruses.
  - New research suggests that some epididymitis might be due to postinfectious inflammation as 50% of patients had respiratory symptoms within 1 month of presentation, and presentations appear to peak in concert with rotavirus and enterovirus.
- Bacterial epididymitis: 2–6% of cases and is related to age
  - Due to ascending infection from the urethra or bladder, reflux of infected urine into the vas deferens, or hematogenous dissemination
  - Infants <1 year:
    - Typically due to genitourinary anomalies (73% vs. 21% in children >1)
    - Abnormalities include meatal stenosis, neurogenic voiding dysfunction, urethral stenosis, posterior urethral valves, ectopic ureter.
    - Typical bacteria include *Escherichia coli*, *Klebsiella*, and *Enterococcus*.
    - Postpubertal sexually active boys may have infection with sexually transmitted diseases such as gonorrhea or chlamydia.
- Chemical epididymitis: due to reflux of sterile urine into the vas deferens or drugs (amiodarone)
- Posttraumatic

COMMONLY ASSOCIATED CONDITIONS

- Systemic serositis (familial Mediterranean fever, sarcoidosis, Kawasaki disease)
- Systemic vasculitis (Henoch-Schönlein purpura, polyarteritis nodosa)

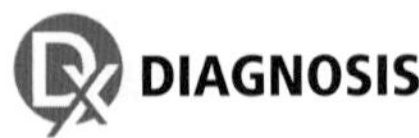

DIAGNOSIS

HISTORY

- It is not always possible to distinguish between testicular torsion, testicular appendage torsion, and epididymitis based on history and physical exam.
- Duration of symptoms is longer than in testicular torsion, typically >12 hours.
- The majority of patients complain of scrotal pain (91–98%), scrotal swelling (83%), and scrotal erythema (74%).
- Patients who have bacterial epididymitis are more likely to have prior urologic history than patients without bacterial epididymitis (73% vs. 0%).
- 16–33% of patients have a fever, almost always in bacterial epididymitis.

PHYSICAL EXAM

Inflamed, swollen scrotum with localized epididymal pain early in the course that can spread to generalized testicular inflammation late in the course

DIFFERENTIAL DIAGNOSIS

Testicular torsion

- Testicular appendage torsion
- Incarcerated inguinal hernia
- Hydrocele
- Systemic vasculitis
- Recent urologic surgery
- Idiopathic scrotal edema
- Testicular tumor
- Appendicitis
- Mumps orchitis

DIAGNOSTIC TESTS & INTERPRETATION

- Urinalysis and urine culture are only positive in a minority of presentations (7% and 1–6% respectively), but they should be sent for all patients to help guide therapy if they are positive for bacterial epididymitis.
- WBC, CRP, and ESR are most elevated in systemic serositis or vasculitis.

- Any sexually active boy or boy with an unclear sexual history should have gonorrhea and chlamydial testing performed.

ALERT
For acute scrotum, perform scrotal ultrasound with Doppler to differentiate between testicular torsion, testicular appendage torsion, or epididymitis.

- Epididymitis typically appears as an enlarged epididymis with hypervascular flow and mixed echogenicity with reactive fluid.

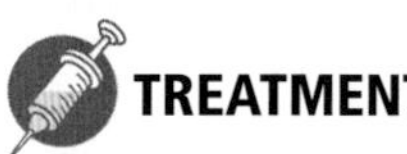

TREATMENT

GENERAL MEASURES

Given that the majority of acute epididymitis is non-bacterial, initial treatment should be supportive with analgesics, nonsteroidal anti-inflammatory drugs, bed rest, scrotal ice packs, and scrotal elevation.

MEDICATION

- Any children <1 year of age or with pyuria should be empirically begun on antibiotics based on a local antibiogram.
- If a child has culture-proven bacterial epididymitis, they should be started on culture-sensitive antibiotics for a 2-week course.

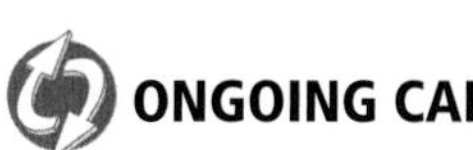

ONGOING CARE

FOLLOW-UP RECOMMENDATIONS

- Schedule for follow-up appointment in 2 to 4 weeks to ensure resolution of epididymitis.
- Recommend referral to pediatric urology.
- Children <1 year of age and any child with a positive urine culture should be evaluated with a renal bladder ultrasound to rule out genitourinary anomalies.

ADDITIONAL READING

- Cappèle O, Liard A, Barret E, et al. Epididymitis in children: is further investigation necessary after the first episode? *Eur Urol*. 2000;38(5):627–630.
- Cristoforo TA. Evaluating the necessity of antibiotics in the treatment of acute epididymitis in pediatric patients: a literature review of retrospective studies and data analysis [published online ahead of print January 17, 2017]. *Pediatr Emerg Care*. doi:10.1097/PEC.0000000000001018
- Halachmi S. Inflammation of the gonad in prepubertal healthy children. Epidemiology, etiology, and management. *ScientificWorldJournal*. 2006;6:1081–1085.
- Mäkelä E, Lahdes-Vasama T, Rajakorpi H, et al. A 19-year review of paediatric patients with acute scrotum. *Scand J Surg*. 2007;96(1):62–66.
- Somekh E, Gorenstein A, Serour F. Acute epididymitis in boys: evidence of a post-infectious etiology. *J Urol*. 2004;171(1):391–394.
- Tekgul S, Riedmiller E, Gerharz P. *Guideline on Paediatric Urology*. Philadelphia, PA: European Society for Paediatric Urology; 2008:15–17.

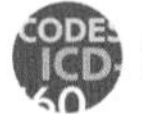

CODES

ICD10

- N45.1 Epididymitis
- N45.3 Epididymo-orchitis
- N45.4 Abscess of epididymis or testis

FAQ

- Q: What is the best empiric antibiotic?
- A: Empiric antibiotic choice should be based on local antibiogram. Typically reasonable choices include Keflex, Bactrim, or a fluoroquinolone.
- Q: What should be done if the epididymitis has not resolved after 2 weeks?
- A: The child should have repeat urinalysis and urine culture to ensure they have not developed a resistant bacterial infection and repeat scrotal ultrasound to ensure they have not developed an abscess.
- Q: What is a Prehn sign?
- A: A Prehn sign (named after Douglas T. Prehn, MD) is a historical diagnostic maneuver that was previously used to help diagnose epididymitis. This maneuver is inferior to Doppler ultrasound. To conduct the Prehn maneuver, elevate the testicles from below. The elevation of the testes should decrease pain if it is due to epididymitis; however, it does not theoretically relieve pain due to testicular torsion.

EPIGLOTTITIS

Sanyukta Desai, MD • Erin E. Shaughnessy, MD, MSHCM

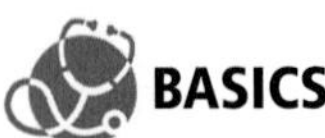

BASICS

DESCRIPTION

Acute life-threatening bacterial infection consisting of cellulitis and edema of the epiglottis, aryepiglottic folds, arytenoids, and hypopharynx, resulting in narrowing of the glottic opening and airway obstruction; also known as supraglottitis

EPIDEMIOLOGY

- Epiglottitis caused by *Haemophilus influenzae* type B occurs most often between the ages of 1 and 7 years (overall range: infancy to adulthood).
- Epiglottitis and other invasive disease secondary to *H. influenzae* type B have been reduced by 99% since the introduction of the conjugate vaccines in 1987 (approved for use at 15 months) and 1990 (approved for use at 2, 4, and 6 months).
- Nontypeable *H. influenzae* now appears to be a more common cause of invasive disease than type B.
- Year-round occurrence
- All geographic areas
- Can have secondary cases in households or child care centers
- May be more frequent in children with sickle cell anemia, asplenia, immunoglobulin defects, or hematologic malignancies (e.g., leukemia)
- Increasing ratio of adult to pediatric cases

Incidence

- Incidence of pediatric epiglottitis due to any organism has declined in the postvaccine era (0.3 to 0.7/100,000 per year from 3.47 to 6/100,000 per year).
- Incidence in adults has remained steady (1 to 4/100,000 per year).

GENERAL PREVENTION

- Universal immunization with *H. influenzae* type B capsular polysaccharide conjugate vaccines at 2 and 4 months (potential dose at 6 months, depending on the vaccine), with booster at 12 to 15 months
- Control measures:
  - Prophylaxis for *H. influenzae* type B index case and susceptible children in household and child care setting and intimate contacts with the assistance of infection control
  - Rifampin: 20 mg/kg/24 h in single dose for 4 days

PATHOPHYSIOLOGY

- Edema of the supraglottic structures (uvula, aryepiglottic folds, arytenoids, epiglottis, and vocal cords) that reduces the airway aperture
- Respiratory arrest can be caused by airway obstruction, aspiration of oropharyngeal secretions, or mucous plugging.

ETIOLOGY

- *H. influenzae*, nontypeable and type B (type B accounted for up to 90% of cases prior to the introduction of *H. influenzae* type B vaccine)
- *Streptococcus pneumoniae*
- *Streptococcus pyogenes* (group A β-hemolytic *Streptococcus*)
- *Staphylococcus aureus*
- Groups C and G β-hemolytic *Streptococcus*
- *Candida albicans* may be an etiologic agent in immunocompromised patients and those receiving prolonged corticosteroid treatment.
- *Pasteurella multocida* has been implicated in a few cases after exposure to nasopharyngeal secretions from a cat.
- Other rare isolates: *Moraxella catarrhalis*, *Klebsiella pneumoniae*, *Neisseria meningitidis*, *Pseudomonas* species, *Histoplasma*
- Bacterial superinfection of viral infections including herpes simplex, parainfluenza, varicella, Epstein-Barr
- Varicella can cause primary infection or lead to a secondary infection, often with *S. pyogenes*.
- Noninfectious etiologies include thermal injuries, trauma, and caustic ingestions.

DIAGNOSIS

HISTORY

- Abrupt onset of high fever (39–40°C), sore throat, and dysphagia
- Drooling or difficulty handling secretions
- Very limited or no prodrome of mild upper respiratory tract infection (URI)
- "Hot potato" voice (muffled)
- Rapid onset of toxicity and respiratory distress
- Cough and hoarseness usually absent. If present, these are late symptoms.
- Time from onset of symptoms to presentation with progressive respiratory distress is generally <12 hours.

PHYSICAL EXAM

Diagnosis can be suspected on history and observation of child's appearance alone.

- General
  - Extremely anxious appearance
  - Child prefers to remain sitting up.
  - Child often leaning forward with chin hyperextended to maintain airway in a "tripod" position
- Respiratory
  - Slow and labored respiratory effort
  - Inspiratory stridor, retractions, and late cyanosis
- Drooling is seen as a manifestation of dysphagia.

ALERT

Do *not* attempt to examine the throat if epiglottitis is a serious consideration.

DIFFERENTIAL DIAGNOSIS

- Viral laryngotracheobronchitis (croup) with or without secondary bacterial tracheitis
- Severe parainfluenza or influenza infection
- Uvulitis
- Peritonsillar, retropharyngeal, or lingual abscess
- Foreign body aspiration in a child with URI
- URI, including croup, in a child with a congenital or acquired airway problem (e.g., premature infant with subglottic stenosis, laryngeal web, vascular ring, tracheal stenosis)
- Hereditary angioedema (deficiency of complement C1 esterase inhibitor) can present with edema of the airway including the epiglottis.
- Diphtheria: rare in the United States
- Laryngeal infections

DIAGNOSTIC TESTS & INTERPRETATION

Initial Tests (screening, lab, imaging)

- Complete blood count: Elevated white blood cell count with left shift
- Cultures of blood and epiglottis (performed only in the operating room)
- Lateral neck radiography (should not be performed until airway team is in place):
  - Characteristic "thumb sign" of edematous epiglottis, with narrowing of the posterior airway and ballooning of the hypopharynx

Diagnostic Procedures/Other

Definitive diagnosis requires direct visualization of erythematous and edematous epiglottis.

ALERT

- Ensure appropriate airway management prior to any interventions, including intrusive examination components, radiographs, and blood collection.
- A radiograph is indicated only when the diagnosis is in doubt and should not delay airway management.

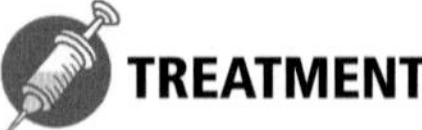

TREATMENT

GENERAL MEASURES

- Maintain child upright, never supine.
- Allow the child to assume his or her most comfortable position (usually in the parent's arms/lap).
- Administer oxygen by mask or blown by face.
- Rapidly assemble a team consisting of an anesthesiologist and otolaryngologist.
- Transport to operating room as soon as possible for anesthesia.
- Personnel experienced in airway management should accompany the child at all times, including during transport and in radiology.

MEDICATION

First Line

- Empiric parenteral antibiotic coverage to include gram-positive cocci and *H. influenzae* (type B and nontypeable)
  - Cephalosporins
    - Cefotaxime: 200 to 225 mg/kg/24 h (max 12 g/24 h) IV divided q4–6h
    - Ceftriaxone: 100 mg/kg/24 h (max 2 g/24 h) IV divided q12 to 24h
    - Cefuroxime: 100 to 200 mg/kg/24 h (max 9 g/24 h) IV divided q6–8h
  - Ampicillin/sulbactam: ampicillin 200 mg/kg/24 h (max 8 g/24 h) IV divided q6h
  - Serious penicillin/cephalosporin allergies
    - Levofloxacin (IV or PO): <5 years: 10 mg/kg/dose twice daily; >5 years: 10 mg/kg/dose once daily; max dose: 750 mg/24 h
- Duration of therapy: 7 to 10 days for all but staphylococcal disease (14 to 21 days)
- Switch may be made to oral medication after extubation and resumption of oral intake.
- Steroids are used commonly but without convincing evidence for their efficacy.

Second Line

- Discuss with infectious disease consultant.
- Chloramphenicol: 50 to 75 mg/kg/24 h (max 4 g/24 h) IV divided q6h; monitor levels
- Ampicillin: 200 to 400 mg/kg/24 h (max 12 g/24 h) IV divided q6h
- Penicillin: 200,000 to 300,000 U/kg/24 h (max 24 million U/24 h) IV divided q6h for streptococcal disease
- Oxacillin: 150 to 200 mg/kg/24 h (max 4 g/24 h) IV divided q4–6h for susceptible staphylococcal disease

ISSUES FOR REFERRAL

Airway should be secured by clinician skilled in airway management (e.g., otolaryngologist, anesthesiologist) while in the operating room.

SURGERY/OTHER PROCEDURES

- Secure airway via direct laryngoscopy and bronchoscopy with intubation.
- Institute IV catheterization and blood collection and culturing of epiglottis only after the airway is secured.
- Perform emergent cricothyrotomy if obstruction occurs prior to controlled airway management.
- Use fluid resuscitation in cases of septic shock.

ADMISSION, INPATIENT, AND NURSING CONSIDERATIONS

- Admit all children with suspicion of epiglottitis to ICU for airway management and close observation.
- Isolation of hospitalized patient: Droplet precautions should be continued for at least 24 hours from the initiation of effective antimicrobial therapy.

ONGOING CARE

FOLLOW-UP RECOMMENDATIONS

Patient Monitoring

- Extubation is usually possible within 24 to 48 hours. Criteria include decreased erythema and edema of the epiglottis on direct inspection and development of an air leak around the endotracheal tube.
- Defervescence is usually prompt after initiation of appropriate antimicrobial therapy.

PROGNOSIS

Mortality is estimated to be 5–10%.

COMPLICATIONS

- Without prompt medical intervention: complete airway obstruction leading to respiratory arrest, hypoxia, and death
- Necrotizing cervical fasciitis, descending necrotizing mediastinitis (rarely)
- Therapeutic complications
  - Aspiration
  - Endotracheal tube dislodgment and extubation
  - Tracheal erosion or irritation
  - Pneumomediastinum
  - Pneumothorax
  - Pulmonary edema
- Complications of *H. influenzae* type B bacteremia:
  - Septic shock
  - Pneumonia
  - Rarely, arthritis, meningitis, and pericarditis

ADDITIONAL READING

- Darras K, Roston A, Yewchuk L. Imaging acute airway obstruction in infants and children. *Radiographics*. 2015;35(7):2064–2079.
- Gorga S, Gilsdorf J, Mychaliska K. *Haemophilus influenzae* serotype f epiglottitis: a case report and review. *Hosp Pediatr*. 2017;7(1):54–56.
- Guardiani E, Bliss M, Harley E. Supraglottitis in the era following widespread immunization against *Haemophilus influenzae* type B: evolving principles in diagnosis and management. *Laryngoscope*. 2010;120(11):2183–2188.
- Rafei K, Lichenstein R. Airway infectious disease emergencies. *Pediatr Clin North Am*. 2006;53(2):215–242.
- Shah RK, Roberson DW, Jones DT. Epiglottitis in the *Hemophilus influenzae* type B vaccine era: changing trends. *Laryngoscope*. 2004;114(3):557–560.
- Shah RK, Stocks C. Epiglottitis in the United States: national trends, variances, prognosis, and management. *Laryngoscope*. 2010;120(6):1256–1262.

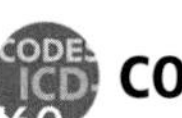

CODES

ICD10

- J05.10 Acute epiglottitis without obstruction
- J05.11 Acute epiglottitis with obstruction

FAQ

- Q: What is the incidence of epiglottitis since the introduction of conjugate vaccines against *H. influenzae* type B?
- A: Because *H. influenzae* type B caused 90% of epiglottitis and the incidence of all invasive disease due to H. influenzae type B has decreased by 99% in children <5 years of age, it is estimated that the incidence of epiglottitis has been reduced by >90%.
- Q: Have there been reports of epiglottitis caused by *H. influenzae* type B after complete vaccination?
- A: Yes. Several cases due to *H. influenzae* type B have been reported in the United States and abroad after partial and complete vaccination. Therefore, even a history of having received a full vaccination series does not necessarily eliminate the possibility of *H. influenzae* type B–associated epiglottitis. In one case series from 2004, 5/6 patients with *H. influenzae* type B epiglottitis had completed the *H. influenzae* type B vaccination series.
- Q: Should a fully vaccinated child who develops invasive disease due to *H. influenzae* type B be tested for an underlying immunodeficiency?
- A: Probably. In one study, about 1/3 of children diagnosed with invasive disease due to *H. influenzae* type B were found to have a previously undiagnosed immunoglobulin deficiency.
- Q: Can epiglottitis recur?
- A: Yes, but rarely.
- Q: Are corticosteroids of any value in the management of epiglottitis?
- A: They are used commonly, but there is no evidence to support their benefit.

E

EPSTEIN-BARR VIRUS (INFECTIOUS MONONUCLEOSIS)

Jessica R. Newman, DO

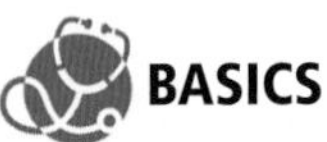

BASICS

DESCRIPTION

Epstein-Barr virus (EBV) is a double-stranded DNA virus implicated as a causative agent for infectious mononucleosis by an infected laboratory worker in 1968.

EPIDEMIOLOGY

- Worldwide distribution
- Humans are the only known reservoir.
- Transmission occurs through saliva and, occasionally, via blood transfusions and solid organ transplant (SOT).
- Incubation period is 4 to 7 weeks.
- Antibodies to EBV are present in up to 90% of adult populations.
- Areas with a high population density or low socioeconomic status usually become primarily infected within the first 3 years of life.

Incidence

In developed countries, acquisition of EBV is biphasic.

- Initial peak in incidence occurs before the age of 5 years.
- Second peak occurs during adolescence, coinciding with an increased frequency of intimate oral contacts.

Prevalence

>90% of adults have demonstrable EBV titers.

GENERAL PREVENTION

- No vaccine is clinically available.
- Standard precautions should be used in the hospitalized patient.
- Restriction of intimate contact with immunosuppressed individuals may be advisable.
- Patients with recent EBV infection, either proven or suspected, should not donate blood or solid organs.

PATHOPHYSIOLOGY

- Enters host via saliva and replicates initially in the oropharyngeal epithelium
- Selective infection of B lymphocytes occurs.
- The clinical syndrome of infectious mononucleosis results from proliferation of cells in the tonsils, lymph nodes, and spleen.
- Nonspecific humoral immune responses include the formation of heterophile antibodies and autoantibodies.
- Specific antibodies to EBV antigens are produced.
- Despite humoral responses, cellular immunity is responsible for controlling EBV infection.
- Latent, lifelong infection of B lymphocytes occurs.
- Latent virus may be reactivated during periods of immunosuppression or cellular stress.

COMMONLY ASSOCIATED CONDITIONS

- Subclinical infection
  - Most EBV infections in children, and even in adolescents, are clinically inapparent.
  - Mild, nonspecific symptoms may include coryza, diarrhea, and/or fever.
  - Immunologic seroconversion does occur.
- Infectious mononucleosis ("glandular fever"): most commonly observed with late primary acquisition of EBV. The classically defined illness is characterized by the following:
  - Fatigue
  - Malaise
  - Fever
  - Tonsillopharyngitis (often exudative)
  - Lymphadenopathy
  - Splenomegaly
  - Usually associated with increased atypical lymphocytes in the peripheral blood
- Rare illnesses of the nervous system have been reported, including the following:
  - Guillain-Barré syndrome
  - Bell palsy
  - Aseptic meningitis
  - Meningoencephalitis
  - Peripheral and/or optic neuritis
- Hematologic complications have been reported in association with EBV:
  - Aplastic anemia
  - Hemolytic anemia
  - Agranulocytosis
  - Hemophagocytic syndrome
- Other illnesses associated with EBV in case reports include the following:
  - Hemolytic uremic syndrome
  - Hepatitis
  - Pancreatitis
  - Myocarditis
  - Mesenteric adenitis
  - Orchitis
  - Genital ulcerative disease
- Lymphoproliferative disorders
  - Burkitt lymphoma
  - Nasopharyngeal carcinoma
  - Lymphoma and non-Hodgkin lymphoma (in immunocompromised children)
  - Lymphomatoid granulomatosis
  - Posttransplant lymphoproliferative disorders (PTLDs)
  - X-linked lymphoproliferative disease (Duncan disease)

DIAGNOSIS

HISTORY

- A prodrome may occur.
  - Most often, lasts 3 to 5 days
  - Malaise, fatigue, with or without fever
- In the acute phase, the following features are common:
  - Fever: begins abruptly, lasts 1 to 2 weeks
  - Fatigue
  - Malaise
  - Anorexia
  - Sore throat
  - "Swollen glands"
  - Rash; more common with associated ampicillin administration
- Young children are more likely to have rash or abdominal pain.

PHYSICAL EXAM

- Tonsillopharyngitis
  - May be exudative and mimic streptococcal pharyngitis
  - Often accompanied by palatal petechiae
- Lymphadenopathy
  - Occurs in 90%
  - Most prominent in cervical chains, including posterior cervical chain
  - May be diffuse
  - Usually nontender, nonerythematous, and discrete
- Hepatosplenomegaly
  - Splenomegaly occurs in more than half the cases.
  - Even if not palpable, splenomegaly may be demonstrated on ultrasound.
  - Most prominent in 2nd to 4th week of illness
  - Hepatomegaly is less common.

DIFFERENTIAL DIAGNOSIS

- Infectious
  - Group A *Streptococcus*
  - Adenovirus
  - Cytomegalovirus
  - *Toxoplasma gondii*
  - Human herpesvirus-6
  - *Mycoplasma pneumoniae*
  - Human immunodeficiency virus
  - Rubella
  - Diphtheria
  - Viral hepatitis (A, B, C)
- Noninfectious
  - Leukemia
  - Lymphoma

DIAGNOSTIC TESTS & INTERPRETATION

Initial Tests (screening, lab, imaging)

- Complete blood count (CBC) with differential
  - Leukocyte count up to 20,000/mm^3
  - Lymphocytosis (>4,500/mm^3)
  - Atypical lymphocytes often constitute >10% of total leukocyte count.
  - Thrombocytopenia may occur.
  - False positives: Atypical lymphocyte counts >10% of the total leukocyte count also occur with cytomegalovirus and toxoplasmosis infections.
- Liver enzymes
  - Mild hepatitis is often found.
  - Jaundice is rare.
- "Monospot" (mononucleosis rapid slide agglutination test for heterophile antibodies)
  - Detects heterophile antibodies (nonspecific IgM antibodies to unrelated antigens)
  - Appears in first 2 weeks of illness, usually slow decline over 6 months
  - Detects 85% of cases in adolescents/adults
  - False positives: infrequent; heterophile antibodies are also produced in serum sickness and neoplastic processes; heterophile antibodies may persist for months after acute infection and be indicative of past illness.

- EBV serology
  - Usually reserved for heterophile-negative patients or children <4 years of age when strong clinical suspicion persists
  - Antibodies are detected by indirect immunofluorescence or enzyme-linked immunosorbent assay techniques.
  - Acute or past infection can usually be detected and differentiated.
  - EBV IgM is consistent with acute infection, whereas EBV nuclear antibody (EBNA) is indicative of past infection.
- EBV polymerase chain reaction (PCR)
  - Sensitivity for detecting EBV DNA in serum of pediatric/young adults with infectious mononucleosis is around 77% with specificity around 98%.
- Other technology
  - Tissue culture of EBV is difficult and, therefore, not clinically useful.
  - Real-time PCR can quantify the amount of EBV genome present, which is useful in patients with PTLD.

ALERT

- Up to 10% of patients with acute EBV infection may have no heterophile response 3 weeks into the illness.
- The heterophile response is less common in infants and children and should not be used in children <4 years of age.

TREATMENT

MEDICATION

- Acetaminophen or ibuprofen reduces fever and provides analgesia.
- Corticosteroids (prednisone 1 mg/kg/24 h PO, maximum of 20 mg/24 h) may reduce swelling of lymphoid tissues (see "FAQ").
  - Indicated for patients with impending airway obstruction
  - May be considered for patients with severe tonsillopharyngitis requiring IV hydration
  - May be considered for patients with rare, life-threatening manifestations of EBV infection, such as hepatitis, aplastic anemia, and central nervous system dysfunction
  - 7-day treatment followed by tapering
- Effectiveness of antiviral agents including acyclovir and valacyclovir is unclear.
  - The quality of available evidence is low.
  - Antiviral agents are sometimes used in cases of active replicating EBV in posttransplant situations.
- Patients with PTLD should have immunosuppression reduced.
- Advise avoidance of contact sports until resolution of symptoms and no further splenomegaly.

ISSUES FOR REFERRAL

- PTLD
- Hemophagocytic syndrome
- EBV in immunocompromised host
- EBV-associated lymphoproliferative disorders
- Considering steroid use as treatment

ADMISSION, INPATIENT, AND NURSING CONSIDERATIONS

- Admission criteria
  - Respiratory distress secondary to airway obstruction
  - Dehydration secondary to severe pharyngitis and poor oral intake
- Discharge criteria
  - Resolved airway obstruction
  - Good oral intake

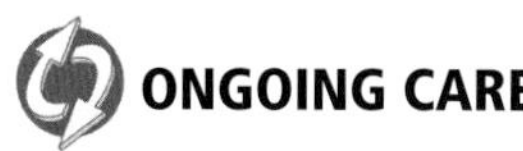

ONGOING CARE

FOLLOW-UP RECOMMENDATIONS

Patient Monitoring

- Immunocompetent individuals usually recover uneventfully in 1 to 4 weeks.
- Recovery is often biphasic, with a worsening of symptoms after a period of improvement.
- Splenomegaly may persist for weeks after primary infection (see "FAQ").
- Fatigue may persist months after recovery.

PROGNOSIS

- Most patients with primary EBV infection will recover uneventfully in 1 to 4 weeks.
- Long-lasting immunity generally ensues.
- Prognosis of patients with unusual manifestations of EBV infection depends on the severity of the illness and the organ system involved.
- Patients with inherited or acquired immunodeficiency are at higher risk of complications and neoplasms.

COMPLICATIONS

- Dehydration
  - Severe pharyngitis often limits fluid intake.
  - Most common problem requiring hospitalization
- Antibiotic-induced rash
  - Morbilliform in appearance
  - Most common after administration of ampicillin or amoxicillin
  - Rare association with penicillin
  - Usually benign; resolves with discontinuation of the aminopenicillin
- Splenic rupture
  - Incidence of ~1 to 2 per 1,000 patients
  - More common in males
  - 50% of the cases of splenic rupture are spontaneous; 50% follow blunt trauma.
- Airway obstruction: may result from massive lymphoid hyperplasia and mucosal edema

ADDITIONAL READING

- Balfour HH Jr, Dunmire SK, Hogquist KA. Infectious mononucleosis. *Clin Transl Immunology*. 2015;4(2):e33.
- Bravender T. Epstein-Barr virus, cytomegalovirus, and infectious mononucleosis. *Adolesc Med State Art Rev*. 2010;21(2):251–264.
- Hurt C, Tammaro D. Diagnostic evaluation of mononucleosis-like illness. *Am J Med*. 2007;20(10): 911.e1–911.e8.
- Luzuriaga K, Sullivan JL. Infectious mononucleosis. *N Engl J Med*. 2010;362(21):1993–2000.
- Macsween KF, Crawford DH. Epstein-Barr virus—recent advances. *Lancet Infect Dis*. 2003;3(3): 131–140.
- Putukian M, O'Connor FG, Stricker P, et al. Mononucleosis and athletic participation: an evidence-based subject review. *Clin J Sport Med*. 2008;18(4):309–315.

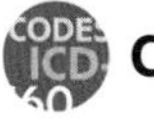

CODES

ICD10

- B27.90 Infectious mononucleosis, unspecified without complication
- B27.99 Infectious mononucleosis, unsp with other complication
- B27.91 Infectious mononucleosis, unspecified with polyneuropathy

FAQ

- Q: Is a monospot test sensitive for diagnosing acute infection?
- A: Heterophile antibodies can be negative in up to 25% of patients in the 1st week of illness, so other diagnostics such as PCR may be necessary to confirm the diagnosis early in the course of illness.
- Q: Should all patients with infectious mononucleosis be given corticosteroids?
- A: No. Symptomatic EBV infection is most often self-limited, and corticosteroids are not indicated. EBV has been linked to certain lymphoproliferative disorders, and theoretic risks to modulating the host immune response with corticosteroids have been proposed.
- Q: How long after infectious mononucleosis may a patient return to athletic activity?
- A: More than half of patients with "mono" will have a boggy, enlarged spleen, which is prone to rupture even if it is not palpable. Athletic activity should be restricted until no evidence exists for a clinically enlarged spleen. Return to contact sports is not advised until >3 weeks after resolution of illness. Some experts recommend ultrasound of the spleen before a return to heavy contact sports such as rugby, football, lacrosse, and hockey.

ERYTHEMA MULTIFORME

Meagan Barrett, MD • Minnelly Luu, MD

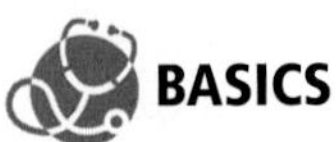

BASICS

DESCRIPTION

- Erythema multiforme (EM) is an acute, self-limited mucocutaneous eruption characterized by distinct targetoid lesions on the skin.
- Although classically defined by the presence of target lesions, at various stages of evolution, EM may appear as erythematous macules, papules, vesicles, or bullae.
- EM is considered an immune-mediated reaction, usually to infectious triggers; numerous additional triggers have been reported in the literature.
- Ranges from relatively mild cutaneous disease (EM minor) to severe forms with significant mucosal involvement (EM major)
- Historically viewed as a spectrum of diseases, most authors now regard EM to be a separate entity from Stevens-Johnson syndrome (SJS) and toxic epidermal necrolysis (TEN). SJS and TEN are distinguished from EM by differing patterns of mucocutaneous involvement, precipitating factors, and prognosis.

EPIDEMIOLOGY

- Predominantly affects healthy young adults but can affect people of all ages, including young children
- Possible seasonal variation with increased frequency in spring and summer. The more severe form has been reported to occur more frequently in winter.
- Recurrences are common.

ETIOLOGY

- ~90% of cases are caused by an infectious agent, most commonly herpes simplex virus (HSV) or *Mycoplasma pneumoniae*.
- <10% of cases are secondary to drug exposure. Common culprits include NSAIDs, sulfonamides, antiepileptics, and antibiotics.
- Reported causes are numerous. Rare precipitants include the following:
  - Chemical and physical exposures
  - Immunizations
  - Autoimmune disease
- Often, the causative factor is not identified.
- HSV is the major cause of recurrent EM.
- *M. pneumoniae* is associated with a distinct phenotype in children, characterized by more severe mucosal involvement, particularly oral and ocular, with less severe cutaneous findings. The term *Mycoplasma*-induced rash and mucositis, (MIRM) has been proposed to describe this particular presentation.

DIAGNOSIS

HISTORY

- A prodrome of fever, malaise, and/or symptoms of HSV, *Mycoplasma*, or other precipitating infections may precede the skin eruption.
- Onset is abrupt with rapid evolution of lesions over the course of 3 to 5 days.
- Although usually appearing at the same time, mucosal lesions occasionally precede or follow cutaneous lesions by a few days.
- Lesions may be associated with pruritus or burning.
- Elicit careful drug (prescription and over-the-counter) and exposure history, including personal and family history of herpetic lesions. Assess for symptoms of mucosal involvement, including dysphagia, dysuria, and ocular symptoms.

PHYSICAL EXAM

- Early lesions are usually round, well-defined erythematous, edematous papules.
- Classically, some of these will evolve to the characteristic target lesion defined by three zones of concentric color change:
  - Dark, dusky center
  - Pale, edematous middle zone
  - Well-defined erythematous outer border
- The center of well-formed lesions will have signs of necrosis: duskiness, blistering, or erosion.
- Atypical target lesions may also be present, defined by only two zones of color change and/or a poorly defined border.
- Lesions may have multiple morphologies including macules, papules, and vesicles/bullae.
- Distribution is typically symmetric and favors acral sites.
- Oral mucosal involvement (labial and buccal mucosa, vermillion lip) is most common, although any mucosal site may be affected, particularly ocular in MIRM.
- Mucosal involvement usually starts with erythema and edema and progresses to painful erosions with hemorrhagic crusting.

DIFFERENTIAL DIAGNOSIS

- SJS/TEN should be considered when a drug is suspected or morphology consists of predominantly atypical targets or dusky, ill-defined macules/patches with or without epidermal detachment.
- Urticaria
- Urticaria multiforme
- Vasculitis/urticarial vasculitis
- Fixed drug eruption
- Atypical hand foot and mouth disease
- Autoimmune blistering disease
- Paraneoplastic pemphigus
- Polymorphous light eruption
- Serum sickness reaction
- Systemic lupus erythematosus (Rowell syndrome)
- Sweet syndrome
- Kawasaki disease
- Varicella (chickenpox)

DIAGNOSTIC TESTS & INTERPRETATION

Initial Tests (screening, lab, imaging)

- Laboratory tests do not establish diagnosis, although they may provide supporting evidence and reveal the underlying cause.
- Eosinophilia may suggest drug as etiology.
- Any lesions suspicious for herpes should be evaluated with culture, direct fluorescent antibody (DFA) testing, or polymerase chain reaction (PCR).
- Consider evaluation for *Mycoplasma* with chest radiograph and cold agglutinins, serology, or PCR.
- Erythrocyte sedimentation rate, white blood cell count, and liver function tests may be elevated in severe EM.

Diagnostic Procedures/Other

- Diagnosis of EM can usually be made on clinical grounds. Biopsy is often not required, although it can help corroborate the clinical diagnosis.
- Of importance, pathology does not reliably distinguish EM from SJS/TEN and thus differentiation between these entities requires clinical correlation.
- Pathologic findings
  - Necrotic keratinocytes
  - Vacuolar basal layer degeneration (liquefactive or hydropic degeneration)
  - Subepidermal blistering may be seen in cases of extensive basal layer degeneration.
  - Perivascular inflammation in the upper and mid-dermis composed mainly of mononuclear cells
  - Spongiosis, papillary dermal edema, and exocytosis of lymphocytes may also be seen.

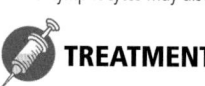

TREATMENT

GENERAL MEASURES

- Treat the underlying cause (e.g., acyclovir for HSV-related cases) or withdraw the offending agent.
- EM minor
  - Care is supportive and symptom-based.
  - White petrolatum +/− topical corticosteroids
  - Oral antihistamines for pruritus
- EM major
  - Skin-directed therapy as above
  - White petrolatum and nonstick dressings for bullous lesions
  - Pain control
  - "Swish and spit" oral preparations composed of diphenhydramine or viscous lidocaine for painful oral lesions.
  - Ophthalmology consultation; consider ENT and urology based on signs and symptoms.
  - Avoid aggressive debridement of crust, which can lead to further scarring.
  - Monitoring of fluid and electrolyte balance and observation for secondary infection
  - The role of systemic corticosteroids is controversial and randomized controlled trials are lacking. Generally thought to be most beneficial when given early in the course of disease. The risks and benefits of corticosteroid therapy must be weighed carefully in the setting of potential infection.

ADMISSION, INPATIENT, AND NURSING CONSIDERATIONS

- Severe mucositis with inability to adequately hydrate
- Atypical progression with suspicion for SJS/TEN or other potentially life-threatening process

ONGOING CARE

PROGNOSIS

- The course of EM is self-limited. Lesions resolve in 2 to 4 weeks with postinflammatory pigment alteration. Severe cases of EM may take longer to heal.
- Recurrences may occur and are often associated with HSV. Prophylactic therapy with acyclovir may be considered with frequent episodes.

COMPLICATIONS

- Complications of the triggering/underlying infection may occur in individual cases.
- EM minor generally heals without significant sequelae.
- In EM major, mucosal involvement may lead to sequelae at individual sites: stricture formation of the oral cavity, trachea, esophagus, and urethra. Ophthalmologic consequences include conjunctivitis, corneal erosions, scarring, and rarely, blindness.
- Skin scarring in severe, ulcerated, or secondarily infected sites

ADDITIONAL READING

- Auquier-Dunant A, Mockenhaupt M, Naldi L, et al. Correlations between clinical patterns and causes of erythema multiforme majus, Stevens-Johnson syndrome, and toxic epidermal necrolysis: results of an international prospective study. *Arch Dermatol*. 2002;138(8):1019–1024.
- Canavan TN, Mathes EF, Frieden I, et al. *Mycoplasma pneumoniae*-induced rash and mucositis as a syndrome distinct from Stevens-Johnson syndrome and erythema multiforme: a systematic review. *J Am Acad Dermatol*. 2015;72(2):239–245.
- Huff JC, Weston WL, Tonnesen MG. Erythema multiforme: a critical review of characteristics, diagnostic criteria, and causes. *J Am Acad Dermatol*. 1983;8(6):763–775.
- Riley M, Jenner R. Towards evidence based emergency medicine: best BETs from the Manchester Royal Infirmary. Bet 2. Steroids in children with erythema multiforme. *Emerg Med J*. 2008;25(9):594–595.
- Sokumbi O, Wetter DA. Clinical features, diagnosis, and treatment of erythema multiforme: a review for the practicing dermatologist. *Int J Dermatol*. 2012;51(8):889–902.

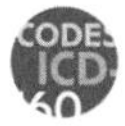

CODES

ICD10

- L51.9 Erythema multiforme, unspecified
- L51.8 Other erythema multiforme
- L51.0 Nonbullous erythema multiforme

ERYTHEMA NODOSUM

Vikash S. Oza, MD

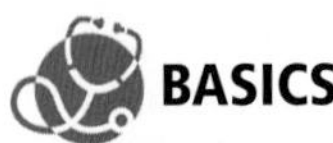

BASICS

DESCRIPTION

Delayed-type hypersensitivity reaction leading to inflammation of the subcutaneous fat (panniculitis) and characterized by red, tender nodules on the shins

EPIDEMIOLOGY

- Girls slightly more frequently affected than boys
- Incidence peaks in adolescence and is rare <2 years of age.

PATHOPHYSIOLOGY

Delayed hypersensitivity immune response to various antigens including bacterial, fungal, viral, and chemical

- Early phase: neutrophilic inflammation
- Late phase: elevated TNF-α production and granuloma formation within lesions

ETIOLOGY

- Idiopathic (~50% of cases)
- Bacterial:
  - β-hemolytic streptococcal infection is the most common trigger in children.
  - Bacterial enteritis (e.g.,*Yersinia*, *Salmonella*, *Campylobacter*)
  - *Mycoplasma*
  - Uncommon: cat-scratch disease, *Chlaymdia trachomatis*, brucellosis, rickettsial infections
- Mycobacterial
  - Tuberculosis
  - Atypical mycobacteria
  - Leprosy
- Viral
  - Epstein-Barr virus
  - HIV
  - Hepatitis B
- Fungal
  - Coccidioidomycosis
  - Histoplasmosis
  - Inflammatory tinea capitis; kerion
- Inflammatory disorders
  - Inflammatory bowel disease (cases with Crohn disease more common than cases with ulcerative colitis)
  - Sarcoidosis
  - Behçet disease
- Pregnancy
- Malignancy (leukemia, lymphoma)
- Medications
  - Oral contraceptives
  - Sulfonamides
  - Phenytoin
  - Bromides and iodides

DIAGNOSIS

HISTORY

- A prodrome of arthralgia, fever, fatigue, malaise, or upper respiratory infection symptoms can precede skin nodules by 1 to 3 weeks.
- Lower extremity pain and swelling is common and can lead to decrease ambulation.
- Important questions to ask:
  - Recent streptococcal infection
  - Medication history (oral contraceptives, sulfonamides, iodides/bromides)
  - Last menses (Erythema nodosum is seen in pregnancy.)
  - History of diarrhea (inflammatory bowel disease or infectious diarrhea)
  - Tuberculosis exposure

PHYSICAL EXAM

- Red, tender nodules on shins, 2 to 6 cm in diameter
- Nodules can occur in other areas with subcutaneous fat such as the thighs, arms, trunk, and face.
- Initially, lesions are slightly elevated, bright to deep red nodules with palpable warmth.
- Later, lesions develop a brownish red or violaceous, bruise-like appearance.
- Exam tips
  - Symmetric distribution
  - Overlying skin is normal except erythema.
  - Usually, no more than six lesions at a time

ALERT

Erythema nodosum never ulcerates or suppurates.

DIFFERENTIAL DIAGNOSIS

- Infection
  - Erysipelas/cellulitis
  - Erythema induratum (nodular vasculitis)
  - Deep fungal infection or Majocchi granuloma
- Sweet syndrome
- Trauma: accidental or from child abuse
- Palmoplantar hidradenitis
- Metabolic
  - Panniculitis secondary to pancreatic disease
  - Pretibial myxedema
- Major insect bite reaction
- Psychosocial (self-injection with foreign material)
- Cutaneous sarcoidosis
- Polyarteritis nodosa
- Granuloma annulare (subcutaneous variant)

DIAGNOSTIC TESTS & INTERPRETATION

Initial Tests (screening, lab, imaging)

- Throat culture and/or antistreptolysin-O titer
- Tuberculin skin test
- CBC
- Erythrocyte sedimentation rate (ESR)
- Stool culture, if history of diarrhea
- Serologic testing, if yersiniosis, rickettsial disease, histoplasmosis, or coccidioidomycosis suspected
- Chest radiograph can help screen for possible tuberculosis or sarcoidosis.

Diagnostic Procedures/Other

- Erythema nodosum is a clinical diagnosis.
- Biopsy for histopathology and culture (bacterial, fungal, mycobacterial) is used if diagnosis is in doubt.
- Pathologic findings
  - Septal panniculitis without primary vasculitis: lymphocytes and neutrophils in the fibrous septa in the subcutaneous fat
  - Older lesions: Histiocytes, giant cells, and occasionally plasma cells can be seen.

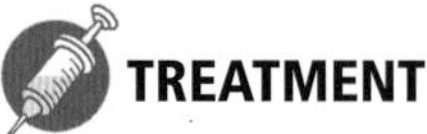

TREATMENT

GENERAL MEASURES

Bed rest and leg elevation

MEDICATION

First Line

Salicylates or other NSAIDs, such as ibuprofen, naproxen, or indomethacin

Second Line

- Potassium iodide 300 mg PO t.i.d. for 3 to 4 weeks, especially for cases diagnosed early in course
- Colchicine
- Corticosteroids (rarely used) for severe cases; courses generally last 2 to 4 weeks.

ONGOING CARE

FOLLOW-UP RECOMMENDATIONS

Patient Monitoring

- Can expect improvement within 1 week
- If lesions recur after cessation of treatment, an underlying infection/inflammatory should be explored.
- If atypical locations or suppurative nodules are present, a biopsy is warranted to rule out a disseminated infection.

PROGNOSIS

- Most individual lesions resolve in 10 to 14 days.
- The course of erythema nodosum typically lasts 3 to 6 weeks with or without treatment unless the underlying cause is a chronic infection or systemic disorder.
- Aching of legs and swelling of ankles may persist for weeks; rarely, symptoms may persist for up to 2 years.

ADDITIONAL READING

- Garty BZ, Poznanski O. Erythema nodosum in Israeli children. *Isr Med Assoc J*. 2000;2(2):145–146.
- González-Gay MA, García-Porrúa C, Pujol RM, et al. Erythema nodosum: a clinical approach. *Clin Exp Rheumatol*. 2001;19(4):365–368.
- Kakourou T, Drosatou P, Psychou F, et al. Erythema nodosum in children: a prospective study. *J Am Acad Dermatol*. 2001;44(1):17–21.
- Labbé L, Perel Y, Maleville J. Erythema nodosum in children: a study of 27 patients. *Pediatr Dermatol*. 1996;13(6):447–450.

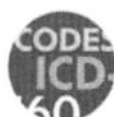

CODES

ICD10

- L52 Erythema nodosum
- A18.4 Tuberculosis of skin and subcutaneous tissue

FAQ

- Q: What is the most common trigger for erythema nodosum in children?
- A: β-hemolytic streptococcal infection
- Q: Will erythema nodosum recur?
- A: In children, the recurrence rate is 4–10% and is often associated with repeated streptococcal infection.
- Q: Will the lesions leave a scar?
- A: In the vast majority of cases, erythema nodosum heals without scarring.

EWING SARCOMA

Steven G. DuBois, MD, MS

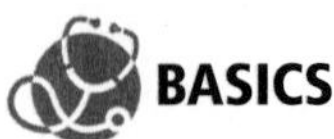

BASICS

DESCRIPTION

- Family of cancers with common biology and treatment:
  - Ewing sarcoma of bone
  - Extraskeletal Ewing sarcoma (arises in soft tissue adjacent to bone)
  - Peripheral neuroectodermal tumor (PNET) of bone or soft tissue
  - Askin tumor (Ewing sarcoma of the chest wall)
- Most common primary tumor sites are as follows:
  - Pelvic bones (26%)
  - Femur (20%)
  - Chest wall (16%)

EPIDEMIOLOGY

- Second most common primary bone cancer of children and young adults after osteosarcoma
- Median age of diagnosis is 15 years, although can occur in any age group.
- Slight male predominance

Incidence

- ~200 to 250 new cases are diagnosed in the United States each year.
- Annual incidence in the United States of 2.7 cases per million children <15 years of age
- Most (~65%) occur in the 2nd decade of life.
- Striking racial difference in incidence: much lower incidence in African American and Asian populations compared to Caucasian population

RISK FACTORS

- Most cases occur sporadically.
- Not associated with familial cancer syndromes
- Only rarely reported as a second malignancy
- One genome-wide association study identified several single nucleotide polymorphisms (SNPs) associated with higher risk.
- Epidemiologic studies suggest higher risk in patients with history of inguinal or umbilical hernia.

GENERAL PREVENTION

There are no known preventive measures.

PATHOPHYSIOLOGY

- Rearrangement of the *EWSR1* gene on chromosome 22 is detected in >95% of cases.
  - 85% of cases have a t(11;22) translocation resulting in a fusion EWS-FLI1 protein.
  - 10% of cases have a t(21;22) translocation between *EWSR1* and *ERG*.
  - Other translocation partners occur in <1% of cases and include other members of the ETS transcription factor family, such as ETV1.
- Fusion proteins thought to play a role as aberrant transcription factor

DIAGNOSIS

HISTORY

- Pain is most common symptom.
- Pain is often attributed to minor injuries that are common in this age group.
- Other presenting symptoms are as follows:
  - Palpable mass
  - Fever
  - Limp
- Systemic symptoms (fever, weight loss) are more common among patients with metastatic disease and more common compared to patients with osteosarcoma.

PHYSICAL EXAM

- Palpable mass (35%)
- Local tenderness (70%)
- Painful movement of joint (35%)
- Fever (30%)
- Regional node involvement uncommon, although more likely with a soft tissue primary tumor

DIFFERENTIAL DIAGNOSIS

- Malignant
  - Osteosarcoma
  - Neuroblastoma
  - Non-Hodgkin lymphoma
  - Undifferentiated sarcoma (Ewing-like sarcoma)
  - Rhabdomyosarcoma
  - Other soft tissue sarcoma
  - Bone metastasis from other malignancy
- Benign
  - Osteomyelitis
  - Tendonitis
  - Trauma
  - Langerhans cell histiocytosis
  - Other benign bone tumor

DIAGNOSTIC TESTS & INTERPRETATION

Initial Tests (screening, lab, imaging)

- CBC as a screen for bone marrow involvement
- Serum lactate dehydrogenase (LDH) is often elevated at diagnosis and may be prognostic.
- Prechemotherapy labs include liver function tests and tests of renal function.
- To evaluate primary site:
  - Plain radiographic findings may include the following:
    - Destructive lesion with "moth-eaten" appearance
    - Periosteal reaction with layers of reactive bone can give an "onionskin" appearance.
    - Raised periosteum may result in a Codman triangle.
    - When arising in long bones, tends to arise from diaphysis rather than metaphysis
- CT or preferably MRI scan in addition to radiograph is essential to fully characterize the extent of the primary tumor (image joint-to-joint to assess for skip lesions).
- 25% have detectable metastases at diagnosis.
  - More common sites of metastases:
    - Lung (50%)
    - Bone (25%)
    - Bone marrow (20%)
  - Less common (<5%) sites of metastases:
    - Lymph nodes and central nervous system
- To evaluate for distant metastases:
  - Chest CT scan
  - Fluorine-18-fluorodeoxyglucose positron emission tomography (FDG PET) or 99m-Tc-diphosphonate bone scan

Diagnostic Procedures/Other

- Biopsy
  - Consultation with a pediatric oncologist and orthopedic oncologist is essential before biopsy.
  - Should be performed by an experienced orthopedic surgeon
  - Avoid contamination of surrounding tissues.
  - Include testing for *EWSR1* translocation, either by fluorescence in situ hybridization (FISH), cytogenetics, reverse transcription-polymerase reaction (RT-PCR), or next-generation sequencing.
  - Small round blue cell tumor with intense membranous CD99 expression
  - PNET shows evidence of neural differentiation.
- Bilateral bone marrow aspirates and biopsies to complete metastatic staging
- Echocardiogram in anticipation of starting chemotherapy

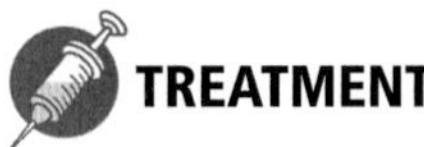

TREATMENT

GENERAL MEASURES

- In addition to systemic treatment with chemotherapy, patients need local control treatment to the site of the primary tumor and metastases (if present) with surgery, radiation, or both.
- The type of local control used depends on the location and extent of the tumor, the morbidity associated with resection, and the presence of tumor cells at the resection margin in those who have surgery.
- The usual sequence of treatment is
  - Neoadjuvant chemotherapy
  - Local control
  - Adjuvant chemotherapy
- Most children are treated on or according to large cooperative group clinical trials.

- Myeloid growth factor (e.g., granulocyte colony-stimulating factor [G-CSF]) is usually given following chemotherapy to shorten the duration of neutropenia.
- Chemotherapy
  - Chemotherapy is essential for cure.
    - Prior to the use of chemotherapy, only 10% of patients survived.
    - Patients with nonmetastatic disease now have an overall survival rate approaching 70% with the use of chemotherapy and appropriate local control.
    - Suggests that patients have small amounts of occult micrometastatic tumor cells that cannot be detected by current technology
  - In North America, standard chemotherapy traditionally includes vincristine, doxorubicin, and cyclophosphamide alternating every 2 weeks with etoposide and ifosfamide.
  - Other agents under investigation include camptothecins (irinotecan and topotecan) as well as IGF-1R inhibitors.

SURGERY/OTHER PROCEDURES

- If surgical local control is pursued, goal is to remove the entire tumor with negative tissue margins.
- Limb salvage surgery is often possible but may not be best in some cases.
- Amputation is less commonly performed given the radiosensitivity of Ewing sarcoma.
- Radiation
  - Definitive radiation provides reasonable local control in cases not amenable to surgical resection.
  - Radiation also used for
    - Attempted surgical resection, but margins positive
    - Treatment of cytology-proven malignant pleural effusions in patients with chest wall tumors
    - Treatment of metastatic disease, including whole lung radiotherapy for patients with lung metastasis
  - Carries risk of second malignancy

ISSUES FOR REFERRAL

Consultation with a pediatric oncologist is essential before any attempt is made at a diagnostic biopsy.

ADDITIONAL THERAPIES

- Physical therapy
  - All patients who receive surgery should be referred to physical therapy following surgery.
  - Patients regardless of surgery may need physical therapy for deconditioning associated with treatment.
- Reproductive endocrinology
  - Given the role of alkylating chemotherapy in the treatment of Ewing sarcoma, all patients should be encouraged to meet with reproductive endocrinology to discuss fertility preservation strategies prior to initiating therapy.

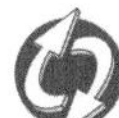

ONGOING CARE

PROGNOSIS

- 5-year overall survival rate for all patients is ~60%.
- Presence of metastases is the most important prognostic factor.
  - Estimated overall survival in those with metastatic disease at diagnosis is <30% at 5 years.
- Other unfavorable prognostic features:
  - Older age (age >18 years)
  - Pelvic primary tumor
  - Large primary tumor
  - Elevated LDH
- Subtype of *EWSR1/FLI1* translocation not prognostic

COMPLICATIONS

- Acute toxicity
  - Alopecia
  - Bone marrow suppression
    - Platelet and packed red blood cell transfusions are usually necessary.
    - Neutropenia: increased risk of bacterial and fungal infections
  - Gastrointestinal side effects
    - Nausea and vomiting
    - Mucositis
  - Kidney and bladder side effects
    - Electrolyte wasting
    - Hemorrhagic cystitis
  - Complications from radiation
    - Skin breakdown and erythema
    - Bone marrow suppression
  - Complications from surgery
    - Wound dehiscence
    - Infection
- Late effects
  - Cardiotoxicity (see "Cancer Therapy Late Effects")
    - Anthracyclines (doxorubicin) can lead to cardiomyopathy and heart failure.
    - Risk depends on cumulative dose of doxorubicin.
    - Radiation to the heart can increase the risk of cardiotoxicity.
    - Patients should have yearly echocardiogram for evaluation.
    - Reduced fertility
  - Second malignancy
    - Sarcomas may occur within the radiation field.
    - Myelodysplastic syndromes and acute myeloid leukemia may occur secondary to chemotherapy.

ADDITIONAL READING

- Grier HE, Krailo MD, Tarbell NJ, et al. Addition of ifosfamide and etoposide to standard chemotherapy for Ewing's sarcoma and primitive neuroectodermal tumor of bone. *N Engl J Med*. 2003;348(8):694–701.
- Postel-Vinay S, Véron AS, Tirode F, et al. Common variants near TARDBP and EGR2 are associated with susceptibility to Ewing sarcoma. *Nat Genet*. 2012;44(3):323–327.
- Rodriguez-Galindo C, Liu T, Krasin MJ, et al. Analysis of prognostic factors in Ewing sarcoma family of tumors: review of the St. Jude Children's Research Hospital studies. *Cancer*. 2007;110(2):375–384.
- Rodriguez-Galindo C, Spunt SL, Pappo AS. Treatment of Ewing sarcoma family of tumors: current status and outlook for the future. *Med Pediatr Oncol*. 2003;40(5):276–287.
- Valery PC, Holly EA, Sleigh AC, et al. Hernias and Ewing's sarcoma family of tumours: a pooled analysis and meta-analysis. *Lancet Oncol*. 2005;6(7):485–490.
- Womer RB, West DC, Krailo MD, et al. Randomized controlled trial of interval-compressed chemotherapy for the treatment of localized Ewing sarcoma: a report from the Children's Oncology Group. *J Clin Oncol*. 2012;30(33):4148–4154.

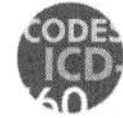

CODES

ICD10

- C41.9 Malignant neoplasm of bone and articular cartilage, unsp
- C41.4 Malignant neoplasm of pelvic bones, sacrum and coccyx
- C40.20 Malignant neoplasm of long bones of unspecified lower limb

FAQ

- Q: At what time point is a child with Ewing sarcoma considered cured?
- A: Most cases of recurrence in Ewing sarcoma occur within 2 years of initial diagnosis. However, late relapses beyond 5 years from initial diagnosis have been seen with Ewing sarcoma.
- Q: Should Ewing sarcoma be completely resected at the time of diagnosis?
- A: Ewing sarcoma tumors are typically large at initial diagnosis. The standard approach is to treat with chemotherapy first, both to reduce the size of the tumor and to treat any distant tumor cells.
- Q: Is surgery or radiation better for local control of the primary tumor in Ewing sarcoma?
- A: This is an area of controversy. Most specialists favor surgical resection when feasible without significantly jeopardizing function, reserving radiation for cases that are less amenable to surgical resection with negative margins.
- Q: Why do Africans and African Americans have such low rates of Ewing sarcoma?
- A: It is not known why these populations are at lower risk for developing Ewing sarcoma, although it suggests a genetic component that influences the risk of developing this disease. Studies are ongoing to investigate this consistent finding.

E

EXCORIATION DISORDER

Carol A. Mathews, MD

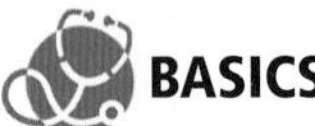

BASICS

DESCRIPTION

Excoriation or skin picking disorder (ExD) is recurrent picking at one's skin to the point of causing skin lesions or recurrent bleeding. Skin picking causes clinically significant distress or functional impairment, is accompanied by repeated efforts to stop or reduce the picking, and is not due to another mental disorder or a general medical or dermatologic condition.

- Skin picking can occur in any region of the body, but the most common sites are the face, arms, and hands. Many individuals pick at multiple sites, which may also vary over time.
- Picking can focus on pimples, scabs, insect bites, or other skin irregularities, but individuals also often pick at healthy unblemished skin.
- Most individuals pick with their fingernails, but instruments such as tweezers, needles, knives, or pins may also be used.
- Squeezing, rubbing or biting of skin, or lancing of pimples of other lesions is also common.
- Some patients experience tension immediately before picking or when attempting to resist the behavior, whereas others experience pleasure or relief when they have picked at a blemish or scab.
- Patients may engage in rituals related to their skin picking, for example, putting the picked scab in the mouth, playing with the extruded material from a pimple.
- Picking and the associated rituals often consume several hours a day.
- Picking may be deliberate (and is often done in front of a mirror) or more automatic or habitual in nature, and is typically not associated with pain.
- Individuals with chronic ExD often attempt to conceal or camouflage the resulting skin lesions with cosmetics, bandages, long sleeves, or other articles of clothing.

EPIDEMIOLOGY

- Although ExD can occur in children <10 years and in adults, the typical onset is in adolescence between ages 13 and 15 years.
- 75% or more of individuals with ExD are female.

RISK FACTORS

ExD is more common in individuals with obsessive-compulsive disorder (OCD) and in their 1st-degree relatives.

Genetics

- A study of >5400 female twins suggests that the heritability of ExD is ~47%, and that it has substantial genetic overlap with trichotillomania (TTM), also known as hair pulling disorder. Approximately 15% of genetic risk for ExD is shared with other obsessive-compulsive and related disorders.
- No specific genes have been implicated for ExD.

COMMONLY ASSOCIATED CONDITIONS

- Localized infections, abscesses and scarring, in severe cases, septicemia can occur.
- Psychiatric comorbidity is common (seen in 20–50% of adolescents with ExD) and includes
  - Mood disorders
  - Anxiety disorders
  - Body dysmorphic disorder
  - OCD
  - Substance abuse
- Skin picking typically begins earlier in childhood than any of the associated psychiatric comorbidities.
- Patients may also engage in nail-biting, hair pulling, or other pathologic grooming behaviors.

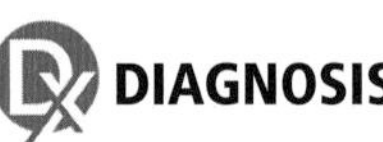

DIAGNOSIS

HISTORY

- Patients may present with multiple open skin lesions or partially healed scabs or with concern regarding picking behavior.
- ExD can be triggered or exacerbated by an underlying dermatologic disorder (e.g., acne, atopic dermatitis); thus treatment resistant cases should be examined for evidence of ExD.
- Use of multiple sources (e.g., parents and children) is preferred, due to secrecy, shame, or lack of insight about behaviors in children.

PHYSICAL EXAM

- Areas with open skin lesions, inflammation, and surrounding lesions
- Infection may be present at sites of severe recurrent picking.
- The scalp is a commonly missed site for skin picking in children.

DIFFERENTIAL DIAGNOSIS

- Skin infestations (e.g., scabies)
- Dermatologic conditions causing pruritus; normative hair removal (e.g., for cosmetic reasons)
- Deliberate self injury
- Psychotic disorders
- Other obsessive-compulsive or related disorders where picking is part of a contamination fear or compulsive ritual
- Body dysmorphic disorder
- Substance-induced picking (e.g., stimulant intoxication)

DIAGNOSTIC TESTS & INTERPRETATION

Diagnostic Procedures/Other

Several instruments are available for clinical use; the Massachusetts General Hospital Skin Picking Scale is one tool commonly used to monitor symptom severity and response to treatment.

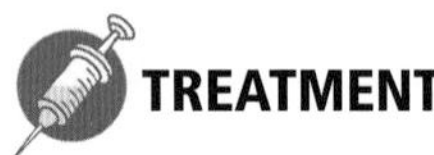

TREATMENT

GENERAL MEASURES

- Triggers should be identified and minimized with a focus on stress management strategies.
- Parent and family education about ExD and associated conditions is essential.
- Cotreatment for any underlying skin disorders can improve treatment outcomes.
- The Trichotillomania Learning Center (www.trich.org) has valuable educational materials for patients, parents, and clinicians as well as a list of mental health providers with experience treating ExD and other grooming disorders.

MEDICATION

Few studies have included children or adolescents. A meta-analysis of published treatment trials shows evidence for behavioral treatments, selective serotonin reuptake inhibitors (SSRIs), and lamotrigine, with good effect sizes.

- SSRIs
  - Six studies were included in the meta-analysis of SSRIs (126 participants total); only fluoxetine was included in more than one study.
  - These studies and the overall meta-analysis indicated a 50–80% response rate for SSRIs, with doses typical of those used in OCD (e.g., higher than MDD doses).
- Lamotrigine
  - Two studies included in the meta-analysis (one open label and one randomized controlled trial [RCT]); 40 participants total
  - Response rates were 44% in the RCT and 67% in the open label trial.
  - Dosing was flexible, up to 300 mg daily as tolerated.

ADDITIONAL THERAPIES

- For mild cases in young children, reward or bandages on fingers may help.
- Behavior modification programs, habit reversal training methods, and cognitive behavioral therapy have all been used.
- Meta-analysis of behavioral therapies had the largest effect size of all forms of treatment.
- Four studies included in the meta-analysis, including one online behavioral treatment study (192 total participants)
- Response rates for these studies were 60–80%.

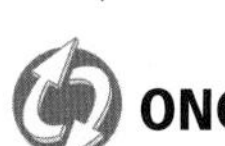

ONGOING CARE

FOLLOW-UP RECOMMENDATIONS

- Patients with ExD should be referred to a mental health professional with training in behavioral therapy and, ideally, with experience treating patients with ExD.
- Online treatments can help in cases where mental health professionals with specific experience are not available.

PROGNOSIS

ExD can wax and wane, with symptoms reemerging or worsening at times of stress or transition.

COMPLICATIONS

- ExD can lead to significant academic, social, and developmental impairment.
  - 40–50% of those with ExD report avoiding social situations due to embarrassment about visible skin lesions.
  - 45% of respondents in one study reported difficulties in studying or other academic activities (e.g., giving speeches in class) due to ExD symptoms.
- Severe and persistent skin picking can lead to infections, abscesses, scarring, and septicemia.

ADDITIONAL READING

- American Psychiatric Association. *Diagnostic and Statistical Manual of Mental Disorders*. 5th ed. Arlington, VA: American Psychiatric Association; 2013.
- Flessner CA, Woods DW. Phenomenological characteristics, social problems, and the economic impact associated with chronic skin picking. *Behav Modif*. 2006;30(6):944–963.
- Grant JE, Odlaug BL, Chamberlain SR, et al. Skin picking disorder. *Am J Psychiatry*. 2012;169(11):1143–1149.
- Keuthen NJ, Wilhelm S, Deckersbach T, et al. The Skin Picking Scale: scale construction and psychometric analyses. *J Psychosom Res*. 2001;50(6):337–341.
- Monzani B, Rijsdijk F, Harris J, et al. The structure of genetic and environmental risk factors for dimensional representations of DSM-5 obsessive-compulsive spectrum disorders. *JAMA Psychiatry*. 2014;71(2):182–189.

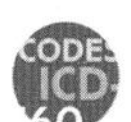

CODES

ICD10

F42.4 Excoriation (skin-picking) disorder

FAQ

- Q: Which patients with skin picking behaviors should be referred for evaluation and treatment?
- A: Patients with recurrent, multiple skin lesions, recurrent localized infections, or who have distress related to their skin lesions or picking behavior should be referred.
- Q: To whom should I refer patients with suspected or diagnosed TTM?
- A: Ideally, a psychologist or other mental health professional with training in behavioral therapy, cognitive behavioral therapy, or exposure-response management therapy. Psychiatrists can also be helpful if behavioral therapy is not available.

E

EXSTROPHY–EPISPADIAS COMPLEX

Timothy S. Baumgartner, FS, MC, Lt Col, USAF • John P. Gearhart, MD

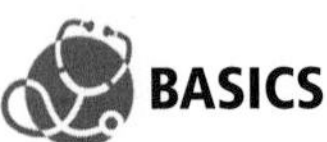

BASICS

DESCRIPTION

The exstrophy–epispadias complex is a rare spectrum of multisystem birth defects involving the genitourinary and gastrointestinal tracts, musculoskeletal system, pelvic floor, and bony pelvis. It is composed of epispadias, bladder exstrophy, and cloacal exstrophy. The latter two conditions present with an open bladder through the anterior abdominal wall.

- The least common variant of the complex, complete epispadias, presents with a closed bladder and a dorsally displaced urethral meatus. The urethra is replaced by a broad mucosal strip on the dorsum, and urinary incontinence is related to the location of the meatus.
- Cloacal exstrophy is the most severe variant, presenting with a large omphalocele, imperforate anus, shortened colon, bladder halves with cecum interposed between, associated cord defects, and multiple upper urinary tract and limb anomalies. All three forms are associated with a pubic diastasis.

EPIDEMIOLOGY

- Bladder exstrophy
  - Male-to-female ratio is between 2:1 and 4:1.
  - Between 1:10,000 and 1:50,000 live births
  - Risk in offspring of individuals with bladder exstrophy and epispadias is 1:70 (500-fold greater than general population).
  - Risk of recurrence in family is approximately 1:100.
- Epispadias
  - Risk of male epispadias: 1:117,000 live births
  - Risk of female epispadias: 1:484,000 live births
- Cloacal exstrophy
  - Male-to-female ratio is between 1:1 and 2:1.
  - Cloacal exstrophy is exceedingly rare, with an incidence between 1:200,000 and 1:400,000 births (decreasing incidence with prenatal diagnosis and termination).

RISK FACTORS

Bladder exstrophy: Only known association is related to offspring of in vitro fertilization pregnancies.

PATHOPHYSIOLOGY

Embryology

- Normal development
  - By week 2 of gestation, the cloacal membrane is located at the caudal end of the infraumbilical abdominal wall.
  - At week 4 of gestation, mesenchyme from the primitive streak migrates between the layers of the cloacal membrane to reinforce the abdominal wall while the cloacal membrane regresses.
- Bladder exstrophy
  - Unclear pathogenesis, but there is an error in embryogenesis
  - The cloacal membrane may overdevelop and prevent mesenchymal migration, which inhibits formation of normal lower abdominal wall.
  - Without reinforcement, the cloacal membrane ruptures. The timing of this rupture determines the variant of the exstrophy–epispadias complex. In bladder exstrophy, rupture of the membrane occurs after the urorectal septum has descended, dividing the genitourinary and gastrointestinal tracts.
- Cloacal exstrophy
  - Abnormally large cloacal membrane ruptures prior to division of the cloaca by the urorectal septum.

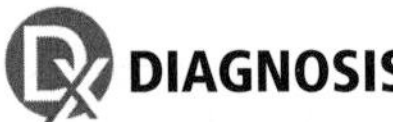

DIAGNOSIS

PHYSICAL EXAM

- Bladder exstrophy
  - All cases have pubic diastasis (mean of 4.8 cm) caused by outward rotation of the innominate bones and iliac wings.
  - The exstrophied bladder and posterior urethra are exposed through a triangular defect in the anterior abdominal wall and are bound by the umbilicus superiorly, the two separated pubic bones laterally, and the anus inferiorly.
  - The anus is anteriorly displaced, shortening the distance between it and the umbilicus.
  - Up to 80% of boys have indirect inguinal hernias that are prone to incarceration because the perineum is short and broad due to the compromised pelvic floor; less common when osteotomy is used
  - Male genital anomalies
    - Penis is 50% shorter and 30% wider than non-exstrophy boys.
    - Corpora cavernosa are short and widely separated secondary to the pubic diastasis.
    - There is a short urethral plate and a marked dorsal chordee causing the penis to curve upward.
    - Epispadias always presents with the lower tract open from the tip of the penis to the dome of the bladder.
  - Female genital anomalies
    - Mons pubis is laterally displaced, with a bifid clitoris secondary to the diastasis.
    - Vagina is short and wide.
    - Vagina and introitus are displaced anteriorly, with the cervix in the anterior vaginal wall.
    - All female patients are at an increased risk for uterine prolapse in adolescent and adult life.
  - Urinary defects
    - Bladder mucosa at birth usually appears normal but may be ectopic or contain polyps.
    - Exstrophic bladder may develop slowly prior to closure.
    - Upper urinary tract usually normal but may observe horseshoe, pelvic, hypoplastic, solitary, or dysplastic kidney.
    - Most children have vesicoureteral reflux requiring correction at the time of their continence procedure.
- Cloacal exstrophy
  - Two halves of the exstrophied bladder are separated by an exstrophied ileocecal bowel segment with various amount of hindgut present.
  - Omphalocele usually present; varies in size
  - Imperforate anus is usually present.
  - Vertebral and neurologic abnormalities (lumbar myelodysplasia, hemivertebrae) are present in >50% of children.
  - Upper urinary tract anomalies (duplicated systems, horseshoe kidney, pelvic kidney) are seen in up to 70% of children.
  - Penis may be duplicate or diminutive.
  - Bifid vagina and uterine abnormalities

DIAGNOSTIC TESTS & INTERPRETATION

Initial Tests (screening, lab, imaging)

- Prenatal sonographic findings (between 15th and 32nd weeks of pregnancy) demonstrating an absence of a normal fluid-filled fetal bladder, an anterior abdominal mass increasing in size, low-set umbilicus, diminutive genitalia, and a wide pubic ramus are suggestive of bladder exstrophy.
- A baseline renal ultrasound and kidneys, ureters, and bladder (KUB) radiograph after birth will demonstrate renal abnormalities and the pubic diastasis, respectively.

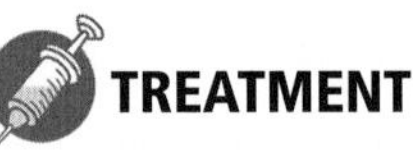

TREATMENT

SURGERY/OTHER PROCEDURES

Goals: Provide urinary continence with a compliant bladder, preserve renal function, and surgically reconstruct the phallus for cosmesis.

- Modern staged repair of bladder exstrophy (MSRE)
  - In the early neonatal period, bladder, posterior urethra, and abdominal wall closure is performed with or without osteotomy.
  - Closure of the urethra occurs at 6 to 12 months of age.
    - Bladder capacity is annually measured with gravity cystogram.
  - If the bladder has adequate capacity and the patient desires continence (between 5 and 9 years of age), a continence procedure, bladder neck reconstruction with or without a continent catheterizable channel, is performed with ureteral reimplantation.
    - Noncandidates or those who fail continence may require bladder neck transection, augmentation cystoplasty, and continent urinary diversion.

- Results and complications: Daytime continence in 60–80% following bladder neck surgery may require clean intermittent catheterization (long-term follow-up); minimal risk for upper urinary tract changes or hydronephrosis
  - Small bladder capacity and failed primary closure are predictors of postsurgical incontinence.
- Complete primary repair of exstrophy (CPRE)
  - Bladder and abdominal wall closure, bladder neck reconstruction, and epispadias repair completed in single procedure; may be performed with or without osteotomy
  - Total penile disassembly dissects the urethral plate from corporal bodies to posteriorly position the bladder neck into the pelvis.
  - Results and complications: daytime continence and volitional voiding in selected patients in up to 20% >5 years of age; additional bladder neck surgery to gain continence is usually required in >75% of patients; >50% require subsequent hypospadias repair and bladder neck fistula rate is up to 40%. Penile disassembly may cause penile soft tissue loss.
- Role of osteotomy and immobilization in all closures
  - Recommended in patients with a diastasis >4 cm who no longer have a malleable pelvis, which usually occurs after 72 hours of age
  - Bilateral transverse anterior innominate and vertical posterior iliac osteotomies performed by pediatric orthopedic surgeon
  - Fixator pins and external fixation devices can be placed and left postoperatively for 4 to 6 weeks.
  - Pelvis immobilized and patient is placed in modified Buck or Bryant traction to increase chance of success.
  - Complications: increased risk of transient nerve and muscle palsies (which typically resolve), need for a blood transfusion, delayed ileal union, and superficial infection at pin sites
- Complications for both types of closure:
  - Dehiscence, bladder prolapse, bladder outlet obstruction, stone formation, hydronephrosis, and vesicocutaneous fistula formation may occur. Patients must be followed carefully.
  - Chance of long-term continence decreases with each additional closure attempt.
  - Failed bladder neck repair in 20–50% may require further reconstruction.
  - 60–95% cosmetic and functional success of epispadias repair with a straight penis with erections
    - Urethral strictures and urethrocutaneous fistula are the most common complications of epispadias repair seen in ≤25% of patients.
  - Adenocarcinoma of the bladder is 400 times more likely than in the normal population. This disease is not reported in adults who have had bladder closure after infancy.
- Fertility and pregnancy
  - Following successful repair, sexual function and libido are normal.
  - Following epispadias repair, up to 87% of boys have erections.
  - Expect retrograde and small-volume ejaculation.
  - Males can have successful impregnation with assisted reproductive techniques.
  - Females can achieve pregnancy, but uterine and cervical prolapse are common following pregnancy. Cesarean section is recommended.

ADMISSION, INPATIENT, AND NURSING CONSIDERATIONS

Postnatal and nursery care:

- Instead of umbilical clamp, tie umbilical cord with 2-0 silk to avoid trauma.
- Cover bladder and other exstrophied bowel/omphalocele with a hydrated gel dressing or apply saline to the surface and cover with plastic wrap to prevent mucosa from sticking to clothing or diapers.
- Until the exstrophied bladder is closed, the patient does not require antibiotics for the genitourinary system. Once the bladder is closed, prophylactic antibiotics are indicated, as all patients will have vesicoureteral reflux.
- Transfer immediately to an appropriate center for evaluation and management by a pediatric urologist, a pediatric orthopedic surgeon, and an experienced team.
- Prophylactic antibiotics should be continued in all children until antireflux procedure or resolution of vesicoureteral reflux.
- Maintain close follow-up with surgeons.

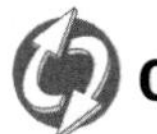

ONGOING CARE

PROGNOSIS

Current treatments preserve the bladder in nearly every patient and allow for continence through the urethra, providing an excellent overall prognosis. There can be favorable long-term outcome with early intervention by a pediatric urologist.

ADDITIONAL READING

- Ebert AK, Reutter H, Ludwig M, et al. The exstrophy-epispadias complex. *Orphanet J Rare Dis*. 2009;4:23.
- Friedlander DA, Di Carlo HN, Sponseller PD, et al. Complications of bladder closure in cloacal exstrophy: do osteotomy and reoperative closure factor in? *J Pediatr Surg*. 2017;52(11):1836–1841.
- Gargollo PC, Borer JG, Diamond DA, et al. Prospective followup in patients after complete primary repair of bladder exstrophy. *J Urol*. 2008;180 (Suppl 4):1665–1670.
- Grady RW, Mitchell ME. Complete primary repair of exstrophy. *J Urol*. 1999;162(4):1415–1420.
- Inouye BM, Massanyi EZ, Di Carlo H, et al. Modern management of bladder exstrophy repair. *Curr Urol Rep*. 2013;14(4):359–365.

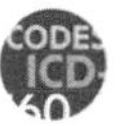

CODES

ICD10

- Q64.0 Epispadias
- Q64.10 Exstrophy of urinary bladder, unspecified
- Q64.12 Cloacal extrophy of urinary bladder

FAQ

- Q: Will a mother be able to hold and nurse a baby with bladder exstrophy after birth?
- A: Yes. A mother will be able to nurse and hold her baby immediately after birth. Once the child undergoes initial closure; however, he/she will be immobilized for approximately 6 weeks. During this time, the baby cannot be picked up. This period of immobilization is critical to achieve a successful closure.
- Q: Will the child have normal sexual function?
- A: Yes. Following a completed, successful repair, the sexual function will be normal.
- Q: Will the child be fertile?
- A: Females commonly achieve pregnancy without the need for in vitro fertilization. Males require in vitro fertilization to impregnate.
- Q: Can an exstrophy patient play sports?
- A: After successfully exstrophy closure, patients are able to play sports.
- Q: Is there risk of recurrence of bladder exstrophy in a family?
- A: Yes. There is a 1:100 chance for bladder exstrophy to recur in a family.

FAILURE TO THRIVE (WEIGHT FALTERING)

Tanya Hinds, MD, FAAP • Allison M. Jackson, MD, MPH

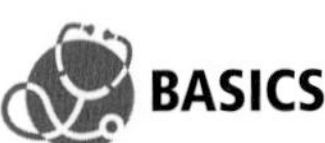

BASICS

DESCRIPTION

Failure to thrive (FTT) or weight faltering describes *a pattern of growth* that is below established standards for age and gender. Anthropometric FTT is defined as any one of the following:

- Weight (or weight for length/height) <2 standard deviations below mean
- Weight deceleration of >2 major percentile lines after a previously established pattern
- Weight <75% of median weight for chronologic age
- Weight <80% of median weight for length
- Weight for chronologic age <5th percentile
- Body mass index for chronologic age <5th percentile
- Length for chronologic age <5th percentile

EPIDEMIOLOGY

- FTT often begins in the first 6 months of life but may not be diagnosed until after 1 year of age.
- It is difficult to accurately determine FTT incidence or prevalence as there is neither consensus on the best definition of FTT nor concordance between definitions. Depending on definition selected, prevalence can range from 1% to 22% based on an analysis of infants from a Danish Birth Registry.

RISK FACTORS

No single risk factor uniformly predicts FTT.

- Substantiated child abuse or neglect is 4 times more likely in FTT children compared to non-FTT children. However, maltreatment is a primary concern in only 4–5% of FTT cases.
- Family poverty was traditionally believed to be an important risk for FTT. However, recent prospective studies of large populations seen in general pediatric clinics have either been equivocal or failed to show poverty to be an important risk factor.
- Maternal mental health vulnerabilities such as depression and other individual and family stressors may play a role in some patients although the research has been equivocal.
- Currently, there is consensus that FTT involves a multiplicity of overlapping dietary, developmental, social, and medical concerns.

GENERAL PREVENTION

Advice should be straightforward, practical, and tailored to specific needs.

- Primary prevention
  - Addresses proper formula and food preparation, feeding quantities and frequencies, community-based nutrition support programs, and mental health resources
- Secondary prevention
  - Involves early identification by regular growth monitoring
- Tertiary prevention
  - Requires creation of an individualized treatment plan that addresses specific factors (dietary, developmental, social, and medical) adversely affecting a child's ability to meet caloric needs
  - Long-term, coordinated multidisciplinary efforts involving home visiting nurses, dietitians, social workers, primary care providers, and medical subspecialists are critical to success.

PATHOPHYSIOLOGY

- Inadequate caloric intake
  - Dietary
    - Breastfeeding difficulties
    - Diluted or inappropriately prepared formula
    - Food fads or restrictions
    - Excessive juice consumption
  - Developmental/neurologic
    - Oral motor difficulties
    - Central nervous system abnormalities
  - Social
    - Unavailability of food
    - Parent–child interaction disorders
    - Mental health or behavioral disorders affecting child's appetite
    - Mental health disorders affecting caregiver's parenting abilities
    - Disorganized meal times
    - Neglect (omitting feeds or creating environment not conducive to feeding)
  - Medical
    - Adenotonsillar hypertrophy
    - Cleft lip and/or palate
    - Dental pain and decay
    - Congenital cardiac disease
    - Gastroesophageal reflux disease
    - Dysphagia
- Inadequate absorption or utilization
  - Food allergies or intolerances
  - Inflammatory bowel disease
  - Gastrointestinal (GI) malformations
  - Pyloric stenosis
  - Hepatitis
  - Cystic fibrosis
  - Parasitic infections
  - Inborn errors of metabolism
- Increased caloric expenditure
  - Hyperthyroidism
  - Chronic infections
  - Chronic immunodeficiencies
  - Malignancy
  - Pulmonary disease
  - Cardiac disease
  - Renal disease

ETIOLOGY

- Historically, FTT was classified as organic (secondary to medical illness) or inorganic (secondary to psychosocial concerns). This categorization is obsolete. It places inordinate emphasis on organic conditions. In outpatient primary care settings, an identifiable organic disease likely contributes to FTT in <18% of children age ≤2 years.
- Children with FTT may eat less. An undemanding child temperament, low appetite, and disinterest in food may either cause or result in FTT.
- FTT children also have significantly fewer positive mealtime interactions with caregivers. Family dysfunction, caregiver incompetence, lack of knowledge about child development, and caregiver mental health vulnerabilities can affect a caregiver–child feeding relationship.

COMMONLY ASSOCIATED CONDITIONS

Severe, chronic FTT may have significant adverse effects on cognition, attention, and behavior.

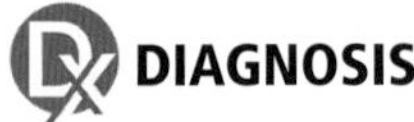

DIAGNOSIS

HISTORY

Responses to questions about the following can help guide evaluation:

- Prenatal
  - Multiple miscarriages (suggesting a genetic disorder)
  - Maternal health and/or medical diagnoses
  - Tobacco, alcohol, or illicit substances
  - Other teratogens or toxins (prescribed medication, radiation exposure)
- Birth
  - Gestational age at delivery
  - Weight, length, and head circumference
  - Asphyxia, infection, other perinatal complications
- Medical
  - Newborn metabolic screening results
  - Medical diagnoses: reflux, cardiac disease, obstructive sleep apnea, respiratory infections, urinary tract infections, other chronic or recurrent conditions
  - Hospitalizations, surgeries, immunizations
  - Event(s) at time of significant loss or gain of weight
- Developmental
  - Personal–social, language, fine and gross motor milestones
  - Loss of previously acquired milestones
- Family
  - Weight, height of biologic parents and siblings
  - Parental history of childhood growth delay
  - Medical, mental, and developmental diagnoses of parents and siblings
  - Maternal depression
  - Caregiver(s) use of illicit substances

- Review of systems
  - Activity level compared to peers
  - Chronic rhinorrhea, congestion, cough
  - Mouth breathing, snoring, frequent awakenings from sleep
  - Difficulty or pain with sucking, chewing, or swallowing
  - Vomiting or excessive spitting up
  - Breathlessness, sweating, or tiring during feeds
  - Frequent, large, bloody, or oily stools
  - Constipation
  - Urinary frequency or dysuria
  - Polyuria, polydipsia, polyphagia
  - Eczema or urticaria exacerbated by select foods
- Psychosocial
  - Difficulty purchasing or preparing food
  - Distractions during feeds/meals
  - Perception of child's behavior during meals
  - Eating habits of siblings when at a similar age as infant/child with FTT
  - Individual and family stressors and strengths
  - Supplemental food and community resources
  - Travel to less developed countries
- Dietary
  - Frequency, duration of active suck
  - Frequency, type, preparation, quantity of typical formula feed
  - Feeding changes at night or on weekends
  - Age of weaning/shift in feeding practices
  - Foods consumed over typical 24 hours
  - Water, juices, sodas over typical 24 hours
  - Food allergies or intolerances
  - Feeding habits and techniques (bottle propping, grazing)
  - Eating habits outside the home (day care, school)
  - Vitamin, herbal, other supplements

PHYSICAL EXAM

- Helps identify chronic illness, syndromes
- Weight, length/height, head circumference
- Vital signs, pain
- General: activity level (lethargic, hyperactive), caregiver–child interactions (eye contact, physical approximation, checking), hygiene, dysmorphic features, lymphadenopathy
- Head: dry, dull, or absent hair; fontanelle size
- Eyes: palpebral fissures, conjunctival pallor, strabismus, cataracts, retinal hemorrhages
- Ears: malposition, otitis
- Mouth, throat: anatomic abnormalities of palate or tongue, glossitis, cheilosis, gum bleeding, thrush, dental abnormalities, enlarged tonsils
- Cardiac: murmur; abnormal femoral pulses
- Chest, lungs: retractions, wheezes, crackles
- GI: distention, masses, hepatomegaly
- Anogenital: malformations; severe rashes; anal fissures, hemorrhoids
- Musculoskeletal: frontal bossing, rachitic rosary, extremity bowing, wrist widening, edema, decreased muscle mass
- Skin: eczema; hives; scaling; spoon-shaped nails; patterned bruises, scars, burns
- Neurologic: cranial nerve palsies, hyper- or hypotonia, retention of primitive reflexes

DIAGNOSTIC TESTS & INTERPRETATION

Initial Tests (screening, lab, imaging)

- CBC: anemia; leukemia
- Comprehensive metabolic panel (CMP), phosphorus: malnutrition; metabolic abnormalities; chronic endocrine, liver, and renal disease
- Thyroid function tests
- UA and culture: renal tubular acidosis, infection

Follow-Up Tests & Special Considerations

- Ferritin
- Lead
- Vitamin D
- Tuberculosis testing
- HIV, hepatitis B and C
- Stool pathogens, *Giardia* antigen
- Stool fat
- Sweat test
- Serum IgA, anti-transglutaminase antibodies: celiac disease
- Karyotype: Turner syndrome

Diagnostic Procedures/Other

- Wrist radiographs: delayed bone age compared with chronological age
- Chest radiograph: cardiac anomalies, cystic fibrosis
- Lateral neck radiograph: adenotonsillar hypertrophy
- Skeletal survey: suspected maltreatment
- Upper GI series, pH probe: anatomic abnormalities, reflux
- ECG

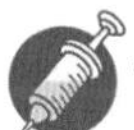

TREATMENT

MEDICATION

- Medications that stimulate appetite and growth hormone therapy have not been extensively studied in FTT.
- Nutritional supplements and calorie-dense foods help promote catch-up growth.

ADDITIONAL THERAPIES

- Community-based nutritional and psychosocial counseling program when no underlying illness
- Multidisciplinary interventions including home nursing visits improve weight gain, parent–child relationships, and cognitive development.
- Goal is catch-up growth (growth faster than normal rate for age).
  - Normal growth rates for age average about 30 g/day until 3 months
  - 20 g/day from 3 to 6 months
  - 10 g/day from 6 to 12 months
  - 8 g/day from 1 to 3 years
- Daily multivitamins, zinc, and iron

ISSUES FOR REFERRAL

Subspecialty consultation

- Minimize risk of refeeding syndrome.
- Genetic syndrome or disease suspected

ADMISSION, INPATIENT, AND NURSING CONSIDERATIONS

Hospitalize when

- FTT persists despite community-based dietary interventions
- Severe malnutrition. Weight for age <60% of median or weight for height <70% of median increases morbidity such as refeeding syndrome.
- Suspicion of abuse or neglect; note, this necessitates mandatory CPS report.

ONGOING CARE

- Monitoring should continue until weight for height deficit is repaired and child no longer needs a specialized diet to maintain normal growth.
- The Centers for Disease Control and Prevention (CDC) suggests World Health Organization growth charts for all children up to age 2 years and CDC growth charts for older children.
- Specialty growth charts for patients with genetic conditions can supplement these charts.

ADDITIONAL READING

- Mash C, Frazier T, Nowacki A, et al. Development of a risk-stratification tool for medical child abuse in failure to thrive. *Pediatrics*. 2011;128(6):e1467–e1473.
- Pulcini CD, Zettle S, Srinath A. Refeeding syndrome. *Pediatr Rev*. 2016;37(12):516–523.
- Rudolf MC, Logan S. What is the long term outcome for children who fail to thrive? A systematic review. *Arch Dis Child*. 2005;90(9):925–931.
- Shields B, Wacogne I, Wright CM. Weight faltering and failure to thrive in infancy and early childhood. *BMJ*. 2012;345:e5931.
- Wright C, Birks E. Risk factors for failure to thrive: a population-based survey. *Child Care Health Dev*. 2000;26(1):5–16.

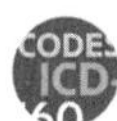

CODES

ICD10

- P92.6 Failure to thrive in newborn
- R63.4 Abnormal weight loss
- R63.3 Feeding difficulties

FAQ

- Q: How should weight gain while hospitalized be interpreted?
- A: Children with and without medical illnesses will grow with sufficient caloric intake. Growth during hospitalization is not diagnostic of FTT.
- Q: What is the likelihood of successful treatment?
- A: Catch-up growth is most likely when FTT does not occur with other forms of maltreatment.

FEEDING DISORDERS

Elizabeth J. Hait, MD, MPH

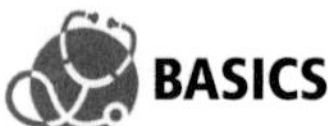

BASICS

DESCRIPTION

- Feeding disorder:
  - Inability to consume by mouth in quantity or quality the nutrition that is developmentally appropriate for that child
- Dysphagia:
  - Disorder of swallowing characterized by difficulty in oral preparation for the swallow or in moving food or liquid from the mouth to the stomach
- Aspiration:
  - Food or fluid enters the trachea and passes through the vocal cords to lungs.
- Penetration:
  - Food or fluid enters the trachea but remains above vocal cord
  - However, food or fluid can be cleared by patient through coughing to prevent aspiration.
- Oral motor disorder:
  - Inability to manipulate an age-appropriate diet
  - Often related to incoordination of facial muscles and/or tongue
- Pharyngeal dysphagia:
  - Inability to protect airway during swallow
  - May be due to anatomic abnormality or neurologic dysfunction
- Avoidant restrictive food intake disorder (ARFID):
  - As defined by the *Diagnostic and Statistical Manual of Mental Disorders* 5th edition (*DSM-5*): a voluntary food or fluid refusal associated with maladaptive interactions at mealtimes; associated with learned fear when foods or textures are advanced before a child is developmentally or medically ready to swallow without dysfunction

RISK FACTORS

- Anatomic deformities (i.e., Pierre Robin sequence, laryngomalacia, tracheotomy, cleft palate)
- Autism spectrum disorder
- Congenital heart disease
- Cystic fibrosis
- Developmental delay/cerebral palsy
- GI disorders: gastroesophageal reflux disease (GERD), eosinophilic esophagitis, celiac disease
- Metabolic disorders
- Neuromotor dysfunction
- Prematurity
- Prolonged tube feeders (>4 weeks)
- Tachypnea (respiratory rate >40 breaths/minute)

GENERAL PREVENTION

- Monitor weight, height, head circumference, weight for height, and BMI percentiles at regular interval office visits to identify changes in nutritional status early, especially in high-risk populations.
- Selective eater: Educate parents on age-appropriate portion sizes and foods.
- Provide vitamin and mineral supplementation or refer to nutritionist for complete assessment if patient is at risk for deficiencies.
- Developmental delay: Evaluate diet and feeding skills to manipulate nutrition provided.
- Ensure that foods offered are matched to developmental readiness rather than to chronologic age.

DIAGNOSIS

HISTORY

- Past and present medical diagnoses
- Personal experience with therapeutic management or procedures in past or at present, especially those aversive to face and upper body (e.g., suctioning, tracheostomy, intubation)
- 24-hour diet: Recall food and fluid consumed over a 24-hour period.
- Previous hospitalizations, especially those involving respiratory illnesses
- Allergies or food intolerances
- Growth history
- Developmental history
- History of snoring or sleep apnea (may indicate adenoidal or tonsillar hypertrophy)
- GI history: stool pattern, vomiting, gagging, spitting up, pain
- Family history: GI disease, allergies, developmental delays, genetic abnormalities
- Failure to thrive
  - Poor linear growth
  - Sucking and swallowing incoordination: Infant should demonstrate 1:1:1 suck, swallow, breathe pattern when sucking from breast or bottle.
  - Recurrent pneumonia
  - Coughing during or after feeding
  - Refractory asthma
  - Drooling
  - Refusal to drink or eat
  - Feeding selectivity
  - Difficulty with texture progression

PHYSICAL EXAM

- HEENT: dysmorphic facial features, shape of head and sutures, facial tone, intact soft and hard palate, shape of mandible, tonsillar size, patency of nares, movement of lips and tongue, presence of stridor, mouth closure, dentition, drooling
- Pulmonary: rate of breathing, use of accessory muscles for respiration, rales
- Cardiac: murmur, rate, and rhythm
- GI: bowel sounds, masses, stool palpable, tenderness, distension
- Neurologic: tone, positioning, cranial nerves, gait, affect, head control
- Extremities: subcutaneous stores, muscle development, adipose tissue
- Skin: rashes, alopecia

DIFFERENTIAL DIAGNOSIS

- Cardiorespiratory
  - Congenital heart disease
    - Infectious pneumonia
    - Bronchopulmonary dysplasia
- Neurologic
  - Diencephalic syndrome
    - Congenital myopathy
    - Arnold-Chiari malformation
    - Hypoxic-ischemic encephalopathy
- GI/nutrition
  - GERD
  - Gastroparesis
  - Eosinophilic esophagitis
  - Failure to thrive
  - Celiac disease
- Metabolic syndromes
- Psychological disorders
  - Behavioral refusal
  - Psychosocial deprivation
  - Anxiety disorder
- Food allergies
- Anatomic
  - Laryngeal cleft
  - Tracheoesophageal fistula
- Genetic disorders
- Developmental disorders:
  - Autistic spectrum disorder
  - Sensory integration disorder

DIAGNOSTIC TESTS & INTERPRETATION

Perform feeding observation: Watch caregiver feed child, preferably through a 1-way observation mirror. Monitor child's behavioral response to placement in the feeding chair and presentation of bottle, breast, or cup and a variety of food types and textures; observe parental reaction to child's behaviors and child's ability to manipulate foods and fluids.

Initial Tests (screening, lab, imaging)

- Tailor labs obtained based on nutritional and/or developmental concerns, including the following:
  - Failure to thrive: celiac panel, CBC, comprehensive metabolic panel, lead, urine analysis, thyroid function; other tests if suspect vitamin or mineral deficiency (i.e., zinc, iron)
  - Developmental and/or genetic concerns: chromosomes, fluorescent in situ hybridization (FISH) test for 22q11 deletion, FISH test for Prader-Willi syndrome, fragile X (males), serum and urine organic acids, lactate, pyruvate, CPK
  - Sweat test if suspected cystic fibrosis: failure to thrive, diarrhea, and/or recurrent pulmonary infections
- Tests indicated based on history and physical
- Suspected pharyngeal dysphagia: modified barium swallow study (MBSS) (videofluoroscopic swallow study) evaluates swallow function and can visualize aspiration during swallow; usually performed by radiologist and speech therapist. Study visualizes function of pharyngeal muscles and structures. See below:
  - Upper GI series (including esophagram and evaluation of upper GI tract) ensures normal anatomy of esophagus, stomach, and duodenum (evaluate for TEF, malrotation).
  - Chest radiograph: determines if infiltrates or atelectasis are present; right upper and/or middle lobe changes may be indicative of aspiration.
  - Gastric emptying scan: Assess gastric emptying potential and whether gastroparesis is present.
  - Salivagram: radionucleotide study to evaluate if patient is aspirating oral secretions
  - Chest CT scan: allows detection of subtle changes from silent aspiration not detectable by pulmonary exam or chest radiograph

Diagnostic Procedures/Other

- MBSS
  - Speech therapist feeds a variety of textures: thin and thickened liquid of honey and nectar consistency, thin and thick purees, and chewable foods to determine safety of oral feeding
  - Allows visualization of oral and pharyngeal phases of swallowing

- Can determine appropriate positioning and type of infant bottles and cups to minimize the risk for aspiration
- Timing of aspiration is evaluated to determine if volume and fatigue result in aspiration; the patient may be safe to drink or eat for short periods of time before the swallow becomes uncoordinated and leads to aspiration.

- Fiberoptic endoscopic evaluation of swallowing (FEES)
  - Usually performed by ENT specialist; direct visualization of airway structures and swallowing mechanism
  - Provides information on pharyngeal phase of swallowing but not oral phase; best used if pharyngeal or laryngeal abnormality is suspected, tracheostomy in place, and there is difficulty managing secretions
  - Can observe food or fluid falling below vocal cords (aspiration)
- Bronchoscopy
  - Visualizes tracheobronchial tree and lungs, sample for lipid-laden macrophages in lungs indicative of aspiration
- Endoscopy
  - To perform esophageal, gastric, and small bowel biopsies to determine presence of eosinophilic esophagitis, celiac disease (positive or inconclusive celiac panel), or presence of GERD

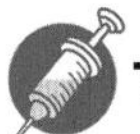

TREATMENT

- Pharyngeal dysphagia: pulmonary referral, oral stimulation program, NPO as indicated by clinical exam and studies, initiate tube feeds; evaluation by speech therapist
- Feeding disorders are complex and should be evaluated and managed by multidisciplinary team involving medical, nutrition, psychology, occupational therapy, and speech therapy.

GENERAL MEASURES

- Calorie counts
- Ensure adequate hydration.

MEDICATION

Medications are administered to treat underlying medical condition (e.g., GERD); refer to specific sections for treatment of identified medical issues resulting in feeding disorder.

ADDITIONAL THERAPIES

- Obtain a list of all supplemental vitamins, minerals, herbs, etc., that the parent may be providing to the patient.
- Investigate if parent is following any special diets (e.g., casein/gluten-free diet in autistic spectrum disorder).

COMPLEMENTARY & ALTERNATIVE THERAPIES

- Speech therapy: Evaluate oral motor skill and safety of swallowing mechanism; perform MBSS when indicated.
- Occupational therapy: Evaluate fine motor skills, sensory processing, and posture to support feeding.
- Psychology: may identify behaviors interfering with food acceptance and recommend strategies to improve oral acceptance
- Nutrition: Perform complete nutritional assessment, including evaluation of growth parameters, identifying patient's nutrition requirements, and adequacy of current diet. A nutritionist may be particularly critical to developing a care plan to meet patient's nutritional requirements, as well as to monitoring their intake and weight gain during hospitalizations.

SURGERY/OTHER PROCEDURES

- Consider gastrostomy tube placement if tube feedings for >3 months are anticipated.
- For GERD not responding to medications, consider bypassing stomach and feeding into intestine with jejunostomy tube or placement of gastrostomy tube in conjunction with Nissen fundoplication.
- Some patients report that blenderized feedings are better tolerated compared to commercial formulas although this is controversial.

ADMISSION, INPATIENT, AND NURSING CONSIDERATIONS

- Prior to initiation of behavioral program, ensure weight gain and growth are adequate.
- Evaluate and treat vitamin and mineral deficiencies.
- If weight-for-height ratio or BMI is <5%, inappropriate weight gain crossing down 2 percentiles on growth chart occurs, or weight loss occurs, consider initiating supplemental nasogastric tube feeds.
- If aspiration pneumonia is suspected, obtain blood cultures, chest x-ray; keep NPO and start IV fluids and antibiotics. Measure oxygen saturation and initiate supplemental oxygen if <95%.

ONGOING CARE

FOLLOW-UP RECOMMENDATIONS

Appointment with multidisciplinary feeding team, if available within reasonable geographic radius

Patient Monitoring

- Patient's weight should be checked within 2 weeks of discharge.
- Pediatrician should monitor patients with respiratory difficulties related to aspiration every 2 weeks until stable.

DIET

- Keep patient NPO if aspiration is suspected until further evaluation (MBSS) can be performed.
- Order diet appropriate for child's current level of feeding skills (i.e., accepts baby food; may trial pureed diet).
- If nutritional intake is inadequate, offer nutritional supplements, monitor calorie counts, and initiate supplemental nasogastric tube feeds if unable to meet nutritional requirements.
- Caregiver education regarding administration of supplemental tube feeds

PROGNOSIS

- Nutritional rehabilitation can be achieved with tube feedings if patient is monitored closely.
- Patients with pharyngeal dysphagia resulting in aspiration may have improvement in their swallow function over time.
- Static or degenerative neurologic conditions resulting in aspiration generally do not resolve.
- Patient demonstrating dysphagia during illness may improve when healthy.

ADDITIONAL READING

- Epp L, Lammert L, Vallumsetla N, et al. Use of blenderized tube feeding in adult and pediatric home enteral nutrition patients. *Nutr Clin Pract*. 2017;32(2):201–205.
- Kral TV, Souders MC, Tompkins VH, et al. Child eating behaviors and caregiver feeding practices in children with autism spectrum disorders. *Public Health Nurs*. 2015;32(5):488–497.
- Mahoney L, Rosen R. Feeding problems and their underlying mechanisms in the esophageal atresia-tracheoesophageal fistula patient. *Front Pediatr*. 2017;5:127.
- Norris ML, Spettigue WJ, Katzman DK. Update on eating disorders: current perspectives on avoidant/restrictive food intake disorder in children and youth. *Neuropsychiatr Dis Treat*. 2016;12:213–218.
- Rudolph CD, Link DT. Feeding disorders in infants and children. *Pediatr Clin North Am*. 2002;49(1):97–112.
- Williams KE, Field DG, Seiverling L. Food refusal in children: a review of the literature. *Res Dev Disabil*. 2010;31(3):625–633.

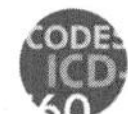

CODES

ICD10

- R63.3 Feeding difficulties
- R13.10 Dysphagia, unspecified
- T17.928A Food in resp tract, part unsp causing oth injury, init

FAQ

- Q: What is the difference between aspiration and penetration in a swallowing disorder?
- A: Penetration occurs when food or fluid enter the trachea but remains above the vocal cords. Aspiration occurs when the food or fluid falls below the vocal cords and enters the lungs.
- Q: How is a MBSS used to evaluate dysphagia?
- A: A speech therapist, in conjunction with the radiologist, feeds the patient a variety of textures, including thin and thickened liquids, thin honey and nectar, thick purees, and chopped food if indicated, and visualizes the pathway during swallowing to determine if the food bolus moves safely into the esophagus without entering the airway. The speech therapist also will engage in therapeutic endeavors, such as repositioning the patient, to determine if they can eliminate aspiration.

F

FETAL ALCOHOL SYNDROME

Tracey A. McLean, MD • Seth J. Bokser, MD, MPH

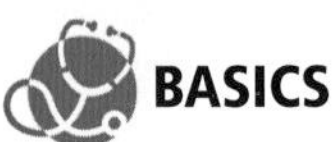

BASICS

DESCRIPTION

- The four major features of classic fetal alcohol syndrome (FAS) are as follows:
  - CNS neurodevelopmental abnormalities
  - Facial dysmorphisms
  - Growth retardation
  - Maternal alcohol use during pregnancy
- First described in 1973; classic FAS has since been recognized as one of the fetal alcohol spectrum disorders (FASDs), which include the following:
  - FAS, partial FAS (pFAS), alcohol-related neurodevelopmental disorder (ARND), and alcohol-related birth defects (ARBD)
  - Taken together, FASDs are 3 times more common than classic FAS, and the effects range from very mild symptoms to very severe.

EPIDEMIOLOGY

Incidence

- Classic FAS: 0.5 to 2 per 1,000 live births
- FASDs: 10 per 1,000 live births in the United States; 23 in 1,000 live births globally

RISK FACTORS

- Binge drinking historically has been noted to be the primary risk factor, although not all authors agree.
- The highest prevalence of reported alcohol use during pregnancy is among those who are aged 35 to 44 years, African-American, college graduates, or employed.
- Poor maternal nutrition appears to increase risk in the presence of maternal binge drinking.
- Other risk factors include low educational attainment, history of multiple miscarriages and stillbirths, social isolation, history of physical or sexual abuse, and current interpersonal violence.
- Maternal polymorphisms of the alcohol dehydrogenase gene (*ADH*): The presence of the *ADH1B*3* allele appears to protect the fetus.
- Concordance of FAS is higher in monozygotic than in dizygotic twins.

GENERAL PREVENTION

- Women who are pregnant or may become pregnant should avoid alcohol. No "safe" level of alcohol consumption has been determined during pregnancy.
- Women with alcohol addiction who are or may become pregnant should enter a treatment program.
- According to the Centers for Disease Control and Prevention (CDC), 7.6% of pregnant women reported alcohol use during the month prior to being surveyed and 1.4% reported binge drinking.
- The highest risk for FAS occurs in children whose mothers consume ≥4 drinks per occasion per week (peak blood alcohol level is more important than a lower sustained blood alcohol level).
- In the United States, the Alcoholic Beverage Labeling Act passed in 1988 requires health warning labels, including risk of alcohol consumption during pregnancy.

PATHOPHYSIOLOGY

- Alcohol and its metabolite acetaldehyde are teratogens.
- Alcohol causes malformation of the developing brain, as well as abnormal brain functioning in multiple regions of the brain.
- Epigenetic changes caused by alcohol can disrupt normal gene expression.
- Abnormalities can occur with alcohol consumption across all gestational ages.

DIAGNOSIS

HISTORY

- Neurodevelopmental and behavioral symptoms:
  - No specific neurobehavioral pattern has been defined.
  - See below for examples of age-specific presentations.
- Fine motor function abnormalities may be present.
- Birth and subsequent growth deficit (weight, height, head circumference)
- Maternal history of alcohol use (binge drinking, average number of drinks per day, timing in pregnancy) and other drug use
- Family history
  - Neurobehavioral abnormalities may not be typical of other family members who were not exposed to alcohol prenatally.
- Neurobehavioral problems in infancy:
  - May or may not have alcohol withdrawal as newborn
  - Irritability, irregular sleep, poor feeding, hypotonia, delayed motor function
- Neurobehavioral problems in preschool and school age:
  - Hyperactivity
  - Slow verbal learning
  - Slow visual–spatial learning
  - Poor abstract thinking (planning and organizing)
  - Perseveration (inability to abandon ineffective strategies)
  - Attention problems
  - Difficulty with peer interactions
- Neurobehavioral problems in adolescence and adulthood:
  - Substance abuse
  - Criminal behavior
  - Inability to work
  - Inability to live independently

PHYSICAL EXAM

- Birth weight (≤10th percentile)
- Birth length (≤10th percentile)
- Microcephaly at birth (≤10th percentile)
- Postnatal growth deficiency persists throughout life.
- Facial manifestations include the following:
  - Short palpebral fissures (measurement from inner to outer canthus of eyes)
  - Long and smooth philtrum (area from nasal septum to vermillion border of lip)
  - Thin vermillion border (upper lip)
- Ptosis, epicanthal folds, and flat face are also common in FAS.

DIFFERENTIAL DIAGNOSIS

- By physical features
  - Normal variant
  - Aarskog syndrome
  - Williams syndrome
  - Noonan syndrome
  - Cornelia-De Lange syndrome
  - Dubowitz syndrome
  - Fetal valproate syndrome
  - Fetal hydantoin syndrome
  - Maternal phenylketonuria fetal effects
  - Toluene embryopathy
  - Velocardiofacial syndrome
  - Duplication 15q syndrome
- By neurobehavioral features
  - Fragile X syndrome
  - 22q11 deletion syndromes
  - Turner syndrome
- Opitz syndrome

DIAGNOSTIC TESTS & INTERPRETATION

Initial Tests (screening, lab, imaging)

- Simple IQ tests cannot distinguish children with FAS from those with other developmental disabilities.
- No laboratory marker exists for FAS.
- No specific neurobehavioral phenotype yet defined
- Testing and diagnosis are complex and best done utilizing a multidisciplinary approach.

Diagnostic Procedures/Other

Classic FAS diagnosis requires three findings:

- Facial anomalies, including:
  - Short palpebral fissures (≤10th percentile)
  - Thin vermilion border upper lip (score of 4 or 5 on the lip/philtrum guide [see Astley reference])
  - Smooth philtrum (4 or 5 on lip/philtrum guide)
- Prenatal and/or postnatal growth deficiency
- Height or weight ≤10th percentile at any time in patient's history

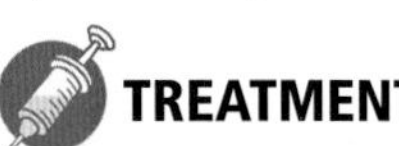

TREATMENT

GENERAL MEASURES

- The role of the pediatrician is early identification, appropriate referrals, and development of a multidisciplinary case plan, including the pediatrician, specialists, early intervention providers, psychologists, and social and educational resources in the community to support family and child.
- Specific medical referrals should include
  - Comprehensive neuropsychological evaluation (IQ, achievement, executive function, memory, adaptive function, language, reasoning and judgment, behavior)
  - Ophthalmologic exam (consider routine screening prior to school and then every 2 years)
  - Hearing test (consider brainstem auditory evoked response [BAER] at 6 to 12 months)
- Parents and caregivers should be counseled on the neurobehavioral challenges to promote understanding that the child's symptoms are not the result of willful misbehavior.
- The primary pediatrician should provide a medical home; help caregivers develop appropriate expectations; provide resources; determine risk for child abuse, neglect, and violence in the family.

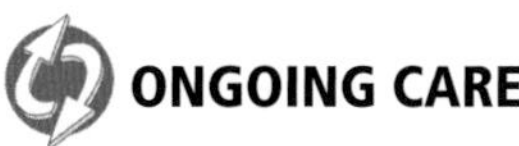

ONGOING CARE

FOLLOW-UP RECOMMENDATIONS

Patient Monitoring

- Growth and nutrition in infancy: Failure to thrive is a common problem.
- Regular evaluations of vision and hearing: Problems occur at a high rate.
- As indicated by other medical/psychological problems

PROGNOSIS

- 50% have intellectual disability (IQ <70). Average IQ in individuals with FAS is in the 60s (mild mental retardation); however, a wide range of IQ exists, from 16 to 115.
- 62% have severe behavioral problems, even if a normal IQ exists.
- The major disabilities of FAS caused by the neurocognitive/neurobehavioral effects can lead to poor academic performance, legal problems, employment difficulties, and secondary mental health problems.
- 35% develop an alcohol or drug problem.
- Many are unable to live independently as adults.

ADDITIONAL READING

- American Academy of Pediatrics. Fetal alcohol syndrome and alcohol-related neurodevelopmental disorders. *Pediatrics*. 2000;106(2 Pt 1):358–361.
- American Academy of Pediatrics Fetal Alcohol Spectrum Disorders Toolkit. Common definitions. http://www.aap.org/en-us/advocacy-and-policy/aap-health-initiatives/fetal-alcohol-spectrum-disorders-toolkit/Pages/Common-Definitions.aspx. Accessed April 10, 2017.
- Astley SJ, Clarren SK. Diagnosing the full spectrum of fetal alcohol-exposed individuals: introducing the 4-digit diagnostic code. *Alcohol Alcohol*. 2000;35(4):400–410.
- Bertrand J, Floyd RL, Weber MK, et al; National Task Force on Fetal Alcohol Syndrome and Fetal Alcohol Effect. *Fetal Alcohol Syndrome: Guidelines for Referral and Diagnosis*. Atlanta, GA: Centers for Disease Control and Prevention; 2004. http://www.cdc.gov/ncbddd/fasd/documents/FAS_guidelines_accessible.pdf. Accessed February 14, 2015.
- Bertrand J, Floyd RL, Weber MK, et al; National Task Force on Fetal Alcohol Syndrome and Fetal Alcohol Effect. *Fetal Alcohol Syndrome: Guidelines for Referral and Diagnosis*. 3rd rev ed. Atlanta, GA: Centers for Disease Control and Prevention; 2005.
- Hoyme HE, Kalberg WO, Elliott AJ, et al. Updated clinical guidelines for diagnosing fetal alcohol spectrum disorders. *Pediatrics*. 2016;138(2):e20154256.
- Hoyme HE, May PA, Kalberg WO, et al. A practical clinical approach to diagnosis of fetal alcohol spectrum disorders: clarification of the 1996 Institute of Medicine criteria. *Pediatrics*. 2005;115(1):39–47.
- National Institute on Alcohol Abuse and Alcoholism. *Fetal Alcohol Exposure and the Brain. Alcohol Alert no. 50*. Bethesda, MD: National Institutes of Health; 2000.
- Riley EP, Infante MA, Warren KR. Fetal alcohol spectrum disorders: an overview. *Neuropsychol Rev*. 2011;21(2):73–80.
- Sampson PD, Streissguth AP, Bookstein FL, et al. Incidence of fetal alcohol syndrome and prevalence of alcohol-related neurodevelopmental disorder. *Teratology*. 1997;56(5):317–326.

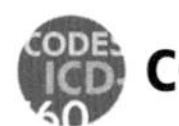

CODES

ICD10

- Q86.0 Fetal alcohol syndrome (dysmorphic)
- P04.3 Newborn affected by maternal use of alcohol

FAQ

- Q: What is pFAS?
- A: pFAS is diagnosed when a person does not meet full diagnostic criteria for FAS but has a history of prenatal alcohol exposure, some of the facial findings, and a growth problem or CNS abnormality.
- Q: What is ARND?
- A: Patients do not have abnormal facial features or growth problems but do have problems with neurocognitive development, adaptive functioning, or behavior regulation, in addition to confirmed prenatal alcohol exposure.
- Q: How much alcohol does it take to produce damage?
- A: The highest risk for FAS occurs in children whose mothers consume ≥4 drinks per occasion at least once per week. However, NO minimum safe level of alcohol consumption has been determined.
- Q: Do most children with FAS have ADHD?
- A: Although hyperactivity appears to be common in FAS, many of these children are misdiagnosed as having ADHD. Instead of difficulty focusing and sustaining attention, children with FAS often have difficulty shifting attention from one task to another. Use of stimulant medication is not routinely supported, although a small proportion may respond to stimulant medication in educational settings.

FEVER AND PETECHIAE

Angela M. Statile, MD, MEd • Craig H. Gosdin, MD, MSHA

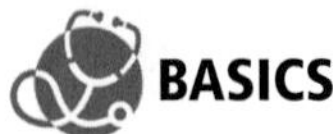

BASICS

DESCRIPTION

- Petechiae
  - Small hemorrhages (<3 mm in size) into the superficial layers of the skin
  - Manifest as a reddish purple, macular, nonblanching skin rash
- Purpura
  - Larger skin hemorrhages (>3 mm in size)
  - Often macular but may be raised or tender

EPIDEMIOLOGY

- Most patients (70–80%) presenting with fever and petechiae have defined or presumed viral infections, which are often caused by enteroviruses, adenovirus, or parvovirus B19.
- A minority of children presenting with fever and petechiae have an invasive bacterial disease, most commonly *Neisseria meningitidis*.
  - Infants and toddlers are at greatest risk of having an invasive bacterial infection with fever and petechiae.
  - Teenagers and young adults are most commonly affected by outbreaks of meningococcemia, presenting with fever and petechiae.
- Streptococcal pharyngitis may cause fever and petechiae in a well-appearing child.
- Other etiologies, such as acute leukemia, idiopathic thrombocytopenic purpura (ITP), and Henoch-Schönlein purpura (HSP), are responsible for a minority of cases of fever and petechiae.

GENERAL PREVENTION

- Vaccine recommendations
  - All children should complete the *Streptococcus pneumoniae* and *Haemophilus influenzae* type B immunization series that begins at 2 months of age.
  - Routine childhood immunization with quadrivalent meningococcal conjugate vaccine (protects against serogroups A, C, Y, and W) is recommended for all children at 11 to 12 years of age and a booster dose at 16 to 18 years of age.
  - Infants and children at high risk for meningococcal disease, such as those with asplenia or terminal complement deficiencies, should receive meningococcal conjugate vaccine as early as 2 months of age.
  - Children ≥10 years at high risk for meningococcal disease should also receive a serogroup B vaccine, which is approved for ages 10 to 25 years and is administered in a 2 or 3 dose schedule depending on the formulation.
  - Annual immunization against influenza viruses is recommended for all children >6 months of age.
- Chemoprophylaxis is recommended for close contacts of patients with meningococcal disease. Ideally, treatment should begin within 24 hours; rifampin is the drug of choice in most children (dosing <1 month of age: 5 mg/kg PO every 12 hours × 2 days, ≥1 month of age: 10 mg/kg [maximum 600 mg] PO every 12 hours × 2 days). Alternatives include ciprofloxacin, ceftriaxone, and azithromycin.

PATHOPHYSIOLOGY

Petechiae may result from several different mechanisms:

- Disruption of vascular integrity—due to infections, vasculitis, or trauma
- Platelet deficiency or dysfunction—typically thrombocytopenia due to sepsis, disseminated intravascular coagulation (DIC), ITP, or leukemia
- Factor deficiencies, although these are more likely to manifest as ecchymoses or deep bleeding

ETIOLOGY

Petechiae, when accompanied by fever, most often have an infectious cause. Multiple organisms are associated with fever and petechiae. Less commonly, fever and petechiae may be caused by other entities such as acute leukemia, ITP, HSP, and bacterial endocarditis.

- Bacterial
  - *N. meningitidis*
  - *S. pneumoniae*
  - *H. influenzae* type B
  - *Staphylococcus aureus*
  - *Streptococcus pyogenes*
  - *Escherichia coli*
- Viral
  - Enterovirus
  - Adenovirus
  - Influenza
  - Parainfluenza
  - Parvovirus B19
  - Epstein-Barr virus (EBV)
  - Rubella
  - Respiratory syncytial virus
  - Hepatitis viruses
- Rickettsial diseases
  - *Rickettsia rickettsii*
  - Ehrlichiosis

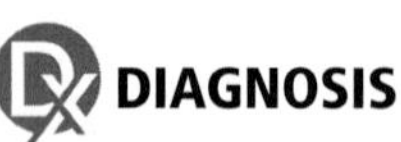

DIAGNOSIS

ALERT

Unsuspected invasive bacterial disease is the most common pitfall in the differential diagnosis of fever and petechiae. A thorough history and physical exam accompanied by laboratory testing, a period of close observation, and empiric antimicrobial therapy may minimize missed serious diagnoses.

HISTORY

Important historical factors to obtain include the following:

- Age of the child
- Underlying immunodeficiency
- Immunizations received
- Exposure to infectious contacts, particularly *N. meningitidis*
- Duration and height of fever
- Duration and progression of rash
- Excessive coughing or vomiting
- Pallor or other bleeding
- Level of activity, excess fatigue
- Travel or recent tick bites
- History of trauma in location of rash

PHYSICAL EXAM

- Important components of exam:
  - Vital signs, noting tachycardia, hypotension, or delayed capillary refill
  - Mental status
  - Meningismus/nuchal rigidity
  - Character of rash: petechiae or purpura, body distribution, number of lesions, progression during observation time
- Important findings suggesting specific diagnoses:
  - **Finding:** pallor, adenopathy, organomegaly
  - *Significance*: may suggest leukemia, EBV infection
  - **Finding:** mucous membrane bleeding
  - *Significance*: may suggest thrombocytopenia, such as ITP
  - **Finding:** headache, myalgias, centripetal rash distribution
  - *Significance*: may suggest Rocky Mountain spotted fever

DIFFERENTIAL DIAGNOSIS

- Viral infections (see "Etiology")
- Invasive bacterial infections
  - Most commonly *N. meningitidis*
  - Less often *S. aureus* or other bacteria (see "Etiology")
- Streptococcal pharyngitis—due to *S. pyogenes*
- Rickettsial infections: diagnosis aided by season, history of tick bite accompanied by fever, petechiae, headache, and myalgias
- Petechiae above the nipple line may be noted after significant coughing or vomiting.
- Coining or other traumatic causes
- Acute leukemias: diagnosis aided by clinical findings of pallor, adenopathy, hepatosplenomegaly, and laboratory findings
- ITP: diagnosis aided by findings of mucous membrane bleeding and isolated thrombocytopenia on laboratory testing
- HSP: diagnosis aided by clinical findings of palpable purpura on dependent areas such as the buttocks and lower extremities, as well as abdominal pain; may be noted without fever
- Endocarditis: diagnosis aided by bacteremia and a history of congenital heart disease, cardiac surgery, or rheumatic fever

DIAGNOSTIC TESTS & INTERPRETATION

Most children with fever and petechiae require laboratory testing. Consider obtaining complete blood count with differential, C-reactive protein (CRP), and blood culture even in non–toxic-appearing children.

- Consider rapid antigen testing for group A *Streptococcus* and throat culture if signs of pharyngitis.
- Children who are ill-appearing may warrant lumbar puncture for cerebrospinal fluid (CSF) studies and coagulation studies, including prothrombin time (PT) and partial thromboplastin time (PTT).
- Viral testing, including cultures, serology, and antibody immunofluorescence, is not routinely required and may be ordered at the discretion of the managing practitioner based on exposures, need for specific therapeutic interventions, admission to the hospital, and severity of illness.
- Although no one factor is 100% sensitive in identifying children with invasive bacterial disease, a constellation of factors is useful in identifying children with fever and petechiae in whom invasive bacterial disease is unlikely:
  - Multiple studies have demonstrated that well-appearing children with a normal WBC count (between 5,000 and 15,000/mm^3), a normal absolute neutrophil count (between 1,500 and 9,000 cells/mm^3), an absolute band count <500 cells/mm^3, and petechiae limited to above the nipple line are exceedingly unlikely to have an invasive bacterial infection. A CRP <6 mg/L has also been shown to have a high negative predictive value for ruling out invasive bacterial infection.

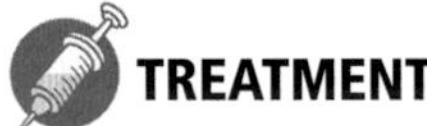

TREATMENT

MEDICATION

- Empiric antibiotic use should be decided on a case-by-case basis. Due to the high morbidity and mortality of *N. meningitidis*, the most likely bacterial pathogen in this circumstance, empiric ceftriaxone should be strongly considered in children with fever and petechiae who are not low risk for bacterial infection.
- 3rd-generation cephalosporins such as ceftriaxone and cefotaxime are effective against most bacterial pathogens causing fever and petechiae.
- Doxycycline should be administered if rickettsial disease is considered.
- Vancomycin should be added to the regimen for children with suspected bacterial meningitis to cover penicillin and cephalosporin-resistant strains of *S. pneumoniae*.

ADMISSION, INPATIENT, AND NURSING CONSIDERATIONS

- The management of children who are ill-appearing and have meningismus or purpura consists of a full sepsis evaluation, admission to the hospital with parenteral antibiotics, and fluids and vasoactive infusions to maintain normal hemodynamics.
- Because sporadic as opposed to epidemic cases of meningococcemia appear to occur in children in the first 2 years of life and these children have less competent immune systems in fighting encapsulated organisms, full sepsis evaluation and admission for all children in this young age group are recommended.
- The well-appearing child with fever and petechiae and a positive streptococcal antigen test and an illness compatible with streptococcal pharyngitis may be treated as an outpatient with antistreptococcal antibiotics.
- After a several-hour period of observation, children who remain well-appearing, are not tachycardic, have no progression of petechiae, and have normal lab studies may be considered for outpatient management.

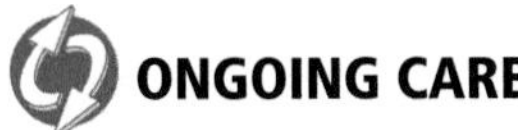

ONGOING CARE

FOLLOW-UP RECOMMENDATIONS

Patient Monitoring

- Children managed as outpatients:
  - Give instructions to return immediately for progression of rash or worsening illness.
  - Follow-up in 12 to 18 hours
  - Monitor cultures closely.
- Most children with viral causes have little progression of their petechiae and are clinically better within several days with the resolution of fever.

PROGNOSIS

- Depends on the underlying cause
- Because most cases of fever and petechiae are caused by viral infections, particularly enteroviruses and adenovirus, the prognosis is excellent.
- Case fatality rate of meningococcemia is 10–14%.

COMPLICATIONS

- Related to the underlying cause
- Most common complications of invasive bacterial disease causing fever and petechiae include sepsis and meningitis.
- Serious sequelae from *N. meningitidis* occur in 11–19% of patients and include neurologic deficits such as hearing loss, digit or limb loss, and skin scarring.

ADDITIONAL READING

- American Academy of Pediatrics. Meningococcal Infections. In: Kimberlin DW, Brady MT, Jackson MA, Long SS, eds. *Red Book: 2015 Report of the Committee on the Infectious Diseases*. Elk Grove Village, IL: American Academy of Pediatrics; 2015:547–558.
- Brayer AF, Humiston SG. Invasive meningococcal disease in childhood. *Pediatr Rev*. 2011;32(4):152–161.
- Klinkhammer MD, Colletti JE. Pediatric myth: fever and petechiae. *CJEM*. 2008;10(5):479–482.

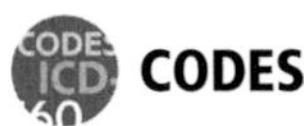

CODES

ICD10

- R50.9 Fever, unspecified
- R23.3 Spontaneous ecchymoses
- D69.2 Other nonthrombocytopenic purpura

FAQ

- Q: What are the most common causes of fever and petechiae in children?
- A: Viruses are the most common overall cause of fever and petechiae in children. The most common invasive bacterial disease causing fever and petechiae in children is *N. meningitidis*.
- Q: Is there ever a role for outpatient management of children with fever and petechiae?
- A: Practitioners may consider outpatient management in well-appearing children >2 years of age with the following criteria after a period of close observation in which they have normal vital signs and no progression of petechiae:
  - A normal WBC count (between 5,000 and 15,000 cells/mm^3)
  - A normal absolute neutrophil count (between 1,500 and 9,000 cells/mm^3)
  - An absolute band count <500 cells/mm^3
  - A CRP <6 mg/L

FEVER OF UNKNOWN ORIGIN

Samir S. Shah, MD, MSCE

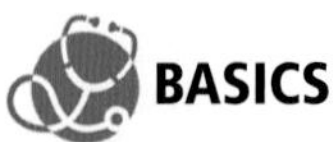

BASICS

DESCRIPTION

Fever of unknown origin (FUO) implies
- A febrile illness (38.3°C on multiple occasions)
- Present for >14 days
- No apparent source despite careful history taking, physical exam, and preliminary lab studies

ETIOLOGY

- Etiology has changed as the use of more sensitive tests (e.g., MRI, polymerase chain reaction [PCR] tests) permits earlier detection of many conditions that caused FUO in the past.
- Fever resolves in 40–60% of children without identification of a specific cause.
- FUO in the pediatric population is more often an unusual presentation of a common disease than a common presentation of an unusual disease.
- Common infectious causes
  - Respiratory infections (otitis media, mastoiditis, sinusitis, pneumonia, pharyngitis, peritonsillar/retropharyngeal abscess)
  - Systemic viral syndrome
  - Infectious mononucleosis (Epstein-Barr virus [EBV], cytomegalovirus [CMV])
  - Urinary tract infection (UTI)
  - Bone or joint infection
  - Enteric infection (*Salmonella*, *Yersinia enterocolitica*, *Yersinia pseudotuberculosis*, *Campylobacter jejuni*)
  - Cat-scratch disease
- Less common infectious causes
  - Tuberculosis (TB)
  - Lyme disease
  - Rickettsial disease (Rocky Mountain spotted fever, ehrlichiosis, anaplasmosis)
  - Malaria
  - CNS infection (bacterial or viral meningoencephalitis, intracranial abscess)
  - Dental or periodontal abscess
  - Subacute bacterial endocarditis (SBE)
  - HIV infection
  - Human herpes viruses
  - Acute rheumatic fever
- Other infectious causes
  - Q fever
  - Brucellosis
  - Toxoplasmosis
  - Syphilis
  - Parvovirus B19
  - Endemic fungi (histoplasmosis, blastomycosis, coccidioidomycosis)
  - Psittacosis
  - Typhoid (*Salmonella* spp.)
  - Chronic meningococcemia
- Possible noninfectious causes
  - Collagen vascular disease (systemic juvenile idiopathic arthritis [JIA], systemic lupus erythematosus, dermatomyositis, sarcoidosis, vasculitis syndrome)
  - Malignancy
  - Kawasaki syndrome
  - Inflammatory bowel disease (IBD)
  - Drug fever
  - Hyperthyroidism
  - Factitious fever or Munchausen syndrome by proxy
  - Centrally mediated fever
  - Periodic fever syndromes
  - Kikuchi-Fujimoto disease (histiocytic necrotizing lymphadenitis)

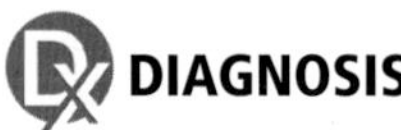

DIAGNOSIS

Approach to the patient
- Phase 1
  - Document fever.
  - Thorough history and physical exam
  - Determine whether constitutional symptoms (e.g., growth failure, developmental arrest) suggest a serious underlying disease.
  - Create broad differential diagnosis.
  - Begin initial laboratory evaluation while tailoring the cadence of evaluation to patient's severity of illness.
- Phase 2
  - Begin invasive studies to seek rarer forms of fever, such as lymphoma, brucellosis, and SBE, only if clinically indicated.
- Phase 3
  - Reexamine patient, consider additional testing, and reconsider causes such as systemic JIA, sarcoidosis, and factitious fever.
- Repeat history and physical exam combined with the results of previous testing should guide the subsequent evaluation.

HISTORY

- **Question**: Temperatures and how they were measured (tympanic, oral, axillary, rectal)?
- *Significance*:
  - As many as 50% of children referred for evaluation of FUO have multiple unrelated infections, parental misinterpretation of normal temperature variation, or complete absence of fever at time of evaluation.
  - Parents are sometimes told to add a 1 to 2°F "correction" onto a temperature measured in the axilla to better approximate the core temperature. Such practices may further cloud the evaluation of the febrile child.
- **Question**: Ethnicity?
- *Significance*: Some hereditary periodic fever syndromes have ethnic predilection. Consider familial Mediterranean fever (Armenian, Arab, Turkish, Sephardic Jew), hyper-IgD syndrome (Dutch, French), and tumor necrosis factor receptor–associated periodic fever syndrome (TRAPS) (Irish, Scottish).
- **Question**: Exposure to animals?
- *Significance*:
  - Household exposures including pets and rodents
  - Recreational activities (e.g., hunting)
  - Household contacts with occupational exposure to animals
  - Consider cat-scratch disease, brucellosis, tularemia, leptospirosis, and lymphocytic choriomeningitis virus (from mice).
- **Question**: Ingestion of raw meat, fish, or unpasteurized milk?
- *Significance*: trichinosis, brucellosis, listeriosis, *Mycobacteria bovis*, salmonellosis, giardiasis, or shiga-toxin producing *Escherichia coli*
- **Question**: Travel history, including past residence?
- *Significance*: malaria, endemic fungi (e.g., coccidioidomycosis in Southwest, blastomycosis in Southeast, histoplasmosis in Midwest), typhoid (Indian subcontinent), TB
- **Question**: Pica or dirt ingestion?
- *Significance*: *Toxocara canis* or *Toxoplasma gondii* infection
- **Question**: Change in behavior or activity?
- *Significance*: brain tumor, TB, EBV, Rocky Mountain spotted fever
- **Question**: Pattern of fever?
- *Significance*:
  - May correlate with underlying cause. A fever diary kept by the parent or caretaker may provide more objective documentation of the fever pattern than simple recall.
  - Need to distinguish continuous fever versus recurrent fever
- **Question**: Medications (including over-the-counter [OTC] medications and eyedrops)?
- *Significance*: drug fever, atropine-induced fever, methylphenidate, anticonvulsants, ranitidine, and antibiotics (especially penicillin, cephalosporins, and sulfonamides)
- **Question**: Well-water ingestion?
- *Significance*: giardiasis

PHYSICAL EXAM

- **Finding:** Impaired weight gain or linear growth?
- *Significance*: collagen vascular disease, malignancy, IBD
- **Finding:** Toxic appearance?
- *Significance*: Kawasaki syndrome

- **Finding:** Conjunctivitis?
- *Significance*: Kawasaki syndrome (limbic sparing), adenovirus, measles
- **Finding:** Ophthalmologic exam?
- *Significance*: Papilledema—consider CNS mass lesion; uveitis—consider TB, systemic lupus erythematosus, Kawasaki syndrome, and sarcoidosis.
- **Finding:** Sinus tenderness, nasal discharge, or halitosis?
- *Significance*: sinusitis
- **Finding:** Pharyngitis?
- *Significance*: Kawasaki syndrome, EBV, CMV
- **Finding:** Tachypnea?
- *Significance*: SBE, pneumonia
- **Finding:** Rales?
- *Significance*: histoplasmosis, sarcoidosis, coccidioidomycosis
- **Finding:** Cardiac murmur, gallop, or friction rub?
- *Significance*: SBE, acute rheumatic fever, pericarditis
- **Finding:** Hepatosplenomegaly?
- *Significance*: hepatitis, EBV, CMV, ehrlichiosis, anaplasmosis
- **Finding:** Rectal abnormalities?
- *Significance*: pelvic abscess, IBD
- **Finding:** Arthritis?
- *Significance*: JIA, IBD, acute rheumatic fever
- **Finding:** Bony tenderness?
- *Significance*: JIA, leukemia, osteomyelitis

DIAGNOSTIC TESTS & INTERPRETATION

The laboratory evaluation for a child with FUO should be directed toward the most likely diagnostic possibilities. Consider the following initial studies.

Initial Tests (screening, lab, imaging)

- **Test:** CBC with differential and careful examination of WBC morphology
- *Significance*: Kawasaki syndrome, cyclic neutropenia, malignancy, ehrlichiosis, anaplasmosis (morulae in WBC cytoplasm), and babesiosis
- **Test:** ESR, C-reactive protein (CRP), or procalcitonin
- *Significance*: collagen vascular disease, IBD, occult infection. ESR and CRP are generally normal in drug fever and central fever. Elevated procalcitonin (>0.25 ng/mL) may indicate bacterial infection.
- **Test:** blood cultures
- *Significance*: endocarditis, salmonellosis, other bloodstream infections
- **Test:** urinalysis and urine culture
- *Significance*: UTI, Kawasaki syndrome (sterile pyuria)
- **Test:** tuberculin skin test (by purified protein derivative)
- *Significance*: TB
- **Test:** stool bacterial culture and examination for ova and parasites
- *Significance*: *Salmonella*, *Giardia*
- **Test:** specific antibody testing
- *Significance*: Depending on clinical suspicion, consider the following:
  - First line: streptococcal enzyme titers (antistreptolysin O, anti-DNase B); EBV; CMV; cat-scratch disease; Lyme disease; hepatitis A, B, or C; or HIV (by PCR)
  - Second line: Rocky Mountain spotted fever; ehrlichiosis/anaplasmosis, toxoplasmosis, brucellosis, Q fever, leptospirosis, tularemia, dengue fever
- **Test:** viral testing of nasopharyngeal aspirates
- *Significance:* systemic viral syndrome (adenovirus)
- **Test:** chest radiograph
- *Significance:* TB, endemic fungi, pneumonia, malignancy

Follow-Up Tests & Special Considerations

Additional testing should be guided by history, physical examination, epidemiologic factors, and results of initial testing; indiscriminate use of laboratory testing and imaging is not likely to be helpful.

- **Test:** evaluation for immune deficiency
- *Significance*: underlying predisposition
- **Test:** bone marrow examination and culture
- *Significance: Salmonella* infection, mycobacteria, histoplasmosis, brucellosis, malignancy
- **Test:** lumbar puncture
- *Significance:* CNS infection
- **Test:** ophthalmology exam
- *Significance:* Uveitis can be present with Behçet disease, Kawasaki disease, TB, syphilis, sarcoidosis, IBD, or poly- or pauciarticular juvenile arthritis.
- **Test:** sinus CT
- *Significance:* sinusitis
- **Test:** chest radiograph
- *Significance:* TB, endemic fungi, pneumonia
- **Test:** chest and/or abdominal CT scan
- *Significance:* TB, liver abscess, hepatosplenic cat-scratch disease
- **Test:** pelvic or extremity MRI
- *Significance:* osteomyelitis, pyomyositis
- **Test:** gallium or bone scan
- *Significance:* multifocal osteomyelitis, malignancy

TREATMENT

Treatment depends on cause of fever.

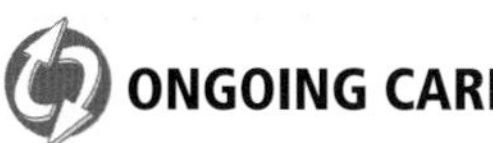

ONGOING CARE

PROGNOSIS

Prognosis depends on cause of fever.

- Most children with FUO who lack a specific diagnosis fare well with resolution of fever and few or no recurrent episodes.
- Occasionally, evolution or progression of symptoms facilitates diagnosis of a specific condition.

ADDITIONAL READING

- Chow A, Robinson JL. Fever of unknown origin in children: a systematic review. *World J Pediatr*. 2011;7(1):5–10.
- Chusid MJ. Fever of unknown origin in childhood. *Pediatr Clin North Am*. 2017;64(1):205–230.
- Drenth JPH, van der Meer JWM. Hereditary periodic fever. *N Engl J Med*. 2001;345(24):1748–1757.
- Gattorno M, Caorsi R, Meini A, et al. Differentiating PFAPA syndrome from monogenic periodic fevers. *Pediatrics*. 2009;124(4):e721–e728.
- Jacobs RF, Schutze GE. Bartonella henselae as a cause of prolonged fever and fever of unknown origin in children. *Clin Infect Dis*. 1998;26(1):80–84.
- Talano JM, Katz BZ. Long-term follow-up of children with fever of unknown origin. *Clin Pediatr (Phila)*. 2000;39(12):715–717.

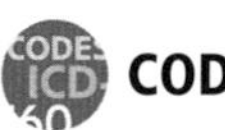

CODES

ICD10

R50.9 Fever, unspecified

FAQ

- Q: Do all of the mentioned tests need to be performed?
- A: A "shotgun" approach to testing is rarely useful in making the diagnosis, and unanticipated abnormalities (e.g., false-positives) may lead to additional invasive tests with potential for harm.
- Q: Is hospitalization required for the diagnosis of FUO?
- A: Many tests, including MRI, can now be performed in the outpatient setting. Hospitalization is not routinely required for diagnosis but should be considered in patients who appear ill, have progression of symptoms, or when the presence of fever needs to be documented.
- Q: How is cat-scratch disease acquired?
- A: Cat-scratch disease, caused by *Bartonella henselae*, can be acquired through cat (usually kittens or young cats) scratches or licks. Rarely, dogs may transmit the organism. If the family does not own a kitten or young cat, remember to ask about other sources of exposure (e.g., friends, family, school trips).

FLOPPY INFANT SYNDROME

Graeme A.M. Nimmo, MBBS, MSc • Ronald D. Cohn, MD, FACMG

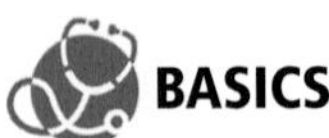

BASICS

DESCRIPTION

- "Floppy infant" refers to the newborn/infant presenting at birth or early in life with hypotonia, a symptom of diminished tone of skeletal muscles associated with decreased resistance of muscles to passive stretching.
- Hypotonia can be caused by abnormalities of the CNS (central hypotonia), peripheral neuromuscular system (peripheral hypotonia), or combined abnormality involving both (combined hypotonia).
- Nonspecific transient hypotonia occurs in nonneurologic conditions and may suggest gastrointestinal (GI), cardiac, pulmonary, infectious, renal, or endocrine disease.

EPIDEMIOLOGY

No comprehensive prevalence known, owing to presence of hypotonia as a feature of many distinct disorders; overall, central hypotonia is more common than peripheral hypotonia.

RISK FACTORS

Genetics

Substantial proportion (>50%) of infantile hypotonia cases accounted for by genetic-metabolic disorders.

ETIOLOGY

Causes may be divided into two major categories:

- Central: hypotonia with decreased alertness, developmental delay, and lack of (or minimal) weakness; caused by upper motor neuron defect
- Peripheral: hypotonia with weakness, paucity of antigravity movements, decreased or absent deep tendon reflexes (DTRs), and visual alertness; caused by lower motor neuron defect (i.e., disorders of anterior horn cell, peripheral nerve, neuromuscular junction, or skeletal muscle)

COMMONLY ASSOCIATED CONDITIONS

- Respiratory problems (apnea/hypoventilation)
- Feeding/swallowing difficulties
- Hip dislocation/contractures/joint laxity
- Seizure disorder
- Cognitive/developmental delay
- Hypersomnolence

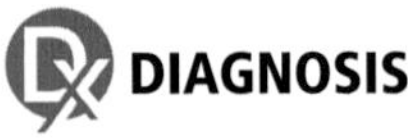

DIAGNOSIS

History and physical exam findings used to categorize patients as having central, peripheral, or combined hypotonia.

HISTORY

- Pregnancy and delivery
  - Pregnancy
    - Maternal illness (especially myasthenia gravis)
    - Drug or teratogen exposure
    - Abnormalities on prenatal ultrasound
    - Polyhydramnios (poor prenatal swallow)
    - Reduced fetal movements (neuromuscular disorders)
  - Delivery
    - Gestational age and presentation
    - Birth trauma, anoxia, or complications
    - Shortened umbilical cord
    - Low Apgar scores
    - Maternal perinatal infection
- Medical history
  - Seizures
  - Apnea
  - Feeding difficulties
  - Review of systems for associated malformations or health conditions
  - Delayed motor milestones
  - Delayed social, fine motor, or language milestones point to CNS defect.
- Course of hypotonia
  - Age at onset
  - Improved or worsened
  - Daily fluctuation
- Family history
  - Parental consanguinity
  - Three-generation pedigree specifically inquiring about history of neuromuscular disease, birth defects, intellectual disability, and recurrent infantile deaths

PHYSICAL EXAM

Exam findings will help determine if hypotonia is suggestive of an upper motor neuron versus a lower motor neuron problem or both. Perform the following:

- General physical exam
  - Dysmorphic features (may lead to particular syndromic diagnosis)
  - Alertness: Infants with neuromuscular disease are typically alert.
  - Poor spontaneous movements
  - Abnormal head size and/or shape
  - Tongue fasciculations (anterior horn cell)
  - Large tongue (storage disorders)
  - Ophthalmologic exam: cataracts (peroxisomal disorders), pigmentary retinopathy (peroxisomal disorders), cherry red spot (storage disorders), lens dislocation (sulfite oxidase/molybdenum cofactor deficiency)
  - Abnormal fat pads, inverted nipples (congenital disorders of glycosylation)
  - Cardiac enlargement and signs of cardiac failure (Pompe disease)
  - Visceral enlargement (storage disorders)
  - Arthrogryposis (central, neuromuscular, or connective tissue disorders)
  - Hip dislocation (intrauterine hypotonia)
  - Joint laxity (connective tissue disorders)
- Neurologic exam
  - Strength
    - Absence of antigravity movement (strongest predictor of peripheral etiology)
    - Low-pitched or progressively weaker cry
    - Poor suck
    - Paucity of facial expression ("myopathic" facies) indicates facial weakness (myotonic dystrophy, congenital muscular dystrophy, congenital myopathies).
    - Ptosis and external ophthalmoplegia (congenital myasthenic syndromes, congenital myopathies, and congenital muscular dystrophies)
    - Regional strength differences: Spinal muscular atrophy (SMA) spares diaphragm, face muscles, and pelvic sphincters. Neuropathies present with distal limb weakness and proximal sparing. Myasthenic syndromes affect bulbar and oculomotor muscles.
  - Muscle tone
    - Abnormal resting posture (abducted, externally rotated legs, flaccid arms) and prominent head lag with pull-to-sit
    - Fisting indicates spasticity.
    - Abnormal posture and tone in supine position, ventral and horizontal suspension, and traction
    - Elbow may easily extend beyond midsternum (scarf sign).
    - Generalized hypotonia with increased tone in thumb adductors, wrist pronators, and hip adductors: early cerebral palsy
    - Fatigability: cardinal feature of myasthenic syndromes but may occur in other neuromuscular diseases
  - DTRs (difficult to elicit in neonates)
    - Hyperreflexia implies central dysfunction.
    - Diminished DTRs in proportion to degree of weakness in myopathic diseases
    - Absent DTRs in setting of minimal weakness typical of neuropathic disease
- Examination of the mother
  - Signs of myotonia (myotonic dystrophy)
    - Handgrip myotonia (inability to release handgrip quickly)
    - Percussion (thenar) and tongue myotonia (slowed relaxation following tapping with reflex hammer)
    - Action myotonia (delayed muscle relaxation after voluntary contraction)

DIFFERENTIAL DIAGNOSIS

- Generalized nonneurologic conditions including the following:
  - Acute systemic disorders
    - Sepsis
    - Trauma
    - Malnutrition
    - GI obstruction or bleed
    - Toxic (hyperbilirubinemia, maternal sedative, analgesic, and/or anesthetic exposure)
- Chronic systemic disorders
  - Congenital heart disease
  - Endocrinopathies (hypothyroidism, rickets, hypercalcemia)
  - Renal tubular acidosis
  - Cystic fibrosis
  - Malabsorption
  - Connective tissue disorders
    - Ehlers-Danlos syndrome
    - Marfan syndrome
    - Loeys-Dietz syndrome
    - Osteogenesis imperfecta
    - Chondrodysplasia
- Neurologic diagnoses including the following:
  - Central hypotonia
    - Disorders involving cerebral cortex, cerebellum, and brainstem
      - Structural brain abnormalities (lissencephaly, holoprosencephaly)
      - Hypoxic-ischemic encephalopathy
      - Intracranial hemorrhage
      - Infections (meningitis, encephalitis)
    - Chromosomal disorders
      - Down syndrome
      - Williams syndrome
      - Prader-Willi syndrome
      - Angelman syndrome
    - Single-gene disorders
      - Fragile X syndrome
      - Rett/Rett-like syndrome
      - PTEN-related disorders
      - Smith-Lemli-Opitz syndrome
      - Peroxisomal disorders (Zellweger syndrome, infantile Refsum, neonatal adrenoleukodystrophy)
      - Congenital disorders of glycosylation
      - Creatine deficiency disorders
      - Neurotransmitter disorders
      - Purine/pyrimidine metabolism disorders
    - Disorders of spinal cord
      - Myelodysplasias (meningomyeloceles, diplomyelia, diastematomyelia)

- Peripheral hypotonia
  - Disorders of anterior horn cell including the following:
    - SMA
    - SMA with respiratory distress (SMARD)
    - Pompe disease (glycogen storage type II)
    - Neonatal poliomyelitis
    - Amyoplasia congenita (suspected vascular origin)
  - Disorders of peripheral nerve
    - Dejerine-Sottas disease
    - Guillain-Barré syndrome
    - Charcot-Marie-Tooth disease
    - Riboflavin transporter deficiencies
    - Familial dysautonomia
  - Disorders of neuromuscular junction
    - Myasthenia gravis (congenital, transient)
    - Infantile botulism
    - Toxic (hypermagnesemia, antibiotics [especially aminoglycosides], nondepolarizing neuromuscular blockers)
  - Disorders of muscle
    - Congenital myotonic dystrophy
    - Congenital muscular dystrophies
    - Congenital structural myopathies: central core, nemaline, centronuclear myopathy
    - Metabolic myopathies (mitochondrial and storage disorders)
    - Organic aciduria (Barth syndrome)
    - Fatty acid oxidation disorders
- Combined hypotonia
  - Dystroglycanopathies
  - Leukodystrophies (Canavan disease, Pelizaeus-Merzbacher disease)
  - Marinesco-Sjögren syndrome
  - Mitochondrial encephalomyopathies

DIAGNOSTIC TESTS & INTERPRETATION

Initial Tests (screening, lab, imaging)

- General laboratory:
  - Electrolytes (including Ca and Mg)
  - Thyroid function tests
  - Creatine kinase (normal in central, may be high in peripheral or combined cases)
  - Arterial blood gas
- Toxoplasmosis, other viruses, rubella, cytomegalovirus, or herpes (TORCH) screen; blood, urine, and CSF cultures (infection)
- Screen for inborn error of metabolism:
  - Ammonia (high in urea cycle defects, organic acidemias, fatty acid oxidation disorders)
  - Lactate in blood, urine, CSF (high in carbohydrate metabolism and mitochondrial disorders)
  - Quantitative amino acid analysis in blood and urine (aminoacidopathies)
  - Plasma acylcarnitine profiles and urine organic acid analysis (organic acidemias, fatty acid oxidation defects)
  - Plasma very-long-chain fatty acids (peroxisomal disorders)
  - Uric acid (low in molybdenum cofactor deficiency)
  - Transferrin isoelectric focusing (abnormal pattern seen in congenital disorders of glycosylation)
  - 7-dehydrocholesterol (high in Smith-Lemli-Opitz syndrome)
  - WBC lysosomal enzyme assays
  - Urine GAA/creatine (creatine deficiency disorders)
  - Urine purine/pyrimidine (purine/pyrimidine metabolism disorders)
  - CSF neurotransmitters
  - Stools for *Clostridium* toxin when botulism suspected (endemic in Pennsylvania, some northwestern states)
- Genetic testing
  - Rapid aneuploidy test (Down syndrome)
  - Microarray/SNP array (microdeletion/microduplication syndromes)
  - DNA methylation/MS-MLPA (Prader-Willi/Angelman syndrome)
  - DNA-based molecular testing (for a specific condition or gene panel testing)
  - Whole exome sequencing
- MRI for structural brain abnormalities; CT for intracranial calcifications
- Magnetic resonance spectroscopy (MRS): assesses neuronal integrity (*N*-acetylaspartate [NAA] peaks), intracerebral accumulation of unusual metabolites (lactate, glycine), or deficiency of a key metabolite (creatine)
- Muscle MRI: specific patterns of muscle involvement in various myopathies
- Abdominal/pelvic ultrasound: assesses other organ involvement

Diagnostic Procedures/Other

- Evaluation of vision and hearing
- Echocardiography
- Anticholinesterase administration in suspected myasthenia may be diagnostic.
- Electromyography (EMG) and nerve conduction velocity: useful tools to assess the lower motor unit and localize involved site
- EEG: if seizures are suspected
- Skin biopsy: lysosomal enzyme assay in fibroblasts and electron microscopy for abnormal organelles, inclusions, or storage material (Pompe disease)
- Muscle biopsy: for histopathology, electron microscopy, respiratory chain studies (congenital myopathies, storage myopathies [Pompe disease], or muscular dystrophies)

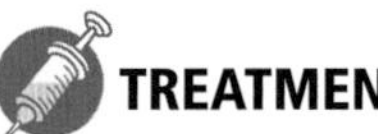

TREATMENT

MEDICATION

- Anticholinesterase inhibitors and 3,4-diaminopyridine in congenital myasthenic syndromes
- IV immunoglobulin and plasmapheresis have been used in treatment of infants with Guillain-Barré syndrome.

ADDITIONAL THERAPIES

- Address apnea, hypoventilation, hypoxia:
  - Intubation or positive pressure devices may be required.
  - Chest physiotherapy, antibiotics, bronchodilators, and oxygen may be needed.
  - Hypermagnesemia can cause apnea.
  - Weak infants in car seats may be at risk for acute respiratory problems.
- Underlying toxic or metabolic causes should be addressed and treated appropriately.
- Physical therapy
  - May help maintain maximum muscle function and reduce secondary deformities
  - Orthopedic consultation to evaluate hips and contractures
- Occupational therapy
- Speech therapy

SURGERY/OTHER PROCEDURES

Surgical intervention in later childhood to correct primary as well as secondary deformities may be indicated.

ADMISSION, INPATIENT, AND NURSING CONSIDERATIONS

Criteria for admission include respiratory insufficiency, feeding intolerance, failure to thrive, and/or metabolic abnormalities.

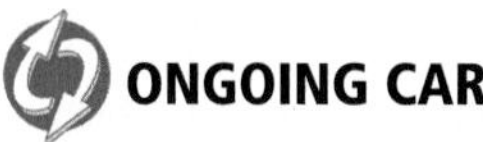

ONGOING CARE

FOLLOW-UP RECOMMENDATIONS

Individualized multidisciplinary care including specialists in neurology, pulmonology, orthopedics, development, physiotherapy, and nutrition; attention to vision and hearing should be considered as well as psychosocial support to caregivers/families.

DIET

Feeding and swallowing difficulties may necessitate nutritional supplementation and/or feeding tube placement.

PROGNOSIS

Many of the paralytic hypotonias are quite variable in their clinical course. Severity of disease depends on underlying cause and associated respiratory and nutritional factors.

COMPLICATIONS

- Respiratory insufficiency/recurrent pneumonia
- Orthopedic deformities
- Poor nutritional status

ADDITIONAL READING

- Bodensteiner JB. The evaluation of the hypotonic infant. *Semin Pediatr Neurol*. 2008;15(1):10–20.
- Harris SR. Congenital hypotonia: clinical and developmental assessment. *Dev Med Child Neurol*. 2008;50(12):889–892.
- Lisi E, Cohn R. Genetic evaluation of the pediatric patient with hypotonia: perspective from a hypotonia specialty clinic and review of the literature. *Dev Med Child Neurol*. 2011;53(7):586–599.
- Prasad A, Prasad C. Genetic evaluation of the floppy infant. *Semin Fetal Neonatal Med*. 2011;16(2):99–108.

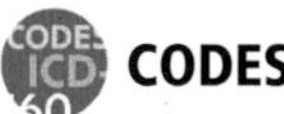

CODES

ICD10

P94.2 Congenital hypotonia

FAQ

- Q: What is the meaning of "benign congenital hypotonia"?
- A: It is an antiquated term used to describe patients in whom hypotonia resolved before 18 months. This designation should be avoided; it is important to find an underlying diagnosis as it may have implications for the child and future pregnancies.
- Q: What is the best test for Prader-Willi syndrome?
- A: DNA methylation analysis detects >99%. Targeted FISH and microarray analysis will be normal for patients with uniparental disomy or imprinting center defects (approximately 25% of children with PWS).
- Q: What clinical sign can help distinguish between SMA and infantile botulism?
- A: Tongue fasciculations are seen in SMA. Decreased pupillary light reflex is seen in botulism.

F

FOLLOW-UP OF NICU GRADUATES

Rebecca A. Dorner, MD • Vera Joanna Burton, MD, PhD • Marilee C. Allen, MD

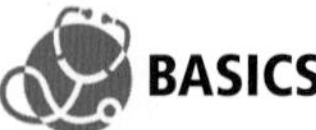

BASICS

DESCRIPTION

Neonatal intensive care unit (NICU) graduates (former premature infants), who have an increased risk for neurodevelopmental disabilities (NDD), require close follow-up and serial cognitive, sensory, and motor monitoring.

EPIDEMIOLOGY

- In the United States, 78 of 1,000 births are admitted to NICUs; admission rates increase with decreasing gestational age (GA).
- Prematurity: In 2016, the U.S. preterm birth rate increased for the 1st time in 8 years to 9.6%.
- Hypoxic ischemic encephalopathy (HIE): 1 to 3/1,000 births should be admitted to the NICU within 6 hours for therapeutic hypothermia.
- Respiratory failure: deficiency of oxygenation with insufficient ventilation; mechanical ventilation required in 18/1,000 births; associated with many comorbidities and up to 15% mortality
- Congenital anomalies (3% of U.S. births) account for 20% infant deaths; most common is congenital heart disease (CHD) in 1%; neural tube defects in 3 to 4/10,000; genetic syndromes

RISK FACTORS

- Prematurity—deficits generally correlate with GA, birth weight (BW); preterm birth associated with injuries to many organ systems due to:
  - Factors that precipitate preterm delivery (infection, inflammation)
  - Physiologic instability after birth
  - Required use of immature organ systems
  - Insufficient endogenous protective factors (thyroxin, cortisol, surfactant)
  - Side effects of treatment
- Brain injury—intraventricular hemorrhage (IVH), HIE, stroke, encephalomalacia, periventricular leukomalacia (PVL), hydrocephalus, seizures
- Congenital/postnatal infections—CMV, HSV, HIV, bacterial sepsis, Zika virus
- Congenital anomalies increase risk for later NDD.
- CHD: higher rates of brain malformations, microcephaly, prolonged hypoxemia with cardiopulmonary bypass/arrest
- Neonatal abstinence syndrome—higher risk with polydrug exposure
- Respiratory failure/chronic lung disease (CLD) intermittent hypoxia and acidosis; poor growth
- Intrauterine growth restriction (IUGR)
- Genetic syndromes
- Severe neonatal illness—sepsis, necrotizing enterocolitis (NEC, especially requiring surgery), retinopathy of prematurity (ROP, grades 4 to 5)

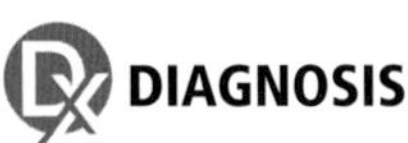

DIAGNOSIS

HISTORY

- BW, GA, NICU complications
- Neuroimaging
- Length of intubation and oxygen need
- Receipt of ototoxic medications
- Umbilical lines—umbilical venous and arterial lines increase risk for hypertension secondary to renal artery or vein stenosis/thrombosis.
- Discharge medications with weaning plans
- Feeding plan

PHYSICAL EXAM

- Vital signs (including blood pressures)
- Growth parameters—height, weight, head circumferences (especially in children with history of hydrocephalus/shunts; lack of head growth concerning as well as rapid growth)
- General physical examination focusing on muscle tone and motor function

DIAGNOSTIC TESTS & INTERPRETATION

- Regular American Academy of Pediatrics (AAP) developmental screening
  - Clinicians should not watch and wait when delay is suspected for these high-risk children.
- NICU follow-up clinics should perform detailed cognitive and motor assessments.
- Use age corrected for degree of prematurity (corrected age) when assessing preterm infants until at least 2 years chronologic age.

Diagnostic Procedures/Other

Immunizations

- Use same chronologic age as term infants.
- See American Academy of Pediatrics (AAP) Guidelines for LBW/preterm infants.
- Palivizumab—use based on AAP guidelines.

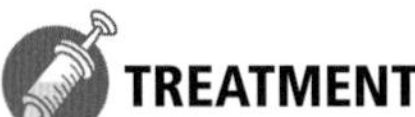

TREATMENT

GENERAL MEASURES

- Prompt referral to early intervention programs for infants and toddlers (Part C of the Individuals with Disabilities Education Act [IDEA])
- Individualized family service plan (IFSP, before 3 years), individualized education plan (IEP)/504 Plan between ages 4 and 7 years of age
- Continue close follow-up for at 2 years (even if the child does not qualify for NICU clinic) due to risk for ongoing school and learning problems.
- Home visits/home nursing: if available, can improve motor development index and interactions between parents and infant

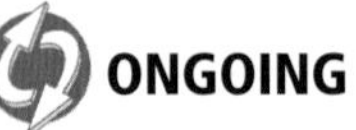

ONGOING CARE

FOLLOW-UP RECOMMENDATIONS

- Cerebral palsy (CP):
  - Definition: nonprogressive motor coordination and planning disorder due to injury or malformation of developing brain
  - Risk factors for CP: IUGR, sepsis, surgery, high-frequency ventilation, postnatal steroids, abnormal neonatal neuroimaging (white matter injury, ventriculomegaly, severe IVH, bilateral cystic, PVL), HIE, GA
  - CP rates increase with decreasing GA.
    - Full term 0.1%
    - 34 to 36 weeks 0.3%
    - 31 to 33 weeks 2%
    - 28 to 30 weeks ~5%
    - 23 to 27 weeks ~5–15%
    - <25 weeks 10–30%
  - Rates of CP in HIE: ~20–30%
  - Most common type in preterm infants is spastic diplegia.
- Minor neuromotor dysfunction
  - Definition: mild motor impairments such as early marked hand preference, overflow movements, poor handwriting, visuospatial, and sensorimotor integration problems
  - Preterm children at increased risk
  - Can also adversely affect child's self-help skills and self-esteem
- Intellectual disability
  - Defined as performance >2 SDs below mean on intelligence + adaptive function tests
  - Increases with decreasing GA
    - ~10% children born at GA <32 weeks
    - Up to 40–50% in children born at GA <26 weeks
  - Higher rates with neuroimaging abnormalities (severe IVH, hydrocephalus, white matter injury)
  - Prematurity generally shifts IQ baseline down by 10 points; IQ scores decrease by 1 to 2 points for every week <33 weeks.
  - Strongly affected by environment (parental education, socioeconomic status), genetics
- Visual impairment
  - Most common causes of pediatric visual impairment in the United States: cortical visual impairment (CVI), ROP, optic nerve hypoplasia
  - 37% of significant visual impairments in children attributable to prematurity
  - CVI—often underdiagnosed visual processing disorder; associated with occipital cortex injury; improves with specific visual/educational interventions
  - ROP—presents at 32 weeks, peaks at 38 to 40 weeks, regresses at 46 weeks
  - 84% of children born at GA <28 weeks have some degree of ROP; 40% of those born at <26 weeks require laser surgery.
  - Can lead to retinal detachment/blindness
  - Other visual problems: reduced visual acuity, amblyopia, strabismus, myopia
  - Follow-up eye exam at 12 months corrected for degree of prematurity if GA <32 weeks
- Hearing impairment
  - 10- to 20-fold higher among NICU infants versus term infants; higher risk with prolonged oxygen use
    - ~3% mild to moderately severe hearing loss
    - ~2% profound loss
  - Sensorineural hearing loss most common
    - 1/2 congenital; 1/2 acquired (i.e., due to gentamicin, furosemide), ECMO (up to 37%), CNS disease, craniofacial defects
  - If high risk, recheck hearing every 6 months for 3 years, as hearing loss onset delayed (previously normal ABR) in 10%; 28% have progressive loss between tests.
  - Early identification/treatment (American Sign Language, hearing aids, cochlear implants) critical for language development

- Language
  - Preterm infants have high risk of language delay and language-based learning disability.
  - 1st year: problems with early speech perception/auditory discrimination (i.e., discriminate native vs. non-native phonemes); fewer vocalizations; delay in babbling, less phonologic complexity, smaller receptive lexicon
  - 12 to 24 months—smaller expressive lexicon
- Behavioral spectrum
  - ADHD-like behaviors are 2 to 6 times higher in premature infants; more often correlating with inattention and slower processing
  - Increased risk for comorbid internalizing disorders (anxiety, depression)
  - Poorer social and communication skills
  - Autism rate higher: 4–8% in children born at GA <28 weeks
  - Important to keep in mind that premature children have higher rates of false positives on screens due to co-occurring brain injury, sensory, or neurodevelopmental impairments
- Executive function
  - Definition: cognitive control used to plan and organize approach to tasks
  - Former preterm children have lower scores on visual and working memory, cognitive flexibility, sustained attention, response inhibition, fluency, and planning.
- Specific learning disabilities (SLD)
  - Definition: low scores on tests of reading, writing, spelling, mathematics in setting of normal IQ, adequate education
  - Higher rates in preterm children for math (highest), reading, and spelling, most in GAs <31 weeks but present in late preterm
  - ELBW rates of ~20–60% for each type SLD versus general population rates ~5–15%
  - Higher rates of SLD and special education use with moderate to severe HIE, respiratory failure, IUGR, congenital infections
- Osteopenia of prematurity
  - Increased risk with low GA, prolonged IV nutrition, long-term ventilation, furosemide, steroids, antibiotics, anticonvulsants
  - The AAP recommends all breast/formula-fed infants with <1,000 mL of vitamin D-fortified milk per day should be supplemented with 400 IU vitamin D daily; premature babies may need up to 1,000 IU daily.
  - Elevations of alkaline phosphatase >650 U/L—consider adding calcium, phosphorus.
- Anemia of prematurity
  - Preterm infants have low iron stores at birth, high requirements due to rapid growth rates.
  - Iron is important for brain development (synapse function and brain myelination).
  - 2 mg/kg/24 h of iron until 1 year corrected; formula-fed babies get in iron in formula, breast-fed babies should be supplemented.
  - Preterm infants have earlier and lower physiologic nadir, with hemoglobin (HgB) 6 to 7 mg/dL at 3 to 7 weeks of age versus term babies—HgB 9 to 10 mg/dL at 6 to 8 weeks of age
  - Iron deficiency anemia occurs earlier, check HgB every 6 months; if <11 mg/dL after nadir, increase supplementation to 3 to 5 mg/kg/24 h.
- Feeding challenges
  - Integration of sucking, swallowing, and breathing can be delayed in preterm infants (later than 33 to 36 weeks postmenstrual age).
  - Late preterm infants—poorer state organization, sleepier, latch challenges
  - The risk of poor feeding outcomes increases with medical problems (CLD, NEC).
  - High rates of feeding problems at 2 years in infants with BW <1,000 g; up to 33% may need gastrostomy.
- Seizures
  - Follow-up with neurologist; drug blood level within 1 month of discharge
  - Seizures in neonatal period do not necessarily predict later childhood seizures but predict increased risk of NDD.
- Dental
  - Premature infants should be seen within 18 months—increased risk for enamel hypoplasia/discoloration, intubation can affect alveolar ridge/palate
- Parental stress
  - NICU parents have high rates of perinatal mood disorders including postpartum depression, post traumatic stress disorder (PTSD), anxiety disorders, obsessive-compulsive disorders (OCD).
  - All have been shown to affect children's developmental trajectory.

DIET

- Preterm formula:
  - Provides increased protein, calcium, phosphorus, zinc, vitamins, trace elements
  - Preterm (vs. term) formula increases 12- to 18-month weight, length, head circumference.
  - Typically, continue premature fortified human milk/preterm formula at minimum 22 kcal/oz until 12 months for infants born <28 weeks GA; consider term formula at 6 to 9 months if good growth.
- No consensus on the length of time milk should be fortified
  - Goals: all feeds taken orally, growing well, no nutritional deficiencies (alkaline phosphatase, calcium/phosphorus, albumin normal)

PATIENT EDUCATION

- Frequent tummy time (2 to 3 times a day for at least 5 minutes) on a firm surface while awake
- Safe sleep recommendations
  - "Back to sleep"
  - Remove soft bedding, blankets, toys, pillows, and bumper pads out of baby's sleep area.
  - Room sharing, but *not* bed sharing, is recommended.
- Avoid standing activities until infant pulls to stand on furniture.
- Hand toys to each hand even if the child has a preference.
- Talking and reading to the infant

ADDITIONAL READING

- Allen MC, Cristofalo E, Kim C. Outcomes of preterm infants: morbidity replaces mortality. *Clin Perinatol*. 2011;38: 441–454.
- Andrews B, Pellerite M, Myers P, et al. NICU follow-up: medical and developmental management age 0 to 3 years. *NeoReviews*. 2014;15:e123–e132.
- Browne JV, Ross ES. Eating as a neurodevelopmental process for high-risk newborns. *Clin Perinatol*. 2011;38(4):731–743.
- de Vries L, Jongmans MJ. Long-term outcome after neonatal hypoxic-ischaemic encephalopathy. *Arch Dis Child Fetal Neonatal Ed*. 2010;95(3):F220–F224.
- Doyle LW, Anderson PJ, Battin M, et al. Long term follow up of high risk children: who, why and how? *BMC Pediatr*. 2014;14:279.
- Johnson S, Marlow N. Growing up after extremely preterm birth: lifespan mental health outcomes. *Semin Fetal Neonatal Med*. 2014;19(2):97–104.
- Mahle WT, Wernovsky G. Long-term developmental outcome of children with complex congenital heart disease. *Clin Perinatol*. 2001;28(1):235–247.
- Repka MX. Ophthalmological problems of the premature infant. *Ment Retard Dev Disabil Res Rev*. 2002;8(4):249–257.
- Robertson CM, Howarth TM, Bork DL, et al. Permanent bilateral sensory and neural hearing loss of children after neonatal intensive care because of extreme prematurity: a thirty-year study. *Pediatrics*. 2009;123(5):e797–e807.

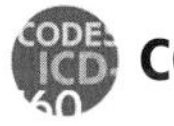

CODES

ICD10

Z09 Encounter for follow-up examination after completed treatment for conditions other than malignant neoplasm

FAQ

- Q: What growth curves should we use for tracking NICU graduates?
- A: Fenton growth curves accurately reflect intrauterine accretion and are used in NICU but are poorer for children >36 weeks GA. WHO growth charts are best adjusted for age once 4 to 8 weeks postterm.
- Monitor growth every 1 to 2 weeks for 2 months; continue close monitoring if the child's growth is ≤3%, if that child has chronic disease, or is falling off curve.
- Q: How long do I account for "catch up" growth for a premature infant?
- A: For any baby born <32 weeks, corrections for GA should be made for weight up to 24 months of age, stature to 40 months of age, and head circumference to 18 months of age. Poor gains in head circumference in first 8 months after birth indicate poor long-term outcomes.

F

FOOD ALLERGY

Jackie P-D. Garrett, MD • Terri Brown-Whitehorn, MD

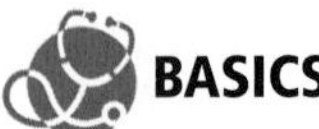

BASICS

DESCRIPTION

Food allergy has recently been defined as "an adverse health effect arising from a specific immune response that occurs reproducibly on exposure to a given food." Most commonly, the protein component of the food is responsible for the adverse immunologic response. An exception is the delayed reaction to meat, which is associated with IgE against the carbohydrate moiety, α-galactose.

- Classifications of food allergies:
  - IgE mediated, including
    - Anaphylaxis
    - Acute urticaria
    - Oral allergy syndrome
    - Galactose-α-1,3-galactose allergy
  - Non–IgE mediated (cell mediated), including
    - Food protein–induced enterocolitis syndrome (FPIES)
    - Food protein–induced allergic proctocolitis
  - Mixed IgE and non–IgE mediated, including
    - Atopic dermatitis
    - Eosinophilic gastroenteropathies (eosinophilic esophagitis, eosinophilic gastroenteritis)
- Most common IgE-mediated food allergies:
  - Children
    - Milk
    - Egg
    - Soy
    - Peanut
    - Wheat
    - Fish
    - Shellfish
    - Sesame
  - Adults
    - Peanuts
    - Tree nuts
    - Fish
    - Shellfish
- Most common non–IgE-mediated food allergies associated with food protein enterocolitis and proctocolitis:
  - Milk
  - Soy
  - Rice
  - Oat
  - Wheat
  - Barley
  - Chicken

EPIDEMIOLOGY

Food-induced anaphylaxis is the most common cause of anaphylactic reactions treated in emergency departments in the United States. The prevalence of food allergy has increased over the past 10 to 20 years.

Prevalence

- 5% of children <5 years of age, 4% of teens and adults
- Milk allergy is the most common childhood food allergy affecting nearly 2.5% of infants during 1st year of life (half of cases are thought to represent GI diseases); approximately 50% outgrow by 5 years of age and 79% outgrow by 16 years of age.
- Egg allergy affects 1.6% of patients.
  - Majority diagnosed by 2.5 years of age
  - Most common food allergy diagnosed in infants with atopic dermatitis
  - 50% outgrow by 6 years of age.
  - 65% outgrow by 12 years of age.
- 0.6% of U.S. population have peanut allergy, 20% may outgrow over time.
- 37% of children <5 years of age with moderate to severe atopic dermatitis have a food allergy.
- 34–49% of children with food allergy have asthma.
- 33–40% of children with food allergy have allergic rhinitis.
- Fatal and near-fatal reactions are associated with uncontrolled asthma and delayed use of epinephrine.

RISK FACTORS

- Timing of food introduction
- Genetic
- Family history
- Presence of atopic dermatitis
- Other unknown factors suspected

GENERAL PREVENTION

- Recent studies have found that delaying introduction of food in babies increases risk of IgE-mediated reactions.
- Current recommendations are to begin adding solid foods between 4 and 6 months of age.
- High-risk infants (those with severe atopic dermatitis and IgE-mediated food allergy to egg) should be evaluated by allergist prior to peanut introduction (otherwise recommended to add into diet between 4 and 11 months of age).

ETIOLOGY

- Oral tolerance to food proteins believed to develop through T-cell anergy or induction of regulatory T cells. Food hypersensitivity develops when oral tolerance fails to develop or breaks down.
- IgE mediated: T cells induce B cells to produce IgE antibodies that initially bind on the surface of mast cells and basophils; when reexposed, the food protein binds to IgE antibodies, leading to degranulation of those cells and release of histamine and other chemical mediators.
- Non–IgE mediated (cell mediated): T cells react to protein-inducing proinflammatory cytokines, leading to inflammatory cell infiltrates and increased vascular permeability. These factors lead to subacute and chronic responses primarily affecting the GI tract.
- Mixed IgE and non–IgE mediated: Eosinophilic esophagitis and eosinophilic gastroenteropathy are characterized by eosinophilic infiltration of intestinal wall, occasionally reaching to serosa.

COMMONLY ASSOCIATED CONDITIONS

- Asthma (4-fold more likely)
- Allergic rhinitis (2.4-fold more likely)
- Atopic dermatitis (1/3 of patients with severe atopic dermatitis has a food trigger.)

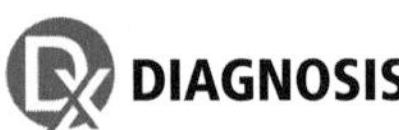

DIAGNOSIS

Varies depending on the individual and the type of food hypersensitivity

- IgE mediated
  - Urticaria
  - Angioedema
  - Immediate GI reactions: abdominal pain (common in pediatrics), nausea, vomiting, diarrhea; typically within minutes of ingestion but up to 2 hours
  - Rhinitis, coughing, wheezing
  - Anaphylaxis (>2 organ systems, hypotension, dyspnea, angioedema, vomiting, sense of impending doom)
  - Oral allergy syndrome: itchy mouth/tongue associated with uncooked fruits/vegetables that resolves when cooked
  - Galactose-α-1,3 galactose allergy (Delayed anaphylaxis is often seen.)
- Mixed IgE and non–IgE (cell mediated)
  - Eosinophilic gastroenteritis
    - Weight loss (key feature), abdominal pain, emesis, failure to thrive (FTT), anorexia
    - Some infants have a large protein-losing enteropathy component causing low serum albumin and hypogammaglobulinemia.
  - Eosinophilic esophagitis
    - Gastroesophageal reflux, heartburn, and regurgitation do not respond to reflux medication (specifically proton pump inhibitor).
    - Intermittent vomiting
    - Food refusal
    - Dysphagia and food impaction (more in adolescents)
    - Abdominal pain
    - FTT (although may present with normal weight or obese)
- Non–IgE mediated
  - Food protein enterocolitis: acute
    - Severe vomiting 2 hours after ingestion; may be followed by profuse diarrhea
    - Shock due to fluid/electrolyte loss (15%)
    - Very ill-appearing
  - Food protein enterocolitis: chronic
    - Intermittent vomiting
    - Abdominal pain
    - Abnormal stools (mucous, diarrhea, blood in stool)
  - Food protein proctocolitis
    - Blood in stool in otherwise healthy infant
    - Abdominal pain
    - Seen in breast-fed infants
  - Food protein–induced enteropathy
    - Diarrhea, bloating, FTT, anemia
    - Abdominal pain

PHYSICAL EXAM

- IgE mediated
  - Hives/angioedema (However, in 12% of patients with anaphylaxis, there are no skin findings and often these are the most severe cases.)
  - Coughing, stridor, wheezing/dyspnea
  - Hypotension/tachycardia
  - Vomiting, abdominal tenderness
  - Ill-appearing
- Mixed IgE mediated, non–IgE mediated:
  - Eosinophilic esophagitis: abdominal tenderness (variable), growth concerns (in some)
  - Eosinophilic gastroenteropathy
    - Abdominal tenderness
    - Weight loss
- Cell mediated
  - Food protein–induced enterocolitis
    - Acute: severe dehydration (may present in shock)
    - Chronic: FTT, abdominal tenderness/distension

DIAGNOSTIC TESTS & INTERPRETATION

Initial Tests (screening, lab, imaging)

Depend on clinical presentation and patient symptoms, may include

- CBC with differential
  - Anemia in patients with enteropathy
  - Eosinophilia may be seen in patients with eosinophilic gastroenteritis, enteropathy, and, on occasion, eosinophilic esophagitis (but cannot be used to monitor therapy).
  - In acute FPIES reactions, elevated WBC count with neutrophilia
- Serum IgE: may be elevated in
  - IgE-mediated hypersensitivities
  - Eosinophilic esophagitis, eosinophilic gastroenteritis

- Albumin: low in
  - Protein-losing enteropathies
  - Non–IgE-mediated protein enterocolitis (chronic version)
  - Eosinophilic gastroenteritis
- Tryptase: may be elevated in anaphylaxis; obtain within 4 hours of initial reaction.
- ImmunoCAP® assay may be helpful in IgE-mediated illness.
  - ImmunoCAP® has many false positives (do not send food allergy panels).
  - Galactose-α-1,3-galactose level if suspected allergy

Diagnostic Procedures/Other

- Skin prick testing
  - Used in conjunction with clinical history for IgE-mediated food allergies
  - 50% positive predictive value; 95% negative predictive value
- Food challenges
  - Gold standard for diagnosis of food allergy is double-blind placebo-controlled challenge but impractical in many clinical settings.
  - Most sites use single-blind or open food challenge.
  - Used to confirm food allergy in patients when unsure of diagnosis or to assess whether someone has outgrown food allergy (either IgE-mediated or food protein–induced enterocolitis)
  - Challenge must be performed in setting equipped to treat severe allergic reactions.
- Endoscopy with biopsies of esophagus, stomach, and small bowel
  - Patients should be on proton pump inhibitor prior to endoscopy if there are concerns for eosinophilic esophagitis, as GERD may also lead to eosinophils in esophagus.
  - Pathologic findings: increased eosinophils in eosinophilic gastroenteropathy
- Colonoscopy
  - If lower GI symptoms are present
- Elimination diets
  - Should be conducted with care
  - May lack critical nutrients
  - Oral rechallenge should be carefully planned because a more severe reaction may ensue after a food has been temporarily removed.

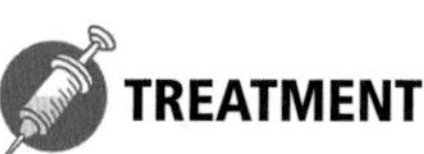

TREATMENT

GENERAL MEASURES

- Avoidance of food allergen
- Education
- Anaphylaxis management plan along with epinephrine autoinjector in event of future reaction
- FPIES acute management plan
- Nutrition evaluation depending on number of foods, type of food, or family needs
- Elemental formula for infants/children with severe or multiple food allergies

MEDICATION

First Line

- Anaphylaxis
  - Epinephrine for severe allergic reaction or anaphylaxis
    - 1st-line of treatment
    - May be repeated every 5 minutes if needed
    - Maximum 3 to 4 doses but should consider epinephrine infusion for severe anaphylaxis
  - H_1 antihistamines (diphenhydramine or cetirizine)
  - H_2 antihistamines may be given in conjunction with H_1 antihistamines (may help with persistent skin and/or abdominal symptoms).
  - Systemic corticosteroids
  - Bronchodilator (in addition to epinephrine if needed)
  - Glucagon in patients on β-blocker if epinephrine does not work
  - Trendelenburg positioning: helps decrease risk of empty ventricle syndrome

ALERT

Once patient's symptoms improve, there is no literature to support >24 hours of corticosteroids/antihistamines.

- Acute FPIES reaction
  - IVF bolus
  - Ondansetron administered IV
  - Removal of offending food
- Chronic FPIES reaction
  - Removal of offending food
  - Ensure adequate growth.
- Eosinophilic esophagitis
  - Dietary restrictions (elemental diet, removal of most common food[s], i.e., milk and/or wheat)
  - "Swallowed" corticosteroids
    - Refers to use of corticosteroid inhaler (no spacer) or nebulized steroid medication made into a slurry and swallowed
    - Patient instructed to avoid eating, drinking, rinsing, or brushing teeth for 30 minutes after use
  - Systemic corticosteroids (briefly)
- Eosinophilic gastroenteritis
  - Dietary restrictions (less successful than in eosinophilic esophagitis)
  - Corticosteroids

ISSUES FOR REFERRAL

Allergy/immunology and/or gastroenterology and/or nutrition follow-up needed for most patients for diagnosis and long-term management

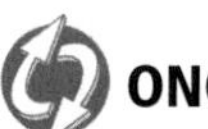

ONGOING CARE

DIET

- Nonanaphylactic and anaphylactic food allergies: removal of the offending food agent from diet
- Nutrition evaluation

PATIENT EDUCATION

- Epinephrine self-administration, if anaphylaxis
- Education regarding specific food avoidance and label reading

PROGNOSIS

- Generally good after offending food antigens are removed from diet and adequate nutrients are ensured
- Tolerance to food allergens may develop over time.
- Current research trials to help induce tolerance in IgE-mediated food allergy are underway (oral immunotherapy, sublingual immunotherapy, and epicutaneous immunotherapy).
- IgE-mediated disease may persist longer than non–IgE mediated.
- Eosinophilic esophagitis and eosinophilic gastroenteritis are considered chronic illnesses.

COMPLICATIONS

- Food allergy
  - Poor growth
  - Feeding disorder
  - Micro- and/or macronutrient deficiency
- Eosinophilic esophagitis
  - Strictures
  - Hiatal hernia concerns
  - Poor growth
  - Feeding disorder
  - Food impaction
  - Micro- and/or macronutrient deficiency

ADDITIONAL READING

- Boyce JA, Assa'ad A, Burks AW, et al; and NIAID-Sponsored Expert Panel. Guidelines for the diagnosis and management of food allergy in the United States: report of the NIAID-sponsored expert panel. *J Allergy Clin Immunol*. 2010;126(Suppl 6):S1–S58.
- Caubet JC, Szajewska H, Shamir R, et al. Non-IgE-mediated gastrointestinal food allergies in children. *Pediatr Allergy Immunol*. 2017;28(1):6–17.
- Cianferoni A, Spergel JM. Food allergy: review, classification and diagnosis. *Allergol Int*. 2009;58(4):457–466.
- Du Toit G, Roberts G, Sayre PH, et al; for LEAP Study Team. Randomized trial of peanut consumption in infants at risk for peanut allergy. *N Engl J Med*. 2015;372(9):803–813.
- Fleischer DM, Perry TT, Atkins D, et al. Allergic reactions to foods in preschool-aged children in a prospective observational food allergy study. *Pediatrics*. 2012;130(1):e25–e32.
- Nwaru BI, Erkkola M, Ahonen S, et al. Age at the introduction of solid foods during the first year and allergic sensitization at age 5 years. *Pediatrics*. 2010;125(1):50–59.
- Perkin MR, Logan K, Marrs T, et al. Enquiring about tolerance (EAT) study: feasibility of an early allergenic food introduction regimen. *J Allergy Clin Immunol*. 2016;137(5):1477–1486.e8.
- Sampson HA, Aceves S, Bock SA, et al. Food allergy: a practice parameter update—2014. *J Allergy Clin Immunol*. 2014;134(5):1016–1025.e43.
- Savage J, Sicherer S, Wood R. The natural history of food allergy. *J Allergy Clin Immunol Pract*. 2016;4(2):196–204.
- Sicherer SH, Sampson HA. Food allergy: recent advances in pathophysiology and treatment. *Annu Rev Med*. 2009;60:261–277.

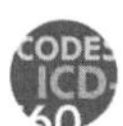

CODES

ICD10

- T78.1XXA Oth adverse food reactions, not elsewhere classified, init
- T78.00XA Anaphylactic reaction due to unspecified food, init encntr
- L27.2 Dermatitis due to ingested food

FAQ

- Q: What are the most common food allergens leading to IgE-mediated allergic reactions in childhood?
- A: Milk, egg, soy, wheat, and peanut are most common food allergens.
- Q: What is the most important medication used to treat anaphylaxis?
- A: Epinephrine given intramuscularly is the 1st-line medication in anaphylaxis.
- Q: What are the new recommendations for food introduction in babies?
- A: New recommendations are to begin adding foods into babies diet between 4 and 6 months of age including "higher risk" foods (milk, egg, soy, wheat, and peanut). Infants at high risk (those with severe atopic dermatitis and/or IgE-mediated food allergy) should be seen by allergist for testing prior to peanut introduction.
- Q: Can food allergies be outgrown?
- A: Yes, many children may outgrow milk, egg, wheat, and soy allergy. Smaller percentages of children may outgrow peanut and tree nut allergies. Newer research focusing on desensitization to foods may offer patients hope.

FOOD HYPERSENSITIVITY (NON-IGE-MEDIATED, GASTROINTESTINAL)

Kirsten M. Kloepfer, MD, MS

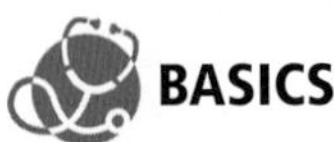

BASICS

DESCRIPTION

- A non–IgE-mediated reaction to a food protein that involves the gastrointestinal (GI) tract
- Previously referred to as milk protein intolerance
- Includes the following:
  - Food protein–induced proctocolitis
  - Food protein–induced enteropathy
  - Food protein–induced enterocolitis syndrome (FPIES)

EPIDEMIOLOGY

- Proctocolitis: >60% of infants with rectal bleeding have proctocolitis.
- Enteropathy: may occur after infectious gastritis
- FPIES
  - Slight male predominance (60%)
  - 30% of infants with FPIES have atopic disease(s).
  - Family history of atopy present in 40–80%

RISK FACTORS

- Proctocolitis
  - 40% react to both milk and soy.
  - 50–60% of infants are breastfed and react to milk and/or soy in mom's diet.
- Enteropathy: usually formula-fed and given intact cow's milk prior to 9 months of age
- FPIES: Exclusive breastfeeding appears to protect against FPIES, but a few cases have been reported.
- Currently, no reports that non–IgE-mediated GI food hypersensitivities are inherited.

PATHOPHYSIOLOGY

- Unclear
- Assumed to be a cell-mediated reaction due to delayed onset

ETIOLOGY

- Cow's milk is the most common cause of proctocolitis, enteropathy, and FPIES, followed by soy, egg, and wheat.
- FPIES: can also react to solid foods thought to be hypoallergenic (rice, oat, barley, chicken, turkey, peanut, potato, corn, fruit protein, fish, and mollusks)

DIAGNOSIS

HISTORY

- Proctocolitis
  - Occurs between 1 and 6 months of age (usually between 2 and 8 weeks)
  - Specks or streaks of blood (± mucus) in the stool of an otherwise healthy infant
  - Absence of vomiting and diarrhea
  - Blood-tinged stools resolve with elimination of offending food protein.
  - Rare in older children
- Enteropathy
  - Occurs between 2 and 24 months of age
  - Persistent diarrhea (rarely bloody)
  - Intermittent vomiting
  - Abdominal pain
  - Failure to thrive (FTT) with hypoproteinemia and anemia
  - Usually formula-fed
  - Do not experience an acute reaction with reexposure
- FPIES
  - Can begin anytime from within a few days of life through 12 months of age
  - FPIES due to solid food usually begins when solids are first introduced (rice cereal).
  - Profuse protracted emesis 1 to 3 hours after exposure to offending food protein
  - Profuse diarrhea 4 to 8 hours after food ingestion in 25% of cases
  - May appear acutely ill with 15% of cases presenting with dehydration and shock
- All non–IgE-mediated GI food hypersensitivities resolve when offending food protein removed from diet.

PHYSICAL EXAM

- Proctocolitis: usually healthy-appearing child with normal physical exam
- Enteropathy
  - Diffuse abdominal pain with distention
  - Weight loss
- FPIES
  - Profuse vomiting and watery diarrhea with signs of dehydration
  - Lethargy, may appear septic

DIFFERENTIAL DIAGNOSIS

- Proctocolitis
  - Anal fissures
  - Vascular malformations
  - Intussusception
  - Meckel diverticulum
- Enteropathy
  - Lactose intolerance
  - Celiac disease
  - Inflammatory bowel disease (IBD)
- FPIES
  - Anaphylaxis
  - Sepsis
  - Necrotizing enterocolitis (NEC)
  - GI infection
  - Reflux
  - Metabolic disorder
  - Surgical abdomen

DIAGNOSTIC TESTS & INTERPRETATION

Diagnostic Procedures/Other

- All non–IgE-mediated GI food hypersensitivities are as follows:
  - Diagnosed clinically
  - No laboratory test available to diagnose hypersensitivity
  - Serum-specific IgE testing and skin testing often negative
- Proctocolitis
  - No endoscopy unless prolonged rectal bleeding, anemia, and/or FTT
  - Eosinophils and lymphoid nodular hyperplasia may be present in the colon.
- Enteropathy
  - Endoscopy shows villous injury with increase in crypt length and villous atrophy.
- FPIES
  - Labs may also show anemia, leukocytosis, eosinophilia, neutrophilia, thrombocytosis, and hypoalbuminemia.
  - If reaction to food is severe, patient may have metabolic acidosis.
  - May see methemoglobinemia in up to 35% of cases that require hospitalization
  - Stool may contain blood, mucus, leukocytes, eosinophils, and/or increased carbohydrate content due to malabsorption.
  - Abdominal x-ray may show intramural gas (may be confused with NEC or ileus).
- With FPIES, if the offending food is discontinued and restarted, the patient will experience vomiting and diarrhea within a few hours (not recommended to be performed at home).

TREATMENT

GENERAL MEASURES

- Proctocolitis
  - Exclusively breastfed infant: Continue breast-feeding with mom eliminating all forms of dairy including casein and whey in packaged food.
  - Symptoms should improve within 72 hours, but it may take up to 2 weeks to completely resolve.
  - If no improvement, eliminate soy in mom's diet, followed by egg.
  - If the infant is formula-fed, consider changing formula to a hydrolysate formula (e.g., Pregestimil®, Nutramigen®, Alimentum®) because many patients are sensitive to both milk and soy protein.
  - If bleeding continues, consider changing formula to an amino acid–based formula (e.g., Neocate®, PurAmino®, EleCare®).
- Enteropathy
  - Eliminate milk from diet.
  - Symptoms should improve in 1 to 3 weeks.
- FPIES
  - Acute episodes should be treated with IV fluids, methylprednisolone (1 mg/kg) to decrease possible cell-mediated intestinal inflammation, plus vasopressors, epinephrine, and/or bicarbonate for shock and possible metabolic acidosis.
  - Long-term management involves strict avoidance of trigger food(s).
  - Stop cow's milk or soy formula and start hydrolysate formula due to possible intolerance to both milk and soy protein.
  - For solid food FPIES:
    - Eliminate trigger food and allow the patient to continue eating foods previously tolerated.
    - Consult allergist for future solid food introduction.

ALERT

If suspect FPIES (patient with vomiting, acute dehydration, lethargy and acidosis), fluid resuscitation and refeeding should be performed in the hospital.

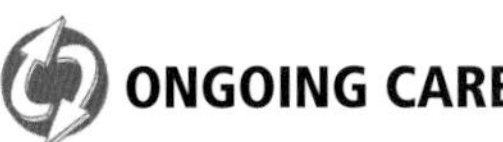

ONGOING CARE

FOLLOW-UP RECOMMENDATIONS

- Proctocolitis
  - 95% tolerate reintroduction of food(s) at 9 months of age. Patient can reintroduce offending food at home 4 to 6 months after beginning protein elimination diet.
  - Prognosis: excellent. Nearly all infants tolerate cow's milk and soy products by 12 months of age.
  - Proctocolitis is not inherited; therefore, subsequent children should not be started on hydrolysate or amino acid formula.
- Enteropathy
  - Most cases resolve spontaneously by 2 years of age.
  - Food can be reintroduced at home 1 to 2 years after beginning protein elimination diet.
- FPIES
  - The trigger food may be reintroduced 12 to 18 months after the last reaction, preferably under the supervision of a physician.
  - Cow's milk and soy FPIES resolve in most patients by 3 years of age.
  - Patients with solid food FPIES may experience protracted courses.
  - Nutritional counseling may be helpful for children with multiple non–IgE-mediated reactions to food.
  - Because close follow-up is needed to determine if tolerance has developed and if an oral food challenge can be performed, an allergy consult is warranted when FPIES is suspected.

ADDITIONAL READING

- Boyce JA, Assa'ad A, Burks AW, et al. Guidelines for the diagnosis and management of food allergy in the United States: summary of the NIAID-sponsored expert panel report. *J Allergy Clin Immunol*. 2010;126(6):1105–1118.
- Caubet JC, Szajewska H, Shamir R, et al. Non-IgE-mediated gastrointestinal food allergies in children. *Pediatr Allergy Immunol*. 2017;28(1):6–17.
- Elizur A, Cohen M, Goldberg MR, et al. Cow's milk associated rectal bleeding: a population based prospective study. *Pediatr Allergy Immunol*. 2012;23(8):766–770.
- Järvinen KM, Nowak-Węgrzyn A. Food protein-induced enterocolitis syndrome (FPIES): current management strategies and review of the literature. *J Allergy Clin Immunol Pract*. 2013;1(4):317–322.
- Lake AM. Food-induced eosinophilic proctocolitis. *J Pediatr Gastroenterol Nutr*. 2000;30(Suppl):S58–S60.
- Mehr S, Kakakios A, Frith K, et al. Food protein-induced enterocolitis syndrome: 16-year experience. *Pediatrics*. 2009;123(3):e459–e464.
- Sampson HA, Anderson JA. Summary and recommendations: classification of gastrointestinal manifestations due to immunologic reactions to foods in infants and young children. *J Pediatr Gastroenterol Nutr*. 2000;30(Suppl):S87–S94.
- Sicherer SH, Eigenmann PA, Sampson HA. Clinical features of food protein-induced enterocolitis syndrome. *J Pediatr*. 1998;133(2):214–219.
- Walker-Smith JA. Cow milk-sensitive enteropathy: predisposing factors and treatment. *J Pediatr*. 1992;121(5 Pt 2):S111–S115.
- Xanthakos SA, Schwimmer JB, Melin-Aldana H, et al. Prevalence and outcome of allergic colitis in healthy infants with rectal bleeding: a prospective cohort study. *J Pediatr Gastroenterol Nutr*. 2005;41(1):16–22.

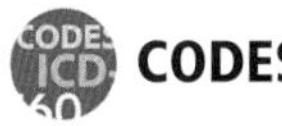

CODES

ICD10

- Z91.011 Allergy to milk products
- E73.9 Lactose intolerance, unspecified
- K90.4 Malabsorption due to intolerance, not elsewhere classified

FAQ

- Q: Will my child outgrow this?
- A: For proctocolitis, most children outgrow milk and/or soy intolerance by 12 months of age. For enterocolitis, symptoms resolve within 1 to 2 years. For FPIES, symptoms may resolve within 1 to 2 years; however, they may persist which is why food challenges are important to determine if symptoms have improved and the food can be safely reintroduced into the diet.
- Q: Should I refer the patient to an allergist?
- A: Infants with suspected FPIES should be referred to an allergist for both evaluation and future food challenges. A patient with proctocolitis or enteropathy that resolves with formula change does not need to be seen by a specialist unless symptoms persist despite a strict elimination diet.
- Q: Can my child have FPIES and an IgE-mediated food allergy?
- A: Although not as common as FPIES alone, there are reports of children with FPIES and elevated food-specific IgE levels. These children tend to have a more protracted course of FPIES and are at increased risk of developing IgE-mediated immediate-type symptoms when challenged. This supports the recommendation to refer children with suspected FPIES to an allergist for further evaluation.

F

FOOD POISONING OR FOODBORNE ILLNESS

Christina R. Hermos, MD

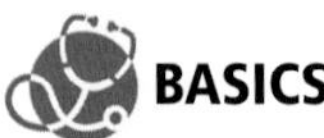

BASICS

DESCRIPTION

Any illness resulting from the ingestion of food or drink contaminated with an infectious organism or associated toxin

EPIDEMIOLOGY

- Highest incidence in children <5 years
- Hospitalizations and death more common in persons >64 years
- See Appendix, Table 8 regarding epidemiologic aspects by organism.

GENERAL PREVENTION

- Vaccination
  - Oral rotavirus vaccine
  - Hepatitis A vaccine
- Preventive strategies
  - Hand washing (soap and water)
  - Avoidance of contaminated water and raw foods (seeded fruits and vegetables)
  - Proper food handling (adequate cooking and refrigeration)
  - Avoidance of unpasteurized dairy products and juices
  - Avoidance of raw or undercooked eggs, meat, and shellfish
  - Avoidance of honey in children <1 year old

PATHOPHYSIOLOGY

- Gastroenteritis
  - Viral epithelial invasion/replication or ingestion of preformed elaborated toxin
- Noninflammatory diarrhea
  - Selective destruction of absorptive cells in mucosa, leaving secretory cells intact
  - Toxin elaboration (secretory diarrhea)
  - Impairment of brush border enzymes and lactose intolerance (osmotic diarrhea)
- Inflammatory diarrhea/dysentery
  - Direct mucosal invasion of intestinal epithelial cells (colon)
  - Toxin elaboration
  - Inflammatory infiltration destroys villous cells and transporters and leads to exudation of mucus/protein/blood into gut.
- Local/remote invasion (bacteremia, meningitis, hepatitis, septic arthritis, osteomyelitis)
- Immune-mediated extraintestinal manifestations (hemolytic uremic syndrome (HUS), reactive arthritis, Guillain-Barré syndrome [GBS])

ETIOLOGY

- Viruses
  - Most common cause of foodborne illness
  - Caliciviruses (norovirus, sapovirus)
  - Rotavirus (infant/child)
  - Astrovirus
  - Enteric adenovirus
  - Hepatitis A
- Bacteria
  - *Salmonella typhi*, *Salmonella paratyphi*, nontyphoidal *Salmonella*
  - *Campylobacter jejuni*, *Campylobacter coli*
  - *Shigella sonnei*, *Shigella flexneri*, *Shigella boydii*
  - *Escherichia coli*
    - Enterohemorrhagic *E. coli* (EHEC) including Shiga toxin–producing *E. coli* (STEC)
    - Enteropathogenic *E. coli* (EPEC)
    - Enterotoxigenic *E. coli* (ETEC)
    - Enteroinvasive *E. coli* (EIEC)
    - Enteroaggregative *E. coli* (EAEC)
  - *Vibrio cholerae*, *Vibrio parahaemolyticus*, *Vibrio vulnificus*
  - *Listeria monocytogenes*
  - *Brucella* spp.
  - *Yersinia enterocolitica*
- Toxin mediated
  - *Clostridium perfringens*
  - *Staphylococcus aureus*
  - *Bacillus cereus*
  - *Clostridium botulinum*
- Parasites
  - *Entamoeba histolytica*
  - *Giardia intestinalis*
  - *Cryptosporidium*
  - *Cyclospora cayetanensis*
  - *Toxoplasma gondii*
  - *Trichinella spiralis*

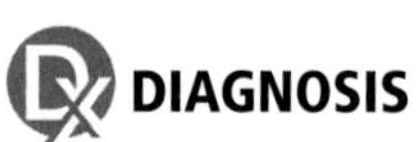

DIAGNOSIS

Signs and symptoms

- Gastroenteritis
  - Sudden onset vomiting
  - Fever and diarrhea may also be present.
  - Consider: viral etiology, preformed toxin ingestion
- Noninflammatory diarrhea
  - Acute watery diarrhea, abdominal pain, without fever/dysentery
  - Some may present with fever.
  - Consider: ETEC, viral or parasitic etiology
- Inflammatory diarrhea
  - Bloody stool, abdominal pain and fever
  - Consider: *Shigella*, *Campylobacter*, *Salmonella*, EIEC, EHEC, STEC O157:H7, EAEC, *V. parahaemolyticus*, *Y. enterocolitica*, *Entamoeba*
- Chronic diarrhea >14 days
  - 3 or more unformed stools per day
  - Consider: *Giardia*, other parasitic etiology
- Neurologic manifestations
  - Paresthesias, respiratory depression, bronchospasm, cranial nerve palsies, GBS
  - Consider: *C. botulinum* toxin, organophosphate, fish toxin poisons, *C. jejuni*
- Systemic illness
  - Fever, weakness, jaundice, arthritis, osteomyelitis
  - Consider: *Listeria*, *Brucella*, *Trichinella*, *Toxoplasma*, *V. vulnificus*, hepatitis A, *S. typhi*, *S. paratyphi*

HISTORY

- Incubation period from suspected exposure
- Duration of illness
- Predominant symptoms
- Similarly exposed persons with related symptoms
- Type of food ingested and type of exposure (location of exposure, pet contact, travel, occupation, institutional/daycare)
- See Appendix, Table 9 regarding clinical symptoms by organism.

PHYSICAL EXAM

- Neurologic examination
- Assessment of dehydration status (examination of mucous membranes, skin turgor)
- Assessment for disseminated disease (sepsis, septic arthritis, osteomyelitis)
- Abdominal examination
- Assessment for liver involvement (hepatomegaly, jaundice, icterus)

DIFFERENTIAL DIAGNOSIS

- Appendicitis, peritonitis, pyelonephritis, pelvic inflammatory disease
- Irritable bowel syndrome
- Inflammatory bowel disease (IBD)
- Malignancy
- Medication adverse effect
- *Clostridium difficile* enterocolitis
- Malabsorption syndromes (celiac disease, cystic fibrosis, malnutrition)
- Food intolerance or allergy
  - Cow's milk (protein allergy)
  - Carbohydrate intolerance (e.g., lactose)
- Dietary manipulations
  - Hyperosmolar formulas
  - Food additives (dyes, processing materials, coloring)
  - Caffeine
  - Overfeeding
  - Excessive fluids
  - Munchausen by proxy
- Ingestion of noninfectious foodborne illness (contaminated seafood, mushroom poisoning, chemical poisoning)

DIAGNOSTIC TESTS & INTERPRETATION

Initial Tests (screening, lab, imaging)

- Routine bacterial stool culture
  - *Salmonella* and *Shigella* species and *C. jejuni/coli*
  - Cultures for *Vibrio* and *Yersinia*, EC O157:H7, and other *Campylobacter* require additional media or incubation conditions and may require communication with laboratory if suspected.
  - Toxin testing, serotyping, and molecular techniques may only be available from large commercial or public health labs.
- Blood/CSF cultures as clinically indicated
- Serology (hepatitis A, *Brucella*, toxoplasmosis, *Trichinella*)
- Ova/parasite examination
- Direct antigen testing/DFA (*Giardia*, *Cryptosporidium*, *Entamoeba*, *Rotavirus*)

- Polymerase chain reaction (PCR) identification is most sensitive (norovirus and increasing availability for other pathogens).
- Careful monitoring of patients with hemorrhagic colitis during illness and 5 to 10 days after resolution of diarrhea to detect HUS (oliguria/hematuria, edema, pallor; evaluate with CBC with smear, BUN/Cr)

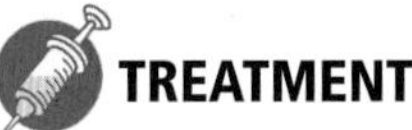

TREATMENT

GENERAL MEASURES

- Gastroenteritis
  - Treat dehydration with oral rehydration solution (ORS):
    - Standard ORS contains 75 to 90 mEq of sodium and 74 to 111 mmol/L of glucose.
    - Alternative ORS, including rice-based carbohydrate or amylase-based solutions, may be more effective for *V. cholerae* infections.
  - Transition rapidly (after 3 to 4 hours of ORS tolerance) to regular diet (see below)
  - Continue breastfeeding infants if possible.
  - PO/nasogastric hydration preferable but IV fluids for indications below
- Botulism
  - Continuous cardiac and respiratory monitoring may need assisted ventilation.

MEDICATION

Use of antibiotics:

- Always indicated
  - *Brucella*
  - *L. monocytogenes* (invasive disease)
  - Invasive *S. typhi*, *S. paratyphi*, nontyphoidal *Salmonella*
  - *Vibrio* spp.
  - *C. cayetanensis*
  - *Trichinella*
  - *E. histolytica*
- Sometimes indicated
  - *E. coli* (severe ETEC in a traveler in resource-limited country)
  - *Shigella* (severe cases and immunocompromised hosts)
  - *Campylobacter* (in severe cases, early treatment limits duration, shortens duration of shedding)
  - Nontyphi *Salmonella*
    - Treatment indicated to reduce risks of bacterial translocation in select populations: patients <3 months old, immunocompromised, hemoglobinopathy, chronic GI condition (IBD)
    - Other patients should not be treated, as antibiotics prolong organism shedding in the stool and promote disease spread.
  - *Y. enterocolitica* (neonates, immunocompromised and invasive disease)
  - *T. gondii* (pregnant and immunocompromised patients)
  - *G. intestinalis*
  - *Cryptosporidium* (severe disease, immunocompromised host)
- Contraindicated
  - *C. botulinum* (aminoglycosides potentiate paralytic effects)
  - EHEC
  - Antimotility agents are contraindicated in children with inflammatory or bloody diarrhea.

ADDITIONAL THERAPIES

Botulism: For suspected infant botulism cases, human-derived antitoxin, BabyBIG (human botulism immune globulin, BIG-IV), may be obtained from the Infant Botulism Treatment and Prevention Program, California Department of Public Health (24-hour line: 510-231-7600).

COMPLEMENTARY & ALTERNATIVE THERAPIES

Supplements with specific probiotic strains (e.g., *Lactobacillus GG*) may reduce duration of less severe, nonrotaviral diarrhea and hospital stays.

ADMISSION, INPATIENT, AND NURSING CONSIDERATIONS

If patient is unable to be rehydrated via oral route (because of ileus, circulatory failure, CNS complications) or if >10% dehydration

ONGOING CARE

Reporting requirements

- Foodborne diseases and conditions generally notifiable at the national level include the following:
  - Botulism, brucellosis, cholera, STEC O157:H7, HUS, listeriosis, salmonellosis (other than *S. typhi*), shigellosis, typhoid fever (*S. typhi and S. paratyphi* infections), hepatitis A, cryptosporidiosis, cyclosporiasis, giardiasis, trichinellosis
- Additional reporting requirements may be mandated by state and territorial laws and regulations: Full reporting instructions are available:
  - 1-800-CDC-INFO (1-800-232-4636)
  - http://www.cdc.gov/foodsafety/fdoss/reporting/how-to-report.html

DIET

Balanced, varied diet; providing easily digestible, complex carbohydrates will promote improved stool consistency.

PROGNOSIS

- Most gastroenteritis is mild and self-limited.
- Recovery is complete in 2 to 5 days in most individuals.
- In the very young, prognosis is more guarded because these patients can become dehydrated quickly.
- After the patient has survived the paralytic phase of botulism, the outlook for complete recovery is excellent.

ADDITIONAL READING

- Centers for Disease Control and Prevention. Diagnosis and management of foodborne illnesses: a primer for physicians and other health care professionals. *MMWR Recomm Rep*. 2004;53(RR-4):1–33.
- Centers for Disease Control and Prevention. *Surveillance for Foodborne Disease Outbreaks, United States, 2014, Annual Report*. Atlanta, GA: US Department of Health and Human Services, CDC; 2016.
- Davidson G, Barnes G, Bass D, et al. Infectious diarrhea in children: working group report of the First World Congress of Pediatric Gastroenterology, Hepatology, and Nutrition. *J Pediatr Gastroenterol Nutr*. 2002;35(Suppl 2):S143–S150.
- Huang JY, Henao OL, Griffin PM, et al. Infection with pathogens transmitted commonly through food and the effect of increasing use of culture-independent diagnostic tests on surveillance—Foodborne Diseases Active Surveillance Network, 10 U.S. Sites, 2012–2015. *MMWR Morb Mortal Wkly Rep*. 2016;65(14):368–371.
- Scallan E, Hoekstra RM, Angulo FJ, et al. Foodborne illness acquired in the United States—major pathogens. *Emerg Infect Dis*. 2011;17(1):7–15.

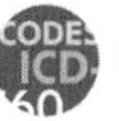

CODES

ICD10

- T62.91XA Toxic effect of unsp noxious sub eaten as food, acc, init
- A05.9 Bacterial foodborne intoxication, unspecified
- A02.0 Salmonella enteritis

FAQ

- Q: What are the most common causes of food poisoning?
- A: Viruses, particularly norovirus, are the leading cause of foodborne illnesses. The most common bacterial causes include *Salmonella* (nontyphi), *C. perfringens*, and *C. jejuni*. The most common parasitis infection is *Giardia*.
- Q: How are the signs and symptoms of food poisoning different from those of a viral gastroenteritis?
- A: The signs and symptoms of food poisoning and gastroenteritis are similar in that the patient displays diarrhea, vomiting, and fever. Historically, food poisoning is distinguished by its association with a common food that affects multiple individuals who consumed it.
- Q: Which foods are most likely to be contaminated?
- A: Poorly cooked foods (e.g., eggs, meats, fish, shellfish), unpasteurized milk and juices, inadequately washed fresh produce, home canned goods, soft unpasteurized cheeses

FRAGILE X SYNDROME

Chad R. Haldeman-Englert, MD • Marni J. Falk, MD

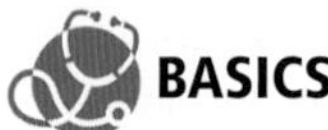

BASICS

DESCRIPTION
- Most common cause of inherited intellectual disability (ID)
- Caused by mutations in the *FMR1* gene on chromosome Xq27.3

EPIDEMIOLOGY
- Affects ~1 in 4,000 to 6,000 males; prevalence in females is ~1/2 than in males.
- Carrier prevalence in females for *FMR1* premutation is 1:382 and for intermediate allele(s) is 1:143.

RISK FACTORS
Genetics
- Caused by loss-of-function mutations in the *FMR1* gene on chromosome Xq27.3
- >99% of affected individuals have a trinucleotide (CGG) repeat expansion (>200 repeats) within the 5′ untranslated region of the *FMR1* gene.
- Repeat size categories (based on guidelines from the American College of Medical Genetics):
  - Normal number of repeats: 5 to 44
  - Intermediate ("gray zone"): 45 to 54
  - Premutation: 55 to 200
  - Full mutation: >200
- Other *FMR1* gene mutations may rarely occur (<1% cases).
- Fragile X syndrome is inherited in an X-linked manner.
- Fragile X is a CGG trinucleotide repeat disorder that shows anticipation, in which the phenotype can be more severe in subsequent generations due to an expansion in the number of CGG repeats.
- Expansion only may occur in the germline of mothers who carry a premutation range repeat allele of *FMR1*.
  - Expansion does not always occur in offspring of female premutation carriers. In general, the larger the number of CGG repeats (>50), the higher the probability that expansion to a full mutation will occur.
- A male with a premutation will pass on the premutation to 100% of his daughters and none of his sons.
- Females with a full mutation are typically less severely affected than males because their second *FMR1* allele is typically normal and, assuming random X-inactivation occurs, produces variable amounts of fragile X mental retardation protein (FMRP).
- Males with mosaicism for the *FMR1* full mutation (some cells with the full mutation and other cells with the premutation) are generally less severely affected (average IQ 60) relative to males with the full mutation in all the cells.
- Patients with larger chromosomal deletions involving *FMR1* and other nearby genes typically have a more severe phenotype

GENERAL PREVENTION
- Prenatal diagnosis by chorionic villus sampling (~10–12 weeks' gestation) or amniocentesis (~16–20 weeks' gestation) is possible for at-risk pregnancies.
- Preimplantation genetic diagnosis in the setting of in vitro fertilization is possible for at-risk couples when a familial *FMR1* mutation is known.

PATHOPHYSIOLOGY
Residual FMRP protein levels directly correlate with the severity of fragile X syndrome manifestations:
- Absence of FMRP results in characteristic craniofacial, neurologic, and connective tissue abnormalities.
- Decreased FMRP levels may cause long-term depression of hippocampal synaptic transmission via specific glutamate receptors, with resulting behavioral and neuronal phenotypes.

COMMONLY ASSOCIATED CONDITIONS
Other *FMR1*-related disorders include fragile X–associated tremor/ataxia syndrome (FXTAS) and premature ovarian insufficiency (POI):
- FXTAS can be seen in older (age >50 years) male and female premutation carriers. Clinical features include intention tremors, abnormal gait with frequent falling, cerebral atrophy, and memory deficits.
- POI can be seen in 20–25% of female premutation carriers, with menopause occurring prior to age 40 years.

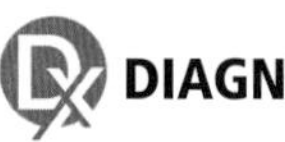

DIAGNOSIS

HISTORY
- Birth/neonatal history
  - Normal to increased birth weight
  - May have large head circumference at birth
  - Feeding problems and frequent emesis due to gastroesophageal reflux may occur but improves with growth.
  - Irritability may result from sensory integration difficulties and tactile defensiveness.
- Past medical history
  - Strabismus and hyperopia occur in 40%
  - Frequent ear infections in ~60%: Conductive hearing loss is possible.
  - Mitral valve prolapse (MVP) and aortic root dilation can occur, typically in adults.
  - Seizures occur in 14–44% of children and may resolve by adolescence.
  - Gastrointestinal problems (diarrhea, gastroesophageal reflux) in ~10%
  - Periventricular heterotopia seen on magnetic resonance imaging (MRI)
  - Pes planus
  - Scoliosis
  - Sleep issues: problems falling asleep, awakening at night, early waking, parasomnias, obstructive sleep apnea
- Developmental/behavioral history
  - Motor delay due to hypotonia
  - Speech may be absent to minimally affected.
  - Autism (60% of males with full mutation)
  - Severe ID in males (average IQ of males with the full mutation is 41, with range of 30 to 55)
  - Borderline or mild ID in 50% of females with the full mutation (IQ range 70 to 85)
  - Tantrums occur around age 2 years.
  - Hyperactivity can be severe.
  - Obsessive and compulsive behaviors
  - Often requires routine for daily activities
  - Social anxiety: Patients are shy and easily overwhelmed by noisy environments.
- Family history
  - Fragile X syndrome
  - ID or autism, especially in males related through the maternal side
  - Tremors or ataxia developing >50 years
  - POI in females <40 years
  - No male–male transmission

PHYSICAL EXAM
- Growth parameters
  - Height, weight, and head circumference
- Characteristic facial features
  - Large head, prominent forehead
  - Long face
  - Large and protruding ears
  - High palate
  - Prominent chin (after puberty)
- Murmur or midsystolic click (MVP)
- Large testicles (after puberty)
- Joint hypermobility, pes planus, scoliosis
- Skin often feels soft and smooth

DIFFERENTIAL DIAGNOSIS
- In early childhood, the symptoms of fragile X syndrome are often nonspecific.
- Other genetic syndromes with overlapping features include the following:
  - Fragile XE syndrome (FRAXE): Patients have a milder degree of ID as well as less specific physical characteristics compared to patients with typical fragile X syndrome (FRAXA). Mutations of *FMR2* on Xq28 are associated with FRAXE.
  - Sotos syndrome: Patients have overgrowth (macrocephaly), ID, behavioral abnormalities, and cardiac and renal defects. Mutations or deletions of *NSD1* are causative of this syndrome.
  - Abnormal parent-specific imprinting of chromosome 15q11 to q13:
    - Paternal chromosome affected: Prader-Willi syndrome—infantile hypotonia, obesity, hyperphagia, developmental delay, cognitive deficits, and behavioral abnormalities
    - Maternal chromosome affected: Angelman syndrome—severe developmental delay or ID, minimal to no speech development, gait ataxia and/or tremulousness of the limbs, and inappropriate happy demeanor that includes frequent laughing, smiling, and excitability
  - A range of other genes is now recognized to cause syndromic autism and X-linked ID. *PTEN* mutations can be associated with macrocephaly and autism. Clinical diagnostic testing either individually, through gene panels, or exome sequencing is available (www.genetests.org).

DIAGNOSTIC TESTS & INTERPRETATION

Initial Tests (screening, lab, imaging)

- Consider *FMR1* mutation testing in the following:
  - Males or females with features of autism, developmental delays, or ID
  - Males or females with clinical findings consistent with fragile X syndrome
  - Family history of fragile X syndrome, recurrent ID or autism, especially in affected males through the maternal side
  - Males or females with tremor and/or ataxia developing age >50 years
  - Females with POI age <40 years
- Polymerase chain reaction (PCR)–based analysis is typically the 1st-line genetic test to determine if there is a repeat expansion and define the number of CGG repeats within the *FMR1* gene. Southern blot analysis can also be performed if PCR testing is not available or results are unclear.

Follow-Up Tests & Special Considerations

- Methylation status can be determined by using a restriction enzyme that selectively cuts nonmethylated DNA or by methylation-sensitive PCR techniques. This may be considered for higher functioning males with a full mutation to establish their degree of *FMR1* methylation.
- Standard karyotype analysis will typically not be able to detect the repeat expansion.
- If the patient has many clinical features of fragile X syndrome and Southern blot analysis is normal, consider further molecular techniques to detect point mutations or whole/partial *FMR1* gene deletions.

Diagnostic Procedures/Other

- Echocardiogram if cardiac exam is consistent with MVP (usually in adults)
- Aortic root dilation may be seen but typically does not progress or require specific treatment.
- Evaluate for hypertension.
- Assess for seizure activity.
- Evaluate GERD if symptomatic.
- Developmental evaluations
  - Feeding assessment in infants
  - Education planning
    - Speech and language
    - Hearing assessment
    - Occupational and physical therapy
    - Behavioral/neuropsychological testing

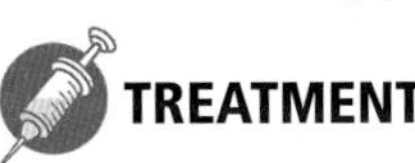

TREATMENT

GENERAL MEASURES

- Treatment is aimed at supportive measures.
- Per American Academy of Pediatrics (AAP) guidelines, routine evaluation for ocular, ENT, skeletal, and neurologic abnormalities. Refer to appropriate specialists as needed.
- Early developmental services
  - Physical therapy for joint laxity/hypotonia
  - Occupational therapy
  - Speech and language therapy
  - Social integration therapy
- Some patients do well in a mainstream school with appropriate support, whereas others require a school for children with special needs.
- Behavioral therapies involve avoidance of overstimulation and providing positive reinforcement.

MEDICATION

- No specific medications are available.
- Some medications are used to treat specific symptoms in individual patients:
  - Medications for hyperactivity (e.g., methylphenidate, clonidine, others)
  - Selective serotonin reuptake inhibitors (SSRIs) (e.g., fluoxetine) for obsessive and compulsive behaviors, social phobia, anxiety, and depression
  - Atypical antipsychotic medications (e.g., risperidone) for psychosis or paranoia
  - Valproic acid or carbamazepine for seizures and/or mood stabilization, lamotrigine can be used as a 2nd-line treatment for seizures.
  - Melatonin and/or clonidine for sleep

ADDITIONAL THERAPIES

- Experimental therapies
  - Glutamate receptor antagonists, γ-aminobutyric acid (GABA) receptor agonists, SSRIs, minocycline, carnitine, valproic acid, and lovastatin have shown some improvement in some of the neurologic and behavioral symptoms.
- Surgery/other procedures
  - Myringotomy tubes if with frequent ear infections and/or conductive hearing loss
  - Inguinal hernia repair, if present
  - Strabismus repair, if necessary
  - Corrective lenses for refractive errors

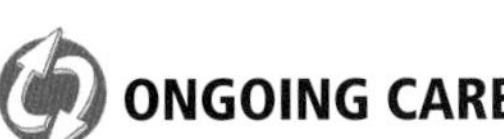

ONGOING CARE

FOLLOW-UP RECOMMENDATIONS

Patient Monitoring

- Regular follow-up with a behavioral and developmental pediatrician as well as a psychiatrist/psychologist is recommended for patients with behavioral problems.
- Hypertension can occur in adults with fragile X syndrome. Therefore, annual blood pressure and cardiac exam should be performed. Hypertension can be treated with typical medications used in the general population. If hypertension is refractory to treatment, evaluate for other causes of high blood pressure (e.g., renal).

DIET

No specific dietary requirements

PROGNOSIS

Most patients generally have a normal lifespan.

ADDITIONAL READING

- American Academy of Pediatrics. Health supervision for children with fragile X syndrome. *Pediatrics*. 2011;127(5):994–1006.
- Ligsay A, Hagerman RJ. Review of targeted treatments in fragile X syndrome. *Intractable Rare Dis Res*. 2016;5(3):158–167.
- Lozano R, Azarang A, Wilaisakditipakorn T, Hagerman RJ. Fragile X syndrome: a review of clinical management. *Intractable Rare Dis Res*. 2016:5(3):145–157.
- Monaghan KG, Lyon E, Spector EB; for American College of Medical Genetics. ACMG standards and guidelines for fragile X testing: a revision to the disease-specific supplements to the standards and guidelines for Clinical Genetics Laboratories of the American College of Medical Genetics and Genomics. *Genet Med*. 2013;15(7):575–586.
- National Fragile X Foundation: www.fragilex.org
- Online Mendelian Inheritance in Man. Fragile X mental retardation syndrome. http://www.omim.org/entry/300624. Accessed December 3, 2014.
- Saul RA, Tarleton JC. FMR1-related disorders. In: Pagon RA, Adam MP, Ardinger HH, et al., eds. GeneReviews® [Internet]. Seattle (WA): University of Washington, Seattle; 1993–2017. https://www.ncbi.nlm.nih.gov/books/NBK1384/.

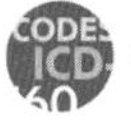

CODES

ICD10

Q99.2 Fragile X chromosome

FAQ

- Q: Why is it called "fragile X syndrome"?
- A: Early cytogenetic studies of male patients with ID identified a site on the X chromosome that would appear constricted when the patient's cells were grown with special culture techniques to induce "fragile" sites.
- Q: How many CGG repeats are necessary to cause the full mutation resulting in fragile X syndrome?
- A: >200 repeats
- Q: What are typical facial features seen in patients with fragile X syndrome?
- A: Prominent forehead, long face, protruding ears, and a prominent chin
- Q: When does the macroorchidism associated with fragile X syndrome typically develop?
- A: After puberty

F

FROSTBITE

Susan Fuchs, MD

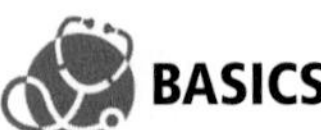

BASICS

DESCRIPTION

- Localized injury of epidermis and underlying tissue resulting from exposure to extreme cold or contact with extremely cold objects
- Distal extremities and unprotected areas (i.e., fingers, toes, ears, nose, and chin) most commonly affected
- Feet and hands account for 90% of frostbite injuries.
  - Severity of injury is based on findings after rewarming (see "Physical Exam").

RISK FACTORS

- Alcohol use
- Arthritis
- Atherosclerosis
- Constricting clothing
- Diabetes mellitus
- High altitude
- Hypothermia
- Immobilization
- Improper use of halogenated hydrocarbons (e.g., Freon®, carbon dioxide fire extinguisher)
- Medications: β-blockers, neuroleptics, sedating drugs
- Previous cold injury
- Smoking tobacco
- Trauma
- Vasoconstrictive drugs
- Body parts most affected:
  - Fingers
  - Toes
  - Nose
  - Cheeks
  - Ears
  - Male genitalia
- Groups at risk:
  - Mentally ill patients
  - Patients with impaired circulation
  - Winter sports enthusiasts and fans
  - Homeless persons
  - Very thin individuals
  - Malnourished people
  - Outdoor laborers
  - Military personnel, especially those of African American and Afro-Caribbean descent, exposed to cold, wet climates
  - Elderly people
  - Infants

GENERAL PREVENTION

- Avoid prolonged cold exposure whenever possible.
- Maintain adequate nutrition and hydration when spending time in cold weather.
- Dress appropriately for cold weather:
  - Dress in layers: Clothing should be made of material that absorbs perspiration and prevents heat loss, such as polypropylene, polyester or synthetic wool, and inner insulation layer such as fleece or wool, and outerwear should be windproof and water repellent but also allow for ventilation and moisture transfer.
  - Cover head, ears, and neck.
  - Mittens help to conserve heat better than gloves.
  - Footwear should be water-repellent and insulated.

PATHOPHYSIOLOGY

- Direct cellular damage can occur from frostbite, as temperature of freezing tissue approaches −2°C.
- Tissue damage and cell death result from initial freeze injury and inflammatory response that occurs with rewarming.
- The prefreeze phase consists of tissue cooling, vasoconstriction, and ischemia.
- In the freeze-thaw phase, ice crystals can form extracellularly (slow freeze) or intracellularly (rapid freeze). This process causes cellular electrolyte shifts, cellular dehydration, cell membrane lysis, and cell death.
- The thawing phase involves ischemia-reperfusion injury and inflammatory response.
- In vascular stasis phase, blood vessels constrict and dilate, blood can leak from vessels or coagulate within them.
- Late ischemic phase involves progressive ischemia and infarction, including the release of inflammatory mediators, especially prostaglandin F2, thromboxane A2, bradykinins, and histamine. There is intermittent vasoconstriction of vessels, emboli production, and thrombi formation, leading to cell death.
- Most severe injuries are seen in tissues that freeze, thaw, and freeze again.

DIAGNOSIS

- Based on a history of cold exposure
- Assessment of skin perfusion should occur after rewarming. This includes skin color, temperature, sensation, pulses and capillary refill.
- The classification systems listed below can assess severity of injury and guide therapy, but return of sensation as below is also helpful.
  - Superficial, 1st degree: transient tingling, stinging, and burning followed by throbbing and aching with possible hyperhidrosis (excess sweating)
  - Superficial, 2nd degree: numbness, with vasomotor disturbances in more severe cases
  - Deep, 3rd degree: no sensation initially, followed by shooting pains, burning, throbbing, and aching
  - Deep, 4th degree: absence of sensation

HISTORY

- Was there prolonged exposure to cold environment? In frostbite, history of prolonged cold exposure is typical.
- Was there contact with a cold object, especially metal? Metal will drain heat from skin through conduction and increase the risk of frostbite.
- Was there immersion in cold water, as this increases the rate of cooling?
- What was the timing and duration of exposure?
- Was there any treatment prior to presentation?
- Does the patient have any underlying medical conditions or behaviors that put him or her at risk?
  - Peripheral vascular disease, medications, smoking, etc.

PHYSICAL EXAM

- 1st degree: numbness and erythema. A white plaque surrounded by erythema and edema develops within 24 hours.
- 2nd degree: blister formation with clear or milky fluid, surrounded by erythema and edema within 24 hours
- 3rd degree: death of skin and subcutaneous tissues resulting in hemorrhagic blisters
- 4th degree: tissue necrosis to muscle and bone. Initially, body part is hard, cold, white, and numb postrewarming.
- Another classification system can be used for hands and feet, based on the level of the skin lesions after rewarming, as surrogate markers for amputation risk.
  - Grade 1: no cyanosis to the extremity = no bone amputation
  - Grade 2: cyanosis of distal phalanx = moderate risk of amputation
  - Grade 3: cyanosis to intermediate and proximal phalangeal joints = high risk of amputation
  - Grade 4: cyanosis over carpal or tarsal bones = 100% bone amputation
- To simplify classification after rewarming, there is a two-tier classification scheme:
  - Superficial—no or minimal anticipated tissue loss, corresponding to 1st- and 2nd-degree injury
  - Deep-deeper injury and anticipated tissue loss corresponding to 3rd- and 4th-degree injury

DIFFERENTIAL DIAGNOSIS

- Frostnip: mild form of cold injury with pallor and painful, tingling sensation. Warming of cold tissue results in no tissue damage.
- Hypothermia
- Thermal injury: easily excluded based on history but can result from warming techniques

DIAGNOSTIC TESTS & INTERPRETATION

Initial Tests (screening, lab, imaging)

- Labs usually not necessary but may be indicated when infection is suspected
- No diagnostic studies done immediately after rewarming can accurately predict amount of nonviable tissue
- Standard or digital subtraction angiography or triple-phase bone scanning with technetium (99m-Tc) can be used to identify candidates for thrombolytic therapy. It is also useful to predict the long-term viability of affected tissue. MRI and MRA are being advocated by some as superior techniques for severe frostbite. They allow for direct visualization of occluded vessels and tissue, giving a more clear-cut demarcation of ischemic tissue injury, which may allow for earlier surgical intervention, but experience is limited.

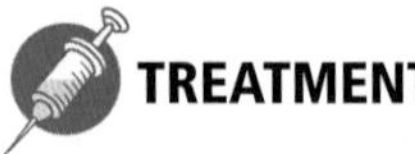

TREATMENT

GENERAL MEASURES

- Check core temperature to rule out hypothermia, which would need to be addressed first.
- Remove wet clothing.
- Remove constrictive clothing and jewelry.
- Rapid rewarming in warm water (37–39°C) for 20 to 45 minutes, ideally in a whirlpool, but if not available, gentle active motion of the extremity while rewarming may help.
  - Do not rewarm slowly.
  - Do not rub while rewarming.
  - Rewarming is complete when skin is soft and sensation returns.
  - Usually all that is needed for superficial, 1st-degree frostbite
- Do not rewarm with direct heat.
- Allow to air dry then apply dry, sterile, bulky dressings loosely to affected areas and between frostbitten toes and fingers.
- Intact, nontense clear blisters should be left in place and wrapped with loosely applied dry gauze dressings. Rupturing may increase the risk of infection.
- Tense or hemorrhagic blister may be carefully aspirated, but this increases the risk for infection.
- Ruptured blisters should be debrided and covered with antibiotic ointment and nonadhesive dressings.
- Elevate affected parts to minimize edema.
- Warm IV fluids (0.9 normal saline) in small boluses if dehydrated

- Daily hydrotherapy. Some advocate for hexachlorophene or povidone-iodine added to water.
- Topical application of aloe vera (for its antiprostaglandin effect) to debrided blisters and intact hemorrhagic blisters to minimize further thromboxane synthesis with every dressing change

ALERT
- Prohibit nicotine use because of its vasoconstrictive properties.
- Full extent of injury may not be apparent at presentation. Close observation is important.

MEDICATION
- Tetanus prophylaxis: dT, dTap, or DT/DTaP, depending on age, and tetanus immunoglobulin if patient not fully immunized
- Ibuprofen 12 mg/kg/24 h PO divided twice a day (or aspirin)
- Analgesics (opiates): as indicated
- Antibiotics: for those with significant trauma, other potential infection sources or signs of cellulitis or sepsis only
- Tissue plasminogen activator (tPA) given intra-arterial or intravenously is being used by frostbite specialists within 24 hours for deep frostbite, for those without contraindications (stroke or persistent neurologic impairment, recent GI bleeding intracranial trauma, recent surgery). It is useful when microvascular thrombosis has already developed. Studies show it can significantly reduce digital amputation rates. It must be given in a hospital experienced in giving tPA and intensive care monitoring. It is given concurrently with IV heparin.
- Iloprost, a prostacyclin analog with vasodilatory properties, given intravenously, has shown benefit if given within 48 hours, with reduced amputation rates for deep injuries, but the IV formulation is not approved by the U.S. Food and Drug Administration or available in the United States.

SURGERY/OTHER PROCEDURES
- Conservative surgical intervention: recommended because it usually takes 6 to 8 weeks for injured tissue to declare viability
- Escharotomy: performed on digits with impaired circulation or movement
- Fasciotomy: performed if significant edema causes compartment syndrome
- Early amputation and debridement with closure of wound site: necessary for uncontrolled infection
- Debridement of mummified tissue: performed after 1 to 3 months

ADMISSION, INPATIENT, AND NURSING CONSIDERATIONS
- Hospital admission is determined on an individual basis; factors such as severity of the injury, comorbidities, and the need for hospital-based interventions (tPA).
- Ongoing excellent wound care: daily hydrotherapy, monitoring blisters (if present), edema, signs of infection
- Surgical consultation as needed

ONGOING CARE

PROGNOSIS
- Depends on degree of cold injury
- Superficial, 1st-degree frostbite heals in a few weeks.
- Favorable indicators: sensation in affected area, healthy-looking skin color, blisters filled with clear fluid
- Unfavorable indicators: cyanosis, blood-filled blisters, unhealthy-looking skin color
- Significant swelling should prompt an evaluation for compartment syndrome.
- Early rehabilitation often needed for functional recovery
- Long-term follow-up for 6 to 12 months to monitor for sequelae
- Education to avoid reexposure and reinjury

COMPLICATIONS
- Arthritis
- Changes in skin color
- Chronic numbness
- Chronic pain
- Cold hypersensitivity
- Digital deformities
- Gangrene
- Growth plate abnormalities (only in children)
- Hyperesthesias
- Increased risk of frostbite
- Neuropathy
- Premature closure of the physis (in children)
- Reduced sensitivity to touch and position
- Rhabdomyolysis
- Squamous cell carcinoma (rare)
- Tetanus
- Tissue loss
- Vasospasm
- Wound infection

ADDITIONAL READING

- Cauchy E, Davis CB, Pasquier M, et al. A new proposal for management of severe frostbite in the austere environment. *Wilderness Environ Med*. 2016;27(1):92–99.
- Fudge J. Preventing and managing hypothermia and frostbite injury. *Sports Health*. 2016;8(2):133–139.
- Handford C, Buxton P, Russell K, et al. Frostbite: a practical approach to hospital management. *Extrem Physiol Med*. 2014;3:7.
- Handford C, Thomas O, Imray CHE. Frostbite. *Emerg Med Clin North Am*. 2017;35(2):281–299.
- Heil K, Thomas R, Robertson G, et al. Freezing and non-freezing cold weather injuries: a systematic review. *Br Med Bull*. 2016;117(1):79–93.
- McIntosh SE, Opacic M, Freer L, et al. Wilderness Medical Society practice guidelines for the prevention and treatment of frostbite: 2014 update. *Wilderness Environ Med*. 2014;25(Suppl 4):S43–S54.
- Poole A, Gauthier J. Treatment of severe frostbite with iloprost in northern Canada. *CMAJ*. 2016;188(17–18):1255–1258.

CODES

ICD10
- T33.90XA Superficial frostbite of unspecified sites, init encntr
- T34.90XA Frostbite with tissue necrosis of unsp sites, init encntr
- T33.829A Superficial frostbite of unspecified foot, initial encounter

FAQ
- Q: Can protective emollients prevent frostbite if used on the face and exposed areas while skiing?
- A: No. Research has shown that the use of "protective" emollients and creams leads to a false sense of safety and leads to an increased risk of frostbite. This is thought to be due to the failure to use more efficient protective measures when the emollients and creams are used.
- Q: If my child has had frostbite in the past, can she get it again?
- A: Yes. Children who have had a previous frostbite injury are at increased risk for repeat injury, especially in the location of previous damage. Appropriate clothing and limitation of cold exposure should be strictly enforced.
- Q: To prevent frostbite, is there a temperature below which I should not let my child go out to play?
- A: The risk for frostbite is a combination of both the ambient temperature and the wind speed. Time to frostbite is reduced as wind speed increases. A wind chill chart provides an approximate frostbite time. Several agencies use −20°F as a no-start temperature for races. If the temperature is this low, encourage indoor play.
- Q: How can I tell if my child has frostbite or just cold fingers?
- A: Cold fingers are red and may be painful but do not become numb or white. Frostbitten fingers are painful, white, and waxy prior to rewarming and turn red with rewarming.
- Q: If I suspect frostbite in my child and we are outdoors without access to warm water, are there any options for treatment?
- A: If there is a delay in reaching shelter, you can start to thaw your child's body part by using your body as a warmer by placing the exposed body part under your armpit or against your abdomen and keeping it there until further care can be initiated. Before starting the rewarming process, you must be sure refreezing will not recur.
- Q: When should I call the doctor or seek emergency care?
- A: The doctor should be called if, after rewarming, the skin is not soft and/or sensation does not return to normal. Go to the emergency department immediately if the skin is discolored and cold, blisters develop during rewarming, or there are signs of infection, such as the appearance of red streaks leading from the affected area, pus accumulation, or fever.
- Q: We are going on a winter vacation this year and expect to spend a lot of time outside skiing and sledding. What types of clothing should I pack for my children?
- A: It would be a good idea to pack a few pairs of waterproof mittens, a ski suit or ski pants which is wind and water repellent, waterproof boots, polypropylene socks, glove liners, and cotton thermal under garments, a warm hat which covers the ears. Try to make sure your child stays dry and warm. Take frequent breaks indoors to warm up and check your child for any early signs of cold injury.
- Q: What is frostnip?
- A: Frostnip is the mildest form of cold injury, which commonly occurs on exposed parts of the body, such as the fingers, nose, and ears. The symptoms of frostnip are numbness and pallor of the involved body parts. Warming of these areas is the only treatment that is needed, and there is no associated tissue damage.

F

FUNCTIONAL DIARRHEA OF INFANCY (TODDLER'S DIARRHEA)

Roberto Gugig, MD

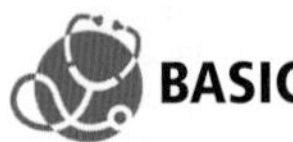

BASICS

DESCRIPTION

- Benign chronic diarrhea in a toddler or a preschool child who appears healthy and is normally active and who is growing, without evidence of systemic illness, infection, malabsorption, or malnutrition
- Also known as chronic nonspecific diarrhea of childhood, toddler's diarrhea, and irritable bowel of childhood

EPIDEMIOLOGY

- The typical age is 12 to 36 months, but range is 6 months to 5 years.
- Prevalence 6–7%

RISK FACTORS

Genetics

Family members often report nonspecific GI complaints or functional bowel disorders.

GENERAL PREVENTION

- Limit the consumption and delay the introduction of sorbitol or fructose-rich fruit juices to the infant diet.
- In the treatment of acute gastroenteritis, parents should be instructed to give an oral rehydration solution (ORS) and resume normal feeding early, avoiding diet restrictions.
- Avoid restrictive diets that may cause caloric deprivation.

PATHOPHYSIOLOGY

- Carbohydrate malabsorption
  - Diarrhea is often preceded by acute gastroenteritis or other viral infection that results in dietary restrictions. Increased oral fluids, including juices, are used to compensate for stool losses and to prevent dehydration.
  - Capacity of the small intestine to absorb fructose is limited. Foods that contain equivalent amounts of fructose and glucose are more readily absorbed because of the additive effect of a glucose-dependent fructose cotransport mechanism.
  - Excessive consumption of juices high in sorbitol (which inhibits fructose absorption) and those with a high fructose-to-glucose ratio (e.g., apple juice) result in fructose malabsorption and increased intraluminal gas caused by fermentation. The end result is abdominal distension, excessive flatulence, and diarrhea.
  - Colonic function: possibly, disruption of colonic ability to ferment unabsorbed carbohydrates into short-chain fatty acids (SCFAs), which maintain colonic function and prevent colon-based diarrhea
- Disturbed motility: short mouth-to-anus transit time
  - Persistence of immature bowel motility pattern; failure of initiation of normal postprandial delayed gastric emptying
  - Low-fat meals. Meals with high dietary fat delay gastric emptying.
  - Excess fluid intake. Infant's colon already operates in high efficiency (in children, higher volume of fluids reach the cecum). Excessive fluids can lead to diarrhea.
  - Low-fiber diet. Dietary fiber serves as a bulking agent.
  - Excessive fecal bile acids. Rapid transit resulting in excess conjugated bile salt entering the colon. Bacterial degradation produces unconjugated bile salts, which decrease net water absorption in the colon.

ETIOLOGY

- Nutritional factors: excessive consumption of fruit juice; high-carbohydrate, low-fat, and low-fiber diet
- Disordered intestinal motility (i.e., variant of irritable bowel syndrome of infancy) with rapid transit

DIAGNOSIS

There is no definitive diagnostic test. The diagnosis is primarily clinical based on age of onset, the history, symptoms, clinical course, and limited number of laboratory tests. Usually, it is an evident condition and not a diagnosis of exclusion.

- Diagnostic criteria (Rome III):
  - Daily, painless, recurrent passage of ≥3 large unformed stools
  - Symptoms that last >4 weeks
  - Onset of symptoms that begins between 6 and 36 months of age
  - Passage of stools that occurs during waking hours
  - There is no failure to thrive (FTT) if caloric intake is adequate.

HISTORY

- Nutritional history is essential, with attention to the 4 Fs (fiber, fluid, fat, and fruit juices) and dietary changes.
- Diarrhea
  - For a toddler, it may not be abnormal to have >3 soft and occasionally loose stools a day with visible food remnants.
  - Children, typically, have intermittent symptoms and are often diagnosed with recurrent viral gastroenteritis.
- Stool characteristics
  - Stools that smell foul and contain undigested food particles. Presence of blood or mucus suggests another diagnosis.
- Timing of diarrhea
  - No stools passed at night, and typically, the first stool of the day is large and has firmer consistency than those occurring later on in the day.
- Recent enteric infection
  - Presence of other affected family members, history of travel, day care, and infectious contacts suggest infectious cause.
- Signs and symptoms:
  - Thorough history is required because all illnesses in the differential diagnosis are associated with morbidity if diagnosis is delayed.

PHYSICAL EXAM

- Normal: Children look healthy, eat well, and are growing normally according to serial plots on the growth chart.
- There are no signs of malnutrition or malabsorption. Weight might be influenced by the dietary measures.
- Fecal mass(es) found on abdominal palpation may signal constipation.

DIFFERENTIAL DIAGNOSIS

- All causes of chronic diarrhea should be considered.
- Common conditions that may cause diarrhea without FTT:
  - Constipation
  - Lactose intolerance
  - Persistent infective diarrhea
- Constipation-related diarrhea
  - Frequently overlooked
  - Consider constipation if diarrhea alternates with hard stools.
- Infection:
  - Bacterial
  - Viral
  - Parasite (giardiasis, cryptosporidiosis)
- Celiac disease
- Malabsorption:
  - Postinfectious secondary lactose intolerance
  - Sucrase-isomaltase deficiency
- Pancreatic:
  - Cystic fibrosis
  - Shwachman-Diamond syndrome
  - Johanson-Blizzard syndrome
  - Chronic pancreatitis
- Bile acid disorders:
  - Chronic cholestasis
  - Terminal ileum disease
  - Bacterial overgrowth
- Immunologic:
  - Cow's milk and soy protein intolerance
  - Food allergy
  - Immunodeficiency
- Food allergies
- Miscellaneous:
  - Antibiotic-associated diarrhea
  - Laxatives
  - Fecal retention constipation
  - UTI
  - Abetalipoproteinemia
  - Inflammatory bowel disease
  - Short-bowel syndrome
  - Hormone-secreting tumors
  - Munchausen by proxy

DIAGNOSTIC TESTS & INTERPRETATION

- The following tests would be helpful only if indicated by history and physical exam:
  - Cystic fibrosis: sweat test, stool for pancreatic enzymes, and genetic testing
  - Celiac disease is common and warrants a serologic testing (antiendomysial antibodies, tissue transglutaminase antibodies with IgA serum levels).

- CBC, iron studies, vitamin levels, serum albumin
- Allergy testing for suspected food proteins (commonly milk, soy, egg, and wheat)
- Inflammatory markers

- Diarrhea as the sole symptom of malabsorption in a normally thriving child is rare.

Initial Tests (screening, lab, imaging)

- Stool tests and culture: negative for white blood cells, blood, fat, and pathogens including ova, parasites, and *Giardia* antigen
- Serum electrolytes normal: no dehydration
- Celiac serology: negative
- CBC normal: no anemia
- Food allergen testing: negative
- Imaging usually unnecessary: Plain abdominal radiograph may demonstrate colonic fecal retention.

Diagnostic Procedures/Other

- A trial of lactose and fruit juice–free diet done separately is practical and diagnostic.
- Breath hydrogen test has limited benefit and is inferior to a trial of milk avoidance.
- Small bowel biopsy is rarely indicated unless strong evidence suggests another cause (e.g., positive celiac serology).

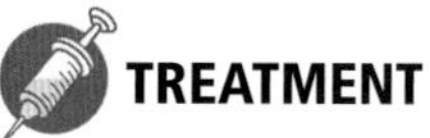

TREATMENT

GENERAL MEASURES

Daily diet and defecation diary may document a specific food responsible for loose stools.

MEDICATION

- Medications are unwarranted for a condition primarily caused by food that does not hamper growth.
- Metronidazole may be beneficial for patients with undetected giardiasis.
- Loperamide is effective in normalizing bowel patterns but should not be used routinely and is only effective for duration of therapy; contraindicated in infectious or inflammatory conditions
- Studies have shown that certain probiotic strains such as *Lactobacillus rhamnosus GG* (LGG) and *Saccharomyces boulardii* may be effective at reducing symptoms, including lowering the incidence of acute diarrhea in healthy children (16–20%) and decreasing the duration of episodes (from 8 days down to 4.2 days).

ISSUES FOR REFERRAL

- Failure of response to diet
- Weight loss despite adequate intake
- Presence of red flag symptoms (e.g., anorexia, irritability, fever, vomiting)
- Fat, blood, and mucus in the stool

ADDITIONAL THERAPIES

In otherwise healthy growing children with no red flag symptoms and a negative appropriate workup, it is important to reassure parents that there is no underlying GI disease, infection, or inflammation.

ONGOING CARE

FOLLOW-UP RECOMMENDATIONS

- Improvement with dietary changes confirms the diagnosis and reassures the parents.
- Follow up phone call to parents within a few days of instituting diet. If no improvement within 2 weeks despite good compliance with dietary recommendations, then reconsider diagnosis; consider more diagnostic tests and referral to a specialist.

Patient Monitoring

- Follow growth parameters.
- Monitor symptoms indicating nonfunctional illness.

DIET

- The child's feeding pattern should be normalized according to the 4 Fs:
  - Overconsumption of *fruit juices* should be discouraged, especially those that contain sorbitol and a high fructose-to-glucose ratio (e.g., apple juice, pear nectar).
    - Cloudy apple juice or white grape juice may be safe as alternatives.
  - *Fiber intake* should be normalized by introduction of whole-grain bread and fruits.
  - Increase *dietary fat* to at least 35–40% of total energy intake. Substitution of low-fat milk with whole milk may be sufficient.
  - Restrict *fluid intake* to <90 mL/kg/24 h if history is significant for fluid consumption >150 mL/kg/24 h.
- Improvement occurs within a few days to a couple of weeks after initiating the earlier discussed therapy.
- Avoid elimination diets as may cause caloric deprivation.

PROGNOSIS

- Good
- Symptoms resolve by school age.
- Long-term benefit of low-carbohydrate diet: contributes to balanced nutrition and the prevention of obesity

COMPLICATIONS

Although children tend not to suffer from the symptom of frequent, loose or soft stools, parents are often worried and frustrated and require frequent reassurance.

ADDITIONAL READING

- Hoekstra JH. Toddler diarrhoea: more a nutritional disorder than a disease. *Arch Dis Child*. 1998;79(1):2–5.
- Huffman S. Toddler's diarrhea. *J Pediatr Health Care*. 1999;13(1):32–33.
- Hyman PE, Milla PJ, Benninga MA, et al. Childhood functional gastrointestinal disorders: neonate/toddler. *Gastroenterology*. 2006;130(5):1519–1526.
- Judd RH. Chronic nonspecific diarrhea. *Pediatr Rev*. 1996;17(11):379–385.
- Kneepkens CM, Hoekstra JH. Chronic nonspecific diarrhea of childhood: pathophysiology and management. *Pediatr Clin North Am*. 1996;43(2):375–390.
- Lloyd-Still JD. Chronic diarrhea of childhood and the misuse of elimination diets. *J Pediatr*. 1979;95(1):10–13.
- Moukarzel AA, Lesicka H, Ament ME. Irritable bowel syndrome and nonspecific diarrhea in infancy and childhood—relationship with juice carbohydrate malabsorption. *Clin Pediatr (Phila)*. 2002;41(3):145–150.
- Oberhelman RA, Gilman RH, Sheen P, et al. A placebo-controlled trial of *Lactobacillus* GG to prevent diarrhea in undernourished Peruvian children. *J Pediatr*. 1999;134(1):15–20.
- Pedone CA, Bernabeu AO, Postaire ER, et al. The effect of supplementation with milk fermented by *Lactobacillus casei* (strain DN-114 001) on acute diarrhoea in children attending day care centres. *Int J Clin Pract*. 1999;53(3):179–184.
- Vernacchio L, Vezina RM, Mitchell AA, et al. Characteristics of persistent diarrhea in a community-based cohort of young US children. *J Pediatr Gastroenterol Nutr*. 2006;43(1):52–58.

CODES

ICD10

- K59.1 Functional diarrhea
- K90.4 Malabsorption due to intolerance, not elsewhere classified

FAQ

- Q: How do I know that my toddler's diarrhea is not serious?
- A: Growth is usually normal and your child looks and feels well. His or her activity and development seem unaffected by the diarrhea. The change of diet results in improvement.
- Q: What are the components of a successful treatment plan?
- A: Attention to the 4 Fs in the diet: decreased fruit juice intake, increased fat intake, decreased fluid, and increased fiber intake
- Q: Are probiotics useful in the treatment of toddler's diarrhea?
- A: There is no adequate data to support such a recommendation, but evidence is emerging that specific probiotic strains may be effective in treating "irritable bowel syndrome like diarrhea and bloating."
- Q: When should care by a pediatric gastroenterologist be sought?
- A: If no response after 2 weeks of compliance with dietary therapy, if growth is delayed, or if other GI or systemic complaints are present, seek a pediatric gastroenterologist's care.
- Q: Did my child get diarrhea because he goes to child care or because he is not clean?
- A: No. Functional diarrhea is not caused by infection.

FUNGAL SKIN INFECTIONS (DERMATOPHYTE INFECTIONS, CANDIDIASIS, AND TINEA VERSICOLOR)

Sonal D. Shah, MD • Renee M. Howard, MD

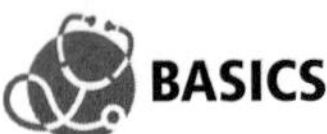

BASICS

DESCRIPTION

Superficial fungal infections of the skin, hair, and nails are characterized by erythema, scaling, pruritus, and change in coloration.

EPIDEMIOLOGY

- Dermatophyte infections:
  - Tinea capitis:
    - Most common fungal infection in pediatric population
    - Occurs mainly in prepubescent children (between ages 3 and 7 years)
    - Asymptomatic carriers are common and contribute to spread.
  - Tinea corporis usually seen in younger children or in young adolescents with close physical contact to others (i.e., wrestlers).
  - Onychomycosis: Overall prevalence is 0–2.6% in children, often occurs with concomitant tinea pedis, or in 1st-degree relatives with infection.
- Candidiasis: majority of infants colonized with *Candida albicans*
- Tinea versicolor: seen in adolescents and young adults

GENERAL PREVENTION

- Measures should be taken to avoid transmission between hosts, including no sharing of combs, brushes, hats, etc.
- Hair utensils and hats should be washed in hot, soapy water at onset of therapy.
- Pets should be watched and treated early for any suspicious lesions.
- In patients in whom appropriate therapy has not led to improvement in symptoms, siblings and close contacts should be examined and fungal cultures performed.
- Isolation of hospitalized patient is unnecessary.

PATHOPHYSIOLOGY

- Fungal elements (arthroconidia) adhere to stratum corneum or hair shaft. Proteases work to degrade keratin, which allows for invasion of dermatophytes.
- Predisposing factors may include moisture, macerated skin, and immunocompromised.
- Host immune response is usually able to contain infection.
- Inflammatory response is variable; highly inflammatory forms may lead to pustular lesions and kerion (large inflammatory mass) formation.

ETIOLOGY

- Varies by geographic region
- Dermatophyte infections:
  - Tinea capitis: >90% caused by *Trichophyton tonsurans* in North America—spread from human to human (anthropophilic); increasing incidence of *Microsporum canis* infection spread from animals such as cats and dogs to humans (zoophilic)
  - Tinea corporis: preadolescent children: *M. canis, Microsporum audouinii*; older children: *Trichophyton rubrum, Trichophyton mentagrophytes, T. tonsurans*
  - Onychomycosis: *T. rubrum, T. mentagrophytes*
- Candidiasis: usually *C. albicans*
- Tinea versicolor: *Malassezia furfur*

DIAGNOSIS

HISTORY

- Determine onset and duration.
- Elicit signs and symptoms such as expanding areas of erythema, scaling, or color change with associated pruritus.
- Determine contacts, including exposure to pets.
- Determine if patient is immunocompromised.
- List of medications previously tried

PHYSICAL EXAM

- Dermatophyte infections:
  - Tinea capitis: may have various presentations:
    - Round patches of alopecia with erythema or black dots (broken hair shafts at surface of skin) and fine scaling
    - Diffusely dry scalp with scaling
    - Follicular pustules resembling bacterial folliculitis
    - Boggy, tender red plaque with follicular pustules or purulent discharge (kerion): represents exaggerated immune response
    - Cervical or occipital lymphadenopathy
  - Tinea corporis:
    - One or more, asymmetrically distributed, annular, well-demarcated erythematous scaling plaques with central clearing
    - Inflammatory forms may be frankly pustular or vesicular at the borders.
    - Lesions may occur anywhere on the body.
  - Onychomycosis:
    - *Distal subungual* type: invasion of the underlying nail bed and inferior portion of the nail plate, which leads to detachment of the nail plate from the nail bed, and subungual thickening and debris with yellowing of the plate
    - *Proximal subungual* type: invasion of the nail unit at the proximal nail fold (most common in HIV patients)
    - *White superficial* type: superficial infection of the nail plate, with white plaques on the dorsal nail plate
- Candidiasis:
  - Diffuse erythema (often "beefy" red) with sharp, marginated border
  - Pinpoint satellite pustules at edge of erythema
  - Prefers warm, moist environments; favors skin folds/creases (axillae, groin, below breasts, and in infants, diaper area)
- Tinea versicolor:
  - Scaling, discrete oval patches that are either hypo- or hyperpigmented
  - Distributed on upper trunk, neck, and proximal arms in areas where there is high amount of sebum and free fatty acids, which the organism requires; occasionally on face

DIFFERENTIAL DIAGNOSIS

- Dermatophyte infections:
  - Dermatologic conditions:
    - Tinea capitis:
      - Seborrheic dermatitis
      - Psoriasis
      - Alopecia areata
      - Trichotillomania
      - Folliculitis
      - Impetigo
      - Atopic dermatitis
    - Tinea corporis:
      - Herald patch of pityriasis rosea
      - Nummular dermatitis
      - Psoriasis
      - Contact dermatitis
      - Granuloma annulare
    - Onychomycosis:
      - Psoriasis
      - Nondermatophyte infection
  - Systemic diseases:
    - Cutaneous T-cell lymphoma
    - Histiocytosis
    - Sarcoidosis
- Candidiasis:
  - Contact dermatitis
  - Seborrheic dermatitis
  - Inverse psoriasis
  - Atopic dermatitis
  - Bacterial infection
- Tinea versicolor:
  - Pityriasis alba
  - Postinflammatory hypopigmentation
  - Vitiligo
  - Seborrheic dermatitis
  - Pityriasis rosea

DIAGNOSTIC TESTS & INTERPRETATION

Initial Tests (screening, lab, imaging)

- KOH preparation:
  - Clean area with alcohol.
  - Using a No. 15 scalpel blade, gently scrape the outer edge of the active border, broken hairs or clip hairs, and gather subungual debris.
  - Place material flat on a glass side in a single layer. Apply coverslip on top.
  - Place a few drops of 10–20% KOH to edge of coverslip until space between slide and coverslip is filled, and apply mild pressure.
  - Warm slide gently or let sit for 30 minutes.
  - Examine slide under microscope at low power under low light.
    - Dermatophytes: arthrospores around or within hair shaft; long, branching fungal hyphae with septations.
    - Candidiasis: budding yeast, pseudohyphae
    - Tinea versicolor: short hyphae and clusters of spores ("spaghetti and meatballs")
- Fungal culture:
  - Obtain specimen with scalpel blade from outer active edge of scaling.
  - For scalp, gently rub a wet sterile toothbrush, cytobrush, or damp cotton swab over the area of scaling and then plate on fungal medium.
  - Results can take up to 4 weeks.
  - Some laboratories provide drug susceptibility testing as well as identification of fungus.

Diagnostic Procedures/Other

Wood lamp examination (~360-nm wavelength of ultraviolet light): Infected hairs may fluoresce (not useful in skin or nail infections).

- Examine in completely darkened room.
- Ectothrix infections (organisms outside of hair shaft): bright green fluorescence (*M. canis* and *M. audouinii*); endothrix infections (organisms inside hair shaft): do not fluoresce (*T. tonsurans*)
- Tinea versicolor: yellow, copper, or bronze fluorescence

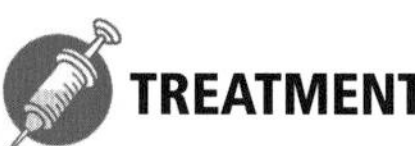

TREATMENT

MEDICATION

First Line

- Dermatophyte infections:
  - Tinea capitis: systemic therapy warranted to penetrate hair shaft
    - Oral griseofulvin: 20 to 25 mg/kg/24 h (max dose: 1 g/24 h) once daily or divided b.i.d. of microsize griseofulvin for 6 to 8 weeks (10 to 15 mg/kg/24 h [max dose: 750 mg/24 h] once daily or divided b.i.d., if ultramicrosize form is used), taken with high-fat food (e.g., milk or ice cream) for 6 to 12 weeks. In addition, topical therapy of 2.5% selenium sulfide or ketoconazole shampoo twice weekly suppresses viable spores. Laboratory monitoring is not needed.
  - Tinea capitis with kerion:
    - Treat for tinea capitis.
    - Systemic steroids may be needed to treat significant inflammatory.
  - Tinea corporis:
    - Topical azole antifungals (1% clotrimazole, 2% ketoconazole) or 1% terbinafine cream applied twice daily for 2 to 4 weeks
  - Onychomycosis:
    - Oral terbinafine 3 to 6 mg/kg/dose (max 250 mg) once daily for 6 to 12 weeks. Can be associated with hepatic failure; avoid use in patients with liver disease. Check liver enzymes before and during treatment.
    - Oral itraconazole (adolescent and adult) in weekly pulses for 3 to 4 months; 200 mg twice daily for 7 days and then off for 3 weeks
- Candidiasis: topical nystatin cream or ointment 3 to 4 times daily for 7 to 10 days
- Tinea versicolor: selenium sulfide 2.5% applied to affected skin for 10 minutes. Wash off thoroughly. Apply daily for 7 to 10 days. Monthly applications may help prevent recurrences.

Second Line

- Dermatophyte infections:
  - Tinea capitis:
    - Itraconazole: 3 to 5 mg/kg once daily for 4 to 6 weeks. May also use oral terbinafine 3 to 6 mg/kg/dose (max 250 mg) once daily for 4 weeks or oral fluconazole 5 mg/kg once daily for 4 to 6 weeks. All of these may be associated with hepatic failure and should be avoided in patients with liver disease. Liver enzymes should be checked before and during treatment.
  - Tinea corporis:
    - Oral griseofulvin microsize 15 to 25 mg/kg/24 h once daily or divided b.i.d. for 4 weeks for persistent or extensive involvement
- Candidiasis:
  - Oral fluconazole:
    - 6 mg/kg on day 1 and then 3 mg/kg/24 h for 2 weeks if poor response to topical therapy
- Tinea versicolor:
  - Topical azole antifungals (ketoconazole 2% shampoo applied daily for 3 days) or clotrimazole cream daily till clear
  - Oral ketoconazole (adolescent and adult) 200 to 400 mg once daily for 5 to 10 days or itraconazole (adolescent and adult) 200 mg once daily for 5 to 7 days if severe, recurrent, or persistent

ONGOING CARE

FOLLOW-UP RECOMMENDATIONS

Patient Monitoring

- Monitor for secondary bacterial infection.
- Highly inflammatory lesions (kerion) may require concomitant systemic steroids.
- Repeated infection may indicate a source that needs to be diagnosed and treated (e.g., family member or pet).

DIET

Griseofulvin is better absorbed with a fatty meal and should be taken with foods such as milk, eggs, or ice cream.

PROGNOSIS

- Dermatophyte: Inflammation improves within several days but may take several weeks to completely resolve; nail infections take 6 to 12 months to show improvement and are prone to recurrence.
- Areas with significant inflammatory component may become scarred and permanently alopecic.
- Candidal skin lesions improve within 24 to 48 hours and resolve by 1 week.
- Tinea versicolor: Resolution of dyspigmentation may take months to occur.
- Relapses and recurrences are common.

COMPLICATIONS

- Dermatophyte infections:
  - Secondary bacterial infection
  - Kerion formation can lead to permanent alopecia and scarring.
- Candidiasis:
  - Scarring in severe disease
  - Fungemia in immunocompromised host

ADDITIONAL READING

- Ameen M. Epidemiology of superficial fungal infections. *Clin Dermatol*. 2010;28(2):197–201.
- Andrews MD, Burns M. Common tinea infections in children. *Am Fam Physician*. 2008;77(10):1415–1420.
- Baldo A, Monod M, Mathy A, et al. Mechanisms of skin adherence and invasion by dermatophytes. *Mycoses*. 2012;55(3):218–223.
- Elewski BE, Cáceres HW, DeLeon L, et al. Terbinafine hydrochloride oral granules versus oral griseofulvin suspension in children with tinea capitis: results of two randomized, investigator-blinded, multicenter, international, controlled trials. *J Am Acad Dermatol*. 2008;59(1):41–54.
- Gupta AK, Ryder JE, Nicol K, et al. Superficial fungal infections: an update on pityriasis versicolor, seborrheic dermatitis, tinea capitis, and onychomycosis. *Clin Dermatol*. 2003;21(5):417–425.
- Shemer A. Update: medical treatment of onychomycosis. *Dermatol Ther*. 2012;25(6):582–593.

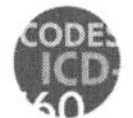

CODES

ICD10

- B35.9 Dermatophytosis, unspecified
- B35.4 Tinea corporis
- B37.2 Candidiasis of skin and nail

FAQ

- Q: What is the role of combination topical antifungals and corticosteroids in the treatment of superficial fungal infections of the skin?
- A: Combination products containing high-potency topical steroids antifungals should be avoided. High potency topical steroids may lead to a decrease in inflammation; however, they can mask the clinical features of tinea infection (so called tinea incognito) and can allow for rapid expansion of tinea infection. In addition, prolonged use of high-potency topical steroids used particularly in intertriginous areas can lead to side effects such as striae formation and atrophy of the skin.
- Q: What can be done to prevent recurrent tinea versicolor infection?
- A: *M. furfur* is a normal part of skin flora and lives in lipid-rich areas of skin. Tropical climates, humid environments, and excessive sweating result in infection in adolescents and young adults. Recurrences are common and can be prevented by regular application of selenium sulfide 2.5%. In addition, itraconazole has been shown to be effective in prevention of tinea versicolor. In one study, the recurrence of tinea versicolor was prevented in 88% of patients over a 6-month period using itraconazole 200 mg b.i.d., 1 day per month.
- Q: How can a clinician adequately assess for complete clearance when treating tinea capitis?
- A: At the end of treatment course, a repeat fungal culture should be performed to ensure complete clearance of spores.

F

GASTRITIS

Richard A. Lirio, MD

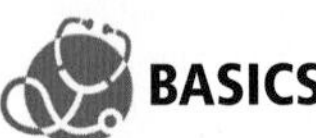

BASICS

DESCRIPTION

Macro or microscopic inflammation of mucosa of stomach

EPIDEMIOLOGY

- 8 out of every 1,000 people are estimated to have gastritis.
- >2% of ICU patients have heavy bleeding secondary to gastritis.

ETIOLOGY

- Common causes
  - Physiologic stress (e.g., chronic disease, CNS disease, overwhelming sepsis, ICU patients)
  - Peptic disease
  - Drug-induced (e.g., NSAIDs, steroids, valproate; more rarely, iron, calcium salts, potassium chloride, antibiotics)
  - Infection
    - *Helicobacter pylori* (children more likely to have more severe gastritis, specifically located in antrum of stomach)
    - Tuberculosis
    - Cytomegalovirus
    - Parasites
  - Celiac disease: lymphocytic gastritis
  - Major surgery; severe burns; renal, liver, respiratory failure; severe trauma
  - Caustic ingestions (e.g., lye, strong acids, pine oil)
  - Protein sensitivity (e.g., cow's milk-protein allergy), allergic enteropathy
  - Eosinophilic gastroenteritis
  - Crohn disease:
    - Up to 40% of Crohn patients have gastroduodenal involvement.
    - Gastric Crohn disease may manifest itself as highly focal, non-*H. pylori*, nongranulomatous gastritis.
  - Direct trauma (nasogastric tubes)
  - Ethanol
  - Idiopathic
- Less common causes:
  - Radiation induced
  - Hypertrophic gastritis (Ménétrier disease)
  - Autoimmune gastritis
  - Collagenous gastritis
  - Zollinger-Ellison syndrome
  - Vascular injury

DIAGNOSIS

HISTORY

- Complaints of epigastric pain
- Abdominal indigestion
- Nausea
- Vomiting postprandially
- Vomiting blood or coffee ground–like material
- Diarrhea
- Dark or black stools (or bright red blood from rectum, if bleeding is brisk and intestinal transit time is short)
- Irritability
- Poor feeding and weight loss
- Less often: chest pain, hematemesis, melena

PHYSICAL EXAM

- Epigastric tenderness is physical finding that most closely correlates with gastritis on endoscopy.
- Normal bowel sounds

DIFFERENTIAL DIAGNOSIS

- Gastroesophageal reflux with esophagitis
- Peptic ulcer disease
- Biliary tract disorders
- Pancreatitis
- Inflammatory bowel disease
- Genitourinary pathology (renal stones, infection)
- Nonulcer dyspepsia
- Functional pain
- Allergic enteropathy

DIAGNOSTIC TESTS & INTERPRETATION

Initial Tests (screening, lab, imaging)

- CBC
  - Evaluate for anemia with other signs of chronic blood loss (e.g., microcytosis, low reticulocyte count).
- Heme testing stool may be helpful.
- *H. pylori* identification
  - Noninvasive *H. pylori* antigen tests for active disease, from stool or urea breath test (UBT)
    - Note: Presence of *H. pylori* antibody (in serum, whole blood, saliva, or urine) may not be indicative of active disease; hence serologic testing, although more widely available, is not currently recommended.
  - Rapid urease test from gastric biopsy specimen for *H. pylori*
- Upper GI radiography may be useful to identify thickened gastric folds, filling defects.
- Chest radiograph may detect free abdominal air secondary to perforation.
- Upper endoscopy with biopsies
  - Greatest sensitivity and specificity for gastritis
  - Possible gross findings:
    - Erythema, granularity, edema, small ulcerations
    - Thickened hyperemic mucosa
    - Atrophic mucosa
    - Antral micronodules (represent lymphoid follicles) commonly seen in children with *H. pylori* infection
    - Antral and prepyloric edema with retained gastric secretions
  - Biopsies will show chronic and/or active inflammation.
    - Can order special staining for *H. pylori* (silver Warthin-Starry stain, Genta stain, modified Giemsa stain, cresyl violet stain, or immunohistochemical staining)
    - Can consider culture and sensitivities of homogenized gastric biopsy for persistent *H. pylori*, which may indicate drug resistance. However, this is difficult to perform and may be limited to research settings.

TREATMENT

MEDICATION

- Proton pump inhibitors (PPIs): drug of choice as 1st-line therapy. May be helpful for both acid-mediated and acid-exacerbated conditions. Can also use antacids or H_2 blockers. Goal is to maintain gastric pH >4 to 5.
  - Ranitidine: 2 to 3 mg/kg/dose b.i.d.–t.i.d. in children
  - Famotidine: 0.5 to 2 mg/kg/24 h divided b.i.d.
  - Omeprazole, lansoprazole, rabeprazole, or esomeprazole: 1 to 2 mg/kg/24 h divided b.i.d.
  - Interactions and side effects:
- Cimetidine is less effective and can increase toxicity when given to patients receiving other medicines metabolized by cytochrome P450 system (e.g., theophylline).
- PPIs can also interfere with the absorption of other medicines and may interact with other medicines metabolized by specific cytochrome P450 isoenzymes.

- Misoprostol
  - Synthetic prostaglanin E1 (PGE1)
  - May reduce risk of progression of gastritis to ulcers in patients taking NSAIDs
  - Concerns exist for increased cardiovascular events in adults when using misoprostol.
- Discontinue NSAIDs.
- Treatment of *H. pylori*:
  - Triple therapy with PPI and two antibiotics (e.g., omeprazole, amoxicillin, and clarithromycin)
  - If eradication unsuccessful, quadruple therapy is recommended for 7 to 14 days, including the following:
    - Bismuth (of note, may need to avoid bismuth subsalicylate and choose instead bismuth subcitrate)
    - Metronidazole
    - A PPI
    - Another antibiotic (either amoxicillin, clarithromycin, or tetracycline)
  - Drug regimens change frequently; clarithromycin resistance becoming increasingly problematic

ALERT

- Antacids are not palatable to children and can lead to diarrhea or constipation. Prolonged use of large doses of aluminum hydroxide–containing antacids may lead to phosphate depletion and aluminum-related CNS toxicity (particularly in patients with renal disease).
- If *H. pylori* eradication is attempted, important to use a tested regimen. Untested substitutions in the triple or quadruple regimens should be avoided.
- Caution if PPI to be used. Recent concern for a number of potential associations with long-term use including acute interstitial nephritis, mineral abnormalities, and increased risk for *Clostridium difficile*.

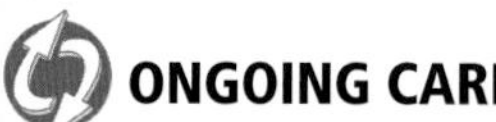

ONGOING CARE

FOLLOW-UP RECOMMENDATIONS

Patient Monitoring

- For stress gastritis with hemorrhage, provide vigilant supportive care with close monitoring of hemodynamics, fluids, and electrolytes.
- Monitor for hemoccult-positive stools.
- Follow CBCs.
- May elect to repeat endoscopy in severe cases
- Once stabilized and gastritis resolved, review ongoing needs for acid suppression and develop plan to discontinue medications when no longer needed.

DIET

- Benefit of changes in diet to managing etiologies or symptoms of gastritis is inconclusive.
- Eliminate alcohol, tobacco, and caffeine, as well as NSAIDs.

PROGNOSIS

Significant gastritis relapse rates for children who remain infected with *H. pylori*

COMPLICATIONS

- Bleeding (from mild to hemorrhagic)
- When gastritis caused by acid/alkali ingestions, outlet obstruction may result from prepyloric strictures (4 to 8 weeks after ingestion).

ADDITIONAL READING

- Aanpreung P, Atisook K. Hematemesis in infants induced by cow milk allergy. *Asian Pac J Allergy Immunol*. 2003;21(4):211–216.
- Drumm B, Koletzko S, Oderda G. *Helicobacter pylori* infection in children: a consensus statement. European Paediatric Task Force on *Helicobacter pylori*. *J Pediatr Gastroenterol Nutr*. 2000;30(2):207–213.
- Hino B, Eliakim R, Levine A, et al. Comparison of invasive and non-invasive tests diagnosis and monitoring of *Helicobacter pylori* infection in children. *J Pediatr Gastroenterol Nutr*. 2004;39(5):519–523.
- Muriithi AK, Leung N, Valeri AM, et al. Biopsy-proven acute interstitial nephritis, 1993–2011: a case series. *Am J Kidney Dis*. 2014;64(4):558–566.
- Pashankar DS, Bishop WP, Mitros FA. Chemical gastropathy: a distinct histopathologic entity in children. *J Pediatr Gastroenterol Nutr*. 2002;35(5):653–657.
- Vesoulis Z, Lozanski G, Ravichandran P, et al. Collagenous gastritis: a case report, morphologic evaluation, and review. *Mod Pathol*. 2000;13(5):591–596.
- Weinstein WM. Emerging gastritides. *Curr Gastroenterol Rep*. 2001;3(6):523–527.
- Zheng PY, Jones NL. Recent advances in *Helicobacter pylori* infection in children: from the petri dish to the playground. *Can J Gastroenterol*. 2003;17(7):448–454.
- Zimmermann AE, Walters JK, Katona BG, et al. A review of omeprazole use in the treatment of acid-related disorders in children. *Clin Ther*. 2001;23(5):660–679, discussion 645.

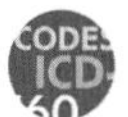

CODES

ICD10

- K29.70 Gastritis, unspecified, without bleeding
- K29.71 Gastritis, unspecified, with bleeding
- K29.60 Other gastritis without bleeding

FAQ

- Q: Will a bland diet help to resolve gastritis?
- A: Dietary changes have not been shown to affect the natural course of gastritis.
- Q: What is *H. pylori*?
- A: *H. pylori* is a bacterium frequently found in the gastric mucosa of patients with gastritis and peptic ulcer disease. It can be diagnosed by a variety of means, often including a combination of upper endoscopy and UBTs. Relapse rates for gastritis secondary to *H. pylori* are high when the infection is left untreated.
- Q: Is it appropriate to treat cases of gastritis with antibiotics not proven to be *H. pylori*?
- A: No. It is important to treat only confirmed *H. pylori* infections, not to treat on suspicion of infection, especially with increasing issues with antibiotic resistance.
- Q: If a patient is treated for *H. pylori* and they still have symptoms and a positive stool *H. pylori* antigen, what would be the next course of action?
- A: Consider retreating with a PPI, amoxicillin, and metronidazole, as clarithromycin resistance in *H. pylori* infection is an increasingly frequent cause for treatment failure.
- Q: What are newly recognized complications of treating patients with PPIs?
- A: Some adult studies show hypomagnesemia, interstitial nephritis, increased risk of pneumonia, hip fracture, and *C. difficile* infection to be associated with PPI use, particularly if it is long term.

GASTROESOPHAGEAL REFLUX

Ninfa M. Candela, MD

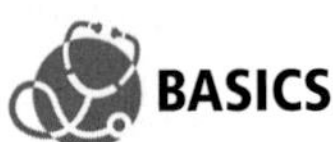

BASICS

DESCRIPTION

- Effortless regurgitation of gastric contents; occurs physiologically, with episodes typically brief and asymptomatic
- Divided into physiologic and pathologic processes:
  - Some degree of physiologic gastroesophageal reflux (GER) is normal at all ages.
  - Physiologic infant GER is very common. Symptoms peak around 4 months of age and generally have resolved by 1 year of age.
  - Pathologic reflux or GER disease (GERD) is defined by troublesome symptoms or complications of GER.
  - Complications of GERD may include reflux esophagitis, bleeding, esophageal stricture, failure to thrive, chronic/recurrent respiratory tract disease, or vomiting.

EPIDEMIOLOGY

Pathologic GERD occurs in 5% of adults; 1–4% of children

RISK FACTORS

- Neurologic disorders (cerebral palsy/quadriplegia)
- Congenital esophageal disorders
- Midgut or diaphragmatic defects
- Cystic fibrosis
- Asthma
- Gastroparesis
- Hiatal hernia

PATHOPHYSIOLOGY

- Transient relaxation of the lower esophageal sphincter during episodes of increased abdominal and gastric pressure
- GERD is a multifactorial process that is mediated by the number and frequency of reflux events, relative acidity, potential for esophageal clearance, delay in gastric emptying, effectiveness of mucosal barriers, degree of visceral hypersensitivity, and airway responsiveness.

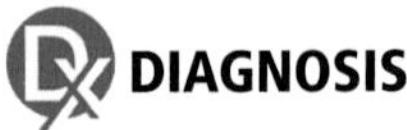

DIAGNOSIS

HISTORY

- General symptoms of GERD:
  - Vomiting or regurgitation
  - Irritability
  - Chest/abdominal pain
  - Heartburn
  - Hematemesis, melena
  - Blood loss
  - Dysphagia
  - Food refusal or prolonged feeding
  - Cough, wheezing
  - Obstructive apnea
  - Dysphonia
  - Aspiration pneumonia
  - Posturing (Sandifer syndrome)
- GERD may be asymptomatic and still carry risk of complications.
- Infant
  - Many common conditions in infancy such as physiologic GER, infant colic, milk protein allergy, or multifactorial feeding difficulties/aversion can present with symptoms that can be difficult to distinguish from GERD and history should also assess for these conditions.
  - Pay attention to feeding volume and frequency in addition to weight gain, failure to thrive, and irritability in association with regurgitation events.
  - Identify episodes of pneumonia, obstructive apnea, chronic cough, stridor, wheezing.
  - Identify additional signs/symptoms that suggest food protein allergy (hematochezia, rash, diarrhea, irritability, failure to thrive).
  - Evaluate for evidence of bowel obstruction (forceful emesis, polyhydramnios during pregnancy).
  - If vomiting is atypical or associated with other signs/symptoms, rule out infection, metabolic disease, anatomic abnormality, or neurologic disease.
  - Special questions:
    - Presence of polyhydramnios or bilious emesis?
    - Family history of metabolic disease?
    - Family history of allergies/atopy?
    - Perinatal asphyxia (and other neurologic disorders)?
    - History of prematurity?
- Older child
  - Identify typical adult GERD complaints (chest pain, heartburn, regurgitation, dysphagia), but recognize that children describe discomfort poorly (often isolated abdominal pain).
  - Identify episodes of pneumonia, choking, chronic cough, laryngitis, stridor, and wheezing (may need to assess swallowing function).
  - Assess for solid food dysphagia (more common with eosinophilic esophagitis).
  - Evaluate for presence of nocturnal GERD symptoms.
  - Special questions:
    - Family history of GERD?
    - Family history of allergies/atopy?
    - Family history of eosinophilic esophagitis or other chronic GI disease such as celiac disease or inflammatory bowel disease?

PHYSICAL EXAM

- May be normal
- Growth failure
- Reactive airway disease and other manifestations of pulmonary complications
- Anemia or blood in stool (uncommon)
- Erosive dental disease (possibly linked to GERD but common unrelated finding)

DIFFERENTIAL DIAGNOSIS

- Toxin
  - Lead
  - Fe
  - Medications
- Renal
  - Obstructive uropathy
  - Uremia
- Infection
  - Gastroenteritis
  - *Candida* esophagitis
  - *Helicobacter pylori*
  - Urinary tract infection
  - Sepsis
  - Pneumonia
  - Hepatitis
  - Otitis media
  - Pancreatitis
  - Cholecystitis
- Neurologic
  - Meningitis/encephalitis: intracranial injury
  - Brain tumor
  - Hydrocephalus
  - Subdural hematoma
- Metabolic
  - Urea cycle defects
  - Aminoacidopathies (phenylketonuria, maple syrup urine disease)
  - Adrenal hyperplasia
  - Galactosemia, fructosemia
- Allergy/food intolerance
  - Milk/soy protein allergy
  - Eosinophilic esophagitis
  - Celiac disease
  - Hereditary fructose intolerance
- Anatomic malformation
  - Diaphragmatic hernia
  - Gastric outlet obstruction
  - Esophageal atresia
  - Pyloric stenosis
  - Antral/duodenal web
  - Volvulus/malrotation
  - Meconium ileus
  - Enteral duplications
  - Intussusception
  - Trichobezoar
  - Foreign body
  - Incarcerated hernia
- Drugs that affect lower esophageal sphincter pressure:
  - Nitrates
  - Nicotine
  - Narcotics
  - Caffeine
  - Theophylline
  - Anticholinergic agents
  - Estrogen
  - Somatostatin
  - Prostaglandins
- Other:
  - Pregnancy
  - Cyclic vomiting syndrome

DIAGNOSTIC TESTS & INTERPRETATION

Diagnosis of GERD is frequently made clinically.

Initial Tests (screening, lab, imaging)

- Testing is typically only needed to evaluate for other conditions, evaluate questionable cases, potential causes, complications, or symptom-reflux correlations. Evaluation may include the following:
  - Common screening laboratories (CBC, routine chemistries, transaminases)
  - Allergen testing (i.e., milk, soy, egg, etc.)
  - Celiac serology
  - Stool occult blood
  - Stool *H. pylori* antigen
- Upper GI contrast study: Evaluate anatomy.
- Chest radiograph: Evaluate for recurrent pneumonia (if warranted by respiratory symptoms).
- Modified barium swallow: Evaluate swallowing function and for aspiration.
- Gastric-emptying study (gastric scintigraphy): Evaluate gastric motility and/or pulmonary aspiration.

Diagnostic Procedures/Other

- Empiric, 4-week trial of medication
- pH probe study
  - To quantify and correlate esophageal acid exposure with symptoms over a 24-hour period (commonly performed off of acid blockade therapy)
  - Wireless pH monitoring (disposable probe placed endoscopically and clipped to esophageal mucosa)

- Combined pH/multichannel intraluminal impedance (MII):
  - Allows detection of both acid and nonacid GER events; may detect more pathologic reflux than pH probe alone (can be performed on or off of acid blockade)
- Esophagogastroduodenoscopy with biopsies
- Laryngoscopy
- Bronchoscopy
- Esophageal manometry
- Antroduodenal manometry
- Pathologic findings
  - Evidence of reflux esophagitis, allergic esophagitis, Barrett esophagus, adenocarcinoma, stricture

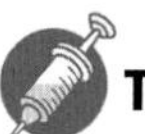

TREATMENT

Treatment should be individualized, and cost effectiveness should be considered.

GENERAL MEASURES

- Parental reassurance and education, especially in otherwise healthy infants with physiologic GER
- Small, frequent infant feedings
- Encourage burping in infants.
- Reassure parents that infant GER/GERD is not associated with sudden infant death syndrome.
- Thickening of infant feedings (1 tablespoon cereal per ounce of formula): may help with volume of regurgitation, does not stop GER
- Positioning: keeping infant upright after feeds, head elevation in bed of older children only; prone positioning not recommended

MEDICATION

First Line

H_2 blockers: good for intermittent or PRN dosing; can be used for maintenance of chronic GERD in some patients and/or promote mucosal healing

- Ranitidine (PO)
  - <1 month: 6 mg/kg/24 h divided t.i.d.
  - ≥1 month to 16 years of age: 5 to 10 mg/kg/24 h divided b.i.d.–t.i.d. (max 300 mg/24 h)
  - Adults 150 mg b.i.d. or 300 mg nightly
- Famotidine (PO)
  - <3 months: 0.5 mg/kg daily
  - 3 months to 1 year: 0.5 mg/kg b.i.d.
  - 1 to 12 years: 1 mg/kg/24 h divided b.i.d. (max 80 mg/24 h)
  - 12 years to adults: 20 mg b.i.d.

Second Line

Proton pump inhibitors (PPI):

- Demonstrated to be more effective at blocking gastric acid as compared to H_2 blockers; can be used for symptoms as well as mucosal injury, refractory to H_2 blockers; may be appropriate for short-term empiric trial of medication
  - Omeprazole (PO)
    - <1 year: 1 to 2 mg/kg/24 h (daily or divided b.i.d.); multiple studies demonstrate no improvement of clinical symptoms (crying, irritability).
    - >1 year: 1 to 2 mg/kg/24 h (daily or divided b.i.d.) to adult dose range
    - >20 kg: 20 mg once or twice daily
    - Up to 3.5 mg/kg/24 h have been used.
  - Lansoprazole (PO)
    - <1 year: 0.4 to 1.8 mg/kg/24 h (daily or divided b.i.d.); multiple studies demonstrate no improvement of clinical symptoms (crying, irritability).
    - 1 to 11 years: <10 kg 7.5 mg/24 h
    - 10 to 30 kg: 15 mg/dose daily up to b.i.d.
    - >30 kg: 30 mg/dose daily up to b.i.d.
  - Several other PPIs are available.
  - Side effects of PPIs may include headache, abdominal pain, and diarrhea.
  - Recent reports of increased risk for acute gastroenteritis, *Clostridium difficile* infection, and pneumonia in children. Adult studies report increased risk of osteopenia and bone fracture associated with higher dose and long-term use. Benefits should outweigh risks, especially for long-term use.
- Prokinetics: as adjunctive therapy for more severe GERD complications and hypomotility
  - No single drug has optimal prokinetic effect without significant side effects.
  - Not recommended as routine therapy
  - Erythromycin (PO)
    - 3 to 4 mg/kg/dose b.i.d.–t.i.d. (used in lower dose than for antibiotic purposes for gastric prokinetic effect)
    - Can prolong QT interval
    - Can develop tachyphylaxis
    - Short-term use can be considered for treatment of GERD symptoms seen in postinfectious gastroparesis which typically resolves spontaneously.
  - Metoclopramide (Reglan®)
    - Dosage is significantly less for GERD indication as compared to the antiemetic indication.
    - Side effects: may cause dystonia or oculogyric crisis, FDA black box warning regarding risk of tardive dyskinesia
- Calcium and aluminum/magnesium-containing antacids
  - Offers short-term symptom relief, requires multiple dosing
  - Side effects: carry risk of diarrhea and aluminum toxicity
  - Interactions: may lead to malabsorption of other medications
- Mucosal protective agents: sucralfate (Carafate®) for erosive esophagitis; maximally effective at pH 4 and on mucosal lesions

SURGERY/OTHER PROCEDURES

- Fundoplication (open or laparoscopic)
  - To increase lower esophageal sphincter tone by wrapping portion of gastric fundus around lower esophagus
  - Variations may include addition of a gastric emptying procedure (i.e., pyloroplasty).
  - Indications: failure of aggressive medical management and/or persistent, life-threatening complications (i.e., esophageal stricture; intestinal metaplastic changes as in Barrett esophagus), presence of large hiatal hernia, poor airway protection leading to aspiration of gastric contents (i.e., severe neurodevelopmental delay)
- Fundoplication complications include the following:
  - Gas bloating syndrome
  - Intractable retching
  - Bowel obstruction
  - Dumping syndrome
  - Dysphagia
  - Paraesophageal hernia
  - Wrap failure with recurrent GERD (up to 6% failure at 48 months)
  - Limited long-term clinical effectiveness
- Greater morbidity may be associated with fundoplication in children with severe physical and mental disabilities.

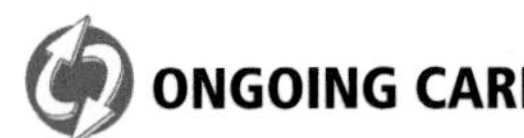

ONGOING CARE

FOLLOW-UP RECOMMENDATIONS

May be appropriate to recommend repeat endoscopy for evidence of pathologic changes of esophagus

DIET

Dietary modifications in older child: Avoid large high-fat meals, especially before bedtime. Avoid caffeine, chocolate, acidic/spicy food, peppermint, but recent adult studies show this is on an individual basis only.

ADDITIONAL READING

- Baird DC, Harker DJ, Karmes AS. Diagnosis and treatment of gastroesophageal reflux in infants and children. *Am Fam Physician*. 2015;92(8):705–714.
- Colletti RB, Di Lorenzo C. Overview of pediatric gastroesophageal reflux disease and proton pump inhibitor therapy. *J Pediatr Gastroenterol Nutr*. 2003;37(Suppl 1):S7–S11.
- Craig WR, Hanlon-Dearman A, Sinclair C, et al. Metoclopramide, thickened feedings, and positioning for gastro-oesophageal reflux in children under two years. *Cochrane Database Syst Rev*. 2004;(4):CD003502.
- El-Serag HB, Gilger M, Carter J, et al. Childhood GERD is a risk factor for GERD in adolescents and young adults. *Am J Gastroenterol*. 2004;99(5):806–812.
- Lightdale JR, Gremse DA; for Section on Gastroenterology, Hepatology, and Nutrition. Gastroesophageal reflux: management guidance for the pediatrician. *Pediatrics*. 2013;131(5):e1684–e1695.
- Lobe TE. The current role of laparoscopic surgery for gastroesophageal reflux disease in infants and children. *Surg Endosc*. 2007;21(2):167–174.
- Thakkar K, Boatright RO, Gilger MA, et al. Gastroesophageal reflux and asthma in children: a systematic review. *Pediatrics*. 2010;125(4):e925–e930.
- Vandenplas Y, Rudolph CD, Di Lorenzo C, et al. Pediatric gastroesophageal reflux clinical practice guidelines: joint recommendations of the North American Society for Pediatric Gastroenterology, Hepatology, and Nutrition (NASPGHAN) and the European Society for Pediatric Gastroenterology, Hepatology, and Nutrition (ESPGHAN). *J Pediatr Gastroenterol Nutr*. 2009;49(4):498–547.

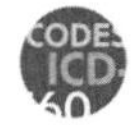

CODES

ICD10

- K21.9 Gastro-esophageal reflux disease without esophagitis
- K21.0 Gastro-esophageal reflux disease with esophagitis
- P78.83 Newborn esophageal reflux

FAQ

- Q: How long will my baby suffer with GERD?
- A: Most infant reflux resolves by 9 to 12 months of age, but symptoms may persist up to 24 months. If GERD continues after 2 to 3 years, it is more likely to behave clinically like adult GERD and require chronic management.
- Q: Should all babies with reflux be treated with medication?
- A: No. Often infant reflux is physiologic and education is all that is needed. Conservative treatments such as thickened feedings, frequent small feedings, and postprandial upright positioning can be tried first, especially as data do not support acid blockade therapy in children <12 months. It is often helpful to explain to parents that physiologic infant reflux tends to worsen from 1 to 3 months of age then typically starts to improve when children can sit upright at 6 to 7 months of age.

G

GERM CELL TUMORS

Cheryl A. C. Peretz, MD • James H. Feusner, MD

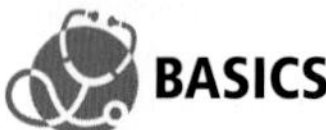

BASICS

DESCRIPTION

Germ cell tumors (GCTs) are a heterogeneous group with a suspected common cell of origin, the primordial germ cell.

- Their location can be gonadal or extragonadal.
- The numerous histologic subtypes are broadly classified as mature or immature teratomas and malignant GCTs.
- See "Brain Tumor" chapter for primary CNS GCT.

EPIDEMIOLOGY

The incidence has a bimodal distribution with a smaller peak in early infancy and a larger peak in adolescence.

- In neonates, most extracranial GCTs are benign midline teratomas.
  - Despite being nonmalignant, they confer high morbidity secondary to hydrops fetalis and premature delivery.
- In children <15 years of age, GCTs occur at a rate of 2.4 cases per million children, and they account for 2–3% of all malignancies.
- In children 15 to 19 years, extracranial GCTs account for approximately 14% of cancer diagnoses; most GCTs in this age group are germinomas.
- Sacrococcygeal teratomas account for 50% of childhood teratomas.
  - They are most prevalent in infants (1:40,000 live births); with a female predominance (4:1)

RISK FACTORS

- GCTs are thought to result from altered intrauterine events; potential risk factors include fetal chemical or hormone exposures or congenital abnormalities, primarily of sex chromosomes or sexual differentiation.
- In boys, increased risk of testicular or mediastinal GCT with cryptorchidism and Klinefelter syndrome respectively
- Approximately 50% of adolescent mediastinal GCTs are associated with Klinefelter syndrome.
- Disorders of sexual differentiation including Turner syndrome with any portion of Y chromosomal material, Frasier syndrome, Swyer syndrome, other androgen insensitivity syndromes, Denys-Drash syndrome are all associated with increased GCT in streak gonads.
- Streak gonads particularly associated with gonadoblastoma

Genetics

Familial GCT has been described in 1.5–2% of adult GCTs and a similar contribution to adolescent GCTs is presumed.

GENERAL PREVENTION

- Prophylactic gonadectomy is recommended for streak gonads in the specific syndromes mentioned above because of the increased risk of developing GCTs.
- Guidelines on the management of cryptorchidism recommend the following to decrease the future risk of testicular GCT:
  - Orchidopexy by 18 months of age
  - Consideration of orchiectomy of an undescended testis in all boys with a normal contralateral testis when orchidopexy is not feasible
  - Consider orchiectomy or biopsy in a postpubertal boy with cryptorchidism.
  - Counsel all men with a history of cryptorchidism and/or their parents regarding the long-term risk of testicular cancer.

ETIOLOGY

- GCTs arise from primordial germ cells with molecular defects.
  - Germinomas (testicular seminomas and ovarian dysgerminomas) originate directly from undifferentiated primordial germ cells.
  - Embryonal carcinomas have early embryonic differentiation, so produce teratomas with all three germ layers (endoderm, ectoderm, mesoderm).
  - Yolk sac tumors and choriocarcinomas originate from primordial germ cells with extra-embryonic differentiation.
  - Mixed malignant GCTs contain various histologies.
- Primordial germs cells migrate through the midline from the yolk sac to the gonadal ridge; disruption of this migration likely explains the midline propensity of extragonadal GCTs.
- Certain oncogenic miRNAs (miR-371-373 and miR-302/367 clusters) are overexpressed in all malignant GCTs.
  - These are detectable in serum at time of diagnosis and should respond to treatment; this is more sensitive and specific than traditional biomarkers.
- Genetic profiles are different in children than adults, even for same histologic subtypes, suggesting gene expression may be driven, at least partially, by pubertal hormonal changes.
- Gain of short arm of chromosome 12, isochromosome 12p [or i(12)p] is present in >80% postpubertal GCTs.
- Malignant GCTs in children <4 years often contain cytogenetic abnormalities in chromosomes 1, 3, 6, 11 and others.
  - Deletion of 1q36 is present in 80–100% of infantile malignant GCTs in testicular as well as extragonadal sites.
  - Infantile yolk sack tumors include alterations including loss of 6q24-qter or 1p, gain of 20q and 1q, and c-myc or n-myc amplification.
- Single nucleotide polymorphisms (SNPs) in genes involved in KIT/ KITLG signaling, male germ cell development, increased telomerase activity, defective microtubules, and DNA damage repair pathways are implicated in GCT development.
- Epigenetics may also contribute to GCT development.
  - Yolk sac tumors have increased methylation.

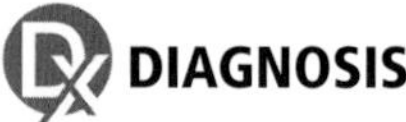

DIAGNOSIS

HISTORY

- GCT diagnosis should be considered for any midline tumor.
- A history of abnormal sexual development may be an indication of an underlying sex chromosome abnormality associated with an increased risk of a GCT.
- Acute or chronic abdominal pain is the presenting symptom in up to 80% of ovarian GCTs.
  - Vaginal bleeding, amenorrhea, and constipation may also be present.
- Pediatric testicular tumors typically present as nontender scrotal masses.
- Sacrococcygeal teratomas typically present with swelling.
  - Pregnancies may be associated with polyhydramnios or high-output cardiac failure.
  - Other congenital anomalies are seen in up to 18% of patients.
- Mediastinal tumors can present with respiratory compromise in younger children, whereas adolescents may have a more insidious presentation.

PHYSICAL EXAM

- A palpable abdominal mass may be present with an ovarian GCT.
- A palpable nontender testicular mass is typical of testicular GCT.
- Sacrococcygeal GCTs can present with a palpable abdominal or perineal mass or signs of spinal cord compression.
- Especially in younger children, a mediastinal GCT may present with potentially critical respiratory compromise or superior vena cava syndrome.
- Inappropriate absence or presence of sexual development may be seen with hormonally active GCTs.

DIFFERENTIAL DIAGNOSIS

- Sacrococcygeal:
  - Pilonidal cyst
  - Meningocele
  - Lipomeningocele
  - Hemangioma
  - Abscess
  - Epidermal cyst
  - Chondroma
  - Lymphoma
  - Ependymoma
  - Neuroblastoma
  - Glioma

- Abdominal:
  - Wilms tumor
  - Neuroblastoma
  - Lymphoma
  - Rhabdomyosarcoma
  - Hepatoblastoma
  - Retained twin fetus
- Vaginal:
  - Rhabdomyosarcoma (sarcoma botryoides)
  - Clear cell carcinoma
- Ovarian:
  - Cyst
  - Appendicitis
  - Pregnancy
  - Pelvic infection
  - Hematocolpos
  - Sarcoma
  - Lymphoma
  - Other ovarian tumors
- Testicular:
  - Epididymitis
  - Testicular torsion
  - Orchitis
  - Hernia
  - Hydrocele
  - Hematocele
  - Rhabdomyosarcoma
  - Lymphoma
  - Leukemia
  - Other testicular tumors
- Mediastinal:
  - Hodgkin and non-Hodgkin lymphoma
  - Leukemia
  - Thymoma

DIAGNOSTIC TESTS & INTERPRETATION

Initial Tests (screening, lab, imaging)

- Serum tumor markers include AFP and β-hCG help to diagnose, monitor, and stage GCTs.
  - AFP and β-HCG vary with age.
  - Elevated AFP: teratoma, embryonal carcinoma and/or yolk sac
  - Elevated β-HCG: germinoma, embryonal carcinoma and/or choriocarcinoma
  - Other tumor markers, including inhibin or sex hormones, are useful for differentiating testicular or ovarian sex cord tumors.
- Other workup should include a CBC and differential, chemistry panel, liver function tests, uric acid, and LDH to evaluate for other malignancies or organ dysfunction.
- Plain radiograph: may reveal mature calcified tissues, such as bone or teeth, within tumor
- Chest radiograph: shows mediastinal mass
- CT scan: necessary to evaluate the primary site and regional disease
- Transscrotal ultrasound: Initial imaging of testicular mass can reveal calcifications or heterogenous features.
- Prenatal MRI: helpful for prenatal counseling and preoperative planning of fetal sacrococcygeal teratomas
- Chest CT and bone scan: indicated to evaluate for metastatic disease when malignancy is suspected

Diagnostic Procedures/Other

- Tissue is mandatory because histology is essential to the classification of GCTs.
- Pathologic findings
  - GCTs are broadly classified as teratomas or malignant GCTs.
  - Teratomas contain elements of all three germ cell layers (ectoderm, mesoderm, and endoderm).
    - They can be mature, immature, or immature with malignant elements.
  - Major malignant histologic subtypes include yolk sac tumor, embryonal carcinoma, gonadoblastoma, choriocarcinoma, and mixed malignant GCT.
    - Histologic subtype does not necessarily correlate with tumor biology, patient age, site of origin, or patient prognosis.

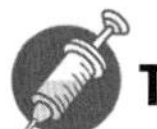

TREATMENT

MEDICATION

- The administration of chemotherapy is based on malignant potential, local tumor extent, surgical outcomes, and the patient's medical history.
- The typical 1st-line chemotherapy regimen for malignant GCTs includes cisplatin or carboplatin, etoposide, and bleomycin (PEB).
  - Current trials are investigating carboplatin compressed PEB cycles for poor risk patients, and carboplatin versus cisplatin regimens for standard risk patient.
  - Cisplatin is associated with a risk of ototoxicity and nephrotoxicity.
  - Bleomycin is associated with a risk of pulmonary toxicity.
  - PEB therapy is associated with a risk of secondary myelodysplasia or acute myeloid leukemia.

SURGERY/OTHER PROCEDURES

- Every effort should be made to preserve fertility in gonadal teratomas.
  - An experienced pediatric–gynecology oncologic surgeon is critical.
- Sacrococcygeal teratoma
  - A complete surgical resection including the coccyx is curative.
  - Close postoperative follow-up should include monitoring of tumor markers.
  - Fetal surgery should be considered if signs of hydrops are seen.
- Mature teratoma
  - Full surgical excision, irrespective of site, is curative in prepubescent patients.
  - Postpubescent patient with testicular teratoma (mature or immature) is at risk for retroperitoneal metastatic recurrence, so adjuvant chemotherapy and retroperitoneal lymph node resection are additional treatment considerations.
- Immature teratoma
  - Complete surgical resection is therapy of choice; close observation and tumor marker evaluation for normalization
  - In cases of elevated AFP and incomplete surgical resection, chemotherapy should be offered given risk of microscopic foci of endodermal sinus tumor.
- Malignant GCT
  - Surgery plus chemotherapy with etoposide, cisplatin or carboplatin, and bleomycin
  - Patients with residual disease should have additional surgery and additional chemotherapy if total resection is not possible.
  - High-dose chemotherapy with autologous stem cell support and radiation are reserved for salvage therapy in recurrent disease.

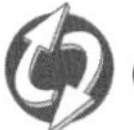

ONGOING CARE

- Serial physical exams and imaging studies of primary site
- Tumor markers (AFP or β-hCG) if elevated at diagnosis
- If chemotherapy or radiation therapy used, need to monitor for secondary malignancies
  - Long term (see "Cancer Therapy Late Effects" chapter)
  - Short term, need to monitor blood counts, chemistries, renal function, and audiology

ADDITIONAL READING

- Isaacs H Jr. Perinatal (fetal and neonatal) germ cell tumors. *J Pediatr Surg*. 2004;39(7):1003–1013.
- Murray MJ, Halsall DJ, Hook CE, et al. Identification of microRNAs from the miR-371-373 and miR-302 clusters as potential serum biomarkers of malignant germ cell tumors. *Am J Clin Pathol*. 2011;135(1):119–125.
- Olson TA, Murray MJ, Rodriguez-Galindo C, et al. Pediatric and adolescent extracranial germ cell tumors: the road to collaboration. *J Clin Oncol*. 2015;33(27):3018–3028.
- Shaikh F, Murray MJ, Amatruda JF, et al. Paediatric extracranial germ-cell tumours. *Lancet Oncol*. 2016;17(4):e149–e162.

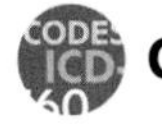

CODES

ICD10

- C80.1 Malignant (primary) neoplasm, unspecified
- D48.0 Neoplasm of uncertain behavior of bone/artic cartl
- C38.3 Malignant neoplasm of mediastinum, part unspecified

FAQ

- Q: What is the chance of cure for immature/malignant teratomas?
- A: With current chemotherapy as outlined earlier, overall survival is 85–97% (dependent on disease stage).
- Q: Can a benign tumor recur? If so, can it then be malignant?
- A: Yes. If there is residual tissue left behind, the tumor can recur. If there were unrecognized areas of malignancy, the recurrence can be a malignant teratoma. The greatest risk for the latter is with the immature teratomas.

GERMAN MEASLES (THIRD DISEASE, RUBELLA)

Michael J. Smith, MD, MSCE

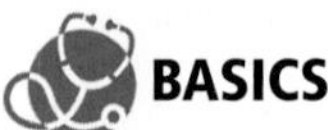

BASICS

DESCRIPTION

- *Rubella* derived from Latin, meaning "little red."
- Disease initially considered variant of measles
- Viral infection characterized by mild symptoms (often subclinical), with an erythematous rash progressing from head to toes
- Congenital rubella syndrome can be devastating.

EPIDEMIOLOGY

- Spread person to person via airborne transmission; worldwide infection
- Infection most contagious when rash is erupting. However, virus may be shed beginning 7 days before rash to 14 days after.
- Infants with congenital rubella syndrome may shed virus for up to 1 year.
- In temperate regions, peaks in late winter and early spring
- Infection occurs equally in following age groups: <5 years, 5 to 19 years, and 20 to 39 years.
  - In prevaccine era, annual incidence of infection in the United States was ~58 per 100,000 population.
  - 2004: no longer endemic in the United States
  - 2004 to 2012: 79 reported cases, mostly in unvaccinated individuals born overseas
- Congenital rubella syndrome
  - 1964: 20,000 newborns
  - 1980s: reported rarely, with <5 cases annually
  - 1990 to 1991: ~30 cases reported annually
  - 2004 to 2012: total of 6 cases reported to Centers for Disease Control and Prevention (CDC), only 1 with mother born in the United States

GENERAL PREVENTION

- Prevention of congenital rubella syndrome is main objective of vaccination programs.
- Rubella vaccine
  - Current strain of vaccine (RA 27/3, developed at the Wistar Institute in Philadelphia) was licensed in 1979 and has replaced all other strains.
  - Given as part of MMR vaccine at 12 to 15 months and again at 4 to 6 years
  - Immunity occurs in 95% of those vaccinated and is thought to be lifelong.
  - Important to ensure full vaccination for preschool-aged children
  - Vaccine virus is not communicable: Pregnant women and persons who are immunodeficient (except asymptomatic HIV infection) should not receive vaccine, but household contacts should.
- Isolation
  - Pregnant women should avoid contact with source patient.
  - Postnatal: Droplet precautions and/or school exclusion is indicated for 7 days after onset of rash.
  - Congenital: contact isolation until first birthday or until two nasopharyngeal and urine cultures consecutively negative

PATHOPHYSIOLOGY

- Respiratory transmission
- Replication in nasopharynx and regional lymph nodes
- Viremia 5 to 7 days after exposure, with spread of virus throughout body
- In congenital rubella syndrome, transplacental infection of fetus occurs during viremia.

ETIOLOGY

Rubella virus

- Classified as a *Rubivirus* in the Togaviridae family
- RNA virus with single antigenic type
- First isolated in 1962 by Parkman and Weller

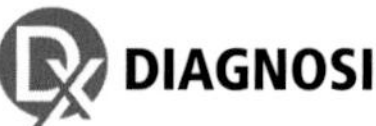

DIAGNOSIS

If rubella is suspected, case should be reported to local public health authorities.

HISTORY

- In children, prodrome is not often recognized.
- In adults, a 1- to 5-day prodrome of low-grade fever, malaise, and cervical adenopathy may precede rash.
- Inquire about immunizations and exposures.

PHYSICAL EXAM

- Rash
  - Begins on face and then progresses to trunk and extremities
  - Does not usually coalesce
  - Lasts for 3 days
- Adenopathies, especially postauricular, posterior cervical, and suboccipital, are commonly noted along with conjunctivitis.
- Arthralgia/arthritis may be seen in adolescents and adults.

DIFFERENTIAL DIAGNOSIS

Infections that are sometimes confused with rubella include the following:

- Modified measles
- Scarlet fever
- Roseola
- Erythema infectiosum (fifth disease, parvovirus B19 infection)
- Enteroviral infections
- Infectious mononucleosis
- Drug eruptions

DIAGNOSTIC TESTS & INTERPRETATION

- Congenital infection
  - Serologic testing should be performed on both mother and infant.
  - Rubella-specific IgM in infant is highly suggestive.
  - Viral isolation from throat or nasal specimen can confirm diagnosis. Blood, urine, and CSF samples may also be diagnostic.
  - Diagnosis is difficult to verify after neonatal period.
- Postnatally acquired
  - Rubella-specific IgM or a ≥4-fold rise in rubella-specific IgG antibodies between acute and convalescent titers is diagnostic.

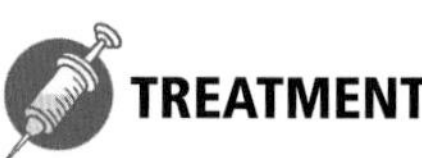

TREATMENT

Supportive care

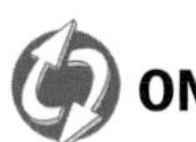

ONGOING CARE

PROGNOSIS

- Quite good; as many as 50% of infections are asymptomatic.
- Rubella infection in a pregnant woman can be devastating for the infant (see "Complications").

COMPLICATIONS

- Tend to occur in adults; most are uncommon.
- Arthritis or arthralgia
  - Occurs in 70% of adult women, lasting up to 1 month
  - Usually affects small joints
- Encephalitis
  - 1 in 5,000 cases
  - May be associated with mortality
- Bleeding
  - 1 in 3,000 cases
  - Occurs in children more than in adults
- Thrombocytopenia: commonly noted
- Orchitis and neuritis: rare
- Congenital rubella syndrome
  - Rubella infection in early gestation can lead to fetal death, premature delivery, and congenital defects.
  - Severity of defects is worse the earlier in gestation the infection occurs.
  - 85% of infants are affected if infection occurs in first trimester.
  - Defects are rare if infection occurs after 20th week.
  - Common defects of congenital rubella syndrome:
    - Deafness: most common defect
    - Ophthalmologic defects: cataracts, glaucoma, microphthalmia
    - Cardiac defects: patent ductus arteriosus, ventricular septal defect, pulmonic stenosis, coarctation of aorta
    - Neurologic defects: mental retardation, microcephaly
  - Some manifestations of congenital rubella syndrome (diabetes mellitus, progressive encephalopathy) may be delayed for years.

ADDITIONAL READING

- American Academy of Pediatrics. Rubella. In: Kimberlin DW, Brady MT, Jackson MA, et al, eds. *Red Book: 2015 Report of the Committee on Infectious Diseases*. 30th ed. Elk Grove Village, IL: American Academy of Pediatrics; 2015:688–695.
- Atkinson W, et al. *Epidemiology and Prevention of Vaccine-Preventable Diseases*. 2nd ed. Bethesda, MD: Centers for Disease Control and Prevention; 1995.
- Gran GB, Reef SE, Dabbagh A, et al. Global progress toward rubella and congenital rubella syndrome control and elimination—2000–2014. *MMWR Morb Mortal Wkly Rep*. 2015;64(37):1052–1055.
- Papania MJ, Wallace GS, Rota PA, et al. Elimination of endemic measles, rubella, and congenital rubella syndrome from the Western hemisphere: the US experience. *JAMA Pediatr*. 2014;168(2):148–155.

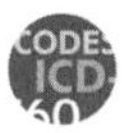

CODES

ICD10

- B06.9 Rubella without complication
- P35.0 Congenital rubella syndrome
- B06.89 Other rubella complications

FAQ

- Q: Although pregnancy is a contraindication to rubella vaccination, if a pregnant woman is inadvertently vaccinated, will there be harm to the fetus?
- A: Data collected since 1979 by the CDC show no evidence of congenital rubella syndrome in 321 susceptible women who were vaccinated while pregnant. Therefore, inadvertent vaccination is not an indication for termination of pregnancy.
- Q: Is there any evidence that the MMR vaccine causes autism spectrum disorder?
- A: No. Multiple epidemiologic studies have shown no difference in the rates of autism spectrum disorder in children who received the MMR vaccine versus those who did not. The original paper that suggested a link between vaccines and autism was retracted in 2010.

GIARDIASIS

Christina R. Hermos, MD

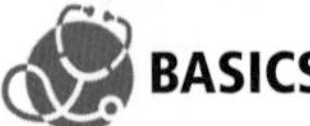

BASICS

DESCRIPTION

Diarrheal illness caused by small intestine (duodenum and jejunum) and biliary tract infection with flagellated protozoan *Giardia intestinalis* (also *Giardia lamblia* and *Giardia duodenalis*)

EPIDEMIOLOGY

- *Giardia* is the most common parasitic enteric pathogen diagnosed across the world and the United States.
- Higher rates in developing countries
- Affects all age groups but peaks at 1 to 4 years, followed by 5 to 9 years, and then 45 to 49 years of age
- Transmission:
  - Acquired by ingestion of cysts directly from infected person (rarely animals) or ingestion of fecally contaminated water or food
  - Cysts infectious for as long as person excretes them (weeks to months), and infectious dose is low (10 cysts).
  - Incubation period 1 to 3 weeks
  - Person-to-person transmission accounts for the high prevalence rates in institutions, day care centers, and family contacts.
  - Waterborne transmission is an important source of endemic or epidemic spread, especially when water is supplied by surface source such as streams and reservoirs (outdoor recreation and international travel).
  - Foodborne infection is less common and generally occurs from foods (e.g., lettuce) that have been washed with a contaminated water source.

Incidence

U.S. average is 5.8 to 6.4 cases per 100,000 and approximately 16,000 cases are reported each year.

Prevalence

- In the U.S., nondysenteric diarrheal stool specimens range from 5% to 7%, with rates up to 15% in children.
- Highest prevalence in early summer through early fall and among residents of the Northwestern U.S.

RISK FACTORS

- Day care attendance (increases risk of exposure to inadequate fecal–oral hygiene)
- Travel to endemic areas
- International adoption
- Contact with recreational fresh water during backpacking, camping, swimming (swallowing water)
- Contact with some animal species
- Sexual practices exposing to fecal flora
- Hypochlorhydria (previous gastric surgery)
- Hypogammaglobulinemia, immunodeficiency
- Cystic fibrosis (CF)

GENERAL PREVENTION

- Handwashing all surfaces with soap and water for 20 seconds after toileting, changing diapers, handling animal waste, gardening, tending to a person with diarrheal illness, and prior to preparing food
- Exclusion from child care and pool/recreational water during acute diarrheal illnesses. Excluding asymptomatic carriers is not recommended.
- Avoiding potentially contaminated water (recreational/drinking) and food
- Examining water sources in endemic areas
- Boiling (1 minute), chemical disinfection or filtration (National Sanitation Foundation [NSF] Standard 53 or 58) of suspect water sources
- Preventing contact with feces during sex
- Administering vitamin A to children in developing countries has been shown to improve host defenses against *Giardia* infection.

ETIOLOGY

Giardia intestinalis has a two-form life cycle: cyst (transmission) and trophozoite (infection)

- Gastric acid and pancreatic enzymes initiate excystation of ingested cysts.
- Trophozoites divide asexually and adhere to brush border of proximal small bowel enterocytes.
- Cyst formation (encystation) occurs in the colon and is passed into the environment.

PATHOPHYSIOLOGY

Trophozoite causes direct damage to intestinal brush border and mucosa (but does not invade mucosa), which leads to the following:

- Disruption of tight junctional zonula occludens of intestinal mucosal cells
- Increased permeability of mucosal cells via myosin light chain kinase-dependent phosphorylation of F-actin
- Induction of epithelial apoptosis
- Induction of host immune response that results in secretion of fluid and damage to the gut
- Secondary lactase deficiency

DIAGNOSIS

- Many (50–75%) infected individuals are asymptomatic.
- Clinical presentation (acute):
  - Sudden-onset watery, foul-smelling diarrhea without blood/pus/mucus
  - Malaise
  - Bloating/flatulence
  - Steatorrhea
  - Abdominal cramps
  - Anorexia/nausea
  - Dyspepsia
  - 25–50% self-limiting, lasting 7 to 10 days
- Clinical presentation (chronic):
  - Loose, semiformed stool >14 days
  - Steatorrhea
  - Profound malaise
  - Abdominal distention
  - Weight loss/failure to thrive
  - Anorexia
  - Anemia
  - Flatulence
  - Depression
  - Alternation of diarrhea/constipation until spontaneous resolution or treatment begun
- Malabsorption syndrome may include the following:
  - Steatorrhea
  - Deficiencies of iron, D-xylose, vitamins A, B_{12}, E
  - Protein-losing enteropathy

HISTORY

- Exposures:
  - Habitation in or travel to endemic area
  - Attendants of child care centers or inhabitants of institutions
  - Camping or hiking near fresh water and/or recreational water exposure
  - Exposure to infected individual
- Recurrent infections and/or failure to thrive (may also indicate primary immunodeficiency)
- Gastric surgery

PHYSICAL EXAM

- Abdominal distention
- Aphthous ulcers in oral mucosa
- Urticaria
- Arthralgia/arthritis

DIFFERENTIAL DIAGNOSIS

- Other infectious diarrhea
- Celiac disease
- CF
- Lactose intolerance

- Irritable bowel syndrome
- Inflammatory bowel disease
- Nonulcer dyspepsia

DIAGNOSTIC TESTS & INTERPRETATION

Initial Tests (screening, lab, imaging)

- Blood testing for enzyme immunoassay (EIA) and direct fluorescent antibody (DFA); faster and more sensitive than stool microscopy
- Stool microscopy for identification of trophozoites or cysts (multiple [three] ova/parasite [O/P] samples provide 90% sensitivity)
- Real-time polymerase chain reaction (PCR) is most sensitive, if available.
- If immunodeficiency is suspected, evaluate for humoral immunodeficiency.
- CBC generally not revealing: WBC usually normal and eosinophilia absent

Diagnostic Procedures/Other

- Direct duodenal aspiration or string test (enterotest) if clinical suspicion is high and routine testing is negative
- Duodenal biopsy rarely indicated
- Pathologic findings
  - Mucosal lesions vary from normal to subtotal villous atrophy, with crypt hyperplasia and proliferation of intraepithelial and lamina propria lymphocytes. Trophozoites may be seen on biopsies.

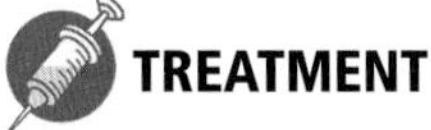

TREATMENT

MEDICATION

- Metronidazole (not indication approved by FDA)
  - 15 mg/kg/24 h divided t.i.d. PO for 5 to 10 days
  - Efficacy 80–100%
  - Poor palatability
- Tinidazole (approved for children ≥3 years)
  - 50 mg/kg, max 2 g; single oral dose
  - Available in tablet form only
  - Fewer adverse effects than metronidazole
  - Median efficacy 91%
- Nitazoxanide (approved for ages 1 to 11 years)
  - Similar efficacy to metronidazole
- Paromomycin (symptomatic infection in pregnant women in the second and third trimesters)
- Asymptomatic giardiasis, in absence of risk factors, should not be treated.
- Treatment of asymptomatic carriers in households of patients with CF or hypogammaglobulinemia may be considered.
- Treatment failures:
  - High-dose courses of original agent
  - Combination of nitroimidazole plus quinacrine for at least 2 weeks

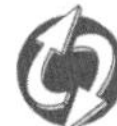

ONGOING CARE

FOLLOW-UP RECOMMENDATIONS

Patient Monitoring

- Symptom recurrence can be attributable to reinfection, secondary lactose intolerance, insufficient treatment, or drug resistance.
- Detailed exposure history and repeat testing with recurrence of symptoms
- If reinfection suspected, a repeat course of the same drug often effective or an alternative agent if resistance suspected
- If symptoms persist, with negative diagnostic studies, consider alternative etiology or enteropathogen.

DIET

Consider lactose avoidance to prevent bloating and diarrhea for 1 month after treatment.

PROGNOSIS

- Good
- Higher risk of refractory course in immunocompromised patients

COMPLICATIONS

- Lactose deficiency
- Malabsorption syndrome
- Steatorrhea
- Deficiencies of iron, folic acid, and vitamins A, B_{12}, and E
- Protein-losing enteropathy
- Urticaria
- Arthralgia
- In pediatric patients:
  - Growth retardation
  - Failure to thrive
  - Lower IQ
  - Urticaria

ADDITIONAL READING

- Ali SA, Hill DR. *Giardia intestinalis*. *Curr Opin Infect Dis*. 2003;16(5):453–460.
- American Academy of Pediatrics. *Giardia intestinalis* (formerly *Giardia lamblia* and *Giardia duodenalis*) infections. In: Kimberlin DW, Brady MT, Jackson MA, et al, eds. *Red Book: 2015 Report of the Committee on Infectious Diseases*. 30th ed. Elk Grove Village, IL: American Academy of Pediatrics; 2015:353–355.
- Centers for Disease Control and Prevention. Giardia. https://www.cdc.gov/parasites/giardia/index.html. Accessed April 11, 2018.
- Huang DB, White AC. An updated review on *Cryptosporidium* and *Giardia*. *Gastroenterol Clin North Am*. 2006;35(2):291–314.
- Lima AA, Soares AM, Lima NL, et al. Effects of vitamin A supplementation on intestinal barrier function, growth, total parasitic, and specific *Giardia* spp infections in Brazilian children: a prospective randomized, double-blind, placebo-controlled trial. *J Pediatr Gastroenterol Nutr*. 2010;50(3):309–315.
- Painter JE, Gargano JW, Collier SA, et al; for Centers for Disease Control and Prevention. Giardiasis surveillance—United States, 2011–2012. *MMWR Suppl*. 2015;64(3):15–25.
- Yoder JS, Gargano JW, Wallace RM, et al; for Centers for Disease Control and Prevention. Giardiasis surveillance—United States, 2009–2010. *MMWR Surveill Summ*. 2012;61(5):13–23.

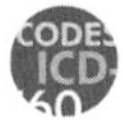

CODES

ICD10

A07.1 Giardiasis [lambliasis]

FAQ

- Q: How is *G. intestinalis* likely contracted?
- A: Direct person-to-person contact via fecal–oral transmission. Most community-wide epidemics occur from a contaminated water supply (drinking water), as well as person-to-person transmission in child care and institutional settings. Food and food handler–associated outbreaks are less often reported.
- Q: What do I do if I suspect *Giardia*, but the stool sample is negative?
- A: Three O/P samples are needed and should optimally be done every other day on a diarrheal stool specimen with an EIA or DFA to increase diagnostic sensitivity. Stool samples should be examined as soon as possible or placed immediately in a preservative, such as neutral buffered 10% formalin or polyvinyl alcohol. In endemic areas, it may be appropriate to treat empirically. If stool testing is negative and the diagnosis is strongly suspected, you can consider ordering a commercially available string test (designed to obtain bile-stained mucus from duodenum to reveal trophozoites on wet mount) or refer to a pediatric gastroenterologist, who can perform endoscopy with duodenal aspiration and biopsy.

GINGIVITIS

Ray J. Jurado, DDS

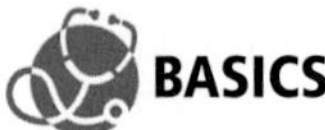

BASICS

DESCRIPTION

- Gingivitis and periodontitis are both classified under periodontal disease.
  - Gingivitis is inflammation limited to the gingiva and not resulting in periodontal ligament (PDL) attachment and bone loss.
  - Periodontitis is inflammation of the gingiva and adjacent connective tissue attachment, characterized by loss of PDL, connective tissue, and alveolar bone.
- Gingivitis can be localized to a limited area or generalized, involving the entire gingiva.
- Depending on etiology, gingivitis can also present as acute or chronic.

EPIDEMIOLOGY

- Gingivitis occurs in 50% of children with mild, marginal gingivitis being the most common form.
- Severe gingivitis is relatively uncommon in healthy children.
- The prevalence of gingivitis increases with age, with a peak at puberty, likely due to hormonal influences and inconsistent oral hygiene.

RISK FACTORS

- General risk factors
  - Increased dental plaque formation—inconsistent brushing and flossing, frequent carbohydrate intake
  - Local areas of plaque accumulation—erupting teeth, crowded teeth, orthodontic appliances/bands/brackets, poor brushing technique
  - Decreased saliva (self-cleaning effect) leading to dry mouth/xerostomia—mouth breathing, many pediatric medications
  - Increase gingival inflammatory response—immunodeficient conditions, chronic illnesses, certain medications
- Specific risk factors
  - Medications: antiepileptics, cyclosporine, calcium channel blockers
  - Hormonal changes: puberty, pregnancy
  - Immunologic deficiencies: HIV, Chédiak-Higashi, cyclic neutropenia
  - Chronic illnesses: diabetes mellitus, chronic renal failure, histiocytosis X, scleroderma, secondary hyperparathyroidism
  - Neurologic problems: developmental delay, cerebral palsy, other conditions where oral hygiene is difficult
  - Behavioral factors: smoking, stress, alcohol consumption
  - Miscellaneous: malnutrition, viral illnesses

GENERAL PREVENTION

- Prevention of gingivitis is directed toward effective removal of dental plaque on a daily basis:
  - Infants: washcloth to remove plaque after feeding; toothbrush using baby toothpaste (nonfluoridated)
  - Children: assistance with brushing with a small amount of toothpaste after meals
  - Older children and adolescents: Brush teeth after meals with fluoridated toothpaste in addition to daily flossing.
  - Children/adolescents with high-risk factors must brush and floss consistently.
- The American Academy of Pediatrics (AAP) recommends that children at high risk for dental caries should establish routine dental care by their first birthday. Children should then continue routine dental checkups at a minimum of every 6 months.

ETIOLOGY

- Gingivitis most often occurs in response to bacterial biofilm/plaque at the gingival margin (gingiva covering the necks of the teeth).
- Accumulation of dental bacterial plaque is a direct cause of gingival inflammation. Plaque accumulation can be caused by:
  - Inconsistent brushing and flossing
  - Local areas that are difficult to access and clean
  - Decreased saliva/xerostomia
- Increased gingival inflammatory response
  - Normal/abnormal hormone fluctuations
  - Alterations in insulin levels in patients with diabetes
  - Vitamin deficiencies (e.g., vitamin C deficiency)
- Infectious diseases leading to gingival inflammation/ulceration
  - Herpes simplex virus (HSV) type I
  - *Candida albicans*
  - HIV
- Medications promoting gingival overgrowth
  - Phenytoin
  - Cyclosporine
  - Nifedipine
  - Oral contraceptive pills
- Trauma

DIAGNOSIS

HISTORY

- Assess medical history for chronic illnesses, bleeding disorders, immunodeficiencies, etc.
- Assess home oral hygiene practice, focusing on brushing/flossing frequency. Review hygiene technique if practical.
- Assess the diet, including carbohydrate intake/frequency, and possible nutritional deficiencies.
- Review medications, taking note of any that may increase risk of gingival inflammation/enlargement.
- Review any intraoral complaints:
  - Bleeding gums on brushing or spontaneously
  - Gingival pain on brushing, eating, or spontaneous
  - Gingival swelling
  - Review when symptoms arose, how often, etc.

PHYSICAL EXAM

- Mild signs are usually gingival erythema and bleeding with brushing or flossing.
- Moderate to severe signs include swelling, ulceration, and tenderness.
- Examine the head and neck for signs of swelling, erythema, warmth, enlarged maxillary lymph nodes, as well as right/left symmetry.
- Examine the gingival tissue for erythema, swelling, ulceration, fluctuance, or drainage.
- Assess whether gingival inflammation is localized to an area (local factor) or generalized, involving the entire upper and lower gingiva (systemic factor/medication).
- Assess for pain or sensitivity on palpation.
- Assess oral hygiene, noting plaque buildup, crowding, carious teeth, abscesses.
- Take note of any orthodontic appliances that may decrease effectiveness of brushing and flossing.
- Evaluate the teeth for caries, fractures, looseness, malocclusion, pain, and plaque.

DIFFERENTIAL DIAGNOSIS

- Localized gingivitis
  - Poor hygiene technique: Check routine.
  - Food impaction: Check diet.
  - Orthodontic appliances
  - Pregnancy tumor (pyogenic granuloma)
  - Abscess: Check for caries.
  - Trauma: Check history.
  - Self-inflicted injury—unusual location and history
- Generalized gingivitis—healthy presentation
  - Extremely poor or no oral hygiene
  - Diet high in carbohydrates
- Generalized gingivitis—systemic manifestations
  - Herpetic gingivostomatitis—fever; malaise
  - Neutrophil disorders
  - Leukemia
  - HIV
  - Graft-versus-host disease (infiltrative gingivitis)
  - Vitamin C deficiency
  - Behçet disease
- Generalized gingivitis—bleeding
  - Hemophilia (factor VIII or IX deficiency)
  - Thrombocytopenia
- Generalized gingivitis—overgrowth
  - Gingival hyperplasia due to medication
  - Gingival hyperplasia due to hormone fluctuation
- Generalized gingivitis—severe, rapid
  - Acute necrotizing ulcerative gingivitis (ANUG)—painful gingivitis associated with rapid onset and tissue ulceration and necrosis
    - Peaks in adolescence and young adulthood
    - Related to high oral concentrations of spirochetes and/or *Prevotella intermedia*

DIAGNOSTIC TESTS & INTERPRETATION

Initial Tests (screening, lab, imaging)

- Most patients do not need laboratory evaluation to assess causes of gingivitis. Biopsy may be necessary to confirm or narrow differential diagnoses but is usually performed by a periodontist or oral surgeon.
- If there is a concern for excessive bleeding, a CBC with differential, PT, and PTT may be helpful to rule out thrombocytopenia, pancytopenia, or a clotting disorder.

- If there is concern for sepsis, blood culture may be necessary.
- Direct fluorescent antibody testing for HSV-1: If herpes is suspected (stomatitis is usually present), swab the base of a stoma/vesicle and smear on a slide. HSV culture is the gold standard.
- Panoramic or intraoral radiographic imaging by a pediatric dentist may be necessary to assess severity of inflammation and possible loss of alveolar bone.

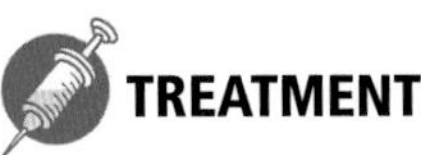

TREATMENT

GENERAL MEASURES

- A consistent oral hygiene regime directed at minimizing plaque buildup is essential to prevent or manage gingivitis.
  - Brushing after breakfast and prior to bedtime allows for consistent clearance of food and keeps plaque manageable.
  - Mechanical/sonic toothbrushes allow for more effective plaque removal.
  - Toothpaste with fluoride when child can expectorate
  - Flossing if teeth are in tight contact and not spaced apart
  - Regular visits to a pediatric dentist for examination and thorough cleaning/scaling every 4 to 6 months
- For moderate to severe gingivitis, possible risk factors should be assessed and additional measures implemented.
  - Mouth rinses for plaque inhibition using 0.12% chlorhexidine gluconate oral rinse
  - More frequent dental visits for reassessment and thorough cleanings/scalings
  - Gingivectomy to allow for more access to plaque
  - Antibiotics to cover mouth flora in more severe cases when bacterial superinfection is suspected.

MEDICATION

- Mouth rinses for plaque inhibition are prescribed when daily oral hygiene is insufficient to control plaque.
  - The most commonly used rinse is 0.12% chlorhexidine gluconate oral rinse.
  - Chlorhexidine gluconate is prescribed as a temporary measure in children to stabilize inflammation as the source of inflammation is controlled.
- Antibiotics are rarely prescribed for mild or moderate gingivitis.

ISSUES FOR REFERRAL

- It is important for providers to evaluate the oral health of all children. When gingival inflammation is noted, the patient should be referred to a pediatric dentist for assessment and management.
- For severe cases of gingivitis, a periodontist should be consulted to provide timely assessment and aggressive management. The pediatric dentist may consult after first assessment.
- Generalized cases of gingivitis may need referral to a pediatric specialist to assess for systemic causes or medications that may be manifesting orally.

SURGERY/OTHER PROCEDURES

In cases of gingival hypertrophy, localized or generalized gingivectomy by a periodontist may be necessary to remove excess gingival tissue, allowing for more effective plaque access and removal.

ONGOING CARE

FOLLOW-UP RECOMMENDATIONS

- Regular dental visits for professional cleanings and plaque removal is recommended for all children and adults.
- Children with moderate to severe gingivitis will need more frequent dental visits until gingivitis is controlled; most dentists recommend every 3 months.

Patient Monitoring

- Children with moderate to severe gingivitis will need more frequent dental visits to assess extent of inflammation and modify office/home management until gingivitis is under control.
- Periodic intraoral radiographs may be necessary to monitor extent of bone loss.

DIET

- Minimize amount and frequency of high–sugar content food and beverages.
- Xylitol-containing chewing gum can improve oral hygiene by reducing plaque adherence to the gum line.

PATIENT EDUCATION

- Establish a daily oral hygiene routine involving a moderate diet, brushing, and flossing.
- Brushing after breakfast and prior to bedtime allows for consistent clearance of food and keeps plaque manageable.
- Mechanical/sonic toothbrushes allow for more effective plaque removal.
- Toothpaste with fluoride when child can expectorate
- Flossing if teeth are in tight contact and not spaced apart
- Regular visits to a pediatric dentist reassessment and thorough cleaning/scaling every 4 to 6 months

PROGNOSIS

- Timely assessment, management, and consistent home oral hygiene may reverse mild to moderate gingivitis within several months.
- Periodontal disease may not be reversible; therefore, prevention is essential.

COMPLICATIONS

- Pain leading to detrimental changes in hygiene, diet, behavior, and daily routine
- Irreversible periodontitis
- Premature tooth loss
- Osteomyelitis
- Subacute bacterial endocarditis (SBE)

ADDITIONAL READING

- American Academy of Pediatric Dentistry. Guideline on periodicity of examination, preventive dental services, anticipatory guidance, and oral treatment for children, and adolescents. http://www.aapd.org/media/Policies_Guidelines/G_Periodicity7.pdf. Accessed May 19, 2017.
- American Academy of Pediatric Dentistry. Endorsement. Periodontal diseases of children and adolescents. http://www.aapd.org/media/Policies_Guidelines/E_PeriodontalDisease1.pdf. Accessed May 19, 2017.
- American Academy of Pediatric Dentistry. Endorsement. Guideline for periodontal therapy. http://www.aapd.org/media/Policies_Guidelines/E_PerioTherapy1.pdf. Accessed May 19, 2017.
- American Academy of Pediatric Dentistry. Endorsement. Treatment of plaque-induced gingivitis, chronic periodontitis, and other clinical conditions. http://www.aapd.org/media/Policies_Guidelines/E_Plaque1.pdf. Accessed May 19, 2017.

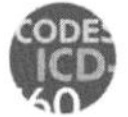

CODES

ICD10

- K05.10 Chronic gingivitis, plaque induced
- K05.00 Acute gingivitis, plaque induced
- A69.1 Other Vincent's infections

G

FAQ

- Q: Are there differences among toothpastes and prevention of gingivitis?
- A: Yes. A stabilized stannous fluoride toothpaste is effective in preventing gingivitis. When essential oil mouthwashes (e.g., Listerine®) are added, there is additional reduction in the amount of gingivitis noted.
- Q: What dietary changes may improve gingival health?
- A: Avoiding frequent carbohydrate intake may reduce gingivitis. Carbonated beverages, sugared chewing gum, and candy often adhere to teeth. When daily dental care is inconsistent, plaque formation is increased and gingivitis is much more likely.
- Q: Why do children generally not have the significant periodontal disease that adults get?
- A: No one knows for sure; however, it is known that the gingiva of the primary dentition is rounder and thicker and contains more blood vessels and less connective tissue than the gingival seen later in life. Whether these differences mask disease or are helpful is unclear.
- Q: How do intraoral piercings impact gum health?
- A: In addition to fractured teeth, gingival recession and gingivitis are complications of the trauma inflicted by a foreign body in the oral cavity.
- Q: Why is smoking associated with gingival disease?
- A: Nicotine inhibits phagocyte and neutrophil function, reduces bone mineralization, impairs vascularization, and reduces antibody production. Smokers do not respond as well as nonsmokers to surgical and nonsurgical treatments.

GLAUCOMA–CONGENITAL

Nazlee Zebardast, MD, MSc • Courtney L. Kraus, MD

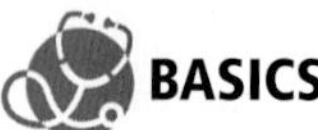

BASICS

DESCRIPTION

- Elevation of intraocular pressure (IOP) and associated damage to the optic nerve
- Subdivided into primary and secondary glaucomas
- Primary congenital glaucomas (PCGs) can present at birth or before age 1 month (neonatal), before age 2 years (infantile), or later in life.
- PCG can occur in isolation or in association with systemic disorders and other anterior segment anomalies.
- >75% of childhood glaucoma presents in the 1st year of life.

EPIDEMIOLOGY

- PCG accounts for ~1/2 of all cases of childhood glaucoma.
- 1:10,000 births in the United States
- Worldwide, ranges from 1:1,250 in Slovakian Romas to 1:18,500 in Great Britain
- Consanguinity increases risk.
- Male > female (3:2)
- ~80% bilaterally affected

Genetics

- Most PCG is sporadic but 10–40% are familial.
- Autosomal recessive with variable penetrance is most common.
- PCG is associated with mutations in cytogenic locations 2p22.2 (*GLC3A*), 1p36.2-p36.1 (*GLC3B*), 14q24.3 (*GLC3C*), and 14q24.2-q24.3 (*GLC3D*).
- Two identified genes for PCG include *CYP1B1* (cytochrome P450 1B1) and *LTBP2*.

ALERT
PCG is a rare disease. Secondary glaucomas are far more common. All children who presents with glaucoma at birth or in infancy should be referred to a geneticist.

PATHOPHYSIOLOGY

- PCG is caused by development anomaly of the anterior chamber angle (junction of iris and cornea) resulting in increased outflow resistance through the trabecular meshwork.
- Secondary glaucoma is mostly due to damage or alteration of the trabecular meshwork.

ETIOLOGY

- Aqueous humor is produced by the ciliary body at the posterior base of the iris, passes through the pupil and exits through the trabecular meshwork and Schlemm canal, which are located at the junction of the cornea and iris.
- Outflow blockage of aqueous humor causes pressure to build in eye.
- The blockage may be microscopic (open-angle glaucoma) or due to obstruction of the outflow by the iris (angle-closure glaucoma).
- High IOP in young children leads to enlargement of eye and destruction of fibers of the optic nerve.

COMMONLY ASSOCIATED CONDITIONS

- Sturge-Weber syndrome
- Neurofibromatosis type 1
- Oculocerebrorenal (Lowe) syndrome
- Marfan syndrome
- Rubinstein-Taybi syndrome
- Stickler syndrome
- Walker-Warburg syndrome
- Hepatocerebrorenal syndrome (Zellweger)
- Pierre Robin syndrome
- Homocystinuria
- Rubella
- Trisomy 13
- Trisomy 21 (Down syndrome)
- Axenfeld-Rieger syndrome
- Ocular anomalies
  - Aniridia
  - Peters anomaly
  - Sclerocornea
  - Congenital iris ectropion syndrome
  - Congenital cataract

ALERT
Intraocular neoplasms such as retinoblastoma can cause glaucoma. Other causes of secondary glaucoma include ocular surgery (cataract extraction), trauma, chronic uveitis, steroid response, and retinopathy of prematurity.

DIAGNOSIS

HISTORY

- Classic triad of symptoms that develop from corneal edema caused by increased IOP
  - Epiphora (excessive tearing)
  - Blepharospasm (squeezing of eyelids)
  - Photophobia (light sensitivity)
- Fussiness/poor feeding
- Parents may note or describe
  - Cloudy corneas
  - Red eyes (can be mistaken for conjunctivitis)
  - Large eyes

PHYSICAL EXAM

- Unlike adult glaucoma, PCG presents with physical changes due to high IOP.
- High IOP results in stretching of immature eye collagen until age 3 to 4 years resulting in:
  - Buphthalmos (ocular enlargement)
  - Corneal enlargement or asymmetry
  - Corneal haze from edema and/or scarring
  - Myopic shift in refractive error
- Usually presents insidiously due to gradual change in pressure; however, rapid changes in IOP can present with redness and pain.
- Nystagmus may be present if corneal haze occurs early, leading to a sensory deficit.
- Common to develop amblyopia and strabismus from insult on developing visual system
- Signs of many systemic syndromes are associated with glaucoma (i.e., neurofibromatosis, Sturge-Weber syndrome).

DIFFERENTIAL DIAGNOSIS

- Excessive tearing
  - Nasolacrimal duct obstruction in neonates
  - Ocular inflammation
  - Corneal abrasion or inflammation
- Large cornea
  - High myopia
  - Contralateral microphthalmia
  - Megalocornea (usually x-linked)
- Corneal haze
  - Birth trauma, forceps
  - Congenital corneal dystrophies
  - Mucopolysaccharidoses, cystinosis, sphingolipidoses
  - Intrauterine inflammation (rubella, syphilis)
  - Corneal malformations (sclerocornea, Peters anomaly)
  - Chemical injury
- Photophobia
  - Uveitis
  - Retinal cone dystrophy
- Enlarged optic nerve cupping
  - Physiologic cupping
  - Optic atrophy from hydrocephalus can look similar to glaucomatous damage.

DIAGNOSTIC TESTS & INTERPRETATION

Initial Tests (screening, lab, imaging)

Ultrasound: axial length measurement using A-scan

- Abnormally long eye for age
- Asymmetry in axial length
- Longitudinal data useful in determining progression of glaucoma

Diagnostic Procedures/Other

- IOP measurement
  - An awake, cooperative child is ideal; use bottle or breast to quiet, along with low lighting.
  - If examination under anesthesia is needed, check IOP as soon as possible after induction, as IOP decreases with anesthetic agents.
  - IOP >20 mm Hg or asymmetry >5 mm Hg is suspicious for glaucoma.
- Corneal inspection
  - Diameter measured with calipers
  - Normal newborn: 10 to 10.5 mm; increases by 0.5 to 1 mm in first year
  - Diameter >11 mm at birth or >12 mm in the 1st year of life is suspicious.
  - Watch for asymmetry.
  - Corneal haze may be due to edema or breaks in the Descemet membrane (Haab striae) as the corneal stretches.
- Optic disc evaluation
  - Increase in cupping of the optic nerve head is early sign.
  - May reverse with good IOP control in the very young
- Refractive error
  - Myopic shift from enlargement of the eye
  - Anisometropia (difference in refractive error between the two eyes)
  - Astigmatism from change in ocular shape or corneal scar
  - Early signs of glaucoma and useful office test for monitoring control of glaucoma
- Gonioscopy: evaluation of anterior chamber angle
  - Helps differentiate among various types of glaucoma and influence surgical plan
  - In PCG, the iris inserts anteriorly into the corneoscleral angle and is often flat or concave.
  - Secondary glaucomas can present with angle-closure: apposition of iris on cornea
- Pachymetry: measurement of corneal thickness to assess corneal edema

TREATMENT

ALERT
Left untreated, congenital glaucoma uniformly results in blindness. However, if detected early and managed promptly, good outcomes can be expected.

GENERAL MEASURES

- Surgery is considered definitive therapy.
- Medical treatment for glaucoma in children is usually a temporizing measure or adjunctive therapy.
  - Involves use of the same medications as those used in adults such as β-blockers, adrenergic agents, and carbonic anhydrase inhibitors

MEDICATION

ALERT
Topical α-adrenergic agonists are contraindicated in infants and young children, as they can cause CNS suppression leading to apnea, sedation, and fatigue.

- Carbonic anhydrase inhibitors: decrease aqueous production. Side effects include metabolic acidosis, growth retardation, loss of appetite, paresthesias, polyuria, diarrhea, and nausea.
  - Systemic
    - Acetazolamide (10 mg/kg/24 h PO divided t.i.d.)
    - Methazolamide
  - Topical
    - Brinzolamide
    - Dorzolamide
- β-Blockers, topical: decrease aqueous production. Side effects include bronchospasm, apnea, and bradycardia.
  - Timolol 0.25% and levobunolol 0.25% are most commonly used.
  - Other options include betaxolol, metipranolol, and carteolol.
- Prostaglandins, topical: increase uveoscleral outflow. Side effects include iris and eyelid pigmentation and growth of lashes.
  - Latanoprost
  - Bimatoprost
  - Travoprost

ALERT
Side effects of topical ocular medications can be decreased by limiting systemic absorption through nasolacrimal duct occlusion.

SURGERY/OTHER PROCEDURES

- Goniotomy/trabeculotomy:
  - Procedure of choice in PCG, success rate as high as 90% reported
  - Both procedures open portions of Schlemm canal into anterior chamber, allowing easier outflow of aqueous humor (goniotomy approaches the Schlemm canal from inside the eye and trabeculotomy from the outside).
- Filtration surgery:
  - Usually procedure of choice in secondary childhood glaucomas
  - Carries 1–2% annual risk of infection
  - Trabeculectomy: creates a sclerotomy covered with a partial-thickness scleral flap to create a controlled outflow that bypasses the Schlemm canal and trabecular meshwork. Fluid drains in the sub-Tenon space.
- Glaucoma drainage implants: various drainage devices placed in subconjunctival space with tube inserted into the anterior chamber, allowing free flow of aqueous humor from eye
- Cyclodestructive procedures:
  - Usually employed when other methods of IOP control have failed
  - Procedures involving destruction of the ciliary body, which produces aqueous humor, can be done internally or externally.
- Iridectomy: If the mechanism of glaucoma is angle closure (limited outflow of aqueous humor due to anatomic blockage with iris), then creating a window in the iris allows bypass for aqueous humor to access the anterior chamber.

ONGOING CARE

FOLLOW-UP RECOMMENDATIONS

- Early postoperative
  - Postoperative steroids and cycloplegic drops to decrease pain and prevent adhesions due to inflammation
  - Corneal edema clears slowly, but IOP falls quickly if surgery is successful.
  - Adjusting pressure-lowering medications based on the success of the surgery
- Longer term
  - Follow-up is needed throughout life.
  - Examination under anesthesia may be required frequently during the first 3 to 4 years of life to ensure adequate control of IOP.
  - Even after IOP control, should be monitored for other causes of visual compromise including amblyopia, refractive error, corneal scarring, cataract, strabismus, and recurrence of glaucoma
  - Due to high risk of severe, lifelong, preventable vision loss, poor parental compliance with appointments, medications, glasses, and other recommendations is cause to contact social services.

PATIENT EDUCATION

Children and parents must understand that glaucoma may recur at any point and that continued, long-term surveillance is essential.

PROGNOSIS

- Newborn PCG has the worst prognosis likely due to greater abnormality of the anterior chamber angle; >50% progress to legal blindness.
- Prognosis worse if diagnosed after 1 year of age due to development of amblyopia
- Lifelong follow-up is necessary to monitor for recurrence of glaucoma, surgical complications, and occurrence of other vision-threatening conditions.

ALERT
Amblyopia treatment must undertaken rigorously even after IOP is controlled as there is still at high risk for visual impairment.

COMPLICATIONS

- Severe visual impairment or blindness due to optic nerve damage likely if glaucoma is undetected or uncontrollable
- Corneal edema and decompensation requiring corneal transplant especially secondary to glaucoma drainage implants
- Development of cataract
- If glaucoma is controlled, the following are relatively common:
  - Unrecognized and untreated amblyopia (most serious threat to child's vision)
  - High degrees of myopia
  - Anisometropia (eyes with different refractive power)
  - Buphthalmos (enlargement of the eyeball) and corneal scarring

ADDITIONAL READING

- Beck AD. Diagnosis and management of pediatric glaucoma. *Ophthalmol Clin North Am*. 2001;14(3):501–512.
- Bejjani B, Edward D. Primary congenital glaucoma. In: Pagon RA, Adam MP, Ardinger HH, et al, eds. *Gene Reviews [Internet]*. Seattle, WA: University of Washington, Seattle; 2007.
- De Silva DJ, Khaw PT, Brookes JL. Long-term outcome of primary congenital glaucoma. *J AAPOS*. 2011;15(2):148–152.
- Kipp MA. Childhood glaucoma. *Pediatr Clin North Am*. 2003;50(1):89–104.
- Mandal AK, Gothwal VK, Bagga H, et al. Outcome of surgery on infants younger than 1 month with congenital glaucoma. *Ophthalmology*. 2003;110(10):1909–1915.
- Papadopoulos M, Khaw PT. Advances in the management of paediatric glaucoma. *Eye (Lond)*. 2007;21(10):1319–1325.
- Yeung HH, Walton DS. Clinical classification of childhood glaucomas. *Arch Ophthalmol*. 2010;128(6):680–684.

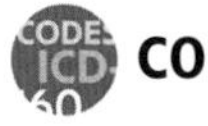

CODES

ICD10

Q15.0 Congenital glaucoma

FAQ

- Q: Can glaucoma be painful?
- A: If the ocular pressure rises quickly (hours), pain occurs frequently. Very high IOPs may be present without pain if they occur slowly (months to years). However, most patients with glaucoma are asymptomatic until they have advanced vision loss.
- Q: Can glaucoma occur after eye trauma?
- A: Yes. This is a very common cause of glaucoma and may be asymptomatic, thus requiring periodic follow-up ophthalmic examinations for early detection and treatment.
- Q: Can infantile glaucoma be inherited?
- A: Yes. Both primary infantile glaucoma and glaucoma related to systemic or ocular syndromes may be inherited. Siblings and children of affected individuals should be examined for glaucoma.
- Q: Can glaucoma be associated with ocular neoplasms?
- A: Yes. Intraocular neoplasms such as retinoblastoma, juvenile xanthogranuloma, leukemia, and melanomas can all lead to secondary forms of childhood glaucomas.

GLOMERULONEPHRITIS

Nadine M. Khouzam, MD • Kevin V. Lemley, MD, PhD

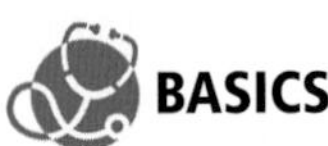

BASICS

DESCRIPTION

- Glomerulonephritis presents with the nephritic syndrome: hematuria with RBC casts, hypertension, variable azotemia, and edema. Proteinuria and oliguria may also be present.
- Acute glomerulonephritis is associated with inflammation and cell proliferation in the glomerular tuft. It may be rapidly progressive.
- Chronic glomerulonephritis indicates permanent damage has occurred.

EPIDEMIOLOGY

- Postinfectious glomerulonephritis can occur after any infection; ~80% of cases are secondary to a streptococcal infection.
- Acute poststreptococcal glomerulonephritis (APSGN) can occur in anyone >2 years but is most frequently found in boys 5 to 15 years old. It can be sporadic or epidemic.
- Incidence of APSGN has declined over the last 2 decades.
- Chronic glomerulonephritis occurs more often at the end of the 1st decade of life and in adults.

RISK FACTORS

Exposure to nephritogenic streptococci

Genetics

Genetic predisposition: hereditary nephritis (e.g., X-linked Alport syndrome); C3 glomerulopathy, atypical HUS (complement regulation disorders)

ETIOLOGY

Can be categorized based on serum complement levels and presence of renal-limited versus systemic disease

- Low serum complement level: systemic diseases
  - Vasculitis and autoimmune disease (e.g., systemic lupus erythematosus [SLE])
  - Subacute bacterial endocarditis (SBE)
  - Shunt nephritis
  - Cryoglobulinemia
- Low serum complement level: renal diseases
  - APSGN
  - Membranoproliferative glomerulonephritis, C3 glomerulopathy
- Normal serum complement level: systemic diseases
  - Microscopic polyangiitis (MPA)
  - Granulomatosis with polyangiitis (GPA)
  - Henoch-Schönlein purpura (HSP)
  - Hypersensitivity vasculitis
  - Anti-GBM disease (Goodpasture syndrome)
- Normal serum complement level: renal diseases
  - IgA nephropathy
  - Idiopathic rapidly progressive glomerulonephritis
  - Pauci-immune glomerulonephritis (renal-limited ANCA vasculitis)
  - Immune-complex disease

DIAGNOSIS

HISTORY

- Macroscopic hematuria (tea-colored urine) in many
- Reduced urine output, edema
- Dyspnea, fatigue, lethargy
- Headache
- Seizures (hypertensive encephalopathy)
- Symptoms of a systemic disease such as fever, rash (especially on the buttocks and legs, posteriorly), arthralgia, and weight loss
- Preceding sore throat, upper respiratory infection (7 to 14 days), *or* preceding impetigo (14 to 28 days) suggests APSGN.
- An upper respiratory infection in the few days prior to macroscopic hematuria may suggest IgA nephropathy.

PHYSICAL EXAM

- Hypertension
- Signs of volume overload (e.g., edema, jugular venous distention, hepatomegaly, rales, a gallop rhythm)
- Impetigo or pyoderma
- Signs of vasculitis such as rash, Raynaud phenomenon, and vascular thrombosis
- Signs of other systemic disorder (e.g., SLE: malar rash, swollen tender joints, pericardial friction rub)
- Signs of chronic kidney disease (CKD), such as short stature, pallor, sallow skin, edema, pericardial friction rub, pulmonary rales, breath that smells of urine, clonus

DIFFERENTIAL DIAGNOSIS

- Acute postinfectious glomerulonephritis (nephritogenic strains of group A β-hemolytic streptococci, *Pneumococcus*, *Staphylococcus*, *Mycoplasma*, Epstein-Barr virus)
- Infection-related (hepatitis B and C, syphilis)
- IgA nephropathy
- Membranoproliferative glomerulonephritis (idiopathic)
- Autoimmune glomerulonephritis (e.g., SLE)
- Immune-complex glomerulonephritis
- Hereditary glomerulonephritis
- Tubulointerstitial nephritis
- Hemolytic uremic syndrome
- Pyelonephritis
- HSP (presents with dependent purpuric rash, normal or elevated platelet count, abdominal pain, arthralgia)
- ANCA-associate vasculitis (GPA, MPA, or Churg-Strauss syndrome)

DIAGNOSTIC TESTS & INTERPRETATION

Initial Tests (screening, lab, imaging)

- Urine
  - Microscopy of the urine for dysmorphic erythrocytes and erythrocyte casts: hallmark of nephritis
  - Proteinuria
- Evidence of prior strep infection
  - Throat culture for β-hemolytic *Streptococcus* (result is positive in only 15–20% with sporadic APSGN)
  - Antistreptolysin O and anti-DNAse B titers: positive result in patients with preceding acute poststreptococcal infection
  - Streptozyme test: A mixed antigen test for β-hemolytic *Streptococcus* (ASO, anti-DNAse, anti-streptokinase, anti-hyaluronidase, etc.) has 85–90% sensitivity and specificity; sensitivity is increased by serial testing.
- Complement C3 serum level will be low in APSGN and in several other causes of acute glomerulonephritis.
- Blood work
  - Can be normal in acute glomerulonephritis
  - Serum creatinine generally <1.5× normal in uncomplicated APSGN
  - In chronic glomerulonephritis, serum chemistries will reflect the degree of CKD (i.e., raised serum urea and creatinine). The serum potassium and phosphate levels may be elevated, and the calcium level decreased.
  - In CKD: normocytic, normochromic, or hypochromic microcytic anemia
  - Obtain PTH and 25-OH vitamin D if CKD suspected.
- Chest radiograph to look for pulmonary edema and determine cardiac size if severe edema or respiratory symptoms are present
- Renal and bladder ultrasound if presentation or course not typical of APSGN. The ultrasound is to assess the size and parenchymal texture and to evaluate for nephrolithiasis and lesions of the bladder that may also cause hematuria.

Diagnostic Procedures/Other

- Electrocardiogram to assess ventricular size and for T-wave changes in cases of hyperkalemia
- Indications for renal biopsy: nephrotic-range proteinuria, significant or progressive renal impairment, sustained hypertension
- Pathologic findings
  - APSGN, light microscopy reveals enlarged, swollen glomerular tufts and mesangial and endothelial cell proliferation, with polymorphonuclear leukocyte infiltration. There is granular deposition of C3 and IgG on immunofluorescence, and electron-dense subepithelial deposits or humps are seen on electron microscopy. The histology varies in chronic glomerulonephritis and depends on the cause. Rapidly progressive glomerulonephritis is associated with crescent formation.

TREATMENT

Aimed toward treating hypertension, renal failure, and the underlying cause of glomerulonephritis. Careful attention to fluid balance and electrolyte abnormalities; may require fluid restriction in case of oliguria

GENERAL MEASURES

- APSGN is typically a self-limited disease. Acute supportive therapy is usually sufficient.
- Dietary salt restriction
- The therapy of chronic glomerulonephritis depends on the underlying disease process; it may include immunosuppressive medications and, ultimately, the management of CKD.

MEDICATION

The following may be required:

- Loop diuretics (furosemide) for volume, BP, and potassium control
- Antihypertensive agents; vasodilators such as calcium channel blockers (e.g., nifedipine, isradipine, amlodipine) as 1st-line agents; IV hydralazine, labetalol, nicardipine, or nitroprusside may be required to treat severe refractory hypertension or posterior reversible encephalopathy syndrome (PRES). Avoid ACE inhibitors or angiotensin receptor blockers (ARBs) in case of hyperkalemia or acute kidney injury (AKI).
- Serum potassium-lowering agents (sodium polystyrene sulfonate [Kayexalate®], furosemide, bicarbonate, insulin/glucose, β-agonists). IV calcium is used to stabilize the myocardium in severe hyperkalemia (with T-wave changes); dialysis in severe renal failure with significant hyperkalemia
- Phosphate binders (calcium carbonate, sevelamer)
- Immunosuppressive agents such as prednisone, cyclophosphamide, mycophenolate mofetil, and rarely rituximab or eculizumab are used in the treatment of vasculitis-associated glomerulonephritis, membranoproliferative glomerulonephritis, rapidly progressing glomerulonephritis, or disorders of complement regulation. Plasmapheresis may be used to treat rapidly progressing glomerulonephritis, especially with multisystem (pulmonary, CNS) involvement or severe acute renal failure requiring dialysis.
- Penicillin is used in active poststreptococcal glomerulonephritis to prevent rheumatic fever and the spread of nephritogenic strains but generally does not affect the course of the renal disease. It may be indicated in exposed individuals in epidemic APSGN and household contacts of sporadic cases.

ADMISSION, INPATIENT, AND NURSING CONSIDERATIONS

- Treat hypertensive encephalopathy and life-threatening electrolyte disturbances immediately.
- Admission criteria
  - Hypertension
  - Severe edema, pulmonary edema
  - AKI (rise in serum creatinine, oligoanuria)

ONGOING CARE

FOLLOW-UP RECOMMENDATIONS

In APSGN, improvement usually occurs within 3 to 7 days, hypertension is not sustained, and macroscopic hematuria is transient. Watch for ongoing oliguria, unresolved hypertension, increasing proteinuria, or progressive azotemia. Complement levels return to normal within 6 to 8 weeks of the initial presentation.

ALERT

- Microscopic hematuria may be present up to 2 years after an episode of poststreptococcal glomerulonephritis.
- Recurrent gross hematuria calls the diagnosis of APSGN into question.
- If complement levels do not return to normal after presumed APSGN, consider SLE or MPGN and refer to nephrology for further evaluation.

Patient Monitoring

- To control seizures, treat the hypertension; anticonvulsants play a secondary role.
- Look for and treat hyperkalemia.
- Monitor the degree of AKI.
- Home testing: BP monitoring may be required.
- Be certain to recognize fluid overload.
- Be certain to recognize the type of renal failure: acute versus chronic.
- Long-term monitoring for hypertension and/or progressive proteinuria may be indicated in some populations (5–10% may develop progressive proteinuria and CKD within 20 years).

DIET

Restrictions of intake of fluid, sodium, potassium, and phosphate are initially required.

PROGNOSIS

- Prognosis is excellent in APSGN and variable for other causes of glomerulonephritis in childhood.
- APSGN rarely recurs.

COMPLICATIONS

- Hypertension
- Acute renal failure
- Hyperkalemia
- Volume overload (e.g., congestive cardiac failure, pulmonary edema, hypertension)
- CKD

ADDITIONAL READING

- Ahn SY, Ingulli E. Acute poststreptococcal glomerulonephritis: an update. *Curr Opin Pediatr*. 2008;20(2):157–162.
- Lau KK, Wyatt RJ. Glomerulonephritis. *Adolesc Med*. 2005;16(1):67–85.
- Ornstein BW, Atkinson JP, Densen P. The complement system in pediatric systemic lupus erythematosus, atypical hemolytic uremic syndrome, and complocentric membranoglomerulopathies. *Curr Opin Rheumatol*. 2012;24(5):522–529.
- Pan CG. Evaluation of gross hematuria. *Pediatr Clin North Am*. 2006;53(3):401–412.
- Wong W, Morris MC, Zwi J. Outcome of severe acute post-streptococcal glomerulonephritis in New Zealand children. *Pediatr Nephrol*. 2009;24(5):1021–1026.

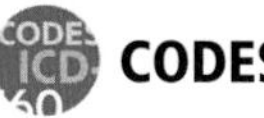

CODES

ICD10

- N05.9 Unsp nephritic syndrome with unspecified morphologic changes
- N00.9 Acute nephritic syndrome with unsp morphologic changes
- N03.9 Chronic nephritic syndrome with unsp morphologic changes

FAQ

- Q: When do serum complement levels return to normal in APSGN?
- A: Serum complement levels (C3) return to normal within a 6- to 8-week period in APSGN. Persistently low C3 levels suggest a cause other than APSGN, and renal biopsy should be considered with persistent urinary abnormalities (hematuria and/or proteinuria).
- Q: What are the indications for renal biopsy in acute glomerulonephritis?
- A: Patients in whom there is sustained hypertension, ongoing or progressive azotemia, or persistent proteinuria of >1 mg/mg creatinine should be biopsied.

GLUCOSE-6-PHOSPHATE DEHYDROGENASE DEFICIENCY

Kandace L. Gollomp, MD • Michele Puszkarczuk Lambert, MD, MSTR

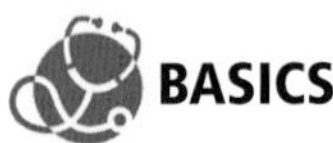

BASICS

DESCRIPTION

Deficiency of the enzyme glucose-6-phosphate dehydrogenase (G6PD) that leads to increased RBC vulnerability to oxidative stress and may cause hemolytic anemia. Several types of genetic mutations result in either deficient enzyme production or diminished enzyme activity.

- Although most patients with this deficiency are never anemic and have mild to no hemolysis, the classic manifestation is acute hemolytic anemia in response to oxidative stress.
- World Health Organization classification of G6PD variants:
  - Class 1: congenital nonspherocytic hemolytic anemia: rare. Chronic hemolysis without exposure to oxidative stressors—splenomegaly in 40%. Affected individuals tend to be white males of Northern European background.
  - Class 2: severe deficiency (1–10% enzymatic activity): oxidative stress–induced hemolysis. Prototype is G6PD-Mediterranean.
  - Class 3: mild deficiency (10–60% enzymatic activity): most common type. Acute hemolytic anemia uncommon occurs only with stressors.
  - Class 4: nondeficient variant (60–100% enzymatic activity): no symptoms, even during oxidant stressors (e.g., G6PD A+ [variant with normal activity]); 20–40% allelic frequency in Africans
  - Class 5: >150% of normal activity
- Deficient neonates may have hyperbilirubinemia out of proportion to their anemia.
  - May, in part, account for increased prevalence of bilirubin encephalopathy in African Americans. In the United States, ~20% of kernicterus is G6PD related.
  - Should be considered in the evaluation of neonatal hyperbilirubinemia in infants of appropriate ethnicity

GENERAL PREVENTION

- Avoid drugs and toxins known to cause hemolysis (see "Pathophysiology" section).
- Prompt follow-up with febrile illness and signs of hemolysis.

EPIDEMIOLOGY

Prevalence

- Most common of all clinically significant enzyme defects, affecting approximately 400 million people worldwide. ~7.5% of the world's population carries one or two genes for G6PD deficiency.
- X linked (Xq28) with almost 400 allelic variants
- Frequency of different mutations varies by population:
  - Africans: 20–40% of X chromosomes are G6PD A+ (mutant enzyme with normal activity).
  - Sardinians (some regions): 30% have G6PD-Mediterranean (variant with 1–10% enzymatic activity)
  - Saudi Arabians: 13% have G6PD deficiency.
  - African Americans: 10–15% have G6PD A– (mutant enzyme with <30% normal activity).
- High incidence of mutant genes in some regions may relate to survival advantage against malarial infection (*Plasmodium falciparum and Plasmodium vivax*).

Genetics

Gene is on the X chromosome (Xq28).

- Males express the enzyme (mutant or normal) from their single X chromosome (hemizygotes).
- Female homozygotes (rare) are more severely affected than female heterozygotes.
- Heterozygote females show variable intermediate expression because of random X inactivation leading to somatic cell mosaicism.

PATHOPHYSIOLOGY

- G6PD catalyzes the production of NADPH that protects RBCs from oxidative damage.
- Normal G6PD activity is 7 to 10 IU/g hemoglobin. Following exposure to oxidative stress, G6PD-deficient RBCs are destroyed by intravascular hemolysis resulting in hemolytic anemia.
- Oxidant stressors include infections and chemicals (e.g., mothballs, antimalarials, some sulfonamides, rasburicase, methylene blue). RBCs lose G6PD activity throughout their lifespan; therefore, older cells are more prone to oxidative hemolysis.
- Normal RBC lifespan of ~120 days is unaffected in unstressed states, even with severe enzyme deficiency but may be shortened during oxidant stress.
- Hemolysis usually follows stressor by 1 to 3 days, and the nadir occurs 8 to 10 days postexposure.
- Favism: severe hemolytic anemia in patients with more severe forms of G6PD deficiency that occurs after fava bean ingestion

DIAGNOSIS

HISTORY

- Symptoms of anemia include fatigue, irritability, and malaise.
- Dark urine (cola or tea colored) may follow moderate to severe hemolysis; may develop jaundice (particularly scleral icterus)
- Patient may have required phototherapy in newborn period for hyperbilirubinemia.
- Recent drug, chemical, or food (fava bean) exposures may precipitate moderate to severe hemolysis.
- Family history of intermittent jaundice, splenectomy, cholecystectomy, or blood transfusion may indicate an inherited condition.
- Ethnicity may help determine type/severity of disease.

PHYSICAL EXAM

- Tachycardia, a flow murmur, or pallor: signs of anemia
- Jaundice or scleral icterus: signs of hemolysis

DIFFERENTIAL DIAGNOSIS

Intravascular hemolysis is very rare in children, but other causes include the following:

- Acute hemolytic transfusion reactions (Coombs test is positive.)
- Microangiopathic hemolytic disease, such as hemolytic uremic syndrome, thrombotic thrombocytopenic purpura, and prosthetic cardiac valves
- Physical trauma (e.g., march hemoglobinuria); severe burns (uncommon)
- Other inherited RBC enzyme deficiencies
- Paroxysmal nocturnal hemoglobinuria
- Extravascular hemolysis can also be confused with G6PD deficiency and includes the following:
  - Hereditary spherocytosis (spherocytes on smear)
  - Autoimmune hemolysis and delayed hemolytic transfusion reactions (both Coombs positive)
  - Hemoglobinopathies
  - Hypersplenism
  - Severe liver disease
  - Gilbert disease

DIAGNOSTIC TESTS & INTERPRETATION

Initial Tests (screening, lab, imaging)

- CBC
  - Usually reveals a normochromic normocytic anemia with appropriate reticulocytosis
  - Hemoglobin can drop precipitously; should be monitored closely until stable or trending upward; checking a single hemoglobin the day of exposure to the stressor is not sufficient.
- Peripheral blood smear
  - Often shows bizarre RBC morphology with marked anisocytosis and poikilocytosis
  - Can see schistocytes, hemighost cells (uneven distribution of hemoglobin), bite cells, blister cells, and occasional Heinz bodies (RBC inclusions composed of denatured hemoglobin visible with supravital staining)
- Hemoglobinemia: seen as plasma (pinkish red supernatant) or measured as free serum hemoglobin
- Hemoglobinuria:
  - Occurs when hemoglobin-binding sites in the plasma (haptoglobin and hemopexin) are saturated
  - May be visible as dark urine—heme positive on dipstick and no RBC on microscopy
- Free haptoglobin levels decrease.
- Direct and indirect Coombs tests
  - Must be done to exclude autoimmune hemolytic anemia
  - Should be negative in G6PD deficiency
- Other:
  - Plasma indirect bilirubin, lactate dehydrogenase, and aspartate aminotransferase may be elevated; hemosiderin may be found in the urine several days after hemolysis.
  - Liver function tests should be normal.

- Renal function assessment can help rule out thrombotic thrombocytopenic purpura and hemolytic uremic syndrome:
  - Rapid screening tests for G6PD activity in RBCs are qualitative; will miss some female heterozygotes with measurable but low enzyme levels
  - Necessary to confirm a deficiency or to diagnose a suspected heterozygote with a test to quantify G6PD activity
  - Normal activity: 7 to 10 IU/g hemoglobin
    - Accurately detects deficiency in males and homozygous females with no recent hemolysis
    - Helpful with heterozygous women
- Newborn screening for G6PD deficiency
  - Included in some panels of genetic screening tests performed on newborns
  - Typically performed by DNA-based methods that detect a few of the most common variants in U.S. populations
  - Does not screen for all G6PD variants and can miss severe but rare variants
  - Results may be reported in terms of predicted enzyme levels but not a true measurement of enzymatic activity.

ALERT

- Following episodes of hemolysis, screening tests may be falsely negative because younger RBC present in higher concentrations due to rapid red cell turnover (reticulocytosis), contain higher levels of G6PD.
- Most cost-effective approach: Defer screening until 1 to 2 weeks after resolution of hemolysis. Smear may be normal during steady state.

- Heterozygote female detection:
  - Two RBC populations exist because of mosaicism from random X inactivation.
  - On average, 50% are normal and 50% are deficient, but there may be variability.

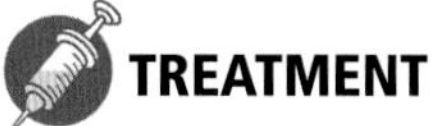

TREATMENT

GENERAL MEASURES

- Removal of the oxidant stressor is of primary importance:
  - Discontinue the suspected drug and/or treat the infection.
    - In class 3 and 4 patients, essential drug therapy may be continued while monitoring for signs of severe hemolysis.
    - Transfusion may be necessary (especially in some class 1 and 2 deficiencies), but any patient who is symptomatic with anemia or has a low hemoglobin and signs of ongoing brisk hemolysis should be transfused immediately with packed RBCs.
- Supportive care, evaluation of renal function (risk of acute tubular necrosis with brisk hemolysis), and monitoring degree of anemia and ongoing hemolysis are important.
- For the affected neonate:
  - Monitor the bilirubin closely and start phototherapy early.
    - If necessary, exchange transfusion should be carried out.
    - Phenobarbital may decrease bilirubin level.
    - Early discharge is not recommended in newborn infants with jaundice and concern for G6PD deficiency.

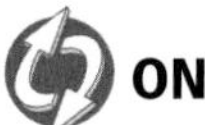

ONGOING CARE

FOLLOW-UP RECOMMENDATIONS

- Most deficient individuals remain asymptomatic.
- When hemolysis does occur, it tends to be self-limited and resolves spontaneously, with a return to normal hemoglobin levels in 2 to 6 weeks.
- Development of renal failure is extremely rare in children, even with massive hemolysis and hemoglobinuria.

DIET

Avoid fava beans (*Vicia faba*). Fava beans have a variety of names in different cultures (e.g., faba bean, broad bean, tick bean, field bean, bell bean, bakela [Ethiopia], faviera [Portugal], ful masri [Sudan], winter field bean [United Kingdom]).

PROGNOSIS

- For those with the milder forms, the prognosis is excellent.
- Can cause significant morbidity, but rarely mortality, in those with the more severe forms

COMPLICATIONS

Neonates can be at risk for hyperbilirubinemia, requiring treatment. Kernicterus has been reported in infants with G6PD deficiency.

ADDITIONAL READING

- Cappellini MD, Fiorelli G. Glucose-6-phosphate dehydrogenase deficiency. *Lancet*. 2008;371(9606):64–74.
- Frank JE. Diagnosis and management of G6PD deficiency. *Am Fam Physician*. 2005;72(7):1277–1282.
- Luzzatto L, Nannelli C, Notaro R. Glucose-6-phosphate dehydrogenase deficiency. *Hematol Oncol Clin North Am*. 2016;30(2):373–393.
- Nkhoma ET, Poole C, Vannappagari V, et al. The global prevalence of glucose-6-phosphate dehydrogenase deficiency: a systematic review and meta-analysis. *Blood Cells Mol Dis*. 2009;42(3):267–278.
- Santucci K, Shah B. Association of naphthalene with acute hemolytic anemia. *Acad Emerg Med*. 2000;7(1):42–47.
- Watchko JF. Hyperbilirubinemia in African American neonates: clinical issues and current challenges. *Semin Fetal Neonatal Med*. 2010;15(3):176–182.
- Youngster I, Arcavi L, Schechmaster R, et al. Medications and glucose-6-phosphate dehydrogenase deficiency: an evidence-based review. *Drug Saf*. 2010;33(9):713–726.

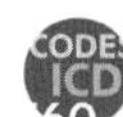

CODES

ICD10

D55.0 Anemia due to glucose-6-phosphate dehydrogenase deficiency

FAQ

- Q: Do I need to follow a special diet or avoid medications if I have G6PD deficiency?
- A: Although most patients will have no symptoms of their disease, certain medications may cause transient hemolytic anemia and these should be avoided. When prescribing medications, your physician and pharmacist should know about your G6PD, but most necessary medications are safe and well tolerated. People with severe variants of the deficiency should also avoid fava beans, but otherwise no dietary restrictions are necessary.
- Q: What are medications that should be avoided?
- A: Medications that create oxidative stress include, but are not limited to: dapsone, mafenide cream, methylene blue (used for treatment of methemoglobinemia) nalidixic acid, nitrofurantoin, primaquine, rasburicase, sulfacetamide, and sulfamethoxazole.
- Q: Why should mothball exposure be avoided for patients with G6PD deficiency?
- A: Mothballs typically contain naphthalene, a polycyclic aromatic hydrocarbon. After naphthalene is absorbed and metabolized by the liver, the naphthalene metabolites provoke an oxidative stress.
- Q: Do I need to know which variant of G6PD I have?
- A: It may be clear which variant you are likely to have based on your clinical symptoms and ethnic background.
- Q: Should my family be screened if someone has G6PD deficiency?
- A: In families of patients with G6PD, screening members may help provide meaningful genetic counseling to female carriers and affected but asymptomatic males.
- Q: How does G6PD affect sickle cell anemia and vice versa?
- A: Having sickle cell disease is somewhat protective in patients with G6PD A deficiency because their RBC population is young and, therefore, has higher enzymatic activity. On the other hand, G6PD has no effect on the clinical characteristics of sickle cell disease.

GOITER

Melissa Schoelwer, MD

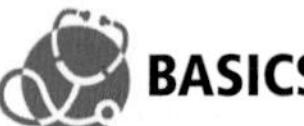

BASICS

DESCRIPTION

A goiter is an enlarged thyroid gland (also known as thyromegaly). A simple or colloid goiter is one that is not associated with thyroid dysfunction, autoimmune thyroid disease, or a neoplastic process. Goiters can be classified by size and by the presence or absence of nodules.

EPIDEMIOLOGY

- The incidence of goiter in school-age children ranges from 1.9% to 6.8%.
- The prevalence of goiter in the United States is 3–7%, although it is much higher in regions of iodine deficiency (15.8% globally).
- Prevalence in childhood peaks during adolescence with females more affected than males.
- Thyroid cancer is a rare cause of pediatric goiter and makes up 0.5–1.5% of all malignancies in children and adolescents.

RISK FACTORS

- Family history
- Female gender
- Autoimmune disease such as type 1 diabetes
- Tobacco smoke
- Radiation
- Iodine deficiency
- Excessive maternal ingestion of iodine during pregnancy can lead to congenital goiter.

Genetics

- Mutations in the following genes can result in a simple goiter:
  - Thyroid peroxidase
  - Sodium iodide symporter
  - Thyroglobulin
  - Thyroid-stimulating hormone (TSH) receptor
- Multinodular goiter (MNG) loci have been identified on chromosome 14q and on chromosome Xp22 and 3q26.
- Germline mutations in *DICER1* (chromosome 14q31) have been found in familial MNG-1.
- Germline mutation in thyroid transcription factor-1 (TITF-1/NKX2.1) has been found in patients with papillary thyroid carcinoma and a history of MNG.
- Thyroid cancers are usually sporadic. Medullary carcinoma can be familial (autosomal dominant), as part of multiple endocrine neoplasia (MEN) type 2A and 2B, or as isolated malignancy. The genetic mutation is in the RET gene.

GENERAL PREVENTION

Iodine administration reduces the incidence of endemic goiter.

PATHOPHYSIOLOGY

- Stimulation of the thyrotropin receptor (either by TSH or TSH-receptor antibodies) results in thyromegaly.
- Thyroid enlargement can also develop due to inflammation, as seen in thyroiditis, or infiltration.
- The pathogenesis of euthyroid simple goiter remains unclear.

ETIOLOGY

- The most common cause of pediatric goiter in the United States is chronic lymphocytic thyroiditis (Hashimoto thyroiditis).
- Genetic etiologies as listed above

COMMONLY ASSOCIATED CONDITIONS

- Pendred syndrome (autosomal recessive): congenital sensorineural deafness and goiter due to a mutation in pendrin which transports iodide into the thyroid follicular lumen
- MEN2A: medullary thyroid cancer, pheochromocytoma, parathyroid adenoma
- MEN2B: medullary thyroid cancer, pheochromocytoma, mucosal neuromas, marfanoid habitus
- Autoimmune polyglandular syndrome (APS): Consider other autoimmune diseases such as type 1 diabetes, Addison disease, and pernicious anemia.

DIAGNOSIS

HISTORY

- Signs/symptoms of hypothyroidism:
  - Decreased linear growth
  - Weight gain
  - Fatigue
  - Constipation
  - Cold intolerance
  - Dry skin and/or hair
  - Hair loss
  - Irregular menses
- Signs/symptoms of hyperthyroidism:
  - Weight loss
  - Hyperactivity
  - Irritability
  - Difficulty concentrating or focusing in school
  - Hyperphagia
  - Diarrhea
  - Heat intolerance, increased sweating
  - Insomnia/poor sleep
  - Tremor
  - Eye symptoms
- Signs/symptoms of compression due to goiter:
  - Stridor
  - Dysphagia
  - Vocal changes, hoarseness
- Careful dietary and medication history
- History of head, neck, or chest irradiation is associated with increased risk of carcinoma.
- Family history of autoimmune thyroid disease, thyroid carcinoma, or MEN syndrome

PHYSICAL EXAM

Inspect, palpate, and auscultate the neck:

- Neck extension aids inspection.
- Can have patient swallow or drink water (thyroid gland moves on swallowing which differentiates it from other neck structures)
- Palpation can be done by standing behind the child or facing the child:
  - Determine if the thyroid is diffusely enlarged or asymmetric, evaluate gland firmness, and assess for any nodularity.
  - Check for cervical lymphadenopathy.
  - Pain on palpation suggests acute inflammation.
- Auscultate with the stethoscope diaphragm (while patient holds his or her breath) for a bruit, which indicates hyperthyroidism-associated hypervascularity.
- Careful examination for signs of hypothyroidism or hyperthyroidism
  - Linear growth and weight pattern
  - Pulse and BP (elevated in hyperthyroidism)
  - Exophthalmos
  - Premature sexual development
  - Deep tendon reflexes
  - Tremor/tongue fasciculations
  - Skin: dry or sweaty
  - Strength (+ milk maid's sign in hyperthyroidism)

DIFFERENTIAL DIAGNOSIS

- Fat neck
  - Adipose tissue
  - Large sternocleidomastoid muscles
- Thyroglossal duct cysts
- Nonthyroidal neoplasms: lymphoma, teratoma, hygroma, ganglioneuroma
- Immunologic
  - Chronic lymphocytic thyroiditis
  - Graves disease
  - Amyloid deposition (familial Mediterranean fever, juvenile rheumatoid arthritis)
- Infectious
  - Acute suppurative thyroiditis (most often *Streptococcus pyogenes*, *Staphylococcus aureus*, and *Streptococcus pneumoniae*)
  - Subacute thyroiditis (often viral)
- Environmental
  - Goitrogens: iodide, lithium, amiodarone, oral contraceptives, perchlorate, cabbage, soybeans, cassava, thiocyanate in tobacco smoke
  - Iodine deficiency (exacerbated by pregnancy)
- Neoplastic
  - Thyroid adenoma/carcinoma
    - Benign follicular adenoma
    - Follicular, papillary, or mixed carcinoma
    - Medullary carcinoma
  - TSH-secreting adenoma
- Congenital
  - Ectopic gland
  - Unilateral agenesis of gland
  - Dyshormonogenesis
  - T_4 resistance
- Miscellaneous:
  - Simple colloid goiter
  - MNG

DIAGNOSTIC TESTS & INTERPRETATION

Initial Tests (screening, lab, imaging)

- Thyroid function tests: Total T_4 (or Free T_4) and TSH are the best screens for hypothyroidism or hyperthyroidism.
- Total T_3 should be obtained in cases of suspected hyperthyroidism.
- In cases of suspected chronic lymphocytic thyroiditis: antithyroglobulin and antimicrosomal (antiperoxidase) antibodies
- In cases of suspected Graves disease: thyroid-stimulating immunoglobulins (TSI) or TSH-receptor antibodies
- A thyroid ultrasound is *not* routinely recommended as part of the initial workup of suspected goiter due to autoimmune thyroid disease.

Follow-Up Tests & Special Considerations

- If thyroid function and antibodies are negative or if exam findings are concerning (lymphadenopathy, thyroid asymmetry, palpable nodule), imaging with a neck ultrasound should be performed.
- Ultrasound is the best imaging to determine the number, size, and nature (cystic, solid, or mixed) of nodules.
  - Heterogeneity and micronodules are frequently seen in the setting of autoimmune thyroid disease.

- If the TSH is suppressed in the setting of a nodule and negative antibodies, thyroid scintigraphy should be done to determine if the nodule is hyperfunctioning.
  - "Cold" nodules (no uptake) are suggestive of neoplasia and require immediate evaluation by a pediatric endocrinologist and surgeon.
- Calcitonin: elevated in 75% of patients with medullary thyroid carcinoma
- Urinary iodine concentration is the best measure of the adequacy of iodine intake.

Diagnostic Procedures/Other

- Fine-needle aspiration under ultrasound guidance should be considered for evaluation of thyroid nodules >1 cm or those with suspicious features on ultrasound.
- Barium swallow studies can reveal a fistulous tract between the left piriform sinus and the left thyroid lobe in children with recurrent acute suppurative thyroiditis which are amenable to surgical resection.

ALERT

- Work-up suspicious solitary thyroid nodules aggressively. Remember: Incidence of malignancy in these nodules in children is 15–40%, which is higher than adults.
- Malignancy is more likely in euthyroid pediatric patients with nodules that have palpable lymph nodes, compressive signs, microcalcifications, intranodular vascularization, and lymph node alterations.
- Differentiated thyroid carcinoma in prepubertal children, compared to pubertal adolescents, has a more aggressive presentation and more frequently a family history of thyroid carcinoma.

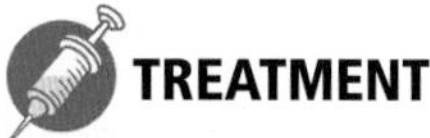

TREATMENT

MEDICATION

- First line for a goiter due to autoimmune hypothyroidism:
  - Levothyroxine (weight-based dosing is dependent on the age of the patient)
    - Interactions: Soy and iron affect absorption.
    - Should not be given in liquid form, rather, the tablet should be crushed and mixed with a small amount of water for those who cannot swallow pills
- First line for a goiter due to autoimmune hyperthyroidism:
  - Methimazole: initial dosing up to 1 mg/kg/24 hr divided b.i.d. or t.i.d.
    - Often used with β-blocker (atenolol or propranolol) for symptomatic control while thyroid levels normalize
    - Adverse reactions: rash, arthralgia, pancytopenia/agranulocytosis, hepatitis, jaundice
  - Radioactive iodine ablation (^{131}I)
    - Generally not used in younger children (<8 years) due to concerns of radiation exposure
    - Results in permanent hypothyroidism
  - Surgery (near-total or total thyroidectomy) may be considered, although is generally considered a 2nd-line therapy.
    - Results in permanent hypothyroidism
- First line for idiopathic nontoxic diffuse goiter: observation and reassurance
  - The use of levothyroxine to decrease TSH to the low normal range in order to reduce the size of nontoxic goiters is generally not recommended.

ALERT

The FDA issued a black box warning against propylthiouracil (PTU) use in treating Graves disease owing to risk of severe liver injury including life-threatening acute liver failure.

SURGERY/OTHER PROCEDURES

- Surgery solely to decrease size of goiter is indicated only if adjacent structures are compressed.
- Surgery (lobectomy) is 1st-line treatment for a hyperfunctioning nodule.
- Potential complications of thyroid surgery include laryngeal nerve damage and hypoparathyroidism.
- Cancer
  - If cancer is confirmed following surgery, radioiodine therapy with ^{131}I can be administered to treat any residual tissue or metastases.
  - Suppressive doses of exogenous thyroid hormone are then given to maintain TSH levels <0.2 mIU/L.
  - Thyroglobulin is a useful tumor marker in those with papillary/follicular carcinoma, and calcitonin serves as tumor marker for medullary carcinoma.

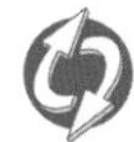

ONGOING CARE

FOLLOW-UP RECOMMENDATIONS

- Children with newly diagnosed Hashimoto thyroiditis who have a TSH >100 and children with newly diagnosed Graves disease should urgently be evaluated by a pediatric endocrinologist and will likely be followed in clinic every 3 to 6 months.
- A patient with a goiter who is clinically and biochemically euthyroid still requires careful follow-up for the detection of the early signs of developing thyroid dysfunction.
  - Patients who are euthyroid but have positive antibodies should have their thyroid function evaluated yearly.
- If surgery is performed, close monitoring of calcium is required to detect hypoparathyroidism postoperatively.
- Benign thyroid nodules should be followed with ultrasonography every 6 to 12 months to determine if change occurs.
- Long-term follow-up of patients with thyroid cancer is recommended, as disease can recur decades after initial diagnosis and therapy.

DIET

- No restrictions, although soy and iron can affect the absorption of levothyroxine and should not be given at the same time
- Incidence of iodine deficiency has greatly declined since the addition of potassium iodide to table salt.
- Iodide can also be added to communal drinking water or administered as iodized oil in isolated rural areas.

PROGNOSIS

- Depends on the cause of the goiter
- Potential for goiter regression depends on its cause. Goiters associated with chronic lymphocytic thyroiditis and Graves disease may or may not decrease in size with treatment.
- Idiopathic nontoxic diffuse goiters regress spontaneously in up to 60% of children, and another 5–10% develop autoimmune thyroiditis (chance of developing antibodies increases if there is a positive family history).
- Thyroid cancer usually follows an indolent course with excellent prognosis. Mortality is most common in medullary and undifferentiated carcinomas, which are relatively rare in children.

COMPLICATIONS

- Depending on gland size, goiters can produce a mass effect on midline neck structures. If the goiter is intrathoracic, it may cause pleural effusions or chylothorax.
- Typically, the child is euthyroid, but clinical hypothyroidism or hyperthyroidism may result from certain types of goiters.
- Surgery and radioactive iodine ablation as treatment for cancer or Graves disease will likely induce permanent hypothyroidism.

ADDITIONAL READING

- Francis G, Waguespack S, Bauer A, et al. Management guidelines for children with thyroid nodules and differentiated thyroid cancer. *Thyroid*. 2015;25(7):716–759.
- Gopalakrishnan S, Chugh P, Chhillar M, et al. Goitrous autoimmune thyroiditis in a pediatric population: a longitudinal study. *Pediatrics*. 2008;122(3):e670–e674.
- Kambalapalli M, Gupta A, Prasad U, et al. Ultrasounds characteristics of the thyroid in children and adolescents with goiter: a single center experience. *Thyroid*. 2015;25(2):176–182.
- Kim S, Lee Y, Jung H, et al. Pediatric goiter: can thyroid disorders be predicted at diagnosis and in follow-up? *J Pediatr*. 2016;170:253–259.e2.
- Krohn K, Führer D, Bayer Y, et al. Molecular pathogenesis of euthyroid and toxic multinodular goiter. *Endocr Rev*. 2005;26(4):504–524.

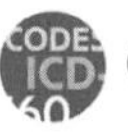

CODES

ICD10

- E04.9 Nontoxic goiter, unspecified
- E04.2 Nontoxic multinodular goiter
- E06.3 Autoimmune thyroiditis

FAQ

- Q: Do all goiters cause thyroid dysfunction?
- A: Goiters can be euthyroid, hypothyroid, or hyperthyroid, depending on the cause.
- Q: Will the goiter decrease in size with treatment?
- A: This depends on the cause of the goiter.
- Q: How does pediatric thyroid cancer usually present?
- A: It usually presents as a solitary, hard, painless nodule in a euthyroid patient. Patients with a history of goiter or benign nodules/adenomas have an increased risk of developing thyroid cancer.
- Q: Is there an increased risk of thyroid cancer from diagnostic radiographs (chest radiographs, lateral neck films)?
- A: Routine diagnostic radiographs should fall well below the levels of radiation thought to increase risk of thyroid neoplasia. During more prolonged radiologic procedures that might expose the thyroid to higher doses of radiation, a lead neck shield is used.
- Q: Should prophylactic thyroidectomy be performed in children identified genetically as having familial medullary carcinoma?
- A: Yes, as these situations have a poorer prognosis.

GONOCOCCAL INFECTIONS

Angela M. Statile, MD, MEd • Samir S. Shah, MD, MSCE

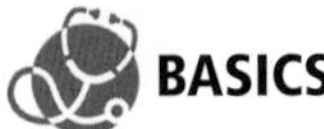

BASICS

DESCRIPTION

Neisseria gonorrhoeae, an aerobic gram-negative diplococcus, is the etiologic agent of gonorrhea.

EPIDEMIOLOGY

- Gonorrhea is the second most common sexually transmitted infection (STI) in the United States.
- Coinfection with *Chlamydia trachomatis* commonly occurs in sexually active patients.
- Less than half of all infections are estimated to be detected or reported.

Incidence

- In the United States, there are >800,000 new cases of gonorrhea each year. Rates of infection are highest among adolescents and young adults.
- Racial and sexual behavior disparities are present, with a disproportionately high incidence in ethnic minorities and males who have sex with males.

RISK FACTORS

- Vaginal delivery to an infected mother is a risk factor for neonatal disease.
- Sexual abuse should be considered in all prepubertal children presenting with gonorrhea.
- Risk factors for sexually active adolescents include
  - Multiple sexual partners
  - Inconsistent or lack of condom use
  - Inconsistent screening by health care providers
- Transmission risk
  - The risk of male-to-female transmission is 50% per episode of vaginal intercourse.
  - The risk of female-to-male transmission is ~20% per episode.
  - Rectal intercourse is also a mode of transmission.

GENERAL PREVENTION

- Ophthalmia neonatorum:
  - Prophylactic ophthalmic ointment is mandatory in the United States regardless of method of delivery.
  - Instillation of 0.5% erythromycin ophthalmic ointment in both eyes occurs immediately after birth.
- Maternal infection:
  - Routine screening cervical cultures should be performed at the first prenatal visit.
  - Repeat in the third trimester if high risk.

PATHOPHYSIOLOGY

- Incubation period is 2 to 7 days.
- Transmission results from contact with infected mucosa and secretions, usually through vaginal delivery, sexual activity, and (rarely) household contact in prepubertal children.
- In prepubertal children, genital infection is mild; ascending or disseminated infection rarely occurs. In adolescents, estrogenization protects the vagina from infection and instead serves as a conduit for cervical exudate.
- Immunity is not induced by infection.

COMMONLY ASSOCIATED CONDITIONS

Pediatric gonococcal infections can be categorized by age group: neonates, prepubertal children, and sexually active adolescents.

- Neonatal gonococcal diseases include ophthalmia neonatorum, scalp abscess (complication of fetal scalp monitoring), and, rarely, disseminated disease.
- Prepubertal gonococcal disease usually occurs in the genital tract. Vaginitis is the most common manifestation. Pelvic inflammatory disease (PID), perihepatitis (Fitz-Hugh–Curtis syndrome), urethritis, proctitis, and pharyngitis rarely occur. Consider sexual abuse.
- Gonococcal diseases in sexually active adolescents resemble those found in adults and may be asymptomatic.
  - Both sexes: pharyngitis, anorectal infection, tenosynovitis-dermatitis syndrome, or arthritis
  - Females: Genital tract infection may cause urethritis, vaginitis, and endocervicitis. Ascending genital tract infection may lead to PID and perihepatitis.
  - Males: Acute urethritis is the predominant manifestation. Epididymitis also occurs.

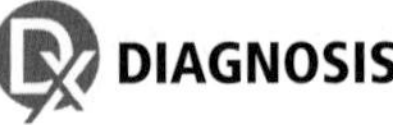

DIAGNOSIS

HISTORY

- In neonates, assess for risk factors such as premature or prolonged membrane rupture, presence of fetal scalp monitoring, or maternal history of infection.
- Onset of eye findings in ophthalmia neonatorum is usually between 2 and 5 days of age but ranges from 1 day to several weeks.
- Sexual history should be thoroughly reviewed with all adolescents.
- Vaginal itching and discharge may indicate vaginitis.
- Purulent urethral discharge and dysuria without urgency or frequency may indicate urethritis.
- Abdominal pain
  - Ascending infection is characterized by diffuse lower quadrant abdominal pain, including discomfort with ambulation.
  - Low back pain, dyspareunia, and abnormal vaginal bleeding occasionally occur.
  - Fever, chills, nausea, and vomiting may be present.
  - Acute perihepatitis causes right upper quadrant pain and results from direct extension of infection from the fallopian tube to the liver capsule.
- Symptoms of extragenitourinary disease including sore throat, joint pain, or rash

PHYSICAL EXAM

- Ophthalmia neonatorum
  - Bilateral eyelid edema, chemosis, and copious purulent discharge
- Neonatal scalp abscess
- PID:
  - Cervical motion tenderness, pelvic adnexal tenderness (usually bilateral), and lower or right upper quadrant abdominal pain (with perihepatitis)
  - May also have mucopurulent cervical discharge
- Cervicitis or urethritis: purulent vaginal or penile discharge
- Rash: classically discrete, tender, necrotic pustules on distal extremities, although macules, papules, and bullae occasionally occur
- Joint findings: tenosynovitis, migratory arthritis

DIFFERENTIAL DIAGNOSIS

- Ophthalmia neonatorum: Other causes of neonatal conjunctivitis include infection with *C. trachomatis*, *Staphylococcus aureus*, *Streptococcus pneumoniae*, *Haemophilus* species, chemical conjunctivitis, and herpes simplex virus (HSV).
- Scalp infection: Gonococcal scalp abscesses may be difficult to distinguish from abscesses caused by staphylococcal species, group B *Streptococcus*, *Haemophilus influenzae*, Enterobacteriaceae, and HSV.
- Vaginitis: In the prepubertal child, other causes include chemical or environmental irritants, pinworms, foreign body, and infections (i.e., streptococci, *Trichomonas vaginalis*). In cases of sexual abuse, consider *C. trachomatis* and syphilis.
- Genitourinary tract infection: In adolescents, other causes include *C. trachomatis*, syphilis, and *T. vaginalis*.
- Arthritis: other bacterial causes of septic arthritis, Reiter syndrome, and reactive arthritis
- Abdominal pain: ectopic pregnancy, appendicitis, cholecystitis, UTI/pyelonephritis, and ovarian torsion

DIAGNOSTIC TESTS & INTERPRETATION

Initial Tests (screening, lab, imaging)

- Gram stain (low sensitivity) and culture of infected exudate or body fluid
  - Intracellular gram-negative diplococci on Gram stain. Confirmation depends on isolation of *N. gonorrhoeae* from culture. Specimens are immediately inoculated onto Thayer-Martin or chocolate–blood agar–based media at room temperature and incubated in an enriched CO_2 environment.
  - In cases of suspected sexual abuse, collect genital, rectal, and pharyngeal cultures.
- Nonculture gonococcal tests
  - Nucleic acid amplification tests (NAATs) for urine specimens (freshly voided specimens), male urethral, and female endocervical or vaginal (self-administered introital) swabs are highly sensitive and specific and allow for easy testing in a variety of clinical settings. NAATs should not be used in investigations of possible sexual abuse (possibility of false-positive results).
  - NAATs cannot provide antimicrobial susceptibility test results.

- STI panel
  - Test for other STIs including *C. trachomatis*, *Treponema pallidum* (syphilis), *T. vaginalis*, and HIV in children in whom sexual abuse is suspected or when evaluating sexually active adolescents.
- CBC, ESR, C-reactive protein, and blood culture may be obtained to evaluate for inflammation and disseminated disease.
- Synovial fluid cell count and culture in patients with joint swelling (cell count often >50,000 WBC/μL with differential of >90% PMNs)
- Synovial fluid cultures are positive in 50% with purulent gonococcal arthritis; blood cultures are positive less often, whereas cultures from other sites (e.g., cervix, urethra) are frequently positive.
- Pelvic ultrasound
  - May detect ectopic pregnancy
  - In PID, may reveal thick, dilated fallopian tubes or tuboovarian abscess.

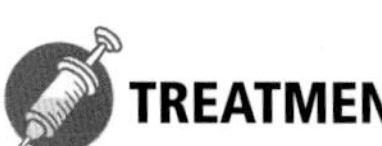

TREATMENT

MEDICATION

- Changing resistance patterns in the United States led to extended-spectrum cephalosporin as initial therapy.
- Neonates
  - Ophthalmia neonatorum: ceftriaxone 25 to 50 mg/kg IV or IM (single dose; maximum, 125 mg); alternate agent for infants with hyperbilirubinemia is cefotaxime 100 mg/kg IV or IM (single dose).
  - Neonates with gonococcal ophthalmia also require eye irrigation with sterile saline at presentation and at frequent intervals until mucopurulent drainage has ceased.
  - Disseminated infection: ceftriaxone or cefotaxime for 7 days for bacteremia, 10 to 14 days for meningitis
- Older children and adolescents
  - Uncomplicated gonococcal infection (including cervicitis, epididymitis, or pharyngeal infection): Cefixime is no longer recommended as 1st-line treatment. Give a single IM dose of ceftriaxone 250 mg. Follow with a treatment regimen for *C. trachomatis*.
  - If ceftriaxone is not available, give single-dose cefixime 400 mg orally, along with *C. trachomatis* treatment. In cases of severe cephalosporin allergy, give single-dose azithromycin 2 g. Alternative regimens to ceftriaxone require tests of cure in 1 week.
  - PID: See pediatric *Red Book* or most recent CDC guidelines for treatment regimens.
  - Complicated gonococcal infection: ceftriaxone or cefotaxime for 7 days (arthritis and septicemia), 10 to 14 days (meningitis), or ≥28 days (endocarditis). Include concomitant *C. trachomatis* therapy.
  - Pursue empiric treatment of sexual partners.

ADMISSION, INPATIENT, AND NURSING CONSIDERATIONS

- Neonates: Hospitalize and obtain appropriate cultures (conjunctivae, blood, CSF, or those from any other site of infection).
- Prepubertal children: Hospitalize if safety concerns are present or for complicated disease.
- Sexually active adolescents: Hospitalize for PID with inability to tolerate oral antibiotics, complicated disease requiring further monitoring.

ONGOING CARE

FOLLOW-UP RECOMMENDATIONS

- Provide risk reduction education.
- Sexual contacts (including a newborn's mother and her partner[s]) of patients with gonorrhea should be counseled and treated.
- Evaluate for concurrent infection with other sexually transmitted diseases, including *C. trachomatis*, syphilis, *T. vaginalis*, hepatitis B, and HIV. Patients whose age has progressed beyond the neonatal period should be treated presumptively for *C. trachomatis* infection.
- All cases of gonorrhea must be reported to public health officials.
- Standard precautions are recommended for all hospitalized patients with gonococcal disease, including newborns with ophthalmia neonatorum.
- Evaluate prepubertal children for abuse.

ALERT

Pitfalls

- Failure to consider the diagnosis of sexual abuse in a prepubertal child with a gonococcal infection. Cases of transmission via nonsexual contact have been reported (i.e., from freshly infected towels/fomites, childhood sexual play, or by digital transmission from an infected caregiver), but such mode cannot be assumed without first excluding sexual abuse.
- Failure to use culture to diagnose infection in cases of suspected abuse
- Failure to differentiate *N. gonorrhoeae* by culture from other *Neisseria* species, especially in prepubertal children, given concern for sexual abuse
- Failure to consider acute gonococcal perihepatitis/ Fitz-Hugh–Curtis syndrome in females with right upper quadrant pain

PROGNOSIS

Prognosis has been improved by treating all forms of infection with a 3rd-generation cephalosporin.

COMPLICATIONS

- Gonococcal infection during pregnancy is associated with spontaneous abortion, preterm labor, and perinatal infant mortality.
- Ophthalmia neonatorum may rapidly progress to corneal ulceration and perforation, with subsequent scarring and blindness.
- PID
  - Endometritis, salpingitis, tuboovarian abscess, and pelvic peritonitis occur as a consequence of untreated vaginal disease.
  - Scarring secondary to salpingitis can cause sterility.
  - Risk of ectopic pregnancy increases 7-fold after one episode of PID.
- In males, rare complications include periurethral abscess, acute prostatitis, seminal vesiculitis, and urethral strictures.
- Disseminated disease
  - Consider evaluation for complement deficiency in those with multiple episodes.
  - In neonates, arthritis is the most frequent systemic manifestation; symptoms develop 1 to 4 weeks after delivery. Involvement of multiple joints is typical, and most infants do not have ophthalmia neonatorum.
  - In older children and adolescents, septic arthritis (one joint) and a characteristic poly–arthritis-dermatitis syndrome are possible manifestations.
  - Gonococcal meningitis, endocarditis, and osteomyelitis are rare in children.
- Gonococcal infection can serve as a cofactor in increasing HIV infection and transmission.

ADDITIONAL READING

- American Academy of Pediatrics. Gonococcal infections. In: Kimberlin DW, Brady MT, Jackson MA, Long SS, eds. *Red Book: 2015 Report of the Committee on Infectious Diseases*. 30th ed. Elk Grove Village, IL: American Academy of Pediatrics; 2015:356–367.
- Comkornruecha M. Gonococcal infections. *Pediatr Rev.* 2013;34(5):228–234.
- Workowski KA, Bolan GA. Centers for Disease Control and Prevention: sexually transmitted diseases treatment guidelines, 2015. *MMWR Recomm Rep.* 2015;64(RR-03):1–137.

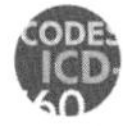

CODES

ICD10

- A54.9 Gonococcal infection, unspecified
- P39.8 Other specified infections specific to the perinatal period
- P39.1 Neonatal conjunctivitis and dacryocystitis

FAQ

- Q: What are the advantages of the NAATs for making a diagnosis?
- A: The transcription-mediated amplification (TMA) test of urine samples, approved by the FDA for women, can be used to simultaneously test for *C. trachomatis* and *N. gonorrhoeae*.
- Q: When is this test not approved?
- A: For rectal and pharyngeal swabs and for cases of suspected abuse

GRAFT-VERSUS-HOST DISEASE

Valerie I. Brown, MD, PhD

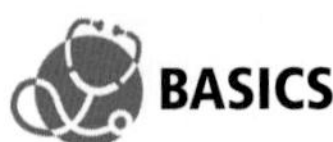

BASICS

DESCRIPTION

Graft-versus-host disease (GVHD) is a multiorgan inflammatory process that develops when immunologically competent T lymphocytes from a histoincompatible donor are infused into an immunocompromised host unable to reject them; divided into acute and chronic, historically based on time of presentation but best delineated by clinicopathologic findings

- Acute:
  - Develops within 100 days after allogeneic hematopoietic stem cell transplant (HSCT)
  - Affects skin, GI tract, and/or liver
  - Graded from I to IV based on organ involvement, percent of body surface area involved (skin), volume of diarrhea (gut), and/or elevation of serum bilirubin (liver)
- Chronic:
  - Develops 100 days after allogeneic HSCT
  - Presents with diverse features resembling autoimmune syndromes; affects multiple organ systems
  - Chronic subtypes
    - Progressive: extension of acute GVHD
    - Quiescent: after resolution of acute GVHD
    - De novo: no prior acute GVHD

EPIDEMIOLOGY

- Acute GVHD (grades II to IV): 10–80% of patients receiving T-cell–replete HSCT
  - 35–45% for human leukocyte antigen (HLA)–identical related donor bone marrow
  - 60–80% if 1-antigen HLA-mismatched unrelated donor bone marrow or peripheral stem cells
  - 35–65% if 2-antigen HLA-mismatched unrelated umbilical cord blood
- Chronic GVHD: most common cause of late morbidity and mortality of allogeneic HSCT
  - 15–25% if HLA-identical related marrow
  - 40–60% if HLA-matched unrelated marrow
  - 54–70% if HLA-matched unrelated peripheral stem cells
  - 20% if unrelated umbilical cord blood
- Flare-ups triggered by infection (usually viral)

RISK FACTORS

- HLA disparity (both major and minor antigens)
- Older donor or recipient age
- Stem cell source and dose
  - Highest risk: with peripheral stem cells
  - Lowest risk: with umbilical cord blood
- Donor leukocyte infusions
- Reactivation of viruses (e.g., HHV-6, CMV)
- T-cell depletion decreases incidence.
- Acute GVHD-specific
  - Higher intensity conditioning regimen
  - Prior pregnancies in female donors
  - Use of total body irradiation
- Chronic GVHD specific
  - Severity of acute GVHD
  - Malignancy as indication for transplantation
  - Gender mismatch (female donor, male recipient)
  - Type of immunosuppressive prophylaxis

Genetics

- HLA gene complex on chromosome 6; inherited as haplotype
- Full siblings: 25% chance HLA identical
- Minor histocompatibility antigen differences likely account for GVHD in HLA-identical sibling stem cell transplants.

GENERAL PREVENTION

- Transfusion: irradiation of all cellular blood products for patients at risk
- Stem cell transplantation
  - Selection of a histocompatible donor
  - Immunosuppression (gold standard): cyclosporine or tacrolimus with a short course of methotrexate
  - Other options: corticosteroids, sirolimus, mycophenolate mofetil, and post-HSCT cyclophosphamide
  - Donor T-cell depletion with anti–T-cell antibodies ex vivo in graft or in vivo in recipient

PATHOPHYSIOLOGY

- Acute GVHD: interaction of donor and host innate and adaptive immune responses
  - Severity related to degree of HLA mismatch
  - Three phases ending in "cytokine storm"
    - Tissue damage by conditioning regimen
    - Priming and activation of donor T cells
    - Infiltration of activated T cells into skin, GI tract, and liver resulting in apoptosis
- Chronic GVHD: findings similar to autoimmune disorders: donor T cells directed against host antigens, donor T-cell alloreactivity, B-cell dysregulation, regulatory T-cell deficiency; marked collagen deposition in target organs and lack of T-cell infiltration

ETIOLOGY

- HSCT
- Transfusion of nonirradiated blood products to immunodeficient hosts: caused by viable donor lymphocytes engrafting in the recipient
- Transfusion of nonirradiated blood from a donor homozygous for one of the recipient's HLA haplotypes (1st- or 2nd-degree relative)
- Intrauterine maternal–fetal transfusions and exchange transfusions in neonates
- Solid organ grafts: contain immunocompetent T cells, into immunosuppressed recipient

DIAGNOSIS

HISTORY

- Acute GVHD
  - Rash: usually first manifestation; pruritus or burning sensation can precede rash.
  - Diarrhea, abdominal pain, and intestinal bleeding: unusual to precede skin disease
  - Anorexia, nausea, vomiting, and dyspepsia
  - Jaundice (liver involvement)
- Chronic GVHD
  - Dry eyes and/or dry mouth, blurry vision, eye irritation, photophobia, eye pain
  - Difficulty swallowing or retrosternal pain
  - Sensitivity to spicy or acidic foods
  - Wasting syndrome: malabsorption, weight loss, failure to thrive, poor performance status, early satiety, dysphagia
  - Nausea, vomiting, diarrhea, crampy abdominal pain
  - Dyspnea, wheezing, cough, activity intolerance, fatigue
  - Poor wound healing, especially posttrauma
  - Joint stiffness and pain, muscle cramps
- Infections: pneumococcal sepsis, *Pneumocystis jiroveci*, fungal infections

PHYSICAL EXAM

- Acute/transfusion-associated GVHD
  - Skin (most common site)
    - Maculopapular rash of palms, soles; can become confluent erythroderma
    - Severe form: bullae formation, to even full-thickness necrosis
  - GI tract: weight loss; profuse, watery, often green, and often bloody diarrhea
  - Liver: jaundice; atypical findings: painful hepatomegaly, ascites, rapid weight gain
- Chronic GVHD
  - Skin (involved in almost every patient)
    - Hyper- or hypopigmentation, xerosis (skin dryness), pruritus, scaling, patchy erythema, poikiloderma, skin atrophy; lichenoid, eczematous, and/or sclerodermatous changes
    - Advanced scleroderma: thickened, tight, and fragile skin
  - Eyes: pseudomembrane formation; keratitis
  - Hair: thin, fragile; premature graying
  - Scalp: dry or seborrheic
  - Nails: dystrophic, fragile; vertical ridging and splitting of nail bed; entire nail loss
  - Mouth: xerostomia, mucositis, ulcers; whitish, lacy plaques on tongue and buccal surfaces, may be painful; tight oral aperture
  - Esophageal strictures, stenosis, webs
  - Blood: thrombocytopenia, anemia, eosinophilia, autoantibodies, hypo- or hypergammaglobulinemia
  - Joints: stiffness, contractures, swelling
  - Muscles: eosinophilic fasciitis, myositis
  - Lung: bronchiolitis obliterans syndrome (obstructive), bronchiolitis obliterans organizing pneumonia (restrictive), pleural effusions
  - Cardiac: pericardial effusion, pericarditis, cardiomegaly
  - Hepatic: jaundice
  - Other: nephrotic syndrome, peripheral neuropathy, genital ulceration, fasciitis, myositis

DIFFERENTIAL DIAGNOSIS

- Acute GVHD
  - Skin: drug reaction, chemoradiotherapy, viral exanthema, engraftment syndrome; TEN for grade IV skin GVHD
  - Liver: hepatic veno-occlusive disease, total parenteral nutrition, drug toxicity, bacterial sepsis, or viral infection
  - GI: diarrhea secondary to transplant conditioning regimen, infectious causes (e.g., *Clostridium difficile*, CMV, adenovirus), or opiate withdrawal
- Chronic GVHD
  - Skin: keratosis pilaris, eczema, psoriasis
  - Oral: candidiasis

DIAGNOSTIC TESTS & INTERPRETATION

Diagnosis is often established based on clinical grounds.

Initial Tests (screening, lab, imaging)

- Complete blood count with differential and Coombs test: autoimmune thrombocytopenia (most common), hemolytic anemia, and neutropenia; eosinophilia resolves with treatment.
- Blood smear: Howell-Jolly bodies due to functional asplenia of chronic GVHD
- Elevated ALT/AST with or without hyperbilirubinemia
- Vitamin D: often low; risk for osteoporosis
- Urinalysis: may show protein, glucose, blood
- Immunoglobulin subsets
- Schirmer test: decreased tear production
- Pulmonary function tests: decreased FEV1
- Echocardiogram/electrocardiogram
- Fluorescein microscopy: punctate keratopathy
- High-resolution chest CT: bronchiolitis obliterans
- Barium swallow: strictures, webs

Follow-Up Tests & Special Considerations

Comprehensive physical and occupational therapy evaluation for chronic GVHD of the joints to improve range of motion and mobility

Diagnostic Procedures/Other

- Endoscopy or colonoscopy with biopsy: apoptosis and loss of villi; GI tract GVHD
- Skin biopsy: localized epidermal atrophy; may show absence of hair follicles and sweat glands
- Liver biopsy: bile duct damage reminiscent of primary biliary cirrhosis
- Rule out viral/fungal infections.
- Analysis of pleural, pericardial fluid

ALERT

- In chronic GVHD, do not give live vaccines; may lead to symptomatic infection
- Sudden high fevers may indicate bacterial sepsis, may be overwhelming. Chronic GVHD patients often functionally asplenic; have profoundly impaired immune function

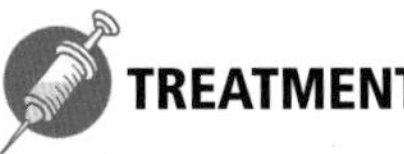

TREATMENT

GENERAL MEASURES

- Prophylaxis for *P. jiroveci* pneumonia and pneumococcal infection
- Antifungal coverage if on multiple immunosuppressive agents
- Hypogammaglobulinemia: IVIG
- Monitor closely for viral reactivation.
- Skin care: Lubricate dry skin with petroleum jelly. Protect skin from injury. Avoid sunburn.
- Correct electrolyte imbalances for muscular aches and cramps.
- Nails: apply clear nail polish to strengthen and prevent breakage

MEDICATION

- Acute GVHD (grades II to IV)
  - First line: systemic steroids (methylprednisolone or prednisone) at 2 mg/kg/24 h for 7 to 14 days then quick taper; cyclosporine or tacrolimus if not taking as prophylaxis
  - Second line: mycophenolate mofetil, sirolimus (rapamycin), antithymocyte globulin, etanercept (experimental), and daclizumab (experimental)
  - Infliximab: steroid-refractory GI disease
  - Visceral organ involvement requires urgent start of 2nd-line therapy.
  - For isolated, mild skin GVHD, topical tacrolimus ointment and triamcinolone
- Chronic GVHD
  - Steroids alone or with cyclosporine, tacrolimus, sirolimus, or mycophenolate mofetil
  - Goal: steroids <0.5 mg/kg alternating days; with cyclosporine or tacrolimus
- Steroid-refractory GVHD
  - Mycophenolate mofetil, sirolimus, pentostatin (investigational), ruxolitinib (experimental)
  - Other options many off-label: antithymocyte globulin, rituximab, low-dose methotrexate in liver GVHD, thalidomide, hydroxychloroquine imatinib, low-dose cyclophosphamide, etanercept, alefacept, alemtuzumab: high infection risk
- Oral rinses with dexamethasone: oral GVHD
- Ursodeoxycholic acid: hepatic GVHD

ALERT

If chronic GVHD persists past 2 to 3 months or prednisone is needed at 1 mg/kg/24 h, alternative therapy should be used.

ADDITIONAL THERAPIES

- Extracorporeal photophoresis: very effective for chronic skin GVHD; lower response rate if visceral organs involved
- Psoralen plus ultraviolet A is of some benefit in skin GVHD (lichenoid, not sclerotic).
- Mesenchymal stem cells (experimental)
- Artificial tears for sicca syndrome
- Physical therapy/range-of-motion exercises to prevent contractures
- Inhaled corticosteroids and azithromycin (experimental) for bronchiolitis obliterans syndrome

ADMISSION, INPATIENT, AND NURSING CONSIDERATIONS

Hospitalization may be required for hydration, nutritional support, IV medications, monitoring, treatment of infections, and other supportive care.

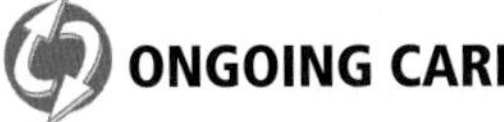

ONGOING CARE

FOLLOW-UP RECOMMENDATIONS

Patient Monitoring

- Corticosteroids: osteoporosis, diabetes
- Calcineurin inhibitors: hypertension, renal dysfunction, hypomagnesemia
- Sirolimus: hyperlipidemia, leukopenia, microangiopathic hemolytic anemia
- Mycophenolate mofetil: GI discomfort, diarrhea, leukopenia

DIET

Nutrition consults for malnutrition and wasting

PROGNOSIS

Prognosis of GVHD is based on severity.

- Acute GVHD: The higher the grade, the lower the long-term survival. Grade I survival is the same as for patients without GVHD; grade II, 60%; grade III, 25%; grade IV, 5–15%.
- Acute GVHD: 50–60% of patients respond to corticosteroids plus cyclosporine or tacrolimus.
- Poor prognosis for survival: extensive skin involvement (lichenoid skin changes), progressive onset, GI involvement, persistent severe thrombocytopenia, weight loss, and low Karnofsky performance status (<70%), bilirubin <1.2 ng/dL (40–60% survival)
- 50% of patients still require therapy 5 years after diagnosis of chronic GVHD.

COMPLICATIONS

- Chronic GVHD is the most common cause of late nonrelapse death and disability.
- Mortality from GVHD after HSCT is usually related to infection.
- Quality of life can be greatly impacted by chronic GVHD.
- In transfusion-associated GVHD, death is usually from bone marrow aplasia with destruction of the host's marrow by donor lymphocytes.

ADDITIONAL READING

- Carpenter PA, Macmillan ML. Management of acute graft-versus-host disease in children. *Pediatr Clin North Am*. 2010;57(1):273–295.
- Dhir S, Slatter M, Skinner R. Recent advances in the management of graft-versus-host disease. *Arch Dis Child*. 2014;99(12):1150–1157.
- Jacobsohn DA. Optimal management of chronic graft-versus-host disease in children. *Br J Haematol*. 2010;150(3):278–292.
- Jagasia MH, Greinix HT, Arora M, et al. National Institutes of Health consensus development project on criteria for clinical trials in chronic graft-versus-host disease: I. The 2014 diagnostic and staging working group report. *Biol Blood Marrow Transplant*. 2015;21(3):389–401.e1.
- Schlomchik WD. Graft-versus-host disease. *Nat Rev Immunol*. 2007;7(5):340–352.
- Wolff D, Schleuning M, von Harsdorf S, et al. Consensus conference on clinical practice in chronic GVHD: second-line treatment of chronic graft-versus-host disease. *Biol Blood Marrow Transplant*. 2011;17(1):1–17.

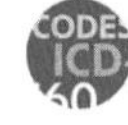

CODES

ICD10

- D89.813 Graft-versus-host disease, unspecified
- D89.810 Acute graft-versus-host disease
- D89.811 Chronic graft-versus-host disease

FAQ

- Q: Do all patients with acute GVHD get chronic GVHD?
- A: No. ~30% of patients <10 years of age who receive HLA-identical sibling HSCT will get acute GVHD, whereas only 13% will develop chronic GVHD. Chronic GVHD can develop in a patient who did not have acute GVHD; the prognosis is much more favorable than for the progressive form.
- Q: Do all severe chronic GVHD patients die?
- A: No. Occasionally, the GVHD will "burn out." This outcome is rare, and the process by which it happens is not understood.
- Q: How does chronic GVHD impact quality of life?
- A: Chronic GVHD can profoundly impact quality of life, and patients with chronic GVHD need to be screened for sleep disturbances and depression.

GRAVES DISEASE

Adda Grimberg, MD

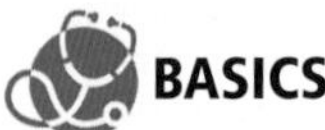

BASICS

DESCRIPTION
Multisystem autoimmune disorder that presents with the classic triad of hyperthyroidism (goiter), exophthalmos, and dermopathy (rare in children)

EPIDEMIOLOGY
- Female > male (4 to 5:1)
- 10–15% of all childhood thyroid disorders
- Incidence increases with age, peaking in adolescence and in the 3rd to 4th decades.
- Rising incidence of pediatric cases in several countries over the past 15 years
- Higher prevalence of thyrotoxicosis among non-Hispanic blacks in the United States, age 12 to 49 years

RISK FACTORS
Genetics
- No simple hereditary pattern (i.e., genetic susceptibility plus environmental factors)
  - Up to 60% of patients have a family history of autoimmune thyroid disease (hyperthyroidism or hypothyroidism).
  - Concordance rates of Graves disease: 17% in monozygotic twins (of note, another 17% had chronic lymphocytic thyroiditis and 10% had other nonthyroid autoimmune conditions), 2% in dizygotic twins, 4% of 1st-degree relatives
- Often associated with HLA-DR3
- Increased incidence in genetic syndromes
  - Down syndrome: presents at a younger age, no female predominance unlike the general population; usually milder course
  - Turner syndrome

PATHOPHYSIOLOGY
- Autoimmune process that includes production of immunoglobulins against antigens in the thyroid, orbital tissue, and dermis
- IgG1 anti–thyroid-stimulating hormone (TSH) receptor autoantibody and thyroid-stimulating immunoglobulin (TSI) activates the TSH receptor, causing constitutive stimulation, leading to increased thyroid follicular cell production and release of thyroid hormone.

COMMONLY ASSOCIATED CONDITIONS
- Increased risk for celiac disease, associated with HLA-DQ2 haplotype, early onset of Graves disease, and family history of autoimmune disorders
- Prevalence of hyperthyroidism is higher among children <18 years with type 1 diabetes than without.

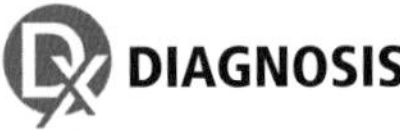

DIAGNOSIS

ALERT

Thyroid storm can constitute an endocrinologic medical emergency.

HISTORY
- Growth acceleration that can be associated with precocious puberty (Hyperthyroidism can accelerate the bone age.)
- Declining school performance, mind racing, difficulty concentrating; may be mistaken for ADHD
- Symptoms of hyperthyroidism and their duration (if child complains of these symptoms, evaluate for possible hyperthyroidism):
  - Restlessness, emotional lability, nervousness
  - Fine tremor
  - Disturbed sleep pattern and insomnia; may result in daytime fatigue
  - Weight loss despite increased appetite
  - Palpitations or chest pain with minimal exertion or at rest; low exercise tolerance
  - Heat intolerance
  - Increased urination and diarrhea
  - Muscle weakness (proximal)
  - Plummer nails (separation of nail from bed)
  - Menstrual irregularities
- Thyroid gland enlargement: Graves disease can present with goiter. Tenderness suggests infectious cause.
- Exophthalmos (bulging of the eyes), increased staring, change in vision or in facial appearance: Exophthalmos due to retro-orbital immune depositions is a hallmark of Graves disease.
- Familial history: increased incidence of Graves disease in families with thyroid disease

PHYSICAL EXAM
- Accelerated growth or height above expected genetic potential due to bone age advancement
- Symmetrically enlarged, smooth, nontender goiter in >95% of cases
- Auscultate the thyroid gland for bruit while patient holds his or her breath (glandular hyperperfusion is associated with hyperthyroidism).
- Resting tachycardia with widened pulse pressure; hyperdynamic precordium: cardiac effects of excessive thyroid hormone
- Slightly elevated temperature: Thyroid hormone controls basal metabolic rate and upregulates catecholamine-induced thermogenesis.
- Lid lag/stare; exophthalmos and proptosis: Severe ophthalmopathy is rare.
- Fine tremor, especially visible in hands and tongue in ~60% of children with Graves disease
- Proximal muscle weakness is common but seldom severe.
- Exaggerated deep tendon reflexes are variable.
- Skin warmth and moisture: heat intolerance and excessive sweating in >30% of children

DIFFERENTIAL DIAGNOSIS
- Infectious
  - Acute suppurative thyroiditis (i.e., transient thyroxine elevations)
  - Subacute thyroiditis after viral illness (also transient)
- Environmental
  - Thyroid hormone ingestion
  - Ingestion of excess iodine (escape from Wolff-Chaikoff block due to impaired autoregulation)
- Tumors (all rare in childhood)
  - TSH-producing pituitary adenoma
  - Thyroid adenoma/hyperfunctioning autonomous thyroid nodule (Most pediatric patients are euthyroid; incidence of nodule hyperfunctioning rises with patient age.)
  - Thyroid carcinoma (rarely presents with hyperthyroidism)
- Congenital
  - Neonatal Graves disease (transplacental antibody transfer from mothers with Graves disease or chronic thyroiditis)
- Genetic and developmental
  - Pituitary resistance to thyroid hormones (dominant negative thyroid-receptor gene mutations causing loss of pituitary negative feedback loop and inappropriately elevated TSH concentrations; can be isolated, with clinical hyperthyroidism, or associated with peripheral thyroid resistance and clinical euthyroidism or hypothyroidism)
  - TSH-receptor gene mutations (rare; germline activating TSH-receptor mutations cause autosomal dominant nonautoimmune hereditary hyperthyroidism)
  - McCune-Albright syndrome: Activating G-protein mutation can lead to indolent hyperthyroidism in addition to the classic features of this syndrome.
  - Ectopic thyroid tissue
- Other causes of hyperthyroidism: See "Goiter."

DIAGNOSTIC TESTS & INTERPRETATION
Initial Tests (screening, lab, imaging)
- Total or free thyroxine: elevated
- Triiodothyronine assessment by radioimmunoassay: elevated (triiodothyronine radioimmunoassay, as direct measurement of triiodothyronine, and not triiodothyronine resin uptake, which indirectly evaluates thyroid hormone–binding capacity)
- TSH: significantly suppressed or undetectable
- TSI titer: positive in 90% of children
- False-positive test results: Elevated total thyroxine levels can also be caused by increased protein binding and so are not necessarily diagnostic for hyperthyroidism: Increased estrogen states (e.g., pregnancy and oral contraceptive use) lead to augmented hepatic thyroxine-binding globulin (TBG) production. Familial dysalbuminemic hyperthyroxinemia: Mutation affecting thyroxine binding affinity leads to increased protein-bound pool.
- I^{123} scan: not needed to diagnose Graves disease. If done, shows diffuse increased uptake at 6 and 24 hours. If palpation suggests nodule, scan may reveal a hot nodule within a suppressed gland.
- ^{99m}Tc uptake assessment is a good second-line test for hyperthyroidism of unclear etiology and negative TSI.

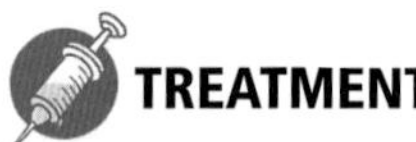

TREATMENT

GENERAL MEASURES
Avoid caffeine.

MEDICATION

ALERT
- Antihistamines and cold medications may worsen sympathetic nervous system symptoms.
- Stopping antithyroid drugs because of low thyroxine values when TSH is still suppressed, reflecting continued TSI activity, will likely result in relapse. Antithyroid medication dosage should be decreased, or L-thyroxine should be added.
- FDA issued a black box warning (June 4, 2009) against propylthiouracil (PTU) use in treating Graves disease owing to risk of severe liver injury including life-threatening acute liver failure.

First Line
- Drug therapy is the first-line choice in children. Antithyroid medications (thiourea derivatives): 65–95% effective: Medications block thyroid hormone synthesis but not the release of existing hormone.
  - Methimazole
  - PTU: Note black box warning. Limited, short-term use of PTU may be considered for patients requiring antithyroid medication (neither I^{131} ablation nor prompt surgery are options) or after a toxic reaction to methimazole. PTU is preferred during first trimester of pregnancy (teratogenic effects of methimazole).

- Propranolol and atenolol block adrenergic symptoms; should be used with antithyroid medications at start of treatment and whenever cardiac symptoms are prominent
- Duration of treatment:
  - Antithyroid medications can be tapered and potentially discontinued after 2 to 3 years of therapy, depending on the patient's course.
  - β-Blockers: Continue until thyroxine and triiodothyronine are under control (~6 weeks).
  - If remission not achieved in 1 to 2 years, ablation with I^{131} or total or subtotal thyroidectomy may be considered.

ISSUES FOR REFERRAL

Treatment for severe ophthalmopathy: must refer patient to an ophthalmologist:

- Three options: high-dose glucocorticoids, orbital radiotherapy, or surgical orbital decompression
- Rehabilitative surgery for eye muscles or eyelids is often needed after the ophthalmopathy has been treated.

SURGERY/OTHER PROCEDURES

- Radiotherapy: I^{131} ablation therapy
  - 90–100% effective; safe and definitive, with predictable outcome
  - Results in permanent hypothyroidism requiring lifelong thyroxine replacement
  - Adequate dose should be used (>150 μCi/g of thyroid tissue) to prevent residual tissue that would be at risk of developing thyroid cancer.
  - Current recommendations advise avoiding I^{131} ablation in children <5 years of age owing to theoretical concerns relating radiation exposure and cancer risks.
  - Radioiodine ablation may exacerbate ophthalmopathy, but this effect can be prevented with concomitant glucocorticoid administration.
- Total or near-total thyroidectomy
  - Effective, rapid, and definitive (vs. 30% recurrence rate for subtotal thyroidectomy)
  - Lifelong thyroxine replacement needed
  - Surgical complication rates higher for children <6 years and for children treated in lower volume centers

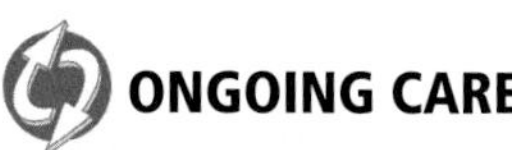

ONGOING CARE

PATIENT EDUCATION

Stop exercising immediately if palpitations develop; patients may need letters for their physical education teachers or coaches.

PROGNOSIS

- Good, if adherent with treatment
- Mortality in severe thyrotoxicosis is possible from cardiac arrhythmias or cardiac failure.
- Spontaneous remission occurs in 20–30% of children after 1 to 2 years but can relapse in 30%. Large thyroid gland size (by ultrasound) and high titers of TSH-receptor antibody (TRAb) predict lower chance of remission.
- Neonatal hyperthyroidism remits by 48 weeks and more commonly by 20 weeks.
- Propranolol or atenolol should result in rapid relief of symptoms of sympathetic hyperactivity.
- 4 to 6 weeks of medical treatment should result in normalization of thyroxine and triiodothyronine concentrations, although TSH levels may remain suppressed owing to persistent underlying activity of the thyroid-stimulating Ig.
- Persistent suppression of TSH is associated with pretreatment presence of thyrotropin-binding inhibitory Ig, severity of thyrotoxicosis, and time to recovery of thyroid hormone levels.
- Duration and type of treatment depend on patient age and remission and relapse pattern.

COMPLICATIONS

- Endocrine disturbances: delayed/early puberty, menstrual irregularity, hypercalcemia
- Ophthalmologic: 3–5% of patients develop severe ophthalmopathy, including eye muscle dysfunction and optic neuropathy, requiring specific treatment by an ophthalmologist. Pediatric ophthalmologic findings (lid lag, soft tissue involvement, and proptosis) are more common but usually less severe than in adults.
- Bone: low bone mineral density for age/sex common at diagnosis due to high bone turnover. Corrects with Graves disease therapy and return to euthyroid status. Osteoporosis and pathologic fractures may occur in undiagnosed hyperthyroidism.
- Fetal/neonatal: intrauterine growth retardation (IUGR), nonimmune hydrops fetalis, craniosynostosis, intrauterine death, goiter that complicates labor and can cause life-threatening airway obstruction at delivery, hyperkinesis, failure to thrive, diarrhea, vomiting, cardiac failure and arrhythmias, systemic and pulmonary hypertension, hepatosplenomegaly, jaundice, hyperviscosity syndrome, thrombocytopenia
- Medication side effects: agranulocytosis (in 0.2–0.5% of patients), rash (most common side effect), gastrointestinal upset, headache, transient transaminitis/hepatitis and life-threatening liver failure with PTU, vasculitis with PTU (frequently associated with perinuclear antineutrophil cytoplasmic antibody [p-ANCA] titers)

ADDITIONAL READING

- Aversa T, Valenzise M, Salerno M, et al. Metamorphic thyroid autoimmunity in Down syndrome: from Hashimoto's thyroiditis to Graves' disease and beyond. *Ital J Pediatr*. 2015;41:87.
- Bahn RS, Burch HB, Cooper DS, et al; for American Thyroid Association, American Association of Clinical Endocrinologists. Hyperthyroidism and other causes of thyrotoxicosis: management guidelines of the American Thyroid Association and American Association of Clinical Endocrinologists. *Endocr Pract*. 2011;17(3):456–520.
- Baskaran C, Misra M, Levitsky LL. Diagnosis of pediatric hyperthyroidism: technetium 99 uptake versus thyroid stimulating immunoglobulins. *Thyroid*. 2015;25(1):37–42.
- Correia MF, Maria AT, Prado S, et al. Neonatal thyrotoxicosis caused by maternal autoimmune hyperthyroidism. *BMJ Case Rep*. 2015;2015:bcr2014209283. doi:10.1136/bcr-2014-209283.
- Harvengt J, Boizeau P, Chevenne D, et al. Triiodothyronine-predominant Graves' disease in childhood: detection and therapeutic implications. *Eur J Endocrinol*. 2015;172(6):715–723.
- Havgaard Kjær R, Smedegård Andersen M, Hansen D. Increasing incidence of juvenile thyrotoxicosis in Denmark: a nationwide study, 1998–2012. *Horm Res Paediatr*. 2015;84(2):102–107.
- Hodax JK, Reinert SE, Quintos JB. Autonomously functioning thyroid nodules in patients <21 years of age: the Rhode Island Hospital experience from 2003–2013. *Endocr Pract*. 2016;22(3):328–337.
- Marcocci C, Marinò M. Treatment of mild, moderate-to-severe and very severe Graves' orbitopathy. *Best Pract Res Clin Endocrinol Metab*. 2012;26(3):325–337.
- Matheis N, Lantz M, Grus FH, et al. Proteomics of orbital tissue in thyroid-associated orbitopathy. *J Clin Endocrinol Metab*. 2015;100(12):E1523–E1530.
- McLeod DS, Cooper DS, Ladenson PW, et al. Race/ethnicity and the prevalence of thyrotoxicosis in young Americans. *Thyroid*. 2015;25(6):621–628.
- Nandi-Munshi D, Taplin CE. Thyroid-related neurological disorders and complications in children. *Pediatr Neurol*. 2015;52(4):373–382.
- Okawa ER, Grant FD, Smith JR. Pediatric Graves' disease: decisions regarding therapy. *Curr Opin Pediatr*. 2015;27(4):442–447.
- Sarezky MD, Corwin DJ, Harrison VS, et al. Hyperthyroidism presenting with pathologic fractures. *Pediatrics*. 2016;137(2):e20150169.
- Srinivasan S, Misra M. Hyperthyroidism in children. *Pediatr Rev*. 2015;36(6):239–248.
- Wilhelm SM, McHenry CR. Total thyroidectomy is superior to subtotal thyroidectomy for management of Graves' disease in the United States. *World J Surg*. 2010;34(6):1261–1264.
- Zirilli G, Velletri MR, Porcaro F, et al. Hyperthyroidism in childhood: peculiarities of the different clinical pictures. *Acta Biomed*. 2015;86(3):220–225.

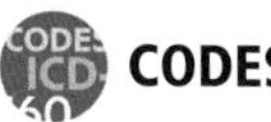

CODES

ICD10

- E05.00 Thyrotoxicosis w diffuse goiter w/o thyrotoxic crisis
- E05.01 Thyrotoxicosis w diffuse goiter w thyrotoxic crisis or storm
- P72.1 Transitory neonatal hyperthyroidism

FAQ

- Q: Does Graves disease lead to thyroid cancer?
- A: No, although controversy surrounds the role of TSH and the closely related TSH-receptor antibodies of Graves disease in thyroid cancer's incidence and aggressiveness. There is an increased incidence of benign thyroid adenoma from 0.6% to 1.9% after therapy involving I^{131} ablation.
- Q: Does hyperthyroidism affect long-term growth or final adult height?
- A: No. Hyperthyroidism can cause tall stature and acceleration of skeletal maturity but does not typically affect final adult height.
- Q: Should WBC counts be monitored routinely while patients are on antithyroid medications?
- A: No. Routine monitoring is not cost-effective because agranulocytosis is rare and sudden in onset. WBC counts should be checked when a patient on antithyroid medication develops fever.
- Q: Will the ophthalmopathy correct with antithyroid treatment?
- A: Not necessarily. It may require specific intervention by an ophthalmologist.
- Q: Can a mother breastfeed while being treated for Graves disease?
- A: Yes. PTU has a lower milk/serum concentration ratio than methimazole (0:1 and 1:0, respectively). In one study, 3 of 11 infants exclusively breastfed by women on 300 to 750 mg daily PTU had high levels of TSH; of these 3, 1 was just above the normal range and the other 2 completely corrected while the mother was still being medicated.

GROWTH HORMONE DEFICIENCY

Paul L. Hofman, FRACP

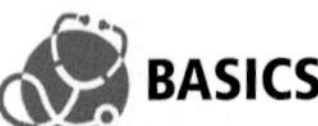

BASICS

DESCRIPTION

- Growth hormone deficiency (GHD) is a rare cause of growth failure due to a lack of growth hormone action caused by a defect in GH synthesis (insufficient hormone) or release.
- GHD can be associated with other pituitary hormone deficiencies.

EPIDEMIOLOGY

- Prevalence in the United States is approximately 1:4,000.
- Males are more commonly diagnosed than females.
- Two peak ages of diagnosis:
  - Infancy (<1 year of age) usually because of associated hypoglycemia
  - Childhood at >4 years of age, usually because of poor linear growth

RISK FACTORS

Genetics

- The majority of cases are either isolated GH deficiency with no clear genetic cause or occur as the result of nonspecific hypothalamic/pituitary damage from etiologies including infection, inflammation, tumors and their treatment (especially radiation therapy).
- Neuromigrational defects such as septo-optic-dysplasia (SOD) are also associated with hypopituitarism. They can be associated with genetic causes (e.g., *HESX1*, *SOX2*, *SOX3*, and *OTX2* mutations for SOD); however, most are usually sporadic, not associated with genetic conditions.
- Autosomal recessive and autosomal dominant forms occur with mutations in the GH gene (*GH1*) and in the GH-releasing hormone receptor (GHRHR) gene.
- X-linked forms also occur and can be associated with immunodeficiency (e.g., *BTK*).

PATHOPHYSIOLOGY

GH has a number of anabolic actions, but its principal one is increasing linear growth. This occurs both from direct GH action on the growth plate and indirectly via stimulation of hepatic and growth plate insulin-like growth factor 1 (IGF-I).

ETIOLOGY

- Idiopathic: probably the commonest diagnosis but only made after exclusion of conditions causing GH deficiency that require further management
- Congenital
  - Congenital malformation of the pituitary can be associated with the following:
    - Holoprosencephaly
    - Septo-optic dysplasia
    - Midline defects: cleft lip, cleft palate, central maxillary incisor
    - Ectopic posterior pituitary, small anterior pituitary, and/or hypoplastic infundibulum
  - Genetic mutations
    - Familial multiple anterior pituitary hormone deficiency (e.g., *HESX1*, *SOX2*, *SOX3*, *LHX3*, *LHX4*, *GHRHR*, *POU1F1*, *PROP1*)
    - *GH1* gene mutations (Type Ia, Ib, II, III)
- Acquired idiopathic
  - CNS tumors: craniopharyngioma, germinoma, medulloblastoma, glioma, pinealoma
  - Pituitary or hypothalamic irradiation
  - Trauma: child abuse or closed head injury
  - Surgical resection/damage of pituitary gland/stalk
  - Birth injury/perinatal insult
  - Infection: viral encephalitis, bacterial or fungal infection, tuberculosis
  - Vascular: pituitary infarction or aneurysm
  - Infiltration affecting pituitary gland or sella turcica: histiocytosis, sarcoidosis
  - Hypophysitis

DIAGNOSIS

HISTORY

- The diagnosis of GH deficiency requires evidence of poor growth (a growth velocity of <25th percentile), usually secondary short stature and biochemical evidence of GH deficiency).
- Two clinical situations do not require biochemical evidence of GH deficiency:
  - Neonatal GH deficiency associated with symptomatic hypoglycemia
  - Children with poor growth, an anatomic pituitary defect, and at least one other pituitary hormone deficiency
- Family history
  - Parental consanguinity
  - Parental heights and a family history of short stature. Rarely autosomal dominant GH deficiency will manifest in family history.
  - Autosomal recessive GH deficiency may manifest in other siblings.
- Birth history
  - Severe neonatal asphyxia, intraventricular or intracerebral hemorrhage
  - Infants with congenital GHD are generally not low birth weight or short at birth but will grow poorly over the next few years.
- Past history of an intracranial tumor, especially when radiotherapy was involved. Intracranial radiation of >10 Gy to the pituitary region can cause GH deficiency, but this may manifest years after treatment so follow-up is essential.

PHYSICAL EXAM

- Measure accurate weight and height with wall-mounted stadiometer. Perform a sitting height and arm span if possible.
- Neurologic examination, including visual fields and funduscopic examination for evaluation of brain tumors
- Assess for signs of Turner syndrome in girls:
  - Cubitus valgus, low posterior hair line, abnormal dentition, abnormal ears, and/or shortened 4th metacarpals suggest Turner syndrome.
  - Turner syndrome is the most common pathologic cause of short stature in girls, and short stature may be the only manifestation.
- Midline facial defects such as submucosal cleft, cleft lip and palate are associated with hypopituitarism.
- Tanner stage
  - Micropenis is associated with congenital hypopituitarism.
  - Delayed puberty suggests constitutional delay but may also be indicative of panhypopituitarism.
- Cherubic facies with frontal bossing, thin hair, high-pitched voice, and relative truncal obesity with adiposity are seen in GHD.

DIFFERENTIAL DIAGNOSIS

Other causes of short stature:

- Abnormal body proportions:
  - Skeletal dysplasia (e.g., hypochondroplasia, achondroplasia)
- Normal skeletal proportions with prenatal growth failure (birth weight <10th percentile):
  - Small for gestational age
  - Congenital infection
  - Maternal drug use (tobacco, alcohol, etc.)
  - Chromosomal short stature (Turner, Down syndrome, etc.)
  - Syndromes (Noonan, Prader-Willi, Russell-Silver, etc.)
- Normal skeletal proportions with postnatal growth failure (birth weight >10th percentile):
  - Constitutional delay of growth and adolescence
  - Familial short stature
  - Malnutrition
  - Renal failure
  - Inflammatory bowel disease
  - Celiac disease
  - Congenital heart disease
  - Hypothyroidism
  - Hypercortisolism
  - Metabolic disorders
  - Rickets
  - Psychosocial deprivation

ALERT

- Children with constitutional growth delay or pubertal delay show poor growth when peers are going through their pubertal growth spurts and have a delayed bone age, mimicking GH deficiency.
- GH-provocative testing may yield false-positive or false-negative results:
  - 30% of normal children will fail at least one GH-provocative test.
  - Hypothyroidism blunts the normal GH release and needs treating (if present) before testing.
  - Obese but otherwise normal children are more likely to fail GH-provocative testing.
  - When GH testing is done in a child at high risk for GHD or if the growth pattern is concerning, the predictive value of GH testing is markedly improved. Assessing growth velocity over a 6- to 12-month period is essential unless there is already proven pituitary or hypothalamic disease.
- Malnutrition can cause low IGF-1.
- Psychosocial deprivation mimics GHD. Such deprived patients may have low growth factors and respond poorly to GH-provocative testing.

DIAGNOSTIC TESTS & INTERPRETATION

Initial Tests (screening, lab, imaging)

- Assessment of a short child who is growing poorly requires a broad range of investigations to exclude occult illness. These include CBC and ESR/CRP, hepatic and renal function tests, celiac screen, urinalysis, and a karyotype in girls.
- When GH deficiency is suspected, other pituitary function should be assessed.
  - Thyroid function tests (thyroid-stimulating hormone [TSH] and either a T_4 or a free T_4)

ALERT

With hypothalamic and pituitary defects, the TSH may be inappropriately normal (rather than low) with a low T_4/free T_4 level.

  - Normal thyroid function is a prerequisite for normal GH secretion. A diagnosis of GH deficiency cannot be made using GH provocation testing unless thyroid function is normal, and it should always be checked prior to testing.
  - Early morning cortisol
  - Prolactin
  - IGF-1 and IGF-binding protein-3 (IGFBP-3) production is regulated directly by GH. However, there is a poor correlation with GH deficiency. IGF-1 values are low early in life and in conditions such as hypothyroidism, diabetes, renal failure, in undernutrition, and in leaner children.
- GH-provocative testing (should be performed by or in consultation with an endocrinologist)
  - A random GH level is of no value in diagnosing GHD beyond the neonatal period.
  - GH stimulation is used as GH is mostly secreted in brief nocturnal pulses that are usually missed with random tests.
  - Although there are a number of provocation tests that are recognized and acceptable, including insulin, clonidine, arginine, glucagon, and L-Dopa, there is no "gold standard" test.
  - It is recommended that two GH provocation tests are used.
  - The diagnosis of GH deficiency in the United States is generally considered a GH level <5 mcg/mL on both tests. However, in normally growing children, 10% will also fail both tests and up to 30% of children would fail any one GH provocation test.
  - Thus, to make a diagnosis of GH deficiency, there should also be evidence of growth failure.
- Bone age: radiography of left hand and wrist to assess skeletal maturation
- If provocative testing shows GH deficiency, obtain MRI with contrast of the pituitary and hypothalamus to look for central nervous system tumor or anomaly of the hypothalamus/pituitary.

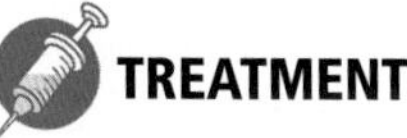

TREATMENT

MEDICATION

- Recombinant human growth hormone (rhGH) was approved by the U.S. Food and Drug Administration (FDA) for use in 1985 by SQ injection daily.
- Daily recommended dosing is between 0.16 and 0.24 mg/kg/week SQ for Genotropin® or Omnitrope® product. Check specific product information for recommended dosages of other growth hormone products.
- Duration of therapy (in children and adolescents)
  - Until growth velocity drops to below 2.5 cm/year
  - When puberty is complete (defined as a bone age >14 years in a girl and >16 years in a boy)
  - Poor growth can be due to occult illness, nonadherence or the use of other medications (especially glucocorticoids). If growth declines and the bone age suggests there is still growth potential, it is essential to investigate the potential causes of growth failure including a screen for occult illness and an IGF-I level which is generally a good assessment of adherence.
  - GH-deficient adults may benefit from lifelong rhGH therapy due to its effects on body composition, lipids, bone density, and general sense of well-being.
  - Before adult GH is initiated, adult patients should undergo repeat GH-provocative testing in all instances, as GH testing can normalize even with known central structural lesions.

ALERT

- rhGH is associated with idiopathic intracranial hypertension (pseudotumor cerebri). This side effect is usually transient and often reverses without cessation of therapy.
- rhGH is usually not given in cancer patients until 1 year has elapsed without recurrence.
- In patients with hypopituitarism, increased doses of hydrocortisone and L-thyroxine will likely be needed after starting rhGH therapy.
- Carefully evaluate any limp or hip or knee pain in patients on rhGH therapy because these symptoms may be associated with slipped capital femoral epiphysis (SCFE); SCFE necessitates orthopedic consultation.
- The spine should be examined regularly after starting rhGH therapy as worsening scoliosis can occur, although this is more likely reflects faster growth than a direct effect on the spine.

ONGOING CARE

FOLLOW-UP RECOMMENDATIONS

Every 3 months by an endocrinologist

- When to expect improvement:
  - Immediate effect on hypoglycemia
  - Growth velocity improves within 3 to 6 months.
- Signs to watch for:
  - Pseudotumor cerebri (headache, vision problems)
  - SCFE
  - Scoliosis
  - In adults, edema and carpal tunnel syndrome, but uncommon in children
  - The risk of malignancy is generally *not* increased in children receiving GH therapy, although there may be a small increased risk of a secondary malignancy in those already who have previously survived a malignancy.

PROGNOSIS

Response to GH therapy is excellent in truly GH-deficient patients. Those who are not GH-deficient have a variable but generally positive growth response. The main cause of poor growth in all children receiving GH therapy, however, is nonadherence. In one national study, 66% of patients missed at least one injection per week, and this lack of adherence affected growth.

COMPLICATIONS

- Short stature
- Lack of self-esteem because of short stature
- Increased truncal adiposity and reduced lean mass
- Delay in pubertal changes (sexual characteristics and growth spurt) due to delayed bone age
- Hypoglycemia (in the newborn period)
- Osteopenia

ADDITIONAL READING

- Clayton PE, Cohen P, Tanaka T, et al. Diagnosis of growth hormone deficiency in childhood. On behalf of the Growth Hormone Research Society. *Horm Res*. 2000;53(Suppl 3):30.
- Cutfield WS, Derraik JGB, Gunn AJ, et al. Non-compliance with growth hormone treatment in children is common and impairs linear growth. *PLoS One*. 2011;6(1):e16223.
- Grimberg A, DiVall SA, Polychronakos C, et al. Guidelines for growth hormone and insulin-like growth factor-I treatment in children and adolescents: growth hormone deficiency, idiopathic short stature, and primary insulin-like growth factor-I deficiency. *Horm Res Paediatr*. 2016;86:361–397.
- Pitukcheewanont P, Desrosiers P, Steelman J, et al. Issues and trends in pediatric growth hormone therapy—an update from the GHMonitor observational registry. *Pediatr Endocrinol Rev*. 2008;5(Suppl 2):702–707.
- Richmond E, Rogol AD. Current indications for growth hormone therapy for children and adolescents. *Endocr Dev*. 2010;18:92–108.
- Wit JM, Kiess W, Mullis P. Genetic evaluation of short stature. *Best Pract Res Clin Endocrinol Metab*. 2011;25(1):1–17.

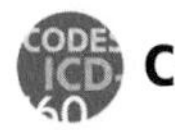

CODES

ICD10

- E23.0 Hypopituitarism
- Q89.2 Congenital malformations of other endocrine glands

FAQ

- Q: Does GH improve the body composition in patients with GH deficiency?
- A: Not only is growth impressive in these patients but also there is a normalization of body composition with a loss of fat and increased muscle mass due to the lipolytic and anabolic effects of growth hormone therapy.
- Q: Will GH use cause long-term safety issues?
- A: Although a study from France suggested increased long-term mortality, several similar studies have refuted this observation. Currently, there is no credible evidence suggesting there are long-term safety issues with GH treatment.

G

GUILLAIN-BARRÉ SYNDROME

Sharon O. Wietstock, MD, MSc • Brett J. Bordini, MD

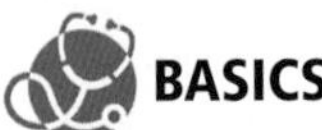

BASICS

DESCRIPTION

Guillain-Barré syndrome (GBS) is a collection of clinically related disorders characterized by acute-onset monophasic inflammation of the peripheral nervous system. Affected individuals typically present with ascending weakness and loss of reflexes over days to weeks. Paresis or even plegia may involve the limbs, face, eyes, or respiratory muscles. Autonomic and sensory disturbances, including numbness and pain, are frequently present. Neurologic deficits usually peak by 4 weeks. Presentations include the most common form, acute inflammatory demyelinating polyradiculoneuropathy (AIDP), as well as acute motor axonal neuropathy, Miller Fisher syndrome, and other variants.

EPIDEMIOLOGY

Incidence

GBS is the most common cause of acute or subacute flaccid weakness worldwide. The annual incidence is as high as 1.34 cases per 100,000 in individuals <15 years of age, with a slight male predominance. AIDP is the most common form, accounting for up to 90% of cases in North America, with Miller Fisher syndrome being the next most common variant presentation.

RISK FACTORS

- Up to two thirds of cases are preceded by a mild upper respiratory or gastrointestinal tract illness in the weeks prior to the onset of symptoms.
- *Campylobacter jejuni* enteritis is the most common bacterial infection associated with developing GBS.
- Viral exposures associated with the development of GBS include cytomegalovirus (CMV), Epstein-Barr virus, varicella-zoster virus, acute HIV infection, influenza A, H1N1 influenza, enterovirus, Zika virus, and others.
- Pregnancy, certain cancers, and recent surgery or vaccination have also been associated with GBS.
- Often, no precipitating exposure can be identified.

Genetics

Polymorphisms in the immunoglobulin Kappa light chains and in TNF-α have been associated with a higher rate of GBS in the setting of antecedent infection with *C. jejuni*. The majority of GBS cases do not demonstrate a clear genetic inheritance pattern. *PMP22* gene (601097) on chromosome 17 was identified in a single family with the acute (AIDP) and chronic (CIDP) forms of inflammatory demyelinating polyneuropathy.

PATHOPHYSIOLOGY

Inflammatory cell–mediated and humoral-mediated immune mechanisms play a role in segmental demyelination on nerve biopsy; lymphocytes and macrophages participate in myelin destruction. Axonal variants of GBS feature axonal degeneration without demyelination. Circulating antiganglioside antibodies (e.g., GM1, GD1a, GM2, GQ1b) found in particular subtypes suggest a molecular mimicry mechanism stimulated by infection. Some variants (e.g., Bickerstaff encephalitis) involve central and peripheral demyelination.

ETIOLOGY

Molecular mimicry is believed to underlie cases of GBS associated with a preceding infection.

COMMONLY ASSOCIATED CONDITIONS

- GBS most commonly affects previously healthy individuals.
- GBS is seen in a higher than expected rate in patients with sarcoidosis, systemic lupus erythematosus, lymphoma, HIV infection, Lyme disease, and solid tumors.

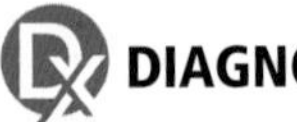

DIAGNOSIS

HISTORY

- GBS has a variety of clinical presentations; a high index of suspicion is critical. Typical features are distal sensory changes followed by progressive motor weakness and areflexia.
- Common presentations include decreased ambulation or crawling in infants, unsteady gait which may be due to sensory ataxia, facial weakness, diplopia, leg or back pain, or sensory changes in the extremities.
- Paresthesia and pain typically occur in a stocking/glove distribution, frequently early in the course.
- Most patients first note leg weakness or gait instability that progresses over days to weeks. 60% are unable to walk at the peak of symptoms.
- Patients may also report shortness of breath, palpitations, light-headedness, constipation, or urinary retention secondary to respiratory and autonomic involvement.
- Two thirds of patients will report an infectious illness 2 to 3 weeks prior to symptom onset. Consider direct infection (e.g., poliomyelitis, West Nile virus) if fever is present at symptom onset.

PHYSICAL EXAM

- Characteristic findings include muscular weakness and sensory changes, most often symmetric with distal greater than proximal involvement. Proximally, predominant symptoms do not preclude the diagnosis but rather may indicate radicular involvement.
- Deep tendon reflexes are usually diminished or absent within 1 week of symptom onset.
- Respiratory muscle weakness may make assessment of respiratory insufficiency or failure, difficult on physical examination. Careful physical assessment, combined with diagnostic procedures such as measurement of vital capacity or maximum inspiratory pressure, are essential, as upper airway or ventilatory compromise may progress rapidly.
  - Respiratory failure leads to intubation in up to 20% of patients. Bulbar weakness and poor airway protection may also necessitate intubation.
  - Impending respiratory failure can often be unpredictable, and hypercarbia on blood gas and desaturation are late findings.
- Bilateral facial weakness occurs in up to 50% of cases.
- Ophthalmoplegia, ataxia, and areflexia are the characteristic features of Miller Fisher syndrome.
- Neonates and infants may (rarely) present as floppy infants.

DIFFERENTIAL DIAGNOSIS

- Myasthenia gravis
- Intoxication (e.g., heavy metals, organophosphates)
- Infection: poliomyelitis, West Nile virus, CMV, HIV, Lyme disease, diphtheria, botulism
- Myopathy/myositis
- Acute cerebellar ataxia (sometimes associated with neuroblastoma)
- Transverse myelitis
- Chronic inflammatory demyelinating polyneuropathy (CIDP)
- Vasculitic neuropathy
- Severe vitamin B_{12} deficiency
- Metabolic abnormalities: hypermagnesemia, hypophosphatemia
- Porphyric neuropathy
- Acute presentations of inherited peripheral neuropathies
- Tick paralysis
- Conversion, psychogenic weakness, astasia/abasia

DIAGNOSTIC TESTS & INTERPRETATION

Initial Tests (screening, lab, imaging)

- In atypical cases, consider heavy metal screening, HIV testing, Lyme testing, porphyria screening, and acetylcholine receptor antibodies (myasthenia gravis).
- IgA level should be considered, particularly if there is a history of frequent pulmonary infections, as IgA deficiency can be associated with a higher risk of anaphylaxis to intravenous immunoglobulin (IVIG) therapy.
- MRI of the spine (with gadolinium enhancement), as spinal nerve root enhancement on MRI can support the diagnosis of GBS

Diagnostic Procedures/Other

- Lumbar puncture may demonstrate an albuminocytologic dissociation with an elevated protein and normal cell count after the 1st week of symptoms. Minimal pleocytosis (<50 cells/mL), largely mononuclear leukocytes, may occur but should prompt consideration of alternative etiology.
- Electrodiagnosis:
  - Nerve conduction studies (NCS) and electromyography (EMG) can confirm diagnosis of GBS and are helpful when clinical, imaging, or CSF findings are ambiguous. NCS and EMG are abnormal in 50% of patients in the first 2 weeks and in 85% of patients afterward.
  - Initially, needle EMG may be normal; consider serial studies if initially nondiagnostic.

ALERT

- Initially, gait instability may mistakenly be interpreted as being psychogenic.
- Reflexes may be preserved in early stages of illness.
- Proximal symptoms may predominate early on.
- Check for reflexes in patients with bilateral Bell palsy.

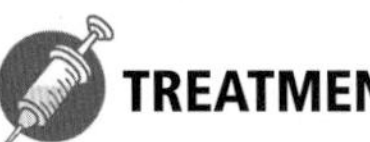

TREATMENT

ALERT

- Respiratory failure necessitating intubation and mechanical ventilation may occur in up to 20% of affected children, may develop quickly, and is of a neuromuscular, rather than obstructive, nature. As such, work of breathing may not appear to be increased.
- Treat hypertension cautiously; catastrophic refractory hypotension may ensue.

GENERAL MEASURES

- Regular monitoring of vital capacity and maximum inspiratory pressure, initially every 4 hours or more frequently if indicated. Consider ICU monitoring for patients with poor or declining respiratory function; strongly consider intubation if vital capacity reaches <50% of normal.
- Frequent heart rate and blood pressure assessments to monitor for autonomic dysregulation
- Bowel regimen and assessment for urinary retention
- Deep venous thrombosis (DVT) prophylaxis
- Swallowing evaluation

MEDICATION

A combination of supportive therapy and immunotherapy is the mainstay of treatment for patients with GBS.

- IVIG and plasmapheresis are equally effective as 1st-line immunotherapy and are well-tolerated. Combining both therapies is not more effective than monotherapy. Complications and discontinuation of therapy are less common with IVIG.
- IVIG dosing:
  - 2 g/kg of body weight, typically given as 0.4 g/kg/24 h for 5 consecutive days
  - Alternate dosing regimens of 1 g/kg/24 h for 2 consecutive days or 2 g/kg as a single dose may be used.
- Plasmapheresis regimen:
  - Total plasma exchange volume of 200 to 250 mL/kg divided in 3 to 5 treatments over 7 to 14 days
  - Therapy initiation is recommended within 4 weeks of symptom onset for patients who cannot walk and within 2 weeks for patients who can.
  - Plasmapheresis may be performed peripherally in children big enough for large-bore peripheral IV lines but requires placement of a central catheter in others.
- Corticosteroids are not helpful and are not recommended.
- Pain from nerve root inflammation is common in GBS and should be treated aggressively. Agents such as gabapentin can be useful.

ISSUES FOR REFERRAL

Neurology follow-up typically 4 to 6 weeks after discharge

ADDITIONAL THERAPIES

Physical therapy: Avoid contractures with lower extremity splinting and early passive range of motion. Aggressive physical and occupational therapy are essential for good outcomes.

ADMISSION, INPATIENT, AND NURSING CONSIDERATIONS

- Hospitalization is often required to monitor for or manage progressive respiratory insufficiency, autonomic dysregulation, or neuropathic pain.
- Hospitalize patients whose symptoms progress over hours to days, who have any respiratory or bulbar complaints, or who are nonambulatory.
- Particular attention should be paid to preventing aspiration, skin breakdown, contractures, DVT, and secondary compressive neuropathies.
- Discharge criteria: completion of immunotherapy and stabilization of symptoms
- Consider intensive inpatient rehabilitation depending on the degree of neurologic impairment.

ONGOING CARE

FOLLOW-UP RECOMMENDATIONS

- Improvement typically begins 2 to 3 weeks after onset of symptoms up to 2 months in some patients.
- Improvement continues for up to 2 to 3 years.

PATIENT EDUCATION

Parent Internet information: Guillain-Barré Syndrome GBS/CIDP Foundation International: http://www.gbs-cidp.org/

PROGNOSIS

- Most individuals recover, although 25% may have residual symptoms; ultimate functional recovery depends on the degree of axonal injury. Follow-up electrodiagnostic studies can be helpful in some cases.
- Early prognosticators include fulminant onset and the severity of weakness at the disease nadir.
- Overall prognosis in children is better than in adults.

COMPLICATIONS

- Complications include respiratory failure, blood pressure dysregulation (hypotension and/or hypertension), urinary retention, aspiration, pain syndromes, DVT with or without pulmonary embolism, and infection.
- Death occurs in up to 6% of cases, typically from early respiratory failure or autonomic instability.

ADDITIONAL READING

- Bordini BJ, Monrad P. Differentiating familial neuropathies from Guillain-Barré syndrome. *Pediatr Clin North Am*. 2017;64(1):231–252.
- Chevret S, Hughes RA, Annane D. Plasma exchange for Guillain-Barré syndrome. *Cochrane Database Syst Rev*. 2017;(2):CD001798.
- Devos D, Magot A, Perrier-Boeswillwald J, et al. Guillain-Barré syndrome during childhood: particular clinical and electrophysiological features. *Muscle Nerve*. 2013;48(2):247–251.
- Hughes RA, Brassington R, Gunn AA, et al. Corticosteroids for Guillain-Barré syndrome. *Cochrane Database Syst Rev*. 2016;(10):CD001446.
- Hughes RA, Swan AV, van Doorn PA. Intravenous immunoglobulin for Guillain-Barré syndrome. *Cochrane Database Syst Rev*. 2014;(9):CD002063.
- Hughes RA, Wijdicks EF, Barohn R, et al; for Quality Standards Subcommittee of the American Academy of Neurology. Practice parameter: immunotherapy for Guillain-Barré syndrome: report of the Quality Standards Subcommittee of the American Academy of Neurology. *Neurology*. 2003;61(6):736–740.
- Korinthenberg R. Acute polyradiculoneuritis: Guillain-Barré syndrome. *Handb Clin Neurol*. 2013;112:1157–1162.
- Lawn ND, Fletcher DD, Henderson RD. Anticipating mechanical ventilation in Guillain-Barré syndrome. *Arch Neurol*. 2001;58(6):893–898.
- Lin JJ, Hsia SH, Wang HS, et al. Clinical variants of Guillain-Barré syndrome in children. *Pediatr Neurol*. 2012;47(2):91–96.
- Pritchard J, Hughes RA, Hadden RD, et al. Pharmacological treatment other than corticosteroids, intravenous immunoglobulin and plasma exchange for Guillain-Barré syndrome. *Cochrane Database Syst Rev*. 2016;(11):CD008630.
- Tekgul H, Serdaroglu G, Tutuncuoglu S. Outcome of axonal and demyelinating forms of Guillain-Barré syndrome in children. *Pediatr Neurol*. 2003;28(4):295–299.

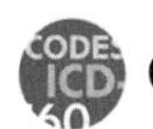

CODES

ICD10

G61.0 Guillain-Barre syndrome

FAQ

- Q: Is GBS contagious?
- A: No.
- Q: Will I get GBS again?
- A: Recurrent attacks occur in up to 5% of patients. Treatment-related fluctuations (worsening after completion of immunotherapy) occur in up to 16% of patients in the first 2 months. Finally, up to 5% of patients ultimately diagnosed with CIDP will present acutely and can be indistinguishable from GBS initially.
- Q: Do all cases require hospitalization and immunomodulatory treatment?
- A: Some youngsters with mild, nondisabling symptoms may be observed as outpatients (≤10%).

G

GYNECOMASTIA

Chirag R. Kapadia, MD • Zoe M. González-García, MD

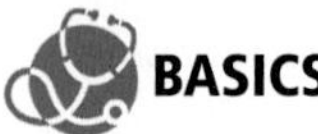

BASICS

DESCRIPTION

Visible or palpable proliferation of unilateral or bilateral breast glandular tissue in a male

EPIDEMIOLOGY

- Two age distribution peaks: neonatal, pubertal
- Neonatal gynecomastia occurs in 60–90% of all newborns.
- Peak incidence for pubertal gynecomastia in males is 14 years of age (range: 10 to 16 years). Onset usually at 5- to 10-mL testicular size and pubic hair Tanner III or IV.
- ~40% of pubertal boys develop transient gynecomastia (measuring ≥0.5 cm). This percentage varies greatly in studies, perhaps due to examination techniques.

RISK FACTORS

Any state that leads to an increase in the net effect of estrogen relative to androgens on breast glandular tissue, such as the following:

- Increased endogenous estrogen
- Increased exogenous estrogen or estrogen-like compounds in commercial products
- Increased sensitivity of breast tissue to estrogen action
- Decreased androgen concentrations
- Androgen receptor defects
- Pharmacologic or commercial product interference with androgen receptors
- Increased aromatase action. Aromatase converts androgens to estrogens. This can be intrinsic as in aromatase excess syndrome or as a result of tumors or hyperthyroidism.
- Elevated leptin concentrations, which may increase aromatase enzyme activity, stimulate growth of mammary cells or increase breast receptor sensitivity to estrogens.
- High serum gonadotropin concentrations altering sex steroid production ratios
- Increased sex hormone–binding globulin, which reduces free testosterone levels
- Hyperthyroidism, which increases aromatization of androgens to estrogens
- Hyperprolactinemia interfering with gonadotropin production, thus altering sex steroid production
- Obesity: may increase leptin concentrations and may increase aromatization. Obesity correlates with true gynecomastia in some studies only. Other studies find obesity correlates with pseudogynecomastia but not true ductal breast tissue development.

ETIOLOGY

- Physiologic
  - Neonatal: Transient palpable breast tissue develops in newborns, owing to elevated estrogen levels in the fetoplacental unit; resolves as estrogen levels decline
  - Pubertal: benign transient gynecomastia occurring in otherwise healthy males. In this setting, breast tissue measuring <5 cm in diameter has a high likelihood of spontaneous regression.
  - Involutional: Breast enlargement occurs in elderly men.
  - Physiologic gynecomastia usually is bilateral.
- Pathologic
  - Drug-induced
    - Hormones: estrogen, androgens, gonadotropins, growth hormone, antiandrogens, commercial products containing estrogenic or antiandrogenic compounds
    - Anti-infective agents: can cause gynecomastia through antiandrogenic properties; ethionamide, isoniazid, ketoconazole, metronidazole, antiretrovirals
    - Antiulcer drugs: usually cause gynecomastia through antiandrogenic properties; cimetidine, ranitidine, omeprazole
    - Chemotherapeutic agents: usually cause gynecomastia by causing hypogonadism; alkylating agents, methotrexate, vinca alkaloids
    - Cardiovascular agents: spironolactone—androgen receptor blocker; unknown mechanism of action: amiodarone, captopril, digitoxin, diltiazem, enalapril, methyldopa, nifedipine, reserpine, verapamil
    - Psychotropic agents: may act by increasing prolactin levels or decreasing androgen levels: diazepam, risperidone, haloperidol, phenothiazines, antidepressants
    - Drugs of abuse: alcohol, heroin, amphetamines, marijuana, methadone
    - Miscellaneous: metoclopramide, phenytoin, penicillamine, theophylline, gabapentin, clonidine, pregabalin
- Hypogonadism/acquired testicular failure
- Infectious: breast abscess
- Tumors: testicular (including Sertoli cell and germ cell), adrenal, ectopic tumors that produce human chorionic gonadotropin
- Chronic disease: renal failure, liver cirrhosis, malnutrition with refeeding, HIV infection
- Congenital disorders causing gonadal hypofunction, androgen receptor issues, or increased aromatization: Klinefelter syndrome, vanishing testes syndrome, androgen resistance syndromes, ovotesticular disorder of sex development
- Late-onset congenital adrenal hyperplasia—elevated androgens converted to estrogen
- Spinal cord injury leading to testicular failure over the long term
- Neoplasms: breast carcinoma, neurofibroma, lymphangioma, lipoma, neuroblastoma metastasis
- Trauma: hematoma
- Peutz-Jeghers syndrome: prepubertal gynecomastia
- Miscellaneous masses: dermoid cyst

DIAGNOSIS

ALERT

- Do not mistake pseudogynecomastia (i.e., fatty enlargement of the breasts in obesity) for true gynecomastia.
- Do not overlook drug-related causes. Drug-related gynecomastia is usually reversible if diagnosed during year of onset.

HISTORY

- Family history: 1/2 of adolescents with gynecomastia have positive family history.
- Time of onset relative to puberty: onset usually at testicular size 5 to 10 mL and Tanner stage III or IV pubic hair
- Prepubertal more concerning than pubertal
- Unilateral more concerning than bilateral
- Rate of progression
  - Rapidly enlarging, painful gynecomastia with acute onset is of more concern than long-standing enlargement.
- Drug exposures, including alcohol, marijuana, and heroin, along with exposure to exogenous estrogen and commercial products containing estrogens, lavender, tea tree oil, phthalates, ginseng, and others
- Symptoms suggestive of hyperthyroidism
- Symptoms suggestive of liver disease, such as cirrhosis
- Symptoms suggestive of renal failure
- Symptoms suggestive of neoplastic disease
- Symptoms suggestive of hypogonadism, such as decreased libido, erectile dysfunction, or infertility, may indicate an abnormal estrogen-to-androgen ratio.

PHYSICAL EXAM

- Assess for malnourishment: may result in hepatic dysfunction causing higher estrogen-to-androgen ratio
- Perform a complete breast exam:
  - With patient supine, grasp breast between thumb and forefinger and move digits toward the nipple: Look for a firm, rubbery, mobile, discoid mound of glandular tissue arising concentrically below the nipple and areola. Measure diameter of the disk. Asymmetry and tenderness are common.
  - Check for galactorrhea, which can be a sign of drug ingestion or hyperprolactinemia.
  - Masses not concentric around the areola; that are hard, firm, fixed; that are unilateral, or have any skin dimpling, nipple retraction, nipple bleeding, or discharge are concerning for carcinoma. This is very rare in male adolescents.
  - Check for pseudogynecomastia (fatty enlargement): If present, no glandular disk will be palpable under areola.
  - If disk diameter is >5 cm, regression is very unlikely.
- Thyroid exam: Goiter may indicate hypothyroidism.
- Testicular exam: Consider testicular tumors with masses or significant asymmetry of testes. Consider gonadal failure for small, firm testes; gynecomastia more likely to be pathologic if testes <5 mL (in this case, not defined as pubertal gynecomastia).

DIFFERENTIAL DIAGNOSIS

See "Etiology."

DIAGNOSTIC TESTS & INTERPRETATION

Initial Tests (screening, lab, imaging)

- Benign presentations do not need extensive workup. Neonatal gynecomastia can be monitored without workup for regression by 1 year of age. Bilateral pubertal gynecomastia arising after pubertal onset, <5 cm in diameter can be monitored as well for further growth.
- In other cases, direct workup to suspected causes based on history and exam:
  - LH for pituitary function
  - FSH to rule out testicular failure
  - Prolactin for hyperprolactinemia
  - TSH for hyperthyroidism
  - Testosterone for gonadal function
  - Estrogen for aromatization excess, estrogen excess, or estrogen-secreting tumors (Although in some cases, local aromatase activity can cause gynecomastia without high circulating estrogen.)
  - Dehydroepiandrosterone sulfate (DHEA-S) for adrenal tumors
  - hCG for germ cell tumors (Note that this specific lab is to be ordered, not a qualitative pregnancy test.)
  - Karyotype to rule out Klinefelter syndrome (only indicated in suspicious cases via history or exam or those with proven testicular failure via high FSH)
  - Most of these labs are best done in the morning if possible.
- None indicated for benign presentations.
- Testicular ultrasound in cases with concerns for testicular tumor via asymmetric exam, elevated estradiol or hCG, or pubertal level testosterone with suppressed LH
- Abdominal/adrenal CT or MRI
  - To rule out adrenal neoplasm, if estradiol elevated, DHEA-S elevated, or in cases concerning for testicular tumor that turn out to have negative testicular ultrasound
  - Consider chest CT in such cases as well.
- Brain MRI or CT, with and without contrast: if pituitary tumor is suspected
- Bone age can be an adjunct evaluation in cases with concerns for estrogen excess; estrogen results in bone age advance.

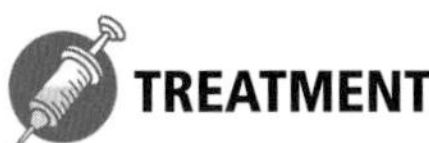

TREATMENT

MEDICATION

- Generally, drug therapy should proceed under the guidance of an endocrinologist.
- Tamoxifen and aromatase inhibitors in off-label use have shown some benefit in benign pubertal gynecomastia if started within 1 year of onset.
- If hypogonadal, replace testosterone.
- If gynecomastia has been present for >1 year, pharmacologic therapy is of little benefit because of an increase in fibrosis of the tissue.

ISSUES FOR REFERRAL

Consider surgical consultation in patients with >5-cm diameter glandular tissue near the end of puberty. Surgery prior to completion of puberty may increase risk of recurrence.

ADDITIONAL THERAPIES

- Reassurance for patients with pubertal gynecomastia measuring <5 cm
- Discontinue drugs or commercial products known or suspected to induce gynecomastia and follow-up in 1 to 2 months.
- Reexamine at 3- to 6-month intervals for size change.
- For gynecomastia >5 cm, consider surgical consultation once history, exam, and lab evaluation for pathology (along with imaging in indicated cases) have been conducted.

SURGERY/OTHER PROCEDURES

- Surgery is therapy of choice for macrogynecomastia or persistent gynecomastia refractory to medical therapy, although obtaining insurance coverage may be difficult.
- Obesity should not preclude surgical intervention.
- Surgical options include periareolar incision with adjunctive liposuction or glandular tissue removal through two incisions in the anterior axillary regions and ultrasound-assisted liposuction.
- Orange-peel excision of the gland has recently emerged as a new surgical technique.

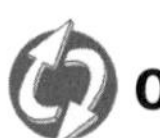

ONGOING CARE

FOLLOW-UP RECOMMENDATIONS

- Reexamine every 3 to 6 months for size and characteristics.
- Watch for signs of psychological stress.
  - Significant issue in some male adolescents and should not be dismissed.
  - Reassure that eventually they shall be referred for treatment.
  - In those with significant psychological stress, referral before completion of puberty may result in repeat surgery later, but this can be considered after discussion with patient and family.

PROGNOSIS

- In benign cases, prognosis is good.
- Neonatal gynecomastia usually resolves within the 1st year of life.
- Pubertal gynecomastia <5 cm: 50–75% disappear spontaneously within 2 years; 90% within 3 years; if size >5 cm, regression unlikely
- Medical therapy effective only if treatment initiated within a year of onset

COMPLICATIONS

In benign cases

- Pain (may interfere with sports)
- Psychological stress
- Embarrassment
- Skin erosion of the nipple owing to rubbing against clothing

ADDITIONAL READING

- Goldman RD. Drug-induced gynecomastia in children and adolescents. *Can Fam Physician*. 2010;56(4):344–345.
- Lapid O, van Windergen JJ, Perlemuter L. Tamoxifen therapy for the management of pubertal gynecomastia: a systematic review. *J Pediatr Endocrinol Metab*. 2013;26(9–10):803–807.
- Ma NS, Geffner ME. Gynecomastia in prepubertal and pubertal men. *Curr Opin Pediatr*. 2008;20(4):465–470.
- Mauras N, Bishop K, Merinbaum D, et al. Pharmacokinetics and pharmacodynamics of anastrazole in pubertal boys with recent-onset gynecomastia. *J Clin Endocrinol Metab*. 2009;94(8):2975–2978.
- Narula HS, Carlson HE. Gynaecomastia—pathophysiology, diagnosis, and treatment. *Nature Rev Endocrinol*. 2014;10(11):684–698.
- Nordt CA, DiVasta AD. Gynecomastia in adolescents. *Curr Opin Pediatr*. 2008;20(4):375–382.
- Rosen H, Webb ML, DiVasta AD, et al. Adolescent gynecomastia: not only an obesity issue. *Ann Plast Surg*. 2010;64(5):688–690.

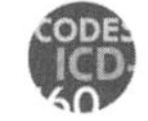

CODES

ICD10

- N62 Hypertrophy of breast
- P83.4 Breast engorgement of newborn

FAQ

- Q: When should a neonate with gynecomastia be referred to a specialist?
- A: For male neonates, if galactorrhea persists at 3 months of age or the gynecomastia not resolved by 1 year of age.
- Q: When should a nonneonatal, but prepubertal, male with gynecomastia be referred to a specialist?
- A: Gynecomastia in a prepubertal boy is rare and concerning. Urgent referral should be made to an endocrinologist.
- Q: When should a pubertal adolescent with gynecomastia be referred to a specialist?
- A: If gynecomastia is unilateral; if size is >5 cm; if size is <5 cm but with visible enlargement ongoing within 1 year of onset of problem; if started before onset of puberty; if nipple bleeding, discharge or retraction. Also, if testes are <5 mL or testicular mass present; if abnormal hormonal workup or imaging study
- Q: How can gynecomastia be distinguished from breast cancer?
- A: Breast cancer usually presents as a unilateral, eccentric hard or firm mass fixed to underlying tissues. Location usually outside the nipple–areolar complex. Associated findings can include dimpling of the skin, retraction of the nipple, nipple discharge, and/or axillary lymphadenopathy. Breast cancer in the pediatric population is extremely rare: <0.1% of all breast cancers occur in patients <20 years of age. Benign tumors, such as fibroadenomas, much more common than malignant tumors. If differentiation between gynecomastia and breast carcinoma cannot be made by physical exam alone, patient should undergo diagnostic mammography.
- Q: Has the incidence of gynecomastia increased?
- A: As the prevalence of childhood and adolescent obesity has increased, the presence of *pseudogynecomastia* has also increased. Pseudogynecomastia is best treated with diet and exercise.

G

HAND, FOOT, AND MOUTH DISEASE

Ross Newman, DO, MHPE

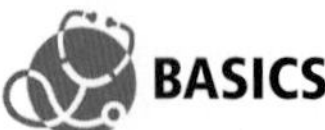

BASICS

DESCRIPTION

Hand, foot, and mouth disease is a viral illness with the characteristic clinical features of the following:

- Vesiculoulcerative stomatitis
- Papular or vesicular exanthem on the hands and/or the feet
- Constitutional symptoms such as fever and malaise

EPIDEMIOLOGY

- In temperate climates, hand, foot, and mouth disease is most common in the summer and fall (a pattern common to many of the enterovirus infections).
- In tropical climates, disease is present year-round.
- Incubation period is 3 to 6 days.
- Highly contagious, afflicting up to 50% of those exposed
- Close household contacts are particularly susceptible.
- Most common in children <5 years but may affect adults
- May occur as an isolated case or in an epidemic distribution

GENERAL PREVENTION

- Frequent hand washing, especially after changing diapers, and good personal hygiene are the most useful means to prevent spread of enteroviral illnesses.
- Contact precautions should be maintained with all hospitalized patients.
- The prodromal and enanthem periods appear to be the most contagious; however, some may shed virus in the stool up to 3 months after infection.

PATHOPHYSIOLOGY

- Enteroviruses are acquired primarily from oral–fecal contamination, but respiratory secretions may also transmit the virus.
- Lymphatic invasion leads to viremia and spread to secondary sites.
- Viremia ceases with antibody production.
- Direct inoculation of the extremities from oral lesions has been hypothesized with regard to hand, foot, and mouth disease.

ETIOLOGY

Coxsackie A16 virus is the most common causative agent. Other enterovirus serotypes commonly associated include:

- Coxsackieviruses A5, A7, A9, A10, A16, B1, and B3
- Enterovirus 71
- Echoviruses

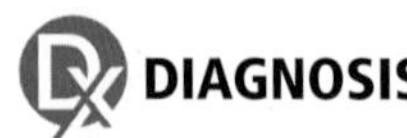

DIAGNOSIS

HISTORY

- History of ill contacts
  - Family members or close contacts are often similarly affected.
  - Incubation period 3 to 6 days
- Any fever, pain, or other symptoms
  - A mild prodrome occasionally precedes the characteristic enanthem and exanthem by 1 or 2 days.
  - Low-grade fever (usually near 101°F [38.3°C])
  - Malaise, sore mouth, anorexia, coryza, diarrhea, abdominal pain
- Lesions in mouth
  - Oral lesions typically occur shortly before the hand and foot manifestations.
- Hydration status
  - Determine quality and amount of oral intake, quality and amount of urine output, recent weight loss, duration of symptoms.

PHYSICAL EXAM

- Enanthem
  - Oral lesions begin as small, red papules.
  - Papules quickly evolve to small vesicles on an erythematous base.
  - Lesions progress to ulcerations.
  - Tongue, buccal mucosa, palate, gingiva, uvula, and/or tonsillar pillars may be involved.
  - Typically 2 to 10 lesions that may persist up to 1 week
- Exanthem
  - Less consistently present than oral lesions occurring in 1/4 to 2/3 of patients
  - Maculopapular eruptions progress to vesicles.
  - Rarely tender or pruritic
  - Most frequent on the dorsal aspects of fingers and toes
  - May also occur on the palms, soles, arms, legs, buttocks, and face
- Adenopathy
  - Enlarged anterior cervical or submandibular nodes are present in 1/4 of cases.
- Other
  - Attention should be given to the patient's vital signs; general appearance; and respiratory, cardiac, and neurologic functioning to help identify the rare patient with a threatening complication of hand, foot, and mouth disease.

DIFFERENTIAL DIAGNOSIS

Few infectious diseases have such characteristic clinical findings. Oral ulcerations followed by lesions on the distal extremities are virtually pathognomonic. The most difficult diagnostic dilemmas may occur early in the disease course when isolated oral lesions predominate:

- Herpangina
  - Also caused by coxsackie A viruses
  - Associated with higher fever
  - Usually limited to the posterior oropharynx
- Herpetic gingivostomatitis
  - Most common cause of stomatitis in children
  - Associated with higher fever
  - More frequently associated with lymphadenopathy
  - Gingival involvement severe
- Aphthous ulcers
  - Can occur without fever or upper respiratory symptoms
  - Does not occur in outbreaks
  - No seasonal predilection
- Stevens-Johnson syndrome
  - Ulcerations frequently coalesce.
  - Usually affects other mucous membranes
  - Often appears with separate cutaneous manifestations
- The Boston exanthem
  - Caused by echovirus 16
  - Mild febrile illness with a macular rash on the palms and soles occurring at time of or after defervescence
  - Oral lesions absent

DIAGNOSTIC TESTS & INTERPRETATION

Initial Tests (screening, lab, imaging)

- Hand, foot, and mouth disease has unique clinical features and a relatively benign course. Laboratory confirmation of the diagnosis is seldom needed or indicated.
- Culture
  - Causative viruses may be cultured from many sites:
    - Oral ulcers
    - Cutaneous vesicles
    - Nasopharyngeal swabs
    - Stool (Isolation of an enterovirus from the stool does not confirm it to be the cause of disease because the virus can be shed for many weeks after infection.)
    - Cerebrospinal fluid (CSF) (in cases where meningoencephalitis is suspected). Reverse transcription-polymerase chain reaction (RT-PCR) can be used and is more sensitive than culture in the CSF.

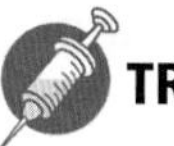

TREATMENT

GENERAL MEASURES

- Hand, foot, and mouth disease is usually self-limited and uncomplicated, resolving within 7 to 10 days.
- No specific therapy is indicated or usually necessary. Most cases are mild and only require parental reassurance.
- Symptomatic relief from particularly painful oral ulcers may be accomplished by application of a topical antihistamine or anesthetic directly to the sores.
- Dehydration should be treated when present. IV fluids may be required in the more severe cases, especially in infants and young children.
- Good supportive care is generally sufficient to treat most complications.

MEDICATION

Acetaminophen may relieve malaise and minor discomfort associated with the oral ulcers. It also may be used as an antipyretic in those children with fever.

ADMISSION, INPATIENT, AND NURSING CONSIDERATIONS

- Admission criteria include dehydration and inability to maintain adequate oral hydration.
- Discharge criteria include rehydration and good oral intake.

ONGOING CARE

FOLLOW-UP RECOMMENDATIONS

Small children must be followed closely for signs of dehydration.

DIET

Dietary adjustments often improve oral intake from painful oral lesions and prevent or relieve dehydration:

- Avoid spicy or acidic foods.
- Provide cool or iced liquids in small quantities frequently.

PROGNOSIS

- In nearly all instances, hand, foot, and mouth disease will resolve quickly, usually within 1 week after diagnosis, requiring only supportive care.
- Careful history and examination should distinguish those patients with rare complications.
- Rare cases may recur at intervals for up to 1 year.

COMPLICATIONS

- Dehydration is the most frequent complication:
  - Oral ulcerations are painful and interfere with feeding.
  - Infants and children are at highest risk.
- Rare complications include the following:
  - Neurologic complications such as aseptic meningitis, encephalitis, and acute flaccid paralysis
  - Pneumonia
  - Myocarditis
  - A possible association with 1st-trimester spontaneous abortions in previously infected women

ADDITIONAL READING

- American Academy of Pediatrics. Enterovirus (nonpoliovirus). In: Kimberlin DW, Brady MT, Jackson MA, et al, eds. *Red Book: 2015 Report of the Committee on Infectious Diseases*. Itasca, IL: American Academy of Pediatrics; 2015:333–336.
- Robinson CR, Doane FW, Rhodes AJ. Report of an outbreak of febrile illness with pharyngeal lesions and exanthem: Toronto, summer 1957; isolation of group A coxsackie virus. *Can Med Assoc J*. 1958;79(8):615–621.
- Ruan F, Yang T, Ma H, et al. Risk factors for hand, foot, and mouth disease and herpangina and the preventive effect of hand-washing. *Pediatrics*. 2011;127(4):e898–e904.
- Scott LA, Stone MS. Viral exanthems. *Dermatol Online J*. 2003;9(3):4.
- Slavin KA, Frieden IJ. Picture of the month. Hand-foot-and-mouth disease. *Arch Pediatr Adolesc Med*. 1998;152(5):505–506.

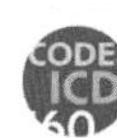

CODES

ICD10

- B08.4 Enteroviral vesicular stomatitis with exanthem
- B34.1 Enterovirus infection, unspecified

FAQ

- Q: What is in the "magic mouthwash" often used to relieve the pain of stomatitis?
- A: Many health care providers will prescribe a magic mouthwash for symptomatic relief of oral ulcers, pharyngitis, and teething pain. The most common such treatment consists of an aluminum hydroxide/magnesium hydroxide gel suspension and diphenhydramine elixir (12.5 mg/5 mL) in a 1:1 formulation. It can be applied directly to the sores with a cotton swab or a small syringe before meals. Note: Some people will have a reaction to topical diphenhydramine.
- Q: Should lidocaine be used topically or in suspension with magic mouthwash for symptomatic relief of oral ulcers?
- A: The routine use of lidocaine in this situation is not recommended. Lidocaine is an effective topical anesthetic and comes in a 2% viscous suspension. In practice, the pain relief is short lived, which encourages frequent administration. Lidocaine is absorbed from the mucous membranes (bypassing 1st-pass liver metabolism) and has been frequently reported to cause poisoning of the cardiovascular and central nervous systems. Both pediatric and adult fatalities have occurred. Topical viscous lidocaine should be reserved for use by physicians knowledgeable about its proper dosage and potential side effects and by educated, compliant parents or caregivers.
- Q: When may children with hand, foot, and mouth disease return to school?
- A: Good hygiene will greatly reduce viral transmission. Isolation from school or day care contacts should occur while fever remains and/or while the enanthem persists. As mentioned, some patients may shed the virus in their stool for weeks after symptoms have resolved (again stressing the need for good personal hygiene).

HEAD BANGING

Ana Catarina Garnecho, MD • Yvette E. Yatchmink, MD, PhD

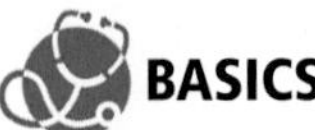

BASICS

DESCRIPTION

- Head banging (HB) is defined as the hitting of head on solid object such as a wall, side of crib, mattress, or floor.
- Tend to hit the front or side of the head
- Usually last for 15 minutes but can go on for >1 hour
- Regular rhythm of 60 to 80 bpm
- Can be seen along with body rocking or head rolling

EPIDEMIOLOGY

- Age
  - Average age of onset is 9 months; usually extinguished by 3 years of age
  - Older patients with HB are more likely to have a developmental delay or other medical problems.
- More common in boys than girls (3:1)
- Occurs in 3–15% of typically developing children
- Estimated that 2–3% of kids with intellectual disability have stereotypic movement disorder (SMD) (HB) and 5% of kids with Tourette syndrome have SMD (HB)

ETIOLOGY

- Can be comforting and be a part of other self-soothing activities such as body rocking or head rolling
- Can be seen during a temper tantrum secondary to frustration or anger
- Can be seen with typically developing children as an expression of happiness or as a method of self-stimulation (sometimes secondary to sensory deprivation)
- Need to rule out medical causes specifically if HB occurs suddenly and is associated with other symptoms
- Can be part of a sleep rhythmic disorder called *Jactatio capitis nocturna* (partial arousal during light, non-REM sleep); HB occurs when drowsy or falling asleep.
- Can be described as SMD, which is a repeated, rhythmic, purposeless movement or activity; these usually cause self-injury or severely interfere with normal activities. These are most prevalent in adolescence and tend to occur in clusters of symptoms. Diagnosis requires 4 weeks of duration.

COMMONLY ASSOCIATED CONDITIONS

- Medical causes:
  - Teething (pain)
  - Ear infection
  - Seizures
  - Meningitis
  - Headaches
  - Drug use (cocaine, amphetamines)
- SMD associated with:
  - Cerebral palsy
  - Intellectual disability
  - Schizophrenia
  - Autism spectrum disorders
  - Down syndrome
  - Lesch-Nyhan syndrome
  - Blindness
  - Deafness
- Tic disorder or Tourette syndrome
- Rule out child abuse if significant scalp laceration, skull fracture, or intracerebral or subdural hemorrhage.

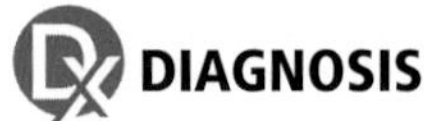

DIAGNOSIS

- Dependent on multiple factors
- Determine factors associated with behavior, including age of child, degree of parental concern, location of behavior, associated behaviors, motivations of the child, benefits to the child, etc.
- Determine if a medical cause exists, particularly if sudden onset.
- Determine if psychological factors are involved.

DIAGNOSTIC TESTS & INTERPRETATION

- Usually, no laboratory testing is needed for diagnosis.
- Physical examination to look for bruising, swelling, scratches, or minor lacerations
- If swelling or blood loss is involved, brain imaging may be necessary to rule out damage.
- If severe and persistent HB is reported, an ophthalmology exam is warranted to rule out complications.
- Developmental screening to rule out possible developmental delay
- If developmental delay is suspected, formal psychoeducational testing can be recommended.

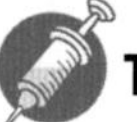

TREATMENT

- Typically developing children will outgrow the habit by age 3 years.
- Older children may need psychological/developmental follow-up to determine delay/cognition status and to determine if behavioral modification therapy could be beneficial in decreasing symptomatology.
- If severe, HB can lead to ophthalmologic complications, including cataracts, glaucoma, or retinal detachment. Referral to ophthalmologist is recommended.
- For patients with particularly violent movements of *Jactatio capitis nocturna*, trials with clonazepam and citalopram have shown some success.
- For patients with SMD, medications may help, including antipsychotics, tricyclic antidepressants, selective serotonin reuptake inhibitors (SSRIs), and benzodiazepines. These should be closely monitored.

ONGOING CARE

PROGNOSIS

- Normally disappears by age 3 to 4 years
- *Jactatio capitis nocturna* is usually benign and resolves by age 5 years.
- SMD usually peaks in adolescence and then declines.

ADDITIONAL READING

- Harris KM, Mahone EM, Singer HS. Nonautistic motor stereotypies: clinical features and longitudinal follow-up. *Pediatr Neurol*. 2008;38(4):267–272.
- Leekam S, Tandos J, McConachie H, et al. Repetitive behaviours in typically developing 2-year-olds. *J Child Psychol Psychiatry*. 2007;48(11):1131–1138.
- Miller JM, Singer HS, Bridges DD, et al. Behavioral therapy for treatment of stereotypic movements in nonautistic children. *J Child Neurol*. 2006;21(2):119–125.
- Sallustro F, Atwell CW. Body rocking, head banging, and head rolling in normal children. *J Pediatr*. 1978;93(4):704–708.
- Vinson R, Gelinas-Sorell D. Head banging in young children. *Am Fam Physician*. 1991;43(5):1625–1628.

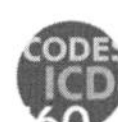

CODES

ICD10

- F98.4 Stereotyped movement disorders
- G47.69 Other sleep related movement disorders

FAQ

- Q: Can HB lead to serious head injury or neurologic damage?
- A: Typically developing children rarely bang their heads hard enough to cause bleeding or fracture. Children with significant cognitive delays or other developmental disorders may bang their heads more severely and can cause neurologic sequelae.
- Q: What can a parent do to prevent injury or diminish HB behavior?
- A: Remove sharp or breakable objects from child's environment to avoid accidental injury.
  - Place a rubber pad on the floor or a thick rug.
  - Secure the crib to the wall to decrease noise and vestibular input to the child.
  - Pad crib with bumpers.
  - If behavior occurs during temper tantrums, ignore the behavior once safety is established. Reward the child for appropriate behaviors.

H

HEADACHE AND MIGRAINE

Christopher B. Oakley, MD

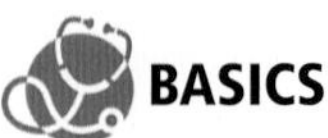

BASICS

DESCRIPTION

- Primary headache: headache without an identifiable underlying etiology; includes but not limited to migraine, tension headache, cluster headache, and other trigeminal autonomic cephalgias; may be episodic or chronic in nature
- Secondary headache: headache attributed to an identifiable underlying etiology
- Other: unusual headaches, especially in children, that include various cranial neuralgias and central and primary facial pain

EPIDEMIOLOGY

- Headache prevalence can approach 30–50% by school age, 60–80% by early adolescence, and as high as 85–90% by adulthood.
- Tension-type headache is most common type of headache, with migraine second.
- Mean age of onset for migraine is 7 years for boys and 11 years for girls. Migraine precursors such as abdominal migraine, cyclic vomiting syndrome, and benign paroxysmal vertigo of childhood can be seen even younger. These may transform into migraines by puberty.
- Overall migraine reported prevalence ranges between 8% and 23%. Suspicion is that migraine prevalence may be as high as 30–35% due to underreporting. Prevalence of chronic daily headache in younger children is 2–4% and 4–5% in adolescence/adulthood.
- Until puberty, migraines more common in males (55–60%), postpuberty in females (75%)

RISK FACTORS

Ethnicity plays a role, with majority of reported chronic migraine sufferers being Caucasian.

Genetics

Genetics plays a role with some reports of 90% family history noted. Genes have been identified for some migraine subtypes including familial hemiplegic migraine and migraine with brainstem aura.

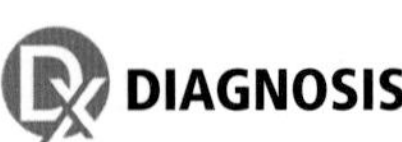

DIAGNOSIS

- Migraine in children is classified into the following groups:
  - Migraine without aura:
    - "Common" migraine
    - Represents most cases
  - Migraine with aura:
    - "Classic" migraine must include aura, a reversible focal neurologic symptom that gradually develops over 5 to 20 minutes and typically resolves within 1 hour.
  - Migraine with brainstem aura
    - Up to 20% of childhood migraines
    - Often with occipital pain and must include two of the following: dysarthria, vertigo, tinnitus, hyperacusis, diplopia, ataxia, and decreased consciousness as well as one common aura symptom (visual, sensory, speech/language)
  - Childhood periodic syndromes that are precursors to migraine:
    - Benign paroxysmal vertigo of childhood
    - Cyclic vomiting
    - Abdominal migraine
    - Benign paroxysmal torticollis
    - Infantile colic and alternating hemiplegia of childhood are being investigated as a possible migraine precursor.
  - Hemiplegic migraine:
    - Migraine with aura, with symptoms that must include motor weakness along with one of the following: sensory symptoms, visual symptoms, dysphasic speech
  - Others:
    - "Alice in Wonderland syndrome" has distortions of vision, space, and/or time.
    - Confusional migraine has impaired sensorium, agitation, and lethargy.
- General migraine diagnostic criteria set by the *International Classification of Headache Disorders*, 3rd edition, beta (*ICHD III*, beta) in children/adolescents
  - Five attacks not attributed to another condition
    - Lasting 2 to 72 hours
    - Two of the following:
      - Unilateral or bilateral pain
      - Moderate to severe pain
      - Pulsating quality
      - Aggravated by routine activity
    - One of the following:
      - Photophobia and phonophobia (may be inferred)
      - Nausea or vomiting
  - Aura has separate criteria.
- Tension-type headache differs from migraine as follows:
  - More episodes typically seen
  - Lasts 30 minutes to 7 days
  - Typically described as bilateral pain, pressing/tightening quality, mild to moderate intensity
  - Not worse with activity
  - Not associated with sensitivity to light or sound
  - Not associated with nausea or vomiting

HISTORY

The history should help clarify the type of headache and help guide workup and treatment.

- The following questions should be asked:
  - Is there >1 type of headache?
  - Have headaches gotten worse?
  - How often do they occur?
  - Where is the pain located?
  - What is the quality of the pain?
  - Do the headaches occur at any special time of day?
  - What associated symptoms are present?
  - Is there a warning sign or aura noted?
  - What triggers a headache?
  - What helps the headache feel better?
  - Any symptoms present between episodes?
  - What treatments have been tried? (Ask about dose, duration, and outcome.)
  - Any migraine precursors noted or other common comorbidities such as motion sickness or psychiatric concerns?
- "Red flags":
  - Age of onset <3 years of age (Some would say 6 years of age as no set age in the practice parameters or guidelines.)
  - First or worst headache
  - Occipital location
  - Recent headache onset
  - Increasing severity or frequency
  - Headache in the morning associated with vomiting
  - Headache causing awakening from sleep
  - Headache worse with straining
  - Change in mood, mental status, or school performance
  - Presence of underlying neurocutaneous syndrome or other neurologic concern
- Lifestyle considerations that affect headaches
  - Amount and quality of sleep
  - Hydration status
  - Consistent diet/meals
  - Caffeine consumption
  - Level of fitness and amount of cardiovascular exercise
  - Presence of stress or anxiety

PHYSICAL EXAM

- Vital signs
  - Blood pressure, heart rate, and weight
  - Consider orthostatic blood pressure and pulse for dizziness or syncope.
  - If patient is obese, consider pseudotumor or sleep apnea syndrome.
- Skin changes consistent with neurocutaneous syndrome
- Sinus tenderness, limitation of jaw excursion, or occipital trigger points
- Complete neurologic exam
  - Include vision screen and funduscopic exam: should be normal in primary headaches
  - Exception is during aura; exam may show temporary deficit.
- Basic depression and psychiatric screen
- Any abnormality on exam warrants further investigation, as it may suggest secondary headache with possible underlying etiology.

DIFFERENTIAL DIAGNOSIS

The pattern of headache can help clarify the differential. There are five patterns.

- Acute, first severe headache
  - CNS infection, cocaine or other substance abuse, medication (methylphenidate, steroids, psychotropic drugs, analgesics, cardiovascular agents), hypertension (usually secondary), hydrocephalus, pseudotumor cerebri (idiopathic intracranial hypertension), post-lumbar puncture (LP), CNS hemorrhage, ventriculoperitoneal shunt malfunction, sinus thrombosis, migraine, other infection including upper respiratory, somatization
- Acute recurrent headache
  - Much of what is listed above in acute, first severe headache can be recurrent as well. Additional consideration would include migraine and variants, cluster, and tension.
- Chronic progressive headache
  - Brain tumor; chronic CNS infection including abscess, hydrocephalus, vascular malformation, hematoma, sinus thrombosis, idiopathic intracranial hypertension, depression or other psychiatric condition, anemia, rheumatologic diseases
- Chronic nonprogressive or daily headache
  - Much of what is listed above in chronic progressive headache can be nonprogressive as well. Additional consideration would include medication overuse, substance abuse including caffeine, chronic infection such as sinusitis, occipital neuralgia, temporomandibular joint syndrome, orthostatic headache, post-LP, other systemic disease, posttraumatic, sleep disorder, tension headache, fibromyalgia.

- Mixed headache
  - Migraine-superimposed tension headache with broad differential including much of what is listed above

DIAGNOSTIC TESTS & INTERPRETATION

Practice parameters were established in 2002 for the evaluation of children and adolescents with recurrent headaches. The guidelines address laboratory evaluation, ancillary testing, and imaging.

Initial Tests (screening, lab, imaging)

- Neuroimaging studies (CT or MRI): generally not recommended if neurologic exam is normal and no red flags. If exam is abnormal or red flags are present, imaging should be obtained with determining which study to obtain based on clinical concern and situation.
  - CT if there is any suspicion for any acute process such as hemorrhage, but otherwise, MRI is preferred
  - Consider risk of imaging (e.g., younger children require anesthesia for MRI; radiation exposure with CT).
  - Consider magnetic resonance angiography (MRA)/magnetic resonance venography (MRV) if vascular cause/etiology in differential diagnosis.
- Neuroimaging guidelines are based on multiple studies with >600 images reviewed. Only 3% of those images obtained led to specific treatments geared toward imaging findings, and in all those who had abnormal imaging that required treatment, their neurologic exams were found to be abnormal.

Diagnostic Procedures/Other

- EEG: no role for EEG in routine testing of patients with headache
- Laboratory investigation: generally not recommended in primary headaches
- LP: not recommended unless concern for secondary headache or underlying etiology such as infection, hemorrhage, sinus thrombosis, pseudotumor cerebri, and low-pressure headache. Imaging should be done first to ensure it is safe to perform LP.

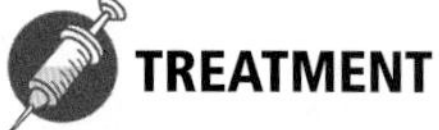

TREATMENT

MEDICATION

Practice parameters were established in 2004 for the pharmacologic treatment of migraine in children and adolescents. The guidelines addressed acute and prophylactic medical management.

- Acute treatment: generally most effective if given early in the acute headache/migraine
  - First line is ibuprofen (10 mg/kg PO).
  - Acetaminophen (10 to 15 mg/kg PO)
  - Naproxen sodium 5.5 to 7.7 mg/kg PO per dose: longer acting NSAID than ibuprofen
  - Sumatriptan nasal spray can be first line in adolescent migraine.
  - Many options noted to have not enough data.
- Additional acute treatments often used especially in refractory patients
  - Antiemetics (prochlorperazine, metoclopramide, ondansetron) also enhance effectiveness of analgesics and may abort migraines. Prochlorperazine has best evidence of this class, with up to 95% improvement noted in some studies.
  - Triptans: generally safe but only four of the seven available triptans are U.S. Food and Drug Administration (FDA)-approved for children or adolescents—almotriptan (≥12 years), rizatriptan (≥6 years), sumatriptan (nasal spray or in combination with naproxen ≥12 years), zolmitriptan (nasal spray ≥12 years). The seven triptans are available in various forms, including tablet, nasal spray, dissolvable, and injection.
  - Any agent that may lead to vasoconstriction such as triptans and ergotamines are not recommended in brainstem aura, hemiplegic, or any migraine with vascular risk factors.
  - Most over-the-counter or prescription pain/headache/migraine medications may cause rebound headaches.
  - Aspirin-containing products should be avoided or used with caution in children and adolescents due to liver concerns and Reye syndrome.
  - Narcotics and barbiturates should not be used to treat headaches of any kind.
- Status migrainosus
  - Migraine lasting >72 hours but <90 days
  - General treatment involved a combination of medications/treatments.
  - Not well studied, but some evidence that the following combinations are successful:
    - Fluids, triptan if used successfully prior, NSAID (ibuprofen/naproxen/ketorolac), antidopaminergic (prochlorperazine [Compazine®] with best evidence), and Benadryl® if needed (helps with possible side effects of the antidopaminergic agents and facilitates sleep)
    - Valproic acid can be used as second tier.
    - No definitive evidence for steroids or magnesium despite often being used
  - Dihydroergotamine (D.H.E. 45) noted to be highly effective in small studies; can be IV, IM, or intranasal; given with combination of treatments including antiemetic
  - Narcotics are not recommended.
- Prophylaxis
  - When to start is controversial, but generally if there is >1 day per week with disability or dysfunction, daily medication is recommended.
  - Goal is reduction in headache frequency or severity by ≥50%. There is no cure for headaches/migraines. Keeping realistic expectations is key to treatment.
  - Start at a low dose and titrate as needed while being mindful of adverse effects.
  - Can take 2 to 6 months for effects to be seen
  - Choose a drug that may address comorbidities or have positive side effects. Be careful to avoid drug classes that may exacerbate other medical conditions (e.g., β-blockers in asthma patients).
  - Practice parameters from 2004 very limited: flunarizine (not available in United States) only prophylactic medication with any recommendation
  - Amitriptyline and topiramate (anticonvulsant) most commonly used and studied options in children. Topiramate is the only FDA-approved headache/migraine prophylactic available—it is approved for ≥12 years.
  - Cyproheptadine (antihistamine) frequently used first line in younger children as well as for migraine precursors and GI symptoms
  - Other options would include the following but are off-label:
    - Calcium channel blockers: verapamil
    - β-Blockers: propranolol, nadolol
    - Tricyclic agents: nortriptyline, imipramine
    - Selective serotonin and norepinephrine reuptake inhibitors (SNRI): venlafaxine, duloxetine
    - Anticonvulsants: valproic acid, gabapentin, carbamazepine (neuralgias), and oxcarbazepine (neuralgias)

COMPLEMENTARY & ALTERNATIVE THERAPIES

- Physical therapy, exercise (aerobic, yoga, Pilates), massage therapy, relaxation techniques (meditation, progressive muscle relaxation, self-hypnosis), stress management, cognitive behavioral therapy, biofeedback, and acupuncture may be beneficial in treating acute headaches and migraines as well as reducing the overall frequency.
- Some evidence for vitamins, supplements, and herbs for migraine prophylaxis include butterbur (50 to 75 mg b.i.d.), coenzyme Q10 (150 to 300 mg daily), feverfew (50 to 150 mg daily), magnesium oxide (200 to 250 mg b.i.d.), melatonin (3 mg nightly), riboflavin (200 to 400 mg daily). Of note, supplements and vitamins are not regulated by the FDA. Butterbur has been removed from some foreign markets or not approved in some foreign markets due to safety and purification concerns. Melatonin as low as 3 mg nightly is reported to be as effective as low-dose amitriptyline.

ADDITIONAL READING

- Abu-Arafeh I, Razak S, Sivaraman B, et al. Prevalence of headache and migraine in children and adolescents: a systematic review of population-based studies. *Dev Med Child Neurol.* 2010;52(12):1088–1097.
- Lewis D. Pediatric migraine. *Pediatr Rev.* 2007;28(2):43–53.
- Lewis DW, Ashwal S, Dahl G, et al. Practice parameter: evaluation of children and adolescents with recurrent headaches: report of the Quality Standards Subcommittee of the American Academy of Neurology and the Practice Committee of the Child Neurology Society. *Neurology.* 2002;59(4):490–498.
- Lewis DW, Ashwal S, Hershey A, et al. Practice parameter: pharmacological treatment of migraine headache in children and adolescents: report of the American Academy of Neurology Quality Standards Subcommittee and the Practice Committee of the Child Neurology Society. *Neurology.* 2004;63(12):2215–2224.
- Powers SW, Coffey CS, Chamberlin LA, et al; for CHAMP Investigators. Trial of amitriptyline, topiramate, and placebo for pediatric migraine. *N Engl J Med.* 2017;376(2):115–124.
- Termine C, Ozge A, Antonaci F, et al. Overview of diagnosis and management of paediatric headache. Part II: therapeutic management. *J Headache Pain.* 2011;12(1):25–34.

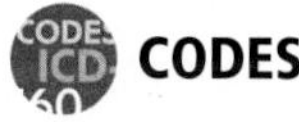

CODES

ICD10

- R51 Headache
- G43.909 Migraine, unsp, not intractable, without status migrainosus
- G44.209 Tension-type headache, unspecified, not intractable

HEAT STROKE AND RELATED ILLNESS

Emily A. Hartford, MD, MPH • George A. (Tony) Woodward, MD, MBA

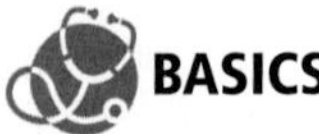

BASICS

DESCRIPTION

- Heat stroke occurs during imbalance in heat production, absorption, and dissipation. It can result from excessive body heat generation and storage without appropriate dissipation, high ambient temperature, low radiation or convective heat loss, decreased evaporation, or inadequate fluid/electrolyte replacement in response to losses through sweat or GI disturbance.
- Two forms of heat stroke exist:
  - Exertional heat stroke (EHS), which occurs during periods of intense exertion with exposure to high temperatures in otherwise healthy individuals
  - Nonexertional or classic heat stroke (NEHS), in which the body is unable to compensate for an increase in ambient temperature; more common in very young and elderly, chronic illness, and during heat waves

EPIDEMIOLOGY

- In the United States, 658 deaths per year from heat illness; recognized as a leading cause of death in athletes, especially football early in the season
- Recent heat waves associated with increase in heat related illness, EHS, NEHS, and deaths

RISK FACTORS

- Environmental: high ambient temperature, humidity, lack of wind or shade, heat waves, overheated indoor environment, lack of air conditioning, social isolation, inability to care for self, or entrapment in closed space (i.e., car, trunk; internal automobile temperature in sunlight with poor ventilation can reach 131–172°F; the sharpest temperature increase occurs within first 15 minutes)
- Medical: obesity, low fitness level, cardiac disease, previous episode of heat illness, lack of sleep, concurrent febrile illness, diabetes mellitus or insipidus, diarrhea, hyperthyroidism, dehydration, vascular disease, sweat gland dysfunction, sunburn, viral illness, sickle cell, history of malignant hyperthermia
- Drugs/medications:
  - Anticholinergics
  - Antihistamines
  - Stimulants
  - β-Blockers
  - Calcium channel blockers
  - Diuretics
  - Psychiatric medications
  - Recreational drugs and alcohol
- Behaviors:
  - Lack of recognition of risk factors or warning signs
  - Overexertion with inadequate or majority hypotonic fluid intake
  - Inappropriate clothing; heavy, dark, tight-fitting, overbundling
  - Lack of acclimatization and conditioning (early in athletic season)
  - Children left in vehicles

GENERAL PREVENTION

- Avoid enclosed spaces; never leave a child in a car.
- In high ambient temperatures: Reduce activity levels, keep cool, frequent breaks, use shaded areas.
- Allow adaptation to warmer climates which may take 8 to 10 exposures of 30 to 45 minutes each daily or every other day; promote gradual conditioning over 10 to 14 days.
- Air conditioning or fans during hot weather
- Cool or tepid baths
- Increase fluid intake before, during, and after scheduled exercise or strenuous activity (up to 200 to 300 mL q10–20min); do not wait until thirsty.
- Precooling using external (cold water immersion, cooling vests) or internal (drinking cold liquid/ice) may improve performance before endurance events in heat.
- Loose, light-colored clothing, protective hat
- Liberal dietary sodium:
  - Avoid NaCl tablets (possible hypernatremia, potassium depletion, gastric irritation, delayed gastric emptying).
- Frequently flex leg muscles when standing.
- Avoid prolonged standing in hot environments.
- Avoid caffeine and alcohol.

PATHOPHYSIOLOGY

- Heat production increases by 10 to 20 times with strenuous exercise.
- When environmental temperature is greater than body temperature, body gains heat by conduction and radiation and can only lose heat by evaporation and convection (limited by humidity and lack of air movement).
- Children have greater body surface-to-mass ratio, higher metabolic rate, inability to increase cardiac output, decreased sweat production, and inability to independently change environments compared to adults.
- Severe disease is a result of thermal injury to tissues which causes a systemic inflammatory response.
  - Dehydration results in loss of sweating, hence decreased evaporation.
  - >40°C, cell volume, membrane integrity, metabolism, acid–base balance is affected.
  - Extreme core temperatures >42°C can uncouple oxidative phosphorylation and allow enzyme systems to cease functioning.

COMMONLY ASSOCIATED CONDITIONS

Heat illness is on a continuum of severity, including the following:

- Miliaria rubra (prickly heat): Heat rash, usually caused by obstruction of sweat glands by clothes or lotions, produces an erythematous papular rash; usually self-limited
- Heat cramps/spasms: exercise-induced muscle spasms during or immediately after exercise; related to poor conditioning and water and sodium depletion
- Heat tetany: progression of heat cramps into paresthesias and carpopedal spasm
- Heat syncope: alteration of consciousness (i.e., dizziness, syncope) at end of strenuous or upright event
- Heat edema: swollen feet and ankles due to peripheral vasodilation, vascular leak, and orthostatic pooling
- Heat exhaustion: relatively insidious onset. Associated with water and/or salt depletion. Copious perspiration with headache, nausea, vomiting, malaise, myalgias, pallor, light-headedness, visual disturbances, syncope, temperature 38–40°C, dehydration, electrolyte imbalance, hemoconcentration; can persist or evolve into heat stroke
- Heat stroke: core body temperature exceeding 40°C with altered mental status ranging from confusion, disorientation, and incoherent speech to delirium, decerebrate posturing, seizure, and coma. May have acute, sudden onset (80%) or slower onset (minutes to hours, 20%). Classic (NEHS) heat stroke is associated with dry skin and prolonged exposure to elevated temperatures at rest. EHS may present with anhidrosis or profuse sweating.

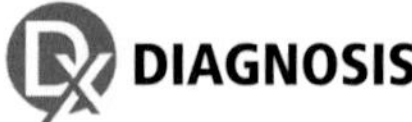

DIAGNOSIS

HISTORY

- Heat exhaustion:
  - Weakness, lethargy, thirst, malaise, diminished ability to work or play, headache, nausea, vomiting, myalgias, pale skin, dizziness
- Heat stroke:
  - History of CNS dysfunction and elevated temperature (>40) in environment consistent with, or predisposing conditions conducive to, development of heat-related illness should suggest heat stroke. In EHS, athlete may suddenly collapse.

PHYSICAL EXAM

- Heat exhaustion:
  - Visual disturbances, syncope, mild CNS dysfunction, impaired judgment, cramps, vertigo, hypotension, tachycardia, hyperventilation, paresthesias, agitation, ataxia, psychosis, temperature 38–40°C, sweating, environmental exposure, and activity; no coma or seizures
- Heat stroke:
  - Temperature >40°C (may be cooler after prehospital interventions)
  - Altered level of consciousness (confusion, drowsiness, irritability, neurologic deficits, euphoria, combativeness, obtundation), ataxia, posturing, incontinence, seizures, coma, purpura, or petechiae; 2/3 with constricted pupils; may have muscle rigidity with tonic contractions and dystonia that mimic seizures

– Shock: tachycardia, hypotension, widened pulse pressure, tachypnea
– Hot, dry (classic), or clammy (exercise-induced) skin, pink or ashen color
– Weakness, nausea, vomiting, anorexia, headache, dizziness
- Temperature measurement (continuous best):
  – Core temperature monitoring by esophageal or rectal thermometry is a good approximation.
  – Tympanic, oral, axillary, temporal artery temperatures are less accurate measures of core temperature.

DIFFERENTIAL DIAGNOSIS

- Heat cramps: rhabdomyolysis, tetany
- Heat edema: thrombophlebitis, lymphedema, congestive heart failure
- Heat stroke: CNS process with fever (cerebrovascular stroke, meningitis, encephalitis), other infections, anticholinergic poisoning (dilated pupils), drug/medication induced, temperature rise, severe dehydration. Chills suggest febrile illness, not heat stroke.
- Neuroleptic malignant syndrome
- Serotonin syndrome
- Malignant hyperthermia

DIAGNOSTIC TESTS & INTERPRETATION

Initial Tests (screening, lab, imaging)

Lab tests may support the diagnosis of EHS or NEHS, evaluate the extent of injury, or rule out other processes, but diagnosis is largely clinical:

- Heat cramps: decreased levels of serum and urine sodium and chloride; BUN level normal or slightly increased
- Heat exhaustion: may see hyponatremia or hypernatremia (free water loss), hypochloremia, low urine sodium, and chloride hemoconcentration; normal LFTs
- Heat stroke:
  – Electrolytes abnormalities: sodium, chloride level normal or high, hypokalemia, elevated BUN/creatinine; hypoglycemia
  – Hematologic: hemoconcentration, leukocytosis, thrombocytopenia
  – Prerenal azotemia
  – Elevated AST/ALT
  – Metabolic acidosis: lactate high, especially with EHS
  – Coagulopathy
- Others: creatine phosphokinase (rhabdomyolysis), arterial blood gases (classic heat stroke: respiratory alkalosis and hypokalemia early; lactic acidosis later; EHS; lactic acidosis), urinalysis (casts, brownish color proteinuria, microscopic hematuria, myoglobinuria), CSF, EKG, chest radiograph

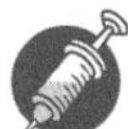

TREATMENT

GENERAL MEASURES

- Heat stroke: Cooling is the mainstay of treatment; the remainder is supportive. Prehospital providers should remove clothing, start cooling during transport as able. Maintain airway, breathing, and circulation including securing airway as indicated, provide supplemental oxygen.
  – Active cooling: cold water immersion (15–16°C) bath preferred, cool water by sponge or spray with a fan, ice packs to groin and axillae, cold water forearm immersion, may do all of the above
  – Additional cooling: cold to room temperature IV fluids, cool water lavage, massage with ice
  – Stop active cooling when patient's temperature reaches 38–39°C to achieve optimal endpoint.
  – Fluid replacement: IV 0.9% normal saline (NS) or LR solution. Rule out hypoglycemia.
  – Ionotropic support as needed
  – Miscellaneous therapies:
    ○ Foley catheter to monitor urine output
    ○ Nasogastric tube
    ○ Myoglobinuria therapy (mannitol, bicarbonate, dialysis if necessary)
    ○ Electrolyte replacement if symptomatic from hypokalemia or hypocalcemia
    ○ Fresh frozen plasma for disseminated intravascular coagulation (DIC)
- Specific therapies by type of heat illness:
  – Heat cramps: rest, salt, and water replacement
  – Heat syncope: self-limited as return to horizontal position is treatment; rest, oral rehydration solution
  – Heat exhaustion: Clinical findings (heart rate, BP, orthostatic changes, urine output) should direct therapy. Most treated as outpatient with rapid rehydration, cooling; mild case with oral electrolyte solution. If nausea, vomiting, inability to drink: IV (0.45% [similar to sweat losses] to 0.9%) NS solution; avoid rapid overcorrection of hypernatremia (treat as with hypernatremic dehydration); if hyponatremic seizures, treat with 3% saline at 3 to 5 mL/kg.

MEDICATION

- Antipyretics not useful because an intact hypothalamus is required for action
- Avoid anticholinergic drugs, which inhibit sweating.
- May require inotropic support
- Chlorpromazine may improve peripheral vasodilatation and prevent shivering.
- Benzodiazepine for shivering during cooling, sedation and/or seizures
- Dantrolene not shown to be effective (unless there is overlap with malignant hypertension)

ADMISSION, INPATIENT, AND NURSING CONSIDERATIONS

- Patients with symptoms suggestive of heat stroke require immediate cooling and should then be closely observed.
- Patients with evidence of multisystem disease (altered mental status, electrolyte imbalances, renal injury, hematologic abnormalities) should be admitted until such issues are resolved.
- Patients with respiratory or hemodynamic instability may require intensive care.

ONGOING CARE

PROGNOSIS

- Heat-related illness (e.g., heat rash, edema, cramps, tetany, syncope, exhaustion): rapid recovery with supportive care
- Heat stroke: poor prognosis if not recognized and aggressively managed; morbidity and mortality directly proportional to how rapidly core temperature is reduced

ADDITIONAL READING

- Gaudio F, Grissom C. Cooling methods in heat stroke. *J Emerg Med*. 2016;50(4):607–616.
- Leon L, Bouchama A. Heat stroke. *Compr Physiol*. 2015;5(2):611–647.
- Pryor RR, Roth RN, Suyama J, et al. Exertional heat illness: emerging concepts and advances in prehospital care. *Prehosp Disaster Med*. 2015;30(3):297–305.
- Santelli J, Sullivan JM, Czarnik A, et al. Heat illness in the emergency department: keeping your cool. *Emerg Med Pract*. 2014;16(8):1–22.

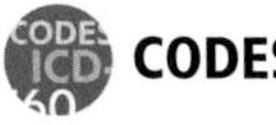

CODES

ICD10

- T67.0XXA Heatstroke and sunstroke, initial encounter
- T67.1XXA Heat syncope, initial encounter
- L74.0 Miliaria rubra

FAQ

- Q: How can one distinguish between heat exhaustion and heat stroke?
- A: Heat stroke involves temperature >40°C with CNS dysfunction, whereas heat exhaustion refers to fatigue and weakness with inability to continue exercise and an elevated temperature (38–40°C).
- Q: What is the best initial treatment for heat stroke?
- A: Rapid cooling by cold water immersion with continuous core body temperature monitoring
- Q: Does the presence or absence of sweating helps with the diagnosis of heat exhaustion versus heat stroke?
- A: No. Sweating will be present with heat exhaustion and may or may not be present with heat stroke.
- Q: Are children at increased risk of heat illness?
- A: Yes. They have a number of predisposing factors: Greater surface area-to-body mass ratio than adults, higher metabolic rate, slower rate of sweating than adults, temperature when sweating starts is higher, lower cardiac output at a given metabolic rate than adults, rate of acclimatization is slower, thirst response is blunted, and access to fluids may be limited.

HEMANGIOMAS AND OTHER VASCULAR LESIONS

Katherine B. Püttgen, MD

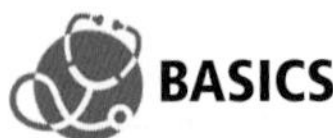

BASICS

DESCRIPTION

- Vascular tumors: proliferative neoplasms of the vasculature include:
  - Infantile hemangioma (IH)
  - Congenital hemangiomas: noninvoluting congenital hemangioma (NICH) and rapidly involuting congenital hemangioma (RICH)
  - Tufted angioma (TA)
  - Kaposiform hemangioendothelioma (KHE)
  - Pyogenic granuloma
- Vascular malformations (VaM): inborn errors of vascular morphogenesis; relatively static
  - Capillary malformations (CM) (e.g., salmon patch, port-wine stain, nevus flammeus)
  - Venous malformations (VM)
  - Arterial malformations: arteriovenous malformations (AVM) or arteriovenous fistula (AVF)
  - Lymphatic malformations (LM) (macrocystic and microcystic)
  - Combined malformations (e.g., capillary-venous-lymphatic)
- Other types of VaM may occur in any part of the body and may be associated with soft tissue or bony overgrowth of the involved part.

EPIDEMIOLOGY

- IHs
  - 4–5% of infants
  - Approximately 10% of Caucasian infants by age 12 months
- CM occurs in 0.3–0.5% of newborns.

RISK FACTORS

- Increased incidence in low-birth-weight and premature infants
- Other demographic risk factors include
  - White non-Hispanic race
  - Female sex
  - Multiple gestation pregnancy
  - Advanced maternal age
  - Chorionic villus sampling during pregnancy
  - Positive family history

COMMONLY ASSOCIATED CONDITIONS

- IHs
  - PHACE(S)
    - Segmental hemangioma (usually facial) associated with other developmental anomalies (posterior fossa malformations; hemangiomas; arterial anomalies; cardiac anomalies, including aortic coarctation; eye abnormalities; sternal defects/supraumbilical raphe)
    - Cerebral malformations occur in >50% and cerebrovascular anomalies in 33%.
  - LUMBAR
    - Lower body hemangiomas; urogenital anomalies; ulceration; myelopathy; bony deformities; anorectal malformations; arterial anomalies; renal anomalies
    - PHACE-like syndrome of the lower body with associated GI and GU anomalies
  - Segmental
    - Commonly located on the face and involving a developmental unit (segment) and frequently associated with complications, even without meeting full PHACE criteria
    - Segmental IH are much more likely to have complications and to receive treatment than focal IH.
- KHE
  - Kasabach-Merritt phenomenon (consumptive coagulopathy, severe thrombocytopenia)
- VaM
  - CM may be present as part of syndromes (e.g., Sturge-Weber, CM-AVM [RASA-1 mutations associated with fast-flow VaM], von Hippel-Lindau, Rubinstein-Taybi, Beckwith-Wiedemann, Cobb syndrome).
  - VM can be inherited autosomal dominantly due to *TIE2/TEK* gene mutations.
  - PIK3CA-related overgrowth spectrum (PROS): VaM due to postzygotic somatic mutation in PIK3CA gene pathway with associated overgrowth of multiple tissues
  - Generalized LM and lymphedema have been associated with multiple mutations including *VEGFR3*, *VEGFC*, *FOXC2*, *SOX18*.

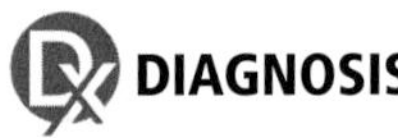

DIAGNOSIS

HISTORY

- Onset of lesions and timing of changes
- IHs are often inapparent at birth or present with nascent telangiectatic patches followed by a rapid proliferative growth phase.
  - Proliferative phase: During the first 2 months of life, nearly all IHs double in size.
  - Most rapid period of growth occurs between 5.5 and 7.5 weeks of age; majority of rapid growth phase is in the first 8 weeks of life.
  - Most IHs reach 80% of their maximum size by 3 to 5 months of age.
  - Involution starts in earnest by age 1 year, and >90% of natural regression occurs between 3.5 and 4 years of age.
- Segmental and deep IH grow longer.
- Congenital hemangiomas (RICH and NICH) are present fully formed at birth.
- VaM are present (although may not be noticed) at birth. Most slowly enlarge over time.
- Past medical history for IH
  - Low birth weight, twin or other multiple gestation, prematurity
- Family history
  - Present in up to 15% of IH
  - CM-AVM and hereditary hemorrhagic telangiectasia (HHT) are autosomal dominantly inherited.
  - Most VaM are due to postzygotic somatic mutations with no family history.

PHYSICAL EXAM

- IHs
  - Neonate: flat pale patch, superficial telangiectasia with halo border
  - Superficial IH: raised red, partially compressible, nontender plaque or nodule with well-demarcated borders. Overlying skin is usually intact, although sometimes ulceration may be present.
  - Deep IH: raised soft mass with bluish-purplish discoloration with smooth, intact, overlying skin
  - Mixed IH: Lesions will have both superficial and deep components.
  - Morphology may be localized (most common), segmental (occupies a "geographic" plaque-like area), indeterminate (looks "sub"-segmental), or multifocal (>5 IH).
  - Ulceration occurs in up to 25% in a referral setting; risk of ulceration peaks by age 4 months.
  - Involuting lesion: flat, atrophic pale or gray center with surrounding raised reddish border with stippled texture
  - The presence of large numbers of small- to moderate-sized IH may indicate a rare condition called multifocal IH—with or without extracutaneous disease (replaces the old term "diffuse neonatal hemangiomatosis"). Internal organ involvement (liver, lungs, GI tract, CNS) may be present.
- VaM
  - Salmon patches (nevus simplex)
    - CM most notable at birth as pinkish-red macules that often blanch and are most commonly found at the nape of the neck, glabella, and upper eyelids
    - Frequently, all three locations are involved in an individual newborn.
    - Nevus simplex on the face disappear, usually by age 3 years, but persist lifelong on posterior scalp.
  - Port-wine stains (nevus flammeus)
    - CM easily seen at birth and are deep pink to red-purplish, nonblanching macules with well-demarcated borders
    - Most commonly located on the face and often cover a large area
    - Mature port-wine stains are deeper in color and frequently develop raised nodules and vascular blebs in adulthood.
    - If an extremity is heavily involved, there may be underlying bony and soft tissue overgrowth with limb hypertrophy.
  - AVM
    - Raised pulsating lesions with bruits audible by stethoscope if large in size
    - Smaller lesions may vary in appearance from macular erythema to thin vascular plaques.
    - Signs of cardiac compromise (i.e., tachycardia, gallop rhythm, shortness of breath, hepatomegaly) may be associated with very large AVMs.
  - VM
    - Most common VaM, most commonly present on the head and neck
    - Deep blue to purplish, soft, fleshy compressible nodules in the skin; may be surrounded by superficial venules
    - The drainage pattern is generally obvious upon inspection.
    - Mature lesions may include small calcifications (phleboliths).
  - LM
    - Present differently depending on size
    - Large lesions are rubbery, skin-colored, massive nodules with ill-defined borders, most often located in the head, neck, axilla, or chest (cystic hygromas in older, less preferred nomenclature).
    - Cervicofacial LM may be associated with airway compromise.
    - Microcystic LM present as nodules or plaques, sometimes in clusters, with overlying skin changes such as discoloration. Complicated lesions may be hemorrhagic or leak translucent lymph fluid.

DIAGNOSTIC TESTS & INTERPRETATION

Diagnosis is usually made by recognition of the typical physical exam findings.

Initial Tests (screening, lab, imaging)

- Most IH do not require imaging, but infants with segmental IH at risk for PHACE require MRI/MRA of brain/head/neck/aortic arch and echocardiogram; workup for LUMBAR requires MRI/MRA of pelvis and lumbosacral spine.
- Occasionally helpful in distinguishing vascular tumors like IH from VaM but primarily useful in determining subtype and extent of VaM for treatment planning
- For multifocal IH, abdominal ultrasound to rule out hepatic involvement should be ordered.
- Preoperative MRI/MRA, CT angiography, or venography aids in treatment planning of VaM.

Diagnostic Procedures/Other

- Biopsy: rarely required but may be helpful to differentiate lesions suspicious for malignancy; should be avoided if lesion is highly suspected to be vascular, as significant bleeding may ensue
- IH stain positive for GLUT1 on histopathology, differentiating them from other vascular tumors and VaM
- Other diagnostic tests should be considered if concerns for syndromes or other complications (e.g., cardiac or respiratory compromise) exist.

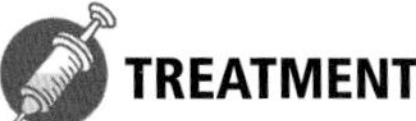

TREATMENT

GENERAL MEASURES

- IHs
  - Most patients will not need treatment, as lesions will spontaneously involute without complications. Anticipatory guidance for caregivers about natural history is key.
  - Consider treatment for IH interfering with critical organ functions, such as vision or breathing or lesions at risk for destruction of anatomic landmarks (e.g., nasal cartilage) or permanent disfigurement.
  - Timing of surgical treatment of IH should be carefully determined to minimize the risk of undesirable cosmetic outcome. Surgery during the proliferative phase in infancy is rarely required. Most surgery is performed between 3 and 6 years of age.
  - Propranolol, given orally at 2 mg/kg/24 h in divided doses (range 1 to 3 mg/kg/24 h) is now United States Food and Drug Administration-approved for IH therapy and is 1st-line therapy for IH.
  - Oral corticosteroids (generally given as prednisolone at 2 to 3 mg/kg/24 h), the prior standard of care, are now 2nd-line treatment.
  - Topical timolol maleate 0.5% gel-forming solution or solution (ophthalmic dosage forms used topically) typically prescribed as 1 drop to IH surface b.i.d. is useful for thin superficial or small IH.
  - Interferon may be useful in refractory or severe lesions. The development of spastic diplegia in up to 20% of treated infants (highest risk group is <12 months of age) is a known complication and has drastically limited modern use of this therapy.
  - Vincristine is another 3rd-line therapy and is rarely used.
  - For ulcerated IH, petrolatum, zinc oxide paste, and topical dressings are used; pulse dye laser (PDL) may be used. Propranolol has been shown to speed ulcer healing.
- VaM
  - PDL
    - The treatment of choice for port-wine stains and other superficial VaM
    - Serial treatments over several years are generally necessary. Large lesions may not completely respond. Most CM become 50–90% lighter after PDL. Redarkening over years can occur, and repeat treatments may be needed.
    - Better outcomes are noted in children treated in infancy and early childhood.
  - Sirolimus has shown recent promise in treating severe, complicated VaM and vascular tumors including KHE, LM, some VM, and combined malformations. It does not appear to be effective for AVM.
  - Sclerotherapy or surgery may be appropriate for complicated, symptomatic VaM.

ISSUES FOR REFERRAL

Consider referral to specialty services if the following conditions are present:

- Lesions in locations where function may be impacted such as periorbital, ear canal, tip of nose, lips, or anogenital areas
- Lesions distributed in a "beard-like" distribution, which may be associated with airway IH
- Presence of numerous cutaneous lesions increasing the likelihood of visceral involvement (including the GI tract, liver, CNS, lungs)
- Lesions causing or likely to cause significant disfigurement
- Lesions located over the lumbosacral spine, which may be associated with spinal dysraphism
- Lesions located in a segmental distribution about the head and face
- Large AVMs impacting circulation and cardiac function (e.g., resulting in high-output heart failure)
- Presence of dysmorphic features along with vascular lesions
- Lesions that are ulcerating or bleeding
- Suspected VaM of unknown type or extent

ONGOING CARE

PATIENT EDUCATION

- Hemangioma Education (www.hemangiomaeducation.org)
- Boston Children's Vascular Anomalies Center (www.childrenshospital.org)

PROGNOSIS

- IHs
  - All IHs undergo spontaneous involution. By 3.5 to 4 years of age, 90% will have completed involution. >85% will resolve without need for treatment.
  - Residual areas of skin atrophy, scarring, and/or discoloration occur in up to 50%.
  - Complicated lesions marked by ulceration result in scarring.
- VaM
  - VaM do not generally involute or resolve.
  - Salmon patches fade over time and generally are not a cosmetic problem.
  - Port-wine stains may darken and become nodular with age; bleeding can occur.
  - Larger VaM can be associated with excessive growth of the involved body area resulting in hypertrophy.
  - Malignant transformation is rare.

COMPLICATIONS

- IHs
  - Bleeding, ulceration, superinfection
  - Interference with function of important organs (including vision, airway, GI tract, CNS)
  - Disfigurement
  - Severe hypothyroidism may occur with large hepatic hemangiomas associated with multifocal IH that stimulate increased breakdown of thyroid hormone.
  - KHE and TA may be associated with Kasabach-Merritt phenomenon with severe thrombocytopenia (due to platelet trapping, consumptive coagulopathy, and microangiopathic hemolytic anemia).
- VaM
  - High-output cardiac failure due to circulatory "steal" associated with AVMs
  - Skeletal and soft tissue overgrowth of the involved limb can occur with disfigurement and orthopedic complications.
  - Limitation of movement and pain from localized ischemia
  - Localized intravascular coagulopathy is common in VM.
  - Problems associated with lymphedema
  - Airway compromise from constriction by large neck lesions

ADDITIONAL READING

- Adams DM, Trenor CC III, Hammill AM, et al. Efficacy and safety of sirolimus in the treatment of complicated vascular anomalies. *Pediatrics*. 2016;137(2):e20153257.
- Darrow DH, Greene AK, Mancini AJ, et al; for Section on Dermatology, Section on Otolaryngology—Head and Neck Surgery, Section on Plastic Surgery. Diagnosis and management of infantile hemangioma. *Pediatrics*. 2015;136(4):e1060–e1104.
- Drolet BA, Frommelt PC, Chamlin SL, et al. Initiation and use of propranolol for infantile hemangioma: report of a consensus conference. *Pediatrics*. 2013;131(1):128–140.
- Wassef M, Blei F, Adams D, et al. Vascular anomalies classification: recommendations from the International Society for the Study of Vascular Anomalies. *Pediatrics*. 2015;136(1):e203–e214.

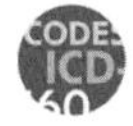

CODES

ICD10

- D18.00 Hemangioma unspecified site
- Q27.9 Congenital malformation of peripheral vascular system, unsp
- Q27.30 Arteriovenous malformation, site unspecified

FAQ

- Q: When will the IH go away?
- A: Growth in nearly all IH stops by 12 months of age. Regression occurs over a period of years, with approximately 90% of involution occurring by age 4 years.
- Q: Is the risk of bleeding in IH significant?
- A: No. Risk of significant bleeding is <1%. Even with ulceration, bleeding is more of an "ooze."

H

HEMATURIA

Stephanie Nguyen, MD, MAS • Jennifer H. Yang, MD

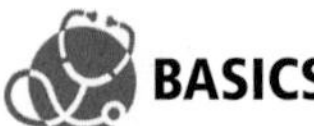

BASICS

DESCRIPTION

- Hematuria is defined as ≥3 to 5 RBCs per high-power field (HPF) using a standard urinalysis technique on a centrifuged sample.
- Persistent hematuria: hematuria on >2 separate examinations
- Macroscopic or gross hematuria: hematuria visible to the naked eye
- Microscopic hematuria: hematuria detected by urinalysis or microscopy only

EPIDEMIOLOGY

- Prevalence of asymptomatic microscopic hematuria in school-aged children is 3–6% on single urine sample and ≤1% on two or more urine samples.
- Gross hematuria: 0.13% children in walk-in clinic
- Gross hematuria is more common in boys.

RISK FACTORS

Nephrogenic causes of hematuria, hypercalciuria, nephrolithiasis, and nephritis can be inherited.

PATHOPHYSIOLOGY

Hematuria can occur from anywhere along the urinary tract or kidney. Causes of hematuria can be divided into glomerular and nonglomerular causes. In glomerular hematuria, RBCs cross the glomerular basement membrane (GBM) into the urinary space. Urine with dysmorphic red cells, proteinuria, and urinary casts suggest a glomerular origin.

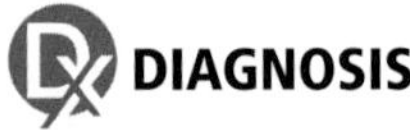

DIAGNOSIS

- No identifiable cause is found in the majority (up to 80%) of children with asymptomatic microscopic hematuria and in up to 30% of children with a single episode of gross hematuria.
- Approach to patient
  - Evaluate all children with gross hematuria and those children with microscopic hematuria confirmed on two of three consecutive samples over several weeks:
    - **Phase 1:** Determine if the pigment in urine is from blood or another source. Are RBCs present on microscopy?
    - **Phase 2:** Determine the source of bleeding: glomerular or nonglomerular, upper or lower urinary tract?
    - **Phase 3:** Select those who will require referral versus those who will simply require follow-up.

HISTORY

- **Question:** Blood on voiding?
- *Significance*: Glomerular or renal source will be constantly bloody; urethral bleeding is more likely at initiation or end of stream.
- **Question:** Prior episodes of gross hematuria or abnormal urinalyses?
- *Significance*: chronic versus acute process
- **Question:** Antecedent infection, streptococcal pharyngitis, or impetigo?
- *Significance*: suggests postinfectious glomerulonephritis (GN)
- **Question:** Concurrent upper respiratory infection (URI) or gastroenteritis?
- *Significance*: suggests IgA nephropathy
- **Question:** Any precipitating factors (trauma, exercise)?
- *Significance*: renal contusion, exercise hematuria, or myoglobinuria
- **Question:** Voiding symptoms, dysuria, urgency, frequency?
- *Significance*: suggests bacterial or viral (adenovirus) hemorrhagic cystitis
- **Question:** Renal colic or other pain?
- *Significance*: suggests stones or other obstructive process
- **Question:** Drops of blood or spotting in underwear after or between voiding in prepubertal boys?
- *Significance*: suggests benign urethrorrhagia
- **Question:** Fever, rash, arthritis?
- *Significance*: signs or symptoms of systemic illness or immune-mediated process
- **Question:** Bleeding from any other source (i.e., gums, GI tract)?
- *Significance*: suggests coagulopathy
- **Question:** Symptomless "terminal" hematuria?
- *Significance*: suggests trigonitis, hemorrhagic cystitis
- **Question:** Medications and diet?
- *Significance*: food or drug pigment, drug nephrotoxicity
- **Question:** Sexually active? STI?
- *Significance*: urethritis, epididymitis
- **Question:** Family history of hematuria or kidney disease?
- *Significance*:
  - Hematuria in family members: Familial hematuria, kidney failure, or premature deafness suggests Alport syndrome.
  - Sickle cell disease or trait in child or family members suggests sickle nephropathy, papillary necrosis, or hemoglobinuria.
  - Renal stone disease in family members suggests renal stones, hypercalciuria, or metabolic disease.
  - Cystic kidney disease in family members: autosomal recessive or autosomal dominant polycystic kidney disease

PHYSICAL EXAM

- **Finding:** Head, ears, eyes, nose, throat (HEENT) exam (periorbital edema)?
- *Significance*: GN, renal failure, volume overload
- **Finding:** Cardiovascular exam (hypertension, tachycardia, murmur, gallop)?
- *Significance*: GN, renal failure, volume overload
- **Finding:** Abdominal exam (ascites, organomegaly, tenderness, or masses)?
- *Significance*: volume overload, tumor, polycystic or hydronephrotic kidneys, venous thrombosis
- **Finding:** Back exam (flank tenderness)?
- *Significance*: pyelonephritis, renal calculi, large cysts
- **Finding:** Genital exam (blood at urethral meatus, normal urethral opening)?
- *Significance*: urethral trauma, meatal stenosis
- **Finding:** Perineal exam (skin breakdown, irritation)?
- *Significance*: external source of bleeding or infection
- **Finding:** Extremities (pretibial edema, arthritis)?
- *Significance*: GN, volume overload, systemic illness
- **Finding:** Skin and mucosal exam (petechial, vasculitic rash, ulcerations)?
- *Significance*: systemic illness (lupus, Henoch-Schönlein purpura [HSP])

DIFFERENTIAL DIAGNOSIS

Nonglomerular causes are more common than glomerular causes.

- Factitious causes: Urine appears bloody, but no RBCs are present.
  - Endogenous pigments
    - Myoglobin (rhabdomyolysis)
    - Hemoglobin (hemolysis)
    - Porphyria
    - Bile pigments
    - Urate crystals (pink diaper syndrome)
  - Exogenous pigments
    - Food and beverage dyes
    - Beets, blackberries
    - Drugs that cause urinary discoloration:
      - Phenazopyridine (Pyridium®)
      - Senna (Ex-Lax®)
      - Rifampin
      - Isoniazid
      - Others
  - *Serratia marcescens*
- Glomerular causes
  - Common:
    - Strenuous exercise
    - Acute postinfectious GN
    - IgA nephropathy
    - Thin basement membrane disease (benign familial hematuria)
  - Uncommon:
    - Alport syndrome, hereditary nephritis
    - Membranoproliferative GN
    - Nephritis of systemic disease (HSP, systemic lupus erythematosus, or other vasculitis)
- Nonglomerular causes
- Upper urinary tract
  - Common:
    - Pyelonephritis
    - Hypercalciuria/nephrolithiasis/nephrocalcinosis
    - Renal trauma (contusion or laceration)
    - Ureteropelvic junction obstruction
    - Hemoglobinopathies (sickle cell disease, sickle cell trait)
  - Uncommon:
    - Drug-induced interstitial nephritis (penicillins, cephalosporins, NSAIDs, phenytoin, cimetidine, omeprazole)
    - Cystic disease (simple cyst, polycystic kidney disease)
    - Neoplasm: Wilms tumor, renal cell carcinoma
    - Coagulopathy
    - Renal venous thrombosis, renal arterial thrombosis
    - "Nutcracker" phenomenon, compression of the left renal vein between the aorta and proximal superior mesenteric artery

- Lower urinary tract
  - Common:
    - Traumatic Foley catheterization
    - Cystitis (bacterial, viral, occasionally chemical)
    - Benign urethrorrhagia
    - Meatal stenosis
    - Urethritis
    - "Terminal hematuria" syndrome (trigonitis)
    - Epididymitis
  - Uncommon:
    - Bladder tumor
    - Arteriovenous malformation
    - Polyp
    - Urethral or bladder trauma
    - Foreign body or calculus in bladder or urethra
    - Schistosomiasis
- External causes of "hematuria"
  - Menstrual contamination
  - Diaper rash, perineal irritation

DIAGNOSTIC TESTS & INTERPRETATION

Initial Tests (screening, lab, imaging)

A positive test for blood on urine dipstick should be followed with repeated urinalyses with microscopy to look for RBCs in the urinary sediment. Heme-positive urine without RBC should be investigated for factitious causes.

- **Test:** repeated urinalysis to confirm persistent microscopic hematuria
- *Significance*:
  - Patient should be told not to exercise before the urine collection.
  - Two of three positive specimens over several weeks should be documented in an otherwise well child before diagnostic testing is initiated.
- **Test:** gross and microscopic analyses of fresh urine specimen
- *Significance*:
  - Absence of RBCs suggests factitious hematuria from pigments such as myoglobin as seen in rhabdomyolysis or hemoglobin as seen in hemolysis.
  - Dysmorphic RBCs suggest glomerular source.
  - Eumorphic RBCs suggest nonglomerular source/collecting system etiology.
  - RBC casts: diagnostic for GN
  - WBCs suggest cystitis.
  - WBC casts suggest pyelonephritis.
- **Test:** screening of the family members for occult hematuria
- *Significance*: familial benign hematuria or Alport syndrome
- **Test:** Testing for hypercalciuria (random urine calcium/creatinine ratio >0.2 mg/mg in children >6 years; >0.6 mg/mg in children 6 to 12 months; >0.8 mg/mg in children <6 months)
- *Significance*: if elevated, 24-hour urine calcium collection >4 mg/kg/day in children >2 years of age: hypercalciuria
- **Test:** culture
- *Significance*: bacterial, viral—cystitis, *S. marcescens*, adenovirus
- **Test:** serum electrolytes, BUN, and creatinine levels
- *Significance*: Impaired renal function suggests inflammation, infection, or obstruction.
- **Test:** evaluation for GN
- *Significance*:
  - Hematuria with RBC casts in combination with proteinuria, edema, hypertension, and/or impaired renal function
  - Streptococcal serology (ASO titer, streptozyme): acute postinfectious GN
  - Complement studies (C3,C4): hypocomplementemic GN—immune complex–mediated (lupus nephritis, postinfectious GN, membranoproliferative GN)
  - Antinuclear antibody (ANA) titer or anti–double-stranded DNA if hypocomplementemic or signs of systemic vasculitis: vasculitis (lupus)
  - Quantitation of proteinuria and serum albumin concentration
    - 3 to 4+ proteinuria, urine protein/creatinine ratio >2 mg/mg, and hypoalbuminemia suggest glomerular disease/nephrosis.
    - 24-hour urine protein ≥ 1 g/day
- **Test:** CBC with platelets, coagulation times
- *Significance*: may suggest hemolysis, clotting disorder, or systemic illness
- **Test:** Hemoglobin electrophoresis should be considered in African American patients.
- *Significance*: Sickle cell disease or sickle trait may cause hematuria.
- Rarely, additional studies, such as voiding cystourethrogram, renal angiography, cystoscopy, and renal biopsy will be required with an appropriate referral to urology or nephrology.
- Audiometry and ophthalmologic exam may be indicated if hereditary (Alport) nephritis is suspected; should be performed on boys with familial hematuria
- Every child with gross hematuria should have imaging of the kidneys and urinary tract. It may or may not be indicated in children with microscopic hematuria.
  - Ultrasound of kidneys and bladder: urinary tract obstruction, congenital malformation, cysts, stones, nephrocalcinosis, malignancy
  - Abdominal CT scan: after trauma if there are >50 RBCs/HPF; if mechanism (deceleration injury, multiple organ injury) or signs or symptoms (flank pain or ecchymosis) are significant, even if <50 RBC/HPF
  - Helical CT without contrast: study of choice for the visualization of stones; however, must consider radiation exposure risk. Ultrasound with KUB is a reasonable first test for stones.

TREATMENT

GENERAL MEASURES

- For children with microscopic hematuria, in the absence of other clinical, laboratory, or imaging findings, no specific treatment is indicated besides routine follow-up.
- For children with glomerular hematuria, treatment depends on the histopathologic diagnosis, clinical features, renal function, and degree of proteinuria.
- For children with an anatomic/structural etiology, treatment is specific to abnormality.

ISSUES FOR REFERRAL

- Nephrology: recurrent gross hematuria, proteinuria, RBC casts, nephrosis, edema, hypocomplementemia, hypertension, azotemia, cysts, hypercalciuria, family history of renal failure, hereditary nephritis, deafness, or cystic kidney disease
- Urology: congenital anomaly of urinary tract, uncontrollable bleeding after trauma, recurrent, symptomatic or large stones, recurrent urinary infections
- Hematology: bleeding secondary to coagulopathy or sickle cell disease papillary necrosis

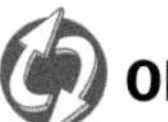

ONGOING CARE

FOLLOW-UP RECOMMENDATIONS

Patient Monitoring

A healthy child with asymptomatic isolated hematuria and a negative workup should be reassessed annually with a complete physical exam, measurement of BP, and urinalysis. If hematuria is persistent, periodic assessment of renal function should also be performed. The development of significant proteinuria, hypertension, elevated creatinine, family history of renal failure, or other concerns should prompt evaluation by a pediatric nephrologist.

PROGNOSIS

- Most children with asymptomatic isolated microscopic hematuria detected on a well-child examination, without proteinuria, hypertension, or azotemia, will NOT be found to have serious underlying pathology and will simply require longitudinal follow-up.
- Many children with hematuria will not have an identifiable cause; however, long-term prognosis is still generally good.
- Children with asymptomatic microscopic or gross hematuria combined with proteinuria have a higher likelihood of glomerular disease.
- Children with a history of stones or hypercalciuria are at increased risk of developing renal stones in the future.
- Familial hematuria secondary to thin GBM disease is a diagnosis of exclusion. Although it often has a benign prognosis, in some families, it can progress to chronic kidney disease. Children should be examined yearly for the development of proteinuria or hypertension.

ADDITIONAL READING

- Bergstein J, Leiser J, Andreoli S. The clinical significance of asymptomatic gross and microscopic hematuria in children. *Arch Pediatr Adolesc Med*. 2005;159(4):353–355.
- Cohen RA, Brown RS. Clinical practice. Microscopic hematuria. *N Engl J Med*. 2003;348(23):2330–2338.
- Diven SC, Travis LB. A practical primary care approach to hematuria in children. *Pediatr Nephrol*. 2000;14(1):65–72.
- Feld LG, Meyers KE, Kaplan BS, et al. Limited evaluation of microscopic hematuria in pediatrics. *Pediatrics*. 1998;102(4):E42.
- Patel HP, Bissler JJ. Hematuria in children. *Pediatr Clin North Am*. 2001;48(6):1519–1537.
- Vivante A, Afek A, Frenkel-Nir Y, et al. Persistent asymptomatic isolated microscopic hematuria in Israeli adolescents and young adults and risk for end-stage renal disease. *JAMA*. 2011;306(7):729–736.
- Youn T, Trachtman H, Gauthier B. Clinical spectrum of gross hematuria in pediatric patients. *Clin Pediatr (Phila)*. 2006;45(2):135–141.

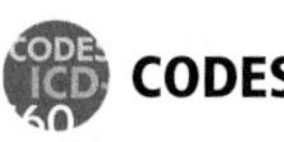

CODES

ICD10

- R31.9 Hematuria, unspecified
- R31.1 Benign essential microscopic hematuria
- R31.0 Gross hematuria

HEMOLYSIS

Julie W. Stern, MD

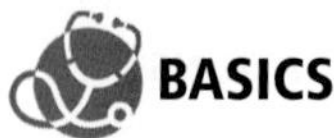

BASICS

DESCRIPTION

Premature destruction of RBCs, either intravascularly or extravascularly, leading to a shortened red cell survival time. The premature destruction can be caused by intrinsic factors (defects within the RBC itself) or extrinsic factors (factors outside the RBC leads to premature destruction).

RISK FACTORS

- Acquired (extrinsic): ABO and/or Rh incapability is a risk factor in the newborn period.
- Hereditary (intrinsic): Although many hereditary disorders are autosomal dominant, 20% of these patients represent new spontaneous mutations and have no affected family members.

Genetics

- Hemoglobinopathies are generally autosomal recessive or the result of compound heterozygosity.
- RBC membrane defects and enzyme defects may be autosomal dominant, recessive, or X-linked.

GENERAL PREVENTION

- Acquired (extrinsic): Most causes of acquired, non–transfusion-related hemolytic disease are not preventable.
- Hereditary (intrinsic): Although there is no way to prevent hereditary forms of hemolysis, newborn screening can help identify and allow proper management of some conditions. Patients with glucose-6-phosphate dehydrogenase (G6PD) deficiency should be counseled to avoid triggers such as fava beans, broad beans, and mothballs.

PATHOPHYSIOLOGY

- Intravascular hemolysis occurs within the circulation as a direct result of trauma, complement fixation, and cellular destruction.
- Extravascular hemolysis generally occurs in the spleen (or liver) as misshaped and/or older red cells are recognized and destroyed by the RE system.

ETIOLOGY

- Extrinsic or acquired disorders
  - Infectious
  - Drug-induced
  - Immune mediated
  - Microangiopathic
- Intrinsic or hereditary disorders
  - Hemoglobinopathies
  - RBC membrane and enzyme defects

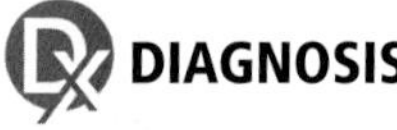

DIAGNOSIS

HISTORY

- Pallor, fatigue, and jaundice may occur with either intravascular or extravascular hemolysis.
- Hemoglobinuria is a sign of intravascular hemolysis.
- General goal is to establish existence of hemolysis rather than other causes of anemia, such as blood loss and hypoproduction.
- Determine acuity and severity of the anemia and hemolysis:
  - With acute onset, there will be evidence of unstable vital signs and possibly heart failure.
  - Parents may give a history of a rapid deterioration of the child's physical and/or mental state.
  - Patients with chronic anemia that has progressed slowly may have a low hemoglobin yet be well compensated with fairly normal vital signs (except for tachycardia).
  - CBC with a corrected reticulocyte count will help determine if there is an appropriate bone marrow response to the level of anemia and, therefore, whether the process is hypoproductive or hemolytic.
- Determine the cause of hemolysis. Treatment approaches will vary depending on the underlying etiology.
- **Question:** History of anemia, splenectomy, or early cholecystectomy in multiple family members?
- *Significance*:
  - Although many hereditary membrane defects and enzyme deficiencies are autosomal dominant, some are autosomal recessive or X-linked. Thus, a negative familial history does not always rule out these diagnoses.
  - In some cases, the diagnosis of hereditary spherocytosis (HS) has not been made, yet multiple family members have had their gallbladders removed at an early age, which may indicate the presence of this defect.
  - Thalassemia (especially β-thalassemia) and sickle cell anemia may present in early childhood with chronic hemolysis with or without a familial history.
- **Question:** History of travel?
- *Significance*: Malaria is endemic to Africa, India, and parts of Central America.
- **Question:** Recent medications, transfusions or new food exposures?
- *Significance*:
  - Specifically ask about exposure to fava beans, mothballs, and antibiotics. Drugs can themselves cause hemolysis or can induce hemolysis if there is an underlying disorder such as G6PD deficiency.
  - Delayed hemolytic transfusion reactions are rare but can be seen days to a week or so later.
- **Question:** Age at first signs and symptoms of hemolysis (pallor or jaundice)?
- *Significance*:
  - Hereditary causes of hemolysis are most often chronic or recurrent, although the diagnosis may be delayed until the child is older if the process is mild.
  - Acute, acquired hemolytic disorders may also recur.

PHYSICAL EXAM

Hemolysis that is a secondary problem (e.g., related to infection, tumors) may be found incidentally during evaluation of the primary process.

- **Finding:** Acute processes such as autoimmune hemolytic anemia (both warm and cold antibody mediated) may present with a child in extremis.
- *Significance*:
  - Tachycardia is a common finding in nearly all cases of acute hemolysis.
  - Hypotension is a late finding.
- **Finding:** More chronic processes, such as HS, G6PD, PK deficiencies, thalassemia intermedia, and sickle cell disease, may be picked up at well visits or by laboratory examination.
- *Significance*: These children often appear well (except for jaundice) but may become more anemic with an acute illness.
- **Finding:** Splenomegaly (often impressive) and hepatomegaly are common findings in extravascular hemolysis.
- *Significance*:
  - Hepatomegaly may be more pronounced if the child is in heart failure due to acute, severe anemia.
  - Splenomegaly may be either the cause of or, more frequently, a result of a hemolytic process.
  - If significant lymphadenopathy is present, look for an underlying cause such as lymphoproliferative disorders or malignancy.
- **Finding:** skin changes
- *Significance*:
  - Pallor is nearly a universal finding in acute hemolysis and in exacerbations of chronic hemolysis.
  - Jaundice is more common in intravascular hemolysis.
  - Presence of ecchymoses or petechiae suggests DIC or thrombocytopenia.

DIFFERENTIAL DIAGNOSIS

- Acquired (extrinsic)
  - Allergic/inflammatory/immune
    - Autoimmune hemolytic anemia
      - Warm antibody mediated
      - Cold antibody mediated
      - Hemolytic transfusion reaction
  - Congenital/anatomic
    - ABO blood type incompatibility and Rh incompatibility between infant and mother
    - Cardiac lesions with turbulent flow; left-sided more common than right-sided
    - Prosthetic heart valve (especially aortic)
    - Kasabach-Merritt syndrome
    - Hypersplenism
  - Infectious
    - Congenital infections with syphilis, rubella, cytomegalovirus, and toxoplasmosis
    - Malaria
    - Bartonellosis
    - *Clostridium perfringens* (via a toxin)
    - *Mycoplasma pneumoniae*
    - HIV
    - Hemolytic uremic syndrome
  - Toxic, environmental, drugs
    - Immune complex "innocent bystander" mechanism
      - Quinidine
      - Acetaminophen
      - Amoxicillin
      - Cephalosporins
      - Isoniazid
      - Rifampin
    - Immune complex drug adsorption mechanism
      - Penicillin
      - Cephalosporins
      - Erythromycin
      - Tetracycline
      - Isoniazid
    - Drug-induced autoimmune hemolytic anemia: α-methyldopa
    - Toxic drug–induced hemolysis: ribavirin (generally mild and not clinically significant)
    - Snake and spider venoms
    - Extensive burns
  - Mechanical hemolysis
    - Cardiac hemolysis
    - Abnormal microcirculation
      - Thrombotic thrombocytopenic purpura (TTP)
      - Disseminated intravascular coagulation (DIC)
      - Malignant hypertension
      - Eclampsia
      - Hemangiomas
      - Renal graft rejection
    - March hemoglobinuria (prolonged physical activity)
  - Tumor
    - Lymphomas
    - Thymoma
    - Lymphoproliferative disorders

- Hereditary (intrinsic)
  - Genetic/metabolic
    - RBC membrane defects
      - HS
      - Hereditary elliptocytosis
      - Pyropoikilocytosis
      - Paroxysmal nocturnal hemoglobinuria (can be acquired)
    - Enzyme defects
      - PK deficiency
      - G6PD deficiency
    - Thalassemias (β-Thalassemia major is the most severe.)
    - Hemoglobinopathies
      - Sickle cell anemia (Hgb SS and SC variants)
      - Unstable hemoglobins

DIAGNOSTIC TESTS & INTERPRETATION

Initial Tests (screening, lab, imaging)

- CBC with differential and reticulocyte count
  - Interpret level of anemia and the reticulocyte count together. Chronic hemolysis in HS, for example, may have a nearly normal hemoglobin count but usually has an increased reticulocyte count.
  - With a rapid fall in hemoglobin, as in acute autoimmune hemolytic anemia, the reticulocyte count may be low at the start, rise in response to anemia, and fall during recovery.
  - Thrombocytopenia should raise suspicions about TTP or hemolytic uremic syndrome.
- Peripheral blood smear
  - Fragmented RBCs, schistocytes, and helmet cells are seen in DIC, TTP, hemolytic uremic syndrome, and cardiac valve hemolysis.
  - Helmet or bite cells are nearly pathognomonic for G6PD deficiency.
  - Other findings on the smear that may be helpful are spherocytes (HS and warm autoimmune hemolytic anemia), target cells (hemoglobin C and thalassemias), and acanthocytes (anorexia nervosa).
- Bilirubin
  - Total and unconjugated bilirubins are elevated in most cases.
- Urinalysis
  - Hemoglobinuria is present in intravascular hemolysis; established by a urine dipstick positive for heme with no intact red cells microscopically
  - Myoglobinuria can also give this picture.
- Coombs test
  - Direct Coombs test (direct antiglobulin test) detects antibodies or complement fragments present on the patient's RBCs.
  - Indirect antiglobulin test detects antibodies in the patient's serum that can bind normal RBCs.
  - Direct antiglobulin test provides direct evidence of immune-mediated hemolysis.
  - Warm antibody autoimmune hemolytic anemia is caused by an IgG antibody that coats RBCs, which are subsequently removed by the spleen.
  - Cold antibody autoimmune hemolytic anemia is caused by an IgM antibody that binds RBCs, fixes complement, and can cause both extravascular and intravascular hemolysis.
- Haptoglobin, hemopexin, and lactate dehydrogenase (LDH)
  - In intravascular hemolysis, haptoglobin levels may be undetectable, hemopexin is reduced, and LDH increased.
  - In extravascular hemolysis, haptoglobin is decreased (but detectable) and LDH may be increased but not to the level seen in intravascular hemolysis.
- Chest radiograph to assess cardiomegaly and evidence of pulmonary edema

Follow-Up Tests & Special Considerations

- Blood for diagnostic RBC enzyme, RBC membrane, or hemoglobinopathy studies must be drawn prior to transfusion to assure only the patient's red cells are studied.
- Bone marrow aspiration is rarely indicated, but if done, erythroid hyperplasia may be seen.

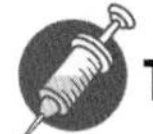

TREATMENT

GENERAL MEASURES

- Avoid triggers of hemolysis (i.e., foods, medications, etc.) for patients with known G6PD deficiency.
- Extended cross-match for minor red cell antigens prior to transfusions in patients with hemoglobinopathies to decrease risk of delayed hemolysis.

MEDICATION

Depends on cause and severity of hemolysis and anemia

First Line

Supportive care with fluids, oxygen, etc.

Second Line

- Red cell transfusion may be indicated for symptomatic anemia regardless of cause: Rate and volume of blood to be transfused will depend on severity of anemia and speed of onset (generally slower transfusion rate needed in chronic anemia).
- Plasmapheresis for TTP
- Withdrawal of inducing drug/agent (G6PD)
- Corticosteroids (Solu-Medrol® 1 to 2 mg/kg/dose q6–12h) may be indicated for hemolytic transfusion reactions and/or immune-mediated hemolysis.

ALERT

Factors that constitute an emergency:

- Hemoglobin <5 g/dL, especially with signs of cardiovascular compromise
  - Attempts to stabilize cardiovascular compromise with volume should be undertaken with care because hemodilution may occur.
  - Transfusion may be riskier in autoimmune hemolysis because of potential problems with cross-matching.
- Renal failure may accompany severe hemolysis in TTP or hemolytic uremic syndrome.
- Hemolysis in the neonatal period secondary to ABO or Rh incompatibility may require exchange transfusion either for anemia or for hyperbilirubinemia.

ISSUES FOR REFERRAL

- Most patients with severe, acute hemolysis or an underlying chronic hemolytic disorder will need to be evaluated by a hematologist.
- Suspected RBC membrane and enzyme defects, as well as hemoglobinopathies, should be referred for initial evaluation.

ADMISSION, INPATIENT, AND NURSING CONSIDERATIONS

Unstable vital signs with acute hemolysis, significant exacerbation of chronic hemolysis

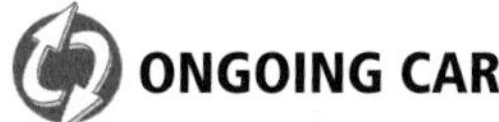

ONGOING CARE

FOLLOW-UP RECOMMENDATIONS

Patient Monitoring

- May need ICU for unstable vital signs
- Inpatient care may be required until acute hemolysis slowed or stopped.
- Monitor CBC, reticulocyte, LFTs every 3 to 7 days until at baseline.

DIET

Avoid food triggers of hemolysis for G6PD-deficient patients.

PATIENT EDUCATION

Sign and symptoms of hemolysis, splenic palpation; learn to identify and avoid triggers of hemolysis.

PROGNOSIS

Generally excellent with early recognition and intervention when warranted

COMPLICATIONS

- Severe, especially if acute, hemolysis may cause cardiovascular insufficiency and/or compromise.
- Chronic hemolysis may lead to gallstones, acute cholecystitis, and require cholecystectomy and/or splenectomy.
- TTP may recur although frequency is hard to predict.

ADDITIONAL READING

- Gallagher PG. Update on the clinical spectrum and genetics of red blood cell membrane disorders. *Curr Hematol Rep*. 2004;3(2):85–91.
- Lo L, Singer ST. Thalassemia: current approach to an old disease. *Pediatr Clin North Am*. 2002;49(6):1165–1191.
- Maisels MJ, Kring E. The contribution of hemolysis to early jaundice in normal newborns. *Pediatrics*. 2006;118(1):276–279.
- Old JM. Screening and genetic diagnosis of haemoglobin disorders. *Blood Rev*. 2003;17(1):43–53.
- Perkins SL. Pediatric red cell disorders and pure red cell aplasia. *Am J Clin Pathol*. 2004;122:S70–S86.
- Shah S, Vega R. Hereditary spherocytosis. *Pediatr Rev*. 2004;25(5):168–172.

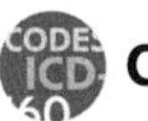

CODES

ICD10

- D58.2 Other hemoglobinopathies
- D59.1 Other autoimmune hemolytic anemias
- P58.9 Neonatal jaundice due to excessive hemolysis, unspecified

FAQ

- Q: When are blood transfusions indicated in patients with active hemolysis?
- A: Patients with severe, acute hemolysis that is causing cardiovascular compromise may require a transfusion if the process cannot be stopped with standard therapy (e.g., steroids for warm autoimmune hemolytic anemia, plasmapheresis for TTP). Transfusions must be given slowly if the hemolytic process has been chronic and the patient's blood volume is expanded.
- Q: Can hemolysis always be identified on a peripheral blood smear?
- A: No. Schistocytes, fragments, spherocytes, targets, and other morphology may provide clues to specific diagnoses but are not always present. The presence of a hemolytic process is inferred from a fall in hemoglobin, rise in the reticulocyte count, and elevation of the bilirubin and LDH levels.

HEMOLYTIC DISEASE OF THE FETUS AND NEWBORN

Maureen M. Gilmore, MD

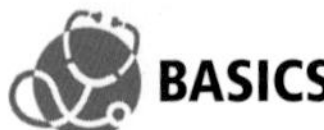

BASICS

DESCRIPTION

- Hemolytic disease of a fetus or newborn (HDFN) occurs due to the destruction of fetal and newborn red blood cells (RBCs) by maternal antibodies passively transferred across the placenta.
- Primarily related to rhesus (Rh) and less often ABO blood group isoimmunization

EPIDEMIOLOGY

- Rh incompatibility
  - Incidence of Rh hemolytic disease: 6 to 7/1,000 live births
  - Prevalence of RhD-positive (RhD+) fetus in RhD-negative (RhD−) mother: 15%
  - RhD− status in 15% of white, 7–8% of black and Hispanic, and 2% of Asian persons
  - 48–55% are heterozygous (Dd)
  - 35–45% are homozygous (DD)
  - Of all Rh-sensitized pregnancies:
    - 9% require intrauterine transfusion
    - 10% are delivered early and require newborn exchange transfusion
    - 31% require treatment after a full-term delivery
    - 50% require no treatment
- ABO incompatibility
  - Occurs in 12% of first pregnancies
  - Only 10–20% become significantly jaundiced, requiring phototherapy.

RISK FACTORS

- RhD− mother becomes pregnant with an RhD+ fetus; D-antigen is inherited from the father.
- Omitted or failed RhIG (anti-D) prophylaxis
- Type O mother pregnant with a type A, type B, or type AB fetus
- Only a fraction of women at risk develop antibodies.

GENERAL PREVENTION

- Rh incompatibility: RhIG is given to an RhD− woman after any exposure to RhD+ blood.
  - Given at 28 weeks, 34 weeks (prophylaxis), and within 72 hours of birth, or following maternal event, for example, amniocentesis, abortion, antepartum bleeds
- No prophylaxis for HDFN caused by other blood group incompatibilities

PATHOPHYSIOLOGY

- Isoimmunization—general principles:
  - Passage of fetal RBCs into maternal circulation occurs as a result of asymptomatic transplacental hemorrhage.
  - Initial sensitization of mother from fetomaternal hemorrhage can occur with placental abruption, abortion, ectopic pregnancy, or procedures (chorionic villus sampling, amniocentesis, or cordocentesis).
  - Exposure triggers maternal immune response (anti-D antibodies).
  - Maternal IgG antibodies cross the placenta and bind to fetal RBCs. Coated RBCs are then destroyed in the reticuloendothelial system, primarily the spleen.
  - Isoimmunization may lead to hyperbilirubinemia, severe anemia, and potentially hydrops.
  - Extramedullary hematopoiesis in the fetal liver and spleen is a response to severe fetal anemia, leading to hepatosplenomegaly.
- Rh isoimmunization
  - Passage of RhD+ fetal RBCs which cross the placenta into the circulation of an Rh− mother
  - RhD− state is the absence of D antigens on RBCs.
  - Decreased risk of RhD sensitization of mother if fetus is also ABO incompatible (<2%) versus ABO compatible (∼16% risk).
  - Rh isoimmunization rarely occurs in first pregnancy.
- ABO isoimmunization
  - Occurs in type O mothers with a type A or B fetus; clinically a milder hemolysis compared to Rh incompatibility and rarely requires intervention
  - 1% of type O mothers have high titers of IgG antibodies against both A and B that cross the placenta and cause HDFN.
  - Hemolysis due to anti-A is more common.
  - Hemolysis due to anti-B can be more severe and may require exchange transfusion in the newborn.

ETIOLOGY

- Fetomaternal hemorrhage, usually asymptomatic, with maternal immune response to foreign fetal RBC antigens
- Most common systems involved: RhD antigens, with more severe HDFN, and ABO blood group antigens, with milder anemia, jaundice
- 1% of cases involve other RBC antigens, such as Kell, Kidd, Duffy, or MNS blood groups.

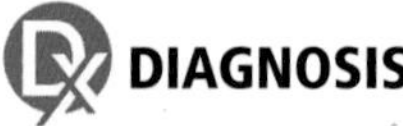

DIAGNOSIS

HISTORY

- Maternal exposure to incompatible blood products
- Previous stillbirths and/or abortions
- Neonatal hyperbilirubinemia requiring exchange transfusion in previous pregnancy
- RhIG not given after previous pregnancy or abortion

PHYSICAL EXAM

- Milder cases—hyperbilirubinemia only
- Minimal jaundice at birth but rapidly develops within 24 hours
- Pallor, tachycardia, tachypnea due to congestive heart failure (CHF) secondary to severe anemia
- Generalized edema and massive hepatosplenomegaly in cases with severe anemia and hydrops

DIFFERENTIAL DIAGNOSIS

Hydrops fetalis

- Hematologic: α-thalassemia, severe G6PD deficiency, twin-to-twin transfusion
- Cardiac: hypoplastic left heart syndrome, myocarditis, endocardial fibroelastosis, heart block
- Congenital infections: parvovirus, syphilis, cytomegalovirus (CMV), rubella
- Renal: renal vein thrombosis, urinary tract obstruction, nephrosis
- Placental: umbilical vein thrombosis, true knot of umbilical cord
- Genetic: trisomy 13, 18, 21; triploidy; aneuploidy
- Other: diaphragmatic hernia

DIAGNOSTIC TESTS & INTERPRETATION

Initial Tests (screening, lab, imaging)

- Antenatal
  - ABO and Rh blood typing of all mothers at first prenatal visit
  - Indirect Coombs test: detects anti-D antibodies in maternal serum
  - Father's ABO and Rh type and zygosity (DD or Dd)
  - Fetal blood group typing from amniotic fluid or fetal cord blood
  - Fetal serial Doppler ultrasounds of the peak systolic velocity in the middle cerebral artery to detect fetal anemia
- Neonatal
  - Cord blood or neonate's RBCs for ABO and Rh types
  - Hemoglobin (Hgb), hematocrit (Hct), bilirubin (direct and indirect), reticulocyte count
  - Direct Coombs test: detects maternal anti-D antibodies already bound to fetal/newborn RBCs
  - Kleihauer-Betke test or flow cytometry: estimates proportion of fetal RBCs in maternal circulation
  - Peripheral smear: nucleated RBCs (spherocytes in ABO disease)
- Fetal ultrasound (estimate fetal size, weight, and organomegaly)
- Doppler ultrasonography of fetal middle cerebral artery: peak systolic velocity

Diagnostic Procedures/Other

- Fetal cordocentesis (for fetal anemia)
- Amniocentesis
- Quantitative polymerase chain reaction, for paternal RhD zygosity
- Pathologic findings
  - Kernicterus
  - Extramedullary hematopoiesis
  - Hepatosplenomegaly

TREATMENT

GENERAL MEASURES

- Antenatal
  - Serial fetal monitoring
  - Intrauterine RBC transfusion: for severely affected fetuses (fetal Hct <25–30%) where early delivery is not possible; usually performed after 20 weeks' gestation
  - Early delivery and neonatal resuscitation may be required if with severe HDFN.
    - For high-risk fetus after amniocentesis or history of a prior stillbirth or hydrops
- Neonatal
  - Phototherapy, IV hydration, and serial bilirubin monitoring begins immediately.
  - Exchange transfusion: removes sensitized fetal RBCs and circulating bilirubin, and also
    - Corrects anemia in severely anemic infants
    - Removes circulating antibodies
- Indications for early exchange transfusion:
  - Cord blood bilirubin >3 mg/dL and Hgb <13 g/dL
  - Bilirubin rising at rate >1 mg/dL/h despite optimal phototherapy
  - Indirect bilirubin ≥20 to 25 mg/dL or rising to reach that level
  - Hgb 11 to 13 g/dL and bilirubin rising at rate >0.5 mg/dL/h despite optimal phototherapy
  - Lower indirect bilirubin triggers are used in preterm or high-risk infants.
- In hydropic infants, immediate partial exchange may be needed to correct anemia and CHF.
- Double-volume exchanges may be needed for hyperbilirubinemia.
- Selection of blood for exchange transfusion:
  - Fresh, washed, CMV-safe, and irradiated, Hgb S negative
  - For Rh disease: type O, Rh− cross-matched against mother's blood
  - For ABO disease: type O, Rh− or Rh compatible cross-matched against mother or infant's serum
  - For other antibodies: antigen-negative RBCs selected to avoid the clinically significant antibody. ABO type–specific blood can be used if baby's type confirmed.
- Risks of exchange transfusion include prolonged neutropenia, thrombocytopenia, hypocalcemia, arrhythmias, thrombosis, late anemia, and death.
- Some infants with milder Rh isoimmunization may have only exaggerated late physiologic anemia at 8 to 12 weeks.
- Most infants with ABO incompatibility require either no treatment or phototherapy only.
- Avoid drugs that interfere with bilirubin metabolism or its binding to albumin (e.g., sulfonamides, caffeine, and sodium benzoate).

ISSUES FOR REFERRAL

Late anemia: Infants who had significant HDFN are at risk due to reticulocytopenia related to persistent high titers of circulating maternal antibody. Small-volume RBC transfusion may be required.

ADDITIONAL THERAPIES

- Intravenous immunoglobulin (IVIG): in some studies shown to diminish hemolysis and may prevent the need for exchange transfusion
- Oral iron supplementation
- Erythropoietin, with iron, may be used to support infants at high risk for late anemia.
- Recombinant Rh immune globulin is in development.

ONGOING CARE

FOLLOW-UP RECOMMENDATIONS

Patient Monitoring

- Hgb/Hct and reticulocyte count every 1 to 2 weeks for first 2 to 3 months, especially for infants who had exchange transfusion, due to risk of late anemia at 8 to 12 weeks
- Assess for neurodevelopmental delays or neurologic injury.

PROGNOSIS

- ~50% of affected infants have minimal anemia and hyperbilirubinemia and require either no treatment or phototherapy only.
- ~25% with severe HDFN will require exchange transfusions.
- Data suggest normal neurologic outcome in 94% of cases following intrauterine transfusion
- Hydropic infants have a ~30% mortality rate.

COMPLICATIONS

- Hydrops fetalis
- Stillbirths
- Kernicterus—bilirubin encephalopathy

ADDITIONAL READING

- Garabedian C, Rakza T, Drumez E, et al. Benefits of delayed cord clamping in red blood cell alloimmunization. *Pediatrics*. 2016;137(3):e20153236.
- Hendrickson JE, Delaney M. Hemolytic disease of the fetus and newborn: modern practice and future investigations. *Transfus Med Rev*. 2016;30(4):159–164.
- Louis D, More K, Oberoi S, et al. Intravenous immunoglobulin in isoimmune haemolytic disease of newborn: an updated systematic review and meta-analysis. *Arch Dis Child Fetal Neonatal Ed*. 2014;99(4):F325–F331.
- Moise KJ Jr, Argoti PS. Management and prevention of red cell alloimmunization in pregnancy: a systematic review. *Obstet Gynecol*. 2012;120(5):1132–1139.
- Ross MB, de Alarcon P. Hemolytic disease of the fetus and newborn. *Neoreviews*. 2013;14:e83–e88.

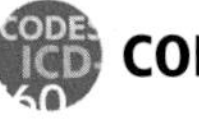

CODES

ICD10

- P55.1 ABO isoimmunization of newborn
- P55.0 Rh isoimmunization of newborn
- P55.8 Other hemolytic diseases of newborn

FAQ

- Q: Why does the Rh isoimmunization become worse with each pregnancy?
- A: Most sensitizing fetomaternal hemorrhages occur at delivery. In the first exposure, mother produces IgM antibodies, which does not cross the placenta; IgG antibodies slowly develops. In second or subsequent pregnancies, repeat exposure to even small amounts of fetal RhD causes rapid production of IgG anti-D, which crosses the placenta and attacks fetal RBCs. Other antibodies, such as Kell, may result in severe HDFN even in a first pregnancy.
- Q: Can maternal blood be used to transfuse the affected baby?
- A: Washed maternal blood may be used, but donor infectious disease testing protocols would need to be followed so it would not be routinely available in an emergency situation.
- Q: How does IVIG work, and does it decrease the need of an exchange transfusion?
- A: The mechanism of action for IVIG is not completely clear. HDFN occurs by destruction of RBCs via an antibody-dependent cytotoxic mechanism mediated by Fc receptors of the neonatal reticuloendothelial system. One possibility is that IVIG nonspecifically blocks these Fc receptors, decreasing hemolysis. However, there may be other ways in which IVIG provides immunomodulation as well.
- Q: How might delayed cord clamping (DCC) following delivery impact neonatal RBC alloimmunization?
- A: In a 2016 single-center study of neonates who required in utero transfusions for fetal anemia, Garabedian et al. found that the DCC group had a higher Hgb and less anemia at birth and were less likely to require a postnatal exchange transfusion compared to the immediate cord clamping group.

H

HEMOLYTIC UREMIC SYNDROME

Erica Winnicki, MD • Marsha May Lee, MD

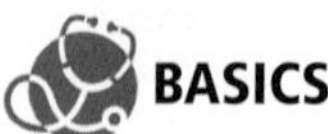

BASICS

DESCRIPTION

- Hemolytic uremic syndrome (HUS) is characterized by the triad of acute kidney injury, thrombocytopenia, and hemolytic anemia with fragmentation of erythrocytes (schistocytes noted on peripheral smear).
- Kidney dysfunction may manifest as hematuria and/or proteinuria and/or azotemia.
- The term "atypical HUS" (aHUS) is used for non-Shiga toxin–producing *Escherichia coli* (STEC) HUS and specifically refers to familial complement-mediated HUS (does not include the sporadic causes listed below).
- aHUS generally has a worse outcome than STEC-HUS.

EPIDEMIOLOGY

- HUS is one of the leading causes of acute kidney injury in infants and young children.
  - Approximately 90% of childhood cases are associated with STEC-HUS, or typical HUS, and follow a diarrheal prodrome. *Shigella dysenteriae* is also a well-recognized infectious cause.
  - Other sporadic causes of HUS include:
    - Malignancy
    - Bone marrow and solid organ transplantation drugs (such as calcineurin inhibitors and antiplatelet agents)
    - Malignant hypertension
    - Autoimmune disorders (such as SLE and antiphospholipid syndrome)
    - Certain infections (*Streptococcus pneumoniae*, influenza, HIV)
- STEC-HUS
  - Tends to occur in the summer months and may be sporadic or occur in epidemic outbreaks
  - Occurs mainly in older infants and young children between 6 months and 5 years of age
- aHUS
  - Has no seasonal variation and can occur at any age (including early infancy); may be sporadic or familial

GENERAL PREVENTION

- STEC is primarily found in the intestine of ruminants, particularly cattle, and can be transmitted by undercooked beef, unpasteurized milk, or by contamination of water and produce.
- For adequate prevention, practice good hand hygiene, wash food well, and cook food, especially meat, thoroughly.

PATHOPHYSIOLOGY

- Vascular endothelial cell injury is central to the pathogenesis of all forms of HUS.
- STEC colonize colonic mucosa, adhere to mucosal villi, and release Shiga toxin (Stx).
- Stx enters the systemic circulation, where it causes endothelial cell injury via inflammation, upregulation of chemokine and cytokine production, and by binding to endothelial cell surface receptors (Gb_3) and interrupting protein synthesis.
- Endothelial cell injury exposes the thrombogenic basement membrane, causing platelet activation and local intravascular thrombosis.
- In vitro studies show that glomerular endothelial cells and proximal tubular epithelial cells have receptors with very high affinity for Stx.
- aHUS is caused by dysregulation of the alternate complement pathway.

ETIOLOGY

- STEC-HUS: Most cases are caused by the O157:H7 strain of *E. coli*.
  - STEC most commonly infects children from 6 months to 5 years of age in the summer and the fall. The primary reservoir is cattle.
  - A negative stool culture in a patient who has HUS does not rule out STEC.
  - 10–15% of children who contract STEC^{+} *E. coli* O157:H7 gastroenteritis develop HUS.
- aHUS: Mutations of complement regulatory proteins are identifiable in ~60% of cases, with either an autosomal dominant or recessive inheritance. Reported mutations include complement factor H (most frequent), I, and B; membrane cofactor protein; and C3. Autoantibodies to complement factor H have also been reported as a cause of aHUS.
- One of the common causes of sporadic non-STEC-HUS is *S. pneumoniae* infection.

DIAGNOSIS

HISTORY

- GI prodrome: STEC-HUS typically develops 5 to 13 days after the onset of diarrhea (usually bloody). There can be associated vomiting and fever.
- Symptoms of pneumonia or meningitis: *S. pneumoniae*–associated HUS is associated with severe disease.
- Consumption of undercooked meat, particularly hamburger; consumption of unpasteurized milk, cheese, or juice; consumption of raw seed sprouts
- Direct animal contact (petting zoos)
- Family history of HUS (reported in up to 20% of patients with aHUS)
- Note that aHUS may be triggered by mild infections; presence of diarrhea does not exclude the diagnosis of aHUS.

PHYSICAL EXAM

- Pallor and petechiae
- Dehydration secondary to gastroenteritis
- Edema
- Pulmonary edema (volume overload)
- Hypertension
- Irritability
- Behavioral changes

DIAGNOSTIC TESTS & INTERPRETATION

- CBC
  - Anemia (Coombs negative), thrombocytopenia (<150,000/mm^3), leukocytosis (often seen in typical HUS)
- Blood smear: schistocytes
- Markers of hemolysis:
  - Elevated LDH, circulating free hemoglobin, decreased haptoglobin, elevated unconjugated bilirubin, increased reticulocyte count
- Renal function: elevated BUN and serum creatinine
- Serum electrolytes
  - Hyperkalemia (hypokalemia can be observed with severe GI involvement), metabolic acidosis, hyponatremia, hypocalcemia, hyperphosphatemia
- Serum albumin: usually low due to enteral losses and/or hypercatabolic state
- Amylase/lipase: elevated with pancreatic involvement
- Stool culture
  - Should be screened for *E. coli* O157:H7
  - Preferably <6 days after the onset of diarrhea
  - The local health department should be notified of any isolates.
- Identification of Stx from stool
- If Stx negative and/or aHUS suspected, it is recommended to rule out thrombotic thrombocytopenic purpura (TTP) by excluding ADAMTS13 deficiency, and send specific complement activity levels and genetic testing to evaluate for alternative pathway dysregulation.
- Plain film of the abdomen often demonstrates colonic distension and may show evidence of bowel perforation.
- Barium enema may show "thumb-printing" secondary to bowel wall edema and submucosal bleeding.
- Pathologic findings
  - Renal biopsy shows thrombotic microangiopathy: hyaline thrombi involving the glomerular capillaries and afferent arterioles with swelling of endothelial cells.

DIFFERENTIAL DIAGNOSIS

- Sepsis
- Diffuse intravascular coagulation
- Vasculitis
- TTP
- HELLP syndrome
- Malaria

TREATMENT

GENERAL MEASURES

- Treatment of STEC-HUS is generally supportive. The mainstay of therapy involves the following:
  - Strict fluid balance
  - Nutritional support
  - Control of hypertension
  - Treatment of seizures
- Of note, patients with significant gastroenteritis may present with significant hypovolemia and benefit from fluid resuscitation despite renal failure and oliguria.

MEDICATION

- Antihypertensives
  - Vasodilators, such as calcium-channel blockers or hydralazine, are useful in the acute phase.
  - After recovery, if a patient persists with hypertension and/or proteinuria, then angiotensin converting enzyme (ACE) inhibitors are indicated.
- In patients with seizures, diazepam or lorazepam is preferred. In patients with recurrent seizures or cerebral infarcts, long-term anticonvulsant therapy is indicated.
- Treatment with insulin may be needed in patients with pancreatic necrosis.
- Antibiotics are not indicated for treatment of STEC but would be indicated for patients with invasive bacterial infections or abscesses.
- Avoid antiperistaltic agents for treatment of colitis.

ADDITIONAL THERAPIES

- Renal replacement therapy
  - Indicated for severe acidosis, fluid overload, electrolyte imbalance, or uremia (required in ~2/3 of patients with STEC-HUS)
  - Mode of renal replacement therapy (intermittent or continuous hemodialysis or peritoneal dialysis) depends on patient condition.
- Treatment of severe anemia
  - Packed RBCs are transfused slowly if the hemoglobin decreases below 6 g/dL (BP can increase during transfusion).
- Platelet transfusion
  - Indicated only if there is active bleeding and severe thrombocytopenia or the patient needs surgery or invasive procedure (as platelet transfusion can contribute to microthrombi formation)
- Eculizumab, a humanized anti-C5 monoclonal antibody that inhibits complement activation, is approved for treatment of aHUS and is considered 1st-line therapy. Patients on this medication are at increased risk of serious bacterial infections, including meningococcal infection. Meningococcal vaccinations and prophylactic antibiotics are recommended for patients receiving eculizumab.
- In some situations and when eculizumab is not immediately available, plasma exchange should be initiated for aHUS.
- Patients with typical or atypical forms of HUS who progress to end-stage renal disease should be considered for kidney transplant. Eculizumab treatment is continued for those with aHUS after kidney transplant. For those with aHUS due to mutations of complement factors synthesized in the liver, liver transplant is curative although not without significant risks.

SURGERY/OTHER PROCEDURES

Some patients can have extensive bowel necrosis requiring resection.

ADMISSION, INPATIENT, AND NURSING CONSIDERATIONS

- Any fluid deficit should be corrected, and additional fluids should be limited to ongoing losses (insensible water loss plus urine and/or GI losses).
- Patients generally require ICU-level care. Along with frequent laboratory monitoring and assessment of fluid balance, frequent neurologic assessments should be performed.

ONGOING CARE

FOLLOW-UP RECOMMENDATIONS

- Resolution is usually heralded by a rise in platelet count and a gradual decrease in the frequency of blood transfusions.
- Pancreatic insufficiency may persist, requiring long-term insulin therapy beyond resolution of acute illness.

DIET

- Adequate nutritional support is important due to the hypercatabolic state of these patients.
- Enteral feeding should be trialed if GI symptoms are not severe, and total parenteral nutrition is used in patients with severe GI involvement.
- Close attention should be paid to fluid, sodium, potassium, and phosphorus intake.
- Some patients can have pancreatic involvement with subsequent exocrine or endocrine pancreatic insufficiency.

PROGNOSIS

- Patients with STEC-HUS can be mildly or severely affected. ~25% of survivors demonstrate long-term renal sequelae such as proteinuria, hypertension, and/or chronic kidney disease.
  - Mildly affected patients do not develop anuria, almost never have seizures, are rarely hypertensive, do not require dialysis, and have an excellent outcome.
  - Severely affected patients develop anuria and require dialysis, develop hypertension, and may have seizures.
  - Overall mortality is 3–5%.
  - 3% of patients progress to end-stage renal disease.
  - Recurrence after kidney transplantation is very uncommon.
- aHUS is associated with a poor prognosis, although prognosis is improved with early initiation of eculizumab.

COMPLICATIONS

- GI
  - Acute colitis is usually transient.
  - Rectal prolapse, toxic megacolon, bowel wall necrosis, intussusception, perforation, and stricture
  - Pancreatic involvement may result in pancreatitis or insulin-dependent diabetes mellitus.
- CNS
  - CNS involvement occurs in 20–25% of patients and may be acutely life-threatening.
  - Most patients have mild CNS symptoms that include irritability, lethargy, and behavioral changes.
  - Major symptoms such as stupor, coma, seizures, cortical blindness, posturing, and hallucinations may also occur. Thrombotic or hemorrhagic stroke may occur.
- Cardiac: Cardiomyopathy may occur.
- Musculoskeletal: rarely, rhabdomyolysis

ADDITIONAL READING

- Joseph C, Gattineni J. Complement disorders and hemolytic uremic syndrome. *Curr Opin Pediatr*. 2013;25(2):209–215.
- Loirat C, Fakhouri F, Ariceta G, et al. An international concensus approach to the management of atypical hemolytic syndrome in children. *Pediatr Nephrol*. 2016;31(1):15–39.
- Noris M, Remuzzi G. Atypical hemolytic-uremic syndrome. *N Engl J Med*. 2009;361(17):1676–1687.
- Pennington H. *Escherichia coli* O157. *Lancet*. 2010;376(9750):1428–1435.
- Scheiring J, Andreoli S, Zimmerhackl LB. Treatment and outcome of Shiga-toxin-associated hemolytic uremic syndrome (HUS). *Pediatr Nephrol*. 2008;23(10):1749–1760.
- Trachtman H, Austin C, Lewinski M, et al. Renal and neurological involvement in typical Shiga toxin-associated HUS. *Nat Rev Nephrol*. 2012;8(11):658–669.

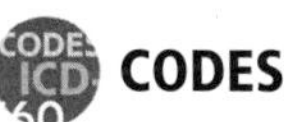

CODES

ICD10

D59.3 Hemolytic-uremic syndrome

FAQ

- Q: What factors should raise concern for aHUS?
- A: Age <6 months at presentation, insidious onset, relapsing disease, or failure to identify STEC or Stx in the stool
- Q: How many patients with gastroenteritis from *E. coli* O157:H7 will develop HUS?
- A: 10–15%
- Q: What should the family tell the day care staff and neighbors?
- A: If the patient has enteropathic HUS, contacts should be informed that any episodes of gastroenteritis merit close follow-up for evidence of anemia, thrombocytopenia, and kidney injury. No prophylaxis is indicated. Exclusion of infected children from day care centers until two consecutive stool cultures are negative for *E. coli* O157:H7 has been shown to prevent additional transmission.

HEMOPHILIA

Char M. Witmer, MD, MSCE

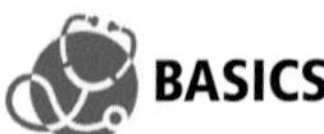

BASICS

DESCRIPTION

- Hemophilia A is factor VIII deficiency, and hemophilia B is factor IX deficiency.
- Deficiency or absence of factor VIII or factor IX leads to a delay and disruption of blood clotting that results in prolonged bleeding.
- The severity of bleeding depends on the baseline percentage of clotting activity that is genetically determined.

EPIDEMIOLOGY

- Most common severe inherited bleeding disorder
- Distribution
  - Hemophilia A: 80–85%
  - Hemophilia B: 10–15%
- No geographic or ethnic associations

Incidence

- Hemophilia A: 1 per 5,000 male births
- Hemophilia B: 1 per 30,000 male births

RISK FACTORS

Genetics

- X-linked recessive disorder
- Daughters of fathers with hemophilia are obligate carriers for the hemophilia gene mutation. An obligate carrier has a 50% chance of passing the hemophilia gene mutations to her offspring.
- Carrier status and prenatal testing available
- Hemophilia A
  - The intron 22 inversion mutation in the factor VIII gene is found in ~40–50% of patients with severe hemophilia A.
- Hemophilia B
  - Most factor IX gene defects are single base pair changes that result in missense, frameshift, or nonsense mutations. Mutations have been detected in all regions of the factor IX gene.

GENERAL PREVENTION

- Prophylaxis: the regularly scheduled infusion of clotting factor concentrate with the goal of preventing bleeding episodes; primarily used in patients with severe disease
- Anticipatory guidance and prevention
  - Good dental hygiene
  - Immunizations: no intramuscular injections; give subcutaneously with a small-gauge needle and apply direct pressure.
  - Rapid treatment of hemarthrosis to avoid chronic joint damage
  - Avoidance of contact sports (e.g., football, hockey, rugby)
  - Encourage physical fitness to ensure strong muscles to maintain joint health and prevent joint bleeding.
  - Head trauma precautions

PATHOPHYSIOLOGY

- Both factors VIII and IX are crucial for normal thrombin generation via the intrinsic pathway. The absence or decrease in activity of either protein severely impairs the ability to generate thrombin and fibrin.
- Hemophilia patients do not bleed more rapidly; rather, there is delayed formation of an abnormal clot resulting in prolonged bleeding.

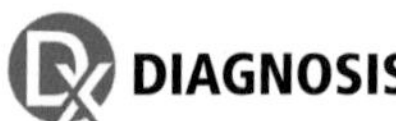

DIAGNOSIS

HISTORY

- Family history
  - Familial history of hemophilia in male offspring of female blood relatives is present in only 70% of cases.
- Excessive bleeding in a male neonate
  - Excessive bleeding with circumcision may be an initial presentation of hemophilia, although only 50% of patients with hemophilia will bleed with circumcision.
  - Muscle bleeding from intramuscular injections (e.g., vitamin K or immunizations); presents as increasing swelling at the site of injection
  - Prolonged bleeding from a torn frenulum, venipuncture, or heel puncture can be seen.
  - 3.5–4% of neonates with hemophilia may present with an intracranial hemorrhage.
- Pattern of bleeding in severe hemophilia
  - Characterized by easy, excessive, and palpable bruising with normal activity, spontaneous joint and muscle hemorrhages, and prolonged hemorrhage after trauma or surgery
- Age of onset of bleeding
  - Bleeding events occur frequently when the child begins to crawl and walk or with the eruption of teeth.
  - Patients with mild hemophilia may not present until they are older.
- Location of hemarthroses
  - Large weight-bearing joints are most often involved: knees, ankles, and hips.
  - Other non–weight-bearing joints can be involved including elbows and shoulders.
- Early symptoms of a hemarthroses:
  - Aura of tingling or warmth, visible swelling
  - Followed by increasing pain and decreasing range of motion (ROM) and inability to bear weight

PHYSICAL EXAM

Joint exam

- Acute hemarthrosis: limitation and pain with ROM, warmth, swelling, tenderness
- Chronic joint changes: crepitus, decreased ROM, synovial hypertrophy, bony abnormalities, and proximal muscle weakness
- Intramuscular hemorrhage: may not have external bruising; pain with motion and swelling; discrepancy in limb circumference
- Distal extremity neurovascular compromise can be a sign of compartment syndrome from bleeding into the forearm.

DIFFERENTIAL DIAGNOSIS

- Isolated prolonged aPTT associated with increased bleeding tendency:
  - von Willebrand disease
  - "Acquired hemophilia" owing to an inhibitory antibody to factor VIII or IX (extremely rare in children)
  - Hereditary factor deficiency of either VIII, IX, or XI
- Prolonged aPTT without increased bleeding tendency:
  - Factor XII deficiency
  - High-molecular-weight kininogen deficiency
  - Prekallikrein deficiency
  - Antiphospholipid antibody
  - Heparin artifact
  - Underfilling of the specimen tube

DIAGNOSTIC TESTS & INTERPRETATION

ALERT

- Neonates have a normal physiologic reduction in the vitamin K–dependent factors, including factor IX, making a determination of the degree of factor IX deficiency difficult in the neonatal period. The factor IX level must be confirmed after 6 months of age.
- When interpreting coagulation testing in a neonate, neonatal normal values for the PT and aPTT are different from those in adults.

Initial Tests (screening, lab, imaging)

Patients with hemophilia either A or B will have a normal PT and a prolonged aPTT. Assay for factor VIII and factor IX levels:

- <1%: severe hemophilia, characterized by spontaneous bleeding, hemarthroses, and deep tissue hemorrhages
- 1–5%: moderate hemophilia; bleeding following mild to moderate trauma; seldom spontaneous hemorrhage
- 5–30%: mild hemophilia; bleeding only from trauma

TREATMENT

GENERAL MEASURES

- Joint hemorrhage
  - Factor replacement
  - Immobilization: splints, casts, crutches, and/or bed rest (24 to 48 hours)
  - Prolonged immobilization may reduce recovery of joint ROM.
  - Initiation of physical therapy with factor coverage may be recommended, particularly after joint surgery.
- Special bleeding situations
  - Intracranial hemorrhage
    - Significant bleeding can occur despite a minor mechanism of head injury and the absence of external bruising.
    - In severe hemophilia, spontaneous intracranial bleeding can occur.
    - Factor replacement to 100% should be administered immediately followed by the diagnostic evaluation.
  - Major surgery
    - Factor replacement to 100% preoperatively and postoperatively
    - Regular dosing of factor for a minimum of 1 week postoperatively, even in mild hemophilia
  - Compartment syndrome
    - Bleeding within the fascial compartments of muscles
    - Most often occurs in the forearm
    - Neurovascular compromise can lead to shortening of the forearm muscles and clawlike deformity of the hand (Volkmann contracture).
  - Iliopsoas bleed
    - Lower abdominal or upper thigh pain may be the first symptom.
    - Exam is notable for inability to extend hip with preservation of internal and external rotation (allows distinction from hemarthrosis of hip joint).
    - Diagnosis confirmed by ultrasound or CT scan
    - Treat with factor replacement and bed rest.
  - Oral bleeding/epistaxis
    - Constant pressure for 15 to 20 minutes
    - Aminocaproic acid or tranexamic acid
    - Topical thrombin directly to the site of bleeding
    - Factor replacement if these measures don't work
  - Dental care
    - Factor replacement is required for significant dental procedures like tooth extraction or procedures that require a mandibular block.
    - Factor replacement is not required for routine teeth cleaning.
  - Lacerations
    - Factor replacement is necessary at time of placement and removal of the sutures.
  - Hematuria
    - Increased fluid intake and bed rest as initial treatment
    - If hematuria persists 24 to 48 hours, 30–40% factor replacement
    - Antifibrinolytics are contraindicated in the setting of hematuria because of the concern of obstructive uropathy from excessive clot formation.
- Patients should be followed regularly at a comprehensive hemophilia treatment center.

MEDICATION

Acute bleeding episodes:

- Factor replacement
  - Factor VIII replacement products
    - Recombinant, non–plasma-derived factor VIII
    - Plasma-derived, monoclonal antibody–purified factor VIII concentrate; heat or solvent detergent treated for viral inactivation
    - Cryoprecipitate (rarely used)
  - Factor IX replacement products
    - Recombinant, non–plasma-derived factor IX
    - Plasma-derived, immunoaffinity-purified factor IX concentrate; heat or solvent detergent treated for viral inactivation
    - Fresh frozen plasma (rarely used)
- Calculation of dose for pediatrics:
  - Recombinant factor VIII dosing (units) = % desired rise in plasma factor VIII × body weight (kg) × 0.5
  - Recombinant factor IX dosing (units) = % desired rise in plasma factor IX level × body weight (kg) × 1.4
- Target factor levels:
  - Joint bleed: 30–50% for 24 to 48 hours
  - Large muscle bleed: 70–100% for 24 to 48 hours
- CNS bleeding: 80–100% maintained for 10 to 14 days
- Desmopressin (dDAVP)
  - Synthetic vasopressin analog that stimulates release of endogenous factor VIII and von Willebrand factor
  - Only suitable for patients with mild or moderate factor VIII deficiency who have shown a response to dDAVP in a trial
  - Tachyphylaxis (unresponsiveness) may occur with repeated dosing.
  - Hyponatremia may also occur. Fluid restriction is recommended after each dose; should not be used in neonates
- Antifibrinolytic therapy (aminocaproic acid or tranexamic acid)
  - Antifibrinolytic therapy is used to stabilize a clot by inhibiting the normal process of clot lysis by the fibrinolytic system.
  - Used for the treatment of oral hemorrhages and to minimize bleeding from dental and some surgical procedures

ADMISSION, INPATIENT, AND NURSING CONSIDERATIONS

Life-threatening hemorrhages

- Prompt therapy with clotting factor concentrate should start immediately and prior to any diagnostic procedures.
- CNS bleeding
- Bleeding into and around the airway
- Exsanguinating hemorrhage

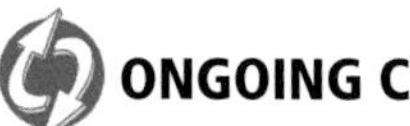

ONGOING CARE

COMPLICATIONS

- Complications of disease:
  - Hemophilic arthropathy: Repeated joint hemorrhages lead to synovial thickening and joint cartilage erosion. Joint space becomes narrowed and eventually fuses. Patients can develop joint contractures, limited ROM, and chronic pain.
- Complications of therapy:
  - Inhibitors: antibodies against factor VIII or IX, which can inactivate infused factor. This is currently the most significant complication in hemophilia and is associated with significant morbidity and decreased quality of life. Bleeding episodes are treated with less effective bypassing agents (activated prothrombin complex concentrates or activated recombinant factor VIIa).
  - Anaphylaxis: seen primarily with infusions of factor IX

ADDITIONAL READING

- Ljung RC. Intracranial haemorrhage in haemophilia A and B. *Br J Haematol*. 2008;140(4):378–384.
- Pruthi RK. Hemophilia: a practical approach to genetic testing. *Mayo Clin Proc*. 2005;80(11):1485–1499.
- Raffini L, Manno C. Modern management of haemophilic arthropathy. *Br J Haematol*. 2007;136(6):777–787.
- Witmer C, Young G. Factor VIII Inhibitors in hemophilia A: rationale and latest evidence. *Ther Adv Hematol*. 2013;4(1):59–72.
- Zimmerman B, Valentino LA. Hemophilia: in review. *Pediatr Rev*. 2013;34(7):289–294.

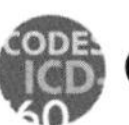

CODES

ICD10

- D66 Hereditary factor VIII deficiency
- D67 Hereditary factor IX deficiency
- D68.1 Hereditary factor XI deficiency

FAQ

- Q: Are there any medications contraindicated in a child with hemophilia?
- A: Aspirin should not be given as it interferes with platelet function. NSAIDs cause a milder effect on platelets and should also be avoided when possible. Patients with hemophilia should use acetaminophen for fever or pain.
- Q: Can immunizations be given to a child with hemophilia?
- A: To prevent bleeding from immunizations, they can be given SC (instead of IM) with the smallest gauge needle available. Pressure should be held postimmunization. Ice or cold packs should be applied to the area to minimize hematoma formation.

HEMOPTYSIS

Stamatia Alexiou, MD • Suzanne E. Beck, MD

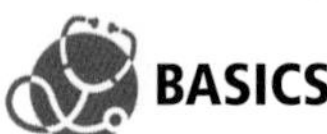

BASICS

DESCRIPTION

- Hemoptysis is the expectoration of blood from the respiratory tract. The term comes from the Greek words *haima*, meaning blood, and *ptysis*, meaning spitting.
- Bleeding from the respiratory tract can range from blood-streaked sputum to massive hemoptysis from the lung. The amount and nature of bleeding should be characterized by taking a careful history.
- The source of bleeding can be anywhere in the respiratory tract, from the nose to the alveolus.
- Consequences of hemoptysis may include exsanguination, hypoxemia, and anemia or there may be none.

EPIDEMIOLOGY

Large series of pediatric patients with massive hemoptysis have not been described.

PATHOPHYSIOLOGY

- Related to the underlying pulmonary or cardiac disease
- Vascular origin of hemoptysis is from two locations:
  - Pulmonary arteries: higher volume, lower pressure
  - Bronchial arteries: lower volume, higher pressure

ETIOLOGY

- More common causes:
  - Infection (pneumonia, bronchitis, viral illnesses)
  - Bronchiectasis leading to erosion into a bronchial artery
  - Trauma (pulmonary contusion, bronchoscopy, airway manipulation)
  - Foreign body aspiration
  - Cystic fibrosis
  - Congenital heart disease with collateral vessels or pulmonary hypertension
  - Tracheostomy-related complications
- Less common causes:
  - Cavitary infections (e.g., tuberculosis, abscess, histoplasmosis)
  - Factitious hemoptysis
  - Congenital vascular or airway lesions (pulmonary arteriovenous malformation, hemangioma, bronchogenic cyst, pulmonary sequestration)
  - Hemorrhagic diathesis, including anticoagulant therapy
  - H-type tracheoesophageal fistula
  - Pulmonary embolism
  - Pulmonary hemosiderosis
  - Tumors (teratomas, lymphomas)
  - Immune mediated: Henoch-Schönlein purpura, Goodpasture syndrome, Anti-neutrophil cytoplasmic antibody (ANCA)-associated granulomatous vasculitis, polyarteritis nodosa, systemic lupus erythematosus, Heiner syndrome
  - Sarcoidosis

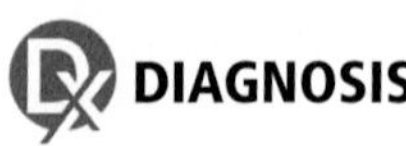

DIAGNOSIS

HISTORY

- Associated symptoms vary and may include cough, chest pain, rhinorrhea, or dyspnea; anemia; failure to thrive; or there may be none.
- Distinguish the source of bleeding: nose, mouth, gastrointestinal (GI) tract versus lungs:
  - Bleeding from the nose and mouth may be associated with recurrent episodes, recent trauma, or pain at the site and is usually self-limited.
  - Bleeding from the GI tract may be associated with vomiting, history of gastritis, or abdominal pain.
  - Bleeding from the lungs may be associated with chest discomfort or sensations, shortness of breath, or coughing.
  - Blood from the GI tract is often darker and acidic, whereas blood from the airway tends to be bright red and alkaline or pink and frothy.
- Determine amount of bleeding:
  - *Massive*: >240 cc in 24 hours or >100 cc per day for several days
  - *Minor*: smaller volumes
  - Life-threatening hemoptysis is typically defined as >8 cc/kg/day
- Determine associated symptoms/conditions:
  - Familial history of pulmonary disease or bleeding disorder
  - Systemic symptoms (weight loss, may indicate tumor)
  - Exposure to environmental toxins (mold or flood-damaged homes)
  - Exposure to tuberculosis
  - Medication/drug use: cocaine, marijuana, propylthiouracil
  - Recurrent episodes of cough associated with blood-tinged sputum or hemoptysis suggests underlying bronchiectasis or chronic pulmonary infection.
  - Acute pleuritic chest pain raises the possibility of pulmonary embolism with infarction or other pleural lesion.

PHYSICAL EXAM

- Respiratory distress or hypoxemia: indicates significant ventilation–perfusion mismatch due to airspace disease, shunt due to pulmonary embolism, or acidosis due to hypovolemia from blood loss
- Pallor indicates anemia or poor perfusion.
- Pleural friction rub: may be associated with pulmonary embolism
- Loud second heart sound suggests primary pulmonary hypertension, mitral stenosis, or Eisenmenger syndrome.
- Localized wheeze over a major lobar airway suggests an intramural lesion such as hemangioma, foreign body, or carcinoma.
- Presence of a murmur over the lung fields: may suggest pulmonary arteriovenous malformation
- Clubbing: indicates the presence of underlying pulmonary disease such as cystic fibrosis, congenital cardiovascular disease, bronchiectasis, or liver disease

DIFFERENTIAL DIAGNOSIS

- Infections
  - Pneumonia
  - Pulmonary abscess
  - Tuberculosis
  - Bronchitis
- Pulmonary disease
  - Cystic fibrosis
  - Bronchiectasis
  - Foreign body aspiration
  - Arteriovenous malformation
  - Congenital lung malformation
  - Pulmonary emboli
  - Pulmonary hemosiderosis
  - Alveolar capillaritis
  - Aspiration
  - Isolated unilateral pulmonary agenesis
  - Bronchogenic cysts
- Cardiovascular disease
  - Congenital heart malformations
  - Pulmonary hypertension
- Collagen vascular disease
  - Systemic lupus erythematosus
  - Vasculitis
  - Goodpasture disease
  - ANCA-associated granulomatous vasculitis
  - Heiner syndrome
- Trauma
- Coagulation disorder
- Other
  - Munchausen syndrome
  - Pseudohemoptysis (red-colored sputum secondary to *Serratia marcescens* production of red pigment)
  - Neoplasms
  - Hemangiomas

DIAGNOSTIC TESTS & INTERPRETATION

Initial Tests (screening, lab, imaging)

- Complete blood count (CBC), reticulocyte count, and coagulation profile: may indicate the degree of blood loss or evidence of a bleeding diathesis
- Comprehensive metabolic panel (CMP): to determine hepatic and renal function, acid–base status
- Sputum for bacterial culture, Gram stain, and acid-fast bacilli
- Purified protein derivative (PPD) testing
- Drug screen: if appropriate
- Electrocardiogram: to determine presence of right ventricular hypertrophy
- Erythrocyte sedimentation rate (ESR) and C-reactive protein (CRP) can help identify the chronicity of the bleed.
- Antinuclear antibodies (ANAs), antineutrophil cytoplasmic antibody (ANCA), and anti–double stranded DNA (anti-dsDNA) can help identify an immune-mediated etiology.
- Chest radiograph, both anteroposterior and lateral
  - Can identify cavitary lesions, foreign bodies, or consolidations
  - May help localize the site of bleeding
  - Fleeting alveolar infiltrates suggest pulmonary hemorrhage.
- Computed tomography (CT)
  - Useful when chest radiographs and fiberoptic bronchoscopy are normal
  - Imaging of choice for bronchiectasis
  - Can identify an extrapulmonary source of bleeding
  - Should be performed with contrast if an arteriovenous malformation or pulmonary arterial bleed is suspected
- Ventilation–perfusion scans: helpful if a pulmonary embolism or infarct is suspected

Diagnostic Procedures/Other

- Flexible fiberoptic bronchoscopy
  - Usually performed to localize the site of bleeding; preferred over rigid bronchoscopy to identify a distal or alveolar bleed
  - If a bronchoalveolar lavage is performed; the presence of hemosiderin-laden macrophages can help identify the time of onset.
  - Hemosiderin-laden macrophages appear 48 hours after the onset of bleeding and can remain present for up to several weeks following the event.
- Rigid bronchoscopy is preferred for removal of foreign objects or masses in the proximal airway. The wide lumen provides airway stabilization and a means to ventilate the patient during the procedure.

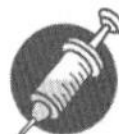

TREATMENT

GENERAL MEASURES

- Initial management is supportive and should be aimed at identifying the underlying cause.
- Blood loss should be replaced using colloidal solutions until red blood cells become available.
- Methods used to stop localized bleeding:
  - Tamponade with balloon-tipped catheter
  - Ice water lavage
  - Local instillation of epinephrine
  - Catheter-directed umbilication
  - IV vasopressin
  - Bronchial artery embolization
  - Surgical resection is usually reserved for the most difficult cases such as extensive collateralization of bronchial arteries or arteriovenous malformations unresponsive to embolization.
  - Other techniques include endoscopic instillation of fibrinogen/thrombin and endobronchial argon plasma coagulation.

MEDICATION

First Line

- Antibiotics, antifungals, or antituberculous agents should be initiated targeting the specific etiology.
- High-dose corticosteroids are often used for acute bleeds in those with autoimmune disorders or idiopathic pulmonary hemosiderosis.

Second Line

Immunosuppressive agents (e.g., azathioprine, rituximab, hydroxychloroquine, low-dose prednisone) can be used for long-term management.

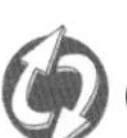

ONGOING CARE

PROGNOSIS

- Depends on the etiology and severity of hemoptysis
  - Massive hemoptysis is fatal in 50–100% of patients receiving conservative treatment.
- Immediate airway management reduces morbidity and mortality.

COMPLICATIONS

- Asphyxiation
- Hypovolemic shock
- Acute airway obstruction
- Anemia
- Pneumonia
- Death

ADDITIONAL READING

- Gaude GS. Hemoptysis in children. *Indian Pediatr.* 2010;47(3):245–254.
- Hurt K, Bilton D. Haemoptysis: diagnosis and treatment. *Acute Med.* 2012;11(1):39–45.
- Salih ZN, Akhter A, Akhter J. Specificity and sensitivity of hemosiderin-laden macrophages in routine bronchoalveolar lavage in children. *Arch Pathol Lab Med.* 2006;130(11):1684–1686.
- Susarla SC, Fan LL. Diffuse alveolar hemorrhage syndromes in children. *Curr Opin Pediatr.* 2007;19(3):314–320.

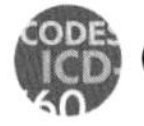

CODES

ICD10

- R04.2 Hemoptysis
- P26.9 Unsp pulmonary hemorrhage origin in the perinatal period

FAQ

- Q: What is the most common cause of hemoptysis in children?
- A: Lower respiratory tract infections are the most common cause, accounting for about 40% of all cases.
- Q: What initial steps should be taken in a stable patient who presents with hemoptysis but without a history of bronchiectasis or a tracheostomy?
- A: A physical exam should be performed to evaluate for a source of bleeding. If no source is identified, a chest radiograph looking for infiltrates should be the next step. If infiltrates are present, lab work to determine the severity of anemia and pinpoint an etiology should be sent. Some of these include a CBC with reticulocyte count, ESR, CRP, CMP, ANA, ANCA, UA, D-dimer, vWF, antiphospholipid antibodies, lupus anticoagulant, anti-GBM antibody. If no opacities are seen on the radiograph, a nasopharyngolaryngoscopy should be performed to evaluate for an upper airway bleed. Further imaging and interventions may be indicated depending on initial findings.

HENOCH-SCHÖNLEIN PURPURA

Amit Thakral, MD, MBA • Pareen Shah Thakral, MD

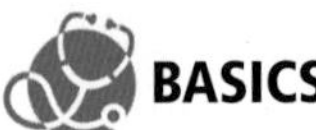

BASICS

DESCRIPTION

- Henoch-Schönlein purpura (HSP), also called immunoglobulin A vasculitis, is an immunologically mediated, purpuric, nonthrombocytopenic, and systemic vasculitis involving the small blood vessels of the skin, gastrointestinal (GI) tract, joints, and kidneys.
- Diagnosis is defined by the presence of at least two of the following classification criteria:
  - Palpable purpura (not related to thrombocytopenia)
  - Age ≤20 years at onset
  - Abdominal pain
  - Biopsy showing granulocytic infiltrates in the walls of arterioles or venules

EPIDEMIOLOGY

- One of the most common acute vasculitides in childhood
- Occurs most frequently between the ages of 3 and 15 years
- Incidence of 13.5 cases per 100,000 children per year
- Male predominance
- Seasonal variation, with most cases occurring primarily in the winter

RISK FACTORS

Genetics

Preliminary studies suggest that certain human leukocyte antigen types may be associated with an increased risk of HSP and nephritis. Patients with complement deficiencies and IgA-related disorders may be predisposed to HSP.

PATHOPHYSIOLOGY

- Predominantly an IgA-mediated immune response to antigen and operates through the alternative complement pathway
- There is a characteristic vascular deposition of IgA in affected organs.
- IgA immune deposits affect the small vessels, predominantly capillaries, arterioles, and venules.
- Studies suggest that renal injury in HSP is due to galactose-deficient IgA1 that is recognized by antiglycan antibodies, leading to the formation of circulating immune complexes and their mesangial deposition
- Renal biopsy shows proliferative glomerulonephritis with an increase in endothelial and mesangial cells, ranging from focal and segmental lesions to severe crescentic disease.

ETIOLOGY

- Genetically predisposed hosts may be susceptible to the following associations and triggers.
- Many cases are preceded by an upper respiratory tract infection (URI), particularly β-hemolytic streptococci.
- Other infectious associations include viral infections (varicella, rubella, rubeola, hepatitis A and B), *Mycoplasma pneumoniae*, *Bartonella henselae*, and *Helicobacter pylori*.
- Vaccinations, drug exposure, and insect bites have been implicated as possible triggers.

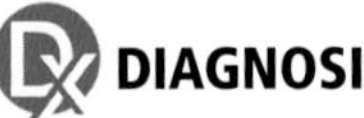

DIAGNOSIS

HISTORY

- Onset is often acute, appearing over several days to weeks.
- Recent history of illness especially URI or streptococcal infection
- Purpuric rash and joint pain are usually the presenting symptoms.
- Purpuric rash:
  - Most prominent in dependent surfaces, especially lower extremities and buttocks

ALERT

Purpuric rash can be preceded by urticarial, nodular, or maculopapular lesions.

- Arthritis or arthralgia:
  - Occurs in >50% of patients
  - Large joints are more commonly affected, although small joints may be involved.
  - Transient, sometimes migratory
  - Arthritis may precede the rash by 1 or 2 days.
- GI manifestations
  - Occurs in 2/3 of children
  - Colicky abdominal pain is the most common GI symptom.
  - Other symptoms include emesis, melena, hematemesis, and GI bleeding.
  - Currant jelly stools

ALERT

Recurrent colicky abdominal pain can suggest intussusception.

- Subcutaneous edema involving the dorsum of the hands and feet, periorbital area, forehead, and scalp
- Scrotal pain and swelling can occur.
- Presence of gross hematuria can suggest renal disease.

PHYSICAL EXAM

- Vital sign abnormalities can include low-grade fever and hypertension.
- Rash initially begins as an erythematous macular or urticarial lesions that evolve into petechiae, palpable purpura, or ecchymoses.
- Palpable purpura appear in crops and progress in color from red to purple to brown.
- Ulcerations can develop in areas of ecchymoses.
- Arthritis has characteristic findings including periarticular swelling and tenderness with considerable pain and limitation of motion. Erythema and warmth are not commonly seen.
- Abdominal pain can be periumbilical without rebound tenderness. Serial abdominal exams are essential to evaluate for progression of complications such as intussusception or GI hemorrhage.
- Subcutaneous edema is typically seen in younger children.
- Unilateral testicular or scrotal swelling can be seen with pain and tenderness. The testicular pain may mimic testicular torsion.
- Neurologic exams should be performed to evaluate for CNS involvement suggested by symptoms including headaches, seizures, or coma.
- Other rare clinical findings include ocular involvement and parotitis.

DIFFERENTIAL DIAGNOSIS

- Idiopathic thrombocytopenic purpura (ITP)
- Hemolytic uremic syndrome (HUS)
- Acute poststreptococcal glomerulonephritis
- Leukemia
- Disseminated intravascular coagulation (DIC)
- Septicemia
- Familial Mediterranean fever
- Meningococcemia
- Coagulopathies
- Rocky Mountain spotted fever
- Systemic lupus erythematosus (SLE)
- Juvenile idiopathic arthritis
- Rheumatic fever
- Granulomatosis with polyangiitis
- Polyarteritis nodosa
- Berger disease (IgA nephropathy)
- Infantile acute hemorrhagic edema

DIAGNOSTIC TESTS & INTERPRETATION

There are no diagnostic laboratory findings.

Initial Tests (screening, lab, imaging)

- CBC
  - Normal or elevated platelet count, which differentiates purpura caused by thrombocytopenia
  - Hemoglobin is typically normal. Normochromic anemia could suggest GI blood loss.
  - Moderate leukocytosis
- Prothrombin time (PT) and partial thromboplastin time (PTT) are normal.
- ESR may be elevated.
- IgA is elevated in the acute phase of illness, with a normal or increased IgM.
- C3 and C4 are typically normal. Hypocomplementemia may be seen in patients with recent poststreptococcal infections.

- Antinuclear antibody (ANA), rheumatoid factor (RF), and antineutrophil cytoplasmic autoantibodies (ANCA) are negative and usually do not need to *checked*.
- von Willebrand factor antigen is elevated due to endothelial cell damage.
- Elevated BUN, elevated creatinine, or hypoalbuminemia may suggest renal disease.
- Urinalysis
  - If abnormal, microscopic hematuria and mild proteinuria are most commonly seen.
  - RBCs, WBCs, proteinuria, and cellular casts suggest renal involvement.
  - When urine dip is abnormal, first morning urine for spot protein to creatinine ratio is helpful to more accurately evaluate proteinuria.
- Positive stool guaiac examinations are commonly seen in patients with abdominal pain.
- Consider throat swab for group A β-hemolytic streptococci.
- Abdominal radiograph may show dilated loops of bowel consistent with dilated loops of bowels.
- Abdominal ultrasound to diagnose intussusception which is typically ileoileal in HSP
- Testicular ultrasound if testicular torsion is suspected or to further evaluate for subcutaneous scrotal swelling or epididymitis

Diagnostic Procedures/Other

- Renal biopsy with severe renal involvement
- If diagnosis is unclear, consider skin biopsy with direct immunofluorescence for IgA.

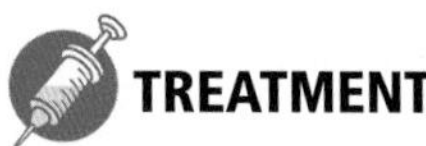

TREATMENT

MEDICATION

- HSP is generally self-limiting with supportive care including adequate oral hydration.
- Pain control with analgesics like acetaminophen
- Typically, NSAIDs should be avoided to prevent exacerbation of abdominal symptoms.
- Glucocorticoids are not typically indicated unless there are severe manifestations including severe abdominal pain, ulcerative rash, scrotal edema, or inability to walk.
- For outpatient management, consider oral prednisone.
- For patients who cannot tolerate oral medications and/or require hospitalization, consider IV methylprednisolone to increase absorption in patients with bowel inflammation.
- In some studies, oral prednisone has shown to decrease the duration of abdominal symptoms.
- Glucocorticoids should be slowly tapered per patient response to therapy.
- In patients with severe renal manifestations, consider early and aggressive glucocorticoids and immunosuppressive agents such as cyclosporine, azathioprine, and IV immunoglobulin.
- Very severely affected patients may require plasma exchange or renal transplant.
- Treat underlying hypertension if present.

ONGOING CARE

FOLLOW-UP RECOMMENDATIONS

Patient Monitoring

- Majority of patients who progress to renal involvement evolve in the first 2 months.
- Urinalysis and blood pressure and monitoring:
  - Weekly or biweekly for the first 2 months
  - Then monthly for the next 4 months (until 6 months from onset)
  - Every other month for the next 6 months (until 1 year from time of onset)

PROGNOSIS

- Excellent prognosis
- Majority of patients have resolution of symptoms within 4 weeks of onset.
- One third of patients can have recurrence of symptoms in the first 4 months from initial presentation.
- Better prognosis and shorter course in younger children
- Short-term morbidity and mortality is due to GI complications.
- Long-term morbidity and mortality is associated with nephritis.
- The development of major renal disease in the first 6 months after the onset is associated with a poor prognosis.

COMPLICATIONS

- Intussusception
- End-stage kidney disease
- Recurrence of disease
- Persistent hypertension
- Bowel perforations, ischemia, and infarctions
- GI bleeding
- Pancreatitis
- Hydrops of the gallbladder
- Protein-losing enteropathy
- Guillain-Barré syndrome
- Skin necrosis
- Pulmonary hemorrhage
- Testicular torsion and torsion of the appendix testis
- Coma

ADDITIONAL READING

- Gedalia A, Cuchacovich R. Systemic vasculitis in childhood. *Curr Rheumatol Rep*. 2009;11(6):402–409.
- Jauhola O, Ronkainen J, Koskimies O, et al. Renal manifestations of Henoch-Schonlein purpura in a 6-month prospective study of 223 children. *Arch Dis Child*. 2010;95(11):877–882.
- Peru H, Soylemezoglu O, Bakkaloglu SA, et al. Henoch Schonlein purpura in childhood: clinical analysis of 254 cases over a 3-year period. *Clin Rheumatol*. 2008;27(9):1087–1092.
- Piram M, Mahr A. Epidemiology of immunoglobulin A vasculitis (Henoch-Schönlein): current state of knowledge. *Curr Opin Rheumatol*. 2013;25(2):171–178.
- Prais D, Amir J, Nussinovitch M. Recurrent Henoch-Schönlein purpura in children. *J Clin Rheumatol*. 2007;13(1):25–28.
- Sinclair P. Henoch-Schönlein purpura—a review. *Curr Allergy Clin Immunol*. 2010;23(3):116–120.
- Watson L, Richardson AR, Holt RC, et al. Henoch Schönlein purpura—a 5-year review and proposed pathway. *PLoS One*. 2012;7(1):e29512.
- Zaffanello M, Fanos V. Treatment-based literature of Henoch-Schönlein purpura nephritis in childhood. *Pediatr Nephrol*. 2009;24(10):1901–1911.
- Zegers RH, Weigl A, Steptoe A. The death of Wolfgang Amadeus Mozart: an epidemiologic perspective. *Ann Intern Med*. 2009;151(4):274–278.

CODES

ICD10

D69.0 Allergic purpura

FAQ

- Q: When will the rash disappear?
- A: The rash may appear uncomfortable. It is generally painless and nonpruritic. Patient should have complete resolution in 4 to 6 weeks.
- Q: When should a patient with HSP be hospitalized?
- A: Patients with HSP can generally be managed in an outpatient setting. However, consider admission for the following indications: inability to tolerate oral hydration or medications, inability to ambulate, severe abdominal pain, GI bleeding, hypertension, aggressive renal involvement.
- Q: What are other names for HSP?
- A: IgA vasculitis, anaphylactoid purpura, allergic purpura, and purpura rheumatic
- Q: Did Wolfgang Amadeus Mozart (1756 to 1791) die due to HSP?
- A: Mozart's cause of death was officially listed was "*hitziges Frieselfieber*" (fever and rash). Different retrospective analyses of the circumstances, description, and timing of Mozart's death have included many theories. These theories include renal failure, trichinosis, poisoning, endocarditis, or acute nephritic syndrome caused by poststreptococcal glomerulonephritis, as well as HSP. Prior to his death, he contracted a strep infection and subsequently developed anaphylactoid purpura in his lower limbs and polyarthritis.
- Q: Who are Henoch and Schönlein?
- A: The clinical finding of joint pain associated with purpura was named "purpura rheumatica" in 1837 by Schönlein. Henoch, a student of Schönlein's, later described the association of GI tract and renal involvement. However, the first report was by Heberden in 1801.

H

HEPATOMEGALY

Sivan Kinberg, MD, MS, MA • Sarah S. Lusman, MD, PhD

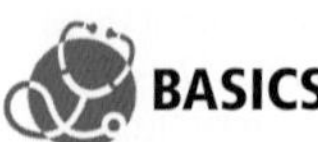

BASICS

DESCRIPTION

Hepatomegaly is enlargement of the liver beyond age-adjusted normal values. It can be due to intrinsic liver disease or associated with systemic diseases seen in infants and children.

- Normal liver size
  - Depends on age, gender, and body size
  - Average liver span is 4.5 to 5 cm (neonates), 6 to 6.5 cm (12-year-old girls), 7 to 8 cm (12-year-old boys), and up to 16 cm (adults).

RISK FACTORS

- Cardiac disease
- Metabolic disorders

PATHOPHYSIOLOGY

- Inflammation (hepatitis)
- Excessive storage
- Infiltration
- Vascular congestion
- Biliary obstruction

ETIOLOGY

- Inflammation (hepatitis)
  - Infections
    - Viral infections
      - Hepatitis types A to E
      - Epstein-Barr virus (EBV)
      - Cytomegalovirus (CMV)
      - Coxsackievirus
    - Congenital infections
    - Bacterial infections
      - Hepatic abscess
      - Tuberculosis
      - Sepsis
    - Parasitic infections
      - Amebiasis
      - Flukes
      - Schistosomiasis
      - Malaria
    - Fungal diseases
      - Candidiasis
      - Histoplasmosis
    - STDs
      - Gonococcal perihepatitis
      - Syphilis
      - HIV
    - Zoonotic diseases
      - Brucellosis
      - Leptospirosis
      - *Bartonella henselae*
      - *Pasteurella multocida*
  - Toxic, metabolic, drugs
    - Acetaminophen
    - Alcohol
    - Corticosteroids
    - Erythromycin
    - Hypervitaminosis A
    - Iron
    - Isoniazid
    - Nitrofurantoin
    - Oral contraceptives
    - Phenobarbital
    - Valproate
  - Autoimmune
    - Autoimmune hepatitis
    - Sarcoidosis
    - Systemic lupus erythematosus
- Storage disorders
  - Glycogen
    - Glycogen storage disease
    - Diabetes mellitus
    - Total parenteral nutrition (TPN)
  - Lipids
    - Wolman disease
    - Niemann-Pick disease
    - Gaucher disease
  - Fat
    - Nonalcoholic fatty liver disease
    - Cystic fibrosis
    - Fatty acid oxidation defect
    - Mucopolysaccharidoses
    - Reye syndrome
  - Iron
    - Hemochromatosis
  - Copper
    - Wilson disease
  - Abnormal proteins
    - α_1-Antitrypsin deficiency
- Infiltration
  - Tumors
    - Benign tumors
      - Hemangioma
      - Hemangioendothelioma
      - Mesenchymal hamartoma
      - Focal nodular hyperplasia
      - Adenoma
    - Malignant tumors
      - Hepatoblastoma
      - Hepatocellular carcinoma
    - Metastatic tumors
      - Leukemia
      - Lymphoma
      - Neuroblastoma
      - Wilms tumor
      - Histiocytosis
  - Cysts
    - Choledochal cysts
    - Parasitic cysts
    - Polycystic liver disease
  - Amyloidosis
  - Granulomatous disease
  - Hemophagocytic syndromes
  - Extramedullary hematopoiesis
- Vascular congestion
  - Intrahepatic
    - Veno-occlusive disease
    - Budd-Chiari syndrome (hepatic vein thrombosis)
  - Suprahepatic
    - Congestive heart failure (CHF)
    - Pericardial disease
    - Suprahepatic web
- Biliary obstruction
  - Biliary atresia
  - Alagille syndrome
  - Choledochal cyst
  - Cholelithiasis
  - Tumors
  - Primary sclerosing cholangitis

DIAGNOSIS

HISTORY

Obtain a detailed history to identify potential risk factors for liver disease and to evaluate for underlying systemic disease.

- **Question:** Prenatal history suggesting possible congenital infection or HIV infection?
- *Significance*: Infections may cause hepatomegaly.
- **Question:** Prolonged hyperbilirubinemia after 2 weeks of age?
- *Significance*: Could suggest biliary atresia, cystic fibrosis, α_1-antitrypsin deficiency
- **Question:** Developmental delay or poor growth?
- *Significance*: Could suggest a metabolic disorder
- **Question:** Age of onset?
- *Significance*: Early age could suggest congenital infection or metabolic disorder.
- **Question:** Family history of early infant death or hepatic, neurodegenerative, or psychiatric disease?
- *Significance*: Could suggest a metabolic disorder
- **Question:** Sexual activity, IV drug use, tattoo?
- *Significance*: Risk factors for hepatitis B and C infections and HIV; also consider gonococcal perihepatitis (Fitz-Hugh–Curtis syndrome) and syphilis.
- **Question:** Foreign travel?
- *Significance*: Parasitic infection or liver abscess
- **Question:** Pruritus?
- *Significance*: Can be a subtle sign of cholestasis
- **Question:** Contaminated shellfish?
- *Significance*: Source of large outbreaks of hepatitis A
- **Question:** Previous TPN?
- *Significance*: Can lead to cholestasis, bile duct proliferation, fatty infiltration, and early cirrhosis
- **Question:** Medications, supplements, and recreational drug use?
- *Significance*: Many commonly used medications can be hepatotoxic; ask about vitamin A, alcohol, and certain mushroom species.
- **Question:** Other chronic illnesses?
- *Significance*:
  - Heart disease: liver enlargement from CHF
  - Cystic fibrosis: related liver disease
  - Diabetes mellitus: increased glycogen secretion
  - Severe anemia: extramedullary hematopoiesis
  - Inflammatory bowel disease: increased likelihood of primary sclerosing cholangitis
  - Obesity: nonalcoholic fatty liver disease

PHYSICAL EXAM

Perform a careful physical exam to look for clues to etiology and for signs of chronic liver disease.

- **Finding:** Liver edge?
- *Significance*:
  - Children <2 years: can be normal up to 3.5 cm below costal margin; however, if >2 cm, further workup or referral may be indicated.
  - Children >2 years: normal up to 2 cm
  - Verify all suspected cases of hepatomegaly by checking the liver span.

- **Finding:** Signs of chronic liver disease?
- *Significance*:
  - Liver is usually firm and enlarged; can decrease in size with advanced disease
  - Splenomegaly, ascites, caput medusae, spider angiomas, esophageal varices, and hemorrhoids suggest portal hypertension.
  - Also look for signs of occult bleeding or bruising due to vitamin K deficiency.
- **Finding:** Tender liver?
- *Significance*: May indicate hepatitis or acutely congested liver secondary to right-sided heart failure or Budd-Chiari syndrome
- **Finding:** Splenomegaly?
- *Significance*:
  - In the context of chronic liver disease, implies portal hypertension
  - In the context of other signs of viral illness, suggests acute viral hepatitis
  - In the absence of these signs, suggests storage disease or malignancy
- **Finding:** Coarse facial features?
- *Significance*: Suggests mucopolysaccharidoses
- **Finding:** Kayser-Fleischer rings or cataracts?
- *Significance*: Suspect Wilson disease

DIFFERENTIAL DIAGNOSIS

- Normal anatomic variations of the liver may be confused with hepatomegaly.
  - Riedel lobe: an extended, tongue-like, right lobe of the liver
  - Beaver tail liver: Large left hepatic lobe extends laterally to contact and surround the spleen.
- Disorders that result in the liver being displaced caudally into the abdomen may result in physical findings that are mistaken for hepatomegaly.
  - Pulmonary hyperinflation
  - Right pleural effusion
  - Congenital diaphragmatic hernia
  - Subdiaphragmatic abscesses
  - Retroperitoneal mass lesions
  - Scoliosis
  - Rib cage anomalies

DIAGNOSTIC TESTS & INTERPRETATION

Initial tests: All patients with hepatomegaly should have a laboratory evaluation. History and physical exam should direct laboratory and further testing.

Initial Tests (screening, lab, imaging)

- CBC with differential
  - Thrombocytopenia may suggest portal hypertension.
- Comprehensive metabolic panel
  - Elevated aspartate aminotransferase (AST) and alanine aminotransferase (ALT) can reflect the amount of damage to hepatocytes. Elevations >1,000 IU/L indicate severe damage. ALT is more liver-specific.
  - Albumin assesses synthetic function.
  - Hyperbilirubinemia suggests cholestasis (direct hyperbilirubinemia) or hemolytic disease (indirect hyperbilirubinemia).
- Prothrombin time (PT)
  - Assesses synthetic function
  - Prolongation can occur with an acute injury or illness.
  - Can also be prolonged due to vitamin K deficiency
- γ-glutamyl transferase (GGT) and alkaline phosphatase
  - Elevation of GGT out of proportion to elevation in aminotransferases can indicate an obstructive or infiltrative process.
  - If an elevated GGT is associated with elevations in bilirubin, cholesterol, and alkaline phosphatase, an obstructive process is more likely.
- Ammonia level
  - Important to send on ice
  - Increasing ammonia levels, with prolonged PT, can suggest liver failure.
- Viral hepatitis serology
  - Hepatitis A IgM, hepatitis B surface antigen, hepatitis B surface antibody, hepatitis B core antibody, hepatitis C antibody
  - Should be obtained in patients with suggestive prodromal illness
- EBV and CMV IgM/IgG
- Monospot
  - Nonspecific heterophile antibody test for EBV infection; can be predictive in association with an elevation of atypical lymphocytes
  - High false-negative rate in children <4 years
- α-Fetoprotein and carcinoembryonic antigen
  - Tumor markers for hepatoblastoma and hepatocellular carcinoma, respectively
- "TORCH" titers
  - Consider toxoplasmosis, syphilis, rubella, CMV, and HIV.
  - Consider in newborns with hepatomegaly.
- Autoimmune markers
  - Serum immunoglobulins, antinuclear antibody, anti–smooth muscle antibody, anti-liver/kidney microsomal antibody, soluble liver antigen
- Ceruloplasmin and urinary copper excretion
  - Wilson disease: decreased ceruloplasmin and increased urinary copper excretion
  - Consider for patients with unexplained liver disease and neurologic symptoms.
- Iron, total iron-binding capacity (TIBC), ferritin
  - To assess for hemochromatosis
- α_1-Antitrypsin phenotype
  - To look for α_1-antitrypsin deficiency
  - Only send if no blood transfusion in last month
- Abdominal ultrasound with Doppler
  - Most helpful initial study
  - Perform in all patients with acholic stools, asymmetric liver enlargement or mass.
  - Can measure liver size and consistency, masses, cysts, abscesses, biliary tree abnormalities, and venous blood flow
- CT or MRI can be done for further evaluation.
- Echocardiogram to assess heart function
- Liver biopsy is often needed for definitive diagnosis.

ALERT

Indications for immediate hospitalization:
- Persistent anorexia and vomiting
- Mental status changes
- Worsening jaundice
- Relapse of symptoms after initial improvement
- Known exposure to a liver toxin
- Rising PT/INR
- Rising ammonia level
- Bilirubin >20 mg/dL
- AST >2,000 IU/L
- Development of new ascites
- Hypoglycemia
- Leukocytosis and thrombocytopenia
- Hematemesis

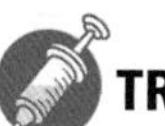

TREATMENT

Depends on underlying etiology of hepatomegaly

ALERT

Refer to gastroenterologist or hepatologist if
- Unexplained or persistent elevation of liver enzymes
- Decreased synthetic function or signs of portal hypertension

ADDITIONAL READING

- Clayton PT. Diagnosis of inherited disorders of liver metabolism. *J Inherit Metab Dis*. 2003;26(2–3):135–146.
- Clemente M, Schwarz K. Hepatitis: general principles. *Pediatr Rev*. 2011;32(8):333–340.
- Diehl-Jones WL, Askin DF. The neonatal liver part II: assessment and diagnosis of liver dysfunction. *Neonatal Netw*. 2003;22(2):7–15.
- Fishbein M, Mogren J, Mogren C, et al. Undetected hepatomegaly in obese children by primary care physicians: a pitfall in the diagnosis of pediatric nonalcoholic fatty liver disease. *Clin Pediatr (Phila)*. 2005;44(2):135–141.
- Wolf AD, Lavine JE. Hepatomegaly in neonates and children. *Pediatr Rev*. 2000;21(9):303–310.

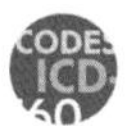

CODES

ICD10

- R16.0 Hepatomegaly, not elsewhere classified
- B19.9 Unspecified viral hepatitis without hepatic coma
- K76.1 Chronic passive congestion of liver

FAQ

- Q: Why does cholestasis cause pruritus?
- A: This phenomenon probably reflects an abnormal accumulation of bile acids in the skin.
- Q: Do patients with chronic liver disease have any different nutritional needs?
- A: Yes. Patients may have impaired fat absorption and therefore may have deficiencies of fat-soluble vitamins A, D, E, and K, which can lead to visual disturbances, rickets, pathologic fractures, neuropathy, hemolytic anemia, or bleeding. Consider supplementing the diet with medium-chain triglycerides, which are more easily absorbed.
- Q: What causes TPN-associated cholestasis?
- A: It is likely multifactorial. TPN components act as toxins; bacterial endotoxins and lack of enteral feeding also play significant roles.
- Q: How is liver span determined by physical exam?
- A: Measure the distance between the upper edge, determined by percussion, and the lower edge, determined by percussion, palpation, or auscultation in the midclavicular line. Can use the "scratch test": with the stethoscope placed below the xiphoid, the examiner should gently scratch superiorly, starting in from the right lower quadrant, and listen for sound enhancement as the finger passes over the liver edge.

HEREDITARY ANGIOEDEMA (C1 ESTERASE DEFICIENCY)

Barry J. Pelz, MD • Anna B. Fishbein, MD, MSc

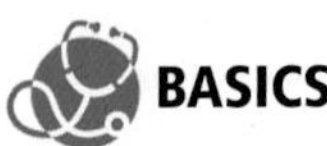

BASICS

DESCRIPTION

Hereditary angioedema (HAE) is an autosomal dominant condition characterized by recurrent, unpredictable, and potentially life-threatening swelling. The swelling results from excess production of bradykinin which is a potent vasodilator. Most commonly, this production results from a deficiency or dysfunction of C1 esterase inhibitor (C1-INH) which leads to unregulated activation of complement and plasma kinin–forming pathways and angioedema. There are three main classifications of HAE and one additional category of acquired angioedema:

- Type I HAE: deficiency of C1-INH (~85% of patients)
- Type II HAE: dysfunction of C1-INH (~15%)
- HAE with normal C1-INH (previously called type III HAE): unclear mechanism (very rare)
- Acquired angioedema, ACE inhibitor–induced angioedema, and idiopathic angioedema (These are not HAE and will be minimally discussed here.)

EPIDEMIOLOGY

- HAE type I or II
  - Prevalence between 1 in 10,000 and 1 in 150,000
  - All genders and races affected equally
  - Onset before puberty in ~50% of patients
  - Symptoms tend to worsen during puberty and persist into adulthood.
- HAE with normal C1-INH
  - Only a few families described, mostly women of childbearing age

RISK FACTORS

Genetics

- HAE type I or II
  - Autosomal dominant, high penetrance
  - 25% spontaneous mutations (may have family history negative for the disease)
  - Mutations on chromosome 11 in *SERPING1* gene which codes for C1-INH
- HAE with normal C1-INH
  - Autosomal dominant, low penetrance
  - Some patients with mutations in coagulation factor XII gene

PATHOPHYSIOLOGY

- Deficiency/dysfunction of C1-INH leads to unopposed activation of the classical complement pathway and conversion of prekallikrein to kallikrein.
- Kallikrein increases formation of bradykinin, which produces angioedema.
- Histamine and other mast cell mediators are NOT involved.

COMMONLY ASSOCIATED CONDITIONS

Mildly increased risk of autoimmunity

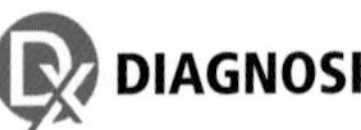

DIAGNOSIS

- Decide if symptoms consistent with HAE; if so, laboratory testing should be used to confirm the diagnosis.
- Any of the following symptoms may be present:
  - Recurrent "attacks" of angioedema worsening in first 24 hours, lasting 2 to 5 days
  - Tingling sensation as prodrome to symptoms
  - Abdominal pain (with possible nausea, vomiting, diarrhea) even without angioedema
  - Laryngeal edema (tightness in throat, dyspnea is a late sign)

HISTORY

- Ask about potential triggers of attacks: minor trauma, emotional distress, surgery, infections, stress, menstruation, and/or pregnancy.
- Explore recurrent nature of symptoms which can be intermittent or more chronic.
- Inquire about family history of angioedema.

PHYSICAL EXAM

- Angioedema, nonpruritic, nonpitting
- 30% with transient serpiginous rash, erythema marginatum, on trunk/medial extremities
- Swelling of face, lips, larynx, gastrointestinal tract, genitals, and/or extremities
- Abdominal tenderness

ALERT

Be aware of laryngeal swelling in absence of facial swelling; can be severe enough to lead to asphyxiation

DIFFERENTIAL DIAGNOSIS

- Allergic reactions and anaphylaxis:
  - IgE-mediated allergic reactions to drug, food, or stinging insects
  - Transfusion reactions
  - Idiopathic anaphylaxis
  - Exercise-induced anaphylaxis
- Drug-induced angioedema (particularly to angiotensin converting enzyme (ACE) inhibitors or NSAIDs)
- Idiopathic angioedema—typically involves urticaria and not posterior oropharynx
- Allergic contact dermatitis
- Rheumatologic diseases (low C3 + low C4)
- Superior vena cava syndrome
- Oncologic diseases such as head and neck tumors or lymphomas
- Physical urticarias such as cold-induced urticaria, cholinergic urticaria, aquagenic urticaria, solar urticaria, pressure urticaria (or angioedema), or vibratory angioedema
- Psychological or psychosomatic disorders
  - Panic attacks
  - Globus sensation
  - Vocal cord dysfunction
- Presence of C4 null alleles can cause low C4 levels.
- Improper lab processing is common, resulting in low C4.

DIAGNOSTIC TESTS & INTERPRETATION

- HAE type I or II: C4 (natural substrate for C1-INH) can be used as a screening test.
  - Will be very low or absent in at least 90% of patients with HAE even at baseline
- HAE type I
  - C1-INH antigen (protein) level will be low.
  - C1-INH function will be low (<50% of normal value) largely because the protein level is deficient.
- HAE type II
  - C1-INH function will be low (<50% of normal value) because, although present, the protein is dysfunctional.
  - Genetic testing available, not required to confirm diagnosis, helpful in children <1 year of age where complement levels usually are less than adult norms
  - Lab testing should be repeated (ideally at least 1 month later) to confirm results.
  - Labs preferably drawn during attacks but usually abnormal in-between episodes as well
  - Parents and siblings should be screened with C4 once proband diagnosis made
- HAE with normal C1-INH
  - Positive family history of angioedema
  - Normal C4, C1-INH level and function (when drawn during an attack)
  - Consider factor XII gene mutation analysis.
- Acquired angioedema
  - No family history of angioedema
  - Low C4, C1-INH level and function usually low
  - Low C1q (<50% normal)
- Imaging rarely necessary
- Abdominal CT scan or ultrasound might demonstrate bowel wall edema in abdominal attacks.

TREATMENT

GENERAL MEASURES

- Assessment and protection of the upper airway is most important in the setting of an acute attack.
- Patients may require intubation if airway patency cannot be maintained.

MEDICATION

First Line

- C1-INH replacement protein (C1INHRP). There are two types derived from purified pooled human plasma (Berinert® and Cinryze®) and a third type which is a recombinant protein derived from rabbits (Ruconest®). In addition to HAE treatment, these therapies can be used for other types of angioedema.
  - Berinert®
    - FDA-approved for acute attacks
    - IV dose suggested for ≥6 years but used for all ages: 20 U/kg or ≤50 kg = 500 U, >50 to 100 kg = 1,000 U, ≥100 kg = 1,500 U, up to 3 doses per attack
  - Cinryze® for prophylaxis
    - ≥6 years: 1,000 U IV q3–4d
- Recombinant C1-INH: Ruconest® (Rhucin®)
  - A rabbit-derived protein approved in Europe and the United States
  - ≥12 years: 50 U/kg (max dose: 4,200 U per dose) IV × 1
- Bradykinin receptor antagonist
  - Icatibant (Firazyr®)
    - ≥18 years: 30 mg SQ q6h up to 3 doses per 24 hours (studies ongoing in pediatrics)
- Recombinant plasma kallikrein inhibitor
  - Ecallantide (Kalbitor®)
    - Rare risk of anaphylaxis so needs to be given under medical observation
    - ≥12 years (limited data with efficacy and no adverse events reported in children <12 years): 30 mg SQ × 1; if attack persists, an additional dose may be administered within a 24-hour period.

Second Line

- Plasma: Solvent-/detergent-treated plasma or fresh frozen plasma (FFP) may be used in the setting of an acute attack if the above medications are not available.
- Historically, attenuated androgens such as danazol or stanozolol were used for prophylactic treatment.
- Plasmin inhibitors (β-aminocaproic acid or tranexamic acid) also were tried.
- These classes have fallen out of favor, as the landscape of treatment has dramatically changed in the past 1 to 2 decades, and they have serious side effects.
- HAE symptoms do not respond to epinephrine, corticosteroids, or antihistamines.
- Short-term prophylaxis
  - Medications may be given prior to dental procedures, intubations, or other anticipated traumas or stressors.
  - None of the therapies confer complete protection from HAE attacks, so procedures should be performed in a setting where emergency intubation can be performed.
- Long-term prophylaxis
  - May be indicated for patients who have
    - Frequent and severe attacks
    - Rapid progression of attacks
    - Poor access or response to on-demand therapy for acute attacks
    - History of intubation(s) due to HAE
    - Excessive absences from work or school
    - Significant decrease in quality of life due to HAE

ISSUES FOR REFERRAL

- Any patient with angioedema should be referred to a physician with experience managing HAE.
- An allergist/immunologist can help with the evaluation, treatment, and management of these patients.

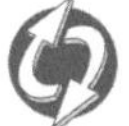

ONGOING CARE

FOLLOW-UP RECOMMENDATIONS

- Patients should be seen at least annually.
- Education should be provided to the patient and patient's family regarding the disease.
- Testing family members should be considered.
- Care should include identification and avoidance of triggers when possible and plan in the event of an acute attack.
  - Medical identification band or wallet card
  - Add emergency information to cell phone.
  - A written emergency action plan should outline treatment during an acute attack.
- Follow-up should include the following:
  - Review of triggers
  - Prospective genetic counseling
  - Review of attacks during the previous year
  - Reconsideration of the need for prophylaxis
  - Review of an emergency plan
- Increased risk for autoimmunity

PATIENT EDUCATION

- General education provided by physician
- Support groups, handouts, ID bands
- www.haea.org
- www.haei.org

PROGNOSIS

Variable. Once attacks begin, they generally persist throughout the patient's life, although the frequency and severity can change during puberty and at other times. Therapy dramatically improves attacks.

COMPLICATIONS

- Upper airway obstruction may be life-threatening and/or lead to asphyxiation.
- Severe abdominal pain may be mistaken for a surgical abdomen.
- Diagnosis may be delayed.
- Patients may be frustrated by the nature of the recurrent attacks and the significant impact on quality of life.

ADDITIONAL READING

- Frank MM, Zuraw B, Banerji A, et al. Management of children with hereditary angioedema due to C1 inhibitor deficiency. *Pediatrics*. 2016;138(5):e20160575.
- Hofman ZL, Relan A, Zeerleder S, et al. Angioedema attacks in patients with hereditary angioedema: local manifestations of a systemic activation process. *J Allergy Clin Immunol*. 2016;138(2):359–366.
- Morgan BP. Hereditary angioedema—therapies old and new. *N Engl J Med*. 2010;363(6):581–583.
- van den Elzen M, Go MF, Knulst AC, et al. Efficacy of treatment of non-hereditary angioedema [published online ahead of print September 27, 2016]. *Clin Rev Allergy Immunol*.

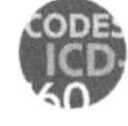

CODES

ICD10

D84.1 Defects in the complement system

FAQ

- Q: What is a good screening test for HAE?
- A: C4 is a good screening test. C1 inhibitor functional and quantitative assays are readily available from commercial labs and are the definitive tests of choice for HAE.
- Q: What is the mode of inheritance in HAE?
- A: Autosomal dominant
- Q: What is one of the most severe complications for patients with HAE?
- A: Airway angioedema can be life-threatening and may require intubation.

H

HEREDITARY SPHEROCYTOSIS

Kandace L. Gollomp, MD • Michele Puszkarczuk Lambert, MD, MSTR

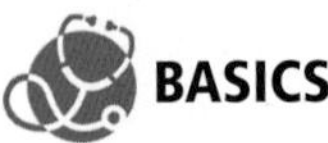

BASICS

DESCRIPTION

- Hereditary spherocytosis (HS) is the most common red blood cell (RBC) membrane disorder causing hemolytic anemia.
- Hemolytic anemia with shortened RBC lifespan due to an inherent defect in RBC membrane proteins leading to selective destruction of RBCs in the spleen
- Gradual membrane loss with preserved intracellular volume results in spherocytosis with decreased RBC deformability and increased osmotic fragility.
- Pathophysiologically related to hereditary elliptocytosis and hereditary ovalocytosis
- Severity related to degree of membrane loss
  - Mild (20% of patients)
    - Hemoglobin near normal
    - Slight reticulocytosis (<6%)
    - Compensated hemolysis, mild splenomegaly
    - Often not diagnosed until adulthood due to gallstones
  - Moderate (60% of patients)
    - Hemoglobin 8 to 12 mg/dL
    - Reticulocytes generally >6%
    - >50% patients have splenomegaly.
  - Moderately severe (10%)
    - Hemoglobin 6 to 8 mg/dL
    - Reticulocytes >10%
    - Intermittent transfusions
  - Severe (3–5%)
    - Life-threatening anemia requiring regular transfusions
    - Almost always recessive

EPIDEMIOLOGY

Most common inherited anemia in individuals of Northern European descent (~1:2,500)

RISK FACTORS

Genetics

- ~75% of cases are inherited in an autosomal dominant pattern.
- The other 25% are autosomal recessive forms, dominant disease with reduced penetrance, or new mutations.

PATHOPHYSIOLOGY

- The most common abnormality is a deficiency of ankyrin and subsequent decrease in spectrin, two major proteins of the erythrocyte membrane skeleton (50–60% Northern European descent; 5–10% Japan).
  - Spectrin deficiency alone accounts for 20% of HS.
  - Mutations in other erythrocyte surface proteins also occur, including the following:
    - β-Spectrin (typically mild to moderately severe), α-spectrin (severe HS)
    - Band 3 (15–20% generally mild to moderately severe)
    - Protein 4.2 (<5% HS, recessive and results in almost complete absence)
    - Rh antigen (<10% mild to moderate hemolytic anemia)
- The membrane skeletal defect causes RBC membrane fragility, resulting in membrane loss.
- The sequelae are as follows:
  - Loss of cell surface area relative to volume (spherocytosis) causes a decrease in cellular deformability.
  - The spleen detains and "conditions" the nondeformable spherocytic RBC.
  - Conditioning of cells involves depletion of adenosine 5′-triphosphate (ATP), increased glycolysis, increased influx and efflux of sodium, and loss of membrane lipid.
- Ultimately, these events lead to premature RBC destruction.

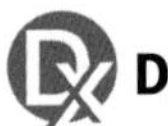

DIAGNOSIS

HISTORY

- Fatigue (symptom secondary to anemia)
- Jaundice, scleral icterus, dark urine (signs of hemolysis)
- Phototherapy required in newborn period (50% of cases): hyperbilirubinemia due to hemolysis
- Positive familial history (for disease, gallstones, or splenectomy) is significant because of autosomal dominant inheritance.

PHYSICAL EXAM

- Splenomegaly is present in a majority of older patients with HS and may worsen with intercurrent illness.
- Icterus/jaundice and pallor are present with increased hemolysis.
- Linear growth, weight gain, and sexual development may be delayed. Delayed growth is indication for splenectomy.

DIFFERENTIAL DIAGNOSIS

- Hemolysis secondary to intrinsic RBC defects
  - Membrane defects secondary to inherited disorders of membrane skeleton (HS and elliptocytosis) and RBC cation permeability and volume (stomatocytosis and xerocytosis)
  - Enzyme defects: Embden-Meyerhof pathway (i.e., pyruvate kinase deficiency) and hexose monophosphate pathway (i.e., glucose-6-phosphate dehydrogenase deficiency)
  - Hemoglobin defects
    - Congenital erythropoietic porphyria
    - Qualitative hemoglobin S (sickle cell), Hgb C, Hgb H, Hgb M
    - Quantitative: thalassemias
  - Congenital dyserythropoietic anemias
- Hemolysis secondary to extracorpuscular RBC defects
  - Immune-mediated (important in differential because spherocytes are present on smear and can give increased osmotic fragility if sent): isoimmune (e.g., hemolytic disease of the newborn, blood group incompatibility) and autoimmune (e.g., cold agglutinin disease, warm autoimmune hemolytic anemia)
  - Non–immune-mediated: idiopathic and secondary to underlying disorder (e.g., hemolytic uremic syndrome, thrombotic thrombocytopenic purpura)

ALERT

- A patient with HS may become extremely anemic during an aplastic crisis, hyperhemolysis episode, or folic acid deficiency, requiring transfusion.
- False-negative osmotic fragility tests can occur in several situations; therefore, index of suspicion must be high to follow the clinical course and repeat test (e.g., in neonatal period, during megaloblastic crisis, and recovery from aplastic crisis after transfusion when cells are youngest and least spherocytic).
- 20–25% of HS patients have normal unincubated osmotic fragility (incubated test almost always positive; therefore, it may be necessary to conduct both tests).
- Spherocytes are often present in immune-mediated hemolysis.

DIAGNOSTIC TESTS & INTERPRETATION

Initial Tests (screening, lab, imaging)

- CBC
  - Mild to moderate anemia
  - Mean corpuscular volume (MCV) usually normal
  - Mean corpuscular hemoglobin concentration (MCHC) elevated (useful screening test with high specificity)
  - Reticulocyte count may only be slightly elevated.
  - The RBC distribution width (RDW) is increased in most patients.
  - Indirect hyperbilirubinemia: present in 50–60% of cases
  - Peripheral smear: microspherocytes, polychromasia; bizarre RBC morphology with severe hemolysis
- Coombs test: negative
  - Important differential test in a patient with hemolytic anemia and spherocytes
- Urinalysis
  - Hemoglobinuria
  - Increased urobilinogen

- Special tests:
  - Osmotic fragility (most useful test in diagnosis but can be normal in 10–20% of patients)
    - Spherocytes are less resistant to osmotic stress and therefore lyse more readily than normal RBCs in saline.
    - False-negative results are common, especially in newborns whose RBCs may be more dehydrated and with high fetal hemoglobin.
    - Any anemia that results in spherocytes will give increased osmotic fragility (especially autoimmune hemolytic anemia) and must be excluded.
  - Eosin-5-maleimide (EMA) binding
    - Flow cytometric analysis with much higher sensitivity and specificity for HS
    - Reduced EMA binding to band 3 and Rh-related proteins in the RBC membrane leading to decreased fluorescent intensity
    - Now the test of choice for diagnosis but not available at all centers
  - Testing for RBC membrane protein mutations is now commercially available.

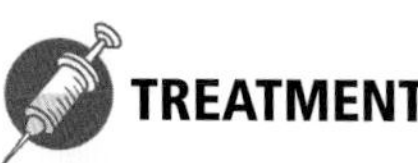

TREATMENT

GENERAL MEASURES

- Folic acid supplement
- Penicillin prophylaxis (if splenectomized)
- Pneumococcal, meningococcal, and *Haemophilus influenza* B vaccines (prior to splenectomy)

SURGERY/OTHER PROCEDURES

- Splenectomy: high response rate (most patients normalize their blood counts):
  - Indications: moderate to severe anemia with significant hemolysis resulting in transfusion dependence, decreased exercise tolerance, skeletal deformities, or delayed growth
  - Complications: risk of postsplenectomy sepsis, emerging data on increased risk of later pulmonary hypertension, and increased risk of thrombosis
- Cholecystectomy
  - Indications: symptomatic gallbladder disease; sometimes done simultaneous with splenectomy if gallstones evident by ultrasound
  - Complications: morbidity of surgical procedure and postoperative period

ONGOING CARE

- Physical exam
  - Check for splenomegaly.
  - Follow growth curves closely.
- CBC with reticulocyte count as needed: if patient develops fatigue, pallor, or increased jaundice especially in setting of viral illness
- Penicillin prophylaxis after splenectomy

PROGNOSIS

Severity of disease is extremely variable, ranging from an incidental diagnosis in adulthood to severe anemia requiring transfusions.

COMPLICATIONS

- Gallstones
  - Most common complication of HS
  - Pigment stones can lead to cholecystitis and/or biliary obstruction.
- Cholelithiasis in HS manifests in 2nd and 3rd decades of life.
- Aplastic crises
  - Can result in severe life-threatening anemia; often caused by parvovirus B19 infection
  - Epstein-Barr virus (EBV), influenza, and cytomegalovirus (CMV) can also cause worsening anemia and reticulocytopenia.
- Hyperhemolysis
  - Increased RBC destruction
  - Often precipitated by infection
- Postsplenectomy sepsis
  - Lower risk of infection if postponed until 4 to 5 years of age and immunized with pneumococcal vaccine
  - Partial splenectomy may be considered in younger children and infants with severe anemia.
  - 50–70% of sepsis caused by *Streptococcus pneumoniae*
- Folate deficiency
  - Caused by insufficient dietary intake of folic acid or increased bone marrow requirement
  - Can result in megaloblastic crisis
- Pulmonary hypertension
  - Long-term complication of splenectomy due to recurrent small vessel thrombosis in the lungs (either local clot or thromboembolic events)
  - Weighs against splenectomy in patients with mild or well-compensated disease
- Other rare complications
  - Gout
  - Indolent leg ulcers
  - Chronic erythematous dermatitis on legs

ADDITIONAL READING

- Barcellini W, Bianchi P, Fermo E, et al. Hereditary red cell membrane defects: diagnostic and clinical aspects. *Blood Transfus*. 2011;9(3):274–277.
- Bolton-Maggs PH, Stevens RF, Dodd NJ, et al; for General Haematology Task Force of the British Committee for Standards in Haematology. Guidelines for the diagnosis and management of hereditary spherocytosis. *Br J Haematol*. 2004;126(4):455–474.
- Christensen RD, Yaish HM, Gallagher PG. A pediatrician's practical guide to diagnosing and treating hereditary spherocytosis in neonates. *Pediatrics*. 2015;135(6):1107–1114.
- Da Costa L, Galimand J, Fenneteau O, et al. Hereditary spherocytosis, elliptocytosis, and other red cell membrane disorders. *Blood Rev*. 2013;27(4):167–178.
- Gallagher PG. Abnormalities of the erythrocyte membrane. *Pediatr Clin North Am*. 2013;60(6):1349–1362.
- Shah S, Vega R. Hereditary spherocytosis. *Pediatr Rev*. 2004;25(5):168–172.

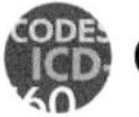

CODES

ICD10

D58.0 Hereditary spherocytosis

FAQ

- Q: Will my child require blood transfusions?
- A: It depends on the clinical severity of your child's disease.
- Q: If a parent has HS, how should the newborn be followed?
- A: The infant has a 50% chance of having HS. In infants with HS, the CBC is usually normal in the first 72 hours of life but then drops because of an inability to mount an appropriate erythropoietic response to increased destruction. Therefore, infants at risk should have a CBC with reticulocyte count after 72 hours. These infants also need to be monitored closely for hyperbilirubinemia.
- Q: What are the risks and benefits of splenectomy?
- A: Splenectomy is almost always successful in ameliorating anemia but adds the risk of postsplenectomy infections and later risks for pulmonary hypertension and possible increased risk of thrombosis and/or cardiovascular disease. The risks and benefits need to be carefully weighed and, in patients with mild, well-compensated hemolysis, splenectomy is not indicated.

HERPES SIMPLEX VIRUS

Paul K. Sue, MD, CM • W. Christopher Golden, MD

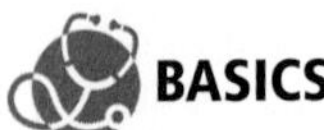

BASICS

DESCRIPTION

Herpes simplex virus (HSV) is an enveloped double-stranded DNA virus. It exists as two distinct subtypes, HSV-1 and HSV-2, and is responsible for a wide spectrum of illness ranging from fever blisters to genital ulcers and fatal encephalitis. It establishes lifelong latency and can lead to interval episodes of asymptomatic shedding and disease recurrence.

EPIDEMIOLOGY

- HSV-1 infects 40–80% of the U.S. population by young adulthood.
- HSV-2 incidence increases during adolescence and adulthood, infecting 20–35% of U.S. adults by age 40 years.
- In the United States, approximately 1,500 cases of neonatal HSV (1:3,200 live births) occur every year, primarily due to HSV-2.
- Following the neonatal period, HSV-1 infections predominate among children.

GENERAL PREVENTION

- Perinatal infection
  - The majority of neonatal HSV infections (85%) occur through contact with maternal HSV shed within the birth canal. A smaller proportion (5%) of infections occur in utero.
  - The majority (60–80%) of mothers of infected infants have no symptoms of HSV infection at the time of delivery.
  - Children born to mothers with primary genital HSV infection at time of delivery are at highest risk (up to 60%). In contrast, the risk of neonatal infection with recurrent maternal genital herpes is significantly lower (2–5%).
  - In the setting of active genital herpes (lesions or pain), cesarean delivery is recommended, preferably within 4 hours of rupture of membranes. However, infections may still occur despite cesarean delivery and intact amniotic membranes.
  - Cesarean delivery is not recommended for mothers with a history of genital HSV in the absence of lesions or symptoms.
  - Fetal scalp monitors should be avoided in women with suspected genital HSV.
  - The use of antiviral therapy (acyclovir or valacyclovir) after 36 weeks' gestation decreases viral shedding and reactivation of genital lesions in mothers with a history of genital HSV, although breakthrough infections may still occur.
- Postnatal infection (neonates and children)
  - Secretions of active HSV lesions are highly infectious, and asymptomatic viral shedding is common. 10% of neonatal HSV infections are contracted postpartum through direct contact with infectious fluids.
  - Standard universal precautions are appropriate in caring for recurrent/localized lesions in immunocompetent persons.
  - Contact precautions should be considered in neonates, immunocompromised persons with active lesions, and in severe primary mucocutaneous HSV.
  - Contact with genital/cutaneous HSV lesions (e.g., sexual intercourse, wrestling) should be avoided until lesions resolve.

PATHOPHYSIOLOGY

- Spread occurs typically via contact with abraded skin or mucous membranes.
- The incubation period for primary infection is approximately 2 to 12 days.
- Viral replication begins at the portal of entry (epithelia) and commences within sensory ganglia. Migration occurs back to the site of inoculation, with subsequent destruction of epithelial cells.
- Following initial infection, the virus remains latent in sensory neural ganglia and can be reactivated by UV exposure, trauma, stress, hormonal changes, or immunosuppression.
- Viral dissemination occurs most often in neonates, pregnant women, or immunosuppressed patients.
- HSV antibodies provide a degree of cross protection across serotypes; previous infection with one HSV serotype (e.g., HSV-1) can decrease the severity of infection with the alternate serotype (e.g., HSV-2).
- HSV antiviral resistance is rare among healthy individuals but can develop in immunocompromised hosts and in the setting of herpetic keratitis.

RISK FACTORS

- Risk factors for HSV-1 and HSV-2 infection include older age and lower socioeconomic status.
- Additional risk factors for HSV-2 include number of lifetime sexual partners and female gender.

COMMONLY ASSOCIATED CONDITIONS

- Gingivostomatitis
- Encephalitis
- Herpes gladiatorum
- Herpetic whitlow
- Eczema herpeticum
- Erythema multiforme

DIAGNOSIS

- The majority of primary HSV infections are asymptomatic in healthy individuals.
- Infections "above the waist" are classically due to HSV-1, whereas HSV-2 most commonly causes genital infection. However, both serotypes can cause genital and/or mucocutaneous infection.
- Recurrent infections, due to reactivation of latent virus, usually are less severe than primary infections.
- Neonatal infection
  - Neonates may present with classic skin lesions or with nonspecific findings of irritability, fever, temperature instability, and poor feeding with or without a rash.
  - Skin, eye, and/or mouth (SEM) disease (40–45% of neonatal HSV) presents in the 1st to 2nd week of life with rash, chorioretinitis, or keratitis. Roughly 85% of patients have visible skin lesions.
  - Disseminated neonatal HSV disease (25% of neonatal HSV) presents with a sepsis-like syndrome in the 1st to 2nd week of life, commonly involving the lungs, liver, adrenals, and the central nervous system (CNS). Approximately 60% have visible skin lesions.
  - HSV CNS disease (30–35% of neonatal HSV) usually presents in the 2nd to 3rd week of life with seizures, fever, and/or temperature instability.
- Oropharyngeal infection
  - Primary infection is characterized by fever, irritability, and severe pain/burning of the oral mucosa, with vesicular and ulcerative lesions on the lips, gingiva, and tongue.
  - Pharyngitis is also common in older children and adolescents.
  - Illness lasts for 2 to 3 weeks, with viral shedding continuing for several weeks.
- Genital infection
  - Infection is characterized by genital pain and itching, associated with tender inguinal adenopathy, fever, malaise, and rash.
  - Lesions begin as vesicles and progress to ulcers before crusting over by 2 to 3 weeks.
- Keratoconjunctivitis (ocular infection)
  - Presents as unilateral or bilateral conjunctivitis with preauricular adenopathy, associated eyelid edema, photophobia, tearing, and/or chemosis
- Eczema herpeticum
  - Infection is characterized by vesiculopustular eruption along with fever, malaise, and lymphadenopathy in the setting of preexisting eczema or other dermatitis.
- Encephalitis (CNS infection)
  - Infection is characterized by fever, headache, altered mental status, focal neurologic symptoms, and seizures.
- Disseminated HSV infection
  - Infection presents with fever or temperature instability and a sepsis-like syndrome with end-organ involvement (e.g., lungs, liver).
  - Neonates, pregnant women, transplant recipients, and other immunocompromised hosts are at increased risk for disseminated infection.

PHYSICAL EXAM

- The "classic" HSV rash consists of vesicles on an erythematous base, which subsequently ulcerate, become friable, and bleed easily.
- Lesions may not be readily apparent, particularly in cases of disseminated disease and CNS infection.

DIFFERENTIAL DIAGNOSIS

- Neonatal HSV disease should be distinguished from severe enteroviral and bacterial sepsis, especially in the first 4 to 6 weeks of life.
- Intrauterine HSV should be considered in newborns born with microcephaly, intracranial calcifications, chorioretinitis, hepatosplenomegaly, and/or skin lesions and must be distinguished from other congenital viral infections (such as cytomegalovirus [CMV] and rubella).
- Oropharyngeal HSV should be distinguished from enteroviral (e.g., coxsackie) herpangina.
- Genital HSV should be distinguished from chancroid and syphilis. Syphilis lesions are usually nonpainful, indurated ulcers. Chancroid lesions are painful, purulent ulcers due to *Haemophilus ducreyi* infection.
- Ocular HSV should be distinguished from other infectious causes of conjunctivitis (adenovirus, *Haemophilus influenzae*, *Staphylococcus aureus*, *Streptococcus pneumoniae*) and rheumatologic or traumatic etiologies.

DIAGNOSTIC TESTS & INTERPRETATION

- Neonatal infection
  - Newborn conjunctival, oropharyngeal, nasal, and rectal samples should be sent for viral culture approximately 24 hours after birth (sooner if suspicious lesions are present).
  - Suspicious vesicles should be unroofed and the vesicle base thoroughly swabbed for viral culture.
  - Cerebrospinal fluid (CSF) should be sent for cell count, differential, chemistries, and HSV-polymerase chain reaction (PCR), in addition to evaluation (blood, urine, CSF) for bacterial and other viral infections.
  - Repeat HSV CSF PCR testing may be required, as false negatives of the CSF can occur early in the disease course.

– HSV blood PCR (where available) and liver function tests (specifically alanine aminotransferase [ALT]) should be sent in cases of suspected disseminated HSV.
– Additional testing (ophthalmoscopy, electroencephalogram [EEG], CNS imaging [MRI], chest radiograph) is recommended in cases of disseminated, CNS, or ophthalmologic disease.
– In asymptomatic neonates of women with genital lesions, maternal serologic status should be used to assess the risk of neonatal herpes and should, along with clinical findings, guide subsequent testing and therapy.

- Oropharyngeal HSV infection is typically diagnosed based on history and clinical exam. Viral culture and polymerase chain reaction (PCR) are recommended to test questionable lesions.
- Genital herpes lesions should be diagnosed using both viral culture and HSV PCR, as the sensitivity of viral culture alone may be as low as 27% in genital ulcers and recurrent lesions.
- Encephalitis
  – CSF PCR is the diagnostic test of choice. Samples should be sent to a reliable laboratory with a low rate of false-positive results.
  – In HSV encephalitis, CSF analysis reveals a lymphocytic, progressive pleocytosis (average 100 WBCs/mm^3) and rising protein (median 80 mg/dL), although these may be normal in 5–10% of early disease.
  – EEG can reveal a characteristic pattern of periodic unilateral or bilateral focal spikes.
  – MRI of the brain in neonates may show temporal lobe enhancement, deep gray matter involvement, and ischemic changes in watershed distribution areas.
- HSV keratoconjunctivitis
  – Ophthalmology referral is recommended.
  – Characteristic dendritic corneal ulcerations with linear branching pattern are observed on slit-lamp examination.
  – Viral culture and HSV PCR are highly sensitive but often unnecessary.
- Disseminated HSV
  – HSV serum PCR is useful in detecting viremia in disseminated infection.
  – CNS involvement is noted in up to 70% of cases.
- Novel multiplex CSF PCR assays may be used for the diagnosis of HSV infection, although clinical data in use in children is limited.

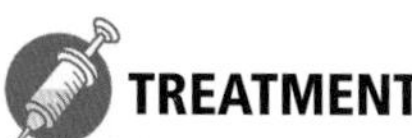

TREATMENT

MEDICATION

- Neonatal disease
  – IV acyclovir (20 mg/kg/dose every 8 hours). The recommended minimum duration of therapy is 14 days (if the disease is limited to the skin, eye, and mouth) or 21 days (for encephalitis or disseminated disease).
  – Newborns with ocular HSV should also receive topical antiviral therapy (trifluridine 1%) in addition to parenteral therapy.
  – Neonates with HSV infection (without proven disease), should receive IV acyclovir (20 mg/kg/dose every 8 hours) for 10 days.
  – Acyclovir prophylaxis (300 mg/m^2/dose orally 3 times per day) for 6 months following initial treatment improves infant neurodevelopmental outcomes and prevents recurrent skin outbreaks.
- Oropharyngeal herpes
  – Symptomatic treatment with antipyretics and analgesia is recommended. IV hydration is sometimes needed in cases of decreased oral intake.
  – Oral acyclovir (15 mg/kg/dose 5 times per day for 7 to 10 days; max 200 mg per dose) may decrease the duration of illness if started within 72 hours at the onset of symptoms.
- Genital herpes
  – Patients ~12 years old with primary genital HSV infection should receive oral acyclovir (400 mg/dose 3 times per day), valacyclovir (1 g/dose twice per day), or famciclovir (250 mg/dose 3 times per day) for 7 to 10 days or until resolution of lesions, whichever is longer. Topical therapy is not recommended.
  – Early treatment of recurrent herpes lesions (within 24 hours) with short-course acyclovir, valacyclovir, or famciclovir can reduce symptom severity and duration.
  – Suppressive oral therapy with acyclovir (400 mg/dose twice per day) or valacyclovir (500 to 1,000 mg once daily) has been shown to reduce recurrence of genital HSV. Patients should be reassessed after 1 year of therapy to determine if ongoing suppression is needed.
  – Suppressive therapy (valacyclovir [500 mg/dose twice per day] or acyclovir [400 mg/dose 3 times per day]) should be offered to pregnant women with a history of genital herpes from 36 weeks' gestation to delivery.
- Encephalitis
  – IV acyclovir (15 to 20 mg/kg/dose every 8 hours if <12 years old, otherwise 10 mg/kg/dose every 8 hours) for 14 to 21 days is recommended for treatment of HSV encephalitis.
- HSV keratoconjunctivitis
  – Topical antiviral therapy: trifluridine 1% (every 2 hours while awake; max 9 drops/24 h), ganciclovir ophthalmic gel 0.15% (every 3 hours while awake), until resolution of lesions
  – Oral acyclovir (100 to 400 mg/dose, 3 times per day; max child dose: 80 mg/kg/24 h) may be considered if topical therapy is not feasible. Oral suppression may be necessary to prevent recurrences.
- Immunocompromised patients and severe cutaneous disease (e.g., eczema herpeticum)
  – HSV lesions should be treated with oral acyclovir 200 mg/dose 5 times per day (patients 2 years old; max child dose: 80 mg/kg/24 h) OR IV acyclovir (750 to 1,500 mg/m^2/24 h divided every 8 hours) for 7 to 14 days.
  – IV acyclovir should be considered initially in patients who are immunocompromised, have severe disease (e.g., eczema herpeticum), or cannot tolerate oral therapy.
- Acyclovir-resistant HSV should be suspected if lesions persist despite 7 to 10 days of antiviral therapy
  – Viral culture should be sent for resistance testing, particularly in the immunocompromised host.
  – Acyclovir-resistant HSV can be treated with IV foscarnet (40 to 80 mg/kg per dose every 8 hours), or IV cidofovir (5 mg/kg per dose once weekly), for 7 to 14 days or until clinical resolution. Imoquod (2.5%-5% cream applied once daily) can also be used for topical disease.

ALERT

- Use of acyclovir in therapeutic and suppressive doses has been associated with neutropenia in infants. Monitoring of the patient's absolute neutrophil count (ANC) is recommended.
- Common side effects of acyclovir therapy in children include diarrhea, nausea, and headache. Rare, but serious side effects of acyclovir therapy may include acute renal failure, hemolytic uremic syndrome, and thrombotic thrombocytopenic purpura.
- Foscarnet and cidofovir use are associated with renal impairment in the majority of individuals. Close monitoring of renal function (creatinine) is necessary, and may require dose adjustment.

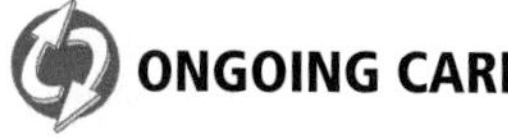

ONGOING CARE

PROGNOSIS

- Despite antiviral therapy, mortality is approximately 30% among infants with disseminated HSV disease.
- Among neonates with encephalitis, mortality is around 5% with treatment, although 70% will have neurodevelopmental sequelae.
- HSV encephalitis mortality outside the neonatal period is 70% without therapy. With treatment, mortality declines to 19%, with 38% of patients returning back to normal neurologic function.
- Herpes simplex keratoconjunctivitis frequently recurs, leading to corneal ulceration and permanent scarring.

COMPLICATIONS

Major morbidities in survivors of HSV disease include neurodevelopmental abnormalities, seizures, visual impairment, and other neurologic dysfunction.

ADDITIONAL READING

- American Academy of Pediatrics. Herpes simplex. In: Kimberlin DW, Brady MT, Jackson MA, et al, eds. *Red Book: 2015 Report of the Committee on Infectious Diseases*. 30th ed. Elk Grove Village, IL: American Academy of Pediatrics; 2015:432–444.
- Corey L, Wald A. Maternal and neonatal herpes simplex virus infections. *N Engl J Med*. 2009;361(14): 1376–1385.
- Kimberlin DW, Whitley RJ, Wan W, et al; for National Institute of Allergy and Infectious Diseases Collaborative Antiviral Study Group. Oral acyclovir suppression and neurodevelopmental after neonatal herpes. *N Engl J Med*. 2011;365(14):1284–1292.
- Liu S, Pavan-Langston D, Colby KA. Pediatric herpes simplex of the anterior segment: characteristics, treatment, and outcomes. *Ophthalmology*. 2012;119(10):2003–2008.
- Pinninti SG, Angara R, Feja KN, et al. Neonatal herpes disease following maternal antenatal antiviral suppressive therapy: a multicenter case series. *J Pediatr*. 2012;161(1):134–138.e3.
- Pinninti S, Kimberlin D. Maternal and neonatal herpes simplex virus infections. *Am J Perinatol*. 2013;30(2):113–119.
- Piret J, Boivin G. Antiviral resistance in herpes simplex virus and varicella-zoster infections: diagnosis and management. *Curr Opin Infect Dis*. 2016;29(6):654–662.
- Vossough A, Zimmerman RA, Bilaniuk LT, et al. Imaging findings of neonatal herpes simplex virus type 2 encephalitis. *Neuroradiology*. 2008;50(4):355–366.
- Workowski KA, Bolan GA; for Centers for Disease Control and Prevention. Sexually transmitted diseases treatment guidelines, 2015. *MMWR Recomm Rep*. 2015;64(RR-03):1–137.

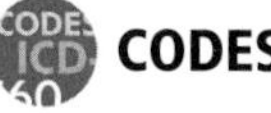

CODES

ICD10

- B00.9 Herpesviral infection, unspecified
- A60.00 Herpesviral infection of urogenital system, unspecified
- B00.1 Herpesviral vesicular dermatitis

HICCUPS (SINGULTUS)

Bethany Woomer, MD • Bradley J. Monash, MD

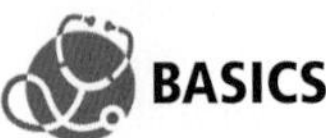

BASICS

DESCRIPTION

- The hiccup (or hiccough) is an onomatopoeic name stemming from the sound made by the abrupt glottic closure following involuntary contraction of the diaphragm and intercostal muscles.
- The medical term for hiccup is singultus, which stems from the Latin *singult*, originally used to describe the sharp intake of breath associated with prolonged sobbing.
- Usually a benign, yet recurrent nuisance
- Prolonged bouts of hiccups can be indicative of an underlying or serious condition.

EPIDEMIOLOGY

- Fetal hiccups are common in pregnancy and are frequently felt in the third trimester.
- Hiccups are a physiologic movement in newborns, who may spend as much as 2.5% of their time hiccupping, which decreases in infancy.
- There is no seasonal, geographic, racial, or socioeconomic predilection.
- Persistent (>48 hours) and intractable (>1 month) hiccups more commonly occur in men and adults.

GENERAL PREVENTION

Avoid precipitating factors (e.g., eating rapidly, carbonated beverages, alcohol, tobacco).

PATHOPHYSIOLOGY

- A hiccup reflex arc has been elucidated through the study of pathologic hiccups.
  - Afferent limb: receptors in the distal esophagus, stomach, and abdominal side of the diaphragm; signals travel through the phrenic nerve, vagus, and sympathetic (T6–T12) chain branches.
  - Central component: the middle and dorsolateral medulla; independent from the respiratory center, the hypothalamus, and the phrenic nerve nuclei
  - Efferent limb: phrenic nerve to the diaphragm; accessory nerves to the intercostal and scalene muscles, glottis structures, and the esophagus
- Hiccups are often unilateral, involving the left hemidiaphragm.

ETIOLOGY

- Environmental
  - Associated with a change in the ambient or internal temperature
  - Examples: cold showers, hot/cold beverages
- Central nervous system
  - Examples: neuromyelitis optica, migraine aura, brainstem lesion, hydrocephalus, VP shunt, meningitis, brain abscess
- Peripheral nervous system
  - Due to irritation or stimulation of phrenic or vagal nerves
  - GI: aerophagia, gastric insufflation, Gastroesophageal reflux disease (GERD), GI malignancies
  - Thoracic: asthma, goiter, pneumonia
  - CV: pericarditis, pericardial effusion, central catheter migration
- Toxic-metabolic
  - Examples: alcohol, tobacco, uremia, electrolyte imbalance, thrush
- Psychogenic
  - Examples: excitement, stress, conversion disorder, anorexia nervosa, secondary gain
- Medications
  - Examples: opioid, benzodiazepines, chemotherapy, anesthetic agents

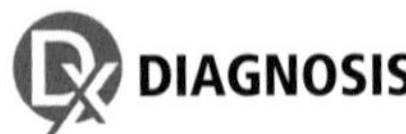

DIAGNOSIS

HISTORY

- Hiccups are typically discernible by their classic appearance.
- Ascertain the onset, duration, potential triggers, and any adverse sequelae of hiccups.
- Obtain a complete medical and surgical history, including a thorough review of systems.
- Inquire about prescription and nonprescription medications, tobacco, alcohol, and illicit drug use.
- Screen for anxiety, depression, and other psychiatric disorders.
- Hiccups persisting during sleep signal an organic cause.

PHYSICAL EXAM

- Head and neck exam may reveal evidence of trauma, foreign body in the ear canal, nuchal rigidity, lymphadenopathy, or goiter.
- Assess the chest for evidence of pneumonia, bronchitis, or pericarditis.
- Examine the abdomen for evidence of an inflammatory process or masses.
- Perform detailed neurologic examination, including cranial nerve assessment.

DIFFERENTIAL DIAGNOSIS

Hiccups present uniquely and are not often mistaken for another entity.

DIAGNOSTIC TESTS & INTERPRETATION

Hiccup bouts are common and do not routinely require extensive investigations. The history and physical examination will often identify the etiology.

ALERT

Persistent (>48 hours) and intractable (>1 month) hiccups require a thorough evaluation.

Initial Tests (screening, lab, imaging)

- CBC
- Electrolytes (e.g., Na, K, Ca)
- Glucose
- Renal function (BUN and Cr)
- Liver function tests, amylase/lipase
- Toxicology screen
- Additional testing should be guided by the patient's history, physical examination, and laboratory findings:
  - Chest radiograph to evaluate for pulmonary, cardiac, and mediastinal abnormalities
  - Chest or abdominal ultrasound or other advanced imaging (e.g., CT, MRI) to assess for occult tumor, infection, or other pathology
  - EKG to assess for pericarditis or ischemia
  - EGD or esophageal manometry if patient has dysphagia or other esophageal symptoms
  - Brain MRI +/− LP to assess for tumor, CNS lesions, stroke, or infection

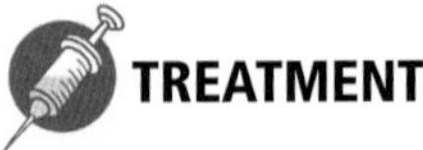

TREATMENT

GENERAL MEASURES

- Treat the underlying cause if identified (e.g., discontinue potential culprit medication).
- Physical maneuvers often serve as the 1st-line treatment for hiccups. Consider potential harmful effects prior to trying any intervention:
  - Interruption of normal respiratory function: sneezing, coughing, breath-holding
  - Disruption of phrenic nerve transmission: tapping over the 5th cervical vertebra, ice applied to the skin over the area of the phrenic nerve
  - Nasopharyngeal or uvula stimulation: traction on the tongue, stimulating the pharynx with a cotton swab, lifting the uvula with a spoon, sipping ice water, gargling, swallowing a teaspoon of granulated sugar
  - Increased vagal stimulation: applying a bag of ice to the face; Valsalva maneuver
  - Combining physical maneuvers (e.g., plugging both ears tightly, pushing both right and left tragus, while drinking a glass of water through a straw without pause and without releasing the pressure over the ears)

MEDICATION

- Pharmaceutical intervention is rarely recommended for children and should be reserved for severe or refractory cases.
- There are limited high-quality data supporting any particular medication or intervention for hiccups. Most treatments stem from case series and case reports, primarily involving adult patients. A recent Cochrane review found insufficient evidence to recommend any particular treatment for hiccups.
- When trialed, medications should target the underlying cause if possible:
  - Chlorpromazine is the only FDA-approved intervention for hiccups in adults and can be given in low doses PO or IV if no response.

- A variety of other medications have been used. Careful attention should be paid to the potential adverse effects of a medication prior to initiating pharmacotherapy:
  - Muscle relaxants: baclofen, cyclobenzaprine
  - Anticonvulsants: gabapentin, phenytoin, valproic acid, carbamazepine
  - Promotility: metoclopramide
  - Antipsychotics: chlorpromazine, haloperidol, olanzapine
  - CNS stimulants: methylphenidate
  - Antiarrhythmics: quinidine sulfate
  - Antidepressants: sertraline, amitriptyline
  - Anesthetics: nebulized, oral, and IV lidocaine; dexmedetomidine
  - Antihypertensives: nifedipine, nimodipine, carvedilol
  - Other: amantadine
- For refractory cases, combination therapy has been used.

SURGERY/OTHER PROCEDURES

- Surgical treatment is rarely performed.
- Success has been reported with phrenic nerve blockade, percutaneous phrenic nerve pacing, vagus nerve stimulation, and short-term positive pressure ventilation but mostly in adults and in those with underlying chronic illnesses.

COMPLEMENTARY & ALTERNATIVE THERAPIES

- Acupuncture
- Behavioral modification
- Hypnosis
- Suboccipital release

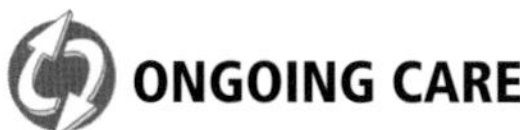

ONGOING CARE

FOLLOW-UP RECOMMENDATIONS

- Frequency of follow-up depends on the underlying etiology of the hiccups.
- Patients should be monitored for adverse effects of any medications trialed.
- Successful interventions can usually be stopped the day after hiccups subside.
- If a medication is ineffective after 7 to 10 days, an alternative treatment should be considered.

PROGNOSIS

- Usually self-limited and resolve within hours
- Persistent (>48 hours) and intractable (>1 month) hiccups may indicate underlying disease and may lead to complications.

COMPLICATIONS

- Adverse effects that have been associated with intractable hiccups:
  - Vomiting
  - Malnutrition and dehydration
  - Insomnia
  - Fatigue
  - Psychological distress
- Rare complications:
  - Reflux esophagitis
  - Wound dehiscence
  - Pulmonary edema
  - Cardiac dysrhythmia
  - Death

ADDITIONAL READING

- Becker D. Nausea, vomiting, and hiccups: a review of mechanisms and treatment. *Anesth Prog*. 2010;57(4):150–157.
- Buyukhatipoglu H, Sezen Y, Yildiz A, et al. Hiccups as a sign of chronic myocardial ischemia. *South Med J*. 2010;103(11):1184–1185.
- Caloro M, Pucci D, Calabrò G, et al. Development of hiccup in male patients hospitalized in a psychiatric ward: is it specifically related to the aripiprazole-benzodiazepine combination? *Clin Neuropharmacol*. 2016;39(2):67–72.
- Chang FY, Lu CL. Hiccup: mystery, nature and treatment. *J Neurogastroenterol Motil*. 2012;18(2):123–130.
- Chaudhry P, Friedman DI. Hiccups as a migraine aura. *Cephalalgia*. 2015;35(9):831–834.
- El-Tahan MR, Doyle DJ, Telmesani L, et al. Dexmedetomidine suppresses intractable hiccup during anesthesia for cochlear implantation. *J Clin Anesth*. 2016;31:208–211.
- Hantoushzadeh S, Sheikh M, Shariat M, et al. Maternal perception of fetal movement type: the effect of gestational age and maternal factors. *J Matern Fetal Neonatal Med*. 2015;28(6):713–717.
- Howes D. Hiccups: a new explanation for the mysterious reflex. *Bioessays*. 2012;34(6):451–453.
- Kremer L, Mealy M, Jacob A, et al. Brainstem manifestations in neuromyelitis optica: a multicenter study of 258 patients. *Mult Scler*. 2014;20(7):843–847.
- Lierz P, Felleiter P. Anesthesia as therapy for persistent hiccups. *Anesth Analg*. 2002;95(2):494–495.
- Moretto EN, Wee B, Wiffen PJ, et al. Interventions for treating persistent and intractable hiccups in adults. *Cochrane Database Syst Rev*. 2013;(1):CD008768.
- Orivoli S, Facini C, Pisani F. Paroxysmal nonepileptic motor phenomena in newborn. *Brain Dev*. 2015;37(9):833–839.
- Pearce JMS. A note on hiccups. *J Neurol Neurosurg Psychiatry*. 2003;74(8):1070.
- Petroianu G, Hein G, Stegmeier-Petroianu A, et al. Gabapentin "add-on therapy" for idiopathic chronic hiccup (ICH). *J Clin Gastroenterol*. 2000;30(3):321–324.
- Rizzo C, Vitale C, Montagnini M. Management of intractable hiccups: an illustrative case and review. *Am J Hosp Palliat Care*. 2014;31(2):220–224.
- Roberts H. Bloodletting and miraculous cures. *BMJ*. 2006;333:1127.
- Takahashi T, Miyazawa I, Misu T, et al. Intractable hiccup and nausea in neuromyelitis optica with anti-aquaporin-4 antibody: a herald of acute exacerbations. *J Neurol Neurosurg Psychiatry*. 2008;79(9):1075–1078.
- Tanaka Y, Koga Y, Takada H. Pilocytic astrocytoma at the medulla oblongata dorsal surface presenting as intractable hiccups. *Pediatr Neurol*. 2015;52(2):254–255.
- Viera AJ, Sullivan SA. Remedies for prolonged hiccups. *Am Fam Physician*. 2001;63(9):1684, 1686.
- Wilcox SK, Garry A, Johnson MJ. Novel use of amantadine: to treat hiccups. *J Pain Symptom Manage*. 2009;38(3):460–465.
- Woelk CJ. Managing hiccups. *Can Fam Physician*. 2011;57(6):672–675.

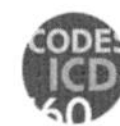

CODES

ICD10

- R06.6 Hiccough
- F45.8 Other somatoform disorders

FAQ

- Q: Why do we hiccup?
- A: The true physiologic function is unknown, although hiccups have recently been postulated as a mechanism to remove air from the stomachs of young suckling mammals. Despite extensive activation of the muscles of respiration, hiccups serve no known respiratory function.
- Q: How good is the evidence supporting the treatment of hiccups?
- A: Most treatments are based on observational studies, case reports, and small case series involving adults. A recent Cochrane review found insufficient evidence to recommend any particular treatment for hiccups.
- Q: Does rebreathing into a paper bag work?
- A: As a fall in P_{CO_2} may increase the frequency of hiccups, rebreathing air may increase P_{CO_2} and thus terminate hiccups. However, this intervention runs the risk of causing hypoxia.
- Q: Will hiccups harm my baby?
- A: Hiccups are usually harmless and are very common in babies. They can be caused by a variety of stimuli, including the swallowing of air or exposure to cold. If they are persistent, intractable, or disrupt sleep, they may lead to adverse effects and warrant an evaluation.

H

HIRSCHSPRUNG DISEASE

Lusine Ambartsumyan, MD

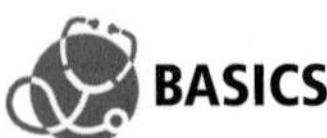

BASICS

DESCRIPTION

- Congenital motor disorder of the gut characterized by lack of ganglion cells in the distal bowel beginning at the anal verge and extending proximally to varying lengths
- Lack of internal anal sphincter (IAS) relaxation and failure of relaxation of the aganglionic segment during peristalsis, producing a functional obstruction

EPIDEMIOLOGY

Incidence

- Most common cause of lower intestinal obstruction in neonates: 1 in 5,000 births
- Involves the rectum and sigmoid in 75%, descending colon in 14%, total colon in 8%, and small bowel in 3%
- There is familial incidence in total colonic (15–21%) and total intestinal aganglionosis (50%).

Prevalence

- Male predominance with short segment disease ranging from 3:1 to 4:1
- Gender predominance <1:1 in long segment disease.
- Syndromic and nonsyndromic Hirschsprung disease (HD): In the former, there are other congenital anomalies (30% of cases), whereas in the latter, it occurs as an isolated trait.

RISK FACTORS

Genetics

- Genes associated with HD: *RET, GDNF, NRTN, SOX10, EDNRB, EDN3, ECE1, ZFHX1B, PHOX2B, KIAA1279, TCF4*
- *RET* proto-oncogene is the major susceptibility gene; mutations of *RET* account for 1/2 of familial and 1/3 of sporadic cases.
- ~5% of patients with HD have mutations in endothelin signaling pathways.

PATHOPHYSIOLOGY

- Defects in and failure of caudal migration of the neural crest cells result in congenital absence of distal enteric nervous system (ENS).
- Basic histologic findings are the absence of ganglion cells in the Meissner and Auerbach plexuses as well as hypertrophied nerve bundles between the circular and the longitudinal muscles and in the submucosa.

COMMONLY ASSOCIATED CONDITIONS

- Isolated trait in 70% (nonsyndromic HD)
- Associated malformations in 30% (syndromic HD)
  - Chromosomal abnormalities (12%): The most common is trisomy 21 (2–10% of trisomy 21 have HD).
  - Congenital birth anomalies (18%): cardiac, limb, sensorineural deafness, central nervous system, genitourinary, and gastrointestinal malformations (anal stenosis, imperforate anus, and small/large bowel atresias)
- Syndromes associated with HD:
  - Waardenburg syndrome type 4
  - Congenital central hypoventilation syndrome
  - MEN2A
  - Smith-Lemli Opitz
  - Mowat-Wilson
  - Cartilage-hair hypoplasia
  - Familial dysautonomia
  - Goldberg-Shprintzen megacolon

DIAGNOSIS

HISTORY

- 80% of patients present in the neonatal period.
- 15% diagnosed in 1st month, 40–50% within 3 months, 60% within 1 year, and 85% within 4 years
- Adult diagnosis of HD reported in 2% of population
- Presentation varies with age:
  - Neonatal period: delay in passage of meconium (>48 hours of life); bilious emesis, abdominal distention, intestinal obstruction, bowel perforation
  - Infancy: constipation associated with abdominal distention and vomiting, fecal impactions, growth failure, vomiting, and/or episodes of enterocolitis
  - Childhood to adulthood: chronic severe constipation refractory to medications, associated episodes of abdominal distention and vomiting, recurrent fecal impactions
- Neonates usually have normal weight, but growth retardation may occur when the disease is severe.
- Children with HD generally have small-volume and small-diameter stools. Some may have overflow diarrhea as well.
- Enterocolitis (chronic infectious colitis of the colon) is primary presentation in up to 17% of patients.

PHYSICAL EXAM

- On rectal exam, the sphincter tone is usually normal.
- Removal of the finger may be followed by explosive diarrhea. In most instances, especially in older children, the rectum is empty.

DIFFERENTIAL DIAGNOSIS

- Mechanical obstruction
- Meconium ileus
- Meconium plug syndrome
- Neonatal small left colon syndrome
- Malrotation with volvulus
- Intestinal atresia
- Intussusception
- Necrotizing enterocolitis
- Functional obstruction
- Intestinal neuronal dysplasia
- Sepsis
- Metabolic disorders (e.g., uremia, hypothyroidism)
- Disorders of intrinsic enteric nerves (diabetes or dysautonomia)
- Disorders of smooth muscle function
- Electrolyte disturbances
- Severe chronic constipation
- Allergic colitis (e.g., milk protein allergy in infants)

DIAGNOSTIC TESTS & INTERPRETATION

Initial Tests (screening, lab, imaging)

- CBC: anemia, leukocytosis in the presence of enterocolitis
- Plain film of abdomen
  - May show distended intestinal loops
  - Air–fluid levels
  - Diffuse intestinal pneumatosis has been reported as a rare presentation.
- Barium enema
  - May be suggestive or supportive but not diagnostic (sensitivity 70%, specificity 50–80%)
  - Normal barium enema does not exclude HD.
  - Transition zone is a funnel-shaped area of intestine with normal distal area and dilated proximal area.
  - Reveals large intestinal mucosal pattern, prominently thickened folds, and irregular margins secondary to ulceration
  - Significant delay in excretion of barium should also raise one's suspicion for HD.
  - Normal barium enema is commonly seen in the neonate (<30 days old).

Diagnostic Procedures/Other

- Anorectal manometry
  - Sensitivity (91%) and specificity (94%)
  - Safe and noninvasive way to exclude HD in patients >3 months of age
  - Lack of IAS relaxation with rectal balloon distention is suggestive of HD.
  - Abnormal study must be confirmed with rectal biopsies.
- Rectal suction biopsy
  - Sensitivity (93%) and specificity (98%)
  - Should be obtained 1, 2, and 3 cm from the dentate line
  - Biopsies must capture adequate submucosa to examine for ganglion cells.
  - The presence of ganglion cells on histology excludes HD.
  - If the suction biopsies are not conclusive, a full-thickness rectal biopsy (gold standard) is mandatory.
- Histologic findings
  - Absence of ganglion cells
  - Hypertrophy of preganglionic cells
  - Increased acetylcholinesterase staining in the lamina propria
  - Normal calretinin staining (newer staining technique)
- Pathologic findings
  - Aganglionic segment and transition zone
  - Hypoganglionosis proximal to aganglionic segment
  - Incomplete maturation of enteric nerve plexus
  - Hypertrophy of nonmyelinated nerve fibers within bowel wall (abnormal extrinsic innervation)

ALERT

Early recognition is of utmost importance in reducing the morbidity and mortality of HD.

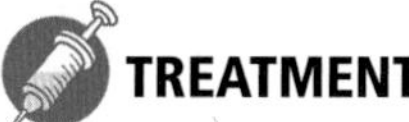

TREATMENT

Surgical resection of the aganglionic segment and subsequent pull-through of the ganglionic segment to the anus

GENERAL MEASURES

Stabilizing treatment if child presents with suspected enterocolitis or obstruction:

- Rectal decompression via rectal tube and irrigations with saline enemas
- Fluid and electrolyte resuscitation
- Nasogastric decompression
- Broad-spectrum antibiotics

SURGERY/OTHER PROCEDURES

- Initial operation
  - Defunctionalizing colostomy or ileostomy for total colonic aganglionosis or if child presents with obstruction not relieved by rectal irrigations
  - Performed to avoid the hazards of enterocolitis
- Definitive surgery
  - Performed 6 months to 1 year after the initial colostomy
  - May be performed as initial procedure in stable, nonobstructed child
- Most common surgical procedures are Swenson (rectosigmoidectomy), Soave (endorectal pull-through), and Duhamel (retrorectal transanal pull-through).
- Recent advances include the following:
  - Transanal surgery
  - Laparoscopic surgery
  - Single-stage operations

ALERT

Clinicians must have *high* suspicion for enterocolitis both *before* and *after* definitive pull-through.

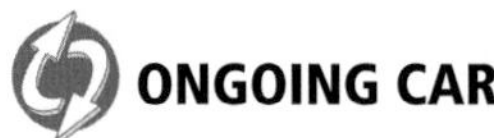

ONGOING CARE

FOLLOW-UP RECOMMENDATIONS

- Followed on a regular basis for the 1st decade after surgery
- Close monitoring for poor growth, fecal incontinence, obstructive symptoms (constipation, abdominal distention, difficulty stooling), recurrent enterocolitis

COMPLICATIONS

- Enterocolitis (chronic infectious colitis of the colon) with initial presentation
  - Mortality rates between 20% and 50%
  - Develops in 15–50% of patients
- Early (<4 weeks postoperation, usually related to technical issues)
  - Anastomotic leak
  - Cuff abscess and retraction of pull-through segment
  - Disturbance of micturition
  - Wound infection, intra-abdominal adhesions
- Late
  - Normal bowel function reported in ~68.7% (45–89%)
  - Defecation disorders present in >50–60%
  - Poor bowel control in total colonic HD and patients with trisomy 21
  - Obstructive symptoms (~11–42%): bloating, constipation, abdominal distention, vomiting, difficulty passing stool, fecal impactions
    - Anatomic: anal stenosis, anastomotic strictures, twisting of pull-through bowel, obstructive Soave cuff
    - Residual aganglionosis or transition zone
    - Functional: IAS dysfunction (high pressures), colonic dysmotility
  - Fecal incontinence (3–53%): "overflow" fecal incontinence and stool impactions, rapid transit in normal or short colon, hypermotile colon, abnormal sensation (disrupted dentate line), iatrogenic injury to the external anal sphincters
  - Enterocolitis (preop: 15–32%, postsurgically in 2–42%)
  - Voiding dysfunction: urinary incontinence, recurrent urinary tract infections
  - Sexual dysfunction due to dissection around pelvic nerve plexus
- Enterocolitis is major cause of morbidity and mortality:
  - Can occur both before and after definitive pull-through (25–45%)
  - Clinicians must have *high* suspicion; can be rapidly progressive and fatal
  - Secondary to obstruction causing an increase in intraluminal pressure and decreased intramural capillary blood flow
  - Affects the protective mucosal barrier, enabling fecal breakdown products, bacteria, and toxins to enter the bloodstream and cause sepsis and systemic inflammatory response syndrome (SIRS)
  - Usually presents with abdominal distention, explosive diarrhea, fever, vomiting

ADDITIONAL READING

- Chumpitazi B, Nurko S. Defecation disorders in children after surgery for Hirschsprung disease. *J Pediatr Gastroenterol Nutr*. 2011;53(1):75–79.
- Dasgupta R, Langer JC. Evaluation and management of persistent problems after surgery for Hirschsprung disease in a child. *J Pediatr Gastroenterol Nutr*. 2008;46(1):13–19.
- de Lorijn F, Boeckxstaens GE, Benninga MA. Symptomatology, pathophysiology, diagnostic work-up, and treatment of Hirschsprung disease in infancy and childhood. *Curr Gastroenterol Rep*. 2007;9(3):245–253.
- Langer JC. Hirschsprung disease. *Curr Opin Pediatr*. 2013;25(3):368–374.
- Langer JC, Rollins MD, Levitt M, et al. Guidelines for the management of postoperative obstructive symptoms in children with Hirschsprung disease. *Pediatr Surg Int*. 2017;33(5):523–526.
- Niramis R, Watanatittan S, Anuntkosol M, et al. Quality of life of patients with Hirschsprung's disease at 5–20 years post pull-through operation. *Eur J Pediatr Surg*. 2008;18(1):38–43.
- Rangel S, de Blaauw I. Advances in pediatric colorectal surgical techniques. *Semin Pediatr Surg*. 2010;19(2):86–95.
- Rintala RJ, Pakarinen MP. Long-term-outcomes of Hirschsprung's disease. *Semin Pediatr Surg*. 2012;21(4):336–343.

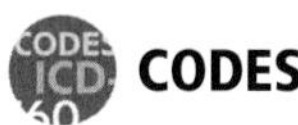

CODES

ICD10

Q43.1 Hirschsprung's disease

FAQ

- Q: What is the likelihood that a newborn with a diagnosis of HD will have normal bowel function after surgery?
- A: There is a good likelihood, but it may take a number of years: A review of 178 patients over a 20-year period demonstrated that bowel habits and continence improve with age: 52.2% were successful at 5 to 10 years postsurgery, 68% at 10 to 15 years postsurgery, and 88.9% at 15 to 20 years postsurgery.
- Q: How will the bowel movements change after surgery and over time?
- A: Patients report 3 to 5 stools per day following pull-through that decreases to 1 to 3 stools per day over time at long-term follow-up. However, up to 50% may have a defecation disorder. Patients must be closely monitored for constipation, fecal incontinence, and recurrent enterocolitis.
- Q: Are laxatives required after surgery?
- A: In ~20% of children, some sort of laxative therapy or rectal irrigation may be required. If the patient is nonresponsive to laxative therapy and/or rectal irrigations are required on a regular basis, then the patient should be evaluated for other possible etiologies of obstructive symptoms.

HISTIOCYTOSIS

Michelle L. Hermiston, MD, PhD

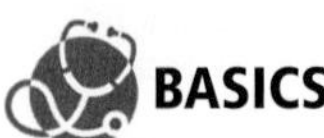

BASICS

DESCRIPTION

- Histiocytic disorders are derived from mononuclear phagocytic cells and dendritic cells. They are divided into three groups.
  - Dendritic cell disorders (e.g., Langerhans cell histiocytosis [LCH], juvenile xanthogranuloma [JXG], Erdheim-Chester disease)
  - Macrophage-related disorders (e.g., hemophagocytic lymphohistiocytosis [HLH], macrophage activation syndrome [MAS], Rosai-Dorfman disease)
  - Malignant histiocytosis (lymphoma subtype)
- LCH (the focus of this chapter) results from the clonal proliferation of immature myeloid dendritic cells that share similar morphologic expression to skin LCH cells.
- Other names include the following (Langerhans cell histiocytosis is the preferred terminology):
  - Histiocytosis X, Hand-Schüller-Christian syndrome, Letterer-Siwe disease, eosinophilic granuloma
  - Hashimoto-Pritzker syndrome: infant dermatologic involvement, often self-limited

EPIDEMIOLOGY

- 2 to 10 cases per million children
- LCH may occur at any age. Median age is 30 months.
- Single-system disease in 55% of patients; multisystem disease is more common in children 1 to 3 years of age.
- Male-to-female ratio approximately 1
- May be more common in whites of northern European descent than African Americans

RISK FACTORS

Genetics

- No evidence that relatives of LCH patients are at increased risk of disease.
- Very rare reports of recurrence within families
- Specific HLA alleles associated with disease phenotype in some case series

PATHOPHYSIOLOGY

- Single-system LCH: limited to one organ system; most commonly bone, followed by skin
- Multisystem LCH involves two or more organs/systems with or without risk organs.
- Risk organs include hematopoietic system, liver, and/or spleen and portend a worse prognosis. Lungs are no longer considered a risk organ.
- CNS risk lesions: Lesions in the facial or anterior or middle cranial fossa bones are associated with 3 times increased risk of CNS involvement.
- CNS lesions can include mass lesions, pituitary stalk involvement, or neurodegenerative disease.

ETIOLOGY

LCH etiology is incompletely understood. *BRAFV600E* mutations are found in ~60% of cases but are not prognostic. Activation of the RAS/MAPK/MEK/ERK pathway is common regardless of *BRAF* mutation status. Inflammatory infiltrates and abnormal cytokine production in lesions are common, although role in disease remains unclear.

DIAGNOSIS

HISTORY

- Signs and symptoms:
  - Wide variation in presenting signs and symptoms depending on affected organ systems
  - Single-system skeletal disease may be asymptomatic, with incidental discovery of lesions on radiographs obtained for other reasons (e.g., trauma).
- Swelling, pain, or pathologic fracture from soft tissue or bone lesion
- Proptosis
- Persistent otorrhea
- Early loss of teeth; persistent oral ulcers
- Erythematous or brown papular rash
- Persistent seborrheic dermatitis
- Gait disturbance
- Failure to thrive
- Diarrhea, possibly bloody
- Fever of unknown origin
- Headache
- Abdominal pain
- Jaundice
- Polydipsia or polyuria (diabetes insipidus [DI])
- School/cognitive problems
- Dyspnea or persistent cough
- History of spontaneous pneumothorax

PHYSICAL EXAM

- Growth or pubertal delay
- Skin: brownish-red papules often involving intertriginous areas, seborrheic dermatitis (cradle cap), purpura, petechial rash especially at areas of skin contact (e.g., top of diaper); rash may become ulcerated, crusted, or scaly.
- Ears: otorrhea, hearing loss
- Skeleton: swelling or mass; may be painless or very tender to palpation; skull, axial skeleton, long bones more often affected than hands or feet
- Teeth: gingivitis, "floating teeth," oral ulcers
- Eyes: orbital swelling, cranial nerve palsies
- Lungs: tachypnea, intercostal retractions
- GI: hepatosplenomegaly, ascites, edema, jaundice; stool with blood or mucus
- Neurologic: ataxia, cognitive difficulties

DIFFERENTIAL DIAGNOSIS

- Broad differential, depending on constellation of presenting symptoms
- Bone/soft tissue lesions
  - Sarcoma (especially osteogenic sarcoma, Ewing sarcoma, or rhabdomyosarcoma)
  - Benign bone lesion (e.g., osteoma, bone cyst)
  - Infection
  - Metastatic tumor (e.g., neuroblastoma, leukemia/lymphoma)
- Skin lesions
  - Seborrheic dermatitis
  - Otitis externa
  - Tinea infection
  - Viral exanthem (especially herpes simplex virus [HSV] in neonates)
- CNS lesions
  - Teratoma or malignant germ cell tumor
  - Craniopharyngioma
  - Primary CNS tumor
  - Neurodegenerative disorder
- Pulmonary involvement
  - Infection
  - Emphysema (e.g., α_1-antitrypsin deficiency)
- Fever, lymphadenopathy (nontender, nonerythematous)
  - Lymphoma
  - Lymphadenitis (especially large DNA viruses)
  - Granulomatous (e.g., fungal, cat-scratch disease) infections
  - Rosai-Dorfman or Castleman disease
  - Rheumatologic disease
  - HLH
- Hepatic involvement
  - Infections
  - Congenital hepatic and storage diseases
  - HLH
  - Tumor infiltration (e.g., leukemia)
  - Primary sclerosing cholangitis
- Cytopenias
  - Leukemia or other tumor infiltration
  - Aplastic anemia
  - HLH
  - Myelofibrosis or storage diseases

DIAGNOSTIC TESTS & INTERPRETATION

Initial Tests (screening, lab, imaging)

- Routine diagnostic evaluation
  - CBC with differential to evaluate for marrow involvement
  - Liver function tests (LFTs), prothrombin time (PT), partial thromboplastin time (PTT) to evaluate liver function
  - Morning urine specific gravity; urine and serum osmolality to evaluate for DI
- Other investigations
  - Pulmonary involvement: pulmonary function tests
  - Suspected DI (polydipsia/polyuria): endocrine evaluation including water deprivation test and evaluation of anterior pituitary hormone production
  - Auricular involvement: audiogram; ear, nose, and throat evaluation
- Bone involvement: biopsy of lesions unless diagnosis of LCH already established
- Chest radiograph and skeletal survey (bone scan not as sensitive in most patients but may be better for infants; whole-body MRI may also be used)
- Liver/spleen ultrasound

- High-resolution chest CT if pulmonary involvement suspected
- If neurologic involvement or signs of DI, MRI of brain with contrast, including detailed evaluation of sella turcica
- Dental radiographs if teeth are involved
- CT/MRI of lytic-appearing lesions often obtained prior to diagnosis to evaluate potential malignancy; classic "punched out" lesions may not require imaging beyond plain films.

Diagnostic Procedures/Other

- Biopsy of lesion to establish diagnosis
- Cytopenias or other high-risk organ involvement: bone marrow aspirate and biopsy
- Liver dysfunction: liver biopsy to evaluate for sclerosing cholangitis
- GI involvement: endoscopic biopsy of small and large intestine
- Pulmonary involvement: bronchoalveolar lavage (BAL) or lung biopsy to evaluate for infection if diagnosis of LCH not already established or if CT appearance is atypical
- Pathologic findings
  - Proliferation of immature myeloid dendritic with surrounding inflammatory infiltrate
  - LCH cells are CD1a and CD207 positive and contain Birbeck granules on electron microscopy.
  - *BRAFV600E* mutation can be detected by immunohistochemical or molecular methods.
  - If negative, consider whole exome or targeted sequencing for RAS/MAPK/MEK/ERK pathway mutations.

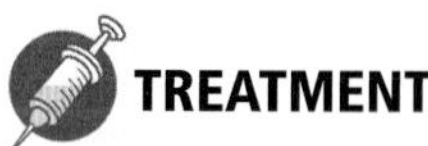

TREATMENT

GENERAL MEASURES

- Site and extent of disease determine therapy.
- A multidisciplinary approach is imperative to ensure the best therapy. Patients should be enrolled on a clinical trial whenever possible.
- Duration: 12 months of therapy associated with decrease in reactivation from 50% to 30%
- Type of therapy depends primarily on
  - Number of organ systems affected
  - Number of bone lesions if single system
  - Involvement of "risk organs" associated with morbidity or mortality: liver, spleen, and bone marrow
- Single-system LCH (most often bone, skin)
  - Observation of isolated lesions; often remain stable or spontaneously resolve
  - Local therapy
    - Isolated bone or lymph node: excision or biopsy often curative
    - Confirmed skin-only LCH: topical steroids, nitrogen mustard, or tacrolimus
  - Systemic therapy if multiple or refractory lesions
    - Low-dose chemotherapy for some multifocal bone disease or multiple recurrent single-bone lesions; superior results with multiagent regimens
    - Reduces risk of later DI in patients with skull, vertebral, or CNS lesions
- Multisystem LCH
  - Chemotherapy
    - Steroid, vinblastine, plus antimetabolites depending on extent of disease and risk organ involvement
  - Limited response by 6 weeks merits intensification (e.g., 6-mercaptopurine [6MP], 2-chlorodeoxyadenosine [2-CdA] + AraC).
  - Limited experience with allogeneic stem cell transplantation for very high-risk refractory disease
- Treatment of disease-related morbidity
  - Lifelong intranasal desmopressin acetate often needed for the management of DI; posterior pituitary dysfunction is rarely reversible.
  - Organ transplantation may be necessary for high-risk patients with organ dysfunction.

MEDICATION

- Frontline: corticosteroids and vinblastine; addition of antimetabolites (6MP, methotrexate) if multisystem disease and risk organ involvement
- Cladribine has been used in case series for CNS mass lesions. For neurodegenerative disease, case series report variable responses (generally stabilization) to dexamethasone, cytarabine, cladribine, vincristine, IVIG, and retinoic acid.
- Bisphosphonates is being tested for isolated bone lesions.
- Confirmed skin-only disease: topical steroids, tacrolimus, or nitrogen mustard; systemic cotrimoxazole
- Refractory disease: 2-CdA ± cytarabine, clofarabine, etoposide, thalidomide, hydroxyurea, or BRAF inhibitors (e.g., vemurafenib)

ISSUES FOR REFERRAL

Multidisciplinary care involving several specialties may be required for coordination of chemotherapy and management of orthopedic, endocrinologic, hepatic, hematologic, or pulmonary complications.

ADDITIONAL THERAPIES

Radiotherapy rarely used; reserved for refractory or critical bone lesions (e.g., spinal cord compression)

SURGERY/OTHER PROCEDURES

- Initial biopsy for diagnosis: often curative for solitary bone lesions even without clean margins
- Excision of isolated bone or lymph node lesions

ONGOING CARE

FOLLOW-UP RECOMMENDATIONS

- Evaluation at regular intervals for recurrence of lesions or new high-risk organ involvement
- Because of variable course, patients should be followed closely at centers with LCH expertise.
- Patients with CNS risk lesions should be monitored for neurodegeneration with detailed neurologic examination, evaluation of school performance, and an annual MRI for 10 years postdiagnosis.

Patient Monitoring

- Laboratory and imaging follow-up as described for initial evaluation, with focus on previously affected and high-risk organ systems
- Routine follow-up typically includes history, physical exam, CBC, LFTs, and skeletal imaging.

DIET

Maintain fluid and electrolyte intake if DI is present.

PROGNOSIS

- Prognosis is linked to extent and location of disease. Single-system or bone/skin disease carries low risk of morbidity. Overall survival for patients with high-risk disease is 84%.
- Often, disease will "burn out" by the end of childhood. ~5% of patients will continue to have exacerbations as adults.
- Survival in neonates and younger children with high-risk disease may be poorer. Response to therapy at 6 weeks is the most important prognostic factor.

COMPLICATIONS

- Most common long-term morbidities include orthopedic problems, DI, and neurodegenerative disease.
- Smoking is strongly associated with development of pulmonary disease in LCH patients.
- Chronic disabilities with multisystem disease include pulmonary fibrosis, hepatic fibrosis, deafness, orthopedic problems, short stature, permanent ataxia, neurocognitive deficits, and poor dentition.

ADDITIONAL READING

- Badalian-Very G, Vergilio JA, Fleming M, et al. Pathogenesis of Langerhans cell histiocytosis. *Annu Rev Pathol*. 2013;8:1–20.
- Filipovich A, McClain K, Grom A. Histiocytic disorders: recent insights into pathophysiology and practical guidelines. *Biol Blood Marrow Transplant*. 2010;16(Suppl 1):S82–S89.
- Gadner H, Grois N, Pötschger U, et al; for Histiocyte Society. Improved outcome in multisystem Langerhans cell histiocytosis is associated with therapy intensification. *Blood*. 2008;111(5):2556–2562.
- Minkov M, Grois N, McClain K, et al. Langerhans cell histiocytosis: Histiocyte Society evaluation and treatment guidelines. April 2009. http://www.histiocytesociety.org/document.doc?id=290. Accessed February 14, 2015.
- PDQ Pediatric Treatment Editorial Board. Langerhans cell histiocytosis treatment (PDQ). https://www.ncbi.nlm.nih.gov/books/NBK65799/. Accessed June 20, 2017.

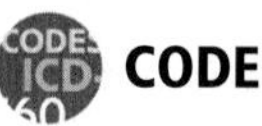

CODES

ICD10

- C96.6 Unifocal Langerhans-cell histiocytosis
- C96.0 Multifocal and multisystemic Langerhans-cell histiocytosis

FAQ

- Q: Is LCH a cancer?
- A: Historically, there has been controversy as to whether LCH was a cancer or an inflammatory disease. The discovery of *BRAFV600E* mutations has led to the conclusion that LCH is a clonal neoplastic disorder.
- Q: Is LCH contagious?
- A: There is no evidence that LCH is caused by an infection or that it is contagious.

H

HISTOPLASMOSIS

Dylan C. Kann, MD

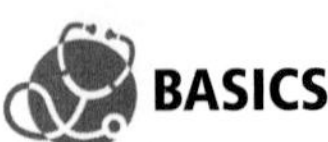

BASICS

DESCRIPTION

- Histoplasmosis (a.k.a., Ohio Valley disease, spelunker's lung, cave disease, Darling disease, Appalachian Mountain disease, and reticuloendothelial cytomycosis) is the most prevalent endemic mycosis in United States.
- Dimorphic fungus *Histoplasma capsulatum* var. *capsulatum* in United States (African var. is *duboisii*, which affects skin, lymph nodes, and bone)
- Forms include acute, chronic, primary, reactivation, and the affected disease areas (pulmonary, extrapulmonary, disseminated)

EPIDEMIOLOGY

- Endemic in central and southeastern states, classically Ohio and Mississippi River valleys; also prominent in Central America but occasionally in Europe, Asia, and Africa
- Mold form at <35°C (whereas yeast form in tissue above 37°C) grows best in soil environments: warm, moist, and rich in nitrogen (bird/bat guano); found in caves, under roosting trees, abandoned buildings
- Occasional cluster infections usually with soil disruptions (spelunking, building demolition)
- Sporadic cases with some activities: gardening, roofing, installing air-conditioning/heating, cleaning older homes, playing in hollow trees
- Only mammals can be infected (birds do not carry the organism).
- No human or animal-to-human transmission except for one case of vertical transmission in infant with co-HIV infection
- Incubation typically 3 to 17 days but up to 5 months
- Total infections: estimated 500,000 per year
  - Chronic pulmonary infection: 1:100,000 cases
  - Disseminated infection: 1:2,000 cases

Prevalence

Skin test reactivity as high as 50–80% by age 18 years in most highly endemic areas

RISK FACTORS

- Males slightly more at-risk than females
- Infections more common in 30s to 40s but all ages affected
- Disseminated disease risk factors: immature cellular immunity (<2 years of age), large inoculum, acquired immunodeficiency (including TNF-α inhibitors), malnutrition

GENERAL PREVENTION

- Avoid areas/dust with likely mold.
- Spray water, oil, or 3% formalin in areas with dust/dirt if work planned.
- Wear cover apparel and face mask able to filter particles >1 millimicron (e.g., N95).
- Prophylaxis for certain populations

PATHOPHYSIOLOGY

- Inhaled mold spores germinate in lungs to yeast form; rarely enter via skin
- Once germinated, some lymphatic and hematologic dissemination even in self-limited disease
- Immune system takes several weeks to respond, involves T lymphocytes, IL-12, IFN-γ, and TNF-α; macrophages kill fungus.

ETIOLOGY

Infectious mold spores are microconidia of *H. capsulatum*.

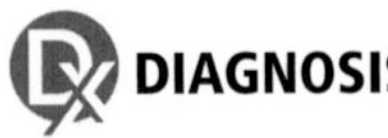

DIAGNOSIS

HISTORY

- Of 5% who develop symptoms, most (60–90%) have pulmonary symptoms and/or flu-like illness lasting days to 2 weeks for acute.
  - Most common complaints: headache, fatigue, fever, cough, myalgias, chest pain, which can be pleuritic
  - Pharyngitis, rhinorrhea, and congestion are unusual.
- 5% of symptomatic patients have more prolonged course with additional anorexia, weight loss, arthralgia, and night sweats lasting >2 weeks.
  - "Severe" symptoms: dyspnea and hypoxemia
  - Cavitary form can have tuberculosis (TB)-like symptoms (e.g., hemoptysis) but rare in children.
- Progressive disseminated histoplasmosis (PDH) (usually <2 years of age or immunocompromised) symptoms: fever, weight loss, hepatosplenomegaly, failure to thrive (in infants) often without respiratory symptoms

PHYSICAL EXAM

- For acute pulmonary disease, exam is usually normal, aside from fever and occasionally crackles or decreased breath sounds; wheezing has been reported.
- More severe or diffuse pulmonary disease can present with weight loss, hypoxia, and dyspnea.
- Erythema nodosum (especially adolescent patients)
- Disseminated findings: hepatosplenomegaly, extrapulmonary lymphadenopathy and/or granulomas, oral or skin lesions, adrenal or intestinal masses, multifocal choroiditis, meningitis (60% of PDH of infancy), endocarditis, parotitis, arthritis, signs of disseminated intravascular coagulation (DIC)
- Other findings could include the following:
  - Pericardial effusion (10% of symptomatic pediatric patients) with potential cardiac rub
  - Pleural effusion
  - Chylothorax
  - Biliary obstruction
  - Superior vena cava syndrome

DIFFERENTIAL DIAGNOSIS

- Pulmonary histoplasmosis
  - TB and other mycobacteria
  - Pneumonia (atypical)
  - Other fungal lung infections (blastomycosis, sporotrichosis, and coccidioidomycosis)
  - *Pneumocystis jirovecii* (can mimic PDH symptoms)
  - *Nocardia* and *Actinomyces*
- Mediastinal lymphadenopathy
  - Malignancy
  - Sarcoidosis
- PDH
  - Malignancy
  - Sepsis
  - Opportunistic infections (Coinfection is common in immunodeficiency.)
  - Hemophagocytic lymphohistiocytosis/macrophage activation syndrome (MAS) (can be sequelae of PDH as well)
  - Brucella, Q-fever, leishmaniasis

DIAGNOSTIC TESTS & INTERPRETATION

Initial Tests (screening, lab, imaging)

- Culture is the definitive method of diagnosis.
  - Sterile site (blood, bone marrow, CSF, tissue biopsy) or nonsterile site (sputum/bronchoalveolar lavage [BAL])
  - Can take from 1 to 6 weeks to grow
  - Culture sensitivity varies with site and host (sputum 10% positive in acute pulmonary, 60% positive in cavitary disease, 90% in BAL from HIV patients).
- Antigen tests using quantitative enzyme immunoassay (often 1st-line test +/− serologic testing below)
  - Urine along with blood most common sources for testing (less sensitive but can be done on BAL, CSF)
  - 92% sensitivity: disseminated infection
  - 80% sensitivity: severe pulmonary disease
  - 34% sensitivity: self-limited pulmonary disease
  - 14% sensitivity: chronic pulmonary disease
  - Used to monitor fungal burden
  - Cross-reactivity rarely with *Paracoccidioides brasiliensis*, *Blastomyces dermatitidis*, *Coccidioides immitis*, *Coccidioides posadasii*, and *Penicillium marneffei*
- Serologic: immunodiffusion (ID) and complement fixation (CF) antibody tests
  - Most common test for localized pulmonary disease but often negative in acute period
  - Best tests for chronic meningitis
  - Less sensitive in immunocompromised patients
  - Antibody appears 4 to 8 weeks after infection, can become negative after 12 to 18 months.
  - ID usually 1st-line serologic test (specific test with only 5% cross-reactivity but only 80% sensitive)
    - Tests for M and H bands; H bands more suggestive of acute infection
    - H bands positive in 23%, M bands positive in 76% of acute pulmonary
  - CF usually 2nd-line serologic test, as more sensitive but less specific (18% cross-reactivity)
    - Cross-reacts with *Blastomyces*, *Paracoccidioides*, and *Coccidioides*
    - 4-fold increase or single 1:32 or greater is presumptive of active/recent infection.
    - Titers 1:8 and 1:16 unclear significance
- Molecular methods
  - Presently used for confirmation or identification of culture isolates or histopathologic findings
    - *Histoplasma*-specific polymerase chain reaction (PCR)
    - Broad-range fungal PCRs/sequencing
- Microscopy
  - Noncaseating granulomas
  - Intracellular yeast form in tissue, blood, bone marrow, or BAL
  - Usually examined with silver stain
- Other lab findings:
  - Mild anemia, elevated ferritin, hypercalcemia, elevated ESR/C-reactive protein
  - PDH: pancytopenia, coagulopathy, elevated liver enzymes
  - Meningitis: CSF lymphocytic pleocytosis, protein elevation, and low glucose
- Skin test: not clinically used; only used for epidemiologic studies

- Chest radiograph
  - Majority are normal in self-limited disease, and 40–50% of cases of PDH are normal.
  - Positive findings can include hilar adenopathy, infiltrates, pleural effusions (5% of children), pericarditis (10% of children), mediastinal granuloma, mediastinal fibrosis (rare in children), mass effect, calcifications.
- Chest CT
  - Miliary nodules and calcifications more easily seen
  - Can be diffuse parenchymal consolidation
- CNS imaging
  - Leptomeningeal enhancement (often basilar), focal brain or spinal cord lesions, strokes, and encephalitis

ALERT

- Most children will not require treatment for *H. capsulatum* pulmonary disease.
- Arthritis, pericarditis, and erythema nodosum do not necessitate antifungals.
- Children with PDH should be screened for HIV and immunodeficiency.
- Alert lab of any specimen suspected of *Histoplasma* (lab hazard if grown).

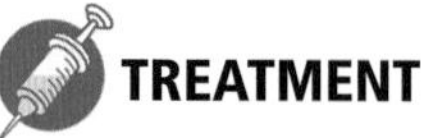

TREATMENT

GENERAL MEASURES

Standard precautions adequate for hospital isolation

MEDICATION

- Immunocompetent patients with primary acute uncomplicated (nonsevere) pulmonary histoplasmosis <4 weeks' duration do not require treatment.
- Therapy indicated for severe/complicated pulmonary disease, after high inoculum, PDH, infection in immunocompromised
- When itraconazole used, oral liquid suspension preferred for more consistent absorption
- Pulmonary disease (moderate but >1 month)
  - PO itraconazole 5 to 10 mg/kg/24 h divided b.i.d. × 6 to 12 weeks (max 400 mg daily)
- Pulmonary disease (severe)
  - Amphotericin B lipid formulation (unless renal involvement) 3 to 5 mg/kg/24 h depending on formulation (lipid complex vs. liposomal) or deoxycholate 1 mg/kg daily IV × 1 to 2 weeks followed by PO itraconazole 5 to 10 mg/kg/24 h divided b.i.d. (max 400 mg daily) for 12 weeks
  - Methylprednisolone (controversial in children) 1 to 2 mg/kg daily IV during first 1 to 2 weeks for patients with worsened hypoxemia or distress
- Disseminated (without HIV infection)
  - Amphotericin B lipid formulation (as above) × 4 to 6 weeks. Alternative: lipid formulation of amphotericin B (as above) for 2 to 4 weeks followed by itraconazole PO 5 to 10 mg/kg/24 h divided b.i.d. for 3 to 6 months until urine antigen concentration <2 mcg/mL
- Disseminated (with HIV infection)
  - Liposomal amphotericin B 5 mg/kg/24 h IV × 2 to 6 weeks followed by oral itraconazole for at least 1 year to life 5 to 10 mg/kg/24 h divided b.i.d. (max of 400 mg/24 h)
  - If highly active antiretroviral therapy (HAART) given for 6 months, CD4 >150 cells/mm^3, antifungal taken for 1 year, and antigen levels low, can consider stopping secondary prophylaxis
- Meningitis
  - Liposomal amphotericin B 5 mg/kg/24 h IV × 4 to 6 weeks then oral itraconazole 5 to 10 mg/kg/24 h divided b.i.d. × 12 months and then until resolution of CSF profile; monitor antigen levels.
- Mediastinitis (rare)
  - Amphotericin B × 1 to 2 weeks then oral itraconazole for 6 months
- Fibrosing mediastinitis (rare)
  - Itraconazole for 3 months
  - May not have any effect on fibrosis
- Pericarditis/rheumatologic manifestations
  - Pericardiocentesis if severe tamponade
  - NSAID (usually indomethacin) for 2 to 12 weeks
  - Consider oral prednisone (1 mg/kg/24 h).
- Compression by granulomatous disease
  - Consider surgery and corticosteroid with concurrent use of itraconazole.
- Vertical transmission in newborn
  - Amphotericin B (lipid formulation)
- Although the Infectious Diseases Society of America (2007) guidelines state that lipid preparations of amphotericin are "not preferred" in children (except HIV patients) as nonlipid preparations are well tolerated, lipid formulations are most often used due to overall favorable side effect profile.
- Salvage therapy can be done with posaconazole and/or voriconazole; fluconazole is inferior to itraconazole.
- Prophylaxis for CD4 <150 cells/μL, in hyperendemic areas or solid organ transplant recipients, those scheduled to receive TNF inhibitors, or those undergoing intensive chemotherapy with a history of histoplasmosis in the past 2 years: oral itraconazole 5 mg/kg/24 h divided b.i.d. (max 200 mg/24 h)

ADMISSION, INPATIENT, AND NURSING CONSIDERATIONS

Patients receiving amphotericin may need prolonged IV access.

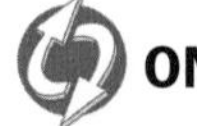

ONGOING CARE

FOLLOW-UP RECOMMENDATIONS

Patient Monitoring

- In PDH, follow antigen levels monthly during therapy and 12 months posttherapy.
- Itraconazole blood levels should be measured after >2 weeks of therapy (goal serum level >1 mcg/mL but ideally 2 mcg/mL at steady state).
- On itraconazole measure liver function tests (LFTs) monthly
- On amphotericin, follow CBC, LFTs, BUN/Cr, and potassium and magnesium.

PROGNOSIS

- Overall good prognosis except for untreated PDH disease, which is highly fatal
- Self-limited pulmonary patients recover in 2 to 3 weeks.
- Most treated PDH patients have significant improvement after 2 weeks of IV antifungals.

COMPLICATIONS

- Lymphatic, GI, esophageal, vascular, and biliary obstruction
- Renal stones
- Multifocal choroiditis
- Calcified nodules
- Fibrosis
- Pleural effusion
- Pericarditis
- Chylothorax
- Superior vena cava syndrome
- Hydrocephalus
- MAS

ADDITIONAL READING

- Azar MM, Hage CA. Laboratory diagnostics for histoplasmosis. *J Clin Microbiol*. 2017;55(6):1612–1620.
- Fischer GB, Mocelin H, Severo CB, et al. Histoplasmosis in children. *Paediatr Respir Rev*. 2009;10(4):172–177.
- Hage CA, Knox KS, Wheat LJ. Endemic mycoses: overlooked causes of community acquired pneumonia. *Respir Med*. 2012;106(6):769–776.
- Kauffman CA. Histoplasmosis: a clinical and laboratory update. *Clin Microbiol Rev*. 2007;20(1):115–132.
- Montenegro BL, Arnold JC. North American dimorphic fungal infections in children. *Pediatr Rev*. 2010;31(6):e40–e48.
- National Institute for Occupational Safety and Health, National Center for Infectious Diseases. *Histoplasmosis: Protecting Workers at Risk*. Washington, DC: U.S. Department of Health and Human Services. http://www.cdc.gov/niosh/docs/2005-109/pdfs/2005-109.pdf. Accessed September 1, 2017.
- Smith JA, Kauffman CA. Pulmonary fungal infections. *Respirology*. 2012;17(6):913–926.
- Wheat LJ, Freifeld AG, Kleiman MB, et al. Clinical practice guidelines for the management of patients with histoplasmosis: 2007 update by the Infectious Diseases Society of America. *Clin Infect Dis*. 2007;45(7):807–825.

CODES

ICD10

- B39.9 Histoplasmosis, unspecified
- B39.4 Histoplasmosis capsulati, unspecified
- B39.2 Pulmonary histoplasmosis capsulati, unspecified

FAQ

- Q: What are the most common clinical presentations of histoplasmosis?
- A: Asymptomatic, mild primary pulmonary disease. Moderate to severe pulmonary, disseminated, and cavitary are uncommon.
- Q: How is histoplasmosis best diagnosed?
- A: Isolation or identification of the organism is definitive. Antigen testing of urine or blood is used for acute infections, especially severe infections. Serologic testing can be helpful but lacks sensitivity and specificity. Skin tests are not useful.
- Q: Does histoplasmosis need to be treated with antifungal therapy?
- A: For mild primary disease in an immunocompetent patient, no treatment is necessary. More severe or disseminated disease is treated.

HODGKIN LYMPHOMA

Elizabeth Robbins, MD

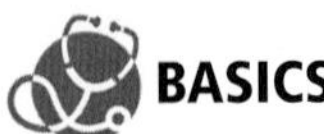

BASICS

DESCRIPTION

B lineage malignant lymphoid neoplasm. Typically presents with painless lymphadenopathy, often cervical (70–80%) or supraclavicular (25%). Mediastinal mass present in 50%. Constitutional symptoms (e.g., fatigue, fever, night sweats, weight loss, cough, pruritus) may or may not be present. Constitutional symptoms sometimes precede development of lymphadenopathy.

EPIDEMIOLOGY

- Represents 7% of childhood cancer
- 11.7 cases/million/y age <20 years
- Most common cancer for ages 15 to 19 years
- Rarely seen in children age <5 years
- M > F age <15 years
- F > M age 15 to 19 years
- Bimodal age distribution in adults: early peak mid/late 20s; late peak age >50 years

RISK FACTORS

- Few known risk factors include the following:
  - Immune deficiency (e.g., HIV infection)
  - Autoimmune disorders
  - Lower socioeconomic status for childhood form (age 14 years or younger)
  - Higher socioeconomic status for young adult form
- Decreased risk if
  - Multiple older siblings
  - Exposure to common infections in preschool

Genetics

- Familial Hodgkin lymphoma (HL) rare, accounting for 4.5% of cases
- Familial cases may reflect
  - Genetic influences, including inherited immunodeficiency states
  - Environmental factors
  - Exposure to viruses

PATHOPHYSIOLOGY

- Reed-Sternberg cells, a clonal population of large binucleate cells arising from B cells, are the malignant cells in HL. Surface antigen expression includes CD30 but not CD20.
- Only 1% of cells in involved nodes are Reed-Sternberg cells and morphologic variants; the rest are inflammatory cells: lymphocytes, macrophages, fibroblasts, plasma cells, eosinophils.
- Two clinically distinct subtypes of HL recognized:
  - Classical HL (90–95% of cases)
    - Nodular sclerosing
    - Mixed cellularity
    - Lymphocyte depleted
    - Lymphocyte rich
  - Nodular lymphocyte predominant (5–10% of cases; treated differently from classical HL. See National Comprehensive Cancer Network (NCCN) guidelines for treatment recommendations.)

ETIOLOGY

- Cause unknown
- Association between Epstein-Barr virus (EBV) infection and HL: 20–50% of patients with classical HL have monoclonal or oligoclonal proliferation of EBV-infected cells.

DIAGNOSIS

HISTORY

- Painless lymphadenopathy slowly increasing in size. Lymphadenopathy often present for weeks to months before presentation. Cervical or supraclavicular sites most common.
- Constitutional ("B") symptoms: One or more occur in 20% of children.
  - Fever >38°C, not otherwise explained
  - Weight loss >10% within 6 months preceding diagnosis, not explained
  - Drenching night sweats
- Other constitutional symptoms include fatigue, pruritus, cough, and orthopnea.
- Patients with large mediastinal mass may have symptoms of superior vena cava syndrome: dyspnea, facial swelling, cough, orthopnea, headache.

PHYSICAL EXAM

- General appearance: Patients with advanced disease may be tired-appearing and cachectic.
- Fever, if present, is usually intermittent.
- Lymph nodes:
  - Nodes >1 cm are considered abnormal.
  - Cervical, supraclavicular (especially left), and axillary nodes are most common. Other sites include epitrochlear, inguinal, and femoral.
  - Lymph nodes are usually firm, rubbery, nontender, and sometimes matted.
- Lungs: Decreased breath sounds or rhonchi may be noted in patients with large mediastinal mass; some patients unable to lie flat due to respiratory distress
- Abdomen: Splenomegaly may be present; hepatomegaly is less common.
- Skin: Pallor due to anemia may be present. Erythematous and excoriated areas may be present in patient with pruritus. Bruises and petechiae rare. Icteric sclera and/or jaundice may be noted in cases with autoimmune hemolytic anemia (rare).

DIFFERENTIAL DIAGNOSIS

- Other malignant process (lymph nodes usually nontender to palpation)
  - Non-HL
  - Anaplastic large cell lymphoma
  - Soft tissue sarcoma, germ cell tumor
  - Metastatic adenopathy—soft tissue sarcoma, nasopharyngeal carcinoma
- Infection (Lymph nodes may be tender to palpation.)
  - EBV
  - Atypical *Mycobacterium*
  - Histoplasmosis
  - Toxoplasmosis
  - Tuberculosis
  - Cat-scratch disease
  - *Staphylococcus aureus*, *Streptococcus*
- Drug reaction (e.g., phenytoin)

DIAGNOSTIC TESTS & INTERPRETATION

Initial Tests (screening, lab, imaging)

- No specific lab assay is diagnostic of HL.
- Erythrocyte sedimentation rate (ESR): useful as tumor marker if elevated at diagnosis
- CBC with differential and platelets
- Bilateral bone marrow biopsy is not usually indicated but is performed in selected cases, for example, if there are cytopenias and negative PET. In cases where PET/CT shows multifocal (three or more) skeletal lesions, marrow is assumed to be involved and bone marrow is not necessary for staging.
- Comprehensive metabolic panel, lactate dehydrogenase, and liver function test
- Thyroid function (if radiation planned)
- Pregnancy test for women of childbearing age
- Baseline echocardiogram for ejection fraction (pre-doxorubicin)
- Pulmonary function tests (pre-bleomycin)
- To evaluate extent of disease at diagnosis for staging and to follow response to treatment
  - Chest radiograph (posterior-anterior and lateral) to evaluate for mediastinal mass
  - PET/CT: Functional imaging with PET has replaced previous staging modalities such as splenectomy, lymphangiogram, and gallium scan; used at diagnosis and to follow response to therapy
  - CT scan, IV contrast-enhanced, of neck, chest, abdomen, pelvis (not needed if PET/CT has been obtained)
  - Ultrasound of cervical or other adenopathy—is sometimes helpful as an initial approach to lymphadenopathy
  - Ann Arbor staging criteria:
    - Stage I—involvement of a single lymph node region (I) or of a single extralymphatic organ or site (I_E)
    - Stage II—involvement of two or more lymph node regions on the same side of the diaphragm (II) or localized involvement of an extralymphatic organ or site and one or more lymph node regions on the same side of the diaphragm (II_E)
    - Stage III—involvement of lymph node regions on both sides of the diaphragm (III), which may be accompanied by involvement of the spleen (III_S) or by localized involvement of an extralymphatic organ or site (III_E) or both (III_{SE})
    - Stage IV—diffuse or disseminated involvement of one or more extralymphatic organs or tissues with or without associated lymph node involvement
    - Modifiers: A/B—presence of one or more B symptoms (see "History") is designated by the suffix B; A denotes absence of B symptoms.

Diagnostic Procedures/Other

- Biopsy
  - Fine-needle aspiration or core needle biopsy, along with immunohistochemistry, may occasionally be adequate for diagnosis provided typical Reed-Sternberg cells can be identified
  - Excisional/incisional biopsy of lymph node is usually necessary for diagnosis.
- Biopsy tissue studies include the following:
  - Flow cytometry (classic HL usually CD30+)
  - Cytogenetics
  - Culture for aerobic, anaerobic, and acid-fast bacilli if indicated
- Fertility preservation options include:
  - Sperm cryopreservation
  - Ovarian tissue or oocyte cryopreservation
  - Oophoropexy (if abdominal radiation planned)

ALERT

General anesthesia is usually contraindicated in patients with mediastinal mass or tracheal deviation because of the possibility of airway collapse from loss of smooth muscle tone during anesthesia.

TREATMENT

MEDICATION

- Long-term survival in pediatric patients with HL is >90%. Recent treatment strategies have therefore focused on decreasing intensity of therapy to minimize late effects. Chemotherapy combined with radiation therapy has been the standard approach historically, but HL is increasingly being treated with chemotherapy alone. Response to treatment as measured by PET serves to guide treatment decisions; patients whose disease is no longer PET-avid after 2 to 4 courses of chemotherapy are often treated with chemotherapy alone.
- Chemotherapy regimens for classical HL (these do not apply to nodular lymphocyte predominant HL):
  - ABVD: doxorubicin (Adriamycin®), bleomycin, vinblastine, dacarbazine; standard 1st-line regimen for adults. Treatment duration depends on stage, response as measured by PET scan after 2 to 4 courses
  - ABVE-PC: doxorubicin, bleomycin, vincristine, etoposide, prednisone, cyclophosphamide; Children's Oncology Group regimen for advanced stage disease
  - COPP/ABV: cyclophosphamide, vincristine (Oncovin), procarbazine, prednisone, doxorubicin (Adriamycin®), bleomycin, vinblastine
  - VAMP: vinblastine, doxorubicin (Adriamycin®), methotrexate, prednisone
  - BEACOPP: bleomycin, etoposide, doxorubicin (Adriamycin®), cyclophosphamide, vincristine (Oncovin®), prednisone, procarbazine; efficacy similar to ABVD but with more acute toxicities, risk of secondary leukemia, nearly universal infertility
  - OEPA/COPDAC: vincristine (Oncovin®), etoposide, prednisone, doxorubicin (Adriamycin®)/cyclophosphamide, vincristine, prednisone, dacarbazine; German regimen for advanced stage disease
- New agents
  - Nivolumab: anti–PD-1 monoclonal antibody (checkpoint inhibitor). Used alone or in combination in recurrent disease
  - Brentuximab vedotin: antibody-drug conjugate that targets cell membrane protein CD30. Used alone or in combination in recurrent disease. Current trial in adults replaces bleomycin with brentuximab vedotin in ABVD regimen. Current trial in Children's Oncology Group replaces bleomycin with brentuximab vedotin in ABVE-PC regimen.

ADDITIONAL THERAPIES

- Radiation therapy
  - Used in combination with chemotherapy
  - Provides effective local control for areas of bulky disease, defined as a mediastinal mass >1/3 the thoracic diameter measured at the dome of the diaphragm on a PA CXR or a large nodal aggregate >10 cm (6 cm by Children's Oncology Group criteria)
  - Radiation doses and fields have been reduced over the past decade, but late effects including cardiac disease and secondary malignancies including breast cancer are still significant.
- Radiotherapy is commonly employed in the following:
  - Patients with bulky disease (some treated with chemotherapy alone)
  - Patients whose disease is responding poorly to chemotherapy
  - As part of a combined modality treatment strategy with lower dose radiation and less intense alkylator therapy (e.g., Stanford V or recent COG regimens)
  - Salvage therapy for relapsed disease
- Long-term survival ~50% for patients with recurrence. Specific salvage therapy based on remission duration and initial therapy. Typical salvage includes reinduction followed by high-dose chemotherapy and autologous stem cell transplant. Radiation may also be used.

ONGOING CARE

FOLLOW-UP RECOMMENDATIONS

Patient Monitoring

- Patients are monitored for evidence of disease recurrence and for long-term toxicity from chemotherapy/radiation therapy. Two thirds of recurrences occur within the first 2 years of diagnosis.
- Monitoring for disease recurrence includes the following:
  - History, physical exam q3–6mo during first 2 years off therapy; q6–12mo during 3rd year off therapy; and then annually
  - Lab studies including ESR if elevated at diagnosis; CBC
  - Imaging: Scheduled surveillance imaging in asymptomatic patients is not usually undertaken in HL. National adult guidelines advise against routine surveillance PET scans because of the risk of false positives. Some treatment protocols require periodic off-therapy CT scans; MRI scans are sometimes substituted to avoid radiation exposure. Detecting recurrence by imaging, presumably earlier than clinically, may not result in improved survival. PET/CT scan is indicated if recurrence suspected.
  - Periodic CXR: Some providers follow CXR first 1 to 2 years off therapy if mediastinal disease.
  - Monitoring for late effects depends on the patient's treatment.
  - Cardiac: periodic echocardiogram, EKG if anthracycline therapy or mediastinal radiation
  - Pulmonary: periodic pulmonary function tests if bleomycin or mediastinal radiation
  - Reproductive: hormonal testing (LH, FSH, estradiol/testosterone) beginning at puberty or by age 12 years
  - Thyroid: annual thyroid function (T_4, TSH) if radiation
  - Secondary malignancies
    - Breast: monthly breast self-exam; yearly mammogram with adjunct MRI beginning 8 years after radiation or age 25 years, whichever is later
    - Thyroid: yearly thyroid exam if radiation
    - Colon: colonoscopy q5y beginning age 35 years if radiation
    - Leukemia: yearly CBC, platelets, differential for 10 years after exposure to etoposide, alkylating agents, anthracyclines

PROGNOSIS

Overall 5-year survival >90% regardless of stage. Prognosis for 5-year disease-free survival depends on stage at diagnosis:

- >90% for low-stage disease (stage I, II, non-bulky, no B symptoms)
- 65–90% for advanced disease (stage III, IV)

COMPLICATIONS

- Acute complications of treatment:
  - Chemotherapy
    - Hair loss, nausea, vomiting, cytopenias resulting in infection, bleeding
- Late complications of treatment:
  - See "Cancer Therapy Late Effects" chapter.
  - Chemotherapy
    - Cardiomyopathy, decreased pulmonary function, pulmonary fibrosis, decreased fertility, secondary leukemia
  - Radiation therapy
    - Breast cancer, other secondary malignant neoplasm, cardiomyopathy, coronary artery disease with myocardial infarction, pericarditis, accelerated atherosclerosis with increased stroke risk, pulmonary fibrosis, hypothyroidism, impaired growth of bones and soft tissue

ADDITIONAL READING

- Cote GM, Canellos GP. Can low-risk, early-stage patients with Hodgkin lymphoma be spared radiotherapy? *Curr Hematol Malig Rep.* 2011;6(3):180–186.
- Kelly KM, Hodgson D, Appel B, et al. Children's Oncology Group's 2013 blueprint for research: Hodgkin lymphoma. *Pediatr Blood Cancer.* 2013;60(6):972–978.
- Meyer RM, Hoppe RT. Point/counterpoint: early-stage Hodgkin lymphoma and the role of radiation therapy. *Blood.* 2012;120(23):4488–4495.
- National Comprehensive Cancer Network. NCCN guidelines for treatment of cancer by site, Hodgkin lymphoma. www.nccn.org. Accessed April 14, 2018.
- O'Brien MM, Donaldson SS, Balise RR, et al. Second malignant neoplasms in survivors of pediatric Hodgkin's lymphoma treated with low-dose radiation and chemotherapy. *J Clin Oncol.* 2010;28(7):1232–1239.
- Radford JR, Illidge T, Counsell N, et al. Results of a trial of PET-directed therapy for early-stage Hodgkin's lymphoma. *N Engl J Med.* 2015;372(17):1598–1607.
- Schaapveld M, Aleman MD, van Eggermond AM, et al. Second cancer risk up to 40 years after treatment for Hodgkin's lymphoma. *N Engl J Med.* 2015;373(26):2499–2511.

CODES

ICD10

- C81.90 Hodgkin lymphoma, unspecified, unspecified site
- C81.91 Hodgkin lymphoma, unsp, lymph nodes of head, face, and neck
- C81.92 Hodgkin lymphoma, unspecified, intrathoracic lymph nodes

HUMAN IMMUNODEFICIENCY VIRUS INFECTION

David C. Griffith, MD • Allison L. Agwu, MD, ScM

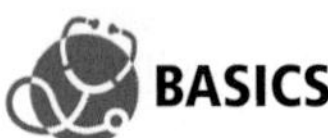

BASICS

DESCRIPTION

- HIV is the etiologic agent of AIDS. HIV suppresses CD4+ T cells leading to impaired cell-mediated immunity.
- HIV-1 is more common worldwide, whereas HIV-2 is mainly prevalent in West Africa.
- An acute phase with flulike symptoms develops 2 to 4 weeks after acquiring infection, followed by a long asymptomatic period (5 to 15 years in adults, shorter in children), followed, if untreated, by development of nonspecific signs and symptoms (weight loss, adenopathy, hepatosplenomegaly, failure to thrive) and clinical immunodeficiency.
- AIDS is the advanced stage of untreated HIV when the infected individual will experience progressive immunologic deterioration and eventually become susceptible to opportunistic infections and cancers.

EPIDEMIOLOGY

- As of 2015, there were an estimated 36.7 million people living with HIV worldwide, and as of 2013, 1.3 million in the United States. The highest prevalence of HIV is in Sub-Saharan Africa.
- In 2015, there were 39,513 new HIV diagnoses in the United States, 120 in those <13 years of age and 8,737 in those between the ages of 13- to 24 years Centers for Disease Control and Prevention (CDC).
- In 2015, approximately 90% of new diagnoses among 13 to 24-year-old men had male-to-male sex as the primary risk factor.
- African American individuals made up approximately 55% of new diagnoses in 2015 among those 13 to 24 years old.

RISK FACTORS

- Sexual contact
  - Unprotected orogenital, vaginal, or anal sex: Anal receptive sex is highest risk.
- Exposure to infected blood or body fluids
  - Needle sharing (injection drug use)
  - Occupational exposure (i.e., needle stick): Risk of transmission from an HIV-contaminated needle is 1:300.
  - Blood transfusion: All donated blood in the United States is screened for HIV.
  - Mucous membrane exposure to infected blood or fluids
- Perinatal infection can occur either in utero or during labor and delivery.
  - Risk of an HIV-infected mother (not on treatment) giving birth to an infected infant is ~20% (in the absence of breastfeeding), with increased rate of transmission for women with low CD4 counts or higher viral titers. Vaginal delivery, especially with rupture of membranes >8 hours, appears to increase the risk of infant infection.
  - Risk of perinatal transmission if mother is effectively treated (undetectable viral load) is <2%.
  - Presence of untreated sexually transmitted infections (STIs), chorioamnionitis, and prematurity all increase the risk of mother-to-child transmission of HIV.
- Breast milk
  - Overall risk of breastfeeding is ~15%.
  - In countries where breastfeeding is the norm, up to 30% of perinatally acquired HIV infections occur through breastfeeding.
  - Breastfeeding is not recommended in the United States.
- HIV is not believed to be transmitted by the following:
  - Bites
  - Sharing utensils, bathrooms, bathtubs
  - Exposure to urine, feces, vomitus (except where these fluids may be grossly contaminated with blood, and even then transmission is rare, if it happens at all)
  - Casual contact at home, school, or day care center

GENERAL PREVENTION

- Prevention of mother-to-child transmission: All pregnant women should be offered HIV testing at the first prenatal visit. In areas of high incidence, repeat testing should be done at 36 weeks of gestation. Women not tested before or during labor should undergo expedited HIV testing.
  - Antenatal three-drug antiretroviral therapy (ART) for all HIV-positive pregnant women
  - Delivery via elective cesarean section for selected cases
  - Postnatal ART prophylaxis for infants:
    - 4-week course of zidovudine for low-risk mothers (on ART with suppressed viral load)
    - For high-risk mothers (not on ART or on ART but with elevated viral load) combination ART with two to three drugs is recommended. One regimen consists of zidovudine for 6 weeks, plus nevirapine given in 3 doses (at birth, 48 hours after the first dose, and 96 hours after second dose). Some experts recommend a three-drug regimen with the addition of lamivudine to zidovudine and nevirapine. However, the optimal duration of nevirapine and lamivudine is not known with guidelines stating a range of 2 to 6 weeks.
- Postexposure prophylaxis
  - ART initiated after possible HIV exposure: unprotected sex or sexual assault, needle sharing, occupational exposure
  - Consists of three-drug ART for 28 days
  - Must be initiated within 72 hours of exposure
- Preexposure prophylaxis
  - Daily tenofovir/emtricitabine approved by the U.S. Food and Drug Administration (FDA) for patients 18 years and older
  - Recommended for high-risk individuals: men who have sex with men or heterosexual men/women with HIV-positive partners, multiple sexual partners, recent STI, and injection drug users who share injection equipment
- General measures: condom use, avoidance of needle sharing, no breastfeeding

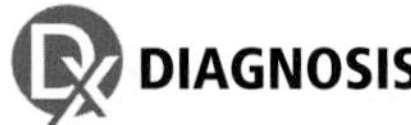

DIAGNOSIS

HISTORY

Clinical signs, symptoms, and scenarios in which HIV testing should be performed:

- Infants with maternal HIV status that is unknown or positive
- All adolescents (particularly those endorsing sexual activity), at least annually
- Patients who use drugs (injectable or noninjectable)
- History of STIs, especially syphilis
- Patients presenting with opportunistic infections (i.e., *Pneumocystis jiroveci* pneumonia, recurrent or resistant thrush, especially after 12 months of age)
- Infants with congenital syphilis, acquired microcephaly, progressive encephalopathy, loss of developmental milestones, failure to thrive, delayed puberty
- Patients with recurrent/chronic diarrhea, recurrent/chronic parotid gland enlargement, generalized lymphadenopathy

PHYSICAL EXAM

- Perinatally acquired HIV
  - May be normal in the 1st months of life
  - 90% have exam findings by 2 years of age.
  - Most common findings are generalized adenopathy, hepatosplenomegaly, failure to thrive, recurrent/resistant thrush, (especially after 1 year of age).
  - Recurrent or chronic parotitis
- Nonperinatally acquired HIV
  - Generally nonspecific: lymphadenopathy, weight loss, evidence of opportunistic infection

DIFFERENTIAL DIAGNOSIS

- Neoplastic disease
  - Lymphoma
  - Leukemia
  - Histiocytosis X
- Infectious
  - Congenital/perinatal cytomegalovirus
  - Toxoplasmosis
  - Congenital syphilis
  - Acquired Epstein-Barr virus
- Congenital immunodeficiency syndromes
  - Wiskott-Aldrich syndrome
  - Chronic granulomatous disease

DIAGNOSTIC TESTS & INTERPRETATION

- Infants with perinatal HIV exposure
  - Virologic testing using HIV RNA and DNA polymerase chain reaction (PCR) tests are recommended at birth, 14 to 21 days, 1 to 2 months (preferably 2 to 4 weeks after cessation of antiretroviral prophylaxis), and 4 to 6 months.
    - Negative testing in a nonbreastfed infant is defined as two or more negative virologic tests with one obtained at >1 month and one at >4 months or two negative antibody tests obtained >6 months of age.
    - Both HIV RNA and DNA PCR have sensitivities and specificities >95% after 2 weeks of age.
    - By 1 month of age, 95% of HIV-infected infants will have positive HIV DNA PCR.
    - Residual maternal antibodies may be detected up to 24 months.

- For those >2 years of age
  - HIV-1/HIV-2 antigen/antibody combination qualitative immunoassay simultaneously detects presence of HIV p24 antigen and HIV-1/HIV-2 antibodies.
    - p24 antigen component allows for detection 2 to 3 weeks after infection and can help identify patients with acute HIV infection.
- CD4 counts
  - Obtained at diagnosis and routinely
  - Results need to be evaluated based on age-adjusted normal values. Absolute CD4 counts are elevated in childhood, with normal median values >3,000/mm^3 in the 1st year of life, which then gradually decline with age, reaching values comparable with adult levels (800 to 1,000/mm^3) by age 7 years.
  - For children <5 years of age, CD4% should be used instead of absolute CD4 count.
- Quantitative viral RNA PCR assays
  - Termed "viral loads," results are reported in a range from undetectable, usually <20 copies/mL (cpm) to upper values of >10 million cpm.
  - Viral loads that remain >100,000 are associated with poor short-term (2 to 5 years) outcomes.
  - Also used as a marker of efficacy of treatment; goal is to suppress viral replication to the undetectable range for as long as possible.
  - Test is done at time of diagnosis to establish baseline and routinely to assess treatment adherence/efficacy.
- Other frequent lab abnormalities include thrombocytopenia, anemia, and elevated liver enzymes.

ALERT

Failure to screen for HIV infection during pregnancy results in inability to offer ART during pregnancy, which may lead to failure of preventing infant infection, as well as the inability to prescribe *Pneumocystis jiroveci* pneumonia prophylaxis to infected newborns.

TREATMENT

GENERAL MEASURES

- Active immunizations
  - All infected children receive standard childhood immunizations, including the pneumococcal conjugate vaccine.
  - Infected children should receive yearly influenza A/B immunizations and 23-valent pneumococcal vaccine at age 2 years.
  - Symptomatic children should not receive the varicella vaccine, and those with severely low CD4 counts should not receive measles-mumps-rubella vaccination.
- Prophylaxis: One of the major advances has been the ability to offer prophylaxis against the most common opportunistic infections.
  - Prophylaxis against *Pneumocystis* pneumonia with TMP-SMX is indicated for all HIV-infected infants between 4 to 6 weeks and 12 months of age, for those 1 to 6 years of age with CD4 count <500 cells/mm^3 or <15%, and for children >6 years of age with CD4 <200 cells/mm^3 or <15%.
  - Prophylaxis against toxoplasmosis and *Mycobacterium avium* complex is indicated in children with severe immune suppression.

MEDICATION

ART

- Specific combination ART prolongs life, delays progression of illness, promotes improved growth, and improves neurologic outcome.
- Standard of care now involves the administration of combination therapy (usually three or more drugs), termed highly active antiretroviral therapy (HAART). There are now five different drug classes and as multiple multiclass combination pills.
- Given the complexities of therapy, ART should always be prescribed in consultation with a specialist in pediatric/adolescent HIV infection.
- Adherence to prescribed schedules is critical. When patients miss even 10–20% of doses, the durability of response is short.

ONGOING CARE

FOLLOW-UP RECOMMENDATIONS

- Family psychosocial support is critical.
- All infected patients should be comanaged with an HIV specialty care site.
- Patients should be seen every 1 to 3 months to monitor adherence, immune status (CD4 counts), virologic suppression (quantitative plasma viral RNA), and medication safety.

PROGNOSIS

Due to HAART, morbidity and mortality have both greatly decreased:

- Median survival is now into adulthood.
- Incidence of new opportunistic infections (AIDS-defining illnesses) has decreased greatly, as have hospital admissions.

COMPLICATIONS

Complications of untreated HIV include:

- *Pneumocystis jiroveci* pneumonia
  - Most common early fatal illness in HIV-infected children (peak age 3 to 9 months); mortality is 30–50%. A high index of suspicion is necessary for prompt diagnosis (by lavage) and initiation of therapy.
- Lymphocytic interstitial pneumonitis
  - Chronic respiratory disorder that causes a distinctive diffuse reticulonodular pattern on chest radiographs, usually diagnosed between 2 and 4 years of age
- Recurrent invasive bacterial infections
  - Bacterial pneumonia, sinusitis, and otitis media are common.
- Progressive encephalopathy
  - Diagnosed between 9 and 18 months of age, the hallmark is progressive loss of milestones or neurologic dysfunction.
- Disseminated *M. avium* intracellulare
  - Older children, usually >5 years of age, with severe immunodeficiency (CD4 ≤100 cells/mm^3)
  - Symptoms include prolonged fevers, abdominal pain, anorexia, and diarrhea.
- *Candida* esophagitis:
  - Older children with severe immunodeficiency usually present with dysphagia or chest pain and oral thrush.
- Disseminated cytomegalovirus disease
  - Retinitis less common in HIV-infected children than in adults
  - Cytomegalovirus may also cause pulmonary disease, colitis, and hepatitis.
- HIV-related cancers
  - Non–Hodgkin lymphoma most common cancer, with primary site usually located in the CNS
- Other organ dysfunction associated with HIV-infection in children: cardiomyopathy, hepatitis, renal disease, thrombocytopenia, idiopathic thrombocytopenic purpura

ADDITIONAL READING

- American Academy of Pediatrics. Human immunodeficiency virus infection. In: Kimberlin DW, Brady MT, Jackson MA, et al, eds. *Red Book: 2015 Report of the Committee on the Infectious Disease*. 30th ed. Elk Grove Village, IL: American Academy of Pediatrics; 2015.
- Panel on Antiretroviral Guidelines for Adults and Adolescents. Guidelines for the use of antiretroviral agents in adults and adolescents living with HIV. https://aidsinfo.nih.gov/contentfiles/lvguidelines/adultandadolescentgl.pdf. Accessed April 15, 2018.
- Panel on Antiretroviral Therapy and Medical Management of Children Infected with HIV. Guidelines for the use of antiretroviral agents in pediatric HIV infection. http://aidsinfo.nih.gov/contentfiles/lvguidelines/pediatricguidelines.pdf. Accessed April 15, 2018.
- Panel on Treatment of Pregnant Women with HIV Infection and Prevention of Perinatal Transmission. Recommendations for the use of antiretroviral drugs in pregnant women with HIV infection and interventions to reduce perinatal HIV transmission in the United States. http://aidsinfo.nih.gov/contentfiles/lvguidelines/PerinatalGL.pdf. Accessed April 15, 2018.
- Rakhmanina N, Phelps BR. Pharmacotherapy of pediatric HIV infection. *Pediatr Clin North Am*. 2012;59(5):1093–1115.
- U.S. Public Health Service. Preexposure prophylaxis for the prevention of HIV infection in the United States—2014. https://www.cdc.gov/hiv/pdf/prepguidelines2014.pdf. Accessed April 15, 2018.

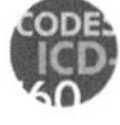

CODES

ICD10

- B20 Human immunodeficiency virus [HIV] disease
- Z21 Asymptomatic human immunodeficiency virus infection status
- R75 Inconclusive laboratory evidence of human immunodef virus

FAQ

- Q: Should HIV-positive mothers breastfeed?
- A: The recommendation for HIV-positive mothers in resource-rich areas is to NOT breastfeed, as breastfeeding poses continued risk of exposure and infection with HIV to the infant. In areas where there are no affordable and safe substitutes of breastfeeding, exclusive breastfeeding is advised.
- Q: What are the recommendations for HIV screening in adolescents?
- A: The CDC recommend routine HIV testing for individuals aged 13 to 65 years. As part of anticipatory guidance, the American Academy of Pediatrics recommends offering HIV testing for adolescents aged 16 to 18 years of age at least once if prevalence of HIV in the area is >0.1%. Continued HIV screening is also recommended for youth with high-risk behavior and those undergoing STI evaluations.

H

HUMAN PAPILLOMAVIRUS

Camille Sabella, MD

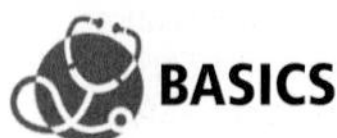

BASICS

DESCRIPTION

- Members of the Papillomaviridae family, the human papillomaviruses (HPV), which cause warts of the skin and mucous membranes
  - Exophytic venereal warts or condylomata acuminata are primarily caused by HPV types 6 and 11.
  - Warts can be found on the external genitalia and the urethra, vagina, cervix, anus, and mouth. HPV types 6 and 11 are also associated with squamous cell carcinoma of the external genitalia.
  - Virus types 16, 18, 31, 33, and 35 typically cause subclinical infection in the anogenital region and have been associated with intraepithelial genital carcinomas.
- HPV can also cause recurrent respiratory papillomatosis (RRP) in infants and young children. RRP primarily impacts the larynx but can also cause lesions anywhere along the respiratory tract.
- Increasing evidence that HPV may play a role in squamous cell carcinomas of the oropharynx

EPIDEMIOLOGY

- General
  - HPV is the most common viral sexually transmitted infection (STI).
  - Genital warts and HPV infection are diseases of young adults 16 to 25 years of age.
  - Cervical cancer is the 3rd most common female cancer worldwide.
- Genital HPV
  - Peak prevalence among women 18 to 24 years of age
  - At least 40% of sexually active adolescents are infected with HPV.
  - <1% of adolescents develop genital warts.
  - 500,000 new cases of cervical cancer diagnosed each year internationally
- RRP
  - RRP impacts 4.5 per 100,000 children, mostly those age 2 to 3 years.
  - 67% of children with RRP are born to mothers who had condyloma during pregnancy.

RISK FACTORS

- Infants
  - Primarily vertical transmission at birth
- Adolescents
  - Behavioral risks, including young age at first coitus, multiple partners, cigarette use, and having older male partners
  - Biologic risk in adolescent girls secondary to cervical anatomy

GENERAL PREVENTION

- 9-valent HPV vaccine (HPV9 [types 6, 11, 16, 18, 31, 33, 45, 52, and 58]) is licensed by the FDA for use in females ages 9 through 26 years and in males ages 9 through 15 years. Condom use may diminish transmission.
- Examine partners; treat those infected.
- Pap smear in adult women to assess for cervical dysplasia
- HPV infection is not a reportable disease.

PATHOPHYSIOLOGY

- Transmission
  - Primarily through sexual contact
  - Can also be acquired during the birth process
  - Transmission from nongenital sites is rare.
- The incubation period is variable and ranges from 3 months to several years.
- The virus is trophic for epithelial cells and infects the basal layer of actively dividing cells.
- Infection results in koilocytosis and nuclear atypia. Genital infections may progress to severe dysplasia and carcinoma in situ (CIS).
- Spontaneous regression of clinical disease occurs in 90% of low-risk types and 75% of high-risk types.
- Recurrence is common.

COMMONLY ASSOCIATED CONDITIONS

- Epidermodysplasia verruciformis
- Other STIs

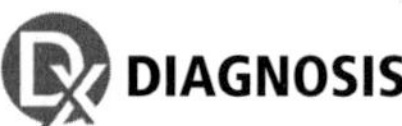

DIAGNOSIS

HISTORY

- Genital HPV
  - Most patients have no symptoms.
  - Presence of warts, often painless
  - Vaginal, urethral, or anal discharge; bleeding; local pain
  - Dysuria
  - Pruritus
- RRP
  - Infants have hoarse or weak cry, stridor, and failure to thrive.
  - Older children have hoarseness, stridor, dysphonia, and obstructive sleep apnea.

PHYSICAL EXAM

- Genital HPV
  - Warts appear as soft, sessile tumors with surfaces ranging from smooth to rough with many finger-like projections.
  - HPV may also cause flat keratotic plaques that project only slightly with a hyperpigmented surface and are difficult to identify without the addition of acetic acid.
  - Subclinical infection is common, causing many foci of epithelial hyperplasia invisible to the examiner.
  - In males, infection is found on the penis, urethra, scrotum, and perianal areas.
  - In females, infection involves the urethra, vagina, cervix, and perianal area.
  - Diagnosis is made by visual inspection of the anogenital region. Cervical dysplasia is not clinically apparent on exam.
- RRP
  - Often normal exam but, on visualization of trachea, multiple verrucous, polypoid growths on vocal rods, subglottic region, and trachea can be seen.

DIFFERENTIAL DIAGNOSIS

- Genital HPV
  - Condyloma lata (syphilis infection)
  - Molluscum contagiosum
  - Pink pearly papules or hypertrophic papillae of the penis
  - Lipomas
  - Fibromas
  - Adenomas
- RRP
  - Croup
  - Vocal cord paralysis
  - Other forms of nasal, laryngeal, pharyngeal, or tracheal obstruction

DIAGNOSTIC TESTS & INTERPRETATION

Initial Tests (screening, lab, imaging)

- Application of 3–5% acetic acid for 5 minutes causes lesions to appear white and thus more readily apparent and can help with the detection of cervical disease.
- Tissue specimens may show koilocytosis typical for HPV infection.
- Pap smear with liquid cytology to assess for evidence of cervical dysplasia resulting from HPV infection
- Colposcopy aids the diagnosis of cervical lesions.
- Polymerase chain reaction is commercially available for HPV typing and is used in patients >21 years with abnormal Pap smears.

Diagnostic Procedures/Other

- Genital HPV
  - Pap smear or colposcopy to screen for cervical dysplasia
- RRP
  - Direct visualization of the airway through laryngoscopy

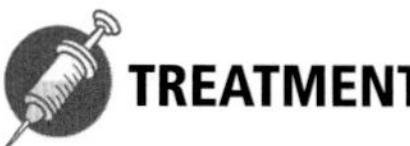

TREATMENT

GENERAL MEASURES

- To date, no therapy exists that eradicates the virus. As a result, recurrences are likely.
- Most patients require a course of therapy rather than a single treatment.
- Genital HPV
  - Lesions on mucosal surfaces respond better to topical treatments.
  - All available therapies have equal efficacy in eradicating warts, ranging from 22% to 94%, with the significant rate of relapse of 25% within 3 months (see Medication):
    - Consider size, location, number of warts, previous treatment, and patient preference.
    - Also consider patient preference, expense, and side effects.
    - Patients with extensive lesions should be referred to physicians who routinely treat these lesions.
  - Treatment:
    - External: See Medication.
    - Meatal: cryotherapy or podophyllin
    - Anal: cryotherapy or trichloroacetic acid (TCA)
    - Vaginal: TCA
    - Cervical: Refer to an expert.
- RRP
  - Primarily surgical excision; may regress after puberty

MEDICATION

Treatment for external warts

- Podofilox 0.5%
  - Patient applies podofilox with a cotton swab b.i.d. for 3 days.
  - After 4 days, podofilox is repeated as necessary for 4 cycles.
  - The area for treatment should not exceed 10 cm^2, and total drug should not exceed 0.5 mL/24 hr.
- Imiquimod 5% cream
  - Patient applies cream at bedtime 3 times per week for up to 16 weeks.
  - It is washed off after 6 to 10 hours.
- Podophyllin 10–25%
  - A practitioner applies a small amount to each wart and allows it to air dry. It is washed off 1 to 4 hours later.
  - Dose is limited to 0.5 mL per treatment to avoid systemic toxicity.
  - Dose may be repeated once weekly up to 4 doses; external lesions only
  - Contraindicated during pregnancy
- TCA 80–90%
  - The practitioner applies TCA sparingly to each wart directly. Talc is applied to remove unreacted acid. It is washed off after 4 hours.
  - Can be used on mucosal lesions

SURGERY/OTHER PROCEDURES

- Laser surgical excision
  - Requires special equipment and training; often requires general anesthesia; controlled tissue destruction
- Cryotherapy
  - Liquid nitrogen or cryoprobe is used every 1 to 2 weeks by a specially trained provider.

ONGOING CARE

FOLLOW-UP RECOMMENDATIONS

Patient Monitoring

- Follow-up should continue until the warts have disappeared.
- Latent infection and recurrent disease are common.
- United States Preventive Services Task Force (USPSTF), American Cancer Society (ACS), and American College of Obstetrics and Gynecology (ACOG) recommend initial Pap smear at 21 years of age.
- Pap smears may be indicated in sexually active patients >21 years of age if they have HIV, solid-organ transplantation, or chronic immunosuppression.

PROGNOSIS

Therapy will not eradicate the virus; thus, HPV causes recurrent disease.

ADDITIONAL READING

- American Academy of Pediatrics. Human papillomaviruses. In: Kimberlin DW, Brady MT, Jackson MA, Long SS, eds. *Red Book: 2015 Report of the Committee on Infectious Diseases*. 30th ed. Elk Grove Village, IL: American Academy of Pediatrics; 2015:576–583.
- Gunter J. Genital and perianal warts: new treatment opportunities for human papillomavirus infection. *Am J Obstet Gynecol*. 2003;189(Suppl 3):S3–S11.
- Hathaway JK. HPV: diagnosis, prevention, and treatment. *Clin Obstet Gynecol*. 2012;55(3):671–680.
- Markowitz LE, Dunne EF, Saraiya M, et al; for Centers for Disease Control and Prevention. Human papillomavirus vaccination: recommendations of the Advisory Committee on Immunization Practices (ACIP). *MMWR Recomm Rep*. 2014;63(RR-05):1–30.
- Workowski KA, Bolan GA; for Centers for Disease Control and Prevention. Sexually transmitted diseases treatment guidelines, 2015. *MMWR Recomm Rep*. 2015;64(RR-03):1–137.

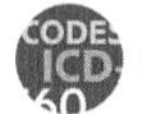

CODES

ICD10

A63.0 Anogenital (venereal) warts

FAQ

- Q: What treatment is indicated during pregnancy?
- A: Most experts recommend surgical removal if necessary. Podophyllin is absolutely contraindicated.
- Q: Should partners of patients with genital warts be referred for examination?
- A: Recurrence is due to reactivation of the virus; reinfection plays no role. Partner may benefit from an examination to evaluate for the presence of warts and for education and counseling. There is no information regarding prophylaxis to prevent infection, so treatment for this is not indicated. Most partners have subclinical infection. Female partners should follow the routine recommendations for Pap smear screening.
- Q: Are genital warts in children always indicative of sexual abuse?
- A: No. The HPV virus has an incubation period of many months. Thus, warts transmitted to infants at the time of birth may not become clinically apparent for 1 to 2 years. Whether the incubation period can be longer than this time period remains unknown. Thus, maternal history and, potentially, examination are both important factors. However, all children with anogenital warts should be evaluated by a clinician experienced in child abuse evaluations. It is possible that caregivers may transmit the virus to children through close but nonsexual contact; thus, this history is also important in older children.
- Q: Will young women still need to get Pap smears if they have received the HPV vaccine?
- A: Yes. The vaccine does offer good protection against the strains most commonly associated with genital warts and cervical cancer, 6, 11, 16, and 18. However, these strains are not the only ones that can cause infection or lead to cervical cancer. It is important to continue regular screening to ensure that one has not been exposed to other strains that may cause cervical dysplasia.

HYDROCELE

Adam B. Hittelman, MD, PhD, FACS

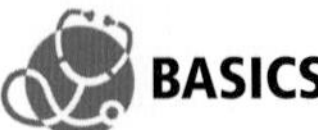

BASICS

DESCRIPTION

A hydrocele is the accumulation of fluids around the testicle, within the tunica vaginalis or processus vaginalis.

- Communicating hydrocele: fluid passing from peritoneal cavity into patent processus vaginalis
- Noncommunicating hydrocele: fluid confined within the processus vaginalis (hydrocele of the cord) or tunica vaginalis
- Abdominal-scrotal hydrocele: fluid collection within processus vaginalis, extending into retroperitoneum
- Reactive hydrocele (noncommunicating): accumulation of fluid within tunica vaginalis caused by infection, trauma, or other inflammatory conditions

EPIDEMIOLOGY

- 2–5% of male neonates have hydrocele.
- Male more common than female
  - Female: "cyst" or "hydrocele" in the canal of Nuck; may be communicating or noncommunicating
- Right more common than left
- Majority asymptomatic
- Simple (noncommunicating): commonly seen at birth, frequently bilateral, may be large
  - Majority spontaneously resolve in 12 to 24 months.
- Persistent hydroceles beyond 24 months and those presenting after birth more likely to be communicating
- Age >12 years old: majority noncommunicating
- Adolescent/adult hydroceles are generally acquired (reactive) and idiopathic in origin.

RISK FACTORS

- Similar to inguinal hernia
- Prematurity, low birth weight, gestational progestin use, connective tissue anomalies, cystic fibrosis, cryptorchidism, posterior urethral valves, and other syndromic disorders
- Trauma or infection
- Lymphatic obstruction (i.e., varicocelectomy, filariasis, pelvic radiation, malignancy)

PATHOPHYSIOLOGY

- Communicating hydrocele can become indirect inguinal hernia, with potential for incarceration.
- Noncommunicating hydrocele generally thought to be low clinical concern.
- Potential damage in large, tense hydroceles
  - Raised intrascrotal temperature can cause potential testicular harm.
  - Tense hydrocele may cause pressure atrophy.
  - Increased resistive index observed in subcapsular artery and absent testicular diastolic flow indicate risk for permanent damage.

ETIOLOGY

- Communicating hydrocele similar to indirect inguinal hernia (defined by contents entering through patent processus vaginalis: peritoneal fluid versus fat or visceral organ)
- In testicular descent, lip of peritoneum descends with testicle, the processus vaginalis, and covers testicle, tunica vaginalis.
- Patent processus in girls (canal of Nuck) related to descent of round ligament to labia, female equivalent of gubernaculum
- Related to delayed closure of processus vaginalis
  - Complete closure on both side in 18% of newborns
  - 40% close in first 2 months of life
  - 60% close by 2 years
  - Patent processus vaginalis commonly associated with undescended testicles
  - Adult autopsy data demonstrate 15–30% patent.
- Reactive (acquired) hydrocele is imbalance between fluid production and absorption.
  - Majority are idiopathic.
    - Defective lymphatic drainage
    - Aspirated fluid similar protein content to lymphatic fluid
  - Result of inflammation from trauma, testicular torsion, torsion of testicular appendage, epididymo-orchitis
  - Postvaricocelectomy second most common cause

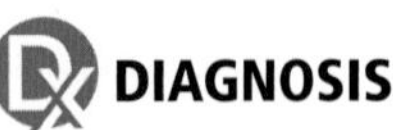

DIAGNOSIS

HISTORY

- Inguinal or scrotal/labial swelling
- Age of onset
  - Birth, after birth, >12 years old
- Laterality
- Fluctuation in size: smaller in morning and larger over day in response to activity and upright position; change with crying/straining
  - May be preceded by constipation, upper respiratory infection, vomiting
- Undescended testicle
- Infection, trauma, torsion
- Pain/discomfort
- History of varicocele or other inguinal surgery

PHYSICAL EXAM

Palpate scrotal/labial swelling.

- Soft or tense
- Compressible/reducible
- Palpate testicle.
  - Confirm descent.
  - Rule out mass, trauma, infection.
- Bowel contents—rule out hernia. Transillumination of scrotum to confirm fluid; not diagnostic

DIFFERENTIAL DIAGNOSIS

- Indirect hernia
- Varicocele
- Spermatocele/epididymal cyst
- Epididymo-orchitis
- Hematocele
- Scrotal lymphedema
- Nephrotic syndrome

DIAGNOSTIC TESTS & INTERPRETATION

Initial Tests (screening, lab, imaging)

- Urine analysis and culture if concerns for epididymo-orchitis
- Tumor markers (hCG, α-fetoprotein [AFP]) if concern for testicular mass
- Imaging not required in an uncomplicated scrotal hydrocele with palpable testicle
- Transscrotal ultrasound if testicle difficult to palpate or concerns for concomitant problem
  - Assess testicle for pathology, blood flow, and inflammation/infection.
  - Differentiate bowel loops (hernia) from fluid.
  - Fluid tracking to peritoneal cavity can differentiate communicating versus noncommunicating.
  - Fluid tracking to abdominal component (retroperitoneal collection) demonstrates abdominoscrotal hydrocele.

ALERT

If palpation of testicle is limited by tense hydrocele, transscrotal ultrasound is important to assess for testicular location, viability, and potential pathology.

TREATMENT

GENERAL MEASURES

- Conservative management for babies presenting at birth with noncommunicating hydrocele (no fluctuation in size) for 24 months
  - Consider surgical intervention if persistent >24 months.
  - Fluid aspiration discouraged in babies due to risk of infection
- Initial conservative management of infantile communicating hydrocele
  - Some surgeons advocate observation up to 12 to 18 months for potential spontaneous resolution.
    - 84–89% spontaneous resolution (most by 6 months; none after 18 months)
    - No difference in resolution rates between preterm versus term babies
  - Surgical intervention for development of inguinal hernia (7% of infantile hydroceles)
- Treatment for communicating hydrocele presenting in children >1 year old is essentially same as for inguinal hernia.
- Reactive hydrocele managed conservatively
  - Antibiotics for epididymo-orchitis
  - Surgery reserved for pain or patients self-conscious regarding size/appearance

SURGERY/OTHER PROCEDURES

- Inguinal approach for communicating hydrocele
  - Concomitant orchiopexy (undescended testicle) or orchiectomy (testis mass) when clinically indicated
- Controversial whether to explore or assess contralateral side with laparoscope for patent processus vaginalis
  - Visualization of a contralateral processus vaginalis (internal ring) does not always correlate with metachronous development of a contralateral inguinal hernia or communicating hydrocele.
- Transscrotal approach for reactive hydroceles in adolescent (>12 years old) and adult
  - Consider surgical intervention if persistent >24 months or very large.
- Transscrotal aspiration, with or without sclerosing agent, reserved for postoperative hydroceles

ONGOING CARE

FOLLOW-UP RECOMMENDATIONS

- Serial physical exam (q4–6mo in babies; annual for adolescent) for nonoperative management
  - Consideration of ultrasound for very tense hydrocele, preventing palpation of testicle
- Postoperative visit within weeks of surgery and subsequent visit to confirm healthy testicle, free of recurrent hydrocele

ADDITIONAL READING

- Cimador M, Castagnetti M, De Grazia E. Management of hydrocele in adolescent patients. *Nat Rev Urol.* 2010;7(7):379–385.
- Clarke S. Pediatric inguinal hernia and hydrocele: an evidence-based review in the era of minimal access surgery. *J Laparoendosc Adv Surg Tech A.* 2010;20(3):305–309.
- Hall NJ, Ron O, Eaton S, et al. Surgery for hydrocele in children—an avoidable excess? *J Pediatr Surg.* 2011;46(12):2401–2405.
- Koski ME, Makari JH, Adams MC, et al. Infant communicating hydroceles—do they need immediate repair or might some clinically resolve? *J Pediatr Surg.* 2010;45(3):590–593.
- Merriman LS, Herrel L, Kirsch AJ. Inguinal and genital anomalies. *Pediatr Clin North Am.* 2012;59(4):769–781.
- Naji H, Ingolfsson I, Isacson D, et al. Decision making in the management of hydroceles in infants and children. *Eur J Pediatr.* 2012;171(5):807–810.
- Osifo OD, Osaigbovo EO. Congenital hydrocele: prevalence and outcome among male children who underwent neonatal circumcision in Benin City, Nigeria. *J Pediatr Urol.* 2008;4(3):178–182.

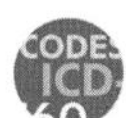

CODES

ICD10

- N43.3 Hydrocele, unspecified
- N43.2 Other hydrocele
- P83.5 Congenital hydrocele

FAQ

- Q: Do hydroceles need to be corrected?
- A: Noncommunicating hydroceles can be managed conservatively and commonly will resolve within the first 12 to 24 months of life. Watchful waiting is recommended in this age group. Persistent hydroceles after age 2 years are assumed to be communicating hydroceles. Communicating hydroceles are managed similarly to indirect inguinal hernias. Some surgeons advocate monitoring asymptomatic communicating hydrocele for 6 to 12 months to see if they resolve. Hydroceles progressing to inguinal hernia require surgical intervention. Reactive hydroceles are treated if patient is symptomatic, self-conscious of size, or testicle is difficult to palpate.
- Q: What are the potential consequences of leaving hydrocele untreated?
- A: There are no clear long-term adverse consequences on fertility for leaving a noncommunicating hydrocele untreated. Potential concerns raised for testicular growth and function, though, may be alleviated with hydrocele repair. However, hydroceles may continue to grow in size, causing discomfort and distress. Untreated communicating hydrocele may progress to inguinal hernia.
- Q: Are there risks of a hydrocele developing on the other side?
- A: Similar to inguinal hernia, communicating hydroceles have risk of metachronous development of hydrocele on contralateral side. Inguinal hernia will present on other side 8.5–15% of time, although this rate is not clearly defined in communicating hydrocele. Visualization of a contralateral patent processus vaginalis does not always correlate with metachronous development of a contralateral inguinal hernia or communicating hydrocele.
- Q: What are the risks of hydrocele repair?
- A: Risks of the surgery are similar to inguinal hernia repair and include anesthetic risks, injury to testicle or spermatic cord structures (gonadal vessels, vas deferens), injury to ilioinguinal nerve, subsequent atrophy of the testicle, and recurrent hydrocele.

HYDROCEPHALUS

Rebecca A. Dorner, MD • Shenandoah Robinson, MD • Vera Joanna Burton, MD, PhD

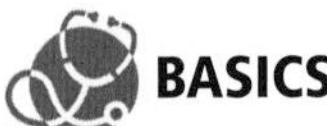

BASICS

DESCRIPTION

- Active distension of the ventricular system resulting from inadequate passage of cerebral spinal fluid (CSF) from its point of production to point of absorption
- CSF compartment progressively enlarged at the expense of brain and/or spinal tissue

EPIDEMIOLOGY

Pediatric prevalence estimated at 1:1,000 children

RISK FACTORS

- Intraventricular hemorrhage (IVH)
- Maternal medications (isotretinoin)
- Megalencephaly
- VACTERL association

Genetics

X-linked mutation in *L1CAM* gene most common genetic cause, accounting for 10% males with idiopathic isolated hydrocephalus, may also be associated with congenital muscular dystrophies/neuronal migrational defects (Walker-Warburg and muscle-eye-brain phenotypes)

PATHOPHYSIOLOGY

- CSF originates from choroid plexus and interstitial fluid of brain/spinal cord and travels via both unidirectional bulk flow and pulsatile flow from cardiac cycle; starts in lateral ventricles → foramina of Monro → 3rd ventricle → aqueduct of Sylvius → 4th ventricle → foramina of Luschka and Magendie → subarachnoid space → into either arachnoid villi to venous system or to lymphatic sinuses
- Hydrocephalus results from obstruction to flow, impaired reabsorption, or rarely overproduction of CSF.
- Obstructive hydrocephalus: Blockage of flow or impaired absorption can necessitate urgent evaluation.
  - Acute (hours) (i.e., direct ventricular obstruction) → surgical emergency
  - Subacute/progressive (weeks to months) → increased ventricle size/interstitial edema = if not treated can cause brain herniation/arrest
  - Chronic (years) (i.e., late-onset aqueductal stenosis) → ventricles and skull slowly increase in size = slow loss of brain volume
- Communicating hydrocephalus—no morphologic obstruction to CSF, less time sensitive
  - May be secondary to arachnoid pathology or impaired elasticity of spinal dura

ETIOLOGY

Hydrocephalus is a heterogeneous condition with varying classification systems, organized here as "congenital," present at birth, or "acquired," occurring after birth, although some conditions may fit into both groups.

- Congenital hydrocephalus
  - Aqueductal stenosis—most common cause of congenital hydrocephalus (~10% cases); stenosis of aqueduct of Sylvius (passageway between 3rd and 4th ventricles)
  - Neural tube defect–associated—that is, myelomeningoceles and Chiari II malformation (cerebellum and brainstem extend into foramen magnum)
  - Arachnoid cysts—most often located in posterior fossa, 3rd ventricle/suprasellar
  - Dandy-Walker malformation—4th ventricle enlarged/cystic as either outlet obstruction or failure of cerebellar development
  - Craniosynostosis/skeletal dysplasias—that is, achondroplasia, FGF mutations
  - Other associated syndromes—that is, trisomies 13, 18, 21, mucopolysaccharidoses (type II [Hunter], type VI [Maroteaux-Lamy]), Apert and Crouzon syndromes, NF1
- Acquired
  - IVH—most in setting of prematurity. Posthemorrhagic hydrocephalus develops secondary to meningeal adhesions, clots, and granular ependymitis in 35% of all neonates surviving IVH; worse prognosis when associated with moderate/severe ventriculomegaly, echolucencies, or white matter injury
  - Infection (meningitis) can lead to leptomeningeal adhesions and granulations that block reabsorption of CSF (high-risk infections include enterovirus, CMV, lymphocytic choriomeningitis virus [LCMV], toxoplasmosis; may also occur intrauterine).
  - Brain tumors—in children, most often posterior fossa tumors compressing 4th ventricle
  - Head injury—blood from ruptured vessels may cause inflammation, scarring of meninges, or clot.

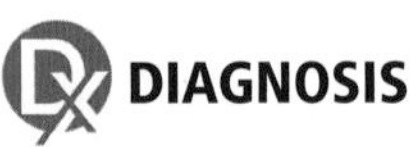

DIAGNOSIS

PHYSICAL EXAM

- Prenatally diagnosed
  - Hydrocephalus may be diagnosed on prenatal ultrasound; when encountered on ultrasound subsequent fetal MRI can help to identify additional brain/spinal cord pathology.
  - Genetic testing via amniocentesis may be performed.
- Infants/children <2 years:
  - Exam: rapidly enlarging infant occipital frontal circumference (OFC) (>2 cm/week), macrocephaly (OFC >2 SDs above mean for age, sex, gestational age), increased splaying of cranial sutures, frontal bossing, full/tense fontanelle with dilated scalp veins, paralysis of upward gaze or setting sun sign, lateral gaze palsy, nystagmus, ptosis, impaired pupillary response, lower extremity spasticity
  - ROS: worsening of apnea/bradycardia, lethargy/excessive fussiness, feeding intolerance
  - Cushing triad (hypertension, reflex bradycardia, respiratory irregularities) not generally seen in infants prior to fusion of cranial sutures
- Older children >2 years
  - Exam: papilledema (although may not be present in chronic hydrocephalus), new-onset diplopia or extraocular movement abnormality, (especially CN VI palsy), strabismus, spasticity of lower > upper extremities, gait ataxia, hypothalamic-pituitary dysfunction from compression of hypothalamus/pituitary stalk by 3rd ventricle → diabetes insipidus, obesity, hypothyroidism, etc.
  - ROS: can have symptoms of increased intracranial pressure (ICP) (early-morning headache, vomiting, double vision, somnolence, behavioral changes) or focal deficits prior to changes in head size

DIFFERENTIAL DIAGNOSIS

Other causes of macrocephaly:

- Chronic subdural hematomas secondary to abusive head trauma
- "Benign" enlargement of subarachnoid spaces—enlargement of subarachnoid space with normal ventricles
- Familial megalencephaly
- Metabolic conditions (i.e., glutaric aciduria type 1) resulting in enlargement of subarachnoid spaces
- Pericerebral effusions
- Congenital anomalies of intracerebral or extracerebral veins (including AVMs)
- Tumors, intracranial cysts
- Head-sparing intrauterine growth retardation (relative macrocephaly)
- Rapid catch-up growth following prolonged malnutrition
- Variety of other causes: fragile X, autism spectrum disorders, Cowden syndrome, leukodystrophies (Alexander disease, Canavan disease, megalencephalic leukoencephalopathy), lysosomal storage disorders (Tay-Sachs, mucopolysaccharidoses, and gangliosidoses), organic acid disorders

DIAGNOSTIC TESTS & INTERPRETATION

- Prenatal anatomy ultrasound and fetal MRI
  - Fetal MRI has superior soft tissue resolution versus ultrasound; can better study maturational, migrational, myelinating processes in high-resolution, ultrafast, single-shot T2-weighted sequences; compared with ultrasound, more sensitive evaluation of the fetal cortex, gray, and white matter structures
  - Fetal MRI does not reach the high sensitivity and specificity that postnatal MRI offers.
- Postnatal head ultrasound
  - Standard screening test for premature infants and neonates with suspected hydrocephalus or IVH
  - Anterior fontanelle must be patent.
  - Demonstrates ventricular size, presence of blood, echolucencies, and additional brain anomalies
- MRI
  - Standard MRI is definitive test in hydrocephalus to describe brain anatomy and white matter injury; should be first choice for elective studies
  - Rapid brain MRI protocols (i.e., FIESTA/HASTE/ultrafast sequences) for urgent shunt obstruction evaluation are replacing CT at some institutions; <1% of children need sedation for this sequence.
  - Rapid MRI detection of shunt malfunction: sensitivity 51–59%, specificity 89–93%
  - Note: Magnetic field may reset programmable valve; test should be done in location where can be reprogrammed by trained provider afterwards.
- Shunt series
  - AP and lateral plain radiographs to evaluate entire length of CSF catheter
  - Poor sensitivity (4–26%) but high specificity (92–98%) for detection of malfunction; should not be used as 1st-line diagnostic test

- Noncontrast CT of the brain (request low-radiation protocol)
  - Traditional test used to assess ventriculomegaly, shunt placement in children with closed anterior fontanelles
  - Better visualization of 4th ventricle/brainstem
  - Detection of shunt malfunction: sensitivity 53–92%, specificity 76–93%

ALERT

When imaging to diagnose shunt malfunction, it is important to consider the lifetime cumulative radiation exposure for each child and use CT cautiously. In addition, up to 20% of shunt malfunctions will have no change in ventricular size noted on either MRI or CT of the brain.

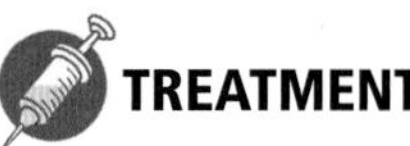

TREATMENT

ADDITIONAL THERAPIES

Temporary treatment options (to be done with neurosurgery/neurology guidance)

- Oral medications (acetazolamide/furosemide)—temporizing measure in older children with CSF disorders like pseudotumor cerebri
  - Not indicated for preterm children—increase the likelihood of death and disability
- Serial lumbar punctures (LPs)
  - Early serial LPs in neonates may decrease need for surgical intervention.

SURGERY/OTHER PROCEDURES

- Indications for surgical intervention
  - Acute symptomatic hydrocephalus
  - Progressive hydrocephalus despite above interventions
- Contraindications
  - Active infection
  - Acute hemorrhage
  - Overall poor prognosis
- Temporary surgical treatment
  - Delays insertion of permanent shunt for premature infants
  - Allows infant to gain weight (goal 2.5 kg for ventriculoperitoneal [VP] shunt) and for blood products to dissipate; placement associated with fewer revisions versus initial VP shunt
    - Ventricular reservoir (ventricular access device): allows for intermittent removal of CSF via serial taps
    - Ventriculosubgaleal shunt: continuous CSF diversion; forms subgaleal collection that deforms skin over scalp; skin deformation will resolve with placement of VP shunt.
- Permanent shunt
  - VP shunt—primary mode of CSF diversion in pediatrics
  - Shunt parts: proximal ventriculostomy catheter, pressure-sensitive valve, distal catheter
  - Peritoneum most common distal endpoint as CSF efficiently absorbed by peritoneum; other possible locations include the pleura, ureter, right atrium.
- Endoscopic third ventriculostomy or 3rd ventricle fenestration
  - Effective for obstructive hydrocephalus in children with space-occupying lesions
  - Less effective for children <1 year

ONGOING CARE

FOLLOW-UP RECOMMENDATIONS

- When etiology of macrocephaly is unclear, it is important to follow children closely:
  - NICU patients should have weekly OFCs at baseline and more frequent measurements and serial head ultrasounds if concern for macrocephaly.
  - OFCs should be closely followed for 6 months as outpatient for resolution of growth in cases of isolated enlargement of subarachnoid spaces.
  - Familial macrocephaly should be diagnosis of exclusion after imaging performed, other genetic diagnoses considered, and parental OFCs analyzed.
- Children with confirmed hydrocephalus of varying etiologies are at high risk for developmental delay and should be screened per most frequent AAP recommendations.
- Referrals as appropriate for physical therapy, occupational therapy, orthopedic therapies for spasticity, interdisciplinary cerebral palsy (CP), and NICU follow-up clinics

PATIENT EDUCATION

National Hydrocephalus Foundation: http://www.nhfonline.org

PROGNOSIS

- Chronic hydrocephalus: increased risk for developmental delay in all domains but outcome varies widely depending on cause and severity of hydrocephalus, presence of comorbid neurologic disorders, or risk factors such as prematurity, neurologic imaging abnormalities
- Commonly encountered issues:
  - Visuospatial challenges (cortical visual impairment, myopia)
  - Motor challenges—CP, spasticity of lower > upper extremities, fine motor coordination problems
  - Hypothalamic-pituitary dysfunction
  - Higher rates of intellectual disability
  - Higher rates of ADHD/attentional disorders

COMPLICATIONS

- Acute hydrocephalus from shunt malfunction or acute progression of hydrocephalus resulting in fatal herniation syndrome
  - Shunt malfunction: due to obstruction of lumen (proximal obstruction most common cause of malfunction in first 2 years of life), overdrainage, pressure valve or reservoir malfunction, catheter damage/disconnection, catheter migration, catheter infection
  - 40% shunts require operative revision within 1 year of placement; 80% need revision within decade. Late shunt failure may occur years after placement, often due to fracture of tubing.
- Other serious complications of shunt placement and revisions include infection (rate of ~10% per shunt manipulation, most within 6 months, commonly *Staphylococcus epidermidis*), CSF leak, neurologic deficits, extraparenchymal hemorrhage.
- Children with ventricular shunts require urgent evaluation for symptoms of possible obstruction or infection: lethargy, headache, low-grade fever, erythema of overlying skin.

ADDITIONAL READING

- Boyle TP, Nigrovic LE. Radiographic evaluation of pediatric cerebrospinal fluid shunt malfunction in the emergency setting. *Pediatr Emerg Care*. 2015;31(6):435–440.
- Boyle TP, Paldino MJ, Kimia AA, et al. Comparison of rapid cranial MRI to CT for ventricular shunt malfunction. *Pediatrics*. 2014;134(1):e47–e54.
- Browd SR, Gottfried ON, Ragel BT, et al. Failure of cerebrospinal fluid shunts: part II: overdrainage, loculation, and abdominal complications. *Pediatr Neurol*. 2006;34(3):171–176.
- Browd SR, Ragel BT, Gottfried ON, et al. Failure of cerebrospinal fluid shunts: part I: obstruction and mechanical failure. *Pediatr Neurol*. 2006;34(2):83–92.
- Huisman TA. Fetal magnetic resonance imaging of the brain: is ventriculomegaly the tip of the syndromal iceberg? *Semin Ultrasound CT MR*. 2011;32(6):491–509.
- Robinson S. Neonatal posthemorrhagic hydrocephalus from prematurity: pathophysiology and current treatment concepts: a review. *J Neurosurg Pediatr*. 2012;9(3):242–258.
- Tully HM, Dobyns WB. Infantile hydrocephalus: a review of epidemiology, classification and causes. *Eur J Med Genet*. 2014;57(8):359–368.

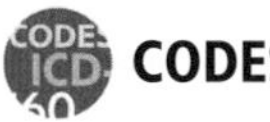

CODES

ICD10

- G91.9 Hydrocephalus, unspecified
- G91.0 Communicating hydrocephalus
- G91.1 Obstructive hydrocephalus

FAQ

- Q: When does an infant need a head ultrasound?
- A: Any infant whose OFC increases by more than a quartile on the growth chart or >2 cm/week, needs a head ultrasound. Preterm infants below a certain gestational age or birth weight (varies from hospital to hospital) should receive screening head ultrasounds while in the NICU.
- Q: What is the workup for shunt obstruction and shunt infection?
- A: Signs and symptoms of increased ICP should lead to an urgent neurosurgical evaluation; the most useful studies to evaluate obstruction include preferably MRI (rapid MRI if available, head CT if no MRI available) +/− shunt series. Fever is the most important indication for a shunt infection evaluation (shunt tap with CSF cell count, protein, glucose, Gram stain, and culture). Vigilance and caution warranted as shunt infection may present similarly to other pediatric viral illnesses with low-grade fever, vomiting, etc.
- Q: Is hydrocephalus inherited?
- A: X-linked hydrocephalus associated with stenosis of the aqueduct of Sylvius is the most common heritable form, thought to account for 10% of males with isolated idiopathic hydrocephalus. Mutations in the *L1CAM* gene are the main genetic cause and often occur within abnormalities of the corpus callosum, hypoplasia or aplasia of the corticospinal tracts, adducted thumbs on exam. *L1CAM* testing should be strongly considered in all males with unexplained hydrocephalus but should be regarded as mandatory for those with a family history of hydrocephalus or adducted thumbs.

H

HYDRONEPHROSIS

J. Christopher Austin, MD • Michael C. Carr, MD, PhD

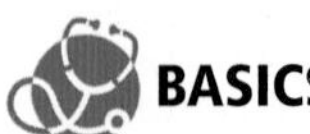

BASICS

DESCRIPTION

- Hydronephrosis: dilation of the renal pelvis (pelviectasis) and calyces (caliectasis) due to excess urine in the collecting system of the kidney
- Hydroureteronephrosis: dilation of the renal collecting system and the ureter to the level of the bladder

EPIDEMIOLOGY

- Incidence of hydronephrosis noted on routine prenatal ultrasound is 0.4–5%.
- 10–30% of fetuses with hydronephrosis are due to ureteropelvic junction obstruction.
- Posterior urethral valves and triad syndrome account for 1–2% of cases.

ETIOLOGY

- Ureteropelvic junction obstruction
  - Partial obstruction at the region where the renal pelvis drains into the ureter
- Megaureter
  - Partial obstruction due to an intrinsic narrowing or an aperistaltic segment of distal ureter at the ureterovesical junction
- Vesicoureteral reflux
  - In primary reflux (grades I to V depending on the severity), it is due to an insufficient flap valve–type mechanism at the ureterovesical junction which allows urine to flow retrograde from the bladder up into the ureters.
  - Hydroureteronephrosis is usually seen only with higher grades of reflux (grades III to V) or secondary reflux (reflux in the presence of an abnormal bladder, in which the reflux is often due to high storage or voiding pressures within the bladder). Secondary reflux is not graded.
- Ureterocele
  - Hydroureteronephrosis secondary to obstruction of the ureter from a cystic dilation of the intravesical portion of the distal ureter
  - Most often associated with the upper pole ureter in duplicated collecting system; less frequently associated with a single system
  - Ureterocele is further classified as intravesical (contained completely within the bladder) or ectopic (extending down the bladder neck and often into the urethra).
- Ectopic ureter
  - A ureter that drains into an abnormal location outside of the bladder
  - The hydroureteronephrosis can be the upper pole ureter of a duplicated collecting system or a single system.
  - Ectopic ureters can drain at various sites along the lower urinary tract depending on the sex of the child. In boys, they can drain into the bladder neck, prostatic urethra, vas deferens, seminal vesicle, or epididymis. In girls, they can drain into the bladder neck, urethra, introitus, and vagina.
  - The ectopic locations often require passage through the bladder neck or urogenital diaphragm, which produces obstruction of the distal ureter.
- Urolithiasis
  - Obstructing calculi often produce dilation of the urinary tract proximal to its location.
  - Stone disease is rare in infancy except in preterm infants who receive furosemide.
  - The hydronephrosis is usually associated with renal colic.
- Posterior urethral valves
  - Hydroureteronephrosis: nearly always bilateral, produced by outflow obstruction of the bladder from an obstructing membrane in the prostatic urethra
  - Because both kidneys are affected, there is a significant risk of chronic kidney disease and eventual progression to end-stage renal disease.
- Triad syndrome
  - Hydroureteronephrosis, often with massively dilated ureters and a large bladder
  - Also known as prune belly syndrome or Eagle-Barrett syndrome
  - These boys have a triad of hypoplastic abdominal wall musculature (leading to a prunelike appearance), bilateral undescended testes, and a dilated urinary tract.
  - May have associated urethral atresia, imparting worse renal function prognosis
  - Significant risk of renal insufficiency and bladder dysfunction in these patients

DIAGNOSIS

HISTORY

- Newborns
  - Antenatal hydronephrosis: presence of hydronephrosis or hydroureteronephrosis
  - If unilateral, severity of hydronephrosis and the status of contralateral kidney
  - If bilateral, presence of bladder wall thickening, bladder enlargement, bladder emptying, or a dilated posterior urethra (keyhole sign) may indicate posterior urethral valves or triad syndrome.
  - If oligohydramnios is present, pulmonary hypoplasia is a concern. The presence of oligohydramnios, increased renal echogenicity, and cystic changes in the kidneys are indicators of poor renal function and dysplasia.
- Older children
  - History of urinary tract infections or gross hematuria
  - General health and growth (poor growth due to chronic kidney disease)
  - Daytime incontinence, poor urinary stream, or symptoms of voiding dysfunction may be an indicator of bladder dysfunction due to posterior urethral valves.
  - History of episodic abdominal (which may not lateralize well), flank, or back pain in the presence of hydronephrosis is often due to symptomatic ureteropelvic junction obstruction (see topic "Ureteropelvic Junction Obstruction").

PHYSICAL EXAM

- Neonate
  - Signs of oligohydramnios (Potter facies, lateral patellar dimples, clubfeet, and other limb deformities) and respiratory distress
  - Palpable abdominal mass
  - Palpable walnut-sized bladder (posterior urethral valves)
  - Patent urachus
  - Ascites
  - Development of abdominal wall musculature (wrinkled prunelike appearance in triad syndrome)
- Older children
  - Presence of abdominal mass
  - Abdominal or flank tenderness

DIFFERENTIAL DIAGNOSIS

- Cystic renal tumor
  - Most commonly Wilms tumor
  - Distinguished from hydronephrosis by ultrasound or CT scanning
- Multicystic dysplastic kidney
  - Can be difficult to distinguish from severe hydronephrosis with marked parenchymal thinning
  - Renal scan will show no function or perfusion with multicystic dysplastic kidney.

DIAGNOSTIC TESTS & INTERPRETATION

- Newborn
  - Hydronephrosis or hydroureteronephrosis with a normal contralateral kidney does not require any immediate laboratory testing.
  - If both kidneys are affected or a solitary kidney is affected, there is a need for serial assessments of renal function (serum electrolytes and creatinine).
- Older children
  - Urinalysis to detect hematuria or pyuria; culture if infection suspected
  - In cases where both kidneys are affected or there is a solitary kidney, renal function should be evaluated.
- Infants with antenatally detected hydronephrosis may be evaluated with three imaging studies:
  - Renal/bladder ultrasound
  - Voiding cystourethrogram
  - Renal scan
- A recent consensus of pediatric radiologists, urologists, nephrologists, and perinatologists have developed a new classification for urinary tract dilation (UTD).
  - The UTD is classified base on the presence or absence of central versus peripheral calyceal dilation, normal or abnormal renal parenchyma, degree of dilation of the renal pelvis, and associated abnormalities of the bladder and ureters.
  - They are reported for postnatal hydronephrosis as UTD—UTD P1 (low risk), UTD P2 (intermediate risk), and UTD P3 (high).
  - Follow-up studies, timing, and prophylactic antibiotic recommended based on the risk stratification groups. This classification system is being adopted at many centers as it gives a uniform system for the classification of prenatal and postnatal hydronephrosis.
- The timing for evaluation can be elective for unilateral hydronephrosis with a normal contralateral kidney, but if both kidneys are affected or a solitary kidney is involved, prompt evaluation of the newborn should be undertaken.
- Renal/bladder ultrasound
  - Because of a period of relative oliguria of a newborn in the first 24 to 48 hours of life, an ultrasound may underestimate the degree of hydronephrosis during this time and thus should be postponed until the infant is at least 48 hours old and having good urine output.

- This should not preclude evaluating an infant during this time as long as a normal study is repeated after 48 hours of life and <1 month of age.
- In cases where both kidneys were affected or there is a solitary affected kidney, the evaluation should not be delayed.
- Ultrasound of the kidneys should reveal the severity of dilation of the renal pelvis and calyces, changes in the amount and echogenicity of the parenchyma, and presence of cortical cysts.
- Evaluation of the full bladder is important as well. It will show dilated distal ureters, which may indicate ureterovesical junction obstruction, vesicoureteral reflux, or hydroureteronephrosis from posterior urethral valves or triad syndrome.

- Voiding cystourethrogram
  - Evaluates presence of vesicoureteral reflux and grading of the severity
  - Bladder shape, presence of diverticulum, and trabeculations may indicate hypertrophy from posterior urethral valves, neurogenic bladder dysfunction, or voiding dysfunction (in older children).
  - Test can be delayed until after discharge from nursery unless there is concern about posterior urethral valves, in which case it should be done in the early postnatal period.
  - The Society for Fetal Urology consensus statement on the evaluation and management of antenatal hydronephrosis states that there is no clear evidence to support or to avoid postnatal imaging for vesicoureteral reflux. The overall incidence of vesicoureteral reflux is up to 30% in children with antenatal hydronephrosis, and currently, it remains unproven whether the identification and treatment of children with vesicoureteral reflux confers any clinical benefit. Without the presence of ureteral dilation on the ultrasound, an argument can be made to defer performing a voiding cystourethrogram study.
- Renal scan
  - Can quantify the differential renal function or the amount each kidney contributes to overall renal function (The normal differential function is 50% ± 5% for each kidney.)
  - The two most commonly used radionuclides are mercaptoacetyltriglycine-3 (MAG-3) and diethylenetriamine pentaacetic acid (DTPA). MAG-3 is the best choice for infants and babies.
  - In addition to the ability to detect diminished function, if there is poor drainage of the affected kidney, furosemide is given to wash out the radiotracer. The duration for washing out 1/2 of the accumulated radiotracer ($T_{1/2}$) is often given in the report. A prompt $T_{1/2}$ (<10 minutes) is indicative of a nonobstructed kidney. A slower $T_{1/2}$ may be indicative of obstruction when it is >20 minutes. A 10- to 20-minute $T_{1/2}$ is indeterminate for obstruction. Many factors affect the $T_{1/2}$, making it less reliable for indicating obstruction. These factors include the hydration status, presence of vesicoureteral reflux, and overall kidney function (very poorly functioning kidneys have a poor response to diuretics).
- CT scan
  - Most commonly done in cases where the hydronephrosis is symptomatic
  - Noncontrast spiral CT is the most sensitive way to detect stones, as even stones radiolucent on plain films (uric acid) will be detected by CT.
- Magnetic resonance urography is being used more widely in the evaluation of hydronephrosis which avoids the use of ionizing radiation. Refinements in the technique and comprehensive automated functional analysis are now available. Ongoing issues remain concerning the use of sedation, need for a Foley catheter, and the overall expense of the study which continue to limit its overall applicability.

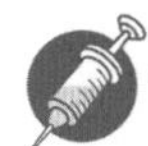

TREATMENT

GENERAL MEASURES

Neonates with severe hydronephrosis or high-risk findings such as a ureterocele or ectopic ureter are started on prophylactic antibiotics of amoxicillin (10 to 15 mg/kg daily). When the baby is 2 months old, the antibiotic can be changed to trimethoprim (2 mg/kg daily), trimethoprim/sulfamethoxazole (2 mg/kg of trimethoprim daily), or nitrofurantoin (12 mg/kg daily).

ONGOING CARE

FOLLOW-UP RECOMMENDATIONS

- Ureteropelvic junction obstruction
  - After initial evaluation, infants are usually followed with serial studies, either ultrasound or renal scans, depending on the degree of functional impairment, the severity of the hydronephrosis, and the pattern of drainage on the renal scan.
  - For more information, see topic "Ureteropelvic Junction Obstruction."
- Ureterovesical junction obstruction
  - After initial evaluation, children are followed with serial studies as with ureteropelvic junction obstruction.
  - These lesions are much less common than ureteropelvic junction obstruction, and most of the time, the affected kidneys have normal function and can be followed conservatively.
  - If the function of the kidney is significantly diminished (differential function of 35–40%), surgical treatment of the obstruction is indicated.
- Vesicoureteral reflux
  - Infants with high-grade reflux are kept on prophylactic antibiotics.
  - In the absence of breakthrough infections, they are reevaluated annually.
  - If persistent high-grade reflux continues or breakthrough infections are a problem, surgical correction is carried out.
  - For more information, see topic "Vesicoureteral Reflux."
- Ureterocele/ectopic ureter: Because these are obstructive lesions, they are generally treated surgically early in life at the time of diagnosis.
- Posterior urethral valves
  - Full-term infants undergo cystoscopic valve ablation, whereas preterm infants may require a temporary vesicostomy until endoscopic treatment is feasible.
  - These boys require careful follow-up from a pediatric urologist and nephrologist through adolescence.
  - For more information, see topic "Posterior Urethral Valves."
- Triad syndrome: Typically, these boys will undergo bilateral orchiopexy with or without an abdominoplasty depending on the severity of abdominal wall hypoplasia during the first 6 to 12 months of life. They need regular follow-up for the hydronephrosis and bladder dysfunction.

PROGNOSIS

- Perinatal mortality associated with hydronephrosis most strongly correlates with the presence of chromosomal abnormalities, multiple system abnormalities, detection earlier in gestation, oligohydramnios, severe bilateral presentation, and evidence of infravesical obstruction.
- For most children with hydronephrosis, there is a very low risk of renal failure or significant chronic kidney disease and a normal life expectancy.

ADDITIONAL READING

- Darge K, Higgins M, Hwang TJ, et al. Magnetic resonance and computed tomography in pediatric urology: an imaging overview for current and future daily practice. *Radiol Clin North Am*. 2013;51(4):583–598.
- Khrichenko D, Darge K. Functional analysis in MR urography—made simple. *Pediatr Radiol*. 2010;40(2):182–199.
- Nguyen HT, Benson CB, Bromley B, et al. Multidisciplinary consensus on the classification of prenatal and postnatal urinary tract dilation (UTD classification system). *J Pediatr Urol*. 2014;10(6):982–998.
- Nguyen HT, Herndon CD, Cooper C, et al. The Society for Fetal Urology consensus statement on the evaluation and management of antenatal hydronephrosis. *J Pediatr Urol*. 2010;6(3):212–231.

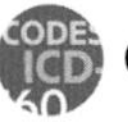

CODES

ICD10

- N13.30 Unspecified hydronephrosis
- N13.39 Other hydronephrosis
- Q62.0 Congenital hydronephrosis

FAQ

- Q: If my baby has hydronephrosis affecting only one kidney, will he need a kidney transplant?
- A: In the absence of oligohydramnios and bilateral hydroureteronephrosis, it would be very rare that a child would develop renal failure requiring transplantation.
- Q: My unborn baby has hydronephrosis in only one kidney, and the other kidney is normal. What are the chances that it is a ureteropelvic junction obstruction?
- A: The chances are ~45% that isolated hydronephrosis is due to a ureteropelvic junction obstruction.
- Q: My male unborn baby has bilateral hydronephrosis but a "normal" bladder. Is there still a chance that he has posterior urethral valves?
- A: Yes. Although it is less likely to be due to posterior urethral valves than if a thick-walled, enlarged, poorly emptying bladder were seen, prenatal ultrasonography is operator dependent. Ultrasound can miss dilated ureters or bladder abnormalities.

H

HYPERCALCEMIA

Philippe F. Backeljauw, MD

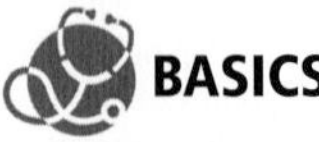

BASICS

DESCRIPTION
Hypercalcemia represents an elevation in ionized and total calcium concentrations.

EPIDEMIOLOGY
- Less common than hypocalcemia
- Less common in children than in adults
- Adults: >90% caused by hyperparathyroidism (HPT) or malignancy
- Children: more diverse etiologies dependent on age of presentation

RISK FACTORS
- Family history of hypercalcemia
- Family history of renal stones
- Chronic renal failure
- Immobilization
- Certain genetic syndromes
- Certain malignancies
- History of neck irradiation
- Gestational maternal hypocalcemia

PATHOPHYSIOLOGY
- Increased calcium influx from the intestinal tract or the skeleton
- Increased renal tubule calcium reabsorption

ETIOLOGY

ALERT

The first step in the determination of an etiology of hypercalcemia is measurement of an intact serum parathyroid hormone (intact PTH) concentration.

- Hypercalcemia with *increased PTH*
  - Familial isolated primary HPT
    - Autosomal dominant (AD)
    - Parathyroid hyperplasia or adenoma(s)
    - *MEN1*, *HRPT2*, *HRPT3* mutations
  - Multiple endocrine neoplasia (MEN)
    - MEN1 (AD)
      - MEN1-inactivating mutation
      - Parathyroid tumors in 90%
      - Pancreatic and pituitary tumors
    - MEN2A (AD)
      - RET proto-oncogene mutations
      - Parathyroid tumors in 20%
      - Medullary thyroid carcinoma and pheochromocytoma
  - Sporadic parathyroid adenoma
    - *Cyclin D1/PRAD1*
    - MEN1 mutations
  - Parathyroid carcinoma (rare)
  - Hyperparathyroidism-jaw tumor syndrome (HPT-JT)
    - *HRPT2* inactivating mutations
    - Parathyroid tumors may present in adolescence.
    - Mandibular, maxillary, and renal tumors may occur.
  - Neonatal severe HPT (NSHPT)
    - Homozygous inactivating calcium-sensing receptor (*CaSR*) mutations (AR)
  - Neonatal HPT (NHPT)
    - Heterozygous inactivating CaSR mutations or dominant/negative (less severe presentation)
- Hypercalcemia with *normal PTH*
  - Familial benign hypercalcemia or familial hypocalciuric hypercalcemia (FHH)
    - Heterozygous inactivating CaSR mutations (AD)
    - Typically asymptomatic
    - Mild hypercalcemia
    - PTH is usually normal (slightly elevated in 15–20%).
    - Fractional calcium excretion <1%
- Hypercalcemia with *low PTH*
  - Williams syndrome
    - 15% with (neonatal, transient) hypercalcemia
    - Hypercalcemia usually resolves after infancy.
    - Caused by a hemizygous microdeletion of up to 28 genes in chromosome 7q11.23, involving the gene encoding the transcription factor TFII-I. TFII-I negatively regulates cellular calcium entry. Without TFII-I, transient receptor potential C3 (TRPC3) channels are overexpressed in kidneys and intestine, leading to hypercalcemia.
    - Associated features: supravalvular aortic stenosis, cognitive impairment, "elfin facies," poor growth
  - Jansen metaphyseal chondrodysplasia
    - Heterozygous mutations in *PTHR1* lead to constitutive activation of PTH/PTHrP receptor.
    - Short-limbed short stature
  - Idiopathic hypercalcemia of infancy
    - Some cases due to loss of function mutations in *CYP24A1*, resulting in impaired inactivation of $1,25(OH)_2$-vitamin D
    - Some patients with a mutation in *SLC34A1*, encoding the renal sodium-phosphate cotransporter 2A (NaPi-IIa), leading to renal phosphate wasting
    - Infants have failure to thrive, vomiting, dehydration, and nephrocalcinosis.
- Other causes of hypercalcemia (mostly PTH-independent):
  - Medications:
    - Thiazides, antifungals, lithium, vitamin A and D
  - Malignancy
    - Local osteolysis (PTHrP, cytokine production, chemotherapy)
    - Humoral hypercalcemia of malignancy (HHM) (PTHrP)
    - Ectopic $1,25(OH)_2$-vitamin D production (lymphomas)
    - Ectopic PTH production
  - Granulomatous disease
    - Sarcoidosis, tuberculosis, cat-scratch disease
    - Increased $1,25(OH)_2$-vitamin D production due to dysregulated 1-α hydroxylase expression in monocytes/macrophages
  - Renal disease
    - Chronic renal failure may lead to secondary and tertiary HPT.
  - Endocrine disorders:
    - Thyrotoxicosis, acute adrenal insufficiency
  - Inborn errors of metabolism:
    - Blue diaper syndrome (defect in tryptophan metabolism)
    - Congenital lactase deficiency
    - Infantile hypophosphatasia (deficiency of tissue nonspecific alkaline phosphatase)
  - Immobilization
    - More common in adolescence
    - Spinal cord injury, quadriplegia
    - May see low serum alkaline phosphatase, hypercalciuria
  - Subcutaneous fat necrosis (SCFN)
    - After complicated delivery
    - Often a history of birth asphyxia
    - Excessive $1,25(OH)_2$-vitamin D production
  - Other
    - Trisomy 21, SHORT syndrome (**s**hort stature, **h**yperextensibility of joints/[inguinal] hernia, **o**cular depression, **R**ieger anomaly, **t**ooth eruption delay), and inflammatory bowel disease, phosphate depletion in severe prematurity

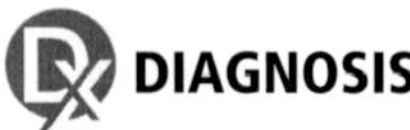

DIAGNOSIS

HISTORY
- Clinical presentation is dependent on age of child, degree of hypercalcemia, and the underlying disorder.
- Mild hypercalcemia (10 to 12 mg/dL)
  - Patients often asymptomatic
  - Failure to thrive
  - Hematuria
  - Nephrolithiasis
  - Nephrocalcinosis
- Moderate hypercalcemia (12 to 14 mg/dL)
  - Constipation
  - Anorexia
  - Abdominal pain
  - Weakness
  - Hematuria
  - Polyuria
  - Dehydration (in infants)
- Severe hypercalcemia (>14 mg/dL)
  - Nausea, vomiting
  - Dehydration
  - Encephalopathy
  - Psychological changes,
  - Poor feeding, hypotonia, and apnea (in newborns)

PHYSICAL EXAM
- Usually normal—unless syndromic
- Parathyroid mass usually not palpable
- Hypertension
- Dehydration
- Soft tissue calcifications uncommon

DIAGNOSTIC TESTS & INTERPRETATION

Initial Tests (screening, lab, imaging)

- Confirm hypercalcemia and obtain intact PTH, serum phosphate, and magnesium, plus electrolyte panel.
- Collect urine to measure calcium excretion and evaluate calcium-to-creatinine ratio:
  - Normal spot urine calcium to creatinine varies by age (<7 months of age, <0.86 mg/mg; 7 to 18 months of age, <0.60 mg/mg; 19 months to 6 years, <0.45 mg/mg; >6 years to adults, <0.22 mg/mg).
  - In children with low muscle mass, can use urine calcium-to-osmolality ratio instead
- Hypercalcemia + low or inappropriately normal urinary calcium indicate FHH (or NSHPT).
- Hypercalcemia, hypophosphatemia, and hyperphosphaturia, plus increased PTH, indicate primary HPT.
- Hypercalcemia, hypophosphatemia, and hyperphosphaturia, with a decreased PTH, indicate HHM if PTHrP is elevated.
- Hypercalcemia/hypercalciuria with normal or increased phosphate points toward other causes (vitamin D or A excess, endocrine disorders, drugs).
- Radiography may show soft tissue calcifications in skin, subcutaneous soft tissues, and gastric mucosa.
- Radiography may show subperiosteal resorption (distal phalanges), tapering of the distal clavicles, "salt and pepper" appearance of the skull, bone cysts and "brown tumors," called osteitis fibrosa cystica (in prolonged hypercalcemia due to HPT).
- Renal ultrasound may show nephrocalcinosis/nephrolithiasis.
- Doppler ultrasound or sestamibi scintigraphy for preoperative assessment of parathyroid adenomas

Diagnostic Procedures/Other

Electrocardiogram may show shortened QTc interval.

ALERT

- In hypoalbuminemia, measured calcium should be corrected for the abnormality in albumin.
- Corrected calcium = measured calcium (in mg/dL) + 0.8 (4.0 − albumin [in g/dL])
- Some prefer to measure ionized calcium in such situations.

TREATMENT

GENERAL MEASURES

- Management depends on the etiology and the severity of hypercalcemia.
- Prompt therapy is needed for severe hypercalcemia (calcium >14 mg/dL).
- In mild/asymptomatic hypercalcemia, no treatment may be needed (FHH).

ALERT

Important to diagnose FHH and distinguish it from other forms of hypercalcemia to avoid unnecessary drug therapy and unwarranted parathyroid surgeries

- General principles
  - Rehydration
  - Increase urinary calcium excretion.
  - Inhibit bone resorption.
  - Decrease intestinal absorption:
    - Depending on cause of hypercalcemia, consider low-calcium diet.

MEDICATION

- Hydration therapy (saluresis)
  - Isotonic saline 3,000 mL/m^2 over 24 to 48 hours intravenously
- Promote calciuresis (only *after* hydration):
  - Furosemide 1 mg/kg every 6 hours intravenously
  - Only use after rehydration because volume contraction and hypokalemic metabolic alkalosis may be further exacerbated
- Decrease bone resorption:
  - For persistent moderate to severe hypercalcemia
  - Acutely: calcitonin 4 U/kg subcutaneously every 12 hours
  - The administration of calcitonin plus isotonic saline usually leads to substantial improvement of hypercalcemia in 1 to 2 days.
  - Bisphosphonate therapy (pamidronate 0.5 to 1 mg/kg, up to 90 mg intravenously over 4 to 6 hours)
  - The bisphosphonate effect will be noticeable after 2 to 4 days.
- Glucocorticoids
  - Inhibit 1-α hydroxylase and reduce intestinal absorption
  - Prednisone 1 to 2 mg/kg/24 h
- Calcimimetics (cinacalcet) increase the sensitivity of the CaSR and suppress PTH secretion:
  - At this time, caution in using cinacalcet in children given pediatric death in a research study using this drug. Denosumab, a monoclonal antibody to nuclear factor-κ ligand (RANKL) can be used for the treatment of giant cell tumor of the bone in adolescents who have completed growth.

SURGERY/OTHER PROCEDURES

- Dialysis: last resort for resistant, life-threatening hypercalcemia
- Surgery (for primary HPT): to be done by experienced thyroid/parathyroid surgeon; rapid perioperative PTH measurement can be helpful to assess if parathyroidectomy was effective in correcting HPT.

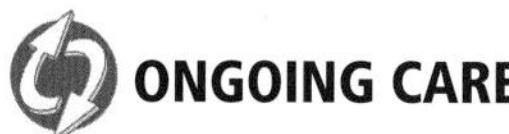

ONGOING CARE

FOLLOW-UP RECOMMENDATIONS

Postsurgical hypocalcemia is common after parathyroidectomy—especially after severe HPT ("hungry bone syndrome"), and requires calcium and phosphate supplementation, and sometimes calcitriol treatment.

PROGNOSIS

- Depends on cause
- Permanent hypoparathyroidism may result from total parathyroidectomy.

ADDITIONAL READING

- Allgrove J. Classification of disorders of bone and calcium metabolism. *Endocr Dev*. 2015;28:291–318.
- Baroncelli GI, Bertelloni S. The use of bisphosphonates in pediatrics. *Horm Res Paediatr*. 2014;82(5):290–302.
- Davies JH. Approach to the child with hypercalcaemia. *Endocr Dev*. 2015;28:101–118.
- Hendy GN, D'Souza-Li L, Yang B, et al. Mutations of the calcium-sensing receptor (CASR) in familial hypocalciuric hypercalcemia, neonatal severe hyperparathyroidism, and autosomal dominant hypocalcemia. *Hum Mutat*. 2000;16(4):281–296.
- Letavernier E, Rodenas A, Guerrot D, et al. Williams-Beuren syndrome hypercalcemia: is TRPC3 a novel mediator in calcium homeostasis? *Pediatrics*. 2012;129(6):e1626–e1630.
- Schlingmann KP, Kaufmann M, Weber S, et al. Mutations in *CYP24A1* and idiopathic infantile hypercalcemia. *N Engl J Med*. 2011;365(5):410–421.

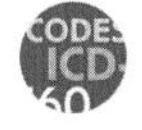

CODES

ICD10

- E83.52 Hypercalcemia
- P71.8 Other transitory neonatal disord of calcium & magnesium metab
- E21.3 Hyperparathyroidism, unspecified

FAQ

- Q: When should vitamin D or vitamin A levels be measured?
- A: If there is a history of alternative medicine, over-the-counter drugs, or supplements
- Q: When should one consider bisphosphonate therapy?
- A: In hypercalcemia, mainly due to mobilization of calcium from bone (e.g., severe HPT, immobilization, tumor)
- Q: When should one consider glucocorticoids?
- A: In hypervitaminosis D or A and in excessive 1,25(OH)$_2$-vitamin D production

HYPERIMMUNOGLOBULINEMIA E SYNDROME

Rachel G. Robison, MD

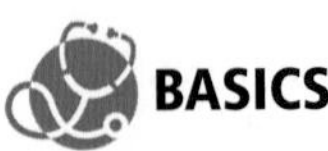

BASICS

DESCRIPTION

Hyperimmunoglobulinemia E syndrome (HIES) is a primary immunodeficiency with markedly elevated serum IgE associated with recurrent skin abscesses, pulmonary infections, and eczematoid dermatitis.

EPIDEMIOLOGY

- Rare
- True incidence and prevalence is unknown; affects equal numbers of males and females

RISK FACTORS

Genetics

- Autosomal dominant cases (AD-HIES) are caused by mutations in signal transducer and activator of transcription 3 (STAT3).
- Autosomal recessive cases (AR-HIES) have mutations in the dedicator of cytokinesis-8 gene (*DOCK8*).
- AR-HIES can also be secondary to tyrosine kinase 2 (TYK2) signaling alterations and phosphoglucomutase 3 (PGM3) mutations.
- AR-HIES patients differ in phenotype from AD-HIES patients.
- Sporadic cases occur.

PATHOPHYSIOLOGY

- *STAT3* is integral in secretion and signaling of multiple cytokines involved in proinflammatory and anti-inflammatory responses.
- A failure of Th17 cell differentiation and failure of IL-17 secretion makes patients susceptible to *Candida* infections.
- Deficiency in IL-11 signaling results in tooth abnormalities and craniosynostosis.
- *DOCK8* deficiency results in failure of dendritic cells to migrate to lymph nodes and affects long-term memory B cells and viral-specific CD8+ T cells.

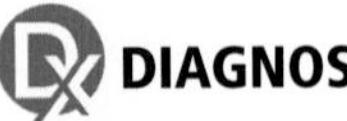

DIAGNOSIS

HISTORY

- Recurrent infections
  - Skin
    - Abscesses
    - Furuncles
    - Cellulitis
    - Lymphadenitis
  - Sinopulmonary infections
    - Pneumonia with aberrant healing, forming pneumatoceles and bronchiectasis
  - Fungal infections: mostly mucocutaneous candidiasis
  - Typical organisms: *Staphylococcus aureus*, *Streptococcus pneumoniae*, *Haemophilus influenzae*
  - Opportunistic infections with *Pneumocystis jiroveci* pneumonia
  - Those with AR-HIES have viral skin infections, including molluscum, warts, and/or recurrent herpes.
- Rash
  - Present in newborn period
  - Can resolve or become eczematoid
- Retention of primary teeth
  - Delayed exfoliation of three or more teeth in 70% of patients
- Vascular anomalies
  - Tortuosity, dilation, and aneurysms of medium-sized vessels

PHYSICAL EXAM

- Facial features are noted in late childhood to early adolescence, including:
  - Asymmetric facies
  - Prominent forehead/chin
  - Wide-set eyes
- Dermatitis
- Skeletal anomalies
  - Scoliosis
  - Craniosynostosis
  - Hyperextensible joints
  - Osteopenia leading to resultant bone fractures from minor trauma
- Hard palate anomalies, high-arched palate

DIFFERENTIAL DIAGNOSIS

- Atopic dermatitis
- Wiskott-Aldrich syndrome
- Severe combined immunodeficiency (SCID)
- Omenn syndrome
- Immune dysregulation, polyendocrinopathy, enteropathy X-linked (IPEX) syndrome
- Netherton syndrome

DIAGNOSTIC TESTS & INTERPRETATION

- Total serum IgE of >2,000 IU/mL
  - Elevation may not be present in newborns.
  - Can decline to normal levels in adult years
  - Level does not correlate with disease severity.
- Lymphopenia with low T cells. B and NK cells are noted, often with impaired function in AR-HIES.
- Peripheral eosinophilia
  - Does not correlate with IgE
  - Present in >90% of patients
- Immunoglobulin levels
  - IgG and IgM are usually normal.
  - IgA may be normal or low.
  - IgM is often decreased in *DOCK8* AR-HIES.
- Specific antibody response is variable.
- Reduced CD45RO+ memory T cells and memory B cells with normal total lymphocyte counts in AD-HIES
- Neutropenia may be present in a subset of patients and with infection.
- CT of the lungs if history of pneumonia to look for bronchiectasis and/or pneumatoceles

TREATMENT

GENERAL MEASURES

- Implement good management of dermatitis with regular hydration and emollient use.
- Control pruritus with antihistamines.
- Dilute bleach baths to decrease staphylococcal skin colonization.
- Promptly and aggressively treat all infections.
- Physical therapy for joint pain related to hyperextensibility

MEDICATION

- Prophylactic antibiotics, typically trimethoprim/sulfamethoxazole, for prevention of staphylococcal infection
- Immunoglobulin replacement therapy in the case of concomitant hypogammaglobulinemia
- Consideration of antifungal prophylaxis if recurrent/chronic *Candida* infections

ADDITIONAL THERAPIES

Hematopoietic stem cell transplantation has been performed in AD-HIES with varying success, may be more successful in *DOCK8* AR-HIES

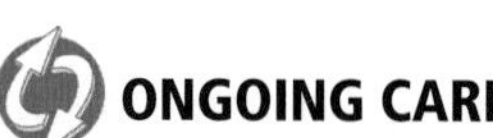

ONGOING CARE

FOLLOW-UP RECOMMENDATIONS

Patient Monitoring

Blood pressure monitoring in patients, especially those with known vascular anomalies, as hypertension is common

PROGNOSIS

Pulmonary complications are the leading cause of death in patients with AD-HIES, followed by lymphoma.

COMPLICATIONS

- Parenchymal lung changes from aberrant healing. Pulmonary surgery to correct these is associated with an increased risk of further complications.
- Increased chance of malignancy, most commonly lymphoma

ADDITIONAL READING

- Buckley RH. The hyper-IgE syndrome. *Clin Rev Allergy Immunol*. 2001;20(1):139–154.
- Davis SD, Schaller J, Wedgwood RJ. Job's syndrome. Recurrent, "cold", staphylococcal abscesses. *Lancet*. 1966;1(7445):1013–1015.
- Freeman AF, Holland SM. Clinical manifestations of hyper IgE syndromes. *Dis Markers*. 2010;29(3–4):123–130.
- Hagl B, Heinz V, Schlesinger A, et al. Key findings to expedite the diagnosis of hyper-IgE syndromes in infants and young children. *Pediatr Allergy Immunol*. 2016;27(2):177–184.
- Yong PF, Freeman AF, Engelhardt KR, et al. An update on the hyper-IgE syndromes. *Arthritis Res Ther*. 2012;14(6):228.

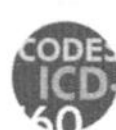

CODES

ICD10

D82.4 Hyperimmunoglobulin E [IgE] syndrome

FAQ

- Q: How do AD-HIES and AR-HIES differ?
- A: Aside from arising from different mutations, AD-HIES has more skeletal and facial anomalies, whereas AR-HIES is more often associated with viral skin infections and has a higher chance of malignancy.
- Q: Will HIES patients show signs typical of infection?
- A: HIES patients may lack classical signs of infection such as warmth and redness. Skin infections have been referred to as "cold" abscesses.
- Q: What are the other names for HIES?
- A: HIES has been referred to as Buckley syndrome, Job-Buckley syndrome, and Job syndrome in the literature. In the initial 1966 case series, Davis and colleagues wrote that the "appearance of these patients and the history of recurrent abscesses and skin infections makes the name 'Job's syndrome' seem suitable." The reference is to the Biblical character Job, who was smote "with sore boils from the sole of his foot unto his crown" (Job, Chapter 2; Verse 7).

H

HYPERLEUKOCYTOSIS

Katie Carlberg, MD • Caroline Hastings, MD

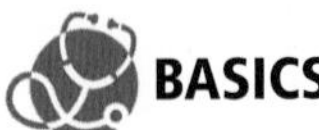

BASICS

DESCRIPTION

Hyperleukocytosis is a total white blood cell (WBC) count of ≥100,000/μL.

RISK FACTORS

- Presentation with hyperleukocytosis depends on the type of leukemia.
- Percent with hyperleukocytosis
  - Chronic myeloid leukemia (CML) especially in blast crisis ~100%
  - Acute myeloid leukemia (AML) especially in infants 5–25%
  - Acute lymphoblastic leukemia (ALL) especially with mediastinal mass 8–13%
- Factors associated with more severe clinical course:
  - Coagulopathy
  - Metabolic derangements
  - Mortality associated more with clinical symptoms (CNS or respiratory) than with WBC

ALERT

Children with trisomy 21 (Down syndrome) have an increased risk of developing transient leukemoid reactions and have an increased risk of developing acute leukemia, more commonly ALL.

PATHOPHYSIOLOGY

The primary mechanism for symptoms is leukostasis due to increased viscosity and impaired blood flow. Contributory factors other than number of leukemic cells include their shape and size, which increases viscosity, as well as endothelial cell damage, which further impedes microcirculation.

- WBCs lack the concave shape that enables reversible deformability characteristic of red blood cells (RBCs) allowing passage through the microvasculature. As compared to normal WBCs, blasts are much larger with less deformability.
- Myeloblasts are twice the size of lymphoblasts, which are 25% larger than mature neutrophil granulocytes. Monoblasts are larger than myeloblasts. Aggregates of these large, undeformable cells cannot pass through capillaries.
- In addition to increased cell-to-cell adhesions, leukemic blasts have increased adhesion to the damaged endothelium, which promote additional cell aggregates through endothelial toxin and cytokine release.
- Leukemic cells have a hypersensitive response to cytokines, which may account for clinical leukostasis at lower peripheral blast counts.
- Leukostasis impairs blood flow and exacerbates hypoxemia; as expected, leukemic blasts have increased oxygen consumption due to a high rate of cell division.

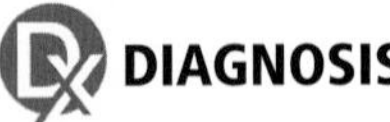

DIAGNOSIS

HISTORY

- Symptoms and signs of hyperleukocytosis relate to the organ involved. Clinical evidence of leukostasis is most apparent in the CNS, lungs, retina, and penis.
- CNS
  - Headache
  - Confusion
  - Blurred vision
  - Tinnitus
  - Paresis
  - Nausea/vomiting
- Pulmonary
  - Dyspnea
  - Shortness of breath
  - Chest pain
- Genitourinary (males)
  - Anuria/oliguria
  - Priapism
- Retina
  - Decreased visual acuity

PHYSICAL EXAM

- CNS
  - Coma
  - Somnolence
  - Altered mental status
  - Agitation
  - Seizures
  - Papilledema
  - Sluggish pupils
- Pulmonary
  - Hypoxia
  - Tachypnea
- Hematologic
  - Hemorrhage
  - Thrombosis
- Reticuloendothelial system
  - Hepatomegaly
  - Splenomegaly
  - Enlarged lymph nodes
- Genitourinary (males)
  - Priapism

ALERT

Symptomatic hyperleukocytosis as a result of leukostasis represents an oncologic emergency. Confused and/or hypoxic patients are at risk for severe late effects or death and require emergent intervention.

DIFFERENTIAL DIAGNOSIS

- Hyperleukocytosis occurs primarily in the setting of malignancy but may be seen with a leukemoid reaction secondary to infection or physiologic stress.
- Malignancy
  - ALL
  - AML
  - CML
  - Transient myeloproliferative disorder (TMPD) is primarily associated with Down syndrome.
- Leukemoid reaction
  - Leukemoid reactions are WBC counts >50,000/μL and consist of myeloid precursor cells in the peripheral blood at all stages of maturity rather than proliferation of an immature WBC clonal population characteristic of malignancies.
  - Infectious causes: *Bordetella pertussis*, *Clostridium difficile*, *Shigella*, EBV, CMV
  - Leukemoid reactions reflect a physiologic bone marrow response to cytokine secretion prompted by external stimuli such as infection or inflammation.
  - Nucleated RBCs (also seen in malignancy)

DIAGNOSTIC TESTS & INTERPRETATION

Initial Tests (screening, lab, imaging)

- Peripheral blood analysis with morphology and flow cytometry aid in immediate diagnosis of acute leukemia.

ALERT

Confirm presence of leukemic blasts. Automated counting machines may mistake leukemic blasts for atypical/reactive lymphocytes or even monocytes.

- Confirmation may require a manual differential and a pathologist or oncologist to review the peripheral smear.
- Evaluate other cell lines. Concurrent presence of anemia and/or thrombocytopenia supports an underlying marrow disorder and may require interventions such as transfusions.
- Tumor lysis syndrome (TLS):
  - Laboratory TLS: occurrence (within same 24-hour period) of two or more of three metabolic derangements (hyperkalemia, hyperphosphatemia, hyperuricemia)
  - Clinical TLS: presence of laboratory TLS plus one or more of the following: increased creatinine, cardiac arrhythmia, seizure, or death
- Obtain chest radiograph (CXR), even if asymptomatic.
  - Evaluate for mediastinal mass.
  - Evaluate for pulmonary infiltrates.
- If clinically indicated, obtain MRI or CT.

Diagnostic Procedures/Other
Bone marrow aspirate may be required per clinical trial criteria, which includes cytogenetics for future prognostic/therapeutic decision making.

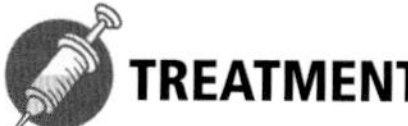

TREATMENT

- The goal of treatment is to quickly make a correct diagnosis and implement definitive therapy while simultaneously identifying and addressing the potential complications of leukostasis secondary to hyperleukocytosis.
- Leukoreduction refers to interventions that result in a rapid decline of the WBC. Leukoreduction is an absolute indication if a patient shows symptoms or signs of leukostasis. It is a relative indication in an asymptomatic patient with a WBC count $\geq$100,000 to 300,000/μL (depending on type of leukemia). Controversy exists about its impact on decreasing morbidity, risk of CNS hemorrhage, or mortality.
- Induction chemotherapy
  - This is the definitive therapy for hyperleukocytosis secondary to malignancy.
  - Initiate chemotherapy as soon as malignant diagnosis is confirmed.
- Management
  - Aggressive hydration at 2 to 4 times maintenance
  - Identify and correct metabolic abnormalities.
    - TLS
    - Hyperuricemia, indication for allopurinol or rasburicase
  - Identify and correct coagulopathies.
  - Transfuse for cytopenias.
    - Do not transfuse packed RBCs if hemodynamically stable due to increased blood viscosity.
    - Do not exceed hemoglobin 10 g/dL.
    - Transfuse platelets to maintain platelets >10,000/μL; will not affect blood viscosity
- Cytoreduction
  - Leukapheresis
    - *Benefit*: Each pheresis session decreases the circulating WBC count by 20–50%. During pheresis, FFP may be administered to reduce risk of hemorrhage.
    - *Limitation*: availability of equipment, trained personnel, and anticoagulation
    - *Caution*: Leukapheresis only transiently decreases blast counts until definitive treatment can be initiated.
  - Exchange transfusion, including partial
    - *Benefit*: This technique is preferred over leukapheresis when (i) patient is an infant or <10 kg and (ii) there is concurrent severe anemia and/or (iii) need for concurrent administration of coagulation factors (i.e., FFP to treat CNS hemorrhage). Partial exchanges minimize volume overload and hyperviscosity.
    - *Limitation*: higher risk of infection
    - *Caution*: Patients are at high risk for TLS.
  - Hydroxyurea
    - *Mechanism of action*: This antimetabolite inhibits ribonucleoside diphosphate reductase, which halts cells in the G_1 phase and interferes with DNA repair.
    - *Dose*: 20 to 30 mg/kg/24 h
    - *Benefit*: Hydroxyurea is an oral medication and easily administered. It may be dissolved in water for NGT/OGT administration. Time to peak onset is only 1 to 4 hours.
    - *Caution*: may also worsen thrombocytopenia

ISSUES FOR REFERRAL
Obtain immediate oncology consult.

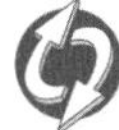

ONGOING CARE

PROGNOSIS
- Patients usually require treatment in a pediatric intensive care unit because they require rapid and continuous monitoring at presentation and during early phase of therapy due to complications of leukostasis and TLS as well as need for meticulous monitoring of fluid status.
- Presence of organ failure or coagulopathy correlates with poor prognosis, specifically death, during induction chemotherapy, despite supportive care.

ALERT
The CNS and lungs are the two most common organs damaged by leukostasis. Early deaths are primarily due to intracranial and pulmonary complications.

ADDITIONAL READING

- Blum W, Porcu P. Therapeutic apheresis in hyperleukocytosis and hyperviscosity syndrome. *Semin Thromb Hemost*. 2007;33(4):350–354.
- Cairo M, Coiffier B, Reiter A, et al; for TLS Expert Panel. Recommendations for the evaluation of risk and prophylaxis of tumour lysis syndrome (TLS) in adults and children with malignant diseases: an expert TLS panel consensus. *Br J Haematol*. 2010;149(4):578–586.
- Jain R, Bansal D, Marwaha RK. Hyperleukocytosis: emergency management. *Indian J Pediatr*. 2013;80(2):144–148.
- Majhail N, Lichtin A. Acute leukemia with a very high leukocyte count: confronting a medical emergency. *Cleve Clin J Med*. 2004;71(8):633–637.
- Nguyen R, Jeha S, Zhou Y, et al. The role of leukapheresis in the current management of hyperleukocytosis in newly diagnosed childhood acute lymphoblastic leukemia. *Pediatr Blood Cancer*. 2016;63(9):1546–1551.
- Porcu P, Cripe LD, Ng EW, et al. Hyperleukocytic leukemias and leukostasis: a review of pathophysiology, clinical presentation and management. *Leuk Lymphoma*. 2000;39(1–2):1–18.
- Sung L, Aplenc R, Alonzo TA, et al; and AAML0531/PHIS Group. Predictors and short-term outcomes of hyperleukocytosis in children with acute myeloid leukemia: a report from the Children's Oncology Group. *Haematologica*. 2012;97(11):1770–1773.

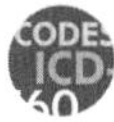

CODES

ICD10
- D72.829 Elevated white blood cell count, unspecified
- C91.00 Acute lymphoblastic leukemia not having achieved remission
- C92.10 Chronic myeloid leukemia, BCR/ABL-positive, not having achieved remission

FAQ

- Q: Is there a linear relationship between the WBC count and the presence/severity of clinical disease and complications?
- A: No. Clinically significant hyperleukocytosis usually occurs at WBC $\geq$200,000/μL or $\geq$300,000/μL in patients with AML or ALL and CML in blast crisis, respectively; however, symptoms may present with a WBC as low as 50,000/μL.
- Q: Is there a linear correlation between the WBC count and presence of TLS?
- A: Yes. Risk increases as the tumor burden increases. With high WBC counts and rapid cell turnover, the lysis/death of malignant cells release by-products, leading to electrolyte and metabolic abnormalities known as TLS. TLS is more common in ALL patients as compared to AML or CML. Components of TLS include hyperkalemia, hyperphosphatemia, hyperuricemia and hyperuricosuria, and hypocalcemia.
- Q: Because transfusions for other cytopenias increase total blood viscosity, what are the current guidelines for transfusions?
- A: For anemia, if hemodynamically unstable, transfuse to maintain hemoglobin 8 to 9 g/dL. Do not exceed hemoglobin levels >10 g/dL as increasing hematocrit increases blood viscosity. For thrombocytopenia, transfuse to maintain platelet >20,000/μL because platelet transfusions minimally increases blood viscosity. If CNS hemorrhage is present, maintain platelets at 75,000 to 100,000/μL.

HYPERLIPIDEMIA

Zeina M. Nabhan, MD

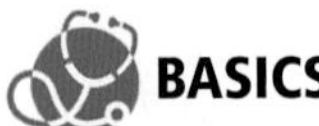

BASICS

DESCRIPTION

Hyperlipidemia is an elevation of serum lipids. These lipids include cholesterol, cholesterol esters (compounds), phospholipids, and triglycerides. Lipids are transported as part of large molecules called lipoproteins.

- Five major families of lipoproteins:
  - Chylomicrons
  - Very-low-density lipoproteins (VLDLs)
  - Intermediate-density lipoproteins (IDLs)
  - Low-density lipoproteins (LDLs)
  - High-density lipoproteins (HDLs)
- Normal serum lipid concentrations:
  - Total cholesterol: 170 mg/dL (borderline, 170 to 199 mg/dL)
  - LDL cholesterol: $<$110 mg/dL (borderline, 110 to 129 mg/dL)
  - HDL cholesterol: $\geq$45 mg/dL (low $<$40 mg/dL)
  - Total triglycerides: 100 mg/dL (borderline, 100 to 140 mg/dL)
  - Non-HDL: $<$120 mg/dL (borderline, 120 to 144 mg/dL)
    - Non-HDL cholesterol is a significant predictor of the presence of atherosclerosis in children and as powerful as any other lipoprotein cholesterol measure. It can be measured nonfasting and should be added as a screening tool for dyslipidemia.
  - More detailed age- and gender-specific values are available (refer to Table 2 of *Lipid Screening and Cardiovascular Health in Childhood*).
- Primary hypercholesterolemia or hypertriglyceridemia: elevation in serum cholesterol or triglyceride as a result of an inherited disorder of lipid metabolism (i.e., familial hypercholesterolemia [FH])
- Secondary hypercholesterolemia or hypertriglyceridemia: elevation in serum cholesterol or triglyceride as a result of another disease process (e.g., diabetes mellitus)

EPIDEMIOLOGY

- The prevalence of homozygous FH is 1 in 1,000,000; the prevalence of the heterozygous state is 1 in 500.
- Overall, hypercholesterolemia and/or hypertriglyceridemia of unknown causes occur in 2% of the pediatric population.
- National Health and Nutrition Exam Surveys (NHANES I to III) provide information about normal pediatric serum cholesterol concentrations.
  - For all children 4 to 17 years, the 95th percentile for serum total cholesterol is 216 mg/dL and the 75th percentile is 181 mg/dL.
  - The average total and LDL cholesterol levels before puberty are significantly higher in girls than they are in boys.
  - The mean total cholesterol level for all children from 4 to 11 years old peaks at age 9 to 11 years and then gradually decreases until mid to late adolescence.

RISK FACTORS

Genetics

- FH: dominantly inherited defect of LDL receptor
- Familial combined hyperlipidemia (FCHL): dominantly inherited lipid disorder, polygenic
- Familial hypertriglyceridemia (FHTG): autosomal recessive disorder due to defects in lipoprotein lipase

GENERAL PREVENTION

- Fat intake is generally unrestricted prior to 2 years of age. After age 2 years, two complementary approaches are recommended:
  - Diet and lifestyle guidelines to promote:
    - Consumption of an overall healthy diet
    - A healthy body weight (BMI between the 5% and 85% for age and sex, in adults 18.5 to 24.9 kg/m^2)
- Recommended lipid levels:
  - LDL cholesterol $<$110 mg/dL
  - HDL cholesterol $>$50 mg/dL in women, $>$40 mg/dL in men
  - Triglycerides $<$150 mg/dL
- Normal BP (age appropriate)
- Normal blood glucose (fasting blood glucose $\leq$100 mg/dL)
- Being physically active
- Avoiding use of and exposure to tobacco products

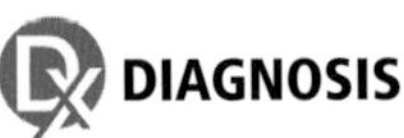

DIAGNOSIS

HISTORY

- Family history of premature heart disease or dyslipidemia:
  - Almost all cases of primary hyperlipidemia are of dominantly inherited.
- Smoking:
  - Smoking reduces HDL cholesterol levels and increases the risk of vascular disease.
- Use of oral contraceptives:
  - Birth control pills elevate lipoprotein levels and, when coupled with baseline elevated lipid levels, can increase the risk of atherosclerosis.
- Diet:
  - Children with increased intake of fat, carbohydrates, sugar added drinks, and fast foods are likely to be overweight/obese.
- Obesity:
  - Obese children are more likely to have abnormal serum lipids.

PHYSICAL EXAM

- Eye exam:
  - Arcus corneae: cholesterol deposits resulting in a thin, white circular ring located on the outer edge of the iris
- Skin exam:
  - Tendon xanthomas: thickened tissue surrounding Achilles and extensor tendons
  - Xanthelasma: yellowish deposits of cholesterol surrounding the eye
  - Palmar xanthomas: pale lines in the palmar creases
  - Eruptive xanthomas: characteristic of hypertriglyceridemia; papular yellowish lesions with a red base that occur on the buttocks, elbows, and knees
  - Enlarged tender liver may present in association with fatty liver.

DIAGNOSTIC TESTS & INTERPRETATION

Initial Tests (screening, lab, imaging)

- Starting age 2 to 8 years: Screen children and adolescents who have:
  - A positive family history of dyslipidemia or premature cardiovascular disease (CVD) ($\leq$55 years old for men, $\leq$65 years old for women), such as coronary atherosclerosis, documented myocardial infarction (MI)
  - Unknown family history
  - Obesity (BMI $\geq$95th percentile) or overweight (BMI $\geq$85th to $<$95th percentile)
  - Cigarette smoking exposure
  - Hypertension
  - Diabetes mellitus
- Screen using a fasting lipid profile (FLP): total cholesterol, HDL cholesterol, LDL cholesterol, and triglycerides
  - If FLP is within normal range, repeat test in 3 to 5 years.
- Age 9 to 11 years: NHLBI-AAP recommends universal screening.
  - Non-FLP: if non-HDL $>$145 mg/dL, then repeat FLP
  - Non-HDL = total cholesterol-HDL
- Age 12 to 16 years: Screen children and adolescents with risk factors like 2 to 8 years group.
- If hyperlipidemia identified, subsequent labs to include
  - Chemistry panel (glucose, ALT, AST, bilirubin, BUN, creatinine, urinalysis):
    - Screening test for diabetes, liver, and kidney disease
  - Thyroid evaluation for hypothyroidism (thyroxine [total T_4], thyroid-stimulating hormone [TSH]):

ALERT

- Serum total cholesterol is inaccurate when serum triglycerides are $>$400 mg/dL.
- Hypertriglyceridemia is associated with falsely lowered serum Na.

DIFFERENTIAL DIAGNOSIS

- Hypercholesterolemia:
  - Primary hypercholesterolemia (see above)
  - Hypothyroidism
  - Nephrotic syndrome
  - Liver disease (cholestatic)
  - Renal failure
  - Anorexia nervosa
  - Acute porphyria
  - Medications (antihypertensives, estrogens, steroids, microsomal enzyme inducers, cyclosporine, diuretics)
  - Pregnancy
  - Dietary: excessive dietary intake of fat, cholesterol, and/or calories
- Hypertriglyceridemia:
  - Primary hypertriglyceridemia (see above)
  - Acute hepatitis
  - Nephrotic syndrome
  - Chronic renal failure
  - Medications (diuretics, retinoids, oral contraceptives)
  - Diabetes mellitus
  - Alcohol abuse
  - Lipodystrophy
  - Myelomatosis
  - Glycogen storage disease
  - Dietary: excessive dietary intake of fat and/or calories

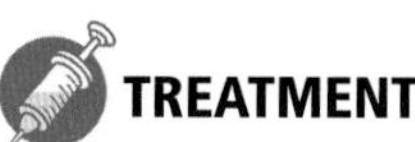

TREATMENT

GENERAL MEASURES

- Outpatient management unless secondary hyperlipidemia caused by liver or renal failure, which necessitates inpatient management of primary illness. Note: The cause of secondary hyperlipidemia should be treated with disease-specific therapy to reduce elevated lipid levels.
- Risk assessment and treatment:
  - Population approach: general emphasis on healthy lifestyle to prevent dyslipidemia development. Recommendations include increasing intake of fruits, vegetables, fish, whole grains, and low-fat dairy products and reducing intake of fruit juice, sugar-sweetened beverages, and food.
  - Individual approach: focuses on patients who are high risk. Initial intervention is focused on changing diet, but patients often require pharmacologic intervention.

MEDICATION

- Drug therapy should be considered only for children ≥8 years of age after an adequate trial of diet therapy (for 6 to 12 months) and if they have one of the following:
  - LDL cholesterol level remains >190 mg/dL
  - LDL cholesterol level remains >160 mg/dL and there is a family history of premature CVD (≤55 years of age for men, ≤65 for women) or ≥2 other risk factors are present (obesity, hypertension, cigarette smoking).
  - Diabetes and LDL ≥130 mg/dL
- Physicians caring for overweight and obese children with lipid disorders should emphasize the importance of diet and exercise rather than drug therapy for most of their patients.
- Statins (1st-line drug therapy): decrease endogenous cholesterol synthesis and increase clearance of circulating LDL
  - Similar safety and efficacy in the treatment of lipid disorders in children as in adults
  - Side effects include hepatitis and myositis.
- Bile acid–binding resins: bind cholesterol in bile acids in intestine and prevent reuptake into enterohepatic circulation
  - Associated with GI discomfort
  - Very poor compliance in children
- Niacin: lowers LDL and triglycerides while increasing HDL; however, poorly tolerated in children due to side effects occurring in >50%, including flushing, itching, and elevated hepatic transaminases
- Drugs needing further pediatric studies: cholesterol absorption inhibitors and fibrates

ADDITIONAL THERAPIES

Activity:

- 60 minutes of moderate to vigorous play or physical activity daily
- Reduce sedentary behaviors (e.g., watching TV, playing videogames, using computers).
- Participation in organized sports

ONGOING CARE

FOLLOW-UP RECOMMENDATIONS

Patient Monitoring

- For patients with primary hyperlipidemia off medication, follow-up should be performed every 1 to 2 years with lipoprotein profile. For those patients on medication, follow-up should be conducted every 3 to 6 months.
- For all other patients with risk factors and normal lipid profile, a monitored lifestyle and diet changes should be strongly recommended at every office visit.

DIET

- Dietary modification is safe in the treatment of hyperlipidemia in children >2 years of age:
  - Restrict saturated fat to <7% daily calories.
  - Restrict dietary cholesterol to 200 mg/24 h.
  - Limit trans fatty acids to <1% daily calories.
  - Supplemental fiber at goal dose of child's age + 5 g/24 h (up to 20 g/24 h)
- Consider use of reduced fat milk for children between 12 months and 2 years of age who are overweight, who are obese, or have a family history of dyslipidemia or CVD.

PROGNOSIS

- FH:
  - Homozygotes: coronary artery disease in 1st or 2nd decade of life
  - Heterozygotes: 50% of males develop premature heart disease by age 50 years (females, age 60 years).
- FCHL: occurs in 1–2% of the population and accounts for 10% of all premature heart disease. A reduction of LDL cholesterol by 1% reduces risk by 2%.
- Children and adolescents with high cholesterol levels are more likely than the general population to have high cholesterol levels as adults.

COMPLICATIONS

- Hypercholesterolemia:
  - Premature heart disease
  - Stroke
  - Vascular disease
- Hypertriglyceridemia:
  - Pancreatitis

ADDITIONAL READING

- Daniels SR, Greer FR; for Committee on Nutrition. Lipid screening and cardiovascular health in childhood. *Pediatrics*. 2008;122(1):198–208.
- Gidding SS, Dennison BA, Birch LL, et al; for American Heart Association, American Academy of Pediatrics. Dietary recommendations for children and adolescents: a guide for practitioners: Consensus statement from the American Heart Association. *Circulation*. 2005;112(13):2061–2075.
- Kavey RE, Allada V, Daniels SR, et al. Cardiovascular risk reduction in high-risk pediatric patients. *Circulation*. 2006;114(24):2710–2738.
- Lichtenstein AH, Appel LJ, Brands M, et al. Diet and lifestyle recommendations revision 2006: a scientific statement from the American Heart Association Nutrition Committee. *Circulation*. 2006;114(1):82–96.
- McCrindLe BW, Urbina EM, Dennison BA, et al. Drug therapy of high-risk lipid abnormalities in children and adolescents. *Circulation*. 2007;115(14):1948–1967.

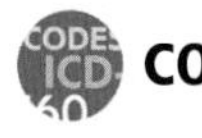

CODES

ICD10

- E78.5 Hyperlipidemia, unspecified
- E78.0 Pure hypercholesterolemia
- E78.1 Pure hyperglyceridemia

HYPERTENSION

Stephanie Nguyen, MD, MAS

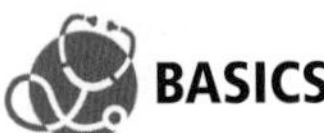

BASICS

DESCRIPTION

- Hypertension: average systolic and/or diastolic blood pressure (BP) at or above the 95th percentile for age, gender, and height percentile or ≥130/80 mm Hg in adolescents ≥13 years of age
- Elevated BP: BP between the 90th and 95th percentile or BP 120–129/<80 mm Hg in adolescents ≥13 years of age
- Stage 1 hypertension: BP ≥95th percentile to 95th percentile plus 12 mm Hg or BP 130–139/80–89 mm Hg in adolescents ≥13 years of age
- Stage 2 hypertension: BP ≥95th percentile plus 12 mm Hg or ≥BP 140/90 mm Hg in adolescents ≥13 years of age
- Primary (essential) hypertension: hypertension for which there is no underlying cause
- Secondary hypertension: hypertension for which an underlying cause can be identified
- White coat hypertension: elevated BP readings in a medical setting with normal BP on ambulatory blood pressure monitoring (ABPM)
- Masked hypertension: normal BP readings in a medical setting with elevated BP readings on ABPM

EPIDEMIOLOGY

- Primary hypertension is now frequently identified in children and adolescents and is associated with overweight status, metabolic syndrome, and family history of hypertension.
- The prevalence of hypertension is increasing due to the epidemic of youth obesity and the metabolic syndrome.
- Hypertension in the pediatric population is estimated to be between 1% and 4%.
- 30% of children with body mass index (BMI) >95% have prehypertension or hypertension.

RISK FACTORS

- Primary hypertension: obesity, sedentary lifestyle, low birth weight, smoking, alcohol use, hyperlipidemia, family history, stress, sodium intake, sleep apnea
- Secondary hypertension: renal or urologic disease, transplant, congenital heart disease, umbilical artery catheterization, urinary tract infection (UTI), diabetes mellitus, elevated intracranial pressure, or medications known to raise BP

Genetics

- The genetic basis of primary hypertension is polygenic but more likely to develop in individuals when there is a strong family history.
- The genetics of secondary causes depend on the underlying condition, for example:
  - Polycystic kidney disease: autosomal dominant, autosomal recessive
  - Neurofibromatosis: autosomal dominant
  - Glucocorticoid-remediable aldosteronism: autosomal dominant

GENERAL PREVENTION

Avoidance of excess weight gain and regular physical activity can prevent obesity-related hypertension.

ETIOLOGY

Secondary causes

- Renal: acute glomerulonephritis, chronic renal failure, polycystic kidney disease, reflux nephropathy
- Renovascular: fibromuscular dysplasia, neurofibromatosis, vasculitis
- Cardiac: coarctation of the aorta
- Endocrine: pheochromocytoma, hypo/hyperthyroid, neuroblastoma, glucocorticoid-remediable aldosteronism, Conn syndrome, apparent mineralocorticoid excess, congenital adrenal hyperplasia, Liddle syndrome, Gordon syndrome
- Neurologic: increased intracranial pressure
- Drugs: corticosteroids, oral contraceptives, sympathomimetics, illicit drugs (cocaine, phencyclidine)
- Other: pain, burns, traction
- Reduced nephron number secondary to premature birth, low birth weight, or postnatal insults are associated with hypertension.

PATHOPHYSIOLOGY

BP is a product of cardiac output and total peripheral vascular resistance. Increases of either or both of these products lead to hypertension. The various causes of hypertension alter BP through different mechanisms such as volume overload (sodium retention, excess sodium intake), volume distribution, renin-angiotensin excess, sympathetic activation, insulin, and endothelin.

DIAGNOSIS

- Hypertensive emergency: severely elevated BP with evidence of target organ injury (encephalopathy, seizures, renal damage)
- Hypertensive urgency: severely elevated BP with no evidence of secondary organ damage

HISTORY

- Headache, blurry vision, epistaxis, unusual weight gain or loss, chest pain, flushing, fatigue
- UTIs can be associated with reflux nephropathy and hypertension.
- Gross hematuria, edema, and fatigue may suggest renal disease.
- Birth history: umbilical artery catheterization, history of prematurity
- Medications: corticosteroids, cold preparations, oral contraceptives, illicit drugs
- Family history: hypertension, diabetes, obesity, familial endocrinopathies, renal disease
- Trauma: arteriovenous (AV) fistula, traction
- Review of symptoms: sleep apnea, obesity

PHYSICAL EXAM

- BP
  - Children >3 years of age should have their BP measured during a health care episode or younger if they have any risk factors for hypertension.
  - Child should be seated quietly for 5 minutes, feet on the floor with the right arm supported at the level of the heart. Routine BPs are measured in the right arm.
  - Use the proper cuff size. The inflatable bladder should completely encircle the arm and cover ~80–100% of the upper arm. A cuff that is inappropriately small will artificially increase the measurement.
  - Elevated BPs obtained by oscillometric devices should be repeated by auscultation.
  - When hypertension is confirmed, BP should be measured in both arms and in a leg. Normally, BP is 10 to 20 mm Hg higher in the legs. If leg BP is lower than arm, consider coarctation of the aorta.
- Tachycardia in hyperthyroidism, pheochromocytoma
- Body habitus: thin, obese, growth failure, virilized, stigmata of Turner or Williams syndromes
- Skin: café au lait spots, neurofibromas, rashes, acanthosis, malar rash
- Head/neck: moon facies, thyromegaly
- Eyes: funduscopic changes, proptosis
- Lungs: rales
- Cardiovascular: rub, gallop, murmur, femoral pulses
- Abdomen: mass, hepatosplenomegaly, bruit
- Genitalia: ambiguous, virilized
- Neurologic: Bell palsy

DIFFERENTIAL DIAGNOSIS

The initial objective after diagnosing hypertension in children is distinguishing primary from secondary causes. Generally, the younger the child and the more elevated the BP measurements, the greater likelihood of a secondary cause.

DIAGNOSTIC TESTS & INTERPRETATION

Initial Tests (screening, lab, imaging)

- The laboratory evaluation to determine the cause of hypertension should proceed in a stepwise fashion. In adolescents with stage 1 hypertension, it is reasonable to evaluate for white coat hypertension using ABPM as a first step before other testing.
- Additional tests may include urinalysis, serum electrolytes, blood urea nitrogen, creatinine, calcium, cholesterol, CBC, ECG, echocardiogram (the most sensitive study to monitor end-organ changes), renal ultrasound, retinal exam.
- Further evaluation is based on history, physical exam, and/or to prove secondary causes: voiding cystourethrogram, DMSA renal scan, 3D CT angiogram, MRA, urine or plasma for catecholamines and metanephrines, plasma renin activity, aldosterone levels.
- More invasive studies include renal angiogram, renal vein renin concentrations, meta-iodobenzylguanidine (MIBG) scan, renal biopsy, genetic studies to identify rare causes of hypertension.

Diagnostic Procedures/Other

- Ambulatory BP monitoring refers to a procedure in which a portable BP device, worn by the patient, records repeated BP measurements over a specified period, usually 24 hours.
- Ambulatory BP monitoring may be helpful in cases in which the diagnosis of hypertension is uncertain (e.g., white coat hypertension) or in assessing the effectiveness of antihypertensive agents. ABPM may also be useful in assessing children at high risk of cardiovascular disease (e.g., diabetes mellitus, labile hypertension, chronic kidney disease).
- Systolic hypertension on ABPM is a better predictor for the development of left ventricular hypertrophy (LVH) when compared to office BP measurements.

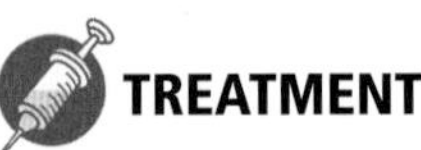

TREATMENT

GENERAL MEASURES

- If BP is >95th percentile, it should be repeated on two more occasions.
- If BP is >99th percentile plus 5 mm Hg, prompt referral for evaluation and therapy should be made.

- If the patient is symptomatic, immediate referral and treatment are indicated.
- Mild primary hypertension may be managed with nonpharmacologic treatment: weight reduction, exercise, sodium restriction, avoidance of certain medications such as pseudoephedrine.
- Pharmacologic therapy should be directed to the cause of secondary hypertension when this is known or for severe, sustained hypertension.
- Medications may be needed in children with mild to moderate hypertension if nonpharmacologic therapy has failed or if end-organ changes, kidney disease, or diabetes is present.

MEDICATION

- Classes of antihypertensive agents include α- and β-blockers, diuretics, vasodilators (direct and calcium channel blockers), ACE inhibitors, and angiotensin receptor blockers (ARBs).
- Therapy should be initiated with a single drug.
- Avoid multiple medications with the same mechanism of action.
- Elicit a history of adverse effects and adjust medications accordingly.
- There are no trials with clinical significant outcomes to support a preferential class of antihypertensive medications in pediatric essential hypertension. Specific classes should be used with concurrent medical conditions:
  - ACE inhibitors or ARBs in children with diabetes and microalbuminuria or proteinuric renal diseases
  - β-blockers or calcium channel blockers with migraine headaches
- Certain classes of medication should be avoided in patients with specific conditions, such as:
  - Asthma and diabetes (β-blockers)
  - Bilateral renal artery stenosis (ACE inhibitors)
- ACE inhibitors are associated with congenital malformations and are contraindicated during pregnancy; calcium channel blockers and β-blockers are alternatives.

ADDITIONAL THERAPIES

- For overweight adolescents, a DASH-type diet: 8 servings of fruits and vegetables, 3 servings of low-fat dairy, and <2 servings of DASH unfriendly foods (>3 g of fat and >480 mg of sodium per serving)
- Regular aerobic physical activity (30 to 60 minutes at least 5 days a week)
- Limitation of sedentary activities to <2 hours per day
- Patients with uncontrolled stage 2 hypertension should be restricted from high-static competitive sports until the BP is in normal range.

SURGERY/OTHER PROCEDURES

- Dialysis may be needed for hypertension in chronic renal failure.
- Surgical correction of renovascular hypertension and coarctation of the aorta. Percutaneous transluminal angioplasty has been used for renal artery stenosis.

ADMISSION, INPATIENT, AND NURSING CONSIDERATIONS

- Hypertensive emergencies should be treated with IV BP medications, aiming to decrease the BP by 25% over the first 8 hours and gradually normalizing BP over 24 to 48 hours.
- Hypertensive urgencies can be treated by either IV or PO antihypertensives depending on symptomatology.
- Hypertensive emergencies should be admitted to the ICU if indicated.
- Hypertensive urgencies should be admitted to the hospital.

ONGOING CARE

FOLLOW-UP RECOMMENDATIONS

Patient Monitoring

- The reduction of BP with medication should be gradual to avoid side effects.
- Ongoing monitoring is required for medication side effects, such as exercise intolerance (β-blockers), headaches (vasodilators), renal insufficiency or hyperkalemia (ACE inhibitors), or hypokalemia (diuretics).
- Regular monitoring for development of LVH (echocardiogram or ECG) is recommended.
- Patients with white coat hypertension require ongoing monitoring, as they are at risk for developing true hypertension.

DIET

- Dietary increase in fresh vegetables, fresh fruits, potassium, fiber, and nonfat dairy
- Restriction of sodium, calories, saturated fat, and refined sugar
- Low-sodium (DASH) diet: <2.3 g of sodium per day for adolescents

PATIENT EDUCATION

- Diet
  - Increase in fresh vegetables, fresh fruits, fiber, and nonfat dairy
  - Restriction of sodium and calories
- Activity
  - Regular aerobic physical activity (30 to 60 minutes at least 5 days a week)
  - Limitation of sedentary activities to <2 hours per day
- Prevention
  - Avoidance of excess weight gain, smoking, and alcohol use; regular physical activity

PROGNOSIS

The patient's prognosis depends on the underlying cause of the hypertension. It is excellent if the BP is well-controlled.

COMPLICATIONS

- LVH and heart failure
- Renal failure
- Encephalopathy
- Retinopathy

ADDITIONAL READING

- Feld LG, Corey H. Hypertension in childhood. *Pediatr Rev*. 2007;28(8):283–298.
- McCambridge TM, Benjamin HJ, Brenner JS, et al; for Council on Sports Medicine and Fitness. Athletic participation by children and adolescents who have systemic hypertension. *Pediatrics*. 2010;125(6):1287–1294.
- McCrindle B. Assessment and management of hypertension in children and adolescents. *Nat Rev Cardiol*. 2010;7(3):155–163.
- Flynn JT, Kaelber DC, Baker-Smith CM, et al. Clinical practice guideline for screening and management of high blood pressure in children and adolescents. *Pediatrics*. 2017;140(3):e20171904.
- Suresh S, Mahajan P, Kamat D. Emergency management of pediatric hypertension. *Clin Pediatr (Phila)*. 2005;44(9):739–745.
- Urbina E, Alpert B, Flynn J, et al; for American Heart Association Atherosclerosis, Hypertension, and Obesity in Youth Committee. Ambulatory blood pressure monitoring in children and adolescents: recommendations for standard assessment: a scientific statement from the American Heart Association Atherosclerosis, Hypertension, and Obesity in Youth Committee of the Council on Cardiovascular Disease in the Young and the Council for High Blood Pressure Research. *Hypertension*. 2008;52(3):433–451.

CODES

ICD10

- I10 Essential (primary) hypertension
- I15.9 Secondary hypertension, unspecified
- I15.1 Hypertension secondary to other renal disorders

FAQ

- Q: What is the value of ambulatory BP monitoring?
- A: This device is similar to a Holter monitor and repeatedly measures BPs over a 24-hour period while the patient is awake and asleep. By reviewing the BPs, one can determine if a significant proportion of readings are elevated and whether or not the normal dip in BP during sleep is seen. Thus, conditions such as white coat hypertension and/or masked hypertension can be verified or discounted.
- Q: What are the indications for invasive studies, such as angiography?
- A: This decision should be individualized and based on the severity of the hypertension, response to medication, the clinical presentation (e.g., neurofibromatosis), and results of other studies. In general, young children and all children with severe, unexplained hypertension should be completely evaluated.
- Q: Can adolescents with elevated BP compete in sports?
- A: Adolescents with hypertension should be encouraged to participate in athletics if their BP is well-controlled. The use of stress testing in this population is controversial.
- Q: Do I need to worry about isolated systolic hypertension?
- A: Studies in adults have shown that sustained systolic hypertension may be just as important as diastolic hypertension.

HYPOCALCEMIA

Mary Scott Ramnitz, MD • Alison Boyce, MD

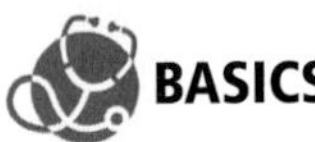

BASICS

DESCRIPTION

- Hypocalcemia refers to calcium levels below the normal range for age.
- The severity of hypocalcemia varies from mild and asymptomatic to acutely life-threatening.
- Identifying the etiology of hypocalcemia is important for appropriate long-term management.

EPIDEMIOLOGY

- The prevalence of hypocalcemia varies depending on the patient's age and underlying etiology.
- Approximately one third of preterm infants and most very low-birth-weight infants will develop low serum calcium concentrations during the first 2 days of life.
- The most common genetic cause of hypocalcemia is 22q11.2 deletion (DiGeorge) syndrome, which occurs in 1 in 4,000 to 5,950 live births.

GENERAL PREVENTION

- Adequate dietary calcium intake
- Vitamin D supplements should be given to breastfed infants and high-risk individuals.

PATHOPHYSIOLOGY

- Calcium is essential for many critical physiologic functions (i.e., nerve action potentials, muscle contractions), and its extracellular concentrations must be maintained within a narrow range.
- There are three circulating forms of calcium in serum: protein bound (40%), complexed with serum anions (15%), and ionized form (45%). Calcium homeostasis involves intestinal, bone, and renal handling mediated by parathyroid hormone (PTH) and 1,25-dihydroxyvitamin D.
- Clinical symptoms of hypocalcemia result from lowered thresholds to nerve conduction and muscle action potentials, and range from mild to severe.

ETIOLOGY

- Neonatal hypocalcemia
  - Early transient hypocalcemia (within 72 hours of life): exaggeration of the normal decline in calcium concentrations after birth
    - Maternal factors: diabetes mellitus, toxemia, severe vitamin D deficiency, anticonvulsants, hyperparathyroidism
    - Neonatal factors: prematurity, low birth weight, perinatal stress/asphyxia, sepsis, respiratory distress syndrome
  - Late transient hypocalcemia (5 to 10 days of life): due to relative PTH resistance of immature renal tubules
    - May be exacerbated by high phosphate intake from cow's milk–based formula
  - Persistent hypocalcemia: Cases of early or late neonatal hypocalcemia that fail to resolve should be investigated for additional etiologies (below).
- Hypocalcemia with elevated PTH levels
  - Insufficient calcium intake: malnutrition, malabsorption
  - Hypovitaminosis D
    - Insufficient dietary intake and/or sun exposure
    - Malabsorption
    - Defects in vitamin D metabolism: liver or renal disease, hereditary resistance to vitamin D (*VDR*)
  - Decreased vitamin D production: 1-α-hydroxylase deficiency
  - PTH insensitivity: End-organ resistance results in appropriately high PTH in the setting of hypocalcemia and hyperphosphatemia.
    - Pseudohypoparathyroidism types IA (*GNAS*), IB (*GNAS*, *STX16*), and 2 (*PRKAR1A*)
- Hypocalcemia with low or inappropriately normal PTH levels: hypoparathyroidism
  - Parathyroid gland dysgenesis:
    - 22q11.2 deletion (DiGeorge) syndrome. Hypocalcemia may present in the neonatal period or later in life. Additional features include thymic aplasia, cardiac defects, and developmental delay (see "22q11.2 Deletion Syndrome [DiGeorge Syndrome, Velocardiofacial Syndrome]" chapter).
    - Hypoparathyroidism-retardation-dysmorphism, Kenny-Caffey, Sanjad-Sakati syndromes
    - Mitochondrial disorders (Kearns-Sayre; Pearson; mitochondrial encephalopathy, lactic acidosis, stroke-like episodes [MELAS])
  - Reduced parathyroid hormone secretion:
    - Autosomal dominant hypocalcemic hypercalciuria (*CaSR*, *GNA11*)
  - Autoimmune disorders:
    - Autoimmune polyendocrinopathy-candidiasis-ectodermal dystrophy (*AIRE1*)
  - Acquired causes:
    - Postsurgical (parathyroidectomy, thyroidectomy)
    - Iron overload (hemochromatosis, thalassemia, chronic transfusions)
    - Copper deposition (Wilson disease)
    - Granulomatous invasion (amyloidosis, sarcoidosis)
- Miscellaneous
  - Hypomagnesemia: impairs PTH release and decreases end-organ responsiveness to PTH action
  - Hyperphosphatemia: decreases serum calcium availability due to calcium-phosphate precipitation in the tissues
    - Tumor lysis syndrome, rhabdomyolysis
    - Phosphate-containing enemas
  - Hungry bone syndrome: mobilization of calcium from the serum during rapid bone remineralization
  - Acute and critical illness (sepsis, acute pancreatitis, shock)
  - Drug mediated:
    - Bisphosphonates
    - Bicarbonate
    - Loop diuretics
    - Denosumab
    - Citrated blood products
  - Hypoalbuminemia: Decreased protein-bound calcium in the circulation results in "pseudohypocalcemia," where total serum calcium levels are low, whereas ionized calcium levels are normal.

RISK FACTORS

- Premature infants, low birth weight, or intrauterine growth restriction
- Perinatal illness, asphyxia
- Infants of mothers with diabetes
- Inadequate nutrition, prolonged breastfeeding without vitamin D supplementation
- Malabsorption

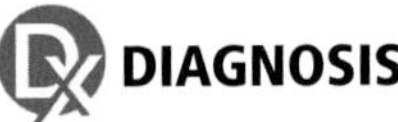

DIAGNOSIS

HISTORY

- For neonates and infants: detailed maternal and birth history
- Dietary history (particularly calcium, vitamin D intake)
- History of neck surgery/radiation
- Family history of calcium disorders
- Feeding problems, nausea, vomiting
- Psychiatric manifestations
- Apnea, jitteriness, irritability
- Cardiac abnormalities or recurrent infections
- Muscle cramps, twitching, or spasms
- Circumoral or distal paresthesias
- Seizures

PHYSICAL EXAM

- Neuromuscular irritability
  - Tetany: perioral numbness, paresthesias of the hands and feet, muscle cramps or spasm
  - Irritability, jitteriness, tremulousness
  - Hyperreflexia
    - Chvostek sign: twitching of the orbicularis oris muscle with light tapping of the facial nerve at the anterior external auditory meatus
    - Trousseau sign: carpopedal spasm when BP cuff maintained 20 mm Hg above SBP for 3 minutes
  - Laryngospasm, apnea
  - Focal or generalized seizure
- Rickets
  - Widening at the wrists, knees, and/or ankles
  - Bowing of the extremities
- Features associated with genetic causes of hypocalcemia
  - Dysmorphic features
  - Hearing loss
  - Congenital heart disease
  - Mucocutaneous candidiasis, ectodermal dysplasia

DIAGNOSTIC TESTS & INTERPRETATION

Initial Tests (screening, lab, imaging)

- Total and ionized calcium, albumin, phosphorus, magnesium, alkaline phosphatase, creatinine
- If hypoalbuminemia present, calculate corrected calcium: [0.8 (4 − albumin) + serum total calcium]
- Intact PTH
- 1,25-dihydroxyvitamin D
- 25-hydroxyvitamin D
- Urine calcium, creatinine, and urinalysis
- 12-lead ECG: evaluates for QTc interval prolongation

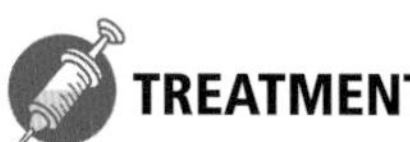

TREATMENT

- Acute symptomatic hypocalcemia (all calcium doses expressed in respective salt amounts unless specified):
  - Calcium gluconate (preferred) 100 to 200 mg/kg/dose (max 1 to 2 g/dose) IV over 5 to 10 minutes with cardiac monitoring
  - Calcium chloride 20 mg/kg/dose (max 2 g/dose) can alternatively be given if readily available.
  - IV calcium should not be infused more rapidly due to risk of cardiac dysfunction.
  - Bolus should be immediately followed by a continuous infusion of calcium gluconate: 500 to 800 mg/kg/24 h or an intermittent infusion of calcium chloride of 10 to 20 mg/kg/dose (max 1 g/dose) q4–6h PRN.
  - Calcium gluconate can be given via peripheral IV, but calcium chloride should only be given via central line due to risk of tissue necrosis with extravasation. Follow respective calcium salt product maximum concentration and rates for IV administration.
  - Continue the IV infusion or intermittent doses until patient is on an effective oral regimen.
  - Oral calcium 25 to 50 mg/kg/24 h elemental calcium (max 1 g elemental calcium per 24 hours) divided 3 to 4 times daily
  - For patients with hypoparathyroidism, calcitriol should be initiated as soon as possible: infants 0.04 to 0.08 mcg/kg/24 h divided twice daily, >1 year 0.25 mcg/24 h and increase as needed up to a maximum of 2 mcg/24 h
  - Magnesium supplements should be given as needed to correct hypomagnesemia.
  - For patients with vitamin D deficiency, treat with high-dose oral cholecalciferol (vitamin D_3) over 8 to 12 weeks (goal total of ~200,000 to 400,000 IU).
    - Infants <1 month: 1,000 IU daily
    - Infants and children 1 month to 5 years: 1,000 to 2,000 IU daily
    - Children 5 years to adult: 5,000 to 6,000 IU daily
- Mild asymptomatic or chronic hypocalcemia
  - Oral calcium and calcitriol supplementation is preferred (see above).

ISSUES FOR REFERRAL

Consult endocrinology for suspected hypoparathyroidism and/or genetic causes of hypocalcemia.

ADMISSION, INPATIENT, AND NURSING CONSIDERATIONS

- Admission criteria
  - Hypocalcemia can be managed in the outpatient setting; however inpatient admission should be considered if:
    - Symptoms of carpopedal spasm, tetany, or seizures
    - Prolonged QTc interval
    - Acute decrease in total corrected calcium to ≤7.5 mg/dL in asymptomatic patient
- Discharge criteria
  - Stable laboratory values
  - Normalization in mental status and neurology exam

ONGOING CARE

FOLLOW-UP RECOMMENDATIONS

Patient Monitoring

- Regular serum and urine monitoring during initial therapy and dose adjustments
- Ongoing monitoring as indicated depending on the etiology of hypocalcemia and risk factors for recurrence

PROGNOSIS

Hypocalcemia typically improves with treatment; however, the long-term prognosis depends on the underlying etiology and risk factors for recurrence.

COMPLICATIONS

- Tetany and seizures
- Laryngospasm, apnea
- Cardiac arrhythmia
- If overtreated, patients can develop hypercalcemia and hypercalciuria that if unaddressed can lead to nephrocalcinosis, nephrolithiasis, and renal insufficiency.

ADDITIONAL READING

- Liamis G, Milionis HJ, Elisaf M. A review of drug-induced hypocalcemia. *J Bone Miner Metab*. 2009;27(6):635–642.
- Lima K, Abrahamsen TG, Wolff AB, et al. Hypoparathyroidism and autoimmunity in the 22q11.2 deletion syndrome. *Eur J Endocrinol*. 2011;165(2):345–352.
- Ross AC, Manson JE, Abrams SA, et al. The 2011 report on dietary reference intakes for calcium and vitamin D from the Institute of Medicine: what clinicians need to know. *J Clin Endocrinol Metab*. 2011;96(1):53–58.
- Shoback D. Clinical practice. Hypoparathyroidism. *N Engl J Med*. 2008;359(4):391–403.
- Tafaj O, Jüppner H. Pseudohypoparathyroidism: one gene, several syndromes. *J Endocrinol Invest*. 2017;40(4):347–356.

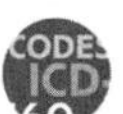

CODES

ICD10

- E83.51 Hypocalcemia
- P71.1 Other neonatal hypocalcemia
- P71.0 Cow's milk hypocalcemia in newborn

FAQ

- Q: How can the phosphorus concentration help establish the cause of hypocalcemia?
- A: In addition to increasing serum calcium, PTH results in renal phosphate wasting. Therefore, in settings of increased PTH secretion such as dietary calcium or vitamin D deficiency, the serum phosphorus will be low or in the normal range. However, in settings of PTH deficiency/resistance, the phosphorus level will be elevated.

Hormonal Problems	Serum Calcium	Serum Phosphate
Calcium/vitamin D deficiency	Low	Normal/low
Parathyroid hormone deficiency/resistance	Low	High

- Q: When should patients be treated with parenteral versus oral calcium supplements?
- A: Acute symptomatic hypocalcemia such as seizures or tetany should be treated with parenteral calcium bolus followed by continuous infusion. In addition, individuals who are unable to tolerate enteral feeding or have active malabsorption issues should be treated with parenteral calcium. The remainder of patients can be treated with oral calcium supplements and calcitriol if needed.
- Q: What are the recommendations for calcium intake in infants and children?
- A: Recommended calcium dietary allowances by age (mg/24 h):
  - 0 to 6 months: 200
  - 6 to 12 months: 260
  - 1 to 3 years: 700
  - 4 to 8 years: 1,000
  - 9 to 18 years: 1,300

HYPOGAMMAGLOBULINEMIA

Rachel G. Robison, MD

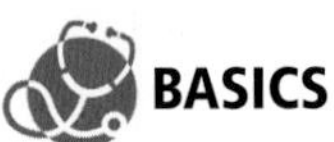

BASICS

DESCRIPTION

- A disorder of the humoral immune system characterized by deficient or absent immunoglobulins and the inability to produce specific antibody
- Subtypes include primary immunodeficiency and secondary deficiency due to other extrinsic disease (i.e., malignancy).

EPIDEMIOLOGY

Incidence and prevalence depends on underlying defect or cause. Antibody deficiency syndromes represent ~70% of primary immune deficiencies.

RISK FACTORS

Genetic defects have been identified in many cases (see "Differential Diagnosis").

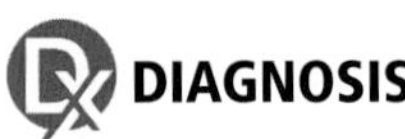

DIAGNOSIS

HISTORY

- Recurrent upper and lower respiratory tract infections (otitis media, pneumonia, and sinusitis)
- Infections with encapsulated bacteria such as *Streptococcus pneumoniae*, *Haemophilus influenzae*
- May have diarrhea, infections with *Giardia*
- Chronic cough and chronic rhinitis may be present.
- Family history of hypogammaglobulinemia, need for immune replacement therapy or history, or of consanguinity

PHYSICAL EXAM

- May be normal if an infection is not present
- Evaluate for growth delay and failure to thrive.
- Patients with X-linked agammaglobulinemia (XLA) may have absent or minimal tonsillar tissue.
- Digital clubbing may be present in cases with history of severe infections.

DIFFERENTIAL DIAGNOSIS

- Primary defects in antibody production
  - Selective IgA deficiency
    - Most common cause of hypogammaglobulinemia
    - Low to undetectable levels of IgA with normal other immunoglobulin classes
    - Prevalence of 1/300 to 1/800 in Caucasians
    - Most are asymptomatic; a proportion may have recurrent infections (upper and lower respiratory infections), risk of giardiasis, and GI infections.
    - May develop anaphylactic reactions to blood products due to presence of antibodies to IgA
  - Common variable immunodeficiency
    - The second most common cause of hypogammaglobulinemia
      - Peaks in 1st and 3rd decades of life
      - Affects both sexes equally; incidence of 1/20,000 to 1/100,000
    - Characterized by decreased IgG (2 *SD* below the age-adjusted mean) and impaired humoral response to polysaccharide antigens
    - Risk of development of malignancy such as non-Hodgkin lymphoma, gastric cancer
    - Can be associated with autoimmunity in up to 25% (i.e., rheumatoid arthritis, idiopathic thrombocytopenic purpura, autoimmune hemolytic anemia)
    - Genetic defects have been identified in the transmembrane activator and calcium-modulating cyclophilin ligand interactor (TACI), inducible T-cell costimulator (ICOS), B-cell-activating factor belonging to the TNF family receptor (BAFF-R), and CD19, although only 10% have a family history of disease.
  - XLA
    - X-linked mutation in Bruton tyrosine kinase (Btk) gene leading to a defect in B cell maturation
    - Reported in 1/379,000 U.S. births
    - Patients often present with infections after waning of maternal IgG after 3 months of age.
    - Labs reveal low serum immunoglobulin levels and <2% circulating B cells.
    - Patients are susceptible to viral infections such as enterovirus.
    - Autosomal recessive agammaglobulinemia occurs in ~15% without Btk mutations and can occur in females; has a similar phenotype
  - Transient hypogammaglobulinemia of infancy
    - Prolongation of the "physiologic" hypogammaglobulinemia of infancy, which is normally observed during the first 3 to 6 months of life
      - IgG levels should be at least 2 *SD* below the mean age-matched controls.
      - Typically recover by 9 to 15 months of age and have normal immunoglobulin levels by 2 to 4 years
      - Must be diagnosed in retrospect after immune recovery and patients should be followed with serial immunoglobulin levels
    - Etiology remains unknown.
    - Antibiotic prophylaxis and/or immunoglobulin replacement should be considered in those with severe recurrent infections.
  - Disorders of immunoglobulin class-switch recombination (Ig-CSR)
    - CD40L mutation: X-linked hyper IgM (HIGM) syndrome
      - Also known as HIGM1
      - Estimated frequency of 1 in 500,000 live male births
      - Due to a mutation in the CD40 ligand gene
      - IgM may be elevated or normal. IgG, IgA, and IgE levels are low to absent.
      - Affects T-cell priming and antigen-specific T-cell responses, in addition to defective antibody production
      - Chronic diarrhea and failure to thrive are present.
      - In addition, can have opportunistic infections, particularly with *Pneumocystis*, *Cryptosporidium*, and *Histoplasma* organisms
      - May have lymphadenopathy and hepatosplenomegaly on exam
      - Treatment includes allogeneic hematopoietic cell transplantation.

- Autosomal recessive hyper IgM (AR-HIGM) syndromes
  - Includes mutations in the following:
    - CD40 (HIGM3)
    - Activation-induced cytidine deaminase (AID) (HIGM2): the most common AR-HIGM; AD mutations in AID are also described.
    - Uracil-N-glycosylase (UNG) (HIGM5)
  - CD40 mutations present similarly to X-linked HIGM.
  - AID and UNG mutations have less incidence of opportunistic infections and neutropenia and are associated with lymph node hyperplasia.
- Secondary defects in antibody production
  - Increased loss: Loss of protein can occur via the kidneys, intestinal tract, lymphatic system, or skin.
    - Protein-losing enteropathy
      - Intestinal lymphangiectasia can be congenital.
      - Post-Fontan procedures with resultant hypogammaglobulinemia
    - Nephrotic syndrome
  - Decreased production
    - Malignancy
      - Chronic lymphocytic leukemia
      - Lymphoma
      - Multiple myeloma
    - Medications
      - Sulfasalazine
      - Systemic steroids
      - Anticonvulsants (phenytoin, carbamazepine)
      - Androgen replacement
      - Rituximab

DIAGNOSTIC TESTS & INTERPRETATION

- CBC with differential
  - Can rule out associated anemia, thrombocytopenia, and neutropenia
- Quantitative immunoglobulins: IgG, IgM, IgA, and IgE
  - Look for low or absent isotypes.

ALERT

Normal immunoglobulin levels vary by age. Maternal immunoglobulin is still present in early infancy until the child is producing their own IgG by 3 to 4 months of age.

- Qualitative antibody titers specifically to tetanus, *H. influenzae* type B, *S. pneumoniae* postvaccination
  - Absent response after vaccination can identify specific antibody deficiencies.
- Evaluate for presence of isohemagglutinins (primary IgM antibodies to the main blood groups) in unvaccinated children.
- Flow cytometry to evaluate B cell numbers
- Chest radiography, CT chest and/or sinus
  - To evaluate for acute disease and if with history of multiple infections, to look for chronic parenchymal changes such as bronchiectasis

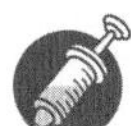

TREATMENT

MEDICATION

- Appropriate antimicrobial therapy at first sign of infection. Prompt initiation of therapy is recommended.
- Select patients may benefit from prophylactic antibiotics.
- Regular replacement therapy with gammaglobulin in either IV or SC forms; usually 300 to 600 mg/kg every 3 to 4 weeks IV or every 1 to 2 weeks SC
- Trough levels of 700 to 800 mg/dL are now preferred compared to previous recommendations of >300 mg/dL.
- Side effects of immunoglobulin therapy can include:
  - Fever
  - Muscle aches
  - Headaches (aseptic meningitis)
- Patients may require switching their replacement product brand or premedication with acetaminophen, ibuprofen, corticosteroids, and/or saline.

ONGOING CARE

FOLLOW-UP RECOMMENDATIONS

Patient Monitoring

Patients on immunoglobulin replacement should have trough IgG levels followed regularly as well as CBCs with differential and metabolic panels to look for hemolytic processes and side effects of replacement.

PROGNOSIS

In most cases (except transient hypogammaglobulinemia of infancy), it requires lifelong therapy.

ADDITIONAL READING

- Conley ME. Genetics of hypogammaglobulinemia: what do we really know? *Curr Opin Immunol*. 2009;21(5):466–471.
- Jolles S. The variable in common variable immunodeficiency: a disease of complex phenotypes. *J Allergy Clin Immunol Pract*. 2013;1(6):545–557.
- Qamar N, Fuleihan RL. The hyper IgM syndromes. *Clin Rev Allergy Immunol*. 2014;46(2):120–130.
- van der Burg M, van Zelm MC, Driessen GJ, et al. New frontiers of primary antibody deficiencies. *Cell Mol Life Sci*. 2012;69(1):59–73.
- Yong PF, Chee R, Grimbacher B. Hypogammaglobulinaemia. *Immunol Allergy Clin North Am*. 2008;28(4):691–713.

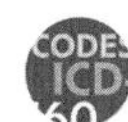

CODES

ICD10

- D80.1 Nonfamilial hypogammaglobulinemia
- D80.0 Hereditary hypogammaglobulinemia
- D80.2 Selective deficiency of immunoglobulin A [IgA]

FAQ

- Q: When should I check immunoglobulin levels?
- A: Immunoglobulins and antibody responses to vaccinations may be considered in any patient with a history of recurrent sinopulmonary infections.
- Q: I have a 2-month-old male patient with a family history of XLA. His IgG level is normal. Do I need to recheck it in the future?
- A: At 2 months of age, most infants still have maternal IgG present. Levels tend to wane and the infant will start to produce his or her own IgG in the 3- to 4-month range. Rechecking after this time is recommended.

HYPOGLYCEMIA

Katherine Lord, MD • Diva D. De León, MD, MSCE

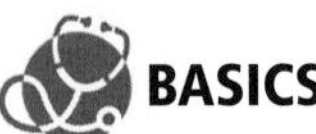

BASICS

DESCRIPTION

Hypoglycemia can be defined as a plasma glucose concentration low enough to impair brain function. Evaluation should be undertaken in infants and young children with documented plasma glucose <60 mg/dL and in older children who demonstrate Whipple triad (see below).

EPIDEMIOLOGY

- Low-plasma glucose is frequent in the first few hours after birth with 19% of neonates having plasma glucose concentrations of <45 mg/dL.
- By 72 hours of life, plasma glucose concentrations in neonates are similar to those in older infants, children, and adults.
- Up to 50% of high-risk neonates (small for gestational age [SGA], intrauterine growth restricted, infants of diabetic mothers) have persistent hypoglycemia due to transient hyperinsulinism (HI).
- Congenital hypoglycemia disorders are less frequent. Of these, congenital HI is the most common.

Incidence

Congenital HI

- Annual incidence estimated at ~1:40,000 to 50,000 live births in United States
- May be as high as 1:2,500 in select populations (Saudi Arabians, Ashkenazi Jews)

PATHOPHYSIOLOGY

- In response to fasting, insulin secretion is suppressed, and counterregulatory hormones (glucagon, cortisol, growth hormone, epinephrine) increase.
- These hormonal changes result in hepatic release of glucose through glycogenolysis and gluconeogenesis. Additionally, activation of lipolysis and ketogenesis leads to an increase in free fatty acids (FFA) and ketone bodies. The brain uses ketones as an alternative source of energy as glucose stores are depleted.
- Disruption of these fasting systems results in hypoglycemia.
- Autonomic symptoms (sweating, tremors, hunger) appear when plasma glucose falls <55 mg/dL.
- Brain dysfunction (confusion, seizures, coma) can result when plasma glucose is <50 mg/dL.

ETIOLOGY

- HI
  - Due to dysregulated insulin secretion
  - Congenital HI is caused by genetic defects in the β-cell insulin secretion pathways (10 identified genes). Most common types include:
    - K_{ATP}HI: Inactivating mutations in K_{ATP} channel genes *ABCC8* and *KCNJ11* (on 11p15) cause the most common and severe forms of HI. Two distinct histologic types:
      - Diffuse HI: mutations inherited in an autosomal recessive or less commonly, autosomal dominant manner, which result in abnormal insulin secretion in all β cells throughout the pancreas (40% of cases)
      - Focal HI: A paternally inherited recessive mutation of K_{ATP} channel gene (*ABCC8* or *KCNJ11*) or a loss of maternal alleles on the imprinted chromosome region 11p15 leads to paternal uniparental disomy; results in focal adenomatous lesion (60% of cases)
    - Glucokinase (GCK) HI: autosomal dominant–activating *GCK* mutations, which result in a lower glucose threshold for insulin secretion and persistent hypoglycemia
    - Glutamate dehydrogenase (GDH) HI: autosomal dominant–activating mutations of GDH, encoded by *GLUD1*; known as HI/ hyperammonemia (HI/HA) syndrome; characterized by fasting and protein-induced hypoglycemia, plus elevated ammonia levels
  - Stress-induced HI is associated with severe perinatal stress (SGA, maternal hypertension, precipitous delivery, or hypoxia); resolves by 3 to 6 months of life
  - HI is also associated with certain syndromes (Beckwith-Wiedemann syndrome [BWS], Turner, Kabuki).
- Insuminoma
  - Insulin-producing islet cell tumors; 5–10% malignant
  - Rare in pediatric populations
  - Associated with multiple endocrine neoplasia (MEN) type 1 (inherited disorder due to mutations in the MEN1 gene associated with tumors of the pituitary, parathyroid glands, and pancreas)
- Glycogen storage disease (GSD)
  - Heterogeneous group of disorders due to defects in glycogen synthesis or degradation
  - Hepatic glycogenoses result in various degrees of ketotic hypoglycemia and hepatomegaly
    - Glycogen synthase deficiency (type 0): characterized by postprandial hyperglycemia and fasting ketotic hypoglycemia
    - Glucose-6-phosphatase deficiency (type I): impaired gluconeogenesis and glycogenolysis. Fasting results in severe lactic acidosis, hypoglycemia, hypertriglyceridemia, and hyperuricemia. Complications include nephropathy, hepatic adenomas, and neutropenia (type Ib).
    - Debrancher enzyme deficiency (type III): significant hepatomegaly, fasting ketotic hypoglycemia, hyperlipidemia, elevated transaminases, myopathy, and cardiomyopathy
    - Liver phosphorylase (type VI) and phosphorylase kinase (type IX): hepatomegaly, fasting ketotic hypoglycemia, growth retardation, elevated transaminases; milder than GSD I and III
- Hormone deficiencies
  - Deficiency of counterregulatory hormones results in ketotic hypoglycemia
    - Adrenal insufficiency: in infants due to hypopituitarism. Addison (autoimmune adrenalitis associated with 21-hydroxylase antibodies) is most common in children.
    - Growth hormone deficiency (GHD): Hypoglycemia occurs primarily in infants.
    - Neonatal panhypopituitarism: mimics HI in neonates with low ketones and positive response to glucagon
- Fatty acid oxidation disorders (FAODs)
  - Due to defects in fatty acid transport and β-oxidation
  - Variable presentation and severity
  - Prolonged fasting provokes hypoketotic hypoglycemia, seizures, cardiac and liver dysfunction, HA.
- Idiopathic ketotic hypoglycemia
  - Children, typically 1 to 4 years old, with fasting hypoglycemia but no identifiable metabolic or endocrine abnormality
  - Commonly presents in the setting of illness and decreased oral intake
  - Resolves by school age
- Other
  - Munchausen and Munchausen by proxy
    - Hypoglycemia from surreptitious insulin or oral hypoglycemic agent administration
    - Consider in patients with abrupt onset of severe, unpredictable hypoglycemia.
  - Liver failure
  - Infections
    - Sepsis
    - Malaria
  - Postprandial hypoglycemia
    - Occurs in infants following fundoplication surgery or other gastrointestinal surgeries and results in hypoglycemia 1 to 2 hours after bolus feed or meal
    - Due to excessive incretin response to a meal that triggers exaggerated insulin secretion

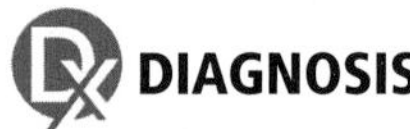

DIAGNOSIS

HISTORY

- Symptoms of hypoglycemia in the infant and young child:
  - Poor feeding
  - Lethargy
  - Irritability
  - Tremors
  - Seizure
- Older children and adolescents demonstrate Whipple triad:
  - Autonomic and neuroglycopenic symptoms
    - Sweating
    - Palpitations
    - Hunger
    - Weakness
    - Altered mental status
    - Seizure
  - Documented low-plasma glucose concentration
  - Resolution of symptoms with normalization of plasma glucose concentration
- Children with HI may have high IV glucose infusion requirements (>10 mg/kg/min).

ALERT

Infants with severe hypoglycemia may be asymptomatic.

PHYSICAL EXAM

- Large for gestational age
  - Suggests K_{ATP}HI
- SGA
  - Suggests transient HI
- Macroglossia, umbilical hernia (or omphalocele), hemihypertrophy
  - Suggest BWS
- Hepatomegaly and growth failure
  - Suggests GSD
- Midline defects (cleft palate, micropenis, umbilical hernia)
  - Suggest hypopituitarism or GHD

DIAGNOSTIC TESTS & INTERPRETATION

Initial Tests (screening, lab, imaging)

- Obtain critical sample at time of hypoglycemia (laboratory plasma glucose <50 mg/dL [2.8 mmol/L]).
  - Insulin and C-peptide
  - Growth hormone
  - Cortisol
  - β-hydroxybutyrate (BOHB)

- FFA
- Lactate
- Ammonia
- Comprehensive metabolic panel (CMP; including liver function tests [LFTs])
- Acylcarnitine profile
- Free and total carnitines
- Urine organic acids

- HI or insulinoma: evidence of insulin excess
  - Detectable insulin (any)
  - Suppressed BOHB (<1.8 mmol/L) and FFA (<1.7 mmol/L)
  - Glycemic response to 1 mg glucagon (Plasma glucose rise ≥30 mg/dL in 40 minutes.)
- Exogenous insulin: detectable insulin, undetectable C-peptide
- Hormone deficiency: Low cortisol and growth hormone at time of hypoglycemia is not diagnostic of adrenal insufficiency/GHD.
  - Perform appropriate stimulation tests to confirm.
- GSD I: elevated lactate, triglycerides, uric acid
- GSD III, VI, IX: elevated BOHB, LFTs
- FAOD: abnormal acylcarnitine profile, high FFA, and low BOHB

ALERT

Insulin levels may not be elevated or detectable at time of hypoglycemia in some persons with HI. Base diagnosis on other evidence of insulin excess.

- ^{18}F-DOPA positron emission tomography (PET) scans at specialized HI centers
  - Identify and to localize focal HI lesions
  - Traditional imaging studies such as ultrasound (US), CT scan, and MRI are not helpful in identifying focal lesions.
- Abdominal US
  - Screen for hepatic adenomas in GSD I.
  - Screen for abdominal tumors in BWS (until age 8 years).
- Brain MRI
  - Hypopituitarism or GHD
- Localization of insulinoma typically requires multiple modalities including abdominal MRI, endoscopic US, and ^{18}F-DOPA PET scan.
- Pathologic findings
  - Two major forms of pancreatic histology in children with HI due to K_{ATP} channel mutations:
    - Diffuse HI: abnormally enlarged islet cell nuclei found throughout the pancreas
    - Focal HI: discrete area of islet cell hyperplasia surrounded by normal pancreas

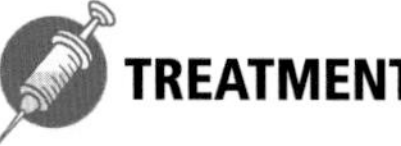

TREATMENT

GENERAL MEASURES

- Major goal is prevention of brain damage.
- IV dextrose infusions should be given to stabilize plasma glucose acutely.
  - For an acute hypoglycemic event, give a bolus of 2 to 3 mL/kg of 10% dextrose (0.2 to 0.3 g/kg).
  - Use dextrose infusion to maintain blood glucose >70 mg/dL.
  - Patients with HI may require central line to administer higher concentrations of dextrose and to avoid fluid overload.
- Frequent oral feeds are not sufficient as treatment for hypoglycemia due to HI.

MEDICATION

- Diazoxide, a K_{ATP} channel agonist, at 5 to 15 mg/kg/24 h PO divided q12h; 1st-line agent for HI
  - Most K_{ATP}HI patients do not respond.
  - Patients with HI/HA or transient HI typically respond well.
  - Diuretic is necessary to prevent fluid retention.
- Octreotide, a somatostatin analog, at 5 to 20 mcg/kg/24 h divided q6–8h; 2nd-line agent for patients with HI who are ≥8 weeks
  - Tachyphylaxis and hyperglycemia may occur.
  - Increased risk of necrotizing enterocolitis in neonates
- Glucagon, at 1 mg/24 h by continuous IV infusion, may stabilize blood glucose in infants with HI awaiting surgery; IM/SQ rescue forms used for severe hypoglycemia in children with diabetes
- Cornstarch at 1 to 2 g/kg/dose at bedtime for GSD or children with idiopathic ketotic hypoglycemia and abbreviated fasting tolerance
- For patients with hormone deficiencies, treatment with physiologic dosing of growth hormone or hydrocortisone leads to resolution of hypoglycemia.

SURGERY/OTHER PROCEDURES

- Pancreatectomy in children with diffuse HI refractory to medical therapy or in those with focal lesions. Near total pancreatectomy with gastrostomy tube for those with diffuse disease; resection of pancreatic adenomatous lesion for focal disease
- For focal HI, surgery is curative.
- Gastrostomy tube for administration of enteral dextrose in patients with GSD I, III, and some HI forms

ONGOING CARE

FOLLOW-UP RECOMMENDATIONS

- Up to 30–48% of HI and 20% of GSD patients can have neurodevelopmental abnormalities due to hypoglycemia.
- Patients who undergo near total pancreatectomy are at very high risk of developing diabetes later in life.

Patient Monitoring

- Home blood glucose monitoring, especially with longer fasts or intercurrent illnesses
- Hospitalizations for IV glucose infusions may be necessary during intercurrent illnesses with vomiting or poor oral intake.
  - Patients with GSD I are at risk of life-threatening lactic acidosis if fasting longer than 3 to 4 hours.
- Follow-up fasting studies may be needed to evaluate safety and/or disease resolution.
- Diazoxide may cause fluid retention, hypertrichosis, and bone marrow suppression. Monitor CBC, CMP.
- Octreotide can suppress growth hormone and TSH secretion, so close observation of linear growth is necessary. Thyroid function tests should also be monitored. Can also cause transaminitis and gallstones; LFTs and right upper quadrant (RUQ) US should be followed.
  - Neonates treated with octreotide should be closely monitored for evidence of necrotizing enterocolitis.
- Formal neurodevelopmental assessments are recommended for all patients with hypoglycemic disorders.

DIET

- Avoidance of long fasts
- Avoidance of protein loads in those with HI/HA and K_{ATP}HI, as high-protein diets may stimulate insulin secretion
- Avoidance of fructose, sucrose, galactose in GSD I

COMPLICATIONS

- Severe refractory hypoglycemia
- Cognitive deficits
- Seizures
- Coma
- Permanent brain damage
- Glucose intolerance or frank diabetes mellitus after near total pancreatectomy for HI
- Pancreatic exocrine insufficiency after near total pancreatectomy for HI
- Excessive weight gain in patients with GSD due to use of cornstarch and frequent meals

ADDITIONAL READING

- Ferrara C, Patel P, Becker S, et al. Biomarkers of insulin for the diagnosis of hyperinsulinemic hypoglycemia in infants and children. *J Pediatr*. 2016;168:212–219.
- Laje P, States LJ, Zhuang H, et al. Accuracy of PET/CT scan in the diagnosis of the focal form of congenital hyperinsulinism. *J Pediatr Surg*. 2013;48(2):388–393.
- Lord K, De León DD. Monogenic hyperinsulinemic hypoglycemia: current insights into the pathogenesis and management. *Int J Pediatr Endocrinol*. 2013;2013(1):3.
- Thornton PS, Stanley CA, De Leon DD, et al; for Pediatric Endocrine Society. Recommendations from the Pediatric Endocrine Society for evaluation and management of persistent hypoglycemia in neonates, infants, and children. *J Pediatr*. 2015;167(2):238–245.
- Wolfsdorf JI, Weinstein DA. Glycogen storage diseases. *Rev Endocr Metab Disord*. 2003;4(1):95–102.

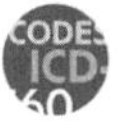

CODES

ICD10

E16.1 Other hypoglycemia

FAQ

- Q: How low can glucose go and for how long before brain damage occurs?
- A: The definition of hypoglycemia has been the subject of controversy in pediatrics, but activation of glucose counterregulatory systems occurs when plasma glucose levels reach the 65- to 70-mg/dL range; symptoms of hypoglycemia present at the 50- to 55-mg/dL level, and cognitive dysfunction occurs when plasma glucose levels are in the 45- to 50-mg/dL range. Taking these data into account, plasma glucose concentration should be maintained >70 mg/dL. The duration of hypoglycemia necessary for brain damage to occur is unknown.
- Q: How frequently should patients with hypoglycemia monitor blood glucose at home?
- A: It depends on the severity of the disorder. In general, patients should check after the longest period of fasting and before 1 to 2 feeds or meals per day. With illness or hypoglycemia, they should check more frequently. Home glucose meters have limited accuracy. Any glucoses <70 mg/dL should be repeated for confirmation prior to treatment.
- Q: What is the chance of HI in the sibling of an affected child?
- A: 25% in the autosomal recessive type; 50% in the autosomal dominant type; <1% for siblings of children with focal HI

HYPOKALEMIA

Onur Cil, MD, PhD • Elaine Ku, MD, MAS

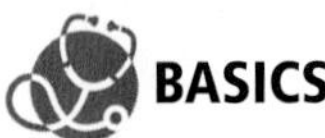

BASICS

DESCRIPTION

- Potassium (K^+) is the major intracellular cation and is important for all electrical activities in the body.
- Majority of K^+ (98%) is located intracellularly and high intracellular K^+ levels are required for normal metabolism and growth.
- Serum K^+ levels are tightly regulated within a narrow range (generally 3.5 to 5 mEq/L in children and 4 to 5.5 mEq/L in infants depending on the lab), and even small changes in serum K^+ levels can have significant effects on excitability of cells.
- Hypokalemia is defined as serum K^+ <3.5 mEq/L and is graded according to level:
  - Mild hypokalemia (3 to 3.5 mEq/L)
  - Moderate hypokalemia (2.5 to 3 mEq/L)
  - Severe hypokalemia (<2.5 mEq/L)
- Hypokalemia usually asymptomatic until serum K^+ is <3 mEq/L, or unless there is a rapid fall in serum K^+.
- Pseudohypokalemia can be seen due to uptake of K^+ in cells when blood samples are inappropriately kept in warm conditions for several hours before processing. This issue is in particular important in primary care setting if samples are being shipped without processing.

EPIDEMIOLOGY

Hypokalemia is common in the inpatient setting, and prevalence was reported to be as high as 40% in critically ill children.

RISK FACTORS

- Malnutrition (more important in developing countries)
- Eating disorders (particularly anorexia nervosa, especially when in conjunction with laxative or diuretic abuse)
- Conditions associated with increased stool losses (diarrhea, vomiting, loss of gastrointestinal [GI] fluid via surgical or tube drainage) increase the risk of developing hypokalemia

Genetics

There are a few causes of hypokalemia that are secondary to monogenic disorders including:

- Bartter syndrome
- Gitelman syndrome
- Liddle syndrome
- Syndrome of apparent mineralocorticoid excess
- Hypokalemic periodic paralysis
- Some types of congenital adrenal hyperplasia
- Congenital chloride diarrhea
- Cystic fibrosis

GENERAL PREVENTION

Prevention of malnutrition and checking serum K^+ levels in high-risk patients (GI fluid losses, malnutrition, eating disorders) is the most important step in prevention of severe hypokalemia.

PATHOPHYSIOLOGY

- There are three major mechanisms affecting serum K^+ levels: intake, excretion, and transcellular shifts.
- Hypokalemia can develop due to the following reasons:
  - Reduced intake
  - Increased losses (GI, renal or skin)
  - Transcellular shifts (β_2-adrenergic receptor stimulation, insulin, alkalosis)

ETIOLOGY

- The most common reason for hypokalemia in children is extrarenal causes including diarrhea, laxatives, vomiting, nasogastric suctioning, pyloric stenosis, ileostomy, congenital chloride diarrhea, excessive sweating.
- The conditions associated with reduced intake include malnutrition and anorexia nervosa.
- Hypokalemia due to renal losses is divided into two major groups according to the presence or absence of hypertension:
  - Renal etiologies associated with *normal* blood pressure: renal tubular acidosis (RTA), diabetic ketoacidosis (due to osmotic diuresis), medications (diuretics, amphotericin B, aminoglycosides, cisplatin), Bartter syndrome, Gitelman syndrome, cystic fibrosis, hypomagnesemia, toluene intoxication
  - Renal etiologies associated with *high* blood pressure: congenital adrenal hyperplasia (17-α hydroxylase or 11-β hydroxylase deficiency), primary hyperaldosteronism (tumors), syndrome of apparent mineralocorticoid excess (11-β hydroxysteroid dehydrogenase deficiency), Cushing syndrome, Liddle syndrome, renal artery stenosis, medications/herbs (mineralocorticoids, glucocorticoids, inhibition of 11-β hydroxysteroid dehydrogenase by licorice)
- Hypokalemia due to transcellular shifts: β_2 agonists (albuterol), insulin, theophylline, alkalosis (metabolic or respiratory), hyperthyroidism, hypokalemic periodic paralysis, refeeding syndrome

DIAGNOSIS

HISTORY

- Patients may present with fatigue, muscle weakness, paralysis, myalgia, muscle cramps, polyuria (due to impaired urine concentrating ability), polydipsia, and constipation.
- Ask patients and/or caregivers about extrarenal losses (diarrhea, vomiting), medication use (diuretics, β_2 agonists, insulin), dietary history (for malnutrition and eating disorders), signs of hyperthyroidism (palpitations, anxiety, weight loss, tremor, heat intolerance, diarrhea).
- History of previous hypokalemic episodes and/or failure to thrive may suggest an underlying chronic pathology. Some forms of Bartter syndrome can present in the neonatal period with dehydration and severe electrolyte abnormalities, whereas classic form can present later in life with polyuria and failure to thrive.
- Antenatal history is particularly important in infants (polyhydramnios is usually present in neonatal Bartter syndrome and congenital chloride diarrhea).
- Family history of periodic muscle weakness can suggest hypokalemic periodic paralysis, especially if hypokalemia is triggered by events that cause increased sympathetic tone (carbohydrate-rich meal, stress, exercise).

PHYSICAL EXAM

- Muscle strength should be examined in all patients.
- Vital signs are particularly important. Heart rate and rhythm abnormalities can be signs of arrhythmias in severe hypokalemia. Hypertension can guide physician toward a renovascular or endocrine problem.
- Anthropometric measures can guide physicians toward a specific diagnosis. Failure to thrive can be seen in RTA and Bartter syndrome. Cachexia can be seen in malnutrition, anorexia nervosa, and chronic diarrhea.
- Abdominal bruit can be a sign of renal artery stenosis.
- Signs of virilization can be seen in congenital adrenal hyperplasia.

DIAGNOSTIC TESTS & INTERPRETATION

Initial Testing (screening, lab, imaging)

- In children with mild hypokalemia and clear causes for hypokalemia (GI losses, medications), further workup is not indicated.
- However, in other patients with no clear cause for hypokalemia, further workup should be done which includes:
  - Serum sodium, K^+, chloride, calcium, magnesium, creatinine, urea, glucose, osmolality, venous blood gas
  - Urinalysis (including pH on a fresh specimen with limited contact with air), urine sodium, chloride, K^+, phosphorus, calcium, creatinine, osmolality
- If there are no signs of extrarenal potassium losses, transtubular potassium gradient (TTKG) and fractional excretion of potassium (FE_K) should be calculated by analyzing simultaneous serum and urine samples. TTKG >4 and FE_K >40% in a hypokalemic patient with normal glomerular filtration rate suggest renal potassium wasting.

Follow-Up Tests & Special Considerations

- If there is suspicion for an endocrine cause of hypokalemia; consider measurement of plasma renin activity (PRA), plasma aldosterone concentration (PAC), serum cortisol or other steroid metabolites.
- In patients with hypokalemia and hypertension PRA and PAC should be measured. In these patients renal ultrasound (US) with Doppler should be done to rule in/out renal artery stenosis.
- If there is suspicion for renal potassium wasting renal US should be done which can demonstrate nephrocalcinosis which is typical for distal RTA or Bartter syndrome.
- Electrocardiogram (EKG) should be done in all symptomatic patients or patients with severe hypokalemia.
- In patients with muscle weakness and severe hypokalemia, creatine kinase levels should be measured to assess presence of rhabdomyolysis.

Test Interpretation

- Hypokalemia can cause various EKG changes and severe hypokalemia can cause giant U waves created by T and U-wave fusion. Tachyarrhythmia and rarely atrioventricular block may also develop.
- Presence of acid–base abnormalities provides valuable information about etiology:
  - If there is concomitant metabolic acidosis anion gap should be checked. Increased anion gap is seen in diabetic ketoacidosis, whereas normal anion gap is seen in RTA.
  - If there is concomitant metabolic alkalosis urine Cl^- measurement should be the next step. In normotensive children, low urine Cl^- (<10 mEq/L) suggests extrarenal losses (vomiting, gastric suction, congenital chloride diarrhea, cystic fibrosis), whereas high urine Cl^- (>20 mEq/L) along with high PRA and PAC suggest renal salt wasting tubulopathies (Bartter/Gitelman syndromes).
  - In patients with renal potassium wasting in the absence of acid–base disorders hypomagnesemia or osmotic diuresis are potential other etiologies.

- In hypertensive patients PRA and PAC results are particularly important:
  - Low PRA and high PAC suggest primary hyperaldosteronism.
  - High PRA and high PAC with PAC/PRA ratio <10 suggests secondary hyperaldosteronism (children with nephrotic syndrome, cirrhosis with hypoproteinemia, and severe heart failure). High PRA and PAC are also seen in renal artery stenosis, coarctation of aorta, hyperthyroidism, pheochromocytoma and renin-secreting tumors.
  - Low PRA and low PAC suggest a nonaldosterone mineralocorticoid excess as seen in syndrome of apparent mineralocorticoid excess, congenital adrenal hyperplasia, licorice ingestion, and Liddle syndrome.
  - Cushing syndrome is usually associated with normal PRA and PAC levels.
  - Clinicians should be cautious while interpreting PRA results as medications (angiotensin converting enzyme inhibitors, angiotensin 2 receptor blockers, aldosterone antagonists, β-blockers) and dietary salt intake can affect results.

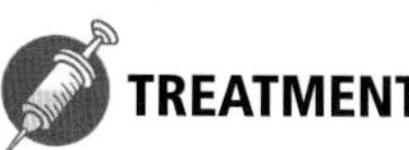

TREATMENT

GENERAL MEASURES

- Hypokalemia can be life-threatening and management primarily depends on the etiology, severity of hypokalemia, ongoing losses, and presence of symptoms. In severe hypokalemia treatment should be started immediately while workup is pending.
- Mild/moderate hypokalemia due to transcellular shift may not require potassium supplementation as correction of the underlying problem will resolve hypokalemia.
- If there is mild hypokalemia due to a medication, the first step should be stopping the medication when possible.
- Mild hypokalemia can be managed by consuming potassium-rich foods (see "Diet").
- Patients who are symptomatic and/or have moderate-severe hypokalemia (serum K^+ <3) require pharmacologic therapy.
- The preferred route for potassium repletion is enteral which has similar efficacy and fewer side effects compared to the IV route.
- IV repletion should be done for patients who have symptomatic hypokalemia (arrhythmias, muscle weakness, paralysis) or in patients whom enteral supplementation is not possible (intestinal obstruction, ileus, loss of consciousness). Continuous EKG monitoring should be done during IV potassium infusion.
- The most important point in hypokalemia treatment is avoiding hyperkalemia due to overrepletion and thus gradual supplementation should be done while rechecking K^+ levels and repleting more as needed.

MEDICATION

First Line

- Potassium salts (potassium chloride, citrate, phosphate, bicarbonate) are the mainstay of therapy.
- Potassium chloride is the most commonly used preparation with both enteral and parenteral formulations available and is associated with faster rises in serum K^+.
- Usual dosing range for oral potassium chloride is 2 to 5 mEq/kg/24 h in 2 to 4 divided doses (do not exceed 2 mEq/kg in a single dose).
- Recommended potassium dose for IV repletion is 0.5 to 1 mEq/kg/dose (do not exceed 20 to 40 mEq) to infuse at 0.3 to 0.5 mEq/kg/h (maximum rate 1 mEq/kg/h). Serum K^+ level should be rechecked 1 h after IV repletion is completed and redosing can be done if patient has persistent severe hypokalemia.
- The concentration of potassium chloride in a peripheral line should not exceed 40 mEq/L due to risk of pain and phlebitis.
- IV repletion should be avoided in oliguric/anuric patients and in patients with chronic kidney disease as it may cause severe hyperkalemia due to impaired excretion.
- Potassium citrate or bicarbonate can be used in patients with metabolic acidosis and hypokalemia as seen in RTA and diarrhea.
- Potassium phosphate is in particular useful in patients with concomitant hypokalemia and hypophosphatemia as seen in proximal tubular dysfunction and diabetic ketoacidosis.

ISSUES FOR REFERRAL

- Patients with eating disorders, malnutrition, and chronic diarrhea should be referred to specialists after acute treatment is completed.
- Patients with hypertension, metabolic acidosis/alkalosis, abnormalities in urinalysis (glucosuria, proteinuria), concomitant abnormalities in other electrolytes (hypomagnesemia, hypophosphatemia, hypernatremia), and failure to thrive should be referred to a pediatric nephrologist.

ADDITIONAL THERAPIES

- In patients with hypomagnesemia, magnesium repletion should be performed because hypomagnesemia can cause or worsen hypokalemia.
- Patients with Bartter and Gitelman syndromes can benefit from indomethacin or amiloride.
- Patients with hyperaldosteronism may benefit from spironolactone.

SURGERY/OTHER PROCEDURES

In patients with a tumor causing hypokalemia, removal of the tumor can be curative depending on the extent of disease.

COMPLEMENTARY & ALTERNATIVE THERAPIES

Patients with chronic hypokalemia can be recommended to consume potassium-rich foods (see "Diet") in addition to supplementation.

ADMISSION, INPATIENT, AND NURSING CONSIDERATIONS

- Patients with severe or symptomatic hypokalemia should be admitted for monitoring and careful repletion of K^+.
- Patients with severe malnutrition should be admitted because they are at risk for refeeding syndrome.

ONGOING CARE

FOLLOW-UP RECOMMENDATIONS

- In children with mild hypokalemia and clear cause of hypokalemia (such as GI losses or medications), further follow-up is not needed once serum K^+ levels return to normal.
- Patients with other conditions should be investigated and monitored by specialists.

Patient Monitoring

- Patients with mild/moderate hypokalemia or those at risk for refeeding syndrome can be monitored in a nonintensive care unit (ICU) setting.
- Severe hypokalemia especially when associated with arrhythmias, muscle weakness, or rhabdomyolysis should be monitored in the ICU due to risk of life-threatening arrhythmias and respiratory muscle weakness.

DIET

Consuming potassium-rich foods (beans, potatoes, bananas, avocados, apricots, orange juice, yogurt) can help hypokalemia management.

PATIENT EDUCATION

Patients should be educated for signs of hypokalemia, and adherence to medical therapy should be reinforced in chronic cases. They should also be informed about conditions with increased risk of hypokalemia (diarrhea, vomiting) and should be instructed to come back to hospital in these situations.

PROGNOSIS

The prognosis is excellent in patients with acute mild/asymptomatic hypokalemia due to GI losses. Prognosis of severe or symptomatic hypokalemia depends on presence of cardiac abnormalities, respiratory depression, and rhabdomyolysis.

COMPLICATIONS

Severe hypokalemia can cause life-threatening arrhythmias, rhabdomyolysis, and respiratory depression that can necessitate intubation/mechanical ventilation.

ADDITIONAL READING

- Gumz ML, Rabinowitz L, Wingo CS. An integrated view of potassium homeostasis. *N Eng J Med.* 2015;373(1):60–72.
- Palmer BF. Regulation of potassium homeostasis. *Clin J Am Soc Nephrol.* 2015;10(6):1050–1060.
- Zieg J, Gonsorcikova L, Landau D. Current views on the diagnosis and management of hypokalaemia in children. *Acta Pediatr.* 2016;105(7):762–772.

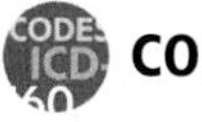

CODES

ICD10

E26.81 Bartter's syndrome

FAQ

- Q: Should I be worried that hypokalemia will recur?
- A: In patients with hypokalemia due to vomiting and diarrhea the problem is usually resolved once vomiting/diarrhea is resolved. Hypokalemia can recur in those who have kidney or endocrine problems causing the problem.
- Q: What are potassium-rich foods?
- A: Beans, potatoes, bananas, avocados, apricots, orange juice, and yogurt are foods rich in K^+.
- Q: Are there spurious laboratory causes of hypokalemia.
- A: Yes, in some conditions inappropriate processing of blood can result in uptake of K^+ by cells in vitro, leading to pseudohypokalemia.

HYPONATREMIA

Paul R. Brakeman, MD, PhD

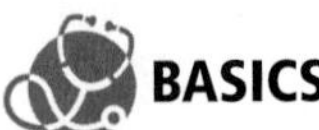

BASICS

DESCRIPTION

- Sodium cation (Na^+) is the major extracellular cation and is important osmole in the extracellular space.
- A positive Na^+ balance is required for growth.
- Serum Na^+ levels reflect extracellular Na^+ and are tightly regulated within a narrow range (generally 135 to 145 mEq/L).
- Approximately 2/3 of body mass is Na^+-containing extracellular fluid space.
- Hyponatremia is defined as serum Na^+ <135 mEq/L and is graded according to level:
  - Mild hyponatremia (130 to 135 mEq/L)
  - Moderate hyponatremia (125 to 129 mEq/L)
  - Severe hyponatremia (<125 mEq/L)
- Even mild hyponatremia (130 to 135 mEq/L) has measurable effects on cognitive function, and severe hyponatremia can lead to seizures, brain edema, and death.
- Hyponatremia can be factitious in the setting of significantly elevated glucose.

EPIDEMIOLOGY

Hyponatremia is common in the inpatient setting, and incidence for moderate to severe hyponatremia (<130 mEq/L) is ~1% hospitalized pediatric patients and mild hyponatremia (<135 mEq/L) is present in up to 45% of pediatric patients admitted for community-acquired pneumonia.

RISK FACTORS

- Conditions associated with syndrome of inappropriate antidiuretic hormone secretion (SIADH) including nausea, hypotension, hypovolemia, reduced circulatory volume (congestive heart failure [CHF], nephrosis, and cirrhosis), asthma, pneumonia, mechanical ventilation, fever, stress, pain and specific medications (narcotics, nonsteroidal anti-inflammatory drugs, serotonin reuptake inhibitors, Cytoxan® and vincristine)
- Conditions associated with increased stool losses (diarrhea, vomiting, loss of gastrointestinal [GI] fluid—surgical or tube drainage) increase the risk of developing hyponatremia.
- Excessive water intake such as in polydipsia or incorrectly mixed formula
- Decreased water excretion such as acute kidney injury

Genetics

There are a few causes of hyponatremia that are secondary to monogenic disorders including congenital adrenal hypoplasia, also known as adrenal hypoplasia congenita (AHC).

GENERAL PREVENTION

Providing adequate Na^+ intake and checking serum Na^+ levels in high-risk patients (GI fluid losses and high risk for SAIDH) is the most important step in prevention of severe hyponatremia.

ALERT

Due to the high rate of SIADH in hospitalized pediatric patients, isotonic saline solution should be used for maintenance IVF therapy specifically in the postoperative setting and in children with central nervous system (CNS) or pulmonary disease.

PATHOPHYSIOLOGY

- There are three major mechanisms affecting serum Na^+ levels: intake, excretion, and total body water. Hyponatremia can develop due to following reasons:
  - Reduced intake of Na^+
  - Increased losses (GI, renal, or skin)
  - Increased total body water
- Hyponatremic encephalopathy results from hypo-osmolality in the extracellular space and the influx of water into the intracellular space down the concentration gradient, resulting in parenchymal brain swelling and resulting symptoms.

ETIOLOGY

- Hyponatremia is usually divided into three classifications: (i) hypovolemic hyponatremia, (ii) euvolemic hyponatremia, and (iii) hypovolemic hyponatremia.
- The most common reason for hyponatremia in hospitalized patients is SIADH.
- The most common cause in the general pediatric population is extrarenal losses including diarrhea and vomiting.

DIAGNOSIS

HISTORY

- Patients may present with fatigue, muscle weakness, confusion, altered mental status, seizure, headache, nausea, and/or vomiting.
- Determine current medications.
- Identify extrarenal losses (diarrhea, vomiting).
- Define recent intake of fluid and Na^+.
- Determine total body water status (edema, weight loss/gain, sunken eyes).
- Determine recent urine volume.
- Past medical history (history of previous hyponatremia episodes, failure to thrive) may suggest an underlying chronic pathology.
- Family history of primary tubular syndromes such as Bartter or Gitelman syndromes or extrarenal conditions that alter water loss such as cystic fibrosis

PHYSICAL EXAM

- Vital signs are particularly important. Heart rate and blood pressure can help determine volume status.
- Cardiac and pulmonary exam to identify causes of SIADH including pneumonia and CHF
- Abdominal exam for signs of liver failure (hepatosplenomegaly)
- Signs of virilization can be seen in AHC.
- Skin turgor (low total body water)
- Neurologic exam: confusion, altered consciousness, agitation

DIFFERENTIAL DIAGNOSIS

Usually, hyponatremia is detected during blood tests for other conditions (diarrhea, vomiting). Some symptoms of hyponatremia can be seen in other neurologic conditions, but severe hyponatremia accompanied by neurologic abnormalities (seizure, change in mental status) should be assumed to be the primary cause of neurologic abnormalities and corrected appropriately.

DIAGNOSTIC TESTS & INTERPRETATION

Initial Tests (screening, lab, imaging)

- In children with mild hyponatremia and clear causes for hyponatremia (GI losses), further workup is not indicated. However in other patients with no clear cause for hyponatremia, further workup should be done which include:
  - Serum Na^+, potassium, chloride, calcium, magnesium, creatinine, urea, glucose, osmolality, venous blood gas
  - Urinalysis (including pH), urine Na^+, chloride, potassium, creatinine, osmolality
- If there are no signs of extrarenal Na^+ losses or if hyponatremia is out of proportion to losses, fractional excretion of Na^+ (FE_{Na}) should be calculated by analyzing simultaneous serum and urine samples.

Follow-Up Tests & Special Considerations

If there is suspicion about an endocrine cause of hyponatremia, consider measurement of plasma renin activity (PRA), plasma aldosterone concentration (PAC), serum cortisol, or other steroid metabolites.

Test Interpretation

- Random urine Na^+ concentration should be <25 mEq/L, and FE_{Na} should be low for patients with reduced effective intravascular volume and hyponatremia.
- Urine Na^+ >25 mEq/L with reduced effective intravascular volume indicates hypoaldosteronism, cerebral salt wasting, and/or diuretic use.
- Euvolemic patients with SIADH will routinely have urine Na^+ >25 mEq/L. SIADH is defined as urine osmolality > serum osmolality and serum Na^+ <130 mEq/L.
- Rarely, a patient with reduced effective intravascular volume, significant metabolic alkalosis, and hyponatremia can have obligate Na^+ losses in the urine accompanying the bicarbonaturia and thus have a urine Na^+ >25 mEq/L.
- Clinicians should be cautious when interpreting PRA results as medications (angiotensin-converting enzyme inhibitors, angiotensin II receptor blockers, aldosterone antagonists, β-blockers), and dietary salt intake can affect results.

TREATMENT

GENERAL MEASURES

- Hyponatremia can be life-threatening and management primarily depends on the etiology, severity of hyponatremia, ongoing losses, and presence of symptoms. In severe and/or symptomatic hyponatremia, treatment should be started immediately while more advanced workup is pending.
- For suspected hyponatremic encephalopathy, patients should receive a 2 mL/kg bolus of 3% NaCl with a maximum of 100 mL immediately to reduce cerebral edema before other measures and evaluation are undertaken. Repeat bolus 1 to 2 times as needed until symptoms improve, with a goal to increase in serum Na^+ 5 to 6 mEq/L in first 1 to 2 hours.

ALERT

- For patients with chronic hyponatremia (>48 hours), Na^+ should be given to increase serum Na^+ no faster than 6 to 8 mEq/L/24 h. The rate of repletion of Na^+ can be calculated using the volume of distribution of Na^+ (0.66) and the desired change in serum Na^+ (rate of Na^+ repletion per hour = [0.66 × weight in kg] × desired rise in serum Na^+ plus Na^+ losses per hour). It is worth noting the large unknown in this equation which is the rate of Na^+ losses which can sometimes be estimated by the volume of GI losses (emesis, ostomy output, diarrhea).
- If SIADH is identified in a euvolemic patient, then the primary treatment is fluid restriction. Fluid restriction should not be applied expectantly to postoperative children as it leads to dehydration; rather, isotonic saline solution should be used postoperatively at a standard rate to replace urine and insensible losses.
- Alternatively, SIADH can be treated by giving extra Na^+ and then driving salt and water excretion with furosemide if total body water increases with salt supplementation (edema).
- If there is mild hyponatremia due to a medication, the therapeutic benefit of the medication can be weighed against the risks of hyponatremia, although Na^+ <130 mEq/L should generally lead to stopping a medication.
- If severe hyponatremia (<120 mEq/L) has resulted from the use of desmopressin acetate (DDAVP®), then the safest approach is to continue the DDAVP® to maintain consistent renal water excretion, and use 3% NaCl boluses to correct the serum Na^+.

MEDICATION

First Line

- For excessive losses, oral or IV Na^+ chloride is the mainstay of treatment.
- IV repletion should be avoided in mild-moderate asymptomatic oliguric/anuric patients with hyponatremia due to total body water excess.

Second Line

In situations of low urine output such as CHF and cirrhosis, vasopressin receptor inhibition (tolvaptan) may be beneficial.

ISSUES FOR REFERRAL

- Patients with chronic diarrhea should be referred to specialists after acute treatment is completed.
- Patients with recurrent or chronic hyponatremia should be referred to a pediatric nephrologist or endocrinologist.

SURGERY/OTHER PROCEDURES

In patients with a tumor causing SIADH and hyponatremia, removal of the tumor can be curative depending on the extent of disease.

ADMISSION, INPATIENT, AND NURSING CONSIDERATIONS

- Patients with severe and/or symptomatic acute hyponatremia should be admitted for monitoring and careful repletion of Na^+ usually in the intensive care unit (ICU) setting.
- Patients with stable, asymptomatic yet severe chronic hyponatremia may require PICU admission to allow for frequent and adequate monitoring to prevent over-rapid correction.

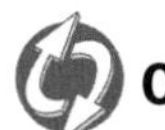

ONGOING CARE

FOLLOW-UP RECOMMENDATIONS

- In children with mild hyponatremia and clear cause of hyponatremia (such as GI losses SIADH with a clear self-limited cause such as pneumonia or surgery), further follow-up is not needed once serum Na^+ levels return to normal.
- Patients with other conditions should be investigated and monitored by specialists.

Patient Monitoring

- Patients with mild/moderate hyponatremia can be monitored on the floor.
- Severe hyponatremia, especially when associated altered mental status, seizure, or severe dehydration, should be monitored in the ICU due to risk of life-threatening arrhythmias and respiratory muscle weakness.

DIET

Consuming Na^+-rich foods can help hyponatremia management in cases of ongoing chronic losses.

PATIENT EDUCATION

Patients should be educated for signs of hyponatremia, and adherence to medical therapy and/or fluid and Na^+ intake goals should be reinforced in chronic cases. They should also be informed about conditions with increased risk of hyponatremia (diarrhea, vomiting) and should be instructed to come back to hospital in these situations.

PROGNOSIS

Prognosis is excellent in patients with acute mild/asymptomatic hyponatremia due to GI losses. Prognosis of severe or symptomatic hyponatremia depends on rate of correction.

COMPLICATIONS

- Severe hyponatremia can cause life-threatening seizure and changes in mental status with respiratory depression that can necessitate intubation/mechanical ventilation.
- Over-rapid correction can lead to cerebral demyelination. Risk factors for cerebral demyelination include chronic hyponatremia combined with liver disease, malnutrition, hypoxia, and/or increase in serum Na^+ >25 mEq/L in 48 hours.

ADDITIONAL READING

- Lavagno C, Milani GP, Uestuener P, et al. Hyponatremia in children with acute respiratory infections: a reappraisal. *Pediatr Pulmonol*. 2017;52(7):962–967.
- Moritz ML, Ayus JC. New aspects in the pathogenesis, prevention, and treatment of hyponatremic encephalopathy in children. *Pediatr Nephrol*. 2010;25(7):1225–1238.
- Padua AP, Macaraya JR, Dans LF, et al. Isotonic versus hypotonic saline solution for maintenance intravenous fluid therapy in children: a systematic review. *Pediatr Nephrol*. 2015;30(7):1163–1172.

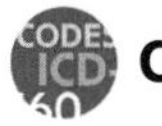

CODES

ICD10

E87.1 Hypo-osmolality and hyponatremia

FAQ

- Q: What is the primary mechanism for developing hyponatremia in hospitalized children?
- A: Excessive ADH in the setting of stress, pneumonia, respiratory distress, CNS disease, and/or postoperative state
- Q: What is the best first therapy for suspected hyponatremic encephalopathy?
- A: 2 mL/kg bolus of 3% NaCl with a maximum of 100 mL to increase serum Na^+ rapidly to decrease cerebral edema
- Q: Are there spurious laboratory causes of hyponatremia?
- A: Yes, significant hyperlipidemia and very high–serum protein levels can decrease the measured serum sodium by interfering with measurement by flame-photometric and indirect ion-selective electrode assays. Hyperglycemia causes the shift of water out of cells and into the extracellular space, thus decreasing measured sodium, albeit without measurement error.

HYPOPHOSPHATEMIC DISORDERS

Erik A. Imel, MD, MS • Peter Tebben, MD

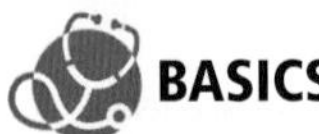

BASICS

DESCRIPTION

Hypophosphatemia is defined by serum phosphorus values below the age-appropriate normal range. Hypophosphatemia may be acute or chronic. Effects on various body systems depend on the severity and duration of hypophosphatemia. Symptoms and signs are nonspecific, most commonly involving generalized muscle weakness and fatigue but can include severe neurologic, cardiovascular, and respiratory compromise with acute severe hypophosphatemia, whereas with chronic hypophosphatemia, patients develop rickets and osteomalacia.

ALERT

- Normal phosphorus concentrations in infants and children are significantly higher than in adults.
- Hypophosphatemia can be missed if an adult normal range is used for pediatric patients.

EPIDEMIOLOGY

- Acute hypophosphatemia is a common laboratory finding in the hospital, especially in the intensive care unit (ICU) setting, resulting from a variety of mechanisms.
- Chronic hypophosphatemia is less common but is clinically important as an etiology of rickets.
  - Vitamin D deficiency may cause hypophosphatemia and remains the most common form of rickets around the world, even in industrialized nations.
  - X-linked hypophosphatemic (XLH) rickets is the most common inherited cause of rickets (prevalence ≈1 in 20,000).
  - Other genetic forms of rickets are more rare.
- Isolated dietary phosphate deficiency is rare; dietary phosphate deficiency usually involves generalized malnutrition or inadequate phosphate availability in parenteral or enteral nutrition formulations.

RISK FACTORS

- Nutritional
  - Vitamin D deficiency
  - Malnutrition/refeeding syndrome
  - Chronic diarrhea
  - Amino-acid based elemental enteral formulas
- Medications affecting phosphate absorption
  - Antacids
  - Sevelamer
  - Lanthanum carbonate
  - Excess calcium salts
- Other:
  - Medications affecting renal phosphate transport
  - Medications or toxins causing generalized proximal renal tubulopathy
  - Treatment of diabetic ketoacidosis (DKA)
  - Acute respiratory alkalosis
  - Post renal transplant
  - Hungry bone syndrome with hypocalcemia after parathyroidectomy for hyperparathyroidism

Genetics

Genetic forms are less common than acquired forms:

- *PHEX* (XLH, X-linked dominant)
- *FGF23* (fibroblast growth factor 23, autosomal dominant hypophosphatemic rickets [ADHR])
- *DMP1* (autosomal recessive [AR] hypophosphatemic rickets [ARHR])
- *ENPP1* (ARHR, generalized arterial calcification of infancy [GACI])
- *FAM20C* (AR hypophosphatemia, Raine syndrome)
- *SCL34A3* (NPT2c, AR hereditary hypophosphatemic rickets with hypercalciuria [HHRH]; nephrolithiasis also occurs in heterozygotes)
- *CYP27B1* (1α-hydroxylase deficiency, AR)
- *VDR* (vitamin D receptor, AR)
- Somatic mutations sometimes associated with hypophosphatemia:
  - *GNAS* (McCune-Albright syndrome [MAS], fibrous dysplasia, somatic activating mutations)
  - *HRAS/NRAS* (somatic activating mutations causing epidermal nevus syndrome)
- Others, including various genetic causes of renal Fanconi syndrome

PATHOPHYSIOLOGY

- Decreased nutritional intake or malabsorption
- Redistribution of extracellular phosphate into the intracellular compartment (causes acute hypophosphatemia only)
  - Insulin mediated (during treatment of DKA)
  - Refeeding syndrome
  - Acute respiratory alkalosis
- Increased renal phosphate loss
  - FGF23-mediated
  - Parathyroid hormone (PTH)-mediated
  - Medications altering phosphate transport
  - Primary proximal renal tubulopathies

ETIOLOGY

See genetic causes and "Differential Diagnosis."

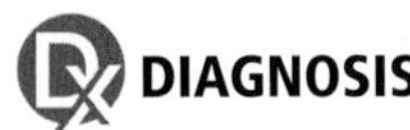

DIAGNOSIS

HISTORY

- Family history of hypophosphatemia or rickets
- Medications
- Known disease affecting phosphate metabolism (see "Differential Diagnosis")
- Nutritional history
  - Vitamin D intake, phosphate sources
  - Anorexia or other malnutrition
  - Parenteral or enteral nutrition formulation
- Duration of symptoms (acute vs. chronic)
- Dental abnormalities
  - Abscessed teeth associated with XLH
- Gastrointestinal symptoms
  - Chronic diarrhea
- Cardiovascular, respiratory, or neurologic symptoms (may accompany acute severe hypophosphatemia, usually in a hospital setting)
- Myalgia or weakness
- Bowed legs, short stature
- Bone pain or stress fractures/pseudofractures
- Precocious puberty, café au lait macules, fibrous dysplasia—due to MAS

PHYSICAL EXAM

- Height, rate of growth
- Rachitic features
  - Frontal bossing
  - Delayed closure of fontanelle
  - Rachitic rosary
  - Harrison sulcus (groove corresponding to the rib insertion site of the diaphragm)
  - Widened wrists or ankles
  - Valgus, varus, or windswept deformity of the legs
- Craniofacial or other bony deformities suggesting fibrous dysplasia
- Dental abscesses
- Muscle weakness
- Signs of precocious puberty (MAS)
- Café au lait macules (MAS)
- Other skin lesions (epidermal nevus syndromes)

DIFFERENTIAL DIAGNOSIS

- Nutritional- or absorption-related
  - Low phosphorus intake
  - Amino-acid based elemental enteral formulas
  - Premature infants
  - Chronic diarrhea
  - Short-bowel syndrome
  - Vitamin D deficiency
    - Nutritional, lack of sun exposure
    - 1α-hydroxylase deficiency
    - VDR mutation
  - Medications
    - Antacids
    - Sevelamer
    - Lanthanum carbonate
    - Excess calcium salts
- Redistribution of phosphate into the intracellular compartment
  - Insulin therapy for DKA
  - Acute respiratory alkalosis
  - Refeeding syndrome
- Phosphate uptake by bone
  - Hungry bone syndrome (after parathyroidectomy for primary hyperparathyroidism)
- Increased renal phosphate loss
  - Medications (glucocorticoids, diuretics)
  - Primary hyperparathyroidism
  - FGF23-dependent (FGF23 excess)
    - XLH
    - ADHR (may present during childhood, or after childhood with new-onset hypophosphatemia)
    - ARHR
    - Tumor-induced osteomalacia (TIO) (primarily diagnosed in adults, but cases reported in children). Consider ADHR if thinking of TIO.
    - Fibrous dysplasia of bone/MAS
    - Postrenal transplant phosphate wasting
    - Elevated FGF23 following some iron infusion formulations in severely iron-deficient patients (Consider in patients with hypophosphatemia developing shortly after iron infusions, or in patients getting repeated iron infusions.)
  - FGF23-independent
    - Renal Fanconi syndrome
      - Familial/genetic
      - Medication-induced
      - Associated with other disorders (cystinosis, multiple myeloma, and others)
    - HHRH (rare—mutations impairing NPT2c)

DIAGNOSTIC TESTS & INTERPRETATION

Initial Tests (screening, lab, imaging)

- Confirm laboratory diagnosis before treating (unless unstable).
- Serum phosphorus concentration—below age-appropriate normal range (ideally fasting)
- Normal ranges by age

– 0 to 1 month	4.8 to 8.2 mg/dL
– 1 to 4 month	4.8 to 8.1 mg/dL
– 4 months to 1 year	4.8 to 6.8 mg/dL
– 1 to 5 years	3.6 to 6.5 mg/dL
– 5 to 10 years	3.4 to 5.5 mg/dL
– 10 to 20 years	2.6 to 5.2 mg/dL
– >20 years	2.5 to 4.9 mg/dL

- Serum calcium
  - Normal in most primary renal phosphate wasting disorders
  - Elevated in primary hyperparathyroidism
  - Low or low normal in vitamin D deficiency rickets
- PTH concentration
  - Can be elevated if chronic hypophosphatemia is due to vitamin D deficiency or to XLH (pre- or posttreatment). However, elevated PTH concurrent with hypercalcemia indicates primary hyperparathyroidism.
- Alkaline phosphatase
  - Elevated in rickets and many patients with hyperparathyroidism
- Serum creatinine
- 25-hydroxyvitamin D
  - Low in vitamin D deficiency rickets
- 1,25-dihydroxyvitamin D
  - Variable (low, normal, or high) in vitamin D deficiency
  - Low in 1α-hydroxylase deficiency
  - Elevated in VDR mutations and nutritional phosphate deficiency
  - Low or inappropriately normal in FGF23-mediated causes of hypophosphatemia
- Urine phosphorus and creatinine in a fasted morning 2-hour collection, or second morning void; should be obtained at the same time as serum phosphorus and creatinine
  - Use to determine tubular maximum phosphate reabsorption per glomerular filtration rate (T_mP/GFR or TP/GFR)
  - T_mP/GFR = serum phosphorus − [(urine phosphorus × serum creatinine)/urine creatinine]
  - T_mP/GFR is normal or high in vitamin D–mediated hypophosphatemia and nutritional deficiency.
  - T_mP/GFR is low in renal phosphate wasting disorders.
- FGF23 (a phosphaturic hormone)—may be helpful in renal phosphate wasting disorders
  - Elevated in many forms of inherited rickets (XLH, ADHR, ARHR)
  - Elevated in most patients with TIO due to FGF23-secreting tumors
  - Low in nutritional phosphate deficiency, malabsorption, Fanconi syndrome or HHRH
- Knee/wrist radiographs to evaluate for signs of rickets
- Skeletal survey in patients suspected of fibrous dysplasia of bone
  - Bone scan is also very sensitive in evaluating for fibrous dysplasia.
- Rare: other imaging to identify TIO
  - These rare tumors can be very difficult to localize.
  - MRI, CT, octreotide scan, whole body sestamibi scan, FDG-positron-emission tomography (PET)/CT, Ga68-DOTATAE PET/CT

Diagnostic Procedures/Other

Genetic studies, when appropriate

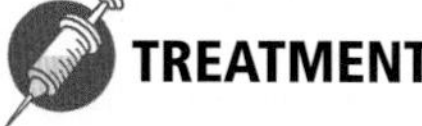

TREATMENT

MEDICATION

- Acute hypophosphatemia
  - Oral phosphate supplementation preferred route
  - IV phosphate may be required for severe hypophosphatemia but should be used with caution (see "Alert").
    - High doses require central venous catheter.
  - Replete vitamin D if needed (this will not acutely increase serum phosphorus levels)

ALERT

IV phosphate infusions can cause severe life-threatening hypocalcemia:
- Avoid in patients who are already hypocalcemic.
- Infuse slowly.
- Monitor calcium.
- Telemetry recommended due to possible arrhythmias

- Chronic hypophosphatemia
  - If dietary deficiency or malabsorption: oral phosphate and vitamin D repletion
  - If renal phosphate wasting is the cause, referral to a specialist in these disorders is recommended for management.
  - If renal phosphate wasting is due to an FGF23-mediated cause:
    - Phosphate 20 to 40 mg/kg/24 h divided in 3 to 5 doses
      - Start therapy with low doses and then increase gradually to reduce risk of diarrhea.
    - Calcitriol 20 to 30 ng/kg/24 h in 2 divided doses (may require higher doses)
    - Burosumab, monoclonal anti-FGF23 antibody, approved in 2018 specifically for XLH:
      - *Stop* calcitriol and phosphate 1 week before starting burosumab.
      - Starting doses: children: 0.8 mg/kg subcutaneously every 2 weeks, adults 1 mg/kg subcutaneously every 4 weeks
  - Non–FGF23-mediated renal phosphate wasting with elevated 1,25-dihydroxyvitamin D (HHRH)
    - Phosphate 20 to 40 mg/kg/24 h divided in 3 to 5 doses
    - Do not use burosumab in this situation.

ADDITIONAL THERAPIES

- Chronic hypophosphatemic disorders resulting in skeletal deformity (especially inherited causes) may require surgical intervention to correct valgus or varus deformities of the lower extremities.
  - Adequate medical therapy should be initiated first, as it may reduce the need for surgery.
- Routine dental care at least twice per year (especially for patients with inherited rickets)
  - Dental abscess common in some genetic forms of hypophosphatemia
  - Consider dental sealants.
- Audiology evaluation in patient with inherited hypophosphatemic rickets
  - Increased risk of hearing loss
- Some children with chronic hypophosphatemic disorders may develop craniosynostosis.
- For the rare cases of TIO, complete surgical removal of the offending tumor is curative.

ONGOING CARE

FOLLOW-UP RECOMMENDATIONS

- For acute hypophosphatemia
  - Telemetry if severe and/or treating intravenously
  - Careful laboratory monitoring until resolution (laboratory measures may be needed multiple times a day depending on severity and mode of treatment)
    - Calcium
    - Phosphorus
    - Creatinine
- For chronic hypophosphatemia
  - Frequent laboratory monitoring is mandatory if long-term phosphate and calcitriol therapy is needed (every 3 to 4 months).
    - Calcium
    - Phosphorus
    - Creatinine
    - Alkaline phosphatase
    - PTH
    - Urine calcium, creatinine, and phosphorus
  - The goal is *not* to normalize serum phosphate in chronic renal phosphate wasting disorders if using calcitriol and phosphate, as this may lead to secondary or tertiary hyperparathyroidism and/or nephrocalcinosis.
  - Monitor labs monthly for the first 3 months of burosumab and then at least every 3 months.
  - Decrease or stop doses if hyperphosphatemic.
  - Monitor growth and leg bowing.
  - Periodic radiographic studies
    - Annual renal ultrasound to evaluate for nephrocalcinosis
    - Periodic radiograph of knees/wrists to evaluate response to treatment

ALERT

Treating chronic hypophosphatemia, especially renal phosphate wasting disorders, carries risks of:
- Hyperparathyroidism
- Nephrocalcinosis

PROGNOSIS

- Hypophosphatemia due to nutritional deficiency
  - Hypophosphatemia resolves with adequate replacement of nutritional deficiencies or discontinuation of phosphate-binding agents.
- Acute hypophosphatemia (typically seen in the hospital setting) can be life-threatening and requires careful monitoring and treatment but resolves when underlying condition addressed.
- Chronic renal phosphate wasting disorders have a variable response to treatment. Some have radiographic healing of rickets, correction of varus/valgus deformity, and normalization of alkaline phosphatase, whereas others have an incomplete response to therapy.
- Short stature is a common result of chronic hypophosphatemia.
- Hypophosphatemia resolves with removal of the offending tumor in patients with TIO, but long-term monitoring for recurrence is necessary, as hypophosphatemia may recur years later.

ADDITIONAL READING

- Carpenter TO, Imel EA, Holm IA, et al. A clinician's guide to X-linked hypophosphatemia. *J Bone Miner Res*. 2011;26(7):1381–1388.
- Carpenter TO, Whyte MP, Imel EA, et al. Burosumab therapy in children with X-linked hypophosphatemia. *N Engl J Med*. 2018;378(21):1987–1998.
- Imel EA, Econs MJ. Approach to the hypophosphatemic patient. *J Clin Endocrinol Metab*. 2012;97(3):696–706.

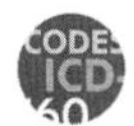

CODES

ICD10

- E83.39 Other disorders of phosphorus metabolism
- E72.09 Other disorders of amino-acid transport
- E83.31 Familial hypophosphatemia

FAQ

- Q: What are dietary phosphate sources?
- A: Phosphate sources are ubiquitous; examples include processed meats, dairy, legumes, nuts, whole grains, citrus, and colas. Phosphates are used as a preservative in processed foods.

H

HYPOPITUITARISM

Craig A. Alter, MD • Shana E. McCormack, MD, MTR

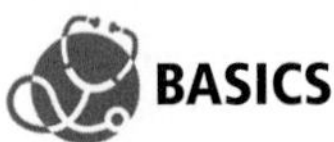

BASICS

DESCRIPTION

Hypopituitarism refers to deficiencies of one or more pituitary hormones.

- "Panhypopituitarism" (*pan* meaning "all") technically requires deficiency of all eight pituitary hormones; however, the term is often used for deficiencies of >1 pituitary hormone.

EPIDEMIOLOGY

- Congenital forms affect both sexes equally and are diagnosed early in childhood.
- The epidemiology of acquired or secondary forms depends on the underlying cause.

RISK FACTORS

Genetics

There is increasing understanding of the genetic etiology of familial and/or congenital forms of hypopituitarism. Patterns of inheritance include autosomal recessive, autosomal dominant, X-linked, and digenic forms; can occur in the setting of other complex medical syndromes

PATHOPHYSIOLOGY

- Pathology is based on specific deficiency or deficiencies.
- Adrenocorticotropic hormone (ACTH): hypocortisolism
- Thyroid-stimulating hormone (TSH): hypothyroidism
- Growth hormone (GH): GH deficiency, which can manifest as hypoglycemia in newborns and poor growth in patients >6 to 12 months
- Luteinizing hormone (LH)/follicle-stimulating hormone (FSH): hypogonadism
- Antidiuretic hormone (ADH): diabetes insipidus (DI)
- Note: prolactin (PRL): Hyperprolactinemia can accompany hypothalamic causes of hypopituitarism.

ETIOLOGY

- Idiopathic
- Congenital
  - Absence of the pituitary (empty sella syndrome is a risk)
  - Pituitary malformations (ectopic posterior pituitary, hypoplastic infundibular stalk, hypoplastic pituitary)
  - Rathke cleft cyst
  - Genetic disorders due to mutations in genes important for CNS development, including transcription factors can be associated with de novo or familial forms (*POUF1, HESX1, LHX3, LHX4, OTX2, SOX2, SOX3, PTX2, PROP1*, etc.).
  - Antenatal exposures/insults may precipitate.
- Mechanical
  - Birth trauma or perinatal insult
  - Surgical resection of the gland or damage to the stalk
  - Traumatic brain injury
- Infiltrative
  - Hypophysitis (inflammation of the pituitary gland)
  - Iron deposition secondary to chronic transfusion therapy (e.g., β-thalassemia)
  - Histiocytosis
  - Sarcoidosis
- Infection
  - Viral encephalitis
  - Bacterial or fungal infection
  - Tuberculosis
- Vascular
  - Pituitary infarction
  - Pituitary aneurysm
- Cranial irradiation
- Tumors
  - Craniopharyngioma
  - Germinoma
  - Glioma
  - Pinealoma
  - Primitive neuroectodermal tumor (medulloblastoma)

COMMONLY ASSOCIATED CONDITIONS

- Midline defects such as cleft lip/palate, hypotelorism, single central maxillary incisor
- Septo-optic dysplasia (de Morsier syndrome)
- Holoprosencephaly

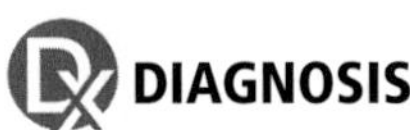

DIAGNOSIS

HISTORY

- Birth history
  - Infants with hypopituitarism are usually normal or small for gestational age, in contrast to hyperinsulinemic infants, who are typically large for gestational age.
  - Documented or symptoms of hypoglycemia, which include poor feeding, lethargy, irritability, or seizures
  - Prolonged hyperbilirubinemia: may be first sign of hypothyroidism and/or hypopituitarism
- Complications during pregnancy or delivery:
  - Birth trauma may be associated with pituitary injury.
  - Breech delivery or vacuum extraction has been associated.
- History of surgeries and previous diseases:
  - Congenital hypopituitarism is often associated with midline facial defects, such as a single central incisor, bifid uvula, or cleft palate, which require repair.
- Growth pattern:
  - Plot previous lengths/heights and look for growth pattern.
  - GH deficiency usually manifests as poor linear growth by the end of the 1st year of life.
- Delayed puberty
  - Children with delayed puberty show further growth failure in adolescence.
  - Sense of smell should be assessed to rule out Kallmann syndrome (isolated central hypogonadism and anosmia).
- Increased thirst and urination: Children with hypothalamic disorders may present with symptoms of DI.
- Complaints of headache and/or a visual defect: can be symptoms of a brain tumor. Focal neurologic symptoms are highly suggestive of CNS pathology.

PHYSICAL EXAM

- Height and weight
  - Patients with panhypopituitarism have normal to small size in the newborn period.
  - May have poor linear growth after 6 to 12 months of life
- Micropenis in male newborns: Neonatal penis should be ≥2.5 cm in length; micropenis suggests gonadotropin and/or GH deficiency.
- Delayed puberty if no breast development by 13 years of age in girls, and no testicular enlargement by 14 years of age in boys.
- May have other anatomic midline defects
- Physical exam pearls:
  - Penile and testicular size: Measure stretched phallic length (from pubic ramus to glans) with patient lying supine and phallus at 90 degrees to the body; use Prader beads to assess testicular volume.
  - Midline defects: Palpate for submucosal cleft palate and look for single central incisor.
  - Visual field testing: Visual field defects suggest a brain tumor.

DIFFERENTIAL DIAGNOSIS

- Hyperinsulinism (HI) in newborns
- Isolated hormone deficiency, such as GH deficiency in newborns
- Constitutional growth delay

DIAGNOSTIC TESTS & INTERPRETATION

Initial Tests (screening, lab, imaging)

- ACTH deficiency: basal serum cortisol: Draw at 8 a.m. in children with a normal diurnal rhythm.
- ACTH deficiency: Cortrosyn stimulation test: more helpful in the diagnosis of primary adrenal insufficiency than secondary (adrenocorticotropic hormone) or tertiary (corticotropin-releasing hormone) deficiency
- ACTH deficiency: metyrapone or corticotropin-releasing hormone stimulation test
  - Tests for ACTH or corticotropin-releasing hormone deficiency
  - Must be performed by a pediatric endocrinologist
- TSH deficiency: liver function tests (LFTs): LFTs in newborns with congenital hypopituitarism are often elevated and accompanied by conjugated hyperbilirubinemia, as opposed to simple congenital hypothyroidism, in which unconjugated hyperbilirubinemia exists.
- TSH deficiency: thyroid function tests: total and free T_4 will be low, but TSH may be low, normal, or elevated.
- GH deficiency: serum insulin-like growth factor-1 (IGF-1) and insulin-like growth factor–binding protein-3 (IGFBP-3): may be low, but normal growth factors do not exclude GH deficiency in children with brain tumors. IGF-1 may be low due to poor nutrition.
- GH stimulation tests: should be performed by a pediatric endocrinologist
- LH/FSH deficiency: estradiol, testosterone, ultrasensitive LH, and FSH: Measure concentrations in first 6 months of life and again after age 11 years; best measured in the morning
- DI: water deprivation test
  - Measurement of water intake and urine output over 24 hours at home can help diagnosis of DI.
  - Definitive test for ADH deficiency (DI)
  - Should be performed by a pediatric endocrinologist
- Overall comments on testing:
  - Baseline serum tests (PRL, 8-a.m. cortisol, T_4, free T_4, IGF-1, IGFBP-3, serum and urine osmolality, testosterone, estradiol, ultrasensitive LH, and FSH) can all be done in a nonfasting state.
  - Stimulation tests must be performed by a pediatric endocrinologist.

- Bone age: typically significantly delayed in GH deficiency and/or hypothyroidism
- MRI with contrast of brain with fine cuts through the hypothalamus and pituitary
  - Look for not only tumors but also size of pituitary, infundibulum, and presence of normal "bright spot" in posterior pituitary.
  - Absence of the "bright spot" is highly associated with central DI of any etiology, although can be present in normal infants.
  - Ectopic pituitary consistent with GH deficiency and other anterior pituitary deficiencies.

ALERT

- If adrenocorticotropic hormone deficient, stress dosing of glucocorticoids is necessary.
- Replacing thyroid hormone in a child with untreated adrenal insufficiency can precipitate adrenal crisis.
- A patient with DI who does not have an intact thirst mechanism and access to free water is at high risk for acute hypernatremia.
- Large volumes of obligate fluids (e.g., IV boluses) in a child receiving DDAVP can precipitate hyponatremia.

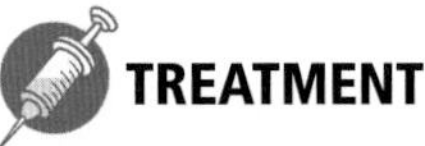

TREATMENT

GENERAL MEASURES

Patients should have clear instructions available to first responders in case of emergency.

MEDICATION

- Hydrocortisone
  - Replacement doses if needed: 8 to 15 mg/m^2/24 h PO, divided b.i.d. or t.i.d.
  - In stress circumstances such as fever, severe illness, vomiting, or surgery, doses increased to 50 to 100 mg/m^2/24 h PO.
  - If dosed IV, provide a loading dose of 50 to 100 mg/m^2 IM or IV followed by 50 to 100 mg/m^2/24 h divided q4h; oral stress doses should be divided q8h.
  - To calculate hydrocortisone dose, estimate body surface area (BSA) using a nomogram or the following formula: BSA (m^2) = square root of (height [cm] × weight [kg] / 3,600).
- Levothyroxine (LT$_4$) PO: 25 to 200 mcg daily, based on weight, age, and free T$_4$ levels
- TSH levels not useful in monitoring therapy for central hypothyroidism, even after treatment is initiated
- Recombinant human GH (rhGH) by SC injection daily: 0.15 to 0.3 mg/kg/week
- Estrogen/testosterone: started at puberty at low doses and slowly increased over ~2 years to mimic endogenous secretion of sex steroids
  - Infants with micropenis may be given monthly testosterone for 3 doses to aid penile enlargement.
- Estrogen given as topical or oral forms to girls, whereas testosterone initially given as injection to boys every month
- Desmopressin acetate (DDAVP®): available in oral and intranasal formulations. Rarely given subcutaneously. Dose is variable. Increasing dose increases duration of action.
  - Acute hypernatremia may be managed with DDAVP®, IV vasopressin, or fluids alone.
  - Some infants with DI can be managed initially with thiazide diuretics.
- Duration: long-term therapy: monitored by a pediatric endocrinologist
  - Hydrocortisone: replacement dose based on individual's need; stress dose coverage for life
  - LT$_4$ for life
  - rhGH: in children and adolescents: until growth velocity drops to 2.5 cm/year; puberty is complete.
  - GH-deficient adults may benefit from lifelong rhGH because of the GH impact on body composition, lipid profile, and cardiac function.
  - Patient may require repeat GH provocative testing off rhGH therapy to determine if adult treatment is necessary.
  - Sex steroids: Begin around age 12 years; may be continued for lifetime
  - DDAVP®: for life, as needed to control symptoms of polyuria/polydipsia

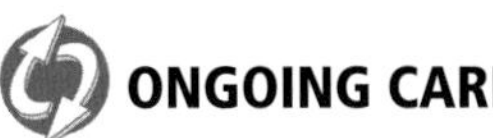

ONGOING CARE

FOLLOW-UP RECOMMENDATIONS

- Initially, every 3 months by a pediatric endocrinologist
- When pituitary hormones are replaced, expect the following:
  - ACTH deficiency: hydrocortisone (daily and stress-dose) steroids are adjusted according to symptoms, growth
  - T$_4$ levels should normalize within 4 to 6 weeks, LT$_4$ is adjusted accordingly.
  - GH: immediate resolution of hypoglycemia and improved growth velocity within 3 to 6 months
  - Possible side effects of GH therapy: headache, vision problems, pseudotumor cerebri syndrome, hyperglycemia, changes in activity level, limp, knee or hip pain
  - Children with DI with intact thirst, typically have one or two "breakthroughs" (diureses) per day and drink to thirst.

PROGNOSIS

- For congenital forms, the prognosis is excellent with endocrine replacement.
- DI in infants can be challenging to manage because infants get nutrition from fluids.
- For secondary forms, the overall prognosis depends on the primary disease.

COMPLICATIONS

- Hypoglycemia in the newborn period
- Adrenal crisis
- Short stature
- Dehydration/hypernatremia
- Evolving understanding of risk for cardiometabolic disease and osteoporosis

ALERT

- Diagnosis of panhypopituitarism must be considered in patients with hypoglycemic seizures.
- TSH levels are generally not helpful when evaluating pituitary/hypothalamic causes of hypothyroidism. The unbound free T$_4$ level (by equilibrium dialysis) is the most useful test both to establish the diagnosis and to monitor L-thyroxine replacement therapy.
- 20% of normal children will fail a single GH provocative test.
- rhGH therapy can be associated with idiopathic intracranial hypertension (pseudotumor cerebri).
- rhGH deficiency/therapy can also be associated with slipped capital femoral epiphysis (SCFE). Carefully evaluate any limp or knee or hip pain in patients on rhGH therapy. SCFE mandates orthopedic consultation.
- The family and the patient must understand the importance of taking stress doses of steroid appropriately (e.g., with surgery, vomiting, or febrile illnesses).

ADDITIONAL READING

- Ascoli P, Cavagnini F. Hypopituitarism. *Pituitary*. 2006;9(4):335–342.
- Di Iorgi N, Napoli F, Allegri AE, et al. Diabetes insipidus—diagnosis and management. *Horm Res Paediatr*. 2012;77(2):69–84.
- Fleseriu M, Hashim IA, Karavitaki N, et al. Hormonal replacement in hypopituitarism in adults: an Endocrine Society Clinical Practice Guideline. *J Clin Endocrinol Metab*. 2016;101(11):3888–3921.
- Grimberg A, DiVall SA, Polychronakos C, et al; for Drug and Therapeutics Committee and Ethics Committee of the Pediatric Endocrine Society. Guidelines for growth hormone and insulin-like growth factor-1 treatment in children and adolescents: growth hormone deficiency, idiopathic short stature, and primary insulin-like growth factor-1 deficiency. *Horm Res Paediatr*. 2016;86(6):361–397.
- Grossman AB. Clinical review: the diagnosis and management of central hypoadrenalism. *J Clin Endocrinol Metab*. 2010;95(11):4855–4863.
- Mostoufi-Moab S, Seidel K, Leisenring WM, et al. Endocrine abnormalities in aging survivors of childhood cancer: a report from the childhood cancer survivor group. *J Clin Oncol*. 2016;34(27):3240–3247.

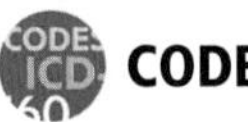

CODES

ICD10

E23.0 Hypopituitarism

FAQ

- Q: When do I give stress doses of steroid and for how long?
- A: Whenever the patient has fever, vomiting, serious illness, or surgery. Continue until 24 hours after stress resolves (e.g., the day after fever breaks or vomiting stops).
- Q: Is it acceptable to replace thyroid hormone while the evaluation of other pituitary hormones is pending?
- A: You must ensure the patient is adrenally sufficient; if not, glucocorticoids must be initiated prior to thyroid hormone replacement.
- Q: Do all state newborn screens detect central hypothyroidism?
- A: No. Many states initially screen only for elevated TSH levels. TSH is often not elevated in central hypothyroidism.

HYPOPLASTIC LEFT HEART SYNDROME

Laura Mercer-Rosa, MD, MSCE • Jie Tang, MD, MS

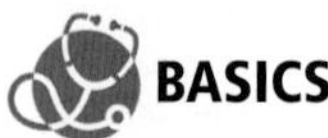

BASICS

DESCRIPTION

Hypoplastic left heart syndrome (HLHS) is a continuum of congenital cardiac defects resulting from severe underdevelopment of the structures of the left side of the heart (left atrium, mitral valve, left ventricle, aortic valve, and ascending aorta).

EPIDEMIOLOGY

- 0.16 to 0.36 per 1,000 live births
- 8% of congenital heart disease (CHD); 3rd most common cause of critical CHD in the newborn
- 23% of all neonatal mortality from CHD
- Male predominance (67%)

RISK FACTORS

Genetics

Familial inheritance: Sibling recurrence risk ranges from 8% to 21%, with higher recurrence observed when cardiovascular malformations are present in either parent. In addition, rare kinships have a frequency approaching autosomal dominant transmission.

COMMONLY ASSOCIATED CONDITIONS

- Increased mortality when associated with definable genetic disorders, which comprise 10–28% of HLHS patients:
  - Turner syndrome, Noonan syndrome, Smith-Lemli-Opitz syndrome, Holt-Oram syndrome
  - Trisomy 13, 18, 21, or microdeletion syndromes
- Major extracardiac anomalies (diaphragmatic hernia, omphalocele)

PATHOPHYSIOLOGY

- The etiology appears multifactorial, most likely resulting from an in utero reduction of left ventricular inflow or outflow (mechanisms postulated include premature closure of the foramen ovale and fetal cardiomyopathy).
- As a result, the right ventricle (RV) must supply both the pulmonary and systemic circulations (via the ductus arteriosus) before and after birth.
- The reduction in pulmonary vascular resistance that occurs with lung expansion at birth reduces the proportion of RV output to the systemic circulation. If the ductus arteriosus closes, shock occurs.

DIAGNOSIS

HISTORY

- In the current era, HLHS is often diagnosed prenatally.
- Postnatal signs and symptoms:
  - Respiratory distress (tachypnea, grunting, flaring, retractions)
  - Cyanosis
  - Cardiovascular collapse and profound metabolic acidosis when the ductus arteriosus closes

PHYSICAL EXAM

- Congestive heart failure (CHF) secondary to pulmonary overcirculation (e.g., tachycardia, hepatomegaly, gallop)
- Normal S_1 and single S_2 (A_2 absent); a murmur of tricuspid regurgitation may be auscultated.
- Varying degrees of cyanosis
- Decreased perfusion and weak peripheral pulses

DIFFERENTIAL DIAGNOSIS

- Cardiac: Other causes of circulatory collapse in the neonate include critical aortic stenosis and coarctation of the aorta, cardiomyopathy (infectious, metabolic, or hypoxic), persistent supraventricular tachycardia, obstructive cardiac neoplasms, and large arteriovenous fistulae.
- Noncardiac: neonatal septicemia, respiratory distress syndrome, inborn errors of metabolism

DIAGNOSTIC TESTS & INTERPRETATION

- Chest radiograph:
  - Varying degrees of cardiomegaly with increased pulmonary vascular markings
  - If the atrial septum is intact or highly restrictive, lungs will appear hazy with a pulmonary venous obstructive pattern.
- Electrocardiogram:
  - Right axis deviation (+90 to +210 degrees)
  - RV hypertrophy with a qR pattern in the right precordial leads, decreased left ventricular forces with an rS pattern in the left precordial leads
- Echocardiogram:
  - Varying degrees of hypoplasia or atresia of the mitral valve, left ventricle, aortic valve, ascending aorta, and aortic arch; patent ductus arteriosus with right-to-left shunt in systole and diastolic flow reversal
  - Retrograde flow in the ascending and transverse aorta; atrial septal defect with left-to-right flow
- Cardiac catheterization:
  - No longer routinely performed
  - Similar findings as with echocardiography

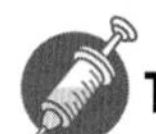

TREATMENT

- Initial stabilization
  - During initial resuscitation and stabilization of a newly diagnosed infant:
    - Prostaglandin E_1 therapy should be initiated as soon as possible to maintain ductal patency.
    - Avoid using oxygen despite low pulse oximetry saturation. Increasing FiO_2 will lower pulmonary vascular resistance, preferentially shunting cardiac output away from the systemic circulation toward the lungs, thereby worsening systemic perfusion.
    - Should invasive ventilation be required, avoid hyperventilation.
      - Permissive hypercapnea is preferred due to the secondary increase in pulmonary vascular resistance and subsequent improvement in systemic perfusion.
      - Maintain mildly elevated $Paco_2$ levels (40 to 50 mm Hg).
- Supportive care
  - Although surgical intervention has become the medical standard, supportive measures can be considered an alternative, especially when multiple noncardiac congenital anomalies exist or when severe multiorgan system damage is present.
  - The preoperative goal is to balance the systemic and pulmonary circulations provided by the RV to a Qp/Qs (ratio of pulmonary to systemic blood flow) of ~1:1, usually achieved with a pulse oximetry measurement of 75%.
  - Alprostadil (prostaglandin E_1) IV infusion: 0.025 to 0.1 mcg/kg/min
  - Aggressive treatment of hypocalcemia with calcium boluses, avoidance of metabolic acidosis with fluid boluses, consider sodium bicarbonate
  - 21% FiO_2, goal Pao_2 of 35 to 40 mm Hg
  - Careful use of small amounts of inotropic agents in cases of sepsis or RV failure. Aggressive use of inotropic agents (alpha effect) may worsen systemic perfusion.

SURGERY/OTHER PROCEDURES

- Palliative surgery is generally performed in three stages:
  - Stage I Norwood palliation (performed in the first few days of life or soon after presentation):
    - Transection of the main pulmonary artery with anastomosis of the augmented aortic arch to the pulmonary valve stump to form a neoaortic valve and arch, placement of an aorta-to-pulmonary artery shunt (modified Blalock-Taussig shunt), and often an atrial septectomy.
    - The RV provides both systemic and pulmonary blood flows with postoperative saturations of ~75%.
  - Stage I Sano modification:
    - Developed in 2003 as an alternative to the Norwood procedure
    - The Sano modification replaces the modified Blalock-Taussig shunt with an RV to pulmonary artery conduit, with the RV continuing to supply both pulmonary and systemic circulations.
  - Hybrid procedure:
    - An additional alternative to the Norwood procedure that combines surgical and catheter-based interventions while avoiding cardiopulmonary bypass.
    - Through cardiac catheterization, the ductus arteriosus is stented to allow the RV to continue to supply the systemic circulation.
    - Bilateral pulmonary artery bands are placed via median sternotomy to protect the pulmonary vascular bed from overcirculation.
  - Stage II/Hemi-Fontan or bidirectional Glenn procedure:
    - Involves anastomosis of the superior vena cava to the pulmonary artery, resulting in volume unloading of the RV
    - All prior shunts are usually removed.
    - The oxygen saturations after this procedure are usually 80–90%.
  - Stage III/modified Fontan procedure:
    - The inferior vena cava is baffled to the pulmonary artery with placement of a small fenestration in the baffle, permitting a small residual right-to-left shunt.
    - The RV is now supplying only systemic blood flow.
    - The oxygen saturations after this procedure are usually 85–95%.
- There are many surgical modifications to these three procedures. In addition, these procedures may be performed at different ages based on an institution's experience. Our approach has been to perform the stage II operation at 4 to 6 months of age and the Fontan operation at 18 months to 2 years of age.
- Orthotopic heart transplantation may be performed either as an initial approach or after a stage I palliation.

ONGOING CARE

FOLLOW-UP RECOMMENDATIONS

The admission for the first operation usually lasts for about 3 to 4 weeks after birth. Patients are watched to ensure stable oxygen saturation and weight gain. Nutritional needs often require nasogastric tube or gastrostomy tube feed supplementation.

Patient Monitoring

Interval evaluations should include careful consideration of growth parameters, cardiovascular symptoms, and developmental milestones. Examinations should focus on the presence or absence of cyanosis, edema, pleural effusions, diarrhea, ascites, and arrhythmias.

- For patients after staged palliation, frequent echocardiograms and intermittent cardiac catheterizations may be needed to assess for the following:
  - RV dysfunction
  - Residual or recurrent aortic arch obstruction
  - Branch pulmonary artery narrowing
  - Venous collateral formation causing increased right-to-left shunting and cyanosis
  - Protein-losing enteropathy
  - Sinus node dysfunction
  - Atrial arrhythmias
- For patients treated alternatively with heart transplantation, other lifelong issues should be addressed:
  - Graft rejection and/or coronary vasculopathy
  - Infection
  - Hypertension
  - Lymphoproliferative disease
- Follow-up medications:
  - Lifelong subacute bacterial endocarditis (SBE) prophylaxis
  - Diuretics such as furosemide are generally administered until the stage II procedure.
  - Afterload reduction (i.e., angiotensin-converting enzyme inhibitors) may be used to reduce the workload on the heart at any stage.
  - Antiplatelet (aspirin) and anticoagulant (warfarin) therapies are used by most physicians after stage 1, and later to prevent thrombosis in the setting of the low-flow state of the cavopulmonary connection.
- For transplant patients, immunosuppressive regimens are managed differently according to institution preferences.

PROGNOSIS

- Fatal if untreated (95% mortality within the 1st month of life)
- Improved outcomes may result from early diagnosis and prevention of the presentation as neonatal shock.
- 90% early survival after stage I palliation if treated in a timely fashion at experienced institutions. Some institutions have reported that addition of a home monitoring program (daily surveillance of weight and saturations by parents, with support from a local cardiologist and monitoring team) between the stage I and stage II operations has reduced mortality during this period to as low as 0–3%.
- 5% mortality at stage II hemi-Fontan or bidirectional Glenn procedure
- Recently, 1% mortality at Fontan operation (with the addition of a fenestration to allow right-to-left shunting)
- Excluding infants who die waiting for a donor organ, the 5-year actuarial survival for either staged palliation (Fontan) or heart transplantation is similar, ~75%.

COMPLICATIONS

At time of neonatal presentation:

- Circulatory collapse with resultant metabolic acidosis
- Multiorgan system failure (i.e., necrotizing enterocolitis, renal failure, liver failure, brain injury)

ADDITIONAL READING

- Alsoufi B, Bennetts J, Verma S, et al. New developments in the treatment of hypoplastic left heart syndrome. *Pediatrics*. 2007;119(1):109–117.
- Grossfeld P. Hypoplastic left heart syndrome: new insights. *Circ Res*. 2007;100(9):1246–1248.
- Mahle WT, Clancy RR, McGaurn SP, et al. Impact of prenatal diagnosis on survival and early neurologic morbidity in neonates with the hypoplastic left heart syndrome. *Pediatrics*. 2001;107(6):1277–1282.
- McClure CD, Johnston JK, Fitts JA, et al. Postmortem intracranial neuropathology in children following cardiac transplantation. *Pediatr Neurol*. 2006;35(2):107–113.
- Pigula FA, Vida V, Del Nido P, et al. Contemporary results and current strategies in the management of hypoplastic left heart syndrome. *Semin Thorac Cardiovasc Surg*. 2007;19(3):238–244.
- Stamm C, Friehs I, Mayer JE Jr, et al. Long-term results of the lateral tunnel Fontan operation. *J Thorac Cardiovasc Surg*. 2001;121(1):28–41.
- Tabbutt S, Dominguez TE, Ravishankar C, et al. Outcomes after the stage I reconstruction comparing the right ventricular to pulmonary artery conduit with the modified Blalock Taussig shunt. *Ann Thorac Surg*. 2005;80(5):1582–1591.
- Tworetzky W, McElhinney DB, Reddy VM, et al. Improved surgical outcome after fetal diagnosis of hypoplastic left heart syndrome. *Circulation*. 2001;103(9):1269–1273.
- Wernovsky G, Ghanayem N, Ohye RG, et al. Hypoplastic left heart syndrome: consensus and controversies in 2007. *Cardiol Young*. 2007;17(Suppl 2):75–86.

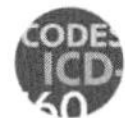

CODES

ICD10

- Q24.8 Other specified congenital malformations of heart
- Q96.9 Turner's syndrome, unspecified
- Q87.1 Congenital malform syndromes predom assoc w short stature

FAQ

- Q: What is the significance of an intact or restrictive atrial septum during the initial stabilization of a neonate with HLHS?
- A: In HLHS patients, restriction to left-to-right flow across the atrial septum causes pulmonary venous congestion as well as hypoxia due to inadequate delivery of oxygenated blood to the systemic circulation. These patients may require urgent balloon atrial septostomy shortly after birth.
- Q: What should the differential diagnosis include when an infant with HLHS who has undergone stage I palliation presents with cyanosis and respiratory distress?
- A: Modified Blalock-Taussig shunt thrombosis, anemia, intercurrent lower respiratory tract infection leading to V/Q mismatch, low cardiac output state, sepsis. Of note, infants with HLHS status after stage I palliation are solely dependent on the modified Blalock-Taussig shunt for pulmonary blood flow. This synthetic tube graft ranges from 3.5 to 4 mm in diameter and is prone to thrombosis, especially during periods of illness, which lead to dehydration (gastroenteritis), poor nutrition, or systemic inflammation.
- Q: After the stage II or stage III procedures, what are some particular diagnoses to consider in a patient who presents with respiratory symptoms such as cough, hemoptysis, cyanosis, and infiltrates on chest radiograph?
- A: After stage II, patients are prone to the formation of pulmonary arteriovenous malformations (AVMs), which may at a later time cause hemoptysis if they rupture or erode into the airways. Another diagnosis to consider is plastic bronchitis, which results from high venous pressures and disturbance to lymphatic drainage as a result of the cavopulmonary anastomosis. In this condition, lymphatic fluid leaks into the airways and solidifies into rubbery casts, which then cause significant airway obstruction. Immediate management is with therapies that promote expectoration of the casts, including bronchodilators, mucolytics, chest wall oscillation, and bronchoscopy.
- Q: Should there be a specific concern if a patient with HLHS who has completed the 3-stage palliation with Fontan procedure presents with complaints of unremitting diarrhea, crampy abdominal pain, ascites, and peripheral edema?
- A: Yes. Protein-losing enteropathy (PLE) is a poorly understood disease process affecting patients with single ventricle physiology after Fontan operation, and is associated with significant morbidity and mortality. PLE is defined as the abnormal loss of serum proteins into the lumen of the gastrointestinal tract and occurs in up to 11% of patients after Fontan palliation. Diuretic therapy and nutritional supplementation are often insufficient management strategies, often requiring the addition of somatostatic analogs (octreotide), sildenafil, and/or the creation of a fenestration in the Fontan circuit to palliate potentially elevated Fontan pressures.

HYPOSPADIAS

Ming-Hsien Wang, MD, FAAP

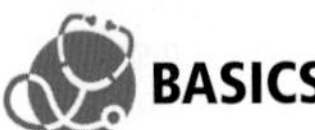

BASICS

DESCRIPTION

Hypospadias is one of the most common congenital anomalies of the male external genitalia. It is characterized by a urethral meatus that opens proximally on the ventral surface of the penis, scrotum, or the perineum. Classification is based on the position of the meatus relative to the penile shaft or surrounding structures (distal, middle, proximal). Although the ventral foreskin is incomplete in the vast majority of cases, the megameatus variant is characterized by an intact foreskin.

EPIDEMIOLOGY

- 1/200 to 1/300 live male births
- Concordance rates among twins: 18–77%
- Megameatus variant: 5% of cases
- Incidence is likely not increasing over time. Although there have been some data suggesting an increasing incidence over time, the majority of published studies in the U.S. population indicate a stable incidence.

RISK FACTORS

- In vitro fertilization
- Maternal exposures to substances such as pesticides, hormones, phthalates, and phytoestrogens that can act as endocrine disruptors during penile development
- Associated with maternal preexisting diabetes mellitus, placental insufficiency, and low birth weight
- More common among Caucasians

Genetics

- Likely polygenic
- Familial clustering: 7% of affected boys have an affected 1st- or 2nd-degree relative.
- Equally maternally and paternally transmitted
- Associated with genetic mutations in several genes involved in the androgen pathway and external genitalia development, including homeobox, fibroblast growth factor, and sonic hedgehog genes

ETIOLOGY

- Due to incomplete fusion of the urethral folds during penile development, which is an androgen-driven process that occurs during weeks 8 to 16 of gestation
- Likely multifactorial with environmental and genetic interplay
- Defects in urethral development are usually accompanied by foreskin developmental defects (an incomplete ventral foreskin and dorsal hooded foreskin), except in the megameatus variant

COMMONLY ASSOCIATED CONDITIONS

- Usually idiopathic and isolated
- Less commonly associated with certain chromosomal abnormalities and ~200 syndromes, including disorders of sexual differentiation (DSD)
- Hypospadias, particularly proximal hypospadias, can be associated with an increased risk of other genitourinary (GU) malformations.
- The most commonly associated GU malformations include the following:
  - Chordee
  - Cryptorchidism
  - Inguinal hernia

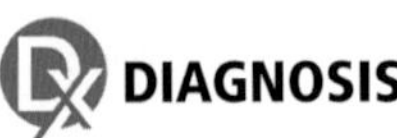

DIAGNOSIS

HISTORY

Important to inquire about the following:

- Family history of hypospadias, congenital anomalies, or genetic disorders
- Patient history of genetic disorder and/or DSD
- GU symptoms
- Maternal history of fertility treatments
- Maternal exposures during pregnancy
- Birth history
- For older patients
  - Painful erections
  - Infertility or difficulties with intercourse
  - Difficulty urinating while standing
  - Deflected urinary stream
  - Urinary tract infections

PHYSICAL EXAM

Assess for hypospadias in all male newborns with complete GU exam, paying particular attention to the following:

- Any sign of incompletely formed foreskin or dorsal hooded foreskin
- Any phallus curvature
- Location of the meatus
- Presence of rugated scrotum
- Location of the testes

DIFFERENTIAL DIAGNOSIS

DSD such as congenital adrenal hyperplasia or partial androgen insensitivity syndrome

DIAGNOSTIC TESTS & INTERPRETATION

- No tests are needed for isolated hypospadias.
- If testes are not palpable bilaterally with proximal hypospadias, consider workup for DSD.
- Additional workup for DSD as needed based on level of concern
- Imaging not usually indicated
- If there is a question of DSD, consider genetic, urology consult, and possible genitogram with pelvic ultrasound.

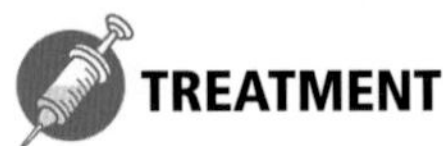

TREATMENT

GENERAL MEASURES

- Preferably refer to pediatric urologist within the first few weeks of life.
- Preoperative stimulation with parenteral testosterone may be required for severe hypospadias.
- Cases of mild, distal hypospadias may be observed.

ALERT
- For newborn circumcision, retract the foreskin (megameatus variant requires foreskin retraction for detection). If any abnormalities noted, abort the circumcision and refer to a pediatric urologist.
- In cases of hypospadias, circumcision is absolutely contraindicated because foreskin is used in hypospadias repair.
- Bilateral impalpable testes and hypospadias during newborn period must be worked-up to rule out DSD.

SURGERY/OTHER PROCEDURES
- Surgical repair
  - Outpatient procedure
  - May be accompanied by chordee repair if needed
  - Performed at age 6 months to 1 year pending on anesthesia concerns
  - Complex cases may require staged repair.
  - Perioperative care may include the following:
    - Antibiotics (no standard course duration)
    - Pain management (generally with a caudal nerve block)
  - Type of repair performed is based on patient's anatomy and surgeon preference.
  - May involve temporary urethral stent placement
- Types of repair include the following:
  - Urethromeatoplasty
  - Meatal advancement and glanuloplasty (MAGPI)
  - Adjacent tissue transfer
  - Glans approximation procedure
  - Thiersch-Duplay
  - Transverse incised plate or Snodgrass procedure
- Most common complications include the following:
  - Urethrocutaneous fistula
  - Urethral diverticulum
  - Urethral or meatal stenosis with associated obstructive symptoms, UTIs
  - Dehiscence

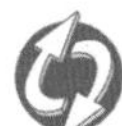

ONGOING CARE

FOLLOW-UP RECOMMENDATIONS

Patient Monitoring
- Surgical dressings are variable and surgeon dependent.
- Postoperative clinic visit (surgeon dependent)
- If urethral stent is placed, removal usually occurs on postoperative days 7 to 10 at clinic visit.
- Antibiotics may be continued postoperatively.

PROGNOSIS
Success rate is generally high, although dependent on the type of repair, degree of hypospadias, and patient's overall medical condition.

ADDITIONAL READING

- Ewalt D. *Pediatric Hypospadias Repair: A New Consensus Document on Coding*. Linthicum, MD: American Urological Association; 2015.
- Kalfa N, Liu B, Klein O, et al. Genomic variants of ATF3 in patients with hypospadias. *J Urol*. 2008;180(5):2183–2188.
- Kalfa N, Liu B, Klein O, et al. Mutations of CXorf6 are associated with a range of severities of hypospadias. *Eur J Endocrinol*. 2008;159(4):453–458.
- Kalfa N, Philibert P, Baskin LS, et al. Hypospadias: interactions between environment and genetics. *Mol Cell Endocrinol*. 2011;335(2):89–95.
- Madhok N, Scharbach K, Shahid-Saless S. Hypospadias. *Pediatr Rev*. 2009;30(6):235–237.
- Moriyama M, Senga Y, Satomi Y. Klinefelter's syndrome with hypospadias and bilateral cryptorchidism. *Urol Int*. 1988;43(5):313–314.
- van der Zanden LF, van Rooij IA, Feitz WF, et al. Aetiology of hypospadias: a systematic review of genes and environment. *Hum Reprod Update*. 2012;18(3):260–283.
- Wang MH, Baskin LS. Endocrine disruptors, genital development, and hypospadias. *J Androl*. 2008;29(5):499–505.
- White PC, Speiser PW. Congenital adrenal hyperplasia due to 21-hydroxylase deficiency. *Endocr Rev*. 2000;21(3):245–291.
- Zaontz M, Long CJ. Management of distal hypospadias. *AUA Update Series*. 2013;32(Lesson 5):1–51.

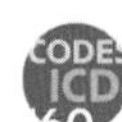

CODES

ICD10
- Q54.9 Hypospadias, unspecified
- Q54.1 Hypospadias, penile
- Q54.3 Hypospadias, perineal

FAQ
- Q: Does the patient with hypospadias routinely have other urinary tract abnormalities?
- A: No. Hypospadias is usually an isolated anomaly, and most patients have no other anatomic problems.
- Q: Should a newborn circumcision be performed if there are concerns with the meatal opening?
- A: Circumcision should be delayed, and the patient should be evaluated by a pediatric urologist.
- Q: Are there any medical alternatives to surgical repair?
- A: No. Surgery is the only treatment of hypospadias, but very mild cases may not warrant surgical repair.

HYPOTHYROIDISM, ACQUIRED

Adda Grimberg, MD

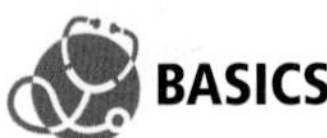

BASICS

DESCRIPTION

Hypothyroidism that occurs after the neonatal period

EPIDEMIOLOGY

- May develop at any age
- Autoimmune thyroid disorders occur more frequently in children and adolescents with type 1 diabetes and other autoimmune conditions.
- Chronic lymphocytic thyroiditis prevalence correlates with iodine intake; countries with the highest dietary iodine also have the highest prevalence.
- Subclinical hypothyroidism (TSH concentration between the upper limit of normal reference range and 10 mIU/L, with normal free thyroxine level) found in 7–23% of obese children and 0.3–2% of normal weight controls. It seems to be a consequence rather than cause of the obesity and can normalize with weight loss.

RISK FACTORS

Genetics

- Family history of thyroid disease or other autoimmune endocrinopathies increases risk.
- Genetic predisposition in patients with chronic lymphocytic thyroiditis; 30–40% of patients have a family history of thyroid disease, and up to 50% of their 1st-degree relatives have thyroid antibodies.
- Weak associations of chronic lymphocytic thyroiditis with certain human leukocyte antigen haplotypes; also associated with genotypes of cytotoxic T lymphocyte–associated 4 (*CTLA4*) and interleukin-18 (*IL-18*) genes.
- Autoimmune thyroid disease may be part of type II autoimmune polyglandular syndrome (Schmidt disease).
- Genetic syndromes associated with higher incidence of autoimmune thyroiditis:
  - Down syndrome
  - Turner syndrome (especially those with isochromosome Xq)

ETIOLOGY

- Myriad causes (see "Differential Diagnosis")
- Can result from thyroid gland dysfunction (primary hypothyroidism) or from pituitary/hypothalamic dysfunction leading to understimulation of the thyroid gland (secondary and tertiary hypothyroidism)

COMMONLY ASSOCIATED CONDITIONS

- Type 1 diabetes
- Other autoimmune conditions
- Pernicious anemia
- Vitiligo
- Alopecia areata
- Obesity

DIAGNOSIS

HISTORY

- Linear growth failure can be the first sign of thyroid dysfunction.
- Declining school performance is a sensitive marker for lethargy and reduced focus.
- Radiation exposure, history of type 1 diabetes, family history of other autoimmune disorders
- Signs and symptoms:
  - Early primary hypothyroidism can be asymptomatic.
  - Hypothyroid-related symptoms indicate progression from compensated to uncompensated hypothyroidism.
  - Hypothyroidism may be preceded in some cases by temporary hyperthyroidism (Hashitoxicosis).
  - Goiter may be the presenting sign of acquired hypothyroidism; tenderness suggests an infectious process.

PHYSICAL EXAM

- Bradycardia: Thyroid hormone has cardiac effects.
- Short stature (or fall-off on growth curve) and increased upper/lower segment ratio: Euthyroidism is required to maintain normal growth.
- Goiter: Note consistency, symmetry, nodularity, signs of inflammation:
  - May give a clue regarding cause of hypothyroidism
  - May provide a clinical marker to follow during therapy
- Myxedema (water retention) is not limited to subcutaneous tissue; it may also lead to cardiac failure, pleural effusions, and coma.
- Muscle hypertrophy, yet muscle weakness
  - Most obvious in arms, legs, and tongue
  - Hypothyroidism causes disordered muscle function.
- Delayed relaxation phase of deep tendon reflexes due to slowed muscle contraction
- Pale, cool, dry, carotenemic (yellow-colored) skin due to decreased cell turnover
- Increase in lanugo hair in children; can be reversed with treatment
- Sexual development is an important factor; hypothyroidism may be associated with either
  - Delayed puberty (due to low thyroid hormone levels)
  - Precocious puberty and galactorrhea (due to elevated TSH)

DIFFERENTIAL DIAGNOSIS

- Immunologic
  - Chronic lymphocytic thyroiditis (Hashimoto thyroiditis)
  - Autoimmune polyglandular syndrome type II (Schmidt syndrome)
- Infectious
  - Postviral subacute thyroiditis
  - Associated with congenital infections
    - Rubella
    - Toxoplasmosis
- Environmental
  - Goitrogen ingestion
    - Iodides
    - Expectorants
    - Thioureas
  - Exposure to polybrominated diphenyl ethers (PBDEs; flame retardants) was associated with an increased prevalence of hypothyroidism in Canadian women.
  - Low selenium intake
- Iatrogenic
  - Following surgical thyroidectomy for thyroid cancer, hyperthyroidism, or extensive neck tumors
  - Following radioiodine ablative therapy for hyperthyroidism or thyroid cancer
  - Following head or neck irradiation for cancer treatment
  - Medications: lithium, amiodarone, iodine contrast dyes, tiratricol (an over-the-counter fat-loss supplement)
- Metabolic
  - Cystinosis
  - Histiocytosis X
- Congenital
  - Late-onset congenital, large ectopic gland
- Genetic syndromes
  - Down syndrome
  - Turner syndrome
- Secondary or tertiary hypothyroidism
  - Hypothalamic or pituitary disease
- Consumptive hypothyroidism
  - Due to increased type 3 iodothyronine deiodinase activity in hemangiomas

DIAGNOSTIC TESTS & INTERPRETATION

Initial Tests (screening, lab, imaging)

- T_4 (low) and TSH (elevated): Elevated TSH with normal T_4 indicates compensated (subclinical) primary hypothyroidism.
- Free T_4: the most sensitive marker for secondary/tertiary hypothyroidism (TSH elevation lost; total T_4 may still be low normal)
- Thyroglobulin antibodies and thyroid peroxidase (microsomal) antibodies are markers for chronic lymphocytic thyroiditis.
- The following conditions may test false-positive for acquired hypothyroidism:
  - Thyroid-binding globulin deficiency: low total T_4 but normal free T_4 and TSH
  - Peripheral resistance to thyroid hormone: normal/high total T_4
  - "Euthyroid sick" syndrome: low T_4 and T_3; normal/low TSH; increased shunting to reverse T_3
- The following tests may be affected in acquired hypothyroidism:
  - Serum creatinine: elevated due to reduced glomerular filtration rate
  - LDL cholesterol level: elevated due to decreased LDL receptor expression
  - Creatine kinase: increased; hypothyroidism is a rare cause of rhabdomyolysis.
- Head MRI for cases of suspected secondary/tertiary hypothyroidism or pituitary or hypothalamic lesion

TREATMENT

GENERAL MEASURES

Weight loss may normalize subclinical hypothyroidism seen in obese children.

MEDICATION

L-Thyroxine (synthetic thyroid hormone) replacement

- Indicated for the treatment of overt or compensated hypothyroidism
- 10 to 15 mcg/kg PO once daily
- Monitor T_4 and TSH and titrate dose to maintain normalized thyroid function tests.
- Duration of therapy:
  - Lifetime
  - In 30% of the cases, children with chronic lymphocytic thyroiditis will undergo spontaneous remission.
  - Need for treatment can be reassessed after growth is completed.

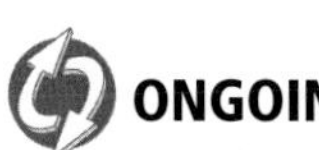

ONGOING CARE

FOLLOW-UP RECOMMENDATIONS

Patient Monitoring

- Whenever starting medication or adjusting dose, check T_4 and TSH at 4- to 6-week intervals to assess adequacy of the new dose; need to wait this long to reach equilibrium given to long half-life of T_4 (5 to 7 days)
- Once dose established, 6 monthly monitoring until linear growth completed; annually thereafter
- Monitor response to treatment by measuring T_4 and TSH levels to assess adequacy of therapy and compliance.

PATIENT EDUCATION

- Pharmacies in recent years have been recommending that L-thyroxine be administered on an empty stomach.
- The Drugs and Therapeutics Committee of the Pediatric Endocrine Society recommended that consistency in administration, coupled with regular dose titration based on thyroid function laboratory tests, is more important than improving absorption by restricting intake to only times of empty stomach.

PROGNOSIS

- If patients are adherent, prognosis is excellent.
- Adherence to L-thyroxine is lower in pubertal than prepubertal children and in children self-administering their medication than those administered by their parents.
- Treated patients often resume growth at a rate greater than normal (catch-up growth).
- In children in whom treatment has been delayed, catch-up growth may not fully normalize height to predicted values.
- Other signs and symptoms resolve at a variable rate.
- Goiters in chronic lymphocytic thyroiditis may not completely regress with treatment (enlargement due to persistent inflammation does not correct, although TSH-mediated hypertrophy will).

COMPLICATIONS

- Most significant complication is impaired linear growth.
- Puberty can also be affected.
- Myxedema coma may occur.
- Encephalopathy of varied clinical presentation has been associated with high titers of thyroid antibodies, especially antimicrosomal; this condition responds well to corticosteroid treatment.

ADDITIONAL READING

- Ban Y, Tomer Y. Genetic susceptibility in thyroid autoimmunity. *Pediatr Endocrinol Rev*. 2005;3(1):20–32.
- Child CJ, Blum WF, Deal C, et al. Development of additional pituitary hormone deficiencies in pediatric patients originally diagnosed with isolated growth hormone deficiency due to organic causes. *Eur J Endocrinol*. 2016;174(5):669–679.
- Haugen BR. Drugs that suppress TSH or cause central hypothyroidism. *Best Pract Res Clin Endocrinol Metab*. 2009;23(6):793–800.
- Lollert A, Gies C, Laudemann K, et al. Ultrasound evaluation of thyroid gland pathologies after radiation therapy and chemotherapy to treat malignancy during childhood. *Int J Radiat Oncol Biol Phys*. 2016;94(1):139–146.
- Lu MC, Chang SC, Huang KY, et al. Higher risk of thyroid disorders in young patients with type 1 diabetes: a 12-year nationwide, population-based, retrospective cohort study. *PLoS One*. 2016;11(3):e0152168.
- Monzani A, Prodam F, Rapa A, et al. Endocrine disorders in childhood and adolescence. Natural history of subclinical hypothyroidism in children and adolescents and potential effects of replacement therapy: a review. *Eur J Endocrinol*. 2012;168(1):R1–R11.
- Nandi-Munshi D, Taplin CE. Thyroid-related neurological disorders and complications in children. *Pediatr Neurol*. 2015;52(4):373–382.
- Nebesio TD, Wise MD, Perkins SM, et al. Does clinical management impact height potential in children with severe acquired hypothyroidism? *J Pediatr Endocrinol Metab*. 2011;24(11–12):893–896.
- Niranjan U, Wright NP. Should we treat subclinical hypothyroidism in obese children? *BMJ*. 2016;352:i941.
- Radetti G, Maselli M, Buzi F, et al. The natural history of the normal/mild elevated TSH serum levels in children and adolescents with Hashimoto's thyroiditis and isolated hyperthyrotropinaemia: a 3-year follow-up. *Clin Endocrinol (Oxf)*. 2012;76(3):394–398.
- Stathatos N, Wartofsky L. Perioperative management of patients with hypothyroidism. *Endocrinol Metab Clin North Am*. 2003;32(2):503–518.
- Zeitler P, Solberg P; for Pharmacy and Therapeutics Committee of the Lawson Wilkins Pediatric Endocrine Society. Food and levothyroxine administration in infants and children. *J Pediatr*. 2010;157(1):13.e1–14.e1.
- Zirilli G, Velletri MR, Porcaro F, et al. In children with Hashimoto's thyroiditis the evolution over time of thyroid status may differ according to the different presentation patterns. *Acta Biomed*. 2015;86(2):137–141.

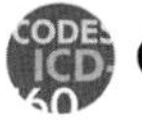

CODES

ICD10

- E03.9 Hypothyroidism, unspecified
- E03.8 Other specified hypothyroidism
- E06.3 Autoimmune thyroiditis

FAQ

- Q: What happens if my child forgets a dose?
- A: Give the dose as soon as you remember. If it is the next day, give 2 doses.
- Q: How long will my child have to take these pills?
- A: Probably for life.
- Q: Are there any side effects from the medication?
- A: No. The medication contains only the hormone that your child's thyroid gland is not making. The hormone is made synthetically, so there is also no infectious risk.
- Q: If my child takes twice the dose, will his or her growth catch up faster?
- A: Your child may grow a little faster but will also have adverse effects from having too much thyroid hormone.
- Q: Does the medication have to be taken at any particular time of day?
- A: No, but consistently choosing the same time of day helps to remember to take it. Do not take simultaneously with soy products, iron-containing medication, calcium supplements, or raloxifene (an antiestrogen medication) because they can cause malabsorption of levothyroxine.
- Q: What if my child needs surgery?
- A: Treatment of hypothyroidism such that the patient is euthyroid (normal thyroid status) prior to surgery is preferable whenever possible (only exception is ischemic heart disease requiring surgery). Euthyroid sick syndrome, which is common in very ill patients, should not be treated.

H

HYPOTHYROIDISM, CONGENITAL

Ari Wassner, MD

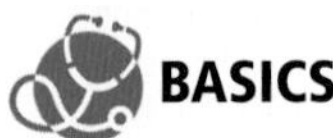

BASICS

DESCRIPTION

Primary thyroid failure present at birth

EPIDEMIOLOGY

- Increasing incidence worldwide
  - Due to stricter newborn screening thresholds, changing demographics
  - Overall incidence: about 1 in 2,000 births
  - Severe congenital hypothyroidism: 1 in 3,000 to 4,000 births
- Male-to-female ratio is 1:2 to 1:3 among severe cases but 1:1 among mild cases.
- 70% dysgenesis; 30% dyshormonogenesis

RISK FACTORS

Genetics

- Dysgenesis is usually sporadic.
  - Familial occurrence in 2–5%
  - Mutations have been found in the TSH receptor (TSHR) and in thyroid transcription factors *PAX8*, *NKX2.1*, and *FOXE1*.
- Dyshormonogenesis is often inherited in autosomal recessive fashion, but many cases do not have a defined genetic cause.
  - Most commonly mutated genes are thyroglobulin (TG), thyroperoxidase (TPO), *DUOX2*, and *TSHR* (relative distribution depends on ethnicity).
  - Pendred syndrome: Mutations in *SLC26A4* cause a common syndromic form of deafness, as well as a mild iodine organification defect that can cause hypothyroidism, usually later in childhood.

ETIOLOGY

- Dysgenesis: failure of normal thyroid gland formation. Includes:
  - Agenesis—absent thyroid gland
  - Ectopy—failure to descend to normal position
  - Abnormally formed (e.g., hypoplastic) thyroid
- Dyshormonogenesis
  - Defects in thyroxine (T_4) synthesis, including in iodide transport and organification
- Transient hypothyroidism
  - Maternal treatment with antithyroid drugs (methimazole, propythiouracil)
  - Transplacental transfer of maternal TSH receptor-blocking antibodies
  - Iodine deficiency or exposure to high levels of iodine (e.g., topical antiseptics, radiographic contrast)
  - Mild forms of dyshormonogenesis

COMMONLY ASSOCIATED CONDITIONS

- Infants with trisomy 21 have a significantly increased incidence of congenital hypothyroidism.
- Newborns with congenital hypothyroidism have a slightly increased risk for congenital heart and kidney malformations.
- Higher incidence of congenital hypothyroidism in infants with low birth weight (<2,500 g), preterm birth (<37 weeks)

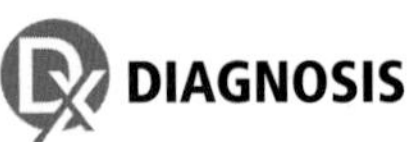

DIAGNOSIS

HISTORY

- Birth history
- Newborn screening results (including hearing test)
- Maternal use of antithyroid drugs
- Maternal iodine ingestion (e.g., iodine supplements, seaweed)
- Family history of thyroid disorders
  - Autoimmune thyroid disease in mother
  - "Mild hypothyroidism" characterized by low total T_4 with normal TSH; free T_4 not requiring treatment may be found in families with thyroxine-binding globulin deficiency.
- Symptoms of hypothyroidism:
  - Most neonates are *asymptomatic* in the first few weeks of life.
  - Symptoms may include
    - Prolonged jaundice (unconjugated hyperbilirubinemia)
    - Poor feeding
    - Constipation
    - Poor linear growth

PHYSICAL EXAM

- Signs of hypothyroidism:
  - Hypothermia
  - Large fontanelles (especially posterior)
  - Coarse facial features, including macroglossia
  - Hoarse cry
  - Hypotonia
  - Delayed relaxation of deep tendon reflexes
  - Distended abdomen
  - Umbilical hernia
  - Edema
- Examine for possible goiter
  - In supine position on exam table, gently elevate shoulders to slightly extend the neck; inspect and palpate for goiter between the sternal notch and cricoid cartilage. A palpable thyroid in a neonate is abnormally enlarged.
  - Inspect base of tongue for ectopic (lingual) gland.

DIFFERENTIAL DIAGNOSIS

- Developmental
  - Transient hypothyroxinemia (low T_4) in the first weeks of life in preterm or low birth weight infants
- Metabolic
  - Sick euthyroid syndrome in severely ill neonates
- Central hypothyroidism
  - Multiple pituitary hormone deficiencies (present in 75% of congenital central hypothyroidism)
  - Isolated central hypothyroidism (mutations in TSH β-subunit, TRH receptor, *IGSF1*)
  - Central hypothyroidism due to maternal hyperthyroidism during pregnancy (presumably caused by altered maturation of the hypothalamic–pituitary–thyroid axis during fetal hyperthyroidism)
- Genetic
  - Thyroxine-binding globulin deficiency (X-linked recessive)
- Environmental
  - Maternal treatment with antithyroid drugs (persists 7 to 10 days until drug is cleared)
  - Iodine excess (e.g., topical antiseptics, radiographic contrast, excessive maternal iodine intake)
  - Iodine deficiency (Pregnant and lactating women should take prenatal vitamins containing 150 mcg of iodine daily.)
- Immunologic
  - Transplacental transfer of maternal TSH receptor–blocking antibodies (persists 1 to 3 months until antibodies are cleared)

DIAGNOSTIC TESTS & INTERPRETATION

- Neonatal screening (whole blood on filter card)
  - Most patients are diagnosed by neonatal screening.
  - Methods vary by state (may screen for T_4, TSH, or both).
  - Abnormal newborn screen results should prompt *immediate* confirmatory serum tests and examination (within 24 hours).
  - To avoid false-negative results, rescreening at 2 weeks of age should be considered in:
    - Preterm or low birth weight infants
    - Same-sex twins
    - Infants initially screened before 24 hours of life
  - Screening should be performed prior to transfer between units or hospitals to be sure it is not overlooked.
- Confirmatory tests:
  - Serum TSH and free T_4 (preferable to repeating newborn screen)
  - If abnormalities in binding are suspected, check thyroxine-binding globulin level and free T_4 concentration or triiodothyronine (T_3) resin uptake.
  - Low free T_4 with normal or low TSH may indicate central hypothyroidism (due to a hypothalamic or pituitary defect).
- Antenatal tests
  - Fetal goiter can be detected by prenatal ultrasound.
  - Reference ranges for third trimester amniotic fluid concentrations of TSH and total and free T_4 are established for diagnosis of fetal hypothyroidism among those with goiters. Otherwise, cordocentesis is needed.
- Imaging rarely affects initial management but may inform prognosis (distinguish permanent vs. possibly transient disease).
- Ultrasonography can evaluate thyroid anatomy to diagnose dysgenesis and does not require deferral of treatment.
- ^{123}I or technetium thyroid scan can define thyroid anatomy (including ectopic gland).
  - Dependent on iodide uptake (which is absent in defects of TSH receptor function)
  - Must be obtained before beginning treatment. If scan would delay treatment, defer scanning until 3 years of age, when a period off medication is safer for brain development.

ALERT

- False positives
  - Thyroxine-binding globulin deficiency *in males*: normal TSH, low total T_4, and normal free T_4. Diagnose with low thyroxine-binding globulin level and/or high T_3 resin uptake. No treatment is necessary.
  - Blood specimens obtained before 24 hours of life may have elevated TSH as a result of the normal postnatal surge in TSH.
- False negatives
  - Newborn screening has a 5–10% false-negative rate.
  - Screening can be falsely reassuring in babies with congenital central hypothyroidism (especially in primary TSH screens, because TSH is normal or low despite low total and free T_4).
  - Preterm or low birth weight infants may have delayed rise in TSH that is missed on initial screening; rescreening is recommended in these patients.

TREATMENT

MEDICATION

Levothyroxine (LT_4)

- Start treatment immediately if
  - Newborn screen TSH ≥40 mIU/L (draw confirmatory serum tests and start treatment while awaiting results)
  - Serum TSH ≥20 mIU/L
  - Serum TSH 6 to 20 mIU/L *and* low free T_4
  - Consider treatment versus monitoring if serum TSH 6 to 20 mIU/L with normal free T_4.
- Start 10 to 15 mcg/kg PO once daily, *as crushed tablet form only*.
- Recheck TSH and free T_4 in 1 to 2 weeks, and titrate dose to achieve treatment goals.
- Goals of treatment:
  - Normalize free T_4 and TSH within 2 weeks
  - Maintain TSH in normal range, and free T_4 in upper half of normal range.
  - Avoid overtreatment (low TSH or high free T_4).
- 10–30% of infants may have persistently elevated TSH even when free T_4 is high-normal or above normal; this pattern is due to central resistance to thyroid hormone, which usually resolves with age.
- Duration of treatment:
  - Dysgenesis is permanent and requires lifelong treatment.
  - Patients with a normally located thyroid gland may have transient disease; if unclear, may trial off LT_4 after 3 years of age and recheck TSH 4 to 6 weeks off therapy

ISSUES FOR REFERRAL

Patients should follow up with a pediatric endocrinologist as soon as possible after diagnosis.

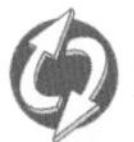

ONGOING CARE

FOLLOW-UP RECOMMENDATIONS

Patient Monitoring

- Serum TSH and free T_4 should be measured.
  - Every 1 to 2 weeks until TSH and free T_4 are normal
  - Every 1 to 3 months until 12 months of age
  - Every 2 to 4 months between 1 and 3 years of age
  - Every 6 months after 3 year of age
  - 4 to 8 weeks after any change in LT_4 dose
- Signs of inadequate treatment include poor growth, elevated TSH, or low T_4. Assess such patients for:
  - Poor adherence to LT_4
  - Interference with LT_4 absorption (administration with calcium, iron, soy formula, or celiac disease)
- Monitoring for neurodevelopmental sequelae:
  - Neurocognitive evaluation should be provided for any developmental concerns.
  - Formal hearing testing should be performed for any hearing concerns.
- Evaluate for heart or kidney malformations if clinically indicated (routine screening is not necessary).

DIET

- No restrictions
- Soy products (e.g., soy formulas), calcium, and iron decrease absorption of LT_4.
- Consistency in administration of LT_4 is more important than taking LT_4 on an empty stomach (as is often recommended by pharmacies).

PATIENT EDUCATION

- The more rapidly thyroid function is normalized and the more consistently it is maintained in the normal range, the less likely neurodevelopmental problems are to occur; however, in severe cases, subtle impairments can still occur even with early and adequate treatment.
- LT_4 tablets should be crushed between 2 spoons and the powder suspended in a small amount of formula or breast milk and given to the baby at the start of a feeding to ensure complete ingestion.
- A forgotten dose of LT_4 should be given as soon as it is remembered. If it is the next day, 2 doses should be given.
- There are no side effects from the medication. The tablet contains only the normal hormone that the child's thyroid is not making.
- When to expect improvement:
  - Most children are asymptomatic at diagnosis.
  - Parents may note increased activity, improved feeding, and increase in bowel movements after starting treatment.

PROGNOSIS

- Excellent if adequate treatment is started early, optimally within the first 2 weeks of life
  - IQ is usually normal.
  - In severe cases, there may be subtle impairments in language, motor skills, attention, memory, or learning despite early and adequate treatment.
  - Low level of T_4 at birth is an important indicator of possible long-term sequelae.
- Permanent versus transient disease
  - Dysgenesis is permanent.
  - Among patients with a normally located thyroid:
    - 35% have transient hypothyroidism.
    - 40% have permanent hypothyroidism.
    - 25% have persistent mild TSH elevation; clinical significance of this is unclear, but treatment is usually recommended.
  - Permanent disease is likely if LT_4 dose is >2 mcg/kg/24 h at age 3 years.

COMPLICATIONS

If untreated:

- Severe cognitive impairment (cretinism)
- Poor motor development
- Poor growth

ADDITIONAL READING

- LaFranchi SH. Approach to the diagnosis and treatment of neonatal hypothyroidism. *J Clin Endocrinol Metab*. 2011;96(10):2959–2967.
- Léger J, Olivieri A, Donaldson M, et al. European Society for Paediatric Endocrinology consensus guidelines of screening, diagnosis, and management of congenital hypothyroidism. *Horm Res Paediatr*. 2014;81(2):80–103.
- Rose SR, Brown RS, Foley T, et al; and Public Health Committee, Lawson Wilkins Pediatric Endocrine Society. Update of newborn screening and therapy for congenital hypothyroidism. *Pediatrics*. 2006;117(6):2290–2303.
- Wassner AJ, Brown RS. Congenital hypothyroidism: recent advances. *Curr Opin Endocrinol Diabetes Obes*. 2015;22(5):407–412.

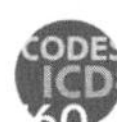

CODES

ICD10

- E03.1 Congenital hypothyroidism without goiter
- E03.0 Congenital hypothyroidism with diffuse goiter

FAQ

- Q: What causes congenital hypothyroidism?
- A: Most cases are caused by failure of the thyroid gland to form correctly (dysgenesis). Almost all of these cases are sporadic, and the underlying cause is unknown. In a minority of cases, an anatomically normal thyroid cannot produce thyroid hormone normally (dyshormonogenesis). Although around 20–60% of such cases are genetic, the cause of the remainder is unknown. Overall, an underlying cause is evident in fewer than 80% of cases.
- Q: Will the patient be developmentally normal?
- A: In most cases, patients with congenital hypothyroidism have normal neurodevelopment as long as they are diagnosed early, receive prompt treatment, and consistently maintain euthyroidism. However, in the most severe cases (particularly those with very low T_4 at diagnosis), subtle deficits may occur in spite of apparently optimal treatment, presumably due to adverse effect of fetal hypothyroidism.
- Q: Will the patient require lifelong LT_4 therapy?
- A: If the thyroid did not form correctly (dysgenesis), hypothyroidism is permanent and requires lifelong therapy. Among patients with an anatomically normal thyroid gland, about 35% have transient disease and can successfully stop treatment after 3 years of age. In patients with a normally placed thyroid, the degree of TSH elevation at diagnosis does not predict the likelihood of having permanent disease.
- Q: Should thyroid imaging be performed?
- A: Although thyroid imaging rarely alters management in the neonatal period, many experts recommend imaging for several reasons. Identification of thyroid dysgenesis confirms the permanence of the condition and provides diagnostic certainty for families who are asked to commit their newborn to lifelong medication. Identification of a normally placed thyroid suggests some chance of transient disease (35%) and may motivate investigation for specific etiologies (e.g., TSH receptor–blocking antibodies). Imaging can also facilitate counseling of parents about recurrence risk in future children, which is very low in dysgenesis but may be 25% in autosomal recessive forms of dyshormonogenesis.

IDIOPATHIC INTRACRANIAL HYPERTENSION (PSEUDOTUMOR CEREBRI)

Sabrina E. Smith, MD, PhD

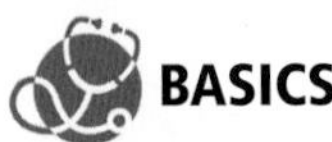

BASICS

DESCRIPTION

Diagnostic criteria of idiopathic intracranial hypertension (IIH) include the following:

- Signs and symptoms of increased intracranial pressure (e.g., headache, vomiting, ocular manifestations, and papilledema)
- Elevated cerebrocranial fluid pressure but otherwise normal cerebrospinal fluid (CSF)
- Normal neurologic exam except for papilledema (occasional abducens or other motor cranial neuropathy)
- Normal neuroimaging study (or incidental findings only)

EPIDEMIOLOGY

- Boys and girls are affected equally in childhood; in adolescence and adulthood, more women than men are affected.
- IIH has been reported in patients as young as 4 months of age, with a median age of 9 years.

Incidence

- Estimated to be 0.71/100,000 cases per year for children <17 years old, with increasing incidence with age and weight
- Annual incidence is estimated to be 4.18 per 100,000 in obese boys ages 12 to 15 years and 10.7 per 100,000 in obese girls ages 12 to 15 years.

RISK FACTORS

Genetics

Sporadic, no clear genetic predisposition, unless related to an underlying hormonal, toxic, or inflammatory condition; no data are available in children.

PATHOPHYSIOLOGY

Pathogenesis unknown but may involve decreased CSF absorption owing to arachnoid villi dysfunction or elevated intracranial venous pressure. For example, obesity may lead to increased intra-abdominal, intrathoracic, and cardiac filling pressure, leading to elevated intracranial venous pressure.

ETIOLOGY

Numerous precipitants of IIH have been reported. In adolescents, it is clearly associated with obesity and weight gain but not clearly linked to obesity in children <11 years of age. Many weaker associations may be due to chance.

COMMONLY ASSOCIATED CONDITIONS

- Exposure to exogenous steroids
- Corticosteroid withdrawal
- Lead exposure
- IIH is often linked to minocycline, tetracycline, sulfonamides, isotretinoin, and thyroid replacements.
- Also linked to vitamin A deficiency or intoxication, chronic anemia, and hypothyroidism

DIAGNOSIS

HISTORY

- Headache
- Blurred vision
- Transient visual darkening
- Stiff neck
- Pulsatile tinnitus
- Dizziness
- Infants and young children may present with irritability, somnolence, or ataxia.
- IIH should be considered in any child with chronic headache or unexplained visual changes.
- Directed history for signs of associated endocrinopathy, exposure to antibiotics or steroids, sinus infection, abnormal clotting, or familial tendency for thrombosis or visual disturbance

PHYSICAL EXAM

- Examination of the fundi is essential.
- Recording baseline visual acuity and visual fields in older children is essential.
- Papilledema is almost always present in older children with IIH.
- Most infants have some degree of papilledema, even with open fontanelles and split sutures.
- 6th cranial nerve (abducens) palsies are common in children with IIH; they were found in 29 of 68 patients in one series.
- Facial or other cranial nerve deficits rare

DIFFERENTIAL DIAGNOSIS

Some conditions may cause increased intracranial pressure and be confused with IIH, but the clinical picture and CSF analysis usually permit their distinction.

- Chronic meningitis (e.g., CNS Lyme disease), encephalitis, or cerebral edema (may show minimal changes on neuroimaging with elevated CSF protein levels and little evidence of pleocytosis)
- Cerebral venous sinus thrombosis
- Chronic headache (common) with pseudopapilledema (optic nerve disc drusen)

DIAGNOSTIC TESTS & INTERPRETATION

Initial Tests (screening, lab, imaging)

- CSF exam including opening pressure; cell count, glucose, and protein are essential and should be normal in IIH.
- CBC and thyroid function tests should be obtained because anemia, hypothyroidism, and hyperthyroidism have rarely been associated with IIH.
- The following may be useful in selected cases:
  - ANA test
  - ESR
  - Urine cortisol
  - Serum lead level
  - Serologic testing for Lyme disease
- Cranial CT or MRI should be normal. MRI is recommended because of superior imaging of brainstem, posterior fossa, and venous sinuses. Magnetic resonance venography is strongly suggested to evaluate for venous sinus thrombosis, which can be difficult to distinguish from IIH.

Diagnostic Procedures/Other

- Lumbar puncture manometry, with the patient in a relaxed lateral decubitus position, should show an opening pressure >280 mm H_2O.
- Goldmann perimeter visual field testing or computerized visual fields are useful in children >5 years of age to document field deficits and monitor response to therapy.

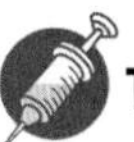

TREATMENT

MEDICATION

First Line

- For patients with mild to moderate visual loss, acetazolamide, a carbonic anhydrase inhibitor that decreases CSF production, is the drug of choice.
  - The pediatric dosage is 25 to 100 mg/kg/24 h divided b.i.d.–q.i.d. for the standard form and b.i.d. for the long-acting form (Diamox Sequels®).
  - The initial adult dose is 250 mg q.i.d. or 500 mg b.i.d., increased to 750 mg q.i.d. or 1,500 mg b.i.d. if tolerated.
- If visual loss, papilledema, and symptoms of pressure resolve, acetazolamide dosage can be tapered after 2 months of therapy.

Second Line

Furosemide can be used if acetazolamide is ineffective or has intolerable adverse effects.

ISSUES FOR REFERRAL

Follow-up and tapering of acetazolamide should be done in conjunction with a neurologist, ophthalmologist, or neuro-ophthalmologist.

SURGERY/OTHER PROCEDURES

- Serial lumbar punctures are not recommended as standard therapy, although the initial puncture can be useful to relieve symptoms quickly.
- Surgical therapy (e.g., optic nerve sheath fenestration, lumboperitoneal shunt) is indicated for progressive visual loss despite medical therapy and may also be considered as an urgent intervention at presentation depending on degree of visual loss. Optic nerve sheath fenestration may be the preferred surgical treatment, especially in children, because of the high failure rates of lumboperitoneal shunting. High-dose IV steroids and acetazolamide therapy may be used while awaiting surgical therapy.
- Recent studies of stenting in adults with transverse sinus stenosis and a pressure gradient on angiography demonstrated some improvement in visual symptoms and papilledema with variable effects on headache. However, this intervention is controversial and may not be technically feasible in children because of the smaller caliber of their vasculature.

ADMISSION, INPATIENT, AND NURSING CONSIDERATIONS

- The urgency of diagnosis and treatment depends on the severity of visual loss. Severe visual loss may progress rapidly, warranting close initial (weekly) tracking of vision and prompt consideration of surgical treatment (see below).
- For patients with no visual loss, removal of possible causative agents may be the only intervention needed, along with treatment of associated conditions (e.g., obesity, anemia, thyroid disease). Consider treatment with acetazolamide (Diamox Sequels®). Headache can be treated symptomatically if needed.

ONGOING CARE

FOLLOW-UP RECOMMENDATIONS

Patient Monitoring

- Initially, patients should have visual acuity, visual fields, and fundi evaluated weekly or biweekly.
- If vision is stable, monthly visits may be adequate for 3 to 6 months.
- More frequent follow-up is required for any signs of progressive visual loss.
- IIH can recur. In one pediatric series, nearly 1/4 of patients had recurrence.
- Pitfalls: Children are not exempt from permanent visual loss as a consequence of IIH. Ophthalmologic follow-up is important. Occasional patients, especially adolescents, may experience headache weeks or months after resolution of objective signs of IIH (i.e., even though intracranial pressure has returned to normal).
- IIH may be diagnosed erroneously if
  - Pseudopapilledema is mistaken for papilledema. (Pseudopapilledema is apparent optic disc swelling that simulates papilledema but is usually secondary to an underlying benign process. It can be differentiated by an experienced ophthalmologist or neurologist.)
  - CSF abnormalities (i.e., isolated increase in protein) are overlooked.
  - Clinician fails to identify underlying cerebral venous sinus thrombosis.

COMPLICATIONS

Visual loss due to optic nerve pressure

ADDITIONAL READING

- Avery RA, Licht DJ, Shah SS, et al. CSF opening pressure in children with optic nerve head edema. *Neurology*. 2011;76(19):1658–1661.
- Matthews YY, Dean F, Lim MJ, et al. Pseudotumor cerebri syndrome in childhood: incidence, clinical profile and risk factors in a national prospective population-based cohort study. *Arch Dis Child*. 2017;102(8):715–721.
- Rook BS, Phillips PH. Pediatric pseudotumor cerebri. *Curr Opin Ophthalmol*. 2016;27(5):416–419.
- Soiberman U, Stolovitch C, Balcer LJ, et al. Idiopathic intracranial hypertension in children: visual outcome and risk of recurrence. *Childs Nerv Syst*. 2011;27(11):1913–1918.

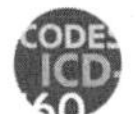

CODES

ICD10

G93.2 Benign intracranial hypertension

FAQ

- Q: What are the side effects of acetazolamide?
- A: Side effects of acetazolamide include GI upset, paresthesias, loss of appetite, drowsiness, metabolic acidosis, and renal stones. An alternative is furosemide.
- Q: If IIH occurs on tetracycline, can the patient take penicillin?
- A: Penicillins/cephalosporins have not been reported as a significant cause of IIH.
- Q: Are there any limitations on physical activity?
- A: Activity can be graded entirely according to the child's symptoms.

IMMUNE DEFICIENCY

Kathleen E. Sullivan, MD, PhD

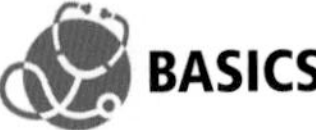

BASICS

DESCRIPTION

Immunodeficiencies generally represent a defect in host defense. Less common deficiencies represent defects in the regulation of immune function. Congenital and acquired forms exist.

- Defects in antibody production: often characterized by frequent sinopulmonary infections with typical organisms
  - X-linked agammaglobulinemia
    - Onset of symptoms after 6 months of age; sinopulmonary infections with typical bacterial pathogens
    - Markedly decreased immunoglobulins (Ig) and B cells. Tonsils are absent.
  - Hyper-IgM syndromes: several forms
    - Usually present with recurrent bacterial infections in infancy; *Pneumocystis jiroveci* is seen; intermittent neutropenia is common.
    - Decreased IgG, IgE, IgA with normal or increased IgM
  - Common variable immunodeficiency (CVID)
    - Usually presents with recurrent bacterial infections; most commonly arises in the 2nd or 3rd decade (but seen at all ages)
    - Ig levels and function gradually decline; autoimmunity is common.
  - IgA deficiency
    - Most common congenital immunodeficiency (1:600); most are asymptomatic.
    - Symptoms seen at any age; typically sinopulmonary infections; increased risk of allergy, autoimmune disease, and reactions to blood products
  - Transient hypogammaglobulinemia of infancy
    - A developmental delay of Ig production; function is intact; typically resolves between 1 and 2 years of age
- T-cell defects: most often characterized by persistent viral infections or opportunistic infections
  - Severe combined immunodeficiency (SCID)
    - Most common presentation is a respiratory virus that fails to clear or chronic diarrhea.
    - Failure to thrive, thrush, and *P. jiroveci* pneumonia are also common.
    - Many states now have SCID newborn screening; patients identified have no symptoms.
  - Combined immune deficiencies
    - Several forms
    - Children exhibit increased severity of a broad range of infections, opportunistic infections, and unusual autoimmunity.
  - Chromosome 22q11.2 deletion syndrome
    - See "DiGeorge Syndrome."
  - Chronic mucocutaneous candidiasis
    - Multiple forms of this disorder
    - One form is also called autoimmune polyendocrinopathy candidiasis ectodermal dystrophy (APECED) and has an association with polyendocrinopathies and ectodermal dysplasia.
    - The other types are more likely to have an associated T-cell defect. Infants have extensive or recurrent *Candida* infections; modest predisposition to other infections
  - IPEX (immunodeficiency, polyendocrinopathy, enteropathy, X-linked syndrome)
    - Diarrhea associated with villous atrophy and a T-cell infiltrate, progressive autoimmune destruction of endocrine organs
    - Infections can be severe, but the autoimmune manifestations predominate.
- Neutrophil defects: *Staphylococcus*, *Pseudomonas*; unusual bacterial or fungal infections are characteristic.
  - Autoimmune neutropenia of infancy
    - Most common neutrophil defect of childhood; usually detected at ~6 to 12 months of age
    - Often resolves by 2 years of age
  - Congenital neutropenia
    - Infections may be skin infections or sinopulmonary.
    - Patients have either persistently absent or markedly low neutrophil counts.
    - Some patients will have 21-day cycles of neutropenia—cyclic neutropenia.
  - Leukocyte adhesion deficiency
    - ~10% have delayed separation of the umbilical cord.
    - Most common presentations are recurrent skin ulcers and periodontitis.
    - Spontaneous peritonitis occurs.
  - Chronic granulomatous disease (CGD)
    - Recurrent skin abscesses common, deep hepatic abscesses, and pulmonary infections
    - Typical organisms are *Staphylococcus aureus*, *Burkholderia*, *Serratia*, *Nocardia*, mycobacteria, *Aspergillus*, and *Candida*.
    - Age of onset is usually 1 to 3 years.
- Innate defects in signaling: typically present with severe bacterial or viral infections in early infancy
  - IRAK4 and MyD88 deficiencies
    - Associated with staphylococcal, streptococcal, or pseudomonal sepsis/meningitis
    - Clostridial infections are also seen.
  - Herpes simplex encephalitis is associated with several gene defects.
- Macrophage activation defects
  - Associated with atypical mycobacteria. *Salmonella* is also seen.
  - Biopsies may reveal poorly formed granulomas.
- Complement deficiency
  - Deficiencies of C5 to C9 are associated with *Neisseria* infections.
  - Deficiencies of C1, C2, and C4 are associated with lupus and recurrent bacterial infections.
  - C3 deficiency associated with glomerulonephritis and severe recurrent infections
  - Defects in complement regulatory proteins are associated with atypical hemolytic uremic syndrome (HUS) or hereditary angioedema.
- Immunodeficiency syndromes
  - Ataxia telangiectasia
    - Progressive cerebellar ataxia during infancy; ocular telangiectasias at about 5 to 15 years of age
    - Recurrent sinopulmonary infections; α-fetoprotein is elevated; IgA and IgG2 are diminished.
  - Wiskott-Aldrich syndrome
    - Clinical triad of eczema, thrombocytopenia, and recurrent infections
    - Ig levels are variable but responses to vaccines often poor; small platelets and thrombocytopenia
  - Hyper-IgE syndrome
    - Recurrent infections of the skin and lungs; *S. aureus* is a major cause of infection, and pulmonary infections typically heal with pneumatoceles.
  - X-linked lymphoproliferative syndrome
    - Four main types of presentation and two genetic types: acute Epstein-Barr virus infection with hemophagocytosis, lymphoma, hypogammaglobulinemia, and aplastic anemia
    - Family history is key to diagnosis.
  - Chédiak-Higashi syndrome
    - Pigmentary dilution, progressive neuropathy, and frequent infections; associated with a hemophagocytic process
    - Neutrophil counts are low, and neutrophils have giant inclusions.
  - Familial hemophagocytic lymphohistiocytosis
    - Multiple defects in cytotoxic function; presents with fever, pancytopenia, and hepatosplenomegaly; usually <5 years of age
  - Ectodermal dysplasia with immune deficiency
    - Two forms. Variable ectodermal dysplasia and variable immune deficiency. Ig levels are variable as are responses to vaccines.
    - Susceptibility to mycobacteria, *Pneumocystis*, and common bacterial pathogens
- Secondary immunodeficiencies include the following:
  - HIV infection
  - Malignancy
  - Viral suppression
  - Nephrotic syndrome
  - Protein-losing enteropathy
  - Malnutrition
  - Medications
  - Splenectomy
  - Complex cardiac anomalies

EPIDEMIOLOGY

Primary immune deficiencies range from the common (1:600) to the very rare (1:1,000,000).

- 1:600 for IgA deficiency in Caucasians
- 1:3,000 for chromosome 22q11.2 deletion syndrome
- 1:20,000 for common variable immune deficiency
- 1:50,000 for SCID
- 1:200,000 for CGD

RISK FACTORS

Genetics

- The immunodeficiencies are generally autosomal recessive, although there are several important exceptions.
- X-linked
  - Properdin deficiency, X-linked agammaglobulinemia, X-linked hyper-IgM, X-linked SCID, X-linked CGD, X-linked lymphoproliferative syndrome (two types), IPEX, Wiskott-Aldrich syndrome, NF-kappa B Essential Modulator (NEMO) deficiency. All of these have autosomal recessive phenocopies or may be seen in females with altered X inactivation.
- Autosomal dominant
  - Hyper-IgE syndrome, chromosome 22q11.2 deletion syndrome, some macrophage activation defects
- Polygenic
  - IgA deficiency and CVID

DIAGNOSIS

HISTORY

- **Question:** Family history?
- *Significance*: X-linked disorders are common.
- **Question:** Number and duration of infections?
- *Significance*: to determine whether the problem is one of clearance or frequency
- **Question:** Types of infections?
- *Significance*: Infections of skin are frequently due to neutrophil problems, whereas recurrent infections of a single site imply an anatomic problem. Opportunistic infections are associated with both neutrophil defects (unusual bacteria and fungi) and T-cell defects (opportunistic viruses).
- HIV risk factors

PHYSICAL EXAM

Examination should be directed at defining organ damage as a result of infection, the presence of any current infections, syndromic features, signs of autoimmune disease, and the characterization of accessible lymphoid organs, liver, and spleen.

DIFFERENTIAL DIAGNOSIS

- Chronic inflammation of mucous membranes such as that due to reflux or allergies can lead to recurrent infections.
- Immunocompromised status due to chemotherapy and immunosuppressive drugs
- Malnutrition
- Intercurrent viral infections such as Epstein-Barr virus and cytomegalovirus
- Medications such as antiseizure drugs and corticosteroids can cause IgA deficiency or hypogammaglobulinemia.
- Inborn errors of metabolism
- Chromosomal syndromes
- Protein loss can be associated with hypogammaglobulinemia.
- HIV infection

DIAGNOSTIC TESTS & INTERPRETATION

- **Test:** IgG, IgA, IgM, IgE levels, and responses to vaccines such as diphtheria and tetanus
- *Significance*: Recurrent sinopulmonary infections with typical organisms are associated with defects in antibody production.
- **Test:** evaluation of T-cell production and function—T-cell enumeration and lymphocyte proliferation studies
- *Significance*: T-cell defects will often have low T-cell numbers.
- **Test:** evaluation of neutrophil numbers and function—a CBC with differential, morphologic exam of neutrophils, and a measure of respiratory burst
- *Significance*: Neutropenia is the most common type of neutrophil defect followed by CGD.
- **Test:** special studies designed to test the function of the toll-like receptor signaling complex
- *Significance*: Innate defects, such as IRAK4, MyD88, and NEMO deficiencies, can be detected.
- **Test:** a CH50
- *Significance*: A CH50 will detect most of the structural component deficiencies. Special studies are needed for defects of the alternative pathway and the regulatory proteins.
- **Test:** CBC with differential; IgG, IgA, and IgM levels; and diphtheria and tetanus titers
- *Significance*: In certain patients, it may be difficult to differentiate between viral processes and bacterial processes. In these cases, a CBC with differential; IgG, IgA, and IgM levels; and diphtheria and tetanus titers are a useful screen to evaluate for the most common immunodeficiencies.

TREATMENT

Prophylactic antimicrobials

- Chronic mucocutaneous candidiasis
- Hyper-IgE syndrome
- CGD

GENERAL MEASURES

- Suspected SCID requires isolation, cytomegalovirus-negative/irradiated blood products, and a prompt evaluation for hematopoietic stem cell transplant (HSCT).
- Ig replacement (either IV or SC)
  - X-linked agammaglobulinemia
  - Hyper-IgM
  - CVID
- Specific strains of probiotic supplements may be useful for antibiotic-associated diarrhea.
- Hand washing to prevent infections
- Prophylactic antibiotics can be useful.

SURGERY/OTHER PROCEDURES

- Hematopoietic stem cell transplantation
  - SCID
  - Wiskott-Aldrich syndrome
  - X-linked lymphoproliferative syndrome
  - Chédiak-Higashi syndrome
  - Familial hemophagocytic lymphohistiocytosis
  - Selected cases of hyper-IgM, CGD, macrophage activation defects
- Thymus transplantation
  - Severe chromosome 22q11.2 deletion syndrome (DiGeorge syndrome)

ONGOING CARE

PROGNOSIS

- Most antibody deficiencies have an excellent prognosis. Transient or developmental deficiencies of IgG or IgG subclasses typically resolve by 2 years of age.
- Some patients with CVID can develop malignancy or autoimmune disease, and this defines the prognosis.
- The treatment of neutrophil disorders remains problematic; most children with CGD will not have full life expectancy. HSCT can be curative.
- Patients with T-cell disorders for whom bone marrow transplantation is not performed can do well if the defect is mild and if they do not suffer from autoimmune disease, malignancy, or recurrent infections.

COMPLICATIONS

- Bronchiectasis
- Deafness
- Autoimmune disease
- Lymphoreticular malignancies occur in patients with T-cell disorders.
- Live viral vaccines administered to patients with significant T-cell dysfunction can result in disease.
- Oral polio vaccine administered to patients with agammaglobulinemia can cause meningo-encephalitis.

ADDITIONAL READING

- Ballow M. Approach to the patient with recurrent infections. *Clin Rev Allergy Immunol*. 2008;34(2):129–140.
- Fischer A. Human primary immunodeficiency diseases. *Immunity*. 2007;27(6):835–845.
- Immunodeficiency Search. www.immunodeficiencysearch.com. Accessed June 8, 2018.
- Picard C, Al-Herz W, Bousfiha A, et al. Primary immunodeficiency diseases: an update on the classification from the International Union of Immunological Societies expert committee for primary immunodeficiency 2015. *J Clin Immunol*. 2015;35(8):696–726.
- Slatter MA, Gennery AR. Primary immunodeficiency syndromes. *Adv Exp Med Biol*. 2010;685:146–165.

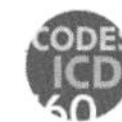

CODES

ICD10

- D84.9 Immunodeficiency, unspecified
- D80.9 Immunodeficiency with predominantly antibody defects, unspecified
- D83.9 Common variable immunodeficiency, unspecified

FAQ

- Q: Does a child with thrush require evaluation?
- A: A child with severe thrush in the absence of risk factors should have an evaluation for T-cell dysfunction, HIV, and the possibility of chronic mucocutaneous candidiasis of childhood. Moderate thrush or recurrent simple thrush does not require evaluation unless it is occurring in an older child.
- Q: A newborn in my practice still has his umbilical cord attached at 6 weeks of age. Is that abnormal, and does it require an evaluation for leukocyte adhesion deficiency?
- A: A completely healthy-appearing cord at 6 weeks of age does not require any evaluation. If there is clinical suspicion of leukocyte adhesion deficiency, a CBC can be performed to identify neutrophilia.
- Q: Which immunodeficiencies are associated with absent tonsils and adenoids?
- A: Boys with X-linked agammaglobulinemia and X-linked hyper-IgM have absent tonsils and adenoids.
- Q: Which immunodeficiency is associated with abscesses that are not painful?
- A: Children and adults with hyper-IgE syndrome develop abscesses that are not painful.

IMMUNE THROMBOCYTOPENIC PURPURA

L. Charles Bailey, MD, PhD

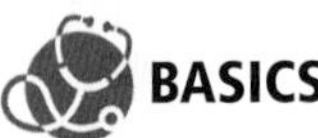

BASICS

DESCRIPTION

- Immune thrombocytopenic purpura (ITP) is an autoimmune syndrome characterized by the following:
  - Isolated thrombocytopenia (platelet count formally <100,000/mm^3, typically <20,000/mm^3)
  - Shortened platelet survival
  - Increased number of megakaryocytes in the bone marrow
- Primary ITP implies absence of other causes for thrombocytopenia; it often follows a viral infection.
- Secondary ITP indicates other immune dysregulation associated with thrombocytopenia.
- Phases of ITP
  - Newly diagnosed (acute) ITP: within 3 months of initial diagnosis
  - Persistent ITP: transient improvement or continued thrombocytopenia for 3 to 12 months
  - Chronic ITP: persistent thrombocytopenia >12 months after initial presentation

EPIDEMIOLOGY

- Most common acquired platelet disorder in childhood
- Incidence is 5/100,000 children per year (<15 years of age).
- Often follows viral syndrome by a few weeks; this may be associated with higher likelihood of spontaneous recovery.
- Males and females are equally affected in childhood ITP but mild male predominance in younger children
- Female-to-male ratio is 3:1 in adult and chronic ITP.
- Median age at diagnosis is 4 years. Children <1 year or >10 years are more likely to develop chronic ITP.
- >70% of childhood ITP resolves within 6 months.
- Risk of severe bleeding is <5% and of intracranial bleeding is <0.5%.

PATHOPHYSIOLOGY

- Thrombocytopenia due to increased destruction of antibody-coated platelets in the reticuloendothelial system, particularly the spleen
- Hypothesized that antibodies generated in response to foreign antigen or drug cross-react with platelet membrane glycoproteins (most commonly IIb/IIIa and Ib/IX)
- Other mechanisms of immune dysregulation have been implicated, including possible inhibition of thrombocytopoiesis, limiting ability to compensate for destruction.
- Typical bone marrow aspirate shows increased numbers of immature megakaryocytes.

COMMONLY ASSOCIATED CONDITIONS

- In younger children, primary ITP is the most common presentation of ITP.
- Secondary ITP is seen with autoimmune disorders (e.g., systemic lupus erythematosus [SLE], autoimmune lymphoproliferative syndrome [ALPS]).
- HIV

DIAGNOSIS

HISTORY

- Presents with increased bruising (with minor or no trauma, or in uncommon locations such as torso, neck, face), petechiae, epistaxis, prolonged bleeding with minor trauma, gingival bleeding, hematuria, or hematochezia
- Acute onset in an otherwise well child
- Not associated with pallor, fatigue, adenopathy, bone pain, weight loss, or persistent fevers
- A majority of cases are preceded by a viral infection 1 to 3 weeks before onset (particularly varicella; also Epstein-Barr virus, cytomegalovirus).
- Associated with recent measles-mumps-rubella (MMR) vaccination in younger children; possibly hepatitis A vaccine, Tdap in older children
- Ascertain history of other autoimmune diseases (e.g., rheumatologic disorders, thyroid disease, hemolytic anemia).
- Obtain medication history, focusing on drugs with antiplatelet effects or associated with thrombocytopenia (e.g., valproate, heparin).
- Family history is usually negative for bleeding disorders. Ask about family autoimmune disease.
- Screen for bleeding, headache, abdominal or back pain, and any focal neurologic change.

PHYSICAL EXAM

- Clusters of petechiae or large or purple bruises readily apparent on skin or mucosae
- Hematomas or persistent slow bleeding on mucosal surfaces or from minor trauma
- Absence of lymphadenopathy, hepatosplenomegaly (HSM), masses, bone pain
  - Mild splenomegaly seen in 5–10% of patients with ITP
- Screen for nonobvious bleeding (neurologic and funduscopic exam, abdominal or muscular tenderness); these events are rare.

DIFFERENTIAL DIAGNOSIS

- Consider malignancy if persistent fever, weight loss, adenopathy, bone pain, or organomegaly is present.
- Other destructive thrombocytopenias
  - Secondary ITP: infection, drug induced, posttransfusion purpura, autoimmune hemolytic anemia (when coexistent with ITP is called Evans syndrome), lymphoproliferative disorders, SLE
  - Nonimmunologic: microangiopathic hemolytic anemia (including TTP, HUS), disseminated intravascular coagulation (DIC), Kasabach-Merritt syndrome (hemangioma), cardiac defects (left ventricular outflow obstruction, prosthetic heart valves), malignant hypertension
- Impaired or ineffective production
  - Marrow-infiltrative processes (leukemias, other tumor metastases, myelofibrosis, osteopetrosis, storage diseases)
  - Drug- or radiation-induced thrombocytopenia or aplastic anemia
  - Nutritional deficiency states (iron, folate, vitamin B_{12})
  - Infection-associated suppression: typically viral (e.g., hepatitis, Epstein-Barr virus, HIV, parvovirus B19), also severe or neonatal sepsis
  - Congenital disorders: thrombocytopenia absent radii (TAR) syndrome, dyskeratosis congenita, Fanconi anemia, trisomies 13 and 18, Bernard-Soulier syndrome, Wiskott-Aldrich syndrome, May-Hegglin anomaly, other inherited thrombocytopenias (X linked or autosomal dominant), metabolic disorders (e.g., methylmalonic acidemia)

DIAGNOSTIC TESTS & INTERPRETATION

- Thrombocytopenia (typically <20,000/mm^3) with normal WBC and hemoglobin (Hb) (or mild anemia in proportion to amount of blood loss)
- Mean platelet volume may be increased.
- Peripheral blood smear will be otherwise normal, with no red cell fragmentation, no spherocytes, and no blasts. Review also rules out pseudothrombocytopenia from platelet aggregation.
- Prothrombin time/INR and partial thromboplastin time are normal. Bleeding time will be prolonged, but testing is unnecessary.
- Direct antiglobulin (Coombs) test to exclude coexisting autoimmune hemolysis (Evans syndrome)
- HIV testing if risk factors are identified
- Limited role for antinuclear antibody (ANA) and other immunologic tests in subset of patients at higher risk for other autoimmune disease
- Bone marrow exam is needed only if unexplained anemia, abnormal WBC, blasts on peripheral smear, organomegaly, jaundice, or lymphadenopathy is present. It is safe to perform with a low platelet count.
- There is controversy over whether to obtain a marrow aspirate before giving corticosteroids, with little evidence to support it.
- Marrow shows normal to increased numbers of megakaryocytes with otherwise normal morphology and cellularity.
- Assays for platelet-associated antibodies (direct or indirect) are not sensitive and not routinely indicated.
- Demonstration of platelet-associated IgG may be useful in more complicated patients in whom chronic ITP is a possible diagnosis.
- Consider head US in younger infants with suspected ITP.
- Consider head CT in evaluation of significant head trauma in a patient with ITP and low platelet counts.
- Otherwise, only as indicated by symptoms, primarily to identify hemorrhage not otherwise apparent on physical exam, such as:
  - Stat head CT for severe headache, vision change, or focal neurologic change
  - Abdominal US, MR, or CT for significant abdominal pain
  - Renal US for significant hematuria
  - Musculoskeletal US for painful swelling or pain with motion of extremities

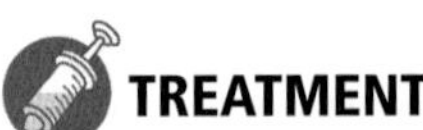

TREATMENT

- Because severe hemorrhage is rare and ITP resolves spontaneously in 90% of pediatric cases, most children without severe bleeding will not require treatment.
- Treatment slows antibody-mediated platelet clearance and raises platelet counts acutely but does not alter long-term course.
- Patients with a platelet count <10,000/mm^3 are at higher risk for bleeding, but platelet count alone is not an indication for treatment.
- Observation alone is acceptable for children without serious bleeding and with adequate supervision and assured follow-up; may be preferable to repeated treatment in clinically well children with chronic ITP
- Treatment decision should include foreseeable risk of bleeding (e.g., nonelective surgical procedures) as well as current symptoms.

GENERAL MEASURES

Platelet transfusions are generally ineffective because transfused platelets are rapidly destroyed. Role is limited to emergent support for critical hemorrhage.

ALERT

Emergency treatment of severe bleeding requires a combination of measures including platelet transfusions, rapid-acting medical therapies (e.g., IVIG), and longer acting medical therapies (e.g., corticosteroids).

MEDICATION

First Line

- IVIG: 94–97% will have an increase in platelet count >20,000/mm^3 by 72 hours. The usual dose is 0.8 to 1 g/kg. Response typically peaks after 1 week and lasts 3 to 4 weeks.
  - Advantages: faster time to platelet increase (24 hours), helps confirm diagnosis
  - Disadvantages: high cost, long infusion time, allergic reactions; 10–30% have evidence of aseptic meningitis with severe headache and stiff neck; headache, nausea, vomiting, or fever more common
  - Scheduled acetaminophen and diphenhydramine for 24 hours after infusion may reduce acute side effects.
  - Subcutaneous administration has been used successfully as an alternative to IV.
- Corticosteroids: 80% respond with platelet counts >20,000/mm^3 by 72 hours (faster with high-dose pulse therapy). Oral prednisone at 2 mg/kg/24 h tapered over 2 to 4 weeks is typical.
  - Advantages: ease of dosing, low cost, often longer duration of response
  - Disadvantages:
    - Short-term side effects: mood changes, increased appetite and weight gain, hypertension, insulin resistance
    - Long-term side effects with chronic use: adrenal suppression, osteopenia, growth delay
- Anti-Rh D immunoglobulin—(patient must be Rh[+], nonsplenectomized, and not have hemolysis or hemorrhage): 80% respond with platelet counts >20,000/mm^3 after 72 hours. Dose is 50 to 75 mcg/kg IV over 3 to 5 minutes. If Hb 8 to 10 mg/dL, give 25 to 40 mcg/kg. Not recommended if Hb <8 mg/dL. 1 mcg = 5 IU of drug. Response lasts ~5 weeks.
  - Advantages: less expensive than IVIG but more costly than steroids; lower rate of allergic side effects (10%) than with IVIG and does not cause aseptic meningitis; amenable to outpatient administration
  - Disadvantages: fever/chills, mild hemolysis (Hb decrease of 1 to 3 g/dL) in all patients; rare reports of catastrophic hemolysis; subcutaneous route may ameliorate risk.
- Any of these therapies may be repeated if responsive patient later develops recurrent thrombocytopenia.

Second Line

- Rituximab (anti-CD20 monoclonal antibody) induces response in many refractory patients (after median 5 weeks); duration is often limited (median 12 months).
- Thrombopoietin receptor agonists (e.g., eltrombopag, romiplostim) have been shown in trials to improve platelet counts and bleeding risk in patients with chronic ITP. Cost, concerns about adverse effects including myelofibrosis and rare thrombosis, and paucity of long-term follow-up data limit use. Periodic bone marrow examination for developing myelofibrosis is indicated while receiving a thrombopoietin receptor agonist.
- Cytotoxic drugs (e.g., vincristine) or immunosuppression (e.g., cyclosporine A or mycophenolate mofetil) is effective in some patients refractory to other therapy and splenectomy.

ISSUES FOR REFERRAL

Consider hematology referral for patients with complex presentation, platelet count <50,000/mm^3, or prolonged course.

SURGERY/OTHER PROCEDURES

Splenectomy: 70–80% respond with complete remission.

- No reliable presurgical predictors of response have been found.
- Generally deferred until >12 months from diagnosis to allow for spontaneous remission or medical response
- Advantages: response in patients refractory to medical therapy
- Disadvantages: surgical morbidity; risk of sepsis with encapsulated organisms (immunize preoperatively against *Haemophilus influenzae*, pneumococcus, and meningococcus and consider penicillin prophylaxis)
- Role unclear given improvements in 2nd-line medical therapies

ADMISSION, INPATIENT, AND NURSING CONSIDERATIONS

- Life-threatening hemorrhage: The goal is to stop bleeding rapidly. Platelet transfusion, IVIG, and steroids (after emergent marrow exam, if indicated) should be given concomitantly.
- Given high transient response rates, consider treatment prior to nonemergent major invasive procedures, where these cannot be delayed to allow recovery or in patients with chronic ITP.

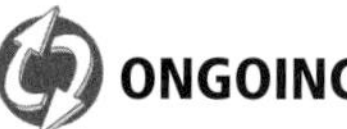

ONGOING CARE

FOLLOW-UP RECOMMENDATIONS

Patient Monitoring

- Platelet count 1 to 2 times weekly when <20,000/mm^3, biweekly when <50,000/mm^3 or after treatment, except in stable chronic ITP. More frequent monitoring is needed earlier in course; when stable pattern has been established, frequency of monitoring may decrease.
- Platelet counts may fall transiently with intercurrent illnesses prior to resolution of ITP.
- Discontinue monitoring when no symptoms and normal platelet count for >3 months.

PATIENT EDUCATION

- Avoid medications that affect platelet function, such as aspirin, ibuprofen, most other NSAIDs, and anticoagulants.
- Educate patients/parents about signs and symptoms of intracranial hemorrhage and GI bleeding.
- Avoid activities with significant fall, collision, or other trauma risk while thrombocytopenic.

PROGNOSIS

- Acute ITP: In 3 months, 60% of children will have a platelet count >100,000/mm^3; at 1 year from diagnosis, 90%. Recurrence is rare.
- Chronic ITP: Platelet count tends to be higher, at 40,000 to 80,000/mm^3. Remissions can occur many years after diagnosis (predicted spontaneous remission rate 61% after 15 years).
- Not yet possible to prospectively distinguish patients with self-limited ITP from those who will persist with chronic ITP
- Patients with chronic ITP should be periodically reevaluated for secondary ITP.
- If patient has received first but not second MMR vaccine, and vaccine titers show full immunity, consider deferring second dose.

COMPLICATIONS

- The incidence of significant bleeding-related morbidity and mortality is low (<5%).
  - Intracranial hemorrhage is rare (<0.5%).
  - May occur without prior trauma
- Retinal hemorrhage is rare.
- Mucosal bleeding from nose, gums, lower GI tract, or kidneys is not uncommon. Hematemesis and melena are rare.
- Significant menorrhagia may occur.

ADDITIONAL READING

- Arnold DM. Bleeding complications in immune thrombocytopenia. *Hematology Am Soc Hematol Educ Program*. 2015;2015:237–242.
- Eberl W, Dickerhoff R; for Pediatric Committee of Society of Thrombosis and Hemostasis Research. Newly diagnosed immune thrombozytopenia—German guideline concerning initial diagnosis and therapy. *Klin Padiatr*. 2012;224(3):207–210.
- Neunert CE, Buchanan GR, Imbach P, et al; for Intercontinental Cooperative ITP Study Group Registry II Participants. Bleeding manifestations and management of children with persistent and chronic immune thrombocytopenia: data from the Intercontinental Cooperative ITP Study Group (ICIS). *Blood*. 2013;121(22):4457–4462.
- Neunert CE, Lim W, Crowther M, et al; for American Society of Hematology. The American Society of Hematology 2011 evidence-based practice guideline for immune thrombocytopenia. *Blood*. 2011;117(16):4190–4207.

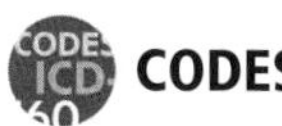

CODES

ICD10

- D69.3 Immune thrombocytopenic purpura
- D69.41 Evans syndrome

FAQ

- Q: Do children with ITP and very low platelet counts (<10,000/mm^3) require prophylactic treatment?
- A: Although there is some evidence that bleeding risk is higher with platelet counts <10,000/mm^3, incidence of severe bleeding remains low even in this group, and most children can be managed by observation alone.
- Q: How can one predict the duration of ITP?
- A: The time to recovery of normal platelet counts varies widely in 80% of children whose ITP resolves spontaneously. Shorter durations are more common in younger children overall, with some studies reporting improvement in a majority of children by 90 days. However, no good predictor of duration for a specific patient currently exists.
- Q: What level of activity is safe for a child with ITP?
- A: There is wide variation in current practice among hematologists regarding activity recommendations. Little evidence exists to suggest increased risk with low-impact activities (e.g., swimming, walking) or noncontact sports. When platelet counts are <30 to 50,000/mm^3, avoiding activities with significant collision or fall risks is prudent.
- Q: Is ITP associated with vaccinations?
- A: A mild increase in ITP incidence following MMR is documented, but the relative risk is significantly lower than the risk of clinical infections. A large retrospective review found no increase in ITP following any other early childhood vaccinations; a possible increased risk in 11- to 17-year-olds following Tdap, hepatitis A virus (HAV), and varicella zoster virus (VZV) vaccinations was also noted. The only recommended modification in current guidelines is deferral of a second MMR in fully-immune patients.

I

IMMUNOGLOBULIN A DEFICIENCY

Nashmia Qamar, DO, MSc • Ramsay L. Fuleihan, MD

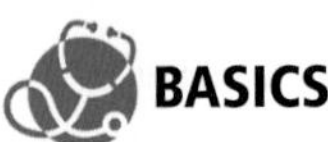

BASICS

DESCRIPTION

Selective IgA deficiency is the most common primary antibody deficiency; diagnosed by:

- Increased susceptibility to infection
- Autoimmune manifestations
- Serum IgA <7 mg/dL and a normal serum IgG and IgM in patients >4 years of age
- Exclusion of secondary causes of hypogammaglobulinemia
- Exclusion of T-cell defect

RISK FACTORS

Genetics

- Exact pattern of inheritance remains unclear; however, the following associations may occur:
  - Mutations in genes affecting cellular and humoral immunity (e.g., *JAK3*, *RAG1*)
  - Combined immunodeficiencies with syndromic features (e.g., ataxia telangiectasia, Wiskott-Aldrich syndrome)
  - Antibody deficiencies (e.g., *BTK*)
  - Phagocytic defects (e.g., *RAC2*)
  - Immune dysregulation (e.g., *IFIH1*, X-linked inhibitor of apoptosis [XIAP])
  - Defects in intrinsic and innate immunity
  - Complement deficiencies (e.g., C3)
- IgA deficiency is associated with
  - Trisomy 21
  - 22q11.2 deletion syndrome
  - 18q syndrome
  - Monosomy 22
  - Monosomy 4p
  - Trisomy 8
  - Trisomy 10p
- Partial deletions in the long or short arm and ring forms of chromosome 18 and 17p11.2 deletions
- The presence of HLA-A1, HLA-A2, B8, DR3, DQ2 (8.1), and Dw3
- Also associated with non–MHC-associated genes involved in autoimmunity including *IFIH1* on chromosome 2q24, *CLEC16A* on chromosome 16

PATHOPHYSIOLOGY

- Unknown, however presumed to be a failure of B lymphocyte differentiation into plasma cells producing IgA
- Defect may be due to
  - Abnormal T-cell regulation (T-helper cells such as Tregs)
  - Antigen-presenting cells
  - Intrinsic B-cell defects
  - Impairment in cytokine networks including IL-21, IL-4, IL-6, IL-7, or IL-10

COMMONLY ASSOCIATED CONDITIONS

Increased association with the following:

- Atopy
- Recurrent sinopulmonary infections
- Gastrointestinal (GI) infections (especially *Giardia lamblia*)
- GI disease:
  - Celiac disease most common, incidence 2–3% of patients with IgA deficiency
  - Inflammatory bowel disease (Crohn disease and ulcerative colitis)
- Nodular lymphoid hyperplasia
- Malignancy, particularly adenocarcinoma of stomach and lymphoma usually of B-cell origin
- Autoimmune illnesses
  - Systemic lupus erythematosus
  - Immune endocrinopathies (e.g., Graves disease, type 1 diabetes)
  - Autoimmune hematologic conditions
  - Chronic active hepatitis

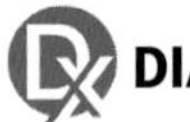

DIAGNOSIS

HISTORY

- Patients with IgA deficiency
  - Can have recurrent sinopulmonary infections
  - Can have frequent GI infections
  - Tend to have atopic disease such as allergic rhinitis, allergic conjunctivitis, urticaria, eczema, food allergy, asthma
  - Have an increased incidence of autoimmune diseases such as Graves disease, type 1 diabetes mellitus, rheumatoid arthritis, thyroiditis, systemic lupus erythematosus, autoimmune hemolytic anemia, and celiac disease
- Patients with concomitant IgG subclass deficiency are more likely to have recurrent sinopulmonary infections caused by extracellular encapsulated bacteria.
- Patients with low switched memory B cells exhibit more severe clinical features including pneumonia, autoimmune disease, bronchiectasis, hepatosplenomegaly, and specific antibody and IgG subclass deficiencies.
- Approximately 30% of patients with IgA deficiency are completely healthy.

PHYSICAL EXAM

- Look for signs of recurrent infection and atopy.
- Allergic rhinoconjunctivitis is associated with IgA deficiency. Signs include the following:
  - Cobblestoning of the conjunctiva
  - Allergic shiners
  - Pale and/or boggy nasal mucosa
- Serous otitis media may be the result of recurrent ear infections or persistent fluid:
  - Increased ear infections can be seen in IgA deficiency.
  - Persistent fluid can be secondary to allergic rhinoconjunctivitis.
- Pain on palpation of the sinuses
  - Recurrent sinus infections are associated with IgA deficiency.
- Lung examination
  - An increased frequency of pneumonia is associated with IgA deficiency.
  - Pay particular attention for signs of bronchiectasis.
- Swollen joints:
  - An increased frequency of autoimmune disease is associated with IgA deficiency.

DIFFERENTIAL DIAGNOSIS

- Toxic, environmental, drugs
  - Penicillamine and anticonvulsants can induce IgA deficiency.
- Cyclosporine A has been reported to cause permanent IgA deficiency.
- Genetic/metabolic
  - X-linked agammaglobulinemia (Bruton)
  - Common variable immunodeficiency (CVID)
  - Severe combined immunodeficiency
  - Ataxia telangiectasia
  - DiGeorge syndrome
  - Chronic mucocutaneous candidiasis
  - Nezelof syndrome
  - Selective IgG2 deficiency
- Miscellaneous: Patients may be completely healthy, and IgA deficiency may be an incidental finding.

ALERT

Factors that may alert you to request a referral include the following:

- Suggestion that IgA deficiency may be part of a more complex immune deficiency: An allergist/immunologist can assist with an appropriate immunologic evaluation.
- Suggestion of associated autoimmune disease: Evaluation and treatment by a rheumatologist is indicated.
- Patient likely to need a blood transfusion: An allergist/immunologist can help select appropriate blood products.

DIAGNOSTIC TESTS & INTERPRETATION

The general goal is to decide whether the patient's complaints are consistent with IgA deficiency (frequent upper respiratory and GI infections or allergies).

- Measure serum IgA level
  - Patient is considered deficient if the serum IgA level is <7 mg/dL.
  - If the patient is IgA deficient, exclude other conditions associated with IgA deficiency.
- Total immunoglobulins
  - If normal, helps rule out X-linked agammaglobulinemia (Bruton), CVID, and severe combined immunodeficiency
- IgG subclasses
  - Helps rule out an associated IgG subclass deficiency
- Lymphocyte stimulation to mitogens
  - A functional lymphocyte study
  - If normal, helps rule out CVID, severe combined immunodeficiency, ataxia telangiectasia, DiGeorge syndrome, and Nezelof syndrome
- Lymphocyte stimulation to *Candida* antigen
  - No response to *Candida* in vivo is consistent with chronic mucocutaneous candidiasis.
- Specific antibody responses to polysaccharide and protein antigens: to evaluate for an associated specific antibody deficiency
- Evaluate for signs/symptoms of bronchiectasis in cases of recurrent sinopulmonary infections.
- Screening for celiac disease
  - Should include IgG antibodies against gliadin and tissue transglutaminase because IgA isotype may not be detected

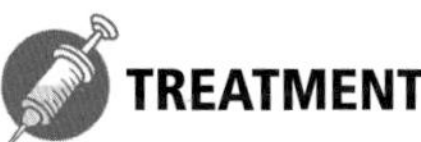

TREATMENT

GENERAL MEASURES

- There is no specific drug therapy.
- Recurrent infections should be treated aggressively with broad-spectrum antibiotics.
- Antibiotic prophylaxis to prevent recurrent sinopulmonary infections is often indicated.
- Vaccination with polyvalent pneumococcal vaccines may be considered to increase immunity.
- IV gammaglobulin is generally not indicated unless there is evidence of an associated specific antibody deficiency or in the severe phenotype of IgA deficiency (recurrent, persistent, invasive infections).

ALERT

Patients with no detectable IgA may develop antibodies against IgA in transfused blood products. These patients are at risk for allergic reactions including anaphylactic (or anaphylactoid) transfusion reactions on subsequent exposure. It should be noted, however, that life-saving products should not be withheld in emergent situations. In the nonurgent setting, to avoid potential allergic reactions, patients may receive the following:

- Packed RBCs (only if these cells have been washed 3 times)
- Plasma products from IgA-deficient donors
- Autologous banked blood

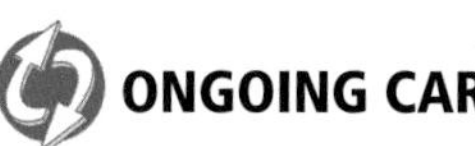

ONGOING CARE

FOLLOW-UP RECOMMENDATIONS

- Patients should be observed for the following:
  - Sinopulmonary infections, particularly signs/symptoms of bronchiectasis
  - GI infections
  - Autoimmune diseases
  - Inflammatory bowel disease
  - Malignancy typically of lymphoid origin
- It is important to manage infectious complications aggressively and to intervene promptly if associated conditions develop.
- It is also known that IgA deficiency may progress to CVID in some cases, typically in adolescence or young adulthood.

PATIENT EDUCATION

- IgA deficiency can be induced by some anticonvulsants and by penicillamine.
- IgA-deficient patients should wear medical alert bracelets. These patients can have anaphylaxis if administered blood products containing IgA. In an emergent situation, this is important information for caregivers to know. However, this is not very common and does not occur with the first blood product infusion/transfusion.

PROGNOSIS

Survival into the 7th decade is common; however, it is also known that some patients may progress to CVID.

COMPLICATIONS

Increased incidence of the following:

- Sinopulmonary infections
- GI tract infections
- Atopy
- Autoimmune diseases
- Malignancy

ADDITIONAL READING

- Burrows PD, Cooper MD. IgA deficiency. *Adv Immunol*. 1997;65:245–276.
- Janzi M, Kull I, Sjöberg R, et al. Selective IgA deficiency in early life: association to infections and allergic diseases during childhood. *Clin Immunol*. 2009;133(1):78–85.
- Smith CA, Driscoll DA, Emanuel BS, et al. Increased prevalence of immunoglobulin A deficiency in patients with the chromosome 22q11.2 deletion syndrome (DiGeorge syndrome/velocardiofacial syndrome). *Clin Diagn Lab Immunol*. 1998;5(3):415–417.
- Stiehm RE. The four most common pediatric immunodeficiencies. *Adv Exp Med Biol*. 2007;601:15–26.
- Wang N, Hammarström L. IgA deficiency: what is new? *Curr Opin Allergy Clin Immunol*. 2012;12(6):602–608.
- Yazdani R, Azizi G, Abolhassani H, et al. Selective IgA deficiency: epidemiology, pathogenesis, clinical phenotype, diagnosis, prognosis and management. *Scand J Immunol*. 2017;85(1):3–12.
- Yel L. Selective IgA deficiency. *J Clin Immunol*. 2010;30(1):10–16.

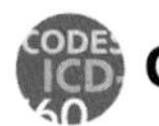

CODES

ICD10

D80.2 Selective deficiency of immunoglobulin A [IgA]

FAQ

- Q: Should patients with IgA deficiency be monitored for the development of progressive immunodeficiency?
- A: Patients with IgA deficiency should be monitored for progression to CVID, as this is associated with a poorer prognosis and would require treatment with IV gammaglobulin.
- Q: Should IgA-deficient patients wear medical alert bracelets?
- A: Yes. These patients can have anaphylaxis if they are given blood products containing IgA. In an emergent situation, this is important information for caregivers to know.

IMMUNOGLOBULIN A NEPHROPATHY

Maha N. Haddad, MD • Lavjay Butani, MD, MACM

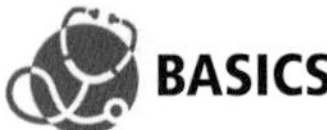

BASICS

DESCRIPTION

Primary immune complex–mediated glomerulonephritis

EPIDEMIOLOGY

- Most common chronic glomerulonephritis worldwide
- Prevalence varies considerably across countries; more common in Caucasians and Asians compared to African Americans
- Because reported prevalence is based on biopsy-confirmed diagnosis and therefore does not account for mild or asymptomatic cases, reported data grossly underestimate "true" prevalence.
- Represents 2–10% of all biopsy-confirmed primary glomerular diseases in adults in the United States
- No robust epidemiologic data in children

RISK FACTORS

- Typically sporadic
- Familial cases have been described suggesting that genetic factors influence susceptibility to and severity of disease.
- Reported in children with history of perinatal HIV-1 infection
- Increased risk of IgA nephropathy in adult patients with celiac disease, cirrhosis, inflammatory bowel disease, and HIV infection

PATHOPHYSIOLOGY

- Etiology and pathogenesis remain uncertain.
- Substantial evidence that IgA nephropathy is a systemic immune complex–mediated disease as it recurs after transplantation
- Multiple studies have found abnormal glycosylation patterns of the IgA1 molecule (galactose deficiency), suggesting the following hypotheses:
  - Glycan-specific IgG antibodies form immune complexes with galactose-deficient IgA1.
  - Complexes deposit in the glomerular mesangium
  - Activated mesangial cells proliferate and secrete extracellular matrix, cytokines, and chemokines with resulting renal injury.
- Majority of patients have elevated galactose-deficient IgA1 in the serum.

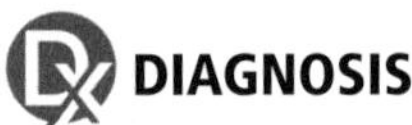

DIAGNOSIS

HISTORY

- Clinical presentation varies widely in constellation of signs and symptoms and also in severity.
- Patients may be completely asymptomatic.
- In children, the most common presentation is recurrent gross hematuria.
  - Triggered by acute upper respiratory tract infection in about half of the patients
  - In IgA nephropathy, in contrast to postinfectious glomerulonephritis, the hematuria presents at the same time ("synpharyngitic") or within a few days after the onset of the respiratory illness.
- Other presentations include the following:
  - Microscopic hematuria found on routine urinalysis (UA)
  - Hematuria (gross or microscopic) and variable levels of proteinuria
  - Acute nephritic syndrome (hematuria, proteinuria, edema, impaired renal function, and hypertension). Rarely, this may be rapidly progressive or accompanied by pulmonary inflammation/hemorrhage.
  - Nephrotic syndrome: edema, hypoalbuminemia, and nephrotic range proteinuria

PHYSICAL EXAM

- Hypertension: usually absent in mild disease; variably present depending on severity
- Edema: found in patients with heavy proteinuria and acute nephritic syndrome

DIFFERENTIAL DIAGNOSIS

- Thin basement membrane disease, Alport syndrome, or idiopathic hypercalciuria in mild cases presenting with hematuria
- Other forms of glomerulonephritis must be considered in the setting of a more acute presentation, including the following:
  - Postinfectious glomerulonephritis
  - Lupus nephritis
  - Membranoproliferative glomerulonephritis (MPGN)
  - Pauci-immune glomerulonephritis
  - Other vasculitides
  - Henoch-Schönlein purpura nephritis has similar biopsy findings as IgA nephropathy but has additional nonrenal manifestations such as skin rash, abdominal pain, and periarthritis.

DIAGNOSTIC TESTS & INTERPRETATION

Initial Tests (screening, lab, imaging)

- UA: RBCs, RBC casts, and protein
- Spot urine protein/creatinine ratio or 24-hour urine collection to quantify proteinuria
- Comprehensive metabolic panel
  - Kidney function tests (blood urea nitrogen and serum creatinine), serum electrolytes, and albumin are normal in mild disease.
  - Variably abnormal based on severity of disease
- In patients presenting with rapidly progressive glomerulonephritis, check complement levels, antinuclear antibody (ANA), antineutrophil cytoplasmic antibody (ANCA), and anti-glomerular basement membrane (GBM) antibodies to rule out other diseases.
- Serum IgA levels have very low sensitivity and specificity and are not recommended.
- Kidney ultrasound findings are nonspecific and either normal or, in more severe cases, may demonstrate increased echogenicity of the renal parenchyma.

Diagnostic Procedures/Other

- Kidney biopsy is required for a definitive diagnosis.
- Hallmark of the diagnosis is the presence, on immunofluorescence staining, of IgA deposits in the mesangium, either alone or with C3 (in children), IgM and IgG, or both (in adults).
- Biopsy is generally not required in mild cases as it does not affect the management or prognosis in the absence of proteinuria.
- Biopsy findings are variable on light microscopy:
  - Main finding is diffuse or focal mesangial proliferation with mesangial expansion.
  - Other possible findings include segmental or global endocapillary hypercellularity with segmental crescents and segmental necrosis.
  - Glomerulosclerosis in advanced disease
  - Tubulointerstitium is usually normal with varying degree of atrophy and fibrosis in chronic cases.
  - Electron microscopy: immune complex deposits in the mesangium
  - Several histologic classifications have been developed with the purpose of predicting clinical course, prognosticating, and in guiding therapy.
  - The Oxford classification is one such example, based on a constellation of findings such as mesangial cellularity score, segmental glomerulosclerosis, endocapillary hypercellularity, and tubular atrophy/fibrosis.

ALERT

May be progressive and lead to end-stage renal disease (ESRD) in moderate to severe cases. Refer to a nephrologist if persistent proteinuria, abnormal creatinine, gross hematuria, or hypertension.

TREATMENT

- Weak evidence base and mostly derived from expert opinion
- Varies based on severity of renal impairment, amount of proteinuria, and whether or not the course is rapidly progressive with associated crescents on biopsy. Higher amounts and persistence of proteinuria are associated with greater risk of disease progression.

GENERAL MEASURES

- Clinical presentation: Treat hypercholesterolemia associated with nephrotic syndrome. Address factors that modulate progression of chronic kidney disease (CKD)—obesity, smoking, hypertension.
- Optimize blood pressure control using angiotensin-converting enzyme inhibitor (ACEI) when possible.

MEDICATION

- Control of proteinuria and blood pressure
  - Protein excretion 0.5 to 1 g/1.73 m^2/24 h: ACEI or angiotensin receptor blockers (ARBs). Increase dose to effect as long as symptomatic hypotension or hyperkalemia do not develop.
  - Protein excretion $>$1 g/1.73 m^2/24 h despite optimum blood pressure control and the use of ACEI or ARB and when GFR is $>$50 mL/min/1.73 m^2: Consider alternate day oral glucocorticoids for 6 months (limited evidence-based).
- Rapidly progressive glomerulonephritis and/or crescents on biopsy: IV (followed by oral) glucocorticoids and consider additional immunosuppression such as cyclophosphamide or azathioprine or even plasmapheresis (Strength of evidence is poor for immunosuppression other than ACEI/ARB and glucocorticoids.)

ADDITIONAL THERAPIES

- Fish oil suggested when proteinuria is persistent $>$1 g/1.73 m^2/24 h despite optimal supportive care.
- Mycophenolate mofetil: multiple studies with conflicting conclusions
- Tonsillectomy: limited and low quality data which currently do not support this as a useful treatment option

ADMISSION, INPATIENT, AND NURSING CONSIDERATIONS

- Admission should take place under the care of pediatric nephrologist.
- Admission maybe needed based on the clinical presentation or complications of IgA nephropathy: such as to establish the diagnosis if the presentation was severe or to treat complications including acute kidney injury (AKI), severe hypertension, CKD, or nephrotic syndrome
- Nursing considerations vary based on the reason for the admission as the acuity of care would vary: In general, close monitoring of blood pressure, weight, and intake/output are of great importance.

ONGOING CARE

FOLLOW-UP RECOMMENDATIONS

IgA nephropathy may be a progressive disease. Patients should be monitored periodically for the following:

- Kidney function tests
- Level of proteinuria
- Blood pressure
- Intensity and frequency of monitoring depends on severity. Patients presenting with microscopic hematuria and minimal proteinuria should be monitored with UA at least every 6 months to assess for progression of proteinuria.

PROGNOSIS

- Variable depending on severity of clinical presentation and renal histopathologic score
- 15–40% of adult patients with IgA nephropathy eventually progress to ESRD.
- Although some reports suggest that children are more likely to have a benign course and have better prognosis than adults, other studies have reported similar outcomes for adults and children.
- In one series, renal survival rates in Japanese children were 95% at 10 years and 80% at 20 years.
- Patients who present with microscopic hematuria and minimal proteinuria have an excellent prognosis.
- Clinical predictors associated with poor outcome include severe persistent proteinuria, hypertension, and impaired renal function at presentation.
- The strongest predictive factor is the amount and persistence of proteinuria.
- Histopathologic features associated with poor outcome include mesangial hypercellularity score, endocapillary hypercellularity, tubular atrophy, and glomerular crescents.

ADDITIONAL READING

- Edström Halling S, Söderberg MP, Berg UB. Predictors of outcome in paediatric IgA nephropathy with regard to clinical and histopathological variables (Oxford classification). *Nephrol Dial Transplant*. 2012;27(2):715–722.
- Gutiérrez E, Zamora I, Ballarín JA, et al; for Grupo de Estudio de Enfermedades Glomerulares de la Sociedad Española de Nefrología. Long-term outcomes of IgA nephropathy presenting with minimal or no proteinuria. *J Am Soc Nephrol*. 2012;23(10):1753–1760.
- Hogg RJ, Fitzgibbons L, Atkins C, et al; for North American IgA Nephropathy Study Group. Efficacy of omega-3 fatty acids in children and adults with IgA nephropathy is dosage-and size-dependent. *Clin J Am Soc Nephrol*. 2006;1(6):1167–1172.
- Purswani MU, Chernoff MC, Mitchell CD, et al. Chronic kidney disease associated with perinatal HIV infection in children and adolescents. *Pediatr Nephrol*. 2012;27(6):981–989.
- Radhakrishnan J, Cattran DC. The KDIGO practice guideline on glomerulonephritis: reading between the (guide)lines—application to the individual patient. *Kidney Int*. 2012;82(8):840–856.
- Rauen T, Eitner F, Fitzner C, et al; for STOP-IgAN Investigators. Intensive supportive care plus immunosuppression in IgA nephropathy. *N Engl J Med*. 2015;373(23):2225–2236.
- Ronkainen J, Ala-Houhala M, Autio-Harmainen H, et al. Long-term outcome 19 years after childhood IgA nephritis: a retrospective cohort study. *Pediatr Nephrol*. 2006;21(9):1266–1273.
- Shima Y, Nakanishi K, Hama T, et al. Validity of the Oxford classification of IgA nephropathy in children. *Pediatr Nephrol*. 2012;27(5):783–792.
- Suzuki H, Kiryluk K, Novak J, et al. The pathophysiology of IgA nephropathy. *J Am Soc Nephrol*. 2011;22(10):1795–1803.
- Wang T, Ye F, Meng H, et al. Comparison of clinicopathological features between children and adults with IgA nephropathy. *Pediatr Nephrol*. 2012;27(8):1293–1300.
- Welander A, Sundelin B, Fored M, et al. Increased risk of IgA nephropathy among individuals with celiac disease. *J Clin Gastroenterol*. 2013;47(8): 678–683.

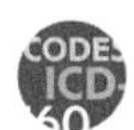

CODES

ICD10

- N02.8 Recurrent and persistent hematuria w oth morphologic changes
- N02.5 Recurrent and perst hematur w diffuse mesangiocap glomrlneph
- N02.2 Recurrent and perst hematur w diffuse membranous glomrlneph

FAQ

- Q: Will my child ever outgrow IgA nephropathy?
- A: No. The etiology and pathogenesis of IgA nephropathy remain uncertain. IgA nephropathy is a chronic condition, but sometimes it can go into spontaneous remission. Spontaneous remission is reported to occur in 59% of children with mild disease. More severe cases can also go into remission with medications.
- Q: My child has had a kidney transplant. Can IgA nephropathy recur in the graft?
- A: Yes. Recurrence of the condition can develop in 33% of patients. Depending on the published series, recurrence rates vary between 9% and 66%. However, even if it does come back, it can usually be controlled/treated with medications.
- Q: My child has microscopic hematuria and proteinuria. He has normal kidney function and blood pressure. His kidney biopsy was consistent with the diagnosis of IgA nephropathy. What is the strongest predictor for progression?
- A: The amount and persistence of proteinuria. Children with no or mild proteinuria usually have good long-term prognosis, whereas those with high amounts of protein in the urine are more likely to progress and develop long-term kidney damage.

IMPERFORATE ANUS

Lusine Ambartsumyan, MD

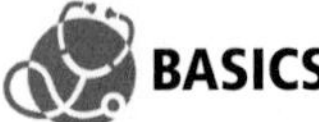

BASICS

DESCRIPTION

- Imperforate anus (IA) is a congenital abnormality in which the bowel fails to perforate or only partially perforates the pelvic muscular floor.
- IA may also perforate the epidermal covering of the pelvic muscular floor (anal membrane).
- Spectrum of anorectal malformations that range in severity from imperforate anal membrane to complete caudal regression
- IA has been classically subcategorized into low or high anomalies.
  - In a low lesion, the colon remains close to the skin and there may be a stenosis of the anus, or the anus may be missing altogether, with the rectum ending in a blind pouch.
  - In a high lesion, the colon is higher up in the pelvis, with a fistula connecting the rectum and the bladder, urethra, or the vagina.
- More recently, classification of IA is based on the presence or absence of fistula and the type of fistulous connection (perineal, bladder, urethra, vagina).

EPIDEMIOLOGY

- Prevalence is estimated to be in the range of 1:4,000 to 1:5,000.
- High lesions are more common in males (2:1).
- Low lesions occur with equal frequency in both sexes.

RISK FACTORS

Genetics

- An isolated defect (~1/3) or part of a syndrome or association (~2/3)
- Chromosomal abnormalities in 4.5–11%. Most common anomaly is trisomy 21 where patients typically have IA without fistula.
- Increased risk in 1st-degree relatives; reports of familial inheritance
- Can be part of omphalocele-exstrophy of the bladder-IA-spinal defects (OEIS) complex or cloacal exstrophy (EC)
- Genes implicated in animal studies: *SHH*, *Wnt5a*, and *Skt*

PATHOPHYSIOLOGY

- During the 6th week of fetal development, the hindgut comes into contact with the cloacal membrane. The hindgut is divided into a ventral urogenital and dorsal rectal component. By the 8th week, the dorsal 1/2 perforates to the exterior. In IA, the process is arrested during this critical period.
- There is a wide spectrum of anatomic variants of IA; commonly associated with urologic and spinal defects
- Classification of anatomic variants is based on the relationship between the rectum and the puborectalis muscle: supralevator (high) and translevator (low) malformations
- Cloaca is a complex defect, where the rectum, urethra, and the vagina drain into a common channel that communicates with the perineum.
- A fistula communicating from the rectum to the external opening (perineal fistula) or to the urogenital system is present in 90% of cases.
- In females, the most common defect is a rectovestibular fistula where the rectum opens into the vestibule.
- In males, the most common defect is a rectourethral fistula from the rectum to lower posterior urethra (bulbar) or upper posterior urethra (prostatic).

COMMONLY ASSOCIATED CONDITIONS

- Anomalies present in 50–67% of patients with IA
- VACTERL is the most common associated anomaly and includes vertebral, cardiac, tracheoesophageal fistula, and renal and limb anomalies.
- Associated organ-specific anomalies:
  - Genitourinary (33–50%): vesicoureteral reflux, renal agenesis, horseshoe kidney, multicystic kidney, ectopic kidney, obstruction, hypoplasia/dysplasia, and chronic renal failure (2–6%).
  - Spine/sacrum (33–50%): tethered cord (most common 20–30%), hypoplastic sacrum, sacral agenesis, presacral mass, vertebral defects formation/fusion, myelomeningocele
  - Gastrointestinal (5–10%): tracheoesophageal atresia and esophageal atresia; others include malrotation, omphalocele, annular pancreas.
  - Gynecologic (~7–17%): vaginal atresia, absent vagina/cervix/uterus, septate vagina, and duplicate uterus
  - Cardiovascular defects (10–30%): atrial and ventricular septal defects
- Other associated syndromes:
  - Currarino (sacral agenesis, presacral mass, and IA)
  - Trisomy 21
  - Townes-Brock syndrome
  - Fragile X
  - McKusick-Kaufman
  - Johanson-Blizzard
  - Opitz-Kaveggia

DIAGNOSIS

HISTORY

- May be diagnosed prenatally (dilated colon, oligohydramnios) especially in setting of associated anomalies
- Most children are diagnosed during a routine neonatal examination.
- Failure to pass meconium, constipation, and/or signs of intestinal obstruction (abdominal distention and bilious vomiting) should mandate reexamination of the perianal area.
- Approximately 13–25% may present beyond the neonatal period; late diagnosis is associated with higher morbidity (19–35%) and mortality (4–10%).

PHYSICAL EXAM

- Placement of the anus: lack of anal opening, anterior or abnormal anal position
- In females, critical to ensure the presence of anal, vaginal, and urethral opening. A single perineal opening indicates likely cloaca.
- Decreased or abnormal radial corrugations of anus
- Abnormal rectal caliber (stenosis)
- Poor anal tone or patulous anal opening
- Absent, asymmetric, or abnormal location of anal wink
- Spinal dimples or tufts
- Flat buttocks, abnormal gluteal crease, lack of midline grove
- Abnormal genitourinary or neurologic examination
- Associated cardiac, vertebral, or limb anomalies

DIFFERENTIAL DIAGNOSIS

- No disorders can mimic IA.
- Neonates may present with failure to pass meconium and intestinal obstruction.
- Older patients may present with intractable constipation and fecal impaction.
- A meticulous perineal examination is critical.
- Upon identification of IA, primary goal is to define the location of the termination of the bowel and the opening of the fistula.

DIAGNOSTIC TESTS & INTERPRETATION

Initial Tests (screening, lab, imaging)

- Screening and exclusion of potential serious associated anomalies (VACTERL screening)
- Classification of the malformation and surgical plan (diverting colostomy or a primary repair) must be formulated within 24 hours to prevent complications.
- Prone cross-table lateral and invertogram:
  - After sufficient time for a transit of gas (>12 hours after birth), the child is placed in an upside-down position for 5 minutes.
  - After which a lateral view of the pelvis is obtained to identify level of obstruction (low or high).
- Nasogastric tube placement and chest x-ray should be obtained to evaluate for esophageal atresia and tracheoesophageal fistula (commonly associated).
- Echocardiogram
- Lumbosacral films to evaluate for vertebral anomalies and sacral integrity (calculation of sacral ratio)
- Ultrasound (US) of the spine to assess for tethered cord. MRI of the spine and pelvis should be considered in a child greater than 3 months to look for a tethered cord and evaluate the pelvic anatomy.
- Renal US to evaluate the kidneys and the urinary system for hydronephrosis, megaureter
- Pelvic US to evaluate for hydrocolpos
- Abdominal US to rule out duodenal atresia

- Voiding cystourethrogram and IV pyelogram can be used if urinary tract anomalies are highly suspected.
- Postsurgically: colostogram after formation of colostomy and prior to final repair to evaluate the fistula and the rectum. In older children, a water contrast enema may be needed to evaluate the anatomy: rectosigmoid caliber and for remnant genitourinary fistulas.

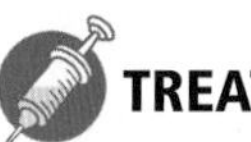

TREATMENT

SURGERY/OTHER PROCEDURES

- Surgery should be performed by an experienced surgeon.
- High lesions require an emergent and protective diverting colostomy, followed by pull-through procedure with posterior sagittal anorectoplasty (PSARP) at 3 to 9 months of age. Colostomy is closed after the anoplasty has healed and any necessary secondary dilations have been completed.
- Laparoscopy-assisted PSARP may be performed in those with complex and high lesions.
- Posterior sagittal anorectal-vaginal-urethral plasty with total urogenital mobilization or with laparotomy is performed for cloaca abnormalities.
- After surgery, follow-up with anal dilatation helps minimize the risk of stricture formation, as well as for the newly constructed canal to become functional.
- Complications of surgery may include: wound infections, anal strictures, rectal prolapse, femoral nerve injury, neurogenic bladder, rectourinary fistula, urologic injuries, vaginal stenosis

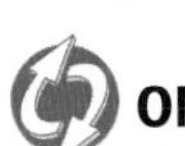

ONGOING CARE

PATIENT EDUCATION

- Prognosis for bowel and urine continence depends on the type of anorectal malformation, degree of associated defects, presence of spinal abnormalities, and sacral integrity.
- In general, children with low malformations have better functional outcomes of bowel and bladder and better bowel and bladder control.
  - However, low malformations also have increased incidence of megacolon and subsequent constipation and "overflow" incontinence.
- High malformations have poor bowel and bladder control and subsequent fecal and urinary incontinence. They also have increased associated defects and organ specific complications.

PROGNOSIS

- Prognostic factors: type of malformation, sacral integrity, spinal anomalies, and length of the cloaca common channel
- Sacral integrity described to be the most important prognostic indicator of bowel control
- Good prognostic indicators of bowel control:
  - Normal sacral integrity
  - No presacral mass
  - Two well-formed buttocks and midline groove
  - Low anorectal malformations (rectal atresia, rectoperineal fistula, rectobulbar urethral fistula, cloaca with common channel <3 cm, and IA without fistula)
- Poor prognostic indicators of bowel control:
  - Abnormal sacral integrity
  - Myelomeningocele
  - High anorectal malformations (rectoprostatic urethral fistula, rectobladder neck fistula, EC cloaca, >3 cm common channel, complex defects)
- Experienced centers report
  - ~75% have voluntary bowel movements after age 3 years, of which 50% continue to have intermittent fecal incontinence.
  - In their cohort, ~25% have fecal incontinence despite treatment.
- Continence can be attained in 80–90% of patients who have low lesions.
- <50% of patients with high lesions are continent before school age, but most continue to improve and achieve continence by adolescence.
- Many patients will need a comprehensive bowel management program where they may require high-volume daily enemas or an appendicostomy to prevent or reduce constipation (megacolon) and achieve fecal continence.
- Patients with poor prognostic indicators and associated genitourinary abnormalities need to be monitored for urinary incontinence and renal complications (chronic kidney disease, ESRD). Those with cloaca and high malformations may require clean intermittent catheterizations or urinary diversion for continence.
- Gynecologic evaluation and monitoring for abnormal menstruation and introitus stenosis during puberty
- Sexual function is greatly preserved in patients who have undergone PSARP and the subsequent modern surgical techniques.
- Fertility data are lacking.

ADDITIONAL READING

- Bischoff A, Levitt MA, Peña A. Update on the management of anorectal malformations. *Pediatr Surg Int*. 2013;29(9):899–904.
- Bischoff A, Martinez-Leo B, Peña A. Laparoscopic approach in the management of anorectal malformations. *Pediatr Surg Int*. 2015;31(5):431–437.
- Di Lorenzo C, Benninga MA. Pathophysiology of pediatric fecal incontinence. *Gastroenterology*. 2004;126(1 Suppl 1):S33–S40.
- Herman RS, Teitelbaum DH. Anorectal malformations. *Clin Perinatol*. 2012;39(2):403–422.
- Khalil BA, Morabito A, Bianchi A. Transanoproctoplasty: a 21-year review. *J Pediatr Surg*. 2010;45(9):1915–1919.
- Lane VA, Skerritt C, Wood RJ, et al. A standardized approach for the assessment and treatment of internationally adopted children with a previously repaired anorectal malformation (ARM). *J Pediatr Surg*. 2016;51(11):1864–1870.
- Levitt M, Kant A, Peña A. The morbidity of constipation in patients with anorectal malformations. *J Pediatr Surg*. 2010;45(6):1228–1233.
- Levitt M, Peña A. Update on pediatric faecal incontinence. *Eur J Pediatr Surg*. 2009;19(1):1–9.
- Pakarinen M, Rintala R. Management and outcome of low anorectal malformations. *Pediatr Surg Int*. 2010;26(11):1057–1063.
- Peña A, Hong A. Advances in the management of anorectal malformations. *Am J Surg*. 2000;180(5):370–376.
- Rintala RJ, Pakarinen MP. Imperforate anus: long- and short-term outcome. *Semin Pediatr Surg*. 2008;17(2):79–89.
- van der Steeg HJ, Schmiedeke E, Bagolan P, et al. European consensus meeting of ARM-Net members concerning diagnosis and early management of newborns with anorectal malformations. *Tech Coloproctol*. 2015;19(3):181–185.
- Wang C, Li L, Cheng W. Anorectal malformation: the etiological factors. *Pediatr Surg Int*. 2015;31(9):795–804.

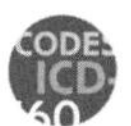

CODES

ICD10

- Q42.3 Congenital absence, atresia and stenosis of anus without fistula
- Q42.2 Congenital absence, atresia and stenosis of anus with fistula

FAQ

- Q: Is IA an isolated defect in my child?
- A: IA is often associated with multiple other anomalies. In particular, renal and vertebral anomalies must be excluded.
- Q: What is the genetic basis for this defect?
- A: IA can be associated with chromosomal anomalies or can be an isolated problem.
- Q: How likely is it that my child will ever be able to be toilet trained successfully?
- A: Successful toilet training will depend on what type of IA defect your child has: Children with high lesions may have more difficulty becoming toilet trained than children with low lesions. All children should improve over time but will need specialist treatment and a comprehensive bowel management program for many years to prevent or reduce constipation and fecal incontinence.

IMPETIGO

Maribeth Chitkara, MD

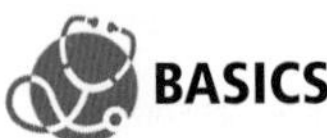

BASICS

DESCRIPTION

- Impetigo is a superficial skin infection seen frequently in children.
  - It is one of the most common skin and soft tissue infections observed in pediatrics.
  - Pyoderma and impetigo contagiosa are synonyms for impetigo.
- Classification
  - Primary impetigo: direct bacterial invasion of previously normal skin
  - Secondary impetigo: infection at sites of minor skin trauma or underlying conditions
- Types of impetigo
  - Nonbullous impetigo
    - Most common form, >70% of cases
    - Lesions begin as papules that progress to vesicles surrounded by erythema.
    - Subsequently, the papules mature into pustules that enlarge and break down to form thick, adherent, golden crusts.
  - Bullous impetigo
    - Vesicles enlarge to form bullae containing clear yellow fluid, which become darker and more turbid.
    - Ruptured bullae leave a honey-colored crust.
  - Ecthyma
    - An ulcerative form of impetigo
    - Lesions extend through the epidermis and deep into the dermis.

EPIDEMIOLOGY

- Location
  - Most frequently in tropical or subtropical regions
  - Also prevalent in northern climates during summer months
- Age:
  - Found most commonly in children aged 2 to 5 years
  - Can spread rapidly through child care centers and schools

RISK FACTORS

- Poverty, overcrowding
- Poor hygiene
- Underlying scabies infection
- Eczema

ETIOLOGY

- *Staphylococcus aureus*: most common etiologic agent. Toxin-producing strains cause cleavage in superficial skin layer.
- Impetigo due to community-associated methicillin-resistant *S. aureus* (CA-MRSA) has occurred in a minority of cases.
- β-Hemolytic streptococci (primarily group A, but serogroups C and G have been implicated in some cases)

DIAGNOSIS

HISTORY

- Patients with impetigo may report a history of minor trauma, insect bites, scabies, herpes simplex virus infection, varicella infection, or eczema before the development of the infection. Lesions are usually present for a few days to weeks before the patient seeks medical attention.
- Lesions may be described as itchy but are usually painless.
- Additional symptoms such as fever, respiratory distress, vomiting, or diarrhea are rare and perhaps indicative of another diagnosis.
- Outbreaks commonly occur in families and child care centers as well as among sports team members.

PHYSICAL EXAM

- Nonbullous impetigo
  - Usually occurs on exposed areas of body, most frequently the face and extremities
  - Lesions first begin as papules or thin-walled vesicles on an erythematous base. The lesions gradually enlarge, may coalesce, and break down over the course of 4 to 6 days. After rupture, their serum is released, which dries and forms a thick brown, "honey-colored" crust.
  - As the lesions resolve with treatment, the crusts slough from the affected areas and may leave hypopigmented areas.
  - Lymphadenopathy is rare.
- Bullous impetigo
  - Lesions may form on grossly normal or previously traumatized skin.
  - Appear initially as superficial vesicles that rapidly enlarge to form flaccid bullae, filled with clear yellow liquid that gradually becomes more turbid and sometimes purulent.
  - After the lesions rupture, a thin, light brown crust remains.
  - Lymphadenopathy is rare.
- Ecthyma
  - The lesion is a vesicle or pustule overlying an inflamed area of skin that deepens into a dermal ulceration. "Punched-out" ulcers are covered with yellow crust, surrounded by raised violaceous margins.
  - Ecthyma heals slowly and commonly produces a scar.
  - Regional lymphadenopathy may occur, but systemic symptoms are usually absent.

DIFFERENTIAL DIAGNOSIS

- Varicella
- Staphylococcal scalded-skin syndrome
- Erythema multiforme
- Herpes simplex virus infection
- Burns (thermal and chemical)
- Contact dermatitis
- Atopic dermatitis
- Tinea corporis
- Insect bites
- Scabies
- Lice

DIAGNOSTIC TESTS & INTERPRETATION

Initial Tests (screening, lab, imaging)

- Impetigo is a clinical diagnosis, and no laboratory workup is routinely indicated.
- Culture of pus or exudates from skin lesions is recommended to help identify whether *S. aureus* or β-hemolytic *Streptococcus* is the cause.
  - Swabs of intact skin are not helpful.
  - If systemic symptoms are present, a CBC and blood culture should be considered to evaluate for other possible causes of infection.
- Skin biopsy may be useful if diagnosis is unclear.

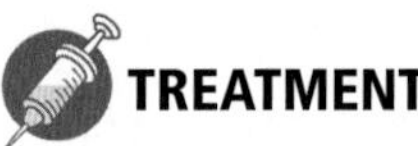

TREATMENT

GENERAL MEASURES

- Clipping fingernails short to minimize effects of scratching is recommended.
- Hand washing is important for reducing spread among children, as is covering the lesions.
- Treatment is important for reducing spread of infection to self and others.
- Cleansing and debriding the lesions are unnecessary.
- Crusted lesions can be cleansed gently with soap and water.

MEDICATION

- Topical therapy can be used for both bullous and nonbullous impetigo.
  - Mupirocin
    - 2% ointment or cream
    - Children >2 months old
    - Applied to affected areas 3 times daily for 5 days
  - Retapamulin
    - 1% ointment
    - Children >9 months old
    - Applied to affected area (up to 2% body surface area[BSA]) twice daily for 5 days
  - Emerging therapies
    - Ozenoxacin 1% cream
    - Clary sage (*Salvia sclarea*) oil
  - Although the components of over-the-counter triple antibiotic ointments (bacitracin, neomycin, polymyxin B) have some activity against the organisms causing impetigo, they are not considered effective for treatment.
- Oral therapy
  - Oral antibiotic therapy should be used for impetigo when the lesions are numerous or in outbreaks affecting multiple people to help decrease further transmission of infection.
  - Methicillin-sensitive *S. aureus* (MSSA) or β-hemolytic streptococci
    - Cephalexin 25 to 50 mg/kg/24 h PO in 3 to 4 divided doses
    - Erythromycin 40 mg/kg/24 h PO in 3 to 4 divided doses
    - Clindamycin 20 mg/kg/24 h PO in 3 divided doses
    - Amoxicillin/clavulanic acid 25 mg/kg/24 h PO in 2 divided doses
  - When MRSA is suspected
    - Clindamycin 20 mg/kg/24 h PO in 3 divided doses
    - Trimethoprim-sulfamethoxazole: trimethoprim 8 to 12 mg/kg and sulfamethoxazole 40 mg/kg daily PO in 2 divided doses (has activity against MRSA but not against streptococci)

ONGOING CARE

FOLLOW-UP RECOMMENDATIONS

- Duration of therapy
  - The duration of antimicrobial therapy should be tailored to clinical improvement.
  - 7 days of treatment is usually adequate.
  - Children should be excluded from out-of-home child care until 24 hours after treatment has been initiated.
- Signs of incomplete therapy
  - Recurrent infection may indicate incomplete therapy, reinfection, or an *S. aureus* carrier state.
  - Development of fever is unusual and may indicate a more serious infection and/or the presence of cellulitis or an abscess.
- Prevention of recurrence
  - Impetigo frequently spreads among close contacts and family members.
    - Patients and family members should wash their hands frequently.
    - Keep clothes and bedding clean.
    - Do not share towels and other personal care items.
  - Underlying skin conditions (e.g., eczema) and infestations (e.g., scabies) should be treated appropriately to decrease the likelihood of the development of impetigo.

COMPLICATIONS

- Cellulitis
- Lymphangitis
- Suppurative lymphadenitis
- Staphylococcal scalded-skin syndrome
- Poststreptococcal glomerulonephritis
  - Most cases are believed to be caused by a preceding streptococcal impetigo rather than streptococcal pharyngitis.
  - Deposition of group A β-hemolytic streptococci (GABHS) nephrogenic antigens induce immune complex formation in kidneys.
  - Latent period is 3 to 6 weeks following skin infection.
- Scarlet fever, osteomyelitis, septic arthritis, pneumonia, septicemia, and rheumatic fever have also been observed in patients with impetigo.

PROGNOSIS

The lesions of impetigo usually heal without significant scarring. Overall, the infection is highly curable, but the condition often recurs in young children.

ADDITIONAL READING

- Koning S, van der Sande R, Verhagen AP, et al. Interventions for impetigo. *Cochrane Database Syst Rev*. 2012;(1):CD003261.
- Stevens DL, Bisno AL, Chambers HF, et al. Practice guidelines for the diagnosis and management of skin and soft tissue infections: 2014 update by the Infectious Diseases Society of America. *Clin Infect Dis*. 2014;59(2):147–159.
- Todd JK. Staphylococcal infections. *Pediatr Rev*. 2005;26(12):444–450.

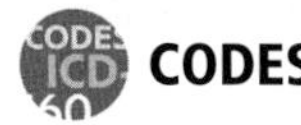

CODES

ICD10

- L01.00 Impetigo, unspecified
- L01.01 Non-bullous impetigo
- L01.09 Other impetigo

FAQ

- Q: Which is the more effective treatment for impetigo—oral or topical antibiotics?
- A: In general, if there are a few localized lesions, topical therapy is preferred. If there is more diffuse involvement, systemic symptoms, or an outbreak in multiple patients, a course of oral antibiotics is recommended.
- Q: Can a child with impetigo attend school or child care?
- A: The child should be excluded from child care until 24 hours after treatment has been initiated. Once the lesions begin to improve, the child may resume his or her activities without restrictions.
- Q: How does one help prevent impetigo from spreading?
- A: Gently wash the affected areas with mild soap and running water, use the antibiotics (topical or oral) as directed, and then cover lesions with bandages. Wear gloves when applying any antibiotic ointment to the patient's lesions and endorse thorough hand washing afterward. Do not share clothes, linens, or towels used by the affected individual until the infection has cleared.

INFANTILE SPASMS

John R. Mytinger, MD

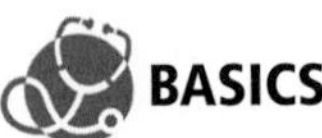

BASICS

DESCRIPTION

- Infantile spasms (IS) are seizures commonly associated with West syndrome—a severe infantile epileptic encephalopathy often with poor developmental outcome.
  - IS are characterized by sudden flexion, extension, or mixed flexion-extension of the neck, trunk, arms, and or legs.
  - IS can be subtle such as a mild contraction of the abdominal muscles or subtle movements of the head, shoulder, or eyes.
  - IS can occur singly, but the clustering (often on awakening) is helpful for diagnosis.
- IS are commonly dismissed as "normal" movements or misdiagnosed as reflux/colic.
- West syndrome is classically the triad of (i) IS, (ii) developmental delay, and (iii) hypsarrhythmia—a chaotic and high amplitude EEG background disrupted by frequent multifocal spikes.

EPIDEMIOLOGY

- The onset occurs in the 1st year of life in >90%, typically 3 to 12 months of age (peak onset 4 to 8 months, mean 6 months).
- Spasms rarely occur after 18 months of age.
- Given that spasms can occur outside the infantile period, the preferred inclusive terminology for this seizure type is *epileptic spasm*.

Incidence

The incidence is 2 to 3.5/10,000 live births.

PATHOPHYSIOLOGY

- Unknown
- In 70–80% of cases, a specific condition is associated with IS; however, this does not necessarily suggest a direct cause-and-effect relationship with IS.

RISK FACTORS

Genetics

There is an expanding list of IS-associated genes: *CDKL5* (more girls than boys), *STXBP1*, *ARX* (boys), *ALG13*, *DOCK7*, *DNM1*, *FOXG1* (duplications), *GABRB1*, *GABRB3*, *GNAO1*, *GRIN1*, *GRIN2A*, *GRIN2B*, *MAGI2*, *MEF2C*, *NEDDL4*, *NDP*, *NRXN1*, *PIGA*, *PLCB1*, *PTEN*, *SCA2*, *SCN1A*, *SETBP1*, *SIK1*, *SLC25A22*, *SLC35A2*, *SPTAN1*, *ST3Gal3*, *TBC1D24*, *TCF4*, *WWOX*.

COMMONLY ASSOCIATED CONDITIONS

- Hypoxic-ischemic encephalopathy (HIE)
- Chromosomal disorders such as trisomy 21
- Brain malformation such as holoprosencephaly, malformations of cortical development (such as pachygyria or lissencephaly [including Miller-Dieker syndrome with deletion of 17p13.3], hemimegalencephaly, schizencephaly, heterotopia, and focal cortical dysplasia)
- Stroke
- Intraventricular/intraparenchymal hemorrhage
- Periventricular leukomalacia
- Tuberous sclerosis complex (TSC)
- Other neurocutaneous conditions such as neurofibromatosis type 1 (NF1), incontinentia pigmenti achromians (hypomelanosis of Ito)
- Disorders of X-linked inheritance such as Aicardi syndrome (Consider in girls with agenesis of the corpus callosum and chorioretinal lacunae.)
- Hydrocephalus of various causes
- Trauma (any but often nonaccidental)
- Progressive encephalopathy with edema, hypsarrhythmia, and optic atrophy syndrome
- Infections: meningitis/encephalitis, congenital infections (e.g., toxoplasmosis, rubella, cytomegalovirus, HIV)
- Inborn errors of metabolism such as Menkes disease, disorders of amino acid metabolism (such as phenylketonuria and maple syrup urine disease), pyruvate dehydrogenase complex deficiency, mitochondrial disorders (such as Leigh syndrome), pyridoxine-dependent seizures, glucose transporter protein type 1 (GLUT1) deficiency, and uncommonly, organic acidurias (such as methylmalonic aciduria)

DIAGNOSIS

HISTORY

- A description of spells including the timing of onset (single IS can precede clustering)
- Prenatal and perinatal history including complications of pregnancy or delivery, gestational and maternal ages, place of birth (for access to newborn screening)
- History of HIE (perinatal, cardiac arrest, near drowning, near-miss SIDS)
- History of miscarriages, early infant death, family members with birth marks or seizures (A family history of IS is rare but can occur.)
- Developmental history including any loss of skills (loss of visual tracking or social smile)

PHYSICAL EXAM

- Head circumference
- Dysmorphisms (such as Down syndrome or Miller-Dieker syndrome)
- Cardiac murmur (rhabdomyoma in TSC)
- Skin abnormalities
  - Hypopigmented macules (may be present at birth in TSC and highlighted by the Wood lamp)
  - Café au lait spots (NF1)
- Hepatomegaly (inborn errors of metabolism)
- Retinal evaluation (for metabolic disease and chorioretinal lacunae in Aicardi syndrome)
- Social smile, tracking, strength (head lag and axial slipping with the child held underarm in vertical suspension), tone, and reflexes

DIFFERENTIAL DIAGNOSIS

- Normal movements confused with IS:
  - Moro reflex and similar-appearing startle/arousal responses
  - Normal sleep myoclonus and hypnagogic/hypnic jerks
- Nonepileptic movement disorders confused with IS:
  - Benign myoclonus of early infancy
  - Posturing
  - Hyperekplexia
  - Colic and gastroesophageal reflux (Sandifer syndrome)
- Epileptic syndrome confused with IS:
  - benign myoclonic epilepsy of infancy
- Neonatal epileptic encephalopathies that may include or evolve to IS:
  - Early infantile epileptic encephalopathy (Ohtahara syndrome)
  - Early myoclonic epilepsy
- Childhood epileptic encephalopathy that may include or evolve from IS: Lennox-Gastaut syndrome (LGS)

DIAGNOSTIC TESTS & INTERPRETATION

- Although nearly all children with IS have an abnormal EEG background, there is poor inter-rater reliability in the determination of hypsarrhythmia. So the presence or absence of hypsarrhythmia will depend on the EEG reader. Only about 60% have hypsarrhythmia (or one of its variants) at diagnosis. Thus, the presence of hypsarrhythmia is *not* required for the diagnosis or treatment of IS.
- The diagnosis is made with a video EEG to characterize the spell and EEG abnormalities.
- An epilepsy protocol brain MRI to determine the etiology is strongly recommended.
- Early diagnosis and effective treatment can improve developmental outcome.
- The diagnostic and posttreatment EEG should include sleep as EEG abnormalities are most often present during non-REM sleep.
  - IS begins with an initial phasic contraction lasting 1 to 2 seconds, sometimes followed by a tonic contraction that can last 2 to 10 seconds.
  - Most IS are clinically symmetric, but asymmetric spasms can occur and may indicate a focal brain lesion.
  - The EEG background is typically high voltage and disorganized; the background is typically disrupted by frequent multifocal spikes.
  - The EEG correlate of IS is often a slow wave or sharp, then slow wave followed by an electrodecrement (i.e., voltage attenuation).
- A 100-mg pyridoxine infusion during the EEG to assess for background improvement may help diagnose pyridoxine-dependent seizures.

Initial Tests (screening, lab, imaging)

- Testing should emphasize those conditions with a specific treatment:
  - Ammonia level
  - Serum lactic acid
  - Biotinidase assay (assess newborn screen) or biotin level
  - Serum amino acids (assess newborn screen)
  - Copper/ceruloplasmin (for Menkes disease)
  - Consider lumbar puncture (LP) for GLUT1 deficiency (compare CSF to serum glucose).
  - Urine organic acids (uncommon etiology, assess new born screen)
- Any metabolic, chromosomal, genetic, and CSF studies must be considered on an individual basis: karyotype and or microarray analysis (especially with dysmorphisms), IS-associated gene/panel testing, whole exome sequencing.
- Epilepsy protocol brain MRI is recommended.
- Consider a PET scan to assess for or better define a lesion that may be correctable with surgery.

Diagnostic Procedures/Other

Consider LP for neurotransmitter and folate metabolites, tetrahydrobiopterin, and lactic acid.

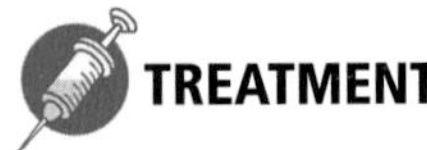

TREATMENT

MEDICATION

First Line

- Generally accepted 1st-line medical treatments include adrenocorticotropic hormone (ACTH), high-dose oral corticosteroids (HOC), and vigabatrin.

- The etiology may determine the initial treatment: epilepsy surgery (such as tumor, hydrocephalus), ketogenic diet (such as GLUT1 deficiency, pyruvate dehydrogenase complex deficiency), vigabatrin (TSC).
- One study showed that in patients with no known etiology, developmental outcomes are superior for patients initially treated with hormone therapy when compared to patients initially treated with vigabatrin.
- The approach should focus on an early "all or none" electroclinical remission with early changes in treatment if needed.
  - If no clinical remission by 2 weeks, consider changing or adding treatment.
  - If there is clinical remission, confirm absence of the epileptic encephalopathy with video EEG (e.g., 1-hour duration 14 to 21 days after the start of treatment).
  - A prolonged video EEG (e.g., overnight) is recommended by some experts to assure electroclinical remission (especially if subtle spasms are a concern); clinically apparent IS can convert to subtle IS with treatment.
  - If there is evidence of an ongoing epileptic encephalopathy or IS on video EEG, consider changing or adding treatment.
- ACTH
  - High rates of electroclinical remission have been reported with high-dose regimens (see Baram et al, 1996, for published regimen).
  - However, one study of high-dose (150 IU/m^2/24 h) versus low-dose (20 to 30 IU/24 h) ACTH found no difference in electroclinical remission rates.
  - Short-course ACTH may limit side effects.
  - Side effect profile
    - Common: weight gain (increased appetite/fluid retention), irritability, poor sleep, hypertension
    - Less common: hyperglycemia, electrolyte abnormalities (hypokalemia), hypertrophic cardiomyopathy, immunosuppression, gastritis/gastric ulcer, reduced bone mineral density, adrenal insufficiency/failure
    - Rare: death most typically due to immunosuppression with infection
  - Inpatient admission is often performed for initiation of treatment and caregiver education.
  - Monitoring during treatment
    - Gastric acid suppression to avoid gastritis/gastric ulceration is typical.
    - $\geq$1 time weekly during treatment: blood pressure, urine glucose, and stool guaiac
    - 1 time weekly during treatment: electrolytes
    - Treatment of hypertension may be needed.
- High-dose oral corticosteroids
  - High-dose regimens are recommended (see Lux et al, 2004, for published regimen).
  - The side effects, initial hospital admittance, and monitoring are the same as for ACTH.
- Vigabatrin
  - Initially, 50 mg/kg/24 h (divided twice daily) and increased by 50 mg/kg/24 h every 3 days to a maximum dose of 150 to 200 mg/kg/24 h (divided twice daily); faster titration schedules have been used.
  - If there is no response in 2 weeks, use an alternative treatment and taper vigabatrin off.
  - With electroclinical remission, the dose can be continued for about 6 months and then weaned.
  - Risk of permanent peripheral visual field loss
  - The incidence of clinically relevant visual changes with short courses of vigabatrin (e.g., 6 months) are unknown but appear to be low.
  - In one study, electroretinogram changes, a marker of retinal toxicity, occurred in 5.3% of children treated for 6 months and in 13.3% in those treated for 12 months.
  - The short-term rates of clinical remission appear to be superior with hormone treatment (ACTH or HOC) compared to vigabatrin, and this may impact later developmental outcome (at least for those with an unknown etiology).
- Combined treatment with a hormone treatment and vigabatrin
  - In one study, combining these 1st-line treatments significantly improved the rate of remission (72% remission with combined treatment vs. 57% with hormone therapy alone). However, there was no difference in remission rates between groups if only patients at high risk of developmental impairment were considered.
  - It remains unclear if initial combined therapy is superior (in regard to developmental outcome) to tandem treatment (i.e., a 1st-line treatment that fails to achieve remission followed by an alternative 1st-line treatment).
  - Other concerns with initial combined treatment include potentially unnecessary drug-related adverse events and drug cost (the latter is especially concerning in the United States where both ACTH and vigabatrin are exceptionally expensive).

Second Line

- Ketogenic diet: treatment of choice for some conditions and can be effective for others
- Zonisamide (5 to 15 mg/kg/24 h divided twice daily)
- Valproic acid: Consider *POLG* mutation analysis before starting (15 to 45 mg/kg/24 h in 2 to 3 divided doses).
- Oral pyridoxine: Some cases of pyridoxine-dependent seizures require longer treatment trials (e.g., 10 mg/kg/24 h for several weeks).
- Topiramate: not a 1st-line treatment due to the low-response rates but commonly used and occasionally effective (10 to 30 mg/kg/24 h divided twice daily)

SURGERY/OTHER PROCEDURES

Can be effective and should be considered early (generally after failed 1st-line treatment)

- Examples: functional hemispherectomy for stroke and hemimegalencephaly, shunting of hydrocephalus, and resection of a tumor and/or focal cortical dysplasia

ADMISSION, INPATIENT, AND NURSING CONSIDERATIONS

After the ABCs, consider metabolic stabilization and treatment of convulsive seizures if presenting with IS (IS themselves are typically not life-threatening).

ONGOING CARE

PROGNOSIS

- Prognosis depends on the underlying etiology and associated conditions.
- The best prognosis is typically for those with unknown etiology and normal development before diagnosis.
- About 1/3 die early (most from underlying disease and rarely from treatment).
- Spontaneous remission of IS can occur (cumulative rate of 25%, 1 year from onset).
- Regardless of treatment, IS typically remits (persisting beyond 7 years of age in only 8%).
- Early, successful, and sustained electroclinical remission, as well as a short time-lag to treatment, is necessary for optimal outcome.
- About 1/3 with electroclinical remission will experience a relapse requiring treatment.
- Neither zonisamide nor topiramate are helpful in preventing a relapse of IS after initial remission.
- About 1/2 have other seizure types (occurring before, after, or at the time of IS onset).
- 1/5 to 1/2 will evolve to LGS.
- 1/5 to 1/4 will have a favorable outcome (normal or slightly impaired intelligence).
- About 1/3 will have autism (common in TSC).
- About 2/5 will have cerebral palsy.

COMPLICATIONS

For hormone treatment: There is no consensus on any modified vaccine schedules. The issue is a balance between safety and adequate immunity after vaccination. At minimum, live vaccines should not be given <1 month after stopping hormone therapy. In the absence of evidence, one approach is to hold nonlive vaccines for 2 months and live vaccines for 6 months.

ADDITIONAL READING

- Baram TZ, Mitchell WG, Tournay A, et al. High-dose corticotropin (ACTH) versus prednisone for infantile spasms: a prospective, randomized, blinded study. *Pediatrics*. 1996;97(3):375–379.
- Lux AL, Edwards SW, Hancock E, et al. The United Kingdom Infantile Spasms Study comparing vigabatrin with prednisolone or tetracosactide at 14 days: a multicentre, randomised controlled trial. *Lancet*. 2004;364(9447):1773–1778.
- Pellock JM, Hrachovy R, Shinnar S, et al. Infantile spasms: a U.S. consensus report. *Epilepsia*. 2010;51(10):2175–2189.

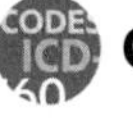

CODES

ICD10

- G40.822 Epileptic spasms, not intractable, w/o status epilepticus
- G40.824 Epileptic spasms, intractable, without status epilepticus

FAQ

- Q: Should I prescribe an abortive medication for longer clusters of IS?
- A: Generally, No. IS do not typically respond acutely to benzodiazepines.
- Q: My patient has IS and an abnormal EEG but no hypsarrhythmia. Should I treat him?
- A: Yes. Treat the seizures with 1st-line therapy; only about 60% will have hypsarrhythmia.
- Q: Caregivers report that IS has resolved with treatment. Do I need the EEG?
- A: Yes. You must have evidence of EEG background improvement. In addition, IS can be subtle (or convert from overt to subtle spasms with treatment) making them difficult to detect without video EEG.

INFLUENZA

Kristen A. Feemster, MD, MPH, MSHP

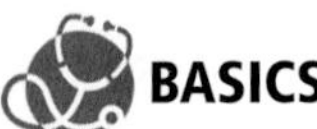

BASICS

DESCRIPTION

An acute febrile illness characterized by fever, malaise, and respiratory symptoms

EPIDEMIOLOGY

- Although influenza affects people of all ages, the highest morbidity and mortality occur in young children <2 years old, the geriatric population, and those with high-risk conditions.
- Influenza epidemics occur almost exclusively during winter months, peak ~2 weeks after the index case, and last 4 to 8 weeks.
- Attack rates are highest among school-aged children (range 10–40%).
- An estimated 10–20% outpatient visits among children <5 years old attributable to influenza
- Transmission of influenza virus occurs via large respiratory droplets or contact with contaminated surfaces.
- After an incubation period of 1 to 4 days, viral shedding starts 24 hours before symptom onset and usually continues for 7 days.
  - Prolonged shedding in young children and immunocompromised individuals

RISK FACTORS

High-risk conditions for severe disease include the following:

- Chronic pulmonary disease (i.e., asthma)
- Hemodynamically significant cardiac disease
- HIV and other immunodeficiencies
- Chronic immunosuppressive therapy
- Hemoglobinopathies (i.e., sickle cell disease)
- Long-term salicylate use
- Chronic renal dysfunction
- Chronic metabolic disease, morbid obesity
- Neuromuscular disorders

GENERAL PREVENTION

- Vaccination
  - Routine influenza vaccination for ALL individuals ≥6 months old
- Prioritize vaccination for those at highest risk for influenza complications and their close contacts, including (see Risk Factors):
  - Young children ages 6 to 59 months
  - Older adults ≥50 years, adults, and children with certain chronic diseases and high-risk conditions
  - Long-term care facility residents
  - American Indians/Alaska Natives
  - Pregnant women
  - Health care professionals
  - Out-of-home caregivers
  - Household contacts of all children <5 years old OR children 5 to 18 years old with high-risk conditions
- Vaccine types
  - Trivalent inactivated influenza vaccine (TIV) Afluria® (Seqirus) for ages ≥9 years and Fluvirin® (Seqirus) for ages ≥4 years
  - Quadrivalent influenza vaccines newly available for 2013 to 2014 season and beyond; include second influenza B strain
    - Inactivated: Fluarix® (GlaxoSmithKline) for ages ≥3 years, Fluzone® (Sanofi Pasteur), and Flulaval® (Seqirus) for ages ≥6 months
    - Live-attenuated influenza vaccine (LAIV) FluMist® (MedImmune), Fluzone® (Sanofi Pasteur); for healthy nonpregnant 2- to 49-year-olds; administered as an intranasal spray
    - Cell culture–based inactivated vaccine Flucelvax® (Seqirus) for ages ≥4 years
  - Recombinant trivalent hemagglutinin vaccine Flublok® (Protein Sciences) for ages ≥18 years; egg-free
  - High-dose (Fluzone® High-Dose, Sanofi Pasteur) and adjuvanted (Fluad®, Seqirus) trivalent-inactivated vaccines available for older adults ≥65 years
- Special vaccination considerations:
  - There is no preferential recommendation for one vaccine product over another for children who are eligible for more than one available vaccine.
  - Children ≤8 years old receiving seasonal influenza vaccination for the first time should receive 2 doses of vaccine at least 4 weeks apart.
- LAIV not recommended for individuals with high-risk conditions, young children (ages 2 to 4 years) with history of wheezing in past year, contacts of severely immunocompromised persons (such as contacts of BMT patients in a protected environment), or children receiving chronic aspirin therapy
- Contraindications to vaccination: history of severe allergic reaction to any vaccine component or after previous influenza vaccine dose
  - Precautions: Those with history of Guillain-Barré syndrome within 6 weeks of previous influenza vaccination should consult a physician before receiving the vaccine.
- Influenza vaccines can be safely administered to children with history of egg allergy (see https://www.cdc.gov/flu/protect/vaccine/egg-allergies.htm#algorithm for specific recommendations).
- Postexposure chemoprophylaxis
  - Indicated for high-risk children who are unvaccinated or were vaccinated within 2 weeks of exposure, immunocompromised patients who have a poor vaccine response, or to control outbreaks in institutions housing high-risk people
  - Chemoprophylaxis should begin within 48 hours of exposure to be most effective.

ETIOLOGY

- Orthomyxoviruses influenza types A, B, and C. Influenza C virus has not been reported as a cause of influenza epidemics.
- Influenza A subtypes defined by two surface antigens: hemagglutinin and neuraminidase
  - Currently circulating subtypes include pH1N1 (pmd09) and H3N2.
- Mild variation, or antigenic drift, for both A and B viruses results in seasonal epidemics; antigenic shift occurs only with A viruses and results in pandemics.

DIAGNOSIS

Clinical case definition of influenza-like illness is fever (≥100°F) AND cough and/or sore throat but may look similar to other respiratory illnesses.

- Positive predictive value of these symptoms for influenza lower (~65%) among children <5 years old
- Clinical presentation varies with age:
  - Infants and young children are less likely to present with typical symptoms but may have higher fever and more severe respiratory symptoms.

HISTORY

- Abrupt onset of illness, beginning with chills, headache, malaise, and dry cough
- Subsequent increase in respiratory tract symptoms that can range from mild cough to severe respiratory distress (infants)
- Other symptoms: fever, anorexia, myalgias, sore throat, irritability
- Younger children may have GI complaints including vomiting, diarrhea, and severe abdominal pain.
- Children may also present with otitis media.

PHYSICAL EXAM

- Cough is the predominant respiratory sign. Infants and small children may exhibit a "barky" cough (croup).
- Nasal congestion with conjunctival and pharyngeal injection
- Cervical adenopathy, especially in children
- Neonates may appear septic with apnea, circulatory collapse, or petechiae.
- A generalized macular or maculopapular rash is sometimes observed.

DIFFERENTIAL DIAGNOSIS

- Viral infections including but not limited to respiratory syncytial virus, parainfluenza, adenovirus
- *Streptococcus pyogenes*, *Mycoplasma pneumoniae*, or *Legionella* spp. infection
- Bacterial sepsis in young infants

DIAGNOSTIC TESTS & INTERPRETATION

Laboratory testing can confirm diagnosis, provide surveillance data, and help guide treatment and infection control decisions because clinical symptoms alone may not accurately identify all influenza cases. However, during periods of high influenza activity when the likelihood of infection is high and a child has symptoms consistent with influenza, testing may not be indicated.

- Gold standard: reverse transcription polymerase chain reaction (RT-PCR) or viral culture
  - RT-PCR preferred: most accurate and sensitive; results within 3 to 8 hours
  - Only viral culture can be used to measure subtype and antiviral resistance of circulating strains but requires 3 to 10 days.
- Direct fluorescent antibody (DFA) and indirect immunofluorescence antibody (IFA) tests
  - Have moderate sensitivity (60–70%) and excellent specificity (>95%); completed within 2 to 4 hours
  - Predictive value greatly affected by prevalence of circulating influenza
- Rapid antigen testing (RIDT)
  - Available for diagnosing influenza A and B
  - Results available in ~15 minutes but with wide range of sensitivities (22–77% in community settings), which may limit their usefulness
  - A negative test result should not guide management, especially when community prevalence is high.
- Serology:
  - Look for 4-fold rise in serum antibody titers between acute and convalescent samples (at least 10 to 14 days apart).
  - Not helpful for clinical decision making
- Special considerations for laboratory testing:
  - The false-positive rate for DFA, IFA, and rapid antigen testing may be as high as 20% (influenza A) and 40% (influenza B).
  - Nasopharyngeal aspirates rather than swabs may reduce false-positive rate by 5–10%.
- Tests most sensitive <4 days of symptom onset

- Ancillary laboratory data
  - Leukocyte count may be high, low, or normal with a variable differential.
  - Arterial blood gas analysis or pulse oximetry to evaluate oxygenation in severe cases of influenza infection. Infants without radiologic evidence of lower respiratory tract infection can experience apnea or rapid decrements in pulmonary function.
  - May see elevated creatine phosphokinase (CPK) with benign acute viral myositis. If with myoglobinuria, consider acute viral rhabdomyolysis, which can damage the kidneys; may require hospitalization and hydration
- Chest radiograph
  - May be normal despite significant respiratory involvement
  - Radiographs of patients with lower airway disease are indistinguishable from those in patients with other viral lower respiratory infections.

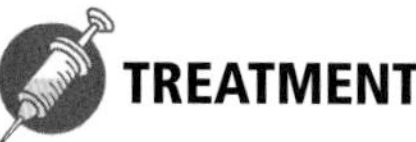

TREATMENT

GENERAL MEASURES

- Most patients with influenza infection require supportive oral hydration, antipyresis, and routine decongestant therapy.
- With the exception of young infants, previously healthy children with influenza infection rarely require emergency treatment.
- Humidified air, with oxygen as needed, is helpful to most patients with respiratory symptoms.
- Airway maneuvers, including endotracheal intubation, may be required for severe laryngotracheitis or patients with hypoxia that is unresponsive to high-flow oxygen administration.

MEDICATION

- Antiviral treatment is recommended for any patient who
  - Is hospitalized
  - Has severe or progressive illness
  - Is at high risk for complications
- Treatment most effective when initiated <2 days after symptom onset but may still reduce morbidity and mortality for hospitalized patients or patients with severe disease if started up to 5 days after symptom onset
- Treatment of healthy children with suspected or confirmed influenza in the outpatient setting is at the clinician's discretion but should be initiated <2 days after symptom onset.
- Neuraminidase inhibitors: the recommended antiviral medications for both treatment of and chemoprophylaxis against influenza A and B
- Zanamivir is approved for treatment in children ≥7 years and prophylaxis in children ≥5 years of age.
  - Treatment: two 10-mg inhalations b.i.d. × 5 days
  - Prophylaxis: two 10-mg inhalations once per day × 10 days
  - Can cause bronchospasm so should not be used in patients with history of chronic pulmonary diseases such as asthma
- Oseltamivir is approved for treatment in children ≥2 weeks of age and prophylaxis in children ≥1 year of age; however, use of oseltamivir for chemoprophylaxis is recommended by Advisory Committee on Immunization Practices (ACIP) for infants 3 months to 1 year.
  - Dose depends on age and weight (<1 year: 3 mg/kg/dose; >1 year and <15 kg: 30 mg; 15 to 23 kg: 45 mg; >23 to 40 kg: 60 mg; >40 kg: 75 mg), twice per day × 5 days for treatment, and once daily × 10 days for prophylaxis.
  - May cause nausea and vomiting
- IV peramivir is approved for adults 18 years and older for treatment of acute uncomplicated influenza. It is not indicated for chemoprophylaxis.
- Amantadine hydrochloride and rimantadine: approved for treatment of influenza A in children >1 year of age but NOT recommended for either treatment or prophylaxis due to increasing resistance; neither effective against influenza B
- Resistance to neuraminidase inhibitors <1% among currently circulating influenza strains
- Investigational parenteral medications: zanamivir
  - For severely ill high-risk patients with suspected or confirmed oseltamivir-resistant infection
  - Available through emergency investigational new drug protocol only
- Consider longer course of therapy if patient remains severely ill after 5 days.
- Preexposure prophylaxis can be considered for very high-risk patients who cannot be protected through other means when there is high risk of exposure to influenza cases.
  - Duration depends on expected duration of exposure but 4 to 6 weeks has been well tolerated.
- Chemoprophylaxis should not be given within 14 days after LAIV receipt as the vaccine strains are susceptible to the antiviral medications.

ONGOING CARE

FOLLOW-UP RECOMMENDATIONS

Patient Monitoring

- Signs to watch for:
  - Clinical signs of secondary bacterial infection
  - Deteriorating mental or respiratory status after initial improvement
  - Myoglobinuria in the face of muscle pain
- When to expect improvement:
  - Fever associated with influenza infection usually lasts up to 5 days. Recrudescence of fever does not necessarily signify the onset of a secondary bacterial infection.
  - Cough may last up to 2 weeks.
  - Lethargy or malaise may persist for up to 2 weeks.
  - Influenza A infection usually lasts longer than influenza B or influenza C infection.

COMPLICATIONS

- Secondary bacterial infections including pneumonia (pneumococcal or staphylococcal)
- Otitis media (24%)
- Sinusitis
- Primary progressive viral pneumonia
- Pulmonary hemorrhage
- Acute myositis during convalescence
  - More common with influenza B
  - Marked by extreme muscle tenderness, especially in the calf muscles
- Rhabdomyolysis/myoglobinuria
- Elevated transaminase levels
- Reye syndrome:
  - Fatty degeneration of the liver and diffuse encephalopathy
  - Associated with aspirin use during acute illness
  - More commonly associated with influenza B but may also occur with influenza A
- Febrile convulsions
- Drug toxicity: Influenza infection may result in increased serum levels of certain medications that are metabolized by the liver.
- Rare sequelae in severe cases of influenza infection:
  - Focal and diffuse myocarditis
  - Diffuse cerebral edema
  - Mediastinal lymph node necrosis
  - Sudden death
  - Guillain-Barré syndrome
  - Encephalitis

ADDITIONAL READING

- Chung EY, Huang L, Schneider L. Safety of influenza vaccine administration in egg-allergic patients. *Pediatrics*. 2010;125(5):e1024–e1030.
- Dawood FS, Chaves SS, Pérez A, et al; for Emerging Infections Program Network. Complications and associated bacterial coinfections among children hospitalized with seasonal or pandemic influenza, United States, 2003–2010. *J Infect Dis*. 2014;209(5):686–694.
- Fiore AE, Fry A, Shay D, et al. Antiviral agents for the treatment and chemoprophylaxis of influenza—recommendations of the Advisory Committee on Immunization Practices (ACIP). *MMWR Recomm Rep*. 2011;60(1):1–24.
- Grohskopf LA, Sokolow LZ, Broder KR, et al. Prevention and control of seasonal influenza with vaccines. *MMWR Recomm Rep*. 2016;65(5):1–54
- Stebbins S, Stark JH, Prasad R, et al. Sensitivity and specificity of rapid influenza testing of children in a community setting. *Influenza Other Respir Viruses*. 2011;5(2):104–109.

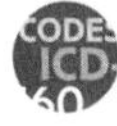

CODES

ICD10

- J11.1 Influenza due to unidentified influenza virus with other respiratory manifestations
- J10.1 Flu due to oth ident influenza virus w oth resp manifest
- J11.00 Flu due to unidentified flu virus w unsp type of pneumonia

FAQ

- Q: When is it safe for a child with influenza to return to day care or school?
- A: Older children with influenza may shed the virus in nasal secretions for up to 7 days from onset of symptoms and younger children even longer. Therefore, older children with influenza may return to school 1 week after onset of symptoms, and infants and toddlers should remain home for 10 to 14 days.
- Q: Can a child on chronic steroid therapy be immunized against influenza?
- A: Children who require maintenance steroid therapy for their underlying illness should still receive influenza immunization. If possible, immunize while the child is on the lowest possible dose of steroids.
- Q: Is chemoprophylaxis an acceptable alternative for protecting children against influenza?
- A: In general, chemoprophylaxis should not be used as a substitute for vaccination. Specific recommendations and indications for chemoprophylaxis can be found at www.cdc.gov/flu/professionals/antivirals/summary-clinicians.htm.

INGUINAL HERNIA

Nora M. Fullington, MD • Jeremy T. Aidlen, MD

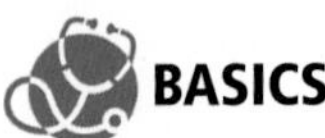

BASICS

DESCRIPTION

Inguinal hernia is a protrusion of abdominal contents (intestine, omentum) into, and often through, the inguinal canal.

EPIDEMIOLOGY

- Inguinal hernia is the most frequent problem requiring elective surgical intervention in children.
- Significantly more common in boys (90% of cases)
- Has a familial tendency
- Laterality
  - Because of later descent of right testis and subsequently delayed obliteration of right processus vaginalis, inguinal hernia presents more frequently on the right side.
  - Clinical presentation is on the right side in 60% of cases, on the left side in 30%, and bilateral in 10%.
- Frequency varies with age and ranges from 3–5% in full-term babies to 10–30% in preterm infants.

RISK FACTORS

- Prematurity
- Urologic conditions:
  - Cryptorchidism
  - Hypospadias
  - Epispadias
  - Bladder exstrophy
- Abdominal wall defects:
  - Gastroschisis
  - Omphalocele
  - Eagle-Barrett syndrome
- Conditions that increase intra-abdominal pressure (e.g., ascites, peritoneal dialysis, ventriculoperitoneal shunt)
- Cystic fibrosis
- Connective tissue disease:
  - Marfan syndrome
  - Ehlers-Danlos syndrome
- Mucopolysaccharidoses
- Family history

PATHOPHYSIOLOGY

- Indirect inguinal hernia
  - During the 7th month of male gestation, the testes begin their descent from the peritoneal cavity through the inguinal canal into the scrotum.
  - Between the 7th and 9th months of gestation, after the testes reach the scrotum, the path of peritoneum through which the testicle passed (processus vaginalis) begins to obliterate spontaneously, leaving only a small potential space adjacent to the testes (tunica vaginalis).
  - In girls, although the ovaries do not leave the abdomen, the round ligament (part of the gubernaculum) travels through the inguinal ring into labium majus. When the processus vaginalis remains open, it is identified as the canal of Nuck.
  - Incomplete obliteration of the processus vaginalis leaves a sac of peritoneum extending all the way from the internal inguinal ring to the scrotum or labium majus, through which an inguinal hernia may develop.
- Direct inguinal hernia
  - Uncommon in children
  - Results from either a congenital or acquired/traumatic weakness or tear in abdominal wall fascia
- Other types of inguinal hernias
  - Sliding hernia occurs when one wall of the hernia is composed of abdominal viscera (bladder, colon, adnexa).
  - Richter hernia results from the herniation of only a part of the bowel wall. If this hernia is incarcerated/strangulated, it may progress to bowel perforation without obstruction.
  - Hernia of Littre includes a Meckel diverticulum within the hernia sac.
  - Amyand hernia is an inguinal hernia in which the appendix is included within the hernia sac.

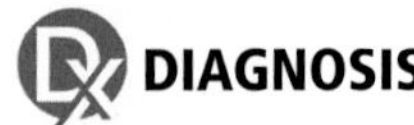

DIAGNOSIS

HISTORY

- Most common presentation is complaint of swelling or bulge in the inguinal area.
- Intermittently appearing
  - Present during times of increased intra-abdominal pressure such as crying or straining
  - A picture taken by the caregiver while the hernia is out may be helpful.
- Reducible hernias are not generally painful.
- If bulge is painful, incarcerated inguinal hernia must be suspected, and other etiologies (e.g., testicular torsion) should be excluded.

PHYSICAL EXAM

- Examine the child in the supine and upright positions.
- If the bulge is apparent in the standing position but disappears when the child is supine, presence of a hernia is strongly suggested.
  - Reduction of hernia contents through the inguinal ring is confirmatory.
  - If the bulge is not readily apparent, perform maneuvers that increase intra-abdominal pressure (gently press on his or her abdomen, have him or her cough, or strain or jump around).
- Transillumination
  - Can be an unreliable finding, particularly in babies
  - Some inguinal hernias (which usually do not transilluminate) can be differentiated from hydroceles (which usually do transilluminate).
- Silk glove sign
  - When empty hernia sac is palpated over the cord structures, sensation is similar to rubbing two layers of silk together: thick tissue that slides over cord structures
- Tender scrotal mass: Consider incarcerated hernia, testicular torsion, epididymitis, orchitis, or trauma.

DIFFERENTIAL DIAGNOSIS

- Lymphadenopathy
- Hydrocele
- Retractile testis
- Undescended testis

- Varicocele
- Testicular torsion
- Testicular tumor

DIAGNOSTIC TESTS & INTERPRETATION

- In cases where incarceration is suspected, such as presentation with a hard, painful, swelling in the groin, CBC and chemistry should be checked. Leukocytosis or acidosis should increase concern for compromised bowel.
- Genetic testing
  - Karyotype is necessary when a testis is discovered during hernia repair in a phenotypic female. Biopsy of the gonad is also typically performed.
  - 1% of full-term females with bilateral inguinal hernias have a disorder of sexual development—complete androgen insensitivity.
- Diagnosis is usually based on history and physical exam. However, use of scrotal or inguinal ultrasonography is indicated in cases involving:
  - Scrotal tenderness
    - Suggestion of torsion (Use duplex ultrasound to evaluate blood flow.)
    - Scrotal trauma and concern for testicular rupture
  - Mass along the spermatic cord or testicular tumor

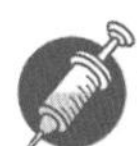

TREATMENT

GENERAL MEASURES

- Try to reduce the hernia with the child in the supine and/or head-down position so that gravity assists the maneuver.
- Many suggest application of pressure to hernia that is directed toward the inguinal canal.
- Gentle traction of the sac away from the canal and toward the contralateral knee is sometimes more effective if constant pressure is applied to the hernia sac contents.
  - The neck of the hernia is elongated by the traction and placed in line with the inguinal canal.
  - As edema is squeezed out, contents slip back into the abdomen.
- It is typical to feel a "pop" at the internal ring once the hernia is completely reduced. This can lead to immediate relief of symptoms.

SURGERY/OTHER PROCEDURES

Inguinal hernia will not resolve spontaneously and must be treated surgically to avoid incarceration.

- Complication rate after elective inguinal hernia repair is low (1–2%).
- Hernia incarceration commonly occurs in the 1st year of life (>50% of cases occur within the first 6 months of life) and is associated with markedly increased complication rate at repair (20%). To avoid this risk, repair is recommended soon after diagnosis of an inguinal hernia.
- Surgeons will often wait 24 to 48 hours after reduction of an incarcerated hernia to operate in order to allow edema to resolve.
- Routine contralateral inguinal exploration in children with unilateral hernia continues to be a topic of debate. Some surgeons perform diagnostic laparoscopy to evaluate for a contralateral patent processus vaginalis at the time of unilateral herniorrhaphy.
- Laparoscopic inguinal hernia repair can be performed safely in children of all ages, with a variety of techniques.

ADMISSION, INPATIENT, AND NURSING CONSIDERATIONS

There is no consensus regarding the optimal timing for hernia repair in hospitalized infants. The risk of incarceration must be balanced against the potential risks of operative and anesthetic complications.

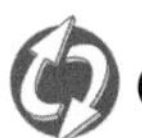

ONGOING CARE

PATIENT EDUCATION

- Preoperative: Parents should consult a physician immediately if signs of incarceration are present (firm or tender lump, pain, or emesis).
- Postoperative: Avoidance of major physical activity for 1 week is recommended.

COMPLICATIONS

- Incarceration
- Bowel obstruction: secondary to incarcerated loop of small intestine
- Strangulation: incarceration with progression to ischemia
- Intestinal infarction: can lead to perforation and peritonitis
- Testicular/ovarian ischemia or infarction: Ovaries are less likely to suffer ischemic insult given narrow vascular pedicle.

ADDITIONAL READING

- Sarpel U, Palmer SK, Dolgin SE. The incidence of complete androgen insensitivity in girls with inguinal hernias and assessment of screening by vaginal length measurement. *J Pediatr Surg*. 2005;40(1):133–137.
- Wang KS; for Committee on Fetus and Newborn, American Academy of Pediatrics, Section on Surgery, American Academy of Pediatrics. Assessment and management of inguinal hernia in infants. *Pediatrics*. 2012;130(4):768–773.
- Yang C, Zhang H, Pu J, et al. Laparoscopic vs open herniorrhaphy in the management of pediatric inguinal hernia: a systemic review and meta-analysis. *J Pediatr Surg*. 2011;46(9):1824–1834.

CODES

ICD10

- K40.90 Unil inguinal hernia, w/o obst or gangr, not spcf as recur
- K40.20 Bi inguinal hernia, w/o obst or gangrene, not spcf as recur
- K40.30 Unil inguinal hernia, w obst, w/o gangr, not spcf as recur

FAQ

- Q: When should a pediatric surgeon be consulted for a suspected inguinal hernia?
- A: Inguinal hernias do not resolve and require repair to avoid the complications associated with incarceration and strangulation. A pediatric surgeon should be consulted at the time of diagnosis in order to plan for elective herniorrhaphy. Findings suspicious at the time of presentation for incarceration or strangulation, such as a painful, swollen mass in the inguinal area, should result in immediate pediatric surgical consultation as urgent intervention may be required.
- Q: At what age is a patient most at risk for incarceration of an inguinal hernia?
- A: Incarceration of an inguinal hernia most often occurs within the first 6 months of life.

INTELLECTUAL DISABILITY

Rita Panoscha, MD

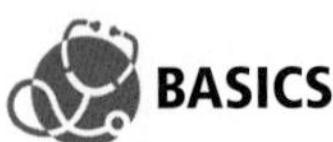

BASICS

DESCRIPTION

- Intellectual disability (formerly called mental retardation) is characterized by a slow rate of learning or slow cognitive-processing abilities. By definition, there are significant cognitive and adaptive delays first evident in childhood. Significant cognitive delays are defined as 2 standard deviations below the population mean on a standard cognitive or IQ test.
  - Usually indicates an IQ score of <70 to 75
- Adaptive skills are the functional skills of everyday life, including communication, social skills, daily living/self-care skills, and the ability to safely move about the home and community.
- Intellectual disability is typically subdivided into mild, moderate, severe, and profound categories, depending on the severity of the delays. A definition by the American Association on Intellectual and Developmental Disabilities (AAIDD) puts more emphasis on the level of functioning and the amount of support required by an individual.

ALERT

- Children with behavioral problems may also be masking cognitive delays.
- Hearing impairment may present as a delay in development.
- Children with mild intellectual disability may not be diagnosed as having a problem until they are having difficulties keeping up in elementary school.

EPIDEMIOLOGY

Found in both sexes and all racial and socioeconomic groups

Prevalence

- Prevalence of intellectual disability is generally listed as 2–3% of the population.
- Of the different subcategories of intellectual disability, the mild form is the most prevalent, at 85% of those with intellectual disability.
  - Profound intellectual disability is least prevalent, at ~1% of this group.

GENERAL PREVENTION

- There is no specific prevention, but prevention of some underlying causes may be possible.
- Immunization programs, early detection of metabolic disorders, and education programs for head injury/asphyxia prevention may be useful in some cases.
- Avoidance of alcohol and some drugs during pregnancy may also decrease the likelihood of some specific brain insults.

ETIOLOGY

The cause of the intellectual disability is usually an insult to the brain or abnormal development of the CNS but is not evident in many cases. The following represent potential causes.

- Genetic/familial/metabolic
  - Fragile X syndrome
  - Trisomy 21 (Down syndrome) and other chromosomal abnormalities
  - Tuberous sclerosis
  - Neurofibromatosis
  - Phenylketonuria (PKU)
  - Other inborn errors of metabolism
- Nervous system anomalies
  - Hydrocephalus
  - Lissencephaly
  - Seizures
- Endocrinologic
  - Congenital hypothyroidism
- Infectious
  - Prenatal cytomegalovirus, rubella, toxoplasmosis, HIV
  - Postnatal bacterial meningitis, neonatal herpes simplex
- Environmental toxins
  - Heavy metal poisoning such as lead
  - In utero drug or alcohol exposure, including fetal alcohol syndrome
- Traumatic
  - Closed-head trauma
  - Asphyxia

COMMONLY ASSOCIATED CONDITIONS

- Associated findings are more common in the more severe forms of intellectual disability.
- Intellectual disability has many associated findings, including seizures, autism, cerebral palsy, communication disorders, failure to thrive, sensory impairments, and psychiatric disorders.
- Behavioral disorders can be seen, including attention-deficit/hyperactivity disorder and self-injurious and self-stimulating behaviors.
- Families often face additional stressors when caring for a child with intellectual disability.

DIAGNOSIS

HISTORY

Complete information regarding the following:

- Pregnancy history
  - Maternal age and parity
  - Maternal complications (including infections and exposures)
  - Medications/drugs used
  - Tobacco or alcohol used, along with quantities
  - Fetal activity
- Birth history
  - Gestational age
  - Birth weight
  - Route of delivery
  - Maternal or fetal complications/distress
  - Apgar scores
- General health
  - Significant illnesses, hospitalizations, or surgeries
  - Accidents or injuries
  - Hearing and vision status
  - Medications used
  - Known exposures to toxins
  - Any new or unusual symptoms
- Developmental history
  - Current developmental achievement in each stream of development
  - Age when developmental milestones were achieved
  - Any loss of skills
  - Where parents think their child is functioning developmentally
- Educational history
  - Type of schooling and services received, if any
  - Any previous educational/developmental testing
- Behavioral history
  - Any perseverative or stereotypical behaviors
  - Interaction skills
  - Attention and activity levels
- Family history
  - Family members with developmental delays, neurologic disorders, syndromes, inherited disorders, or consanguinity

PHYSICAL EXAM

A complete physical exam including growth parameters is needed looking for etiology. Key features to include are the following:

- Observation of interactions and behavior
  - Atypical behaviors and general impressions
- Head circumference
  - Macro- or microcephaly
- Skin exam
  - Neurocutaneous lesions
- Major or minor dysmorphic features
  - Indication of a syndrome or anatomic malformation
- Neurologic exam
  - Assess for cranial nerve deficits, neuromuscular status, reflexes, balance and coordination, and any soft signs.

DIFFERENTIAL DIAGNOSIS

The differential can include several other developmental diagnoses, including the following:

- Borderline cognitive abilities
- Developmental language disorder
- Autism spectrum disorder
- Specific learning disability
- Cerebral palsy
- Significant visual or hearing impairment
- Degenerative disorders

DIAGNOSTIC TESTS & INTERPRETATION

Initial Tests (screening, lab, imaging)

- There is no specific laboratory test battery for intellectual disability.
- Testing must be tailored to the individual situation based on history and physical exam. A high index of suspicion should be maintained for any associated findings and delays in the other streams of development. Listed below are some of the more common studies.
  - Genetic testing
    - For any dysmorphic features or a family history of delays or genetic disorder, a karyotype and fragile X DNA testing should be considered, particularly for significant cognitive delays, although the comparative genomic hybridization (CGH) microarray is now recommended as a 1st-line genetic test.
  - Metabolic tests
    - Quantitative plasma amino acid, quantitative urine organic acid, lactate, pyruvate, or ammonia levels should be considered if there is any loss of skills, indication of a metabolic disorder, or if no newborn metabolic screen was done.
    - Additional metabolic tests may be indicated depending on symptoms.
  - Thyroid function tests
    - Most infants will have had screening for hypothyroidism shortly after birth. This should be rechecked if symptoms indicate.
  - Head MRI: Consider for head abnormalities; significant neurologic findings; loss of skills; or for workup of a specific disorder, such as trauma or leukodystrophy.

Diagnostic Procedures/Other

- When developmental delays are present and intellectual disability is suspected, more formal developmental screening or testing should be done.
- The pediatrician can do some in office developmental screening, but the diagnosis needs to be made based on standardized tests, usually done by a clinical psychologist. Such standardized testing might involve the Stanford-Binet Intelligence Scale, the Wechsler Adult Intelligence Scale, and the Vineland Adaptive Behavior Scale.
- Audiologic testing
  - For any child with speech and language and/or cognitive delays
- EEG
  - An EEG should be considered if there is any concern about seizures.

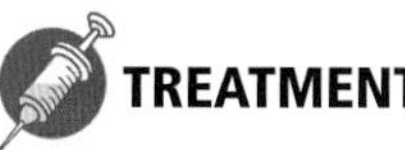

TREATMENT

GENERAL MEASURES

- There is no specific cure for intellectual disability. The ultimate goal of all therapies is to help the child reach his or her full potential.
- Therapy should consist of appropriate treatment for any underlying or associated medical condition.
- Early intervention and special education programs are available for an individualized education program based on the child's needs and abilities.
- Behavior management programs or selected use of medications is available for patients with severe behavioral problems.

ISSUES FOR REFERRAL

- A referral is made to a clinical psychologist for the formal diagnosis.
- Subspecialists
  - Referral to other medical specialists may also be indicated.
  - These specialists may include developmental pediatrics, neurology, genetics, or ophthalmology.

ONGOING CARE

FOLLOW-UP RECOMMENDATIONS

Patient Monitoring

- Children with intellectual disability will need regular pediatric preventive care in addition to management of any underlying medical conditions.
- Ongoing monitoring of the educational programs, to ensure that it is still meeting the child's needs, is important.
- The family will also need ongoing counseling and support in dealing with a child having special needs.

PROGNOSIS

- The prognosis for longevity varies with the associated findings and overall health, but individuals with intellectual disability can live to adulthood and old age.
- An individual's level of functioning is variable depending on the level of retardation, special individual skills, and family or community supports. In general, the following applies:
  - Mild intellectual disability (IQ 55 to 70): formerly called educable. May be in school with extra help and may achieve roughly a 4th to 6th grade level in reading and math. May be employed in an unskilled to semiskilled job; may live in a group home or independently
  - Moderate intellectual disability (IQ 40 to 54): may learn to recognize basic words and learn basic skills. May work in a sheltered workshop or with supported employment in an unskilled job; may live with family or in a group home doing much of their own care
  - Severe intellectual disability (IQ 25 to 39): may live with family or in a group home or institution. Some may be in a sheltered workshop; may be able to do some daily self-care or chores with supervision
  - Profound intellectual disability (IQ <25): live with family, in a group home, or in institution; usually require full-time care

ADDITIONAL READING

- Battaglia A. Neuroimaging studies in the evaluation of developmental delay/mental retardation. *Am J Med Genet C Semin Med Genet*. 2003;117C(1):25–30.
- Battaglia A, Carey JC. Diagnostic evaluation of developmental delay/mental retardation: an overview. *Am J Med Genet C Semin Med Genet*. 2003;117C(1):3–14.
- Gropman AL, Batshaw ML. Epigenetics, copy number variation, and other molecular mechanisms underlying neurodevelopmental disabilities: new insights and diagnostic approaches. *J Dev Behav Pediatr*. 2010;31(7):582–591.
- Jeste SS. Neurodevelopmental behavioral and cognitive disorders. *Continuum (Minneap Minn)*. 2015;21(3):690–714.
- Moeschler JB, Shevell M; for American Academy of Pediatrics Committee on Genetics. Clinical genetic evaluation of the child with mental retardation or developmental delays. *Pediatrics*. 2006;117(6):2304–2316.
- Shea SE. Intellectual disability (mental retardation). *Pediatr Rev*. 2012;33(3):110–121.
- Shevell M. Global developmental delay and mental retardation or intellectual disability: conceptualization, evaluation, and etiology. *Pediatr Clin North Am*. 2008;55(5):1071–1084.
- Stankiewicz P, Beaudet AL. Use of array CGH in the evaluation of dysmorphology, malformations, developmental delay, and idiopathic mental retardation. *Curr Opin Genet Dev*. 2007;17(3):182–192.
- Walker WO Jr, Johnson CP. Mental retardation: overview and diagnosis. *Pediatr Rev*. 2006;27(6):204–212.

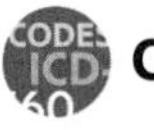

CODES

ICD10

- F79 Unspecified intellectual disabilities
- F70 Mild intellectual disabilities
- F71 Moderate intellectual disabilities

FAQ

- Q: Will my child be "normal" by adulthood?
- A: Generally, intellectual disability is considered a lifelong condition. Some individuals, usually with the milder form of intellectual disability, can function well in the community, especially when given added supports.
- Q: Can my child learn?
- A: Except for the most severe forms of intellectual disability, children do learn. This learning may not be as rapid or as extensive as that of a typically developing child.
- Q: But my child looks fine and has had appropriate motor development. How can he or she be mentally retarded?
- A: Mental retardation or intellectual disability is a slowed rate of cognitive development. Many children with intellectual disability do not have obvious dysmorphic features. Other streams of development, such as gross motor skills, may be reached on time or nearly so; yet, the cognitive developmental streams can be significantly delayed.

INTESTINAL OBSTRUCTION

Nora M. Fullington, MD • Jeremy T. Aidlen, MD

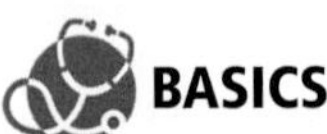

BASICS

DESCRIPTION

- Blockage of normal flow of air and other contents through the intestine
  - May be partial or complete, mechanical or functional
  - May arise from intrinsic abnormalities (e.g., meconium ileus, intestinal atresia) or extrinsic abnormalities (e.g., adhesions, bands, or volvulus)
  - May also be caused by neuromotor dysfunction of the gastrointestinal (GI) tract (i.e., hypomotility or paralysis of the intestine)
  - Most commonly involves the small bowel
- Untreated, obstruction can lead to intestinal ischemia.

PATHOPHYSIOLOGY

- Pathophysiology depends on the mechanism of the obstruction.
- Functional obstruction (paralytic ileus)
  - Failure of intestinal motor function without mechanical obstruction
    - Common after abdominal surgery, following extensive manipulation of the bowel
    - Other causes: infection (pneumonia, gastroenteritis, urinary tract infection, peritonitis, systemic sepsis), drugs (e.g., opiates, loperamide, vincristine), metabolic abnormalities (hypokalemia, hypomagnesemia, uremia, myxedema, and diabetic ketoacidosis)
- Mechanical obstruction
  - Intestinal dilation proximal to site of obstruction as the bowel fills with intestinal contents and air
  - Buildup of intestinal contents results in further distention, nausea, and vomiting.
  - Internal and external losses result in hypovolemia, oliguria, and azotemia.
  - Bacteria proliferate in the small bowel and its contents can become feculent.
  - "Closed loop" obstruction occurs when contents cannot get in or out of an intestinal segment.
- Ischemic obstruction
  - Occurs secondary to occlusion of intestinal blood supply
  - Causes
    - Twisting/kink of feeding blood vessels
    - Increased intramural pressure in the setting of bowel distention can result in decreased perfusion to the affected area.
  - With progression, gangrene, peritonitis, and perforation may occur.
  - Damage to the normal gut barrier may enable bacteria, bacterial toxins, and inflammatory mediators to enter the circulation, causing sepsis.

ETIOLOGY

May be congenital (e.g., atresia, duplication, malrotation), acquired (e.g., neoplastic, inflammatory), or iatrogenic (e.g., adhesions, radiation stricture); etiology varies by age:

- Neonates
  - Intestinal atresia (most common cause in neonates)
  - Obstructive meconium disorders (associated with cystic fibrosis)
    - Meconium ileus
    - Meconium plug syndrome
    - Meconium peritonitis
  - Duodenal atresia (associated with Down syndrome)
  - Annular pancreas
  - Anorectal malformation/imperforate anus
  - Necrotizing enterocolitis
  - Hirschsprung disease
- Infants
  - Pyloric stenosis (age: 1 to 2 months)
  - Intussusception (age: 2 months to 2 years)
  - Postoperative adhesions
  - Incarcerated inguinal hernia
  - Hirschsprung disease
  - Duplications
  - Meckel diverticulum
- Older children
  - Postoperative or postinfectious intestinal adhesions (e.g., perforated appendicitis)
  - Inflammatory bowel disease (IBD)
  - Malrotation with or without midgut volvulus
  - Annular pancreas
  - Meckel diverticulum
  - Superior mesenteric artery syndrome
  - Corrosive injury
  - Foreign body ingestion
  - Juvenile polyposis and related syndromes
  - Distal intestinal obstruction syndrome (cystic fibrosis)
  - Roundworm (*Ascaris lumbricoides*)
  - Gastric and intestinal bezoars
  - Colonic volvulus secondary to aerophagia and constipation (more common in neurodevelopmentally impaired)
  - Cancer-related intestinal obstruction and radiotherapy-induced adhesions

DIAGNOSIS

- Presentation may be acute and dramatic or chronic and subtle.
- Chronic or intermittent obstruction can be more challenging to diagnose.
- Careful history, physical examination, and consideration of age-related etiology will usually identify the specific cause.

HISTORY

- The classic symptoms of intestinal obstruction include vomiting, abdominal distention, colicky abdominal pain, and failure to pass flatus/stool (vomiting will be bilious if obstruction is distal to ampulla of Vater). Closed loop obstruction may present with pain and retching without emesis.
- Neonates
  - History of maternal polyhydramnios and aspiration of >20 mL gastric fluid after birth may suggest high intestinal obstruction.
  - Failure to pass meconium within 48 hours of birth is suggestive of a distal obstruction.
- Older children
  - Commonly present with pain which can be poorly localized, colicky visceral pain, or sharp peritoneal pain
  - Nausea and vomiting: High intestinal obstruction results in bilious emesis; distal obstruction may lead to feculent emesis.
  - Passage of blood or mucus per rectum may be a sign of intestinal ischemia or mucosal sloughing (e.g., intussusception and volvulus).

ALERT

Due to potentially delayed diagnosis and reduced functional reserve, neonates with unrecognized intestinal obstruction deteriorate rapidly, with increased morbidity, mortality, and surgical complications.

PHYSICAL EXAM

- General assessment and vital signs, signs of dehydration, sepsis, or malnutrition
- Palpation typically reveals abdominal distention. It may also reveal the presence of a hernia, a mass, fecal impaction, or intussusception.
- Tenderness denotes inflammation, significant distention, or ischemia. As a result, tenderness should raise concern for bowel compromise.
- Guarding and rigidity result from full-thickness bowel wall involvement or perforation/peritonitis.
- Bowel sounds are unreliable.
  - Bowel sounds may be initially increased in hyperperistaltic obstructed loops; however, they may also become decreased, occasional, or even absent.
  - Absent sounds are typically associated with ileus.
- Anal inspection excludes anorectal malformation. Rectal examination reveals, at times, a palpable polyp or intussusceptum and blood (overt, occult, or "currant jelly," typical of intussusception).
- Fever, tachycardia, signs of peritonitis, and severe pain that persists after nasogastric decompression may indicate a need for surgical intervention.

DIFFERENTIAL DIAGNOSIS

Other causes of abdominal pain and vomiting should be considered and ruled out by history and physical examination:

- Appendicitis
- Torsion of testis or ovary
- Lower lobe pneumonia
- Pancreatitis
- Sickle cell crisis

- Henoch-Schönlein purpura
- Biliary colic
- Lead poisoning
- Acute adrenal insufficiency
- Diabetic ketoacidosis
- Acute intermittent porphyria

ALERT
There is no spontaneous resolution of inguinal hernia. Surgery should be scheduled before incarceration occurs. Inguinal hernias have 10–28% risk for incarceration.

DIAGNOSTIC TESTS & INTERPRETATION

Initial Tests (screening, lab, imaging)

- No laboratory studies are diagnostic, but CBC, electrolytes, and blood gas should be obtained to help optimize supportive treatment.
- Assess for hypochloremic, hypokalemic metabolic alkalosis.
- Bowel infarction may lead to marked leukocytosis, thrombocytopenia, and metabolic acidosis.
- Serum amylase and lipase should be determined to evaluate for pancreatitis (may be mildly elevated in intestinal obstruction).
- Plain abdominal radiographs: supine and erect or decubitus views may identify the classic features: gasless abdomen or air–fluid levels and distended loops of intestine
  - In small bowel obstruction: dilated small bowel, air–fluid levels without gas in the colon
  - Paralytic ileus: distended loops of bowel throughout
  - Duodenal obstruction: "double-bubble" sign
  - Pneumoperitoneum: indicates intestinal perforation
  - Peritoneal calcifications: seen with meconium peritonitis
  - Right lower quadrant ground-glass appearance: consistent with meconium ileus
  - High small bowel obstruction or ischemic obstruction (midgut volvulus) may present with normal or nearly normal radiographs.
- Ultrasonography: may identify a mass or phlegmon (e.g., perforated appendix), pyloric stenosis, malrotation (orientation of vessels), intussusception ("target sign" or "doughnut sign"), or pelvic pathology in adolescents
- CT or MRI: localize the obstruction "transition zone"; diagnosis of strangulation-ischemic segment does not perfuse with contrast; may demonstrate ileus—absence of transition zone, Crohn disease—terminal ileitis or stricture, and neoplasms
- Contrast enema: to confirm/treat intussusception or to evaluate for Hirschsprung; may show "microcolon" of disuse in neonatal small bowel obstruction
- Upper GI series: for malrotation with or without volvulus
- Water-soluble, low osmolarity materials should be preferred (risk of perforation). Effort should be made to minimize radiation exposure.

ALERT
Evaluation for associated congenital anomalies is mandatory in some surgical conditions, as some are life-threatening. The most frequent are cardiac and renal abnormalities.

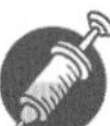

TREATMENT

GENERAL MEASURES

- Paralytic ileus is usually self-limiting and resolves with supportive treatment.
- Nasogastric decompression and fluids alone initially for adhesions. Adhesive postoperative obstruction is less likely to resolve without surgery in a child age <1 year old.
- In intussusception, hydrostatic or air enema reduction is successful in 90% of cases.
- Anti-inflammatory medication (e.g., steroids) for inflammatory obstruction of IBD; persistent strictures may require resection.
- Contrast enemas and direct enteral installation of *N*-acetylcysteine for uncomplicated meconium ileus
- Manual reduction of incarcerated inguinal hernias followed by repair
- Colonic volvulus may be treated with endoscopic decompression followed by elective surgery.
- Endoscopic removal of foreign bodies

ADDITIONAL THERAPIES

Nonoperative management with decompression by nasogastric tube (NGT) and IV fluids is the 1st-line approach in

- Early postoperative, partial, and recurrent adhesive obstructions
- Necrotizing enterocolitis
- Meconium ileus
- Duodenal hematomas
- Superior mesenteric artery syndrome
- Crohn disease

SURGERY/OTHER PROCEDURES

- Surgery may be required for definitive correction of bowel obstruction.
- Exceptions to this rule may include the above-mentioned conditions managed conservatively.
- In all situations: If no improvement within 12 to 24 hours, surgery is advisable.
- Additionally, bowel obstruction without a definitive causal diagnosis requires surgery.
- The surgical procedure is individualized according to the specific type, site, anatomy of the obstruction, and associated conditions.
- Laparoscopic surgery can be used for the diagnosis and repair of select intestinal obstructions and for adhesiolysis.

ADMISSION, INPATIENT, AND NURSING CONSIDERATIONS

- Hold oral intake.
- Decompress the stomach using an NGT.
- Administer IV fluids, correct electrolyte imbalance, and ensure adequate urine output.
- Obtain cultures and administer broad-spectrum antibiotics (covering gram-negative aerobes and anaerobes) if any concerns for sepsis or perforation/peritonitis.
- Identify etiology of obstruction.

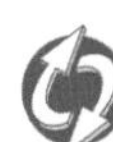

ONGOING CARE

PROGNOSIS

- Varies with different causes of intestinal obstruction, age of the patient, and associated conditions
- Extensive bowel resection or multiple repeat bowel resections can lead to short bowel syndrome, which is associated with significant morbidity and mortality.

COMPLICATIONS

May result from delayed operation

- Dehydration, azotemia, renal failure
- Intestinal ischemia with sepsis and shock
- Bowel perforation and peritonitis
- Short-bowel syndrome

ADDITIONAL READING

- McAteer JP, Kwon S, LaRiviere CA, et al. Pediatric specialist care is associated with a lower risk of bowel resection in children with intussusception: a population-based analysis. *J Am Coll Surg*. 2013;217(2):226–232.
- Reid JR. Practical imaging approach to bowel obstruction in neonates: a review and update. *Semin Roentgenol*. 2012;47(1):21–31.
- Young J, Kim DS, Muratore CS, et al. High incidence of postoperative bowel obstruction in newborns and infants. *J Pediatr Surg*. 2007;42(6):962–965.

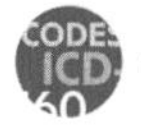

CODES

ICD10

- K56.60 Unspecified intestinal obstruction
- P76.0 Meconium plug syndrome
- Q41.9 Congen absence, atresia and stenosis of sm int, part unsp

FAQ

- Q: When should I consult a pediatric surgeon?
- A: If there is concern for bowel obstruction, a pediatric surgical consultation should be obtained early. In some cases, emergency surgery is necessary, whereas other times, it is more reasonable to place an NGT, administer IV fluids, and monitor for gradual resolution of the obstruction by clinical exam and radiographs.
- Q: Why are NGTs used in the treatment of intestinal obstruction?
- A: Tube decompression of the stomach allows for some symptomatic relief of nausea. In addition, it decreases the amount of fluid in obstructed intestine which may speed recovery. NGT output volume and character can guide management.
- Q: Is my child likely to have recurrent episodes of intestinal obstruction?
- A: It depends on the cause of the obstruction. Conditions associated with recurrence include intussusception, inflammatory conditions, and postoperative adhesions.

INTOEING–TIBIAL/FEMORAL TORSION

George D. Gantsoudes, MD

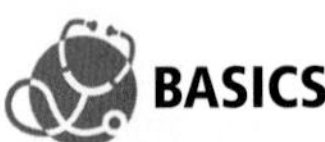

BASICS

DESCRIPTION

- Intoeing, as a presumptive diagnosis, results in numerous orthopedic consultations.
- Causes of intoeing are most frequently one or more of the following: metatarsus adductus, internal tibial torsion, and femoral anteversion.
- Definitions:
  - Version: normal variation in axial alignment
  - Torsion: any variation beyond two standard deviations of normal
- Clear explanation of the difference between physiologic variations and pathologic anatomy will allow the treating physician to effectively manage expectations.

EPIDEMIOLOGY

Very common; one of the most common reasons for a "well child" to visit an orthopedist

RISK FACTORS

Genetics

No strong evidence, but in some cases, a history of "intoeing that didn't resolve" is reported

PATHOPHYSIOLOGY

- Most are self-limiting issues but when paired together, can cause significant issues.
- Excessive femoral anteversion and external tibial torsion can result in the so-called "miserable malalignment," known to cause significant patellofemoral issues.

ETIOLOGY

- In utero, fetuses are subjected to forces that mold feet and tibiae into adductus and internal torsion, respectively.
- Most children are born with a relatively increased femoral anteversion (approximately 45 degrees).
  - Tends to resolve and "unwind" as the child develops
  - Usually resolves by age 8 to 10 years to the normal adult anteversion of 10 to 20 degrees

COMMONLY ASSOCIATED CONDITIONS

May be more common in first-born children (especially metatarsus adductus) as part of the "packaging disorders" such as developmental dysplasia of the hip and torticollis

DIAGNOSIS

HISTORY

- Varies based on age of presentation
- The most common reasons for malalignment visits in the preambulatory infant are either intoeing due to metatarsus adductus/internal tibial torsion or due to an external hip rotation contracture that all children have, which results in an obligatory and physiologic outtoeing.
- The ambulatory toddler will commonly come in with either intoeing or "bowleggedness" as a complaint.
  - The bowleggedness is almost always physiologic or related to the illusion of genu varum due to the child externally rotating their hips to prevent tripping over their internally rotated feet.
  - Internal tibial torsion is a common reason for consultation in the toddler age group.
- Intoeing in an older child is most often due to femoral anteversion, which is slightly slow to "unwind."
- The most common complaints are as follows:
  - Frequent tripping
  - Motor delay that is slower than peers or other relatives
  - Family member observation (e.g., an older relative who insists "something is wrong")
- There may be also an adult family member with similar issues who did not "grow out of it," prompting an early evaluation.

ALERT

Functional limitations (such as tripping and falling frequently) may suggest other diagnoses, such as mild cerebral palsy, especially if abnormal birth history, abnormal developmental milestones, and physical findings consistent with cerebral palsy. All children should also be evaluated for reflexes, Gowers, etc.

PHYSICAL EXAM

- Goal to rule out significant pathologies that could cause the relatively benign complaints
  - For example, any male child with a history of clumsiness must get a Gowers test and deep tendon reflexes to rule out muscular dystrophy.
- If possible, observe the child exploring the room before starting the physical exam. The examiner may gain more information here than at any other point in your exam.
- Watch the child walk and run in the hallway.
  - Ask the child to toe walk, heel walk, and use tandem gait (walk in a straight line touching the heel of one foot to the toes of the other foot) to further explore levels of coordination and function.
  - Look at the foot progression angle (angle formed between axis of foot and axis of forward progression of gait; this varies by age). An abnormal angle should be explainable by looking at rotation of other parts of leg during gait (hip rotation, thigh-foot angle, and/or foot abnormalities). If something does not add up, ask the child to walk again.
  - Gait can be too complex to observe all at once. If necessary, focus on one level (hips, knees, feet) at a time and have the child walk back and forth numerous times.
  - A "quick hint" is to watch the patella when evaluating the knees; they should always be roughly collinear with the feet.
- All children should have a thorough hip exam to rule out hip dysplasia as a cause.
  - All children have their hip abduction checked; any asymmetry is further evaluated with pelvis radiographs.
  - Children <2 years: Get a Barlow/Ortolani to check for hip instability.
    - Barlow: Adduct hip (thigh toward midline) applying light pressure on knee and direct force posteriorly; positive sign if femoral head dislocates
    - Ortolani: Flex hip to 90 degrees, use index fingers to place anterior pressure on greater trochanters, and abduct the legs using thumbs. Positive sign is "clunk" as femoral head relocates in acetabulum.
- The usefulness of a prone hip rotation exam far outweighs that of the supine exam. The spine can also be easily examined in this position.
- When examining for tibial torsion, there are a few different methods to evaluate the angle.
  - Thigh-foot axis
    - With the patient prone and the knee flexed 90 degrees, measure the difference between the axis of the foot and the axis of the femur.
    - The angle of the foot should be approximately 15 degrees externally rotated.

- Transmalleolar axis
  - With the patella facing the ceiling, the axis between the floor and a line drawn through the malleoli is measured.
  - 20 degrees external is normal.
- 2nd toe test
  - With the patient prone, the 2nd toe is rotated until it is perpendicular to the floor.
  - The femur is then held in place, and the knee is flexed 90 degrees.
  - The angle of the tibia to the vertical should be roughly 20 degrees.

- Metatarsus adductus is assessed by looking at the sole of the foot and drawing a bisecting line from the center of the heel distal. The line should travel through the 2nd and 3rd webspace. The further lateral the bisector line exits the foot, the more severe the adductus.
  - Spontaneous correction of the adducted forefoot is a positive sign and is assessed by gently stroking the lateral border of the foot.
- Assess for limb length differences.
- Assess deep tendon reflexes.

DIFFERENTIAL DIAGNOSIS

- Almost always the diagnosis is that of physiologic alignment.
- Correlate the findings to the normal values established by Staheli et al; a child that is >2 standard deviations from the mean is considered to have pathologic torsion and may warrant further follow-up or surgical treatment.
- The examiner must rule out cerebral palsy, muscular dystrophy, hip dysplasia, etc.

DIAGNOSTIC TESTS & INTERPRETATION

Initial Tests (screening, lab, imaging)

- Lab ever useful for simple torsion
- Imaging almost never ordered for run-of-the-mill torsional exams
- Order AP and frog pelvis films if there is a high suspicion of hip dysplasia.
- A standing (or supine) AP limb alignment radiograph can be a useful tool to examine for frontal plane abnormalities; taken from pelvis to ankles
  - Should be standardized at each institution with patellae facing the beam
- In the event of significant torsion, advanced imaging (e.g., CT or MRI) can be ordered to discover the true anatomic axes. This has been shown to have high inter- and intra-observer variability and has not been demonstrated to be better than a good physical exam.

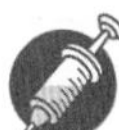

TREATMENT

- The younger child (<8 years) should spontaneously resolve minor internal torsion of the tibia and femur.
- Corrective shoes, Denis-Browne bars, twister cables, stretching, and formal physical therapy are no more effective than observation. In addition, there is evidence of poor self-esteem in those patients prescribed with braces.
- Observation is the rule.
  - There are no restrictions to activity; in fact, the children should be encouraged to be active.
- Recalcitrant torsion in the older patient may be an indication for osteotomy to derotate the limbs; only very rarely recommended
- Managing family expectations is crucial.
  - It may be helpful to have a handout to give to families, to both explain the issues and to show the frequency with which the diagnosis shows up in the office.
  - Get comfortable with a standard explanation of the normal physiology; use terms that are easy to understand.
  - Families may be reassured by data suggesting positive correlation with intoeing and elite-level sprinting.

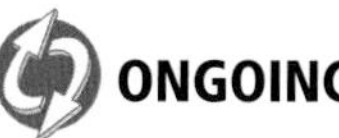

ONGOING CARE

PROGNOSIS

- Most patients are discharged with follow-up "as needed" with instructions to return if the problem hasn't improved over a period of 2 years or if the problem acutely worsens.
- Patience is strongly encouraged, as the "unwinding" of the limbs takes years to occur.
- The publications by Staheli et al contain numerous figures/graphs that can be beneficial in explaining this to concerned parents.
- The overall prognosis is excellent.
  - This is a very common reason for an orthopedic visit and a very rare reason to go the operating room.
  - Cosmetics and clumsiness are relative indications for surgery, but this is controversial.

COMPLICATIONS

Many patients will come in already having seen practitioners (podiatry, physical therapy, chiropractic, orthotists) who will associate torsion with degenerative arthritis and as a cause of more proximal issues (hips, spine). There is no evidence to support this association. In fact, a recent publication by Weinberg et al showed that there is no causal relationship between torsion and arthritis of the hip or knee.

ADDITIONAL READING

- Craig CL, Goldberg MJ. Foot and leg problems. *Pediatr Rev*. 1993;14(10):395–400.
- Fuchs R, Staheli LT. Sprinting and intoeing. *J Pediatr Orthop*. 1996;16(4):489–491.
- Schoenecker PL, Rich MM. The lower extremity. In: Morrissy RT, Weinstein SL, eds. *Lovell and Winter's Pediatric Orthopaedics*. 6th ed. Philadelphia, PA: Lippincott Williams & Wilkins; 2005:1157–1212.
- Staheli LT. Lower positional deformity in infants and children: a review. *J Pediatr Orthop*. 1990;10(4):559–563.
- Staheli LT, Corbett M, Wyss C, et al. Lower-extremity rotational problems in children. Normal values to guide management. *J Bone Joint Surg Am*. 1985;67:39–47.
- Weinberg DS, Park PJ, Morris WZ, et al. Femoral version and tibial torsion are not associated with hip or knee arthritis in a large osteological collection. *J Pediatr Orthop*. 2017;37(2):e120–e128.

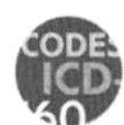

CODES

ICD10

Q68.4 Congenital bowing of tibia and fibula

FAQ

- Q: Are special shoes or braces ever indicated for tibial torsion?
- A:There is no convincing evidence that any of these treatments truly alter the natural history of the condition. The situation will improve without treatment in most children.
- Q: Can torsional pathology be a source of knee pain?
- A: Children may have increased femoral anteversion with associated external tibial torsion (i.e., an external rotation of the tibia that matches and, in effect, balances the internal rotation of the femur). This can be diagnosed by observing the rotational profile and by noting an increased Q-angle of the knee. This situation is sometimes a "setup" for patellofemoral pain. It has been called "miserable malalignment."

INTRACRANIAL HEMORRHAGE

Sarah Lee, MD

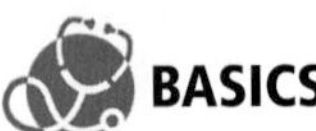

BASICS

DESCRIPTION

Intracranial hemorrhage (ICH) is defined as the pathologic accumulation of blood into the epidural, subdural, subarachnoid, intraparenchymal, or intraventricular space within the cranium due to loss of blood vessel integrity or coagulopathy. The term "hemorrhagic stroke" refers to nontraumatic, spontaneous, intraparenchymal, intraventricular, or subarachnoid hemorrhage.

EPIDEMIOLOGY

- Isolated intraventricular hemorrhage is rare beyond the newborn period.
- Trauma: most common cause of ICH in children
- Arteriovenous malformations (AVMs): most common cause of nontraumatic ICH in children

Incidence

Incidence of hemorrhagic (nontraumatic) stroke is 1.1 per 100,000 person years.

RISK FACTORS

- Trauma is the number one cause of ICH in children.
- Ruptured vascular malformations are the most common cause of nontraumatic ICH in children.
- Additional risk factors include:
  - Hereditary disorders of coagulation
  - Congenital heart disease
  - Cancer
  - Hypertension

Genetics

- Multiple cerebral cavernomas may be associated with autosomal dominant trait with *CCM1*, *CCM2*, and *CCM3*.
- Hereditary hemorrhagic telangiectasia (HHT) is an autosomal dominant condition associated with cerebral and visceral AVMs, frequent nosebleeds, and mucocutaneous telangiectasias.

GENERAL PREVENTION

- Automobile seat belts
- Bicycle, skating, and skateboarding helmets
- Child abuse prevention
- Diving safety practices
- Preventing falls
- Maintaining safe driving speeds
- Keeping children away from firearms
- Hematologic monitoring for those at risk for hemorrhage due to bleeding disorders
- Drug abuse prevention

PATHOPHYSIOLOGY

- Epidural hematoma (blood between the skull and the dura mater) is typically the result of a middle meningeal artery tear following temporal bone fracture; may also arise from dural venous sinus laceration.
- Subdural hematoma (blood between the dura mater and the arachnoid membrane) is frequently venous, from stretching and tearing of bridging cortical veins from trauma or coagulopathy.
- Subarachnoid hemorrhage (blood between the arachnoid membrane and brain) can be caused by a ruptured intracranial aneurysm, AVM, or trauma.
- Intraparenchymal hemorrhage can be a result of trauma, infections (herpes simplex encephalitis, bacterial endocarditis), coagulopathy, brain tumors, Moyamoya arteriopathy, venous sinus thrombosis, or hemorrhagic conversion of ischemic stroke.
- Intraventricular hemorrhage (IVH): may occur in isolation (more frequent in preterm infants <36 weeks' gestation) or in a mixed pattern with intraparenchymal or subarachnoid hemorrhage. In term infants, rule out venous sinus thrombosis (especially in patients with accompanying thalamic hemorrhage).
- Four grades of neonatal IVH:
  - Grade I: IVH isolated to 1 or both germinal matrices
  - Grade II: IVH without ventricular dilatation
  - Grade III: IVH with ventricular dilatation (hydrocephalus)
  - Grade IV: IVH with ventricular dilatation and extension into the periventricular white matter

ETIOLOGY

- Vascular
  - Congenital vascular anomalies: AVM, aneurysm, cavernous hemangioma, arteriovenous fistula, vein of Galen malformation
  - Developmental vasculopathy: Ehlers-Danlos syndrome type IV, Moyamoya arteriopathy, sickle cell disease
  - Acquired vasculopathy: hypertension, posterior reversible encephalopathy syndrome, reversible vasoconstricition syndrome, mycotic aneurysm, vasculitis (cocaine, inflammatory diseases), cerebral venous sinus thrombosis, hemorrhagic conversion of ischemic stroke, brain tumor
- Hematologic abnormalities: thrombocytopenia, hemophilia, sickle cell disease, liver failure, disseminated intravascular coagulation, iatrogenic (ECMO or anticoagulation therapy), hypercoagulability of malignancy
- Traumatic
  - Accidental injury
  - Nonaccidental injury

ALERT

ICH, especially in young infants and children without an obvious etiology, should raise the suspicion of nonaccidental trauma.

COMMONLY ASSOCIATED CONDITIONS

- Prematurity
- Hemophilia (prevalence of ICH 3–12%)
- Sickle cell disease (250-fold increased risk of ICH)
- Bacterial endocarditis
- Venous infarction
- Arterial infarction
- Alcohol, cocaine, and other sympathomimetics

DIAGNOSIS

HISTORY

- Delivery complications
- Head trauma
- Infection
- Cardiac disease
- High-output cardiac failure
- Patient or family history of coagulopathy
- Drug use
- Cerebral venous sinus thrombosis: dehydration, coagulopathy, polycythemia, sepsis, asphyxia (especially in newborns)
- Arterial aneurysms: polycystic kidney disease, coarctation of the aorta, fibromuscular dysplasia, connective tissue disease
- Vein of Galen malformation: presents as failure to thrive, hydrocephalus, seizures, high-output cardiac failure
- Clinical presentation of ICH: headache ("thunderclap headache" classically associated with subarachnoid hemorrhage due to aneurysm rupture or reversible vasoconstriction syndrome), neck pain or stiffness, vomiting, irritability, altered level of consciousness ("lucid interval" with epidural hematoma), seizures, visual problems (diplopia, blurred vision), focal neurologic deficits, epistaxis (may occur if skull fracture is present)
- Posterior fossa bleed: dysconjugate gaze, ataxia, and rapid deterioration to coma

ALERT

Increasing intracranial pressure from hemorrhage or hydrocephalus is life-threatening.

PHYSICAL EXAM

- Signs of increased intracranial pressure or herniation such as Cushing triad (hypertension, bradycardia, abnormal respiratory pattern); papilledema; fixed, dilated pupil; ophthalmoparesis
- In infants, increased intracranial pressure may result in a bulging fontanelle, splayed sutures, restricted upgaze, and/or increasing head circumference.
- Low-grade fever
- Meningeal signs
- In setting of trauma:
  - Leakage of CSF from the ear or nose
  - Battle sign: bruising over the mastoid process suggestive of basilar skull fracture
  - Raccoon eyes: periorbital ecchymosis suggestive of basilar skull fracture
  - Retinal hemorrhages

DIFFERENTIAL DIAGNOSIS

- Ischemic stroke/transient ischemic attack
- Brain tumor
- Headache (migraine, primary thunderclap)
- Metabolic derangements (hyper/hyponatremia, hypoglycemia)
- Encephalitis
- Meningitis
- Seizure with postictal Todd paralysis

DIAGNOSTIC TESTS & INTERPRETATION

Initial Tests (screening, lab, imaging)

- CBC
- Metabolic profile
- INR, prothrombin time (PT), activated partial thromboplastin time (aPTT)
- Fibrinogen
- Factors VIII, IX, XI
- von Willebrand factor antigen

- Urine toxicology screen
- Blood cultures
- Echocardiogram (for evaluation of cardiac disease or endocarditis)
- Lumbar puncture: Lumbar puncture will show RBCs, reduced glucose, and xanthochromia. Consider spinal fluid evaluation if CT negative.
- Imaging initial approach
  - STAT noncontrast CT of the head
    - The most important study to obtain when suspecting ICH because of its relative convenience, speed, and low false-negative rate
    - Acute intracerebral blood is bright (hyperdense) on CT; between 1 and 6 weeks becomes isodense with adjacent brain parenchyma. Acute ICH may appear isodense if hemoglobin <8 to 10 g/dL.
    - Epidural hemorrhage: biconvex, lens-shaped hemorrhage, displacing gray-white matter
    - Subdural hemorrhage: crescent-shaped hemorrhage; bilateral subdural hemorrhage frequent in nonaccidental injury
  - Contrast-enhanced CT: Contrast extravasation within the hematoma ("spot sign") may identify patients at high risk of ICH expansion.
  - MRI sequences are helpful for timing acute, subacute, and chronic hemorrhage or identifying underlying mass or abnormal shunting pattern on ASL sequences.

Follow-Up Tests & Special Considerations

- Consult neurosurgery emergently once intracranial hemorrhage is identified on imaging.
- Repeat neuroimaging (CT or MRI) 4 to 6 hours after initial scan to ensure bleed stability.
- CT/MR/conventional cerebral angiography and venography may be warranted to look for underlying vascular malformation, vasculopathy, or venous sinus thrombosis.
- Head ultrasound: Intraventricular hemorrhage in infants warrants serial head ultrasounds to rule out hydrocephalus.

ALERT

Early subarachnoid hemorrhage may not be apparent on initial CT and may require lumbar puncture (if safe to perform) or serial CT evaluation while the patient is under clinical observation.

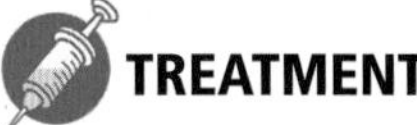

TREATMENT

GENERAL MEASURES

- Temperature management: Maintain normothermia; fever associated with worse neurologic outcome in adults
- Maintain normoglycemia and euvolemia.
- Urgent neurosurgical consultation
- Management of elevated ICP: head of bed elevated to 30 degrees, maintain adequate analgesia and sedation, consider invasive ICP monitoring and aggressive therapies (mannitol, hypertonic saline, hyperventilation) in consultation with neurosurgery and PICU on a case-by-case basis.
- Consider continuous EEG monitoring for seizures.

MEDICATION

- Correction of coagulopathy (suggested by PT, PTT, platelet abnormalities) should be done promptly and may require hematology evaluation. Therapies include vitamin K, fresh frozen plasma, cryoprecipitate, or platelet infusion. Monitor for fluid overload, especially in patients with cardiac disease.
- Management of elevated blood pressure: Blood pressure should be maintained within normal parameters for age with a general target of 50th to 95th percentile according to age and height. Nicardipine drip (1 mcg/kg/min) or labetalol (0.2 mg/kg IV push over 2 to 3 minutes, repeat every 15 minutes PRN)
- Management of seizures: fosphenytoin or levetiracetam 20 mg/kg IV load + maintenance for clinical or electrographic seizures; no evidence for seizure prophylaxis in ICH
- Acyclovir therapy if herpes simplex type 1 encephalitis is suspected
- Consider antibiotics if concern for bacterial endocarditis.
- Recombinant factor VIIa is FDA-approved in children with hemophilia who have systemic bleeding and are resistant to factor VIII therapy.
- Corticosteroids NOT recommended; may result in harmful hyperglycemia

ADDITIONAL THERAPIES

Physiotherapy, occupational therapy, speech therapy as required.

SURGERY/OTHER PROCEDURES

- Elevated intracranial pressure may necessitate surgical hematoma evacuation or decompressive hemicraniectomy.
- Aneurysms or AVMs may require urgent neurosurgical or neurointerventional treatment.

ADMISSION, INPATIENT, AND NURSING CONSIDERATIONS

- Initial stabilization
  - Admission to pediatric/neurointensive care unit
  - Consultation with neurosurgery and neurology
  - Urgent management of coagulopathy, hypertension, seizures, elevated ICP as listed earlier
- Admission criteria
  - Patients with altered mental status to monitor for elevated ICP
  - Patients with focal neurologic deficits for workup, management, and rehabilitation
  - Patients with seizures for continuous EEG monitoring and anticonvulsant management
  - Patients with hypertension for management
  - Patients with coagulopathy for correction
  - Patients requiring neurosurgical or neurointerventional management
  - Patient with ICH expansion on repeat scan
- IV fluids
  - Avoid D5 and excessive fluid.

ONGOING CARE

FOLLOW-UP RECOMMENDATIONS

Patient Monitoring

Long-term follow-up for signs of injury: cognitive deficits, focal weakness, seizures

PROGNOSIS

- Children may develop long-term focal or cognitive deficits or seizures; however, good neurologic recovery is possible.
- Predictors of poor neurologic outcome: infratentorial location, GCS ≤7 at admission, aneurysm, age <3 years, underlying hematologic disorder
- Pediatric ICH score:
  - Assess ICH volume ≥4% of total brain volume (2 points) or 2–3.99% (1 point); acute hydrocephalus (1 point), herniation (1 point), and infratentorial location (1 point).
  - Score ≥1 predicts moderate disability with 75% sensitivity; score ≥2 predicts severe disability or death with 90% sensitivity and specificity.

COMPLICATIONS

- Increased intracranial pressure and brain herniation syndromes
- Hydrocephalus
- Vasospasm secondary to blood and breakdown products of erythrocytes
- Seizures
- Motor, visual, and cognitive deficits
- Death (5–54%, pooled data 25%)

ADDITIONAL READING

- Beslow LA, Ichord RN, Gindville MC, et al. Pediatric intracerebral hemorrhage score: a simple grading scale for intracerebral hemorrhage in children. *Stroke*. 2014;45(1):66–70.
- Jordan LC, Hillis AE. Hemorrhagic stroke in children. *Pediat Neurology*. 2007;36(2):73–80.
- Lo WD, Lee J, Rusin J, et al. Intracranial hemorrhage in children: an evolving spectrum. *Arch Neurol*. 2008;65(12):1629–1633.
- Proust F, Toussaint P, Garniéri J, et al. Pediatric cerebral aneurysms. *J Neurosurg*. 2001;94(5):733–739.
- Roach ES, Golomb MR, Adams R, et al; for American Heart Association Stroke Council, Council on Cardiovascular Disease in the Young. Management of stroke in infants and children: a scientific statement from a special writing group of the American Heart Association Stroke Council and the Council on Cardiovascular Disease in the Young. *Stroke*. 2008;39(9):2644–2691.
- Squier W. Shaken baby syndrome: the quest for evidence. *Dev Med Child Neurol*. 2008;50(1):10–14.

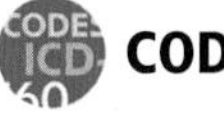

CODES

ICD10

- I62.9 Nontraumatic intracranial hemorrhage, unspecified
- S06.300A Unsp focal TBI w/o loss of consciousness, init
- Q28.2 Arteriovenous malformation of cerebral vessels

FAQ

- Q: What is the annual risk of hemorrhage in children with known AVM?
- A: The estimated annual hemorrhagic risk is 2–4%. In 25% of patients, the hemorrhage is fatal.
- Q: How often should an asymptomatic child at risk for AVM be screened, and with what imaging modality?
- A: Depending on the risk of aneurysm in a given condition, screening with magnetic resonance angiography every 1 to 5 years is reasonable.

I

INTUSSUSCEPTION

Alejandro V. Garcia, MD

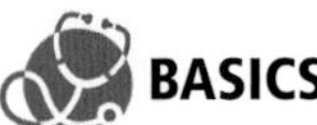

BASICS

DESCRIPTION

The invagination or telescoping of a proximal portion of bowel (the intussusceptum) into a distal segment of bowel (the intussuscipiens) which can result in ischemia and obstruction

EPIDEMIOLOGY

- Worldwide prevalence of 74 per 100,000 children <1 year of age
- Male-to-female ratio: 2:1
- Generally occurs in patients 3 months to 3 years of age
- Peak age: from 5 to 9 months
- The most frequent cause of bowel obstruction in infancy and second most common cause of abdominal pain (next to constipation)

RISK FACTORS

- Children <3 years:
  - Usually idiopathic (95%) or due to an enlarged Peyer patch (from infection), which is circumferential in distal ileum (common location of condition)
- Children ≥3 years:
  - Higher incidence of a pathologic lead point (4%): Meckel diverticulum, polyps, and lymphomas are most common.
  - Other common etiologies include Henoch-Schönlein purpura (HSP), Peutz-Jeghers syndrome, intestinal duplications, inflammatory bowel disease, appendix, and tumors.
- Postoperative (<1%):
  - Can occur in children who have had large retroperitoneal tumors removed (usually within 1 week of surgery)
- Recent vaccination
  - Increased incidence after administration of the RotaShield® rotavirus vaccine (no longer available)
  - Current vaccines (RotaTeq® or Rotarix®) present a small but significant increase in risk 1 to 7 days after first dose of the vaccine.

PATHOPHYSIOLOGY

- The invagination or telescoping of a proximal portion of bowel (the intussusceptum) into a distal segment of bowel (the intussuscipiens)
  - Can be unremitting (80%) or transient (20%)
  - 85% are ileocolic; ileoileal and colocolic types also occur.
  - Telescoping of the bowel occurs over a "lead point"—a lesion or defect in the bowel wall.
- Telescoping of the bowel causes diminished venous blood flow and bowel wall edema, which can result in ischemia and obstruction.
  - Over time, arterial blood flow is inhibited and infarction of the bowel wall occurs, which results in hemorrhage or perforation.
  - If untreated, can lead to death
- Bowel necrosis can occur within 48 to 72 hours after onset.
- Clinical presentation can vary but usually includes the following:
  - "Paroxysms of pain": episodes of calmness interspersed with fussiness
  - Persistent vomiting
  - "Currant jelly stools" which represent mucosal sloughing

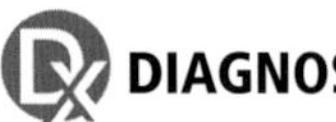

DIAGNOSIS

HISTORY

- Common to have recent history (prodrome) of a viral upper respiratory illness or gastroenteritis
- Classic triad
  - Involves the acute onset of severe intermittent (colicky) abdominal pain (98%), vomiting (70%), and bloody stool (35%)
  - The pain is characterized by drawing the legs up to the abdomen with crying lasting 2 to 10 minutes.
  - The child may appear asymptomatic between paroxysms of pain that recur in <24 hours.
  - Classical presentation only occurs in 7.5–65% of patients mostly in children <1 year of age.
- Young infants during episodes may demonstrate
  - Hyperextension
  - Writhing
  - Breath holding
  - Listlessness
  - Lethargy
- Emesis
  - Nonbilious emesis initially
  - Becomes bilious or feculent with progressive obstruction
- Currant jelly stools
  - Sloughed mucosa, blood, and mucous
  - Appear in 35% of cases
  - Should be considered a late finding suggestive of a longer prodrome due to vascular compromise and bowel ischemia

PHYSICAL EXAM

- Lethargic with intermittent colicky abdominal pain
- Palpable abdominal mass
  - Usually in right upper quadrant
  - Tubular or "sausage" shaped
- Can develop right lower quadrant (RLQ) tenderness with progressive obstruction
- Dance sign:
  - Abdominal retraction or absence of bowel contents in RLQ
- Abdominal distention or prolapse (late findings)
- Rectal exam:
  - Blood-tinged mucous or currant jelly stool
- May develop tachycardia from dehydration and tachypnea from metabolic acidosis
- Symptoms and signs of peritonitis from perforation

DIFFERENTIAL DIAGNOSIS

- Infectious
  - Gastroenteritis
  - Enterocolitis
  - Parasites
- Immunologic
  - HSP
- Gastrointestinal
  - Gastroesophageal reflux disease (GERD)
  - Food allergy
  - Inflammatory bowel disease
  - Celiac disease
- Miscellaneous
  - Appendicitis
  - Peutz-Jeghers syndrome
- Obstruction
  - Adhesions
  - Hernias
  - Volvulus
  - Stricture
  - Foreign body
  - Polyp
  - Tumor

DIAGNOSTIC TESTS & INTERPRETATION

Initial Tests (screening, lab, imaging)

- CBC, electrolytes
- Abdominal radiograph
  - May show paucity of gas in RLQ, air–fluid levels
  - "Meniscus sign" is indicative of a mass in the colon (25–45%).

- Abdominal ultrasound
  - Primary diagnostic modality
  - Highly sensitive and specific with experienced radiologist
  - "Target sign" or "pseudokidney sign" with presence of several concentric rings of bowel
  - Can sometimes indicate the pathologic lead point
- CT and MRI may demonstrate "target" or "doughnut" sign but are not part of routine evaluation.
- Contrast enema
  - Diagnostic and therapeutic with reduction often achieved (95%)
  - Air enema preferred over barium enema (more effective with less radiation and good chance of success with low risk of perforation)

ALERT

- Only 7.5–65% of patients present with the classical triad of abdominal pain, vomiting, and currant jelly stool, so high clinical suspicion is necessary.
- Patients should always have an IV placed and be undergoing fluid resuscitation prior to imaging or procedures.

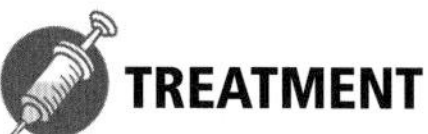

TREATMENT

GENERAL MEASURES

- Prompt recognition and reduction is imperative.
- Spontaneous reduction occurs in 5–20%.
- IV insertion, fluid therapy, and surgical consultation should be obtained once diagnosis is entertained.
- A fluid bolus of 10 to 20 ml/kg of normal saline can be administered depending on duration of symptoms and severity of dehydration.
- Broad-spectrum antibiotics if perforation, peritonitis, or bacterial translocation due to a compromised gastrointestinal mucosa is suspected
- Radiologic, pneumatic reduction with air contrast enema is mainstay of therapy.
- Absolute contraindications to reduction by enema:
  - Peritonitis
  - Shock
  - Perforation
- Multiple attempts may be made at reduction if initially unsuccessful or patient transferred to tertiary care facility after failed attempt.
- Perforation during reduction occurs in <1% of cases and requires immediate operative intervention.

SURGERY/OTHER PROCEDURES

- If patient presents with generalized peritonitis, persistent hypotension, and/or signs of perforation, they should immediately go to the operating room (OR).
- Unsuccessful attempts at pneumatic reduction
- Open surgery involves milking the intussusceptum out of the intussuscipiens and rarely involves resection.
- Laparoscopic surgery has gained more traction with better cosmesis, less pain, and shorter length of stay.

ADMISSION, INPATIENT, AND NURSING CONSIDERATIONS

- Initiation of IV fluids with normal saline should occur, with close monitoring for adequate urine output.
- New onset of pain could represent recurrence and should be followed by repeat ultrasound.
- Diet usually can resume 6 hours following reduction, with discharge after 24 hours following adequate PO intake.

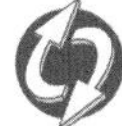

ONGOING CARE

FOLLOW-UP RECOMMENDATIONS

Some centers may discharge home after emergency department (ED) observation versus admission.

PATIENT EDUCATION

- Parents should be counseled that a 10% recurrence risk exists after nonsurgical reduction in the first 24 hours.
- Recurrences may require repeat pneumatic reduction and/or ultimate operative intervention.

PROGNOSIS

- Timely diagnosis results in a highly favorable prognosis with no effects on the bowel.
- Recurrences or failed reduction in children >3 years old may require workup for pathologic lead point.

COMPLICATIONS

- Bowel necrosis and perforation secondary to local ischemia
- Gastrointestinal bleeding
- Sepsis, shock, death

ADDITIONAL READING

- Daneman A, Navarro O. Intussusception. Part 1: a review of diagnostic approaches. *Pediatr Radiol*. 2003;33(2):79–85.
- Daneman A, Navarro O. Intussusception. Part 2: an update on the evolution of management. *Pediatr Radiol*. 2004;34(2):97–108.
- Glass RI, Parashar UD. Rotavirus vaccines—balancing intussusception risks and health benefits. *N Engl J Med*. 2014;370(6):568–570.
- McCollough M, Sharieff GQ. Abdominal surgical emergencies in infants and young children. *Emerg Med Clin North Am*. 2003;21(4):909–935.
- Pepper VK, Stanfill AB, Pearl RH. Diagnosis and management of pediatric appendicitis, intussusception, and Meckel diverticulum. *Surg Clin North Am*. 2012;92(3):505–526.

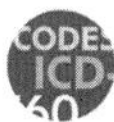

CODES

ICD10

K56.1 Intussusception

FAQ

- Q: Can my child have a recurrent intussusception?
- A: Yes, if your child has had a nonsurgical reduction via air (or barium) enema. However, the risk is considered low (<10%). If the lead point has been removed surgically, recurrence is very unlikely. The greatest risk for recurrence is in the first 24 hours after reduction.
- Q: What are common ages for presentation with intussusception?
- A: 3 months to 3 years is the age range associated with the greatest risk of intussusception, but the condition may occur at any age. The prevalence of intussusception being a sign of an underlying pathologic condition rises with age.
- Q: Could an infant have intussusception and not be crying in pain?
- A: Yes. Infants often present without the classical manifestations of intussusception. It is critical to have a high index of suspicion in any infant presenting with acute onset of emesis, especially bilious emesis and lethargy.
- Q: What should be done if the intussusception is only partially reduced by enema?
- A: One or two additional attempts at pneumatic reduction can be performed if the patient does not demonstrate signs of perforation or sepsis. Some recommend repeat attempts only if progress is made with each attempt, with each one being done 2 to 4 hours apart.

IRON DEFICIENCY ANEMIA

Irina B. Pateva, MD

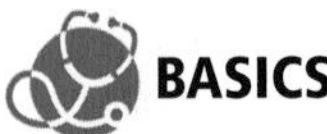

BASICS

DESCRIPTION

A reduction in hemoglobin production due to an insufficient supply of iron that results in a microcytic, hypochromic anemia

EPIDEMIOLOGY

- Iron deficiency is the most common nutritional deficiency of children.
- Leading cause of anemia among infants and children in the United States
- Most commonly seen in children ages 9 months to 3 years and in teenage girls

Prevalence

- Prevalence is variable depending on socioeconomic status, availability of iron-fortified formulas, and prevalence and duration of breastfeeding.
- Prevalence of iron deficiency anemia in United States is generally between 1% and 5% of children.

RISK FACTORS

- Low socioeconomic status
- Certain ethnic groups (e.g., Southeast Asian) may be at increased risk due to dietary practices.
- History of prematurity

GENERAL PREVENTION

- Maintain breastfeeding for the first 5 to 6 months of life if possible.
  - Breast milk has lower iron concentration than formula, but iron in breast milk is more bioavailable (50% vs. 10%).
- Iron supplementation
  - 1 mg/kg/24 h for infants who are exclusively breastfed beyond 4 months
  - 2 mg/kg/24 h by 1 month of life for low-birth-weight and premature infants who are breastfed because of poor iron stores and increased growth rate
  - Iron-fortified formula for the first 12 months of life for infants who are not breastfed
  - Encourage iron-enriched cereal when infants are started on solid food.
- Screen hemoglobin level at periodic intervals.
  - The American Academy of Pediatrics (AAP) recommends screening at 12 months, 1 to 3 years old, and adolescents as well as annually in menstruating females.
  - Centers for Disease Control and Prevention (CDC) recommends screening high-risk groups annually between ages 2 and 5 years and all menstruating women every 5 to 10 years.

PATHOPHYSIOLOGY

- Iron is required for oxygen transport by hemoglobin.
- Iron absorption and distribution is regulated by hepcidin, a peptide hormone secreted by liver, macrophages, and adipocytes.
- Iron is absorbed primarily in the duodenum.
- Iron deficiency develops because of an inadequate supply or increased demand for iron or a combination of these.
- Sequential stages of iron deficiency
  - Depletion of iron stores: reflected by low serum ferritin and absent bone marrow stores
  - Iron-deficient erythropoiesis: near-normal number of red blood cells (RBCs) produced, but they have abnormal hemoglobin synthesis with wide distribution in RBC size
  - Iron deficiency anemia: microcytosis evident

ETIOLOGY

- Causes of inadequate supply include dietary deficiency and malabsorption.
  - Dietary deficiency in infants and young children results from introduction of cow's milk prior to age 12 months, exclusive breastfeeding beyond age 6 months without iron supplementation, and excessive cow's milk intake (>24 oz/24 h).
  - Malabsorption results from surgical resection of intestine or celiac disease.
  - Certain foods impair iron absorption (tannins in tea and coffee, phytates).
- Causes of increased demand include rapid growth and blood loss.
  - Periods of rapid growth include infancy (especially low-birth-weight and premature infants) and adolescence.
  - GI blood loss is most common and includes cow's milk enteropathy (seen in infants), inflammatory bowel disease (IBD), and bleeding from Meckel diverticulum.
- Other etiologies of blood loss include perinatal loss, menorrhagia, pulmonary hemosiderosis, and hematuria.
- Several studies showed an association of obesity and iron deficiency; exact pathophysiologic mechanisms for this association are still under investigation.

DIAGNOSIS

HISTORY

- Evaluate dietary intake of iron, including breast or formula feeding and type of formula (iron fortified or low iron).
- Age at introduction of cow's milk
- Daily intake of cow's milk
- Birth history for prematurity or blood loss
- Lead exposure
- Blood loss from urine, stool, menorrhagia
- Iron deficiency anemia often develops slowly and no symptoms may be present. When present, signs and symptoms include the following:
  - Irritability and behavioral disturbances
  - Fatigue, exercise intolerance
  - Pallor
  - Headache
  - Pica or pagophagia (chewing ice)

PHYSICAL EXAM

- Often normal
- Pallor, irritability
- Tachycardia, flow murmur if anemia is more severe
- Koilonychia (spoon nails)
- Glossitis or stomatitis

DIFFERENTIAL DIAGNOSIS

- Recent infection
- Lead poisoning
- Thalassemia trait
- Anemia of chronic inflammation (e.g., juvenile rheumatoid arthritis, IBD)
- Sideroblastic anemias

DIAGNOSTIC TESTS & INTERPRETATION

Initial Tests (screening, lab, imaging)

- Hemoglobin level <2 standard deviations below the age-specific mean defines anemia.
- Low MCV (red cell volume) and MCH (hemoglobin concentration) for age
- High red cell distribution width (RDW)
  - Measures the variation in red cell size
  - Normal is <14.5%.
  - Often increased before anemia is present
- Low serum ferritin (≤12 ng/mL) reflects reduced tissue iron stores.
  - Earliest laboratory abnormality
  - May be normal or increased with concurrent infection or inflammation
  - Higher cutoff improves sensitivity of the test.
  - Ferritin ≤30 ng/mL has sensitivity of 92% and PPV of 83% for iron deficiency anemia versus sensitivity of 25% for ferritin ≤12 ng/mL.
- Low serum iron
- Increased total iron-binding capacity
- Low transferrin saturation; measures the iron available for hemoglobin synthesis
- Increased soluble transferrin receptor (sTfR)
  - Indicator of increased tissue iron demand
  - Also increased in thalassemia syndromes but not in anemia of chronic inflammation
  - sTfR/log(ferritin) <1 suggests anemia of chronic inflammation.
  - sTfR/log(ferritin) >2 suggests iron deficiency anemia.
- Decreased reticulocyte hemoglobin content: This test is an early indicator of iron deficiency because reticulocytes have a short (1 to 2 days) lifespan before becoming mature red cells.
- Increased free erythrocyte protoporphyrin, a precursor molecule in hemoglobin synthesis; also high in lead poisoning and chronic inflammation
- Thrombocytosis (can approach 1 million/dL)
- Peripheral blood smear with microcytosis, hypochromia, poikilocytosis (varying shapes), pencil forms, and anisocytosis (varying sizes)
- Test for occult blood in stool often positive with GI blood loss
  - However, the test can be positive with oral iron supplementation.
- Iron absorption test can assess adequacy of PO iron supplementation. 3 mg/kg elemental iron should increase serum iron >100 mcg/dL within 4 hours of ingestion.

Diagnostic Procedures/Other

Bone marrow examination: shows decreased iron stores by Prussian blue staining; it is the gold standard to determine iron stores but rarely needed to establish diagnosis.

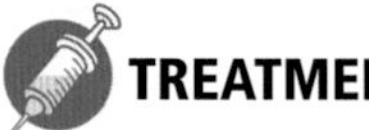

TREATMENT

- Iron supplementation
- Family education regarding age-appropriate diet and iron-containing foods
- Specific treatment if underlying condition causing blood loss is found (e.g., hormonal therapy for menorrhagia, medications for IBD)
- May require initial inpatient observation in cases of severe anemia
- Red cell transfusion only if evidence of cardiovascular compromise (rarely indicated)

MEDICATION

First Line

Oral replacement with ferrous iron, 3 to 6 mg/kg/24 h of elemental iron divided into 2 or 3 doses

- Iron should be given on an empty stomach or with a vitamin C–containing juice to increase absorption. Ascorbic acid increases oral absorption of iron by ~30%.
- Side effects (in 10–20%) include nausea, constipation, GI upset, and vomiting. Iron suspensions can stain teeth temporarily.

Second Line

- Parenteral iron formulations are used more frequently in the last few years because of their favorable side effect profile and quicker effect on hematologic response.
  - They are indicated when poor compliance, poor tolerance for oral preparations, malabsorption, or if ongoing loss exceeds absorption capacity.
  - Administration may be associated with infusion reactions or anaphylaxis, less common with newer preparations such as ferric gluconate and iron sucrose.
- Some products like ferric carboxymaltose can be given as a short infusion in a single dose which appears to be efficacious and cost effective.

ISSUES FOR REFERRAL

- Evaluation for source of GI blood loss
- Unexplained recurrence after treatment
- Failure to improve with iron supplementation

ADMISSION, INPATIENT, AND NURSING CONSIDERATIONS

- Admission criteria
  - Active bleeding
  - Severe anemia (hemoglobin level <6 g/dL) especially if symptoms or ongoing blood loss
  - Tachycardia, S_3 gallop, or other signs of congestive heart failure (CHF)
- Discharge criteria
  - No signs of CHF
  - If blood loss, bleeding is controlled
  - Stable hemoglobin level
  - Parent demonstrates ability to administer oral iron therapy to young children and demonstrates adequate knowledge about dietary modifications.
  - Adequate follow-up ensured

ONGOING CARE

FOLLOW-UP RECOMMENDATIONS

Patient Monitoring

- Reticulocyte count increases in 3 to 4 days.
- Absolute reticulocyte count and reticulocyte hemoglobin content predict good early hematologic response to iron supplements after 1 week of therapy.
- Hemoglobin concentration should rise by at least 1 g/dL in 2 to 3 weeks.
- Continue iron for 2 months beyond correction of anemia to replenish body stores.
- Causes of poor response to oral iron supplementation include the following:
  - Nonadherence (most common)
  - Ongoing blood loss
  - Insufficient duration of therapy
  - High gastric pH
  - Concurrent lead intoxication
  - Other diagnosis: Thalassemia trait and anemia of chronic disease are not iron responsive.

DIET

- Milk should be restricted to <24 oz daily or eliminated in those with milk protein enteropathy.
- Bottle should be discontinued after 12 months.
- Diet should include foods rich in iron: meats, beans, iron-fortified cereal, strawberries, spinach.

PATIENT EDUCATION

- Activity: Usually, no activity restriction is needed. Those with severe anemia resulting in CHF should have limited activity until the anemia is corrected.
- Diet: A diet containing iron-rich foods should be encouraged. Limit milk intake to <24 oz daily.
- Prevention: Prevention of iron deficiency is preferable. Anticipatory guidance about diet, prolonged bottle use, etc., should be given.

PROGNOSIS

- Anemia is readily corrected with iron replacement.
- Developmental delay may be long lasting or irreversible.

COMPLICATIONS

- Impaired cognitive and motor development as well as behavioral changes in infants and toddlers
- Short-term memory impairment and poor exercise performance in adolescents

ADDITIONAL READING

- Baker RD, Greer FR; for Committee on Nutrition American Academy of Pediatrics. Diagnosis and prevention of iron deficiency and iron-deficiency anemia in infants and young children (0–3 years of age). *Pediatrics*. 2010;126(5):1040–1050.
- Centers for Disease Control and Prevention. Iron deficiency—United States, 1999–2000. *MMWR Morb Mortal Wkly Rep*. 2002;51(40):897–899.
- Grandone A, Marzuillo P, Perrone L. et al. Iron metabolism dysregulation and cognitive dysfunction in pediatric obesity: is there a connection? *Nutrients*. 2015;7(11):9163–9170.
- Mantadakis E. Advances in pediatric intravenous iron therapy. *Pediatr Blood Cancer*. 2016;63(1):11–16.
- McCann JC, Ames BN. An overview of evidence for a causal relation between iron deficiency during development and deficits in cognitive or behavioral function. *Am J Clin Nutr*. 2007;85(4):931–945.
- Powers JM, Buchanan GR. Diagnosis and management of iron deficiency anemia. *Hematol Oncol Clin North Am*. 2014;28(4):729–745.
- Wu AC, Lesperance L, Bernstein H. Screening for iron deficiency. *Pediatr Rev*. 2002;23(5):171–178.

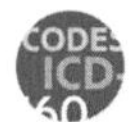

CODES

ICD10

- D50.9 Iron deficiency anemia, unspecified
- D50.8 Other iron deficiency anemias
- D50.0 Iron deficiency anemia secondary to blood loss (chronic)

FAQ

- Q: What dietary changes can help prevent the recurrence of iron deficiency?
- A: Limit milk to 24 oz/24 h to improve appetite for iron-containing foods. Heme iron, found in meats, fish, and poultry, is absorbed better than nonheme iron and enhances absorption of nonheme iron. Other foods that have iron are raisins, dried fruit, sweet potatoes, lima beans, chili beans, green peas, peanut butter, and enriched foods. Give iron on an empty stomach along with an ascorbic acid–containing juice to increase absorption. Foods that decrease absorption include bran, vegetable fiber, tannins found in tea, and phosphates. Antacids may also decrease iron absorption.
- Q: What are the side effects of iron therapy?
- A: Iron may cause temporary staining of the teeth, which can be decreased by diluting the iron with a small amount of juice. Iron will also change the color of bowel movements to greenish black. Constipation may occur.
- Q: What are the most important tests to do to establish the diagnosis of iron deficiency?
- A: For patients with a history of dietary deficiency or known blood loss, a CBC that shows a low hemoglobin and MCV and an elevated RDW is very suggestive of iron deficiency. A therapeutic trial of iron without further laboratory testing is an appropriate next step. A rise in the hemoglobin concentration of ≥1 g/dL after 1 month of therapy confirms the diagnosis. Otherwise, further laboratory testing is necessary, and other diagnoses should be considered.
- Q: How does a concurrent infection affect the diagnosis of iron deficiency?
- A: Common childhood infections may be associated with a mild microcytic anemia that resembles iron deficiency. Laboratory tests to diagnose iron deficiency may be misleading while a child is acutely ill. Acute infection is associated with a shift of iron from serum to storage sites, causing a decrease in serum iron and an increase in ferritin. It is more helpful to test a child for iron deficiency 3 to 4 weeks after an acute infection.

IRON POISONING

Jessica L. Perniciaro, MD • Todd P. Chang, MD, MAcM

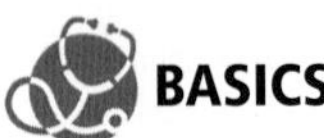

BASICS

DESCRIPTION

- Iron poisoning is a common and potentially fatal ingestion.
- Toxicity depends on the amount of elemental iron ingested, although tolerable and lethal concentrations are not firmly established.
- Doses of <20 mg/kg of elemental iron are generally not symptomatic, of 20 to 60 mg/kg are variably symptomatic, and of >60 mg/kg are severely toxic and potentially fatal.

EPIDEMIOLOGY

- Accounts for about 2–4% of all exposures in children and adolescents
- Can be divided into unintentional (younger children) and intentional (adolescents)
- Incidence: almost 11,000 iron exposures per year in children <6 years old in United States, based on the 2015 American Association of Poison Control Centers Annual Report
- Many factors contribute to the incidence of iron ingestion:
  - High-iron preparations such as prenatal vitamins are readily available (prenatal vitamins contain the highest amount of iron per tablet).
  - Many preparations are attractive and candy-like.
  - Caregivers often fail to appreciate the danger of overdose from vitamins and pure iron preparations.
- Although vitamin ingestions are increasing, the incidence of fatal iron ingestions has declined since the 1990s, perhaps due to changes in package labels and child-resistant packaging.

RISK FACTORS

- Birth of a sibling, including up to 1 year after (increased availability of prenatal vitamins)
- Among unintentional ingestion, almost all serious mortality and morbidity is in children <5 years of age (ingestion of adult iron formulations).

GENERAL PREVENTION

- Parental education: Keep all medications and vitamins out of reach in child-resistant packaging.
- In 1997, federal regulations required unit-dose packaging (blister packs) for all iron preparations with >30 mg of elemental iron per dose.
- Significant decrease in iron ingestion–related deaths after regulations
- The United States Food and Drug Administration (FDA) removed regulations in 2003, although many manufacturers voluntarily continue this type of packaging.

PATHOPHYSIOLOGY

- Iron directly damages cells, interfering with aerobic respiration. The primary systems affected by iron are the gastrointestinal (GI) tract, including the liver, and the cardiovascular system.
- There are five classic stages of iron poisoning:
  - Stage I (GI phase)
    - Occurs up to 6 hours post ingestion
    - Characterized by GI mucosal injury, leading to abdominal pain, vomiting, diarrhea, and GI bleeding (hematemesis or hematochezia)
    - Metabolic acidosis may be present, and death may be caused by capillary leakage and hypovolemic shock.
  - Stage II (latent)
    - 6 to 24 hours after ingestion
    - Relative stability and temporary resolution of GI symptoms
    - Does not always occur
    - Although there may be improvement of symptoms, there is continued cellular toxicity and metabolic acidosis.
  - Stage III (shock)
    - 12 to 24 hours after ingestion (can occur earlier with high dose ingestions)
    - Systemic symptoms: hemodynamic instability, shock, metabolic acidosis
    - Coagulopathy is common and worsens GI bleeding (can occur even without hepatotoxicity).
    - Vasodilation can lead to hypovolemia, and myocardial injury can lead to cardiogenic shock.
  - Stage IV (hepatotoxicity)
    - Within 48 hours after ingestion
    - May result in liver failure
  - Stage V (late)
    - 2 to 8 weeks post ingestion
    - Gastric injury may result in strictures, leading to vomiting and potentially gastric outlet obstruction.

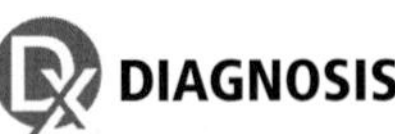

DIAGNOSIS

HISTORY

- Witnessed or suspected iron product ingestion
- Determine the amount of elemental iron ingested and the time of ingestion.
- Determine formulation (iron salt, vitamin with iron, delayed release).
- The percentage of elemental iron by iron salt is
  - ferrous fumarate, 33%
  - ferrous chloride, 28%
  - ferrous sulfate, 20%
  - ferrous gluconate, 12%

ALERT

Strongly consider the diagnosis of acute iron poisoning in a lethargic, hypotensive toddler.

PHYSICAL EXAM

- Evaluate for poor perfusion:
  - Hypotension
  - Decreased capillary refill
  - Pallor
  - Tachycardia
- Evaluate for GI injury:
  - Abdominal tenderness
  - Occult or apparent GI bleeding
- Evaluate for cardiac injury:
  - Distant heart sounds
  - Poor pulses
  - Mottled skin
  - Distended jugular veins
  - Pulmonary edema
- CNS depression (lethargy or coma)

DIFFERENTIAL DIAGNOSIS

- Ingestions
  - Acetaminophen
  - Salicylate
  - Methanol
  - Propylene glycol
  - Ethanol
  - Ethylene glycol
- GI bleeding
  - Perforation
  - Intussusception
  - Gastritis
  - Esophageal inflammation or tear
  - Vascular malformation
- Other
  - Serious bacterial infection: sepsis, meningitis
  - Trauma (including child abuse)
  - Diabetic ketoacidosis

DIAGNOSTIC TESTS & INTERPRETATION

Initial Tests (screening, lab, imaging)

- Serum iron level (most useful diagnostic test)
  - Measure on presentation and every 1 to 2 hours.
  - The serum iron level peaks at 4 to 6 hours postingestion and can help determine the severity of overdose. Iron levels 300 to 500 mcg/dL: usually mild to moderate GI toxicity; 500–1,000 mcg/dL: serious toxicity; >1,000 mcg/dL: severe and life-threatening toxicity
- Supplemental labs
  - Blood gas (metabolic acidosis)
  - Complete blood count (leukocytosis)
  - Glucose/electrolytes (hyperglycemia)
  - Renal function
  - Liver function and coagulation studies

- Total iron-binding capacity (TIBC) not recommended (may be inaccurate in toxicity)
- Abdominal radiograph
  - May reveal iron pills. The absence of findings does not exclude iron toxicity (liquid preparations and multivitamins are not radiopaque).
  - GI decontamination may be recommended if undissolved tablets are confirmed.

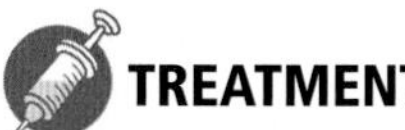

TREATMENT

GENERAL MEASURES

- Contact local Poison Control Center (1-800-222-1222) for specific recommendations.
- All intentional iron ingestions should be evaluated at a medical facility, regardless of dose.
- Generally, asymptomatic patients >6 hours after ingestion or ingestions of <20 mg/kg elemental iron with mild symptoms require no treatment and can be observed at home.
- Symptomatic patients with persistent or severe GI symptoms, or ingestion with >40 mg/kg elemental iron, should be evaluated in a health care facility.

ADDITIONAL THERAPIES

- GI decontamination
  - Whole-bowel irrigation is the GI decontamination method of choice for heavy metals.
    - Decreases GI transit time
    - Especially useful when a significant number of pills are seen on radiographs
    - Use osmotically neutral solution such as polyethylene glycol solution.
    - By nasogastric tube until rectal effluent clear
    - Recommended rates: 500 mL/h for children 9 months to 6 years; 1,000 mL/h for 6 to 12 years; 2,000 mL/h for 13 years and older (Consultation with a specialist or regional poison control center is recommended.)
  - Gastric lavage is not routinely recommended (may consider if early after ingestion and suspect a large iron load).
  - Activated charcoal is not recommended (iron binds poorly).
  - Syrup of ipecac is not recommended.
  - Rarely, endoscopy or gastrotomy may need to be performed to remove embedded pills.
- Iron chelation with deferoxamine
  - Deferoxamine binds with free iron and is excreted by the kidneys.
  - It is indicated for systemic signs of toxicity, metabolic acidosis, or peak iron concentration >500 mcg/dL.
  - Administered parenterally via continuous infusion at initial rate of 15 mg/kg/h. (Consultation with a specialist or regional poison control center is recommended.)
  - Chelation can be discontinued with clinical improvement and resolution of metabolic acidosis.
  - Side effects of chelation include hypotension, renal failure, ARDS, and *Yersinia* sepsis.
  - Ferrioxamine complex created by the binding of deferoxamine and free iron is excreted by the kidneys and gives urine "vin rosé" color.
  - Although iron cannot be dialyzed, the ferrioxamine complex after chelation can be, and dialysis may be indicated in the setting of acute renal failure.

ADMISSION, INPATIENT, AND NURSING CONSIDERATIONS

- Initial goals: Evaluate and stabilize shock; volume resuscitation important in early management
- Intubation should be considered in a lethargic patient to facilitate GI decontamination.
- Consider admission for patients with mild but persistent symptoms after 6 hours or ingestion with >40 mg/kg (recommend consultation with a specialist or poison control center).
- Symptomatic patients with significant toxicity or shock should be treated in an intensive care setting by specialists skilled in management of pediatric ingestions.
- Can discharge from inpatient admission if stable hemodynamic status and resolution of metabolic acidosis (Recommend consultation with a specialist or poison control center.)

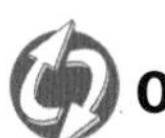

ONGOING CARE

FOLLOW-UP RECOMMENDATIONS

Monitor for possible late complications, such as strictures of the GI tract (can occur up to 2 months post ingestion).

PATIENT EDUCATION

Encourage families to secure iron-containing vitamins and supplements out of reach of children.

PROGNOSIS

- Iron ingestions rarely result in serious injury.
- Shock and ingestion of elemental iron >1,000 mcg/dL associated with mortality

COMPLICATIONS

- GI and hepatic infarction and necrosis
- Gastric or intestinal scarring and strictures
- Metabolic acidosis
- Shock (hypovolemic, hemorrhagic, cardiogenic)
- Coagulopathy
- Pulmonary edema
- *Yersinia enterocolitica* infection or sepsis (Chelation can encourage bacterial growth.)
- Death

ADDITIONAL READING

- Chang T, Rangan C. Iron poisoning: a literature-based review of epidemiology, diagnosis, and management. *Pediatr Emerg Care*. 2011;27(10):978–985.
- Fine JS. Iron poisoning. *Curr Probl Pediatr*. 2000;30(3):71–90.
- Henretig FMI. Acute iron poisoning. In: Shaw LM, Kwong TC, eds. *The Clinical Toxicology Laboratory: Contemporary Practice of Poisoning Evaluation*. Washington, DC: AACC Press; 2001:401–409.
- Manoguerra AS, Erdman AR, Booze LL, et al. Iron ingestion: an evidence-based consensus guideline for out-of-hospital management. *Clin Toxicol (Phila)*. 2005;43(6):553–570.
- Tenenbein M. Unit-dose packaging of iron supplements and reduction of iron poisoning in young children. *Arch Pediatr Adolesc Med*. 2005;159(6):557–560.

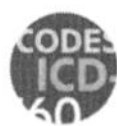

CODES

ICD10

- T45.4X1A Poisoning by iron and its compounds, accidental, init
- T56.891A Toxic effect of other metals, accidental (unintentional), initial encounter

FAQ

- Q: Why isn't activated charcoal recommended for GI decontamination?
- A: Because charcoal binds poorly to iron and so is not effective in GI decontamination. There is also the risk of vomiting and aspiration in the patient with severe poisoning.
- Q: What is the recommendation regarding observation of a patient for development of symptoms with iron ingestion of an unknown quantity?
- A: Observe for 6 hours. Those who are asymptomatic 6 hours after ingestion are not likely to exhibit systemic illness.
- Q: What is the recommendation regarding nonintentional ingestion of children's vitamins with iron, carbonyl iron formulations, or polysaccharide iron complex formulations?
- A: These ingestions are generally deemed to contain low levels of iron, and the American Association of Poison Control Centers recommends against emergency room referral for nonacute patients with adequate home supervision. Even patients with mild diarrhea and emesis can be safely observed in the home following these ingestions, although consultation with a physician and poison control hotline is still advised.

IRRITABLE BOWEL SYNDROME

Laurie N. Fishman, MD

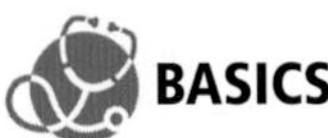

BASICS

DESCRIPTION

- Irritable bowel syndrome (IBS) is a common functional GI tract disorder where defecation is disordered and associated with abdominal discomfort.
- IBS is characterized by abdominal pain, bloating, diarrhea, or constipation
- Symptoms of IBS do not result from inflammatory, infectious, metabolic, or anatomic causes. However, there can be overlap with other conditions.
- Symptoms typically exacerbated by stress or particular foods (i.e., spices, fatty foods, caffeine, certain carbohydrates, etc.).

EPIDEMIOLOGY

- 10–15% of the general population is affected to some degree by IBS.
  - Prevalence estimates vary based on whether the study is community-based or practice-based.
  - Higher estimates in the community reflect the fact that many people do not seek medical care for their IBS symptoms.
  - Prevalence is also based on whether Manning, Rome II, or Rome III criteria are used.
- More common in females
- IBS occurs in children.
  - 6% of middle school students
  - 14% of high school students

RISK FACTORS

- Prior history of bacterial enteritis
- History of abuse or trauma

PATHOPHYSIOLOGY

- IBS considered a disorder of GI function relating to motility, sensation, and/or perception
- Best model is a biopsychosocial construct with dysregulation of the gut-brain homeostasis affected bidirectionally by both peripheral and central factors.
- The pathogenesis of IBS is believed to be multifactorial and include the following:
  - Abnormal gut motility
  - Genetics
  - Bacterial overgrowth
  - Visceral hypersensitivity
  - Behavioral response
  - Microscopic inflammation
  - Dysregulation of brain-gut axis
  - Malabsorption

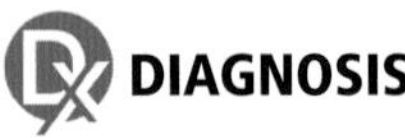

DIAGNOSIS

- IBS is not a diagnosis of exclusion.
- Diagnosis is based on careful history with particular attention to characteristics of pain, precipitating factors, and defecation pattern.

HISTORY

- Symptoms that support constipation-predominant IBS (IBS-C) include the following:
  - <3 stools per week
  - Hard or lumpy stools
  - Straining with defecation
- Symptoms that support diarrhea-predominant IBS (IBS-D) include the following:
  - >3 stools per day
  - Loose or mushy stools
  - Urgency
- All IBS types may have the following:
  - Sense of incomplete evacuation
  - Mucus in stools
  - Abdominal bloating
- Symptoms may not only intensify with known stressors (such as school exams, sports competitions) but also with positive emotionally charged events (such as parties, amusement park trips, dates, school prom, etc.).

DIFFERENTIAL DIAGNOSIS

- *Giardia* infection
- Lactose intolerance
- Fructose intolerance
- Celiac disease
- Inflammatory bowel disease
- Constipation with overflow
- Endometriosis
- Medication effects
- Psychiatric disorder (especially anxiety, depression, posttraumatic stress disorder, or school avoidance)

DIAGNOSTIC TESTS & INTERPRETATION

Initial Tests (screening, lab, imaging)

- There is no laboratory testing that confirms IBS. Tests are done solely to rule out other conditions.
- Selective testing:
  - CBC, ESR, or CRP
  - Stool for occult blood
  - Stool for parasites (*Giardia*)
  - Total IgA, tissue transglutaminase (IgA)
  - Thyroid-stimulating hormone (TSH)
  - Stool lactoferrin or calprotectin
  - Consider albumin.
  - Consider lactose testing.
- More testing needed if "red flags" present the following:
  - Weight loss (>5 to 10 lb)
  - Bloody stool
  - Fever
  - Anemia
  - Family history of inflammatory bowel disease or GI cancer
- There is no imaging that can be used to diagnose IBS. Imaging studies should be performed if indicated to evaluate for other conditions.

Diagnostic Procedures/Other

- In severe IBS, with weight loss and diarrhea resulting in incontinence or nocturnal stooling, colonoscopy may be required to rule out colitis.
- If history and empiric restriction do not clarify whether lactose intolerance is a contributing factor, can perform lactose breath testing to objectively see if low lactase activity.

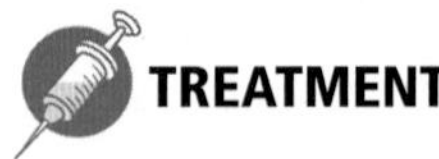

TREATMENT

GENERAL MEASURES

- The aims of IBS treatment are to:
  - Improve a global sense of well-being.
  - Reduce specific symptoms.
- It is important to remind patients that treatment will not cure their IBS.
- Comprehensive treatment consists of the following:
  - Education about IBS
  - Dietary changes
  - Soluble fiber
  - Probiotics/antibiotics
  - Pharmacology
  - Herbal and natural products
  - Complementary techniques
  - Psychological techniques
  - Continued provider relationship
- Generally speaking, eating small, regular meals and avoiding insoluble fiber, fatty foods, and caffeine is helpful, along with increased exercise, high-quality sleep (minimum 8 hours, minimal screen time), and stress reduction, for alleviating symptoms.
- For patients with mild symptoms of IBS, reassurance, education, and lifestyle changes such as avoiding identified triggers may be adequate for management.
- In patients with more severe or complex symptoms, a multidisciplinary approach including pharmacotherapy and psychosocial intervention may be needed.

MEDICATION

- Antibiotics can be used intermittently for gassiness and bloating symptoms:
  - Neomycin, rifaximin (nonabsorbed)
  - Metronidazole, norfloxacin (systemic)
- Bile acid malabsorption has been postulated as a trigger in IBS-D (even in absence of liver or ileal disease). Potential medications include cholestyramine (Questran®), colesevelam.
- Symptomatic relief for diarrhea:
  - Consider loperamide (μ-opioid receptor agonist).
  - Side effects include constipation.
- Symptomatic relief for constipation:
  - Consider magnesium, polyethylene glycol, senna, or bisacodyl; however, these therapies are not well-studied for this indication.

- Lubiprostone
  - Can be used at 8 mcg b.i.d. for general IBS discomfort or 24 mcg b.i.d. for constipation
  - Nausea is a frequent side effect.
- Linaclotide
  - Guanylate cyclase receptor agonist
  - Recently approved for patients >18 years of age with IBS-C
  - Minimal side effects as not absorbed systemically
- Antispasmodics (dicyclomine, hyoscyamine)
  - Can be used on a regular basis or as needed
  - It can be very reassuring to the patient to have a medication available when needed.
- Belladonna/phenobarbital is also described as useful but is not available in United States.
- Low-dose antidepressants (amitriptyline, citalopram)
  - Can be very useful for the treatment of abdominal pain
  - It is important to explain the rationale for using these medications to avoid the misperception by the patient that the diagnosis is a psychiatric disease.
- Placebo rates in IBS are often >40% in studies. Effectiveness of known placebos for patients with migraine may also be helpful in patients with IBS.

COMPLEMENTARY & ALTERNATIVE THERAPIES

- Probiotics
  - Current literature suggests mixed results from clinical trials.
  - Different individual and combinations of specific probiotic strains of *Bifidobacterium*, *Lactobacillus*, and *Saccharomyces* have been used.
  - 3 to 4 weeks of treatment are considered adequate trial.
- Herbal products
  - Chamomile, in the form of warm tea, can be helpful for spasms.
  - Peppermint, either tea or capsules of peppermint oil, will relax the smooth muscle via the calcium channel; can cause heartburn
  - Less commonly cited remedies have been reported such as artichoke leaf extract, turmeric, and natural clay powder.

ISSUES FOR REFERRAL

- Psychological therapies such a cognitive behavioral therapy (CBT) and psychodynamic therapy are helpful.
  - Acquiring CBT skills can help lower stress, address comorbid anxiety or depression, and often have lasting effect.
- Hypnotherapy requires trained provider but has proven benefits lasting 6 to 12 months.

ONGOING CARE

FOLLOW-UP RECOMMENDATIONS

Patient Monitoring

- The provider–patient relationship is an important component of therapy, and ongoing visits can help monitor symptoms.
- Planned medical follow-up also provides a sense of well-being, helps patients to anticipate flares, and prevent repeated evaluations.

DIET

- Have patients systematically look at typical dietary triggers:
  - Spicy foods
  - Fatty or fried foods
  - High-sugar foods
  - Beans/legumes
  - Sugar-free gum, candy, or drinks
  - Lactose
- Try gluten withdrawal (after testing to rule out celiac), as some patients can have non-celiac gluten sensitivity.
- In conjunction with a nutritionist, consider trying elimination of FODMAP foods (fermentable oligosaccharides, disaccharides, monosaccharides, and polyols). However, it is important to add back foods to avoid potential nutritional deficiencies.
- Fiber
  - Gradually increase to goal of 10 g (adults) or age +5 g (child)
  - Fiber can help with global symptoms and constipation; less helpful for pain
  - Soluble fibers (psyllium or ispaghula, calcium polycarbophil) improve symptoms, whereas insoluble (bran, corn) worsen symptoms.
  - Adequate trial of any particular fiber is at least 3 to 4 weeks; may need to try multiple types

PATIENT EDUCATION

- Establish a positive diagnosis:
  - It is important that patients perceive that their MD "knows they have IBS" rather than the MD has "ruled everything else out so the diagnosis must be IBS."
- Reassurance about overall health
- Explain there are many interventions (diet, medication, techniques) that will improve, although not cure, symptoms.
- Reassure patients that you will not abandon them but continue to help.

COMPLICATIONS

- Patients with moderate to severe IBS can have significantly lower quality of life, absenteeism from school/work.
- IBS can also lead to frequent physician visits, unnecessary medical testing, and high health care costs.

ADDITIONAL READING

- Bijkerk CJ, de Wit NJ, Muris JW, et al. Soluble or insoluble fibre in irritable bowel syndrome in primary care? Randomised placebo controlled trial. *BMJ*. 2009;339:b3154.
- Bijkerk CJ, Muris JW, Knottnerus JA, et al. Systematic review: the role of different types of fibre in the treatment of irritable bowel syndrome. *Aliment Pharmacol Ther*. 2004;19(3):245–251.
- Chogle A, Mintjens S, Saps M. Pediatric IBS: an overview on pathophysiology, diagnosis and treatment. *Pediatr Ann*. 2014;43(4):e76–e82.
- Cristofori F, Fontana C, Magista A, et al. Increased prevalence of celiac disease among pediatric patients with irritable bowel syndrome: a 6-year prospective cohort study. *JAMA Pediatr*. 2014;168(6):555–560.
- Dorn SD, Morris CB, Hu Y, et al. Irritable bowel syndrome subtypes defined by Rome II and Rome III criteria are similar. *J Clin Gastroenterol*. 2009;43(3):214–220.
- Ford AC, Lacy BE, Talley NJ. Irritable bowel syndrome. *N Engl J Med*. 2017;376(26):2566–2578.
- Halmos EP, Power VA, Shepherd SJ, et al. A diet low in FODMAPs reduces symptoms of irritable bowel syndrome. *Gastroenterology*. 2014;146(1):67–75.e5.
- Spiegel BM, Farid M, Esrailian E, et al. Is irritable bowel syndrome a diagnosis of exclusion?: a survey of primary care providers, gastroenterologists, and IBS experts. *Am J Gastroenterol*. 2010;105(4):848–858.

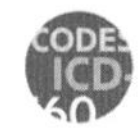

CODES

ICD10

- K58.9 Irritable bowel syndrome without diarrhea
- K58.0 Irritable bowel syndrome with diarrhea

FAQ

- What is the low-FODMAP diet?
- The low-FODMAP diet involves the exclusion of foods that are more likely to be "fermentable" by bacteria in the colon, including those with "oligosaccharides, disaccharides, monosaccharides, and polyols." Following the FODMAP diet has been shown to provide relief for patients with IBS. However, it also can be deficient in some micronutrients, including fiber, calcium, iron, zinc, folate, vitamin B, vitamin D, and natural antioxidants.

I

JAUNDICE

Andrew J. Wehrman, MD • Kathleen M. Loomes, MD

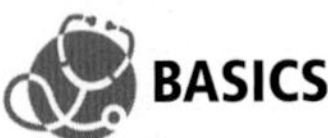

BASICS

DESCRIPTION

- Jaundice: a yellow or green/yellow hue to the skin, sclerae, and mucous membranes which can be appreciated at serum bilirubin levels >2 mg/dL. Intensity of color is directly related to the serum bilirubin level.
- Unconjugated bilirubin: 80% is due to hemoglobin turnover and 20% is from degradation of hepatic and renal heme proteins. It is a hydrophobic compound that must be carried to the liver by albumin for processing.
- Conjugated bilirubin: conjugated to glucuronic acid in the liver, a water-soluble derivative that helps lipid emulsification and absorption
- Direct bilirubin: conjugated bilirubin plus bilirubin that is covalently bound to albumin (delta fraction)
- Direct bilirubin is higher than a measured conjugated bilirubin and has a longer half-life.
- Conjugated hyperbilirubinemia (direct hyperbilirubinemia): a conjugated bilirubin of >2 mg/dL or >20% of the total bilirubin

EPIDEMIOLOGY

The most common causes of pathologic jaundice are as follows:

- Newborn period: biliary atresia, idiopathic neonatal hepatitis, α_1-antitrypsin deficiency, infection
- Older child: autoimmune hepatitis, viral hepatitis, Wilson disease, biliary obstruction

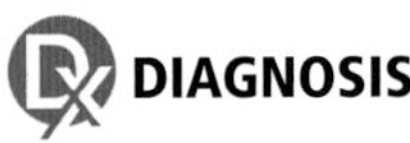

DIAGNOSIS

Approach to patient

- **Phase 1:** Determine if hyperbilirubinemia is unconjugated or conjugated.
- **Phase 2:** if unconjugated hyperbilirubinemia
  - Obtain CBC and indices.
  - Reticulocyte count
  - Coombs test: If test is positive, the diagnosis is isoimmune; if test is negative, then consider polycythemia, extravascular bleed, or RBC structural or enzyme defects.
  - Peripheral smear
- **Phase 3:** if conjugated hyperbilirubinemia
  - Alanine aminotransferase (ALT), aspartate aminotransferase (AST), γ-glutamyltranspeptidase (GGT)
- PT/PTT/international normalized ratio (INR)
  - Ultrasound of the liver/pancreas/gallbladder and biliary tree
  - Rule out those etiologies of conjugated hyperbilirubinemia that may adversely affect the outcome if diagnosis is delayed (biliary atresia, tyrosinemia, galactosemia, inborn error of bile acid synthesis, hereditary fructose intolerance, panhypopituitarism, and others).

HISTORY

- **Question:** Unexplained itching?
- *Significance*: cholestatic liver disease (conjugated hyperbilirubinemia)
- **Question:** History of poor school performance, change in mental status, handwriting?
- *Significance*: Wilson disease
- **Question:** History of other family members having prolonged jaundice, hepatic failure, or sudden death in infancy?
- *Significance*: Suggests an underlying inborn error of metabolism such as tyrosinemia, galactosemia, or a fatty acid oxidation defect
- **Question:** History of IV drug abuse or exposure to blood or blood products, especially prior to 1992?
- *Significance*: The patient may have transfusion-associated viral hepatitis (e.g., hepatitis C).

PHYSICAL EXAM

- **Finding:** Scratch marks?
- *Significance*: pruritus secondary to cholestasis
- **Finding:** Spider angioma, palmar erythema?
- *Significance*: chronic liver disease
- **Finding:** Petechiae, purpura, microcephaly, thrombocytopenia?
- *Significance*: congenital TORCH infection
- **Finding:** Heart murmur?
- *Significance*: Alagille syndrome (peripheral pulmonic stenosis)
- **Finding:** Splenomegaly?
- *Significance*: suggests acute hemolysis (in unconjugated hyperbilirubinemia) or chronic liver disease and portal hypertension (conjugated hyperbilirubinemia)
- **Finding:** Ascites?
- *Significance*: suggests portal hypertension
- **Finding:** Acholic stool?
- *Significance*: severe cholestasis or biliary obstruction
- **Finding:** Xanthomata?
- *Significance:* cholesterol deposits that can be seen in chronic liver disease

DIFFERENTIAL DIAGNOSIS

- Unconjugated hyperbilirubinemia
  - Congenital/anatomic
    - Placental dysfunction/insufficiency resulting in polycythemia (e.g., infants of diabetic mothers)
    - Upper GI tract obstruction (e.g., pyloric stenosis, duodenal web, atresia)
    - Congenital hypothyroidism
  - Infectious
    - Sepsis
  - Trauma/delivery complications
    - Cephalohematoma/bruising
    - Delayed cord clamping, twin–twin transfusion, maternal–fetal transfusion leading to polycythemia
    - Intrauterine hypoxia (secondary to cocaine abuse, high altitude) resulting in polycythemia
    - Induction of labor with oxytocin
    - Prematurity
  - Genetic/metabolic
    - Inherited red cell enzyme, membrane defects (e.g., spherocytosis, glucose-6-phosphate dehydrogenase [G6PD] deficiency, phosphokinase deficiency, elliptocytosis)
    - Hemoglobinopathies (sickle cell anemia, thalassemia)
    - Defect in hepatic bilirubin conjugation (e.g., Crigler-Najjar types I and II, Gilbert)
    - Inborn errors of metabolism
  - Allergic/inflammatory/immunologic
    - Isoimmunization (ABO, Rh, Kell, other incompatibility)
  - Functional
    - Physiologic jaundice
    - Breastfeeding-associated jaundice
    - Swallowed maternal blood
    - Increased bilirubin load due to infant bleeding from a clotting disorder
    - Familial benign unconjugated hyperbilirubinemia in mother and neonate (Lucey-Driscoll syndrome)
- Conjugated hyperbilirubinemia
  - Extrahepatic
    - Extrahepatic biliary atresia
    - Choledochal cysts and other abnormalities of the choledochopancreatic ductal junction
    - Compression of bile duct from mass (malignancy, adenoma, focal nodular hyperplasia, or extrahepatic mass)
    - Spontaneous perforation of the bile duct
    - Bile or mucous plug or biliary sludge
    - Gallstones
  - Infectious etiologies
    - Bacterial: gram-negative sepsis, urinary tract infection
    - Viral: cytomegalovirus; echovirus; herpes simplex virus; rubella; Epstein-Barr virus; HIV; hepatitis A, B, C, D, and E
    - Toxoplasmosis
    - *Pneumocystis carinii*
    - *Entamoeba histolytica*
    - *Mycobacterium tuberculosis*
    - *Mycobacterium avium*-intracellulare
    - Syphilis
  - Toxic, environmental, drugs
    - Post shock or post-asphyxia (ischemic injury to liver)
    - Drugs: acetaminophen, valproate, chlorpromazine, Amanita toxin, and others
    - Hyperalimentation (total parenteral nutrition)
  - Neoplastic
    - Neuroblastoma, hepatic, biliary, pancreatic, duodenal, peritoneal
    - Infiltrative processes such as HLH
    - Langerhans cell histiocytosis
  - Genetic/metabolic
    - Arteriohepatic dysplasia (Alagille syndrome)
    - Progressive familial intrahepatic cholestasis (including FIC1, BSEP, and MDR3 deficiency)
    - Benign recurrent intrahepatic cholestasis
    - Defects in bile acid metabolism
    - Defects in amino acid metabolism: tyrosinemia
    - Defects in lipid metabolism: Wolman disease, Niemann-Pick disease, Gaucher disease
    - Defects in carbohydrate metabolism: galactosemia, hereditary fructose intolerance, glycogenosis type IV
    - Defects in fatty acid oxidation
    - Defects in mitochondrial DNA and respiratory chain defects
    - α_1-antitrypsin deficiency
    - Cystic fibrosis
    - Wilson disease (older children)
    - Inherited noncholestatic conjugated jaundice syndromes (e.g., Dubin-Johnson and Rotor syndrome)
    - Hereditary cholestasis with lymphedema (Aagenaes syndrome)
  - Inflammatory/immunologic/endocrine:
    - Idiopathic neonatal hepatitis
    - Congenital alloimmune hepatitis
    - Idiopathic panhypopituitarism
    - Autoimmune hepatitis (children and adolescents)
    - Sclerosing cholangitis (children and adolescents, unless neonatal form)

DIAGNOSTIC TESTS & INTERPRETATION

- Percutaneous liver biopsies: Liver pathology—in infants with cholestasis, the most common patterns are giant cell hepatitis, bile duct proliferation, and bile duct paucity. A pattern of duct proliferation, bile plugs, portal expansion, and fibrosis suggests biliary obstruction, most likely biliary atresia.
- Intraoperative cholangiogram is indicated for infants with a liver biopsy suggestive of biliary obstruction and possible biliary atresia. If the cholangiogram is consistent with biliary atresia, the surgeon will perform the Kasai portoenterostomy.
- **Test:** Total bilirubin with fractionation into unconjugated, conjugated, and delta fractions
- *Significance*: direct versus indirect hyperbilirubinemia
- If unconjugated hyperbilirubinemia, investigation is initiated with the following:
  - **Test:** CBC with indices, reticulocyte count, and peripheral blood smear for RBC morphology
  - *Significance*: polycythemia in neonate, hemolysis, or other conditions associated with increased destruction of red cells
  - **Test:** Coombs test
  - *Significance*: isoimmune and autoimmune hemolytic anemia
  - **Test:** PT/PTT/INR, platelet count
  - *Significance*: coagulopathy associated with hemorrhage that causes an increased bilirubin load
- If neonatal conjugated hyperbilirubinemia, investigation is initiated with the following:
  - **Test:** serum aminotransferases (ALT, AST)
  - *Significance*: ongoing liver inflammation
  - **Test:** alkaline phosphatase and GGT
  - *Significance*: biliary tree obstruction, bile duct injury, or cholestasis
  - **Test:** PT/INR, PTT, serum albumin, fibrinogen
  - *Significance*: liver synthetic function
  - **Test:** sepsis evaluation (blood and urine and spinal fluid)
  - *Significance*: Sepsis can impair conjugation and excretion of bilirubin.
  - **Test:** free T_3, T_4, and thyroid-stimulating hormone
  - *Significance*: congenital hypothyroidism
  - **Test:** α_1-antitrypsin serum levels and PI phenotype
  - *Significance*: Serum α_1-antitrypsin levels will be low in inherited protease inhibitor deficiency.
  - **Test:** urine dipstick for glucose and reducing substances
  - *Significance*: Positive reducing substances are seen in galactosemia and hereditary fructose intolerance.
  - **Test:** urine for bile acid analysis
  - *Significance*: Inborn error of bile acid metabolism
  - Metabolic workup may be performed depending on clinical setting, including plasma amino acids, urine organic acids, succinylacetone, lactate, pyruvate, and other tests as indicated.
  - In an older child presenting with conjugated hyperbilirubinemia, the most common causes are biliary obstruction due to gallstones, viral hepatitis, and autoimmune hepatitis.
- Ultrasound
  - A noninvasive method to examine the overall liver appearance, size, and density
  - Allows for examination of the biliary tree and gallbladder to rule out choledochal cysts, sludge/stones, and ductal dilatation indicating possible obstruction
  - Infants with biliary atresia/splenic malformation syndrome may have other findings including polysplenia, asplenia, and preduodenal portal vein with azygous continuation.
- Hepatobiliary scintigraphy (HIDA scan): Tracer secretion into the duodenum is evidence against biliary atresia or extrahepatic biliary obstruction.

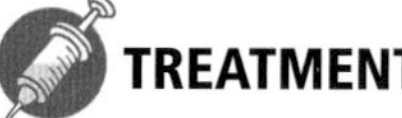

TREATMENT

GENERAL MEASURES

- Treatment largely depends on etiology of jaundice.
- In infants with confirmed biliary atresia, Kasai portoenterostomy is performed.
- Ursodeoxycholic acid is an exogenous bile acid that can help improve cholestasis and is frequently used in children with chronic cholestasis and jaundice.
- Treat Crigler-Najjar syndrome promptly with phototherapy and/or phenobarbital to prevent kernicterus.
- Autoimmune hepatitis in older children and teenagers is treated with immunosuppression, often azathioprine and prednisone.
- Older children with Wilson disease may present with profound hemolysis and may have predominantly unconjugated hyperbilirubinemia with severe parenchymal liver disease and fulminant liver failure.

ISSUES FOR REFERRAL

- Any infant with jaundice beyond 10 to 14 days of age should have a fractionated bilirubin sent.
- Any infant with conjugated hyperbilirubinemia should be referred immediately to a pediatric gastroenterologist for further workup.
- Kasai portoenterostomy is more successful in treating infants with biliary atresia if performed at <8 weeks of age (prompt referral to pediatric gastroenterology is imperative).

ADMISSION, INPATIENT, AND NURSING CONSIDERATIONS

Admission criteria

- Any infant >2 months of age with jaundice should be admitted for biliary atresia evaluation.
- Outcomes of Kasai procedure are improved when completed before 60 days of age.
- Any child with biliary atresia and fever should be admitted for IV antibiotics due to increased risk of sepsis and/or ascending cholangitis.
- Patients with biliary atresia and fever must have blood culture prior to starting antibiotics.
- Limit IV fluids in children with chronic liver disease and portal hypertension.
- If fluids are necessary, use hypotonic fluids to minimize ascites.
- Daily weights are important in determining fluid status in children with chronic liver disease.
- Infants with newly diagnosed biliary atresia who underwent Kasai procedure will be discharged once tolerating feeds and recovered from surgery.
- Jaundice can take up to 3 months to resolve after Kasai procedure.
- Children admitted for fever and antibiotics can be discharged once cultures are negative; labwork is improving and source of fever is identified and patient is tolerating oral antibiotics

ADDITIONAL READING

- American Academy of Pediatrics Subcommittee on Hyperbilirubinemia. Management of hyperbilirubinemia in the newborn infant 35 or more weeks of gestation. *Pediatrics*. 2004;114(1):297–316.
- Brumbaugh D, Mack C. Conjugated hyperbilirubinemia in children. *Pediatr Rev*. 2012;33(7):291–302.
- Cohen RS, Wong RJ, Stevenson DK. Understanding neonatal jaundice: a perspective on causation. *Pediatr Neonatol*. 2010;51(3):143–148.
- Fawaz R, Baumann U, Ekong U, et al. Guideline for the evaluation of cholestatic jaundice in infants: joint recommendations of the North American Society for Pediatric Gastroenterology, Hepatology, and Nutrition and the European Society for Pediatric Gastroenterology, Hepatology, and Nutrition. *J Pediatr Gastroenterol Nutr*. 2017;64(1):154–168.
- Kelly DA, Davenport M. Current management of biliary atresia. *Arch Dis Child*. 2007;92(12):1132–1135.
- Mack CL, Feldman AG, Sokol RJ. Clues to the etiology of bile duct injury in biliary atresia. *Semin Liver Dis*. 2012;32(4):307–316.
- Maisels MJ, McDonagh AF. Phototherapy for neonatal jaundice. *N Engl J Med*. 2008;358(9):920–928.
- Watchko JF. Hyperbilirubinemia in African American neonates: clinical issues and current challenges. *Semin Fetal Neonatal Med*. 2010;15(3):176–182.

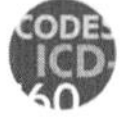

CODES

ICD10

- R17 Unspecified jaundice
- P59.9 Neonatal jaundice, unspecified
- P59.0 Neonatal jaundice associated with preterm delivery

FAQ

- Q: Are there any findings in neonatal jaundice that are specifically concerning?
- A: These findings are concerning until proven otherwise:
  - Jaundice before 36 hours of life
  - Persistent jaundice beyond 10 days of life
  - Serum bilirubin concentration >12 mg/dL
  - Elevation of direct bilirubin >2 mg/dL or 20% of total bilirubin at any time
- Q: Are there any specific factors associated with higher bilirubin levels in neonates?
- A: Factors that have been associated with high serum bilirubin levels are low birth weight, certain ethnic groups (Asian, Native American, Greek), delayed meconium passage after birth, and breastfeeding. G6PD deficiency has also been associated with a higher risk of neonatal jaundice. Factors that have been associated with lower serum levels in neonates include maternal smoking and certain drugs such as phenobarbital. Of note, African American neonates have a lower risk of jaundice overall but are overrepresented in the U.S. Kernicterus Registry. This finding is due partially to a higher incidence of G6PD deficiency in males.
- Q: What is the difference between direct bilirubin and conjugated bilirubin?
- A: Direct bilirubin includes conjugated bilirubin plus bilirubin covalently bound to albumin (delta fraction). Because the half-life of albumin is 20 to 30 days, direct bilirubin can often stay elevated longer than conjugated bilirubin due to the delta fraction.
- Q: Where does the term "jaundice" come from?
- A: Jaundice is derived from the French word jaune, which means "yellow."

JAUNDICE ASSOCIATED WITH BREASTFEEDING

Jennifer A. F. Tender, MD, IBCLC • Sahira A. Long, MD, IBCLC, FABM

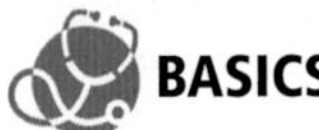

BASICS

DESCRIPTION

The three major categories of unconjugated hyperbilirubinemia associated with breastfeeding:

- Physiologic jaundice:
  - Occurs between 1 and 7 days of life
  - Peaks at 3 to 5 days
- Suboptimal intake jaundice (SIJ):
  - Currently, there is no consensus for the terminology for jaundice associated with suboptimal intake in a breastfed infant or SIJ.
  - The term "breastfeeding jaundice" has been used historically but this is inaccurate because these infants are not jaundiced because they are breastfeeding; they are jaundiced because their intake of breast milk is not adequate. Until a consensus is reached, this chapter uses SIJ.
  - SIJ occurs in the first 1 to 2 weeks.
- Prolonged jaundice associated with breast milk feeding or prolonged unconjugated hyperbilirubinemia (PUH):
  - Occurs between 1 and 12 weeks in thriving human milk-fed infants
  - "Breast milk jaundice" has been used historically, yet researchers question this terminology.

EPIDEMIOLOGY

Prevalence

- Physiologic jaundice: 40–60% of infants
- SIJ: 10% of breastfed infants
- PUH: 0.5–2% of breastfed infants

RISK FACTORS

- Jaundice in first 24 hours (pathologic)
- Elevated total serum bilirubin prior to nursery discharge
- Blood type incompatibility
- Glucose-6-phosphate dehydrogenase (G6PD) deficiency
- Gilbert syndrome
- Gestational age <36 weeks
- Previous sibling receiving phototherapy
- Cephalohematoma or significant bruising
- Exclusive breastfeeding
- Eastern Asian race

PATHOPHYSIOLOGY

- Normal physiology:
  - Bilirubin is a breakdown product of hemoglobin. Unconjugated bilirubin is bound to albumin, transported to the liver, and conjugated by the hepatic enzyme uridine diphosphate glucuronosyl transferase 1A1 (UGT1A1).
  - Conjugated bilirubin is transported into the small intestines via the bile ducts, where it is modified and excreted in stool.
  - If stooling is delayed, bilirubin is deconjugated by intestinal enzymes and returned to the liver via the portal circulation (enterohepatic circulation).
- Physiologic jaundice: Bilirubin levels are elevated in newborns due to several factors:
  - Increased hematocrit and red blood cell volume
  - Increased red blood cell lysis due to shorter red blood cell lifespan
  - Impaired bilirubin excretion because of an immature hepatic UGT1A1 enzyme and increased enterohepatic circulation
- SIJ: Lack of effective breastfeeding causes inadequate milk and calorie intake and results in decreased stooling and increased enterohepatic circulation. Infants may also be dehydrated.
- PUH: unclear etiology and probably multifactorial. No causative agent has yet been found in breast milk. One theory is that breast milk may unmask underlying genetic disorders such as G6PD deficiency and/or Gilbert syndrome.

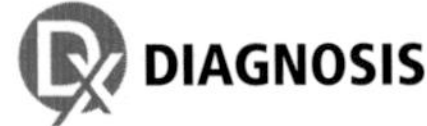

DIAGNOSIS

HISTORY

- SIJ
  - Weight loss: Infants should not lose >8% of their birth weight. Infants should gain 15 to 30 g/24 h after maternal copious milk production (around day 4 or 5).
  - Frequency and duration of breastfeeding: Breastfed infants should suckle at least 8 to 12 times per 24 hours.
  - Pain with breastfeeding may indicate poor latch and therefore decreased milk transfer.
  - Urination per 24 hours: urinates 1 time for each day of life until copious milk production
  - Stooling: changes from meconium to transitional to yellow seedy by 4 to 5 days of life
  - Maternal causes of decreased milk production: prior breast surgery, hypothyroidism, retained placenta, insufficient glandular tissue, few medications, obesity, and infertility
- PUH
  - Infants should be in good health, gaining at least 15 to 30 g/24 h and nursing well.
  - Family history of neonatal jaundice may indicate a genetic propensity for developing jaundice.
  - Screen for G6PD deficiency.
  - Screen for risk factors associated with pathologic jaundice:
    - Jaundice in the first 24 hours of life
    - Direct hyperbilirubinemia
    - Congenital hypothyroidism
    - Maternal blood type to screen for Rh or ABO incompatibility
    - Inherited hemolytic diseases (hereditary spherocytosis). Ask about family history of severe neonatal jaundice, anemia, or splenectomy.
    - Infection: maternal group B strep infection, maternal chorioamnionitis or intrapartum fever, prolonged rupture of membranes, infant fever ≥100.4°F rectally, decreased infant feeding, increased infant sleepiness or fussiness

PHYSICAL EXAM

- Infant
  - General: thin, not thriving infant in 1st week associated with SIJ. Well appearing, thriving older infant associated with PUH. An ill-appearing, grunting, tachypneic, sleepy, or fussy infant not interested in nursing should be evaluated for infection. Sleepy infants may be or become dehydrated.
  - Mucous membranes: dry mucous membranes associated with dehydration
  - Skin: Jaundice (and bilirubin levels) generally progresses from head to toe, but bilirubin levels estimated visually may be inaccurate. Infants with dark skin tones are especially difficult to assess.
  - Cephalohematomas and bruising are associated with increased red blood cell breakdown.
  - Abdomen: Hepatosplenomegaly is associated with metabolic or hemolytic process or biliary obstruction. Abdominal distension may be a result of intestinal obstruction.
- Direct observation of a feeding is crucial:
  - Lips should be everted and mouth wide open approaching a 180-degree angle.
  - As much of the areola as possible should be in the infant's mouth.
  - The infant should have deep movement of the jaw and suck/swallow/breathe rhythmically with milk visible in infant's mouth.

DIFFERENTIAL DIAGNOSIS

- Increased bilirubin production
  - Hematologic
    - ABO or Rh isoimmunization
    - Erythrocyte enzyme defects (e.g., G6PD deficiency)
    - Erythrocyte membrane defects (e.g., hereditary spherocytosis)
    - Polycythemia
- Impaired bilirubin conjugation
  - Gilbert syndrome
  - Crigler-Najjar syndrome
- Decreased bilirubin excretion
  - Biliary obstruction
  - Biliary atresia
  - Choledochal cyst
  - Dubin-Johnson syndrome
  - Rotor syndrome
- Intestinal obstruction
  - Meconium ileus
  - Hirschsprung disease
- Congenital: transient familial neonatal hyperbilirubinemia
- Metabolic
  - Hypothyroidism
  - Galactosemia
- Miscellaneous
  - Dehydration
  - Sepsis
  - Cephalohematoma
  - Maternal oxytocin use

DIAGNOSTIC TESTS & INTERPRETATION

Initial Tests (screening, lab, imaging)

- All mothers should be screened for blood and Rh type. Infants of mothers with blood type O or Rh negative need their cord blood tested for blood type and Coombs to identify risk for hemolytic anemia. These infants are at greater risk for kernicterus and need to be treated at lower total serum bilirubin levels.
- Infants should have a predischarge either total serum bilirubin or transcutaneous bilirubin level.
  - Bilirubin levels are interpreted based on age in hours/days and risk factors (blood incompatibility, preterm, illness). Use of a nomogram tool (such as www.bilitool.com) stratifies the infants' risk based on the American Academy of Pediatrics (AAP) bilirubin guidelines.
- Generally, minimal laboratory evaluation is needed in a healthy breastfed infant with mild jaundice in the absence of risk factors. However, SIJ and PUH are diagnoses of exclusion. The following tests should be considered, depending on the clinical presentation:
  - Conjugated/unconjugated (direct/indirect) bilirubin level interpreted based on age and risk factors
    - May guide treatment
    - Must be measured in all infants with very early jaundice $<$24 hours of age
    - Recommended in all infants with persistent jaundice
  - Conjugated or direct serum bilirubin: Elevated level ($>$1 mg/dL or 10% of total serum bilirubin) may indicate infection, biliary obstructive disease, cholestasis, metabolic disease, or severe hemolysis.
  - Thyroid tests
  - CBC and smear:
    - Look for polycythemia or anemia.
    - Smear may assist with diagnosing hemolysis.
    - Decreases in hematocrit over time may reflect ongoing hemorrhage or hemolysis.
    - A mean corpuscular hemoglobin concentration (MCHC) of $>$36.0 g/dL may suggest hereditary spherocytosis.
    - Abnormal white cell count may indicate infection.
  - Electrolytes (especially sodium) in infant, if concern for dehydration
  - G6PD quantitative test
    - G6PD deficiency may cause an increase in bilirubin later than other hemolytic disease and has been associated with an increased risk of kernicterus.

TREATMENT

- SIJ
  - Evaluate and treat for insufficient milk intake. Assess latch, position, and milk transfer. Consult a lactation expert if needed.
  - Increase frequency of effective breastfeeding to 8 to 12 times per 24 hours.
  - Supplement with pumped breast milk, donor breast milk or formula if weight loss $>$10%; clinical signs or laboratory results suggest dehydration.
  - Phototherapy if serum bilirubin levels meet or exceed the AAP recommended threshold levels for phototherapy based on infant's age in hours, gestational age, and neurotoxicity risk factors.
  - Consider home phototherapy in low-risk infants if bilirubin levels close to threshold. Home phototherapy poses less of an obstruction to breastfeeding.
  - Monitor serum bilirubin levels closely until they are acceptable. Check levels after stopping phototherapy.
  - Phototherapy may contribute to dehydration; it is essential to monitor hydration status.
  - Use the AAP exchange transfusion guidelines and nomograms to assist with decisions about exchange transfusions. Exchange transfusions should be performed only by trained personnel in a neonatal intensive care unit with full monitoring and resuscitation capabilities.
- PUH:
  - Encourage and support exclusive breastfeeding for almost all cases of PUH.
  - Phototherapy if indicated
  - Bilirubin levels approaching 17 to 20 mg/dL are rare ($\leq$1% of 7- to 14-day old infants). It is essential to exclude other causes (such as G6PD and/or Gilbert syndrome). Different strategies exist for managing PUH when bilirubin levels approach 17 to 20 mg/dL.
    - Strategy 1: Stop breastfeeding for 24 hours and give either donor milk or a casein hydrolysate formula.
    - Strategy 2: Continue breastfeeding and replace two feedings a day with a casein hydrolysate formula for 48 hours.
    - Strategy 3: Continue breastfeeding exclusively without interruption and follow bilirubin levels closely. Consider above strategies when bilirubin $\geq$20 mg/dL.
    - With strategy 1 or 2, mothers should pump or express their breast milk to maintain their milk supply and consider supplementing with a feeding method other than a bottle, such as a cup or supplemental nursing device.

ONGOING CARE

FOLLOW-UP RECOMMENDATIONS

- Follow up 2 to 3 days after discharge, earlier if infant at high risk for jaundice. Weight check, physical exam, assessment of hydration, and observation of feeding; bilirubin level if clinically indicated
- Close follow-up 1 to 2 days later if concern about milk intake or jaundice
- Patient education: Mother should be assisted with latch and positioning and be taught signs/symptoms of adequate milk intake, dehydration, illness, and jaundice.
- Late preterm/near-term infants need especially close follow-up as they have increased risk of poor milk intake.
- Visual assessment of jaundice may be inaccurate. Consider an objective measure of jaundice (e.g., total serum bilirubin or transcutaneous bilirubin level) for follow-up assessment.

ADMISSION, INPATIENT, AND NURSING CONSIDERATIONS

If a breastfed infant is hospitalized for jaundice, encourage continued breastfeeding if possible. For infants with SIJ, consult a lactation expert to evaluate cause for insufficient milk intake and assist with positioning and latch. The mother may need a hospital grade double electric pump to increase her milk supply.

COMPLICATIONS

- Bilirubin-induced neurologic dysfunction (BIND) is when bilirubin crosses the blood–brain barrier and binds to the brain.
  - Acute bilirubin encephalopathy: Acute manifestations of BIND include lethargy, hypotonia, opisthotonus, seizures, high-pitched cry.
  - Kernicterus: Chronic and permanent symptoms of BIND include sensorineural hearing loss, upward gaze palsy, dental enamel dysplasia, cerebral palsy, cognitive impairment.
- Unnecessary cessation of breastfeeding
- Parental and health care provider anxiety

ADDITIONAL READING

- Academy of Breastfeeding Medicine. Clinical protocols. Guidelines for management of jaundice in the breastfeeding infant equal to or greater than 35 weeks' gestation. http://www.bfmed.org/Resources/Protocols.aspx. Accessed February 20, 2017.
- American Academy of Pediatrics Subcommittee on Hyperbilirubinemia. Management of hyperbilirubinemia in the newborn infant 35 or more weeks of gestation. *Pediatrics*. 2004;114(4):297–316.
- Gourley GR, Li Z, Kreamer BL, et al. A controlled, randomized, double-blind trial of prophylaxis against jaundice among breastfed newborns. *Pediatrics*. 2005;116(2):385–391.
- Lauer BJ, Spector ND. Hyperbilirubinemia in the newborn. *Pediatr Rev*. 2011;32(8):341–349.

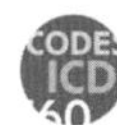

CODES

ICD10

- P59.3 Neonatal jaundice from breast milk inhibitor
- P59.8 Neonatal jaundice from other specified causes
- P59.9 Neonatal jaundice, unspecified

FAQ

- Q: Will jaundice cause my baby to have developmental or neurologic problems?
- A: If hyperbilirubinemia is appropriately monitored and treated, it should not cause any developmental problems.
- Q: What can be done to prevent SIJ?
- A: Early, frequent, and effective breastfeeding at least 8 to 12 times in 24 hours can decrease the risk of SIJ. Do not supplement unless recommended by a health care provider. Get help from a breastfeeding expert if you have pain or if the infant is not latching on and/or nursing well.
- Q: Should I stop breastfeeding if my baby is jaundiced?
- A: The frequency and effectiveness of breastfeeding should be increased and appropriate lactation consultation obtained for SIJ. Supplementation may be necessary. Most infants with PUH should continue to breastfeed. If bilirubin levels approach 17 to 20 mg/dL, may consider 48 hours of supplementation or 24 hours of cessation of breastfeeding with pumping and/or hand expression to maintain your milk supply.

KAWASAKI DISEASE

Rebecca Reindel, MD • Stanford T. Shulman, MD

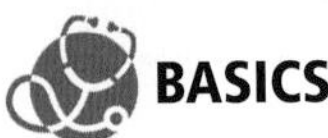

BASICS

DESCRIPTION

- Kawasaki disease (KD) is a medium-sized vessel arteritis of early childhood with a predilection for the coronary arteries, which can result in dilatation, aneurysms, thrombosis, and stenosis.
- No diagnostic test exists, and incomplete presentations are common. Prompt recognition and treatment can reduce risk of coronary artery involvement from 25% to 5%.

EPIDEMIOLOGY

- Worldwide with highest incidence in Japan
- Peak of hospitalizations December to March
- Approximately 80% of children with KD are <5 years old.

Incidence

- U.S. hospitalization data (2003, 2006, 2009, and 2012) demonstrate an annual incidence of 18 to 20.8/100,000 children aged <5 years and 6.11 to 6.64/100,000 children aged 0 to 19 years.
- KD is more common in boys than girls. In 2012, the U.S. hospitalization rate for boys was 7.24/100,000 versus 5.11/100,000 in girls.
- More common in Asian/Pacific Islanders, with highest rates in Japan
  - Ethnic predisposition persists in different geographic locations, with highest incidence in the United States in Asian/Pacific Islander children (10.3/100,000).
  - Rates are higher in black and Hispanic children compared to Caucasian children, but most KD patients in the United States are Caucasian.

Prevalence

5,033 reported cases of KD in the United States in 2012

RISK FACTORS

- Patients of Asian/Pacific Islander descents are at higher risk of KD.
- Patients who are younger and/or refractory to standard therapy are at higher risk of coronary artery disease.

Genetics

- Siblings have 10- to 30-fold higher risk of KD.
- Genome-wide linkage studies suggest polymorphisms in multiple genetic loci involved in immune response may confer susceptibility to KD.

PATHOPHYSIOLOGY

- Generalized arteritis with early neutrophilic infiltrate, with later transition to lymphocyte infiltration, and lastly to luminal myofibroblastic proliferation
- Can very rarely result in destruction of the endothelium through to the adventitia resulting in aneurysms and the rare possibility of rupture

ETIOLOGY

- Etiology is unknown.
- Infectious cause suggested by the following:
  - Abrupt onset and resolution of symptoms, usually without recurrence
  - Clusters and epidemics
  - Age of affected patients
  - Seasonal predominance
  - Oligoclonal IgA plasma cells noted in KD tissues, which bind to cytoplasmic inclusion bodies found in affected tissues
- Data suggest that KD is caused by a previously unrecognized ubiquitous RNA virus that causes disease in a genetically susceptible population.
  - No supporting evidence for multiple proposed etiologic agents: toxic shock toxin, rug shampoo, retrovirus, bocavirus, coronavirus, mercury, Epstein-Barr virus (EBV)/cytomegalovirus (CMV)

DIAGNOSIS

- KD is a clinical diagnosis.
- Current diagnostic criteria: fever for ≥5 days and ≥4 of 5 clinical findings, which need not be present at the same time
  - Extremity changes (erythema of palms, soles, and/or edema of hands, feet)
  - Polymorphous exanthema (frequently in perineal region with early desquamation)
  - Nonexudative bilateral bulbar conjunctivitis (with limbic sparing)
  - Mucosal changes (erythema of lips and oropharyngeal mucosa, strawberry tongue, cracked/swollen lips)
  - Unilateral cervical lymphadenopathy (>1.5 cm in diameter)
- Incomplete KD
  - If patient has characteristics consistent with KD along with fever for ≥5 days with two or three clinical criteria and CRP ≥3 and/or ESR ≥40, obtain echocardiogram (ECHO). If patient with ≥3 supplemental lab criteria, treat for KD.
  - Supplemental lab criteria for incomplete KD: albumin ≤3 g/dL, platelets (after 7 days) ≥450,000/μL, WBC ≥15,000/μL, urine ≥10 WBC/HPF, anemia for age, ALT elevation

ALERT
Young infants with KD often present with few, if any, clinical characteristics of KD. Maintain a high index of suspicion for KD in young infants with prolonged fever.

HISTORY

- High-spiking fevers usually >39°C can persist up to 3 to 4 weeks (mean 11 days).
- In addition to the clinical criteria above, the following complaints are sometimes seen:
  - Irritability
  - Abdominal pain/emesis/diarrhea
  - Refusal to ambulate or pain with ambulation
  - Poor appetite

PHYSICAL EXAM

- Extremity changes with palmar/plantar erythema and/or hand/foot swelling
  - Periungual desquamation of hands and feet within 2 to 3 weeks of fever onset
  - Beau lines (transverse grooves across nails) within 1 to 2 months of fever onset
- Polymorphous rash
  - Usually, diffuse maculopapular rash
  - Often, perineal rash with desquamation
  - Also seen: erythema multiforme, erythroderma, urticaria, scarlatiniform rash
  - Not vesicular or bullous
- Bilateral nonexudative conjunctivitis
  - Bulbar, with limbic sparing
  - Painless
  - Anterior uveitis/iridocyclitis can be seen.
- Mucosal changes
  - Cracked, red, swollen lips
  - Strawberry tongue with erythema and prominent papillae
  - Buccal mucosa erythema

ALERT
In a patient with ongoing fever and nonsuppurative lymphadenitis despite adequate antibacterial therapy, consider KD.

- Unilateral cervical lymphadenopathy of one or more nodes that are >1.5 cm in diameter
  - Can be misdiagnosed as bacterial lymphadenitis
  - Usually without overlying erythema
  - Least common clinical finding in KD
- Other clinical findings
  - Myocarditis with tachycardia, gallop, innocent flow murmur
  - Shock and hypotension
  - Arthritis and arthralgias (early can be multiple joints, later is usually weight-bearing joints)
  - Urethritis, meatitis
  - Transient hearing loss (rare)

DIFFERENTIAL DIAGNOSIS

- Viral infections
  - Measles, adenovirus, EBV, CMV
- Bacterial infections
  - Scarlet fever
  - Streptococcal or staphylococcal toxic shock
  - Staphylococcal scalded-skin syndrome
  - Leptospirosis
  - Cervical lymphadenitis
- Rheumatologic conditions
  - Juvenile idiopathic arthritis, especially systemic onset
  - Autoinflammatory conditions (periodic fever syndromes) such as tumor necrosis factor receptor associated periodic syndrome (TRAPS) or neonatal onset multisystem inflammatory disease (NOMID)
- Drug reactions
  - Stevens-Johnson syndrome
- Mercury hypersensitivity

DIAGNOSTIC TESTS & INTERPRETATION

- No definitive diagnostic test
- The presence of ancillary lab findings can support diagnosis of KD and be helpful in identifying those patients with incomplete KD.
- Elevated ESR (>40 mm/h) and/or CRP (>3 mg/dL or 30 mg/L)

ALERT
ESR is artifactually elevated and not useful after administration of IV immunoglobulin (IVIG).

- CBC
  - WBC normal to elevated with left shift
  - Anemia (normocytic/normochromic)
  - Platelets usually normal in the 1st week of illness and increase over the next 2 to 3 weeks, sometimes to >1,000,000/mm^3
- Chemistries
  - Hypoalbuminemia
  - Hyponatremia
  - Transaminitis and elevated GGT
  - Hyperbilirubinemia
- Aseptic meningitis with mild to moderate CSF pleocytosis
- Sterile pyuria

- Synovial fluid leukocytosis
- Chest radiograph
  - Interstitial pneumonitis may be present.
- ECHO
  - Aneurysms or ectasias of the epicardial coronary arteries that evolve over time
    - Z-score corrects for variations in body surface area among children.
    - Larger aneurysms with higher risk of thrombosis and death
  - Decreased myocardial contractility
  - Mitral or aortic (rare) regurgitation
  - Pericardial effusion
  - Rarely, aneurysms of other medium-sized vessels, including iliac and axillary
- Abdominal ultrasound
  - Hydrops of the gallbladder

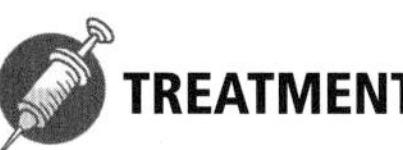

TREATMENT

GENERAL MEASURES

- Rapid diagnosis and treatment can decrease the risk of coronary artery aneurysms.
- Close follow-up and monitoring for the development of aneurysms after discharge

MEDICATION

- Combination therapy with IVIG and aspirin
  - Proven efficacy in reducing coronary artery aneurysms when given by 10th day of illness
  - Clinical benefit to therapy after 10th day, although prevention of coronary aneurysms unclear
  - IVIG dose: 2 g/kg given over 10 to 12 hours
  - Aspirin dose: 80 to 100 mg/kg/24 h PO divided q6h until acute-phase reactants normalize and patient defervesces or until 14th day of illness, at which time the dose is reduced to 3 to 5 mg/kg *once daily*
- Primary adjunctive corticosteroid therapy appears to reduce the incidence of coronary artery disease in a subset of high-risk Japanese patients.
  - Scoring systems used to identify high-risk patients in Japan do not appear effective in U.S. populations; no accepted scoring system currently in use in the United States
  - Optimal dose, duration, and formulation of steroids for adjunctive use has not been established.
- Treatment of refractory KD
  - 10–20% of patients do not respond to the first dose of IVIG.
  - 70–80% of nonresponders will respond to a second dose of IVIG.
  - Limited evidence to support a treatment recommendation for those not responding to second IVIG dose, but salvage therapy with a third dose of IVIG, IV corticosteroids, infliximab, cyclosporine, cyclophosphamide, and methotrexate has been reported
  - Consider consultation with a KD expert for refractory patients.
- Antithrombotic therapy for aneurysms
  - Consider addition of antiplatelet therapy or anticoagulation in consultation with cardiology depending on size and extent of aneurysms.

ADDITIONAL THERAPIES

Interventional therapy for life-threatening aneurysms

- Coronary artery bypass
- Percutaneous angioplasty
- Heart transplantation (rarely)

ADMISSION, INPATIENT, AND NURSING CONSIDERATIONS

- Admission criteria
  - Prolonged fever and clinical and laboratory findings suggestive of KD
- Nursing
  - Frequent vital signs and monitoring during IVIG administration
  - Patient and caregiver education
- Discharge criteria
  - Resolution of fever for 24 hours after completion of IVIG administration
  - Substantial decline or normalization of CRP levels
  - Improvement in clinical symptoms
  - Patients should have ECHO completed and interpreted prior to discharge, with additional therapy, monitoring, and prolonged hospital stay as indicated.

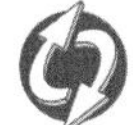

ONGOING CARE

FOLLOW-UP RECOMMENDATIONS

- Low-dose aspirin should be continued until follow-up ECHO at 2 weeks and 6 to 8 weeks after discharge are normal.
- Some centers perform ECHO at 6 to 12 months after discharge.
- Inflammatory markers and CBC should be followed until normalized.

Patient Monitoring

- More frequent follow-up, monitoring, and cardiac imaging for those with coronary abnormalities; advise to monitor for emesis, irritability, and nonspecific symptoms of myocardial ischemia.
- Assessing the risk for myocardial ischemia in long-term follow-up involves consideration of the Z-score for coronary artery luminal dimension and the current and maximum degree of coronary involvement.
- The intensity and frequency of follow-up visits and imaging and the need for additional medications (anticoagulant/antiplatelet therapy, β-blockers, statins) can be determined by assessing the individual risk of a patient, as per American Heart Association recommendations.

PROGNOSIS

- The process of resolution of aneurysms is incompletely understood. Some histopathologic changes in the arterial wall and lumen likely persist despite angiographic regression and may result in stenosis.
- Smaller aneurysms are more likely to resolve by echocardiography and angiography than larger aneurysms.
- Resolution of aneurysms (by angiography) is reported in ~50–67% of vessels.
- Improved prognosis with age <1 year, fusiform rather than saccular aneurysm, distal location
- Giant aneurysms with worst prognosis: higher likelihood of thrombosis and stenosis
- Cause of death usually myocardial infarction due to thrombosis
- Long-term implications for cardiovascular health appear positive, but some uncertainty remains, even when there are no coronary aneurysms.

COMPLICATIONS

- Aneurysmal rupture (very rare)
- Myocardial infarction
- Coronary artery stenosis years after onset
- Rare association with hemophagocytic syndrome
- Recurrence rate <1%, higher in Asian populations

ADDITIONAL READING

- Burns JC, Glodé MP. Kawasaki syndrome. *Lancet*. 2004;364(9433):533–544.
- Freeman AF, Shulman ST. Refractory Kawasaki disease. *Pediatr Infect Dis J*. 2004;23(5):463–464.
- Holman RC, Belay ED, Christensen KY, et al. Hospitalizations for Kawasaki syndrome among children in the United States, 1997–2007. *Pediatr Infect Dis J*. 2010;29(6):483–488.
- Kawasaki T. Acute febrile mucocutaneous syndrome with lymphoid involvement with specific desquamation of the fingers and toes in children. *Arerugi*. 1967;16(3):178–222.
- Kawasaki T, Kosaki F, Okawa S, et al. A new infantile acute febrile mucocutaneous lymph node syndrome (MLNS) prevailing in Japan. *Pediatrics*. 1974;54(3):271–276.
- Kobayashi T, Saji T, Otani T, et al; for RAISE Study Group Investigators. Efficacy of immunoglobulin plus prednisolone for prevention of coronary artery abnormalities in severe Kawasaki disease (RAISE study): a randomised, open-label, blinded-endpoints trial. *Lancet*. 2012;379(9826):1613–1620.
- Newburger JW, Sleeper LA, McCrindle BW, et al; for Pediatric Heart Network Investigators. Randomized trial of pulsed corticosteroid therapy for primary treatment of Kawasaki disease. *N Engl J Med*. 2007;356(7):663–675.
- Newburger JW, Takahashi M, Gerber MA, et al. Diagnosis, treatment, and long-term management of Kawasaki disease: a statement for health professionals from the Committee on Rheumatic Fever, Endocarditis, and Kawasaki Disease, Council on Cardiovascular Disease in the Young, American Heart Association. *Pediatrics*. 2004;114(6):1708–1733.
- Okubo Y, Nochioka K, Sakakibara H, et al. National survey of pediatric hospitalizations due to Kawasaki disease and coronary artery aneurysms in the USA. *Clin Rheumatol*. 2017;36(2):413–419.
- Pinna GS, Kafetzis DA, Tselkas OI, et al. Kawasaki disease: an overview. *Curr Opin Infect Dis*. 2008;21(3):263–270.
- Rowley A. Kawasaki disease: novel insights into etiology and genetic susceptibility. *Annu Rev Med*. 2011;62:69–77.
- Rowley A, Shulman ST. Pathogenesis and management of Kawasaki disease. *Expert Rev Anti Infect Ther*. 2010;8(2):197–203.
- Shulman ST, Rowley A. Kawasaki disease: insights into pathogenesis and approaches to treatment. *Nat Rev Rheumatol*. 2015;11(8):475–482.

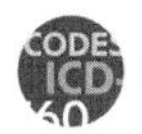

CODES

ICD10

M30.3 Mucocutaneous lymph node syndrome [Kawasaki]

FAQ

- Q: Who first described KD?
- A: Tomisaku Kawasaki, MD is a pediatrician and graduate of the Chiba University School of Medicine. He noted his first case of the disease while working in the Department of Pediatrics at the Red Cross Hospital in Hiroo, Tokyo in January 1961. In 1967, he first described a series of 50 patients with "acute febrile mucocutaneous lymph node syndrome." The first English description of the syndrome was published in 1974.

K

KNEE PAIN, ANTERIOR/PATELLOFEMORAL MALALIGNMENT SYNDROME

Theodore J. Ganley, MD • Matthew Grady, MD, CAQSM

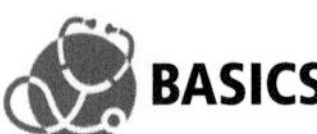

BASICS

DESCRIPTION

- Condition characterized by discomfort at the anterior aspect of the knee that is generally associated with activities, especially those that involve running, jumping, and climbing stairs
- Has also been called "miserable malalignment syndrome"

PATHOPHYSIOLOGY

- Predisposing factors for patellofemoral malalignment syndrome include the following:
  - Femoral anteversion
  - Genu valgus
  - Pes planus
- These three anatomic features have been commonly referred to as a terrible triad contributing to anterior knee pain. Because the entire kinetic chain is linked in function, malalignment at one area can lead to secondary stresses at a distant location.
- Excess femoral anteversion, as well as marked pes planus, can contribute to increased lateral pull on the patella and subsequent patellofemoral pain.
- Further contributing factors include a wider pelvis and a more laterally positioned tibial tubercle, both of which also contribute to altered biomechanics at the knee.
- Weak hip abductors and quadriceps muscles and tight hamstrings, iliotibial band, Achilles tendons, and quadriceps can lead to increased forces across the patellofemoral joint.

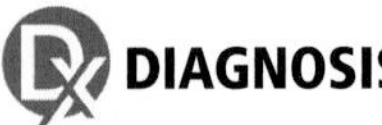

DIAGNOSIS

HISTORY

- Pain under and around the kneecap with activities including squatting, sitting for prolonged periods with the knees bent, and going up or down stairs or hills: These activities increase patellofemoral contact stress.
- Recent history of direct trauma to the kneecap: A blunt trauma to the kneecap can cause soft tissue or subchondral contusion that may exacerbate this condition.

PHYSICAL EXAM

- Assess one-legged squat for weak hip abductors—knee will go into valgus.
- Palpate medial and lateral patellar facets for areas of pain due to increased contact forces.
- Cracking noises from the front of the knee with flexion and extension
  - Cracking can be a sign of softening of the undersurface of the patella.
  - Chondromalacia is patellar articular cartilage pathologic change, which ranges from mild cracking attributed to softening to locking and catching attributed to cartilage disruption.
- There is no single angulation or rotation profile that is universal for all anterior knee pain patients. However, many have femoral anteversion, genu valgus, and pes planus. Weak hip abductors and tight hamstrings or quadriceps may also be found.

DIFFERENTIAL DIAGNOSIS

- Osgood-Schlatter disease
  - Tenderness not at the patella but at the anterior tibial tubercle
  - A self-limiting inflammation of the apophysis that tends to occur in growing teenagers and preteens
  - Irregularity and fragmentation of the apophysis are seen on lateral radiographs.
- Meniscus tear
  - Disruption of the crescent-shaped fibrocartilaginous tissue adjacent to the tibial and femoral articular surfaces
  - Most commonly presents as posteromedial or posterolateral hemijoint tenderness with knee hyperflexion and rotation
- Distal iliotibial band tendonitis
  - Irritation of distal iliotibial band as it rubs over the lateral condyle before attaching on lateral tibia (Gerdy tubercle)
  - Common in runners or those with weak hip abductors
- Prepatellar bursitis
  - An inflammation of the fluid-filled bursa sac beneath the SC tissue and immediately anterior to the patella
  - More common in patients who kneel for extended periods of time and has been called "carpet layer's knee"
  - Swelling and tenderness immediately anterior to the patella; does not primarily present with deeper tenderness in the medial and lateral parapatellar regions found in patellofemoral syndrome

ALERT
Patients with a traumatic effusion, locking, catching, instability to ligamentous stress testing, multiple joint effusions, or night waking should be evaluated for other traumatic or medical conditions.

DIAGNOSTIC TESTS & INTERPRETATION

- Anterior and posterior, lateral, Merchant plain radiographs of the knee
  - The Merchant kneecap view shows the shape of the patella within the trochlea.
  - Patients will frequently be found to have lateral patellar tilt, as well as an abnormally shaped patella with excessive elongation of the lateral portion of the patella/lateral patellar facet.
- MRI: not a 1st-line study for patellofemoral syndrome; however, it may be performed to rule out associated pathology in patients with recalcitrant pain and unusual clinical presentations.

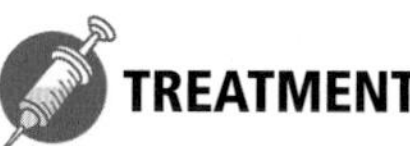

TREATMENT

GENERAL MEASURES

- A progressive exercise program is the main focus of treatment.
- Strength and flexibility exercises are needed to improve the mechanics of the patellofemoral joint.
- Strengthening should include hip abductors, hip extensors, hamstrings, and the quadriceps muscles.
  - This strengthening can be performed several times each day as a home exercise program or formally with physical therapy in more recalcitrant cases.
- Stretching should include quadriceps, hamstrings, iliotibial band, and tendoachilles stretches as indicated by the physical examination (PE).
- Patients can be advanced from low-resistance exercises such as swimming, stationary bike, and elliptical trainers to higher level running activities.
- Activity restriction in the initial acutely symptomatic stage is instituted to eliminate high-impact sports, including especially those that involve running and jumping.

ADDITIONAL READING

- Collado H, Fredericson M. Patellofemoral pain syndrome. *Clin Sports Med*. 2010;29(3):379–398.
- Crossley KM, Stefanik JJ, Selfe J, et al. 2016 Patellofemoral pain consensus statement from the 4th International Patellofemoral Pain Research Retreat, Manchester. Part 1: terminology, definitions, clinical examination, natural history, patellofemoral osteoarthritis and patient-reported outcome measures. *Br J Sports Med*. 2016;50(14):839–843.
- Crossley KM, van Middelkoop M, Callaghan MJ, et al. 2016 Patellofemoral pain consensus statement from the 4th International Patellofemoral Pain Research Retreat, Manchester. Part 2: recommended physical interventions (exercise, taping, bracing, foot orthoses and combined interventions). *Br J Sports Med*. 2016;50(14):844–852.

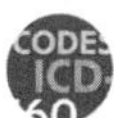

CODES

ICD10

- M25.569 Pain in unspecified knee
- M22.2X9 Patellofemoral disorders, unspecified knee
- M22.40 Chondromalacia patellae, unspecified knee

FAQ

- Q: Is it acceptable to play sports, or is this condition too dangerous?
- A: Patients with a history of patellofemoral syndrome who have regained their strength and flexibility are permitted to return to their activities, provided that they do not have pain and limping during their activities. A history of catching, locking, or knee effusions may be a sign of further biomechanical intra-articular pathology that should be addressed.
- Q: Is bracing indicated?
- A: Some patients with anterior knee pain respond to neoprene sleeves, and those with a component of increased lateral translation may benefit from neoprene sleeves with lateral patellar supports. Bracing, however, is not a substitute for strength and conditioning program.
- Q: Is chondromalacia patella the same as patellofemoral syndrome?
- A: No. Chondromalacia is a classification of the anatomic pathologic changes of the undersurface of the patella. Patellofemoral syndrome is the clinical condition encompassing the patient's history, physical, and radiographic elements of anterior knee pain.

K

LACRIMAL DUCT OBSTRUCTION

Bethlehem Abebe-Wolpaw, MD

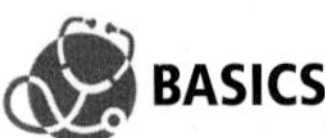

BASICS

DESCRIPTION

A congenital blockage identified in infants from failure of canalization, most commonly at the distal portion, of the nasolacrimal duct. Epiphora (constant tearing) is the most common presentation followed by discharge unresponsive to treatment. Less commonly, the blockage is an acquired condition.

EPIDEMIOLOGY

- Most common lacrimal system abnormality
- Affects up to 6% of newborns
- Spontaneous resolution occurs in 80–90% of cases within 1 year.
- Most common cause of pediatric epiphora

RISK FACTORS

Incidence is higher in infants with craniofacial malformations and Down syndrome.

PATHOPHYSIOLOGY

- Congenital obstruction most commonly occurs at the caudal end of the duct at the level of the valve of Hasner where there is an imperforate membrane as it enters the nose.
- Obstruction is usually due to a persistence of a membrane but can also be a bony obstruction or narrowing of the inferior meatus abutting the nasal mucosa.
- Acquired obstructions are rare in children but do occur as a result of chronic inflammation and scar tissue occluding the duct. Causes include infection (i.e., ethmoidal sinusitis), inflammation, malignancy, and trauma.

ETIOLOGY

Canalization of the duct is usually complete by the 7th month of gestation, but a persistent membrane can remain and may represent the embryologic basis of lacrimal duct obstruction.

COMMONLY ASSOCIATED CONDITIONS

- Acute dacryocystitis
  - Strongly suggestive of the presence of obstruction
  - Unclear whether obstruction is the primary cause leading to secondary infection from accumulation of tears and cellular debris or that dacryocystitis is the primary event with an acquired obstruction from fibrosis and inflammation
- Dacryocystocele (distention of the lacrimal sac)
  - A rare variant of lacrimal duct obstruction seen in 0.1% of infants with the disorder
  - There is the typical distal obstruction as well as a proximal obstruction at the junction of the common canaliculus and the lacrimal sac presenting as a bluish mass.
  - Can be associated with infection (i.e., dacryocystitis) as well as respiratory distress because of cystic expansion protruding into the nose
- Anisometropic amblyopia and refractive error have been found to have a higher incidence in those with lacrimal duct obstruction.
- Craniofacial malformations or Down syndrome

DIAGNOSIS

HISTORY

- Congenital obstruction presents in first few weeks of life once tear production matures usually by 6 weeks after birth.
- Frequency and duration
- Symptoms can be either unilateral or bilateral.
- Chronic tearing
- Increased tear meniscus
- Mucoid discharge
- Crusting on eyelids and/or eyelashes
- Acquired obstruction is associated with chronic eye infections or a history of trauma (i.e., naso-orbito-ethmoidal fractures, lid laceration).
- Tearing is worse in the cold, wind, or when child has an upper respiratory tract infection.

PHYSICAL EXAM

- Discharge and/or crusting on the eyelashes
- Eyelid excoriation
- May have lower lid skin changes (red, chafed) because of the chronic epiphora
- Compression or digital massage of lacrimal sac reveals mucoid discharge and/or tears expressed through the punctum.
- Absence of conjunctival injection
- Usually absence of pain, discomfort, or photosensitivity
- Bluish firm mass below the medial canthus suggests presence of dacryocystocele.

DIFFERENTIAL DIAGNOSIS

- Neonatal conjunctivitis
- Acute dacryocystitis
- Agenesis or imperforation of the lacrimal puncta or canaliculi
- Congenital lacrimal fistula
- Congenital dacryocystocele
- Excess tear production
  - Congenital glaucoma
  - Corneal abrasion
  - Abnormal eyelid position (entropion, epiblepharon)
  - Functional epiphora
  - Dacryoadenitis
  - Ophthalmia neonatorum
  - Trichiasis
  - Foreign body
  - Blepharitis
  - Keratitis
  - Uveitis
  - Allergies

DIAGNOSTIC TESTS & INTERPRETATION

Usually, patients are diagnosed without imaging and testing. If symptoms are intermittent and diagnosis is unclear, imaging and tests may be done.

Initial Tests (screening, lab, imaging)

- Bacterial cultures are not a reliable indicator of the presence of obstruction or infection thus is not indicated for diagnostic purposes. If concerns for ophthalmia neonatorum, consider chlamydial cultures.
- Radionuclide dacryocystography (also known as dacryoscintigraphy) helps evaluate the functioning of the lacrimal system by taking pictures as a radioisotope passes through the lacrimal system.
  - Technically difficult to perform in children so is rarely done
  - Does not allow for visualization of surrounding bony structures
- CT scan is useful for trauma or to assess bony obstruction resulting from craniofacial malformations or presence of dacryocystocele or other masses.

Diagnostic Procedures/Other

Fluorescein dye disappearance test

- Preferred tool for diagnosis of congenital obstruction if symptoms are intermittent and diagnosis is unclear based on history and physical examination
- 90% sensitive and 100% specific for nasolacrimal duct obstruction
- Fluorescein strip is placed in the lower conjunctival cul-de-sac, and the patient is observed for 5 minutes preferably with a cobalt blue light.
- If there is no obstruction, most of the fluorescein drains into the nose and minimal amount of fluorescein is noted in the eye.
- If there is an obstruction, fluorescein will be seen in the eye with an increased tear meniscus with likely overflow of tears onto the cheeks.
- If dacryocystocele is suspected, nasal endoscopy is recommended. Application of a topical decongestant such as oxymetazoline hydrochloride to the nasal mucous membranes enhances visualization.

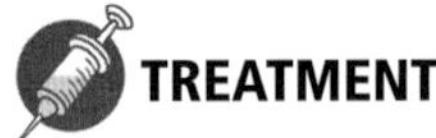

TREATMENT

GENERAL MEASURES

- Primary treatment for congenital obstruction is lacrimal sac massage or compression in a downward fashion (Crigler maneuver).
- Encourage parents to massage. This may increase the chance of resolution.
- Crigler maneuver can be effective in rupturing the membranous obstruction.
- Topical antibiotics are added as needed for a 3- to 5-day course if signs of conjunctivitis.
- Recent studies suggest that more than half of patients age 6 to 10 months will resolve within 6 months of nonsurgical management.

MEDICATION

- Topical ophthalmic antibiotics are used in congenital obstruction when there is an increase in discharge, purulent discharge, or findings consistent with conjunctivitis. Topical antibiotics of choice include erythromycin, tobramycin, or sulfacetamide.
- Steroid use is discouraged.

ISSUES FOR REFERRAL

- Referral to a pediatric ophthalmologist is indicated if symptoms persist beyond 6 to 12 months of age with the application of conservative measures. Depending on severity and preference of the ophthalmologist, probing is done or conservative measures are continued.
- Early referral is warranted in cases of acute dacryocystitis and dacryocystocele.
- Cases of acquired obstruction should be referred for surgical treatment.
- Recent studies suggest higher risk of having amblyopia in cases persisting beyond age 12 months. Referral to ophthalmology for both evaluation and possible intervention of the lacrimal duct obstruction and for orthoptic examination is indicated.

SURGERY/OTHER PROCEDURES

- Probing and irrigation are generally recommended if symptoms persist after 6 to 12 months of age.
  - Timing of surgical management is controversial. Some ophthalmologists prefer to perform the procedure prior to 12 months of age, and some continue with conservative measures until 15 to 18 months of age.
  - Failed probing is usually noted within 6 weeks of procedure with return of symptoms.
  - Failed in office probing is more likely in bilateral obstruction versus unilateral obstruction.
  - Probing may be repeated, although with increasing age, repeated probing may be less successful.
  - Probing and irrigation is less successful as primary treatment when done beyond age 3 years.
- Additional procedures may be done at the time of repeat probing that may increase the success rate, including the following:
  - Balloon catheter dilatation. Some experts advocate that this can be considered as a primary treatment in place of probing.
  - Nasal endoscopy allows visualization of the probe entering the nose, helping to avoid false passage; also allows diagnosis and management of any associated intranasal pathology
  - Silicone tube intubation helps prevent formation of granulation tissue and can aid in dilating stenotic segments of the lacrimal outflow system. Tube is left in place for 2 to 6 months, but success has been seen with removal as early as 6 weeks in patients <2 years.
  - Some advocate silicone tubing on initial probing, but this requires general anesthesia.
- Dacryocystorhinostomy
  - Indicated when aforementioned procedures have failed and in cases of chronic dacryocystitis, bony obstruction, or dacryocystocele.
  - Creates a passage through a bony ostium between the lacrimal sac and the nasal cavity providing an alternate pathway for lacrimal flow
  - Should be avoided until the child is 2 to 5 years old to avoid disturbing bone growth except in cases of emergency
- Primary conjunctivodacryocystorhinostomy (CDCR)
  - Creates a direct bypass tract between the medial canthus and the nose
  - Limited reports on this technique being used in children
- Surgery is typically performed on patients with acquired obstructions and congenital anomalies of the upper lacrimal system.

ADMISSION, INPATIENT, AND NURSING CONSIDERATIONS

- Neonates with dacryocystocele with an associated intranasal cyst obstructing their airway causing significant respiratory distress need to be admitted for airway management.
- Acute dacryocystitis should be admitted for parenteral antibiotic therapy with ophthalmology involved in the plan of care; may need surgery to drain the collection

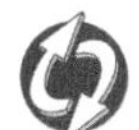

ONGOING CARE

FOLLOW-UP RECOMMENDATIONS

Patient Monitoring

- Conservative measures are appropriate for infants with congenital obstruction, although at 6 to 12 months of age, referral to ophthalmology should be considered for possible probing and irrigation.
- Children with a history of lacrimal duct obstruction need close follow-up for anisometropic amblyopia.

PATIENT EDUCATION

- Conservative measures usually result in resolution.
- Review lacrimal sac massage and topical antibiotic use with parents (see "General Measures").

PROGNOSIS

- About 90% of cases of congenital obstruction resolve by 12 months of age.
- Success rate of initial probing when performed at 12 months of age is about 80–90%.
- Probing is less successful after age 3 years.

COMPLICATIONS

- Infections such as bacterial conjunctivitis, acute and chronic dacryocystitis, and orbital cellulitis
- Respiratory distress in neonates with dacryocystocele that have an associated intranasal cyst at the valve of Hasner that obstructs their airway
- If surgical probing is undertaken, improper passage of the probe may create a false passage resulting in persistence of symptoms and potential scarring.

ADDITIONAL READING

- Kamal S, Ali MJ, Gupta A, et al. Lacrimal and nasal masquerades of congenital nasolacrimal duct obstructions: etiology, management, and outcomes. *Int Ophthalmol*. 2015;35(6):807–810.
- Mataftsi A, Malamaki P, Tsinopoulos IT, et al. Fifteen-minute consultation: congenital nasolacrimal duct obstruction. *Arch Dis Child Educ Pract Ed*. 2014;99(2):42–47.
- Miller AM, Chandler DL, Repka MX, et al. Office probing for treatment of nasolacrimal duct obstruction in infants. *J AAPOS*. 2014;18(1):26–30.
- Olitsky SE. Update on congenital nasolacrimal duct obstruction. *Int Ophthalmol Clin*. 2014;54(3):1–7.
- Örge FH, Boente CS. The lacrimal system. *Pediatr Clin North Am*. 2014;61(3):529–539.
- Pediatric Eye Disease Investigator Group. Resolution of congenital nasolacrimal duct obstruction with nonsurgical management. *Arch Ophthalmol*. 2012;130(6):730–734.
- Schnall BM. Pediatric nasolacrimal duct obstruction. *Curr Opin Ophthalmol*. 2013;24(5):421–424.
- Takahashi Y, Kakizaki H, Chan WO, et al. Management of congenital nasolacrimal duct obstruction. *Acta Ophthalmol*. 2010;88(5):506–513.

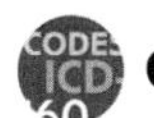

CODES

ICD10

- H04.559 Acquired stenosis of unspecified nasolacrimal duct
- H04.539 Neonatal obstruction of unspecified nasolacrimal duct
- Q10.6 Other congenital malformations of lacrimal apparatus

FAQ

- Q: Why not fix the obstruction upon diagnosis?
- A: Studies have shown that about 90% of cases of congenital obstruction resolve by 12 months of age using conservative measures consisting of massage with occasional addition of topical antibiotics for infection that can occur concurrently with obstruction.
- Q: When is the optimal age for probing and irrigation?
- A: This is controversial. Most studies suggest conservative measures are preferred in children <12 months of age. After 12 months of age, continued conservative measures or probing are selected based on severity of symptoms. Recent studies indicate that probing becomes less successful as a primary treatment in patients around age 3 years. This may be due to factors other than increasing age, including severe symptoms, canalicular stenosis, and nonmembranous obstruction.
- Q: Does probing and irrigation require general anesthesia?
- A: Sometimes probing is performed as an in-office procedure without general anesthesia if done when child is <12 months of age. When child is >12 months of age, probing is ideally performed under general anesthesia to ensure procedure is controlled and safe as well as allowing for direct visualization with endoscopy.

L

LACTOSE INTOLERANCE

Elizabeth J. Hait, MD, MPH

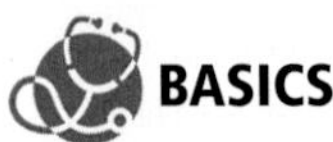

BASICS

DESCRIPTION

- Lactose intolerance is defined as the inability to digest the ingested disaccharide lactose, secondary to a deficiency of the intrinsic enzyme lactase, resulting in clinical symptoms.
- Lactase deficiency is an intrinsic low level of lactase production which may or may not be associated with clinical symptoms.
- Lactose is a disaccharide composed of glucose and galactose.
- Lactose is important as a source of energy; it is the major carbohydrate in human and other mammalian milks; promotes the absorption of calcium, phosphorus, and iron; and has a probiotic effect on the gut flora.
- Four types of lactase deficiency
  - Congenital lactase deficiency
    - Extremely rare
    - Presents during the newborn period
    - Will cause severe diarrhea and failure to thrive and risk the newborn's life
  - Primary lactase deficiency (adult-type hypolactasia)
    - Due to relative or absolute absence of lactase
    - Develops during childhood at different ages in different racial groups
    - Most common cause of lactose intolerance
  - Secondary lactase deficiency
    - Results from small bowel injury (acute gastroenteritis, persistent diarrhea, small bowel bacterial overgrowth, chemotherapy)
    - Can present at any age, more common in infancy
  - Developmental lactase deficiency
    - A relative lactase deficiency observed in premature infants <34 weeks' gestation

EPIDEMIOLOGY

Prevalence

- ~70% of the world's population is prone to developing primary lactase deficiency by adulthood.
  - The prevalence of primary lactase deficiency in northern Europeans, who have a diet rich in dairy, is 2%.
  - In Hispanic populations, the prevalence of primary lactase deficiency is 50–80%.
  - In Ashkenazi Jewish and African American populations, the prevalence is 60–80%.
  - In Asian populations, the prevalence of primary lactase deficiency is nearly 100%.
- Nearly 20% of children <5 years from Hispanic, Asian, or African American descent have lactase deficiency and lactose malabsorption.
- Caucasian children usually do not develop symptoms until after 5 years of age.

RISK FACTORS

Genetics

- Posttranslational regulatory mechanisms in primary lactase deficiency or adult-type hypolactasia
- Correlation between the genetic polymorphism of mRNA and persistence of lactase activity with early loss at 1 to 2 years in Thai children and late loss at 10 to 20 years in Finnish children

PATHOPHYSIOLOGY

- Symptoms depend on the amount of lactose ingested.
- Malabsorbed lactose creates an osmotic load that draws fluid and electrolytes into the bowel lumen, leading to an osmotic diarrhea.
- Nonabsorbed lactose acts as a substrate for intestinal bacteria.
- In the colon, bacteria metabolize lactose, producing volatile fatty acids and gases leading to flatulence, bowel distension, pain, and low pH.

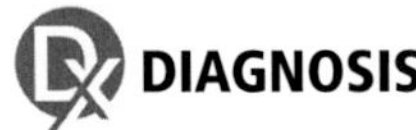

DIAGNOSIS

HISTORY

- Classic symptoms include bloating, gaseousness, colicky abdominal pain, and diarrhea after digestion of lactose-containing meal.
- Dietary intake history provides important information.
- Association with milk ingestion may not be evident.
- Symptoms vary in severity with dose of lactose ingested.
- Detailed history of symptoms:
  - Blood or mucus in the stools, weight loss, poor growth, fat malabsorption, or any extraintestinal symptoms strongly suggest different causes.

PHYSICAL EXAM

- Height and weight should be measured and plotted against age-appropriate norms; any deviation should not be attributed to lactose intolerance alone.
- Abdomen percussion: Abdomen may be distended and tympanitic.
- Lactose intolerance does not cause gastrointestinal bleeding or blood to appear in the stool.

DIFFERENTIAL DIAGNOSIS

- Infection
  - Viral and bacterial infections can cause secondary lactose intolerance due to villous injury.
  - Most common pathogen is rotavirus.
  - Parasitic infections can mimic lactose intolerance (giardiasis).
- Inflammatory conditions
  - Small intestinal Crohn disease
  - Celiac disease
- Congenital
  - Other carbohydrate enzyme deficiencies can mimic lactose intolerance. These include sucrase–isomaltase deficiency or glucose–galactose malabsorption.
  - Cystic fibrosis

- Shwachman-Diamond syndrome (SDS): Primary features include the following:
  - Bone marrow insufficiency
  - Pancreatic insufficiency
  - Skeletal abnormalities
  - Short stature
- Allergic/immune
  - Food protein allergies
  - Oral medications containing lactose: common in tablets

DIAGNOSTIC TESTS & INTERPRETATION

Initial Tests (screening, lab, imaging)

- Stool-reducing substances and fecal acidity
  - A pH <6.0 or reducing substances >0.5% should be interpreted as positive results.
  - Positive results indicate malabsorption of carbohydrates.
- Lactose hydrogen breath test
  - Noninvasive and highly sensitive
  - A rise of breath H_2 concentration of ≥20 ppm over baseline has been shown to correlate with enzyme deficiency.
  - However, there is poor association between symptoms of lactose intolerance and breath H_2 excretion, which underscores the need for caution in the interpretation of the clinical significance of the breath hydrogen test.
  - False-positive test results can occur if inadequate fasting before the test, rapid intestinal transit, toothpaste, smoking, and bacterial overgrowth.
  - False-negative results occur with diarrhea, hyperventilation, recent antibiotic exposure, and delayed gastric emptying. In addition, up to 10% of the population is colonized with bacteria unable to produce hydrogen, which can lead to a falsely negative result.
- Lactase activity measurement from endoscopically obtained duodenal tissue biopsies (invasive and expensive)
- The small bowel intestinal histology will often be normal in primary lactase deficiency (unless the reason is insult/damage to the small bowel mucosa).

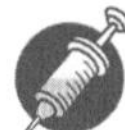

TREATMENT

GENERAL MEASURES

- Removal of lactose from the diet is effective in eliminating symptoms.
- However, it is important to recognize that a milk-free diet is associated with calcium deficiency.
- Predigestion of lactose can be done by the addition of commercially available enzyme supplementation (extrinsic lactase). Multiple products are available over the counter. Liquid preparations, capsules, and chewable tablets can be obtained.
- Acquired deficiencies, particularly those associated with infection, may resolve over time or with specific treatment. Many patients with lactose intolerance do not recover the ability to digest lactose.
- Specific strains of supplemental probiotics may improve symptoms of lactose intolerance.

MEDICATION

- Oral lactase replacement capsules
- Calcium supplements to ensure daily recommended intake levels despite dairy restriction

ONGOING CARE

DIET

- Lactose-free formula, lactase-containing milk
- Cow milk substitutes (e.g., rice or soy milk)
- Yogurt and aged cheeses, which generally have smaller content of lactose

PROGNOSIS

- Prognosis of lactase deficiency and clinical intolerance is excellent with lactose reduction or elimination as well as enzyme replacements are possible.
- Lactose intolerance secondary to disease processes should be recognized and treated appropriately.

ADDITIONAL READING

- Heyman MB; for Committee on Nutrition. Lactose intolerance in infants, children, and adolescents. *Pediatrics*. 2006;118(3):1279–1286.
- Levitt M, Wilt T, Shaukat A. Clinical implications of lactose malabsorption versus lactose intolerance. *J Clin Gastroenterol*. 2013;47(6):471–480.
- Mattar R, de Campos Mazo DF, Carrilho FJ. Lactose intolerance: diagnosis, genetic, and clinical factors. *Clin Exp Gastroenterol*. 2012;5:113–121.
- Rezaie A, Buresi M, Lembo A, et al. Hydrogen and methane-based breath testing in gastrointestinal disorders: The North American Consensus. *Am J Gastroenterol*. 2017;112(5):775–784.
- Usai Satta P, Congia M, Schirru E, et al. Genetic testing is ready to change the diagnostic scenario of lactose malabsorption. *Gut*. 2008;57(1):137–138.

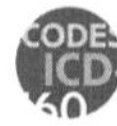

CODES

ICD10

- E73.9 Lactose intolerance, unspecified
- E73.0 Congenital lactase deficiency
- E73.8 Other lactose intolerance

FAQ

- Q: When is the usual time for presentation of lactose intolerance?
- A: In Caucasians, the age of presentation is after 5 years of age. In African Americans, 2- to 3-year-old children may present with clinical signs and symptoms. The differential diagnosis must distinguish primary from secondary causes.
- Q: Does lactose intolerance prevent a child from ever eating lactose?
- A: No. The patient can take smaller amounts of lactose in the diet or have the enzyme supplemented.
- Q: Does this problem ever get better?
- A: No. It is a lifelong problem, but seems to become less symptomatic for adults, in light of their individual desire to tolerate symptoms. Secondary lactose intolerance may improve with time or treatment of the primary disorder.

L

LEAD POISONING

Julie S. O'Brien, MD, MS • Kent R. Olson, MD

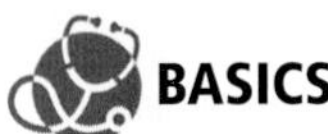

BASICS

DESCRIPTION

- Lead poisoning is one of the most common pediatric environmental health problems, most often involving systemic intoxication with inorganic lead. Lead poisoning is an older term that is less specific than an actual blood lead level (BLL).
- The Centers for Disease Control and Prevention (CDC) considers an elevated BLL to be ≥5 mcg/dL.
  - This "reference value" is based on the 97.5th percentile for lead levels of children aged 1 to 5 years collected for the National Health and Nutrition Examination Survey (NHANES).
  - This replaced the previous "level of concern" terminology for levels ≥10 mcg/dL based on the Advisory Committee on Childhood Lead Poisoning Prevention (ACCLPP) recommendations in light of many studies demonstrating cognitive and behavioral effects at BLL <10 mcg/dL.

EPIDEMIOLOGY

There are >500,000 U.S. children 1 to 5 years of age with BLLs >5 micrograms per deciliter (mcg/dL).

- 24 million housing units have hazards from lead-based paint.
- In 2015, lead poisoning became national news when the water supply in Flint, Michigan was found to have significantly elevated lead levels. Due to the change in water source, the percentage of Flint children with elevated BLLs may have risen from about 2.5% in 2013 to as much as 5% in 2015.
- Racial income disparities persist due to disparities in housing quality, nutrition, and access to health care.

RISK FACTORS

- Young children with more oral behaviors
- Children with developmental delays/mental retardation
- Children with pica
- Residence in older homes with flaking or deteriorating lead-based paint
- Renovation or remodeling of older homes without lead hazard controls in place
- Recent immigration from countries where ambient lead contamination is high (i.e., where leaded gasoline is still used)
- Use of lead-glazed ceramic pottery
- Use of traditional therapies containing lead (e.g., azarcon, some Ayurvedic and Chinese medicines)
- Ingestion of lead-containing candies from Mexico

GENERAL PREVENTION

- Primary prevention: removal of potential environmental lead hazards prior to exposure
  - The ACCLPP focuses on primary prevention as it emphasizes that there is no "safe" level of lead and the effects of lead are likely irreversible.
  - Clinicians should provide anticipatory guidance to all parents about lead exposure pathways and the prevention of exposures.
- Secondary prevention: screening for elevated BLLs
  - Minimum screening recommendations: blood lead test for children at 1 and 2 years and for those 36 to 72 months old who have not had previous screening
  - Screening children immigrating from other countries and screening pregnant and lactating women and their neonates and infants for lead exposure prior to or during pregnancy and lactation
- Tertiary prevention: case management and environmental remediation for children with lead poisoning
- Control measures
  - Abatement of building-based (residential) lead hazards by removal, encapsulation, or enclosure of lead-containing structures
  - Control of environmental lead dust exposure and ingestion by good housekeeping (wet dusting and mopping of household dust); personal hygiene (cleaning of child's hands, toys, personal items, wiping feet on mats prior to entering the home), and hiring certified renovators who are United States Environmental Protection Agency (EPA)-approved to perform renovations that may disrupt lead-based paint
  - Removal of any other known lead source from the child's environment

PATHOPHYSIOLOGY

- Lead adversely affects many organ systems including neurologic, hematologic, GI, renal, and reproductive.
  - Many toxic effects result from inhibition of enzymes involved in heme biosynthesis, as the electropositive metal binds to negatively charged sulfhydryl groups on active sites of δ-aminolevulinic acid dehydratase (ALAD), ferrochelatase, porphobilinogen synthase, coproporphyrinogen oxidase, and other enzymes.
  - Divalent lead also acts competitively with calcium in various biologic systems.
- Children absorb lead more efficiently from the GI tract and are more likely than adults to ingest lead through hand-to-mouth activities.
- Because the developing, immature CNS is susceptible to toxic effects of lead, the neuropsychological effects of lead poisoning on fetuses/young children are of particular concern. Even relatively low BLLs are associated with IQ deficits, attention-related behaviors, and poor academic achievement.

DIAGNOSIS

HISTORY

- It is important to assess for risk factors for exposure, as most children are asymptomatic.
- Etiology/common sources of lead:
  - Ingestion of lead-based paint or contaminated dust or soil through residence in or visitation of older (pre-1980), deteriorated housing
  - A parental occupation or hobby involving lead exposure (e.g., construction or battery plant work, stained glass window or pottery making)
  - Use of remedies, cosmetics, pottery, toys, or consumer products containing lead
  - Ingestion of contaminated water, food, or beverages
- Typical symptoms:
  - Most children are asymptomatic; many clinical manifestations are nonspecific. A cluster of complaints including anorexia, intermittent abdominal pain, constipation, sporadic vomiting, change in mental status (e.g., irritability or lethargy), decreased play activity, and change in developmental status (e.g., regression of developmental milestones) may herald this condition.
- Lead encephalopathy
  - Can present with change in consciousness, ataxia, persistent vomiting, seizures, and coma
  - Often presents after a prodrome of symptoms mentioned above

PHYSICAL EXAM

As patients are generally asymptomatic, physical exam is not generally helpful at lower lead levels.

- Symptomatic and/or encephalopathic patients may have acute GI, neurologic, hematologic, and systemic manifestations.
- Assess for developmental delay.

DIFFERENTIAL DIAGNOSIS

Consider lead poisoning as the etiology for the following diagnoses:

- Seizures, altered mental status, and/or coma
- Anemia

ALERT

Failure to diagnose results from the following:

- Delay in checking a blood lead test in the presence of clinical signs, symptoms of lead poisoning, or neuropsychological disorders
- Failure to inquire about lead exposure possibilities

DIAGNOSTIC TESTS & INTERPRETATION

Initial Tests (screening, lab, imaging)

- Blood lead test, either venous or capillary (but must be drawn in lead-free tube):
  - Results may be reportable to local health authorities.
  - The test result is a measure only of recent lead exposure and does not indicate total body burden of lead.
  - Capillary testing is associated with more false-positive results. If abnormal, a venous lead should be sent.
  - A confirmed elevated BLL is defined as a child with a venous blood sample ≥5 mcg/dL.
- CBC: to assess for anemia
  - Iron deficiency anemia is often seen concomitantly.
  - Anemia related to lead toxicity is typically normocytic and normochromic; a microcytic, hypochromic anemia may be seen with a mixed etiology.
  - Basophilic stippling is sometimes seen on peripheral blood smear.
- Free erythrocyte protoporphyrin
  - Marker of lead-induced inhibition of heme synthesis
  - Can be useful clinically to follow the recovery from heme synthesis inhibition during management
- Abdominal radiograph: Look for radiopaque foreign material suggestive of ingestion of lead paint chips or other lead-containing foreign body, when ingestion of such is suspected in the history or with very high BLLs.
- Long bone radiographs are not recommended for routine screening.

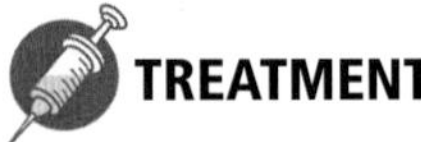

TREATMENT

Treatment for most individuals is focused on environmental management to prevent further lead exposure. Medications are only required at higher BLLs.

GENERAL MEASURES

- Environmental management
  - Remove children from the lead source(s).
  - Should occur when venous lead levels are recurrently 10 mcg/dL (CDC class IIA) and higher; could be done for lower BLLs as resources allow
- Reduction of lead levels in the household
  - Consultation with a qualified lead abatement contractor is advised.

MEDICATION

- Chelation therapy
  - Should complement environmental management in all children with venous levels of ≥45 mcg/dL using parenteral calcium disodium ethylenediaminetetraacetate (Ca-EDTA; calcium disodium versenate) or oral agents such as meso-2,3-dimercaptosuccinic acid (DMSA, succimer, Chemet®)
  - Chelation of children with levels <45 mcg/dL is not recommended, as evidence suggests it does not reverse or diminish neuropsychological effects of lead.
  - Outpatient therapy can take place if a lead-safe environment has been identified and compliance is expected.
  - Succimer is given at 10 mg/kg (or 350 mg/m^2) PO q8h for 5 days and then q12h for 14 more days. Weekly monitoring for neutropenia, platelet abnormality, and increased liver enzymes is recommended.
- Children with symptomatic lead poisoning or with levels of ≥70 mcg/dL should be admitted immediately to a hospital for parenteral chelation with both IM dimercaprol (British anti-Lewisite, BAL) and IV or IM calcium disodium EDTA. Because there are many issues involved with administration of both chelating agents, consultation with a clinician experienced in lead toxicity treatment is advised.
- Children with encephalopathy constitute a medical emergency and should receive the preceding treatment in an intensive care setting with attentive neurosurgical support.
- Ingested lead-containing foreign bodies should be evacuated with whole-bowel irrigation using a polyethylene glycol electrolyte solution.

ISSUES FOR REFERRAL

- Close communication with the local health department is essential before, during, and after admission.
- Referral may be made to early intervention or development assessment programs, social workers, therapists, neurologists, or other specialists, as needed.

ADMISSION, INPATIENT, AND NURSING CONSIDERATIONS

- Admit all symptomatic children, those with BLLs ≥70, and those with BLLs ≥45 for which one cannot ensure a lead-safe environment and/or compliance with oral medication.
- Consider discharge when symptoms have resolved, BLL has significantly declined, and a lead-safe discharge environment has been identified.

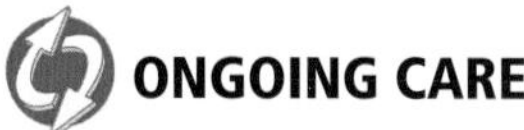

ONGOING CARE

FOLLOW-UP RECOMMENDATIONS

Patient Monitoring

- Prompt environmental follow-up of current lead exposure situations and investigation for additional exposure (e.g., with family moves, visitation of new residences) should occur.
- Follow-up venous lead levels should be performed for those with BLLs ≥5 mcg/dL about every 1 to 3 months, with less frequent follow-up after levels decline.
- Follow-up venous levels should be performed 1 to 3 weeks following chelation therapy, with frequent monitoring thereafter until levels have decreased significantly and no new lead exposure is apparent. BLLs will increase from the nadir level immediately after treatment to rebound to a level between this and the pretreatment level.

DIET

- Nutritional support with calcium and iron supplementation should be given if intake is inadequate; deficiencies of these increase lead absorption from the gastrointestinal (GI) tract.
- The recommendation for adequate intake of calcium is 500 mg/day, which can typically be achieved through a regular healthy diet.
  - There is currently no evidence that supplementation of calcium beyond the recommended "adequate intake" is beneficial for children with elevated BLLs.
- Iron repletion should be initiated with 3 mg/kg of elemental iron for those children who are found to be iron deficient.
  - Iron supplementation should be withheld during chelation therapy.
- Additionally, it is recommended to consume at least two servings daily of foods high in vitamin C, such as fruits, vegetables, and juices.

PROGNOSIS

There is an increased risk for long-term neuropsychological sequelae, which increases with lead exposure and absorption that is more intense, of longer duration, and begins at an early age when the CNS is still developing.

- Recurrent episodes of symptomatic lead poisoning increase the risk for permanent sequelae.
- Subtle effects may be missed until school entry.

COMPLICATIONS

- Acute encephalopathy
- Seizures
- Coma
- Death (predominantly owing to cerebral edema)
- Mental retardation
- Cognitive, behavioral, attentional, and neurodevelopmental impairment
- Anemia
- Fanconi syndrome
- Abdominal colic
- Adverse reproductive outcomes

ADDITIONAL READING

- Advisory Committee on Childhood Lead Poisoning Prevention of the Centers for Disease Control and Prevention. *Low Level Lead Exposure Harms Children: A Renewed Call for Primary Prevention*. Atlanta, GA: U.S. Department of Health and Human Services, Centers for Disease Control and Prevention; 2012.
- American Academy of Pediatrics Committee on Environmental Health. Lead exposure in children: prevention, detection, and management. *Pediatrics*. 2005;116(4):1036–1046.
- Bellinger DC. Very low lead exposures and children's neurodevelopment. *Curr Opin Pediatr*. 2008;20(2):172–177.
- Binns HJ, Campbell C, Brown MJ. Interpreting and managing blood lead levels of less than 10 microg/dL in children and reducing childhood exposure to lead: recommendations of the Centers for Disease Control and Prevention Advisory Committee on Childhood Lead Poisoning Prevention. *Pediatrics*. 2007;120(5):e1285–e1298.
- Canfield RL, Henderson CR Jr, Cory-Slechta DA, et al. Intellectual impairment in children with blood lead concentrations below 10 microg per deciliter. *N Engl J Med*. 2003;348(16):1517–1526.
- Centers for Disease Control and Prevention. *CDC response to Advisory Committee on Childhood Lead Poisoning Prevention Recommendations in "Low Level Lead Exposure Harms Children: A Renewed Call for Primary Prevention."* Atlanta, GA: Centers for Disease Control and Prevention; 2012.
- Centers for Disease Control and Prevention. *Guidelines for the Identification and Management of Lead Exposure in Pregnant and Lactating Women*. Atlanta, GA: Centers for Disease Control and Prevention; 2010.
- Evens A, Hryhorczuk D, Lanphear B, et al. The impact of low-level lead toxicity on school performance in the Chicago Public Schools: a population-based retrospective cohort study. *Environ Health*. 2015;14:21.
- Lanphear BP, Hornung R, Khoury J, et al. Low-level environmental lead exposure and children's intellectual function: an international pooled analysis. *Environ Health Perspect*. 2005;113(7):894–899.
- Lanphear BP, Matte TD, Rogers J, et al. The contribution of lead-contaminated house dust and residential soil to children's blood lead levels. *Environ Res*. 1998;79(1):51–68.
- McLaine P, Navas-Acien A, Lee R, et al. 2013. Elevated blood lead levels and reading readiness at the start of kindergarten. *Pediatrics*. 2013;131(6):1081–1089.
- Raymond J, Brown MJ. Childhood blood lead levels in children aged <5 years—United States, 2009–2014. *MMWR Surveill Summ*. 2017:66(3);1–10.

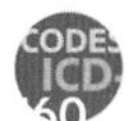

CODES

ICD10

- T56.0X4A Toxic effect of lead and its compounds, undetermined, init
- T56.0X1A Toxic effect of lead and its compounds, accidental, init

FAQ

- Q: What is lead abatement?
- A: Lead abatement is removal of a lead hazard from the environment either by replacing it (e.g., installing a new window), enclosing the area with the lead source (e.g., installing paneling), removing the lead-based paint from a surface (burning or dry sanding methods should never be used), or encapsulating the area (placement of a specific coating over the lead-containing surface, which prevents access to the lead hazard).
- Q: Is lead abatement permanent?
- A: Often, lead paint that is chipping or peeling is removed from a home. Any areas with intact lead-based paint may become deteriorated with aging, leading to new lead hazards, although ongoing maintenance and repair may prevent this.
- Q: Why didn't my child's brother and sister get lead poisoning at the same age although they lived in the same house?
- A: Children are different; some do much more hand-to-mouth activity than others, which is the main way that children get lead into their bodies. Also, your home may not have had the same lead dangers (hazards) when the siblings were younger.

L

LEARNING DISABILITIES

Monica Dowling, PhD • Jeffrey P. Brosco, MD, PhD

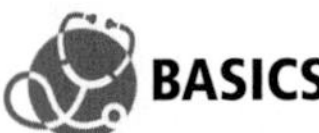

BASICS

DESCRIPTION

Learning disabilities (LD) are a group of disorders characterized by unexpected and sustained difficulties acquiring and applying academic skills, including reading accuracy, reading fluency, reading comprehension, written expression, mathematic calculations, and mathematic problem-solving.

- LD comprise one category within the classification of Neurodevelopmental Disorders (NDDs) in the *Diagnostic and Statistical Manual of Mental Disorders*, 5th edition (DSM-5, 2013) and the *International Classification of Diseases, Code Book 10* (ICD-10, 1992).
- Academic achievement must be substantially below the level expected for age and not attributable to intellectual disability (ID), neurologic or motor disorders, lack of schooling, psychosocial factors, economic disadvantage, or major sensory problems.
- LD have neurobiologic and genetic roots.
- Reading disability is the most frequently diagnosed type of LD and is typically characterized by impairments in phonologic processing and/or orthographic coding skills that impact word reading and fluency. Poor comprehension is associated with language difficulties and executive dysfunction. Children with math disability show procedural, retrieval, and number sense deficits.
- The role of the pediatrician is to screen for LDs, advocate for a child with LD to obtain early intervention, interpret predisposing factors in child's developmental and medical history, and offer scientific interpretation of the range of theories and interventions.

EPIDEMIOLOGY

The lifetime prevalence of LD in U.S. children is 9.7%.

RISK FACTORS

- LD are familial and moderately heritable.
- Risk loci and genes have been identified for reading and language disorders.
- Hypothesized pathophysiology includes neuronal migration, cell adhesion, axonal guidance, neurometabolites, gray and white matter, activation, adaptation, and connectivity.
- Genetic contribution increases with a high level of parent education (a bioecologic gene by environment interaction).
- Environmental factors include prematurity, low birth weight, prenatal nicotine or alcohol exposure, infections, toxins, anesthesia and TBI.

GENERAL PREVENTION

- High-quality developmentally appropriate preschool experiences
- Early literacy initiatives (e.g., Reach Out and Read)
- Early intervention for speech, language, motor difficulties
- Evidence-based reading curricula and ongoing academic progress monitoring beginning in kindergarten
- Supplemental instruction for children who show early signs of learning problems

COMMONLY ASSOCIATED CONDITIONS

- Language disorders
- Speech sound disorders
- Auditory processing disorders
- Developmental coordination disorder
- ADHD/executive function deficits

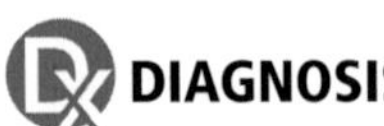

DIAGNOSIS

- Many learning problems respond to appropriate educational interventions, regardless of specific etiology, and failure to respond to intervention is part of the diagnostic process for specific LD.
- It is the role of the educator to (i) monitor academic progress of all students, (ii) provide educational intervention and frequent progress monitoring to struggling students, and (iii) conduct a psychoeducational assessment of students who do not respond to initial intervention.
- Once a child presents with learning problems, it is the role of the pediatrician to
  - Help the family obtain timely and evidence-based educational interventions. LD Navigator (http://www.ncld.org) provides health care professionals with resources.
  - Identify and treat underlying medical problems.
  - Identify and help treat underlying psychosocial issues:
    - Psychosocial stresses may exacerbate learning difficulties or be a primary etiologic factor.
    - School attendance is a particularly important factor in learning.
  - Identify and treat comorbid psychiatric disorders, especially ADHD.

HISTORY

- **Question:** Do you have any concerns about how your child is learning?
- *Significance*:
  - Screening question at well-child care visits; can also review report card with child and family
  - Formal screening for LD done in schools
- **Question:** When and how does the child have difficulties in his or her daily academic pursuits?
- *Significance*:
  - LD typically impact only school activities and are often limited to one skill area such as reading or math.
  - Children with ADHD typically show problems in multiple settings (school, home, extracurricular, peers).
  - Children with ID usually have a history of developmental concerns.
- **Question:** Is decline in school performance recent and/or abrupt?
- *Significance*: If abrupt, consider pathophysiologic processes such as vision or hearing impairment, side effect from medication, neurodegenerative disorders (rare), or recent psychosocial issue.
- **Question:** Past medical history, medications, review of systems, psychosocial stresses?
- *Significance*:
  - School attendance (illness vs. avoidance)
  - Early development and behavior
  - Family history of learning problems
  - Sleep patterns (apnea, insomnia)

PHYSICAL EXAM

- **Finding:** Subtle dysmorphology?
- *Significance*: may suggest the presence of a genetic syndrome or a pattern of malformation resulting from teratogenic fetal exposures (e.g., alcohol, phenytoin)
- **Finding:** Skin lesions?
- *Significance*: may suggest underlying genetic syndromes such as tuberous sclerosis
- **Finding:** Enlarged tonsils?
- *Significance*: may cause sleep disturbance that affects learning and/or behavior
- **Finding:** Abnormal neurologic examination?
- *Significance*:
  - Any focal signs demand additional evaluation.
  - Slow rapid alternating finger movements (neuromaturational signs) are often present in children with LD but are generally not helpful clinically.

DIFFERENTIAL DIAGNOSIS

- ID
  - Borderline intellectual functioning or mild ID may not be evident in early childhood.
- ADHD
  - Especially when inattentive and distractible, symptoms are greater than hyperactive symptoms.
  - Comorbidity is approximately half of diagnosed cases of LD.
- Sensory impairments
  - Hearing or vision impairments
  - School screening results should be confirmed by the pediatrician in children with academic problems.
- Neurologic etiologies
  - Absence seizures and other nonconvulsive epileptic disorders
  - Neurodegenerative disorders such as Niemann–Pick disease, adrenoleukodystrophy, ceroid lipofuscinosis, and subacute sclerosing panencephalitis may rarely present as school-age learning problems.
  - CNS trauma
- Genetic syndromes
  - Some genetic syndromes may show subtle dysmorphology that is not noted until learning problems arise. Examples include the following:
    - Sex chromosome aneuploidies
    - Fragile X syndrome
    - Neurofibromatosis
    - Tuberous sclerosis
    - Velocardiofacial/DiGeorge syndrome

- Hypothyroidism
- HIV infection
- Lead intoxication
- Chronic malnutrition
- Iron deficiency
- Iatrogenic interventions
  - Some medications (e.g., antiepileptic drugs) affect cognition.
  - Cancer treatment
- Psychosocial issues
  - Issues related to family stress, peer relationships, illness, school absence, or adolescence may present as academic difficulty.
  - Conversely, behavior problems at home or at school always should prompt evaluation of school functioning.
- Psychiatric comorbidity
  - Adjustment disorders, anxiety, mood disorders, oppositional defiant disorder, conduct disorder, tic disorders, substance abuse, and other behavior problems may precede or follow the presentation of LD.

DIAGNOSTIC TESTS & INTERPRETATION

- Physician
  - Audiology and vision screening
  - Standardized questionnaires (e.g., Teachers and Parent Vanderbilt, Shaywitz Dyslexia Screen)
  - Consider other screening tools for depression, anxiety, family dysfunction, parental depression, and substance abuse.
  - Genetic, neurologic evaluation if indicated by history or physical exam
- Educator
  - Teacher-administered measures or computer-administered tests to monitor progress. Standardized achievement tests can be administered yearly to measure current functioning and review progress.
- Psychologist
  - Testing must be performed individually and include intellectual and academic functioning at a minimum.
  - Federal law requires schools to provide comprehensive evaluations on written request by the parents. Specific information for each state is available from the National Dissemination Center for Children with Disabilities (800-695-0285; http://www.nichcy.org).
  - University- and hospital-based centers outside the school system also conduct evaluations of children with LD.
  - For children who do not respond to educational interventions, or if the psychoeducational evaluation is inconclusive, neuropsychological testing may identify specific cognitive factors that are helpful in developing an effective educational plan.

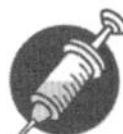

TREATMENT

- Discourage a "wait and see" approach to decision making. Early intervention using evidence-based reading programs improves outcomes.
- Begin evidence-based interventions as soon as problems are evident; children who do not respond require more thorough etiologic workup.
- Academic or attention difficulties may lead to spiraling psychological problems from depression or damaged self-esteem to conduct disorder and school dropout.

GENERAL MEASURES

- Physician
  - Must be alert to signs and symptoms of LD, such as poor grades and behavior concerns in school
  - Responsible for ensuring early reading intervention
  - Treat underlying medical diagnoses.
  - Ensure appropriate treatment of psychiatric problems with pharmacologic therapy and behavioral therapy (family therapy, social skills training, cognitive behavioral therapy) as needed.
- School
  - Educational treatment varies with the age and educational level of the child and should utilize a multitier system of increasing intensity:
    - Tier 1: For patients displaying poor academic achievement, begin with extra support (e.g., homework clinic, tutoring) in the regular educational program (assuming culturally and linguistically appropriate instruction).
    - Tier 2: If academic problems disrupt classroom participation and impede progress, refer to school-based child study team and provide intensive assistance as part of general curriculum, such as summer school or specialized materials.
    - Tier 3: If child is >1 year behind or has shown minimal response to Tier 2 interventions, refer for a comprehensive psychoeducational evaluation to identify specialized interventions, typically provided under the umbrella of special education.
  - Specialized instruction is at the center of treatment, often within the regular classroom (inclusion) with supplemental instruction through either a consultant special teacher or a resource room.
  - Children may also benefit from classroom accommodations such as preferential seating, extra time for test taking, word processors and computer applications, text-to-speech programs, calculators, note-takers, and modified instructions.
  - Treatment is most effective when it uses a team approach, including parents, teachers, and other therapists.
  - Grade retention has not been shown to be effective and should be discouraged.

ONGOING CARE

Children with LD require continued monitoring of academic progress. Even when the initial learning problems are resolved, later difficulties may arise in writing, note-taking, composition, organization, or with more abstract academic subjects.

PROGNOSIS

- In most cases, prognosis is quite good with treatment, although LD never go away.
- Prognosis varies with intensity, timing, and appropriateness of intervention.
- Early diagnosis and treatment is essential for minimizing impact and to take advantage of typical developmental progression.
- Current brain imaging research shows remedial instruction alters brain functioning if provided during critical window of development (<8 to 10 years) for both reading and math.

ADDITIONAL READING

- American Psychiatric Association. *Diagnostic and Statistical Manual of Mental Disorders*. 5th ed. Arlington, VA: American Psychiatric Association; 2013.
- McArthur G, Castles A. Helping children with reading difficulties: some things we have learned so far. *npj Science of Learning*. 2017;2:7.
- Norton ES, Beach SD, Gabrieli JD. Neurobiology of dyslexia. *Curr Opin Neurobiol*. 2015;30:73–78.
- Olulade OA, Napoliello EM, Eden GF. Abnormal visual motion processing is not a cause of dyslexia. *Neuron*. 2013;79(1):180–190.
- World Health Organization. *International Statistical Classification of Diseases and Related Health Problems, 10th Revision (ICD-10)*. Geneva, Switzerland: World Health Organization; 1992.

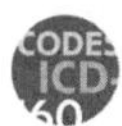

CODES

ICD10

- F81.9 Developmental disorder of scholastic skills, unspecified
- F81.0 Specific reading disorder
- F81.2 Mathematics disorder

FAQ

- Q: What is the evidence that visual training will improve reading?
- A: Despite anecdotal reports of value, there is strong evidence that visual dysfunction is not causal to reading disability; there is insufficient evidence to recommend vision therapy.
- Q: Can brain imaging diagnose LD?
- A: Brain imaging is a research tool. No brain imaging technology has been validated for clinical use and cannot replace psychoeducational evaluations.

L

LEUKOCYTOSIS

Katie Carlberg, MD • Caroline Hastings, MD

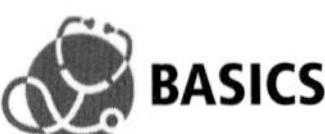

BASICS

DESCRIPTION
Leukocytosis refers to a total white blood cell (WBC) count above the normal range for age.

RISK FACTORS
- Very low-birth-weight neonates
- Immunodeficiencies or immunocompromised states
- Inflammatory disorders
- Autoimmune disorders

ALERT
Children with trisomy 21 (Down syndrome) have an increased risk of developing transient myeloproliferative disorder (TMD) or leukemoid reactions.

PATHOPHYSIOLOGY
Leukocytosis results from increased marrow production, demargination, prolonged cell survival, and/or defective extravascularization in response to external stimuli or, less commonly, from an underlying marrow disorder.

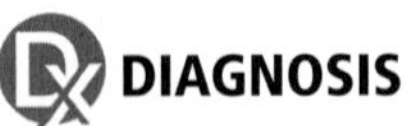

DIAGNOSIS

HISTORY
- Evaluate for history or signs of infection.
  - Acute infection is the most common cause of leukocytosis.
  - Fever is nonspecific and may be present in infectious, inflammatory, rheumatoid, or malignant diseases.
- Obtain thorough past medical history.
  - Down syndrome: TMD occurs in ~10% infants and spontaneously resolves in 1 month, although 20–30% of these patients progress to acute myeloid leukemia (AML). This is a medical emergency if there is organomegaly with cardiopulmonary compromise.
  - Hereditary neutrophilia: autosomal dominant disorder with heterozygous mutation in the *CSF3R* gene on chromosome 1p34
  - Leukocyte adhesion deficiency (LAD): rare autosomal recessive disorder characterized by recurrent bacterial infections
  - Sickle cell anemia: Leukocytosis likely reflects chronic inflammation and may be associated with increased vasoocclusive events.
- Comprehensive review of symptoms may indicate malignancy.
  - B symptoms include fever, drenching night sweats, and weight loss of ≥10% over 6 months.
  - Persistent bone pain may indicate leukemia and be initially diagnosed as growing pains or worked up for osteomyelitis or juvenile idiopathic arthritis (JIA).
- Do not forget to obtain history of travel or unusual exposures.
  - Shigellosis enteritis may be seen after travel to areas with suboptimal sanitation and present with leukocytosis and even seizures.
  - Nursing home residents, incarcerated individuals, and health care professionals are at higher risk for developing and transmitting mycobacterium tuberculosis (TB).
  - Reptiles commonly carry *Salmonella* and rodents commonly carry *Hantavirus*.
- Obtain complete family history.
  - Family histories positive for autoimmune disorders may raise suspicion for inflammatory bowel disease (IBD), JIA, hypereosinophilic syndrome (HES), thyroid disease, vasculitis, etc.

PHYSICAL EXAM
- Cardiopulmonary
  - A careful lung examination is necessary, as pneumonia is a common cause of leukocytosis.
  - A new murmur or gallop may be an early sign of bacterial endocarditis.
- Abdominal/lymph
  - If hepatosplenomegaly and/or lymphadenopathy is present, consider acute viral hepatitis, infectious mononucleosis from either Epstein-Barr virus (EBV) or cytomegalovirus (CMV), malignancy, malaria, or lysosomal storage disease.
- Musculoskeletal/dermatologic
  - Arthritis or joint pain and/or rashes may be one manifestation in a constellation that may suggest JIA, rheumatic fever, or Lyme disease.

DIFFERENTIAL DIAGNOSIS
- Atopy
  - Allergies
  - Asthma
  - Eczema
  - Psoriasis
- Congenital/genetic
  - Down syndrome
  - Hereditary neutrophilia
  - LAD
  - Sickle cell anemia
- Hemolysis
  - Hemolytic anemia
  - Transfusion reaction
- Infectious
  - Bacterial
    - *Brucella*
    - *Bartonella*
    - *Bordetella pertussis*
    - *Clostridium difficile*
    - *Francisella tularensis*
    - *Haemophilus*
    - *Mycobacterium tuberculosis* (TB)
    - *Neisseria*
    - *Rickettsia*
    - *Streptococcus pneumoniae*
    - *Staphylococcus aureus*
  - Viral
    - CMV
    - EBV
    - *Hantavirus* (*Hantavirus* pulmonary syndrome)
    - Hepatitis
    - Respiratory syncytial virus
  - Parasitic
    - *Toxocara canis*
    - *Toxoplasma*
    - *Trichinella*
    - *Plasmodium* spp.
  - Fungal
    - Coccidioidomycosis
  - Spirochetal
    - *Treponema pallidum*
- Immunologic/inflammatory/reactive
  - Appendicitis
  - Addison disease
  - Asplenia
  - Chronic granulomatous disease
  - HES
  - IBD
  - JIA
  - Löffler syndrome
  - Sarcoidosis
  - Smoking
  - Thyrotoxicosis
  - Vasculitis including Kawasaki disease
- Malignancy
  - Acute leukemias
  - Chronic leukemias
  - Lymphomas
  - Solid tumors

- Medications
  - Antiepileptics
  - β-Agonists
  - Corticosteroids
  - Epinephrine
  - All-trans retinoic acid
  - Granulocyte or granulocyte–macrophage colony-stimulating factor
  - Heparin
  - Lithium
  - Minocycline
  - Prostaglandin
- Myeloproliferative disorders
  - Polycythemia vera
  - Essential thrombocytopenia
  - Myelofibrosis (but more often associated with cytopenias)
- Poisons
  - Lead
- Stress
  - Anesthesia
  - Anxiety
  - Emotional stress
  - Overexertion
  - Heat stroke
  - Seizures
- Trauma
  - Acute hemorrhage
  - Severe burns
  - Nonaccidental trauma

DIAGNOSTIC TESTS & INTERPRETATION

Initial Tests (screening, lab, imaging)

- Step 1: Confirm that the leukocytosis is real.
  - Etiologies of spurious leukocytosis by automated analyzers of whole blood include nucleated or partially lysed RBCs, cryoglobulin or cryofibrinogen, or platelet clumps.
  - Confirmation includes review of peripheral smear via consultation of a pathologist or hematologist.
- Step 2: Obtain a differential of the WBC count.
  - A manual differential may be required.
  - Distinguishing between myeloid and lymphoid or even blasts contributes to identifying the correct etiology.
  - Myeloid leukocytosis include (i) neutrophilia, which commonly results from bacterial infections; (ii) monocytosis; (iii) eosinophilia, typically reactive; (iv) basophilia, which is rare and suggestive of myeloproliferative neoplasms; and (v) increased blasts, concerning for underlying marrow abnormality.
  - Lymphoid leukocytosis results from viral infections.

ALERT

Beware of any differential that has a high percentage of monocytes or atypical lymphocytes, whether machine generated or manual. Leukemic blasts can be mistaken for these cell types.

- Step 3: Distinguish between reactive and clonal populations.
  - Reactive leukocytosis is heterogeneous—pleomorphic, polyclonal, and/or large granular cells are present.
  - Neoplasms such as leukemia/lymphoma are homogenous.
  - May need to use flow cytometry with immunophenotyping and/or cell receptor gene rearrangements to rule out malignancy, especially in lymphoproliferative disorders
- Step 4: Evaluate other cell lines.
  - Concurrent presence of anemia and/or thrombocytopenia suggests an underlying marrow disorder such as leukemia.
  - Leukocytosis and thrombocytosis may be associated with iron deficiency anemia, sickle cell anemia, LAD type III, and pregnancy.
- Step 5: Use this information in clinical context.
- Imaging
  - Although universal vaccination with Prevnar (pneumococcal conjugate vaccine [PCV]) has decreased the incidence of pneumonia, clinicians should still strongly consider chest radiography in young, highly febrile children with leukocytosis and no obvious source of infection.

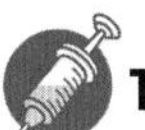

TREATMENT

GENERAL MEASURES

- Isolated leukocytosis may be monitored without intervention.
- If ill-appearing, age-appropriate empiric antibiotics are indicated
- Consultation with other subspecialties may be necessary.
- Prognosis depends on diagnosis.

ONGOING CARE

In the setting of bacterial infection with appropriate microbial coverage, anticipate resolution of leukocytosis within 4 days.

ALERT

If malignancy is in the differential, consult hematology/oncology prior to initiating steroids.

ADDITIONAL READING

- Abramson N, Melton B. Leukocytosis: basics of clinical assessment. *Am Fam Physician*. 2000;62(9):2053–2060.
- Cerny J, Rosmarin AG. Why does my patient have leukocytosis? *Hematol Oncol Clin North Am*. 2012;26(2):303–319.
- George TI. Malignant or benign leukocytosis. *Hematology Am Soc Hematol Educ Program*. 2012;2012:475–484.

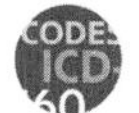

CODES

ICD10

- D72.829 Elevated white blood cell count, unspecified
- D72.0 Genetic anomalies of leukocytes
- D72.828 Other elevated white blood cell count

FAQ

- Q: Does the degree of leukocytosis correlate to the severity of infection?
- A: Just as the height of fever does not always correlate to the severity of infection, the same is true for the degree of leukocytosis. Even a normal WBC does not rule out bacteremia.
- Q: What is a leukemoid reaction?
- A: A leukemoid reaction is a physiologic response to a stress or infection and is characterized by a WBC of $\geq 50 \times 10^9$/L with peripheral blood myeloid precursors at all stages of maturity rather than proliferation of an immature WBC clonal population, which is characteristic of malignancies.
- Q: When is an elevated WBC a clinical emergency?
- A: Leukocytosis or hyperleukocytosis is a clinical emergency when the patient is symptomatic from leukostasis. Hyperleukocytosis is a total WBC count of $\geq 100 \times 10^9$/L. Clinically significant hyperleukocytosis usually occurs at WBC $\geq 200 \times 10^9$/L or $\geq 300 \times 10^9$/L in patients with acute myeloid or lymphoblastic leukemia and chronic myeloid leukemia in blast crisis, respectively; however, symptoms may present with a WBC as low as 50×10^9/L. Refer to "Hyperleukocytosis" chapter for more information.

LICE (PEDICULOSIS)

Daniel Newman, MD • Linda Y. Fu, MD, MS

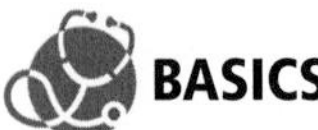

BASICS

DESCRIPTION

Infestation of the head, body, or anogenital region by parasitic, wingless insects that feed exclusively on human blood

EPIDEMIOLOGY

- Head lice
  - Spread by head-to-head contact
  - Most common among children 3 to 12 years old
  - Associated with female gender, crowded living conditions
  - Less common among African Americans
  - Point prevalence estimates range from <1% in some places to >90% in others.
  - In the United States, seasonal peak of prescriptions for treatment are filled in July to September coinciding with the back-to-school period.
- Body lice
  - Spread by close physical contact with infested persons, clothing, or bedding
  - Associated with poor sanitation, cool climates, homelessness, war, disasters, refugee camps
  - No racial or gender differences
- Pubic lice
  - Usually sexually transmitted
  - Can also spread through contact with clothing or bedding recently used by infested person
  - Most common among young adults

Incidence

- Varies widely with location and living conditions
- Estimated 6 to 12 million cases of head lice per year in the United States among children ages 3 to 11 years

GENERAL PREVENTION

Humans are the only host for all three types of lice. Recurrences are common and may be prevented by examining and treating close contacts, especially bedmates.

- Head lice
  - Avoid head-to-head contact with infested persons; don't share brushes, hats, or hair ties.
  - Avoid lying on pillows, furniture, or stuffed toys used by infested persons within last 2 days.
  - Wash clothing and bedding used by infested persons with hot water (≥130°F) and set dryer to highest heat setting. Items may also be dry-cleaned or sealed in a plastic bag for 2 weeks.
  - Treatment of furniture, upholstery, and carpets is not necessary because lice only survive for a short while away from host, making transmission via textiles extremely unlikely.
  - Environmental insecticide is not helpful.
  - Treatment of pets is not necessary.
  - "No-nit" school policies do not control head lice transmission and are not recommended.
- Body lice
  - Regularly wash clothes.
  - Avoid using clothing or bedding used by infested persons.
- Pubic lice
  - Avoid close body contact or sharing clothes with infested persons.
  - Not prevented by condom use

PATHOPHYSIOLOGY

- Lice bites are painless.
- To facilitate the blood meal, lice inject enzymes, anticoagulant, and vasodilators. These provoke host inflammatory response causing pruritus.
- Bites cause intradermal hemorrhage with infiltrates of eosinophils and lymphocytes.
- Excoriation can introduce secondary infections.
- Vector-borne pathogens (body lice only) can cause chronic bacteremia, angiomatosis, or endocarditis.

ETIOLOGY

- Head lice (*Pediculus humanus capitis*)
  - Adult lice are white to gray, 2- to 4-mm long, have six legs, and no wings. They crawl quickly away from threat or bright light and cannot jump or fly. If removed from host, lice will die within 2 days.
  - Females lay up to eight eggs (also called "nits") per day over a 2- to 3-week lifespan, attaching nits to base of hair shafts with adhesive.
  - Nymphs hatch from nits in 7 to 12 days, leaving behind empty white nit casings on hair.
  - Emerging nymphs die without a blood meal within a few hours. Nymphs molt 3 times over 9 to 11 days to become nit-laying adults.
  - Typical infestation includes lice in all stages of development.
- Body lice (*Pediculus humanus corporis*)
  - Morphology and life cycle are similar to head lice, but adults are slightly larger.
  - Live and lay eggs on clothing and only come to the skin to feed 4 to 5 times per day
  - Able to live longer off host than head lice
  - Nits hatch in 6 to 10 days
- Pubic lice (*Phthirus pubis*)
  - Crab-like appearance with larger talus adapted to coarser hair
  - Predilection for pubic hair; may also infest axillary hair, perianal area, eyelashes, beard, and rarely scalp

COMMONLY ASSOCIATED CONDITIONS

- Body lice
  - May act as a vector for epidemic typhus (*Rickettsia prowazekii*), relapsing fever (*Borrelia recurrentis*), trench fever (*Bartonella quintana*), or plague (*Yersinia pestis*)
- Pubic lice
  - Commonly occurs with other sexually transmitted infections
  - Although pubic lice on children's eyelashes usually result from close contact with infested parent, must also consider sexual abuse

DIAGNOSIS

HISTORY

- Chief complaint is most often pruritus; however, the majority of patients are asymptomatic.
- Pruritus is an immune-mediated process and may not begin until 1 to 4 weeks after initial infestation or sooner if repeat infestation.
- May complain of disrupted sleep
- Ask about exposure to others with similar symptoms, crowded living conditions, and previous similar episodes.
- Review details of previous treatments to differentiate improper or incomplete treatment from reinfestation or resistance to pediculicide.

PHYSICAL EXAM

- General points
  - Definitive diagnosis requires visualization of live lice, not just nits.
  - Bright light and magnification are helpful.
- Head lice
  - Wetting hair with conditioner and then combing with a fine-tooth nit comb slows movement of lice for diagnosis.
  - Use comb to lift and separate hair to visualize scalp and base of hair shafts.
  - Live lice, nits, and empty nit casings are most commonly found at the temples, behind ears, on back of head, and nape of neck.
  - Typical case involves 5 to 10 live lice.
  - Nits are firmly affixed at a characteristic angle to the hair shaft (unlike dandruff or dried hairspray).
  - Nits within 1 cm of scalp suggest active infestation.
  - Nits beyond 1 cm from scalp are likely empty casings.
  - May see excoriations, oozing, matted hair, or lymphadenopathy with secondary infection
- Body lice
  - Skin exam may reveal erythematous macules and papules from bites; rarely live lice
  - Live lice and nits may be found along seams on inside of clothing, especially near axillae, inguinal areas, waistband, or collar.
  - In long-standing infestations, may find epidermal thickening, hyperpigmentation, or scaly plaques
  - If lice have transmitted secondary bacterial infection, may find adenopathy, fever, and malaise
- Pubic lice
  - Live lice and nits may be found in pubic hair or perianal region; be sure also to check axillae, beard, and eyelashes.
  - May find brownish clumps of louse fecal matter
  - With heavy infestation, may find maculae cerulean—that is, 0.5- to 1-mm bluish macules on the lower abdomen, thighs, or buttocks
  - Eyelash infestation may cause blepharitis or conjunctivitis.

DIFFERENTIAL DIAGNOSIS

- Seborrheic (dandruff), contact, or atopic dermatitis
- Impetigo
- Scabies
- Xerosis with excoriation
- Dried hair spray or other debris
- Infestation with other insects

DIAGNOSTIC TESTS & INTERPRETATION

Diagnostic Procedures/Other

- Diagnosis of head lice is made by direct visualization of live lice or under magnification.
  - Lice will stick to cellulose tape applied to infested area, and tape can then be affixed to glass slide for microscopy.
  - Lice and nits fluoresce yellow green under Wood lamp.
- Misdiagnosis of head lice is common.
- Wet combing is more sensitive and specific for diagnosing active infestation with head lice than visualization alone.

TREATMENT

GENERAL MEASURES

- Head lice: Synchronized treatment of all infested persons (i.e., family, play group, other close contacts) is key to preventing reinfestation.
- Because different pediculicides have variable mechanisms of action and potential to cause adverse effects, careful adherence to manufacturers' instructions is essential (repreparation of hair, duration of application, posttreatment rinsing, combing and reapplication).
- Conditioner or excess water on hair can interfere with pediculicide efficacy.
- Pediculicides can irritate mucous membranes and may be toxic if taken internally.
- Enough product must be used to coat all hair and scalp, especially areas behind ears and along hairline at back of neck. After treatment, a nit comb should be used to remove visible lice and nits.
- Use of pediculicides (kill live lice) that are not ovicidal (kill nits) requires repeat treatment in 7 to 10 days—after new lice hatch from nits but before they lay new nits.
- Treatment may leave residue on hair that will continue to kill lice over the next few days. Use a nit comb to remove dead and any remaining live lice.
- Meticulous wet combing alone to remove nits and live lice may be helpful when medication is ineffective or as an alternative to pediculicides.

MEDICATION

- Head lice
  - Permethrin lotion 1% (over-the-counter [OTC])
    - Minimum age: 2 months
    - Some forms (e.g., shampoo) must be used on dry hair. Other forms (e.g., lotion) must be used on damp hair. Follow manufacturer's instructions.
    - 10-minute application and then shampoo out. Reapply in 7 to 10 days.
    - Not ovicidal
    - Despite development of significant resistance, often still the primary initial treatment choice due to low cost, easy access, and proven safety profile
  - Pyrethrin 1% with piperonyl butoxide (OTC)
    - Minimum age: 2 years
    - 10-minute application to dry hair and then rinse out with water. Reapply in 9 to 10 days.
    - Not ovicidal
    - Avoid if allergic to chrysanthemums.
  - Malathion lotion 0.5% (Rx)
    - Minimum age: 6 years
    - 8- to 12-hour application to dry hair and then shampoo out. Reapply in 7 to 10 days if live lice persist.
    - Pediculicidal and partially ovicidal
    - Highly flammable, so avoid hair dryers, smoking, and irons during treatment
    - Organophosphate with theoretical risk of respiratory depression if swallowed
    - Resistance common in many countries but not in the United States where product contains the complimentary agent terpineol
  - Benzyl alcohol lotion 5% (Rx)
    - Minimum age: 6 months
    - Dosing is by hair length; see manufacturer's instructions.
    - 10-minute application to dry hair and then rinse out with water. Reapply in 7 days.
    - Not ovicidal
  - Spinosad topical suspension 0.9% (Rx)
    - Minimum age: 6 months
    - 10-minute application to dry hair and then rinse out with water. Reapply in 7 days if live lice persist.
    - Pediculicidal and ovicidal
    - Formulation also contains benzyl alcohol (combination prevents resistance).
  - Ivermectin lotion 0.5% (Rx)
    - Minimum age: 6 months
    - 10-minute application to dry hair and then rinse out with water; single treatment only
    - Wait 24 hours before applying shampoo to hair and scalp.
    - Not ovicidal, but newly hatched lice are not viable.
  - Controversial and untested treatments:
    - Occlusion: Olive oil, mayonnaise, and petroleum jelly do not asphyxiate lice but may slow their movement and facilitate removal with nit comb.
    - Dimethicones (synthetic silicone oils): popular treatment outside of the United States but no data available to support the effectiveness or safety in the United States
    - Shaving: can be effective but not necessary and may not be cosmetically acceptable
    - Ivermectin: oral; single dose of 200 μg/kg, repeated in 10 days has shown to be effective; not FDA-approved for this use; not for use in weight <15 kg
    - Trimethoprim-sulfamethoxazole: oral; 10-day course; may enhance cure rate of topical permethrin; not FDA-approved for this use
    - Essential oils (e.g., tea tree oil): may have some activity against live lice and nits but are unregulated and may be toxic
    - Hot air: Several mechanical devices deliver hot air to the scalp to desiccate live lice and nits, but efficacy is questionable.
    - Lindane shampoo 1%: no longer recommended due to neurotoxicity and increased resistance
- Body lice
  - Pediculicides are usually not needed if infested clothing and other fomites are appropriately laundered, treated with pediculicide, or destroyed. Oral ivermectin has been used effectively during epidemics.
- Pubic lice
  - The same OTC pediculicides are used for head lice and pubic lice; resistance is less common.
  - It is important to treat all infested areas and sexual contacts.
  - For eyelash infestation, apply petroleum jelly twice daily for 10 days. Remove nits with tweezers.

ALERT

- Pediculicides are oculotoxic. Do not use on eyelashes or eyebrows. If pediculicide gets in eyes, immediately flush with water.
- Pregnancy risk category varies for pediculicides. Check package insert.

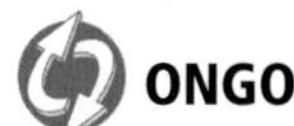

ONGOING CARE

COMPLICATIONS

Head lice

- Intense pruritus can disrupt sleep.
- Stigma associated with infestation can lead to social isolation, teasing, or bullying.
- Days lost from school or work due to inappropriate "no-nit" policies impact on academic performance and worker productivity.
- Secondary bacterial infections can result in pyoderma and lymphadenopathy.

ADDITIONAL READING

- Centers for Disease Control and Prevention. Lice. http://www.cdc.gov/parasites/lice. Accessed February 3, 2017.
- Devore CD, Schutze GE; and Council on School Health and Committee on Infectious Diseases, American Academy of Pediatrics. Head lice. *Pediatrics*. 2015;135(5);e1355–e1365.
- Koch E, Clark JM, Cohen B, et al. Management of head louse infestations in the United States—a literature review. *Pediatr Dermatol*. 2016;33(5): 466–472.
- Feldmeier H. Treatment of pediculosis capitis: a critical appraisal of the current literature. *Am J Clin Dermatol*. 2014;15(5):401–412.

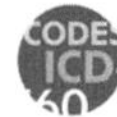

CODES

ICD10

- B85.2 Pediculosis, unspecified
- B85.0 Pediculosis due to Pediculus humanus capitis
- B85.1 Pediculosis due to Pediculus humanus corporis

FAQ

- Q: Are people with long hair more likely to get head lice?
- A: No, longer hair is not associated with greater likelihood of getting head lice. However, removing lice and nits is easier when hair is shorter.
- Q: How long should children with head lice be excluded from school?
- A: The risk of transmission decreases enough to allow children to return to school once they have been treated with a single pediculicide application.
- Q: How significant is resistance to OTC pyrethrin and permethrin?
- A: Recent studies in the United States have shown a decline in effectiveness of these medications from 90–100% in the 1990s to ~25% in the 2000s.
- Q: Given evolving resistance patterns, should we stop using OTC treatments and use prescription products instead?
- A: Resistance of head lice to pediculicides varies widely by community. Currently, permethrin 1% remains the initial treatment of choice. Prescription products are more expensive and have greater potential for toxicity. Careful adherence to manufacturers' directions and simultaneous treatment of close contacts (especially bedmates) decrease the likelihood of treatment failure and reinfestation.
- Q: How can health professionals allay anxiety and decrease the social stigma of head lice?
- A: Emphasize that head lice infestation is not a sign of poor housekeeping or hygiene. Point out that the benefits of close friendships outweigh the minimal health risks related to head lice. Encourage open communication to facilitate treatment of close contacts.
- Q: Can head lice transmit diseases as body lice have been found to do?
- A: A recent study found that head lice can in fact transmit *R. prowazekii* and *B. quintana*. The clinical implications of these findings are still uncertain.

LONG QT SYNDROME

Akash R. Patel, MD, CEPS, FHRS

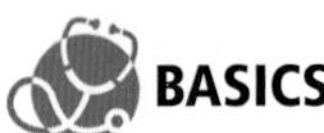

BASICS

DESCRIPTION

Long QT syndrome (LQTS) is characterized by prolongation of the QT interval on the surface electrocardiogram (EKG) that can result in symptomatic ventricular arrhythmias. The symptoms can include palpitations, syncope, and sudden cardiac arrest. The prolonged QT interval reflects abnormal ventricular repolarization associated with cardiac ion channel dysfunction that results in electrical instability.

EPIDEMIOLOGY

- Prevalence of LQTS is estimated to be approximately 1 in 2,500.
- Cardiac events occur in ~50% of congenital LQTS patients; most occur in preteens, adolescents, and young adults.

RISK FACTORS

Genetics

- Autosomal dominant (Romano-Ward syndrome)
- Autosomal recessive, sometimes associated with congenital bilateral sensorineural hearing loss (Jervell and Lange-Nielsen syndrome)
- Genetic studies have demonstrated that nearly 500 genetic mutations among 15 cardiac ion channel genes account for nearly 80% of congenital LQTS.
- Genotype-phenotype–based research studies have identified gene-specific electrocardiographic profiles, gene-specific arrhythmia triggers, gene-directed treatment strategies, and gene-specific risk stratification.

GENERAL PREVENTION

- Preventive measures focus on targeted screening for the electrocardiographic abnormality, especially in individuals who appear to be at risk of having the diagnosis based on symptoms and family history.
- Patients with LQTS should avoid exposure to stimulants; medications that are known to prolong the QT interval or provoke ventricular arrhythmias; and situations such as exercise, emotional stress, or auditory stimuli that may aggravate abnormalities in ventricular repolarizations resulting in ventricular arrhythmias, in particular torsades de pointes.

PATHOPHYSIOLOGY

Two hypotheses have been proposed to explain the pathogenesis of congenital LQTS syndrome:

- An abnormality or imbalance in sympathetic innervation to the heart, which helps explain the findings of sinus bradycardia, abnormal repolarization, adrenergic dependence of arrhythmias, and response to adrenergic antagonist medications (i.e., β-blockers) associated with the syndrome
- Intrinsic cardiac ion (potassium, sodium, or calcium) channel defects are also responsible for cardiac repolarization abnormalities and abnormal cardiac myocyte excitability. These genetic mutations alter cardiac ion channel proteins resulting in gain or loss of function mutations that lead to altered cardiac ion flows into and out of cardiac cells.

DIAGNOSIS

HISTORY

- Notable findings include the following:
  - Palpitations
  - Presyncope
  - Syncope
  - Cardiac arrest
- These symptoms may be a result of provocative stimuli, especially emotional or physical stress.
- Concomitant use of medications that prolong the QT interval should be noted.
- Most importantly, a thorough family history for arrhythmia, syncope, seizures, cardiac arrest, or sudden unexplained death should be obtained.

PHYSICAL EXAM

Findings are usually normal, but sinus bradycardia may be present. Rare types of congenital LQTS can be associated with syndromes with noncardiac findings such as bilateral congenital deafness, facial dysmorphism, hand/foot abnormalities, neurodevelopmental delay, and muscle weakness.

DIFFERENTIAL DIAGNOSIS

- Vasovagal syncope: Recurrent and atypical syncope should raise suspicion and warrants an EKG.
- Seizure disorder: Recurrent and nonepileptic seizures should raise suspicion and warrants an EKG.
- Sudden infant death syndrome (SIDS): Some studies have demonstrated the presence of cardiac ion channelopathies that result in LQTS.
- Acquired LQTS
  - Electrolyte abnormalities: hypokalemia, hypocalcemia, hypomagnesemia, and metabolic acidosis
  - Toxins: organophosphates
  - Central nervous system trauma
  - Malnutrition: anorexia
  - Primary myocardial disease: myocarditis, ischemia, cardiomyopathy
  - Medication
    - Cardiac medications: quinidine, procainamide, disopyramide, sotalol, and amiodarone
    - Antibiotics/antifungals: erythromycin, clarithromycin, ciprofloxacin (and other fluoroquinolones), trimethoprim sulfa, pentamidine, ketoconazole, fluconazole
    - Psychotropic medications: tricyclic antidepressants, phenothiazines, haloperidol
    - Antihistamines: terfenadine, astemizole, diphenhydramine
    - Gastrointestinal: cisapride, ondansetron, granisetron

DIAGNOSTIC TESTS & INTERPRETATION

Initial Tests (screening, lab, imaging)

- A resting EKG with calculation of the corrected QT interval
  - Generally, a QTc >480 msec is considered abnormal, although some clinicians allow a slightly longer QTc for infants <6 months of age.
  - QT interval prolongation may be subtle such that ~10% of affected patients may have a normal result on routine EKG and ~40% may have only borderline prolongation of the QT interval (QTc >450 msec).
- Exercise stress testing may be helpful in identifying ventricular arrhythmias and/or prolongation of the QT interval during recovery.
- Since 2004, genetic testing has been available as a commercial diagnostic test. Unfortunately, only ~80 of all genetic causes of LQTS have been identified, so false-negative genetic testing is possible.
- Clinical scoring systems may help stratify patients into high, moderate, and low probability of having the diagnosis, based on symptoms, family history, and EKG findings

Diagnostic Procedures/Other

- Echocardiogram
  - Usually demonstrates normal cardiac structure and function and used to exclude other cardiac etiologies
- 24-hour ambulatory Holter monitoring
  - May disclose asymptomatic ventricular ectopy or arrhythmias, T-wave alternans, or variability in the QTc interval during different periods of the day

Follow-Up Tests & Special Considerations

- 2:1 atrioventricular block can be seen on the EKG in infants with relatively rapid heart rates and P waves that occur during the prolonged repolarization period (QT interval) of ventricular refractoriness.
- Ambulatory Holter monitoring and exercise testing can be used for arrhythmia surveillance and medication efficacy/compliance.

Test Interpretation

EKG—baseline or exercise stress testing

- The QT interval measurement should be taken in lead II or V5 without significant sinus arrhythmia.
- The QT interval is corrected for heart rate using the Bazett formula; QTc = QT/(square root of prior RR interval)
- Some clinicians believe that the QTc should not be corrected at heart rates <60 bpm.
- Children frequently have a prominent U wave. It should generally be included in the measurement of the QTc if it exceeds 1/2 the amplitude of the T wave.
- A single measured prolonged QTc interval does not confirm the diagnosis of LQTS.
- T-wave alternans on an electrocardiographic recording can be seen.

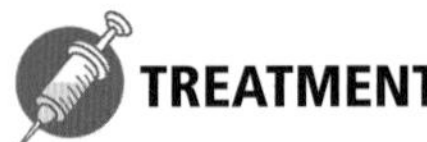

TREATMENT

GENERAL MEASURES

- Patients are usually treated based on symptoms and the clinical severity of the disease; avoidance of QT-prolonging medications and avoidance of provoking situations
- Automated external defibrillator (AED) availability at school and home may be considered.

MEDICATION

First Line

- β-Blockers—most commonly propranolol or nadolol. Metoprolol and atenolol may be less effective for this diagnosis.
- Class Ib antiarrhythmic medications (e.g., mexiletine) are also used in patients with congenital LQTS due to sodium ion channel dysfunction, especially in those with documented ventricular arrhythmia.
- Antiarrhythmic medications generally do not help treat patients with acquired LQTS, but the administration of magnesium sulfate may be beneficial.

ISSUES FOR REFERRAL

- Based on presenting symptoms and QT prolongation, initial evaluation may occur as inpatient cardiology consult or elective outpatient cardiology referral.
- Annual follow-up with a pediatric cardiologist or pediatric electrophysiologist is typical.
- Syncope while on treatment requires urgent evaluation.

SURGERY/OTHER PROCEDURES

- A permanent pacemaker is indicated occasionally based on the theory that the tachyarrhythmias (e.g., torsades de pointes) are dependent on bradycardia and/or pauses. Rarely, pacemaker implantation may be necessary to support the low heart rate that occurs as a result of β-blocker therapy. Newborns and infants with a very prolonged QT interval, atrioventricular block, and low ventricular rates are historically treated with a pacemaker.
- An implantable cardioverter-defibrillator (ICD) may be recommended for patients thought to be at higher risk of sudden cardiac death due to significant symptoms (i.e., syncope on treatment), documented ventricular arrhythmias, or other significant risk factors.
- A left stellate ganglionectomy is performed to potentially eliminate the hyperactive left sympathetic ganglion output that has been proposed as a mechanism of ventricular arrhythmias. This treatment option is not universally accepted and is used most often as adjunctive therapy in severe cases.

ADMISSION, INPATIENT, AND NURSING CONSIDERATIONS

- Most clinicians treat diagnosed asymptomatic children with medications because of a high incidence of sudden death that occurs as the first symptom.
- Inpatient admission for patients with LQTS typically occurs for evaluation of unexplained syncope or cardiac arrest, procedural interventions, or noncardiac reasons.
- Cardiac rhythm monitoring should be performed during hospitalizations.
- Avoidance of QT-prolonging medications should be adhered to.

ONGOING CARE

FOLLOW-UP RECOMMENDATIONS

Patient Monitoring

- Follow-up outpatient appointments should review new or recurrent symptoms, including palpitations, near syncope or syncope, and the efficacy and adverse effects of medical therapy.
- EKG may demonstrate a normal or prolonged QTc.
- Follow-up 24-hour ambulatory Holter monitor recordings and exercise stress tests may help assess the adequacy of β-blocker therapy and identify ventricular arrhythmias.
- All 1st-degree family members of the patient should have an EKG as a minimum screening measure.
- Potassium supplementation may be required in congenital LQTS in the setting of hypokalemia.

PATIENT EDUCATION

Pediatric patients should avoid potential triggers as outlined.

PROGNOSIS

- Children have a higher incidence of sudden death than adults, which may reflect an inherent bias because adult patients have already survived childhood. The risk of cardiac events is higher in boys before puberty and in women during adulthood.
- Pediatric patients with greatest risk for sudden death are those with QTc >550 msec. Gender, environmental factors, genotype, and therapy are other factors that influence the clinical course.
- A particular clinical phenotype may be caused by different genetic substrates, whereas a single gene can cause very different phenotypes, even within the same family, by acting through different pathways.
- Without treatment, mortality is 21% within 1 year from the first syncope. With proper treatment, mortality has been estimated at 1% during 15-year follow-up. β-Blocker therapy has been shown to reduce the incidence of sudden death.
- Current research may lead to the development of therapy specific to the precise ion channel defect.

COMPLICATIONS

- Complications, especially in untreated patients, include the following:
  - Ventricular tachyarrhythmias, specifically torsades de pointes
  - Syncope
  - Sudden death
- In patients with the congenital and inherited form of the condition, asymptomatic family members may be affected.

ADDITIONAL READING

- Ackerman MJ. Genotype-phenotype relationships in congenital long QT syndrome. *J Electrocardiol*. 2005;38(Suppl 4):64–68.
- Hedley PL, Jørgensen P, Schlamowitz S, et al. The genetic basis of long QT and short QT syndromes: a mutation update. *Hum Mutat*. 2009;30(11):1486–1511.
- Morita H, Wu J, Zipes DP. The QT syndromes: long and short. *Lancet*. 2008;372(9640):750–763.
- Priori SG, Napolitano C, Vicentini A. Inherited arrhythmia syndromes: applying the molecular biology and genetic to the clinical management. *J Interv Card Electrophysiol*. 2003;9(2):93–101.
- Priori SG, Schwartz PJ, Napolitano C, et al. Risk stratification in the long-QT syndrome. *N Engl J Med*. 2003;348(19):1866–1874.
- Roden DM. Clinical practice. Long-QT syndrome. *N Engl J Med*. 2008;358(2):169–176.
- Schwartz PJ, Crotti L, Insolia R. Long-QT syndrome: from genetics to management. *Circ Arrhythm Electrophysiol*. 2012;5(4):868–877.

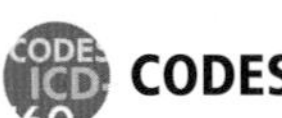

CODES

ICD10

I45.81 Long QT syndrome

FAQ

- Q: Should activity be restricted in patients with congenital LQTS?
- A: Because sudden rises in serum catecholamine levels may precipitate symptoms, it is appropriate to initially restrict competitive and vigorous athletics. However, recent data suggests that with appropriate precautions and treatment, liberalization of activities can be considered in a select group. Symptomatic patients may require greater restrictions. Documentation of appropriate β-blockade by a lower maximal heart rate at peak exercise on follow-up exercise stress test may be helpful.
- Q: If someone is identified as having LQTS, should family members be evaluated?
- A: Yes, with a high degree of suspicion. Most cases of congenital LQTS are inherited in an autosomal dominant pattern, so that each child of an affected parent has a 50% chance of having the gene. This finding does not predict severity of symptoms, but parents, all siblings, and children of patients should be examined initially with an EKG and cascade genetic testing if a pathogenic mutation is identified. Additional evaluation, including Holter monitoring and exercise stress testing may be required.
- Q: Are ICD always needed?
- A: No, in fact the majority of patients with LQTS do not require an ICD. Medical management with β-blocker therapy is very effective in reducing the risk of significant cardiac events and is the mainstay of treatment.

LOWER GI BLEEDING

Michael A. Manfredi, MD

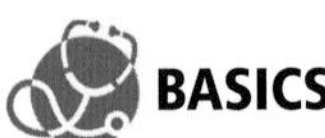

BASICS

DESCRIPTION

Lower gastrointestinal bleeding (LGIB) is defined as bleeding that occurs distal to the ligament of Treitz. The classic clinical symptom is hematochezia. However, always keep in mind that severe upper gastrointestinal bleeding can present with hematochezia. Melena and maroon-colored stools can be seen with small bowel bleeding.

EPIDEMIOLOGY

Incidence

- The incidence of GI bleeding in children is not well established in the general population.
- In a population study of LGIB based on 40,000 admissions to a tertiary care pediatric emergency department, LGIB was seen in 0.3% of all admissions.
- Few patients have severe life-threatening LGIB.

ETIOLOGY

Causes of LGIB vary by age:

- Neonatal period (birth to 1 month)
  - Allergic colitis
  - Anorectal fissure
  - Necrotizing enterocolitis
  - Enteric infections
  - Upper GI source
  - Duplication cyst
  - Hirschsprung disease enterocolitis
  - Meckel diverticulum
  - Malrotation with volvulus
  - Hemorrhagic disease of the newborn
- Infancy (1 month to 2 years)
  - Allergic colitis
  - Anorectal fissure
  - Enteric infections
  - Intussusception
  - Meckel diverticulum
  - Malrotation with volvulus
  - Lymphonodular hyperplasia
  - Upper GI source
  - Duplication cyst
  - Enterocolitis with Hirschsprung disease
  - Vascular malformation
- Preschool age (2 to 5 years)
  - Anorectal fissure
  - Enteric infections
  - Polyps
  - Parasites
  - Meckel diverticulum
  - Intussusception
  - Lymphonodular hyperplasia
  - Inflammatory bowel disease
  - Hirschsprung disease enterocolitis
  - Hemolytic uremic syndrome
  - Henoch-Schönlein purpura (HSP)
  - Vascular malformation
  - Volvulus
  - Rectal prolapse/rectal ulcer
  - Child abuse
  - Perianal streptococcal cellulitis
- School age (5 to 13 years)
  - Anorectal fissure
  - Enteric infections
  - Inflammatory bowel disease
  - Intussusception
  - Meckel diverticulum
  - Polyps
  - HSP
  - Hemolytic uremic syndrome
  - Intestinal ischemia
  - Neutropenic colitis (typhlitis)
  - Parasites
  - Child abuse
  - Vascular malformations
  - Perianal streptococcal cellulitis
- Adolescent (>13 years)
  - Anorectal fissure
  - Hemorrhoids
  - Parasites
  - Enteric infections
  - Inflammatory bowel disease
  - Hemolytic uremic syndrome
  - Intussusception
  - Midgut volvulus
  - Intestinal ischemia
  - Neutropenic colitis (typhlitis)
  - Polyps
  - Vascular malformations
  - Lymphonodular hyperplasia

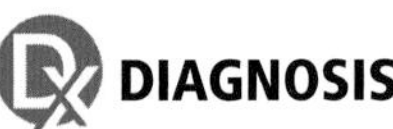

DIAGNOSIS

The initial evaluation of patients presenting with GI bleeding focuses on assessment of vital signs, history of present illness, focused medical history, physical examination, and lab testing.

- General goals: Determine if patient is bleeding, the location of the bleeding and cause. In parallel, assess hemodynamic status and begin stabilization if necessary.
- Phase 1: Determine if there is blood or other cause of bright red or black stools.
- Phase 2: Assess patient to determine etiology using history, physical exam, and laboratory assessments.
- Phase 3: Assess and stabilize patient, determine if bleeding is acute or chronic condition, decide if emergency treatment is needed; decide if outpatient referral is required.

HISTORY

- Obtain a detailed history and note if any recently ingested foods resemble blood.
- Evaluate the color of blood:
  - Bright red, then site of bleeding is probably in left colon, rectosigmoid, or anal canal
  - Darker red stool, then from right colon
  - If melena or maroon, then bleeding is proximal to ileocecal valve
- Location of blood in the stool:
  - In colitis, the blood will be mixed with stool.
  - With an anal fissure/constipation, it will be in streaks on the outer aspect of the stool.
- Consistency of the stool:
  - Diarrhea, more likely consistent with colitis
  - Hard stool, more likely consistent with fissure/constipation
- Painful stools suggest anal fissure, local proctitis, or ischemic bowel.
- Painless rectal bleeding is associated with polyps, Meckel diverticulum, nodular lymphoid hyperplasia of colon, intestinal duplication, intestinal submucosal mass (GIST), or vascular anomaly.
- Abdominal pain can be seen with inflammatory bowel disease, other causes of colitis, or a surgical abdomen.
- Obtain past medical history for any underlying or known GI disease, such as previous GI surgery, past history of colitis, Hirschsprung disease, necrotizing enterocolitis.
- Evaluate for history of jaundice, hepatitis, liver disease, neonatal history: suggestive of portal vein thrombosis (sepsis, shock, exchange transfusion, omphalitis, IV catheters), portal hypertension, and variceal bleeding
- Familial history of inflammatory bowel disease, intestinal polyps, and bleeding diathesis: von Willebrand disease, hemophilia
- Medication history: Screen for use of NSAIDs or anticoagulants (i.e., heparin or warfarin). In addition, a history of medications in the house should also be obtained due to possible accidental ingestion in younger children.
- Associated symptoms:
  - Mouth ulcers
  - Weight loss
  - Joint pains
  - Fevers
  - Rashes
  - Petechiae
  - Renal insufficiency
  - History of ingestion of unpasteurized juice or uncooked meat, consider hemolytic uremic syndrome.
  - Purpuric rash, consider HSP.

PHYSICAL EXAM

ALERT

Assess hemodynamic stability immediately.

- Heart rate: Tachycardia may be an early sign of intravascular volume depletion.
- Blood pressure (BP): Hypotension is a late sign and may not be present even with significant blood loss, as vasoconstriction can maintain BP until decompensation occurs.
- In the setting of normal BP readings, be sure to obtain orthostatic BP.
- Capillary refill: Delayed capillary refill suggests intravascular volume depletion.
- Oxygen saturation: may be decreased due to decreased oxygen-carrying capacity
- Evaluate for signs of shock:
  - Vitals signs listed above
  - Cool clammy extremities
  - Poor mentation

- Skin:
  - Petechiae or purpura: HSP or coagulopathy
  - Ecchymosis: coagulopathy
  - Hemangiomas: vascular anomaly
  - Spider angioma: liver disease or portal hypertension
  - Caput medusa: liver disease or portal hypertension
  - Palmar erythema: liver disease or portal hypertension
  - Jaundice: liver disease or portal hypertension
- HEENT
  - Freckles on buccal mucosa: Peutz-Jeghers syndrome
  - Telangiectasias on buccal mucosa: Osler-Weber-Rendu syndrome
  - Mouth ulcers: Crohn disease
  - Icteric sclera: portal hypertension
- Abdomen:
  - Hepatosplenomegaly, ascites: liver disease or portal hypertension
  - Isolated splenomegaly: cavernous transformation of the portal vein
- Rectal examination:
  - Evidence of any perianal disease (e.g., perirectal tags, fistulae): inflammatory bowel disease
  - Polyps: may be felt on rectal examination
  - Hemorrhoids: chronic constipation, portal hypertension

DIAGNOSTIC TESTS & INTERPRETATION

Initial Tests (screening, lab, imaging)

- NG tube lavage
  - Should be performed for decompression and/or patient comfort only
  - No longer required as diagnostic test in patients with suspected upper or LGIB, or useful for determining prognosis, or aiding visualization or therapeutic effect
- Stool guaiac
  - If possible, check stool for blood.
- CBC
  - Initial hemoglobin values may be unreliable because a delay in hemodilution may falsely produce near normal values; therefore, hemoglobin should be measured serially.
  - Leukopenia, anemia, and thrombocytopenia: Consider chronic liver disease and portal hypertension.
  - Anemia with normal RBC indices: truly an acute cause for bleeding
  - RBC indices indicate iron-deficiency anemia: Consider mucosal lesion or diffuse injury (e.g., as in colitis due to inflammatory bowel disease) causing chronic blood loss.
  - Thrombocytopenia: Consider hemolytic uremic syndrome.
- Coagulation profile (PT/PTT/INR): abnormal in liver disease or disseminated intravascular coagulation with sepsis
- Liver function tests (AST/ALT/ALB): abnormal in chronic liver disease
- Renal function tests (BUN, creatinine, urine analysis): abnormal in hemolytic uremic syndrome, HSP, acute bleed
- ESR or C-reactive protein (CRP): abnormal in inflammatory disorders or infectious colitis
- Stool tests:
  - Stool culture (*Salmonella*, *Shigella*, *Campylobacter*, *Yersinia*, *Aeromonas*, *Escherichia coli*, *Klebsiella*)
  - Stool for *Clostridium difficile* toxin A and B
  - Three stool samples for ova and parasites (amoebae)
  - Stool smears for WBCs (not always positive in colitis) and eosinophils (not always positive in allergic colitis)
  - Stool CMV: Consider for immunocompromised patients.
- Abdominal radiograph
  - Helpful in surgical abdomen (dilated bowel, air–fluid levels, perforation), constipation (presence of excessive stool), colitis (edematous bowel, thumb-printing), pneumatosis intestinalis, and toxic megacolon
- Ultrasound
  - Can show bowel wall thickening and Meckel diverticulum
  - Diagnostic of intussusception
- Barium tests:
  - Air-contrast enema is diagnostic and therapeutic in intussusception and diagnostic in mucosal lesions (polyps).
  - Upper GI series with small bowel follow-through is helpful in evaluating anatomy and inflammatory bowel disease.
  - CT scan can show evidence of intestinal inflammation and evidence of bowel obstruction.
- Nuclear medicine
  - Meckel scan: Technetium-99m pertechnetate can detect a Meckel diverticulum when it contains gastric mucosa.
  - Bleeding scan: useful in a patient with significant bleeding that precludes endoscopy or in whom endoscopy is undiagnostic. Technetium-99m–tagged erythrocyte scan detects rapid bleeding at a rate of 0.1 to 0.5 mL/min; can be performed at 30-minute intervals for up to 24 hours

Diagnostic Procedures/Other

- Endoscopy:
  - Upper endoscopy and colonoscopy has become the prime diagnostic and therapeutic tool for upper and LGIB. Endoscopy will accurately delineate the bleeding site and determines the specific cause. It is 90–95% sensitive at locating bleeding site.
  - Upper endoscopy diagnostic in massive upper GI bleeding presenting with hematochezia or melena
  - Upper endoscopy and colonoscopy should be performed when the suspicion is high for inflammatory bowel disease.
  - Colonoscopy should be performed when there is a suspicion for polyps.
- Video capsule endoscopy
  - Capsule endoscopy has become 1st-line treatment in adults and children to diagnose obscure causes of GI bleeding in the small intestine.
  - Limiting factor in capsule endoscopy can be the ability of the patient to swallow capsule.
  - The capsule can be placed endoscopically into the small intestine in younger children.
- Enteroscopy:
  - Enteroscopy (either via push, single balloon or double balloon technique) involves the passage of a special endoscope to evaluate the length of the small intestine. In general, enteroscopy is performed if a lesion is seen on capsule endoscopy and there is a need for endoscopic therapy.
- Angiography
  - Useful in detecting vascular causes of upper GI bleeding
  - Can also be therapeutic (i.e., injection of coils into a vascular malformation may occlude it)
  - Requires bleeding rate of 0.5 to 1 mL/min

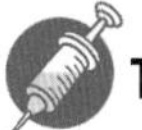

TREATMENT

GENERAL MEASURES

- Initial management of significant LGIB with hemodynamic instability:
  - Patients should be made NPO.
  - Achieve stable IV access.
  - Obtain blood type, and cross-match RBCs.
  - Stabilize the patient with IV fluids and blood products, as necessary (target hemoglobin ≥7 g/dL).
  - Target INR <2.5
- Disease-specific therapy
  - Anal fissure: Treat the underlying constipation (mineral oil, lactulose, MiraLax, high-fiber diet, increased water intake). Local therapy consists of sitz baths, local emollient creams, and steroid suppositories.
  - Polyp: colonoscopy with polypectomy
  - Intussusception: Air-contrast enema permits confirmation and hydrostatic reduction.
  - Parasites: antiparasitic drugs
  - Inflammatory bowel disease: referral to pediatric gastroenterologist for therapy

ISSUES FOR REFERRAL

Refer the following patients to a specialist:

- Any patient with significant acute LGIB after initial stabilization
- Patients with less acute bleeding for whom an easily identifiable cause has not been found or patients with chronic or recurrent LGIB.

SURGERY/OTHER PROCEDURES

In cases of massive or persistent bleeding with no identifiable site, exploratory laparotomy with intraoperative endoscopic evaluation of the entire bowel to identify mucosal lesions may be required.

ADMISSION, INPATIENT, AND NURSING CONSIDERATIONS

Emergency care

- If patient is critical, stabilize with IV fluids and blood products.
- Order laboratory tests: CBC, PT/PTT, disseminated intravascular coagulation screen, liver function tests, blood type, and cross-match
- Monitor patient's vital signs and hemoglobin.
- Make appropriate diagnosis and institute appropriate therapy (e.g., abdominal x-ray, cross-sectional imaging, nuclear medicine bleeding scans, and/or pediatric gastroenterology consultation for colonoscopy).

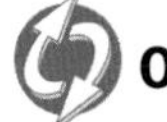

ONGOING CARE

FOLLOW-UP RECOMMENDATIONS

Patient Monitoring

- Monitor hemoglobin in the hospital until patient's condition is stable.
- For patients with LGIB that is chronic in nature and hemodynamically stable, they can be referred to specialist for further workup once initial blood and stool studies are sent.

DIET

Introduce extensively hydrolyzed protein formula in infants with suspected cow's milk protein allergy.

ADDITIONAL READING

- Boyle JT. Gastrointestinal bleeding in infants and children. *Pediatric Rev*. 2008;29(2):39–52.
- Cohen SA, Klevens AI. Use of capsule endoscopy in diagnosis and management of pediatric patients, based on meta-analysis. *Clin Gastroenterol Hepatol*. 2011;9(6):490–496.
- Fox V. Gastrointestinal bleeding in infancy and childhood. *Gastroenterol Clin North Am*. 2000;29(1):37–66.
- Leung AK, Wong AL. Lower gastrointestinal bleeding in children. *Pediatr Emerg Care*. 2002;18(4):319–323.
- Liu K, Kaffes AJ. Review article: the diagnosis and investigation of obscure gastrointestinal bleeding. *Aliment Pharmacol Ther*. 2011;34(4):416–423.

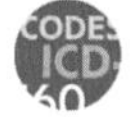

CODES

ICD10

- K92.2 Gastrointestinal hemorrhage, unspecified
- K92.1 Melena
- K52.2 Allergic and dietetic gastroenteritis and colitis

FAQ

- Q: What is the most common cause of LGIB in an infant?
- A: Allergic colitis
- Q: What common foods cause stools to be red?
- A: Raspberries, cranberries, Kool-Aid, artificial coloring in cereal
- Q: What common foods cause stools to be black?
- A: Bismuth, spinach, blueberries, licorice

LUPUS ERYTHEMATOSUS

Elizabeth Candell Chalom, MD

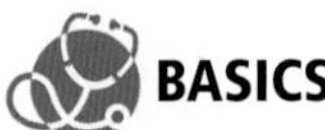

BASICS

DESCRIPTION

Systemic lupus erythematosus (SLE) is a multisystem autoimmune disease characterized by production of antibodies to various components of the cell nucleus and tissues, in conjunction with a variety of clinical manifestations.

EPIDEMIOLOGY

- Age: 20% of lupus begins in childhood, but it is very rare in <5 years old.
- Female-to-male ratio: between 3 to 5:1 (prepubertal) and 9 to 10:1 (postpubertal)
- SLE occurs about 3 times more often in African Americans than Caucasians. It is also more common in Hispanic, Asian, and Native Americans.

Incidence

- Peak incidence: between ages 15 and 40 years
- Incidence in children is from 10 to 20 cases per 100,000 children per year.

Prevalence

5,000 to 10,000 children in the United States

RISK FACTORS

Genetics

- Increased frequency in 1st-degree family members of patients with SLE
- 10% of patients have ≥1 affected relative.
- Concordance rate of 25–50% in monozygotic twins and 5% in dizygotic twins
- Some major histocompatibility complex antigens are associated with increased incidence of lupus, such as HLA-DR2 and DR3 in whites and DR2 and DR7 in blacks.

ETIOLOGY

Lupus is an autoimmune disease, with multiple genetic, environmental, and hormonal factors playing a role.

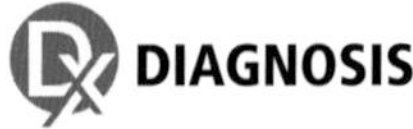

DIAGNOSIS

- Classification criteria are used for research purposes but when met, have high sensitivity and specificity for diagnosis of lupus.
- 4 of the following 11 criteria, developed by the American College of Rheumatology (ACR), must be met to classify a patient as having SLE:
  - Malar (butterfly) rash
  - Discoid rash
  - Photosensitivity
  - Oral or nasal ulcers
  - Arthritis
  - Cytopenia
    - Anemia, leukopenia (<4,000/mm^3), lymphopenia (<1,500/mm^3), or thrombocytopenia (<100,000/mm^3)
  - Neurologic disease: seizures or psychosis
  - Nephritis: >0.5 g/24 h proteinuria or cellular casts
  - Serositis: pleuritis or pericarditis
  - Positive immunoserology (revised 1997): antibodies to double-stranded DNA or Smith nuclear antigen, false-positive serologic test for syphilis, lupus anticoagulant, or antiphospholipid (APL) antibodies
  - Positive antinuclear antibody (ANA)
- Classification criteria used by the Systemic Lupus International Collaborating Clinics (SLICC) have recently been validated.
  - In addition to the ACR criteria, SLICC criteria include nonscarring alopecia, hypocomplementemia, and positive direct Coombs test.
  - Photosensitivity is not included.

HISTORY

- History of photosensitivity or malar rash common but not necessary
- Many patients have systemic complaints, such as fever, fatigue, and malaise.
- Many patients complain of joint pain, Raynaud phenomenon, or alopecia.
- Chest pain from pericarditis or pleural effusions may be present.
- Signs and symptoms:
  - Immune complex–mediated vasculitis, which can occur in almost any organ system
  - Cutaneous lesions: very variable; include
    - Erythematous malar or "butterfly" rash
    - Maculopapular rashes (can occur anywhere on body)
    - Discoid rashes
    - Periungual erythema
    - Mucosal membrane vasculitis
  - Arthritis: can affect large and small joints; usually symmetric and nonerosive
  - Hematologic pathology includes the following:
    - Hemolytic anemia
    - Anemia of chronic disease
    - Leukopenia
    - Lymphopenia
    - Thrombocytopenia
  - Neurologic symptoms include the following:
    - Headaches
    - Psychosis
    - Depression
    - Seizures
    - Organic brain syndromes
    - Peripheral neuropathies
  - Renal pathology
    - Present in up to 75% children with SLE
    - Includes mesangial changes and glomerulonephritis (focal, diffuse proliferative, or membranous)
    - First signs of renal disease in lupus patients are often proteinuria and active urine sediment.
    - Hypertension, nephrotic syndrome, and renal failure can also occur.
  - Serositis: usually seen as pericarditis or pleuritis but peritonitis can also occur
  - Constitutional symptoms are very common: fatigue, weight loss, fever.

PHYSICAL EXAM

- Rash: may be malar, discoid, or vasculitic. Periungual erythema may also be seen.
- Oral or nasal ulcers (usually on hard or soft palate) that are painless and often go unnoticed by patients
- Arthritis of large and small joints
- Pericardial friction rub if patient has pericarditis
- Edema may be present secondary to renal disease.
- CNS changes such as personality changes, psychosis, or seizures

DIFFERENTIAL DIAGNOSIS

- Systemic-onset juvenile idiopathic arthritis
- Oncologic disease (leukemia, lymphoma)
- Viral or other infectious illness
- Other vasculitic disorders
- Dermatomyositis
- Fibromyalgia
- Drug-induced lupus

ALERT

Avoid overdiagnosis; positive ANA in the absence of clinical signs or symptoms of SLE is not lupus.

DIAGNOSTIC TESTS & INTERPRETATION

- ANA
  - Found in >95% of patients with SLE, but a positive ANA can occur in many diseases and in up to 20% of normal population
- Anti–double-stranded DNA and anti–Smith nuclear antigen
  - Very specific to lupus, but not all patients with lupus have these autoantibodies. In many patients, anti-DNA levels vary with activity of disease.

- CBC
  - Anemia, leukopenia, lymphopenia, and/or thrombocytopenia may be seen.
- Urinalysis
  - May show proteinuria or active urinary sediment if there is renal dysfunction
- Complement levels
  - Can fall very low during a lupus flare (C3 and C4)
- PTT
  - Patients may also have prolonged PTT, as result of APL antibodies, often seen in SLE.
  - Patients with APL antibodies are at increased risk for thrombotic events, such as deep venous thrombosis, stroke, and fetal loss during pregnancies.

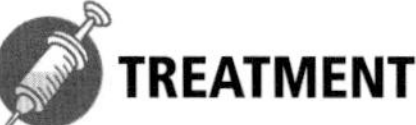

TREATMENT

GENERAL MEASURES

Avoid excessive sun exposure and use sunscreen liberally.

MEDICATION

- NSAIDs
  - May be used for musculoskeletal and mild systemic complaints, although ibuprofen has been noted to cause aseptic meningitis in a small number of patients with SLE
  - NSAIDs can also exacerbate renal disease in lupus.
- Hydroxychloroquine often used to help control cutaneous manifestations and to help minimize the chance of lupus flares; helps improve lipid profile as well
- Corticosteroids often necessary to control systemic and renal manifestations
- Patients with renal disease often need immunosuppressive agents such as cyclophosphamide (usually given as monthly IV boluses). Mycophenolate mofetil, cyclosporine, or azathioprine may also be used.
- Patients with mainly arthritic symptoms may be treated with weekly methotrexate, PO or SC.
- Patients with APL antibodies can be treated with a baby aspirin daily. If they have already had a significant clotting event, they need stronger anticoagulation.
- Angiotensin-converting enzyme (ACE) inhibitors are often used to help prevent renal damage from proteinuria.
- Patients with abnormal lipid profiles that do not respond to diet may need statins.
- Rituximab (anti-CD20 antibody) causes B-cell depletion and is used in SLE, especially for thrombocytopenia.
- Belimumab, a B-lymphocyte stimulator (BLyS) inhibitor, has been used for mild-to-moderate SLE.
- Antibodies to CD40 and C5 are also being studied.
- Plasmapheresis and IVIG have been used as well.

ADDITIONAL THERAPIES

For very severe lupus, bone marrow immunoablation or transplantation are options.

ONGOING CARE

PROGNOSIS

- Extremely variable. Renal disease and CNS involvement are poor prognostic signs, whereas systemic complaints and joint findings are not.
- 10-year survival in children presenting with SLE is >90%.
- Most deaths related to infection, renal, CNS, cardiac, and pulmonary disease

COMPLICATIONS

- End-stage renal disease
- Infections secondary to treatments used to control disease
- Atherosclerosis and myocardial infarctions at a young age
- Libman-Sacks endocarditis, which increases risk of subacute bacterial endocarditis
- Neonatal lupus
  - Neonatal lupus erythematosus (NLE) is due to maternal autoantibodies (usually SSA or SSB antibodies) that cross the placenta and can cause rashes, congenital heart block, cytopenias, and/or hepatitis in the newborn.
  - Most symptoms of NLE resolve by 6 months of age, but heart block, if it occurs, is permanent.
  - Many mothers of babies with NLE are asymptomatic and unaware that they have these autoantibodies.
  - The rash, erythema annulare, can begin a few days after delivery or within the first few weeks of life.
  - Topical steroids can minimize skin lesions.
  - Congenital heart block is due to damage of the conducting system of the developing fetal heart.
  - Bradycardia may be noted by 22 weeks' gestation, and CHF with nonimmune hydrops fetalis may ensue.

ADDITIONAL READING

- Brunner HI, Huggins J, Klein-Gitelman MS. Pediatric SLE—towards a comprehensive management plan. *Nat Rev Rheumatol*. 2011;7(4):225–233.
- Gottlieb BS, Ilowite NT. Systemic lupus erythematosus in children and adolescents. *Pediatr Rev*. 2006;27(9):323–330.
- Macdermott EJ, Adams A, Lehman TJ. Systemic lupus erythematosus in children: current and emerging therapies. *Lupus*. 2007;16(8):677–683.
- Malattia C, Martini A. Paediatric-onset systemic lupus erythematosus. *Best Pract Res Clin Rheumatol*. 2013;27(3):351–362.
- Yildirim-Toruner C, Diamond B. Current and novel therapeutics in the treatment of systemic lupus erythematosus. *J Allergy Clin Immunol*. 2011;127(2):303–312.

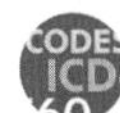

CODES

ICD10

- L93.0 Discoid lupus erythematosus
- M32.9 Systemic lupus erythematosus, unspecified
- L93.2 Other local lupus erythematosus

FAQ

- Q: If a patient has a positive ANA but no clinical signs of SLE, how often should the ANA be followed?
- A: A positive ANA test will usually remain positive indefinitely, but it has no real significance in the absence of clinical or other laboratory disturbances. Up to 20% of the normal population may have a positive ANA, so there is no need to repeat the test.
- Q: Can SLE patients with end-stage renal disease obtain renal transplants?
- A: Yes, and SLE usually does not recur in the new kidney.

LYME DISEASE

Elizabeth Candell Chalom, MD

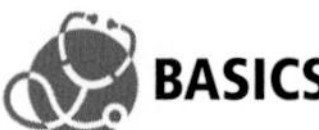

BASICS

DESCRIPTION

Multisystem illness caused by the spirochete *Borrelia burgdorferi*, carried by the deer tick

EPIDEMIOLOGY

- Can affect people of all ages, but 1/3 to 1/2 of all cases occur in children and adolescents
- Male/female ratio: 1:1 to 2:1
- Onset most often in summer months
- Although Lyme disease can be found anywhere, the majority of the cases in the United States are found in Southern New England and the mid-Atlantic states. It is also seen frequently in California, Minnesota, and Wisconsin.
- The most common tick-borne disease in the United States, with incidence in 2015 of 8.9/100,000.
  - However, incidence varies significantly in different parts of the country and 95% of all cases reported were found in 14 states: Connecticut, Delaware, Maine, Maryland, Minnesota, New Hampshire, New Jersey, New York, Pennsylvania, Rhode Island, Vermont, and Virginia.
  - Outside of those states, Lyme disease remains rare.

RISK FACTORS

Genetics

Chronic Lyme arthritis seems to be associated with increased incidence of HLA-DR4 and less so with HLA-DR2.

PATHOPHYSIOLOGY

- *B. burgdorferi* is injected into skin with saliva during bite of Ixodes tick.
- Spirochetes first migrate within skin, forming the typical rash, erythema migrans.
- Spirochetes then spread hematogenously to other organs, including heart, joints, and nervous system.

ETIOLOGY

The tick-borne spirochete *B. burgdorferi*

COMMONLY ASSOCIATED CONDITIONS

The same ticks that transmit Lyme disease can also transmit *Ehrlichia* and *Babesia*, so infections with those spirochetes can occur simultaneously.

DIAGNOSIS

HISTORY

- Tick bite
  - History of tick bite can only be elicited in 1/3 of patients with Lyme disease.
  - Most people with tick bites do not develop Lyme disease.
  - Even in endemic areas, risk of developing Lyme disease after tick bite is <5%.
- Rash
  - 50–80% will have or will recall the typical often target-shaped erythema migrans rash.
  - Rash is not painful or pruritic but feels warm.
- Other symptoms
  - Many patients will complain of fatigue, headaches, fevers, chills, myalgias, and conjunctivitis early on.
- Joint pain
  - Many patients will complain of painful joints early on and later will develop joint swelling.
- Signs and symptoms
  - Skin: erythema migrans (typical rash)
    - Starts as red macule or papule and then expands to annular lesion up to 30 cm in diameter with partial central clearing
    - The lesion is usually painless and lasts 4 to 7 days.
  - Musculoskeletal
    - Early on, patient may experience myalgias, migratory joint pain (often without frank arthritis), and painful tendons and bursae.
    - Weeks to months later, 60% of untreated patients will develop monoarticular or oligoarticular arthritis of large joints, especially knees.
    - Joint fluid can have WBC count anywhere from 500 to 110,000 cells/mm^3, and cells are mostly neutrophils.
  - Neurologic
    - Several weeks after initial rash, 14% of untreated patients will develop neurologic symptoms including aseptic meningitis, cranial nerve palsies (especially facial nerve palsies), mononeuritis, plexitis, or myelitis.
    - Months to years later, chronic neurologic symptoms may occur, including a subtle encephalopathy: memory, mood, and sleep disturbances.
    - Significant fatigue can occur early or late in the course of Lyme disease.
  - Cardiac
    - Several weeks after initial rash, ~5% of untreated patients develop cardiac disease.
    - Most common cardiac lesion is atrioventricular block (primary, secondary, or complete).
  - Pericarditis, myocarditis, or pancarditis can also develop.

PHYSICAL EXAM

- May be completely normal early in course of disease
- Rash of erythema migrans, if seen, is virtually pathognomonic for Lyme disease.
- If patient does not have the rash, no physical finding exists that gives definitive diagnosis of Lyme disease.
- Patient may have arthritis, Bell palsy, a cranial nerve palsy, conjunctivitis, or an irregular heartbeat.

DIFFERENTIAL DIAGNOSIS

- Viral arthritis/arthralgias
- Septic arthritis
- Juvenile idiopathic arthritis
- Postinfectious arthritis
- Fibromyalgia syndrome
- Systemic lupus erythematosus

ALERT

Many patients with vague systemic complaints (e.g., fatigue, headaches, arthralgias) are incorrectly diagnosed with Lyme disease, even though their Lyme tests are negative (or enzyme-linked immunosorbent assay [ELISA] mildly positive and Western blot negative).These patients are then treated with multiple courses of oral antibiotics; if they do not respond, they are often treated with IV antibiotics, sometimes for prolonged periods. This situation delays diagnosing true problem and subjects patients to unnecessary risks of long-term antibiotic use and occasionally of central venous lines.

DIAGNOSTIC TESTS & INTERPRETATION

- ELISA
  - Can detect antibodies to *B. burgdorferi* several weeks after tick bite. However, it has relatively high false-positive rate and occasionally false-negative results. It remains positive for years after treatment.
- Western blot analysis
  - Much more specific. After 4 to 8 weeks of infection, ≥5 of the following IgG bands must be present for test to be positive: 18, 21, 28, 30, 39, 41, 45, 58, 66, and 93 Kd. During first 2 to 4 weeks of infection, two IgM bands may establish diagnosis, but false-positive IgM blots are common.

- Positive ELISA with negative Western blot:
  - Usually means patient does not have Lyme disease and ELISA was a false positive, but false-positive IgM blots are common.
- Polymerase chain reaction (PCR)
  - PCR testing may be done with synovial tissue or fluid or with CSF. Positive PCR indicates active disease, but negative result does not rule out Lyme disease.
  - Urine tests for Lyme disease have been shown to be very inaccurate and should not be used.

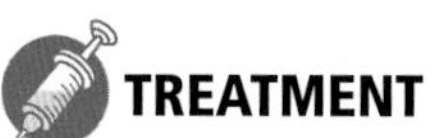

TREATMENT

MEDICATION

- Oral antibiotics
  - Initial therapy for early Lyme disease
  - Specific therapies
    - Patients >8 years old: Doxycycline is drug of choice.
    - Younger children or people who do not tolerate tetracyclines: Amoxicillin or cefuroxime is preferred, but penicillin V is also acceptable.
    - Penicillin-allergic patients: Erythromycin may be used but is less effective.
    - Duration of therapy for patients with only skin rash: 10 to 21 days of oral antibiotics usually sufficient
    - If other symptoms present: 21 to 28 days recommended
  - Of note: It is not uncommon for patients with Lyme arthritis to develop a Jarisch-Herxheimer reaction within the first 10 days of antibiotic treatment. This may look like an allergic reaction to the antibiotic, with a rash (nonpruritic, not palpable) and significant joint pain, but it is not.
- IV antibiotics
  - Become necessary for
    - Persistent arthritis unresponsive to oral medications
    - Severe carditis
    - Neurologic disease (other than an isolated 7th nerve palsy)
  - Specific IV therapies
    - Ceftriaxone: drug of choice
    - Penicillin V: may also be used
  - Duration of therapy: 14 to 21 days
- Prevention
  - Some studies suggest that a single dose of doxycycline after tick bite will prevent Lyme disease.
  - Protective clothing, tick repellant (containing N, N-Diethyl-meta-toluamide [DEET]), and checking daily for ticks are good preventive measures.

ONGOING CARE

PROGNOSIS

- In general, prognosis is much better for children than for adults. Only 2% of children have chronic arthritis at 6 months.
- Most of the cardiac manifestations will disappear with or without treatment in a short time (3 to 4 weeks) but may later recur. Severe cardiac involvement rarely may be fatal.

COMPLICATIONS

- Chronic arthritis occurs in ~2% of children.
- Other complications arise from treatment, such as cholecystitis secondary to treatment with ceftriaxone or infections from indwelling catheters used for IV antibiotics.
- Some patients develop what is thought to be a post–Lyme disease syndrome. This syndrome is not well defined and is very controversial. It often consists of arthralgias and fatigue but may include paresthesias and cognitive complaints. Prolonged antibiotics have not been shown to be helpful. Some of these patients present with a fibromyalgia-like syndrome and improve with physical therapy.

ADDITIONAL READING

- Bunikis J, Barbour AG. Laboratory testing for suspected Lyme disease. *Med Clin North Am*. 2002;86(2):311–340.
- Feder HM Jr. Lyme disease in children. *Infect Dis Clin North Am*. 2008;22(2):315–326.
- Nachman SA, Pontrelli L. Central nervous system Lyme disease. *Semin Pediatr Infect Dis*. 2003;14(2):123–130.
- Shapiro ED. *Borrelia burgdorferi* (Lyme disease). *Pediatr Rev*. 2014;35(12):500–509.
- Shapiro ED. Clinical practice. Lyme disease. *N Engl J Med*. 2014;370(18):1724–1731.
- Steere AC, Strle F, Wormser GP, et al. Lyme borreliosis. *Nat Rev Dis Primers*. 2016;2:16090.
- Weinstein A, Britchkov M. Lyme arthritis and post-Lyme disease syndrome. *Curr Opin Rheumatol*. 2002;14(4):383–387.

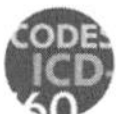

CODES

ICD10

- A69.20 Lyme disease, unspecified
- A69.23 Arthritis due to Lyme disease
- A69.21 Meningitis due to Lyme disease

FAQ

- Q: What does the deer tick look like?
- A: The deer tick is flat, very small (about the size of a pin head), and has eight legs. The adult male is black, and the female is red and black. They can grow to 3 times their normal size when they are engorged with blood.
- Q: Do all bites from infected deer ticks cause Lyme disease?
- A: No. Even infected ticks will not cause Lyme disease if they are attached to the skin for a short period of time. If the tick is attached for <24 hours, the chances of transmitting the disease are exceedingly low. The longer the tick is attached, the higher the probability of disease transmission.
- Q: Should all patients be retested for Lyme disease after a full course of treatment?
- A: No. Lyme titers and the Western blot will remain positive for years after adequate treatment for Lyme disease. If the patient's symptoms have resolved, there is no point in rechecking the titer. If the patient is still symptomatic, titers and a Western blot may be checked before starting IV antibiotic therapy to look for a rising titer and to be sure the patient truly has Lyme disease. If symptoms remain after IV therapy, other diagnoses should be considered.
- Q: Should patients with nontraumatic Bell palsy be tested for Lyme disease?
- A: Bell palsy is seen in association with Lyme disease infections. It is a reasonable indication for testing for Lyme disease.

LYMPHADENOPATHY

Lauren A. Sanchez, MD • Morna J. Dorsey, MD, MMSc

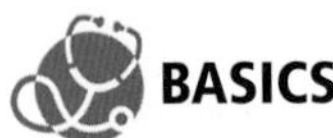

BASICS

DESCRIPTION

- Term used to describe ≥1 enlarged lymph nodes >10 mm in diameter (for inguinal nodes, >15 mm; for epitrochlear nodes, >5 mm)
- Any palpable supraclavicular and popliteal lymph node is considered abnormal.

EPIDEMIOLOGY

Incidence

Depends on the underlying process that causes lymph node enlargement

Prevalence

Palpable nodes are present in up to 50% of neonates (cervical, axillary, inguinal), infants, and older children (all areas except epitrochlear, supraclavicular, and popliteal).

PATHOPHYSIOLOGY

- Lymph nodes are often palpable in normal, healthy children.
  - Normal lymph nodes: generally <10 mm
  - They are present from birth, peak in size between 8 and 12 years of age, and then regress during adolescence.
- Lymph nodes drain contiguous areas.
  - Cervical nodes drain head and neck area (up to 15% of biopsied nodes are malignant).
  - Axillary nodes drain arm, thorax, and breast.
  - Epitrochlear nodes drain forearm and hand.
  - Inguinal nodes drain leg and groin.
  - Supraclavicular nodes drain thorax and abdomen.
- Lymphatic flow from adjacent nodes or inoculation site brings microorganisms to lymph nodes.
- Lymph node enlargement may occur via any of the following mechanisms:
  - Nodal cells may replicate in response to antigenic stimulation (e.g., Kawasaki disease) or malignant transformation (e.g., lymphoma).
  - Lymphocyte proliferation due to immune defect (e.g., primary immunodeficiency disease [PIDD])
  - Large number of reactive cells from outside node (e.g., neutrophils or metastatic cells) may enter node.
  - Foreign material may be deposited into node by lipid-laden histiocytes (e.g., lipid storage diseases).
  - Vascular engorgement and edema may occur secondary to local cytokine release.
  - Suppuration secondary to tissue necrosis (e.g., *Mycobacterium tuberculosis*)
- Many systemic infections (e.g., HIV) cause hepatic or splenic enlargement in addition to generalized lymphadenopathy.

ETIOLOGY

- Usually determined by performing a thorough history and physical exam
- Infectious etiology more likely in a child <5 years old (i.e., *Staphylococcus aureus, Streptococcus pyogenes*).

COMMONLY ASSOCIATED CONDITIONS

Many systemic infections, malignancy, and lymphoproliferative disorders cause hepatic or splenic enlargement in addition to generalized lymphadenopathy.

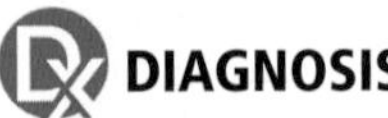

DIAGNOSIS

HISTORY

- Preceding symptoms (e.g., URI symptoms preceding cervical lymphadenopathy)
- Localizing signs or symptoms (e.g., stomatitis may be associated with submandibular lymphadenopathy)
- Duration
  - Acute (<3 weeks)
  - Subacute (3 to 6 weeks)
  - Chronic (>6 weeks)
- Constitutional or associated symptoms (e.g., fever, night sweats, or weight loss)
- Exposures
  - Cat exposure (cat-scratch disease)
  - Uncooked meat (toxoplasmosis)
  - Tick bite (Lyme disease)
  - Flea bite (*Yersinia*)
- Medications (e.g., phenytoin or isoniazid) or prior treatments
- Travel to or residence in an endemic area should raise suspicion for tuberculosis and Lyme disease.
- Vaccination history (e.g., measles or rubella in an unimmunized child)
- History of recurrent, deep seated, or opportunistic infections, family history of PIDD
- Signs and symptoms
  - Localized lymphadenopathy: involves enlarged nodes in any one region
  - Generalized lymphadenopathy: involves ≥2 noncontiguous regions secondary to a systemic process, such as EBV infection
  - Supraclavicular nodes seen with malignancy: Right-sided supraclavicular node is associated with mediastinal malignancy; left-sided node suggests abdominal malignancy.

PHYSICAL EXAM

- Complete physical exam is imperative to look for signs of systemic disease such as skin, oropharyngeal, or ocular findings or hepatosplenomegaly.
- The child's weight should also be checked to be sure there has been no weight loss.
- If localized lymphadenopathy is suspected, examine the area that the lymph node drains for pathology. For example, an arm papule may be associated with axillary lymphadenopathy in cat-scratch disease.
- Cervical, axillary, and inguinal nodes, as well as liver and spleen, must be palpated to help determine if signs of systemic disease or infection are present.
- Characterize nodes. Be sure to note the following:
  - Location: Be as exact as possible (see above).
  - Size: Specify dimensions.
  - Consistency: soft, firm, solid, cystic, fluctuant, rubbery. Firm, rubbery nodes may be associated with lymphomas, whereas soft nodes are generally palpated with reactive lymphadenopathy.
  - Fixation: normally freely mobile; infection or malignancy may cause adherence to surrounding tissues or nodes.
  - Tenderness: suggests inflammation

DIAGNOSTIC TESTS & INTERPRETATION

Initial Tests (screening, lab, imaging)

Consider the following tests if ≥1 node is persistently enlarged, has increased in size, has changed in consistency or mobility, or if systemic symptoms are present:

- CBC with differential: Consider in generalized lymphadenopathy; leukocytosis (acute bacterial or viral infection), leukopenia (malignancy), lymphopenia (HIV, PIDD) can be seen.
- ESR or CRP: increased with infection or inflammation
- Lactate dehydrogenase (LDH), uric acid, and liver enzymes: Consider if history and physical exam raise concern for malignancy or hepatomegaly.
- Throat culture: if concern for group A β-hemolytic streptococcal (GAS) pharyngitis
- EBV/cytomegalovirus (CMV) titers: Consider with persistent generalized adenopathy.
- *Bartonella henselae* titers: Consider with persistently enlarged unilateral node and/or history of cat exposure.
- Purified protein derivative (PPD) testing: Consider with persistently enlarged node (2 to 4 weeks) or travel to areas where tuberculosis is endemic.
- HIV testing: Consider with persistent generalized lymphadenopathy and failure to thrive.
- Antinuclear antibody (ANA): if other signs of systemic disease to rule out systemic lupus erythematosus (SLE)
- Consider STD testing in adolescents (e.g., syphilis).
- Other infectious workup as dictated by history and physical findings (e.g., Lyme titers for bull's eye rash)
- Chest radiograph: helpful with supraclavicular nodes, systemic symptoms, cough, wheezing, or if positive PPD
- Ultrasound: may help differentiate cystic from solid masses, evaluate for congenital neck mass
- CT: may help delineate anatomy or extent of the lesion; iliac lymphadenopathy is abnormal.

Diagnostic Procedures/Other

- Biopsy should be considered if
  - Nodes are persistently enlarged, especially if accompanied by signs of systemic disease such as hepatosplenomegaly, weight loss, and exanthema.
  - Nodes are fixed to underlying skin.
  - Ulcerations or skin changes are present.
  - Not responsive to conventional therapy
  - Node is supraclavicular, nontender, or increasing in size or firmness.
- Fine-needle aspiration: cost-effective but sometimes nondiagnostic (e.g., unable to assess architecture, high false-negative rate); may result in fistulous tract
- Open biopsy: Consider early if concern for malignancy; often diagnostic but requires general anesthesia

DIFFERENTIAL DIAGNOSIS

Must be carefully differentiated from lymphadenitis, defined as lymph node enlargement with signs of inflammation (including erythema, tenderness, induration, warmth); often treated with antibiotics

- Localized lymphadenopathy
  - Generally occurs as reactive adenopathy in response to local infection
  - Differential diagnosis for localized adenopathy varies depending on affected site.
    - Cervical adenopathy includes cystic hygroma, branchial cleft cyst, thyroglossal duct cyst, thyroid nodule, epidermoid cyst.
    - Inguinal adenopathy: lower extremity infection (e.g., osteomyelitis) or perineal disease
- Generalized lymphadenopathy: may be seen in many systemic illnesses
  - Viral infections: EBV, CMV, adenovirus, HSV, HIV, enterovirus, rubella, measles virus, varicella virus, viral hepatitides
  - Bacterial infections: *S. aureus*, *B. henselae*, GAS, *Yersinia*, brucellosis, tularemia, *M. tuberculosis*, atypical mycobacterium, *Mycoplasma pneumoniae*, rickettsiae
  - PIDDs: common variable immunodeficiency disease, X-linked lymphoproliferative syndrome, autoimmune lymphoproliferative syndrome, hyper-IgM syndrome
  - Malignancy: lymphoma, neuroblastoma, leukemia
  - Autoimmune disorders: SLE, juvenile rheumatoid arthritis
  - Other infections: parasites (e.g., Chagas disease) or fungal infections
  - Medications can cause drug-induced hypersensitivity syndromes (e.g., DRESS): aromatic anticonvulsants, sulfonamides, allopurinol
  - Miscellaneous: PFAPA (periodic fever, aphthous stomatitis, pharyngitis, and cervical adenitis syndrome). Kawasaki disease, Castleman disease, Kikuchi-Fujimoto disease (histiocytic necrotizing lymphadenitis), Gianotti-Crosti syndrome (papular acrodermatitis), sarcoidosis, lipid storage diseases (Niemann-Pick, Gaucher, Wolman, Faber diseases), autoimmune lymphoproliferative syndromes

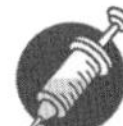

TREATMENT

GENERAL MEASURES

- Treat underlying disease.
- Close observation, unless history and physical suggest malignancy or lymphadenitis

MEDICATION

Acute lymphadenitis should be treated with antibiotics directed against *Streptococcus* and *Staphylococcus*.

First Line

- Dicloxacillin 50 to 100 mg/kg/24 h PO in 4 divided doses; max 4 g/24 h *OR*
- Amoxicillin-clavulanic acid 45 mg/kg/24 h PO in 2 divided doses, children >40 kg adult dosing
- Consider using clindamycin 30 mg/kg/24 h PO in 3 divided doses OR trimethoprim-sulfamethoxazole (TMP–SMX) 8 to 10 mg TMP/kg/24 h PO/IV in 2 divided doses in areas with a high prevalence of methicillin-resistant *S. aureus* (MRSA) in the community.
- Penicillin-allergic patients: clindamycin 30 mg/kg/24 h PO in 3 divided doses or erythromycin 50 mg/kg/24 h PO in 4 divided doses

Second Line

Consider broader antibiotic coverage for *B. henselae* and atypical mycobacterium: oral: azithromycin 10 mg/kg dose on day 1, followed by 5 mg/kg divided once for 4 more days

ISSUES FOR REFERRAL

Refer to surgery or otolaryngology if biopsy or excision required.

SURGERY/OTHER PROCEDURES

Excision for special, prolonged cases

ONGOING CARE

FOLLOW-UP RECOMMENDATIONS

Patient Monitoring

- Localized lymphadenopathy: Observe for several weeks or treat with antibiotics if indicated.
- Serial observation if nodes are persistently enlarged

PROGNOSIS

- Depends on underlying diagnosis
- Excellent for reactive lymphadenopathy

COMPLICATIONS

- Lymphadenitis
- Local infection (e.g., cellulitis)
- Lymph node abscess
- Sepsis via hematogenous spread of inadequately contained infection
- Fistula (e.g., with atypical mycobacteria)
- Fibrosis secondary to purulence or lymphadenitis
- Stridor secondary to enlarged cervical lymph nodes
- Wheezing secondary to enlarged parabronchial mediastinal lymph nodes

ADDITIONAL READING

- Albright JT, Pransky SM. Nontuberculous mycobacterial infections of the head and neck. *Pediatr Clin North Am.* 2003;50(2):503–514.
- Bamji M, Stone RK, Kaul A, et al. Palpable lymph nodes in healthy newborns and infants. *Pediatrics.* 1986;78(4):573–575.
- Brook I. Microbiology and antimicrobial management of head and neck infections in children. *Adv Pediatr.* 2008;55:305–325.
- Friedmann AM. Evaluation and management of lymphadenopathy in children. *Pediatr Rev.* 2008;29(2):53–60.
- Gosche JR, Vick L. Acute, subacute, and chronic cervical lymphadenitis in children. *Semin Pediatr Sur.* 2006;15(2):99–106.
- Nield LS, Kamat D. Lymphadenopathy in children: when and how to evaluate. *Clin Pediatr (Phila).* 2004;43(1):25–33.
- Rajasekaran K, Krakovitz P. Enlarged neck lymph nodes in children. *Pediatr Clin North Am.* 2013;60(4):923–936.
- Twist CJ, Link MP. Assessment of lymphadenopathy in children. *Pediatr Clin North Am.* 2002;49(5):1009–1025.

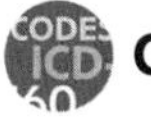

CODES

ICD10

- R59.1 Generalized enlarged lymph nodes
- R59.0 Localized enlarged lymph nodes
- P37.1 Congenital toxoplasmosis

FAQ

- Q: When should there be concern about malignancy in a child with lymphadenopathy?
- A: Malignancy should be considered in any child who has lymphadenopathy that does not improve in spite of antibiotic therapy, that has a location of concern (e.g., supraclavicular) or physical exam features of concern (hard, large size [>2 cm]) that persistently enlarges, or if the child shows signs of systemic disease.
- Q: When should a workup of a well child with localized lymphadenopathy be pursued?
- A: As long as the lymph nodes are soft, mobile, and nontender, the lymphadenopathy is likely to be self-limited. If the cause is unclear, then children should be observed for a couple of weeks. Further workup is needed if the nodes persist or enlarge, if the location is worrisome (e.g., supraclavicular), or if there are signs of systemic disease (e.g., hepatomegaly or weight loss).
- Q: When should a child with lymphadenopathy be referred to a specialist?
- A: Most cases of lymphadenopathy in children are self-limited and can be observed for a few weeks and/or treated with antibiotics, if appropriate. Referral to a surgeon should be considered in any child with persistently enlarged lymphadenopathy (>4 weeks) or immediately if there are signs of malignancy. If there is a history of recurrent or opportunistic infections, referral to an immunologist or infectious disease specialist is warranted.

LYMPHEDEMA

Heidi Engel, PT, DPT • Cynthia Burke, NNP-BC

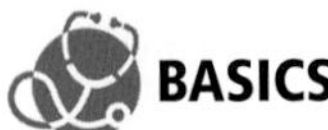

BASICS

DESCRIPTION

- Lymphedema is a chronic progressive swelling in subcutaneous tissues, typically in an extremity or the genitals, due to protein-rich accumulation of interstitial fluid from disruption of the lymphatic system. It can be of primary or secondary origin.
- Primary lymphedema has three forms, all of which stem from a developmental abnormality of lymphatic flow. Not all primary lymphedemas are clinically evident at birth.
  - Congenital lymphedema, due to anomalous development of lymph system
    - Present at birth
    - Lower to upper extremity ratio: 3:1
    - 2/3 of cases are bilateral.
    - May improve with age
  - Lymphedema praecox (65–80% of primary lymphedema)
    - Usually becomes evident at puberty but may appear between infancy and age 35 years
    - 70% unilateral lower extremity (L > R)
  - Lymphedema tarda: presents at age 35 years or older
- Secondary lymphedema is from an acquired abnormality of lymphatic flow, an injury to the lymphatic system.
  - Common causes in children include the following:
    - Postsurgical obstruction
    - Burns
    - Insect bites
    - Infection
    - Scar tissue from radiation
    - Neoplasm
    - Trauma
- Classification: There are several systems for grading the severity of lymphedema.
  - The International Society of Lymphology (ISL) describes lymphedema using skin consistency and outcome.
    - Stage 0: dormant condition where a patient might describe their extremity as heavy
    - Stage I (mild): soft tissue that may pit, no dermal fibrosis; improves with elevation of extremity
    - Stage II (moderate): evolving dermal fibrosis that does not pit; no improvement with limb elevation
    - Stage III (severe): Tissue is swollen and thick; there may be peeling, discoloration, or trophic changes.
  - The American Physical Therapy Association (APTA) describes lymphedema by measurement between the affected and unaffected extremity.
    - Mild: girth difference <3 cm
    - Moderate: girth difference of 3 to 5 cm
    - Severe: girth difference of >5 cm

EPIDEMIOLOGY

- Most lymphedemas in childhood are primary (or idiopathic) lymphedema (96%).
- Congenital lymphedema comprises 10–25% of primary lymphedema cases; lymphedema praecox, 65–80%; and lymphedema tarda, 10%.
- Affected males—most likely congenital and bilateral; affected females—most likely unilateral lymphedema praecox
- Secondary lymphedema is more common in adults and rare in children. In the United States, it is commonly from breast cancer; worldwide, due to filariasis
- Affects 1.15 of 100,000 in children <20 years

RISK FACTORS

Genetics

- Milroy disease
  - Also known as hereditary lymphedema type IA
  - A rare, autosomal dominant condition that affects lymphatic function
  - Associated with mutations in the *FLT4* gene that encodes vascular endothelial growth factor receptor 3
- Meige disease
  - Hereditary lymphedema type II—familial lymphedema praecox
- Fabry disease
  - A serious, X-linked inborn error of glycosphingolipid catabolism associated with progressive renal failure, cardiovascular disease, neuropathy, and angiokeratosis
- Lymphedema-distichiasis
  - An autosomal dominant condition that presents with lymphedema and double rows of eyelashes
  - The condition is associated with mutations in the *FOXC2* gene.
- Other genetic conditions prone to lymphedema: Down, Turner, Noonan, yellow nail, Klippel-Trenaunay-Weber, and pes cavus

PATHOPHYSIOLOGY

- Abnormal accumulation of interstitial fluid due to the lymphatic load overwhelming the transport capacity of lymph vessels
- Lymph flow occurs under a low pressure system; unlike generalized edema, capillary filtration remains normal in patients with lymphedema.
- Initially, edema is pitting, whereas chronic edema is generally nonpitting as a result of fibrosis.

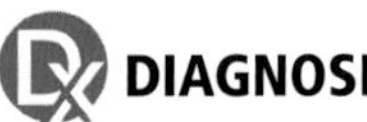

DIAGNOSIS

History and physical exam are primary source for diagnosis.

HISTORY

- Unilateral, heavy, often aching lower extremity edema in healthy pubertal female strongly suggests lymphedema praecox.
- Heavy, aching pitting edema distal to site of extremity surgery or trauma suggests secondary lymphedema.
- Sites of previous cellulitis, infection, or insect bites can be associated with secondary lymphedema.

PHYSICAL EXAM

- Heavy, aching pitting edema in unilateral limb is suggestive of lymphedema.
- Lymphedema responds to elevation.
- Risk factors include obesity and inflammatory arthritis.
- Primary lymphedema sites:
  - Extremities, usually legs, rare in upper limbs
  - The foot is always involved in lower extremity lymphedema.
- Chronic inflammation leads to fibrosis and nonpitting or "woody" edema with induration.
- Hair loss and hyperkeratosis of the affected limb develop over time.
- Intense sharp pain in affected limb is uncommon and suggests secondary lymphedema due to thrombophlebitis, cellulitis, or reflex sympathetic dystrophy.
- Global edema suggests other disease states.
- Red streaking of extremity, fever, chills, or nodal enlargement suggests development of cellulitis or lymphangitis.

DIFFERENTIAL DIAGNOSIS

- Infection
  - Cellulitis
  - Lymphangitis
  - Herpes simplex virus type 2
- Tumors
  - Pelvic mass
  - Multiple enchondromatosis
- Metabolic
  - Cushing disease
  - Hyperthyroidism
  - Lipedema
- Anatomic
  - Venous stasis
  - Deep vein thrombosis
  - Hemihypertrophy
  - Arteriovenous fistula or malformation
  - Popliteal arterial aneurysm
  - Popliteal cyst (Baker cyst)
- Miscellaneous
  - Heart failure
  - Glomerulonephrosis
  - Cirrhosis
  - Hypoproteinemia
  - Reflex sympathetic dystrophy

DIAGNOSTIC TESTS & INTERPRETATION

Initial Tests (screening, lab, imaging)

- Not usually necessary but may be useful to rule out other causes of edema
  - Urinalysis for proteinuria as seen with glomerulonephrosis
  - Serum total protein and albumin to rule out hypoproteinemia
  - Liver function tests to assess functional status
  - Pregnancy test
- Usually unnecessary to make diagnosis but may help to plan or evaluate therapy
  - Lymphangiography is no longer used because related dyes caused inflammation and worsening of lymphatic obstruction.
  - Radionuclide lymphoscintigraphy, when indicated, is the preferred method of imaging to define anatomy and to evaluate lymph flow and obstruction.
  - CT and MRI may be valuable if a malignancy is suspected or to differentiate subcutaneous from adipose swelling.
  - Doppler ultrasound may be helpful if deep vein thrombosis is suspected.

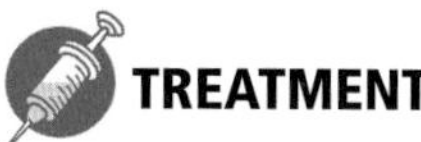

TREATMENT

GENERAL MEASURES

- Therapy should be instituted as soon as possible and before fibrosis develops.
- Goals of therapy are to minimize or decrease edema and to prevent infection, fibrosis, and skin changes.
- Compression garments (e.g., Jobst® stockings or elastic wraps) is recommended long term, but compliance can be a challenge.
- Extremity elevation, especially at night
- Exercise, stay active for a lifetime; muscle contraction assists lymph flow and does not exacerbate swelling.
- Weight control
- Diligent skin care and appropriately fitting shoes to avoid infection
- Manual massage decompression can be helpful for digital edema and for infants who may not tolerate compression garments.
- Automated intermittent pneumatic compression machines shown to facilitate home regimen compliance
- Psychological effects of cosmesis are prominent and should not be overlooked.
- Patient education and support groups can be found through the National Lymphedema Network.

MEDICATION

- Diuretics: not generally used in children and adolescents; efficacy for adults is debated.
- Prophylactic antibiotic use is indicated for patients with recurrent cellulitis or lymphangitis.

ADDITIONAL THERAPIES

- Complex decongestive physiotherapy (CDP) is part of a specialized treatment with an initial reductive phase 1 and a maintenance phase 2 provided by a licensed physical therapist or occupational therapist certified in the treatment of lymphedema.
- Treatment is time sensitive and should be instituted as soon as possible to prevent fibrosis developing.
- Phase 1 consists of manual lymph-drainage therapy, compression therapy specialized bandaging, fitting for appropriate tailored compression garment, and detailed skin and nail care.
- Phase 2 consists of self-management for drainage techniques, skin care, use and care of compression garments, and exercise advice.

SURGERY/OTHER PROCEDURES

- Microsurgical treatment has been proven to show excellent outcomes in carefully selected patient populations via lymphatic-venous anastomoses or lymphatic-venous-lymphatic anastomoses.
- Traditional surgery has one of two goals: removal of excess edematous tissue or attempts to restore lymph drainage.
  - Both may decrease the rate of infections but have poor cosmetic results.
  - Recommended only for those with uncontrolled swelling with significant disability

ONGOING CARE

DIET

In children with chylous reflux syndromes, a diet low in long-chain triglycerides may be of benefit.

PROGNOSIS

- Edema persists throughout life.
- Lymphedema can be staged and monitored via circumferential measurements. Guidelines have been established by the APTA.
- Natural history: plateau in severity of edema after an initial few years of progression in 50%, slow constant progression in 50%

COMPLICATIONS

- Cellulitis and lymphangitis are the most common complications and are treated with antibiotics; published series showed 24% of cases developed infection and half of these required hospitalization.
- Poor long-term compliance with compression garments due to uncomfortable nature of therapy
- Lymphangiosarcoma (rare)
- Psychological problems
- Physical limitations
- Chronic inflammation and edema ultimately lead to fibrosis and induration of the involved area.

ADDITIONAL READING

- Gary DE. Lymphedema diagnosis and management. *J Am Acad Nurse Pract*. 2007;19(2):72–78.
- International Society of Lymphology. The diagnosis and treatment of peripheral lymphedema: 2013 Consensus Document of the International Society of Lymphology. *Lymphology*. 2013;46(1):1–11.
- Kerchner K, Fleischer A, Yosipovitch G. Lower extremity lymphedema update: pathophysiology, diagnosis, and treatment guidelines. *J Am Acad Dermatol*. 2008;59(2):324–331.
- Mayrovitz HN. The standard of care for lymphedema: current concepts and physiological considerations. *Lymphat Res Biol*. 2009;7(2):101–108.
- Rockson SG. Current concepts and future directions in the diagnosis and management of lymphatic vascular disease. *Vasc Med*. 2010;15(3):223–231.
- Schook CC, Mulliken JB, Fishman SJ, et al. Differential diagnosis of lower extremity enlargement in pediatric patients referred with a diagnosis of lymphedema. *Plast Reconstr Surg*. 2011;127(4):1571–1581.
- Zuther JE. *Lymphedema Management: The Comprehensive Guide for Practitioners*. 2nd ed. New York, NY: Thieme; 2009.

CODES

ICD10

- I89.0 Lymphedema, not elsewhere classified
- Q82.0 Hereditary lymphedema
- I97.89 Oth postproc comp and disorders of the circ sys, NEC

FAQ

- Q: Is the swelling going to go away?
- A: It depends if it is due to a primary or secondary cause. A mild to moderate secondary cause may be reversible with therapy. A chronic, primary cause will require long-term management.
- Q: Could this have been prevented?
- A: No, primary lymphedema is typically due to abnormal embryologic development.
- Q: If the lymph channels have been abnormal since birth, why does the swelling present during adolescence?
- A: No one really knows; hormones may play a role in lymphedema.

L

LYMPHOPROLIFERATIVE DISORDERS

David T. Teachey, MD

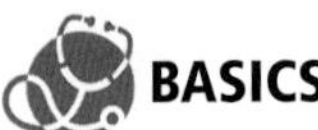

BASICS

DESCRIPTION

- Lymphoproliferative disorders are a class of non-malignant diseases characterized by uncontrolled growth of lymphoid tissues (spleen, bone marrow, liver, lymph nodes).
- Can be congenital or acquired
- Based on recent advances in next generation sequencing technology, new disorders are defined constantly.
- Most common in children include
  - Autoimmune lymphoproliferative syndrome (ALPS)
  - Castleman disease (CD)
  - Rosai–Dorfman disease (RDD)
  - EBV-associated lymphoproliferative disorder (ELD)
  - X-linked lymphoproliferative syndrome (XLP)
- Rarer disorders (not discussed in detail)
  - Angioimmunoblastic lymphadenopathy
  - Caspase-8 deficiency syndrome (CEDS)
  - Dianzani autoimmune lymphoproliferative disease
  - Kikuchi-Fujimoto syndrome
  - Lymphomatoid granulomatosis
  - Lymphomatoid papulosis
  - Ocular adnexal lymphoid proliferation
  - RAS-associated leukoproliferative disorder (RALD)
  - *p110δ* activating mutation causing senescent T cells lymphadenopathy and immunodeficiency (PASLI)
  - *CTLA-4* haploinsufficiency with autoimmune infiltration (CHAI)
  - *LRBA* deficiency with autoantibodies, regulatory T-cell defects, autoimmune infiltration and enteropathy (LATAIE)
  - X-linked immunodeficiency with magnesium defect, EBV infection, and neoplasia (X-MEN)
  - Interleukin-2-inducible T-cell kinase (ITK) deficiency

EPIDEMIOLOGY

All uncommon

RISK FACTORS

Often multifactorial with inherited genetic defect and acquired infection

Genetics

- ALPS (80% of patients have identifiable mutation)
  - 60–70% germline mutation in *FAS* (*TNFRSF6*)
  - 10% somatic mutation in *FAS*
  - 2% germline mutation in *CASP10*
  - <1% germline mutation in *FASL*
- XLP
  - Majority of cases mutation in *SH2DIA*
  - XLP-like syndrome caused by X-linked inhibitor of apoptosis protein (XIAP) mutations

PATHOPHYSIOLOGY

- ALPS
  - Defective FAS-mediated apoptosis leads to abnormal lymphocyte survival with subsequent lymphoproliferation, autoimmunity, and cancer.
- CD
  - Largely unknown but can be triggered by HHV-8 infection, especially in immunocompromised patients
- ELD
  - EBV triggered lymphoproliferative disorder found in patients on chronic immune suppression typically after organ or bone marrow transplant (posttransplant lymphoproliferative disorder [PTLD]) or with inherited immune deficiency
- XLP
  - Mutation in *SH2D1A* leads to abnormal production of SAP protein in NK and T cells, leading to defective SAP-SLAM signaling and inability to appropriately respond to EBV infection.

DIAGNOSIS

HISTORY

- ALPS
  - Typically presents at young age (average 18 months) with massive lymphadenopathy and splenomegaly
  - Many patients develop secondary autoimmune disease.
  - Most often, autoimmune destruction of blood cells (80% of patients); can be mild to severe
  - Destruction of platelets: See chapter on "Idiopathic Thrombocytopenic Purpura."
  - Destruction of erythrocytes: See chapter on "Autoimmune Hemolytic Anemia."
  - Destruction of neutrophils: See chapter on "Neutropenia."
  - Can have autoimmune involvement of any organ system, similar to systemic lupus erythematosus
  - In young adult years, 10–20% develop lymphoma.
  - Lymphoproliferation can improve or worsen with infection; often progresses through teenage years and improves in adulthood
  - Autoimmune disease is less likely to improve with older age.
- CD
  - Two variants
    - Hyaline vascular: presents with enlarged single lymph node or chain of nodes; >90% with no other symptoms; rarely can have fever, weight loss, fatigue
    - Plasma cell: presents with enlarged single lymph node or chain (unicentric) or diffuse adenopathy (multicentric); often with constitutional symptoms (fever, sweats, lethargy, rashes, neuropathy, arthritis)
- RDD
  - Massive, painless bilateral cervical lymphadenopathy with or without other involved nodal groups
  - Fever
  - Snoring common
  - Can have extranodal invasion of almost any organ (25% of patients have extranodal disease) and signs and symptoms depend on involved organ
- ELD/PTLD
  - Can be mild, with lymphadenopathy, fever, and/or diarrhea, or severe, with massive lymphadenopathy, high fever, night sweats, rash, and pruritus, and organ compression from involved nodes
- XLP
  - Can present as fulminant infectious mononucleosis or aplastic anemia or lymphoma or hemophagocytic syndrome
  - Often critically ill in the setting of EBV infection
  - Patients with XLP2 (*XIAP*) often have less fulminant presentation and can present with inflammatory bowel disease at a young age.
  - Patients with X-MEN (*MAGT1* mutations) and ITK deficiency can have similar clinical presentation.

PHYSICAL EXAM

- ALPS
  - Massive lymphadenopathy (90% of patients): can compress vital organs including trachea (rare). Most common site of adenopathy is anterior cervical. Nodes are hard but mobile.
  - Splenomegaly (90% of patients)
  - Hepatomegaly (50% of patients)
  - Other physical exam findings as expected with autoimmune destruction of blood cells and/or end-organ autoimmune disease
- CD
  - Hyaline vascular: single enlarged lymph node or chain; most often cervical or mediastinal; may have shotty diffuse nonpathologic adenopathy
  - Plasma cell: single or multiple pathologically enlarged lymph nodes; abdominal nodes most common; hepatosplenomegaly common. Peripheral edema, ascites, and pleural effusions may be present.
- RDD
  - Massive bilateral anterior cervical lymphadenopathy (90% of patients). Other physical exam findings can vary based on extranodal disease.
  - Hepatosplenomegaly (10% of patients)
- ELD/PTLD
  - Similar to other lymphoproliferative disorders (see "Epstein-Barr virus [Infectious Mononucleosis]" chapter)
- XLP
  - Similar to other lymphoproliferative disorders, however, far more acutely ill (see also "Epstein–Barr virus [Infectious Mononucleosis]" chapter and "Aplastic Anemia" chapter)

DIFFERENTIAL DIAGNOSIS

- Other lymphoproliferative disorders
- Lymphoma
- Infection:
  - EBV
  - CMV
  - Toxoplasmosis
  - HIV
  - TB
- Evans syndrome
- Rheumatologic disease

DIAGNOSTIC TESTS & INTERPRETATION

Initial Tests (screening, lab, imaging)

- Complete blood and reticulocyte count for anemia, thrombocytopenia, and neutropenia
- Direct antiglobulin test (DAT) to check for autoimmune destruction of red blood cells
- Serum chemistries, uric acid, phosphorus to look for cell turnover (usually normal in lymphoproliferative disorders)
- Liver function tests, PT, PTT, and fibrinogen to measure liver function and for coagulopathy
- EBV, PCR and titers, CMV-PCR
- If acutely ill, consider ESR or CRP and ferritin.
- Quantitative immunoglobulins: often elevated in lymphoproliferative disorders
- Mandatory criteria for ALPS
  - Chronic (>6 months) nonmalignant lymphoproliferation (lymphadenopathy) and/or splenomegaly
  - Elevated peripheral blood double-negative T cells (DNTs): T cells that are CD3+, TCR alpha/beta+, CD4−, and CD8−. DNTs are usually rare in peripheral blood (<1% of total lymphocytes or <2.5% of total T cells). DNTs are elevated and often markedly elevated in ALPS. Slight elevation in DNTs can be found in other autoimmune disorders.
- Major (primary) criteria for ALPS
  - Genetic mutation in ALPS causative gene (germline or somatic) in *FAS*, *FASL*, or *CASP10*
  - In vitro evidence of defective FAS-mediated apoptosis. This assay requires growing blood cells from patient in culture for weeks and exposing to anti-Fas monoclonal antibody to see if T cells are resistant to death; only performed in a few labs

- Minor (secondary) criteria for ALPS
  - (1) Elevated vitamin B_{12} (>1,500 ng/L)
  - (2) Elevated IL-10 (>20 pg/mL)
  - (3) Elevated IL-18 (>500 pg/mL)
  - (4) Elevated sFASL (>200 pg/mL)
  - (5) Classic histopathologic findings on lymph nodes or spleen biopsy
  - (6) Autoimmune cytopenias AND elevated serum IgG
  - (7) Positive family history
- Diagnosis of ALPS
  - Definitive: both mandatory and one major criteria
  - Probable: both mandatory and one minor criteria (Probable ALPS should be treated the same as definitive ALPS but only after known ALPS-like disorders ruled out by genetic testing.)
- Diagnostic tests for CD
  - Castleman syndrome diagnosed by histopathology
  - Hypergammaglobulinemia, anemia, high ESR, high IL-6, HHV-8, PCR+
- Diagnostic tests for RDD
  - RDD diagnosed by histopathology
  - Hypergammaglobulinemia, anemia, high ESR, leukocytosis with neutropenia, hematologic autoantibodies
- Diagnostic tests for ELD/PTLD
  - PTLD after bone marrow graft
  - Persistent EBV infection (positive EBV PCR or abnormal seroconversion by titers) in setting of immune suppression or immune compromise
  - Diagnosis confirmed with imaging and/or histopathology
- Diagnostic tests for XLP
  - Persistent EBV infection (positive EBV PCR or abnormal seroconversion on titers)
  - Inverted CD4/CD8 ratio
  - High IgM and IgA, low IgG
  - Defective NK activity
  - Secondary hemophagocytic syndrome (elevated ferritin, high triglycerides, low fibrinogen, cytopenias, high fever, splenomegaly, poor NK function, elevated s-IL-2R-alpha, and hemophagocytosis on marrow or node biopsy)
  - Diagnosis confirmed by genetic testing for mutations in *SH2D1A* and *XIAP* genes and/or SAP and XIAP protein expression by flow cytometry
- CT scans of head, neck, chest, abdomen, and pelvis with IV contrast is important for all lymphoproliferative disorders at initial diagnosis to define extent of disease.
- It is *important* to obtain plain chest radiograph on initial presentation in patient with diffuse lymphadenopathy before CT scan to ensure a large mediastinal mass is not present. If present, it may be unsafe to lie patient flat and/or sedate for CT scan.
- Most lymphoproliferative disorders are very PET-avid.

Diagnostic Procedures/Other

- ALPS and PTLD can be diagnosed without histopathology; however, most patients have a lymph node biopsy.
- Other lymphoproliferative disorders typically require tissue for diagnosis (biopsy, not fine needle aspirate).
- Consider bone marrow aspirate and/or biopsy to rule out marrow disease or other disease processes.
- Genetic testing is needed as there is considerable phenotypic overlap between many lymphoproliferative diseases. For many of these disorders, targeted therapies now exist.
- Pathological findings
  - ALPS: DNTs in lymph node and spleen
  - CD: hyaline vascular (shrunken germinal centers with eosinophilic expansion of mantle zones with and vessel hyalinization); plasma cell (extensive plasma cell infiltrate in interfollicular regions)
  - RD: emperipolesis (lymphophagocytosis)—hallmark of disease on biopsy; presence of histiocytes
  - XLP/PTLD/ELD: EBV-encoded small RNA (EBER)+

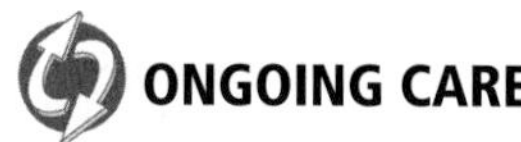

TREATMENT

MEDICATION

First Line

- For ALPS: corticosteroids or IVIG for acute flares
- For CD localized disease
  - Surgical resection or focal radiation. Steroids may be used to shrink lesions prior to surgery.
- For CD multicentric disease
  - Multiagent therapy (vincristine, prednisone, rituximab, cyclophosphamide, doxorubicin)
- For RD
  - May self-resolve (20% of patients)
  - If not, consider prednisone, or vinblastine plus prednisone, or mercaptopurine plus methotrexate, or 2CdA.
- For ELD/PTLD
  - Reduce immune suppression or convert immune suppression to sirolimus, if possible.
  - Consider rituximab, adoptive transfer of EBV-specific cytotoxic T cells.
  - If fails, systemic disease, or clonal malignancy consider multiagent chemotherapy. Most commonly used regimen includes corticosteroids, cyclophosphamide, and rituximab.
- For XLP
  - If hemophagocytosis or aplasia: rituximab, etoposide, steroids
  - Hematopoietic stem cell transplant is the only cure. Patients with XIAP may not need stem cell transplant.

Second Line

For ALPS

- Sirolimus or mycophenolate mofetil for chronic disease
- Sirolimus (rapamycin): pros: improves autoimmune disease and lymphoproliferation and eliminates DNTs. Cons: drug–drug interactions; requires therapeutic drug monitoring; 10% of patients develop mouth sores (most common in first month).
- Mycophenolate mofetil (CellCept®): pros: no drug–drug interactions, no mouth sores, no therapeutic drug monitoring. Cons: not as effective; does not help lymphoproliferation or lower DNTs; GI upset
- Recommended treatment: mild autoimmune disease without significant lymphoproliferation, start with mycophenolate and transition to sirolimus if poor response or side effects; moderate to severe autoimmune disease or clinically significant lymphoproliferation, start with sirolimus.
- For ALPS-like disorders including PASLI, CHAI, LATAIE, and RALD seek expert consultation. Some of these have newly identified targeted therapies, and some patients need stem cell transplant.

Third Line

For ALPS

- Combination therapy: stem cell transplant
- Relative contraindications (AVOID, if possible)
  - Splenectomy: high incidence of pneumococcal sepsis even with antibiotic prophylaxis and immunization
  - Rituximab: can lead to lifelong hypogammaglobulinemia (5–10% of patients)

ONGOING CARE

FOLLOW-UP RECOMMENDATIONS

Recommended follow-up imaging varies among institutions. Most physicians will repeat imaging if patient's history changes OR to determine response to therapy.

PROGNOSIS

- Prognosis is good to fair for most lymphoproliferative disorders.
- Prognosis is poor in XLP and advanced CD.

ADDITIONAL READING

- Dharnidharka VR, Webster AC, Martinez OM, et al. Post-transplant lymphoproliferative disorders. *Nat Rev Dis Primers*. 2016;2:15088.
- George LA, Teachey DT. Optimal management of autoimmune lymphoproliferative syndrome in children. *Paediatr Drugs*. 2016;18(4):261–272.
- Oliveira JB, Bleesing JJ, Dianzani U, et al. Revised diagnostic criteria and classification for the autoimmune lymphoproliferative syndrome (ALPS): report from the 2009 NIH International Workshop. *Blood*. 2010;116(14):e35–e40.
- Schulte KM, Talat N. Castleman's disease—a two compartment model of HHV8 infection. *Nat Rev Clin Oncol*. 2010;7(9):533–543.
- Veillette A, Pérez-Quintero LA, Latour S. X-linked lymphoproliferative syndromes and related autosomal recessive disorders. *Curr Opin Allergy Clin Immunol*. 2013;13(6):614–622.

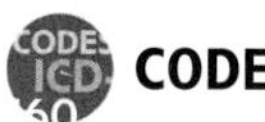

CODES

ICD10

- D47.9 Neoplasm of uncertain behavior of lymphoid, hematopoietic and related tissue, unspecified
- D89.82 Autoimmune lymphoproliferative syndrome [ALPS]
- D47.Z1 Post-transplant lymphoproliferative disorder (PTLD)

L

MALABSORPTION

Ninfa M. Candela, MD

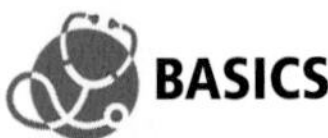

BASICS

DESCRIPTION

- Malabsorption is characterized as a syndrome, as opposed to a disease entity, and is defined as any state in which there is a disturbance of digestion and/or absorption of nutrients across the intestinal mucosa.
- The classical symptoms of malabsorption include chronic diarrhea, abdominal distention, and failure to thrive.
- Malabsorption is caused by either a congenital or acquired disorder.

EPIDEMIOLOGY

Depends on the underlying disease causing malabsorption

ETIOLOGY

The most common causes of malabsorption in developed countries are as follows:

- Celiac disease: most common inherited malabsorption syndrome; documented prevalence of 1%
- Cystic fibrosis
- Post enteritis syndrome
- Cow's milk protein intolerance
- Giardiasis
- Inflammatory bowel disease (IBD)

PATHOPHYSIOLOGY

- Differs depending upon which nutrient is malabsorbed
  - Carbohydrate
    - Monosaccharide: congenital glucose-galactose deficiency, fructose intolerance
    - Disaccharide: lactase deficiency (congenital or acquired), sucrase-isomaltase deficiency
    - Polysaccharide: amylase deficiency (congenital or acquired)
  - Fat
    - Bile salt deficiency: cholestasis, resection of terminal ileum
    - Exocrine pancreatic insufficiency: cystic fibrosis, chronic pancreatitis
    - Inadequate surface area: celiac disease, flat villous lesions
  - Protein
    - Protein-losing enteropathy: intestinal lymphangiectasia, congenital heart failure
    - Exocrine pancreatic insufficiency: cystic fibrosis, Shwachman-Diamond syndrome
    - Inadequate surface area: celiac disease
- Differs according to location of alteration in absorptive function of gut
  - Mucosal abnormality
    - Anatomic: postenteritis syndrome, celiac disease, IBD
    - Functional: disaccharidase deficiencies
  - Luminal abnormality
    - Exocrine pancreatic insufficiency: cystic fibrosis, Shwachman-Diamond syndrome
    - Bile salt insufficiency: biliary cholestatic liver disease, ileal resection
  - Anatomic abnormality
    - Short gut: surgical resection
    - Motility disturbance: intestinal pseudo-obstruction

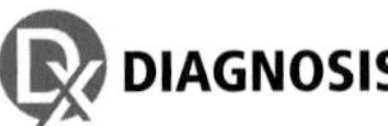

DIAGNOSIS

HISTORY

- GI symptoms
  - Common in patients with malabsorption syndromes
  - Range from mild abdominal gaseous distention to severe abdominal pain and vomiting
  - Chronic or recurrent diarrhea is by far the most common symptom.
  - Abdominal distention and watery diarrhea, with or without mild abdominal pain associated with skin irritation in the perianal area, are characteristics of carbohydrate malabsorption syndromes.
  - Fat malabsorption can present with bulky, foul-smelling stools that are oily and thus float in water. Abdominal distention, increased gas, weight loss, and increased appetite are also seen.
  - Periodic nausea, abdominal distention, pain, and diarrhea are common in patients with chronic *Giardia* infections.
  - Vomiting, with moderate to severe abdominal pain and bloody stools, is characteristic of enterocolitis associated with protein sensitivity.
  - Abdominal pain or irritability, distension, and constipation (particularly seen in celiac disease)
- Stool characteristics
  - Frequent loose watery stools may indicate carbohydrate intolerance.
  - Bulky, greasy, or loose foul-smelling stools indicate fat malabsorption.
  - In protein malabsorption, stools may be normal or loose.
  - Bloody and/or mucousy stools are seen in patients with cow's milk protein allergy, infection, and IBD.
- Other symptoms
  - Failure to thrive caused by malabsorption of carbohydrates, fats, or proteins
  - Anemia, with weakness and fatigue, due to inadequate absorption of vitamin B_{12}, iron, and folic acid
  - Edema, due to decreased protein absorption and hypoalbuminemia
  - Muscle cramping due to decreased vitamin D causing hypocalcemia and decreased potassium levels

PHYSICAL EXAM

- Malabsorption syndromes should be considered during the workup for failure to thrive, malnutrition, poor weight gain, or delayed puberty.
- In particular, they should be suspected in infants with weight loss or little weight gain since birth and in infants with low weight and weight-for-height percentiles.
- Signs of malnutrition, including reduced subcutaneous fat, paleness, angular cheilitis, and muscle weakness
- Abdominal distention, increased bowel sounds
- Rash around mouth and/or perianal erythema are commonly seen.

DIFFERENTIAL DIAGNOSIS

- Pancreatic disorders
  - Cystic fibrosis
  - Shwachman syndrome
  - Johanson-Blizzard syndrome
- Chronic cholestasis
  - Biliary atresia
  - Vitamin E deficiency
  - Alagille syndrome
- Infectious diarrhea
  - Giardiasis
  - Cryptosporidiosis
- Mucosal injury
  - Celiac disease
  - Crohn disease
  - Postinfectious diarrhea
- Congenital brush border enzyme deficiencies
  - Glucose-galactose transporter deficiency
  - Sucrase-isomaltase deficiency
  - Microvillus inclusion disease
- Abnormal intestinal lymphatic drainage
  - Primary intestinal lymphangiectasia
  - Secondary intestinal lymphangiectasia

DIAGNOSTIC TESTS & INTERPRETATION

Initial Tests (screening, lab, imaging)

- Stool analysis
  - The presence of reducing substances and pH <5.5 indicates that carbohydrates have not been properly absorbed.
  - The level of quantitative stool fat and the amount of fat intake in the diet should be measured and monitored for 3 days using special stains; a coefficient of fat absorption is calculated using the following equation:

$$\frac{\text{Ingested fat (g)} - \text{fat in stool (g)}}{\text{Ingested fat (g)}} \times 100$$

  - Normal values for the coefficient of fat absorption: >93% in children and adults, >85% in infants, >67% in premature infants
    - Moderate fat malabsorption ranges from 60% to 80%.
    - Fat absorption of <50% indicates severe malabsorption.
  - The presence of large serum proteins in the stool, such as α_1 antitrypsin, indicates leakage of serum protein. A 24-hour stool collection for α_1 antitrypsin (along with a serum level) serves as a screening test for protein-losing enteropathy.
  - Exam of the stool for ova and parasites or testing for the stool antigen may reveal the presence of *Giardia* species; stool *Clostridium difficile* PCR and stool culture for infectious bacterial pathogens
  - If bile acid malabsorption is suspected, quantitative conjugated and unconjugated bile acids may be measured in stool, although this test is not commonly available or used.
- Other laboratory studies
  - Serologic studies for celiac disease (tissue transglutaminase IgA and a total IgA level are best tests for screening)
  - CBC
    - May reveal anemia in patients with iron, folate, and vitamin B_{12} malabsorption
    - Neutropenia is seen in patients with Shwachman-Diamond syndrome.
  - Total serum protein and albumin levels
    - May be lower than reference range in syndromes in which protein is lost or not absorbed, particularly in protein-losing enteropathy and pancreatic insufficiency
  - With fat malabsorption or ileal resection, fat-soluble vitamin levels in the serum are low.
  - With bile acid malabsorption, levels of LDL cholesterol may be low.
  - Serum calcium may be low due to vitamin D and amino acid malabsorption.
  - Serum vitamin A, E, and carotene may be low due to bile salt deficiency and impaired fat absorption.
  - Other studies must be performed when a specific disease is suspected (e.g., mucosal biopsy for celiac disease, sweat test for cystic fibrosis, or appropriate workup for IBD).
  - Urine analysis should be done to rule out proteinuria in patients with low albumin levels.
  - An upper GI radiographic series and/or a barium enema for anatomical abnormalities and to look for small bowel dilation due to bacterial overgrowth
  - Breath hydrogen testing preferred for the investigation of lactose malabsorption or bacterial overgrowth (lactulose breath test); also, sucrose or fructose malabsorption can be evaluated.
  - Genetic testing may be performed for identification of inherited malabsorption syndromes.
  - If tissue samples are acquired through a biopsy, ultrastructural analysis may be performed using electron microscopy; mucosal enzyme determination

TREATMENT

- Overall, nutritional support is paramount.
- Specific treatment depends on etiology, for example, gluten-free diet for celiac disease, metronidazole for *Giardia* infection, or elimination diet of the offending agent in a case of food intolerance.
- Evidence supports restriction of fermentable oligosaccharides, disaccharides, monosaccharides and polyols (i.e., following a low-fermentable, oligo-, di-, monosaccharides, and polyols [FODMAP] diet) in functional disorders presenting with malabsorption.

ONGOING CARE

COMPLICATIONS

- Complications of malabsorption syndromes vary according to etiology, but malnutrition and other consequences of malabsorption will almost always become progressively worse if the cause is not determined and appropriate treatment prescribed.
- Frequent complications of malabsorption and malnutrition include growth failure, vitamin and micronutrient deficiency (zinc, magnesium, calcium), bone disease, hypoproteinemia and edema, essential fatty acid deficiency, perianal dermatitis, immune dysfunction, and anemia.

ADDITIONAL READING

- Ali SA, Hill DR. Giardia intestinalis. *Curr Opin Infect Dis*. 2003;16(5):453–460.
- Chumpitazi BP, Shulman RJ. Dietary carbohydrates and childhood functional abdominal pain. *Ann Nutr Metab*. 2016;68(Suppl 1):8–17.
- Crittenden RG, Bennett LE. Cow's milk allergy: a complex disorder. *J Am Coll Nutr*. 2005; 24(Suppl 6):582S–591S.
- Dodge JA, Turck D. Cystic fibrosis: nutritional consequences and management. *Best Pract Res Clin Gastroenterol*. 2006;20(30):531–546.
- Fasano A, Catassi C. Coeliac disease in children. *Best Pract Res Clin Gastroenterol*. 2005;19(3): 467–478.
- Pietzak MM, Thomas DW. Childhood malabsorption. *Pediatr Rev*. 2003;24(6):195–206.

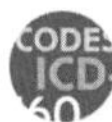

CODES

ICD10

- K90.9 Intestinal malabsorption, unspecified
- K90.4 Malabsorption due to intolerance, not elsewhere classified
- K90.0 Celiac disease

FAQ

- Q: Why do patients with malabsorption become anemic?
- A: Patients with malabsorption can become deficient in vitamin B_{12}, iron, and folic acid and in turn can become anemic.
- Q: Why do patients with celiac disease develop symptoms of malabsorption?
- A: Celiac disease causes an autoimmune-mediated inflammation of the small bowel mucosa that is characterized by villous atrophy, which decreases the absorptive capacity of the bowel.

MALARIA

Samina S. Bhumbra, MD • Chandy C. John, MD, MS

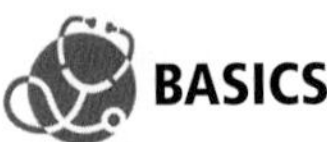

BASICS

DESCRIPTION

- Malaria is a febrile illness caused by the *Plasmodium* species of protozoan parasites, transmitted by the *Anopheles* mosquito vector.
- Five *Plasmodium* strains infect humans: *Plasmodium falciparum*, *Plasmodium vivax*, *Plasmodium malariae*, *Plasmodium ovale*, and *Plasmodium knowlesi*. *P. falciparum* and *P. vivax* cause the majority of disease.
- Classic symptoms include stages of chills, followed by high fevers, and then sweating. However, this classic symptom pattern is less likely to be seen in children. Children may manifest initially with only fever as a complaint.

EPIDEMIOLOGY

- High-risk areas of endemic malaria include Africa, parts of Central and South America, Oceania, and tropical regions of Asia.
- *P. falciparum* is the major species in sub-Saharan Africa. Both *P. falciparum* and *P. vivax* are found in India, Southeast Asia, Oceania, and Central and South America, and *P. vivax* is present in some areas of Africa. *P. ovale* is usually found in West Africa.
- *P. falciparum* causes more deaths in children <5 years of age than any other organism.
- The World Health Organization (WHO) reports that 70% of malaria deaths occur in children <5 years of age. Pregnant women are also at high risk.
- Mortality has decreased by 35% from 2010 to 2015 for children <5 years old.

Incidence

- Worldwide, in 2015, an estimated 212 million cases of malaria occurred, and 430,000 deaths were due to malaria.
- ~1,500 to 2,000 cases of malaria are imported into the United States annually. In 2013, 1,700 cases of malaria were imported into the United States. This is a 35% increase in cases >10 years.

RISK FACTORS

Genetics

- Sickle cell trait is known to provide protection against malaria.
  - The risk of death of severe falciparum malaria is 60–70% less in children with Hb AS than those with Hb AA.
- Thalassemias, other hemoglobinopathies (C+E), ovalocytosis, and G6PD deficiency also provide some protection against malaria.
- Individuals with a Duffy-negative blood type lack receptors for *P. vivax* merozoite invasion and are typically resistant to *P. vivax*, although recently, cases of *P. vivax* in Duffy-negative individuals have been reported.

GENERAL PREVENTION

- Personal protective measures against mosquito bites are extremely important.
  - Remain in well-screened areas.
  - Wear protective clothing, including pants and long-sleeved shirts.
  - Use insect repellents containing *N*,*N*-Diethyl-meta-toluamide (DEET).
  - Use insecticide-treated bed nets.
- Chemoprophylaxis is strongly advised for travelers to endemic areas.
  - In areas with chloroquine-sensitive parasites only, chloroquine may be used (5 mg/kg base [8.3 mg/kg salt] once a week—max 300 mg base/500 mg salt).
  - In chloroquine-resistant areas, effective options are atovaquone-proguanil (Malarone®), mefloquine, or doxycycline.
    - Malarone® can be used in all areas but is contraindicated in severe renal impairment and pregnancy, or mothers breastfeeding infants <5 kg.
      - Dosing: 5 to 8 kg: 1/2 pediatric tab daily; 8 to 10 kg: 3/4 pediatric tab daily; 10 to 20 kg: 1 pediatric tab (62.5/25) daily; 20 to 30 kg: 2 pediatric tabs daily; 30 to 40 kg: 3 pediatric tabs daily; ≥40 kg: 1 adult tab (250/100) daily
  - Mefloquine resistance is present in parts of Asia. Contraindications to mefloquine include seizure disorder, major psychiatric illness, or cardiac disease. It is safe in pregnancy and for young infants.
    - Dosing: ≤9 kg: 4.6 mg/kg weekly; 9 to 19 kg: 1/4 tablet weekly; 19 to 30 kg: 1/2 tab weekly; 30 to 45 kg: 3/4 tab weekly; >45 kg: 1 tab weekly
  - Doxycycline is contraindicated if <8 years of age and in pregnancy; dosing: 2.2 mg/kg daily (max 100 mg/day)
- Chloroquine and mefloquine are started 1 and 2 weeks respectively before travel, continued during the period of exposure and for 4 weeks after leaving the endemic region. Malarone is started 2 days prior to travel and continued 1 week after return. Doxycycline is started 2 days before travel and continued for 4 weeks after return.

ETIOLOGY

- Infection is typically transmitted by the bite of the female *Anopheles* mosquito, but it can also be transmitted through contaminated blood transfusions or acquired congenitally.
- The majority of human disease is caused by *P. falciparum* and *P. vivax*.
  - *P. vivax* and *P. ovale* can cause relapsing disease because of the persistent hepatic (hypnozoite) stage of the infection.
  - Asymptomatic carriage for years may occur with *P. malariae*.
  - *P. knowlesi* is a primate parasite that can cause severe disease in humans. To date, it has occurred in humans only in Southeast Asia.

COMMONLY ASSOCIATED CONDITIONS

- Severe malaria is most commonly caused by *P. falciparum*; however, severe cases caused by *P. vivax* have been reported.
- Severe malaria is defined as parasitemia >5%, shock, acidosis, severe anemia or signs of CNS or other end-organ involvement such as renal failure, pulmonary edema, respiratory distress (acidotic/irregular breathing), impaired consciousness, seizures, hemoglobinuria, disseminated intravascular coagulation (DIC), or hypoglycemia.
- Cerebral malaria is a serious consequence of malaria infection, defined as coma in conjunction with *P. falciparum* parasitemia.
  - Occurs most often in children age 1 to 6 years in Africa but often occurs in adolescents and adults in Southeast Asia
- Severe anemia is common and can be severe, especially with *P. falciparum*. This is due to high parasitemia, hemolysis, sequestration and bone marrow suppression.
- Respiratory distress has high mortality, particularly if combined with impaired consciousness.
- Blackwater fever is a complication associated with falciparum malaria. It occurs due to massive hemolysis with resulting hemoglobinuria and acute renal failure.
- Pulmonary edema, renal failure, distributive shock, and progression to coma or death can occur.
- Acute kidney injury is common in children with severe malaria but rarely requires dialysis.
- Hyperreactive malarial splenomegaly is seen with chronic exposure to malaria in endemic areas. High levels of malaria IgM are present, and massive hepatosplenomegaly is seen.
- Splenic rupture may occur due to splenomegaly.
- *P. malariae* can cause nephrotic syndrome.

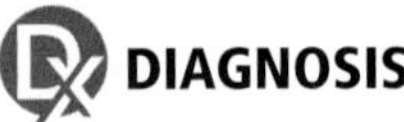

DIAGNOSIS

HISTORY

- History of travel to malaria endemic region
- Poor compliance with or lack of malaria prophylaxis
- Signs and symptoms
  - High fevers, headache, chills, and sweats are classic symptoms.
  - Periodicity of fever depends on the *Plasmodium* species and is less commonly seen in young children and travelers.
  - GI symptoms are common in children. Irritability, anorexia, vomiting, abdominal pain, cough, and arthralgias may be seen.
  - 95% of malaria cases occur within 30 days of return from travel, but malaria may occur as late as months after return.
  - Malaria can cause altered mental status, increased intracranial pressure, seizures, and coma.

ALERT

A high index of suspicion is necessary for the diagnosis of malaria, as failure to diagnose malaria has led to death in some instances. Fever may be the only sign in infants and young children.

PHYSICAL EXAM

- Fever, malaise, ill appearance
- Pallor or jaundice
- Hepatosplenomegaly may be present.
- In severely ill patients, respiratory distress with acidotic, deep breathing may be seen.
- Coma in cerebral malaria

DIFFERENTIAL DIAGNOSIS

- Malaria should be considered in any febrile traveler from an endemic area.
- Other causes of fever in travelers should be considered based on the region of travel are as follows:
  - Dengue
  - Typhoid fever

- Yellow fever
- Hepatitis A
- Influenza
- Measles
- Leptospirosis
- Chikungunya
- Common causes of fever such as pneumonia and viral illnesses should also be considered.

DIAGNOSTIC TESTS & INTERPRETATION

Initial Tests (screening, lab, imaging)

- Hemolytic anemia is commonly seen, with severe malarial anemia most common with *P. falciparum*.
- Thrombocytopenia is common.
- Hypoglycemia may occur with *P. falciparum*.
- Peripheral blood smear
  - Thick and thin peripheral smears are required for definitive diagnosis (thick smears provide better sensitivity if the parasitemia is low; thin smears provide for species identification).
  - If initial smears are negative, repeated specimens should be obtained q12–24 h over 72 hours to confirm a truly negative result with three smears.
  - A parasitemia of >2% of red blood cells, altered mental status, or other organ involvement makes the diagnosis of severe malaria and requires more intensive therapy.
- Rapid diagnostic tests
  - Rapid tests for antigen detection show excellent sensitivity for *Plasmodium* species, require a small amount of blood for testing, and provide results in <20 minutes.
  - Rapid tests should complement but not replace microscopy testing, as they do not provide an estimate of parasite density. They can remain positive up to 1 week following treatment.
- Polymerase chain reaction (PCR)
  - PCR is highly sensitive and can be useful for determining the *Plasmodium* species if it is unclear by blood smear. It is typically not available rapidly, so can be used to confirm a diagnosis, but treatment should not await PCR results.

ALERT
Consider malaria when a patient with fever has a history of travel.

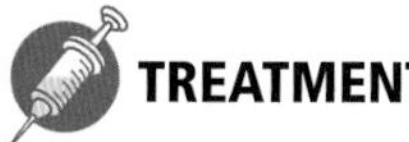

TREATMENT

MEDICATION

- Uncomplicated malaria
  - For known chloroquine-susceptible *P. falciparum* and *P. vivax* and for all *P. ovale*, *P. malariae*, and *P. knowlesi* infections, chloroquine can be used for known chloroquine-susceptible *P. falciparum* and *P. vivax* and for all *P. ovale*, *P. malariae*, and *P. knowlesi* infections.
    - Chloroquine is dosed at 10 mg/kg base PO (max 600 mg) and then 5 mg/kg base PO at 6, 24, and 48 hours (max 300 mg/dose); 10 mg chloroquine base = 16.6 mg chloroquine phosphate
    - Chloroquine-susceptible areas include Central America west of Panama Canal, Haiti, Dominican Republic, and parts of the Middle East.
  - For chloroquine-resistant *P. falciparum* or if species is unidentified, options are as follows:
    - Atovaquone-proguanil (Malarone®). Malarone® (mg atovaquone/mg proguanil) is given as 1 dose daily for 3 days; 5 to 8 kg: 2 pediatric tabs (62.5/25) per dose; 9 to 10 kg: 3 pediatric tabs per dose; 11 to 20 kg: 1 adult tab (250/100) per dose; 21 to 30 kg: 2 adult tabs per dose; 31 to 40 kg: 3 adult tabs per dose; ≥40 kg: 4 adult tabs per dose
    - Artemether-lumefantrine (Coartem®). Coartem® is given for a 6-dose course. The second dose is given 8 hours after the first, and then b.i.d. 5 to <15 kg: 1 tablet (20 mg artemether/120 mg lumefantrine) per dose. 15 to <25 kg: 2 tabs per dose; 25 to <35 kg: 3 tabs per dose; ≥35 kg: 4 tabs per dose
    - Mefloquine. Mefloquine is dosed at 15 mg/kg (max 750 mg) PO, followed by 10 mg/kg (max 500 mg) PO 6 to 12 hours later.
    - Quinine sulfate (10 mg salt/kg PO t.i.d.) plus doxycycline or clindamycin for 3 days (malaria acquired outside Southeast Asia) or 7 days (malaria acquired in Southeast Asia)
  - For chloroquine-resistant *P. vivax*, options are Malarone, mefloquine, or quinine + doxycycline, all in addition to primaquine.
  - Primaquine is used for the prevention of *P. vivax* and *P. ovale* relapses, in addition to primary treatment. It should not be used in patients with G6PD deficiency or in pregnancy.
  - Resistance to artemisinin is currently found in Southeast Asia (Cambodia, Laos, Thailand, Myanmar, Vietnam, and the Yunnan Province, China). Artemisinin-based combination therapies (ACT) for 6 days is currently recommended.
- Severe malaria
  - Quinidine gluconate, 10 mg salt/kg IV initial dose (max 600 mg) over 2 hours followed by 0.02 mg salt/kg/min infusion + doxycycline or clindamycin
  - In 2011, WHO guidelines made artesunate the drug of choice for children with severe malaria worldwide. Artesunate IV is available from the Centers for Disease Control and Prevention (CDC) under an investigational protocol for severe malaria in the United States but is available currently only if quinidine is not available or there is a contraindication to quinidine use.
  - Change to an oral agent once parasite density <1% and the patient can take oral medication. The use of exchange transfusion for patients with hyperparasitemia is controversial, as no controlled trial has shown a clear benefit to this treatment.

ADMISSION, INPATIENT, AND NURSING CONSIDERATIONS

Nonimmune travelers diagnosed with malaria infection should be managed as inpatients under standard precautions.

ONGOING CARE

PATIENT EDUCATION

- Consultation with a travel clinic is advised prior to travel to a malaria-endemic region.
- Chemoprophylaxis and mosquito bite prevention methods are both essential.

PROGNOSIS

- The prognosis depends on the severity of illness, *Plasmodium* species, underlying health conditions, and age of the patient.
- Infants with *P. falciparum* infection account for most of the mortality due to malaria.
- In African children, highest risk of death occurs in children with impaired consciousness and respiratory distress.
- If treated promptly, *P. falciparum* malaria typically responds well to treatment.

COMPLICATIONS

- Cerebral malaria and severe malarial anemia can cause long-term neurocognitive impairment.
- Severe malarial anemia is frequent due to *P. falciparum*. However, death rates with adequate treatment are low.
- Chronic relapses can occur from *P. vivax* and *P. ovale* infections.
- Pregnant women are at higher risk for complications from malaria infection.

ADDITIONAL READING

- Agarwal D, Teach SJ. Evaluation and management of a child with suspected malaria. *Pediatr Emerg Care*. 2006;22(2):127–133, quiz 134–136.
- Bangirana P, Opoka RO, Boivin MJ, et al. Severe malarial anemia is associated with long-term neurocognitive impairment. *Clin Infect Dis*. 2014; 59(3):336–344.
- Freedman DO. Clinical practice. Malaria prevention in short-term travelers. *N Engl J Med*. 2008;359(6): 603–612.
- Kiang KM, Bryant PA, Shingadia D, et al. The treatment of imported malaria in children: an update. *Arch Dis Child Educ Pract Ed*. 2013;98(1):7–15.
- White NJ, Pukrittayakamee S, Hien TT, et al. Malaria. *Lancet*. 2014;383(9918):723–735.

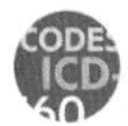

CODES

ICD10

- B54 Unspecified malaria
- B50.9 Plasmodium falciparum malaria, unspecified
- B51.9 Plasmodium vivax malaria without complication

FAQ

- Q: What drugs are acceptable choices for treatment of malaria in pregnancy?
- A: Options for uncomplicated malaria treatment in pregnant women in the United States include chloroquine (if sensitive), mefloquine, or quinidine + clindamycin.
- Q: Is there a vaccine available to prevent malaria?
- A: No vaccination is commercially available; however, antimalarial vaccines are currently in clinical trials.
- Q: How can I determine if the area my patient is traveling to has chloroquine-resistant malaria?
- A: The CDC Web site at www.cdc.gov/malaria has extensive information for travelers, including parasite sensitivity patterns and treatment recommendations. A malaria hotline is also available for clinician questions at 770-488-7788.

MALNUTRITION

Amanda Posner, MD • Patrika M. Tsai, MD, MPH

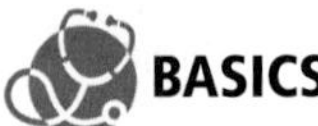

BASICS

DESCRIPTION

- Globally, the World Health Organization (WHO) identifies malnutrition in many forms, including undernutrition, inadequate intake of vitamins and minerals (micronutrients), and overweight/obesity. Undernutrition includes low weight-for-height (wasting), low height-for-age (stunting), and low weight-for-age (underweight). Obesity is addressed in a separate chapter.
- In 2013, a comprehensive definition of pediatric malnutrition was put forth by the American Society for Parenteral and Enteral Nutrition (ASPEN) guidelines, which incorporates the chronicity, etiology, and severity of malnutrition, as well as the pathogenic mechanism of nutrient imbalance, association with inflammatory state, and impact on functional outcomes such as growth, development, neurocognition, lean body mass, muscle strength, and immune function. "Pediatric malnutrition (undernutrition) is defined as an imbalance between nutrient requirement and intake, resulting in cumulative deficits of energy, protein, or micronutrients that may negatively affect growth, development, and other relevant outcomes."
- This definition of pediatric malnutrition considers the etiology of energy, protein, and/or micronutrient imbalance as either "illness-related malnutrition" (secondary to disease/injury) or "non–illness-related malnutrition" (secondary to environmental/behavioral factors). Malnutrition may also be classified as either acute (<3 months in duration) or chronic (>3 months in duration).
- In the United States, this issue has become very important in the setting of pediatric critical care, as children with malnutrition have increased mortality.
- The older term "protein-energy malnutrition" describes a general state of undernutrition and deficiency of multiple nutrients and energy.
- Malnutrition is much more common in areas that are resource poor with high levels of mortality age <5 years.
- There are two clinical presentations of severe malnutrition: kwashiorkor and marasmus.
  - Kwashiorkor (edematous malnutrition) is characterized by hypoproteinemia, pitting edema, varying degrees of wasting and/or stunting, dermatosis, and fatty infiltration of the liver.
  - Marasmus is characterized by wasting, fatigue, and apathy and thought to be from deficiency of energy and protein, especially total calories.
  - The distinction between kwashiorkor and marasmus is frequently blurred, and many children present with features of both conditions as marasmic kwashiorkor.
- Moderate to severe acute malnutrition is associated with 3 to 9 times higher mortality than well-nourished children.

RISK FACTORS

- Undernutrition can be attributed to increased nutritional needs in a chronic disease setting or decreased intake in the setting of underresourced areas with endemic gastrointestinal (GI) and lower respiratory infections.
- Lack of sanitation, poor hygiene, economic deprivation, and food insecurity are contributing factors. Availability of resources and design for allocation as determined by social, cultural, and political factors also affect undernutrition in less developed countries.
- In developed nations, symptoms of kwashiorkor have been described in chronic malabsorptive conditions such as cystic fibrosis, but such cases have become increasingly rare as novel treatments for both underlying diseases and direct causes of malabsorption (e.g., pancreatic enzyme replacement) have become standard of care.
- In the United States, a few cases of kwashiorkor unrelated to chronic illness have been described. This is usually due to severe neglect or previously undiagnosed chronic disease.
- Consumption of a protein-deficient milk alternative, sugar water, or fruit juice can be due to poor caregiver knowledge about nutrition, a perceived milk or formula intolerance or adherence to food fads.
- Consumption of a low-protein health food milk alternative, such as rice milk, secondary to a history of chronic eczema and perceived milk intolerance, has occurred in the United States.

EPIDEMIOLOGY

- Undernutrition underlies 45% of childhood mortality <5 years of age worldwide.
- The WHO estimates that 52 million children <5 years old have wasting, of whom 17 million have severe acute malnutrition globally.
- Moreover, 293 million children and 190 million of all preschoolers have iron deficiency anemia and vitamin A deficiency, respectively.
- 2/3 of children with acute malnutrition live in South Asia, and 1/4 live in Africa.
- The MAL-ED study follows eight global cohorts of children in Africa, Asia, and South America to identify environmental exposures including infection, nutrition, and socioeconomic factors and their impact on growth and development with several publications on nutritional status, stunting, environmental enteropathy, and diarrheal illness. As undernutrition is corrected, children and adolescents can have higher risk for obesity.

PATHOPHYSIOLOGY

- Temperature regulation is impaired, leading to hypothermia in a cold environment and hyperthermia in a hot environment.
- Increase in total-body sodium and decrease in total-body potassium
- Hypophosphatemia is associated with malnutrition and can result in high mortality, especially upon refeeding.
- Protein synthesis is reduced, particularly albumin, transferrin, and apolipoprotein B. Decreased ability to transport fat leads to fatty infiltration of the liver.
- Gluconeogenesis is reduced, which increases risk of hypoglycemia during infection.
- Reduced cardiac output leads to low blood pressure, compromised tissue perfusion, and a reduction in renal blood flow and glomerular filtration rate.
- Diminished inspiratory and expiratory pressures and vital capacity
- Reduction of gastric and pancreatic secretions
- Reduced intestinal motility
- Intestinal mucosa atrophy resulting in malabsorption of carbohydrates, fats, and fat- and water-soluble vitamins
- Low circulating insulin levels
- Growth hormone secretion is increased, whereas somatomedin activity is reduced.
  - Glucagon, epinephrine, and cortisol levels are increased.
  - Serum T_3 and T_4 levels are reduced.
- Immune system
  - T-cell immune function is diminished in malnutrition, thereby increasing susceptibility to infection.
  - Serum immunoglobulins are typically normal or increased, although enteral IgA is known to be decreased in experimental models of severe acute malnutrition.
  - Delayed wound healing may be seen owing to nutritional deficiencies.

ETIOLOGY

- Several theories have been proposed regarding the etiology of kwashiorkor with its characteristic edema, but more recent studies have suggested that protein deficiency and oxidant stress with free radical damage may be sequelae rather than causes.
- Studies are suggesting a link between the gut microbiome and poor diet resulting in kwashiorkor. There is a hierarchy of causes of undernutrition operating at different levels and interacting with one another: from food scarcity, infection, malabsorption, and neglect; to poverty and social disadvantage; to drought, war, or civil disturbance.
- The multiplicity of causes of undernutrition necessitates a multidisciplinary approach to its treatment and prevention.

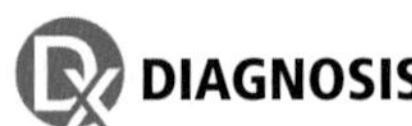

DIAGNOSIS

HISTORY

- Dietary history:
  - Diet before current illness episode
  - Adequacy of protein and total calories
  - Food and fluids taken in past few days
  - Special diets or use of health food milk alternatives, such as rice milk
  - Cultural beliefs and practices regarding infant and childhood feeding
- Duration and frequency of emesis or diarrhea
- Loose stools with evidence of malabsorption are common. Stools may be watery and/or tinged with blood.
- Any death of siblings
- Growth records: decreased growth velocity commensurate with poor protein intake
- History of chronic disease
- Recent immigration from a country where undernutrition is endemic (e.g., war-stricken areas or low-income countries)
- Recent international adoption

PHYSICAL EXAM

- Weight and length/height
  - Growth failure always occurs to some extent.
  - Wasting is also typical, although it may be masked by the presence of edema.
  - The current WHO and ASPEN standards vary slightly, but both now use z-scores as part of their guidelines when interpreting weight-for-height, BMI-for-age, height-for-age, and mid-upper arm circumference (MUAC). Generally, the z-score cutoffs for moderate malnutrition are between −2 and −3 and for severe malnutrition below −3.
  - Weight gain velocity, weight loss, and deceleration in weight-for-length/height z-score are useful if two data points are available.
- MUAC can be used as an indicator of lean body mass and is a useful screening tool in mass settings. For children 6 to 60 months, the cutoff for severe acute malnutrition is 115 mm, and for moderate is 115 to 124 mm.

- Triceps skinfold thickness (TSF) can be used to monitor changes in body fat and provides a useful estimate of energy stores.
- Hypothermia or hyperthermia
- General appearance
  - Affected child is usually apathetic and/or irritable.
  - Child is usually unsmiling and prefers to remain in one position.
- There is some degree of edema in all cases of kwashiorkor:
  - Peripheral edema usually begins in the feet and ascends up the legs.
  - The hands and face may become edematous.
  - Hair lacks luster, and color may change to brown or reddish-brown and is easily pluckable.
  - Bands of discolored hair, representing periods of malnutrition, are termed the "flag sign."
  - Dermatosis often develops in areas of friction or pressure.
  - Hypo- or hyperpigmented patches may appear, which subsequently desquamate in scales or sheets, exposing atrophic ulcers resembling burns.
- Additional clinical signs of undernutrition:
  - Signs of B-vitamin deficiency, such as perioral lesions
  - Signs of vitamin A deficiency, such as xerosis and/or xerophthalmia
  - Pale, cold, and cyanotic extremities: decreased vascular volume secondary to decreased protein concentration
  - Abdomen is frequently protuberant secondary to poor peristalsis, leading to distended stomach and intestinal loops.
  - Respiratory: Look for signs of pneumonia or heart failure.
  - Tanner stage
  - Handgrip strength using a handheld dynamometer

DIFFERENTIAL DIAGNOSIS

- Nephrotic syndrome
- Liver failure
- Disordered eating, restrictive type
- Hookworm anemia
  - May cause edema alone; commonly seen in association with kwashiorkor
  - It is not associated with the kwashiorkor-related dermatologic findings.
- Chronic dysentery or commonly environmental enteropathy in underresourced countries
- Protein-losing enteropathy (e.g., celiac disease and inflammatory bowel disease)
- Pellagra

DIAGNOSTIC TESTS & INTERPRETATION

- Metabolic profile, with frequent checks of potassium, magnesium, and phosphorus to monitor for refeeding syndrome
- Albumin to assess for hypoalbuminemia and possible inflammation and protein loss rather than as a marker for nutritional status as half-life is 2 to 3 weeks
- Hemoglobin and hematocrit and iron studies
- Vitamin B12 and folate
- Vitamin A, E, and D
- PT/INR to evaluate vitamin K status
- Zinc and carnitine
- Prealbumin is used in select cases, but it is a negative acute phase reactant and falls during times of inflammation. It is not a reliable indicator of nutritional status during injury or illness. C-reactive protein should be checked concurrently to identify the presence of inflammation and validity of a prealbumin level.
- UA with microscopy to evaluate for proteinuria or urinary tract infection
- Infectious stool studies
- Fecal elastase to check for pancreatic insufficiency
- Stool reducing substances and stool pH to evaluate for carbohydrate malabsorption; stool alpha-1-antitrypsin (A1AT) to look for GI protein loss

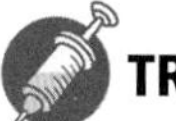

TREATMENT

WHO guidelines:

- Prevent and treat the following:
  - Hypoglycemia
  - Hypothermia
  - Dehydration
  - Electrolyte imbalances
  - Infection
  - Micronutrient deficiencies
- Provide specially tailored feeds for the following stages of recovery:
  - Initial stabilization (requires frequent monitoring for refeeding syndrome)
  - Providing catch-up growth
  - Maintenance
- Where guidelines have been fully implemented, mortality has been reduced by at least half.

GENERAL MEASURES

- Whenever possible, a dehydrated child with malnutrition should be rehydrated orally or by nasogastric tube.
- IV infusion should be avoided except when it is essential (e.g., severe dehydration and shock).
- Hypoglycemia is an important cause of death in the first 2 days of treatment.
- Suspected hypoglycemia should be treated with 10% glucose by mouth, nasogastric tube, or intravenously.
- Severely malnourished children have high levels of sodium and are deficient in potassium. Standard WHO oral rehydration salts (ORS) does not meet the special electrolyte requirements of the severely malnourished child.
- ReSoMal is a modified ORS that contains less sodium and more potassium than the standard WHO ORS and is sometimes recommended ORS for severely malnourished children under inpatient medical supervision

ALERT

Rapid and inappropriate refeeding of malnourished individuals may result in the refeeding syndrome, which is manifested as hypophosphatemia, hypomagnesemia, and hypokalemia. Cardiac dysfunction, edema, and neurologic changes, due to shifts in fluid and electrolytes following aggressive introduction of nutrients, are associated with refeeding syndrome. Refeeding syndrome can be fatal when not managed appropriately.

ONGOING CARE

PROGNOSIS

- Treatment corrects the acute signs of the disease, but catch-up growth in height may never be achieved.
- Mortality rate in kwashiorkor can be as high as 40%, but adequate treatment can reduce it to <10%.
- Some of the factors that indicate poor prognosis:
  - Age <6 months
  - Infections
  - Dehydration and electrolyte abnormalities
  - Persistent tachycardia, signs of heart failure
  - Total serum protein <3 g/100 mL
  - Elevated serum bilirubin
  - Severe anemia with hypoxia
  - Hypoglycemia and/or hypothermia

COMPLICATIONS

Several longitudinal studies have demonstrated associations between early childhood stunting and later cognitive function and academic attainment.

ADDITIONAL READING

- Becker PJ, Nieman Carney L, Corkins MR, et al. Consensus statement of the Academy of Nutrition and Dietetics/American Society for Parenteral and Enteral Nutrition: indicators recommended for the identification and documentation of pediatric malnutrition (undernutrition). *J Acad Nutr Diet*. 2014;114(12):1988–2000.
- Darby WJ. Cicely D. Williams, her life and influence. *Nutr Rev*. 1973;31:331–333.
- Ghosh-Jerath S, Singh A, Jerath N, et al. Undernutrition and severe acute malnutrition in children. *BMJ*. 2017;359:j4877.
- MAL-ED Network Investigators. Childhood stunting in relation to the pre- and postnatal environment during the first 2 years of life: the MAL-ED longitudinal birth cohort study. *PLoS Med*. 2017;14(10):e1002408.
- Mehta N, Corkins M, Lyman B, et al. Defining pediatric malnutrition: a paradigm shift toward etiology-related definitions. *JPEN J Parenter Enteral Nutr*. 2013;37(4):460–481.
- Mehta N, Skillman HE, Irving SY, et al. Guidelines for the provision and assessment of nutrition support therapy in the pediatric critically ill patient: Society of Critical Care Medicine and American Society for Parenteral and Enteral Nutrition. *JPEN J Parenter Enteral Nutr*. 2017;41(5):706–742.
- Terán G, Cuna W, Brañez F, et al. Differences in nutritional and health status in school children from the highlands and lowlands of Bolivia. *Am J Trop Med Hyg*. 2018;98(1):326–333.

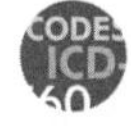

CODES

ICD10

- E46 Unspecified protein-calorie malnutrition
- E40 Kwashiorkor
- E41 Nutritional marasmus

FAQ

- Q: What are some common causes of severe undernutrition in the United States that may present as kwashiorkor?
- A: Chronic malabsorptive conditions (e.g., cystic fibrosis), autoimmune disease, and consumption of protein-deficient milk substitutes such as rice milk, fruit juices, and so forth.
- Q: Can a child be both overweight and stunted?
- A: Yes, a child can be stunted and overweight. Some children can suffer from more than one type of malnutrition. There is no data to show the prevalence of these particular coexisting diseases. This condition was recognized as an increasing problem in the *Joint child malnutrition estimates—Levels and trends* (2017 edition) released by UNICEF-WHO-The World Bank Group.
- Q: What is the etiology of the term "kwashiorkor"?
- A: Cicely Delphine Williams, BM, ChB introduced the name "kwashiorkor" in 1935 in a classic description of her observations of the Ga tribe on the Gold Coast of Africa (currently Ghana). "Kwashiorkor" in the Ga language is translated as "the disease of the deposed child (deposed from the breast) when the next baby is born."

MAMMALIAN BITES

Erin Dunbar, MD, MSc • Margaret S. Wolff, MD

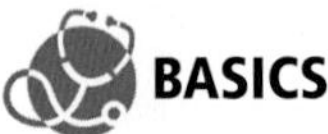

BASICS

DESCRIPTION

A bite to the human skin and/or subcutaneous tissues by another mammal causing local, and in some cases systemic, effects

EPIDEMIOLOGY

- Animal bites
  - Approximate frequency
    - Dogs: 80–90%
    - Cats: 5–15%
    - Rodents or rabbits: 1%
    - Raccoons and other animals: 1%
  - The offending animals are often well known to the victim.
  - Children are the most common victims:
    - Boys are more likely than girls to be bitten by dogs.
    - Girls are more likely to be bitten by cats.
- Human bites
  - Third most common cause of all bites seen in ED
  - Younger children more often present with occlusion bites (which generally compress tissue causing ecchymoses).
  - Children >10 years old are more likely to present due to accidental injury during sports activities or intentionally during altercations or abusive situations. These are more likely to be due to clenched fist/fight bites (puncture wounds when fist hits teeth).

Incidence

- An estimated 4.5 million dog bites and 400,000 cat bites occur annually in the United States.
- The incidence of human bites is unknown due to underreporting.

GENERAL PREVENTION

- Ensure that children receive routine immunizations against tetanus and hepatitis and that family pets are immunized against rabies.
- Never leave small children alone with pets.
- Encourage children to avoid contact with wild animals and dead animals.

PATHOPHYSIOLOGY

- Injury associated with bite types:
  - Dog
    - Younger children more often have head and neck bites; older children more often extremities are affected.
    - Crush and tear injuries
    - May involve bone
  - Cat
    - Puncture-type wounds
    - Penetrate deeper and carry a higher risk of infection (think osteomyelitis, septic arthritis)
  - Human
    - Generally only violate skin
    - However, clenched fist/fight bites tend to be worse due to the possibility of penetrating injury.
    - Penetration into joint and tendon sheath spaces can occur (especially bites overlying the metacarpal-phalangeal areas).
- Infection
  - Animal bites are considered grossly contaminated.
  - Infections are most commonly polymicrobial with both aerobic and anaerobic organisms.
  - Infected dog and cat bites
    - *Pasteurella* species are the most frequent isolates.
    - Dog: *Pasteurella canis*, new emerging bacteria *Capnocytophaga species* (can cause endocarditis, meningitis, sepsis)
    - Cat: *Pasteurella multocida* and *Pasteurella septica*
    - Common anaerobes include *Fusobacterium*, bacteroides, *Porphyromonas*, and *Prevotella*.
  - Infected human bites
    - *Streptococcus anginosus*
    - *Staphylococcus aureus*
    - *Eikenella corrodens*
    - *Fusobacterium* species
    - *Prevotella* species

ALERT

Bites that are high risk of infection:

- Bite on the hand or face
- Cat bites or any deep puncture wound
- Crush injuries
- Patient with diabetes, asplenia, or immunosuppression
- Delayed presentation
  - >6 to 12 hours for arm or leg
  - >12 to 24 hours for face

DIAGNOSIS

HISTORY

- Animal bites
  - Type of animal
  - Apparent health of the animal
  - Provocation for the attack
  - Timing of the bite
  - Location of the bite or bites
  - Availability of animal for undergoing observation (i.e., known animal as opposed to a stray or wild animal)
  - Rabies immunization status of the animal
- Past medical history
  - Tetanus immunization status of the child
  - Hepatitis B immunization status of child
  - Is patient immunocompromised or asplenic?

PHYSICAL EXAM

- Carefully assess neurovascular integrity.
- Location of bite
  - If bite is located over a joint, assess for violation of joint capsule.
- Examine entire patient to ensure that all wounds are identified and treated.
- Older wounds
  - Assess for signs of infection such as erythema, induration, purulence, regional adenopathy, and elevated temperature.

DIAGNOSTIC TESTS & INTERPRETATION

Initial Tests (screening, lab, imaging)

- Blood culture if fever or systemic toxicity is noted
- Aerobic and anaerobic cultures from infected wounds (but not helpful in fresh bites without signs of infection)
- In penetrating injuries overlying bones or joints, consider radiography to evaluate for presence of fracture, foreign body (e.g., tooth), and air within joint.

Diagnostic Procedures/Other

No tests routinely done

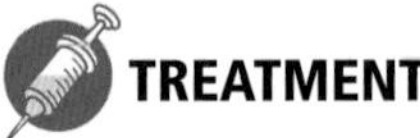

TREATMENT

GENERAL MEASURES

- Wound care:
  - Copious irrigation with normal saline or tap water to remove visible debris
  - Do not use antimicrobial solutions to irrigate.
  - Cleanse but do not irrigate puncture wounds.
- Human bites over metacarpals (clenched-fist injuries) require orthopedic evaluation for possible surgical exploration and irrigation.
- Debride devitalized tissue.
- The increased risk of infection associated with suturing a potentially contaminated wound must be weighed against the cosmetic effect due to nonclosure:
  - Primary closure of larger wounds or significant facial wounds may be indicated unless wound is old or has evidence of infection.
- Hand wounds may be an exception, due to high propensity for infection.
- Avoid tissue adhesives for wound closure.

MEDICATION

- Antibiotics: Data are often contradictory. In general, treat all high-risk individuals or bites requiring closure and consider in average risk individuals (see "Alert" section).
  - Amoxicillin–clavulanic acid PO is drug of choice (50 mg amoxicillin/kg/24 h divided b.i.d. or t.i.d. for 5 days).
  - An alternative antibiotic regimen for penicillin-allergic patients is trimethoprim–sulfamethoxazole plus clindamycin.
  - Infected wounds should be treated for at least 10 days.
- IV antibiotics and hospitalization should be considered for patients with signs of systemic involvement or infected-appearing wounds to face and hands.
  - Ampicillin/sulbactam IV 150 mg ampicillin/kg/24 h in 4 divided doses
  - For penicillin-allergic patients, 3rd-generation cephalosporin
- Tetanus prophylaxis if indicated
- Rabies prophylaxis if indicated
  - Unknown dog or cat; dogs or cats with unknown immunization status that cannot be observed for 10 days
  - Bites from wild animals, including raccoons, bats, skunks, foxes, coyotes
  - Because bat bites may go undetected, especially by a sleeping child, rabies prophylaxis is recommended after exposure to bats in a confined setting.
  - Rabies is unlikely if the child was bitten by an immunized dog, cat, or other pet (e.g., hamsters, guinea pigs, gerbils).
  - Rabies is unlikely if the child was bitten by a small rodent (squirrels, mice, or rats) or rabbit.
  - The regimen for patients who have not been vaccinated previously should include both human rabies vaccine (a series of 4 doses administered IM on days 0, 3, 7, and 14; immunocompromised patients should receive a fifth dose on day 28) and rabies-immune globulin (20 IU/kg) administered as much as possible into the wound, the remainder given IM at a site distant from the site used for vaccine administration.
- HIV postexposure prophylaxis (PEP)
  - There are case reports describing transmission of HIV by human bites; however, the risk of transmission due to biting is unknown. It is estimated to be extremely small. Bites with saliva containing no visible blood have no associated risk for transmission and, therefore, are not considered exposures.
  - HIV PEP requires a multidrug regimen administered over 28 days that can be associated with significant toxicity.
  - Decisions to initiate PEP are best made in consultation with local experts or by contacting the National Clinicians Post-Exposure Prophylaxis hotline at 888-448-4911.
  - Hepatitis B has been transmitted from nonbloody saliva. Check the vaccination status of the bitten (or biter if necessary) to consider PEP. Unvaccinated children should begin the hepatitis B vaccine series.
  - The transmission rate of hepatitis C via human bites is unknown, and no regimen for PEP currently exists.

ALERT

A bite with a break in the skin is considered low risk, and a bite with intact skin is felt to pose no risk.

ISSUES FOR REFERRAL

- Human bites over metacarpals (clenched-fist injuries) require orthopedic evaluation for possible surgical exploration and irrigation.
- Local regulations dictate the reporting of animal bites to health departments.

ONGOING CARE

FOLLOW-UP RECOMMENDATIONS

Patient Monitoring

- Signs and symptoms of infection
- All patients with significant bites should receive follow-up 48 hours after bite.

PROGNOSIS

Most injury from animal bites is trivial, but infections, and rarely deaths, do occur.

COMPLICATIONS

Human bites over metacarpals (clenched fist) can penetrate tendon sheaths, become infected, and result in a tenosynovitis.

ADDITIONAL READING

- American Veterinary Medical Association. Dog bite prevention. https://www.avma.org/public/Pages/Dog-Bite-Prevention.aspx. Accessed March 5, 2018.
- Aziz H, Rhee P, Pandit V, et al. The current concepts in management of animal (dog, cat, snake, scorpion) and human bite wounds. *J Trauma Acute Care Surg*. 2015;78(3):641–648.
- Havens PL; for American Academy of Pediatrics Committee on Pediatric AIDS. Postexposure prophylaxis in children and adolescents for nonoccupational exposure to human immunodeficiency virus. *Pediatrics*. 2003;111(6 Pt 1):1475–1489.
- Medeiros I, Saconato H. Antibiotic prophylaxis for mammalian bites. *Cochrane Database Syst Rev*. 2001;(2):CD001738.
- Rupprecht CE, Briggs D, Brown CM, et al. Use of a reduced (4-dose) vaccine schedule for postexposure prophylaxis to prevent human rabies: recommendations of the advisory committee on immunization practices. *MMWR Recomm Rep*. 2010;59(RR-2):1–9.
- Wu PS, Beres A, Tashjian DB, et al. Primary repair of facial dog bite injuries in children. *Pediatr Emerg Care*. 2011:27(9):801–813.

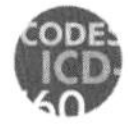

CODES

ICD10

- S61.459A Open bite of unspecified hand, initial encounter
- S01.85XA Open bite of other part of head, initial encounter
- S61.259A Open bite of unsp finger without damage to nail, init encntr

FAQ

- Q: What are the clinical features of *Pasteurella* infections?
- A: Infections caused by *Pasteurella* tend to progress rapidly, usually over a 12- to 24-hour period, and are characterized by tenderness and purulent drainage. The rapid progression of these infections tends to distinguish them from wounds that are infected with *S. aureus* and other pathogens.
- Q: Why are cat bites often more severe than dog bites?
- A: Cat bites are associated with puncture-type wounds and are more likely to involve *Pasteurella* infection, which is generally more aggressive than other organisms. However, dog bite infections may also be caused by *Pasteurella*.

M

MASTOIDITIS

Sadiqa Kendi, MD, FAAP • Frances M. Nadel, MD, MSCE

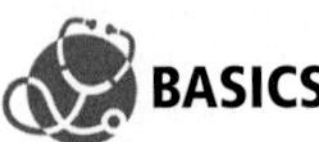

BASICS

DESCRIPTION

Infection of the mastoid air cells characterized clinically by protrusion of the pinna and erythema/tenderness over the mastoid process; can range from an asymptomatic illness to a severe life-threatening disease. Acute mastoiditis is defined as the presence of symptoms for <1 month. Masked mastoiditis is a persistent middle ear and mastoid infection with bony destruction.

EPIDEMIOLOGY

- Most patients are between 6 and 24 months old.
- It is unusual to see mastoiditis in young infants because of incomplete pneumatization of the mastoid air cells.

Incidence

- Incidence varies greatly in the literature, from 1.88 to 12/100,000 children per year.
- Although some single-site reports have suggested that mastoiditis is on the rise, larger population-based studies demonstrate a stable incidence.

RISK FACTORS

- Age <2 years of age
- Acute otitis media
- Recurrent otitis media

GENERAL PREVENTION

- Appropriate treatment of otitis media and timely follow-up to identify treatment failures
- Avoid factors that predispose to otitis media, including caretaker smoking and bottlefeeding.
- Pneumococcal vaccination may help decrease the occurrence of otitis media.
- Delayed antibiotic treatment for antecedent otitis media does not increase the risk of more severe mastoiditis.

PATHOPHYSIOLOGY

- The mastoid process is the posterior portion of the temporal bone and consists of interconnecting air cells that drain superiorly into the middle ear. Because these mastoid air cells connect with the middle ear, all cases of acute otitis media are associated with some mastoid inflammation.
- Acute mastoiditis develops when the accumulation of purulent exudate in the middle ear does not drain through the eustachian tube or through a perforated tympanic membrane but spreads to the mastoid.
- Acute mastoiditis can progress to a coalescent phase after the bony air cells are destroyed and may then progress to subperiosteal abscess or to chronic mastoiditis.

ETIOLOGY

- Acute mastoiditis is generally caused by an extension of the inflammation and infection of acute otitis media into the mastoid air cells. However, 20–50% of patients may present without evidence of preceding otitis media.
- The bacteria isolated from middle ear drainage or from the mastoid are usually *Streptococcus pneumoniae*, *Streptococcus pyogenes*, and *Staphylococcus aureus*. Many patients' cultures are sterile which may be related to antibiotic use prior to retrieval of fluid.
  - *S. pneumoniae* is the most frequently isolated cause of mastoiditis. Isolates highly resistant to penicillin has decreased since the introduction of the 13-valent pneumococcal vaccine.
  - *Pseudomonas* infection should be suspected if the child has been on antibiotics recently or has a history of recurrent otitis media.
- Chronic mastoiditis is usually caused by *S. aureus*, anaerobic bacteria, enteric bacteria, *Pseudomonas aeruginosa,* or multiple-organism infection.
- *Fusobacterium necrophorum* should be considered in younger children and those with complications such as osteomyelitis, bacteremia, and Lemierre syndrome.
- Unusual agents of chronic mastoiditis include *Mycobacterium tuberculosis*, nontuberculous mycobacteria, *Nocardia asteroides*, and *Histoplasma capsulatum*.
- Cholesteatomas may contribute to the development of mastoiditis by impeding mastoid drainage or erosion of underlying bone.

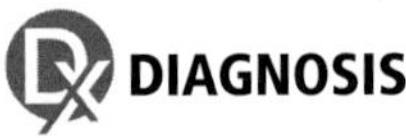

DIAGNOSIS

HISTORY

- May include a recent or a chronic history of treatment for otitis media
- Sign and symptoms
  - May include fever, otalgia, otorrhea, and postauricular swelling
  - Children who are already on antibiotics or have masked mastoiditis may present with more subtle findings.
  - Intracranial extension should be suspected if there is lethargy, a stiff neck, headache, focal neurologic symptoms, seizures, visual changes, or persistent fevers despite appropriate antibiotic treatment.

PHYSICAL EXAM

- The ear may protrude away from the scalp:
  - In children <2 years old, the ear protrudes out and is displaced down. In older children, the ear is displaced up.
- The external ear canal may be edematous or sagging.
- The tympanic membrane often is hyperemic, with decreased mobility, or perforated:
  - The tympanic membranes of children on antibiotics may have a normal appearance.
- The mastoid process is tender, with soft tissue swelling:
  - The overlying skin may be warm and erythematous, with posterior auricular fluctuance.
- In chronic mastoiditis, the fever and posterior auricular swelling are often not present, and the patient presents with ear pain, persistent drainage, or hearing loss.

DIFFERENTIAL DIAGNOSIS

- Parotitis
- Posterior auricular lymphadenopathy or cellulitis
- Otitis externa or an ear canal furuncle
- Perichondritis of the auricle
- Neoplastic disease
  - Leukemia
  - Lymphoma
  - Rhabdomyosarcoma
  - Langerhans cell histiocytosis
- Branchial cleft anomaly
- Tuberculosis

DIAGNOSTIC TESTS & INTERPRETATION

Initial Tests (screening, lab, imaging)

- CBC with differential: nonspecific
  - May be normal or show a leukocytosis with a neutrophil predominance
- ESR/CRP: nonspecific
  - May be elevated in acute mastoiditis but is usually normal in the chronic stage; more often elevated in complicated mastoiditis
- Purified protein derivative (PPD)
  - Should be done if tuberculosis is suspected
- Middle ear aspirate
  - Gram stain and cultures for aerobic and anaerobic bacteria
  - There is some correlation between middle ear bacterial cultures and mastoid cultures.
  - If possible, drainage prior to antibiotic administration is more helpful in making a microbiologic diagnosis.
- Radiographs
  - Reveal haziness of the mastoid air cells and can show bony destruction in more advanced disease
  - Are unreliable and can be falsely normal, as well as falsely abnormal

- Contrast-enhanced temporal bone and cranial CT
  - Helpful in the confirmation of the diagnosis, identification of coalescence or a subperiosteal abscess, and evaluation for concomitant intracranial complications
- Ultrasound
  - May be helpful in evaluating for subperiosteal abscess
- MRI
  - Best for evaluating for intracranial complications

Diagnostic Procedures/Other

Lumbar puncture must be performed in any child with symptoms of meningitis once the patient is stabilized.

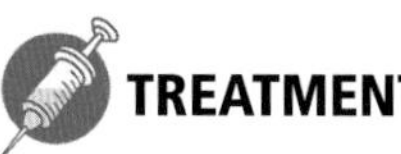

TREATMENT

GENERAL MEASURES

Middle ear drainage is essential; therefore, a myringotomy with or without tube placement should be performed early.

MEDICATION

- Parenteral antibiotics are chosen based on the most likely organisms, regional bacterial resistance patterns, and the child's condition.
- IV antibiotics are given for at least 7 to 10 days followed with oral antibiotics for a total duration of 4 weeks of therapy.
- A 3rd- or 4th-generation cephalosporin such as ceftriaxone or cefotaxime or cefepime is often used with or without vancomycin for empiric treatment.
- Subsequent antibiotic choice should be tailored to antimicrobial sensitivities of the ear aspirate.
- If *M. tuberculosis* is suspected, then antituberculosis therapy should be started.

SURGERY/OTHER PROCEDURES

- Indications for further surgical intervention include the following:
  - Subperiosteal abscess
  - Coalescence
  - Meningitis
  - Intracranial abscess
  - Venous thrombosis
  - Persistent symptoms despite adequate antibiotic treatment
- In the preantibiotic era, mastoidectomy was the treatment of choice for mastoiditis. Currently, this therapy is generally reserved for cases complicated by the aforementioned indications.
- Neurosurgical consultation for treatment of intracranial complications may be necessary.

ADMISSION, INPATIENT, AND NURSING CONSIDERATIONS

Admit for IV antibiotics and for otolaryngology (ENT) evaluation for surgical drainage and to ensure response to antibiotics and to rule out complications.

ONGOING CARE

FOLLOW-UP RECOMMENDATIONS

Patient Monitoring

- If patients respond quickly to parenteral therapy, they can complete a 3- to 4-week course with oral antibiotics and weekly follow-up visits.
- Audiograms should be performed later to screen for hearing loss.

PROGNOSIS

- Mastoiditis has a good prognosis generally. However, intracranial extension of mastoiditis can lead to permanent neurologic deficits and death.
- Chronic mastoiditis can lead to irreversible hearing loss.

COMPLICATIONS

- The proximity of the mastoid to many important structures can result in serious complications from extension of infection or as a response to the inflammatory process.
- Complication rates may be as high as 16%.
- Intracranial complications include meningitis and extradural, subdural, or brain parenchymal abscesses.
- Venous sinus thrombophlebitis results from extension of disease to the sigmoid or lateral sinus:
  - Sepsis, increased intracranial pressure, or septic emboli may result.
- Facial nerve palsy is usually unilateral and can be permanent.
- Labyrinthitis, petrositis, or osteomyelitis may result from extension of the infection into adjacent bones.
- Subperiosteal abscess
- Hearing loss can occur from destruction of the ossicles or from labyrinthine damage.
- Bezold abscess is a deep neck abscess along the medial sternocleidomastoid muscle that develops when the infection erodes through the tip of the mastoid bone and dissects down tissue planes.
- Gradenigo syndrome (or Gradenigo-Lannois syndrome)—triad of CNVI palsy, retro-orbital pain, and otorrhea
- Death is uncommon but has been reported (0.03% incidence)

ADDITIONAL READING

- Bilavsky E, Yarden-Bilavsky H, Samra Z, et al. Clinical, laboratory, and microbiological differences between children with simple or complicated mastoiditis. *Int J Pediatr Otorhinolaryngol*. 2009;73(9):1270–1273.
- Grossman Z, Zehavi Y, Leibovitz E, et al. Severe acute mastoiditis admission is not related to delayed antibiotic treatment for antecedent acute otitis media. *Pediatr Infect Dis J*. 2016;35(2):162–165.
- Groth A, Enoksson F, Hultcrantz M, et al. Acute mastoiditis in children aged 0-16 years—a national study of 678 cases in Sweden comparing different age groups. *Int J Pediatr Otorhinolaryngol*. 2012;76(10):1494–1500.
- Kaplan SL, Center KJ, Barson WJ, et al. Multicenter surveillance of *Streptococcus pneumoniae* isolates from middle ear and mastoid cultures in the 13-valent pneumococcal conjugate vaccine era. *Clin Infect Dis*. 2015;60(9):1339–1345.
- Kaplan SL, Mason EO Jr, Wald ER, et al. Pneumococcal mastoiditis in children. *Pediatrics*. 2000;106(4):695–699.
- Marom T, Roth Y, Boaz M, et al. Acute mastoiditis in children: necessity and timing of imaging. *Pediatr Infect Dis J*. 2016;35(1):30–34.
- Minks DP, Porte M, Jenkins N. Acute mastoiditis—the role of radiology. *Clin Radiol*. 2013;68(4):397–405.
- Pang LH, Barakate MS, Havas TE. Mastoiditis in a paediatric population: a review of 11 years experience in management. *Int J Pediatr Otorhinolaryngol*. 2009;73(11):1520–1524.
- Pritchett CV, Thorne MC. Incidence of pediatric acute mastoiditis: 1997–2006. *Arch Otolaryngol Head Neck Surg*. 2012;138(5):451–455.
- Psarommatis IM, Voudouris C, Douros K, et al. Algorithmic management of pediatric acute mastoiditis. *Int J Pediatr Otorhinolaryngol*. 2012;76(6):791–796.

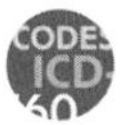

CODES

ICD10

- H70.90 Unspecified mastoiditis, unspecified ear
- H70.009 Acute mastoiditis without complications, unspecified ear
- H70.099 Acute mastoiditis with other complications, unspecified ear

FAQ

- Q: Do all children with mastoiditis need a CT scan of the head if mastoiditis is suspected?
- A: No. In general, if the child with mastoiditis has mild swelling, no fluctuance of the mastoid, and responds to therapy, no CT scan is needed. A patient who appears toxic or fails to respond to appropriate antibiotic therapy or one who may be a surgical candidate should undergo additional imaging studies.
- Q: Should all children with mastoiditis be admitted to the hospital?
- A: Yes. In general, admission with IV antibiotics and ENT evaluation/drainage is warranted to ensure response to antibiotics and rule out complications.

M

MEASLES (RUBEOLA)

Jeffrey S. Gerber, MD, PhD

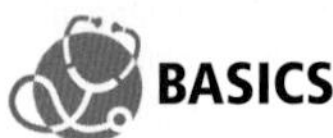

BASICS

DESCRIPTION

- An exanthematous disease that has a relatively predictable course, making clinical diagnosis possible
- Because it is rare, cases are often initially misdiagnosed as a nonspecific viral exanthema, drug eruption, or Kawasaki disease.
- Types of measles include the following:
  - Typical measles (outlined below)
  - Modified measles
    - A mild form of measles can occur in children with passive immunity to the virus.
    - This setting includes babies with maternal-acquired antibody and children who have received immune globulin.
    - Some of the classic symptoms and signs may be absent.

EPIDEMIOLOGY

- Measles is one of the most *highly contagious* of all infectious diseases.
- Patients are contagious from 1 to 2 days before onset of symptoms (3 to 5 days before rash) until 5 days after the appearance of the rash. The incubation period is generally 8 to 12 days from exposure to onset of symptoms and ~14 days until the appearance of rash.
- Hospital or clinic waiting rooms, especially pediatric emergency department waiting rooms, have been identified as a major risk, accounting for up to 45% of known exposures. With adequate immunization (2 doses = 99% effective), measles could be eliminated as a disease.
- Although no longer endemic in the United States, networks of intentionally unvaccinated children have led to several recent U.S. outbreaks originating from measles virus imported from abroad.
- Because 20 million cases of measles, resulting in 150,000 deaths, occur globally per year, it is critical to maintain high levels of vaccination coverage.

Incidence

- Before the 1963 licensure of vaccine, an estimated 3 to 4 million people acquired measles in the United States each year, including 4,000 cases of encephalitis and 500 deaths; by 1983, there were only 0.7 cases per 100,000 population.
- Delays in immunization facilitated large outbreaks in the United States from 1989 to 1991, peaking in 1990 when 27,672 cases were reported, 89 of which were fatal.
- From 2001 to 2012, the median annual number of measles cases reported in United States was 60.
- From January to August 2013, 159 U.S. cases were reported, including the largest U.S. outbreak since 1996 (58 cases). The majority of cases occurred in underimmunized individuals and imported from abroad (including U.S. travelers).
- In 2014, 667 measles cases from 23 outbreaks occurred in the United States, including a single outbreak of 383 cases, primarily among unvaccinated Amish communities in Ohio.
- In 2015, a large, multistate measles outbreak was linked to an amusement park in California.

GENERAL PREVENTION

- Vaccine recommendations
  - Routine vaccination against measles, mumps, and rubella (MMR) for children begins at 12 to 15 months of age, with a second MMR vaccination at age 4 to 6 years.
  - With the recent resurgence of measles, aggressive employee immunization programs should be pursued for all health care workers.
  - Health care workers born after 1956 who have no documentation of vaccination or evidence of measles immunity should be vaccinated at the time of employment and revaccinated ≥28 days later.
- Infection control measures
  - Any inpatient suspected of having measles should be in a negative-pressure respiratory isolation room; health care workers must wear masks, gloves, and gowns (airborne and contact precautions).
  - Isolation is required for 4 days after the first appearance of the rash; immunocompromised patients require isolation for the course of the illness.
  - All suspected cases of measles should be reported immediately to the local health department.

PATHOPHYSIOLOGY

Transmission of measles occurs through direct contact with infectious droplets, less commonly by airborne spread.

ETIOLOGY

Measles is an RNA virus (paramyxovirus, genus *Morbillivirus*) with only one serotype.

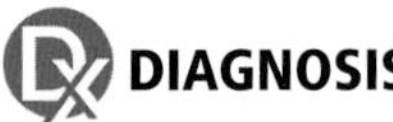

DIAGNOSIS

- Case definition from the Centers for Disease Control and Prevention (CDC) includes the following:
  - Generalized rash lasting ≥3 days
  - A temperature of ≥38.3°C (101°F)
  - Cough, coryza, or conjunctivitis
  - Positive testing or epidemiologic linkage to known case
- The mean incubation period is 10 days (range: 8 to 21 days).

HISTORY

- The disease involves fever, cough, conjunctivitis, and coryza with an erythematous rash, which has a characteristic progression:
  - The rash appears on the face (often the nape of the neck, initially) and abdomen 14 days after exposure. The rash is erythematous and maculopapular and spreads from the head to the feet, often becoming confluent at more proximal sites.
- The prodrome of measles lasts 2 to 4 days and begins with symptoms of upper respiratory infection, fever up to 104°F, malaise, conjunctivitis, photophobia, and increasing cough.
- Fever usually resolves by the 4th day of rash.

PHYSICAL EXAMINATION

- During the prodrome, Koplik spots (white spots on the buccal mucosa) appear on most people.
- Following this prodrome, the rash appears on the face, often initially at the hairline, and abdomen 14 days after exposure. The rash is erythematous and maculopapular and spreads from the head to the feet.
- After 3 to 4 days, the rash begins to clear, leaving a brownish discoloration and fine scaling.
- Pharyngitis, cervical lymphadenopathy, and splenomegaly may accompany the rash.

DIFFERENTIAL DIAGNOSIS

With a careful history and physical exam, it is usually possible to diagnose measles. The differential diagnosis includes the following:

- Stevens-Johnson syndrome
- Kawasaki disease
- Other viral exanthem
- Meningococcemia
- Rocky Mountain spotted fever (RMSF)
- Toxic shock syndrome

DIAGNOSTIC TESTS & INTERPRETATION

- When measles is suspected, laboratory confirmation is important.
- The course of typical measles follows a predictable pattern; therefore, laboratory studies to confirm infection in known contacts might not be required.
- Serum measles-specific IgM titer (simplest)
  - Sensitivity may be diminished if assay performed <72 hours from onset of rash; repeat if negative; IgM detectable for at least 1 month from onset of rash
- A comparison of IgG titers obtained during the acute and convalescent stages can be done. Blood samples must be taken at least 7 to 10 days apart.
- Culture or RNA (RT-PCR) testing of nasopharyngeal, throat, blood, or urine

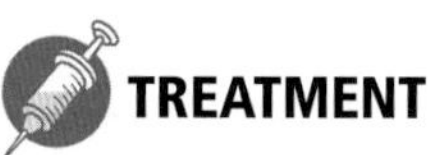

TREATMENT

GENERAL MEASURES

- No specific therapy; supportive care
- Ribavirin is active in vitro but not approved by FDA for treatment of measles.
- Vitamin A treatment of children with measles in developing countries has been associated with decreases in both morbidity and mortality.
  - The World Health Organization recommends vitamin A for all children with measles worldwide.
  - Vitamin A is given once daily for 2 days:
    - 200,000 IU for children ≥12 months of age
    - 100,000 IU for infants 6 to 11 months of age
    - 50,000 IU for infants <6 months of age
  - The higher dose may be associated with vomiting and headache for a few hours.
  - For children with signs/symptoms of vitamin A deficiency, a third dose at 4 weeks is indicated.
  - Vitamin A is available in 50,000 IU/mL injectable solution and may be given orally.

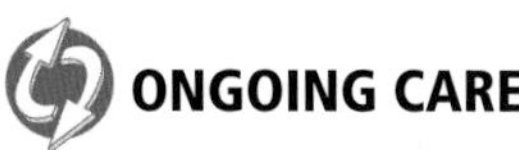

ONGOING CARE

FOLLOW-UP RECOMMENDATIONS

In uncomplicated measles infection, clinical improvement and fading of rash typically occur on the 3rd or 4th day.

PROGNOSIS

- Mortality in the modern outbreak of 1989 to 1990 occurred in 3 of every 1,000 cases in the United States.
- Case fatality rates are increased in immunocompromised children.

COMPLICATIONS

- Complication rate in 1989 to 1990 outbreaks that occurred throughout the country was 23% and included diarrhea (9%), otitis media (7%), pneumonia (6%), and encephalitis (0.1%):
  - Encephalitis, which can lead to permanent neurologic sequelae, occurs in 1 of every 1,000 cases reported in the United States.
  - Croup, myocarditis, pericarditis, and disseminated intravascular coagulation (black measles) can also occur.
- In 1990, ~18–20% of patients required hospitalization, many for either dehydration or pneumonia.
- In patients with poor nutrition, most common in developing countries, mortality is higher.
- Subacute sclerosing panencephalitis (SSPE) occurs in 1 per 100,000 children with naturally occurring measles:
  - After an incubation period of several years (mean 10.8), a progressive, usually fatal, encephalopathy develops among unvaccinated children.
  - Patients with SSPE are not infectious.

ADDITIONAL READING

- American Academy of Pediatrics. Measles. In: Kimberlin DW, Brady MT, Jackson MA, et al, eds. *Red Book: 2015 Report of the Committee on Infectious Diseases*. 30th ed. Elk Grove Village, IL: American Academy of Pediatrics; 2015:535–547.
- Bester JC. Measles and measles vaccination: a review. *JAMA Pediatr*. 2016;170(12):1209–1215.
- Centers for Disease Control and Prevention. Global measles mortality, 2000–2008. *MMWR Morb Mortal Wkly Rep*. 2009;58(47):1321–1326.
- Clemmons NS, Gastanaduy PA, Fiebelkorn AP, et al; for Centers for Disease Control and Prevention. Measles—United States, January 4–April 2, 2015. *MMWR Morb Mortal Wkly Rep*. 2015;64(14):373–376.
- Duke T, Mgone CS. Measles: not just another viral exanthem. *Lancet*. 2003;361(9359):763–773.
- Farizo KM, Stehr-Green PA, Simpson DM, et al. Pediatric emergency room visits: a risk factor for acquiring measles. *Pediatrics*. 1991;87(1):74–79.
- Fiebelkorn AP, Redd SB, Gallagher K, et al. Measles in the United States during the postelimination era. *J Infect Dis*. 2010;202(10):1520–1528.
- Gastañaduy PA, Budd J, Fisher N, et al. A measles outbreak in an underimmunized Amish community in Ohio. *N Engl J Med*. 2016;375(14):1343–1354.
- Imdad A, Mayo-Wilson E, Herzer K, et al. Vitamin A supplementation for preventing morbidity and mortality in children six months to five years of age. *Cochrane Database Syst Rev*. 2017;(3):CD008524.
- Mulholland EK, Griffiths UK, Biellik R. Measles in the 21st century. *N Engl J Med*. 2012;366(19):1755–1757.
- Rall GF. Measles virus 1998–2002: progress and controversy. *Annu Rev Microbiol*. 2003;57:343–367.
- Sugerman DE, Barskey AE, Delea MG, et al. Measles outbreak in a highly vaccinated population, San Diego, 2008: role of the intentionally undervaccinated. *Pediatrics*. 2010;125(4):747–755.

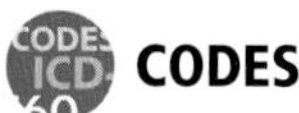

CODES

ICD10

- B05.9 Measles without complication
- B05.3 Measles complicated by otitis media
- B05.2 Measles complicated by pneumonia

FAQ

- Q: If a health care worker has had a natural measles infection or measles immunization, should one be concerned about infection following exposure?
- A: Those persons born before 1957 who had wild-type measles virus infection are usually immune from reinfection. However, in a report in 1993, four health care workers who were previously vaccinated with positive pre-illness measles antibody levels developed modified measles following exposure to infected patients. Therefore, all health care workers should observe respiratory precautions in caring for patients with measles.
- Q: During an outbreak of measles, should children <12 months of age be vaccinated?
- A: In an outbreak of measles, public health officials may recommend vaccination of infants ages 6 to 11 months with a single-antigen measles vaccine; children initially vaccinated before their first birthday should be revaccinated at 12 to 15 months of age. A second dose should be administered during the early school years.

MECKEL DIVERTICULUM

T. Matthew Shields, MD

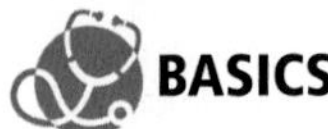

BASICS

DESCRIPTION

- Meckel diverticulum (MD) is the most common congenital abnormality of the gastrointestinal (GI) tract.
- Derives from remnants of the omphalomesenteric duct
- The most common clinical presentation of MD is painless rectal bleeding.
- Classically characterized by "Rule of 2's"
  - Present in approximately 2% of the population
  - Male-to-female ratio 2:1
  - Within 2 feet of the ileocecal valve
  - Can be up to 2 inches in length
  - Symptoms usually present by 2 years of age.

EPIDEMIOLOGY

- MD as an anomaly occurs in ~2% of the population, but only ~4% of patients with MD develop symptoms over their lifetime.
- MD is more common in patients with other malformations including anorectal atresia, esophageal atresia, omphalocele, and cardiac abnormalities.
- MD is considered to be more common in males, with a male-to-female ratio of 2:1.
- Males also more likely to have symptomatic diverticula.

PATHOPHYSIOLOGY

- Diverticula with ectopic tissue are more likely to be symptomatic.
- Ectopic tissue in MD is often of gastric origin; can also be comprised of pancreatic, duodenal, or colonic tissue
- Bleeding occurs when gastric mucosa is present, resulting in peptic ulcerations of the small bowel downstream from the diverticulum (90% of cases).
- Alkaline secretions from ectopic pancreatic tissue can also cause ulcerations with bleeding.
- Obstruction can occur when the diverticulum acts as a lead point for intussusception, when the diverticulum becomes inflamed with subsequent lumen narrowing, or when the diverticulum induces a volvulus.

ETIOLOGY

- True diverticulum (contains all three layers of the bowel wall)
- Originates from the antimesenteric border of the bowel in the region of the terminal ileum and proximal to the ileocecal valve
- Remnant of the omphalomesenteric (vitelline) duct which fails to involute completely during the 5th to 6th week of gestation as the placenta replaces the yolk sac as the source of fetal nutrition
- MD accounts for 90% of the vitelline duct anomalies. Other anomalies include the following:
  - Omphalomesenteric fistula
  - Omphalomesenteric cyst
  - Fibrous band

COMMONLY ASSOCIATED CONDITIONS

- MD has also been associated with several other congenital anomalies that include the following:
  - Anorectal atresia (affects 11% of patients with MD)
  - Esophageal atresia (12%)
  - Minor omphalocele (25%)
  - Cardiac malformations
  - Exophthalmos
  - Cleft palate
  - Annular pancreas
  - Some central nervous system malformations
- Malignancies have also been reported in association with MD.
  - Can be present within the diverticulum and can cause obstructive symptoms or can be found incidentally
  - Sarcomas are the most common malignancy associated with MD, followed by carcinoids and adenocarcinomas.

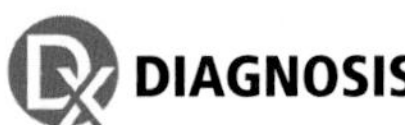

DIAGNOSIS

HISTORY

- Rectal bleeding
  - In children, the most common presentation is with painless rectal bleeding, which may range from occult blood to frank bright red blood and hemodynamic instability.
  - The bleeding tends to be self-limiting because of constriction of the splanchnic vessels secondary to hypovolemia.
  - Bleeding is most commonly seen in children <5 years of age.
- Obstruction
  - Partial or complete small bowel obstruction
  - The clinical symptoms in this setting include recurrent abdominal pain, abdominal distention, nausea, and vomiting.
  - Most common type of presentation in adults and can occur in up to 40% of pediatric patients
  - Intraperitoneal bands, volvulus, or internal herniation may also lead to an obstructive presentation.
- Inflammation/fever
  - Another common presentation for symptomatic MD is inflammation or diverticulitis, which can occur in 12–40% of cases.
  - Patients often present with signs and symptoms consistent with appendicitis, and the diagnosis is made at the time of surgical exploration.
  - In a subset of this group (~1/3), the diverticulum may perforate from infarction or ulceration and lead to a more acute and toxic presentation.

PHYSICAL EXAM

Physical exam may be normal but will often reflect the type of presenting complication:

- Bleeding
  - Tachycardia
  - Hypotension
  - Blood in the stool
  - Hyperactive bowel sounds

- Obstruction
  - Abdominal pain
  - Vomiting
  - Bilious emesis
  - Abdominal distention
- Inflammation (i.e., diverticulitis, ruptured diverticulum with peritonitis)
  - Fever
  - Abdominal tenderness
  - Symptoms more consistent with acute abdomen

DIFFERENTIAL DIAGNOSIS

- Allergic colitis
- Appendicitis
- Infectious colitis
- Polyps
- Inflammatory bowel disease
- Angiodysplasia
- Constipation/anorectal fissure
- Coagulopathy
- Henoch-Schönlein purpura
- Intussusception
- Lymphonodular hyperplasia
- Intestinal duplication

DIAGNOSTIC TESTS & INTERPRETATION

- The diagnosis of symptomatic MD is difficult to make and requires a high index of suspicion.
- This diagnosis should be considered in any patient with recurrent unexplained abdominal pain, nausea and vomiting, or rectal bleeding.

Initial Tests (screening, lab, imaging)

- The diagnosis of MD cannot be made with laboratory evaluation or plain radiography alone.
- Laboratory analysis may be helpful to determine the degree of bleeding, with a hemoglobin count and a coagulation profile to rule out an underlying coagulopathy.
- Plain radiographs may show evidence of obstruction but are not diagnostic of MD.
- Meckel scan (technetium-99m pertechnetate scan)
  - Evaluates for ectopic gastric mucosa within the diverticulum
  - Sensitivity 85%, specificity 95% in children; considerably lower in adults
  - Cimetidine can be used to increase retention of isotope within ectopic gastric mucosa.
- Mesenteric arteriography
- RBC scan with severe bleeding

Diagnostic Procedures/Other

- Surgery
  - In situations in which the Meckel scan is nondiagnostic or in patients with nonbleeding symptoms (but when there is a high index of suspicion for MD), exploratory laparoscopy may be indicated.
- Capsule endoscopy and balloon enteroscopy can establish the diagnosis but are not routinely used.

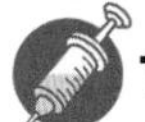

TREATMENT

The treatment for MD that are symptomatic and identified is surgical removal. Surgery involves diverticulectomy or partial bowel resection.

SURGERY/OTHER PROCEDURES

- Initial management should include supportive care.
- Correct any electrolyte abnormalities.
- Initiate proton pump inhibitor (PPI) for GI bleeding (PPI will not affect the results of the Meckel scan).
- Nasogastric tube placement for decompression of bowel obstruction
- Surgical intervention of an incidentally found MD is controversial.
  - If it is found during surgical exploration, intervention depends on the size of the diverticulum, age of the patient, and whether fibrous bands are present.
  - If it is found incidentally during radiologic imaging, symptoms should be monitored closely, but most do not recommend elective surgery.

ADMISSION, INPATIENT, AND NURSING CONSIDERATIONS

- Bleeding
  - Address issues of anemia and volume status based on vital signs and blood tests.
- Obstruction
  - Evaluate the need for acute management (surgical) and decompression.

ADDITIONAL READING

- McCollough M, Sharieff GQ. Abdominal surgical emergencies in infants and young children. *Emerg Med Clin North Am*. 2003;21(4):909–935.
- Mendelson KG, Bailey BM, Balint TD, et al. Meckel's diverticulum: review and surgical management. *Curr Surg*. 2001;58(5):455–457.
- Ruscher KA, Fisher JN, Hughes CD, et al. National trends in the surgical management of Meckel's diverticulum. *J Pediatr Surg*. 2011;46(5):893–896.
- Shalaby RY, Soliman SM, Fawy M, et al. Laparoscopic management of Meckel's diverticulum in children. *J Pediatr Surg*. 2005;40(3):562–567.
- Snyder CL. Current management of umbilical abnormalities and related anomalies. *Semin Pediatr Surg*. 2007;16(1):41–49.
- Tseng YY, Yang YJ. Clinical and diagnostic relevance of Meckel's diverticulum in children. *Eur J Pediatr*. 2009;168(12):1519–1523.
- Uppal K, Tubbs RS, Matusz P, et al. Meckel's diverticulum: a review. *Clin Anat*. 2011;24(4):416–422.
- Wong C, Dupley L, Varia H, et al. Meckel's diverticulitis: a rare entity of Meckel's diverticulum. *J Surg Case Rep*. 2017;2017(1).

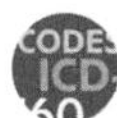

CODES

ICD10

Q43.0 Meckel's diverticulum (displaced) (hypertrophic)

FAQ

- Q: What is the reason for bleeding due to a MD?
- A: Bleeding is most commonly due to excessive acid production from ectopic gastric tissue causing mucosal breakdown in intestine downstream from the diverticulum. It is not typically from the diverticulum itself.
- Q: What is the most common type of ectopic tissue present in MD?
- A: Gastric
- Q: What is the most common presentation of a MD?
- A: Intermittent, painless rectal bleeding

M

MECONIUM ASPIRATION SYNDROME

Hussnain S. Mirza, MD, FAAP • Thomas E. Wiswell, MD

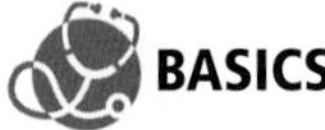

BASICS

DESCRIPTION

Meconium aspiration syndrome (MAS) is a clinical diagnosis defined as respiratory distress in a newborn delivered through meconium-stained amniotic fluid (MSAF) with no other explanation for clinical symptoms. Severity of MAS can be (i) mild: requiring $<$0.4 FiO_2 for $<$48 hours; (ii) moderate: requiring $\geq$0.4 FiO_2 for $>$48 hours with no air leak; and (iii) severe: requiring assisted ventilation or if associated with persistent pulmonary hypertension of the newborn (PPHN).

EPIDEMIOLOGY

- Frequency of MSAF: 10–15% of all pregnancies
  - MSAF is rare in premature infants and almost nonexistent before 31 weeks' gestation.
  - 2–9% infants born through MSAF develop MAS (0.2–1.4% of all live births).
- MAS accounts for 10% cases of respiratory failure in all newborns.

RISK FACTORS

- Fetal hypoxia (in utero aspiration)
- Postmature gestation
- Thick consistency of meconium
- 1- and 5-minute Apgar $<$6
- Small for gestational age (SGA)
- Chorioamnionitis
- African American or South Asian ethnicity

PATHOPHYSIOLOGY

Meconium aspiration creates ventilation/perfusion (V/Q) mismatch by the following variable effects on the airways, leading to hypoxemia, hypercarbia, acidosis, and cardiopulmonary failure.

- Mechanical obstruction of airways
  - Complete (atelectasis +/− consolidation)
  - Partial (patchy atelectasis and hyperinflation)
  - Air leaks (due to the ball-valve phenomenon)
- Meconium-associated pulmonary inflammation
- Inactivation of existing surfactant
- Decreased production of surfactant
- Meconium-induced lung apoptosis
- Coexisting pulmonary hypertension

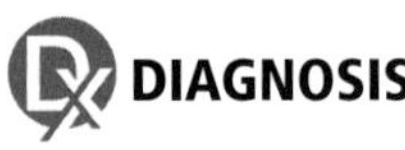

DIAGNOSIS

HISTORY

- Term or postterm gestation
- Abnormal fetal heart rate
- Evidence of MSAF
- Low Apgar score at 1 and 5 minutes
- Respiratory distress at or shortly after birth

PHYSICAL EXAM

- Meconium staining (vocal cords, skin, nails, and/or umbilical cord)
- Respiratory distress (tachypnea, retractions, grunting, cyanosis, and flaring)
- Barrel-shaped chest (air trapping or air leak)
- Rales and rhonchi
- Systolic murmur (tricuspid regurgitation) due to pulmonary hypertension
- Preductal oxygen saturation $\geq$10% higher than postductal value
- Signs of encephalopathy, particularly if associated with perinatal asphyxia
- Signs of hypoxemia (cyanosis, poor perfusion, hypotension)
- Rarely, green color urine (meconium metabolites may appear in urine)

DIFFERENTIAL DIAGNOSIS

- Transient tachypnea of newborn (TTN)
- Congenital pneumonia
- Neonatal sepsis
- Persistent pulmonary hypertension
- Congenital heart defects
- Congenital surfactant deficiency
- Amniotic aspiration syndrome

DIAGNOSTIC TESTS & INTERPRETATION

Initial Tests (screening, lab, imaging)

- CBC with differential count
  - Leukocytosis with left shift can help to identify secondary infection or congenital pneumonia; however, a left shift is also common with MAS.
- Peripheral blood culture
  - May help to identify secondary infection, sepsis, or congenital pneumonia
- Arterial blood gases (ABGs)
  - Can identify respiratory failure or hypoxemia and guide the need for respiratory support
  - An ABG is also used to calculate an oxygenation index (OI) if the infant is mechanically ventilated.
- Initial chest radiograph
  - Radiographic appearance lags behind clinical symptoms.
  - Frequently, there is no direct correlation between the extent of radiographic abnormalities and the severity of disease.
  - Initial radiograph can be normal or may have some streaky, linear densities.
- Follow-up chest radiograph
  - As the disease progresses, there can be diffuse patchy densities, hyperinflation, flattening of the diaphragm, pleural effusion, alternating areas of atelectasis, hyperinflation, and consolidation.
  - Significant air leaks can be noted in 10–30% of infants with MAS.

Diagnostic Procedures/Other

- Pre- and postductal SpO_2 gradient
  - $>$10% may be associated with PPHN.
- OI
  - OI = (FiO_2 × mean airway pressure × 100) / PaO_2
  - After optimizing mechanical ventilation, OI $>$40 on two serial ABGs performed 4 hours apart is an indication for extracorporeal membrane oxygenation (ECMO).
- Echocardiography
  - To rule out congenital heart disease and to evaluate for PPHN

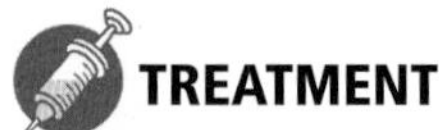

TREATMENT

GENERAL MEASURES

- Neonatal ICU care
  - For SpO_2 and continuous cardiopulmonary monitoring, to provide optimal thermal environment, and to ensure minimal handling
- Chest percussion or physiotherapy is generally not recommended.
- IV fluids
  - Required for maintenance of hydration and prevention of hypoglycemia
  - IV fluid bolus may be required for hypovolemia or hypoperfusion.
- Cardiotropic therapy
  - May be required to support the systemic perfusion especially if cardiac output is low due to left ventricular (LV) dysfunction (hypoxia or acidosis), severe PPHN, or decreased venous return
- Sedation
  - May be helpful to decrease agitation, optimize ventilation, and minimize right-to-left shunting. However, routine use of paralysis or muscle relaxants is controversial, as they may increase the risk for atelectasis and V/Q mismatch.
- Feeding
  - During acute phase of severe illness, enteral feedings are discouraged to protect the underperfused gut from ischemic injury.
- Preventive measures
  - Prevention of fetal hypoxia
    - Optimal obstetric care is the key for prevention of MAS. The decreased incidence of MAS in the last decade has been attributed to the reduction in postterm delivery and aggressive management of abnormal fetal heart tracings.
  - Amnioinfusion: not recommended
  - Intratracheal suctioning in the delivery room is also recommended only if clinical findings of airway obstruction are present.
  - Gastric suctioning: no clinical benefit to prevent or decrease the severity of clinical symptoms or feeding intolerance associated with MAS
  - Contraindicated procedures:
    - Attempts to prevent deep inspiration prior to oropharyngeal or endotracheal suctioning by mechanical means (e.g., cricoid pressure, manual blockage of the airway, and thoracic compression)

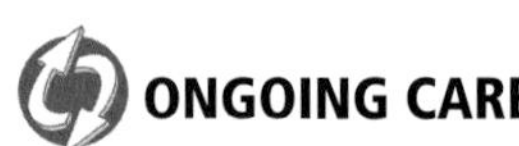

ONGOING CARE

FOLLOW-UP RECOMMENDATIONS

- Long-term consequences include increased bronchial reactivity and wheezing among the survivors of MAS.
- Infants with severe MAS are at risk for adverse neurodevelopmental outcomes. We recommend developmental follow-up for infants with severe MAS.

PROGNOSIS

- Severity of lung injury is related to the consistency of meconium (thick meconium is high risk for severe disease) and to the degree of hypoxia and acidosis present at birth.
- Generally, 1/3 of infants with MAS need mechanical ventilation, 15–20% develop PPHN, and 10–30% can have air leaks.
- In spite of appropriate management and clinical care, up to 10% of infants with severe MAS may die.

COMPLICATIONS

- Respiratory failure
  - One third of infants with MAS develop respiratory failure and require mechanical ventilation.
- Air leaks
  - Up to 10% infants with MAS may develop pneumothorax or pneumomediastinum in spite of appropriate management strategies.
- Pulmonary hemorrhage
  - Occurs in $<1\%$ infants with MAS and can occasionally cause severe destabilization and hypoxemia
- Birth depression
  - Occurs in 20–33% of infants born through MSAF
  - These infants can have neurologic manifestations of hypoxic ischemic encephalopathy (HIE) and need appropriate management.
- SIADH
  - More likely to occur among infants with a history of perinatal asphyxia or air leaks
- PPHN
  - Occurs in 15–20% of infants with MAS
  - PPHN in these infants may be caused by (i) pulmonary vasoconstriction secondary to pulmonary inflammation, hypoxia, hypercarbia, and acidosis and (ii) pulmonary vascular remodeling as a result of chronic intrauterine hypoxia.
- Secondary lung infection
  - Meconium provides an excellent growth medium for microorganisms. Meconium may also inhibit polymorphonuclear cells.
- Reactive airway disease
  - Up to 50% of infants who survive severe MAS are at risk to develop reactive airway disease during infancy and beyond.

MEDICATION

- IV antibiotics
  - In the early stage of the disease, it is difficult to differentiate between MAS and congenital pneumonia. Many clinicians treat empirically while awaiting the results of cultures.
  - Prophylactic antibiotic treatment does not prevent secondary infection in MAS.
- Surfactant bolus treatment
  - Bolus surfactant therapy may decrease the severity of illness and need for ECMO and should be considered for all intubated infants with MAS requiring $F_{IO_2} > 0.4$.
  - Small clinical trials of surfactant lung lavage showed some benefit. However, additional larger trials are needed to confirm the benefit of this therapy.
- Steroid therapy
  - Limited clinical data indicate possible benefits of both systemal and inhalational steroids.
  - More data are needed before steroid therapy can be recommended for routine use in MAS.
- Inhaled nitric oxide (iNO)
  - iNO is used to treat PPHN associated with MAS.

ADDITIONAL THERAPIES

- Oxygen therapy
  - Keep peripheral Sp_{O_2} between 92% and 98% or Pa_{O_2} between 60 and 80 torr (8 to 10.7 kPa) for infants without pulmonary hypertension.
  - If MAS is complicated by PPHN, maintain higher Pa_{O_2} (80 to 100 mmHg) and Sp_{O_2} (95–99%).
  - Oxygen can be provided via oxyhood or nasal cannula. However, if >0.5 F_{IO_2} is required to achieve the above-mentioned goal, consider additional respiratory support like mechanical ventilation, surfactant, and nitric oxide.
- Continuous positive airway pressure (CPAP)
  - Due to the possible complications (i.e., air trapping, hyperinflation, and air leaks), many clinicians prefer to avoid CPAP. However, CPAP can be cautiously used if air trapping or air leak is not a major issue.
- Conventional ventilation
  - Most common form of mechanical ventilation to manage respiratory failure among infants with MAS
  - No specific mode has been proven superior.
  - Most clinicians prefer low positive end-expiratory pressure (PEEP), low rate and higher inspiratory to expiratory time ratio (I:E) to prevent hyperinflation, air trapping, and air leaks.
- High-frequency oscillatory ventilation (HFOV):
  - HFOV is used as a rescue treatment. No clinical trial has demonstrated clear benefits of HFOV over conventional mode in the initial management of MAS.
  - Indications for transitioning to HFOV include ongoing hypoxemia, high F_{IO_2}, and respiratory acidosis. In infants with significant atelectasis, adequate lung recruitment may require considerably higher mean airway pressure.
- High-frequency jet ventilation (HFJV):
  - HFJV is an alternative choice when high-frequency ventilation is required. No clinical study to date has been conducted to compare the benefits of HFOV or HFJV for infants with MAS.
  - Anecdotally, some infants with intractable hypoxemia and/or respiratory acidosis do show improvements after transition from HFOV to HFJV.
  - On HFJV, a significantly higher I:E ratio is possible (up to 1:12) by using low JET frequency (240 bpm) and standard inspiratory time (0.02 seconds) that is desirable especially for infants with air leak or air trapping.
- ECMO
  - Indicated for severe respiratory failure manifested by an OI >40 on two serial ABGs performed 4 hours apart while on optimal mechanical ventilation
  - Veno-arterial or veno-venous ECMO can be considered in the absence of any vital organ failure, significant congenital anomaly, genetic syndrome, or intraventricular hemorrhage.

ADDITIONAL READING

- Chettri S, Adhisivam B, Bhat BV. Endotracheal suction for nonvigorous neonates born through meconium stained amniotic fluid: a randomized controlled trial. *J Pediatr*. 2015;166(5):1208.e1–1213.e1.
- Dargaville PA. Respiratory support in meconium aspiration syndrome: a practical guide. *Int J Pediatr*. 2012;2012:965159.
- Mokra D, Calkovska A. How to overcome surfactant dysfunction in meconium aspiration syndrome? *Respir Physiol Neurobiol*. 2013;187(1):58–63.
- Natarajan CK, Sankar MJ, Jain K, et al. Surfactant therapy and antibiotics in neonates with meconium aspiration syndrome: a systematic review and meta-analysis. *J Perinatol*. 2016;(36 Suppl 1):S49–S54.
- Swarnam K, Soraisham AS, Sivanandan S. Advances in the management of meconium aspiration syndrome. *Int J Pediatr*. 2012;2012:359571.

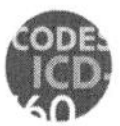

CODES

ICD10

- P24.01 Meconium aspiration with respiratory symptoms
- P24.00 Meconium aspiration without respiratory symptoms

FAQ

- Q: What is the composition of meconium?
- A: Meconium is a variable mixture of intestinal epithelial debris, gastrointestinal secretions, bile, mucus, pancreatic juice, blood, swallowed vernix caseosa, and lanugo.
- Q: How to manage infants born through MSAF?
- A: Asymptomatic infants should be managed like normal newborns. We recommend observing depressed infants for any signs of respiratory distress for at least 24 hours following birth.
- Q: What are the changes in the recommendations for intratracheal suctioning of meconium-stained infants at delivery?
- A: The *Neonatal Resuscitation Program* (7th edition) no longer recommends routine delivery room intubation in depressed meconium-stained infants. The procedure is only recommended if there are clinical signs of airway obstruction. It is believed that attention to ventilation and oxygenation is of upmost importance.
- Q: Meconium-stained amniotic fluid was reported for an infant with severe respiratory distress born at 30 weeks' gestation; what differential diagnosis shall be considered?
- A: Chorioamnionitis (especially secondary to the *Listeria monocytogenes*) is possible if a history of meconium-stained amniotic fluid is given for a preterm infant. Meconium aspiration is extremely rare prior to 34 weeks' gestation.
- Q: A nurse in the neonatal intensive care unit taking care of an infant with MAS noted green color urine in the diaper. What is the likely explanation?
- A: Green urine may be observed in newborns with MAS. Meconium pigments can be absorbed by the lungs, enter the systemic circulation, and be excreted in urine.

MEDIASTINAL MASS

Michelle L. Hermiston, MD, PhD

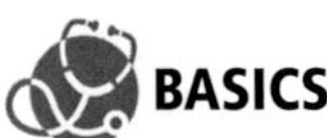

BASICS

DESCRIPTION

Space-occupying lesion of the mediastinum

- Anterior mediastinum includes the thymus and other structures anterior to the pericardium.
- Middle mediastinum contains the heart, great vessels, ascending aorta, and aortic arch, as well as lymph nodes.
- Posterior mediastinum contains the tracheobronchial tree, esophagus, descending aorta, and neural structures.

PATHOPHYSIOLOGY

Morbidity is due to compression of adjacent normal structures, particularly large airways, heart, and great vessels.

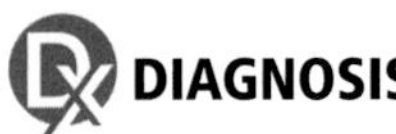

DIAGNOSIS

Goal is to quickly establish diagnosis and begin treatment as indicated, as condition may rapidly progress and become life-threatening. If malignancy is suspected, the child should be immediately referred to an oncologist.

HISTORY

- **Question:** Systemic symptoms (fever, weight loss, night sweats, fatigue)?
- *Significance*: may be associated with infection or malignancy
- **Question:** Cough, wheeze, dyspnea on exertion, orthopnea?
- *Significance*: may indicate early airway compromise
- **Question:** Face/neck swelling?
- *Significance*: suggests superior vena cava syndrome

PHYSICAL EXAM

Focused attention for signs of respiratory distress or cardiovascular compromise. Check for signs and symptoms noted below.

- **Finding:** Edema/suffusion of face and neck, jugular venous distension, conjunctival injection, headache, altered mental status?
- *Significance*: superior vena cava syndrome
- **Finding:** Cough (nonproductive), orthopnea or dyspnea, stridor, or wheezing?
- *Significance*: airway compression
- **Finding:** Quiet heart sounds, hypotension, narrowed pulse pressure, or pulsus paradoxus?
- *Significance*: cardiac tamponade/diastolic dysfunction secondary to mass effect
- **Finding:** Lymphadenopathy or hepatosplenomegaly?
- *Significance*: malignancy or infection; low cervical, posterior, or supraclavicular adenopathy particularly concerning for malignancy
- **Finding:** Pallor, ecchymoses, petechiae, and/or mucosal bleeding?
- *Significance*: suggest anemia and thrombocytopenia, which are seen in malignant conditions also infiltrating the bone marrow
- **Finding:** Horner syndrome
- *Significance*: posterior mediastinal mass, most commonly a neuroblastoma

DIFFERENTIAL DIAGNOSIS

- Congenital/anatomic
  - Large normal thymus in neonate (anterior)
  - Bronchogenic, pericardial, or foregut cyst (middle)
  - Aortic aneurysm and other vascular anomalies (middle)
  - Thoracic meningocele (posterior)
- Infectious (may cause mediastinal adenopathy and/or pulmonary nodules) (middle/posterior)
  - Tuberculosis
  - Histoplasmosis
  - Aspergillosis
  - Coccidioidomycosis
  - Blastomycosis
- Foreign body in the trachea or esophagus
- Sarcoidosis
- Tumor
  - Benign
    - Thymoma (anterior)
    - Teratoma/dermoid cyst (anterior)
    - Thyroid (goiter) (anterior/superior)
    - Lymphangioma/cystic hygroma (middle/posterior)
    - Hemangioma (middle/posterior)
    - Ganglioneuroma (posterior)
    - Neurofibroma (posterior)
  - Malignant
    - Malignant germ cell tumor (anterior)
    - Hodgkin lymphoma (anterior/middle)
    - Non-Hodgkin lymphoma or leukemia (anterior/middle)
    - Thyroid cancer (anterior/superior)
    - Neuroblastoma (posterior)
    - Ganglioneuroblastoma (posterior)
    - Ewing sarcoma or osteogenic sarcoma (anterior/posterior)
    - Pheochromocytoma (posterior)
    - Neurofibrosarcoma (posterior)
    - Rhabdomyosarcoma or pleuropulmonary blastoma (any)

DIAGNOSTIC TESTS & INTERPRETATION

Initial Tests (screening, lab, imaging)

- **Test:** CBC with differential
- *Significance*: anemia, thrombocytopenia, and neutropenia noted in malignant diseases infiltrating bone marrow. Circulating blasts frequently noted in leukemia or lymphoma; leukocytosis in infection
- **Test:** lactate dehydrogenase, uric acid, electrolytes, calcium, phosphate, creatinine
- *Significance*: tumor lysis screen
- **Test:** purified protein derivative (PPD) skin test
- *Significance*: tuberculosis
- **Test:** urine vanillylmandelic acid (VMA) and homovanillic acid (HVA)
- *Significance*: elevated in 90% of children with neuroblastoma
- **Test:** α-fetoprotein and β-hCG
- *Significance*: can be elevated in germ cell tumors
- **Test:** other assays for specific pathogens based on history of exposure
- *Significance*: For a patient with a large mass or potential cardiopulmonary compromise, goal is rapid diagnosis using least invasive/painful procedure, to minimize need for sedation/anesthesia.
- **Test:** pulmonary function test
- *Significance*: may be useful to assess pulmonary reserve
- **Test:** bone marrow aspiration/biopsy
- *Significance*: simplest procedure if CBC is suspicious
- **Test:** lymph node biopsy
- *Significance*: if adenopathy at easily accessible site
- **Test:** biopsy of mass
- *Significance*: Consider radiologically guided fine-needle biopsy.
- **Test:** pleurocentesis, pericardiocentesis, or excision of isolated mass
- *Significance*: may have both diagnostic and therapeutic roles
- **Test:** lumbar puncture
- *Significance*: may be combined with other procedures if meningitis or hematologic malignancy is suspected

ALERT

Recumbent positioning, sedation, or positive pressure ventilation may lead to catastrophic respiratory or cardiovascular collapse in patients with partial compromise.

- Imaging of airway and consultation with anesthesiologist, surgeons, and critical care specialists should be obtained prior to any sedation.
- Procedures may need to be done with local anesthesia only with patient sitting upright.
- If patient develops acute airway compromise, place prone to decrease pressure of mass on airway.
- Chest radiograph (lateral film required) to establish size and location of mass
- CT of the chest (if patient can tolerate semirecumbent positioning)
  - To define size, location, and consistency of mass
  - To assess large blood vessels and airways
  - To assess safety for anesthesia or oral sedation/pain medications
- Echocardiogram to assess diastolic filling and vascular patency

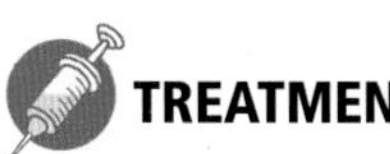

TREATMENT

GENERAL MEASURES

- Close monitoring of cardiorespiratory status
- With cardiorespiratory compromise, avoid positive-pressure ventilation, if feasible.
- Definitive therapy will be based on the diagnosis.

MEDICATION

First Line

- Steroids may be given after diagnosis is established to treat hematologic malignancies or decrease edema/inflammation.
- If leukemia/lymphoma, diagnostic lumbar puncture should be performed prior to steroid treatment if possible.
- Additional therapy depends on diagnosis (e.g., chemotherapy, antibiotics).

ADDITIONAL THERAPIES

Radiotherapy

- May be indicated for emergent management of malignancies

ALERT

- Do not treat a patient with wheezing who has no history of asthma with steroids without obtaining a chest radiograph to confirm that there is no mediastinal mass.
- If symptoms are progressing rapidly or there is evidence of superior vena cava syndrome, tracheal compression or spinal cord compression, emergent steroids, or radiation may be required, following rapid diagnostic procedures if possible.

SURGERY/OTHER PROCEDURES

- May be required for diagnostic biopsy
- Excision may relieve acute compression and may be primary therapy for isolated benign mass.

ONGOING CARE

ADMISSION, INPATIENT, AND NURSING CONSIDERATIONS

- Admission criteria
  - All patients with significant mass, until cardiopulmonary risk defined
  - All patients with evidence of significant airway or vascular compression
  - All patients with evidence of significant tumor lysis syndrome
- Discharge criteria
  - Resolution/resection of mass or clear evidence of cardiopulmonary stability through all activities of daily living (ADLs), including sleep

COMPLICATIONS

- Superior vena cava syndrome
- Tracheal compression
- Spinal cord compression
- Pleural and pericardial effusions
- Secondary infection
- Horner syndrome: ptosis, miosis, and anhidrosis resulting from compression of the cervical sympathetic nerve trunk
- Esophageal narrowing or erosion: may result in feeding difficulty or bleeding
- Tumor lysis syndrome with electrolyte disturbances, kidney failure

ADDITIONAL READING

- Franco A, Mody NS, Meza MP. Imaging evaluation of pediatric mediastinal masses. *Radiol Clin North Am*. 2005;43(2):325–353.
- Gothard JW. Anesthetic considerations for patients with anterior mediastinal masses. *Anesthesiol Clin*. 2008;26(2):305–314.
- Pearson JK, Tan GM. Pediatric anterior mediastinal mass: a review article. *Semin Cardiothorac Vasc Anesth*. 2015;19(3):248–254.
- Pizzo PA, Poplack DG, eds. *Principles and Practice of Pediatric Oncology*. 7th ed. Philadelphia, PA: Lippincott Williams & Wilkins; 2015.

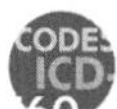

CODES

ICD10

- R22.2 Localized swelling, mass and lump, trunk
- Q34.1 Congenital cyst of mediastinum
- D15.2 Benign neoplasm of mediastinum

FAQ

- Q: What should be done if the child is asymptomatic and a mediastinal mass is an incidental finding on chest radiograph?
- A: Careful history and physical exam with specific attention to pulmonary, cardiac, and hematologic systems.
  - Vital signs to include temperature and pulse oximetry
  - CBC with differential, ESR, tumor lysis labs
  - PPD, anergy panel if high risk for tuberculosis or initial evaluation is negative
  - CT of chest
  - Referral to oncologist, surgeon, or infectious disease specialist pending above results
- Q: When should an oncologist be consulted?
- A: With any of the following:
  - Rapidly enlarging mass
  - Signs and symptoms of tracheal compression, superior vena cava syndrome, or spinal cord compression
  - Hepatomegaly, splenomegaly, lymphadenopathy, bruises, or petechiae on physical examination
  - Anemia, thrombocytopenia, or leukocytosis suggesting bone marrow involvement
  - Malignant histology demonstrated with biopsy
  - When help is needed in establishing diagnosis

M

MEGALOBLASTIC ANEMIA

Tiffany F. Lin, MD

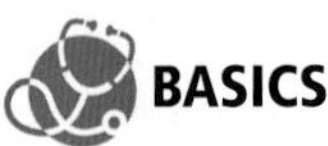

BASICS

DESCRIPTION

- Macrocytosis refers to a blood condition in which red blood cells (RBCs) are larger than normal. It is reported in terms of mean corpuscular volume (MCV). Normal MCV values range from 80 to 100 fL and vary by age and reference laboratory.
- No complications arise from macrocytosis itself as an isolated finding; however, its presence can suggest an underlying pathologic state.
- Macrocytosis with associated anemia (macrocytic anemia) can be broadly classified as megaloblastic or nonmegaloblastic anemia.
- Megaloblastic anemia describes an anemic state characterized by the presence of abnormally large RBCs (macro-ovalocytes) and hypersegmented neutrophils in the peripheral blood and bone marrow.

EPIDEMIOLOGY

- The incidence and prevalence is unknown, although is significantly less common than iron deficiency anemia.
- The most frequent causes of megaloblastic anemia are disorders resulting from vitamin B_{12} (cobalamin) or folate deficiency.

PATHOPHYSIOLOGY

- Megaloblastic anemia is a direct result of ineffective or dysplastic erythropoiesis caused by a defect in DNA synthesis that interferes with cellular proliferation and maturation.
- When vitamin B_{12} or folate is deficient, RBC proliferation and maturation result in large erythroblasts with nuclear/cytoplasmic asynchrony. The erythroblasts become large, oval shaped, and contain a characteristic immature, lacy nucleus. These bone marrow features are called "megaloblastic."
- Nonmegaloblastic anemia are associated with accelerated erythropoiesis or increased red cell membrane phospholipid production.

ETIOLOGY

- The most common etiologies of megaloblastic anemia are vitamin B_{12} or folate deficiencies.
- Medications or severe copper deficiencies are another less common cause of megaloblastic anemia.
- Pernicious anemia
  - Common cause of megaloblastic anemia in adults but rare in children
  - A type of vitamin B_{12} deficiency anemia and is caused by a decrease in the secretion of intrinsic factor (IF) by gastric parietal cells in the setting of autoimmune atrophic gastritis. IF is a protein essential for absorption of vitamin B_{12} in the ileum.
- Nonmegaloblastic macrocytic anemias can be due to
  - Alcohol intake
  - Liver disease (with normal vitamin B_{12} and folate),
  - Diamond-Blackfan anemia
  - Myelodysplastic syndrome

DIAGNOSIS

HISTORY

- Pallor, fatigue, poor appetite, irritability caused by anemia
- Malabsorption/diarrhea, steatorrhea, weight loss can be signs of gastrointestinal (GI) acute infections or chronic inflammatory disease that can contribute to vitamin B_{12} or folic acid loss
- Neurologic symptoms primarily seen in vitamin B_{12} deficiency:
  - Paresthesias, altered gait, impaired vision, psychiatric symptoms
- Diet history
  - General malnutrition
  - Personal history of strict veganism without milk, cheese, or egg intake (vitamin B_{12} deficiency)
  - Infants with vegan mothers (vitamin B_{12} deficiency)
  - Infants fed goat's milk (folic acid deficiency)
- Family history of pernicious anemia or autoimmune diseases
- Surgical history of partial or total gastrectomy, ileal resection, splenectomy
- Drug history
  - Anticonvulsants
  - Chemotherapy agents, particularly antimetabolites
  - HIV antiretrovirals
  - Metformin
  - Aminosalicylates
  - Nitrous oxide, use and abuse

PHYSICAL EXAM

- Pallor, pale conjunctiva
- Glossitis: smooth, tender tongue (associated with vitamin B_{12} deficiency)
- Neurologic findings (associated with vitamin B_{12} deficiency)
  - Muscular weakness
  - Peripheral neuropathy
  - Abnormal position and vibratory sensation
  - Ataxia
  - Positive Babinski test
  - Psychiatric and cognitive changes

DIFFERENTIAL DIAGNOSIS

The differential diagnosis for megaloblastic anemia is large and should include other causes of macrocytic anemia:

- Vitamin B_{12} deficiency
- Folate deficiency
- Bone marrow disorders (e.g., myelodysplastic syndrome)
- Marked reticulocytosis during marrow recovery from microcytic or normocytic anemia (can cause high RDW with high MCV because of increased size of reticulocytes)
- Chronic alcohol abuse
- Chronic liver disease
- Hypothyroidism
- Chronic lung disease with hypoxia
- Heavy smoking
- Pregnancy
- Medications (as listed in "History")
- Arsenic poisoning

DIAGNOSTIC TESTS & INTERPRETATION

Initial Tests (screening, lab, imaging)

- Complete blood count with differential
  - Decreased hemoglobin
  - Increased MCV
  - May have normal or decreased white blood cell count and platelets depending on degree of megaloblastosis
- Peripheral blood smear in megaloblastic anemia
  - Macro-ovalocytes
  - Hypersegmented neutrophils
  - Poikilocytosis: abnormally shaped RBCs
  - Anisocytosis: abnormal variation in size of RBCs
- Reticulocyte count: low
- Increased homocysteine levels

- Serum vitamin B_{12} level:
  - <100 pg/mL: vitamin B_{12} deficiency
  - 100 to 400 pg/mL: borderline result; check serum methylmalonic acid (MMA) and homocysteine levels to help differentiate between vitamin B_{12} deficiency and folate deficiency.
  - >400 pg/mL: Vitamin B_{12} deficiency is unlikely; check RBC folate level.
- RBC folate level: low in folate deficiency
- If the above testing does not reveal an obvious diagnosis, consider further testing:
  - Comprehensive metabolic panel to look for liver and kidney disease, hemolysis, hematologic malignancies or disorders
  - Thyroid-stimulating hormone to look for thyroid disorders
  - Bone marrow examination to check for myelodysplastic syndrome or Diamond-Blackfan anemia
  - Testing for orotic aciduria

ALERT

Coexistent microcytic anemias due to iron deficiency, thalassemias, and chronic disease can obscure the diagnosis of megaloblastic anemia by lowering the MCV. Hypersegmented neutrophils will still persist in the peripheral blood smear and aid in diagnosis.

- Diagnostic imaging with a barium study may be needed to rule out GI anomalies.

Diagnostic Procedures/Other

- Consider a referral to a hematologist for a bone marrow examination if the diagnosis remains unclear.
- Diagnostic testing for pernicious anemia may include the following:
  - Serum anti-IF antibodies, gastric parietal cell antibodies, pepsinogen (PG) I and II, gastrin
  - Schilling test

TREATMENT

ALERT

It is imperative that vitamin B_{12} deficiency is diagnosed correctly. Treatment of undiagnosed vitamin B_{12} deficiency with folate replacement will not improve the neurologic deficits and may worsen the condition while improving the hematologic parameters.

ALERT

Hypokalemia associated with vitamin B_{12} repletion can be life-threatening. For severe anemia, a lower initial dose of cyanocobalamin of 0.2 mcg/kg/dose IM or SQ for 2 days followed by the above regimen(s) has been recommended. The clinician should anticipate this complication and provide a potassium supplement.

MEDICATION

- Folate deficiency
  - Folic acid 1 to 5 mg PO daily for 1 to 4 months or until complete hematologic recovery occurs
  - Long-term treatment is not warranted except in certain cases of malnutrition or ongoing hemolysis.
- Several forms and administration regimens exist for vitamin B_{12} deficiency:
  - Cyanocobalamin 1,000 mcg/24 h IM or SQ for 2 to 7 days based on clinical response, followed by 100 mcg weekly for 1 month and then monthly maintenance doses thereafter
  - Hydroxocobalamin 1,000 mcg IM every 1 to 3 months is also an effective therapy due to its long half-life in the tissues.
  - Oral cyanocobalamin 1,000 to 2,000 mcg/24 h for 1 month, followed by 125 to 150 mcg/24 h with option to taper to less frequent dosing
  - In some cases, nasal and sublingual cyanocobalamin may also be useful in replenishing vitamin B_{12} stores.
  - In the majority of patients (e.g., pernicious anemia), treatment is usually lifelong due to abnormal absorption.

FOLLOW-UP RECOMMENDATIONS

Patient Monitoring

- Metabolic abnormalities begin to normalize within the first 1 to 2 days following treatment with parenteral vitamin B_{12}.
- Reticulocytosis occurs about 3 to 4 days, peaking at 1 week, followed by a rise in hemoglobin within 10 days and a fall in MCV. The hemoglobin will normalize by 8 weeks. A delayed response suggests the presence of an additional abnormality or an incorrect diagnosis.
- Hypersegmented neutrophils disappear at 10 to 14 days.
- During this period, the patient might note an improved feeling of well-being, long before there are any changes in the degree of anemia.
- Dementia and depression often respond to therapy, whereas other neurologic abnormalities improve gradually over a period of 6 months and may not return to normal.

PROGNOSIS

- In cases of dietary deficiencies, the prognosis is good.
- Inborn errors of metabolism with associated megaloblastic anemia generally has a poor outcome.

COMPLICATIONS

- Patients with severe anemia may have accompanying heart failure because of the anemia itself and myocardial hypoxia. However, due to its insidious onset, this is a rare finding in megaloblastic anemias.
- Neurologic complications from vitamin B_{12} deficiency
- Concomitant folate deficiency can complicate the diagnosis of vitamin B_{12} deficiency.

ADDITIONAL READING

- Aslinia F, Mazza JJ, Yale SH. Megaloblastic anemia and other causes of macrocytosis. *Clin Med Res.* 2006;4(3):236–241.
- Kaferle J, Strzoda CE. Evaluation of macrocytosis. *Am Fam Physician.* 2009;79(3):203–208.
- Wickramasinghe SN. Diagnosis of megaloblastic anaemias. *Blood Rev.* 2006;20(6):299–318.

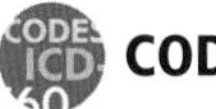

CODES

ICD10

- D53.1 Other megaloblastic anemias, not elsewhere classified
- D75.89 Other specified diseases of blood and blood-forming organs
- D51.8 Other vitamin B12 deficiency anemias

FAQ

- Q: What are the common dietary sources of vitamin B_{12}?
- A: Red meat, liver, seafood, chicken, dairy products, eggs
- Q: What are the common dietary sources of folate?
- A: Vegetables (especially green, leafy ones), legumes/beans, peanuts, liver. Since 1998, many grain food products have been fortified with folate in the United States and Canada, including breads, cereals, flours, pastas, and rice.

M

MENINGITIS

Ross Newman, DO, MHPE

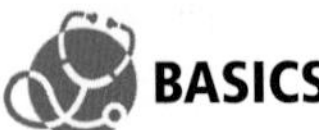

BASICS

DESCRIPTION

Inflammation of the membranes of the brain or spinal cord, usually caused by viruses or bacteria and, rarely, fungi or parasites

EPIDEMIOLOGY

- Bacterial meningitis
  - Most common agents in children of all ages include *Streptococcus pneumoniae* and *Neisseria meningitidis*.
  - Underlying host factors, age, exposure, and geographic location alter incidence and pathogen.
- Viral meningitis
  - Most common agent in all age groups
  - Most common isolated viruses are enteroviruses that tend to occur in outbreaks in summer and early fall.
- Fungal meningitis
  - *Cryptococcus neoformans* is a budding encapsulated yeast-like organism found in soil and avian excreta; associated with immunocompromised patients (especially AIDS), rare cases in healthy children
  - *Candida* species occurs in immunocompromised patients and ill premature infants.
- Tuberculous meningitis
  - *Mycobacterium tuberculosis* (TB) meningitis occurs in 0.5% of untreated primary TB infections.
  - Most common in children aged 6 months to 4 years
  - In ~50% of cases, miliary TB is accompanied by meningitis.

GENERAL PREVENTION

- *Haemophilus influenzae* type b (Hib) vaccine has significantly reduced the incidence of meningitis and other invasive Hib infections by up to 99%.
- 13-valent pneumococcal conjugate vaccine (PCV13) for use in all infants given at 2, 4, 6, and 12 to 15 months of age
- Quadrivalent meningococcal vaccine for serogroups A, C, Y, and W is recommended for all patients ≥11 years of age and select at-risk populations <11 years. A booster dose is recommended for all patients who receive the first dose of the vaccine between 11 and 15 years of age.
- Children with anatomic or functional asplenia or persistent complement deficiency should be considered for meningococcal serogroup B vaccines.

ETIOLOGY

- Bacterial
  - Cause differs depending on age:
    - <1 month old: group B *Streptococcus*, gram-negative pathogens (*Escherichia coli*, *Citrobacter koseri*, *Cronobacter sakazakii*, *Serratia marcescens*, and *Salmonella* species), *Listeria monocytogenes*, *S. pneumoniae*
    - 1 to 3 months old: group B *Streptococcus*, *E. coli*, *S. pneumoniae*, Hib
    - 3 months to 5 years old: *S. pneumoniae*, *N. meningitidis*, Hib
    - >5 years old: *S. pneumoniae*, *N. meningitidis*
    - Consider Hib in unvaccinated patients of any age.
- Viral
  - Herpes simplex virus (HSV) in the neonatal population
  - Enteroviruses: ~70 different strains that include polioviruses, coxsackie A, coxsackie B, and echoviruses. Recently discovered enteroviruses are not placed in these four groups but are numbered (e.g., enterovirus 68).
  - Other, less common: arboviruses (e.g., West Nile virus), mumps
- Fungal
  - Fungi most commonly isolated include *Candida* species, *Coccidioides immitis*, *C. neoformans*, and *Aspergillus* species.
- Aseptic meningitis
  - Agents not easily cultured in the viral or microbiology laboratory can cause meningitis and include *Borrelia burgdorferi* (Lyme disease) and *Treponema pallidum* (syphilis).
- Tuberculous meningitis
- Unusual pathogens more likely in immunocompromised patients

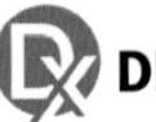

DIAGNOSIS

HISTORY

- Bacterial meningitis
  - Older children may complain of classic meningeal inflammation signs including neck pain, headache, or back pain as well as photophobia, anorexia, and myalgias.
  - Nausea and vomiting are common.
  - In younger children, symptoms are often nonspecific, including fever, hypothermia, irritability, and poor feeding as well as signs of increased intracranial pressure, including seizures and apnea.
  - Attention should be noted to the patient's immunization status, birth history, travel history, trauma, health status, geographic location, and exposure to high-risk contacts.
  - Common chief complaints by the infants' caregivers include the following:
    - Irritable or "sleeping all the time"
    - "Won't take to bottle"
    - "Not acting right"
    - "Cries when moved or picked up"
- Viral meningitis
  - Headache and fever may precede signs of meningitis, such as stiff neck, vomiting, and photophobia.
  - Duration 2 to 6 days
- Fungal meningitis
  - Cryptococcal meningitis is often indolent, with complaints of worsening headaches and vomiting for days to weeks.
  - Exposure to pigeon or other bird droppings can be a valuable clue.
- Tuberculous meningitis
  - Symptoms are often nonspecific initially, with personality changes, fever, nausea, and vomiting progressing to anorexia, irritability, and lethargy (stage I disease).
  - Stage II disease is characterized by focal neurologic signs (most often involving the cranial nerves III, VI, and VII).
  - Stage III disease is characterized by coma and papilledema.

PHYSICAL EXAM

- Stiff neck in older children. Infants have poor neck muscle tone and this finding is commonly absent.
- Brudzinski and Kernig signs may be present.
  - Brudzinski sign: With the patient supine, flexion of the neck elicits involuntary flexion of the hips or knees.
  - Kernig sign: With the patient supine, the legs are flexed 90 degrees at the hip, extensions of the lower legs are unable to be accomplished beyond 135 degrees.
  - Negative Brudzinski or Kernig sign does not rule out meningitis.
- Younger children may not have nuchal rigidity and Kernig and/or Brudzinski signs.
- Any infant presenting with a sepsis-like picture needs to have meningitis as a consideration.
- Classically, there may be "paradoxical" crying—crying that increases when child is picked up.
- Signs of increased intracranial pressure, including papilledema, asymmetric pupils, bulging fontanelle, diplopia
- Skin exam for erythema migrans from borreliosis (Lyme disease), petechiae, or purpura with invasive meningococcal disease or vesicles in an infant <6 weeks old with HSV

DIFFERENTIAL DIAGNOSIS

- Encephalitis
- Toxic encephalopathy
- Epidural abscess
- Cerebral abscess

DIAGNOSTIC TESTS & INTERPRETATION

Initial Tests (screening, lab, imaging)

- CSF analysis (cell count with differential, protein measurement, glucose concentration, and measurement of pressure)
- CSF Gram stain and culture
- Blood culture
- CBC, platelet count, electrolytes, BUN, creatinine, serum glucose
- Consider prothrombin time (PT), partial thromboplastin time (PTT), liver function tests, arterial blood gas

Diagnostic Procedures/Other

- Lumbar puncture
  - Contraindicated with cardiopulmonary compromise, uncorrected coagulopathy, signs of increased intracranial pressure, or focal neurologic findings until head imaging can be obtained
- If no etiology is discovered after the first lumbar puncture and the child is not responding to therapy, repeat lumbar puncture at 36 to 48 hours.
- Opening pressure: Normal is <200 mm H_2O in lateral recumbent position.

- Depending on the presentation, age, history, and physical exam findings, some or all of the following tests should be requested for CSF analysis:
  - Cell count with differential and Gram stain
    - Bacterial meningitis is characterized by CSF pleocytosis (>$1.0 \times 10^3/\mu L$) with predominance of neutrophils. Culture is the gold standard for diagnosis.
    - Viral meningitis typically has a lower CSF cell count (0.05 to $0.50 \times 10^3/\mu L$) compared to bacterial meningitis with a predominance of lymphocytes.
  - Glucose: Compare with serum glucose; normal is >40 mg/dL or 1/2 to 2/3 of the serum glucose.
  - Protein: Normal is 5 to 40 mg/dL except in newborns, who may have protein levels of 150 to 200 mg/dL.
    - >1.0 g/dL in bacterial meningitis and normal to slightly elevated in viral meningitis
  - Cultures for bacteria, fungi, virus, and mycobacteria
    - 80% of blood cultures are positive in children with bacterial meningitis.
  - Polymerase chain reaction (PCR) analysis for enterovirus, TB, HSV, Epstein-Barr virus
    - *B. burgdorferi* PCR for CSF samples has a diagnostic yield as low as 17%. Antibody studies for neuroborreliosis are recommended.

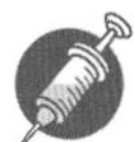

TREATMENT

GENERAL MEASURES

- Ensure adequate ventilation and cardiac function.
  - Circulation, airway, breathing (CABs)
- Initiate hemodynamic monitoring and support by achieving venous access and treat shock syndrome, if present.
- Prompt initiation of appropriate antimicrobials
  - If a lumbar puncture cannot be obtained or is contraindicated, a blood culture should be obtained and antimicrobials initiated immediately.
- Monitor serum sodium concentrations because syndrome of inappropriate ADH secretion (SIADH) is a frequent complication during the first 3 days of treatment.
- Steroids should be used in the initial therapy of TB meningitis along with anti-TB medication.
- Steroids are indicated for Hib meningitis and can be considered in *S. pneumoniae* meningitis; has been shown to decrease hearing loss and neurologic sequelae but not overall mortality. Consult ID expert for use.
  - If giving steroids, use dexamethasone 0.6 mg/kg/24 h divided into 4 doses and given for 4 days. The first dose should be given before or with the first dose of antibiotic.

MEDICATION

- Antimicrobial agents
  - <1 month of age: ampicillin IV 200 to 300 mg/kg/24 h divided q6–12h based on postnatal age and weight. If <7 days of age, 200 mg/kg/24 h divided q8h; if >7 days of age, ampicillin 300 mg/kg/24 h divided q6h and cefotaxime IV 200 to 300 mg/kg/24 h divided q6h
  - >1 month of age: vancomycin IV 60 to 80 mg/kg/24 h divided q6h; cefotaxime IV 300 mg/kg/24 h divided q6h or ceftriaxone 100 mg/kg/24 h divided q12h (should not be used in infants <2 months of age)
  - Vancomycin IV 60 to 80 mg/kg/24 h divided q6h should be considered in a patient of any age suspected of *S. pneumoniae*.
  - Alternative therapy for penicillin- or cephalosporin-allergic patients can include carbapenem or a quinolone in addition to vancomycin. Infectious disease specialist input should be considered.
- Fungal meningitis
  - Amphotericin B with or without 5-flucytosine
- Tuberculous meningitis
  - Treatment is generally with four drugs for 2 months followed by two drugs for 10 months.
  - Initially, treat with isoniazid, rifampin, pyrazinamide, and streptomycin.
- Viral meningitis
  - Enterovirus: supportive care
  - HSV: acyclovir 60 mg/kg/24 h IV divided q8h

ALERT

- Remember that in tuberculous meningitis, up to 50% of children will not react to the 5-tuberculin unit Mantoux tests. Therapy should be started if suspicious; do not rely on the skin testing.
- With the potential for resistant *S. pneumoniae*, vancomycin and cefotaxime or ceftriaxone should be used until antibiotic susceptibility data are available.

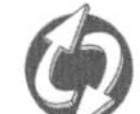

ONGOING CARE

FOLLOW-UP RECOMMENDATIONS

- Neonatal HSV meningitis should be evaluated with a repeat CSF HSV DNA PCR at day 21 and therapy extended if the PCR remains positive.
- Prophylaxis in Hib:
  - Oral rifampin (20 mg/kg/dose, maximum 600 mg/24 h for 4 days) should be given to all household contacts if one member is <4 years of age and is unvaccinated.
- Prophylaxis in *N. meningitidis*:
  - Oral rifampin (10 mg/kg/dose, maximum 600 mg b.i.d. for 2 days) for all household contacts, day care contacts, and other persons with close contact 7 days prior to onset of illness

Patient Monitoring

- Most children with bacterial meningitis become afebrile by 7 to 10 days after starting therapy, with gradual improvement in activity with less irritability.
- Evaluation for neurologic sequelae, such as hearing and vision testing, is essential.

PROGNOSIS

- Bacterial meningitis
  - Fatality approaches 100% if untreated.
  - ~500 to1,000 deaths each year or 5–10% of cases
  - Hearing deficits and neurologic damage may occur in up to 30% of children.
- Viral meningitis
  - Prognosis for enteroviral meningitis is good.
- Aseptic meningitis
  - Lyme disease: Prognosis with diagnosis and treatment is good.
- Tuberculous meningitis
  - The long-term prognosis in children with tuberculous meningitis depends on the stage of disease in which treatment is begun.
  - Complete recovery occurs in 94% of those whose treatment was started in stage I but only 51% and 18% for those whose treatment began in stage II or stage III, respectively.

COMPLICATIONS

- Bacterial meningitis
  - Acute complications: SIADH and seizures occur in up to 1/3 of patients; focal neurologic signs occur in 10–15%.
  - Long-term complications: neurocognitive defects, hearing defects (most common morbidity among survivors)
- Viral meningitis
  - Acute complications: SIADH in 10%
  - Long-term complications: Complications from viral meningitis are rare. However, neonates (<1 month of age) may develop severe enterovirus disease and older agammaglobulinemic children may develop chronic enterovirus meningoencephalitis.
- Tuberculous meningitis
  - Acute complications: Most common are cranial nerve findings, especially 6th cranial nerve palsy affecting the eyes; hydrocephalus
  - Long-term complications: many, including blindness, deafness, and mental retardation

ADDITIONAL READING

- Brouwer MC, McIntyre P, Prasad K, et al. Corticosteroids for acute bacterial meningitis. *Cochrane Database Syst Rev*. 2013;(6):CD004405.
- Kestenbaum LA, Ebberson J, Zorc JJ, et al. Defining cerebrospinal fluid white blood cell count reference values in neonates and young infants. *Pediatrics*. 2010;125(2):257–264.
- Maconochie IK, Bhaumik S. Fluid therapy for acute bacterial meningitis. *Cochrane Database Syst Rev*. 2016;(11):CD004786. doi:10.1002/14651858.CD004786.pub5.
- Mann K, Jackson MA. Meningitis. *Pediatr Rev*. 2008;29(12):417–429.

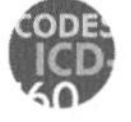

CODES

ICD10

- G03.9 Meningitis, unspecified
- G00.9 Bacterial meningitis, unspecified
- A87.9 Viral meningitis, unspecified

FAQ

- Q: Is a lumbar puncture required before starting antibiotics in the patient with suspected meningitis with unstable vital signs requiring resuscitation?
- A: No. In the unstable patient, it is contraindicated to perform a lumbar puncture. Appropriate IV antibiotics should be started. When resuscitated, a lumbar puncture should be performed.

M

MENINGOCOCCEMIA

Eimear Kitt, MB, BCh, BAO (NUI) • Andrew P. Steenhoff, MBBCh, DCH

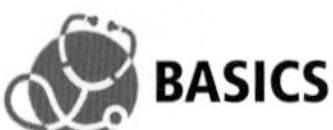

BASICS

DESCRIPTION

A systemic infection caused by the relatively fastidious gram-negative diplococcus *Neisseria meningitidis*. Despite treatment with appropriate antibiotics, this disease may have a fulminant course (i.e., significant complications within hours of presentation) with a high likelihood of mortality.

EPIDEMIOLOGY

- The rates of meningococcal disease in the United States have been declining since the 1990s. In 2015, there were 375 cases with an annual incidence of 0.18 cases per 100,000.
- In North America, infants and children are most often affected, with a secondary peak occurring in adolescents, who are the population predominantly responsible for disease carriage. Indeed, it has been shown that 23.7% of adolescents carry meningococcus in their nasopharynx.
- The disease occurs most commonly in winter and spring months.
- Increased disease activity may follow an influenza A outbreak.
- 13 serogroups have been described on the basis of capsular polysaccharide antigens.
  - In the United States, serogroup B causes approximately 60% of cases in children <5 years of age.
  - Serogroups C, Y, or W cause approximately 2/3 cases of meningococcal disease among persons 11 years old and older.

RISK FACTORS

- Patients with asplenia, deficiencies of properdin C3, or a terminal complement component (C5 to C9), and HIV are at increased risk for invasive and recurrent disease.
- People who take eculizumab for treatment of atypical hemolytic uremic syndrome or paroxysmal nocturnal hemoglobinuria are also at increased risk.
- Other risk groups include microbiologists who are routinely exposed to isolates of *N. meningitidis*, military recruits, college students living in residence halls, and those traveling to a country where meningococcal disease is endemic.
- Organism virulence factors, such as differences in the bacterial cell wall lipopolysaccharide, play a role in disease severity. Less virulent organisms are more likely in chronic meningococcemia, which has a favorable prognosis.

Genetics

- Inherited deficiency of terminal complement may be found in 5–10% of patients during epidemics. The frequency increases to 30% in patients with recurrent disease.
- A number of other immune function–related genes associated with either susceptibility or protection from infection have been identified.

GENERAL PREVENTION

- Exposed contacts, including household, day care, and nursery school, should receive the following:
  - Rifampin, 10 mg/kg (maximum 600 mg) PO q12h for 4 doses
  - Contacts <1 month of age should receive rifampin 5 mg/kg PO q12h for 4 doses.
  - Alternatively, ceftriaxone is also effective prophylaxis for contacts ≤15 years of age; a single dose of 125 mg IM is recommended.
  - For contacts >15 years old, ceftriaxone 250 mg IM is recommended. Its safety profile is preferred for pregnant women.
- Medical personnel should receive prophylaxis only if they had close contact with respiratory secretions.
- Vaccines for types A, B, C, W, and Y are available and produce an immune response in 10 to 14 days.
- A tetravalent conjugate meningococcal vaccine, MCV4, is licensed for use in people in the age range of 2 to 55 years. It is recommended in all unimmunized 11- to 12-year-old adolescents, with a booster dose at age 16 years.
- Serotype B vaccine was recently approved by the U.S. Food and Drug Administration (FDA) and is licensed for use in people 10 to 25 years of age. The Centers for Disease Control and Prevention (CDC) recommends that:
  - All adolescents and young adults aged 16 to 23 years *may* be vaccinated, ideally at aged 16 to 18 years, to give protection during this stage of increased risk.
  - Certain adolescents and young adults *should* receive this vaccine. This includes those identified at increased risk at times of an outbreak and those with medical conditions, including complement deficiencies and functional or anatomic asplenia.
- The CDC continues to recommend routine adolescent immunization with the exception of persons with a history of Guillain-Barré syndrome (GBS) who are not in a high-risk group for invasive meningococcal disease. An updated fact sheet on GBS and MCV4 is available at: https://www.cdc.gov/vaccinesafety/concerns/history/gbs-menactra-faqs.html. Two large studies published in 2012 did not support an association between GBS and MCV4 vaccination.

PATHOPHYSIOLOGY

- Fulminant disease is signified by diffuse microvascular damage and disseminated intravascular coagulation (DIC); see "Diagnosis" section.
- Death results from effects of endotoxic shock, including circulatory collapse and myocardial dysfunction.

ETIOLOGY

- Colonization and infection of the upper respiratory tract occurs after inhalation of, or direct contact with, the organism, usually in oral secretions.
- Disseminated disease occurs when the organism penetrates the nasal mucosa and enters the bloodstream, where it replicates.

COMMONLY ASSOCIATED CONDITIONS

- Terminal complement deficiencies
- Asplenia
- HIV disease

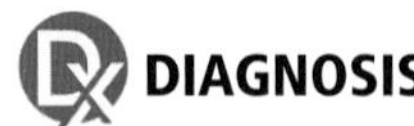

DIAGNOSIS

HISTORY

- Fever
- Malaise
- Rash
- Bacteremia without sepsis presents with fever, malaise, myalgias, and headache. Patients may clear the infection spontaneously, or it may invade meninges, joints, lungs, and so forth.
- Meningococcemia without meningitis occurs after initial bacteremia with systemic sepsis. A rash erupts, which may be nonspecific maculopapular, morbilliform, or urticarial. Progression to petechiae or purpura signifies evolution of disease.
- Fulminant disease can manifest within 1 to 2 hours of onset of signs or symptoms and is signified by hypotension, oliguria, DIC, myocardial dysfunction, and vascular collapse.

PHYSICAL EXAM

- Tachycardia
- Delayed capillary refill
- Petechiae
- Abnormal mental status
- Physical examination of a child with fever should include careful evaluation of the skin for petechiae and signs of early shock (tachycardia, delayed capillary refill, abnormal mental status, etc.).
- Nuchal rigidity, lethargy, and irritability should be carefully but expeditiously evaluated.

DIFFERENTIAL DIAGNOSIS

- Meningitis due to *N. meningitidis* is indistinguishable from that of other causes, except for 1/3 of children who have a petechial rash.
- Sepsis from other microbial causes (e.g., *Streptococcus*, Rocky Mountain spotted fever, viruses) may have a very similar clinical presentation, including the petechiae or purpuric rash.

DIAGNOSTIC TESTS & INTERPRETATION

The organism can be cultured from blood, CSF, and skin lesions.

Initial Tests (screening, lab, imaging)

- Gram stain of CSF or scraped petechial lesion (pressed against a glass slide) revealing gram-negative diplococci will give a presumptive diagnosis.
- Culture of *N. meningitidis* (e.g., from blood or CSF, remains the gold standard)
- CBC
  - One study showed that 94% of children show abnormalities in one or more of the following parameters: abnormalities in absolute neutrophil count ($\leq$1,000/mm^3 or $\geq$10,000/mm^3), immature neutrophil count ($\geq$500/mm^3), and/or immature-to-total neutrophil ratio ($\geq$0.20).

Diagnostic Procedures/Other

Lumbar puncture: antigen detection although culture remains the gold standard

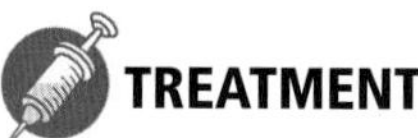

TREATMENT

GENERAL MEASURES

- Because of the rapidly progressing nature of meningococcemia in some, patients with acute onset of petechial rash and fever should receive a prompt initial dose of antibiotics (if possible and practical, after blood culture or lumbar puncture).
- Patients require close clinical monitoring, often in an intensive care unit (ICU) setting.

MEDICATION

- Cefotaxime or ceftriaxone can be initiated as presumptive therapy. After sensitivity is confirmed, penicillin is preferred.
- After isolate is proven sensitive to penicillin, treatment of choice is aqueous penicillin G IV at a dose of 300,000 IU/kg/24 h q4–6h (max, 12 million U/24 h) for 5 to 7 days.
- In penicillin-allergic patients, 3rd-generation cephalosporins, or chloramphenicol are acceptable alternatives.

ALERT

All suspected cases or outbreaks should be promptly reported to state or local health departments.

ADMISSION, INPATIENT, AND NURSING CONSIDERATIONS

- Patients with meningococcemia require respiratory isolation until 24 hours after initiation of appropriate antibiotic therapy.
- Health care personnel with direct exposure to respiratory secretions require antibiotic prophylaxis.
- Close monitoring of vital signs and clinical status is necessary, with prompt transfer to an ICU setting, if deemed clinically appropriate.

ONGOING CARE

FOLLOW-UP RECOMMENDATIONS

Patient Monitoring

Patients with bacterial meningitis should have a hearing test as a follow-up.

PROGNOSIS

- Fatality rate of meningococcemia is 15–20%, even when recognized and treated.
- Fatality rate of meningococcal meningitis is 5%. The most severe cases often have a rapid progression from onset of symptoms to death over a matter of hours. At the time of hospital admission, the following signs predict poor survival:
  - Lack of meningitis
  - Shock
  - Coma
  - Purpura
  - Neutropenia
  - Thrombocytopenia
  - DIC
  - Myocarditis

COMPLICATIONS

- Complications may result directly from the infection or be classified as allergic immune complex mediated.
- Approximately 10–20% of survivors have significant sequelae, including hearing loss in 5–10% and other neurologic complications such as subdural effusions and cranial nerve palsies.
- Meningococcemia may also be complicated by
  - Myocarditis
  - Arthritis
  - Hemorrhage
  - Pneumonia
  - Digit or limb amputation
  - Skin scarring
- Immunologic complications include
  - Arthritis
  - Vasculitis
  - Pericarditis
  - Episcleritis

ADDITIONAL READING

- Banzhoff A. Multicomponent Meningococcal B vaccination (4CMenB) of adolescents and college students in the United States. *Ther Adv Vaccines*. 2017;5(1):3–14.
- Brouwer MC, Spanjaard L, Prins JM, et al. Association of chronic meningococcemia with infection by meningococci with underacylated lipopolysaccharide. *J Infect*. 2011;62(6):479–483.
- Centers for Disease Control and Prevention. Update: Guillain-Barré syndrome among recipients of Menactra meningococcal conjugate vaccine—United States, June 2005–September 2006. *MMWR Morb Mortal Wkly Rep*. 2006;55(41):1120–1124.
- Christensen H, May M, Bowen L, et al. Meningococcal carriage by age: a systematic review and meta-analysis. *Lancet Infect Dis*. 2010;10(12):853–861.
- Demissie DE, Kaplan SL, Romero JR, et al. Altered neutrophil counts at diagnosis of invasive meningococcal infection in children. *Pediatr Infect Dis J*. 2013;32(10):1070–1072.
- MacNeil JR, Rubin L, Folaranmi T, et al. Use of serogroup B meningococcal vaccines in adolescents and young adults: recommendations of the Advisory Committee on Immunization Practices, 2015. *MMWR Morb Mortal Wkly Rep*. 2015;64(41):1171–1176.
- Pathan N, Faust SN, Levin M. Pathophysiology of meningococcal meningitis and septicaemia. *Arch Dis Child*. 2003;88(7):601–607.
- Welch SB, Nadel S. Treatment of meningococcal infection. *Arch Dis Child*. 2003;88(7):608–614.

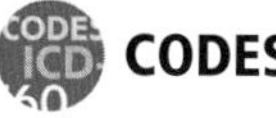

CODES

ICD10

- A39.4 Meningococcemia, unspecified
- A39.3 Chronic meningococcemia
- A39.2 Acute meningococcemia

FAQ

- Q: How long should antibiotic therapy be given to a patient with septic shock?
- A: 7 days
- Q: Should my patient receive both MCV4 and serotype B vaccine?
- A: MVC4 is recommended in all unimmunized 11- to 12-year-old adolescents, with a booster dose at age 16 years. Serotype B vaccine *should* be given to those in areas of known outbreaks and patients with significant risk factors, including complement deficiencies and asplenia. The CDC also states that this vaccine *may* be given to adolescents aged 16 to 23 years, ideally at age 16 to 18 years.
- Q: How does one approach MCV4 immunization of adolescents who previously received MPSV4?
- A: If 3 to 5 years have elapsed since their MPSV4 vaccination, then MCV4 immunization is indicated.
- Q: When should one test for complement deficiency?
- A: In patients with recurrent disease
- Q: Which hospital personnel should receive prophylaxis?
- A: Only those with direct exposure to index patient's secretions require prophylaxis.

MESENTERIC ADENITIS

Adrienne M. Scheich, MD

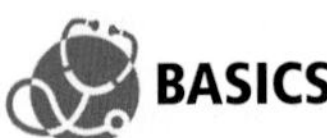

BASICS

DESCRIPTION

Mesenteric adenitis is defined as inflammation of the mesenteric lymph nodes. The inflamed nodes are usually clustered in the right lower quadrant (RLQ) small bowel mesentery or are located ventral to the psoas muscle.

EPIDEMIOLOGY

- Age related, most common in patients <15 years of age
- Affects males and females equally
- History of recent sore throat or upper respiratory tract infection found in 20–30% of subjects
- Most common cause of acute abdominal pain in young adults and children
- Self-limiting condition
- Most common cause of inflammatory adenopathy (more common than tuberculosis)
- Mesenteric adenitis in childhood is related to a decreased risk of ulcerative colitis in adulthood.

PATHOPHYSIOLOGY

- Lymph nodes involved are those draining the ileocecal area. Lymph nodes absorb toxic products or bacterial products secondary to stasis.
- Nodes are enlarged up to 10 mm; discrete, soft, and pink; and with time, become firm. Calcification and suppuration are rare.
- Cultures of the nodes are negative.
- Reactive hyperplasia: Adenitis results from a reaction to some material absorbed from the small intestine, reaching the intestine from the blood or lymphatic system.
- Hypersensitivity reaction to a foreign protein

ETIOLOGY

- Viral
  - Adenovirus
  - Echovirus 1 and 14
  - Coxsackieviruses
  - Epstein-Barr virus (EBV)
  - Cytomegalovirus (CMV)
  - HIV
- Bacterial
  - Tuberculosis
  - *Streptococcus* species
  - *Staphylococcus* species
  - *Escherichia coli*
  - *Yersinia enterocolitica*
  - *Bartonella henselae* (cat-scratch disease)

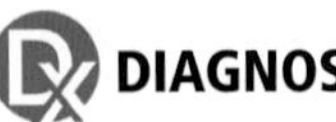

DIAGNOSIS

Can be difficult to differentiate from acute appendicitis clinically, and many patients may undergo laparotomy before diagnosis

HISTORY

- Abdominal pain
  - Dull ache as well as colicky pain occurs due to stretch on the mesentery.
  - May initially be in the upper abdomen/RLQ or generalized
  - If generalized, eventually becomes localized to RLQ
  - Patients often have difficulty localizing the exact point of the most intense pain, in contrast to appendicitis, where pain is often localized to RLQ.
- Intermittent spasms: Between spasms, the patient feels well.
- Signs and symptoms:
  - Abdominal pain (RLQ)
  - Anorexia and fatigue are common.
  - Nausea and vomiting usually precede abdominal pain.
  - Fever
  - Diarrhea

PHYSICAL EXAM

- Often febrile to >38°C (100.4°F)
- May have associated upper respiratory tract infection symptoms, such as rhinorrhea or hyperemic pharynx
- Presence of peripheral lymphadenopathy
- Abdominal examination
  - Tenderness of the RLQ: may be a little higher, more medial, and less severe than acute appendicitis
  - Point of maximal tenderness may vary from one examination to the next.
  - Voluntary guarding with or without rebound tenderness and without rigidity
- Rectal tenderness

DIFFERENTIAL DIAGNOSIS

- Infection
  - Acute appendicitis: 20% of patients treated for possible acute appendicitis had mesenteric adenitis.
  - Infectious mononucleosis: associated lymphadenopathy more generalized
  - Associated splenomegaly: can screen for positive EBV titers
  - Tuberculosis: associated intestinal involvement, positive purified protein derivative (PPD) test, elevated erythrocyte sedimentation rate (ESR)
  - Pelvic inflammatory disease: should be considered in sexually active adolescents, and pelvic exam may be helpful
  - Urinary tract infections/pyelonephritis: Urinalysis and urine culture are helpful.
  - Abscess: related to missed acute appendicitis or inflammatory bowel disease (IBD)
  - *Y. enterocolitica* infection: bloody diarrhea, arthropathy present; stool culture is diagnostic.
  - Typhlitis: Transmural inflammation of the cecum is seen in patients with neutropenia.
- Tumors
  - Lymphoma: Adenopathy can be more generalized.
  - CT scan of the abdomen and/or laparotomy to confirm the diagnosis
- Trauma
  - Hematomas of the abdominal wall and intestines
  - History of trauma
- Metabolic
  - Acute intermittent porphyria
  - Cyclic episodes of acute abdominal pain and vomiting
  - Appropriate metabolic workup diagnostic

- Congenital
  - Duplication cysts: may present with abdominal pain due to rupture, bleeding, intussusception, or volvulus
  - Meckel diverticulum: may present with diverticulitis or act as a lead point for intussusception
- Miscellaneous
  - Crohn disease: associated mesenteric adenitis and intestinal involvement
  - Intussusception: acute abdominal pain with "currant jelly" stools; barium/air enema is diagnostic and therapeutic.
  - Ovarian cysts: may need abdominal/pelvic ultrasound to differentiate between the two
  - Chronic mesenteric ischemia

DIAGNOSTIC TESTS & INTERPRETATION

- Mesenteric adenitis is a diagnosis of exclusion.
  - It can only be diagnosed accurately at laparoscopy or laparotomy.
  - Ultrasound or CT scan may demonstrate enlarged mesenteric lymph nodes.
- See "Differential Diagnosis."

Initial Tests (screening, lab, imaging)

- Complete blood count and C-reactive protein may be increased but are not specific.
- Abdominal ultrasound
  - Differentiates acute appendicitis, pelvic inflammatory disease, ovarian pathology, and mesenteric adenitis
- Contrast-enhanced CT scan of the abdomen and pelvis shows enlarged mesenteric lymph nodes, with possible ileal or ileocecal wall thickening, normal appendix.
- MRI

Diagnostic Procedures/Other

- Laparoscopic surgery
- Laparotomy

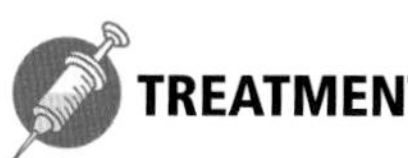

TREATMENT

Most patients recover completely without any specific treatment.

ONGOING CARE

FOLLOW-UP RECOMMENDATIONS

Patient Monitoring

Watch for

- Increasing abdominal pain
- Vomiting
- Fevers
- Toxic appearance
- Severe tenderness that is persistent
- Guarding
- Rigidity
- Decreasing bowel sounds

PROGNOSIS

- Most patients recover completely without any specific treatment.
- When to expect improvement: Acute symptoms may take days to resolve and generally persist after associated viral symptoms have resolved.

COMPLICATIONS

- Suppuration
- Intussusception (Enlarged lymph nodes can be a lead point for intussusception.)
- Rupture of lymph nodes
- Abscess formation
- Peritonitis
- Death (very rare) from abscess and peritonitis

ADDITIONAL READING

- Carty HM. Paediatric emergencies: non-traumatic abdominal emergencies. *Eur Radiol*. 2002;12(12): 2835–2848.
- Frisch M, Pedersen BV, Andersson RE. Appendicitis, mesenteric lymphadenitis, and subsequent risk of ulcerative colitis: cohort studies in Sweden and Denmark. *BMJ*. 2009;338:b716.
- Karmazyn B, Werner EA, Rejaie B, et al. Mesenteric lymph nodes in children: what is normal? *Pediatr Radiol*. 2005;35(8):774–777.
- Lucey BC, Stuhlfaut JW, Soto JA. Mesenteric lymph nodes seen at imaging: causes and significance. *Radiographics*. 2005;25(2):351–365.
- Macari M, Balthazar EJ. The acute right lower quadrant: CT evaluation. *Radiol Clin North Am*. 2003;41(6):1117–1136.
- Macari M, Hines J, Balthazar E, et al. Mesenteric adenitis: CT diagnosis of primary versus secondary causes, incidence, and clinical significance in pediatric and adult patients. *AJR Am J Roentgenol*. 2002;178(4):853–858.
- Toorenvliet B, Vellekoop A, Bakker R, et al. Clinical differentiation between acute appendicitis and acute mesenteric adenitis in children. *Eur J Pediatr Surg*. 2011;21(2):120–123.
- Zeiter DK, Hyams JS. Recurrent abdominal pain in children. *Pediatr Clin North Am*. 2002;49(1):53–71.

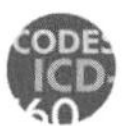

CODES

ICD10

I88.0 Nonspecific mesenteric lymphadenitis

FAQ

- Q: Can one differentiate clinically between acute appendicitis and nonspecific mesenteric adenitis?
- A: Yes, but the differences can be subtle. Patients with nonspecific mesenteric adenitis generally cannot localize the exact point of the most intense pain, unlike patients with appendicitis, who can localize their pain to the RLQ. Abdominal examination in patients with mesenteric adenitis is characterized by increased tenderness of the RLQ that is a little higher, more medial, and less severe than that in acute appendicitis. Point of maximal tenderness may vary between examinations in patients with nonspecific mesenteric adenitis. There is no rigidity on abdominal examination in patients with nonspecific mesenteric adenitis. However, it is clinically difficult to differentiate the two entities.
- Q: Which investigations can be diagnostic for RLQ pain?
- A: An ultrasound or CT scan of the RLQ can differentiate between acute appendicitis, ovarian pathology, and lymphadenopathy. An upper gastrointestinal series with small bowel follow-through or a magnetic resonance enterography study can be diagnostic for IBD.

METABOLIC DISEASES IN ACIDOTIC NEWBORNS

Noura Al Dhaheri, MBBS • Hilary Vernon, MD, PhD • Leah R. Fleming, MD

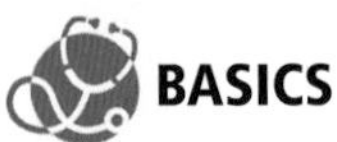

BASICS

DESCRIPTION

- Metabolic acidosis is a common acute presentation of an inborn error of metabolism (IEM), particularly in the presence of elevated anion gap. Acidosis can also be seen as a result of hypoperfusion, congenital heart disease, sepsis, liver failure, toxic ingestion, and diabetic ketoacidosis (DKA).
- IEMs are generally defects of protein, fat, or carbohydrate metabolism or of the mitochondrial respiratory chain that result in either accumulation or deficiency of a metabolite.
- IEMs should be considered early in the workup of a child with metabolic acidosis in order to detect those conditions that are treatable prior to development of permanent neurologic sequelae. Sequelae can be related to duration and severity of exposure. Basic evaluation for IEMs should be undertaken concurrently with other diagnostic evaluations.

ALERT

Infants with IEMs are at increased risk for decompensation and acute presentation in cases of infection, fever, fasting, or other causes of catabolism.

RISK FACTORS

Genetics

Generally autosomal recessive, with the exception of pyruvate dehydrogenase deficiency (X-linked dominant), ornithine transcarbamylase (X-linked), and some diseases of the mitochondrial genome (maternally inherited)

GENERAL PREVENTION

- Avoid propofol if possible (anecdotal increase in pancreatitis).
- Avoid prolonged fasting or nutritional deprivation.
- Avoid use of systemic steroids whenever possible (steroids may increase the metabolic demands).

PATHOPHYSIOLOGY

Metabolic acidosis is often a downstream effect of the primary metabolic abnormality. A block in normal metabolism can result in dysfunction of the mitochondrial respiratory chain, buildup of toxic intermediates, disordered or reduced energy production, buildup of waste nitrogen in the form of ammonia and specific amino acids, and through conjugation of the acids with carnitine, lead to carnitine depletion. These events can lead to multiorgan dysfunction including the following:

- CNS toxicity: edema, neurologic effects of hypoglycemia, toxic encephalopathy
- Cardiac: arrhythmias, left ventricular noncompaction cardiomyopathy
- Liver: hepatosplenomegaly, elevation of liver function tests, prolonged hyperbilirubinemia
- Hematologic: bone marrow suppression
- Renal: proximal tubule dysfunction, kidney failure (typically later onset)

ETIOLOGY

Multifactorial. Primary metabolic disease is typically due to a genetic defect that causes a block in metabolism resulting in buildup of toxic intermediates or absence/reduction of necessary downstream products.

COMMONLY ASSOCIATED CONDITIONS

- Maternal hemolysis, elevated liver enzymes, low platelets (HELLP), fatty liver of pregnancy, preeclampsia: associated with specific fetal disorders of fatty acid oxidation
- Metabolic stroke: stroke affecting the basal ganglia (not ischemic or hemorrhagic in character)

DIAGNOSIS

HISTORY

- Pregnancy history: maternal HELLP syndrome; acute fatty liver of pregnancy; preeclampsia; reduced fetal movements; intrauterine growth retardation (IUGR); fetal bradycardia
- Family history of consanguinity, siblings with unexplained severe childhood illness, hypoglycemia, sudden infant death syndrome (SIDS), developmental delay, Reye syndrome, or death
- Deterioration after a symptom-free interval (typically at least several days required for toxic metabolic buildup)
  - Classic presentation is of poor feeding, vomiting, and alterations in neurologic status (irritability, hypotonia, encephalopathy).
  - Without treatment, this will progress to lethargy, temperature instability, seizure, coma, and death.
- Diet history including frequency of feeds, vigor, whether breast milk or formula and, if formula, the type of formula (Low protein may delay onset of symptoms.)
- Fits, cycling movements
- Associations with IEMs
  - Gram-negative sepsis (galactosemia)
  - Cerebral or pulmonary hemorrhage (urea cycle disorder)
  - Severe, prolonged, unexplained hypoglycemia in term neonate (suggests organic acidemia or defect of gluconeogenesis)
  - Mild respiratory alkalosis (hyperammonemia)
  - Ketosis (organic acidemia, congenital lactic acidosis)
  - Coagulopathy, jaundice (mitochondrial, hemochromatosis, fatty acid oxidation disorders, hereditary fructose intolerance, tyrosinemia, galactosemia)

PHYSICAL EXAM

- Vital signs: tachypnea, hypotension. Assess for Cushing triad.
- General
  - Dysmorphic features (may be present in mitochondrial and peroxisomal disorders and some fatty acid oxidation disorders)
- HEENT: bulging fontanelle (cerebral edema), maple syrup urine disease (MSUD)
- Eye: cataracts, dislocated lens, corneal clouding, retinal changes
- Skin: jaundice, rashes
- Cardiac
  - Cardiomyopathy (fatty acid oxidation, propionic acidemia), pericardial effusion (congenital disorder of glycosylation), cardiomegaly
- Respiratory: tachypnea, Kussmaul breathing, apnea
- Hepatosplenomegaly (disorders of gluconeogenesis, storage disorders, galactosemia)
- Neurologic: reflexes, tone, seizure
- Odor
  - Sweet: MSUD (urine and ear cerumen)
  - Sweaty feet: isovaleric acidemia
  - Fruity: methylmalonic acidemia, propionic acidemia
  - "Tomcat" urine odor: multiple carboxylase deficiency
- Growth parameters
  - Typically normal in newborn period but may have IUGR or delayed return to birth weight (BW)

DIFFERENTIAL DIAGNOSIS

- In neonates, IEMs present with similar symptoms and can easily be confused with other serious diseases.
  - Sepsis
  - Birth asphyxia
  - Ductal-dependent congenital heart disease
  - Neonatal withdrawal syndrome
  - Endocrine abnormalities (adrenal insufficiency)
- IEM resulting in metabolic acidosis can be divided into the lactic acidoses, those that cause a ketoacidosis, and the organic acid disorders.
  - Lactic acidosis
    - Pyruvate dehydrogenase deficiency
    - Pyruvate carboxylase deficiency
    - Phosphoenolpyruvate carboxykinase deficiency
    - Defects in tricarboxylic acid cycle enzymes
    - Mitochondrial diseases or other conditions affecting oxidative phosphorylation
    - Severe disorders of gluconeogenesis (e.g., glucose-6-phosphatase deficiency)
    - Multiple carboxylase deficiency, biotinidase deficiency
    - Disorders of fatty acid oxidation
  - Ketoacidosis
    - Disorders of ketone use (e.g., β-ketothiolase deficiency)
    - Ketosis can also occur in lactic acidosis syndromes (above) and organic acidemias (below).
  - Other organic acid disorders
    - MSUD
    - Branched-chain organic acidurias (methylmalonic acidemia, propionic acidemia, isovaleric acidemia)
- Others: In some cases, other abnormalities (e.g., lethargy, hyperammonemia) may occur prior to severe acidosis.

DIAGNOSTIC TESTS & INTERPRETATION

Initial Tests (screening, lab, imaging)

- Initial evaluation (concurrently with sepsis evaluation)
  - Complete blood count with differential
  - Blood gas including pH and lactate
  - Serum urea, creatinine, glucose, electrolytes (anion gap), AST, ALT
  - Ammonia (place on watery ice, run immediately)
  - Creatine kinase
  - Urinalysis, urine-reducing substance
  - Obtain copy of newborn screen (NBS) report.
- CSF: if obtained in course of complete sepsis evaluation
  - Consider freezing a tube for later use.
  - May send lactate, lactate-to-pyruvate ratio
- Should be sent for definitive diagnosis:
  - Plasma amino acids (PAA), acylcarnitines, urine organic acids, urine orotic acid (if ammonia is elevated), urine ketones

- Treatment should not be delayed in the case of presumptive IEM.
- Echocardiogram to evaluate for structural heart disease and cardiac function
- Consider head ultrasound (ventriculomegaly seen in pyruvate dehydrogenase complex deficiency).

Diagnostic Procedures/Other

- Ammonia (>200 μmol/L) very strongly implies metabolic disease. Up to 65 to 100 μmol/L is normal in a healthy neonate.
- Calculate anion gap: High anion gap implies excessive acid production or retention.
- If not previously performed, secondary testing should include acylcarnitine profile, free fatty acids and 3-hydroxybutyrate, osmolality, PAA, lactate and pyruvate ratio, and urine organic acids.
- Ophthalmology exam
- Confirmatory testing is by specific enzyme analysis or genetic testing.
- In case of death, obtain the following:
  - Urine: deep frozen
  - Blood: ethylenediaminetetraacetic acid (EDTA) for DNA analysis
  - Skin: sterile, for fibroblast culture; store at 4–8°C
  - Liver, muscle: snap frozen
  - CSF if possible (for amino acids and neurotransmitters)
  - Plasma: heparinized
  - Blood spot: for acylcarnitine profile

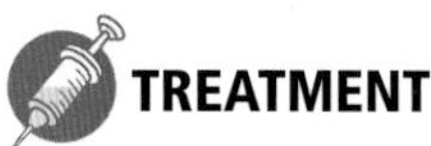

TREATMENT

GENERAL MEASURES

- Stop feeding.
- Provide 6 to 10 mg/kg/min dextrose (typically as D10 at 1.5 to 2 times maintenance rate).
  - If considering pyruvate dehydrogenase deficiency, use lower dextrose infusion rate, typically D5.
- Admit to intensive care unit.
- Consult biochemical genetics team.
- Consider early continuous venovenous hemodialysis to remove toxin and decrease ammonia. Peritoneal dialysis is less effective but can be used.
- Correct hypothermia, dehydration, electrolyte disturbance, etc.
- Consider sodium bicarbonate.
  - Start at 1 mEq/kg.
  - Often, the patient will require large doses due to ongoing acid production.
- Insulin as needed for iatrogenic hyperglycemia
- Resume nutritionally complete feeding as soon as possible under guidance of biochemical genetics team. This may include specialized iTPN or formula.

ADDITIONAL THERAPIES

- Nitrogen scavenger such as sodium benzoate and sodium phenylacetate if urea cycle overwhelmed or primary urea cycle disorder; carbamylglutamate (Carbaglu) used for patients with NAGS deficiency
- Carnitine promotes excretion of organic acids. Administer 50 mg/kg/dose IV every 6 hours. Use is controversial in disorders of fatty acid oxidation; not to be used in LCHAD (theoretical arrhythmia risk)
- Specific supplementation
  - Biotin (holocarboxylase synthetase deficiency) 10 mg PO/NG
  - Hydroxocobalamin (cobalamin-responsive methylmalonic acidemia) 1 mg IM
  - Pyridoxine (pyridoxine-dependent seizure)
  - Pyridoxal phosphate (pyridoxine-5′-phosphate oxidase deficiency)
  - Glycine (isovaleric acidemia)
  - Nitisinone (tyrosinemia)
  - Arginine (urea cycle)
  - Thiamine (MSUD, some forms of congenital lactic acidosis) 50 mg PO/NG daily to b.i.d. (Dose varies based on responsiveness.)

ADMISSION, INPATIENT, AND NURSING CONSIDERATIONS

- Initial stabilization
  - Treatment may differ for specific IEMs. However, the overall goal for acute management is primarily focused on:
    - Immediate life support/electrolyte balance/ sample procurement
    - Reduce the formation of toxic metabolites (preventing the production of toxic endogenous metabolites and preventing further catabolism): by stopping all oral intake (Eliminate protein, galactose, fructose.)
    - Promoting anabolism: by providing calories through IV dextrose containing fluids or special formula depending on diagnosis
    - Removal of toxic substances and supplementation of substrates/cofactors (i.e., ammonia scavengers or hemodialysis for hyperammonemia)
    - Treatment of coexisting/precipitating factors (e.g., infection, dehydration)
  - IV fluids typically, are started for initial stabilization to provide additional calories, which will help promote anabolism and prevent further catabolism.
    - IV fluids can be in the form of dextrose-containing electrolyte solution (6 to 10 mg/kg/min dextrose; typically, D10 at 1.5 to 2 times maintenance rate).
  - Intralipids can also be considered (if fatty acid oxidation defect is not suspected).
- Admission criteria:
  - Almost all patients with suspected or known IEMs will need admission for initial stabilization according the aforementioned goals.
  - Other criteria for admission include inability to tolerate oral/tube feeding, active GI losses and dehydration, neurologic symptoms such as lethargy.
- Discharge criteria:
  - Patient can be discharged if he/she has stable electrolytes, is afebrile, is tolerating feeding regimen, and has no evidence of catabolism.
  - Specific lab monitoring (per biochemical genetics consultant's recommendation) is based on underlying diagnosis (e.g., PAA, ammonia).

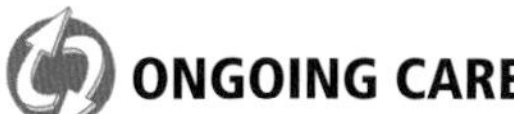

ONGOING CARE

FOLLOW-UP RECOMMENDATIONS

Patient Monitoring

- Refer to a biochemical genetics team for ongoing evaluation and management.
- Generally, patients will require frequent monitoring in the newborn period and throughout life; however, this need varies with the diagnosis.
- Specific treatment is required based on correct diagnosis of IEM.

COMPLICATIONS

- Prognosis varies based on disease.
- For some disorders, appropriate treatment dramatically improves morbidity and mortality (especially the fatty acid oxidation disorders and vitamin responsive disorders); for others, there is improved survival but still significant morbidity.
- Long-term complications are becoming better understood with improved survival (e.g., risk of pancreatitis and renal failure in the branch chain acidurias).
- As in other chronic pediatric illnesses, such as diabetes, recurrent episodes are often triggered by stress, noncompliance, or illness and may increase in frequency during the teen years.
- Severity of neurologic complications increases with frequency and duration of episodes of metabolic decompensation and/or frequency and duration of elevated ammonia. Neurologic complications can include metabolic stroke (basal ganglia), herniation, seizure disorder, and intellectual impairment.
- There may be progressive impairment of the heart, liver, or kidney; chronic bone marrow suppression; as well as effects of malnutrition and hyperglycemia (due to frequent D10 infusions).

ADDITIONAL READING

- Burton BK. Inborn errors of metabolism in infancy: a guide to diagnosis. *Pediatrics*. 1998;102(6):E69.
- Cook P, Walker V. Investigation of the child with an acute metabolic disorder. *J Clin Pathol*. 2011;64(3):181–191.
- Leonard J, Morris A. Diagnosis and early management of inborn errors of metabolism presenting around the time of birth. *Acta Paediatr*. 2006;95(1):6–14.
- Saudubray JM, Sedel F, Walter JH. Clinical approach to treatable inborn metabolic diseases: An introduction. *J Inherit Metab Dis*. 2006;29(2–3):261–274.

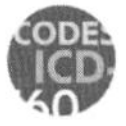

CODES

ICD10

- P74.0 Late metabolic acidosis of newborn
- E88.89 Other specified metabolic disorders
- E72.29 Other disorders of urea cycle metabolism

FAQ

- Q: What factors determine developmental outcome in children with IEMs?
- A: The specific diagnosis and patient mutation, how rapidly appropriate therapy is initiated, frequency of decompensating, and compliance with chronic management all contribute to developmental outcome.
- Q: If the NBS was normal, can the infant still be affected by an IEM?
- A: Many IEMs are not included on the NBS and there can also be false negatives.
- Q: Do IEMs only affect infants?
- A: No. An individual can present with an IEM at any point in his or her life, depending on the level of enzyme deficiency/threshold for catabolic stress.
- Q: Why is a blood gas measurement helpful in addition to a comprehensive metabolic panel (CMP) in evaluating acid/base status?
- A: The blood gas can be used to determine the etiology of the pH abnormality (respiratory vs. metabolic).

METABOLIC DISEASES IN HYPERAMMONEMIC NEWBORNS

Tamanna R. Roshan Lal, MBChB • Ada Hamosh, MD, MPH

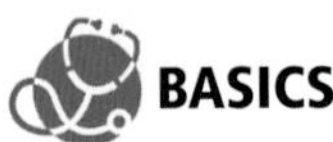

BASICS

DESCRIPTION

- Inborn errors of metabolism are inherited defects in biosynthesis, catabolism, or transport of lipids, amino acids, or carbohydrates. The first presentation of an inborn error of metabolism can be at any age, with most cases manifesting during states of metabolic catabolism and/or increased dietary intake of an offending metabolite.
- Clinical findings can range from acute life-threatening crises to milder, nonspecific clinical episodes of malaise, emesis, lethargy, anorexia, or even acute neuropsychiatric abnormalities.
- Some inborn errors of metabolism present with elevated levels of ammonia (>100 μM/L). Ammonia is highly neurotoxic, and elevated levels can lead to encephalopathy and death. Maintaining a high degree of clinical suspicion in sick neonates is essential.

EPIDEMIOLOGY

- Incidence and prevalence vary among different types of inborn errors of metabolism. Collectively, approximately 1 in 500 newborns are affected by one of the various inborn errors of metabolism.
- Estimated incidence of urea cycle defects is 1:18,000. Incidence of organic acidemias is 1:1,000 and of medium-chain acyl-CoA dehydrogenase (MCAD) deficiency ranges from 1:4,900 to 1:17,000.

RISK FACTORS

Genetics

- Inheritance of most inborn errors of metabolism is autosomal recessive.
- Ornithine transcarbamylase (OTC) deficiency (the most common urea cycle defect) is X-linked.

PATHOPHYSIOLOGY

- Nitrogen is an essential building block of amino acids and a major source of ammonia from protein degradation.
  - Ammonia is highly toxic, especially to the central nervous system (CNS).
  - A major mechanism for ammonia detoxification is the urea cycle, which converts ammonia in the liver to water-soluble urea. Urea is then excreted by the kidneys.
- Inborn errors of metabolism causing hyperammonemia interfere with urea cycle function, either directly through primary enzymatic defects of the urea cycle or indirectly caused by liver failure, decreased production, increased use, or defective transport of a urea cycle intermediate as seen in aminoacidopathies, organic acidemias, fatty acid oxidation defects, and defective carbohydrate metabolism.

ETIOLOGY

Any biochemical defect that alters the amount of ammonia or that interferes with the detoxification of ammonia

DIAGNOSIS

HISTORY

- Evidence of systemic disease: A variety of systemic newborn illnesses, including sepsis, can be complicated by secondary hyperammonemia.
- Family history of poorly explained pediatric death, developmental disability, or neuropsychiatric disorders should raise suspicion for a genetic disorder, such as an inborn error of metabolism; diagnoses to ask about:
  - Sepsis or recurrent infections (opportunistic organism or no organism identified)
  - Sudden infant death syndrome
  - Cardiomyopathy
  - Uncontrollable seizures
  - Coma
  - Liver failure
- Current diet and feeding schedule: In urea cycle defects, hyperammonemia is exacerbated by protein intake.
- Failure to wake and feed spontaneously is a sign of CNS dysfunction in neonates.
- Perinatal hypoxia can cause temporary liver dysfunction and reduced urea cycle capacity. Relative immaturity of the urea cycle can cause hyperammonemia in premature infants.

PHYSICAL EXAM

- ABCs and vital signs: Cushing triad (apnea, bradycardia, hypertension) should prompt immediate evaluation for elevated intracranial pressure, a complication of hyperammonemia.
- Head, eyes, ears, nose, and throat: macrocephaly, bulging fontanelle (elevated intracranial pressure)
- Cardiac: dilated or hypertrophic cardiomyopathy in some organic acidemias and fatty acid oxidation defects
- Respiratory: hyperpnea (rapid deep breathing that will lead respiratory alkalosis which is different from the rapid shallow breathing of transient tachypnea of the newborn)
- GI: Hepatomegaly occurs in some of these disorders (argininosuccinate lyase deficiency, fatty acid oxidation, galactosemia).
- Skin: Jaundice is not typical in urea cycle defects but occurs in other inborn errors of metabolism associated with hepatotoxicity.
- Neurologic: extrapyramidal signs, encephalopathy, myoclonic jerks, hyper-/hypotonia, obtundation, and coma

DIFFERENTIAL DIAGNOSIS

- Neonatal hyperammonemia not caused by inborn errors of metabolism
  - Sepsis or other severe illness
  - Liver failure (drugs, toxins, others)
  - Transient neonatal hyperammonemia (e.g., open ductus venosus)
  - Perinatal depression/hypoxia
  - Iatrogenic (valproic acid, asparaginase)
- Inborn errors of metabolism
  - Urea cycle defects: *N*-acetylglutamate (NAG) synthetase deficiency, carbamoyl phosphate synthetase deficiency, OTC deficiency, argininosuccinate synthetase deficiency, argininosuccinate lyase deficiency
  - Organic acidemias (i.e., isovaleric acidemia, propionic acidemia, methylmalonic acidemia)
  - Fatty acid oxidation defects (i.e., MCAD deficiency)
  - Hyperornithinemia, hyperammonemia, homocitrullinuria (HHH) syndrome
  - Pyruvate carboxylase deficiency
  - Hepatopathy (due to galactosemia, hereditary fructose intolerance)
  - Hyperinsulinism-hyperammonemia syndrome (HIHA; glutamate dehydrogenase deficiency)
  - Tyrosinemia type 1
  - Mitochondrial disorders
  - Citrin deficiency leading to citrullinemia type II and neonatal intrahepatic cholestasis caused by citrin deficiency

DIAGNOSTIC TESTS & INTERPRETATION

Initial Tests (screening, lab, imaging)

- Initial labs for a presumptive diagnosis in a patient with hyperammonemia:
  - Dextrose stick
  - Electrolytes, BUN, creatinine
  - CBC, blood culture, serum ketones
  - Blood gas with lactate
  - Liver function tests and PT/PTT
  - Urinalysis for ketones, reducing substances
  - Frequent ammonia levels (q4–12h), obtain as free-flowing samples, placed on wet ice and immediately transport to the lab for processing
  - Review state newborn screen.
- Suspected disorders and follow-up testing:
  - Urea cycle defects: plasma amino acids and urine orotic acid
  - Organic acidemias: urine organic acids, plasma amino acids, and acylcarnitine profile
  - Fatty acid oxidation defects: creatine phosphokinase, urine organic acids, plasma acylcarnitine profile
  - Galactosemia: urine galactitol, red blood cell galactose-1-phosphate uridyltransferase (GALT) activity
  - Open ductus venosus: low urea and glutamine
  - Definitive diagnosis may require enzyme testing or mutation analysis.
- Brain MRI/CT may show demyelination; circumscribed brain atrophy; cerebellar hypoplasia or aplasia, symmetric and/or fluctuation; and abnormalities of brainstem, basal ganglia, thalamus, and/or hypothalamus, especially in "cerebral" organic acidurias.

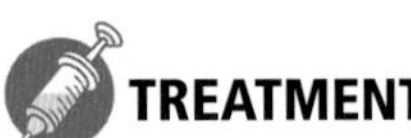

TREATMENT

Presumptive treatment should not await a definitive diagnosis but should be based on clinical suspicion and initial labs. Delays in treatment can be fatal and will cause brain damage.

GENERAL MEASURES

- Many patients will require admission to an intensive care unit and may require ventilator support.
- Obtain IV access.
- Promote renal ammonia excretion through increased maintenance fluids.
- Immediately discontinue exogenous protein intake, which exacerbates ammonia production.

- Enhance anabolism with calories from high-rate dextrose infusion (10 mg/kg/min) with insulin (0.1 to 1 IU/kg/h) and intralipids (0.5 to 1 g/kg/24 h) (exclude long-chain fatty acid disorder).
- Nitrogen-scavenging agents enable ammonia to bind to amino acids, which yield products that can be excreted in the urine:
  - Sodium benzoate (250 mg/kg/24 h)
  - Sodium phenylacetate (250 mg/kg/24 h) intravenously when ill
  - Sodium phenylbutyrate (400 to 600 mg/kg/24 h) orally when well. Note that high levels (or serum concentrations) of sodium benzoate and sodium phenylbutyrate can be toxic, >2 mmol/L and >4 mmol/L, respectively. Monitor sodium and potassium levels when using these scavengers.
- Arginine (180 to 360 mg/kg) or citrulline therapy to supplement residual urea cycle function
- L-Carnitine supplementation (100 to 200 mg/kg/24 h) to support mitochondrial metabolism (unless urea cycle defect is identified as the cause)
- Administration of *N*-carbamyl-L-glutamic acid (Carbaglu®) (100 to 200 mg/kg/24 h, PO) has been shown to reduce ammonia levels in NAG synthetase deficiency, carbamoyl phosphate synthetase (CPS) I deficiency, and the organic acidemias.
- Antiemetics (e.g., ondansetron)
- Metronidazole (10 to 20 mg/kg/24 h PO/IV for 10 days every month) to decrease bacterial gut flora as a major source of ammonia and propionate
- Dialysis in severe hyperammonemia (>250 μmol/L) if unresponsive to IV scavengers
- Monitor ammonia, electrolytes, and neurologic status closely during a crisis.
- Consider introducing total parenteral nutrition or semisynthetic amino acid formulas once patient is stable—typically within 24 to 48 hours.

ADMISSION, INPATIENT, AND NURSING CONSIDERATIONS

- Admission criteria
  - New onset hyperammonemia
    - Any newborn with an elevated ammonia level for age with or without neurologic deficits will need to be admitted for further workup and management.
  - Recurrent hyperammonemia
    - Elevated ammonia not controlled by medication and diet
    - Inability to tolerate feeds
    - Dehydration
    - Altered mental status
    - Neurologic deficits
    - Fever
    - Lethargy
    - Vomiting and diarrhea
- Discharge criteria
  - Ammonia levels have normalized
  - Resolution of underlying illness causing the metabolic crises
  - Fully fed and able to tolerate feeds
  - Able to control ammonia levels with oral medication
  - Treatment plan to prevent future episodes understood by the parent or guardian
  - Follow-up with metabolic specialist and dietitian has been arranged.

ONGOING CARE

- Specific therapies are best carried out under the supervision of a metabolic specialist and a metabolic nutritionist. Goal of every long-term treatment is to achieve a protein-sparing anabolic effect of an optimal diet that limits the episodes of acute crises and promotes adequate growth.
- Adjust diet to underlying metabolic defect by restricting metabolites prior to their respective enzymatic block and/or their precursors from the diet, for example:
  - Urea cycle defects
    - Restrict natural protein; protein elimination during times of stress during illness/stress; avoid fasting.
    - Chronic therapy with nitrogen-scavenging agents
    - Amino acid supplements when indicated (e.g., citrulline in OTC deficiency; arginine in citrullinemia, argininosuccinate lyase deficiency)
    - Long-term therapy may involve an orthotopic liver transplant.
  - Fatty acid oxidation disorders
    - Low-fat, high-carbohydrate diets with frequent feeds; avoid fasting.
  - Organic acidemias
    - Protein restriction, semisynthetic amino acid formulas lacking the offending amino acid; protein elimination during times of stress during illness/stress; and avoidance of fasting; intermittent metronidazole in propionic acidemia to eliminate intestinal propionate production; liver and/or kidney transplant
  - Growth and nutrition
    - Provide vitamins, minerals, trace elements, cofactors, and calories in accordance to the recommended daily allowance (RDA) to promote adequate growth and an anabolic state because catabolism may trigger acute crises, especially in urea cycle defects and organic acidemias.
    - To assess adequate nutritional therapy, measure height, weight, and head circumference
    - Obtain CBC, plasma protein and albumin, plasma amino acids, iron and ferritin, lipid panel, renal and hepatic function test, as well as calcium and phosphorus levels frequently.
  - Dietary protocol for treatment of intercurrent illness at home
  - Emergency letter/protocol and bracelet
  - Early treatment of infection
  - Routine vaccination

COMPLICATIONS

- Recurrent episodes of hyperammonemia
- Malnutrition → growth retardation, osteoporosis
- Elevated intracranial pressure
- Intellectual disability
- Vision loss due to optic neuropathy
- Nephropathy, cardiomyopathy
- Coma, metabolic strokes, early death

ADDITIONAL READING

- Champion MP. An approach to the diagnosis of inherited metabolic disease. *Arch Dis Child Educ Pract Ed*. 2010;95(2):40–46.
- Ficicioglu C, Bearden D. Isolated neonatal seizures: when to suspect inborn errors of metabolism. *Pediatr Neurol*. 2011;45(5):283–291.
- Häberle J. Clinical practice: the management of hyperammonemia. *Eur J Pediatr*. 2011;170(1):21–34.
- Häberle J, Boddaert N, Burlina A, et al. Suggested guidelines for the diagnosis and management of urea cycle disorders. *Orphanet J Rare Dis*. 2012;7:32.
- Kasapkara C, Ezgu F, Okur I, et al. N-carbamylglutamate treatment for acute neonatal hyperammonemia in isovaleric acidemia. *Eur J Pediatr*. 2011;170(6):799–801.
- Machado MC, Pinheiro da Silva F. Hyperammonemia due to urea cycle disorders: a potentially fatal condition in the intensive care setting. *J Intensive Care*. 2014;2(1):22.
- New England Consortium of Metabolic Programs. Neonate/infant/child with hyperammonemia. http://newenglandconsortium.org/for-professionals/acute-illness-protocols/urea-cycle-disorders/neonate-infant-child-with-hyperammonemia. Accessed March 24, 2017.

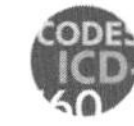

CODES

ICD10

- E88.89 Other specified metabolic disorders
- E72.20 Disorder of urea cycle metabolism, unspecified
- E72.4 Disorders of ornithine metabolism

FAQ

- Q: Can females have OTC deficiency?
- A: OTC is an X-linked gene, and females are generally asymptomatic carriers. However, due to "skewed" X inactivation of the OTC gene, affected female may exhibit symptoms after increased protein intake or states of catabolism.
- Q: Can any hyperammonemia disorders present outside of the newborn period?
- A: Disease severity depends in large part on a patient's enzyme activity. Therefore, hyperammonemia can occur at any age during a period of metabolic stress.
- Q: What determines developmental outcome in children with inborn errors of metabolism?
- A: Outcome depends on prompt diagnosis, residual enzyme activity, early treatment, and compliance with long-term treatment.
- Q: How often should ammonia levels and amino acid levels be monitored?
- A: This should be determined by the metabolic specialist. Depending on the severity of the disease and the age of child, this can vary from weekly to several times a year.

METABOLIC DISEASES IN HYPOGLYCEMIC NEWBORNS

Tamanna R. Roshan Lal, MBChB • Ada Hamosh, MD, MPH

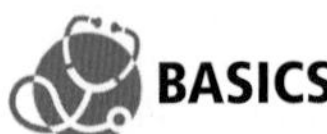

BASICS

DESCRIPTION

- Hypoglycemia is a frequent finding in the neonatal period, which results from the imbalance between carbohydrate intake, endogenous glucose production, and tissue usage.
- Neonates stabilize their serum glucose levels by about 12 hours after birth to 45 mg/dL (2.6 mmol/L). In a healthy state, glucose homeostasis underlays tight regulation through glucose-lowering hormones (insulin) and counterregulatory, glucose-mobilizing hormones (cortisol, growth hormone, and others) by acting on glycolysis, gluconeogenesis, glycogenolysis, and many other metabolic pathways involved in the biosynthesis, catabolism, or transport of carbohydrates, lipids, and amino acids.
- Hence, many inborn errors of metabolism can present with episodes of hypoglycemia during metabolic crises, which can be life threatening if not treated promptly.
- First presentation of an inborn error of metabolism can be at any age, with most cases presenting during times of metabolic stress or transition, as in infancy, illness, and dietary changes. Therefore, it is prudent to quickly establish a tentative diagnosis and initiate treatment in a sick neonate.

EPIDEMIOLOGY

- Incidence of hypoglycemia is estimated at 1 to 3/1,000 live births.
- Incidence of inherited forms is estimated at 1/50,000 live births in sporadic populations and higher in Ashkenazi Jews.
- The incidence of medium-chain acyl-CoA dehydrogenase (MCAD) deficiency ranges from 1:4,900 to 1:17,000 live births.
- Incidence of familial hyperinsulinism is 1 in 2,500 live births.

RISK FACTORS

Genetics

- Almost all inborn errors of metabolism causing hypoglycemia are autosomal recessive.
- Congenital hyperinsulinism can be autosomal dominant or recessive.
- Glycerol kinase deficiency is X-linked.

PATHOPHYSIOLOGY

- Through glycolysis and oxidative phosphorylation, glucose is a major source of cellular energy (ATP). Failure to produce ATP is probably the main source of hypoglycemia-associated tissue dysfunction.
- The brain preferentially uses glucose metabolism to produce energy and is particularly sensitive to hypoglycemia.
- A long list of metabolic disturbances in a variety of pathways can result in hypoglycemia.
- Neonates are at particular risk for hypoglycemia because they use glucose more rapidly than adults and have immature ability to obtain energy from other sources (glycogen, muscle protein, adipose tissue).

ETIOLOGY

- Inherited defects in biochemical pathways affecting metabolism of fats, amino acids, or carbohydrates
- Mutations in genes known to be involved in glucose metabolism, for example, congenital hyperinsulinism (*ABCC8, KCNJ11, GLUD1, CAK, HADH, SLC16A1, HNF4A*) and Fanconi-Bickel syndrome (*GLUT2, SCLA2*)

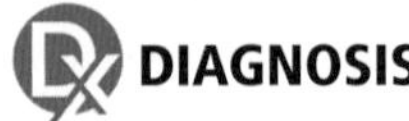

DIAGNOSIS

HISTORY

- Family history: Because inborn errors of metabolism are genetic disorders, patients may have a family history of poorly explained pediatric death. Diagnoses to ask about include the following:
  - Sepsis (was an organism identified?)
  - Sudden infant death syndrome
  - Cardiomyopathy
  - Uncontrollable seizures
  - Coma
  - Liver failure
- Unexplained developmental delay or hypoglycemia in older siblings
- First hypoglycemia after introducing different foods (e.g., milk, fruits)
- Complications with the pregnancy:
  - Maternal diabetes
  - Certain disorders of fatty acid oxidation are associated with fatty liver of pregnancy or HELLP (hemolysis, elevated liver enzymes, low platelets) syndrome.
  - Small for gestational age/intrauterine growth retardation/prematurity: may present with transient hypoglycemia
- Results of newborn screen: Children are tested for a variety of inborn errors of metabolism through newborn screening programs. Some of these disorders predispose to hypoglycemia and have specific therapies.
- Current diet and feeding schedule: Timing of hypoglycemia helps form differential diagnosis:
  - Hypoglycemia occurring shortly after feeding (0 to 4 hours) is suggestive of hyperinsulinism or inability to process carbohydrates (hereditary fructose intolerance).
  - Hypoglycemia between 2 and 10 hours after feeding is concerning for glycogen storage diseases, defects in gluconeogenesis, or counterregulatory hormone deficiencies.
  - Hypoglycemia after fasting (>6 hours) is suggestive of ketotic hypoglycemia, defects in gluconeogenesis, or fatty acid oxidation defects.

PHYSICAL EXAM

- ABCs and vital signs: Tachycardia, irritability, and weakness are commonly seen in hypoglycemia.
- Facies: Decreased interpupillary diameter or other midline anomalies occur in association with abnormalities of the pituitary.
- Skin: Diaphoresis is an effect of the catecholamine surge that accompanies hypoglycemia.
- CVS: cardiomyopathy (fatty acid oxidation defects, glycogen storage disorders, organic acidemias)
- Respiratory: Tachypnea may be the result of either respiratory compensation of metabolic acidosis or hyperammonemia.
- Hepatomegaly
- Occurs in many inborn errors of metabolism causing hypoglycemia and is a key feature in differentiating possible diagnoses
- May be due to abnormal accumulation of lipid (e.g., in fatty acid oxidation defects) or glycogen (e.g., glycogen storage disease)
- Renal: nephropathy/tubulopathy (organic acidemias, Fanconi-Bickel syndrome)
- GU:
  - Virilization in congenital adrenal hyperplasia
  - Micropenis in hypopituitarism
- Neurologic: Every neonate with a suspected inborn error of metabolism needs a complete neurologic exam to evaluate for level of consciousness, tone, unusual movements, and reflexes. Symptoms of neuroglycopenia include the following:
  - Tremulousness
  - Polyphagia
  - Seizures
  - Irritability
  - Weakness
  - Hypotonia
  - Stupor and coma occur if hypoglycemia is not reversed.
- Growth parameters:
  - Infants with Beckwith-Wiedemann syndrome, familial hyperinsulinism, or infants of diabetic mothers may be large for gestational age.
  - Beckwith-Wiedemann syndrome may also present with additional physical stigmata (hemihypertrophy, visceromegaly, macroglossia, abdominal wall defects) and hyperinsulinism.

DIFFERENTIAL DIAGNOSIS

Hypoglycemia is caused by increased glucose use or decreased glucose availability. Examples of disorders causing each:

- Increased glucose use
  - Sepsis increases metabolic demand and is a leading cause of neonatal hypoglycemia.
  - Familial hyperinsulinism: suspect when required glucose infusion rate (GIR) >10 to 20 mg/kg/min to maintain normoglycemia
  - Increased insulin production: Beckwith-Wiedemann syndrome, congenital hyperinsulinism
  - Decreased insulin counterregulatory hormones (glucagon, cortisol, growth hormone) due to adrenal insufficiency, hypopituitarism
- Decreased glucose availability/production
  - Infants of diabetic mothers
  - Small for gestational age: low energy stores, immaturity of glucose-regulating pathways
  - Liver failure/disease from ingested carbohydrates: galactosemia, hereditary fructose intolerance
  - Glycogen storage diseases
  - Glycerol kinase deficiency, glycerol intolerance

- Decreased gluconeogenesis: phosphoenolpyruvate carboxykinase deficiency, fructose-1, 6-diphosphatase deficiency, pyruvate carboxylase deficiency
- From decreased efficiency of pathways providing alternate energy sources: organic acidemias, fatty acid oxidation defects
- Disorders of glucose transporter:
  - GLUT1 or 2 deficiency
  - SGLT1 or 2 deficiency
- Various toxins or medications interfere with pathways needed to maintain glucose homeostasis, including salicylates, valproate, β-blockers, ethanol, and exogenous insulin.

DIAGNOSTIC TESTS & INTERPRETATION

Initial Tests (screening, lab, imaging)

The goal of the initial lab evaluation is to make a presumptive diagnosis. In many cases, definitive diagnosis requires specialized and time-consuming tests.

- Initial labs for a presumptive diagnosis in patient with hypoglycemia:
  - Dextrose stick
  - Urine dipstick: glucosuria (glucose transporter defects)
  - Electrolytes, BUN, creatinine, anion gap
  - CBC, blood culture
  - Serum and urinary ketones
  - Arterial blood gas with lactate
  - Liver function tests and PT/PTT
  - Urinalysis for reducing substances: positive in fructose intolerance, galactosemia
  - Plasma ammonia levels (obtained as free-flowing samples without tourniquet): Sample must be placed on wet ice and immediately transported to the lab for processing.
  - Review state newborn screen.
- Suspected disorders and follow-up testing:
  - Familial hyperinsulinism: high insulin levels, low/absent serum/urinary ketones
  - Adrenal insufficiency, hypopituitarism: low cortisol, growth hormone, epinephrine/norepinephrine levels
  - Defects of fatty acid oxidation or ketogenesis: plasma acylcarnitine profile, free fatty acids + 3-hydroxybutyrate/ketones (low)
  - Organic acidemias: urine organic acids, acylcarnitine profile
  - Factitious hypoglycemia/Munchausen syndrome by proxy: elevated C-peptide levels, toxicology screen: sulfonylureas, ethanol
  - Urea cycle defects: plasma amino acids, urine orotic acid
  - Galactosemia: urine galactitol, red blood cell galactose-1-phosphate uridyltransferase (GALT) activity, total galactose
  - Defects of gluconeogenesis/glycogen storage disease: arterial blood gas with lactate (lactic acidosis), +/− elevated creatine kinase (CK), specific enzyme testing or mutation analysis
  - Prolonged fasting: elevated free fatty acids + 3-hydroxybutyrate
  - Gene testing for specific disorders (Beckwith-Wiedemann syndrome)

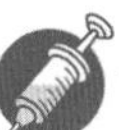

TREATMENT

Presumptive treatment should not await a definitive diagnosis but should be based on clinical suspicion and initial labs.

GENERAL MEASURES

- A well-appearing neonate with a low dextrose stick should be fed immediately. If feeds are contraindicated or not tolerated, obtain IV access.
- In children with associated physical or laboratory findings consistent with an inborn error of metabolism or other serious illness (e.g., vital sign instability, lethargy, acidosis), IV access should be obtained.
- A dextrose bolus (e.g., 5 cc/kg D10) rapidly corrects hypoglycemia in most cases. Infants requiring high GIR to maintain normoglycemia are suspicious for hyperinsulinism.

ADDITIONAL THERAPIES

Specific therapies vary according to the diagnosis and are best carried out by metabolic specialists:

- Hyperinsulinism
  - May require continuous glucose administration of 7 to 10 mg/kg/min (IV or via continuous gastric feeds)
  - Medical therapies including diazoxide and octreotide
  - Pancreatectomy
- Deficiencies in counterregulatory hormones: hormone supplementation
- Elimination of dietary lactose and galactose for those with galactosemia
- Elimination of dietary fructose for those with hereditary fructose intolerance
- Fatty acid oxidation disorders, glycogen storage disease type I, defects in gluconeogenesis: frequent feeds, fasting avoidance, increase caloric intake during stress. Some children may benefit from cornstarch supplementation before bedtime to prevent nocturnal hypoglycemia.

ADMISSION, INPATIENT, AND NURSING CONSIDERATIONS

- Admission criteria
  - Persistent or recurrent hypoglycemic episodes
  - Neurologic deficits
  - Unknown etiology of hypoglycemia requiring further workup
- Discharge criteria
  - Hypoglycemic episodes have resolved.
  - Full neurologic recovery
  - Fully fed and able to tolerate feeds
  - No major comorbid conditions that require hospital admission
  - Cause of the episode identified and addressed
  - Treatment plan to prevent future episodes understood by the parent or guardian
  - Follow-up with relevant specialist or physician has been arranged.

ONGOING CARE

COMPLICATIONS

Recurrent and severe hypoglycemic episodes affect neurocognitive development.

ADDITIONAL READING

- Datye KA, Bremer AA. Endocrine disorders in the neonatal period. *Pediatr Ann*. 2013;42(5):67–73.
- Hoe FM. Hypoglycemia in infants and children. *Adv Pediatr*. 2008;55:367–384.
- Stanley CA. Hypoglycemia in the neonate. *Pediatr Endocrinol Rev*. 2006;4(Suppl 1):76–81.
- Thornton PS, Stanley CA, De Leon DD, et al; for Pediatric Endocrine Society. Recommendations from the Pediatric Endocrine Society for evaluation and management of persistent hypoglycemia in neonates, infants, and children. *J Pediatr*. 2015;167(2):238–245.

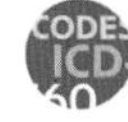

CODES

ICD10

- P70.4 Other neonatal hypoglycemia
- E88.9 Metabolic disorder, unspecified
- E88.89 Other specified metabolic disorders

FAQ

- Q: Why is hypoglycemia dangerous?
- A: Glucose is a crucial source of rapidly available energy for many tissues, especially the brain. Prolonged hypoglycemia causes CNS damage.
- Q: Why are the critical labs so important?
- A: In some metabolic disorders, the biochemical disturbance is apparent only during hypoglycemic episodes. Collecting this panel of informative labs during an episode greatly increases the chance of making a diagnosis.
- Q: If an infant dies before a diagnosis is made, what can be done to provide information for family members regarding future pregnancies?
- A: A postmortem exam can be helpful. A skin biopsy can yield fibroblasts for genetic and biochemical assays to investigate defects in specific pathways, and a muscle biopsy can be used to investigate mitochondrial disorders. Follow specific protocol for obtaining biopsies.
- Q: How soon after an infant dies should a skin biopsy be obtained?
- A: The skin biopsy does not need to be done immediately. Skin fibroblasts can grow if obtained up to 24 hours postmortem.

METABOLIC SYNDROME

Michele Mietus-Snyder, MD • Sheela N. Magge, MD, MSCE

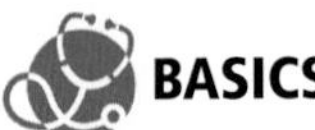

BASICS

DESCRIPTION

- A systemic disorder of energy regulation associated with ectopic fat deposition, immune activation, insulin resistance, and increased risk for cardiovascular disease (CVD) and type 2 diabetes mellitus (T2DM)
- Recognized by central adiposity, dyslipidemia, hypertension, and abnormal glucose tolerance
- These metabolic parameters change with age, gender, race, and ethnicity, so no established pediatric thresholds have been defined.
- Extrapolation from adult criteria permits diagnosis when ≥3 of the following five elements are present (approximate levels):
  - Waist circumference >90th percentile (waist to height ratio ≥0.5)
  - Low high-density lipoprotein cholesterol (HDL-c) <10th percentile (<40 mg/dL)
  - High triglycerides (TG) >90th percentile (≥90 mg/dL to age 9 years and then ≥110 mg/dL)
  - Hypertension: systolic and/or diastolic blood pressure (BP) ≥95th percentile for age, height, and gender
  - Elevated fasting blood sugar (>99 mg/dL) in youth with insulin resistance; hyperinsulinemia is more common than hyperglycemia.

EPIDEMIOLOGY

- Uncommon in children of normal weight
- Up to 60% of obese children meet criteria for the metabolic syndrome.
- Rates correlate with visceral and other ectopic fat depots.
- Highest rates in Native Americans > Hispanics > non–Hispanic (NH) Whites ~ Asians > NH Blacks
- More prevalent with age and in males than females

RISK FACTORS

- Prenatal and postnatal stressors
- Family history of T2DM and/or early CVD
- Diet high in processed foods, added sugars, trans fats
- Sedentary lifestyle
- Smoking or passive smoke exposure

Genetics

Sequence and epigenetic modification of genes involved in energy regulation have been implicated in disease progression, including adipose tissue differentiation, insulin signaling, and circadian clock genes as well as the mitochondrial genome.

PATHOPHYSIOLOGY

- Subcutaneous adipose capacity (which varies in individuals for both genetic and environmental reasons) is exceeded.
- Deposition of fat in hypertrophied adipose cells within nonadipose depots, notably visceral, hepatic, and muscular
- Triglyceride-engorged adipocytes trigger major histocompatibility complex (MHC) II response and immune activation. Antigen presentation may be endotoxin from microbial translocation.
- Stimulated monocyte/macrophage infiltration into ectopic adipose depots release tumor necrosis factor-α (TNF-α), interleukin-6 (IL-6), and monocyte chemotactic protein-1 (MCP-1).
- Chronic low level inflammation
- Mitochondrial dysfunction and excessive intracellular oxidative stress
- Insulin resistance and systemic consequences

ETIOLOGY

- Decreased mitochondrial reserve with age and physical inactivity
- Excessive caloric load, particularly a diet high in refined carbohydrate and/or trans fat
- Genetic and epigenetic predisposition

COMMONLY ASSOCIATED CONDITIONS

- Nonalcoholic fatty liver disease (NAFLD)
- Disordered sleep ± obstructive sleep apnea (OSA)
- Polycystic ovary syndrome (PCOS)
- Low 25-OH vitamin D level

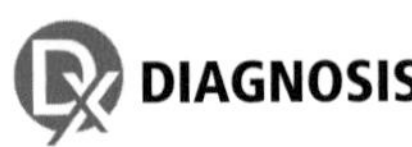

DIAGNOSIS

HISTORY

- Prenatal stress
  - Small or large for gestational age
  - Maternal gestational diabetes or eclampsia
  - Maternal or pregnancy-related overweight
- History of accelerated weight gain
  - Age at which weight gain started (physiologic insulin resistance of peripubertal years is a common trigger)
  - Previous difficulty losing weight (difficult to lose weight if insulin resistant)
- Psychosocial stressors: adverse childhood experiences, food insecurity, teasing
- Family history: early CVD and T2DM
- Lifestyle
  - Eating behavior
    - Sugared beverage consumption
    - Frequent processed snacks
    - Low fruit, vegetable, and whole grain intake
    - Aberrant eating patterns (skipping breakfast, lack of balanced meals)
  - Physical activity
    - Increased hours of screen time
    - Decreased moderate to vigorous physical activity
  - Poor sleep hygiene
- Parenting skills
  - Ability to set boundaries
  - Lifestyle role modeling
- Smoke exposure and smoking history
- Signs and symptoms
  - Obese patients with metabolic syndrome are usually asymptomatic but may have
    - Easy and rapid weight gain
    - Excessive hunger, carbohydrate craving
    - Snoring, gasps during sleep (OSA)
    - Fatigue, disinterest in activity
    - Headaches (may be symptom of OSA or pseudotumor cerebri)
    - Thickened, darkened skin in flexures, notably at the nape of the neck and axillae (suggestive of acanthosis nigricans) and skin tags
    - Polydipsia, polyuria, nocturia (concerning for diabetes)
    - Depression, anxiety, low self-efficacy
    - Abnormal menses, hirsutism, acne (concerning for PCOS)

PHYSICAL EXAM

A complete physical exam should be done on all patients. Special attention should be paid to the following:

- Weight, height, and BMI
- Waist circumference and waist to height ratio
- BP
- Papilledema
- Tanner stage
- Abdominal striae
- Hepatomegaly
- Acanthosis nigricans and skin tags
- Hirsutism, acne
- Affect, mood

DIFFERENTIAL DIAGNOSIS

The full cardiometabolic constellation of findings is unique to this syndrome, but individual features may present in other conditions:

- Familial combined hyperlipidemia
- Hereditary hypertriglyceridemia
- Essential hypertension
- Type 1 or 2 diabetes mellitus
- Lipodystrophies, complete or partial

DIAGNOSTIC TESTS & INTERPRETATION

Initial Tests (screening, lab, imaging)

Cardiometabolic screening (preferably fasting specimens) should be done on all obese patients:

- Fasting lipid profile: total cholesterol, HDL-c, and TG. Metabolic syndrome is a condition of hypertriglyceridemia not increased cholesterol. LDL-c is typically unremarkable; but in the presence of high TG, LDL particles are smaller and less well cleared so they are more numerous, whereas HDL particles, also smaller, are less stable and decreased in number and thus HDL-c is low. TG/HDL-c >3.0 predicts small LDL particles.
- Nonfasting lipid profile: non–HDL-c elevation
- Fasting glucose and insulin: Compensatory hyperinsulinism suggests (although not definitive) insulin resistance; homeostasis model assessment of insulin resistance (HOMA-IR) = (fasting insulin × FBG)/405: measure of insulin resistance in nondiabetics
- Hemoglobin A1c (HbA1c): may be indicative of chronic nonfasting sugar elevation; considered a screen for prediabetes and diabetes
- Liver function tests (LFTs): ALT and AST elevation are nonsensitive indicators of NAFLD.
- Thyroid function tests: may find mild elevations of TSH with normal T4
- 25-OH vitamin D level: often low
- 2-hour oral glucose tolerance test (OGTT): if fasting blood sugar >99 mg/dL, +/− HbA1c >5.6% (use clinical judgment), and/or symptoms of diabetes (polydipsia, polyuria, nocturia) to assess for impaired glucose tolerance and T2DM
- Abnormal lab tests should be repeated after a trial of weight management.
- Patients with hypertension should have an ECG to evaluate for LVH; consider ambulatory BP monitoring.
- Patients with elevated ALT or AST (particularly ALT) could have a 2D echo to assess for NAFLD.
- MRI is currently the gold standard for ectopic/visceral fat evaluation, although typically reserved for research.
- A history of disordered sleep and heavy snoring, especially with pauses in breathing, warrants a sleep study (polysomnogram).

TREATMENT

GENERAL MEASURES

Comprehensive behavioral modification through both improved diet and increased physical activity is the 1st-line treatment for metabolic syndrome. It decreases body weight, improves body composition and insulin sensitivity, and can positively affect CVD risk factors even if weight loss is not achieved, due to redistribution of fat from ectopic to subcutaneous depots and/or a favorable shift to lean muscle weight. The first 7–10% of weight lost comes preferentially from ectopic depots.

- Physical activity: ≥60 minutes per day of moderate to vigorous physical activity (can be in short intervals) defined as a level of effort that increases heart rate and produces heavier than at-rest breathing
- Diet: upgrade carbohydrate and fat quality
  - Avoid/limit sugar-sweetened beverages, specifically soda and juice. Limit sugar substitutes. Encourage water.
  - Dairy or dairy-free low-fat or fat-free unflavored milks for 2 to 21 years olds
  - Increase fiber intake.
    - ≥5 servings of whole fruits and vegetables per day
    - Increase whole grains in diet; avoid grains with <3 g fiber/serving.
  - Limit foods containing high-fructose corn syrup; limit added sugars; aim for total sugar to fiber ratio <5, ideally <3.
  - Fat content
    - Total fat, 30% of daily kcal/estimated energy requirement (EER)
    - Saturated fat, 8–10% of daily kcal/EER
    - Avoid trans fat.
    - Monounsaturated and polyunsaturated fat (PUFA) up to 20% of daily kcal/EER
    - Favor omega-3 PUFA
    - Cholesterol <300 mg/day
- Sedentary activity/screen time
  - Includes television, video games, texting, or computer not related to school
  - Limit screen <6 years and set consistent limits for children >6 years per AAP recommendations.
    - *See* Family Media Planning Tool: https://www.healthychildren.org/English/media/Pages/default.aspx
  - No TV in bedroom or screens after bedtime
- Smoking
  - Explicitly counsel about the dangers of smoking and advocate smoking cessation.
  - Counsel to avoid secondhand smoke.

MEDICATION

There are no pharmacologic treatments approved for the treatment of metabolic syndrome as a whole. Medications can be used to treat individual components. See "Additional Therapies."

ADDITIONAL THERAPIES

For individual elements of the metabolic syndrome

- Dyslipidemia: ≥10 to 21 years of age
  - LDL-c will not exceed 190 mg/dL with metabolic syndrome alone.
  - LDL-c >160 mg/dL unusual in metabolic syndrome, but hypercholesterolemia may coexist (See "Hyperlipidemia" chapter.)
  - LDL-c 130 to 159 mg/dL + 2 high-level risk factors OR 1 high-level + ≥2 moderate-level risk factors OR clinical CVD
    - Risk factor algorithm helps identify risk for small dense LDL and a higher LDL particle burden.
    - HMG-CoA reductase inhibitors (statins)—pravastatin or rosuvastatin preferred. Note side effects; needs monitoring. Counsel to use contraceptive methods to avoid pregnancy.
  - TG ≥110 to 499, non–HDL-c ≥145 (mg/dL)
    - Restrict refined carbohydrate intake.
    - Consider daily fish oil over-the-counter preparations with ~400 mg DHA + EPA.
  - TG >500 to 700 mg/dL and >10 years of age
    - Consider adjunct fibrate (off label).
  - TG ≥1,000 mg/dL
    - Not likely in metabolic syndrome alone; rule out primary hypertriglyceridemia
- Hypertension: stage 1 with no response to lifestyle changes × 3 to 6 months and stage 2
  - Rule out primary renal etiology (check U/A, BUN, creatinine, renin)
  - Angiotensin converting enzyme (ACE) inhibitors, angiotensin receptor blockers, diuretics, and vasodilators are used most commonly in pediatrics. Note side effects; needs monitoring
- T2DM
  - OGTT: fasting blood glucose ≥126 mg/dL or 2-hour ≥200 mg/dL or HbA1c ≥6.5%
    - Metformin or metformin ER are the only oral agents approved for the treatment of T2DM in children.
      - To minimize GI distress, titrate up over 2 to 4 weeks to 1,000 mg PO b.i.d. with meals.
      - Common side effects: nausea, bloating, diarrhea, and gas, which often resolve within 2 weeks
      - Rare side effects: lactic acidosis (increased risk with coexisting renal disease), megaloblastic anemia due to vitamin B_{12} deficiency; follow CBCs or prophylaxis with a daily multivitamin; follow LFTs.
      - Discontinue 48 hours prior to and after contrast administration or surgery.
      - Counsel to use contraceptive methods to avoid pregnancy.
  - Insulin injections—refer to endocrinology.
- Prediabetes
  - Impaired fasting glucose: 100 to 125 mg/dL
  - Impaired glucose tolerance: 2-hour glucose on OGTT: 140 to 199 mg/dL
  - HbA1c, 5.7–6.4%
    - Consider OGTT to rule out diabetes.
    - No consensus on the use of metformin in prediabetic states but some evidence of efficacy

ISSUES FOR REFERRAL

- Referral to pediatric lipid specialist for LDL-c ≥130 and/or TG ≥150 mg/dL and/or TG/HDL-c ≥3.0
- Referral to pediatric endocrinologist for diabetes, prediabetes, or PCOS
- Referral to pediatric gastroenterologist for ALT >2 times normal to rule out NAFLD
- Referral to pediatric hypertension specialist for stage 1 hypertension not responsive to lifestyle or stage 2 hypertension
- Consider referral to multidisciplinary pediatric weight management clinic for intensive lifestyle counseling.
- Consider psychological/behavioral counseling to overcome mood-related and motivational barriers to lifestyle therapy.

SURGERY/OTHER PROCEDURES

Bariatric surgery is a potential weight loss treatment for extreme obesity with cardiometabolic complications in older adolescents, with potential for significant insulin sensitization. Refer to a pediatric center experienced in bariatric surgery.

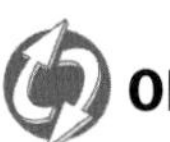

ONGOING CARE

FOLLOW-UP RECOMMENDATIONS

Patient Monitoring

- Ongoing weight management
- Children ≥10 years of age with BMI from 85th to 94th percentile: Check lipid profile at least every 2 years until normalized; if other risk factors are present, include fasting glucose and LFTs.
- Children ≥10 years of age with BMI ≥95th percentile: Check fasting lipid panel, glucose, and AST/ALT at least every 2 years and other tests as indicated.

PROGNOSIS

Multiple studies have shown that without aggressive intervention, cardiometabolic risk factors track from childhood to adulthood, increasing lifetime risk for T2DM and CVD.

ADDITIONAL READING

- Bremer AA, Mietus-Snyder M, Lustig RH. Toward a unifying hypothesis of metabolic syndrome. *Pediatrics*. 2012;129(3):557–570.
- D'Adamo E, Santoro N, Caprio S. Metabolic syndrome in pediatrics: old concepts revised, new concepts discussed. *Curr Probl Pediatr Adolesc Health Care*. 2013;43(5):114–123.
- Expert Panel on Integrated Guidelines for Cardiovascular Health and Risk Reduction in Children and Adolescents; National Heart, Lung, and Blood Institute. Expert panel on integrated guidelines for cardiovascular health and risk reduction in children and adolescents: summary report. *Pediatrics*. 2011;128(Suppl 5):S213–S256.
- Khoury M, Manlhiot C, McCrindle BW. Role of the waist/height ratio in the cardiometabolic risk assessment of children classified by body mass index. *J Am Coll Cardiol*. 2013;62(8):742–751.
- Magge SN, Goodman E, Armstrong SC; and the Committee on Nutrition, Section on Endocrinology, Section on Obesity. The metabolic syndrome in children and adolescents: shifting the focus to cardiometabolic risk factor clustering [published online ahead of print July 24, 2017]. *Pediatrics*. doi:10.1542/peds.2017-1603.

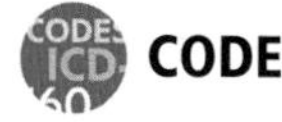

CODES

ICD10

E88.81 Metabolic Syndrome

FAQ

- Q: Why is it important to diagnose metabolic syndrome?
- A: Although obesity increases metabolic risk, not everyone who is obese develops complications; those at the greatest cardiometabolic risk need additional screening and intervention.
- Q: Do children with the metabolic syndrome have it when they become adults?
- A: If children with the metabolic syndrome do not use diet and exercise to treat it, they will likely have it as adults.
- Q: Does cardiovascular risk improve if these children lose weight?
- A: Yes, 7–10% body weight loss can result in improvement of CVD risk factors due to preferential weight loss from the ectopic visceral fat depot.

METHEMOGLOBINEMIA

Kevin C. Osterhoudt, MD, MS

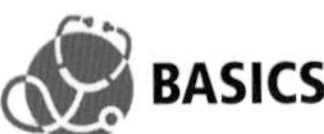

BASICS

DESCRIPTION

- Methemoglobin is dysfunctional hemoglobin in which the deoxygenated heme moiety has been oxidized from the ferrous (Fe^{2+}) to the ferric (Fe^{3+}) state.
- Methemoglobinemia is an undue accumulation of methemoglobin within the blood.

EPIDEMIOLOGY

- Toxic methemoglobinemia, resulting from exposure to oxidant chemicals or drugs, is the most common cause of methemoglobinemia among children >6 months of age.
- Enteritis-associated methemoglobinemia is the most common cause among children <6 months of age:
  - As many as 2/3 of infants with severe diarrhea have methemoglobinemia.

PATHOPHYSIOLOGY

- Hemoglobin in the allosteric configuration of methemoglobin cannot carry oxygen.
- Methemoglobin increases the oxygen affinity of normal heme moieties in the blood and results in impaired oxygen delivery to tissues.
- NADH-dependent cytochrome b5 methemoglobin reductase is the major source of physiologic reduction of methemoglobin.
- A normally dormant NADPH-dependent methemoglobin reductase is the site of action for antidotal methylene blue therapy.

ETIOLOGY

- Toxic methemoglobinemia
  - Dietary or environmental chemicals:
    - Chlorates
    - Chromates
    - Copper sulfate fungicides
    - Naphthalene
    - Nitrates
    - Nitrites
  - Industrial chemicals: aniline and other nitrogenated organic compounds
  - Drugs (e.g., amyl nitrite, benzocaine, dapsone, metoclopramide, nitric oxide, nitroprusside, phenazopyridine, prilocaine)
  - Methemoglobinemia is a common iatrogenic complication of drug therapy.
- Illness/enteritis-associated methemoglobinemia is multifactorial in origin:
  - Intestinal nitrate and nitric oxide promotes methemoglobin formation.
  - Innate enzymatic methemoglobin reduction systems may be underdeveloped during infancy.
  - Acidemia further inhibits enzymatic methemoglobin reduction systems.
  - Methemoglobinemia is also reported with nitrite-producing bacterial infections of the intestines or urinary tract.
- Congenital methemoglobinemia (rare)
  - Hemoglobin M: Heterozygotes for autosomal dominant hemoglobin M will exhibit lifelong cyanosis.
  - NADH-dependent methemoglobin reductase deficiency: Homozygotes for this autosomal recessive enzyme will have lifelong cyanosis; heterozygotes may have increased susceptibility to oxidative hemoglobin injury.

COMMONLY ASSOCIATED CONDITIONS

- Heinz body hemolytic anemia
  - Oxidant stress on the globin protein may cause hemolysis.
- Sulfhemoglobinemia
  - Oxidant stress on the hemoglobin porphyrin ring may cause sulfhemoglobinemia.

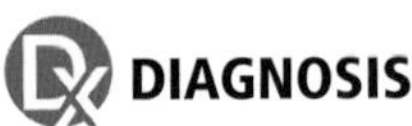

DIAGNOSIS

HISTORY

- Age of onset
  - New onset of cyanosis in children >6 months of age is unlikely to be due to congenital or enteritis-associated methemoglobinemia.
- Source of water
  - Well water may be contaminated with nitrates.
- Drug or chemical exposure
  - May suggest a source of toxic methemoglobinemia
- Diarrhea
  - May suggest enteritis-associated methemoglobinemia

PHYSICAL EXAM

- Cyanosis
  - Cyanosis becomes apparent in the presence of 1.5 g/dL of methemoglobin (in contrast to 4 to 5 g/dL of deoxyhemoglobin).
- Heart murmur
  - May suggest right-to-left intracardiac shunting rather than methemoglobinemia
- Abnormal lung auscultation:
  - May suggest cyanosis due to pulmonary disorder
- Signs and symptoms
  - Malaise
  - Fatigue
  - Dyspnea
  - Tachycardia
  - Cyanosis

DIFFERENTIAL DIAGNOSIS

- Environmental hypoxia
- Cardiovascular disease
- Pulmonary disease
- Sulfhemoglobinemia
- Factitious skin discoloration

DIAGNOSTIC TESTS & INTERPRETATION

Initial Tests (screening, lab, imaging)

- Oxygen saturation
  - Oxygen saturation measured by pulse oximetry is artificially low, but oxygen saturation calculated from arterial blood gas is normal (a "saturation gap").
- Co-oximetry
  - Multiple-wavelength co-oximetry is the standard for quantifying methemoglobin in the blood.
- Hemoglobin quantitation
  - The percent methemoglobin concentration must be considered in relation to the total hemoglobin.
  - Anemia may suggest concurrent hemolysis.
- Serum bicarbonate
  - Metabolic acidosis is relatively mild in cases of <40% toxic methemoglobinemia.
  - Metabolic acidosis is typically profound in cases of enteritis-associated methemoglobinemia.
- Glucose-6-phosphate dehydrogenase (G6PD) assay
  - G6PD deficiency does not predispose to methemoglobinemia and should not be routinely ordered.
  - G6PD deficient patients develop hemolysis in face of oxidant stress.

- Hemoglobin electrophoresis
  - Hemoglobin M is rare; it can be suspected if methemoglobinemia is chronic and does not respond to therapy.
  - This test should not be routinely ordered.
- Methemoglobin reductase deficiency quantitation
  - Homozygous enzyme deficiency may be suspected if methemoglobinemia is congenital and chronic and does respond to therapy.
  - This test should not be routinely ordered.

Diagnostic Procedures/Other

- Pulse oximetry may be inaccurate in the setting of methemoglobinemia or methylene blue therapy; suspect methemoglobinemia if frank cyanosis is noted with pulse oximetry measurement of 84–90%.
- Blood may have a "chocolate brown" appearance despite exposure to air.

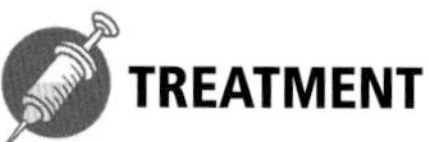

TREATMENT

GENERAL MEASURES

- Acquired methemoglobinemia
  - Administer 100% oxygen.
  - Decontaminate or remove from toxic source of oxidative stress.
  - Alleviate enteritis with IV fluids or elemental formulas.
  - Treat identified bacterial infections.
  - Exchange transfusion is a consideration of last resort.
- Congenital methemoglobinemia
  - No beneficial therapy exists for hemoglobin M.
  - Oral methylene blue or ascorbic acid may provide alternative reduction pathways for patients with NADH-dependent reductase deficiencies.

MEDICATION

- Consider administration of 1% methylene blue.
  - Dose: 1 to 2 mg/kg IV >5 minutes, repeated as necessary (consider alternative therapy if resolution does not occur after 2 doses; caution above 4 to 7 mg/kg total)
  - Indications: signs of tissue hypoxia, CNS depression, >30% methemoglobinemia
  - Contraindications (relative): known, severe G6PD deficiency
  - Consider alternative therapy after 2 doses without resolution.
- Methylene blue therapy may be ineffective if
  - Patient is G6PD deficient.
  - Ongoing drug or chemical absorption or biotransformation leads to continuing methemoglobin formation.
  - Sulfhemoglobin is present.
  - Hemoglobin M is present.
  - High doses of methylene blue add to, rather than ameliorate, the oxidant stress.

ONGOING CARE

FOLLOW-UP RECOMMENDATIONS

- Toxic methemoglobinemia
  - Consider consultation with a medical toxicologist.
  - May require environmental investigation
- Enteritis-associated methemoglobinemia
  - Careful formula rechallenge warranted if possibility exists for milk protein allergy or other dietary intolerance
- Congenital methemoglobinemia
  - Consider consultation with a hematologist and or metabolism specialist.

PROGNOSIS

- Toxic methemoglobinemia
  - Full recovery with recognition, removal of oxidant stress, and appropriate therapy
- Enteritis-associated methemoglobinemia
  - Methemoglobinemia may be prolonged and relapsing until enteritis healed.
- Congenital methemoglobinemia
  - Lifelong cyanosis expected

COMPLICATIONS

- >10% methemoglobinemia
  - Cyanosis
- >30% methemoglobinemia
  - Malaise, fatigue, dyspnea, tachycardia
- >50% methemoglobinemia
  - Somnolence, tissue ischemia
- 60% methemoglobinemia
  - Potential lethality

ADDITIONAL READING

- Canning J, Levine M. Case files of the medical toxicology fellowship at Banner Good Samaritan Medical Center in Phoenix, AZ: methemoglobinemia following dapsone exposure. *J Med Toxicol*. 2011;7(2):139–146.
- D'sa SR, Victor P, Jagannati M, et al. Severe methemoglobinemia due to ingestion of toxicants. *Clin Toxicol (Phila)*. 2014;52(8):897–900.
- Skold A, Cosco DL, Klein R. Methemoglobinemia: pathogenesis, diagnosis, and management. *South Med J*. 2011;104(11):757–761.

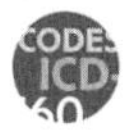

CODES

ICD10

- D74.9 Methemoglobinemia, unspecified
- D74.8 Other methemoglobinemias
- D74.0 Congenital methemoglobinemia

FAQ

- Q: Can methemoglobinemia be diagnosed by the color of the blood?
- A: The "chocolate brown" blood of methemoglobinemia is most easily noted when compared to "control" blood on a white filter paper background. In contrast to deoxygenated blood from patients with cardiopulmonary disease, methemoglobin-darkened blood does not redden on exposure to room air.
- Q: Is methemoglobin responsible for the profound metabolic acidosis often found in diarrheal infants?
- A: Benzocaine-induced methemoglobinemia rarely causes acidosis in infants. In contrast, infants with enteritis-associated methemoglobinemia often have a profound acidemia with a relatively narrow anion gap. Acidosis should be considered a contributing or coexisting factor, rather than a result, of methemoglobinemia among infants with diarrhea.

M

MICROCYTIC ANEMIA

Tannie Huang, MD • James N. Huang, MD

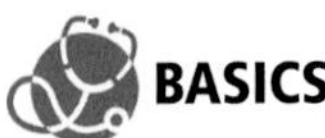

BASICS

DESCRIPTION

Microcytic anemia is defined as a hemoglobin 2 standard deviations (*SD*) below the mean associated with an abnormally low mean corpuscular volume (MCV). Use of age-based norms for both indices is critical.

EPIDEMIOLOGY

- In pediatrics, the most common cause of microcytic anemia is iron deficiency anemia (IDA).
- IDA incidence by age:
  - 1 to 2 years, 14%
  - Adolescent females, 9%
- Hemoglobinopathies causing microcytic anemia are common in Mediterranean countries, Southeast Asia, China, Africa, and India. Incidence in the United States is currently increasing due to increasing immigration.

RISK FACTORS

- Prematurity, breastfeeding, lower socioeconomic class, and overweight infants are more likely to have IDA.
- Certain ethnic groups such as African Americans and Hispanics have higher rates of iron deficiency. These groups also have a higher incidence of hemoglobinopathies, which can complicate the clinical picture.
- Exposures to lead-based products can cause microcytic anemia resulting from lead poisoning.

PATHOPHYSIOLOGY

- Iron homeostasis in the body is primarily regulated through mechanisms of iron absorption.
- Iron is absorbed through duodenal enterocytes and then transported to the liver. Hepcidin is synthesized by the liver and is the major regulator of iron absorption. The amount of dietary iron that is absorbed is relatively low but varies depending on the patient's iron stores.
- The body loses about 1 to 2 mg/day of iron through loss of intestinal epithelia. This amount is higher in menstruating females.
- IDA usually develops from absorption that is inadequate to compensate for excretion and the demands required for growth (in children).
- Hemoglobin is made up of two alpha globin chains and two beta globin chains. Abnormalities in the production of these chains can lead to microcytic anemia. Anemia can develop either through inadequate production of one of these chains or through increased clearance of red blood cells (RBCs) with mutated globin chains
- Disturbed iron utilization results from lead poisoning or sideroblastic anemia.

ETIOLOGY

- The most common cause of microcytic anemia is iron deficiency.
- Hemoglobinopathies are the next most common cause in childhood. Of the hemoglobinopathies, hemoglobin E and α- and β-thalassemias most commonly cause microcytic anemia.
- Rarely, disorders of heme synthesis such as dyserythropoietic anemias and sideroblastic anemia can be a cause of microcytic anemia.
- Anemia of chronic disease can occasionally be microcytic, although more frequently is normocytic.

DIAGNOSIS

HISTORY

- Age of onset: Iron deficiency is most common in infancy and menstruating females. An adolescent male with IDA should be a red flag and an alert to look for ongoing occult blood loss.
- Ethnic background
- Dietary history, including
  - Breast- versus formula-fed in infancy
  - Daily milk consumption of >24 oz is associated with IDA.
  - Lack of red meat consumption
  - Pica (including geophagia and pagophagia)
  - Restrictive eating (anorexia)
- Lead exposure (often paint in older homes, mini blinds, ceramic dishware, or toys)
- GI symptoms including diarrhea/constipation
- Blood loss (can be from GI, urinary, epistaxis, menstruation, and rarely pulmonary causes)
- Weight loss/fever/malaise or other symptoms of systemic disease
- Family members who have needed transfusions. In pubertal females, a maternal menstrual history may be informative.
- Special questions: Children with behavioral problems, including breath-holding spells, have higher rates of iron deficiency.

PHYSICAL EXAM

- Most children with iron deficiency are well appearing with a normal physical exam. They may be somewhat irritable.
- Frontal bossing or malocclusion of the teeth can be seen in children with thalassemia due to expansion of the bone marrow compartment.
- Pallor is the most common finding.
  - Evaluate in the face, conjunctiva, gums, and nail beds. Palmar crease becomes pale with a hemoglobin <7 g/dL.
- Eyes
  - Blue sclera can be occasionally observed in iron deficiency.
  - Scleral icterus may be seen in patients with hemoglobinopathies.
- Glossitis may be seen in patients with chronic iron deficiency.
- Cardiovascular examination
  - Auscultate for tachycardia and flow murmurs. However, often, children with chronic IDA may not have tachycardia.
  - Cardiac instability is rare but does occur.
- Splenomegaly: The spleen enlarges in some patients with thalassemia as a site of extramedullary hematopoiesis. This is a rare finding in IDA, although it has been reported.
- Nail abnormalities: Spoon nails (koilonychia) can be seen in long-standing iron deficiency.

DIFFERENTIAL DIAGNOSIS

- Iron deficiency
- Hemoglobinopathies
- Chronic lead poisoning
- Anemia of chronic disease
- Sideroblastic anemia

DIAGNOSTIC TESTS & INTERPRETATION

- No single test identifies all the causes of microcytic anemia. Children are often identified through routine screening at well-child exams.
- CBC: low hemoglobin level and low MCV for age (lower limit of normal can be estimated by 70+ age in years)
  - Red cell distribution width (RDW) is increased in IDA and normal in thalassemia.
  - RBC count is elevated in thalassemia. Mentzer index: MCV/RBC count in millions: <13 points, toward thalassemia; >13 points, toward IDA
  - Reticulocyte count: reticulocytopenia in IDA, reticulocytosis in hemoglobinopathies
  - Thrombocytosis is often seen in IDA (can appear prior to microcytosis). In severe, prolonged iron deficiency, thrombocytopenia eventually develops.
  - Peripheral blood smear
    - Hypochromia and bizarre forms in IDA
    - Target cells are seen in patients with thalassemia.
    - Basophilic stippling with lead poisoning
- Iron studies: Ferritin, serum iron, transferrin saturation, and TIBC must be interpreted together. In the face of iron deficiency, the body's iron stores are first mobilized. It is only once these iron stores are depleted that microcytosis develops.
  - Ferritin
    - Decreased in iron deficiency
    - Most sensitive index for iron deficiency. A ferritin of less than 30 is over 90% sensitive and specific for IDA.
    - As a measure of iron stores in the liver, it is one of the earliest indices to change in IDA.
    - May be elevated out of proportion to iron stores because it is an acute-phase reactant and will rise with infection, inflammation, malignancy, or liver disease
    - Can be increased in patients with thalassemia who have not received transfusion because ineffective erythropoiesis leads to increased GI absorption of iron

- Serum iron
  - Fluctuates with daily iron intake
  - Normal in thalassemia (unless chronically transfused, which leads to increased iron levels)
  - Normal or reduced in infection or inflammatory states
- TIBC
  - Elevated in IDA but can be normal to decreased in anemia of chronic disease
  - Oral contraceptives can increase TIBC.
  - Liver disease and malnutrition can decrease TIBC.
- Transferrin saturation
  - Calculated value (serum iron/TIBC × 100)
  - Low in IDA
- Soluble transferrin receptor
  - Newer test used to determine iron status. It is increased in IDA and also in thalassemia syndromes but not with the anemia of chronic disease.
  - Unlike ferritin, it is not an acute phase reactant and does not increase with inflammation or infection.
  - Should not be used routinely in patients in the evaluation of IDA but only in patients with other illnesses that make the interpretation of ferritin levels difficult
- Lead level and free erythrocyte protoporphyrin (FEP) are both elevated in lead intoxication. Lead poisoning and IDA can exist together.

ALERT

Results of hemoglobin electrophoresis are only reliable in patients with normal iron stores.
If patients have abnormal iron studies, repeat hemoglobin electrophoresis after adequate period of iron supplementation

- Hemoglobin electrophoresis (quantitative)
  - Decreased hemoglobin A and increased hemoglobin A2 in β-thalassemia trait
  - Normal hemoglobin electrophoresis in patients with one (silent carrier) and two (trait) alpha-globin thalassemic mutations
  - Hemoglobin H consists of tetramers of beta globin chains and is seen in patients with three alpha-globin mutations.
- If a patient has been transfused or labs cannot be drawn, labs on the parents may be helpful. A CBC, peripheral smear, and a hemoglobin electrophoresis are usually sufficient.

Diagnostic Procedures/Other

- Bone marrow aspirate is rarely indicated but can be performed if malignancy or disorders of heme synthesis are in the differential.
- Recurrent iron deficiency despite treatment raises suspicion for ongoing blood loss. Guaiac test stools to look for occult GI bleeding, common in children with milk protein allergy. Urinalysis for evidence of renal RBC loss. Pulmonary hemosiderosis can present as recurrent pneumonias.

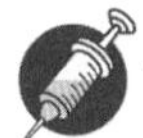

TREATMENT

Depends on cause of microcytic anemia

GENERAL MEASURES

- Many patients are identified on routine well-child screening. Consider therapeutic trial of iron supplementation without further workup if history is suspicious.
- Encourage intake of iron-rich foods and elimination of milk. Oral iron supplementation and altered dietary practices improves anemia in almost all patients.
- For adolescent females, oral hormones can help control ongoing blood losses through menstruation.
- Parents should be able to report seeing dark black iron in the stool. Iron can cause nausea, GI discomfort, and constipation. Stool softeners can help.
- Transfusion of RBCs is rarely indicated and is only needed in patients with cardiovascular instability.
- Treatment of lead poisoning is achieved through chelation and removal of environmental exposures. Discuss with local health department.
- In patients with microcytic anemia from hemoglobinopathies, but normal iron indices, iron therapy is not indicated.
- Hematology referral and genetic counseling for patients with hemoglobinopathies

MEDICATION

- For patients with iron deficiency (see "Iron Deficiency Anemia" chapter for details) ferrous sulfate or ferrous gluconate at 6 mg/kg of elemental iron per day in divided doses
  - Iron salts should be taken with orange juice, as ascorbic acid increases absorption. It should *not* be taken with milk. Patients on proton pump inhibitors may have decreased absorption.
  - For patients who do not tolerate iron salts because of GI side effects, an alternative oral regimen using polysaccharide-iron complexes may be considered. Dosing is the same as iron salts (6 mg/kg/24 h of elemental iron).
  - IV iron is generally reserved for patients with malabsorption. Iron sucrose, ferric gluconate, and iron dextran are available in the United States. Anaphylaxis is the primary adverse reaction; iron sucrose and ferric gluconate have lower rates of anaphylaxis.
- For patients with lead poisoning, chelation therapy may be necessary (see "Lead Poisoning" chapter).

ONGOING CARE

FOLLOW-UP RECOMMENDATIONS

- Repeat laboratory evaluation can be done in 1 month. Reticulocyte count is the first laboratory value to change and begins to increase within a week after the initiation of iron therapy. Hemoglobin levels take at least 2 to 3 weeks to respond. MCV is the last index to improve.
- Poor adherence to therapy is the most common cause of treatment failure.
- Children with IDA are more likely to have more difficulties with learning and behavioral problems.
- Children with other hemoglobinopathies should be referred to a hematologist. They do not need further treatment with iron.

ADDITIONAL READING

- Borgna-Pignatti C, Zanella S. Pica as a manifestation of iron deficiency. *Expert Rev Hematol*. 2016;9(11):1075–1080.
- Higgs DR, Engel JD, Stamatoyannopoulos G. Thalassemia. *Lancet*. 2012;379(9813):373–383.
- Janus J, Moerschel SK. Evaluation of anemia in children. *Am Fam Physician*. 2010;81(12):1462–1471.
- McCann JC, Ames BN. An overview of evidence for a causal relation between iron deficiency during development and deficits in cognitive or behavioral function. *Am J Clin Nutr*. 2007;85(4):931–945.
- Walters MC, Abelson HT. Interpretation of the complete blood count. *Pediatr Clin North Am*. 1996;43(3):599–622.
- Wang B, Zhan S, Gong T, et al. Iron therapy for improving psychomotor development and cognitive function in children under the age of three with iron deficiency anaemia. *Cochrane Database Syst Rev*. 2013;(6):CD001444.

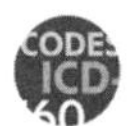

CODES

ICD10

- D50.9 Iron deficiency anemia, unspecified
- D58.2 Other hemoglobinopathies
- D50.8 Other iron deficiency anemias

MILIA

Danielle G. Dooley, MD, MPhil, FAAP

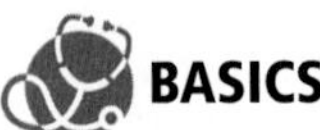

BASICS

DESCRIPTION

- Small (<3 mm) benign, keratin-filled cysts that present as white papules most typically on the face but may occur elsewhere on the body (palate, gingiva, genitals)
- Subtypes include primary and secondary milia.
  - Primary: spontaneous
  - Secondary: secondary to trauma, medications, or another disease
- Milia en plaque is a rare type of primary milia which typically occurs in the posterior auricular area as an erythematous plaque.
- Multiple eruptive milia (MEM) occurs in children and adults when milia erupt in a large number; may be spontaneous, familial, or associated another disease

EPIDEMIOLOGY

- Congenital milia is the most common form of primary milia.
  - 40–50% of newborns have milia.
  - Less common in premature infants
  - No gender or racial predilection
- Secondary milia can occur in all age groups.

RISK FACTORS

- Full-term newborns
- Any bullous condition increases the risk of secondary milia, particularly epidermolysis bullosa and porphyria.

Genetics

- No known genetic predisposition for primary congenital milia, the most common type of milia encountered in pediatrics
- Milia may be a major feature of rare genetic diseases of the skin.
  - Loeys-Dietz syndrome
  - Oral-facial-digital syndrome type 1
  - Rombo syndrome
  - Bazex-Dupré-Christol syndrome

GENERAL PREVENTION

There are no known preventative measures for primary milia.

PATHOPHYSIOLOGY

Retention of keratin and sebaceous material within the sebaceous collar surrounding fine vellus hair (primary milia) or eccrine sweat duct (secondary milia)

ETIOLOGY

- Most commonly spontaneous in newborns
- May be related to trauma or blistering conditions in older children

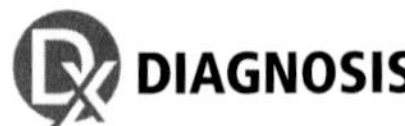

DIAGNOSIS

HISTORY

- Primary congenital milia
  - Asymptomatic
  - Typically present at birth or in the first few days of life
  - Parents may report oral findings.
- Secondary milia
  - Ask about recent trauma, burns, skin grafts or peels, laser treatment, medications.
  - History of blistering diseases

PHYSICAL EXAM

- 1 to 2 mm pinpoint, white, pearly smooth papules without surrounding erythema or inflammation
- Congenital milia distribution is most often on nose, cheeks, chin, and forehead in congenital milia.
- Benign primary milia distribution is most often eyelids and cheeks in children and adults.
- Other places to consider
  - Oral mucosa: Epstein pearls on midline palate, Bohn nodules, and gingival cysts on gums
  - Glans penis cysts
  - Nasal crease

DIFFERENTIAL DIAGNOSIS

Other considerations in the newborn period are as follows:

- Sebaceous gland hyperplasia:
  - Secondary to exposure to maternal hormones
  - Lesions are yellowish, follicular papules typically on nose, cheeks, upper lip, and forehead.
- Neonatal acne:
  - Inflammatory, erythematous, papulopustular rash on the face and scalp
  - Usually appears after 1 to 2 weeks of life, although it may be present at birth
- Erythema toxicum:
  - Benign rash in the neonatal period
  - It is characterized by erythematous macules, often with a central pustule or vesicle.
- Other considerations in children:
  - Seborrheic keratosis
  - Congenital melanocytic nevi
  - Calcinosis cutis

DIAGNOSTIC TESTS & INTERPRETATION

The diagnosis of milia can be made by history and physical exam alone. No further diagnostic testing is needed.

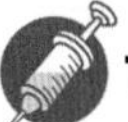

TREATMENT

- Primary congenital milia require no treatment. Milia are benign, asymptomatic, and self-limiting in this condition.
- Treatment may be indicated in the following settings:
  - Diffuse or persistent milia in older children
  - Milia in areas of trauma or burn leading to cosmetic concern
- Treatment could include topical retinoid, electrocautery, or manual extraction.

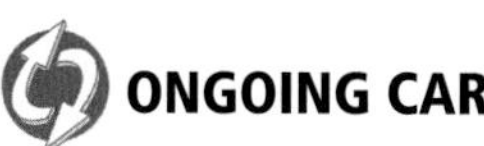

ONGOING CARE

FOLLOW-UP RECOMMENDATIONS

No specific monitoring or follow-up is necessary in congenital milia.

PROGNOSIS

- Natural history of primary congenital milia is that the majority of cases will resolve spontaneously within a few weeks to months without scarring or recurrence.
- In infants or children with diffuse or persistent milia, consider further evaluation for genodermatoses. Such conditions include Loeys-Dietz syndrome, oral-facial-digital syndrome type 1, Rombo syndrome, or Bazex-Dupré-Christol syndrome.

COMPLICATIONS

Cosmetic concerns based on location of milia are usually the only complicating factor.

ADDITIONAL READING

- Berk DR, Bayliss SJ. Milia: a review and classification. *J Am Acad Dermatol*. 2008;59(6):1050–1063.
- Connelly T. Eruptive milia and rapid response to topical tretinoin. *Arch Dermatol*. 2008;144(6):816–817.
- Leong T, Torres A, Macknet KD Jr, et al. Pronounced secondary milia precipitated by a superficial traumatic abrasion in a 4-year-old boy. *J Pediatr*. 2010;156(5):854.
- Wang AR, Bercovitch L. Congenital milia en plaque. *Pediatr Dermatol*. 2016;33(4):e258–e259.
- Link to images
  - Aby J. Photo gallery, professional education. Stanford School of Medicine Newborn Nursery at Lucille Packard Children's Hospital Web site. http://newborns.stanford.edu/PhotoGallery/Milia1.html. Published 2013. Accessed January 31, 2017.

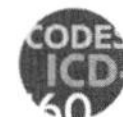

CODES

ICD10

- L70.2 Acne varioliformis
- L85.1 Acquired keratosis [keratoderma] palmaris et plantaris
- K09.8 Other cysts of oral region, not elsewhere classified

FAQ

- Q: Are milia painful or pruritic?
- A: No. Milia are asymptomatic. If there is pain, pruritus, fever, or other constitutional symptoms, the diagnosis of milia should be reconsidered.
- Q: Are milia contagious?
- A: No, they are not transmitted from person to person. In the case of congenital milia of the newborn, the parent should be reassured that the lesions are not infectious.
- Q: Are milia and miliaria the same condition?
- A: No. Both are benign skin conditions of childhood. However, miliaria is a disorder of the eccrine sweat glands, not of the pilosebaceous duct. Miliaria is characterized by sweat retention and subsequent vesicle formation, usually after prolonged perspiration. Miliaria is thought to occur because of sweat duct obstruction.

MORPHEA (LOCALIZED SCLERODERMA)

Lisa M. Arkin, MD • Kaveh Ardalan, MD, MS

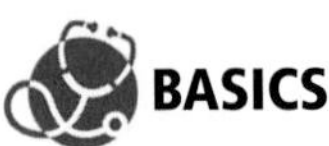

BASICS

DESCRIPTION

- The term for localized scleroderma is morphea, which is derived from the Greek word for "form" or "structure." Fibrosis is characteristic and may involve the skin, subcutaneous (SC) fat, cartilage, muscle, and bone.
- Morphea must be differentiated from systemic sclerosis, which is a systemic vasculopathy that carries a poorer prognosis. Both are clinical, rather than laboratory diagnoses, because the skin histopathology is identical for both diseases. Clinical hallmarks to differentiate these diagnoses include:
  - Progressive systemic sclerosis: begins with symmetric distal acral sclerosis with sclerodactyly, Raynaud phenomenon, dilated nailfold capillary loops with dropout (All are stigmata of vasculopathy.)
  - Morphea: *spares* the distal finger tips and toes but may involve the dorsal hands and feet, absence of Raynaud and abnormal nailfold capillary loops, no true visceral fibrosis
- Padua classification for morphea:
  - Circumscribed: localized indurated plaques
  - Generalized: ≥4 plaques, >3 cm, >2 body sites
  - Linear: linear plaques face, scalp, extremity, or trunk
    - Affecting trunk or limbs
    - Affecting head: includes en coup de sabre (epidermal change) and Parry-Romberg syndrome (hemifacial atrophy)—these are thought to exist on a spectrum.
  - Pansclerotic: confluent full-thickness sclerodermoid plaques, generally *spares* the distal fingertips and toes
  - Mixed: more than one subtype
  - Any subtype can have a deep component.

EPIDEMIOLOGY

- Linear morphea is the most frequent subtype (~50–65%), followed by circumscribed morphea (~25%), generalized morphea (5–8%), and pansclerotic (1–2%) morphea.
- Many patients (15–20%) present with more than one subtype of morphea (mixed morphea).
- Localized scleroderma is approximately 10 times more common than systemic sclerosis in childhood. The annual age and sex adjusted incidence is 2.7 cases per 100,000.

PATHOPHYSIOLOGY

- Speculated to share common pathophysiology with systemic sclerosis despite differing clinical presentations
- Early: T-cell mononuclear cell population, with CD4 > CD8 predominance, and Th1/Th17 activation inducing inflammation with clinical evidence of erythema, induration, and lesional enlargement
- Late: T-cell associated cytokines stimulate fibroblasts and endothelial cells to produce transforming growth factor β (TGF-β) and connective tissue growth factor (CTGF), which are main stimulators of tissue fibrosis and increased collagen production. Skewing to immunologic Th2 axis leads to permanent disease damage including late fibrosis and atrophy.

DIAGNOSIS

PHYSICAL EXAM

- General concepts:
  - Fibrosis limited to skin, SC tissue, muscle, and bone
  - Systemic features including Raynaud phenomenon and true visceral fibrosis should prompt reconsideration of diagnosis.
  - Extracutaneous manifestations in 25–40% strongly correlate with subtype:
    - Linear morphea on the face: increased risk of ocular findings (episcleritis, uveitis) and CNS disease including T1 and T2 hyperintensities on MRI that may mimic imaging findings in multiple sclerosis; symptoms including seizures, migraines, headaches, and difficulty concentrating
    - Linear morphea that traverses a joint: increased risk of joint contractures and limb length discrepancy if involvement of the epiphyseal plate. Inflammatory arthritis can occur; may not always correspond to site of skin lesion; musculoskeletal complications reported in 30–50%
    - Pansclerotic morphea: rapidly progressive deep fibrosis with joint contractures, muscle atrophy, and ulceration. Risk for development of squamous cell carcinoma in chronic ulcerations; restrictive lung disease from fibrosis of the chest wall
- Differentiating disease activity and damage has important implications for therapy.
  - Signs of disease activity:
    - Inflammatory lymphoplasmacytic infiltrate on histopathology
    - Clinically purple to violaceous patches with a lilac halo
    - Lesional expansion
    - Pruritus
    - Early yellow sclerosis
  - Signs of disease damage:
    - Thickened collagen bundles in the dermis and subcutis
    - Decreased elastic fibers on histopathology
    - Increasing skin thickness
    - Ivory colored sclerotic change
    - Atrophy: ranges from "cliff-drop appearance," venous prominence, to visible concavities
    - Hyperpigmentation
- All forms of morphea can be associated with genital lichen sclerosus, and risk is highest in those with generalized morphea.

DIFFERENTIAL DIAGNOSIS

- Stiff skin syndrome
- Radiation fibrosis
- Scleromyxedema
- Nephrogenic systemic fibrosis
- Systemic sclerosis

DIAGNOSTIC TESTS & INTERPRETATION

Initial Tests (screening, lab, imaging)

- Lab testing: no specific diagnostic tests
- Nonspecific lab tests:
  - 40–80% with positive ANA
  - In linear morphea only: Autoantibodies may predict greater severity of disease including functional limitation (+histone Ab, ssDNA) and greater BSA (+ANA, +ssDNA).
- Imaging:
  - For linear morphea on the face, consider MRI with and without contrast if neurologic symptoms are present. Imaging findings do not always correlate with symptoms but may be useful to quantitate disease response to therapy.
  - For linear morphea that traverses a joint, consider MRI with and without contrast to evaluate for extent and depth of musculoskeletal involvement.
  - In refractory cases or to evaluate for inflammatory arthritis, consider repeat imaging to quantitate disease activity to guide treatment decisions.

- Doppler US: experimental utility to evaluate for disease activity (tissue echogenicity and vascularity) and response to therapy
- Thermography: experimental utility to evaluate for tissue heat as a marker for disease activity
- Skin biopsy:
  - Biopsy can be useful to confirm the diagnosis but will not differentiate systemic sclerosis.
  - Histology varies by stage of disease:
    - Early: perivascular infiltrate of lymphocytes, plasma cells, and eosinophils in the deep dermis with thickened collagen bundles, decreased elastic fibers, and enlarged endothelial cells
    - Later: homogenized collagen with atrophic eccrine glands and hair follicles

Diagnostic Procedures/Other
The Localized Scleroderma Cutaneous Assessment Tool (LoSCAT) is a validated tool to quantitate disease activity and damage in localized scleroderma and can be used to measure response to therapy.

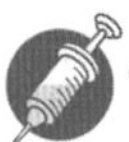

TREATMENT

ALERT
Differentiating disease activity (inflammation) and damage (fibrosis) has important implications for therapy: Disease activity responds to therapy but longstanding disease damage does not.

GENERAL MEASURES
Physical therapy
- Helps retard development of contractures and muscle atrophy
- Pitfall: insufficient physical therapy resulting in permanent joint contractures

MEDICATION
- Disease modification: Many agents have been tried; however, there are few controlled trials, and no proven treatment exists. Medications include the following:
  - Circumscribed morphea
    - Imiquimod, calcipotriene ointment, topical calcineurin inhibitors, topical steroids, psoralen ultraviolet A (PUVA) light, UVA therapy, methotrexate, mycophenolate mofetil, and others
- Linear, generalized, mixed morphea:
  - Consensus treatment plan (CTP) for moderate to severe morphea published by the Childhood Arthritis and Rheumatology Research Alliance (CARRA) gives treating physicians three treatment pathways:
    - CTP A: methotrexate + oral prednisone
    - CTP B: methotrexate + IV pulse steroids
    - CTP C: methotrexate monotherapy

ALERT
Avoid excessive use of immunosuppressive therapy late in disease course when active inflammatory phase has resolved.

ISSUES FOR REFERRAL
- Symptom-based evaluation with referral to collaborating subspecialists including rheumatology, dermatology, occupational therapy, physical therapy, and orthopedic surgery
- For morphea crossing a joint, early referral to physical therapy/occupational therapy with consideration for orthopedic surgery consultation if there are contractures or other abnormal joint findings

ADDITIONAL THERAPIES
Surgical correction of SC atrophy:
- No consensus on optimal timing of surgery—most experts recommend waiting until disease activity has resolved.
- Risk of disease relapse from surgical trauma

ONGOING CARE

FOLLOW-UP RECOMMENDATIONS
Patient Monitoring
- Once systemic immunosuppressive therapy is initiated, disease activity typically begins to resolve within months, and features of damage may also improve.
- Ongoing periodic assessment is important after the period of initial improvement, because early weaning of immunosuppression can result in relapse.
- Physical exam for joint mobility, muscle bulk, and growth
- Photographic documentation of lesions every 3 to 6 months to follow disease activity/damage, with consideration of LoSCAT scoring at visits to quantitate response to therapy

PROGNOSIS
- In localized forms, natural course includes several phases:
  - Initial: inflammation
  - Late: sclerosis
  - Occasional regression over 3 to 5 years, but a significant subset continue to have relapsing disease into adulthood
- Contractures and limb size difference can persist with linear scleroderma.
- A recent study found a 28% rate of relapse after mean treatment duration of 2.4 years.
- Predictors of relapse included older age at disease onset and extremity involvement.

COMPLICATIONS
- Skin thickening
- Joint contractures
- Leg length discrepancies
- Neurologic signs/symptoms for linear morphea on the face

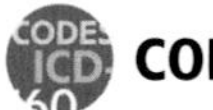

CODES

ICD10
L94.0 Localized scleroderma [morphea]

ADDITIONAL READING

- Li SC, Torok KS, Pope E, et al; and Childhood Arthritis and Rheumatology Research Alliance (CARRA) Localized Scleroderma Workgroup. Development of consensus treatment plans for juvenile localized scleroderma: a roadmap toward comparative effectiveness studies in juvenile localized scleroderma. *Arthritis Care Res (Hoboken)*. 2012;64(8):1175–1185.
- Kelsey CE, Torok KS. The Localized Scleroderma Cutaneous Assessment Tool: responsiveness to change in a pediatric clinical population. *J Am Acad Dermatol*. 2013;69(2):214–220.
- Mirsky L, Chakkittakandiyil A, Laxer RM, et al. Relapse after systemic treatment in paediatric morphoea. *Br J Dermatol*. 2012;166(2):443–445.
- Zulian F. New developments in localized scleroderma. *Curr Opin Rheumatol*. 2008;20(5):601–607.
- Zulian F, Athreya BH, Laxer R, et al. Juvenile localized scleroderma: clinical and epidemiological features in 750 children. An international study. *Rheumatology (Oxford)*. 2006;45(5):614–620.
- Zulian F, Vallongo C, Woo P, et al. Localized scleroderma in childhood is not just a skin disease. *Arthritis Rheum*. 2005;52(9):2873–2881.

FAQ

- Q: Is a biopsy necessary?
- A: Biopsy is often useful primary to evaluate for the extent of disease activity (lymphoplasmacytic infiltrate) versus damage (homogenized collagen and fibrosis) and to exclude mimics.

MULTICYSTIC DYSPLASTIC KIDNEY

Kelly A. Benedict, MD

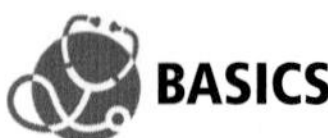

BASICS

DESCRIPTION

- Multicystic dysplastic kidney (MCDK) disease is the most severe type of cystic renal dysplasia and is characterized by multiple, noncommunicating cysts which are divided by dysplastic tissue.
- In general, there is no functioning renal tissue in a MCDK.
- Involutes over time (usually within the first 5 years)

EPIDEMIOLOGY

- Incidence is 0.3 to 1 in 1,000 live births
  - Most cases are detected antenatally.
- Affects boys > girls
- Left kidney > right kidney
  - Usually unilateral but can be bilateral

PATHOPHYSIOLOGY

- Initial growth of the ureteric bud is normal; then renal development halts at a later stage.
- Histology shows disordered renal tissue with areas of undifferentiated mesenchymal cells, abnormal differentiation (i.e., cartilage), rare nephrons.
- Etiology unknown; recent studies suggest genetic cause.

COMMONLY ASSOCIATED CONDITIONS

Associated anomalies of contralateral GU tract include the following:

- Vesicoureteral reflux (VUR), most common, occurs in ~25%.
- Renal hypoplasia
- Ureterocele
- Ureteropelvic junction (UPJ) obstruction
- Genital anomalies

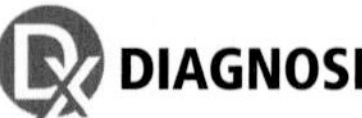

DIAGNOSIS

HISTORY

- Commonly diagnosed by antenatal ultrasound
- May present as abdominal or flank mass

PHYSICAL EXAM

- Blood pressure at each visit to monitor for hypertension
- Evaluate height and weight.
- Neonates: Palpable flank mass may be present.

DIFFERENTIAL DIAGNOSIS

Hydronephrotic kidney with poor function

DIAGNOSTIC TESTS & INTERPRETATION

Initial Tests (screening, lab, imaging)

- Creatinine
  - If unilateral kidney is hypertrophied, then serum creatinine likely will be normal.
  - One strategy is to monitor serum creatinine at 1 month, 18 months, 5 years, and when growth complete to detect reduced function in remaining kidney.
- Urinalysis to check for proteinuria to evaluate for hyperfiltration in remaining kidney
- Urinalysis and urine culture, if the patient has any symptoms of UTI or unexplained fever
- Renal ultrasound
  - To confirm diagnosis of MCDK and evaluate the contralateral kidney
  - Usually no detectable Doppler flow to affected kidney
  - Useful to follow involution of MCDK and hypertrophy of contralateral kidney
  - 50% will have complete involution by 5 years and 74% by 10 years of age.
  - Should be done after birth and at 1 month, 2 years, 5 years, and 10 years of life
- Voiding cystourethrogram (VCUG)
  - To evaluate for urinary reflux is controversial.
  - Although rate of VUR is high, most is low-grade and would not require prophylactic antibiotics.
  - Patients with febrile UTI should have a VCUG.
- Mercaptoacetyl-triglycine (Mag3) scan
  - To confirm diagnosis and rule out a kidney with severe hydronephrosis

ALERT

If contralateral kidney is abnormal, renal function should be evaluated, and the patient will require ongoing nephrology follow-up.

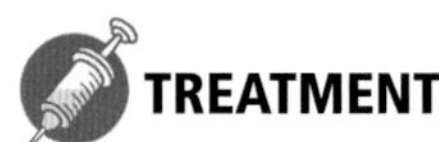

TREATMENT

GENERAL MEASURES

- No specific treatment is needed for MCDK.
- Previously, nephrectomy was treatment of choice; however, given low risk of hypertension and malignancy, currently, routine nephrectomy of MCDK is not recommended.

MEDICATION

- Generally, none
- Occasionally, these patients may require:
  - Antihypertensive medication
  - ACE-inhibitor for proteinuria
  - Prophylactic antibiotics if they suffer from severe VUR or recurrent UTI

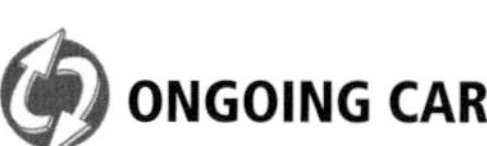

ONGOING CARE

FOLLOW-UP RECOMMENDATIONS

- Blood pressure monitoring
  - Anecdotally, these patients were thought to be at risk for hypertension.
  - However, more recent studies show no increased risk.
- Patients may be at increased risk for developing Wilms tumor in MCDK.
  - Monitored with periodic renal ultrasound and abdominal exam
- Periodic urinalysis to evaluate for proteinuria and serum creatinine to monitor renal function

PROGNOSIS

- Patients with contralateral anomalies are at greater risk for developing chronic kidney disease (CKD).
- Patients with normal contralateral kidneys may have hyperfiltration (~30%) and proteinuria (~10%).
- Risk of developing Wilms tumor
  - May be as high as 3 to 10 times higher than the general population (1 in 10,000)
  - This estimate is controversial, however, as a systematic review of 1,041 children with unilateral MCDK found no cases of Wilms tumor.

ADDITIONAL READING

- Aslam M, Watson AR; for Trent & Anglia MCDK Study Group. Unilateral multicystic dysplastic kidney: long term outcomes. *Arch Dis Child*. 2006;91(10):820–823.
- Gaither TW, Patel A, Patel C, et al. Natural history of contralateral hypertrophy in patients with multicystic dysplastic kidneys. *J Urol*. 2018;199(1):280–286.
- Mansoor O, Chandar J, Rodriguez M, et al. Long-term risk of chronic kidney disease in unilateral multicystic dysplastic kidney. *Pediatr Nephrol*. 2011;26(4):597–603.
- Onal B, Kogan B. Natural history of patients with multicystic dysplastic kidney—what follow-up is needed? *J Urol*. 2006;176(4 Pt 1):1607–1611.
- Weinstein A, Goodman TR, Iragorri S. Simple multicystic dysplastic kidney disease: end points for subspecialty follow-up. *Pediatr Nephrol*. 2008;23(1):111–116.
- Xi Q, Zhu X, Wang Y, et al. Copy number variations in multicystic dysplastic kidney: update for prenatal diagnosis and genetic counseling. *Prenat Diagn*. 2016;36(5):463–468.

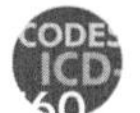

CODES

ICD10

- Q61.4 Renal dysplasia
- Q61.3 Polycystic kidney, unspecified

FAQ

- Q: What can be done to preserve contralateral renal function?
- A: Well-controlled blood pressure, treatment of proteinuria, and quick treatment of UTI may decrease the progression of CKD.
- Q: Are patients with MCDK at an increased risk for developing a UTI?
- A: Risk of UTI is ~5%, consistent with general pediatric population. However, if a patient with MCDK has a febrile UTI, a VCUG is recommended to evaluate for VUR.
- Q: Can patients with unilateral MCDK live a normal life?
- A: Yes, if the contralateral kidney is normal. Patients should be encouraged to live a healthy lifestyle. If the patient has hypertension or diabetes, they should be tightly controlled.
- Q: How is this different than polycystic kidney disease (PKD)?
- A: PKD tends to affect both kidneys and is a progressive disorder. Infants with PKD such as autosomal dominant PKD (ADPKD) may have relatively normal kidneys at birth, and cystic disease develops over time. MCDK is not progressive and usually affects only one kidney. ADPKD is an inherited condition, whereas MCDK is usually not inherited.

MUMPS/PAROTITIS

Camille Sabella, MD

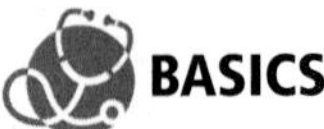

BASICS

DESCRIPTION

Centers for Disease Control and Prevention (CDC) clinical case definition for mumps: illness with acute onset of unilateral or bilateral, tender, self-limited swelling of the parotid or other salivary gland, lasting ≥2 days, without other apparent cause

EPIDEMIOLOGY

- In the prevaccine era, 90% of all children contracted mumps virus infection by 14 years of age.
- Incidence of this once very common disease has declined dramatically since the advent of universal childhood immunization.
- Outbreaks, however, continue to occur, and cases in the United States have ranged from several hundred to several thousand cases annually.
- Since 2014, >1,000 cases per year have been reported in the United States, with >6,000 cases reported in 2016.
- Most outbreaks have been linked to being in a close crowded environment and intense exposures, such as universities, sports teams, and close-knit religious communities.
- Outbreaks can occur in highly vaccinated communities, particularly in very close-contact settings such as college dormitories and camps.
- High vaccination rate helps limit the severity, size, and duration of mumps outbreaks.

GENERAL PREVENTION

- Two combination mumps vaccine are used:
  - MMR: measles, mumps, rubella
  - MMRV: measles, mumps, rubella, varicella
- A single 0.5-mL SC injection of live mumps vaccine (MMR or MMRV) is recommended at 12 to 15 months.
- A second vaccination is recommended between 4 and 6 years of age.
- The efficacy of 2 doses of vaccines is estimated at approximately 80–90%.
- Primary vaccine failure and waning vaccine-induced immunity have been reported.
- During mumps outbreaks, a third dose of vaccine may be recommended by public health authorities for targeted populations in conjunction with CDC guidance. Studies indicate no increase in adverse effects after a third vaccine dose and improved control of mumps outbreak.
- The first dose of MMR vaccine can be associated with fever and rash:
  - These symptoms occur 7 to 12 days after immunization.
  - Measles component is usually the culprit.
- Both MMRV and MMR vaccines, but not varicella vaccine alone, are associated with increased outpatient fever visits and seizures 5 to 12 days after vaccination in 12- to 23-month-olds, with MMRV vaccine increasing fever and seizure twice as much as the MMR + varicella vaccine.
- Vaccine should not be administered to children who are immunocompromised by disease or pharmacotherapy, as well as to pregnant women.
- If a child has recently received immune globulin (IG), administration of MMR vaccine should be delayed (for 3 to 11 months depending on the dose of immune globulin).
- Children with HIV infection who are not severely immunocompromised (age-specific CD4+ T-lymphocyte percentages of 15% or greater) should be immunized with the MMR vaccine.
- One attack of mumps (clinical or subclinical) usually confers lifelong immunity.
- Links of the MMR vaccine to autism by Andrew Wakefield in a 1998 *Lancet* publication have now been exposed as fraudulent, and multiple studies have documented no association between MMR vaccine and autism.

ETIOLOGY

- Epidemic parotitis is caused by mumps, an RNA virus in the Paramyxoviridae family.
- Other viral causes of parotitis include Epstein-Barr virus, cytomegaloviruses, influenza, parainfluenza, and enteroviruses.
- Parotid enlargement can be an initial sign in HIV-infected children.
- Bacterial cases are usually secondary to *Staphylococcus aureus* (suppurative parotitis).
- Streptococci, gram-negative bacilli, and anaerobic infections are also possible.
- Rare childhood cases may be secondary to an obstructing calculus, foreign body (sesame seed), tumors, sarcoid, Sjögren syndrome, or various drugs (antihistamines, phenothiazines, iodine-containing drugs/contrast media).

PATHOPHYSIOLOGY

- The virus is spread by contact with respiratory secretions.
- The mumps virus enters via the respiratory tract, and a viremia ultimately ensues.
- The virus spreads to many organs, including the salivary glands, gonads, pancreas, and meninges.
- Period of communicability: 7 days before to 9 days after onset of parotid swelling
- Most communicable period: 2 to 3 days before to 5 days after onset of parotid swelling
- Incubation period: 12 to 25 days after exposure (16 to 18 days most common)
- Humans are the only known host for mumps.

COMMONLY ASSOCIATED CONDITIONS

- Salivary adenitis
  - Most common manifestation of mumps
  - 1/3 of cases occur subclinically.
- Epididymoorchitis
  - Up to 35% of adolescent mumps cases are complicated by orchitis.
  - Orchitis develops within 4 to 10 days of the onset of the parotid swelling.
  - Sterility is uncommon.
- Aseptic meningitis
- Pancreatitis
  - Mild inflammation is common.
  - Serious involvement is rare.

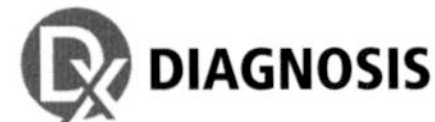

DIAGNOSIS

HISTORY

- Prodromal symptoms uncommon but may include the following:
  - Fever
  - Anorexia
  - Myalgia
  - Headache
- Onset usually pain and swelling in front of and below ear
- Swelling
  - Usually starts on one side of the face, then progresses to the other
- Mild fever
  - Usually accompanies parotid swelling
- Dysphagia and dysphonia are common.
- Testicular pain and swelling, along with constitutional symptoms, occurs in postpubertal males usually 1 week after parotid swelling but occasionally simultaneously or alone.
- Epigastric pain and constitutional symptoms with pancreatic involvement
- Fever, headache, and stiff neck with meningitis
- Behavioral changes, seizures, and other neurologic abnormalities are rare.
- Other symptoms are analogous to the particular organ involved.

PHYSICAL EXAM

- Nonerythematous, tender parotid swelling (erythema suggests suppurative parotitis)
- Swelling ultimately obscures the mandibular ramus.
- The ear is displaced upward and outward.
- Importantly, up to 30% of symptomatic cases of mumps are not associated with parotitis.
  - These may manifest only with upper respiratory tract symptoms.
- Submaxillary and sublingual glands also may be swollen.
- Inflammation may be noted intraorally at the orifice of Stensen duct.
- Presternal edema is occasionally noted.
- Mumps are infrequently associated with truncal rash.
- Tender, edematous testicle in mumps orchitis (usually unilateral)
- Ask the patient if the pain (at the parotid) intensifies with the tasting of sour liquids:
  - Have the patient suck on a lemon drop or lemon juice and note any discharge from Stensen duct.

DIFFERENTIAL DIAGNOSIS

- Mumps parotitis can be distinguished from the other viral causes by clinical presentation along with specialized laboratory studies.
- Cases of tuberculous and nontuberculous (atypical) mycobacterial parotitis are rare but have been reported.
- Salivary calculus can be diagnosed by sialogram.
- Recurrent childhood parotitis, also known as juvenile recurrent parotitis
  - Rare, recurrent swelling of parotids
  - Seen in children 3 to 6 years old
  - Not associated with suppuration or external inflammatory changes
  - Largely a diagnosis of exclusion
- Cervical or preauricular adenitis
  - May simulate parotitis
  - Close anatomic localization should be diagnostic.
- Infectious mononucleosis and cat-scratch disease are other considerations.
- Drug-induced parotid enlargement occasionally occurs.
- Malignancies of the parotid are extremely rare.
- Sjögren syndrome is rare but reported in children.
- Pneumoparotitis is seen in those with a history of playing a wind instrument, glass blowing, scuba diving, and even general anesthesia.

DIAGNOSTIC TESTS & INTERPRETATION

- Uncomplicated parotitis
  - Mild leukopenia with lymphocytosis
- Suppurative parotitis and mumps orchitis
  - Leukocytosis
- Pancreatic involvement
  - Hyperamylasemia and elevated serum lipase
- Salivary adenitis without pancreatic involvement
  - Isolated hyperamylasemia
- Gram stain and culture of pus expressed from Stensen duct is diagnostic in suppurative parotitis.
- CDC lab criteria for mumps diagnosis
  - Isolation of mumps virus from clinical specimens: blood, urine, buccal swab (Stensen duct exudates), throat washing, saliva, or CSF
  - Detection of mumps virus nucleic acid by reverse transcriptase PCR
  - Obtain specimens for culture and PCR as soon as possible after onset of symptoms, particularly in vaccinated individuals.
  - Positive serologic test for mumps IgM
  - Significant rise between acute and convalescent titers in mumps IgG levels by any standard assay (complement fixation, neutralization, hemagglutination inhibition, or enzyme immunoassays)
  - For detailed information regarding collection and interpretation of laboratory studies and mumps case reporting, see http://www.cdc.gov/mumps/.
- Sialography is useful to evaluate for stones or strictures but is contraindicated in acute infection.
- Lumbar puncture if meningitis is suspected: CSF pleocytosis (predominately mononuclear)

ALERT

- Mumps IgM may be negative in MMR-vaccinated individuals who develop mumps disease. A negative IgM test in these patients does not rule out mumps.
- Paired acute and convalescent serum titers may not show a rise in IgG levels in MMR-vaccinated individuals with mumps disease.

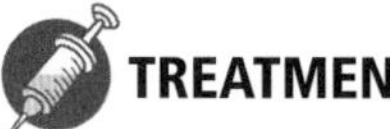

TREATMENT

GENERAL MEASURES

- Supportive therapy is all that is required in mumps parotitis.
- Antibiotics directed against *S. aureus* should be used in cases of suppurative parotitis.

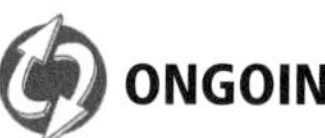

ONGOING CARE

FOLLOW-UP RECOMMENDATIONS

- Most children have resolution of glandular swelling by ~1 week.
- Disappearance of testicular pain and swelling can be expected 4 to 6 days after onset.
- Testicular atrophy is common, although infertility is rare.
- Markedly elevated pancreatic enzymes should be monitored until they improve.
- Children should not return to school until at least 5 days after the onset of parotid swelling.
- Isolation: standard precautions; droplet precautions for 5 days after onset of parotid swelling

PROGNOSIS

Complete recovery in 1 to 2 weeks is the rule.

COMPLICATIONS

- Meningitis
  - >50% have a CSF pleocytosis.
  - This "aseptic meningitis" is usually benign.
- Encephalitis: rarely causes permanent sequelae
- Cerebellitis
- Facial nerve palsy
- Oophoritis, nephritis, thyroiditis, myocarditis, mastitis, arthritis, transient ocular involvement, deafness, and sterility (all rare)

ADDITIONAL READING

- Albertson JP, Clegg WJ, Reid HD, et al. Mumps Outbreak at a University and Recommendation for a Third Dose of Measles-Mumps-Rubella Vaccine—Illinois, 2015–2016. *MMWR Morb Mortal Wkly Rep.* 2016;65(29):731–734.
- American Academy of Pediatrics. Mumps. In: Kimberlin DW, Brady MT, Jackson MA, et al, eds. *Red Book: 2015 Report of the Committee on Infectious Diseases.* American Academy of Pediatrics; 2015:564–568.
- Barskey AE, Schulte C, Rosen JB, et al. Mumps outbreak in Orthodox Jewish communities in the United States. *N Engl J Med.* 2012;367(18):1704–1713.
- Cardemil CV, Dahl RM, James L, et al. Effectiveness of a third dose of MMR vaccine for mumps outbreak control. *N Engl J Med.* 2017;377(10):947–956.
- Dayan GH, Quinlisk MP, Parker AA, et al. Recent resurgence of mumps in the United States. *N Engl J Med.* 2008;358(15):1580–1589.
- Klein NP, Fireman B, Yih WK, et al; for Vaccine Safety Datalink. Measles-mumps-rubella-varicella combination vaccine and the risk of febrile seizures. *Pediatrics.* 2010;126(1):e1–e8.
- McLean HQ, Fiebelkorn AP, Temte JL, et al; for Centers for Disease Control and Prevention. Prevention of measles, rubella, congenital rubella syndrome, and mumps, 2013: summary recommendations of the Advisory Committee on Immunization Practices (ACIP). *MMWR Recomm Rep.* 2013;62(RR-04):1–34.
- Ogbuanu IU, Kutty PK, Hudson JM, et al. Impact of a third dose of measles-mumps-rubella vaccine on a mumps outbreak. *Pediatrics.* 2012;130(6):e1567–e1574.
- Quinlisk MP. Mumps control today. *J Infect Dis.* 2010;202(5):655–656. doi:10.1086/655395.
- Senanayake SN. Mumps in the United States. *N Engl J Med.* 2008;359(6):654.

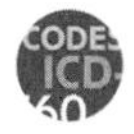

CODES

ICD10

- B26.9 Mumps without complication
- B26.89 Other mumps complications
- B26.0 Mumps orchitis

FAQ

- Q: Should immunization be deferred in children with intercurrent illness?
- A: No. Children with minor illnesses, even with fever, should be vaccinated.
- Q: Should vaccination be withheld in children living with immunocompromised hosts?
- A: No. Vaccinated children do not transmit mumps vaccine virus.
- Q: Is immune globulin effective in controlling mumps outbreaks?
- A: No. Postexposure prophylaxis for mumps with immune globulin is not effective.

MUNCHAUSEN SYNDROME BY PROXY (MEDICAL CHILD ABUSE)

Christopher C. Stewart, MD

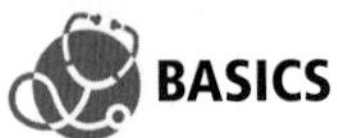

BASICS

DESCRIPTION

- The term medical child abuse (MCA) focuses on potential or real harm to a child, regardless of the caretaker's motivations. MCA is the preferred term for the spectrum of caretaker behaviors that includes the term Munchausen by proxy.
  - Often involves lying or providing false information in the medical setting
  - Results in symptoms of illness in a child that are exaggerated, fabricated, or induced by the actions of a caretaker. There is usually no underlying health disorder in the child.
  - Leads to harm to the child victim directly from a caretaker's actions or through resulting repeated interactions with the medical care system, including unnecessary tests, medications, and surgeries
  - Symptoms often will decrease when the child is separated from the perpetrator.
- MCA presents as a spectrum and can be categorized as mild, moderate, or severe.
  - Mild:
    - Excessive visits despite reassurance resulting in unnecessary tests or antibiotics
  - Moderate:
    - Disruptions in the life of a child from insistence by parent for medications, tests or exams despite negative workups
    - Child's life not placed in danger but long-term negative consequences possible
  - Severe:
    - Potentially life-threatening to the child from parent-induced illness or interventions based on fabricated symptoms
    - Example: a mother smothering her child to produce cyanosis and altered consciousness
- Known by many names, including the following:
  - "Pediatric condition falsification"
  - "Caregiver-fabricated illness in a child"
  - Doctor shopping
  - "Factitious disorder by proxy"
- All refer to harm to children through medical care due to the actions of a caregiver.

EPIDEMIOLOGY

- Rare, with estimated annual incidence of 0.4 to 1.2 per 100,000 in children <16 years of age although data lacking for less extreme or complex cases
- Most victims are <5 years of age, but victims may often be older children.
- Sometimes a true disability or medical condition may be present.
- The mother is usually the perpetrator.
- Often multisymptom presentations
- The most commonly described symptoms include apnea, seizures, factitious fevers, feeding and GI problems, failure to thrive, behavioral problems, bleeding, and sepsis.
- Presenting symptoms may present along a spectrum of severity from mild to fatal.
- Symptoms may be present for years before factitious illness is considered and diagnosed.
- Morbidity is significant; cases may be fatal, especially those involving surreptitious administration of medications, poisoning, or inducing apnea.

ETIOLOGY

- The parent, most commonly the mother, exaggerates, fabricates, or induces the illnesses.
- Caretaker often has somatoform or factitious disorders, as well as often having a history of criminal activity, substance abuse, self-harm, abuse.
- The term Munchausen syndrome by proxy refers to specific instances where the caregiver is motivated by a desire for self-aggrandizement. As such, it only defines a subset of factitious illnesses.
- There is no single clear profile of perpetrator, thus medical providers are advised to concentrate on the specific harm done and the patient's safety rather than on the caregiver's motives.

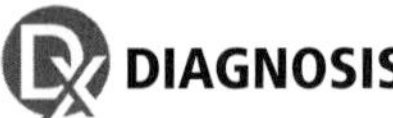

DIAGNOSIS

HISTORY

MCA should be considered when

- Symptoms and signs described are incongruous with patient's appearance or are seen only when the caregiver is present.
- Diagnostic tests fail to confirm the diagnosis.
- Usual medical treatment is ineffective in alleviating the presenting symptom(s).
- If the child has a specific diagnosis, it may be extremely rare, although a chronic illness or disability may be present.
- Caregiver seems unusually knowledgeable or aggressive in suggesting particular medical interventions.
- "Red flags":
  - Frequent housing location changes
  - Siblings who have either died or had unusual medical illnesses
  - Seeking care at a variety of facilities
  - Multiple: office visits/exams, tests, interventions/procedures, specialists involved
  - Reluctance to accept less severe diagnoses
  - Signs or symptoms only begin in the presence of the caregiver.

PHYSICAL EXAM

- Examinations are usually normal.
- When symptoms have been exaggerated, findings are less than expected (e.g., mild asthma or hyperactive behavior).
- When symptoms have been inflicted, findings are often atypical for the medical condition being considered.
- Failure to thrive or obesity is common.
- Patient may have evidence of additional injuries, including old fractures or scars.

DIAGNOSTIC TESTS & INTERPRETATION

Diagnostic Procedures/Other

- For diagnosis, the medical provider must recognize that the caregiver is exaggerating, fabricating, or inducing illness in a child, and that workup or treatments are causing harm.
- Careful documentation of provider's history is important.
- Comparison with other documented histories and with clinical findings and/or test results can help raise the possibility of diagnosis.
- Testing or procedures solely based on history should be avoided. Workup is dictated by the presenting complaint with least invasive means to confirm or exclude medical illness (e.g., EEG for seizures, cardiac monitors for syncope, pneumogram for apnea).
- When the workup is consistently normal and symptoms are still described, the differential diagnosis should include MCA.
- Input from other observers (e.g., other family members, day care providers, or teachers) can frequently confirm the physician's suspicions that the initial history is not true.
- Compile a table that chronologically lists the date and site of all medical care since birth, the treating physician, chief complaint, and summary of medical findings; treatment can help identify MCA.
- If bleeding is the major presentation, identify the blood as the patient's blood (as opposed to that of the perpetrator or an animal).
- A toxicology screen may be helpful for unusual presentations of poisoning.
- Repeated blood or urine cultures with multiple organisms suggest intentional contamination of the specimen or of the patient.
- Special care must be taken to prevent the caregiver from tampering with diagnostic testing.
- If separating the perpetrator from the patient results in disappearance of symptoms, this "test" may suggest the diagnosis.
- Covert video monitoring of a patient's room may demonstrate the perpetrator harming the child.
- Sometimes reviewing public social media information can provide information helpful to the diagnosis.

DIFFERENTIAL DIAGNOSIS

MCA patients may have underlying medical disease and be subject to other forms of abuse. Comorbid abusive conditions include failure to thrive, intentional injury, inappropriate administration of medications, and child neglect. But the abuse in MCA cases comes from medical interventions. Fabricated symptoms often mimic difficult-to-diagnose diseases:

- Apnea/apparent life-threatening event
- Asthma
- Seizures
- Intermittent fevers
- Genitourinary or GI bleeding
- Unexplained abnormalities in electrolytes

- Feeding problems, chronic diarrhea, or vomiting
- Infections with multiple organisms found in blood or urine culture

ALERT

Diagnosis is often delayed and may take months. There are often impediments:

- Physicians and nursing personnel may be reluctant to suspect the parent because of their own relationship to the family.
- It can be difficult to acknowledge that the child has been harmed by well-intentioned but unnecessary medical procedures or investigations.
- It is often necessary to review records from multiple institutions covering months or years of care. These are often unsuspected and may be difficult to obtain.

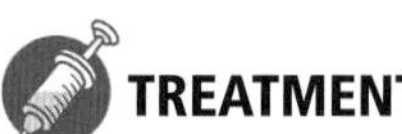

TREATMENT

- Mild:
  - Recommended consultation with a child abuse specialist to help differentiate from a case of simply an anxious parent. The physician should avoid giving in to irrational demands for testing or treatment.
  - If the parent's continued presentations for care become detrimental to the well-being of the child (e.g., frequent absences from school) or lead to unnecessary health care being provided, then moderate child abuse may be occurring, and consultation with a multidisciplinary child abuse team and a report to child protection services is indicated.
- Moderate:
  - Requires consultation with a multidisciplinary child abuse team and child protection involvement
  - Unnecessary medical care should be stopped. It is prudent to stop the most dangerous medical care first:
    - Cancel scheduled but unnecessary surgery.
    - Take out unnecessary vascular access (e.g., peripheral or central venous catheters).
    - Stop the medications that can have the worst potential side effects such as cancer or seizure medications.
  - A multispecialty case conference should be arranged so there is consensus among treating health care providers. Then an informing session should be arranged which should include the health care team, government agencies, and the caretakers to describe the diagnosis, plan, and agreement going forward. If the caretaker cannot agree, action by protective services may be required. Mental health services should be available for the caretaker and child (if appropriate).
- Severe:
  - Same as moderate but requires urgent consultation with a multidisciplinary child abuse team and child protection services notification
  - If a crime has been committed, police notification may be made. Temporary removal of the child from the care of the perpetrator may be necessary with legal intervention.

GENERAL MEASURES

- Effective care requires that medical providers work closely with other professionals in the community, both to gather information and to ensure the patient's eventual safety.
- Child protective services, mental health services, and law enforcement agencies each have a role to play. Evaluations must be multidisciplinary.
- Education of these agencies may be required, with an emphasis on the child abuse, rather than on possible mental illness of the caretaker. The physician should avoid speculation about motivation of the perpetrator or the need for them to receive a psychological evaluation.
- A variety of interventions may be appropriate depending on the severity of the presentation, from counseling to foster care to criminal prosecution.
- Some damage caused by MCA can be reversed by stopping the unnecessary care. Medication side effects may resolve. Appetite and energy levels may return to baseline. Rarely, interventions may require operative reversal such as removal of gastric tubes.

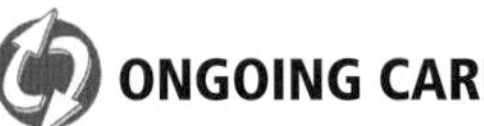

ONGOING CARE

FOLLOW-UP RECOMMENDATIONS

- Psychological treatment for caretaker and child if appropriate
- Long-term follow-up is necessary for both victim and caregiver.
- Watch for recurrence of original presentation or unusual new symptoms, with special attention to the child's self-image.

PROGNOSIS

- If undiagnosed, morbidity and mortality may be significant.
- Children can experience increased incidence of anxiety, depression, and posttraumatic stress disorder (PTSD) symptoms, similar to the emotional effects of other types of child maltreatment.
- Better outcomes for the family are associated with:
  - An identifiable stressor present at the time of the abuse
  - Perpetrator admission to the false reporting and/or induction of illness
  - Perpetrator working cooperatively with child protection, pediatric, and psychiatric services
  - Long-term multidisciplinary child protection, social work, medical, and psychiatric follow-up being in place for the child and perpetrator

ADDITIONAL READING

- Bass C, Glaser D. Early recognition and management of fabricated or induced illness in children. *Lancet*. 2014;383(9926):1412–1421.
- Brown P, Tierney C. Munchausen syndrome by proxy. *Pediatr Rev*. 2009;30(10):414–415.
- Flaherty E, Macmillan H; for Committee on Child Abuse and Neglect. Caregiver-fabricated illness in a child: a manifestation of child maltreatment. *Pediatrics*. 2013;132(3):590–597.
- Hall DE, Eubanks L, Meyyazhagan LS, et al. Evaluation of covert video surveillance in the diagnosis of Munchausen syndrome by proxy: lessons from 41 cases. *Pediatrics*. 2000;105(6):1305–1312.
- Pankratz L. Persistent problems with the Munchausen syndrome by proxy label. *J Am Acad Psychiatry Law*. 2006;34(1):90–95.
- Roesler TA, Jenny C. *Medical Child Abuse: Beyond Munchausen Syndrome by Proxy*. Elk Grove Village, IL: American Academy of Pediatrics; 2009.
- Schreier H. Munchausen by proxy defined. *Pediatrics*. 2002;110(5):985–988.
- Sheridan MS. The deceit continues: an updated literature review of Munchausen syndrome by proxy. *Child Abuse Negl*. 2003;27(4):431–451.
- Souid AK, Keith DV, Cunningham AS. Munchausen syndrome by proxy. *Clin Pediatr (Phila)*. 1998;37(8):497–503.

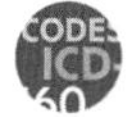

CODES

ICD10

- F68.12 Factitious disorder w predom physical signs and symptoms
- F68.13 Factitious disord w comb psych and physcl signs and symptoms
- F68.11 Factitious disorder w predom psych signs and symptoms

FAQ

- Q: When should MCA be reported to child abuse authorities?
- A: When there is reasonable suspicion (note: not certainty) that a child is coming to harm due to the actions of a caregiver. When suspicion exists, it is important to involve community agencies in the investigation.
- Q: Is it legal to use video surveillance or to separate the parent from the patient?
- A: Yes, if done properly. When suspicions of MCA are high and other diagnostic tests are negative, diagnostic surveillance may be required. Hospital administration and/or risk management should be consulted on how to proceed. However, sometimes the diagnosis for the purposes of child protection can be made without use of diagnostic surveillance. A child abuse specialist can be helpful and may arrange a multidisciplinary meeting to decide the appropriate course of action.

MUSCULAR DYSTROPHIES

Jessica Rose Nance, MS, MD

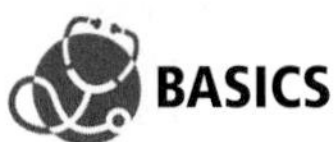

BASICS

DESCRIPTION

- Muscular dystrophies (MDs) are a heterogeneous group of disorders characterized by a slow degeneration of muscle with consequent weakness and contracture deformity. Cardiac muscle can be involved in some forms.
- MDs with childhood onset can be divided into five groups:
  - Dystrophinopathies (i.e., Duchenne MD [DMD], Becker MD [BMD])
  - Limb-girdle MD (LGMD)
  - Congenital MD (CMD)
  - Facioscapulohumeral MD (FSH-MD)
  - Emery-Dreifuss MD (EDMD)
- Types of MDs can be differentiated by their clinical features (i.e., pattern of muscle weakness, joint contractures), age of onset, genetic test results, and/or muscle biopsy.

EPIDEMIOLOGY

- Dystrophinopathies
  - DMD: 1 per 3,500 boys (most common)
  - BMD: 1 per 30,000 boys
- LGMD (childhood onset): 5 to 10 per million
- CMD (all types): 1 to 10 per 100,000
- FSH-MD: 1 per 20,000
- EDMD: 1 per 300,000

RISK FACTORS

Genetics

Genetic testing is clinically available for most MDs:

- Dystrophinopathies (DMD/BMD): X linked
  - DMD exon duplication/deletion in 70% cases
  - DMD point mutation in almost 30% cases
  - New mutations of the dystrophin gene are common, and hence, most cases have no affected relatives despite X-linked recessive inheritance. New mutations in the dystrophin gene are found frequently in the mothers of affected boys.
- LGMD: Most childhood-onset LGMDs are autosomal recessive.
  - Sarcoglycanopathies (LGMD2C–F) make up roughly 70% of childhood-onset LGMD.
  - LGMD2I (FKRP): 5% childhood-onset LGMD
- CMD: most autosomal recessive (12 genes)
  - Nonsyndromic (*LAMA2, COL6A1 to COL6A3*)
  - Syndromic (e.g., *POMT1, POMGT1, FKRP*)
- FSH-MD: autosomal dominant (*D4Z4* deletion)
- EDMD: X linked (*EMD* or *FHL1* mutations) or autosomal dominant (*LMNA* mutation)

PATHOPHYSIOLOGY

- Deficient or defective muscle fiber proteins causing fiber dysfunction and/or increased membrane fragility
- Muscle biopsy: increased variability in muscle fiber size (i.e., degenerating, regenerating, and necrotic fibers), split muscle fibers and increased internal nuclei, fibrosis. Immunohistochemistry may note decreased/absent sarcolemmal proteins (e.g., DMD, LGMD, CMD).

DIAGNOSIS

HISTORY

- Neonatal hypotonia, feeding difficulty (CMD)
- Gross motor delay/regression
- Global developmental delay (syndromic CMD) or learning disorders (DMD)
- Exercise intolerance/cramping
- Myalgia (BMD, DMD, FSH-MD)
- Seizures: merosin-negative and syndromic CMD
- DMD
  - Onset typically <5 years old with gross motor delays, increasing falls, toe walking, and proximal muscle weakness (e.g., difficulty climbing stairs, rising from floor)
  - Dependence on wheelchair for mobility usually between 8 and 12 years of age
  - Calf pseudohypertrophy is common.
  - Serum creatine kinase (CK) levels are markedly elevated (often >50× normal). Serum transaminases may be elevated (muscle origin).
  - Higher incidence of learning difficulties, ADHD, autism, OCD. Loss of ambulation occurs around 13 to 16 years old. Incidence of cardiomyopathy increases with age, although respiratory muscle weakness (e.g., ineffective cough, hypoventilation, and eventual respiratory failure) is the cause of death in about 75% of DMD boys.
- BMD
  - Milder version of DMD phenotype; onset typically >8 years old
  - Boys remain ambulatory into their 20s.
  - Higher incidence of myalgia, cramps, and myoglobinuria in BMD (vs. DMD)
  - Rarely, cardiomyopathy may be sole or presenting feature.
- LGMD
  - Proximal muscle weakness (neck flexors, hip flexors, shoulder girdle)
  - Onset and progression highly variable
  - Sarcoglycanopathies (LGMD2C–F) can mimic DMD (including calf pseudohypertrophy).
  - Patients are cognitively normal.
- CMD
  - Hypotonia, gross motor delay, weakness, and feeding difficulty typically noted from birth
  - Two main groups of CMDs: (i) nonsyndromic CMD due to defective structural proteins (e.g., merosin-negative CMD, Ullrich/Bethlem MD) and (ii) syndromic CMD due to defective glycosylation (e.g., Fukayama MD, muscle-eye-brain disease, Walker-Warburg syndrome)
    - Most children with nonsyndromic CMD are cognitively normal. Seizures may occur in merosin-negative CMD (20–30%). Ullrich MD shows characteristic proximal contractures and distal joint hyperlaxity (fingers, toes). Bethlem MD shows proximal muscle weakness and distal contractures.
    - Syndromic CMD shows variable severity, often associated with intellectual disability, eye manifestations, and brain anomalies (e.g., neuronal migration disorders, seizures, hydrocephalus).
- FSH-MD
  - Onset typically <20 years old with facial weakness, scapular winging, and humeral (biceps, triceps) weakness
  - Relative sparing of deltoid strength is seen.
  - Rare infantile-onset cases have been reported.
  - Retinal vasculopathy (Coates disease) and sensorineural hearing loss can occur.
  - Cardiac arrhythmia is occasionally noted (<10%).
- EDMD
  - Onset typically in 1st decade
  - Patients initially present with joint contractures (neck, elbow, and ankles) disproportionate to degree of weakness.
  - Muscle weakness and wasting develop in biceps, triceps, spinates muscles, and (later) tibialis anterior and peroneal muscles.
  - Cardiac arrhythmias are common by 2nd decade.
  - Pseudohypertrophy is not seen.

PHYSICAL EXAM

- Facial weakness (FSH-MD)
- Pattern of muscle weakness and atrophy
- Scapular winging (FSH-MD)
- Pattern of joint contractures (EDMD) or joint hypermobility (Ullrich MD)
- Pattern of muscle pseudohypertrophy (e.g., calf muscles in DMD, BMD, LGMD)
- Reflexes normal to mildly decreased (except for joints with contractures). Reflexes are not lost until late in disease course.
- Normal sensory exam
- Scoliosis: rapid progression if nonambulatory
- Gower maneuver (when arising from sitting to standing position, patient must put his hand on his knees and "climb up himself")
- Gait abnormalities (e.g., toe walking, exaggerated lumbar lordosis, Trendelenburg gait)
- Cardiomyopathy (tachycardia, hypotension)
- Respiratory weakness (weak cough)

DIFFERENTIAL DIAGNOSIS

- Inflammatory myopathy (e.g., dermatomyositis)
- Metabolic myopathy
- Congenital myopathy
- Anterior horn cell disease (e.g., SMA)
- Polyneuropathy (e.g., CIDP)
- Myotonic dystrophy (different pathology)

DIAGNOSTIC TESTS & INTERPRETATION

Initial Tests (screening, lab, imaging)

Serum CK

- Markedly elevated in DMD, BMD, some LGMD, and CMD (e.g., Fukayama MD)
- CK may be normal late in disease owing to severe muscle atrophy.
- CK is typically normal in FSH-MD and some CMDs (e.g., Ullrich MD). Normal to mild CK elevation is seen in EDMD.

Diagnostic Procedures/Other

- Nerve conduction study: Merosin-negative CMD may show mild conduction velocity slowing.
- EMG: nonspecific myopathic changes

- MRI muscle: signal change noted reflecting muscle atrophy and fatty infiltration. May guide site of optimal muscle biopsy. Pattern of muscle involvement maybe helpful in diagnosis.
- MRI brain: Merosin-negative CMD shows diffuse white matter signal abnormalities (typically visible by 6 months old).
- Muscle biopsy can be used to confirm dystrophy (see "Differential Diagnosis"), whereas immunohistochemistry can help in diagnosis of nondystrophic MDs (e.g., LGMD) if DMD genetic testing is normal.

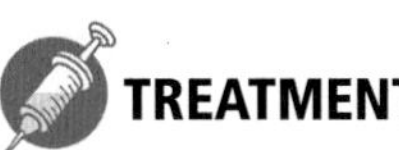

TREATMENT

GENERAL MEASURES

- Supportive care (e.g., routine immunizations)
- Psychological and/or school support
- Night splinting (DMD, LGMD) to prevent progression of joint contractures
- Physiotherapy: passive stretching
- Orthopedic evaluation: scoliosis surveillance and/or management of joint contractures
- Genetic counseling
- Ophthalmology (retinal) evaluation (FSH-MD), cataract surveillance (DMD patients on steroids)

MEDICATION

- Early attention should be directed to prevention of deformity that encumbers function with weakness and prevention of obesity.
- For DMD
  - Oral corticosteroids (prednisone [0.75 mg/kg/24 h] or deflazacort [0.9 mg/kg/24 h]): Improve muscle strength, prolong independent ambulation (mean = 2.5 years), delay onset of cardiomyopathy and scoliosis, and improve pulmonary function testing. Patients must be monitored for adverse effects of steroid therapy (weight gain, bone demineralization, behavior issues).
  - Eteplirsen: FDA-approved genetic therapy for 13% of DMD boys with mutations amenable to antisense-oligonucleotide-mediated skipping of exon 51
- All other MDs: no treatment

ADDITIONAL THERAPIES

Several potential therapies for DMD are being studied (e.g., gene replacement, DMD nonsense mutation read-through therapy, myostatin inhibitor therapy, stem cell therapy). These therapies remain experimental and are not commercially available in North America or Europe.

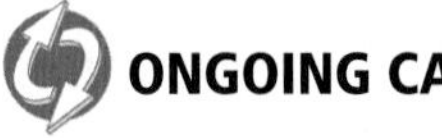

ONGOING CARE

FOLLOW-UP RECOMMENDATIONS

Patient Monitoring

- Respiratory surveillance
  - Baseline pulmonary evaluation (DMD, CMD) with periodic pulmonary function test (PFT) surveillance, incentive spirometry, and/or cough assist devices
  - Monitor for decline in PFT scores (especially forced vital capacity [FVC]) and/or clinical evidence of nocturnal hypoventilation (e.g., morning headache/nausea, daytime somnolence, orthopnea). If noted, obtain sleep study to evaluate for potential need for nocturnal bilevel positive airway pressure (BiPAP).
  - Monitor kyphoscoliosis.
- Orthopedic surveillance
  - When progressive scoliosis is evident, treatment with spinal fusion is indicated to prevent deteriorating quality of life associated with severe deformity.
  - Following loss of ambulation in DMD, affected boys are at high risk for progressive, collapse-type scoliosis and should be screened at 6- to 12-month intervals until young adult years.
- Cardiology surveillance
  - Cardiomyopathy is well documented for many MDs, necessitating periodic echocardiogram and ECG surveillance studies for DMD, BMD, LGMD1B, LGMD2C–F (20–30% risk), LGMD2I (30–60% risk), merosin-negative CMD, and EDMD.
  - American Academy of Pediatrics (AAP) guidelines recommend DMD patients receive complete cardiac evaluation every 2 years until age 10 years and annually thereafter.
  - Cardiac arrhythmia surveillance is required for EDMD, LGMD1B, and FSH-MD (<10% risk); also consider for any MD patient showing echocardiogram evidence of a cardiomyopathy
  - Cardiac transplantation should be considered for BMD patients with severe cardiomyopathy, particularly if they have relatively minor skeletal muscle involvement.

PROGNOSIS

- DMD:
  - Life expectancy into late 20s, death typically from respiratory failure
  - Life expectancy is improving with advances in care and realistic hope for specific therapies.
- BMD:
  - Life expectancy into mid-40s
  - Death typically due to cardiomyopathy
- LGMD: variable
  - Sarcoglycanopathies may show a DMD-like progression.
  - Autosomal dominant LGMD later onset with slow progression
- FSH-MD:
  - Normal life expectancy

ADDITIONAL READING

- American Academy of Pediatrics Section on Cardiology and Cardiac Surgery. Cardiovascular health supervision for individuals affected by Duchenne or Becker muscular dystrophy. *Pediatrics*. 2005;116(6):1569–1573.
- Bönnemann CG. Limb-girdle muscular dystrophy in childhood. *Pediatr Ann*. 2005;34(7):569–577.
- Bönnemann CG, Wang CH, Quijano-Roy S, et al. Diagnostic approach to the congenital muscular dystrophies. *Neuromuscul Disord*. 2014;24(4):289–311.
- Bushby K, Finkel R, Birnkrant DJ, et al; for Duchenne Muscular Dystrophy Care Considerations Working Group. Diagnosis and management of Duchenne muscular dystrophy, part 1: diagnosis, pharmacological and psychosocial management. *Lancet Neurol*. 2010;9(1):77–93.
- Bushby K, Finkel R, Birnkrant DJ, et al; for Duchenne Muscular Dystrophy Care Considerations Working Group. Diagnosis and management of Duchenne muscular dystrophy, part 2: implementation of multidisciplinary care. *Lancet Neurol*. 2010;9(2):177–189.
- El-Bohy A, Wong B. The diagnosis of muscular dystrophy. *Pediatr Ann*. 2005;34(7):525–530.
- Guglieri M, Straub V, Bushby K, et al. Limb-girdle muscular dystrophies. *Curr Opin Neurol*. 2008;21(5):576–584.
- Hermans MCE, Pinto YM, Merkies IS, et al. Hereditary muscular dystrophies and the heart. *Neuromuscul Disord*. 2010;20(8):479–492.
- Kirschner J, Bönnemann C. The congenital and limb-girdle muscular dystrophies: sharpening the focus, blurring the boundaries. *Arch Neurol*. 2004;61(2):189–199.
- Tawil R, Van Der Maarel SM. Facioscapulohumeral muscular dystrophy. *Muscle Nerve*. 2006;34(1):1–15.

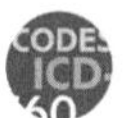

CODES

ICD10

- G71.0 Muscular dystrophy
- G71.2 Congenital myopathies

FAQ

- Q: What test should be ordered first in a boy with suspected DMD?
- A: After confirmation that CK is elevated, 1st-line testing is *DMD* duplication/deletion analysis (detects 70% cases). If negative, *DMD* gene should be sequenced. Muscle biopsy is typically reserved for patients with negative genetic testing (i.e., LGMD) or if there is clinical suspicion for inflammatory myopathy (e.g., dermatomyositis). Nerve conduction—electromygraphy studies can help differentiate neurogenic disorders (i.e., SMA, polyneuropathy) but show nonspecific myopathic changes in MDs.
- Q: What is the recurrence risk in DMD?
- A: About 2/3 of mothers of males with DMD are carriers. If a female DMD carrier has a son, that boy has a 50% chance of having DMD. If she has a daughter, that girl has a 50% chance of becoming a DMD carrier. Males with DMD or BMD will transmit the mutated gene to all daughters (who become carriers). The sons of DMD males will not be affected (X linked).
- Q: Can female DMD carriers be symptomatic?
- A: Yes. Owing to the random nature of X-chromosome inactivation, roughly 10% of female DMD heterozygotes may develop cardiomyopathy and/or proximal muscle weakness. The AAP recommends female carriers receive a cardiac evaluation in early adulthood and every 5 years after 25 to 30 years old.

MYASTHENIA GRAVIS

Diana X. Bharucha-Goebel, MD • Melissa L. Cirillo, MD • Vamshi K. Rao, MD

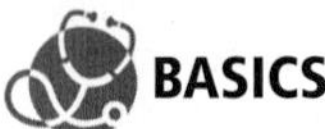

BASICS

DESCRIPTION

- A neuromuscular (NM) disease presenting with varying weakness that worsens with exercise and improves with rest
- Three types of myasthenia gravis seen in childhood:
  - Neonatal transient
    - 10–20% of infants born to mothers with autoimmune myasthenia
  - Congenital myasthenia
    - Rare; represents <10% of all childhood myasthenia
    - Weakness usually starts within first 2 years of life.
    - Caused by inherited disorder in NM transmission
    - Classified by mutation site (presynaptic, postsynaptic) or by molecular genetics
  - Juvenile myasthenia
    - Relatively rare: one new diagnosis per million per year
    - Average age of onset 10 to 13 years, with a female predominance of 2:1 or 4:1
    - Autoimmune disorder similar to adult-onset, autoimmune myasthenia gravis; mostly due to production of antibodies against the acetylcholine receptor (AChR)

EPIDEMIOLOGY

- Rare: incidence 4 to 6 per million per year
- Prevalence: 40 to 80 per million
- Children account for 10–15% of cases of myasthenia gravis annually in North America.

RISK FACTORS

Genetics

- Congenital type: generally autosomal recessive (check for consanguinity)
- Occasional family history

PATHOPHYSIOLOGY

- Caused by a disruption in signal transmission from the motor neuron to the muscle. Sensory or cognitive symptoms are absent.
  - The motor nerve terminal lies in close proximity to the end plate, a region of the muscle cell membrane with a high concentration of AChR.
  - Normally, when stimulated, the motor nerve terminal releases acetylcholine that binds receptors, causing muscle contraction. The cleft contains acetylcholinesterase (AChE), an enzyme that breaks down acetylcholine and helps terminate muscle contractions.
- Autoimmune form (juvenile myasthenia or juvenile myasthenia gravis [JMG])
  - Autoantibody blocks AChR activity → increased rate of receptor breakdown → fewer receptors are present → leads to decreased muscle contraction
  - AChR antibody accounts for ~85% of JMG.
  - Thymic pathology is believed to be central to pathogenesis of autoimmune myasthenia; however, thymic pathology (e.g., hyperplasia) is present in <1/3 of children who undergo thymectomy.
  - Of JMG patients without elevated AChR antibody, some are positive for antibodies to muscle-specific kinase (MuSK).
  - A small percentage of autoimmune JMG patients do not have an identified antibody.
- Neonatal (transient) myasthenia: Infants are born with weakness and hypotonia.
  - Due to maternal–fetal transmission of antibodies against AChR
  - Severity of maternal symptoms does NOT predict likelihood that infant will be affected. Occasional arthrogryposis (joint contractures) reflects decreased fetal movement in utero.
  - High levels of maternal antibodies against fetal form of AChR pose an increased risk of disease.
  - Previous pregnancy with affected infant places future child at much higher risk.
  - In rare cases, mother is asymptomatic despite placentally transmitted antibody.
- Congenital myasthenic syndromes: group of genetic disorders of NM junction; classified by site of NM transmission defect and more recently by molecular genetics
  - Includes presynaptic defects, synaptic defect (due to end plate AChE deficiency), postsynaptic defects (primary AChR deficiency, primary AChR kinetic abnormality, or perijunctional skeletal muscle sodium channel mutation)

COMMONLY ASSOCIATED CONDITIONS

- In juvenile myasthenia, other autoimmune disorders may occur:
  - Hyperthyroidism in 3–9% of patients
  - Small increase in incidence of type 1 diabetes
- Screening for thymoma at initial diagnosis by chest CT or MRI scan is appropriate:
  - Children appear to have lower incidence of thymic tumor or pathology than adults with autoimmune myasthenia.

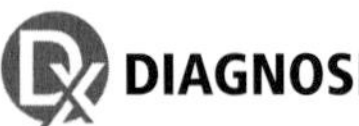

DIAGNOSIS

Most patients present with fluctuating ptosis that often alternates and diplopia alone or in combination with swallowing difficulties, dysphonia, and generalized weakness.

HISTORY

- Neonatal transient: mother with known autoimmune myasthenia or history of weakness, ptosis, or dysphagia
- Congenital myasthenia
  - Usually presents in first 1 to 2 years of life (rarely later) with hypotonia, poor feeding, ptosis, and delayed motor milestones
  - Possible family history of similar weakness
  - No response to thymectomy or immunosuppressant medications
- Juvenile myasthenia
  - Gradual onset of fatigable weakness over weeks, months, or even years
  - Symptoms are worse after prolonged activity or late in the day.
  - Intermittent ptosis, diplopia, dysphagia, and dysphonia are common.
  - Ocular myasthenia gravis: a subset of 10–15% of patients with myasthenia who have isolated ptosis and ophthalmoplegia (weakness in extraocular muscles) in absence of systemic or bulbar symptoms

PHYSICAL EXAM

- Neonatal transient: from birth, hypotonic infant with weak suck, weak cry, and ptosis
- Congenital and juvenile myasthenia
  - Weakness of neck flexion
  - Reflexes often preserved
  - Ptosis, ophthalmoplegia, and variable feeding problems often are earliest findings.
  - Generalized weakness in limbs may be asymmetric. Weakness is more pronounced with endurance tasks.
  - Shallow, rapid respirations and/or vital capacity <50% predicted (in older children) suggest impending respiratory failure.
  - Check for scoliosis.

DIFFERENTIAL DIAGNOSIS

- Generalized botulism
  - In endemic areas, may cause generalized weakness in infants; caused by *Clostridium* toxin that blocks release of acetylcholine from nerve terminal
- Guillain-Barré syndrome or acute inflammatory demyelinating polyneuropathy
  - Frequent cause of rapidly progressive generalized weakness
  - Unlike myasthenia, patients often have sensory symptoms, and hyporeflexia or areflexia occurs even with minimal weakness.
- Acute spinal cord compression
  - Can present as generalized (but not variable) weakness of extremities
  - Look for sparing of facial and extraocular muscles, a sensory level, bowel or bladder dysfunction, and initially hyporeflexia or areflexia, followed by hyperactive reflexes.
- Tick paralysis
  - Due to a neurotoxin
  - Ascending paralysis
  - Hyporeflexia or areflexia
  - Can cause ophthalmoplegia and bulbar palsy
  - Treatment involves removal of the entire tick and supportive care.
- Organophosphate ingestion
  - Can cause profound weakness
  - Symptoms of parasympathetic hyperactivity are usually present: hypersalivation, miosis, diarrhea, and bradycardia.
  - Penicillamine used to treat autoimmune disorders can induce autoantibodies that bind AChR, causing myasthenia gravis.

DIAGNOSTIC TESTS & INTERPRETATION

- Juvenile myasthenia
  - Nerve conduction and electromyography studies: Repetitive stimulation of nerve shows diagnostic decremental response due to decreased AChR. May be normal in some patients; normal study doesn't exclude diagnosis.
  - Single-fiber electromyography measures variability in firing rates of two muscle fibers innervated by different branches of the same motor neuron. Large variability suggests higher threshold for activation. This test is more sensitive than repetitive nerve stimulation but is technically more challenging and often requires sedation.

- Edrophonium chloride (Tensilon®) is a fast-acting AChE-blocking agent (no longer widely used diagnostically).
  - Patients with myasthenia often show immediate, transient improvement in muscle strength after IV infusion.
  - Measurable weakness should be present prior to testing.
  - Although risk of hyperreactive cholinergic response with muscle weakness and bradycardia is low, atropine should always be available, and vital signs should be closely monitored during test; contraindicated in patients with heart disease
  - Measurable cranial nerve dysfunction, such as ptosis, is often responsive to edrophonium.
  - Children receive 20% of 0.2 mg/kg dose (0.04 mg/kg) of Tensilon® over 1 minute; if no response after 45 seconds, the rest of the dose (0.16 mg/kg) is given, up to a maximum of 10 mg. Have atropine and epinephrine readily available.
- AChR antibody levels (most specific): elevated in ~80% of patients with generalized myasthenia and ~50% of patients with isolated ocular myasthenia
- Antibodies are less commonly present in prepubertal children.
- Second most common antibody is to muscle-specific kinase antibody (MuSK-Ab). Antibodies to striated muscle protein and low-density lipoprotein receptor–related protein are also described but are rare and not yet commercially available.

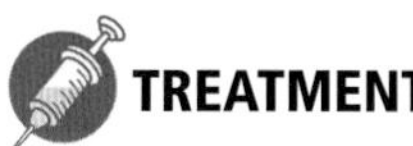

TREATMENT

Treat respiratory failure, a rare but serious complication of JMG.

GENERAL MEASURES

- Neonatal myasthenia
  - Severity of disability should be used to guide aggressiveness of therapy.
  - Respiratory or swallowing impairment: pyridostigmine syrup, 60 mg/5 mL, 1 mg/kg/dose q4h up to a daily maximum of 7 mg/kg/24 h divided 5 to 6 doses; 1 mg IM = 30 mg PO dose
- Juvenile myasthenia
  - Most patients benefit from pyridostigmine bromide (Mestinon®) given 3 to 4 times per day. A long-acting formulation prior to bedtime may alleviate obstructive hypoventilation during sleep.
  - Pyridostigmine blocks AChE activity and results in increased acetylcholine.
  - Usual starting dosage is ~1 mg/kg/24 h. Dosage is slowly titrated upward, following symptoms, at several-day intervals to a maximum dose of ~7 to 8 mg/kg/24 h. Absolute maximum daily dose is 300 mg/24 h for older children; common side effects: hypersalivation, blurry vision, and diarrhea
  - Glycopyrrolate (1 mg PO) may decrease diarrhea.
  - Prednisone
    - Consider in patients with disabling symptoms and inadequate response to pyridostigmine.
    - Watch for transient worsening within weeks in up to 50% of patients.
    - Start daily dose at 2 mg/kg, watch for improvement in 3 to 6 weeks, and taper toward 1.5 mg/kg/24 h on alternate-day schedule for 4 months. Taper slowly thereafter by 5 mg/week.
    - Monitor for side effects, including growth stunting.
    - Calcium every-other-day dosing may limit bone loss from chronic steroids.
  - Rituximab
    - MuSK Ab–positive patients are often refractory to other treatments (pyridostigmine, steroids, IVIG) with incomplete or short-lived benefit.
    - Rituximab has induced sustained benefit in patients with refractory disease via B-cell depletion in MuSK Ab–positive patients; however, large controlled studies in this population have not been performed.
  - Azathioprine
    - Induces remission in 30%; significant improvement in another 25–60%
    - Useful adjunct to steroids and thymectomy; however, requires 3 to 12 months for benefits to occur
    - Mycophenolate mofetil, cyclosporine, and methotrexate have also been used, but controlled studies are lacking and reports are anecdotal.
- Juvenile myasthenics with profound weakness and respiratory failure (myasthenic crisis) should undergo immediate therapy to decrease the number of circulating antibodies:
  - Plasmapheresis or IV immunoglobulin can help within days by decreasing AChR antibodies.
  - Steroids diminish antibody production over weeks to months.

SURGERY/OTHER PROCEDURES

Thymectomy

- In adults, 20–60% remission; another 15–30% show marked improvement (somewhat less in pediatric patients).
- Thymectomy earlier in the course of illness appears to produce a higher rate of remission.

ONGOING CARE

- The following medications can exacerbate myasthenia gravis:
  - Corticosteroids may worsen symptoms.
  - Aminoglycosides
  - Ciprofloxacin
  - β-Adrenergic blocking agents, including eye drops
  - Lithium
  - Procainamide
  - Quinidine
  - Phenytoin
- Prolonged recovery after exposure to nondepolarizing NM blocking agents
- Always start new medications cautiously.

FOLLOW-UP RECOMMENDATIONS

Patient Monitoring

- Watch for transient worsening of symptoms.
- Monitor for side effects of corticosteroids, including growth stunting.
- Medication effects: GI upset due to AChE inhibitors

PROGNOSIS

- Neonatal transient
  - Self-limited disorder that resolves spontaneously over weeks or months of life as maternal antibodies disappear
  - Infant may require ventilator and nutritional support during first few months of life.
  - Infants with arthrogryposis multiplex congenita (born to mothers with antibodies against the fetal form of AChR) may gain some mobility over time and with passive range-of-motion therapy.
- Congenital myasthenia
  - Prognosis depends on specific defect.
  - Autosomal recessive disorders tend to be more severe than dominant disorders. Weakness shows variable response to cholinesterase inhibitors.
  - Immunosuppressants are not helpful. In general, these are indolent disorders.
  - Ptosis and fatigability resemble the juvenile type but are more stable over time.
- Juvenile myasthenia
  - Most patients do extremely well with treatment; patient selection for early thymectomy requires experience and may improve outcome.
  - Longitudinal studies suggest rate of spontaneous remission ~2% per year.
  - Patients with generalized weakness slightly less likely to experience remission.
  - Mortality rate from myasthenia is near that of the general population in patients <50 years old.

COMPLICATIONS

Respiratory failure, nocturnal hypoventilation, visual disturbance, thymic cancer (more common in adults, rare in pediatrics), other autoimmune disorders

ADDITIONAL READING

- Castro D, Derisavifard S, Anderson M, et al. Juvenile myasthenia gravis: a twenty-year experience. *J Clin Neuromuscul Dis*. 2013;14(3):95–102.
- Harper CM. Congenital myasthenic syndromes. *Semin Neurol*. 2004;24(1):111–123.
- Liew WK, Kang PB. Update on juvenile myasthenia gravis. *Curr Opin Pediatr*. 2013;25(6):694–700.
- Parent internet information: Myasthenia Gravis Foundation of America, Inc. Living with MG. http://www.myasthenia.org/LivingwithMG.aspx. Accessed March 26, 2017.
- Pineles SL, Avery RA, Moss HE, et al. Visual and systemic outcomes in pediatric ocular myasthenia gravis. *Am J Ophthalmol*. 2010;150(4):453–459.e3.
- Sanders DB, Wolfe GI, Benatar M, et al. International consensus guidance for management of myasthenia gravis: executive summary. *Neurology*. 2016;87(4):419–425.
- VanderPluym J, Vajsar J, Jacob FD, et al. Clinical characteristics of pediatric myasthenia: a surveillance study. *Pediatrics*. 2013;132(4):e939–e944.

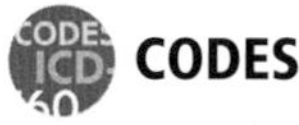

CODES

ICD10

- G70.00 Myasthenia gravis without (acute) exacerbation
- P94.0 Transient neonatal myasthenia gravis
- G70.01 Myasthenia gravis with (acute) exacerbation

MYOCARDITIS

Jason F. Goldberg, MD, FAAP • Javier J. Lasa, MD, FAAP

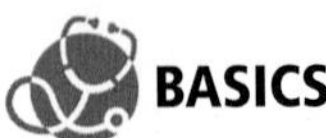

BASICS

DESCRIPTION

Myocarditis is defined as an inflammatory disease of heart muscle, diagnosed by histologic and/or immunologic examination. The associated myocardial dysfunction can cause varying clinical manifestations, ranging from minimal cardiac symptoms to severe heart failure, arrhythmias, and sudden death.

EPIDEMIOLOGY

- Prevalence of clinical myocarditis is estimated at 5.5 per 10,000 adults, with further estimates difficult to ascertain given variation in clinical severity with subacute presentation, as well as various etiologies and underdiagnosis.
- There is a bimodal age distribution with highest rates of diagnosis in infants <1 year of age and in ages 14 to 18 years.

RISK FACTORS

- Exposure to infectious agents (mainly viruses), drugs, toxins, and systemic diseases
- Autoimmune disease
- Systemic disease

PATHOPHYSIOLOGY

- Pathophysiology of myocarditis may vary based on cause (see "Etiology").
- Viral myocarditis is best characterized and involves a complex interaction among the virus, host immune response, and environmental factors. Three stages include (i) viral injury and innate immune response, (ii) acquired host immune response, and (iii) recovery or chronic cardiomyopathy.
- Inflammatory response from innate and acquired immune response may result in significant damage to the myocardium and conduction system.
- Development of autoantibodies may also play a key role in acute and chronic myocardial damage.
- Virus may cause direct damage to the myocardium independent of inflammation, secondary to cleavage of structural proteins.
- Pathogenesis of nonviral myocarditis is poorly understood.
- Regardless of the cause, symptom severity increases with worsening ventricular function and/or with worsening arrhythmias.
- Fulminant myocarditis may be characterized by both severe systolic and diastolic dysfunction.
- Progressive left ventricular systolic dysfunction may lead to hypotension, acidosis, and end-organ dysfunction.
- Left ventricular diastolic dysfunction may result in elevated left ventricular end diastolic pressures, leading to pulmonary venous and arterial hypertension, with concomitant pulmonary edema and right-sided heart failure.

ETIOLOGY

- Causes include infection, toxins, drugs, autoimmune disease, and systemic disease.
- Infectious causes include viral, bacterial, rickettsial, fungal, helminthic, spirochetal, and protozoal agents.
- Viral infection is the most common in developed countries including enteroviruses (e.g., coxsackievirus), erythroviruses (e.g., parvovirus B19), adenoviruses, herpes viruses (e.g., human herpesvirus 6 [HHV-6], Epstein-Barr virus [EBV], cytomegalovirus [CMV]), as well as hepatitis C. Both RNA and DNA viruses have been implicated. The last 20 years has seen a shift in viral etiology: from more cases with enteroviruses and adenoviruses to more frequent parvovirus and HHV-6.
- Nonviral infectious causes are far less common but must be considered especially in endemic areas, such as Central and South America where Chagas disease is prevalent.
- Nonviral myocarditis may be secondary to exposure to chemicals (arsenic and hydrocarbons), alcohol, radiation, drugs (chemotherapeutics), as well as drug hypersensitivity, autoimmune disease such as systemic lupus erythematosus, or systemic disease such as Churg-Strauss or sarcoidosis.
- Giant cell myocarditis is a very rare form of myocarditis in children that is associated with autoimmune disease and drug hypersensitivity. These patients respond poorly to typical care and frequently require cardiac transplantation.

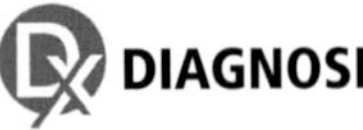

DIAGNOSIS

Signs and symptoms

- Prodrome (may occur a few weeks before presentation)
  - Antecedent flulike illness
  - Gastroenteritis
  - Fever
- Heart failure symptoms
  - Tachypnea, dyspnea
  - Gastrointestinal symptoms: anorexia, early satiety, abdominal pain, vomiting
  - Easy fatigability
  - Exercise intolerance
  - Orthopnea
  - Swelling of abdomen/lower extremities
  - Chest pain
  - Tachycardia, palpitations
  - Syncope

ALERT

Often multiple visits to medical care occur before the diagnosis of myocarditis is made. Consider myocarditis when respiratory or gastrointestinal symptoms in infants and young children persist without clear etiology or worsen acutely.

HISTORY

- Duration of symptoms
- Travel history
- Family history of myocarditis, cardiomyopathy, sudden death, or heart attacks at a young age

PHYSICAL EXAM

Any of the following may be present:

- Pulmonary
  - Rales
  - Tachypnea
  - Retractions
- Cardiovascular
  - Jugular venous distention
  - Normal to hyperdynamic precordium with or without right ventricular heave
  - Lateral displacement of the point of maximal impulse (PMI)
  - Tachycardia: sinus tachycardia or arrhythmia (atrial and/or ventricular ectopy may be present)
  - Heart sounds: accentuation of second heart sound (secondary to pulmonary artery hypertension), murmur (mitral and/or tricuspid insufficiency), gallop, and/or rub
- Abdomen: hepatomegaly, splenomegaly, ascites
- Extremities
  - Lower extremity edema
  - Weak pulses
  - Poor capillary refill
  - Cool extremities

DIFFERENTIAL DIAGNOSIS

- Severe left-sided obstructive heart lesions
  - Mitral stenosis
  - Valvular aortic stenosis
  - Coarctation of the aorta
- Congenital coronary artery anomalies
  - Anomalous left coronary artery from the pulmonary artery and other coronary variants
- Incessant arrhythmias
  - Incessant supraventricular tachycardia
  - Ventricular tachycardia
- Metabolic disorders including mitochondrial disease
- Drug use
  - Cocaine or other stimulants
- Acquired disease
  - Kawasaki disease
  - Coronary artery disease
- Genetic syndromes
  - Neuromuscular disease
  - Genetically triggered cardiomyopathies

DIAGNOSTIC TESTS & INTERPRETATION

- Electrocardiogram findings may be supportive of the diagnosis:
  - Highly variable findings may include sinus tachycardia, low voltage QRS, ST segment depression/elevation, flattening or inversion of the T wave, conduction system disease including complete heart block, prolongation of the QT interval, and arrhythmias (premature atrial contractions/supraventricular tachycardia or premature ventricular contractions/ventricular tachycardia).
- Despite limited sensitivity and specificity, endomyocardial biopsy (EMB) remains the gold standard for confirming the diagnosis of acute myocarditis.
  - The Dallas criteria examine the presence of inflammatory cellular infiltrate and myocyte necrosis. A more recent technique includes the use of immunohistochemistry to evaluate inflammation in biopsy samples. These methods are limited in that they provide information with regard to inflammation but do not assess for the presence of viral pathogens.
  - Current approaches indicate benefit in analyzing the tissue for viral DNA by polymerase chain reaction (PCR).
  - EMB has inherent problems, including sample selection bias, as tissue is only obtained from the right ventricular endocardium, as well as the possible morbidity and mortality associated with an invasive procedure. Biopsy is not indicated in all cases of suspected myocarditis.

Initial Tests (screening, lab, imaging)

- White blood cell count, erythrocyte sedimentation rate, and C-reactive protein level may be elevated.
- Creatine kinase MB fraction and troponin T and I levels may be elevated.
- B-type natriuretic peptide (BNP) may be elevated and can assist with distinguishing a cardiac from a noncardiac cause of respiratory symptoms.
- Cultures (bacterial, viral, fungal) of blood, urine, stool, and nasopharyngeal swabs may be considered.
- Viral PCR analysis of tissue including myocardium, blood, or sputum may be considered.
- Acute and convalescent serologic studies may be considered for selected pathogens.
- Chest radiograph
  - Cardiomegaly
  - Varying degrees of pulmonary edema
  - Possible pleural effusions
- Echocardiography
  - Depressed systolic function (may be biventricular with normal to mildly dilated chamber sizes)
  - Depressed diastolic function (stiff myocardium with abnormal relaxation)
  - Focal wall motion abnormalities are possible.
  - Valvular insufficiency
  - Pericardial effusion
- Cardiac magnetic resonance imaging (MRI)
  - Assessment of chamber size and systolic function
  - Fibrosis by delayed enhancement
  - The Lake Louise cardiac MRI criteria can be used to diagnose myocardial edema and myocarditis by analyzing early enhancement on T1 images and delayed enhancement on T2 images.

TREATMENT

- Initial management should be based on the clinical presentation. These include the following: bed rest and limited activity (during acute phase).
- Standard medical regimens for acute care should be based on appropriate heart failure therapies and may include the following:
  - Inotropic support should be considered for patients with evidence of low cardiac output. Milrinone and/or dobutamine are used as 1st-line rescue therapy, with epinephrine used with refractory hypotension and poor end-organ perfusion.
  - Diuretics (e.g., furosemide and hydrochlorothiazide)
  - Afterload reduction may be considered if volume overload exists with preserved cardiac output (e.g., nitroprusside).
  - Antiarrhythmics may be used in cases of hemodynamically significant arrhythmias.
  - Mechanical ventilation in patients with respiratory failure secondary to myocardial failure
  - Mechanical circulatory support (left ventricular or biventricular assist devices [VAD/BiVADs], extracorporeal membrane oxygenation [ECMO]) should be considered in patients with rapidly progressing, severe heart failure as temporary rescue modality or as bridge to long-term VAD and/or cardiac transplantation.
- Standard medical regimens for chronic care should be based on appropriate heart failure therapies and may include the following:
  - Angiotensin-converting enzyme inhibitors (ACE inhibitors)
  - β-blockers
  - Angiotensin receptor blockers
  - Diuretics (e.g., spironolactone to assist in ventricular remodeling)
  - Anticoagulation with unfractionated or low-molecular-weight heparin acutely and aspirin and/or warfarin chronically for patients with severe myocardial depression and ventricular dilation
  - Implantable devices may be considered for patients with conduction system disease (pacemaker) or those at risk for sudden cardiac death (implantable cardioverter-defibrillator).

MEDICATION

- Intravenous immunoglobulin (IVIG): The use of IVIG is highly controversial with differing results in multiple trials. However, given evidence of immune suppression with this therapy, it is still often used in the treatment of myocarditis.
- Steroids, azathioprine, calcineurin inhibitors, cyclosporine, cyclophosphamide, and other immunosuppressive medications have all been proposed as effective agents, although insufficient evidence of therapeutic benefit is currently available to recommend routine use.
- Antiviral therapy does not currently have an accepted role in myocarditis management.

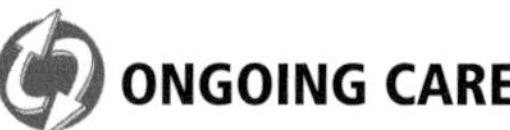

ONGOING CARE

FOLLOW-UP RECOMMENDATIONS

Patient Monitoring

- Ongoing surveillance for heart failure signs and symptoms
- Monitoring for life-threatening arrhythmias
- Effects of the illness on other systems
  - Nutritional status
  - Growth
  - Development
  - Comorbid illnesses

PROGNOSIS

- Prognostic data are limited by the lack of complete ascertainment of all cases of acute myocarditis, with many patients likely exhibiting mild symptoms, which spontaneously resolve.
- Prognosis is often dictated by clinical presentation and underlying etiology. However, if treated appropriately early in the course, outcome can be favorable, with >50% of patients achieving echocardiographic normalization within the first 3 years after diagnosis and a relatively low mortality rate of 7–15%.
- The long-term prognosis of diagnosed myocarditis is significantly better than that of idiopathic cardiomyopathy.
- Worse outcomes are associated with:
  - Younger age at presentation
  - Significant left ventricular dilation
  - Fulminant myocarditis (severe biventricular dysfunction)
  - Requirement of mechanical circulatory support
- Giant cell myocarditis represents a unique subgroup with a particularly poor prognosis, unless transplanted.

COMPLICATIONS

- Acidosis and electrolyte abnormalities
- End-organ hypoperfusion and resultant dysfunction
- Pulmonary venous and arterial hypertension
- Pulmonary edema
- Conduction system disease including heart block
- Arrhythmias

ADDITIONAL READING

- Canter CE, Simpson KE. Diagnosis and treatment of myocarditis in children in the current era. *Circulation*. 2014;129(1):115–128.
- Foerster SR, Canter CE, Cinar A, et al. Ventricular remodeling and survival are more favorable for myocarditis than for idiopathic dilated cardiomyopathy in childhood: an outcomes study from the Pediatric Cardiomyopathy Registry. *Circ Heart Fail*. 2010;3(6):689–697.
- Ghelani SJ, Spaeder MC, Pastor W, et al. Demographics, trends, and outcomes in pediatric acute myocarditis in the United States, 2006 to 2011. *Circ Cardiovasc Qual Outcomes*. 2012;5(5):622–627.
- Kirk R, Dipchand AI, Rosenthal DN, et al. The International Society for Heart and Lung Transplantation Guidelines for the management of pediatric heart failure: executive summary. [Corrected]. *J Heart Lung Transplant*. 2014;33(9):888–909.
- Sagar S, Liu PP, Cooper LT Jr. Myocarditis. *Lancet*. 2012;379(9817):738–747.
- Singh RK, Humlicek T, Jeewa A, et al. Pediatric Cardiac Intensive Care Society 2014 consensus statement: pharmacotherapies in cardiac critical care immune therapy. *Pediatr Crit Care Med*. 2016;17(3 Suppl 1): S69–S76.

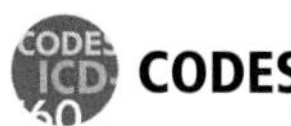

CODES

ICD10

- I51.4 Myocarditis, unspecified
- B33.22 Viral myocarditis
- I40.9 Acute myocarditis, unspecified

M

NARCOLEPSY

Jessica R. Litwin, MD

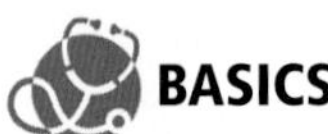

BASICS

DESCRIPTION

- Lifelong neurologic disorder that often initially manifests in childhood or adolescence and can cause significant functional impairment and disability
- Excessive daytime sleepiness (EDS) and inappropriate transitions from wakefulness into rapid eye movement (REM) sleep
- Narcolepsy may occur with or without cataplexy.
- Other associated features include hypnagogic hallucinations, sleep paralysis, and nighttime sleep fragmentation.

GENERAL PREVENTION

- Narcolepsy is not preventable.
- Narcolepsy is underrecognized, especially in children.
- Physicians should screen for sleep dysfunction and excessive sleepiness as part of anticipatory guidance.

EPIDEMIOLOGY

- Prevalence in the United States is reported to range from 25 to 50 per 100,000; prevalence may be higher in the Japanese population.
- An estimated 200,000 Americans have narcolepsy, but fewer than 50,000 of these individuals have been diagnosed with the disorder.
- Approximately half of patients with narcolepsy have symptoms before age 15 years and <10% with symptoms <age 5 years, but often, diagnosis may lag 10 to 15 years after onset of symptoms.
- Cataplexy is present in 50–70% of adult patients and perhaps at least as many pediatric patients but may be initially sporadic or difficult to identify.

RISK FACTORS

- 1st-degree relatives of patients with narcolepsy with cataplexy have a 1–2% risk (which is 10- to 40-fold more than the general population) of developing narcolepsy.
- Both genetic and environmental factors may be involved in the development of narcolepsy.
- There is an association between narcolepsy with cataplexy and human leukocyte antigens (HLAs) subtypes, specifically DQB1*0602 in 85–95% and DR2 antigens. About 40% of cases of narcolepsy without cataplexy are also DQB1*0602 positive.
- Increased risk of narcolepsy after H1N1 vaccination or infection has been a topic of interest.

PATHOPHYSIOLOGY

- Hypocretin (also known as orexin) is a neuropeptide produced by neurons in the perifornical area of the lateral hypothalamus that is supplied to several areas of the brain that promote wakefulness. It may also inhibit REM sleep. It mediates appetite.
- To better reflect pathophysiology, the American Academy of Sleep Medicine has categorized narcolepsy into type 1 and type 2.
  - Type 1 involves hypocretin deficiency, such as would be detected in cerebrospinal fluid (CSF) via lumbar puncture or manifested clinically by the presence of cataplexy.
  - Type 2 does not involve hypocretin deficiency, and in the absence of CSF testing would be the presumptive diagnosis for a patient who had not manifested cataplexy.
  - Onset of cataplexy would herald a change in diagnosis from type 2 to type 1.
- Narcolepsy type 1 is caused by selective loss of the hypocretin-producing neurons in the hypothalamic region.
- The association between narcolepsy and specific HLA antigens has suggested autoimmune pathogenesis; however, this has yet to be definitively established.

COMMONLY ASSOCIATED CONDITIONS

- Secondary narcolepsy may be seen with CNS trauma, strokes, brain tumors, and demyelinating diseases, particularly involving the lateral and posterior hypothalamus, midbrain, and the pons.
- Genetic syndromes associated with secondary narcolepsy include:
  - Prader-Willi syndrome
  - Myotonic dystrophy
  - Niemann-Pick type C

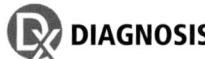

DIAGNOSIS

HISTORY

- EDS starting with recurrence of naps may be early signs of disease.
- In adults, naps tend to be restorative but are more likely to be described as "unrefreshing" in children.
- Cataplexy, the abrupt loss of muscle tone provoked by laughter or strong emotions such as surprise, sadness, or anger, is almost pathognomonic for narcolepsy. Loss of muscle tone can range from sagging of face, eyelids, or jaw; blurred vision; and knee buckling to complete collapse but with preserved consciousness.
- Hypnagogic (on sleep onset) and hypnopompic (on awakening) hallucinations involve vivid auditory or visual hallucinations during transitions between sleep and wakefulness. Such hallucinations can also be experienced infrequently by normal individuals.
- Sleep paralysis is the inability to move or speak for a few seconds or minutes at sleep onset or offset. Normal individuals can also experience sleep paralysis, often in the context of sleep deprivation.
- The classic tetrad of EDS, cataplexy, hypnagogic hallucinations, and sleep paralysis is often not recognizable in the early stages of the disorder and may gradually appear over time; this may contribute to delays in diagnosis.

PHYSICAL EXAM

- Normal in most idiopathic cases; children with narcolepsy are often overweight/obese.
- Vertical gaze palsy, confusion, poor memory, developmental regression, impaired thermoregulation, and signs of endocrine dysfunction may be present in cases of secondary narcolepsy.

DIFFERENTIAL DIAGNOSIS

- Chronic insufficient sleep
- Poor sleep hygiene (particularly nighttime electronics use)
- Delayed sleep phase disorder (manifesting as daytime sleepiness)
- Idiopathic CNS hypersomnia (without cataplexy, sleep-onset REM periods [SOREMPs], or other REM intrusion phenomena in wakefulness or sleep)
- Primary sleep disorders such as obstructive sleep apnea, restless legs syndrome, periodic limb movement disorder

- Kleine-Levin syndrome (cyclical episodes of hypersomnolence, classically also with overeating and hypersexuality lasting days to weeks with normal intervals in between)
- Psychiatric disorders/depression
- Medication side effects, drug/alcohol abuse
- Atonic drop attacks associated with childhood epilepsy syndromes such as Lennox-Gastaut syndrome
- Cataplexy can be associated with Coffin-Lowry syndrome or Norrie syndrome, both rare and involving other deficits including intellectual disability.

DIAGNOSTIC TESTS & INTERPRETATION

Initial Tests (screening, lab, imaging)

- Levels of CSF hypocretin ≤110 pg/mL (30% of mean control value) are strongly indicative of narcolepsy with cataplexy. CSF testing is usually reserved for complicated or ambiguous cases.
- HLA antigen typing with HLA DQB1*0602 and DR2 are strongly associated with narcolepsy with cataplexy but also present in 12–38% of the normal population. A negative result can be helpful in ruling out the condition, and HLA testing should be considered supportive rather than diagnostic.
- Brain MRI is indicated with sudden onset of sleepiness, recent head injury, or an abnormal neurologic exam.

Diagnostic Procedures/Other

- Overnight polysomnography (PSG) and multiple sleep latency test (MSLT) are considered standard of care for diagnosis.
- MSLT is a protocol consisting of four or five 20-minute nap opportunities 2 hours apart after an overnight PSG to determine mean sleep latency (MSL) and SOREMPs within 15 minutes of falling asleep. PSG is performed to ensure adequate nighttime sleep and exclude other sleep disorders that could cause daytime sleepiness. On MSLT, MSL <8 minutes and ≥2 SOREMPs are diagnostic of narcolepsy. SOREMP at the beginning of the preceding night's PSG can now be substituted for a SOREMP on the MSLT. Two or more SOREMPs tend to be specific for narcolepsy, whereas up to 30% of the general population may have MSL <8 minutes. Other factors influencing sleepiness such as chronic sleep deprivation or sedating medications must provide context for test interpretation.

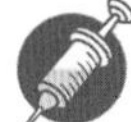

TREATMENT

MEDICATION

- Daytime sleepiness
  - Methylphenidate, 5 to 30 mg/24 h (max 60 mg/24 h). Consider other long-acting formulations such as Concerta®, Ritalin LA®, Metadate CD®, Focalin XR®, etc.
  - Dextroamphetamine (Dexedrine®) 5 to 40 mg/24 h (max 60 mg/24 h)
  - Mixed amphetamine salts (Adderall XR®) 10 to 30 mg/24 h
  - Modafinil (Provigil®), 100 to 400 mg/24 h. FDA Pediatric Advisory Committee warning; recommends use only if 1st- and 2nd-line treatments have failed and the benefits outweigh the risks of serious dermatologic and psychiatric side effects
- Cataplexy
  - Sodium oxybate (Xyrem®): treats both hypersomnia and cataplexy. Dose is given at bedtime while in bed and again 2 1/2 to 4 hours later due to profound sedating effects.
  - Venlafaxine (Effexor®) starting at 12.5 to 25 mg
  - Selective serotonin reuptake inhibitors: fluoxetine (Prozac®) 5 to 30 mg/24 h or sertraline (Zoloft®) 25 to 100 mg/24 h
  - Clomipramine (Anafranil®) 25 to 100 mg/24 h
  - Imipramine (Tofranil®) 25 to 75 mg/24 h

ADDITIONAL THERAPIES

- Regular sleep schedule
- Short scheduled naps
- Regular physical exercise

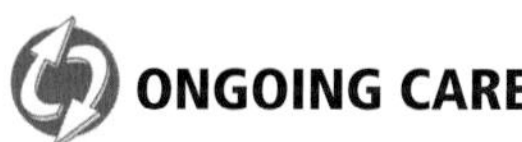

ONGOING CARE

PROGNOSIS

Children with narcolepsy can be expected to have normal life expectancy and normal intellectual functioning. Lifestyle and medication treatments to reduce sleepiness and cataplexy improve academic performance, quality of life, and ability to participate.

ADDITIONAL READING

- Babiker MO, Prasad M. Narcolepsy in children: a diagnostic and management approach. *Pediatr Neurol*. 2015;52(6):557–565.
- Lecendreux M. Pharmacological management of narcolepsy and cataplexy in pediatric patients. *Paediatr Drugs*. 2014;16(5):363–372.
- Postiglione E, Antelmi E, Pizza F, et al. The clinical spectrum of childhood narcolepsy. *Sleep Med Rev*. 2018;38:70–85.

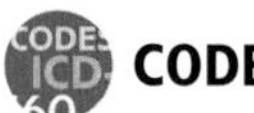

CODES

ICD10

- G47.419 Narcolepsy without cataplexy
- G47.411 Narcolepsy with cataplexy
- G47.429 Narcolepsy in conditions classified elsewhere w/o cataplexy

FAQ

- Q: What is the chance that a sibling of the patient may develop narcolepsy?
- A: There is a 1% possibility that siblings and offspring could be affected.
- Q: Will a patient with narcolepsy be able to drive a car?
- A: Patients with narcolepsy can legally drive, provided they are on the appropriate medications to keep them from falling asleep at the wheel.
- Q: Is there a cure for narcolepsy?
- A: No. Treatment is symptomatic.

NECK MASSES

Nicholas Tsarouhas, MD

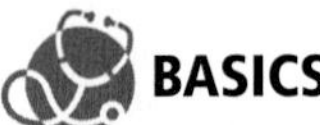

BASICS

DESCRIPTION

A mass in the tissues of the neck; cervical adenopathy is defined as a neck node >1 cm.

ETIOLOGY

Varies depending on underlying condition

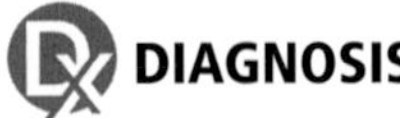

DIAGNOSIS

To diagnose and appropriately manage neck masses, one must combine the history with a careful examination of the mass. The major task of the differential diagnosis is to distinguish infections from congenital and malignant causes.

HISTORY

- Fever: infection, Kawasaki disease (KD), malignancy, "PFAPA" (periodic fever, aphthous stomatitis, pharyngitis, and cervical adenitis) syndrome
- Intercurrent infection: reactive hyperplasia, mononucleosis, abscess, congenital cyst
- Subacute or chronic cervical lymphadenitis: cat-scratch disease, toxoplasmosis, Epstein-Barr virus (EBV), and mycobacterial infection
- Increasing size: infection, newly infected congenital lesion, malignancy (less common)
- Sore throat: mononucleosis, peritonsillar or retropharyngeal abscess
- Swallowing problems: retropharyngeal or peritonsillar abscess, thyroglossal duct cyst
- Cat contact: cat-scratch disease, toxoplasmosis
- Recurrently infected mass: infected congenital cyst (thyroglossal duct, branchial cleft)
- Mass noticed neonatally: cystic hygroma, hemangioma, sternocleidomastoid tumor of infancy
- Weight loss, cough, chronic constitutional symptoms: malignancy, tuberculosis
- Hypothyroid or hyperthyroid symptoms: thyroglossal duct cyst, thyroidal diseases

PHYSICAL EXAM

- Tender, erythematous, indurated mass may indicate cervical adenitis, infected congenital lesion, or cat-scratch disease.
- Nontender, enlarged lymph nodes suggest reactive hyperplasia or malignancy.
- Fluctuant mass may indicate adenitis with abscess or cystic hygroma.
- Drainage suggests adenitis with abscess, atypical mycobacterial disease, infected thyroglossal duct, or branchial cleft cyst.
- Regional adenopathy: reactive hyperplasia, cat-scratch disease, or malignancy
- Exudative pharyngitis: mononucleosis
- Asymmetric soft palate with uvular deviation suggests peritonsillar abscess.
- Pulmonary findings: tuberculosis, malignancy
- Midline mass suggests thyroglossal duct or dermoid cyst or thyroidal disease.
- If mass moves with tongue protrusion, thyroglossal duct cyst may be present.
- Sinus opening may indicate thyroglossal duct, branchial cleft, or dermoid cyst.
- Multiloculated mass that transilluminates suggests cystic hygroma.
- Matted-down mass may indicate malignancy.
- Mass posterior to sternocleidomastoid muscle may be malignancy or infection.
- Inferior deep cervical nodes (scalene and supraclavicular) suggest malignancy.
- Generalized adenopathy suggests malignancy.
- Hepatosplenomegaly may indicate malignancy or infectious mononucleosis.
- Skin discoloration suggests trauma, abscess, or atypical mycobacterial disease.
- A skin papule is a clue to cat-scratch disease.
- Conjunctivitis, oral mucositis, extremity changes, rash, and adenopathy, in the context of fever: Suspect KD.
- Torticollis in a neonate suggests sternocleidomastoid (pseudo) tumor of infancy.

DIFFERENTIAL DIAGNOSIS

- Infectious
  - Reactive hyperplasia: self-limited, enlargement of bilateral minimally tender nodes; usually viral
  - Bacterial lymphadenitis
    - Usually staphylococcal or streptococcal infection of unilateral, tender, swollen, warm, erythematous node
    - Cellulitis-adenitis syndrome in neonates caused by group B *Streptococcus*
  - Cat-scratch disease
    - A usually self-limited, although sometimes protracted, illness (2 to 4 months)
    - Caused by the gram-negative bacillus *Bartonella henselae*
    - Starts as a papule at a cat-scratch site; progresses to regional adenopathy, 5 to 50 days later (median, 12 days)
    - Axillary adenopathy is most common; cervical nodes second most common
    - Adenopathy for weeks to months
  - Tuberculosis: acute or insidious onset of fever and firm, nontender adenopathy in children exposed to adult infected with acid-fast bacillus *Mycobacterium tuberculosis*
  - Atypical mycobacterial disease
    - Infection usually caused by *Mycobacterium avium* complex or *Mycobacterium scrofulaceum* (ubiquitous agents found in the soil)
    - Rapidly enlarging mass of firm, nontender nodes in young children with no known exposure to tuberculosis
    - Nodes often occur with overlying skin discoloration and thinning; some spontaneously drain.
  - Infectious mononucleosis: EBV infection most commonly seen in older children who present with fever, exudative pharyngitis, adenopathy, and hepatosplenomegaly
  - Toxoplasmosis
    - Parasitic disease caused by *Toxoplasma gondii* which presents with cervical adenopathy, rash, fever, malaise, and hepatosplenomegaly
    - Acquired from contact with cat feces or inadequately cooked meat
  - Retropharyngeal abscess
    - Suppurative adenitis of the retropharyngeal nodes that presents in children <5 years of age
    - These children often have fever, neck stiffness, dysphagia, respiratory distress, drooling, and stridor.
  - Peritonsillar abscess: suppurative sequela of a severe tonsillopharyngitis, usually caused by group A β-hemolytic *Streptococcus* (GABHS); commonly presents in older children and adolescents with trismus, "hot potato" voice, and uvular deviation from a bulging palatal abscess
  - Ludwig angina
    - Rapidly expanding, diffuse inflammation of the submandibular/sublingual spaces
    - May compromise the airway
    - Often occurs with dental infections
- Congenital
  - Branchial cleft cyst: common congenital neck lesion (usually a remnant of the 2nd branchial cleft) which presents as a nontender (unless infected) cyst at the anterior border of the sternocleidomastoid
  - Thyroglossal duct cyst: common congenital neck mass which is a remnant of the embryonic thyroglossal sinus and presents as a nontender (unless infected), mobile, anterior midline mass near the hyoid bone
  - Cystic hygroma (lymphangioma): complex, multiloculated mass of lymphatic tissue, which presents in the 1st year of life as a large, soft, compressible mass in the posterior triangle of the neck; may cause airway obstruction
  - Dermoid cyst: small, firm, nontender mass, usually high in the midline, which typically move with the overlying skin
  - Hemangioma: bluish purple, blanching mass characterized by rapid growth in the 1st year of life, then slow regression
  - Sternocleidomastoid (pseudo) tumor of infancy (congenital muscular torticollis): benign perinatal fibromatosis, often associated with difficult deliveries or abnormal uterine positioning, that results in a hard, immobile, fusiform mass in the sternocleidomastoid
  - Laryngocele: cystic dilation of the laryngeal saccule; presents as an air-filled cyst or as a foreign body sensation with coughing
  - Cervical wattle: benign pedunculated congenital anomaly on lateral neck with a core of elastic cartilage
  - Cervical bronchogenic cyst: cervical neck mass in the anteromedial neck (superior to the sternal notch), resulting from abnormal development of the tracheobronchial tree
  - Thymic cyst: ectopic thymic mass resulting from abnormal development of pharyngeal pouches and branchial clefts
  - Teratoma: malformation of all three germ layers that can cause significant airway obstruction as well as feeding dysfunction
  - Ranula: a mucocele created by obstruction of the sublingual salivary glands; usually a painless, slowly accumulating mass
  - Pilomatrixoma: benign neoplasm of the follicular matrix presenting as firm, solitary papule or nodule, often with a faintly blue hue
- Malignant
  - Hodgkin lymphoma: slowly enlarging, unilateral, firm, nontender neck malignancy; usually presents in previously well adolescents
  - Non-Hodgkin lymphoma: presents in young adolescents as a painless, rapidly growing, firm collection of lymph nodes

- Leukemia: most common tumor associated with cervical adenitis in first 6 years of life
- Neuroblastoma: commonly presents in infants/young children as a large, nontender abdominal mass; associated with a myriad of signs and symptoms due to its propensity for metastasis
- Rhabdomyosarcoma: head and neck malignancy that usually presents as a rapidly enlarging mass
- Melanoma: an increasingly identified cause of neck malignancy in pediatrics

- Thyroid
  - Chronic lymphocytic thyroiditis (Hashimoto thyroiditis): autoimmune childhood goiter that may be eu-, hypo-, or hyperthyroid
  - Thyrotoxicosis (Graves disease): clinically hyperfunctioning thyroid caused by circulating thyroid cell–stimulating antibodies
  - Thyroiditis: painful bacterial infection of the thyroid caused by *Staphylococcus* or *Streptococcus*
- Miscellaneous
  - KD
    - Idiopathic vasculitis distinguished by prolonged fever (5 days or more), conjunctivitis, oral mucositis, extremity changes, rash, and unilateral cervical node >1.5 cm
    - Cervical node: least common feature seen
    - Classic KD defined by fever and four of five above criteria, although "incomplete" KD requires fewer.
  - PFAPA syndrome
    - PFAPA
    - Idiopathic, periodic, benign, febrile syndrome most commonly seen in young children
  - Sinus histiocytosis with massive lymphadenopathy (Rosai–Dorfman disease); benign form of histiocytosis that presents as massive, painless enlargement of cervical nodes
  - Hematoma: secondary to trauma
  - Hypersensitivity reaction: secondary to bites, stings, or other allergens
  - Drugs: Notably, phenytoin and isoniazid may be associated with lymphadenopathy.
  - Immunization: Adenopathy may follow DPT or polio immunization.

DIAGNOSTIC TESTS & INTERPRETATION

- CBC
  - Infections: leukocytosis
  - Mononucleosis: atypical lymphocytosis
  - Kawasaki: thrombocytosis after 1st week, along with elevation in other inflammatory markers
  - Neck malignancies: usually normal initially
  - Pancytopenia with blast cells suggests leukemia.
- Complete metabolic panel with lactate dehydrogenase (LDH) and uric acid when malignancy is suspected
- "Mono spot" (mononucleosis) test: less reliable in children <4 years old; EBV titers more useful
- Indirect fluorescent antibody titers for *Bartonella*: confirms cat-scratch disease
- Purified protein derivative: negative or weakly positive in atypical mycobacterial infections
- Chest radiograph: important in all evaluations when malignancy is a possibility; adenopathy seen in malignancies and tuberculosis; cavitary lesions and infiltrates in tuberculosis
- Lateral neck radiograph: prevertebral soft tissue space at C2–C3 abnormally wide (>1/2 adjacent vertebral body diameter) in cases of retropharyngeal abscess
- Ultrasound
  - 1st-line imaging modality in neck masses
  - Provides immediate, noninvasive information on location, size, and composition of mass (cystic vs. solid)
  - Doppler adds information about vascularity.
- CT or MRI scan: useful in evaluating deep neck infections and complex neck masses
  - CT advantages: more readily available; shorter study; less need for sedation
  - MRI advantages: no ionizing radiation; better soft tissue resolution
  - MRI is the imaging study of choice when a vascular malformation is suspected.
- Thyroid scintigraphy: useful when malignancy is a concern for midline neck masses
- Gram stain and culture of specimen after needle aspiration or incision and drainage (I&D): diagnostic and therapeutic with infections
- Histologic evaluation after fine-needle aspiration or biopsy: diagnostic for malignant versus congenital versus infectious causes

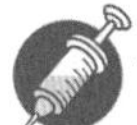

TREATMENT

GENERAL MEASURES

- Infectious neck masses often benefit from warm compresses.
- Sternocleidomastoid tumor of infancy: massage, range of motion, and stretching

MEDICATION

- Infectious
  - Antibiotics directed at the causative organism
  - Empiric coverage for skin and soft tissue infections usually includes antibiotics with antistaphylococcal and antistreptococcal activity.
  - Local resistance patterns, as well as the presence of abscess, often define the need for coverage versus methicillin-resistant *Staphylococcus aureus* (MRSA).
  - Other antibiotics depending on most likely suspected bacteria
- Malignancy: oncologic referral for evaluation, then possible chemotherapy

ALERT

Corticosteroids should not be given to neck mass patients until malignancy has been excluded, except in dire conditions of airway compromise.

- Thyroidal: endocrine referral for pharmacotherapy
- KD: IVIG and aspirin therapy are effective in preventing most cases of coronary artery aneurysms; some high-risk populations are also treated with prednisone.
- PFAPA syndrome: A single dose of prednisone is often efficacious in aborting fever attacks.

SURGERY/OTHER PROCEDURES

- Abscesses require I&D.
- I&D can often be performed in the primary care or emergency care setting.
- Surgical referral may be necessary in some cases.
- ENT surgeons will often wait for antibiotics to "quiet down" infections prior to surgical excision.
- Possible oncologic masses should be referred for consideration of radiation or excision.
- Cardiology referral is mandatory for consideration of echocardiography in suspected KD cases to rule out coronary artery aneurysms.
- Some studies have shown tonsillectomy to be an effective treatment for PFAPA.

ONGOING CARE

Close follow-up is essential for all neck masses; consider referral for biopsy in the following cases:

- Nodes not responding to antibiotics
- Toxic illness/systemic symptoms
- Clinical signs of malignancy (weight loss, peripheral adenopathy, hepatosplenomegaly)
- Firm, nontender nodes fixed to deep tissues
- Nodes posterior to the sternocleidomastoid or in the lower cervical/supraclavicular regions
- Bilateral nodes >2 cm

ADDITIONAL READING

- Cohen E, Sundel R. Kawasaki disease at 50 years. *JAMA Pediatr*. 2016;170(11):1093–1099.
- Friedman ER, John SD. Imaging of pediatric neck masses. *Radiol Clin North Am*. 2011;49(4):617–632.
- Geddes G, Butterly MM, Patel SM, et al. Pediatric neck masses. *Pediatr Rev*. 2013;34(3):115–124.
- Lantto U, Koivunen P, Tapiainen T, et al. Long-term outcome of classic and incomplete PFAPA (periodic fever, aphthous stomatitis, pharyngitis, and adenitis) syndrome after tonsillectomy. *J Pediatr*. 2016;179:172–177.e1.
- Meier JD, Grimmer JF. Evaluation and management of neck masses in children. *Am Fam Physician*. 2014;89(5):353–358.

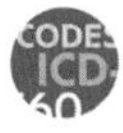

CODES

ICD10

- R22.1 Localized swelling, mass and lump, neck
- R59.0 Localized enlarged lymph nodes
- L02.11 Cutaneous abscess of neck

FAQ

- Q: How should nodes respond to therapy?
- A: Consider referral for biopsy if increasing size after 2 weeks, no decrease in size >2 to 4 weeks, or not back to normal >8 to 12 weeks.
- Q: Do all external neck abscesses need antibiotic therapy after drainage?
- A: Many experts believe that antibiotics are not always necessary if I&D is done appropriately.
- Q: Is antibiotic coverage for community-acquired MRSA (CA-MRSA) necessary?
- A: As CA-MRSA is increasingly common, an antibiotic agent with MRSA coverage is indicated; clindamycin is a common choice.

NECROTIZING ENTEROCOLITIS

May W. Chen, MD • Susan W. Aucott, MD • David J. Hackam, MD, PhD, FACS

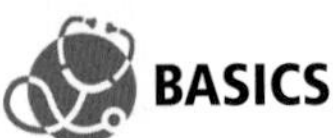

BASICS

DESCRIPTION

Necrotizing enterocolitis (NEC) is a life-threatening gastrointestinal (GI) emergency that occurs in the newborn period and consists of diffuse necrotic injury to the bowel, which can result in perforation or subserosal collections of gas. The entire GI tract is susceptible, but the most frequently involved areas are the distal small bowel and proximal colon. Lesions vary from being diffuse areas of patchy necrosis to more isolated focal disease. Systemic signs and symptoms related to the inflammatory GI injury are accompanied by characteristic radiographic findings of pneumatosis.

EPIDEMIOLOGY

- NEC typically has an onset at 2 to 5 weeks of life (3 to 20 days after the initiation of enteral feedings). The more premature the infant, the longer the child is at risk for developing NEC, with cases reported as late as 3 months of age.
- NEC affects mostly premature infants, but up to 10% of cases occur in term infants.
- The incidence of NEC is variable and ranges from 1% to 7% of all neonatal intensive care unit admissions or 1 to 3 per 1,000 live births.
- Preterm infants account for the vast majority of total NEC cases; the risk increases with decreasing gestational age and birth weight.
- Prevalence in very-low-birth-weight (VLBW) infants (birth weight <1,500 g) is 7%.
- Highest risk is in infants with birth weights between 500 and 750 g (15%).

RISK FACTORS

The greatest risk factor for NEC is prematurity. Additional risk factors for both preterm and full-term infants include the following:

- Enteral feeding with formula
- Cardiovascular instability
- Respiratory compromise resulting in recurrent or prolonged hypoxia
- Cyanotic heart disease
- Polycythemia
- Exchange transfusions
- Gastroschisis
- Perinatal asphyxia
- Small size for gestational age
- Maternal preeclampsia
- Antenatal cocaine abuse
- Prolonged use of IV antibiotics
- Gastric acid suppression with H_2 blockers

GENERAL PREVENTION

- Exclusive maternal breast milk feeding has been advocated. When maternal breast milk is unavailable, use of donor milk may decrease the risk of developing NEC when compared to formula.
- Standardized feeding protocols with early initiation of trophic feeds (<10 mL/kg/24 h) for several days prior to advancing feeding volumes may stimulate maturation of the GI tract with resultant improvement in feeding tolerance. A rapid rate of feeding advancement (>20 mL/kg/24 h) may increase the risk of NEC in infants <1,500 g.
- Minimizing prolonged use of empiric antibiotics immediately after birth
- Specific probiotic strains may decrease the incidence for VLBW infants. Concern has been raised regarding lack of quality standards and an increased risk of sepsis when using probiotics.
- Immunonutrient supplementation with agents such as arginine, glutamine, lactoferrin, and omega-3 polyunsaturated fatty acids is being investigated, but there is currently insufficient evidence to make any recommendations for their use.

PATHOPHYSIOLOGY

- Exact mechanism of injury in NEC is unclear, but research suggests a multitude of factors in an immature host lead to activation of the inflammatory cascade with subsequent tissue injury and necrosis.
- Components of the innate immune system, such as toll-like receptors (TLRs), play a role.
  - Specifically, TLR type 4 (TLR4) activation by pathologic bacteria inhibits the body's ability for intestinal repair and increases the release of inflammatory cytokines causing epithelial injury.
  - In preterm infants, expression of TLR4 is elevated leading to an increased risk for overactivation, intestinal injury, and NEC.
- The most common sites for NEC include the terminal ileum, ileocecal region, and ascending colon.
  - 50% of infants have both colonic and small intestine disease, with the other 50% divided between isolated ileal and colonic involvement.

ETIOLOGY

- The etiology of NEC is unknown but thought to be a multifactorial process.
- Various factors that cause direct and indirect mucosal disruption, which in turn may lead to an increased permeability in the gut of agents that lead to injury, include the following:
  - Hypoxia/ischemia leading to mucosal injury
  - GI tract immaturity
  - Immature host defense
  - Enteral feedings
  - Decreased diversity of bacteria within the GI lumen
  - It is noteworthy that each of these factors can increase expression of immune receptors including TLR4 in the gut.
- Enteral alimentation
  - Because 95% of infants who develop NEC have been enterally fed, initiation of feedings has been implicated as an important contributor to the etiology of NEC.
  - The composition of the formula (osmolarity), the rate of volume increase, and the immaturity of the mucosa have all been implicated as factors.
- Because of the frequent report of epidemic, cluster-type episodes, a variety of microorganisms has been implicated in the development of NEC, although there is no single causative organism.
  - Blood cultures may be positive in 20–30% of cases, often gram-negative organisms.
- Immaturity of the GI mucosal defense system, including factors such as reduced levels of defensins and impaired mucin production, may impair defense against invading organisms, leading to NEC.
- Medications may cause direct mucosal injury.

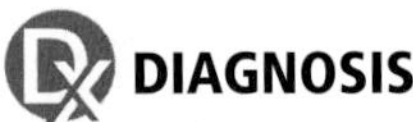

DIAGNOSIS

ALERT

Delay in making the correct diagnosis of NEC and instituting appropriate therapy may lead to a rapid progression of symptoms and often a worse outcome.

PHYSICAL EXAM

- The triad of abdominal distention, bloody stools, and feeding intolerance is frequently seen 3 to 10 days after initiating enteral feedings.
- The clinical spectrum varies dramatically from nonspecific symptoms of feeding intolerance to severe abdominal distention, sepsis, and shock. A staging system ranks the disease into three categories based on severity of the clinical signs and symptoms, aiding formulation of individual treatment plans.
  - Stage I (suspected NEC)
    - Temperature instability
    - Apnea
    - Bradycardia
    - Lethargy
    - Cyanosis
    - Glucose instability
    - Increased gastric residuals
    - Emesis (may be bilious)
    - Abdominal distention
    - Heme-positive stools
  - Stage II (definitive NEC): stage I plus
    - Mild metabolic acidosis
    - Mild thrombocytopenia
    - Poor perfusion
    - Severe abdominal distention
    - Absent bowel sounds
    - Abdominal tenderness
    - Grossly bloody stools
    - Possible abdominal wall erythema from necrotic bowel, cellulitis, fullness/mass
    - Ascites
  - Stage III (advanced NEC): stage I and II plus
    - Shock/deterioration of vital signs
    - Metabolic acidosis
    - Thrombocytopenia
    - Disseminated intravascular coagulation (DIC)
    - Significant abdominal tenderness/peritonitis
    - Respiratory compromise
    - Neutropenia

DIFFERENTIAL DIAGNOSIS

- Systemic
  - Sepsis with ileus
  - Pneumothorax causing a pneumoperitoneum
  - Hemorrhagic disease of the newborn
  - Swallowed maternal blood
- GI tract
  - Volvulus
  - Malrotation
  - Hirschsprung colitis
  - Intussusception
  - Spontaneous bowel perforation
  - Stress gastritis
  - Meconium ileus
  - Milk protein allergy

DIAGNOSTIC TESTS & INTERPRETATION

Initial Tests (screening, lab, imaging)

No single laboratory feature is diagnostic of NEC. Obtaining a blood culture and monitoring serial complete blood counts (CBCs) and blood gases are essential for monitoring patients with NEC to assess for the following:

- Thrombocytopenia
- Acidosis, metabolic
- Anemia
- Leukopenia/neutropenia
- DIC
- Abdominal radiographs are essential for the diagnosis and staging of NEC:
  - Obtain both an anterior-posterior radiograph and a left lateral recumbent film (to evaluate for free air).
  - Stage I: mild dilatation of bowel loops, intestinal ileus
  - Stage II
    - Dilated loops, which may be fixed
    - Pneumatosis intestinalis (presence of submucosal or subserosal air in the intestinal wall)
    - Possible portal venous gas
  - Stage III: likely pneumoperitoneum, free air
    - "Football" sign on anterior-posterior radiograph
- Abdominal ultrasonography is currently being investigated as a noninvasive diagnostic modality for NEC.

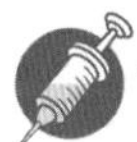

TREATMENT

The best therapy for NEC is prevention. When present, early recognition and rapid medical management of infants with NEC are critical to minimize the progression of this aggressive disease. There is no specific cure for NEC.

GENERAL MEASURES

- Length of therapy and reinstitution of feedings are based on the severity of the episode and on clinical, laboratory, and radiologic abnormalities.
- If there are no laboratory or radiographic abnormalities, feedings may be started 24 to 72 hours after the episode.
- If mild abnormalities are present and the infant is only mildly ill, a 7-day course of therapy is considered.
- When laboratory and radiologic abnormalities include pneumatosis intestinalis, acidosis, and/or thrombocytopenia, a 10- to 14-day course is indicated.

SURGERY/OTHER PROCEDURES

- 1st-line therapy for NEC is medical management and is successful in 50–75% of infants.
- Surgical intervention is required in 25–50% of all cases.
- Indications for surgery include the following:
  - Pneumoperitoneum
  - Cellulitis of the anterior abdominal wall, abdominal mass
  - Suspicion of intestinal infarction with a fixed loop of dilated bowel on radiography
  - Metabolic acidosis secondary to bowel necrosis unresponsive to medical therapy
  - Persistent sepsis and abdominal x-rays showing persistent ileus or a fixed loop, in the setting of progressive thrombocytopenia
- The goal of surgery is to remove all necrotic bowel and to preserve as much bowel length as possible. The most widely accepted procedure is laparotomy with resection of gangrenous intestine and exteriorization of all viable ends as stomas.
- Peritoneal drains placed at the bedside were developed as a palliative procedure to decrease surgical morbidity and mortality in infants weighing <1,000 g, decompressing the peritoneal cavity of gas, necrotic debris, and stool. There may be a role for peritoneal drainage as a definitive surgery. However, studies have not shown a benefit of drainage over laparotomy with additional concerns for increased adverse neurodevelopmental outcomes.
  - An ongoing multicenter randomized trial is comparing the effectiveness of laparotomy versus drainage in ELBW infants with a focus on neurodevelopmental outcomes.

ADMISSION, INPATIENT, AND NURSING CONSIDERATIONS

- Therapy is based on the severity and progression of the symptoms.
- Initial management of all patients with suspected or proven NEC
  - NPO status
  - IV fluids
  - Nasogastric (NG) tube placement for decompression
  - IV antibiotics: broad spectrum
  - Total parenteral nutrition (TPN) to ensure adequate nutrition and growth
  - Severely ill patients may require hemodynamic support, acid–base regulation, and respiratory support as clinically appropriate.
- Evaluate every 6 hours to once a day, depending on the severity of the episode:
  - Blood cultures
  - CBC, electrolytes, and blood gas
  - Fluid status
  - Abdominal radiograph

ONGOING CARE

FOLLOW-UP RECOMMENDATIONS

Despite early recognition and intervention, NEC is associated with a significant morbidity and mortality.

DIET

- During acute illness, NPO and TPN
- On resolution of illness, slow reintroduction of feeds is necessary, as the infant is at risk for recurrent NEC.

PROGNOSIS

- Overall mortality for infants with NEC is between 20% and 40% but can be as high as 60% in patients with stage III NEC.
- Infants who survive the acute stage of NEC have a good long-term survival with 80–95% survival to discharge. However, hospitalization is 20 days longer on average than similar infants without NEC.
- As many as 50% of infants recovering from NEC have neurodevelopmental delays.

COMPLICATIONS

- Acute complications that may occur with NEC include GI perforation, DIC, sepsis, shock, fluid and electrolyte imbalance, and respiratory failure.
- Long-term complications occur in 10–30% of infants and include the following:
  - Intestinal strictures
  - Acquired short bowel syndrome if the patient undergoes lengthy surgical resection of bowel
  - Enterocolic fistulas or anastomotic leaks
  - Malabsorption
  - Failure to thrive
  - Cholestasis
  - Liver failure from prolonged TPN
- Most common complication (10–35%) is intestinal stricture: occurs mainly in the left colon

ADDITIONAL READING

- Christensen RD, Lambert DK, Baer VL, et al. Necrotizing enterocolitis in term infants. *Clin Perinatol*. 2013;40(1):69–78.
- Fallon EM, Nehra D, Potemkin AK, et al. A.S.P.E.N. Clinical Guidelines: nutrition support of neonatal patients at risk for necrotizing enterocolitis. *JPEN J Parenter Enteral Nutr*. 2012;36(5):506–523.
- Lin PW, Stoll BJ. Necrotising enterocolitis. *Lancet*. 2006;368(9543):1271–1283.
- Neu J, Walker WA. Necrotizing enterocolitis. *N Engl J Med*. 2011;364(3):255–264.
- Niño DF, Sodhi CP, Hackam DJ. Necrotizing enterocolitis: new insights into pathogenesis and mechanisms. *Nat Rev Gastroenterol Hepatol*. 2016;13(10):590–600.
- Rao SC, Basani L, Simmer K, et al. Peritoneal drainage versus laparotomy as initial surgical treatment for perforated necrotizing enterocolitis or spontaneous intestinal perforation in preterm low birth weight infants. *Cochrane Database Syst Rev*. 2011;(6):CD006182.
- Rees CM, Pierro A, Eaton S. Neurodevelopmental outcomes of neonates with medically and surgically treated necrotizing enterocolitis. *Arch Dis Child Fetal Neonatal Ed*. 2007;92(3):F193–F198.

CODES

ICD10

- P77.9 Necrotizing enterocolitis in newborn, unspecified
- P77.1 Stage 1 necrotizing enterocolitis in newborn
- P77.2 Stage 2 necrotizing enterocolitis in newborn

FAQ

- Q: What are the most common complications of NEC?
- A: Mortality, poor growth, prolonged hospitalization, and the development of intestinal strictures
- Q: Is NEC preventable?
- A: The development of NEC is not clearly preventable, but cautious feedings in extremely premature infants with gradual advancement and use of breast milk decrease the risk of NEC.
- Q: Is NEC exclusively a process that occurs in the premature infant?
- A: Approximately 10% of cases occur in full-term infants with underlying risk factors (i.e., polycythemia, congenital heart disease, opioid withdrawal).
- Q: How is spontaneous intestinal perforation (SIP) different from NEC?
- A: SIP represents a perforation not associated with pneumatosis, inflammation, or ischemia (all hallmarks of NEC) and occurs in infants that often have not yet been fed. Risk factors include extreme prematurity and early steroid use, particularly in combination with indomethacin in the 1st week of life.
- Q: Do red blood cell transfusions cause NEC?
- A: There has been an association reported between red blood cell transfusions and NEC, but recent evidence suggests that transfusions do not cause NEC.
- Q: If an infant requires surgery for NEC with ostomy creation, when does the child undergo reanastomosis?
- A: There is typically at 6-week minimum waiting period before consideration of ostomy reversal.

NEONATAL ABSTINENCE SYNDROME

Cheryl A. Harrow, DNP, FNP-BC, MS, RNC-LRN, IBCLC • Maureen M. Gilmore, MD

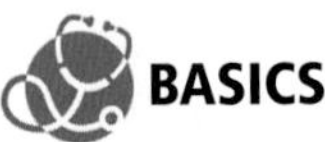

BASICS

DESCRIPTION

- Neonatal abstinence syndrome (NAS) occurs due to intrauterine exposure to maternal opioid medications (whether the mother is on maintenance opioid therapy, using illicit opioids, or abusing licit opioids), causing a postnatal withdrawal syndrome.
- Signs of NAS include gastrointestinal (GI) tract dysfunction, central nervous system (CNS) irritability, and autonomic overreactivity following birth secondary to a lack of maternal drug supply.
- Iatrogenic drug withdrawal syndrome may be seen in infants and children treated with opioids (following severe illness or surgery with similar symptoms) but is not the focus of this chapter.

EPIDEMIOLOGY

Incidence

- NAS symptoms occur in 55–94% of neonates with intrauterine opioid exposure.
- Marked rise from 1.5 cases per 1,000 live births in 1999 to 6 cases per 1,000 live births in 2013

RISK FACTORS

Maternal: Chronic pain, medication-seeking behaviors, opioid maintenance therapy, report of drug abuse, multidrug use (e.g., nicotine, benzodiazepines, trazodone, SSRIs), homelessness, history of sexual abuse, or domestic violence

- 4.5% of pregnant women age 15 to 44 years reported recent use of illicit drugs.
- 6% of mothers reported use of prescription opioids for >1 month of pregnancy.

GENERAL PREVENTION

- Prenatal education and counseling of at-risk women
- Prenatal treatment—opioid maintenance therapy
- Prevention of abrupt drug cessation during pregnancy

PATHOPHYSIOLOGY

- Opiates are low-molecular-weight, water soluble, lipophilic compounds that easily cross placenta, increasingly as gestation progresses.
- Opioids easily cross fetal blood–brain barrier.
- Opioid receptors are extensive in CNS as well as the peripheral nervous system, GI tract, and other organ systems.
- Opioids have a prolonged half-life in fetus.
- Neonatal neurobehavioral dysregulation is the major manifestation of NAS.

ETIOLOGY

Intrauterine exposure to maternal licit or illicit opioid use, with cessation of the exposure at clamping and cutting of the umbilical cord

COMMONLY ASSOCIATED CONDITIONS

- Premature birth
- Placental abruption
- Poor intrauterine growth and/or small for gestational age
- Feeding problems
- Seizures (uncommon)
- Birth defects (rare)

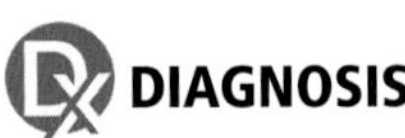

DIAGNOSIS

HISTORY

- Obtain maternal history with a nonjudgmental attitude.
- Document maternal opioid maintenance therapy, use of illicit drugs, or abuse of prescription medications.
- Validate prescription medications with treating physician or drug counselor (with mother's permission).

PHYSICAL EXAM

- Complete neonatal exam with full neurologic assessment
- Symptoms

Tremors (trembling)	Vomiting
Irritability (with consoling)	Diarrhea
Sleep problems	Dehydration
High-pitched crying	Poor feeding and suck
Tight muscle tone	Excoriation (chin, cheeks)
Hyperactive reflexes	Mottling
Seizures	Fever
Yawning	Tachypnea
Sneezing, stuffy nose	Weight loss >10%
Sweating	Unable to self-console

DIFFERENTIAL DIAGNOSIS

- Sepsis
- Hypoglycemia
- Hypocalcemia
- Hyperthyroidism
- Seizures not related to drug withdrawal (i.e., due to intracranial hemorrhage, brain malformation)

DIAGNOSTIC TESTS & INTERPRETATION

Initial Tests (screening, lab, imaging)

- Urine toxicology screen—mother and infant
- NAS scoring tool (e.g., modified Finnegan scoring system)

Follow-Up Tests & Special Considerations

- Meconium toxicology—testing is reliable until stool transitions. Check testing availability in hospital setting.
- Umbilical cord toxicology. Check testing availability in hospital setting.

Test Interpretation

Toxicology screening panels do not always include methadone and buprenorphine. If exposure to these drugs is suspected or known, an order for specific testing may be needed.

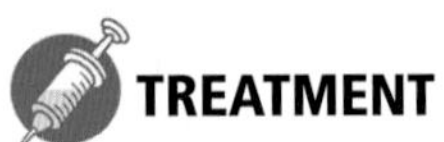

TREATMENT

GENERAL MEASURES

- Nonpharmacologic interventions—that is, positioning, swaddling, side-lying, sucking, swaying, "shh"-ing, skin to skin, gentle touch; avoid overstimulation.
- Environmental controls—for example, quiet/low noise setting, ambient light
- Avoid sedating medications (i.e., phenobarbital).
- Avoid alcohol-based medications.

MEDICATION

First Line

- Oral morphine
  - For symptom-based dosing, start at 0.04 mg every 3 to 4 hours, escalate by 0.02 to 0.04 mg or more based on symptoms.
  - For weight-based dosing, start at 0.04 mg/kg every 3 to 4 hours, escalate by 0.04 mg/kg/dose.
  - Titrate to effect based on NAS scoring performed every 3 to 4 hours.
- IV morphine: Dosing conversion is 1:1 oral to IV.

Second Line

- Clonidine 6 to 12 mcg/kg/24 h divided every 4 to 6 hours may reduce total morphine dosing required.
- Benzodiazepines—consider in setting of known benzodiazepine exposure or polysubstance exposure in utero.

ISSUES FOR REFERRAL

- Social work for positive toxicology noted in mother and/or baby
- Child Protective Services: mandates differ in various states; should be coordinated with social work referral
- Infant and toddler early intervention and assessment
- Inpatient occupational therapy (OT) and/or physical therapy (PT), for feeding difficulty. Outpatient therapy may be necessary.

ADMISSION, INPATIENT, AND NURSING CONSIDERATIONS

- Nonpharmacologic interventions taught to parents and environmental controls should be taught to parents in house in preparation for home discharge (if approved by Child Protective Services/social work).
- Rooming-in should be promoted to encourage bonding with parents, guardians, or adoptive parents.
- Cluster exams, feedings, and nursing cares may be necessary.
- Neonatal abstinence scoring should be done every 3 to 4 hours, beginning at 2 hours of age until discharged.
- Vital signs should be monitored every 3 to 4 hours with cares/feedings.
- Pulse oximetry, if ordered
- Minimum 4-day observation for methadone and buprenorphine exposure
- Minimum 3-day observation for opiate exposure

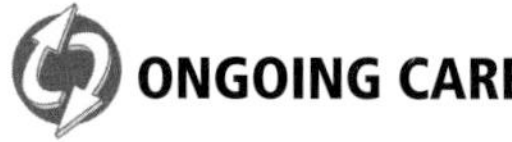

ONGOING CARE

FOLLOW-UP RECOMMENDATIONS

- Early follow-up with pediatrician/primary care provider
- Family/caregiver support

Patient Monitoring

Expect ongoing low-level signs of opiate withdrawal after complete weaning from medication, especially with long-acting opiate (i.e., methadone) exposure.

DIET

- Breastfeeding should be considered if negative maternal toxicology screen and no reported use (>90 days of abstinence).
- Team consult to discuss breastfeeding (including drug treatment therapist) if the mother is abstinent >30 days but <90 days
- If the mother is <30 days abstinent, breastfeeding is not recommended.
- Breastfeeding is approved with methadone and buprenorphine in any dose.
- Infants may require higher calorie formula due to increased metabolic demand.

PATIENT EDUCATION

Parents/caregivers should receive education on:

- Nonpharmacologic interventions
- Environmental controls
- Assistive feeding techniques
- Ongoing lactation support

COMPLICATIONS

- Babies may be rehospitalized for vomiting, poor feeding, poor weight gain, inability to sleep.
- Babies undergoing withdrawal are at increased risk for abuse by parent/caregiver.

ADDITIONAL READING

- American Congress of Obstetricians and Gynecologists Committee on Health Care for Underserved Women, American Society of Addiction Medicine. Committee Opinion No. 524: opioid abuse, dependence, and addiction in pregnancy. *Obstet Gynecol*. 2012;119(5):1070–1076.
- Agthe AG, Kim GR, Mathias KB, et al. Clonidine as an adjunct therapy to opioids for neonatal abstinence syndrome: a randomized, controlled trial. *Pediatrics*. 2009;123(5):e849–e856.
- Hudak ML, Tan RC; for Committee on Drugs, Committee on Fetus and Newborn, American Academy of Pediatrics. Neonatal drug withdrawal. *Pediatrics*. 2012;129(2):e540–e560.
- Jansson LM, Choo RE, Harrow C, et al. Concentrations of methadone in breast milk and plasma in the immediate perinatal period. *J Hum Lact*. 2007;23(2):184–190.
- Reece-Stremtan S, Marinelli KA. ABM Clinical Protocol #21: guidelines for breastfeeding and substance use or substance use disorder, revised 2015. *Breastfeed Med*. 2015;10(3):135–141.

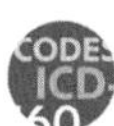

CODES

ICD10

- P96.1 Neonatal withdrawal symptoms from maternal use of drugs of addiction
- P96.2 Withdrawal symptoms from therapeutic use of drugs in newborn

FAQ

- Q: If a mother is treated with methadone, should her infant also be treated with methadone?
- A: Methadone has a long half-life, whereas morphine has a short half-life. Dosing adjustments and weaning can occur according to the infant's symptoms and weaning tolerance when morphine is used as treatment.
- Q: An infant's mother is breastfeeding and taking methadone. Will the infant have withdrawal symptoms if she stops breastfeeding?
- A: The amount of methadone in breast milk ranges from 21 to 314 ng/dL, far less than the 10% dose applied to most medications in breast milk. It is recommended that weaning from breastfeeding be done gradually to prevent the possibility of withdrawal.
- Q: Maternal drug treatment with buprenorphine is on the rise. How does this impact NAS in neonates?
- A: Neonates who were exposed to buprenorphine in utero may still undergo NAS. In small studies, the buprenorphine-exposed infants were found to require a lower total dose of morphine, had a shorter duration of treatment, and a shorter length of stay.
- Q: Are preterm newborns affected by NAS to the same degree as full-term newborns?
- A: For preterm newborns, the incidence and severity of NAS are less. Several factors which may explain this presentation include decreased total in utero exposure, less placental transmission due to preterm delivery, decreased morphine clearance, hepatic and renal immaturity of liver and kidneys, decreased fatty tissue in preterm infants (where drug accumulates), and fewer and less sensitive opioid receptors.

NEONATAL ALLOIMMUNE THROMBOCYTOPENIA

Anne M. Marsh, MD • Alison T. Matsunaga, MD

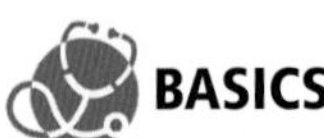

BASICS

DESCRIPTION

Neonatal alloimmune thrombocytopenia (NAIT) is one of the major causes of severe thrombocytopenia in the newborn.

- Analogous to ABO/Rh incompatibility but involves platelets instead of RBCs
- Presents with bleeding complications including petechiae, bruising, mucosal bleeding, and/or intracranial hemorrhage (ICH) that can occur in utero

EPIDEMIOLOGY

1:1,000 live births

GENERAL PREVENTION

In pregnancies known to be at risk of NAIT, maternal treatment with IVIG in the antenatal period can be considered.

PATHOPHYSIOLOGY

Antibody-mediated platelet destruction

ETIOLOGY

Maternal IgG antibodies, directed against paternally inherited platelet-specific antigens in the fetus, cross the placenta, enter the fetal circulation, and attack fetal platelets.

- HPA-1a (formerly PLA-1) incompatibility is by far the most common cause of NAIT in those of Caucasian ancestry, accounting for ~75% of cases. The disease happens when the mother is HPA-1a negative (HPA 1b/1b) and father is HPA-1a positive (HPA 1a/1a or 1a/1b). If the fetus inherits HPA-1a from father, maternal exposure to HPA-1a–positive fetal platelets during pregnancy causes mother to generate anti–HPA-1a IgG antibodies. Anti–HPA-1a antibodies crosses the placenta and causes platelet destruction.
- Other common antigens implicated in NAIT include HPA-2, HPA-3, HPA-5, HPA-9, and HPA-15.
- HPA-4 incompatibility accounts for the majority of cases in Asian populations.
- At least 23 other low-frequency antigens have been reported in a small fraction of cases.
- HPA-1a–negative mothers who are HLA-DRB3*0101 positive are far more likely to develop antibodies than those who are DRB3 negative.
- The role of HLA platelet antigens in NAIT is controversial.

DIAGNOSIS

HISTORY

- NAIT is suspected in a non–ill-appearing neonate who presents shortly after birth with clinical signs of bleeding and documented thrombocytopenia.
- Patient may have a history of mild easy bruising and bleeding symptoms.
- Maternal history of previous births with thrombocytopenia, NAIT, ICH, or fetal losses?
- Maternal history of thrombocytopenia or idiopathic thrombocytopenic purpura (ITP)?
- Is current maternal platelet count normal?
- Family history of thrombocytopenia or bleeding disorders?
- Symptoms suggestive of an infection in the mother or infant?
- Medications used during pregnancy or in the newborn period

ALERT

Maternal platelet count in NAIT should be normal. Thrombocytopenia in the mother and/or a history of maternal ITP should prompt you to consider alternative diagnoses such as autoimmune thrombocytopenia (i.e., antibodies directed toward maternal platelets, passively transfer into the fetal circulation and destroy fetal platelets).

PHYSICAL EXAM

- General:
  - Most neonates with NAIT are well and nonseptic appearing.
  - Evaluate for evidence of a congenital disorder (e.g., dysmorphic features).
- Head/neck: Exclude presence of full fontanelle and cephalohematoma.
- Abdomen: Exclude presence of organomegaly and mass.
- Extremities: Exclude presence of radial-thumb defects.
- Neurologic exam:
  - Evaluate for irritability, lethargy, seizure, and focal neurologic deficits.
  - If severely affected, may develop ICH
- Skin:
  - Evaluate for pallor, petechiae, ecchymoses, hemangiomas, and vascular lesions.
  - Evaluate for bleeding from phlebotomy sites, heel sticks, circumcision, and the umbilical cord.
- If congenital anomalies, hepatosplenomegaly, abdominal mass, or skeletal defects are present, consider alternative diagnoses.

DIFFERENTIAL DIAGNOSIS

- Infection
  - Bacterial or viral (e.g., rubella, cytomegalovirus [CMV], herpes simplex virus)
- Congenital
  - Thrombocytopenia absent radius
  - Amegakaryocytic thrombocytopenia
  - Wiskott-Aldrich syndrome: triad of immunodeficiency, eczema, and thrombocytopenia (small platelet size)
  - May-Hegglin anomaly: Döhle bodies in WBCs (large platelet size)
- Immunologic
  - Autoimmune thrombocytopenia (i.e., maternal ITP): The degree of thrombocytopenia in autoimmune thrombocytopenia tends to be much less severe than in NAIT.
- Hematologic
  - Disseminated intravascular coagulation (DIC): increased platelet consumption (e.g., sepsis, necrotizing enterocolitis)
  - Thrombosis: for example, renal vein thrombosis, catheter-associated thrombosis
  - Hemangioma with Kasabach-Merritt syndrome
- Oncologic
  - Leukemia
  - Neuroblastoma
  - Down syndrome—transient myeloproliferative disorder (TMD)
- Metabolic
  - Methylmalonic acidemia
  - Isovaleric acidemia

DIAGNOSTIC TESTS & INTERPRETATION

Initial Tests (screening, lab, imaging)

- CBC
  - Isolated thrombocytopenia: Platelets are often $<50,000/\mu L$ at birth.
  - May see anemia if the infant has suffered severe bleeding complications
- Screening coagulation studies
  - PT, PTT, thrombin time, and fibrinogen should be normal.

- Maternal platelet count: should be normal
- NAIT testing: HPA incompatibility between mother and child needs to be identified. Testing can be performed on mother and father to avoid collecting blood samples on the infant.
  - Serologic testing: Maternal serum containing platelet-reactive antibodies is tested against a panel of platelet glycoproteins, including HPA-1a, to look for incompatibility.
  - Platelet cross-matching: Maternal serum containing platelet-reactive antibodies is tested against washed paternal platelets to look for incompatibility.
  - Testing also against washed maternal platelets can exclude "autoantibodies" as seen in ITP.
  - Platelet antigen genotyping: DNA-based testing of the platelet glycoprotein genotype of both parents can be performed in only a few laboratories but can reveal potential incompatibilities (i.e., specifically HPA-1 through HPA-6, HPA-9, and HPA-15).
- Head ultrasound to rule out ICH

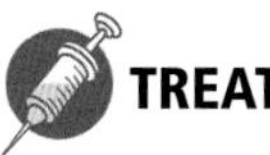

TREATMENT

GENERAL MEASURES

- Daily platelet counts should be obtained until there is documentation of improvement without treatment/intervention.
- Close monitoring for any evidence of bleeding complications, especially ICH
- Avoidance of any invasive procedures (e.g., arterial or lumbar punctures) until platelet count is in a more stable range
- Platelet count $<30 \times 10^9$/L is generally accepted as a threshold for therapeutic intervention. Much higher thresholds are used if ICH is present.
- Treatment is platelet transfusion (10 mL/kg).

ALERT

All blood products administered should be treated appropriately for a neonate (i.e., irradiated, CMV negative, ABO compatible, volume reduced, and washed if indicated).

- Potential sources of platelets for transfusion
  - HPA-1b/1b (i.e., HPA-1a negative) platelets
    - An excellent first choice but not always readily available
    - It is *not* appropriate to await HPA-matched platelets for transfusion, especially if the infant has clinically significant bleeding.
  - Random donor platelets
    - Most readily available but not ideal, given that 98% of the population is HPA-1a positive
    - Will usually elevate the platelet count transiently until a more suitable blood product can be obtained
  - Maternal apheresis platelets
    - Ideal source for platelets but can take days to obtain
    - Do *not* wait for maternal platelets if the infant has clinically significant bleeding.
    - *Important*: Maternal platelets must be washed or volume reduced to remove antibody-containing maternal plasma.
    - Failure to wash or volume reduce maternal platelets may result in prolongation of the fetal thrombocytopenia.
  - HPA-specific platelets
    - If an incompatibility other than HPA-1a is identified, consult your blood bank to see if HPA-specific platelets are available.
- IVIG is another potential therapeutic agent.
- May be used concurrently with platelet transfusions when the platelet count is $<30 \times 10^9$/L, especially when clinical signs of bleeding are present
- Consider use as monotherapy when the platelet count is $<50 \times 10^9$/L. Dose of IVIG is 1 g/kg. Multiple doses may be required.

ONGOING CARE

FOLLOW-UP RECOMMENDATIONS

- Given the implications for future pregnancies, NAIT testing should be considered in all infants with thrombocytopenia ($<50 \times 10^9$/L), even if there is another likely etiology.
- If diagnosis of NAIT is confirmed, family counseling regarding management of future pregnancies is strongly recommended. Consultation with a high-risk obstetrician and perinatologist should be made for any future pregnancy at risk for NAIT.

PROGNOSIS

- Overall prognosis is fair to good. Most patients will experience little morbidity or mortality. ICH may lead to very significant morbidity and/or mortality.
- Most cases will resolve in 1 to 4 weeks.

COMPLICATIONS

- ICH: incidence ~20%, most occur antenatal
- Bleeding from umbilical stump, phlebotomy sites, and/or circumcision
- Petechiae and ecchymoses
- Cephalohematoma
- GI or GU bleeding

ADDITIONAL READING

- Crighton GL, Scarborough R, McQuilten ZK, et al. Contemporary management of neonatal alloimmune thrombocytopenia: good outcomes in the intravenous immunoglobulin era: results from the Australian neonatal alloimmune thrombocytopenia registry. *J Matern Fetal Neonatal Med*. 2017;30(20):2488–2494.
- Curtis BR. Recent progress in understanding the pathogenesis of fetal and neonatal alloimmune thrombocytopenia. *Br J Haematol*. 2015;171(5):671–682.
- Peterson JA. Neonatal alloimmune thrombocytopenia: pathogenesis, diagnosis and management. *Br J Haematol*. 2013;161(1):3–14.
- Winkelhorst D, Murphy MF, Greinacher A, et al. Antenatal management in fetal and neonatal alloimmune thrombocytopenia: a systematic review. *Blood*. 2017;129(11):1538–1547.

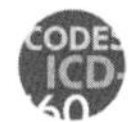

CODES

ICD10

- P61.0 Transient neonatal thrombocytopenia
- D69.42 Congenital and hereditary thrombocytopenia purpura

FAQ

- Q: Can an infant with NAIT safely receive maternal breast milk (MBM)?
- A: Colostrum and MBM contain immunoglobulins that are passively transferred to an infant. In a pregnancy affected by NAIT, this may include antiplatelet antibodies. The amount of antiplatelet antibodies transferred in MBM is probably minor and there are no reports of adverse consequences in infants with NAIT who have received MBM. The use of MBM in infants with NAIT therefore appears to be safe and should not be discouraged.
- Q: What is the HPA-1a–negative (homozygous HPA-1b/1b) mother's risk of having other affected newborns?
- A: It depends on the genotype of the father.
  - If the father is homozygous for HPA-1a (HPA 1a/1a), all offspring will be heterozygous HPA 1a/1b positive and at great risk for developing NAIT.
  - If the father is heterozygous for HPA-1a (HPA 1a/1b), 50% of offspring will be at risk for developing NAIT.
- Q: Can NAIT happen in a first pregnancy?
- A: Unlike hemolytic disease of the newborn due to Rh incompatibility, NAIT can occur even in 1st-born offspring and tends to become more severe with each subsequently affected pregnancy.

NEONATAL APNEA

Kalpashri Kesavan, MD • Zankhana Master, MD • Estelle B. Gauda, MD

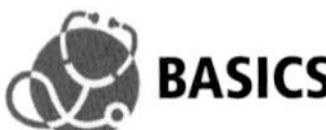

BASICS

DESCRIPTION

- Apnea of infancy
  - An unexplained episode of cessation of breathing for 20 seconds or longer or a shorter respiratory pause associated with bradycardia, cyanosis, pallor, and/or marked hypotonia in infants with gestational age (GA) of 37 weeks or more at the onset of apnea
- Apnea of prematurity (AOP)
  - The cessation of breathing for >20 seconds or if <20 seconds is accompanied by oxygen desaturation or bradycardia in infants born <37 weeks GA.
- Periodic breathing
  - A normal neonatal breathing pattern, defined by ≥3 pauses, each ≥3 seconds, with <20 seconds of regular respiration between pauses
- Classification of apnea based on respiratory effort and airflow
  - Central apnea
    - No evidence of obstruction to airflow but absent chest wall motion
    - Caused by decreased central nervous system (CNS) stimuli to respiratory muscles
  - Obstructive apnea
    - Characterized by absent airflow but persistent chest wall motion
    - Often caused by pharyngeal instability, neck flexion, or nasopharyngeal occlusion
  - Mixed apnea (most frequent in preterm infants)
    - Obstructive apnea preceding (usually) or following central apnea

EPIDEMIOLOGY

- Apnea and bradycardia occur in ~2% of all healthy term infants.
- AOP is inversely correlated to GA. It occurs in <10% of neonates 34 to 35 weeks GA and in almost all neonates <28 weeks GA at birth.

RISK FACTORS

- Prematurity is the most common cause of apnea.
- Risk factors common to both AOP and apnea of infancy are as follows:
  - Maternal medications, such as magnesium sulfate, prostaglandins, or narcotics
  - Age (first 30 days of life)
  - Infections: upper respiratory tract infections
  - Gastroesophageal reflux disease (GERD)
  - Anemia
  - Cardiac arrhythmias
  - CNS insult (hemorrhage, seizure, tumors)
  - Immunizations (after DTaP injection)

PATHOPHYSIOLOGY

- Immature respiratory control in neonates
  - Immature structural development of central respiratory network in the brainstem
  - Enhanced sensitivity to inhibitory neurotransmitters (such as γ-aminobutyric acid [GABA]) and neuromodulators (such as adenosine, serotonin, and prostaglandin) that can lead to apnea
  - Low functional residual capacity predisposing to hypoxia when short apneas occur
- Hypoxic ventilatory depression
  - Increased peripheral chemoreceptor sensitivity, leading to more unstable breathing (such as periodic breathing) *or* decreased sensitivity, which prolongs apnea when it does occur
- Impaired hypercapnic ventilatory response
  - Prolonging expiratory time (but not increasing frequency or overall tidal volume) may lead to less minute volume as well as uncoordinated movements of respiratory muscles in response to hypercapnia, resulting in apnea.
- Laryngeal chemoreflex
  - Activation of laryngeal chemoreceptors (via superior laryngeal nerve afferents) as seen in GERD can result in apnea, bradycardia, and hypotension.
- Sleep state
  - Neonates spend majority of their time in active sleep. Apneas are more common during active sleep when breathing is irregular and chest wall and upper airway muscles are inactivated.
- Upper airway obstruction
  - Hypotonic pharynx in preterm infants with additional loss of upper airway tone during active sleep

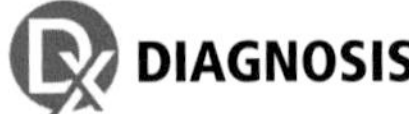

DIAGNOSIS

HISTORY

- Immaturity of respiratory control is the primary cause for AOP, but many coexisting factors can potentiate or worsen apnea.
- Apnea of infancy is uncommon and should warrant a thorough evaluation.
- Most important part of the evaluation is a thorough and appropriately tailored history.
- Detailed review of the event including
  - Time
  - Duration
  - Surrounding circumstances
  - Relation to feeds
  - Appearance of the infant
  - Need for stimulation or resuscitation efforts
  - Extent of stimulation and resuscitation
- Thorough details of past medical history including prenatal, birth, and neonatal course; history of prematurity, lung disease, previous brief, resolved, unexplained events (BRUEs)
- Evaluate for recent illness, exposure to infection, feeding difficulties, medications, or vaccines.
- Significant family history includes smoke exposure, previous infant deaths, genetic disorders, and cardiac/respiratory disorders.
- Probe for evidence or suspicion of child maltreatment.

PHYSICAL EXAM

- Detailed physical examination, including vital signs, with particular attention to cardiorespiratory and neurologic system is very crucial in determining any underlying condition.
- Examine for signs of child abuse.

DIFFERENTIAL DIAGNOSIS

- Respiratory
  - Nasal or airway obstruction
  - Foreign body aspiration
  - Tracheomalacia/laryngomalacia
  - Chest masses or malformations
  - Pulmonary hypoplasia
  - Pneumonia
- Neurologic
  - Seizure
  - Intracranial hemorrhages
  - CNS malformations, tumors
  - Neuromuscular disorders
  - Postgeneral anesthesia
  - Stroke
- Infectious
  - Sepsis
  - Viral respiratory infection—RSV
  - Bacterial respiratory infection—pneumonia
  - Urinary tract infection
  - CNS infection—meningitis, encephalitis
- Cardiovascular
  - Congenital heart disease
  - Patent ductus arteriosus
  - Cardiomyopathy
  - Arrhythmias—prolonged QT, heart block, Wolff-Parkinson-White syndrome
  - Myocarditis
- Gastrointestinal
  - GERD
  - Dysphagia
  - Intussusception
  - Necrotizing enterocolitis (NEC)
  - Malrotation +/− volvulus
- Pharmacologic
  - Sedatives
  - Seizure medications
  - Pain medications
  - Magnesium exposure
- Hematologic
  - Anemia
  - Polycythemia
- Genetic
  - Congenital central hypoventilation syndrome
  - Craniofacial anomalies
  - Down syndrome
  - Prader-Willi syndrome
- Metabolic
  - Inborn errors of metabolism
  - Hypoglycemia
  - Electrolyte disturbances
- Environmental
  - Suffocation
  - Traumatic head injury
  - Hypothermia/hyperthermia

DIAGNOSTIC TESTS & INTERPRETATION

- Routine screening tests for various etiologies without historical risk factors or suggestive physical exam findings is a very low-yield process.
- Testing should be based on clinician judgment depending on history and physical exam findings.

Initial Tests (screening, lab, imaging)

- Workup to rule out infection as indicated: CBC/differential, CRP, blood culture, urine culture, CSF culture, and viral cultures
- Serum electrolytes, glucose if concerned about electrolyte abnormalities
- Blood gas if respiratory compromise is noted

- Ammonia, plasma amino acids, and urine organic acids if there are concerns for metabolic syndrome
- Chest radiograph to evaluate for infection or cardiac disease
- Skeletal survey if child abuse is suspected
- Head CT or head ultrasound (if <6 months old) in suspected trauma or elevated intracranial pressure
- Head MRI, if indicated, to evaluate for congenital malformations

Diagnostic Procedures/Other

- EKG/Holter monitoring to evaluate for arrhythmias or conduction problems
- Lumbar puncture if sepsis/meningitis is in the differential diagnosis
- EEG to rule out seizures
- A pH probe or modified barium swallow if event is associated with feeding
- Sleep study for evaluation of different types of apnea
- Genetic testing for *PHOX2B* mutations (congenital central hypoventilation syndrome)
- Ophthalmologic exam to identify retinal hemorrhages if child abuse is suspected

ALERT

Preterm infants with a high frequency of apnea associated with chronic intermittent hypoxia need prolonged respiratory support, take longer to achieve oral feeds, have a greater incidence of retinopathy of prematurity, and have greater risk of adverse neurodevelopmental outcomes.

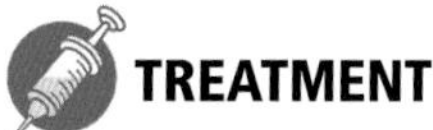

TREATMENT

GENERAL MEASURES

- Back-to-sleep positioning
- Avoid extreme flexion or extension of neck.
- Provide stable thermoneutral environment.
- Smoke-free environment

MEDICATION

- AOP:
  - Methylxanthines (caffeine citrate or theophylline) are used in hospital settings.
  - Caffeine is preferred due to better absorption, less toxicity, a wider therapeutic window, and half-life that allows once-daily dosing.
  - Caffeine citrate IV/PO
    - Load: 20 mg/kg
    - Maintenance: 5 to 10 mg/kg (q24h)
    - Monitor heart rate, apnea, serum caffeine levels if appropriate.
  - Theophylline PO
    - Load: 5 to 6 mg/kg
    - Maintenance: 2 to 6 mg/kg/24 h (divided q8–12h)
    - Monitor respiratory rate, heart rate, apnea, serum theophylline levels.
- Usually, AOP resolves by 36 to 40 postmenstrual weeks; however, in more immature infants, born at <28 weeks' gestation, apnea may continue until 40 to 43 weeks postmenstrual age (PMA).
- Once caffeine is discontinued, it is recommended to watch the infant for 5 to 7 days for recurrence of apnea.

ADDITIONAL THERAPIES

- Oxygen
  - Provide supplemental oxygen via nasal cannula (NC) to maintain saturations (90–95% in premature neonates; >94% in term infants), as hypoxia can lead to apneic episodes.
  - Use heated humidified air to prevent crusting of nasal secretion and maintain nasal patency while administering oxygen via NC.
- Noninvasive respiratory support:
  - Continuous positive airway pressure (CPAP) splints open the upper airway and improves oxygenation by increasing functional residual capacity.
  - CPAP may be used to treat mixed and obstructive apnea.
- Positive pressure ventilation (nasal or endotracheal) may be needed for severe or persistent apnea.

ONGOING CARE

FOLLOW-UP RECOMMENDATIONS

- Infants born before 37 weeks should pass a car seat test prior to discharge after birth.
- Caregivers should be instructed on back-to-sleep, crib safety measure, and avoidance of tobacco smoke exposure and trained in cardiopulmonary resuscitation.
- Home cardiorespiratory monitoring
  - May be considered for infants with chronic lung disease (especially those requiring oxygen supplementation or ventilator)
  - Home monitoring should be used in infants with a tracheostomy or with neurologic, genetic, or metabolic conditions affecting respiratory control.
  - Parents should be appropriately counseled about the purpose, stresses, end point, and proper usage.
  - Parents should be made aware that use of home monitoring does not reduce the risk for sudden infant death.
- Follow-up of the infant with a health care practitioner is recommended within 48 hours after discharge.

PROGNOSIS

- Premature infants have 3–5% increased risk for sudden infant death syndrome (SIDS).
- AOP has not been found to be precursor or predictor of SIDS.

ADDITIONAL READING

- Di Fiore JM, Martin RJ, Gauda EB. Apnea of prematurity—perfect storm. *Respir Physiol Neurobiol*. 2013;189(2):213–222.
- Di Fiore JM, Poets CF, Gauda E, et al. Cardiorespiratory events in preterm infants: etiology and monitoring technologies. *J Perinatol*. 2016;36(3):165–171.
- Di Fiore JM, Poets CF, Gauda E, et al. Cardiorespiratory events in preterm infants: interventions and consequences. *J Perinatol*. 2016;36(4):251–258.
- Eichenwald E; for Committee on Fetus and Newborn, American Academy of Pediatrics. Apnea of prematurity. *Pediatrics*. 2016;137(1):e20153757.
- Thompson JM, Mitchell EA; for New Zealand Cot Death Study Group. Are the risk factors for SIDS different for preterm and term infants? *Arch Dis Child*. 2006;91(2):107–111.

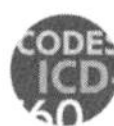

CODES

ICD10

- P28.4 Other apnea of newborn
- P28.3 Primary sleep apnea of newborn
- G47.31 Primary central sleep apnea

FAQ

- Q: Should infants on caffeine for AOP be discharged home?
- A: It is not universal practice that infants with AOP are discharged home on caffeine and home monitoring. It is more common to discharge the infant home 5 to 7 days after caffeine has been discontinued.
- Q: What should be the end point of home monitoring?
- A: For AOP, if no true events are detected for several weeks and the infant is >43 weeks PMA and off of all respiratory stimulants for 7 days. For infants who are born at 23 to 25 weeks, apnea could persist beyond 43 weeks PMA. For monitoring in other cases, it would depend on the frequency and severity of the events.
- Q: What is the role of antireflux medication in the treatment of apnea?
- A: Controversy exists regarding the role of GERD in causing apnea in premature infants. If there is a clear relationship between the apneic event and reflux, then a trial of antireflux precautions and medication is recommended. However, if there is no clinical improvement, it should be discontinued. There may be increase in incidence of NEC with routine use of H_2 blockers in hospitalized premature infants.
- Q: Should parents of former premature infants be worried about SIDS in their child?
- A: Infants with a history of AOP have been noted to have alteration in the autonomic function for the first several months, similar to infants who have died of SIDS. The resolution of AOP is generally seen around 44 weeks, and SIDS in extremely premature infants occurs later, ~47 weeks PMA; thus, AOP and SIDS are not considered to be related. Although there is no direct causal relationship between AOP and SIDS, the autonomic immaturity and dysfunction seen in premature infants who have had persistent AOP could explain the increased risk of SIDS in these infants and is an important consideration for both the clinician and the families caring for former preterm infants.

NEONATAL CHOLESTASIS

Irini D. Batsis, MD • Wikrom Karnsakul, MD

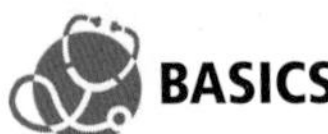

BASICS

DESCRIPTION

- Neonatal cholestasis is defined as elevated conjugated bilirubin levels that occur in the newborn period and often extends during the infancy. It typically indicates hepatobiliary dysfunction.
- Further studies are needed on any infant who is jaundiced beyond 2 weeks old (or 3 weeks if breastfed).
- Biochemical definition: serum conjugated bilirubin >20% of the total bilirubin (TB) concentration or direct bilirubin >2 mg/dL

EPIDEMIOLOGY

- Full-term infants: Most common causes in the 1st month are extrahepatic biliary atresia (EHBA), idiopathic neonatal hepatitis, α_1-antitrypsin deficiency, and progressive familial intrahepatic cholestasis (PFIC).
- Premature infants: must consider sepsis and total parenteral nutrition (TPN)-associated cholestasis
- Incidence of neonatal cholestasis is 1 in 2,500 live births (excluding infants with history of parenteral nutrition).

RISK FACTORS

Genetics

Causes of biliary atresia (BA), neonatal hepatitis, and most other etiologies of neonatal cholestasis remain unknown. Known genetic causes include the following:

- α_1-Antitrypsin deficiency
  - Autosomal codominant expression
  - Mutations in *SERPINA1* gene
  - 10–15% of individuals develop hepatic disease.
  - Two alleles most commonly associated with liver disease: Z and M
- Alagille syndrome
  - Autosomal dominant, variable expressivity
  - Mutations in *JAG1* and *NOTCH2* gene
- PFIC and bile acid synthetic defects (BASDs)
  - Group of familial cholestatic disorders: PFIC1, PFIC2, and PFIC3. Note PFIC1, PFIC2, and some types of BASD have low γ-glutamyl transpeptidase (GGT) values.
  - Autosomal recessive
  - Caused by mutations in *FIC1*, *ATP8B1*, *ABCB11*, and *ABCB4* genes
- Cystic fibrosis (CF)
  - Autosomal recessive
  - *CFTR* gene mutations, most common ΔF508 deletion (causes 70% of cases in United States)
- Citrin deficiency: neonatal-onset type II
  - *SLC25A13* gene mutation
  - Transient cholestasis, diffuse fatty liver with hepatic fibrosis
  - Almost exclusively Asian infants
- Arthrogryposis-renal dysfunction-cholestasis (ARC) syndrome
  - Autosomal recessive: *VPS33B* gene mutation
  - Multiple joint contractures, renal dysfunction, bleeding tendency, affected infants die during infancy
  - Normal GGT
- Aagenaes syndrome
  - Autosomal recessive
  - Congenital hypoplasia of lymph vessels
    - Lymphedema of legs, cholestasis, hepatic cirrhosis

PATHOPHYSIOLOGY

- Neonatal cholestasis is jaundice secondary to elevated conjugated bilirubin levels in the newborn period.
- Typically, infants are not jaundiced at birth but develop cholestasis within days to weeks of life. In utero, the placenta and maternal liver perform the necessary hepatic functions for the infant. The liver slowly matures throughout the 1st year of life to reach full hepatic metabolism potential.
- Neonatal cholestasis can be caused by a variety of mechanisms of hepatobiliary dysfunction that results in poor bile flow or excretion. In addition, there is inefficient enterohepatic circulation in the newborn period, which contributes to bilirubin accumulation.

ETIOLOGY

Most likely etiologies in infant <2 months of age:

- Obstructive: BA, gallstones/sludge, inspissated bile, choledochal cyst, neonatal sclerosing cholangitis, congenital hepatic fibrosis/Caroli disease, Alagille syndrome
- Idiopathic: idiopathic neonatal hepatitis
- Infection: UTI, sepsis, cytomegalovirus (CMV), herpes simplex virus (HSV), syphilis, parvovirus B19, adenovirus, enterovirus
- Metabolic/genetic: α_1-antitrypsin deficiency, tyrosinemia, PFIC, CF, galactosemia, lipid storage disease, bile acid synthesis defects, mitochondrial hepatopathy, peroxisomal disorders, neonatal/infantile intrahepatic cholestasis caused by citrin deficiency (NICCD)
- Endocrine: hypothyroidism, panhypopituitarism
- Toxic: parenteral nutrition–associated cholestasis, drug-induced
- Immune mediated: gestational alloimmune liver disease (GALD)
- Miscellaneous: hypoperfusion/shock

COMMONLY ASSOCIATED CONDITIONS

- 10% of infants with BA also have another major congenital defect (other than laterality defects, see below).
- Biliary atresia splenic malformation (BASM): syndromic form of BA with laterality defects
  - Situs inversus
  - Polysplenia or asplenia
  - Malrotation
  - Congenital heart disease
- Alagille syndrome
  - Syndromic appearance (triangular face, deep set eyes, broad nose)
  - Cardiac anomalies, typically pulmonic stenosis
  - Butterfly vertebrae
  - Ophthalmologic findings: posterior embryotoxon
- Panhypopituitarism
  - Persistent hypoglycemia
  - Septooptic dysplasia and optic nerve hypoplasia

DIAGNOSIS

HISTORY

- Pregnancy and birth history
- History of consanguinity
- Family history/racial background
- Infectious exposure
- TPN exposure, prolonged history of NPO status
- Presence/absence of extrahepatic manifestations
- Signs and symptoms:
  - Jaundice
  - Hepatomegaly
  - Pale-colored stools
  - Dark-colored urine
  - For specific diagnoses:
    - Alagille syndrome: typical facies, heart murmur
    - Congenital infections: low birth weight, microcephaly, rash, chorioretinitis
    - Metabolic disorders: irritability, hypoglycemia, poor feeding, lethargy

PHYSICAL EXAM

- Jaundice/scleral icterus: In newborn, scleral icterus may not be obvious if TB <5 mg/dL requiring bright light in exam room; some cholestasis like PFIC may not manifest early with jaundice.
- Hepatomegaly
- Splenomegaly: in young newborn <2 to 4 weeks, may suggest hemolysis or infection, otherwise may indicate portal hypertension from significant hepatic fibrosis/cirrhosis
- Cardiac murmurs
- Dysmorphic facial features
- Abnormal eye exam: wandering eye movements in panhypopituitarism, cataracts in TORCH (toxoplasmosis, other agents, rubella, CMV, herpes simplex) infections and galactosemia
- Tone abnormalities in neurologic/muscular disorders
- Abnormal extremities (arthrogryposis, lymphedema)
- Abnormal genitalia (micropenis in panhypopituitarism)
- Abnormal stool color: Stool color cards or other promising equivalent tools or technologies may improve early detection of hepatobiliary disease at a low cost.
- Skin rash in TORCH infections ("blueberry muffin" for congenital rubella)

DIFFERENTIAL DIAGNOSIS

See "Etiology." The provider must be able to distinguish neonatal cholestasis from physiologic or breast milk jaundice in infancy.

DIAGNOSTIC TESTS & INTERPRETATION

Initial Tests (screening, lab, imaging)

Clinical scenario must be taken into consideration to determine which of the following are appropriate:

- Fractionated serum bilirubin (total and direct)
- ALT, AST, alkaline phosphatase
- GGT
- Serum albumin
- Prothrombin time/INR
- Glucose
- CBC
- Urine culture +/− blood culture

- Urine-reducing substances
- Serum α_1-antitrypsin level and phenotype
- Serologies for infectious disorders: hepatitis B surface antigen, TORCH, Epstein-Barr virus, parvovirus B19, human herpesvirus 6, HIV, enterovirus
- Red blood cell galactose-1-phosphate uridyltransferase
- Cortisol, TSH, T_4
- Infant metabolic screen
- Urine succinylacetone (tyrosinemia)
- Fat-soluble vitamin levels: vitamin A and retinol-binding protein, D, and E
- Newborn metabolic screen
- Plasma amino acids, urine organic acids, lactate/pyruvate, and ammonia (if having urea cycle dysfunction or liver failure)
- Genetic testing for Alagille syndrome, PFIC (1 to 3), α_1-antitrypsin deficiency, CF
- Serum and urine bile acids (It is essential that ursodeoxycholic acid is discontinued for 7 days for urine specimen.)
- Abdominal ultrasound (dilated intrahepatic bile ducts indicating downstream obstruction such as choledochal cyst, bile duct stricture, stones; other findings to evaluate include presence/absence of gallbladder, asplenia, polysplenia, annular pancreas, portal vein/hepatic artery, and hepatic vein flow)
- Spine radiograph (for butterfly vertebrae or hemivertebrae with Alagille syndrome)
- Hepatobiliary scintigraphy (HIDA scan) is particularly performed in infants when suspected EHBA is suspected after phenobarbital administrations for 5 days. (HIDA scan neither is a diagnostic test for EHBA nor excludes EHBA because EHBA is an evolving disease during the first few months of life; if there is high suspicion for EHBA, consider repeating the test after a few weeks or proceeding with liver biopsy or intraoperative cholangiogram.)
- Radiographs of skull and long bones (for congenital infections and peroxisomal disorders)

Diagnostic Procedures/Other

- Liver biopsy for histology, routine viral culture, immunohistochemistry, and electron microscopy as indicated
- Sweat chloride analysis
- Magnetic resonance cholangiopancreatography (MRCP)
- Ophthalmologic exam (for posterior embryotoxon in Alagille syndrome, chorioretinitis, cataracts), septooptic dysplasia, and optic disc atrophy in panhypopituitarism
- Intraoperative cholangiogram (gold standard for EHBA diagnosis)
- Echocardiogram (pulmonic stenosis in Alagille syndrome)

ALERT

Most causes of neonatal cholestasis require expedited diagnosis and intervention:
- BA
- Choledochal cyst or other obstructed common bile duct
- Infections (sepsis, DIC, HSV, enterovirus)
- Metabolic disorders (e.g., galactosemia)
- Endocrine disorders (e.g., hypothyroidism, hypopituitarism)

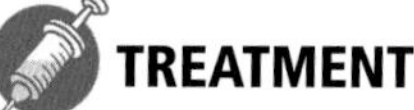

TREATMENT

MEDICATION

- Ursodeoxycholic acid (improvement in hepatic function and absorption of fat-soluble vitamins)
- Cholic or chenodeoxycholic acid for BASD
- Antihistamines (for pruritus associated with cholestasis)
- Antibiotics and antivirals (when appropriate)
- ADEK vitamins (if fat-soluble vitamin deficiencies)

ISSUES FOR REFERRAL

All neonates with cholestasis as defined earlier should have referrals to a pediatric gastroenterologist for further evaluation and management. If the provider suspects BA or metabolic disease, referral to the appropriate subspecialist should be prompt such as geneticists, infectious disease specialists, endocrinologists, and pediatric general surgeons.

ADDITIONAL THERAPIES

- Consider the need for speech therapy, occupational therapy, or physical therapy when appropriate.
- Nutritional support

SURGERY/OTHER PROCEDURES

- Liver biopsy (via percutaneous route by GI, or open wedge by general surgeon, or transjugular route by interventional radiologist)
- Intraoperative cholangiogram if suspect BA
- Kasai procedure (hepatoportoenterostomy) for BA
- Surgical referral for removal of choledochal cyst, common bile duct stones, bile duct strict, and sclerosing cholangitis
- Biliary diversion for severe pruritus associated with Alagille syndrome and PFIC
- Liver transplantation
- Other subspecialty consults as indicated

ADMISSION, INPATIENT, AND NURSING CONSIDERATIONS

- Sepsis must be identified and treated.
- Hypopituitarism may cause hypoglycemia during stress, that is, during/after procedures (liver biopsy), which should be monitored closely and treated.
- Metabolic genetic syndromes should be investigated by metabolic or genetic services.
- Obstructed common bile duct will require surgical intervention.
- Coagulopathy (prolonged INR) should be treated with vitamin K, especially in significant cholestasis.

ONGOING CARE

DIET

- Nutritional support needed. Typically, an elemental formula with high content medium-chain triglycerides is better absorbed in cholestasis.
- Consider need for nasogastric tube feeds.
- Special diets
  - Supplementation with pancreatic enzymes (CF)
  - Galactose-free (galactosemia)

PROGNOSIS

Varies based on underlying diagnosis. BA remains the most common indication for pediatric liver transplantation.

COMPLICATIONS

- End-stage liver disease (ascites, coagulopathy) and portal hypertension requiring liver transplantation
- Infection
- Failure to thrive
- Poor bone health
- Developmental delay

ADDITIONAL READING

- Bakshi B, Sutcliffe A, Akindolie M, et al. How reliably can paediatric professionals identify pale stool from cholestatic newborns? *Arch Dis Child Fetal Neonatal Ed*. 2012;97(5):F385–F387.
- Benchimol EI, Walsh CM, Ling SC. Early diagnosis of neonatal cholestatic jaundice: test at 2 weeks. *Can Fam Physician*. 2009;55(12):1184–1192.
- Emerick KM, Whitington PF. Neonatal liver disease. *Pediatr Ann*. 2006;35(4):280–286.
- Fawaz R, Baumann U, Ekong U, et al. Guideline for the evaluation of cholestatic jaundice in infants: joint recommendations of the North American Society for Pediatric Gastroenterology, Hepatology, and Nutrition and the European Society for Pediatric Gastroenterology, Hepatology, and Nutrition. *J Pediatr Gastroenterol Nutr*. 2017;64(1):154–168.
- Moerschel SK, Cianciaruso LB, Tracy LR. A practical approach to neonatal jaundice. *Am Fam Physician*. 2008;77(9):1255–1262.

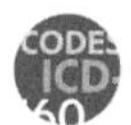

CODES

ICD10

- K83.1 Obstruction of bile duct
- Q44.2 Atresia of bile ducts
- P59.20 Neonatal jaundice from unspecified hepatocellular damage

FAQ

- Q: What information in the patient's history can be used to identify neonatal cholestasis?
- A: Direct observation of urine color along with stool color, as acholic stools and dark urine suggest the presence of cholestasis and conjugated hyperbilirubinemia. Note that even experienced physicians often do not recognize stool color associated with biliary obstruction. Stool color cards or other promising technologies are being developed to improve early detection of hepatobiliary disease at a low cost.
- Q: If my patient has an abnormal HIDA scan, does that mean he or she has BA?
- A: A HIDA scan can be abnormal in obstructive causes of cholestasis other than BA. A surgical evaluation via an intraoperative cholangiogram is the gold standard to diagnose BA.
- Q: What vitamin deficiencies are most common in infants with cholestasis?
- A: Infants with cholestasis often have malabsorption of fat-soluble vitamins (A, D, E, and K) and require supplementation.

NEONATAL ENCEPHALOPATHY

Raul Chavez-Valdez, MD • Johana Diaz, MD • Frances J. Northington, MD

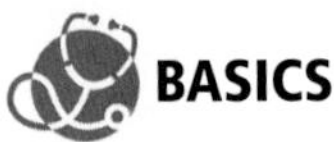

BASICS

DESCRIPTION

Neurologic dysfunction in infants >35 weeks of gestation notable for depressed level of consciousness, altered muscle tone and reflexes (with or without seizures) along with difficulty in initiation or maintenance of breathing and low Apgar scores. This nonspecific condition has many etiologies, most commonly hypoxic ischemic encephalopathy (HIE).

EPIDEMIOLOGY

- Represents approximately 20% of all neonatal death worldwide
- Incidence in developed countries 2 to 9 per 1,000 live births
- $>50\%$ of cases secondary to HIE

RISK FACTORS

- Maternal risk factors:
  - Advanced age
  - Obesity
  - Diabetes
  - Severe preeclampsia
  - Infertility treatments
  - Thyroid disease
  - Seizures or neurologic disorder
  - Placental abnormalities
- Fetal factors: intrauterine growth restriction
- Intrapartum factors:
  - Sentinel event (placental abruption, uterine rupture, cord accident, among others)
  - Shoulder dystocia
  - Emergency cesarean delivery

PATHOPHYSIOLOGY

- Hypoxic ischemic event leading to brain injury with energy failure and ongoing secondary injury leading to encephalopathy and possibly seizures
- Ongoing injury involves excitotoxic glutamate accumulation in synaptic space, alterations in cellular calcium management, free radical production and nitrosative/oxidative damage, mitochondrial failure, activation of proteases, and other cell death cascades with both acute and delayed cytokine production and neuroinflammation.
- Other etiologies include various metabolic disorders, hypoglycemia, kernicterus, nonketotic hyperglycinemia, intracranial infection, perinatal arterial ischemic stroke (PAIS), and sinovenous thrombosis.

DIAGNOSIS

HISTORY

- Sentinel event (uterine rupture, placental abruption, cord accident, cardiorespiratory arrest in delivery room)
- Apgar scores <5 at 5 and 10 minutes
- Advanced resuscitation required in delivery room (intubation, chest compressions, medications)

PHYSICAL EXAM

- Altered level of consciousness (hyperalert or lethargic/obtunded)
- Altered muscle tone
- Weak or absent reflexes
- Decerebrate posturing
- Distal flexion, complete extension
- Abnormal autonomic nervous system:
  - Constricted or unreactive pupils
  - Deviated/dilated pupils
  - Bradycardia
  - Periodic breathing/apnea
- Possible seizure activity: Importantly, seizures may present as or continue as subclinical (electrical only) after loading dose of an antiepileptic drug (AED).
- Dysmorphic features: may suggest metabolic disorders/genetic disorders

DIFFERENTIAL DIAGNOSIS

- HIE
- Metabolic disorder
- Intracranial hemorrhage or PAIS
- Hypoglycemia
- Kernicterus
- Nonketotic hyperglycinemia
- Epileptic syndromes/seizure disorder
- Infection (meningitis, encephalitis)

DIAGNOSTIC TESTS & INTERPRETATION

Initial Tests (screening, lab, imaging)

- Umbilical artery cord and/or neonatal blood gas (looking at pH and base deficit [HIE])
- Glucose (hypoglycemia)
- Electrolytes, including phosphorus and magnesium (metabolic abnormalities)
- Bilirubin (kernicterus)
- Lactate and ammonia (HIE and metabolic abnormalities)
- Plasma amino acids and urine organic acids (metabolic abnormalities)
- Head ultrasound (cerebral edema associated with HIE, intracranial hemorrhage)
- MRI with diffusion weighting (DW-MRI; structural anomalies, stigmata of various encephalopathies, stroke, intracranial hemorrhage, HIE) and MRS (increased lactate/NAA ratio in HIE and PAIS)

Diagnostic Procedures/Other

- EEG (seizures, electrographic background—specifically discontinuity, burst suppression patterns)
- Amplitude-integrated EEG (if available)
- Lumbar puncture (cell count/HSV PCR for infection, metabolic workup including neurotransmitters)
- Placenta pathology (infection, infarcts/embolism, abruption)

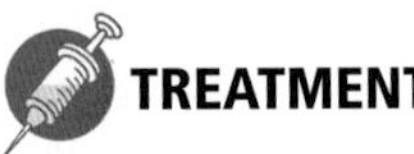

TREATMENT

GENERAL MEASURES

- Control seizures
  - Phenobarbital, fosphenytoin, and/or levetiracetam, depending on clinical preference. Multiple other AED (lorazepam, lidocaine) are used based on clinical experience and preference. Consider pyridoxine deficiency if no response to AED.
- Maintenance of adequate:
  - Fluid (restriction)/electrolytes/glucose/pH
  - Ventilation/oxygenation, avoid hypocapnia and hyperoxia
  - Perfusion of the brain and other end organs

ADDITIONAL THERAPIES

- Therapeutic hypothermia (TH) for moderate to severe neonatal encephalopathy (significantly decreases risk of death or moderate to severe disability)
- Criteria for initiation of TH in newborns:
  - <6 hours of age, ≥ 35 weeks' gestation, and $\geq 1,800$ g
  - Umbilical cord artery or infant (<1 hour of life) pH ≤ 7.0 or base deficit ≥ 16 mmol/L AND moderate to severe encephalopathy
  - Umbilical cord artery or infant (<1 hour of life) pH between 7.01 and 7.15 or base deficit between 10 and 15.9 mmol/L AND
    - 10-minute Apgar score <5 OR
    - Need for assisted ventilation at birth with continuation by 10 minutes AND
  - Moderate to severe encephalopathy (1 to 3 of the following present in the newborn)
    - Consciousness:
      - Lethargy (moderate)
      - Stupor/coma (severe)

- Activity:
  - Decreased (moderate)
  - Absent (severe)
- Posture:
  - Distal flexion, complete extension (moderate)
  - Decerebrate posture (severe)
- Tone:
  - Hypotonia (moderate)
  - Flaccidity (severe)
- Abnormal primitive reflexes:
  - Weak/incomplete Moro, suck (moderate)
  - Absent (severe)
- Abnormal autonomic nervous system
  - Pupils:
    - Constricted (moderate)
    - Unreactive/deviated/dilated (severe)
  - Bradycardia and periodic breathing/apnea

- Specific management of metabolic disorder or electrolyte/glucose abnormality
  - Time of appearance of symptoms in relationship to birth and presence or absence of a perinatal sentinel event often provides important clues to presence of a metabolic disorder.
  - Immediate recognition and treatment of hypoglycemia; electrolyte disturbances with further investigation into causality and prevention of recurrence
  - Recognition of hyperammonemia is emergent.
  - Lactate/pyruvate ratios, plasma amino acids, urine organic acids, and possibly CSF neurotransmitter levels are often helpful and diagnostic.
  - EEG combined with pyridoxine supplementation can be diagnostic as well.
  - DW-MRI may reveal important diagnostic clues for metabolic encephalopathies.

ONGOING CARE

FOLLOW-UP RECOMMENDATIONS

- Developmental pediatrician
- Pediatric neurologist
- Geneticist (if applicable)

PROGNOSIS

- Widely variable depending on etiology, severity (if HIE), and treatment
- Of patients with moderate to severe HIE treated with TH: at 6 to 7 years of age, death, or an IQ score below 70, 47%; death, 28%; death or severe disability, 41%; moderate or severe disability, 35%; attention–executive dysfunction, 4%; visuospatial dysfunction, 4%
- Perinatal arterial stroke: cerebral palsy (58%), epilepsy (39%), language delay (25%), and behavioral abnormalities (22%)

ADDITIONAL READING

- Executive summary: neonatal encephalopathy and neurologic outcome, second edition. Report of the American College of Obstetricians and Gynecologists' Task Force on Neonatal Encephalopathy. *Obstet Gynecol*. 2014;123:896–901.
- Lee J, Poretti A, Perin J, et al. Optimizing cerebral autoregulation may decrease neonatal regional hypoxic-ischemic brain injury. *Dev Neurosci*. 2017;39(1–4):248–256.
- Raju TN, Nelson KB, Ferriero D, et al; for NICHD-NINDS Perinatal Stroke Workshop Participants. Ischemic perinatal stroke: summary of a workshop sponsored by the National Institute of Child Health and Human Development and the National Institute of Neurological Disorders and Stroke. *Pediatrics*. 2007;120(3):609–616.
- Sarnat HB, Sarnat MS. Neonatal encephalopathy following fetal distress. A clinical and electroencephalographic study. *Arch Neurol*. 1976;33(10):696–705.
- Shankaran S, Laptook AR, Ehrenkranz RA, et al. for National Institute of Child Health and Human Development Neonatal Research Network. Whole-body hypothermia for neonates with hypoxic-ischemic encephalopathy. *N Engl J Med*. 2005;353(15):1574–1584.
- Shankaran S, Laptook AR, McDonald SA, et al; for Eunice Kennedy Shriver National Institute of Child Health and Human Development Neonatal Research Network. Acute perinatal sentinel events, neonatal brain injury pattern, and outcome of infants undergoing a trial of hypothermia for neonatal hypoxic-ischemic encephalopathy. *J Pediatr*. 2017;180:275–278.
- Volpe JJ. Neonatal encephalopathy: an inadequate term for hypoxic-ischemic encephalopathy. *Ann Neurol*. 2012;72(2):156–166.
- Weeke LC, Boylan GB, Pressler RM, et al; NEonatal seizure treatment with Medication Off-patent (NEMO) Consortium. Role of EEG background activity, seizure burden and MRI in predicting neurodevelopmental outcome in full-term infants with hypoxic-ischaemic encephalopathy in the era of therapeutic hypothermia. *Eur J Paediatr Neurol*. 2016;20(6):855–864.

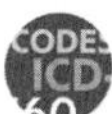

CODES

ICD10

- P91.60 Hypoxic ischemic encephalopathy [HIE], unspecified
- P91.61 Mild hypoxic ischemic encephalopathy [HIE]
- P91.62 Moderate hypoxic ischemic encephalopathy [HIE]

FAQ

- Q: Is neonatal encephalopathy secondary to HIE always associated with an acute perinatal event?
- A: No. Neonatal encephalopathy may be secondary to an ongoing process in utero and not associated with an acute event. There may be signs prenatally such as decreased fetal movement or abnormalities in fetal heart tracings.
- Q: Does the infant have to be <6 hours old to be a candidate for hypothermia therapy?
- A: Yes. Current research has shown that in order to prevent the secondary energy failure and further brain injury, TH should be initiated as soon as possible and within 6 hours of birth. If there is concern for encephalopathy in the delivery room, according to the Neonatal Resuscitation Program, the radiant warmer may be turned off and the infant may be passively cooled until further evaluation can be performed. If applicable, consultation with a referral center that provides TH should be performed as soon as possible. Research trials will determine if there is any value in a more delayed application of the therapy.
- Q: Are there any other therapies available to treat for neonatal encephalopathy?
- A: No. Currently the only available treatment for neonatal encephalopathy is TH; however, multicenter trials using TH combined with erythropoietin (HEAL) or xenon (CoolXenon3) are ongoing.
- Q: What are the best noninvasive technologies available to provide early prognosis in survivors of neonatal encephalopathy?
- A: Currently, EEG and MRI have the best positive predictive values to detect future neurodevelopmental disabilities. Other technologies such as near-infrared spectroscopy to evaluate alterations in cerebral autoregulation and early biomarkers are under investigation.

NEPHROTIC SYNDROME

Nadine M. Khouzam, MD • Kevin V. Lemley, MD, PhD

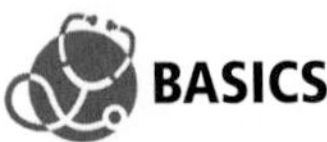

BASICS

DESCRIPTION

Nephrotic syndrome (NS) is defined by nephrotic-range proteinuria, hypoalbuminemia, edema, and hypercholesterolemia. Nephrotic-range proteinuria is typically found when there is 3 to 4+ protein on the urine dipstick and is defined as >40 mg/m^2/h or a spot protein-to-creatinine ratio >2 mg protein/mg creatinine.

EPIDEMIOLOGY

- Minimal change nephrotic syndrome (MCNS) is the most frequent cause of NS in younger children:
  - Occurs mainly between 2 and 8 years of age, with a peak at 3 years
  - Boys are more commonly affected than girls (3:2).
- Focal segmental glomerulosclerosis (FSGS) is the 2nd most frequent cause of NS in childhood:
  - Children with FSGS are more likely than children with MCNS to have steroid-resistant nephrotic syndrome (SRNS).
- Less common than MCNS and FSGS are congenital NS (<3 months) and infantile NS (3 to 12 months).

Prevalence

- 2 to 7 per 100,000 in children <16 years
- 16 cases per 100,000 in children <16 years
- African American and Hispanic children have a higher prevalence of FSGS than Caucasian and Asian children.

PATHOPHYSIOLOGY

- Disruption of podocyte architecture composing the glomerular filtration barrier leads to proteinuria, hypoalbuminemia, and subsequently edema.
- Hypercholesterolemia occurs due to increased liver production of cholesterol in response to hypoalbuminemia as well as to loss of lipoprotein lipase in urine.
- MCNS pathology
  - Minimal histologic changes on light microscopy
  - The glomerular tuft size is normal.
  - Mesangial expansion is absent or minimal.
  - Immunofluorescence is usually negative, although mild staining for C3, IgM, and IgA may occasionally be found.
  - Electron microscopy reveals diffuse effacement of the podocyte foot processes.

ETIOLOGY

- Most pediatric cases are primary; 5–10% are secondary to other diseases.
- The most common primary cause of NS in childhood is MCNS.
- Other causes of primary NS include FSGS, membranous nephropathy, and membranoproliferative glomerulonephritis (GN).
- Secondary causes of NS include infections, vasculitis, diabetes, drugs (e.g., NSAIDs), and hereditary disorders.
- Examples of congenital NS include Finnish type caused by *NPHS1* mutations, diffuse mesangial sclerosis (DMS), and infections (toxoplasmosis, rubella, cytomegalovirus, herpes simplex virus, HIV, syphilis).
- NS can be caused by inherited mutations in proteins involved in the podocyte cytoskeleton, which often results in SRNS and FSGS (up to 20–30% of SRNS).

COMMONLY ASSOCIATED CONDITIONS

- Atopy and MCNS have an association.
- Syndromes associated with NS include Denys-Drash, nail-patella, Lowe, Galloway-Mowat, Frasier, and Pierson.

DIAGNOSIS

HISTORY

- Inquire about atopy or food sensitivity.
- Inquire about drug exposure (especially NSAID agents).
- Inquire about any recent infections.
- Try to establish recent nonedematous weight.
- Signs and symptoms:
  - Fatigue and general malaise
  - Reduced appetite
  - Weight gain
  - Puffy eyes and facial swelling
  - Abdominal swelling or pain
  - Foamy urine
  - Diarrhea
  - Trouble breathing
  - Pitting, dependent edema
  - Scrotal swelling

PHYSICAL EXAM

- Assess for edema.
  - Locations: periorbital, legs, lumbar spine, scrotum/labia
  - Tends to be around the eyes in the morning and in the most dependent parts of the body at the end of the day
- Abdomen: Assess for ascites.
- Decreased breath sounds at lung bases (effusion)
- Mild hypertension (10–20% of patients)

DIFFERENTIAL DIAGNOSIS

- Edema without proteinuria
  - CHF
  - Liver failure
  - Protein-losing enteropathy
  - Protein-energy malnutrition (kwashiorkor)
- Idiopathic NS:
  - MCNS
  - FSGS
  - Membranous GN
  - Membranoproliferative GN
  - Diffuse mesangioproliferative GN
- NS associated with systemic disease (e.g., systemic lupus erythematosus [SLE])

DIAGNOSTIC TESTS & INTERPRETATION

Initial Tests (screening, lab, imaging)

- The urine dipstick usually shows 2,000 mg/dL (4+) of protein:
  - In small children with NS, the urine dipstick may show <4+.
- Timed or spot urine protein collection
  - Timed urine shows >40 mg/m^2/h.
  - Spot urine protein-to-creatinine ratio >2 mg/mg
- Microscopic hematuria is present in 10–20% of cases.
- Serum creatinine usually normal
- Serum albumin usually <2.5 g/dL
- Total cholesterol elevated, usually >200 mg/dL but can be as high as 500 mg/dL
- High hematocrit suggests decreased intravascular volume.
- In complicated cases, renal ultrasound to evaluate for kidney size, parenchymal architecture, and renal venous thrombosis
- Consider chest radiograph for suspected pleural effusion.

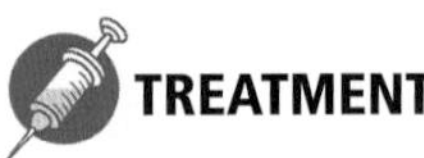

TREATMENT

GENERAL MEASURES

- PPD, interferon-gamma-release (IGRA), and/or chest radiograph at initial presentation prior to starting corticosteroids if risk factors for tuberculosis are present
- Low-salt diet

MEDICATION

First Line

Corticosteroids are 1st-line therapy in suspected MCNS.

- On presentation: prednisone 2 mg/kg/24 h (maximum: 60 mg) for 6 weeks, then prednisone 1.5 mg/kg on alternate days (maximum: 40 mg) for 6 weeks with tapering off of the dose by 0.25 mg/kg weekly thereafter
- On relapse: prednisone 2 mg/kg/24 h until urine protein test results are negative or trace for 3 consecutive days, then prednisone 1.5 mg/kg on alternate days for at least 4 weeks
- Inadequate duration of corticosteroid therapy is associated with increased risk of relapse.

Second Line

Steroid-dependent NS or SRNS

- Alkylating agents (cyclophosphamide, chlorambucil)
- Mycophenolate mofetil (MMF)
- Calcineurin inhibitors (cyclosporine A, tacrolimus)

- Rituximab
- Supportive medications
  - Diuretics (often with 25% albumin infusion as an inpatient) to reduce discomfort from swelling
  - ACE inhibitors or angiotensin receptor blockers
  - Statins for hypercholesterolemia in persistent NS

ALERT

- Live vaccines are contraindicated while daily corticosteroids or alkylating agents are being given.
- Children in relapse, on corticosteroids, or on alkylating agents and who are nonimmune and exposed to varicella should receive VZIG. NS patients require admission and acyclovir if they develop varicella.
- Albumin and/or furosemide must be used cautiously to prevent pulmonary edema from rapid fluid shifts or intravascular dehydration.

ISSUES FOR REFERRAL

- Refer to pediatric nephrology.
- Consider hospitalization during initial episode for teaching.

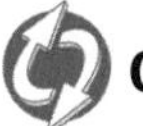

ONGOING CARE

- Influenza vaccination yearly
- Full pneumococcal vaccination with PCV13 when needed and 23-valent pneumococcal vaccine

FOLLOW-UP RECOMMENDATIONS

- When to expect improvement: Remission usually occurs 2 to 4 weeks after starting corticosteroids in MCNS.
- Home testing: The first morning urine is tested for protein with urine dipsticks daily during illnesses.
- Signs to watch for:
  - Fever
  - Abdominal pain
  - Oliguria
  - Respiratory distress
  - Asymmetry; one extremity larger than the other.
  - Recognize situations in which hypovolemia may occur and trigger thrombosis and/or acute kidney injury.
- Monitor for complications of glucocorticoid therapy:
  - Growth failure
  - Cataracts
  - Hypertension
  - Osteopenia
  - Steroid-induced gastritis
  - Increased infection risk
  - Myopathy
  - Striae, skin thinning
  - Mood changes
  - Weight gain
  - Cushingoid appearance
  - Hirsutism

DIET

Restrict salt intake while in relapse or on daily corticosteroids.

PATIENT EDUCATION

Educate the family about urine testing, complications, diet, and prognosis.

PROGNOSIS

- The prognosis for MCNS is excellent, with a mortality rate of <1%:
  - 80–90% of MCNS are steroid-sensitive.
  - 70% of those who respond to steroids will have a relapse.
  - 40% of MCNS become steroid-dependent or frequent relapsers.
  - Remaining 30–40% MCNS have infrequent relapses.
- Patients with FSGS, genetic forms of NS, or other secondary causes are more likely to be steroid-resistant and may progress to develop chronic kidney disease and renal failure.

COMPLICATIONS

- Risk factors for hypovolemia in NS:
  - Severe relapse, GI illness, diuretic use
- Risk factors for thrombosis in patients with NS:
  - Hypovolemia, polycythemia, thrombocytosis; urinary losses of proteins C/S and antithrombin III
- Risk factors for acute kidney injury in patients with NS:
  - Hypovolemia, bilateral renal vein thrombosis, diuretics, or ACE inhibitors
- Risk factors for infection with NS:
  - Defective opsonization
  - Decreased serum complement levels
- Spontaneous bacterial peritonitis (SBP) is a rare but important and potentially life-threatening complication of NS.
  - Symptoms include fever, abdominal pain, vomiting, and diarrhea.
  - Diagnosis is confirmed by ascitic fluid polymorphonuclear cell count of $\geq$250 cells/mm^3 and positive bacterial culture.
  - Rapid institution of antibiotic therapy is crucial in any patient with NS and suspected SBP.
- Diarrhea and vomiting may result in rapid, severe hypovolemia.
- Venous thrombosis may occur with NS in relapse, especially if hypovolemia is present (lower extremities, IVC, renal veins, cerebral sinuses, and pulmonary emboli).
- Viral infections (measles, varicella) may be life-threatening in immunocompromised patients.
- Acute reversible renal failure is an uncommon complication of NS of childhood.

ADDITIONAL READING

- Eddy AA, Symons JM. Nephrotic syndrome in childhood. *Lancet*. 2003;362(9384):629–639.
- Gipson DS, Massengill SF, Yao L, et al. Management of childhood onset nephrotic syndrome. *Pediatrics*. 2009;124(2):747–757.
- Hodson EM, Knight JF, Willis NS, et al. Corticosteroid therapy for nephrotic syndrome in children. *Cochrane Database Syst Rev*. 2005;(1):CD001533.
- Hogg RJ, Portman RJ, Milliner D, et al. Evaluation and management of proteinuria and nephrotic syndrome in children: recommendations from a pediatric nephrology panel established at the National Kidney Foundation conference on proteinuria, albuminuria, risk, assessment, detection, and elimination (PARADE). *Pediatrics*. 2000;105(6):1242–1249.
- Lombel RM, Gipson DS, Hodson EM; for Kidney Disease: Improving Global Outcomes. Treatment of steroid-sensitive nephrotic syndrome: new guidelines from KDIGO. *Pediatr Nephrol*. 2013;28(3):415–426.
- Van Husen M, Kemper MJ. New therapies in steroid-sensitive and steroid-resistant idiopathic nephrotic syndrome. *Pediatr Nephrol*. 2011;26(6):881–892.

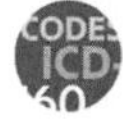

CODES

ICD10

- N04.9 Nephrotic syndrome with unspecified morphologic changes
- N04.0 Nephrotic syndrome with minor glomerular abnormality
- N05.1 Unsp neph syndrome w focal and segmental glomerular lesions

FAQ

- Q: Will the MCNS recur?
- A: The clinical course tends to be one of multiple remissions and relapses. Relapses usually improve around the time of puberty.
- Q: Can the NS return in adult life?
- A: Yes.
- Q: Is macroscopic hematuria ever found with MCNS?
- A: Gross hematuria suggests a renovascular event or a diagnosis other than MCNS. Microscopic hematuria occurs in ~10–20% of cases.

NEURAL TUBE DEFECTS

Eric B. Levey, MD • Sarah A. Korth, MD

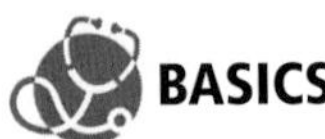

BASICS

DESCRIPTION

Neural tube defects (NTDs): CNS malformations due to abnormalities of neural tube closure during early embryonic development that can be either open or closed defects. *Spina bifida* (SB) is a term referring to a subset of NTDs involving the spinal cord and means "spine split in two."

- *Anencephaly*: due to failed closure of rostral neural tube with total or partial absence of cranial vault and cerebral hemispheres
- *Encephalocele*: partial failure of rostral neural tube closure
  - Abnormal brain tissue protrudes through a skull defect usually covered by skin.
  - 70–80% are occipital; 20% are frontal.
  - 10–20% of occipital defects are meningoceles and contain no brain tissue.
- Open SB: Exposed neural tissue and membranes protrude through a bony defect.
  - Due to failure of primary neural tube closure during the 3rd and 4th weeks after fertilization
  - Includes myelomeningocele (MMC) and myeloschisis
  - MMC: open NTD of the spine, most common type of SB, and characterized by herniation of dysplastic spinal cord and meninges through a posterior vertebral column defect
- Closed SB: Often referred to as occult spinal dysraphism (OSD). Theorized to be due to defects of secondary neurulation; less common than open NTDs
  - Often not diagnosed at birth
  - Skin-covered lesions
  - Wide spectrum of defects including *lipomyelomeningocele, dermal sinus tracts, diastematomyelia* (split cord malformations), *myelocystocele*, other tumors and cysts of the cord, and *congenital spinal cord tethering*

EPIDEMIOLOGY

- NTDs affect ~1 in 1,000 established pregnancies worldwide, with significant geographic variation.
- In the United States, birth prevalence has been decreasing due to periconceptional supplementation with folic acid, food fortification, as well as prenatal diagnosis and termination of pregnancy.
- Centers for Disease Control and Prevention (CDC) data from 2004 to 2006 showed 0.64 NTDs per 1,000 births (~2,660 cases per year), with 54% classified as SB, 32% anencephaly, and 13% encephalocele.

RISK FACTORS

Most NTDs are due to the interaction of genetic, environmental, and dietary risk factors.

- Variants of multiple genes probably confer some increased genetic susceptibility.
- Maternal nutrition and dietary factors, including inadequate maternal folic acid intake
- Maternal diabetes mellitus
- Maternal obesity
- Maternal use of valproic acid (10 times risk), carbamazepine, or alcohol during pregnancy
- Maternal exposure to hyperthermia during early pregnancy (e.g., sauna, hot tub, fever)
- Prior pregnancy with NTD

Genetics

- A specific genetic cause is not found for most NTDs.
- Positive family history in ~5% NTD cases
- After one child with an NTD, the recurrence rate is 2–5% for subsequent pregnancies.
- A chromosomal or cytogenetic abnormality found only in ~10% of isolated NTDs; higher percentage in those with multiple congenital anomalies
- NTDs are common in trisomy 13 and 18 and can be seen with duplications and deletions.
- Found in single gene disorders or syndromes (e.g., Meckel, Waardenburg, 22q11 deletion syndromes)
- A number of candidate risk factor genes have been studied; the most implicated are those in the folate one-carbon metabolic pathway.
  - A homozygous 677C > T mutation of the methylenetetrahydrofolate reductase (MTHFR) gene in mother or child is associated with ~1.8 times increased risk.

GENERAL PREVENTION

- Periconceptual folic acid supplementation has the potential to reduce NTDs by 50–70%.
- Because many pregnancies are not identified until after neural tube closure occurs and because >50% of pregnancies are unplanned, the CDC recommends that all women of childbearing age receive a minimum of 0.4 mg (400 mcg) of folic acid daily.
- Women at high risk (prior pregnancy with NTD, on valproic acid, etc.) should take high-dose folic acid (4 mg daily), starting 1 month before and through the first 3 months of pregnancy.
- If taking valproic acid, consider switching to alternative medication during pregnancy.

COMMONLY ASSOCIATED CONDITIONS

- MMC is virtually always associated with some malformation of the brain.
- Most children with MMC have a Chiari II (Arnold-Chiari) malformation, small posterior fossa with elongation of the cerebellum, and herniation through the foramen magnum.
  - Chiari II malformation often causes obstructive hydrocephalus.
  - Historically, about 80% of children with MMC required a CSF shunt.
- Callosal dysgenesis, cortical dysplasia, and subependymal heterotopias are also common.
- MMC is commonly associated with nonverbal learning disabilities and executive dysfunction.
- Open and closed SB impairments from spinal cord dysfunction:
  - Paraparesis and sensory loss usually correlating with the level of the lesion
  - Neurogenic bladder dysfunction
  - Neurogenic bowel dysfunction
- Congenital foot deformities (club foot) and hip dysplasia are common with NTDs.

DIAGNOSIS

HISTORY

- Anencephaly, occipital encephaloceles, and open forms of SB are usually diagnosed prenatally and are obvious at birth.
- Occult frontal encephaloceles may come to attention because of developmental delays, seizures, or focal neurologic signs.
- OSDs can present with progressive neurogenic bowel and bladder dysfunction, lower extremity (LE) weakness and/or sensory loss, gait abnormalities, foot deformities, and (rarely) recurrent meningitis.

PHYSICAL EXAM

- Serial head circumferences (HC) are used to monitor infants for progressive hydrocephalus.
  - Macrocephaly strongly suggests increased intracranial pressure (ICP).
  - Normal HC but, with increasing percentiles over time, may indicate hydrocephalus
- Dysmorphic features may indicate a syndrome.
- Cranial nerve palsies (strabismus, vocal cord paresis, facial asymmetry), upper extremity (UE) weakness, and abnormal muscle tone can be seen with Chiari II malformation.
- OSD often signaled by a dimple, sinus tract, lipoma, hemangioma, or tuft of hair in the lumbosacral area.
- Functional motor level correlates with ambulatory potential in patients with SB.
- Flaccid paralysis is usually seen below the SB lesion; however, spasticity can be seen.
- Sensory level may not correspond to motor level.
- Signs/symptoms of tethered cord syndrome include worsening LE weakness, spasticity, and/or positional back pain.
- Limb growth may be asymmetric with shorter limb on more affected side (especially in OSD).
- Orthopedic exam should focus on hips, feet/ankles, and spine.
- Skin exam is important for identifying pressure ulcers in areas of impaired sensation.

DIAGNOSTIC TESTS & INTERPRETATION

Initial Tests (screening, lab, imaging)

- Maternal:
  - Maternal serum α-fetoprotein (MSAFP) testing, routinely done at 16 to 18 weeks' gestation, is usually elevated with open NTDs.
  - Elevated MSAFP should prompt referral for high-resolution ultrasound.
  - Genetic testing including chromosomal microarray is often done to look for cause.
- Child:
  - Annual evaluations of renal function with serum creatinine (cystatin C also being used, as it is not dependent on muscle mass)
  - Annual vitamin D 25-OH levels given risk of deficiency and fractures
- Prenatal ultrasound
  - Identifies >99% of cases of anencephaly and 90% of cases of MMC
- Postnatal neuroimaging
  - CT: often used to evaluate hydrocephalus: for initial newborn scan and older children when acute shunt malfunction suspected
  - Ultrasound: useful before anterior fontanel closes, especially to monitor hydrocephalus
  - MRI: gold standard for evaluating congenital anomalies of the spine and brain
    - For most patients with MMC, MRI is not necessary in the newborn period.
    - MRIs are better for defining the Chiari II malformation and other brain anomalies.
    - Spine MRI is used to evaluate tethered cord or syringomyelia.
- Evaluation for suspected OSD
  - Spine ultrasound may be useful for ruling out OSD or tethered cord in newborn or young infant.
  - MRI is used to diagnose and define OSD in infants >6 months of age.
    - Lumbosacral MRI will identify most lesions.
    - However, consider MRI of brain and entire spine to evaluate for higher associated CNS anomalies

(e.g., syringomyelia, diastematomyelia, Chiari malformation).
- OSD is common incidental finding on imaging.
- Isolated OSD can be found in ~10% of the general population at autopsy.
- OSD is usually asymptomatic but should be vigilant for signs/symptoms of neurologic involvement.
- Further imaging is usually not necessary.

- Renal imaging is commonly done in children with MMC or other types of SB.
  - Ultrasound of kidneys and bladder is used to evaluate urinary tract in newborns and on regular basis in older children to monitor for hydronephrosis, hydroureter, and stones.
  - Voiding cystourethrogram (VCUG) is used to evaluate bladder emptying and vesicoureteral reflux in newborns and later as needed.
  - Nuclear medicine studies can be useful for evaluating kidney function and scarring from previous pyelonephritis.

Diagnostic Procedures/Other

- Urodynamic studies (cystometrograms) are used to evaluate bladder function and identify those at high risk for hydronephrosis as well as for objective data that can be used in conjunction with history and physical examination to evaluate for neuropathic changes as a result of tethered cord.
- EEG for suspected seizures

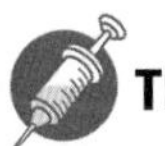

TREATMENT

GENERAL MEASURES

- Route of delivery
  - For most NTDs with vertex presentation, no clear benefit of cesarean section (CS)
  - Infants who undergo fetal surgery delivered by CS
- Clean intermittent catheterization (CIC):
  - Commonly used for neurogenic bladder dysfunction
  - CIC started in newborns with hydronephrosis, high-grade reflux, or high postvoid residuals
  - In addition to above, CIC used in older children just to achieve continence
- Latex precautions: avoidance of natural rubber latex to prevent development of latex allergy

MEDICATION

- Anticholinergic medications (e.g., oxybutynin, tolterodine) are used to relax the spastic bladder and increase capacity.
- Prophylactic antibiotics used for significant vesicoureteral reflux or recurrent urinary tract infections (UTIs)

ADDITIONAL THERAPIES

- Infants with SB are generally referred to their state's early intervention program.
- Older children typically receive therapy in school but may benefit from additional therapy through the health care system.

SURGERY/OTHER PROCEDURES

- Open encephalocele and SB: neurosurgical closure usually done within first few days of life to prevent infection and protect brain/spinal cord from injury. A moist, sterile dressing is applied to the defect until it is closed.
- Hydrocephalus often develops after an open NTD is closed (stopping leakage of CSF).
- CSF shunts (usually ventriculoperitoneal [VP]) are placed to treat progressive hydrocephalus.
- Open fetal closure of MMC has been associated with reduced risk of hydrocephalus and improved developmental and motor outcomes in one prospective randomized trial.
- Fetal surgery for MMC should be considered in select patients prior to 26 weeks' gestation and is considered a new standard of care option at select fetal surgery centers; long-term follow-up studies still needed
- OSD: Neurosurgical exploration and untethering of the spinal cord is usually done after diagnosis.
- Multiple urologic and orthopedic procedures are used to treat the complications of SB. Extensive discussion is beyond the scope of this chapter.

ONGOING CARE

Children with symptomatic SB ideally should be followed in a multidisciplinary SB clinic that includes neurosurgery, urology, and orthopedics as well as a medical generalist (pediatrics, physiatry, or neurology) with experience evaluating and treating children with SB.

- Other important specialties include:
  - Physical therapy (mobility, LE function, bracing)
  - Occupational therapy (ADLs, UE function, including self-catheterization)
  - General psychology, neuropsychology, and/or behavioral psychology (cognitive and executive function, addressing increasing independence)
  - Social work (coping, adjustment to chronic illness, linkage to resources)
  - Ophthalmology (can identify increased ICP when imaging is equivocal)

PROGNOSIS

- Anencephaly: 75% are stillborn; the remainder do not survive beyond the neonatal period.
- Encephalocele: Prognosis depends on the size of the defect, the amount of brain tissue involved, development of hydrocephalus, and the extent of associated brain malformation.
- MMC
  - Most survive into adulthood.
  - Most have IQ in normal range, and almost all of remainder have mild intellectual disability. However, nonverbal learning disabilities and executive dysfunction are very common.
  - Risk of epilepsy ~15%; corresponds to degree of intellectual disability
- SB (open and closed types)
  - Prognosis for ambulation depends on the functional level of the lesion:
    - Sacral level: Most are community ambulators without assistive devices.
    - Low lumbar (L4–L5): Most will walk, but many require bracing and some require crutches or other assistive devices.
    - Midlumbar (L3): often require bracing of the knee (and sometimes hip) to walk with crutches or a walker
    - High lumbar (L1–L2) and thoracic: usually walk in therapy only and use wheelchair as primary means of mobility

COMPLICATIONS

- Encephalocele: Hydrocephalus, intellectual disability, motor deficits, and epilepsy are common.
- MMC
  - VP shunt infection or malfunction
  - Symptomatic Chiari II malformation
    - Infants: feeding difficulties/aspiration, hoarse cry or stridor (due to vocal cord paralysis), and central apnea
    - Older children: cranial nerve palsies, occipital headaches, UE weakness, sleep-disordered breathing, increasing tone over time
  - Syringomyelia
  - Strabismus
- SB (open and closed types)
  - Neurogenic bladder: UTI, hydronephrosis, stones, incontinence, risk of CKD
  - Neurogenic bowel: constipation, impaction, incontinence
  - Orthopedic deformities: scoliosis, hip dysplasia, ankle/foot deformities
  - Tethered spinal cord syndrome
  - Latex allergy
  - Pressure ulcers
  - Osteoporosis and pathologic fractures
  - Deep venous thrombosis
  - Obesity (especially nonambulatory patients)
  - Sexual dysfunction

ADDITIONAL READING

- Adzick NS, Thom EA, Spong CY, et al; for MOMS Investigators. A randomized trial of prenatal versus postnatal repair of myelomeningocele. *N Engl J Med*. 2011;364(11):993–1004.
- Copp AJ, Stanier P, Greene ND. Neural tube defects: recent advances, unsolved questions, and controversies. *Lancet Neurol*. 2013;12(8):799–810.
- Dennis M, Barnes MA. The cognitive phenotype of spina bifida meningomyelocele. *Dev Disabil Res Rev*. 2010;16(1):31–39.
- Liptak GS, Dosa NP. Myelomeningocele. *Pediatr Rev*. 2010;31(11):443–450.
- Sandler AD. Children with spina bifida: key clinical issues. *Pediatr Clin North Am*. 2010;57(4):879–892.

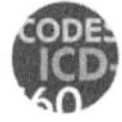

CODES

ICD10

- Q00.0 Anencephaly
- Q01.9 Encephalocele, unspecified
- Q76.0 Spina bifida occulta

FAQ

- Q: Are neural defects genetic?
- A: Genetic factors are definitely involved, but in most cases, a single genetic cause is not found.
- Q: What is the chance of having another child with an NTD?
- A: Recurrence risk with each subsequent pregnancy is about 2–5%.
- Q: How can someone reduce their risk of having a child with an NTD?
- A: Take 400 mcg of folic acid daily (or 4 mg if prior pregnancy with NTD), preferably starting 1 month prior to conception, and avoid alcohol and drugs that can increase risk (especially valproic acid).
- Q: What are examples of reasons to initiate CIC for management of a neurogenic bladder?
- A: To avoid kidney damage as a result of high transmitted pressures from the bladder; to reduce risk of UTIs; to achieve continence

NEUROBLASTOMA

Lars M. Wagner, MD

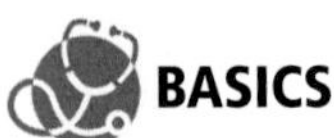

BASICS

DESCRIPTION

- Neuroblastoma is a "small round blue cell tumor" of childhood which arises from developing neural crest cells in the sympathetic nervous system.
- The clinical behavior of neuroblastoma is amazingly diverse. Some tumors undergo maturation into benign ganglioneuroma or even spontaneously regress without therapy, whereas others inexorably progress despite intensive treatment.
- Behavior of neuroblastoma tumors can often be predicted by combining clinical features (age, stage) with pathologic/molecular features (histologic characteristics, tumor ploidy, *MYCN* amplification, 1p, and 11q23 status).
- Integrating clinical and molecular features allows for appropriate risk stratification so that treatment can be tailored to the risk of recurrence. Current risk stratification identifies three separate groups of patients with different prognoses and treatment strategies:
  - Low-risk patients: localized tumors and/or favorable clinical and molecular features
  - Intermediate-risk patients: more extensive primary tumor or regional disease or unfavorable clinical and molecular features
  - High-risk patients: patients >18 months with metastatic disease or unfavorable molecular features

EPIDEMIOLOGY

- The median age at diagnosis is 19 months, with 89% of cases diagnosed <5 years of age. Fewer than 5% of patients are diagnosed >10 years of age.
- The male-to-female ratio is 1.1:1.
- The majority of tumors arise in the retroperitoneum, with the adrenal gland being the single most common location.

Incidence

About 800 new cases per year in the United States (10 per million children per year)

Prevalence

- Accounts for 8–10% of all childhood cancer, making it the most common extracranial solid tumor and the most common cancer overall during the first 2 years of life
- Accounts for 15% of all pediatric cancer deaths
- Occurs in 1 per 7,000 live births

RISK FACTORS

Genetics

- Most cases arise spontaneously. 1% are familial (autosomal dominant) and are usually associated with *ALK* mutations.
- Patients with associated congenital central hypoventilation syndrome often have *PHOX2B* mutations.
- Low-risk patients usually have hyperdiploid tumors with increased chromosome number, whereas high-risk patients more often have segmental chromosome abnormalities such as *MYCN* amplification and are either near diploid or near tetraploid.

PATHOPHYSIOLOGY

Tumor growth can cause symptoms in multiple ways:

- Neurologic: nerve or cord compression from paraspinal tumors, such as the development of Horner syndrome from a posterior mediastinal mass
- Hypertension: from renal artery distortion or occasionally from excessive catecholamine release
- Pain: from metastatic bone disease or abdominal distension
- Hematologic: pancytopenia from marrow disease
- Skeletal: proptosis or periorbital ecchymosis from skull metastases
- Dermatologic: subcutaneous bluish skin nodules seen in infants

ETIOLOGY

No known etiology or causative environmental exposures

COMMONLY ASSOCIATED CONDITIONS

May occur along with other disease that have dysregulation of the peripheral nervous system, such as neurofibromatosis type I, Hirschsprung disease, or central congenital hypoventilation syndrome

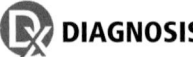

DIAGNOSIS

HISTORY

- Patients with low-risk disease often appear well, and the tumor is discovered incidentally on exam or imaging studies for other reasons.
- High-risk patients often are ill-appearing with obvious symptoms related to tumor location:
  - Abdominal pain or distension
  - Painful bone metastases causing limp
  - Orbital bone metastases causing swelling or discoloration (raccoon eyes)
  - Paraspinal tumors causing weakness, pain, or bowel/bladder symptoms
- Marrow involvement causing pallor and fatigue, petechiae
- Some patients may have paraneoplastic syndromes causing opsoclonus/myoclonus/ataxia related to antineuronal antibodies or excessive diarrhea related to vasoactive intestinal peptide (VIP) secretion.

PHYSICAL EXAM

- Exam findings depend on primary tumor site and extent of dissemination.
- Patients with disseminated disease often have fever and/or worsening nutritional status.
- Patients with abdominal disease may have bulky firm abdominal mass, and hypertension may occur from renal artery distortion or rarely catecholamine release. The liver may be massively enlarged, particularly in patients with stage 4S/MS disease in the 1st year of life.
- Patients with thoracic tumors may have Horner syndrome, and occasionally, respiratory symptoms from airway compression.
- Patients with paraspinal tumors with invasion into the spinal canal may have weakness and/or radicular pain.
- Bone metastases may have associated proptosis, soft tissue swelling, or discoloration from venous stasis.
- Regional or distant nodes may be enlarged, particularly in the supraclavicular region.
- Bluish firm skin nodules may be seen in infants.
- Pallor or petechiae from marrow metastases

DIFFERENTIAL DIAGNOSIS

- Abdominal masses: Wilms tumor, germ cell tumor, hepatoblastoma, abdominal sarcoma, or lymphoma
- Thoracic masses: lymphoma, leukemia, germ cell tumor
- "Small round blue cell tumors of childhood": non-Hodgkin lymphoma, rhabdomyosarcoma, Ewing sarcoma/primitive neuroectodermal tumor (PNET)

DIAGNOSTIC TESTS & INTERPRETATION

Initial Tests (screening, lab, imaging)

- CBC
  - Decreased hemoglobin, platelets, and/or WBC may indicate marrow involvement.
- Lactic dehydrogenase (LDH)
  - Often elevated with large or metastatic tumors
- Urine catecholamines (homovanillic acid [HVA], vanillylmandelic acid [VMA])
  - Can be done on spot urine samples
  - Elevated in 90% of patients
- CT or MRI
  - To evaluate primary tumor site
  - Calcification quite common in neuroblastoma
- Metaiodobenzylguanidine (MIBG)
  - Most specific test for neuroblastoma
  - Uptake seen in primary tumor and metastases in 90% of patients
- Bone scan done if tumor is not avid on MIBG
- Alternatively, fluorodeoxyglucose-18 positron emission tomography (FDG-PET) scan may also identify tumor in MIBG-negative patients.

Diagnostic Procedures/Other

- Tumor biopsy is usually required, unless there is metastatic tumor in bone marrow coupled with elevated urine HVA/VMA.
  - Tumor tissue usually expresses neuroendocrine markers (synaptophysin, neuron-specific enolase [NSE]) and often contains neuropil.
  - The determination of favorable versus unfavorable histology is made based on degree of differentiation, presence of stroma, mitotic/karyorrhectic index, and age of patient.
- Neuroblastomas are immature; ganglioneuroblastomas have some maturity but are still malignant, whereas ganglioneuromas are fully mature and benign.
- Bilateral bone marrow aspirates and biopsies help complete staging.

- The International Neuroblastoma Staging System (INSS) is the traditional surgical staging system:
  - Stage 1: completely resected localized tumor
  - Stage 2: incompletely resected localized tumor (2A) or with regional node involvement (2B)
  - Stage 3: unresectable tumor crossing midline or contralateral regional lymph node involvement
  - Stage 4: dissemination to nodes, bone marrow, liver, skin (except 4S)
  - Stage 4S: <1 year old, with stage 1 to 2 primary tumor and metastases limited to liver, skin, or bone marrow
- The International Neuroblastoma Risk Group Staging System is a preoperative system using image-defined risk factors (IDRFs) that can be applied at the time of diagnosis:
  - Stage L1—localized tumor not involving vital structures and confined to one body compartment
  - Stage L2—locoregional tumor with presence of one or more IDRF
  - Stage M—distant metastatic disease (except MS)
  - Stage MS—metastatic disease in children <18 months with metastases confined to skin, liver, and/or bone marrow

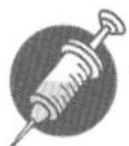

TREATMENT

- Treatment is based on risk stratification using age 18 months, stage, DNA ploidy, favorable versus unfavorable histology, and genomic features (presence or absence of segmental copy number aberrations such as *MYCN* amplification).
- Low-risk tumors
  - Treatment is surgery alone, generally without adjuvant chemotherapy.
  - Certain patients with stage 4S/MS disease spontaneously regress and may never even require surgery or chemotherapy and may be closely observed without therapy.
- Intermediate-risk tumors
  - Treatment generally uses 2 to 8 cycles of outpatient chemotherapy, performing surgical resection when appropriate.
  - Chemotherapy includes carboplatin, etoposide, doxorubicin, and cyclophosphamide.
  - Selected patients may also receive topotecan or cis-retinoic acid.
- High-risk tumors
  - Treatment involves multiple cycles of intense induction chemotherapy, with surgical resection of primary tumor done when appropriate.
  - Treatment is then consolidated with high-dose chemotherapy and autologous peripheral blood stem cell transplant.
  - Following recovery, they receive irradiation to the primary tumor site as well as any metastatic sites that were slow to respond to induction therapy. Finally, patients receive multiple cycles of cis-retinoic acid and immunotherapy with the anti-GD2 antibody dinutuximab, which targets the GD2 protein that is ubiquitously expressed on neuroblastoma cells.
  - Chemotherapy used during induction consists of vincristine, doxorubicin, cyclophosphamide, cisplatin, and etoposide. High-dose chemotherapy often involves carboplatin, etoposide, and melphalan. Newer regimens are testing the use of busulfan and melphalan and the use of therapeutic ^{131}I-MIBG for consolidation.
- Relapsed/refractory neuroblastoma
  - Prognosis is very poor; consider investigational therapy options.

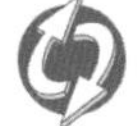

ONGOING CARE

FOLLOW-UP RECOMMENDATIONS

Referral to a pediatric oncologist is essential before any diagnostic procedures or therapeutic interventions.

Patient Monitoring

- On therapy
  - Laboratory monitoring for myelosuppression and organ function
  - Disease reevaluation with imaging and bone marrow testing prior to surgery and stem cell transplant
- Off therapy
  - Close follow-up for disease recurrence up to 5 years after completion of therapy, using imaging and urine catecholamine measurement
  - Monitoring for late effects of cancer therapy, especially in young growing children

PROGNOSIS

- Adverse prognostic factors
  - Age >18 months
  - Advanced stage
  - *MYCN* gene amplification
  - Unfavorable histology
  - Diploid tumor genome (primarily infants)
  - Loss of heterozygosity (LOH) at chromosome arms 1p or 11q
- Expected outcomes with current therapy
  - Low-risk disease: >90% 3-year event-free survival
  - Intermediate-risk disease: approximately 85–95% 3-year event-free survival
  - High-risk disease: approximately 40–50% 3-year event-free survival
  - Relapse: <10% survival

COMPLICATIONS

Treatment-related complications (see "Cancer Therapy Late Effects" chapter)

- Growth delays
- Renal insufficiency
- Hearing loss
- Hypothyroidism
- Second malignancy
- Cardiac dysfunction
- Infertility

ADDITIONAL READING

- Bagatell R, Cohn SL. Genetic discoveries and treatment advances in neuroblastoma. *Curr Opin Pediatr*. 2016;28(1):19–25.
- Maris JM. Recent advances in neuroblastoma. *N Engl J Med*. 2010;362(23):2202–2211.
- Park JR, Eggert A, Caron H. Neuroblastoma: biology, prognosis, and treatment. *Hematol Oncol Clin North Am*. 2010;24(1):65–86.

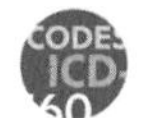

CODES

ICD10

- C74.90 Malignant neoplasm of unsp part of unspecified adrenal gland
- C48.0 Malignant neoplasm of retroperitoneum
- C38.3 Malignant neoplasm of mediastinum, part unspecified

FAQ

- Q: Are siblings of children with neuroblastoma at increased risk for neuroblastoma compared with the general population?
- A: No, except in rare families with a known history of neuroblastoma (<1%).
- Q: Can neuroblastoma spontaneously regress?
- A: Yes, but this is usually seen only in children <1 year of age with lower stage disease or in infants with stage 4S disease.
- Q: What are the biggest risks during therapy?
- A: As with all intensive chemotherapy regimens, the risk of infection is high. This is especially true during the autologous stem cell transplant phase.
- Q: What therapy is available to patients who either fail to go into remission or relapse following aggressive therapy?
- A: There is no curative therapy after disease recurrence in high-risk neuroblastoma. However, some patients can have meaningful stabilization of disease with therapeutic MIBG administration or other experimental therapies.
- Q: Is screening of asymptomatic infants by testing urine HVA and VMA levels helpful?
- A: Current data do not support neuroblastoma screening in well infants, as this practice did not reduce mortality nor identify high-risk patients.
- Q: Should all neonates with adrenal masses undergo surgical resection?
- A: Recent data from a cooperative group study show that expectant observation alone in select patients with small adrenal masses led to excellent outcomes while avoiding surgery in over three-fourths of patients.

NEUROFIBROMATOSIS-1

Robert Listernick, MD

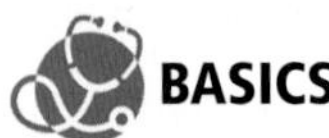

BASICS

DESCRIPTION

- Neurofibromatosis type 1 (NF-1) is an autosomal dominant tumor suppressor gene disorder.
- NF-1 is diagnosed based on the presence of any two of the following National Institutes of Health (NIH) Consensus Conference diagnostic criteria:
  - Six or more café au lait spots, at least 1.5 cm in diameter in postpubertal individuals or 0.5 cm in diameter in prepubertal individuals
  - Inguinal or axillary freckling
  - Two or more cutaneous neurofibromas or one plexiform neurofibroma
  - Two or more iris Lisch nodules
  - Optic nerve glioma
  - Osseous lesions, including sphenoid wing dysplasia, dysplasia of a long bone (most commonly tibia)
  - A 1st-degree relative (parent, sibling, or offspring) with NF-1

ALERT

Note: Neurofibromatosis type 2 (NF-2) is a rare distinct autosomal dominant tumor suppressor gene disorder characterized by bilateral vestibular schwannomas as well as schwannomas of cranial and peripheral nerves, meningiomas, and ependymomas. It is caused by mutations in the *NF2* gene, which codes for a protein known as merlin. This chapter focuses on NF-1.

EPIDEMIOLOGY

Incidence

- NF-1: 1 in 3,000 live births
- NF-2: 1 in 33,000 live births

Prevalence

- NF-1: 1 in 4,000 to 5,000
- NF-2: 1 in 60,000

RISK FACTORS

Genetics

- Autosomal dominant
  - 50% of the cases are inherited; others occur as sporadic mutations.
  - Penetrance is complete; however, expression is variable even between family members who have same mutation.
  - *NF1* gene, which codes for neurofibromin, is located on chromosome 17q11.2.
- No known ethnic predisposition
- Course impossible to predict except in two circumstances
  - Deletion of whole *NF1* gene leads to early appearance and large numbers of cutaneous neurofibromas, severe cognitive impairment, and dysmorphic features.
  - Three base pair in-frame deletion of exon 17 leads to multiple café au lait spots and intertriginous freckling but no other NF-1 manifestations.

DIAGNOSIS

HISTORY

- Growth
  - Accelerated linear growth may be first sign of precocious puberty and presence of optic pathway tumor (OPT).
- Vision
  - OPTs generally occur before 7 years of age; young children rarely complain of visual loss.
- Development
  - Speech delay, motor incoordination, learning problems, and attention-deficit/hyperactivity disorder (ADHD)
- Headache
  - Common; hydrocephalus due to obstructing tumor may occur.
- Family history
  - 1st-degree relative may have unrecognized NF-1.

PHYSICAL EXAM

- Growth
  - Assess growth chart with attention to possible accelerated linear growth as early sign of precocious puberty, rarely growth hormone excess.
  - Assess head circumference for macrocephaly.
- Café au lait spots
  - Collections of heavily pigmented melanocytes of neural crest origin in the epidermis
  - 53% of children with NF-1 will have six or more by 3 years; 97% by 6 years
- Axillary and inguinal freckling
  - Present in 80% of children by 6 years
- Discrete neurofibromas
  - Benign nerve sheath tumors that appear as discrete masses arising from peripheral nerve
  - Cutaneous neurofibromas protrude just above the skin surface or lie just under the skin often with an overlying violaceous hue.
  - Subcutaneous neurofibromas are generally much harder.
- Plexiform neurofibromas
  - Benign peripheral nerve sheath tumors which involve single or multiple nerve fascicles, often arising from branches of major nerves
  - "Wormy" sensation on palpation often with overlying hyperpigmentation or hypertrichosis
  - Most external plexiform neurofibromas are present at birth or become apparent during the first several years of life.
  - May lead to disfigurement, blindness (secondary to amblyopia, glaucoma, or proptosis), or loss of limb function
  - Thoracic or abdominal plexiform neurofibromas may have no external manifestations but may lead to invasion or compression of vital structures (e.g., ureters, bowel, and spinal cord).
- Lisch nodules
  - Best assessed with slit lamp
  - Slightly raised, well-circumscribed melanocytic hamartomas of the iris thought to be virtually pathognomonic of NF-1
  - Increase with age; present in only 30% of children <6 years but >95% of adults
- OPTs
  - Are present in 15% of children with NF-1, although only half are symptomatic and 40% of those will require treatment
  - Complete yearly eye exams are mandatory for NF-1 patients <10 years.
  - Ophthalmologic signs include afferent papillary defect, optic nerve atrophy, papilledema, strabismus, or defects in color vision.
  - 40% of children who have chiasmal tumors develop precocious puberty.
- Bony dysplasias
  - Sphenoid wing dysplasia may lead to enophthalmos or pulsating exophthalmos.
  - Tibial dysplasia, congenital thinning and bowing; failure of primary union following fracture results in pseudarthrosis.
- Hypertension
  - In children, most commonly due to fibromuscular dysplasia of renal artery
  - Pheochromocytoma rare in children
- Complete neurologic exam
  - Assess for signs of intracranial or intraspinal tumors.
- Scoliosis
  - Assess for idiopathic juvenile scoliosis which generally becomes manifest at onset of puberty; short-segment dystrophic scoliosis present at birth

DIFFERENTIAL DIAGNOSIS

- Legius syndrome, mutation in *SPRED1*, manifested by multiple café au lait spots, intertriginous freckling, and macrocephaly but no other manifestations of NF-1, for example, neurofibromas, Lisch nodules, bony dysplasias
- Some individuals with Noonan syndrome may have multiple café au lait spots or intertriginous freckling. Alternately, some individuals with NF-1 have phenotypic manifestations of Noonan syndrome (e.g., abnormal facies, pectus excavatum, pulmonic stenosis).
- McCune-Albright syndrome has large café au lait spots with irregular margins, polyostotic fibrous dysplasia, and autonomous endocrine hyperfunction (e.g., precocious puberty, Cushing syndrome, hyperthyroidism).

DIAGNOSTIC TESTS & INTERPRETATION

Initial Tests (screening, lab, imaging)

- *NF1* gene mutation
  - Can be identified in >98% of individuals with clinical diagnosis of NF-1
  - However, gene testing is not necessary in vast majority of cases.
  - Gene testing may be useful for:
    - Very young children who do not meet diagnostic criteria
    - Prenatal testing in familial cases
    - Children with unusual or very mild manifestations of NF-1 (e.g., to distinguish from Legius or Noonan syndromes)
- "Screening neuroimaging" of asymptomatic children not recommended
- Brain MRI recommended for signs of increased intracranial pressure or focal neurologic deficits, abnormal visual exam, or accelerated growth suggestive of precocious puberty
- Unidentified bright objects ("UBOs")
  - Regions of increased signal intensity on T2-weighted images found in the internal capsule, basal ganglia, cortex, cerebellar hemispheres, optic tract, or brainstem
  - Disappear with age
  - UBOs don't enhance or cause mass effect.
  - Significance unknown; may be associated with cognitive impairment or learning disabilities

Diagnostic Procedures/Other

A biopsy of plexiform neurofibroma looking for malignancy (malignant peripheral nerve sheath tumor) is necessary if there are signs of rapid growth, new onset pain, or neurologic dysfunction.

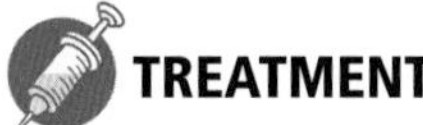

TREATMENT

GENERAL MEASURES

- Treatment of NF-1 should be performed in a multidisciplinary setting.
- All 1st-degree relatives should be examined for the cutaneous manifestations of NF-1 and should undergo slit-lamp examination to ascertain presence of Lisch nodules.
- Available consultants should include experts in orthopedics, oncology, ophthalmology, genetics, endocrinology, surgery, neurosurgery, plastic surgery, and psychiatry.

ONGOING CARE

FOLLOW-UP RECOMMENDATIONS

- Yearly visits allow the physician to identify early NF-1 complications while providing counseling and dissemination of information regarding NF-1.
- All children with NF-1 who are ≤10 years old should have complete yearly ophthalmologic examinations looking for signs of an OPT.
- Blood pressure taken at each visit
- Vigilance/anticipatory care regarding common psychological and developmental issues, such as speech delay, incoordination, ADHD, and learning disabilities
- Early educational assessment and interventions may improve developmental outcome.

COMPLICATIONS

- Cognitive impairment
  - Mean IQ ~95
  - 60% incidence of learning disabilities/ADHD; visual/perceptual disabilities common
- Malignancies
  - Malignant peripheral nerve sheath tumor (7–13% lifetime incidence); almost all arise in preexisting plexiform neurofibromas.
  - Acute lymphocytic leukemia
  - Juvenile myelomonocytic leukemia
  - Rhabdomyosarcoma
  - Gastrointestinal stromal tumors
  - Pheochromocytoma
- Skeletal
  - Pseudarthrosis
  - Scoliosis
  - Osteoporosis
- Vasculopathy
  - May involve any arterial vessel
  - Renal artery stenosis, hypertension
  - Moyamoya disease—poststenotic capillary proliferation in cerebral vasculature may lead to cerebral infarct; treatment by encephaloduroarteriomyosynangiosis (EDAMS) procedure
  - Intermittent claudication of an extremity
- Endocrine
  - Precocious puberty due to chiasmal glioma
  - Pheochromocytoma (rare in children)
  - Growth hormone excess (also rare)

ADDITIONAL READING

- Avery RA, Fisher MJ, Liu GT. Optic pathway gliomas. *J Neuroophthalmol*. 2011;31(3):269–278.
- Brossier NM, Gutmann DH. Improving outcomes for neurofibromatosis 1-associated brain tumors. *Expert Rev Anticancer Ther*. 2015;15(4):415–423.
- Hirbe AC, Gutmann DH. Neurofibromatosis type 1: a multidisciplinary approach to care. *Lancet Neurol*. 2014;13(8):834–843.
- Hoa M, Slattery WH III. Neurofibromatosis 2. *Otolaryngol Clin North Am*. 2012;45(2):315–332.
- Lehtonen A, Howie E, Trump D, et al. Behaviour in children with neurofibromatosis type 1: cognition, executive function, attention, emotion, and social competence. *Dev Med Child Neurol*. 2013;55(2):111–125.
- Listernick R, Ferner RE, Liu GT, et al. Optic pathway gliomas in neurofibromatosis-1: controversies and recommendations. *Ann Neurol*. 2007;61(3):189–198.
- Messiaen L, Yao S, Brems H, et al. Clinical and mutational spectrum of neurofibromatosis type 1-like syndrome. *JAMA*. 2009;302(19):2111–2118.
- Rosser T, Packer RJ. Intracranial neoplasms in children with neurofibromatosis 1. *J Child Neurol*. 2002;17(8):630–637, 646–651.
- Stevenson DA, Little D, Armstrong L, et al. Approaches to treating NF1 tibial pseudarthrosis: consensus from the Children's Tumor Foundation NF1 Bone Abnormalities Consortium. *J Pediatr Orthop*. 2013;33(3):269–275.

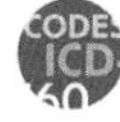

CODES

ICD10

- Q85.01 Neurofibromatosis, type 1
- L81.3 Cafe au lait spots

FAQ

- Q: My child has NF-1. What specialists must he see?
- A: Your child should have annual follow-up with a physician familiar with the issues of NF, ideally in an NF-1 multidisciplinary clinic.
- Q: Does my child with NF-1 need any radiographs?
- A: Radiographs or MRI scans need only be done if your child has signs or symptoms suggestive of a particular complication of NF-1.
- Q: Is my child going to die because of NF-1?
- A: Although a very small minority of children with NF-1 has life-threatening complications, almost all individuals with NF-1 live long, productive lives.

NEUTROPENIA

Kristin A. Shimano, MD

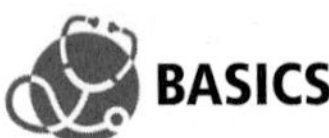

BASICS

DESCRIPTION

A decrease in the number of circulating neutrophils (both segmented and band forms), strictly defined as an absolute total neutrophil count (ANC) of <1,500/μL in children >1 year of age, <1,000/μL in children <1 year of age, and <5,000/μL in the 1st week of life

- To calculate ANC, multiply the total WBC count by the percentage of segmented neutrophils and band forms.
- For example: WBC count 5,200/μL with 15% segs/polys, 4% bands, 76% lymphocytes, 5% monocytes: ANC = 5,200 × (0.15 + 0.04) = 988
- Severe neutropenia is defined as an ANC <500/μL.

EPIDEMIOLOGY

- Normal values for total WBC counts and ANC vary with age and race.
  - Children of some ethnic groups, including African and Middle Eastern groups, have lower total WBC counts and lower ANCs than do Caucasian children.
  - Lower end of normal range for ANC may be 800/μL in 30% of African Americans and does not represent an increased risk for infection.
- Infants have a higher total WBC count and a higher percentage of lymphocytes in their differential counts.
- Prevalence of congenital and idiopathic neutropenia: 2.1 cases per million in the United States
- Incidence of neonatal alloimmune neutropenia: 2 per 1,000 live births

RISK FACTORS

Genetics

- A number of mutations causing severe congenital neutropenia have been identified.
  - Autosomal recessive: *HAX1* (Kostmann syndrome), *G6PC3*, *SBDS* (Shwachman-Diamond syndrome), others
  - Autosomal dominant: *ELANE*, *GFL1*, *GATA2*, others
  - X-linked: *WASP*, *TAZ* (Barth syndrome), others
- Cyclic neutropenia: autosomal dominant or sporadic (*ELANE*)

PATHOPHYSIOLOGY

Decreased phagocytic activity due to decreased numbers of neutrophils

ETIOLOGY

- Decreased production of neutrophils
  - Viral suppression
  - Marrow suppression by drugs, chemotherapy, or radiation
  - Nutritional deficiencies
  - Primary disorders of myelopoiesis
- Increased destruction of neutrophils
  - Immune-mediated destruction
  - Increased use (usually with overwhelming infection)
  - Sequestration in the spleen

DIAGNOSIS

HISTORY

- Recent or current viral infection
- Current or recurrent fever, skin abscesses, infections, or oral ulceration
- Temporal pattern of symptoms
- Symptoms of malabsorption, such as diarrhea or failure to thrive
- Delayed cord separation
- Medication use or toxin exposure
- Diet: evidence of nutritional deficiency
- Developmental history
- Ethnicity
- Family history of neutropenia, recurrent infection, or early death; consanguinity
- Review prior CBC with differential results: Prior normal WBC count and ANC essentially rule out severe congenital neutropenia.

PHYSICAL EXAM

- Growth curve
- Oral ulceration or gingival irritation
- Phenotypic abnormalities (thumb anomalies, dwarfism, partial albinism)
- Hepatosplenomegaly or lymphadenopathy
- Bruises, petechiae, pallor
- Birthmarks (café au lait spots)
- Neurologic exam
- Signs of infection
  - Fever (Temperature should not be taken rectally.)
  - Tachycardia or hypotension
  - Pharyngitis or thrush
  - Cellulitis, perirectal or labial abscesses
  - Signs of local infection (such as inflammation, pus) may be diminished due to lack of neutrophils.

DIFFERENTIAL DIAGNOSIS

- Neutropenia associated with infection
  - Viral suppression is a very common cause of transient neutropenia.
  - Viral: hepatitis A and B, parvovirus B19, respiratory syncytial virus (RSV), influenza A and B, rubeola, rubella, varicella, cytomegalovirus (CMV), Epstein-Barr virus (EBV), HIV
  - Bacterial: group B streptococcal disease, tuberculosis, brucellosis, tularemia, typhoid, paratyphoid
  - Other: malaria, visceral leishmaniasis, scrub typhus, sandfly fever
- Drug-induced
  - Antibiotics: sulfonamides (trimethoprim/sulfamethoxazole is a common offender), penicillin, chloramphenicol (may be irreversible)
  - Chemotherapy agents: alkylating agents, antimetabolites, anthracyclines
  - Antipyretics: aspirin, acetaminophen (uncommon)
  - Sedatives: barbiturates, benzodiazepines
  - Phenothiazines: chlorpromazine, promethazine
  - Antirheumatic agents: gold, penicillamine, phenylbutazone
- Immunologic
  - Benign neutropenia of childhood: very common cause of chronic neutropenia; immune-mediated; onset usually <2 years of age; typically a benign course with resolution within several years
  - Isoimmune neonatal neutropenia: due to transplacental transfer of maternal antibodies against paternal antigens
  - Manifestation of an autoimmune disease: systemic lupus erythematosus, autoimmune lymphoproliferative syndrome (ALPS), Felty syndrome (neutropenia, splenomegaly, and rheumatoid arthritis), others
- Congenital
  - Severe congenital neutropenia
  - Cyclic neutropenia: regular oscillations in the number of circulating neutrophils (periodicity, every 7 to 36 days; duration of neutropenia, 3 to 10 days)
- Marrow failure syndromes
  - Shwachman-Diamond syndrome: neutropenia and exocrine pancreatic insufficiency
  - Part of evolving aplastic anemia: acquired (idiopathic), Fanconi anemia, dyskeratosis congenital, Diamond-Blackfan anemia
- Primary immunodeficiencies
  - Cartilage/hair hypoplasia: neutropenia, dwarfism, abnormal cellular immunity
  - Reticular dysgenesis
  - Chédiak-Higashi syndrome: oculocutaneous albinism, platelet dysfunction, leukocyte inclusions
  - Other abnormalities in T and B lymphocytes
- Bone marrow infiltration
  - Malignancy: leukemia or solid tumors metastatic to bone marrow
  - Osteopetrosis
  - Gaucher disease (lysosomal storage disorder)
- Metabolic
  - Nutritional: malnutrition, copper deficiency, zinc deficiency, megaloblastic anemia secondary to folate or vitamin B_{12} deficiency
  - Inborn errors of metabolism: Barth syndrome (skeletal myopathy, dilated cardiomyopathy, neutropenia), glycogen storage disease I, others
- Miscellaneous
  - Hypersplenism
  - Radiation injury

DIAGNOSTIC TESTS & INTERPRETATION

Initial Tests (screening, lab, imaging)

- Repeat CBC with differential
  - Neutropenia due to viral suppression is extremely common, and counts may normalize on repeat exam.
  - Hemoglobin and platelets are important as well; can help determine if this is an isolated neutropenia or pancytopenia
- Serial CBCs, twice weekly for 6 weeks, to rule out cyclic neutropenia

- Evaluation of exocrine pancreatic function if Shwachman-Diamond syndrome is a consideration
- Immunologic evaluation (immunoglobulins, lymphocyte subsets) to rule out immunodeficiency
- Cross-typing maternal serum and paternal neutrophils in evaluation of neonatal alloimmune neutropenia
- Genetic testing for certain disorders
- Antineutrophil antibodies: can often be detected in autoimmune neutropenia if multiple methods of testing are used; not routinely recommended, however, given imperfect sensitivity and specificity

Diagnostic Procedures/Other

- Bone marrow aspirate and biopsy indicated in severe chronic neutropenia, pancytopenia, or when there is other concern for a marrow disorder or malignancy
- Biopsy may be normal or may reveal a decrease in the number of myeloid precursors or a maturational arrest of the myeloid line (usually in the later stages), depending on the cause of neutropenia.

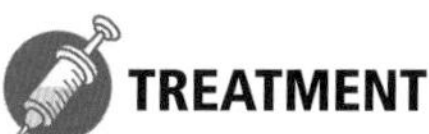

TREATMENT

GENERAL MEASURES

- Correction of underlying cause of neutropenia (discontinue drug, treat infection, correct nutritional deficiency)
- Treatment of fever and suspected infection when neutropenic: Initially, broad-spectrum antibiotics are indicated; after the diagnosis has been established, this may not always be necessary (i.e., individuals with chronic benign neutropenia). Follow institution-specific practices for fever and neutropenia in oncology patients.
- Prophylactic antibiotics are not usually beneficial and may predispose to systemic fungal infection.
- Stool softeners may be helpful in the profoundly neutropenic patient at risk for constipation to prevent development of a perirectal abscess.
- No therapy may be required if neutropenia is not severe and there are no serious or recurrent infections (often the case in chronic benign neutropenia).

MEDICATION

Granulocyte colony–stimulating factor (G-CSF)

- Indicated for severe congenital neutropenia and cyclic neutropenia (decreases infections and mortality)
- May be used in some patients with neutropenia due to other causes

ISSUES FOR REFERRAL

- Chronic or profound neutropenia
- History of recurrent unusual or severe infections
- When bone marrow examination is indicated

ADDITIONAL THERAPIES

- Stem cell transplant may be indicated in some patients with severe congenital neutropenia or neutropenia due to other causes (such as bone marrow failure syndromes).
- Granulocyte transfusion are generally discouraged as they are associated with significant morbidity and do not seem to affect the risk of death. However, they can be considered in patients with overwhelming infections and with expectation of neutrophil count recovery.

ADMISSION, INPATIENT, AND NURSING CONSIDERATIONS

- "Neutropenic precautions": Standard hand hygiene is sufficient (no need for masks/gowns/gloves).
- Depending on etiology of neutropenia, patients will often require admission for IV antibiotics for treatment of fever and neutropenia.

ONGOING CARE

FOLLOW-UP RECOMMENDATIONS

Management of febrile episodes (depends on etiology of neutropenia)

- Prompt evaluation by a physician.
- Obtain CBC with differential and blood culture.
- Treat with IV antibiotics.
- Hospitalize if ill-appearing or high-risk for infection.
- Monitor daily CBC with differential.

Patient Monitoring

- CBCs and physical exams at regular intervals while the patient is neutropenic
- Depending on the etiology of the neutropenia, annual bone marrow biopsy surveillance for leukemia or myelodysplastic syndrome (MDS)

PROGNOSIS

- Duration of neutropenia depends on diagnosis.
  - Neutropenia resulting from infection or drug-related marrow suppression is usually short lived.
  - Autoimmune neutropenia (benign neutropenia of childhood) typically resolves within 2 years.
  - Congenital neutropenia syndromes may result in chronic lifelong neutropenia.
- Likelihood of infection depends on severity of neutropenia (higher risk if $<500/\mu L$) and cause of neutropenia (higher risk in disorders of neutrophil production).

COMPLICATIONS

- Systemic infections, including pneumonia and sepsis
- Localized infections such as cellulitis, labial abscesses, perirectal abscesses, oral mucosal ulceration, thrush, otitis media, stomatitis, or gingivitis
- Typical pathogens:
  - Bacterial: staphylococci, streptococci, enterococci, *Pseudomonas*, gram-negative bacilli
  - Fungal: *Candida* or *Aspergillus*
- Transformation to leukemia or MDS

ADDITIONAL READING

- Fioredda F, Calvillo M, Bonanomi S, et al. Congenital and acquired neutropenia consensus guidelines on diagnosis from the Neutropenia Committee of the Marrow Failure Syndrome Group of the AIEOP (Associazione Italiana Emato-Oncologia Pediatrica). *Pediatr Blood Cancer*. 2011;57(1):10–17.
- Lehrnbecher T, Phillips R, Alexander S, et al; for International Pediatric Fever and Neutropenia Guideline Panel. Guideline for the management of fever and neutropenia in children with cancer and/or undergoing hematopoietic stem-cell transplantation. *J Clin Oncol*. 2012;30(35):4427–4438.
- Pascual C, Trenchs V, Hernández-Bou S, et al. Outcomes and infectious etiologies of febrile neutropenia in non-immunocompromised children who present in an emergency department. *Eur J Clin Microbiol Infect Dis*. 2016;35(10):1667–1672.
- Walkovich K, Boxer LA. How to approach neutropenia in childhood. *Pediatr Rev*. 2013;34(4):173–184.

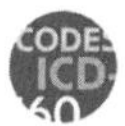

CODES

ICD10

- D70.9 Neutropenia, unspecified
- D70.0 Congenital agranulocytosis
- D70.4 Cyclic neutropenia

FAQ

- Q: Do all patients with neutropenia require G-CSF?
- A: No. Patients with severe congenital neutropenia have fewer infections when treated with G-CSF. Patients with benign neutropenia generally do not need G-CSF.
- Q: Can a neutropenic patient receive vaccinations?
- A: Yes, if neutropenia is the only immunologic abnormality.
- Q: Should a child with neutropenia be kept in isolation?
- A: No. Neutropenic patients may go to school and do not need to wear masks.

NON-HODGKIN LYMPHOMA

Michelle L. Hermiston, MD, PhD

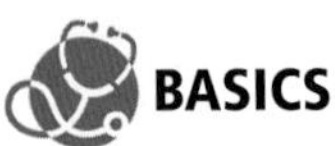

BASICS

DESCRIPTION

- Non-Hodgkin lymphoma (NHL) arises from the malignant proliferation of developing or mature B or T lymphocytes.
- Extent of disease is determined using the Murphy staging system:
  - Stage I: single tumor (extranodal) or single nodal area, excluding mediastinum or abdomen
  - Stage II: single tumor with regional nodal involvement, two or more tumors or nodal areas on the same side of the diaphragm, or a primary GI tract tumor (resected) with or without regional node involvement
  - Stage III: tumors or lymph node (LN) areas on both sides of the diaphragm, any primary intrathoracic or extensive intra-abdominal disease (unresectable), or any paraspinal or epidural tumors
  - Stage IV: bone marrow or CNS disease regardless of other sites; marrow involvement defined as 0.5–25% malignant cells

EPIDEMIOLOGY

- Third most common childhood malignancy (~12% cancers in individuals <20 years of age in developed countries)
- Number of cases is increasing in adolescents and young adults.
- Male-to-female ratio: 3:1

Incidence

- 10 to 20 cases per 1 million children per year
- Higher frequency of endemic Burkitt-type in equatorial African countries (10 to15 per 100,000 children <5 to 10 years)
- Incidence increases steadily with age; in children, usually seen in 2nd decade of life (unusual in those <3 years of age)

RISK FACTORS

Environmental factors

- Drugs: immunosuppressive therapy and diphenylhydantoin
- Radiation: atomic bomb survivors and ionizing radiation
- Viruses: Epstein-Barr virus (EBV) present in >95% of cases of endemic Burkitt versus <20% cases of sporadic; HIV

Genetics

Genetic predisposition: increased risk in patients with immunologic defects (e.g., Bruton agammaglobulinemia, ataxia telangiectasia, Wiskott-Aldrich, severe combined immunodeficiency [SCID], X-linked lymphoproliferative syndrome [XLP])

PATHOPHYSIOLOGY

- Unlike adults, low- and intermediate-grade NHL is uncommon in children (~7% of cases).
- NHL in children and adolescent can be divided into three major categories according to the National Cancer Institute (NCI):
  - Mature B-cell NHL (Burkitt and Burkitt-like lymphoma, diffuse large B-cell lymphoma [DLBCL], primary mediastinal B-cell lymphoma)
    - 50% of childhood NHL
    - Express mature B-cell markers (CD20, surface immunoglobulin [Ig])
    - Terminal deoxynucleotidyl transferase (TdT) negative
    - Burkitt lymphoma has characteristic t(8;14), rarely t(8;22) or t(2;8); all chromosomal translocations involve the c-myc proto-oncogene.
    - DLBCL usually of the germinal center B-cell phenotype. Unlike adults, the t(14:18) translocation is rare.
  - Lymphoblastic lymphomas (LL)
    - 30% of childhood NHL
    - In children, 90% T-cell and 10% B-cell origin
    - Morphologically identical to acute lymphoblastic leukemia. TdT positive; express early T (CD5, CD7, cytoplasmic CD3) or B (CD19, CD10) cell markers. Bone marrow involvement of >25% blasts is considered leukemia.
    - Early thymic progenitor (ETP) subtype arises earlier in T-cell ontogeny. Most recent studies indicate it has a slower response to therapy but does not have a worse prognosis.
  - Anaplastic large cell lymphoma (ALCL) (mature T-cell or null-cell lymphomas):
    - 10% of childhood NHL
    - Express CD30 (Ki-1)
    - Contain chromosomal rearrangement involving the *ALK* gene (85% t2;5)
- Immunodeficiency-associated NHL usually of B-cell origin

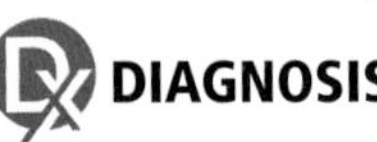

DIAGNOSIS

HISTORY

- Mature B-cell lymphomas
  - Systemic manifestation (e.g., fever, weight loss, anorexia, fatigue) if disseminated; less likely if tumor localized
  - Abdominal mass with pain, swelling, change in bowel habits, nausea, or vomiting
  - Lump in neck unresponsive to antibiotics
- T-cell LL
  - Mediastinal mass symptoms include cough, hoarseness, dyspnea, orthopnea and chest pain, anxiety, confusion, lethargy, headache, distorted vision, syncope, and/or a sense of fullness in the ears.
  - Marrow involvement: bleeding and/or bruising, bone pain, pallor, fatigue
- B-cell LL
  - Tender or painless swelling in neck, axilla, groin, or extremities
  - Symptoms of marrow involvement
- ALCL
  - Painless swelling in neck, axilla, groin
  - B type symptoms: fever, night sweats, weight loss

PHYSICAL EXAM

- Mature B-cell NHL
  - Intra-abdominal mass (90%)
    - Involving ileocecal region, appendix, ascending colon, or a combination
    - Lymphadenopathy may be present in inguinal or iliac region.
    - Hepatosplenomegaly may be present.
    - Acute abdomen with intussusception, peritonitis, ascites, and acute GI bleeding
    - Lymphoma is the most frequent cause of intussusception in children >6 years of age.
  - Other sites: testis, unilateral tonsil hypertrophy, peripheral LNs, parotid gland, skin, bone, CNS, and marrow
  - In endemic Burkitt lymphoma, jaw tumors are the most frequent. Infants often have orbital involvement.
- LL
  - T-LL: mediastinal mass (50–70%), possibly pleural effusion present with decreased breath sounds, rales, and cough with or without superior vena cava (SVC) syndrome or superior mediastinal syndrome (SMS):
    - Signs include swelling, plethora, and cyanosis of the face, neck, and upper extremities; diaphoresis; stridor; and wheezing.
  - Lymphadenopathy (50–80%); primarily above diaphragm
  - Abdominal involvement uncommon: likely to involve only liver, spleen, or kidneys
  - Cranial nerve involvement: rare
  - B-LL: firm mass in extremity, enlarged LN
- ALCL
  - Sites: mediastinum, bone, inguinal nodes, skin
  - Bone marrow and CNS involvement: rare at diagnosis

DIFFERENTIAL DIAGNOSIS

- Abdominal mass (see chapter)
  - Newborn: hydronephrosis, renal cysts, Wilms tumor, or neuroblastoma
  - Older children: constipation, full bladder, hamartoma, hemangioma, cysts, leukemic or lymphomatous involvement of the liver and/or spleen, Wilms tumor, or neuroblastoma
- Mediastinal mass (see "Mediastinal Mass" chapter)
  - Anterior: masses of thymic origin, teratomas, angiomas, lipomas, or thyroid tumors
  - Middle: metastatic or infectious lesions involving the LNs, pericardial or bronchogenic cysts, esophageal lesions, or hernias
  - Posterior: neurogenic tumors (e.g., neuroblastoma, ganglioneuroma, neurofibroma), enterogenous cysts, thoracic meningocele, or hernias

DIAGNOSTIC TESTS & INTERPRETATION

A diagnosis needs to be made expeditiously, as pediatric lymphomas generally have a rapid growth rate.

- Bone marrow aspirate and biopsy may establish the diagnosis without further testing.
- Fluid from ascites in patients with abdominal disease or pleural fluid should be obtained for cytology, immunophenotyping, and cytogenetics.
- Fine-needle aspirate or biopsy of an enlarged LN

Initial Tests (screening, lab, imaging)

- CBC with differential
- Liver and renal function studies
- Tumor lysis labs: serum lactate dehydrogenase (LDH), potassium, calcium, phosphate, uric acid
- Ascitic, CSF, or pleural fluid
  - Cytology
  - Immunophenotyping
  - Cytogenetics
- Abdominal ultrasound
- Chest radiographs: posteroanterior and lateral
- CT scan of chest, abdomen, and pelvis
- PET/CT scan
- MRI (especially for bone involvement)

Diagnostic Procedures/Other
- Adequate fine needle aspiration or excisional biopsy
- Bone marrow aspirate and biopsy
- Lumbar puncture with CSF cytology

ALERT
Recumbent positioning, sedation, or positive pressure ventilation may lead to catastrophic respiratory or cardiovascular collapse in patients with partial compromise due to a mediastinal mass. Imaging of airway and consultation with anesthesia, surgeons, and critical care specialists should be obtained prior to any sedation. Procedures may need to be done with local anesthesia only.

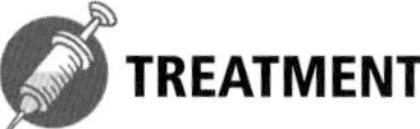

TREATMENT

GENERAL MEASURES
- Pathologic diagnosis, site, and extent of disease determine therapy.
- A multidisciplinary approach is imperative to ensure the best therapy.
- Patients should be enrolled on clinical trials whenever possible.
- Prechemotherapy management
  - Tumor lysis can be present even before initiation of chemotherapy.
  - Allopurinol, hydration, and alkalinization of urine to promote uric acid excretion; may use rasburicase for uric acid >8 mg/dL
  - Monitor uric acid, BUN, calcium, creatinine, potassium, and phosphate levels closely.
  - Consider fertility preservation prior to start of chemotherapy.
- Duration: mature B-cell lymphomas and ALCL, 1 to 8 months; LL, 24 months

MEDICATION
- Chemotherapy
  - Histology and stage determine therapy.
  - Because of a high conversion rate of lymphomas to leukemias, prophylactic CNS treatment is given (except in patients with totally excised intra-abdominal tumor); drugs: cyclophosphamide, vincristine, methotrexate (IV and intrathecal [IT]), prednisone, dexamethasone, daunorubicin, asparaginase, cytarabine, thioguanine, hydrocortisone, doxorubicin, mercaptopurine, etoposide, vinblastine
  - ALCL: crizotinib (a kinase inhibitor that blocks NPM-ALK fusion protein activity)
  - Common side effects: hair loss, myelosuppression with transfusions required, nausea/vomiting
- Immunotherapy
  - Rituximab
    - A chimeric monoclonal antibody to the CD20 antigen, which is almost universally expressed in B-cell NHL
    - Few overlapping side effects with the combination of rituximab and conventional chemotherapeutic agents
  - Brentuximab vedotin
    - Antibody drug conjugate to CD30 that is expressed on all ALCL; currently in clinical trials in children
  - Chimeric antigen receptor T cells (CAR-T)
    - Patient's own T cells are genetically modified to recognize CD19 or other cell surface epitope on malignant cells.
    - Efficacy has been shown in pediatric acute lymphoblastic leukemia and in adult DLBCL.
    - Efficacy in pediatric NHL unknown
- Management of relapse
  - Relapse indicates extremely poor prognosis.
  - No uniform approach to rescue therapy; different chemotherapy and immunotherapy combinations may induce a new response.
  - For patients with chemosensitive relapse, salvage therapy followed by high-dose therapy with stem cell support

ADDITIONAL THERAPIES
Radiotherapy
- Adds no therapeutic benefit in children with limited disease; may be indicated in mediastinal DLBCL
- Used occasionally as emergent treatment for SVC obstruction or CNS or testicular involvement
- Cranial radiotherapy given for CNS-positive children with LL
- Increases short- and long-term toxicity

SURGERY/OTHER PROCEDURES
- Avoid extensive surgery in patients with NHL.
- Performed in mature B-cell NHL if total resection can be achieved
- Additional indications: intussusception, intestinal perforation, suspected appendicitis, or serious GI bleeding

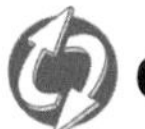

ONGOING CARE

FOLLOW-UP RECOMMENDATIONS
- Patient monitoring weekly to monthly with CBC and physical examination
- Radiologic imaging at intervals during and off therapy

Patient Monitoring
Late effects from therapy:
- Cardiomyopathy from anthracyclines
- Impaired reproductive function or infertility from alkylating agents or radiation
- Second malignant neoplasms from etoposide and alkylators
- Psychological consequences of severe illness

PROGNOSIS
- Important prognostic factors for outcome include tumor burden at presentation.
- Favorable
  - Stages I and II with primary site head and neck (nonparameningeal), peripheral nodes, or abdomen (≥90% 2-year survival)
  - Burkitt: >90% 2-year survival
- Less favorable
  - Stage III or IV disease; ALCL, LL
  - Parameningeal stage II
  - Stage IV with CNS involvement
  - Incomplete initial remission within 2 months (50–80% 2-year survival)

COMPLICATIONS
- Tumor lysis syndrome
  - Combination of hyperuricemia, hyperkalemia, and hyperphosphatemia with hypocalcemia, resulting in uric acid nephropathy that leads to renal failure
- GI obstruction, perforation, bleeding, intussusception
- Inferior vena cava obstruction and venous thromboembolism
- Neurologic (e.g., paraplegia, increased intracranial pressure)
- SVC syndrome and SMS: associated with LL that invade the thymus and nodes surrounding the vena cava and airways
- Massive pleural effusion
- Cardiac tamponade or arrhythmia

ADDITIONAL READING

- Abramson SJ, Price AP. Imaging of pediatric lymphomas. *Radiol Clin North Am*. 2008;46(2):313–338.
- Bollard CM, Lim MS, Gross TG; for COG Non-Hodgkin Lymphoma Committee. Children's Oncology Group's 2013 blueprint for research: non-Hodgkin lymphoma. *Pediatr Blood Cancer*. 2013;60(6):979–984.
- Childhood Non-Hodgkin Lymphoma Treatment (PDQ®) Cancer Information Summaries [Internet]. Bethesda, MD: National Cancer Institute (US); 2002–2017. https://www.ncbi.nlm.nih.gov/books/NBK65738/. Accessed April 29, 2018.
- Hochberg J, Waxman IM, Kelly KM, et al. Adolescent non-Hodgkin lymphoma and Hodgkin lymphoma: state of the science. *Br J Haematol*. 2009;144(1):24–40.
- Lange J, Lenz G, Burkhardt B. Mature aggressive B-cell lymphoma across age groups—molecular advances and therapeutic implications. *Expert Rev Hematol*. 2017;10(2):123–135.

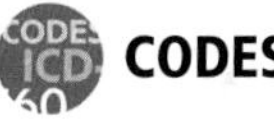

CODES

ICD10
- C85.90 Non-Hodgkin lymphoma, unspecified, unspecified site
- C85.10 Unspecified B-cell lymphoma, unspecified site
- C83.70 Burkitt lymphoma, unspecified site

FAQ
- Q: Did I do something to cause this?
- A: No. Most cases are sporadic and not associated with diet, underlying immune dysfunction, or viral illness.
- Q: Is this contagious?
- A: No. Siblings may have slightly higher inherent risk than the general population, but they are not at risk from the affected child.

NONTUBERCULOUS MYCOBACTERIAL INFECTIONS (ATYPICAL MYCOBACTERIAL INFECTIONS)

Yalda Serena Dastmalchi, MD • Rebecca Schein, MD

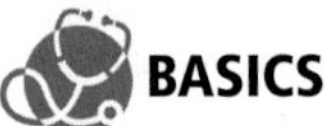

BASICS

DESCRIPTION

Nontuberculous mycobacteria (NTMB) are mycobacteria other than the *Mycobacterium tuberculosis* complex bacteria (*M. tuberculosis, Mycobacterium africanum, Mycobacterium bovis, Mycobacterium canettii*, and *Mycobacterium microti*) or *Mycobacterium leprae* capable of causing disease in humans.

- NTMB are classified based on growth rate in culture media as "rapid" or "slow" growers.
- Runyon classification was used priorly to classify NTMB and still may be referenced in literature.
- Disease from these infections most commonly presents as cervical lymphadenitis in children.
  - Pulmonary, disseminated skin or soft tissue diseases are other possible forms of NTMB infections present in adolescents.
- NTMB's biofilm-forming capabilities within aqueous environments contributes not only to its transmission but also to its increased difficulty of eradication.
- NTMB may also be referred to as mycobacteria other than tuberculosis (MOTT).

EPIDEMIOLOGY

- NTMB are ubiquitous in nature and may be found in soil, food, water, and animals.
  - Both fresh and tap water sources are NTMB reservoirs as well with the later serving as the most common source for humans.
- Although more than 130 species of mycobacteria have been identified, not all have been shown to cause disease in humans.
- Each species has a different level of virulence, and many species are associated with specific reservoirs or geographic areas. For example, *Mycobacterium marinum* is found in fish tanks and *Mycobacterium malmoense* is found in Northern Europe.
- Health care–related infections can occur, typically due to rapid-growing *Mycobacterium abscessus* or *Mycobacterium fortuitum*.
- NTMB can gain entry through a person's skin via various modes of exposure.
  - Some examples include following a pedicure, punch biopsies, surgical procedure, tattoos, injections, or piercing as well as from an open or contaminated wound.

RISK FACTORS

- Factors that are associated with an increased risk of NTMB disease are as follow:
  - Cystic fibrosis
  - Primary ciliary dyskinesia
  - Immune deficiency, especially HIV
  - Tympanostomy tubes
  - Foreign bodies or medical hardware
  - Interleukin-12 receptor deficiency
  - Interferon-γ receptor defects
  - Immunosuppressive therapies
- Factors that are associated with a decreased risk of NTMB disease are as follows:
  - Bacillus Calmette–Guérin (BCG) vaccination
    - Children vaccinated with BCG have shown a decreased risk of *Mycobacterium avium* complex (MAC) cervical adenitis.

GENERAL PREVENTION

- Discourage cleaning of open or contaminated wound with tap water.
- Recommended sterilization guidelines followed for disinfection of surgical equipment

PATHOPHYSIOLOGY

- Dirty wounds and breaks in oral, respiratory, or gastrointestinal mucosa are the common portals of entry.
- Infection is usually localized near the inoculation site and related regional lymph nodes.
- No evidence of person-to-person spread

ETIOLOGY

- Rapid growers include the *M. fortuitum* and *Mycobacterium chelonae/abscessus* groups. These rapid growers show significant growth on culture media in 3 to 7 days.
- Slow-growing mycobacteria, such *as* MAC and *Mycobacterium kansasii*, take >7 days and typically 4 to 6 weeks to grow in culture.
- Cervical adenitis is the most common presentation in healthy children 1 to 5 years of age. In the United States, 80% of these cases are due to *M. avium-intracellulare* (MAI).
- In healthy adults, pulmonary disease is the most common illness, typically caused by MAI, *M. kansasii, Mycobacterium xenopi*, or *M. malmoense*.
- Other presentations may include skin and soft tissue infections, bone and joint infections, chronic ear infections, catheter-associated infections, and pneumonia.
- Disseminated disease is seen primarily with MAI in patients with advanced HIV.

COMMONLY ASSOCIATED CONDITIONS

- Coexisting primary or structural lung disease
- Scoliosis
- Pectus excavatum
- Diabetes mellitus

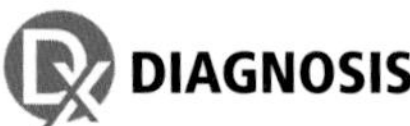

DIAGNOSIS

HISTORY

- Travel history and area of residence
- Fever history and systemic complaints
- Length of symptoms: Longer history is characteristic.
- Water and animal exposures
- Trauma history
- Recent surgery or hardware

PHYSICAL EXAM

- Lymphadenitis is typically gradually growing, unilateral, and minimally tender with possible rupture and sinus tract formation.
  - The submandibular followed by the preauricular lymph nodes are primarily affected.
  - Typically affects the toddler age group
- Skin disease is usually an ulcer, a localized cellulitis, a draining abscess, or a persistent nodule.
  - Nodules of a violet coloration may be noted over the pathogen's cutaneous entry point.
- Pulmonary disease may be associated with cough, fever, weight loss, and fatigue.
  - Mediastinal and hilar lymphadenopathy are common.
  - Lung findings are nonspecific.
- Otitis media in children with tympanostomy tubes presents with chronic drainage unresponsive to antibiotics.
- Disseminated disease is rare; findings include fever, night sweats, abdominal pain, and wasting.

DIFFERENTIAL DIAGNOSIS

- *M. tuberculosis* complex
- Dimorphic fungi: *Histoplasma capsulatum*, *Coccidioides* species, *Blastomyces dermatitidis*, *Sporothrix schenckii*
- Malignancy typically leukemia/lymphoma
- *Bartonella henselae*: cat-scratch disease
- Viral or bacterial adenitis
- Congenital neck mass or cyst

DIAGNOSTIC TESTS & INTERPRETATION

- Definitive diagnosis requires isolation of NTMB in culture.
- Special media and laboratory facilities are required.
- Contamination of nonsterile sites can occur and may require two or more cultures to confirm diagnosis.
- Any growth from a draining wound is clinically significant the majority of the time.
- A tuberculin skin test may be positive as cross-reactivity occurs but is not diagnostic.
- PCR for identification of specific NTMB is becoming more readily available and may facilitate quicker diagnosis.

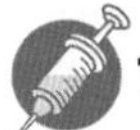

TREATMENT

Treatment is variable depending on the site of infection and the specific mycobacterium isolated. In general, complete surgical excision of infected lymph nodes is curative.

MEDICATION

- MAI is treated orally with a macrolide (clarithromycin or azithromycin) plus ethambutol or rifampin. Azithromycin is used as prophylaxis in patients with AIDS.
- Other slow growers such as *M. kansasii*, *M. marinum*, and *Mycobacterium ulcerans* are treated with rifampin-based regimens in combination with ethambutol, macrolides, trimethoprim-sulfamethoxazole, doxycycline, and/or aminoglycosides.
- For rapid growers (*M. fortuitum*, *M. abscessus*, and *M. chelonae*), serious diseases are treated intravenously with an aminoglycoside plus meropenem or cefoxitin depending on susceptibilities. Milder disease or subsequent oral therapy is treated with clarithromycin, doxycycline, trimethoprim-sulfamethoxazole, or ciprofloxacin based on susceptibility testing.
- Combination therapy is indicated in immunocompromised hosts.

SURGERY/OTHER PROCEDURES

- Isolated lymphadenitis is treated with complete surgical excision. Typically, antimicrobials are not beneficial in this situation.
  - Incision and drainage not recommended as a treatment option due to persistent wound drainage after such procedures
  - If adolescent experiences incomplete resection or recurrence following surgery, use of clarithromycin or azithromycin in addition to ethambutol, rifampin, or rifabutin may be considered.
- Any infected hardware should be removed and serious localized disease debrided.

ONGOING CARE

FOLLOW-UP RECOMMENDATIONS

- Medical treatment is typically for a minimum of 3 to 6 months.
- Follow-up should last 1 year after completion of therapy.

PATIENT EDUCATION

- Chemoprophylaxis for patients with CD4 count <50 cells/μL
- Avoid tap water contamination of central lines.

PROGNOSIS

For localized disease and adenitis, prognosis is excellent.

COMPLICATIONS

- Chronic draining wounds can occur and treatment is typically long-term antimicrobials in combination with surgical debridement.
- Disseminated disease—occurs in immunocompromised patients

ADDITIONAL READING

- American Academy of Pediatrics. Diseases caused by nontuberculous mycobacteria. In: Kimberlin DW, Brady MT, Jackson MA, et al, eds. *Red Book: 2015 Report of the Committee on Infectious Diseases*. Itasca, IL: American Academy of Pediatrics; 2015:831–839.
- Cruz AT, Ong LT, Starke JR. Mycobacterial infections in Texas children: a 5-year case series. *Pediatr Infect Dis J*. 2010;29(8):772–774.
- Griffith DE, Aksamit T, Brown-Elliott BA, et al; for ATS Mycobacterial Diseases Subcommittee, American Thoracic Society, Infectious Disease Society of America. An official ATS/IDSA statement: diagnosis, treatment, and prevention of nontuberculous mycobacterial diseases. *Am J Respir Crit Care Med*. 2007;175(4):367–416.
- Hypolite T, Grant-Kels JM, Chirch LM, et al. Nontuberculous mycobacterial infections: a potential complication of cosmetic procedures. *Int J Womens Dermatol*. 2015;1(1): 51–54.
- Iseman MD, Buschman DL, Ackerson LM. Pectus excavatum and scoliosis. Thoracic anomalies associated with pulmonary disease caused by *Mycobacterium avium* complex. *Am Rev Respir Dis*. 1991;144(4):914–916.
- Lindeboom JA, Kuijper EJ, Bruijnesteijn van Coppenraet ES, et al. Surgical excision versus antibiotic treatment for nontuberculous mycobacterial cervicofacial lymphadenitis in children: a multicenter, randomized, controlled trial. *Clin Infect Dis*. 2007;44(8):1057–1064.
- Starke JR. Management of nontuberculous mycobacterial cervical adenitis. *Pediatr Infect Dis J*. 2000;19(7):674–675.

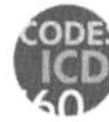

CODES

ICD10

- A31.9 Mycobacterial infection, unspecified
- A31.1 Cutaneous mycobacterial infection
- A31.8 Other mycobacterial infections

FAQ

- Q: When should I worry about NTMB?
- A: NTMB should be on the differential for any child with persistent lymphadenitis or a chronically draining wound.
- Q: When should NTMB be considered as a cause of lymphadenitis?
- A: Most lymphadenitis is due to an acute viral or bacterial infection and will improve with time or respond to a short course of antibiotics. NTMB should be suspected in a healthy toddler (age 1 to 5 years) who presents with a subacute or chronic lymphadenitis. Other considerations should include cat-scratch disease, malignancy, and tuberculosis.
- Q: If infected node is excised, should I treat with antibiotics?
- A: Surgical excision is the treatment of choice of NTMB adenitis. Most studies show that antibiotics are not beneficial after complete surgical excision.

NOSEBLEEDS (EPISTAXIS)

Bethlehem Abebe-Wolpaw, MD

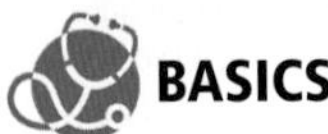

BASICS

DESCRIPTION

- Epistaxis: bleeding from the nostril, nasal cavity, or nasopharynx
- Classified as either anterior or posterior
  - Anterior epistaxis is from the anterior nasal septum, usually is venous from an area known as Kiesselbach plexus.
  - Posterior epistaxis occurs through the nasopharynx typically arising from the sphenopalatine artery.

EPIDEMIOLOGY

- At least 75% of children will experience at least one episode of epistaxis, commonly occurs between the ages of 3 and 8 years.
- Rarely seen in children <2 years
- Up to 9% of children may have recurrent epistaxis, but the majority grows out of it.
- Anterior epistaxis more common in children
- Occurs more frequently in the cold winter months when there is low humidity and when upper respiratory tract infections are more frequent
- Dry air from indoor heating likely increases the incidence during winter months.

RISK FACTORS

- Mucosal dryness (also known as rhinitis sicca) is a frequent precursor to episodes of epistaxis as are upper respiratory tract infections.
- Children with allergic rhinitis are more prone to epistaxis because the nasal mucosa is more friable and inflamed.
- Children with recurrent epistaxis are more likely to have nasal colonization with *Staphylococcus aureus*.

GENERAL PREVENTION

- Keeping nasal passages moist with the use of humidifiers, saline nasal sprays and emollients (e.g., Vaseline®) help reduce mucosal irritation, dryness and thus friability.
- Ensure fingernails are short and nasal trauma (i.e., nose picking, foreign body) is discouraged.
- Use appropriate protective athletic equipment to avoid trauma.

PATHOPHYSIOLOGY

- Blood supply to the nasal cavity contains multiple anastomoses that originate from both the internal and external carotid arteries.
- Kiesselbach plexus is located under a thin mucosal lining in the anteroinferior aspect of the nasal septum and is the most common site of bleeding in children.
- The thin mucosal surface of the nasal septum and the lateral nasal walls are fragile and thus prone to inflammation, drying, and excoriation.

ETIOLOGY

- Most episodes of epistaxis in the younger age group are due to digital trauma as well as local inflammation:
  - Upper respiratory tract infections, allergic rhinitis, rhinosinusitis, nasal vestibulitis, colonization of nasal cavity with *S. aureus*.
  - Digital trauma, facial trauma, foreign body insertion, inhalants/irritants (intranasal corticosteroids, cocaine, heroin)
  - <2 years, must consider trauma (nonaccidental or accidental) or a serious systemic disease (leukemia)
- In the pediatric population, epistaxis is less likely a sign of systemic illness:
  - Acquired or congenital bleeding disorders: von Willebrand disease, hemophilia, idiopathic thrombocytopenic purpura, hematologic malignancies
  - Coagulopathy secondary to systemic infection, hepatic disease, renal failure, antiplatelet agents (i.e., aspirin), NSAID use
- Local structural/vascular abnormalities
  - Septal deviation, rhinitis sicca, spurs, nasal polyps
  - Telangiectasias (Osler-Weber-Rendu disease also known as hereditary hemorrhagic telangiectasia [HHT])
  - Nasal neoplasms: juvenile angiofibroma (consider in adolescent boys), papillomas, hemangiomas

COMMONLY ASSOCIATED CONDITIONS

- Frequently associated with viral upper respiratory tract infections, allergic rhinitis, digital trauma
- >90% of children with epistaxis do not have an underlying systemic cause.

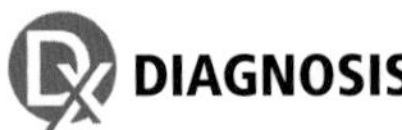

DIAGNOSIS

HISTORY

- Frequency and duration
- Laterality of the nosebleed
- Local trauma (nose picking, foreign body)
- Upper respiratory tract infection
- Allergies
- Obstruction
- Discharge
- Medications or drug use
  - NSAIDs, aspirin, anticoagulants, cocaine, intranasal corticosteroids
  - Alternative medicines: garlic, ginkgo, ginseng
- Personal or family history of bleeding disorders, easy bruising, significant bleeding from minor wounds
- Menstrual history, if applicable

PHYSICAL EXAM

- Vital signs
- Use a good light source to perform direct visualization and inspection of nasal mucosa, nasal cavity, nasopharynx, and oropharynx.
  - In children >6 years, exam of the nose may be facilitated by application of a topical vasoconstricting agent (e.g., oxymetazoline or phenylephrine) with a topical anesthetic agent (e.g., lidocaine) to enhance view and slow any current bleeding.
- General exam with particular attention to the skin (bruising, petechiae, purpura, icterus, pallor), lymph nodes, liver, and spleen

DIFFERENTIAL DIAGNOSIS

Epistaxis is a common occurrence in healthy children unless <2 years. A detailed history and physical exam should help identify children with systemic causes for epistaxis, including bleeding disorders and malignancies.

DIAGNOSTIC TESTS & INTERPRETATION

- Most episodes are minor and do not require intervention or medical evaluation.
- If history and physical exam are reassuring, diagnostic evaluation is not warranted in healthy children with easily controlled anterior epistaxis.
- If suspicious findings on history or physical exam or child has chronic recurrent epistaxis, laboratory evaluation including complete blood count with platelet count and coagulation panel are indicated.
- Children <2 years presenting with epistaxis should have laboratory evaluation and consideration of trauma (nonaccidental and accidental) as part of their evaluation.
- Studies suggest that 5–10% of children with chronic recurrent nosebleeds may have mild undiagnosed von Willebrand disease so consider laboratory evaluation to include plasma von Willebrand factor (VWF) antigen, VWF activity, and factor VIII activity.
- Persistent unilateral bleeding warrants nasal endoscopy to rule out neoplasm.

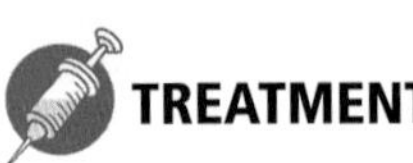

TREATMENT

GENERAL MEASURES

- Acute
  - Elevate the head forward.
  - Direct pressure, applied by gently squeezing the nostrils for 5 to 15 minutes, is usually sufficient to stop most nosebleeds.
  - Vasoconstricting agents intranasally (1% phenylephrine, 0.05% oxymetazoline, 1:1,000 epinephrine, or 1–5% cocaine) will help reduce bleeding as well as improve visualization and can be used in children >6 years.

- Absorbable hemostatic agents, such as Floseal, a bovine-derived gelatin matrix, can also be used for refractory bleeding.
- Epistaxis generates distress and anxiety among patients and parents so parental reassurance is an important, but often neglected, aspect of therapy.
- Chronic
  - Aggressive moisturization including nasal saline spray, emollients such as Vaseline® applied with a Q-tip®, and humidified air are important for prevention.
  - Avoidance of trauma such as repetitive digital manipulation

ISSUES FOR REFERRAL

Otorhinolaryngologic consultation may be needed for:

- Severe nosebleeds
- Unstable hemodynamics
- Significant facial trauma
- Suspicion for nonaccidental trauma
- Posterior bleeding
- Difficulty identifying bleeding source
- When surgery or embolization is required

SURGERY/OTHER PROCEDURES

- Silver nitrate cautery
  - Can be performed selectively on prominent vasculature on the anterior septum known as Kiesselbach plexus when the site of bleeding is clearly visible.
  - This procedure should only be done unilaterally to avoid the risk of septal perforation. If adequate time is given for healing (4 to 6 weeks), cautery can be performed on the contralateral side.
  - If silver nitrate cautery is undertaken, 75% is more effective and causes less pain than 95% silver nitrate.
  - Antiseptic nasal cream (chlorhexidine-neomycin) may provide added benefit after successfully performing silver nitrate cautery.
- For persistent bleeding despite silver nitrate cautery, more powerful cauterization such as Bovie electrocautery can be performed.
  - This procedure is generally not tolerated in patients without general anesthesia.
  - Intraoperative bipolar electrocautery is less likely to result in recurrent epistaxis compared to those treated with silver nitrate within 2 years of treatment. Benefit is lost 2 years after treatment. Major disadvantage is the need for general anesthesia.
- In rare cases that do not respond to cautery, vessel embolization by an interventional radiologist or surgical vessel ligation may be required.
- Nasal packing is rarely indicated in children.

ONGOING CARE

FOLLOW-UP RECOMMENDATIONS

- Nosebleeds are easily controlled and self-limited in most cases.
- Referral to an otorhinolaryngologist is indicated for patients with specific local abnormalities, such as polyps, tumors, or vascular malformations, or severe nosebleeds, recurrent nosebleeds, and/or posteriorly located nosebleeds.
- Identification of systemic illness may require referral to the appropriate specialist (i.e., hematologist).

Patient Monitoring

- Blood clots in the nasopharynx should be removed to enhance visualization.
- Failure to detect a posterior location within the nasal cavity as the source of bleeding may interfere with measures to control bleeding.
- If nasal packing is needed, it is essential to examine the oropharynx to confirm adequate hemostasis.
- Absorbable-type packing should be used, if required, in patients with bleeding disorders. Removable packings are prone to rebleeding on removal.
- Impregnation of nasal packings with antibiotic ointment reduces the risk of toxic shock syndrome.

PATIENT EDUCATION

- Families should be given instructions in basic first aid and instructed on appropriate way to control nosebleeds.
- Minor insults, such as sneezing or minor trauma, may cause nosebleeds to recur.

PROGNOSIS

- Uncomplicated epistaxis is most often self-limited and resolves with simple direct pressure techniques.
- Refractory or recurrent epistaxis may require more specialized techniques by an otorhinolaryngologist.

COMPLICATIONS

- Usually uncomplicated
- Rare complications: significant blood loss, hemodynamic instability, airway obstruction, aspiration, and vomiting

ADDITIONAL READING

- Béquignon E, Teissier N, Gauthier A, et al. Emergency department care of childhood epistaxis. *Emerg Med J.* 2017;34(8):543–548.
- Davies K, Batra K, Mehanna R, et al. Pediatric epistaxis: epidemiology, management & impact on quality of life. *Int J Pediatr Otorhinolaryngol.* 2014;78(8):1294–1297.
- DeLaroche AM, Tigchelaar H, Kannikeswaran N. A rare but important entity: epistaxis in infants. *J Emerg Med.* 2017;52(1):89–92.
- Johnson N, Faria J, Behar P. A comparison of bipolar electrocautery and chemical cautery for control of pediatric recurrent anterior epistaxis. *Otolaryngol Head Neck Surg.* 2015;153(5):851–856.
- Kasperek ZA, Pollock GF. Epistaxis: an overview. *Emerg Med Clin North Am.* 2013;31(2):443–454.
- Melia L, McGarry GW. Epistaxis: update on management. *Curr Opin Otolaryngol Head Neck Surg.* 2011;19(1):30–35.
- Patel N, Maddalozzo J, Billings KR. An update on management of pediatric epistaxis. *Int J Pediatr Otorhinolaryngol.* 2014;78(8):1400–1404.
- Qureishi A, Burton MJ. Interventions for recurrent idiopathic epistaxis (nosebleeds) in children. *Cochrane Database Syst Rev.* 2012;(9):CD004461.

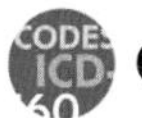

CODES

ICD10

R04.0 Epistaxis

FAQ

- Q: How should I explain to a child to stop a nosebleed that occurs at home?
- A: The child or parent should apply pressure by compressing the lateral cartilaginous surface of the external nose together for at least 5 minutes. It is important to keep the head elevated and forward but not hyperextended to avoid aspiration of the blood. This can be accomplished either by sitting or standing while bending forward slightly at the waist. Avoid lying down or tilting the head backward. Avoid checking prior to 5 minutes to see if bleeding has ceased.
- Q: When should I work-up a patient to ensure there is not an underlying systemic cause for epistaxis?
- A: Most children do not require laboratory evaluation. If the history or physical is concerning or the child has chronic recurrent epistaxis, initial laboratory evaluation may include complete blood count with platelets and coagulation panel. In addition, you can consider checking for von Willebrand disease because data suggests that up to 5–10% of children with chronic recurrent epistaxis may have a mild form of the disease. Children <2 years warrant a workup given how rare it is to have epistaxis <2 years.

OBESITY

Susma Vaidya, MD, MPH • Nazrat Mirza, MD, ScD

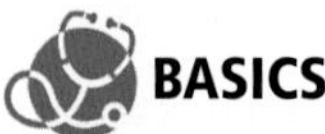

BASICS

DESCRIPTION

Excess adiposity correlates closely with increased health risk for multiple medical and psychological disorders. Body mass index (BMI) is an easily obtained clinical measure to assess for increased body fat and concomitant health risks. BMI is calculated as weight in kilograms divided by height in meters squared. In children, age- and sex-specific percentiles define obesity.

- Children ≥2 years of age
  - BMI 85–94%: overweight
  - BMI 95–98% or BMI ≥30 kg/m^2: obese
  - BMI ≥99%: severe obesity. Severe obesity has also been defined as BMI ≥120% of the 95th%.
- BMI reference standards are not available for children <2 years of age. In this age group, overweight is defined as weight-for-length ≥95% for age and sex.

EPIDEMIOLOGY

Prevalence

National Health and Nutrition Examination Survey (NHANES), 2011 to 2014 data:

- 2 to 19 years of age: 17%
- 2 to 5 years of age: 8.9% obese
- 6 to 11 years of age: 17.5% obese
- 12 to 19 years of age: 20.5% obese
- No difference in prevalence by gender
- Highest rates among black and Hispanic youth
- Severe obesity: 5.8%

RISK FACTORS

- Obesity is most often a multifactorial condition with several risk factors:
  - Parental obesity
  - Maternal obesity in pregnancy
  - Maternal history of gestational diabetes
  - Intrauterine growth retardation
  - Rapid weight gain in first 6 months of life
  - Low socioeconomic status
- Genetics
  - Obesity with developmental delay and/or dysmorphic features: Bardet- Biedl syndrome, Cohen syndrome, Prader-Willi syndrome
- Endocrine
  - Obesity with poor linear growth: Cushing syndrome, hypothyroidism

GENERAL PREVENTION

- Encourage exclusive breastfeeding at prenatal visit and support breastfeeding throughout the 1st year of life.
- In formula-fed infants, watch for signs of overfeeding and rapid weight gain in 1st year of life. Educate families on the difference between hunger and oral suck reflex. Avoid rice cereal in the bottle.
- Recognize parental obesity as a significant risk.
- Incorporate early nutrition and activity counseling.
- Careful attention to BMI (and weight-for-length for children <2 years) with intensive counseling for children crossing percentiles
- Stress importance of portion size and nutrient-rich foods (fruits and vegetables) as infants transition to a solid diet
- Daily physical activity; limit screen time.

PATHOPHYSIOLOGY

Complex interaction between genetics, hormones, environment, and behavior

- Short-term energy regulation: adaptation of meal size in response to energy needs. Hypothalamic neurons modulate sensitivity of nucleus tractus solitarius (NTS) neurons to satiety signals adjusting for changes in body fat mass.
- Long-term energy regulation: Hypothalamus senses and integrates energy balance signals including hormones such as insulin, leptin, ghrelin, and nutrients such as fatty acids, amino acids, and glucose.
  - Leptin
    - A negative feedback regulator—plays an important role in energy homeostasis.
    - Communicates to hypothalamus changes in energy balance and fuel stored as fat
    - Increased fat mass results in increased leptin signaling which limits energy intake and supports energy expenditure.
    - Decreased leptin promotes increased food intake, positive energy balance, and fat accumulation.
  - Ghrelin
    - Derived from the stomach, it is the only known peripherally acting orexigenic hormone. It stimulates appetite.
    - All other gut-derived hormones are anorectic and limit food, optimize digestion and absorption, and avoid overfeeding.
  - Adiponectin
    - Insulin sensitizing, anti-inflammatory, and antiatherogenic
    - Increased visceral fat results in reduced levels of adiponectin and increased proinflammatory milieu leading to insulin resistance and endothelial dysfunction. This predisposes to metabolic syndrome, diabetes, and atherosclerosis.

ETIOLOGY

Energy imbalance

- Excessive caloric intake: calorie-rich foods and beverages consumed preferentially over nutrient-rich foods. Portion size is inappropriately large for age.
- Low-caloric expenditure: excessive sedentary time with TV, computers, video games, and handheld devices; limited daily physical activity

COMMONLY ASSOCIATED CONDITIONS

- Endocrine
  - Type 2 diabetes mellitus
  - Metabolic syndrome
  - Polycystic ovarian syndrome (PCOS)
  - Low vitamin D level
- Cardiovascular
  - Hypertension
  - Dyslipidemia
- Respiratory
  - Sleep apnea
  - Asthma
- Gastrointestinal
  - Nonalcoholic fatty liver disease (NAFLD)
  - Nonalcoholic steatohepatitis (NASH)
  - Gallstones
  - Gastroesophageal reflux (GER)
- Orthopedic
  - Slipped capital femoral epiphysis (SCFE)
  - Blount disease (tibial bowing)
- Skin conditions
  - Acanthosis nigricans
  - Hirsutism
- CNS: pseudotumor cerebri
- Psychiatric
  - Binge-eating disorder
  - Mood disorder: anxiety and depression
  - Low self-esteem

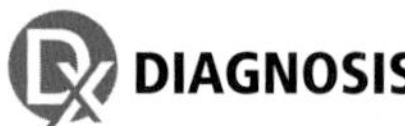

DIAGNOSIS

HISTORY

- Birth history: birth weight, maternal gestational weight gain, gestational diabetes
- Growth history: weight trajectory and age where percentiles were crossed
- Medical and/or social stressors
- Medical history: asthma, medications, obesity comorbidities
- Motivation
  - Parental concern and desire for change and willingness to modify family's behavior
  - Child's concern and motivation (as age appropriate)
- Family history
  - Obesity
  - Diabetes
  - Cardiovascular disease
  - Dyslipidemia
  - Eating disorders
- Dietary history
  - Sugar-sweetened beverages consumed
  - Frequency of fruits and vegetables
  - Frequency and type of snack foods
  - Frequency of fast food
- Eating behavior
  - Family meals
  - TV viewing during meals
  - Recognition of satiety
  - Binge eating with or without loss of control
- Physical activity
  - Total screen time including phone and handheld devices
  - Duration, intensity, and frequency of physical activity
- Sleep duration and pattern
- Previous attempts at weight loss
  - Medication use (prescribed and over-the-counter [OTC])
  - Weight loss programs
- Review of systems
  - Headache: pseudotumor cerebri
  - Snoring/pauses in breathing, daytime somnolence: obstructive sleep apnea (OSA)
  - Abdominal pain: reflux, gallstones

- Joint pains: hip pain (SCFE)
- Social isolation, emotional eating, behavior difficulties: depression
- Skin color changes (acanthosis nigricans)
- Irregular menses/amenorrhea: PCOS
- Polydipsia, polyuria: diabetes

PHYSICAL EXAM

- Anthropometrics: weight, height, BMI, and BMI percentile
- Blood pressure for age, sex, and height percentile
- General physical findings suggestive of endocrine or genetic condition
  - Short stature
  - Dysmorphic facies
  - Developmental delay
- Head, ears, eyes, nose, throat (HEENT)
  - Papilledema
  - Tonsillar hypertrophy and narrow pharyngeal opening
- Cardiopulmonary
  - Poor aeration, wheezing
  - Heart murmur
- Abdomen
  - Hepatomegaly
  - Abdominal pain
- Genitourinary: Tanner stage
- Musculoskeletal
  - Range of motion at hips
  - Abnormal curvature of lower leg
  - Limp
- Skin
  - Acanthosis nigricans
  - Hirsutism
  - Striae
  - Hidradenitis suppurativa
- Psychological
  - Mood: Assess for evidence of depression.
  - Bullying, social isolation

DIAGNOSTIC TESTS & INTERPRETATION

Initial Tests (screening, lab, imaging)

- BMI 85th to 94th percentile without risk factor: fasting lipid profile
- BMI 85th to 94th percentile age ≥10 years with risk factors: fasting lipid profile, ALT, AST, fasting glucose
- BMI ≥95th percentile age ≥10 years: fasting lipid profile, ALT, AST, fasting glucose, other tests as indicated by health risks

Diagnostic Procedures/Other

- Polysomnogram: history of snoring with pauses in breathing, narrow pharyngeal airway, or tonsillar hypertrophy (OSA)
- AP and frog-leg views of the hips: knee pain or hip pain, limitation or pain with internal rotation of hip (SCFE)
- Knee and lower extremity radiographs: abnormal curvature of the lower extremities, especially asymmetry (Blount disease)
- Echocardiogram: hypertension (LVH)
- Ambulatory blood pressure monitoring: elevated blood pressure/hypertension
- Abdominal ultrasound: elevated LFTs or abdominal pain (NAFLD, gallstones)
- Head CT: headache and papilledema on ocular exam (pseudotumor cerebri)

Test Interpretation

Abnormal results

- Lipid panel: Obese children often have elevated LDL and triglycerides and low HDL.
  - High LDL ≥130 mg/dL
  - High triglyceride:
    - 0 to 9 years old ≥100 mg/dL
    - 10 to 19 years old ≥130 mg/dL
  - Low HDL <40 mg/dL
- ALT value >2 times normal or >60 IU/L merits gastroenterology consult.
- Fasting glucose ≥126 mg/dL or random glucose ≥200 mg/dL supports a diagnosis of diabetes and warrants endocrinology consult.
  - HgbA1c ≥6.5% diagnostic of diabetes
  - Fasting glucose ≥100 mg/dL or HgbA1c ≥5.7% and ≤6.4% indicates impaired fasting glucose and a prediabetic state.

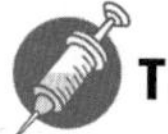

TREATMENT

GENERAL MEASURES

- Prevention and treatment include healthy lifestyle behavior: Goal is to start with small incremental changes in lifestyle.
  - Eliminate consumption of sugar-sweetened beverages including juice and sports drinks.
  - Encourage nonfat milk and water.
  - Increase servings of nutrient-rich foods such as fruits and vegetables with every meal and for snacks.
  - Avoid skipping meals.
  - Reduce eating out or takeout foods.
  - Encourage family meals.
  - Educate families about portion size as soon as solids are started and in early childhood.
  - Advise 1 hour per day of moderate physical activity.
  - Limit screen time to <2 hours a day.
- Weight loss goals
  - Weight maintenance may be appropriate in younger children, as BMI will improve with increase in height.
  - Older children and severely obese children should aim to lose up to 2 lb a week.

MEDICATION

Orlistat: an intestinal lipase inhibitor that is the only United States Food and Drug Administration (FDA)-approved medication for obesity in children ≥12 years

- Limits nutrient absorption
- Side effects: abdominal pain, oily stools, flatulence, fat-soluble vitamin deficiencies; self-limited success, poor compliance
- 5% weight loss, similar to placebo
- Not recommended for routine use

SURGERY/OTHER PROCEDURES

Bariatric surgery indication

- Adolescents with a BMI ≥40 kg/m^2 or BMI ≥35 kg/m^2 with concomitant comorbidities such as diabetes and hypertension
- Lack of sustained weight loss on supervised weight-reduction program for 6 to 12 months
- Physical, emotional, and cognitive maturity

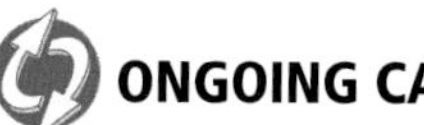

ONGOING CARE

FOLLOW-UP RECOMMENDATIONS

- Assess BMI monthly and achievement of dietary and physical activity goals.
- Follow patient more frequently with weight gain and/or refer for nutrition counseling or a weight management program at a tertiary care center.
- Refer to subspecialist with diagnosis of accompanying comorbidities.

PROGNOSIS

- Success is greater in younger children and children with lower BMIs.
- Better success if whole family is involved in healthy lifestyle change
- Better success with self-monitoring
- Less success with severe obesity
- Poor prognosis if untreated mental health issues and/or lack of motivation

ADDITIONAL READING

- Barlow SE; for Expert Committee. Expert committee recommendations regarding the prevention, assessment, and treatment of child and adolescent overweight and obesity: summary report. *Pediatrics*. 2007;120(Suppl 4):S164–S192.
- Daniels SR. Complications of obesity in children and adolescents. *Int J Obes (Lond)*. 2009;33(Suppl 1): S60–S65.
- Ogden CL, Carroll MD, Fryar CD, et al. Prevalence of obesity among adults and youth: United States, 2011–2014. *NCHS Data Brief*. 2015;(219):1–8.
- Spear BA, Barlow SE, Ervin C, et al. Recommendations for treatment of child and adolescent overweight and obesity. *Pediatrics*. 2007;120(Suppl 4): S254–S288.

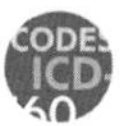

CODES

ICD10

- E66.9 Obesity, unspecified
- E66.3 Overweight
- R63.5 Abnormal Weight Gain

FAQ

- Q: How do I broach such a sensitive topic with families?
- A: Review growth charts at every well-child visit and discuss any concerning increase in BMI. Describe in terms of healthy weight and the need to avoid comorbidities which become more likely with increasing BMI.
- Q: How do I counsel a family not interested in making lifestyle changes?
- A: Discuss the risk that an unhealthy BMI poses for the child. Describe small simple changes the family can make to alleviate this risk. Avoid assigning blame. Abnormal lab values may motivate a family to make changes.

OBSESSIVE-COMPULSIVE DISORDER

Holly H. Martin, MD • Manisha Punwani, MD

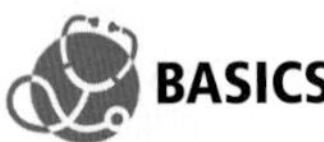

BASICS

DESCRIPTION

- Obsessive-compulsive disorder (OCD) is a psychiatric illness manifested by recurrent and persistent obsessions and compulsions.
- Obsessions are defined as intrusive, unwanted thoughts, images, or impulses that cause the patient distress, and attempts are made to ignore or suppress these thoughts.
- Compulsions are repetitive actions that patient feels driven to perform in response to an obsession. The behaviors are aimed at preventing or reducing anxiety or distress or preventing some dreaded event or situation.
  - It is not necessary that children recognize these thoughts or behaviors to be excessive or unreasonable.
  - The obsessions or compulsions cause marked distress, are time consuming (>1 hour daily), and cause impairment in daily functioning.
  - Not attributed to physiologic effects of a substance nor are explained by another mental disorder
  - Specified as "with good or fair insight," "with poor insight," "with absent insight/delusional beliefs," or tic-related

EPIDEMIOLOGY

- OCD can start at any time from preschool to adulthood.
- Although OCD does occur at earlier ages, there are generally two age ranges when OCD first appears. The first range is between ages 10 and 12 years and the second between the late teens and early adulthood.

RISK FACTORS

- Familial heritability pattern
- Moderate genetic component based on twin studies
- Acute streptococcal infection (pediatric autoimmune neuropsychiatric disorders associated with streptococcal infections [PANDAS])

COMMONLY ASSOCIATED CONDITIONS

- Depression
- Anxiety disorders
- Tourette syndrome
- Trichotillomania

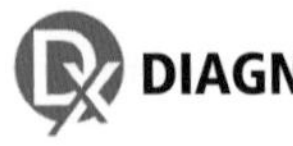

DIAGNOSIS

HISTORY

- The diagnostic evaluation should entail gathering data through separate interviews with the child/adolescent and the parents.
- Current symptoms should be elicited within attention to severity, duration, and level of functional impairment.
- Core symptoms should be elicited concerning the content of obsessions and the nature of compulsions. These are most frequently checking behaviors, repetition rituals, or a focus on symmetry and organization.
- Sensitivity in assessing violent or sexually intrusive thoughts is necessary, as children may be uncomfortable disclosing these.
- Compulsions may manifest in physical action or in mental repetition.
- Assess the amount of functional impairment by estimating the time spent occupied by obsession and compulsions and how it interferes with their daily lives.
- Explore their level of insight into the irrationality of the symptoms. Diagnostically, children do not have to recognize the symptoms to be excessive. Assess any parental accommodation of the ritualized behaviors, such as excessive cleaning.
- Determine if the onset was acute, severe, and temporally associated with symptoms of a streptococcal infection.

PHYSICAL EXAM

No pertinent findings

DIFFERENTIAL DIAGNOSIS

- Pervasive developmental disorders
- Delusional disorder
- Obsessive-compulsive personality disorder
- Body dysmorphic disorder
- Anorexia nervosa
- Trichotillomania
- Tourette syndrome
- Schizophrenia
- Sydenham chorea
- PANDAS

DIAGNOSTIC TESTS & INTERPRETATION

Initial Tests (screening, lab, imaging)

- No pathognomonic laboratory findings
- If onset is acute, severe, and associated with symptoms of a streptococcal infection, consider obtaining an ASO titer.

Diagnostic Procedures/Other

Diagnostic scales: Children's Yale-Brown Obsessive Compulsive Scale (CY-BOCS)

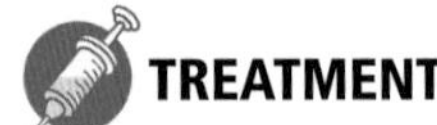

TREATMENT

GENERAL MEASURES

There are two types of treatment for OCD, psychosocial treatment and pharmacotherapy.

- Cognitive behavioral therapy (CBT) is recommended as the most effective and well-studied psychosocial treatment:
  - Selective serotonin reuptake inhibitors (SSRIs) are the 1st-line agents for medication management.
  - Start intervention with CBT alone and add medication if treatment response is limited.
- Emphasis is placed on graduated exposure with response prevention.
- Parental education is an important aspect of treatment adherence.

- Pitfalls
  - Failing to use appropriate psychosocial treatments especially school-based modifications
  - Not identifying the extent of the functional impairment
- It is important to recognize
  - The child's fear of the internal thoughts he or she is having
  - The parents' desire to have a "normal" child and thus their tendency to minimize/reassure the child who has concerns

MEDICATION

- SSRIs (1st-line) once-daily oral dosing; initiate one half the starting dose for children with anxiety disorders:
  - Fluoxetine (Prozac®) (10 to 60 mg)
  - Sertraline (Zoloft®) (25 to 200 mg)
  - Fluvoxamine (Luvox®) (25 to 200 mg)
  - Side effects include GI upset, headaches, dizziness, and agitation.

ALERT

A black box warning by the United States Food and Drug Administration (FDA) indicates that all antidepressants may increase suicidal thinking and behavior in children and adolescents.

- Close monitoring is recommended (see next section).
- Tricyclic antidepressants (TCAs) are 2nd-line agents:
  - Clomipramine (Anafranil®) (25 to 250 mg PO once daily)
  - Side effects include dizziness, xerostomia, blurred vision, postural hypotension, tachycardia, sedation, and constipation; rare sudden cardiac death (get EKG prior to initiating med)

ONGOING CARE

FOLLOW-UP RECOMMENDATIONS

Patient Monitoring

- Monitoring of response to psychosocial treatment should be performed routinely every 2 to 3 months.
- If medication is initiated, close monitoring on a weekly basis is recommended for the first 4 weeks, followed by monthly monitoring.
- CBT is performed on a weekly or twice weekly regimen.
- Monitoring of any emerging comorbidities is suggested.
- The obsessions may change or evolve over time.

PROGNOSIS

- OCD is a chronic condition. Treatments have been demonstrated to show significant response, but permanent remission of symptoms is rare.
- Childhood onset is a poor prognostic indicator.

ADDITIONAL READING

- Coskun M, Zoroglu S, Ozturk M. Phenomenology, psychiatric comorbidity and family history in referred preschool children with obsessive-compulsive disorder. *Child Adolesc Psychiatry Ment Health*. 2012;6(1):36.
- O'Neill J, Gorbis E, Feusner JD, et al. Effects of intensive cognitive-behavioral therapy on cingulate neurochemistry in obsessive-compulsive disorder. *J Psychiatr Res*. 2013;47(4):494–504.
- Pediatric OCD Treatment Study Team. Cognitive-behavior therapy, sertraline, and their combination for children and adolescents with obsessive-compulsive disorder: the Pediatric OCD Treatment Study (POTS) randomized controlled trial. *JAMA*. 2004;292(16):1969–1976.
- Robinson S, Turner C, Heyman I, et al. The feasibility and acceptability of a cognitive-behavioural self-help intervention for adolescents with obsessive-compulsive disorder. *Behav Cogn Psychother*. 2013;41(1):117–122.

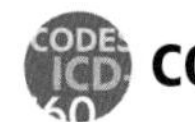

CODES

ICD10

- F42 Obsessive-compulsive disorder
- F63.3 Trichotillomania
- R46.81 Obsessive-compulsive behavior

FAQ

- Q: Is OCD inherited?
- A: Although no specific genes for OCD have been identified, there appears to be familial relationship to its inheritance.
- Q: What causes OCD?
- A: There is no proven cause of OCD. Research suggests that OCD involves problems in communication between the front part of the brain (the orbital cortex) and deeper structures (the basal ganglia).
- Q: Is there a cure?
- A: OCD is a chronic condition, but effective treatments are available.

OMPHALITIS

Jessica P. Clarke-Pounder, MD • W. Christopher Golden, MD

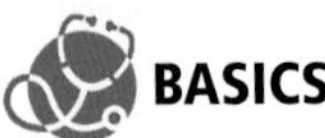

BASICS

DESCRIPTION

Omphalitis, a bacterial infection of the umbilical stump, begins in the neonatal period as a superficial cellulitis but may track along umbilical vessels and progress to systemic illness.

EPIDEMIOLOGY

- Episodes of omphalitis are usually sporadic.
- Mean age of onset is 5 to 9 days in term infants and 3 to 5 days in preterm infants.
- Omphalitis is rare in developed countries, with an incidence of approximately 1 out of 1,000 live births, but in developing countries, incidence may be upward of 8–22% of infants, depending on risk factors.

RISK FACTORS

- Low birth weight
- Prior umbilical catheterization
- Septic delivery
- Home birth
- Prolonged rupture of membranes
- Chorioamnionitis/funisitis

GENERAL PREVENTION

- There are multiple methods used for umbilical cord care, including dry cord care, triple dye, 4% chlorhexidine, and 70% alcohol solution.
- Clean, dry cord care is recommended by the American Academy of Pediatrics (AAP) and World Health Organization (WHO) for infants born in a hospital setting in developed countries.
- Aseptic delivery and hygienic cord care, including cutting the cord in a sterile manner (with gloves and sterile instruments), are key to preventing infection.
- There is significant evidence to support the use of topical 4% chlorhexidine in infants born at home in settings with high neonatal mortality (>30 deaths per 1,000 live births).
- There is no evidence that application of an antiseptic to the umbilical cord is better than clean, dry cord care in a hospital setting.

PATHOPHYSIOLOGY

- Once the umbilical cord is cut after birth, the stump dries and falls of within 5 to 15 days.
- The umbilical stump is colonized by microorganisms soon after birth, both pathogenic and nonpathogenic.
- Pathogenic bacteria may invade the umbilical stump, leading to omphalitis.
  - The type of organisms present varies depending on the birth setting and quality of cord care.
  - In high-resource settings, gram-positive organisms are most likely, and gram-negative organisms are more common in low-resource settings.
- Omphalitis may present in varying severity:
  - Funisitis/umbilical discharge—abnormal-appearing umbilical cord and purulent, malodorous discharge
  - Omphalitis with associated cellulitis—periumbilical erythema and tenderness in addition to cord discharge
  - Omphalitis with systemic signs of infection
  - Omphalitis with necrotizing fasciitis—crepitus, bullae, and evidence of involvement of superficial and deep fascia, often associated with septic shock
- Unhygienic cord care, as well as the application of harmful substances to the umbilical cord, can lead to an increased incidence of omphalitis in developing countries.
- Established aerobic bacterial infection, necrotic tissue, and poor blood supply facilitate the growth of anaerobic organisms.

ETIOLOGY

- The most common causative organisms are gram-positive cocci, including *Staphylococcus aureus* (MSSA and methicillin-resistant *S. aureus* [MRSA]), group A and group B streptococci.
- Gram-negative pathogens include *Escherichia coli*, *Klebsiella pneumoniae*, *Pseudomonas* species, and *Proteus mirabilis*.
- Gram-positive organisms predominate; however, antistaphylococcal cord care has led to an increase in colonization and infection with gram-negative organisms.
- Anaerobic bacteria, including *Bacteroides fragilis* and *Clostridium perfringens*, are most likely in cases complicated by necrotizing fasciitis or myonecrosis.
- *Clostridium tetani* and *Clostridium sordellii* are seen primarily in developing countries when unhygienic instruments may be used to cut the cord and/or cow dung is used in cord care.

COMMONLY ASSOCIATED CONDITIONS

- Leukocyte adhesion deficiency (LAD)
  - Omphalitis may be the initial manifestation of one of the LADs.
  - LADs are rare, autosomal recessive immunologic disorders affecting leukocyte adhesion to blood vessel walls.
  - Cord separation requires the influx of leukocytes; therefore, this deficiency causes delayed separation and can cause concomitant omphalitis.
  - Infants also may present with leukocytosis, absence of pus formation, impaired wound healing, and recurrent infections localized to the skin and mucosal surfaces.
  - Treatment involves prompt recognition of infection and use of appropriate antibiotics. Severe cases may need hematopoietic stem cell transplantation.
- Neutropenia
  - Omphalitis complicated by sepsis can be associated with neutropenia.
  - Other syndromes of neonatal neutropenia may present initially with omphalitis.
    - Neonatal alloimmune neutropenia: Maternal IgG antibodies cross the placenta and cause immune-mediated destruction of fetal neutrophils bearing antigens differing from mother's.
    - Other causes of neutropenia: autoimmune neutropenias, X-linked agammaglobulinemia, hyper-IgM immunodeficiency syndromes, HIV, glycogen storage disease type IB, or disorders of amino acid metabolism
- Anatomic abnormalities
  - Patent urachus:
    - The urachus, a tubular structure connecting the bladder to the umbilicus, should obliterate by the fifth gestational month.
    - If it remains patent, a continuous, significant amount of urine can drain from the umbilicus.
  - Persistent omphalomesenteric duct:
    - Congenital malformation where a communication exists between the umbilicus and the gut
    - Drainage consists of intestinal secretions.
  - Excessive granulation tissue:
    - Results from delayed healing of cord stump
    - Drainage is serosanguinous and pink.
- Considerations in preterm infants:
  - Preterm infants are more susceptible secondary to immature immune defenses (including the skin) and possible umbilical catheterization.
  - These infants are more likely to present with omphalitis at an earlier age and with low neutrophil counts.

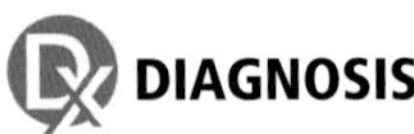

DIAGNOSIS

HISTORY

- Identify risk factors such as prolonged membrane rupture and septic delivery.
- Symptoms such as fever, irritability, lethargy, respiratory distress, or feeding intolerance may indicate systemic dissemination of the infection.
- A history of urine or stool discharge from the umbilicus suggests an underlying anatomic abnormality.
- Family history may reveal individuals with metabolic disorders or recurrent infections.

PHYSICAL EXAM

- Varies with the extent of disease
- Localized infection
  - Abdominal tenderness
  - Periumbilical edema and erythema
  - Purulent or malodorous discharge from the umbilical stump
- Indications of more extensive local disease, such as necrotizing fasciitis or myonecrosis:
  - Periumbilical ecchymoses or gangrene
  - Abdominal wall crepitus
  - Progression of cellulitis despite antimicrobial therapy
- Signs of systemic disease are nonspecific and include thermodysregulation and evidence of multiorgan dysfunction:
  - Fever or temperature instability
  - Tachycardia, hypotension, poor perfusion
  - Respiratory distress
  - Abdominal distention, diminished bowel sounds
  - Cyanosis, petechiae, jaundice
  - Lethargy, hypotonia

DIFFERENTIAL DIAGNOSIS

- The characteristic clinical picture of omphalitis allows diagnosis on clinical grounds.
- Determine the presence of associated complications, such as systemic infection, abscess, necrotizing fasciitis, or myonecrosis.
- Consider an underlying immunologic or metabolic disorder.

DIAGNOSTIC TESTS & INTERPRETATION

Initial Tests (screening, lab, imaging)

- Umbilical stump Gram stain and culture for aerobic and anaerobic organisms
  - Identify potential organisms and antimicrobial susceptibility patterns. Cultures of umbilical discharge may reflect only colonization of the stump and are not proof of an etiologic role in the underlying process. If myonecrosis is suspected, muscle specimens should be cultured.
- Blood culture
  - Identifies systemic dissemination of infection
- CBC with differential
  - Identifies neutropenia or leukocytosis
  - An immature-to-total neutrophil ratio >0.2 is suggestive of systemic infection.
  - Thrombocytopenia may be present.
- D-dimers, prothrombin time, partial thromboplastin time, and fibrinogen
  - Indicated for sepsis or disseminated intravascular coagulation
- Radiographs (case dependent)
  - Abdominal radiographs
    - Intestinal ileus may indicate systemic spread of infection; free air, portal venous air, or intramural air requires immediate surgical consultation.
  - Abdominal CT
    - Confirms involvement of fascia and muscle and delineates the extent of infection
    - May identify anatomic abnormalities
  - Voiding cystourethrogram
    - Reveals patent urachus

Diagnostic Procedures/Other

Lumbar puncture: for any neonate with signs of focal/systemic illness or a positive blood culture

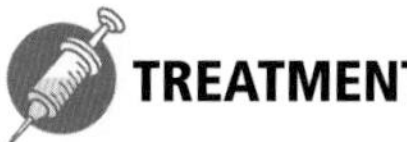

TREATMENT

GENERAL MEASURES

Antibiotics and supportive care

MEDICATION

Empiric coverage

- Antistaphylococcal agent (oxacillin, vancomycin) plus an aminoglycoside (e.g., gentamicin) or cefepime
- Consider local antibiotic susceptibility patterns when choosing antibiotics, paying particular attention to hospital and community incidence of MRSA.
- Add anaerobic coverage (e.g., metronidazole or clindamycin) with necrotizing fasciitis or myonecrosis.
- Duration of therapy is typically 7 to 14 days.

ISSUES FOR REFERRAL

If systemic illness is present, infants may need referral to a tertiary care center and consultation by a pediatric infectious disease specialist or pediatric surgeon.

SURGERY/OTHER PROCEDURES

- Early and complete surgical debridement of affected tissue and muscle is important.
- Delay in diagnosis or surgical intervention allows local progression of infection and worsening systemic toxicity.

ADMISSION, INPATIENT, AND NURSING CONSIDERATIONS

Emergency care: Immediate evaluation, IV antimicrobial therapy, and supportive care are essential to survival.

ONGOING CARE

FOLLOW-UP RECOMMENDATIONS

Infants developing associated portal venous thrombosis require follow-up for complications owing to portal hypertension.

PROGNOSIS

- The outcome of infants with uncomplicated omphalitis is generally good.
- The mortality rate among all infants with omphalitis, including those who develop complications, is 7–15%.
- The mortality rate is significantly higher (38–87%) with necrotizing fasciitis or myonecrosis.

COMPLICATIONS

- Much more common in resource-poor settings
- Systemic sepsis (up to 13% of cases)
  - Evidenced by temperature instability, abdominal distension, respiratory distress, and/or hypotension
- Abscess
  - Retroperitoneal, pelvic, cutaneous, hepatic
- Peritoneal complications
  - Peritonitis can occur if the umbilical vein is involved in infection and is evidenced by poor feeding, bilious vomiting, and signs of systemic illness.
  - Portal vein thrombosis or hepatic abscess can occur with transmission via the umbilical vein.
  - Adhesive small bowel obstruction may be seen as a late complication.
- Myonecrosis
  - Infectious involvement of the muscle
  - Requires surgical treatment with resection
- Necrotizing fasciitis (8–16% of cases)
  - Bacterial infection of the subcutaneous fat and superficial and deep fascia
  - Characterized by rapidly spreading infection and systemic toxicity
- Evisceration
  - Spontaneous evisceration of bowel through the umbilical stump may develop, requiring surgical evaluation and treatment.

ADDITIONAL READING

- Ameh E, Nmadu P. Major complications of omphalitis in neonates and infants. *Pediatr Surg Int*. 2002;18(5–6):413–416.
- Anderson J, Philip A. Management of the umbilical cord: care regimens, colonization, infection, and separation. *Neoreviews*. 2004;5:155–163.
- Evens K, George J, Angst D, et al. Does umbilical cord care in preterm infants influence cord bacterial colonization or detachment? *J Perinatol*. 2004;24(2):100–104.
- Fraser N, Davies BW, Cusack J. Neonatal omphalitis: a review of its serious complications. *Acta Paediatr*. 2006;95(5):519–522.
- Gras-Le Guen C, Caille A, Launay E, et al. Dry care versus antiseptics for umbilical cord care: a cluster randomized trial. *Pediatrics*. 2017;139(1):e20161857.
- Güvenç H, Aygün AD, Yaşar F, et al. Omphalitis in term and preterm appropriate for gestational age and small for gestational age infants. *J Trop Pediatr*. 1997;43(6):368–372.
- Imdad A, Bautista R, Senen K, et al. Umbilical cord antiseptics for preventing sepsis and death among newborns. *Cochrane Database Syst Rev*. 2013;(5):CD008635.
- Osrin D, Colbourn T. No reason to change WHO guidelines on cleansing the umbilical cord. *Lancet Glob Health*. 2016;4(11):e766–e768.
- Stewart D, Benitz W; for Committee on Fetus and Newborn. Umbilical cord care in the newborn infant. *Pediatrics*. 2016;138(3):e20162149.
- van de Vijver E, van den Berg TK, Kuijpers TW. Leukocyte adhesion deficiencies. *Hematol Oncol Clin North Am*. 2013;27(1):101–116.

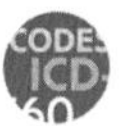

CODES

ICD10

- P38.9 Omphalitis without hemorrhage
- B95.0 Streptococcus, group A, causing diseases classd elswhr
- 95.8 Unsp staphylococcus as the cause of diseases classd elswhr

FAQ

- Q: Do all infants require antiseptic treatment of the umbilical cord?
- A: No. Infants born in a hospital setting can be treated with clean, dry cord care. In developing countries or in a circumstance of septic birth (i.e., unplanned home birth), 4% chlorhexidine solution may be used for umbilical cord antisepsis.
- Q: Do infants need to be hospitalized with omphalitis?
- A: Yes. Infants require treatment with IV antibiotics. If not treated appropriately, the infection may spread systemically, causing significant morbidity and mortality.
- Q: What are the warning signs of more severe infection?
- A: Periumbilical tenderness, temperature instability, respiratory distress, abdominal crepitus, or bullae may indicate systemic spread of infection beyond the umbilical stump.

OPIOID INTOXICATION

Pamela D. Fazzio, MD • Jeannine Del Pizzo, MD

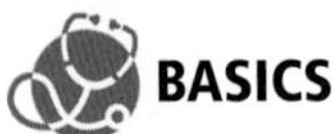

BASICS

DESCRIPTION

- Opioids are a group of natural and synthetic substances used both illicitly and for prescription analgesia.
- Opioids include:
  - Opiates—naturally occurring in the opium poppy (e.g., codeine, morphine)
  - Semisynthetic derivatives (e.g., hydromorphone, nalbuphine, oxycodone, heroin)
  - Synthetic compounds (e.g., fentanyl, meperidine, methadone, tramadol, and various "designer" opioids)
- Complications of opioid use include acute intoxication, dependence/abuse, and withdrawal.
- Opioid use disorder is a *DSM-5* diagnosis.
- Please see related chapter, "Neonatal Abstinence Syndrome," for special considerations of opioid intoxication and withdrawal in the neonate.

EPIDEMIOLOGY

- Prescription opioids are the most commonly abused and lethal opioids in the United States.
- Poison control centers received reports of 188,468 prescription opioid exposures among children aged <20 years from 2000 to 2015.
- Children who suffer an opioid overdose are more likely to have a mother who was prescribed opioids and antidepressants.
- Hospitalizations for methadone intoxications and adolescent heroin intoxications are rising.
- Strongest risk factor for heroin addiction is addiction to prescription opioids.
  - 45% of heroin users are addicted to prescription opioids.
  - Prescription opiate-drug era associated with shorter time from first illicit drug use to injection

Incidence

- Between 1997 and 2012, in children aged 1 to 19 years, hospitalizations for opioid intoxication rose to 3.71 per 100,000 children, representing a 165% increase; 1.3% of these children died during hospitalization.
- In 2013, 169,000 people aged ≥12 years used heroin for the first time within the previous year.

Prevalence

- Difficult to estimate, based on National Survey on Drug Use and Health (NSDUH) data
- 3.8 million people in the United States aged ≥12 years reported past month misuse of a prescription pain medication in 2015.

PATHOPHYSIOLOGY

- Exposure:
  - Young children with opioid intoxication typically ingest opioids found in the home.
  - Adolescents most commonly become intoxicated through intentional ingestion for recreational use or intent to self-harm.

ALERT
Round-the-clock dosing of opioids can produce opioid dependence within 5 days.

- Routes for use: oral, intranasal, inhalation, or injection (IV, IM, or SC)
- Well absorbed from gastrointestinal (GI) tract, nasal mucosa, pulmonary capillaries, and injection sites
- Metabolized by liver
- Receptor types
  - Mu (a.k.a., OP3, MOP)
    - Location: CNS, GI tract, and sensory nerve endings
    - Effect: analgesia, euphoria, respiratory depression, physical dependence, GI dysmotility, miosis, pruritus, bradycardia
  - Kappa (a.k.a., OP2, KOP)
    - Location: CNS
    - Effect: analgesia, miosis, diuresis, dysphoria
  - Delta (a.k.a., OP1, DOP)
    - Location: CNS
    - Effect: spinal analgesia, modulation of mu receptors/dopaminergic neurons
- Metabolites excreted by kidneys
- Death:
  - Typically, from respiratory depression
  - Anaphylaxis (rare)

DIAGNOSIS

HISTORY

- Neonate: maternal history of drug use
- Young child: opioids present in home
- Adolescents:
  - Recreational drug use
  - Depression/suicidality
  - Involvement with law enforcement (ingestion as attempt to conceal drugs)

PHYSICAL EXAM

- Frequent use: nasal septum damage, scarred veins (track marks)
- Intoxication/overdose
  - Classic toxidrome: depressed level of consciousness, decreased respiratory effort, miotic pupils
  - Other symptoms: decreased bowel sounds, flushing, pruritus, muscle rigidity/rhabdomyolysis
  - More severe overdose: bradycardia, hypotension, hypothermia, noncardiogenic pulmonary edema
- Withdrawal
  - Early signs (8 to 24 hours): craving, anxiety, restlessness, insomnia, yawning, rhinorrhea, lacrimation, diaphoresis, increased bowel sounds, mydriasis
  - Late signs (up to 3 days): tremor, muscle spasms, piloerection, vomiting, diarrhea, hypertension (from agitation) or hypotension (from vomiting and diarrhea causing volume depletion), tachycardia, seizures

DIFFERENTIAL DIAGNOSIS

- Presume coinjection from other substance abuse and/or impure opioids (e.g., heroin laced with benign or toxic substances)
- Other pharmacologic agents
  - Clonidine, sedative hypnotics, barbiturates, antipsychotics, γ-hydroxybutyrate
- Organophosphate poisoning
- Hypoglycemia
- Hypothermia
- Hypoxia
- Sepsis
- Heat stroke
- Intussusception
- Trauma: intracranial hemorrhage or spinal cord injury

DIAGNOSTIC TESTS & INTERPRETATION

Initial Tests (screening, lab, imaging)

- Intoxication and withdrawal are clinical diagnoses.
- Therapy should not be withheld pending laboratory results.

ALERT
Consultation with a toxicologist is recommended for assistance treating opioid intoxication or withdrawal:
- American Association of Poison Control Centers: (800) 222-1222

- Urine toxicology screen
  - Detects morphine and heroin metabolites
  - Typically detected for up to 4 days from exposure
- Serum toxicology screen for acetaminophen, salicylates, and alcohol levels, etc. Expect polydrug ingestion.
- Serum tests to rule out other causes if needed (e.g., glucose)
- Blood gas
- EKG (Methadone prolongs QTc.)
- Chest radiograph to evaluate for pulmonary edema
- Basic metabolic panel, CK, and urinalysis to evaluate for rhabdomyolysis
- Neonates: urine testing in neonates and mothers
- Meconium, hair, and cord blood testing have also been used.

TREATMENT

GENERAL MEASURES

Intoxication/overdose

- ABCDEs (airway, breathing, circulation, disability, exposure)
- Support respiratory failure with bag-mask ventilation and 100% FiO_2, escalate to intubation to protect airway as needed.
- Manage other vital sign derangements as indicated (e.g., crystalloid boluses for hypotension, warm blankets for hypothermia, etc.).
- Evaluate for other complications of opioid intoxication (see "Ongoing Care: Complications").

MEDICATION

- Intoxication/overdose
  - Naloxone (Narcan®), an opioid antagonist, is antidote.
    - Consider naloxone as diagnostic challenge.
    - Onset 1 minute when given IV, highly lipophilic, moves rapidly into CNS
    - Route of administration
      - IV preferred (can be given via an intraosseous needle)
      - Can also be administered intramuscularly, subcutaneously, intranasally, endotracheally
    - Dosing
      - 0.1 mg/kg IV; max dose is 2 mg.
      - If suspect dependence in an adolescent, start with lower dose (0.4-mg flat dose) to avoid iatrogenic withdrawal.
      - Dose may be repeated up to every 2 to 3 minutes and given as an infusion if needed.
    - Loses efficacy in 20 to 40 minutes
    - Main adverse effect is withdrawal syndrome in opioid-dependent patients.
    - Neonates: Use caution. Naloxone can precipitate seizures in opioid-dependent neonates.
- Withdrawal
  - Treatment depends on if withdrawal is from opioid discontinuation or administration of an opioid antagonist.

First Line

Methadone for withdrawal symptoms from opioid discontinuation. Methadone is not indicated in withdrawal from an opioid antagonist because opioids will not overcome the antagonist and may lead to later intoxication.

- Blocks euphoria and prevents withdrawal symptoms
- Patients generally treated in established methadone maintenance programs
- Breastfeeding is not recommended in mothers using heroin but is recommended during opioid-replacement treatment.
- Clonidine decreases withdrawal symptoms.
  - Hourly until symptoms resolve
  - Monitor for hypotension.

Second Line

- Benzodiazepines, antiemetics, antidiarrheals, and nonopioid pain medications such as NSAIDs are adjuncts.
- Consultation with a specialist is indicated for detoxification and rehabilitation programs.

ISSUES FOR REFERRAL

- Child protective services to assess safety of home, access to drugs, and possible abuse
- Referral to substance abuse program
- Mental health referral
- Consider referral for testing for HIV and hepatitis B and C if IV drug use.

ADMISSION, INPATIENT, AND NURSING CONSIDERATIONS

- Most patients with overdose, those that receive naloxone, and those that are suicidal will warrant hospitalization.
- Discuss observation time and management with poison control and/or toxicology.

ONGOING CARE

PROGNOSIS

- Intoxication/overdose
  - With adequate early treatment, patients with uncomplicated overdoses do well—key is to prevent respiratory arrest.
  - 33,000 deaths from opioids, including prescription opioids and heroin, in 2015 (record high)
- Withdrawal: Iatrogenic withdrawal (from an opioid antagonist) can be fatal.
- Addiction
  - Dependent on involvement in other risky behaviors (polydrug use, high-risk sexual practices, school failure, delinquency, etc.)
  - Longer treatment likely produces a better outcome.
  - Most relapses require lifetime of therapy.

COMPLICATIONS

- Intoxication/overdose
  - Respiratory arrest
  - Noncardiogenic pulmonary edema
  - CNS depression/coma
  - Hypotension
  - Aspiration pneumonia
  - Rhabdomyolysis (from lying immobile)
  - Trauma such as motor vehicle collision
  - High-risk sexual behavior and sexually transmitted infections (STIs)
  - Death
- Infection from IV opioid use: cellulitis or abscess at injection site, endocarditis, osteomyelitis, hepatitis, and HIV

ADDITIONAL READING

- Compton WM, Jones CM, Baldwin GT. Relationship between nonmedical prescription-opioid use and heroin use. *N Engl J Med*. 2016;374(2):154–163.
- Finkelstein Y, Macdonald EM, Gonzalez A. Overdose risk in young children of women prescribed opioids. *Pediatrics*. 2017;139(3):e20162887.
- Gaither JR, Leventhal JM, Ryan SA, et al. National trends in hospitalizations for opioid poisonings among children and adolescents, 1997 to 2012. *JAMA Pediatr*. 2016;170(12):1195–1201.
- Galinkin J, Koh JL; for Committee on Drugs, Section On Anesthesiology and Pain Medicine, American Academy of Pediatrics. Recognition and management of iatrogenically induced opioid dependence and withdrawal in children. *Pediatrics*. 2014;133(1):152–155.
- Jordan AE, Blackburn NA, Des Jarlais DC, et al. Past-year prevalence of prescription opioid misuse among those 11 to 30 years of age in the United States: a systematic review and meta-analysis. *J Subst Abuse Treat*. 2017;77:31–37.
- Substance Abuse and Mental Health Services Administration. *Results from the 2013 National Survey on Drug Use and Health: Summary of National Findings*. NSDUH Series H-48, HHS Publication No. (SMA) 14-4863. Rockville, MD: Substance Abuse and Mental Health Services Administration; 2014.

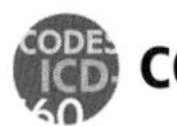

CODES

ICD10

- F11.929 Opioid use, unspecified with intoxication, unspecified
- F11.23 Opioid dependence with withdrawal
- P96.1 Neonatal w/drawal symp from matern use of drugs of addiction

FAQ

- Q: What causes false-positive and false-negative urine drug screens?
- A: Opiates are typically detected in the urine up to 1 to 4 days after exposure. A dilute sample decreases test sensitivity. Rifampin, fluoroquinolones, and poppy seeds can cause false-positive tests. Urine drug screens usually detect morphine (a metabolite of heroin and codeine) *not* synthetic and semisynthetic opioids.
- Q: What are "designer" opioids?
- A: "Designer" opioids are high potency synthetic opioids. Examples include α-methylfentanyl ("China White"), 1-methyl-4-phenyl-4-propionoxypiperidine (MPPP) ("new heroin" or "designer heroin"), and U-47700 ("pink" heroin).

OSTEOGENESIS IMPERFECTA

Eric T. Rush, MD, FAAP, FACMG

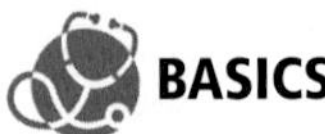

BASICS

DESCRIPTION

Osteogenesis imperfecta (OI) is a genetic disorder primarily affecting bones and connective tissues.

- Clinical severity variable and dependent in part on the nature of the molecular lesion
- Typical findings can include recurrent fracture, bone and/or spine deformities, short stature, blue or grey sclerae dentinogenesis imperfecta (DI), and joint hypermobility.

EPIDEMIOLOGY

Incidence

1 in 10,000 births

Prevalence

6 to 8:100,000 persons

RISK FACTORS

Genetics

- Most cases (~85%) are due to variants in genes encoding type I collagen, *COL1A1*, and *COL1A2* inherited in an autosomal dominant manner
- Traditionally, OI has been classified by clinical severity. The Sillence criteria are the most widely used, and they have been modified to accommodate expansion of phenotypically or genotypically distinct forms of OI. (Note: A second classification system from the International Consortium of Skeletal Dysplasia [ICSD] is also used and indicated in parentheses in the list of types below when relevant):
  - Type I (mild nondeforming OI): usually normal stature, fracture frequency is variable, and usually lessens after puberty. No bowing of long bones. Blue sclerae are frequent. Hearing loss is frequent, but hearing loss onset before adulthood is uncommon.
  - Type II (perinatally lethal OI): death in perinatal period due to pulmonary hypoplasia; intrauterine fractures, shortened long bones, and blue sclerae common
  - Type III (progressively deforming OI): severely shortened stature, severe deformities of long bones, prevalent vertebral fractures, scoliosis, chest deformities; characteristic triangular face
  - Type IV (common variable OI): DI common, short stature, bowing of long bones, vertebral fractures, scoliosis, and joint laxity. Patients are usually ambulatory.
- Other clinical forms of OI
  - Type V (OI with calcification of the interosseous membranes and/or hypertrophic callus): Patients frequently develop hyperplastic calluses in long bones after fracture causing tender, firm swellings over bones. Patients also will develop calcification in the interosseous membrane between the radius and ulna, which limits supination and pronation. Caused by variants in *IFITM5* gene; inherited in an autosomal dominant manner
  - Type VI: rhizomelic shortening of extremities with less prominent bowing than appreciated in other patients with moderate severity OI. Caused by variants in *SERPINF1* gene and inherited in an autosomal recessive manner; bone histology with a characteristic lamellar fish-scale appearance
  - Type VII/VIII/XI: moderate to lethal OI caused by variants in one of the three subunits of the prolyl hydroxylase enzyme encoded by *CRTAP*, *P3H1*, and *PPIB* genes and inherited in an autosomal recessive manner. These three OI types have a similar phenotype including prominent rhizomelic shortening, significant early fractures, and short stature.
  - Type X and XI: moderate to severe OI, which has been mostly seen in consanguineous families; due to defects in chaperone proteins, caused by variants in the *SERPINH1* or *FKBP10* genes and inherited in an autosomal recessive manner
  - Type XII: one case report with moderately severe disease from a consanguineous family; caused by homozygous deletion in the *SP7* gene
  - Type XIII: A few cases have been reported with generally severe disease; caused by variants in the *BMP1* gene and inherited in an autosomal recessive manner
  - Type XIV: described in several consanguineous families and appears to be of variable severity; caused by variants in the *TMEM38B* gene and inherited in an autosomal recessive manner
  - Type XV: moderate severity OI caused by variants in the *WNT1* gene; inherited in an autosomal recessive manner
  - Type XVI: described in a handful of families with variable severity of OI and caused by deletions in the *CREB3L1* gene. It is inherited in an autosomal recessive manner, but carriers can present with mild phenotype of blue sclerae and hypermobility.
  - Type XVII: described cases of moderate severity with multiple fractures but normal stature; caused by variants in the *SPARC* gene and inherited in an autosomal recessive manner

PATHOPHYSIOLOGY

- Truncating *COL1A1* mutations cause haploinsufficiency of the α-1 peptide causing a quantitative collagen defect resulting in type I OI.
- Missense mutations in *COL1A1* or *COL1A2* alter triple-helical collagen structure leading to abnormal collagen fibrils and result in types II, III, or IV OI.
- Recessive OI is caused by defects in genes whose products interact with type I collagen in several different fashions including posttranslational modification, cellular trafficking and chaperone, mineralization, and cellular fate.
- Osteoblasts: increased osteoblast cellularity; however, reduction in differentiated cells capable of making mineralized matrix
  - Decreased bone formation during remodeling
- Osteoclasts: increased osteoclast number to remove defective matrix
- The etiology of short stature is incompletely understood but is suggested to result from disruption of balance between bone formation and resorption, which is more pronounced during periods of rapid linear growth.

ETIOLOGY

- Abnormality of procollagen I production, modification, and extracellular trafficking
- Defect of osteoblast development resulting in collagen I insufficiency

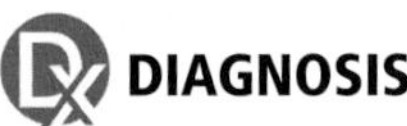

DIAGNOSIS

HISTORY

- Widely varied; may include recurrent fractures including fractures with little or no predisposing trauma
- May have positive family history. Proportion of people who have OI and have a family history is higher in mild compared to severe OI.

PHYSICAL EXAM

- Prenatal findings
  - Intrauterine and perinatal fractures, most common in moderate and severe forms
  - Limbs variably bowed and shortened
  - Undermineralization and compressibility of the skull (caput membranaceum)
  - Small thorax and pulmonary hypoplasia leads to respiratory insufficiency postnatally.
- Postnatal findings:
  - General: short stature of variable severity. Often, patients with type I OI will have normal stature but below expected for family height.
  - Facies: typically, macrocephaly with temporal bossing, pointed chin, premaxillary hypoplasia
  - Eyes: blue or grey sclerae in some patients. Absence of this feature should never be used, however, to exclude of OI as a diagnosis. Additionally, some normal babies will have blue/grey sclerae that lighten with age.
  - Ears: hearing loss common in adulthood and can be conductive, sensorineural, or mixed
  - Teeth: DI can be present. Deciduous teeth more severely affected than permanent teeth, enamel normal, teeth easily broken with secondary caries but not clear that there is an inherent risk of caries; malocclusion is also common and may be severe.
  - Spine and thorax: kyphoscoliosis, pectus carinatum or excavatum. Compression fractures are seen most frequently located in the midthoracic and lumbar region.
  - Pelvis: Protrusio acetabuli is common and can be associated with significant constipation.
  - Extremities: bowing of long bones, coxa vara, and joint hypermobility

DIFFERENTIAL DIAGNOSIS

- In utero
  - Hypophosphatasia
  - Thanatophoric dysplasia
  - Campomelic dysplasia
  - Achondrogenesis
  - Collagen II-opathies
- Infancy and childhood
  - Nonaccidental trauma
  - Juvenile idiopathic osteoporosis
  - Osteoporosis-pseudoglioma syndrome
  - Cole-Carpenter syndrome
  - Hajdu-Cheney syndrome
  - Bruck syndrome: Patients have congenital bone fragility, congenital joint contractures, and pterygia. Bruck syndrome is caused by variants in the *FKBP10* or *PLOD2* genes and is inherited in an autosomal recessive manner.
  - Hypophosphatasia
  - Immobilization
- Hyperplastic callus formation in OI type V may be confused with osteogenic sarcoma.

DIAGNOSTIC TESTS & INTERPRETATION

Initial Tests (screening, lab, imaging)

- Serum calcium and phosphorus levels
  - Normal
- Alkaline phosphatase
  - May be elevated after a fracture
- Type I collagen *N*-telopeptide normalized to urinary creatinine (uNTx/uCr) or other markers of bone resorption may correspond to severity of disease.
- Diagnosis typically confirmed by sequencing of genes implicated in OI by NGS (or Sanger sequencing if limited to *COL1A1/COL1A2*)
- Deletion/duplication analysis by MLPA or array-based platform important for some types of OI
- Biochemical collagen analysis on fibroblasts seldom required, less informative, and increasingly difficult to obtain
- Imaging
  - Bone mineral density (total body less head; lumbar spine): low for age
  - Plain radiographs
    - Skull
      - Wormian bones: detached portions of primary ossification centers in adjacent membranous bones; can be seen in other conditions
    - Spine
      - Scoliosis
      - "Codfish vertebrae" due to compression fractures
      - Atlantoaxial subluxation
      - Spondylolisthesis
    - Long bones
      - Fractures: varying stages of healing
      - Apparently low bone mineralization for age
      - Bowing deformity
      - Protrusio acetabuli
      - Popcorn calcifications, particularly in severe forms of OI

Diagnostic Procedures/Other

Once diagnosis is established

- Formal audiology assessment, although it is not clear what age serial audiometric assessment is required
- Dental evaluation if DI present
- Imaging for basilar invagination is indicated if symptomatic, but utility is unclear in asymptomatic patients.
- Bone densitometry by dual-energy x-ray absorptiometry (DEXA) at baseline is indicated, particularly if treatment with antiresorptive medications is contemplated.

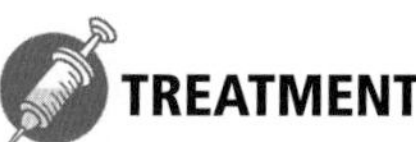

TREATMENT

GENERAL MEASURES

- Intramedullary rodding with or without osteotomies:
  - Often performed as early as 18 months of age, but timing depends on several considerations including size of the patient/bone size
  - Rehabilitation postsurgically is crucial to maximizing postsurgical function.
  - Correction of long bone bowing may improve mobility and likelihood of ambulation.
- Spinal deformities
  - Seen in ~90%
  - Management per orthopedics for monitoring/treatment of scoliosis
- Fracture treatment
  - Bone mineral density can decline after fracture while immobilized, particularly in weight-bearing bones.
  - Postfracture physiotherapy critical

MEDICATION

- Antiresorptive agents (bisphosphonates)
  - Widely used in clinical practice
  - Preponderance of evidence suggests that they improve bone mineral density, pain, and mobility.
  - Probably lessens fracture risk in children; improvement in fracture with treatment in adults with OI is uncertain.
  - Most common side effects: flu-like syndrome during initial treatment; hypocalcemia
  - Delayed osteotomy healing has been reported with some centers delaying treatment after osteotomy.
  - Long-term side effects unknown
  - Theoretically could be associated with atypical fractures and jaw osteonecrosis, although no cases reported in pediatric patients with OI
- Adequate calcium (varies with age) and vitamin D intake (to achieve serum 25[OH]D levels of 32 to 50 ng/mL)
- Anabolic agents (growth hormone, insulin-like growth factor 1 [IGF-1], parathyroid hormone [PTH]) are not considered routine treatment options.
- PTH (1 to 34) has black box warning for pediatric indications.

ADMISSION, INPATIENT, AND NURSING CONSIDERATIONS

Emergency care

- For unstable fractures, such as femur fractures
- For control of pain in fractures, such as with compression fractures

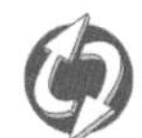

ONGOING CARE

FOLLOW-UP RECOMMENDATIONS

Patient Monitoring

Multidisciplinary approach

- Pediatric endocrinologist, geneticist, or other metabolic bone specialist
  - Medical management of OI
- Pediatric orthopedic surgeon
  - Fracture repair, rodding, osteotomies, spinal fusion
- Physiotherapist/occupational therapist
  - Postoperative rehabilitation, orthotics, physical therapy to improve mobility and stability of bones, increase muscle strength, and increase hand strength and endurance
- Psychologist/social worker
  - Adjustments and accommodations at school
  - Issues regarding self-esteem
- Pediatric dentist
  - Patients with OI should have a dental home for hygiene, monitoring for caries, and assessment of dental eruption and occlusion.
  - Those patients with significant DI may also require dental rehabilitation including capping of teeth.

PATIENT EDUCATION

- Techniques for safe handling, protective positioning, and safe movement should be taught to parents.
- Physical education at school should be strongly encouraged, but children should not participate in contact sports. An individualized program is required.

PROGNOSIS

- Largely depends on severity of OI
- In general, the earlier the fractures occur, the more severe the disease.
- Tendency toward improvement in adolescence with fewer fractures is commonly seen.

COMPLICATIONS

- Repeated fractures with secondary deformity
- Scoliosis
- Cardiorespiratory problems (restrictive lung disease in severe cases with severe kyphoscoliosis, aortic dissection, mitral valve prolapse, aortic regurgitation)
- Hearing loss
- Short stature
- Basilar invagination: descent of the skull on the cervical spine; may progress to brainstem compression or obstructive hydrocephalus

ADDITIONAL READING

- Forlino A, Marini JC. Osteogenesis imperfecta. *Lancet*. 2016;387(10028):1657–1671.
- Glorieux FH, Moffatt P. Osteogenesis imperfecta, an ever-expanding conundrum. *J Bone Miner Res*. 2013;28(7):1519–1522.
- Marom R, Lee YC, Grafe I, et al. Pharmacological and biological therapeutic strategies for osteogenesis imperfecta. *Am J Med Genet C Semin Med Genet*. 2016;172(4):367–383.

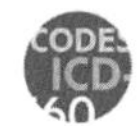

CODES

ICD10

Q78.0 Osteogenesis imperfecta

FAQ

- Q: What is the typical life expectancy for persons with OI?
- A: Infants with perinatal/lethal (type II) OI do not survive the perinatal period and often die within the first 48 hours of life. For mild and moderate OI, life expectancy is normal. Life expectancy for patients with severe (type III) OI is widely variable and can be shortened by kyphoscoliosis contributing to restricted lung disease.
- Q: How is OI inherited?
- A: OI is often inherited in an autosomal dominant manner. New mutations are not uncommon, and this often provides the explanation for lethal cases of OI in families with no history of OI. More recently, autosomal recessive forms of OI (mainly severe and lethal) have been described, and for those families, a one in four recurrence risk should be communicated.
- Q: How is OI differentiated from nonaccidental trauma?
- A: The family history and physical examination can often provide clues to help differentiate OI from nonaccidental trauma. Usually, in patients with moderate or severe OI, the diagnosis is less problematic. However, it can be difficult in cases of mild OI as those patients may not have typical facial characteristics of OI and may have normal growth.
- Q: How does one decide to use bisphosphonates in patients with OI?
- A: There are no evidence-based guidelines for which patients should receive these medications, but it is suggested that the patient should have significant enough disease to experience a potentially tangible benefit (i.e., improvement in fracture rate, lessening pain, improvement in mobility).
- Q: Are there good patient resources for persons living with OI?
- A: The OI foundation (www.oif.org) is an excellent resource for information for patients and their physicians.

OSTEOMYELITIS

Blanca E. Gonzalez, MD

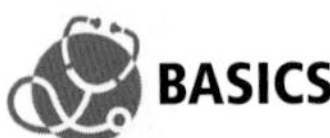

BASICS

DESCRIPTION

- Infection of any bone
- Most commonly occurs in the metaphysis of a long bone (especially the distal femur or proximal tibia)

EPIDEMIOLOGY

- One of the most common invasive bacterial infections in children, accounting for 1% of all pediatric hospitalizations
- One third occurs in children <2 years of age, and ~50% of cases occur in children ≤5 years of age.
- A history of minor trauma to the affected site is common but of unclear significance.
- Boys are more commonly affected than girls (2:1 ratio).

PATHOPHYSIOLOGY

- Hematogenous spread is most common in children (inoculation of bone during an episode of bacteremia). The infecting organism enters the bone via a nutrient artery and then is deposited in the metaphysis due to its rich vascular supply. The organism replicates in metaphyseal capillary loops, causes local inflammation, spreads through vascular tunnels, and adheres to the bone matrix. Increased pressure in the metaphysis allows pus to perforate through the cortex and lift the periosteum.
- In newborns and young infants, rupture of pus into the adjacent joint space is more common because blood vessels connect the metaphysis and epiphysis.
- Local spread from a contiguous focus of infection and direct inoculation (e.g., penetrating injury) are less common mechanisms of infection.

RISK FACTORS

- Sickle hemoglobinopathy
- Primary or acquired immunodeficiency, especially chronic granulomatous disease (CGD), and HIV
- Bone trauma (open fractures, puncture wounds, bites, surgical manipulation)
- Implanted orthopedic devices or indwelling vascular catheters
- Pressure ulcers

ETIOLOGY

- *Staphylococcus aureus* is responsible for 70–90% of osteomyelitis in all age groups, with MRSA an increasingly common problem.
- *Streptococcus pyogenes* accounts for ~10% of osteomyelitis and is more common in preschool and early school–aged children.
- *Streptococcus pneumoniae* causes ~10% of osteomyelitis in children <3 years old, although a decline in pneumococcal infections has been seen with widespread vaccination. Conversely, *S. pneumoniae* remains an important cause of osteomyelitis in children infected with HIV.
- *Kingella kingae*, a gram-negative organism found in the respiratory tract, is an important pathogen in children age <3 years, especially in those that attend day care centers.
- Group B *Streptococcus*, gram-negative enterics, and *Candida* spp. are important causative organisms in neonates.
- *Salmonella* spp. can be the cause in children with sickle cell disease and in patients from or traveling to tropical countries.
- *Pseudomonas aeruginosa* is a common cause following puncture wounds to the foot.
- There has been a significant decline in the incidence of *Haemophilus influenzae* type b (Hib) osteomyelitis since immunization with the Hib conjugate vaccine became widespread.
  - Prior to widespread vaccination, this organism was an important cause of bone and joint infection in children and infants <2 years.
- Other more unusual pathogens may be seen in patients with specific risk factors (e.g., coagulase-negative staphylococci in the presence of prosthetic material, anaerobes after animal or human bites, *Aeromonas* after injuries sustained in fresh water settings).
- In a significant percentage of cases, a definitive causative microorganism is not identified. The use of antibiotic prior to collection of samples, presence of fastidious organisms, low inoculum, or inappropriately collected samples, may be a factor in culture-negative osteomyelitis.
- Infections after open fractures or puncture wounds may be polymicrobial.

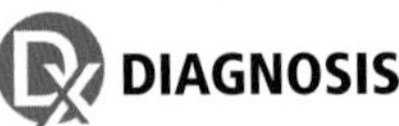

DIAGNOSIS

HISTORY

- Persistent, increasing pain and tenderness over the affected bone
- Restricted use of the involved limb (pseudoparalysis may be the only sign in a neonate), refusal to bear weight, or limp
- Fever, malaise, anorexia, irritability
- Children with vertebral and pelvic osteomyelitis may complain of poorly localized pain for several weeks, often resulting in delay in the diagnosis and treatment.
- In some patients, osteomyelitis will have an indolent, subacute presentation with the development of a minimally symptomatic abscess within the bone, eponymously known as a "Brodie abscess."

PHYSICAL EXAM

- Swelling, warmth, and erythema of the soft tissues over the affected bone may be noted.
- Exaggerated immobility/pain with micromotion of an adjacent joint suggests pyogenic arthritis (alternatively or in addition to osteomyelitis).
- Multifocal osteomyelitis may be seen in neonates and in children with *S. aureus* sepsis syndrome.

DIFFERENTIAL DIAGNOSIS

- Trauma
- Cellulitis
- Soft tissue abscess
- Pyomyositis or fasciitis
- Septic arthritis
- Congenital syphilis
- Aseptic bone necrosis or bone infarction (sickle cell disease)
- Tumor (e.g., Ewing sarcoma, osteoid osteoma, eosinophilic granuloma)
- Acute leukemia, neuroblastoma with bone invasion
- Chronic recurrent multifocal osteomyelitis (CRMO)
- Inflammatory arthritis or juvenile idiopathic arthritis
- Transient synovitis
- Bone cyst

DIAGNOSTIC TESTS & INTERPRETATION

Initial Tests (screening, lab, imaging)

- The white blood cell count may be normal or elevated.
- Erythrocyte sedimentation rate (ESR) and C-reactive protein (CRP) levels are usually elevated, although in certain cases, such as puncture wounds, they may be normal.
- Blood cultures are positive in ~50% of patients.
- Bone needle aspiration cultures are positive in ~60–70% of cases.
- Some uncommon bacteria-causing osteomyelitis are fastidious and difficult to culture; they may require molecular methods to establish the diagnosis (e.g., polymerase chain reaction).
- Plain radiographs may show deep soft tissue swelling early in the course of infection and may help to suggest or exclude alternative diagnoses. Evidence of bone destruction and periosteal elevation are not typically seen until 10 to 14 days after the onset of symptoms.
- MRI is sensitive and specific and offers superior anatomic resolution, making it a more useful modality for surgical planning and for identification of intraosseous, subperiosteal, and soft tissue abscesses.
- Bone scans are useful if the site of infection is poorly localized or if there is concern for multifocal osteomyelitis. However, they may be positive in other illnesses that cause osteoblastic activity.

Diagnostic Procedures/Other

- Biopsy or aspiration of the infected bone (or an associated abscess) for Gram stain and culture is useful for determining the etiologic organism. Inoculating a portion of an aspirated sample into a blood culture bottle enhances yield for *K. kingae*.
- If a plan is in place to rapidly obtain a bone culture in a clinically stable patient, it is reasonable to defer initiation of antibiotic therapy until after the culture specimen is secured.
- Biopsy may help differentiate osteomyelitis from noninfectious bone pathology.

TREATMENT

MEDICATION

- Empiric antibiotics should cover the most likely pathogens considering patient age, history of presentation, physical findings, and underlying medical conditions.
- Empiric therapy should always include an agent directed against *S. aureus*, usually nafcillin, oxacillin, or a 1st-generation cephalosporin. However, in areas where the rate of methicillin resistance among community *S. aureus* isolates exceeds 10%, an antibiotic effective against community-acquired MRSA should be selected (i.e., clindamycin or vancomycin).
- When clindamycin is considered for treatment of an identified MRSA isolate, the D-test (to exclude inducible macrolide, lincosamide, and streptogramin B resistance) should be performed by the clinical microbiology laboratory.
- Clindamycin and vancomycin are also usually effective against *S. pneumoniae* and *S. pyogenes* but are not effective in vitro against *K. kingae*. The latter organism is usually susceptible to most β-lactam antibiotics (penicillins and cephalosporins).
- In addition to antistaphylococcal coverage, a 3rd-generation cephalosporin, such as ceftriaxone or cefotaxime, should be used to cover *Salmonella* spp. in patients with sickle cell disease.
- Gram-negative coverage should also be added to the empiric regimen for neonates.
- If the patient recently had a foot puncture wound, coverage for *P. aeruginosa* should be considered.
- If an organism is isolated and susceptibilities determined, antibiotic therapy should be modified based on the susceptibility profile.

ISSUES FOR REFERRAL

The treatment of osteomyelitis should be done in consultation with an infectious disease specialist.

SURGERY/OTHER PROCEDURES

- If an intraosseous, subperiosteal, or soft tissue abscess is present, surgical debridement may be necessary in addition to antibiotic therapy.
- Surgical debridement is important in the management of osteomyelitis that is secondary to a puncture wound.

ADMISSION, INPATIENT, AND NURSING CONSIDERATIONS

- Traditionally, 4 to 6 weeks of antibiotics have been recommended. Newer data is emerging suggesting that for non-MRSA hematogenous osteomyelitis, 20 days of therapy may be sufficient. However, this may require the use of more frequent dosing schedules as well as higher doses.
- Total treatment duration should be individualized based on the extent of infection, the promptness and completeness of surgical debridement (when indicated), the rate of clinical response, the presence or absence of distant foci of infection, and the patient's underlying risk factors and comorbid conditions.
- After an initial period of parenteral antibiotic administration, many patients can be transitioned to an oral regimen to complete therapy (assuming the availability of an oral antibiotic with an appropriate spectrum of activity and adequate bone penetration as well as patient's ability to adhere to and absorb an oral regimen). This sequential IV–oral approach reduces the risk of complications (e.g., catheter-associated bloodstream infection, catheter malfunction, and thrombosis) associated with the prolonged presence of a central venous catheter.
- The decline in CRP alongside improvement in clinical signs may be a good indicator of when it is safe to transition to oral therapy.

ONGOING CARE

FOLLOW-UP RECOMMENDATIONS

- Most children who receive appropriate treatment have no long-term sequelae.
- Inflammatory markers (ESR and CRP) are typically measured serially until they normalize during the course of antibiotic therapy.
- Patients should be followed to ensure medication compliance, adequacy of treatment, side effects of therapy, and continued growth of the involved extremity.

COMPLICATIONS

- Septic arthritis
- Recurrence or progression to chronic osteomyelitis in ~5% of patients
- Disturbances of bone growth, limb length discrepancy
- Arthritis
- Pathologic fractures

ADDITIONAL READING

- Arnold JC, Cannavino CR, Ross MK, et al. Acute bacterial osteoarticular infections: eight-year analysis of C-reactive protein for oral step-down therapy. *Pediatrics*. 2012;130(4):e821–e828.
- Dodwell E. Osteomyelitis and septic arthritis in children: current concepts. *Curr Opin Pediatr*. 2013;25(1):58–63.
- Harik NS, Smeltzer MS. Management of acute hematogenous osteomyelitis in children. *Expert Rev Anti Infect Ther*. 2010;8(2):175–181.
- Kaplan SL. Osteomyelitis in children. *Infect Dis Clin North Am*. 2005;19(4):787–797.
- Keren R, Shah SS, Srivastava R, et al. Comparative effectiveness of intravenous vs oral antibiotics for postdischarge treatment of acute osteomyelitis in children. *JAMA Pediatr*. 2015;169(2):120–128.
- Pääkkönen M, Peltola H. Bone and joint infections. *Pediatr Clin North Am*. 2013;60(2):425–436.
- Peltola H, Pääkkönen M, Kallio P, et al. Short- versus long-term antimicrobial treatment for acute hematogenous osteomyelitis of childhood: prospective, randomized trial on 131 culture-positive cases. *Pediatr Infect Dis J*. 2010;29(12):1123–1128.
- Yagupsky P. *Kingella kingae*: from medical rarity to an emerging paediatric pathogen. *Lancet Infect Dis*. 2004;4(6):358–367.
- Zaoutis T, Localio AR, Leckerman K, et al. Prolonged intravenous therapy versus early transition to oral antimicrobial therapy for acute osteomyelitis in children. *Pediatrics*. 2009;123(2):636–642.

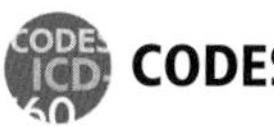

CODES

ICD10

- M86.9 Osteomyelitis, unspecified
- M86.00 Acute hematogenous osteomyelitis, unspecified site
- M86.10 Other acute osteomyelitis, unspecified site

FAQ

- Q: Can children with osteomyelitis present without fever and with normal CBCs and inflammatory markers?
- A: Fever along with leukocytosis and elevated inflammatory markers (CRP and ESR) are common in children who have acute hematogenous osteomyelitis. However, children with subacute or chronic osteomyelitis and with other forms of osteomyelitis, such as puncture wound osteochondritis, may not exhibit these findings.
- Q: What is the imaging modality of choice in a child suspected of having acute hematogenous osteomyelitis?
- A: MRI is the most sensitive and specific imaging study to detect acute osteomyelitis. Plain films do not reveal periosteal elevation for at least 10 to 14 days after infection. A bone scan is less specific than MRI and does not reveal extraosseous features of infection.

OSTEOSARCOMA

Sheila Thampi, MD • Steven G. DuBois, MD, MS

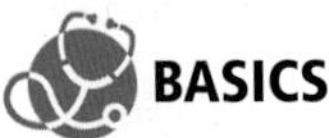

BASICS

DESCRIPTION
Osteosarcoma is a malignant tumor of the bone and arises from mesenchymal cells. The malignant cells are usually pleomorphic spindle cells that lay down abnormal bone (osteoid formation).

EPIDEMIOLOGY
- Osteosarcoma is the most common pediatric primary bone cancer.
- In the United States, there are about 4.4 cases per million children and adolescents.
- Approximately 400 new pediatric cases of osteosarcoma are diagnosed each year in the United States, which is about 2% of all childhood cancers.
- A bimodal distribution is noted with the first peak in adolescence (median, age 16 years) and second peak during the 7th and 8th decade of life.
- Incidence of osteosarcoma parallels skeletal growth and is more frequently noted in tall individuals.
- Males are more commonly affected than females.

RISK FACTORS
- Radiation exposure
- Hereditary retinoblastoma, in which patients with germline *Rb* gene mutation have increased risk of osteosarcoma with or without radiation exposure
- Li-Fraumeni syndrome, in which patients have germline *TP53* gene mutation and increased risk of a range of sarcomas, among other malignancies
- Rothmund-Thomson syndrome
- Bloom syndrome
- Enchondromatosis
- Hereditary multiple exostoses
- Fibrous dysplasia
- Paget disease of the bone, although less relevant to pediatric populations

PATHOPHYSIOLOGY
- The histologic hallmark of osteosarcoma is the presence of osteoid formation.
- Most cases of pediatric osteosarcoma are high-grade cancers, although lower grade variants are seen.
- No single genetic change, although karyotypes are typically highly abnormal
- At diagnosis, 80% of patients will have localized disease and 20% will have metastatic disease.
- In >80% of tumors, the metaphysis of long bones will be involved, such as the femur, tibia, and humerus, with distal femur the most common primary site. Less common primary sites include the pelvis, facial bones, and scapula.
- The most common sites of metastatic disease are lungs and bone. Regional lymph node or extraosseous involvement is rare.

ETIOLOGY
- The etiology of most cases is unknown.
- Abnormal p53 and/or Rb function implicated in laboratory studies of osteosarcoma
- Radiation exposure is a known cause of osteosarcoma and usually presents 10 to 20 years after exposure.

DIAGNOSIS

HISTORY
- Pain and palpable mass are the most common clinical symptoms.
- Pain is often described as dull or aching at the tumor site.
- Pain is often initially attributed to an injury in active children or adolescents, but there is no convincing evidence to support an association between trauma and osteosarcoma.
- Symptoms of pain can vary prior to presenting to medical attention but warrant further investigation if present for several weeks to months and if it disrupts sleep.
- Presence of bone metastasis may result in pain at sites distant from the primary tumor.
- Systemic symptoms, such as fever and weight loss, are unusual.

PHYSICAL EXAM
- Presence of a firm, often tender mass
- Swelling at the tumor location
- Depending on location of the tumor, one can have a loss of function, limp, or decreased range of motion.

DIFFERENTIAL DIAGNOSIS
- Benign tumors
  - Unicameral bone cyst
  - Aneurysmal bone cyst
  - Osteoblastoma
  - Langerhans cell histiocytosis (eosinophilic granuloma)
  - Osteochondroma
  - Fibrous dysplasia
- Malignant tumors
  - Ewing sarcoma
  - Undifferentiated (Ewing-like) sarcoma
  - Chondrosarcoma
  - Fibrosarcoma
  - Metastatic lesions
- Infection
  - Osteomyelitis
  - Septic arthritis
- Trauma: fracture with or without hematoma

DIAGNOSTIC TESTS & INTERPRETATION

Initial Tests (screening, lab, imaging)
- 30% of patients will have an elevated lactate dehydrogenase (LDH).
- An elevated erythrocyte sedimentation rate (ESR) can be seen.
- May see an elevated alkaline phosphatase (AP), particularly with metastatic disease
- Leukocytosis may suggest osteomyelitis.
- Conventional x-ray may show
  - Osteolytic and sclerotic lesion
  - Periosteal reaction including Codman sign (shadow from a lifted periosteum), onion-skinning as new layers of periosteum are laid down, and sunburst appearance reflecting calcified bone beyond periosteum
  - Pathologic fracture
- An MRI from joint to joint of involved bone will show full extension of the tumor and involvement of surrounding structures as well as potential for skip lesions.
- Nuclear medicine scan (bone scan or FDG-PET) can show areas of intense primary tumor uptake and screen for bone metastasis.
- A chest CT should be performed to evaluate for pulmonary metastasis.

Follow-Up Tests & Special Considerations
- Children with a suspected malignant bone tumor should be immediately referred to a children's hospital with expertise in these tumors.
- Multidisciplinary teams include pediatric oncologists, orthopedic oncologists, pediatric surgeons, nurses, pharmacists, physical therapists, and social workers.

Diagnostic Procedures/Other
The diagnosis of osteosarcoma is based on tissue diagnosis.

ALERT
Biopsy should be performed at the center that will provide definitive treatment for the patient with a suspected primary malignant bone tumor. The placement of biopsy is critical to the planning of surgical local control and inappropriate biopsy could lead to adverse outcomes.

Test Interpretation
Pathology consists of malignant cells, which are usually pleomorphic spindle with abnormal osteoid formation. Major subtypes of osteosarcoma include osteoblastic, chondroblastic, fibroblastic, telangiectatic, and small cell.

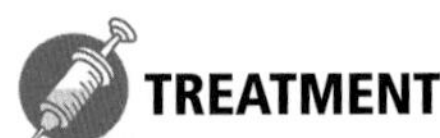

TREATMENT

MEDICATION
- Prior to the 1970s, overall survival for high-grade osteosarcoma was poor, as treatment primarily consisted of surgical resection allowing for relapse with metastatic disease. With the addition of both neoadjuvant and adjuvant chemotherapy, survival has improved.
- Neoadjuvant chemotherapy (before definitive surgery) allows for treatment of micrometastases and shrinkage of the primary tumor mass prior to resection.

- Neoadjuvant chemotherapy also allows time for complex endoprostheses to be constructed prior to planned limb salvage procedures.
- Response to neoadjuvant chemotherapy (percent of tumor that is necrotic at the time of complete resection) has proven to be an important prognostic factor.
- Most children and adolescents with high-grade osteosarcoma are treated based on or according to cooperative group chemotherapy protocols.

First Line

In North America, the standard backbone of treatment is high-dose methotrexate, doxorubicin, and cisplatin. Treatment duration is usually 9 months depending on the individual protocol, response to therapy, and tumor extent at diagnosis.

Second Line

Clinical trials in patients with newly diagnosed disease have investigated the role of ifosfamide and etoposide. Given lack of improved survival with upfront ifosfamide and etoposide, these agents are now used for relapsed or refractory osteosarcoma. The addition of interferon with chemotherapy did not improve survival.

ISSUES FOR REFERRAL

- Treatment for osteosarcoma involves a multidisciplinary team and patients will be followed as an outpatient by pediatric oncology and orthopedics.
- After surgery, patients will require physical therapy and may require prosthetic support.
- As approximately 10% of patients with osteosarcoma may harbor a cancer predisposition germline mutation, referral to a cancer risk clinic should be considered.

ADDITIONAL THERAPIES

- Osteosarcoma is not a radiation-sensitive tumor, although radiation has been used for palliative purposes to treat unresectable primary or metastatic lesions.
- Physical therapy is critical after either amputation or limb-sparing procedures.

SURGERY/OTHER PROCEDURES

- Complete surgical resection with wide margins is necessary for cure.
- Surgical options for osteosarcomas of the extremities include the following:
  - Amputation
  - Limb salvage with local resection and reconstruction of the limb
  - Rotationplasty for tumors at the knee
- Surgical resection alone is curative in low-grade osteosarcoma.
- Surgical resection of lung metastases at presentation or at relapse also plays an important role in management.

ADMISSION, INPATIENT, AND NURSING CONSIDERATIONS

- Patients with suspected malignant bone tumors are often admitted to the hospital to facilitate an expedited workup with labs, imaging, consultations, surgical biopsy, and initiation of treatment.
- Chemotherapy administration is often given in the hospital due to supportive care requirements for these drugs.
- As a side effect of chemotherapy, patients can develop fever and neutropenia and require inpatient hospitalization for antibiotics.

ONGOING CARE

FOLLOW-UP RECOMMENDATIONS

Patient Monitoring

- Patients should be followed by a pediatric oncologist with serial imaging of the primary site (MRI and/or radiographs) and lungs (chest CT or chest radiograph) to monitor for recurrence.
- Once therapy is complete, patients will be followed at least every 3 to 6 months for the first few years of therapy to monitor for relapse.
- Long-term survivors will be followed annually and monitored for long-term side effects/complications of therapy, ideally within the context of a survivorship clinic.

PATIENT EDUCATION

- During therapy and while a central line is in place, patients are counseled to call for all fevers as this symptom requires an examination, laboratory evaluation with a CBC and blood culture, and systemic antibiotics administered through the central line.
- After surgery, patients will be instructed on physical limitations (i.e., nonweight bearing) and when they can resume normal activity.

PROGNOSIS

- Patients with localized disease have an estimated 5-year overall survival of 60–80%, with better outcomes seen with good response to neoadjuvant chemotherapy. Patients with metastatic disease have an estimated 5-year overall survival of 20–30%.
- Key adverse prognostic factors are as follows:
  - Axial primary tumor location
  - Metastatic disease
  - Histologic necrosis <90% after neoadjuvant chemotherapy
  - Inability to achieve wide surgical margins during resection

COMPLICATIONS

- Orthopedic
  - Surgical site wound infections
  - Limb length discrepancy after surgical treatment in growing children
  - Phantom leg pain after amputation
- Acute chemotherapy toxicity
  - Myelosuppression
  - Ototoxicity and tinnitus
  - Mucositis
  - Renal dysfunction
- Late effects
  - Cardiomyopathy from doxorubicin
  - Hearing loss and nephrotoxicity from cisplatin
  - Reduced fertility from ifosfamide
  - Secondary malignancy from radiation or chemotherapy

ADDITIONAL READING

- Bielack SS, Carrle D, Hardes J, et al. Bone tumors in adolescents and young adults. *Curr Treat Options Oncol*. 2008;9(1):67–80.
- Bielack SS, Smeland S, Whelan JS, et al; for EURAMOS-1 investigators. Methotrexate, doxorubicin, and cisplatin (MAP) plus maintenance pegylated interferon alfa-2b versus MAP alone in patients with resectable high-grade osteosarcoma and good histologic response to preoperative MAP: first results of the EURAMOS-1 good response randomized controlled trial. *J Clin Oncol*. 2015;33(20):2279–2287.
- Gill J, Ahluwalia MK, Geller D, et al. New targets and approaches in osteosarcoma. *Pharmacol Ther*. 2013;137(1):89–99.
- Heare T, Hensley MA, Dell'Orfano S. Bone tumors: osteosarcoma and Ewing's sarcoma. *Curr Opin Pediatr*. 2009;21(3):365–372.
- Marina NM, Smeland S, Bielack SS, et al. Comparison of MAPIE versus MAP in patients with a poor response to preoperative chemotherapy for newly diagnosed high-grade osteosarcoma (EURAMOS-1): an open-label, international, randomised controlled trial. *Lancet Oncol*. 2016;17(10):1396–1408.

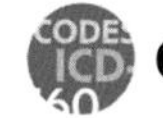

CODES

ICD10

- C41.9 Malignant neoplasm of bone and articular cartilage, unsp
- C40.20 Malignant neoplasm of long bones of unspecified lower limb
- C40.00 Malig neoplasm of scapula and long bones of unsp upper limb

FAQ

- Q: How can we differentiate between malignant osteosarcoma and benign tumors?
- A: An experienced radiologist can look for defining features on imaging of malignant osteosarcoma that are not found with benign tumors. However, only a biopsy can confirm a diagnosis of osteosarcoma.
- Q: What are long-term survival rates of patients who relapse after treatment?
- A: Unfortunately, patients who relapse after treatment do poorly and long-term survival is poor at 10–20%. Late relapses (>24 months after completion of treatment), relapsed disease that can be fully resected, and unilateral lung involvement at relapse appear to be more favorable.
- Q: Do siblings of children with osteosarcoma need to be evaluated?
- A: If there is suspicion for a genetic risk factor (i.e., Li-Fraumeni syndrome), then siblings and families should be evaluated by a geneticist to determine if the risk factor is present. This will provide education for families and siblings. Otherwise, siblings of children with osteosarcoma that are asymptomatic do not need evaluation for osteosarcoma.
- Q: What are the differences between Ewing sarcoma and osteosarcoma?
- A: The two sarcomas are the most common malignant bone tumors in pediatrics and both require multimodal therapy, although the chemotherapy regimens are different. Ewing sarcoma can have both bone or soft tissue involvement and presence of different histologic features will allow differentiation from osteosarcoma.

OTITIS EXTERNA

Melissa Long, MD

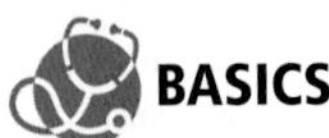

BASICS

DESCRIPTION

- Diffuse inflammation of external auditory canal with or without infection
- Also known as "swimmer's ear"
- May be categorized as acute, chronic, or malignant
  - Acute: rapid onset, usually bacterial
  - Chronic: lasting longer than 4 weeks or occurring 4 or more times in 1 year, usually due to nonbacterial causes such as atopic or allergic contact dermatitis from contact with metal, plastic, or chemicals
  - Malignant or necrotizing: extension of infection to osteomyelitis of the base of the skull; more common in immunocompromised patients (e.g., HIV, diabetes)

EPIDEMIOLOGY

- Peaks in children ages 5 to 14 years
- Uncommon in children age <2 years
- Peaks in summer months in temperate climates; occurs year-round in warm/humid climates

Incidence

Annual incidence is 8.1/1,000 in the general population.

Prevalence

Affects 3–5% of the population

RISK FACTORS

- Prolonged exposure to water (e.g., frequent swimming, shampooing, long showers, excessive sweating) leading to impaired natural defense mechanisms in external ear
- Microfissures from trauma
- Debris from dermatologic conditions (e.g., atopic or seborrheic dermatitis)
- Use of external devices (e.g., hearing aids or ear plugs)
- Obstruction of ear canal (e.g., by impacted cerumen, foreign body, sebaceous cyst)
- Chronic otorrhea or purulent otorrhea from otitis media
- Drainage from tympanostomy tubes
- Hairy ear canal
- Anatomic abnormalities
  - Stenosis of ear canal
  - Exostoses (abnormal bone growth within the ear canal)
- History of radiotherapy leading to damaged epithelium, desquamation, and diminished cerumen production

GENERAL PREVENTION

- Elimination of predisposing factors when feasible is the key to prevention.
- Avoid exposure to excessive moisture.
  - There are no randomized trials evaluating preventive strategies. It may be helpful to instruct swimmers to keep their ears as dry as possible by toweling off, tilting the head to assist with drainage, and using a hair dryer to the ear canal on the lowest setting.
  - Some experts also recommend the use of ear plugs, although this strategy is controversial because it may lead to cerumen impaction, predisposing to otitis externa (OE).
  - Use of a 1:1 alcohol-to-vinegar solution before and after swimming and again before bedtime also may decrease the rate of recurrence.
- Avoid trauma to the ear canal—in particular, avoid cotton-tip swabs or other cleaning devices.
- Manage underlying dermatologic conditions.

PATHOPHYSIOLOGY

- The ear canal is lined with apocrine and sebaceous glands that produce cerumen.
- Cerumen serves as a barrier to excessive moisture and may help prevent infection due to lysozyme activity and a slightly acidic pH that helps inhibit the growth of pathogenic bacteria.
- With prolonged exposure to water, cerumen may be washed away and no longer be able to serve this barrier function.
- Too much cerumen can also lead to entrapment of debris and water retention, thus predisposing to infection.
- In certain dermatologic conditions, the integrity of the keratin layer may be affected by excessive desquamation.
- Local trauma to the external canal may also predispose to infection.

ETIOLOGY

- In the United States, bacterial agents are implicated in >90% of cases and most commonly include *Pseudomonas aeruginosa* and *Staphylococcus aureus*.
- May be polymicrobial in up to 30% of cases
- Fungal causes include *Aspergillus niger* and *Candida* and are more likely in cases of chronic OE or after antibiotic treatment of OE.
- Viral infections (in particular, varicella-zoster leading to Ramsay Hunt syndrome) account for a minority of cases.

DIAGNOSIS

HISTORY

- Symptoms are rapid in onset (generally within 48 hours) and include otalgia (70%), pruritus (60%), a sense of fullness (22%), drainage (32%), and occasionally impaired hearing.
- 90% of cases are unilateral.
- May have a low-grade fever, but temperature >101°F (38.3°C) suggests more serious infection and likely extension beyond the external ear canal
- Ask about potential predisposing factors including swimming, dermatologic conditions, or trauma.
- Important to know status of immune system (e.g., history of diabetes, HIV infection)

PHYSICAL EXAM

- Examine external canal, tympanic membrane (TM), regional lymph nodes, and skin for dermatologic conditions.
- Signs of inflammation include tenderness or pain with manipulation of the pinna and with pressure on the tragus, erythema and edema of the external auditory canal, and otorrhea.
- More severe forms of OE may involve regional lymphadenopathy or frank lymphadenitis, cellulitis extending beyond the external canal, and/or perichondritis.
- May be difficult to visualize TM due to edema and debris
  - Can clear debris with ear curette or suction
  - Avoid lavage until TM is known to be intact.
  - Pneumatic otoscopy to assess for TM mobility and/or tympanometry can aid in the diagnosis of otitis media.
- Although rare in children, consider malignant OE if there is necrosis of the skin of the canal, exposed bone or granulation tissue, severe pain, and/or cranial nerve palsy.
- Consider viral infection (Ramsay Hunt syndrome) if there are vesicular lesions with facial paralysis, loss of taste, and decreased lacrimation on the affected side.

DIFFERENTIAL DIAGNOSIS

- Important to rule out life-threatening causes of otalgia and otorrhea
  - Clear persistent fluid may occur after traumatic head injury, leading to cerebrospinal fluid otorrhea.
  - Purulent otorrhea could be due to acute otitis media associated with mastoiditis, brain abscess, or venous sinus thrombosis.
  - With bloody drainage, must consider traumatic perforation of the TM, barotrauma leading to hemotympanum, or a tumor
- Other infections
  - Furunculosis in the external auditory canal (also known as localized OE)
  - Otomycosis
  - Infected sebaceous cyst
  - Acute otitis media
  - Chronic suppurative otitis media with ruptured TM
  - Drainage through tympanostomy tubes
- Miscellaneous
  - Foreign body
  - Cholesteatoma
  - Contact dermatitis (e.g., to metal, plastics)

DIAGNOSTIC TESTS & INTERPRETATION

- In uncomplicated OE, testing is generally not indicated.
- Consider bacterial culture of drainage with Gram stain and/or fungal culture in cases of severe illness or treatment failure.
- Consider viral testing if vesicular lesions are present.
- If concerned for malignant OE by history or exam, consider lab work (including erythrocyte sedimentation rate) and imaging (MRI generally preferred over CT scan).

TREATMENT

GENERAL MEASURES

- Pain management
  - For mild to moderate pain, acetaminophen or ibuprofen and application of heat or cold packs often will suffice.
  - For severe pain, a short course of narcotics may be required because pain may intensify during first 48 hours of treatment.
  - There is no data to suggest that benzocaine otic drops are effective for pain management, and in fact, they may limit the effectiveness of the topical antibiotic by interfering with its contact with the epithelium of the ear canal and may mask progression of OE.
- Clearing aural debris
  - In moderate to severe cases of OE when thick drainage obstructs the view of the TM, it may be necessary to clear debris with light suction or manual removal.
  - Do not use irrigation until you have confirmed the TM is intact.
  - May need to refer to ear, nose, and throat (ENT) physician for aural toilet under microscopic guidance
- Edema
  - In cases in which edema has progressed to cause >50% narrowing of the canal, a medication wick may be necessary (e.g., 1/4-inch ribbon gauze or compressed cellulose) to ensure adequate delivery of antimicrobial therapy directly to the epithelium.
  - Do not use a cotton ball because it could fall apart and pieces could become trapped in the canal.
  - The wick may fall out on its own as edema resolves or may be removed by clinician.
- Keep the area dry and refrain from swimming for the duration of treatment or at least until symptoms resolve.
- Refrain from using hearing aids until symptoms resolve.

MEDICATION

- For uncomplicated OE, topical antibiotics are the treatment of choice, as they are both effective and well tolerated.
- A 2010 Cochrane review found no difference among topical antibiotic preparations in terms of clinical or microbiologic cure rates. There was also insufficient evidence to suggest that the addition of corticosteroids to topical antibiotic preparations leads to improved outcomes.
- Choice of topical antibiotic therapy should be guided by the following:
  - Effectiveness
  - Consideration of potential adverse effects
  - Patency of the TM
  - Expected adherence
  - Risk of developing drug resistance
  - Cost and availability
- Aminoglycoside preparations (e.g., neomycin) should be avoided when the patency of the TM cannot be confirmed because of the associated middle ear ototoxicity. Neomycin can also cause an allergic contact dermatitis. It is often combined with polymyxin B for antipseudomonal coverage and with hydrocortisone.
- Fluoroquinolone preparations are safe to use in cases of nonintact TM and are dosed once or twice daily, which may increase adherence.
- Tips for medication administration
  - Consider warming the ototopical agent to body temperature prior to administration to decrease likelihood of dizziness from caloric stimulation.
  - Preferable for parent to administer treatment, even for older children
  - Patient should lie with affected ear upward.
  - Drops should fill the canal.
  - Manipulate the pinna/tragus to help disperse the medication.
  - Remain in that position for 3 to 5 minutes.
  - Leave canal open to dry (do not insert cotton ball).
- Duration of treatment is usually 7 to 10 days, with expected improvement of symptoms within 2 to 3 days and resolution by 6 days.
- For those with symptoms persisting beyond the 7- to 10-day period, treatment should continue until symptoms resolve to a maximum of 14 days, at which point, treatment failure should be considered. At that time, a culture may guide further antimicrobial therapy.
- Oral antibiotics should be considered only in the following situations:
  - Complicated OE (coexisting acute otitis media, lymphadenitis, or facial cellulitis)
  - OE in an immunocompromised individual who is at higher risk for developing necrotizing or malignant OE
  - Inability to deliver topical therapy despite aural toilet

ISSUES FOR REFERRAL

Referral to an otolaryngologist may be indicated for aural cleaning, severe disease, treatment failure, or suspicion of malignant OE.

ONGOING CARE

FOLLOW-UP RECOMMENDATIONS

- Reevaluate if symptoms do not improve within 2 to 3 days of initiating treatment, progression of symptoms despite treatment, or severe illness.
- Immunocompromised patients should be followed closely due to risk for developing malignant OE.

PROGNOSIS

- Excellent in uncomplicated OE with symptom improvement in 2 to 3 days and resolution of symptoms in 6 days
- Recurrence is common if steps are not taken to address predisposing factors.

COMPLICATIONS

- Stenosis of the ear canal, cellulitis, lymphadenitis, chondritis, parotitis, chronic OE (rare in children)
- Malignant OE in immunocompromised patients (also rare in children)
- Reaction to antibiotic preparation (pruritus, local reaction, rash, discomfort, otalgia, dizziness, vertigo)

ADDITIONAL READING

- Conover K. Earache. *Emerg Med Clin North Am.* 2013;31(2):413–442.
- Ely JW, Hansen MR, Clark EC. Diagnosis of ear pain. *Am Fam Physician.* 2008;77(5):621–628.
- Kaushik V, Malik T, Saeed SR. Interventions for acute otitis externa. *Cochrane Database Syst Rev.* 2010;(1):CD004740.
- Rosenfeld RM, Schwartz SR, Cannon CR, et al. Clinical practice guideline: acute otitis externa. *Otolaryngol Head Neck Surg.* 2014;150(Suppl 1):S1–S24.
- Schaefer P, Baugh R. Acute otitis externa: an update. *Am Fam Physician.* 2012;86(11):1055–1061.

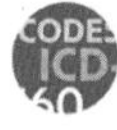

CODES

ICD10

- H60.90 Unspecified otitis externa, unspecified ear
- H60.339 Swimmer's ear, unspecified ear
- H60.509 Unsp acute noninfective otitis externa, unspecified ear

FAQ

- Q: How should I clean my child's ear?
- A: The external ear can be cleaned with a washcloth. Cotton swabs or other objects should not be inserted into the ear canal, as they may cause trauma or lead to impaction of cerumen. If there is concern for impacted cerumen causing symptoms such as ear fullness, pain, or hearing loss, then a physician should be consulted for discussion of methods for removal.
- Q: Is there a role for oral antibiotics in the treatment of OE?
- A: In uncomplicated OE where the infection is limited to the external canal, topical antibiotics are sufficient. If infection extends beyond the external canal (e.g., otitis media or cellulitis), then an oral antibiotic is advised.
- Q: How should treatment of OE differ if one cannot visualize the TM due to accumulated debris and/or edema?
- A: In cases where the TM cannot be confirmed to be intact, do not perform lavage. Debris can be removed by curette in the primary care physician's office, or the patient may be referred to an otolaryngologist for removal under microscopic guidance. Choose a topical antimicrobial agent other than an aminoglycoside due to its toxic effects on the middle ear. Depending on the certainty of your diagnosis of OE, consider whether the history suggests a coexisting acute otitis media necessitating presumptive treatment with oral antibiotics.

OTITIS MEDIA

C. Matthew Stewart, MD, PhD • Rosalyn W. Stewart, MD, MS, MBA

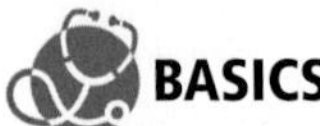

BASICS

DESCRIPTION

Otitis media is a general term for middle ear inflammation with or without symptoms. It can be acute or chronic.

- Two specific diagnoses
  - Otitis media with effusion, middle ear effusion (MEE)
  - Acute otitis media (AOM)
    - Uncomplicated/nonsevere
    - Severe
    - Recurrent

EPIDEMIOLOGY

- Most common condition for which antibacterial agents are prescribed for children in the United States
- Peak incidence between 6 and 12 months of age
- By age 3 years, 50–85% of children have had AOM.

RISK FACTORS

- Age <2 years
- Gender: male > female
- Family history of AOM
- Anatomic differences, craniofacial abnormalities
- Environmental tobacco smoke exposure
- Exposure to large numbers of other children
  - Day care
  - Siblings in home

GENERAL PREVENTION

- Breastfeeding for at least 3 to 6 months
- Decreasing pacifier use after 6 months
- Vaccines
  - Pneumococcal conjugate vaccine
  - Influenza vaccine
- Reduction in secondhand smoke
- Reduction of day care crowding

PATHOPHYSIOLOGY

- Eustachian tube dysfunction leads to MEE. If effusion is not cleared by the mucociliary system, bacteria and viruses have a good environment for growth.
- Severe eustachian tube dysfunction occurs during 66% of upper respiratory infections (URIs) in school-aged children and in 75% of URIs in day care–aged children.

ETIOLOGY

- Nontypeable *Haemophilus influenzae*: 35–50%
- *Streptococcus pneumoniae*: 25–40%
- *Moraxella catarrhalis*: 5–10%
- Viruses: 40–75%
  - High rate of coinfection with bacteria
  - Without bacterial coinfection: 5–22%
- Group A *Streptococcus* (3%)
- *Staphylococcus aureus* (2%)
- Gram-negative organisms such as *Pseudomonas aeruginosa*: 1–2%
  - More common in neonatal AOM

DIAGNOSIS

HISTORY

- Recent abrupt onset of signs and symptoms of middle ear inflammation and MEE
- Ear pain for <48 hours
- New-onset otorrhea not caused by acute otitis externa
- Fever
- Irritability
- Past medical history, including underlying disorders (e.g., cleft palate, Down syndrome), immune deficiency, and previous history of otitis media
- Recent treatment with antibiotics
- Exposure to large numbers of children (school, child care, large family)

PHYSICAL EXAM

- Look for other causes of fever and irritability in children: URIs, pharyngitis, lymphadenitis, meningitis, urinary tract infection, and bone and joint infections.
- Physical exam is best done with pneumatic otoscopy:
  - The patient should be adequately restrained if uncooperative.
  - Cerumen should be removed if view of tympanic membrane (TM) is inadequate.
  - Visualize TM at rest and with gentle positive and negative pressure via pneumatic otoscopy.
- The presence of an MEE is determined by the characteristics of the TM:
  - Contour: normal, retracted, full, or bulging; associated bulla(e)
  - Color: gray, pink, yellow, white, or red; hemorrhagic
  - Translucency: translucent or opaque
  - Mobility: normal, decreased, or absent
- Middle ear inflammation is indicated by the following:
  - Erythema of the TM
  - Otalgia
- MEE is indicated by the following:
  - Bulging of the TM
  - Limited or absent mobility of the TM
  - Air–fluid level behind the TM
  - Otorrhea
- A diagnosis of AOM is suggested if an MEE is present along with ear pain, fever, erythema, fullness, or bulging of TM.
- The concomitant presence of conjunctivitis (otitis media–conjunctivitis syndrome) suggests the presence of *H. influenzae* or a virus as a causative organism.
- AOM should not be diagnosed when pneumatic otoscopy and/or tympanometry do not show MEE.

DIFFERENTIAL DIAGNOSIS

- MEE: TM may appear dull with a diffuse light reflex, fluid bubbles may be visible, and mobility may be decreased.
- Otitis externa
- Auricular lesions like a furuncle or laceration
- Other causes of fever, including viral URIs, pharyngitis, pneumonia, meningitis, UTIs, and bone and joint infections
- Pharyngitis and dental pain may be mistaken for otalgia.

DIAGNOSTIC TESTS & INTERPRETATION

Diagnostic Procedures/Other

- Tympanometry
  - Easily performed by office personnel
  - Provides information on middle ear pressure and TM compliance
  - Sensitive in detecting MEE but poor positive predictive value
- Tympanocentesis
  - For episodes of AOM that are resistant to antibiotic therapy, tympanocentesis and culture and sensitivity of the middle ear fluid may help guide antibiotic therapy.
- Tympanocentesis or myringotomy may also be required as part of the treatment of suppurative complications.

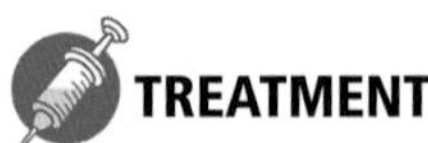

TREATMENT

GENERAL MEASURES

- Do not use prophylactic antibiotics to reduce frequency of episodes of AOM in children with recurrent AOM.
- AOM management should include pain evaluation and treatment.
- Adjunctive therapy for pain management
  - Fever relief with acetaminophen or ibuprofen
  - Pain may be treated with acetaminophen or ibuprofen
  - Pain may be briefly treated with topic anesthetic drops (benzocaine, procaine, or lidocaine) in children >5 years old.

MEDICATION

- Antibiotic therapy for AOM in children ≥6 months of age with severe signs or symptoms (moderate or severe otalgia or otalgia of 48 hours or temperature ≥39°C [102.2°F])
- Antibiotic therapy for bilateral AOM in children 6 to 23 months of age without severe signs or symptoms
- Antibiotic therapy or observation with close follow-up including joint decision-making with caregiver for unilateral AOM in children 6 to 23 months of age without severe signs or symptoms
  - Observation and follow-up and antibiotic therapy if child worsens or fails to improve in 48 to 72 hours
- Initial treatment
  - Amoxicillin (80 to 90 mg/kg/24 h PO divided b.i.d.)
    - When child has not received amoxicillin in past 30 days
    - Does not have concurrent purulent conjunctivitis
    - Not allergic to penicillin
  - Amoxicillin-clavulanate (90 mg/kg/24 h amoxicillin using formulations suited for b.i.d administration which contain either 7:1 or 14:1 amoxicillin:clavulantate ratio)
    - Has received amoxicillin in the last 30 days
    - Concurrent purulent conjunctivitis
    - History of recurrent AOM unresponsive to amoxicillin
- Initial oral antibiotic treatment if penicillin allergy
  - Cefdinir (14 mg/kg/24 h once daily or divided b.i.d.)
  - Cefuroxime (30 mg/kg/24 h divided b.i.d.)
  - Cefpodoxime (10 mg/kg/24 h divided b.i.d.)
  - Ceftriaxone (50 mg/kg IM or IV per day for 1 or 3 days)
- Treatment after 48 to 72 hours of no improvement after initial antibiotic therapy
  - Amoxicillin-clavulanate PO (90 mg/kg/24 h PO of amoxicillin using formulations suited for b.i.d. administration which contain either 7:1 or 14:1 amoxicillin:clavulantate ratio)
  - Ceftriaxone (50 mg/kg IM or IV per day for 1 or 3 days)
  - Clindamycin (30 to 40 mg/kg/24 h PO divided t.i.d.), with or without 3rd-generation cephalosporin

ISSUES FOR REFERRAL

Consider otolaryngology referral:

- Tympanostomy tubes for recurrent AOM if
  - Three episodes in 6 months
  - Four episodes in 1 year with one episode in the preceding 6 months
  - Persistent and/or recurrent otitis with abnormal hearing and/or speech

ONGOING CARE

FOLLOW-UP RECOMMENDATIONS

- Expect symptomatic improvement within 48 to 72 hours of treatment; may need to switch antibiotic and/or evaluate for complications
- Follow-up exam should be scheduled 3 to 4 weeks after completion of antibiotic therapy to ensure resolution of AOM.
- If effusion is present, follow up monthly. For persistent effusions of >3 months' duration, a hearing evaluation is recommended.

PROGNOSIS

- Symptoms of acute infection (fever and otalgia) are relieved within 48 to 72 hours in most patients.
- Treatment failures are more likely with increased severity of disease and younger age.
- Development of another infection within 30 days usually represents a recurrence caused by a different organism rather than a relapse.
  - Recurrences are frequent and more common in younger children and if initial episode is severe.
- 30–70% of treated children will have an effusion at 2 weeks.
  - MEE may persist for weeks to months.

COMPLICATIONS

- Hearing loss
  - Acute conductive hearing loss is common and usually resolves as the effusion resolves.
  - Fluid of long-standing duration may lead to permanent conductive hearing loss.
  - Sensorineural hearing loss may result from spread of infection into the labyrinth.
- TM perforation
- Chronic suppurative otitis media
- Tympanosclerosis
- Cholesteatoma
- Acute mastoiditis
- Petrositis
- Labyrinthitis
- Facial nerve paralysis
- Bacterial meningitis
- Subdural empyema
- Brain abscess
- Lateral sinus thrombosis

ADDITIONAL READING

- Coker TR, Chan LS, Newberry SJ, et al. Diagnosis, microbial epidemiology, and antibiotic treatment of acute otitis media in children: a systematic review. *JAMA*. 2010;304(19):2161–2169.
- Gould JM, Matz PS. Otitis media. *Pediatr Rev*. 2010;31(3):102–116.
- Hoberman A, Paradise JL, Rockette HE, et al. Treatment of acute otitis media in children under 2 years of age. *N Engl J Med*. 2011;364(2):105–115.
- Lieberthal AS, Carroll AE, Chonmaitree T, et al. The diagnosis and management of acute otitis media. *Pediatrics*. 2013;131(3):e964–e999.
- Rosenfeld RM, Shin JJ, Schwartz SR, et al. Clinical practice guideline: otitis media with effusion (update). *Otol Head Neck Surg*. 2016;154(Suppl 1):S1–S41.
- Spiro DM, Tay KY, Arnold DH, et al. Wait-and-see prescription for the treatment of acute otitis media: a randomized controlled trial. *JAMA*. 2006;296(10):1235–1241.
- Takata GS, Chan LS, Morphew T, et al. Evidence assessment of the accuracy of methods of diagnosing middle ear effusion in children with otitis media with effusion. *Pediatrics*. 2003;112(6, Pt 1):1379–1387.

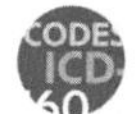

CODES

ICD10

- H66.90 Otitis media, unspecified, unspecified ear
- H65.199 Other acute nonsuppurative otitis media, unspecified ear
- H65.499 Other chronic nonsuppurative otitis media, unspecified ear

FAQ

- Q: When should children with AOM be treated?
- A: Antibiotic therapy for AOM in children ≥6 months of age with severe signs or symptoms; antibiotic therapy for bilateral AOM in children 6 to 23 months of age without severe signs or symptoms
- Q: What is the antibiotic of choice for initial therapy of AOM?
- A: The initial therapy is amoxicillin. The antibiotic treatment after 48 to 72 hours of no improvement is amoxicillin-clavulanate. Ceftriaxone and clindamycin are alternatives.
- Q: When is it acceptable to offer observation with close follow-up for AOM?
- A: Observation can be offered, with joint decision making from the care provider, in unilateral AOM in children 6 to 23 months without severe signs or symptoms and in children ≥24 months without severe signs or symptoms.
- Q: What are severe signs and symptoms of AOM
- A: A toxic-appearing child, with moderate or severe otalgia for >48 hours or temperature >39°C (102.2°F) in past 48 hours
- Q: What can be done to prevent the development of AOM in an individual child?
- A: The following can be done to prevent the development of AOM in an individual child:
  - Pneumococcal conjugate vaccine
  - Annual influenza vaccine
  - Encourage breastfeeding for at least 6 months.
  - Encourage avoidance of tobacco smoke exposure.

PALLOR

David T. Teachey, MD

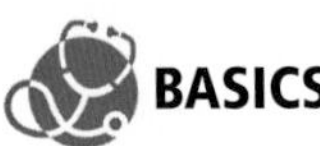

BASICS

DESCRIPTION

- Pallor is defined as paleness of the skin and may be a reflection of anemia or poor peripheral perfusion.
- The normal range for hemoglobin is age-dependent.
- Anemia can be defined functionally as the inability of hemoglobin to meet cellular oxygen demand.
- Parents often fail to notice pallor of gradual onset.
  - Grandparents or others who see the child less often may be the first to suspect pallor.

RISK FACTORS

- Ages between 6 months and 3 years or adolescent females
  - Peak age ranges for iron deficiency
- Gender
  - Some red cell–enzyme X-linked defects such as glucose-6-phosphate dehydrogenase (G6PD) and phosphoglycerate kinase deficiencies are sex linked.
- Race
  - African: hemoglobins S and C, α- and β-thalassemia trait, G6PD deficiency
  - Southeast Asian: hemoglobin E and α-thalassemia
  - Mediterranean descent: β-thalassemia and G6PD deficiency

Genetics

Familial history: Some of the congenital hemolytic anemias are autosomal dominant.

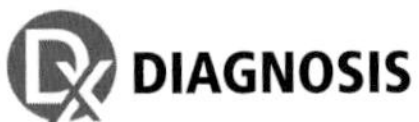

DIAGNOSIS

- Determine first that the child appears pale, not simply fair skinned. Second, decide if there is a medical emergency associated with circulatory failure. If not, the goal is to investigate the etiology and intervene appropriately.
  - **Phase 1**: Assess for signs of shock.
    - If present, initiate emergency procedures as required to stabilize the patient, such as airway, breathing, and circulation.
  - **Phase 2**: If patient is stable, perform history, physical examination, and CBC with reticulocyte count to establish time of onset of pallor, associated symptoms, and level of anemia.
  - **Phase 3**: Follow specific diagnostic workup based on findings in phase 2.
- Signs and symptoms
  - Pallor
  - Other signs and symptoms dependent on etiology

HISTORY

- Acute versus chronic onset
  - Helps with differential diagnosis
- Associated symptoms: weight loss, fever, night sweats, cough, and/or bone pain
  - Suggest an underlying systemic illness, such as leukemia, infection, or rheumatologic disorder
- Jaundice, scleral icterus, dark urine
  - Suggest hemolysis
- Age <6 months
  - May represent a congenital anemia or isoimmunization
- Premature infant
  - Increased risk of both iron and vitamin E deficiency
  - Exaggerated hyperbilirubinemia can be the presenting symptom of isoimmune hemolytic or other congenital hemolytic anemia.
- Pica
  - Often associated with plumbism and iron deficiency
- Medications
  - Can cause bone marrow suppression and/or hemolysis
- Milk intake
  - Introduction of cow's milk at <12 months of age is associated with iron deficiency.
  - Drinking a lot of cow's milk (>24 oz/24 h) puts a toddler at risk for iron deficiency.
- Recent trauma and/or surgery
  - Blood loss can result in iron deficiency.
- Recent infection
  - Can be associated with hemolysis or bone marrow suppression
  - Most common form of mild anemia in childhood
- Family history
  - Familial history of splenectomy and/or early cholecystectomy can be a clue for a previously undiagnosed hemolytic anemia.

PHYSICAL EXAM

- Pallor varies with patient's natural skin color. Conjunctiva and oral mucosa examinations are essential to assess pallor.
- Rapid respiratory rate, decreased BP, weak pulses, slow capillary refill
  - Indications of uncompensated anemia and/or shock
- Frontal bossing and prominence of the malar and maxillary bones
  - Extramedullary erythropoiesis
- Enlarged spleen
  - Hemolytic anemias, malignancy, infection
- Glossitis
  - Vitamin B_{12} deficiency
  - Iron deficiency
- Scleral icterus or jaundice
  - May indicate hemolysis
- Systolic flow murmur
  - Anemia
- Bruits
  - May indicate vascular malformations
- Petechiae and bruising
  - May indicate an associated thrombocytopenia, coagulopathy, or vasculitis
- Dysmorphic features
  - Diamond-Blackfan and Fanconi anemia are associated with other congenital defects, including thumb abnormalities, short stature, and congenital heart disease.

DIAGNOSTIC TESTS & INTERPRETATION

Initial Tests (screening, lab, imaging)

- CBC with red cell indices
  - Establishes the diagnosis of anemia, distinguishes by size: normocytic, macrocytic, microcytic
- Reticulocyte count
  - Distinguishes between decreased production and increased destruction of red cells
- Coombs test and antibody screen
  - Identifies immune-mediated red cell destruction
  - Can have false positives and false negatives
- Peripheral blood smear
  - Specific morphologic findings can be diagnostic.
- Iron studies: iron-binding capacity, serum iron, ferritin, transferrin
  - Iron deficiency anemia or anemia of chronic disease
- Hemoglobin electrophoresis with quantification
  - Hemoglobinopathy
- Lead studies: serum lead, free erythrocyte protoporphyrin
  - Plumbism
- Stool guaiac
  - Occult blood loss
- Osmotic fragility
  - Red cell membrane defects (spherocytosis)
  - Any spherocytic anemia may be positive.
- Quantitative red cell–enzyme assays
  - Inherited RBC enzyme deficiencies
- Serum folate, RBC folate, and serum vitamin B_{12} levels
  - Deficiency

P

Diagnostic Procedures/Other
Bone marrow aspiration and biopsy: if malignancy or bone marrow failure syndrome suspected

DIFFERENTIAL DIAGNOSIS
- Congenital
  - Hemoglobinopathies: sickle cell syndromes, thalassemia syndromes, other unstable hemoglobins
  - Erythrocyte membrane defects: hereditary spherocytosis, elliptocytosis, stomatocytosis, pyropoikilocytosis, infantile pyknocytosis
  - Erythrocyte enzyme defects: G6PD deficiency, pyruvate kinase deficiency
  - Diamond-Blackfan anemia: congenital pure red cell aplasia (rare)
  - Fanconi anemia: constellation of varied cytopenias, multiple congenital anomalies, abnormal bone marrow chromosomal fragility
- Infectious
  - Septic shock
  - Can get mild anemia after mild infections in childhood (anemia of inflammation)
  - Infection-related bone marrow suppression: parvovirus B19 infection
  - Infection-related hemolytic anemias: Epstein-Barr virus, influenza, coxsackievirus, varicella, cytomegalovirus, *Escherichia coli*, *Pneumococcus* species, *Streptococcus* species, *Salmonella typhi*, *Mycoplasma* species
- Nutritional/toxic/drugs
  - Iron deficiency anemia: common cause of anemia in children, especially those <3 years of age and in female adolescents
  - Plumbism: anemia usually due to coexisting iron deficiency; very high lead levels associated with altered heme synthesis
  - Vitamin B_{12} and/or folate deficiency: results in a megaloblastic anemia
  - Medication-induced bone marrow suppression: chemotherapy; antibiotics, especially trimethoprim-sulfamethoxazole
  - Drug-related hemolytic anemia: antibiotics, antiepileptics, azathioprine, isoniazid, nonsteroidal anti-inflammatory drugs
- Trauma
  - Acute blood loss
- Tumor
  - Leukemia with bone marrow infiltration
  - Metastatic tumors with bone marrow infiltration
- Genetic/metabolic
  - Metabolic derangements: severe electrolyte disturbance, pH disturbance, inborn errors
  - Shwachman-Diamond syndrome: marrow hypoplasia with associated pancreatic insufficiency and associated failure to thrive
- Other
  - Transient erythroblastopenia of childhood: acquired pure RBC aplasia
  - Aplastic anemia: bone marrow failure syndrome with at least two of the three blood cell lines eventually affected
  - Systemic diseases: anemia of chronic disease, chronic renal disease, uremia
  - Hypothyroidism
  - Sideroblastic anemia: defective iron use within the developing erythrocytes
  - Autoimmune and isoimmune hemolytic anemias
  - Microangiopathic hemolytic anemias: thrombotic thrombocytopenic purpura (TTP), hemolytic uremic syndrome (HUS), disseminated intravascular coagulation (DIC)
  - Mechanical destruction: vascular malformation, abnormal or prosthetic cardiac valves

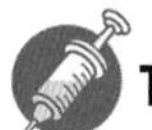

TREATMENT

GENERAL MEASURES
- Treat underlying cause.
- Consider packed RBC transfusion if in extremis or severe anemia and low likelihood of recovery in near future.
- Consider emergent plasmapheresis if with microangiopathic hemolytic anemia.
- Consider immunosuppressive medications (corticosteroids, intravenous immunoglobulin [IVIG]) if with autoimmune hemolytic anemia.
- Iron deficiency anemia
  - Elemental iron

MEDICATION
Elemental iron for patients with iron deficiency
- 4 to 6 mg/kg/24 h PO divided b.i.d.–t.i.d.
- Absorbed best with acidic drinks, including orange juice; dairy products decrease absorption.
- Reticulocyte should improve 72 hours after starting iron therapy; the hemoglobin may take a week to rise.
- Iron should be continued for at least 3 months to replenish iron stores.

ISSUES FOR REFERRAL
- Severe or unexplained anemia
- Anemias other than dietary iron deficiency or thalassemia trait
- Recurrent iron deficiency
  - May suggest ongoing bleeding or iron malabsorption
- All bone marrow failure or infiltrative processes

ADMISSION, INPATIENT, AND NURSING CONSIDERATIONS
- Severe anemia of unclear etiology with hemodynamic instability
  - Transfuse with packed RBCs cautiously.
  - In an autoimmune hemolytic process, the child is at risk for a transfusion reaction and there may be delay in obtaining cross-matched blood.
  - Obtain blood for diagnostic studies before transfusion if possible.
- Circulatory failure without anemia
  - Requires intensive monitoring and access to critical care in an emergency department or intensive care unit
  - Fluid resuscitation and/or inotropic pressor support as needed
- Acute blood loss
  - Treat circulatory failure as described.
  - Transfuse with packed RBCs, platelets, and fresh frozen plasma as needed.
- Malignancies
  - Emergency care should be directed toward treatment of circulatory failure and possible associated infection and then to rapid diagnosis and treatment of the malignancy.
  - Consultation with an oncologist should be sought as soon as possible.

ADDITIONAL READING

- Baker RD, Greer FR; for Committee on Nutrition American Academy of Pediatrics. Diagnosis and prevention of iron deficiency and iron-deficiency anemia in infants and young children (0–3 years of age). *Pediatrics*. 2010;126(5):1040–1050.
- Glader BE. Hemolytic anemia in children. *Clin Lab Med*. 1999;19(1):87–111.
- Graham EA. The changing face of anemia in infancy. *Pediatr Rev*. 1994;15(5):175–183.
- Monzon CM, Beaver BD, Dillon TD. Evaluation of erythrocyte disorders with mean corpuscular volume (MCV) and red cell distribution width (RDW). *Clin Pediatr (Phila)*. 1987;26(12):632–638.
- Segel G, Hirsh M, Feig S. Managing anemia in a pediatric office practice: part 2. *Pediatr Rev*. 2002;23(4):111–122.
- Sills RH. Indications for bone marrow examination. *Pediatr Rev*. 1995;16(6):226–228.

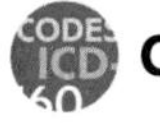

CODES

ICD10
R23.1 Pallor

PANCREATIC PSEUDOCYST

Amit S. Grover, MB BCh BAO, MSc

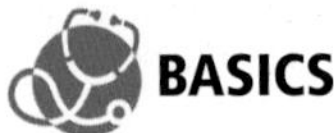

BASICS

DESCRIPTION

- A pancreatic pseudocyst is a peripancreatic (or intrapancreatic) fluid collection associated with a history of pancreatitis, that is surrounded by a well-defined inflammatory wall and that has no solid component.
  - The term "pseudocyst" is often incorrectly used to define various types of fluid collections associated with pancreatitis. As a result, medical literature on pseudocysts is not consistent in its descriptions or its findings.
  - An important distinction between "fluid collections" associated with pancreatitis is that some consist of fluid alone, whereas others arise from necrosis of pancreatic parenchyma and/or peripancreatic tissues. The latter type of fluid collection involves a solid component (with variable amounts of fluid), which distinguishes them from pseudocysts.
- Types of fluid collections:
  - Acute peripancreatic fluid collection (APFC)
    - A fluid collection that develops in the early phase of interstitial edematous acute (typically mild) pancreatitis
    - Lack a well-defined wall on CT scan
    - Not associated with necrotizing pancreatitis
    - Remains sterile and usually resolves without intervention
    - If APFC persists beyond 4 weeks, likely to develop into a pancreatic pseudocyst, although this is considered a rare outcome
  - Pancreatic pseudocyst
    - Refers specifically to a peripancreatic (or less commonly, an intrapancreatic) fluid collection
    - Surrounded by a well-defined inflammatory wall and containing *no* solid material
    - Pancreatic pseudocysts develop >4 weeks after the onset of interstitial pancreatitis.
  - Acute necrotic collection (ANC)
    - A collection of *both* variable amounts of fluid and solid (necrotic) material related to pancreatic and/or peripancreatic necrosis
    - Occur within the first 4 weeks of disease and can resemble an APFC in the first few days of acute pancreatitis
    - As necrotizing pancreatitis develops and necrosis evolves, solid component become evident.
    - May be multiple and may involve the pancreatic parenchyma alone, the peripancreatic tissue alone, or most commonly both
    - May be infected or sterile
    - Generally associated with more severe sequelae of acute pancreatitis
  - Walled-off necrosis (WON)
    - Collection of varying amounts of liquid and solid material surrounded by a mature, enhancing wall of reactive tissue
    - Represents a mature, encapsulated ANC
    - Develops no earlier than 4 weeks after episode of necrotizing pancreatitis
    - May be multiple and present at sites distant from the pancreas
    - May be sterile or infected

PATHOPHYSIOLOGY

- Pseudocysts occur when there is disruption in the pancreatic ductular system, or its intrapancreatic branches, without any evidence of pancreatic or peripancreatic necrosis.
- This results in the extravasation of pancreatic enzymes evoking an inflammatory response.
- The inflammatory reaction leads to a fluid collection that is rich in pancreatic enzymes (APFC).
- If the duration of the fluid collection is >4 weeks, becomes localized (intrapancreatic or extrapancreatic), and develops a fibrin capsule, it becomes a pseudocyst.
- A pseudocyst does not have a true epithelial lining.
- If there is communication between the pseudocyst and the pancreatic duct, the enzyme level in the fluid remain elevated; if there is no communication, the enzyme level falls with time.

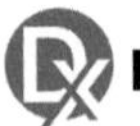

DIAGNOSIS

HISTORY

Acute or chronic pancreatitis

- Suspect pancreatic pseudocyst in patients recovering from acute pancreatitis, or in the patient with chronic pancreatitis, who has recurrent/persistent abdominal pain, a palpable abdominal mass, or persistently elevated serum pancreatic enzymes.

PHYSICAL EXAM

- Abdominal tenderness
- Abdominal mass
- Nausea and vomiting
- Weight loss
- Jaundice
- Abdominal distention
  - Mass/ascites
- In many situations, no clinical signs are seen.
- Clinical signs may be secondary to complications:
  - Jaundice in hepatobiliary obstruction
  - Lower limb edema in compression of inferior vena cava
  - Ascites in peritonitis
  - Pleural effusion
  - Early satiety from compression on stomach

DIFFERENTIAL DIAGNOSIS

- Congenital/genetic
  - Congenital cysts
  - Polycystic disease
  - Von Hippel-Lindau disease
  - Cystic fibrosis
- Infections
  - Pancreatic abscess
  - Echinococcal (hydatid) cyst
  - *Taenia solium* cyst
- Tumor
  - Serous cystadenoma
  - Mucinous cystadenoma
  - Cystic islet cell tumors
  - Teratoma
  - Pancreatoblastoma
  - Cystadenocarcinoma
  - Frantz tumor
  - Angiomatous cystic neoplasms
  - Lymphangiomas
  - Hemangioendothelioma
- Miscellaneous:
  - Splenic cyst
  - Adrenal cyst
  - Enterogenous cyst
  - Duplication cysts
  - Endometriosis

DIAGNOSTIC TESTS & INTERPRETATION

- Serum pancreatic enzyme levels:
  - Persistently elevated enzymes in blood can be a clue but is not an absolute indicator.
  - Elevated enzymes in fluid drained from a peripancreatic or intrapancreatic fluid collection with no solid component is consistent with a pancreatic pseudocyst.
- CT scan
  - Reveals pseudopancreatic cyst; can also be used to gauge size of pseudocyst and its relationship to adjacent organs
- Ultrasonography
  - Visualizes pancreatic pseudocysts
  - Can be used to follow cyst size over time
- Endoscopic ultrasound (EUS)
  - Common modality in adult patients and increasingly used in pediatrics
  - Can be used to diagnose presence and size of pseudocyst; can also be used to guide peroral fluid aspiration and drainage
- Endoscopic retrograde cholangiopancreatography (ERCP)
  - Used in some cases to delineate the pancreatic ductular system before drainage to distinguish ductal stenosis, disruption, stones, and other obstructions

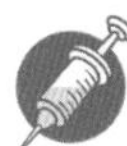

TREATMENT

GENERAL MEASURES

- Medical management:
  - Most cases resolve with supportive care.
  - If eating precipitates pain, short-term nasojejunal feedings or parenteral nutrition may be warranted.
  - Follow up with ultrasound or CT scan to make sure there are no complications.
  - >60% have complete resolution by the end of 1 year.
  - Usually, no medications are used for managing pseudocysts.
  - Somatostatin analogue (octreotide) has been reported to be used to decrease fluid collection along with drainage.
  - Antibiotics are used in situations of infected pseudocyst.
- Drainage
  - Most often used in the setting of WON or symptomatic pseudocyst
  - Indications: infection, rupture with cardiopulmonary compromise, biliary and gastric outlet obstruction, persistent symptoms, rapid enlargement, failure of large pseudocysts (>6 cm) to shrink after 6 weeks
  - Modalities:
    - Percutaneous drainage (aspiration or catheter drainage) is done in cases in which the pseudocyst has a less mature wall.
    - Percutaneous aspiration has a high recurrence rate of 63% and failure rate of 54%.
    - Continuous drainage has a recurrence rate of 8% and a failure rate of 19%.
    - Endoscopic procedures are becoming the 1st-line drainage modality, as they are less invasive than surgery.
    - Endoscopic procedures include transmural cystenterostomies and transpapillary route procedures such as stent placement for pseudocysts that communicate with the main pancreatic duct.
    - Endoscopic procedures in experienced hands report success rates of 82–89%, complication rates of 10–20%, and recurrence rates of 6–18%.

SURGERY/OTHER PROCEDURES

- Reserved for failed endoscopic procedures, difficult to access areas of WON and multiple WONs
- Includes internal drainage (cystogastrostomy, cystoduodenostomy, and Roux-en-Y cystojejunostomy), resection, and external drainage
- Success rate is 85–90%.
- Recurrence rate is 0–17%.
- Mortality rate is between 3% and 5%.

ONGOING CARE

PROGNOSIS

Majority of pseudocysts resolve without intervention.

COMPLICATIONS

- Perforation/rupture
  - Cardiopulmonary compromise secondary to pleural effusion and ascites
  - Peritonitis and ascites, which can be fatal
- Hemorrhage
  - Erosions of vessels lining the cyst cause intracystic bleeding and rapid increase in the cyst size.
  - Bleeding may occur directly into stomach, duodenum (clinically manifesting as GI bleeding), or peritoneal cavity.
- Obstruction
  - Biliary obstruction: jaundice
  - Portal obstruction: portal hypertension
  - Gastric outlet obstruction
  - Inferior vena cava obstruction: peripheral edema
  - Urinary obstruction
  - Colonic obstruction
- Infection of pseudocysts is rare in children compared to adults:
  - Associated with high mortality rate for children and adults
  - Management usually requires surgical drainage.

ADDITIONAL READING

- Law NM, Freeman ML. Emergency complications of acute and chronic pancreatitis. *Gastroenterol Clin North Am*. 2003;32(4):1169–1194.
- Reber HA. Surgery for acute and chronic pancreatitis. *Gastrointest Endosc*. 2002;56(Suppl 6):S246–S248.
- Sarr MG, Banks PA, Bollen TL, et al. The new revised classification of acute pancreatitis 2012. *Surg Clin North Am*. 2013;93(3):549–562.
- Vidyarthi G, Steinberg SE. Endoscopic management of pancreatic pseudocysts. *Surg Clin North Am*. 2001;81(2):405–410.
- Weckman L, Kylänpää ML, Puolakkainen P, et al. Endoscopic treatment of pancreatic pseudocysts. *Surg Endosc*. 2006;20(4):603–607.

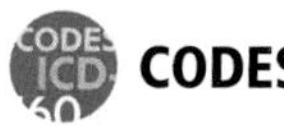

CODES

ICD10

K86.3 Pseudocyst of pancreas

PANCREATITIS

Amit S. Grover, MB BCh BAO, MSc

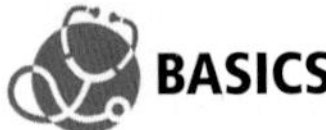

BASICS

DESCRIPTION

- Inflammation within the pancreas characterized by three phases: (i) early trypsin activation within acinar cells; followed by (ii) surrounding intrapancreatic inflammation; and finally, (iii) extrapancreatic inflammation with systemic inflammatory responses
- Classified into acute and chronic
  - Acute pancreatitis (AP)
    - *Variable* presentation; most often characterized by acute onset of abdominal pain, nausea, and vomiting with elevation of pancreatic enzymes
    - Nonverbal children may present with irritability; infants may present with lethargy and fever.
    - Often self-limited, with reversible changes but can progress if not appropriately managed
    - Severe AP is rare in children; however, a high suspicion should always be maintained, as severe disease can progress rapidly and result in significant morbidity and mortality.
  - Chronic pancreatitis (CP)
    - Characterized by irreversible morphologic changes and fibrotic replacement of the pancreatic parenchyma
    - Clinically characterized by recurrent abdominal pain or evidence of exocrine and/or endocrine insufficiency
    - Often the result of a persistent and continued pancreatic inflammation secondary to acute attacks

ETIOLOGY

- Biliary tract disease
  - Gallstones
- Medications
  - L-asparaginase, azathioprine/6-MP, mesalamine, sulfonamides, thiazides, furosemide, tetracyclines, valproic acid, corticosteroids, estrogens, procainamide, ethacrynic acid, and others
- Toxins
  - Alcohol, organophosphates, scorpion poison, snake poison
- Trauma
  - Bicycle handle injuries
  - Motor vehicle collisions
  - Child abuse
  - Postoperative
    - Endoscopic retrograde cholangiopancreatography (ERCP)
- Systemic disease
  - Shock/hypoxemia/sepsis
  - Inflammatory bowel disease (IBD)
  - Cystic fibrosis
- Idiopathic
- Less common
  - Infections
    - Bacterial: typhoid, mycoplasma
    - Viral: measles, mumps, Epstein-Barr virus, coxsackie B, rubella, influenza, echovirus, hepatitis A and B
    - Parasites: *Ascaris lumbricoides*, *Echinococcus granulosus*, *Cryptosporidium parvum*, *Plasmodium falciparum*
  - Metabolic diseases:
    - Hyperlipidemia
    - Hypercalcemia
    - Diabetic ketoacidosis
    - Uremia
    - Inborn errors of metabolism
  - Systemic diseases:
    - Hemolytic uremic syndrome (HUS)
    - Celiac disease
    - Diabetes mellitus
    - Vasculitis: systemic lupus erythematosus (SLE), Henoch-Schönlein purpura, Kawasaki disease
- Rare causes:
  - Autoimmune pancreatitis: rare condition divided into two subtypes
    - Type I often grouped with IgG4-related disease and systemic manifestations.
    - Type II does not have IgG4 association, however, is more common in younger patients and associated with IBD.
  - Congenital anomalies:
    - Pancreatic divisum
    - Annular pancreas
    - Anomalous pancreaticobiliary junction
    - Biliary tract malformations
    - Duplication cyst of the duodenum/gastropancreatic/common bile duct (CBD)
  - Gene mutations
    - *PRSS1*: trypsinogen
    - *SPINK1*: serine protease inhibitor of Kazal type 1
    - *CFTR*: cystic fibrosis transmembrane regulator
    - *CTRC*: chymotrypsin C
    - *CASR*: calcium-sensing receptor

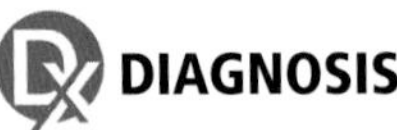

DIAGNOSIS

HISTORY

- Pain
  - Onset, location, and severity can be variable in children.
  - Aggravated by food intake
  - Nonverbal patients (i.e., younger age, developmental delay) may present with increased irritability.
- Vomiting
  - May or may not always be present
  - May be bilious
  - May present as feeding intolerance
- Trauma
  - Even trivial abdominal trauma should be a red flag.
  - Evaluate for evidence of child abuse.
- Family history
  - Hereditary pancreatitis
  - Hypertriglyceridemia (I, IV, or V)
  - CFTR mutations/FH of CF
- Prior history of, or risk factors for, cholelithiasis
- Toxic exposures (i.e., EtOH, pesticides)
- Review of systems:
  - Associated fever may suggest infectious etiology.
  - Diminished urine output raises concern for 3rd-space losses.
  - Shortness of breath raises concern for pulmonary involvement (i.e., effusions).

PHYSICAL EXAM

- General exam
  - Growth parameters (weight and height), vital signs, capillary refill, pulse oximetry, pallor, jaundice, edema, and clubbing
  - Abnormal vital signs (heart rate, respiratory rate, and blood pressure) can be indicative of the systemic inflammatory response syndrome (SIRS), a poor prognostic sign.
  - Clubbing can be an indicator of cystic fibrosis.
- GI
  - Mouth: Presence of aphthous lesions raises possibility of Crohn disease.
    - Inspection: abdominal distention or flank fullness (ascites or pseudopancreatic cyst); bluish discoloration of the flanks (Grey Turner sign) and periumbilical region (Cullen sign) in hemorrhagic pancreatitis
    - Palpation: for liver, gall bladder, spleen, and masses. Patients will have guarding, tenderness, and rebound tenderness, especially in the epigastric region and/or upper abdomen; palpable mass could be a pancreatic pseudocyst.
  - Percussion: dullness and fluid thrill consistent with ascites
  - Auscultation: bowel sounds decreased in ascites or absent in paralytic ileus
- Rectal exam
  - Perianal region for skin tags, fistulas, abscesses, or healed scars, which could be indicative of IBD; perirectal exam for mass, melena, or occult blood
  - Hematochezia can be suggestive of IBD.
- GU
  - Assess urinary output.
  - High specific gravity suggestive of reduced intravascular volume, result of 3rd-space losses
- Respiratory system
  - Pleural effusion and acute respiratory distress syndrome (ARDS)
  - Diffuse respiratory findings could be indicative of cystic fibrosis.
- CNS
  - Stupor or coma

DIAGNOSTIC TESTS & INTERPRETATION

- CBC
  - Hemoglobin may be decreased in hemorrhagic pancreatitis.
  - Leukocytosis may be present in infectious pancreatitis.
  - Hemoconcentration: elevated HCT
- Basic metabolic panel
  - Hemoconcentration due to 3rd-space losses and intravascular depletion (elevated BUN, Cr)
  - Calcium may be elevated (etiology) or decreased (sequelae).
  - Glucose may be transiently elevated.
  - Bicarbonate may be low secondary to acidosis.
- Liver function tests:
  - Elevated transaminase levels suggest biliary cause.
  - Elevated bilirubin level, GGT, alkaline phosphatase suggestive of gallstone pancreatitis
- Amylase level
  - 3-fold elevation of amylase levels increases specificity for the diagnosis of pancreatitis.
  - Starts rising 2 to 12 hours after the insult and remains elevated for 3 to 5 days

- Degree of elevation does not have any correlation to the severity or the course of the illness.
- Other causes of elevated amylase levels include bowel obstruction, acute appendicitis, biliary obstruction, salivary duct obstruction, diabetic ketoacidosis, cystic fibrosis, pneumonia, salpingitis, ruptured ectopic pregnancy, ovarian cyst, cerebral trauma, burns, renal failure, and macroamylasemia.

- Lipase level
  - Lipase levels are more specific than amylase for the diagnosis of pancreatitis.
  - Starts rising 4 to 8 hours after the insult and remains elevated for 8 to 14 days
  - 3-fold increase in the level is very sensitive and specific for pancreatitis.
  - Levels do not correlate with severity or with clinical outcome.
  - Other causes of elevated lipase levels include intestinal perforation, intestinal obstruction, appendicitis, mesenteric infarction, cholecystitis, diabetic ketoacidosis, renal failure, and macrolipasemia.
- Urinalysis
  - Urine specific gravity is a simple indicator of intravascular volume.
    - Elevated specific gravity can suggest 3rd-space losses and is associated with severe disease.
- Abdominal radiographs:
  - Sentinel loop: distended small intestinal loop near the pancreas
  - Colon cutoff sign: absence of gas shadow in the colon distal to the transverse colon
  - Multiple fluid levels in paralytic ileus
  - Calcification or stones in pancreas or gallbladder
  - Diffuse haziness: ascites
- Chest radiograph
  - Pleural effusion or ARDS
  - Diaphragmatic involvement
- US abdomen
  - Best initial test
  - Will demonstrate pancreatic size; echogenicity; associated fat stranding; ductal diameter/disruption; and calcifications, cholelithiasis, CBD dilation, ascites, and free fluid within abdomen
  - Can consider contrast enhanced US if equipment, and radiologist with expertise in this modality is available
  - Limited by obesity and bowel gas
  - Endoscopic US (EUS) is more useful than the transabdominal US study but is difficult in children and requires anesthesia.
- CT scan
  - May be used if history of trauma to look at extent of injury to pancreas and other intra-abdominal structures
  - Best to show evidence of pancreatic necrosis with AP from any cause, however, not sensitive within the first 48 to 72 hours
  - Reveals pathology in the pancreaticobiliary system in most instances
  - Involves exposure to radiation
- Magnetic resonance cholangiopancreatography (MRCP)
  - Good for ductal visualization (especially if secretin stimulated)
  - Can reveal anatomic abnormalities/obstructive lesions, that is, pancreatic divisum, abnormal pancreaticobiliary junction
  - Can mitigate need for therapeutic procedures (i.e., ERCP), unless there is concern for choledocholithiasis +/− ascending cholangitis
  - Good for distinguishing pseudocyst versus walled-off necrosis
  - No exposure to radiation; however, may require anesthesia if needed in a young child
- ERCP
  - Indicated in persistent/CP for delineation of pancreatic ducts and for therapeutic interventions (i.e., sphincterotomy, stricture dilation, and/or stent placement)
  - Risk of post-ERCP pancreatitis in 10–20% of cases
    - In adults, administration of rectal indomethacin has been shown to reduce this risk.

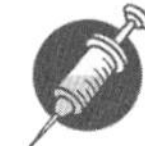

TREATMENT

Fluid resuscitation

- Aggressive volume resuscitation with isotonic solutions is the cornerstone of therapy for AP.
- Adult data supports the use of lactated Ringer solution (has not been studied in pediatrics).
- Under-resuscitation is associated with increased risk of mortality from AP.
- Targeted approach involving bolus (20 mL/kg), followed by continuous infusion at 1.5 to 2 times maintenance (contraindicated if presence of fluid-sensitive cardiac disease)
- Perform serial monitoring of fluid status q6–8h (measure strict ins/outs; urine specific gravity).

MEDICATION

- Antibiotics
  - No evidence to support the routine use of antibiotics in patients with acute necrotizing pancreatitis *unless*:
    - Sepsis is suspected.
    - An extrapancreatic infection (bacteremia, pneumonia, UTI) is present.
    - Patient is on chemotherapy and/or is neutropenic.
- Pain management
  - Effective analgesia should be a priority.
  - Combination of intermittent IV narcotics +/− PCA

ADDITIONAL THERAPIES

Nutrition

- Initially (i.e., first 24 hours), patient typically remains NPO and is aggressively fluid resuscitated.
- Extensive evidence in adult literature has demonstrated that early enteral nutrition has been shown to improve outcomes in patients with severe AP.
- Postpyloric feeds can be considered if initial trial of enteral feeding fails.
- If prolonged NPO course and failure of postpyloric feeds, consider parenteral nutrition.

SURGERY/OTHER PROCEDURES

- If gallstone impaction with choledocholithiasis, should consider ERCP + sphincterotomy +/− stent
- Severe third spacing can lead to abdominal compartment syndrome, necessitating surgical decompression.
- Development of walled-off necrosis with persistent pain or symptoms may benefit from necrocystectomy (endoscopic or surgical).

ONGOING CARE

PROGNOSIS

AP is usually a self-limiting disorder in children.

COMPLICATIONS

- Pancreatic edema
- Peripancreatic fat necrosis
- Acute pancreatic fluid collections
- Pancreatic necrosis
- Pancreatic pseudocyst or walled-off necrosis
- Pancreatic ductal strictures
- Pancreatic ductal dilatation
- Systemic complications:
  - Shock and multiorgan failure
- GI and hepatobiliary
  - Paralytic ileus
  - Ascites, peritonitis
  - Stress ulcer
  - Intestinal hemorrhage
  - Portal vein thrombosis/splenic vein thrombosis/obstruction
  - Bile duct obstruction
- Pulmonary
  - Atelectasis, pleural effusion, pneumonitis, ARDS
- Cardiovascular
  - Hypotension/circulatory collapse
  - Pericarditis/pericardial effusion
  - EKG changes
- Sudden death

ADDITIONAL READING

- Bai HX, Lowe ME, Husain SZ. What have we learned about acute pancreatitis in children? *J Pediatr Gastroenterol Nutr*. 2011;52(3):262–270.
- Banks PA, Bollen TL, Dervenis C, et al; for Acute Pancreatitis Classification Working Group. Classification of acute pancreatitis—2012: revision of the Atlanta classification and definitions by international consensus. *Gut*. 2013;62(1):102–111.
- Forsmark CE, Baillie J; for AGA Institute Clinical Practice and Economics Committee, AGA Institute Governing Board. AGA Institute technical review on acute pancreatitis. *Gastroenterology*. 2007;132(5):2022–2044.
- Tenner S, Baillie J, DeWitt J, et al; for American College of Gastroenterology. American College of Gastroenterology guideline: management of acute pancreatitis. *Am J Gastroenterol*. 2013;108(9):1400–1415.

CODES

ICD10

- K85.9 Acute pancreatitis, unspecified
- K86.1 Other chronic pancreatitis
- K85.8 Other acute pancreatitis

PARVOVIRUS B19 (ERYTHEMA INFECTIOSUM, FIFTH DISEASE)

Camille Sabella, MD

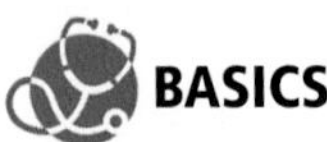

BASICS

DESCRIPTION

Parvovirus B19 (B19) is a small, single-stranded DNA virus of the family *Parvoviridae*. There are three major genetic variants (1 to 3). B19 is a common infection in humans, most often associated with the childhood exanthem, erythema infectiosum, also known as fifth disease.

EPIDEMIOLOGY

- B19 infections are ubiquitous worldwide, occurring most often in school-aged children.
- Humans are the only hosts.
- Incubation period is 4 to 14 days (up to 21 days).
- Attack rates: 15–60% of susceptibles (i.e., seronegative) will become infected upon exposure.
- Modes of transmission
  - Contact with respiratory secretions
  - Percutaneous exposure to blood or blood products (10^{11} virions/mL of serum in patients with hereditary hemolytic anemias)
  - Vertical transmission from mother to fetus

Prevalence

Seroprevalence of B19 IgG antibodies

- >5 years old: 2–9%
- 5 to 18 years old: 15–35%
- Adults: 50%
- Elderly: 90%

GENERAL PREVENTION

- B19 transmission can be decreased through routine infection prevention practices, including hand hygiene and appropriate disposal of contaminated facial tissues.
- For hospitalized children with suspected aplastic crisis, immunocompromised patients with chronic infection and anemia, and patients with papular purpuric gloves and socks syndrome (PPGSS) secondary to B19, droplet precautions in addition to standard precautions are recommended.
- No additional preventive measures are needed for normal hosts with rash.
- Due to the potential risks to the fetus from B19 infections, pregnant health care workers should adhere to strict infection control procedures and avoid contact with immunocompromised hosts with B19 infection or those with aplastic crisis.
- Due to high prevalence of B19 in the community, routine exclusion of pregnant women from the workplace where B19 infections are suspected (e.g., schools, child care) is not recommended.

PATHOPHYSIOLOGY

- Parvovirus B19 inhibits erythropoiesis by lytically infecting red blood cell (RBC) precursors in the bone marrow.
- It is associated with a number of clinical manifestations, ranging from benign to severe.

COMMONLY ASSOCIATED CONDITIONS

- Erythema infectiosum, or fifth disease, is the most common form of infection caused by B19 and occurs in up to 35% of school-aged children.
- Asymptomatic infection may occur in ~20% of children and adults.
- Transient aplastic crisis secondary to B19 infection may cause severe anemia in patients with hereditary hemolytic anemias or any condition that shortens the RBC lifespan, such as sickle cell disease or spherocytosis.
- Polyarthropathy syndrome (symmetric joint pain and swelling, typically of the hands, knees, and feet) is seen in up to 80% of adults, especially women. Arthralgias and arthritis occur infrequently in children. When present, arthritis in children most often involves the knees.
- Hydrops fetalis may develop after maternal B19 infection with intrauterine involvement (typically within the first 20 weeks of pregnancy).
- Chronic anemia/pure red cell aplasia due to persistent B19 infection has been reported in immunocompromised patients.
- PPGSS consists of painful and pruritic papules, petechiae, and purpura localized to the hands and feet and is often associated with fever.
- B19 is one of the most common viruses identified in cases of myocarditis, although its role in pathogenesis is unclear.
- Reports of neurologic manifestations (including meningitis, encephalitis, and peripheral neuropathy), hemophagocytic syndrome, hepatitis, and Henoch-Schönlein purpura have also been associated with B19 infection, although the precise role of the virus in these conditions is unclear.

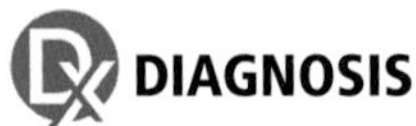

DIAGNOSIS

Diagnosis depends on recognition of typical symptoms and the results of laboratory testing.

HISTORY

- Erythema infectiosum (fifth disease)
  - Characterized by an erythematous facial rash with a distinctive "slapped cheek" appearance, often accompanied by circumoral pallor
  - A brief, mild prodrome of systemic symptoms, including headache, sore throat, myalgias, and low-grade fevers, often precedes the appearance of rash by 7 to 10 days.
  - The child is usually well appearing and remains active and playful.
- Aplastic crisis
  - Prodromal symptoms in B19-infected children with sickle cell disease or other hereditary hemolytic anemias are nonspecific and consist of fever, malaise, and headache. Rash is usually absent.
  - Symptoms are usually self-limited, lasting 7 to 10 days.
  - Severe anemia, CHF, stroke, and acute splenic sequestration have also been associated.
- Chronic anemia/pure red cell aplasia
  - In immunocompromised patients, B19 infection may persist for months, leading to chronic anemia with B19 viremia.
  - Low-grade fever and neutropenia may accompany anemia.

PHYSICAL EXAM

Fifth disease

- Characterized by an erythematous facial rash with a distinctive "slapped cheek" appearance, often accompanied by circumoral pallor
- A symmetric, macular, often lace-like rash occurs on the trunk, spreading outward to the rest of the body and extremities. The rash is often pruritic and may intensify with exposure to sunlight, heat, or exercise. It occasionally involves the palms and soles. Rarely, the rash can be papular, vesicular, or purpuric. It may last for ~7 days but can persist >20 days.
- Child usually well appearing

DIFFERENTIAL DIAGNOSIS

B19 infection should be considered in all patients with arthritis or viral exanthems with a consistent history and exam.

DIAGNOSTIC TESTS & INTERPRETATION

- There is no practical in vitro system for isolation or culture of the virus.
- Antibodies
  - Detection of parvovirus B19-specific IgM or IgG antibodies as determined by EIA or radioimmunoassay
  - The presence of B19-specific IgM antibodies is diagnostic in patients with symptoms of erythema infectiosum or aplastic crisis. IgM- and IgG-specific antibodies are detected in 90% of such patients by 3 to 7 days of illness.
  - B19-specific IgG antibodies persist for life, whereas specific IgM antibodies begin to decrease 30 to 60 days after onset of illness.
- Polymerase chain reaction (PCR) techniques
  - B19 DNA can be detected by PCR in serum for up to 9 months following the initial viremic phase. B19 DNA has also been shown to persist in solid tissues following primary infection, even in healthy individuals. Thus, identification of B19 DNA does not necessarily signify acute infection.
  - Immunocompromised patients with chronic marrow suppression may be unable to produce B19-specific IgG or IgM antibodies. In such cases, PCR for B19 viral DNA is the diagnostic method of choice.
  - PCR may also be used to detect virus in the fetus.
- Hematocrit and reticulocyte count in patients with aplastic crisis
  - Laboratory studies reveal reticulocytopenia, usually with counts of <1%. During the illness, the patient's hematocrit may fall as low as 15%.

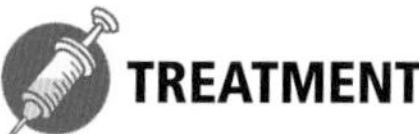

TREATMENT

GENERAL MEASURES

- There is no specific antiviral therapy for B19 infection.
- Most patients require supportive care only.
- Transfusions may be required for treatment of severe anemia in patients with aplastic crisis.
- IV immunoglobulin (IVIG) therapy has been given with some success to patients with chronic marrow suppression secondary to B19 infection.
- Cases of hydrops fetalis caused by B19 have been treated with intrauterine transfusions.

ONGOING CARE

FOLLOW-UP RECOMMENDATIONS

Expected course of illness

- The rash of erythema infectiosum in a child or adult may last up to 20 days. It may, at times, fade and/or intensify, depending on sunlight exposure, exercise, or body surface temperature changes (e.g., bathing).
- During aplastic crisis secondary to B19, the reticulocyte count usually remains low (often <1%) for several days before spontaneous recovery.

PROGNOSIS

- The prognosis is quite good for all manifestations of B19 infections.
- Most patients recover spontaneously and require only supportive care.

COMPLICATIONS

- Parvovirus B19 during pregnancy
  - 30–50% of pregnant women are susceptible to B19 infection.
  - Fetal loss, intrauterine growth retardation, or hydrops fetalis may result from maternal infection with B19 during pregnancy. Fetal death occurs in 2–6% of cases.
  - B19 has not been proven to cause congenital anomalies.
  - The greatest risk for B19 infection affecting the fetus exists in the first 20 weeks of gestation.
  - The risk of fetal death after exposure, if antibody status is unknown, is <1.5%.
- Arthritis/arthropathy
  - Although most cases of polyarthritis resolve within 2 weeks, persistent symptoms for months to even years (rarely) have been reported.

ADDITIONAL READING

- American Academy of Pediatrics. Parvovirus B19. In: Kimberlin DW, Brady MT, Jackson MA, et al, eds. *Red Book®: 2015 Report of the Committee on Infectious Diseases*. Elk Grove Village, IL: American Academy of Pediatrics; 2015:593–596.
- Douvoyiannis M, Litman N, Goldman DL. Neurologic manifestations associated with parvovirus B19 infection. *Clin Infect Dis*. 2009;48(12):1713–1723.
- Lamont RF, Sobel JD, Vaisbuch E, et al. Parvovirus B19 infection in human pregnancy. *BJOG*. 2011;118(2):175–186.
- Molina KM, Garcia X, Denfield SW, et al. Parvovirus B19 myocarditis causes significant morbidity and mortality in children. *Pediatr Cardiol*. 2013;34(2):390–397.
- Smith-Whitley K, Zhao H, Hodinka RL, et al. Epidemiology of human parvovirus B19 in children with sickle cell disease. *Blood*. 2004;103(2):422–427.
- Young NS, Brown KE. Parvovirus B19. *N Engl J Med*. 2004;350(6):586–597.

CODES

ICD10

B08.3 Erythema infectiosum [fifth disease]

FAQ

- Q: When may children with B19 infection return to school?
- A: Children are contagious only during the prodromal phase of illness, which is often unrecognized. Once the rash appears, they are no longer infectious and may return to school or day care.
- Q: What can be done to reduce risk of fetal infection?
- A: Because B19 infections during pregnancy may result in fetal death and B19 infections often occur in community outbreaks, fetal risks following maternal exposure to persons with recognized B19 infection are a frequent concern. Risk to the fetus appears to be greatest if the infection occurs prior to the 20th week of gestation. Among pregnant women of unknown antibody status, the risk of fetal death after exposure to B19 is estimated to be <1.5%. Routine exclusion of pregnant women from the workplace when B19 infection is suspected is not recommended.

PATENT DUCTUS ARTERIOSUS

Alexander Lowenthal, MD

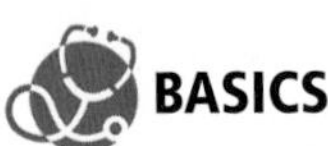

BASICS

DESCRIPTION

- Patent ductus arteriosus (PDA) is the persistence into postnatal life of the normal fetal vascular conduit between the central pulmonary and systemic arterial systems. Normally, the ductus arteriosus (DA) functionally closes within the first 1 to 3 days of life. Structural closure is usually completed by the 3rd week of life. If the DA remains patent beyond 3 months of life, it is considered abnormal and is unlikely to close spontaneously (spontaneous closure rate 0.6% per year).
- In the infant with a normal left aortic arch, the DA connects the main pulmonary artery (MPA) at the origin of the left pulmonary artery to the descending aorta, distal to the origin of the left subclavian artery.
- Many variations can occur, although they are less common. The main, proximal right, or proximal left pulmonary artery may be connected to virtually any location on the aortic arch or proximal portions of the brachiocephalic vessels.
- Five distinct clinical conditions are associated with PDA:
  - Isolated cardiovascular lesion in premature infants
  - Isolated cardiovascular lesion in otherwise healthy term infants and children
  - Incidental finding associated with more significant structural cardiovascular defects
  - Compensatory structure in cases of neonatal pulmonary hypertension without congenital heart disease (CHD)
  - Critical compensatory structure in some cyanotic or left-sided obstructive lesions

EPIDEMIOLOGY

- As an isolated defect, PDA is the 6th most common congenital cardiovascular lesion.
  - Represents 5% of all types of CHD
  - 1 per 2,000 live births
  - If "silent" PDA are included, the rate may be as high as 1:500 live births.
- Female-to-male ratio: 2:1

RISK FACTORS

- Prematurity
  - Increases with the degree of prematurity (50–80% in preterm infants <26 weeks' gestation)
  - 60–70% of preterm infants of <28 weeks' gestation receive medical or surgical therapy for a PDA.
- Incidence of PDA varies significantly depending on environmental factors (altitude), management style (e.g., amount of maintenance fluid prescribed, surfactant administration), and presence of coexisting diseases (e.g., respiratory distress syndrome, hypoxemia, fluid overload, necrotizing enterocolitis, sepsis, hypocalcemia).
- Higher rate of PDA in babies with
  - Trisomy 21
  - Wolf-Hirschhorn syndrome (4p deletion)
  - Char syndrome
  - Carpenter syndrome
  - Holt-Oram syndrome
  - Incontinentia pigmenti

PATHOPHYSIOLOGY

- The PDA is derived from the distal portion of the left 6th embryonic arch, connecting the left pulmonary artery to the descending aorta.
  - The PDA is formed by the 8th week of fetal life.
  - It is necessary for fetal circulation throughout the remainder of gestation.
- Fetal blood flows from the MPA to the DA to the aorta, thus bypassing the pulmonary vascular bed and supplying systemic blood flow. With the first postnatal breaths, the pulmonary vascular resistance falls abruptly, the DA constricts, and pulmonary blood flow is directed into the lungs.
- With a PDA, excessive blood flow will continue from the aorta into the pulmonary artery, causing increased pulmonary blood flow and volume overloading of the left side of the heart.
- In premature infants and term infants with pulmonary hypertension, delayed closure represents an impaired developmental process, whereas in the healthy full-term infant, PDA probably reflects an anatomic abnormality of the ductal tissue.

ETIOLOGY

- Prematurity
- Rubella infection in the first trimester
- Genetic or familial factors
- High altitude
- Idiopathic

DIAGNOSIS

HISTORY

- Premature infants
  - Variable: ranging from asymptomatic to complete cardiovascular collapse
  - Increased ventilatory support, pulmonary hemorrhage, respiratory or metabolic acidosis from low cardiac output, and excessive pulmonary blood flow
  - Tachypnea, feeding intolerance, apnea, bradycardia, necrotizing enterocolitis, and decreased urine output
- Infants and older children
  - Small PDA: usually asymptomatic, with incidental heart murmur found on routine exam
  - Moderate PDA: possible congestive heart failure (CHF), poor feeding, and poor weight gain
  - Large PDA: symptoms as above and recurrent respiratory infections

PHYSICAL EXAM

- Premature infants
  - Tachypnea, rales, tachycardia ($\pm S_3$ gallop)
  - Hyperdynamic precordium and bounding pulses with wide pulse pressure (due to diastolic "runoff" from the aorta to the pulmonary artery)
  - The typical PDA murmur in a premature infant is a pansystolic murmur audible at the left upper or midsternal border.
  - With a large PDA and equalization of pressure between the MPA and the aorta, no murmur may be heard.
  - Hepatomegaly may exist with heart failure (late sign).
- Infants and older children: Findings vary with size of shunt.
  - Small PDA
    - Pansystolic murmur may be heard at the 2nd left intercostal space.
    - Murmur becomes continuous (i.e., extends into diastole), as the pulmonary vascular resistance decreases over the 1st months of life.
  - Moderate or large PDA
    - The murmur is louder, has a harsh quality, and acquires a machine-like quality often being heard posteriorly. In that case, a systolic thrill may be felt at the left upper sternal border.
    - Tachycardia, bounding pulses with a wide pulse pressure, and a mid-diastolic low-frequency rumbling murmur may be audible at the apex with a large PDA.
    - With severe left ventricular failure, the classic PDA signs may disappear, but there will be findings consistent with CHF (tachycardia, S_3 gallop at the apex, hepatomegaly, tachypnea, rales).
    - In extreme cases, pulmonary hypertension may occur, with the murmur shortening, the diastolic component disappearing, and S_2 becoming accentuated. At advanced stages of irreversible pulmonary vascular disease, cyanosis begins to appear, often more pronounced in the lower limbs, with reversal of shunting.

DIFFERENTIAL DIAGNOSIS

- Aortopulmonary window
- Systemic or pulmonary arteriovenous communications
- Ruptured sinus of Valsalva
- Coronary artery fistula
- Truncus arteriosus
- Aortic insufficiency
- Innocent venous hum in older children
- Pulmonary atresia with collaterals
- Ventricular septal defect with aortic regurgitation
- Ventricular septal defect in infancy

DIAGNOSTIC TESTS & INTERPRETATION

- ECG
  - Usually normal with a small PDA
  - Left atrial enlargement and left ventricular hypertrophy with moderate and large PDA
  - Biventricular hypertrophy in later stages
- Chest radiograph
  - Usually normal with a small PDA, although prominence of main and peripheral pulmonary arteries may be seen
  - In moderate and large PDAs, these findings become more pronounced, along with an enlarged heart. Increased pulmonary vascular markings are proportionate to the left-to-right shunt. Pulmonary edema can be seen if CHF develops. In premature infants with respiratory distress syndrome, there is evidence of deteriorating lung disease with unclear cardiac borders.
- Echocardiogram
  - Delineates the PDA and assesses the size of the left atrium and the left ventricle
  - Doppler techniques assess the ductal flow pattern and may be useful for estimating the pulmonary artery pressure.
- Cardiac catheterization
  - Most often not essential for diagnosis
  - Indicated for suspected concomitant pulmonary hypertension
  - Can be performed for treatment via transcatheter closure techniques

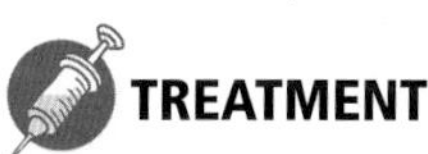

TREATMENT

GENERAL MEASURES

- Premature infant
  - Supportive treatment (careful use of oxygen, respiratory assistance, correction of metabolic acidosis)
  - Management of CHF with fluid restriction and diuretics
  - If PDA persists or patient is symptomatic, closure of PDA is indicated.
  - Medical closure: Indomethacin is most often used; ibuprofen is as effective. Meta-analysis of controlled and uncontrolled studies has demonstrated an efficacy of paracetamol (acetaminophen) comparable with that reported for ibuprofen.
    - Contraindications to medical management with nonsteroidal medications include renal failure (creatinine >1.8 mg/dL), thrombocytopenia (platelets <100,000), and associated conditions (necrotizing enterocolitis, intraventricular hemorrhage). Paracetamol appears to be a suitable alternative.
  - Surgical closure is indicated if medical treatment fails or use of indomethacin is contraindicated.
- Infants and older children
  - Medical management of CHF with diuretics and afterload reduction
  - PDA is no longer a stated indication for subacute bacterial endocarditis (SBE) prophylaxis, but clinical practice may vary.
  - Spontaneous closure rate is low, and closure with indomethacin is not usually effective in this group of patients.
  - Closure is indicated whenever a symptomatic or hemodynamically significant PDA exists.
  - For asymptomatic audible PDA, closure can be performed electively and is primarily performed to reduce the risk of endocarditis. Recommendations for closure of an asymptomatic, incidentally found ("silent" ductus) PDA are not standard.
  - Most infants and children can have a PDA safely and effectively closed during cardiac catheterization, obviating the need for a surgical procedure.

SURGERY/OTHER PROCEDURES

Surgical closure of PDA can be achieved by one of three techniques:

- Open surgical ligation and division: mostly in premature infants
- Video-assisted thoracoscopic ligation: depends on the institution
- Transcatheter occlusion with coils or other devices

ONGOING CARE

PROGNOSIS

- Outcome in treated premature infants is generally good but depends mostly on the degree of prematurity and the presence of associated conditions.
- Outcome in term infants and older children is excellent if no complications have occurred.
- PDA among adults may be associated with significant mortality with or without surgery.
- After closure of PDA, no endocarditis prophylaxis is needed if complete obliteration of flow is achieved. Most cardiologists continue prophylaxis for 6 months after the procedure that closed the PDA if closed by a coil or device.

COMPLICATIONS

- Pulmonary edema and CHF
- Pulmonary hemorrhage
- Pulmonary vascular obstructive disease
- Increased chronic lung disease
- Failure to thrive
- Recurrent respiratory infections
- Lobar emphysema or collapse
- Infective endarteritis
- Thromboembolism of cerebral arteries
- Aneurysm of the ductus
- Intracranial hemorrhage
- Necrotizing enterocolitis
- Renal dysfunction

ADDITIONAL READING

- Anilkumar M. Patent ductus arteriosus. *Cardiol Clin.* 2013;31(3):417–430.
- Clyman RI, Chorne N. Patent ductus arteriosus: evidence for and against treatment. *J Pediatr.* 2007;150(3):216–219.
- Clyman RI, Couto J, Murphy GM. Patent ductus arteriosus: are current neonatal treatment options better or worse than no treatment at all? *Semin Perinatol.* 2012;36(2):123–129.
- El-Khuffash A, Weisz DE, McNamara PJ. Reflections of the changes in patent ductus arteriosus management during the last 10 years. *Arch Dis Child Fetal Neonatal Ed.* 2016;101(5):F474–F478.
- Hamrick SE, Hansmann G. Patent ductus arteriosus of the preterm infant. *Pediatrics.* 2010;125(5):1020–1030.
- Noori S. Pros and cons of patent ductus arteriosus ligation: hemodynamic changes and other morbidities after patent ductus arteriosus ligation. *Semin Perinatol.* 2012;36(2):139–145.
- Schneider DJ. The patent ductus arteriosus in term infants, children, and adults. *Semin Perinatol.* 2012;36(2):146–153.
- Prescott S, Keim-Malpass J. Patent ductus arteriosus in the preterm infant: diagnostic and treatment options. *Adv Neonatal Care.* 2017;17(1):10–18.
- Terrin G, Conte F, Oncel MY, et al. Paracetamol for the treatment of patent ductus arteriosus in preterm neonates: a systematic review and meta-analysis. *Arch Dis Child Fetal Neonatal Ed.* 2016;101(2):F127–F136.

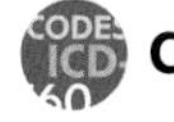

CODES

ICD10

Q25.0 Patent ductus arteriosus

FAQ

- Q: How long would you wait before pronouncing a DA persistent?
- A: 3 months
- Q: Is lifelong follow-up of patients who have undergone transcatheter occlusion with coils or other devices needed?
- A: No studies have been performed, although it is customary to follow patients until somatic growth has ceased.
- Q: Is paracetamol treatment for PDA as good as treatment with nonsteroidal medications?
- A: Paracetamol has fewer side effects and similar efficacy, but more data on safety and long-term outcomes are needed.

PELVIC INFLAMMATORY DISEASE

Maria Trent, MD, MPH

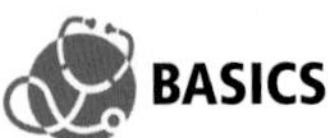

BASICS

DESCRIPTION

- Pelvic inflammatory disease (PID) refers to a spectrum of upper female genital tract inflammatory disorders, including endometritis, salpingitis, tubo-ovarian abscess (TOA), and peritonitis.
- Definitive diagnosis of PID can be made by laparoscopy; however, diagnosis is usually made based on clinical findings.
- Centers for Disease Control and Prevention (CDC) guidelines state that empiric PID therapy should be initiated in sexually active young women with pelvic or lower abdominal pain if no other cause for the symptoms can be identified and the patient has the following:
  - Uterine tenderness, *OR*
  - Adnexal tenderness, *OR*
  - Cervical motion tenderness
- Additional criteria enhance diagnostic specificity but not required:
  - Oral temperature >38.3°C (101°F)
  - Abnormal cervical or vaginal discharge
  - Abundant WBCs on vaginal secretion wet mount
  - Elevated ESR or C-reactive protein (CRP)
  - Laboratory-documented evidence of infection with *Neisseria gonorrhoeae* or *Chlamydia trachomatis*
- Definitive diagnostic criteria:
  - Histopathologic evidence of endometritis on endometrial biopsy
  - Transvaginal sonography or MRI showing thickened fluid-filled tubes with or without free pelvic fluid or TOA
  - Laparoscopic abnormalities consistent with PID

EPIDEMIOLOGY

- Estimated 750,000 cases annually in United States
- In 2011, 90,000 initial visits to physician offices for PID:
  - Visits for PID declined between 2002 and 2011
  - Increased screening and treatment of chlamydia likely led to this decline.
- Cases disproportionately higher among adolescent girls and racial minorities

RISK FACTORS

- Factors that increase PID risk include the following:
  - Multiple sexual partners
  - Intercourse with a partner who has multiple sexual partners
  - Prior history of sexually transmitted infection (STI) or PID
  - Intercourse without condoms
  - Douching
  - Recent (within past 20 days) insertion of intrauterine device (IUD)
- PID cases are highest among the following:
  - Sexually active adolescents and young women age <25 years
  - Women in communities with high prevalence of gonorrhea and chlamydia
  - Patients presenting to STD clinics

GENERAL PREVENTION

- Consistent condom use
- Regular STI screening
- Partner screening for STIs
- Limit number of sexual partners.
- Avoid douching.

PATHOPHYSIOLOGY

- Ascending infection spreading from vagina/cervix to upper genital tract by the following:
  - Migration
  - Sperm transport
  - Refluxed menstrual blood flow
- Up to 75% of cases occur within 7 days of menses.

ETIOLOGY

- Polymicrobial origin
- Many cases associated with *N. gonorrhoeae* and *C. trachomatis*
- *Mycoplasma genitalium* and *Ureaplasma urealyticum* have been associated with laparoscopic PID and infertility.
- Other vaginal, enteric, and respiratory flora associated with PID include the following:
  - *Gardnerella vaginalis*, *Escherichia coli*, *Bacteroides* species, *Haemophilus influenzae*, group B to D streptococci, *Streptococcus pneumoniae*, and group A *Streptococcus*

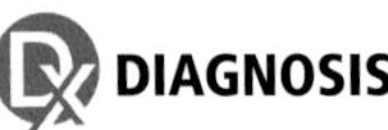

DIAGNOSIS

ALERT

- Clinical criteria for PID are designed to have high sensitivity because consequences of untreated PID are significant.
- If PID suspected based on clinical presentation and examination, treatment should be initiated prior to results of other supportive testing.

HISTORY

- Should be taken from the patient in a private interview:
  - Confidentiality policies should be reviewed with the patient in advance of history.
- Abdominal or pelvic pain is a common presenting complaint:
  - "Classic" presentation of shuffling gait or "chandelier sign" is rare.
- Some cases may be mild with relatively few symptoms:
  - Subclinical or "silent" PID can result in infertility and chronic pelvic pain.
- Other presenting symptoms may include the following:
  - Vaginal discharge
  - Abnormal vaginal bleeding
  - Dyspareunia
  - Dysuria
  - Right upper quadrant pain
- Complete history should be taken including past medical, gynecologic, gastrointestinal, and urinary history.
- Sexual history should be elicited in a sensitive manner and should include:
  - Number of partners
  - New partners
  - Condom use
  - Contraceptive method use
  - History of sexual assault

PHYSICAL EXAM

- Evaluate the patient for signs of general discomfort.
- Review vital signs for fever, tachycardia.
- Careful abdominal exam to evaluate for tenderness, rebound, or guarding
  - Evaluate right upper quadrant for tenderness associated with perihepatitis.
- Pelvic exam is essential to PID diagnosis and must be performed for any sexually active female with abdominal pain or genital complaints.
- External genital exam should assess for external lesions, inguinal adenopathy.
- Speculum exam should note vaginal discharge or lesions, signs of cervical friability or discharge.
  - Collect vaginal swabs for pH and wet prep.
  - Collect cervical swabs for STI testing.
  - Collect swab for Gram stain if materials and equipment available.
- Bimanual exam to evaluate for cervical motion tenderness, uterine tenderness, and adnexal tenderness or fullness

DIFFERENTIAL DIAGNOSIS

- Pelvic pain may be the presenting complaint for a variety of disease processes.
- Gynecologic
  - Ectopic pregnancy
  - Intrauterine pregnancy
  - Endometriosis
  - Hemorrhagic ovarian cyst
  - Ovarian cyst
  - Ovarian tumor
  - Ovarian torsion
  - Tubal torsion
  - Septic abortion
  - Vaginal foreign body
  - Hematometrocolpos
  - Chemical irritants
- Urinary
  - Urinary tract infection
  - Acute pyelonephritis
- Gastrointestinal
  - Acute appendicitis
  - Acute cholecystitis
- Heme/vascular
  - Pelvic thrombophlebitis
- Other:
  - Functional abdominal pain
  - Sexual assault
  - Sexual abuse

DIAGNOSTIC TESTS & INTERPRETATION

Initial Tests (screening, lab, imaging)

- Urine β-hCG
- Vaginal pH (pH >4.5 is abnormal.)

- Wet mount and KOH (>10 WBC/HPF is suggestive of infection.)
- Nucleic acid amplification test for *N. gonorrhoeae*, *C. trachomatis*, and *Trichomonas vaginalis*
  - If the patient reports sexual assault or abuse at the time of evaluation, bacterial cultures should also be obtained.
- Urinalysis and culture
- Consider collecting CBC, CRP to support diagnosis.
- Testing for other STIs including HIV and syphilis should also be done.
- In patients with adnexal fullness or other signs suggestive of TOA, obtain transvaginal ultrasound.
- Signs of PID on imaging include the following:
  - Thickened or fluid-filled fallopian tubes
  - Free pelvic fluid
  - TOA

Diagnostic Procedures/Other

- Laparoscopy
- Endometrial biopsy
- These tests can provide definitive evidence of PID but are not routinely used.

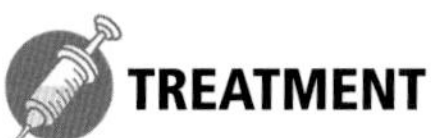

TREATMENT

ALERT

- All CDC-recommended regimens for PID require 14-day treatment duration.
- Fluoroquinolones not recommended for PID treatment because of *N. gonorrhoeae* resistance
- Metronidazole treatment should be initiated among women who have evidence of bacterial vaginosis, active infection with *T. vaginalis* on wet prep, and/or reside in communities with high rates of *T. vaginalis*.

MEDICATION

- Recommended parenteral treatment regimens:
  - Cefotetan 2 g IV q12h OR cefoxitin 2 g IV q6h PLUS
    - Doxycycline 100 mg PO b.i.d. × 14 days
    - May add metronidazole 500 mg PO b.i.d. × 14 days for severe cases or suspected anaerobes, OR
  - Clindamycin 900 mg IV q8h PLUS
    - Gentamicin loading dose IV or IM (2 mg/kg), followed by a maintenance dose (1.5 mg/kg) q8h
- Alternate regimen:
  - Ampicillin/sulbactam 3 g (ampicillin) IV q6h PLUS
    - Doxycycline 100 mg PO b.i.d. × 14 days
- Recommended oral treatment regimens:
  - Ceftriaxone 250 mg IM (single dose) PLUS
    - Doxycycline 100 mg PO b.i.d. × 14 days
    - May add metronidazole 500 mg PO b.i.d. × 14 days, OR
  - Cefoxitin 2 g IM (single dose) PLUS
    - Probenecid 1 g PO (single dose) PLUS
    - Doxycycline 100 mg PO b.i.d. × 14 days
    - May add metronidazole 500 mg PO b.i.d. × 14 days
- Alternate regimen:
  - Other parenteral 3rd-generation cephalosporin PLUS
    - Doxycycline 100 mg PO b.i.d. × 14 days
    - May add metronidazole 500 mg PO b.i.d. × 14 days

ADDITIONAL THERAPIES

- Criteria for hospitalization:
  - Surgical emergency
  - Pregnancy
  - Lack of response to outpatient therapy
  - Inability to tolerate or follow outpatient regimen
  - Severe illness (e.g., fever, nausea/vomiting)
  - Suspected or confirmed TOA
- Strong consideration of hospitalization should be given for early and middle adolescents who may require additional supports for optimal management.
- Patients should be counseled to:
  - Abstain from intercourse for at least 14 days.
  - Notify their partners for STI testing and treatment.
  - Use condoms consistently and correctly.
  - Limit number of sexual partners.
  - Consider contraception if not currently using and not desiring pregnancy.
  - Return if worsening symptoms or not able tolerate the prescribed treatment.

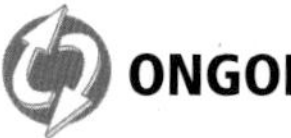

ONGOING CARE

FOLLOW-UP RECOMMENDATIONS

- All patients diagnosed with PID should have follow-up within 72 hours to assess the following:
  - Treatment tolerance/adherence
  - Symptom improvement
- If patients are not improving, additional evaluation may be necessary including:
  - Bimanual examination
  - Pelvic imaging
  - Hospitalization
- Return for repeat STI testing in 3 months.

PROGNOSIS

- Dependent on treatment adherence and number of episodes of PID
- Women with documented *N. gonorrhoeae* or *C. trachomatis* infection have higher rates of reinfection within 6 months of treatment.
- Each additional episode of PID increases risk of infertility and chronic pelvic pain.

COMPLICATIONS

- Short term
  - Perihepatitis (in 15% of patients)
  - Periappendicitis
- Long term
  - Ectopic pregnancy
  - Infertility (10–15% of cases of PID)
  - Chronic pelvic pain

ADDITIONAL READING

- Butz AM, Gaydos C, Chung SE, et al. Care-seeking behavior after notification among young women with recurrent sexually transmitted infections after pelvic inflammatory disease. *Clin Pediatr (Phila)*. 2016;55(12):1107–1112.
- Centers for Disease Control and Prevention. 2015 Sexually transmitted diseases treatment guidelines: pelvic inflammatory disease (PID). https://www.cdc.gov/std/tg2015/pid.htm. Accessed May 3, 2018.
- Savaris RF, Teixeira LM, Torres TG, et al. Comparing ceftriaxone plus azithromycin or doxycycline for pelvic inflammatory disease: a randomized controlled trial. *Obstet Gynecol*. 2007;110(1):53–60.
- Trent M. Status of adolescent pelvic inflammatory disease management in the United States. *Curr Opin Obstet Gynecol*. 2013;25(5):350–356.
- Trent M, Haggerty CL, Jennings JM, et al. Adverse adolescent reproductive health outcomes after pelvic inflammatory disease. *Arch Pediatr Adolesc Med*. 2011;165(1):49–54.

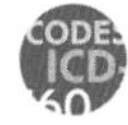

CODES

ICD10

- N73.9 Female pelvic inflammatory disease, unspecified
- N71.9 Inflammatory disease of uterus, unspecified
- N70.93 Salpingitis and oophoritis, unspecified

FAQ

- Q: My patient has negative testing for *N. gonorrhoeae* and *C. trachomatis*, should I have her discontinue the medications if she has clinically improved?
- A: No. PID is a polymicrobial infection and the patient's improvement is likely secondary to broad-spectrum antibiotic treatment to also treat organisms for which testing is not usually performed. The patient should continue antibiotics as prescribed.
- Q: My patient has problems with adherence, could I use directly observed doses of azithromycin in the office?
- A: Although use of azithromycin is not considered a standard and/or recommended therapy by the CDC, ceftriaxone 250 mg and azithromycin 1 g at baseline and then repeated the dose in 1 week has shown effectiveness in a single randomized controlled trial (RCT). These results have not been replicated, and the CDC currently recommends that metronidazole 500 mg b.i.d. × 14 days be administered with azithromycin to improve anaerobic coverage.
- Q: My patient is 6 weeks pregnant. Can she really have PID?
- A: PID is less common during pregnancy given the bactericidal protection afforded by the cervical mucous plug. However, it is possible for sperm to transport bacteria into the uterus during fertilization, infection to occur in the interim between implantation and full establishment of the mucous plug, and early loss of the mucus plug later in pregnancy. Caution should be used in caring for pregnant patients with PID because fetal wastage can occur due to infection. As such, the CDC recommends that these women be hospitalized for initial treatment.

PENILE AND FORESKIN PROBLEMS

Benjamin M. Whittam, MD, MS • Richard C. Rink, MD • Mark P. Cain, MD

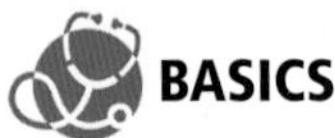

BASICS

DESCRIPTION

- Penile problems:
  - Buried penis
    - Hidden or concealed penis, poor skin fixation at the penoscrotal/penopubic junction resulting in buried or hidden appearance
    - May be normal in obese children with large suprapubic fat pad
  - Penile curvature (chordee)
    - Bending of the penis with erection, can be lateral, ventral (most common), or dorsal curve
    - Chordee is usually associated with abnormal foreskin.
    - Often associated with an abnormal or wandering median raphe
  - Webbed penis
    - Penoscrotal webbing or poor separation of penile skin from scrotum, obscuring penoscrotal angle
  - Balanitis
    - Inflammation of the glans
    - Probably overdiagnosed owing to drainage of smegma or urea dermatitis from failure to retract foreskin during voiding in toilet-trained boys
    - When infections present, there can be significant cellulitis of the penis, edema, and fever.
    - Most commonly caused by gram-positive organisms. Yeast is another causative organism.
- Foreskin problems:
  - Balanoposthitis
    - Inflammation of glans and prepuce (foreskin)
    - Seen in 4% of uncircumcised boys age 2 to 5 years
    - See balanitis.
  - Phimosis/penile adhesions
    - Physiologic attachment of prepuce to glans, which it protects and gradually separates to allow retraction of the foreskin
    - Ring of fibrotic scar tissue that prevents the foreskin from being retracted
  - Paraphimosis
    - When narrow prepuce is retracted behind the glans, constricting penile shaft causing glanular and foreskin edema and preventing replacement of prepuce over glans
- Postcircumcision problems:
  - Penile adhesions
    - Attachments of the foreskin back to the glans after circumcision
    - Penile skin bridges are dense scar adhesions that cannot be separated.
  - Meatal stenosis
    - Urethral meatus narrowing
    - Significant meatal narrowing will produce an upwardly deflected urine stream, which is narrow and strong; in severe cases causes straining and prolonged voiding
  - Epidermal inclusion cysts
    - Small, enlarging white lesions growing subcutaneously along the scar from circumcision

ETIOLOGY

- Buried/webbed penis
  - Scrotal attachments attending along ventral penile surface to varying degrees
  - Penis tethered by abnormal attachments of dartos tissue
- Penile curvature (chordee)
  - Asymmetry in tunica albuginea of corporal bodies and compliance of corpora cavernosa
- Balanoposthitis/balanitis
  - Unclear etiology: possible infection, mechanical trauma, contact irritation, and contact allergies
- Phimosis
  - Physiologic phimosis: inability to retract foreskin due to natural adhesions between prepuce and glans: Epithelial debris (smegma) over time separates foreskin from glans, normal.
  - Pathologic phimosis: probably results from recurrent bouts of foreskin irritation from improper hygiene habits such as voiding through the foreskin or repetitive forceful retraction
- Penile adhesions
  - Physiologic adhesions: The prepuce has adhered down to the glans after circumcision.
  - Surgical adhesions (skin bridges): adherence between the scar of the circumcision and the glans due to healing of the crushed tissue where the foreskin was removed and the glans
- Meatal stenosis
  - Narrowing of the urethral meatus secondary to recurrent irritation of the meatus, likely from rubbing against moist diapers; occurs almost exclusively in circumcised boys
- Epidermal inclusion cysts
  - Caused by small islands of epithelium buried beneath the skin surface that progressively accumulate desquamated skin cells

RISK FACTORS

Genetics

Epidermal inclusion cysts may occur from congenital rests of skin cells buried during development, but these are rare and occur along the median raphe of the penis or scrotum.

GENERAL PREVENTION

Some penile and foreskin problems may be prevented with proper hygiene and caretaker education.

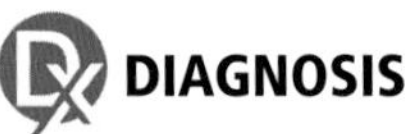

DIAGNOSIS

HISTORY

- Issues with newborn circumcision
- Ability to retract foreskin
- Retraction of foreskin in uncircumcised males during voiding
- Penis straight with erection
- Character of urinary stream
- Ballooning of the foreskin with voiding
- Straining to void
- Presence of fever
- Penile discharge
- In older boys, inquire about sexual activity.

PHYSICAL EXAM

- Circumcised males
  - Size and position of meatus
  - Redundancy of preputial skin
  - Presence of adhesions to the glans and whether they involve the scar line between the shaft skin and the inner preputial skin
  - Lesions or erythema of glans or shaft
  - Watch patient void if meatal stenosis is suspected, usually upward deviated stream.
- Uncircumcised males
  - Ability to retract foreskin with gentle retraction
  - Presence of phimotic ring
  - Lesions or erythema of prepuce

ALERT

- Do not try to forcefully retract the foreskin in an infant or young child. It can take 3 to 5 years before the foreskin can be retracted, but no definite time exists when it is normal to retract foreskin.
- Do not circumcise infants with a buried or webbed penis, asymmetric foreskin, or those with a significantly deviated penile raphe.
- Never circumcise an infant with an abnormally located meatus (hypospadias, epispadias).
- Never circumcise an infant with bilaterally undescended testes until evaluation for disorder of sexual development ruled out.
- Always replace the foreskin back over the glans after retraction (for cleaning, voiding, or examination) to prevent paraphimosis.
- Paraphimosis is an emergency. The sooner it is diagnosed, the easier it is to treat and reduce without surgical intervention.

DIAGNOSTIC TESTS & INTERPRETATION

- In cases of balanitis with drainage, cultures may be taken by spreading foreskin (with hemostat) and sending drainage for culture.
- In sexually active males, if urethral discharge is present, culture for gonorrhea and chlamydia

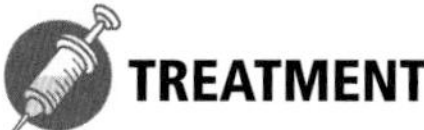

TREATMENT

GENERAL MEASURES

- Phimosis
  - Physiologic: no need for intervention
  - Good hygiene practices should be encouraged such as pulling the foreskin back to expose the meatus when voiding and not voiding through the foreskin.
  - The foreskin should always be placed back over the glans after voiding (or any retraction) to prevent paraphimosis.
  - Pamphlets or information on websites that explain the care of the penis for uncircumcised males are helpful to provide to the parents.
  - If there is a fibrotic ring of scar tissue preventing the retraction of the foreskin, a trial of betamethasone cream 0.05–0.01% applied to the foreskin t.i.d. for 4 to 6 weeks with daily gentle retraction may soften the scar tissue enough to resolve the phimosis. Use small amounts of cream only in the constrictive ring and do not use occlusive dressings.
  - In cases where conservative measures fail, a circumcision may be indicated.
- Penile adhesions
  - Physiologic: Practices in the past have included separation using anesthetic cream (lidocaine 2.5% and prilocaine 2.5% [EMLA®]). If there is redundancy of the foreskin or a prominent suprapubic fat pad that can tend to hide the penis in infants, adhesions often recur or require constant application of barrier creams or ointments to the penis and manual retraction of the redundant foreskin by the parents to prevent recurrence:
    - In many cases, no treatment is necessary, as the adhesions will break down over a period of years.
    - If there are extensive adhesions with significant foreskin redundancy, consideration should be given to revision of the circumcision if the adhesions are to be treated.
  - Surgical (skin bridges)
    - These are due to scar tissue formation between the raw cut edge where the foreskin was removed and the glans.
    - As this represents true scarring and not two epithelial surfaces stuck together, the surfaces cannot be simply pulled apart like physiologic adhesions. They will not resolve with time, and if left in place, with growth, penile skin will be transferred to the glans, resulting in discoloration, especially in patients with darker skin tones.
    - These adhesions need sharp division either in the office with EMLA® cream anesthesia or under general anesthesia if they are extensive.
- Meatal stenosis
  - When the narrowing at the meatus is producing an upwardly deflected, narrow stream (which can make aiming into the toilet difficult) or is causing straining and prolonged voiding, treatment is indicated.
  - A meatotomy can be done in the office using EMLA® anesthesia or as an outpatient surgical procedure.
- Epidermal inclusion cysts
  - These subcutaneous islands of skin cells will progressively enlarge over time.
  - Complete excision is generally curative.
- Balanitis
  - When the inflammation and irritation seem to be from chronic dampness and exposure to urine, treat with barrier creams or ointments.
  - Keeping the area clean and dry will help prevent future episodes.
  - If there are small whitish plaques (not smegma), associated with redness, yeast may be present, and an antifungal cream such as 1% clotrimazole can be used to help speed the healing.
  - Antibiotics as necessary (see "Medication")
  - In cases where there is purulent drainage and cellulitis of the penis, which can often be rapidly spreading over 24 hours, treatment with antibiotics is recommended.
  - Genital infections of this nature should be taken quite seriously, and if treatment as an outpatient is attempted, close follow-up (return visit in 24 to 48 hours) is prudent.

MEDICATION

Balanitis/balanoposthitis

- If child is afebrile, oral antibiotics such as a 1st-generation cephalosporin would be the first line of treatment.
- If the child develops fever or there is progression of cellulitis, then treat with IV antibiotics (cefazolin, clindamycin).

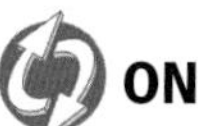

ONGOING CARE

PATIENT EDUCATION

- It is important that all parents of uncircumcised boys teach them proper hygiene habits during toilet training.
- Guidance for parents:
  - Do not forcibly retract the foreskin.
  - Gently clean with warm water during baths and dry after.
  - Retract the skin when voiding in toilet-trained boys.
  - Always place the foreskin back over glans after voiding or retraction of foreskin.

ADDITIONAL READING

- Blalock HJ, Vemulakonda V, Ritchey ML, et al. Outpatient management of phimosis following newborn circumcision. *J Urol*. 2003;169(6):2332–2334.
- Orsola A, Caffaratti J, Garat JM. Conservative treatment of phimosis in children using a topical steroid. *Urology*. 2000;56(2):307–310.
- Van Howe RS. Incidence of meatal stenosis following neonatal circumcision in a primary care setting. *Clin Pediatr (Phila)*. 2006;45(1):49–54.

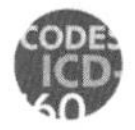

CODES

ICD10

- Q55.64 Hidden penis
- Q54.4 Congenital chordee
- Q55.69 Other congenital malformation of penis

FAQ

- Q: The foreskin is stuck down to my son's penis. Does that mean he needs another circumcision?
- A: Not necessarily. If there is minor redundancy and a small physiologic adhesion, then no treatment is needed.
- Q: My uncircumcised son had some thick white drainage from his foreskin. Is that from an infection?
- A: Probably not. The thick white material is probably shed skin cells, which have been slowly separating the foreskin from the glans, this is also known as smegma (Greek for soap).
- Q: At what age is it normal to be able to completely retract my son's foreskin?
- A: There is no definite "normal" time, some literature reports ages from 5 to 10 years, but the foreskin should slowly retract with intermittent erections.

PERICARDITIS

Hythem M. Nawaytou, MBBCh, MSc

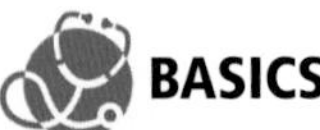

BASICS

DESCRIPTION

Inflammation of the pericardium, usually resulting in the accumulation of fluid in the pericardial space between the visceral (serosal tissue intimately related to the myocardium) and parietal (fibrous layer composed of elastic fibers and collagen) pericardium. Pericarditis may be serous, fibrinous, purulent, hemorrhagic, or chylous.

EPIDEMIOLOGY

- Infectious pericarditis is more frequently seen in children <13 years of age, with predominance in children <2 years of age.
- 2 to 3/1,000 hospitalized children have pericarditis.
- Adolescent males constitute the majority of children hospitalized with idiopathic or viral pericarditis.
- Postpericardiotomy syndrome occurs in ~5–10% of children following uncomplicated cardiac surgery, particularly when the atrium has been entered.

PATHOPHYSIOLOGY

- Fine deposits of fibrin develop next to the great vessels, leading to altered function of the membranes of the pericardium, including changes in oncotic and hydrostatic pressure with subsequent accumulation of fluid in the pericardial space.
- Effusion is defined as excessive pericardial contents secondary to inflammation, hemorrhage, exudates, air, or pus.
- In postpericardiotomy syndrome, there appears to be a nonspecific hypersensitivity reaction to the direct surgical entrance into the pericardial space.

ETIOLOGY

- Infectious
  - Viral: coxsackievirus, echovirus, mumps, varicella, Epstein-Barr, adenovirus, influenza, HIV
  - Bacterial: *Streptococcus*, pneumococcus, *Staphylococcus* (most common cause of bacterial pericarditis), meningococcus, *Mycoplasma*, tularemia, *Haemophilus influenzae* type B, *Pseudomonas aeruginosa, Listeria monocytogenes, Pasteurella multocida, Escherichia coli*
  - Tuberculosis, atypical mycobacterium
  - Fungal: candidiasis, histoplasmosis, actinomycosis
  - Parasitic: toxoplasmosis, *Echinococcus*, *Entamoeba histolytica*, *Rickettsia*
- Rheumatologic/inflammatory
  - Acute rheumatic fever
  - Rheumatoid arthritis
  - Systemic lupus erythematosus
  - Systemic sclerosis
  - Sarcoidosis
  - Dermatomyositis
  - Kawasaki disease
  - Familial Mediterranean fever
  - Inflammatory bowel disease
- Metabolic/endocrine
  - Hypothyroidism
  - Uremia (chemical irritation)
  - Gout
  - Scurvy
- Neoplastic disease
  - Lymphoma
  - Lymphosarcoma
  - Leukemia
  - Sarcoma
  - Metastatic disease to the pericardium
  - Radiation therapy–induced
- Postoperative
  - Postpericardiotomy syndrome (after cardiac surgery)
  - Chylopericardium
- Other
  - Trauma
  - Drug-induced (hydralazine, isoniazid, procainamide)
  - Aortic dissection
  - Postmyocardial infarction
  - Idiopathic

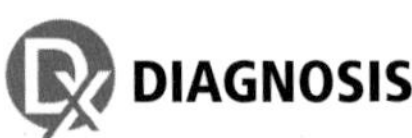

DIAGNOSIS

HISTORY

- Symptoms:
  - Most common symptoms:
    - Sharp precordial chest pain: increasing with inspiration and cough and often relieved if the child sits leaning forward
    - Fever
    - Cough
    - Shoulder pain aggravated by changes in position
  - Rapid accumulation of fluid may lead to the following:
    - Dyspnea
    - Change in mental status/loss of consciousness
  - Slow, chronic accumulation may be associated with no symptoms at all until tamponade develops.
  - Other symptoms depend on the etiology of the pericarditis.
- Recent upper respiratory infection or gastroenteritis (viral pericarditis)
- Sepsis or other source of bacterial infection
- Recent cardiac surgery, usually in the past month
- Symptoms of rheumatic disease
- Known thoracic neoplasm

PHYSICAL EXAM

- Pericardial friction rub is the pathognomonic finding.
- Pericardial effusion:
  - Quiet precordium, tachycardia, hypotension; muffled heart sounds may be heard when there is a large amount of fluid and/or tamponade.
- Cardiac tamponade:
  - Respiratory distress, tachycardia, poor peripheral perfusion, hypotension
  - Evidence of right-sided heart failure: peripheral edema, jugular venous distention, and hepatomegaly
  - Pulmonary edema: rare
  - Pulsus paradoxus: an exaggerated decrease in systolic blood pressure (BP) with inspiration
  - Kussmaul sign: paradoxical rise in jugular venous pressure during inspiration, often considered diagnostic of tamponade physiology

DIFFERENTIAL DIAGNOSIS

- Acute myopericarditis
  - History, physical examination, and EKG findings of acute pericarditis with elevated cardiac enzymes
  - Echocardiogram reveals normal cardiac function.
  - Management as pericarditis with excellent prognosis regardless of troponin level
- Acute myocarditis
  - History, physical examination, and laboratory findings of acute pericarditis can be quite similar to those found in acute myocarditis.
  - In addition, myocarditis can be associated with pericardial disease.
  - Echocardiogram reveals diminished cardiac function and evidence of myocarditis.
- Restrictive cardiomyopathy
- Other causes of chest pain
- Myocardial infarction

DIAGNOSTIC TESTS & INTERPRETATION

Initial Tests (screening, lab, imaging)

- Electrocardiogram
  - Early: diffuse ST segment elevation
  - Later: ST segment normalizes followed by T wave flattening then inversion.
  - Low QRS voltage or electrical alternans can be seen with large effusions.
- Chest radiograph
  - Heart size maybe normal in acute pericarditis.
  - Often shows enlargement of the cardiac silhouette ("water bottle sign"), usually in association with normal pulmonary vascular markings with a pericardial effusion
  - Calcification may be seen in constrictive pericarditis.
- Echocardiogram
  - Most sensitive and specific test for pericardial thickening and fluid in the pericardial space
  - In the presence of a large effusion, the heart may appear to swing within the pericardial cavity.
  - In tamponade, diastolic collapse of the right atrium may be seen. Collapse of the left atrium and right ventricle occur in severe cases.
  - Tamponade can be diagnosed using Doppler inflow patterns of the tricuspid and mitral valves. In tamponade, mitral inflow E-wave velocity decreases by >30% during inspiration, whereas the tricuspid inflow E-wave velocity increases by >50% during inspiration.
- Computed tomography (CT)
  - CT can also demonstrate calcification of the pericardium with excellent sensitivity.
- Cardiac MRI (cMRI)
  - cMRI is diagnostic in constrictive pericarditis and can differentiate between constrictive pericarditis and restrictive cardiomyopathy.

P

Diagnostic Procedures/Other

Diagnostic pericardiocentesis is performed only when the etiology of the effusion is in question.

- Fluid obtained should be sent to the lab for cell count, cytology, and culture (including bacteria, viruses, *Mycobacterium tuberculosis*, and fungi).
- Complications include myocardial puncture, coronary artery/vein laceration, hemopericardium, and pneumothorax.
- Echocardiogram or fluoroscopic guidance is useful for this procedure.

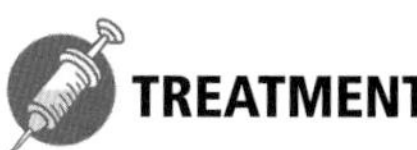

TREATMENT

GENERAL MEASURES

- Treatment should be directed toward the etiology of the disease. However, no matter the cause, pericardiocentesis is required if there is an effusion that causes hemodynamic compromise. It may also be life-saving in patients with bacterial pericarditis.
- Pericardiocentesis is indicated in moderate- and large-sized pericardial effusion not responding to medical management.
- Echocardiogram or fluoroscopic guidance is useful for pericardiocentesis but is not required if there is impending cardiovascular collapse.
- Pericardial window: removal of part or most of the pericardium in cases of chronic pericardial effusion
- Viral pericarditis usually resolves spontaneously in 3 to 4 weeks with bed rest and analgesics (NSAIDs).
- Bacterial pericarditis is potentially life-threatening and requires immediate decompression of the pericardial space (often with open drainage and pericardial window creation), IV antibiotic therapy for at least 4 weeks, and supportive therapy for sepsis/septic shock (i.e., volume expansion, inotropes).
- Rheumatologic causes of pericardial inflammation usually respond to corticosteroids and/or NSAIDs and rarely require pericardiocentesis.
- Uremic pericarditis usually responds to dialysis, but pericardiotomy (surgical removal of the pericardium) may be necessary in chronic situations.
- Neoplastic pericarditis is addressed by treating the primary disease. Pericardiocentesis is indicated only for diagnostic and/or hemodynamic reasons.
- Hemorrhagic pericarditis with effusion accumulation secondary to trauma should be drained because of the risk of subsequent development of constrictive pericarditis.
- Constrictive pericarditis is treated with complete stripping of the pericardium (pericardiectomy). Often, immediate clinical improvement is not seen because there has been myocardial damage. However, eventual full recovery is the norm.
- Postpericardiotomy syndrome occurs 1 to 4 weeks after cardiac surgery accounting for 1% of readmissions after cardiac surgery.
  - Treat with bed rest and anti-inflammatory drugs. Resistant cases may respond to steroids or colchicine.

ONGOING CARE

- Most forms of pericarditis resolve on their own or with anti-inflammatory medication, over the course of several weeks.
  - Follow-up is necessary to ensure that effusions have resolved and to assess for recurrence (up to 30% relapse).
  - Patients with bacterial pericarditis require long-term antibiotic therapy and close follow-up to assess for the development of constrictive pericarditis.
- Signs to watch for include the following:
  - Postpericardiotomy syndrome: All cardiac surgical patients need an evaluation 2 to 4 weeks after surgery to assess for postpericardiotomy syndrome, with treatment and follow-up as necessary.
  - Signs of low cardiac output and right-sided heart failure indicate impending cardiac tamponade.
  - Constrictive pericarditis may present with signs or symptoms of right-sided heart failure and a rapidly decreasing cardiac silhouette, calcifications on chest radiograph.

PROGNOSIS

- Most children recover fully from pericarditis.
  - However, there is significant morbidity and mortality associated, especially in young infants, when the diagnosis is delayed and/or when *Staphylococcus aureus* is the etiologic agent.
- Pericarditis can also recur in as many as 15–30% of patients.
- Prognosis varies with the cause of pericarditis but generally is related directly to the primary disease.

COMPLICATIONS

- Cardiac tamponade
  - Intrapericardial pressure increases at a rapid rate secondary to intrapericardial fluid accumulation with decreased compliance of the pericardial membranes, resulting in restriction of ventricular filling and eventual decrease in stroke volume and cardiac output.
  - The compliance of the pericardium is influenced by the disease process itself (i.e., the pericardium is thickened and stiff in bacterial and tuberculous pericarditis).
  - During cardiac tamponade, ventricular end-diastolic, atrial, and venous pressures are all equal.
  - In acute pericarditis, tamponade may occur with small amounts of fluid because of a rapid increase in the intrapericardial pressure. In contrast, large amounts of fluid may be tolerated if the accumulation is a chronic, slow process.
- Constrictive pericarditis
  - Thick, fibrotic, and often calcified pericardium is seen, usually a late result of purulent or tuberculosis pericarditis; it can occur months to years after the initial infection. It can also be seen in oncology patients with direct invasion of tumor into the pericardium or after significant radiation to the chest.
  - Poor compliance of the pericardium leads to diminished diastolic filling of the ventricle. Patients may complain of exercise intolerance and fatigue. Additionally, they may have signs of right-sided heart failure.
  - This entity may be difficult to distinguish from restrictive cardiomyopathy.
  - cMRI is helpful in making the diagnosis.
- Recurrent pericarditis
  - Occurs in 15–30% of cases
  - Treatment includes NSAIDs, corticosteroids, colchicine, immunosuppressive therapy, biologic agents (e.g., interleukin-1 receptor antagonist [Anakinra]).

ADDITIONAL READING

- Alabed S, Pérez-Gaxiola G, Burls A. Colchicine for children with pericarditis: systematic review of clinical studies. *Arch Dis Child*. 2016;101(10):953–956.
- Elias MD, Glatz AC, O'Connor MJ, et al. Prevalence and risk factors for pericardial effusions requiring readmission after pediatric cardiac surgery. *Pediatr Cardiol*. 2017;38(3):484–494.
- Shakti D, Hehn R, Gauvreau K, et al. Idiopathic pericarditis and pericardial effusion in children: contemporary epidemiology and management. *J Am Heart Assoc*. 2014;3(6):e001483.

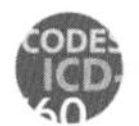

CODES

ICD10

- I31.9 Disease of pericardium, unspecified
- I30.9 Acute pericarditis, unspecified
- I30.1 Infective pericarditis

FAQ

- Q: How does cardiac tamponade present?
- A: Patients with impending tamponade appear quite ill, with tachycardia, chest pain, and signs of right-sided heart failure including jugular venous distention, hepatomegaly, ascites, and peripheral edema. They may also have signs of poor systemic perfusion secondary to low cardiac output. Chest radiograph may or may not show an enlarged cardiac silhouette, depending on how acutely the process occurs. It takes much less fluid to cause tamponade in an acute process than in a chronic process. Echocardiography is the standard diagnostic tool, and pericardiocentesis is the treatment.
- Q: What is pulsus paradoxus and how does one measure it?
- A: Pulsus paradoxus is an exaggerated response of the systolic BP to the normal respiratory cycle. Normally with inspiration, the systolic BP drops <5 mm Hg secondary to the increased capacitance of the pulmonary veins from the increased systemic venous return. In tamponade, this response becomes more profound (>10 mm Hg), most likely secondary to diminished filling of the left heart. Pulsus paradoxus can also be seen in patients with severe respiratory distress associated with asthma and emphysema.
- To assess for pulsus paradoxus, measure the systolic BP first in expiration and then allow it to fall to the place where it is heard equally well in inspiration and expiration. A difference of >10 mm Hg is considered abnormal.

PERIODIC BREATHING

Richard M. Kravitz, MD

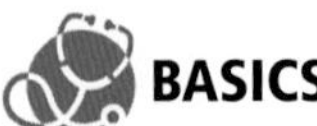

BASICS

DESCRIPTION

- A respiratory pattern consisting of regular oscillations in breathing amplitude
- Typically, a respiratory pattern in which ≥3 apneas lasting ≥3 seconds occur, separated by <20 seconds of respiration

ALERT

Don't confuse periodic breathing with obstructive and/or central apnea.

EPIDEMIOLOGY

- Usually absent in the first 48 hours of life
- More frequent during rapid eye movement (REM or active) sleep versus non-REM (quiet) sleep
- Less common in prone versus supine position
- In full-term infants
  - Amount of periodic breathing usually <4% of total sleep time
  - Amount gradually decreases through the 1st year of life.
  - By 1 year of age, the mean amount of periodic breathing is <1% of total sleep time.
- In premature infants
  - Amount of periodic breathing is higher than in full-term infants.
  - Amount correlates inversely with gestational age.

PATHOPHYSIOLOGY

- No common pathologic finding
- Abnormalities, when they exist, are related to the underlying disorder causing the periodic breathing.

ETIOLOGY

- Periodic breathing can be seen in healthy infants, children, and adults.
- Abnormalities, in any component of the breathing control system, may result in an increased amount of periodic breathing.
- Possible etiologies
  - A delay in detecting changes in blood gas values by the chemoreceptors
  - Increased chemoreceptor gain

COMMONLY ASSOCIATED CONDITIONS

- Periodic breathing in infants is associated with the following:
  - Apnea of prematurity or infancy
  - Familial history of sudden infant death syndrome (SIDS)
  - Anemia of prematurity
  - Hypoxemia
  - Hypochloremic alkalosis
- Periodic breathing with adults is associated with the following:
  - Cardiac abnormalities (especially congestive heart failure [CHF])
  - Neurologic dysfunction (meningitis, encephalitis, brainstem dysfunction)
  - Exposure to high altitudes

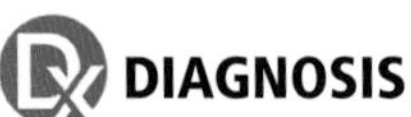

DIAGNOSIS

HISTORY

- In most cases, parents notice periodicity in the child's respiratory pattern.
- A brief resolved unexplained event (BRUE; previously described an "apparent life-threatening event" [ALTE]) might precipitate an evaluation in which periodic breathing is documented.
- In otherwise healthy premature or term infants, there are no other symptoms.

PHYSICAL EXAM

In otherwise healthy premature or term infants, the physical exam is normal.

DIFFERENTIAL DIAGNOSIS

- Other forms of apnea:
  - Central apnea
  - Mixed apnea
  - Obstructive apnea (or hypopnea)
- Other forms of periodic breathing:
  - Cheyne-Stokes respirations
  - Biot breathing
  - Kussmaul respirations
- Normal irregular respiration seen in infants

DIAGNOSTIC TESTS & INTERPRETATION

Initial Tests (screening, lab, imaging)

Chest radiography: usually normal findings

Diagnostic Procedures/Other

- Polysomnography
  - Assesses the extent of periodic breathing episodes
  - Determines if there is accompanying hypoxemia, hypercarbia, or bradycardia with the events
  - Distinguishes between periodic breathing and obstructive and/or central apnea
  - Useful for following response to treatment (i.e., normalization of polysomnography)
- pH probe done in combination with the polysomnogram (if gastroesophageal reflux is suspected): Record for a minimum of 6 hours.
- 2-channel pneumogram
  - Gives less information than polysomnography
  - Can document periodic breathing, but it may miss episodes of obstructive apnea
  - Monitors heart rate and respiratory effort (If oxygen saturation monitoring is desired, an additional channel is required.)

TREATMENT

GENERAL MEASURES

- Therapy should be directed at treating the underlying primary disease:
  - If periodic breathing is associated with apnea, hypoxemia, and/or other sleep disturbances, appropriate treatment of the underlying etiology should be instituted.
  - In cases secondary to CHF, appropriate cardiac interventions need to be instituted.
  - In cases associated with high altitude, treatment options include the following:
    - Acclimation (if tolerated)
    - Descent to lower altitude, then gradual ascent
    - Medication (acetazolamide most commonly used)
- Duration of therapy
  - Depends on the underlying cause of the periodic breathing
  - Treatment does not change the natural course of periodic breathing in otherwise healthy infants.
  - Therapy should continue until the periodic breathing resolves or is no longer clinically significant.

MEDICATION

Stimulants

- Caffeine IV or PO (based on caffeine base; multiply dosage by two for caffeine citrate salt)
  - Loading dose: 10 mg/kg
  - Maintenance dose: 2.5 mg/kg/24 h
  - Therapeutic level: 5 to 20 mg/L
- Theophylline PO (if using aminophylline IV, divided dosage by 0.79)
  - Loading dose: 4 to 5 mg/kg
  - Maintenance dose: 3 to 5 mg/kg/24 h divided t.i.d.
  - Therapeutic level: 6 to 10 mg/L

ADDITIONAL THERAPIES

- Supplemental oxygen: useful if periodic breathing is secondary to hypoxemia
- Nasal continuous positive airway pressure (CPAP): very effective in eliminating periodic breathing
- Home monitoring should be considered (although not absolutely indicated) in the following cases:
  - Significant amount of periodic breathing
  - Accompanying apnea
  - Associated hypoxia and/or bradycardia
  - History of a significant BRUE
  - Parental anxiety

ONGOING CARE

FOLLOW-UP RECOMMENDATIONS

- Time to improvement depends on the underlying cause of the periodic breathing.
- Improvement is anticipated as the infant ages.
- When treatment is started, a decrease in the amount of periodic breathing should be seen almost immediately.

PROGNOSIS

- Excellent in otherwise healthy premature or term infants
- Governed by primary process in patients with an underlying cardiac or neurologic disorder

COMPLICATIONS

Relationship between periodic breathing and SIDS is controversial.

ADDITIONAL READING

- Carroll JL, Agarwal A. Development of ventilatory control in infants. *Paediatr Respir Rev*. 2010;11(4):199–207.
- Horemuzova E, Katz-Salamon M, Milerad J. Breathing patterns, oxygen and carbon dioxide levels in sleeping healthy infants during the first nine months after birth. *Acta Paediatr*. 2000;89(11):1284–1289.
- Hunt CE, Corwin MJ, Lister G, et al. Longitudinal assessment of hemoglobin oxygen saturation in healthy infants during the first 6 months of age. Collaborative Home Infant Monitoring Evaluation (CHIME) Study Group. *J Pediatr*. 1999;135(5):580–586.
- Miano S, Castaldo R, Ferri R, et al. Sleep cyclic alternating pattern analysis in infants with apparent life-threatening events: a daytime polysomnographic study. *Clin Neurophysiol*. 2012;123(7):1346–1352.
- Poets CF. Apnea of prematurity: what can observational studies tell us about pathophysiology? *Sleep Med*. 2010;11(7):701–707.
- Schechter MS; for Section on Pediatric Pulmonology, Subcommittee on Obstructive Sleep Apnea Syndrome. Technical report: diagnosis and management of childhood obstructive sleep apnea syndrome. *Pediatrics*. 2002;109(4):e69.
- Sterni LM, Tunkel DE. Obstructive sleep apnea in children: an update. *Pediatr Clin North Am*. 2003;50(2):427–443.

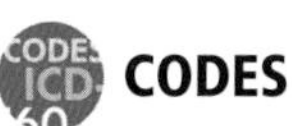

CODES

ICD10

R06.3 Periodic breathing

FAQ

- Q: What is the risk of the patient dying of SIDS?
- A: The relationship between periodic breathing and SIDS is not clear, although most studies have not found a higher frequency of SIDS among patients with periodic breathing.

PERIORBITAL CELLULITIS

Aaron E. Kornblith, MD • Christine S. Cho, MD, MPH, MEd

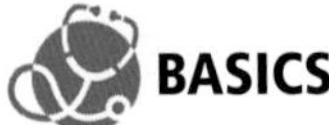

BASICS

DESCRIPTION
- Periorbital or preseptal cellulitis is an acute infection characterized by pain, erythema, and edema to the anterior eyelid and surrounding tissue.
- The infection lies superficial to the orbital septum, a thin fascial layer forming the anterior boundary of the orbital compartment.
- In contrast, orbital cellulitis (postseptal disease) is a deep space infection involving the deeper structures of the orbit and requires emergent intervention.

EPIDEMIOLOGY
- Often occurs in young children, commonly <5 years of age but can occur at any age
- Periorbital cellulitis is at least 3 times more common than orbital cellulitis.

RISK FACTORS
- Predisposing factors that may lead to periorbital cellulitis include local skin trauma (e.g., insect bite, scratch, eczema) and lacrimal/eyelid injury.
- There is a slight increase incidence of orbital cellulitis in winter months.

GENERAL PREVENTION
- *Haemophilus influenzae* type b vaccine has decreased the incidence of *H. influenzae*-associated periorbital cellulitis.
- Pneumococcal conjugate vaccine may decrease streptococcal disease.

PATHOPHYSIOLOGY
- Often, extension from an external source including trauma (insect bite, recent surgery, foreign body) or adjacent infection (sinusitis, dacryocystitis, hordeola, dental abscess)
- In contrast, orbital cellulitis is often caused by paranasal sinus disease.

ETIOLOGY
Variable depending on mechanism
- Most common pathogens are from skin flora including
  - *Staphylococcus aureus* (increasingly methicillin-resistant)
  - Group A *Streptococcus*
  - *Streptococcus pneumoniae*
  - Other streptococci species
- Anaerobic infections can extend from dental source.
- *H. influenzae* type b was historically the most common pathogen; consider in unimmunized child <5 years of age.

COMMONLY ASSOCIATED CONDITIONS
Rarely associated with bacteremia; however, consider this condition in children <3 years of age or in immunocompromised patients.

DIAGNOSIS

HISTORY
- Onset, time course of symptom progression, and any predisposing factors
- A history of trauma is suggestive of periorbital cellulitis.
- A history of prolonged sinus disease suggests orbital cellulitis.
- The presence of pain supports cellulitis, whereas complaints of pruritus are more suggestive of an allergic etiology.
- Diplopia, proptosis, and visual changes are more suggestive of orbital cellulitis.
- Quantify systemic symptoms such as fever and lethargy.
  - These indicate a more severe, disseminated infection.

PHYSICAL EXAM
- Superficial orbital tissues and lids will be edematous, erythematous, warm to the touch, and typically tender on palpation.
  - Often unilateral, the findings can start in one eyelid, but both the upper and lower eyelids may be involved.
  - Evaluate for signs of previous trauma, cutaneous injury, insect bite, and so forth.
- Children with *H. influenzae* preseptal cellulitis are usually febrile and ill-appearing.
- Occasionally, the eyelids are so swollen that it is difficult to examine the globe. To do so, place anesthetic eyedrops on the eye and use ocular speculum or fashion a paperclip into a lid retractor to lift the eyelid.
- The globe should be carefully examined.
  - In periorbital cellulitis, the ocular exam is often normal. The sclera is usually white, although patients can have some conjunctival erythema but rarely chemosis.
  - Any change in vision, pupillary function, or limitations in eye motility suggests orbital involvement.
- The presence of proptosis and/or pain with eye movement suggests orbital involvement.
- Neurologic findings, such as cranial nerve deficit, are suggestive of deep space involvement.
- Evaluate for signs of fever, respiratory infection, and sepsis.

DIFFERENTIAL DIAGNOSIS
- Infectious
  - Early orbital cellulitis
  - Dacryocystitis
  - Stye
  - Severe viral conjunctivitis
- Allergic
  - Periocular allergic reaction: insect bite, angioedema, contact dermatitis

- Other
  - Periocular trauma
  - Rhabdomyosarcoma
  - Idiopathic orbital inflammatory syndrome (IOIS)
  - Cavernous venous thrombosis
  - Hypoproteinemia (e.g., nephrotic syndrome)

ALERT
Orbital cellulitis is an ophthalmologic emergency and requires prompt therapy and specialist consultation.

DIAGNOSTIC TESTS & INTERPRETATION

- Lab tests are usually not helpful or indicated.
- CBC is warranted only if bacteremia is suspected.
  - Leukocytosis has no value in differentiating periorbital and orbital cellulitis.
- For bilateral periorbital edema, obtain a urine dipstick to rule out proteinuria, which would suggest nephrotic syndrome.
- Skin cultures and blood cultures have a low yield.
  - Blood cultures are obtained only when the child is febrile or appears septic.
  - Wound cultures can be obtained if there is an abscess.
- Periorbital cellulitis is a clinical diagnosis, and radiologic confirmation is only indicated if the diagnosis is unclear. Imaging may be required in the following circumstances:
  - If orbital cellulitis is suspected
  - Cases that do not respond to medical treatment
  - Neurologic symptoms are present.
- Computed tomography (CT) with contrast is the preferred imaging choice for evaluating orbital cellulitis.
- Serial CT scanning should be done only if the child is not improving with treatment.

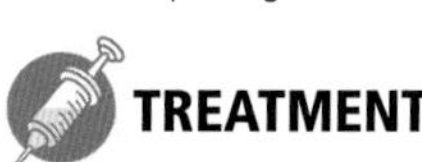

TREATMENT

GENERAL MEASURES

- Simple periorbital cellulitis should be empirically treated based on local prevalence of *Staphylococcus* and *Streptococcus* species.
  - Consider methicillin-resistant *Staphylococcus aureus* (MRSA).
  - Examples include 2nd-generation cephalosporins or β-lactamase–resistant penicillins.
- There is no evidence to suggest that IV antibiotics are better than oral antibiotics; however, younger children need close observation and/or follow-up.
- For children <1 year of age, strongly consider hospitalization for IV therapy and very close observation.
- Children between the ages of 1 and 5 years should be either hospitalized or followed-up closely after initiating antibiotics.
- Children >5 years of age can usually be treated with an oral regimen as long as they do not appear toxic or have orbital involvement.
- Any patient with symptoms suggestive of deep space involvement or hematogenous involvement should be hospitalized.

MEDICATION

- In nontoxic children, oral antibiotics: Amoxicillin/clavulanate, cephalexin, clindamycin (if MRSA is a concern) are started on an outpatient basis; the child should be seen again within 24 to 48 hours.
- Consider admission for IV antibiotics (clindamycin, ampicillin/sulbactam) for those patients are <1 year of age, are ill appearing, have bacteremia, or have symptoms suggestive of orbital involvement.

SURGERY/OTHER PROCEDURES

- For preseptal disease, surgical intervention is usually required when an abscess or a foreign body is present.
- Treatment of orbital disease should be under the guidance of a specialist.

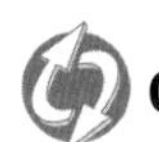

ONGOING CARE

FOLLOW-UP RECOMMENDATIONS

Patient Monitoring

- Watch patients closely for signs of orbital extension, bacteremia, or other forms of disseminated infection.
- Neonates and infants can become septic quickly, so they need to be closely monitored.
- Patients should have close follow-up 24 to 48 hours after initiating outpatient treatment.
- Patients who do not improve after close follow-up should be admitted for IV antibiotics and possible imaging.
- Patients should be seen on a daily basis until a definite improvement is noted.

PROGNOSIS

Excellent, with minimal incidence of long-term sequelae, unless a complication is encountered

COMPLICATIONS

- Orbital extension
- Skin abscess (8%)
- Eyelid necrosis (1–2%)
- Sepsis
- Intracranial extension (2–3%)

ADDITIONAL READING

- Bedwell J, Bauman N. Management of pediatric orbital cellulitis and abscess. *Curr Opin Otolaryngol Head Neck Surg*. 2011;19(6):467–473.
- Foster JA, Katowitz JA. Pediatric orbital and periocular infections. In: Katowitz JA, ed. *Pediatric Oculoplastic Surgery*. New York, NY: Springer-Verlag; 2001:407–420.
- Georgakopoulos CD, Eliopoulou MI, Stasinos S, et al. Periorbital and orbital cellulitis: a 10-year review of hospitalized children. *Eur J Ophthalmol*. 2010;20(6):1066–1072.
- Hauser A, Fogarasi S. Periorbital and orbital cellulitis. *Pediatr Rev*. 2010;31(6):242–249.
- Wald ER. Periorbital and orbital infections. *Pediatr Rev*. 2004;25(9):312–320.

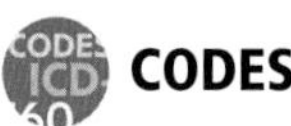

CODES

ICD10

- H05.019 Cellulitis of unspecified orbit
- H00.039 Abscess of eyelid unspecified eye, unspecified eyelid

PERIRECTAL ABSCESS

Naamah Levy Zitomersky, MD

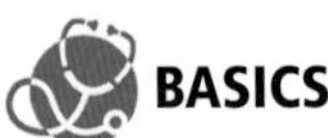

BASICS

DESCRIPTION

- Abscess in the perirectal area
- May be associated with fistula-in-ano
- Classification of the abscess is based on the location in relation to the levator and sphincteric muscles of the pelvic floor.
- Classification by decreasing frequency: perianal, ischioanal, intersphincteric, and supralevator

EPIDEMIOLOGY

- May occur at any age
- More common in males 2:1
- In children, more common in those <2 years

PATHOPHYSIOLOGY

- Most often originates from an occluded anal gland with subsequent bacterial overgrowth and abscess formation
- Infection from within the anal glands, penetrates through the internal sphincter, and ends in the intersphincteric space
- Chronic infection and inflammation may result in the formation of fistula-in-ano. This occurs in up to 50% as a result of persistent anal sepsis or an epithelialized tract.
- Also can be associated with transmural inflammation and fistulization of the rectosigmoid mucosa due to Crohn disease

COMMONLY ASSOCIATED CONDITIONS

- Nonspecific anal gland infection
- Crohn disease
- Immune deficiency (e.g., neutropenia, diabetes mellitus, AIDS)
- Perforation by a foreign body
- External trauma
- Tuberculosis
- Chronic granulomatous disease (CGD)
- Tumor (e.g., carcinoma, rhabdomyosarcoma)

DIAGNOSIS

Signs and symptoms

- General
  - Constant anal or perianal pain that often precedes local findings
  - Localized swelling, erythema, and fluctuance
  - Painful defecation or ambulation
  - Constitutional symptoms (e.g., fever or malaise)
- Perianal abscess
  - Result of distal vertical spread of the infection to the anal margin
  - Presents as tender, fluctuant mass
  - Most common type of perianal abscess
- Ischiorectal abscess
  - Secondary to horizontal spread of infection across the external anal sphincter into the ischiorectal fossa
  - Infection may track across the internal anal sphincter into the anal canal.
  - Presents as diffuse, tender, indurated, fluctuant area
  - Patients may have pain and fever prior to visible swelling.
- Intersphincteric abscess
  - Limited to the intersphincteric space between the internal and external sphincters; therefore, often does not cause perianal skin changes
  - Associated with painful defecation
  - Accounts for only 2–5% of all anorectal abscesses
- Supralevator abscess
  - May arise from two different sources
    - Proximal vertical spread from the gland through the intersphincteric space to the supralevator space
    - Pelvic inflammation or infection (e.g., Crohn disease)
  - Presents with pelvic or anorectal pain, fever, and, at times, urinary retention
  - Rectal exam usually reveals an indurated swelling above the anorectal ring.
  - Imaging may be necessary to establish the diagnosis.
- Horseshoe abscess
  - Secondary to abscessed anal gland located in the posterior midline of the anal canal
  - Due to presence of anococcygeal ligament, the infection is forced laterally into the ischiorectal fossae and is therefore known as "horseshoe."
  - May be unilateral or bilateral
  - Presents with pain

DIFFERENTIAL DIAGNOSIS

- Pilonidal infection
- Bartholin abscess
- Presacral epidermal inclusion cyst
- Hidradenitis suppurativa
- Rectal duplication cyst

DIAGNOSTIC TESTS & INTERPRETATION

Initial Tests (screening, lab, imaging)

- CBC
- Abscess culture
- Magnetic resonance imaging (MRI)
  - Preferred modality, as it provides excellent spatial and contrast resolution
  - Enables comprehensive evaluation of the entire peritoneum and lower pelvis
- Computed tomography (CT) scan
  - Has limited soft tissue contrast resolution which makes distinguishing perineal musculature and fistula tracts difficult, although organized fluid collections larger than 1 cm are generally seen
  - This modality also uses ionizing radiation, which is less desirable in the pediatric population.

- Ultrasound (US)
  - Endoscopic and transperineal US have been used but do not always show the full extent of inflammation.
  - Deeper structures may not be visualized, owing to the lack of sound wave penetration.
  - Endoscopic US may be used to diagnose, characterize, and monitor rectal abscesses.

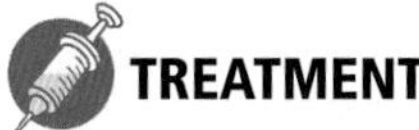

TREATMENT

GENERAL MEASURES

- Lack of fluctuation should not delay treatment.
- Abscess should be drained with placement of a seton or drainage catheter.
- Abscess should be cultured at time of drainage to direct therapy in the case antibiotics are needed.
- Antibiotics are reserved for situations in which the infection does not appropriately respond to drainage infections with adjacent cellulitis, of infections secondary to an enteric organism on culture. Antibiotics are also indicated for infection in an immunocompromised patient, a patient with abnormal cardiac valves, or a patient with Crohn disease.
- Sitz baths may be helpful with drainage.

SURGERY/OTHER PROCEDURES

- Drainage may be performed either with conservative incision and drainage or with judicious probing for fistulae.
- It is a matter of debate as to whether a fistulotomy or fistulectomy should be performed at the time of drainage for an accompanying fistula.

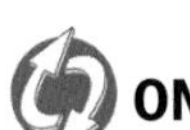

ONGOING CARE

- If abscess recurs, consider other associated conditions (e.g., neutropenia, HIV, diabetes mellitus, Crohn disease, rectal duplication cyst).
- Exploration for fistula-in-ano is recommended to prevent recurrence.

PROGNOSIS

- Prognosis is good if there is early detection and drainage of abscesses.
- Patients typically recover well after surgical drainage without the need for antibiotics.

COMPLICATIONS

- Sepsis
- Fistula formation

Special Considerations

- Crohn disease should be considered in patients with perirectal abscess with or without fistula-in-ano.
- Signs and symptoms that increase suspicion for Crohn disease include weight loss or poor growth, chronic diarrhea, or abdominal pain.

ADDITIONAL READING

- Caliste X, Nazir S, Goode T, et al. Sensitivity of computed tomography in detection of perirectal abscess. *Am Surg*. 2011;77(2):166–168.
- Chang HK, Ryu JG, Oh JT. Clinical characteristics and treatment of perianal abscess and fistula-in-ano in infants. *J Pediatr Surg*. 2010;45(9):1832–1836.
- Hammer MR, Dillman JR, Smith EA, et al. Magnetic resonance imaging of perianal and perineal Crohn disease in children and adolescents. *Magn Reson Imaging Clin N Am*. 2013;21(4):813–828.
- Huang A, Abbasakoor F, Vaizey CJ. Gastrointestinal manifestations of chronic granulomatous disease. *Colorectal Dis*. 2006;8(8):637–644.
- Lejkowski M, Maheshwari A, Calhoun DA, et al. Persistent perianal abscess in early infancy as a presentation of autoimmune neutropenia. *J Perinatol*. 2003;23(5):428–430.
- Malik AI, Nelson RL, Tou S. Incision and drainage of perianal abscess with or without treatment of anal fistula. *Cochrane Database Syst Rev*. 2010;(7):CD006827.
- Marcus RH, Stine RJ, Cohen MA. Perirectal abscess. *Ann Emerg Med*. 1995;25(5):597–603.
- Niyogi A, Agarwal T, Broadhurst J, et al. Management of perianal abscess and fistula-in-ano in children. *Eur J Pediatr Surg*. 2010;20(1):35–39.
- Rosen NG, Gibbs DL, Soffer SZ, et al. The nonoperative management of fistula-in-ano. *J Pediatr Surg*. 2000;35(6):938–939.
- Whiteford MH, Kilkenny J III, Hyman N, et al; for The Standards Practice Task Force. Practice parameters for the treatment of perianal abscess and fistula-in-ano (revised). *Dis Colon Rectum*. 2005;48(7):1337–1342.

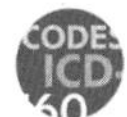

CODES

ICD10

- K61.1 Rectal abscess
- K60.3 Anal fistula
- K61.3 Ischiorectal abscess

FAQ

- Q: What are complications of this problem?
- A: Fistula formation is seen in up to 50% of patients, with a predilection for males.
- Q: What are the most common organisms of the abscess?
- A: *Staphylococcus* species
- Q: What other disease may perirectal abscess be associated with?
- A: Crohn disease. If there has been exposure, tuberculosis should also be excluded.
- Q: What treatments can be done other than surgery?
- A: Sitz baths and warm compresses may be able to help with smaller more superficial abscess.

PERITONITIS

Sarah S. Lusman, MD, PhD • Arunjot Singh, MD, MPH

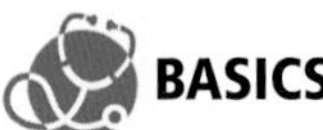

BASICS

DESCRIPTION

- Inflammation of the peritoneal cavity in reaction to infection or chemical irritation by organic fluids (e.g., intestinal contents, bile, blood, or urine)
- Infectious peritonitis can be classified as follows:
  - Primary or spontaneous bacterial peritonitis (SBP), which occurs without an obvious source or a break in continuity of the intestinal lumen
  - Secondary peritonitis occurs with visceral disruption from bowel perforation, abscess formation, ischemic necrosis, or penetrating abdominal injury; typically polymicrobial
  - Tertiary peritonitis is recurrent infection of the peritoneal cavity after presumed adequate treatment for primary or secondary peritonitis.

EPIDEMIOLOGY

Rates of peritonitis vary based on the underlying abdominal processes but classically occurs in association with cirrhosis, nephrotic syndrome, and malignancy.

Incidence

- In children on peritoneal dialysis, SBP incidence increases with duration, but majority suffer episode in first 6 months.
- Age may have inverse relationship on incidence rates: 0.79 peritoneal infections per year (in patients <1 year of age) versus 0.57 infections in children >12 years.

Prevalence

In children with chronic liver disease–related ascites, prevalence of SBP ranges from 19% to 56%.

RISK FACTORS

- End-stage liver disease
- Serum albumin <1.5 g/dL
- Low serum levels of complement factors C3 and C4
- Nephrotic syndrome (inability to clear organisms, most common is *Streptococcus pneumoniae*)
- Splenectomy (encapsulated organisms: group A streptococci, *Escherichia coli*, *S. pneumoniae*, *Bacteroides* sp.)
- Peritoneal dialysis
- Presence of gastrointestinal hemorrhage
- Prematurity
- Proton pump inhibitor use

GENERAL PREVENTION

- Children with chronic liver disease should receive all recommended childhood vaccinations.
- Children with functional asplenia due to portal hypertension should receive the meningococcal and pneumococcal conjugate vaccines as early as possible.
- Oral antibiotic prophylaxis reduces occurrence of SBP and improves short-term survival in adults with cirrhosis.

PATHOPHYSIOLOGY

- When bacteria or chemicals reach the peritoneal cavity, a local peritoneal and systemic host defense response is initiated:
  - Mechanical clearance of bacteria via lymphatics: Entrance of bacteria and bacterial products into the bloodstream contributes to the systemic response.
  - Phagocytosis and destruction of bacteria
  - Sequestration and walling off of bacteria with delayed clearance by phagocytic cells
  - Initial response is characterized by hyperemia, exudate of fluid into peritoneal cavity, and influx of macrophages followed by neutrophils.
  - Mesothelial cells secrete cytokines after stimulation (interleukins [IL-6, IL-8], tumor necrosis factor-α [TNF-α]). IL-6 stimulates T- and B-cell differentiation, and IL-8 is a selective chemoattractant for neutrophils.
  - Cytokines promote local resolution and compartmentalization through fibrin deposition.
- In SBP, pathogenic bacteria are cultured from peritoneal fluid without any apparent intra-abdominal surgical treatable source of infection; recognized as a complication in patients with ascites as a result of cirrhosis of any etiology
  - Generalized bacteremia and translocation of organisms from the gut (*E. coli*, *Klebsiella* sp.) into the portal veins or lymphatics or, less likely, directly into the ascitic fluid may account for the source of the infection.
  - Clearance of bacteria from the bloodstream may be impaired in patients with cirrhosis and ascites.
    - Poor clearance is due to diminished phagocytic activity of the hepatic reticuloendothelial system secondary to cellular functional defects or shunting of blood away from the liver.
  - Complement, necessary for the opsonization of bacteria and ultimately clearance by phagocytes, is decreased in the ascitic fluid.
- Infectious organisms include aerobic gram-negative organisms (*E. coli* and *Klebsiella* species) and aerobic gram-positive organisms (*Streptococcus* and *Enterococcus* species).
- In secondary peritonitis, the underlying bacterial infection tends to be a complex polymicrobial infection. Most common isolates are a combination of *E. coli* and *Bacteroides fragilis*.
- In tertiary peritonitis, the recurrence of infection is due to inadequate control of the infectious source or altered host immunity.

ETIOLOGY

- Primary peritonitis: liver cirrhosis or other conditions associated with ascites, such as the following:
  - Budd-Chiari syndrome
  - Congestive heart failure
  - Nephrotic syndrome
  - Systemic lupus erythematosus and other vasculitides
  - Rheumatoid arthritis
- The etiology of secondary peritonitis varies with age.
  - Neonates and infants
    - Meconium peritonitis (begins prenatally)
    - Necrotizing enterocolitis
    - Idiopathic gastrointestinal perforation
    - Perforation due to Hirschsprung disease
    - Spontaneous biliary perforation
    - Omphalitis (common in developing countries due to poor umbilical cord care)
    - Perforation of a urachal cyst
  - Children and adolescents
    - Secondary to appendicitis
    - Perforation of Meckel diverticulum
    - Gastric ulcer perforation
    - Pancreatitis
    - Cholecystitis
    - Traumatic or spontaneous perforation of the intestine
    - Intussusception and other bowel obstruction leading to necrosis
    - Neutropenic enterocolitis (typhlitis)
    - Crohn disease with fistula and abscess formation
    - Toxic megacolon
    - Tuberculosis
    - Salpingitis and pelvic inflammatory disease
    - Toxins

COMMONLY ASSOCIATED CONDITIONS

- Cirrhosis
- Peritoneal dialysis
- Perforated viscus (particularly if trauma/surgery)

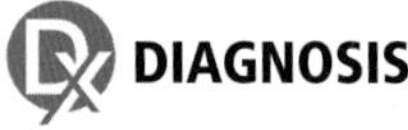

DIAGNOSIS

HISTORY

- Dependent on stage, age, and etiology
- Abdominal pain is the most common symptom.
  - Young children may be unable to verbalize pain.
- Fever, chills, vomiting, diarrhea
- ~10% of SBP cases are entirely asymptomatic; presentation may be subtle.
- Infants may present with poor feeding and lethargy.
- Other less common findings include the following:
  - Hypothermia
  - Hypotension
  - Increasing ascites despite diuretics
  - Worsening encephalopathy
  - Unexplained decrease in renal function

PHYSICAL EXAM

- Abdominal distension
- Rebound tenderness
- Decreased bowel sounds
- Evidence of chronic liver disease
- Evidence of ascites

DIFFERENTIAL DIAGNOSIS

- Liver disease
  - Hepatitis
  - Decompensated cirrhosis
- Pyelonephritis
- Cystitis

- Appendicitis
- Pericarditis
- Pneumonia
- Acute intestinal obstruction (volvulus, intussusception)
- Pancreatitis
- Cholecystitis
- Abdominal abscess
- Cellulitis

DIAGNOSTIC TESTS & INTERPRETATION

Initial Tests (screening, lab, imaging)

- Blood: leukocytosis, elevated CRP. There may be leukopenia and thrombocytopenia in cases of sepsis.
- Urinalysis to exclude renal diseases which may mimic peritonitis
- Abdominal radiograph may show evidence of ileus, obstruction, or perforation.
- Abdominal ultrasound or CT shows ascites, thickening of bowel wall, and abscesses.

Diagnostic Procedures/Other

- Paracentesis is diagnostic and should be performed in cases of new-onset ascites and when SBP suspected.
- Cell count including absolute neutrophil count suggestive of SBP
- Inoculate blood culture bottles with 10 mL of fluid immediately at the bedside. A separate tube is sent for Gram stain; fluid chemistries: albumin, total protein, glucose, LDH, amylase, bilirubin
- Serum-ascites albumin gradient = serum albumin − fluid albumin. Difference >1.1 indicates portal hypertension.
- Diagnostic criteria for secondary peritonitis: positive ascitic fluid culture, neutrophil count of $\geq$250/mm^3, and surgically treatable source of infection

Test Interpretation

- Positive peritoneal fluid culture is confirmatory of SBP but only positive in ~25–50% of SBP cases.
- Elevated neutrophil count of $\geq$250/mm^3 in ascitic fluid is the most important laboratory indicator of SBP.

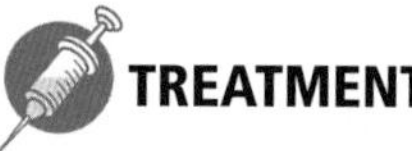

TREATMENT

GENERAL MEASURES

- Fluid resuscitation with isotonic saline, 20 mL/kg boluses up to 60 mL/kg, or albumin if large amounts of fluid are required to restore intravascular volume
- Decompression with nasogastric tube
- Patients at significant risk for SBP will benefit from selective intestinal decontamination with fluoroquinolones, trimethoprim-sulfamethoxazole, or rifaximin as an effective preventive measure.
- Timely diagnosis and treatment are key to improving survival—maintain a high index of suspicion.

MEDICATION

Empiric antibiotic coverage should be initiated early and directed primarily toward enteric gram-negative aerobes and gram-positive cocci.

- After the organism is identified, antibiotic coverage may be optimized.
- First line: 3rd-generation cephalosporin (i.e., cefotaxime) is drug of choice for SBP in pediatrics.
- Consider adding metronidazole for secondary SBP.
- Quinolones may also be used in areas with low resistance.
- Carbapenems for severe nosocomially acquired cases

SURGERY/OTHER PROCEDURES

In secondary peritonitis, surgery is the primary management tool:

- Control of the underlying source of infection by closing, diverting, or resecting the affected bowel
- Intraoperative peritoneal lavage and debridement of loculations and abscesses decrease bacterial inoculum and help prevent recurrent sepsis.
- Older studies in adults show benefit of antibiotic peritoneal lavage; controversial, as it may impair the local response and promote adhesions
- Catheters may be placed to drain a well-defined abscess cavity, form a controlled fistula, or provide access for continuous postoperative peritoneal lavage.

ADMISSION, INPATIENT, AND NURSING CONSIDERATIONS

- Acute peritonitis typically warrants inpatient admission.
- Volume resuscitation and fluid status are critical.
- Correction of albumin may decrease mortality in patients with renal/hepatic dysfunction.

ONGOING CARE

FOLLOW-UP RECOMMENDATIONS

Patient Monitoring

- Normalization of vital signs to mark clinical improvement and effective intervention
- Serial abdominal exams to assess change in tenderness, ascites, and volume status
- Reduction in leukocytosis or inflammatory markers
- If follow-up paracentesis performed, evaluate clearance of peritoneal fluid culture, reduction in absolute neutrophil count.

DIET

- NPO, total parenteral nutrition as necessary while treatment is initiated and patient stabilized
- Resume enteral feeding as tolerated if normal bowel function. Consider sodium restriction to reduce reaccumulation of ascitic fluid.

PROGNOSIS

- SBP in adults has inpatient mortality of 10–50%.
  - SBP markedly worsens the prognosis in patients with cirrhosis.
- Recurrence is common: 60% of patients who survive the first episode develop one or more recurrences.
- Severe secondary peritonitis in adults has a mortality rate of 30–55%.

COMPLICATIONS

- Hypovolemia from reduced fluid intake, vomiting, and 3rd-space fluid extravasation
- Liver failure, encephalopathy, coagulopathy
- Sepsis, adrenal insufficiency, renal failure
- Abdominal compartment syndrome
- Intra-abdominal abscess
- Long-term: adhesions

ADDITIONAL READING

- Haecker FM, Berger D, Schumacher U, et al. Peritonitis in childhood: aspects of pathogenesis and therapy. *Pediatr Surg Int*. 2000;16(3):182–188.
- Pericleous M, Sarnowski A, Moore A, et al. The clinical management of abdominal ascites, spontaneous bacterial peritonitis and hepatorenal syndrome: a review of current guidelines and recommendations. *Eur J Gastroenterol Hepatol*.2016;28(3):e10–e18.
- Saab S, Hernandez JC, Chi AC, et al. Oral antibiotic prophylaxis reduces spontaneous bacterial peritonitis occurrence and improves short-term survival in cirrhosis: a meta-analysis. *Am J Gastroenterol*. 2009; 104(4):993–1002.
- Srivastava A, Malik R, Bolia R, et al. Prevalence, clinical profile, and outcome of ascitic fluid infection in children with liver disease. *J Pediatr Gastroenterol Nutr*. 2017;64(2):194–199.
- Wong CL, Holroyd-Leduc J, Thorpe KE, et al. Does this patient have bacterial peritonitis or portal hypertension? How do I perform a paracentesis and analyze the results? *JAMA*. 2008;299(10):1166–1178.

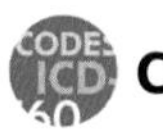

CODES

ICD10

- K65.9 Peritonitis, unspecified
- K65.2 Spontaneous bacterial peritonitis
- P78.1 Other neonatal peritonitis

FAQ

- Q: Is peritonitis common in children with ascites?
- A: Despite the frequency of ascites from many different causes, peritonitis occurs rarely. In the setting of children with chronic liver disease and ascites, SBP may occur in about 30% of patients.
- Q: What are the most useful laboratory aids for this diagnosis?
- A: Paracentesis and analysis of the fluid neutrophil count provides the most useful information regarding the diagnosis of peritonitis. Fluid culture is not required for diagnosis but helps to guide therapy.

PERITONSILLAR ABSCESS

Nicholas Tsarouhas, MD

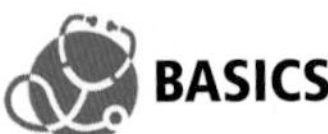

BASICS

DESCRIPTION

Infectious complication of tonsillitis or pharyngitis resulting in an accumulation of purulence in the tonsillar fossa; also referred to as "quinsy"

EPIDEMIOLOGY

- Most common deep space infection of head and neck
- Seen most commonly in adolescents but occasionally in younger children

RISK FACTORS

- Tonsillitis
- Pharyngitis

GENERAL PREVENTION

Abscess formation can often be prevented if appropriate antimicrobial therapy is initiated while the infection is still at the cellulitis stage.

PATHOPHYSIOLOGY

- Infectious tonsillopharyngitis progresses from cellulitis to abscess.
- The infection starts in the intratonsillar fossa, which is situated between the upper pole and the body of the tonsil and eventually extends around the tonsil.
- The abscess is a suppuration outside the tonsillar capsule, in proximity to the upper pole of the tonsil, involving the soft palate.
- Purulence usually collects within one tonsillar fossa but it may be bilateral.
- The pterygoid musculature may become irritated by pus and inflammation, which leads to the clinical finding of trismus.
- Tonsillar and peritonsillar edema may lead to compromise of the upper airway.

ETIOLOGY

- Most abscesses are polymicrobial.
- Group A β-hemolytic streptococci (GABHS) is the most common bacterium isolated.
- α-Hemolytic streptococci is the second most common bacterium reported in most studies.
- *Staphylococcus aureus*
- Anaerobic bacteria play an important role:
  - *Prevotella*
  - *Porphyromonas*
  - *Fusobacterium*
  - *Peptostreptococcus*
- Possible synergy between anaerobes and GABHS
- Gram-negatives such as *Haemophilus influenzae* and, more rarely, *Pseudomonas* species may be isolated.

COMMONLY ASSOCIATED CONDITIONS

- Tonsillitis or pharyngitis usually precedes its development.
- Peritonsillar cellulitis is often associated with infectious mononucleosis.

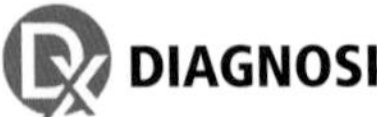

DIAGNOSIS

HISTORY

- Fever and sore throat
  - Most common initial complaints
- Trouble swallowing, pain with opening the mouth (trismus), muffled ("hot potato") voice
  - Classic presenting symptoms
- Unilateral neck or ear pain
  - Other common presenting symptoms

PHYSICAL EXAM

- Unilateral peritonsillar fullness or bulging of the posterior, superior, soft palate
  - Diagnostic finding
- Uvular deviation
  - Classic finding, although it may be *absent* in the more rare bilateral peritonsillar abscess
- Palpable fluctuance of palatal swelling
  - Calls for urgent aspiration
- Erythematous, edematous pharynx, with enlarged and exudative tonsils
  - Coexisting tonsillopharyngitis is common.
- Cervical adenopathy
  - Common
- Drooling
  - Often present
- Torticollis
  - Sometimes seen

DIFFERENTIAL DIAGNOSIS

- Peritonsillar cellulitis
  - Most common diagnostic consideration
  - Also referred to as "phlegmon"
  - Can be distinguished by the lack of classic peritonsillar abscess findings: peritonsillar space fullness, uvular deviation, and trismus
- Retropharyngeal abscess
  - Minimal to no peritonsillar findings
  - Widened prevertebral space on lateral neck radiograph
  - This airway-compromising disease usually occurs in preschool children, not adolescents.
- Epiglottitis
  - This life-threatening airway emergency presents abruptly with fever, stridor, increased work of breathing, and drooling.
  - Usually occurs in toxic-appearing children 3 to 7 years old
  - Rare entity in children since the advent of the *H. influenzae* type b vaccine
- Other infectious causes of severe tonsillopharyngitis:
  - EBV (infectious mononucleosis), coxsackievirus (herpangina), *Corynebacterium diphtheriae,* and *Neisseria gonorrhoeae*

DIAGNOSTIC TESTS & INTERPRETATION

- WBC count
  - Not a mandatory part of the workup
  - Usually elevated with prominent left shift
- Rapid streptococcal throat antigen studies
  - Helpful to diagnose GABHS infection
- Gram stain and culture of aspirate specimen
  - Confirms causative microorganism
- Aerobic bacteria may be more commonly reported due to laboratory/collection/culture media factors.
- Monospot/EBV antibody titers
  - Not a mandatory part of the workup
  - Infectious mononucleosis is both in the differential diagnosis and may coexist in some cases of peritonsillar abscess.
- Radiographic studies are rarely necessary, as this is clinical diagnosis.
- Intraoral ultrasound or computed tomography (CT) (with contrast):
  - Sometimes useful if clinical distinction of peritonsillar cellulitis from peritonsillar abscess is difficult
  - CT scan is most useful if patient cannot open mouth secondary to trismus.
  - CT scan is also important if deep neck extension is suspected.
- MRI
  - MRI may be more precise than CT in detecting multiple space involvement and, of course, is devoid of radiation exposure.
  - Pediatric use is limited by need for longer acquisition time and greater need for patient cooperation.
  - In younger children, the need for sedation for MRI introduces additional logistical challenges and potential airway risks.

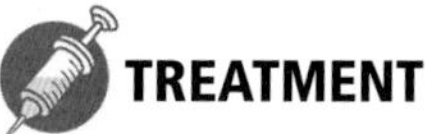

TREATMENT

GENERAL MEASURES

Treating an abscess without surgical drainage is inadequate and can have airway-threatening implications.

- Abscesses should be urgently/emergently drained via either needle aspiration or surgical incision and drainage (I&D).
- Appropriate analgesia and adequate hydration should be ensured in all cases.

MEDICATION

First Line

- Clindamycin or ampicillin/sulbactam are the most commonly used 1st-line antibiotics, owing to their efficacy versus GABHS, *Staphylococcus*, and anaerobes.
- As methicillin-resistant *S. aureus* isolates continue to increase, clindamycin is becoming more popular as drug of choice.
- Some initiate therapy with high-dose IV penicillin—in the presence of a positive strep antigen or throat culture study.
- The combination of piperacillin/tazobactam is used by some clinicians for broader coverage.

Second Line

- Nafcillin, oxacillin, and cefazolin are acceptable antibiotic alternatives.
- Steroids: Some experts recommend steroids to decrease swelling, pain, and trismus.
  - Most evidence from adult rather than pediatric studies
  - Methylprednisolone, dexamethasone, and prednisone all have been used.
  - A single dose of corticosteroids appears to be both safe and effective in peritonsillar abscess.

ISSUES FOR REFERRAL

Peritonsillar abscess: Otorhinolaryngology consultation is imperative both for acute and chronic management.

SURGERY/OTHER PROCEDURES

- As mentioned earlier, either needle aspiration or surgical I&D is mandatory in the acute setting for true abscesses.
- Most surgeons currently prefer interval tonsillectomy after the acute infection has been managed with antibiotics and an acute drainage procedure (needle aspiration or I&D).
- Surgical drainage with tonsillectomy is considered in children not responding to parenteral antibiotics within 24 to 48 hours.
- Acute or "hot" tonsillectomy (also "quinsy tonsillectomy") is advocated by some.

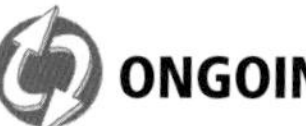

ONGOING CARE

FOLLOW-UP RECOMMENDATIONS

- Patients may be discharged on oral antibiotics to complete a 10- to 14-day course when afebrile and peritonsillar swelling has subsided.
- Recurrent peritonsillar abscess is more common in patients with recurrent tonsillitis.
- Early tonsillectomy (a.k.a. quinsy tonsillectomy or interval tonsillectomy) should be considered in patients with recurrent or severe peritonsillar abscesses, as well as patients with extraperitonsillar spread on CT.

PROGNOSIS

- Complete recovery with appropriate therapy.
- Recurrence of the abscess may occur.

COMPLICATIONS

- Upper airway obstruction is the most feared complication.
- Dehydration from decreased oral intake is the most common complication, however.
- Abscesses left untreated can rupture spontaneously into the pharynx, leading to aspiration and pneumonia.
- Other serious complications include parapharyngeal abscess, jugular vein suppurative thrombophlebitis (Lemierre syndrome), cavernous sinus thrombosis, sepsis, brain abscess, meningitis, and dissection into the internal carotid artery.
- Even after appropriate drainage, a small number (10–15%) of peritonsillar abscesses may reform.
- Most studies quote the overall recurrence rate of peritonsillar abscess from 9% to 22%.
- Risk factors for recurrent peritonsillar abscess includes history of previous peritonsillar abscess and extraperitonsillar spread on CT.

ADDITIONAL READING

- Chung JH, Lee YC, Shin SY, et al. Risk factors for recurrence of peritonsillar abscess. *J Laryngol Otol*. 2014;128(12):1084–1088.
- ENT Trainee Research Collaborative—West Midlands. National prospective cohort study of peritonsillar abscess management and outcomes: the Multicentre Audit of Quinsies study. *J Laryngol Otol*. 2016;130(8):768–776.
- Plum AW, Mortelliti AJ, Walsh RE. Microbial flora and antibiotic resistance in peritonsillar abscesses in Upstate New York. *Ann Otol Rhinol Laryngol*. 2015;124(11):875–880.
- Powell J, Wilson JA. An evidence-based review of peritonsillar abscess. *Clin Otolaryngol*. 2012;37(2):136–145.
- Shaul C, Koslowsky B, Rodriguez M, et al. Is needle aspiration for peritonsillar abscess still as good as we think? A long-term follow-up. *Ann Otol Rhinol Laryngol*. 2015;124(4):299–304.
- Stoner MJ, Dulaurier M. Pediatric ENT emergencies. *Emerg Med Clin North Am*. 2013;31(3):795–808.
- Tagliareni JM, Clarkson EI. Tonsillitis, peritonsillar and lateral pharyngeal abscesses. *Oral Maxillofac Surg Clin North Am*. 2012;24(2):197–204, viii.

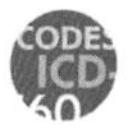

CODES

ICD10

J36 Peritonsillar abscess

FAQ

- Q: Are radiographs necessary to make the diagnosis of peritonsillar abscess?
- A: No. The physical examination is diagnostic. A lateral neck radiograph, ultrasound, CT, or MRI is indicated only if the diagnosis is in question or to delineate extent of disease or additional complications.
- Q: Is surgical consultation necessary in cases of peritonsillar abscess?
- A: Yes. Otorhinolaryngology consultation is indicated for both acute and chronic management.

PERSISTENT PULMONARY HYPERTENSION OF THE NEWBORN

Jennifer J. Miller, MD • Temitope Akinmboni, MBBS

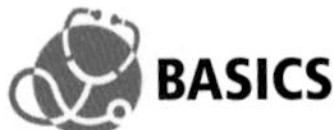

BASICS

DESCRIPTION

Clinical syndrome characterized by hypoxia and respiratory failure in a neonate due to a failure of the pulmonary vascular resistance (PVR) to decrease after birth, resulting in high pulmonary arterial pressures which causes intracardiac right to left shunting

EPIDEMIOLOGY

- Incidence of 1.8 per 1,000 live newborns, with a higher incidence in late preterm infants (5.4 per 1,000 births) than term infants (1.6 per 1,000 births)
- Typically occurs in newborns >34 weeks' gestation, owing to the presence of the muscular layer of pulmonary arterioles, the risk of uteroplacental insufficiency, and the potential for the passage of meconium in utero
- Meconium aspiration is the leading cause of persistent pulmonary hypertension of the newborn (PPHN).
- Males are affected more often than females.
- Mortality from PPHN is currently estimated at 7–15%.

RISK FACTORS

Genetics

- Alveolar capillary dysplasia is a rare, inheritable cause of PPHN in which there is abnormality in the air–blood interface, with increased distance between the alveolar epithelium and capillaries.
- Surfactant B deficiency has also been implicated, but it is a rare, lethal, autosomal recessive disorder.
- Infants with trisomy 21 are at increased risk of PPHN.

PATHOPHYSIOLOGY

- At a neonate's first breath after delivery, PVR normally decreases to redirect ~50% of the cardiac output to the pulmonary circulation. This phenomenon fails to occur in PPHN, hence, the previous name of this condition, "persistent fetal circulation."
- Increased PVR increases right ventricular afterload, causing retrograde blood flow to the right heart. This leads to increased right heart pressures (and subsequent tricuspid regurgitation), which can lead to right ventricular failure.
- Increased pulmonary arterial pressure also causes intracardiac shunting across any patent foramen ovale, ductus arteriosus, or atrioseptal or ventriculoseptal defect that may be present. This shunting causes more deoxygenated blood to go to the left heart and to be pumped to the body. The oxygen saturations postductally are lower than preductally.
- Deoxygenated blood in the left heart can lead to ischemic damage to the heart and right or left ventricular failure.
- If there is no shunting of blood, or the blood cannot get from the right to left heart because of a lack of persistent fetal pathways, a neonate may develop poor systemic perfusion, severe acidosis, shock, right ventricular failure, and even death.
- Hypoxia, acidosis, or stress occurring after birth further increases PVR.

ETIOLOGY

- Abnormal persistence of pulmonary vasculature constriction after birth secondary to underlying disease:
  - Sepsis
  - Pneumonia
  - Meconium aspiration
- Abnormality that has caused hypoplastic vasculature secondary to an anatomic condition:
  - Congenital diaphragmatic hernia
  - Oligohydramnios
  - Pulmonary hypoplasia
  - Alveolar capillary dysplasia
- Other disease states such as hypoxic-ischemic encephalopathy, polycythemia, neonatal leukemia, and hydropis fetalis can all cause PPHN.
- Maternal factors can contribute such as a cigarette smoking, obesity, gestational or pregestational diabetes, and in utero drug exposure (NSAIDs, salicylates, and selective serotonin reuptake inhibitors [SSRIs]).

COMMONLY ASSOCIATED CONDITIONS

Related to the underlying disease or as a complication of treatment

- Pneumothorax or air leak syndrome
- Chronic lung damage
- Long-term developmental delays
- Cerebral palsy
- Sensorineural hearing loss

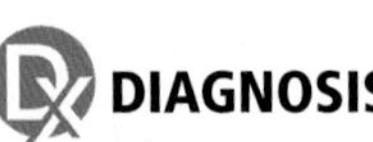

DIAGNOSIS

HISTORY

- Pregnancy history
  - History of oligohydramnios, which may be associated with pulmonary hypoplasia in the neonate
- Problems during labor and delivery
  - Events that can cause fetal distress and/or hypoxia: maternal chorioamnionitis, group B streptococcal infection, difficult delivery, or meconium aspiration
- Initial clinical course
  - Infants with PPHN usually present with mild respiratory distress that worsens in the first minutes to hours of life, progressing to respiratory failure, labile oxygenation with pre- and postductal saturation differences >5%, hypoxia, and poor perfusion.
- Infants with cardiac disease, congenital pulmonary airway malformation, or congenital diaphragmatic hernia are at increased risk of pulmonary hypertension.

PHYSICAL EXAM

- The following physical exam findings suggest a diagnosis of PPHN:
  - Significant respiratory distress with tachypnea, nasal flaring, grunting, and retractions and cyanosis
  - Lung sounds may be clear or coarse.
  - Pale, gray color with poor perfusion
  - Tricuspid regurgitation murmur heard at the left lower sternal border or prominent S_2
- The following physical exam findings suggest diagnoses other than idiopathic PPHN:
  - Barrel chest shape suggests a pneumothorax.
  - Scaphoid abdomen suggests congenital diaphragmatic hernia.

DIFFERENTIAL DIAGNOSIS

- Congenital
  - Cyanotic congenital heart disease
  - Congenital diaphragmatic hernia
  - Congenital pulmonary airway malformation
  - Alveolar capillary dysplasia
  - Surfactant deficiency
- Infectious
  - Pneumonia
  - Sepsis
- Pulmonary
  - Meconium aspiration syndrome
  - Maternal blood aspiration
  - Pneumothorax or air leak syndrome
  - Surfactant deficiency (respiratory distress syndrome [RDS])
  - Pulmonary hypoplasia

DIAGNOSTIC TESTS & INTERPRETATION

Initial Tests (screening, lab, imaging)

- CBC with differential: Leukocytosis, leukopenia, bandemia, or neutropenia suggests bacterial infection.
- Blood culture: should be performed in all cases of PPHN to rule out sepsis
- Frequent arterial blood gases monitoring
  - Helps to determine degree of hypoxia, hypercapnia, acidosis, and illness
  - Helps with management of ventilator support
- Hyperoxia test: While exposed to FiO_2 of 1, a PaO_2 >250 mm Hg almost completely rules out cyanotic heart disease.
- Oxygenation Index (OI)
  - OI = (mean airway pressure × FiO_2 / PaO_2) × 100
  - Used to express severity of respiratory distress and to determine if neonate is a candidate for extracorporeal membrane oxygenation (ECMO)
  - Should be calculated with every blood gas
  - An OI >40 suggests that ECMO should be considered, but specific criteria vary by institution.
- Chest radiograph (chest x-ray [CXR])
  - In idiopathic disease, usually shows clear lung fields
  - CXR will help diagnose pneumothorax, hyperinflation, meconium aspiration, and atelectasis.
  - Assessing cardiac silhouette and pulmonary vascular markings may help rule out certain forms of congenital heart disease.
- Echocardiogram
  - To exclude congenital heart disease
  - To diagnose PPHN with right to left blood flow in the patent ductus arteriosus (PDA)
  - Echocardiography also can estimate pulmonary artery pressure by septal positioning and tricuspid regurgitation.
  - To monitor ventricular function
- Cranial ultrasound
  - Should be obtained prior to initation of ECMO

TREATMENT

GENERAL MEASURES

- All infants should be transferred to a level IV neonatal intensive care unit where high-frequency ventilation (HFV) and inhaled nitric oxide (iNO) are available. If the neonate meets or nearly meets criteria for starting ECMO (OI >40), then ECMO should be available at the receiving institution.
- Support respiratory status.
  - Conventional ventilation or HFV to improve oxygenation and ventilation while minimizing lung damage
  - No set guidelines for ventilator management
  - Most institutions feel that HFV minimizes lung damage when high mean airway pressures (>15 cm H_2O) are needed.
  - Frequent monitoring to keep Pa_{O_2} between 60 and 90 mm Hg, Pc_{O_2} >35 to 45 mm Hg, and OI below ECMO criteria (OI >40)
  - Avoid hyperventilation and alkalosis, which have been associated with poor neurodevelopmental outcome.
  - Avoid acidosis, which can worsen pulmonary vasoconstriction.
- Maintain systemic blood pressure (BP).
  - Systemic hypotension exaggerates right-to-left shunting and reduces pulmonary blood flow.
  - Dopamine can be used to increase systemic BP. However, animal studies have suggested that dopamine increases both systemic and PVR, and that pulmonary arterial pressures should be monitored (by echocardiography) in patients receiving dopamine at >10 mcg/kg/min.
  - Milrinone, a phosphodiesterase 3A (PDE-3A) inhibitor, promotes improved left ventricular function, decreases PVR, and may synergistically act with iNO to improve outcomes in babies with PPHN.
- Lower the PVR and thus promote pulmonary blood flow:
  - Initially, 100% O_2 should be used to keep the Pa_{O_2} >60 to 90 mm Hg and the O_2 saturation around >97%.
  - Hypoxia and hyperoxia (due to oxidative stress) should both be avoided.
  - Keep blood gas pH normal (7.3 to 7.4) while keeping Pa_{CO_2} >35 to 45 mm Hg by ventilator manipulation.
  - Keep systemic BP high (mean BP >45 to 50 mm Hg in a term infant) with volume, transfusions, or medications.
  - Treat acidosis with fluid boluses (albumin, blood crystalloid).
  - iNO, a pulmonary vasodilator, should be used (or trialed) at a maximum dose of 20 parts per million (ppm) if the infant is on 1 FiO_2.
    - iNO has been shown to decrease the need for ECMO in term neonates with hypoxic respiratory failure secondary to PPHN, except for those babies with congenital diaphragmatic hernia.
    - Wean FiO_2 and iNO slowly as the infant improves. If oxygen and iNO are weaned too quickly, the infant can quickly become critically ill.
    - 30% of infants with PPHN do not respond to iNO and will need ECMO.
    - iNO does not reduce mortality or length of hospital stay.
  - Sildenafil and tadalafil, phosphodiesterase-5 inhibitors, have been shown to improve oxygenation and survival in PPHN.
    - Use as an adjunctive therapy when patients are refractory to iNO
- Reduce oxygen demand due to agitation and movement.
  - Sedatives and paralytics may be given to prevent fluctuations in oxygenation during care. Minimize the use of paralytics because they have been shown to increase mortality.
- Treat any underlying lung disease with the following, if applicable:
  - Antibiotics (for presumed pneumonia/sepsis)
  - Surfactant (especially early in the course of disease and especially in meconium aspiration)

ALERT

- Stable vascular access is important for frequent arterial blood gas monitoring and medication administration.
- PPHN is a neonatal emergency and a very labile condition. Neonates can change from being stable to being very sick and emergently needing ECMO.
- ECMO, although lifesaving in some cases of PPHN, is not without risk. Side effects include the following:
  - Repeated exposure to blood products
  - Risk of bleeding
  - Potential for long-term neurologic sequelae
  - Long-term risk of having only one patent carotid artery

ONGOING CARE

PROGNOSIS

- PPHN usually resolves either spontaneously or as the underlying parenchymal lung disease improves.
- Survival rate is good even for neonates who receive ECMO. Survival rate and incidence of long-term sequelae depend on underlying disease and severity of illness.
- Survival rate for all causes of PPHN in patients not requiring ECMO is >90%. ~10–20% has sensorineural hearing loss or an abnormal neurologic exam at follow-up.
- For those requiring ECMO, survival rate is 80% for idiopathic disease, 90% for meconium aspiration syndrome, 80% for disease secondary to sepsis, and 50–60% for patients with congenital diaphragmatic hernia. Roughly 20% of these survivors have sensorineural hearing loss or abnormal neurologic examinations at follow-up.

COMPLICATIONS

- Myocardial dysfunction
- Congestive heart failure (CHF)
- Hypoxic-ischemic insult

ADDITIONAL READING

- Abman SH, Hansmann G, Archer SL, et al. Pediatric pulmonary hypertension: guidelines from the American Heart Association and American Thoracic Society. *Circulation*. 2015;132(21):2037–2099.
- Barrington KJ, Finer N, Pennaforte T. Inhaled nitric oxide for respiratory failure in preterm infants. *Cochrane Database Syst Rev*. 2017;(1):CD000509.
- Danhaive O, Margossian R, Geva T, et al. Pulmonary hypertension and right ventricular dysfunction in growth-restricted, extremely low birth weight neonates. *J Perinatol*. 2005;25(7):495–499.
- Konduri GG, Kim UO. Advances in the diagnosis and management of persistent pulmonary hypertension of the newborn. *Pediatr Clin North Am*. 2009;56(3):579–600.
- Lakshminrusimha S, Konduri GG, Steinhorn RH. Considerations in the management of hypoxemic respiratory failure and persistent pulmonary hypertension in term and late preterm neonates. *J Perinatol*. 2016;36(Suppl 36):S12–S19.
- Steurer MA, Jelliffe-Pawlowski LL, Baer RJ, et al. Persistent pulmonary hypertension of the newborn in late preterm and term infants in California. *Pediatrics*. 2017;139(1):e20161165.

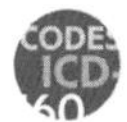

CODES

ICD10

P29.3 Persistent fetal circulation

FAQ

- Q: Does iNO improve outcome in newborns with severe PPHN?
- A: Yes. Although iNO has not been shown to reduce mortality, it has been shown to decrease the need for ECMO by 40% and reduce the length of hospital stay. Evidence suggests that early treatment with iNO (OI >15) is associated with a lower total cost of care.
- Q: Are there any other potential therapies for treating PPHN?
- A: Yes. Prostacyclin (PGI_2) analogs (iloprost, epoprostenol, and treprostinil) and an endothelin receptor antagonist (bosentan) are being studied in enhancing the vasodilatory effects of iNO. In animal models, hydrocortisone has been shown to help restore normal pulmonary vascular function by reducing oxidative.
- Q: Does PPHN occur in preterm infants (<34 0/7 weeks' gestation age at birth) and is the treatment different?
- A: Although the most common type of pulmonary hypertension in premature infants is secondary to chronic lung disease (which typically occurs at >30 days of life), there are case reports of surfactant deficiency and RDS associated with elevated right ventricular pressures in newborn ELBW infants. To date, there is no clear evidence to support iNO for infants <34 weeks' gestational age, and conflicting evidence about whether iNO can increase the risk of intraventricular hemorrhage in these infants.

PERTHES DISEASE

Harry K.W. Kim, MD

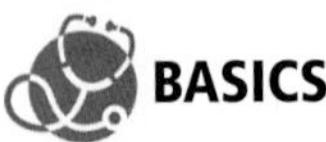

BASICS

DESCRIPTION

Childhood femoral head osteonecrosis of unknown etiology, which can weaken the femoral head and produce a permanent deformity in some patients, predisposing them to early arthritis

EPIDEMIOLOGY

- Incidence varies depending on the region: 0 to 15 per 100,000 children <15 years of age
- In United States and Canada, about 5 per 100,000
- Rare in persons of African descent
- Most frequent in children 4 to 8 years old
- 3 to 5 times more common in boys than girls
- 10–15% develop bilateral disease in asynchronous fashion.
- Associated factors: delayed bone age, hyperactivity, exposure to smoking, genitourinary anomalies (hypospadias, undescended testis, and inguinal hernia)

PATHOPHYSIOLOGY

- A partial or complete disruption of femoral head blood supply produces a partial or total femoral head osteonecrosis.
- Greater the head involvement, worse prognosis
- Bone necrosis and subsequent resorption of necrotic bone weaken the femoral head.
- Weight bearing worsens the femoral head deformity.
- Chronic hip joint synovitis also develops producing pain and restriction of motion.
- Necrotic head goes through four stages of healing over 3 to 5 years:
  - 1. Stage of avascular necrosis: smaller femoral head epiphysis with increased radiodensity
  - 2. Stage of fragmentation: Necrotic epiphysis shows fragmentation. Necrotic bone is resorbed, weakening the head. Most deformity occurs during this stage, which lasts 1 to 2 years.
  - 3. Stage of reossification: New bone begins to fill the epiphysis; longest stage, lasting up to 3 years
  - 4. Healed: Head is completely reossified. Not all heads heal back in round shape, and deformed heads are at risk for developing arthritis later.

ETIOLOGY

- Unknown
- Unlikely genetic transmission, as <5% have family history
- Many theories:
  - Multifactorial (genetic predisposition with environmental trigger)
  - Hyperactivity and subclinical trauma
  - Type II collagenopathy
  - Thrombophilia (factor V Leiden)
  - Smoke exposure

DIAGNOSIS

HISTORY

- Age at onset of symptoms, duration, patient's activity level, and risk factors for osteonecrosis are important.
- Age at onset before 6 years has better prognosis than after 6 years.
- Most common symptoms are limping and pain.
  - Insidious, relatively mild, activity related, able to ambulate (unlike septic hip)
  - Commonly complain of knee or thigh pain and *not* hip or groin pain, which may mislead an unsuspecting physician and delay diagnosis
  - Weeks to months duration with waxing and waning of pain and limping with rest
  - Worse during or after sports activities
- Participation in high-impact activities that involve running and jumping may produce greater symptoms, synovitis, and limping.
- Known causes of osteonecrosis must be ruled out through history: previous hip surgery, corticosteroid use, sickle cell disease, neonatal hip sepsis, coagulopathy, Gaucher disease.
- Obtain family history for Perthes disease, skeletal dysplasia, early arthritis.

PHYSICAL EXAM

- Because pain can be nonspecific (such as knee or thigh pain), careful exam required to localize the pain source
- Gently check hip and knee passive range of motion with patient recumbent:
  - Patients with Perthes will have limited hip rotation and abduction. Knee exam should be normal.
  - The loss of motion may be mild in the early stage and becomes worse during the stage of fragmentation.
  - In severe cases, hip flexion and adduction contractures may be found.
- Assess walking for limping and Trendelenburg gait: head and trunk leaning over to the affected leg as it takes stance.
- Positive Trendelenburg test: Have the patient lift one leg off the ground while standing straight. When the weight is on the normal hip, the pelvis is maintained in a horizontal position. When the weight is on the affected hip, the pelvis drops due to the hip abductor muscle weakness.
- Atrophy of thigh muscles and slight shortening of the affected side are late findings.
- Check face, hands, feet, chest, and spine for signs of skeletal dysplasia.

DIFFERENTIAL DIAGNOSIS

Perthes is a diagnosis of exclusion. Known causes of osteonecrosis along with other conditions that mimic Perthes must be ruled out.

- Transient or toxic synovitis
- Infection: neonatal sepsis, septic arthritis, subacute osteomyelitis, TB of hip
- Chondrolysis
- Juvenile idiopathic arthritis
- Traumatic osteonecrosis secondary to hip fracture or dislocation
- Corticosteroid-associated osteonecrosis: for treatment of leukemia and inflammatory conditions
- Sickle cell disease induced osteonecrosis
- Iatrogenic osteonecrosis: hip surgery for developmental dysplasia of the hip (DDH), hip pinning
- Tumor or tumor-like conditions affecting the proximal femoral epiphysis or acetabulum: osteoid osteoma, chondroblastoma, bone cyst
- Skeletal dysplasias:
  - Multiple epiphyseal dysplasia
  - Trichorhinophalangeal syndrome
  - Spondyloepiphyseal dysplasia
- Gaucher disease
- Hypothyroidism
- Hemophilia

DIAGNOSTIC TESTS & INTERPRETATION

Initial Tests (screening, lab, imaging)

- Labs not required
- May be helpful only if infectious, inflammatory, or metabolic conditions mimicking Perthes are suspected.
- Diagnosis requires imaging.
- Anteroposterior (AP) pelvis and frog-leg lateral views primarily used
- Radiographic findings vary depending on the duration and the stage of the disease.
- Early stage: smaller femoral epiphysis, increased radiodensity, and a widened space between the epiphysis and the medial acetabulum compared to the normal side. In some patients (30%), subchondral fracture or crescent sign is present.
- Fragmentation stage: slight to severe epiphyseal flattening, which is best seen on a lateral view; fragmented appearance of the epiphysis with radiolucent areas (bone resorption); and lateral extrusion or subluxation of the epiphysis
- MRI, especially gadolinium-enhanced MRI, may be helpful in the early stage of the disease when the diagnosis is questionable.

TREATMENT

- Treatment principles:
  - Restore and maintain good hip motion, especially abduction.
  - Prevent collapse and lateral extrusion of the femoral epiphysis.
- Initial treatment for symptomatic patients include rest, activity restriction, weight-relief using crutches, walker, or wheelchair, gentle range of motion exercises, and NSAIDs PRN.
- In general, patients should be referred and followed by a pediatric orthopedic surgeon with expertise in managing Perthes.
- Early recognition and treatment may prevent or minimize the development of the femoral head deformity in older children (age >6 years).

GENERAL MEASURES

- Patients with the onset of disease before age 6 years are treated with nonoperative means:
  - Rest for few days if motion is severely limited.
  - Weight relief of the affect limb using crutches, walker, or wheelchair during the stages of avascular necrosis and fragmentation if severe disease
  - Range of motion exercises
  - Petrie casts (long leg casts with abduction bar) and abduction bracing if unresponsive to above
- Older patients often need surgery to keep the femoral head contained within the acetabulum.

MEDICATION

- NSAIDs should only be used for a short duration (few days to a week) as prolonged use may inhibit bone formation.
- Supplemental calcium and vitamin D if poor diet and inadequate sun exposure

ADDITIONAL THERAPIES

Based on age at onset of the disease, the stage of disease, and the extent of head involvement

SURGERY/OTHER PROCEDURES

- Surgical treatments such as femoral varus osteotomy or pelvic osteotomy are recommended for patients with the onset of disease after age 8 years and greater 50% head involvement.
- For 6- to 8-year-olds, unclear whether surgical treatment is beneficial

ISSUES FOR REFERRAL

Patients with Perthes disease should be referred to a pediatric orthopedic surgeon.

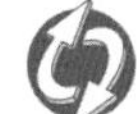

ONGOING CARE

FOLLOW-UP RECOMMENDATIONS

- Patient should be seen every 3 to 4 months to assess disease progression and compliance to treatment during the active phase of disease.
- Activity and weight-bearing restrictions generally continue until patient enters the reossification stage.

Patient Monitoring

Examine for the following:

- Worsening of limping and pain
- Loss of hip motion, especially hip abduction
- Radiographic changes: progression of femoral head collapse, lateral extrusion of the femoral epiphysis, and subluxation

PROGNOSIS

- Depends on the following:
  - Age at onset of the disease (onset before age 6 years is better than after age 6 years)
  - Extent of femoral head involvement; poorer prognosis if >50% head involvement
  - Development of poor prognostic radiographical signs: flattening of the lateral part of the epiphysis (lateral pillar C hip), subluxation of the epiphysis, growth disturbance of the proximal femoral physis producing short, broad femoral neck
- Long-term prognosis depends on the shape of the femoral head at skeletal maturity and how well it fits the acetabulum.

COMPLICATIONS

- 1 to 2 cm limb length discrepancy
- Restricted hip range of motion
- Permanent femoral head deformity
- Overriding greater trochanter with lateral impingement and abductor weakness
- Femoroacetabular impingement and acetabular labral disease
- Early osteoarthritis

ADDITIONAL READING

- Frick SL. Evaluation of the child who has hip pain. *Orthop Clin North Am*. 2006;37(2):133–140.
- Kim HK. Legg-Calvé-Perthes disease. *J Am Acad Orthop Surg*. 2010;18(11):676–686.
- Kim HK. Pathophysiology and new strategies for the treatment of Legg-Calvé-Perthes disease. *J Bone Joint Surg Am*. 2012;94(7):659–669.
- Saran N, Varghese R, Mulpuri K. Do femoral or salter innominate osteotomies improve femoral head sphericity in Legg-Calvé-Perthes disease? A meta-analysis. *Clin Orthop Relat Res*. 2012;470(9): 2383–2393.

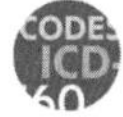

CODES

ICD10

- M91.10 Juvenile osteochondrosis of head of femur, unspecified leg
- M91.11 Juvenile osteochondrosis of head of femur, right leg
- M91.12 Juvenile osteochondrosis of head of femur, left leg

FAQ

- Q: When should I get radiographs?
- A: Diagnosis of Perthes requires radiographic confirmation. AP pelvis and frog-leg lateral radiographs should be obtained when a child presents with intermittent thigh, knee, or groin pain that has been present for weeks and has the finding of decreased hip range of motion but normal knee exam.
- Q: Why do patients with Perthes complain of knee or thigh pain instead of hip pain?
- A: Knee, thigh, and hip regions share the same sensory nerve. Thus, pain originating from one site (for instance hip) can be felt by a child as if its originating from another site (for instance knee). This can cause confusion in localizing the correct source of pain and obtaining appropriate radiographs. Some patients get knee radiographs and MRI before getting hip radiographs because of this misinterpretation of symptoms. Thus, it is important to examine both the hip and knee even if a child complains only of knee pain.

PERTUSSIS

Camille Sabella, MD

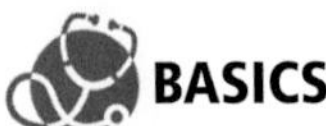

BASICS

DESCRIPTION

Pertussis (whooping cough), classically caused by *Bordetella pertussis*, is a protracted illness characterized by spasms of cough.

EPIDEMIOLOGY

- Pertussis is one of the most highly communicable diseases with attack rates close to 100% in susceptible individuals exposed at close range.
- Humans are the only hosts of *B. pertussis*.
- Route of spread is via large aerosolized respiratory droplets.
- Spread most commonly occurs during the catarrhal stage and first 2 weeks of cough onset.
- Incubation period 5 to 21 days
- Pertussis occurs with seasonal peaks (late summer-autumn) and 3- to 5-year cycles of increased incidence of disease.
- Adolescents and adults serve as major reservoirs and source of pertussis for infants.

Incidence

- Pertussis infection rates have steadily risen since the early 1980s.
  - This is due to the combination of imperfect vaccines, waning immunity, incomplete vaccination, low transplacental protection for infants, and increased detection and reporting.
- Infants <2 months of age have the highest age-related incidence.
- Rates in adolescents have been steadily increasing and now approach rates in infants.
- 10–30% of adolescents and young adults with prolonged cough have pertussis.

GENERAL PREVENTION

- Infection prevention
  - Isolation of hospitalized patient: droplet precautions for 5 days after starting appropriate antimicrobial therapy or for 3 weeks after the onset of cough, if antibiotics were not given
  - Care of exposed people: Exposed individuals (all household contacts, other close contacts, other children in child care) should receive chemoprophylaxis (same agents and doses as treatment; see the following discussion) to limit secondary transmission, regardless of immunization status. Immunization should be given to all unimmunized and underimmunized children and to adolescents and adults who have not yet received the Tdap booster vaccination.
- Immunization
  - All pertussis vaccines available in the United States are acellular vaccines in combination with diphtheria and tetanus toxoids.
  - Universal immunization of all children <7 years of age with DTaP vaccine is recommended as per Centers for Disease Control and Prevention (CDC) and American Academy of Pediatrics (AAP) guidelines.
  - Undervaccinated children ages 7 to 10 years, all adolescents ages 11 to 18 years, adults ages 19 to 64 years, as well as certain adults ages 65 years and older should receive a single dose of Tdap vaccine to help control the rate of infection in infants and young children.
  - Pregnant mothers should be vaccinated with Tdap during each pregnancy to protect their newborn infants; optimal time of vaccination is 27 to 36 weeks' gestation.

PATHOPHYSIOLOGY

- Tropism and replication are limited to the ciliated epithelium of the respiratory tract.
- Biologically active substances such as pertussis toxin (PT), filamentous hemagglutinin, tracheal cytotoxin, adenylate cyclase, and pertactin are responsible for virulence of the organism, including attachment, ciliostasis, impaired leukocyte function, and local epithelial damage.

ETIOLOGY

- *B. pertussis*, a small, nonmotile, fastidious, gram-negative coccobacillus, causes classic pertussis.
- *Bordetella parapertussis* causes a less protracted cough illness.

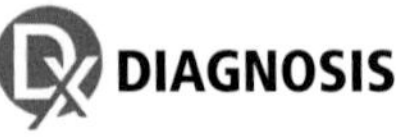

DIAGNOSIS

HISTORY

- History of a cough illness in other family members, including older siblings, parents, and grandparents, is important to elicit.
- Three clinical stages
  - Catarrhal stage (1 to 2 weeks) with symptoms of an upper respiratory infection
  - Paroxysmal stage (≥2 to 4 weeks) characterized by paroxysmal cough with increased severity and frequency producing the characteristic whoop during the sudden forceful inspiratory phase; posttussive vomiting is also observed during this stage.
  - The convalescent stage begins and lasts 1 to 2 weeks, but cough can persist for several months. In the adolescent or adult, long-standing cough of 2 to 3 weeks is the hallmark symptom. Most patients report a paroxysmal or staccato quality to the cough.
- Apnea is a common manifestation in infants <6 months. The characteristic whoop is typically absent. Short catarrhal stage, gasping, and choking are other manifestations in young infants.
- History of fever is typically absent.

PHYSICAL EXAM

- Normal physical examination between paroxysms is supportive of the diagnosis.
- Conjunctival hemorrhage and petechiae on the upper body may be present.
- Cyanosis, apnea, and bradycardia can be observed during the paroxysmal stage in young infants.
- Fever and signs of lower respiratory tract disease are uncommon.

DIFFERENTIAL DIAGNOSIS

- *B. parapertussis*
- Adenoviruses
- *Mycoplasma pneumoniae*
- *Chlamydia trachomatis*
- Bronchiolitis
- Bacterial pneumonia
- Cystic fibrosis
- Tuberculosis
- Foreign body aspiration
- Reactive airway disease

DIAGNOSTIC TESTS & INTERPRETATION

- CBC
  - Leukocytosis (15,000 to 100,000 cells/mm^3) with predominant lymphocytosis is commonly observed at the end of the catarrhal stage and throughout the paroxysmal stage of illness in infants and children; not commonly observed in adolescents and adult
- Culture of *B. pertussis*
  - Achieved using calcium alginate or Dacron® swabs of the nasopharynx and plated onto selective media such as Regan-Lowe and incubated for 10 days
  - Most frequently successful during the catarrhal or early paroxysmal stages and is rarely found beyond the 3rd week of illness
  - Specificity 100%; overall sensitivity is 60–70% but can be lower in previously vaccinated individuals, if antibiotics have already been given, or if beyond the 3rd week of illness.
- Polymerase chain reaction (PCR)
  - Most commonly used diagnostic test
  - Higher sensitivity and more rapid diagnosis than culture in the detection of *B. pertussis* from nasopharyngeal specimens
- Direct immunofluorescent assays (DFA) of nasopharyngeal specimens are no longer recommended for the diagnosis of pertussis.
- Serology
  - Can be helpful later in the course of the illness
  - No commercially available FDA-approved test available and difficult to interpret in previously immunized individuals
  - In the absence of recent immunization, an elevated serum IgG antibody to PT after 2 weeks of onset of cough is suggestive of recent infection. An increasing titer or a single IgG anti-PT value of approximately 100 IU/mL or greater can be used for diagnosis.
- Chest radiograph may reveal perihilar infiltrates, interstitial edema, and atelectasis.

TREATMENT

GENERAL MEASURES

- Patients with more severe disease manifestations (apnea, cyanosis, feeding difficulties) or other complications require hospitalization for supportive care:
  - Infants <6 months of age may develop apnea from fatigue secondary to excessive coughing.
  - Infants need close observation, preferably in the hospital.
- Antibiotics have little effect on the clinical course unless begun early in the disease process (catarrhal phase) but should always be given to prevent spread of the infection.

MEDICATION

- Azithromycin (PO)
  - 10 mg/kg as a single dose on day 1, then 5 mg/kg/24 h as a single daily dose on days 2 to 5 is recommended for ages ≥6 months.
  - For infants <6 months of age, dosage is 10 mg/kg/24 h as a single daily dose for 5 days.
  - For adolescents and adults, dosage is 500 mg as a single dose on day 1, followed by 250 mg as a single daily dose on days 2 to 5.
- Erythromycin ethylsuccinate PO (40 mg/kg/24 h; max dose: 2,000 mg/24 h in 4 doses for 14 days)
  - Erythromycin in infants <4 weeks of age is associated with hypertrophic pyloric stenosis. Thus, azithromycin is the drug of choice for treatment or prophylaxis of pertussis in that age group.
- Clarithromycin PO (15 mg/kg/24 h divided b.i.d. for 7 days; max dose: 1,000 mg/24 h) can be used in children ≥1 month of age.
- Trimethoprim/sulfamethoxazole in children ≥2 months of age, is an alternative agent, although its efficacy is unproven.

ADMISSION, INPATIENT, AND NURSING CONSIDERATIONS

- Young infants (<6 months of age) with concern for apnea or fatigue with coughing should be admitted.
- Patients with severe disease manifestations or complications should be admitted.
- Infants can be discharged when there is no evidence of cardiorespiratory instability and when they are able to self-recover from coughing spells.

ONGOING CARE

FOLLOW-UP RECOMMENDATIONS

The paroxysmal stage can last up to 4 weeks and the convalescent stage up to several months.

PROGNOSIS

Directly related to patient age

- Highest mortality is observed in infants <6 months of age, with a 0.5–1% risk of death.
- In the older child, prognosis is good.

COMPLICATIONS

- The complications of pertussis are more likely to occur in infants <6 months of age:
  - Apnea
  - Pneumonia, which may be primary or secondary to viruses (adenovirus, respiratory syncytial virus) or bacteria (*Streptococcus pneumoniae*, *Staphylococcus aureus*), occurs in 13–25%; the presence of fever or respiratory symptoms in between cough episodes should raise the possibility of secondary bacterial pneumonia.
  - Other pulmonary complications include atelectasis, pneumothorax, pneumomediastinum, and subcutaneous emphysema.
  - Seizures (2%) and encephalopathy (0.5%) have also been observed in infants with pertussis.
- Complications of pertussis in adolescents and adults include:
  - Cough syncope
  - Incontinence
  - Rib fractures
  - Pneumonia

ADDITIONAL READING

- American Academy of Pediatrics. Pertussis (whooping cough). In: Kimberlin DW, Brady MT, Jackson MA, et al, eds. *Red Book: 2015 Report of the Committee on Infectious Diseases*. 30th ed. Elk Grove Village, IL: American Academy of Pediatrics; 2015:608–621.
- Centers for Disease Control and Prevention. Updated recommendations for use of tetanus toxoid, reduced diphtheria toxoid and acellular pertussis (Tdap) vaccine from the Advisory Committee on Immunization Practices, 2010. *MMWR Morb Mortal Wkly Rep*. 2011;60(1):13–15.
- Klein NP, Bartlett J, Rowhani-Rahbar A, et al. Waning protection after fifth dose of pertussis vaccine in children. *N Engl J Med*. 2012;367(11):1012–1019.
- Murray EL, Nieves D, Bradley JS, et al. Characteristics of severe *Bordetella pertussis* infection among infants ≤90 days of age admitted to pediatric intensive care units—Southern California, September 2009–June 2011. *J Pediatr Inf Dis Soc*. 2013;2(1):1–6.
- Tartof SY, Lewis M, Kenyon C, et al. Waning immunity to pertussis following 5 doses of DTaP. *Pediatrics*. 2013;131(4):e1047–e1052.
- Tiwari T, Murphy TV, Moran J; and National Immunization Program, Centers for Disease Control and Prevention. Recommended antimicrobial agents for the treatment and postexposure prophylaxis of pertussis: 2005 CDC guidelines. *MMWR Recomm Rep*. 2005;54(RR-14):1–16.

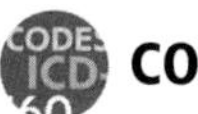

CODES

ICD10

- A37.90 Whooping cough, unspecified species without pneumonia
- A37.00 Whooping cough due to *Bordetella pertussis* without pneumonia
- A37.01 Whooping cough due to *Bordetella pertussis* with pneumonia

FAQ

- Q: Why is the transmission of pertussis difficult to control in the young infant?
- A: Unfortunately, many physicians do not consider pertussis in adolescents or adults because the symptoms can be nonspecific and often are not severe. They also assume that childhood immunization will protect adults against pertussis. Therefore, delays in antimicrobial treatment are common in adults, owing to the lack of index of suspicion of pertussis by their providers. Finally, there was not a universal recommendation for adolescents and adults to receive pertussis boosters until 2005, even though the immunity protection by pertussis vaccination is limited. It is largely adolescents and adults with pertussis who then spread the disease to young infants and children.
- Q: What is the best way to diagnose pertussis in the young infant?
- A: The diagnosis can be made clinically but requires a high index of suspicion. The diagnosis should be considered based on a history of severe cough in any young infant. At the time of presentation, infants usually appear well and have a normal exam. So, the history provided by the parents of the paroxysmal and severe nature of the course, often associated with gagging, posttussive emesis, and exhaustion, should be taken seriously.
- Q: What is the most commonly used diagnostic test to confirm the diagnosis of pertussis?
- A: PCR is now most commonly used because it offers a sensitive and rapid diagnosis. The gold standard for diagnosis is a culture because it has 100% specificity, but culture is not as sensitive as PCR and is laborious.

PHARYNGITIS

Daniel E. Felten, MD, MPD

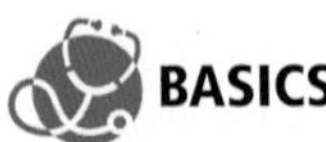

BASICS

DESCRIPTION

Pharyngitis specifically refers to inflammation of the pharynx as indicated by erythema and swelling of the structures in the posterior portion of the oral cavity including the tonsillar pillars, the tonsils, the inferior soft palate, the uvula, and the posterior wall. Pharyngitis is usually caused by viral or bacterial infections.

EPIDEMIOLOGY

- Prevalence and etiology of pharyngitis vary based on age of patient and time of year.
- In preschool-aged children, viral agents are most common and exhibit seasonal variation depending on the specific virus.
- Group A *Streptococcus* (GAS) pharyngitis is most common in children between the ages of 5 and 15 years, is very rare in children age <3 years, and may occur in outbreaks affecting up to 20% of children at risk.
- Pharyngitis caused by *Neisseria gonorrhoeae* occurs primarily in sexually active adolescents.

ETIOLOGY

- Viral
  - Common causes: adenovirus, Epstein-Barr virus (EBV), influenza A and B, enteroviruses (specifically, coxsackievirus A), herpes simplex virus (HSV) (especially in adolescents), and echoviruses
  - Uncommon: measles, rubella, cytomegalovirus, HIV
  - Rhinovirus, coronavirus, parainfluenza virus, and respiratory syncytial virus (RSV) may cause sore throat but not usually pharyngitis.
- Bacterial
  - Common: *Streptococcus pyogenes* (group A β-hemolytic *Streptococcus*)
  - Uncommon: *Mycoplasma pneumoniae*, group C or G streptococci, *N. gonorrhoeae* (more likely in sexually active adolescents), *Arcanobacterium haemolyticum*, *Fusobacterium necrophorum* (Lemierre syndrome), *Corynebacterium diphtheriae* (diphtheria), *Chlamydophila pneumoniae*, *Chlamydophila psittaci*, *Yersinia enterocolitica*, *Treponema pallidum* (syphilis), *Francisella tularensis* (tularemia), oral anaerobes (Vincent angina or trench mouth)
- Fungal: *Candida* species (oral thrush)

GENERAL PREVENTION

- Most infectious agents that cause pharyngitis are spread through contact with respiratory droplets or other body fluids, although many can live for some time outside of the body.
- Careful hand washing and avoiding respiratory secretions are keys to minimizing transmission.
- Return to school/child care
  - Children diagnosed with GAS pharyngitis may return to school the day following initiation of antibiotics.
  - Children with pharyngitis due to presumed viral etiology should be fever-free for 24 hours and have symptoms under control prior to return.

RISK FACTORS

- Children who are immunocompromised and children on chronic inhaled corticosteroids who are otherwise immune competent are at risk for candidiasis of the pharynx.
- Adolescents or sexually abused children engaging in oral sex are at risk for pharyngitis due to gonorrhea or HSV.
- Unvaccinated patients or travelers from certain areas are at risk for vaccine-preventable diseases: diphtheria and measles.

DIAGNOSIS

HISTORY

- Typical: sore throat, fever
- Variable
  - Headache, nausea, vomiting, abdominal pain (suggest GAS pharyngitis)
  - Rhinorrhea, cough, hoarseness, stridor, conjunctivitis (suggest viral etiology)
- Rash: scarlatiniform or nonspecific viral
- Sudden onset of fever and sore throat with difficulty swallowing, headache, stomach pain, nausea, vomiting, or scarlatiniform rash support diagnosis of GAS pharyngitis.
- Pharyngitis associated with rhinorrhea, cough, hoarseness, conjunctivitis, diarrhea, or nonspecific rash is more likely to have a viral cause.
- Significant systemic complaints such as fever and malaise are characteristic of EBV or HIV (acute retroviral syndrome).
- History of oral sex suggests possibility of *N. gonorrhoeae* infection.

PHYSICAL EXAM

- Pharynx and oral cavity
  - Exudative tonsillitis suggestive of GAS but also present in EBV, *N. gonorrhoeae*, *Arcanobacterium*, HSV, adenovirus
  - Palatal petechiae suggest GAS.
  - Ulcers on tonsils or tonsillar pillars seen in coxsackievirus, HSV, echovirus
  - Ulceration or inflammation of buccal mucosa or gums seen in HSV, coxsackievirus
- Lymph nodes
  - Tender anterior lymphadenopathy more common in GAS pharyngitis
  - Diffuse LAD, splenomegaly suggests EBV.
- Rash
  - Scarlatiniform rash (diffuse, erythematous, fine-papular, "sandpapery" rash) key feature of scarlet fever from GAS pharyngitis but can be seen with *A. haemolyticum*, Kawasaki disease, and in some viral illnesses as well
  - Nonspecific, diffuse rash can be associated with viral infection; may be seen shortly after starting antibiotic if underlying etiology is EBV
  - Vesicular lesions on hands, feet, and/or buttocks characteristic of coxsackievirus

DIFFERENTIAL DIAGNOSIS

- Infectious
  - Peritonsillar or retropharyngeal abscess or cellulitis
  - Lemierre syndrome
  - Epiglottitis
  - Kawasaki disease
  - Tularemia
- Ingestions
  - Caustic or irritant ingestions
  - Inhaled irritant
- Tumors
  - Leukemia
  - Lymphoma
  - Rhabdomyosarcoma
- Trauma: vocal abuse from shouting
- Allergy: potnasal drip from allergic rhinitis
- Miscellaneous
  - PFAPA syndrome (periodic fever, aphthous ulcers, pharyngitis, and cervical adenitis)
  - Psychogenic pain (globus hystericus)
  - Vitamin deficiency (A, B complex, C)
  - Dehydration

DIAGNOSTIC TESTS & INTERPRETATION

- Rapid antigen detection test (RADT)
  - Because GAS is the most common bacterial etiology of pharyngitis, most patients who present with sore throat in the absence of symptoms suggesting viral illness should undergo testing for GAS.
  - Use of clinical scoring systems (e.g., Centor) may be helpful in identifying who does not need testing but should not be used to make a diagnosis.
  - RADT is preferred as the initial test for GAS. Sensitivity of RADT varies (55–90%) based on quality of sample obtained. Specificity is more consistent at about 95%.
  - RADT is a good test to rule in GAS, but culture or DNA probe should be used to confirm negative RADTs. Confirmation of positives is not needed.
  - RADT is not recommended when patients present with symptoms that strongly suggest viral etiology (cough, rhinorrhea, hoarseness, oral ulcers).
  - Testing children <3 years old is not indicated, as those children are at very low risk for acute rheumatic fever (ARF). Testing may be considered in this age group if other risk factors are present such as an older sibling with GAS.
  - Testing of asymptomatic household contacts is not recommended.
- Monospot (heterophile antibody) test
  - Detects presence of IgM for EBV, which appears during the first 2 weeks of illness and gradually disappears over 6 months
  - Atypical lymphocytes may also be seen on WBC differential during the 2nd week of EBV infection. >10% atypical lymphocytes plus a positive heterophile antibody test is diagnostic of acute infection.
  - Heterophile antibody is often negative in children <4 years of age with EBV, so it should not be used in this age group.
- Testing for certain bacteria (*N. gonorrhoeae*, *A. haemolyticum*, *F. necrophorum*) requires special handling and processing; confirm appropriate collection medium and alert the laboratory performing the test if any of these agents is suspected.

TREATMENT

GENERAL MEASURES

Treatment is largely supportive for most viral causes of pharyngitis, including pain control and hydration.

MEDICATION

First Line

- Penicillin-resistant GAS has never been documented. Apparent treatment failure (recurrent episode of acute pharyngitis with positive lab tests for GAS) most likely indicates repeat intercurrent viral infection in GAS carrier.
- Oral penicillin V
  - Children: 400,000 U (250 mg) b.i.d. or t.i.d. for 10 days
  - Adolescents/adults: 800,000 U (500 mg) b.i.d. for 10 days or 400,000 U (250 mg) 3 to 4 times per day for 10 days
- Amoxicillin: 50 mg/kg (max dose 1 g) daily divided b.i.d. for 10 days
  - Once-daily dosing may increase adherence.
- IM penicillin G benzathine: ensures compliance, useful in outbreaks
  - Children (>1 month and <27 kg): 600,000 U IM × 1
  - Children (>27 kg) and adults: 1,200,000 U IM × 1
  - Procaine penicillin combinations are less painful.

Second Line

- A 10-day course of a 1st-generation oral cephalosporin is indicated for most penicillin-allergic patients. However, 5–10% of penicillin-allergic patients may also be allergic to cephalosporins, so patients with a type I hypersensitivity to penicillin should not be given a cephalosporin.
- Oral clindamycin 20 mg/kg/24 h (max 1.8 g/24 h) divided t.i.d. may be given to patients with type I hypersensitivity to penicillin.
- Oral azithromycin, clarithromycin, or erythromycin are also acceptable alternatives in penicillin-allergic patients, although cases of ARF have been reported after treatment with these drugs.
  - Azithromycin 12 mg/kg (max 500 mg) daily for 5 days
  - Clarithromycin 15 mg/kg/24 h divided q12h for 10 days or 500 mg extended-release tablets given once a day for 5 days (studied in adolescents ≥12 years of age)
  - Erythromycin ethylsuccinate 40 to 50 mg/kg/24 h in 2 to 4 divided doses. Resistance is rare in the United States (<5% of isolates).
- Tetracyclines and sulfonamides should not be used due to high rates of resistance.
- In patients with *N. gonorrhoeae* infection
  - 250 mg ceftriaxone IM (>45 kg); 125 mg ceftriaxone IM (<45 kg)
  - Coinfection with *Chlamydia trachomatis* is unusual in pharyngitis caused by *N. gonorrhoeae*; however, treatment is recommended: azithromycin 1 g PO in adolescents; in younger children, should confirm infection
- In patients with EBV, antibiotics should not be given; in particular, if amoxicillin or ampicillin is given, a high proportion of patients will develop a nonallergic rash.
- Short-course corticosteroids may be beneficial but can also have significant adverse effects; should only be used in patients with marked tonsillar inflammation and impending airway obstruction. Usual prednisone dose is 1 mg/kg/24 h for 7 days with subsequent tapering.

SURGERY/OTHER PROCEDURES

Tonsillectomy for recurrent pharyngitis is not recommended but may be considered in the rare patient who has frequent symptomatic episodes of pharyngitis in whom no alternative explanation to GAS pharyngitis is found (e.g., recurrent viral infections in a GAS carrier). Benefit is relatively short-lived.

ONGOING CARE

FOLLOW-UP RECOMMENDATIONS

Patient Monitoring

- Most cases of pharyngitis are self-limited; however, patients are at risk for dehydration if PO intake is limited by pain.
- Caregivers should be cautioned to monitor fluid intake and urine output and to return for reassessment if oral intake and/or urine output drops significantly.

COMPLICATIONS

- Streptococcal pharyngitis
  - Suppurative complications include peritonsillar abscess, cervical lymphadenitis, and mastoiditis.
  - Most significant nonsuppurative complication is ARF. This can be prevented if adequate antibiotic treatment is provided within 10 days.
  - Another nonsuppurative complication is poststreptococcal glomerulonephritis.
- Lemierre syndrome:
  - Spread of *F. necrophorum* from peritonsillar abscess caused by GAS to jugular vein causing thrombophlebitis, bacteremia, and thromboembolism
- Pediatric autoimmune neuropsychiatric disorder associated with streptococcal infection (PANDAS): controversial association that has not been demonstrated in prospective studies

ADDITIONAL READING

- Leckman JF, King RA, Gilbert DL, et al. Streptococcal upper respiratory tract infections and exacerbations of tic and obsessive-compulsive symptoms: a prospective longitudinal study. *J Am Acad Child Adolesc Psychiatry*. 2011;50(2):108–118.
- Logan LK, McAuley JB, Shulman ST. Macrolide treatment failure in streptococcal pharyngitis resulting in acute rheumatic fever. *Pediatrics*. 2012;129(3):e798–e802.
- Shulman ST, Bisno AL, Clegg HW, et al. Clinical practice guideline for the diagnosis and management of group A streptococcal pharyngitis: 2012 update by the Infectious Diseases Society of America. *Clin Infect Dis*. 2012;55(10):e86–e102.

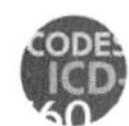

CODES

ICD10

- J02.9 Acute pharyngitis, unspecified
- J02.0 Streptococcal pharyngitis
- B08.5 Enteroviral vesicular pharyngitis

FAQ

- Q: Is there any benefit to starting therapy while waiting for culture results?
- A: Immediate therapy of GAS pharyngitis has been shown to shorten the symptomatic period. However, studies of various clinical criteria have shown that even patients who meet all criteria only have GAS about 50% of the time. Therefore, waiting for culture is appropriate because the goal of treatment is to minimize progression to ARF, and starting treatment within 10 days of onset of symptoms is effective.
- Q: Should all patients with sore throat be swabbed for RADT and/or strep culture?
- A: No. Most cases of sore throat are not due to GAS. However, clinical exam alone is insufficient to diagnose strep throat. Patients with symptoms that highly suggest a viral etiology (rhinorrhea, congestion, cough, conjunctivitis) should not be tested for GAS, as a positive result would most likely indicate carrier status rather than GAS pharyngitis.
- Q: Should contacts of patients with documented GAS pharyngitis be tested for GAS?
- A: Contacts who have recent or current clinical symptoms of GAS infection should undergo appropriate testing. However, carrier rates of contacts are quite high, up to 50% for siblings and 20% for other contacts, so routine testing of asymptomatic contacts is usually not indicated except during outbreaks or when contacts are at increased risk of developing sequelae of infection.

PHIMOSIS AND PARAPHIMOSIS

Kara N. Saperston, MD • Michael DiSandro, MD

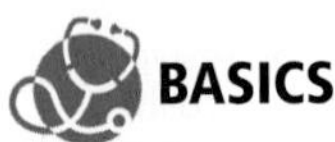

BASICS

DESCRIPTION

- Phimosis is the inability to retract the prepuce (foreskin) after puberty due to a narrow preputial opening.
- Infants and prepubertal children rarely have true phimosis but rather a normal physiologic phimosis.
- Paraphimosis is the entrapment of the prepuce in a retracted position.

EPIDEMIOLOGY

The incidence of phimosis is 0.4 cases per 100 boys per year.

RISK FACTORS

- Phimosis
  - Forced retraction of the prepuce
  - Lichen sclerosis
- Paraphimosis
  - Prolonged retraction of the prepuce

PATHOPHYSIOLOGY

- Phimosis
  - As the constriction of the phimosis worsens, urine is trapped in the foreskin and ballooning of the prepuce occurs. In severe cases, urine will fill the entire preputial space and extend down the shaft.
- Paraphimosis
  - Prolonged retraction of the prepuce around the glans causes edema of the prepuce and the glans. The edema makes it harder to correct the phimosis and causes significant pain for the child.

GENERAL PREVENTION

Boys should be instructed to return the foreskin to covering the glans after cleaning to prevent paraphimosis.

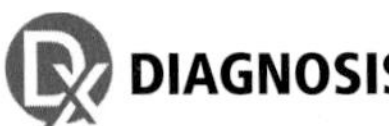

DIAGNOSIS

HISTORY

- Phimosis
  - Parent may report ballooning of the prepuce during voiding.
  - Parent may report having to squeeze the prepuce to clear all the trapped urine.
- Paraphimosis
  - Parent will report cleaning the penis during a diaper change, pulling the foreskin back, and then being unable to return it to its normal position covering the glans.
  - Child may pull the foreskin back and then be unable to return the foreskin to its normal position.

PHYSICAL EXAM

- Phimosis
  - Gentle attempt to retract the foreskin to evaluate the size of the preputial opening
  - A child who cannot retract foreskin after onset of puberty has phimosis.
  - Dry, white patchy areas of the foreskin indicate lichen sclerosis and seen with phimosis 50% of the time.
- Paraphimosis
  - Tender penis with marked edema of the prepuce (foreskin)
  - Tight collar around the glans
  - Long duration of the retracted skin will compromise the blood supply of the prepuce and glans.
  - There are case reports of gangrene.
    - Consider calling child protective services if there is gangrene.

DIAGNOSTIC TESTS & INTERPRETATION

Initial Tests (screening, lab, imaging)

Not needed

Diagnostic Procedures/Other

Not needed

DIFFERENTIAL DIAGNOSIS

Physiologic phimosis

- A child who has not gone through puberty will have a normal physiologic phimosis. This will change as he nears puberty, and the foreskin will be easier to retract over time.
- There may be small lumps of white material under the glans that are desquamated skin cells that are not infection and slowly work their way out of the preputial cavity. This desquamated skin helps with skin separation.

ALERT

Early (before puberty), forced retraction of the foreskin before the foreskin is naturally ready to retract may cause phimosis.

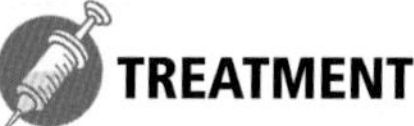

TREATMENT

GENERAL MEASURES

- Phimosis
  - Refer to pediatric urologist if patient fails 2 months of medical management.
- Paraphimosis
  - Refer to pediatric urologist immediately if unable to return the foreskin to covering the glans without sedation.
  - Sedation will most likely be necessary.

MEDICATION

- Phimosis
  - Topical steroids t.i.d. for 6 weeks; use a small bead size amount.
    - Fluticasone propionate, 0.05% (cream)
    - Betamethasone valerate, 0.1% (cream)
    - Triamcinolone cream
  - This also treats lichen sclerosis.
    - Topical tacrolimus is 2nd-line treatment for lichen sclerosis.
- Paraphimosis
  - Should be considered an emergency
  - Sedation and reduction by applying pressure to the glans and prepuce

ADDITIONAL THERAPIES

- Phimosis
  - Circumcision
    - Performed when medical treatment fails
- Paraphimosis
  - Dorsal slit is performed if compression fails.
    - Dorsal incision of the prepuce: under sedation

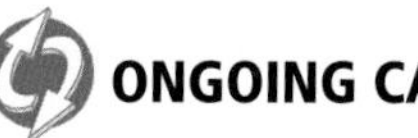

ONGOING CARE

FOLLOW-UP RECOMMENDATIONS

- Phimosis
  - Follow-up in 2 months after use of steroids
- Paraphimosis: if foreskin is back in normal position:
  - Follow up with pediatric urologist in 2 weeks.
  - There should be no retraction of the foreskin in that time frame.
  - Consider use of topical steroids to avoid development of severe phimosis.

PROGNOSIS

- Phimosis
  - Use of steroids is successful 70–90% of the time.
- Paraphimosis
  - High risk of development of severe phimosis
  - May require circumcision in the future

ADDITIONAL READING

- DeVries CR, Miller AK, Packer MG. Reduction of paraphimosis with hyaluronidase. *Urology*. 1996;48(3):464–465.
- Edwards S. 2001 National guideline on the management of balanitis. http://www.pdfdrive.net/2001-national-guideline-on-the-management-of-balanitis-bashh-e7997290.html. Accessed February 15, 2015.
- Gausche M. Genitourinary surgical emergencies. *Pediatr Ann*. 1996;25(8):458–464.
- Moreno G, Corbalán J, Peñaloza B, et al. Topical corticosteroids for treating phimosis in boys. *Cochrane Database Syst Rev*. 2014;(9):CD008973.

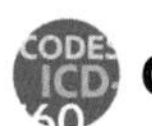

CODES

ICD10

- N47.1 Phimosis
- N47.2 Paraphimosis

FAQ

- Q: Can a child have phimosis as a newborn?
- A: Physiologic phimosis (inability to retract the foreskin) is normal in prepubertal children. It occurs because of incomplete separation of skin between the glans and the inner prepuce. It does not require treatment.

PHOTOSENSITIVITY

Leslie Castelo-Soccio, MD, PhD • Laura E. Kaplan, BA

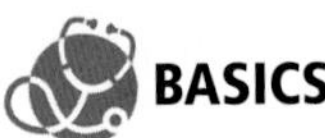

BASICS

DESCRIPTION

Group of disorders where skin reactions are triggered by light. Rare in children, often with different etiologies than adults. Photosensitivities may be classified as:

- Chemical and drug-induced photosensitivity: substances altered by light into toxins
- Genetic disorders: abnormal DNA repair of normal light induced damage, for example, xeroderma pigmentosum
- Photoaggravated dermatoses: skin diseases exacerbated by light, for example, systemic lupus erythematosus (SLE)
- Idiopathic/immunologically mediated photodermatoses: Polymorphous light eruption (PMLE), most common photosensitivity, is thought to have an immunologic basis.
- Photosensitivity resulting from pigment loss: for example, albinism

EPIDEMIOLOGY

- Increased incidence of photosensitivity disorders in some populations, for example, Bloom syndrome in Ashkenazi Jews, actinic prurigo (AP) in American Indians and Hispanics
- Age of onset is variable for each disorder.
- Onset in infancy: congenital erythropoietic porphyria (CEP), neonatal lupus erythematosus
  - Rarely, CEP is discovered when neonates with this disorder are given phototherapy for jaundice and develop severe blistering skin lesions.
- Onset in childhood: albinism, hydroa aestivale, hydroa vacciniforme, certain porphyrias, xeroderma pigmentosum, Hartnup disease, poikiloderma congenitale, Bloom, Rothmund-Thomson, and Cockayne syndromes
- Onset in adults, but can occur in childhood: vitiligo, drug-induced photosensitivities, PMLE, SLE, porphyria cutanea tarda, and pellagra

RISK FACTORS

- Family history
  - Positive in 3–56% of PMLE
- Preexisting skin disease, for example, atopic dermatitis, SLE
- Exposure to plants, drugs, or toxins

Genetics

Genetic disorders include the porphyrias, DNA repair defects, and other biochemical disorders.

- Most genetic disorders are autosomal recessive. The various porphyrias have variable inheritance patterns.

PATHOPHYSIOLOGY

Findings are diverse for the different disorders and rarely diagnostic.

- Photosensitivity may be due to multiple mechanisms.
  - Phototoxicity: Light alters chromophore substances in the skin into a toxic-reactive form. Skin reaction may occur on first exposure.
  - Photoallergy: Light alters substances in the skin to become antigenic. Skin reaction occurs only after multiple exposures.
    - Can be type 1 histamine-mediated and occurs immediately after exposure, for example, solar urticaria (SU)
    - Can be type 4 cellular immune-mediated and occurs hours to days after exposure, for example, PMLE
  - Inability to repair DNA damage, for example, xeroderma pigmentosum
  - Loss of natural ultraviolet (UV) skin protection (melanin), for example, albinism, vitiligo, Hermansky-Pudlak syndrome
- "Hardening"
  - Although light induces the skin abnormalities in photosensitivity, in some instances, repeated light exposure may suppress the skin reaction.
  - This may be due to the immunosuppressive effect of light exposure.
  - Can occur spontaneously. Skin eruption may occur in early spring with first sun exposure but diminish with repeated exposure, for example, juvenile spring eruption (JSE).
  - This phenomenon can be used therapeutically by administering UV light to patients with PMLE and others.

ETIOLOGY

- Combination of sunlight with some abnormality in the skin such as loss of pigment, a chemical agent, a metabolic product, another skin disorder, a genetic disease, or an unknown factor produces a cutaneous abnormality.
- Specific wavelengths of the radiant energy emitted by the sun and reaching the earth are usually responsible for each photosensitivity disorder, most commonly UVB (290 to 320 nm), or UVA (320 to 400 nm). Commercially available sunscreens target these wavelengths. Some disorders, such as the porphyrias, are triggered by visible light (400 to 800 nm), thus are difficult to prevent with sunscreens. β-carotene has been used as a protective agent in some of the porphyrias due to its ability to absorb in the visible light spectrum.

DIAGNOSIS

HISTORY

- Age of onset of rash
- Occurrence
  - Season: spring and summer, for example, JSE
  - Relation to sun exposure: time frame, effect of sun through glass. Ordinary glass blocks most UVB but not UVA.
  - Some children may present with skin pain and sensitivity and develop skin lesions only later, for example, erythropoietic protoporphyria.
- Oral medications
  - May be related to oral contraceptives, tetracyclines (doxycycline in particular), sulfa drugs, iodides/bromides, or phenytoin
- Recent change in perfumes, sunscreens, or moisturizers:
  - Some products contain photoactive chemicals such as citrus oils or musk ambrette.
  - Photosensitivity may occur on neck or places where agents were placed on skin.
- Rash
  - Prior episodes of sun sensitivity or other dermatologic conditions and the distribution
    - Response to previous treatments
- Review of symptoms
  - Chronic abdominal pain can be seen in porphyria, joint pain with SLE (see also "Associated conditions" in the "Physical Exam" section).

PHYSICAL EXAM

This must begin with a complete cutaneous skin exam.

- Distribution of lesions
  - This is the main sign of photosensitivity reactions.
  - Lesions are prominent on sun-exposed skin such as the face, pinnae of the ears, the V of the neck, the nuchal area, and the dorsa of the hands.
    - Malar rash of SLE and heliotropic rash of juvenile dermatomyositis are photodistributed lesions.
  - Often, sparing of the philtrum, the area below the chin, the eyelids, and other covered areas is seen.
  - In phytophotodermatitis, cutaneous exposure to certain plant products followed by light exposure causes dermatitis in a linear or bizarre pattern. For example, if a caregiver has been squeezing limes and has residual citrus oils on his or her hand, then touches a child who is later exposed to sunlight, an erythematous and pigmented hand pattern may occur on the child which can mimic child abuse.
- Lesion characteristics
  - Vary with the particular disease and can include the following:
    - Papules
    - Vesicles: for example, porphyria
    - Plaques: for example, PMLE
    - Sunburn: for example, doxycycline
    - Linear hyperpigmentation: for example, phytophotodermatitis
    - Skin cancers: for example, xeroderma pigmentosum
    - Scarring: for example, hydroa vacciniforme
- Associated conditions
  - Skin conditions, for example, SLE, psoriasis, squamous cell carcinoma, melanoma
  - Cheilitis, for example, AP
  - Hirsutism, for example, porphyrias
  - Neurologic or ophthalmologic conditions, mental disorders, osseous abnormalities may suggest a genetic syndrome.

DIFFERENTIAL DIAGNOSIS

- Chemically induced reactions
  - Topical agents
    - Perfumes containing musk ambrette or citrus oils
    - Plant-associated phytophotodermatitis, for example, lemons, limes, celery, parsnips, carrots, dill, parsley, figs, meadow grass, giant hogweed, mangos, wheat, clover, cocklebur, buttercups, shepherd's purse, and pigweed
    - Blankophors (brighteners in detergents)
    - Sunscreens containing benzophenone, oxybenzone, or butyl methoxydibenzoylmethane (avobenzone)
    - Topical retinoids (e.g., tretinoin, adapalene, tazarotene)
  - Systemic agents
    - Tetracyclines, sulfonamides, nalidixic acid, griseofulvin, phenothiazines, oral hypoglycemic agents, amiodarone, quinine, isoniazid, and thiazide diuretics
- Genetic disorders
  - For example, xeroderma pigmentosum, Rothmund-Thomson, Bloom, and Cockayne syndrome

- Metabolic disorders
  - Porphyrias: disorders of hemoglobin synthesis producing various porphyrins
  - Pellagra: niacin deficiency
- Hartnup disease: autosomal recessive (AR) disorder resulting in a deficiency in tryptophan, a precursor of niacin
- Photoaggravated dermatoses
  - For example, SLE, atopic dermatitis, juvenile dermatomyositis, Darier disease
- Idiopathic/immunologic photosensitivity
  - For example, PMLE, AP, hydroa vacciniforme, JSE, SU
- Photosensitivity resulting from pigment loss
  - For example, albinism, vitiligo, Hermansky-Pudlak syndrome

DIAGNOSTIC TESTS & INTERPRETATION

Phototesting

- Using an artificial source of light can confirm the presence of certain photosensitivities. There are two types of procedures:
  - Phototesting: exposure of skin to increasing doses of UVA and UVB to determine the erythema response (present at lower exposures than usual) and possibly reproduce lesions in certain diseases
  - Photopatch testing: Photoallergic chemicals are applied under patches in duplicate. One set of patches is subsequently to UVA. Patients who have photoallergic contact dermatitis develop a reaction under only the exposed patch.

Initial Tests (screening, lab, imaging)

- Genetic tests: Find labs that perform genetic tests at www.genetests.org and enter disease name:
  - Cell culture: evaluates DNA repair for xeroderma pigmentosum or shows chromosomal breaks in Bloom disease
- Biochemical tests
  - Measurement of specific amino acid and indole excretion patterns in Hartnup disease
  - Helpful for the diagnosis of the porphyrias, with elevated levels of various porphyrins specific to each type in the urine, blood, or stool. Red urine that fluoresces under UV light is another indication.
  - Screening for niacin deficiency
  - Connective tissue disease screening: ANA, anti-Ro, anti-La, skin biopsy, and direct immunofluorescence

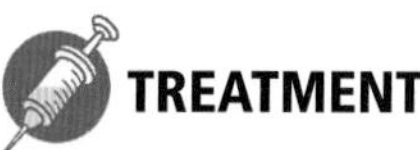

TREATMENT

GENERAL MEASURES

- Protection against sun exposure
  - Avoiding the sun, particularly between 10 a.m. and 3 p.m.
  - Wearing protective clothing is important. Some fabric is not fully sun protective, although specialty clothing with higher UV protection is commercially available.
  - Sunscreens
    - Most effective to those sensitive to UVB; less effective for blocking UVA and therefore less helpful to those patients with sensitivities to longer wavelengths
    - Sunscreens should be water-resistant and reapplied q2h.
    - Sun protection factor (SPF; ratio of minimal erythema dose of sunscreened skin to minimal erythema dose of unprotected skin) >30
  - Sunscreens that contain both UVA- and UVB-blocking capabilities offer better protection than most. These include sunscreens containing avobenzone, titanium dioxide, and zinc oxide.
    - Avobenzone has a relatively short lifespan but is now available in a chemically stabilized form known by the trade names Helioplex® and Active Photobarrier Complex®.
    - Mexoryl is another long-acting broad-spectrum sunscreen that has especially good UVA protection.
  - Opaque formulations such as zinc oxide and titanium dioxide block UV and visible light but may be less cosmetically appealing; however, new formulations made from microfine particles of titanium dioxide or zinc oxide make it more appealing.
  - Patients with severe photosensitivities may have to avoid any significant light exposure. Recall that UVA is not completely filtered by most windows. Window tinting and shades may be helpful.
  - Most patients require chronic protection against sun exposure. However, the problem is generally more acute in spring and summer months.
- Removal of the offending agent is necessary in chemically induced photosensitivities.
  - Any severe and acute eruptions may require a short course of oral prednisone.
- Additional treatment regimens are available for complex or refractory conditions. They require the experience of a specialist. These include:
  - Antimalarials for PMLE, SLE, SU, and porphyria cutanea tarda
  - Immunosuppressives for SU
  - Light therapy including UVB, narrowband (NB)-UVB, psoralen and ultraviolet A (PUVA) for PMLE, SU, AP, hydroa vacciniforme
  - β-Carotene for erythropoietic protoporphyria
  - Calcineurin for atopic dermatitis
  - Thalidomide for AP

ISSUES FOR REFERRAL

If possible, it is important to accurately document the specific wavelength of light and the degree of photosensitivity to accurately advise the patient. This requires phototesting by a specialist. Genetic counseling is appropriate for the genodermatoses. Appropriate referrals to the ophthalmologist and neurologist for treatment of the associated abnormalities in disorders such as albinism and xeroderma pigmentosum are appropriate.

ONGOING CARE

FOLLOW-UP RECOMMENDATIONS

Patient Monitoring

The frequency of skin exams depends on type of photosensitivity; for example, patients with xeroderma pigmentosum need dermatologic exams every 3 to 6 months for prompt detection of malignancy and treatment of premalignant conditions.

PATIENT EDUCATION

Education regarding importance of using proper sunscreen with frequent reapplication, sun protective hats and clothing, and often sunglasses. Patients with severe conditions such as xeroderma pigmentosum may benefit from UV blocking window screens and other measure.

PROGNOSIS

With the exception of chemically induced photosensitivities, most of the conditions are chronic. Hydroa vacciniforme, AP, and JSE may resolve in adulthood.

ADDITIONAL READING

- Chantorn R, Lim HW, Shwayder TA. Photosensitivity disorders in children: part I. *J Am Acad Dermatol*. 2012;67(6):1093.e1–1093.e18.
- Chantorn R, Lim HW, Shwayder TA. Photosensitivity disorders in children: part II. *J Am Acad Dermatol*. 2012;67(6):1113.e1–1113.e15.
- Grossberg AL. Update on pediatric photosensitivity disorders. *Curr Opin Pediatr*. 2013;25(4):474–479.
- Kuhn A, Ruland V, Bonsmann G. Photosensitivity, phototesting, and photoprotection in cutaneous lupus erythematosus. *Lupus*. 2010;19(9):1036–1046.
- Pacha O, Hebert AA. Pediatric photosensitivity disorders. *Dermatol Clin*. 2013;31(2):317–326.
- Ten Berge O, Sigurdsson V, Bruijnzeel-Koomen CA, et al. Photosensitivity testing in children. *J Am Acad Dermatol*. 2010;63(6):1019–1025.
- Yan AC, Castelo-Soccio L. Optimizing sun protection for children: having our day in the sun. *JAMA Pediatr*. 2016;170(4):318–319.

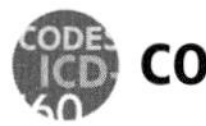

CODES

ICD10

- L56.8 Oth acute skin changes due to ultraviolet radiation
- L59.8 Oth disrd of the skin, subcu related to radiation

FAQ

- Q: What is the best sunscreen to use?
- A: It depends on your particular problem. If you are sensitive to UVB, use a sunscreen with the highest SPF. If you are sensitive to UVA, sunscreens containing avobenzone, titanium dioxide, or zinc oxide are best.
- Q: I have heard that sunscreens with an SPF >15 are not necessary. Is this true?
- A: This is definitely not true for patients with photosensitivities who have abnormal responses to light and require excessive protection. Even for the healthy person, it is often not true. An SPF of 15 suggests that someone may receive 15 times more sun exposure with the sunscreen applied than without and not become sunburned. Some physicians have suggested that this is more than anyone should need. However, this number is calculated by testing in a controlled laboratory. Normal outdoor conditions, such as wind, reflection from water and sand, perspiration, and water exposure can significantly decrease the effectiveness of the sunscreen.
- Q: What is "sun allergy"?
- A: This is a lay term for PMLE, one of the most common photosensitivities, presenting with papules, vesicles, and plaques 1 to 2 days after sun exposure. It usually recurs every spring, and most patients learn to avoid sun exposure. However, ironically, it can improve with slow, gradual sun exposure.
- Q: Can I become allergic to sunscreens?
- A: Certain active agents in sunscreens can produce an allergic response in rare individuals. If the rash recurs with each use, switch to another sunscreen with different ingredients. If the problem continues, consult a specialist for evaluation. Sunscreens can, paradoxically, become sensitizers for photodermatitis in rare instances.

PINWORMS

Terry Kind, MD, MPH • Hope E. Rhodes, MD, MPH, FAAP

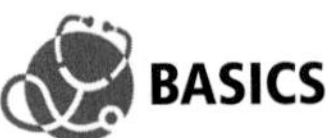

BASICS

DESCRIPTION
- Infection by a small, white nematode (roundworm), typically *Enterobius vermicularis*
- Pinworms may also be caused by *Enterobius gregorii* in Europe, Africa, and Asia.

EPIDEMIOLOGY
- Considered the most common helminthic infection of humans (the only known natural host) and the most common worm infection in the United States
- Occurs predominantly in school-aged children (5 to 10 years) and less commonly in preschool children
- Does occur in adults, usually in those caring for infected children. Some individuals may be predisposed to either heavy or light worm burdens.
- Independent of socioeconomic status

Prevalence
- U.S. infection rates: 5–15%
- Among children, people caring for infected children, and people who are institutionalized, prevalence can reach 50%.
- Occurs worldwide but is more prevalent in temperate climates

GENERAL PREVENTION
- Decontaminate the environment by washing underclothes, bedclothes, bedsheets, and towels.
- Maintain good hand hygiene, including hand washing and proper toileting.
- Keep fingernails short and avoid nail biting.
- Treat family members and close contacts.

PATHOPHYSIOLOGY
- *E. vermicularis* eggs are ingested and hatch in the human's stomach and duodenum. Then the larvae migrate to the ileum and cecum. Adult worms copulate in the cecum.
- The pregnant female pinworm migrates from the cecum to the anus ~5 weeks later and deposits eggs on the perianal skin (at which point the female pinworm usually dies). Thousands of eggs are laid, which may result in hundreds of worms.
- Pruritus is caused by the perianal deposition of eggs and a mucosal mastocytosis response. Other GI symptoms, such as anorexia or abdominal pain, may occur because of the mucosal inflammatory response.
- Granulomas may form if dead worms and eggs invoke an inflammatory response in ectopic locations such as the peritoneal cavity, vulva, cervix, uterus, and fallopian tubes.

ETIOLOGY
- Ingestion of organism via fecal–oral transmission
- Can be spread directly, hand-to-mouth, or via fomites found on toys, bedding, clothing, toilet seats, and baths

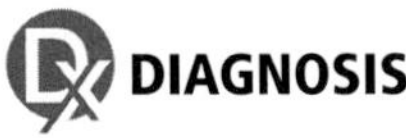

DIAGNOSIS

HISTORY
- Prior pinworms or sibling with pinworms
  - Eggs can survive for several days in the environment, and the incubation period can be 1 to 2 months.
  - Spread can occur between family members.
- Daytime itching
  - Pinworm infections usually cause perianal itching during the night or just before waking in the morning.
  - Daytime perianal or perivulvar itching or irritation is likely due to other causes.
- Fevers, diarrhea, or vomiting
  - Pinworms are highly unlikely to cause systemic symptoms (except in rare cases where they migrate aberrantly).
- Visible worms at night
  - Pinworms may be seen 2 to 3 hours after the child has gone to sleep. Female worms are 8 to 13 mm, and males are 2 to 5 mm.
  - They may be visible as small, white worms in the perianal area at night.

PHYSICAL EXAM
- Exam may be normal, and the child may be well-appearing.
- May have self-inflicted, perianal excoriation
- Pinworms may be visible perianally.
- Infection is characterized by perianal pruritus that occurs at night or just before waking.
- Difficulty sleeping, decreased appetite, and/or abdominal pain may occur.

DIFFERENTIAL DIAGNOSIS
- Infection
  - Other parasites (e.g., *Strongyloides stercoralis*)
  - Nonparasitic vulvovaginitis (due to bacterial, fungal, or viral causes)
- Dermatologic
  - Contact or irritative diaper dermatitis
  - Hidradenitis suppurativa
  - Irritative vulvovaginitis secondary to soaps, bubble baths, or lotions
  - Anal fissures (usually cause pain rather than itching)
- Miscellaneous
  - Behavioral: self-stimulation (normal)
  - Sleep disorders not owing to nocturnal pruritus
  - Hemorrhoids

DIAGNOSTIC TESTS & INTERPRETATION

Initial Tests (screening, lab, imaging)
- Stool or urine samples for ova or parasites
  - Generally not helpful or recommended
  - Very few ova present in stool (even more rare in urine)
- Blood count for eosinophilia
  - Generally not helpful or recommended
  - Eosinophilia is not observed because usually there is no tissue invasion.

Diagnostic Procedures/Other

Transparent tape, Scotch tape test

- In the morning, prior to the child awakening and before defecation or washing, the adhesive side of transparent tape is applied to the perianal area.
- After removal, the tape is applied to a glass slide and examined under light microscopy for pinworm ova.
- Several samples may be necessary to see the pinworms.

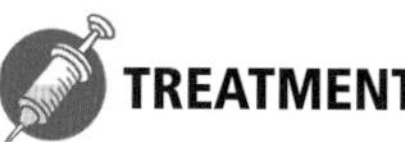

TREATMENT

- Reinfection is common especially if not all close contacts are treated.
- Treat all symptomatic contacts, and consider treating close household contacts, especially if repeated infections have occurred.
- Reinfection can occur if eggs remain on bed linen or clothing.
- Infection may be asymptomatic and transmitted to others.
- Autoreinfection can occur if eggs remain under the nails.

MEDICATION

Single-drug and single-dose therapy with one of the following agents:

- Mebendazole, 100 mg (available as a chewable tablet) PO once, may repeat in 2 weeks if symptoms still present
- Pyrantel pamoate, 11 mg/kg (maximum 1 g) PO once, may repeat in 2 weeks
- Albendazole, 400 mg PO once, may repeat in 2 weeks
- There is limited safety data for the above medications in children <2 years of age. Consider risks and benefits before use.
- Caution in treating pregnant individuals with anthelminthic medications because mebendazole, pyrantel pamoate, and albendazole are all category C and are not recommended in pregnancy.

ONGOING CARE

FOLLOW-UP RECOMMENDATIONS

Patient Monitoring

Watch for signs of reinfection.

PATIENT EDUCATION

- National Library of Medicine's health information site: http://www.nlm.nih.gov/medlineplus/pinworms.html
- Centers for Disease Control and Prevention site: http://www.cdc.gov/healthywater/hygiene/disease/pinworms.html

PROGNOSIS

- Reinfection is common.
- With appropriate treatment, symptoms resolve within a few days.
- Any chronic symptoms are likely due to recurrence rather than chronic infection because the life cycle of the adult worm is short, with eggs being laid by the adult worm within 5 weeks.

COMPLICATIONS

- Intestinal
  - Appendicitis (uncommon)
  - Bacterial superinfection of perianal excoriations
  - Granuloma formation
- Extraintestinal
  - Urethritis
  - Vulvovaginitis
  - Pelvic inflammatory disease

ADDITIONAL READING

- American Academy of Pediatrics. Pinworms infection *(Enterobius vermicularis)*. In: Kimberlin DW, Brady MT, Jackson MA, et al, eds. *Red Book: 2015 Report of the Committee on Infectious Diseases*. 30th ed. Elk Grove Village, IL: American Academy of Pediatrics; 2015.
- Arca MJ, Gates RL, Groner JI, et al. Clinical manifestations of appendiceal pinworms in children: an institutional experience and a review of the literature. *Pediatr Surg Int*. 2004;20(5):372–375.
- Burkhart CN, Burkhart CG. Assessment of frequency, transmission, and genitourinary complications of enterobiasis (pinworms). *Int J Dermatol*. 2005;44(10):837–840.
- Centers for Disease Control and Prevention. Parasites—enterobiasis (also known as pinworm infection). https://www.cdc.gov/parasites/pinworm/health_professionals/index.html. Accessed February 15, 2017.
- Stermer E, Sukhotnic I, Shaoul R. Pruritus ani: an approach to an itching condition. *J Pediatr Gastroenterol Nutr*. 2009;48(5):513–516.

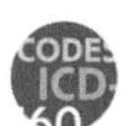

CODES

ICD10

B80 Enterobiasis

FAQ

- Q: Could the child have acquired pinworms from a pet dog or cat?
- A: No. Household pets are not involved in the life cycles of pinworms.
- Q: When can an infected child return to day care?
- A: After receiving the first treatment dose, the child can return to school or day care. It is prudent to bathe the child and to trim and scrub his or her nails prior to school reentry.
- Q: Is it necessary to reevaluate and retest a child once treated?
- A: No. However, reinfection is common.
- Q: Can pinworm eggs survive on bedding, toilet seats, or clothing?
- A: Yes. Eggs can remain infectious in an indoor environment for up to 3 weeks.
- Q: Does pinworm infection cause nocturnal bruxism?
- A: There is no proof of any causal relationship.
- Q: How do the anthelminthic medications work?
- A: They inhibit microtubule function and cause glycogen depletion in the adult worms.

PLAGUE

Amaran Moodley, MD

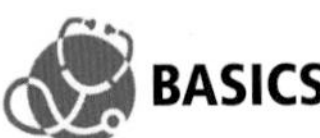

BASICS

DESCRIPTION

Plague is an enzootic disease transmitted by fleas from wild rodents and caused by *Yersinia pestis*. Humans and their pets can enter this cycle, resulting in human plague. Human plague has three main forms:

- Bubonic: 80–85% cases
- Septicemic: 10% cases
- Pneumonic: <5% cases
- Other forms include meningeal, pharyngeal, ocular, and gastrointestinal (GI) plague.

EPIDEMIOLOGY

- Worldwide: enzootic in Africa, Asia, and Americas. Since 2000, 95% of the 22,000 cases reported to the World Health Organization (WHO) have been from countries in sub-Saharan Africa.
- In the United States, most cases occur sporadically or in small clusters in Arizona, New Mexico, California, Colorado, Oregon, and Nevada during spring and summer.
- A median of three cases (range 1 to 17) of plague were reported each year in the United States between 2001 and 2012, with a slight male preponderance.
- No cases of person-to-person transmission of pneumonic plague have been reported in the United States since 1924.

GENERAL PREVENTION

- Reduce rodent shelter and food sources in the immediate vicinity of the home by storing grain and animal food in rodent-proof containers.
- Flea disinfestation of cats and dogs, especially in endemic areas
- Avoid direct contact with ill or dead animals and never feed squirrels, chipmunks, or other wild rodents.
- Hospital isolation precautions:
  - Patients with bubonic or septicemic plague and no evidence of pneumonia: standard precautions; add droplet precautions for first 24 hours of therapy until chest radiograph persistently clear.
  - Patients with pneumonic plague: standard and droplet precautions. Continue droplet precautions until patient has completed 48 hours of appropriate antimicrobial therapy.
- Postexposure management:
  - All persons with exposure to a known or suspected plague source in the previous 6 days should be offered prophylaxis or be told to report illness or fever >38.3° C to their physician.
  - Persons with close (<2 m) contact with a patient with pneumonic plague should receive antimicrobial prophylaxis, but isolation is not necessary.
- Chemoprophylaxis ≥8 years:
  - Doxycycline (PO), *OR*
  - Ciprofloxacin (PO) at treatment doses for 7 days from last exposure
- Chemoprophylaxis <8 years: ciprofloxacin (PO)
- Notify state public health authorities of cases of suspected and proven *Y. pestis* infection.
- A vaccine for plague is no longer available.

PATHOPHYSIOLOGY

- Skin portal of entry
  - *Y. pestis* is transmitted most commonly to humans from fleas via the regurgitation of the organism into the bite during the flea's blood meal (*Y. pestis* blocks the flea foregut, causing regurgitation).
  - Ground squirrels, rats, chipmunks, prairie dogs, deer mice, marmots, rabbits, and occasionally domestic dogs and cats harbor infected fleas and may be reservoirs of infection (enzootic).
  - Direct skin inoculation of organisms from infected animal tissue or blood occurs through breaks in the skin (e.g., cat scratch or during skinning of animals).
  - Lymphatic spread of infection to the regional lymph nodes creates a localized inflammatory response (bubo, bubonic).
  - Subsequent hematogenous spread of the organism to other organs results in high levels of circulating bacterial endotoxin (septicemic plague).
  - By hematogenous spread to lungs, both bubonic and septicemic plague can cause secondary pneumonic plague.
- Respiratory portal of entry
  - Primary pneumonic plague is acquired via inhalation of respiratory tract droplets from a human or animal (e.g., dog or cat) with pneumonic plague.
- Incubation period
  - 2 to 8 days for bubonic or septicemic plague
  - 1 to 6 days for pneumonic plague

ETIOLOGY

Plague is caused by *Y. pestis*, a pleomorphic, bipolar-staining, gram-negative coccobacillus.

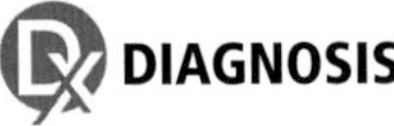

DIAGNOSIS

The diagnosis of plague requires a high index of suspicion and a thorough review of the patient's lifestyle, travel history, and recent activities.

HISTORY

- A thorough travel history (especially to enzootic areas) is imperative to raise the index of suspicion for diagnosing plague.
- Environmental history should include epizootic deaths (die-offs) of rodents, ground squirrels, or prairie dogs in the patient's locale.
- In enzootic areas, a sick household cat or dog is an additional risk factor.
- Plague is characterized by the sudden onset of fever, chills, headache, and malaise accompanied by nausea, vomiting, and abdominal pain.
- Bubonic plague:
  - Initial symptom: pain in the groin or axillae prior to lymph node swelling
  - Lymphadenitis (usually inguinal > axillary > cervical)
  - Fever, chills, prostration
- Septicemic plague:
  - Tachycardia and hypotension without localizing signs or symptoms
  - Abdominal pain, nausea, vomiting, diarrhea
  - Hemorrhage
  - Fever, chills, prostration
- Pneumonic plague:
  - Cough, dyspnea, pleuritic type chest pain, and hemoptysis
  - Systemic manifestations
    - Fever, chills, shock
    - Rapidly progressive and often fatal

PHYSICAL EXAM

- Tachycardic, hypotensive, tachypneic, and toxic-appearing
- Skin lesions at the site of the flea bite are usually not noticeable; however, occasionally eschars, pustules, papules, vesicles, or necrotic lesions may be seen.
- Buboes (swollen lymph nodes) are mostly unilateral, painful, nonfluctuating, and often associated with erythema and edema of overlying skin.
- Flea bite lymphadenitis classically affects inguinal nodes; cat-associated plague affects mostly axillary, cervical, or epitrochlear nodes.
- GI: Abdominal pain, nausea, and diarrhea are common, secondary to inflammatory mediators.
- Neurologic: weakness, delirium, and coma, owing to the effects of the endotoxin of *Y. pestis*
- Heme: disseminated intravascular coagulation with purpura
- Renal: glomerular parenchymal damage
- Rare: meningitis, endophthalmitis, endocarditis, and pleuritis

DIFFERENTIAL DIAGNOSIS

The presence of septicemia and endotoxin-mediated shock includes a large differential diagnosis that includes sepsis owing to other bacteria or viruses as well as distributive shock resulting from toxic ingestion or anaphylaxis.

- Infection
  - Streptococcal and staphylococcal infections (especially between the toes) can result in tender inguinal lymph nodes, fever, shock.
  - Cat-scratch fever (*Bartonella henselae*) can present with a history of cat scratch or bite, regional lymphadenitis, and fever.
  - *Hantavirus* in humans has a clinical presentation similar to septicemic and pneumonic plague and occurs in many of the plague-enzootic areas.
  - Rickettsial diseases: *Rickettsia*, *Orientia*, *Coxiella*, *Ehrlichia*, *Anaplasma* (e.g., Rocky Mountain spotted fever [*Rickettsia rickettsii*] and relapsing tick fever due to *Borrelia* sp. may mimic septicemic or pneumonic plague)
  - Purpura and peripheral gangrene can be confused with meningococcemia.
  - Recent reports of plague-like illnesses have been associated with infections by other organisms such as *Burkholderia pseudomallei* (melioidosis) and *Francisella tularensis* (tularemia).

ALERT

Pitfalls in diagnosis

- Patients who present with a nonspecific febrile illness, tachycardia, and tachypnea, rather than lymphadenitis, are at higher risk for delayed diagnosis and serious sequelae (e.g., septicemic plague, death).
- Failure to consider septicemic plague in the appropriate epidemiologic setting and withholding appropriate antibiotics or using an empiric β-lactam regimen
- Failure to treat suspected bubonic plague with antibiotics while awaiting culture results when needle aspiration of the bubo shows no organisms on direct stain

DIAGNOSTIC TESTS & INTERPRETATION

Initial Tests (screening, lab, imaging)

- Hematology:
  - WBC count usually 10,000 to 20,000/mm^3 but may be as high as 100,000/mm^3, with immature neutrophils
  - Disseminated intravascular coagulopathy and thrombocytopenia may be found.
- Perform Gram, Wayson, Wright-Giemsa, or fluorescent antibody staining on specimens (blood, bubo, CSF, sputum) to look for gram-negative, bipolar-staining organisms.
- *Y. pestis* culture (notify receiving lab)
  - Suspect bubonic plague: needle aspiration of the bubo for stain and culture. Puncture center of bubo with a sterile syringe and inject 1 mL of nonbacteriostatic, sterile saline. Withdraw aspirate vigorously until blood-tinged liquid appears in syringe.
  - Suspect pneumonic plague: sputum for stain and culture
  - Blood cultures are usually positive, even with bubonic plague, and should always be done prior to therapy.
  - Slow grower; may be misidentified as *Yersinia pseudotuberculosis, Pseudomonas luteola*, or *Acinetobacter* sp. by automated bacterial identification systems
- Serology
  - Single positive acute serology *OR*
  - At least a 4-fold increase in antibody titers by passive hemagglutination test between acute and convalescent sera obtained at least 2 weeks apart
- Polymerase chain reaction assay for rapid diagnosis may be available in reference or public health labs.
- Chest radiographs are nonspecific and may reveal consolidation, pleural effusion, cavitation, hilar or mediastinal adenopathy.
- State health departments should be notified immediately when *Y. pestis* is suspected.

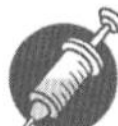

TREATMENT

GENERAL MEASURES

For septic patients in shock, initial attention should be given to airway management and fluid resuscitation, then antibiotics.

MEDICATION

- Immediate antibiotic treatment, even before laboratory confirmation, greatly improves outcomes.
- For children, gentamicin or streptomycin administered intramuscularly or intravenously are equally effective.
- Gentamicin (IV): pediatric dose: 2.5 mg/kg/dose q8h; adult dose: 5 mg/kg/dose q24h
- Streptomycin traditionally has been the drug of choice (IV/IM): peds: 20 to 30 mg/kg/24 h divided q12h; adult: 15 mg/kg/dose q12h to max 1 g q12h
- Meningitis or severe disease: Consider adding chloramphenicol or levofloxacin.
- Alternatives include doxycycline, tetracycline, chloramphenicol, and trimethoprim-sulfamethoxazole; however, the latter has been associated with higher risk of treatment failure.
- Continue antibiotic therapy for 7 to 10 days or until several days after lysis of fever.
- Severely ill patients may require a substantially longer course of therapy.
- Foci (e.g., abscess) are infectious until sufficient appropriate antimicrobial therapy is given.

ONGOING CARE

FOLLOW-UP RECOMMENDATIONS

Resolution of symptoms should begin in the first 3 days after initiation of therapy; however, the rate of clinical improvement depends on the initial severity of illness.

PROGNOSIS

- Untreated plague will often progress to overwhelming sepsis with renal failure, acute respiratory distress syndrome, hemodynamic instability, diffuse intravascular coagulopathy, necrosis of distal extremities, and death.
- In the antibiotic era, mortality has been reduced to approximately 16%.
- Relapse after completion of therapy is rare.

COMPLICATIONS

- Hematologic (disseminated intravascular coagulation)
- Renal (glomerular and parenchymal damage)
- Meningitis is a late complication and is more common in children.
- Untreated bubonic plague: >50% fatal
- Untreated pneumonic plague: nearly 100% fatal

ADDITIONAL READING

- Butler T. Plague into the 21st century. *Clin Infect Dis*. 2009;49(5):736–742.
- Gage KL, Dennis DT, Orloski KA, et al. Cases of cat-associated human plague in the western US, 1977–1998. *Clin Infect Dis*. 2000;30(6):893–900.
- Koirala J. Plague: disease, management, and recognition of act of terrorism. *Infect Dis Clin North Am*. 2006;20(2):273–287.
- Kugeler KJ, Staples JE, Hinckley AF, et al. Epidemiology of human plague in the United States, 1900–2012. *Emerg Infect Dis*. 2015;21(1):16–22.
- Raoult D, Mouffok N, Bitam I, et al. Plague: history and contemporary analysis. *J Infect*. 2013;66(1):18–26.
- Rubini M, Gualdi-Russo E, Manzon VS, et al. Mortality risk factors show similar trends in modern and historic populations exposed to plague. *J Infect Dev Ctries*. 2016;10(5):488–493.
- Runfola JK, House J, Miller L, et al. Outbreak of human pneumonic plague with dog-to-human and possible human-to-human transmission—Colorado, June–July 2014. *MMWR Morb Mortal Wkly Rep*. 2015;64(16):429–434.

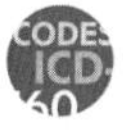

CODES

ICD10

- A20.9 Plague, unspecified
- A20.0 Bubonic plague
- A20.7 Septicemic plague

FAQ

- Q: Can one determine the risks of being exposed to plague during international travel?
- A: Yes. The Centers for Disease Control and Prevention (CDC) provides a service that contains updated information for international travel exposures at www.cdc.gov/travel.
- Q: What are the community risk factors for plague?
- A: Although the mortality rate for plague has decreased with the advent of antibiotic therapy, the community-level risk factors are unchanged. Areas and communities at risk for plague include those communities with poor environmental hygiene, communities with populations that are undernourished, and communities with a weak public health infrastructure and system.
- Q: Does persistent fever during treatment for plague warrant altering the antibiotic regimen?
- A: No. Fever can persist for up to 2 weeks despite appropriate 1st-line antibiotic therapy for *Y. pestis*. However, an evaluation for a focus of infection requiring drainage is recommended under these circumstances.
- Q: What is a bubo?
- A: "Bubo" (plural: buboes) comes from the Greek word for groin. A bubo is a painful, swollen lymph node.

PLEURAL EFFUSION

Richard M. Kravitz, MD

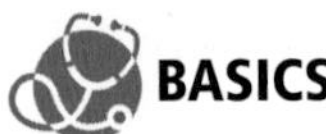

BASICS

DESCRIPTION
Accumulation of fluid in the pleural cavity

PATHOPHYSIOLOGY
- Normally 1 to 15 mL of fluid in the pleural space
- Alterations in the flow and/or absorption of this fluid lead to its accumulation.
- Mechanisms that influence this flow of fluid:
  - Increased capillary hydrostatic pressure (i.e., congestive heart failure [CHF], overhydration)
  - Decreased pleural space hydrostatic pressure (i.e., after thoracentesis, atelectasis)
  - Decreased plasma oncotic pressure (i.e., hypoalbuminemia, nephrosis)
  - Increased capillary permeability (i.e., infection, toxins, connective tissue diseases, malignancy)
  - Impaired lymphatic drainage from the pleural space (i.e., disruption of the thoracic duct)
  - Passage of fluid from the peritoneal cavity through the diaphragm to the pleural space (i.e., hepatic cirrhosis with ascites)
- Two types of pleural effusion:
  - Transudate: Mechanical forces of hydrostatic and oncotic pressures are altered, favoring liquid filtration.
  - Exudate: Damage to the pleural surface occurs that alters its ability to filter pleural fluid; lymphatic drainage is diminished.
- Stages associated with parapneumonic effusions (infectious exudates):
  - See "Appendix, Table 3."
  - Exudative stage
    - Free-flowing fluid
    - Pleural fluid glucose, protein, lactate dehydrogenase (LDH) level, and pH are normal.
  - Fibrinolytic stage
    - Loculations are forming.
    - Increase in fibrin, polymorphonuclear leukocytes, and bacterial invasion of pleural cavity are occurring.
    - Pleural fluid glucose and pH falls, whereas protein and LDH levels increase.
  - Organizing stage (empyema)
    - Fibroblasts grow.
    - Pleural peal forms.
    - Pleural fluid parameters worsen.

DIAGNOSIS

HISTORY
- Underlying disease determines most systemic symptoms.
- Patient may be asymptomatic until the amount of fluid is large enough to cause cardiorespiratory compromise/distress.
- Dyspnea and cough are associated with large effusions.
- Fever (if infectious etiology)
- Pleuritic pain (pneumonia may cause irritation of the parietal pleura, causing pleural pain; as the effusion increases and separates the pleural membrane, the pain may disappear)

PHYSICAL EXAM
- Decreased thoracic wall excursion on the ipsilateral side
- Fullness of intercostal spaces on the ipsilateral side
- Trachea and cardiac apex displaced toward the contralateral side (may produce a mediastinal shift that can reduce venous return and compromise the cardiac output)
- Dull or flat percussion on the ipsilateral side (suggesting the presence of consolidation of pleural effusion)
- Decreased tactile and vocal fremitus
- Decreased whispering pectoriloquy
- Pleural rub during early phase (may resolve as fluid accumulates in the pleural space)
- Decreased breath sounds

DIFFERENTIAL DIAGNOSIS
- Transudate
  - Cardiovascular
    - CHF
    - Constrictive pericarditis
  - Nephrotic syndrome with hypoalbuminemia
  - Cirrhosis
  - Atelectasis
- Exudate
  - Infection
    - *Staphylococcus aureus* (increasing incidence of methicillin-resistant species)
    - *Streptococcus pneumoniae* (increasing incidence of penicillin-resistant species)
    - *Haemophilus influenzae* (decreasing incidence since introduction of *H. influenzae* type b [Hib] vaccine)
    - Group A *Streptococcus*
    - Anaerobes
    - Gram-negative enterics
    - No identified organisms (all cultures sterile)
    - Tuberculous effusion
    - Viral effusions (adenovirus, influenza)
    - Fungal effusions: most not associated with effusions; *Nocardia* and *Actinomyces* are most commonly seen.
    - Parasitic effusions
  - Neoplasm: seen mostly in leukemia and lymphoma; uncommon in children
  - Connective tissue disease
    - Rheumatoid arthritis
    - Systemic lupus erythematosus
    - Wegener granulomatosis
  - Pulmonary embolus
  - Intra-abdominal disease
    - Subdiaphragmatic abscess
    - Pancreatitis
  - Sarcoidosis
  - Esophageal rupture
  - Hemothorax
  - Chylothorax
  - Drugs
  - Chemical injury
  - Postirradiation effusion

DIAGNOSTIC TESTS & INTERPRETATION
- Cytologic exam of pleural fluid
  - Fresh and heparinized specimen should be refrigerated at 4°C (39.2°F) until it can be processed.
  - Fixatives should not be added.
- Pleural fluid parameters to be routinely measured include the following (Appendix, Table 4):
  - pH
  - LDH
  - Protein
  - Glucose
    - Note: Glucose of <40 mg/dL suggests a parapneumonic, tuberculosis, malignant, or rheumatic etiology to the effusion.

Initial Tests (screening, lab, imaging)
Serology values to follow the degree of inflammation and the response to therapy:
- Erythrocyte sedimentation rate (ESR)
- C-reactive protein (CRP)
- Chest radiograph
  - Anteroposterior projection can show >400 mL of pleural fluid.
  - Lateral projection can show <200 mL of pleural fluid.
  - Lateral decubitus film to evaluate for free-flowing pleural fluid can show as little as 50 mL of pleural fluid.
- Ultrasound
  - Reveals small (3 to 5 mL) loculated collections of pleural fluid
  - Useful as a guide for thoracentesis
  - Aids in distinguishing between pleural thickening and pleural effusion
- CT scan
  - Clearly reveals effusions/empyemas, abscess, or pulmonary consolidations
  - Useful for defining the extent of loculated effusions

Diagnostic Procedures/Other
- Thoracentesis
  - Indicated whenever etiology is unclear or if the effusion causes symptoms (e.g., prolonged fever or respiratory distress)
- Pleural biopsy
  - If thoracentesis is nondiagnostic
  - Most useful for diseases that cause extensive involvement of the pleura (i.e., tuberculosis, malignancies)
  - Confirms neoplastic involvement in 40–70% of cases

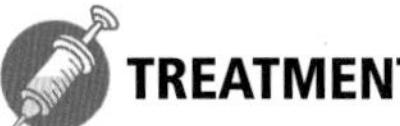

TREATMENT

GENERAL MEASURES

- Supportive measures:
  - Maintain adequate
    - Oxygenation
    - Fluid status
    - Nutritional balance
  - Antipyretic agents when febrile
  - Pain control
- Treat the underlying disease:
  - Antibiotics for infections
  - Cardiac medications for CHF
  - Chemotherapeutic agents for malignancies
  - Anti-inflammatory agents (i.e., steroids) for connective tissue diseases
  - Medium-chain triglycerides and low-fat diet for chylothorax
- Effective drainage of pleural fluid
  - Thoracentesis
  - Chest tube drainage
  - Surgical drainage
- Duration of chest tube drainage
  - Discontinue when patient is asymptomatic (afebrile, no distress) and drainage <50 mL/h.
  - Thick, loculated empyema requires prolonged drainage (and possibly a video-assisted thoracic surgery [VATS] procedure if effusion not improving).

MEDICATION

- Antibiotics
  - Used when effusion is caused by a bacterial infection
  - Specific antibiotics dictated by organism identified
  - If effusion is sterile, broad-spectrum antibiotics are indicated to cover for the usually seen organisms.
  - Clinical improvement usually begins within 48 to 72 hours of therapy.
  - Continue IV antibiotics until afebrile.
  - Complete remainder of therapy on oral antibiotics.
- Duration of antibiotic therapy depends on the infectious organism and the degree of illness:
  - Total duration is controversial.
  - Usually, at least 2 to 4 weeks of total IV and PO

COMPLEMENTARY & ALTERNATIVE THERAPIES

- Thoracentesis
  - For diagnosis purposes
    - To distinguish between a transudate and an exudate
    - For culture material (if infection is suspected)
    - For cytology (if malignancy is suspected)
  - For relief of dyspnea or cardiorespiratory distress
- Chest tube thoracostomy
  - Reduce reaccumulation of fluid.
  - Drain parapneumonic effusion (before loculations develop which will prevent fluid drainage).
- Intrapleural fibrinolytics
  - Adjunct to aid in drainage of complicated (i.e., multiloculated empyema) pleural effusions
  - Streptokinase, urokinase, and tPA are the agents of choice.

SURGERY/OTHER PROCEDURES

- VATS
  - Alternative to more invasive procedures (e.g., open thoracotomy/decortication)
  - Debridement through pleural visualization and lysis of adhesions/loculations
  - Useful when
    - Initial drainage is delayed.
    - Loculations prevent adequate drainage by chest tube alone.
    - Patient is failing more conservative therapy.
- Pleurectomy
  - Chylothorax
  - Malignant effusions
- Pleurodesis
  - For recurrent effusions
  - Chemical agents frequently used include talc, tetracycline, doxycycline, and quinacrine.
  - Surgical methods include the following:
    - Mechanical abrasion
    - Pleurectomy via VATS
    - Open thoracotomy route
  - In cases of malignant effusion:
    - Sclerosing procedures are usually ineffective.
    - Chest tube drainage can create a pneumothorax because the lung is incarcerated by the tumor.

ONGOING CARE

FOLLOW-UP RECOMMENDATIONS

- Clinical improvement usually within 1 to 2 weeks
- With empyemas, the patient may have fever spikes for up to 2 to 3 weeks after improvement is noted.

DIET

When the effusion is a chylothorax:

- Medium-chain triglycerides
- Nutritional replacement
- At least 4 to 5 weeks on this regimen

PROGNOSIS

Depends on underlying disease process:

- Properly treated infectious cause: excellent prognosis
- Malignancy: poor prognosis

COMPLICATIONS

- Hypoxia
- Respiratory distress
- Persistent fevers
- Decreased cardiac function
- Malnutrition (seen in chylothorax)
- Shock (secondary to blood loss in cases of hemothorax)
- Trapped lung

ADDITIONAL READING

- Beers SL, Abramo TJ. Pleural effusions. *Pediatr Emerg Care*. 2007;23(5):330–334.
- Buckingham SC, King MD, Miller ML. Incidence and etiologies of complicated parapneumonic effusions in children, 1996 to 2001. *Pediatr Infect Dis J*. 2003;22(6):499–504.
- Calder A, Owens CM. Imaging of parapneumonic pleural effusions and empyema in children. *Pediatr Radiol*. 2009;39(6):527–537.
- Doski JJ, Lou D, Hicks BA, et al. Management of parapneumonic collections in infants and children. *J Pediatr Surg*. 2000;35(2):265–268.
- Heffner JE. Discriminating between transudates and exudates. *Clin Chest Med*. 2006;27(2):241–252.
- Krenke K, Peradzyńska J, Lange J, et al. Local treatment of empyema in children: a systematic review of randomized controlled trials. *Acta Paediatr*. 2010;99(10):1449–1453.
- Merino JM, Carpintero I, Alvarez T, et al. Tuberculous pleural effusion in children. *Chest*. 1999;115(1):26–30.
- Proesmans M, De Boeck K. Clinical practice: treatment of childhood empyema. *Eur J Pediatr*. 2009;168(6):639–645.
- Rocha G. Pleural effusions in the neonate. *Curr Opin Pulm Med*. 2007;13(4):305–311.

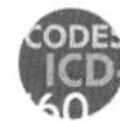

CODES

ICD10

- J90 Pleural effusion, not elsewhere classified
- J86.9 Pyothorax without fistula
- J91.0 Malignant pleural effusion

FAQ

- Q: When will the chest radiograph findings become normal?
- A: They may take up to 6 months (or longer) to return to normal appearance.
- Q: When will the pulmonary function tests normalize?
- A: Depending on extent of effusion, they may take up to 6 to 12 months.

PNEUMOCYSTIS JIROVECI (PREVIOUSLY KNOWN AS *PNEUMOCYSTIS CARINII* PNEUMONIA)

Danna Tauber, MD, MPH

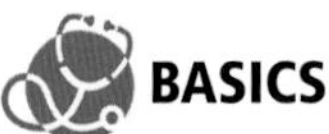

BASICS

DESCRIPTION

Opportunistic lung infection caused by *Pneumocystis jiroveci*. This organism is currently considered a primitive fungus based on DNA sequence analysis. It has two developmental forms (the cysts contain sporozoites that become trophozoites when excised).

- Although previously known as *Pneumocystis carinii* pneumonia (PCP), the acronym PCP is still in use and refers to *Pneumocystis* pneumonia.
- PCP occurs almost exclusively in the immunocompromised host.
- PCP is an AIDS-defining illness. It is the most common opportunistic life-threatening lung infection in infants with perinatally acquired HIV disease.
- *P. jiroveci* causes a diffuse pneumonitis characterized by fever, dyspnea at rest, tachypnea, hypoxemia, nonproductive cough, and bilateral diffuse infiltrates in the roentgenogram. It is a severe condition frequently leading to respiratory failure, necessitating intubation and mechanical ventilation.
- Chemoprophylaxis against this microorganism has proven successful. Therefore, early identification of the HIV-infected mother becomes essential.
- Despite advances in therapy, the infection continues to be associated with significant morbidity and mortality.

EPIDEMIOLOGY

- Ubiquitous in mammals worldwide, particularly rodents
- Growth on respiratory tract surfaces
- Mode of transmission is unknown:
  - Airborne person-to-person transmission is possible, but case contacts are rarely identified.
  - Environmentally acquired
- Asymptomatic infection appears early in life; >70% of healthy individuals have antibodies by age 4 years.
- Primary infection is likely to be the mechanism in infants. Reactivation of latent disease with immunosuppression was proposed as an explanation for disease later in childhood; however, animal models of PCP do not support this proposition.
- PCP in the HIV patient can occur at any time but usually presents during the 1st year of life. The highest incidence is between 3 and 6 months of age.

RISK FACTORS

Immunocompromised host

- Children with congenital or acquired AIDS and recipients of suppressive therapy in the treatment of malignancies or after organ transplantation are at high risk.
- In leukemic patients, the incidence of PCP has been directly related to the degree of immunodeficiency resulting from chemotherapy.
- Epidemics of PCP were reported in premature and malnourished infants and children in resource-limited countries and during times of famine.

GENERAL PREVENTION

- Chemoprophylaxis indications: During high-risk periods, PCP can be effectively prevented in the immunodeficient host by chemoprophylaxis in the following groups:
  - HIV exposed: 4 to 6 weeks to 4 months
  - HIV infected or indeterminate: 4 to 12 months
  - HIV infected: 1 to 5 years if $CD4^+$ T-lymphocyte count is <500 cells/μL or <15%
  - HIV infected: ≥6 years if $CD4^+$ T-lymphocyte count is <200 cells/μL or <15%
  - Severely symptomatic HIV patients or those with rapidly declining CD4 counts
  - HIV patients who have had previous PCP illness
  - Children who have received hematopoietic stem cell transplants (HSCTs)
  - All HSCT recipients with hematologic malignancies (e.g., leukemia, lymphoma)
  - All HSCT recipients receiving intense conditioning regimens or graft manipulation
    - Prophylaxis is initiated at engraftment and administered for 6 months; longer than 6 months in children receiving immunosuppressive therapy or with chronic graft-versus-host disease
- Drug regimen for prophylaxis
  - Trimethoprim-sulfamethoxazole (TMP-SMX) is the drug of choice.
    - 150 mg/m^2 body surface area per day of TMP or 750 mg/m^2 body surface area per day of SMX PO divided into 2 doses on 3 consecutive days per week
    - TMP-SMX can also be given 7 days a week when prevention against other bacterial infections is sought.
  - For patients who cannot tolerate TMP-SMX
    - Dapsone (>1 month of age): 2 mg/kg (maximum 100 mg) PO daily or 4 mg/kg (maximum 200 mg) PO weekly
    - Aerosolized pentamidine (>5 years of age): 300 mg via Respirgard II nebulizer inhaled monthly
    - Atovaquone at age 1 to 3 months and >24 months: 30 mg/kg (maximum 1,500 mg/dose) PO daily; at age 4 to 24 months: 45 mg/kg (maximum 1,500 mg/dose) PO daily

PATHOPHYSIOLOGY

- In the immunodeficient child, the pathologic changes occur predominantly in the alveoli. Cysts and trophozoites are seen adhering to the alveolar lining cells or in the cytoplasm of macrophages.
- As infection progresses, the alveolar spaces are filled with a pink, foamy exudate containing fibrin, abundant desquamative cells, and a large number of organisms. Alveolar septal thickening with mononuclear cell infiltration is also seen.

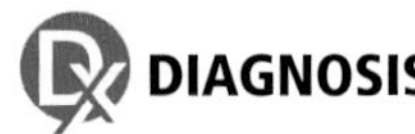

DIAGNOSIS

HISTORY

- In malnourished host
  - Subacute onset with nonspecific manifestations
    - Poor feeding, weight loss, and restlessness
    - Chronic diarrhea
    - Usually without fever
    - After 1 to 2 weeks, the patient develops progressive tachypnea, respiratory distress, and cough.
- In sporadic or immunocompromised host
  - This form has a more abrupt onset, sometimes even fulminant:
    - Fever (>38.5°C)
    - Nonproductive cough
    - Dyspnea at rest
- These subtypes are characterized by general clinical guidelines. Symptoms may be superimposed and can be seen in infants, children, and adolescents.

PHYSICAL EXAM

- Fever and significant tachypnea are characteristic.
- Hypoxemia: early in the course of disease and disproportionate to the auscultatory findings
- Rapidly progressive respiratory distress with cyanosis: respiratory failure early in course
- Absence of crackles is a common initial finding.
- Chest auscultation can reveal decreased breath sounds, crackles, and rhonchi.
- Coryza and wheezing have infrequently been reported.

DIFFERENTIAL DIAGNOSIS

- Viral infections
  - Common viral respiratory pathogens
  - Cytomegalovirus
  - Epstein-Barr virus
- Bacterial infections
  - *Mycobacterium tuberculosis*
  - *Mycobacterium avium-intracellulare*
- Other
  - Lymphocytic interstitial pneumonitis

DIAGNOSTIC TESTS & INTERPRETATION

- Arterial blood gas
  - pH is usually increased.
  - Reduced Pa_{O_2} in room air (<70 mm Hg)
  - Alveolar–arterial oxygen gradient (>35 mm Hg)
- Chest radiograph
  - Most common radiologic presentation is diffuse bilateral alveolar infiltrates:
    - Initially a perihilar distribution that spreads to the periphery
    - Apices are the least affected.
    - Interstitial infiltrates and air bronchograms can be seen.
    - Rapid progression to whole lung consolidation
- Presence of hilar or mediastinal adenopathy may indicate another process such as *M. tuberculosis*, *M. avium-intracellulare*, fungal infections, cytomegalovirus, or lymphoma.
- Other tests
  - Lactate dehydrogenase (LDH) can be elevated in patients with AIDS and PCP, but this finding is nonspecific.
  - White blood cell (WBC) count is usually normal.
- Pathologic findings
  - Definitive diagnosis can be obtained by demonstration of *P. jiroveci* in pulmonary specimens:
    - Induced sputum
    - Bronchoalveolar lavage (BAL) usually through flexible bronchoscopy (90% sensitivity)
    - Open lung or transbronchial biopsy
  - Staining
    - Cysts stain with methenamine-silver, toluidine blue-O stains, calcofluor white, and fluorescein monoclonal antibody
    - Sporozoites and trophozoites are identified with Giemsa stain, modified Wright-Giemsa stain, and fluorescein-conjugated monoclonal antibody stain.
    - Polymerase chain reaction assays of BAL fluid or induced sputum is available and more sensitive for detecting *P. jiroveci* than microscopic methods but is not approved for diagnosis by the U.S. Food and Drug Administration (FDA).

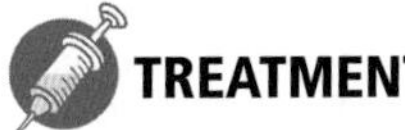

TREATMENT

GENERAL MEASURES

- Supply oxygen as necessary to keep Pa_{O_2} >70 mm Hg.
- Mechanical ventilation must be considered if Pa_{O_2} is <60 mm Hg on FiO_2 of 0.5.

MEDICATION

First Line

- Minimum duration of therapy is 2 weeks; 3 weeks of therapy recommended in patients with AIDS
- Antibiotics
  - TMP-SMX is the drug of choice:
    - TMP (15 to 20 mg/kg/24 h) and SMX (75 to 100 mg/kg/24 h) IV/PO divided q6h
    - Oral therapy is reserved for patients with mild illness who do not have malabsorption or diarrhea.

Second Line

- Minimum duration of therapy is 2 weeks; 3 weeks of therapy recommended in patients with AIDS
- Pentamidine isethionate
  - 3 to 4 mg/kg/dose IV (or intramuscular) given in a single daily dose
  - Used in patients who cannot tolerate TMP-SMX or are unresponsive after 5 to 7 days of therapy
  - If clinical improvement is seen after 7 to 10 days of IV pentamidine, consider oral regimen to complete the 21-day course.
- Atovaquone
  - 1 to 3 months and >24 months of age: 30 mg/kg/24 h PO divided into 2 doses
  - 4 to 24 months of age: 45 mg/kg/24 h PO divided into 2 doses
  - Maximum dose: 750 mg b.i.d.
- Dapsone plus trimethoprim
  - Dapsone: 2 mg/kg PO daily to a maximum of 100 mg daily
  - Trimethoprim: 15 mg/kg/24 h PO divided into 3 doses
- Primaquine plus clindamycin
  - Primaquine: 0.3 mg/kg PO daily to a maximum of 30 mg PO daily
  - Clindamycin: 40 mg/kg/24 h PO divided into 4 doses to a maximum of 600 mg q6h

ADDITIONAL THERAPIES

Corticosteroids

- May be beneficial in HIV patients with moderate to severe PCP
- Not systematically evaluated in children
- Consider when Pa_{O_2} is <70 mm Hg or the alveolar–arterial oxygen gradient is >35 mm Hg.
- In patients >13 years of age, suggested dose is prednisone 40 mg PO b.i.d. for days 1 to 5, 40 mg PO once daily for days 6 to 10, and 20 mg PO once daily for days 11 to 21 with tapering. Doses of methylprednisolone or prednisone at 1 mg/kg given b.i.d.–q.i.d. for 5 to 7 days with a taper over the next 5 days have been suggested.

ONGOING CARE

FOLLOW-UP RECOMMENDATIONS

- After 5 to 7 days of treatment
- If no improvement, TMP-SMX should be replaced with pentamidine.
- Standard precautions are required. Isolation from other immunodeficient patients is recommended.

PROGNOSIS

- 5–40% mortality in treated patients
- Near 100% mortality if patient is untreated
- ~35% of patients will have recurrence unless lifetime prophylaxis is instituted.

COMPLICATIONS

- High rate of respiratory failure necessitating intubation and mechanical ventilation (~60%)
- HIV-infected patients have a higher rate (40%) of adverse reactions to TMP-SMX than the general population. Rash is most common, with fever, neutropenia, anemia, renal dysfunction, nausea, vomiting, and diarrhea occurring as well.
- Prophylactic medication protects the patient as long as the drug is administered. However, this does not eradicate *P. jiroveci*.

ADDITIONAL READING

- King SM; and American Academy of Pediatrics Committee on Pediatric AIDS, American Academy of Pediatrics Infectious Diseases and Immunization Committee. Evaluation and treatment of the human immunodeficiency virus-1–exposed infant. *Pediatrics*. 2004;114(2):497–505.
- Miller RF, Huang L, Walzer PD. Pneumocystis pneumonia associated with human immunodeficiency virus. *Clin Chest Med*. 2013;34(2):229–241.
- Mofenson LM, Brady MT, Danner SP, et al. Guidelines for the prevention and treatment of opportunistic infections among HIV-exposed and HIV-infected children: recommendations from CDC, the National Institutes of Health, the HIV Medicine Association of the Infectious Diseases Society of America, the Pediatric Infectious Diseases Society, and the American Academy of Pediatrics. *MMWR Recomm Rep*. 2009;58(RR-11):1–166.
- Morris A, Wei K, Afshar K, et al. Epidemiology and clinical significance of pneumocystis colonization. *J Infect Dis*. 2008;197(1):10–17.

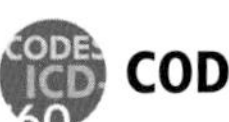

CODES

ICD10

B59 Pneumocystosis

FAQ

- Q: Which are the most common side effects of pentamidine?
- A: They include hypoglycemia, impaired renal or liver function, anemia, thrombocytopenia, neutropenia, hypotension, and skin rashes. These side effects can be expected in 50% of patients.
- Q: How frequently is prophylaxis failure seen?
- A: Adequate TMP-SMX treatment has only a 3% failure rate.
- Q: How are adverse reactions to TMP-SMX during PCP therapy managed?
- A: Continuation of treatment, if the reactions are not severe, is recommended.

PNEUMONIA—BACTERIAL

Erica S. Pan, MD, MPH, FAAP • Dylan C. Kann, MD

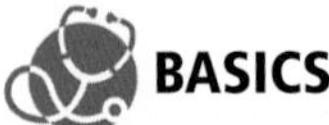

BASICS

DESCRIPTION

- Pneumonia is an infection of the lungs involving the alveoli and distal airways.
- Complicated pneumonia implies pneumonia with: effusion/empyema, abscesses, multilobar disease, necrosis, fistulae, or multisystem infection
- Although viral pneumonias still generally comprise a large proportion of pediatric pneumonia, this chapter focuses on bacterial etiologies and treatment.

EPIDEMIOLOGY

Incidence

- Annual incidence estimated to be 14.9 to 16.5/10,000 children in the United States
- Highest incidence in children <2 years of age (57.6 to 67.1/10,000)

RISK FACTORS

- Immune deficiency
  - Immunocompromised status
  - Sickle cell anemia
- Increased aspiration risk
  - Altered mental status
  - Tracheoesophageal fistula
  - Cerebral palsy
  - Seizure disorder
- Compromised lung function/anatomy
  - Cystic fibrosis
  - Congenital pulmonary malformations
  - Bronchopulmonary dysplasia
  - Asthma
  - Smoke exposure

GENERAL PREVENTION

Routine vaccination (e.g., PCV13, *Haemophilus influenzae* type b [Hib], DTaP)

ETIOLOGY

- Etiology of bacterial pneumonia differs by age:
  - Neonates: group B *Streptococcus*, enteric gram-negative rods (e.g., *Escherichia coli*), *Listeria monocytogenes*, *H. influenzae*, *Bordetella pertussis*
  - 1 to 3 months: neonate organisms + *Staphylococcus aureus*, *Streptococcus pneumoniae*, *Chlamydia trachomatis*
  - 4 months to 4 years: *Streptococcus pneumoniae*, *Staphylococcus aureus*, *Streptococcus pyogenes*, *Mycoplasma pneumoniae*, *H. influenzae*
  - >5 years of age: *Staphylococcus pneumoniae*, *M. pneumoniae*, *Staphylococcus aureus*, *H. influenzae*, *Chlamydophila pneumoniae*, *Mycobacterium tuberculosis*
- Etiology can also differ based on risk factors:
  - Aspiration as etiology increases the risk for oral flora including anaerobes such as *Bacteroides* and *Peptostreptococcus*
  - Ventilator-dependent patients are at increased risk for *Pseudomonas* or *Klebsiella* infections and infection with other gram-negative rods.
  - Cystic fibrosis increases the risk for *Pseudomonas* and other more unusual organisms as well as drug-resistant bacteria.

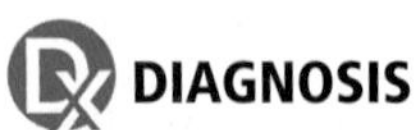

DIAGNOSIS

HISTORY

- Fever and/or chills
- Rapid breathing is a highly sensitive but nonspecific finding in bacterial pneumonia.
- Difficulty breathing or shortness of breath is common (can be associated with difficulty feeding in infants).
- Poor feeding or apnea in young infants
- Cough is often seen in bacterial pneumonia. *B. pertussis* pneumonia often presents after a catarrhal phase with a paroxysmal cough and post-tussive vomiting.
- Pleuritic chest pain
- Abdominal pain and/or vomiting: most often seen with lower lobe pneumonia
- Irritability, lethargy, and/or malaise
- Birth history, including maternal infections (e.g., *C. trachomatis*)
- Immunization status: In a fully immunized child, Hib, *B. pertussis*, and *S. pneumoniae* infections are less common.
- Recent history of upper respiratory tract infection (URI) or respiratory syncytial virus (RSV) can predispose to bacterial pneumonia.
- History of repeated bacterial infections may suggest immunodeficiency or cystic fibrosis.
- Exposure to close contacts with pertussis, tuberculosis, or history of recent travel
- Foreign-born and travelers (for >1 month) to endemic countries and persons working in incarcerated, institutional, or homeless shelter settings are at greater risk for tuberculosis.
- Subacute onset of respiratory symptoms with headache, sore throat, low-grade fever, and/or wheeze are more typical with *M. pneumoniae* or viral etiologies.

PHYSICAL EXAM

- Most common findings: oxygen saturation <95%, elevated respiratory rate, nasal flaring, fever, and ill appearance
- General examination can range from mildly ill-appearing to toxic in appearance.
- Infants may have a paucity of exam findings disproportionate to their appearance and tachypnea.
- Patients may be dehydrated or in shock.
- Most children with bacterial pneumonia have fever. Patients with atypical bacterial or viral pneumonia or pertussis may be afebrile.
- Tachypnea or increased work of breathing: nasal flaring, grunting, and/or retracting
- Decreased oxygen saturation; use pulse oximetry in children with tachypnea or other signs of distress.
- Localized rales, crackles, rhonchi, decreased breath sounds, or wheezing
- With increasing consolidation, dullness to percussion and decreased breath sounds may be noted.
- In patients who are actively wheezing, it may be difficult to distinguish rales from other auscultated sounds.

DIFFERENTIAL DIAGNOSIS

- Infectious (nonbacterial)
  - Sepsis and septic emboli
  - Viral pneumonia (Coinfections with other viruses and sometimes bacteria occur.)
    - Infants: cytomegalovirus (CMV), RSV, human metapneumovirus (HMPV), herpes simplex virus (HSV)
    - From 1 month to 4 years: RSV, rhinovirus, adenovirus, influenza, HMPV, parainfluenza, enterovirus (e.g., D68)
  - Bronchiolitis
  - URI
  - Croup (laryngotracheobronchitis)
  - Fungal infection (if immunodeficiency or exposure history to dimorphic fungal areas)
  - Parasitic infection (if immunodeficiency or exposure history)
- Pulmonary: asthma, atelectasis, pneumonitis (i.e., chemical), pneumothorax, pulmonary edema, pulmonary hemorrhage, or pulmonary embolism
- Congenital: pulmonary sequestration, congenital pulmonary airway malformation
- Genetic: cystic fibrosis
- Tumors: lymphoma, primary lung tumor, metastatic tumor
- Cardiac: CHF (e.g., acute myocarditis)
- GI: gastroesophageal reflux disease
- Foreign body aspiration
- Sarcoidosis

DIAGNOSTIC TESTS & INTERPRETATION

- Generally not indicated for outpatients with uncomplicated pneumonia
- In toxic-appearing infants, consider blood, urine, and CSF cultures (i.e., a sepsis workup).
- Viral testing for RSV, influenza, and other respiratory viruses if readily available can help in management of children who are candidates for outpatient therapy; inpatient viral testing is useful for infection control and may contribute to antibiotic usage and duration decisions.

Initial Tests (screening, lab, imaging)

- Blood culture
  - Not indicated in healthy, immunized children with uncomplicated pneumonia. Routine blood cultures are rarely positive.
  - Should be obtained in children not responding to antibiotic therapy or moderate to severe pneumonia requiring hospitalization
  - Bacteremia has been noted in up to 30% of patients with pneumococcal pneumonia.
- CBC generally only recommended for outpatients with serious disease
- Elevated peripheral WBC or range 15,000 to 40,000/mm^3 is associated with bacterial pneumonia or even higher WBC in pertussis but should not be relied on to distinguish etiology of pneumonia.
- Testing for *M. pneumoniae* antibodies may be considered to guide antibiotic therapy if signs or symptoms of atypical infection present but false positives and false negatives remain problematic. PCR testing may be considered.
- Acute-phase reactants such as ESR, CRP, procalcitonin, or others may provide useful information for clinical management in serious disease but are nonspecific and cannot distinguish between viral and bacterial etiologies.
- Purified protein derivative (PPD) test or an interferon-γ release assay (e.g., quantiFERON®) should be obtained in all patients in whom *M. tuberculosis* is suspected.
- Respiratory sputum culture should be obtained in hospitalized children who can produce it.
- If obtaining pleural fluid, collect cultures, microbiologic PCRs, and other pertinent testing as indicated (see "Pleural Effusion" chapter).
- Chest radiograph (CXR), upright
  - A CXR is not required for diagnosis if clinical symptoms and examination findings are consistent with uncomplicated pneumonia.
  - A CXR (PA and lateral) is recommended if pneumonia is suspected but clinical findings

are unclear, if the patient has hypoxemia or significant respiratory distress, if a pleural effusion is suspected, or if the patient is not responding to treatment.
  - Characteristic CXR patterns include "alveolar or lobar infiltrate" with air bronchograms. "Round" infiltrates may be seen with *S. pneumoniae*. "Diffuse" interstitial infiltrates and hyperinflation may be seen with atypical pneumonia such as *M. pneumoniae* or chlamydial pneumonias.
  - More commonly, CXR cannot be reliably used to distinguish between viral and bacterial disease.
  - An infiltrate may not be seen (negative CXR) if early in disease course or patient dehydrated
- CXR, lateral decubitus: more sensitive than an upright radiograph in detecting pleural effusions or foreign body aspiration
- Ultrasound can be useful for distinguishing dense consolidation from effusion.
- CT scan: not recommended as 1st-line imaging for suspected pneumonia. CT is mainly used as adjunct imaging for patients who are worsening (not improving) despite treatment or have complications.

Diagnostic Procedures/Other

If diagnosis is unclear, consider the following:
- Tracheal aspirates for Gram stain and culture if intubation necessary
- In immunocompetent children, bronchoscopy, bronchoalveolar lavage, percutaneous lung aspiration, or lung biopsy should be reserved for severe pneumonia if initial tests are not diagnostic.

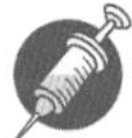

TREATMENT

MEDICATION

Outpatient: empiric treatment
- Nontoxic, uncomplicated pneumonias in patients >3 to 6 months of age and anticipated to comply with antibiotic therapy may be managed as outpatients.
- Courses are 10 days unless otherwise noted.
- Infants and preschool children (<5 years old)
  - Amoxicillin 80 to 100 mg/kg/24 h (max 3 g/24 h) PO divided q8–12h
- School-aged children (≥5 years old)
  - Amoxicillin 80 to 100 mg/kg/24 h (max 3 g/24 h) PO divided q8–12h
- Consider coverage of atypical bacterial pathogens (as primary or additive therapy).
  - Azithromycin 10 mg/kg/dose (max 500 mg) PO × 1 day then 5 mg/kg/dose (max 250 mg) PO once daily × 4 days
  - May consider clarithromycin 15 mg/kg/24 h (max 1 g/24 h) PO divided q12h or doxycycline 4.4 mg/kg/24 h (max 200 mg/24 h) PO divided q12h if >7 years
- If pathogen is known or suspected, use appropriate specific antibiotic therapy.
- For patients with more severe disease, may consider combining β-lactam antibiotic and macrolide
- For amoxicillin allergy: trial of oral cephalosporin, azithromycin, levofloxacin, clindamycin

ALERT

Patients with moderate to severe pneumonia as defined by respiratory distress and hypoxemia (<90%), infants <3 to 6 months of age, children and infants with pneumonia caused by a pathogen with increased virulence (e.g., community-associated methicillin-resistant *Staphylococcus aureus* [MRSA] [CA-MRSA]), and failed outpatient therapy should be hospitalized.

ADMISSION, INPATIENT, AND NURSING CONSIDERATIONS

- Oxygen, intubation, and ventilation support, if clinically indicated
- Empiric antibiotic treatment
- First line:
  - Ampicillin 200 to 400 mg/kg/24 h (max 12 g/24 h) IV divided q6h (or penicillin 250,000 U/kg/24 h [max 24 million U/24 h] IV divided q6h)
- Alternative:
  - Ceftriaxone 50 to 100 mg/kg/24 h (max 2 g/24 h) IV divided q12–24h or cefotaxime 200 mg/kg/24 h (max 12 g/24 h) IV divided q8h
  - Parenteral 3rd-generation cephalosporins should be reserved for severe or ICU-level pneumonia, in under/unimmunized children, or if concern for significant local penicillin resistance levels.
- If atypical pathogens suspected, may add macrolide or use as alternative: azithromycin IV or PO using the same initial empiric dosage regimen from above
- For suspected MRSA coverage, add vancomycin 15 mg/kg/dose IV q6–8h or clindamycin 30 mg/kg/24 h IV/PO divided q8h.
- If aspiration pneumonia, consider ampicillin-sulbactam 200 mg ampicillin /kg/24 h IV divided q6h, or clindamycin 30 mg/kg/24 h IV divided q6–8h.
- May also consider azithromycin, levofloxacin, clindamycin, or linezolid as alternative for β-lactam–allergic patients

ISSUES FOR REFERRAL

- For additional antibiotic guidance for children not improving, consider pediatric infectious disease consultation.
- For management of complicated pneumonia, consider subspecialty consultation and see "Pleural Effusion" chapter for more guidance.

ONGOING CARE

FOLLOW-UP RECOMMENDATIONS

Patient Monitoring

- Children on appropriate therapy should show improvement within 48 to 72 hours.
- If worsening or not responding to treatment, consider repeated or additional diagnostic studies. For example, persistent fever may be due to loculated pleural fluid or an empyema.
- CXR may be abnormal for up to 10 weeks after successful treatment. Consider follow-up CXR only if indicated for severe disease, clinical progression, or suspected complications (e.g., effusion, empyema).
- For children with recurrent bacterial pneumonia, consider an underlying anatomic or immunologic disorder (e.g., abnormal antibody production, cystic fibrosis, tracheoesophageal fistula, pulmonary sequestration).

COMPLICATIONS

- Pleural effusion, empyema, lung abscess, pneumatoceles, pneumothorax
- Bacteremia/sepsis

ADDITIONAL READING

- Bartlett JG. How important are anaerobic bacteria in aspiration pneumonia: when should they be treated and what is optimal therapy. *Infect Dis Clin North Am*. 2013;27(1):149–155.
- Bradley JS, Byington CL, Shah SS, et al. Executive summary: the management of community-acquired pneumonia in infants and children older than 3 months of age: clinical practice guidelines by the Pediatric Infectious Diseases Society and the Infectious Diseases Society of America. *Clin Infect Dis*. 2011;53(7):617–630.
- Jain S, Williams DJ, Arnold SR, et al; for Centers for Disease Control and Prevention Etiology of Pneumonia in the Community Study Team. Community-acquired pneumonia requiring hospitalization among U.S. children. *N Engl J Med*. 2015;372(9):835–845.
- Lee GE, Lorch SA, Sheffler-Collins S, et al. National hospitalization trends for pediatric pneumonia and associated complications. *Pediatrics*. 2010;126(2):204–213.
- Ranganathan SC, Sonnappa S. Pneumonia and other respiratory infections. *Pediatr Clin North Am*. 2009;56(1):135–156.

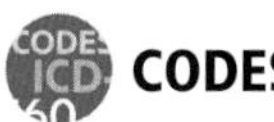

CODES

ICD10

- J15.9 Unspecified bacterial pneumonia
- J15.3 Pneumonia due to streptococcus, group B
- J15.5 Pneumonia due to Escherichia coli

FAQ

- Q: What is the appropriate duration of therapy for bacterial pneumonia?
- A: Empiric treatment courses of 10 days have been studied the most, although shorter courses may be effective in uncomplicated disease. Pneumonias caused by some pathogens (e.g., CA-MRSA) may require longer duration.
- Q: What is the most common causative organism of pulmonary abscess, and what is the appropriate treatment?
- A: *S. aureus* is the most common causative organism. Treatment includes IV vancomycin, IV or PO clindamycin, or PO linezolid. If MSSA is confirmed, use cefazolin or nafcillin.
- Q: Which children are most likely to have systemic complications from community-acquired pneumonia? Local complications?
- A: An analysis of inpatient data from pediatric hospitals from 1997 to 2006 suggests that children <1 year of age are more likely to have systemic complications (e.g., sepsis, acute respiratory failure), whereas patients aged 1 to 5 years are more likely to have local complications (e.g., empyema, abscess).
- Q: What are risk factors for invasive pneumococcal disease?
- A: Conditions associated include congenital immune deficiency (e.g., B- or T-lymphocyte deficiencies), HIV, asplenia/functional hyposplenism, complement deficiency, receipt of immunosuppressive therapy or radiation therapy (including malignancies), and solid organ transplant and chronic cardiac disease.
- Q: What are eligible criteria for discharging a hospitalized child with community-acquired pneumonia?
- A: Documented overall clinical improvement including: afebrile for 12 to 24 hours, oxygen saturations >90% for 12 to 24 hours, normal vital signs and baseline mental status, able to tolerate outpatient medications and oral hydration, and near baseline activity level and appetite

PNEUMOTHORAX

Richard M. Kravitz, MD

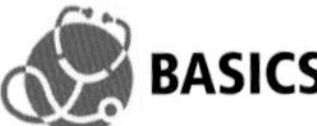

BASICS

DESCRIPTION
Abnormal collection of free air or gas in the pleural space

EPIDEMIOLOGY
Depends on the underlying lung disease

Incidence
- Spontaneous pneumothorax
  - Male > female (1.4 to 10.1:1)
  - Peak incidence: 10 to 30 years
- Pneumothorax with cystic fibrosis (CF)
  - For overall CF population: 3.5–8%
  - CF patients >18 years: 16–20%
  - Risk factors for pneumothorax:
    - More severe disease
    - Decreased pulmonary function (i.e., forced expiratory volume in 1 second [FEV_1] <30–50%)
    - Colonization with *Pseudomonas aeruginosa*, *Burkholderia cepacia*, or *Aspergillus*

RISK FACTORS
- Asthma
- CF
- Pneumonia
- Collagen vascular diseases

PATHOPHYSIOLOGY
- Air can enter the pleural space via the following:
  - Chest wall (i.e., penetrating trauma)
  - Intrapulmonary (i.e., ruptured alveoli)
- Usually, collapse of the lung on the affected side seals the leak.
- If a ball valve mechanism ensues, however, air can accumulate in the thoracic cavity, causing the development of a tension pneumothorax (a medical emergency).

ETIOLOGY
- Spontaneous (secondary to rupture of apical blebs)
- Mechanical trauma
  - Penetrating injury (i.e., knife or bullet wound)
  - Blunt trauma (i.e., auto accident)
- Barotrauma
  - Mechanical ventilation
  - Cough (if severe enough)
  - Vaginal birth
- Iatrogenic
  - Central venous catheter placement
  - Bronchoscopy (especially with biopsy)
- Infection: most common organisms
  - *Staphylococcus aureus*
  - *Streptococcus pneumoniae*
  - *Mycobacterium tuberculosis*
  - *Bordetella pertussis*
  - *Pneumocystis jiroveci*
- Airway occlusion
  - Mucus plugging (asthma)
  - Foreign body
  - Meconium aspiration
- Bleb formation (i.e., idiopathic, secondary to CF)
- Malignancy
- Catamenial

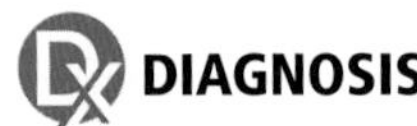

DIAGNOSIS

HISTORY
- May be asymptomatic (pneumothorax discovered on chest film obtained for other reasons)
- Cough
- Shortness of breath
- Dyspnea
- Pleuritic chest pain that is usually sudden in onset and localized to apices (referred pain to shoulders)
- Respiratory distress
- Underlying medical problems which increases risk for pneumothorax
- Activity prior to developing symptoms that might have caused the pneumothorax:
  - Heavy lifting
  - Increased coughing

PHYSICAL EXAM
- May be normal
- Decreased breath sounds on the affected side
- Decreased vocal fremitus
- Hyperresonance to percussion on the affected side
- Tachypnea
- Tachycardia
- Shortness of breath
- Respiratory distress
- Shifting of the cardiac point of maximal impulse away from the affected side
- Shifting of the trachea away from the affected side
- Subcutaneous emphysema
- Cyanosis
- Scratch sign (heard through the stethoscope): A loud scratching sound is heard when a finger is gently stroked over the area of the pneumothorax.

DIFFERENTIAL DIAGNOSIS
- Pulmonary
  - Congenital lung malformations
    - Cysts (i.e., bronchogenic cysts)
    - Cystic adenomatoid malformation
    - Congenital lobar emphysema
  - Acquired emphysema
  - Hyperinflation of the lung
  - Postinfectious pneumatocele
  - Bullae formation
- Miscellaneous
  - Diaphragmatic hernia
  - Infections (i.e., pulmonary abscess)
  - Muscle strain
  - Pleurisy (i.e., pleuritis)
  - Rib fracture

DIAGNOSTIC TESTS & INTERPRETATION

Initial Tests (screening, lab, imaging)
- EKG
  - Diminished amplitude of the QRS voltage
  - Rightward shift of the QRS axis (if left-sided pneumothorax)
- Arterial blood gas
  - Po_2 can frequently be decreased.
  - Pco_2
    - Elevated with respiratory compromise
    - Decreased from hyperventilation
- Pulse oximetry
  - Useful for assessing oxygenation
- Chest radiograph
  - Primary test for establishing the diagnosis
  - Radiolucency of the affected lung
  - Lack of lung markings in the periphery of the affected lung
  - Collapsed lung on the affected side
  - Possible pneumomediastinum with subcutaneous emphysema
- Chest CT
  - Useful for finding small pneumothoraces
  - Can help distinguish a pneumothorax from a bleb or cyst
  - Helpful for locating small apical blebs associated with spontaneous pneumothoraces

Diagnostic Procedures/Other
Pitfalls:
- Not considering the diagnosis in otherwise healthy patients
- Confusing the symptoms with those of an underlying lung disease
- Inserting a needle into a cyst or bleb (can cause a tension pneumothorax with rapid respiratory compromise)

TREATMENT

GENERAL MEASURES

- Stabilization of the patient
- Evacuation of the pleural air
  - Should be done urgently if a tension pneumothorax is suspected
  - In small asymptomatic pneumothoraces, observation of the patient is indicated.
- Treat the underlying condition predisposing for the pneumothorax:
  - Antibiotics for any underlying infection
  - Bronchodilators and anti-inflammatory agents for asthma attacks
- Oxygen
  - Used to keep $Sao_2 \geq 95\%$
  - Breathing 100% oxygen
    - Can speed the intrapleural air's reabsorption into the bloodstream, hastening lung reexpansion
    - Useful for treating smaller pneumothoraces, especially in neonates

SURGERY/OTHER PROCEDURES

- Needle thoracentesis: useful for evacuation of the pleural air in simple, uncomplicated spontaneous pneumothorax
- Chest tube drainage
  - Used for evacuation of the pleural air in recurrent, persistent, or complicated pneumothoraces and cases with significant underlying lung disease
  - Chest tube should be left in (usually 2 to 4 days) until
    - Most air is reabsorbed.
    - No reaccumulation of air is seen on sealing of the chest tube.
- Surgical removal of pulmonary blebs
  - Blebs have a high rate of rupturing with resultant pneumothorax.
  - In patients with established pneumothoraces, the blebs should be removed or oversewn to prevent reoccurrence of the pneumothorax (blebs have a high rate of reoccurrence if not repaired).
  - Thoracotomy versus video-assisted thoracic surgery (VATS)
- Pleurodesis
  - Used to attach the lung to the intrathoracic chest wall to prevent reoccurrence of a pneumothorax
  - Useful in cases of recurrent pneumothorax or if the pneumothorax is unresponsive to chest tube drainage (i.e., CF, malignancy)
  - Mechanism of action: The surface of the lung becomes inflamed and adheres to the chest wall via the formation of scar tissue.
  - Two commonly used methods:
    - Surgical pleurodesis:
      - Mechanical abrasion of part of the lung or pleurectomy
      - Advantages: very effective; low reoccurrence rate; site specific (limits affected area)
      - Disadvantages: requires surgery and general anesthesia; contraindicated if patient is unstable
    - Chemical pleurodesis
      - Chemicals are used to cause inflammation.
      - Chemicals commonly used: talc, tetracycline, minocycline, doxycycline, quinacrine
      - Advantages: requires no surgery or general anesthesia
      - Disadvantages: less effective than surgery; generalized inflammation (rather than site-specific; makes future thoracic surgery more difficult; painful)

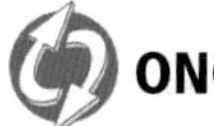

ONGOING CARE

FOLLOW-UP RECOMMENDATIONS

Symptomatic relief within seconds of the air being evacuated

Patient Monitoring

Sign to watch for: inability to remove the chest tube without reaccumulation of air (suggestive of a bronchopulmonary fistula; requires surgical exploration if no improvement in 7 to 10 days)

PROGNOSIS

- Depends on the underlying cause of the pneumothorax
- If simple, spontaneous pneumothorax, recovery is excellent.
- CF: Development of pneumothorax can be associated with increased morbidity and mortality.

COMPLICATIONS

- Pain
- Hypoxia
- Respiratory distress
- Tension pneumothorax
  - Hypoxia
  - Hypercarbia with acidosis
  - Respiratory failure
- Pneumomediastinum with subcutaneous emphysema
- Bronchopulmonary fistula

ADDITIONAL READING

- Baumann MH. Management of spontaneous pneumothorax. *Clin Chest Med*. 2006;27(2):369–381.
- Briassoulis GC, Venkataraman ST, Vasilopoulos AG, et al. Air leaks from the respiratory tract in mechanically ventilated children with severe respiratory disease. *Pediatr Pulmonol*. 2000;29(2):127–134.
- Dotson K, Johnson LH. Pediatric spontaneous pneumothorax. *Pediatr Emerg Care*. 2012;28(7): 715–723.
- Dotson K, Timm N, Gittelman M. Is spontaneous pneumothorax really a pediatric problem? A national perspective. *Pediatr Emerg Care*. 2012;28(4):340–344.
- Flume PA, Strange C, Ye X, et al. Pneumothorax in cystic fibrosis. *Chest*. 2005;128(2):720–728.
- Johnson NN, Toledo A, Endom EE. Pneumothorax, pneumomediastinum, and pulmonary embolism. *Pediatr Clin North Am*. 2010;57(6):1357–1383.
- Noppen M. Management of primary spontaneous pneumothorax. *Curr Opin Pulm Med*. 2003;9(4):272–275.
- Sahn SA, Heffner JE. Spontaneous pneumothorax. *N Engl J Med*. 2000;342(12):868–874.
- Ullman EA, Donley LP, Brady WJ. Pulmonary trauma emergency department evaluation and management. *Emerg Med Clin North Am*. 2003;21(2):291–313.

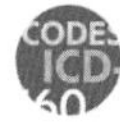

CODES

ICD10

- J93.9 Pneumothorax, unspecified
- J93.11 Primary spontaneous pneumothorax
- S27.0XXA Traumatic pneumothorax, initial encounter

FAQ

- Q: Can a pneumothorax reoccur?
- A: Reoccurrence depends on the underlying cause of the pneumothorax. Spontaneous pneumothorax reoccurrence rates:
  - Observation alone: 20–50%
  - If thoracentesis performed: 25–50%
  - If chest tube drainage performed: 32–38%
  - Overall reoccurrence rate: 16–52%
- Chemical pleurodesis reoccurrence rates:
  - Tetracycline: 25%
  - Talc: 8–10%
- Surgical pleurodesis reoccurrence rates:
  - VATS: 13%
  - Thoracotomy: 3%
  - Thoracotomy with pleurectomy: 0–4%
- CF reoccurrence rates:
  - If no drainage attempted: 68%
  - Thoracentesis alone: 90%
  - Chest tube drainage alone: 72%
  - Chemical pleurodesis:
    - Tetracycline: 42–86%
    - Quinacrine: 12.5%
    - Talc: 8%
  - Surgical pleurodesis: thoracotomy with pleurectomy: 0–4%

POLYARTERITIS NODOSA

Jay Mehta, MD, MS

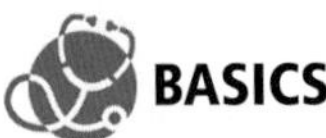

BASICS

DESCRIPTION
An inflammatory process of small- and medium-sized muscular arteries resulting in multi-system organ dysfunction

EPIDEMIOLOGY
Incidence
Extremely rare in childhood

Prevalence
Prevalence equal in boys and girls

PATHOPHYSIOLOGY
Necrotizing arteritis of small- and medium-sized arteries resulting in segmental fibrinoid necrosis

ETIOLOGY
- Idiopathic
- Postinfectious (streptococcal, especially for isolated cutaneous form)
- Hepatitis B association rare in children with widespread vaccination

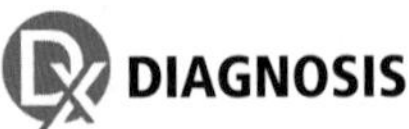

DIAGNOSIS

HISTORY
- Persistent constitutional symptoms
- Bilateral calf pain and other myalgia
- Abdominal pain
- Weight loss
- Unexplained fever
- Headache
- Arthralgia
- Rashes
- Seizures
- Weakness

PHYSICAL EXAM
- Check skin for the following:
  - Livedo reticularis
  - Skin nodules
  - Necrotic digits
- Assess BP and pulses.
- Neurologic exam for findings consistent with neuropathy (mononeuritis multiplex)
- Check testes for tenderness or swelling.
- Check muscles for tenderness, especially calves.

DIFFERENTIAL DIAGNOSIS
- Infection
  - Bacterial endocarditis
  - Brucellosis
  - Influenza B (calf pain)
- Tumors
  - Left atrial myxoma
  - Burkitt lymphoma
- Metabolic
  - Homocystinuria (thromboembolic events)
- Congenital
- Immunologic
  - Systemic necrotizing vasculitis
  - Systemic lupus erythematosus
  - Kawasaki disease
  - Systemic juvenile idiopathic arthritis
  - Granulomatosis with polyangiitis
  - Takayasu arteritis
  - Cryoglobulinemia
  - Antiphospholipid antibody syndrome
  - Thrombotic thrombocytopenic purpura
- Psychologic
  - Munchausen syndrome (factitious skin lesions)
- Miscellaneous
  - Degos disease (malignant atrophic papulosis)

DIAGNOSTIC TESTS & INTERPRETATION
Initial Tests (screening, lab, imaging)
- ESR
  - Usually extremely elevated; leukocytosis and thrombocytosis are seen.
- Urine analysis
  - Proteinuria and hematuria can be present.
- Creatinine and BUN levels
  - May be elevated
- Antinuclear antibodies and rheumatoid factor
  - Usually negative
- Muscle enzymes (creatine kinase, lactate dehydrogenase, aspartate aminotransferase, and aldolase levels)
  - Muscle involvement is common, especially in those with calf pain.
- Antineutrophil cytoplasmic antibodies (ANCAs)
  - Usually negative; if positive, more likely to be granulomatosis with polyangiitis or microscopic polyangiitis
- Streptococcal titers
  - Polyarteritis nodosa may develop after streptococcal infections.
- MRI of tender muscles
  - Short T1 inversion recovery (STIR) images may show edema, so a directed biopsy can be done to avoid false-negative muscle biopsy.
- Magnetic resonance angiography (MRA), CT angiography (CTA), or angiography
  - Aneurysms are characteristic finding; may not be seen on MRA or CTA, as they are insensitive for small vessel disease
  - Conventional angiography gold standard but must weigh risks of procedure/radiation

Diagnostic Procedures/Other
Biopsy of affected tissue/organ: usually skin, kidney, nerve, testicle

TREATMENT

MEDICATION

- Ideally, diagnosis established with angiography or biopsy before beginning treatment
- Corticosteroids are mainstay.
  - Usually start at dose of oral prednisone 1 to 2 mg/kg/24 h and adjust based on response
  - May initially give methylprednisolone 30 mg/kg up to 1 g/24 h IV once daily for 3 days
- Immunosuppressives such as methotrexate, azathioprine, cyclophosphamide, and infliximab may be necessary.
- Hypertension should be managed aggressively.
- Initiation of steroid therapy may bring response in 1 to 2 weeks; however, management of specific organs affected during acute stage is essential.
- May require long-term therapy

ONGOING CARE

FOLLOW-UP RECOMMENDATIONS

Patient Monitoring

- Watch for the following:
  - Rising creatinine and BUN levels
  - Abdominal pain
    - Severe abdominal pain suggests peritoneal bleed.
  - Chest pain or cardiac dysfunction suggestive of coronary involvement
  - Uncontrolled hypertension
- Home testing
  - May wish to have patients monitor BP periodically if renal involvement suspected

DIET

- If renal system involved, diet low in sodium and potassium
- If on high-dose steroids, diet low in sodium
- Possible conflicts with medications

PROGNOSIS

- May be extremely poor over the long term
- Risk is high for renal failure, hypertension, stroke, myocardial infarction, bowel infarction, and death.
- Owing to low incidence/prevalence, precise data are not available.
- Cutaneous polyarteritis nodosa is relatively benign.

COMPLICATIONS

- Hypertension
- Renal failure
- Digital necrosis
- Intestinal infarction
- Stroke

ADDITIONAL READING

- Eleftheriou D, Dillon MJ, Tullus K, et al. Systemic polyarteritis nodosa in the young: a single-center experience over thirty-two years. *Arthritis Rheum*. 2013;65(9):2476–2485. doi:10.1002/art.38024.
- Kawakami T. A review of pediatric vasculitis with a focus on juvenile polyarteritis nodosa. *Am J Clin Dermatol*. 2012;13(6):389–398.
- Khubchandani RP, Viswanathan V. Pediatric vasculitides: a generalists approach. *Indian J Pediatr*. 2010;77(10):1165–1171.
- Morgan AJ, Schwartz RA. Cutaneous polyarteritis nodosa: a comprehensive review. *Int J Dermatol*. 2010;49(7):750–756.
- Ozen S, Anton J, Arisoy N, et al. Juvenile polyarteritis: results of a multicenter survey of 110 children. *J Pediatr*. 2004;145(4):517–522.
- Ting TV, Hashkes PJ. Update on childhood vasculitides. *Curr Opin Rheumatol*. 2004;16(5):560–565.

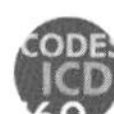

CODES

ICD10

M30.0 Polyarteritis nodosa

FAQ

- Q: When should I consider polyarteritis nodosa in the differential?
- A: There are five major clues to polyarteritis nodosa: (i) prolonged constitutional symptoms without a diagnosis, (ii) multisystem disease, (iii) an unusual patient for the presenting symptom (i.e., myocardial infarction in a teen), (iv) a rash that looks vasculitic, and (v) bilateral calf pain in a sick child.
- Q: Are there any specific lab tests for polyarteritis nodosa?
- A: No. The diagnosis is made on the basis of symptoms, characteristic organ involvement, and either biopsy showing necrotizing arteritis or angiography demonstrating aneurysms.
- Q: Who should manage the patient with polyarteritis nodosa?
- A: Usually, one discipline provides a comprehensive management plan—either the pediatrician or rheumatologist. Subspecialist(s) of the affected organ systems provide management guidelines for specific organ issues.

POLYCYSTIC KIDNEY DISEASE

Paul R. Brakeman, MD, PhD

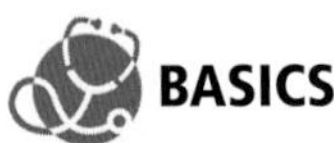

BASICS

DESCRIPTION

Polycystic kidney disease (PKD) is a heritable disorder with diffuse cystic involvement of both kidneys without other dysplastic elements. The term PKD is generally used to describe two genetically distinct syndromes:

- Autosomal dominant polycystic kidney disease (ADPKD)
  - Saccular, epithelial-lined, fluid-filled cysts of various sizes are derived from all segments of the nephron.
  - Cysts progressively enlarge and become disconnected from the tubule of origin.
  - Usually not clinically apparent until the 3rd or 4th decade of life
  - ~2–5% of patients have early-onset disease.
- Autosomal recessive polycystic kidney disease (ARPKD)
  - Fusiform dilations arise from the collecting ducts and maintain contact with the nephron of origin.
  - Associated hepatic abnormalities include biliary dysgenesis, periportal fibrosis (congenital hepatic fibrosis), and portal hypertension. At the histologic level, almost all patients with ARPKD demonstrate some hepatic fibrosis.
  - Renal abnormalities may progress before liver abnormalities in some patients, whereas, in other patients, liver abnormalities predominate early on before kidney pathology progresses.

EPIDEMIOLOGY

- ADPKD
  - One of the most common human genetic disorders; the most common renal inherited disease
  - 3rd leading cause of end-stage renal disease (ESRD) in adults (5% of all cases)
  - Frequency: 1 in 400 to 1,000
- ARPKD
  - Incidence of 1 in 20,000 to 40,000 live births

RISK FACTORS

Genetics

- ARPKD
  - Mutations in the polycystic kidney hepatic disease 1 gene (*PKHD1*, chromosome 6)
  - >300 mutations have been reported in the *PKHD1* gene.
  - There is poor correlation between genotype and phenotype.
- ADPKD
  - Type I ADPKD accounts for 85–90% of cases of ADPKD and is caused by mutations in the *PKD1* gene (chromosome 16).
  - Large genomic deletions may encompass *PKD1* and *TSC2* genes, resulting in early-onset ADPKD with tuberous sclerosis.
  - Type II ADPKD is caused by mutations in the *PKD2* gene (chromosome 4) and accounts for 10–15% of the cases.
- Nephronophthisis (NPHP) refers to a group of autosomal recessive cystic kidney disease disorders with >20 identified causative genes. NPHP occurs as isolated kidney disease but approximately 15% of NPHP patients also have additional extrarenal symptoms affecting other organs.
- Other
  - Presymptomatic genetic screening for ADPKD is not recommended.
  - Normotensive women with ADPKD usually have uncomplicated pregnancies.
  - Higher risk for maternal/fetal complications if there is preexisting hypertension

PATHOPHYSIOLOGY

- Most protein abnormalities that have been associated with cystic kidney disease localize to cilia on epithelial cells.
- Cilia are critical for cell architecture, proliferation, apoptosis, and polarity.
- ADPKD is caused by decreased or loss of function of polycystins:
  - Polycystin-1 is a membrane mechanoreceptor-like protein that forms multiprotein complexes at focal adhesions, cell–cell junctions, and cilia. It is involved in cell polarity, proliferation, cell–matrix interactions, and secretion.
  - Polycystin-2 is a divalent cation channel involved in calcium signaling and intracellular calcium homeostasis and is likely critical for cytoskeletal organization, cell adhesion, migration, and proliferation.
- ARPKD is produced by loss of function of fibrocystin/polyductin:
  - Fibrocystin/polyductin is an integral membrane receptor with extracellular protein-interaction sites that transduce intracellular signals to the nucleus.

ETIOLOGY

- ADPKD is generally an adult-onset, systemic disorder with cystic and noncystic manifestations. Cyst growth begins in utero but only becomes visible by conventional imaging in adolescence or early adulthood. Cysts occur in the kidneys and other epithelial organs (e.g., seminal vesicles, pancreas, and liver):
  - Polycystic liver disease is the most common extrarenal manifestation occurring in ~90% of patients.
  - Intracranial aneurysms occur in 5–10%.
  - Mitral valve prolapse is the most common valvular abnormality (demonstrated in up to 25% of affected individuals).
  - Colonic diverticula in 80% with ESRD
- ARPKD is a renal and hepatic developmental disorder. The hallmark of ARPKD liver disease is congenital hepatic fibrosis and dilation of intrahepatic bile ducts (Caroli disease).
  - Severely affected infants may have the oligohydramnios sequence at birth, and associated pulmonary hypoplasia and respiratory complications convey a high mortality risk.

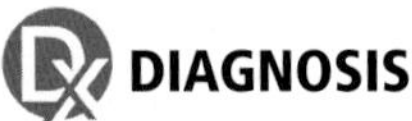

DIAGNOSIS

HISTORY

- ADPKD
  - Detailed family history is essential.
  - Most common presenting complaint in adults is pain.
  - Hypertension, polyuria, gross hematuria, nephrolithiasis, and UTIs are common.
- ARPKD
  - Oligohydramnios sequence in infants
  - Postnatal respiratory insufficiency
  - Renal insufficiency
  - Hypertension (may be severe)
  - Hepatobiliary manifestations include cholestasis, cholangitis, liver failure, portal hypertension, hypersplenism.
- Signs and symptoms
  - ADPKD
    - Children are usually asymptomatic but may present with hypertension, abdominal pain, abdominal mass, gross hematuria after trauma, proteinuria, UTI/cyst infection, renal calculi, or decreased renal function.
  - ARPKD
    - Presentation variable
    - Severely affected infants have "Potter" oligohydramnios sequence.
    - Pulmonary hypoplasia/respiratory insufficiency is a major cause of neonatal mortality.
    - Renal insufficiency
    - Hepatobiliary complications later in course (portal hypertension, hematemesis, hepatosplenomegaly hypersplenism with pallor, petechiae)

PHYSICAL EXAM

- Clinical spectrum variable, particularly in ARPKD
- Hypertension
- Abdominal pain; tenderness at flank or costovertebral angle
- Flank mass or palpable kidneys
- Hepatosplenomegaly, varices, jaundice/icterus, abdominal ascites in ARPKD

DIFFERENTIAL DIAGNOSIS

- Multicystic dysplastic kidney (MCDK)
- Medullary cystic kidney disease
- NPHP
- Acquired cystic disease may occur in patients with ESRD.
- Genetic syndromes with cystic renal dysplasia and one or more other organs affected including, but not limited to, the following:
  - Meckel syndrome
  - Jeune syndrome
  - Ivemark syndrome
  - Zellweger syndrome
  - Bardet-Biedl syndrome
  - Tuberous sclerosis

DIAGNOSTIC TESTS & INTERPRETATION

Initial Tests (screening, lab, imaging)

- Metabolic panel to include BUN, creatinine, electrolytes
- Calcium, phosphorus
- Liver function tests
- CBC
- Urinalysis
- Note: Hyponatremia is often present in the neonatal period in ARPKD.
- Ultrasonography is the preferred screening method and should include liver and Doppler to evaluate for portal hypertension in ARPKD.
- ARPKD
  - Kidneys enlarged with increased echogenicity and loss of corticomedullary differentiation
  - The liver may be normal in infants and young children. Over time, it becomes enlarged and hyperechoic. Dilated intrahepatic biliary ducts may be seen.
  - Prenatal ultrasound after 24 to 30 weeks' gestation may show hyperechoic enlarged kidneys, oligohydramnios, and absence of bladder filling.
- Ultrasound diagnostic criteria for ADPKD
  - $<$40 years should have at least 2 cysts in 1 of the kidneys and 1 cyst in the other kidney or 3 cysts in a single kidney.
  - $\geq$40 and $\leq$59 years of age should have at least 2 cysts in each kidney.
  - $>$60 years should have at least 4 cysts in each kidney.
- CT scan with contrast
  - Has limited use in young children owing to exposure to ionizing radiation
  - It is mostly used in adults with ADPKD because it can distinguish between solid and liquid renal masses.
- MRI with gadolinium
  - Heavy-weighted T2 MRI is the most sensitive method currently available.
  - Can be used in both conditions
  - Particularly useful to evaluate liver involvement in ARPKD
  - Increasing evidence that kidney volume on MRI is a useful tool to follow disease progression and efficacy of therapies in ADPKD
  - Avoid gadolinium in patients with advanced chronic kidney disease.

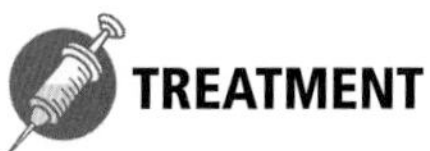

TREATMENT

GENERAL MEASURES

- No currently approved targeted treatments to cure or slow progression
- Medical management is supportive.
- Pain is the most common symptom in ADPKD and can be difficult to treat.

MEDICATION

- Hypertension is common in PKD
  - Patients respond well to diuretics, angiotensin converting enzyme (ACE) inhibitors, or calcium channel blockers.
  - ACE inhibitors or angiotensin-receptor blockers are first line.
- In patients with PKD and nephrolithiasis, thiazide diuretics may be used for hypercalciuria, and potassium citrate supplements if hypocitraturia is found.
- Pyelonephritis in patients with PKD may lead to infected cysts. The treatment should include antibiotics that penetrate into the cysts (quinolones, trimethoprim) and prolonged treatment duration if cephalosporins and aminoglycosides fail to eradicate the infection.

ADDITIONAL THERAPIES

- Patients with PKD should not participate in high-contact athletics in which the abdomen may be traumatized repeatedly.
- Strenuous static exercise should be avoided in hypertensive patients.

ONGOING CARE

FOLLOW-UP RECOMMENDATIONS

A pediatric nephrologist should be involved in the care of children with PKD.

DIET

- In both conditions, dietary changes depend on the degree of renal failure.
- Sodium restriction is indicated in cases of hypertension and/or edema.
- Caffeine should be avoided in cases of ADPKD.

PATIENT EDUCATION

- Emotional support and education of patients with PKD and their families can be obtained through the PKD Foundation (https://pkdcure.org) and the ARPKD/CHF Alliance (http://www.arpkdchf.org).
- Genetic counseling is indicated in these disorders and genetic testing may help families understand future risks.

PROGNOSIS

- ADPKD
  - The probability of being alive and not having ESRD is about 77% at age 50 years, 57% at age 58 years, and 52% at age 73 years. Median onset of ESRD is 53 years (PKD1) versus 69 years (PKD2).
  - Cystic expansion occurs at a consistent rate per individual, although it is heterogeneous in the population.
  - Larger kidneys are associated with more rapid disease progression.
  - *PKD1* mutation is more severe because more cysts develop earlier, not because they grow faster.
- ARPKD
  - Neonatal onset is fatal in up to 50% of infants because of pulmonary hypoplasia with associated respiratory failure.
  - Patients who survive the neonatal period have up to an 80% 10-year survival.
  - Overall, the likelihood of developing ESRD for those surviving infancy is $\sim$60% at 10 years of age.

ADDITIONAL READING

- Dell KM. The spectrum of polycystic kidney disease in children. *Adv Chronic Kidney Dis*. 2011;18(5):339–347.
- Hoyer PF. Clinical manifestations of autosomal recessive polycystic kidney disease. *Curr Opin Pediatr*. 2015;27(2):186–192.
- Patil A, Sweeney WE Jr, Avner ED, et al. Childhood polycystic kidney disease. In: Li X, ed. *Polycystic Kidney Disease*. Brisbane, Australia: Codon Publications; 2015:chap 2.
- Reddy BV, Chapman AB. The spectrum of autosomal dominant polycystic kidney disease in children and adolescents. *Pediatr Nephrol*. 2017;32(1):31–42.
- Sweeney WE Jr, Avner ED. Diagnosis and management of childhood polycystic kidney disease. *Pediatr Nephrol*. 2011;26(5):675–692.
- Sweeney WE Jr, Avner ED. Emerging therapies for childhood polycystic kidney disease. *Front Pediatr*. 2017;5:77.

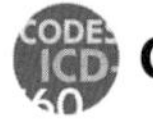

CODES

ICD10

- Q61.3 Polycystic kidney, unspecified
- Q61.19 Other polycystic kidney, infantile type
- Q61.2 Polycystic kidney, adult type

FAQ

- Q: What can be done to slow the progression of renal insufficiency in ADPKD?
- A: Well-controlled BP and rapid treatment of UTIs may decrease the progression of renal failure.
- Q: Should asymptomatic older siblings of an infant with ARPKD be evaluated?
- A: Yes. An older child may have congenital hepatic fibrosis with minimal renal involvement.
- Q: Should one screen ADPKD-affected family members for the presence of cerebral vessel aneurysms if other family members have aneurysms?
- A: Although routine screening is not recommended in childhood, intrafamilial clustering of aneurysms has been reported, and it may be advisable to screen symptomatic adolescents with MRI or cranial CT in families with previous history of ADPKD and aneurysms.

POLYCYSTIC OVARY SYNDROME

Ellen Lancon Connor, MD

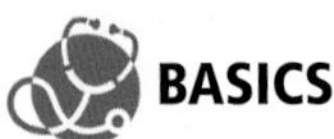

BASICS

DESCRIPTION

- Polycystic ovarian syndrome (PCOS) is a syndrome of hyperandrogenism, altered ovarian morphology, and chronic anovulation with infertility.
- Consensus guidelines recommend that although having two of the three features is enough to make a diagnosis of PCOS in adulthood, all three features of PCOS should be present before diagnosis in an adolescent. Additionally, the menstrual abnormality should have persisted for >2 years.
- Obesity, hyperinsulinemia, and insulin resistance are common but not required for diagnosis.
- Because features of PCOS overlap the androgen effects, ovarian morphology, and menstrual irregularity seen in normal puberty, diagnosis may be suspected but not confirmed in some adolescent girls. Thus, symptoms should be treated after appropriate hormonal investigation and do not require confirmation of PCOS diagnosis.

EPIDEMIOLOGY

- Present in 6–14% of postpubertal women
- Risk factors may be noted in childhood, including low birth weight, premature adrenarche, and earlier menarche.
- Insulin resistance, often with obesity, is a frequent accompanying feature.

RISK FACTORS

Genetics

- Multifactorial heritable syndrome
- Polycystic ovaries appear to be inherited as an autosomal dominant trait.
- PCOS may occur in mothers and sisters and in daughters of fathers with type 2 diabetes (T2D).
- Fibrillin-3 (*FBN-3*), THADA, DENN/MADD domain containing 1A (*DENND1A*), follicle-stimulating hormone (FSH) receptor (*FSHR*), luteinizing hormone (LH) receptor (*LHCGR*), IL-6. TNF-α, GNRHR, FABP1, IL-1β, and IL-1Ra polymorphisms may contribute to the development of PCOS.

PATHOPHYSIOLOGY

- Developmental programming by androgens and/or glucocorticoids
- Prenatal and childhood factors include being small for gestational age (SGA), rapid compensatory weight gain postnatally, and premature adrenarche.
- Epigenetic factors observed in animal models include maternal hyperandrogenism and diabetes.
- Ovarian follicular growth arrests at the antral stage before a dominant follicle occur, leading to chronic anovulation.
- Insulin resistance or sensitivity varies by cell location.
  - Hepatic, adipose, and musculoskeletal insulin resistance
  - Adrenal, ovarian, and hypothalamic insulin sensitivity
- Insulin resistance leads to hyperinsulinism. Hyperinsulinism leads to theca cell androgen production and decreased hepatic sex hormone–binding globulin (SHBG) production with increased free testosterone.
- Obesity can worsen insulin resistance, PCOS symptoms, and risk of T2D.
- 17-hydroxyprogesterone progesterone secretion is hyperresponsive to gonadotropins.
- Decreased suppression of testosterone secretion by dexamethasone may be seen. This suggests ovarian hyperandrogenism.

ETIOLOGY

- Unknown
- Several potential mechanisms may begin neuroendocrine abnormalities, excessive ovarian and adrenal hyperandrogenism, and metabolic dysfunction.
- LH hypersecretion is common in women with PCOS and could be a primary neuroendocrine effect or due to hyperandrogenism.
- Although the molecular mechanisms responsible for insulin resistance and hyperinsulinemia in PCOS are uncertain, improved insulin sensitivity by weight loss or metformin therapy improves PCOS symptoms.

COMMONLY ASSOCIATED CONDITIONS

- Generalized obesity or overweight diagnosis
- Insulin resistance
- Impaired glucose tolerance
- T2D
- Dyslipidemia with low HDL and elevated triglycerides
- Metabolic syndrome
- Endometriosis
- Hypertension (use age/sex tables)
- Increased risk for cardiovascular disease
- Nonalcoholic fatty liver disease
- Sleep apnea
- Depression, anxiety, impaired social functioning

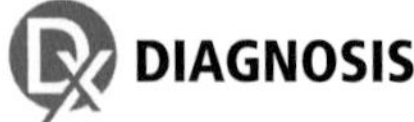

DIAGNOSIS

Signs and symptoms

- Amenorrhea or irregular menses
- Abnormal uterine bleeding
- Hyperandrogenism (clinical or biochemical)
- Hirsutism in context of ethnicity
- Polycystic ovaries on ultrasound or MRI
- Exclusion of other disorders (see "Differential Diagnosis")
- Infertility may occur in adulthood.

HISTORY

- Birth weight, gestational history
- Age at pubertal onset and pattern
- Menstrual history
- Infertility and reproductive history
- Hirsutism, acne, temporal hair loss (more common in older patients)
- Family history of PCOS, hyperandrogenism, T2D, infertility
- Medication history

PHYSICAL EXAM

- BMI ≥95th percentile for age
- Hirsutism (increased androgen-dependent terminal hair)
- Acanthosis nigricans
- Acne that is severe, scarring, and/or early onset
- Hydradenitis suppurativa
- Presence of clitoromegaly

DIFFERENTIAL DIAGNOSIS

- Physiologic adolescent anovulation
- Premature ovarian failure
- Thyroid dysfunction
- Hyperprolactinemia
- Exogenous exposure to androgens
- Androgen-secreting tumors
- Cushing syndrome
- Nonclassical virilizing congenital adrenal hyperplasia

P

DIAGNOSTIC TESTS & INTERPRETATION

- Hormone determinations:
  - LH, FSH
  - Total and free testosterone measured by reliable methods
  - SHBG
  - Morning 17-hydroxyprogesterone
  - Androstenedione
  - Dehydroepiandrosterone sulfate (DHEAS)
  - Prolactin
  - Thyroid function studies (free T_4, TSH)
  - HgbA1c
  - Antimüllerian hormone (AMH)
  - Salivary cortisol (midnight) or 24-hour urinary free cortisol
- Stimulation and tolerance tests:
  - Oral glucose tolerance test to assess for impaired fasting glucose, impaired glucose tolerance, or T2D
  - Consider referral to endocrinologist for evaluation of possible Cushing syndrome, nonclassical congenital adrenal hyperplasia, or androgen-secreting tumor.
- Imaging studies:
  - Ovarian ultrasound or pelvic MRI to assess ovarian volume
  - Follicle count is not recommended in adolescent girls as a criterion.

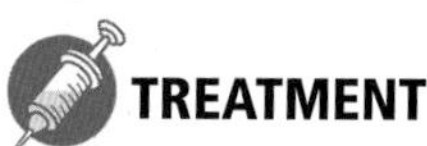

TREATMENT

GENERAL MEASURES

- Treatment should be individualized to reduce hyperandrogenism effects, regulate menses and ovulation, and decrease risk for infertility and comorbidities.
- Lifestyle modification
  - Dietary change for at least 2–5% weight loss
  - Concomitant regular exercise
- Pharmacologic
  - Combined oral contraceptives
  - Metformin (if abnormal glucose tolerance)
  - Spironolactone
  - Antiandrogens (flutamide, finasteride)
  - Statins or other lipid-lowering agents
  - Oral progestins
- Consider longitudinal reevaluation by withdrawing combined oral contraceptives for 3 months (after providing contraceptive counseling) when adolescent is gynecologically mature to determine if hyperandrogenic anovulation is persistent.

SURGERY/OTHER PROCEDURES

- Ovarian surgery is not recommended.
- Bariatric surgery in obese patients may improve fertility and metabolic disease.
- Hirsutism may be further addressed with laser therapy, depilatory, bleaching, threading, or other dermatologic procedure.

ONGOING CARE

COMPLICATIONS

- Impaired glucose tolerance, metabolic syndrome, and T2D
- Infertility
- Increased pregnancy loss
- Gestational diabetes, pregnancy-associated hypertension, and preeclampsia
- Greater endometrial cancer risk
- Impaired self-image, decreased quality of life

ADDITIONAL READING

- Abbott DH, Bacha F. Ontogeny of polycystic ovary syndrome and insulin resistance in utero and early childhood. *Fertil Steril*. 2013;100(1):2–11.
- Carmina E, Oberfield SE, Lobo RA. The diagnosis of polycystic ovary syndrome in adolescents. *Am J Obstet Gynecol*. 2010;203(3):201.e1–201.e5.
- de Melo AS, Dias SV, Cavalli RD, et al. Pathogenesis of polycystic ovary syndrome: multifactorial assessment from the foetal stage to menopause. *Reproduction*. 2015;150(1):R11–R24.
- Javed A, Chelvakumar G, Bonny AE. Polycystic ovary syndrome in adolescents: a review of past year evidence. *Curr Opin Obstet Gynecol*. 2016;28(5):373–380.
- McGee WK, Bishop CV, Bahar A, et al. Elevated androgens during puberty in female rhesus monkeys lead to increased neuronal drive to the reproductive axis: a possible component of polycystic ovary syndrome. *Hum Reprod*. 2012;27(2): 531–540.
- Moran LJ, Pasquali R, Teede HJ, et al. Treatment of obesity in polycystic ovary syndrome: a position statement of the Androgen Excess and Polycystic Ovary Syndrome Society. *Fertil Steril*. 2009;92(6):1966–1982.
- Rosenfield RL. The diagnosis of polycystic ovary syndrome in adolescents. *Pediatrics*. 2015;136(6): 1154–1165.
- Sirmans SM, Pate KA. Epidemiology, diagnosis, and management of polycystic ovary syndrome. *Clin Epidemiol*. 2014;6:1–13.
- Witchel SF, Oberfield S, Rosenfield RL, et al. The diagnosis of polycystic ovary syndrome during adolescence. *Horm Res Paediatr*. 2015;83(6): 376–389.

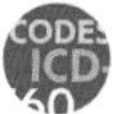

CODES

ICD10

- E28.2 Polycystic ovarian syndrome
- L68.0 Hirsutism

FAQ

- Q: Can PCOS patients get pregnant?
- A: Yes. Women with PCOS should not assume they will always be infertile. Some patients may become pregnant spontaneously, and others can become pregnant with reproductive induction of ovulation.
- Q: What can I do about acne and embarrassing body hair?
- A: Combined oral contraceptives and spironolactone can improve these symptoms over 3 to 6 months. Dermatology intervention may be used when hirsutism treatment has been started or to remove acne scarring.
- Q: Will my daughter inherit this disorder?
- A: Daughters can inherit PCOS. Diagnosis may be suspected in daughters with low birth weight, premature adrenarche, increased BMI, and/or early menarche.
- Q: Will losing weight help with PCOS symptoms?
- A: Some of the PCOS symptoms can result from obesity. These include insulin resistance with hyperinsulinism. Insulin resistance can lead to low SHBG and elevated free testosterone and alter ovarian function. Weight loss of 5% may improve PCOS symptoms.

POLYCYTHEMIA

Benjamin J. Huang, MD • Tannie Huang, MD

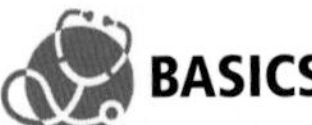

BASICS

DESCRIPTION

Polycythemia (sometimes referred to as erythrocytosis) is defined as an absolute increase in red blood cell (RBC) mass, most commonly suspected in the context of an elevated hemoglobin, hematocrit, or RBC count. Use of age- and gender-based norms is critical, as they fluctuate throughout childhood. Polycythemia can be categorized as follows:

- Primary polycythemia: Defect within erythroid progenitors, resulting in overproduction of RBCs. Serum erythropoietin (EPO) levels are usually low.
- Secondary polycythemia: stimulation of erythrocyte production by an increased level of EPO, which is either elevated appropriately in response to hypoxia or elevated inappropriately due to an EPO-producing tumor or exogenous administration
- Relative polycythemia: elevated hemoglobin, hematocrit, or RBC count without a true increase in RBC mass, often caused by decreased plasma volume in the setting of dehydration

EPIDEMIOLOGY

Primary polycythemias are very rare in children:

- Myeloproliferative neoplasms, including polycythemia vera (PV): Vast majority of cases occur in older adults, but cases of childhood PV have been described.
- Primary familial and congenital polycythemia (PFCP): very rare but presents during infancy or childhood
- The incidence and prevalence of secondary polycythemias depend on the respective underlying conditions.

RISK FACTORS

Genetics

Inherited polycythemias are very rare:

- PFCP: autosomal dominant
- Chuvash polycythemia: autosomal recessive disorder affecting individuals from the Chuvash Republic in Russia
- 2,3-bisphosphoglycerate (2,3-BPG) mutase deficiency: autosomal recessive

GENERAL PREVENTION

There are no preventive measures for conditions of primary polycythemia. Treatment of underlying conditions, such as correction of congenital heart disease, will prevent the development of secondary polycythemia.

PATHOPHYSIOLOGY

- Primary polycythemias:
  - PV: myeloproliferative neoplasm arising from a clonal population of abnormal hematopoietic progenitor cells with EPO-independent proliferation. EPO levels are usually low. The mutation *JAK2* V617F is found in the vast majority of cases.
  - PFCP: Erythroid progenitors are hypersensitive to EPO. Some families have a mutation in the EPO receptor (EPO-R).
- Secondary polycythemias:
  - High altitude: compensation for low atmospheric oxygen pressure
  - Chronic pulmonary disease or hypoventilation: compensation for inadequate oxygenation
  - Cyanotic heart disease and arteriovenous malformations: right-to-left cardiac or extracardiac shunting, resulting in desaturation of arterial blood
  - High oxygen-affinity hemoglobinopathies: mutation in either α- or β-globin chains leading to increased oxygen affinity and decreased oxygen delivery to tissues
  - 2,3-BPG mutase deficiency: rare defect that leads to deficiency of 2,3-BPG and decreased oxygen delivery to tissues
  - Methemoglobinemia: elevated levels of Fe^{3+} hemoglobin, which has an increased affinity for oxygen compared to Fe^{2+} hemoglobin
  - Carboxyhemoglobinemia: Carbon monoxide binds to hemoglobin preferentially compared to oxygen.
  - Hypoxia-sensing pathway defects: Mutations in the gene von Hippel Lindau (VHL) are common in certain ethnic groups (Chuvash polycythemia).
  - EPO-producing tumors: renal cell carcinoma, hepatocellular carcinoma, hemangioblastoma, pheochromocytoma, and uterine fibroids

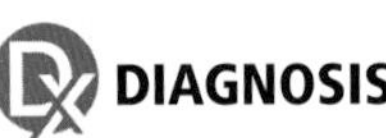

DIAGNOSIS

HISTORY

- Age of onset:
  - Neonates, who are born to mothers with pre-eclampsia or diabetes, are small for gestational age, undergo delayed cord clamping, or have certain chromosomal abnormalities (e.g., Down syndrome), are at increased risk for polycythemia during the neonatal period.
- Weight:
  - Obesity is associated with obstructive sleep apnea.
- Dehydration:
  - Diuretic use or abuse
  - Severe diarrhea
- Hyperviscosity:
  - Headache, dizziness, syncope, transient blindness, history of thrombosis
- Symptoms concerning for congenital heart disease or chronic pulmonary disease:
  - Cyanosis
  - Decreased exercise tolerance
  - Shortness of breath
  - Dyspnea on exertion
- Pruritus:
  - Seen with PV
- Sleep history:
  - Snoring, nocturnal apnea, mouth breathing, excessive daytime sleepiness, behavioral problems concerning for obstructive sleep apnea
- Living situation:
  - High altitude
  - Older house with fuel-burning heaters
  - Cigarette exposure
- Social history:
  - Smoking
  - Drug use including steroids, EPO, diuretics
- Family history:
  - High hematocrit, hyperviscosity, or need for phlebotomy
  - Household members with similar symptoms may also indicate concurrent exposure to carbon monoxide.

PHYSICAL EXAM

Signs and symptoms:

- Pulse oximetry
- Cyanosis
- Plethora
- Clubbing
- Cardiac murmurs or bruits
- Dehydration
- Splenomegaly

ALERT

- Fingerstick hematocrit: Squeezing the finger to collect a specimen may give a falsely elevated hematocrit.
- Capillary hematocrit: often higher than venous hematocrit
- Dehydration during blood draw may result in relative polycythemia due to decreased plasma volume.
- Pa_{O_2} is only interpretable with an arterial blood gas.

DIFFERENTIAL DIAGNOSIS

- Primary polycythemia
  - PV
  - PFCP
- Secondary polycythemia
  - High altitude
  - Chronic pulmonary disease
  - Hypoventilation: obstructive sleep apnea, neuromuscular disorders, severe obesity (Pickwickian syndrome), or congenital central hypoventilation syndrome
  - Right-to-left cardiac shunts
  - Arteriovenous malformations
  - High oxygen-affinity hemoglobinopathies
  - 2,3-BPG mutase deficiency
  - Methemoglobinemia
  - Carbon monoxide poisoning
  - EPO-producing tumors: renal cell carcinoma, hepatocellular carcinoma, hemangioblastoma, pheochromocytoma, uterine fibroids
  - Status—postrenal transplant
  - Exogenous testosterone or EPO: competitive athletes
  - Cobalt poisoning: Homemade beer may contain cobalt.
- Neonatal polycythemia
  - Preeclampsia or gestational hypertension
  - Small for gestational age
  - Gestational diabetes
  - Delayed cord clamping
  - Placental transfusion
  - Twin-to-twin transfusion
- Relative polycythemia
  - Cigarette smoking
  - Dehydration

DIAGNOSTIC TESTS & INTERPRETATION

Initial Tests (screening, lab, imaging)

- Many patients may be asymptomatic with polycythemia noted on routine screening.
- Initial workup should include the following:
  - CBC with differential: Polycythemia may be associated with abnormalities in other lineages.
  - Arterial blood gas with co-oximetry: $Pa{O_2}$ may be low in cardiopulmonary diseases. Co-oximetry allows for evaluation of carboxyhemoglobin and methemoglobin levels. Half-life of carboxyhemoglobin is 4 hours, so testing should be timed to accurately reflect exposures.
  - BUN, serum creatinine, and urinalysis to evaluate renal function
  - Serum EPO may be helpful in distinguishing primary from secondary polycythemia, but there is significant overlap in EPO levels between the two categories.
- Further investigation:
  - Oxygen dissociation p50: the partial pressure of oxygen at which hemoglobin is 50% saturated
  - Hemoglobin electrophoresis: Normal results do not rule out the presence of high oxygen-affinity hemoglobin, as many abnormal hemoglobins can comigrate with normal hemoglobins. If there is a high index of suspicion, consider molecular genetic analysis of globin genes.
  - 2,3-BPG level
  - Testosterone level
  - Genetic testing for *JAK2* V617F mutation
- Chest radiograph: for clinical findings concerning for chronic pulmonary disease
- Abdominal ultrasound: for clinical findings concerning for abdominal tumors

Diagnostic Procedures/Other

- EKG and echocardiogram: for clinical findings concerning for congenital heart disease
- Polysomnography sleep study: for clinical findings concerning for sleep apnea
- If myeloproliferative neoplasm is suspected, bone marrow aspirate and biopsy with cytogenetics should be performed.

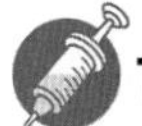

TREATMENT

GENERAL MEASURES

- Most asymptomatic patients with secondary polycythemia require no additional therapy other than management of their underlying condition.
- Pediatric patients with primary polycythemia are managed with phlebotomy alone. Low-dose aspirin may be considered to reduce thrombosis risk.
- In neonatal polycythemia, partial exchange transfusion should be considered based on symptoms and degree of polycythemia.

MEDICATION

Primary polycythemia should be managed by a hematologist. Certain medications, such as hydroxyurea and interferon-α, may be considered.

ISSUES FOR REFERRAL

Unexplained cyanosis, symptoms concerning for hyperviscosity, or persistent elevation in hematocrit that is not related to dehydration or neonatal etiologies

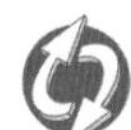

ONGOING CARE

FOLLOW-UP RECOMMENDATIONS

Patient Monitoring

Periodic laboratory follow-up depending on the etiology of polycythemia. Monitor for the following:

- Headache, dizziness, or syncope
- Blurred vision or transient vision loss
- Decreased exercise tolerance, shortness of breath, or dyspnea on exertion
- Stroke or thrombosis

PROGNOSIS

Depends on underlying condition:

- PV: guarded as may progress to acute leukemia
- High oxygen-affinity hemoglobinopathies: excellent
- Other secondary polycythemias: depends on underlying condition

ADDITIONAL READING

- Cario H, McMullin MF, Pahl HL. Clinical and hematological presentation of children and adolescents with polycythemia vera. *Ann Hematol.* 2009;88(8):713–719.
- Messinezy M, Pearson TC. The classification and diagnostic criteria of the erythrocytoses (polycythaemias). *Clin Lab Haematol.* 1999;21(5):309–316.
- Ozek E, Soll R, Schimmel MS. Partial exchange transfusion to prevent neurodevelopmental disability in infants with polycythemia. *Cochrane Database Syst Rev.* 2010;(1):CD005089.
- Prchal JT. Polycythemia vera and other primary polycythemias. *Curr Opin Hematol.* 2005;12(2):112–116.
- Sarkar S, Rosenkrantz TS. Neonatal polycythemia and hyperviscosity. *Semin Fetal Neonatal Med.* 2008;13(4):248–255.
- Tefferi A. Polycythemia vera and essential thrombocythemia: 2012 update on diagnosis, risk stratification, and management. *Am J Hematol.* 2012;87(3):285–293.

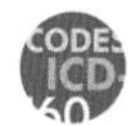

CODES

ICD10

- D45 Polycythemia vera
- D75.1 Secondary polycythemia
- P61.1 Polycythemia neonatorum

FAQ

- Q: What are common causes of polycythemia in the pediatric population?
- A: Secondary polycythemias. In particular, neonates and patients with cyanotic heart disease commonly present with polycythemia.
- Q: What are common causes of relative polycythemia?
- A: Dehydration and heavy cigarette smoking have been associated with decreased plasma volume and relative polycythemia.
- Q: When should a child with polycythemia be referred to a pediatric hematologist?
- A: The child should be referred to a pediatric hematologist if there are symptoms concerning for hyperviscosity or if the elevation in hematocrit is persistent and not clearly due to dehydration or neonatal etiologies.

POLYPS, INTESTINAL

Anthony F. Porto, MD, MPH

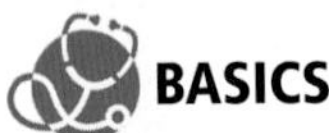

BASICS

DESCRIPTION

- Intestinal polyps are abnormal tissue growths protruding from the intestinal mucosa into the lumen.
  - Most common in children are solitary juvenile polyps, but these may also be multiple in number.
  - May be associated with various polyposis syndromes
- Classified by gross appearance
  - Pedunculated: mushroom-like and attached to mucosa with a narrow stalk
  - Sessile: elevated, flat lesions broadly attached to mucosa
- Types of polyps:
  - Hamartomas
  - Adenomatous
- Hamartomatous polyps
  - Juvenile polyps: usually a solitary polyp
  - Juvenile polyposis syndrome (>3 to 5 juvenile polyps or any number of juvenile polyps with a positive family history)
    - Juvenile polyposis of infancy
    - Juvenile polyposis coli (colonic involvement only)
    - Generalized juvenile polyposis (small bowel and colonic involvement)
  - Peutz-Jeghers syndrome
  - Cowden syndrome
  - Bannayan-Riley-Ruvalcaba syndrome (BRRS)
- Adenomatous polyps
  - Familial adenomatous polyposis (FAP)
    - Severe form and attenuated forms
  - Gardner syndrome (colonic polyps with osteomas and epidermal inclusion cysts)
  - Turcot syndrome (colonic polyps with brain tumors)
- Other polyposis syndromes
  - MUTYH-associated polyposis syndrome
  - Serrated polyposis syndrome

EPIDEMIOLOGY

- Juvenile polyps are the most common childhood polyps:
  - Account for >90% of polyps seen in children
  - 1–2% of asymptomatic children are estimated to have juvenile polyps.
  - Typically present between 2 and 5 years of age
  - Twice as common in boys than girls
  - >5 juvenile polyps should raise clinical suspicion for juvenile polyposis syndrome.
- Adenomatous polyps in FAP may present in early childhood or adolescence with an average age of onset of 16 years.

Prevalence

- Juvenile polyposis syndrome: 1 in 100,000 to 1 in 160,000
- Peutz-Jeghers syndrome: 1 in 25,000 to 1 in 300,000
- FAP: 1 in 5,000 to 1 in 17,000

RISK FACTORS

Family history of polyposis syndrome

Genetics

Different genes and inheritance patterns with various polyposis syndromes:

- Juvenile polyposis syndrome
  - Autosomal dominant with variable penetrance
  - Mutations in *SMAD4* and *BMPR1A* genes, involved in transforming growth factor-β (TGF-β) signal transduction
  - *SMAD4* mutation also associated with hereditary hemorrhagic telangiectasia and arteriovenous malformations
- Peutz-Jeghers syndrome
  - Autosomal dominant
  - Mutations in *STK11/LKB1* tumor suppressor gene are associated.
- Cowden syndrome and BRRS
  - Autosomal dominant
  - Associated with mutations in *PTEN* gene
- FAP
  - Autosomal dominant
  - Mutation in adenomatous polyposis coli (*APC*) tumor suppressor gene

PATHOPHYSIOLOGY

Mutations in tumor suppressor genes likely lead to dysregulation of cell proliferation and apoptosis in polyposis syndromes.

COMMONLY ASSOCIATED CONDITIONS

- Juvenile polyposis syndrome, Cowden syndrome, and BRRS all have juvenile polyps as part of their manifestations.
  - Cowden syndrome is associated with colonic and gastric polyps with extraintestinal symptoms including mucocutaneous lesions, thyroid adenomas and goiter, fibroadenomas and fibrocystic disease of the breast, uterine leiomyomas, and macrocephaly.
  - BRRS is associated with colonic and ileal polyps.
- Peutz-Jeghers syndrome is characterized by multiple gastrointestinal (GI) pedunculated hamartomatous polyps.
- FAP, Gardner, and Turcot syndrome are characterized by multiple adenomatous polyps.

DIAGNOSIS

HISTORY

- Family history of polyps or polyposis syndrome is essential to obtain.
- Presence and amount of blood in stool
- Signs and symptoms:
  - Frequently asymptomatic
  - Painless rectal bleeding is typical presentation.
  - Iron deficiency anemia
  - Prolapsing rectal lesion
  - Abdominal pain or obstruction from intussusception
  - Diarrhea
- History of congenital anomalies, including malrotation, hydrocephalus, Meckel diverticulum, and cardiac defects, seen in 20% of juvenile polyposis syndrome

PHYSICAL EXAM

- Digital rectal exam may identify rectal polyp.
- Pigmentation of skin and mucous membranes consistent with Peutz-Jeghers syndrome. These skin findings typically appear at birth and become lighter by puberty.
- Mucocutaneous lesions such as facial trichilemmoma, oral fibromas, and acral keratosis are seen in Cowden syndrome.
- Mental retardation, macrocephaly, lipomatosis, hemangiomas, and genital pigmentation are seen in BRRS.
- Presence of visible osteomas in the skull, mandible, and tibia in Gardner syndrome
- Congenital hypertrophy of the retinal pigmented epithelium via ophthalmoscopic exam with FAP

DIFFERENTIAL DIAGNOSIS

Because juvenile polyps often present with rectal bleeding, the differential diagnosis for lower GI bleeding should be considered:

- Milk protein allergy (in infants)
- Anal fissure
- Meckel diverticulum
- Infectious enterocolitis
- Inflammatory bowel disease
  - Inflammatory polyps (also known as "pseudopolyps") typically occur in ulcerative colitis more than Crohn disease.
  - These are not true polyps but rather associated with inflammatory infiltrate with distorted mucosa. Grossly resemble adenomatous polyps; as a result, biopsy is recommended to differentiate, although removal is not indicated unless symptomatic. Histology demonstrates normal, regenerating mucosa surrounded by areas of mucosal loss.
- Intussusception
- Vascular malformation
- Hemorrhoids
- Hemolytic uremic syndrome
- Henoch-Schönlein purpura
- Rectal trauma
- Neoplasm

DIAGNOSTIC TESTS & INTERPRETATION

Initial Tests (screening, lab, imaging)

- Stool test for occult blood may be positive.
- CBC can assess degree of anemia and also for baseline hemoglobin before polypectomy.
- PT/PTT should be considered before polypectomy due to risk of bleeding.
- Genetic testing can be considered if a polyposis syndrome is suspected.
- Use of urine and tissue matrix metalloproteinases (MMPs) as biomarkers for the presence of polyps is being researched.
- Radiologic studies are not the most effective methods of identifying polyps but can be used:
  - Barium enema may identify colonic polyps.
  - Upper GI with small bowel study may locate presence of small bowel polyps.
  - Use of CT and MR colonography has been studied mainly in adults.

Diagnostic Procedures/Other

- Full colonoscopy with polypectomy is the preferred test to perform.
- Flexible sigmoidoscopy may miss polyps in proximal colon:
  - 32% of juvenile polyps are located proximal to splenic flexure.
  - 12% of patients with juvenile polyps only have polyps located proximal to splenic flexure.

- Video capsule endoscopy and balloon enteroscopy may be useful to identify small bowel polyps.
- Pathologic findings
  - Polyp pathology cannot be determined by gross visualization; hence polyps must be removed for histologic exam.
  - Juvenile polyps
    - Hamartomatous but occasionally capable of adenomatous changes
    - Potential of malignancy in a solitary juvenile polyp is extremely low but is increased in juvenile polyposis syndrome where there is also an increased risk for other malignancies including gastric, duodenal, and pancreatic cancers.
  - Peutz-Jeghers syndrome
    - Hamartomatous
    - Microscopically have hyperplasia of the smooth muscle layer, extending in an arborizing, tree-like manner
    - Relatively low potential of GI malignancy but increased potential for malignancy in other organs such as breast, pancreas, ovary, testicle, and uterus
  - FAP
    - Adenomatous polyps
    - Lifetime risk for colorectal cancer is 100%.
    - Thousands of polyps are common by adulthood in the severe form of FAP with mean age of colorectal cancer of 35 years if untreated.
    - In attenuated FAP, 20 to 100 colonic polyps are common with mean age of colorectal cancer of 50 to 60 years
    - Associated with gastric, duodenal, and periampullary polyps
    - Increased association with hepatoblastoma, periampullary carcinoma (risk of 5–10%), and desmoid tumors. Gastric polyps have low malignant potential.
    - Desmoid tumors are second most common cause of mortality after colorectal cancer.
    - Other malignancies: liver, extrahepatic biliary tree, adrenals, and thyroid

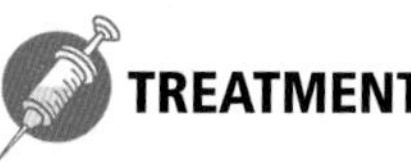

TREATMENT

GENERAL MEASURES

Full colonoscopy with polypectomy is an essential diagnostic and therapeutic tool. Removal of GI polyps can help to control symptoms and reduce the risk of malignancy.

MEDICATION

Administration of some NSAIDs (such as sulindac and celecoxib) may slow progression or reduce the number of adenomatous polyps.

ISSUES FOR REFERRAL

Patients suspected of having a polyp or polyposis syndrome should be referred to a gastroenterologist for evaluation. Patients with polyposis syndromes should be referred to a tertiary care center for genetic counseling.

SURGERY/OTHER PROCEDURES

- When adenomatous polyps are identified in FAP, prophylactic colectomy should be considered.
- Indications for surgery for Peutz-Jeghers syndrome include obstruction, bleeding, or diagnosed cancer because polyps may be found diffusely throughout the colon.
- Colectomy should also be considered in other polyposis syndromes with innumerable polyps or polyps showing premalignant changes.
- The main surgical options include a subtotal colectomy with ileorectal anastomosis (IRA) or a proctocolectomy with ileal pouch–anal anastomosis (IPAA).
- Treatment of Cowden and BRRS is typically dictated by symptoms, and prophylactic colectomy is not recommended.

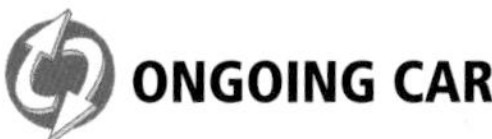

ONGOING CARE

FOLLOW-UP RECOMMENDATIONS

- For solitary juvenile polyps, follow-up with stool guaiac check and CBC 6 months after polypectomy. Repeat colonoscopy is indicated with any abnormalities.
- For polyposis syndromes, screening recommendations differ depending on the syndrome:
  - Typically involve surveillance colonoscopies every 1 to 3 years depending on findings
  - Asymptomatic children with an *APC* mutation for FAP should have annual colonoscopies starting at 10 to 12 years of age with an upper endoscopy to evaluate especially for parapapillary polyps (10–20% malignant risk every 1 to 3 years after the first colonic polyp is found).
  - Patients with juvenile polyposis syndrome should begin screening with colonoscopy when symptomatic or beginning at 15 years old. If colonic polyps are found, annual screening is recommended and screening is recommended every 2 to 3 years if no polyps found.
  - Patients with Peutz-Jeghers syndrome should undergo upper endoscopy, colonoscopy, and upper GI series with small bowel follow-through every 2 years starting at 20 years old. Regular evaluation for other malignancies via physical exam, mammography at 25 years (breast cancer), annual Pap smear (cervical), and transvaginal ultrasound (ovarian) or testicular ultrasound (testicular cancer) should also be done.
  - Published guidelines for follow-up of patients with various polyposis syndromes are available.

ADDITIONAL READING

- Barnard J. Screening and surveillance recommendations for pediatric gastrointestinal polyposis syndromes. *J Pediatr Gastroenterol Nutr*. 2009;48(Suppl 2):S75–S78.
- Chow E, Macrae F. A review of juvenile polyposis syndrome. *J Gastroenterol Hepatol*. 2005;20(11):1634–1640.
- Durno CA. Colonic polyps in children and adolescents. *Can J Gastroenterol*. 2007;21(4):233–239.
- Erdman SH, Barnard JA. Gastrointestinal polyps and polyposis syndromes in children. *Curr Opin Pediatr*. 2002;14(5):576–582.
- Giardiello FM, Trimbath JD. Peutz-Jeghers syndrome and management recommendations. *Clin Gastroenterol Hepatol*. 2006;4(4):408–415.
- Gupta SK, Fitzgerald JF, Croffie JM, et al. Experience with juvenile polyps in North American children: the need for pancolonoscopy. *Am J Gastroenterol*. 2001;96(6):1695–1697.
- Merg A, Howe JR. Genetic conditions associated with intestinal juvenile polyps. *Am J Med Genet C Semin Med Genet*. 2004;129C(1):44–55.
- Shussman N, Wexner SD. Colorectal polyps and polyposis syndromes. *Gastroenterol Rep (Oxf)*. 2014;2(1):1–15.
- Thakkar K, Fishman DS, Gilger MA. Colorectal polyps in childhood. *Curr Opin Pediatr*. 2012;24(5):632–637.

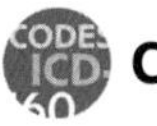

CODES

ICD10

- K63.89 Other specified diseases of intestine
- D12.6 Benign neoplasm of colon, unspecified
- Q85.8 Other phakomatoses, not elsewhere classified

FAQ

- Q: What is the potential of developing cancer from a polyp?
- A: Risk of neoplasia depends on the type of polyp:
  - Patients with solitary juvenile polyps have essentially no increased risk of colorectal carcinoma.
  - Patients with juvenile polyposis syndrome have been reported to have up to a 65% chance of developing GI cancer, with the risk of malignancy commencing from age 20 years.
  - Patients with Peutz-Jeghers syndrome have been reported to have almost a 50% chance of developing cancer in the intestinal tract or another organ systems.
  - Patients with FAP have a 100% lifetime risk of developing colorectal cancer.
- Q: Is a flexible sigmoidoscopy sufficient for the detection of polyps?
- A: No. Approximately 37% of patients with juvenile polyps have polyps proximal to the splenic flexure, and 12% of patients have only proximal colon polyps. A flexible sigmoidoscopy would not identify these polyps, making it necessary to perform a full colonoscopy.
- Q: What is your management recommendation for a patient with painless rectal bleeding that stops on its own?
- A: It is widely believed that pedunculated polyps will autoamputate after outgrowing their blood supply, although there is no objective evidence supporting this process. If there is no family history of a polyposis syndrome, the patient can be followed with stool guaiac checks and a CBC in 6 months. If there is a family history, then referral to a gastroenterologist for full colonoscopy is indicated.
- Q: How many polyps can patients have?
- A: Patients with juvenile polyposis syndrome often have 50 to 200 polyps distributed throughout the colon. Patients with FAP may have a few to over a thousand polyps in the colon.
- Q: When does endoscopic surveillance typically begin for children with FAP?
- A: It is generally recommended that annual endoscopic surveillance begin between 10 and 12 years of age in patients with an *APC* mutation.

PORTAL HYPERTENSION

Pamela L. Valentino, MD, MSc, FRCP(C)

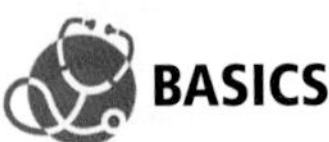

BASICS

DESCRIPTION

- Definition of portal hypertension (P-HTN): elevation of portal pressure (PP) >5 mm Hg
  - Risk of developing complications occurs with "clinically significant P-HTN": PP >10 mm Hg
  - Significant risk of bleeding from esophageal varices (EV) with PP >12 mm Hg
- May be pre-, intra-, or posthepatic in origin
- A major cause of morbidity and mortality in children with chronic liver disease

PATHOPHYSIOLOGY

- P-HTN is secondary to both increases in portal resistance and portal blood flow:
  - Other contributing factors include hyperdynamic circulation, expanded intravascular volume, systemic arteriolar vasodilatation, decreased splanchnic arteriolar tone, and humoral factors (i.e., nitric oxide).
- Portosystemic collaterals develop to decompress the high PPs, leading to a number of sequelae, all with high morbidity and mortality risks, including:
  - Variceal hemorrhage
  - Splenomegaly/hypersplenism
  - Ascites
  - Spontaneous bacterial peritonitis
  - Hepatorenal syndrome
  - Hepatopulmonary syndrome
  - Portopulmonary hypertension
  - Hepatic encephalopathy

ETIOLOGY

- Prehepatic (presinusoidal) causes:
  - Portal vein thrombosis (PVT) with cavernous transformation (increased risk with umbilical vein catheterization, sepsis, dehydration, hypercoagulable state)
  - Splenic vein thrombosis
- Intrahepatic (sinusoidal) causes:
  - Hepatocellular disorders: cirrhosis (secondary to chronic viral hepatitis [e.g., Hep B, Hep C, etc.], α_1-antitrypsin deficiency, autoimmune hepatitis, Wilson disease, glycogen storage disease, tyrosinemia, etc.), schistosomiasis, peliosis hepatitis, vitamin A toxicity
  - Biliary tract disorders: cirrhosis (secondary to biliary atresia, intrahepatic cholestasis syndromes, primary sclerosing cholangitis, cystic fibrosis, etc.), ductal plate malformation/congenital hepatic fibrosis, choledochal cyst
- Posthepatic (postsinusoidal) causes:
  - Budd-Chiari syndrome: occlusion of suprahepatic inferior vena cava or hepatic veins by congenital web, tumor, or thrombus
  - Congestive hepatopathy (cardiac: right-sided heart failure or hypertension, such as post-Fontan procedure; pulmonary hypertension)
  - Sinusoidal obstruction syndrome (veno-occlusive disease of hepatic sinusoids and terminal venules)

DIAGNOSIS

HISTORY

- History of neonatal umbilical catheterization
- History of chronic hepatitis; underlying medical problem such as cystic fibrosis, tyrosinemia, glycogen storage disease, Wilson disease
- History of abdominal trauma, clotting disorder, use of oral contraceptive pills
- Ingestion of excessive amounts of vitamin A
- Hematemesis, hematochezia, or melena: Variceal bleed may be the first sign of long-standing silent liver disease or previously undiagnosed PVT.
- Cyanosis or exercise intolerance (hepatopulmonary syndrome)
- Mental status changes with memory loss, irregular hand writing, poor academic performance (hepatic encephalopathy).

PHYSICAL EXAM

- Growth failure
- Oxygen desaturation (hepatopulmonary syndrome)
- Pallor (GI bleeding and anemia)
- Digital clubbing
- Palmar erythema
- Telangiectasia
- Prominent vascular pattern on the abdomen (caput medusa)
- Hepatomegaly may or may not be present.
- Splenomegaly
- Ascites (distension, fluid wave)
- Scrotal edema in males with ascites
- Hemorrhoids
- Asterixis (hepatic encephalopathy, although uncommon in children)

DIAGNOSTIC TESTS & INTERPRETATION

Initial Tests (screening, lab, imaging)

- Liver enzymes: alanine aminotransferase (ALT), aspartate aminotransferase (AST), alkaline phosphatase, and γ-glutamyl transferase (GGT; may be elevated with cholestasis and bile duct injury)
- Assessment of liver synthetic function: bilirubin (total, direct/conjugated), albumin, PT/INR
- Basic metabolic profile: electrolytes (hyponatremia can occur with cirrhosis), blood urea nitrogen and creatinine (elevated with hepatorenal syndrome)
- Ammonia: elevated with P-HTN and shunting, but may not correlate well with degree of hepatic encephalopathy
- CBC: detects hypersplenism and thrombocytopenia, anemia of chronic disease/GI bleeding
- Abdominal ultrasound with Doppler to evaluate:
  - Liver size, contour, and echogenicity
  - Biliary anatomy
  - Spleen size
  - Renal cysts
  - Presence of ascites
  - Vessel patency and direction of blood flow
  - Presence of EV or splenorenal shunt
- Additional laboratory testing to determine the cause of underlying liver disease, depending on clinical scenario (see chapter on "Chronic Hepatitis" for more details)

Follow-Up Tests & Special Considerations

- Esophagogastroduodenoscopy (EGD) for surveillance of EV. In the setting of acute GI tract bleeding, EGD can identify and treat variceal rupture.
- Abdominal paracentesis to determine etiology of ascites and test for spontaneous bacterial peritonitis
- Bubble (contrast) echocardiogram to assess for hepatopulmonary syndrome in the setting of P-HTN and oxygen desaturation

Diagnostic Procedures/Other

- Liver biopsy: identifies the underlying cause of P-HTN
- CT or MRI angiography to evaluate for PVT or Budd-Chiari syndrome; need to specify the desired venous phases that should be studied (PV/HV)
- Hepatic venous pressure gradient (HVPG) and selective angiography are seldomly used in pediatrics.

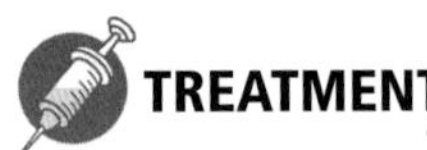

TREATMENT

GENERAL MEASURES

Management of EV:

- Risk of bleeding from EV is increased in setting of P-HTN and the presence of splenomegaly and thrombocytopenia. Surveillance endoscopy and primary prophylaxis (intervention to prevent the first GI bleed) with esophageal band ligation in children with P-HTN is controversial with variations in clinical practice.
- An acute GI bleed from EV is treated with EGD with band ligation.
- Sclerotherapy is used in small children (<10 kg), because endoscopic band ligation is not feasible. However, sclerotherapy is less effective and carries higher complication rates.
- Following acute bleeding from EV, serial EGD and band ligation are performed until varices are eradicated.
- Secondary prophylaxis (prevention of recurrent GI bleeding) can be achieved with endoscopic band ligation or sclerotherapy, β-blockade, portosystemic shunts, and liver transplantation. The approach may depend on the underlying cause of the P-HTN.

MEDICATION

- β-Blockade: Nonselective β-blockers, such as propranolol, have been shown to be effective in preventing both initial (primary prophylaxis) and recurrent (secondary prophylaxis) variceal bleeds in adults. Data are limited on use of β-blockers in children with P-HTN to prevent initial or recurrent variceal bleeding. Use in children for this indication is empiric and mainly based on adult data:
  - Mechanisms include lowering portal blood flow and thus PP by both β_2-blockade, which increases splanchnic tone, and β_1-blockade, which decreases cardiac output.
  - Propranolol, specifically, may also decrease collateral circulation.
  - β-Blocker effect on decreasing cardiac output may blunt an adaptive cardiovascular response (elevated heart rate) in the event of a hemorrhage; these medications should not be used in patients with asthma or diabetes.

- Diuretic therapy (spironolactone, +/− furosemide, +/− chlorothiazide) to treat ascites
- Lactulose is used to treat and prevent hepatic encephalopathy in patients with cirrhosis.

SURGERY/OTHER PROCEDURES

- Portosystemic shunts
  - Splenorenal shunt can decompress the P-HTN; performed preferentially in patients with compensated cirrhosis (Child-Turcotte-Pugh class A—lowest severity of liver disease)
  - The MesoRex bypass (mesenteric to left portal vein shunt) is performed in the setting of cavernous transformation of the portal vein without the presence of advanced liver disease/cirrhosis.
  - Transjugular intrahepatic portosystemic shunt (TIPS) procedure may be an effective bridge to liver transplantation in pediatric patients with progressive liver disease and recurrent variceal bleeds; may worsen hepatic encephalopathy
  - Thrombosis of any of these shunts may occur, so anticoagulation may be used.
- Liver transplantation
  - Referral to a liver transplant center for transplant evaluation is recommended following the first sign of cirrhotic decompensation: GI bleeding, ascites, hepatic encephalopathy, etc.

ADMISSION, INPATIENT, AND NURSING CONSIDERATIONS

Acute management of variceal bleed

- Stabilize the patient and transfer to a hospital with advanced endoscopic capabilities in pediatrics.
- Vital signs: Remember that hemodynamic instability can be masked by β-blockers.
- Fluid resuscitation: two large-bore IV catheters or intraosseous needles; give crystalloid initially and then transfuse pRBC (goal hemoglobin of 7 to 9 g/dL).
- IV fluids with high glucose infusion rate (D10) in setting of cirrhosis and NPO status
- Nasogastric tube placement: Lavage with room temperature saline or sterile water until clear; leave tube in place for evaluation and removal of continued or recurrent bleeding.
- Correction of coagulopathy: parenteral vitamin K (IM), fresh frozen plasma, platelet transfusion if platelets $<50{,}000/\mu L$
- IV antibiotics: Bacterial translocation can precipitate recurrent variceal hemorrhage.
- IV proton pump inhibitor to decrease risk of bleeding from ulcers or erosions
- Pharmacotherapy to control active bleeding
  - Octreotide IV (somatostatin analog with longer half-life) decreases splanchnic blood flow via its inhibition of intestinal vasoactive peptide secretion. In turn, portal blood pressure is decreased. Patient should be NPO while on continuous IV octreotide.
  - Vasopressin decreases splanchnic blood flow via its vasoconstriction effects, but its use is limited owing to systemic vasoconstriction and a poor side effect profile. Nitroglycerin, a venodilator, has been used in conjunction with vasopressin to decrease side effects. However, this combination is not preferred.
- Lactulose to treat hepatic encephalopathy in patients with cirrhosis
- Endoscopy (after stabilization) to determine source of hemorrhage (variceal rupture or other, such as gastric ulcer) and perform therapeutic procedures such as endoscopic band ligation or sclerotherapy for EV versus injection or clip placement for ulcers
- Direct tamponade: Sengstaken-Blakemore tube for severe uncontrollable hemorrhage but high rate of complications such as esophageal rupture; patient must be intubated; seldomly used in pediatrics
- Interventional radiology: variceal embolization, TIPS; seldomly used in pediatrics
- Surgical intervention: portosystemic shunt, esophageal devascularization, and/or transection; in general, last resort
- Referral to a pediatric liver transplant center

ALERT

- The site of bleeding needs to be identified and managed appropriately: Not all GI bleeding in a patient with P-HTN is an upper GI tract source (i.e., hemorrhoids); nasogastric lavage will help to determine if the problem is from the upper tract.
- Phytonadione (vitamin K) can be given IM; anaphylaxis can occur with the IV formulation.

ONGOING CARE

FOLLOW-UP RECOMMENDATIONS

- Patients are followed closely for hepatic decompensation.
- Growth failure, recurrent life-threatening bleeds not controllable with prophylactic intervention, refractory ascites, and poor quality of life are indications for liver transplantation.

DIET

Sodium restriction when ascites is present

PROGNOSIS

- The disease course and prognosis depend on the underlying cause.
- Acute variceal bleeding is associated with a 6-week mortality of up to 30% in adults. The mortality rate in children is much lower.
- Patients with congenital hepatic fibrosis also do very well because the underlying disease is not progressive and bleeding may be easily managed with endoscopic therapy.
- Progressive liver disease has a worse prognosis and often requires liver transplantation.

COMPLICATIONS

- Hemorrhage from varices (esophageal, gastric) may present as hematemesis, hematochezia, or melena.
- Hemorrhoids
- Splenomegaly/hypersplenism
- Malabsorption due to congestion of the intestinal mucosa
- Ascites, spontaneous bacterial peritonitis
- Hepatorenal syndrome
- Hepatopulmonary syndrome (intrapulmonary right-to-left shunting) leads to hypoxemia, shortness of breath, exercise intolerance, and digital clubbing.
- Portopulmonary hypertension can be a life-threatening complication of P-HTN.
- Hepatic encephalopathy

ADDITIONAL READING

- Abd El-Hamid N, Taylor RM, Marinello D, et al. Aetiology and management of extrahepatic portal vein obstruction in children: King's College Hospital experience. *J Pediatr Gastroenterol Nutr*. 2008;47(5):630–634.
- Garcia-Tsao G, Abraldes JG, Berzigotti A, et al. Portal hypertensive bleeding in cirrhosis: risk stratification, diagnosis, and management: 2016 practice guidance by the American Association for the Study of Liver Diseases. *Hepatology*. 2017;65(1):310–335.
- Gugig R, Rosenthal P. Management of portal hypertension in children. *World J Gastroenterol*. 2012;18(11):1176–1184.
- Ling SC. Advances in the evaluation and management of children with portal hypertension. *Semin Liver Dis*. 2012;32(4):288–297.
- Shneider BL, Abel B, Haber B, et al; for Childhood Liver Disease Research and Education Network. Portal hypertension in children and young adults with biliary atresia. *J Pediatr Gastroenterol Nutr*. 2012;55(5):567–573.
- Shneider BL, de Ville de Goyet J, Leung DH, et al. Primary prophylaxis of variceal bleeding in children and the role of MesoRex bypass: summary of the Baveno VI Pediatric Satellite Symposium. *Hepatology*. 2016;63(4):1368–1380.

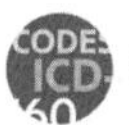

CODES

ICD10

- K76.6 Portal hypertension
- K72.90 Hepatic failure, unspecified without coma
- K76.81 Hepatopulmonary syndrome

FAQ

- Q: What is my child's long-term prognosis?
- A: Disease prognosis of P-HTN depends on the underlying cause. Variceal bleeding associated with prehepatic causes of P-HTN such as PVT typically becomes less problematic as the child ages and may be managed with endoscopic therapy.
- Q: What anticipatory guidance should be provided to patients with P-HTN?
- A: With any hematemesis/GI bleeding, emergent evaluation for variceal bleeding should be obtained and 911 should be called for transportation.
- Q: Are there any medications I should avoid giving my child with P-HTN?
- A: Avoid aspirin and NSAID-containing products such as ibuprofen.

POSTERIOR URETHRAL VALVES

Ryan W. Zipper, MD • Andrew A. Stec, MD

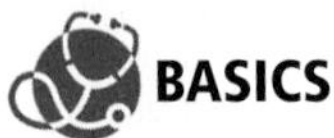

BASICS

DESCRIPTION

- A posterior urethral valve (PUV) is an embryologic remnant of tissue in the urethra that causes obstruction of the lower urinary tract during fetal development.
- This obstruction results in short- and long-term structural abnormalities and physiologic dysfunction in the genitourinary system (kidney, ureter, bladder, and urethra).

EPIDEMIOLOGY

- Most common cause of lower urinary tract obstruction in males
- The incidence is estimated to be between 1:3,000 and 1:8,000 live male births.
- PUVs are the cause of 10% of urinary obstructions diagnosed prenatally.
- Approximately 24–45% of children born with PUV will exhibit renal insufficiency during childhood and approximately 50% progress to end-stage renal disease in 10 years.
- PUV accounts for up to 17% of the cases of children with end-stage renal failure.
- Children with PUVs receive 25% of pediatric renal transplantations.

RISK FACTORS

Genetics

- Majority of cases are isolated and occur sporadically.
- Rarely, cases have been reported in siblings.
- No causative genetic abnormality has yet been found.

PATHOPHYSIOLOGY

- The valve is a leaflet or membrane of thin connective tissue that extends from the anterior urethral lip to the verumontanum posteriorly, obstructing the normal flow of urine through the urethra. This results in an elongated urethra and upstream dilation in the urinary system.
- PUVs exist in a spectrum of severity, from being lethal *in utero* to subtle symptoms late in childhood.
- PUVs are commonly associated with intrinsic renal dysplasia. Studies have demonstrated that dysplastic renal parenchyma at time of birth is permanent.
- Renal injury may be caused by persistent high pressure (reversible) as well as renal dysplasia (irreversible).
- Commonly associated pathophysiologic findings in children with PUV include (i) hydroureteronephrosis, (ii) dilated bladder with trabeculations and/or diverticulum, and (iii) vesicoureteral reflux.
- PUVs may result in early or late bladder dysfunction with decreased compliance and increased voiding pressure that affect both the storage and expulsion of urine. Additionally, PUVs expose the upper tract of the urinary system to increased pressure, which leads to worsening renal function over time.
- Neonates may have respiratory failure (due to pulmonary hypoplasia) and limb and facial malformations (due to oligo- or anhydramnios).

ETIOLOGY

- Multiple theories exist as to the embryologic origin of PUVs.
- Male urethral development is usually complete by 14 weeks' gestation; PUV formation is presumed to occur prior to this point.
- Possible embryologic origin of PUVs include (i) presence of an obstructing membrane in the posterior urethra, (ii) overgrowth or abnormal folding during normal urethral development, (iii) abnormal integration of the wolffian ducts into urethral development, or (iv) abnormal persistence of the urogenital membrane.

COMMONLY ASSOCIATED CONDITIONS

- Genitourinary: hydroureteronephrosis, vesicoureteral reflux, bladder wall thickening and diverticulum, obstructive urinary symptoms, urinary ascites in cases of bladder rupture, perirenal urinoma in cases of renal collecting system rupture, renal dysplasia
- Varying degrees of renal insufficiency may also be present in patients from birth through adulthood.
- PUV has been associated with other congenital anomalies of the genitourinary tract, prune belly syndrome, imperforate anus, and congenital heart disease.

DIAGNOSIS

HISTORY

- PUVs generally present in four ways:
  - Fetal diagnoses by ultrasound (US)
  - Neonates with respiratory distress, abdominal distension, metabolic abnormalities
  - Infants with a febrile urinary tract infection (UTI)/sepsis/poor urinary stream
  - Delayed presentation in children with UTI or voiding difficulties
- Fetal presentation (diagnosis on US)
  - Dilated, thick-walled bladder
  - Bilateral and in some cases unilateral hydroureteronephrosis
  - "Keyhole sign": dilated posterior urethra at the base of the bladder
  - Decreased amniotic fluid/oligohydramnios
- Neonatal presentation
  - Tachypnea/respiratory distress
  - Poor feeding/failure to thrive/abdominal distension
  - Lethargy/acidosis and azotemia
  - Cardiovascular compromise and arrhythmia/hyperkalemia
  - Delayed or infrequent voiding
- Infant/toddler presentation
  - Failure to thrive
  - Abdominal distension
  - Fever of unknown origin
  - Febrile UTI
  - Urosepsis
- Delayed presentation
  - UTI
  - Abnormal or weak urinary stream
  - Urinary complaints such as hesitancy, incomplete emptying, dysuria, straining
  - Urinary incontinence, sometimes with palpable bladder
  - Polyuria and urinary frequency secondary to renal concentrating defect

PHYSICAL EXAM

- A palpable bladder is the most common physical exam finding. In infants, abdominal distension may be present from severe bladder distension and hydroureteronephrosis or urinary ascites.
- Hyperpigmented perigenital skin may also be noted from severe incontinence and urine irritation of the skin.

DIAGNOSTIC TESTS & INTERPRETATION

Initial Tests (screening, lab, imaging)

- Screening
  - Renal and bladder US in any patient with hydronephrosis noted prenatally
- Lab
  - Urinalysis: UTI, proteinuria, low specific gravity
  - Metabolic panel: elevated creatinine, azotemia, acidosis, hyperkalemia, hyponatremia, renal tubular acidosis (RTA) (type IV)
  - CBC: leukocytosis from UTI; anemia in renal insufficiency
- Imaging
  - Renal and bladder US:
    - Dilation of posterior urethra (keyhole sign), distended/thick-walled bladder with possible diverticula and hypertrophied bladder neck, hydroureteronephrosis, echogenic or dysplastic renal parenchyma
    - Diameter of posterior urethra on postnatal US >6 mm (sensitivity 100%, specificity 89%, PPV 88%)
  - Voiding cystourethrogram (VCUG):
    - Diagnostic study of choice
    - Shows dilated posterior urethra with abnormal runoff of urine in the posterior urethra, change in caliber between posterior and anterior urethra (normal ratio 3:1), capacious bladder with possible trabeculations or diverticulum, vesicoureteral reflux
  - Kidney, ureter, and bladder (KUB) radiograph
    - Ground-glass appearance in cases of bladder rupture and urinary ascites
    - Not a diagnostic study for PUV

Follow-Up Tests & Special Considerations

- Metabolic panel: Creatinine nadir is a predictor of long-term renal function.
- US: Hydroureteronephrosis may improve or persist after valve ablation.

Diagnostic Procedures/Other

Operative cystoscopy: Visual evaluation of urethra and bladder provides definitive diagnosis with identification of a valve.

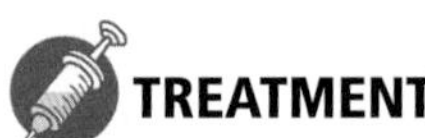

TREATMENT

GENERAL MEASURES

Supportive

- Insertion of a urethral catheter or feeding tube in the neonate to bypass obstruction is the initial treatment.
- Confirm placement of catheter in the bladder by US, as small catheters may coil in the posterior urethra and drain some urine, giving the false impression of being located within the bladder.
- Correction of electrolyte abnormalities with careful observation for postobstructive diuresis
- Monitoring of fluid status
- Prophylactic antibiotics should be started due to an increased risk of UTI.
- UTIs should be treated as complicated.
- Consultation with a pediatric urologist

ISSUES FOR REFERRAL

- Neonates suspected of having PUVs prenatally with abnormal amniotic fluid volume should be delivered at a hospital with pediatric subspecialists.
- Lifelong follow-up is required, as renal insufficiency and bladder dysfunction can occur at any time during infancy, childhood, puberty, or adulthood.

SURGERY/OTHER PROCEDURES

- Resection of the valve (ablation) is the definitive treatment of the primary lesion; typically performed cystoscopically (through the urethra)
- *In utero* drainage of the fetal bladder is performed at some centers. Typically, this procedure is performed on patients with good urine parameters to mitigate pulmonary dysfunction from oligohydramnios. However, no significant improvement has been found in long-term renal outcome compared to valve ablation after delivery.
- If the infant is premature or the urethra is too small for the cystoscope, a vesicostomy may be required.
- Supravesical diversion (of the kidney or ureter) is sometimes performed in select patients who fail to improve after bladder decompression; this procedure is associated with poorer long-term bladder function.
- Following valve ablation, the posterior urethra should have decreasing dilation on VCUG. Improvement in hydroureteronephrosis and vesicoureteral reflux (if it resolves spontaneously) will occur more slowly.

ADMISSION, INPATIENT, AND NURSING CONSIDERATIONS

- Neonates should be monitored in the hospital with NICU level monitoring until metabolic and respiratory derangements have been stabilized. Nurses should document strict intake and output on patients and monitor for respiratory compromise.
- Infants with urosepsis, febrile UTIs, or failure to thrive after surgical intervention should be admitted for evaluation and management.

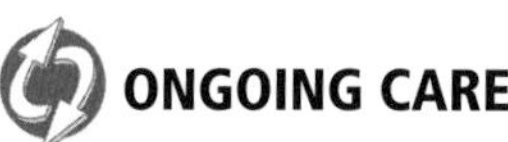

ONGOING CARE

FOLLOW-UP RECOMMENDATIONS

Patient Monitoring

- Careful follow-up through adulthood should be performed.
- Pediatric urology follow-up is required for future reconstructive procedures and monitoring of bladder function, reflux, and hydronephrosis.
- Pediatric nephrology follow-up is recommended for long-term monitoring and mitigation of renal dysfunction.
- Visits should include the following:
  - Imaging (US) to evaluate renal, ureteral, and bladder anatomy
  - Assessment of bladder function (incontinence, UTI, incomplete emptying)
  - Blood pressure monitoring
  - Serial creatinine
  - Urinalyses to asses for proteinuria
  - Assessment of overall linear growth
  - Serum 25-hydroxy vitamin D and intact parathyroid hormone
- Recurrent obstruction following ablation occurs in approximately 10–20% of cases, possibly due to residual valve or from stricture formation. This may require repeat valve ablation or further surgery.
- Patients with persistent incontinence, those who develop incontinence, or those with incomplete bladder emptying may require urodynamic evaluation to evaluate the bladder function/physiology and tailor therapy.

PATIENT EDUCATION

- Families should be educated on the risk of progression of renal dysfunction despite treatment of PUV, and children may progress to need for dialysis or renal transplant.
- Families should be educated on the possibility of delayed obstruction from urethral stricture or incomplete valve resection.
- Patients may have voiding dysfunction such as incontinence, straining, incomplete emptying, and weak urinary stream.
- Any fevers in the patient should prompt consideration of UTI.

PROGNOSIS

- Oligohydramnios during pregnancy is a predictor of worse long-term renal outcomes. More severe issues are typically noted when oligo- or anhydramnios occurs earlier in pregnancy.
- Pulmonary hypoplasia (with concomitant renal dysfunction) accounts for the highest mortality in infants.
- Overall, the prognosis for severe PUV has improved over the past few decades, owing to earlier recognition and improved management of pulmonary hypoplasia and fluid and metabolic derangements.
- The rate of improvement in renal function after the valvular obstruction is relieved is more indicative of prognosis than initial creatinine at presentation.
- A creatinine level of <0.8 mg/dL around 1 year of age has the best long-term renal prognosis in patients treated in infancy.
- A nadir creatinine level <1 mg/dL may still be associated with eventual renal failure as the child ages; monitoring is warranted in all cases.
- Patient may progress to renal failure and require renal transplantation at any point during childhood or adulthood. An abnormal creatinine at 2 years of age carries higher likelihood of end-stage renal progression during adolescence or puberty.
- Children who develop proteinuria have bilateral renal dysplasia and/or bladder dysfunction and are more likely to eventually develop renal insufficiency and hypertension.

COMPLICATIONS

- Intrauterine oligohydramnios in severe cases may result in Potter syndrome and pulmonary hypoplasia.
- Renal dysplasia and parenchymal damage may lead to progressive renal failure, including associated issues, such as anemia, acidosis, fluid and electrolyte abnormalities, and failure to thrive.
- UTIs and vesicoureteral reflux are commonly associated with PUV.
- Urinary incontinence may result from overactive bladder (uninhibited contractions), incomplete emptying (bladder noncompliance), and polyuria.

ADDITIONAL READING

- Chertin B, Cozzi D, Puri P. Long-term results of primary avulsion of posterior urethral valves using a Fogarty balloon catheter. *J Urol*. 2002;168(4, Pt 2):1841–1843.
- Eckoldt F, Heling KS, Woderich R, et al. Posterior urethral valves: prenatal diagnostic signs and outcome. *Urol Int*. 2004;73(4):296–301.
- Hodges SJ, Patel B, McLorie G, et al. Posterior urethral valves. *ScientificWorldJournal*. 2009;9:1119–1126.
- Holmes N, Harrison MR, Baskin LS. Fetal surgery for posterior urethral valves: long-term postnatal outcomes. *Pediatrics*. 2001;108(1):E7.
- Krishnan A, de Souza A, Konijeti R, et al. The anatomy and embryology of posterior urethral valves. *J Urol*. 2006;175(4):1214–1220.
- Radhakrishnan J. Obstructive uropathy in the newborn. *Clin Perinatol*. 1990;17(1):215–239.
- Roth KS, Carter WH Jr, Chan JC. Obstructive nephropathy in children: long-term progression after relief of posterior urethral valve. *Pediatrics*. 2001;107(5):1004–1010.
- Yiee J, Wilcox D. Management of fetal hydronephrosis. *Pediatr Nephrol*. 2008;23(3):347–353.

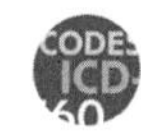

CODES

ICD10

- Q64.2 Congenital posterior urethral valves
- Q64.39 Other atresia and stenosis of urethra and bladder neck
- N28.89 Other specified disorders of kidney and ureter

FAQ

- Q: Do patients with PUV have decreased fertility?
- A: Limited studies suggest that children treated for PUV appear to have similar fertility rates as the general population. Rarely, investigation into causes of infertility of men has found undiagnosed PUVs. Persistent dilatation of the posterior urethra, damage to tissue near the verumontanum, and urethral strictures from valve ablation can affect ejaculation.
- Q: What can be done for children with long-term bladder dysfunction and incontinence?
- A: Patients should be on a comprehensive bowel and bladder regimen due to increased incidence of voiding dysfunction. Additionally, more advance bladder management including intermittent catheterization and pharmacotherapy may be required.
- Q: Are patients with PUVs good candidates for renal transplantation?
- A: PUV patients have a 5-year transplanted kidney survival rate of around 50%, likely resulting from poor bladder function. Therefore, aggressive bladder management and long-term follow-up are prudent in these patients.
- Q: What is "valve-bladder syndrome"?
- A: A valve-bladder is a bladder that is noncompliant and stores urine at high pressure, increasing the incidence of renal damage. It is thought to occur in approximately 20% of PUV patients.
- Q: What is vesicoureteral reflux and unilateral renal dysplasia (VURD) syndrome in PUV patients?
- A: VURD occurs in 13% of PUV patients. A single renal unit has renal dysplasia and severe reflux, thereby allowing the high bladder pressures in PUV to be transmitted to a single kidney, sparing the contralateral (nonrefluxing) kidney from damage.

PRECOCIOUS PUBERTY

Patrick C. Hanley, MD, FAAP • Andrew C. Calabria, MD

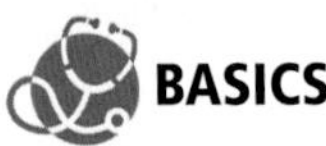

BASICS

DESCRIPTION

- In most populations, the mean ages of onset of puberty are 10.5 years in girls and 11.5 years in boys.
  - Girls: The first sign of puberty is most commonly breast development (thelarche), followed by pubic hair (pubarche), and then menarche, which generally occurs 2 to 3 years after thelarche.
  - Boys: The first sign is usually testicular enlargement, followed by pubarche and penile growth.
- Definitions
  - Precocious puberty has traditionally been defined as physical signs of sexual development before age 8 years in girls and age 9 years in boys (2 to 2.5 standard deviations below the mean age of onset of puberty).
  - Guidelines in 1999 by the Pediatric Endocrine Society proposed lowering the age considered to be normal for sexual development in girls to as young as age 6 years in African American girls and age 7 years in Caucasian girls. These guidelines have not been universally adopted.
- When evaluating precocious puberty, the entire clinical picture must be considered, including the rate of pubertal progression and the presence of any neurologic symptoms.

EPIDEMIOLOGY

- Occurs in ~1 in 5,000 children
- Up to 10 times more common in girls than boys
- In girls: 80–90% of central precocious puberty is idiopathic.
- In boys: Precocious puberty is more likely to be associated with underlying pathology.
- Only ~50% of boys have idiopathic central precocious puberty.
- Racial differences observed in girls: African American girls may enter puberty 1 year sooner on average than Caucasian girls; racial differences not present in males
- Increased incidence in internationally adopted children and in children born premature or small for gestational age

RISK FACTORS

Genetics

Genetic causes include the following:

- Familial male precocious puberty (testotoxicosis): sex-limited, autosomal dominant inheritance of luteinizing hormone (LH) receptor activating mutation
- McCune-Albright syndrome: sporadic, postzygotic, somatic mutation in the stimulatory subunit of G-protein receptor; precocious puberty more common in girls
- More recently mutations in kisspeptin (*KISS1*), kisspeptin receptor (*KISS1R*), and makorin ring finger protein 3 (*MKRN3*) genes have been identified as genetic causes of central precocious puberty.

PATHOPHYSIOLOGY

- Central precocious puberty can be associated with central nervous system (CNS) disorders.
- Peripheral precocious puberty
  - Arises from peripheral sex hormone sources, including gonadal and adrenal disorders, abdominal or pelvic tumors, or exogenous sex steroids
  - Can progress to central precocious puberty due to maturation of the hypothalamic–pituitary axis by sex steroids

ETIOLOGY

- Central precocious puberty (gonadotropin-releasing hormone [GnRH] dependent)
  - Associated with gonadotropin (LH and/or follicle-stimulating hormone [FSH]) levels that are elevated beyond the normal prepubertal range; results from activation of hypothalamic–pituitary–gonadal axis
  - Physical changes are typically those of normal puberty for a child of that sex.
- Peripheral sex hormone effects (peripheral precocious puberty or GnRH-independent; less common)
  - Gonadotropin-independent elevation of sex steroids arising (i) directly from gonads and/or adrenals, (ii) through stimulation of gonads by GnRH-independent mechanism, or (iii) from an exogenous source
  - Physical changes reflect predominant excess hormones (estrogenic or androgenic) and are often markedly discordant from normal pubertal development.

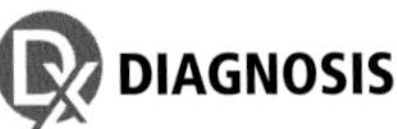

DIAGNOSIS

Signs and symptoms

- Careful history focusing on chronology: physical changes, growth spurt, onset of menses
- Neurologic, visual, or behavioral changes suggest a CNS lesion.

HISTORY

- Family history of early puberty (e.g., menarche before age 10 years) or hyperandrogenic disorders (e.g., congenital adrenal hyperplasia)
- Presence of exogenous sex steroid medications or creams in home

PHYSICAL EXAM

- Plot accurate height (using wall-mounted stadiometer), weight, and growth velocity. Growth acceleration within the past year may be strong evidence for puberty.
- Careful inventory of early estrogenic and androgenic effects
- Estrogenic effects
  - Girls: careful staging of breasts and color of vaginal mucosa
  - Boys: gynecomastia in prepubertal child (Gynecomastia is common and normal part of puberty in pubescent male.)
- Androgenic effects
  - Girls: careful staging of pubic hair, clitoromegaly
  - Boys: careful staging of testicular volume (with Prader orchidometer or by measuring testicular length), penile size, and pubic hair
- Examine skin for acne and café au lait spots.
- Perform comprehensive neurologic evaluation to assess for possible CNS pathology.

DIFFERENTIAL DIAGNOSIS

- Causes of central precocious puberty:
  - Often idiopathic (girls >> boys)
  - Any cause of peripheral precocious puberty
  - CNS tumors:
    - Hypothalamic hamartoma: most common CNS mass causing precocious puberty; benign (nonprogressive) congenital malformation of GnRH-secreting neurons
    - Chiasmatic–hypothalamic glioma: often associated with neurofibromatosis
    - Astrocytoma
    - Ependymoma
  - Post-CNS trauma or damage:
    - Surgery
    - Radiation: may occur after 18-Gy exposure
    - Hydrocephalus/other CNS malformations
    - Infections: brain abscess, meningitis, encephalitis, granuloma. Lesions may result in stimulation or lack of inhibition of GnRH-secreting area of the hypothalamus, resulting in early pituitary activation.
- Mimickers of central precocious puberty:
  - Human chorionic gonadotropin (hCG)-secreting tumors (pineal gland or liver): Ectopic hCG activates testicular LH receptors.
  - Severe, acquired hypothyroidism: Elevated thyroid-stimulating hormone (TSH) may cross-stimulate gonadal FSH and/or LH receptors.
- Causes of peripheral sex hormone effects:
  - Environmental: exogenous estrogens (creams and oral forms) and/or exogenous androgens (anabolic steroids or testosterone formulations)
  - Congenital adrenal hyperplasia: Poorly controlled congenital adrenal hyperplasia can activate the hypothalamic–pituitary–gonadal axis in either gender.
  - McCune-Albright syndrome: triad of precocious puberty, café au lait spots, and polyostotic fibrous dysplasia
  - Familial male precocious puberty (testotoxicosis)
  - Tumors (gonadal and adrenal)
  - Refeeding after severe malnutrition during early development (such as adopted children who had kwashiorkor)
- Incomplete pubertal development
  - Premature thelarche
  - Premature adrenarche
  - Premature menarche

DIAGNOSTIC TESTS & INTERPRETATION

Initial Tests (screening, lab, imaging)

- Labs should be selected based on inventory of estrogenic and/or androgenic effects and drawn in the early morning.
- Estrogenic effects
  - Girls: FSH, LH, (ultrasensitive, pediatric, immunochemiluminometric assays [ICMA] or electrochemiluminescent [ECL]) (LH is most accurate) and estradiol
  - Boys: ultrasensitive LH and FSH, estradiol, hCG level
- Androgenic effects
  - Total testosterone by assay designed to measure low concentrations, adrenal steroids including 17-hydroxyprogesterone (17-OHP) to evaluate for late-onset congenital adrenal hyperplasia and dehydroepiandrosterone sulfate (DHEA-S) to exclude or confirm adrenarche, and ultrasensitive LH to evaluate for central puberty
- Other tests
  - Prolactin: may be elevated with CNS tumors
  - TSH and free thyroxine (free T_4)
  - Avoid lower yield tests, such as total estrogens, nonultrasensitive LH, free testosterone levels (more helpful in adolescent girls with testosterone levels >30 ng/dL), and other adrenal steroids such as 17-hydroxypregnenolone and DHEA.
- Provocative stimulation tests should be done when tests are abnormal or equivocal:
  - GnRH test (typically leuprolide stimulation) for central precocious puberty; prepubertal GnRH response is predominantly FSH, whereas pubertal response is predominantly LH. Estradiol levels drawn 24 hours after leuprolide may improve the sensitivity of GnRH testing.
  - Adrenocorticotropic hormone (ACTH) stimulation test to evaluate adrenal abnormalities. Exogenous corticosteroid therapy will interfere with ACTH test but does not interfere with GnRH test of pituitary–gonadal axis.
- Bone age radiograph of left hand and wrist:
  - If advanced, further studies, guided by history and physical examination, warranted
  - If not advanced, or if only early breast or pubic hair development (but not both), premature thelarche or premature adrenarche, respectively, most likely diagnoses
- MRI of head:
  - In the absence of specific clues to CNS disease, the probability of an intracranial abnormality depends primarily on age of onset of puberty, rate of progression, and the sex of the child.
  - MRI is almost always done in boys because they are less likely than girls to have idiopathic precocious puberty.
- Ultrasound of gonads/adrenals:
  - As indicated by examination and studies
  - Evaluates for tumors in both sexes; in girls, ultrasound can also evaluate ovarian/uterine maturity.

ALERT

- Obese children often have advanced bone ages.
- Palpation of breast tissue (buds) can be difficult due to adiposity.

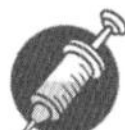

TREATMENT

MEDICATION

- Central precocious puberty: GnRH agonists (leuprolide depot injection or histrelin acetate implant) are treatment of choice. Adjunctive therapy with growth hormone may be needed to optimize final adult height.
- Calcium and vitamin D supplementation may assist bone mass accretion during GnRH agonist therapy.
- Peripheral sex hormone effects: aromatase inhibitors (letrozole or anastrozole) and antiandrogens (spironolactone or ketoconazole), glucocorticoids for congenital adrenal hyperplasia

ONGOING CARE

- When to expect improvement:
  - Depends on cause. For example, sexual changes of McCune-Albright syndrome are due to autonomously functioning ovarian cysts, which regress variably over time.
  - Treatment of central precocious puberty with a GnRH agonist usually results in cessation of menses within 2 months, slowing or nonprogression of pubertal changes over 4 to 6 months, and decreased rate of bone age acceleration within 12 months.
- Typically, GnRH agonists such as leuprolide (Lupron) are administered in a depot form every 28 days. Some children require shortening of the interval, often prompted by incomplete pubertal suppression. A longer acting formulation of leuprolide is sometimes used as an every 3-month injection. A 12-month duration implantable formulation histrelin acetate (Supprelin) is also available; in some children, histrelin may work for up to 2 years before requiring surgical replacement.
- The length of treatment is highly individualized but typically continues until the normal age of pubertal onset.

PROGNOSIS

- With treatment, improvement in predicted height may be achieved. Earlier treatment results in improved final height, but most children do not reach target height predicted by midparental height measurements.
- Treatment may decrease psychosocial distress.
- Long-term effects of central precocious puberty and GnRH agonists on fertility have not been fully elucidated.

COMPLICATIONS

- Short stature
- Psychosocial stresses of early puberty

ADDITIONAL READING

- Carel JC, Eugster EA, Rogol A, et al; for ESPE-LWPES GnRH Analogs Consensus Conference Group. Consensus statement on the use of gonadotropin-releasing hormone analogs in children. *Pediatrics*. 2009;123(4):e752–e762.
- Carel JC, Léger J. Clinical practice. Precocious puberty. *N Engl J Med*. 2008;358(22):2366–2377.
- Herman-Giddens ME, Slora EJ, Wasserman RC, et al. Secondary sexual characteristics and menses in young girls seen in office practice: a study from the Pediatric Research in Office Settings network. *Pediatrics*. 1997;99(4):505–512.
- Kaplowitz PB. Treatment of central precocious puberty. *Curr Opin Endocrinol Diabetes Obes*. 2009;16(1):31–36.
- Kaplowitz PB, Oberfield SE. Reexamination of the age limit for defining when puberty is precocious in girls in the United States: implications for evaluation and treatment. Drug and Therapeutics and Executive Committees of the Lawson Wilkins Pediatric Endocrine Society. *Pediatrics*. 1999;104(4, Pt 1): 936–941.
- Lewis KA, Goldyn AK, West KW, et al. A single histrelin implant is effective for 2 years for treatment of central precocious puberty. *J Pediatr*. 2013;163(4):1214–1216.
- Midyett LK, Moore WV, Jacobson JD. Are pubertal changes in girls before age 8 benign? *Pediatrics*. 2003;111(1):47–51.
- Nathan BM, Palmert MR. Regulation and disorders of pubertal timing. *Endocrinol Metab Clin North Am*. 2005;34(3):617–641.
- Oostdijk W, Rikken B, Schreuder S, et al. Final height in central precocious puberty after long term treatment with a slow release GnRH agonist. *Arch Dis Child*. 1996;75(4):292–297.
- Shin YL. An update on the genetic causes of central precocious puberty. *Ann Pediatr Endocrinol Metab*. 2016;21(2):66–69.
- Sun SS, Schubert CM, Chumlea WC, et al. National estimates of the timing of sexual maturation and racial differences among US children. *Pediatrics*. 2002;110(5):911–919.
- Tanner JM, Davies PS. Clinical longitudinal standards for height and height velocity for North American children. *J Pediatr*. 1985;107(3):317–329.

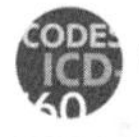

CODES

ICD10

- E30.1 Precocious puberty
- E22.8 Other hyperfunction of pituitary gland
- E30.8 Other disorders of puberty

FAQ

- Q: If my child is treated with a GnRH agonist, will he or she go through puberty when we stop the medication?
- A: Yes. Children on GnRH agonist treatment proceed through normal puberty when the medication is stopped. Effects on fertility have not been fully studied long-term.
- Q: If my child already has some pubertal changes, can they be reversed?
- A: If GnRH agonists are used, menses will cease, and breast tissue and pubic hair will often partially or completely regress.

PREMATURE ADRENARCHE

Patrick C. Hanley, MD, FAAP • Andrew C. Calabria, MD

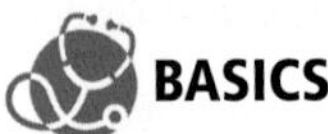

BASICS

DESCRIPTION

- Appearance of pubic hair before age 8 years in girls and age 9 years in boys with elevated adrenal androgens (dehydroepiandrosterone [DHEA] or dehydroepiandrosterone-sulfate [DHEA-S])
- Some data suggest that the age of normal sexual development onset in girls is younger than previously recognized, but lowering of the traditionally accepted limits remains subject to debate.
- Axillary hair, acne, and apocrine sweat gland secretion are not always present with premature adrenarche.
- No other signs of sexual development should be present.
- Presence of breast development in girls or testicular enlargement in boys suggests precocious puberty and not premature adrenarche.
- Occurs independently of hypothalamic–pituitary–gonadal axis activation seen with true puberty

RISK FACTORS

Genetics

- Often sporadic
- Familial patterns suggesting recessive and dominant inheritance have been described.

PATHOPHYSIOLOGY

- Concentrations of adrenal steroids such DHEA or DHEA-S increase earlier than typically seen in normal puberty.
- Note: Zona reticularis of adrenal normally begins to increase androgen secretion at age 6 to 8 years.

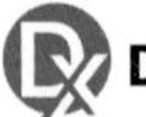

DIAGNOSIS

HISTORY

- Careful attention to presence of any other signs of sexual precocity, as well as rate of progression
- Family history of pubertal development, infertility, irregular menses, hirsutism, polycystic ovarian syndrome (PCOS), and premature male-pattern balding
- Birth weight that is small for gestational age (SGA) may predispose children to development of premature adrenarche.
- Obesity has been associated with an increased incidence of premature adrenarche.
- Girls with premature adrenarche are at increased risk for the development of PCOS.

PHYSICAL EXAM

- Linear growth velocity may be increased.
- The presence of pigmented, curly hairs in the pubic area is consistent with androgenic effect from adrenal steroids.
- In girls, clitoromegaly suggests congenital adrenal hyperplasia or androgen-secreting tumors.
- Acanthosis nigricans suggests that insulin resistance and risk of developing ovarian hyperandrogenism (PCOS) are present.

ALERT

Be careful to differentiate between true pubic hair (curly and short) and vellus or dark lanugo hair (straight, long, fine). An extra light source may be helpful.

DIFFERENTIAL DIAGNOSIS

- For infants with isolated pubic hair: idiopathic pubic hair of infancy
- Idiopathic premature pubarche: premature pubarche (pubic hair) with normal labs and bone age
- Congenital: late-onset (nonclassical) congenital adrenal hyperplasia
- Tumors: Androgen-secreting tumors can arise in the gonads or adrenal glands.
- Miscellaneous:
  - Central precocious puberty
  - Familial male precocious puberty (testotoxicosis)
  - Exogenous male hormone exposure
  - Hypertrichosis

DIAGNOSTIC TESTS & INTERPRETATION

Initial Tests (screening, lab, imaging)

- If predominantly androgenic effects are present, the most useful initial tests are as follows:
  - Total testosterone by pediatric assay
  - Adrenal steroids including 17-hydroxyprogesterone (17-OHP) to evaluate for late-onset congenital adrenal hyperplasia and DHEA-S to exclude or confirm adrenarche
  - Pediatric luteinizing hormone (LH), also listed as immunochemiluminometric (ICMA), electrochemiluminescent (ECL), or ultrasensitive, to evaluate for central puberty
- Adrenal steroids are often elevated for chronologic age but normal for pubertal stage (usually Tanner 2 or 3). However, testosterone and 17-OHP should be in prepubertal range.
- Additional hormone measurements are often lower yield.
  - These include hormones to evaluate for estrogenic effects (e.g., estradiol) when these effects (e.g., thelarche) are not present, adult LH or testosterone assays, and free testosterone levels (more helpful in adolescent girls with testosterone levels >30 ng/dL and with concerns for hyperandrogenism/PCOS).
  - Other adrenal steroids, such as 17-hydroxypregnenolone and DHEA, are typically less useful as 1st-line tests.
- Gonadotropin-releasing hormone (leuprolide) stimulation test: not routinely recommended but would have a normal prepubertal response
- Children with systemic signs of virilization (such as a significantly advanced bone age) or elevated adrenal steroids (17-OHP) should have adrenocorticotropic hormone (ACTH) stimulation testing to exclude congenital adrenal hyperplasia and other hyperandrogenic syndromes.

ALERT
When evaluating labs, be sure to note if correct assays (pediatric, ICMA, ECL, or ultrasensitive noted above) were used when ordering LH to evaluate for central puberty, and be careful to look at both age and pubertal reference ranges when included.

- Bone age may be advanced by 1 to 2 years but correlates with height age.
- Abdominal ultrasound, CT scan, or MRI should be considered if signs of significant virilization are present or if rapid progression has occurred; look for intracranial or intra-abdominal masses, especially if androgens are markedly elevated.

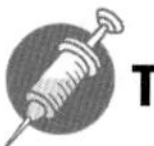

TREATMENT

GENERAL MEASURES

- No treatment
- Reassure parents and children that this is a benign process.
- Reassess every 6 months to look for signs of virilization and/or pubertal progression.

ONGOING CARE

- Regression does not occur.
- Increasing virilization suggests nonclassical congenital adrenal hyperplasia or early PCOS.
- Watch for other signs of puberty, such as breast development, testicular enlargement (≥4 mL), or growth acceleration that suggest onset of true precocious puberty.
- Acanthosis nigricans or signs of insulin resistance have been reported in girls with a history of premature adrenarche.
- Monitor for glucose intolerance or early type 2 diabetes. Fasting glucose and insulin levels or oral glucose tolerance test may be checked if suspicion is high (e.g., obesity, acanthosis nigricans, polyuria, polydipsia).

PROGNOSIS

- Undergo puberty appropriately with normal fertility.
- Ovarian or adrenal hyperandrogenism development during adolescence (also known as "PCOS") is more common in some girls with a history of premature adrenarche.
- Insulin resistance, a common finding in ovarian hyperandrogenism, has been reported in some children and adolescents with a history of premature adrenarche.
- Final adult height is not affected.

COMPLICATIONS

- Can be the first sign of true precocious puberty (i.e., development of breast tissue or testicular enlargement with advancement of bone age) and thus warrants careful observation
- Boys with premature adrenarche and precocious puberty are more likely than girls to have an underlying CNS disorder.

ADDITIONAL READING

- Auchus RJ, Rainey WE. Adrenarche—physiology, biochemistry and human disease. *Clin Endocrinol (Oxf)*. 2004;60(3):288–296.
- Herman-Giddens ME, Slora EJ, Wasserman RC, et al. Secondary sexual characteristics and menses in young girls seen in office practice: a study from the Pediatric Research in Office Settings network. *Pediatrics*. 1997;99(4):505–512.
- Ibáñez L, Jiménez R, de Zegher F. Early puberty-menarche after precocious pubarche: relation to prenatal growth. *Pediatrics*. 2006;117(1):117–121.
- Kaplowitz P. Clinical characteristics of 104 children referred for evaluation of precocious puberty. *J Clin Endocrinol Metab*. 2004;89(8):3644–3650.
- Kaplowitz PB, Oberfield SE. Reexamination of the age limit for defining when puberty is precocious in girls in the United States: implications for evaluation and treatment. Drug and Therapeutics and Executive Committees of the Lawson Wilkins Pediatric Endocrine Society. *Pediatrics*. 1999;104(4, Pt 1):936–941.
- Kousta E. Premature adrenarche leads to polycystic ovary syndrome? Long-term consequences. *Ann N Y Acad Sci*. 2006;1092:148–157.
- Midyett LK, Moore WV, Jacobson JD. Are pubertal changes in girls before age 8 benign? *Pediatrics*. 2003;111(1):47–51.
- Nebesio TD, Eugster EA. Pubic hair of infancy: endocrinopathy or enigma? *Pediatrics*. 2006;117(3): 951–954.
- Neville KA, Walker JL. Precocious pubarche is associated with SGA, prematurity, weight gain, and obesity. *Arch Dis Child*. 2005;90(3):258–261.
- Oberfield SE, Sopher AB, Gerken AT. Approach to the girl with early onset of pubic hair. *J Clin Endocrinol Metab*. 2011:96(6):1610–1622.
- Williams RM, Ward CE, Hughes IA. Premature adrenarche. *Arch Dis Child*. 2012; 97(3):250–254.

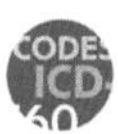

CODES

ICD10

E27.0 Other adrenocortical overactivity

FAQ

- Q: Is there a dietary cause of excess adrenal hormones?
- A: No.
- Q: Does premature adrenarche mean puberty will be early?
- A: The onset of puberty in these children is within the normal range and should follow the familial pattern.
- Q: Can anything be done to reverse the changes?
- A: This is a benign process that does not require treatment. Antiandrogen drugs are available but are not recommended. Girls are at increased risk for the development of PCOS, but most children do not have long-term sequelae from premature adrenarche.

PREMATURE THELARCHE

Patricia Vuguin, MD, MSc

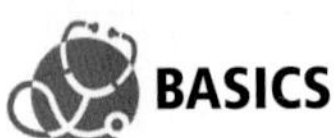

BASICS

DESCRIPTION

- Breast development in girls <8 years of age without evidence of sexual hair development, vaginal mucosa estrogenization, linear growth acceleration, rapid bone maturation, adult body odor, or behavioral changes
- Exaggerated thelarche, a variant of isolated breast development, occurs without axillary or pubic hair but with some acceleration of growth and bone maturation, and increased uterine size.
- Data suggest that African American girls may develop pubertal changes as early as 6 years of age and Caucasian girls as early as 7 years of age. However, caution should be used when evaluating children because signs of puberty at these younger ages may not be considered normal and may be due to pathologic conditions.

EPIDEMIOLOGY

- 60–85% of cases are noted between 6 months and 2 years of age.
- There is no one identifiable group of girls who develops early thelarche.

RISK FACTORS

Unknown

PATHOPHYSIOLOGY

- Transient increases in follicle-stimulating hormone levels causing follicular ovarian development.
- Low levels of estrogen secretion by normal follicular cysts
- Increased sensitivity of breast tissue to low levels of estrogen
- Delay in inhibition of the "minipuberty" of infancy
- Exposure to exogenous estrogen (e.g., cosmetic and hair products, lavender oil, infant formulas containing soy, xenoestrogens, and polybrominated diphenyl ethers)

DIAGNOSIS

HISTORY

- Careful assessment of onset and progression of breast tissue
- Careful assessment of growth (growth velocity changes in height percentiles)
- Family history of early puberty and or early menses
- Exogenous exposure to estrogens (e.g., foods, creams, etc.)

PHYSICAL EXAM

- Palpate carefully to distinguish fat from true breast tissue.
- Areolar hyperpigmentation and/or enlargement is usually not present.
- Galactorrhea is not present.
- Look carefully for other signs of puberty:
  - Menstrual blood
  - Dull, gray-pink, or rugose vaginal mucosa (vs. prepubertal appearance: shiny, bright red, and smooth)
  - Pubic or axillary hair or any other sign of androgen excess
- Inspect skin for birthmarks suggestive of McCune-Albright syndrome (café au lait spots in a "coast of Maine" pattern).
- Evaluate height and assess growth velocity.
- Evaluate for signs of hypothyroidism: goiter, short stature.

DIFFERENTIAL DIAGNOSIS

- Tumors: benign lipomas
- Congenital
  - Neonatal breast hyperplasia in newborn boys or girls that appears shortly after birth and is caused by gestational hormones
  - This form of breast development is normal and usually regresses.
- Severe acquired hypothyroidism
  - High levels of thyroid-stimulating hormone may cross-stimulate gonadal follicle–stimulating hormone and/or luteinizing hormone (LH) receptors.
- Gonadotropin-independent estrogen production
  - McCune-Albright syndrome: triad of precocious puberty, café au lait spots, and polyostotic fibrous dysplasia due to gain of function mutations of G proteins
  - Ovarian or adrenal tumors
- True precocious puberty

DIAGNOSTIC TESTS & INTERPRETATION

Initial Tests (screening, lab, imaging)

- No test is specific.
- Serum follicle-stimulating hormone, inhibin B, sex hormone–binding globulin, and estradiol may be slightly higher than age-matched controls but are not consistently elevated and often not necessary to measure.
- In isolated premature thelarche, serum ultrasensitive LH level is prepubertal.
- Bone age is not significantly or is very mildly advanced (<1 year ahead of chronologic age).
  - Bone age estimates the extent of estrogen stimulation because estrogen promotes bone maturation.
  - Advanced bone age implies significant estrogen effect, suggesting the need for evaluation of true precocious puberty.
  - Exception: Prepubertal obese girls often have advanced skeletal maturation.
- Breast ultrasonography
  - Not needed because its ability to distinguish precocious puberty from premature thelarche is limited
- Pelvic ultrasonography
  - Not generally needed; may demonstrate presence and regression of small ovarian cysts (1 to 15 mm) and a prepubertal-size uterus

ALERT

- It is a concern if a male infant outside of the newborn period or a young prepubertal boy shows breast enlargement.
- Must distinguish fat from breast tissue in obese girls
- Caution should be used when evaluating 6- to 7-year-old girls because signs of puberty at these younger ages may not be considered normal.
- Removal of a breast bud will result in failure of that breast to develop during adolescence.
- Prompt referral is indicated if the breasts increase in size over a 4- to 6-month period (especially if accompanied by growth acceleration) or there is vaginal bleeding.

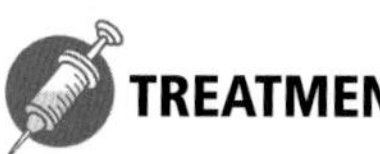

TREATMENT

GENERAL MEASURES

- Observation
- Reassurance for benign processes

ONGOING CARE

- Regression often occurs by 2 years but may occur up to 6 years after onset.
- No specific characteristics assist with prediction of which girls with premature thelarche will go on to have precocious puberty.
- Evidence of pubertal progression should prompt additional evaluation by an endocrinologist:
  - Rapid increase in size of breast tissue
  - Growth acceleration
  - Development of other secondary sexual characteristics
  - Vaginal bleeding

PROGNOSIS

- No known effects on growth, timing of menarche, fertility, or increase risk of breast cancer
- Onset after age 2 years may be associated with increased risk of progression to precocious puberty, if it is accompanied by an increase in growth velocity and basal LH level ≥0.3 IU/L.
- None of the available tests alone will identify which girls will progress to precocious puberty.

COMPLICATIONS

May be the first sign of true precocious puberty or may be associated with other pathologies (e.g., tumors, hypothyroidism, and McCune-Albright syndrome)

PATIENT EDUCATION

- Many newborn male and female infants have breast buds as a result of exposure to maternal estrogen in utero; this resolves quickly.
- Asymmetric breast development is quite common in the early stages of pubertal development.
- Malignant tumors of the breast during childhood are extremely rare.
- Removal of breast tissue prior to or during puberty must be avoided.

ADDITIONAL READING

- Diamantopoulos S, Bao Y. Gynecomastia and premature thelarche: a guide for practitioners. *Pediatr Rev*. 2007;28(9):e57–e68.
- Haber HP, Wollmann HA, Ranke MB. Pelvic ultrasonography: early differentiation between isolated premature thelarche and central precocious puberty. *Eur J Pediatr*. 1995;154(3):182–186.
- Herman-Giddens ME, Slora EJ, Wasserman RC, et al. Secondary sexual characteristics and menses in young girls seen in office practice: a study from the Pediatric Research in Office Settings network. *Pediatrics*. 1997;99(4):505–512.
- Kaplowitz PB, Bloch C; for the Section on Endocrinology, American Academy of Pediatrics. Evaluation and referral of children with signs of early puberty. *Pediatrics*. 2016;137(1).
- Kaplowitz PB, Oberfield SE. Reexamination of the age limit for defining when puberty is precocious in girls in the United States: implications for evaluation and treatment. Drug and Therapeutics and Executive Committees of the Lawson Wilkins Pediatric Endocrine Society. *Pediatrics*. 1999;104(4, Pt 1):936–941.
- Klein K, Mericq V, Brown-Dawson JM, et al. Estrogen levels in girls with premature thelarche compared with normal prepubertal girls as determined by an ultrasensitive recombinant cell bioassay. *J Pediatr*. 1999;134(2):190–192.
- Lebrethon MC, Bourguignon JP. Management of central isosexual precocity: diagnosis, treatment, outcome. *Curr Opin Pediatr*. 2000;12(4):394–399.
- Midyett LK, Moore WV, Jacobson JD. Are pubertal changes in girls before age 8 benign? *Pediatrics*. 2003;111(1):47–51.
- Salardi S, Cacciari E, Mainetti B, et al. Outcome of premature thelarche: relation to puberty and final height. *Arch Dis Child*. 1998;79(2):173–174.
- Sømod ME, Vestergaard ET, Kristensen K, et al. Increasing incidence of premature thelarche in the Central Region of Denmark—challenges in differentiating girls less than 7 years of age with premature thelarche from girls with precocious puberty in real-life practice. *Int J Pediatr Endocrinol*. 2016;2016:4.
- Stanhope R. Premature thelarche: clinical follow-up and indication for treatment. *J Pediatr Endocrinol Metab*. 2000;13(Suppl 1):827–830.

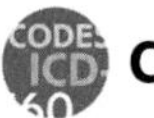

CODES

ICD10

E30.8 Other disorders of puberty

FAQ

- Q: Does premature thelarche predispose the child to later abnormalities in pubertal development?
- A: If onset occurs after age 2 years, the girl may be more likely to enter puberty earlier. However, most girls with premature thelarche will have normal pubertal development and fertility.

PREMENSTRUAL SYNDROME

Ann Bruner, MD

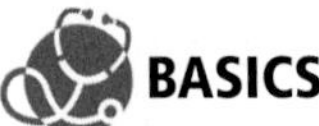

BASICS

DESCRIPTION

- Premenstrual syndrome (PMS), also called late luteal phase disorder, is characterized by psychological and physical symptoms that occur cyclically and consistently during the second half of the menstrual cycle, which negatively impact usual activities of daily living and remit after the onset of menstruation.
- PMS is diagnosed through prospective symptom charting with symptoms present beginning at approximately day 13 of the cycle and resolving within 4 days of menses for two consecutive cycles.
  - At least one of the following symptoms must occur within 5 days of menses onset: breast tenderness, bloating/weight gain, headache, swelling of hands/feet, aches/pains, mood symptoms (depression, anger, irritability, anxiety, social withdrawal), poor concentration, sleep disturbance, or change in appetite.
- Premenstrual dysphoric disorder (PMDD) is the extreme variant of PMS; defined in *DSM-5* as severe psychological symptoms causing significant dysfunctions in activity, which are not an exacerbation of symptoms of a chronic condition; have occurred in most cycles in the previous year; and are confirmed through prospective daily ratings of at least two symptomatic cycles
- Criteria for PMDD: at least five symptoms among the following, present in the final week before menses, and improving within a few days of onset of menses, with at least one of the symptoms being among the first four:
  - Depressed mood: feeling sad, hopeless, or self-deprecating
  - Anxiety or tension: feeling tense, anxious, or "on edge"
  - Affective lability: fluctuating emotions interspersed with frequent tearfulness
  - Irritability or anger: increased interpersonal conflicts
  - Decreased interest in usual activities, which may be associated with withdrawal from social relationships
  - Difficulty concentrating
  - Feeling fatigued, lethargic, or lacking in energy
  - Marked changes in appetite, which may be associated with binge eating or craving certain foods
  - Hypersomnia or insomnia
  - A subjective feeling of being overwhelmed or out of control
  - Physical symptoms such as breast tenderness/swelling, headaches, bloating or weight gain, arthralgias, or myalgias

EPIDEMIOLOGY

- Up to 75% of women experience some PMS symptoms at some time.
- Clinically significant PMS occurs in 3–8% of women.
- 2% of women have symptoms that interfere with their usual activities (PMDD).
- 14–88% of adolescent girls have moderate to severe PMS; one study demonstrated a 5.8% prevalence of PMDD in young women ages 14 to 24 years.

RISK FACTORS

- Age
  - More severe symptoms of PMDD may be seen in younger women.
- Culture
  - PMS/PMDD appear to be more prevalent in Western cultures, possibly due to differences in socialization and symptom expectations.
- Stress
  - PMS and PMDD may be associated with high levels of day-to-day stress and/or a history of stressful events, including sexual abuse.

Genetics

Genetic factors may play a role in the development of PMS/PMDD: Twin studies show a 93% concordance rate in monozygotic twins, with only a 44% rate in dizygotic twins.

PATHOPHYSIOLOGY

- Occurrence of symptoms is related to ovarian function/ovulation:
  - PMS does not occur before menarche, during pregnancy, or after menopause.
  - PMS can occur after hysterectomy but not after bilateral oophorectomy.
  - Symptoms not observed during anovulatory cycles
- Research suggests altered cyclic interactions between sex hormones (particularly progesterone produced by corpus luteum), prostaglandins, and neurotransmitters including serotonin, γ-aminobutyric acid (GABA), and endogenous opioids.
- Women with PMS do not have abnormal serum concentrations of estrogen or progesterone or hormonal imbalance; women with PMS seem to have abnormal responses to normal variations in sex hormones.

ETIOLOGY

Etiology unknown but presumed to be multifactorial

DIAGNOSIS

HISTORY

- Many women report that their PMS symptoms are not taken seriously.
- Complete medical history, including use of medications or illicit substances, cigarettes, dietary evaluation
- Gynecologic history: age at onset of pubertal development, menstrual pattern, sexual activity, contraceptive use, dysmenorrhea
- Psychiatric history: mental health disorders, medications
- Family history: mental health and substance use/abuse
- Psychosocial history: living situation, school/vocational activities and goals, hobbies, peers
- Complete review of systems including both physical and emotional symptoms
  - Physical symptoms: fatigue, breast tenderness/swelling, bloating, edema, weight gain, headache, arthralgias, myalgias, pelvic discomfort, changes in bowel habit, reduced coordination
  - Emotional/psychological symptoms: depression, mood lability, irritability, tension, anxiety, tearfulness, restlessness, reduced concentration, fatigue, altered libido, altered appetite/eating habits, altered sleep
- Chronologic review to determine if symptoms are recurrent with most menstrual cycles, isolated to luteal phase of cycle, and remit with onset of menses

PHYSICAL EXAM

- There are no specific physical findings of PMS.
- Enlarged thyroid gland: may suggest hypothyroidism and need to evaluate for thyroid disease
- Virilization (hirsutism, clitoromegaly): may suggest hyperandrogenism and need to evaluate for adrenal disease, including Cushing syndrome, or other hormonal disorders such as polycystic ovarian syndrome
- Pallor: may suggest anemia
- Orthostatic hypotension: may suggest neurally mediated hypotension

DIFFERENTIAL DIAGNOSIS

- Psychiatric
  - Mood disorder, including major depression, dysthymia, bipolar disorder, postpartum depression, anxiety disorder
  - Substance abuse
  - Physical, sexual, or emotional abuse
  - Somatization disorder
  - Eating disorder
- Endocrinologic
  - Thyroid disease
  - Cushing disease
  - Diabetes mellitus
- Gynecologic
  - Dysmenorrhea (primary or secondary)
  - Pregnancy
  - Endometriosis
  - Hormonal contraceptive use
  - Perimenopause
- Immunologic/hematologic
  - Anemia
  - Fibromyalgia
  - Systemic lupus erythematosus (SLE)
  - Chronic fatigue syndrome
- Neurologic
  - Migraine headache
  - Neurally mediated hypotension

DIAGNOSTIC TESTS & INTERPRETATION

Premenstrual Assessment Form (PAF), Prospective Record of the Impact and Severity of Menstruation (PRISM), or Calendar of Premenstrual Experiences (COPE)

- Prospective symptom calendars can help establish diagnosis and provide information about symptom patterns (recurrence and relation to menses).
- Differences in symptom severity between the follicular and luteal phases (before and after ovulation) may be most diagnostic.

Initial Tests (screening, lab, imaging)

- CBC: Rule out anemia.
- Thyroid-stimulating hormone (TSH) assay: Rule out thyroid disease.

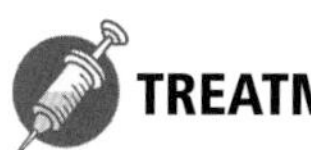

TREATMENT

GENERAL MEASURES

- Treatment goals include reducing both symptom frequency and severity and the impact of symptoms on patients' activities.
- Patient education, counseling, and reassurance may be all that is needed for women with milder symptoms.
- Many pharmacologic and nonpharmacologic modalities have not been formally evaluated.
- Pharmacologic interventions are the mainstay of treatment for patients with moderate to severe PMS and PMDD.
- Activity
  - Increasing physical activity, ensuring adequate and regular sleep, and maintaining a healthy diet are important first steps.
  - Mind/body therapies are frequently used including individual psychotherapy, relaxation techniques, guided imagery, yoga, massage, biofeedback, and group therapy; to date, there is no strong evidence to support their use in PMS.

MEDICATION

- Mild symptoms
  - Many menstrually associated symptoms can be managed with nonsteroidal anti-inflammatory drugs (NSAIDs).
  - NSAIDs (e.g., naproxen sodium 275 to 550 mg PO b.i.d.) relieve the majority of physical symptoms: premenstrual/menstrual cramping, headaches, and myalgias/arthralgias.
  - Side effects include gastrointestinal upset and renal dysfunction.
- Moderate to severe symptoms
  - Oral selective serotonin reuptake inhibitors (SSRIs)
    - First line for moderate to severe PMDD and PMS, especially those with predominantly psychological symptoms
    - SSRIs have been shown to improve mood, decrease irritability, ameliorate physical symptoms such as bloating and breast tenderness, and improve psychosocial function. Continuous and intermittent (during luteal phase) dosing can be used, and symptom amelioration can occur during the first cycle of treatment.
    - Intermittent use includes administration during the last 14 days of the menstrual cycle or treatment begun at expected date of symptom onset. Intermittent/luteal phase therapy is less expensive and may minimize SSRI side effects:
      - Fluoxetine (20 to 60 mg/24 h), sertraline (50 to 150 mg/24 h), paroxetine (20 to 30 mg/24 h), escitalopram (10 to 20 mg/24 h), and citalopram (20 to 30 mg/24 h) are some of the most commonly used SSRIs for PMS/PMDD.
      - Side effects include gastrointestinal upset, insomnia, tremor/agitation, fatigue, dry mouth, and sexual dysfunction. SSRIs recently received a U.S. Food and Drug Administration (FDA) black box warning concerning an increased risk of suicidality among depressed children and adolescents; the warning was for the treatment of depression, not PMS/PMDD.
      - Start with lowest dose and increase as needed; symptom improvement should occur during first cycle of treatment.
      - 60–70% of patients will improve with an SSRI; if there is no improvement try a different SSRI.
  - Hormonal contraceptives (i.e., low-dose oral contraceptive pills, contraceptive patch)
    - Suppress ovulation; formulations with drospirenone may be more effective against hormonally mediated symptoms such as breast swelling/tenderness and bloating.
    - Patients also seeking contraception may prefer to try oral contraceptives as 1st-line therapy instead of SSRIs.
  - Spironolactone (50 mg PO once daily or b.i.d.) is effective for breast tenderness and bloating; potassium levels must be monitored, and spironolactone is contraindicated in patients with abnormal renal function.

ISSUES FOR REFERRAL

A gynecologist/reproductive endocrinologist can assist in the management of severe PMS/PMDD: Other pharmacologic agents that are used include gonadotropin-releasing hormone (GnRH) analogues, danazol, estrogen implants, and androgens.

ONGOING CARE

- Frequent follow-up and the use of a prospective menstrual/symptom calendar are important.
- After the diagnosis of PMS is established and after recommending appropriate lifestyle changes (and possibly NSAIDs), the patient should be reevaluated after 3 months. If there has not been substantial improvement, secondary pharmacologic therapies (SSRIs) may need to be considered. When SSRIs are prescribed as 1st-line therapy for patients with more severe PMS or PMDD, response to SSRIs and any adverse reactions should be assessed at follow-up and dosage adjusted as needed.

COMPLICATIONS

Psychological morbidity includes difficulty with interpersonal relationships (family and friends) and school absence/failure.

ADDITIONAL READING

- American Psychiatric Association. *Desk Reference to the Diagnostic Criteria from DSM-5*. Arlington, VA: American Psychiatric Association; 2013.
- Borenstein J, Chiou CF, Dean B, et al. Estimating direct and indirect costs of premenstrual syndrome. *J Occup Environ Med*. 2005;47(1):26–33.
- Claman F, Miller T. Premenstrual syndrome and premenstrual dysphoric disorder in adolescence. *J Pediatr Health Care*. 2006;20(5):329–333.
- Halbreich U. The etiology, biology, and evolving pathology of premenstrual syndromes. *Psychoneuroendocrinology*. 2003;28(Suppl 3):55–99.
- Halbreich U, Borenstein J, Pearlstein T, et al. The prevalence, impairment, impact, and burden of premenstrual dysphoric disorder (PMS/PMDD). *Psychoneuroendocrinology*. 2003;28(Suppl 3):1–23.
- Nevatte T, O'Brien PM, Bäckström T, et al; and Consensus Group of the International Society for Premenstrual Disorders. ISPMD consensus on the management of premenstrual disorders. *Arch Womens Ment Health*. 2013;16(4):279–291.
- Rapkin AJ, Akopians AL. Pathophysiology of premenstrual syndrome and premenstrual dysphoric disorder. *Menopause Int*. 2012;18(2):52–59.
- Steiner M, Pearlstein T, Cohen L, et al. Expert guidelines for the treatment of severe PMS, PMDD, and comorbidities: the role of SSRIs. *J Womens Health (Larchmt)*. 2006;15(1):57–69.
- Vigod SN, Ross LE, Steiner M. Understanding and treating premenstrual dysphoric disorder: an update for the women's health practitioner. *Obstet Gynecol Clin North Am*. 2009;36(4):907–924.

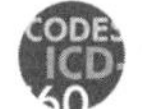

CODES

ICD10

N94.3 Premenstrual tension syndrome

FAQ

- Q: Can adolescent girls have PMS and PMDD?
- A: The incidence of PMS and PMDD in adolescents is not well established. Although ≤50% of cycles are anovulatory during the first 1 to 2 years after menarche, younger patients experience many PMS symptoms, and menstrual problems are some of the most common reasons for school absence. Most experts believe that PMS/PMDD will not develop until a regular ovulatory pattern is established, ~2 to 3 years after menarche.
- Q: Is family history important?
- A: Genetic factors may play a role in the development of PMS/PMDD; twin studies show a 93% concordance rate in monozygotic twins, with only a 44% rate in dizygotic twins.
- Q: Are there any common comorbidities?
- A: The symptoms of PMS/PMDD are also seen with depression, anxiety, and other mood disorders. Psychiatric symptomatology can fluctuate, and symptoms may change in relation to the menstrual cycle. Careful and thorough history taking and prospective symptom diaries can help differentiate PMS/PMDD from another mental health disorder.
- Q: Can oral contraceptives and SSRIs both be used?
- A: Oral contraceptives can be combined with SSRIs in patients who have a partial response to SSRIs or in patients who also desire contraception.

PRIMARY ADRENAL INSUFFICIENCY

Jennifer M. Barker, MD

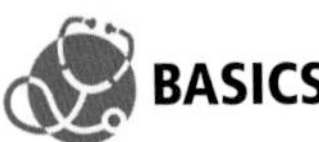

BASICS

DESCRIPTION

Deficiency in the secretion of cortisol and/or aldosterone by the adrenal glands

EPIDEMIOLOGY

- Age
  - Adrenal insufficiency associated with congenital adrenal hyperplasia (CAH) presents in the newborn period (1/10,000 to 15,000 live births).
  - Adrenal hypoplasia congenita presents in infancy or early childhood (1/12,500 live births).
  - Adrenocorticotropic hormone (ACTH) unresponsiveness presents in late infancy or the toddler period (rare).
  - Adrenoleukodystrophy typically presents late in the 1st decade of life with neurologic symptoms. Signs and symptoms of adrenal insufficiency in persons with adrenoleukodystrophy may first present at any age (prevalence 1/20,000 to 60,000).
  - Addison disease is rare in children and usually presents between the ages of 20 and 50 years. In the pediatric population, it is most often seen in late childhood and adolescence (prevalence 1/10,000 adults).
- Sex
  - CAH and ACTH unresponsiveness affect both sexes equally.
  - Adrenal hypoplasia congenita, an X-linked disorder, predominantly affects boys.
  - Adrenoleukodystrophy, an X-linked disorder, predominantly affects boys.
  - Addison disease is more common in females.

RISK FACTORS

Genetics

- CAH: autosomal recessive inheritance associated with a gene defect in one of multiple adrenal steroidogenic enzymes, most commonly *CYP21A2* for the 21-hydroxylase gene
- Adrenal hypoplasia congenita: X-linked mutation in *DAX1* gene
- ACTH unresponsiveness: autosomal recessive ACTH receptor defect
- Adrenoleukodystrophy
  - X-linked recessive disorder of very-long-chain fatty acid metabolism due to *ABCD1* gene mutation
  - An autosomal recessive form of the disease exists which presents during infancy.
- Autoimmune adrenal insufficiency
  - May be isolated or part of autoimmune polyglandular syndromes (APSs)
  - *AIRE1* gene mutations cause APS type 1.
  - APS type 2 is associated with human leukocyte antigens (HLAs) DR3 and DR4.

PATHOPHYSIOLOGY

- CAH: a group of enzymatic disorders of steroid metabolism, of which 21-hydroxylase deficiency is the most common (Appendix, Table 13)
- Adrenal hypoplasia congenita: a defect in adrenal organogenesis
- ACTH unresponsiveness
  - Inherited defect in the ACTH receptor, resulting in isolated glucocorticoid deficiency with hypoglycemia in infancy and hyperpigmentation
- Adrenoleukodystrophies
  - Inherited disorders of impaired peroxisomal degradation of very-long-chain fatty acids, resulting in adrenal insufficiency and progressive neurologic deterioration
- Addison disease
  - Primary hypoadrenalism due to bilateral destruction of the adrenal cortices
  - This can be due to autoimmune destruction (isolated or associated with APS), tuberculosis, hemorrhage, fungal infection, neoplastic infiltration, or AIDS.
- Waterhouse-Friderichsen syndrome:
  - Bilateral adrenal gland hemorrhage classically associated with fulminant meningococcemia
  - Also reported with *Staphylococcus aureus* and *Streptococcus pneumoniae*

COMMONLY ASSOCIATED CONDITIONS

- Adrenal hypoplasia congenita is associated with hypogonadotropic hypogonadism.
- APSs are associated with other autoimmune disorders:
  - APS type 1: mucocutaneous candidiasis, hypoparathyroidism
  - APS type 2: autoimmune thyroid disease, type 1 diabetes
  - Both types can also present in conjunction with multiple other autoimmune disorders (e.g., primary ovarian or testicular insufficiency, celiac disease, pernicious anemia, vitiligo, autoimmune hepatitis).

DIAGNOSIS

HISTORY

Symptoms of primary adrenal insufficiency are nonspecific and similar to those found in many other disease processes. Symptoms may be present for years prior to diagnosis and can include

- Weakness and fatigue
- Anorexia, weight loss
- Headache
- Nausea, vomiting, diarrhea, abdominal pain
- Orthostatic symptoms
- Muscle or joint pains
- Emotional lability
- Salt craving
- Hyperpigmentation
- Decreased axillary or pubic hair in females due to lack of adrenal androgens
- Amenorrhea in females
- Unexplained hypoglycemia, decreasing insulin requirements, and decreasing HgbA1c in patients with type 1 diabetes

PHYSICAL EXAM

- Low BMI
- Hypotension or orthostatic hypotension
- Tachycardia
- Hyperpigmentation, especially on lip borders, buccal mucosa, nipples, and over skin creases (associated with elevated ACTH)
- Vitiligo (autoimmune)
- Thyromegaly (sign of autoimmune thyroid disease)
- Pubertal staging
- Signs of virilization in females (CAH)

DIFFERENTIAL DIAGNOSIS

- CAH
- Adrenal hypoplasia congenita
- ACTH unresponsiveness
- Adrenoleukodystrophy
- Autoimmune adrenal cortical destruction
- Infectious adrenal cortical destruction
  - Tuberculous
  - Fungal
  - HIV
- Adrenal hemorrhage
- Neoplastic adrenal infiltration

DIAGNOSTIC TESTS & INTERPRETATION

Diagnostic Procedures/Other

- Specific
  - Newborn screening (NBS) for 21-hydroxylase deficiency (measurement of 17-hydroxyprogesterone) identifies infants with CAH prior to presentation with adrenal crisis. Abnormal NBS results require follow-up with serum 17-hydroxyprogesterone, plasma renin activity, and/or electrolytes depending on clinical scenario.
  - Random elevated ACTH with low cortisol may be sufficient to diagnose primary adrenal insufficiency.
  - Cosyntropin (Cortrosyn) stimulation test: Administer cosyntropin (synthetic ACTH) 250 mcg IV and measure cortisol at baseline, 30 and 60 minutes.
    - A normal response is a final cortisol >18 mcg/dL. An insufficient cortisol response is diagnostic of adrenal insufficiency.
    - A baseline ACTH >200 pg/mL with inadequate cortisol is seen in primary adrenal insufficiency.
  - Serum adrenal antibodies (21-hydroxylase autoantibodies) may be positive in autoimmune Addison disease.
  - Very-long-chain fatty acids are elevated in adrenoleukodystrophy.
  - Low gonadotropin and sex steroid levels suggesting hypogonadotropic hypogonadism may be seen with adrenal hypoplasia congenita.
  - Adrenal steroid precursors will be elevated in CAH.

- Nonspecific
  - Electrolytes
    - Hyponatremia: result of the mineralocorticoid defect and glucocorticoid deficiency; combination of sodium loss from kidneys and the inability to excrete a water load
    - Hyperkalemia and acidosis: chronic mineralocorticoid deficiency with the inability to excrete potassium and acid
    - Hypercalcemia: most likely a result of increased calcium absorption due to the lack of glucocorticoid effect on the gut
    - Hypoglycemia: Glucocorticoids have permissive effects on gluconeogenesis.
    - Renin levels are elevated when a mineralocorticoid deficiency is present.

ALERT

- Differential above only covers primary forms of adrenal insufficiency; secondary/tertiary forms may also need to be considered (ACTH/CRH deficiency); for these children, evaluation for other pituitary hormone disorders often warranted (see "Hypopituitarism")
- Replacing thyroid hormone in a child with untreated adrenal insufficiency can precipitate adrenal crisis.
- The electrolyte picture of adrenal insufficiency can be seen in renal disorders, obstructive uropathy, and isolated aldosterone deficiency.

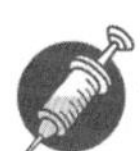

TREATMENT

MEDICATION

- Acute adrenal crisis
  - Hydrocortisone: stress dosage of hydrocortisone: 100 mg/m^2 IV/IM followed by 100 mg/m^2/24 h of hydrocortisone divided q4–6h. Decrease to a physiologic replacement dosage when acute illness has resolved. Note: High-dose hydrocortisone has mineralocorticoid effect.
  - Mineralocorticoid replacement: Florinef 0.1 mg daily when able to take PO
- Chronic adrenal insufficiency
  - Hydrocortisone 10 to 12 mg/m^2/24 h PO divided t.i.d. Increase the dose to 30 to 50 mg/m^2/24 h for stress of fever, illness, or vomiting. Lower doses may sometimes be used, particularly for forms of adrenal insufficiency other than CAH.
  - For major stress (surgery, significant illness), give hydrocortisone 50 to 100 mg/m^2 IV/IM followed by 50 to 100 mg/m^2/24 h IV divided q4–6h. IM hydrocortisone is recommended for emergency home use. In some cases, equivalent doses of prednisone or dexamethasone may be used.
  - Florinef 0.1 to 0.2 mg PO daily
  - May require sodium supplementation (especially infants)

ISSUES FOR REFERRAL

Children and adolescents with adrenal insufficiency should be evaluated and treated by pediatric endocrinologists.

ADMISSION, INPATIENT, AND NURSING CONSIDERATIONS

- Acute adrenal crisis
  - An intercurrent illness or surgical procedure may provoke an episode of hypotension, tachycardia, and shock.
  - Electrolytes reveal decreased serum sodium, elevated potassium, metabolic acidosis, and a decreased or normal glucose.
  - Serum should be drawn and saved to aid in diagnosis, but emergent treatment should not be delayed for a diagnostic ACTH stimulation test.
- Treatment
  - 5% dextrose in normal saline (D5NS) solution for volume repletion and treatment of salt wasting and hypoglycemia
  - Hydrocortisone or other glucocorticoid
  - Mineralocorticoid replacement
- D5NS for volume repletion and treatment of salt wasting

ONGOING CARE

FOLLOW-UP RECOMMENDATIONS

Acute adrenal crisis usually improves rapidly with the administration of fluids and glucocorticoids. Once the acute phase of illness has resolved, steroids can be resumed at physiologic replacement doses.

Patient Monitoring

- Clinical status: blood pressure, heart rate
- Growth
- Reduction in hyperpigmentation
- Electrolytes, ACTH, and renin levels
- Screen for polyautoimmune disorders; very-long-chain fatty acid levels and neurologic function in adrenoleukodystrophy
- Pubertal development
  - Virilization/adrenarche (CAH)
  - Delayed puberty (autoimmune)

PATIENT EDUCATION

- Stress dosing
- Importance of seeking medical attention for significant illness, persistent vomiting, or the inability to take fluids by mouth
- MedicAlert bracelet

PROGNOSIS

- Long-term prognosis of isolated adrenal insufficiency is good, provided adequate hydrocortisone is administered, particularly in times of illness.
- Risk for early mortality related to inappropriately treated adrenal crisis
- Adrenoleukodystrophy carries a poor prognosis.

COMPLICATIONS

- If not diagnosed and/or treated properly, a significant physical stress such as surgery or illness may result in a life-threatening adrenal crisis.
- CAH can cause virilization/ambiguous genitalia in female infants with the disease and can cause salt-wasting crises in infants of both sexes.
- Pubertal delay or hypogonadotropic hypogonadism is seen with adrenal hypoplasia congenita due to *DAX1* mutations.
- Unrecognized ACTH unresponsiveness is associated with recurrent hypoglycemia, seizures, mental retardation, and death.
- Adrenoleukodystrophy results in severe neurologic impairment and death.
- Autoimmune adrenal insufficiency is commonly associated with additional autoimmune disease that can complicate treatment.

ADDITIONAL READING

- Bornstein SR, Allolio B, Arlt W, et al. Diagnosis and treatment of primary adrenal insufficiency: an Endocrine Society Clinical Practice Guideline. *J Clin Endocrinol Metab*. 2016;101(2):364–389.
- Falorni A, Minarelli V, Morelli S. Therapy of adrenal insufficiency: an update. *Endocrine*. 2013;43(3):514–528.
- Hsieh S, White PC. Presentation of primary adrenal insufficiency in childhood. *J Clin Endocrinol Metab*. 2011;96(6):E925–E928.
- Husebye ES, Perheentupa J, Rautemaa R, et al. Clinical manifestations and management of patients with autoimmune polyendocrine syndrome type I. *J Intern Med*. 2009;265(5):514–529.
- Speiser PW, Azziz R, Baskin LS, et al. Congenital adrenal hyperplasia due to steroid 21-hydroxylase deficiency: an Endocrine Society clinical practice guideline. *J Clin Endocrinol Metab*. 2010;95(9):4133–4160.
- White PC, Bachega TA. Congenital adrenal hyperplasia due to 21 hydroxylase deficiency: from birth to adulthood. *Semin Reprod Med*. 2012;30(5):400–409.

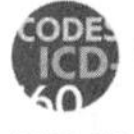

CODES

ICD10

- E27.1 Primary adrenocortical insufficiency
- Q89.1 Congenital malformations of adrenal gland
- E71.529 X-linked adrenoleukodystrophy, unspecified type

FAQ

- Q: What are the indications for stress dosing and how rapidly can the stress hydrocortisone dose be tapered?
- A: Patients will require stress dosing of hydrocortisone for surgical procedures, fever (>37.7°C [100°F]), vomiting, diarrhea, and particularly vigorous exercise. The stress dose is typically given for 24 hours, after which the usual dose is resumed. Should it be necessary to administer the stress dosage for a more prolonged period, the dosage can usually be tapered rapidly to physiologic dosage, once the patient's clinical condition has improved.

PRION DISEASES (TRANSMISSIBLE SPONGIFORM ENCEPHALOPATHIES)

John Bower, MD

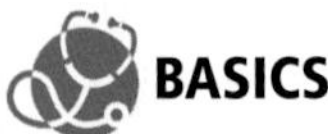

BASICS

DESCRIPTION

- Prion diseases or transmissible spongiform encephalopathies (TSEs) are a family of progressive neurodegenerative diseases of humans and animals that cause irreversible cumulative brain damage and are uniformly fatal.
- Prions are the causative agent for prion disease and are misfolded forms of normally occurring prion protein (PRP^c).
- Human prion diseases include Creutzfeldt-Jakob disease (CJD), variant CJD (vCJD), kuru, Gerstmann-Sträussler-Scheinker syndrome, and fatal familial insomnia (FFI) syndrome.
- Six TSEs in animals have been described: bovine spongiform encephalopathy (BSE, also known as mad cow disease), scrapie in sheep and goats, feline spongiform encephalopathy, transmissible mink encephalopathy, exotic ungulate encephalopathy, and chronic wasting disease of cervids.

EPIDEMIOLOGY

- CJD
  - CJD is the most prevalent form of prion disease in humans and occurs as either a sporadic or a familial disease.
  - ~85% of cases are sporadic with no family history and no known source of transmission. Sporadic CJD occurs throughout the world at a rate 1/1,000,000 people.
  - Familial CJD (fCJD) cases are associated with a gene mutation in the gene (*PRNP*) for making PRP^c and account for ~10–15% of cases. fCJD shows an autosomal dominant inheritance, with >50 mutations in *PRNP* identified.
  - ~1% of CJD cases are iatrogenic, resulting from accidental transmission of the causative agent via contaminated surgical equipment, as a result of cornea or dura mater transplants, or administration of human-derived pituitary growth hormones.
  - No evidence confirms person-to-person transmission among family members via direct contact, droplet, or airborne spread.
  - Disease is characterized by progressive dementia, myoclonus, visual or cerebellar disturbance, pyramidal/extrapyramidal dysfunction, and/or akinetic mutism.
  - Classic sporadic CJD most often occurs between the ages of 50 and 70 years and affects both sexes equally; whites have about a 2-fold higher rate than blacks.
  - Death usually occurs within 1 year of onset of symptoms.
- vCJD
  - First reported in 1994; variant CJD has unique clinical features.
  - In contrast to CJD, vCJD affects younger patients (as young as 11 years of age with an average age of 29 years) and has a longer duration of illness with median of 14 months.
  - Strong epidemiologic evidence links vCJD to BSE:
    - BSE is a TSE that affects cattle; it was first reported in the United Kingdom. The most likely route of exposure is through bovine-based foods derived from BSE-infected cattle.
    - Highest incidence of vCJD is seen in the United Kingdom, the country with the largest potential exposure to BSE.
    - Three cases of vCJD have been confirmed in the United States, although each were likely to have been contracted outside the United States.
  - Clinical features, found early in the illness, include the following:
    - Prominent psychiatric symptoms (e.g., depression, schizophrenia-like psychosis) and ataxia
    - Other neurologic signs (e.g., paresthesia/dysesthesia, chorea, dystonia, myoclonus, and akinetic mutism) develop as the disease progresses.
  - Clinical criteria for the diagnosis of vCJD have been validated in the United Kingdom by autopsy/biopsy-proven cases compared to noncases.
- FFI
  - An autosomal dominant disorder, caused by mutation at codon 178 of *PRNP*, also identified in fCJD. If there are homozygous alleles at codon 129 encoding methionine in conjunction with the codon 178 mutation, FFI ensues. If codon 129 encodes valine in conjunction with the codon 178 mutation, then fCJD develops.
  - Clinical features include insomnia, dysautonomia, ataxia, myoclonus, and late dementia.
  - Pathology reveals minimal vacuolization and no plaques.
- Gerstmann-Sträussler-Scheinker syndrome
  - A disorder with autosomal dominant inheritance
  - Clinical features include ataxia and dementia.
  - Pathology reveals amyloid plaques.

PATHOPHYSIOLOGY

- PRP^c are metal-binding proteins normally found on neuronal cells and other cells throughout the body.
- Infections arise when normal host PRP^c undergoes spontaneous misfolding to yield the abnormal protease-resistant conformers (PRP^{RES} or PRP^{SC} for protease-resistant or scrapie-causing PRPs, respectively).
- Progressive accumulation of PRP^{RES} in the CNS disrupts function, leading to vacuolization and cell death. There is no host-adaptive immune response beyond microglial cell activation involved in the pathologic process.
- Neuropathologic findings include neuronal loss, atrophy, vacuolization or spongiform change, reactive astrogliosis, and cell death.
- PRP^{RES} also accumulate in the reticular endothelial system, mucosa-associated lymphoid tissues, and areas of chronic inflammation throughout the body.
- Newly formed host PRP^{RES} recruit neighboring cellular PRP^C and convert it to the infectious conformer. The exact molecular and cellular mechanisms surrounding propagation of PRP^{RES} remains unknown.

ETIOLOGY

- The majority of prion disease cases develop without explanation (sporadic CJD).
- Genetic forms of prion disease variously arise from a number of missense, nonsense, insertion or deletion mutations in the PRP^c (*PRNP*) gene.
- The etiologic agent for vCJD is BSE and can be transmitted to the CNS by oral, parenteral, or direct inoculation.
- For vCJD, the mechanism of prion transmission to the CNS from oral and parenteral exposure remains uncertain.

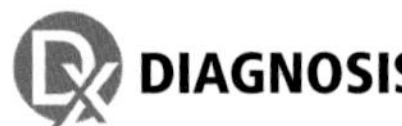

DIAGNOSIS

HISTORY

- Evidence of a familial form of prion disease
- Potential iatrogenic exposures such as administration of human-derived pituitary growth hormones, implantation of dura mater or corneal grafts from humans, epilepsy surgery, or other CNS surgery involving stereotactic electrodes
- Duration of symptoms >6 months
- Afebrile illness
- In vCJD, progressive neuropsychiatric symptoms including:
  - Depression, anxiety, apathy, withdrawal, or delusions
  - Painful sensory symptoms including pain and/or dysesthesia
  - Ataxia
  - Myoclonus, chorea, or dystonia
  - Dementia

PHYSICAL EXAM

- Afebrile
- Abnormal mental status exam with defects in memory, personality, and other higher cortical functions or psychosis
- Neurologic signs include unsteady gait and the presence of involuntary movements.
- Late findings include mutism and complete immobility.

DIFFERENTIAL DIAGNOSIS

- Neurodegenerative disorders—mostly seen in older adults with the exception of Alpers disease
  - Alzheimer disease
  - Parkinson disease
  - Frontotemporal dementia
  - Pick disease
  - Alpers disease (progressive cerebral hemiatrophy)
  - Amyotrophic lateral sclerosis
  - Huntington disease
  - Spinocerebellar ataxia

- Psychiatric disorders—especially when considering vCJD as a diagnosis
  - Depression
  - Schizophrenia
  - Drug-induced psychosis
- Encephalitis, infectious
- Sydenham chorea
- Subacute sclerosing panencephalitis
- Progressive multifocal leukoencephalopathy
- Toxic encephalopathy
- Inborn errors of metabolism
- Hashimoto thyroiditis
- CNS vasculitis
- CNS tumors

DIAGNOSTIC TESTS & INTERPRETATION

Initial Tests (screening, lab, imaging)

- Conventional laboratory tests are of little value in the diagnosis of prion disease.
- Exam of cerebrospinal fluid (CSF) may reveal a mild elevation of protein, but otherwise the CSF is normal.
- CSF studies that may aid in confirming prion disease include assays for surrogate markers such as 14-3-3 protein and tau protein.
- New prion amplification systems for rapid detection of prions in the CSF of acutely affected patients include the real-time quaking-induced conversion (RT-QuIC) test.
- EEG
  - In CJD, generalized slowing is seen early in the disease with progression to periodic burst of biphasic or triphasic sharp-wave complexes.
  - In vCJD, the EEG does not show the waveforms characteristic of sporadic CJD.
  - Although EEG abnormalities are seen in most patients, these findings are not specific.
- MRI
  - In patients with vCJD, abnormally high T2 signal in the bilateral pulvinar regions of the thalamus may be seen.
  - In CJD, hyperintense signals in the basal ganglia are often seen.
  - In later stages of CJD and vCJD, imaging studies such as MRI or CT scan reveal generalized atrophy with large ventricles.

Diagnostic Procedures/Other

- Diagnosis of prion disease in humans can be confirmed only following pathologic exam of the brain.
- Microscopic exam of patients with all types of human prion diseases reveals spongiform change accompanied by neuronal loss and gliosis.
- Amyloid plaques or immunohistochemical demonstration of abnormal PRP in the brain may also be seen.
- "Florid" plaques (amyloid plaques encircled by holes or vacuoles resulting in a daisy-like appearance) are consistently present in patients with vCJD.
- Tonsil biopsy revealing accumulation of PRP^{RES} may be helpful in confirming suspected cases of vCJD.

TREATMENT

GENERAL MEASURES

- No treatment is effective in slowing or stopping the progression of disease. Appropriate supportive care should be provided. Prognosis for patients with human prion diseases is uniformly poor.
- Several compounds and methods have undergone testing in cell-free, tissue, and animal models of prion disease. Some decrease the rate of PRP^{RES} accumulation and allow animals to reach their expected lifespan. None reverses the damage seen in the CNS after plaques have formed.
- Infection control/prevention
  - Standard universal precautions are indicated for infection control.
  - Strict isolation is not necessary.
  - Caution should be used in obtaining CSF and handling tissues obtained at autopsy.
  - Equipment contaminated by high-risk tissue should be soaked in ≥1 N sodium hydroxide solution for at least 1 hour and then autoclaved at 134°C for at least 1 hour.

ADDITIONAL READING

- Aguzzi A, Heikenwalder M. Pathogenesis of prion diseases: current status and future outlook. *Nat Rev Microbiol*. 2006;4(10):765–775.
- Diack AB, Head MW, McCutcheon S, et al. Variant CJD. 18 years of research and surveillance. *Prion*. 2014;8(4):286–295.
- Glatzel M, Stoeck K, Seeger H, et al. Human prion diseases: molecular and clinical aspects. *Arch Neurol*. 2005;62(4):545–552.
- Holman RC, Belay ED, Christensen KY, et al. Human prion diseases in the United States. *PLoS One*. 2010;5(1):e8521.
- Johnson RT. Prion diseases. *Lancet Neurol*. 2005;4(10):635–642.
- Kretzschmar HA. Diagnosis of prion diseases. *Clin Lab Med*. 2003;23(1):109–128.
- Prusiner SB. Shattuck lecture—neurodegenerative diseases and prions. *N Engl J Med*. 2001;344(20):1516–1526.
- Takada LT, Kim MO, Cleveland RW. Genetic prion disease: experience of a rapidly progressive dementia center in the United States and a review of the literature. *Am J Med Genet B Neuropsychiatr Genet*. 2017;174(1):36–69.
- Urwin PJ, Mackenzie JM, Llewelyn CA. Creutzfeldt-Jakob disease and blood transfusion: updated results of the UK Transfusion Medicine Epidemiology Review study. *Vox Sang*. 2016;110(4):310–316.

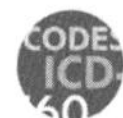

CODES

ICD10

- A81.9 Atypical virus infection of central nervous system, unsp
- A81.00 Creutzfeldt-Jakob disease, unspecified
- A81.81 Kuru

FAQ

- Q: Is transmission of prion disease from human blood possible?
- A: There have been three verified cases of vCJD attributed to transfusion of blood products in the United Kingdom. There have been no cases of transfusion-related vCJD in the United States.
- Q: Is our food supply safe?
- A: No cases of BSE have been recognized in North America. The incidence in the United Kingdom has been low and is not increasing rapidly. Measures have been taken by the World Health Organization (WHO) and the U.S. Food and Drug Administration (FDA) to reduce the risk of TSE, including a ban on the use of ruminant tissues in animal feed and surveillance systems to detect TSE in animals and to prevent any part or product of an animal with suspected TSE to enter the human or animal food chain. The FDA has banned biologic agents of bovine origin produced in countries at risk of BSE. There have been three cases of vCJD in U.S. citizens, but each case was likely contracted outside the United States (United Kingdom and Saudi Arabia).

PROTEINURIA

Stephanie Nguyen, MD, MAS

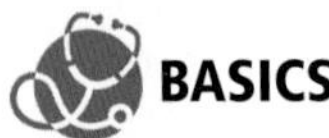

BASICS

DESCRIPTION

- Protein may be found in the urine of healthy children.
- The term proteinuria is used to indicate urinary protein excretion beyond the upper limit of normal (100 mg/m^2/24 h or 4 mg/m^2/h in children and 150 mg/24 h in adults).
  - Nephrotic-range proteinuria >1,000 mg/m^2/24 h or 40 mg/m^2/h
  - Nephrotic syndrome: nephrotic-range proteinuria with edema and hypoalbuminemia (<2.5 g/dL)
  - Microalbuminuria: elevated urinary excretion of albumin (30 to 300 mg/g albumin/creatinine ratio or 30 to 300 mg/24 h); generally used to indicate kidney disease in those with diabetes mellitus
- Classification
  - Persistent or fixed proteinuria
    - Urinary dipstick ≥1+ on the first morning urine specimen on ≥3 samples >1 week apart
    - Requires prompt referral to nephrology
  - Transient proteinuria
    - Proteinuria absent on subsequent urine examinations
    - It is not usually associated with clinically significant underlying renal disease.
    - May be associated with high fever, cold stress, dehydration, and exercise
  - Orthostatic or postural proteinuria
    - Elevated protein excretion when the patient is upright but normalizes when patient is supine
    - The most common cause of fixed or transient proteinuria in childhood and adolescence
    - Rarely exceeds 1 g/m^2/24 h
    - Benign condition and not associated with edema

EPIDEMIOLOGY

Prevalence of asymptomatic proteinuria in school-aged children is 5.4–10.7% on single urine sample and <1% on ≥3 urine samples.

PATHOPHYSIOLOGY

- Normally, ~50% urinary proteins are derived from tissue proteins and proteins from cells lining the urinary tract (i.e., Tamm-Horsfall protein).
- Proteinuria may be the result of glomerular proteinuria or tubular proteinuria.
- Glomerular proteinuria
  - An increased permeability of the glomeruli to the passage of plasma proteins
  - Large amounts of glomerular proteinuria may be found in the context of edema and hypoalbuminemia (nephrotic syndrome).
  - If there is hypertension, abnormal glomerular filtration rate, and hematuria, there may be nephritis as well.
- Tubular proteinuria
  - Decreased reabsorption of low-molecular-weight proteins by the proximal renal tubules
  - Rarely >1 g/24 h and is not associated with edema
  - The major marker is urinary β-2-microglobulin.
  - May be associated with other defects of proximal tubular function (e.g., renal tubular acidosis [RTA], glucosuria, phosphaturia, aminoaciduria) and tubular interstitial processes

DIAGNOSIS

The American Academy of Pediatrics (AAP) no longer recommends screening urinalysis for asymptomatic children due to high false-positive rate, low cost-effectiveness, and lack of treatable disease.

HISTORY

- **Question:** Changes in aspects of the urine?
- *Significance*: foamy (nephrotic syndrome) or red or tea-colored (hematuria)
- **Question:** Recent illness?
- *Significance*: Pharyngitis and upper respiratory infections can trigger postinfectious glomerulonephritis (GN).
- **Question:** Frequent episodes of fever?
- *Significance*: lymphoma, malignancies, vasculitides
- **Question:** Medications or herbal/folk remedies?
- *Significance*: toxins
- **Question:** Illicit drug use and risk factors for STI in adolescent and adults?
- *Significance*: HIV, syphilis, hepatitis
- **Question:** Urinary tract infection in the past?
- *Significance*: reflux nephropathy
- **Question:** Family history of renal diseases or hearing loss?
- *Significance*: hereditary nephritis
- **Question:** Facial swelling (in the morning) and lower limb swelling (in the afternoon)? Weight changes?
- *Significance*: edema related to nephrotic syndrome
- **Question:** Symptoms related to rheumatologic conditions (skin rash, joint pain, joint stiffness)?
- *Significance*: lupus
- **Question:** Cough, shortness of breath?
- *Significance*: vasculitis, infections

PHYSICAL EXAM

- General
  - Hypertension
  - Growth and development
- HEENT
  - Periorbital edema
  - Malar rash
- Chest
  - Pericardial or pleural effusions
- Abdomen
  - Ascites
  - Hepatosplenomegaly
  - Abdominal masses/organomegaly
- Genitalia
  - Scrotal edema
  - Ambiguous genitalia (Denys-Drash syndrome)
- Skin
  - Purpuric (HSP) or petechial rash (leukemia, lymphomas)
  - Pallor (malignancies, chronic renal failure, hemolytic uremic syndrome [HUS])
  - Angiokeratomas (Fabry disease)
- Extremities
  - Pitting edema
  - Arthralgias/arthritis
- Dystrophic nails

DIFFERENTIAL DIAGNOSIS

- Idiopathic nephrotic syndrome
  - Minimal change nephrotic syndrome
  - Focal segmental glomerulosclerosis
  - Membranous nephropathy
  - Mesangial proliferation
- Nephrotic syndrome due to genetic causes
  - Finnish-type congenital nephrotic syndrome
  - Familial focal segmental glomerulosclerosis
  - Diffuse mesangial sclerosis
  - Denys-Drash syndrome (nephropathy, Wilms tumor, and genital abnormalities)
- Chronic kidney disease
- Acquired glomerular disease
  - Idiopathic GN
  - Lupus-associated nephritis
  - IgA nephropathy
  - Systemic vasculitides
  - Subacute bacterial endocarditis
  - Diabetes mellitus
  - Hypertension
  - HUS

P

- Genetic disorders
  - Nail-patella syndrome
  - Alport syndrome
  - Fabry disease
  - Glycogen storage disease
  - Cystic fibrosis
  - Hurler syndrome (mucopolysaccharide type-I)
  - α-1-Antitrypsin
  - Mitochondrial disorders (usually tubular proteinuria)
  - Gaucher disease
  - Dent disease (X-linked nephrolithiasis)
  - Cystinosis
  - Wilson disease
- Oncologic/hematologic
  - Sickle cell disease
  - Renal vein thrombosis
  - Leukemia
  - Lymphoma
- Infectious
  - Poststreptococcal GN
  - HIV-associated nephropathy
  - Hepatitis B and C virus infection
  - Malaria
  - Syphilis (can present as congenital nephrotic syndrome)
  - Pyelonephritis
- Drugs/toxins
  - Bee sting
  - Food allergens
  - Antibiotic-induced interstitial nephritis
  - Penicillamine
  - Sirolimus
  - Gold salts
  - NSAIDs
  - Heavy metals (e.g., mercury, lead)
- Miscellaneous
  - Tubular interstitial nephritis
  - Acute tubular necrosis
  - Reflux nephropathy
  - Hypothyroidism
- Congestive heart failure

DIAGNOSTIC TESTS & INTERPRETATION

- For a first morning urine sample, instruct patient to urinate before bedtime and to collect urine as soon as they awaken and before ambulation.
- Dipstick testing
  - Always to be performed on a first morning urine sample
  - A negative or trace result in a concentrated urine specimen (specific gravity >1.020) is normal.
  - 1+ protein may be normal in very concentrated samples (specific gravity >1.030).
- Spot urine protein and urine creatinine (urine protein/creatinine ratio):
  - Always to be performed on a first morning urine sample
  - Simplest method to quantitate proteinuria
  - Normal values
    - <0.2 mg/mg in children >2 years of age
    - <0.5 mg/mg in children 6 to 24 months old
- 24-hour collection of urine for protein
  - Indicated for quantification of proteinuria and to confirm the diagnosis
  - Normal range: $<100\ mg/m^2/24\ h$ or $<4\ mg/m^2/h$
- Serum albumin
  - To assess for hypoalbuminemia, nephrotic syndrome
- Serum BUN and creatinine levels
  - Impaired renal function suggests inflammation, infection, or obstruction.
- Serum electrolytes and phosphorous levels
  - To screen for RTA and tubular function
- Evaluation for GN
  - Proteinuria with edema, hematuria, hypertension, and/or impaired renal function
  - Streptococcal serology (ASO titer, streptozyme): acute postinfectious GN
  - Complement studies (C3,C4): hypocomplementemic GN—immune complex mediated (lupus nephritis, postinfectious GN, membranoproliferative GN)
  - Antinuclear antibody (ANA) titer or anti–double-stranded DNA, hypocomplementemic or signs of systemic vasculitis: vasculitis (lupus nephritis)

ALERT

- Most pediatric patients with proteinuria will have orthostatic proteinuria that is identified by a first morning urine sample testing negative for protein while samples collected while upright test positive for protein.
- It is important to check the urine sediment for red cell casts; this indicates a glomerular involvement and requires additional studies for nephritis and chronic renal disease.

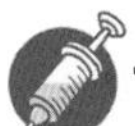

TREATMENT

GENERAL MEASURES

- Treatment is based on the etiology of the persistent proteinuria.
- In general, patients with chronic kidney disease and/or glomerulopathies should be treated with angiotensin-converting enzyme inhibitors or angiotensin receptor blockers to reduce proteinuria, inhibit renal fibrosis, and slow the progression of kidney disease.
- Patients with transient proteinuria or orthostatic proteinuria require no treatment.

ISSUES FOR REFERRAL

Nephrology should be consulted for patients with persistent (or fixed) proteinuria; proteinuria with hypertension, hematuria, or abnormal renal function; as well as patients with a family history of renal diseases with proteinuria.

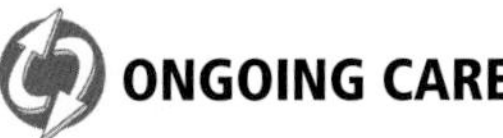

ONGOING CARE

PROGNOSIS

- Prognosis and follow-up is based on the etiology of the persistent proteinuria.
- Transient proteinuria resolves when the associated factor also resolves.
- Orthostatic proteinuria tends to resolve over time; there are no long-term adverse effects on renal function.

ADDITIONAL READING

- Gipson DS, Massengill SF, Yao L, et al. Management of childhood onset nephrotic syndrome. *Pediatrics*. 2009;124(2):747–757.
- Hogg RJ, Portman RJ, Milliner D, et al. Evaluation and management of proteinuria and nephrotic syndrome in children: recommendations from a pediatric nephrology panel established at the National Kidney Foundation Conference on proteinuria, albuminuria, risk, assessment, detection, and elimination (PARADE). *Pediatrics*. 2000;105(6):1242–1249.
- Quigley R. Evaluation of hematuria and proteinuria: how should a pediatrician proceed? *Curr Opin Pediatr*. 2008;20(2):140–144.

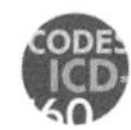

CODES

ICD10

- R80.9 Proteinuria, unspecified
- R80.2 Orthostatic proteinuria, unspecified
- R80.1 Persistent proteinuria, unspecified

FAQ

- Q: When to refer to nephrology?
- A: Patients with one of the following: fixed proteinuria; proteinuria with hypertension, hematuria, or abnormal renal function; and patient with family history of renal diseases with proteinuria
- Q: When are imaging studies indicated?
- A: Patients with abnormal renal function, hematuria, or nephrolithiasis. The best initial study is renal and bladder ultrasound.

PRURITUS

Anubhav Mathur, MD, PhD • Ilona J. Frieden, MD

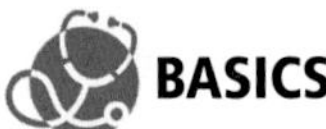

BASICS

DESCRIPTION

Pruritus, or itch, is one of the most frequent dermatologic complaints. It is an unpleasant sensation characterized by the reflexive behavior to scratch and is a symptom associated with numerous inflammatory and infectious skin diseases. However, generalized and persistent pruritus without or with minimal skin changes may be a presenting feature of a variety of systemic diseases.

PATHOPHYSIOLOGY

- Itch-specific peripheral nerves are unmyelinated afferent C-fibers.
- Pruritus is dependent on the complex interplay of neuroinflammatory modulators among peripheral nerves, keratinocytes, and leukocytes as well as central nervous system (CNS) processing.
- There are numerous mediators of pruritus, although histamine is the prototypical pharmacologic target for many patients.

ETIOLOGY

- Dermatologic: arising from skin disease
- Systemic: arising from noncutaneous organ systems including metabolic causes, drugs, and multifactorial disorders
- Neurogenic: arising from disorders of the central or peripheral nervous system
- Psychogenic: arising from primary psychiatric disorders
- Mixed: coexistence of more than one etiology of pruritus
- Idiopathic: pruritus of uncertain etiology

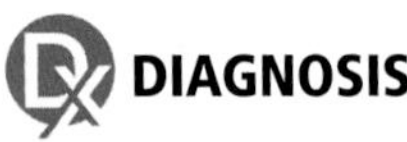

DIAGNOSIS

HISTORY

- Acute versus chronic (>6 weeks) of pruritus
- Location: generalized, scattered spots or localized
- Severity of symptoms
- Presence or absence of a preceding or concurrent rash
- Family members or close contacts with a similar complaint
- Environmental exposures: pets/other animals, poison oak or ivy, skin care products, soaps, shampoos, length and frequency of bathing/showering
- Medications (topical or systemic) or recreational drugs
- History of hematologic, hepatobiliary, renal, metabolic, neurologic, neoplastic, and psychiatric diseases
- Complete review of systems—particularly important for those without obvious skin findings

PHYSICAL EXAM

- Define and differentiate primary morphologies from secondary changes.
- Determine the location of the rash and areas of sparing.
- Evaluate for evidence of secondary cutaneous infections.
- Approach to the patient
  - Most children with pruritus have a primary dermatologic disease.
  - Common conditions include: atopic dermatitis (AD), allergic reactions to insect bites (so-called papular urticaria), fungal infection, scabies, hives, and dermatographism.
  - To develop a differential diagnosis, it is helpful to subdivide patients into one of four groups as below:
    - Generalized pruritus with definite skin disease
    - Generalized pruritus without definite skin disease (minimal or nonspecific skin lesions)
    - Localized pruritus with definite skin disease
    - Localized pruritus without definite skin disease (minimal or nonspecific skin lesions)
  - To identify common patterns of pruritus, consider the questions listed below:
    - **Question 1:** Are the findings characteristic of AD—the most common skin disease in children?
    - *Significance*:
      - Does the patient have a history of severe cradle cap or chronic/intermittent rash involving the face, antecubital or popliteal fossae, ankles or wrists?
      - AD is very common and typically has distinctive sites of predilection.
    - **Question 2:** Are there specific or nonspecific (scratching/rubbing induced) skin lesions present?
    - *Significance*:
      - If there are multiple morphologies, consider scabies.
      - If minimal or mostly secondary skin changes are present, but pruritus is severe, consider either scabies or a systemic cause (see below).
    - **Question 3:** Does the patient have clustered pink excoriated papules on the ankles, mid torso, or legs?
    - *Significance*:
      - This may represent bug bite reactions which are a common cause of pruritus in children.
      - These reactions disproportionately affect young children and may not be evident in their parents/guardians or even siblings.
    - **Question 4:** Does the patient have acute onset of rash with tiny vesicles, linear streaks of erythema on the face, arms, or legs?
    - *Significance*:
      - Poison oak/ivy is common and presents as an acute eczematous or vesiculobullous reaction.
    - **Question 5:** Does the patient have well-defined erythematous and scaling rash involving the scalp, extensor elbows, knees, umbilicus, or gluteal cleft?
    - *Significance*:
      - These findings suggest psoriasis. Although less common in children than AD, and usually less itchy, it has distinct sites of involvement with characteristic morphology.
      - Family history of psoriasis is common in patients who develop it in childhood.
    - **Question 6:** Does the patient have a chronic pruritic scaly rash around the umbilicus?
    - *Significance*:
      - Chronic allergic contact dermatitis from metals, especially to nickel, may present as an isolated itchy rash around the umbilicus due to a belt buckle or pant button.
      - For patients who wear earrings, ear lobes may be affected providing a diagnostic clue.
      - Many patients with nickel dermatitis have fine papules scattered on the arms and legs (so-called "id" reaction) or may have preexisting AD.
    - **Question 7:** Does the patient have any itchy rash involving the cheeks and nose with a rash on the dorsal forearms, sparing the volar arms?
    - *Significance*:
      - This pattern may present photosensitivity and suggests possible polymorphous light eruption or actinic prurigo.
  - For patients with a definite dermatologic cause for pruritus, treat the underlying cause.
  - Consider nondermatologic causes (listed below) for patients with severe generalized pruritus and nonspecific skin lesions—exclude scabies/infestation, dermatographism, and AD.
  - Localized pruritus with minimal or nonspecific skin lesions may suggest neuropathic itch, which is rare in children.

P

DIFFERENTIAL DIAGNOSIS

- Dermatologic diseases
  - Inflammatory skin diseases:
    - Dermatitis (atopic including nummular morphology, allergic contact, irritant contact, other)
    - Urticaria
    - Dermatographism
    - Psoriasis
    - Lichen planus
    - Mastocytosis
    - Dermatitis herpetiformis
    - Bullous pemphigoid
    - Epidermolysis bullosa pruriginosa
    - Polymorphous light eruption
  - Cutaneous infections and arthropod reactions
    - Scabies
    - Tinea/dermatophyte infection
    - Pediculosis
    - Flea bites
    - Mite reactions
    - Bedbug bites
    - Papular urticarial
    - Other arthropod reactions
  - Neoplastic: cutaneous lymphomas
- Systemic diseases
  - Endocrine
    - Thyroid and parathyroid disease
    - Diabetes mellitus
  - Infections
    - HIV
    - Hepatitis B and C
    - Systemic parasitic infections
  - Hematologic
    - Polycythemia vera/aquagenic pruritus
    - Iron deficiency anemia
    - Lymphomas
    - Leukemias
    - Hypereosinophilic syndrome
    - Myelodysplastic syndromes
  - Biliary diseases leading to cholestasis
  - Renal disease: uremic pruritus in chronic kidney disease
  - Malignancies
    - Solid tumors
    - Carcinoid syndrome
- Neurologic diseases
  - CNS malignancies or infections
  - Multiple sclerosis
  - Peripheral nerve injuries from compression or irritation
  - Radiculopathy
  - Polyneuropathy
- Psychiatric diseases
  - Psychogenic excoriations
  - Delusions of parasitosis
  - Somatoform disorders

DIAGNOSTIC TESTS AND INTERPRETATION

- Diagnostic testing is rarely required or helpful, as most children with pruritus have a primary dermatologic cause that can be clinically diagnosed.
- In patients with generalized pruritus without an obvious primary skin disease, the following studies should be considered based on clinical suspicion of the underlying cause for pruritus.

Initial Tests (screening, lab, imaging)

- CBC with differential
- Thyroid function tests (TFTs)
- Parathyroid hormone (PTH)
- HgbA1c
- Liver function tests
- AST, ALT, alkaline phosphatase, total bilirubin
- BUN, creatinine
- HIV 1, HIV 2 enzyme-linked immunosorbent assay (ELISA)
- Hepatitis B surface antigen
- Hepatitis C serology
- Iron studies
- Abdominal ultrasound
- Chest radiograph
- CNS imaging with MRI
- Light microscopy (from skin scrapings): KOH preparation for dermatophyte infections, and mineral oil examination for scabies. Note: must only be done with proper training
- Pathology
  - Skin biopsy specimens for H&E and direct immunofluorescence may be helpful in confirming the suspected dermatologic diagnosis.

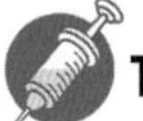

TREATMENT

- Treatment is directed to the underlying cause.
- Supportive measures:
  - Gentle skin care measures—including the use of nonsoap cleansers and gentle emollients
  - Loose cotton clothing
  - Sedating antihistamines in select cases
  - Topical corticosteroids and/or topical calcineurin inhibitors in select cases
- Phototherapy
  - Certain inflammatory conditions including psoriasis and some cases of severe AD may benefit from narrow band ultraviolet B (NBUVB) therapy.
  - Patients with certain systemic causes of pruritus such hepatobiliary or renal pruritus may benefit from NBUVB.

ISSUES FOR REFERRAL

- Severe or recalcitrant cases of pruritus
- Identification of or suspicion for a noncutaneous cause for pruritus

ADDITIONAL READING

- Cassano N, Tessari G, Vena GA, et al. Chronic pruritus in the absence of skin disease: an update on pathophysiology, diagnosis, and therapy. *Am J Clin Dermatol*. 2010;11(6):399–411.
- Charlesworth EN, Beltrani VS. Pruritic dermatoses: overview of etiology and therapy. *Am J Med*. 2002;113(Suppl 9A):25S–33S.
- Greaves MW. Pathogenesis and treatment of pruritus. *Curr Allergy Asthma Rep*. 2010;10(4):236–242.
- Paller AS, Mancini A. *Hurwitz Clinical Pediatric Dermatology*. 4th ed. New York, NY: Saunders; 2011.

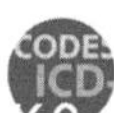

CODES

ICD10

- L29.9 Pruritus, unspecified
- F45.8 Other somatoform disorders
- L23.9 Allergic contact dermatitis, unspecified cause

FAQ

- Q: Which antihistamines work the best to treat itch?
- A: Although evidence is conflicting, sedating antihistamines such as hydroxyzine tend to work better than nonsedating ones for itch. An exception is urticaria, where sedating and nonsedating antihistamines relieve itch and prevent hives.
- Q: How does scratching affect pruritus?
- A: Scratching disrupts the skin barrier. By irritation or secondary infection, inflammatory mediators in the skin can worsen pruritus leading an "itch-scratch-itch" cycle.
- Q: What is gentle skin care?
- A: Gentle skin care is the concept of keeping the skin moist with emollients including creams or ointments thereby "repairing" the skin barrier. Application of an emollient, particularly after bathing, will help to keep the skin moist and reduce pruritus in patients with several inflammatory skin diseases.

PSITTACOSIS

Nicholas Tsarouhas, MD

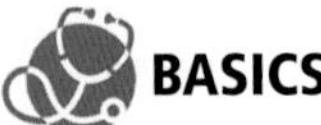

BASICS

DESCRIPTION

- An acute febrile disease characterized by pneumonitis and other systemic symptoms
- The name is derived from the Greek for parrot, *psittakos*; thus, psittacosis is often referred to as "parrot disease."
- Also known as *ornithosis*

EPIDEMIOLOGY

- Birds are the major reservoir of the psittacosis pathogen.
- Nearly all domestic and wild birds may spread this infection.
- Psittacine birds (parakeets, parrots, and macaws) are a major source of disease in the United States, but pigeons and turkeys are also common culprits.
  - Infecting agent is present in bird nasal secretions, urine, feces, feathers, viscera, and carcasses.
  - Inhalation of aerosols of feces, urine, and secretions of infected birds is the most common route of infection.
  - Handling of plumage, bird bites, and mouth-to-beak contact are known to spread infection.
  - Birds may be healthy or sick.
- Most reported cases (70%) are the result of exposure to pet caged birds (especially parrots, parakeets).
- Psittacosis is mainly an occupational disease among workers in poultry plants, duck or goose pluckers, pigeon breeders, pet store employees, and workers on farms and in zoos.
- Most common mammalian source of infection is sheep.
- Person-to-person transmission is so unusual that isolation of the infected patient is likely unnecessary.

Incidence

- Psittacosis is rare in humans.
- Only 100 to 200 total cases reported in United States each year. The Centers for Disease Control and Prevention (CDC) noted 813 cases of psittacosis from 1988 to 1998.
- Very rare disease in young children

RISK FACTORS

Close human contact with birds and, in some cases, sheep

GENERAL PREVENTION

- Epidemiologic investigation is indicated in all suspected cases.
- Birds suspected to be infected should be killed, transported, and analyzed by qualified experts.
- Potentially contaminated living areas where bird was kept should be disinfected and aired.
- Pathogen is susceptible to most household disinfectants (rubbing alcohol, bleach).
- The U.S. Department of Agriculture (USDA) requires veterinary inspection of birds at the first port of entry into the United States and quarantine for a minimum of 30 days at USDA-approved facilities to ensure the birds are free of evidence of communicable diseases.
- In addition, during U.S. quarantine, psittacine birds receive medicated feed containing chlortetracycline for the entire quarantine period as a precautionary measure against avian chlamydiosis.
- Human psittacosis is a nationally notifiable disease and should be reported to public health authorities.

PATHOPHYSIOLOGY

- Inhalation of aerosolized organisms into the respiratory tract
- Incubation period 5 to 14 days; may be longer
- Spreads via bloodstream to lungs, liver, and spleen
- Lymphocytic inflammatory alveolar response

ETIOLOGY

- Infection produced by *Chlamydophila psittaci*, an obligate intracellular parasitic bacterium
- Morphologically, antigenically, and genetically different from *Chlamydia* species

COMMONLY ASSOCIATED CONDITIONS

Pneumonitis (with a severe headache) is a common presentation.

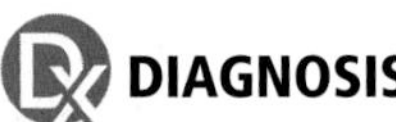

DIAGNOSIS

HISTORY

- Mandatory to question parents about exposure of the patient to any type of bird—wild or domestic
- Signs and symptoms
  - Abrupt onset of symptoms
  - Fever, headache, cough, weakness, chills, muscle aches, and joint pain
  - Nonproductive cough
  - Vomiting, confusion, and photophobia are less common findings.

PHYSICAL EXAM

- Ill-appearance, tachypnea, rales, and splenomegaly are common.
- A relative bradycardia is found in some cases.
- Less common findings
  - Rash
  - Meningismus
  - Pharyngeal injection
  - Cervical adenopathy
  - Hepatomegaly
  - Mental status changes

DIFFERENTIAL DIAGNOSIS

- Psittacosis should be considered in a patient with fever of unknown origin or atypical pneumonitis.
- Differential diagnosis includes the following:
  - *Mycoplasma pneumoniae*
  - *Chlamydophila pneumoniae*
  - *Legionella* spp.
  - *Coxiella burnetii* (i.e., Q fever)
  - Tuberculosis
  - Viral pneumonitis
  - Fungal pneumonitis
  - Pneumococcal pneumonia

DIAGNOSTIC TESTS & INTERPRETATION

- Routine laboratory studies are rarely helpful.
- Psittacosis can be diagnosed by culture, but *C. psittaci* is difficult to grow.
- Due to safety concerns with its isolation, it can only be grown in select laboratories.
- Polymerase chain reaction (PCR) of sputum or bronchial secretions and serology are the cornerstones of microbiologic diagnosis.

- Serologic techniques such as complement fixation test (CFT) and microimmunofluorescence (MIF) are most common.
- CFT (see "FAQ") do not, however, distinguish between the chlamydial infections (*Chlamydia trachomatis*) and the various chlamydophila infections (*C. psittaci*, *C pneumoniae*, and *Chlamydophila pecorum*).
- Chest radiographs are abnormal in 90% of hospitalized cases.
- Chest radiographs often not only demonstrate diffuse interstitial infiltrates but may also have unilateral lower lobe consolidation.

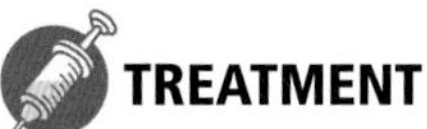

TREATMENT

MEDICATION

First Line

- Tetracycline (40 mg/kg/24 h divided q6h) or doxycycline (100 mg b.i.d.) in children ≥8 years of age
- In patients with severe infection, IV doxycycline (4 mg/kg/24 h, divided into two infusions, maximum 100 mg/dose) may be considered.
- Antibiotic therapy should be for a minimum of 10 days and should continue for 10 to 14 days after fever abates.

Second Line

Azithromycin and erythromycin are alternative agents and are recommended for younger children and pregnant women.

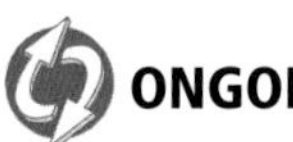

ONGOING CARE

PROGNOSIS

- The mortality rate prior to the advent of antimicrobial treatment was 15–20%, but now <1% with appropriate antibiotic therapy.
- Resolution of fever and most other systemic symptoms can be expected within 48 hours of antibiotic therapy.
- Untreated patients may have severe pulmonary symptoms for 1 to 3 weeks.

COMPLICATIONS

- Hepatitis
- Anemia
- Thrombophlebitis
- Pulmonary embolus
- Adult respiratory distress syndrome
- Arthritis
- Keratoconjunctivitis
- Endocarditis
- Myocarditis
- Pericarditis
- Encephalitis: agitation, delirium, confusion, stupor

ADDITIONAL READING

- American Academy of Pediatrics. Chlamydial infections: *Chlamydophila* (formerly *Chlamydia*) *psittaci* (psittacosis, ornithosis). In: Kimberlin DW, Brady MT, Jackson MA, et al, eds. *Red Book: 2015 Report of the Committee on Infectious Diseases*. 30th ed. Elk Grove Village, IL: American Academy of Pediatrics; 2015:286–287.
- Basarab M, Macrae MB, Curtis CM. Atypical pneumonia. *Curr Opin Pulm Med*. 2014;20(3):247–251.
- Honigsbaum M. In search of sick parrots: Karl Friedrich Meyer, disease detective. *Lancet*. 2014;383(9932):1880–1881.
- Ionescu AM, Khare D, Kavi J. Birds of a feather: an uncommon cause of pneumonia and meningoencephalitis. *BMJ Case Rep*. 2016;2016:bcr2016216879.
- Knittler MR, Sachse K. *Chlamydia psittaci*: update on an underestimated zoonotic agent. *Pathog Dis*. 2015;73(1):1–15.
- Levison M. Diseases transmitted by birds. *Microbiol Spectr*. 2015;3(4):IOL5-0004-2015.
- Spoorenberg SM, Bos WJ, van Hannen EJ, et al. *Chlamydia psittaci*: a relevant cause of community-acquired pneumonia in two Dutch hospitals. *Neth J Med*. 2016;74(2):75–81.

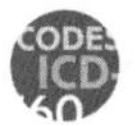

CODES

ICD10

A70 Chlamydia psittaci infections

FAQ

- Q: How is a clinical case confirmed?
- A: A clinically compatible illness with fever, chills, headache, cough, and myalgia with (i) isolation of *C. psittaci* from respiratory tract specimens or blood or (ii) 4-fold or greater increase in immunoglobulin G (IgG) by complement fixation (CF) or MIF against *C. psittaci* between paired acute- and convalescent-phase serum obtained at least 2 to 4 weeks apart. A "probable case" of psittacosis requires a clinically compatible illness and either (i) supportive serologic test results (e.g., *C. psittaci* immunoglobulin M [IgM] ≥32 in at least one serum specimen obtained after onset of symptoms) or (ii) detection of *C. psittaci* DNA in a respiratory tract specimen by PCR assay.
- Q: Does the source bird usually exhibit signs of disease?
- A: No. The bird is often asymptomatic; it may, however, show some signs of illness (e.g., anorexia, ruffled feathers, depression, or watery green droppings).

PSORIASIS

Leslie Castelo-Soccio, MD, PhD • Laura E. Kaplan, BA

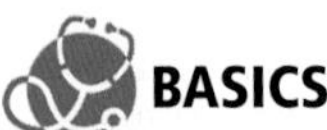

BASICS

DESCRIPTION

- A chronic relapsing skin disease most often characterized by thick white scales over erythematous plaques often involving elbows, knees, and scalp (i.e., psoriasis vulgaris). In children, psoriasis may present with less scaling and more erythema than in adults; may also present as diaper rash.
- Other variants include:
  - Guttate psoriasis—drop like plaques on the chest, back, and limbs; often in children following strep throat
  - Inverse psoriasis—lesions in flexures, also called intertriginous
  - Erythrodermic psoriasis—a severe variant with widespread erythematous skin involvement often accompanied by fever; can be life-threatening
  - Pustular psoriasis—generalized or localized, often affecting palms and soles; potentially lethal
  - Psoriatic arthritis—joint pain can precede skin involvement.

EPIDEMIOLOGY

- Involves both genders equally
- Onset of psoriasis is bimodal, commonly presenting in the 3rd decade with a smaller second peak of onset in the 6th decade; however, it can present at any age. Mean age of onset in children is 8.1 years.
- Earlier onset is associated with more severe disease.

Prevalence

Psoriasis is universal in occurrence, but prevalence varies in different populations. The average prevalence in the United States is ~1–3%.

RISK FACTORS

Genetics

- Although psoriasis has a strong genetic influence, mode of transmission is not defined. It is likely multifactorial with more than one gene involved and is modified by environmental influence.
- 1/3 of patients with psoriasis report a relative with the disease.
- In family studies, 8.1% of children develop psoriasis when one parent is affected.
- When both parents have psoriasis, the affected percentage increases to 41%.
- In twin studies, 65% of monozygotic twins are concordant for the disease, whereas only 30% of dizygotic twins are concordant.

PATHOPHYSIOLOGY

- Plaque-type psoriasis is characterized by a thickened parakeratotic epidermis with an absent granular layer above dermal papillae containing dilated tortuous capillaries.
- Collections of polymorphonuclear leukocytes extend from the dermal papillae into the epidermidis stratum corneum (i.e., Munro microabscesses).
- A mixed perivascular infiltrate is confined to the papillary dermis.

ETIOLOGY

The pathogenesis is unknown, possibly an immune-mediated inflammatory disease. Genetic factors are important. Well-defined trigger factors include the following:

- Trauma—psoriasis can develop in areas of trauma (i.e., isomorphic response, sometimes called the Koebner phenomenon).
- Infections (e.g., upper respiratory infections, *Streptococcus pyogenes*, human immunodeficiency virus)
- Stress
- Winter in colder climates in Northern Hemisphere
- Some drugs (i.e., systemic corticosteroids, lithium, NSAIDs, and antimalarials)

COMMONLY ASSOCIATED CONDITIONS

- Obesity
- Metabolic syndrome
- Hypertension
- Depression
- Anxiety
- Uveitis
- Arthritis
- Rheumatoid arthritis
- Crohn disease
- Diabetes mellitus
- Lymphoma (rare)

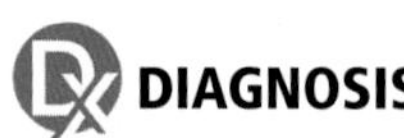

DIAGNOSIS

HISTORY

- Age of appearance of first eruption
- Recent illness, particularly sore throat
- Recent medications, particularly systemic steroids
- Family history of psoriasis
- Rash
  - Areas involved
  - Any appearance of lesions with trauma to skin
  - Improvement with sun exposure
  - Previous treatments and response
- Review of symptoms
  - Joint pain or swelling, nail changes

PHYSICAL EXAM

This must begin with a complete cutaneous skin exam.

- Lesion characteristics
  - Skin has thick, flaky scales over an erythematous base.
  - Psoriasis vulgaris
    - In psoriasis vulgaris, sharply demarcated erythematous plaques with white scale are located most commonly on the elbows, knees, scalp, lumbar area, and umbilicus, but they can cover any surface and large areas of the body.
  - Inverse psoriasis
    - Involves intertriginous regions and the face
    - Minimal or absent scale
    - More common in children
  - Guttate psoriasis
    - Form that more often presents in children and young adults as small papules (0.5 to 1.5 cm), with limited scale over the trunk and proximal extremities; can be symmetrically distributed
    - Frequently associated with a preceeding streptococcal infection
  - Scalp psoriasis
    - May be the first area involved in children
    - Pruritis may be prominent.
    - Occasionally, hair may be matted by thick scales and cause nonscarring alopecia (tinea amiantacea). Hair may return following treatment of psoriasis.
  - Erythrodermic psoriasis
    - Erythema with variable scale involving the majority of the body accompanied by chills is characteristic.
  - Generalized pustular psoriasis
    - Most serious variant
    - Sterile pustules as large as 23 mm arising on erythematous skin over large areas of the body. Usually, such appearance is accompanied by high fever.
  - Note: Classic plaque psoriasis is easily diagnosed, but variants and less virulent cases require careful exam for physical clues.
- Lesions in a linear or geometric pattern corresponding to areas of trauma are suggestive of Koebner phenomenon.
- Removal of scale on plaques produces bleeding points, a feature known as the Auspitz sign.
- Careful examination of the retroauricular portion of the scalp and the perianal region may reveal hidden disease.
- Other potential findings
  - Nails changes including pinpoint pits, hyperkeratosis, and oil spots.
  - Swollen or deformed joints suggest associated psoriatic arthritis. Dactilitis with sausage-shaped fingers may occur in children.
    - Can preceed or follow skin lesions

DIFFERENTIAL DIAGNOSIS

The differential diagnosis varies with the type of psoriasis and includes the following:

- Nummular eczema
- Cutaneous T-cell lymphoma
- Tinea corporis
- Pityriasis rosea
- Pityriasis lichenoides et varioliformis acuta
- Secondary syphilis
- Atopic dermatitis
- Drug eruption
- Candidiasis
- Seborrheic dermatitis

DIAGNOSTIC TESTS & INTERPRETATION

Initial Tests (screening, lab, imaging)

- An elevated uric acid level is a common finding.
- *S. pyogenes* infection is frequent in guttate disease, and throat culture is appropriate.
- Leukocytosis and hypocalcemia are associated with pustular psoriasis.
- Other laboratory values are generally within normal ranges. However, in more severe variants, anemia, elevated ESR, and decreased albumin levels may be found.
- Radiograph may be appropriate for joint involvement.
- Biopsy if uncertain of the diagnosis
  - See "Pathophysiology."

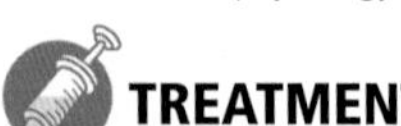

TREATMENT

GENERAL MEASURES

Most treatment regimens for children have not been evaluated in controlled studies and are based on expert opinion rather than evidence based.

- Moisturizers and keratolytics
  - Used as adjuvants
  - Moisturizers decrease itch and can remove scales. They are very well-tolerated.
  - Keratolytics such as salicylic acid, lactic acid, or urea are helpful to remove scales.
    - Salicylates should not be used in patients <2 years old due to systemic absorption.

- Topical
  - Topical corticosteroids
    - Mid- to high-potency topical corticosteroid ointments are applied twice daily.
    - Mid-potency preparations (e.g., 0.025% fluocinolone ointment, 0.1% triamcinolone acetonide) are preferred in children.
    - Low-potency corticosteroids (e.g., 1% and 2.5% hydrocortisone) are used on the face and intertriginous regions to prevent atrophy.
    - Potential side effects include striae, telangiectasia, acneiform dermatitis.
  - Anthralin
    - Used as a "short contact treatment" where high concentrations (0.1–3%) are applied for 10 to 30 minutes and carefully washed off. This diminishes the risk of irritation.
    - Avoid use on the face and intertriginous regions, as staining and irritation are common.
  - Calcipotriene
    - Calcipotriene ointment is a vitamin D_3 derivative.
    - It is applied twice daily, avoiding the face and intertriginous regions because of irritation.
    - Maximum weekly dosage in adults is 100 g or in children 45 g/m^2/week.
    - Not recommended for children <2 years
    - Rare cases of hypercalcemia have been reported.
    - Combination steroid/calcipotriene products exist.
  - Tazarotene gel
    - A topical retinoid
    - Can be irritating when used as monotherapy
    - Often combined with topical steroids as adjunctive therapy
  - Calcineurin (tacrolimus)
    - Good for sensitive sites such as face, flexures, and groin where corticosteroids may cause atrophy.
  - Coal tar
    - A weak therapeutic agent as monotherapy.
    - More effective when combined with UVB phototherapy (Goeckerman therapy)
    - Used in various shampoo preparations as well as in solution that can be added to the bath
- Phototherapy
  - UVB
    - Administered on average 2 to 3 times weekly in a booth with bulbs that emit the appropriate wavelength of UV radiation.
    - Effective for guttate and plaque psoriasis
    - Average treatment time: 3 months, with gradual increases in time of exposure. Sunscreen should be used on the face.
    - Narrow-band UVB represents a form of monochromatic UVB, using 311 nm wavelengths; appears to be a somewhat more effective form of delivering UVB phototherapy using booth or handheld device.
  - PUVA (psoralen and UVB)
    - PUVA and oral medications (e.g., methotrexate, acitretin) should be reserved for severe cases and carefully monitored by a dermatologist.

ALERT

Photosensitizing medication (e.g., tetracyclines, sulfa derivatives, phenothiazines, griseofulvin, among others) should be avoided with phototherapy.

- Systemic agents
  - May be considered when the psoriasis is especially severe or when joint symptoms are prominent
  - Most are not United States Food and Drug Administration (FDA)-approved for psoriasis in children, and potential risks exists. Etanercept was approved in 2016 for children 4 years to 17 years. They should not be prescribed without dermatology or rheumatology consultation.
  - Methotrexate
  - Isotretinoin or acitretin
  - Cyclosporine
  - Biologic agents such as etanercept, adalimumab, ustekinumab
  - Systemic corticosteroids should be avoided because withdrawal from steroids may be accompanied by a pustular psoriasis flare.

ISSUES FOR REFERRAL

- Pustules, a significant increase in degree or extent of erythema, or fever may require hospitalization and systemic therapy.
- Erythrodermic psoriasis may require hospitalization.
- Adult and pediatric patients with psoriasis have an increased prevalence of cardiovascular disease and metabolic syndrome. Patients should be monitored for blood pressure, glucose, weight, and lipids to decrease risk.

ADMISSION, INPATIENT, AND NURSING CONSIDERATIONS

Initial stabilization

- Therapy is delivered by topical medications, phototherapy, or systemic medications.
- Localized disease is treated with topical and more diffuse disease with phototherapy.
- Except in severe cases, therapy for children should be limited to topical medication and UVB phototherapy.
- Systemic medications for resistant cases

ONGOING CARE

FOLLOW-UP RECOMMENDATIONS

- Topical therapy is administered chronically, with breaks to minimize side effects.
- Remissions may occur in summer with sun exposure.
- The average treatment course with UVB therapy is 3 months and may be followed by an average remission period of 5 months.

PROGNOSIS

- Once psoriasis appears, it generally persists throughout life, typically in a chronic relapsing course.
- Spontaneous remissions of variable length and frequency occur but are unpredictable.
- Response depends on potency of medication and frequency of treatment.
- Improvement with topical medication is obvious at 2 weeks and usually peaks at 2 months.
- Scrubbing by the patient to remove scales also irritates the disease.
- Psychological aspects of the disease, particularly in children, should be addressed.

ADDITIONAL READING

- Garber C, Creighton-Smith M, Sorensen EP, et al. Systemic treatment of recalcitrant pediatric psoriasis: a case series and literature review. *J Drugs Dermatol*. 2015;14(8):881–886.
- Gutmark-Little I, Shah KN. Obesity and the metabolic syndrome in pediatric psoriasis. *Clin Dermatol*. 2015;33(3):305–315.
- Napolitano M, Megna M, Balato A, et al. Systemic treatment of pediatric psoriasis: a review. *Dermatol Ther (Heidelb)*. 2016;6(2):125–142.
- Oka A, Mabuchi T, Ozawa A, et al. Current understanding of human genetics and genetic analysis of psoriasis. *J Dermatol*. 2012;39(3):231–241.
- Raaby L, Ahlehoff O, de Thurah A. Psoriasis and cardiovascular events: updating the evidence. *Arch Dermatol Res*. 2017;309(3):225–228.
- Silverberg NB. Update on pediatric psoriasis. *Cutis*. 2015;95(3):147–152.
- Tollefson MM. Diagnosis and management of psoriasis in children. *Pediatr Clin North Am*. 2014;61(2):261–277.

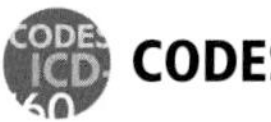

CODES

ICD10

- L40.9 Psoriasis, unspecified
- L40.0 Psoriasis vulgaris
- L40.4 Guttate psoriasis

FAQ

- Q: Will my disease get worse?
- A: It is impossible to predict the course of any patient's disease because it is influenced by both heredity and everyday factors in the environment. Although there is no cure, with treatment, the disease can be kept under control. Remissions do occur and may be for prolonged periods of time.
- Q: When my disease is in remission, what can I do to prevent it from returning?
- A: Avoiding trauma and keeping skin moist are important. In the summer, controlled sun exposure is helpful. You may have to continue other treatments at less frequent intervals. Any cases of sore throat should be cultured and treated if streptococcal disease is present.
- Q: Will my other children get psoriasis?
- A: If neither parent has psoriasis, the chances are <10% that another child will develop the disease; if one parent is affected, the chances increase to 15%; if both parents are affected, the chances are 50%. Therefore, unless both parents are affected, it is more likely that other children will not get psoriasis.
- Q: Does stress make psoriasis worse?
- A: Some studies have suggested that flare-ups of psoriasis are associated with increased stress. It is difficult to evaluate whether stress is the cause or the result of the disease. Do all you can to reasonably relieve stress, but do not focus on this as the cause of your psoriasis.

PUBERTAL DELAY

Angela P. Mojica, MD • Lucy D. Mastrandrea, MD, PhD

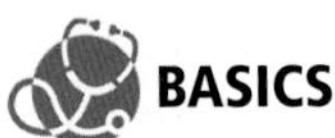

BASICS

DESCRIPTION

- Pubertal delay is the absence of secondary sexual characteristics (testicular enlargement in boys or breast development in girls) by an age that is >2 to 2.5 standard deviations (SD) beyond the population mean.
  - In the United States, this is considered to be ~13 years of age for girls and 14 years of age for boys.
  - Pubic hair development is usually not considered in the definition because adrenarche (adrenal gland maturation) may occur independently of gonadarche.
- Pubertal delay may also occur if progression through puberty stalls or takes >4 years between first signs of puberty and completion.
- Most cases of pubertal delay can be ascribed to constitutional delay of growth and puberty (CDGP); however, missing the presentation of an underlying disease should be avoided.
- CDGP
  - Extreme normal variant of pubertal development
  - Enter puberty late and usually reach normal adult height
  - More common in boys than in girls
  - Strong familial component (50–75%)

GENERAL PREVENTION

- Perform pubertal staging at regular intervals.
- Examine growth charts at routine visits to identify potential problems or changes in growth.
- Begin conversations about pubertal development with both patients and parents in late childhood. Realistic expectations regarding timing can avoid undue stress and unnecessary testing.
- Children with chronic health conditions should receive counseling regarding the effect their illness may have on their puberty. For example, children with cystic fibrosis generally have delayed puberty.

EPIDEMIOLOGY

- Approximately 2.5% of healthy teens will meet criteria for pubertal delay.
- CDGP explains 53–70% of pubertal delay.
- In contrast to boys, in girls, pubertal delay more frequently represents underlying pathology.
- Malnutrition is a risk factor for delayed puberty.

RISK FACTORS

Genetics

- Pubertal timing is highly influenced by genetic factors. This is evidenced by high correlation within ethnic groups, families, and between monozygotic twins.
- 50–80% of variation in timing can be explained by genetics, and in most cases, is due to multiple regulatory genes, rather than single gene mutations.
- CDGP
  - Inheritance is often consistent with an autosomal dominant pattern.
  - No specific causative gene mutations have been identified.
- Hypogonadotropic hypogonadism is associated with mutations in single genes including *GNRHR*, *KAL1*, *FGFR1*, and *GPR54*.
- *GPR54* (a G protein–coupled receptor) and its ligand (kisspeptin) play an important role as a signal for gonadotropin-releasing hormone (GnRH) release. Mutations in the *GPR54* gene have been found in patients with isolated hypogonadotropic hypogonadism (IHH) but not in those with CDGP.
- Pubertal delay due to underlying medical conditions is influenced by the pathophysiology of each disorder.
- Environmental factors
  - Influence pubertal timing through epigenetic mechanisms during neonatal or early postnatal life
  - Chronic disease and malnutrition may lead to delayed puberty.
  - Endocrine disruptors (industrial chemicals, pesticides, and phytoestrogens) influence pubertal timing. These effects likely are mediated through sex steroid receptors.

ETIOLOGY

Deficiency of gonadal sex steroids, estrogen in girls or testosterone in boys, is the underlying cause of delayed puberty. Several pathways to the common etiology exist:

- Hypogonadotropic hypogonadism: delayed puberty as a result of a deficiency in secretion of GnRH or gonadotropins (luteinizing hormone/follicle-stimulating hormone [LH/FSH])
  - Functional: delay or transient decrease in GnRH or gonadotropin secretion; describes CDGP, hypothyroidism, chronic illness
  - Permanent: irreversible deficiency of GnRH, such as in Kallmann syndrome, or gonadotroph abnormalities, as in panhypopituitarism
- Hypergonadotropic hypogonadism: gonadal failure as seen in Turner syndrome, Klinefelter syndrome, and anorchia

DIAGNOSIS

HISTORY

- A thorough history of past medical conditions, past growth patterns, and family history is essential.
- Parental family history of childhood growth patterns and age at pubertal onset (late menarche in the mother or delayed adult height completion in the father)
- A complete review of systems to uncover an underlying chronic disorder, such as inflammatory bowel disease, thyroid disorder, celiac disease, or eating disorder, is necessary.
- Assess nutrition history to evaluate for chronic malnutrition or eating disorder.
- Medication history may be useful (history of chronic glucocorticoid exposure or cytotoxins).
- A history of chemotherapy or radiotherapy may indicate primary gonadal failure.
- Bilateral cryptorchidism or a small penis at birth as well as hyposmia or anosmia may suggest hypogonadotropic hypogonadism.
- Prolactinomas may present as stalled pubertal progression ± galactorrhea.
- Request and examine a long-term growth chart:
  - CDGP will generally exhibit a consistent low percentile of growth throughout childhood, with linear growth deceleration in the peripubertal period. Growth rate is within the prepubertal normal range.
  - Gonadotropin or gonadal causes will generally present with normal growth in childhood but no increase in growth rate during the expected age of pubertal spurt.
- Obtain history of progression of secondary sex characteristics:
  - Adolescents with complete gonadal or gonadotropin deficiencies will not enter puberty unless initiated using exogenous hormones; those with CDGP will progress at a normal rate after initiation of puberty.
  - In CDGP, both adrenarche and gonadarche occur later than average.
  - In IHH, adrenarche usually occurs at a normal age.

PHYSICAL EXAM

A thorough physical exam is essential. Pay particular attention to the following elements:

- Thyroid examination
- Neurologic and funduscopic examinations to check for intracranial pathology
- Genital examination and sexual maturity rating (Tanner staging)
  - Pubic hair
  - Breast exam for girls
  - Penis/testicular exam for boys
  - Internal gynecologic examination for girls with amenorrhea may be indicated.
- The first sign of puberty in boys is when testicular length is >2.5 cm (>4 cc volume).
- The first sign of gonadarche in girls is breast development.
- In girls, determine whether there is marked discordance between pubic hair and breast development (androgen insensitivity).
- Assess for physical signs of Turner syndrome or Klinefelter syndrome.

DIFFERENTIAL DIAGNOSIS

- Increased serum gonadotropins (LH/FSH)
  - Congenital
    - Chromosomal abnormalities
    - Turner syndrome (gonadal dysgenesis)
    - Klinefelter syndrome
    - Disorders of sex development
  - Acquired
    - Primary gonadal failure
    - Cytotoxic chemotherapy or radiotherapy
    - Autoimmune gonadal failure
    - Vanishing testes syndrome
    - Trauma

- Normal or low serum gonadotropins
  - CDGP
  - Congenital
    - Gene defects (e.g., Kallmann syndrome)
    - Syndromes (e.g., Prader-Willi syndrome)
  - Acquired
    - CNS tumors/traumatic brain injury
    - Hypothalamic amenorrhea (strenuous exercise, eating disorders)
    - Chronic illness
    - Malnutrition
    - Primary hypothyroidism
    - Hyperprolactinemia
    - Drug-associated (psychotropics)

DIAGNOSTIC TESTS & INTERPRETATION

Initial Tests (screening, lab, imaging)

- Initial workup: routine screening tests for chronic or systemic disease
  - CBC
  - ESR
  - Electrolytes, renal function
  - Thyroid-stimulating hormone
  - Prolactin
  - Gonadotropin level—FSH and LH
    - Low levels suggest prepuberty or hypothalamic-pituitary failure.
    - High levels suggest gonadal failure or absence.
    - LH is a better marker of pubertal initiation than FSH.
    - In delayed puberty, an FSH value above the upper limit of the normal range for the assay is a sensitive and specific marker of primary gonadal failure.
    - If hypergonadotropic, obtain karyotype:
      - XX is suggestive of ovarian failure.
      - XO or abnormal X chromosome is indicative of Turner syndrome or gonadal dysgenesis.
      - XXY is indicative of Klinefelter syndrome.
- If all of the aforementioned studies are normal and there is no evidence to support CDGP, reevaluate for cryptic chronic illness (including prolactinoma), substance abuse, eating disorder, or ongoing psychosocial stress until puberty progresses or the underlying cause of delay becomes clear.
- No test reliably distinguishes CDGP from IHH. Patients with IHH have lower gonadotropins levels on average, yet there is still overlap with patients with CGDP.
- GnRH stimulation tests have limited diagnostic value for distinguishing IHH from CGDP.
- Inhibin B and anti-müllerian hormone (AMH, also known as Müllerian-inhibiting substance) are indicators of gonadal function and mass. However, absolute levels may not assist in the diagnosis.
- A combination of inhibin B <110 pg/mL and basal LH <0.3 IU/L demonstrated 98.1% specificity for IHH in a small cohort of patients.
- Bone age
  - An essential step in primary workup
  - Plain film of the epiphyseal growth centers in the left hand.
  - Epiphyses change in response to growth hormone, thyroxine, and steroids of adrenal or gonadal origin.
  - Bone age should be reviewed by a practitioner who is experienced in interpreting such radiographs.
  - Comparison to chronologic age can help to differentiate CDGP from organic disorders. A bone age that is >2 years delayed from chronologic age is consistent with CDGP. However, this degree of delay is not specific and can be found with other hypogonadotropic causes of delayed puberty or in gonadal failure.
- Pelvic ultrasound
  - Can be useful in locating intra-abdominal testicular structures or in determination of the presence or absence of müllerian structures
  - Indicated when testes are not palpated in patients with a male phenotype or when müllerian structures cannot be confirmed on physical examination in patients with a female phenotype
- MRI of the brain/pituitary
  - Useful in assessing pituitary or hypothalamic structures, mass lesions, pathologic calcifications, or increased intracranial pressure if a central cause of delayed puberty is suspected
- Full neuroendocrine testing
  - Warranted in patients with hypothalamic-pituitary tumors causing hypogonadotropic hypogonadism
- Imaging in patients with Kallmann syndrome commonly shows olfactory bulb and sulcus aplasia or hypoplasia.

ALERT

- No test can make a definitive diagnosis of CDGP. Eventual pubertal progression remains the primary discriminator between CDGP and IHH.
- Consultation with a specialist or experienced laboratory personnel is recommended before obtaining pituitary stimulation tests, as they may require special conditions.

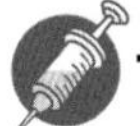

TREATMENT

GENERAL MEASURES

Most patients with pubertal delay do not require pharmacotherapy but may benefit from psychological and social support.

MEDICATION

- In cases of presumed CDGP, estrogen/testosterone therapy can be used to affect hypothalamic maturation, thereby initiating endogenous puberty.
- Referral to an endocrinologist or adolescent specialist is usually recommended before the initiation of hormonal therapy to aid in diagnosis and management.

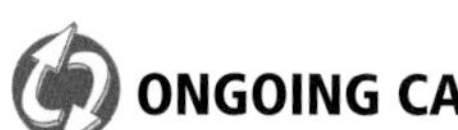

ONGOING CARE

In cases of permanent hypogonadism because of gonadal absence, failure, or gonadotropin deficiency, long-term hormonal therapy is necessary.

ADDITIONAL READING

- Abitbol L, Zborovski S, Palmert MR. Evaluation of delayed puberty: what diagnostic tests should be performed in the seemingly otherwise well adolescent? *Arch Dis Child*. 2016;101(8):767–771.
- Joffe A, Blythe MJ. Abnormalities of growth and development. *Adolesc Med State Art Rev*. 2009;20:434–441.
- Palmert MR, Dunkel L. Clinical practice. Delayed puberty. *N Engl J Med*. 2012;366(5):443–453.
- Pinyerd B, Zipf WB. Puberty-timing is everything! *J Pediatr Nurs*. 2005;20(2):75–82.
- Rosen DS, Foster C. Delayed puberty. *Pediatr Rev*. 2001;22(9):309–315.
- Wei C, Crowne EC. Recent advances in the understanding and management of delayed puberty. *Arch Dis Child*. 2016;101(5):481–488.

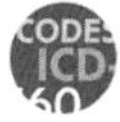

CODES

ICD10

- E30.0 Delayed puberty
- E28.39 Other primary ovarian failure
- E23.0 Hypopituitarism

FAQ

- Q: As ~70% of pubertal delay is constitutional or physiologic, when can I avoid an expensive workup and just observe the patient?
- A: Only the spontaneous onset of puberty confirms the diagnosis of constitutional delay. Anxiety from delayed puberty may preclude waiting. To make a presumptive diagnosis of CDGP, pathology must be ruled out:
  - Physical examination, including genital anatomy and sense of smell, must be normal.
  - There should be no signs or symptoms consistent with chronic disease.
  - History, including nutritional history and review of systems, must be negative.
  - Screening blood work must be negative.
  - Growth is slow for age, but height and growth rate are within prepubertal range.
  - A delay in bone age is characteristic but not diagnostic of CDGP.
- Q: When should patients with pubertal delay be seen by an endocrinologist or adolescent specialist?
- A: Often, the initial workup of pubertal delay can be completed by the primary care provider. For complex stimulation tests, or if help is needed in interpreting test results, referral to an experienced specialist is warranted. If a specific chronic disease is suspected as the underlying cause, then referral should be made to the appropriate subspecialist.

PULMONARY EMBOLISM

Akinyemi Ajayi, MBBS, FAAP, FCCP, FAASM

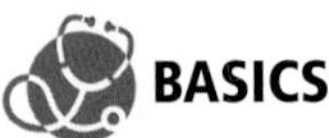

BASICS

DESCRIPTION
Occlusion of a pulmonary vessel by a thrombus

EPIDEMIOLOGY
- Pulmonary embolism (PE) is seen more frequently in adults and tends to occur in postsurgical situations, especially when patients have been bedridden. Two patterns are described in children, classic thromboembolic PE (TE-PE) and in situ pulmonary artery thrombosis (ISPAT).
- Mean age for TE-PE in children is 14.9 years and 51% of cases are male.
- ~10% of adults who present with an acute PE die within 1 hour of onset.
- Increasing incidence is secondary to increased central catheter use.
- Mortality rate can be as high as 30% if diagnosis is delayed.
- The incidence of new cases of PE presenting to a large, urban pediatric emergency department was 2.1 cases per 100,000 visits.

RISK FACTORS
- In children
  - Presence of a central venous catheter
  - Lack of mobility
  - Congenital heart disease
  - Ventriculoatrial shunt
  - Trauma
  - Solid tumors or leukemia
  - After-surgical procedures (especially reparative intervention for scoliosis repair)
  - Hypercoagulable condition
  - Systemic infection
  - Elevated factor VIII or von Willebrand factor levels
  - Protein C deficiency
  - Factor V Leiden deficiency
  - Protein S deficiency
- In adults: most commonly due to the presence of a deep vein thrombosis, usually in the legs or pelvis

PATHOPHYSIOLOGY
- Thromboemboli may develop anywhere in the systemic venous system.
- PE is characterized by the triad of hypoxemia, pulmonary hypertension, and right ventricular failure.
  - Diminished pulmonary perfusion causes a ventilation–perfusion mismatch, resulting in hypoxemia.
  - Hyperventilation occurs secondary to stimulation of proprioceptors in the lung.
  - Hypercapnia is seen with severe occlusion of the pulmonary artery (often not seen with smaller emboli).
- Pulmonary infarction is uncommon due to the presence of collateral pulmonary and bronchial arteries along with the airways providing additional sources of oxygen to the tissues.
- Death occurs with 85% obstruction of the pulmonary artery.

ETIOLOGY
Blood clots appear as a result of deep vein thrombosis or other disease states.

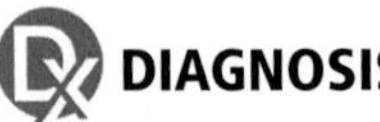

DIAGNOSIS

ALERT

Failure to make the diagnosis is the most common mistake.
- PE must be suspected in critically ill children who have a central venous catheter in place and subsequently develop sudden respiratory failure.
- Because the symptoms of severe lung disease and PE are similar, the diagnosis might be missed if the index of suspicion is low.

Signs and symptoms
- PE should be suspected in children who present with the following:
  - Pleuritic chest pain
  - Shortness of breath
  - Hemoptysis
  - Cough
  - Acute respiratory distress
  - Apprehension or anxiety
  - Syncope
  - Cardiovascular shock
- Symptoms may be nonspecific and indicative of other disorders.

HISTORY
Ask about chest symptoms: The clinician must have a high index of suspicion and recognize risk factors to establish the correct diagnosis.

PHYSICAL EXAM
- Findings on physical examination are nonspecific.
- General
  - Fever
  - Diaphoresis
  - Nervousness or apprehension (Altered mental status is uncommon.)
- Cardiovascular
  - Increased intensity of the pulmonic component of S_2
  - Tachycardia
  - Gallop rhythm
  - New murmur
- Pulmonary
  - Tachypnea
  - Rales
  - Cyanosis (present with 65% obstruction of the pulmonary artery)
  - Pleuritic chest pain
  - Dyspnea
  - Cough
  - Hemoptysis
  - Wheezing (uncommon)
- Extremities
  - Deep venous thrombosis is frequently found in the adult population.
  - Phlebitis
  - Edema

DIFFERENTIAL DIAGNOSIS
- Cardiac
  - Cardiac tamponade
  - Constrictive pericarditis
  - Restrictive cardiomyopathy
- Pulmonary
  - Chronic cough
  - Status asthmaticus
  - Pneumonia with empyema
  - Pneumothorax

DIAGNOSTIC TESTS & INTERPRETATION

Initial Tests (screening, lab, imaging)
- In general, blood tests are nonspecific and of no significant value in making the diagnosis of a PE.
- Arterial blood gases
  - Decreased Pa_{O_2} and Pa_{CO_2}
  - Increased alveolar–arterial (A–a) gradient
- Electrocardiogram
  - Useful in ruling out other conditions
  - May show sinus tachycardia or nonspecific ST-T wave changes
- Echocardiogram
  - Useful for identifying
    - Abnormalities of cardiac anatomy
    - Thrombi on catheter tips
  - If emboli are seen on echocardiogram, mortality rate is 40–50%. Additionally, if signs of right ventricular dysfunction are noted (e.g., right ventricular dilatation, abnormal right ventricular wall motion, or increased tricuspid regurgitation jet velocity), risk of poor outcome is greater.
- Spiral computed tomography (CT)
  - Greater sensitivity than ventilation–perfusion scan in the diagnosis of PE due to the ability to image abnormal pulmonary pathology
- Chest radiograph
  - May be abnormal in 70% of patients with PE
  - Most frequent findings:
    - Parenchymal infiltrates
    - Atelectasis
    - Pleural effusions: seen in 33% of cases, mostly unilateral
    - Hampton hump (pyramidal shape pointing toward the hilum)
- Ventilation–perfusion scan
  - Results of a ventilation–perfusion scan performed to rule out a PE are reported in one of five categories, ranging from high probability to normal.
  - An abnormal ventilation–perfusion scan with normal ventilation and decreased perfusion in the appropriate clinical setting is 90% specific for a PE.
  - A normal result on ventilation–perfusion scan does not completely rule out PE, although if the patient is at low risk, a PE is highly unlikely.
- CT pulmonary angiography
  - Most sensitive and specific test
  - Not done as frequently in children as in adults because of complications associated with the procedure

– With the introduction of newer, improved catheters and safer contrast solutions, this test can now safely be performed in the pediatric population.
– Indicated for cases
  ○ Intermediate-probability ventilation–perfusion scans
  ○ High-probability scans in patients who are poor candidates for anticoagulation, hemodynamically unstable, or require an embolectomy

Diagnostic Procedures/Other

- Pulmonary function testing
  – Results are nonspecific.
- Evaluation of the lower extremities
  – Diagnosing deep vein thrombosis via the following
    ○ Impedance plethysmography
    ○ Doppler technology
    ○ Venography

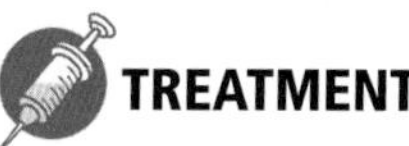

TREATMENT

GENERAL MEASURES

Initial stabilization

- Stabilize patient before anticoagulation or thrombolytic therapy is begun:
  – Improve oxygenation.
  – Correct acidosis.
  – Stabilize blood pressure.
  – Analgesia for severe pleuritic chest pain. Avoid prescribing opiates in cases of cardiovascular collapse.
- Goal of therapy is anticoagulation and/or thrombolysis.
- In patients with an intermediate or high suspicion, begin anticoagulation before investigations.

MEDICATION

- Anticoagulation therapy to prevent further thrombus formation
  – Heparin
    ○ Bolus dose: 100 to 200 U/kg
    ○ Maintenance dose: 10 to 25 U/kg/h
    ○ Keep partial thromboplastin time (PTT) at 55 to 60 seconds.
    ○ Should be given for 7 to 10 days
  – Warfarin
    ○ Warfarin should be started 24 to 48 hours after heparin therapy is begun.
    ○ Maintenance dose: 2.5 to 10 mg/24 h
    ○ Keep prothrombin time (PT) twice normal and maintain the international normalized ratio (INR) between 2 and 3.
    ○ Should be continued for 36 months
- Thrombolytic therapy
  – Agents available
    ○ Urokinase
    ○ Tissue plasminogen activator (TPA): same efficacy as streptokinase and lower incidence of allergic reactions
  – Indications
    ○ Hemodynamically unstable
    ○ Large embolus
- Low-molecular-weight heparin has been used as prophylaxis or as treatment for preexisting conditions in both adults and children.
  – A synthetic, nonthrombocytopenic heparin pentasaccharide with pure antifactor Xa activity is currently being tested.
- Ticlopidine and clopidogrel have been used successfully to prevent thrombotic strokes and arterial thrombotic syndromes.
- Non–vitamin K antagonists (VKAs) have been used for long-term anticoagulant benefit in patients with PE.
- Contraindications to anticoagulation therapy
  – Active internal bleeding
  – Recent cerebrovascular accident
  – Major surgery
  – Recent gastrointestinal bleed

SURGERY/OTHER PROCEDURES

- Embolectomy
  – Indicated when hemodynamic instability persists; reserved for patients who have failed thrombolytic therapy or in whom medical treatment is contraindicated
  – Late results are excellent if the patient has not suffered from a perioperative cardiac arrest, which is associated with early mortality.
- Percutaneous caval filtration
  – Indicated if commencement or continuation of anticoagulation is strongly contraindicated or if full anticoagulation has failed to prevent recurrent emboli
  – This should be considered in patients undergoing venous thrombolysis because up to 20% may develop embolization during treatment.

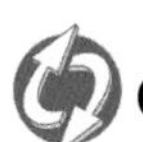

ONGOING CARE

Patients receiving warfarin therapy should have the usual follow-up for those receiving an anticoagulant.

PROGNOSIS

- If treated promptly, prognosis is good.
- If treatment is delayed, especially if the patient is hemodynamically unstable, prognosis is poor.

ADDITIONAL READING

- Agha BS, Sturm JJ, Simon HK, et al. Pulmonary embolism in the pediatric emergency department. *Pediatrics*. 2013;132(4):663–667.
- Biss TT, Brandão LR, Kahr WH, et al. Clinical features and outcome of pulmonary embolism in children. *Br J Haematol*. 2008;142(5):808–818.
- Cohen AT, Dobromirski M, Gurwith MM. Managing pulmonary embolism from presentation to extended treatment. *Thromb Res*. 2014;133(2):139–148.
- Fedullo PF, Tapson VF. Clinical practice. The evaluation of suspected pulmonary embolism. *N Engl J Med*. 2003;349(13):1247–1256.
- Goldhaber SZ, Elliott CG. Acute pulmonary embolism: part I: epidemiology, pathophysiology, and diagnosis. *Circulation*. 2003;108(22):2726–2729.
- Hennelly KE, Baskin MN, Monuteuax MC, et al. Detection of pulmonary embolism in high-risk children. *J Pediatr*. 2016;178:214–218.e3.
- Kalaniti K, Lo Rito M, Hickey EJ, et al. Successful pulmonary embolectomy of a saddle pulmonary thromboembolism in a preterm neonate. *Pediatrics*. 2015;135(5):e1317–e1320.
- Kruip MJ, Leclercq MG, van der Heul C, et al. Diagnostic strategies for excluding pulmonary embolism in clinical outcome studies. A systematic review. *Ann Intern Med*. 2003;138(12):941–951.
- Meister B, Kropshofer G, Klein-Franke A, et al. Comparison of low-molecular-weight heparin and antithrombin versus antithrombin alone for the prevention of symptomatic venous thromboembolism in children with acute lymphoblastic leukemia. *Pediatr Blood Cancer*. 2008;50(2):298–303.
- Monagle P. Diagnosis and management of deep venous thrombosis and pulmonary embolism in neonates and children. *Semin Thromb Hemost*. 2012;38(7):683–690.
- Patocka C, Nemeth J. Pulmonary embolism in pediatrics. *J Emerg Med*. 2012;42(1):105–116.
- Rajpurkar M, Biss T, Amankwah EK, et al. Pulmonary embolism and in situ pulmonary artery thrombosis in paediatrics. A systematic review. *Thromb Haemost*. 2017;117(6):1199–1207.
- Snow V, Qaseem A, Barry P, et al; and Joint American College of Physicians/American Academy of Family Physicians Panel on Deep Venous Thrombosis/Pulmonary Embolism. Management of venous thromboembolism: a clinical practice guideline from the American College of Physicians and the American Academy of Family Physicians. *Ann Fam Med*. 2007;5(1):74–80.
- Zierler BK. Ultrasonography and diagnosis of venous thromboembolism. *Circulation*. 2004;109(12 Suppl 1): I9–I14.

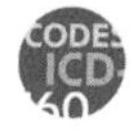

CODES

ICD10

I26.99 Other pulmonary embolism without acute cor pulmonale

FAQ

- Q: Is it safe for children on warfarin to play contact sports?
- A: The general recommendation is that no contact sports should be allowed while children are on warfarin therapy because of the increased risk of bleeding.

PULMONARY HYPERTENSION

Richard M. Kravitz, MD

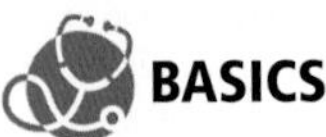

BASICS

DESCRIPTION
Increased pulmonary vascular resistance

EPIDEMIOLOGY
Incidence
Incidence in children is unknown.

PATHOPHYSIOLOGY
- Structural alterations in pulmonary vessel architecture (remodeling)
- Smooth muscle hypertrophy
- Extension of blood vessel's smooth muscle into smaller vessels
- Inflammation

ETIOLOGY
- Hypoxemia-induced pulmonary hypertension
- Chronic lung disease
  - Cystic fibrosis
  - Bronchopulmonary dysplasia
  - Interstitial lung disease
  - Diaphragmatic hernia with secondary pulmonary hypoplasia
- Upper airway obstruction
  - Tonsillar and/or adenoid hypertrophy
  - Obesity
- Hypoventilation
  - Neurologically mediated process
  - Secondary to muscular weakness
- High pulmonary blood flow secondary to left-to-right shunting (seen in congenital heart disease)
  - Patent ductus arteriosus
  - Atrial septal defect
  - Ventricular septal defect
- Left-sided cardiac disorders that increase pulmonary venous pressure
  - Left ventricular failure
  - Mitral valve stenosis
  - Obstructed anomalous pulmonary veins
- Occlusion of pulmonary vessels
  - Sickle cell disease
  - Veno-occlusive disease
  - Thromboembolism
- Pulmonary vasculitis
  - Systemic lupus erythematosus
  - Rheumatoid arthritis
  - Scleroderma
- Persistent pulmonary hypertension of the newborn
- Idiopathic cases (primary pulmonary hypertension)

DIAGNOSIS

HISTORY
- Dyspnea (usually earliest complaint reported)
- Fatigue
  - Seen early in course of illness with exercise or exertion (but not at rest)
  - Seen at rest in the later stages of the illness or in severe cases
- Exercise intolerance
- Feeding intolerance
- Failure to thrive
- Excessive sleeping
- Diaphoresis
- Chest pain
- Syncope
- Palpitations (late finding)
- Signs and symptoms pitfalls:
  - Signs and symptoms of pulmonary hypertension are not specific and can easily be missed.
  - Consider obstructive sleep apnea as a possible cause of pulmonary hypertension (ask about snoring if suspecting pulmonary hypertension in the absence of overt cardiac or pulmonary disease).

PHYSICAL EXAM
- Typically governed by the signs and findings related to underlying lung or heart disease
- Tachypnea
- Arrhythmias
- Narrowed splitting of S_2 heart sound
- Increased P_2 heart sound
- Presence of S_3 and/or S_4 heart sounds
- Murmur of pulmonary or tricuspid insufficiency; tricuspid insufficiency more common
- Jugular venous distention
- Peripheral edema
- Hepatomegaly

DIFFERENTIAL DIAGNOSIS
- Pulmonary
  - Asthma
  - Cystic fibrosis
  - Chronic obstructive pulmonary disease
  - Emphysema
  - Pulmonary arteriovenous malformations
- Miscellaneous
  - Congestive heart failure (CHF)
  - Noncardiogenic pulmonary edema
  - Fatigue
  - Syncope

DIAGNOSTIC TESTS & INTERPRETATION
Initial Tests (screening, lab, imaging)
- Arterial blood gases
  - Measurement of Po_2 assesses degree of hypoxia.
  - Evaluation of Pco_2 determines presence or absence of hypoventilation.
- Chest radiograph
  - Will vary according to the underlying disorder and extent of pulmonary hypertension
  - Degree of pulmonary hypertension correlates poorly with chest radiograph findings.
  - In primary pulmonary hypertension
    - Cardiomegaly
    - Enlarged pulmonary artery
    - Peripheral lung appears underperfused ("pruning" of pulmonary vessels).

Diagnostic Procedures/Other
- EKG
  - Can be normal if cor pulmonale has not yet developed
  - If cor pulmonale present, EKG can demonstrate
    - Right QRS axis deviation
    - Right ventricular hypertrophy
    - Right atrial hypertrophy
- Echocardiogram with Doppler flow
  - Increased pulmonary artery pressure
  - Right ventricular hypertrophy
  - Paradoxical movement of the intraventricular septum
  - Pulmonic and tricuspid valve regurgitation
  - Right-to-left shunting via an open foramen ovale
- Cardiac catheterization
  - Most accurate measurement of pulmonary artery pressure is accomplished by right heart catheterization.
  - Criteria for pulmonary hypertension in children:
    - Mean pulmonary arterial pressure >25 mm Hg (at rest)
    - Mean pulmonary arterial pressure >30 mm Hg (with exercise)
    - Pulmonary vascular resistance >3 U/m^2
    - Systolic pulmonary artery pressure >1/2 systolic systemic pressure
- Pressures should be measured before and after various vasodilators to assess potential reversibility of pulmonary hypertension.
- Caution: In patients with severe disease, catheterization is associated with increased risk of complications.

TREATMENT

GENERAL MEASURES

- Provide for patient stabilization.
- Treat the primary disease process.
- Treat underlying hypoxia (supplemental oxygen).
- Treat underlying hypoventilation:
  - Useful for correcting hypoxia and hypercarbia secondary to hypoventilation
  - Available methods:
    - Noninvasive positive pressure ventilation (bilevel ventilation)
    - Mechanical ventilation (tracheostomy with mechanical ventilation)

MEDICATION

- Oxygen
  - Acts as a vasodilator
  - Keep $Sao_2 \geq 95\%$
  - Supplemental oxygen may prove useful even with normal resting Sao_2 (supplemental oxygen will cover for desaturations associated with exertion, exercise, or illness).
  - Caution: Supplemental oxygen can sometimes cause hypercapnia by blunting the hypoxia-driven respiratory drive.
- Anticoagulation therapy (i.e., Coumadin)
  - Prevents clot formation in the narrowed pulmonary vessels
  - Helpful even in the absence of thromboembolic disease
- Vasodilators
  - Methods of action
    - Decreases pulmonary arterial pressures
    - Improves right-sided cardiac function
  - Available agents
    - Oxygen
    - Calcium channel blocker (i.e., nifedipine)
    - Nitric oxide (continuous inhalation)
    - Prostacyclin (continuous IV infusion) (i.e., epoprostenol)
    - Endothelin receptor antagonist, PO (i.e., bosentan)
    - Phosphodiesterase inhibitor PO (i.e., sildenafil)
  - Caution: Vasodilators should be used under close supervision because of their effect on systemic BP (systemic hypotension can be a significant problem).

SURGERY/OTHER PROCEDURES

- Tonsillectomy and/or adenoidectomy if obstructive sleep apnea is the underlying etiology
- Atrial septostomy may be considered when inadequate right-to-left shunting is present with syncopal episodes and/or right-sided heart failure.
- Transplantation (lung or heart-lung transplantation): reserved for patients with refractory, severe pulmonary hypertension

ONGOING CARE

PROGNOSIS

- Dependent on underlying etiology, but the overall prognosis has been improving with the advent of newer therapies
- In cases of primary pulmonary hypertension, improvement of pulmonary hypertension with administration of vasodilators during initial catheterization is associated with a better survival rate than if no response occurs.
- 10–40% mortality in treated patients
- Near 100% mortality if patient is untreated
- Treatment can be lifelong unless the primary cause of the pulmonary hypertension can be corrected.
- In acute pulmonary hypertension, response to most treatment modalities is almost immediate.
- Oxygen has been shown to reverse hypoxia-related remodeling of the airways after 1 month of therapy.

COMPLICATIONS

- Chronic hypoxia
- Exercise intolerance
- Right-sided heart failure (cor pulmonale)
- Death

ADDITIONAL READING

- Abman SH, Hansmann G, Archer SL, et al; for American Heart Association Council on Cardiopulmonary, Critical Care, Perioperative and Resuscitation; Council on Clinical Cardiology; Council on Cardiovascular Disease in the Young; Council on Cardiovascular Radiology and Intervention; Council on Cardiovascular Surgery and Anesthesia; and the American Thoracic Society. Pediatric pulmonary hypertension: guidelines from the American Heart Association and the American Thoracic Society. *Circulation*. 2015;132(21):2037–2099.
- Barst RJ, Ertel SI, Beghetti M, et al. Pulmonary arterial hypertension: a comparison between children and adults. *Eur Respir J*. 2011;37(3):665–677.
- Berger RMF, Bonnet D. Treatment options for paediatric pulmonary arterial hypertension. *Eur Respir Rev*. 2010;19(118):321–330.
- Chatterjee K, De Marco T, Alpert JS. Pulmonary hypertension: hemodynamic diagnosis and management. *Arch Intern Med*. 2002;162(17):1925–1933.
- Hawkins A, Tulloh R. Treatment of pediatric pulmonary hypertension. *Vasc Health Risk Manag*. 2009;5(2):509–524.
- Klings ES, Farber HW. Current management of primary pulmonary hypertension. *Drugs*. 2001;61(13):1945–1956.
- Mourani PM, Sontag MK, Younoszai A, et al. Clinical utility of echocardiography for the diagnosis and management of pulmonary vascular disease in young children with chronic lung disease. *Pediatrics*. 2008;121(2):317–325.
- Oishi P, Datar SA, Fineman JR. Advances in the management of pediatric pulmonary hypertension. *Respir Care*. 2011;56(9):1314–1340.
- Ravishankar C, Tabbutt S, Wernovsky G. Critical care in cardiovascular medicine. *Curr Opin Pediatr*. 2003;15(5):443–453.
- Rosenzweig EB, Widlitz AC, Barst RJ. Pulmonary arterial hypertension in children. *Pediatr Pulmonol*. 2004;38(1):2–22.
- Schulze-Neick I, Beghetti M. Issues related to the management and therapy of paediatric pulmonary hypertension. *Eur Respir Rev*. 2010;19(118): 331–339.
- Simonneau G, Galiè N, Rubin LJ, et al. Clinical classification of pulmonary hypertension. *J Am Coll Cardiol*. 2004;43(12, Suppl S):5S–12S.
- Widlitz A, Barst RJ. Pulmonary arterial hypertension in children. *Eur Respir J*. 2003;21(1):155–176.
- Yeh TF. Persistent pulmonary hypertension in preterm infants with respiratory distress syndrome. *Pediatr Pulmonol*. 2001;32(Suppl 23):103–106.

CODES

ICD10

- I27.2 Other secondary pulmonary hypertension
- I27.0 Primary pulmonary hypertension
- P29.3 Persistent fetal circulation

FAQ

- Q: How many hours per day should supplemental oxygen be used?
- A: Studies have shown decreased mortality in patients using oxygen 24 hours per day compared with patients using supplemental oxygen for only part of the day.
- Q: Should the dosage of oxygen be adjusted during the day according to the patient's activity?
- A: Increasing supplemental oxygen should be considered for activities that require increased oxygen consumption (i.e., exercise, eating, and sleeping).
- Q: Can an echocardiogram replace the need for a cardiac catheterization?
- A: No. Although an abnormal echocardiogram can confirm the presence of pulmonary hypertension, it does not inform one of its severity or the (acute) response to therapy. Furthermore, a normal study does not rule out pulmonary hypertension (especially mild cases).

PURPURA FULMINANS

Mihir D. Bhatt, MD, FRCPC • Victoria E. Price, MBChB, MSc, FRCPC

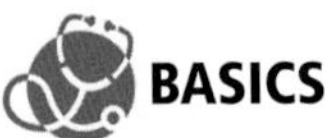

BASICS

DESCRIPTION

- Hematologic emergency characterized by dermal hemorrhagic necrosis and disseminated intravascular coagulation (DIC)
- Associated with a congenital or acquired protein C and/or protein S deficiency
- Life-threatening condition that requires prompt diagnosis and judicious replacement therapy to decrease morbidity and mortality

EPIDEMIOLOGY

- Neonatal purpura fulminans related to homozygous protein C deficiency: 1 in 2 to 4 million births
- Clinical protein C deficiency: 1 in 20,000 individuals
- Homozygous protein S deficiency is exceptionally rare.
- Predicted prevalence of severe protein C deficiency is 1 in 40,000 to 250,000 individuals; significantly less seen in practice, likely due to associated high rate of fetal loss and perinatal mortality

RISK FACTORS

Genetics

- Deficiencies of protein C and protein S are autosomally inherited with variable penetrance.
- >150 different genetic mutations of protein C have been described, leading to both qualitative and quantitative defects of the proteins.
- Homozygous protein C or S deficiency and compound heterozygous states are associated with severe deficiency, <1% normal activity level.
- Neonatal purpura fulminans is associated with a severe protein C or S deficiency.
- Coinheritance with other thrombophilias may also contribute to the risk of developing purpura fulminans.
- Heterozygous protein C and S deficiency are associated with a lifetime increased risk of venous and arterial thrombosis.

PATHOPHYSIOLOGY

Common features of purpura fulminans:

- DIC: Endothelial injury from bacterial endotoxin or other trigger may initiate secretion of inflammatory cytokines or activation of coagulation and complement proteins.
- Purpura: due to perivascular hemorrhage
- Dermal vascular thrombosis: formation of microthrombosis in blood vessels of the skin, leading to hemorrhage in the skin (purpura), necrosis of skin, and gangrene

ETIOLOGY

- Acquired causes
  - Severe acute bacterial or viral infections: *Neisseria meningitidis* most common
  - Postinfectious fulminans: most commonly associated with varicella and *Streptococcus* infections. Caused by cross-reacting IgG antibodies that increase protein S clearance from the circulation. Consider in an otherwise well child with new-onset purpura fulminans and DIC.
  - Warfarin (Coumadin®)-induced skin necrosis
  - DIC
  - Antiphospholipid antibodies
  - Cardiac bypass
  - Severe liver dysfunction
  - Galactosemia
  - Severe congenital heart disease
- Inherited protein C pathway defects
  - Predisposes to a reduced capacity to inhibit thrombin formation and therefore a hypercoagulable state
- Inherited defect of coagulation presenting as neonatal purpura fulminans
  - Protein C slows ("brakes") the coagulation cascade at two steps: by degrading activated factor V and activated factor VIII.
  - Also plays a role in inflammatory cascade
  - Protein S is a cofactor for protein C.

DIAGNOSIS

HISTORY

- Current sepsis: fever, weakness, dizziness, nausea, vomiting, onset of petechial/purpuric rash
- Recent history of febrile illness
- Medications (e.g., warfarin)
- Family history suggestive of hypercoagulable state
- History of consanguinity
- Thromboses at an early age, such as stroke, deep vein thrombosis, pulmonary embolism
- Family members taking warfarin (Coumadin®) or low-molecular-weight heparin or other anticoagulant
- Previous affected child with purpura fulminans or hypercoagulable state

PHYSICAL EXAM

- Signs of sepsis:
  - Fever
  - Hypotension
  - Tachycardia
  - Poor perfusion
  - Cool extremities
  - Decreased pulses
  - Shock
- Nonblanching purpura
- Acral purpura and necrosis: Check fingers, nose, toes, and penis for black areas.
- Skin lesions initially appear dark red and then become purple-black. Lesions may be mistaken as bruising.
- Bullae may form over purpuric skin.
- Skin lesions occur at previous sites of trauma (e.g., IV cannula insertion).
- Skin is frequently tight and shiny proximal to areas of purpura.
- Pain, ischemia, and edema of extremities or internal organ dysfunction may result from deep vein thrombosis or arterial thrombosis, depending on location and severity.
- Severe protein C deficiency is associated with cerebral vessel thrombosis, vitreous hemorrhage, and retinal detachment. These complications may occur in utero.
- Physical exam tip: Depress the purpuric area with a glass slide to determine whether it blanches.

DIFFERENTIAL DIAGNOSIS

- Infection
  - *N. meningitidis*, most common infectious cause of purpura fulminans
  - Streptococci
  - *Haemophilus* species
  - Staphylococci
  - Gram-negative bacteremia: *Escherichia coli, Klebsiella, Proteus, Enterobacter*
  - Rickettsia: Rocky Mountain spotted fever
  - Varicella
  - *Plasmodium falciparum*
- Environmental
  - Warfarin-induced skin necrosis: 1 in 500 to 1,000 individuals starting warfarin therapy develop necrosis in subcutaneous fat.
  - Thought to be caused by relative depletion of anticoagulant protein C (a vitamin K–dependent factor) during the initial phase of warfarin effect
- Malignancy: myeloid leukemia
- Congenital: inherited deficiencies of protein C and protein S
  - Only severe, homozygous, or compound heterozygous (<1% activity) deficiencies of proteins C and S are associated with purpura fulminans.
  - Milder, heterozygous deficiencies of protein C and protein S as well as other prothrombotic defects all give rise to hypercoagulable states but usually not neonatal purpura fulminans.
  - Patients with one or more risk factors for thrombosis may be more likely to develop purpura fulminans with an environmental stimulus.
- Immune mediated: heparin-induced thrombocytopenia: Antibody to heparin–platelet complex causes platelet activation, thrombocytopenia, and microthrombosis, including dermal vessels.
- Postinfectious purpura fulminans: autoimmune-mediated protein S and C deficiency
- Antiphospholipid antibody syndrome: Predisposition to thrombosis can include skin necrosis.
- Miscellaneous
  - Thrombotic thrombocytopenic purpura
  - Paroxysmal nocturnal hemoglobinuria
  - Henoch-Schönlein purpura

DIAGNOSTIC TESTS & INTERPRETATION

Initial Tests (screening, lab, imaging)

- Screening:
  - CBC
    - Platelet count may be low.
    - Hemoglobin may be low.
  - Smear screen: thrombocytopenia, schistocytes (evidence of microangiopathic hemolysis)
  - Prothrombin time and international normalized ratio (INR): prolonged as in DIC
  - Partial thromboplastin time: prolonged as in DIC
  - Fibrinogen: decreased with consumption and fibrinolysis
  - D-dimer: increased fibrinolysis as in DIC
- Etiologic:
  - Prior to initiation of treatment, collection of citrated plasma sample for functional activity assays for an accurate diagnosis. Confirm the assay that is used (chromogenic vs. functional), as the results may be discrepant.

- Protein C and S activity levels are undetectable in homozygotes.
- Protein C and/or S activity levels are low or undetectable in acquired cases.
- Antigen levels may be helpful if interfering factors (e.g., factor V Leiden mutation, antiphospholipid antibodies, direct thrombin inhibitors) are present.
- Genetic testing of the child and family to confirm diagnosis. Initiation of treatment should not depend on the return of these results.
- Protein C activity in patient, parents, and siblings
- Protein S antigen (total and free) in patient, parents, and siblings
- False positives: Protein C and S levels may decrease because of consumption during a thrombotic episode that is not related to an underlying congenital deficiency. Low measurements often need to be repeated at baseline after recovery. Protein C and S levels may be below adult normal ranges for the first 3 to 6 months of life in healthy infants. Pediatric reference ranges should be used.
- Test for antiphospholipid antibodies: usually lupus anticoagulant or anticardiolipin antibody
- Factor V Leiden mutation assay

- Imaging is not usually indicated in acquired cases.
- To document presence and extent of suspected large vessel thrombosis: The most useful imaging strategy depends on location and clinical situation:
  - Ultrasound with Doppler flow study
  - CT scan
  - MRI: better for visualization of vessels
  - Angiography: most invasive; requires vascular injury for access
  - Imaging is potentially useful to
    - Distinguish thrombosis from other pathology
    - Assess clot size prior to anticoagulant or thrombolytic therapy

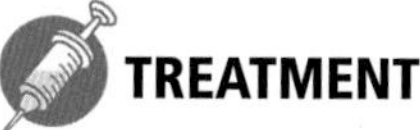

TREATMENT

GENERAL MEASURES

- If classical signs of purpura fulminans, therapy should be commenced emergently.
- Treat underlying cause.
- Anti-infective agents depending on underlying cause
- Manage DIC based on clinical and laboratory findings.

MEDICATION

- There is no protein S concentrate available. Fresh frozen plasma (FFP) 10 to 20 mL/kg every 12 hours or cryoprecipitate is used as replacement therapy.
- Protein C replacement therapy: FFP 10 to 20 mL/kg every 6 to 12 hours until protein C concentrate available. 1 mL/kg of FFP will increase plasma protein C concentrate by 1 IU/dL. Aim for trough protein C level of 10 IU/dL.
- Protein C concentrates (human plasma derived): initial dose of 100 U/kg followed by 50 U/kg every 6 hours. Aim protein C trough level of 50 IU/dL.
- In acquired cases, required dose and frequency of protein C concentrate (to maintain trough level of 50 IU/dL) will decrease overtime as the patient's underlying condition improves.
- Recombinant activated protein C is no longer available.
- Anticoagulation therapy:
  - Start with replacement therapy in the case of severe protein C or S deficiency. Start with unfractionated heparin (UFH) or low-molecular-weight heparin (LMWH). Warfarin should only be started after a few days of UFH/LMWH and overlap to avoid warfarin-induced skin necrosis.
  - In acquired cases, start with UFH/LMWH after 5 to 7 days once the risk of bleeding is decreased. Continue UFH/LMWH for 4 to 12 weeks until the purpura has resolved or stabilized.
- Maintenance therapy for congenital protein C or S deficiency: prophylaxis with warfarin alone (INR target 2.5 to 3.5) or protein C concentrate 30 to 50 IU/kg every 1 to 3 days with warfarin therapy (INR target 1.5 to 2.5)
- LMWH has been used for maintenance anticoagulation therapy (target anti-Xa 0.5 to 1 U/mL). The role of other new anticoagulants has not been defined.
- Venous access is challenging. Long-term SC administration of protein C concentrate is reported.

ONGOING CARE

FOLLOW-UP RECOMMENDATIONS

Patient Monitoring

- When to expect improvement: related to underlying cause of purpura fulminans
- Signs to watch for:
  - Spread of purpura
  - Hypotension
  - Gangrene
- Treatment during the acute phase should continue until all lesions have resolved.
- Referral to ophthalmologist for management and follow-up of ocular lesions
- Monitor INR weekly on maintenance therapy.
- D-dimer can be used as a marker for adequate replacement therapy and anticoagulation. An increasing D-dimer may be the first sign of recurrent purpura fulminans.

DIET

Patients on warfarin therapy may need to avoid foods with high vitamin K content, especially if there is variation in the dose of warfarin required to maintain adequate anticoagulation.

PROGNOSIS

- Related to underlying cause of purpura fulminans
- Overall, poor for homozygous deficiencies of proteins C and S
- For acquired cases, prognosis depends on the commencement of protein C replacement—starting within 4 to 8 hours of onset of purpura has been shown to minimize need for amputations/grafts.
- Report of cure of protein C deficiency by liver transplantation

COMPLICATIONS

- Skin necrosis and gangrene
- Scarring
- Acral amputations, from tips of digits to whole limbs
- Small and large vessel thrombosis
- Death

ADDITIONAL READING

- Goldenberg NA, Manco-Johnson MJ. Protein C deficiency. *Haemophilia*. 2008;14(6):1214–1221.
- Leclerc F, Leteurtre S, Cremer R, et al. Do new strategies in meningococcemia produce better outcomes? *Crit Care Med*. 2000;28(Suppl 9):S60–S63.
- Manco-Johnson MJ, Bomgaars L, Palascak J, et al. Efficacy and safety of protein C concentrate to treat purpura fulminans and thromboembolic events in severe congenital protein C deficiency. *Thromb Haemost*. 2016;116(1):58–68.
- Minford A, Behnisch W, Brons P, et al. Subcutaneous protein C concentrate in the management of severe protein C deficiency—experience from 12 centres. *Br J Haematol*. 2014;164(3):414–421.
- Pathan N, Faust SN, Levin M. Pathophysiology of meningococcal meningitis and septicaemia. *Arch Dis Child*. 2003;88(7):601–607.
- Price VE, Ledingham DL, Krümpel A, et al. Diagnosis and management of neonatal purpura fulminans. *Semin Fetal Neonatal Med*. 2011;16(6):318–322.
- Veldman A, Fischer D, Wong FY, et al. Human protein C concentrate in the treatment of purpura fulminans: a retrospective analysis of safety and outcome in 94 pediatric patients. *Crit Care*. 2010;14(4):R156.

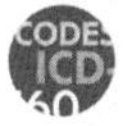

CODES

ICD10

- D65 Disseminated intravascular coagulation
- P54.5 Neonatal cutaneous hemorrhage

FAQ

- Q: What is the risk of a second affected child with protein C or S deficiency?
- A: If the diagnosis is confirmed by family studies that show both parents to be carriers of the deficiency and the affected child to be homozygous, there is a 25% chance that each subsequent infant would have purpura fulminans and a 50% chance that each child would be a carrier. However, other hypercoagulable states have been described that may be risk factors for purpura fulminans.
- Q: Should a child with purpura fulminans be followed by a specialist?
- A: Generally yes, with a pediatric hematologist, to assist in acute management of purpura, establishment of diagnosis, and management of long-term anticoagulation

PYELONEPHRITIS

Christopher E. Bayne, MD • Michael H. Hsieh, MD, PhD

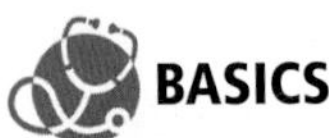

BASICS

DESCRIPTION

- Acute pyelonephritis (APN; or upper urinary tract infection [UTI]) is a clinical diagnosis that may feature fever, positive urine culture, and urinary symptoms (e.g., dysuria, frequency, urgency, and/or flank pain). APN shows renal parenchymal (interstitial) inflammation secondary to bacterial invasion.
- APN and febrile UTI (fUTI) are often used interchangeably. This usage assumes fUTIs always involve the upper tracts and is not accurate as lower tract UTIs may present with fever.
- Chronic pyelonephritis is a term reserved for prolonged or incompletely treated infection of renal parenchyma.

EPIDEMIOLOGY

- UTIs are more likely to involve the upper renal tracts in children <3 years of age.
- UTIs are more common in males ≤12 months of age; thereafter, UTI is more common in females.

Prevalence

- 5–7% of febrile infants <8 weeks
- 1% of school-aged children (0.03% school-aged boys)

RISK FACTORS

- Previous history of UTI (e.g., recurrent UTI [rUTI])
- Female sex, especially sexually active females
- Bladder and bowel dysfunction (BBD)
- Sibling with a history of UTI
- Structural abnormalities or foreign bodies in urinary tract, including stones, catheters, or stents
- Neurologic conditions affecting bladder and bowel
- Vesicoureteral reflux (VUR)
  - Present in ~30–40% of children with fUTIs
  - The majority (>95%) of VUR associated with fUTIs is low or moderate grade (I to III). There is stronger association of fUTI with high-grade (≥IV) VUR
- Uncircumcised boys <12 months
  - Circumcision can reduce risk of UTI by up to 87%.

PATHOPHYSIOLOGY

- Host-related factors:
  - Anatomic abnormalities (e.g., obstruction)
  - Functional abnormalities (e.g., BBD, VUR)
- Pathogen-related factors:
  - Adherence factors (e.g., P and type 1 fimbriae, adhesins)
  - Virulence factors (e.g., lipopolysaccharide, capsular antigen)
  - Antibiotic- and immune clearance–resistant intracellular bacterial pods within urothelium
- Bacterial adhesion to uroepithelium induces cytokine release and subsequent inflammatory response.
- Patchy infiltration of the medullary parenchyma by polymorphonuclear leukocytes and lymphocytes leads to degradation of extracellular matrix, tubular disruption, and interstitial edema.
- Parenchymal scarring may result as a consequence.

ETIOLOGY

- Enterobacteriaceae: *Escherichia coli* most frequent (90% of initial infections and up to 66% of rUTIs); *Proteus, Klebsiella, Enterobacter* spp. are less common.
- Gram-positive organisms cause 10–15% of cases: *Staphylococcus aureus, Staphylococcus epidermidis, Staphylococcus saprophyticus, Enterococci* spp.
- Other organisms: *Pseudomonas, Haemophilus influenzae, Streptococcus* group B

COMMONLY ASSOCIATED CONDITIONS

- Struvite kidney stones: associated with urease-producing bacteria (e.g., *Proteus* and *Klebsiella* spp.)
- Anatomic or physiologic abnormality of the urinary tract are found in up to 50% of infants with APN.

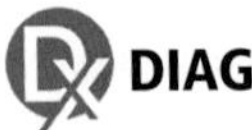

DIAGNOSIS

HISTORY

- Fever may be the only presenting complaint.
- In the neonate, inquire about vomiting, lethargy, poor feeding, irritability, fever, hypothermia, trembling, and jaundice
- Older children are more likely to present with flank pain, dysuria, frequency, urgency, and incontinence.
- Important factors that predispose to development of UTI that should be specifically inquired about:
  - Low oral fluid intake
  - Incorrect toilet training (e,g., wiping incorrectly, hurried [incomplete] emptying)
  - Perineal skin irritation, including phimosis in males
  - Recent antibiotic exposure
  - Personal or family history of UTIs, VUR, urolithiasis, or genitourinary system abnormalities
  - Urine and bowel habits. Symptoms suggestive of BBD include infrequent urination, dysuria, feeling of incomplete voiding leading to frequent urination, urinary urgency, constipation, and hard stools.
  - New incontinence of urine or stool
  - Previous surgery or trauma to back
- Presence of neurologic abnormalities and achievement of appropriate lower motor milestones
- Signs and symptoms:
  - Constitutional: fever, chills
  - Urinary symptoms: dysuria, frequency, urgency
  - Suprapubic or flank pain

PHYSICAL EXAM

- Fever, irritability, rigors, lethargy
- Bimanual palpation of both kidneys to assess costovertebral angle tenderness and kidney size
- Inspection of the lower back for signs of occult spinal abnormalities (e.g., dimple, hair tuft, hemangioma, birth marks, short or asymmetrical gluteal cleft)
- In females, exam includes inspection of urethral meatus and vaginal introitus, pooling of urine in the vaginal vault, discharge, or signs of skin irritation.
- In males, exam includes inspection of foreskin for possible phimosis in the uncircumcised penis, location and caliber of the urethral meatus, and scrotal exam for erythema, swelling, or tenderness.
- Careful neuromuscular exam of lower limbs and back to evaluate for a neurologic abnormality that may be associated with neuropathic bladder.
- Inspect anus and assess rectal tone.

DIFFERENTIAL DIAGNOSIS

- Cystitis (can occasionally present with fever)
- Sterile pyuria
  - Balanitis or vulvovaginitis
  - Systemic viral illness or postvaccination
  - Pregnancy
  - Appendicitis
  - Cystic renal disease
  - Tuberculosis
  - Nonbacterial epididymoorchitis
- Lower lobe pneumonia

DIAGNOSTIC TESTS & INTERPRETATION

Initial Tests (screening, lab, imaging)

- Collect urine using sterile methods (e.g., midstream in toilet-trained children, catheter or suprapubic aspiration for infants).
  - Catheterized specimens have specificity of 83–89% compared with suprapubic aspiration
- Bagged specimens have 75% false-positive rate (positive urine culture in absence of UTI) and are not useful for diagnosing UTI. Negative urinalysis or urine culture for bagged specimens may be helpful in ruling out UTI.
- Urine dipstick for measurement of leukocyte esterase (LE) and nitrites is a rapid screen for UTI.
  - Positive LE is 84% sensitive and 78% specific for UTI. Positive nitrite test is 80–90% sensitive and 60–96% specific. These are upper-end values
  - Positive likelihood ratio (LR+) with positive LE and nitrites = 28.2; negative likelihood ratio (LR−) when dipstick negative for both = 0.2
- Urine microscopy involves either manual or automated methods. Urine is usually centrifuged.
  - WBC casts on urine microscopy are diagnostic.
  - >10 WBC/high power field (hpf) = pyuria
  - Unspun clean-catch urine specimen with bacteria on stained microscopic exam correlates (~80–90%) with urine culture exceeding 100,000 cfu/mL.
  - LR+ positive urine culture when microscopy positive for both pyuria and bacteruria = 37. LR− when microscopy negative for both = 0.11
- Dipstick alone has been shown to be as effective as combined dipstick and UA. Combining tests may increase false positives.
- For children who use clean intermittent catheterization, urine showing *absence* of moderate or large LE on dipstick *and* <10 WBC/hpf on microscopy is usually clinically insignificant.
- Urine for culture and sensitivity: Culture result is generally regarded as positive with a single pathogenic organism of 100,000 cfu/mL in a clean-catch specimen, ≥1,000 cfu/mL in a catheter-acquired specimen, or any growth in a suprapubic specimen.
- CBC with an elevated WBC count and left shift
- Erythrocyte sedimentation rate (ESR),C-reactive protein (CRP), and serum procalcitonin (sPCT) levels are often increased and have been studied to differentiate lower from upper tract UTI.
  - A Cochrane meta-analysis found ESR was not sufficiently accurate. CRP <20 mg/L may be helpful in ruling out APN. sPCT >0.5 ng/mL had a sensitivity of 86% and specificity of 74% for APN.
- Acute imaging in children with fUTI and APN is controversial due to the questionable need to confirm the diagnosis and definitively identify risk factors for rUTI and renal scarring (RS) (e.g., VUR) versus simply screening for these risk factors.
  - Risk factors for rUTI and renal scarring include obstruction, VUR, and other anatomic abnormalities, such as ureterocele, diverticula.
  - See VUR chapter for specific details.
- Imaging studies capable of confirming APN are ^{99m}Tc-dimercaptosuccinic acid (DMSA) renography, magnetic resonance imaging (MRI), and computed tomography (CT). These tests are similar in accuracy. Previous studies showed preference for DMSA, but MRI and CT technology has since improved.

- DMSA involves ionizing radiation and may require sedation in young children. DMSA is very reliable for identifying APN in the acute phase. In the delayed phase, DMSA is the best test for identifying renal scarring.
  - Acute phase DMSA usually performed ≤7 days after fUTI. Photopenic defects suggest APN with 86% sensitivity and 91% specificity.
  - Delayed phase DMSA usually performed ≥5 months after fUTI. Photopenic defects suggest renal scarring.
- MRI avoids ionizing radiation but is expensive and may require sedation in young children.
- In absence of urolithiasis, CT is not practical for the workup of APN due to the ionizing radiation involved.
- Voiding cystourethrogram (VCUG) confirms the presence or absence of VUR and other anatomic abnormalities of the upper and lower tracts (e.g., posterior urethral valve, ureterocele). It involves ionizing radiation and urethral catherization.
  - VCUG can be performed after urine is sterile.
  - Administer antibiotics before VCUG.

Diagnostic Procedures/Other

- According to the American Academy of Pediatrics (AAP), diagnosis of UTI requires UA evidence of infection (e.g., pyuria or bacteruria) and ≥50,000 cfu/mL of a uropathogen cultured from a sterile specimen
- APN is a clinical diagnosis based on findings of UTI and flank tenderness or suggestive imaging.
- Imaging evaluation of the urinary tract after UTI should be individualized based on the child's age, sex, clinical presentation, and risk factors.
- All children <24 months should undergo renal bladder ultrasound (RBUS) to identify hydronephrosis, renal scarring, or other abnormalities. It is controversial whether to routinely perform DMSA or VCUG in children 2 months to 2 years with a first fUTI.
- RBUS can detect hydronephrosis, ureteronephrosis, urolithiasis, and other anatomic abnormalities (e.g., ureterocele, diverticula, suspected renal scarring). It has been proposed as a screening test for rUTI and renal scarrning.
  - The benefit of screening with RBUS is, it does not require ionizing radiation and is not invasive.
  - A notable disadvantage is RBUS, at best, moderately predictive of VUR and renal scarring.
- In children 2 to 24 months with a first fUTI, the AAP recommends RBUS in the acute setting to rule out obstruction and other anatomic abnormalities. VCUG is not routinely recommended after first UTI unless RBUS findings are abnormal (AAP 2016).
  - This guideline is founded on premise VUR is a risk for rUTI, thus children without VUR are less likely to have rUTI. Assuming 90% of children will not have a second UTI (AAP 2011), the guideline uses RBUS and watchful waiting to screen for VUR.
- The National Institute for Health and Clinical Excellence (NICE) recommends RBUS for children of all ages with an "atypical UTI" (e.g., sepsis, poor urine flow, abdominal or bladder mass, elevated serum creatinine, failure to respond to antibiotics, or infection with non-*E. coli* organism) and within 6 weeks for infants <6 months with a first UTI (NICE 2007).
- Separate studies have retrospectively applied the AAP and NICE guidelines to cohorts after UTI to investigate their overall effects. In general, AAP results in the least radiation, and NICE is the least costly (also see "Vesicoureteral Reflux" chapter).

ALERT

- False-positive test results:
  - May be due to nonsterile collection techniques (bagged specimen) or storing unrefrigerated urine
- False-negative test results:
  - False-negative nitrite tests may result from urine residing in bladder <4 hours, non–nitrite-producing bacteria (e.g., Gram-positive or *Pseudomonas*).
  - Urine specimen collection after antibiotic exposure

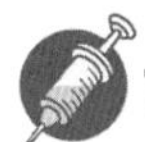

TREATMENT

MEDICATION

- Initiate broad-spectrum antibiotics. Children who appear toxic, dehydrated, <2 months, or vomiting should receive IV antibiotics until afebrile for at least 24 hours, then change to an oral formulation.
- 7 to 14 days of total antibiotic therapy is required.
- Trimethoprim-sulfamethoxazole and amoxicillin-clavulanate are usually appropriate unless patient is on similar agents for continuous antibiotic prophylaxis (CAP).
- 1st- and 2nd-generation cephalosporins are increasingly used due to growing resistances to other agents.
- Nitrofurantoin concentrates in urine and is ineffective in treating parenchymal infection.
- Be familiar with local antibiograms before initiating treatment. This is particularly important when treating hospital-acquired infections.
- Antipyretics (e.g., acetaminophen) and analgesics. Be cautious of using nonsteroidal anti-inflammatory drugs (e.g., ibuprofen) in the setting of renal injury.
- Consider CAP after treatment of APN until imaging evaluation is complete.
- Children with frequent symptomatic rUTI, BBD, and those with VUR grade ≥III may benefit from CAP.

ALERT

- Removing struvite or other infected calculi during active infection may precipitate bacteremia/urosepsis.
- High index of suspicion is required for APN associated with cystic renal disease or renal abscesses as urine cultures may be negative.

ADMISSION, INPATIENT, AND NURSING CONSIDERATIONS

- Patients with underlying anatomic or functional urinary tract abnormality or persistent fever despite antibiotics should be evaluated/treated by a urologist.
- Measure ins and outs. IV fluids may be necessary.

ONGOING CARE

FOLLOW-UP RECOMMENDATIONS

Patient Monitoring

- Educate caregivers on signs, symptoms of UTI, need for sterile urine specimen, and need for urgent medical attention.
- If child has suffered several episodes of APN or has known renal scarring, measure blood pressures at follow-up visits and consider UAs for proteinuria.

PROGNOSIS

- Fever usually resolves ≤48 hours. Persistent fever or pain requires further evaluation to exclude a drug-resistant organism, renal abscess, or obstruction (e.g., stone). Repeat or intensify imaging workup.
- Diagnose and treat underlying BBD and constipation for successful management of UTIs in children.
- Outcome of APN is usually good but may result in renal scarring.
  - The risk of renal scarring after first APN episode is ~5%. Renal scarring risk doubles after second, third episode, then increases sharply. VUR (especially grade ≥III) significantly increases renal scarring risk after APN.
- Pyelonephritis associated with renal stones requires removal of the infectious stones after antibiotic treatment is completed.

COMPLICATIONS

- Acute:
  - Reduced concentrating ability, hyperkalemic renal tubular acidosis (transient mineralocorticoid resistance)
  - Bacteremia: highest risk in young infants (23% of children <2 months)
  - Renal abscess formation
- Chronic:
  - RS, HTN, proteinuria, azotemia, emphysematous and xanthogranulomatous pyelonephritis

ADDITIONAL READING

- Morello W, La Scola C, Alberici I, et al. Acute pyelonephritis in children. *Pediatr Nephrol*. 2016;31(8):1253–1265.
- National Institute for Health and Clinical Excellence. *Urinary Tract Infection in Children*. London, United Kingdom: National Institute for Health and Clinical Excellence; 2007.
- Schmidt B, Copp HL. Work-up of pediatric urinary tract infection. *Urol Clin North Am*. 2015;42(4): 519–526.
- Subcommittee on Urinary Tract Infection. Reaffirmation of AAP Clinical Practice Guideline: the diagnosis and management of the initial urinary tract infection in febrile infants and young children 2–24 months of age. *Pediatrics*. 2016;138(6):e20163026.

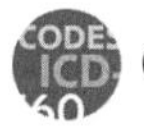

CODES

ICD10

- N12 Tubulo-interstitial nephritis, not spcf as acute or chronic
- N10 Acute tubulo-interstitial nephritis
- N11.9 Chronic tubulo-interstitial nephritis, unspecified

NOTE: The term urosepsis does not exist in ICD10 coding and instead is sepsis secondary to pyelonephritis/UTI.

FAQ

- Q: Should a DMSA scan be used to diagnose APN?
- A: Routine use of the DMSA scan to diagnose APN is controversial because disagreement exists about the therapeutic implications of a positive test, and such routine testing is expensive and involves radiation. Children with hypertension and previous UTIs require a delayed phase DMSA scan to look for renal scarring.
- Q: Does renal scarring occur *without* reflux?
- A: Yes. Up to ~20% of renal scarring may occur in the absence of VUR. The causal relationships between VUR, APN, and RS are complex.

PYLORIC STENOSIS

Pradeep P. Nazarey, MD

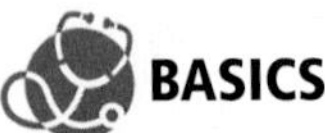

BASICS

DESCRIPTION

Hypertrophy of the muscular layers of the pylorus with elongation and thickening, leading to projectile nonbilious emesis and gastric outlet obstruction

EPIDEMIOLOGY

- Usually presents between the 3rd and 10th week of life
- Male-to-female ratio 4:1, with 1st-born males more affected
- More common in Caucasians

Incidence

~2 to 4 per 1,000 live births in Western populations

PATHOPHYSIOLOGY

- Marked muscle hypertrophy and hyperplasia primarily involving the circular layer and hyperplasia of the underlying mucosa
- Growth of abnormally contorted and thickened nerve fibers and/or lack of neural elements
- Net result is either partial or complete obstruction of the pyloric channel.

ETIOLOGY

- No definitive causative factors have been identified despite considerable research.
- Genetic predisposition evidenced by variability among races, male preponderance, and genetic syndromes with pyloric stenosis
- Children of affected fathers are affected 3–5%, whereas affected mothers are associated with a 7–20% incidence.
- Several growth factors and gastrointestinal (GI) peptides, including gastrin and elevated acid levels, as well as increases in substance P, epidermal growth factor (EGF), transforming growth factor alpha (TGF α), and insulin-like growth factor-1 (IGF-1), have been implicated.
- Erythromycin estolate given for postexposure prophylaxis for pertussis may cause strong gastric and pyloric contractions that induce hypertrophy. Erythromycin exposure to lactating mothers is associated with breastfed infants who have an increased incidence of pyloric stenosis.
- Decreases in nerve differentiation, reduced density of neural elements, and deficiency of nitric oxide–induced muscle relaxation have been implicated.

COMMONLY ASSOCIATED CONDITIONS

Esophageal atresia and malrotation was noted in 5% of infants with pyloric stenosis.

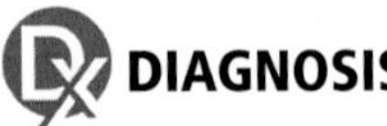

DIAGNOSIS

HISTORY

- Emesis
  - Otherwise healthy full-term infant that initially vomits intermittently
  - Over time (approximately 2 weeks), frequency slowly progresses to emesis with nearly every feeding.
  - Emesis becomes forceful or projectile "across the room."
  - Color of vomitus will resemble the feeds and is nonbilious.
- Infants look well appearing but act hungry.
- There may be a history of prescription of antireflux medications or formula changes that have no effect on symptoms.
- Parents describe a decrease in the frequency of wet diapers.
- As dehydration progresses, infants will become less vigorous and increasingly lethargic.

PHYSICAL EXAM

- Dehydration
  - Infants may have decreased skin turgor, flat fontanelles, and dry mucous membranes.
  - Infants are usually tachycardic and may be hypotensive.
- Abdominal exam
  - Visible peristalsis may be appreciated just after the infant feeds, which is seen as a waveform proceeding from the left upper quadrant toward the pylorus in the right upper quadrant (RUQ).
  - A palpable, hard, mobile, and nontender mass in the epigastrium to the right of the midline, referred to as an "olive" (palpable 45–75% of cases)
  - Palpation should be attempted after the stomach has been emptied and with the infant quiet and comfortable and can take time.

DIFFERENTIAL DIAGNOSIS

- Gastroesophageal reflux
- Gastroenteritis
- Milk protein allergy
- Anatomic considerations
  - Malrotation
  - Webs
  - Pyloric atresia
  - Duplications

DIAGNOSTIC TESTS & INTERPRETATION

- Hypochloremia and metabolic alkalosis
- Hypokalemia
- 2–5% of infants have indirect hyperbilirubinemia associated with jaundice.
- Ultrasound
  - Primary modality for diagnosis
  - Ultrasonography identifies the hypertrophic pyloric musculature and identifies wall thickness and channel length.

- Can see "shoulder sign," which is bulging of hypertrophic muscle into lumen of antrum
- To confirm the diagnosis, muscle thickness should be >3 mm and pyloric length >15 mm.
- GI studies
  - An upper GI study may be an adjunct if qualified ultrasonographer is unavailable.
  - Can see "string sign" of contrast going through narrowed pyloric channel

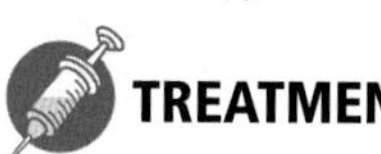

TREATMENT

ADMISSION, INPATIENT, AND NURSING CONSIDERATIONS

- Early identification of electrolyte abnormalities and correction with appropriate IV fluids
- Bolus with 10 to 20 mL/kg of normal saline (NS)
  - Followed by initiation of maintenance fluids of D5W 0.45NS + 2 mEq potassium chloride (KCl)/100 mL at 6 mL/kg/h
  - Goal urine output is >2 mL/kg/h.
- Surgery is definitive treatment but is not emergent or urgent. Electrolyte anomalies and alkalosis must be corrected prior to OR.
- Postoperative feedings usually resume within 4 to 6 hours after surgery, with spitting up or vomiting common.
- Discharge within 1 to 2 days

SURGERY/OTHER PROCEDURES

- Pyloromyotomy (Ramstedt procedure): longitudinal incision and spreading of the antropyloric muscle either through an RUQ or umbilical incision
- Laparoscopic pyloromyotomy is safe, feasible, has been gaining traction, and is favored by many surgeons over an open approach.

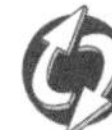

ONGOING CARE

FOLLOW-UP RECOMMENDATIONS

- Vomiting may persist for days after the operation.
- Babies are seen 2 weeks after discharge in clinic.

ALERT

- Alkalosis must be corrected prior to surgery to prevent difficulty with extubation as well as risks of postoperative apnea and death.
- Infants should undergo aggressive fluid resuscitation.

PROGNOSIS

- Morbidity and mortality rates are low.
- Surgery is curative with virtually no recurrence.

COMPLICATIONS

- Dehydration
- Electrolyte abnormalities, primarily hypochloremic, hypokalemic metabolic alkalosis that results from loss of hydrochloric acid and fluid caused by persistent vomiting
- Postoperative complications
  - Incomplete pyloromyotomy
  - Difficult extubation after surgery
  - Postoperative apnea
  - Mucosal injury; may lead to leak and sepsis if not immediately recognized and repaired

ADDITIONAL READING

- Hernanz-Schulman M. Pyloric stenosis: role of imaging. *Pediatr Radiol*. 2009;39(Suppl 2):S134–S139.
- Pandya S, Heiss K. Pyloric stenosis in pediatric surgery: an evidence-based review. *Surg Clin North Am*. 2012;92(3):527–539.
- Panteli C. New insights into the pathogenesis of infantile pyloric stenosis. *Pediatr Surg Int*. 2009;25(12):1043–1052.
- Sola J, Neville H. Laparoscopic vs open pyloromyotomy: a systematic review and meta-analysis. *J Pediatr Surg*. 2009;44(8):1631–1637.

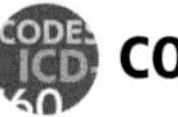

CODES

ICD10

Q40.0 Congenital hypertrophic pyloric stenosis

FAQ

- Q: What is the best initial imaging study to help make the diagnosis?
- A: An abdominal ultrasound is the best initial imaging study to obtain, as the pylorus can be well visualized.
- Q: Why is so much chloride lost?
- A: The chloride loss occurs with the loss of gastric acid, which contains hydrochloric acid.
- Q: What plan should I follow when replacing electrolytes?
- A: Correct the deficiency of fluids with 1.5 to 2 times maintenance fluid volumes. Correct chloride loss with NS, and correct potassium loss with KCl.

RABIES

Sergio E. Recuenco, MD, MPH, DrPH

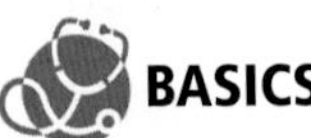

BASICS

DESCRIPTION

Fatal acute viral encephalomyelitis transmitted from animals to humans through bites or exposure to saliva or nervous tissue from a rabid animal. Only mammals are able to contract and transmit the disease.

EPIDEMIOLOGY

- An estimated 59,000 deaths are due to rabies every year in the world, most of them in Asia and Africa. Many of the affected countries do not have proper surveillance systems for rabies.
- Only 1 to 3 human cases reported annually in the United States. Imported cases infected overseas add 1 to 3 more cases annually.
- The dog is the main animal reservoir in most of world. In the United States and most developed countries, canine rabies had been eliminated.
- Wildlife such as bats, raccoons, skunk, and foxes are main reservoirs in North America, with frequent spillover to cats, dogs, and other domestic animals.
- All of the continental United States is enzootic for bat rabies, whereas transmission among terrestrial reservoirs occurs in specific geographic regions such as the Eastern United States (raccoon); south central, north central areas, and the state of California (skunk); south west (fox); Alaska (Arctic fox); and Puerto Rico (mongoose).
- Hawaii is considered rabies-free.

Incidence

- From 2003 to 2015, there were 26 cases of rabies acquired in the United States, 21 of these were associated with bat rabies strains, 3 with raccoon rabies, 1 with mongoose rabies, and 1 of unknown origin.
- 28% of the cases involved patients who were <18 years old.
- A total of five rabies cases were due to organ transplant.
- The real burden of human rabies exposure in the United States is unknown, but 36,000 individuals are estimated to receive postexposure prophylaxis (PEP) every year across the country.
- Wildlife accounts for 92% of all animal rabies cases; raccoons continue as the most frequent species (33%), followed by bats (31%), skunks (28%), foxes (6%), and other wildlife (2%).

RISK FACTORS

- Travel to areas where canine rabies is endemic
- Recent scratch or bite from known animal reservoir species including bats or other wildlife; exposure from an unvaccinated domestic animal (e.g., cat, dog) without the ability for appropriate management
- Transmission from transplanted corneas, vessels, and solid organs has occurred.
- Working with animals (e.g., veterinarians) or working in a laboratory with the virus
- Outdoor occupations and recreational activities that increase contact with high-risk species
- Mass exposures to potentially rabid animals (e.g., bats, cats) may occur in summer camps, county fairs (e.g., rabid goat), petting zoos (e.g., rabid sheep), schools, and public events.

GENERAL PREVENTION

- Targeted to humans and domestic animals
- Immunoprophylaxis: Preexposure rabies prophylaxis (Pre-EP) is offered to those at high risk (e.g., veterinarians, animal handlers, trappers, travelers to high-risk regions).
- Avoid unnecessary contact with wild animals in the United States and overseas.
- Pets should be vaccinated and kept updated on their immunizations.

PATHOPHYSIOLOGY

- Except for rare cases, the rabies virus enters the body through a bite that breaks the skin and introduces infected saliva:
  - From there, the virus gains access to muscle, where it is sequestered.
  - The virus then enters the peripheral nerves, where it moves centripetally to the CNS at a rate of ~3 mm/h.
  - Once in the CNS, infection spreads rapidly throughout many areas of the brain.
  - Neurologic manifestations progress rapidly from sensorial alterations to coma.
  - Leads to autonomic instability, the mechanisms of which are still poorly understood, which leads to acute death
- Average incubation period is 2 to 3 weeks to 2 to 3 months and, in rare cases, is suspected to be several to many years, with the longest documented incubation being 8 years.

ETIOLOGY

- The 14 known members of the *Lyssavirus* genus, rhabdovirus family (rabies virus, Lagos bat virus, Mokola virus, Duvenhage virus, Aravan virus, Irkut virus, Khujand virus, European bat lyssavirus types 1 and 2, West Caucasian bat virus, Australian bat lyssavirus, Shimoni bat virus, Ikoma virus, and Bokeloh virus) are suspected to be capable of causing human rabies death.
- Lyssaviruses are single-stranded RNA viruses and all except Mokola had been associated with bats.
- Most cases are due to the rabies virus, with rare cases due to the other lyssaviruses.

DIAGNOSIS

HISTORY

- Behavior of animal:
  - Although signs of rabies in animals vary greatly, atypical behavior for the animal is the norm (e.g., passive animals become aggressive, nocturnal animals roam in daylight).
  - Excessive salivation and lack of coordination may be present.
- History of animal contact:
  - Probably due to long incubation periods, some human rabies cases lack a history of animal contact.
  - The animal contact may have seemed trivial at the time (i.e., from a small bat).
- Assessment for PEP considers risk of rabies in the species, clinical presentation of the exposing animal, route and severity of exposure, and availability of the animal for observation or testing.
- Signs and symptoms:
  - Prodrome: 2 to 10 days with vague and insidious symptoms (e.g., sore throat, malaise, anxiety, change of behavior, hallucinations, fever). Other prodromal symptoms observed are itching, pain, or tingling at the site of the bite.
  - Acute neurologic phase: furious (80%) versus paralytic (20%) rabies
    - Furious rabies: agitation, hyperactivity, bizarre behavior, nuchal rigidity, sore throat, and hoarseness. The pathognomonic sign is hydrophobia and, at times, aerophobia.
    - Paralytic rabies: Initial finding is flaccid paralysis in the limb that was bitten; subsequently spreads to other limbs. Cranial nerve involvement can give complete lack of facial affect.
    - Coma: Onset follows acute neurologic phase; may persist up to 2 weeks and is followed by death almost universally

PHYSICAL EXAM

- Although neurologic findings can vary, cranial nerve paralysis (e.g., palate, vocal cords) is common. Therefore, hoarseness and stridor may occur.
- Meningismus is also fairly common, along with involuntary movements. Beyond this, findings depend on type of presentation (furious vs. paralytic).
- Imaging (e.g., MRI, CT) is unremarkable or unspecific.

DIFFERENTIAL DIAGNOSIS

- Other causes of encephalitis:
  - Herpes simplex virus
  - Enterovirus
  - West Nile virus
  - Zika and other arbovirus encephalitis
  - Rocky Mountain spotted fever and other rickettsial encephalitis
  - Japanese encephalitis
  - Guillain-Barré syndrome
  - Limbic encephalitis
  - Tetanus
  - Acute disseminated encephalitis
  - *Bartonella* encephalitis
- Other conditions can mimic rabies
  - Delirium tremens
  - Cocaine overdose
  - Amphetamine overdose
  - Acute psychosis
- Case reports of rabies wrongly diagnosed as cerebral malaria exist in countries with high malaria risk.

DIAGNOSTIC TESTS & INTERPRETATION

- Existing diagnostic methods for rabies virus infection are not useful before the onset of clinical signs. However, after signs appear, human antemortem laboratory diagnosis is possible with a set of four samples: serum, CSF, skin biopsy of at the hairline at the back of the neck, and fresh saliva. All four samples need to be taken on the same day and shipped express on dry ice. The following standard methods are used to rule out rabies:
  - Reverse transcription polymerase chain reaction (PCR) for rabies RNA detection in saliva and skin
  - Direct fluorescent antibody test (DFA) on cryostat sections of the skin biopsy
  - Virus-neutralizing antibody detection in CSF and serum with Rapid Fluorescent Foci Inhibition Test (RFFIT)
  - Indirect fluorescent antibody test on CSF and sera to detect IgM and IgG that may bind to rabies virus antigens present in infected cell culture
- Postmortem diagnosis is made by DFA and PCR in samples from brainstem, cerebellum, and sometimes other samples.

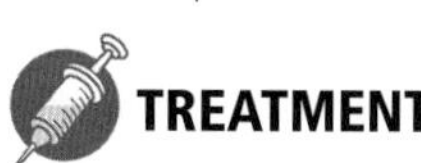

TREATMENT

MEDICATION

- Immunization: Both passive and active immunization should be initiated concurrently when an exposure is identified. Local or state health departments can advise about the risk of specific animal exposures.
- Passive
  - Human rabies immune globulin (HRIG) derived from the plasma of volunteers hyperimmunized with rabies vaccine
  - The present recommendation for HRIG vaccination is 20 IU/kg instilled locally into the tissue at the site of the bite.
    - Remaining HRIG can be given IM, avoiding the arm in which the rabies vaccine (RV) is administered.
    - In cases of multiple wounds, to ensure that all wounds receive an injection of HRIG, dilution in saline (2- to 3-fold) is acceptable.
    - HRIG is only administered the day 0 of the PEP schedule simultaneously to the first dose of RV. In case not available at the same time of first dose of RV, still can be administered until day 7; after that, it is not necessary.
- Active
  - Two RVs are licensed in the United States: human diploid cell rabies vaccine (HDCV) and purified chick embryo cell vaccine (PCEC).
  - For preexposure vaccination, the recommended schedule is 1 mL of RV IM dose in the deltoid area on days 0, 7, and 21 or 28. No HRIG is used.
  - For PEP, the current schedule in the United States is 1 mL of RV IM in the deltoid region on days 0, 3, 7, and 14. For immunocompromised patients, an additional dose on day 28 is given. The anterolateral thigh can be used in infants or young children.
- Discontinue the vaccine series if fluorescent antibody testing of the brain of the biting animal is conducted and result is negative, or if it is a cat, dog, or ferret healthy after a period of 10 days of observation after the bite.

ADMISSION, INPATIENT, AND NURSING CONSIDERATIONS

- Local wound care immediately after bite
  - The first step in preventing infection is washing out the virus mechanically or inactivating it before it has a chance to attach to and enter susceptible cells.
  - The wound should be flushed with copious amounts of soap and water or saline solution.
  - For puncture wounds, insertion of a catheter (i.e., angiocatheter) and irrigation with fluid by means of an attached syringe should be performed. If irrigation is too painful, infiltration of the area with local anesthetic can help.
- For symptomatic patients after incubation period
  - Request antemortem to rule out rabies tests.
  - Palliative and supportive care should be made available in an intensive care unit.
  - Consider experimental therapies (e.g., induced coma) in selected patients (e.g., early rabies confirmation, young age).

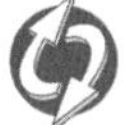

ONGOING CARE

PROGNOSIS

- After the patient CNS is infected with the rabies virus, prognosis is poor. There is no medical therapy available once the encephalitis onset, and after that, PEP is no longer indicated.
- Without PEP before clinical presentation, the disease is fatal with very rare survivors.
- 15% of patient survival had been observed following intensive care and induced coma (see www.mcw.edu/rabies) attempted in about 50 of cases. Six of 10 survivors using this regimen are still alive; the other patients survived the acute illness but died of complications during rehabilitation.

ADDITIONAL READING

- Brown CM, Slavinski S, Ettestad P, et al; and National Association of State Public Health Veterinarians, Compendium of Animal Rabies Prevention and Control Committee. Compendium of animal rabies prevention and control, 2016. *J Am Vet Med Assoc.* 2016;248(5):505–517.
- Feder HM Jr, Petersen BW, Robertson KL, et al. Rabies: still a uniformly fatal disease? Historical occurrence, epidemiological trends, and paradigm shifts. *Curr Infect Dis Rep.* 2012;14(4):408–422.
- Manning SE, Rupprecht CE, Fishbein D, et al; for Advisory Committee on Immunization Practices Centers for Disease Control and Prevention. Human rabies prevention—United States, 2008: recommendations of the Advisory Committee on Immunization Practices. *MMWR Recomm Rep.* 2008;57(RR-3):1–28.
- Monroe BP, Yager P, Blanton J, et al. Rabies surveillance in the United States during 2014. *J Am Vet Med Assoc.* 2016;248(7):777–788.
- Warrell MJ. Current rabies vaccines and prophylaxis schedules: preventing rabies before and after exposure. *Travel Med Infect Dis.* 2012;10(1):1–15.
- World Health Organization. *WHO Expert Consultation on Rabies. Second Report.* Geneva, Switzerland: World Health Organization; 2013. WHO technical report series 982.

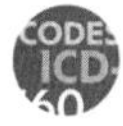

CODES

ICD10

- A82.9 Rabies, unspecified
- Z20.3 Contact with and (suspected) exposure to rabies

FAQ

- Q: Does a wild squirrel or rabbit bite necessitate rabies prophylaxis?
- A: In general, rodents (e.g., squirrels, rats, mice, hamsters, gerbils), lagomorphs (e.g., rabbits and hares), and marsupials are not known to serve as natural rabies reservoirs. They should not be considered rabid unless they exhibit unusual behavior.
- Q: Is there any evidence of human-to-human spread?
- A: No. However, health care workers or others exposed to a patient with known or suspected rabies should receive vaccination if they have suffered a bite wound or if mucosal surfaces or open wounds have been exposed to the patient's body fluids.
- Q: Are there any countries that require "routine rabies vaccination"?
- A: Yes, Nepal. Recently, Peru, Ecuador, and Colombia started mandatory vaccination programs restricted to very high-risk areas in Amazonia.
- Q: What if a severe allergic reaction occurs during postexposure rabies prophylaxis?
- A: The reaction should be treated at the time as you would any systemic anaphylactic reaction. PEP should continue after that using a different RV and taking additional precautions. The two RVs licensed in the United States (PCECV, HDCV) are interchangeable if indicated.
- Q: If a bat is found in the house, should the family members receive immunoprophylaxis?
- A: If a bat is found in the room of a sleeping person, previously unattended child, or mentally compromised person, it should be tested. If the bat escapes, prophylaxis should be considered case by case. The injury inflicted by a bat bite or scratch may not be obvious.

RADIAL HEAD SUBLUXATION (NURSEMAID'S ELBOW)

Meredith C. Laguna, MD, MPH • Steven Bin, MD

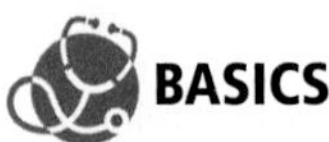

BASICS

DESCRIPTION

- Cause of acute upper extremity immobility and elbow injury in young children that results from axial traction on an extended arm
- Also called "nursemaid's elbow," "babysitter's elbow," "toddler elbow" "pulled elbow," "annular ligament displacement"

EPIDEMIOLOGY

- Most common upper extremity injury among children <6 years of age
- Peak incidence: 2 to 3 years of age
- Age range: 0 to 11 years of age

RISK FACTORS

- Female sex
- Obesity

GENERAL PREVENTION

Avoid pulling child by arm; lift child from axilla.

PATHOPHYSIOLOGY

Annular ligament in young children is more loosely connected to radial head.

ETIOLOGY

"Pull" on the arm or axial traction results in displacement of the annular ligament over the radial head, trapping it in the radiocapitellar joint, causing pain and refusal to move arm.

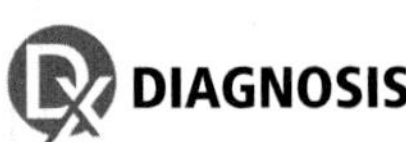

DIAGNOSIS

HISTORY

- Child suddenly not using one arm, frequently with unknown mechanism
- More commonly left arm
- May describe an injury occurring when a caregiver holds the child's arm and the child pulls away, during a tantrum, roughhousing, or swinging child by arms
- Infants may have rolled over onto arm in bed.
- About 50% of cases lack classic mechanism.

PHYSICAL EXAM

- Child usually in no distress and refuses to move arm
- Holds arm close to body with elbow flexed and pronated
- Usually no tenderness nor swelling of arm
- Exam must include palpation of clavicle, humerus, radius, ulna, and wrist to exclude fracture.
- Can ask parent to assist in palpation for anxious toddlers

ALERT

Point tenderness, edema, ecchymosis, neurovascular compromise, trauma, or fall onto outstretched hand suggests fracture rather than nursemaid's elbow.

DIFFERENTIAL DIAGNOSIS

- Fractures: Clavicle, radial neck, lateral condyle, medial epicondyle, supracondylar, and ulnar are most common.
- Soft tissue injury: strain, sprain, contusion
- Osteomyelitis

DIAGNOSTIC TESTS & INTERPRETATION

Initial Tests (screening, lab, imaging)

- No radiographs are needed if history and exam consistent with nursemaid's elbow.
- Obtain AP and lateral elbow radiographs if point tenderness, swelling, high-impact injury, or if concern for fracture.
- Elbow ultrasound may be considered to exclude fracture.

Test Interpretation

- Elbow radiographs are normal in nursemaid's elbow.
- Posterior fat pad on lateral elbow radiograph suggests supracondylar fracture.

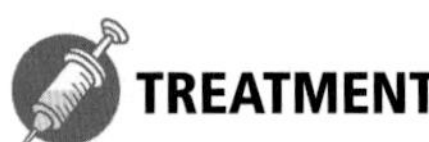

TREATMENT

GENERAL MEASURES

There are two types of reduction maneuvers; both maneuvers can be performed in the office or ED without need for sedation.

- Hyperpronation method:
  - Support the elbow with one hand, with your thumb over the radial head.
  - Use other hand to clasp child's hand or wrist and then hyperpronate the forearm.
  - May be less painful and is significantly more effective in initial reduction
- Supination-flexion method:
  - Support the elbow with one hand, with your thumb over the radial head.
  - Use other hand to fully supinate the forearm, then into full elbow flexion.
- General notes
  - With both methods, a palpable click or pop signals successful reduction but is not always noted.
  - Both methods may be attempted sequentially.
  - Child should begin to use arm normally within 5 to 10 minutes; can encourage by holding out desired item such as a toy
  - Several attempts may be made.
  - If unsuccessful, then obtain radiograph to rule out fracture.

MEDICATION

First Line

Acetaminophen (15 mg/kg) for pain control PRN

ISSUES FOR REFERRAL

If multiple attempts at reduction unsuccessful and no radiographic fracture noted, recommend long arm splint, sling, and referral to orthopedic clinic in 1 to 2 days

SURGERY/OTHER PROCEDURES

Case reports describe open operative reduction of trapped annular ligament, but this is very rare.

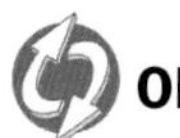

ONGOING CARE

FOLLOW-UP RECOMMENDATIONS

With successful reduction, no routine follow-up required

PATIENT EDUCATION

- Prevention with lifting technique; avoid pulling child's arm.
- Teach caregivers reduction maneuver, although they should be counseled to return if any new symptoms.

PROGNOSIS

- Recurrence occurs in 15–39% of patients.
- Patients who are 2 years old or younger are at greater risk of recurrence.
- Although case reports describe up to 7 or 8 recurrences per patient, generally decrease with age and stop after 4 to 5 years of age

ADDITIONAL READING

- Aylor M, Anderson JM, Vanderford P, et al. Videos in clinical medicine. Reduction of pulled elbow. *N Engl J Med*. 2014;371(21):e32.
- Bexkens R, Washburn FJ, Eygendaal D, et al. Effectiveness of reduction maneuvers in the treatment of nursemaid's elbow: a systematic review and meta-analysis. *Am J Emerg Med*. 2017;35(1):159–163.
- Cohen-Rosenblum A, Bielski RJ. Elbow pain after a fall: nursemaid's elbow or fracture? *Pediatr Ann*. 2016;45(6):e214–e217.
- Rudloe TF, Schutzman S, Lee LK, et al. No longer a "nursemaid's" elbow: mechanisms, caregivers, and prevention. *Pediatr Emerg Care*. 2012;28(8):771–774.

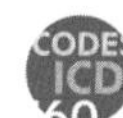

CODES

ICD10

- S53.03 Nursemaid's elbow
- S53.032 Nursemaid's elbow, left elbow
- S53.031 Nursemaid's elbow, right elbow

FAQ

- Q: Are radiographs required if mechanism is unknown prior to performing attempted reduction?
- A: If arm is held in classic position, close to body, minimally flexed at elbow and forearm pronated, with no swelling nor tenderness on physical exam, then closed reduction can be safely performed.
- Q: Does reduction have to be performed by a physician?
- A: No. While one study demonstrated more successful reduction by emergency physicians (97%) than by emergency triage nurses (85%), any trained provider may perform the maneuver. Parents can be also coached to perform reduction over the telephone.
- Q: Why does the condition occur more frequently in the left arm?
- A: The theory is that caregivers use dominant right hand to hold child's left arm, increasing risk.
- Q: Is there a role for splinting in management of the injury?
- A: Unlikely. Although most sources do not routinely recommend it, one study found that with splinting, fewer children had an immediate reinjury. However, at 10 days from reduction, both splinted and unsplinted groups were injury-free, suggesting benefit is modest.
- Q: Will the child's elbow be permanently damaged?
- A: No. Although some children can have recurrence, they grow out of the condition as the annular ligament strengthens, usually by age 5 years.

RECTAL PROLAPSE

Pradeep P. Nazarey, MD

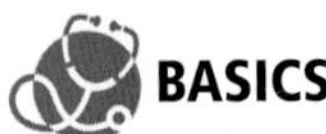

BASICS

DESCRIPTION

There are three types of rectal prolapse:

- Complete: full thickness of rectum prolapses through anus (two layers of rectum with an intervening peritoneal sac, which may contain small bowel)
- Incomplete/mucosal: prolapse limited to only two layers of mucosa
- Concealed: internal intussusception of upper rectum into lower, with no extrusion into the anus

EPIDEMIOLOGY

- Most cases occur in children <4 years of age around time of toilet training; equal incidence in boys and girls
- In older children and adults, strong (6-fold) female predilection
- Common in developing countries, perhaps because of poor nutrition and parasitic infection; less common in industrialized countries

RISK FACTORS

- Cystic fibrosis (CF)
  - Typically presents between 6 months and 3 years of age in patients with CF
  - Presentation in children with CF >5 years of age is rare.
- Chronic constipation
  - About 50% of children with chronic constipation will experience prolapse.

Genetics

- Inheritance patterns depend on associated underlying etiologies.
- No known inheritance pattern for idiopathic rectal prolapse

ETIOLOGY

Exact etiology uncertain

COMMONLY ASSOCIATED CONDITIONS

- Excessive straining with bowel movements from constipation and toilet training (hips and knees flexed) is the most common cause in industrialized countries.
- Diarrhea; may be more of a cause in tropical and subtropical countries
- Infections: hookworms and other parasitic infections
- Malnutrition; can cause loss of the ischiorectal fat pad
- Complication of past surgery, such as imperforate anus repair
- Complete prolapse is rare in children, but when it occurs, it may be related to poor fixation of rectum to sacrum and to weak pelvic and anal musculature.
- CF
- Ulcerative colitis
- Hirschsprung disease
- Ehlers-Danlos syndrome
- Meningomyelocele
- Pertussis
- Rectal polyp
- Pneumonia
- Anorexia
- Rectal neoplasm

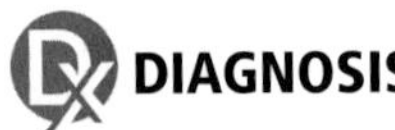

DIAGNOSIS

HISTORY

- Signs and symptoms:
  - Protrusion of rectal layers through anus, usually found during defecation or attempted defecation
  - Although the history of rectal prolapse may be evident, it is often difficult to elicit on examination, and by the time the patient is seen after a prolapse at home, it may already be spontaneously reduced. Thus, the assumption of the diagnosis may have to rest primarily on the parental history.
  - Although usually benign, rectal prolapse is distressing to both the parents and the child.
- Assess for symptoms of CF, risk factors for CF, or for symptoms of other associated conditions (infection, malnutrition, etc.).
- Suggest pictures to be taken by family when it occurs.
- Often reduces spontaneously; if not, can instruct parents to attempt reduction manually
- Rectal prolapse may cause some discomfort during bowel movements.
- Trauma to the recurrently prolapsed mucosa may lead to ulceration and mucus discharge.

PHYSICAL EXAM

- Usually, prolapse is not seen on examination while the patient is at rest, unless it is irreducible (dark or bright red mass protruding from child's anus without discomfort).
- May see poor anal tone and/or large anal orifice, especially within hours after the prolapse
- In complete rectal prolapse, concentric mucosal rings can be seen, whereas incomplete (mucosal) prolapse reveals radial folds.
  - If clinician sees >5 cm of rectum emerging, it is most likely a complete prolapse.
  - Asking the patient to strain may allow the mucosa to prolapse. However, this may be challenging in young patients.
- If prolapsed mucosa visualized, insert a finger around the prolapsing apex of the intussusception, between it and the lining of the anal canal.
- Will appear different from a polyp, which is generally plum-colored and does not involve the entire anal circumference

DIFFERENTIAL DIAGNOSIS

- Tumors
- Prolapsing rectal tumor
- Trauma
- Sexual abuse (e.g., result of trauma from anal penetration)
- Metabolic
- CF: From 10% to 50% of patients diagnosed with CF, >4 years of age have experienced rectal prolapse (either at the time of the diagnosis or as a past event), but few individuals with rectal prolapse have CF.
- Anatomic abnormality (such as absence of Houston valves in infants)
- Solitary rectal ulcer syndrome: An uncommon benign condition usually affecting older children that involves rectal bleeding on defecation is common.
- Prolapsing polyp
- Large hemorrhoids
- Colonic intussusception
- Constipation
- Ehlers-Danlos syndrome
- Hirschsprung disease
- History of imperforate anus
- Pertussis/pneumonia
- Ulcerative colitis
- Meningomyelocele

DIAGNOSTIC TESTS & INTERPRETATION

Initial Tests (screening, lab, imaging)

- Sweat test
  - All children with rectal prolapse should have a sweat test to rule out CF.
  - Complete CF genetic testing can be considered but is more costly.
- Stool cultures for bacterial and parasitic infestations
- Other tests for the aforementioned conditions as clinically indicated
- Evacuation proctography
  - A barium enema is given, and movement of barium is observed under fluoroscopy during defecation.
  - This study may reveal an internal prolapse not easily recognizable on physical examination.
  - This study is not commonly used in children because full cooperation is essential.
- Consider AP/lateral lumbosacral imaging to evaluate for spinal fusion anomalies.

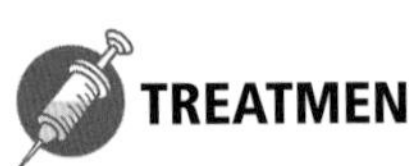

TREATMENT

GENERAL MEASURES

- Rectal prolapse in children <4 years of age has strong tendency to resolve spontaneously over time (90%).
- Patients who develop rectal prolapse at >4 years of age have less certain prognosis.

- Patients who present with a prolapsed rectum should undergo manual reduction in a prone position:
  - Parents should be provided with gloves and lubricant and taught how to reduce the prolapse.
  - The prolapsed bowel may be grasped with lubricated gloved fingers and pushed back in with gentle steady pressure.
  - If the bowel has become edematous, firm steady pressure for several minutes may be necessary to reduce the swelling and allow for reduction.
  - Placing granulated sugar on edematous prolapsed bowel and letting it sit for 15 minutes will also allow for reduction of swelling and potential for successful manual reduction.
  - Digital rectal examination should always follow this procedure to verify complete reduction.
  - If the prolapse immediately recurs, it may be reduced again and the buttocks taped together for several hours.
- The prolapse will resolve more successfully and quickly if the patient is treated for constipation:
  - This should include both dietary manipulations (e.g., increased fiber, hydration) and improved defecation methods.
  - It also will usually require the use of supplemental aids such as laxatives (polyethylene glycol).
- A small child should try to defecate with his or her hips at 90 degrees, his or her buttocks at toilet seat level, and on an appropriately sized toilet.
- In the rare case of stool infection with diarrhea as the underlying etiology, the appropriate therapy for that infection should be instituted.

MEDICATION

- Stool softeners (i.e., docusate, polyethylene glycol) to relieve constipation or medication with the associated condition
- In patients with CF, optimization of pancreatic enzyme supplementation; associated with significant improvement in rectal prolapse in this population

SURGERY/OTHER PROCEDURES

Surgery should be reserved for refractory cases or those children with severe neurologic or musculoskeletal defects. Numerous (>130) approaches have been attempted and advocated with varying degrees of enthusiasm, suggesting that none is perfect. Across all procedures, including as follows, efficacy is higher in older patients >4 years old; most common procedures:

- Delorme procedure: Rectal mucosa is excised, and underlying rectal muscle is plicated with sutures.
- Laparoscopic suture rectopexy: rectal wall is exposed and then sutured to the fascia of the sacral promontory; 5% full-thickness recurrence rate
- Anterior resection rectopexy: resection of the sigmoid loop and upper rectum; good results, but again, high complication rate
- Perineal resection: perineal rectosigmoidectomy with a coloanal anastomosis; good results (Altemeier procedure)
- Circumferential injection procedures (90–100% success rate): injection of phenol, oil, hypertonic saline, dextrose 50% solution (500 g/L), or ethyl alcohol to promote adhesion and stabilization of the rectum

ADMISSION, INPATIENT, AND NURSING CONSIDERATIONS

Palliative

- Reassurance of patient and/or family and caregivers
- Teaching around techniques of manual reduction
- Education regarding pros and cons of surgery, which may appear to offer more definite solution but are not without risk and may lead to further complications. In most cases, it may be more prudent to allow time and medical management to solve the problem.

ONGOING CARE

FOLLOW-UP RECOMMENDATIONS

Patient Monitoring

- Treatment of constipation should continue indefinitely or until the child has demonstrated regular bowel habits on a high-fiber diet on his or her own without evidence of prolapse for at least several months.
- Intermittent parental observation to ensure child is avoiding straining with defecation

DIET

- Increase consumption of liquids.
- Add larger amounts of fiber to diet (goal: 5 g + age in years = total g/day fiber intake).
- Increase amounts of fruits and vegetables.

PROGNOSIS

- 90% of children who develop prolapse will respond to conservative measures with resolution of their symptoms.
- 10% may have symptoms that persist into adulthood.
- With proper medical management, there is an excellent prognosis, defined as resolution without surgery.
- May require months to years on a good dietary and behavioral regimen

COMPLICATIONS

- In some older patients who may also have an overactive external sphincter, the need to generate high rectal pressures to defecate, together with the rectal prolapse, may cause venous congestion and solitary rectal ulcer syndrome.
- Repetitive trauma to mucosa can produce proctitis.
- Surgical complications of repair
- Frequent recurrence

ADDITIONAL READING

- Akkoyun I, Akbiyik F, Soylu SG. The use of digital photos and video images taken by a parent in the diagnosis of anal swelling and anal protrusions in children with normal physical examination. *J Pediatr Surg*. 2011;46(11):2132–2134.
- Antao B, Bradley V, Roberts JP, et al. Management of rectal prolapse in children. *Dis Colon Rectum*. 2005;48(8):1620–1625.
- Chan WK, Kay SM, Laberge JM, et al. Injection sclerotherapy in the treatment of rectal prolapse in infants and children. *J Pediatr Surg*. 1998;33(2): 255–258.
- Laituri CA, Garey CL, Fraser JD, et al. 15-Year experience in the treatment of rectal prolapse in children. *J Pediatr Surg*. 2010;45(8):1607–1609.
- Potter DD, Bruny JL, Allshouse MJ, et al. Laparoscopic suture rectopexy for full-thickness anorectal prolapse in children: an effective outpatient procedure. *J Pediatr Surg*. 2010;45(10):2103–2107.
- Sajid MS, Siddiqui MR, Baig MK. Open vs laparoscopic repair of full-thickness rectal prolapse: a re-meta-analysis. *Colorectal Dis*. 2010;12(6):515–525.
- Siafakas C, Vottler TP, Andersen JM. Rectal prolapse in pediatrics. *Clin Pediatr (Phila)*. 1999;38(2):63–72.

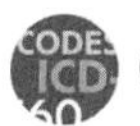

CODES

ICD10

K62.3 Rectal prolapse

FAQ

- Q: What should I do if my child has a rectal prolapse but I cannot reduce it?
- A: You should wrap the prolapse in moist towels and bring your child to the emergency department. Physicians there will try to reduce it. Rarely, if a prolapse is irreducible and left for a period of time, it can cause bowel ischemia and may require surgery.
- Q: My child has rectal prolapse, and now, he is supposed to have a sweat test to determine whether he has CF. Is this very likely?
- A: No. Although it is important to rule out this disease, most patients with rectal prolapse do not have CF. However, many children with CF suffer from rectal prolapse.
- Q: My child, who has rectal prolapse, is in day care. How will I know if he is having the prolapse?
- A: You should inform someone in the school (a teacher or guardian) of his condition, and he or she should check the child for prolapse after a bowel movement. Although, if present, it usually resolves spontaneously, the teacher should inform you so you can do a manual reduction, if necessary.

REFRACTIVE ERROR

Leah G. Reznick, MD • Allison R. Loh, MD

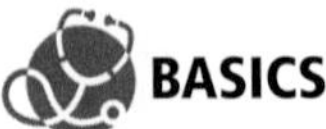

BASICS

DESCRIPTION

- Refractive errors are abnormalities in the optical components of the eyes that cause light not to be focused on the retinal plane. In order for a person to have clear vision, light entering the eye must precisely focus on the retina.
  - Uncorrected refractive errors blur vision in one or both eyes.
  - If left untreated in children, uncorrected refractive errors may cause permanent vision loss from amblyopia and strabismus (see "Amblyopia" and "Strabismus").
- Refractive errors are measured in diopter units.
- Refractive errors can be classified in three groups based on the optic effects (Appendix, Figure 1):
  - Myopia (near-sightedness): Objects are focused in front of the retinal plane. Near vision is clearer, and distance vision is more blurry. Optical correction is with concave lenses (negative power).
  - Hyperopia (farsightedness): Objects are focused behind the retinal plane and optical correction contains convex lens (plus power).
  - Astigmatism: unequal curvature of the cornea causing the cornea to be more curved in one direction than another (aspherical). The shape of the cornea is more like a football than a basketball in astigmatism.
    - Images are blurred at near and far distances.
    - Astigmatism can occur concomitantly with myopia and hyperopia.
- Other terms related to refractive error include the following:
  - Emmetropia: no refractive error. Objects are focused on the retinal plane.
  - Anisometropia: unequal refractive error between the two eyes that increases the risk of amblyopia
- Accommodation: the changing of the shape of the eye's lens to focus clearly at near or all of the time in hyperopes

EPIDEMIOLOGY

Prevalence of refractive errors varies during childhood as the optical components change with development. At birth, usual median refractive error is low hyperopia, approximately +2.00 diopters. In adults, the median is emmetropia; approximately 30% require optical correction.

Prevalence

- In children aged 5 to 17 years, the prevalence of visually significant refractive error varies on type.
  - Myopia = 0.7–5.0%
  - Hyperopia = 4.0–9.0%
  - Astigmatism = 0.5–3.0%
- The prevalence and type of refractive error varies among ethnic groups. For example, people of Native American, Chinese, and Japanese descent have an increased prevalence of myopia.

RISK FACTORS

Genetics

- Both genetic and environmental factors are important in refractive status. ~60% of myopia can be predicted by parental degree of refraction.
- There is an increased prevalence of visually significant refractive errors in individuals with prematurity, autism, and cerebral palsy.
- Some genetic syndromes or medical problems associated with refractive errors include the following:
  - Myopia is associated with Stickler, Marfan, Down, and Ehlers-Danlos syndromes.
  - Hyperopia is associated with Senior-Loken syndrome, WAGR (Wilms tumor, aniridia, genitourinary malformations, mental retardation) syndrome, and Down syndrome.
  - Astigmatism is associated with Down syndrome, craniofacial abnormalities, and albinism.
  - Environmental factors associated with refractive error include prematurity, eye surgery, and trauma.

GENERAL PREVENTION

- Early detection and correction of refractive errors is important to prevent amblyopia and strabismus. A child should be able to perform a visual acuity examination by age 4 years.
- Children with significant refractive errors are often asymptomatic. All children should be screened for visual acuity in each eye.
- Glasses may not improve vision alone because of amblyopia (maldevelopment of the brain's ocular cells). Patients with suspected amblyopia should be rechecked even if wearing glasses.

PATHOPHYSIOLOGY

- The three most important determinants of refractive error include the cornea, lens, and axial length of the eye. The cornea and lens bend light to meet the retina in order to create a sharply focused image. The optical power of the cornea and lens must match the actual eye length (distance from cornea to retina). If the cornea and lens do not bend light to hit the retina, there is a refractive error and can blur the vision.
- Small amounts of hyperopia are normal for children. With small hyperopic errors, a child's eye can easily bring objects into clear focus by adjusting the shape of the lens (accommodation). These children have no problems seeing at far or near distances.
- With larger amounts of hyperopia (>+3.50 diopters), a child's vision may be blurred at distance and near because accommodation may be limited or cause esotropia (see "Strabismus").
- The refractive components evolve as the eye develops over childhood. The cornea, lens, and eye length should simultaneously develop to lead to emmetropia. Factors determining the normal and abnormal growth of eye are not completely understood.
- There are likely genetic and environmental factors determining the growth of the eye. There may be an association with increased level of education and increased incidence of myopia. Epidemiologic data suggest that increased amount of time spent outdoors protects against the development of myopia.

COMMONLY ASSOCIATED CONDITIONS

Refractive errors are frequently associated with other ocular conditions.

- Anisometropia is associated with nasolacrimal duct obstruction.
- Myopia is associated with childhood glaucoma, deprivation amblyopia, retinopathy of prematurity, retinal dystrophies, coloboma, and retinal detachments.
- Hyperopia is associated with esotropia, Leber congenital amaurosis, and aphakia (absence of lens).
- Astigmatism is associated with ptosis, coloboma, glaucoma, retinopathy of prematurity, lid hemangioma, nystagmus, and limbal dermoid.

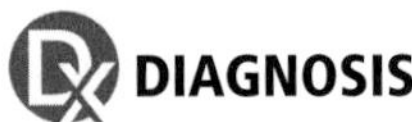

DIAGNOSIS

HISTORY

- Age of onset of vision loss
- History of headaches, squinting, or subjective vision problems
- Associated ocular abnormalities, trauma, injury, or surgery
- History of strabismus, amblyopia
- History of prematurity, genetic disorders
- Family history of strabismus, amblyopia, congenital cataract, ocular or systemic genetic disease

PHYSICAL EXAM

- Age-appropriate vision screening is the most effective diagnostic tool for detecting refractive errors.
- Vision must be tested with each eye separately (patch or occluder over one eye).
- In children <3 years of age:
  - Monocular testing for fixing and following will determine visual behavior for each eye.
  - Brückner (simultaneous red reflex) examination with the direct ophthalmoscope can objectively identify high refractive errors (distorted or darkened red reflex) or anisometropia (asymmetric brightness of red reflex).
- In children age 3 years or older:
  - Subjective visual acuity should be testing with matching or identifying optotypes on a vision chart (Allen figures, HOTV, Lea, or Snellen).
  - A failed vision screening or untestable vision after two attempts warrants a referral to an eye care provider.
- Vision screenings are important at regular intervals throughout childhood to prevent vision loss.
- Strabismus is frequently a secondary sign of refractive error in children and can be detected by cover test, Hirschberg corneal light reflex test, or Brückner test.

DIFFERENTIAL DIAGNOSIS

- Decreased binocular or monocular vision can be caused by a number of structural abnormalities of the eye as well as decreased cortical visual development. In any child with vision loss, refractive error needs to be evaluated as the cause or one of many factors contributing to decreased vision.
- True refractive error needs to be measured by only after instilling cycloplegic eye drops with retinoscopy (objective technique to measure refractive error). Without these drops, a child's lens will accommodate (change shape) and give a false amount of refractive error.

DIAGNOSTIC TESTS & INTERPRETATION

Photoscreening, which uses the principle of red reflex testing, is also effective in detecting high or asymmetric refractive errors.

TREATMENT

GENERAL MEASURES

- Refractive errors are treated by corrective lenses. Young children typically use glasses and teenagers may use contact lenses.
- The following guidelines for prescribing glasses have been developed to improve visual acuity and reduce the risk of amblyopia and strabismus.
  - Myopia: >3.00 diopters for age 2 to 3 years and >1.00 diopter or more in school-age children
  - Hyperopia: +4.50 diopters or more for age 2 to 3 years, +3.00 diopters or more in school-age children, or +1.50 diopters or more anisometropia
  - Astigmatism: >2.00 diopters in age 2 to 3 years or >1.50 diopters in school-age children
- If hyperopic correction is needed for treatment but is not well accepted by the child, a brief period of cycloplegia with topical atropine can increase usage of glasses.
- In suspected amblyopia, vision should be retested to measure visual improvement after glasses have been worn for several weeks
- Hyperopic patients may develop esotropia when their glasses are taken off. Full-time glasses usage will prevent loss of vision and depth perception when children have accommodative esotropia.

MEDICATION

Low-dose atropine (0.01%) eye drops may prevent myopia progression, and continued research is needed before being routinely recommended to all myopic children.

SURGERY/OTHER PROCEDURES

- Routine refractive surgery including laser-assisted in situ keratomileusis (LASIK) and photorefractive keratectomy (PRK) are not approved or recommended for children. In a few circumstances including severe developmental delay or inability to wear corrective glasses, refractive surgery can be considered
- Corneal collagen cross-linking is a technique that uses ultraviolet A light and riboflavin to create a chemical reaction within the corneal stroma that strengthens the cornea and slows or stops the progression of keratoconus. It is routinely used for adults and more recently its use is expanding to children with keratoconus.

ONGOING CARE

Because refractive error depends on the eye's shape and the eye's shape changes as a child grows, the refractive error will evolve over time. Because this process is dynamic, children require at least an annual vision evaluation and refraction to assess whether they need a change in their glasses. They also need to be evaluated for amblyopia and strabismus.

PROGNOSIS

If a child has a significant refractive error, his or her visual acuity will likely improve with optical correction. Refractive error rarely leads to significant functional limitations for daily activities and school. If refractive errors accompany other vision problems such as amblyopia or strabismus, other treatments may be needed to improve visual acuity. Special frames for athletic activities should be considered for children if standard glasses are interfering with those activities.

COMPLICATIONS

In children, the most significant complications of uncorrected refractive errors are strabismus and amblyopia.

- Accommodative esotropia
  - For children with moderate to high hyperopia, their eyes will normally accommodate (change shape of lens) to bring objects into focus.
  - This accommodative process may involuntarily cause overconvergence of the eyes and thus esotropia.
  - Small amounts of convergence normally occur with accommodation so that both eyes can be looking at a near target. But in children with accommodative esotropia, they cannot control the degree of convergence and develop esotropia when focusing at both distance and near.
- Refractive amblyopia is poor cortical visual development resulting from a poorly focused image in one or both eyes.
  - Anisometropia (unequal refractive error) is the most frequent cause of unilateral amblyopia (~35%). The brain learns to see well from the eye that has the least amount of refractive error but does not develop equal vision from the eye that has a higher refractive error.
- Bilateral high refractive errors may cause bilateral amblyopia from chronically poor visual input from both eyes.
- High myopia (>5 diopters) can lead to retinal thinning and eventual retinal detachment. It is also associated with increased risk of glaucoma and cataracts as an adult.

ADDITIONAL READING

- American Academy of Ophthalmology. *Preferred Practice Pattern: Refractive Errors*. San Francisco, CA: American Academy of Ophthalmology; 2013.
- American Academy of Ophthalmology Pediatric Ophthalmology/Strabismus Panel. *Preferred Practice Pattern Guidelines. Pediatric Eye Evaluations*. San Francisco, CA: American Academy of Ophthalmology; 2012.
- Bell AL, Rodes ME, Collier Kellar L. Childhood eye examination. *Am Fam Physician*. 2013;88(4):241–248.
- Donahue SP, Baker CN; for Committee on Practice and Ambulatory Medicine, Section on Ophthalmology, American Academy of Pediatrics, et al. Procedures for the evaluation of the visual system by pediatricians. *Pediatrics*. 2016;137(1).
- Paysse EA, Williams GC, Coats DK, et al. Detection of red reflex asymmetry by pediatric residents using the Brückner reflex versus the MTI photoscreener. *Pediatrics*. 2001;108(4):E74.
- Thorn F. Development of refraction and strabismus. *Curr Opin Ophthalmol*. 2000;11(5):301–305.
- Wen G, Tarczy-Hornoch K, McKean-Cowdin R, et al; and Multi-Ethnic Pediatric Eye Disease Study Group. Prevalence of myopia, hyperopia, and astigmatism in non-Hispanic white and Asian children: multi-ethnic pediatric eye disease study. *Ophthalmology*. 2013;120(10):2109–2116.

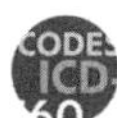

CODES

ICD10

- H52.7 Unspecified disorder of refraction
- H52.10 Myopia, unspecified eye
- H52.209 Unspecified astigmatism, unspecified eye

FAQ

- Q: Will my child always need glasses?
- A: Not necessarily. As children grow, the shape of the eyes change. Because the need for glasses depend on the eye's shape, it is unclear whether the child will continue to need glasses to have normal vision as his or her eye develops. If optical correction remains necessary, contact lenses and refractive surgery are also possible in older children or adults.
- Q: Will wearing glasses weaken my child's eyes?
- A: No. Glasses change the way light enters the eye to focus on the retina and optimize vision. Glasses do not weaken the eyes or vision. Glasses are important to prevent amblyopia and permanent vision loss.
- Q: If my child wears glasses and his or her vision improves, can my child stop wearing glasses?
- A: In the majority of children, they will need to continue to wear glasses to clarify the blur from their refractive error. The glasses are improving their visual acuity.
- Q: Is my child too young for glasses?
- A: If a child needs glasses to improve his or her visual acuity, then a child is never too young to wear them. Small frames are designed for children as young as a few months. If glasses improve vision, a child usually quickly accepts correction.
- Q: My child can see well. Why does he need glasses?
- A: Some children with hyperopia can see charts well, but the accommodation (i.e., focusing) necessary to overcome the refractive error may cause eye strain, fatigue, and esotropia. Others may need glasses for unilateral refractive error and seem to see well with both eyes open. In these children, wearing correction may treat or prevent problems even though they may seem to see well without correction.
- Q: Everyone in my family has needed glasses for myopia in childhood. Is there anything we can do for my child that will prevent the development of myopia?
- A: Unfortunately, few environmental factors have been clearly identified to affect the development of myopia. Reading, particularly at an early age; excessively close visual targets (holding books or toys too close to the face); and light exposure during nighttime have been suggested as factors in myopia development. Increased hours spent outdoors may prevent myopic progression. Avoiding long periods of reading, avoiding intensive near work, using a reasonable reading distance (i.e., 16 to 18 inches), and avoiding use of night lights may reduce some environmental stimuli.

RENAL ARTERY STENOSIS

Danielle Soranno, MD • Michelle Denburg, MD, MSCE

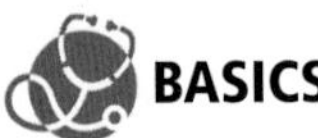

BASICS

DESCRIPTION

Narrowing of one or both renal arteries and/or their more distal branches, resulting in decreased perfusion, increased renin release, increased vascular resistance, and systemic hypertension

EPIDEMIOLOGY

- Hypertension in infants and young children is often secondary to some identifiable cause. Of those with secondary hypertension, most have intrinsic renal disease (e.g., renal scarring, dysplasia, chronic nephritis).
- Up to 5% of adults with hypertension have renal artery stenosis (RAS).
- RAS accounts for ~10% of secondary hypertension in children. Its importance clinically is not its frequency but its potential curability.

RISK FACTORS

- Any condition associated with thromboembolic events (such as a complication of an umbilical artery catheter in newborns)
- Renal trauma including renal artery surgery (e.g., transplantation)
- Extrinsic compression of the renal artery (e.g., Wilms tumor, neuroblastoma, or pheochromocytoma)
- Underlying vascular disease such as midaortic syndrome, Williams syndrome, or Takayasu arteritis

GENERAL PREVENTION

Reduce risk factors, such as thromboembolic events, which can lead to renal artery narrowing.

PATHOPHYSIOLOGY

Arterial narrowing leads to diminished perfusion of the affected kidney, leading to signals in the juxtaglomerular apparatus, which lead to renin release and results in increased vascular resistance, sodium retention, and blood pressure (BP).

ETIOLOGY

- Majority are caused by fibromuscular dysplasia (FMD), a noninflammatory vascular disease of unknown etiology.
  - Primarily affects females and affects up to 4 in 100 adults
  - The renal vasculature is the most common arterial bed affected.
  - FMD can concurrently affect other vascular beds including carotid, vertebral, and intracranial vascular beds.
- Arterial narrowing by atheroma is common in adults but rare in children.

COMMONLY ASSOCIATED CONDITIONS

- Renal artery hypoplasia
- Neurocutaneous disorders (neurofibromatosis [type 1], tuberous sclerosis)
- Vasculitis (granulomatous polyangiitis, polyarteritis nodosa, Kawasaki disease, Takayasu arteritis, moyamoya disease)
- Williams syndrome
- Marfan syndrome
- Alagille syndrome
- Infections (e.g., congenital rubella, fungal infection)
- Nephrotic syndrome may accompany RAS and is probably secondary to it.
- RAS has been associated with multicystic dysplasia in the contralateral kidney.

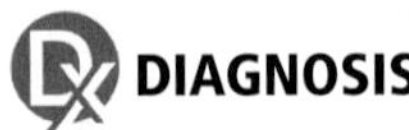

DIAGNOSIS

HISTORY

- Ask about prior BP determinations, family history of hypertension, previous renal disease, symptoms of hypertension, and preexisting conditions associated with RAS.
- Signs and symptoms:
  - Symptoms of hypertension in infants are not specific and include irritability, poor feeding, and vomiting.
  - In children, symptoms include headache, nausea/vomiting, visual disturbance, dizziness, and seizure.
  - Many affected children remain asymptomatic and 1/3 of children with RAS are diagnosed incidentally.

PHYSICAL EXAM

- BP assessment
  - Consider RAS in a child with very high BP readings (i.e., at or above the 99th percentile).
  - Obtain multiple, manual BP readings using an appropriate-size cuff in the right upper extremity with patient relaxed at baseline heart rate and compare to the BP nomogram for age, sex, and length/height percentile.
  - Most accurate readings are obtained with either a mercury column or an aneroid sphygmomanometer.
- Determine the BP in all extremities. A gradient from the upper to lower extremities should prompt evaluation for aortic coarctation or midaortic syndrome.
- Examine the skin for lesions suggestive of vasculitis or neurocutaneous disorder (e.g., café au lait macules).
- Assess the child's facies and habitus for features of associated syndromes.
- View the optic fundi for hypertensive vascular changes.
- Auscultate the lower back and abdomen for the presence of a bruit (suggesting turbulent flow).
- In infancy, signs of heart failure may be present.

DIFFERENTIAL DIAGNOSIS

- RAS should be suspected and investigated in children with severe, progressive, and/or difficult-to-manage hypertension.
- The differential diagnosis consists of other causes of significant hypertension, including increased intracranial pressure, coarctation of the aorta, midaortic syndrome, rapidly progressive glomerulonephritis, vasculitis, and pheochromocytoma.

DIAGNOSTIC TESTS & INTERPRETATION

Echocardiogram to assess for left ventricular hypertrophy and function

Initial Tests (screening, lab, imaging)

- BUN and creatinine to evaluate for renal insufficiency
- Electrolytes to assess possible hyperaldosteronism with hypokalemia and metabolic alkalosis. Hyponatremia may sometimes occur.
- ESR or CRP to screen for vasculitis
- The definitive diagnostic test remains the selective renal arteriogram. If the diagnosis is made, angioplasty may be part of the same procedure. Angiography should not be delayed in any child in whom the diagnosis is strongly suspected.
- Renal ultrasound with Doppler to identify a smaller kidney and/or increased resistance to flow is simple and not invasive, but it is neither sensitive nor specific. Length discrepancy of >1 cm in children can increase suspicion for RAS.
- Contrast-enhanced CT angiography (CTA) or MR angiography (MRA) also is not completely diagnostic and is not therapeutic.
- Nuclear renal scans using dimercaptosuccinic acid (DMSA) or MAG3 enhanced with an angiotensin converting enzyme (ACE) inhibitor, such as captopril (and more recently angiotensin receptor blockers [ARBs]) also are not diagnostic for all children.
- Diagnostic accuracy of various imaging studies

Technique	Sensitivity (%)	Specificity (%)
Ultrasound	73–85	71–92
DMSA with ACE	52–93	63–92
CTA	64–94	62–97
MRA	64–93	72–97

Diagnostic Procedures/Other

- Avoid excessive investigation in children whose BP is minimally or episodically elevated and therefore in whom the diagnosis of RAS is less likely.
- Selective renal vein renin determinations suggest unilateral stenosis if the affected side is 1.5 times the contralateral (normal) side. However, the procedure is invasive and requires catheterization of the femoral vein.
- Random renin determinations have little value and may be misleading. If obtained, renin levels should be interpreted in the context of the urine sodium concentration.
- Pathologic findings
  - FMD is a segmental sclerotic process involving smooth muscle hyperplasia of the media layer of the artery. It is unilateral in 75%.
  - Stenosis is usually distal in the renal artery, at times involving intrarenal branches.
  - The stenotic area(s) of the artery may be associated with distal aneurysms.
  - In neurofibromatosis, arterial narrowing is at the vessel's ostium and usually involves the intimal layer.

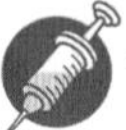

TREATMENT

Treat children who are symptomatic immediately (e.g., severe headaches, seizures, blurred vision, facial palsy).

GENERAL MEASURES

- If RAS is suspected, begin the diagnostic evaluation and pharmacotherapy together, avoiding ACE inhibitors and ARBs until bilateral RAS has been ruled out.
- If BP is very high, use bed rest until BP is better controlled.

MEDICATION

- Hypertension accompanying RAS is often difficult to control and may worsen over time. Multiple medications given in high doses are common until the diagnosis is made and angioplasty can be done.
- Because RAS results in increased renin levels, renin-angiotensin blockade with ACE inhibitor therapy (e.g., enalapril, lisinopril) and/or ARBs (e.g., losartan) is often effective.

ALERT

In children where bilateral RAS is known or suspected, ACE inhibitor and ARB therapy must be avoided to prevent acute renal failure. 50% of children will have bilateral disease. Renal function should be checked before and after initiation of ACE inhibition or ARB therapy.

- If BP is easy to control on monotherapy, may consider medical management alone rather than angioplasty.
- β-Blockers, calcium channel blockers, diuretics, and direct vasodilators (e.g., minoxidil, hydralazine) are all possibly effective.

ISSUES FOR REFERRAL

- Cardiology follow-up for echocardiogram changes, if indicated
- Ophthalmologic follow-up for resolution of vascular changes, if indicated

SURGERY/OTHER PROCEDURES

- Actual surgery on the stenotic renal artery has been replaced by angioplasty, which has been successfully carried out in very young infants. Stents are occasionally used.
- Surgery must sometimes be performed, especially in children with neurofibromatosis where the stenosis is frequently at the renal artery's ostium. Surgical options include bypass or autotransplantation.

ADMISSION, INPATIENT, AND NURSING CONSIDERATIONS

- Initial stabilization
  - If symptomatic, use potent, rapidly acting medications such as labetalol or nicardipine with goal to decrease BP by ~10% over the first 8 to 12 hours.
  - Be prepared to have difficulty adequately controlling the BP using a single medication.
- Admission criteria
  - Children who present with a BP at or above the 99th percentile
  - Children who appear to have symptomatic hypertension
  - Children with progressive renal insufficiency
- Nursing
  - Obtain BP levels frequently and carefully.
  - Notify MD if high or low limits exceeded.
  - Monitor intake of salt, I&O, and weight.
- Discharge criteria
  - BP in the 90th to 95th percentile

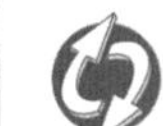

ONGOING CARE

FOLLOW-UP RECOMMENDATIONS

- The child's BP must be followed closely, both before and after the angioplasty. Response to angioplasty may be immediate but may require continued antihypertensive therapy at some level for weeks to months.
- Medical therapy should be monitored closely. Until correction, the need for progressively higher doses and/or additional medications is common.
- Disposition
  - Close follow-up by the primary care provider, mainly for monitoring BP, and a specialist comfortable with the evaluation and treatment of childhood hypertension
  - Patient and/or family must be familiar with medication, exercise program, and diet.

Patient Monitoring

- Long-term follow-up of the BP is most important. If on no medications, the BP should be checked monthly, preferably somewhere the child is comfortable and the correct cuff is employed. Begin to space visits after 6 months.
- Checking renal growth on serial renal ultrasounds is important (e.g., at 6 months postangioplasty and then yearly). If the child is fully grown, check ultrasound at 6 months.
- Check renal function annually.

DIET

Limit salt intake.

PROGNOSIS

Long-term outcome of percutaneous angioplasty is excellent; most children require no long-term antihypertensive medications. Percutaneous angioplasty is less successful in neurofibromatosis than in other causes of RAS.

COMPLICATIONS

- Rate of restenosis of the renal artery, either ipsilateral or contralateral, is 22–39%.
- When RAS causes severe hypertension, it may cause encephalopathy, severe headache, seizures, or stroke.
- If untreated, chronic hypertension may cause end-organ damage, including heart and kidney.
- Angiography may lead to contrast-induced renal failure. The procedure may also cause injury to the kidney and/or renal artery.
- Rare cases of subarachnoid hemorrhage secondary to coexisting intracranial aneurysm may occur.
- Utilization of ACE inhibitors or ARBs in bilateral disease may result in acute kidney injury and hyperkalemia.

ADDITIONAL READING

- König K, Gellermann J, Querfeld U, et al. Treatment of severe renal artery stenosis by percutaneous transluminal renal angioplasty and stent implantation: review of the pediatric experience: apropos of two cases. *Pediatr Nephrol*. 2006;21(5):663–671.
- Meyers KE, Cahill AM, Sethna C. Interventions for pediatric renovascular hypertension. *Curr Hypertens Rep*. 2014;16(4):422.
- Olin JW, Gornik HL, Bacharach JM, et al. Fibromuscular dysplasia: state of the science and critical unanswered questions: a scientific statement from the American Heart Association. *Circulation*. 2014;129(9):1048–1078.
- Rountas C, Vlychou M, Vassiou K, et al. Imaging modalities for renal artery stenosis in suspected renovascular hypertension: prospective intraindividual comparison of color Doppler US, CT angiography, GD-enhanced MR angiography, and digital substraction angiography. *Ren Fail*. 2007;29(3):295–302.
- Sethna CB, Kaplan BS, Cahill AM, et al. Idiopathic mid-aortic syndrome in children. *Pediatr Nephrol*. 2008;23(7):1135–1142.
- Shahdadpuri J, Frank R, Gauthier BG, et al. Yield of renal arteriography in the evaluation of pediatric hypertension. *Pediatr Nephrol*. 2000;14(8–9):816–819.
- Spyridopoulos TN, Kaziani K, Balanika AP, et al. Ultrasound as a first line screening tool for the detection of renal artery stenosis: a comprehensive review. *Med Ultrason*. 2010;12(3):228–232.
- Tullus K. Renal artery stenosis: is angiography still the gold standard in 2011? *Pediatr Nephrol*. 2011;26(6):833–837.
- Vade A, Agrawal R, Lim-Dunham J, et al. Utility of computed tomographic renal angiogram in the management of childhood hypertension. *Pediatr Nephrol*. 2002;17(9):741–747.
- Zhu G, He F, Gu Y, et al. Angioplasty for pediatric renovascular hypertension: a 13-year experience. *Diagn Interv Radiol*. 2014;20(3):285–292.

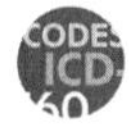

CODES

ICD10

- I70.1 Atherosclerosis of renal artery
- Q27.1 Congenital renal artery stenosis
- I15.0 Renovascular hypertension

RENAL TUBULAR ACIDOSIS

Elaine Ku, MD, MAS

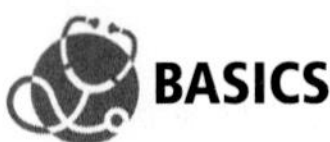

BASICS

DESCRIPTION

- Renal tubular acidosis (RTA) is characterized by hyperchloremic metabolic acidosis in the setting of normal or near-normal glomerular filtration rate (GFR).
- The acidification defect can be localized to the proximal tubule (type II RTA) resulting in incomplete bicarbonate reabsorption or the distal tubule (type I or type IV RTA) resulting in impaired net acid secretion.
- Type I and II RTA are associated with hypokalemia; type IV is associated with hyperkalemia.
- Timing of onset and severity of presentation are variable, depending on the underlying cause of the acidification defect.
- Type I RTA is associated with nephrocalcinosis, osteopenia, rickets, and sometimes hearing loss.
- Four different types of RTA are recognized:
  - Type I (classic, hypokalemic, distal)
  - Type II (proximal)
  - Type III (characteristics of both proximal and distal RTA, rare inherited disorder associated with mental retardation, osteopetrosis, and cerebral calcification)
  - Type IV (hyperkalemic, distal)
    - Associated with aldosterone deficiency or resistance to its renal effect

EPIDEMIOLOGY

RTA is a rare disorder. Increased prevalence is observed in areas where consanguinity is common.

ETIOLOGY

- Genetic causes of proximal RTA:
  - Mutation in carbonic anhydrase II
  - Mutation in sodium bicarbonate cotransporter
- Genetic causes of distal RTA (present in up to ~70% of cases):
  - Mutation in anion exchanger 1 (AE1) in α-intercalated cell
  - Mutation in H^+-ATPase
  - Mutation in carbonic anhydrase II
- Genetic causes of Fanconi syndrome/proximal RTA:
  - Lowe syndrome
  - Dent disease
  - Cystinosis
  - Tyrosinemia
  - Galactosemia
  - Hereditary fructose intolerance
  - Wilson disease
  - Fanconi-Bickel syndrome
  - Mitochondrial disorders
- Acquired causes of proximal RTA:
  - Drugs:
    - Ifosfamide
    - Cisplatin/oxaliplatin
    - Valproic acid
    - Carbonic anhydrase inhibitor (e.g., acetazolamide)
    - Topiramate
    - Aminoglycosides
    - Antiretroviral therapy (tenofovir)
- Acquired causes of distal RTA type I:
  - Autoimmune disorders
  - Drugs:
    - Lithium toxicity
    - Amphotericin
    - Ifosfamide
- Acquired causes of distal RTA type IV:
  - Aldosterone resistance/deficiency
    - Diabetic renal disease
    - Obstructive uropathy
    - Adrenal insufficiency
  - Drugs:
    - Nonsteroidal anti-inflammatory medications
    - Heparin
    - Potassium-sparing diuretics
    - Angiotensin-converting enzyme inhibitor or angiotensin receptor blocker
    - Calcineurin inhibitors (e.g., tacrolimus or cyclosporine)
    - Trimethoprim
    - Pentamidine

PATHOPHYSIOLOGY

- With ingestion of a typical Western diet, healthy adults generate ~1 mEq/kg net acid per day and infants and children ~2 to 3 mEq/kg/day.
- Under physiologic conditions, the proximal tubule is responsible for reclaiming 85–90% of filtered bicarbonate.
  - Bicarbonate reclamation in the proximal tubule is achieved by a sodium–hydrogen ion antiporter, which secretes hydrogen ion into the urine resulting in generation of bicarbonate within the cell.
  - Cellular bicarbonate is then transported into the bloodstream via an $Na\text{-}HCO_3$ transporter on the basolateral membrane.
- The distal tubule normally reclaims the remaining 10–15% of filtered bicarbonate and secretes a net amount of acid, both via hydrogen ion secretion.
  - In the distal tubule, hydrogen ion secretion occurs primarily via H^+-ATPase.
  - Secreted hydrogen ions are buffered in the urinary lumen primarily by ammonia and excreted as ammonium ions.
- In proximal RTA, mutations in the basolateral sodium bicarbonate cotransporter or in carbonic anhydrase prevent adequate bicarbonate reclamation in the proximal tubule.
  - Unreclaimed bicarbonate enters the distal nephron, which has limited capacity for bicarbonate reclamation, resulting in bicarbonaturia and non–anion gap metabolic acidosis (usually serum bicarbonate does not decrease <16 mEq/L).
- In distal RTA, mutations in the basolateral anion exchanger or the H^+-ATPase prevent bicarbonate transport into the bloodstream and hydrogen ion secretion into the lumen, respectively, resulting in impaired net acid secretion and non–anion gap metabolic acidosis.
- Proximal RTA is often associated with Fanconi syndrome in which there is general proximal tubular dysfunction leading to bicarbonaturia, glucosuria, phosphaturia, and tubular proteinuria.
- Distal RTA type I is associated with urine pH >5.5.
- Distal RTA type IV is associated with either low aldosterone levels or aldosterone resistance and presents with hyperkalemic non–anion gap metabolic acidosis.

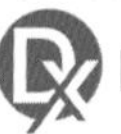

DIAGNOSIS

HISTORY
- Failure to thrive in infants and children
- Polyuria
- Constipation
- Anorexia
- Symptoms of hypokalemia:
  - Muscle weakness
  - Constipation
- Kidney stones
- Intellectual disability
- Propensity for fractures

PHYSICAL EXAM
- Constitutional: failure to thrive
- Head: frontal bossing
- Ears: deafness (associated with some forms of RTA)
- Neurologic: developmental and cognitive delay
- Skin: decreased turgor, prolonged capillary refill

DIFFERENTIAL DIAGNOSIS
- Renal insufficiency (earlier stages)
- Diarrhea
- Urinary diversion via bowel conduits
- Acetazolamide use

DIAGNOSTIC TESTS & INTERPRETATION
- Serum electrolytes
  - To identify metabolic acidosis with normal anion gap, and hypokalemia or hyperkalemia
  - Magnesium level (can be low in Fanconi syndrome)
  - Phosphorus level (can be low in Fanconi syndrome)
- Serum creatinine: to evaluate GFR
- Urine electrolytes
  - Urine anion gap, calculated as (urine sodium + urine potassium − urine chloride): typically >10 in distal RTA (type I or IV)
  - Urine phosphorus: Fractional excretion is high in Fanconi syndrome, resulting in hypophosphatemia.
- Urinalysis
  - Urine pH is high in distal RTA, often >6.8 and can be elevated or normal in proximal RTA.
  - Look for glucosuria in setting of normal serum glucose.
- Urine spot for calcium/creatinine ratio: Look for hypercalciuria (normal values are age dependent).
- 24-hour urine collection for citrate (typically low)
- Renal ultrasound: Evaluate for nephrocalcinosis and kidney stones.
- Long bone films to look for signs of rickets or osteopenia

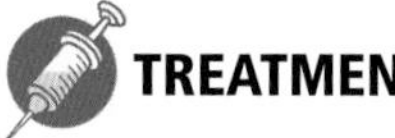

TREATMENT

GENERAL MEASURES
- Vitamin D supplementation as needed
- Phosphorus supplementation as needed (if concurrent Fanconi syndrome)

MEDICATION
- Alkali supplementation given as sodium or potassium bicarbonate or citrate (typically requires 5 to 8 mEq/kg/24 h in distal RTA and 5 to 15 mEq/kg/24 h in proximal RTA)
- Thiazide diuretics (in proximal RTA) to induce volume depletion which can be sensed by the proximal tubule, resulting in increased proximal tubular reabsorption of bicarbonate
- Mineralocorticoid supplementation (for those with select causes of type IV RTA)

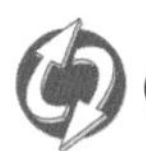

ONGOING CARE

FOLLOW-UP RECOMMENDATIONS
- Frequent monitoring of serum electrolytes
- Close follow-up of linear growth
- Renal ultrasound to monitor for evidence or progression of nephrocalcinosis

PROGNOSIS
- Can rarely progress to chronic kidney disease over time depending on etiology of RTA (as in cystinosis) or if associated with nephrocalcinosis
- May be associated with development of nephrolithiasis

ADDITIONAL READING

- Batlle D, Haque SK. Genetic causes and mechanisms of distal renal tubular acidosis. *Nephrol Dial Transplant*. 2012;27(10):3691–3704.
- Haque SK, Ariceta G, Batlle D. Proximal renal tubular acidosis: a not so rare disorder of multiple etiologies. *Nephrol Dial Transplant*. 2012;27(12):4273–4287.
- Karet FE. Mechanisms in hyperkalemic renal tubular acidosis. *J Am Soc Nephrol*. 2009;20(2):251–254.
- Palazzo V, Provenzano A, Becherucci F, et al. The genetic and clinical spectrum of a large cohort of patients with distal renal tubular acidosis. *Kidney Int*. 2017;91(5):1243–1255.
- Santos F, Ordóñez FA, Claramunt-Taberner D, et al. Clinical and laboratory approaches in the diagnosis of renal tubular acidosis. *Pediatr Nephrol*. 2015;30(12):2099–2107.

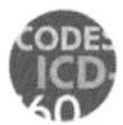

CODES

ICD10
N25.89 Other disorders resulting from impaired renal tubular function

FAQ
- Q: Can RTA be diagnosed in the setting of renal failure?
- A: No. Typically, RTA is diagnosed in the setting of relatively preserved renal function. Renal function associated with non–anion or anion gap acidosis typically occurs when GFR is <30 mL/min/1.73 m^2.
- Q: Does a urine pH <5.5 exclude RTA?
- A: A low urinary pH excludes distal RTA but could still be consistent with a proximal RTA. However, urine pH as tested on urine dipsticks or formal urinalysis can be unreliable depending on duration between time of sample delivery and analysis.
- Q: What are the available forms of alkali supplementation?
- A: Alkali supplementation is best provided as a combination of sodium and potassium citrate or bicarbonate (except in distal RTA type IV, in which potassium alkali is avoided).

RENAL VENOUS THROMBOSIS

Daniel Ranch, MD

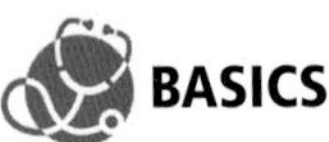

BASICS

DESCRIPTION

- Thrombus formation in renal veins (stellate veins, interlobular veins, ascending vasa recta, arcuate veins, hilar veins, or renal vein)
- Most common non–catheter-related thromboembolism in the neonatal period
- May also be associated with nephrotic syndrome, hypercoagulable states, and oral contraceptive use
- May present with a clinical triad of flank mass, gross hematuria, and thrombocytopenia

EPIDEMIOLOGY

- Most commonly seen in the newborn period
- Slight male predominance
- In neonates, most cases are unilateral (70%), with the left kidney more frequently affected. The left side predominance may be due to the anatomical course of the left renal vein underneath the aorta.

Incidence

- Not well-defined due to lack of data
- Ranges from 0.5 to 2.3 per 100,000 live births

Prevalence

Accounts for 16–20% of thromboembolic events in newborns

RISK FACTORS

- Maternal diabetes mellitus
- Birth asphyxia
- Dehydration/blood loss
- Polycythemia
- Cyanotic heart disease
- Hypercoagulable states
- Nephrotic syndrome
- Venous catheter
- Sepsis
- Oral contraceptive use
- Renal transplant recipient

Genetics

- ~50% of affected neonates have at least one hereditary prothrombotic risk factor.
- Factor V Leiden, protein C/S, and *MTHFR* mutations and lupus anticoagulant

GENERAL PREVENTION

- Maintaining a high index of suspicion in patients at risk (i.e., infant of diabetic mother, child with nephrotic syndrome)
- Counseling regarding the importance of adequate fluid intake and avoidance of dehydration, especially in newborn infants
- Prophylactic anticoagulation may be indicated in certain populations, although conclusive data is lacking.

PATHOPHYSIOLOGY

- Thrombus formation is initiated by endothelial cell injury from hypoxia or other insults.
- In neonates, non–catheter-related renal vein thrombosis (RVT) is believed to originate in the arcuate or interlobular veins, as evidenced by early ultrasound findings.
- Thrombosis may extend to the inferior vena cava (IVC) in 50–60% of cases.
- Neonates also have decreased levels of protein C, protein S, antithrombin, and plasminogen, which may make them more susceptible to thrombosis.
- Lower renal blood flow may also predispose neonates to venous thrombosis.
- In older children, thrombosis may be associated with nephrotic syndrome, hypercoagulable states, or cyanotic heart disease.
- Renal venous thrombosis can result in renal enlargement, decreased renal venous flow, and increased arterial resistive indices.
- Adrenal hemorrhage and left varicocele may also result from renal venous thrombosis.

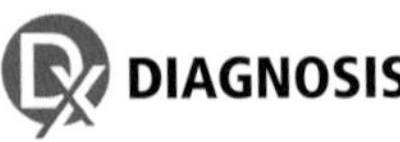

DIAGNOSIS

HISTORY

- More than half of neonatal cases present within 3 days of birth and almost all within the 1st month of life.
- Macroscopic hematuria is seen in about half of affected infants.
- The classic triad of flank mass, gross hematuria, and thrombocytopenia is present in <25% of patients.
- Signs and symptoms:
  - Hematuria (56%)
  - Palpable flank mass (45%)
  - Abdominal/flank pain
  - Dehydration/shock
  - Edema
  - Fever
  - Hypertension
  - Varicocele

PHYSICAL EXAM

- Palpable enlarged kidney can be found in about half of neonates.
- Abdominal/flank tenderness
- Periorbital/peripheral edema
- Left varicocele
- Hypertension

DIFFERENTIAL DIAGNOSIS

- Renal tumors (Wilms, mesoblastic nephroma)
- Pyelonephritis/renal abscess
- Hematoma
- Cystic kidney disease
- Obstructive uropathy
- Thrombotic microangiopathy (hemolytic uremic syndrome [HUS], thrombotic thrombocytopenic purpura [TTP])

DIAGNOSTIC TESTS & INTERPRETATION

- Urinalysis
  - Macroscopic or microscopic hematuria
  - Proteinuria
- Complete blood count
  - Thrombocytopenia is seen in about half of affected neonates.
  - Hemolytic anemia may be present on peripheral blood smear.
- Coagulation tests
  - Prothrombin time and partial thromboplastin time may be prolonged.
  - Fibrin split products may be elevated.
  - Plasma fibrinogen levels may be decreased.
  - Tests for hypercoagulable states, such as factor V Leiden or lupus anticoagulant, should be performed.
- Renal function tests
  - Increased blood urea nitrogen (BUN) and/or creatinine may be present due to acute kidney injury.
  - Electrolyte abnormalities may exist depending on the underlying disease and degree of renal insufficiency.
- Contrast angiography
  - Gold standard for vascular thrombosis but rarely used in the newborn
  - Exposure to radiation and contrast agent
- Ultrasonography
  - Pathognomonic echogenic streaks may be seen with early clot formation.
  - Progresses to renal enlargement and increased parenchymal echogenicity
  - Later findings include loss of corticomedullary differentiation and calcified thrombi in the renal veins.
- Doppler ultrasound
  - Demonstrates decreased or absent renal venous flow
  - May see increased arterial resistive indices

TREATMENT

GENERAL MEASURES

- Treatment of the underlying disease process, if present
- Management of acute kidney injury (i.e., fluid imbalance, electrolyte abnormalities, hypertension)

MEDICATION

The American College of Chest Physicians *Evidence-Based Clinical Practice Guidelines for Antithrombotic Therapy in Neonates and Children* (9th edition) recommend the following:

- For unilateral RVT in the absence of renal impairment or extension into the IVC, either (i) supportive care with radiologic monitoring for extension of thrombosis (if extension occurs, anticoagulation is suggested) or (ii) anticoagulation with unfractionated heparin (UFH)/low-molecular-weight heparin (LMWH) or LMWH in therapeutic doses rather than no therapy; if anticoagulation is used, a total duration of between 6 weeks and 3 months rather than shorter or longer durations of therapy
- For unilateral RVT that extends into the IVC, anticoagulation with UFH/LMWH or LMWH for a total duration of between 6 weeks and 3 months
- For bilateral RVT with evidence of renal impairment, anticoagulation with UFH/LMWH or initial thrombolytic therapy with tissue plasminogen activator (tPA) followed by anticoagulation with UFH/LMWH
- However, the overall evidence supporting these recommendations is weak. Also, no recommendations exist for patients with unilateral RVT and renal impairment or patients with prothrombotic risk factors.

ISSUES FOR REFERRAL

Management should involve a multidisciplinary team that includes neonatologists, radiologists, pediatric hematologists with experience in managing thromboembolism, and pediatric nephrologists.

SURGERY/OTHER PROCEDURES

- Surgery is rarely indicated, except possibly for malignancy-related cases or refractory hypertension or infection.
- Local thrombolytic therapy via an angiocatheter has been reported for severe IVC thrombosis and bilateral RVT causing renal failure.

ADMISSION, INPATIENT, AND NURSING CONSIDERATIONS

- Initial stabilization
  - Supportive therapy for the underlying process, correction of fluid/electrolyte imbalance, and pain control
- Admission criteria
  - Admission for treatment of an underlying cause, if present
  - Renal impairment
  - Pain management
  - Thrombolytic therapy

ONGOING CARE

FOLLOW-UP RECOMMENDATIONS

Patient Monitoring

Long-term monitoring for development of hypertension, renal atrophy, or chronic renal insufficiency

PROGNOSIS

- Treatment with anticoagulants may not change renal outcomes.
- RVT has a low mortality rate but may result in significant complications.
- Patients require long-term follow-up to screen for development of hypertension, renal atrophy, proteinuria, or renal insufficiency.
- Hypertension develops in ~20% of patients with neonatal RVT.
- Kidney atrophy has been reported to develop in up to 71%.
- However, end-stage renal disease is uncommon and is more commonly associated with bilateral RVT.
- Death is uncommon and is usually related to the underlying disease process.
- Certain findings may be linked to worse outcomes, such as the following:
  - Kidney size >6 cm at presentation
  - Decreased overall renal perfusion by Doppler ultrasound
  - Subcapsular bleeding
  - Patchy hypoechogenicity or
  - Irregular pyramids

COMPLICATIONS

- Hypertension
- Renal atrophy
- Proteinuria
- Renal insufficiency

ADDITIONAL READING

- Bidadi B, Nageswara Rao AA, Kaur D, et al. Neonatal renal vein thrombosis: role of anticoagulation and thrombolysis—an institutional review. *Pediatr Hematol Oncol*. 2016;33(1):59–66.
- Brandão LR, Simpson EA, Lau KK. Neonatal renal vein thrombosis. *Semin Fetal Neonatal Med*. 2011;16(6):323–328.
- Kuhle S, Massicotte P, Chan A, et al. A case series of 72 neonates with renal vein thrombosis. Data from the 1-800-NO-CLOTS registry. *Thromb Haemost*. 2004;92(4):729–733.
- Lau KK, Stoffman JM, Williams S; for Canadian Pediatric Thrombosis and Hemostasis Network. Neonatal renal vein thrombosis: review of the English-language literature between 1992 and 2006. *Pediatrics*. 2007;120(5):e1278–e1284.
- Monagle P, Chan AKC, Goldenberg NA, et al. Antithrombotic therapy in neonates and children: Antithrombotic Therapy and Prevention of Thrombosis, 9th ed: American College of Chest Physicians evidence-based clinical practice guidelines. *Chest*. 2012;141(Suppl 2):e737S–e801S.
- Resontoc LP, Yap HK. Renal vascular thrombosis in the newborn. *Pediatr Nephrol*. 2016;31(6):907–915.

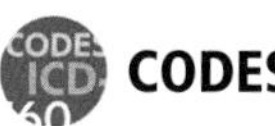

CODES

ICD10

I82.3 Embolism and thrombosis of renal vein

FAQ

- Q: Which population is most susceptible to RVT?
- A: Neonates have the highest risk, especially those with a history of maternal diabetes mellitus, birth asphyxia, or dehydration.
- Q: What is the classic presentation of RVT?
- A: Flank mass, gross hematuria, and thrombocytopenia. However, this "triad" is present in <25% of patients, so a high degree of suspicion must be maintained.
- Q: How is RVT diagnosed?
- A: Renal Doppler ultrasound can show renal enlargement, increased echogenicity, or absent renal venous flow.
- Q: What are the current treatment recommendations for RVT?
- A: Supportive therapy and monitoring is recommended, except for bilateral involvement, IVC extension, or evidence of renal impairment. The role of anticoagulation is otherwise still controversial.

R

RESPIRATORY DISTRESS SYNDROME

Julie M. Nogee, MD • Lawrence M. Nogee, MD

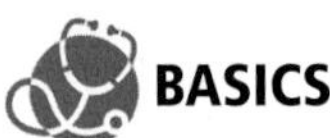

BASICS

DESCRIPTION

Respiratory distress syndrome (RDS) is an acute, developmental lung disease affecting primarily premature infants. Disease is characterized by alveolar collapse due to a lack of pulmonary surfactant owing to lung immaturity that results in increased work of breathing, hypoxemia, and respiratory acidosis. The term hyaline membrane disease (HMD) is often used synonymously.

EPIDEMIOLOGY

- RDS is the most common lung disease in premature infants, affecting approximately 60,000 to 80,000 infants per year in the United States.
- Risk increases with the degree of prematurity; nearly 100% of infants born at <26 weeks' gestation affected
- For near-term infants delivered operatively without benefit of labor, the risk of developing RDS increases roughly 2-fold for every week <39 weeks' gestation.

RISK FACTORS

- Prematurity
- Low birth weight
- Maternal diabetes
- Delivery without labor
- Absence of antenatal steroid administration
- Male gender
- Caucasian race
- Perinatal depression

GENERAL PREVENTION

- Prevention of prematurity
- Maternal antenatal steroids

PATHOPHYSIOLOGY

- Insufficient or dysfunctional surfactant results in alveolar instability and atelectasis, causing hypoventilation and ventilation–perfusion mismatch, leading to hypoxemia and respiratory acidosis.
- The lack of surfactant in conjunction with pulmonary immaturity also leads to transudation of fluid and alveolar edema.
- Surfactant inactivation from transudation of proteins or other substances into the alveolus
- Increased work of breathing generates high negative intrathoracic pressures to overcome alveolar collapse. Retractions result from the highly compliant newborn rib cage combined with poorly compliant lungs.
- Expiratory grunting is due to glottic closure at the end of expiration to prevent end-expiratory atelectasis and maintain functional residual capacity.
- Infants with a well-developed pulmonary arterial muscular bed can develop secondary pulmonary hypertension, with hypoxemia leading to pulmonary vasoconstriction.

DIAGNOSIS

HISTORY

- Gestational age, birth weight
- Lack of antenatal steroids
- Delivery history: maternal diabetes, perinatal asphyxia, route of delivery, absence of labor, 2nd-born twin
- Resuscitation: need for supplemental oxygen, positive pressure, intubation, surfactant

PHYSICAL EXAM

- Assessment of color (cyanosis), grunting, nasal flaring, accessory muscle usage
- Vital signs (including respiratory rate to assess for tachypnea) and pulse oximetry (to assess for hypoxemia)
- Pulmonary exam, including shallow or decreased breath sounds, symmetry of breath sounds, and inspiratory rales

DIFFERENTIAL DIAGNOSIS

- Common
  - Transient tachypnea of the newborn (TTN)
  - Infection (sepsis, pneumonia)
  - Air leak (may also be a complication of RDS)
  - Meconium aspiration syndrome
- Unusual
  - Pulmonary hypoplasia
  - Congenital heart disease
  - Primary ciliary dyskinesia
  - Genetic surfactant dysfunction

DIAGNOSTIC TESTS & INTERPRETATION

Initial Tests (screening, lab, imaging)

- Blood gases (BGs): Arterial BGs allow for accurate determination of pH, $Paco_2$, and Pao_2 to avoid hyperoxia as well as hypoxemia.
- Capillary BGs obtained from appropriately warmed extremities can provide accurate determinations of pH and Pco_2, but poor perfusion to the extremity or inadequate warming may result in inaccurate determinations.
- Oxygenation may be determined noninvasively through pulse oximetry.
- Chest radiography
  - Classic findings include hypoinflation, diffuse reticulogranular or "ground-glass" appearance, and air bronchograms.
  - Lateral films may be helpful for determination of air leak.
- Other imaging modalities (CT, ultrasound) are generally unnecessary for the diagnosis and management of RDS but may be indicated if there is suspicion for other pulmonary pathology.

TREATMENT

GENERAL MEASURES

- Diet
  - Sufficient glucose infusion to prevent hypoglycemia
  - Hydration and nutrition for expected increased caloric needs with early initiation of IV nutrition while working to establish enteral nutrition
- Supportive care
  - Radiant warmer or incubator for warmth. Temperature should be maintained between 36.5° and 37.5°C during stabilization and after admission.
  - Blood pressure support with volume expansion and/or pressors to maintain perfusion and normal blood pressure for gestational age

MEDICATION

- Exogenous surfactant
  - Both modified mammalian-derived surfactants and synthetic surfactants have been shown to reduce morbidity and mortality from RDS.
  - Delivery
    - Exogenous surfactant typically has been delivered directly into the trachea through an endotracheal tube.
    - Alternate methods of delivery such as less invasive surfactant administration (LISA), minimally invasive surfactant therapy (MIST), and laryngeal mask airway (LMA) increasingly are being employed.
    - Any modality of delivery should be performed or supervised by providers experienced with that technique.
  - Timing of surfactant
    - Prophylactic: as soon as infant is stabilized, usually <15 minutes of life, based on the risk for RDS without demonstrating that the infant has disease. Early studies demonstrated reduced mortality with prophylactic surfactant administration in infants <26 weeks' gestation, but such studies predated routine use of antenatal corticosteroids and early continuous positive airway pressure (CPAP) use. Prophylactic use is reserved for those infants at extremely high risk for RDS.
    - Early rescue: after the diagnosis of RDS is established; usually after first hour. INSURE (**in**tubate, **sur**factant, **e**xtubate): intubation for surfactant administration followed by immediate extubation to noninvasive support
    - Additional doses are considered for persistently high Fio_2 requirements (Fio_2 >0.3 to 0.4) or for ongoing need for mechanical ventilation. Consultation with a neonatologist is recommended.

ALERT

- Occasionally, the surfactant material may clog the endotracheal tube, causing acute airway obstruction with resultant hypercapnia and hypoxemia, necessitating suctioning or removal and replacement of the endotracheal tube.
- Surfactant therapy can also result in acute improvements in pulmonary compliance. Monitor physical exam, SpO_2, blood gasses, and tidal volumes to avoid inadvertent overventilation.

- Caffeine citrate
  - Used for apnea of prematurity and may be helpful in RDS if it is able to minimize the duration of mechanical ventilation

ADDITIONAL THERAPIES

- CPAP
  - Can be delivered via nasal prongs or mask either using a ventilator, dedicated apparatus, or through "bubble CPAP"
  - CPAP prevents end-expiratory atelectasis and can be started in the delivery room.
- Humidified high-flow nasal cannula (HFNC)
  - May achieve CPAP benefit with easier handling of the patient and less risk of pressure necrosis of nasal septum
  - Pressure delivery variable
- Nasal intermittent positive pressure ventilation (NIPPV)
  - Nonsynchronized nasal respiratory support through a ventilator with prongs. Combines support of CPAP with additional positive pressure "sigh" breaths; delivers higher mean airway pressure than CPAP alone
- Neurally adjusted ventilator assist (NAVA)
  - Synchronized mode of support titrated to diaphragmatic electrical impulse that can be delivered either noninvasively through nasal prongs or invasively via an endotracheal tube

- Mechanical ventilation
  - May be required for infants with significant respiratory acidosis and hypoxemia; can be initiated following intubation for surfactant delivery
  - Tidal volume guarantee or volume-controlled methods of ventilation may have benefit of reducing preterm infant comorbidities such as bronchopulmonary dysplasia (BPD) or intraventricular hemorrhage compared to pressure-controlled ventilation.
  - High-frequency ventilation (oscillatory or jet) may be valuable in very severe cases or with air leak (jet).

ADMISSION, INPATIENT, AND NURSING CONSIDERATIONS

- A naso- or orogastric tube should be placed in infants on noninvasive positive pressure support in order to avoid overdistension of the stomach and intestines.
- Care should be exercised to maintain equipment essential for delivering noninvasive (prongs, mask) or invasive (endotracheal tube) support in place.

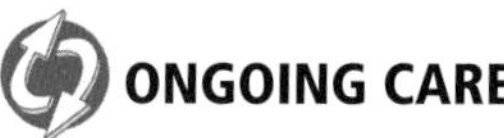

ONGOING CARE

FOLLOW-UP RECOMMENDATIONS

- Very low-birth-weight and extremely low-birth-weight infants should receive follow-up in specialty clinics that can provide for their specialized needs, including neurodevelopmental, pulmonary (for those with BPD), and ophthalmology (for those with retinopathy of prematurity).
- Immunizations are extremely important preventive measures to prevent subsequent respiratory morbidity and mortality. See chapter on "Bronchopulmonary Dysplasia" for recommendations for passive immunization against respiratory syncytial virus with palivizumab (Synagis).

PROGNOSIS

- Natural history: Disease severity worsens over the first 24 to 72 hours, with improvement occurring after 5 to 10 days of age. With antenatal steroids, CPAP, newer modes of mechanical ventilation, and surfactant replacement therapy, more rapid improvement is often seen, and mortality from RDS is rare.
- Outcome is usually related to the degree of prematurity and its related complications.

COMPLICATIONS

- Air leak:
  - Pneumothorax
  - Pneumomediastinum
  - Pulmonary interstitial emphysema
  - Pneumopericardium

ALERT
Emergency treatment of pneumothorax: Acute tension pneumothorax can occur as a complication of RDS and its management and can be life-threatening, even in larger or term infants. Needle aspiration may provide temporary stabilization, and chest tube placement may be necessary.

- Pulmonary hemorrhage:
  - Typically occurs between 1 and 3 days of age with sudden respiratory deterioration
  - Pink or red frothy fluid or bright red blood may be present in the endotracheal tube.
  - Associated with diffuse opacification of the lung fields and marked decrease in pulmonary compliance
- Complications related primarily to prematurity that are often associated with RDS:
  - Patent ductus arteriosus: Pulmonary edema and high-output congestive heart failure may develop as a consequence of left-to-right shunting through the ductus.
  - BPD: a chronic disease of multifactorial etiology involving abnormal lung development and abnormal repair following lung injury due in part to RDS as well as edema, infection, and other factors causing inflammation

ADDITIONAL READING

- Committee on Fetus and Newborn, American Academy of Pediatrics. Respiratory support in preterm infants at birth. *Pediatrics*. 2014;133(1):171–174.
- Finer NN, Carlo WA, Walsh MC, et al; and SUPPORT Study Group of the Eunice Kennedy Shriver National Institute of Child Health and Human Development Neonatal Research Network. Early CPAP versus surfactant in extremely preterm infants. *N Engl J Med*. 2010;362(21):1970–1979.
- Gyamfi-Bannerman C, Thom EA, Blackwell SC, et al. Antenatal betamethasone for women at risk for late preterm delivery. *N Engl J Med*. 2016;374(14):1311–1320.
- Jobe AH. What is RDS in 2012? *Early Hum Dev*. 2012;88(Suppl 2):S42–S44.
- Morley CJ, Davis PG, Doyle LW, et al. Nasal CPAP or intubation at birth for very preterm infants. *N Engl J Med*. 2008;358(7):700–708.
- Polin RA, Carlo WA; and Committee on Fetus and Newborn, American Academy of Pediatrics. Surfactant replacement therapy for preterm and term neonates with respiratory distress. *Pediatrics*. 2014;133(1):156–163.
- Sardesai S, Biniwale M, Wertheimer F, et al. Evolution of surfactant therapy for respiratory distress syndrome: past, present, and future. *Pediatr Res*. 2017;81(1–2):240–248.
- Sweet DG, Carnielli V, Greisen G, et al. European consensus guidelines on the management of respiratory distress syndrome—2016 update. *Neonatology*. 2017;111(2):107–125.

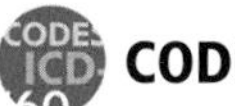

CODES

ICD10

P22.0 Respiratory distress syndrome of newborn

FAQ

- Q: Should all babies with a diagnosis of RDS be started on antibiotics?
- A: It is important to consider sepsis/pneumonia in all infants with a diagnosis of RDS, particularly infection with group B *Streptococcus* (GBS). Risk factors to be considered include maternal GBS colonization, evidence of chorioamnionitis, intrapartum antibiotic use, and route of delivery. Antibiotics may sometimes be held if the risk factors for sepsis are low compared to those for RDS, such as in a baby delivered electively by cesarean section for maternal indications. However, as congenital pneumonia can radiographically appear identical to RDS, it is often common practice to screen for sepsis in all infants with RDS by performing blood cultures and looking for other laboratory evidence of infection including complete blood counts with differentials and acute-phase reactants such as C-reactive protein and start empiric antibiotic therapy with ampicillin or penicillin in combination with an aminoglycoside. Duration of antibiotics is typically 48 hours depending on results of blood cultures as well as the clinical picture and other laboratory data. Therapy may be narrowed if a specific organism is identified.
- Q: What is the most worrisome acute complication of RDS?
- A: Acute air leak (primarily tension pneumothorax) can be life-threatening, even in near-term or full-term infants with RDS, and such infants should be cared for in centers that are prepared to properly handle this emergent situation in a timely fashion (i.e., availability of a provider who can perform an emergent needle aspiration and chest tube placement). In smaller infants, pulmonary hemorrhage can also be life-threatening.
- Q: Because the risk of a baby developing RDS for a baby born at 26 weeks' gestation is high, should such babies automatically receive prophylactic surfactant?
- A: Not necessarily. Early prospective, randomized, placebo-controlled studies demonstrated reduced mortality from RDS with prophylactic surfactant in preterm infants ≤26 weeks' gestation. However, those studies were conducted in an era before widespread use of antenatal steroids and early use of CPAP. Recent prospective, randomized trials of different approaches to extremely low-birth-weight infants in the delivery suite have demonstrated that such infants treated with early and continued CPAP alone may have outcomes comparable to those immediately intubated and treated with surfactant replacement therapy.
- Q: Where should oxygen saturations be maintained for preterm infants being treated for RDS?
- A: The SUPPORT, BOOST, and COT trials were designed to assess effects of targeting oxygen saturations in a lower range (85–89%) compared to a higher range (91–95%). These trials have generated significant controversy regarding targeted oxygen saturations for preterm infants as they reported an association with morbidity and mortality in the lower target range. Rates or retinopathy of prematurity were similar between the two saturation ranges. While there is still significant uncertainty regarding ideal oxygen saturation range, it seems reasonable to target saturations between 90% and 94%.
- Q: As some surfactant preparations are prepared from cow lungs, is there an increased risk that babies receiving such surfactants will develop a protein allergy?
- A: It is very unlikely that surfactant treatment with preparations derived from animal lungs increases the risk of immune responses. The two proteins in replacement surfactants are present in low amounts and are extremely hydrophobic and unlikely to generate an immune response given the limited number of surfactant doses (usually maximum of four) administered.
- Q: You are seeing siblings in your practice for well-child visits whose mother is pregnant and at 34 weeks of gestation. Her previous child was born at 35 weeks of gestation due to preeclampsia and had RDS and spent 2 weeks in the NICU. Her obstetrician plans to deliver this child by repeat cesarean section at 36 weeks because of additional prior maternal uterine surgery and mentioned that she plans on giving her antenatal steroids starting 48 hours before the planned delivery. Is this plan reasonable?
- A: Assuming that the delivery does need to occur at 36 weeks for maternal indications, antenatal steroids are indicated, as their administration has been shown to reduce the likelihood of the child having respiratory disease and needing admission to the NICU. The family history of a late preterm child who had RDS also reinforces this course of action.

R

RESPIRATORY SYNCYTIAL VIRUS (SEE ALSO: BRONCHIOLITIS)

Marie E. Wang, MD, MPH • Alan R. Schroeder, MD

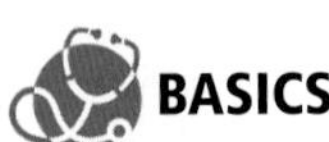

BASICS

DESCRIPTION

- An enveloped, nonsegmented RNA virus of the family Paramyxoviridae and in the subfamily Pneumovirinae along with human metapneumovirus. There are two subgroups, A and B, differentiated by the major attachment G protein, a large surface glycoprotein. The fusion or F protein is relatively homologous between the two subgroups.
- It is the most common cause of bronchiolitis, a lower respiratory tract disease that primarily affects the small airways.

EPIDEMIOLOGY

- Incubation period is 2 to 8 days.
- Virus is detected in secretions 4 days prior to clinical symptoms. Typically shedding of infectious virions is 3 to 8 days but can be as long as 3 to 4 weeks in immunocompromised.
- Transmission occurs by direct contact of nasopharyngeal or ocular mucosa with infected secretions or fomites.
- Nosocomial spread can occur because the virus can survive on surfaces for several hours and hands for 30 minutes or more.
- In the United States, epidemics typically occur between November and April and last for roughly 18 to 20 weeks.
- In tropical climates, respiratory syncytial virus (RSV) seasons are less predictable and can circulate year-round.
- One antigenic strain predominates during any given epidemic, but both subtypes can circulate concurrently.

Incidence

- Peak incidence is the first 2 years of life, and 20–30% of infected infants develop lower respiratory tract disease.
- Annual rate of RSV-associated hospitalization is roughly 3/1,000 in children <5 years of age and 17/1,000 in children <6 months of age.

Prevalence

- 50% of children are infected by their first birthday. 100% of children are infected by age of 2 years.
- Reinfection can occur during the same RSV season and is common during the first few years of life.
- Subsequent infections are typically milder.

RISK FACTORS

Those at greatest risk for severe infection include:

- Children <1 year of age, especially those <6 months of age
- Children born prematurely (<35 weeks' gestation)
- Children with underlying cardiopulmonary disease (e.g., chronic lung disease of prematurity, congenital heart disease)
- Those with primary immune deficits
- Patients on immunosuppressive medications (e.g., transplant patients, oncology patients)

GENERAL PREVENTION

- There is currently no RSV vaccine. A formalin-inactivated RSV vaccine tested in the 1960s caused enhanced illness after reexposure to wild-type RSV likely due to an overexuberant immune response.
- Because RSV can survive on surfaces, strict hand washing can minimize nosocomial spread.
- Contact isolation with routine usage of gowns and gloves has been shown to decrease RSV nosocomial spread.
- Patients with RSV infection should be isolated in private rooms or cohorted.
- Palivizumab, a humanized monoclonal antibody directed against the highly conserved F protein of RSV, is the only product available for the prevention of RSV infection in certain high-risk children.
  - Children who should receive palivizumab:
    - Infants born before 29 weeks' gestation
    - Preterm infants with chronic lung disease of prematurity. In these children, palivizumab should also be given during the 2nd year of life if they are receiving medical therapy (e.g., oxygen, chronic corticosteroids, or diuretics) for chronic lung disease.
  - Children for whom palivizumab should be considered:
    - Infants with hemodynamically significant congenital heart disease, anatomic pulmonary abnormalities, or neuromuscular disease
    - Children <24 months who will be profoundly immunocompromised during RSV season
  - Palivizumab is given IM (15 mg/kg) every 30 days for a maximum of 5 doses during RSV season (usually from October/November to March/April).
  - Palivizumab prophylaxis should be discontinued if a patient experiences a breakthrough RSV hospitalization due to the low likelihood of another RSV hospitalization in the same season.
  - Specific recommendations (last updated in 2014) are available from the American Academy of Pediatrics (AAP).

PATHOPHYSIOLOGY

- The G protein is the major surface glycoprotein responsible for attachment of virus to cells.
- The F protein aids in viral entry in to cells and is responsible for fusion of adjacent cells to form a syncytia.
- Infection is initiated in nasopharynx and then can move to the lower respiratory tract.
- Infection of smaller airways leads to edema and necrosis of epithelial cells and infiltration of inflammatory cells, resulting in airway obstruction and air trapping.
- Severe RSV infection has been associated with recurrent wheezing later in life. It is unclear whether RSV infection causes subsequent wheezing or if patients predisposed to severe wheezing are more likely to have severe RSV disease.

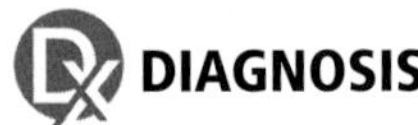

DIAGNOSIS

HISTORY

- Initial symptoms include copious nasal discharge, cough, and fever.
- Cough is the most common symptom typically progressing over 1 to 2 days.
- Concerning findings on history:
  - Apnea, severe coughing with possible cyanotic episodes
  - Poor oral intake
  - Decreased urine output (e.g., fewer wet diapers)
  - Trouble breathing

PHYSICAL EXAM

- Profuse rhinorrhea
- Acute otitis media or otitis media with effusion
- Signs of dehydration (dry mucus membranes, delayed capillary refill time)
- Conjunctivitis
- Varying levels of respiratory distress:
  - Mild: suprasternal retractions, mild tachypnea
  - Moderate: subcostal or intracostal retractions
  - Severe: severe retractions, grunting, RR >60, lethargy
- Air trapping resulting in hyperexpansion of lungs can lead to a barrel-shaped chest, palpable liver, or spleen below the costal margin.
- Pulse oximetry may reveal hypoxemia.

DIFFERENTIAL DIAGNOSIS

- Infection
  - Influenza virus
  - Parainfluenza virus
  - Human metapneumovirus
  - Adenovirus
  - Coronaviruses
  - Human bocavirus
  - Rhinovirus
  - *Mycoplasma pneumoniae*
- Environmental: foreign body in upper airway
- Tumors: mass compressing upper airway
- Congenital: laryngomalacia or tracheomalacia

DIAGNOSTIC TESTS & INTERPRETATION

- Routine viral testing is not recommended for outpatients or inpatients with suspected bronchiolitis.
- Viral testing is recommended in patients receiving palivizumab prophylaxis and may also be useful in high-risk patients and patients with an atypical presentation. Rapid diagnostic antigen assays from nasopharyngeal specimens (e.g., enzyme immunoassay, immunofluorescent assay) can be used for RSV detection, usually with a sensitivity of 80–90%.
- Reverse transcriptase-polymerase chain reaction (RT-PCR) assays are commercially available and have superior sensitivity to rapid antigen testing. However, these assays detect viral RNA that may persist in nasal secretions after patient is no longer shedding infectious virus.
- A definitive diagnosis of RSV can be made by viral culture but requires up to 5 days.

- Because concurrent serious bacterial infections are not common, routine complete blood counts or blood cultures are not indicated.
- Given that published estimates of concurrent urinary tract infections (UTIs) range from 1% to 7%, urinalysis and urine culture can be considered for infants with persistent fever.
- Chest radiographs should not be routinely obtained in children with RSV.
- When obtained, often reveal hyperinflation, increased bronchial markings, and areas of atelectasis/infiltrates, findings which may not alter the treatment plan or may, in some cases, lead to unnecessary antibiotics

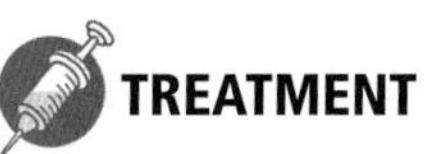

TREATMENT

GENERAL MEASURES

- Supportive care: hydration therapy and supplemental oxygen as needed if oxygen saturation persistently falls <90%
- Cardiorespiratory monitoring and pulse oximetry should be used for infants at risk for apnea and hypoxemia.
- In severe cases, respiratory support with continuous positive airway pressure (CPAP) or mechanical ventilation is required.

MEDICATION

- β-Adrenergic agents: Bronchodilators should not be used routinely. However, there are some data to suggest that they may lead to transient improvement in respiratory scores in some patients, but no data that suggests that this impacts hospitalization rates or length of stay. β-agonists increase heart rate and overall metabolic demand.
- Neither β- or α-adrenergic agonists are recommended by the AAP for routine use.
- Recent studies of nebulized hypertonic saline (HTS) did not demonstrate improvement in length of stay, respiratory score, or readmission rate compared to nebulized normal saline.
- Corticosteroids are not useful in bronchiolitis and should not be used.
- Ribavirin: has in vitro antiviral activity against RSV; however, studies evaluating the effectiveness of inhaled ribavirin have shown mixed results. Ribavirin is not recommended for routine use in bronchiolitis treatment due to conflicting results of efficacy studies, its high cost, and potentially toxic effects in exposed health care workers. Ribavirin may be considered in immunocompromised patients with severe RSV disease.
- Antibiotics are not indicated unless there is a strong evidence of a concurrent bacterial infection (e.g., UTI, bacterial pneumonia).

ADMISSION, INPATIENT, AND NURSING CONSIDERATIONS

Apnea or severe respiratory distress with impending respiratory failure may require intubation and mechanical ventilation.

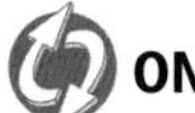

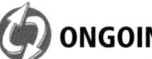

ONGOING CARE

FOLLOW-UP RECOMMENDATIONS

- Lower respiratory tract symptoms usually arise 2 to 3 days after initial symptoms.
- Symptoms usually peak from 5 to 7 days, but 20% of children can have symptoms for 3 weeks.
- Recurrent apneic episodes are rare, and home monitoring is usually not indicated.
- Fever commonly resolves over 2 to 3 days.

Patient Monitoring

Signs to watch for:

- Increased respiratory rate and increased work of breathing
- Lethargy, altered mental status
- Signs and symptoms of dehydration (dry mucous membranes, decreased urine output)

PROGNOSIS

- Most children have a mild to moderate disease course requiring only supportive care.
- Approximately 1–3% of children will require hospitalization. Most children recover with no sequelae.
- Infants born prematurely or with underlying cardiopulmonary disease are at increased risk for more severe and longer duration of disease.
- Reinfections occur throughout life with an incidence of about 5% per year.
- There are some data to suggest that patients with severe RSV bronchiolitis may have more episodes of recurrent wheezing in the 1st year of life. It is unclear whether severe RSV infection causes long-term airway hyperresponsiveness.

COMPLICATIONS

- Dehydration
- Apneic episodes in young infants (can occur in all causes of bronchiolitis, not just RSV)
- Hypoxemia
- Hypercarbia
- Respiratory failure
- Pneumonia, rarely bacterial
- Croup
- Acute otitis media
- Asthma

ADDITIONAL READING

- American Academy of Pediatrics. Respiratory syncytial virus. In: Kimberlin DW, Brady MT, Jackson MA, et al, eds. *Red Book: 2015 Report of the Committee on Infectious Diseases*. 30th ed. Elk Grove Village, IL: American Academy of Pediatrics; 2015:667–676.
- American Academy of Pediatrics Committee on Infectious Diseases, American Academy of Pediatrics Bronchiolitis Guidelines Committee. Updated guidance for palivizumab prophylaxis among infants and young children at increased risk of hospitalization for respiratory syncytial virus infection. *Pediatrics*. 2014;134(2):e620–e638.
- Brooks CG, Harrison WN, Ralston SL. Association between hypertonic saline and hospital length of stay in acute viral bronchiolitis: a reanalysis of 2 meta-analyses. *JAMA Pediatr*. 2016;170(6):577–584.
- Hall CB, Weinberg GA, Iwane MK, et al. The burden of respiratory syncytial virus infection in young children. *N Engl J Med*. 2009;360(6):588–598.
- Ralston SL, Lieberthal AS, Meissner HC, et al. Clinical practice guideline: the diagnosis, management, and prevention of bronchiolitis. *Pediatrics*. 2014;134(5):e1474–e1502. *Pediatrics*. 2015;136(4):782.
- Please also see references from Bronchiolitis chapter.

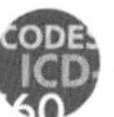

CODES

ICD10

- B97.4 Respiratory syncytial virus causing diseases classd elswhr
- J21.0 Acute bronchiolitis due to respiratory syncytial virus
- J20.5 Acute bronchitis due to respiratory syncytial virus

FAQ

- Q: How did my child get this illness?
- A: RSV bronchiolitis is caused by RSV, an extremely common virus which is passed from one person to another by contact with nasal secretions and through airborne transmission of droplets.
- Q: For how long is my child contagious?
- A: Viral shedding occurs for 24 hours prior to the onset of clinical symptoms and for up to 21 days from the onset of symptoms.
- Q: Will my child develop asthma because of the wheezing that is occurring now?
- A: There is an association between severe RSV bronchiolitis and recurrent wheezing episodes during the 1st year of life. However, it is not clear whether RSV causes asthma later in life.
- Q: How do I prevent my child from being infected with RSV?
- A: Unfortunately, there is no vaccine against RSV. In high-risk infants (infants born prematurely with chronic lung disease, congenital heart disease), palivizumab can be administered during RSV season to prevent severe lower respiratory tract disease.

RETINOBLASTOMA

Sheila Thampi, MD • Bertil Damato, MD, PhD, FRCOphth

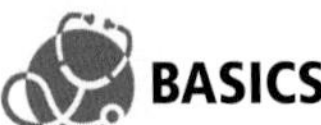

BASICS

DESCRIPTION
Retinoblastoma is a malignant tumor of the retina and is the most common intraocular tumor in children. It is caused by an *RB1* gene mutation at 13q14, which can be germline or somatic.

EPIDEMIOLOGY
- In the United States, retinoblastoma occurs approximately once in every 18,000 live births.
- Approximately 300 new pediatric cases of retinoblastoma are diagnosed each year in the United States, which represents 3% of all childhood cancers.
- 25% of patients will present with bilateral disease at diagnosis, which signifies germline retinoblastoma. 40% of all retinoblastoma cases are germline, which most often presents with not only bilateral disease but also unilateral disease in 15%.
- Median age at diagnosis is 24 months in patients with unilateral disease and 12 months in patients with bilateral tumors.
- There is no association with race, gender, or laterality of eye involvement.
- The greatest disease burden is found in countries with the largest populations and high birth rates, such as Asia and Africa.

RISK FACTORS
- *RB1* gene mutations are inherited in an autosomal dominant pattern.
- Family history of retinoblastoma in parents or siblings warrants early screening and genetic studies to determine the risk of disease.

GENERAL PREVENTION
Although there is no definite way to prevent retinoblastoma, careful eye exams during well-child examinations will allow earlier detection of the disease.

PATHOPHYSIOLOGY
- Tumor development requires loss of function of the *RB1* gene, which is a cell cycle regulator and resides in chromosome 13.
- Constitutional loss of one *RB1* allele predisposes a patient to cancer. Loss of the second allele with other genetic or epigenetic changes in the retinal lesion will initiate formation of retinoblastoma.
- Somatic retinoblastoma has no germline *RB1* mutation and thus requires biallelic inactivation of the *RB1* gene in a single retinal cell.
- Other genetic changes have been described in tumor cells such as *MYCN* oncogene amplification.
- There are three common growth patterns:
  - Intraretinal (growth only in the retina)
  - Endophytic (inner surface of retina to vitreous)
  - Exophytic (outer surface of retina to subretinal space)
  - Tumor cells seeding from the primary mass to grow independently in the vitreous or subretinal space.
- Children with loss of *RB1* with large chromosomal deletions of surrounding genes are at risk for developmental anomalies such as facial dysmorphism and mental and/or motor impairment (13q deletion syndrome).
- Patients with bilateral retinoblastoma are at risk for involvement of the pineal gland, termed "trilateral" retinoblastoma.

ETIOLOGY
Mutations in the *RB1* gene predispose to retinoblastoma, pinealoblastoma, osteosarcoma, and other cancers.

DIAGNOSIS

HISTORY
Parents often report noticing a white color in the pupil, eye(s) turning inward or outward, and poor vision.

PHYSICAL EXAM
- Most common presenting signs include the following:
  - Leukocoria
  - Strabismus
  - Poor vision (poor tracking)
- Proptosis is worrisome for more advanced disease.
- Bone pain should be evaluated for metastatic disease.

DIFFERENTIAL DIAGNOSIS
- Coats disease
- Persistent fetal vasculature
- Vitreous hemorrhage
- Congenital cataract
- Coloboma
- Toxocariasis
- Astrocytic hamartoma
- Retinopathy of prematurity
- Other rare diseases
  - Medulloepithelioma
  - Norrie disease
  - Incontinentia pigmenti
  - Autosomal dominant familial exudative vitreoretinopathy (adFEVR)

DIAGNOSTIC TESTS & INTERPRETATION

Initial Tests (screening, lab, imaging)
- CBC to look for leukopenia, anemia, or thrombocytopenia
  - CBC should be evaluated to determine bone marrow involvement.
  - If cytopenias are noted, then evaluation of the bone marrow is indicated.
- Extraocular spread noted on imaging warrants evaluation of the cerebrospinal fluid.
- Chromosome analysis should be performed, particularly in patients with bilateral eye involvement or developmental delay.
- Brain and orbit MRI
  - Can aid in distinguishing between retinoblastoma and Coats disease and will assess for "trilateral" disease (involvement of the pineal gland) and invasion of the optic nerve
  - CT scan can provide information regarding tumor calcification but due to radiation is used less frequently.
- Ophthalmic ultrasonography to demonstrate retinal masses and calcifications
- Nuclear medicine scan (bone or positron emission tomography [PET] scan)
  - May show primary tumor uptake and screen for bone metastasis
  - Should be performed if concern for metastasis is noted

Follow-Up Tests & Special Considerations
- Children with a suspected retinoblastoma should be immediately referred to a children's hospital with expertise in these tumors.
- Multidisciplinary teams include pediatric oncologists, ocular oncologists, radiation oncologists, nurses, pharmacists, and social workers.

Diagnostic Procedures/Other
- Biopsy is not performed due to risk for dissemination.
- The diagnosis of retinoblastoma is based on ophthalmologic exam.
- An experienced pediatric ocular oncologist should perform the exam under anesthesia (EUA).
- Early involvement of pediatric oncology should be initiated.

Test Interpretation
- EUA consists of a detailed eye exam involving use of ultrasound, photographs, and drawings to document the retinoblastoma location and extent.
- Based on the EUA results, the ocular oncologist will determine the classification and assign a group.
- Initial classification of tumor extent is imperative for assessment of prognosis and outcomes.

- International Intraocular Retinoblastoma Classification (IIRC), also known as the ABC classification system, is predictive of treatment success following systemic chemotherapy and focal laser treatment. However, the older Reese-Ellsworth classification system is still commonly used and was designed to predict outcomes of external beam radiation.
  - IIRC groups eyes from less advanced disease, labeled group A, to most advanced disease, labeled group E.
  - IIRC predicts high-risk retinoblastoma seen in group D or E eyes.
- If a patient undergoes enucleation high-risk features on histology include tumor invasion of the optic nerve and massive choroidal invasion. High-risk features will lead to metastases in about 24% of patients if not treated with systemic chemotherapy as compared to 4% of those treated with systemic chemotherapy.

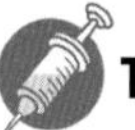

TREATMENT

MEDICATION

- Systemic chemotherapy allows preservation of the globe and prevention of systemic metastasis.
- Systemic chemotherapy is combined with local retinal therapy to enhance local tumor control.
- It has been suggested that systemic chemotherapy may prevent development of trilateral retinoblastoma.
- Most common chemotherapeutic agents used for retinoblastoma include carboplatin, etoposide, and vincristine (CEV).
- Intra-arterial chemotherapy (IAC) is a newer modality for treatment of retinoblastoma and provides direct retinal chemotherapy via the ophthalmic artery. Agents given in this fashion include melphalan, topotecan, and/or carboplatin.
- Less commonly used approaches to deliver chemotherapy include periocular or intravitreal injections.

ISSUES FOR REFERRAL

All children with retinoblastoma should be referred to a pediatric cancer geneticist to rule out germline or mosaic *RB1* mutations.

ADDITIONAL THERAPIES

- Retinoblastoma is a radiosensitive tumor.
- Radiation therapy can be provided by external beam therapy, plaque therapy (brachytherapy), or proton beam therapy and is a useful method to preserve vision.
- Use of radiation is generally avoided due to risk of secondary malignancies, particularly in children with hereditary retinoblastoma.
- Occupational therapy or speech therapy can help children cope with loss of vision or hearing changes that develop due to side effects of chemotherapy.

SURGERY/OTHER PROCEDURES

- Local retinal therapy with cryotherapy or laser photocoagulation is an important modality of treatment.
- Enucleation, removal of the eye, provides definitive treatment for retinoblastoma. Advanced eye conditions (group E) are usually managed with enucleation to prevent metastatic spread.

ADMISSION, INPATIENT, AND NURSING CONSIDERATIONS

As a side effect of chemotherapy, patients can develop fever and neutropenia and require inpatient hospitalization for antibiotics.

ONGOING CARE

FOLLOW-UP RECOMMENDATIONS

Patient Monitoring

- Patients should be followed regularly by an ocular oncologist for EUAs to monitor for reoccurrence and for adjustment for the orbital implant if enucleation occurred.
- Patients should be followed by a pediatric oncologist with serial MRI of the brain and orbit and additional imaging based on sites of disease at presentation.
- Patients should be monitored for long-term side effects/complications of therapy, ideally within the context of a survivorship clinic.

PATIENT EDUCATION

- During therapy and if a central line is in place, patients are counseled to call for all fevers as this symptom requires an examination, laboratory evaluation with a CBC and blood culture, and systemic antibiotics administered through the central line.
- If enucleation occurs, patients will be educated on how to protect the remaining eye.
- Survivors will be counseled on lifestyle modifications to decrease their risk of a second cancer (i.e., avoid unnecessary radiation and carcinogens such as smoking).

PROGNOSIS

- 5-year overall survival in the United States is excellent at >95%.
- All forms of metastatic spread: Leptomeningeal disease, trilateral or pineal involvement, and distant metastases require aggressive therapy and result in poor overall survival.

COMPLICATIONS

- Surgical
  - Surgical site wound infections after enucleation
  - Complications associated with orbital implants (infection, bleeding, conjunctival erosion, wound dehiscence, implant extrusion)
- Acute systemic chemotherapy toxicity
  - Myelosuppression
  - Ototoxicity
  - Infections
  - Renal dysfunction
  - Peripheral neuropathy
- Radiation
  - Skin erythema
  - Risk of cataract development
  - Vascular endothelium damage
  - Vitreous hemorrhage
  - Facial and temporal bone hypoplasia
  - Secondary malignancy
- IAC toxicity
  - Myelosuppression
  - Redness or swelling of the eyelid
  - Vitreous hemorrhage
  - Choroidal atrophy
  - Rare risk of stroke or blindness
- Late effects
  - Hearing loss and nephrotoxicity from carboplatin
  - Secondary malignancy from radiation or chemotherapy (i.e., etoposide)

ADDITIONAL READING

- Abramson DH, Schefler AC. Update on retinoblastoma. *Retina*. 2004;24(6):828–848.
- Dimaras H, Corson TW, Cobrinik D, et al. Retinoblastoma. *Nat Rev Dis Primers*. 2015;1:15021.
- Dimaras H, Kimani K, O Dimba EA, et al. Retinoblastoma. *Lancet*. 2012;379(9824):1436–1446.
- Shields CL, Fulco EM, Arias JD, et al. Retinoblastoma frontiers with intravenous, intra-arterial, periocular, and intravitreal chemotherapy. *Eye (Lond)*. 2013;27(2):253–264.

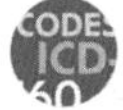

CODES

ICD10

- C69.20 Malignant neoplasm of unspecified retina
- C69.21 Malignant neoplasm of right retina
- C69.22 Malignant neoplasm of left retina

FAQ

- Q: Are children with retinoblastoma at risk for developmental delays?
- A: Children who carry *RB1* gene mutations should be followed closely for developmental delays with speech and/or motor skills. Children with deletions in chromosome 13 have been described to have an array of developmental delays in association with retinoblastoma.
- Q: Do siblings of children with retinoblastoma need to be evaluated?
- A: Given the high possibility of hereditary *RB1* mutations, children of siblings or parents with retinoblastoma should be evaluated at an early age and followed by an ophthalmologist.
- Q: Do I need to worry about other cancers in my child who has retinoblastoma?
- A: Children with the hereditary form of retinoblastoma (*RB1* gene mutation, bilateral disease, or family history) are at increased risk for other cancers such as osteosarcoma. If they have received radiation therapy, their risk of second cancers is significantly increased.
- Q: Is my child with retinoblastoma blind?
- A: The size and location of the tumor(s) will determine your child's vision. Advanced retinoblastoma (group D or E) is more likely to have total retinal involvement and poor vision.

RETINOPATHY OF PREMATURITY

Michael X. Repka, MD, MBA

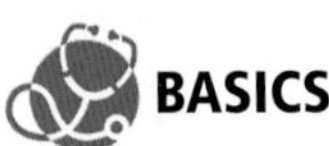

BASICS

DESCRIPTION

Retinopathy of prematurity (ROP) is an abnormal pattern of retinal vascularization of preterm infants leading in some cases to permanent visual loss and blindness as well as many other eye problems.

EPIDEMIOLOGY

- ROP is the leading cause of blindness among children in the developed world:
  - 0.2% of all infants born in the United States
  - 20% of infants born <1,500 g
- 1,300 develop severe disease requiring treatment annually in the United States.
- Birth weight and ROP (frequency of ROP stage 1 or greater)
  - <750 g: 90%
  - 750 to <1,000 g: 78%
  - 1,000 to 1,250 g: 47%
  - >1,250 g: <1%
- Gestational age and ROP (frequency of any ROP stage 1 or greater with BW <1,251 g)
  - ≤27 weeks: 83%
  - 27 to 31 weeks: 55%
  - ≥31 weeks: 29%

RISK FACTORS

- Gestational age
- Hyperoxia
- Hypoxia
- Acidosis
- Hypercarbia
- Apnea
- Bradycardia
- Nutritional deficiencies
- Ambient light
- Intraventricular hemorrhage
- Lower birth weight
- Lower gestational age
- Multiple gestation
- Born at another facility and transferred

PATHOPHYSIOLOGY

- Normal retinal vascularization begins at the optic disc at about 16 weeks postmenstrual age and is typically completed at about term.
- Preterm delivery exposes the actively growing vessels to unusual conditions. These alter production of vascular endothelial growth factors (VEGFs). In some cases, the vascular growth stops and then resumes normally, whereas in other cases, the retinal blood vessels grow abnormally off the surface of the retina.
- The timing for development of acute ROP is related to postmenstrual age and not chronologic age or birth weight. It is rare to see any acute ROP prior to 32 weeks' postmenstrual age.
- Although the incidence of ROP increases with decreasing birth weight, fewer than 10% of babies smaller than 1,250 g birth weight will have ROP sufficiently severe to require treatment.

DIAGNOSIS

HISTORY

- All infants with birth weight <1,500 g or gestational age <30 weeks are at risk.
- Other children with significant oxygen exposure are also referred for retinal evaluations.
- Each nursery needs a protocol to identify and document the infants needing examinations, both initial and follow-up. Reasons for exam deferral should be included in the medical record.

ALERT

A common error in ROP management is failure to perform exams on the required schedule. The most vulnerable time for this lapse is during a transition to another unit or another facility or after discharge to home.

PHYSICAL EXAM

- Requires a retinal examination with pupillary dilation using binocular indirect ophthalmoscopy with a sterile eyelid speculum and scleral depression
  - Topical anesthesia may be used (proparacaine 0.5%).
  - Pupillary dilation is obtained using 1% phenylephrine/0.2% cyclopentolate solution (Cyclomydril®) administered as a single drop to each eye, repeated in 5 to 10 minutes.
    - Administer at least 30 minutes and preferably 1 hour prior to the exam.
    - The dilating eye drops are associated with delay in gastric emptying.
    - Careful monitoring is needed following the drop administration and the eye examination.
    - Bradycardia and emesis are common following mydriatic eye drop administration and eye examination.
- The results of the examination should be recorded in a manner defined by the International Classification of ROP. A retinal drawing is suggested:
  - Zone I: posterior circular area of the retina centered on the optic disc with a radius twice the distance from disc to fovea
  - Zone II: peripheral ring of retina extending from zone I to anterior edge of the nasal retina and estimated temporally
  - Zone III: temporal retina beyond zone II
- Diagnostic retinal examinations and/or imaging should commence unless the infant is too unstable.
  - At 31 weeks for those infants born at 26 weeks postmenstrual age or earlier
  - By 4 weeks postnatal age for infants >26 to 30 weeks postmenstrual age
- Examinations may be requested by neonatology for infants outside the consensus birth weight and postmenstrual age criteria.
- Subsequent examinations are determined by the ophthalmologist.
  - Exams are typically ordered every 2 weeks.
  - When there is prethreshold disease, weekly or even more frequent exams are conducted.
  - When there is zone III disease, the exam interval may be lengthened.
  - Exams continue until retinal vascularization into zone III is recorded.
  - If VEGF inhibitors have been used for treatment of ROP, exams need to be performed substantially past term. Recurrence has been seen as late as 65 to 70 weeks postmenstrual age.
- ROP is typically symmetric, with similar exams in both eyes seen in 85% of infants.
- Eye examinations performed in the office setting may require monitoring depending on the infant's medical status.

DIFFERENTIAL DIAGNOSIS

- Norrie disease
- Incontinentia pigmenti
- Familial exudative vitreoretinopathy
- Trauma
- Stickler syndrome
- Cyanotic congenital heart disease (in rare cases)
- Idiopathic

DIAGNOSTIC TESTS & INTERPRETATION

Initial Tests (screening, lab, imaging)

- Wide-field digital camera with images of posterior pole, as well as superior, inferior, nasal, and temporal retinas, allows documentation and review of the findings as well as remote consultation.
- The images are reviewed using store-forward technology for evidence of referral-warranted ROP, at which time indirect ophthalmoscopy must be performed to determine if the patient has reached the treatment threshold or be monitored.
- Some facilities are using telemedicine as a substitute, rather than a supplement, for a clinical exam.
  - Skilled nursery personnel are needed to handle the camera and obtain useful images.
  - Plan for rapid image review and urgent treatment referral (when needed) needs to be established in advance.

Diagnostic Procedures/Other

Ophthalmic ultrasonography

- If difficult to obtain adequate indirect ophthalmoscopy
- B-mode ultrasound of the eye can be useful to determine progression of ROP to retinal detachment and to monitor the detachment.

TREATMENT

MEDICATION

- Oxygen restriction: Restriction of oxygen to 85–89% saturation (measured by pulse oximetry) was associated with a reduction in the risk of severe ROP but was associated with an increased mortality rate.
- Oxygen supplementation: In the Stop-ROP trial, supplemental oxygen for infants with prethreshold disease appeared to reduce the rate of progression but was associated with increased risk for pulmonary disease.

SURGERY/OTHER PROCEDURES

- Each nursery needs a policy in place for where and how treatment is to be performed.
  - Treatment should be performed within 48 hours if at all possible, although 72 hours is acceptable.
- Treatment is recommended when a particular stage of disease called type 1 occurs. Type 1 is ROP in zone I or II with PLUS characteristics (dilation and tortuosity of retinal arteries and veins), any stage in zone I, and stage 2 or 3 in zone II. Ideally, the treatment is completed within 48 hours, depending on the stability of the infant.
- Standard care treatment of ROP is ablation (destruction) of the peripheral nonvascularized retina using a laser incorporated into a binocular indirect ophthalmoscope.
  - Requires airway management, topical eye drop anesthesia, and either sedation or general anesthesia
  - 25% have unfavorable visual outcomes at 6 years.
  - 9% have unfavorable structural outcomes at 6 years.
  - 83% of treatments performed in infants born at <27 weeks' gestation
- VEGF inhibitors (e.g., bevacizumab)
  - Intravitreal injection of a small dose of one of these drugs is being offered.
  - In a clinical trial, a single dose of bevacizumab was more effective than laser ablation for zone I disease, with similar outcomes for zone II.
  - Reinjections are often necessary. The optimum dose has not been established.
- Cryotherapy of the peripheral retina that has not been vascularized (anterior) has been shown to be effective compared to observation.
  - Used less frequently today because of pain, tissue damage, and difficulty treating more posterior disease
  - Improves the chance of favorable structural outcomes at age 15 years from 48% to 70%
- Vitreoretinal surgery including vitrectomy is performed after retinal ablation or intravitreal injection has failed and the infant has progressed to stage 4 or 5 ROP (retinal detachment).
  - Rarely associated with visual outcome of 20/200 or better (16%)
  - Retinal reattachment occurs in about 30%.

ADMISSION, INPATIENT, AND NURSING CONSIDERATIONS

- Periods of apnea are common after the ROP examination. Discharge on the same day should be carefully evaluated.
- Transfer of a patient with ROP to a different medical unit or team in the hospital is a common cause for missing follow-up examinations, which can be associated with a poor outcome.

ONGOING CARE

FOLLOW-UP RECOMMENDATIONS

- Infants with treated ROP and more severe stages of ROP without treatment typically require lifelong ophthalmologic monitoring.
  - Substantially increased risk for the development of multiple eye conditions
    - Retinal detachment
    - Strabismus
    - Amblyopia
    - Myopia
    - Glaucoma
    - Optic nerve atrophy
    - Cerebral visual impairment
- Infants with prethreshold ROP have moderately increased risk of the ophthalmic conditions mentioned above; referral managed with typical practice
- A history of treatment for ROP is correlated with a high risk of disability on motor, communication–social, self-care, and continence scales on the Functional Independence Measure for Children (Wee-FIM).

PROGNOSIS

If ROP treatment by retinal ablation was required, visual outcomes reported at 15 years are estimated to be:

- 25% with 20/20 to 20/40
- 50% with 20/20 to 20/200
- 33% with <20/200

ADDITIONAL READING

- Carlo WA, Finer NN, Walsh MC, et al; and SUPPORT Study Group of the Eunice Kennedy Shriver National Institute of Child Health and Human Development Neonatal Research Network. Target ranges of oxygen saturation in extremely preterm infants. *N Engl J Med*. 2010;362(21):1959–1969.
- Fierson WM; and American Academy of Pediatrics Section on Ophthalmology, American Academy of Ophthalmology, American Association for Pediatric Ophthalmology and Strabismus, et al. Screening examination of premature infants for retinopathy of prematurity. *Pediatrics*. 2013;131(1):189–195.
- Fierson WM, Capone A Jr; for American Academy of Pediatrics Section on Ophthalmology, American Academy of Ophthalmology, American Association of Certified Orthoptists. Telemedicine for evaluation of retinopathy of prematurity. *Pediatrics*. 2015;135(1):e238–e254.
- Good WV, Hardy RJ, Dobson V, et al; and Early Treatment for Retinopathy of Prematurity Cooperative Group. Final visual acuity results in the early treatment for retinopathy of prematurity study. *Arch Ophthalmol*. 2010;128(6):663–671.
- International Committee for the Classification of Retinopathy of Prematurity. The International Classification of Retinopathy of Prematurity revisited. *Arch Ophthalmol*. 2005;123(7):991–999.
- Mintz-Hittner HA, Kennedy KA, Chuang AZ, et al. Efficacy of intravitreal bevacizumab for stage 3+ retinopathy of prematurity. *N Engl J Med*. 2011;364(7):603–615.
- Palmer EA, Hardy RJ, Dobson V, et al; for Cryotherapy for Retinopathy of Prematurity Cooperative Group. 15-Year outcomes following threshold retinopathy of prematurity: final results from the multicenter trial of cryotherapy for retinopathy of prematurity. *Arch Ophthalmol*. 2005;123(3):311–318.
- The natural ocular outcome of premature birth and retinopathy. Status at 1 year. Cryotherapy for Retinopathy of Prematurity Cooperative Group. *Arch Ophthalmol*. 1994;112(7):903–912.

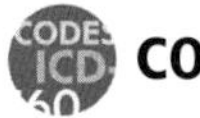

CODES

ICD10

- H35.109 Retinopathy of prematurity, unspecified, unspecified eye
- H35.119 Retinopathy of prematurity, stage 0 unspecified eye
- H35.129 Retinopathy of prematurity, stage 1 unspecified eye

FAQ

- Q: Does intrauterine growth retardation (IUGR) affect the chance for development of ROP?
- A: The chance for development of ROP in an IUGR infant is related more to the baby's postmenstrual birth age rather than birth weight. However, in as much as these infants often are sick, growth restriction could increase the risk of ROP over infants of similar postmenstrual age at birth.
- Q: When should a missed exam be made up?
- A: In most cases, it is safe to wait up to a week unless there has been recent evidence of stage 2 or worse ROP, in which case the exam should be completed as soon as the infant is stable for the dilated exam.
- Q: Does acute ROP ever need to be retreated?
- A: Following ablative therapy, about 10% of eyes will need additional treatment to untreated areas of the retina if the PLUS disease has not begun to diminish. This typically occurs about 10 to 14 days. The rate for retreatment after VEGF inhibitor intravitreal injection is not yet established but is common.
- Q: What are the two most important protocols to have established prior to launching a telemedicine program for ROP?
- A: The quality and timeliness of reading the photos and rapid availability of an ophthalmologist to provide a confirming exam and treatment, if needed.

RETROPHARYNGEAL ABSCESS

Camille Sabella, MD

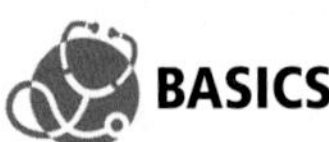

BASICS

DESCRIPTION

A relatively rare but potentially life-threatening infection occurring in the potential space between the posterior pharyngeal wall and prevertebral fascia

EPIDEMIOLOGY

- Winter-spring seasonality
- Children <5 years are at highest risk.
- 4.1 per 100,000 children <20 years old
- Male-to-female ratio 2:1

PATHOPHYSIOLOGY

- Most infections result from pharyngitis or supraglottitis and occur because of suppuration of the retropharyngeal lymph nodes, which lie in two paramedian chains and drain various nasopharyngeal structures and sinuses.
- These lymph gland chains disappear in childhood; thus, retropharyngeal abscesses are most common in infancy and early childhood.
- Cellulitis of the retropharyngeal area leads to formation of a phlegmon, which matures into an abscess.
- Other sources of infection in this space, often seen in older children and adolescents, include penetrating trauma of the posterior pharynx (e.g., foreign object aspiration, dental procedures, attempts at intubation).
- Extension of infection into this space can arise from vertebral body osteomyelitis or a dental abscess.

ETIOLOGY

- Infectious: Cultures often reveal multiple organisms.
- The predominant organisms isolated include the following:
  - *Streptococcus* (group A and others)
  - *Staphylococcus aureus*
  - Various anaerobic species (e.g., *Bacteroides*, *Peptostreptococcus*, *Fusobacterium*)
- Many of the isolates are β-lactamase producers.

DIAGNOSIS

HISTORY

- Symptoms may be present from hours to days before correct diagnosis is established. Many patients will have been taking oral antibiotics for presumed pharyngitis/sinusitis.
- Ask about neck trauma, especially penetrating injuries, recent surgery (especially dental), and history consistent with aspiration of a foreign object.
- Physicians must maintain a high index of suspicion. The presentation of a retropharyngeal abscess can be subtle, with the most frequent initial diagnostic impression usually epiglottitis or severe pharyngitis.
- Signs and symptoms:
  - Most frequent symptoms include sore throat, decreased oral intake, stiff or painful neck, fever, dysphagia, odynophagia, and stridor.
  - Fever
  - Stridor (seen in up to 50% of children in one study but only 5% in a more recent series)
  - A tender cervical neck region/mass and restricted range of motion
  - Classic diagnostic finding of a bulging posterior pharyngeal wall; may be absent or difficult to appreciate in an ill, apprehensive child

PHYSICAL EXAM

- Classic presentation is the young child who develops fever, neck stiffness, torticollis, neck mass, and acute cervical lymphadenitis.
- Infants and children often appear ill, but the manifestations are subacute and may be subtle.
- Other findings may include the following:
  - Muffled voice
  - Drooling
  - Fever
  - Dysphagia
  - Stridor

DIFFERENTIAL DIAGNOSIS

- Pharyngitis
- Peritonsillar or lateral wall abscess
- Epiglottitis/supraglottitis
- Penetrating foreign body
- Cervical osteomyelitis

DIAGNOSTIC TESTS & INTERPRETATION

- CBC may reveal an elevated total leukocyte level, with a significant left shift.
- Lateral neck radiograph
  - Widening of retropharyngeal space and at times an air-fluid level may be visualized
  - Normal plain neck radiograph does not rule out retropharyngeal abscess.
- CT scan (contrast-enhanced) of the neck
  - Superior to plain radiograph
  - Can usually differentiate abscess from local cellulitis/adenitis, although the sensitivity and specificity of this study for defining abscess versus cellulitis are <70%

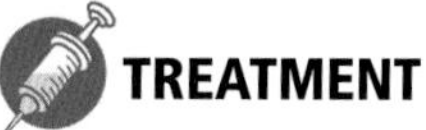

TREATMENT

GENERAL MEASURES

- Urgent consultation with an otolaryngology surgical team is warranted for airway management and possible surgical drainage; a team experienced in pediatric airway management is critical.
- Medical management alone (without surgical drainage) sufficient for about half the cases
- Patients with a well-defined abscess on admission CT are most likely to require surgical intervention.
- Patients treated with antibiotics alone must be followed closely for signs of worsening clinical status.

MEDICATION

- Start empiric broad-spectrum antibiotics, active against *S. aureus*, *Streptococcus pyogenes*, other non–group A streptococci, and anaerobic organisms.
- Ampicillin-sulbactam or clindamycin are good initial choices. Vancomycin may be added for suspected methicillin-resistant *S. aureus* infections in a child with severe infection.
- Antibiotics may be tailored based on microbiologic and susceptibility data.

ISSUES FOR REFERRAL

After diagnosis is confirmed, urgent consultation with experienced surgical staff who have expertise in management of a pediatric airway is mandatory.

SURGERY/OTHER PROCEDURES

- Recent data indicate that more than half the cases do not require surgical drainage.
- Severe respiratory distress and airway compromise is an indication for surgical drainage.
- Transoral approach most common mode of drainage

ONGOING CARE

PROGNOSIS

Excellent with appropriate antibiotics, expectant care, and surgery, if needed, at optimal time

COMPLICATIONS

- Spontaneous rupture with aspiration of infected material, with subsequent asphyxia or overwhelming pulmonary infection
- Hemorrhage from extension into local arteries and/or venous thrombosis from involvement of major neck vessels
- Extension of the infection inferiorly can occur, leading to mediastinitis, a subdiaphragmatic or psoas abscess.

ADDITIONAL READING

- Chang L, Chi H, Chiu NC, et al. Deep neck infections in different age group of children. *J Microbiol Immunol Infect*. 2010;43(1):47–52.
- Elsherif AM, Park AH, Alder SC, et al. Indicators of a more complicated clinical course for pediatric patients with retropharyngeal abscess. *Int J Pediatr Otorhinolaryngol*. 2010;74(2):198–201.
- Gavriel H, Lazarovitch T, Pomortsev A, et al: Variations in the microbiology of peritonsillar abscess. *Eur J Clin Microbiol Infect Dis*. 2009;28(1):27–31.
- Grisaru-Soen G, Komisar O, Aizenstein O, et al. Retropharyngeal and parapharyngeal abscess in children—epidemiology, clinical features and treatment. *Int J Pediatr Otorhinolaryngol*. 2010;74(9):1016–1020.
- Page NC, Bauer EM, Lieu JEC. Clinical features and treatment of retropharyngeal abscess in children. *Otolaryngol Head Neck Surg*. 2008;138(3):300–306.
- Woods CR, Cash ED, Smith AM, et al. Retropharyngeal and parapharyngeal abscesses among children and adolescents in the United States: epidemiology and management trends, 2003–2012. *J Pediatr Infect Dis*. 2016;5(3):259–268.

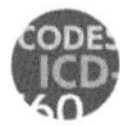

CODES

ICD10

J39.0 Retropharyngeal and parapharyngeal abscess

FAQ

- Q: What is the age group most at risk of having a retropharyngeal abscess?
- A: They are most common in preschool children; the paramedian chains of lymph nodes in the retropharyngeal area regress during childhood and adolescents. Thus, prior to their regression, these nodes filter lymph from the nasopharynx and paranasal sinuses and are responsible for retropharyngeal abscesses.
- Q: Is surgical management indicated in all patients?
- A: No. Recent trends have documented that more than half the cases can be managed with IV antibiotics without surgical drainage. Management with IV antibiotics for 24 to 48 hours in a stable child who does not have airway compromise is appropriate.

R

REYE SYNDROME

Orkun Baloglu, MD

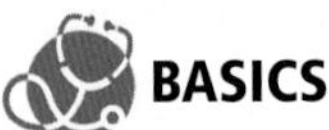

BASICS

DESCRIPTION

- Reye syndrome is described as acute noninflammatory encephalopathy and fatty degeneration of the liver which may be idiopathic or secondary.
- Reye syndrome is associated with aspirin (acetylsalicylic acid) therapy, whereas Reye-like syndromes are due to metabolic disorders or other etiologies that manifest similar to Reye syndrome.
- Patients must meet all of the following criteria of Reye syndrome by Centers for Disease Control and Prevention (CDC).
  - Acute, noninflammatory encephalopathy that is documented clinically by (i) an alteration in consciousness and, if available, (ii) a record of the CSF containing ≤8 leukocytes/mm^3 or a histologic specimen demonstrating cerebral edema without perivascular or meningeal inflammation
  - Acute encephalopathy must be associated with either (i) fatty metamorphosis of liver documented by a liver biopsy or an autopsy or (ii) a 3-fold or greater increase in the levels of the serum alanine aminotransferase (ALT), aspartate aminotransferase (AST), or elevated serum ammonia levels.
  - No more reasonable explanation for the cerebral and hepatic abnormalities

EPIDEMIOLOGY

- Both sexes are affected equally.
- Caucasians represent 93% of all age groups <18 years old affected. African Americans represent only 5%.
- Age: Infants 1 year old are 13.5%, and school-age children 5 to 14 years old are 53.5% of all cases.
- Association with ingestion of aspirin-containing medicines by children with varicella or influenza B infection.
- Reye-like illness is often associated with fatty acid oxidation defects and other inborn errors of metabolism.

Incidence

- Peak incidence of 555 cases in children in the United States in 1980
- In 1980, CDC cautioned physicians and parents about not to use salicylates in children with varicella or influenza-like illness.
- In 1982, the U.S. Surgeon General issued an advisory on the use of salicylates and Reye syndrome.
- Due to increased awareness about association of aspirin and Reye syndrome and improved diagnostic tests for disorders of inborn errors of metabolism (IEM), Reye syndrome incidence dramatically decreased since 1980s.
- From 1994 to 1997, there were no more than two cases of Reye syndrome annually.
- Reye-like illness due to metabolic causes should be suspected now in all cases with this presentation.

PATHOPHYSIOLOGY

- Mitochondrial injury of unknown etiology in a viral-infected host results in dysfunction of oxidative phosphorylation and fatty acid oxidation.
- Mitochondrial toxins, usually salicylates, exacerbate the condition when ingested after mitochondrial injury.
- Postmortem findings:
  - Liver: grossly yellowish-white due to increased triglyceride levels; foamy cytoplasm with increased microvesicular fat, decreased glycogen
  - Brain: marked edema with increased intracellular fluid and loss of neurons
  - Abnormal-looking mitochondria can be detected in many tissues.
  - Multiple organ involvement may be present in fatty acid oxidation or other defects.

DIAGNOSIS

HISTORY

- Typical history includes a viral illness with a remission period of 3 to 5 days followed by acute onset of vomiting and neurologic changes.
- At least one episode prodromal illness was reported in 93% of patients during the 3 weeks before the onset of Reye syndrome.
- Prodromal illness
  - Upper respiratory tract infection (73%)
  - Varicella (21%)
  - Diarrhea (14%)
- Use of salicylates during prodromal illness
- Abrupt onset of vomiting followed by neurologic deterioration
- Recurrent previous similar episodes, family history of disorders of IEM, frequent hypoglycemia, and cardiac enlargement suggest disorders of IEM resulting in Reye-like syndrome.

PHYSICAL EXAM

- Clinical signs of dehydration due to vomiting
- Absence of focal neurologic signs
- Altered mental status result of elevated intracranial pressure (ICP)
- Convulsive seizures
- Neurologic exam varies with stage of disease:
  - Stage 0: alert, wakeful
  - Stage 1: difficult to arouse, lethargic, sleepy
  - Stage 2: delirious, combative, with purposeful or semipurposeful motor responses
  - Stage 3: unarousable, with predominantly flexor motor responses, decorticate
  - Stage 4: unarousable, with predominantly extensor motor responses, decerebrate
  - Stage 5: unarousable, with flaccid paralysis, areflexia, and pupils unresponsive
  - Stage 6: treated with curare (neuromuscular blocker) or equivalent drug and therefore unclassifiable
- 81% of patients had stage 0, 1, or 2 illness at the time of hospital admission.
- Slight liver enlargement without jaundice
- Organomegaly may also be present in Reye-like illness.

DIFFERENTIAL DIAGNOSIS

- It is important to distinguish between Reye syndrome, associated with aspirin (acetylsalicylic acid) therapy, and Reye-like syndromes, often due to metabolic disorders and other causes as mentioned subsequently.
- All cases that present with Reye syndrome should be investigated for metabolic disorders.
- Metabolic diseases:
  - In a report by Hou et al., Reye-like syndrome was secondary to hereditary organic acidemias (n = 13), urea cycle defects (n = 4), mitochondrial disorders (n = 3), fulminant hepatitis (n = 2), tyrosinemia (n = 1), and valproate-associated hepatotoxicity (n = 1).
  - In the United Kingdom, 12% of Reye syndrome cases between 1981 and 1996 were subsequently reclassified as metabolic disorders.
- CNS infections (e.g., meningitis, encephalitis)
- Toxins
- Drug ingestion other than aspirin (e.g., valproate)

DIAGNOSTIC TESTS & INTERPRETATION

Initial Tests (screening, lab, imaging)

- Serum ammonia: may be normal at the onset of disease. However, serum level of ammonia >45 mcg/dL (26 μmol/L) suggests higher mortality.
- Elevated ALT and AST levels >3 times upper normal limits
- Serum bilirubin level may be normal or elevated initially.
- Elevated BUN and creatinine consistent with dehydration
- CSF: ≤8 leukocytes/mm^3
- Hypoglycemia is often present.
- EEG: characteristic of metabolic encephalopathy with generalized slow wave abnormalities
- Head CT/brain MRI: may be normal initially or may show findings consistent with cerebral edema

Diagnostic Procedures/Other

- Metabolic workup: Abnormalities of organic and amino acids may be present if symptoms are caused by a metabolic disorder.
- Cultured fibroblasts for fatty acid oxidation defects

ALERT

Failure to recognize early and control or prevent cerebral edema can be associated with poor outcomes.

TREATMENT

GENERAL MEASURES
- Stabilization of airway, breathing, and circulation should always be priority.
- Frequent assessment of neurologic status, especially signs of elevated ICP is required.

MEDICATION
- No specific treatment is available for Reye syndrome.
- Treatment is largely supportive.
- IV glucose to counteract effects of glycogen depletion
- Hyperammonemia management
- Antiepiletic agents to control seizures

SURGERY/OTHER PROCEDURES
- Intracranial pressure monitoring may be required in addition to central venous catheter and arterial catheter placement for invasive hemodynamic monitoring.
- A case of Reye syndrome with acute liver failure was reported to be treated with liver transplantation.

ADMISSION, INPATIENT, AND NURSING CONSIDERATIONS
All patients should be hospitalized for close clinical observation.

ONGOING CARE

FOLLOW-UP RECOMMENDATIONS

Patient Monitoring
- Admission to pediatric intensive care unit should be considered early in the disease course for close neurologic and cardiopulmonary monitoring.
- Focus is mainly on management of acute liver failure and elevated ICP.
- Multidisciplinary approach including neurologist, gastroenterologist/hepatologist, metabolic disease specialist, and pediatric intensivist should be established.

PROGNOSIS
- Overall mortality was reported as 31%.
- Higher stages of illness at admission were associated with poor prognosis; 17.8% of patients with stage 0 illness at admission died, as compared with 89.6% of mortality with stage 5 illness.
- Age <5 years old and serum ammonia levels >45 mcg/dL (26 μmol/L) are also associated with worse prognosis in terms of mortality and neurologic outcomes.
- Complete recovery was observed in 62% of patients who survived. Rest of them had varying degrees of neurologic sequelae.

COMPLICATIONS
Elevated intracranial pressure secondary to cerebral edema and fulminant liver failure

ADDITIONAL READING

- Altman LK. Tale of triumph on every aspirin bottle. *The New York Times*. May 11, 1999.
- Belay ED, Bresee JS, Holman RC, et al. Reye's syndrome in the United States from 1981 through 1997. *N Engl J Med*. 1999;340(18):1377–1382.
- Cağ M, Saouli AC, Audet M, et al. Reye syndrome and liver transplantation. *Turk J Pediatr*. 2010;52(6):662–664.
- Centers for Disease Control and Prevention. Reye syndrome 1990 case definition. https://wwwn.cdc.gov/nndss/conditions/reye-syndrome/case-definition/1990/. Accessed October 5, 2017.
- Chow EL, Cherry JD, Harrison R, et al. Reassessing Reye syndrome. *Arch Pediatr Adolesc Med*. 2003;157(12):1241–1242.
- Duerksen DR, Jewell LD, Mason AL, et al. Coexistence of hepatitis A and adult Reye's syndrome. *Gut*. 1997;41(1):121–124.
- Glasgow JF. Reye's syndrome: the case for a causal link with aspirin. *Drug Saf*. 2006;29(12):1111–1121.
- Glasgow JF, Middleton B. Reye syndrome—insights on causation and prognosis. *Arch Dis Child*. 2001;85(5):351–353.
- Gosalakkal JA, Kamoji V. Reye syndrome and reye-like syndrome. *Pediatr Neurol*. 2008;39(3):198–200.
- Green CI, Blitzer MG, Shapira E. Inborn errors of metabolism and Reye syndrome: differential diagnosis. *J Pediatr*. 1988;113(1, Pt 1):156–159.
- Hou JW, Chou SP, Wang TR. Metabolic function and liver histopathology in Reye-like illnesses. *Acta Paediatr*. 1996;85(9):1053–1057.
- Orlowski JP, Hanhan UA, Fiallos MR. Is aspirin a cause of Reye's syndrome? A case against. *Drug Saf*. 2002;25(4):225–231.
- Reye RD, Morgan G, Baral J. Encephalopathy and fatty degeneration of the viscera. A disease entity in childhood. *Lancet*. 1963;2 (7311):749–752.
- Schrör K. Aspirin and Reye syndrome: a review of the evidence. *Paediatr Drugs*. 2007;9(3):195–204.
- van Bever HP, Quek SC, Lim T. Aspirin, Reye syndrome, Kawasaki disease, and allergies; a reconsideration of the links. *Arch Dis Child*. 2004;89(12):1178.

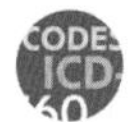

CODES

ICD10
G93.7 Reye's syndrome

FAQ
- Q: Is Reye syndrome fatal?
- A: ~30% of children will die, usually due to cerebral edema. Mortality rates are best predicted by neurologic state at the onset of presentation.
- Q: How can the neurologic findings of Reye syndrome be differentiated from those of meningitis?
- A: Aside from elevated intracranial pressure, the lumbar taps of patients with Reye syndrome are at best unremarkable. Elevated leukocyte count is not seen in these cases.
- Q: What additional recommendations are suggested for children on chronic aspirin therapy?
- A: When annual influenza vaccine supply is limited, according to the CDC, vaccination efforts should focus on delivering vaccination to specific subpopulations, including children "receiving long-term aspirin therapy and who therefore might be at risk for experiencing Reye syndrome after influenza virus infection."
- Q: What makes Reye-like syndrome secondary to disorders of IEM more likely than Reye syndrome in differential diagnosis?
- A: Recurrent previous similar episodes, family history of disorders of IEM, frequent hypoglycemia, and cardiac enlargement.
- Q: Why is Reye syndrome called "Reye syndrome"?
- A: Drs. J. Douglas Reye, Graeme Morgan, and Jim Baral published the first description of the syndrome in 1963 in *The Lancet*. Dr. Reye was a pathologist at the Royal Alexandra Hospital in Sydney, Australia. Beginning in 1951, he had identified 20 similar cases. Drs. Morgan and Baral were trainees (and later coauthors) who encouraged him to publish these observations, as there were no descriptions of the entity in any textbooks or articles. The syndrome was subsequently labeled Reye syndrome.

RHABDOMYOLYSIS

Erica Winnicki, MD • Farzana Perwad, MD

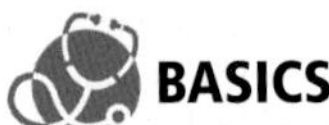

BASICS

DESCRIPTION

- Rhabdomyolysis is defined as skeletal muscle breakdown resulting from injury.
- Injury may result from many causes including trauma, infection, medications, or inherited disorders.
- Classic presentation is with a triad of myalgia, weakness, and dark or reddish brown urine.
- Characterized by elevated creatine kinase (CK) and myoglobinuria
- Release of intracellular contents from damaged muscle cells may cause severe electrolyte disturbances including life-threatening hyperkalemia, hyperphosphatemia, and hypocalcemia.
- The resulting myoglobinuria can cause obstruction of renal tubules and pigment-induced acute kidney injury (AKI), the most serious complication of rhabdomyolysis.

EPIDEMIOLOGY

- Rhabdomyolysis is more common in adults than children, where it is commonly due to illicit or prescription drugs or due to trauma.
- Rhabdomyolysis is a common clinical problem in a catastrophic disaster (e.g., an earthquake).
- Rhabdomyolysis accounts for 7–10% of cases of AKI in the United States.

RISK FACTORS

Genetics

Muscle enzyme deficiencies, muscular dystrophy, and disorders of mitochondrial metabolism increase the risk of rhabdomyolysis.

ETIOLOGY

- The most common causes of rhabdomyolysis in children are:
  - Viral myositis: This is the most common cause for young children. Influenza A and B, Epstein-Barr virus, cytomegalovirus, and HIV have all been associated with rhabdomyolysis.
  - Exercise: This is the most common cause for 9- to 18-year-olds. Exercise which is novel, intense, or prolonged, and especially in the presence of extremely hot weather may cause rhabdomyolysis.
  - Trauma: Muscle trauma may occur from crush injury, compartment syndrome, or electric shock.
  - Autoimmune myopathy: juvenile dermatomyositis or polymyositis
  - Drugs: Illicit drug use including alcohol (alcohol withdrawal syndrome), cocaine, heroin, amphetamines, phencyclidine (PCP), and ecstasy have been associated with rhabdomyolysis.
  - Causative prescription medications include lipid-lowering drugs (statins, fibrates) and antipsychotic medications (due to neuroleptic malignant syndrome).
- Less common causes of rhabdomyolysis in children include the following:
  - Myopathies involving muscle enzyme or energy substrate deficiencies: These include disorders of lipid metabolism (e.g., carnitine palmitoyltransferase II deficiency), disorders of glycogenolysis (e.g., phosphorylase kinase deficiency, McArdle disease), disorders of glycolysis (lactate dehydrogenase deficiency), and mitochondrial deficiency disorders. Usual triggers for rhabdomyolysis in such conditions are fasting, exertion, or viral illness.
  - Dystrophinopathies: Rhabdomyolysis is more likely to occur after exertion in association with all forms of muscular dystrophy.
  - Muscle hypoxia: prolonged immobilization or loss of consciousness; certain metabolic and electrolyte disorders: hypokalemia, hypophosphatemia, hypocalcemia, and hyperosmolar states such as diabetic ketoacidosis
  - Body temperature changes (hyperthermia and hypothermia): Malignant hyperthermia is a rare inherited condition that results in hyperthermia, muscle breakdown, and subsequent rhabdomyolysis on receiving halogenated hydrocarbon–containing anesthetics or muscle relaxants such as succinylcholine.
  - Neuroleptic malignant syndrome: a rare neurologic disorder characterized by hyperthermia, rhabdomyolysis, and autonomic changes in patients receiving neuroleptic or antipsychotic medications
  - Certain toxins: snake bite, spider venom and vespid venoms, quail, and some mushrooms
- The list of causes of rhabdomyolysis above is not exhaustive. Any child with sudden onset of muscle pain, tenderness, or weakness should be suspected of having rhabdomyolysis and any child with dark or reddish brown urine suspected of myoglobinuria.

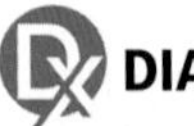

DIAGNOSIS

HISTORY

- Prior history of any illness or insult associated with rhabdomyolysis should be sought. Rhabdomyolysis may follow infections (e.g., influenza), insults (e.g., crush injury, severe exertion), and medications (e.g., statins).
- Symptoms of muscle pain or weakness may result from rhabdomyolysis and help suggest diagnosis if present but its absence does not exclude it.
- Signs of reddish-brown discoloration of the urine may be present, but its absence does not exclude it.

PHYSICAL EXAM

- Palpate muscles for tenderness and, less commonly, swelling or fullness which usually appears after hydration.
- Test for motor strength.
- Elicit reflexes to exclude neuropathy.
- Examine skin and mucous membranes for signs of vasculitis and dehydration.
- Look for signs suggestive of child abuse.
- Examine for signs of a concomitant precipitating illness.
- The clinical picture is generally consistent with volume depletion given the sequestration of fluids in injured muscle tissue.

DIFFERENTIAL DIAGNOSIS

- Consider other causes of reddish brown urine.
  - Hematuria (positive dipstick, supernatant of spun urine is not red, sediment is red, >5 red blood cell [RBC]/HPF)
  - Beet ingestion, porphyria, phenazopyridine use (negative dipstick, supernatant of spun urine is red, sediment is not red, <5 RBC/HPF)
- Consider other causes of muscle pain and/or weakness:
  - Viral illnesses
  - Lyme disease
  - Suppurative myositis
  - Guillain-Barré syndrome
  - Collagen vascular diseases

DIAGNOSTIC TESTS & INTERPRETATION

- Serum CK level, specifically the CK-MM isoenzyme, which is found in skeletal muscle, will be elevated to >4 to 5 times the upper limit of normal.
  - CK levels usually rise within 12 hours of the injury and peak within 2 to 3 days.
  - If the CK levels continue to rise, it should raise suspicion for ongoing muscle damage or development of compartment syndrome.
- Serum electrolytes including calcium and phosphorus must be measured given the potential for severe derangements.
  - Abnormalities may include hyperkalemia, hyperphosphatemia, and/or hypocalcemia.
  - There may be metabolic acidosis with a wide anion gap in those conditions associated with lactate production.
- Creatinine level may be elevated out of proportion to that of BUN, secondary to conversion of liberated muscle creatine to creatinine.
- CBC and smear should be obtained because many of the metabolic disorders causing rhabdomyolysis can cause hemolytic anemia simultaneously.
- Patients with rhabdomyolysis are at increased risk for disseminated intravascular coagulation (DIC) secondary to thromboplastin released from the injured myocytes. Therefore, PT/INR, PTT, platelets, and fibrinogen levels should be obtained.
- Serum uric acid may be elevated from release of purines from muscle cells and may contribute to renal tubule obstruction.

- Other muscle enzyme levels (myoglobin, aldolase, lactate dehydrogenase, AST, ALT) will be elevated secondary to muscle injury but are not necessary for diagnosis.
- Urinalysis
  - Urine may appear brown and test positive for blood on dipstick without RBCs on microscopy (<5 RBC/HPF).
  - Granular pigmented casts are common.
  - Low fractional excretion of sodium (<1%) is found in those with AKI.
- Myoglobin is not generally measured; however, urine myoglobin can be quantitatively measured using an immunoassay. Myoglobin is rapidly cleared and maybe absent in urine despite high CK levels. Serum CK levels are more sensitive to assess the degree of ongoing rhabdomyolysis.
- Other tests
  - EKG may reveal changes associated with acute hypocalcemia (prolonged QTc) or hyperkalemia (peaked T waves, prolongation of PR, absent P wave with prolonged QRS interval, or even ventricular tachycardia/fibrillation in severe untreated hyperkalemia). EKG also helps to rule out myocardial infarction which can cause elevated CK-MM levels.
  - Metabolic and genetic testing if recurrent or otherwise suspected metabolic myopathy
- Imaging is not generally required for the diagnosis. Note that use of radiocontrast in imaging studies as part of diagnostic evaluation can worsen AKI.

Diagnostic Procedures/Other

- Muscle biopsy: necessary to diagnose metabolic myopathies; should wait several weeks after the clinical event to perform. A biopsy will demonstrate immunohistochemical features of myopathy.
- Immunoblotting is helpful in evaluating dystrophinopathies.

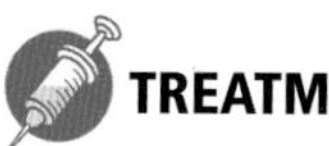

TREATMENT

Aggressive repletion of fluids should be initiated promptly. If an underlying cause is identified, it should be corrected or removed.

GENERAL MEASURES

- Early fluid resuscitation is essential to prevent worsening kidney function. Vigorous hydration with crystalloid IV fluids should be followed by adequate maintenance fluids (e.g., 2 to 3 times maintenance) to provide brisk urine flow (e.g., >2 mL/kg/h or >200 mL/h).
- Alkalinization of the urine is not clearly superior to fluids alone, although risks of alkalinization are minimal.
- Use of diuretics, including furosemide (a loop diuretic), is controversial, and use should be limited to fluid-replete patients. Use of mannitol is not clearly beneficial and may worsen AKI.

MEDICATION

- Administration of sodium bicarbonate (along with fluids) to correct or prevent acidosis is reasonable. Correction of acidosis is also beneficial in the management of hyperkalemia (potassium is shifted intracellularly).
- If alkalinization is initiated, monitor closely for worsening hypocalcemia.
- Use of diuretics is controversial; consider use in fluid-replete patients with AKI to maintain urine output and avoid or treat volume overload (e.g., furosemide 1 to 2 mg/kg/dose IV). Furosemide will also maximize potassium elimination by the kidney.
- Additional treatment for severe hyperkalemia may be necessary and incudes IV calcium gluconate, sodium bicarbonate, insulin and glucose, β_2-agonist drugs, and Kayexalate®.
- Correct hypocalcemia only if symptoms are present or in the setting of severe hyperkalemia in order to prevent the complication of calcium-phosphate deposition and late hypercalcemia.
- Benefit of early initiation of dialysis to remove myoglobin or uric acid to prevent the development of AKI has not been demonstrated.
- In established AKI, when renal replacement therapy is indicated, continuous venovenous hemofiltration or hemodiafiltration may be most effective in removing myoglobin which has a molecular weight of 17 kDa. Indications for dialysis include AKI with the following:
  - Severe hyperkalemia refractory to medical management or rapidly rising potassium levels
  - Severe metabolic acidosis resistant to medical management
  - Volume overload/respiratory distress secondary to pulmonary edema

ONGOING CARE

Close monitoring of labs with serial measurements of CK levels, creatinine, and electrolytes is essential. The patient's fluid status should be monitored closely, and volume repletion should be continued until urine is clear and negative for blood. The patient should also be watched closely for signs of ongoing muscle injury, compartment syndrome, or DIC.

PROGNOSIS

- Prognosis is generally good, with AKI being the major life-threatening complication. With resolution of myoglobinuria, AKI is expected to be reversible.
- Prompt cessation of rhabdomyolysis may be expected when the inciting cause is corrected or resolved.
- Although most children recover promptly, severe muscle injury may cause prolonged muscle weakness and warrant follow-up by physical and occupational therapy.
- Patients are generally safe to be discharged home if AKI is resolved or absent, electrolytes are normal, they are able to maintain excellent oral hydration with brisk urine output, and CK is both downtrending and <3,000 U/L.

COMPLICATIONS

- The insult may lead to muscle cell destruction with release of intracellular contents including proteins and electrolytes and sequestration of fluids by damaged muscle leading to severe hypovolemia.
- Electrolyte release from muscle can lead to severe hyperkalemia, hyperphosphatemia, and secondary hypocalcemia.
- Electrolyte derangement may result in cardiac arrhythmias.
- Rhabdomyolysis leads to AKI by direct toxicity of myoglobin to the renal tubules, renal tubular obstruction, and renal ischemia from hypoperfusion.
- AKI occurs in 13–50% of patients. Risk factors for AKI include higher CK level (>3,000 U/L), concurrent administration of nephrotoxic agents, and volume depletion.
- Compartment syndrome may result from muscle swelling.
- Use of bicarbonate may precipitate symptomatic hypocalcemia.
- Use of calcium therapy for severe hyperkalemia or symptomatic hypocalcemia may result in calcium-phosphate deposition or exacerbate late hypercalcemia.
- Failure to discontinue IV fluids if oligoanuric renal failure develops can produce iatrogenic fluid overload.

ADDITIONAL READING

- Bosch X, Poch E, Grau J. Rhabdomyolysis and acute kidney injury. *N Engl J Med*. 2009;361(1):62–72.
- Elsayed EF, Reilly RF. Rhabdomyolysis: a review, with emphasis on the pediatric population. *Pediatr Nephrol*. 2010;25(1):7–18.
- Mannix R, Tan ML, Wright R, et al. Acute pediatric rhabdomyolysis: causes and rates of renal failure. *Pediatrics*. 2006;118(5):2119–2125.
- Talving P, Karamanos E, Skiada D, et al. Relationship of creatine kinase elevation and acute kidney injury in pediatric trauma patients. *J Trauma Acute Care Surg*. 2013;74(3):912–916.

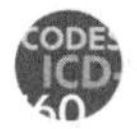

CODES

ICD10

- M62.82 Rhabdomyolysis
- T79.5XXA Traumatic anuria, initial encounter

RHABDOMYOSARCOMA

Amit J. Sabnis, MD • Steven G. DuBois, MD, MS

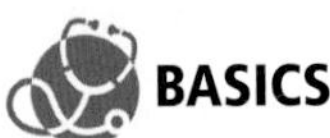

BASICS

DESCRIPTION

A soft tissue cancer with features of skeletal muscle differentiation. Prognostic classification of rhabdomyosarcoma (RMS) currently depends on:

- Anatomic site of disease (stage)
- Extent of resection and spread (group)
- Presence of a *FOXO1* gene fusion (either *PAX3-FOXO1* or *PAX7-FOXO1*). This has supplanted histologic subtype (alveolar vs. embryonal) in North America.

EPIDEMIOLOGY

- The most common pediatric soft tissue sarcomas (tumors of mesenchymal origin)
- Accounts for ~5% of childhood cancer
- Boys at slightly increased risk compared to girls (incidence by gender of 1.5:1)

Incidence

- 4.5 cases per 1 million children per year
- U.S. annual incidence is approximately 350 cases per year.
- Age distribution
  - Peaks in children <7 years, with another smaller peak in late adolescence
  - Median age at diagnosis is 5 years.

RISK FACTORS

Genetics

- About 90% of cases are sporadic.
- Several predisposing conditions:
  - Li-Fraumeni (autosomal dominant)
    - *TP53* mutation leads to cancer predisposition due to inadequate response to DNA damage.
    - Increased risk for soft tissue sarcomas, osteosarcoma, adrenocortical carcinoma, choroid plexus carcinoma, leukemias, breast cancer, and other cancers
  - Beckwith-Wiedemann syndrome (sporadic)
    - Improper epigenetic regulation of 11p15 leads to an overgrowth syndrome.
    - Increased risk of a range of embryonal cancers early in life, including Wilms tumor, hepatoblastoma, and RMS
  - Neurofibromatosis type I and Costello syndrome (autosomal dominant)
    - Mutational activation of *HRAS* (Costello) or loss of the RAS-negative regulator *NF1* (neurofibromatosis) leads to unchecked RAS signaling and increased risk for RMS.

GENERAL PREVENTION

- No standard approach because usually sporadic
- Avoidance of radiation in patients with known predisposing syndromes (e.g., Li-Fraumeni syndrome)

PATHOPHYSIOLOGY

- Chromosomal translocations (most commonly t[2;13] or t[1;13]) create fusion transcription factors *PAX3-FOXO1* and *PAX7-FOXO1*.
  - Fusions are usually found in alveolar histology tumors, but fusion-negative alveolar cases have a superior prognosis.
  - Animal models combining expression of *PAX3-FOXO1* and loss of either *TP53* or *CDKN2A* recapitulate RMS.
- Fusion-negative RMS (~60% of cases) commonly carry mutations in the *RAS* pathway, as well as loss of heterozygosity at 11p15.
  - Animal models of fusion-negative RMS target activating *RAS* mutations to myogenic progenitor cells.
- Distinct histologies include pleomorphic or anaplastic RMS, which harbor poor prognoses.

COMMONLY ASSOCIATED CONDITIONS

- Syndromes listed in "Genetics" section have the highest association.
- Radiation exposure, including a possible connection to in utero exposure.
- Single studies showed an association with high birth weight or incomplete childhood vaccination, respectively.

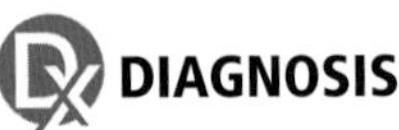

DIAGNOSIS

HISTORY

- Often presents as a firm, painless mass
- Additional symptoms relate to location of primary mass:
  - Orbital (10%): unilateral proptosis, ophthalmoplegia, visual changes
  - Head and neck—parameningeal (16%): sinus pressure, nasal congestion, hypophonation, discharge from the nose or ear, unilateral hearing loss, ophthalmoplegia
    - Parameningeal tumors with intracranial extension can present with headache, vomiting, and cranial nerve palsies.
  - Head and neck—nonparameningeal (10%; includes scalp, buccal mucosa, face): asymmetric facies, palpable mass
  - Extremities (20%): palpable mass, often tender or inflamed
  - Genitourinary (25%): bloody or mucousy vaginal discharge, prolapse of tissue through vagina or urethra, hematuria, urinary retention, constipation, firm testicular mass

PHYSICAL EXAM

- Exam findings correlate with sites of lesion.
  - Orbital: proptosis; tumor may be visible beneath everted palpebrum.
  - Head and neck: visibly asymmetric facies. Tumors arising in the sinuses or pharynx may be visible in the oral or nasal cavity.
  - Extremities: palpable mass, often tender or inflamed; lymph nodes commonly involved
  - Genitourinary: Prolapsed tissue may be visible through urethra (bladder primary) or vagina (vaginal primary); firm scrotal mass (paratesticular primary)
- Abnormal neurologic exam raises suspicion for intracranial extension.
- Evidence of cytopenias (petechiae, pallor) raises suspicion for bone marrow metastases.
- Enlarged lymph nodes suggest regional nodal spread, common in extremity RMS.

DIFFERENTIAL DIAGNOSIS

- Other small, round blue cell tumors
  - Ewing sarcoma (CD99+)
  - Neuroblastoma (synaptophysin+)
  - Non-Hodgkin lymphoma (CD45+)
- Other cancers
  - Non-RMS soft tissue sarcomas
  - Germ cell tumors (especially GU masses)
  - Rhabdoid tumor
- Nonmalignant masses:
  - Trauma
  - Benign growths (lipoma, rhabdomyoma)
  - Abscess or other infectious process

DIAGNOSTIC TESTS & INTERPRETATION

Initial Tests (screening, lab, imaging)

- CBC to provide an estimate of marrow involvement and to help rule out a hematopoietic malignancy
- Electrolytes including calcium and magnesium, liver function tests, and BUN/creatinine prior to initiating therapy
- Tumor lysis labs (uric acid, LDH, and phosphate in addition to chemistries above) may be helpful if other malignancies are diagnostic considerations.
- MRI (preferred) or CT scan of primary site
- Chest CT to rule out pulmonary metastases (most common site of metastatic disease)
- Abdominal and pelvic CT to evaluate for nodal metastases in paratesticular tumors
- ^{99m}Tc bone scan and/or PET scan to evaluate for bone metastasis

Diagnostic Procedures/Other

- Surgical biopsy or upfront resection with negative margins, depending on clinical context. Either should be performed by an experienced oncology surgeon with a high index of suspicion for malignancy and with appropriate precautions to prevent tumor spill.
- Regional lymph node sampling is needed in certain cases, particularly extremity tumors or subsets of paratesticular tumors.

ALERT

Testicular masses should not be biopsied but rather resected along with the spermatic cord through an inguinal approach. It is vital that the performing surgeon is aware of the potential diagnosis of RMS.

- Bilateral bone marrow biopsies to evaluate for metastatic disease in the bone marrow, particularly in subsets at highest risk for bone marrow metastasis
- Lumbar puncture for CSF cytology if intracranial extension is a possibility (parameningeal tumors)
- Echocardiogram to ensure normal cardiac function before administering anthracyclines
- Pathologic findings
  - Small round blue cells are characteristic although may see spindle cell elements.
  - All RMS are considered high-grade tumors.
  - Immunohistochemical stains include positivity for desmin and myogenin and negativity for CD45.
  - *FOXO1* fusions are detected by fluorescent in situ hybridization (FISH) probes (fresh sample required), reverse transcription polymerase chain reaction (RT-PCR), or next generation sequencing-based assays.

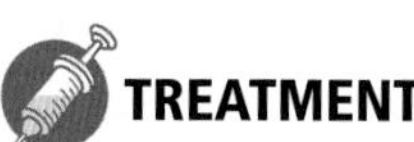

TREATMENT

MEDICATION

- The backbone of RMS chemotherapy in North America is cycles of vincristine and actinomycin D, with or without cyclophosphamide (a.k.a. "VA" or "VAC").
  - Can often be given as outpatient therapy
  - Cyclophosphamide omitted for low-risk patients
- Intermediate-risk patients may alternate between VAC and vincristine/irinotecan (VI), which may be more cost effective and spares high alkylator doses.
- A subset of high-risk patients benefit from intensified therapy including VAC, VI, doxorubicin, ifosfamide, and etoposide.
- Experimental protocols include the mTOR inhibitor temsirolimus based on promising results in patients with relapsed disease.
- Supportive care includes *Pneumocystis jirovecii* (i.e., pneumocystis pneumonia [PCP]) prophylaxis, myeloid growth factors (e.g., G-CSF) to shorten neutropenia antiemetics, and laxatives.

ISSUES FOR REFERRAL

- Referral to an experienced pediatric oncology center is strongly encouraged.
- A pediatric oncologist should be consulted whenever the diagnosis of RMS is suspected prior to any invasive procedures.
- Consider referral to cancer risk clinic.

ADDITIONAL THERAPIES

- In North America, radiation therapy is used for local control in all cases except completely resected fusion-negative RMS.
- Sites of metastatic disease are also typically treated with radiation.

SURGERY/OTHER PROCEDURES

- Surgeons assist in pretreatment staging and in determining a patient's clinical group based on extent of initial surgery.
- Given radiosensitivity of RMS, avoid surgical procedures that will result in significant loss of function.
- If deemed resectable without significant loss of function, the goal should be complete excision with negative margins.

ADMISSION, INPATIENT, AND NURSING CONSIDERATIONS

- Admit patients with severe cytopenias, threat to vision or airway due to mass effect, or for expedited workup if unable to access care.
- Diagnostic workup can often be performed on an expedited outpatient schedule.

ONGOING CARE

FOLLOW-UP RECOMMENDATIONS

- Patients seen regularly by pediatric oncology
- After completion of therapy, follow-up with pediatric oncology is every 3 months for the 1st year and then gradually spaced.
- Patients should continue to receive annual preventive health visits with their primary care provider.
- Vaccinations are deferred during cytotoxic therapy due to limited efficacy, although annual influenza vaccines are recommended.

PATIENT EDUCATION

- Families are reminded that fevers are medical emergencies in children on chemotherapy.
- Families are advised of signs/symptoms that might suggest recurrent disease.

PROGNOSIS

- Overall survival is approximately 70%, with significant differences based on risk group.
- Current risk stratification in North America includes:
  - Stage (based on anatomic site of disease, size, and regional node involvement)
    - Orbital, nonparameningeal head and neck, vaginal, and biliary tract are favorable.
    - Extremity and parameningeal sites are unfavorable.
  - Clinical group (extent of residual disease remaining after initial surgery)
    - Gross residual disease is unfavorable (except in orbital disease).
    - Metastatic disease is very unfavorable.
  - Fusion status:
    - *FOXO1* fusion is unfavorable.
- 5-year event-free survival is estimated to be:
  - >90% for low-risk disease
  - 70–80% for intermediate-risk disease
  - <30% for high-risk disease

COMPLICATIONS

- RMS therapy is intensive and has numerous secondary effects.
- Acute toxicities:
  - Marrow suppression, requiring blood and platelet transfusions and raising the risk of life-threatening sepsis
  - Severe nausea and vomiting
  - Mucosal injury with pain and poor PO intake
  - Neuropathic pain, extremity weakness, and constipation due to vincristine
  - Risk of hemorrhagic cystitis (rare) with cyclophosphamide
  - Hepatic sinusoidal obstructive syndrome
- Late effects (poorly predicted at present):
  - Infertility (related to cyclophosphamide or ifosfamide)
  - Cardiomyopathy (related to doxorubicin)
  - Secondary malignancies (e.g., leukemia from chemotherapy or sarcomas in radiation field)
  - Radiation vasculopathy (increased risk of stroke in patients with CNS radiation, hypertension in those with renal radiation)
  - Long-term monitoring in a Cancer Survivorship program is recommended.

ADDITIONAL READING

- Hayes-Jordan A, Andrassy R. Rhabdomyosarcoma in children. *Curr Opin Ped*. 2009; 21(3):373–378.
- Malempati S, Hawkins DS. Rhabdomyosarcoma: review of the Children's Oncology Group (COG) Soft-Tissue Sarcoma Committee experience and rationale for current COG studies. *Pediatr Blood Cancer*. 2012;59(1):5–10.
- Weigel BJ, Lyden E, Anderson JR, et al. Intensive multiagent therapy, including dose-compressed cycles of ifosfamide/etoposide and vincristine/doxorubicin/cyclophosphamide, irinotecan, and radiation, in patients with high-risk rhabdomyosarcoma: a report from the Children's Oncology Group. *J Clin Oncol*. 2016;34(2):117–122.

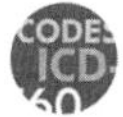

CODES

ICD10

- C49.9 Malignant neoplasm of connective and soft tissue, unsp
- C49.0 Malignant neoplasm of connective and soft tissue of head, face and neck
- C49.5 Malignant neoplasm of connective and soft tissue of pelvis

FAQ

- Q: Are other children in the family at risk for developing RMS?
- A: Familial risk for developing RMS is rare, outside of syndromes addressed in "Genetics."
- Q: Will this child lose his or her hair?
- A: Hair loss is common while receiving therapy but regrows after therapy concludes.
- Q: Does a patient's age influence outcome?
- A: Patients <1 and >10 years of age have poorer outcomes than the majority of RMS patients, who are diagnosed between those ages.

RHEUMATIC FEVER

Shashank P. Behere, MD • David Hehir, MD, MS

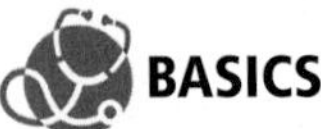

BASICS

DESCRIPTION

- A postinfectious inflammatory disease caused by rheumatogenic strains of group A β-hemolytic *Streptococcus* (GABHS)
- Acute rheumatic fever (ARF) results in a wide range of disease, from mild joint involvement to chronic carditis.
- The most significant socioeconomic impact is caused by its most severe form, rheumatic heart disease (RHD). Although rarely fatal in the acute phase, chronic RHD may result in significant disability and shortened lifespan.

EPIDEMIOLOGY

- Occurs usually following pharyngitis with rheumatogenic GABHS strains
- GABHS strains causing skin infections have also been associated with ARF in the developing world.
- Initial episode of ARF/RHD seen primarily in patients 5 to 15 years of age; chronic RHD presents in young adults.

Incidence

- Incidence of 2 to 14 per 100,000 per year in the United States.
- Global annual incidence of 350,000 in children
- 350,000 deaths annually
- Historically, untreated GABHS infection results in ARF in 0.1–0.3% of cases, with attack rates as high as 3% in endemic areas.
- 40% of patients with RHD did not have recognized ARF.
- Profound decrease in incidence in developed world due to increased use of antibiotics, improved living conditions, nutrition, and changing virulence patterns of GABHS strains

Prevalence

- 33 to 34 million people are affected by RHD worldwide; probable underestimation due to poor data collection in some parts of developing world
- RHD accounts for 25–40% of all cardiac disease worldwide.
- RHD accounts for greatest cardiovascular-related loss of disability-adjusted life years.

RISK FACTORS

Strongly associated with overcrowding and socioeconomic deprivation

Genetics

No specific genetic risk factor identified, although numerous studies have demonstrated polygenic association of ARF with specific human leukocyte antigen (HLA) alleles; concordance risk in twins.

GENERAL PREVENTION

- Primary prevention
  - Interventions to address poverty, crowding, and housing challenges
  - Appropriate and early treatment of GABHS pharyngitis
- Treatment of ARF
  - Antibiotics: full course of penicillin or equivalent to eradicate active infection; does not alter course of carditis
  - Anti-inflammatory: High-dose aspirin is standard; steroids may help for severe carditis but remain controversial.
  - Cardiac support: aggressive support of cardiac function and use of systemic afterload reduction for severe disease
  - Surgical valvuloplasty or valve replacement may be necessary in severe cases.
  - Bed rest: controversial; recommended at times for severe cases
- Surveillance screening for RHD
  - 10 times more RHD can be detected by echocardiography than auscultation.
  - Echocardiographic screening with handheld devices, including by nonexperts needs to be studied further before adoption.
- Secondary prevention of recurrence
  - Ideally administered as penicillin G benzathine as a monthly IM injection, but oral daily penicillin or erythromycin is acceptable in areas of low prevalence
  - Duration is based on clinical presentation and degree of cardiac involvement:
    - ARF without cardiac involvement: 5 years or until age 21 years, whichever is longer
    - ARF with mild or resolved carditis: 10 years or until age 21 years, whichever is longer
    - ARF with RHD: 10 years or until age 40 years, whichever is longer; consider lifelong if high risk.

PATHOPHYSIOLOGY

- GABHS triggers a complex inflammatory host response, affecting the heart, joints, brain, blood vessels, and subcutaneous tissue.
- Classic example of molecular mimicry, in which the host produces antibodies to certain GABHS antigens, which are similar in structure to host proteins such as vimentin (valve protein), myosin, resulting in cross-reactive autoimmune tissue damage
- Aschoff nodules are proliferative lesions noted in the myocardium that may persist for months to years after initiation of disease.
- New recognition of disease causing serotypes other than classical "rheumatogenic strains"

ETIOLOGY

Immune-mediated inflammatory reaction to specific rheumatogenic strains of GABHS

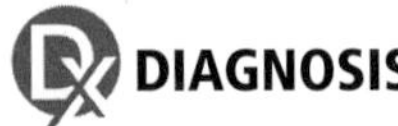

DIAGNOSIS

HISTORY

Diagnosis is based on the modified Jones criteria (updated 2015):

- Evidence of recent GABHS infection PLUS two major OR one major and two minor criteria for initial ARF; as above, OR three minor criteria for recurrent ARF
- Major criteria (% affected)
  - Polyarthritis (70%):
    - Migratory arthritis of major joints; more common in adults
    - Must by polyarthritis in low-risk populations, can also be monoarthritis or polyarthralgia in high-risk populations
  - Carditis (50–65%):
    - 85% of those with carditis have mitral regurgitation, and 54% have aortic valve involvement.
    - Symptoms range from asymptomatic murmur to fulminant heart failure; carditis is more common and more severe in children; usually endocarditis, pericarditis
    - Unclear if myocarditis occurs; can be subclinical carditis based on new echocardiographic criteria
  - Sydenham chorea (15%):
    - Abnormal behavior and/or involuntary, purposeless movements
  - Erythema marginatum (<5%):
    - Evanescent, pink rash with serpiginous borders
  - Subcutaneous nodules (<5%):
    - Painless nodules over extensor surfaces of large joints, the occiput, and/or vertebral processes
- Minor criteria
  - Fever: ≥38.5°C in low risk, ≥38°C in high risk
  - Arthralgia (mild pain without objective findings): must be polyarthralgia in low risk, can be monoarthralgia in high risk
  - Elevated acute-phase reactants: erythrocyte sedimentation rate (ESR), C-reactive protein
  - Prolongation of the PR interval on electrocardiogram (EKG)
- Exceptions to the Jones criteria include the following:
  - Sydenham chorea alone

PHYSICAL EXAM

- Cardiac
  - Murmur of valvulitis: holosystolic mitral regurgitant murmur, Carey-Coombs apical mid-diastolic murmur, or a basal diastolic murmur of aortic insufficiency (major criterion)
  - Pericardial friction rub: pericardial effusion
- Musculoskeletal
  - Pain, limited motion, erythema, warmth of two or more large joints: arthritis (major criterion)
- Neurologic
  - Choreiform movements (must be differentiated from tics, athetosis, and hyperkinesis)
  - Sydenham chorea (major criterion)
- Dermatologic
  - Evanescent, pink rash with pale centers and serpiginous borders on the trunk and proximal extremities: erythema marginatum (major criterion)
  - Firm, painless nodules over the extensor surface of large joints, occiput, and/or spinous processes: subcutaneous nodules (major criterion)

DIFFERENTIAL DIAGNOSIS

- Carditis
  - Viral
  - Bacterial
  - Rickettsial
  - Parasitic
  - *Mycoplasma* myocarditis
  - Kawasaki disease
- Arthritis
  - Poststreptococcal reactive arthritis (PSRA)
  - Serum sickness
  - Septic arthritis (e.g., gonococcal)
  - Lyme disease
- Collagen vascular disease
  - Juvenile rheumatoid arthritis (small joints, not migratory, and not relieved promptly with aspirin)
  - Systemic lupus erythematosus
  - Bacterial endocarditis
- Chorea
  - Congenital choreoathetosis
  - Brain tumors
  - Huntington chorea
  - Wilson disease
  - Pediatric autoimmune neuropsychiatric disorders associated with streptococcus (PANDAS)

- Hematologic disorders with joint involvement
  - Sickle cell anemia
  - Leukemia
- Congenital heart defects: previously undiagnosed valvular heart disease
- Mitral valve prolapse with regurgitation

DIAGNOSTIC TESTS & INTERPRETATION

- Specific tests:
  - No specific diagnostic test is available.
  - Research on biomarkers is ongoing.
- Nonspecific tests.
  - Throat culture: neither sensitive nor specific; false negative in up to 2/3 of affected patients or false positive in patients who are colonized
  - Elevated or rising streptococcal antibody titers, antistreptolysin O, anti-DNase B, and antihyaluronidase may be helpful.
  - ESR and C-reactive protein elevation
- EKG:
  - Prolonged PR interval (minor criterion), junctional rhythm, transient arrhythmias, ST-T wave changes
- Chest radiograph:
  - Cardiomegaly may indicate carditis or pericardial effusion.
  - Pulmonary edema may reflect left heart failure due to valvulitis.
- Echocardiogram:
  - Assess valve involvement, ventricular dilatation, function, and pericardial effusion
  - Able to detect subclinical carditis
  - New consensus criteria on echocardiographic findings included in Jones criteria

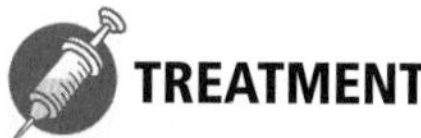

TREATMENT

MEDICATION

First Line

- Anti-inflammatory
  - Aspirin 100 mg/kg/24 h PO divided q6–8h; may be reduced to 60 to 70 mg/kg/24 h when fever and acute-phase reactants have normalized for 6 to 8 weeks
- Antibiotics in ARF
  - Penicillin V potassium
    - Children: 250 mg 2 to 3 times per day PO for 10 days
    - Adolescents, adults: 500 mg 2 to 3 times per day PO for 10 days
- Secondary prophylaxis
  - Penicillin G benzathine IM (600,000 U for weight <27 kg or 1,200,000 U for weight >27 kg) every 3 to 4 weeks

Second Line

- Anti-inflammatory
  - Prednisone 2 mg/kg/24 h PO for 2 weeks, then taper. Recent Cochrane review failed to show benefit of steroids to reduce risk of valvular heart disease.
- Antibiotics in ARF
  - Erythromycin, amoxicillin, 1st-generation cephalosporin
- Secondary prophylaxis
  - Penicillin V potassium 250 mg b.i.d. PO
  - Erythromycin, sulfadiazine

ISSUES FOR REFERRAL

Patients with new murmurs or clinical evidence of heart failure should be referred to a cardiologist.

ADDITIONAL THERAPIES

Treatment of chorea

- Usually supportive
- Phenobarbital and haloperidol are most commonly used; chlorpromazine, diazepam, or valproic acid also used

SURGERY/OTHER PROCEDURES

- Early valve repair for acute mitral regurgitation
- Aortic valve replacement for chronic RHD with aortic stenosis
- Surgical correction with valvotomy, commissurotomy, valve replacement for chronic RHD with mitral stenosis
- Catheter intervention
  - Balloon mitral valvotomy for mitral stenosis

ADMISSION, INPATIENT, AND NURSING CONSIDERATIONS

- Full treatment of streptococcal pharyngitis infection and cardiac support if heart failure present
- Treatment phases include primary prevention, management of ARF, and secondary prevention of recurrence.

ONGOING CARE

FOLLOW-UP RECOMMENDATIONS

- Patients without carditis
  - Close follow-up is needed for 2 to 3 weeks to assess patient's condition for development of acute carditis.
  - Long-term pediatric follow-up is needed to diagnose patients with indolent carditis.
  - Long-term follow-up is needed to evaluate patients who develop chorea.
  - Prophylaxis should be stressed even in patients without carditis.
- Patients with carditis
  - Cardiology follow-up is needed to assess development or evolution of RHD.
  - Symptoms of worsening heart failure suggest progression of valvular or myocardial disease, recurrent ARF, or endocarditis.
  - Secondary prophylaxis and bacterial endocarditis prophylaxis should be stressed.

PROGNOSIS

- 60–65% of patients develop RHD after ARF.
- ARF recurrence rate as high as 36% without prophylaxis
- Chorea may last weeks to months and has a similarly high recurrence rate.
- Carditis may resolve spontaneously (70–80%) or progress. Severity of the initial carditis is a major determinant of progression.

COMPLICATIONS

Long-term complications related to evolution of RHD

- Mitral stenosis
- Mitral regurgitation
- Aortic stenosis
- Aortic regurgitation
- Chronic heart failure

ADDITIONAL READING

- Cilliers A, Manyemba J, Adler AJ, et al. Anti-inflammatory treatment for carditis in acute rheumatic fever. *Cochrane Database Syst Rev*. 2012;(6):CD003176.
- Gewitz MH, Baltimore RS, Tani LY, et al. Revision of the Jones criteria for the diagnosis of acute rheumatic fever in the era of Doppler echocardiography: a scientific statement from the American Heart Association. *Circulation*. 2015;131(20):1806–1818.
- Essop MR, Peters F. Contemporary issues in rheumatic fever and chronic rheumatic heart disease. *Circulation*. 2014;130(24):2181–2188.
- Remenyi B, Carapetis J, Wyber R, et al. Position statement of the World Heart Federation on the prevention and control of rheumatic heart disease. *Nat Rev Cardiol*. 2013;10(5):284–292.
- Webb RH, Grant C, Harnden A. Acute rheumatic fever. *BMJ*. 2015;351:h3443.

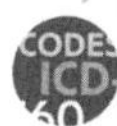

CODES

ICD10

- I00 Rheumatic fever without heart involvement
- I09.9 Rheumatic heart disease, unspecified
- M06.9 Rheumatoid arthritis, unspecified

FAQ

- Q: Does a negative throat culture rule out ARF?
- A: No. Throat cultures may be negative in 2/3 of patients.
- Q: Is there a vaccine available that is effective in preventing ARF?
- A: Not at present. Given that >90 antigenic strains of group A *Streptococcus* have been identified; vaccine development is focused on strains with the greatest virulence.
- Q: What genetic factors predispose to ARF?
- A: Patients with certain HLA-DR antigens are predisposed to ARF. The specific antigen/allele varies with the ethnic group.
- Q: Can EKG evidence of carditis alone be used to diagnose rheumatic fever?
- A: An EKG finding of carditis in the absence of a murmur does not fulfill the Jones criteria. However, many experts would agree to treat subclinical carditis as ARF, especially in areas of high prevalence.
- Q: What is the implication of subclinical carditis compared to clinical carditis on developing chronic RHD?
- A: It is unclear at present but some evidence suggests that echocardiographic evidence of carditis may be a better predictor for progression.
- Q: Who developed the Jones criteria?
- A: Thomas Duckett Jones, MD (1899 to 1954). Dr. Jones received his MD from the University of Virginia. He first presented the criteria in a lecture entitled, "Diagnosis of Rheumatic Fever" in 1944 at the American Medical Association Symposium on Rheumatic Fever in Chicago, Illinois.

RHINITIS, ALLERGIC

Esther K. Chung, MD, MPH

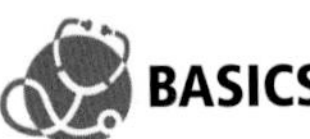

BASICS

DESCRIPTION

- Inflammation of the nasal and sinus mucosae, associated with sneezing, swelling, increased mucus production, and nasal obstruction; may be classified as seasonal, perennial, or a combination
  - Seasonal: periodic symptoms, involving the same season for at least 2 consecutive years; most often due to pollens (e.g., trees, grass, weeds) and outdoor spores
  - Perennial: occurring at least 9 months of the year; may be more difficult to detect because of overlap with viral infections; may be due to multiple seasonal allergies or continual exposure to allergens (e.g., dust mites, cockroaches, molds, and animal dander)
  - Perennial, with seasonal exacerbations
- The Allergic Rhinitis and its Impact on Asthma (ARIA) World Health Organization expert panel prefer the classification for allergic rhinitis of intermittent or persistent, with subclassifications of mild, moderate, or severe.

EPIDEMIOLOGY

Prevalence

Most common allergic disease, affecting approximately 40 million Americans; affects 40% of children and 15–30% of adolescents

RISK FACTORS

Genetics

Increased incidence in families with atopic disease. If one parent has allergies, each child has approximately a 30% chance of having an allergy; if both parents have allergies, each child has a 70% chance of having an allergy.

GENERAL PREVENTION

- Minimize exposure to dust mites: Consider removal of carpets, upholstered furniture, and curtains; wash bedding in hot water (130°F for at least 10 minutes) at least every 1 to 2 weeks; use pillow and mattress covers; use of acaricides to kill dust mites
- Minimize exposure to animal dander and all animals; consider using solutions containing tannic acid, which will denature animal allergens; shampoo pets frequently if they cannot be removed from the household; use air vent filters or air-filtration systems.
- Minimize exposure to pollens: Keep windows closed, use air-conditioning, and avoid leaf raking or lawn mowing.
- Minimize exposure to molds: Keep houseplants out of the bedroom; avoid spending time in the basement; keep humidity at 35–50%.

ETIOLOGY

- Indoor allergens: house dust mite, cockroaches, animal dander, cigarette smoke, hair spray, paint, molds
- Pollens: tree pollens in early spring, grass in late spring and early summer, ragweed in late summer and autumn
- Multiple environmental factors
- Changes in air temperature

COMMONLY ASSOCIATED CONDITIONS

- Asthma
- Allergic conjunctivitis
- Atopic dermatitis (eczema)
- Pollen food allergy syndrome (PFAS)
- Urticaria
- Otitis media with effusion
- Sleep, taste, and/or smell disturbance
- Nasal polyps
- Mouth breathing
- Snoring and sleep-disordered breathing
- Adenoidal hypertrophy
- Decreased appetite
- Delayed speech

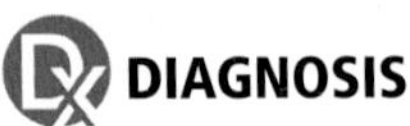

DIAGNOSIS

HISTORY

- Typical symptoms: Patient often reports bilateral stuffy nose, sneezing, itching, runny nose, noisy breathing, snoring, cough, halitosis, and repeated throat clearing. Sensation of plugged ears and wheezing may occur.
- Red and itchy eyes
- Symptom occurrence: seasonal, perennial, or episodic
- Exacerbating factors including pollen, animals, cigarette smoke, dust, molds
- Family history of atopic disease such as asthma or atopic dermatitis
- Any related illnesses: Asthma, urticaria, eczema, ear infections, and delayed speech are commonly associated conditions.

PHYSICAL EXAM

- Allergic shiners
  - Dark discoloration beneath the eyes due to obstruction of lymphatic and venous drainage, chronic nasal obstruction, and suborbital edema
- Dennie-Morgan lines
  - Creases in the lower eyelid radiating outward from the inner canthus; caused by spasm in the muscles of Müller around eye due to chronic congestion and stasis of blood
- Allergic salute
  - A gesture characterized by rubbing the nose with the palm of the hand upward to decrease itching and temporarily open the nasal passages
- Allergic crease
  - Transverse crease near the tip of the nose, secondary to rubbing
- Nasal mucosa may appear pale and/or edematous; mucoid or watery material may be seen in the nasal cavity; check for nasal polyps and septal deviation.

DIFFERENTIAL DIAGNOSIS

- Infection
  - Viral upper respiratory tract infection
  - Bacterial sinusitis
- Environmental
  - Foreign body
  - Temperature
  - Odors
- Tumors
  - Nasal polyps
  - Dermoid cyst
  - Nasal glioma
- Congenital
  - Cystic fibrosis
  - Choanal atresia
  - Ciliary motility disorder (e.g., immotile cilia syndrome)
  - Septal deviation
  - Primary atrophic rhinitis
- Immunologic
  - Sarcoidosis
  - Granulomatosis with polyangiitis
  - Systemic lupus erythematosus
  - Sjögren syndrome
- Miscellaneous
  - Nonallergic perennial rhinitis
  - Idiopathic (vasomotor) rhinitis
  - Drug-induced rhinitis
  - Food-induced rhinitis
  - Rhinitis medicamentosa
  - Rhinitis associated with pregnancy/other hormonal rhinitis
  - Hypothyroidism
  - Idiopathic neonatal rhinitis

DIAGNOSTIC TESTS & INTERPRETATION

Initial Tests (screening, lab, imaging)

- Audiometry and tympanometry when indicated
- Sweat test if cystic fibrosis is suspected or if nasal polyps present
- Nasal cytology
- Specimen of nasal discharge to check for the presence of eosinophils. Have the patient blow his or her nose into a piece of nonporous paper or collect discharge with a cotton swab and transfer the discharge to a glass slide. >10% eosinophils are considered positive for nasal eosinophilia. Note: Use of intranasal steroids may reduce the number of eosinophils found in nasal discharge.
- Radioallergosorbent test (RAST)
  - In vitro test to measure allergen-specific IgE; expensive; useful in patients who do not respond to empiric therapy, when diagnosis is uncertain, or when avoidance of causative allergen is desired. The ImmunoCAP® system (Pharmacia Diagnostics) is the preferred method for specific IgE testing; uses a single blood sample to identify levels of specific IgE to a number of common respiratory allergens (available as a profile specific to the region of the country where the patient resides), food antigens (food allergy profile), or both (childhood allergy profile)
- CBC: may show eosinophilia; not routinely indicated
- Skin testing
  - Skin prick test: qualitative test in which antigen concentrate is placed on the skin of the volar surface of the arm or upper back, and a needle is inserted; high negative predictive value; the skin reaction is graded subjectively from 0 to 4.
  - Intradermal test: qualitative test in which antigen is introduced intradermally (0.02 mL with a 26- to 30-gauge needle); more sensitive than the prick test and often used if prick test is negative or equivocal; the degree of swelling and erythema is graded from 0 to 4.
  - Caution: Skin tests may be difficult to interpret in patients with diffuse eczema and dermatographism.
  - Although positive allergen-specific IgE testing or skin prick testing denote sensitization to an allergen, these tests must be interpreted in the context of the clinical presentation.

Diagnostic Procedures/Other

- Rhinoscopy to assess the nasal turbinates and to look for nasal polyps
- Avoid routine sinonasal imaging.

TREATMENT

GENERAL MEASURES

- Avoidance therapy: Identify and eliminate known/suspected allergens.
- Improve mucociliary flow.
  - Steam inhalation
  - Normal saline drops

MEDICATION

- Antihistamines: particularly useful when sneezing and itching are present; competitively block histamine (H_1) receptors; suppress itching, ocular symptoms, sneezing, and rhinorrhea; not very effective against nasal congestion
- 2nd-generation antihistamines: tend not to cross the blood–brain barrier and therefore do not have CNS side effects such as drowsiness
  - Loratadine (Claritin®): U.S. Food and Drug Administration (FDA)-approved for children as young as 2 years of age. Dose: ages 2 to 5 years, 5 mg/24 h PO; ages ≥6 years, 10 mg/24 h PO
  - Desloratadine (Clarinex®): FDA-approved for children ≥6 months of age. Dose: 6 to 12 months, 1 mg/24 h PO; 12 months to 5 years, 1.25 mg/24 h PO; 6 to 11 years, 2.5 mg/24 h PO; ≥12 years, 5 mg/24 h PO
  - Cetirizine HCl (Zyrtec®): FDA-approved for children as young as 6 months of age. Dose: age 6 months to 5 years, 2.5 mg = 1/2 tsp/24 h (1 mg/mL banana-grape flavored–syrup) PO with maximum dose of 5 mg/24 h (must be divided into 2.5 mg b.i.d. for children <2 years of age); age ≥6 years, 5 to 10 mg/24 h
  - Levocetirizine (Xyzal®): dose: age 6 months to 5 years: 1.25 mg/24 h (1/2 tsp = 2.5 mL); ages 6 to 11 years: 2.5 mg/24 h (half tab or 1 tsp = 5 mL) PO; age ≥12 years: 5 mg/24 h (1 tab or 2 tsp = 10 mL) PO
  - Fexofenadine HCl (Allegra®): ages 2 to 11 years: 1 tsp = 5 mL (30 mg/5 mL) or 30-mg tab b.i.d.; age ≥12 years, 60 mg b.i.d. or 180 mg/24 h PO
- 1st-generation antihistamine side effects include drowsiness, performance impairment, and paradoxical excitement; anticholinergic effects (e.g., dry mouth, tachycardia, urinary retention, and constipation): diphenhydramine (Benadryl®) 5 mg/kg/24 h PO divided q.i.d.
- Intranasal steroids: indicated when symptoms affect quality of life; blunt early-phase reactions and block late-phase reactions; may not be fully effective until several days to 2 weeks following initiation; must be used regularly and best when administered lying down with the head back
  - Beclomethasone (Vancenase®, Beconase®): for use in children ≥6 years of age
  - Flunisolide: for use in children ≥6 years of age
  - Fluticasone propionate (Flonase® 0.05%): for use in children ≥4 years of age
  - Budesonide (Rhinocort®): for use in children ≥6 years of age
  - Triamcinolone acetonide (Nasacort®): for use in children ≥2 years of age
  - Mometasone furoate monohydrate (Nasonex®): for children ≥2 years of age
- Intranasal antihistamines:
  - Azelastine hydrochloride (Astelin®; approved for children ≥2 years; 2 to 5 years [use 0.1% product]: 1 spray to each nostril b.i.d.; 6 to 11 years [0.1% or 0.15% product]: 1 spray to each nostril b.i.d.; ≥12 years [0.1% or 0.15% product]: 1 or 2 sprays to each nostril b.i.d.)
  - Olopatadine (Patanase®; approved for children ≥6 years; 6 to 11 years: 1 spray per nostril b.i.d.; ≥12 years: 2 sprays per nostril b.i.d.) are FDA-approved for use in seasonal allergic rhinitis.
- Combination intranasal antihistamine and corticosteroid: indicated when monotherapy is not effective; azelastine C and fluticasone (Dymista®); approved for children ≥6 years: 1 spray to each nostril b.i.d.
- Topical cromolyn (Nasalcrom®): considered to be alternative therapy; mast cell stabilizer; minimal side effects; t.i.d. to q.i.d. dosing; does not provide immediate relief (may take 2 to 4 weeks to see clinical effect): for use in children ≥2 years of age
- Oral decongestants: α-1 and -2 agonists (e.g., ephedrine, pseudoephedrine, and phenylephrine) act to cause vasoconstriction, decreased blood supply to the nasal mucosa, and decreased mucosal edema. Cardiovascular and CNS side effects include tremors, agitation, hypertension, insomnia, and headaches.
- Topical decongestants: Sympathomimetics such as short-acting phenylephrine (Neo-Synephrine®) and long-acting oxymetazoline (Afrin®) may be useful short-term to open nasal passages to allow for delivery of topical steroids; side effects include drying of the mucosa and burning. Prolonged use may result in rebound vasodilatation and congestion (rhinitis medicamentosa).
- Combined oral decongestants and antihistamines: numerous preparations on the market
- Leukotriene receptor antagonist montelukast (Singulair®): not recommended as primary therapy; for use in children ≥6 months of age. Dose for 6 months to 23 months, one packet 4-mg granules; 2 to 5 years, 1 granule packet (4 mg) or 4-mg chewable tab daily; 6 to 14 years, 5-mg chewable tab daily; age ≥15 years, 10-mg tab daily
- Immunotherapy (i.e., hyposensitization or desensitization): consists of a series of injections with specific allergens with increasing concentrations of allergens, once or twice weekly; recommended for patients who have not responded to pharmacologic therapy; may also consist of repeated use of full or short escalation in dose of sublingual tablets or drops
  - Effective and long lasting. After several months to years of treatment, total serum IgE levels decrease, and the intensity of the early-phase response is reduced.
  - Side effects to injections include urticaria, bronchospasm, hypotension, and anaphylaxis. Side effects to sublingual forms include mouth swelling, throat irritation, tongue/ears/mouth itching, and anaphylaxis.

SURGERY/OTHER PROCEDURES

- Removal of allergic polyps
- Inferior turbinate surgery to reduce the size of the turbinate and relieve obstruction if patients fail medical management
- Endoscopic sinus surgery to relieve obstruction

ONGOING CARE

FOLLOW-UP RECOMMENDATIONS

Patient Monitoring

Fever, prolonged or severe headache, dizziness, pain, or purulent discharge suggests a diagnosis other than allergic rhinitis alone.

PROGNOSIS

Generally good: Complete recovery occurs in 5–10% of patients.

COMPLICATIONS

- Chronic sinusitis
- Recurrent otitis media
- Hoarseness
- Loss of smell
- Loss of hearing
- High-arched palate and dental malocclusion from chronic mouth breathing
- Disorders of learning performance, behavior, and attention

ADDITIONAL READING

- Berger WE, Meltzer EO. Intranasal spray medications for maintenance therapy of allergic rhinitis. *Am J Rhinol Allergy*. 2015;29(4):273–282.
- Brozek JL, Bousquet J, Baena-Cagnani CE, et al. Allergic Rhinitis and its Impact on Asthma (ARIA) guidelines: 2010 revision. *J Allergy Clin Immunol*. 2010;126(3):466–476.
- Nelson H, Cartier S, Allen-Ramey F, et al. Network meta-analysis shows commercialized subcutaneous and sublingual grass products have comparable efficacy. *J Allergy Clin Immunol Pract*. 2015;3(2):256–266.e3.
- Scadding GK. Optimal management of allergic rhinitis. *Arch Dis Child*. 2015;100(6):576–582.
- Seidman MD, Gurgel RK, Lin SY, et al. Clinical practice guideline: allergic rhinitis executive summary. *Otolaryngol Head Neck Surg*. 2015;152(2):197–206.
- Sicherer SH, Wood RA; for American Academy of Pediatrics Section on Allergy and Immunology. Allergy testing in childhood: using allergen-specific IgE tests. *Pediatrics*. 2012;129(1):193–197.
- Wheatley LM, Togias A. Clinical practice. Allergic rhinitis. *N Engl J Med*. 2015;372(5):456–463.

CODES

ICD10

- J30.9 Allergic rhinitis, unspecified
- J30.1 Allergic rhinitis due to pollen
- J30.89 Other allergic rhinitis

FAQ

- Q: How does one minimize exposure to dust mites?
- A: Keep household temperature low; maintain humidity at ~40–50%; wash linens weekly at hot temperatures; use a microfilter when vacuuming; place mattress and box spring in tightly woven casing; use air-conditioning; use high-efficiency particulate air filter units.
- Q: How often are nasal polyps associated with cystic fibrosis?
- A: In up to 40% of children, nasal polyps are associated with cystic fibrosis. <0.5% of children with asthma and rhinitis have nasal polyps.
- Q: When used on a daily basis, are intranasal corticosteroids safe?
- A: Yes. It is generally accepted that inhaled corticosteroids are safe. Growth suppression has been reported in children using certain intranasal steroids; however, this effect does not appear to be an effect of all intranasal steroids. Importantly, one should use the lowest effective dose of intranasal corticosteroids when treating allergic rhinitis.

RICKETS/OSTEOMALACIA

Alison Boyce, MD

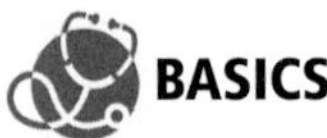

BASICS

DESCRIPTION
- Osteomalacia refers to impaired bone mineralization, caused primarily by deficiencies in vitamin D, calcium, and/or phosphate.
- In children, osteomalacia can lead to growth plate abnormalities, termed rickets.

EPIDEMIOLOGY
- The prevalences of rickets and osteomalacia are very high in many parts of the world.
- Reported with increasing frequency in the United States since the 1980s

GENERAL PREVENTION
- Vitamin D supplements should be provided to breastfed infants and high-risk individuals.
- In the United States and Canada, cow's milk, infant formula, and cereals are fortified with vitamin D.

PATHOPHYSIOLOGY
Rickets arises due to decreased availability of phosphorus and calcium to mineralize the skeletal matrix, leading to growth plate disorganization and accumulation of undermineralized osteoid. This results in growth plate expansion, bone weakening, and skeletal deformities.

ETIOLOGY
Primary causes include the following:
- Nutritional
  - Insufficient vitamin D and/or calcium intakes (common)
  - Insufficient phosphorus intake (rare)
- Deficient sunlight exposure
- Malabsorption
  - Celiac disease
  - Cystic fibrosis
  - Liver disease
- Renal tubular defects
  - Cystinosis
  - Fanconi syndrome
  - Renal tubular acidosis
- Abnormalities in vitamin D metabolism
  - Anticonvulsant use
  - Liver disease
- Genetic forms (see "Table 1")

RISK FACTORS
- Infants born to vitamin D–deficient mothers
- Low birth weight and/or prematurity
- Breastfeeding without vitamin D supplementation
- Poor nutrition
- Increased skin pigmentation
- Higher latitudes and winter months
- Sunscreen use
- Malabsorption
- Renal tubulopathies

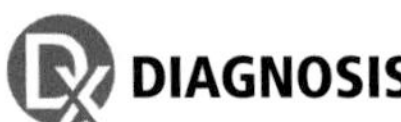

DIAGNOSIS

HISTORY
- Inadequate nutrition
  - Low dietary calcium intake
  - Strict vegan diet without adequate calcium
  - Prolonged breastfeeding without vitamin D supplementation
  - Premature infants taking unfortified formula
  - Parenteral hyperalimentation
- Low levels of sunlight exposure
- Anticonvulsant use
- Bone pain
- Fractures following minimal trauma
- Dental abscesses
- Malabsorption symptoms:
  - Steatorrhea, abdominal pain, weight loss
- Renal tubular dysfunction symptoms:
  - Nephrolithiasis, polyuria
- Irritability
- Generalized muscular weakness
- Delayed gross motor development
- Family history of rickets

PHYSICAL EXAM
- Growth deceleration
- Hypotonia
- Widening at the wrists, knees, and/or ankles
- Bowing of the extremities (varus or valgus deformities)
- Scoliosis
- Waddling gait
- Skull abnormalities
  - Anterior fontanelle widening and/or delayed closure
  - Frontal bossing
  - Craniotabes (softening of the skull)
- Chest deformities
  - Prominent costochondral junctions ("rachitic rosary")
  - Pectus carinatum
  - Horizontal groove along the lower ribs ("Harrison groove")

DIAGNOSTIC TESTS & INTERPRETATION

Initial Tests (screening, lab, imaging)
- 25-vitamin D
  - Major circulating form and most sensitive indicator of vitamin D stores
  - Sometimes reported as D_2 (plant derived) and D_3 (animal derived) forms
  - $D_2 + D_3$ = total available 25-vitamin D
- Serum calcium, phosphorous (make sure age-appropriate norms for phosphorus are used by lab), and alkaline phosphatase
- Intact parathyroid hormone (PTH)
- Spot urine calcium, creatinine, and urinalysis
- If rarer forms of rickets being considered: 1,25-vitamin D, urine phosphorus
- Radiographic findings:
  - Growth plate widening, cupping, and/or fraying
  - Expansion of anterior ribs at the costochondral junctions
  - Long bone bowing
  - Osteopenia
- Knee or wrist films may be used diagnostically and to monitor treatment response.

DIFFERENTIAL DIAGNOSIS
- See Table 1 for primary differential and ways to differentiate these forms of rickets.
- Blount disease
- Chronic recurrent multifocal osteomyelitis
- Metaphyseal chondrodysplasia
- Neurofibromatosis type 1
- Renal osteodystrophy (combines features of rickets, osteomalacia, secondary hyperparathyroidism, and osteoporosis)

Table 1. Biochemical Features of Rickets/Osteomalacia

	Ca	Phos	Alk phos	iPTH	25-(OH)D	$1,25\text{-}(OH)_2D$	Urine Ca/ Cr	TRP
Nutritional/insufficient sunlight	N or ↓	↓	↑	↑	↓	↑	↓	↑
Malabsorption	N or ↓	↓	↑	↑	↓	↑	↓	↑
Renal tubular defects	N or ↓	↓	↑	↑	N	↑	↑	N or ↓
Altered vitamin D metabolism	N or ↓	↓	↑	↑	↓	↑	↓	↑
Genetic forms of rickets								
X-linked, AD, and AR hypophosphatemic rickets	N	↓	↑	N or ↑	N	N or ↑	N or ↓	↓
1α-hydroxylase deficiency	↓	↓	↑	↑	N	↓	↓	↑
Vitamin D receptor mutations (Vitamin D resistance)	↓	↓	↑	↑	N	↑	↓	↑
Hereditary hypophosphatemic rickets with hypercalciuria	N or ↓	↓	↑	↑	N	↑	↑	↓
Hypophosphatasia	N or ↑	N or ↑	↓	N or ↓	N	N or ↓	N or ↑	N

Ca, calcium; Phos, phosphorus; Alk phos, alkaline phosphatase; iPTH, intact parathyroid hormone; 25-(OH)D, 25-vitamin D; $1,25\text{-}(OH)_2D$, 1,25-dihydroxyvitamin D; Ca/Cr, calcium/creatinine ratio; TRP, tubular reabsorption of phosphorus ([1− (U phos × P Cr/U Cr × S Phos)] × 100, normal 85–95%); N, normal; AD, autosomal dominant; AR, autosomal recessive.

Table 2. Dietary Reference Intake for Calcium and Vitamin D

	Calcium			Vitamin D		
Age	Estimated Average Requirement (mg/day)	Recommended Dietary Allowance (mg/day)	Upper Level Intake (mg/day)	Estimated Average Requirement (IU/day)	Recommended Dietary Allowance (IU/day)	Upper Level Intake (IU/day)
0–6 months	200	200	1,000	400	400	1,000
6–12 months	260	260	1,500	400	400	1,500
1–3 years	500	700	2,500	400	600	2,500
4–8 years	800	1,000	2,500	400	600	3,000
9–18 years	1,100	1,300	3,000	400	600	4,000
19–30 years	800	1,000	2,500	400	600	4,000

Adapted from Ross C, Abrams S, Aloia J, et al. *Dietary Reference Intakes for Calcium and Vitamin D*. Washington, DC: National Academies Press; 2011.

R

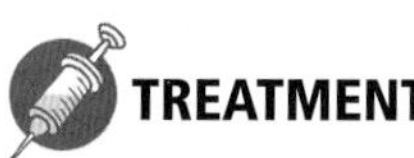

TREATMENT

GENERAL MEASURES

Treatment depends on the underlying etiology.

ADDITIONAL THERAPIES

- Treatment of vitamin D deficiency: high dose repletion with cholecalciferol (vitamin D_3) over 8 to 12 weeks (goal total of ~200,000 to 400,000 IU)
  - Infants <1 month: 1,000 IU daily
  - Infants and children 1 month to 5 years: 1,000 to 2,000 IU daily
  - Children 5 years to adult: 5,000 to 6,000 IU daily or single dose of 150,000 to 300,000 intramuscular
- Following repletion, transition to daily maintenance dose (see "Table 2").
- Supplement with 30 to 75 mg/kg/24 h elemental calcium divided t.i.d. to prevent hungry bone syndrome (hypocalcemia and hypophosphatemia during healing).
- Higher doses of vitamin D often required in patients with malabsorption, altered vitamin D metabolism, and/or obesity
- Optimal serum 25-vitamin D concentrations are controversial; however, concentrations >20 ng/mL (50 nmol/L) are sufficient to prevent rickets in otherwise healthy children.

ISSUES FOR REFERRAL

- Consider endocrinology referral for infants, children with hypocalcemia, severe disease, suspected genetic forms of rickets, and/or lack of radiographic evidence of healing by 3 months.
- Nephrology referral for management of tubular dysfunction
- Orthopedic referral for patients with bowing, scoliosis

ADMISSION, INPATIENT, AND NURSING CONSIDERATIONS

- Rickets can generally be managed in the outpatient setting; however, inpatient admission may be considered if:
  - Severe hypocalcemia with tetany or seizures
  - Lack of response to therapy (suspected nonadherence)
- Discharge criteria
  - Stable laboratory values
  - Normalization in mental status and neurologic exam improvement

ONGOING CARE

FOLLOW-UP RECOMMENDATIONS

Patient Monitoring

- Monitor serum calcium, phosphorus, alkaline phosphatase, PTH, and spot urinary calcium/creatinine ratio every 2 to 4 weeks. Note: Alkaline phosphatase may rise initially with treatment and then decrease gradually.
- Consider follow-up imaging after completion of high-dose vitamin D repletion.
- Patients who continue high-dose vitamin D for longer than prescribed may be at risk for hypercalcemia.

PATIENT EDUCATION

Ensure appropriate vitamin D and calcium intake to prevent recurrence (see "Table 2").

PROGNOSIS

- Rickets generally resolves with appropriate treatment.
- If radiographs and/or biochemical parameters not improving, consider the possibility of poor adherence, other forms of rickets, or alternative diagnoses.

COMPLICATIONS

- Failure to thrive, poor motor development
- Hypocalcemic tetany and seizures
- Bowing and skeletal deformity
- Fractures

ADDITIONAL READING

- Creo AL, Thacher TD, Pettifor JM, et al. Nutritional rickets around the world: an update. *Paediatr Int Child Health*. 2017;37(2):84–98.
- Holick MF, Binkley NC, Bischoff-Ferrari HA, et al; for Endocrine Society. Evaluation, treatment, and prevention of vitamin D deficiency: an Endocrine Society clinical practice guideline. *J Clin Endocrinol Metab*. 2011;96(7):1911–1930.
- Munns CF, Shaw N, Kiely M, et al. Global consensus recommendations on prevention and management of nutritional rickets. *J Clin Endocrinol Metab*. 2016;101(2):394–415.
- National Institutes of Health. Kids and their bones: a guide for parents. https://www.bones.nih.gov/health-info/bone/bone-health/juvenile. Accessed May 20, 2018.
- Ross AC, Manson JE, Abrams SA, et al. The 2011 report on dietary reference intakes for calcium and vitamin D from the Institute of Medicine: what clinicians need to know. *J Clin Endocrinol Metab*. 2011;96(1):53–58.
- Shaw NJ, Mughal MZ. Vitamin D and child health part 1 (skeletal aspects). *Arch Dis Child*. 2013;98(5):363–367.
- Vogiatzi MG, Jacobson-Dickman E, DeBoer MD; for the Drugs and Therapeutics Committee of the Pediatric Endocrine Society. Vitamin D supplementation and risk of toxicity in pediatrics: a review of current literature. *J Clin Endocrinol Metab*. 2014;99(4):1132–1141.

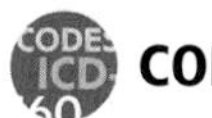

CODES

ICD10

- E55.0 Rickets, active
- E55.9 Vitamin D deficiency, unspecified
- E58 Dietary calcium deficiency

FAQ

- Q: What is the best way to diagnose rickets?
- A: Laboratory evaluation and radiographs are the best ways to make the diagnosis. Radiographic findings are best seen at the distal radius and ulna, and/or the distal femur and proximal tibia.
- Q: What are the recommendations for vitamin D supplementation in infants and children?
- A: The American Academy of Pediatrics (AAP) recommends the following:
  - All breastfed infants should receive 400 IU daily.
  - Nonbreastfed infants ingesting <500 mL/day of vitamin D–fortified formula or milk should receive 400 IU daily.
  - Children who do not get regular sunlight exposure or do not consume at least 500 mL/day of vitamin D–fortified milk should receive 600 IU daily.
- Q: How is rickets/osteomalacia different from osteoporosis?
- A: Osteoporosis in children is defined by a combination of decreased bone mass and fractures. Although bone density is reduced, bone matrix is generally normally mineralized. In rickets/osteomalacia, the primary defect is impaired mineralization of the underlying bone matrix. Osteoporosis and rickets/osteomalacia both result in an increased fracture risk; however, osteoporosis does not generally lead to growth plate and long bone deformities.

RICKETTSIAL DISEASE

Camille Sabella, MD

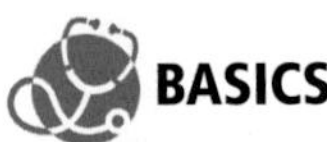

BASICS

DESCRIPTION

- Disorders caused by the *Rickettsiae* family of organisms including those which cause Rocky Mountain spotted fever and other similar tick-borne illnesses, the typhus group, and the organisms that cause ehrlichiosis and anaplasmosis
- All organisms are obligate intracellular gram-negative bacteria and therefore are difficult to grow in culture.
- The diseases caused by each group of organisms are similar, encompassing a syndrome including fever, rash, headache, and capillary leak; all are transmitted via an insect vector.

GENERAL PREVENTION

- Fleas, ticks, and mites should be controlled in endemic areas with the appropriate insecticides.
- Clothing to cover the entire body should be worn in tick-infested areas. In the case of a recognized bite, ticks should be removed from human skin properly, with care not to expel the contents of the tick's stomach into the site of the bite.
- In areas where louse-borne typhus is epidemic, periodic delousing and dusting of insecticide into clothes are recommended.
- Paradoxic effect of rodenticides:
  - Fleas and mites seek alternate hosts (i.e., humans) when mice or rats are not present.
  - Therefore, rodenticides should not be the only preventive measure taken in endemic areas.
- Except for scrub typhus, all rickettsial diseases produce long-term immunity to the etiologic organisms within the same group.

PATHOPHYSIOLOGY

- Spotted fever, typhus, ehrlichiosis, and anaplasmosis groups cause vasculitis as a result of organisms invading the endothelial cells of small blood vessels or white blood cells.
- This vasculitis manifests as rash in cutaneous tissues and systemic illness due to capillary leak throughout other organs.

ETIOLOGY

- Spotted fever group *Rickettsia* and the agents of ehrlichiosis and anaplasmosis (*Ehrlichia* and *Anaplasma* species) are transmitted to humans by ticks.
- Rickettsialpox and scrub typhus are transmitted by mites associated with mice.
- Epidemic typhus is a louse-borne illness, and endemic typhus, also known as murine typhus, is transmitted by fleas.
- The rickettsial diseases that occur in the United States are Rocky Mountain spotted fever, murine typhus, rickettsialpox, epidemic typhus, ehrlichiosis, and anaplasmosis.

DIAGNOSIS

HISTORY

- In general, rickettsial disease should be considered as a diagnosis in a patient with fever, headache, and rash. Progression of rash can be particularly helpful in considering the diagnosis.
- Signs and symptoms:
  - Spotted fever group
    - Illness often begins with fever, myalgia, and headache.
    - Rash occurs 3 to 5 days following onset of symptoms and is typically described as centripetal, beginning on hands and feet and moving toward the trunk. Rash is variable and may not always follow this pattern.
    - Other symptoms include headache, neurologic changes, hypotension, hyponatremia, and consumptive coagulopathy.
    - Fulminant Rocky Mountain spotted fever may cause cardiovascular collapse.
  - Rickettsialpox
    - Similar to spotted fever group, although less severe and with fewer systemic symptoms; rash often includes an inoculation eschar.
  - Typhus group
    - Epidemic typhus is transmitted by the human body louse and causes fever, headache, and rash that can progress to pulmonary symptoms, neurologic disease, and death.
    - Endemic typhus is transmitted by fleas associated with rodents and causes symptoms similar to epidemic typhus although with a less prevalent rash.
    - Scrub typhus is also similar but causes marked neurologic symptoms including mental status changes.
  - Ehrlichiosis/anaplasmosis
    - Spectrum of illnesses including human monocytotropic ehrlichiosis and human granulocytotropic anaplasmosis that cause fever, headache, and myalgias similar to the spotted fever group.
    - Rash is less common as compared to spotted fever and occurs in about 60% of children in ehrlichiosis and very few in anaplasmosis.

PHYSICAL EXAM

- All rickettsial diseases cause fever and the majority cause rash.
- These three findings suggest illness caused by the spotted fever group:
  - Hypotension, cardiovascular instability
  - Hepatosplenomegaly
  - *Tache noire* (French for black spot): The earliest finding in the spotted fever group, this lesion originates at the site of the infecting bite and may form eschar with regional lymphadenopathy related to the eschar. The lesion is usually found on the head in children and on the legs in adults; present in 30–90% of cases
- These three findings suggest illness caused by the typhus group:
  - Impaired level of consciousness
  - Pulmonary and renal involvement
  - Brill-Zinsser disease is actually a recrudescence of a previous infection with epidemic (louse-borne) typhus caused by *Rickettsia prowazekii*; can occur years after the initial infection and is usually less severe than the initial episode of louse-borne typhus

- These findings suggest ehrlichiosis:
  - Acute febrile illness characterized by headache and myalgia
  - Rash in ~60%; spares palms, soles, and face
  - Thrombocytopenia, leukopenia (lymphopenia), hyponatremia, and elevated liver function tests
- These findings suggest anaplasmosis:
  - Acute febrile illness characterized by headache and myalgia
  - Thrombocytopenia, leukopenia (neutropenia), hyponatremia, and elevated liver function tests

DIFFERENTIAL DIAGNOSIS

- Before rash appears, constitutional symptoms associated with the spotted fevers result in a broad differential diagnosis. After rash appears, the diagnoses are more limited.
- Infectious:
  - Measles
  - Meningococcemia
  - Secondary syphilis
  - Coxsackievirus (e.g., hand, foot, and mouth disease)
  - Infectious mononucleosis
  - Enteroviral infection
- Environmental (poisons)
- Drug hypersensitivity reaction (i.e., toxicodermatosis)
- Tumors: leukemia with thrombocytopenia
- Immunologic: idiopathic thrombocytopenia purpura
- Miscellaneous:
  - Leukocytoclastic angiitis
  - Erythema multiforme/Stevens-Johnson syndrome

DIAGNOSTIC TESTS & INTERPRETATION

Initial Tests (screening, lab, imaging)

- Serologic testing has been the standard for laboratory diagnosis of rickettsial disease because the organisms are obligate intracellular bacteria and do not grow in culture.
- Serologic tests are available for all rickettsial organisms. There is some cross-reactivity among similar organisms.
- Serologic testing is often negative at the onset of illness and requires a convalescent (paired) sample done 2 to 3 weeks later for comparison. If the convalescent titer is 4-fold or greater than the acute, it is considered positive.
- Polymerase chain reaction (PCR) tests are becoming more commonly used to diagnose these infections; they appear to be sensitive and offer earlier diagnosis than serology.

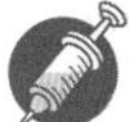

TREATMENT

GENERAL MEASURES

- Fluid resuscitation and respiratory support as indicated
- Antimicrobial therapy should be instituted as soon as the diagnosis is suspected and should not be delayed while awaiting serologic confirmation.
- Patients may require blood product transfusion in the case of consumptive coagulopathy or severe thrombocytopenia.

MEDICATION

- The 1st-line antibiotic treatment for all rickettsial diseases is doxycycline. Therapy is most effective if instituted within the 1st week of illness.
- Antibiotics should be given for 7 to 14 days.
  - Studies have shown that there is little risk of tooth staining in children <8 years old who receive doxycycline.
  - In the case of rickettsial disease, the benefit of giving doxycycline far outweighs the risk of adverse effects.

ONGOING CARE

PROGNOSIS

Improvement in the patient's clinical status usually takes place within 1 to 2 weeks after therapy starts, depending on the severity of illness. This improvement may also be delayed if treatment is begun after the 1st week of illness.

COMPLICATIONS

- Venous thrombosis
- Disseminated intravascular coagulation
- Cardiac injury including endocarditis
- Severe disease is more common in patients with glucose-6-phosphate dehydrogenase (G6PD) deficiency, cardiac insufficiency, or immunodeficiency.

ADDITIONAL READING

- Buckingham SC, Marshall GS, Schutze GE, et al; for Tick-borne Infections in Children Study Group. Clinical and laboratory features, hospital course, and outcome of Rocky Mountain spotted fever in children. *J Pediatr.* 2007;150(2):180–184.e1.
- Chapman AS, Bakken JS, Folk SM, et al; and Tickborne Rickettsial Diseases Working Group, Centers for Disease Control and Prevention. Diagnosis and management of tickborne rickettsial diseases: Rocky Mountain spotted fever, ehrlichioses, and anaplasmosis—United States: a practical guide for physicians and other health-care and public health professionals. *MMWR Recomm Rep.* 2006;55(RR-4):1–27.
- Demma LJ, Holman RC, McQuiston JH, et al. Epidemiology of human ehrlichiosis and anaplasmosis in the United States, 2001–2002. *Am J Trop Med Hyg.* 2005;73(2):400–409.
- Drexler NA, Dahlgren FS, Heitman KN, et al. National Surveillance of Spotted Fever Group Rickettsioses in the United States, 2008–2012. *Am J Trop Med Hyg.* 2016;94(1):26–34.
- Purvis JJ, Edward MS. Doxycycline use for rickettsial disease in pediatric patients. *Pediatr Infect Dis J.* 2000;19(9):871–874.

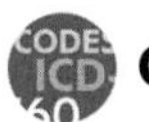

CODES

ICD10

- A79.9 Rickettsiosis, unspecified
- A77.0 Spotted fever due to Rickettsia rickettsii
- A75.9 Typhus fever, unspecified

FAQ

- Q: Should my child receive antibiotics if he is bitten by a tick in an area endemic to rickettsial disease?
- A: There is no role for prophylaxis against rickettsial diseases for patients who have suffered tick bites.
- Q: Are there differences between typhoid and typhus?
- A: Typhoid, or typhoid fever, is a separate entity from typhus. Typhoid is an enteric infection caused by *Salmonella typhi* and is unrelated to the rickettsial diseases.
- Q: If I contract a rickettsial illness, can I get that illness or a similar illness again?
- A: With the exception of scrub typhus, infection with a rickettsial organism confers immunity to other rickettsia within the same group.

R

ROCKY MOUNTAIN SPOTTED FEVER

Carolyn A. Paris, MD, MPH • George A. (Tony) Woodward, MD, MBA

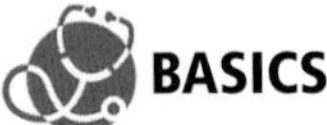

BASICS

DESCRIPTION

- Life-threatening, small vessel vasculitis
- Caused by infection with *Rickettsia rickettsii*, an obligate intracellular gram-negative coccobacillus, predominantly transmitted by *three species of* ticks in the United States
- Member of spotted fever subgroup of rickettsial diseases
- Seasonal endemic disease but may occur in other areas and throughout the year
- Classic symptoms of fever, headache, and rash following tick exposure are often not present.

EPIDEMIOLOGY

- Most common rickettsial disease in the United States
- Seasonal: April to September accounts for 90% of cases.
- Geographic
  - Restricted to countries of Western Hemisphere
  - Cases reported from all states except Alaska and Hawaii
  - Occurs most often in mid-Atlantic and south central regions: 1994 to 2003, >50% of cases in North Carolina, South Carolina, Tennessee, Oklahoma, Arkansas
  - Less often seen in Rocky Mountain states
  - Also occurs in southern Canada, Mexico, and Central and South America
- Single isolated cases most common in United States; clusters are reported infrequently in United States (4.4% familial) but are more typical in certain endemic areas (e.g., Brazil)
- Up to 2/3 of patients are <15 years old.

Incidence

- Annual incidence: 7 cases per million people (2002 to 2007); the highest recorded level in >80 years of national surveillance
- The recent increase in incidence and decrease in case fatality may be due to changes in reporting, diagnostic abilities, and possibly climate change.
- Cyclic (every 30 to 40 years) fluctuations in incidence; 250 to 1,200 cases reported per year
- More often reported in Native American, whites, males, and children; incidence highest in 5- to 9-year-olds
- Fatal outcome reported in 23% of untreated and 5% of treated cases
- Geographic variations in case fatality occur, likely due to different levels of pathogenicity, host factors, and delayed recognition in less endemic regions.
- 15% reported deaths in children <10 years of age

Prevalence

4–22% of children show significant antibody titers in endemic areas, likely representative of subclinical disease.

RISK FACTORS

- *R. rickettsii*–infected tick exposure
- Environment or occupation with increased forest exposure in endemic region

GENERAL PREVENTION

- Avoid tick-infested areas; limit skin exposure with long, light-colored clothing, tucked-in socks, or boots; inspect frequently.
- Use tick repellants or impregnated clothing.
  - N,N-Diethyl-meta-toluamide (DEET) most effective
  - Essential oils that offer natural alternatives considered safe (soybean, lemon eucalyptus, citronella, and clove)
- Remove ticks promptly.
  - Do not crush; may increase transmission
  - Avoid direct contact; remove with tweezers or gloved fingers close to skin.
  - Apply steady upward traction until tick's grip is released.
  - Clean wound.
  - Matches, petroleum jelly, nail polish, and rubbing alcohol are not effective for removal.
- Vaccine not available in the United States; may not prevent disease but does prevent deaths

PATHOPHYSIOLOGY

- Transmission usually occurs from tick bite (reservoir):
  - Usually >4 hours of attachment needed to transmit disease (often 24 hours)
  - Can occur by transfusion or aerosol route
- Incubation period 2 to 14 days, average 7 days
- *R. rickettsii* spreads through the lymphatic system, causing a small vessel vasculitis that affects all organs, especially skin and adrenals; increased vascular permeability and focal areas of endothelial proliferation
- Causes hyponatremia, hypoalbuminemia, edema, and hypotension
- Immunity is conferred following disease.

ETIOLOGY

Wood tick (*Dermacentor andersoni*) in Rocky Mountain States and southwest Canada; dog tick (*Dermacentor variabilis*) in east central region and areas of Pacific coast; *Rhipicephalus sanguineus* in Arizona and Northern Mexico; *Amblyomma cajennense* and *Amblyomma aureolatum* in Central and South America

COMMONLY ASSOCIATED CONDITIONS

- Patients with glucose-6-phosphate dehydrogenase (G6PD) deficiency account for a disproportionate number of deaths.
- Serious biologic weapon threat due to virulence causing severe disease; difficulty establishing diagnosis; low levels of immunity; agent available in nature; high infectivity; and feasibility of propagation, stabilization, and dispersal; thus, development of a cross-protective vaccine against all *Rickettsia* is desirable for biodefense as well as for travel medicine.

DIAGNOSIS

HISTORY

- History: classic triad of fever (high, abrupt onset), headache, and rash seen in ~50% of cases
- Abdominal pain common mainly in children
- Symptoms usually appear 2 to 8 days after tick bite.
- Gradual fever onset to >40°C (104°F), often unresponsive to antipyretics
- Headache: intense, retrobulbar or frontal, persistent and difficult to treat; young children may not describe.
- Cough, dyspnea
- Nausea, vomiting, abdominal pain, diarrhea
- Tick bite is reported in only 50–60% of cases.

PHYSICAL EXAM

- Fever and rash present in 85% of patients.
- Skin
  - Rash: usually appears by illness days 2 to 3, may be >6th day; 10–15% never develop rash, so absence should not delay therapy.
  - Usually, small, irregular, erythematous blanching macules become maculopapular then petechial and confluently hemorrhagic
  - Usually, on wrists and ankles first, spreads within hours to trunk, neck, and face; may involve palms, soles, and scrotum
    - May appear first on trunk or diffusely; can progress to necrosis of ears, nose, scrotum, fingers, or toes
    - Difficult to detect in people with dark skin
- CNS: meningismus, restlessness, irritability, apprehension, confusion, delirium, lethargy, stupor, coma, ataxia, opisthotonos, aphasia, papilledema, seizures, cortical blindness, central deafness, spastic paralysis, cranial nerve palsy
- Cardiac: congestive heart failure (CHF), myocarditis, arrhythmias, hypovolemic vascular collapse
- Pulmonary: pneumonitis, dyspnea, pulmonary edema, hypoxemia, pleural effusions, alveolar infiltrates
- GI: diarrhea, hepatomegaly, splenomegaly, anorexia, jaundice, mild pancreatitis
- Ocular: conjunctivitis, venous engorgement, papilledema, cotton wool spots, retinal hemorrhages, retinal artery occlusion, uveitis
- Other: edema, myalgias (especially calf or thigh), parotitis, orchitis, pharyngitis, polyarticular arthritis

DIFFERENTIAL DIAGNOSIS

- Measles
- Meningococcemia
- Ehrlichiosis
- Typhoid fever
- Leptospirosis
- Rubella
- Scarlet fever
- Disseminated gonococcal disease
- Infectious mononucleosis
- Secondary syphilis
- Rheumatic fever
- Enteroviral infection
- Immune thrombocytic purpura
- Thrombotic thrombocytopenic purpura
- Immune complex vasculitis
- Drug hypersensitivity reaction
- Murine typhus
- Rickettsialpox
- Recrudescent typhus

DIAGNOSTIC TESTS & INTERPRETATION

Presumptive diagnosis based on signs, symptoms, exposure history, and epidemiologic considerations rather than laboratory aids

Initial Tests (screening, lab, imaging)

- Nonspecific
  - CBC: anemia (30%), thrombocytopenia (from consumptive coagulopathy); normal or low leukocytes days 4 to 5, subsequent leukocytosis associated with secondary bacterial disease; bandemia common
  - Electrolytes: hyponatremia

- Elevated BUN, creatinine, liver function tests, bilirubin, creatine kinase
- Screen for disseminated intravascular coagulation (rare), prolonged prothrombin time, decreased fibrinogen (consumption).
- Arterial blood gases: acidosis
- Hypoalbuminemia
- CSF: usually clear (leukocyte count <10), may see pleocytosis in 1/3 and increased protein in 1/2 of patients

- Specific serologic tests
  - No early specific laboratory tests; serologic data reliable by days 10 to 12 of illness; negative results do not exclude diagnosis.
  - All test results normalize with early intervention.
  - Indirect immunofluorescence assay (IFA)
    - Best and most widely available method
    - Two serum samples obtained weeks apart showing 4-fold increase in IgG and IgM anti-*R. rickettsii* antibody titers
    - Positive 6 to 10 days after onset of disease, sensitivity increases to 94% with convalescence serum sample from days 14 to 21 days; specificity 100%
  - Weil-Felix test: oldest specific test but nonspecific and insensitive; no longer recommended
- Polymerase chain reaction (PCR), immunohistochemical staining, and culture are best done on biopsy specimen (of rash site or at autopsy) due to low circulating organism levels.
- Routine hospital blood cultures will not detect; available only at specialty labs
- Chest radiograph, EKG, and echocardiogram are recommended. Distinctive features on MR images (brain and spinal cord) may lead to early diagnosis; CT findings are less often present.

ALERT

Do not exclude diagnosis even if there is no history of a tick bite, no rash present, and/or results of serologic tests are negative. An eschar is rarely present at the site of infection and rash is blanching initially and only later develops petechia and more specific distribution (involvement of palms and soles with sparing of the face common). Treatment should be started presumptively; therapy should not be postponed while awaiting laboratory confirmation or onset of rash.

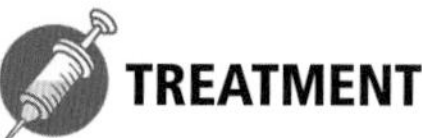

TREATMENT

GENERAL MEASURES

- Treat empirically if clinical suspicion.
- 3rd-generation cephalosporin indicated to treat potential meningococcemia until blood culture results final
- Platelets as indicated for thrombocytopenia
- Vitamin K (IM) for prolonged clotting time
- Manage hyponatremia with fluid restriction; avoid sodium supplements.
- Albumin if indicated
- Report to state health department.

MEDICATION

Treatment should be initiated based on clinical and epidemiologic information, as laboratory confirmation may not be available during acute illness. All agents are rickettsiostatic (hinder replication), not rickettsicidal, so host can eradicate disease. Treat until there is evidence of clinical improvement and at least 3 days without fever; standard duration is 5 to 10 days.

First Line

- Doxycycline (usual tetracycline antibiotic) is the drug of choice at any age:
  - Adults: 100 mg q12h PO/IV
  - Children <45 kg (100 lb): 4.4 mg/kg/24 h PO/IV divided b.i.d.
  - Also treats ehrlichiosis (similar presentation)
  - Side effects: less likely to stain teeth than tetracycline; contraindicated for pregnancy, although can be considered even in pregnancy if the mother's life is in danger and the theoretical concerns on the fetus is discussed
- Chloramphenicol (for severe doxycycline allergy or alternative during pregnancy)
  - 50 to 100 mg/kg/24 h IV divided q6h (max 4 g/24 h)
  - Side effects: peripheral neuropathy, aplastic anemia, "gray baby syndrome" with high dosage, possible association with leukemia, hemolytic anemia with G6PD
  - Not as effective as tetracyclines, or against ehrlichiosis; higher mortality rate in those treated with chloramphenicol than tetracyclines; consider only rarely such as during pregnancy.
  - Oral form no longer available
  - Monitor serum drug concentration.

Second Line

- Quinolones (ciprofloxacin, pefloxacin), macrolide (clarithromycin) with in vitro effect, no clinical evidence of efficacy
- Corticosteroids
  - May be helpful in severe cases, although no controlled studies published
  - Not advised for mild or moderately ill patients

ADMISSION, INPATIENT, AND NURSING CONSIDERATIONS

Initial stabilization: volume, electrolyte support as indicated

ONGOING CARE

FOLLOW-UP RECOMMENDATIONS

Expect improvement in 24 to 36 hours and defervescence in 2 to 3 days with treatment, especially if initiated <5 days after onset of symptoms.

PROGNOSIS

- Related to early recognition of disease and initiation of appropriate therapy
- Case fatality 2–4% if treated <6 days from onset of symptoms
- Case fatality 15–22.9% if treated >6 days from onset of symptoms
  - Higher mortality if <4 years, G6PD deficiency, CNS involvement, renal failure, jaundice, cardiovascular collapse, hepatomegaly, thrombocytopenia, disseminated intravascular coagulation (DIC), GI symptoms, inappropriate antibiotics, late rash, absence of headache, or male gender
  - Death usually between 8th and 15th days (fulminant cases with death in 5 to 6 days)

COMPLICATIONS

- Uncommon with early, appropriate treatment
- Neurologic sequelae
  - Behavioral disturbances, learning disabilities (more common), emotional lability, hyperactivity, memory loss, seizures
- Dermatologic sequelae
  - Gangrene of extremities, end organs, skin necrosis
  - Skin rash usually heals without sequelae.
- Hematologic sequelae: DIC
- GI sequelae
  - Hepatic dysfunction
  - Hypoalbuminemia from hepatic dysfunction, protein loss from damaged vessels
- Cardiac sequelae: can have persistent cardiac findings, CHF, cardiovascular collapse
- Metabolic sequelae: hyponatremia from water shift to intracellular spaces, sodium loss in urine
- Renal sequelae: acute tubular necrosis

ADDITIONAL READING

- Akgoz A, Mukundan S, Lee TC. Imaging of rickettsial, spirochetal, and parasitic infections. *Neuroimaging Clin N Am*. 2012;22(4):633–657.
- Andersen LK, Davis MDP. Climate change and the epidemiology of selected tick-borne and mosquito-borne diseases: update from the International Society of Dermatology Climate Change Task Force. *Int J Dermatol*. 2017;56(3):252–259.
- Buckingham SC, Marshal GS, Schutze GE, et al; for Tick-borne Infections in Children Study Group. Clinical and laboratory features, hospital course, and outcomes of Rocky Mountain spotted fever in children. *J Pediatr*. 2007;150(2):180–184.e1.
- Centers for Disease Control and Prevention. Rocky Mountain spotted fever (RMSF). http://www.cdc.gov/ncidod/dvrd/rmsf/index.htm. Accessed March 27, 2015.
- Chen LF, Sexton DJ. What's new in Rocky Mountain spotted fever? *Infect Dis Clin North Am*. 2008;22(3):415–432, vii–viii.
- Dantas-Torres F. Rocky Mountain spotted fever. *Lancet Infect Dis*. 2007;7(11):724–732.
- Openshaw JJ, Swerdlow DL, Krebs JW, et al. Rocky Mountain spotted fever in the United States, 2000–2007: interpreting contemporary increases in incidence. *Am J Trop Med Hyg*. 2010;83(1):174–182.
- Shapiro R. Prevention of vector transmitted diseases with clove oil insect repellent. *J Pediatr Nurs*. 2012;27(4):346–349.
- Walker DH. The realities of biodefense vaccines against *Rickettsia*. *Vaccine*. 2009;27(Suppl 4):D52–D55.

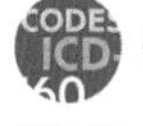

CODES

ICD10

A77.0 Spotted fever due to Rickettsia rickettsii

FAQ

- Q: In which patients should Rocky Mountain spotted fever be considered in the differential diagnosis?
- A: Anyone with a fever during the spring and summer who has been in an endemic area, regardless of presence of rash or history of tick bite. Nonspecific symptoms (e.g., GI, respiratory, rashes) may lead to misdiagnosis and thus delay therapy.
- Q: Should a child with a tick bite receive antibiotic prophylaxis when a tick is discovered?
- A: There is no evidence that prophylaxis is necessary or efficacious in preventing disease. To contract disease, one must be bitten by a tick that carries the disease (low risk), the tick must transmit the *Rickettsia* (low risk, usually requires >6 hours of attachment), and the *Rickettsia* must be pathogenic if inoculated (low risk).

ROSEOLA

Ross Newman, DO, MHPE

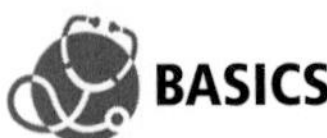

BASICS

DESCRIPTION

Roseola infantum is a common illness in preschool-aged children with a classic presentation of fever lasting 3 to 7 days followed by rapid defervescence and the appearance of a blanching maculopapular rash.

EPIDEMIOLOGY

- Roseola affects children from 3 months to 4 years of age. The peak age is 7 to 13 months.
- 90% of cases occur in the first 2 years of life.
- No gender predilection
- Roseola can occur throughout the year; outbreaks have occurred in all seasons.

GENERAL PREVENTION

- The virus that causes roseola infantum is usually transmitted via respiratory secretions or fecal–oral spread.
- Good hand hygiene is recommended.
- Outbreaks in hospitals have been reported, and standard infection control precautions are recommended.

PATHOPHYSIOLOGY

- Incubation period is 5 to 15 days.
- The typical pattern of rash that appears as the fever disappears may represent virus neutralization in the skin.

ETIOLOGY

- The major causes of roseola are human herpesvirus 6 and 7 (HHV-6 and HHV-7).
  - HHV-6 was first associated with roseola infantum in 1988.
  - HHV-6 and HHV-7 account for 20–40% of unexplained febrile illness in emergency department visits by febrile infants 6 months to 2 years of age.
  - Almost all children will acquire a primary infection and be seropositive for HHV-6 by the age of 4 years.
  - ~30% of children infected with HHV-6 will present with the classic manifestations of roseola.
- Roseola-like illnesses have been associated with a number of different viruses, including:
  - Enterovirus (coxsackievirus A and B, echoviruses)
  - Adenoviruses (types 1, 2, 3)
  - Parainfluenza virus
  - Measles vaccine virus

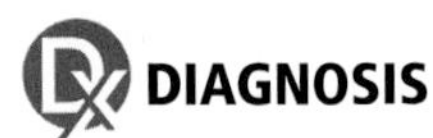

DIAGNOSIS

HISTORY

- Diagnosis is clinical, based on classic features.
- Affected children generally do not look sick.
- Fever, typically >39.5°C, lasting 3 to 7 days
- Mild cough and acute rhinitis may be present.

PHYSICAL EXAM

- Rash
  - Erythematous, blanching, maculopapular
  - First appears on trunk, spreads to face and extremities
  - Appears for 1 to 2 days after fever resolves
- Other findings:
  - Lymphadenopathy
  - Eyelid edema
  - Bulging fontanelle can occur occasionally.

DIFFERENTIAL DIAGNOSIS

- Roseola has a distinctive presentation but does resemble other viral exanthems.
- Antibiotic-associated rash in a child taking oral antibiotics when rash develops after defervescence
- Rubella and enteroviral infections
- Viral exanthems in preschool-aged children are sometimes called roseola even when fever is concomitant with rash.
- Before the development of the classic rash with defervescence, urinary tract infection is typically considered in this age group presenting with fever.

DIAGNOSTIC TESTS & INTERPRETATION

- Labs generally not helpful in diagnosis
  - Polymerase chain reaction (PCR) tests are available for detecting HHV-6 and HHV-7 but generally not needed.
- CBC, if obtained:
  - May show leukopenia with lymphocytosis
  - Thrombocytopenia is likely secondary to viral bone marrow suppression.
  - Leukocytosis >10,000 cells/mm^3 can help differentiate a urinary tract infection from roseola during febrile stage.
- Urine analysis
  - Sterile pyuria has been reported in up to 13% of patients.

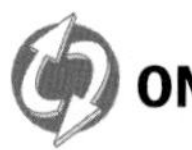

ONGOING CARE

PROGNOSIS

Most children with roseola infantum recover without sequelae.

COMPLICATIONS

- Febrile seizures
  - Most common complication of roseola
  - Between 10% and 15% of children have a generalized tonic–clonic seizure associated with fever.
- Aseptic meningitis with <200 cells, primarily mononuclear cells, have been reported.
- Encephalitis
- Thrombocytopenic purpura

ADDITIONAL READING

- American Academy of Pediatrics. Human herpesvirus 6 (including roseola) and 7. In: Kimberlin DW, Brady MT, Jackson MA, et al, eds. *Red Book: 2015 Report of the Committee on Infectious Diseases*. American 30th ed. Elk Grove Village, IL: American Academy of Pediatrics. 2015:449–452.
- Huang CT, Lin LH. Differentiating roseola infantum with pyuria from urinary tract infection. *Pediatr Int*. 2013;55(2):214–218.
- Jackson MA, Sommerauer JF. Human herpesviruses 6 and 7. *Pediatr Infect Dis J*. 2002;21(6):565–566.
- Leach CT. Human herpesvirus-6 and -7 infections in children: agents of roseola and other syndromes. *Curr Opin Pediatr*. 2000;12(3):269–274.
- Stoeckle MY. The spectrum of human herpesvirus 6 infection: from roseola infantum to adult disease. *Annu Rev Med*. 2000;51:423–430.
- Vianna RA, de Oliveira SA, Camacho LA, et al. Role of human herpesvirus 6 infection in young Brazilian children with rash illnesses. *Pediatr Infect Dis J*. 2008;27(6):533–537.

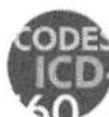

CODES

ICD10

- B08.20 Exanthema subitum [sixth disease], unspecified
- B08.21 Exanthema subitum [sixth disease] due to human herpesvirus 6
- B08.22 Exanthema subitum [sixth disease] due to human herpesvirus 7

FAQ

- Q: When can a child with roseola return to day care?
- A: As soon as fever subsides; there is no infectious risk of spread afterward. The child may return to day care even with the rash visible.
- Q: Will there be long-term sequelae in the child who has a seizure associated with roseola?
- A: In general, these seizures are typical febrile seizures that hold only a slightly higher risk than the general population for long-term neurologic sequelae (e.g., epilepsy).

ROTAVIRUS

John Bower, MD

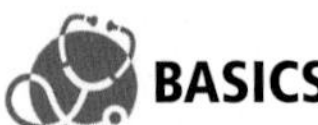

BASICS

DESCRIPTION

Rotavirus is a leading cause of gastroenteritis in the United States and worldwide. Characterized by frequent watery stools, illness ranges from mild diarrhea to disease complicated by severe dehydration, especially in young children.

EPIDEMIOLOGY

- Rotavirus is a major cause of diarrheal disease and accounts for over 200,000 deaths in children <5 years of age worldwide.
- The peak age for infection is between 6 and 24 months of age. Nearly all children acquire the virus by 5 years of age.
- In temperate climates, rotavirus activity peaks during the cold weather months but can appear year round in warmer climates.
- Transmission occurs primarily by the fecal–oral route.
- Rotavirus is highly contagious. This is due to several factors.
  - The virus has a very low inoculum of infection, requiring as few as 10 infectious particles to cause disease.
  - A high density of virus is shed into the stool during acute illness and for 1 to 3 days before and after diarrhea.
  - There is prolonged survival of the virus on a variety of environmental surfaces.
- The incubation period is 1 to 3 days.
- Prior to the rotavirus vaccine, U.S. children <5 years of age with diarrhea had a hospitalization rate of 52/10,000 person-years and an emergency department (ED) visit rate of 185/10,000 person-years.
- After the rotavirus vaccine was introduced in 2006, the hospitalization rate for all U.S. children <5 years with diarrhea fell by nearly 50% and ED visits by 25%.
- Hospitalizations for rotavirus-coded gastroenteritis among vaccinated children fell by >90%, compared to unvaccinated children.
- Rotavirus infection persists among older unvaccinated children and in the adult population.

RISK FACTORS

- Young infants, especially preterm infants, are at higher risk for severe dehydration and gastrointestinal (GI) complications.
- Immunocompromised patients, particularly with primary immunodeficiencies and hematopoietic stem cell transplantation are at higher risk for complications and prolonged shedding.

GENERAL PREVENTION

- Proper hand hygiene and cleaning of contaminated surfaces is essential to reducing person-to-person transmission.
- Contact precautions for hospitalized patients
- Two live oral vaccines are licensed in the United States:
  - Live human/bovine reassortant pentavalent rotavirus (RV5); given as a 3-dose series
  - Live human attenuated monovalent rotavirus (RV1); given as a 2-dose series
- Vaccine administration is contraindicated in patients with a history of intussusception or SCID.
- The first dose of rotavirus vaccine should be administered between 6 weeks and 14 weeks and 6 days of age.

PATHOPHYSIOLOGY

Rotavirus infects and replicates within the enterocytes of the small bowel. Several factors appear to contribute to secretory diarrhea.

- The nonstructural protein (NSP4) acts as an enterotoxin that triggers secretory diarrhea by increasing Cl^- secretion and decreasing Na^+ absorption.
- NSP4 also appears to activate the enteric nervous system, which activates a secretory state that further contributes to intestinal fluid loss.
- NSP1 is capable of inhibiting IFN induction.
- Malabsorption develops due to disruption of microvilli and decreased surface transport of digestive enzymes.

ETIOLOGY

- Rotavirus is an 11-segment double-stranded RNA virus with seven different antigenic groups (A to G).
- Types A, B, and C are responsible for most human infections, with group A being the most common.
- Group A rotavirus is further divided into multiple serotypes based on two outer capsid viral proteins: VP7 (G) and VP4 (P).

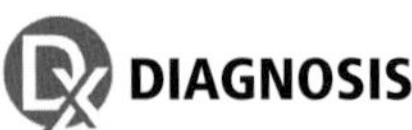

DIAGNOSIS

HISTORY

- Stools are watery and often foul-smelling.
- Gross blood or mucus is usually absent—their presence more often suggests a bacterial pathogen.
- Diarrhea usually lasts 3 to 8 days.
- Stool frequency can range from several to 20 episodes per day.
- Vomiting accompanies diarrhea 85% of the time. Vomiting often precedes diarrhea and resolves in 1 to 2 days.
- Fever can exceed 102°F in 1/3 of patients.
- Two thirds of patients present with diarrhea, vomiting, and fever.
- Family members often have a history of current or recent diarrhea.

PHYSICAL EXAM

Relevant physical findings are targeted to assess for potential dehydration.

DIFFERENTIAL DIAGNOSIS

- Viral pathogens occur in 80–90% of patients with secretory diarrhea. Besides rotavirus, common gastrointestinal viruses include the following:
  - Norovirus
  - Sapovirus
  - Astrovirus
  - Enteric adenovirus

- Bacterial infections may present with secretory diarrhea.
  - *Salmonella*
  - *Shigella*
  - *Campylobacter*
  - *Aeromonas*
  - *Clostridium difficile*
  - *Yersinia*
- Parasitic infections:
  - *Giardia*
  - *Cryptosporidium*
  - *Cyclospora*
  - *Isospora*

DIAGNOSTIC TESTS & INTERPRETATION

- Serum electrolytes, BUN, and creatinine are important in evaluating for dehydration and electrolyte abnormalities secondary to diarrhea.
- Rapid tests for rotavirus
  - By enzyme immunoassay (EIA) or latex agglutination
  - Have an overall sensitivity of 80% and specificity of 99%
  - Sensitivity is highest in the first 4 days of illness.
  - Rapid multiplex polymerase chain reaction (PCR) GI panels, which are increasingly used, include rotavirus and other common parasitic, viral, and bacterial agents of gastroenteritis.
- Fecal leukocyte and stool guaiac testing is not helpful.
- Two thirds of hospitalized children have mild elevations in their transaminases.

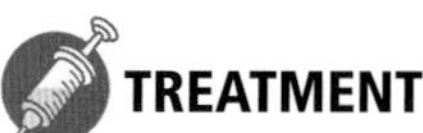

TREATMENT

MEDICATION

- Antimotility agents are generally avoided for all forms of infectious diarrhea in children.
- Several studies suggest that supplementation with a specific probiotic strain, *Lactobacillus rhamnosus* GG, during acute rotavirus gastroenteritis might decrease the duration of diarrhea (mean duration decrease: approximately 1 day).
- Human immune globulin, administered orally, has been used in immunocompromised patients with rotavirus infection to reduce disease severity and the duration of shedding.

ADMISSION, INPATIENT, AND NURSING CONSIDERATIONS

- Provide appropriate IV, nasogastric, or oral fluids for volume replacement and correction of electrolyte abnormalities due to diarrhea.
- Monitor fluid balance and serum electrolytes.
- Place patients in contact precautions.

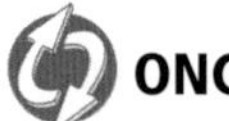

ONGOING CARE

COMPLICATIONS

- Hypernatremia and metabolic acidosis occur more often with rotavirus gastroenteritis than other forms of viral gastroenteritis and may become severe enough to require intensive care management.
- Gram-negative sepsis can occur secondary to mucosal injury.
- Rotavirus gastroenteritis has been associated with necrotizing enterocolitis in preterm infants.
- Diarrhea may be more severe and protracted in immunocompromised hosts.
- Seizures and encephalitis have been associated with rotavirus infection.

ADDITIONAL READING

- Bernstein DI. Rotavirus overview. *Pediatr Infect Dis J*. 2009;28(Suppl 3):S50–S53.
- Cox E, Christenson JC. Rotavirus. *Pediatr Rev*. 2012;33(10):439–447.
- Curns AT, Steiner CA, Barrett M, et al. Reduction in acute gastroenteritis hospitalizations among US children after introduction of rotavirus vaccine: analysis of hospital discharge data from 18 US states. *J Infect Dis*. 2010;201(11):1617–1624.
- Dennehy PH. Treatment and prevention of rotavirus infection in children. *Curr Infect Dis Rep*. 2013;15(3):242–250.
- Kaiser P, Borte M, Zimmer KP, et al. Complications in hospitalized children with acute gastroenteritis caused by rotavirus: a retrospective analysis. *Eur J Pediatr*. 2012;171(2):337–345.
- Leshem E, Moritz RE, Curns AT, et al. Rotavirus vaccines and health care utilization for diarrhea in the United States (2007–2011). *Pediatrics*. 2014;134(1):15–23.
- Madhi SA, Cunliffe NA, Steele D, et al. Effect of human rotavirus vaccine on severe diarrhea in African infants. *N Engl J Med*. 2010;362(4):289–298.
- Tate JE, Burton AH, Boschi-Pinto C, et al. Global, regional, and national estimates of rotavirus mortality in children <5 years of age, 2000–2013. *Clin Infect Dis*. 2016;62(Suppl 2):S96–S105.
- Tate JE, Yen C, Steiner CA, et al. Intussusception rates before and after the introduction of rotavirus vaccine. *Pediatrics*. 2016;138(3):1–6.

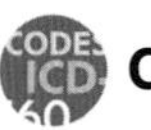

CODES

ICD10

A08.0 Rotaviral enteritis

FAQ

- Q: How long are children contagious following rotavirus infections?
- A: In most children, rotavirus shedding ceases within 7 days of the diarrhea resolving. However, asymptomatic shedding can persist in some children for up to several weeks—and in some cases longer. Young infants with severe diarrhea and immunocompromised patients are more likely to have persistent asymptomatic rotavirus shedding and may pose a risk for spread in the day care and hospital setting.
- Q: Is there a risk for intussusception with rotavirus vaccine?
- A: Postlicensure data for the RV5 and RV1 vaccines do point to a slightly higher risk for intussusception following administration of the first 2 doses of rotavirus vaccine. This infrequent complication, however, is far outweighed by the vaccine's substantial benefits in reducing hospitalization and death, and its worldwide use is strongly recommended.

SALICYLATE (ASPIRIN) POISONING

Kevin C. Osterhoudt, MD, MS

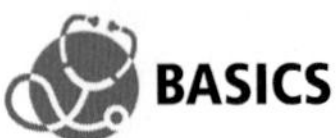

BASICS

DESCRIPTION

- May occur with acute or chronic overdosage of the following:
  - Acetylsalicylic acid (aspirin)
  - Methyl salicylate (oil of wintergreen)
  - Bismuth subsalicylate (Pepto Bismol®)
  - Salicylic acid (a keratolytic)
  - Other salicylate-containing drugs
- The potentially toxic acute oral dose of acetylsalicylic acid is >150 mg/kg.

EPIDEMIOLOGY

- Analgesics are the most common drugs implicated in human exposures reported to U.S. poison control centers.
- Salicylate preparations constitute ~10% of all analgesic poisoning exposures reported to poison control centers.

PATHOPHYSIOLOGY

- Ingested drug is absorbed in stomach and proximal intestine.
- With therapeutic aspirin dosing, serum levels peak in 1 to 2 hours (standard preparations) or 4 to 6 hours (enteric coated).
- After oral overdose, absorption may be prolonged and erratic.
- Acetylsalicylate ingestion may produce gastritis and may trigger centrally mediated vomiting.
- After overdose, the elimination half-life of salicylate becomes prolonged.
- As blood pH falls, the proportion of nonionized salicylate rises, and more salicylate shifts into tissues, including brain.
- Toxic salicylate exposures uncouple mitochondrial oxidative phosphorylation and increase oxygen consumption.
- Direct stimulation of the medullary respiratory center leads to hyperventilation and respiratory alkalosis.
- Multiple metabolic derangements produce a wide anion gap metabolic acidosis.
- Dehydration and electrolyte shifts are common.
- Low cerebral glucose concentrations may exist despite normal serum glucose concentrations.
- Pulmonary and/or cerebral edema may occur.

COMMONLY ASSOCIATED CONDITIONS

- Aspirin is often marketed in combination with other pharmaceuticals, which may complicate drug overdose situations.
- Adolescents frequently overdose on >1 drug preparation.
- Therapeutic use of acetylsalicylic acid among children with influenza has been associated with the occurrence of Reye syndrome.

DIAGNOSIS

HISTORY

- Enteric coating may lead to significantly delayed drug absorption.
- Timing of ingestion allows for proper consideration of the risks versus benefits of gastrointestinal (GI) decontamination.
- Tinnitus frequently associated with serum salicylate levels >25 mg/dL

PHYSICAL EXAM

- Hyperpnea indicates primary central hyperventilation and/or compensation for metabolic acidosis.
- Hyperpyrexia: Presence of "fever" may confuse salicylism with infection.
- Hypoxia: Pulmonary edema complicates therapy of aspirin overdose.
- Hypotension indicates severe dehydration, likely complicated by metabolic acidosis and salicylate-mediated myocardial inefficiency.
- Encephalopathy: Central nervous system (CNS) depression or seizures represent grave toxicity.

DIFFERENTIAL DIAGNOSIS

- Gastroenteritis
- Pneumonia
- Metabolic disease
- Ketoacidosis
- Sepsis
- Meningitis/encephalitis

ALERT

Aspirin poisoning mimics many illnesses, and chronic overdosage often results in delayed diagnosis.

DIAGNOSTIC TESTS & INTERPRETATION

- Serum electrolytes:
  - A wide anion gap metabolic acidosis is common.
  - Hypoglycemia or hyperglycemia may also occur.
- Arterial blood gas: may show mixed respiratory alkalosis/metabolic acidosis
- Salicylate level: Serum salicylate levels >60 to 100 mg/dL (acute) or 30 to 40 mg/dL (chronic) portend serious toxicity.
- Urine pH: allows monitoring of adequacy of urinary alkalinization
- Acetaminophen level: Acetaminophen may be a coingestant.
- Ferric chloride test: A few drops of 10% ferric chloride will turn brown or purple in 1 mL of urine that contains salicylate.

ALERT

- Respiratory acidosis suggests CNS depression and is an ominous sign.
- Salicylate levels after chronic or acute-on-chronic overdose correlate poorly to clinical condition.
- Serial salicylate levels may be necessary to rule out delayed or ongoing drug absorption after overdose.

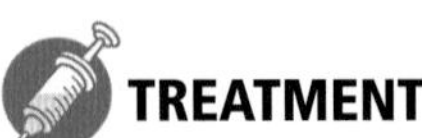

TREATMENT

GENERAL MEASURES

- GI decontamination
  - Activated charcoal (without sorbitol) 1 g/kg (maximum 75 g) may be administered if aspirin is judged to be present in the stomach or proximal intestine.
  - Some authorities suggest a second charcoal dose 2 to 4 hours after the first if salicylate levels continue to rise.
  - Whole-bowel irrigation may reduce drug absorption after large overdoses.

- Fluids/alkalinization
  - Intravascular volume should be repleted with intermittent boluses of 10 to 20 mL/kg of isotonic crystalloid.
  - Altered mentation may imply CNS hypoglycemia and should be treated with dextrose.
  - Acidemia should be treated with sodium bicarbonate to limit salicylate distribution to the brain. Serum pH of 7.5 is reasonable goal.
  - With significant poisoning, an IV infusion of 5% dextrose with 100 to 150 mEq/L of sodium bicarbonate and 20 to 40 mEq/L of potassium chloride should be initiated at 1.5 to 2 times maintenance requirements. Titrate fluid volume to produce urine output of 2 to 3 mL/kg/h. Titrate alkalinization to produce urine pH between 7.5 and 8, which greatly increases the urinary elimination of salicylate via "ion-trapping" effect.

ALERT

- Hypokalemia may interfere with the ability to achieve urinary alkalinization.
- Sedating a salicylate-poisoned patient may lead to respiratory depression and clinical deterioration.
- Endotracheal intubation is dangerous and, if performed, must be accompanied by sodium bicarbonate IV bolus and hyperventilation to prevent worsening acidemia and salicylate distribution to the brain.
- Hemodialysis equipment must be carefully primed to prevent worsening hypovolemia and cardiovascular collapse.
- If hemodialysis is performed, adjust dialysate to maintain alkalemia.
- Pulmonary edema and/or cerebral edema may complicate fluid management.

- Hemodialysis indications
  - Acute serum salicylate level >100 mg/dL
  - Confusion, hypersomnolence, or other neurologic dysfunction
  - Acute respiratory distress syndrome
  - Severe acidosis or severe electrolyte disturbance
  - Progressive clinical deterioration

ALERT

Patients with chronic salicylate overdose, or with renal insufficiency, may warrant hemodialysis at lower blood levels.

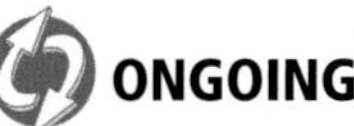

ONGOING CARE

FOLLOW-UP RECOMMENDATIONS

- Drug administration education should be offered to victims of chronic overdose.
- Mental health services should be provided to victims of intentional overdose.

PROGNOSIS

- Chronic therapeutic misuse often leads to delayed diagnosis and has the most serious prognosis.
- Single acute ingestion of >300 mg/kg acetylsalicylic acid should be considered life-threatening.

COMPLICATIONS

- Nausea and vomiting
- Dehydration
- Metabolic acidosis
- Electrolyte abnormalities
- Disorientation, coma, seizures
- Noncardiogenic pulmonary edema
- Renal failure
- Cerebral edema and death

ADDITIONAL READING

- Chyka PA, Erdman AR, Christianson G, et al. Salicylate poisoning: an evidence-based consensus guideline for out-of-hospital management. *Clin Toxicol (Phila)*. 2007;45(2):95–131.
- Juurlink DN, Gosselin S, Kielstein JT, et al. Extracorporeal treatment for salicylate poisoning: systematic review and recommendations from the EXTRIP workgroup. *Ann Emerg Med*. 2015;66(2):165–181.
- Shively RM, Hoffman RS, Manini AF. Acute salicylate poisoning: risk factors for severe outcome. *Clin Toxicol (Phila)*. 2017;55(3):175–180.
- Stolbach AI, Hoffman RS, Nelson LS. Mechanical ventilation was associated with acidemia in a case series of salicylate-poisoned patients. *Acad Emerg Med*. 2008;15(9):866–869.

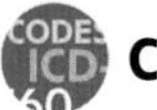

CODES

ICD10

- T39.014A Poisoning by aspirin, undetermined, initial encounter
- E87.2 Acidosis
- T39.011A Poisoning by aspirin, accidental (unintentional), init

FAQ

- Q: What amount of the candy-scented oil of wintergreen is toxic to a toddler?
- A: Oil of wintergreen may contain as much as 98% methyl salicylate. 1 mL of methyl salicylate is the equivalent of 1,400 mg of aspirin. Therefore, one teaspoon of oil of wintergreen represents a very serious "aspirin" overdose.
- Q: Is there a prognostic nomogram for aspirin poisoning similar to that used for acetaminophen overdose?
- A: The Done nomogram is applicable only to ingestion of non–enteric-coated aspirin by children with normal mentation and normal blood pH, and the validity of its prognostication is suspect. Its use is not widely recommended.

S

SALMONELLA INFECTIONS

John Bower, MD

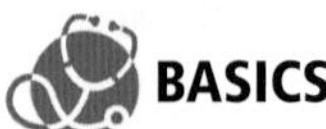

BASICS

DESCRIPTION

Salmonella isolates are broadly divided into the following: (i) nontyphoidal serotypes, with illness ranging from uncomplicated gastroenteritis to meningitis; and (ii) typhoidal serotypes, responsible for typhoid and paratyphoid fever (collectively called enteric fever).

EPIDEMIOLOGY

- *Salmonella* is a leading cause of foodborne infection in the United States and worldwide.
- Reservoirs
  - Nontyphoidal *Salmonella* serotypes are commonly found in agricultural products, particularly cattle, poultry, and eggs. Less common sources include produce, dairy products, and processed foods.
  - Humans may asymptomatically shed the bacteria for weeks, even months.
  - Reptiles are another well-recognized reservoir for infection. Small turtles remain a source of potential *Salmonella* infection despite a 1975 federal ban on their sale.
  - Typhoidal serotypes are found only in humans with acute or chronic infection.
- Transmission
  - Spread occurs via the fecal–oral route. Food and water contamination is the most common mechanism of exposure, followed by direct contact with contaminated surfaces and live animals.
  - *Salmonella* generally requires a high bacterial inoculum to cause infection.
- Age/season: *Salmonella* infections are most common in children <4 years of age and during the summer months.

RISK FACTORS

- Young infants (especially those <3 months of age), children with sickle cell disease (SCD), HIV, malignancy, and other immunocompromised conditions are at higher risk for extraintestinal complications from nontyphoidal *Salmonella* gastroenteritis.
- Travel to underdeveloped countries

GENERAL PREVENTION

- Hand hygiene, particularly when handling foods at risk for *Salmonella* contamination
- Proper cleaning of food preparation surfaces, particularly when handling foods at risk for *Salmonella* contamination
- Foods that frequently harbor *Salmonella*, such as meat, poultry, and eggs, require thorough cooking.
- Children <5 years old, and all those with high-risk conditions, should avoid contact with reptiles (e.g., lizards, snakes, turtles).
- Vaccines for typhoid fever have an efficacy of 50–80% and are recommended for the following: (i) travel to endemic areas and (ii) close contacts of carriers. Available vaccines include the following:
  - Ty21a, live vaccine for children ≥6 years of age; given PO every other day for 4 doses
  - ViCPS, inactivated vaccine for children ≥2 years of age; given as a single IM dose
  - Neither vaccine can be relied on to protect against *Salmonella* serotype paratyphi A and B.

ETIOLOGY

Salmonella is classified into two species: *Salmonella enterica* and *Salmonella bongori*. Species are further divided into 1 of over 2,500 serotypes.

- Common nontyphoidal serotypes include the following: *S. enterica* serotype enteritidis, *S. enterica* serotype typhimurium, *S. enterica* serotype Newport, and *S. enterica* serotype Heidelberg.
- Typhoidal serotypes include the following: *S. enterica* serotype typhi and *S. enterica* serotype paratyphi A, B, and C.

COMMONLY ASSOCIATED CONDITIONS

Following infection of the intestinal epithelium, *Salmonella* strains present with a variety of clinical manifestations.

- Acute gastroenteritis is the most common illness involving nontyphoidal serotypes:
  - Diarrhea is often watery but can be inflammatory with varying amounts of mucus and/or blood.
  - The incubation period is 12 to 48 hours, and illness usually resolves within 3 to 5 days. Asymptomatic shedding is common with a mean duration of 5 weeks—longer in infants. A small percentage of children can have asymptomatic shedding for up to 1 year.
- Transient bacteremia (nontyphoidal)
  - Bacteremia occurs in up to 5% of infected immunocompetent children and in 10% or more of high-risk patients. Young infants are generally at higher risk for bacteremia.
  - The most common serotypes associated with bacteremia include *Salmonella* enteritidis, *Salmonella* Heidelberg, and *Salmonella* typhimurium.
  - Bacteremia can result in localized extraintestinal infection.
- Localized extraintestinal infection (nontyphoidal)
  - Local infections occur in 3–5% of otherwise healthy bacteremic children and in up to 30% of high-risk bacteremic patients.
  - Infections include meningitis, septic arthritis, osteomyelitis, and pneumonia.
  - Infants <3 months of age are at higher risk for complications of bacteremia including meningitis.
- Enteric fever (typhoid and paratyphoid fever)
  - The most important serotypes are *Salmonella typhi*, followed by the less frequent and milder paratyphi A, B, and C strains.
  - Incubation is usually 7 to 10 days but can be 3 to 60 days.
  - The clinical course is often insidious with progression of disease over 3 to 4 weeks.
    - Weeks 1 to 2: Fever, headache, myalgia, abdominal pain, and listlessness are common. Diarrhea occurs in less than half of patients, and constipation is common.
    - Weeks 2 to 3: Fever increases, and rose spots (maculopapular rash) may appear. Splenomegaly and respiratory symptoms may develop.
    - Weeks 3 to 4: Fever gradually improves, however, serious complications, such as intestinal perforation, may develop at this time.

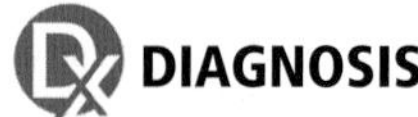

DIAGNOSIS

HISTORY

- Exposure history: nontyphoidal
  - Recent contact with farm animals (e.g., fairs and petting zoos) or reptiles. Reptiles may pose a risk even without direct contact.
  - Recent travel to underdeveloped regions of the world
  - Close contacts with recent gastroenteritis
  - Consumption of raw milk or undercooked eggs
- Exposure history: typhoidal
  - Travel to underdeveloped countries or close contact to persons recently living in, or visiting, endemic regions
- Clinical history: nontyphoidal
  - Vomiting appears in half of infected children.
  - Fever (up to 39°C) and abdominal pain are common complaints.
  - Stools with mucus and/or blood should raise suspicion for *Salmonella* as well as other common bacterial intestinal pathogens. Blood in the stool appears in <1/3 of patients with *Salmonella*.
  - Signs or symptoms indicative of sepsis, meningitis, osteomyelitis, or septic arthritis—especially in young infants and other high-risk patients—should raise suspicion for *Salmonella*.
  - A positive blood culture with a gram-negative rod may precede the diagnosis of *Salmonella* gastroenteritis.
- Clinical history: typhoidal
  - Half of infected patients present with constipation. Only 1/3 of children have diarrhea.
  - Fever ranges from 39°C to 40°C and worsens through the 1st and 2nd week of illness.
  - Rash and mental status changes may be present.
  - In children <5 years, enteric fever may appear as a nonspecific viral illness.
  - Family members who travelled with an index case of *Salmonella* serotype typhi should have stool cultures and be instructed to observe for symptoms of infection.

PHYSICAL EXAM

- Nontyphoidal infections
  - Examine for signs of dehydration.
  - Children with uncomplicated bacteremia may be clinically indistinguishable from nonbacteremic patients.
  - Fever can be absent in children with *Salmonella* bacteremia, especially young infants.
  - Examine for localized signs of infection in bone and joints.
  - Very young infants with *Salmonella* may present with a normal exam, including those with meningitis.
  - When possible, directly inspect stool for gross blood and mucus.
- Enteric fever
  - Patients with high fever may exhibit a relative bradycardia.
  - A coated tongue may be noted.
  - Hepatomegaly and splenomegaly are common.
  - 2- to 4-mm maculopapular lesions (rose spots) appear in up to 25% of patients.
  - Rales and rhonchi can be present.

DIFFERENTIAL DIAGNOSIS

- Illnesses that appear similar to nontyphoidal *Salmonella* infection
  - Acute gastroenteritis caused by *Shigella*, *Escherichia coli*, *Campylobacter*, and *Yersinia* is indistinguishable from *Salmonella*.
  - *Clostridium difficile* causes watery and inflammatory diarrhea, especially in children >2 years of age.
  - Norovirus, rotavirus, *Cryptosporidium*, and *Giardia* are common causes of watery diarrhea.
  - Allergic colitis
  - Inflammatory bowel disease
  - Bone and joint infection due to *Staphylococcus aureus*, group A strep, pneumococcus, and *Kingella*
- Enteric fever from *Salmonella* may appear similar to the following:
  - Appendicitis
  - Brucellosis
  - Dengue fever
  - Malaria
  - Nonspecific viral illness

DIAGNOSTIC TESTS & INTERPRETATION

Testing involves the following:

- Basic blood chemistries may reveal dehydration and electrolyte imbalances.
- WBC counts vary widely and are generally not helpful in diagnosis.
- Bilirubin and serum transaminases may be elevated with enteric fever.
- Stool culture for nontyphoidal gastrointestinal infection. Preliminary culture results reveal nonlactose fermenting, H_2S-producing colonies.
- Rapid multiplex polymerase chain reaction (PCR) GI panels generally include *Salmonella* as well as other common parasitic, viral, and bacterial agents of gastroenteritis.
- Fecal leukocyte and stool guaiac tests have limited sensitivity and specificity for diagnosing bacterial gastroenteritis.
- Blood cultures are positive in up to 5% of nontyphoidal infections and 60–80% of patients with enteric fever.
- Bone marrow aspirations are positive in 80–95% of patients with typhoid fever.
- Routine bacterial culture of urine, CSF, or bone or joint aspirates should be obtained when clinically indicated.

TREATMENT

MEDICATION

- Antimicrobials are not indicated for uncomplicated nontyphoidal gastroenteritis. Antimicrobial use does not shorten the duration of diarrhea and has been associated with prolonged carriage.
- Antimicrobial therapy is indicated for the following:
  - High-risk patients with nontyphoidal gastroenteritis pending blood culture results. These include the following: (i) infants <3 months of age; (ii) children with HIV, SCD; and (iii) those with malignancy and/or receiving immunosuppressive therapy.
  - Patients with known or suspected nontyphoidal bacteremia or localized infection
  - Patients with known or suspected enteric fever
- Antimicrobial choice
  - Ceftriaxone or cefotaxime is the preferred drug for empirical therapy of nontyphoidal and typhoidal infections while awaiting blood culture and sensitivity results. Patients with typhoid fever should receive a full 14-day parenteral course of treatment.
  - If shown to be susceptible, amoxicillin, trimethoprim/sulfamethoxazole (TMP/SMX), or azithromycin may be used in high-risk patients with uncomplicated nontyphoidal gastroenteritis and negative blood cultures.
  - Antimicrobial selection should be based on culture results and local resistance patterns. In the United States, the overall rate of antimicrobial resistance among nontyphoidal strains is 12%, but individual rates of resistance, such as for ampicillin and TMP/SMX, may vary significantly between states.
  - Quinolones are generally active but not approved for patients <18 years of age.
  - Quinolone resistance is increasing among typhoidal strains.
- Corticosteroids may provide benefit to critically ill patients with enteric fever.

ADMISSION, INPATIENT, AND NURSING CONSIDERATIONS

- Patients with dehydration and electrolyte abnormalities require appropriate volume replacement.
- Antimotility agents are generally avoided for all forms of infectious diarrhea in children.
- Consult orthopedics for management of suspected bone and joint infections.
- Administer antimicrobials only for specific clinical indications.
- Contact isolation for any *Salmonella*-infected child in diapers or with diarrhea.
- Contact isolation for any child with typhoid fever until three negative cultures following completion of antimicrobial therapy are documented.

ONGOING CARE

FOLLOW-UP RECOMMENDATIONS

- Acute nontyphoidal gastroenteritis
  - Encourage appropriate oral rehydrating fluids and monitor for signs and symptoms of dehydration.
  - Monitor for invasive complications, especially among high-risk patients.
  - Apprise patients and/or families of the risk for prolonged asymptomatic shedding.
  - Instruct patients and families in proper hand hygiene.
- Enteric fever
  - Fever can persist up to 7 days after starting appropriate antimicrobial therapy.
  - Monitor for serious complications such as intestinal bleeding, even after the patient appears to be improving.
  - Monitor for evidence of relapse.
  - Instruct patients and families in proper hand hygiene.

ALERT

- Serious complications of enteric fever can present as the patient appears to be improving.
- Even with appropriate therapy, patients with enteric fever may relapse 2 to 3 weeks after the initial fever resolves.
- Enteric fever should be considered in any febrile patient following recent travel to Asia, Africa, and South America.

PROGNOSIS

- Noninvasive nontyphoidal gastroenteritis is typically a self-limiting infection.
- Individuals often shed the organism for weeks, and a small number of patients may continue to shed for >1 year.
- Relapse of typhoid fever occurs in 4–20% of patients up to 3 weeks after the fever resolves.

COMPLICATIONS

- Dehydration is the most common complication caused by acute gastroenteritis.
- Nontyphoidal *Salmonella* gastroenteritis may be complicated by the following:
  - Bacteremia, especially in high-risk patients
  - Osteomyelitis and septic arthritis. Patients with SCD are particularly susceptible.
  - Meningitis. The course is frequently severe and may be associated with abscess formation and relapse.
  - Other infectious complications include pneumonia, pyelonephritis, and pericarditis.
- Enteric fever complications include intestinal perforation and hemorrhage, cholecystitis, hepatitis encephalopathy, pneumonia, myocarditis, shock, and disseminated intravascular coagulation.

ADDITIONAL READING

- Bar-Meir M, Raveh D, Yinnon AM, et al. Non-typhi *Salmonella* gastroenteritis in children presenting to the emergency department: characteristics of patients with associated bacteraemia. *Clin Microbiol Infect*. 2005;11(8):651–655.
- Bhutta ZA. Current concepts in the diagnosis and treatment of typhoid fever. *BMJ*. 2006;333(7558):78–82.
- Cheng LH, Crim SM, Cole CR, et al. Epidemiology of infant salmonellosis in the United States, 1996–2008: a Foodborne Diseases Active Surveillance Network Study. *J Pediatric Infect Dis Soc*. 2013;2(3):232–239.
- Christenson JC. *Salmonella* infections. *Pediatr Rev*. 2013;34(9):375–383.
- Geme JW III, Hodes HL, Marcy SM, et al. Consensus: management of *Salmonella* infection in the first year of life. *Pediatr Infect Dis J*. 1988;7(9):615–621.
- Medalla F, Gu W, Mahon BE, et al. Estimated incidence of antimicrobial drug-resistant nontyphoidal *Salmonella* infections, United States, 2004–2012. *Emerg Infect Dis*. 2016;23(1):29–37.
- Shkalim V, Amir A, Samra Z, et al. Characteristics of non-*typhi Salmonella* gastroenteritis associated with bacteremia in infants and young children. *Infection*. 2012;40(3):285–289.

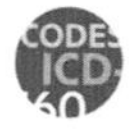

CODES

ICD10

- A02.9 Salmonella infection, unspecified
- A02.0 Salmonella enteritis
- A01.00 Typhoid fever, unspecified

FAQ

- Q: When can children infected with *Salmonella* return to day care or school?
- A: In general, infants and children with nontyphoidal *Salmonella* infection may return to day care or school 24 hours after their diarrhea has resolved. Repeat stool cultures are not recommended because asymptomatic shedding is common, and the risk of spread is low. Health officials may recommend documenting a negative stool culture if there are obvious concerns regarding a child's hygiene or in outbreak settings. Children with *S. typhi* infection who are ≥5 years of age and asymptomatic for over 24 hours, may attend school without repeating stool cultures. For children <5 years of age with *S. typhi*, it is generally required that the child be asymptomatic and have three negative stool cultures before returning to day care. Most health departments adopt this approach.

SARCOIDOSIS

Peter Weiser, MD • Randy Q. Cron, MD, PhD

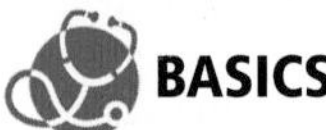

BASICS

DESCRIPTION

A chronic granulomatous disease (CGD) with noncaseating epithelioid giant cell granulomas in multiple organs that has two distinct variants often differentiated by age of onset

EPIDEMIOLOGY

- Early-onset sarcoidosis (EOS)/Blau syndrome
  - Incidence 0.29/100,000/year
  - No gender or geographic predominance
  - Triad of arthritis, uveitis, and dermatitis presenting prior to age 5 years
- Adult-type disease (ATD)
  - Incidence 1.02/100,000/year
  - Likely more common in the southwestern part of the United States
  - More often with systemic symptoms
  - Pulmonary involvement may also occur in older adolescents.
  - CNS involvement (rare): seizures, cranial neuropathy, hypothalamic dysfunction

RISK FACTORS

Genetics

- EOS/Blau
  - Mutation in the *CARD15/NOD2* gene on chromosome 16 (different location than Crohn disease) either spontaneous (EOS) or familial AD (Blau)
- ATD
  - African Americans are more commonly affected than whites.
  - Specific genetic tendencies not identified

ETIOLOGY

- Unknown (possibly an inflammatory response to an unknown antigen—infection)
- EOS/Blau—NOD2 is a bacterial sensor in dendritic cells; mutation is a gain-of-function leading to exuberant inflammation; possibly changes in autophagy
- Possible association with substantial dust inhalation (e.g., collapse of World Trade Center towers in New York City in 2001)

PATHOPHYSIOLOGY

- EOS/Blau—large polycyclic granulomas with dense lymphocytic coronas, $CD68^+$ macrophages, and $CD4^+$ T lymphocytes; abundant inflammatory cytokine expression
- ATD—noncaseating epithelioid granulomas with monocytes/macrophages/epithelioid and multinucleated giant cells in the center surrounded by $CD4^+$ T lymphocytes, plasma cells

DIAGNOSIS

- EOS/Blau—patients have more typical clinical triad presentation; gene mutation testing can confirm diagnosis.
- ATD—presentation is more vague; symptoms are less specific and biopsy confirmation of granulomas might be necessary.

HISTORY

- Systemic symptoms of prolonged malaise, fever, weight loss, especially in ATD
- EOS/Blau: rash and joint swelling; uveitis is initially asymptomatic.
- ATD: organ involvement with rash, painful arthritis, swollen lymph nodes, chronic cough, and hematuria (can be microscopic)

PHYSICAL EXAM

- EOS/Blau
  - Very small round macules to papules, pink to tan, usually raised, can resemble granuloma annulare
  - May note subcutaneous nodules often of lower limbs
  - Polyarticular, symmetrical arthritis of small and large joints with "boggy" synovitis
  - Tendonitis
  - Ophthalmologic exam: granulomatous iridocyclitis and posterior uveitis
- ATD
  - Patients can present with a different constellation of affected organs and symptoms—usually multiple organs are involved, but isolated organ presentation also occurs.
  - Peripheral lymphadenopathy is the most common manifestation.
  - Lung involvement and hilar adenopathy are common.
  - Uveitis can be both anterior and posterior.
  - Bilateral parotid gland enlargement and hepatosplenomegaly may be present.
  - Rash can be diffuse, erythematous, and macular or plaque-like.
  - Erythema nodosum and livedo reticularis can occur.
  - Neurosarcoidosis can present with seizures, cranial neuropathy, hypothalamic dysfunction.
  - Some patients present with Löfgren syndrome: constellation of erythema nodosum, polyarthritis, and hilar adenopathy in adolescence

ALERT

In most cases, uveitis is painful; however, it may also be asymptomatic. Slit-lamp ophthalmologic evaluation is important in all patients with suspected and confirmed sarcoidosis.

DIFFERENTIAL DIAGNOSIS

- Infection
  - Tuberculosis
  - Histoplasmosis/pulmonary mycoses
  - Bacterial sepsis
  - Mumps
  - HIV
  - Gonorrhea
  - Lyme disease
  - Toxocara/Toxoplasma (uveitis)
- Tumors
  - Leukemia
  - Neuroblastoma
  - Lymphoma
- Immunologic
  - Crohn disease
  - Oligoarticular juvenile idiopathic arthritis (for early-onset type)
  - Systemic juvenile idiopathic arthritis
  - Systemic lupus erythematosus
  - Sjögren disease
  - Dermatomyositis
  - Behçet disease
- Immunodeficiency
  - CGD
  - Common variable immunodeficiency
- Skin
  - Granuloma annulare
  - Lupus pernio
  - Cutaneous T-cell lymphoma
  - Psoriasis
  - Erythema nodosum due to *Streptococcus*, hepatitis B, or inflammatory bowel disease (IBD)

ALERT

Consider IBD-related arthritis especially with erythema nodosum. Gene mutations in *CARD15/NOD2* occur in both IBD and Blau syndrome, albeit at different regions of the same gene.

DIAGNOSTIC TESTS & INTERPRETATION

- CBC
  - Mild anemia, leukopenia, lymphopenia
- Erythrocyte sedimentation rate (ESR) elevated

- Angiotensin-converting enzyme (ACE) level
  - Can be elevated but not in all patients
  - Produced in many granulomatous diseases but is useful in cases in which index of suspicion is high
  - Not a perfect screening test; however, can follow levels in response to treatment
  - False positives: may be elevated in
    - Miliary tuberculosis
    - Biliary cirrhosis
- Lysozyme level elevation
  - May be more sensitive than ACE level for detecting sarcoidosis but is mostly correlated with pulmonary involvement
  - May be useful to follow disease activity in proven cases, if ACE levels cannot be used
  - False positives: may be elevated in
    - Lymphoma
- Serum calcium and creatinine levels
  - Important during baseline evaluation
- Urine test for blood
  - Seen in patients with hypercalciuria
- Synovial effusion is typically mildly inflammatory.
- Biopsy of affected organ, such as peripheral lymph node, parotid gland, skin, conjunctivae, minor salivary gland, or synovium, demonstrating noncaseating granuloma is helpful and many times diagnostic.
- Chest radiography
  - May demonstrate hilar adenopathy
- Brain MRI
  - Mass lesions often basilar, leptomeningeal enhancement, multifocal T2 hyperintense lesions in subcortical gray and white matter
- Gallium scan
  - Demonstrates uptake diffusely in lungs (extremely sensitive test)

TREATMENT

Medications are used to treat active disease with clinical symptoms.

- Pitfalls include overtreating asymptomatic lymphadenopathy and not detecting hypercalciuria.

MEDICATION

- Corticosteroids often provide rapid improvement.
- NSAIDs/analgesics for symptom relief
- In cases of chronic disease, immunosuppressive medications such as methotrexate can be used in addition to corticosteroids.
- The tumor necrosis factor inhibitors, specifically antibodies like infliximab and adalimumab, show promising preliminary results and should be considered especially in uveitis.
- In cases of hypercalciuria/hypercalcemia, consider hydration and furosemide.
- Cyclophosphamide for neurosarcoidosis

ONGOING CARE

FOLLOW-UP RECOMMENDATIONS

Patient Monitoring

- Referral to rheumatologist indicated
- Regular ophthalmologic assessment
- Signs to watch for:
  - Rising creatinine levels
  - Shortness of breath
  - Persistent uveal tract inflammation
  - Neurologic deficit

PROGNOSIS

- Variable for EOS/Blau. Severe organ involvement, joint, and eye damage can occur—needs close follow-up.
- Löfgren syndrome can resolve after a couple of years.
- >40% of older children with ATD have persistent pulmonary changes, but only a few will have pulmonary symptoms.

COMPLICATIONS

- In children, usually related to uveitis or from hypercalciuria resulting in renal injury. Lung, CNS, and ocular involvement can bring long-term defects.
- In older adolescents, pulmonary problems, such as restrictive lung disease, as well as severe growth delay, may occur.

ADDITIONAL READING

- Baumann RJ, Robertson WC Jr. Neurosarcoid presents differently in children than in adults. *Pediatrics*. 2003;112(6, Pt 1):e480–e486.
- Blau EB. Familial granulomatous arthritis, iritis, and rash. *J Pediatr*. 1985;107(5):689–693.
- Gedalia A, Khan TA, Shetty AK. Childhood sarcoidosis: Louisiana experience. *Clin Rheumatol*. 2016;35(7):1879–1884.
- Iannuzzi MC, Rybicki BA, Teirstein AS. Sarcoidosis. *N Engl J Med*. 2007;357(21):2153–2165.
- Nathan N, Marcelo P, Houdouin V, et al. Lung sarcoidosis in children: update on disease expression and management. *Thorax*. 2015;70(6):537–542.
- Rosé CD, Pans S, Casteels I, et al. Blau syndrome: cross-sectional data from a multicentre study of clinical, radiological and functional outcomes. *Rheumatology (Oxford)*. 2015;54(6):1008–1016.
- Rosé CD, Wouters CH, Meiorin S, et al. Pediatric granulomatous arthritis: an international registry. *Arthritis Rheum*. 2006;54(10):3337–3344.
- Shetty AK, Gedalia A. Childhood sarcoidosis: a rare but fascinating disorder. *Pediatr Rheumatol Online J*. 2008;6:16.

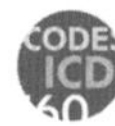

CODES

ICD10

- D86.9 Sarcoidosis, unspecified
- D86.0 Sarcoidosis of lung
- D86.86 Sarcoid arthropathy

S

FAQ

- Q: Why is therapy in childhood sarcoidosis more aggressive compared with adults?
- A: These may be two distinct granulomatous diseases. EOS/Blau is a very aggressive and destructive disease requiring chronic therapy rather than a relatively short course of steroids.
- Q: Does a single negative biopsy (no noncaseating granulomas) rule out sarcoidosis?
- A: No. It may take several biopsies of multiple involved organs to demonstrate noncaseating granulomas consistent with sarcoidosis.
- Q: Besides sarcoidosis, what are some of the other diagnoses to exclude with parotid gland involvement?
- A: Sjögren syndrome, IgG4-related disease, lymphoma, mumps, HIV-1/AIDS, and tuberculosis to name a few
- Q: Who is Blau?
- A: Edward Blau, MD is a pediatrician based in Marshfield, WI. In 1985, he published an article describing 11 family members across four generations who all had "granulomatous disease of the skin, eyes, and joints."

SCABIES

Jessica E. Nash, MD

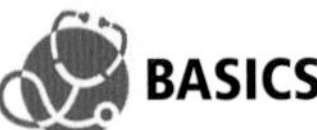

BASICS

DESCRIPTION

- Scabies is a parasitic infection caused by the mite *Sarcoptes scabiei*, which infects the stratum corneum of the skin and results in an intense pruritic rash.
- Crusted scabies is a subtype categorized by a more intense pruritus and rash with a heavier burden of mites.
  - Previously called "Norwegian scabies"
  - More common in immunocompromised (i.e., HIV, long-term steroid use) and debilitated patients with sensory neuropathies and paralysis
- Nodular scabies is a rare clinical subtype presenting with red to brown nodules secondary to hypersensitivity reaction to mites and their by-products.

EPIDEMIOLOGY

- Results from close personal and prolonged contact with another human infected with mites
- Occurs worldwide and is endemic in many countries
- Scabies affects all people from different ethnicities, social economic levels, and gender.

Incidence

Varies worldwide, with cyclical fluctuations for new cases; estimates are 1 to 15 new cases per 1,000 people per year.

Prevalence

Estimated 300 million cases worldwide

GENERAL PREVENTION

- Avoid direct skin-to-skin contact with a person who has scabies and with the clothing/bedding used by a person who has scabies.
- Ensure that any close contacts that have been exposed are treated even if asymptomatic because symptoms can take up to 30 days to develop.
- Everyone in the household should be treated at the same time.
- All bedding and clothing used in the prior 3 days by a person with scabies needs to be washed with hot water and dried in a hot dryer for at least 10 minutes or should be dry-cleaned.
- Furniture and carpets in the household of an infected person should be vacuumed.
- Anything that cannot be washed should be isolated from humans for at least 2 days or, more conservatively, for up to 3 weeks.

PATHOPHYSIOLOGY

- The mite of scabies is a parasite that burrows into the skin and lays eggs. They travel anywhere between 0.5 and 5.0 mm a day. The larvae hatch from the eggs in 2 to 3 days and become adults and then the cycle repeats.
- Papules are not due to the mite itself but due to a hypersensitivity reaction (immune-mediated response) to the mites' saliva, eggs, and feces.
- If the individual has never been exposed, there is an incubation period which can be between 4 and 6 weeks before symptoms manifest.
- Those with prior exposure and thus sensitized can have milder symptoms that occur within 1 to 4 days.
- Crusted scabies subtype has thousands to millions more mites, making infectivity easier even at less contact. The mite is the same as with classic scabies.

ETIOLOGY

S. scabiei var *hominis* adult female mite is about 0.3-mm long with eight legs and barely visible with the naked eye.

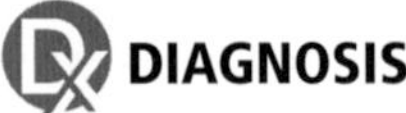

DIAGNOSIS

HISTORY

- Patients usually present with a history of rash that is intensely pruritic and worse at night because mite activity increases at night based on temperature of the human body.
- Rash present on hands and wrist and may also be in genital area
- Children <2 years of age may present with a vesicular rash on face and other regions of body not typical in older children and adults.
- Other family members or household contacts with a similar rash given contact with infected person is needed for transmission.

PHYSICAL EXAM

- Usually presents with a papular (<5 mm) erythematous rash
- One pathognomonic sign is the burrow line, a linear, wavy, S-shaped mark which occurs as the mite burrows into the skin; can be difficult to see because scratching can obliterate the burrow, but it helps with diagnosis if visualized
- To better identify burrows, can use a washable marker on the skin, and then remove markings with water or alcohol. The ink will remain within the burrow, making it easier to see.
- Common sites of rash are interdigital web spaces of hands and feet. Papules can be present in flexor region of wrist, ankles, extensor region of elbows, axillary folds, genital region, and periareolar regions of breast.
- Presentation differs in young children versus older children and adults.
  - Children <2 years of age usually have a more widespread distribution that also includes face, neck, palms, and soles.
  - Rash in infants more likely to be nodules, and young children can have more of a vesicular appearance

DIFFERENTIAL DIAGNOSIS

- Contact dermatitis
- Atopic dermatitis
- Insect bites
- Drug rash
- Infantile acropustulosis
- Impetigo
- Papular urticaria
- Viral exanthem

DIAGNOSTIC TESTS & INTERPRETATION

- Direct visualization
  - Potassium hydroxide preparation of a skin scraping
  - Use a blade to scrape skin, isolate the mite from scrapings, and view scrapings under microscopy.
  - Look for mites and mite fecal matter.
- Visualization of the burrows can be made easier using the "burrow ink test."
  - Use ink to mark areas where scabies are suspected, then wipe away the surface ink with alcohol pad.
  - If ink tracks into the mite burrow, making a grossly visible zigzagged line, the test is positive.
- In atypical cases, skin biopsy can be formed.
- Other more specialized tests are under development such as antigen detection, polymerase chain reaction (PCR) of skin scrapings, or intradermal tests.

TREATMENT

MEDICATION

- Permethrin 5% cream
  - Drug of choice for children and infants >2 months of age
  - Is neurotoxic to the mite
  - The cream is applied from neck to toe, paying special attention to interdigital regions; skinfolds of wrist, elbow, and inguinal creases; and under nails.
  - In young children, include the entire head and neck as well because these aren't spared in this age group.
  - Rinse cream off the body 8 to 14 hours after application.
  - Often, one retreatment 1 week after initial treatment is needed. Some recommend retreating once 4 days later (instead of waiting 7 days).
- Crotamiton 10% cream
  - Not commonly used
  - Not approved in children
  - Apply from chin to toe and reapply 24 hours later, and then remove by a cleansing bath 48 hours after the last application.
- Sulfur 5–10% cream
  - Can be used for infants <2 months and pregnant lactating woman
  - Must be reapplied daily for 3 days
- Ivermectin
  - Oral antiparasitic agent
  - Not recommend for women who are pregnant or lactating
  - Safety profile for children is unknown.
  - Not United States Food and Drug Administration (FDA)-approved for treatment of scabies
- Mild to moderate topical steroids
  - Note, topical steroids have no efficacy in treating the mite infection but can be helpful for the intense pruritus during and just after the scabies infection.
- Lindane 1%
  - Not commonly used due to concern for systemic toxicity
  - Black box warning in United States, banned in other countries
  - Because of safety concerns and availability of other treatments, lindane should not be used as a 1st-line agent for treatment of scabies.
  - Side effects can include seizures, headache, and vertigo.

ONGOING CARE

FOLLOW-UP RECOMMENDATIONS

Patient Monitoring

- Treatment failure occurs but is usually due to incomplete treatment of all contacts at the same time.
- Recommend follow-up 2 weeks after treatment to ensure no new burrows, new papules, or new vesicles have developed, which would most likely indicate inadequate application of treatment.

PROGNOSIS

- Prognosis is great with early identification and treatment.
- Concerns for drug-resistant scabies emerging are more notable in crusted scabies.

COMPLICATIONS

- Secondary bacterial skin infection (i.e., impetigo)
- Postscabies pruritus: Pruritus that occurs for weeks after treatment should not be confused with treatment failure.

ADDITIONAL READING

- American Academy of Pediatrics. Scabies. In: Kimberlin DW, Brady MT, Jackson MA, et al, eds. *Red Book: 2015 Report of the Committee on Infectious Diseases*. 30th ed. 2015. Elk Grove Village, IL: American Academy of Pediatrics.
- Boralevi F, Diallo A, Miquel J, et al; for Groupe de Recherche Clinique en Dermatologie Pédiatrique. Clinical phenotype of scabies by age. *Pediatrics*. 2014;133(4):e910–e916.
- Golant AK, Levitt JO. Scabies: a review of diagnosis and management based on mite biology. *Pediatr Rev*. 2012;33(1):e1–e12.
- Hay RJ, Steer AC, Engelman D, et al. Scabies in the developing world—its prevalence, complications, and management. *Clin Microbiol Infect*. 2012;18(4):313–323.
- Leone P. Scabies and pediculosis pubis: an update of treatment regimens and general review. *Clin Infect Dis*. 2007;44(Suppl 3):S153–S159.
- Mounsey KE, McCarthy JS, Walton SF. Scratching the itch: new tools to advance understanding of scabies. *Trends Parasitol*. 2013;29(1):35–42.
- Strong M, Johnstone P. Interventions for treating scabies. *Cochrane Database Syst Rev*. 2007;(3):CD000320.

CODES

ICD10

B86 Scabies

FAQ

- Q: What do I do with the clothes or cloth items that cannot be washed at this time?
- A: Store them in a plastic bag and put them away for 3 days because the mite cannot live more than 3 days without a human host. Couches and carpet should be vacuumed.
- Q: When will my child no longer be contagious?
- A: If treated properly, children are no longer contagious after one treatment. Although your child may still have pruritus, he or she is no longer considered contagious and can return to school.
- Q: When will the rash resolve?
- A: The rash may take 3 to 4 weeks to resolve after treatment and should not be considered a treatment failure unless a new rash develops.

SCARLET FEVER

Emily C. Borman-Shoap, MD • John S. Andrews, MD

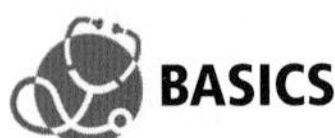

BASICS

DESCRIPTION

- Scarlet fever or "scarlatina" is a manifestation of infection with *Streptococcus pyogenes* (group A β-hemolytic *Streptococcus*) that is characterized by an erythematous "sandpaper" rash. It results from infection with a strain of *S. pyogenes* that elaborates streptococcal pyrogenic exotoxin (SPE).
- Typical presentation is in the setting of streptococcal pharyngitis but may occur with group A streptococcal skin or wound infections.
- Disease is linked to SPE A, B, C, and F. SPE A is associated with more virulent disease.
- A similar syndrome may also be seen in infection with certain enterotoxin-producing strains of *Staphylococcus aureus*, known as staphylococcal scarlet fever.

EPIDEMIOLOGY

Incidence

- Disease is most common between ages 3 and 15 years.
- Peak incidence is during the early school years.
- There is little seasonal variation with slightly increased prevalence in winter and spring.
- Recent studies have documented increasing incidence in certain parts of the world (e.g., United Kingdom, China, South Korea).
- Incubation period is 2 to 5 days for strep pharyngitis and may be up to 10 days for strep skin infections.

Prevalence

- Prevalence is equal in boys and girls.
- By age 10 years, 80% of children have developed toxin-specific antibodies.

RISK FACTORS

- Close contact with a case of scarlet fever
- Crowded living conditions may contribute (schools, daycare centers, military training centers).
- Prior sensitization to *S. pyogenes* is required.
- Susceptible individuals may lack toxin-specific immunity.

GENERAL PREVENTION

- Control measures were ineffective in a school outbreak. These included hygiene advice and exclusion of infected students for 24 hours while initiating penicillin treatment.
- Prompt treatment of infection leads to fewer secondary cases of streptococcal disease.

PATHOPHYSIOLOGY

- Susceptible individuals are thought to lack toxin-specific immunity. This is supported by results of the now seldom-used Dick test, in which a small amount of toxin introduced intradermally produces local erythema in susceptible individuals but no reaction in those with toxin-specific immunity.
- Rash and other toxic manifestations of scarlet fever have been attributed to the development of hypersensitivity to the toxin, which requires prior exposure to the toxin.
- Toxin is produced when viral DNA is introduced into the streptococcal genome by a bacteriophage.
- Histologic examination of affected skin shows dilated blood and lymphatic vessels and engorged capillaries, most prominently around hair follicles.
- Acute, edematous polymorphonuclear inflammatory reaction is seen microscopically within affected tissues.
- Epidermal inflammatory reaction is usually followed by hyperkeratosis, which accounts for scaling during defervescence.

ETIOLOGY

Scarlet fever is a toxin-mediated consequence of infection with group A β-hemolytic *Streptococcus*.

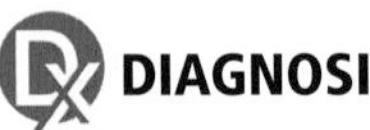

DIAGNOSIS

HISTORY

- Sudden onset of fever up to 40.5°C, sore throat, headache, nausea, vomiting, and toxicity are classic symptoms for group A streptococcal disease.
- Characteristic rash typically occurs 12 to 48 hours after onset of fever.
- Texture of rash (e.g., feels like sandpaper) is more important than appearance.
- Patient may complain of abdominal pain or muscle aches before onset of rash as well as aching in extremities or back.
- There may be close contacts with streptococcal infection.

PHYSICAL EXAM

- Fine maculopapular (sandpaper texture) rash on erythematous background: usually begins on the trunk and spreads to involve almost the entire body within hours to days. Although the rash seen with scarlet fever is generally fine and sandpaper-like, larger papules and petechiae may be seen.
- Rash may be more easily detected by palpation than visual inspection.
- Pastia line: accentuation of erythema in flexor creases (antecubital, axillary, inguinal)
- Circumoral pallor: Area around mouth appears pale in comparison to flushed cheeks.
- Rash blanches with pressure and ultimately desquamates: Desquamation occurs within 7 to 21 days from onset of illness.
- Systemic toxicity may indicate incorrect diagnosis.
- Dorsum of tongue has white coat early in illness with edematous red papillae. White covering desquamates and reveals swollen, red, and mottled strawberry tongue.
- Other findings:
  - Pharynx and tonsils are beefy red and may demonstrate exudate.
  - Hemorrhagic spots on interior pillar of tonsils and soft palate
  - Large, tender anterior cervical nodes

DIFFERENTIAL DIAGNOSIS

- Viral exanthems (measles, rubella, erythema infectiosum)
- Drug eruptions
- Staphylococcal scalded skin syndrome
- Toxic epidermal necrolysis
- Toxic shock syndrome (streptococcal or staphylococcal)
- Kawasaki disease
- Uncommon entities:
  - Infection with *Arcanobacterium hemolyticum*
  - Far East scarlet-like fever (*Yersinia pseudotuberculosis)*
  - Mercury poisoning (acrodynia)
  - Atropine intoxication
  - Boric acid poisoning
  - Rifampin overdose

DIAGNOSTIC TESTS & INTERPRETATION

Initial Tests (screening, lab, imaging)

Rapid streptococcal antigen tests for throat swabs:

- Effective as screening tests; sensitivity = 70–90% and specificity >95%
- Positive rapid tests do not require culture confirmation. A negative rapid test should prompt additional testing with a throat culture to effectively rule out streptococcal infection.

Follow-Up Tests & Special Considerations

- Culture confirmation is not necessary to make the clinical diagnosis of scarlet fever.
- Throat culture: the gold standard with best sensitivity (>90%) for group A β-hemolytic streptococci. A culture should be performed when rapid test is negative.
- In cases where skin infection is suspected as the cause of scarlet fever, wound cultures are not routinely recommended.
- White blood cell count: usually elevated, although may be elevated in viral pharyngitis as well. Low count would be rare with streptococcal infection.
- Eosinophilia (up to 30%): common in the recovery phase

- Dick test: of historic interest; no longer used clinically
- Pitfalls
  - A positive throat culture may represent carriage in some cases of acute pharyngitis that are actually viral (e.g., Epstein-Barr virus).
  - Milder disease is becoming more common and is easy to miss. Rash may involve only the bridge of the nose, face, shoulders, and upper chest. Circumoral pallor and severe exudative pharyngitis are being seen less frequently.

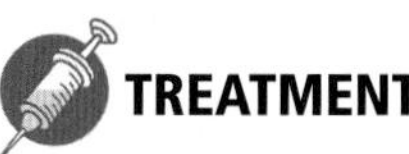

TREATMENT

GENERAL MEASURES

- Treatment for scarlet fever is identical to therapy for streptococcal pharyngitis.
- Therapy started up to 9 days after illness onset is effective for preventing acute rheumatic fever.
- Antibiotic therapy may be withheld until throat culture result is available.

MEDICATION

First Line

Penicillin or amoxicillin remain the drugs of choice to treat streptococcal pharyngitis. Resistance to penicillin has never been documented in the United States.

- Oral penicillin V potassium (10 days)
  - Children: 250 mg twice or 3 times daily
  - Adolescents: 250 mg 4 times daily or 500 mg twice daily
- Oral amoxicillin (10 days)
  - 50/mg/kg once daily (max 1,000 mg/dose)
  - OR 25 mg/kg/dose (max 500 mg/dose) twice daily
- Intramuscular penicillin G benzathine
  - Equally effective as oral penicillin
  - Dose: 600,000 U for children <14 kg (<30 lb); 900,000 to 1,200,000 U for children 14 to 27 kg; and 1,200,000 U for children >27 kg and adults
  - Ensures compliance (only 1 dose needed)
  - Benzathine/procaine penicillin combinations are less painful.

Second Line

- The following medications are options for penicillin-allergic patients:
  - Oral cephalexin (10 days)
    - 20 mg/kg/dose twice daily (max 500 mg/dose)
  - Oral cefadroxil (10 days)
    - 30 mg/kg/dose once daily (max 2 g/dose)
  - Oral azithromycin (5 days)
    - 12 mg/kg/dose once daily (max 500 mg/dose)
  - Oral clarithromycin (10 days)
    - 7.5 mg/kg/dose twice daily (max 500 mg/dose)
- Tetracyclines and sulfonamides should not be used because of resistance by group A streptococci.

ISSUES FOR REFERRAL

Specialty referral is seldom necessary for straightforward scarlet fever. Consultation with an otolaryngologist may be considered for children with repeated episodes of pharyngitis.

ADDITIONAL THERAPIES

Antibiotics are the mainstay of treatment for scarlet fever. Antipyretics and analgesics are helpful adjuncts for symptomatic relief.

SURGERY/OTHER PROCEDURES

Infectious Disease Society of America (IDSA) guidelines do not currently recommend tonsillectomy solely to reduce the frequency of GAS pharyngitis.

COMPLEMENTARY & ALTERNATIVE THERAPIES

There are no well-documented complementary or alternative treatments for streptococcal infection.

ONGOING CARE

FOLLOW-UP RECOMMENDATIONS

Patient Monitoring

- Fever and symptoms usually resolve within 24 to 48 hours of antibiotic treatment.
- Patients with scarlet fever may experience hyperkeratosis. Peeling of the affected skin may also occur 2 weeks after the acute infection.

PROGNOSIS

- Overall prognosis is excellent.
- Few patients suffer suppurative complications.
- Risk of developing acute rheumatic fever in untreated streptococcal infections is ~3% under epidemic conditions (0.3% in endemic situations).
- Acute postinfectious glomerulonephritis is uncommon. Risk may be as high as 10–15% following infections with certain nephritogenic strains.

COMPLICATIONS

- Complications are due to group A streptococcal infections and are not specific to scarlet fever.
- Nonsuppurative complications occur after the acute streptococcal infection has resolved.
  - Acute rheumatic fever may occur an average of 18 days after untreated infection. Effective antibiotic treatment can prevent this complication.
  - Acute postinfectious glomerulonephritis occurs an average of 10 days after infection. The risk of glomerulonephritis is not reduced by treatment with antibiotics.
- Other complications of streptococcal infections worth noting include:
  - Streptococcal toxic shock syndrome is a toxin-mediated complication of streptococcal infection that may be life-threatening.
  - Suppurative complications of streptococcal pharyngitis include the following:
    - Cervical adenitis
    - Peritonsillar abscess
    - Retropharyngeal abscess
    - Sinusitis
    - Otitis media
    - Mastoiditis
    - Meningitis
    - Brain abscess
    - Thrombosis of intracranial venous sinuses

ADDITIONAL READING

- Lamden KH. An outbreak of scarlet fever in a primary school. *Arch Dis Child*. 2011;96(4):394–397.
- Park DW, Kim SH, Park JW, et al. Incidence and characteristics of scarlet fever, South Korea, 2008–2015. *Emerg Infect Dis*. 2017;23(4):658–661.
- Schwartz RH, Kim D, Martin M, et al. A reappraisal of the minimum duration of antibiotic treatment before approval of return to school for children with streptococcal pharyngitis. *Pediatr Infect Dis J*. 2015;34(12):1302–1304.
- Shulman ST, Bisno AL, Clegg HW, et al. Clinical practice guideline for the diagnosis and management of group A streptococcal pharyngitis: 2012 update by the Infectious Diseases Society of America. *Clin Infect Dis*. 2012;55(10):e86–e102.
- Wong SS, Yuen KY. Streptococcus pyogenes and re-emergence of scarlet fever as a public health problem. *Emerg Microbes Infect*. 2012;1(7):e2.

CODES

ICD10

- A38.9 Scarlet fever, uncomplicated
- J02.0 Streptococcal pharyngitis

FAQ

- Q: Is culture confirmation of strep infection necessary to make the diagnosis of scarlet fever?
- A: No. Although laboratory evidence of strep infection is supportive, scarlet fever is a clinical diagnosis.
- Q: Is there any indication for throat culture in asymptomatic individuals (e.g., household contact of infected individual or test of cure in treated individual)?
- A: No. Throat culture of close contacts of highly vulnerable individuals (e.g., those with recurrent rheumatic fever) may be indicated.
- Q: Can scarlet fever occur in the absence of pharyngitis?
- A: Yes. Scarlet fever has been reported after group A streptococcal skin infections.
- Q: How soon can children return to school or child care?
- A: The current standard is return to school or daycare after 24 hours of effective antibiotic therapy. A recent study suggests that a 12-hour interval may be sufficient. The child should also be afebrile and feeling well enough to resume their regular activities.

SCOLIOSIS

Brian P. Hasley, MD

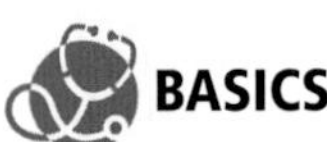

BASICS

DESCRIPTION

Coronal plane deformity (lateral curvature) of spine exceeding 10 degrees on radiographs with associated rotational deformity of the spine

EPIDEMIOLOGY

Adolescent idiopathic scoliosis

- Female-to-male ratios:
  - 1.4:1 for curves 11 to 20 degrees
  - 5.4:1 for curves >20 degrees

Prevalence

- 1–4% of population for curves ≥10 degrees
- 0.3–0.5% of population have curves >20 degrees.

RISK FACTORS

- Positive familial history of idiopathic scoliosis in 30% (not predictive of severity)
- Females have higher prevalences of larger and progressive idiopathic scoliosis.
- Persons with underlying conditions (e.g., Marfan syndrome, spina bifida, cerebral palsy) have increased risk for development of scoliosis.

Genetics

Under investigation: Several candidate genes have been identified.

ETIOLOGY

- Connective tissue disorder
  - Associated with several connective tissue disorders (including Marfan syndrome, Ehlers-Danlos syndrome)
  - Alterations in connective tissue of the spine, paraspinous muscles, and platelets
  - May be related to decreased bone mineral density of vertebral bodies
- Neurologic (equilibrium system)
  - Abnormalities noted in vestibular, ocular, proprioceptive, and vibratory functions
- Hormonal
  - Lower melatonin levels secreted from pineal body in those with adolescent idiopathic scoliosis
  - Growth hormone: more of an influential factor than an etiologic factor in studies
- Vertebral growth abnormalities
  - Asymmetric growth rates between the right and left sides of the spine

DIAGNOSIS

- Idiopathic scoliosis is a diagnosis of exclusion.
- Screening
  - Scoliosis screening recommended for children between 10 and 14 years
  - Many states have school screening programs.
  - Adams forward bend test is used to assess for scoliosis (see below). A scoliometer measurement of 7 degrees or greater warrants further evaluation.

HISTORY

- Onset: Consider when first noted, by whom, rate of worsening, previous treatment, patient recent growth, the physical change of puberty, associated signs or symptoms, familial history, etc.
- Patients with idiopathic scoliosis usually should not have pain, although they might have a discomfort or mild pain.
- Back pain in scoliotic patients is relatively common but should be taken seriously and investigated.
  - Present in 23% at time of initial evaluation (additional 9% during follow-up)
  - Of those with back pain, only ~9% have identifiable cause (e.g., spondylolysis, Scheuermann, syrinx, disc herniation, tumor, tethered cord).
  - If night pain, consider tumor such as osteoid osteoma.

PHYSICAL EXAM

- General inspection to look for skin changes such as café au lait spots, pigmentation, axillary freckling, or other signs of neurofibromatosis; also dysraphic signs (e.g., hairy patches, midline hemangioma, skin dimpling)
- Assess for skeletal maturity, hyperelasticity, contracture, congenital anomalies.
- Evaluate for deformity; asymmetry of spine, shoulders, waist, and trunk, including decompensation; abnormalities of thoracic kyphosis or cervical or lumbar lordosis; torso disfigurement.
- Assess for leg length discrepancy.
- Adams forward bend test used to look for vertebral rotation
  - Patient stands with knees straight and bends forward at the waist with arms dangling until the spine is horizontal.
  - For leg length inequalities, level pelvis with appropriate blocks under the short limb prior to measuring.
  - Scoliometer is used to assess the degree and direction of the spine and/or rib rotation.
- Neurologic exam to include abdominal reflexes. Abnormal reflexes may be associated with underlying spinal cord abnormality (e.g., syrinx).
- Cardiac auscultation is warranted for patients with congenital scoliosis due to associated cardiac abnormalities.

DIFFERENTIAL DIAGNOSIS

- Leg length inequality
- Spinal asymmetry
  - No rib hump or rotation
  - Does not have fixed deformities
  - Disappears with forward bending
  - No progression
- Scheuermann kyphosis—can have mild scoliosis
- Spondylolisthesis—may have long coronal curve associated with this condition

DIAGNOSTIC TESTS & INTERPRETATION

Initial Tests (screening, lab, imaging)

- Radiographs
  - Standing anterior-posterior and lateral scoliosis films on long 3-foot radiograph cassette or 3D low-dose radiation system
    - Assess for any soft tissue and congenital bony abnormalities (wedge vertebrae, bars, hemivertebrae).
    - Coronal plane deformity is measured as an angle (in degrees) using Cobb method.
    - Determine the triradiate cartilage and Risser classification of iliac apophysis ossification.
      - The triradiate cartilage and Risser grade (0 to 5) gives an estimate of how much skeletal growth remains and is correlated with risk of curve progression.
      - Triradiate cartilage usually closes before the iliac apophysis appears (Risser 0).
      - Risser sign is defined by the amount of calcification present in the iliac apophysis and measures the progressive ossification from anterolaterally to posteromedially.
        - Risser grade of 1 signifies up to 25% ossification of the iliac apophysis, proceeding to grade 4, which signifies 100% ossification.
          - A Risser grade of 5 means iliac apophysis has fused to the iliac crest after 100% ossification and indicates full maturity.
  - Curve patterns are classified according to King or Lenke classifications.
  - Bone age of the left hand and wrist
    - Another option to assess skeletal maturity and risk for scoliosis progression
    - Tanner-Whitehouse III RUS score—highly predictive of maturation and curve acceleration phase of growth

- Other diagnostic tests
  - MRI of the spine
    - May be indicated for abnormal neurologic findings or atypical scoliosis deformity (7% prevalence of intraspinal abnormalities found in left thoracic curves)
    - Not routinely necessary for adult idiopathic scoliosis without back pain
    - Indicated prior to spinal surgery for congenital scoliosis
  - Renal ultrasound indicated for evaluation of patient with congenital scoliosis (to assess associated renal abnormalities)
  - Echocardiogram—may be indicated for patient with congenital scoliosis to assess for possible associated cardiac anomalies
  - Labs—not usually helpful unless underlying metabolic condition is suspected

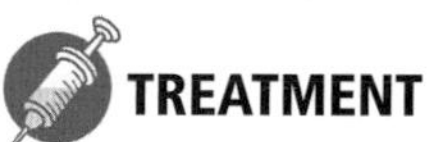

TREATMENT

GENERAL MEASURES

Principles of management are based on severity of deformity and on likelihood of progression.

- Observation
  - Curves <25 degrees
    - Immature patients (Risser 0, 1, 2) should be reevaluated in 4 to 6 months.
    - Skeletally mature patients (Risser 4 or 5) usually do not require ongoing follow-up unless special circumstances exist.
  - Curves 25 to 50 degrees in skeletally mature patients
    - Risser 4 or 5 patients are usually reevaluated in 6 months to 1 year.
    - Mature patients are usually reevaluated annually.
- Bracing
  - Goal—prevent curve progression in a skeletally immature patient.
  - Indications for bracing
    - Curves 25 to 45 degrees (Risser 0, 1, 2). 20- to 25-degree curve may be considered for bracing in skeletally immature patients with documented progression.
    - Continue brace treatment until maturity (2 years postmenarchal and Risser 4 in females, Risser 5 in males).
  - Brace types
    - Thoracolumbosacral orthosis (TLSO): success reported when used >16 to 18 hours per day; significantly improved outcome when compared with natural history
    - Cervicothoracolumbosacral orthosis (CTLSO): seldom needed except for higher thoracic or cervical curves
    - Nighttime bending brace: may be option for isolated lumbar/thoracolumbar curve <35 degrees

SURGERY/OTHER PROCEDURES

- Spinal fusion
- Recommended when curves exceed 45 to 50 degrees
  - Exception: Balanced thoracic and lumbar curves <55 degrees may be observed for progression.
- Thoracic curves and double major curves
  - Posterior segmental fixation instrumentation remains current standard.
  - Anterior spinal instrumentation for selected curves
- Isolated thoracolumbar and lumbar curves
  - Anterior spinal fusion using solid rod segmental constructs or posterior segmental fixation based on surgeon preference

ONGOING CARE

PROGNOSIS

- Overall good for most patients
- Risk of curve progression related to patient's maturity (Risser sign, menarcheal status) and to size of curve
- Curves <20 to 25 degrees have low risk of progression, even if patient is immature.
- Curves 25 to 45 degrees have higher risk of progression, particularly in skeletally immature patients.
- Curves >45 to 50 degrees have much higher risk of progression, regardless of maturity.

COMPLICATIONS

- Reduced pulmonary function for patients with thoracic curves >60 degrees
- Progression of lumbar curves >50 degrees in adult life with degenerative disc disease and pain in some individuals
- Cosmetic and emotional issues
- Complications of brace use include skin irritation, discomfort, and noncompliance.
- Surgical complications are usually more severe, including infection, implant loosening or breakage, neurologic damage, paralysis, blindness, or death.

ADDITIONAL READING

- Dormans JP. Establishing a standard of care for neuromonitoring during spinal deformity surgery. *Spine (Phila Pa 1976)*. 2010;35(25):2180–2185.
- Dunn J, Henrikson NB, Morrison CC, et al. *Screening for Adolescent Idiopathic Scoliosis: A Systematic Evidence Review for the U.S. Preventive Services Task Force*. Evidence Synthesis No. 156. AHRQ Publication No. 17-05230-EF-1. Rockville, MD: Agency for Healthcare Research and Quality; 2018.
- El-Hawary R, Chukwunyerenwa C. Update on evaluation and treatment of scoliosis. *Pediatr Clin North Am*. 2014;61(6):1223–1241.
- Hresko MT. Clinical practice. Idiopathic scoliosis in adolescents. *N Engl J Med*. 2013;368(9):834–841.
- Scoliosis Research Society: www.srs.org
- Sponseller PD, Flynn JM, Newton PO, et al. The association of patient characteristics and spinal curve parameters with Lenke classification types. *Spine (Phila Pa 1976)*. 2012;37(13):1138–1141.
- Sucato DJ. Management of severe spinal deformity: scoliosis and kyphosis. *Spine (Phila Pa 1976)*. 2010;35(25):2186–2192.
- Weinstein SL, Dolan LA, Wright JG, et al. Effects of bracing in adolescents with idiopathic scoliosis. *N Engl J Med*. 2013;369(16):1512–1521.

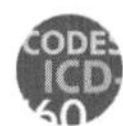

CODES

ICD10

- M41.9 Scoliosis, unspecified
- M40.209 Unspecified kyphosis, site unspecified
- M40.56 Lordosis, unspecified, lumbar region

FAQ

- Q: How long do you observe a patient with spinal asymmetry before ordering a radiograph?
- A: It depends on the presence or absence of abnormalities on the physical exam. If any of the signs mentioned here are seen or significant back pain is present, a radiograph or referral is indicated. The scoliometer is also a useful tool in screening patients.
- Q: How long do you observe a patient with spinal asymmetry before referral to an orthopedic surgeon?
- A: Consider referral if
  - Scoliometer measurement of 7 degrees or more on the Adams forward bend test
  - Cobb angle
    - >20 degrees
    - Progression of >5 degrees
- Q: If a child presents with scoliosis and back pain that occurs especially at night and is promptly relieved with nonsteroidal anti-inflammatory drugs, what diagnosis is suggested?
- A: Scoliosis associated with osteoid osteoma
- Q: What are the current recommendations for routine scoliosis screening from national professional organizations?
- A: Although the United States Preventive Services Task Force (USPSTF) has stated that "the current evidence is insufficient to assess the balance of benefits and harms of screening for adolescent idiopathic scoliosis in children and adolescents," the American Academy of Pediatrics (AAP) has endorsed the American Academy of Orthopaedic Surgeons and Scoliosis Research Society recommendation to screen for scoliosis.

SEBORRHEIC DERMATITIS

Olanrewaju O. Falusi, MD, FAAP

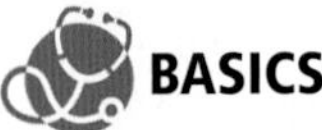

BASICS

DESCRIPTION

- Seborrheic dermatitis (SD) is a common, multifactorial skin disease influenced by both host and environmental factors.
- Involves sebaceous areas of the body
  - Including the scalp, face, back, chest, and intertriginous areas
  - Characterized by greasy, yellow, scaly erythematous lesions
- Usually a self-limited condition in infants but can be a chronic, relapsing condition in adolescents and adults

EPIDEMIOLOGY

- Trimodal distribution: infants, adolescents, and adults >50 years of age
- Highest prevalence between 2 weeks and 3 months of life
- Affects approximately 10% of the general population and up to 70% of infants in the first 3 months of life
- No sex predilection in infants; however, in adolescents and adults, males are affected more commonly than females.
- Seasonal pattern: Prevalence of disease increases in winter months.
- Strong association between *Malassezia* species, a common commensal organism, and SD

RISK FACTORS

- There are no known genetic factors that contribute to disease.
- Hormonal effects: exposure to maternal estrogen in infancy and surge of androgens in puberty
- Use of neuroleptic medications
- Immunocompromised status
  - Impaired cellular immunity may contribute to pathogenesis of disease.
  - Prevalence of SD in immunocompromised patients is significantly higher than in general population.

GENERAL PREVENTION

There are no known preventive measures.

PATHOPHYSIOLOGY

- Unknown, but suspected role of sebum, *Malassezia*, and inflammatory factors
- Androgens stimulate sebaceous glands, causing production of more sebum.
- *Malassezia*
  - A lipophilic yeast that is normally found in sebum-rich areas of the skin
  - Can break down skin sebum lipids, producing potentially inflammatory fatty acids
- In response to the inflammatory fatty acids, keratinocytes produce proinflammatory cytokines.

ETIOLOGY

Not completely known, although it is hypothesized that yeast, androgens, and the local host immune response play a role in SD development.

DIAGNOSIS

HISTORY

- Older children and adolescents: Ask about onset of puberty symptoms.
- Typically asymptomatic or only mildly pruritic
- Children and adolescents: Ask about symptoms and signs of immunocompromised such as frequent infections, failure to thrive, and chronic diarrhea.
- HIV and tuberculosis (TB) history

PHYSICAL EXAM

- Infants: "cradle cap"
  - Yellow, greasy adherent scales on the scalp
  - Lesions may also occur on the forehead, eyebrows, eyelids, postauricular area, nasolabial folds, diaper area, and trunk (usually periumbilical).
  - No excoriations
  - No hepatosplenomegaly
- Adolescents and adults
  - Mild: "dandruff"; dry, flaking scalp or face in areas of facial hair; no surrounding inflammation
  - More severe SD: patchy, orange/yellow, greasy plaques in scalp, nasolabial folds, postauricular area, intertriginous areas, or other regions of increased sebaceous gland activity
  - Blepharitis with erythema and scaling of the eyelid margins may also occur.
  - No excoriations
  - No hepatosplenomegaly

DIFFERENTIAL DIAGNOSIS

- SD can be confused with infectious conditions of the skin, malignancy, or inflammatory disorders.
- Dermatophyte infections
  - *Tinea capitis*, *tinea faciei*, and *tinea corporis* are also scaling lesions. The lesions are scaly but not typically greasy or plaque-like and lack erythema.
  - Microscopic evaluation of lesion can differentiate it from SD by the presence of hyphae in dermatophyte infection.
- Immunologic
  - Atopic dermatitis
    - May present on the face of infants but typically spares the nasolabial folds
    - May also involve the extensor aspects of the extremities
    - Usually is pruritic
  - Psoriasis vulgaris
    - Typically presents as sharply defined plaques, bright red in color with thick silver scales
    - Unlike SD, children with psoriasis may have nail changes such as nail pitting and onycholysis.
- Malignancy/Langerhans cell histiocytosis (LCH)
  - LCH may present with a scaly erythematous lesions in the same distribution as SD.
  - Unlike SD, LCH may have the presence of small reddish-brown crusted papules or vesicles.
  - In addition, there may be organ system involvement such as hepatosplenomegaly.
  - LCH is refractory to typical treatment for SD.

DIAGNOSTIC TESTS & INTERPRETATION

Initial Tests (screening, lab, imaging)

Primarily a clinical diagnosis; there are no specific tests for seborrhea.

Diagnostic Procedures/Other

Skin biopsy should be reserved for unusual or refractory cases of SD to reconsider the diagnosis.

Test Interpretation

Pathologic findings

- Skin biopsy findings
  - Focal parakeratosis in epidermis; more prominent in HIV-infected individuals
  - Predominance of neutrophils in the scale crust at the margins of follicular ostia
  - Yeast cells sometimes are visible within keratinocytes on special stains, but hyphae should not be present in SD.

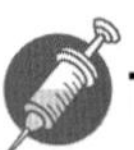

TREATMENT

- Treatment depends on presentation and age of patient.
- For infants, SD usually has a benign and self-limited course. Medications may not be necessary for the treatment of infant SD.

- Physical measures such as the application of emollients followed by the removal of scalp scales with a brush or comb may improve symptoms.
  - Examples of emollients include mineral oil, baby oil, or petroleum jelly.
  - There have been some studies to suggest that the use of organic oils such as olive oil or vegetable oil may provide an excellent media for *Malassezia* overgrowth, potentially worsening SD.
  - Frequent shampooing with a nonmedicated shampoo may also be beneficial.

MEDICATION

- For infants who do not respond to conservative therapy or for older children/adults, medications will likely be necessary.
- Classes of drugs that should be considered are keratolytic, antifungal, and anti-inflammatory medications. At the current time, there is no evidence to support the use of one class of drug versus another.
- Antifungals
  - Azoles: ketoconazole
    - 1% or 2% gel, lotion, or shampoo
    - Shampoo should be used twice per week (at least 3 days between doses) for up to 8 weeks; caution: may cause eye irritation
    - Gel or lotion should be used twice daily for up to 2 to 4 weeks.
    - Oral antifungals have been studied in refractory cases; in clinical practice, the diagnosis should be reconsidered prior to initiating oral treatments.
  - Selenium sulfide
    - Antifungal and keratolytic effect
    - Shampoo. Massage 5 to 10 mL into wet scalp, leave on scalp 2 to 3 minutes, and then rinse thoroughly.
    - Usually, two applications each week for 2 weeks will provide control.
  - Ciclopirox: 1% shampoo
    - Can be used in children ≥16 years old
    - Massage 5 mL into wet scalp, leave on scalp 3 minutes, and then rinse.
    - Use 2 times per week (at least 3 days between doses) for up to 4 weeks.
- Keratolytics: Massage into scalp 2 to 3 times per week, leave on 5 minutes, and then rinse.
  - Salicylic acid
    - Shampoo or lotion
    - No studies on efficacy and safety in infants
  - Coal tar
    - Shampoo
    - Decreases sebum production
  - Pyrithione zinc
    - Most commonly used as a shampoo
    - Also has antifungal properties
- Anti-inflammatory therapies
  - Corticosteroids
    - Shampoo, foam, ointment, creams, or lotions
    - There are multiple options; treatment will depend on severity of inflammation and age of patient.
    - May reduce erythema and scaling more effectively than antifungals
    - Ointments should be considered for more severe cases because skin absorption is improved.
    - Foams can be used in hairy areas because of ease of application.
  - Calcineurin inhibitors: tacrolimus ointment
    - Can be used in children >2 years of age
    - Fungicidal and anti-inflammatory properties
    - Apply thin layer of 0.03% ointment to affected area twice daily until symptoms resolve or up to 6 weeks.

ALERT

FDA black box warning on tacrolimus due to potential increased risk of malignancy. Avoid prolonged use in any age.

COMPLEMENTARY & ALTERNATIVE THERAPIES

- Tea tree oil 5% has been demonstrated to be effective in treating scalp seborrhea.
- Other alternative nutritional therapies that have been considered are probiotics and omega-3 essential fatty acids. However, there are no sufficient data on effectiveness or safety in children.

ONGOING CARE

PATIENT EDUCATION

- Response to treatment will likely occur in the first 2 weeks of therapy; however, long-term intermittent therapy may be required. Adolescents with SD may have a chronic course.
- The intermittent use of an antifungal shampoo can be used to prevent relapses.

PROGNOSIS

- The infantile form will typically self-resolve by the end of the 1st year of life.
- Older children and adolescents may have a more chronic, relapsing course.
- If SD doesn't respond to therapy within approximately 6 weeks, consider alternative diagnoses or underlying conditions such as immunodeficiency.

ADDITIONAL READING

- Borda LJ, Wikramanayake TC. Seborrheic dermatitis and dandruff: a comprehensive review. *J Clin Investig Dermatol*. 2015;3(2):1–22. doi:10.13188/2373-1044.1000019.
- Clark GW, Pope SM, Jaboori KA. Diagnosis and treatment of seborrheic dermatitis. *Am Fam Physician*. 2015;91(3):185–190.
- Dessinioti C, Katsambas A. Seborrheic dermatitis: etiology, risk factors, and treatments: facts and controversies. *Clin Dermatol*. 2013;31(4):343–351.
- Gupta AK, Nicol K, Batra R. Role of antifungal agents in the treatment of seborrheic dermatitis. *Am J Clin Dermatol*. 2004;5(6):417–422.
- Kastarinen H, Oksanen T, Okokon EO, et al. Topical anti-inflammatory agents for seborrhoeic dermatitis of the face or scalp. *Cochrane Database Syst Rev*. 2014;(5):CD009446.
- Satchell AC, Saurajen A, Bell C, et al. Treatment of dandruff with 5% tea tree oil shampoo. *J Am Acad Dermatol*. 2002;47(6):852–855.
- Siegfried E, Glenn E. Use of olive oil for the treatment of seborrheic dermatitis in children. *Arch Pediatr Adolesc Med*. 2012;166(10):967.

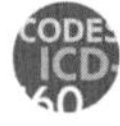

CODES

ICD10

- L21.9 Seborrheic dermatitis, unspecified
- L21.0 Seborrhea capitis
- L21.1 Seborrheic infantile dermatitis

FAQ

- Q: How does one distinguish SD from candidiasis, another common skin finding in infants?
- A: Candidiasis can appear scaly and affect intertriginous areas similar SD but often has a more beefy red and glistening appearance.
- Q: Is there a laboratory test to diagnose SD?
- A: There are no specific laboratory tests. It is a clinical diagnosis. If the diagnosis is unclear or refractory to treatment, consider a skin biopsy.
- Q: Are there seasonal changes in the course of SD?
- A: Some patients report worsening of symptoms in the winter months. Sunlight may improve patients' symptoms. UV therapy is a treatment option for extensive SD.
- Q: Does SD cause permanent hair loss?
- A: SD may cause some hair loss acutely. However, patients can be reassured that it does not cause permanent hair loss.

S

SEIZURES, PARTIAL AND GENERALIZED

Kristen Park, MD • Kelly G. Knupp, MD

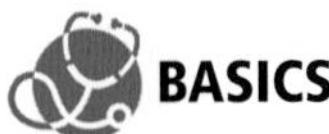

BASICS

DESCRIPTION

Seizures arise from abnormal electrical discharges in the cerebral cortex that lead to alterations of consciousness, behavior, motor activity, sensation, or autonomic function. Epilepsy is a disease defined as (i) two or more seizures without acute provocation, (ii) one seizure and >60% further risk of additional seizures, or (iii) diagnosis of an epilepsy syndrome. Seizures are classified as focal, generalized, unknown, and focal to bilateral based on where the seizure starts.

- Focal seizure types
  - Awareness should be described as focal aware, focal impaired awareness, or awareness unknown.
  - Motor and other symptoms should be described as focal motor seizure and focal nonmotor seizure.
- Aura is not in the updated classification but can still be used to describe a feeling at the beginning of a seizure.
- Generalized seizure types
  - Tonic–clonic, absence, myoclonic, clonic, tonic, atonic
- Unknown onset seizure types: epileptic spasms, behavior arrest
- Focal to bilateral seizure is used to describe a seizure that is focal in onset and evolves into a generalized seizure.

EPIDEMIOLOGY

Incidence

Epilepsy affects 0.5–1% of all children (birth through 16 years). 120,000 children seek care annually in the United States for a seizure. Between 20,000 and 45,000 children per year are diagnosed with epilepsy; highest risk is in the 1st year of life.

Prevalence

4 to 10 per 1,000 children in developed countries have epilepsy.

ETIOLOGY

- Structural
  - Brain tumor
  - Malformations of cortical development
  - Prior stroke
- Genetic
- Infectious
  - Neurocysticercosis
  - Cerebral malaria
- Metabolic
  - Aminoacidopathies
  - Pyridoxine-dependent epilepsy
- Immune
  - *N*-methyl D-aspartate (NMDA) receptor encephalitis
- Unknown cause

RISK FACTORS

Genetics

- Epilepsy is both polygenic and multifactorial.
- There are currently >400 single genes known to be associated with epilepsy in childhood.
- Copy number variations encompassing deletions and duplications of various sizes have also been implicated in the genetics of epilepsy.
- The risk of epilepsy with an affected primary relative increases from the population risk (1–2%) to 4–8%.
- Epilepsy may also be a feature of other genetic disorders such as trisomy 21 and Angelman syndrome or be part of a larger neurodevelopmental presentation.

COMMONLY ASSOCIATED CONDITIONS

- The incidence of childhood-onset epilepsy associated with intellectual disability and cerebral palsy is 15–38%.
- Epilepsy occurs in 8–28% of children with autism.
- Attention deficit hyperactivity disorder (ADHD), depression, and anxiety are more common in children with epilepsy than in the general population.

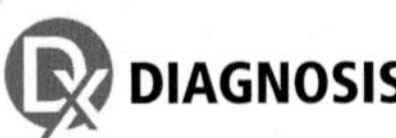

DIAGNOSIS

HISTORY

- Age, family history of seizures, developmental status, birth history
- Health at seizure onset: febrile, ill, sleep deprivation, trauma, toxins, ingestion, head injury
- Current medications and change in antiepileptic medication
- Other neurologic signs: confusion; encephalopathy; weakness; sensory deficits; and change in vision, behavior, balance, or gait
- Detailed history of symptoms during seizure
  - Aura: subjective sensations
  - Behavior: preceding and during seizure
  - Change in consciousness or responsiveness
  - Vocal: cry, gasp, speech
  - Motor: head or eye turning, jerking, posturing, stiffening, automatisms (purposeless repetitive movements such as picking at clothing, lip smacking)
  - Respiration: cyanosis, change in breathing pattern, apnea
  - Autonomic: pupillary dilation, drooling, incontinence, pallor, vomiting, tachycardia
- Symptoms after seizure: amnesia, confusion, sleepiness, transient focal weakness (Todd paresis), headache

PHYSICAL EXAM

- Vital signs: ABCs need to be checked immediately and recurrently; fever, tachycardia, bradycardia, or hypertension
- Signs of head trauma or child abuse: retinal hemorrhages, papilledema, presence of fractures, bruises of different ages
- Head circumference/abnormal head growth
- Signs of systemic infection: meningismus, purpura
- Skin examination: café au lait or ash leaf spots, facial hemangioma (suggesting neurocutaneous disorders)
- Neurologic examination: pupillary reactivity, mental status, focal motor weakness
- Seizures: If there is a question of continuing seizures, proceed with recommendations for "Status Epilepticus."

ALERT

- Attention to adequate airway and breathing and need for oxygenation or ventilatory support is the primary focus.
- If the child continues to have a seizure or has recurrent seizures, an abortive benzodiazepine should be administered either rectally or IV.

DIFFERENTIAL DIAGNOSIS

Nonepileptic events

- Syncope
- Breath-holding spells
- Hyperventilation
- Movements related to gastroesophageal reflux (Sandifer syndrome)
- Sleep disorders: benign sleep myoclonus, night terrors, somnambulism, narcolepsy with cataplexy
- Migraine/headache syndromes, especially complicated migraine
- Nonepileptic movement disorders: startle disease, shuddering spells, paroxysmal dyskinesias, tics, drug-induced dystonia
- Behavioral: stereotypies, self-stimulatory behaviors, inattention/ADHD

DIAGNOSTIC TESTS & INTERPRETATION

Initial Tests (screening, lab, imaging)

- Testing should be based on clinical history.
  - Hyponatremia (<125 mEq/L) was found to be associated with seizures in 70% of infants <6 months of age in one clinical study.
- However, in general, a standard laboratory evaluation (electrolytes, CBC, liver enzymes, calcium, and magnesium) did not show unsuspected abnormalities or contribute to the diagnosis or management in several clinical studies. Toxicology screening should be considered in any child in whom there is a question of drug exposure or substance abuse.
- Blood glucose (fingerstick can be obtained quickly)
- Antiseizure medication (ASM) levels if indicated; few of the newer ASMs have relevant or rapidly available serum levels but may be useful for documenting adherence to a medication regimen.
- Neuroimaging: Evidence-based reviews showed low yields of acute CT or MRI in children presenting with seizures without focal signs or deficits. Current recommendations are as follows:
  - MRI is generally the preferred modality.
  - Emergent neuroimaging should be performed in any child with focal deficit not returning to baseline within several hours.
  - Nonurgent MRI is recommended based on clinical scenario and EEG findings.

Diagnostic Procedures/Other

- EEG
  - Indicated urgently if there is concern that child may be continuing to seize
  - Nonurgent EEGs are indicated for first afebrile seizure.
- Lumbar puncture
  - Should be considered for meningeal signs, infants <6 months of age, or persistent alteration of consciousness; however, it is not routinely recommended.
  - If intracranial hypertension, mass lesion, or hydrocephalus is suspected, defer lumbar puncture until after neuroimaging.

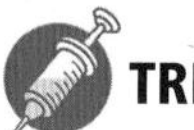

TREATMENT

Seizure first aid

- Assess airway and breathing.
- Turn the patient on their side to allow the tongue to fall forward and saliva to run out.
- Place nothing in the mouth.
- Time the event—a convulsive seizure lasting longer than 5 minutes constitutes a medical emergency. Refer to the guidelines on "Status Epilepticus."

MEDICATION

- Acute treatment of seizures
  - Benzodiazepines should be given for prolonged seizures (>5 minutes) or acute repetitive seizures.
    - Rectal diazepam (0.3 to 0.5 mg/kg/dose; max dose 20 mg), intranasal/buccal midazolam (0.2 mg/kg/dose; max dose 10 mg), or intranasal lorazepam (0.1 mg/kg/dose; max dose: 4 mg, needs refrigeration) can be administered by parents/caregivers.
  - Fosphenytoin 20 mg phenytoin sodium equivalents (PE)/kg IM/IV
  - Phenobarbital 10 to 20 mg/kg IV
  - Levetiracetam 20 mg/kg IV
- Chronic ASM therapy is not indicated after acute symptomatic seizures or after a single unprovoked seizure in a child with normal neurologic examination and EEG.
- Chronic ASM therapy may be considered after first seizure, symptomatic of an acute injury or structural brain lesion (i.e., brain tumor).
- The choice of ASM for long-term management of epilepsy depends on the specific seizure type and epilepsy syndrome. Monotherapy is always preferred.
- Many formulations (liquid, sprinkle caps, and extended-release) are available and should be individualized to the patient. For teenagers, extended-release forms may be recommended for compliance.
- Focal seizures (any type)
  - Oxcarbazepine 20 to 40 mg/kg/24 h
  - Levetiracetam 20 to 60 mg/kg/24 h
  - Lamotrigine: dosing varies with valproate
  - Topiramate 4 to 10 mg/kg/24 h
  - Valproate 15 to 50 mg/kg/24 h
  - Zonisamide 2 to 10 mg/kg/24 h
- Genetic (idiopathic) generalized epilepsies
  - Ethosuximide 15 to 40 mg/kg/24 h: initial ASM for absence seizures
  - Levetiracetam 20 to 90 mg/kg/24 h (limited data)
  - Topiramate 8 to 12 mg/kg/24 h (limited data)

ALERT

- Hyponatremic seizures: serum sodium <120 mEq/dL in infants with gastroenteritis; slow sodium correction indicated
- Apnea and hypoventilation from excessive administration of benzodiazepines and phenobarbital for seizures. Monitor ventilation and oxygenation; avoid large doses.

ISSUES FOR REFERRAL

In general, patients who have not responded to two seizure medications should be evaluated by a neurologist who specializes in epilepsy.

ADDITIONAL THERAPIES

Patients refractory to ASM treatment: other options—ketogenic diet, vagus nerve stimulator, surgical resection

ALERT

A 2-fold risk of increased suicidality has been associated with ASM use, with a U.S. Food and Drug Administration (FDA) black box warning on product labeling. Monitoring for suicidal ideation and mood changes is warranted in all patients taking ASMs.

ONGOING CARE

PATIENT EDUCATION

- Injuries: Rarely, serious injury occurs with brief seizures from loss of consciousness and resultant falls.
- Daily precautions: Few restrictions are needed with the exceptions of driving (see state laws) and dangerous sports.
- Supervision around water is strongly advised; showering is generally safer than bathing.
- Helmets should be worn with all wheeled toys; avoid top bunk beds or locked bedrooms and unprotected heights.
- Sudden unexplained death in epilepsy patients (SUDEP) should be mentioned to all patients at appropriate times.
- Families should be instructed in seizure first aid: Roll patient on the side, place nothing in the mouth, ensure safe environment.

PROGNOSIS

- In a large review of prospective studies, the aggregate risk for recurrence of seizures after the first unprovoked event was 40% within 2 years.
- 80–90% of children who recur do so within the first 2 years after the initial event.
- Various risk factors have been found to increase recurrence risk in studies but concordance is incomplete. The strongest association has been seen with nocturnal seizures, prior neurologic insult, and an abnormal EEG.
- If a second event occurs (separated by at least 24 hours as two seizures within a day is typically considered a single event), the risk for further seizures increases to 61% within 2 years.

COMPLICATIONS

- Brain damage
  - From brief seizures: no convincing evidence
  - From prolonged seizures (>30 minutes): Brain injury may occur secondary to hypoxia.
  - Untreated or poorly controlled epilepsy: increased risk of intractable epilepsy and SUDEP
- Status epilepticus
  - Incidence of 18 to 20/100,000 per year in childhood
  - Mortality in children between 3% and 6%
  - Recurrence risk for status epilepticus is approximately 16% within the 1st year.
- Patient monitoring: depends on treatment and as mentioned earlier

ADDITIONAL READING

- Arthur TM, deGrauw TJ, Johnson CS, et al. Seizure recurrence risk following a first seizure in neurologically normal children. *Epilepsia*. 2008;49(11):1950–1954.
- Epilepsy Foundation. Answer place: parent information on the Internet. http://www.epilepsy.com/learn. Accessed October 30, 2017.
- Berg AT. Risk of recurrence after a first unprovoked seizure. *Epilepsia*. 2008;49(Suppl 1):13–18.
- Hirtz D, Ashwal S, Berg A, et al. Practice parameter: evaluating a first nonfebrile seizure in children: report of the quality standards subcommittee of the American Academy of Neurology, the Child Neurology Society, and the American Epilepsy Society. *Neurology*. 2000;55(5):616–623.
- Hirtz D, Berg A, Bettis D, et al. Practice parameter: treatment of the child with a first unprovoked seizure: report of the Quality Standards Subcommittee of the American Academy of Neurology and the Practice Committee of the Child Neurology Society. *Neurology*. 2003;60(2):166–175.

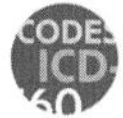

CODES

ICD10

- R56.9 Unspecified convulsions
- G40.209 Local-rel symptc epi w cmplx prt seiz,not ntrct,w/o stat epi
- G40.309 Gen idiopathic epilepsy, not intractable, w/o stat epi

FAQ

- Q: How do I know if my child has epilepsy?
- A: The term "epilepsy" is applied to children with two or more seizures without an acute cause or with a single seizure and a significant risk of more seizures.
- Q: Will my child always have epilepsy?
- A: The likelihood of outgrowing epilepsy depends on the syndrome. In many cases, anticonvulsants can be discontinued if the child has been seizure free for 2 years.
- Q: Why does my child have epilepsy?
- A: There are many different reasons to have epilepsy, including genetic, trauma, and other abnormalities of the brain. About 40% of people with epilepsy never have an identified etiology.

SEIZURES–FEBRILE

Jennifer L. Griffith, MD, PhD • Liu Lin Thio, MD, PhD

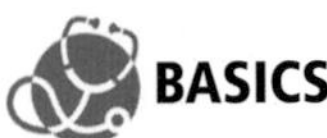

BASICS

DESCRIPTION

- Febrile seizure: seizure in ≤60-month-old child accompanied by a fever (≥100.4°F or 38°C by any method) but without central nervous system infection or prior unprovoked seizure (American Academy of Pediatrics [AAP] guidelines use 6 months as the lower age limit, whereas International League Against Epilepsy uses 1 month.)
- Two types:
  - Simple: febrile seizures that are generalized from the start, last <15 minutes, *AND* do not recur in 24 hours
  - Complex
    - Febrile seizures that are focal (including postictal weakness), last ≥15 minutes, *OR* occur >1 time in 24 hours (simple febrile seizures plus—a proposed new category for those whose only complex feature is >1 seizure in 24 hours)
    - Febrile status epilepticus: one febrile seizure or series of febrile seizures without full recovery in between lasting ≥30 minutes

EPIDEMIOLOGY

- Age
  - Most febrile seizures occur between 6 months and 3 years of age.
  - Peak age is about 18 months.
- Type
  - 65–70% are simple febrile seizures.
  - 20–35% are complex febrile seizures.
  - ~5% are febrile status epilepticus.
- Timing of seizure
  - ~20% before or <1 hour of fever onset
  - ~60% 1 to 24 hours after fever onset
  - ~20% >24 hours after fever onset

Prevalence

- Most common childhood seizure
- Febrile seizures occur in 2–5% of children in the United States and Western Europe, 9–10% of children in Japan, and 14% of children in Guam.

RISK FACTORS

- Positive family history of febrile seizures
- Prior febrile seizure (see "Prognosis" section)

Genetics

Usually multifactorial or polygenic inheritance

GENERAL PREVENTION

- Antipyretics do not reduce the recurrence risk of simple febrile seizures.
- Very low risk of febrile seizure after some vaccinations, for example, DPT, influenza and MMR(V)
  - Nonetheless, routine childhood immunizations are recommended, as the morbidity of vaccine-preventable illnesses outweighs the risk of febrile seizures.
  - Centers for Disease Control and Prevention (CDC) Advisory Committee on Immunization Practices (ACIP) does not list febrile seizures as a contraindication to any commonly used vaccine; seizures ≤3 days after a previous dose of DTP/DTaP is listed as a precaution for future doses.

PATHOPHYSIOLOGY

- Elevated temperatures in developing brain may increase neuronal excitability.
- Fever increases cytokines that may enhance neuronal excitability.
- Genetic factors
- Hyperventilation from fever causes a respiratory alkalosis that may promote seizures.

ETIOLOGY

- Any viral or bacterial infection
  - Human herpesvirus 6 and 7
  - Influenza A
  - Shigellosis
- Vaccines
  - Influenza, DPT, and MMR(V)
  - These may increase the risk of febrile seizures but not epilepsy.

COMMONLY ASSOCIATED CONDITIONS

- Generalized epilepsy with febrile seizures plus (GEFS+)
  - Febrile seizures beyond 6 years of age or afebrile seizures of varying types ranging from mild to severe
  - Multiple genes identified including *SCN1A*, *SCN2A*, *SCN1B*, *GABRG2*, *GABRD*, and *PCDH19*
- Febrile infection–related epilepsy syndrome (FIRES)
  - Catastrophic epileptic encephalopathy of unknown etiology that begins with a febrile illness and refractory status epilepticus
  - High morbidity and mortality

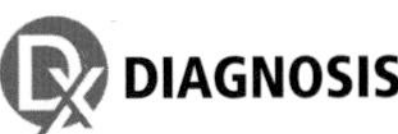

DIAGNOSIS

HISTORY

- Obtain detailed description of spell to determine if it was a seizure.
  - Circumstances in which spell occurred
  - Duration
  - Focal features suggest seizure.
  - Focal postictal weakness suggests seizure.
- Ask about prior seizures/spells.
  - Prior afebrile seizure suggests epilepsy.
  - Prior febrile seizure supports diagnosis.
  - Prior nonepileptic spells
- Determine cause of fever/illness.
  - Duration
  - Height of fever
  - Symptoms: rhinorrhea, diarrhea
- Ask about new neurologic symptoms such as headache or change in gait that would require further evaluation.
- Ask about toxic ingestions.
- Identify seizure risk factors from past medical history.
  - Perinatal complications
  - Prior brain insult: trauma, meningitis
  - Developmental delay
- Ask about medications, including antibiotics that might mask signs/symptoms of meningoencephalitis.
- Family history: ask about family members with
  - Febrile seizures
  - Epilepsy

PHYSICAL EXAM

- Identify fever source.
  - Vital signs, including temperature
  - Assess anterior fontanelle, sutures, and head circumference for increased intracranial pressure, which may occur with meningitis or space-occupying lesion.
  - Assess for signs of meningitis such as nuchal rigidity.
  - Examine ears and throat for infection.
  - Examine skin for rashes and other signs of infection.
  - Examine heart and lungs for infection.
  - Assess for trauma.
- Detailed neurologic exam
  - Assess skin for neurocutaneous syndromes.
  - Assess mental status.
  - Assess for subtle signs of ongoing seizure such as myoclonus or nystagmus.
  - Examine cranial nerves. Include funduscopic exam for papilledema.
  - Examine gait, motor system, sensation, coordination, and deep tendon reflexes for abnormalities and asymmetries.

DIFFERENTIAL DIAGNOSIS

- Acute symptomatic seizure
  - Infection
    - Meningoencephalitis: primary diagnostic consideration; bacterial or viral; consider HSV.
    - Other infection such as gastroenteritis causing hypernatremic dehydration
    - Benign convulsions with mild gastroenteritis
  - Toxic/metabolic
  - Stroke
  - Trauma
- Epilepsy
- Nonepileptic spell
  - Febrile delirium
  - Chills
  - Breath-holding spells

DIAGNOSTIC TESTS & INTERPRETATION

Initial Tests (screening, lab, imaging)

- Simple febrile seizure
  - Serum electrolytes, calcium, phosphorus, magnesium, glucose, and complete blood count are not recommended solely for determining the cause of the seizure.
  - Consider studies to determine fever source.
  - Lumbar puncture
    - Perform when symptoms/signs of meningitis or intracranial infection are present.
    - Consider lumbar puncture if
      - 6- to 12-month-old infant has deficient or unknown immunization status for *Haemophilus influenzae* type b or *Streptococcus pneumoniae*.
      - Pretreated with antibiotics

- Complex febrile seizure
  - Consider studies to identify fever source and as clinically indicated.
  - Indications for lumbar puncture are similar to indications for lumbar puncture for simple febrile seizure but strongly consider for all, especially those with altered mental status.
- Febrile status epilepticus
  - Recommend studies to treat correctable causes of seizures (e.g., hypoglycemia, hyponatremia) and to identify fever source.
  - Lumbar puncture
    - Perform for any suspicion of meningitis or intracranial infection but strongly consider for all especially if first episode or if mental status is altered.
    - It is important to note that febrile status epilepticus *rarely* causes a CSF pleocytosis.
- Imaging
  - Simple febrile seizure: imaging not indicated
  - Complex febrile seizure
    - Acute brain imaging usually unnecessary, especially if the only complex feature is multiple seizures. Recommend acute MRI (CT acceptable) if child has persistently altered mental status, persistent focal neurologic findings, or symptoms/signs of increased intracranial pressure.
    - Recommend routine brain MRI if not done acutely, especially for focal seizure, focal exam findings, or focal EEG abnormality.
  - Febrile status epilepticus
    - Recommend acute brain imaging (MRI preferred but CT acceptable), especially if first episode with abnormal mental status or focal neurologic findings.
    - Recommend routine brain MRI if not done acutely; may show hippocampal injury that may increase risk for developing epilepsy
- Electroencephalogram
  - Simple febrile seizure
    - EEG not indicated; not predictive of febrile seizure recurrence or development of epilepsy
  - Complex febrile seizure
    - Recommend stat EEG if concerned about nonconvulsive status epilepticus.
    - Recommend routine EEG, especially for abnormal neurologic development or exam. Epileptiform abnormalities or focal slowing may increase risk for developing epilepsy.
  - Febrile status epilepticus
    - Recommend stat EEG if concerned about nonconvulsive status epilepticus.
    - Recommend routine EEG; may show temporal slowing or attenuation that correlates with hippocampal abnormality on MRI

TREATMENT

GENERAL MEASURES

Treat infection.

MEDICATION

- Abortive
  - Consider rectal diazepam (0.5 mg/kg) for febrile seizures ≥5 minutes; may cause drowsiness and ataxia; rarely causes respiratory depression
  - See "Status Epilepticus" chapter for treating febrile status epilepticus.
- Preventive
  - In certain clinical circumstances, for parental anxiety, may use oral diazepam (0.33 mg/kg every 8 hours) during a febrile illness until afebrile for 24 hours; may cause drowsiness and ataxia
  - Daily phenobarbital or valproate therapy may prevent febrile seizures, but risks outweigh benefits.

ISSUES FOR REFERRAL

- Simple febrile seizure
  - Routine or as needed follow-up with primary health care provider for underlying infection
- Complex febrile seizure
  - Children with developmental delay, preexisting neurologic findings, focal neurologic findings during or after seizure, abnormal imaging, or abnormal EEG may benefit from follow-up with a pediatric neurologist to evaluate for risk of future epilepsy and an underlying neurologic disorder.

ADMISSION, INPATIENT, AND NURSING CONSIDERATIONS

- Any child who has not returned to baseline following a seizure should, at a minimum, be admitted for observation.
- Parents should be educated about febrile seizures, seizure precautions, and seizure first aid (see FAQ).

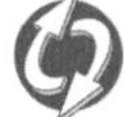

ONGOING CARE

PROGNOSIS

- Febrile seizure recurrence
  - 50% of children <12 months of age at time of first simple febrile seizure have recurrent febrile seizures.
  - 30% of children >12 months of age at time of first febrile seizure have a second.
  - Of children with a second febrile seizure, 50% experience a third.
- Risk for developing epilepsy
  - 6–7% for all febrile seizures
  - 2–7.5% for simple febrile seizures
  - 10–20% for complex febrile seizures
- Mortality
  - 0.85% for all febrile seizures
  - 0% for simple febrile seizures
  - <1.6% for complex febrile seizures with all deaths from febrile status epilepticus
- No evidence that simple febrile seizures increase risk of neurologic or cognitive deficits.

ADDITIONAL READING

- Chungath M, Shorvon S. The mortality and morbidity of febrile seizures. *Nat Clin Pract Neurol*. 2008;4(11):610–621.
- Gupta A. Febrile seizures. *Continuum (Minneap Minn)*. 2016;22(1):51–59.
- Principi N, Esposito S. Vaccines and febrile seizures. *Expert Rev Vaccines*. 2013;12(8):885–892.
- Steering Committee on Quality Improvement and Management, Subcommittee on Febrile Seizures, American Academy of Pediatrics. Febrile seizures: clinical practice guideline for the long-term management of the child with simple febrile seizures. *Pediatrics*. 2008;121(6):1281–1286.
- Subcommittee on Febrile Seizures, American Academy of Pediatrics. Neurodiagnostic evaluation of the child with a simple febrile seizure. *Pediatrics*. 2011;127(2):389–394.

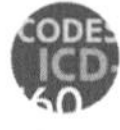

CODES

ICD10

- R56.00 Simple febrile convulsions
- R56.01 Complex febrile convulsions

FAQ

- Q: What should parents be told?
- A: Good neurodevelopmental outcome for simple febrile seizures but relatively high risk for recurrence.
- Q: Can a child die from a febrile seizure?
- A: No. Reported mortality from simple febrile seizures or short complex febrile seizures; low mortality with febrile status epilepticus
- Q: Can a febrile seizure cause brain damage?
- A: Simple febrile seizures do not. Febrile status epilepticus may.
- Q: What should the parents do when the child has a seizure?
- A: Stay calm. Place child in safe place. Turn child on side to keep airway clear. Do not restrain. Do not put anything in mouth. Time seizure. If seizure lasts 5 minutes, call 911 and administer abortive medication such as rectal diazepam if available.
- Q: What precautions should the parents take?
- A: Common sense steps such as no unsupervised baths or swimming and no climbing above head height. Always wear helmet when riding bike or doing other activity with wheels; no driving all-terrain vehicles

S

SEPARATION ANXIETY DISORDER

Julie S. O'Brien, MD, MS • Eva C. Ihle, MD, PhD

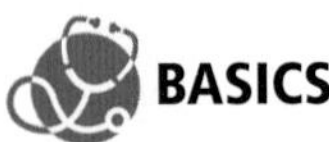

BASICS

DESCRIPTION

Separation anxiety disorder (SAD) is defined as developmentally inappropriate fear and anxiety about being away from home and/or apart from the individuals to whom a child is most attached.

- This diagnosis should be distinguished from developmentally appropriate worries, fears, and responses to stressors.

EPIDEMIOLOGY

- Prevalence estimates range from 4% in children aged 7 to 9 years to 1.6% in adolescents.
- Prevalence is slightly higher in females than males.
- Symptoms tend to peak between 7 and 9 years of age, but the disorder can present at any age.

ETIOLOGY

Studies show that there are genetic and environmental precursors to the development of SAD:

- A temperament of behavioral inhibition in which a child tends to approach unfamiliar situations with distress, restraint, and avoidance has been shown to be associated with development of anxiety disorders.
- Low experience of control over the environment
- Early development of stranger anxiety
- Insecure attachment between parent and child
- Increased parental anxiety
- Parenting style of being excessively controlling and overprotective
- Exposure to negative life events or stressors
- Genetic predisposition with family history of anxiety or depression

COMMONLY ASSOCIATED CONDITIONS

Comorbid conditions are present in up to 80% of children with SAD, most commonly including the following:

- School refusal
- Depression
- Simple phobia
- Social phobia
- Generalized anxiety disorder
- Obsessive-compulsive disorder
- Agoraphobia

DIAGNOSIS

- Anxiety with separation is a normative part of development, typically beginning around 6 or 7 months of age, peaking around 18 months and decreasing after 30 months.
  - Normal separation anxiety at 6 to 7 months manifests as shyness and anxiety with strangers.
  - At 12 to 18 months of age, children may have sleep disturbances, nightmares or nocturnal panic attacks, and oppositional behavior.
- SAD is distinguished by anxiety that becomes maladaptive, interfering with normal functioning, or becomes overly frequent, severe, and persistent.
- *DSM-5* criteria are as follows:
  - Developmentally inappropriate and excessive anxiety concerning separation from home or from those to whom the individual is attached as evidenced by three (or more) of the following:
    - Recurrent excessive distress when separation from home or major attachment figures occurs or is anticipated
    - Persistent and excessive worry about losing, or about possible harm befalling, major attachment figures
    - Persistent and excessive worry that an untoward event will lead to separation from a major attachment figure (e.g., getting lost or being kidnapped)
    - Persistent reluctance or refusal to go to school or elsewhere because of fear of separation
    - Persistent and excessive fears or reluctance to be alone or without major attachment figures at home or without significant adults in other settings
    - Persistent reluctance or refusal to go to sleep without being near a major attachment figure or to sleep away from home
    - Repeated nightmares regarding separation
    - Repeated complaints of physical symptoms (such as headaches, stomachaches, nausea, or vomiting) when separation from major attachment figures occurs or is anticipated
    - Duration of symptoms is at least 4 weeks.
    - Onset is before age 18 years.
    - Disturbance causes clinically significant distress or impairment in social, academic, or other important areas (occupational).

HISTORY

- Ask parents about the specific behaviors/complaints of the child at separation, including protests (tantrums/pleading negotiating), fearfulness, or somatic complaints.
  - Somatic complaints such as stomachaches and headaches are most typical.
- Ask caregivers what situations are impacted. Settings can include the following:
  - Separation for school or social/extracurricular activities
  - When the caregiver leaves the home
  - Being separated within the home (e.g., in another room from caregiver)
  - Bedtime
- Ask if sleep is impacted; specifically, ask about nightmares.
  - Children with SAD often have nightmares about separation, death, kidnapping, or serious accident.
- Ask if school attendance is impacted.
  - Avoidance behaviors such as procrastination during the morning routine before school or refusing to leave the side of a parent is common.
  - School refusal has been reported to occur in approximately 75% of children with SAD.
- Ask about duration.
  - Transient separation fears are common. In SAD, symptoms must last >4 weeks.
- Ask about possible stressors.
  - Symptoms may be precipitated by a stressor in some cases.
- Ask about impact.
  - Interferes with normative development in a number of ways such as difficulty attending school, participating in extracurricular activities, and attending sleepovers
  - Bedtime separation anxiety may result in sleep disruption to child and family.

PHYSICAL EXAM

There are no pertinent findings on physical exam.

DIFFERENTIAL DIAGNOSIS

SAD should be distinguished from normal, developmentally appropriate separation anxiety. Additionally, one should consider possible life stressors or abuse. Alternate anxiety disorders include the following:

- Generalized anxiety disorder
  - Distinguished by anxiety that is generalized and often presents in later adolescence
  - In children, this tends to manifest as excessive concern over the quality of school or athletic performance at school, concern about punctuality, or overzealously seeking approval from authority figures.

- Social anxiety
  - Presents as fear or avoidance of social situations in general or specific situations (e.g., eating in public)
- Specific phobias
  - Occur when anxiety is due to an identifiable object or situation; unlike in adults, children may not recognize their anxiety/fear of the specific item as excessive.

DIAGNOSTIC TESTS & INTERPRETATION

- There are no pertinent findings on lab work.
- There is no standard tool for diagnosis, but some children have increased sensitivity to a challenge of breathing CO_2-enriched air.
- There are a variety of scales that can help in the diagnosis, including the Separation Anxiety Assessment Scale, which has both child and parent versions.

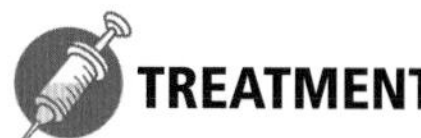

TREATMENT

Initial treatment should include psychoeducation for the caregiver (who will need to implement changes with the child) and cognitive behavioral techniques for the child.

- Psychoeducation for the caregiver includes explanations of the following:
  - The normative nature of anxiety
  - Caregiver response to child's protests and fears can inadvertently reinforce the child's separation behaviors.
- Specific advice to caregivers:
  - Do not prolong a goodbye:
    - Be brief.
    - Let the child know when you will return.
    - Reassure the child that you know that he or she will be ok.
  - Do not let the child see you are upset at the separation.
  - Do not overdo the reunion.
  - If a child is having extreme difficulties:
    - Start with briefer separations.
    - Use incentives and positive reinforcement for success (e.g., sticker charts or points).
    - Gradually build to more significant or longer separations.
- Anxiety workbooks can be used by the caregiver at home to provide activities for relaxation and reducing stress.
- Caregivers may need treatment for anxiety if their own anxiety is heightened by the child's behavior.
- Cognitive behavioral therapy (CBT) with the child is aimed at helping the child evaluate the accuracy of his or her fears and learn helpful skills, like self-talk.

MEDICATION

Psychopharmacology should generally be used for separation anxiety only if behavioral (nonmedication) treatment is insufficient or if there are additional comorbid anxiety diagnoses that are significantly impairing and psychosocial treatments are simultaneously being pursued.

- Selective serotonin reuptake inhibitor (SSRI) medications are the primary choice for anxiety disorders in children.
- Young children (<10 years of age) are at increased risk of side effects with SSRI medications.
  - As a result, slow dosing and frequent monitoring is needed.
  - Side effects include GI upset, headaches, dizziness, and agitation.
- SSRI medications have an FDA black box warning due to an increase in suicidal thinking and behavior in children and adolescents; monitoring recommendations need to be followed.

ISSUES FOR REFERRAL

If improvement is not seen within a month after providing education and guidance to caregiver, a referral to a mental health provider is indicated.

- A referral should be made to a mental health provider before medications would be considered for SAD.
- Treatment is usually brief for uncomplicated SAD. Therapy 1 to 2 times per week may last 6 to 12 weeks.

ONGOING CARE

FOLLOW-UP RECOMMENDATIONS

- If impairing symptoms continue for more than a month, a higher level of intervention may be indicated.
- If medications are started for anxiety in children, monitoring on a weekly basis is needed for at least 4 weeks after the medication is started or increased and monthly thereafter (see United States Food and Drug Administration (FDA) guidelines for specific medications).

PROGNOSIS

Outcomes are good with intervention.

- Children with SAD are at higher lifetime risk for other mental health conditions, particularly panic disorders.
- SAD can continue through childhood and into adulthood; early identification and intervention is important to minimize morbidity.

ADDITIONAL READING

- Brewer S, Sarvet B. Management of anxiety disorders in the pediatric primary care setting. *Pediatr Ann*. 2011;40(11):541–547.
- Ehrenreich JT, Santucci LC, Weiner CL. Separation anxiety disorder in youth: phenomenology, assessment, and treatment. *Psicol Conductual*. 2008;16(3):389–412.
- Eisen AR, Schaefer CE. *Separation Anxiety in Children and Adolescents: An Individualized Approach to Assessment and Treatment*. New York, NY: Guilford Press; 2005.
- Ost L-G, Treffers P. Onset, course and outcome for anxiety disorders in children. In: Silverman W, Cambridge P, eds. *Anxiety Disorders in Children and Adolescents: Research, Assessment and Intervention*. Cambridge, United Kingdom: Cambridge University Press; 2001.

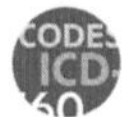

CODES

ICD10

F93.0 Separation anxiety disorder of childhood

FAQ

- Q: How do I know if it is developmentally normal separation anxiety?
- A: When separation anxiety arises after the age of 6 years, it warrants intervention if it lasts for >4 weeks and/or is markedly impacting expected activities. Before the age of 6 years, separation fears are more common but warrant intervention if impairment in normal functioning is seen.
- Q: Can a teenager have SAD?
- A: Yes. SAD can affect a child of any age and can even persist into adulthood.
- Q: What type of mental health provider can treat SAD that does not respond to primary care intervention?
- A: Any master's- or doctorate-level mental health provider with experience in anxiety disorders in children and behavioral techniques such as CBT.

S

SEPSIS

Erik R. Hoefgen, MD, MS • Craig H. Gosdin, MD, MSHA

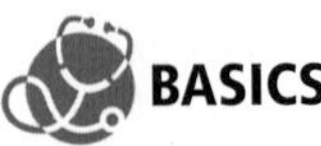

BASICS

DESCRIPTION

- Systemic inflammatory response syndrome (SIRS): nonspecific inflammatory response, defined as at least two of the following four criteria (one of which must be either abnormal temperature OR leukocyte count):
  - Temperature >38.5 or <36°C
  - Tachycardia (mean HR >2 *SDs* above normal for age)
  - Tachypnea (mean RR >2 *SDs* above normal for age), or requiring mechanical ventilation for acute respiratory failure
  - Leukocytosis, leukopenia, or >10% bands
- Sepsis: SIRS in the presence of infection
  - Infection: suspected or proven infection or clinical syndrome associated with high probability of infection
- Severe sepsis: sepsis accompanied by evidence of altered end organ perfusion (cardiovascular dysfunction OR acute respiratory distress syndrome [ARDS] OR two or more other organ dysfunctions)
- Septic shock: sepsis with cardiovascular dysfunction (hypotension, need for vasoactive drug to maintain normal BP, or any combination of altered mental status, unexplained metabolic acidosis, increased arterial lactate, oliguria, prolonged capillary refill, and core-to-peripheral temperature gap)

EPIDEMIOLOGY

Incidence

Estimated overall annual incidence of 0.9 cases per 1,000 children but varies by age

- Newborn infants: 9.7 per 1,000 children
- Non–newborn infants: 2.3 per 1,000 children
- Age 1 to 4 years: 0.5 per 1,000 children
- Age 5 to 14 years: 0.2 per 1,000 children
- Age 15 to 19 years: 0.5 per 1,000 children

Prevalence

Sepsis is among the most common (10–25%) medical diagnoses on admission to pediatric intensive care units (PICUs).

RISK FACTORS

Sepsis may occur in previously healthy children, but children with chronic underlying conditions that render them immunosuppressed or vulnerable to invasive infections are at increased risk, including:

- Neutropenia (neutrophils <1,000/mm^3, especially <500/mm^3)
- Primary or acquired immunodeficiency (e.g., AIDS, severe combined immunodeficiency)
- Malignancy
- Organ transplant recipients
- Chronic use of high-dose systemic steroids
- Indwelling central venous catheters or other invasive devices (e.g., urinary catheter)
- Hyposplenism, either surgical or functional (e.g., sickle cell anemia)
- Neuromuscular disease (e.g., static encephalopathy)
- Extensive burns
- Multiple trauma injuries
- Prematurity
- Unimmunized/underimmunized children
- Severe malnutrition

GENERAL PREVENTION

- Routine vaccination for *Haemophilus influenzae* type b (Hib), *Streptococcus pneumoniae*, and *Neisseria meningitidis* particularly in high-risk patients (e.g., asplenia)
- Antibiotic prophylaxis for household or day care exposure to confirmed cases of Hib or *N. meningitidis*
- Antibiotic prophylaxis for children with asplenia
- Prompt evaluation of fever in immunosuppressed patients
- Aseptic technique for insertion and care of vascular catheters, minimizing duration of use

ETIOLOGY

- Microbial invasion of the bloodstream or release of microbial products/toxins into the bloodstream; stimulates host defense, resulting in activation of proinflammatory mediators and systemic inflammation
- Pathogens vary with age, host immune status, and setting (community or hospital).
- Neonates
  - Group B *Streptococcus*
  - *Escherichia coli*
  - *Staphylococcus aureus*
  - *Listeria monocytogenes*
  - *Enterococcus* spp.
  - Herpes simplex virus
  - Enterovirus
- In neonates with a history of hospitalization, instrumentation, or mechanical ventilation, also consider
  - Coagulase-negative staphylococci
  - Gram-negative bacilli
  - *Candida* spp.
- Otherwise healthy older infants and children
  - *S. pneumoniae*
  - *N. meningitidis*
  - *S. aureus*
  - Group A *Streptococcus*
  - *Salmonella* spp.
  - Rickettsiae
  - Influenza
- Patients with underlying immune defects are also susceptible to a broad range of additional organisms.

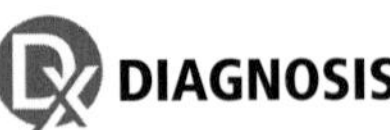

DIAGNOSIS

Requires high suspicion; fever and tachycardia are nonspecific and hypotension is generally a late sign.

HISTORY

- See "Risk Factors."
- Duration of illness before presentation
  - Abrupt onset of symptoms more typical of invasive bacterial infection
- Change in behavior may be initial sign of systemic infection.
  - Irritability, lethargy, and poor feeding are especially important in infants and young children.
- Decreased urine output

PHYSICAL EXAM

All patients with suspected sepsis should have a full set of vital signs (e.g., temperature, pulse, respiratory rate, BP, pulse oximetry).

- Temperature
  - Fever is the hallmark of an infection but may be absent; infants may demonstrate hypothermia.
- General
  - Ill or toxic appearing
- HEENT and neck exam
  - Dehydration: sunken fontanelle, dry mucous membranes, sunken eyes
  - Meningismus or bulging fontanelle
  - Mucocutaneous bleeding
- Cardiovascular exam
  - Tachycardia or bradycardia
  - Hypotension
  - Cold shock: delayed capillary refill; diminished pulses; mottling; and cool, clammy extremities
  - Warm shock: flash capillary refill; bounding pulses; and warm, dry extremities
- Respiratory exam
  - Hypoxia and/or cyanosis
  - Apnea or tachypnea
  - Retractions, flaring or grunting
  - Poor air flow
- Abdominal exam
  - Distension
  - Hepatomegaly, splenomegaly
- Skin exam
  - Presence of petechiae and purpura (associated with meningococcemia and/or disseminated intravascular coagulation)
  - Pallor
- Neurologic
  - Abnormal mental status (somnolence, confusion, agitation, irritability)
  - Seizures
  - Abnormal reflexes or tone

DIFFERENTIAL DIAGNOSIS

- Cardiovascular
  - Congenital heart disease
  - Myocarditis, pericarditis, cardiomyopathy
  - Pericardial effusion
  - Cardiac dysrhythmia
  - Myocardial infarction
  - Pulmonary embolus
- Endocrine
  - Congenital adrenal hyperplasia
  - Adrenal insufficiency
  - Thyrotoxicosis, hypothyroidism
  - Hypoglycemia
  - Diabetic ketoacidosis
- Gastrointestinal
  - Pyloric stenosis
  - Necrotizing enterocolitis
  - Malrotation/volvulus
  - Intussusception
  - Pancreatitis
- Hematology/oncology
  - Severe anemia
  - Neoplasm
  - Hemophagocytic lymphohistiocytosis
  - Macrophage activation syndrome
- Genetic
  - Inborn errors of metabolism
  - Methemoglobinemia
- Other
  - Dehydration
  - Infant botulism
  - Toxic ingestion/poisoning
  - Trauma (accidental or nonaccidental)

DIAGNOSTIC TESTS & INTERPRETATION

ALERT

Diagnosis is primarily clinical; do not delay treatment. Cultures and other diagnostic tests are largely confirmatory.

Initial Tests (screening, labs, imaging)

Patients with suspected sepsis should have

- Blood culture
  - Prior to starting antibiotics when possible
  - Culture yield is related to sample volume.

- CBC with differential
  - Leukocytosis with increased band count or leukopenia may be present.
- Electrolytes, glucose, ionized calcium
  - Metabolic acidosis
  - Hypoglycemia or hyperglycemia
  - Hypocalcemia
- BUN, creatinine:
  - May reflect dehydration
  - Evaluate for acute kidney injury.
- Liver function tests
  - Evaluate for end organ injury.
- Lactate
  - Elevated for inadequate tissue perfusion
- Arterial blood gas (ABG) and lactate
  - Metabolic acidosis and/or hypoxemia
- PT, PTT, fibrinogen, fibrin degradation products, platelets, peripheral smear
  - Screen for disseminated intravascular coagulation (DIC): elevated PT, PTT, INR; decreased fibrinogen; increased fibrin degradation products
- Urinalysis and urine culture
  - Potential source of infection
- Lumbar puncture (when hemodynamically stable)
  - Required for diagnosis of meningitis
- Inflammatory biomarkers (e.g., CRP, procalcitonin) may be helpful.
- Culture other potential sources of infection: abscess, wounds, indwelling devices, sputum, tracheal aspirate
- Diagnostic testing for other potential causative organisms (e.g., HSV, enterovirus, influenza)
- Chest radiograph
- Head CT may be necessary if with altered mental status in presence of coagulopathy.

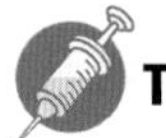

TREATMENT

ALERT

- Rapid recognition of sepsis is critical.
  - Fluid resuscitation targeting cap refill ≤2 seconds, normalized BP for age, normal peripheral pulses, and urine output >1 mL/kg/h within 6 hours from recognition is associated with improved survival (goal directed therapy).
- Continuous monitoring and reassessment of the patient are essential.
- Administer IV antibiotics within 1 hour of recognition of severe sepsis.

GENERAL MEASURES

- Ensure a patent airway, early endotracheal intubation may improve cardiac output.
- Provide supplemental oxygen and assist ventilation (e.g., bag-valve-mask device) as needed.
- Obtain large-bore peripheral IV access (consider central venous line or intraosseous line).
- Hemodynamic support
  - Early fluid resuscitation is imperative.
  - Volume resuscitation: bolus 20 mL/kg of normal saline, repeat as needed; consider blood after 60 to 80 mL/kg of crystalloid and or Hgb <10 g/dL.
  - Consider inotropic agents if hemodynamic instability persists despite adequate fluid resuscitation, see "Medications."
- Correct hypoglycemia and hypocalcemia; drainage or eradication of focus of infection

MEDICATION

- Broad-spectrum IV antibiotics to cover likely causative pathogens should be initiated within 1 hour of recognition of severe sepsis.
- Antibiotic choice dependent on patient age, immune status, need for penetration into certain tissues (e.g., CNS), and whether the infection was community- or nosocomially acquired in empiric choice. In general, bactericidal drugs should be used.
  - Neonates ≤4 weeks: ampicillin (100 mg/kg/dose q6h, max dose 3,000 mg) and gentamicin (3 mg/kg/dose q24h) or ampicillin and cefotaxime (50 mg/kg/dose q6h). Add acyclovir (15 to 20 mg/kg/dose q8h) to either regimen if herpes simplex virus infection is suspected.
  - Infants and children ≥4 weeks: not concerned for meningitis: cefotaxime (50 mg/kg/dose q6–8h) or ceftriaxone (50 mg/kg q12h); concern for meningitis: vancomycin (15 to 20 mg/kg/dose q6–12h based on age) and cefotaxime (50 mg/kg/dose q6h) or ceftriaxone (50 mg/kg q12h)
  - Patients with immunosuppression and/or central venous catheters: vancomycin plus aminoglycoside plus advanced-generation cephalosporin (e.g., cefepime [50 mg/kg/dose q8h])
  - Patients with an intra-abdominal focus of infection: carbapenem; ticarcillin-clavulanate or piperacillin-tazobactam (100 mg/kg/dose q6h); ceftriaxone, cefotaxime, or cefepime plus metronidazole (7.5 mg/kg/dose q6h); ampicillin plus gentamicin plus metronidazole or clindamycin
- Inotropic agents: If hemodynamic instability persists despite fluid resuscitation, start dopamine (begin at 5 mcg/kg/min, titrate up to 10 mcg/kg/min as needed). If fluid refractory/dopamine-resistant shock, start epinephrine (0.05 to 0.3 mcg/kg/min) for cold shock or norepinephrine (0.05 to 1.5 mcg/kg/min) for warm shock to normalize BP and restore perfusion.
- Corticosteroids: stress-dose hydrocortisone (50 mg/m^2/24 h) for catecholamine-resistant hypotension and in patients at risk for adrenal insufficiency

ADMISSION, INPATIENT, AND NURSING CONSIDERATIONS

- Patients with sepsis should be admitted for close monitoring.
- Patients with severe sepsis or septic shock should be admitted to an ICU (e.g., requiring >60 mL/kg fluid resuscitation).

ONGOING CARE

FOLLOW-UP RECOMMENDATIONS

Patient Monitoring

- Admit all patients with suspected sepsis to the hospital; consider ICU admission.
- Continuous BP monitoring for the development of refractory shock
- Serial vital signs and physical exams to monitor response to therapy
- Monitoring for complications of sepsis and the development of multiple organ dysfunction syndrome (MODS)
  - Chest radiograph and serial ABGs for evidence of acute lung injury/ARDS
  - Urine output, BUN, creatinine for acute kidney injury
  - Serial coagulation studies (PT/PTT) and platelets for development of DIC
  - Serial blood glucose levels for hypo- or hyperglycemia
  - Serial liver function tests for evidence of hepatic dysfunction
  - Serial neurologic examinations for evidence of CNS dysfunction
- Reassess antibiotic therapy daily for opportunity to narrow coverage following pathogen identification.

PROGNOSIS

Case fatality rates have improved from nearly 50% to ~9%. With implementation of clinical practice guidelines focused on early reversal of shock, several studies have reduced in-hospital mortality rates to ~4–8% for patients with severe sepsis.

- Mortality is higher in children with chronic illnesses than in previously healthy children.
- Development of ARDS or MODS is associated with increased mortality.

COMPLICATIONS

- Sepsis is one of the leading causes of pediatric mortality and accounts for 7% of deaths.
- The most common complications are those resulting from hypoperfusion of vital organs or from organ injury incurred by the uncontrolled systemic inflammatory response:
  - Acute lung injury
  - Acute kidney injury
  - DIC
  - Hypoglycemia
  - ARDS
  - MODS

ADDITIONAL READING

- Bateman SL, Seed PC. Procession to pediatric bacteremia and sepsis: covert operations and failures in diplomacy. *Pediatrics*. 2010;126(1):137–150.
- Brierley J, Carcillo JA, Choong K, et al. Clinical practice parameters for hemodynamic support of pediatric and neonatal septic shock: 2007 update from the American College of Critical Care Medicine. *Crit Care Med*. 2009;37(2):666–688.
- Czaja AS, Zimmerman JJ, Nathens AB. Readmission and late mortality after pediatric sepsis. *Pediatrics*. 2009;123(3):849–957.
- Dellinger R, Levy M, Rhodes A, et al; for Surviving Sepsis Campaign Guidelines Committee including the Pediatric Subgroup. Surviving Sepsis Campaign: international guidelines for management of severe sepsis and septic shock, 2012. *Intensive Care Med*. 2013;39(2):165–228.
- Hartman M, Linde-Zwirble W, Angus D, et al. Trends in the epidemiology of pediatric severe sepsis. *Pediatr Crit Care Med*. 2013;14(7):686–693.
- Prusakowski M, Chen A. Pediatric sepsis. *Emerg Med Clin N Am*. 2017;35(1):123–138.

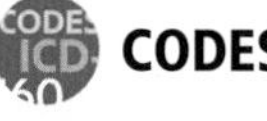

CODES

ICD10

- A41.9 Sepsis, unspecified organism
- R65.10 SIRS of non-infectious origin w/o acute organ dysfunction
- R65.20 Severe sepsis without septic shock

FAQ

- Q: What are the early clinical signs of sepsis?
- A: Vital sign changes such as tachycardia, tachypnea, along with respiratory distress/hypoxia and central nervous system alterations can be early signs of sepsis.

SEPSIS, NEONATAL

Julia Johnson, MD • Azadeh Farzin, MD, MHS

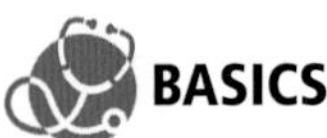

BASICS

DESCRIPTION

- Clinical syndrome characterized by systemic infection occurring within the first 28 days of life
- Early-onset sepsis (EOS) and late-onset sepsis (LOS) occur within and following the first 72 hours of life, respectively.
- Some consider infection within the first 7 days of life early onset, especially in term infants who are not hospitalized.

EPIDEMIOLOGY

- EOS: 1/1,000 live births in the United States. Incidence is much higher among very-low-birth-weight (VLBW) neonates.
- LOS: Among febrile neonates presenting to the emergency department, approximately 12% are diagnosed with a serious bacterial infection. Incidence among hospitalized preterm infants is inversely associated with birth weight.

RISK FACTORS

- Neonates are at increased risk for infection due to their immature immune system (permitting relative immune tolerance) and their developing, underkeratinized cutaneous barrier.
- Maternal factors:
  - Low socioeconomic status
  - Illicit substance use
  - Inadequate or no prenatal care
  - Poor maternal nutrition
  - Intra-amniotic procedures
  - Preterm labor, prolonged or premature rupture of membranes
  - Chorioamnionitis or "intrauterine inflammation, infection, or both" (III, "triple I"; a new term describing the heterogenous conditions labeled previously as chorioamnionitis)
  - Presence of cervical cerclage
  - Septic/traumatic delivery
  - Peripartum infection, including urinary tract infections (UTIs)
  - Group B *Streptococcus* (GBS) colonization
  - Ingestion of contaminated foods during pregnancy (*Listeria*)
- Infant factors:
  - Male sex
  - Prematurity or low birth weight
  - Low Apgar scores
  - Congenital anomalies
  - Compromised skin integrity
  - Galactosemia (*Escherichia coli* sepsis)
  - Invasive procedures,
  - Presence of central line

Genetics

Single nucleotide polymorphisms (SNPs) in genes involved in inflammation have been linked to increased risk of neonatal sepsis.

GENERAL PREVENTION

- Recognition and treatment of maternal peripartum infections and colonization (i.e., GBS)
- General obstetric practices to reduce risk of chorioamnionitis/III and postnatal clean cord care
- Thermoregulation and early breastfeeding
- Hand hygiene, avoidance of fomites

PATHOPHYSIOLOGY

- EOS: primarily vertical transmission, with ante- or intrapartum acquisition of bacteria colonizing the maternal genitourinary tract
- LOS: primarily due to horizontal transmission or nosocomial infection in hospitalized infants

ETIOLOGY

- EOS:
  - GBS is most common (~40%), followed by *E. coli* (~20–30%), other streptococci (~10%).
  - Incidence of GBS disease has decreased since initiation of intrapartum antibiotic prophylaxis (IAP).
  - *E. coli* is the most common pathogen in VLBW infants.
  - Overall incidence of *Listeria* sepsis is low, but it is more common in preterm infants.
  - Viral pathogens, including enteroviruses, may present with EOS.
- LOS:
  - GBS and *E. coli* remain important; consider *Staphylococcus aureus* (up to a quarter methicillin-resistant) and coagulase-negative staphylococci (CoNS), especially in hospitalized infants.
  - *Pseudomonas aeruginosa* carries the highest mortality risk in preterm infants (up to 75%).
  - Yeast infections should be considered, with hospitalized preterm infants at greatest risk.
  - Viral pathogens, including enteroviruses, may present with LOS; viral meningitis is more common in the late-onset period.
  - Perinatally acquired HSV infection should be considered in neonates at any period during the 1st month of age.

COMMONLY ASSOCIATED CONDITIONS

- Meningitis: Up to a quarter of neonates with bacteremia have meningitis.
- Pneumonia
- UTI
- Omphalitis
- Osteomyelitis
- Severe hyperbilirubinemia
- Persistent pulmonary hypertension of the newborn (PPHN)
- Patent ductus arteriosus (PDA)

DIAGNOSIS

HISTORY

- Thorough pregnancy, labor, and delivery history to elicit presence of risk factors
- Change in behavior or level of alertness
- Poor feeding
- Decreased urinary output
- Family history of sibling with GBS sepsis

PHYSICAL EXAM

- Vital signs, including temperature, heart rate, respiratory rate, oxygen saturation, and blood pressure
  - Hypothermia is more likely than fever.
- General exam
  - Lethargy, irritability, poor suck
- HEENT exam
  - Dry mucous membranes, sunken fontanelle
- Respiratory exam
  - Cyanosis, hypoxia, apnea, or tachypnea
  - Increased work of breathing, including nasal flaring, grunting, and retractions
- Cardiovascular exam
  - Tachycardia or bradycardia, flow murmur
  - Hypotension, poor perfusion
- Abdominal exam
  - Distention
  - Purulent discharge or erythema surrounding umbilicus
- Dermatologic exam
  - Pustules, vesicles (HSV), petechiae (DIC)
  - Scalp electrode site, erythema, discharge, rash
  - Jaundice
- Neurologic exam
  - Altered mental status
  - Hyper- or hypotonia
  - Seizures (may present with apnea, abnormal oral movements, "bicycling" as opposed to tonic-clonic activity)

DIFFERENTIAL DIAGNOSIS

- Hypoxic-ischemic encephalopathy (HIE)
- Congenital heart disease
- Meconium aspiration syndrome
- Inborn errors of metabolism
- Congenital adrenal hyperplasia
- Necrotizing enterocolitis (NEC)
- Malrotation/volvulus
- Hypoglycemia
- Trauma

DIAGNOSTIC TESTS & INTERPRETATION

Initial Tests (screening, lab, imaging)

- Blood culture (preferably) prior to antibiotics; however, testing should never delay initiation of treatment.
  - At least 1 mL of blood in an aerobic bottle
  - Cultures obtained from umbilical venous catheter are more likely to be contaminated.
- Arterial blood gas and lactate
- Complete blood count with differential
  - If presenting shortly after birth, consider obtaining at 6 to 12 hours of age to allow for normal transition. Observed abnormalities include leukopenia, leukocytosis, "left shift," thrombocytopenia.
- Comprehensive metabolic panel—electrolytes, liver-associated enzymes
  - Assess for end-organ injury, electrolyte derangements.
- Inflammatory biomarkers
  - C-reactive protein (CRP), procalcitonin
- Lumbar puncture (LP) for cerebrospinal fluid (CSF) cell count, glucose, protein, and culture
  - All neonates <28 days old presenting from community with rectal temperature ≥38°C should have an LP.
  - Among hospitalized neonates, guidelines are less clear. LP should always be considered in infants with high probability of sepsis, neurologic signs, or positive blood culture.
  - Contraindicated in cases of hemodynamic instability, severe thrombocytopenia
  - Care should be taken with LPs in neonates with concern for increased intracranial pressure.
- Urinalysis and urine culture
  - UTIs are less common in neonates <3 days of age.
  - Obtain via catheter or suprapubic tap.
- Chest radiograph (if respiratory symptoms are present)
- Abdominal radiograph (if abdominal distention, bloody stools, or GI findings are present)

Follow-Up Tests & Special Considerations

- For neonates with a positive blood culture, obtain a repeat culture to document clearance.
- Consider MRI of brain in cases of neonatal meningitis, especially if caused by *Citrobacter* spp. or *Cronobacter sakazakii*, which are pathogens associated with brain abscesses.

Diagnostic Procedures/Other

No other specific diagnostic procedures are indicated for sepsis; other diagnostic procedures may be considered if diagnosis is uncertain.

Test Interpretation

- Normal values for white blood cell counts and absolute neutrophil counts are age-dependent.
- Immature to total neutrophil count of <0.3 has a high negative predictive value (NPV) for sepsis. Very low positive predictive value (PPV) should not be used for confirmation.
- CRP is a nonspecific acute phase reactant that peaks at 24 hours after inflammation. This laboratory test is not sensitive enough to withhold antibiotics at initial evaluation nor specific enough to solely justify continuation of antibiotics. Two normal values 24 hours apart effectively rule out sepsis (NPV 99.7%), except in VLBW infants and those with immunosuppression (including infants on systemic steroids and those manifesting severe granulocytopenia).
- CSF cultures may be negative if LP was performed after initiation of antibiotics. Cell counts remain abnormal for days in cases of meningitis.

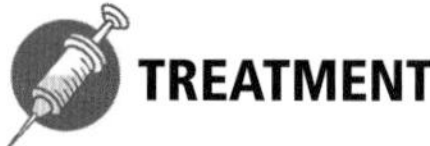

TREATMENT

GENERAL MEASURES

Supportive measures should focus on monitoring and treatment of associated comorbidities, including cardiorespiratory compromise and temperature instability.

MEDICATION

- Goal of antibiotic use before detection of bacteremia is to eradicate harmful organisms as early in course as possible. This aim should be balanced against impact of therapy on the neonatal microbiome and its potential association with various short- and long-term morbidities.
- Empiric antibiotic selection should be guided by infant's risk factors and local epidemiology.
- Parenteral administration is preferred.
- Duration of treatment:
  - >98% of positive cultures have a time to detection ≤48 hours.
  - Antibiotic therapy should be narrowed once an organism is identified.
  - Duration of treatment ranges from 7 days for gram-positive bacteremia without meningitis to 21 days for treatment for gram-negative bacteremia with possible meningitis.
  - In critically ill infants, treatment for "culture-negative sepsis" can be considered, but it is critical to be judicious, as prolonged courses of empiric antibiotics have been associated with increased mortality.

First Line

Ampicillin + gentamicin or cefotaxime

- All GBS isolates in the United States are ampicillin-sensitive; *E. coli* resistance to ampicillin is increasing.
- Gentamicin has poor CSF penetration; select cefotaxime if meningitis is suspected.

ALERT

Ceftriaxone is contraindicated in patients <28 days of age due to risk of hyperbilirubinemia and intravascular precipitation when infused with calcium-containing fluids.

Second Line

- Vancomycin: Consider in neonates with risk of MRSA or CoNS sepsis.
- Acyclovir: Initiate when concerned for HSV.
- Amphotericin B: antifungal therapy of choice if concerned for systemic yeast infection

ISSUES FOR REFERRAL

All neonates with suspected sepsis should be referred to a pediatric specialist for further evaluation and management.

ADDITIONAL THERAPIES

Current evidence on use of probiotics or other immunoprophylactic interventions, including IVIG for prevention of neonatal sepsis, is inconclusive.

SURGERY/OTHER PROCEDURES

May be indicated in instances of occult infections (including osteomyelitis), bowel injury (i.e., malrotation with volvulus, NEC), and abscesses (intracranial, intra-abdominal, pulmonary)

COMPLEMENTARY & ALTERNATIVE THERAPIES

None indicated

ADMISSION, INPATIENT, AND NURSING CONSIDERATIONS

Hospital admission is required for infants <28 days with suspected sepsis.

ONGOING CARE

FOLLOW-UP RECOMMENDATIONS

In cases of end-organ dysfunction, consider additional follow-up with appropriate subspecialty and support services, including a developmental specialist and occupational/physical therapy.

Patient Monitoring

Neonates are at high risk of rapid deterioration and should be monitored closely, especially during early stages of illness.

DIET

- Once infant is able to tolerate enteral nutrition, routine diet can be resumed.
- Human milk provides benefit of intestinal recolonization after treatment with antibiotics.

PATIENT EDUCATION

Educate parents on the importance of breastfeeding, hand hygiene, avoidance of exposure to fomites, and early signs of sepsis.

PROGNOSIS

Mortality risk has changed dramatically, decreasing to 10–15% in recent years. Preterm infants are at highest risk of mortality.

COMPLICATIONS

Infants with gram-negative or GBS meningitis are at highest risk of developing complications, including cognitive and motor disabilities, convulsive disorders, hydrocephalus, hearing loss, and speech delay.

ADDITIONAL READING

- Benitz WE, Wynn JL, Polin RA. Reappraisal of guidelines for management of neonates with suspected early-onset sepsis. *J Pediatr*. 2015;166(4):1070–1074.
- Camacho-Gonzalez A, Spearman PW, Stoll BJ. Neonatal infectious diseases: evaluation of neonatal sepsis. *Pediatr Clin North Am*. 2013;60(2):367–389.
- Higgins RD, Saade G, Polin RA, et al; and Chorioamnionitis Workshop Participants. Evaluation and management of women and newborns with a maternal diagnosis of chorioamnionitis: summary of a workshop. *Obstet Gynecol*. 2016;127(3):426–436.
- Puopolo KM, Draper D, Wi S, et al. Estimating the probability of neonatal early-onset infection on the basis of maternal risk factors. *Pediatrics*. 2011;128(5):e1155–e1163.
- Simonsen KA, Anderson-Berry AL, Delair SF, et al. Early-onset neonatal sepsis. *Clin Microbiol Rev*. 2014;27(1):21–47.

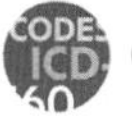

CODES

ICD10

- A41.9 Sepsis, unspecified organism
- P36.9 Bacterial sepsis of newborn, unspecified

FAQ

- Q: Are any decision-making tools available to providers evaluating neonates for sepsis?
- A: In neonates born at ≥34 weeks' gestation, the risk of EOS can be calculated using the Neonatal Sepsis Calculator, a tool which utilizes data on maternal risk factors and clinical appearance of the infant. Based on assessed risk, the calculator provides guidance on laboratory evaluation and antibiotic therapy. The calculator is available online at https://www.dor.kaiser.org/external/DORExternal/research/InfectionProbabilityCalculator.aspx.
- Q: Are infants with EOS at higher LOS risk?
- A: In contrast to adults and older children, infants with EOS are not at increased risk for reoccurrence of sepsis. This suggests a potential immune priming benefit, especially in preterm infants at highest risk for both EOS and LOS.
- Q: Why do the antibiotic recommendations for neonates with suspected sepsis differ between those hospitalized in the NICU as compared to the community setting?
- A: Among community infants presenting with suspected LOS, the higher risk of associated meningitis justifies administering cefotaxime while awaiting confirmatory results. In hospitalized infants, who are often preterm, this approach is counterbalanced by increased future risk of NEC and fungal infection during their prolonged hospital course, which often includes additional episodes of suspected sepsis.

SEPTIC ARTHRITIS

Angela Y. Choe, MD • Joanna E. Thomson, MD, MPH

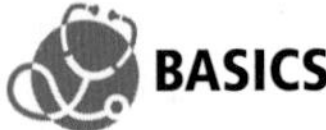

BASICS

DESCRIPTION

Microbiologic infection and inflammation of the usually sterile joint space

EPIDEMIOLOGY

- Most common age: toddler and school age (2 to 6 years)
- Predominant sex: male (2:1 female)
- Most common location: lower extremities (hip, knee, and ankle) and large joints (hip, shoulder, elbow)

PATHOPHYSIOLOGY

- Entry of bacteria into joint space
  - Hematogenous spread (seeding during transient bacteremia) most common
  - Direct inoculation (penetrating trauma or during surgery)
  - Extension from bone infection (mainly in children <1 year old when vessels cross from metaphysis to epiphysis)
- In response to cytokines, influx of inflammatory cells and release of proteolytic enzymes
- Leads to destruction of synovium and cartilaginous structures

ETIOLOGY

- Most common causes by age:
  - Neonates: group B *Streptococcus*, *Staphylococcus aureus*, *Escherichia coli*, and *Candida albicans*
  - Older children: *S. aureus*, group A *Streptococcus*, *Kingella kingae* in toddlers, *Haemophilus influenzae*
- Also consider
  - *Salmonella*: in patients with sickle cell
  - *Neisseria gonorrhoeae*: in sexually active adolescents and in neonates
  - *Neisseria meningitidis*
  - *Mycobacterium tuberculosis*
  - Anaerobes (rare)
  - Rubella
  - Parvovirus
  - Hepatitis B or C
  - Mumps
  - Herpesviruses (Epstein-Barr virus, cytomegalovirus, herpes simplex virus, varicella-zoster virus)
  - Fungal etiologies (e.g., coccidioidomycosis, rarely candida)

COMMONLY ASSOCIATED CONDITIONS

- Sickle cell disease: *Salmonella*
- Immunocompromised patients: *Mycoplasma*, *Ureaplasma*, *Klebsiella*, or *Aspergillus* infection

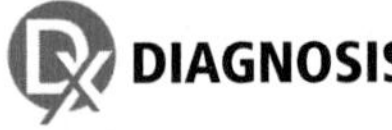

DIAGNOSIS

HISTORY

- Systemic symptoms:
  - Fever (occurs within the first few days of illness in 75% of patients)
  - Malaise
  - Poor appetite
- Joint symptoms:
  - Pain: worsening, does not wax and wane
  - Limp
  - Inability to bear weight, refusal to move joint, positional preferences
  - Typically monoarticular
  - Consider hip involvement when the patient complains of knee or thigh pain.

PHYSICAL EXAM

- Ill-appearing
- Joint
  - Warm, swollen, erythematous
  - Held in "position of comfort" maximizing intracapsular joint volume (e.g., hip held flexed, abducted, externally rotated)
  - "Pseudoparalysis": refusal to move the affected extremity
  - Pain throughout entire range of motion (even passive motion)
- Presentation may be delayed and without external findings in deep joints (hip and shoulder)
- In the frightened or uncooperative child, it is possible to have the parent perform an examination for tenderness and range of motion while observing from a distance.

DIFFERENTIAL DIAGNOSIS

- Infectious
  - Osteomyelitis with or without contiguous spread to proximal joint (concurrent infection 40–70%)
  - Infectious and postinfectious reactive arthritides: *N. meningitidis*, group A *Streptococcus*, *Salmonella*, *Mycoplasma*, *Campylobacter*, *Shigella*, *Yersinia*, *Chlamydia*
  - Cellulitis causing decreased range of motion of joint secondary to inflammation
  - Psoas abscess or retroperitoneal abscess
  - Tuberculous arthritis
  - Lyme arthritis (*Borelia burgdorferi*)
  - Septic bursitis
- Tumors
  - Osteogenic sarcoma (long bone pain spreading to joint space)
  - Leukemia/lymphoma
- Trauma
  - Occult fracture in proximity to growth plate
  - Ligamentous injury (sprain)
  - Foreign body synovitis
  - Traumatic knee effusion/hemarthrosis
- Immunologic/rheumatic
  - Toxic (transient) synovitis: most common mimic; must examine joint aspirate to differentiate from septic arthritis
  - Acute rheumatic fever
  - Systemic lupus erythematosus
  - Juvenile rheumatoid arthritis
  - Henoch-Schönlein purpura
  - Reactive arthritis syndrome (after GI or chlamydial infection): arthritis, uveitis, urethritis
  - Behçet syndrome (iridocyclitis, genital, and oral ulcerations)
  - Serum sickness
  - Inflammatory bowel disease
- Musculoskeletal
  - Knee: apophysitis (e.g., Osgood-Schlatter disease), patellofemoral pain syndrome, osteochondritis dissecans
  - Hip: slipped capital femoral epiphysis

DIAGNOSTIC TESTS & INTERPRETATION

Initial Test (screening, lab, imaging)

- Synovial fluid analysis and culture is critical to diagnosis:
  - WBC count: >50 to 100,000/mm^3 with >75% neutrophils highly suggestive of septic arthritis, although WBC count may be <50,000 in some cases
  - Glucose: <50% that of the serum
  - Gram stain: reveals organism in 40–50% of cases
  - Culture: reveals organism in ~75% of cases (except for gonorrhea)
    - Emerging polymerase chain reaction (PCR) technology may allow higher yield and faster identification of causative organisms, including timely distinction between gram negative and positive organisms.
  - Inoculation of joint fluid into blood culture bottle facilitates recovery of *K. kingae*.
    - Real-time PCR for *K. kingae* toxin from joint fluid provides higher yield than routine Gram stain or culture alone.
- Other supportive blood tests:
  - WBC count: neither sensitive nor specific
  - Erythrocyte sedimentation rate (ESR): elevated (>30 mm/h) in 95% of cases
  - C-Reactive protein (CRP): increased (>1.0 mg/dL). In one study, a CRP <1.0 mg/dL had a negative predictive value of 87%.
  - Blood cultures: positive in 20–40% of cases, sometimes yield pathogen when joint cultures are negative
- Serology for *B. burgdorferi* or PCR of joint fluid may be helpful in differentiating between bacterial arthritis and Lyme disease.
- Algorithm to differentiate septic arthritis from transient synovitis of the hip: Absence of all four factors is strongly associated with absence of septic arthritis.
  - Fever
  - ESR >20 mm/h
  - CRP >1.0 mg/dL
  - WBC >11,000 cells/mL
  - Joint space fluid apparent on plain radiograph
- Radiography (anteroposterior and lateral)
  - May show widening of joint space and/or displacement of normal fat pads
- Ultrasound
  - Delineates amount of fluid within joint capsule
  - Increased blood flow with color Doppler is associated with infection
  - Bilateral effusions suggest transient synovitis.
  - Useful in guiding needle aspiration (especially of deep joints such as the hip)
- MRI and bone scan
  - Should not delay aspiration or antibiotic management
  - Should be considered to identify concomitant osteomyelitis in patients <4 years of age, involvement of the shoulder, or symptoms >6 days
  - MRI: early detection of joint fluid; also will reveal adjacent bone abnormalities to suggest osteomyelitis
  - Bone scan: reveals increased uptake in the perimeter of the joint during the "blood pool" phase of the study

ALERT
- Clinical examination in conjunction with a history of acute onset should raise suspicion for septic arthritis, even in the face of "negative" laboratory screening tests.
- Analysis of the synovial fluid is necessary for diagnosis.
- Some children, especially neonates and young infants, will not manifest signs of systemic disease early in the course of the illness.

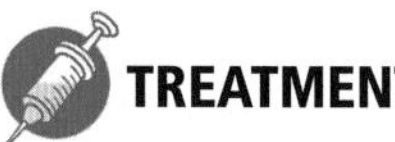

TREATMENT

GENERAL MEASURES
- Orthopedic emergency
- Antibiotic administration
- Immobilization of extremity
- Pain management

MEDICATION
- Should be initiated immediately after blood and fluid cultures obtained
- Target empiric antibiotic therapy toward common organisms in age group; may be aided by Gram stain results
  - Typical first line: anti-staphylococcal penicillin or 1st-generation cephalosporin
  - In areas of methicillin-resistant *S. aureus* (MRSA) high prevalence (>15%), consider vancomycin or clindamycin as 1st-line treatment
- Consider addition of 3rd-generation cephalosporin:
  - In neonates (alternatively could add gentamicin)
  - If gram-negative organism on Gram stain
  - If no organisms on Gram stain
  - High suspicion for *K. kingae*
  - In sexually active adolescents for coverage of *N. gonorrhoeae*
  - In patients with sickle cell for coverage of *Salmonella*
- Narrow coverage once organism is identified and susceptibilities known
- Duration of therapy depends on organism:
  - *S. aureus*: 3 weeks
  - *Streptococcus pneumoniae, K. kingae*, and *N. meningitidis*: 2 to 3 weeks
  - Longer courses may be necessary for unusual organisms and in complicated courses.
  - May be able to transition to oral antibiotics after short course of IV therapy if improving exam and labs (Timing remains controversial.)
- Pain management with analgesics
- Intra-articular injection of antibiotics is not recommended.

ADDITIONAL THERAPIES
Emerging evidence suggests that short courses of IV dexamethasone as an adjuvant to initial antibiotic therapy may improve short-term clinical outcomes, although evidence is insufficient to make treatment recommendation.

ADMISSION, INPATIENT, AND NURSING CONSIDERATIONS
- Early orthopedic surgery consultation and involvement: Drainage of infection should occur as soon as possible (may include aspiration, irrigation, and debridement via arthroscopy or open arthrotomy).
- Parenteral antibiotic administration immediately after joint aspiration is performed and transition to oral regimen if improving exam and labs
- Indications for open surgical drainage and/or irrigation
  - Hip involvement
  - Shoulder involvement (controversial)
  - Thick, purulent, loculated, or fibrinous exudate unable to pass through 18-gauge needle
  - Lack of improvement within 3 days
- Pain management may require parenteral regimen although can transition to oral regimen if improving exam.

ONGOING CARE

FOLLOW-UP RECOMMENDATIONS

Patient Monitoring
- Follow-up with orthopedic surgery
- Physical therapy and rehabilitation services may be useful.
- When to expect improvement:
  - Symptoms typically improve with 2 days of appropriate antibacterial therapy.
  - CRP typically peaks on day 2 of therapy and quickly normalizes within 7 to 10 days.
- Concerning signs:
  - Continued pain, fever, or lack of improvement of range of motion after 3 to 4 days of appropriate antibiotic treatment
  - Rising ESR or CRP in the face of antibiotic treatment
  - Severe cases of septic arthritis may require serial drainage and debridement.

PROGNOSIS
Depends on duration of illness prior to institution of appropriate therapy
- If antibiotic therapy not instituted within first 4 days of illness, increased incidence of residual joint dysfunction

COMPLICATIONS
- Permanent limitation of range of motion due to tissue destruction and scarring
- Growth disturbance if the epiphysis is involved (limb length discrepancy)
- Avascular necrosis of femoral head (due to increased pressure within joint interrupting blood flow)

ADDITIONAL READING

- Farrow L. A systemic review and meta-analysis regarding the use of corticosteroids in septic arthritis. *BMC Musculoskelet Disord*. 2015;16:241.
- Kocher MS, Mandiga R, Murphy JM, et al. A clinical practice guideline for treatment of septic arthritis in children: efficacy in improving process of care and effect on outcome of septic arthritis of the hip. *J Bone Joint Surg Am*. 2003;85-A(6):994–999.
- Montgomery NI, Rosenfeld S. Pediatric osteoarticular infection update. *J Pediatr Orthop*. 2015;35(1):74–81.
- Pääkkönen M, Kallio MJ, Kallio PE, et al. Sensitivity of erythrocyte sedimentation rate and C-reactive protein in childhood bone and joint infections. *Clin Orthop Relat Res*. 2010;468(3):861–866.
- Sultan J, Hughes PJ, Septic arthritis or transient synovitis of the hip in children: the value of clinical prediction algorithms. *J Bone Joint Surg Br*. 2010;92(9):1289–1293.

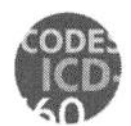

CODES

ICD10
- M00.9 Pyogenic arthritis, unspecified
- M00.859 Arthritis due to other bacteria, unspecified hip
- M00.861 Arthritis due to other bacteria, right knee

S

FAQ
- Q: What is the optimal management of the child with suspected septic arthritis of the hip?
- A: Aspiration of the hip joint is indicated. If purulent fluid is found or analysis of the fluid is suspicious for infection, serial irrigation via arthroscopy or open drainage of the joint must be performed to prevent long-term joint damage. This is a surgical emergency.
- Q: Is MRI necessary in diagnosis of septic arthritis?
- A: This is not necessary in discerning the amount of fluid within the joint capsule and should not delay aspiration or antibiotic management. However, this should be considered to identify concomitant osteomyelitis in patients <4 years of age, involvement of the shoulder, or symptoms >6 days.
- Q: What tools are available to distinguish septic arthritis from transient synovitis of the hip?
- A: In addition to thorough history and physical exam, modified versions of Kocher algorithm can be helpful. Absence of fever in the setting of normal ESR, CRP, and WBC is strongly associated with absence of septic arthritis. Elevated procalcitonin may indicate bacterial infection, but it is not specific to septic arthritis and is not yet validated for routine use.
- Q: Are steroids indicated in management of septic arthritis?
- A: There had been theoretical concern regarding worsening sepsis associated with steroid use in the setting of bacterial infection, but this has not been validated in literature. Emerging evidence suggests short courses of IV dexamethasone as an adjuvant to initial antibiotic therapy may improve short-term clinical outcomes. However, evidence is insufficient to make treatment recommendation at this time.

SERUM SICKNESS

Denise A. Salerno, MD • Amer M. Khojah, MD

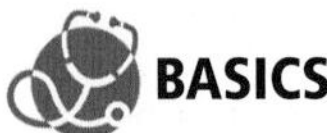

BASICS

DESCRIPTION

- Serum sickness
  - Type III hypersensitivity reaction that occurs 7 to 21 days after injection of foreign protein or serum (e.g., biologics or streptokinase)
  - Immune complexes deposit in the skin, joints, kidneys, and other organs
  - Clinical syndrome consists of skin rash, itching, fever, malaise, proteinuria, edema, joint pain, lymphadenopathy, and vasculitis.
- Serum sickness–like reactions
  - Characterized by fever, rash, lymphadenopathy, and arthralgia
  - Occur 1 to 3 weeks after drug exposure, can be sooner if previously sensitized to the drug
  - Immune complexes, vasculitis, and hypocomplementemia are *absent*.
  - This type of reaction, most commonly associated with medications, is commonly referred to as serum sickness as well.
  - More common than true serum sickness because equine serum antitoxins have been replaced with human antitoxin sera
- Clinically, these entities present and are treated in the same manner.

EPIDEMIOLOGY

- Limited information is available regarding the incidence of adverse drug reactions in children; generally believed to occur less frequently in children than in adults
- >90% of serum sickness cases are drug-induced.
- <5% of serum sickness cases are fatal.

RISK FACTORS

Genetics

People with a genetic predisposition to produce IgE are more susceptible.

GENERAL PREVENTION

- No known way to prevent first occurrence
- Obtain careful history of previous allergic reactions.
- Skin testing prior to antiserum administration will prevent anaphylaxis but not serum sickness.
- When the need for antiserum arises, consider prophylactic antihistamines.

PATHOPHYSIOLOGY

- Serum sickness—type III immune complex, antigen–antibody complement reaction
  - Antibodies form 6 to 10 days after the introduction of foreign material.
  - Antibodies interact with antigens, forming immune complexes that diffuse across the vascular walls.
  - They become fixated in tissue and activate the complement cascade.
  - C3a and C5a are produced, resulting in increased vascular permeability and activated inflammatory cells.
  - Polymorphonuclear cells and monocytes cause diffuse vasculitis.
- Serum sickness–like reaction
  - Abnormal inflammatory reaction in response to defective metabolism of drug by-products

ETIOLOGY

- Common causative agents:
  - Horse antithymocyte globulins
  - Biologics (especially infliximab and rituximab)
  - Human diploid-cell rabies vaccine
  - Streptokinase
  - Insect stings (Hymenoptera venom)
  - Antivenom
  - Penicillins
  - Cephalosporins (especially cefaclor)
  - Sulfonamides
  - Hydralazine
  - Thiouracils
  - Metronidazole
  - Naproxen
  - Dextrans
- Case-reported agents:
  - Minocycline
  - Carbamazepine
  - IVIG
  - Bupropion
  - H1N1 vaccination

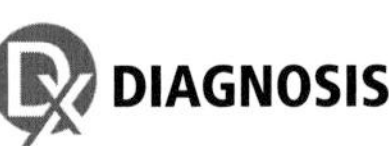

DIAGNOSIS

HISTORY

- Suspect in any patient who has been taking any new drug during the past 2 months and who has an unexplained vasculitic rash.
- Presentation and evolution of rash
  - Typically, the rash first appears on the sides of the fingers, hands, and feet before becoming widespread.
- Previous history of a similar rash
  - Was it associated with any medications in the past?
  - The rash and symptoms of serum sickness will occur sooner on repeat exposure.
- Exposure history
  - Has patient had any drug or antitoxin exposure in the past month?
  - Especially exposures to penicillins, cephalosporins, sulfonamides, hydralazine, thiouracils, streptokinase, metronidazole, naproxen, monoclonal antibodies, or dextrans?
- Timing of the rash and exposure
  - Try to differentiate from simple drug rash; timing of rash after exposure is important in differentiating the two entities.
  - Hypersensitivity reactions occur closer to the time of administration of the offending agent.
- Pruritus is often present.
- Fever
  - Present in 10–20% of cases
  - Usually mild
- Arthritis or arthralgia
  - Present >50% of the time
  - Usually involves the metacarpophalangeal and knee joints
- Associated abdominal pain
  - Some cases may have visceral involvement.
- History of hematuria
  - There can be modest renal involvement, usually presenting as proteinuria and microscopic hematuria.
  - Case reports of renal failure
- Neurologic symptoms
  - Peripheral neuropathy, brachial plexus involvement, and Guillain-Barré syndrome have been reported associations.

PHYSICAL EXAM

- Erythematous purpuric rash starts at the sides of the feet, toes, hands, and fingers and then becomes more widespread.
- Erythema multiforme, maculopapular, purpuric, or urticarial type rash
- Mild to severe fever
- Generalized lymphadenopathy; may be localized to lymph nodes that drain the injection site
- Splenomegaly, occasionally
- Edema of the face and neck
- Joint swelling and tenderness

DIFFERENTIAL DIAGNOSIS

- Erythema multiforme
- Stevens-Johnson syndrome
- Mononucleosis
- Systemic lupus erythematosus
- Rocky Mountain spotted fever
- Systemic juvenile idiopathic arthritis
- Henoch-Schönlein purpura
- Hepatitis B and C infection
- Hypersensitivity syndrome reaction
- Drug-induced pseudoporphyria
- Acute generalized exanthematous pustulosis
- Granulomatosis with polyangiitis (Wegener granulomatosis)

ALERT

- A history of fever, rash, and arthralgias is commonly seen with many infectious childhood illnesses. One must always consider a broad set of differential diagnoses.
- Symptoms may be so minimal that patient does not seek medical attention.
- Often misdiagnosed as simple drug allergy

DIAGNOSTIC TESTS & INTERPRETATION

Laboratory tests are not extremely helpful in establishing diagnosis because no abnormality is universally present; diagnosis usually apparent by classic findings and history of foreign protein or drug exposure:

- Urinalysis: may show proteinuria and/or hematuria
- Complement levels variably reduced before returning to normal
- Leukocytosis or leukopenia with or without eosinophilia
- Erythrocyte sedimentation rate may be slightly elevated.
- Elevated level of circulating immune complexes
- Skin biopsy of rash with direct immunofluorescence is not routinely recommended as part of workup.
  - Shows leukocytoclastic vasculitis with neutrophilic involvement and deposits of IgM and C3 complement in capillary walls

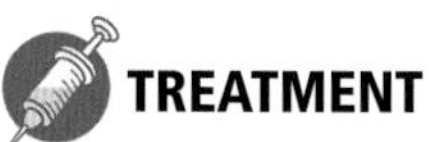

TREATMENT

GENERAL MEASURES

- Stop suspected medication/antigen immediately.
- Topical steroids to relieve itching
- Antihistamines to inhibit the action of vasoactive mediators
- Antipyretics for fever
- NSAIDs to relieve joint pain
- Oral corticosteroids for severe cases
  - Administer and taper over 10- to 14-day period.
  - Shorter course may result in relapse, and recurrent symptoms are more difficult to alleviate.
- Admit if symptoms are severe or diagnosis is unclear.
- Future avoidance of triggering agent if identified

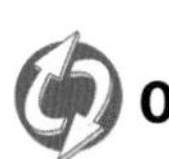

ONGOING CARE

FOLLOW-UP RECOMMENDATIONS

When to expect improvement:

- Usually self-limited illness that resolves in a few days to weeks after stopping the culprit agent
- If symptoms persist for >1 month, reconsider the diagnosis.

PATIENT EDUCATION

- An initial episode of serum sickness cannot be prevented.
- Future episodes can be prevented by avoiding the causative medication (and class of medications) if it has been identified.

PROGNOSIS

Excellent. Most cases are mild and transient with no long-term sequelae.

COMPLICATIONS

- Shock
- Digital necrosis
- Guillain-Barré syndrome (rare)
- Generalized vasculitis (rare)
- Peripheral neuropathy (rare)
- Glomerulonephritis (rare)
- Acute flaccid paralysis (case report)
- Increased risk of anaphylaxis with repeat exposure to precipitating substance
- Fatality (rare, usually due to continued administration of antigen)

ADDITIONAL READING

- Bettge AM, Gross G. A serum sickness-like reaction to a commonly used acne drug. *JAAPA*. 2008;21(3):33–34.
- Bonds RS, Kelly BC. Severe serum sickness after H1N1 influenza vaccination. *Am J Med Sci*. 2013;345(5):412–413.
- Guidry MM, Drennan RH, Weise JW, et al. Serum sepsis, not sickness. *Am J Med Sci*. 2011;341(2):88–91.
- Khan DA. Hypersensitivity and immunologic reactions to biologics: opportunities for the allergist. *Ann Allergy Asthma Immunol*. 2016;117(2):115–120.
- Lawley TJ, Bielory L, Gascon P, et al. A prospective clinical and immunologic analysis of patients with serum sickness. *N Engl J Med*. 1984;311(22):1407–1413.
- McCollom R, Elbe DH, Ritchie AH. Bupropion-induced serum sickness-like reaction. *Ann Pharmacother*. 2000;34(4):471–473.
- Roujeau J, Stern RS. Severe adverse cutaneous reactions to drugs. *N Engl J Med*. 1994;331(19):1272–1285.
- Tolpinrud B, Bunick C, King B. Serum sickness-like reaction: histopathology and case report. *J Am Acad Dermatol*. 2011;65(3):e83–e85.

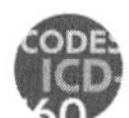

CODES

ICD10

- T80.69XA Other serum reaction due to other serum, initial encounter
- T80.62XA Other serum reaction due to vaccination, initial encounter
- T80.61XA Oth serum reaction due to admin blood/products, init

FAQ

- Q: My child broke out all over her body with an itchy rash and hives a few days after taking cefaclor. Was this serum sickness?
- A: It is more likely that she is allergic to cefaclor. The difference is that drug allergies are type I IgE-mediated hypersensitivity reactions that occur very soon after drug exposure in a previously sensitized individual. Serum sickness is a type III antibody–antigen immune complex and complement amplified hypersensitivity reaction that occurs 1 to 3 weeks after an initial exposure.
- Q: If my child has had serum sickness, is she at risk for getting it again?
- A: Yes, if she receives the same medication or related medications again. The symptoms will occur more quickly, usually in 2 to 4 days, and may be more severe.
- Q: Can the vaccines that my doctor recommends for my child give my child serum sickness?
- A: It is possible but very rare. There have been a few reports of serum sickness–like reactions occurring after receiving vaccines submitted to the Vaccine Adverse Event Reporting System (VAERS).
- Q: Is there any way to prevent my child from getting serum sickness?
- A: Unfortunately, there is no way to predict if your child will have a serum sickness–like reaction to a particular medication. It is extremely important to be aware of your child's exact allergies to medications and to inform all health care providers caring for your child.
- Q: My oldest child had serum sickness after taking cefaclor. Is it true that all my children should now avoid taking cefaclor?
- A: No. There is no known genetic predisposition to serum sickness. Your other children do not need to avoid the medication that caused serum sickness.
- Q: How is the Arthus reaction different from serum sickness?
- A: The Arthus reaction is also a type III hypersensitivity reaction but causes only a local reaction. This phenomenon was first described in 1903 by the French physiologist Nicolas Maurice Arthus. The Arthus reaction is a local vasculitis caused by formation of antigen–antibody complexes in local vessel walls, which then activate the inflammation process. The reaction occurs within hours after an individual is injected intradermally with an antigen against which he or she has been actively immunized.
- Q: My child was diagnosed with serum sickness 1 year ago. He still gets episodes of rash, fever, and joint pain every now and then. How can this be cured?
- A: Serum sickness is a self-limited disease, and as long as the offending agent is stopped, your child will completely recover. If there are continuing symptoms and your child is no longer taking the offending agent, then other causes for these symptoms need to be considered.
- Q: My child's best friend was recently diagnosed with serum sickness. Do I need to be concerned?
- A: No. Serum sickness is not contagious.

SEVERE ACUTE RESPIRATORY SYNDROME (SARS)

Nicholas Tsarouhas, MD

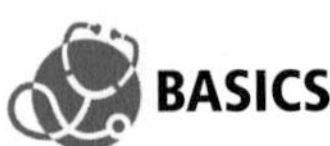

BASICS

DESCRIPTION

- World Health Organization (WHO) clinical criteria (2003):
  - Suspect severe acute respiratory syndrome (SARS) case:
    - A person presenting after November 1, 2002, with high fever (>38°C), and
    - Cough or difficulty breathing, and
    - Close contact with SARS patient or travel criteria to SARS area (see "History")
  - Probable SARS case:
    - A suspect case with radiographic pneumonia or respiratory distress syndrome
    - A suspect case with confirmatory laboratory studies (see "Lab")
    - A suspect case with autopsy findings
- Centers for Disease Control and Prevention (CDC) clinical criteria (2003):
  - Early illness
    - Two or more constitutional symptoms—fever, chills, rigors, myalgia, headache, diarrhea, sore throat, or rhinorrhea
  - Mild to moderate illness
    - Temperature >100.4°F (>38°C)
    - One or more lower respiratory findings—cough, shortness of breath, or difficulty breathing
  - Severe illness
    - Clinical criteria of mild to moderate illness, and
    - One or more of the following—radiographic evidence, acute respiratory distress syndrome, or autopsy findings
- Clinical criteria for SARS must be interpreted in the context of the prevailing epidemiologic laboratory criteria as published by the WHO and the CDC.

EPIDEMIOLOGY

- SARS time line
  - November 2002: A series of severe idiopathic respiratory illnesses begin occurring in Southeast Asian countries (China, Hong Kong, Vietnam, and Singapore).
  - February 2003
    - The Chinese Ministry of Health notifies the WHO that 305 cases of acute respiratory syndrome of unknown etiology have occurred in Guangdong province in southern China.
    - SARS outbreak in Toronto
  - March 2003
    - CDC activates emergency operations center with first confirmed death of SARS patient.
    - CDC implicates a coronavirus (CoV) as the causative SARS agent.
  - May 2003: Deaths dramatically rise—7,761 cases, 623 deaths, 31 countries
  - June 2003: Reported cases slow—over 8,000 cases, >770 deaths, 32 countries
  - July 2003: WHO declares that the SARS epidemic is over.
  - Since July 2003, no further epidemics, but brief reemergence from accidental laboratory exposures in Singapore, Taiwan, and Beijing and from recurrent animal-to-human transmissions in Guangzhou in late 2003 and early 2004
- First emergence of an important human pathogen in the 21st century
- A decade after the emergence of SARS, Middle East respiratory syndrome (MERS) emerged.
- The ease with which SARS coronavirus (SARS-CoV) and MERS-CoV, as well as other respiratory CoVs crossed species to infect humans make it all the more likely that serious CoV outbreaks will continue to emerge.
- Final statistics of SARS epidemics:
  - Worldwide: >8,000 cases, nearly 800 deaths, >30 countries affected
  - United States: 134 suspected cases, 19 probable cases, 8 confirmed cases, no deaths, 17 states affected

RISK FACTORS

Transmission

- Direct or indirect contact of mucous membranes with infectious respiratory droplets or fomites; thus, simple masks and good hand hygiene are important.
- Period of infectivity: most likely during period with active symptoms (fever, cough)
- Incubation period 2 to 14 days but may be as long as 21 days; mean 6 days
- All cases can be traced to contact with individuals from Asian countries or community, spread from an individual whose illness could be traced to Asia.
- There have been no suspected SARS cases among casual contacts of the U.S. cases.
- Many health care workers were infected after providing care to SARS patients.
- No evidence that SARS is transmitted from asymptomatic individuals
- However, health care workers who developed SARS may have been a source of transmission within health care facilities during early phases of illness, when symptoms were mild and not recognized as SARS.
- There is no evidence that SARS can be spread after recovery from the disease.
- Pediatric population
  - Children pose a lower risk of transmission than do adults; only one reported case of transmission of SARS from pediatric patient
  - Vertical transmission of SARS-CoV from infected mothers to their newborns has not been observed.
  - None of the newborns had clinical, laboratory, or radiologic evidence suggestive of SARS-CoV infection.

GENERAL PREVENTION

- As there is no specific treatment, public health and infection control measures including contact tracing and quarantine of close contacts are paramount.
- Hospital infection control precautions:
  - Hospitalized patients meeting SARS case definition should be placed in a negative-pressure, single examination room.
  - Protective equipment appropriate for standard, contact, and airborne precautions (e.g., hand hygiene, gown, gloves, and N95 respirator) in addition to eye protection are recommended for health care workers to prevent transmission of SARS in health care settings.
- Pediatric patients with potential SARS exposure:
  - Children who have been exposed to an ill individual who is suspected of having SARS, or children who have traveled to an area where SARS is occurring, should be evaluated based on the following:
    - If well, parents should self-monitor the child's condition for fever or respiratory tract illness. Attendance at child care or school is not restricted.
    - If the child is not well, parents should contact their physician and the child should be isolated at home.
    - If the child is not well and is experiencing breathing difficulty, he or she should be hospitalized. Health care workers should be informed before the admission so SARS precautions can be initiated.
  - Children who have been exposed to individuals who are not ill but have traveled to areas where SARS is occurring do not require isolation.
- Vaccine
  - No effective human vaccine has been developed.
  - Safety concerns exist for vaccine production workers.

PATHOPHYSIOLOGY

The virus attaches to human receptor cells and initiates a nonspecific acute lung injury response leading to diffuse, severe alveolar damage.

ETIOLOGY

- SARS-CoV, a previously unrecognized single-stranded RNA CoV
- CoVs are a common cause of mild to moderate upper respiratory infections in humans and have occasionally been linked to pneumonia.
- Many believe that the virus originated in an animal species in China and then mutated in such a way that it was able to attach itself to human receptor cells.

DIAGNOSIS

HISTORY
- Recent travel
  - Travel (including transit in an airport) within 10 days of onset of symptoms to an area with recently documented or suspected transmission of SARS is an important epidemiologic criterion for diagnosis.
  - At the height of the SARS epidemic, these areas included China, Hong Kong, Singapore, Taiwan, Toronto, and Hanoi.
- Recent contact with a SARS patient
  - Close contact within 10 days of onset of symptoms with a person known or suspected to have SARS infection is another important epidemiologic criterion.
- The clinical presentation of SARS in children >12 years of age is similar to that of adults.
- Constitutional symptoms, such as fever, chills, rigors, headache, malaise, myalgias, and diarrhea, are common in older patients.
- A meta-analysis of six pediatric series of 135 SARS cases noted the following symptom prevalence: fever (98%), cough (60%), and nausea or vomiting (41%).
- Respiratory symptoms
  - At the onset of illness, most cases have mild respiratory symptoms.
  - After 3 to 7 days, a dry, nonproductive cough begins, often with dyspnea.

PHYSICAL EXAM
- Fever generally heralds the start of the illness.
- Tachypnea, increased work of breathing, or rales are common in adults.
- Adult patients generally present with some evidence of respiratory distress or hypoxemia.
- Importantly, however, although some children present with cough or difficulty breathing, many have remarkably normal examinations.

DIFFERENTIAL DIAGNOSIS
- Bacterial infections
  - *Pneumococcus*
  - *Staphylococcus*
  - *Legionella*
  - *Mycoplasma*
  - *Chlamydophila pneumoniae*
- Viral infections
  - MERS
  - Avian influenza A (H7N9) infection (bird flu)
  - Influenza A and B
  - Respiratory syncytial virus
  - Ebola viral infection

DIAGNOSTIC TESTS & INTERPRETATION

Initial Tests (screening, lab, imaging)
- Detection of SARS-CoV: confirmatory laboratory criteria for the diagnosis of SARS:
  - Antibody by enzyme-linked immunosorbent assay (ELISA) or indirect fluorescent-antibody assay (IFA)
  - RNA by reverse transcriptase-polymerase chain reaction (RT-PCR) assays
  - Viral culture
- SARS virus may be detected in blood, throat, nasopharyngeal aspirates, and stool samples.
- CBC: Hematologic abnormalities are common in children with SARS.
  - Leukopenia (lymphopenia or neutropenia)
  - Thrombocytopenia
- Liver enzymes: elevated transaminases seen
- Raised serum lactate dehydrogenase is also seen.
- The characteristic feature of pulmonary SARS-CoV infection is patchy airspace consolidation, predominantly located at the periphery of the lungs and in the lower lobes.
- Normal chest radiographs also possible

ALERT
- Even during an epidemic of SARS, other diseases should still be considered.
- Microbiologic studies should still be performed to confirm or rule out other infectious diseases.

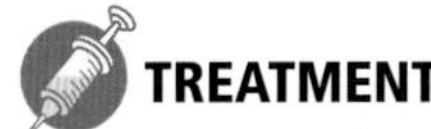

TREATMENT

GENERAL MEASURES
- It is paramount that strict infection control practices be maintained and monitored.
- These are outlined in "General Prevention" above.

MEDICATION
- There is no proven effective treatment.
- CDC recommends that patients with SARS receive the same treatment and supportive care that would be used for any patient with serious community-acquired atypical pneumonia of unknown cause.
- Steroids, interferon, ribavirin, oseltamivir, and other antivirals have been used without consistent success.
- Administration of convalescent plasma, serum, or hyperimmune immunoglobulin may be of clinical benefit for treatment of severe acute respiratory infections (SARIs) of viral etiology; however, this therapy has not been studied in the context of a clinical trial.
- Unfortunately, both SARS-CoV and MERS-CoV have evolved effective immune evasion strategies.

ONGOING CARE

PROGNOSIS
- Patients 12 years of age and younger
  - Milder disease
  - Fewer ICU admits
  - Decreased need for supplemental oxygen
  - No reported pediatric deaths
- Overall fatality rate: 9.5% (all adults)
  - Highest: 27% (Taiwan)
  - Lowest: 0 (United States)
- Very concerningly, MERS has emerged with an even higher mortality rate than SARS.

COMPLICATIONS
- Overall, in 10–20% of cases, the respiratory illness was severe enough to require mechanical ventilation.
- In children, only 5% required admission to an ICU, and <1% required mechanical ventilation.

ADDITIONAL READING

- Braden CR, Dowell SF, Jernigan DB, et al. Progress in global surveillance and response capacity 10 years after severe acute respiratory syndrome. *Emerg Infect Dis*. 2013;19(6):864–869.
- Cheng VC, Chan JF, To KK, et al. Clinical management and infection control of SARS: lessons learned. *Antiviral Res*. 2013;100(2):407–419.
- Li AM, Ng PC. Severe acute respiratory syndrome (SARS) in neonates and children. *Arch Dis Child Fetal Neonatal Ed*. 2005;90(6):F461–F465.
- Mair-Jenkins J, Saavedra-Campos M, Baillie JK, et al; and Convalescent Plasma Study Group. The effectiveness of convalescent plasma and hyperimmune immunoglobulin for the treatment of severe acute respiratory infections of viral etiology: a systematic review and exploratory meta-analysis. *J Infect Dis*. 2015;211(1):80–90.
- Momattin H, Mohammed K, Zumla A, et al. Therapeutic options for Middle East respiratory syndrome coronavirus (MERS-CoV)—possible lessons from a systematic review of SARS-CoV therapy. *Int J Infect Dis*. 2013;17(10):e792–e798.
- Stockman L, Massoudi MS, Helfand R, et al. Severe acute respiratory syndrome in children. *Pediatr Infect Dis J*. 2007;26(1):68–74.
- Vijay R, Perlman S. Middle East respiratory syndrome and severe acute respiratory syndrome. *Curr Opin Virol*. 2016;16:70–76.

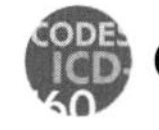

CODES

ICD10
- J12.81 Pneumonia due to SARS-associated coronavirus
- B97.21 SARS-associated coronavirus causing diseases classd elswhr

FAQ
- Q: Is the clinical presentation and course different in children?
- A: Fortunately, younger children tend to have a shorter and milder course, consisting mainly of low-grade fever, cough, and rhinorrhea. Adolescents, conversely, follow a more severe course, similar to that of adults.
- Q: What constitutes close contact with a SARS patient?
- A: Close contact includes having cared for or lived with a person known to have SARS or having a high likelihood of direct contact with respiratory secretions and/or body fluids of a patient known to have SARS.

SEVERE COMBINED IMMUNODEFICIENCY

M. Elizabeth M. Younger, CRND, PhD • Howard M. Lederman, MD, PhD

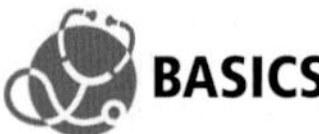

BASICS

DESCRIPTION

Severe combined immunodeficiency (SCID) is a primary immunodeficiency disease characterized by functional defects in both the humoral and cellular immune systems. Most babies present with lymphopenia. Even the suspicion of SCID constitutes a pediatric emergency. Untreated, SCID is universally fatal, usually within the 1st year of life.

EPIDEMIOLOGY

- Estimated to be 1 in 100,000 births but may be underreported because of early infant mortality
- Highest in regions where consanguineous marriages take place
- SCID due to Artemis defects occurs in 1 in 2,500 births in the Navajo and Apache populations because of a founder mutation.

RISK FACTORS

Genetics

- Multiple genetic defects (about 20) can cause SCID.
- Approximately 50% of cases are X-linked (mutation in the IL-2 γ-chain); the others are autosomal recessive mutations.
- Classified by the lymphocyte subsets affected (e.g., T− B+ NK+, T− B− NK+)

ETIOLOGY

SCID is caused by mutations in genes required for T-cell growth and development, purine salvage pathway function (e.g., adenosine deaminase [ADA]), expression of histocompatibility (HLA) antigens, and DNA repair.

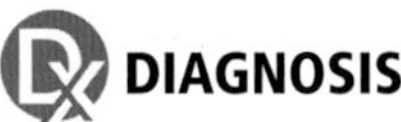

DIAGNOSIS

HISTORY

- Infants who have not been identified with newborn screening tests, usually present in the 1st year of life as their immunity from maternal antibody wanes.
- Failure to thrive
- Chronic diarrhea
- Chronic thrush or candidal diaper rash
- Frequent and/or severe infections with common pathogens
- Rotavirus infection after immunization
- Opportunistic infections
- Consanguinity
- Family history of SCID or unexplained infant deaths

PHYSICAL EXAM

- Emaciated or wasted appearance
- Atypical morbilliform rash
- Absence of lymphoid tissue (small or absent tonsils and lymph nodes)
- Evaluation for infection
  - Thrush or diaper dermatitis
  - Manifestations of graft-versus-host disease (skin rash, conjunctivitis, hepatitis, diarrhea) secondary to transplacentally transferred alloreactive maternal T cells or T cells from unirradiated blood products

DIFFERENTIAL DIAGNOSIS

- HIV infection
- Other syndromes with T lymphopenia
  - DiGeorge (22q11.2 deletion) syndrome
  - Trisomy 21
  - Ataxia-telangiectasia
- Secondary T lymphopenia caused by loss of T lymphocytes such as congenital heart disease and vascular leakage
- Iatrogenic T lymphopenia (e.g., steroid therapy)
- Idiopathic T lymphopenia

DIAGNOSTIC TESTS & INTERPRETATION

- Newborn screening tests:
  - T-cell receptor excision circles (TRECs) assay in newborn screening (currently available in 42 of 50 states in the United States)
  - Identifies most infants with SCID
- CBC with differential
  - To assess for lymphopenia
  - Suspect SCID if absolute lymphocyte count (ALC) $<3{,}000/\mu L$ in the neonatal period or if ALC is $<1{,}000/\mu L$ in any child <3 years of age.
- Lymphocyte subsets (CD4 and CD8 T cells, CD19 B cells, CD16/56 NK cells; CD45RA naïve CD4 and CD8 T cells): All populations are generally decreased, but T cells are almost always severely decreased.
- Serum immunoglobulins (IgG, IgA, IgM):
  - Usually low or absent, but IgG may be normal in first 4 months of life because of transplacental transfer
- TRECs
  - Profoundly low or absent
  - TRECs may be reduced in premature infants or infants with other conditions associated with T lymphopenia such as DiGeorge syndrome or ataxia-telangiectasia.
- Lymphocyte proliferation assay: Cells do not proliferate when stimulated with mitogens or antigens.
- Appropriate cultures to identify pathogens
- Identification of causative mutation is necessary to allow for formulation of treatment plan and genetic counseling.

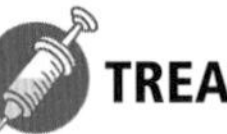

TREATMENT

- Hematopoietic (bone marrow) stem cell transplantation is curative for all types of SCID.
  - Success rates $>70\%$ have been reported and increase to 96% when the transplant is done before the age of 3 1/2 months.
  - Preconditioning is generally not required because of the lack of T-cell function, but reduced intensity conditioning is often done to ensure engraftment.
- In patients with ADA-deficient SCID, enzyme replacement therapy with pegylated ADA (Adagen®) can be given, however this treatment is not curative.
- Gene therapy may be an option for certain forms of SCID.

ONGOING CARE

- Pretransplant supportive care
  - Pneumocystis prophylaxis with trimethoprim/sulfamethoxazole
  - Immunoglobulin replacement therapy (IV every 3 to 4 weeks, subcutaneously every 1 to 2 weeks)
  - Palivizumab during respiratory syncytial virus season
  - Aggressive and early treatment of infections
  - Nutritional support
  - Avoidance of crowds and persons with symptoms of infection (fever, cough, etc.)
  - Routine immunization is unnecessary, as patients are unable to mount antibody responses.
  - Live viral vaccines are absolutely contraindicated.
  - If blood transfusion is required, use only irradiated, CMV negative blood products.
- Posttransplant care
  - Close monitoring for signs of graft-versus-host disease, engraftment failure, infection
  - Immunoglobulin replacement therapy may still be required if B-cell reconstitution is absent or impaired.
  - Genetic counseling for parents

COMPLICATIONS

- Pre- or posttransplant graft-versus-host disease
- Engraftment failure
- Omenn syndrome caused by clonal autoreactive T cells, resembling graft-versus-host disease seen in patients with *RAG1* or *RAG2* mutations
- Increased risk for lymphoreticular cancers
- Radiation sensitivity in patients with SCID caused by DNA repair syndromes (Artemis, ligase 4, DNA-PKcs, Cernunnos)
- Growth failure and hearing impairment in patients with ADA-deficient SCID

ADDITIONAL READING

- Buckley RH. Transplantation of hematopoietic stem cells in human severe combined immunodeficiency: longterm outcomes. *Immunol Res*. 2011;49(1–3):25–43.
- Chinn IK, Shearer WT. Severe combined immunodeficiency disorders. *Immunol Allergy Clin North Am*. 2015;35(4):671–694.
- Diamond CE, Sanchez MJ, LaBelle JL. Diagnostic criteria and evaluation of severe combined immunodeficiency in the neonate. *Pediatr Ann*. 2015;44(7):e181–e187.
- Dorsey MJ, Dvorak CC, Cowan MJ, et al. Treatment of infants identified as having severe combined immunodeficiency by means of newborn screening. *J Allergy Clin Immunol*. 2017;139(3):733–742.
- van der Spek J, Groenwold RHH, van der Burg M, et al. TREC based newborn screening for severe combined immunodeficiency disease: a systemic review. *J Clin Immunol*. 2015;35(4):416–430.

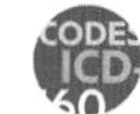

CODES

ICD10

- D81.9 Combined immunodeficiency, unspecified
- D81.1 Severe combined immunodeficiency w low T- and B-cell numbers
- D81.2 Severe combined immunodef w low or normal B-cell numbers

FAQ

- Q: What should I do if I am notified that a newborn screen has identified a low number of TRECs?
- A: As a precaution while the child is being evaluated, prevent the infant's exposure to sick contacts and public places or places with large crowds (day care centers, malls, churches, large family gatherings). Send blood for enumeration of T-cell subsets (CD4 and CD8), B cells (CD19), and NK cells (CD 16/56), and refer the child to a clinical immunologist. Consider the need for pneumocystis prophylaxis and immunoglobulin replacement therapy while the evaluation proceeds.
- Q: What vaccines should be given to a child with SCID or suspected SCID?
- A: Live vaccines of any type (rotavirus, MMR, varicella, and BCG) are absolutely contraindicated. Other vaccines should not be given because they will not be effective.
- Q: What is the chance of another child in the family being affected with SCID?
- A: The answer to this question depends on the cause of SCID. If a child has X-linked SCID, then there is a 50% chance of SCID in any male child born to the mother. In other forms of SCID, the risk is 25% for any male or female. It is crucial that a genetic diagnosis is made for each case of SCID so that families can be given accurate information about recurrence risk, they can be offered prenatal testing, and other affected children can be identified as soon as possible after birth.
- Q: Is SCID a fatal disease?
- A: Untreated, most children with SCID die within the 1st year of life. Hematopoietic stem cell transplantation is usually curative, especially when it is done early in life before an infant has had infections.
- Q: What is the most common reason for a false-positive TREC result (i.e., low TREC number in a baby without SCID)?
- A: Prematurity. One can rely on a normal TREC result to rule out SCID in infants of any gestational age, but TREC counts may be low in premature infants until they reach about 37 weeks postconception.

SEXUAL ABUSE

Mitchell Goldstein, MD, MBA • Courtney W. Mangus, MD

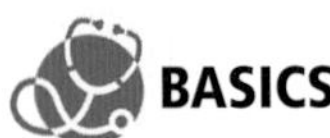

BASICS

DESCRIPTION

Sexual abuse is the involvement of children in sexual activities that they cannot understand, for which they are not developmentally prepared, to which they cannot give informed consent, and/or that violate societal norms.

- Ranges from oral, genital, or anal contact; fondling; child pornography; prostitution; exhibitionism; and voyeurism
- 25% of perpetrators are parents, and 30% are nonparental relatives.
- Most children sexually abused will have no discernible physical injury.

EPIDEMIOLOGY

- ~150,000 substantiated cases per year; most likely underestimate the incidence as these include only those cases reported
- Prevalence rates between 10% and 30%. The National Violence Survey reported 27% of adult women and 16% of adult men reported sexual abuse during childhood.

RISK FACTORS

- Peak age of vulnerability: 7 to 13 years of age
- Girls are victimized more than boys, although abuse of boys is underreported.
- Single-parent households, domestic violence, parental substance abuse, and mental illness are risk factors.
- Children who experience other types of abuse are also more likely to be victimized sexually.
- Race and socioeconomic status do not appear to be risk factors for child sexual abuse.
- Risk factors for revictimization: younger aged children, more severe maltreatment, families with mental health and substance abuse problems and violence histories

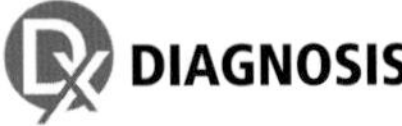

DIAGNOSIS

HISTORY

- Diagnosis is made based on the child's history because abnormal physical findings or lab tests are infrequent.
- Attempt to limit the number of interviews.
- Interview should be detailed enough to know whether a report to child protection or law enforcement is needed.
- If the medical provider is the first person to which the child has disclosed, then that person is an "an outcry witness," and that disclosure can be used in court testimony.
- Answers from the children that are obtained for the medical diagnosis and treatment may be admitted into evidence. Verbatim documentation is recommended if possible.
- The interview should be conducted with the child separate from family members.
- Ask open-ended, nonleading questions.
- Use developmentally appropriate language.
- Specific questions important to the triage of the child include the following:
  - Identity of alleged perpetrator/relationship to child
  - Time of last possible contact
  - Specific types of sexual contact
  - Review of systems including genital pain, bleeding, dysuria, constipation, painful bowel movements, and behavioral changes

PHYSICAL EXAM

- Serves to ensure the overall health of a child after an abusive event and to document any injuries or other forensically relevant evidence
- Most exams are normal.
- Timing
  - An emergency exam is indicated if the most recent assault was within 72 hours or if the patient has complaints of pain, dysuria, or bleeding.
  - Beyond 72 hours, the exam can be scheduled at the local child advocacy center.
- A speculum should not be used for a prepubertal sexual abuse exam unless there is acute bleeding, and its origin must be determined.
  - Use of the techniques of labial separation and labial traction (gently grasping the posterior portion of the labia majora and pulling laterally, down, and toward the examiner) allows for the best visualization of the hymenal edges.
  - Normal hymenal configurations: annular, crescentic, and fimbriated
  - Newborn hymen: thickened, pale, and redundant
  - Prepubertal hymen: thin, less redundant, with sharp well-defined edges
  - Postpubertal hymen: thickened, pale, and redundant
- A few physical findings are diagnostic of abuse:
  - Presence of semen or sperm on the victim
  - Pregnancy
  - Acute genital/anal injuries without an adequate accidental explanation (bruising, lacerations, complete hymenal transaction between 4 and 8 o'clock along hymenal rim)
  - Syphilis and *Neisseria gonorrhoeae* infection (excluding perinatal infection)
  - Chlamydia if the child is >3 years of age
  - Trichomoniasis in a child >1 year of age
- Many genital findings are unlikely to be related to abuse:
  - Normal variants including intravaginal ridges, hymenal mounds, linea vestibularis, diastasis ani
  - Perineal redness
  - Labial adhesions
  - Anal fissures
  - Venous pooling in perianal area
- Any finding on exam thought to be abnormal or diagnostic of child sexual abuse should be reviewed with a child abuse expert for confirmation.
- Photo documentation is recommended as it preserves visual evidence for expert review and legal proceedings.

DIFFERENTIAL DIAGNOSIS

- Sexualized behaviors
  - Normal behaviors for age (e.g., masturbation)
  - Exposure to sexual activity (e.g., media)
- Abnormal GU exam
  - Normal variations in hymenal anatomy (e.g., septate, cribriform, imperforate)
  - Normal variations in perineal anatomy (e.g., hymenal mound, intravaginal ridge, vestibular bands)
  - Linea vestibularis: white streaks that run from inferior hymenal border to posterior commissure
  - Failure of midline fusion: presence of mucosal surface between fossa navicularis and anus that commonly resolves at puberty
  - Irritant, contact, and seborrheic dermatitis
  - Labial adhesions
  - Lichen sclerosus et atrophicus: thinned white atrophic skin in figure-of-8 appearance which may have bruising or petechiae
  - Ureterocele
  - Urethral prolapse
  - Pearly pink papules in males
  - Balanitis in males
  - Phimosis or paraphimosis in males
  - Accidental trauma, including straddle and impaling injuries
  - Accidental tourniquet of genitals by hair
- Abnormal anal exam
  - Diastasis ani: absence of muscle fibers in middle of external anal sphincter
  - Anal skin tags
  - Anal dilatation from constipation or sedation
  - Group A streptococcal perianal cellulitis
- Urethral discharge/bleeding
  - Foreign body
  - UTI
  - Nonspecific vulvovaginitis
  - Group A *Streptococcus*
  - *Haemophilus influenzae*
  - *Staphylococcus aureus*
  - *Mycoplasma hominis*
  - *Gardnerella vaginalis*
  - *Shigella flexneri* (discharge commonly bloody)
- Genital ulcers
  - EBV, herpes simplex virus (HSV)
  - Behçet disease
  - Inflammatory bowel disease
- Genital irritation
  - Pinworms
  - Scabies
  - *Candida albicans*
  - Trauma

DIAGNOSTIC TESTS & INTERPRETATION

Initial Tests (screening, lab, imaging)

- Forensic evidence collection
  - Standard rape kit if the last contact was 72 hours or less
  - Always obtain consent.
  - In prepubertal children, recovery of useful forensic evidence is rare beyond 24 hours.
  - Some experts support forensic evidence recovery up to 5 days from the contact in pubertal children.
  - Most positive forensic evidence comes from clothing and linens.
- Sexually transmitted infection (STI) screening:
  - For adolescents: Universal screening is recommended.
  - For prepubertal children, the Centers for Disease Control and Prevention (CDC) and American Academy of Pediatrics (AAP) recommend STI testing when:
    - Child discloses high-risk sexual contact (genital-genital, anal-genital, or oral-genital).
    - Child's symptoms or physical exam suggest presence of STI or anogenital trauma.
    - Abuser is known to have an STI or be at risk for STI.
    - Abuser is a stranger.
    - Community prevalence of STI is high.
    - Family member is infected with an STI.
    - Patient or family member requests testing.

- Testing for *N. gonorrhoeae* and *Chlamydia trachomatis* may be performed with vaginal/urethral culture or nucleic acid amplification techniques (NAATs).
- Cultures have historically been the gold standard method for diagnosing STIs in prepubertal children. NAATs have proven to be sensitive and specific for *N. gonorrhoeae* and *C. trachomatis* infection in this age group.
- NAATs are not approved for rectal or pharyngeal specimens.
- NAATs have a higher sensitivity than culture.
- If a NAAT is done, then important not to treat empirically because if the NAAT is positive, the clinician will want to repeat with another NAAT or culture to reconfirm
- Trichomoniasis in a child ≥1 year of age is diagnostic of child sexual abuse; can be tested for by wet preparation, culture, or polymerase chain reaction (PCR). In adolescents, NAAT is the preferred test to diagnose trichomoniasis.
- Screen for syphilis and hepatitis B in any case which meets other screening recommendations.
- HIV screening should also be considered.
- Pregnancy testing should be performed in adolescent girls.

Follow-Up Tests & Special Considerations

- Genital warts are not diagnostic of child sexual abuse. Neonatal transmission is common and human papilloma virus (HPV) may remain latent for several years. Children who present after age 3 to 5 years should have a complete medical evaluation for sexual abuse.
- Herpes simplex infections in the genital area are most commonly (but not always) caused by sexual contact. Most mouth infections are caused by HSV-1, and most genital infections are caused by HSV-2, but this distinction is not absolute. Culture or PCR can detect HSV when clinically indicated.
- Any positive NAAT needs to be repeated with a different NAAT for confirmation prior to empiric treatment.
- Any positive syphilis screening test should be confirmed with a treponemal test.
- If serologic testing for HIV, HBV, and syphilis is negative acutely, it should be repeated at 6 weeks, 3 months, and 6 months.

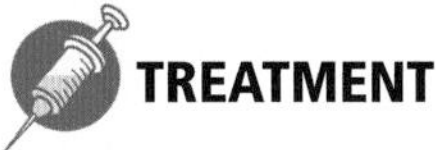

TREATMENT

GENERAL MEASURES

Cases of child sexual abuse require a multidisciplinary approach that includes medical, social services, law enforcement, and states attorney expertise.

MEDICATION

- Empiric prophylactic antibiotics
  - Recommended following sexual abuse/assault in adolescents and adults to prevent *N. gonorrhoeae*, *C. trachomatis*, and *Trichomonas vaginalis*
  - Not recommended in prepubertal victims because of the low likelihood of STI and the importance of establishing the diagnosis
- *N. gonorrhoeae* treatment per CDC guidelines:
  - Adolescents: ceftriaxone 250 mg IM once or cefixime 400 mg PO once + azithromycin 1 g PO once
  - Prepubertal child: ceftriaxone 25 to 50 mg/kg IM once (not to exceed 125 mg)
- *C. trachomatis* treatment per CDC guidelines:
  - Adolescents: azithromycin 1 g PO one time or doxycycline 100 mg PO b.i.d. × 7 days
  - Prepubertal child
    - Weight <45 kg: erythromycin 50/mg/kg/24 h divided into 4 daily doses for 14 days
    - Weight >45 kg but <8 years: azithromycin 1 g PO × 1; age >8 years: azithromycin 1 g PO one time or doxycycline 100 mg PO b.i.d. × 7 days
- Syphilis treatment per CDC guidelines: parenteral penicillin G; dose depends on stage of disease and child age.
- Trichomoniasis treatment: metronidazole 2 g PO once
- HIV postexposure prophylaxis (PEP)
  - Indicated for patients presenting within 72 hours of exposure with high risk of HIV infection (perpetrator with known HIV; high local prevalence of HIV in unknown perpetrator; high-risk sexual contact with anal, vaginal, or oral penetration; or presence of anogenital injuries)
  - Recommend consultation with pediatric infectious disease specialist before initiating PEP to determine appropriate medication regimen.
  - Discuss risk and benefits of treatments with patient/family including treatment duration of 28 days.
  - HIV PEP is not indicated if patient presents >72 hours after the exposure.
- Hepatitis B vaccination for unimmunized patients
- Hepatitis B immune globulin for patients with recent sexual contact with known positive perpetrator
- HPV vaccination for girls ≥9 years who are incompletely immunized or unimmunized
- Consider pregnancy prevention (e.g., emergency hormonal contraceptive) for adolescents after ensuring the patient is not pregnant.
- Tetanus booster for patients with acute, serious genital or other injuries

ADMISSION, INPATIENT, AND NURSING CONSIDERATIONS

Consider hospital admission.

- In children with injuries that require operative care
- In cases where the clinician wants to ensure protection of the child and external forces preclude that assurance
- In cases where there is a significant mental health concern

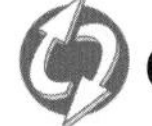

ONGOING CARE

FOLLOW-UP RECOMMENDATIONS

Patient Monitoring

Children should be screened for posttraumatic stress disorder (PTSD) and feelings of self-blame. Most children should be followed by a mental health provider.

PROGNOSIS

Varies greatly depending on specifics of abuse sustained and available support systems

COMPLICATIONS

- PTSD
- Depression
- Domestic violence and revictimization
- Substance abuse
- Chronic pelvic pain
- Males are more likely to have concerns about sexual orientation.

ADDITIONAL READING

- Adams JA, Kellogg ND, Moles R. Medical care for children who may have been sexually abused: an update for 2016. *Clin Pediatr Emerg Med*. 2016;17:255–263.
- Berenson AB, Chacko MR, Wiemann CM, et al. A case-control study of anatomic changes resulting from sexual abuse. *Am J Obstet Gynecol*. 2000; 182(4):820–831.
- Christian CW. Timing of the medical examination. *J Child Sex Abus*. 2011;20(5):505–520.
- Gavril AR, Kellogg ND, Nair P. Value of follow-up examinations of children and adolescents evaluated for sexual abuse and assault. *Pediatrics*. 2012;129(2):282–289.
- Hammerschlag MR. Sexual assault and abuse of children. *Clin Infect Dis*. 2011;53(Suppl 3):S103–S109.
- Williams HN, Letson MM, Tscholl JJ. transmitted infections in child abuse (initials lowercase). *Clin Pediatr Emerg Med*. 2016;17:264–273.
- Workowski KA, Bolan GA; for Centers for Disease Control and Prevention. Sexually transmitted diseases treatment guidelines, 2015. *MMWR Recomm Rep*. 2015;64(RR-03):1–137.

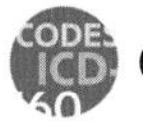

CODES

ICD10

- T74.22XA Child sexual abuse, confirmed, initial encounter
- T76.22XA Child sexual abuse, suspected, initial encounter

FAQ

- Q: How could there have been penetration with a normal physical examination?
- A: The vast majority of child sexual abuse exams are completely normal even with a history of penetration. The healing properties of genital tissues are quick and complete; past injuries are often difficult to detect on physical exam.
- Q: What should I do if I examine a patient with no history of sexual abuse and detect an anatomic abnormality that I think is suggestive of sexual abuse?
- A: Always have exams confirmed by a child abuse expert in your area, as nuances of exams can be hard to discern. Photo documentation can preserve images of findings if a child abuse expert cannot reexamine the patient in a timely manner.
- Q: Is an STI diagnosed in a prepubertal patient always indicative of abuse?
- A: No. All STIs may be transmitted vertically (from mother to infant). The incubation periods of different infections vary, so they are expressed at different ages accordingly. Gonorrhea and syphilis are considered diagnostic of sexual abuse outside of congenital infection. *Chlamydia*, HSV-2, and *Trichomonas* are probably due to sexual abuse and should be reported for evaluation. *Condyloma acuminata* is probably related to sexual abuse in school-aged and older children but may be transmitted to younger children innocently during toileting or diaper changes.
- Q: Why is the physical exam deferred to local child abuse experts if the child presents >72 hours after the exposure?
- A: Unless the child has physical complaints (bleeding, dysuria, pain, etc.), the physical exam can be deferred because its purpose is to collect forensic evidence. In adolescents, beyond 72 hours, the yield for evidence is very low. In prepubertal children, forensic evidence is rarely obtained after 24 hours.

SHORT STATURE

Bhavana Narala, MD • Susanne M. Cabrera, MD

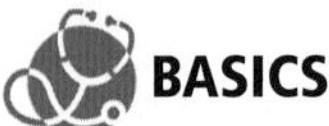

BASICS

DESCRIPTION

- Short stature is height 2 standard deviations (*SD*) or more below mean or <3rd percentile for age and sex of the normal population.
- Growth failure is defined as height 2 *SD* or more, below midparental height (MPH), or height velocity (HV) <10th percentile for age resulting in downward crossing of height percentiles.
- The majority of children with short stature are essentially healthy. Conversely, true growth failure is typically pathologic and requires evaluation.
- Failure to thrive (FTT) is failure of appropriate weight gain (decreasing weight to height ratio); may be accompanied by poor linear growth

RISK FACTORS

- Poor nutrition, systemic chronic illness, certain medications, and psychosocial factors can all contribute to the clinical presentation of short stature or growth failure.
- A family history of short stature or delayed growth and puberty are well-established risk factors for childhood short stature.

PATHOPHYSIOLOGY

- Adequate nutrition and weight gain play major roles in linear growth during childhood.
- Throughout infancy and childhood, growth hormone (GH) and thyroid hormone exert major influences on normal growth.
- Pulsatile GH release stimulates insulin-like growth factor 1 (IGF-1) secretion from the liver and other tissues to promote growth at growth plates.
- The pubertal growth spurt is largely mediated by androgen and estrogen activity at the growth plate as well as enhanced GH release.
- Chronic illnesses can cause growth failure.
- Glucocorticoid excess inhibits growth through downregulation of the GH/IGF-1 axis and suppresses osteogenesis.
- Although boys are more frequently referred for short stature, girls are more likely to have a pathologic reason for short stature.

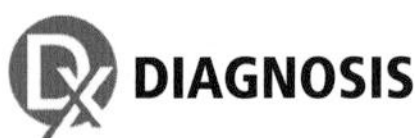

DIAGNOSIS

HISTORY

- **Question:** Have length/height and weight been measured correctly and charted appropriately on the correct growth curve?
- *Significance*: Interpretation of growth depends on *precise* and *accurate* measurements that account for both year and month of age.
- **Question:** Is the child short for his or her MPH?
- *Significance*: Height can only be judged to be inappropriate in the context of the genetic potential as determined by MPH:
  - For boys: [father's height (cm) + (mother's height [cm] + 13)] divided by 2
  - For girls: [(father's height [cm] − 13) + mother's height (cm)] divided by 2
  - MPH target range (± 2 *SD*) is +/− 10 cm.
  - If the child's height percentile is decreased relative to the MPH range, evaluation may be warranted.
- **Question:** HV?
- *Significance*: A normal HV is reassuring, whereas noting a reduced HV for age/gender, *regardless of absolute height*, can result in earlier detection of a growth-slowing disorder.
  - The HV for an interval of at least 6 months (to minimize seasonal variation or measurement error) should be annualized.
  - As a general rule, normal HV is at least >4 cm per year in children (faster prior to age 6 years) and >8 cm per year during pubertal growth spurt.
- **Question:** Birth measurements and gestational age?
- *Significance*: Intrauterine growth restriction (IUGR) and/or small for gestational age (SGA) can be associated with possible maternal disorders, genetic disorders, and intrauterine drug exposure or stress that later impact growth.
- **Question:** Postnatal history including hypoglycemia or prolonged jaundice?
- *Significance*: Birth trauma, prolonged jaundice, and postnatal hypoglycemia can be associated with hypopituitarism.
- **Question:** Family history of short stature or delayed puberty?
- *Significance*:
  - Short stature in family members may suggest a heritable growth disorder.
  - Consider a diagnosis of constitutional delay of growth and puberty.
- **Question:** Dietary and feeding history?
- *Significance*: Low daily intake, difficulty feeding, or inefficient use of calories may point to anorexia or malabsorptive states.
- **Question:** Developmental milestones?
- *Significance*: Delays may signal chromosomal, metabolic, or behavioral syndromes.
- **Question:** Social situation?
- *Significance*: Psychosocial stressors affect growth and development.
- **Question:** Chronic illness or any prior hospitalizations, surgery, or head trauma?
- *Significance*: Growth failure may be the first/only sign of diseases such as rheumatoid arthritis, celiac disease, or inflammatory bowel disease (IBD). Previous hospitalizations, trauma, or surgery may be a sign of underlying or acquired pathology. Head trauma may cause hypopituitarism.
- **Question:** Any medication use?
- *Significance*: Use of oral or inhaled steroids as well as stimulant medications can lead to short stature or growth deceleration.
- The history should be completed by obtaining a full review of systems, specifically inquiring about general development, headache, emesis, vision change, anorexia, fatigue, weight change, bowel irregularities, pubertal development, exercise tolerance, polyuria and polydipsia, activity pattern, sleep hygiene.

PHYSICAL EXAM

- **Finding:** Decreased upper to lower segment ratio?
- *Significance*: suggests scoliosis
- **Finding:** Abnormal trunk-to-arm span ratio?
- *Significance*: suggests skeletal dysplasia
- **Finding:** Low weight-to-height ratio?
- *Significance*: FTT, malnutrition, psychosocial deprivation, stimulant medication, chronic systemic illness, or metabolic disorders
- **Finding:** Proportionate/high weight-to-height ratio?
- *Significance*: if normal/near normal HV, then familial short stature, genetic syndrome, SGA, constitutional delay, mild chronic disease, prior resolved growth-attenuating disorder, or acquired growth limitations; if associated with low HV, suggests endocrine disorder, chronic disease, or growth-affecting medications
- **Finding**: Dysmorphic features?
- *Significance*: primary growth disorders
- **Finding:** Mid-facial hypoplasia, cherubic appearance, truncal fat deposition?
- *Significance*: suggests GH deficiency
- **Finding:** Goiter, edema, slow relaxation of deep tendon reflexes, hair loss, dry skin?
- *Significance*: suggests hypothyroidism
- **Finding:** Abdominal distention or tenderness and gluteal wasting?
- *Significance*: malabsorption and celiac disease
- **Finding:** Webbed neck, increased carrying angle, shield chest, lymphedema, heart murmur?
- *Significance*: Turner or Noonan Syndrome
- **Finding:** Microphallus?
- *Significance*: hypogonadism, GH deficiency
- **Finding:** Abnormal funduscopic or cranial nerve exam? Midline abnormalities?
- *Significance*: CNS pathology ± associated hypopituitarism
- **Finding:** Signs of neglect or abuse?
- *Significance*: psychosocial dwarfism
- **Finding:** Round face, hypocalcemia, short 4th and 5th metacarpals, and mental retardation?
- *Significance*: pseudohypoparathyroidism
- **Finding:** Hypertension, virilization, moon face, buffalo hump, thick violaceous striae?
- *Significance*: glucocorticoid excess
- **Finding:** Delayed pubertal maturation?
- *Significance*: Turner syndrome, constitutional delay, hypogonadism, hypothyroidism, IBD, chronic renal disease
- **Finding:** Leg bowing, widening of wrists, rachitic rosary, frontal bossing?
- *Significance*: rickets, malabsorption

DIFFERENTIAL DIAGNOSIS

- Extremes of normal growth:
  - Familial short stature
    - Normal exam, no systemic illness
    - Height <3rd percentile with normal HV
    - Normal bone age (BA) and onset of puberty
    - Adult height close to MPH
  - Constitutional delay of growth and puberty
    - Family history common
    - Normal exam, no systemic illness
    - Proportionately short; height percentile below MPH
    - Decelerating HV during first 3 years of life with normal to near-normal HV until puberty, when delays in pubertal growth spurt leads to decreased HV compared to peers

- Delayed BA and pubertal maturation
- Adult height commensurate with MPH
- Idiopathic short stature
  - Categorizes otherwise normal patients who cannot be diagnosed with a variant of normal growth or other short stature cause
  - Predicted adult height is >2 *SD* below MPH.
  - Height is <3rd percentile ± delayed BA.
- Primary growth disorders: disorders intrinsic to skeletal system, BA normal
  - Skeletal dysplasia/defects: may lead to disproportionate short stature. Skeletal involvement can be subtle.
    - Skeletal radiographs with typical findings
    - Common forms: achondroplasia, hypochondroplasia, dyschondrosteosis (Leri-Weill and other *SHOX* mutations)
  - Syndromes
    - Usually associated with other abnormalities
    - Clinical findings may be subtle (mosaicism).
    - Common forms: trisomies (13, 18, 21), Turner or Noonan syndrome, Prader-Willi, DiGeorge, neurofibromatosis type 1
  - IUGR and SGA
    - Often due to maternal, fetal, or placental problems and/or exposures, or idiopathic
    - SGA infants have relative GH resistance seen as elevated GH with low IGF-1 levels.
    - 10% of infants with SGA don't have catch-up growth with height *SD* <−2 by 2 years and need endocrine evaluation. GH therapy may be indicated.
  - Primordial dwarfism: inherited intrinsic defect leading to prenatal and postnatal growth failure
- Secondary short stature
  - Malnutrition
    - Most common cause internationally
    - Poor nutrition (caloric, vitamin, mineral)
    - Especially <2 years of age
  - Chronic illness: Poor growth can be presenting symptom.
    - Hematopoietic (anemia, sickle cell)
    - Cardiovascular (congenital heart defect)
    - Pulmonary (severe asthma, cystic fibrosis)
    - GI/liver (IBD, celiac disease, malabsorption syndromes, chronic liver disease)
    - Renal (renal tubular acidosis, Fanconi syndrome, uropathy, congenital anomalies)
    - Metabolic (poorly controlled diabetes mellitus, storage disorders, disorders of calcium and phosphorous metabolism)
    - Infectious/immunologic (HIV)
  - Iatrogenic
    - Medications: glucocorticoids, stimulants
    - Treatment of childhood malignancy, irradiation, chemotherapy
  - Psychosocial growth retardation
    - Emotional deprivation
    - Anorexia
    - Depression
  - Endocrine
    - GH or IGF-1 deficiency/resistance, hypogonadism, hypothyroidism, Cushing syndrome, short stature from earlier accelerated bone maturation (e.g., precocious puberty, hyperthyroidism, congenital adrenal hyperplasia)
    - Among secondary short stature, endocrine causes are *least* frequent.

DIAGNOSTIC TESTS & INTERPRETATION

- **Test:** Radiograph of the left hand and wrist
- *Significance*: BA determination (not reliable in kids <2 years of age)
- **Test:** IgA and anti-tissue transglutaminase IgA
- *Significance*: celiac disease
- **Test:** CBC with differential
- *Significance*: anemia, infection, malignancy, or chronic inflammatory conditions
- **Test:** C-reactive protein (CRP) and/or erythrocyte sedimentation rate (ESR)
- *Significance*: infection, inflammatory conditions
- **Test:** complete metabolic panel
- *Significance*: renal/liver disorders, malnutrition, calcium disorders
- **Test:** urinalysis
- *Significance*: diabetes, renal/metabolic issue
- **Test:** T_4/free T_4 and TSH
- *Significance*: hypothyroidism
- **Test:** karyotype or targeted gene testing
- *Significance*: Turner syndrome in girls, *SHOX* mutation, or other chromosomal disorders
- **Test:** IGF-1 and Insulin-like growth factor-binding protein 3 (IGF-BP3) concentrations, compared to pubertally matched norms
- *Significance*: proxy measurements for GH secretory reserve and screen for GH deficiency; not reliable <3 years of age and IGF-1 can be falsely low in poor nutrition states

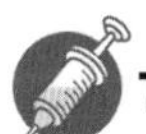

TREATMENT

GENERAL MEASURES

Evaluation warranted if HV low for age or growth pattern deviates significantly from the MPH target.

- In the majority of short children, history and exam are unrevealing, and tests yield equivocal or normal results. These children are then considered to have idiopathic short stature.
- Observation is reasonable for familial short stature or constitutional delay.
- In cases of malnutrition, restoration of adequate nutrition results in HV acceleration.
- In cases of endocrinopathies, replacement of the deficient hormone (thyroid hormone for hypothyroidism, GH for GH deficiency, hydrocortisone for adrenal insufficiency) or removal of excess hormone (glucocorticoids) will normalize the HV.
- Children with short stature or poor predicted adult height, who do not have true GH deficiency, may receive different evaluation and treatment options depending on costs, risks, physician practice, extent of family's concern, and presence of associated psychosocial stressors (e.g., teasing by peers).

ISSUES FOR REFERRAL

- Critical to obtain accurate measurements plotted appropriately to assess growth
- Referrals should be guided by abnormal laboratory evaluations or clinical suspicion (i.e., nephrology referral for elevated creatinine, pulmonary referral for clubbing).
- Endocrine referral warranted if slow HV, growth plateau, delayed bone age with short stature/growth failure, or suggestive labs.
- If poor weight gain, consider nutritional deficiency, malabsorption syndromes; initial referral to gastroenterologist appropriate
- The evaluation of growth failure or short stature best done in outpatient setting

ADDITIONAL READING

- Allen DB, Cuttler L. Clinical practice. Short stature in childhood—challenges and choices. *N Engl J Med*. 2013;368(13):1220–1228.
- Oostdijk W, Grote FK, de Muinck Keizer-Schrama SM, et al. Diagnostic approach in children with short stature. *Horm Res*. 2009;72(4):206–217.
- Rogol AD, Hayden GF. Etiologies and early diagnosis of short stature and growth failure in children and adolescents. *J Pediatr*. 2014;164(Suppl 5):S1–S14.

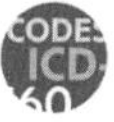

CODES

ICD10

- R62.52 Short stature (child)
- E34.3 Short stature due to endocrine disorder
- E23.0 Hypopituitarism

FAQ

- Q: Does short stature portend worse psychosocial outcomes?
- A: No. The majority of children with idiopathic short stature have normal psychosocial function, peer acceptance, and social behavior. Clinic-based populations may exhibit distress, however, as those seeking treatment have the highest degree of parental concern.
- Q: How much height does a child with idiopathic short stature gain from treatment with recombinant GH?
- A: 1.2 to 2.8 inches in final adult height, at a cost of $10,000 to $60,000 per patient per year. Height gains are much better in other conditions such as true GH deficiency and Turner syndrome, but the cost remains steep.
- Q: What is a reasonable strategy for constitutional delay of growth and puberty?
- A: Observation and reassurance alone are frequently all that is needed. A short course of testosterone or estrogen therapy may be considered if puberty is delayed to "jump start" pubertal changes.
- Q: Should a primary care provider obtain a random GH level in evaluation of short stature?
- A: No. A random serum GH concentration measurement is not helpful in diagnosing GH deficiency because GH secretion is pulsatile and occurs mostly during sleep. Random IGF-1 and IGF-BP3 levels more accurately reflect GH secretion. However, IGF-1 may not be reliable in young children or in cases of inadequate nutrition. IGF-BP3 is a more sensitive marker of GH deficiency in those <10 years of age.

SHORT-BOWEL SYNDROME

Nina N. Sainath, MD • Christina B. Bales, MD • Judith Kelsen, MD

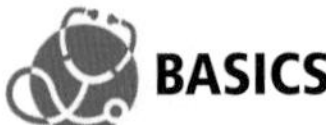

BASICS

DESCRIPTION

Malnutrition, malabsorption, and/or fluid and electrolyte loss after extensive small bowel resection

PATHOPHYSIOLOGY

- Markedly decreased mucosal surface area due to resection
- Loss of trophic hormones
- Loss of peptide hormones that regulate motility
- Abnormal transit
- Malabsorption of protein, fat, carbohydrate, vitamins, electrolytes, and trace elements, depending on site of resected intestine (see "Follow-Up Recommendations"). The patient can lose as much as half of the intestine, if the duodenum, distal ileum, and ileocecal valve (ICV) are present. If the ICV is gone, patients may not be able to tolerate even a 25% loss of intestine without the help of parenteral nutrition (PN).
- Normal bowel length: 150 to 200 cm (26 weeks' gestation); 200 to 300 cm (at birth in full-term infant); 600 to 800 cm (adult)
- Infants have low intestinal reserve and do not tolerate small bowel resection as well as adults. However, long-term prognosis is often better because of hypertrophy and hyperplasia of the intestine.
- Gastric acid hypersecretion occurs soon after intestinal resection but is transient.
- Bowel adaptation can occur over time. Increased surface area due to bowel dilatation, villous hypertrophy, and bowel lengthening can occur. Stimulation of luminal contents is needed for bowel growth, and factors such as glutamine, short-chain fatty acids, tropic hormones, and growth factors may be important for bowel growth.

ETIOLOGY

- Infants: intestinal resection in setting of necrotizing enterocolitis, intestinal atresia, gastroschisis, omphalocele, cystic fibrosis (CF)-associated meconium ileus, and malrotation with volvulus
- Older children: intestinal resection associated with Crohn disease, trauma, pseudoobstruction syndrome, mesenteric ischemia, neoplasms, and radiation enteritis

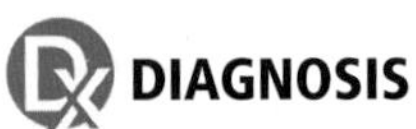

DIAGNOSIS

HISTORY

- Defecation pattern: number, size, nature (watery, bulky, foul smelling), presence of blood and mucous
- Ostomy output: consistency (watery, viscous, thick), volume (≥50 mL/kg/24 h often leads to dehydration and electrolyte imbalance)
- Abdominal pain and characteristics
- Abdominal distention and flatulence
- Vomiting and characteristics
- Intense perianal rashes related to stool acidity and malabsorption of carbohydrates
- Weight loss or gain; gaining length/height
- Diet history: appetite, oral intake, tube feeds, PN
- Central line–associated bloodstream infection (CLABSI) history (if receiving PN)
- Medication history
- Surgical history

PHYSICAL EXAM

- Weight, length, and head circumference measurements (if applicable); try to get previous growth chart if available.
- Look for signs of vitamin deficiencies in examination of mouth, lips, skin, hair, and skeleton and in assessment of healing difficulties.
- Look for signs of liver disease (scleral icterus, jaundice, hepatomegaly, splenomegaly, dilated abdominal veins).
- Look for signs of vascular thrombosis (extremity swelling, dilated veins in neck region).
- Abdominal examination: surgical scars, ostomies, distention, bowel sounds
- Rectal examination: consistency of stool, heme positivity, perianal rash

DIFFERENTIAL DIAGNOSIS

- Infants: necrotizing enterocolitis, volvulus, atresia (jejunal and ileal), gastroschisis, perforated meconium ileus, congenital short-bowel syndrome, aganglionosis of the intestine
- Older children: midgut volvulus (due to malrotation), Crohn disease, adhesions causing intestinal obstruction, strictures, trauma

DIAGNOSTIC TESTS & INTERPRETATION

Initial Tests (screening, lab, imaging)

- Blood tests:
  - CBC: Check for anemia and mean corpuscular volume.
  - Electrolytes: Check for losses and adequacy of replacement.
  - Minerals: calcium, phosphorus, magnesium, iron, zinc; check for losses and adequacy of replacement therapy.
  - Albumin and prealbumin: Check for protein stores and nutritional status.
  - Liver evaluation: Alanine transaminase (ALT), γ-glutamyl transpeptidase (GGT), bilirubin may be elevated in PN-associated liver disease (PNALD).
  - Vitamin levels: vitamin A, 25-hydroxyvitamin D, vitamin E, RBC folate, and vitamin B_{12}; check for adequacy. An elevated methylmalonic acid (MMA) level is a more sensitive marker of B_{12} deficiency but may also be elevated in small bowel bacterial overgrowth. PT/INR indirectly measures vitamin K deficiency. Protein induced by vitamin K absence (PIVKA) is a more sensitive marker of vitamin K deficiency.
  - Carnitine: Check status if on long-term PN and presence of liver disease.
  - Breath tests: lactose and lactulose breath test to check for lactase deficiency and bacterial overgrowth, respectively
- Stool tests:
  - Stool for pH and reducing substances: Check for carbohydrate malabsorption.
  - Stool smear for fat (Sudan stain—qualitative): Check for excessive fat loss.
  - Stool for blood: Check for mucosal damage.
  - Stool elastase: measure of pancreatic insufficiency; may be falsely depressed if watery stools (dilutional effect)
  - Stool calprotectin: Check for GI tract inflammation.
- Tests of absorption:
  - D-xylose absorption test and lactose breath test to check for carbohydrate malabsorption
  - Coefficient of fat absorption: 72-hour quantitative fecal fat collection along with concomitant diet record
  - Carotene levels to check for fat absorption
  - 24-hour stool collection for α_1-antitrypsin clearance to check for protein absorption
- Upper GI series with small bowel follow-through and barium enema to evaluate length, caliber, and location of remaining bowel

Diagnostic Procedures/Other

Endoscopy:

- Upper endoscopy: Look for presence of inflammation that may be contributing to malabsorption; obtain and culture duodenal aspirates to assess for bacterial overgrowth.
- Lower endoscopy: Look for presence of colitis, especially eosinophilic colitis. Evaluate caliber and quality of anastomosis site and presence of anastomotic ulcers.

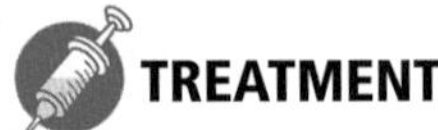

TREATMENT

MEDICATION

- Supplementation of deficient vitamins (E, D, K, A, B_{12}, folic acid)
- Supplementation of deficient minerals (calcium, magnesium, iron, copper, selenium, and zinc)
- H_2-receptor antagonists and proton pump inhibitors decrease gastric acid hypersecretion and reduce gastric secretory volume (particularly in the postoperative period).
- Antidiarrheal drugs: opioid agonists (diphenoxylate, and loperamide) to decrease motility (caution in patients with slow transit or bacterial overgrowth)
- Ion-exchange resins: Cholestyramine binds intraluminal dihydroxy bile acids to limit bile acid–induced diarrhea.
- Octreotide/somatostatin: decreases gastric, pancreatic, and intestinal secretions; slows GI motility. Use with caution, although, as may reduce splanchnic blood flow.
- Glucagon-like peptide 2 (GLP-2) agonist: Teduglutide has been shown to improve intestinal adaptation and allow PN to be weaned in adults, currently being studied for use in pediatric short-bowel syndrome.
- Bacterial overgrowth: Commonly used oral antibiotics are metronidazole, trimethoprim-sulfamethoxazole, ciprofloxacin, vancomycin, and gentamicin.
- Prokinetic agents: erythromycin, metoclopramide to treat delayed gastric emptying. Use with caution given potential side effects.
- Ethanol lock therapy has been successful in reducing CLABSI. Therapy may be associated with an increased risk of central venous catheter thrombosis. Randomized control trials in the pediatric short-bowel population are needed.

- Miscellaneous: sucralfate to treat bile reflux, prebiotics and probiotics to treat bacterial overgrowth, ursodiol for cholestasis, Bicitra® for electrolyte losses, dietary fiber to enhance absorption; caution in infancy and in patients with bacterial overgrowth

SURGERY/OTHER PROCEDURES

- Surgery is useful in patients who develop strictures and partial obstruction or in those who have very short intestine length with one or more significantly dilated segments distal to the duodenum.
- Intestinal interpositions (isoperistaltic or antiperistaltic) historically used to delay gastric emptying, slow intestinal transit, and increase absorption but have largely fallen out of favor
- Intestinal lengthening and tapering procedures, including the Bianchi and serial transverse enteroplasty (STEP) procedures, increase absorptive surface area.
- In patients with extremely short intestines and PN dependency, small bowel transplantation or multivisceral transplantation is considered. Factors favoring consideration include advanced liver disease, recurrent prolonged hospitalizations, life-threatening bloodstream infections, and loss of central venous access sites.

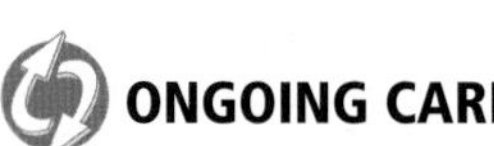

ONGOING CARE

FOLLOW-UP RECOMMENDATIONS

Patient Monitoring

- When to expect improvement: depends on site and extent of bowel resection
- Signs to watch for:
  - Vomiting, diarrhea, weight loss, severe fluid and electrolyte abnormalities, sepsis, bowel dilatation, intestinal obstruction
- Major cause of death: sepsis and cholestatic liver disease

DIET

- Fluid and electrolyte therapy: extremely important in the acute phase immediately after bowel resection. In the chronic phase, it is important to keep up with ongoing losses, especially when enteral feeds are started.
- Oral diet: In those patients who are able to avoid PN or tube feeds, a diet low in simple sugars and high in complex starch, protein, and unsaturated fat (e.g., canola and olive oil) may be well tolerated. Low-oxalate diets are helpful in preventing cholelithiasis.
- Enteral feeds: more successful in the patient with less extensive resection, intact ICV, and colon in continuity
  - Feeds advanced slowly and held for ostomy output exceeding 50 mL/kg/24 h of ostomy output, excessive watery diarrhea, and/or electrolyte imbalance
  - Maternal breast milk preferred in infancy
  - More complex nutrients and long-chain fats promote adaptation.
  - Elemental formulas may be better tolerated but may also contribute to diarrhea due to high osmolarity.
- Development of oral skills and oral feeding should be encouraged when possible as introduction of solid foods with maturity slows transit and improves enteral capacity.
- PN: important in the acute phase postoperatively, when nutrition must be maintained in the face of paralytic ileus; indispensable in the chronic phase when full enteral feeds cannot be instituted and nutrition needs to be maintained
  - Need permanent central access to deliver concentrated PN solutions
  - Balanced solutions of protein, glucose, and fat should be administered.
  - Prophylactic measures to prevent PN-induced liver damage should be instituted (e.g., prevention of overfeeding, early introduction of enteral feeds, cycling of PN when patient is stable, limitation of IV fat emulsion).
- IV fish-based oil emulsion (composed of omega-3 polyunsaturated fatty acids) and Smoflipid (composed of soybean oil, MCT, olive oil, fish oil) have been studied as a preventive measure against PNALD with promising results.

PROGNOSIS

- Contingent on site and amount of bowel resected
- Adaptation is better after jejunal resection than after ileal resection.
- More extensive resection (<50 cm of residual bowel in neonatal period) and loss of the ICV portend a worse prognosis.
- Gastroschisis, care in multiple institutions, and recurrent sepsis portend prolonged PN dependence.

COMPLICATIONS

- Fluid and electrolyte loss, resulting in diarrhea, dehydration, and metabolic acidosis
- Calcium and magnesium deficiency, resulting in bone disease and osteoporosis
- Carbohydrate malabsorption
- Fat malabsorption
- Vitamin A deficiency: visual deficits and increased susceptibility to infections
- Vitamin D deficiency: bone demineralization
- Vitamin E deficiency: hemolytic anemia, impaired immunity, neuromuscular dysfunction
- Vitamin K deficiency: prolonged clotting time, bruising, bleeding
- Vitamin B_{12}: megaloblastic anemia, peripheral neuropathy
- Folic acid: megaloblastic anemia
- Iron deficiency: microcytic anemia
- Copper deficiency: anemia, neutropenia, myelopathy, and neuropathy
- Zinc deficiency: poor wound healing, diarrhea, poor vertical growth
- Essential fatty acid deficiency: increased susceptibility to infection, decreased energy stores, dermatitis
- Gallstones: due to disturbed enterohepatic circulation of bile salts and lithogenic bile formation
- Renal stones: due to fat malabsorption and increased oxalate absorption
- Failure to thrive
- TPN-dependent liver disease: cholestasis, end-stage cirrhosis, and portal hypertension
- Carnitine deficiency: contributes to development of steatosis, hypoglycemia
- Sepsis
- Small bowel bacterial overgrowth and D-lactic acidosis due to stasis, causing ataxia and other neurologic symptoms

ADDITIONAL READING

- Cober PM, Killu G, Brattain A, et al. Intravenous fat emulsions reduction for patients with parenteral nutrition-associated liver disease. *J Pediatr*. 2012;160(3):421–427.
- Cole CR, Kocoshis SA. Nutrition management of infants with surgical short bowel syndrome and intestinal failure. *Nutr Clin Pract*. 2013;28(4): 421–428.
- Fallon EM, Mitchell PD, Nehra D, et al. Neonates with short bowel syndrome: an optimistic future for parenteral nutrition independence. *JAMA Surg*. 2014;149(7):663–670.
- Gosselin KB, Duggan C. Enteral nutrition in the management of pediatric intestinal failure. *J Pediatr*. 2014;165(6):1085–1090.
- Jeppesen PB, Gilroy R, Pertkiewicz M, et al. Randomised placebo-controlled trial of teduglutide in reducing parenteral nutrition and/or intravenous fluid requirements in patients with short bowel syndrome. *Gut*. 2011;60(7):902–914.
- Khan FA, Squires RH, Litman HJ, et al; for Pediatric Intestinal Failure Consortium. Predictors of enteral autonomy in children with intestinal failure: a multicenter cohort study. *J Pediatr*. 2015;167(1):29–34.e1.
- Mercer DF, Hobson BD, Gerhardt BK, et al. Serial transverse enteroplasty allows children with short bowel to wean from parenteral nutrition. *J Pediatr*. 2014;164(1):93–98.
- Pieroni KP, Nespor C, Ng M, et al. Evaluation of ethanol lock therapy in pediatric patients on long-term parenteral nutrition. *Nutr Clin Pract*. 2013; 28(2):226–231.
- Puder M, Valim C, Meisel JA, et al. Parenteral fish oil improves outcomes in patients with parenteral nutrition-associated liver injury. *Ann Surg*. 2009; 250(3):395–402.

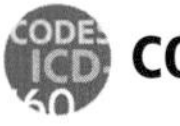

CODES

ICD10

K91.2 Postsurgical malabsorption, not elsewhere classified

FAQ

- Q: What are the favorable prognostic factors in short-bowel syndrome?
- A: Greater length of residual small bowel, jejunal versus ileal resection, maintenance of the ICV, and lack of PNALD. Neonates demonstrate better bowel adaptation than do adults.
- Q: Are elemental formulas better than intact formulas in the management of patients with short-bowel syndrome in patients?
- A: Limited case series suggest that elemental formulas may be associated with a shorter duration of PN dependence than intact formula, which may be related to a higher incidence of food allergy in the short-bowel population. However, elemental formulas have a higher cost and higher osmolarity, which may exacerbate diarrhea. Animal studies demonstrate that intestinal adaptation is improved with nutrient complexity, suggesting that elemental formula may be inferior to intact protein formula in this regard.

SICKLE CELL DISEASE

Tiffany F. Lin, MD

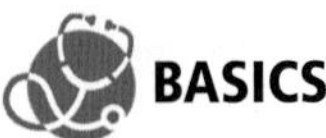

BASICS

DESCRIPTION

Sickle cell disease (SCD) is a disease caused by a homozygous inheritance of a one base pair change leading to an amino acid change in the beta globin gene at the sixth position: glutamic acid to valine on chromosome 11. The mutation leads to undesired polymerization of hemoglobin in the red cell causing membrane distortion which has systemic effects on the host.

EPIDEMIOLOGY

- The incidence of SCD is 1 in 500 African Americans, 1 in 36,000 Hispanics, with a lesser frequency in other ethnic groups. The incidence of sickle cell trait (SCT) in African Americans is 1 in 14.
- There are 70,000 to 100,000 affected individuals with SCD in the United States.

RISK FACTORS

Genetics

- SCD is autosomal recessive.
- The disease can be caused by homozygous inheritance of beta globin with the S mutation or by inheriting the mutated beta globin S with an additional beta globin mutation such as abnormal beta globin causing hemoglobin C, beta thalassemia, or $D^{Los\ Angeles}$, and O^{Arab}.

PATHOPHYSIOLOGY

- Membrane distortion caused by this abnormal hemoglobin leads to: increased adhesion to vascular endothelium, activation of cytokines leading to activation of platelets and leukocytes, and ultimately to vaso-occlusion.
- Extravascular hemolysis causes release of free hemoglobin and subsequent oxidative stress causing vasoconstriction, inflammation and platelet activation.

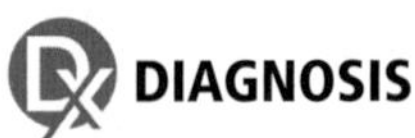

DIAGNOSIS

HISTORY

- Diagnosis:
  - In the United States, diagnosed on newborn screening with hemoglobin electrophoresis showing FSA or FS findings
  - Often asymptomatic in early infancy (<6 months) due to protective effects of residual fetal hemoglobin (HbF) production
  - Family history of trait
- Subsequent to diagnosis, obtain this history:
  - SCD genotype (i.e., sickle cell SS vs. SC vs. sickle beta thalassemia)
  - Obtain history of:
    - Dactylitis (presents in infants and associated with more severe phenotype after infancy)
    - Splenic sequestration
    - Stroke and/or transcranial Doppler (TCD) abnormalities
    - Transfusion history (chronic transfusions vs. PRN transfusions for crises)
    - Hospitalizations, particularly intensive care unit (ICU) admissions
    - Pain (sites and usual therapy)
    - Acute chest syndrome (if exchange transfusion was required)
    - Surgery (splenectomy, cholestectomy)
    - History of iron overload
  - Baseline hemoglobin and pulse oximetry
  - Current medication and therapy

PHYSICAL EXAM

- Pallor of anemia with flow murmur
- Mild scleral icterus
- Splenomegaly in splenic sequestration
- Decreased breath sounds, or wheeze as signs of obstructive lung disease associated with SCD and acute chest
- Decreased range of motion: hip and shoulder avascular necrosis
- Neurologic examination: stroke

DIAGNOSTIC TESTS & INTERPRETATION

Initial Tests (screening, lab, imaging)

- Diagnostic
  - All states have newborn screening. Below are the interpretation of the possible hemoglobin electrophoresis results:
    - F: thalassemia major
    - FA: normal hemoglobin
    - FAS: A > S: SCT
    - FSA: S > A: SCD, S beta plus thalassemia
    - FS: hemoglobin S: sickle cell anemia or sickle beta zero thalassemia
    - FSC: hemoglobin SCD
  - If SCD is found on newborn screen, beta gene analysis should be done for confirmation.
- Monitoring
  - CBC: Degree of anemia depends on genotype, mean corpuscular volume is generally normal but should be elevated with hydroxyurea therapy.
  - Hemoglobin electrophoresis: useful to monitor compliance with hydroxyurea (goal: elevated hemoglobin F%) and transfusion therapy (goal: <30% hemoglobin S)
  - TCD annually: This predicts stroke risk.
  - Screening brain MRI/MRA: abnormal TCD or neurologic findings
  - Echocardiogram: pulmonary hypertension or heart failure in patients with cardiac iron overload
  - Pulmonary function testing: obstructive lung disease seen in patients with acute chest or as follow-up of multiple episodes of acute chest
  - Ophthalmology: Check for retinopathy.
  - Neurocognitive testing: stroke or school delay
  - 25-hydroxyvitamin D level for bone health

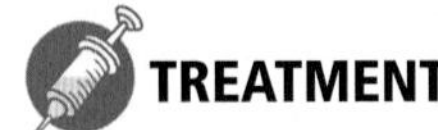

TREATMENT

GENERAL MEASURES

- Teaching regarding fever precautions (for functional asplenia in SCD patients), signs of acute chest, splenic sequestration monitoring, aplastic crises, stroke identification, and home pain management
- Prevention
  - Infection prophylaxis with oral penicillin 125 mg b.i.d. starting at the latest by 2 months of age, 250 mg b.i.d. at 36 months
  - Pneumococcal vaccine (23-valent at 2 and 5 years of age)
  - Meningococcal vaccine
  - Recommended routine immunizations including annual influenza
  - Avoidance of drastic changes in temperature (jumping into a cold pool) which can precipitate vaso-occlusive event
  - Good pulmonary hygiene to prevent acute chest syndrome while hospitalized or if they have concurrent pulmonary disease (asthma)

ALERT

Fluid overload or significant dehydration can precipitate vaso-occlusion such as pain crises or acute chest syndrome so fluid status should be maintained at euvolemic and excessive fluid boluses should be avoided.

- Routine screening with TCDs and brain MRI/MRA if necessary to implement stroke prevention if results are abnormal

ADDITIONAL THERAPIES

- Hydroxyurea: indicated for patients who have two or more acute events leading to hospitalization a year or more frequent pain events not leading to hospitalization
  - Requires monthly monitoring to check for hepatotoxicity and myelosuppression
- Patient adherence to regimen over time is necessary to see improved SCD phenotype. Red cell transfusion can prevent complications, morbidity, and are lifesaving because it immediately decreases %S in the blood but can cause iron overload over time.
  - Using phenotypically matched red cells (for ABO, D, C, c, E, e, Kell) decreases alloimmunization. (Send red cell phenotype soon after birth.)
  - Generally transfuse to hemoglobin levels of 9 to 10 and can perform exchange transfusions to prevent increased viscosity in the setting of acute stroke or severe acute chest syndrome
  - Goal for transfusion is to have percentage of hemoglobin S <30% (i.e., the level of S there is in a SCT patient).
  - Patients at high risk for stroke or with known silent stroke are chronically transfused to prevent overt stroke (TCD levels of >200 cm/s are an indication for chronic transfusion).
  - Transfusion iron overload is an important and common complication related to transfused SCD patients: All patients are monitored (for liver iron deposition and cardiac function) and treated with oral or subcutaneous chelation chronically.

- Stem cell transplant is the only cure for SCD.
  - If patient has full siblings: HLA typing for the patient and the prospective donor
  - Consider cord blood collection for full siblings.
  - Consultation with a transplant physician familiar with transplantation for sickle cell anemia

ADMISSION, INPATIENT, AND NURSING CONSIDERATIONS

- Fever
  - Patients with SCD and fever are presumed septic because of their functional asplenic status presumed due to repeated splenic infarcts from vaso-occlusion.
    - History, physical exam, CBC with reticulocyte count, blood culture, chest radiograph if <3 years or if has any respiratory symptoms, other cultures as indicated
    - Parenteral antibiotic: ceftriaxone until culture negative
    - Children <3 years, admitted to hospital
    - Older children and adolescents with a benign examination, no pulmonary infiltrate, or urinary tract infection: ceftriaxone with follow-up in 24 hours if persistently febrile
- Acute chest syndrome
  - Defined as a new pulmonary infiltrate frequently accompanied by hypoxia, pain, fever, and severe anemia
  - Treat for fever (above) and add a macrolide antibiotic for anti-inflammatory properties and additional antibacterial coverage.
  - Type and cross or screen for possible exchange transfusion or simple transfusion.
  - Transfusion indicated for severe anemia, progressive infiltrate, hypoxia
  - Oxygen to maintain O_2 saturation 95%
  - Fluid overload can exacerbate pulmonary disease; monitor I and O.
  - Chest clearance with incentive spirometry and chest physiotherapy and bronchodilators if indicated as supportive care
- Pain (thought to be due to vaso-occlusion within bones or in the soft tissues)
  - Severe pain is a medical emergency.
  - Hydration: to maintenance, avoid fluid overload.
  - Analgesics
    - Be aware that many SCD patients have acute or chronic pain.
    - Mild pain: NSAIDs and mild oral opioids
    - Moderate pain: may need parenteral therapy with opioids and ketorolac
    - Severe pain: admission with patient-controlled analgesia (PCA) parenteral opioids, may need antihistamine, ketorolac, H_2 blocker with ketorolac
  - Pain assessment after administration of medications and close monitoring of pain, the fifth vital sign
  - Adjunctive therapy: heating pad, visualization, distraction, other therapy
- Aplastic crises
  - Presents with profound, acute anemia
  - Most commonly due to parvovirus B19 infection
    - CBC with reticulocyte count will show an anemia with reticulocytopenia secondary to severe viral suppression and aplasia of red cell production.
    - Type and cross and transfuse for severe anemia causing cardiovascular compromise.
    - Parvoviral B19 PCR is diagnostic.
    - Droplet isolation precautions
- Splenic sequestration
  - Tends to occur in preschool age children with sickle cell SS disease and can occur later in life for patients with sickle cell SCD
  - May present with left upper quadrant (LUQ) pain or sudden anemia
  - Exam with splenomegaly present that can be progressively enlarging
  - Closely monitor hemoglobin (every 6 hours) as hemoglobin can drop quickly.
  - Consider a small volume slow transfusion for anemia. Often, small transfusion opens up venules of spleen allowing sequestered (i.e., trapped); red blood cells to escape and hemoglobin responds significantly compared to what you transfused
  - Splenectomy indicated for life-threatening or repeated episodes. Remember to immunize prior to splenectomy.
- Stroke
  - Diagnosis by history and physical examination
  - Treatment should not be delayed for imaging although imaging should be obtained as well as urgent neurology evaluation.
  - Evidence suggests initial exchange transfusion, to hemoglobin of 9 to 10 g/dL, percent hemoglobin S of <30%, leads to improved long-term outcome.
  - After a stroke, patients are treated with chronic transfusions to prevent reoccurrence of stroke.
- Dactylitis
  - Tends to occur in infants
  - Presents with swelling of the finger/toes or hands and feet
  - Treatment is supportive with NSAID therapy to decrease swelling.
- Priapism
  - Diagnosis: unwanted erection with pain lasting for longer than 1 hour
  - Medical emergency
  - Initial management: pain management, IV hydration
  - Treatment with subcutaneous terbutaline has been used.
  - Definitive treatment: is aspiration and instillation of pseudoephedrine

ONGOING CARE

PROGNOSIS

The prognosis for children with SCD has improved dramatically due to hydroxyurea therapy, increased use of blood transfusion with adequate chelation, and screening for stroke risk factors. Transition to adult care is a priority.

- Chronic complications:
  - Cholecystitis
  - Avascular necrosis (hip and shoulder)
  - Obstructive pulmonary disease
  - Pulmonary hypertension
  - Renal disease (proteinuria)
  - Hyposthenuria (enuresis, dehydration)
  - Retinopathy (increased in SCD)
  - School failure due to hospitalization
  - Cerebral vascular disease/infarcts

ADDITIONAL READING

- Adams RJ, Brambilla D; for Optimizing Primary Stroke Prevention in Sickle Cell Anemia (STOP 2) Trial Investigators. Discontinuing prophylactic transfusions used to prevent stroke in sickle cell disease. *N Engl J Med*. 2005;353(26):2769–2778.
- Aidoo M, Terlouw DJ, Kolczak MS, et al. Protective effects of the sickle cell gene against malaria morbidity and mortality. *Lancet*. 2002;359(9314):1311–1312.
- Ballas SK. New era dawns on sickle cell pain. *Blood*. 2010;116(3):311–312.
- Bernaudin F, Verlhac S, Arnaud C, et al. Impact of early transcranial Doppler screening and intensive therapy on cerebral vasculopathy outcome in a newborn sickle cell anemia cohort. *Blood*. 2011;117(4):1130–1140, quiz 1436.
- Ferreira A, Marguit I, Bechmann I, et al. Sickle hemoglobin confers tolerance to *Plasmodium* infection. *Cell*. 2011;145(3):398–409.
- Thornburg CD, Files BA, Luo Z, et al. Impact of hydroxyurea on clinical events in the BABY HUG trial. *Blood*. 2012;120(22):4304–4310. 2016;128(24):2869.

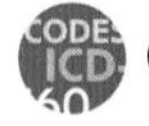

CODES

ICD10

- D57.1 Sickle-cell disease without crisis
- D57.3 Sickle-cell trait
- D57.40 Sickle-cell thalassemia without crisis

FAQ

- Q: When can I stop penicillin prophylaxis?
- A: Most morbidity and mortality from infections in sickle cell anemia occur in the first 5 years of life. The risk of pneumococcal sepsis decreases with age but continues to be a significant risk of morbidity and mortality. Patients with surgical splenectomy need penicillin prophylaxis for life.
- Q: Are phenotypically matched red cells necessary for transfusion?
- A: Historically, the incidence of red cell alloimmunization is 30% for patients with SCD who do not receive phenotypically matched red cells. By providing phenotypically matched red cells, the rate of alloimmunization is significantly decreased.
- Q: Why is the sickle cell gene mutation relatively common?
- A: The sickle cell hemoglobin gene may confer a survival advantage to individuals living in endemic areas of malaria. Hemoglobin S is associated with decreased risk of severe malarial anemia and malarial mortality.

SINUSITIS

Esther K. Chung, MD, MPH

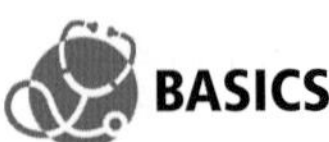

BASICS

DESCRIPTION

- Sinusitis is inflammation of the mucous membranes lining the paranasal sinuses.
- The term is most commonly used to describe bacterial rhinosinusitis, which is a clinical diagnosis made by the presence of upper respiratory tract symptoms that have not improved in 10 days or have worsened after 5 to 7 days. Sinusitis may be classified in a number of ways.
  - Classification based on duration of symptoms:
    - Acute: persistent nasal and sinus symptoms for 10 to 30 days; worsening or new onset of nasal discharge, daytime cough, or fever after initial improvement; or concurrent high fever and purulent nasal discharge for the first 3 to 4 days of an acute upper respiratory infection (URI)
    - Subacute: clinical symptoms for 30 to 90 days
    - Chronic: symptoms lasting >90 days
    - Recurrent: acute sinusitis with 10 days of complete resolution between episodes; three episodes in 6 months or four in 1 year
  - Classification by severity of illness:
    - Persistent acute: >10 to 14 days but <30 days; nasal discharge and/or daytime cough
    - Severe acute: temperature of ≥39°C (102.2°F) with concurrent purulent nasal discharge for ≥3 days and/or facial pain, headache, or periorbital edema

GENERAL PREVENTION

- Avoid allergen exposure and treat allergies if present.
- Improve mucociliary clearance by increasing ambient humidity with a humidifier.

PATHOPHYSIOLOGY

- Normal sinus function depends on patency of paranasal sinus ostia, function of the ciliary apparatus, and secretion quality.
- Secretions accumulate due to ostial obstruction, reduction in ciliary function, and overproduction.
- Viral URIs and/or allergic rhinitis often precede(s) acute bacterial sinusitis.
- Acute bacterial sinusitis is a complication of 5–10% of URIs.

ETIOLOGY

- Viral pathogens (e.g., rhinovirus, parainfluenza virus) are often recovered in respiratory isolates.
- Most illnesses of short duration (<7 days) are thought to be due to viral infection and therefore should not be treated with antibiotics.
- Chronic sinusitis is often secondary to allergic rhinitis, cystic fibrosis, environmental pollutants, or gastroesophageal reflux.
- Most common bacterial pathogens:
  - *Haemophilus influenzae*, nontypeable (with *Streptococcus pneumoniae*, make up 30% of cases)
  - *S. pneumoniae*
  - *Moraxella catarrhalis* (10% of cases)
- Other bacterial pathogens:
  - Group A streptococci
  - Group C streptococci
  - Peptostreptococci
  - Other *Moraxella* species
  - *Streptococcus viridans*
  - *Eikenella corrodens*
  - *Staphylococcus aureus* (infrequent but significant pathogen in orbital and intracranial complications)
  - *Pseudomonas aeruginosa* (in patients with cystic fibrosis)
  - Anaerobic organisms
- Polymicrobial
- Fungal pathogen: *Aspergillus*

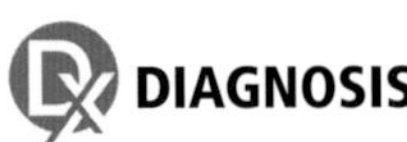

DIAGNOSIS

HISTORY

- Previous sinusitis, previous antibiotic use, allergies, child care attendance
- Key symptoms to differentiate from viral URI:
  - Duration of symptoms >10 days or worsening of symptoms after initial improvement
  - Onset of fever, especially with a duration of ≥3 to 4 days, facial pain, purulent discharge at onset
- Some or all of the following may be present:
  - Nasal discharge: consistency, color. In older patients, nasal discharge may not be the primary complaint, but concurrent rhinitis is a common feature.
  - Postnasal drainage, nasal congestion
  - Fever
  - Recent history of a URI
  - Sore throat from mouth breathing due to nasal obstruction
  - Cough present during the day; may be worse at night
  - Malodorous breath
  - Hyposmia/anosmia
  - Maxillary dental pain
  - Facial swelling
  - Ear pressure or fullness
  - Headache and facial pain are uncommon in young children with sinusitis but may be seen in older children and adolescents.
  - Fatigue
  - Irritability
  - Snoring
  - Hyponasal speech

PHYSICAL EXAM

- Fever may be present.
- Nasal-sounding voice may be present.
- Malodorous breath may be noted but is not a specific indicator of sinusitis.
- Purulent drainage in the nose and/or oropharynx may be appreciated.
- Nasal mucosa may be erythematous, pale, and/or boggy, but these are nonspecific findings.
- Frontal, maxillary, and ethmoid areas may be tender to palpation/percussion.
- Headache and/or facial pain may change with position, increasing in intensity as the patient leans forward.
- Sinus transillumination and percussion are not reliable aids in diagnosis.
- Proptosis, eye swelling, and impaired extraocular movements suggest orbital infection.

DIFFERENTIAL DIAGNOSIS

- Infection: viral URI with or without mucopurulent rhinitis
- Environmental: allergic rhinitis
- Drug-induced: rhinitis medicamentosa
- Tumors
  - Nasal polyps
  - Hypertrophied adenoids
  - Neoplasms
- Trauma: foreign body (e.g., bead, cotton, tissue paper)
- Congenital
  - Septal deviation
  - Unilateral choanal atresia
  - Dysmotile cilia syndrome
- Dental disorder
- Other: vasomotor rhinitis

DIAGNOSTIC TESTS & INTERPRETATION

- Gold standard is culture from sinuses via direct aspiration/endoscopy; not indicated for diagnosis of acute, uncomplicated sinusitis
- For chronic or recurrent sinusitis, consider
  - Sweat chloride test to rule out cystic fibrosis
  - Immunoglobulin levels, IgG subclass levels, complement levels, and testing for HIV infection
  - Mucosal biopsy to assess ciliary function
- Imaging is not recommended in uncomplicated cases of sinusitis.
- Sinus radiographs
  - Of limited value with the exception of the Waters (occipitomental) view for identifying maxillary sinusitis
  - Plain radiographs do not adequately identify ethmoid sinusitis.
  - Findings suggestive of sinusitis include complete sinus opacification, mucosal thickening ≥4 mm, and air–fluid levels.
- CT scan with contrast of the paranasal sinuses:
  - Useful in complicated, recurrent, and chronic sinusitis and/or history of polyposis
- CT scan of the head with contrast:
  - Indicated when sinusitis is accompanied by signs of increased intracranial pressure, meningeal irritation, proptosis, toxic appearance, limited extraocular movements, or focal neurologic deficits or in patients being considered for sinus-related surgery
- MRI of the sinuses:
  - Reserve for complicated cases and in immunocompromised patients in which fungal infection is suspected; will show mucosal thickening and fluid
- MRI with contrast of the head
  - An alternative or adjunct to CT with contrast, when intracranial complications are suspected
- Pitfalls
  - Sinus radiographs may be abnormal in asymptomatic children or those with mild URIs.
  - Studies have shown a relatively high incidence of sinus abnormalities on CT scan in asymptomatic children, especially in infants <12 months of age.
  - Up to 1/3 of patients with symptoms of chronic sinusitis may have normal CT scans.

TREATMENT

GENERAL MEASURES

- Current guidelines support the option of observing children with persistent symptoms, but not those with worsening or severe symptoms, for 3 days before treating with antibiotic therapy.
- If orbital or central nervous system (CNS) infection is suspected by history and examination, antibiotics should be started immediately, and emergency CT studies should be performed.
- Pitfalls
  - Sinusitis is diagnosed with increasing frequency and may result in overuse of antibiotics, given that up to 50% will have spontaneous resolution.

MEDICATION

- Antibiotics
  - Appropriate drug choice depends on local resistance patterns.
  - High-risk children include age <2 years, hospitalization, antibiotic use within 3 months of diagnosis, and child care attendance.
  - 1st-line treatment: amoxicillin 45 mg/kg/24 h or 80 to 90 mg/kg/24 h of amoxicillin if high risk, local pneumococcal resistance >10%, severe symptoms or comorbidity, divided twice daily with a maximum of 2 g/dose
  - For non–type I penicillin allergy (late or delayed, >72 hours) or type I allergy (anaphylaxis) in children age ≥2 years, cefdinir (14 mg/kg/24 h), cefpodoxime (10 mg/kg/24 h), or cefuroxime axetil (30 mg/kg/24 h divided twice daily) may be used.
  - Amoxicillin with clavulanate, with dosing based on the amoxicillin component (see above) considered 1st-line therapy by some experts
  - Ceftriaxone 50 mg/kg IV or IM as a single dose may be used for children unable to tolerate oral medicine or who are vomiting.
  - For type I penicillin allergy in children age <2 years, consider clindamycin combined with cefixime to cover resistant bacteria.
  - Macrolides and trimethoprim-sulfamethoxazole are not recommended due to high resistance rates.
  - Duration of treatment should be for 10 (minimum) to 28 days (and until 7 days beyond symptom resolution).
  - Consider changing antibiotic coverage and/or obtaining a culture if symptoms do not improve after 3 to 5 days of antibiotics, especially in a hospitalized patient.
  - Complicated sinusitis (CNS or orbital involvement) or children with toxic appearance: IV antibiotics and hospitalization; ceftriaxone (100 mg/kg/24 h in 2 doses) or ampicillin-sulbactam (200 to 400 mg ampicillin component/kg/24 h in 4 divided doses); cefotaxime 150 to 225 mg/kg/24 h divided every 6 hours or, if no other alternative, levofloxacin 10 to 20 mg/kg/24 h divided every 12 to 24 hours
  - If a hospitalized, ill child is not improving on the IV antibiotics listed above, consider adding vancomycin (60 mg/kg/24 h divided into 4 doses) for penicillin-resistant *S. pneumoniae* +/− metronidazole (30 mg/kg/24 h divided into 4 doses) for anaerobic coverage.
  - Chronic sinusitis: Consider broad-spectrum antibiotic (amoxicillin/clavulanate [80 to 90 mg/kg/24 h of amoxicillin divided in 2 doses]) for at least 3 weeks and use of adjuvants such as saline irrigation or intranasal steroids; consider culture if no resolution after 1 week of treatment.
- Other pharmaceuticals:
  - Decongestants and antihistamines are not recommended due to side effects and lack of evidence of clinical improvement with use.
  - Mucolytics, such as guaifenesin, may improve mucous clearance.
  - Topical nasal steroids: Some studies show modest reductions in symptoms in acute bacterial sinusitis. Nasal steroids may reduce and prevent mucosal swelling, which can lead to ostial occlusion, in patients with allergic rhinitis.
- Other treatments:
  - Humidifier: may improve mucociliary clearance
  - Normal saline: Although there is no evidence to support its efficacy in acute sinusitis, saline irrigation and or spray is used by some for symptom relief; increases humidity and enhances mucociliary transport; vasoconstricts and improves drainage and ventilation

SURGERY/OTHER PROCEDURES

- Maxillary sinus aspiration: if unresponsive to multiple antibiotics, severe facial pain, and orbital or intracranial complications; should be performed by a trained ear, nose, and throat (ENT) specialist
- Surgery: performed as a last resort after medical therapy attempted and in patients with orbital or CNS complications

ONGOING CARE

FOLLOW-UP RECOMMENDATIONS

Patient Monitoring

- Immediate referral to appropriate specialists—including pediatric neurology, ophthalmology, and otolaryngology—is indicated if there are CNS symptoms, periorbital edema, visual changes, facial swelling, extraocular muscle involvement, or proptosis.
- Radiographic soft tissue changes may last for up to 8 weeks; therefore, reimaging is of limited value.
- Referral to an ENT specialist when sinusitis is chronic and not responsive to medical therapy, recurrent, complicated, or when there is polyposis

PROGNOSIS

- Spontaneous resolution in up to 50% of patients
- Usually improves within 72 hours of initiation of antibiotics
- Excellent for those who are otherwise healthy

COMPLICATIONS

- Periorbital cellulitis
- Orbital cellulitis
- Orbital abscess
- Meningitis
- Intracranial—epidural, subdural, and brain—abscess(es) (in general, infectious intracranial complications seen more commonly in previously healthy adolescent males)
- Optic neuritis
- Cavernous or sagittal sinus thrombosis
- Osteomyelitis of the maxilla
- Osteomyelitis of the frontal bone (Pott puffy tumor)
- Subperiosteal abscess

ADDITIONAL READING

- Brook I. Acute sinusitis in children. *Pediatr Clin North Am*. 2013;60(2):409–424.
- Chow AW, Benninger MS, Brook I, et al; for Infectious Diseases Society of America. IDSA Clinical practice guideline for acute bacterial rhinosinusitis in children and adults. *Clin Infect Dis*. 2012;54(8):e72–e112.
- DeMuri GP, Wald ER. Clinical practice. Acute bacterial sinusitis in children. *N Engl J Med*. 2012;367(12): 1128–1134.
- Leo G, Triulzi F, Incorvaia C. Diagnosis of chronic rhinosinusitis. *Pediatr Allergy Immunol*. 2012; 23(Suppl 22):20–26.
- Rosenfeld EA, Rowley AH. Infectious intracranial complications of sinusitis, other than meningitis, in children: 12-year review. *Clin Infect Dis*. 1994;18(5):750–754.
- Setzen G, Ferguson BJ, Han JK, et al. Clinical consensus statement: appropriate use of computed tomography for paranasal sinus disease. *Otolaryngol Head Neck Surg*. 2012;147(5):808–816.
- Wald ER, Applegate KE, Bordley C, et al. Clinical practice guideline for the diagnosis and management of acute bacterial sinusitis in children aged 1 to 18 years. *Pediatrics*. 2013;132(1):e262–e280.

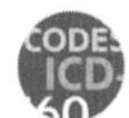

CODES

ICD10

- J32.9 Chronic sinusitis, unspecified
- J01.90 Acute sinusitis, unspecified
- J01.10 Acute frontal sinusitis, unspecified

FAQ

- Q: Are all of the sinuses present at birth?
- A: No. The maxillary and ethmoid sinuses form during the third and fourth gestational months and are present at birth. They continue to enlarge until the preteen years. The sphenoid sinuses are pneumatized by 5 years; isolated sphenoid sinusitis is rare. The frontal sinuses are present at age 7 to 8 years and are not completely developed until late adolescence.
- Q: Does the nasal discharge seen with sinusitis have to be purulent and thick?
- A: No. Although the nasal discharge is often described as purulent and thick, it may also be clear or mucoid, or thick or thin. Multiple studies have shown that a change in color or consistency is not a specific sign of a bacterial infection.
- Q: Are radiographic studies useful in the diagnosis of sinusitis?
- A: There is evidence to suggest that plain radiographs (x-rays) have limited value in the diagnosis of sinusitis and are not recommended in cases of uncomplicated sinusitis. Mucosal thickening may be seen with viral URIs and allergic rhinitis. Studies have shown that x-rays do not correlate well with CT scans in the diagnosis of chronic sinusitis.
- Q: Can one make the diagnosis of sinusitis based on CT scan results alone?
- A: No. Up to 50% of patients who had CT scans performed for other reasons had soft tissue changes in their sinuses. Mucosal thickening and opacification on CT imaging have been seen in large numbers of asymptomatic patients. These findings seem to occur more frequently in infants <12 months of age. Given the poor specificity of CT imaging of the paranasal sinuses, results must be used in the context of the patient's clinical presentation.

S

SLEEP APNEA–OBSTRUCTIVE SLEEP APNEA SYNDROME

Akinyemi Ajayi, MBBS, FAAP, FCCP, FAASM

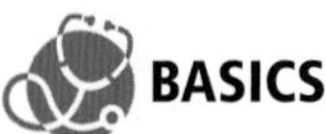

BASICS

DESCRIPTION

- Sleep-disordered breathing encompasses a range of breathing disorders occurring during sleep. These conditions include primary snoring (PS), respiratory events related to arousals (RERA), and obstructive sleep apnea syndrome (OSAS).
- Obstructive apnea is defined as the cessation of airflow at the nose and mouth despite respiratory effort, associated with some gas exchange abnormality and/or loss of regular sleep patterns.

EPIDEMIOLOGY

- 8–10% of children snore.
- 1.3–4% of children have sleep apnea.
- 30% of children with Down syndrome have some degree of sleep apnea by the age of 3 years.

PHYSIOLOGY

- OSAS may be subdivided into mild, moderate, and severe forms.
- Many children with OSAS exhibit partial airway obstruction. This is known as obstructive hypoventilation or hypopnea and is more commonly seen in children than is complete obstruction.
- OSAS is distinct from central apnea (cessation of airflow that is not accompanied by respiratory effort), which indicates brain immaturity or dysfunction.
- Upper airway resistance syndrome is a respiratory disorder characterized by partial airway obstruction and arousals leading to sleep fragmentation and is not associated with gas exchange abnormalities.
- Central apnea up to 20 seconds may be a normal finding in premature or newborn infants during the 1st month of life.
- Periodic breathing: three or more episodes of central apnea lasting at least 3 seconds each, separated by <20 seconds. Periodic breathing may be found in the newborn; however, it should not exceed >4% of sleep time (from a sleep study) and is not associated with bradycardia or hypoxemia.

RISK FACTORS

- In infants, OSAS is uncommon; however, it may exist with craniofacial anomalies, neurologic disorders associated with low muscle tone, laryngomalacia or tracheomalacia, and gastroesophageal reflux.
- Impaired arousal mechanisms also contribute to abnormalities seen in OSAS.
- In older children, OSAS may be associated with obesity. This form may resemble the adult type of OSAS.
- PS or habitual snoring implies snoring that does not lead to abnormalities in gas exchange or sleep fragmentation; however, 20–50% of children with habitual snoring may have OSAS.

Genetics

Several genetic disorders with associated craniofacial anomalies, hypotonia, and obesity may lead to OSAS. These include the following:

- Pierre Robin syndrome
- Treacher Collins syndrome
- Down syndrome
- Mucopolysaccharide disorders
- Arnold-Chiari malformations
- Prader-Willi syndrome
- Hereditary neuromuscular disorders

COMMONLY ASSOCIATED CONDITIONS

- Adenotonsillar hypertrophy
- Craniofacial anomalies including midfacial hypoplasia and mandibular hypoplasia
- Laryngomalacia
- Neurologic and neuromuscular disorders that cause hypotonia may underlie poor ventilation during sleep.
- Gastroesophageal reflux
- Obesity
- Metabolic disorders
- Allergic rhinitis, nasal septum deviation, nasal polyps
- Sedatives, seizure medications, and anesthesia

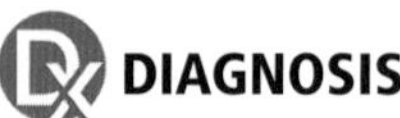

DIAGNOSIS

HISTORY

- Nocturnal symptoms:
  - Difficulty breathing when asleep, snoring, apnea, and restless sleep with frequent arousals
- Daytime symptoms:
  - Excessive sleepiness, frequent upper respiratory/ear infections, conductive hearing loss, mouth breathing, poor appetite, and a hyponasal voice
- Other concerns: attention deficit hyperactivity disorder (ADHD), gastroesophageal reflux, poor school performance, and headaches (especially in the morning and upon awakening)
  - OSAS rarely produces these symptoms acutely but tends to occur over weeks to months.
  - Parents may notice that symptoms worsen with upper respiratory infections.
- The possibility of sleep-disordered breathing or a primary sleep disorder should be considered in children evaluated for ADHD.

PHYSICAL EXAM

- Assessment of the child's growth. In severe cases of OSAS, failure to thrive has been reported.
- Obesity remains a risk factor, especially in older children.
- Assessment of tonsillar size

ALERT

Normal-sized tonsils do not exclude OSAS.

- Presence of mouth breathing, hyponasal speech, adenoidal facies, midfacial hypoplasia, retrognathia, micrognathia, or other craniofacial anomalies may be present at times and may suggest the diagnosis.
- Nasal obstruction due to polyps, nasal septum deviation, turbinate hypertrophy, or congestion
- Tongue size
- Mobility and elevation of the soft palate; hard palate integrity
- In extreme cases, cardiac involvement may lead to cor pulmonale and heart failure. Examination may suggest signs of pulmonary hypertension or congestive heart failure, such as an increased second heart sound.
- A neurologic examination to evaluate general muscle strength, tone, and developmental status, especially in infants and children who do not improve after adenotonsillectomy

DIFFERENTIAL DIAGNOSIS

- PS or habitual snoring
- Upper airway resistance syndrome: This condition is associated with sleep fragmentation and daytime sleepiness.
- Obesity–hypoventilation syndrome: a variant of OSAS
- Central apnea and periodic breathing
- Congenital central hypoventilation syndrome
- Other causes of excessive daytime sleepiness include the following:
  - Disorganized home environment, emotional stress
  - Substance abuse/drug intoxication: psychotropic medications, antihistamines, anticonvulsants, narcotics
  - Narcolepsy: onset typically around adolescence, but cataplexy may occur later and delay the diagnosis
  - Epilepsy: absence spells of unresponsiveness, electroencephalogram changes
- Causes of obstructive apnea include:
  - Any cause of lymphoidal hypertrophy in the upper airway (allergies, viral/bacterial tonsillitis, neoplasm, epiglottitis, retropharyngeal abscess), chronic phenytoin exposure, and excessive storage material in upper airway submucosa
- Causes of abnormal laxity of upper airway soft tissues:
  - Down syndrome, acute polyneuropathy (Guillain-Barré syndrome), chronic neuromuscular disease, Prader-Willi syndrome, myasthenia gravis
- Causes of abnormal control/coordination of upper airway musculature:
  - Almost any cause of diffuse central nervous system (CNS) dysfunction, including cerebral palsy and acquired lesions of the CNS such as stroke and head trauma
- Causes of central apnea:
  - Beyond infancy, most commonly due to drugs that suppress ventilatory drive
  - In premature infants, may be due to nonspecific immaturity of neural ventilatory control mechanism
  - Sepsis, seizures, brainstem compression, brain tumors, Arnold-Chiari type 2 (although increasingly seen with type 1)
- Gastroesophageal reflux may potentiate central apnea and should be investigated.
- Androgen steroids may cause central apnea in adults.

DIAGNOSTIC TESTS & INTERPRETATION

Initial Tests (screening, lab, imaging)

- Polysomnography
  - The gold standard for the diagnosis of OSAS is nocturnal polysomnography to differentiate the type of sleep apnea and to assess severity.
  - Polysomnography is an 8- to 10-hour-long multichannel study performed in a controlled setting to assess respiratory and/or sleep abnormalities.
  - Indices such as oxygenation, ventilation, apnea index (AI), apnea–hypopnea index (AHI), arousal index, arousal awakening index, and periodic limb movements index are determined along with sleep efficiency and sleep stages.
  - Monitoring includes electroencephalogram, electrooculogram, electromyogram, arterial oxygen saturation, end tidal CO_2 tension, airflow, respiratory effort, and electrocardiogram.

- Normative respiratory and sleep variables for children have recently been published and include an AHI of <1 being normal.
- Scoring for pediatric polysomnography differs from that of adults. This includes using two respiratory cycles to define both obstructive apnea and central apnea or two respiratory cycles associated with a 30% decline in airflow and a >4% decline in oxygen level to define hypopnea. Lower AHI values are considered significant in children compared with adults.

- Other studies
  - Validated questionnaires are helpful to screen for OSAS in the office.
  - Routine blood work is generally noncontributory; in severe forms, polycythemia, hypercarbia, and elevated bicarbonate may be noted.
  - Evaluation for gastroesophageal reflux may include pH monitoring during sleep, barium swallow, or radionuclide studies (milk scan).
  - Home testing is not approved for use in children with suspected OSAS, although there are now several articles looking into its use in pediatric patients with high predicted risk of OSAS.
- Lateral neck radiograph is easy to perform to assess adenoid and tonsillar size as well as patency of the nasopharyngeal airway.
- Nocturnal audio- and videotaping, as well as abbreviated nap polysomnography, are useful studies if the results are positive but generally have a poor negative predictive value.
- Upper airway endoscopy as well as bronchoscopy may be performed to evaluate anatomic or dynamic causes for airway obstruction (pharyngeal hypotonia, pharyngeal stenosis, laryngotracheomalacia, vocal cord polyps, papilloma).
- Head or neck computed tomography or magnetic resonance imaging (MRI) should be considered for complex craniofacial anomalies. If central apnea is noted, then MRI studies should also evaluate the brainstem to evaluate for an Arnold-Chiari malformation.
- In severe cases of OSAS, a cardiac evaluation, including electrocardiogram, chest x-ray, and echocardiogram, may be indicated.

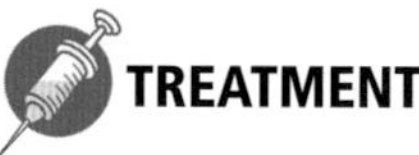

TREATMENT

GENERAL MEASURES

- In most cases, adenotonsillectomy is 1st-line therapy. However, some patients continue to have significant postoperative OSAS that requires further evaluation.
- Noninvasive ventilatory support with continuous positive airway pressure/bilevel positive airway pressure (CPAP/BiPAP) may be helpful.
- Intranasal steroids and leukotriene modifiers have been shown to have a positive effect in children with mild sleep apnea. Duration of use and long-term outcomes remain unclear.
- In complicated cases, when craniofacial malformations are involved, surgical procedures such as tongue reduction, uvulopalatopharyngoplasty, or mandibular or maxillary advancement may be indicated.
- When there is evidence of gastroesophageal reflux, treatment with acid suppression agents and chalasia precautions are indicated.
- Weight loss may be useful in obese children.
- Laser surgery and dental appliances may be useful in adults with mild OSAS, but there is no experience with these approaches in children.
- In extreme cases, a tracheostomy may be indicated, especially when significant craniofacial abnormalities exist.

ALERT

Treatment of gastroesophageal reflux in infants with obstructive apnea may be helpful even in the absence of obvious symptoms of reflux.

ADMISSION, INPATIENT, AND NURSING CONSIDERATIONS

Initial stabilization

- Severe cases may require urgent intervention.
- Severe cases of upper airway obstruction are usually diagnosed during polysomnography or during procedures involving sedation or anesthesia.
  - Ensure adequate ventilation and oxygenation, with quick assessment of the cause.
  - Temporary relief of the obstruction should be undertaken by an experienced team.
  - Transfer to an intensive care unit where the airway can be monitored carefully.
  - Following relief of airway obstruction, pulmonary and airway edema, as well as copious secretion production, may develop.
  - Modalities of care should include placement of a nasopharyngeal airway, noninvasive ventilation with CPAP/BiPAP, or placement of an endotracheal tube for mechanical ventilation.
- Risk factors for postoperative complications in children with OSAS include:
  - Age <3 years
  - Severe OSAS
  - Pulmonary hypertension
  - Obesity
  - Prematurity
  - Failure to thrive
  - Craniofacial or neuromuscular disorders
  - Upper respiratory tract infection

ONGOING CARE

COMPLICATIONS

Complications are due to chronic hypoxemia, hypercarbia, acidosis, as well as impaired sleep and include the following:

- Pulmonary hypertension, later cor pulmonale (rare)
- Systemic hypertension has been reported in adults and a few pediatric cases.
- Congestive heart failure: Arrhythmias are common in adults with underlying coronary artery disease.
- Neurodevelopmental complications: daytime somnolence, poor school performance, hyperactivity, and social withdrawal
- Poor growth and failure to thrive
- Postanesthesia respiratory failure and death have been reported in children with OSAS.

FOLLOW-UP RECOMMENDATIONS

- Clinical improvement is expected soon after adenotonsillectomy. In children <1 year of age with severe forms of OSAS, underlying craniofacial anomalies, or neurologic disorders, repeat overnight polysomnography is indicated 6 to 8 weeks after surgery.
- Regrowth of adenoid tissue may occur months to years after adenoidectomy. Therefore, if clinical symptoms, such as snoring, difficulty breathing while asleep, or a decline in school performance recur, a reevaluation is indicated.

ADDITIONAL READING

- American Academy of Sleep Medicine. *The International Classification of Sleep Disorders: Diagnostic & Coding Manual*. 2nd ed. Westchester, IL: American Academy of Sleep Medicine; 2005.
- American Sleep Apnea Association: http://www.sleepapnea.org
- Baker M, Scott B, Johnson RF, et al. Predictors of obstructive sleep apnea severity in adolescents. *JAMA Otolaryngol Head Neck Surg*. 2017;143(5):494–499.
- D'Andrea LA. Diagnostic studies in the assessment of pediatric sleep-disordered breathing: techniques and indications. *Pediatr Clin North Am*. 2004;51(1):169–186.
- Li Z, Celestin J, Lockey RF. Pediatric sleep apnea syndrome: an update. *J Allergy Clin Immunol Pract*. 2016;4(5):852–861.
- Marcus CL, Brooks LJ, Draper KA, et al; for American Academy of Pediatrics. Diagnosis and management of childhood obstructive sleep apnea syndrome. *Pediatrics*. 2012;130(3):e714–e755.
- Pandit C, Fitzgerald DA. Respiratory problems in children with Down syndrome. *J Paediatr Child Health*. 2012;48(3):E147–E152.
- Rosen CL. Obstructive sleep apnea syndrome in children: controversies in diagnosis and treatment. *Pediatr Clin North Am*. 2004;51(1):153–167.
- Tapia IE, Marcus CL, McDonough JM, et al. Airway resistance in children with obstructive sleep apnea syndrome. *Sleep*. 2016;39(4):793–799.
- Witmans M, Young R. Update on pediatric sleep-disordered breathing. *Pediatr Clin North Am*. 2011;58(3):571–589.

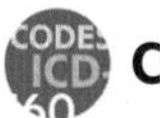

CODES

ICD10

- G47.30 Sleep apnea, unspecified
- G47.33 Obstructive sleep apnea (adult) (pediatric)
- G47.36 Sleep related hypoventilation in conditions classd elswhr

FAQ

- Q: Can my child still have OSAS after adenotonsillectomy?
- A: Yes. At times, the adenoid tissue can grow back again. In addition, some cases of OSAS are related to a small upper airway that is restricted by anatomic or neurologic conditions. In these cases, adenotonsillectomy will not always resolve OSAS.
- Q: Does OSAS cause neurologic problems?
- A: Several studies suggest neurocognitive deficits in children with OSAS. The most common findings include reduced school performance and ADHD.

SLIPPED CAPITAL FEMORAL EPIPHYSIS

Craig J. Finlayson, MD

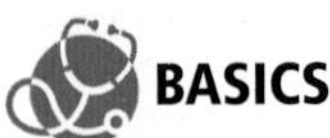

BASICS

DESCRIPTION

Slipped capital femoral epiphysis (SCFE) is displacement of the femoral head (epiphysis) relative to the femoral neck (metaphysis).

EPIDEMIOLOGY

- Most common adolescent hip disorder
- Male > female (3:2)
- Up to 25% bilateral at presentation
- 20–40% have contralateral involvement at some point.

Incidence

- 2 to 7 per 100,000
- Age of onset: males 13 to 15 years; females 11 to 13 years

RISK FACTORS

Genetics

No clear genetic predisposition to SCFE

PATHOPHYSIOLOGY

- Stress across the proximal femoral physis results in slippage of the femoral neck relative to the head.
- Weakening of the perichondrial ring and physis have been implicated.
- The femoral head maintains its position within the acetabulum, whereas the femoral neck displaces anteriorly and more commonly superolaterally (varus).
- In some cases, the neck displaces inferomedially (valgus).

ETIOLOGY

- Stress on the proximal femoral physis from increased body weight, femoral retroversion, or inclination of the physis
- Abnormal bone metabolism secondary to endocrinopathy or renal disorders
- Toxicity to the physis from prior radiation or chemotherapy

COMMONLY ASSOCIATED CONDITIONS

- Obesity
- Endocrine dysfunction
  - Hypothyroidism
  - Hypopituitarism
  - Hyperparathyroidism
- Growth hormone replacement therapy
- Pelvic radiotherapy
- Renal osteodystrophy

DIAGNOSIS

HISTORY

- Pain in the affected hip, thigh, or knee
- Limp

ALERT

Hip pain may be absent. Referred pain to the thigh or knee and/or limp may be the only presenting symptoms.

- Occasional history of trauma, although the level of trauma does not usually explain the slip
- Temporal classification
  - Chronic: most common, onset of symptoms >3 weeks
  - Acute: sudden onset of symptoms <3 weeks
  - Acute-on-chronic: acute exacerbation of symptoms that have been present for >3 weeks; may occur in setting of trauma to previously symptomatic hip
- Stability-based classification (Loder)
  - Stable: able to ambulate, even with an assistive device such as crutches
  - Unstable: unable to ambulate; most common with acute and acute-on-chronic patterns
  - Acute, unstable slips carry the highest risk of complications.

PHYSICAL EXAM

- Limp: antalgic gait with external foot progression
- Hip range of motion:
  - Painful and limited
- Decreased flexion, internal rotation, and abduction due to proximal femoral deformity
- Obligate external rotation: Hip externally rotates spontaneously with passive hip flexion.
- Trendelenburg sign
- In patients presenting with knee pain, the knee examination is unremarkable, although thigh/knee pain may be reproduced with provocative testing of the hip.

DIFFERENTIAL DIAGNOSIS

- Avascular necrosis of the hip
- Legg-Calve-Perthes disease
- Acute physeal or femoral neck fracture
- Septic arthritis
- Transient synovitis
- Inflammatory arthritis

DIAGNOSTIC TESTS & INTERPRETATION

Initial Tests (screening, lab, imaging)

- Diagnosis is made primarily by plain radiographs.
  - Anteroposterior (AP) and frog-leg lateral (cross-table lateral if unable to position due to pain)
  - Include both hips to evaluate for contralateral slip and to serve as an internal control.
- Klein line:
  - Line along superior aspect of the femoral neck intersects the femoral head on AP radiograph of the normal hip.
  - Failure to intersect femoral head indicates SCFE.
  - Valgus slips are the rare exception in which Klein line remains intact.
- Lateral view is most sensitive for early slips: anterior displacement of the neck relative to the head (true for both varus and valgus slips)
- Slip angle: angle between line perpendicular to femoral physis and line parallel to femoral shaft. Measure difference between affected and contralateral hip. For cases of bilateral slip, 12 degrees can be used as normal value.
- Severity classified based on slip angle
  - Mild: slip angle <30
  - Moderate: slip angle 30 to 50
  - Severe: slip angle >50
- Blanch sign: radiodense area in proximal femoral neck due to overlapping density of femoral head
- Epiphyseal plate may appear widened or irregular.

Follow-Up Tests & Special Considerations

ALERT

Patients with "atypical" presentations should be evaluated for associated conditions such as endocrinopathy or renal dysfunction with appropriate lab studies.

- Age <10 years or >16 years
- Weight <50th percentile for age
- Height <10th percentile for age
- Pathologic findings
  - Histologic findings include widening of the physis, disorganization and slippage through the hypertrophic zone of the physis, and callus formation along the anterior and superior neck.

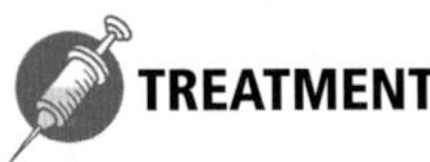

TREATMENT

GENERAL MEASURES

- Prompt surgical consultation to minimize the risk of progressive slippage and associated complications
- Protected weight bearing with crutches or bed rest pending surgical consultation

MEDICATION
Appropriate analgesia for symptoms of hip pain

ISSUES FOR REFERRAL
- Appropriate consultation for evaluation and perioperative management of any associated endocrinopathy or renal dysfunction
- Consider consultation for weight optimization.

SURGERY/OTHER PROCEDURES
- Acute, unstable SCFE should be treated urgently.
- Due to the risk of progressive slip, surgical treatment of stable SCFE should be done with minimal delay.
- The primary goal of initial surgery is to stabilize the physis and prevent further slippage.
- In situ pinning of the affected hip remains the gold standard.
- Aggressive closed manipulation is not recommended for unstable slips as this may increase the risk of avascular necrosis.
- Osteotomy through the physis with debridement of anterior-superior callus; realignment of the femoral head and internal fixation (Dunn osteotomy) is an option for acute, unstable slips, but long-term results are not yet available.
- Prophylactic pinning of the contralateral hip should be considered in patients at increased risk for contralateral slips.
  - Young patients
  - Patients with endocrinopathy, renal dysfunction, or other associated conditions
  - Patients with limited access to follow-up care
- Secondary surgery to address persistent deformity may be indicated based on the degree of deformity and clinical symptoms.
  - Open or arthroscopic osteoplasty of the femoral neck
  - Osteotomy through the femoral neck or intertrochanteric region

ADMISSION, INPATIENT, AND NURSING CONSIDERATIONS
- Consider direct admission or transfer to the emergency department upon diagnosis.
- Acute, unstable slips should be treated urgently.

ONGOING CARE

FOLLOW-UP RECOMMENDATIONS
Patient Monitoring
Patients should be followed radiographically until physeal closure to ensure appropriate healing and to evaluate for contralateral slip.

DIET
Patients with obesity should be evaluated for weight optimization with appropriate diet and exercise.

PATIENT EDUCATION
- Patients should be educated about the early signs and symptoms of contralateral slip to enable prompt treatment.
- Patients should be educated about postoperative activity restrictions to reduce the risk of short-term complications.

PROGNOSIS
- Prognosis depends on stability and severity of slip.
- Acute, unstable SCFE has a much higher risk of complications.
- Satisfactory short-term outcomes associated with in situ fixation of chronic SCFE but may deteriorate over time, especially with greater deformity
- Moderate and severe slips are at high risk for femoroacetabular impingement and degenerative arthritis.

COMPLICATIONS
- Avascular necrosis of the femoral head
  - Up to 25% in unstable slips
  - Due to disruption of epiphyseal blood vessels from acute slip, surgical manipulation, hardware insertion
  - Rare in stable slips
  - Radiographs reveal increased lucency, irregularity, and ultimately collapse of the epiphysis.
- Chondrolysis (acute cartilage necrosis)
  - Etiology unclear, has been associated with hardware penetration into joint
  - Radiographs show joint space narrowing.
- Progressive slip
  - Suboptimal hardware size or placement
  - Rapid growth
  - May require revision pinning or open epiphysiodesis
- Femoroacetabular impingement
  - Residual deformity of the head-neck junction limits hip motion and may cause injury to the acetabular labrum and cartilage with repetitive abutment.

ADDITIONAL READING

- Bittersohl B, Hosalkar HS, Zilkens C, et al. Current concepts in management of slipped capital femoral epiphysis. *Hip Int*. 2015;25(2):104–114.
- Georgiadis AG, Zaltz I. Slipped capital femoral epiphysis: how to evaluate with a review and update of treatment. *Pediatr Clin North Am*. 2014;61(6):1119–1135.
- Larson AN, Sierra RJ, Yu EM, et al. Outcomes of slipped capital femoral epiphysis treated with in situ pinning. *J Pediatr Orthop*. 2012;32(2):125–130.
- Lehmann CL, Arons RR, Loder RT, et al. The epidemiology of slipped capital femoral epiphysis: an update. *J Pediatr Orthop*. 2006;26(3):286–290.
- Loder RT. Controversies in slipped capital femoral epiphysis. *Orthop Clin North Am*. 2006;37(2): 211–221, vii.
- Millis MB, Lewis CL, Schoenecker PL, et al. Legg-Calvé-Perthes disease and slipped capital femoral epiphysis: major developmental causes of femoroacetabular impingement. *J Am Acad Orthop Surg*. 2013;21(Suppl 1):S59–S63.
- Shank CF, Thiel EJ, Klingele KE. Valgus slipped capital femoral epiphysis: prevalence, presentation, and treatment options. *J Pediatr Orthop*. 2010;30(2):140–146.
- Tosounidis T, Stengel D, Kontakis G, et al. Prognostic significance of stability in slipped upper femoral epiphysis: a systematic review and meta-analysis. *J Pediatr*. 2010;157(4):674–680.

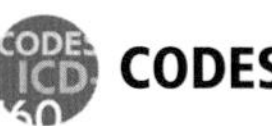

CODES

ICD10
- M93.003 Unspecified slipped upper femoral epiphysis (nontraumatic), unspecified hip
- M93.023 Chronic slipped upper femoral epiphysis (nontraumatic), unspecified hip
- M93.033 Acute on chronic slipped upper femoral epiphysis (nontraumatic), unspecified hip

FAQ
- Q: Is surgical treatment necessary for SCFE?
- A: Yes, without surgical stabilization of the physis, there may be progressive slippage and increasing deformity. A stable slip may also develop acute instability, which increases the risk of complications and poor outcome.
- Q: Does SCFE cause hip arthritis?
- A: SCFE causes deformity of the proximal femur that may result in hip impingement and, ultimately, degenerative arthritis. Prompt diagnosis and treatment of SCFE may help minimize deformity. Complications associated with the underlying disease process and its treatment may also lead to arthritis.
- Q: Should the contralateral hip be stabilized at the time of initial treatment?
- A: The answer varies based on the relative risk of contralateral slip for the patient. Younger patients and those with atypical slips are at higher risk and should be considered for prophylactic pinning. Patients with limited access to health care may also be considered.

SMALLPOX (VARIOLA VIRUS)

Eimear Kitt, MB, BCh, BAO (NUI) • Hamid Bassiri, MD, PhD

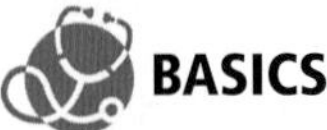

BASICS

DESCRIPTION

- Smallpox is a life-threatening, acute, eruptive, contagious disease caused by variola virus.
- The disease is characterized by a febrile prodrome followed by the development of rash.
- Rash evolves in a characteristic fashion: macules → papules → vesicles → pustules; scabs form and fall off, leaving scars called pockmarks.
- There are two clinical forms of smallpox:
  - Variola minor is a less common and less severe form of disease.
  - Variola major is the more common and serious form of disease, of which there are five types.
    - Ordinary smallpox
    - Modified smallpox
    - Flat smallpox
    - Hemorrhagic smallpox
    - Variola sine eruptione

EPIDEMIOLOGY

- The last documented case of endemic smallpox was in Somalia in 1977.
- The last case in the United States was in the late 1940s.
- Smallpox was declared eradicated by the World Health Organization in 1979.
- Historically, in unvaccinated individuals, ordinary smallpox accounted for 90% of cases, hemorrhagic smallpox for 7% of cases, and flat and modified smallpox for the remainder.
- Modified smallpox was rare in unvaccinated individuals but accounted for 25% of cases of disease in vaccinated individuals.

GENERAL PREVENTION

- Prior to 1972, all U.S. children were vaccinated.
- Vaccines were produced from the vaccinia virus, a closely related orthopoxvirus to variola.
- Historically, the vaccine was prepared from virus grown on the skin of animals, and in some cases, the vaccine was contaminated with animal proteins, bacteria, and other viruses.
- Newer smallpox vaccines are developed from vaccinia clones grown in tissue culture and therefore are free of contamination from bacteria and other viruses.
- Due to concern for use of smallpox as an agent of bioterrorism, the U.S. Strategic National Stockpile still stores smallpox vaccine.
- The only currently U.S. Food and Drug Administration (FDA)-licensed smallpox vaccine, ACAM2000 (which replaced Dryvax®), is used for active immunization of persons determined to be at highest risk for infection.
- The Advisory Committee on Immunization Practices (ACIP) recommends smallpox vaccination for the following:
  - Public health response teams responsible for investigating suspected smallpox cases
  - Hospital-based health care teams responsible for assessing and caring for suspected smallpox cases
  - Laboratory personnel who work with the virus that causes smallpox or other viruses similar to it
- Vaccine efficacy
  - 95% efficacious in preventing disease if given prior to exposure
  - May prevent smallpox or decrease severity if given 1 to 3 days after exposure
  - May decrease severity of disease if given 4 to 7 days after exposure
- Vaccination is estimated to provide protective immunity for 3 to 10 years but may decrease the severity of disease for 10 to 20 years.
- Vaccine administration
  - A skin abrasion is created using a bifurcated needle dipped in vaccine.
  - The vaccinia vaccine is a live vaccine; thus, the vaccine site should be loosely covered to prevent the spread of virus to others.
  - After 3 to 4 days, a red pruritic papule appears at the vaccination site, which evolves into a vesicle followed by a pustule; after a few weeks, a scab forms, which then falls off leaving a scar.
- Contraindications to vaccine:
  - Atopic dermatitis or exfoliative skin disorder
  - Immunosuppression
  - Pregnancy or breastfeeding
  - Close contact of someone who is pregnant, immunosuppressed, or has skin disease
  - Allergy to vaccine component
  - Moderate or severe acute illness
  - Inflammatory eye disease
  - Heart disease (myocardial infarction, stroke, cardiomyopathy, heart failure, or angina) or $\geq$3 risk factors for heart disease
  - Age $<$1 year
  - These contraindications may be reevaluated if smallpox is reintroduced into the population.
- Common adverse reactions to vaccination:
  - Fever, swelling, lymphadenitis, and headache are seen in 2–16% of adults receiving the vaccine for the first time.
  - A mild rash occurs in ~8% of cases.
- Less common vaccine reactions:
  - Vaccinia keratitis and/or vision loss
  - Accidental inoculation with blister formation
  - Moderate to severe generalized rash
  - Eczema vaccinatum
  - Encephalitis
  - Congenital or generalized vaccinia
  - Myopericarditis
  - Progressive vaccinia/vaccinia gangrenosum
  - Bacterial superinfection

PATHOPHYSIOLOGY

- The virus infects the upper respiratory tract and replicates; rarely, primary infections can occur via skin, conjunctival, or placental routes.
- The virus enters the bloodstream (primary viremia) and is taken up by macrophages.
  - Patient is asymptomatic during this time.
- Next, the virus enters the reticuloendothelial system where it continues to replicate.
- Secondary viremia occurs as the virus reenters the bloodstream and infects organs.
  - Can cause epidermal necrosis and swelling
  - Infections of the bone marrow, kidneys, liver, lymph nodes, spleen, and other organs result in coagulopathy and multiorgan system failure.
- Exact mechanisms of viral toxicity are not understood but may involve both viral cytopathic effects and inflammatory pathology.

ETIOLOGY

- Variola virus is a member of the poxvirus family and *Orthopox* genus.
- Variola is a double-stranded DNA virus most commonly transmitted during face-to-face contact via respiratory aerosols or direct contact with infected skin lesions.
- Transmission of the virus via air in enclosed settings or via infected fomites is uncommon.
- Humans are the only vectors.

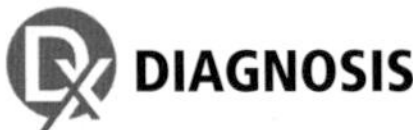

DIAGNOSIS

HISTORY

- Ordinary smallpox
  - Incubation period lasts 7 to 17 days, followed by a 1- to 4-day febrile prodrome characterized by high fever, headache, back pain, chills, abdominal pain, and emesis.
  - Eruptive phase begins with lesions of the mouth, tongue, and oropharynx.
  - The rash
    - Often starts on face and spreads to rest of body within 24 to 48 hours
    - On day 1, rash is macular.
    - On day 2, rash becomes papular.
    - On days 4 and 5, rash becomes vesicular.
    - By day 7, rash becomes pustular.
    - By 2 to 3 weeks, scabs form.
    - Scabs fall off, leaving pockmarks and scars.
- Modified smallpox
  - Occurs in previously vaccinated individuals
  - Milder than ordinary smallpox with shorter incubation period and accelerated course
  - Lesions are not as deep.
  - Fever not typically present with evolution of rash
- Flat-type (malignant) smallpox
  - Occurs more frequently in children
  - Characterized by soft, flat, semiconfluent, or confluent rash that does not evolve to pustules but can still result in significant skin loss
- Hemorrhagic smallpox
  - Occurs more frequently in adults, particularly pregnant women
  - Shorter incubation time
  - Skin becomes dusky and erythematous, followed by bleeding in skin and mucous membranes.
  - Can be difficult to diagnose unless exposure to variola virus is known
- Variola sine eruptione
  - Seen in infants with protective maternal antibodies and in vaccinated individuals
  - May be asymptomatic or cause an influenza-like illness
  - Noncontagious

PHYSICAL EXAM

The Centers for Disease Control and Prevention (CDC) protocol for evaluating patients for smallpox can be used to guide the assessment of a suspicious rash illness. This can be found at: https://emergency.cdc.gov/agent/smallpox/diagnosis/pdf/spox-poster-full.pdf

- If a patient has an acute, generalized rash on the body with vesicles or pustules, use the major and minor criteria to assess the likelihood of smallpox.

- Major criteria
  - Febrile prodrome: 1 to 4 days prior to rash onset, including a temperature ≥101°F and one or more of the following: prostration, headache, backache, chills, vomiting, or severe abdominal pain
  - Classic smallpox lesions are deep-seated, firm/hard, round, well-circumscribed vesicles or pustules that can become umbilicated or confluent as they evolve on any one part of the body; all the lesions are in the same stage of development.
- Minor criteria
  - Centrifugal distribution with greatest concentration of lesions on face and extremities
  - First lesions appear on the oral mucosa, palate, face, or forearms.
  - Patient appears toxic or moribund.
  - Slow evolution: Lesions evolve from macules to papules to pustules over days (each stage lasts 1 to 2 days)
  - Lesions on the palms and soles
- High risk of smallpox
  - Febrile prodrome and classic lesions in same stage of development
- Moderate risk of smallpox
  - Febrile prodrome and either 1 other major criterion or ≥4 minor criteria
- Low risk of smallpox
- No febrile prodrome, or febrile prodrome and <4 minor criteria

DIFFERENTIAL DIAGNOSIS

Multiple rash illnesses, including the following, can be confused with smallpox:

- Varicella and herpes zoster
- Herpes simplex virus
- Measles
- Rubella
- Monkeypox, cowpox, and tanapox
- Viral exanthema including enterovirus
- Disseminated molluscum contagiosum
- Impetigo, insect bites, or scabies
- Postsmallpox vaccine rash (vaccinia)
- Secondary syphilis
- Acne and contact dermatitis
- Drug reactions including erythema multiforme
- Meningococcemia can be confused with hemorrhagic smallpox.

DIAGNOSTIC TESTS & INTERPRETATION

Diagnostic Procedures/Other

- Use the CDC smallpox evaluation protocol to guide testing.
  - If high risk of smallpox:
    - Consult infectious disease and/or dermatology.
    - Public health agency will advise on management and collection of samples.
    - Testing will be performed at an approved laboratory prior to other tests.
  - If moderate risk of smallpox:
    - Consult infectious disease and/or dermatology.
    - Perform testing for varicella and other disorders including herpes simplex virus as indicated.
    - If no diagnosis is made after testing, ensure adequacy of specimen and have consultants reevaluate.
    - If smallpox still cannot be ruled out, then classify case as high-risk case.
  - If low risk of smallpox, and history and physical exam are highly suggestive of varicella, then varicella testing is optional.
  - If low risk of smallpox and diagnosis is uncertain, then testing should be done for varicella and other disorders as indicated.
- Variola testing
  - Should not be performed in low- and moderate-risk cases because of risk of false positives
  - Should only be performed in designated high-containment facilities
  - Lesion specimens (fluid, cells, and scabs) are preferred for testing, but blood, tonsillar swabs, and biopsy specimens may be used.
  - Serologic studies and electron microscopy cannot distinguish between the variola virus and other orthopoxviruses.
  - Polymerase chain reaction (PCR) assays can distinguish variola virus from other orthopoxviruses.
  - Variola virus can be cultured.

ALERT

- Varicella can be confused with smallpox.
- Varicella lesions present in different stages, are superficial, and concentrate on the trunk and face, sparing the palms and soles.
- Smallpox lesions all present in the same stage, are deep, and concentrated on the face and limbs, often involving the palms and soles.

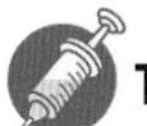

TREATMENT

GENERAL MEASURES

- Suspected cases of smallpox require notification of state and local authorities, in addition to the CDC.
- For patients with acute, generalized vesicular or pustular rash, institute airborne and contact precautions and alert infection control.
  - If high risk, report to state and local public health agency immediately.
- Individuals recently exposed (within 3 to 4 days) to someone with contagious smallpox (e.g., someone with oral or skin lesions) should receive postexposure vaccination, as this offers the potential to limit disease and also provides significant protection from death.
- Individuals with smallpox may be contagious during the febrile prodrome, are contagious during the early rash phase, and remain contagious until all the scabs have fallen off.

MEDICATION

- Patients suspected of having smallpox should be vaccinated against smallpox, especially if they are in the early stages of the disease.
- The efficacy of antiviral drugs are not fully known; however, cidofovir and brincidofovir have shown efficacy in treating animals with diseases similar to smallpox and have been safely used in humans for other viruses.
- Tecovirimat has been tested in both animals and humans with minor side effects only.
- Both cidofovir and tecovirimat are currently stockpiled by the CDC in case of a smallpox outbreak.
- The use of vaccinia immune globulin (VIG) can be considered for complications from vaccinia immunization but not for smallpox therapy or postexposure prophylaxis.

ONGOING CARE

PROGNOSIS

- The mortality rate for variola minor was <1%.
- Historically, the overall mortality rate for variola major was 30% but was close to 100% for the flat and hemorrhagic forms of the disease.
- The highest mortality rates occurred among young children, pregnant women, elderly individuals, and those with immunodeficiency.
- Long-term sequelae include pockmarks, vision loss, and limb deformities.

COMPLICATIONS

- Dehydration and electrolyte abnormalities can occur during the vesicular and pustular stages and should be corrected.
- Secondary bacterial superinfections may require antibiotic treatment.
- Corneal ulcers or keratitis, arthritis, or encephalitis may develop.

ADDITIONAL READING

- Besser JM, Crouch NA, Sullivan M. Laboratory diagnosis to differentiate smallpox, vaccinia, and other vesicular/pustular illnesses. *J Lab Clin Med*. 2003;142(4):246–251.
- Breman JG, Henderson DA. Diagnosis and management of smallpox. *N Engl J Med*. 2002;346(17):1300–1308.
- Hutchins SS, Sulemana I, Heilpern KL, et al. Performance of an algorithm for assessing smallpox risk among patients with rashes that may be confused with smallpox. *Clin Infect Dis*. 2008;46(Suppl 3):S195–S203.
- Moore ZS, Seward JF, Lane JM. Smallpox. *Lancet*. 2006;367(9508):425–435.

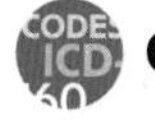

CODES

ICD10

B03 Smallpox

FAQ

- Q: What are my first steps in management should I suspect smallpox in a patient?
- A: If, after reviewing the CDC protocol for evaluation of suspected smallpox and suspicion remains, the patients should be placed in airborne and contact precautions with prompt notification of the local public health department and the CDC.
- Q: How can I differentiate the rash of varicella to that of smallpox?
- A: The rash of varicella will typically appear more superficial than that of smallpox. It will concentrate on the trunk and face with lesions in different stages. Smallpox lesions involve the trunk and face, in addition to the palms and soles, with lesions all in the same stage of evolution.
- Q: Should healthcare workers routinely be vaccinated for smallpox?
- A: At this time, the smallpox vaccine is only recommended for emergency response teams and health care workers investigating and evaluating patients with suspected smallpox, in addition to laboratory personnel who work with the virus that causes smallpox, or other similar viruses.

SNAKE AND INSECT BITES

Mamata V. Senthil, MD • Payal K. Gala, MD

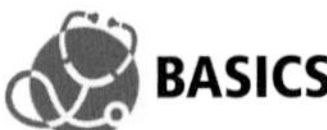

BASICS

DESCRIPTION

- Injury to the human skin and/or subcutaneous tissues caused by bite, envenomation, or sting, causing local but sometimes systemic effects
- Snake bites
  - Crotalinae (pit vipers: cottonmouths, copperheads, and rattlesnakes)
  - Elapidae (coral snakes)
- Spider bites
  - Black widow (*Latrodectus mactans*)
  - Brown recluse (*Loxosceles reclusa*)
- Insect stings: *Hymenoptera*, fire ants (*Solenopsis*), wasps (including hornets and yellow jackets), bees

EPIDEMIOLOGY

- Snake bites
  - Only 15% of all snake bites are from poisonous snakes, and only ~2/3 of those involve true envenomation.
  - Crotaline snakes are the most common cause of venomous snake bites in the United States.
  - Between 2010 and 2013, approximately 1,300 snake bites per year were reported in children and adolescents and about half of those were venomous.
  - Coral snake bites constitute <1% of all snake bites.
- Spider bites
  - The black widow spider is found in most areas of North America but especially in southern New England.
  - The brown recluse spider is found in southern and midwestern states.
- Approximately 3% of the U.S. population is at risk for anaphylaxis from *Hymenoptera* stings.

Incidence

- Annually, ~8,000 people sustain a poisonous snake bite in the United States, 99% of which are from crotaline snakes; 5 to 6 fatalities occur annually.
- The incidence of black widow and brown recluse spider bites are unknown.
- 90 to 100 people die each year from sting anaphylaxis.

PATHOPHYSIOLOGY

- Snake bites
  - Snake venom consists of numerous enzymes and polypeptides that are neurotoxic, cytotoxic, and/or hemotoxic.
  - Pit viper venom produces significant local inflammation and injury to vascular endothelium and may lead to coagulopathy, thrombocytopenia, and shock.
  - The venom of the coral snake is primarily neurotoxic and may produce neuromuscular paralysis and respiratory depression.
- Spider bites
  - Most of the 20,000 species of venomous spiders in the United States lack fangs capable of penetrating human skin or toxin strong enough to produce more than a mild reaction. However, the black widow and brown recluse spiders can cause significant harm.
  - The black widow venom, α-latrotoxin, is a neurotoxin that stimulates myoneural junctions and nerve terminals by increasing synaptic release of acetylcholine and by initiating a massive influx of calcium, causing severe skeletal muscle pain and cramping and autonomic disturbances such as hypertension, tachycardia, and diaphoresis. Pediatric patients are more severely inflicted given the ratio of milligram of venom to kilogram of body weight.
  - The brown recluse venom, mainly sphingomyelinase D and hyaluronidase, acts on erythrocyte membranes, platelets, endothelial cells, and other cells, resulting in tissue infarction and necrosis. Systemic symptoms are more likely to occur in children, presumably because of a smaller ratio of body weight to venom volume. Hemolysis, hemoglobinuria, renal failure, DIC, shock, seizures, and death may occur.
- Insect stings
  - The fire ant bites with its jaws and then swings its head around to inflict multiple stings. The venom has a direct toxic effect on mast cell membranes, causing an immediate urticarial reaction at the bite site.
  - The venoms of the bee and wasp (hornet and yellow jacket) contain antigens that trigger an IgE antibody response, resulting in allergic reactions that vary in severity from mild local effects to anaphylaxis.
  - Cross-reaction between *Hymenoptera* species occurs. Those who react to fire ants may also react to bees and wasps.

DIAGNOSIS

HISTORY

ALERT

- If the snake is brought in for identification, *use caution*. The head of a dead snake can deliver a venomous bite for up to 1 hour after death/decapitation.
- Snake bites
  - Poisonous snakes have triangular-shaped heads, a pit (heat sensor in front of each eye), fangs, slit-like pupils, and a single row of subcaudal plates and may have a rattle.
    - Exception to this rule: Coral snakes have oval heads and round pupils, yet are still poisonous.
  - Nonpoisonous snakes have oval heads, no pits, rows of small teeth, round pupils, a double row of subcaudal plates, and no rattles.
  - In the Elapidae family, the coral snake can be differentiated from the benign king snake by the pattern of the colored bands: "Red on yellow, kill a fellow; red on black, venom lack."
- Spider bites:
  - Identification of spider (rare): The black widow is about the size of a quarter, is glossy black, gray, or brown, with a red, orange, or yellow hourglass-shaped marking on the ventral surface.
  - A single bite can deliver a lethal dose of venom.
  - The brown recluse is small (1 to 1.5 cm), gray, or reddish/brown, with a violin-shaped mark on the dorsum of the cephalothorax.
- Insect bites
  - Identify type of insect (bee, wasp, ant).
  - Assess for history of insect bite allergy.

PHYSICAL EXAM

- Crotalinae (pit viper) bites
  - 25% of Crotalinae bites are "dry bites"—no envenomation occurs and only local tissue irritation develops.
  - Intense local pain/burning occur in the first few minutes, followed by edema and perioral numbness that may extend to the scalp and periphery. Paresthesias may be accompanied by a metallic taste.
  - Local ecchymosis and vesicles appear within the first few hours, and by 24 hours, hemorrhagic blebs are present.
  - Edema and tissue necrosis through the bitten extremity may occur. Compartment syndrome is rare.
  - Systemic symptoms such as nausea, vomiting, diarrhea, weakness, chills, and sweating can also occur.
  - Neuromuscular involvement (e.g., diplopia, dysphagia, lethargy) can develop within several hours.
  - Signs of hypovolemic shock, hemorrhagic diathesis, coagulopathy, and neuromuscular dysfunction may occur in life-threatening envenomations.
- Elapidae (coral snake) bites
  - Mild, often unimpressive local signs and symptoms (pain, swelling), but significant neurologic effects that include extremity paresthesias, weakness, fasciculations, and bulbar dysfunction that can progress to flaccid paralysis and respiratory failure may occur.
  - Inspect bite wound for fang punctures.
  - Carefully assess neurovascular integrity, and consider compartment pressures if severe edema.
- Black widow spider bites
  - Local lesion—pale circular areas with central punctum and surrounded by an erythematous ring
  - Within 8 hours after bite, regional or generalized pain and muscle cramping, fasciculations may occur; abdominal rigidity without tenderness is a hallmark sign.
  - Children often have nausea and vomiting.
  - Respiratory difficulty may occur.
  - Systemic symptoms: hypertension, tachycardia, and cholinergic effects (diaphoresis, salivation, lacrimation, and bronchorrhea)
  - Death may occur from respiratory or cardiovascular collapse, and young children are at higher risk.
  - Syndrome can last 3 to 6 days.
- Brown recluse spider bites
  - Spectrum from minor local reaction to severe necrosis
  - Local reaction: initially painless blister with symptoms typically occurring 2 to 8 hours after the bite including pain, erythema, swelling, and pruritus; classic "bull's eye" lesion or "red-white-and-blue" sign
  - Ischemia and skin necrosis: A bright red papule appears within a few hours of the bite and can evolve within 48 to 72 hours into a hemorrhagic vesicle surrounded by blue discoloration (necrosis) or white blanching (vasospasm): the bull's eye. Shortly after, a firm, purple necrotic lesion appears, and within 7 to 14 days, black eschar is visible. Ulcer healing can take weeks to months, leaving a deep scar.
- Insect bites
  - Small local reactions: painful, pruritic, urticarial lesion at the sting site
  - Large local reaction: edema and erythema, may be several centimeters in diameter
  - Anaphylaxis is rare with fire ants but occurs more frequently with bee stings.

DIFFERENTIAL DIAGNOSIS

- Black widow spider bites: acute abdomen, renal colic, opioid withdrawal, tetanus
- Poisonous snake bites: nonpoisonous snake bite (leaves scratches, not punctures), rodent bites, thorn wounds
- Brown recluse spider bite: other spider bites, insect bites and stings (including Lyme disease), cellulitis, poison ivy/oak, Stevens-Johnson syndrome, toxic epidermal necrolysis, erythema nodosum, chronic herpes simplex, purpura fulminans, diabetic ulcer, gonococcal hemorrhagic lesion, pyoderma

DIAGNOSTIC TESTS & INTERPRETATION

- Snake bites: CBC, platelet count, PT/PTT, fibrinogen, fibrin split products, electrolytes, creatine kinase, creatinine, urinalysis
- Spider bites: CBC, PT/PTT, fibrinogen, electrolytes, creatinine, creatine kinase, urinalysis, Coombs test
- Insect bites: no tests done routinely

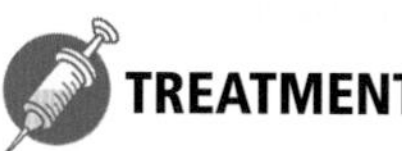

TREATMENT

- Crotalinae (pit vipers) bites
  - Remove constrictive items (jewelry or clothing) and immobilize extremity at the level of the heart. Cryotherapy, arterial tourniquets, incision, excision, oral suctioning are *not* recommended.
  - Focus on rapid transport to medical facility.
  - Address airway, breathing, and circulation.
  - The use of a constrictive band has fallen out of favor as field management because it can worsen local cytotoxic effects. Main indication is for cases of prolonged transport time to a medical facility or rapid progression of systemic symptoms.
  - Pressure immobilization of the involved extremity to theoretically delay systemic absorption of venom is no longer recommended. This first aid measure could potentially worsen local tissue injury and be limb-threatening, while showing no survival benefit in humans.
- Elapidae (coral snakes)
  - Constriction band, suction, and drainage do not prevent coral snake venom absorption.

GENERAL MEASURES

Consider contacting your local poison control center to assist with diagnosis and management. The national phone number for all centers is 1-800-222-1222.

- Crotalinae (pit vipers) bites
  - Wound care: irrigation and dressing
  - Determine if envenomation has occurred via serial exams (q30min) and laboratory studies (q4h).
  - Antivenom: Administration of antivenom should be made in consultation with a toxicologist. General indications include progressive local swelling, pain or ecchymosis, and any systemic signs or symptoms.
  - Crotalidae polyvalent immune Fab (CroFab®) is the Crotalinae antivenom product approved by the U.S. Food and Drug Administration (FDA), and data suggests it is safe and effective with few hypersensitivity reactions. Antivenin (Crotalidae) polyvalent (ACP) was often associated with serum sickness and anaphylaxis and is no longer manufactured. A new $F(ab')_2$ antivenom has been found to be safe and effective in children for the treatment of hematotoxicity and local tissue toxicity from Crotalinae envenomation but will not be available until 2018.
  - Some hospitals (in endemic areas) and many zoos stock antivenoms. The regional poison control center may have access to the Antivenom Index and will be able to help locate the nearest supply.
  - Early administration of Fab within 6 hours is advised. Initial dose is 4 to 6 vials of Fab diluted in 250 mL normal saline infused over 1 hour. Dosing is based on amount of venom injected, not weight of patient.
  - Supportive care: volume replacement, packed red blood cells, platelets, fresh frozen plasma, cryoprecipitate as indicated for hypovolemia and bleeding diathesis. Observe for respiratory and renal failure.
  - Frequent assessment of tissue perfusion and measurement of compartment pressure; fasciotomy only for elevated compartment pressures
  - Empiric antibiotics are controversial but may be indicated in cases of extensive tissue involvement.
  - Analgesia and tetanus prophylaxis
- Elapidae (coral snakes)
  - Crotalinae antivenom is ineffective in treating Elapidae envenomation. Currently, there are only two lots of FDA-approved Elapidae antivenom in the United States, which expire in 2017 and 2018. It is not known when more will be manufactured.
  - Any degree of neurotoxicity or systemic symptoms is an indication for antivenom therapy. Prophylactic therapy should be avoided due to limited supply and need to preserve antivenom.
  - Local wound care, supportive care, analgesia, and tetanus vaccination
- Black widow spider bites
  - Local wound care, tetanus prophylaxis
  - To alleviate muscle pain and cramping, parenteral opioids and benzodiazepines can be administered.
  - Calcium infusions had been used anecdotally but have not proven to be effective.
  - Latrodectus-specific antivenom is available for more severe envenomations given via IV infusion. Specific indications include young age, pregnancy, life-threatening hypertension and tachycardia, respiratory difficulties, or severe symptoms refractory to other treatment measures. Administration of an equine serum preparation has been associated with hypersensitivity reactions and occasionally death. 1 vial is generally sufficient.
- Brown recluse spider bites
  - Most bites can be treated on an outpatient basis with local wound care with Burow solution or hydrogen peroxide and symptom treatment for pain and pruritus.
  - No antivenom is available in the United States.
  - Patients with systemic symptoms, serious infection, or extensive necrosis warrant hospitalization, IV fluids, and aggressive supportive care.
  - Skin grafting or debridement may be warranted for wound management. Surgical excision is no longer indicated.
  - Neither dapsone nor hyperbaric oxygen therapy has proved to be effective; dapsone in children is associated with methemoglobinemia.
- Insect bites or stings
  - Rarely require more than ice and antihistamine for pruritus
  - If stinger remains in skin, remove by pinching with forceps or scraping. Emphasis should be on quick removal to decrease exposure to venom. Do not squeeze venom gland.
  - Life-threatening anaphylaxis should be treated with IM epinephrine (0.01 mL/kg 1:1,000 or 1 mg/mL, max 0.3 mL), methylprednisolone IV/IM (2 mg/kg), and/or diphenhydramine IV/IM (1.25 mg/kg).
- Bacterial superinfection is rare but, if present, can usually be treated with oral and/or topical antibiotics.

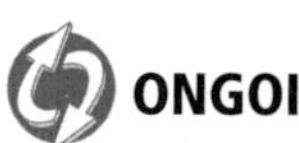

ONGOING CARE

PROGNOSIS

- Snake bites: Because the majority of snake bites are from nonvenomous snakes, and ~1/3 of bites from venomous snakes do not involve envenomation, the majority of bites cause only local injury. However, once serious injury is established, prognosis becomes unclear.
- Spider bites: Children have severe reactions and rare fatalities.
- Insect bites: Most bites and stings cause minimal local effects, although some cause serious systemic reactions and, rarely, death. For those patients with severe anaphylactic reactions, discharge the patient with a subcutaneous epinephrine autoinjector.

ADDITIONAL READING

- American College of Medical Toxicology, American Academy of Clinical Toxicology, American Association of Poison Control Centers, European Association of Poison Control Centres and Clinical Toxicologists, International Society on Toxinology, Asia Pacific Association of Medical Toxicology (2011). Pressure immobilization after North American Crotalinae snake envenomation. *Clin Toxicol (Phila)*. 2011;49(10):881–882.
- Anz AW, Schweppe M, Halvorson J, et al. Management of venomous snakebite injury to the extremities. *J Am Acad Orthop Surg*. 2010;18(12):749–759.
- Lasoff DR, Ruha AM, Curry SC, et al. A new $F(ab')_2$ antivenom for the treatment of crotaline envenomation in children. *Am J Emerg Med*. 2016;34(10):2003–2006.
- Patrick Walker J, Morrison R, Stewart R, et al. Venomous bites and stings. *Curr Probl Surg*. 2013;50(1):9–44.
- Quan D. North American poisonous bites and stings. *Crit Care Clin*. 2012;28(4):633–659.
- Schulte J, Domanski K, Smith EA, et al. Childhood victims of snakebites: 2000–2013. *Pediatrics*. 2016;138(5):e20160491.
- Warrell DA. Venomous bites, stings, and poisoning. *Infect Dis Clin North Am*. 2012;26(2):207–223.

S

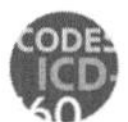

CODES

ICD10

- T63.481A Toxic effect of venom of arthropod, accidental, init
- T63.001A Toxic effect of unsp snake venom, accidental, init
- T63.301A Toxic effect of unsp spider venom, accidental, init

FAQ

- Q: How many patients with crotaline snake bites die from envenomation?
- A: Death is rare even with snake bites and occur in <1% of patients who are bitten. Prognosis is worst for those who are bitten by rattlesnakes, those who have bites in proximal body parts, those who did not receive antivenom therapy, and those who were inappropriately resuscitated.
- Q: What clues may steer you away from the possibility of a spider bite as the cause of a lesion on a patient?
- A: If multiple lesions are present, a spider bite is unlikely. Usually spider bites are one lesion. Also, when multiple household members have lesions similar to the patient, the lesions are not typically caused by spiders.

SOCIAL ANXIETY DISORDER

David K. Becker, MD, MPH, MA, LMFT

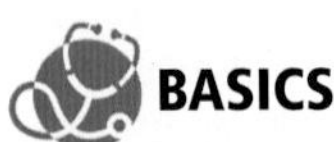

BASICS

DESCRIPTION

- Social anxiety disorder, also known as social phobia, is a psychological condition with developmental and genetic underpinnings. The disorder is characterized by marked and persistent fear of social situations in which the person is exposed to unfamiliar people or possible scrutiny by others.
- *DSM-5* criteria:
  - Marked fear or anxiety of one or more social situations in which the individual is exposed to possible scrutiny by others (in children: anxiety must occur in peer situations, not just in interactions with adults)
  - The individual fears that he/she will act in a way or show anxiety symptoms that will be negatively evaluated.
  - The social situations almost always provoke fear or anxiety and are avoided or endured with intense fear or anxiety.
  - The fear/anxiety is out of proportion to the actual threat posed by the situation/context and is persistent, typically lasting 6 months or more.
  - The fear/anxiety or avoidance causes significant distress or impairment in social, occupational, or other areas of functioning.
  - The fear/anxiety is not attributable to psychological effects of substances, a medical condition, or by another psychiatric diagnosis.

EPIDEMIOLOGY

Approximately 7% of youths suffer from social anxiety disorder. The prevalence is somewhat higher in girls than in boys. Subclinical social anxiety symptoms are much more common and are distinguished by the degree of functional impairment and cultural context.

RISK FACTORS

- Preexisting shyness or social inhibition
- Avoidant temperament
- Behavioral inhibition
- Family history: 1st-degree relatives have 2 to 6 times greater chance of having the disorder.
- Moderate genetic component based on twin studies

COMMONLY ASSOCIATED CONDITIONS

- Anxiety disorders
  - Generalized anxiety disorder
  - Specific phobia
  - Selective mutism
  - Obsessive-compulsive disorder
  - Panic disorder
- Attention deficit hyperactivity disorder (ADHD)
- Depression

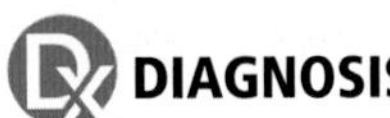

DIAGNOSIS

HISTORY

- The diagnostic evaluation should entail gathering of data through separate interviews with the child/adolescent and the parents.
- Current symptoms should be elicited with attention to severity, duration, and level of functional impairment.
- Core symptoms of marked anxiety in social situations, fear of negative scrutiny by others, and avoidance of these situations should be present.
- Distress can be manifested by physical symptoms such as blushing, palpitations, trembling, or GI upset.
- Younger children may exhibit periods of selective mutism in social situations while having the ability to talk freely while at home.
- Older children may appear oppositional and exhibit school refusal.
- Symptoms may be exacerbated by environmental transitions such as attending a new school or the family moving.

PHYSICAL EXAM

There are no pertinent findings on physical exam.

DIFFERENTIAL DIAGNOSIS

- Normative shyness or subclinical symptoms without significant adverse impact on functioning
- Anxiety disorders
- Depression
- Autistic spectrum disorders

DIAGNOSTIC TESTS & INTERPRETATION

There are no pertinent findings on laboratory studies.

Diagnostic Procedures/Other

Diagnostic scales:

- Multidimensional Anxiety Scale for Children (MASC)—broad anxiety scale (ages 8 to 18 years), self-report
- Social Phobia and Anxiety Inventory for Children (SPAI-C) (ages 8 to 17 years), self-report
- Social Anxiety Scale for Children-Revised (SASC-R) (ages 8 to 14 years) and Adolescents (SAS-A) (ages 13 to 18 years), self-administered
- Liebowitz Social Anxiety Scale for Children and Adolescents (LSAS-A) (ages 13 to 17 years), clinician-administered

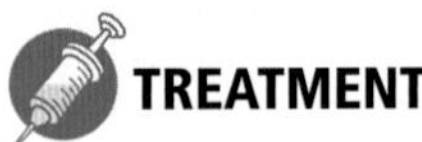

TREATMENT

- General considerations
  - Both psychotherapy and medications have roles in core treatment and symptom alleviation.
  - Additional therapies such as group therapy, individual and family psychoeducation, and/or self-regulation strategies can be considered first line in mild cases or adjuncts for more clinically impairing cases.
  - Combination treatment with selective serotonin reuptake inhibitors (SSRIs) and cognitive behavioral therapy (CBT) may be superior to either treatment alone.
- Psychotherapy
  - The most studied and most supported by structured clinical trials is CBT.
    - Exposure to a hierarchy of avoided situations with concomitant cognitive reframing is core to CBT.
  - Other psychotherapeutic approaches such as play therapy, interpersonal, or psychodynamic therapy may be better suited in some cases.

- Supportive psychosocial treatments can include mind–body strategies to support self-regulation skills. These may include biofeedback, progressive muscle relaxation, self-hypnosis, and/or mindfulness techniques.
- Group therapy may also be helpful.
- Family therapy or collaborative work with parents may be important to decrease parental accommodation or help with other dysfunctional dynamics.

MEDICATION

- SSRIs: first line for symptom control and adjunctive psychopharmacologic support. Begin half the recommended starting dose for children with anxiety disorders.
  - Side effects include GI upset, headaches, dizziness, and agitation.
  - There is a black box warning by the U.S. Food and Drug Administration (FDA) indicating that all antidepressants may increase suicidal thinking and behavior in children and adolescents. It is not clear how this may apply to treatment of social anxiety disorder that presents without depression.
  - Close monitoring is important following initiation of treatment.
    - Fluoxetine (Prozac®) (10 to 60 mg)
    - Sertraline (Zoloft®) (25 to 200 mg)
    - Paroxetine (Paxil®) (10 to 40 mg)
    - Citalopram (Celexa®) (10 to 60 mg)
    - Escitalopram (Lexapro®) (10 to 20 mg)
    - Fluvoxamine (Luvox®) (25 to 200 mg)
- Selective serotonin and norepinephrine reuptake inhibitors (SNRIs): second line
  - Side effects include somnolence, insomnia, dizziness, anxiety, headache, sweating, and tremor.
  - There is a black box warning by the FDA indicating that all antidepressants may increase suicidal thinking and behavior in children and adolescents.
  - Venlafaxine extended release (Effexor XR®) (25 to 225 mg)
- Benzodiazepines: may be considered for short-term symptomatic relief in rare circumstances; not appropriate for long-term therapy
  - Side effects include sedation, dizziness, and weakness.

ONGOING CARE

FOLLOW-UP RECOMMENDATIONS

Patient Monitoring

- Psychotherapy on a weekly or twice weekly regimen
- If medication is initiated, close monitoring on a weekly basis is recommended for the first 4 weeks followed by monthly monitoring.
- The primary care provider should monitor the response to the chosen treatment plan at least every 2 to 3 months.
- Monitoring of any emerging comorbidities is suggested.

PROGNOSIS

- Among patients who come to the attention of clinicians, social anxiety disorder is generally considered a chronic condition that does not significantly improve without intervention.
- Significant comorbidities may develop in adulthood, such as depression and alcohol dependence.

ADDITIONAL READING

- American Psychiatric Association. *Diagnostic and Statistical Manual of Mental Disorder*. 5th ed. Arlington, VA: American Psychiatric Association; 2013.
- Beesdo K, Knappe S, Pine D. Anxiety and anxiety disorders in children and adolescents: developmental issues and implications for DSM-V. *Psychiatr Clin North Am*. 2009;32(3):483–524.
- Beesdo-Baum K, Knappe S, Fehm L, et al. The natural course of social anxiety disorder among adolescents and young adults. *Acta Psychiatr Scand*. 2012;126(6):411–425.
- Beidel DC, Ferrell C, Alfano CA, et al. The treatment of childhood social anxiety disorder. *Psychiatr Clin North Am*. 2001;24(4):831–846.
- Khalid-Khan S, Santibanez MP, McMicken C, et al. Social anxiety disorder in children and adolescents: epidemiology, diagnosis, and treatment. *Paediatr Drugs*. 2007;9(4):227–237.
- Masi G, Pfanner C, Mucci M, et al. Pediatric social anxiety disorder: predictors of response to pharmacological treatment. *J Child Adolesc Psychopharmacol*. 2012;22(6):410–414.
- Scaini S, Belotti R, Ogliari A, et al. A comprehensive meta-analysis of cognitive-behavioral interventions for social anxiety disorder in children and adolescents. *J Anxiety Disord*. 2016;42:105–112.
- Spence SH, Rapee RM. The etiology of social anxiety disorder: an evidence-based model. *Behav Res Ther*. 2016;86:50–67.
- Walkup JT, Albano AM, Piacentini J, et al. Cognitive behavioral therapy, sertraline, or a combination in childhood anxiety. *N Engl J Med*. 2008;359(26):2753–2766.

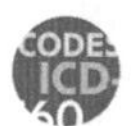

CODES

ICD10

- F40.10 Social phobia, unspecified
- F41.8 Other specified anxiety disorders
- F40.11 Social phobia, generalized

SORE THROAT

Daniel E. Felten, MD, MPD

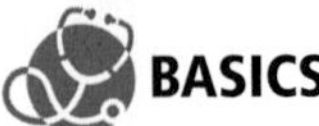

BASICS

DESCRIPTION
Throat pain with swallowing (odynophagia) or without swallowing may be a lone complaint or accompanied by a variety of other complaints. The most likely etiologies are self-limited but must rule out potentially life-threatening causes.

EPIDEMIOLOGY
- Sore throat is a common complaint year-round, but etiology depends on season and age of patient.
- In winter months, viral agents are more active.
- In spring and fall, postnasal drip from allergic rhinitis is a common cause of throat irritation.

GENERAL PREVENTION
- Careful hand washing and avoidance of respiratory secretions are keys to minimizing spread of most infectious agents.
- Noninfectious etiology often triggered by specific exposure, so avoidance of that trigger would limit symptoms

ETIOLOGY
- Infectious
  - Urgent/emergent: epiglottitis, peritonsillar cellulitis/abscess, retropharyngeal abscess, Lemierre syndrome
  - Viral: adenovirus, influenza, coxsackie, parainfluenza, Epstein-Barr virus (EBV), cytomegalovirus (CMV), herpes simplex virus (HSV), human immunodeficiency virus
  - Bacterial: group A β-hemolytic *Streptococcus* (GAS), *Streptococcus pyogenes*, *Mycoplasma pneumoniae*, groups C and G streptococci, diphtheria, *Neisseria gonorrhoeae*, anaerobic bacteria, tularemia, *Arcanobacterium haemolyticum*
  - Fungal: *Candida*
- Allergic/inflammatory
  - Postnasal drip from allergic rhinitis
  - Gastroesophageal reflux disorder (GERD)
  - Eosinophilic esophagitis
- Environmental
  - Tobacco smoke or aerosolized irritant
- Trauma
  - Foreign body: either retained or causing laceration to posterior pharynx
  - Burns: hot liquids/foods
  - Caustic ingestion
  - Voice overuse
- Tumor
  - Acute lymphocytic leukemia (ALL) or T-cell lymphoma can rarely present as sore throat and fever.
- Miscellaneous
  - Kawasaki disease
  - PFAPA: periodic fever, aphthous stomatitis, pharyngitis, adenitis
  - Psychogenic pain
  - Referred pain

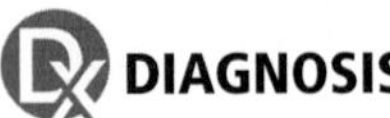

DIAGNOSIS

HISTORY
- Drooling, inability to swallow, rapid progression of symptoms, or respiratory distress may suggest more urgent/emergent problem: epiglottitis, peritonsillar abscess (especially with unilateral symptoms), or retropharyngeal abscess.
- Exposures, ingestions, foreign bodies: need to elicit whether patient was exposed to agent that could cause progression of symptoms
  - Caustic ingestion burns may progress rapidly and require transfer to higher level of care.
  - Foreign body ingestion may require removal or endoscopic visualization.
- Outbreaks in child care setting or school: GAS, influenza, and coxsackie can spread rapidly.
- Sexual activity or concern for sexual abuse: oral sex a risk factor for development of pharyngitis due to *N. gonorrhoeae*
- Children who are immunocompromised or children on chronic inhaled corticosteroids who are otherwise immune competent are at risk for esophageal candidiasis. Throat pain is often chronic and not responsive to other treatments.
- Associated symptoms
  - Fever, headache (HA), stomach pain, absence of viral symptoms: Consider GAS.
  - Fever, HA, rhinorrhea, myalgias, fatigue: Consider influenza.
  - Rhinorrhea, cough, conjunctivitis: more likely viral
  - Runny nose, itchy nose, congestion: Consider postnasal drip from allergic rhinitis.
  - Burning sensation, acid taste in mouth, positional: Consider GERD.

PHYSICAL EXAM

ALERT
- Although rare since the introduction of the vaccine for *Haemophilus influenzae* type b, patients may present with epiglottitis.
- Caution approaching a febrile, toxic-appearing patient who is unable to control secretions and exhibiting any respiratory distress. Defer exam or imaging until patient is in a setting where an emergent airway could be established if epiglottitis is suspected.

- General
  - Ill-appearing, respiratory distress: epiglottitis, retropharyngeal abscess
- Pharynx and oral cavity
  - Exudative tonsillitis: usually GAS but also present in EBV, *N. gonorrhoeae*, *Arcanobacterium*, HSV, adenovirus
  - Vesicles or ulceration on tonsils, tonsillar pillars, or buccal mucosa; inflammation of gums: HSV, coxsackievirus, echovirus
  - Posterior pharyngeal cobblestoning: postnasal drip from allergic rhinitis
  - Asymmetry in tonsil size or deviation of uvula: peritonsillar abscess
  - Burns on lips or tongue: hot liquid or caustic ingestion
- Eyes, ears, nose
  - Conjunctivitis with sore throat: adenovirus
  - Rhinorrhea: viral etiology most likely
  - Boggy nasal turbinates, allergic shiners: postnasal drip from allergic rhinitis
- Neck/lymph nodes
  - Tender anterior cervical lymph nodes: classic for GAS
  - Diffuse lymphadenopathy +/− splenomegaly: EBV, less likely CMV
  - Neck swelling or crepitus: possible perforation due to foreign body ingestion
- Skin
  - Scarlatiniform rash (diffuse, erythematous, fine-papular, "sand-papery" rash): scarlet fever from GAS pharyngitis but can be seen with infections due to *A. haemolyticum* and in Kawasaki disease
  - Vesicular rash, particularly on palms, soles, and/or buttocks: coxsackievirus

DIAGNOSTIC TESTS & INTERPRETATION
- Rapid antigen detection test (RADT)
  - Initial test of choice if GAS pharyngitis suspected
  - High specificity (≥95%), variable sensitivity (55–90%)
  - Need to confirm negatives with culture or DNA probe for GAS
- Heterophile antibody test (monospot)
  - Can be used to confirm EBV infection
  - Not reliable <4 years
- Cultures for other bacteria (e.g., *N. gonorrhoeae*, *A. haemolyticum*) require special handling and specific medium for growth.
- Lateral neck radiograph
  - Do not obtain radiograph in unstable patient.
  - Thumb print sign: enlarged epiglottis
  - Widened prevertebral soft tissue space suggestive of retropharyngeal abscess

- Chest radiograph if foreign body is suspected
  - Must ensure object passes out of esophagus
  - Look for free air indicating perforation.
- CT scan of neck
  - For diagnosis of retropharyngeal abscess in setting of suggestive lateral neck radiograph or peritonsillar abscess if suggested by physical exam

TREATMENT

The treatment of sore throat is primarily supportive, including fluids and pain control. Additional treatment depends on underlying etiology.

MEDICATION

- Pain relievers such as ibuprofen or acetaminophen are generally sufficient to manage pain.
  - Rarely, addition of an opioid may be warranted in patients who are unable to maintain sufficient PO intake.
  - Avoid use of codeine due to variability in metabolism by cytochrome P450 CYP2D6. Patients who are "ultra-rapid metabolizers" of codeine convert up to 15% (vs. 3%) of the drug to morphine, which can lead to toxicity.
  - Alternatively, for less severe pain, topical treatments such as throat lozenges or throat sprays may provide additional comfort with fewer potential side effects.
- GAS pharyngitis: penicillin G benzathine IM (600,000 U <27 kg, 1.2 million U >27 kg as a single dose) or penicillin V potassium PO (250 mg b.i.d. <27 kg, 500 mg b.i.d. >27 kg × 10 days) or amoxicillin (50 mg/kg/24 hr; max 1,000 mg/24 hr) first line
  - 1st-generation cephalosporin for penicillin-allergic patients with nonanaphylactic reactions
  - Clindamycin for patients with type I hypersensitivity to penicillin
  - Macrolides are also acceptable alternatives.
- Some studies have shown steroids (oral or IM) to be of benefit to patients with severe symptoms. However, they should be used only in limited circumstances due to side effects.
- Esophageal candidiasis: fluconazole (6 mg/kg × 1, then 3 mg/kg daily; max 400 mg/24 h) or itraconazole (5 to 10 mg/kg/24 h divided daily or b.i.d.; max 200 mg/24 h) × 14 to 21 days after resolution of symptoms

ISSUES FOR REFERRAL

- Epiglottitis: Exam, airway stabilization, and ongoing management must be done in controlled setting.
- Peritonsillar abscess: often requires drainage either by needle aspiration, incision and drainage, or tonsillectomy
- Presence of foreign body in esophagus: should be removed if signs of airway compromise, if object is button battery or sharp, or if object doesn't pass in 24 hours; may require additional treatment in cases of perforation

ADMISSION, INPATIENT, AND NURSING CONSIDERATIONS

- Patients with signs of airway compromise or respiratory distress may require emergent airway management.
  - Patients suspected to have epiglottitis must have airway stabilized prior to any other treatment or diagnostic testing.
  - If no impending airway obstruction, can undertake diagnostic and therapeutic interventions, including IV placement for fluid administration if patient is not tolerating PO, antibiotics for treatment of abscess or cellulitis, or anesthetic agents if endotracheal intubation becomes necessary
  - Supplemental O_2 as needed
  - Make NPO if surgical intervention is required.
- Patients with conditions causing airway compromise require monitoring until they demonstrate response to treatment.
- Pain control or hydration: Patients with uncontrolled throat pain may be unable to take adequate PO to maintain hydration at home.

ADDITIONAL READING

- Galioto N. Peritonsillar abscess. *Am Fam Physician*. 2008;77(2):199–202.
- Madadi P, Koren G. Pharmacogenetic insights into codeine analgesia: implications to pediatric codeine use. *Pharmacogenomics*. 2008;9(9):1267–1284.
- Sadowitz PD, Page NE, Crowley K. Adverse effects of steroid therapy in children with pharyngitis with unsuspected malignancy. *Pediatr Emerg Care*. 2012;28(8):807–809.
- Schwartz B, Marcy SM, Phillips WR, et al. Pharyngitis—principles of judicious use of antimicrobial agents. *Pediatrics*. 1998;101:171–174.
- Wing A, Villa-Roel C, Yeh B, et al. Effectiveness of corticosteroid treatment in acute pharyngitis: a systematic review of the literature. *Acad Emerg Med*. 2010;17(5):476–483.

CODES

ICD10

- J02.9 Acute pharyngitis, unspecified
- R07.0 Pain in throat
- J02.0 Streptococcal pharyngitis

FAQ

- Q: Are steroids effective adjuvant therapy for sore throat?
- A: Several well-conducted studies have shown that giving steroids to patients with GAS pharyngitis has decreased time to improvement in symptoms on average about 5.2 hours. However, there was no significant difference in pain at 24 hours. In patients with non–GAS-associated sore throat, results are more mixed. One study did show significant decrease in time to improvement in symptoms in patients with severe symptoms. The most recent guidelines from the Infectious Disease Society of America (2012) do not recommend routine use of corticosteroids for treating GAS pharyngitis.
- Q: What is the risk of giving steroids to a patient with sore throat?
- A: None of the studies of steroid use in treatment of acute throat pain reported any significant side effects in the treatment groups. There were some reports of GI upset that often were attributed to concurrent use of antibiotics. However, sore throat plus fever is rarely the presentation of ALL, and it has been shown that steroid administration prior to the diagnosis of ALL has a significant adverse effect of the chance a patient will achieve complete remission. Current children's oncology group protocols may assign children who have received steroids prior to an ALL diagnosis to more intensive treatment depending on time of steroid administration.
- Q: Should antibiotics be given to children with sore throat based on physical exam findings that suggest GAS pharyngitis?
- A: No. Most cases of sore throat in children are due to viruses, and the RADT is a widely available screening test that is easy to administer, with excellent specificity. Patients with a positive RADT should be treated. Negative results should be sent for culture or DNA probe, which may delay treatment by 24 to 48 hours. However, the primary reason for treating GAS pharyngitis with antibiotics is to prevent rheumatic fever, which can be accomplished as long as antibiotics are administered within 10 days of onset of symptoms.

SPEECH DELAY

Maureen C. McMahon, MD

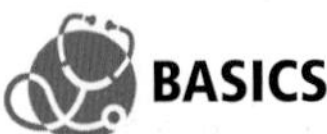

BASICS

DESCRIPTION

- Speech delay is delay in the acquisition of spoken language.
- Language is a system of symbols through which humans communicate thoughts, feelings, and ideas. It has three components—receptive, expressive, and visual language.
  - Receptive language is the ability to process and understand language.
  - Expressive language is the ability to communicate through speech, written, or formal sign language.
  - Visual elements include eye contact, pointing, and gestures.
- Speech delay can be primary, as in specific language impairment (SLI) or developmental language disorder (DLD), or secondary to another condition such as a syndrome or neurologic disorder. SLI is impaired speech/language in an otherwise normally developing child who lacks signs or stigmata of other conditions.
- Constitutional language delay, a retrospective diagnosis, is language delay associated with eventual achievement of normal speech and language milestones by school age. There are no subsequent difficulties with learning to read or write.
- Expressive language disorders include the following:
  - Verbal dyspraxia: little speech produced with great effort, very dysfluent, single words most commonly
  - Speech programming deficit disorder: poorly organized, difficult-to-understand speech
- Mixed receptive and expressive disorders
  - Verbal auditory agnosia: impaired ability to decode speech, resulting in a severe expressive impairment; can often learn language visually
  - Phonologic/syntactic deficit disorder: most common type of DLD. Comprehension exceeds spoken ability. Speech is dysfluent, grammatically incorrect with short utterances.
  - Most frequent causes of speech delay:
    - Hearing loss
    - SLI
    - Autism spectrum disorder
    - Intellectual disability (formerly mental retardation)

EPIDEMIOLOGY

- Up to 15% of 2-year-olds have speech and language delays.
- 5% of school-aged children have speech and language delays.
- 3:1 male-to-female ratio in DLD

RISK FACTORS

- Family history of speech/language delay or disorder
- Male gender
- Low maternal education
- Maternal depression
- Prematurity
- Birth weight <1,000 g

DIAGNOSIS

HISTORY

Does the family note a concern about speech delay or hearing impairment?

- **Question:** Perinatal history?
- *Significance*: prenatal care, maternal illness, neonatal intensive care unit (NICU) admission, hyperbilirubinemia requiring exchange transfusion, treatment with ototoxic drugs such as gentamicin, newborn hearing screen results
- **Question:** Full developmental history?
- *Significance*: to determine if global delay or isolated speech and language delay
- **Question:** Parental concern about delayed expressive language?
- *Significance*: often the presentation of autism
- **Question:** History of feeding, swallowing difficulties, or poor acceptance of textured foods?
- *Significance*: signs of oromotor dysfunction which may indicate a neurologic problem
- **Question:** Family history of speech delay, hearing loss, neurologic disorder, or syndrome?
- *Significance*: may direct further evaluation
- **Question:** Any regression or loss of language milestones?
- *Significance*: should prompt a neurologic and metabolic workup
- **Question:** What is the social interaction of the child?
- *Significance*: Lack of interest in playing is a red flag for autism.
- **Question:** Any concern regarding child abuse or neglect or psychosocial deprivation?
- *Significance*: may have occurred as the result of a parental, genetic, or developmental disorder; drug or alcohol abuse; poverty; child malnutrition; or environmental toxins such as lead
- **Question:** History of frequent acute otitis media or otitis media with effusion and conductive hearing loss?
- *Significance*: may precede speech delay
- **Question:** Visual impairments?
- *Significance*: may impact speech development because interpretation of facial expressions and gestures is a component of infant receptive language development
- **Question:** History of traumatic brain injury?
- *Significance*: Speech delay may occur with a seizure disorder.

PHYSICAL EXAM

Complete examination looking for signs that may be associated with speech delay

- **Finding:** Microcephaly?
- *Significance*: associated with intellectual disability, in utero cytomegalovirus (CMV) infection, or dysmorphic features
- **Finding:** Macrocephaly?
- *Significance*: associated with hydrocephalus, various syndromes
- **Finding:** Dysmorphic features?
- *Significance*: suggestive of a syndrome
- **Finding:** Excess drooling and open-mouth posture?
- *Significance*: signs of poor oral motor control of muscles used for speech production
- **Finding:** Craniofacial abnormalities?
- *Significance*: Articulation difficulty may be due to velopharyngeal insufficiency (VPI) seen with unrepaired cleft lip or palate.
- **Finding:** Scarred tympanic membranes or middle ear fluid?
- *Significance*: may be clue to acquired intermittent or chronic conductive hearing loss
- **Finding:** Macroorchidism?
- *Significance*: fragile X syndrome
- **Finding:** Neurologic exam—hypertonia or hypotonia, abnormal reflexes, other focal findings?
- *Significance*: suggestive of neurologic impairment
- **Finding:** Café au lait spots, hypopigmented macules, shagreen patch, axillary or inguinal freckling?
- *Significance*: skin findings suggestive of a neurocutaneous syndrome

DIFFERENTIAL DIAGNOSIS

- Hearing loss
  - Isolated genetic hearing loss
  - Hearing loss secondary to in utero CMV infection: full syndrome at birth or asymptomatic infection with delayed onset of progressive hearing loss
  - Acquired hearing loss: following head trauma, tumor-associated, complication of bacterial meningitis, end result of frequent acute otitis media, or chronic otitis media with effusion
- Intellectual disability
- Autism spectrum disorder
- SLI
- Constitutional language delay
- Selective mutism
- Environmental
  - Lack of stimulation and/or poor linguistic environment
  - Child abuse or neglect
  - Lead poisoning
- Congenital
  - Cerebral palsy
  - Hydrocephalus
  - Down syndrome
  - Fragile X syndrome
  - 22q11 microdeletion syndrome
  - Fetal alcohol syndrome
  - Turner syndrome
  - Klinefelter syndrome
  - Prader-Willi syndrome
  - Angelman syndrome
  - Muscular dystrophy
  - Tuberous sclerosis
  - Neurofibromatosis
  - Williams syndrome
  - Branchio-oto-renal (BOR) syndrome
  - Craniofacial anomalies such as Treacher Collins and Goldenhar syndromes

- Nutritional
  - Malnutrition
  - Iron deficiency
- Infectious
  - HIV encephalopathy
  - Other in utero viral infection
  - Congenital toxoplasmosis
  - Congenital syphilis

ALERT

- Avoid late referral of congenital hearing loss: Amplification and therapy by 6 months of age can result in near-normal rate of speech/language acquisition.
- Constitutional language delay is a retrospective diagnosis. Do not miss a language disorder if assuming a delayed toddler is a "late bloomer."
- Avoid overlooking fine or gross motor delays.
- Avoid missing a genetic or neurologic diagnosis.

DIAGNOSTIC TESTS & INTERPRETATION

- The American Academy of Pediatrics recommends a specific development screening tool be administered at the 9-, 18-, and 24- or 30-month well-child care visits and an autism-specific tool be administered at the 18- and 24-month visits.
- Office development screening tools
  - Denver Developmental Assessment II
- Early Language Milestone Scale (ELMS)
- Clinical Linguistic and Auditory Milestone Scale (CLAMS)
- Hearing evaluation
  - Most states have mandated universal newborn hearing screening programs.
  - Screening tests: automated auditory brainstem response (AABR) and transient evoked otoacoustic emissions (OAEs)
  - Hearing should be tested in all speech-delayed children, even if the newborn hearing screen was normal.
  - <6 months of age: The definitive test is brainstem auditory evoked response (BAER).
  - >6 months of age in a neurologically normal child: The definitive test is behavioral audiometry, such as visual reinforcement audiometry (VRA), performed by a trained audiologist.
- Selected speech/language milestones
  - 2 months: cooing, response to voice
  - 6 months: babbling
  - 4 to 9 months: turns to sound, responds to name
  - 9 months: dada/mama nonspecific, begins to understand "no"
  - 9 to 12 months: jargon
  - 12 months: dada, mama specific, one additional word, jargon is complex, points to gesture, follows one-step command
  - 18 months: 10 words, knows body parts
  - 2 years: 50 words, two-word phrases, 50% intelligible by strangers, pronouns, can point to specific objects in a picture, may know one color, follows two-step commands
  - 3 years: 300 to 500 words, tells stories, 75% intelligible by strangers
  - 4 years: grammatically correct sentences, 100% intelligible by strangers
- Routine cranial imaging or screening tests for metabolic diseases are not recommended.
- **Test:** full speech and language evaluation
- *Significance*: to delineate the disorder and determine therapy
- **Test:** Individuals with Disabilities Education Act (IDEA) mandates early intervention services from birth to 3 years.
- *Significance*: Children can get a full developmental evaluation and appropriate therapy if sufficient delays are demonstrated.
- **Test:** electroencephalogram (EEG)
- *Significance*: indicated if there is concern for seizures
- **Test:** genetics evaluation
- *Significance*: should be obtained for congenital hearing loss or if there is concern for a syndrome or genetic diagnosis
- **Test:** prolonged sleep EEG
- *Significance*: indicated with loss of language milestones (Consider the diagnosis of Landau-Kleffner syndrome.)

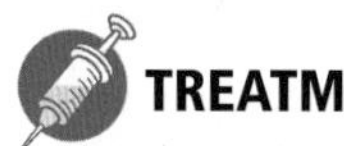

TREATMENT

GENERAL MEASURES

- Congenital hearing loss is managed by a team consisting of an otolaryngologist, audiologist, and speech/language therapist who individualize management. Options are amplification, cochlear implant for the severely impaired, or use of sign language.
- Speech and language therapy can be provided through physician referral or parent-generated referral to early intervention programs.
- Sign language can be used as a bridge to promote communication while the child learns verbal skills. It will not preclude or delay the development of speech.
- Augmentative communication devices such as picture boards or programmed computers with voice synthesizers can be used by children with physical impairments such as cerebral palsy.
- Children with DLD usually speak adequately by school age. Some percentage will go on to have difficulty reading and writing.
- Children with constitutional language delay will achieve normal milestones by school entrance without reading disability or other learning problem.

ADDITIONAL READING

- Agin M. The "late talker"—when silence isn't golden. *Contemp Pediatr*. 2004;21:22–32.
- Campbell T, Dollaghan C, Rockette H, et al. Risk factors for speech delay of unknown origin in 3-year-old children. *Child Dev*. 2003;74(2):346–357.
- Coplan J. Normal speech and language development: an overview. *Pediatr Rev*. 1995;16(3):91–100.
- Feldman H. Evaluation and management of language and speech disorders in preschool children. *Pediatr Rev*. 2005;26(4):131–142.
- Rapin I. Practitioner review: developmental language disorders: a clinical update. *J Child Psychol Psychiatry*. 1996;37(6):643–655.
- Sokol J, Hyde M. Hearing screening. *Pediatr Rev*. 2002;23(5):155–162.

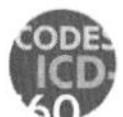

CODES

ICD10

- F80.9 Developmental disorder of speech and language, unspecified
- F80.4 Speech and language development delay due to hearing loss
- F80.1 Expressive language disorder

FAQ

- Q: Do 2nd- and 3rd-born children speak later than 1st-born children?
- A: No. The norms for expected speech/language development are the same regardless of birth order. 2nd- and 3rd-born children should have the same degree of motivation to speak as their 1st-born sibling.
- Q: When should I refer a child for speech/language evaluation?
- A: If the parents or physician have any concern for speech delay, then referral for evaluation is wise. Some speech-delayed children will eventually normalize and meet all milestones. It is difficult to distinguish who is constitutionally delayed from those who have another disorder. There are several indications for a prompt referral: no pointing or babbling by 1 year, no single words by 16 months, no 2-word spontaneous phrases by 2 years, no sentences by 3 years, poor intelligibility for age, child has behavioral "melt downs" or tantrums with efforts to communicate, or any regression in language skills.
- Q: Do children raised in bilingual households have expressive language delay?
- A: No. Living in a bilingual household is not a cause of expressive language delay. However, toddlers who are learning two languages may interchange words in both languages. Total vocabulary and phrase length are typically normal in these children by 2–3 years of age.

SPEECH PROBLEMS

Helen M. Sharp, PhD • Kathryn L. Hillenbrand, MA, CCC-SLP

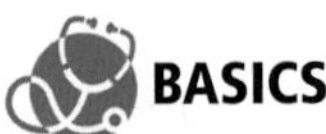

BASICS

DESCRIPTION

- Communication is the exchange of ideas between two or more individuals.
- Language is a systematic means of communication that relies on a socially agreed on set of symbols and rules for combining those symbols. Language includes comprehension, expression, and social-pragmatic rules (e.g., eye contact and turn-taking).
- Speech is produced through vocal and articulatory movements using neuromotor control of respiration, phonation (vocalization), and articulation to shape airflow and vocal sounds into strings of speech sounds (phonemes) to form words and word combinations.
- Articulation refers to the use of oral and pharyngeal structures (lips, tongue, palate, teeth) to shape vocal sounds and airflow into recognizable speech.
- Hearing is the process of transferring sound from the environment to the brain via the outer, middle, and inner ear systems.
- Speech disorders have three general points of origin: (i) neurologic, (ii) structural, or (iii) functional. Functional disorders are those that are unrelated to neurologic or structural disorders. More than one of these causes may be present in the same child.
- Speech disorders can be classified and are described as follows:
  - Articulation or phonologic disorders
    - Disrupt the way a child says one or more speech sounds
    - Simplifications of complex adult speech are often normal very early in speech development but should be evaluated if these changes linger, are atypical, or interfere with socialization.
  - Fluency disorders
    - Disrupt the easy flow of speech production and include the conditions of stuttering and cluttering.
    - Examples of stuttering include repetitions of sounds, syllables, words, or phrases, pauses, blocks, or hesitations.
    - Easy repetitions are common in children ages 2 to 4 years and typically resolve quickly. Persistence, visible struggle, or avoidance of talking warrant referral.
  - Motor speech disorders
    - Disrupt timing, coordination, or the execution of the motor plan for speech
    - Divided into two major categories: (i) dysarthrias, which are most often related to neuromotor weakness or paralysis, and (ii) apraxia, a motor planning disorder in the absence of neuromotor weakness or paralysis
  - Voice disorders
    - Heard as atypical laryngeal quality such as hoarseness (dysphonia) or completely absent voice (aphonia)
  - Resonance disorders
    - Describe speech quality usually described as nasality
    - Hypernasality (excessively nasal quality) is associated with velopharyngeal dysfunction and is atypical.
    - Hyponasality (inadequate nasality) is common in young children in association with acute upper respiratory infection or adenoid hypertrophy.
- Language disorders may occur in receptive, expressive, pragmatic, or some combination of these domains. Language disorders may occur in conjunction with other developmental, sensory, neurologic, or structural concerns but may also be isolated as an area of delay (see "Speech Delay" and "Autism" chapters).

EPIDEMIOLOGY

- The American Speech-Language Hearing Association states that communication disorders occur in 1 of every 8 people in the population.
  - Newborn screening identifies hearing loss or deafness in 1 to 5 per 1,000 newborns, with higher rates in neonatal intensive care.
- Speech sound disorders including articulation, phonologic, and developmental apraxia of speech are considered the most prevalent communication problem diagnosed in 15% of preschoolers and 4–6% of school-aged children.
  - Fluency disorders affect 11% of children by age 4 years.
  - Boys are 3 times more likely to persist in stuttering beyond age 4 years.
- Cerebral palsy affects 1 in 500 children born each year and may include mild to severe motor speech disorders and risk of other communication disorders.
- Voice disorders such as chronic hoarseness are reported in 6–23% of children.

DIAGNOSIS

HISTORY

- Prenatal history
  - Prenatal exposures to alcohol, prescription or non-prescription medications, or infections are known to relate to developmental delay and/or hearing loss.
- Medical history
  - Prematurity, trauma, seizure disorders, major surgeries, and systemic infections are all risk factors for communication disorders.
  - Multiple anomalies may relate to an underlying syndrome.
- Feeding history
  - Neuromotor and structural disorders may be noted in early feeding history.
  - Ask about failure to thrive, frequent pneumonia, prolonged feeding time, or chronic nasal regurgitation.
- Family history
  - Heredity may be a factor associated with stuttering, specific language impairment, autism spectrum disorders, cleft palate, developmental apraxia of speech, hearing loss, deafness, and other speech-language disorders.
- Social history
  - Evaluate for history of abuse, trauma, or neglect.
  - Smoking in the home is a known risk for middle ear infections.
  - Frequent verbal interaction and reading promote speech and language skills.
- Speech and language history
  - Routine screening for speech and language milestones aid early identification.
  - Duration of symptoms for voice and resonance disorders will separate acute infection from true disorders.
  - Regression of speech or language skills may be associated with autism spectrum disorders or trauma.
- Key milestones
  - By 1 year of age
    - Points to (or gazes toward) known person or object name (Where's mama?)
    - Produces at least *one* true word; may not be recognized by all but is consistent
  - By 2 years of age
    - Identifies body parts; follows one-element commands (Get your book.)
    - Uses about 50 expressive words and starts to *combine 2 words* together (up dada)
  - By 3 years of age
    - Follows *two to three element commands*, combines *three-word phrases*, and uses short questions (e.g., Why?)
    - Consistent production of speech sounds "m, p, b, d, n, w, h, and y (in *you*)" and all or most vowel sounds
    - Speech is understood by familiar listeners the majority of the time.
  - By 4 years of age
    - Uses longer sentences and tells short stories/sequences of events
    - Answers who, what, where, and when questions
    - Speech is understood by an unfamiliar listener nearly all the time.
- Speech emerges and becomes more accurate as motor coordination develops. The most complex speech sounds (the late 8) "s," "r, "z," "l," "sh" (in sheep), "th" (ba*th*), "th" in ba*the*), and "zh" (measure) should emerge by age 5 years and be accurate consistently by 7 to 8 years of age. Very early in development, children may omit these sounds or substitute similar sounds.
- Physical and social development
  - Missed physical or social milestones are indicative of overall delay. Delayed or absent social milestones may aid in early identification of autism spectrum disorders.

PHYSICAL EXAM

- Face
  - Evaluate for facial symmetry at rest (structural) and during movement (neurologic).
  - Drooling is typical during early infancy and teething but should resolve by 18 to 24 months.
- Eye color
  - Iris heterotropia together with white forelock frequently associate with hearing loss in Waardenburg syndrome.
- Skin
  - Café au lait spots are associated with neurofibromatosis and hearing loss.
- Head shape and size
  - Microcephaly, macrocephaly, or plagiocephaly or other skull asymmetries may be associated with developmental delay, hypotonia, or craniosynostosis conditions.
- Symmetry, structure, and height of ears
  - Ear tags, atresia, and low-set ears have high association with hearing loss and should prompt audiologic and otolaryngology evaluation.

- Intraoral exam
  - Dental health, palatal shape, and jaw relationships should be noted.
  - Soft palate (velar) elevation should be symmetric on "ah."
  - Bifid uvula, bluish color of velum, or V-shaped notch at the border of the hard and soft palate are indicative of a submucous cleft palate.
  - Absent gag response is not a contraindication to feeding but should be noted.
- Phonation
  - Listen to vocal quality on sustained "ah."
  - Wet voice may indicate swallowing disorder.
  - Rough, hoarse, or strained vocal quality is atypical and requires evaluation.

DIFFERENTIAL DIAGNOSIS

Communication disorders may be associated with other underlying conditions. A diagnosis of speech or language delay should include a process of evaluating the child for underlying causes, which alter the treatment approach:

- Hearing loss. Evaluate for familial or congenital loss, chronic middle ear infection, or acquired loss (e.g., ototoxic medications, systemic infection, underlying syndrome, or noise exposure).
- Developmental delay or autism spectrum disorders. Failure to develop verbal language in the absence of hearing loss should yield examination of physical and social–behavioral milestones to rule out overall delay and/or autism spectrum disorders.
- Neuromotor disorders. Neuromotor disorders may yield low facial/oral tone, weakness, or paralysis that may reduce speech intelligibility. Developmental apraxia of speech requires assessment and may coincide with limb apraxia.
- Vocal overuse or trauma. Evaluate for overuse patterns from habitual screaming, poor singing technique, and cheerleading.
- Structural and dental changes. Dental malocclusion or oral structural anomalies may reduce speech intelligibility for particular speech sounds.
- Sleep apnea. Poor sleep may be the cause of behavioral and learning concerns.
- Selective mutism. Specific situations in which the child will not speak in the absence of evident speech or language disorder; may coincide with social withdrawal, shyness, social anxiety
- Social isolation, neglect, or malnutrition should be ruled out, as these may associate with delays or losses of communication skills.
- Seizure disorders such as Landau-Kleffner syndrome can be associated with loss of language skills.

DIAGNOSTIC TESTS & INTERPRETATION

Initial Tests (screening, lab, imaging)

- Speech-language screening
  - Brief check on domains of communication designed to determine whether to refer child for full speech-language evaluation
  - Results often reported as "Pass/Refer" with minimal or no interpretation
  - May be conducted by speech-language pathologist, audiologist, teacher, or other professional
- Hearing screening
  - Brief assessment that may be conducted for newborns or older children to detect presence or absence of response to sound at a set hearing level across frequencies
  - Results often reported as "Pass/Refer" with minimal or no interpretation
  - Screening may be conducted by an audiologist, speech-language pathologist, nurse, or trained paraprofessional.

Diagnostic Procedures/Other

- Speech-language evaluation
  - Measurement of receptive, expressive, and/or pragmatic language skills; articulatory/phonologic development; and oral structural and physiologic examination with interpretation of findings and recommendations
  - Conducted by speech-language pathologist
- Hearing evaluation
  - Testing to obtain auditory thresholds (in decibels, dB) across sound frequencies (in Hertz, Hz) in both ears
  - If hearing loss is identified, further testing to determine if the source is middle ear (conductive) or inner ear (sensorineural) or mixed (both conductive and sensorineural)
  - Very young children may be tested using auditory brainstem response (ABR) or otoacoustic emissions (OAE).
  - Conducted by an audiologist
- Cognitive evaluation
  - Testing to assess overall cognitive development across verbal and nonverbal domains with results interpreted together with recommendations for interventions and/or school placement
  - Typically conducted by a psychologist
- Genetics evaluation and testing
  - Comprehensive family history, physical exam, metabolic, and/or cytogenetic testing often to identify or rule out specific diagnoses (e.g., fragile X, 22q deletion syndrome, neurofibromatosis, or genes associated with hereditary hearing impairment)
  - Interpretation of findings includes explanation to family of carrier status and recurrence risk.
  - Typically conducted by clinical geneticist or interdisciplinary genetics clinic
- Radiologic or other imaging studies: rarely used to assess underlying cause of speech or language disorders but may be used to rule out or identify related conditions such as intraventricular hemorrhage or swallowing and resonance disorders

TREATMENT

- Direct service
  - In-home services
    - Evaluation and treatment for high-risk infants and toddlers in family-centered, natural environment, with minimal or no expense to family
  - Clinic-based services. Evaluation and individual or group treatment through a medical center, private, or university speech–language–hearing clinic
    - May be needed for specialized services
  - School-based services
    - Evaluation, individual or group treatment usually through special education services that yield an individualized education plan (IEP)
    - Service delivery is often limited to conditions that impact the child's educational performance.
- Related services
  - Interdisciplinary team care
    - Children with complex medical needs should be served by an interdisciplinary team such as a cleft palate/craniofacial, spina bifida, autism, feeding, or multiple disability team clinic.
    - Provides comprehensive physical, functional, and psychosocial care of the child and family in collaboration with primary care providers
  - Otolaryngology. Detailed examination of laryngeal structures, airway, palatal structures, enlarged tonsils, and/or management of otologic concerns

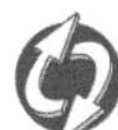

ONGOING CARE

- Early identification of hearing, speech, or language problems is critical and leads to better outcomes.
- Children who have untreated hearing, speech sound, and language disorders are at risk for academic difficulties.
- Many speech problems can be resolved with short-term treatment. Some conditions may require longer term management extending through adolescence.
- Adenoid removal is usually contraindicated for children with cleft palate, including submucous cleft palate. Airway and apnea management may be an exception that requires interdisciplinary decision making.

ADDITIONAL READING

- American Speech-Language-Hearing Association: http://www.asha.org
- Campbell TF, Dollaghan CA, Rockette HE, et al. Risk factors for speech delay of unknown origin in 3-year old children. *Child Dev*. 2003;74(2):346–357.
- Graham SA, Fisher SE. Decoding the genetics of speech and language. *Curr Opin Neurobiol*. 2013;23(1):43–51.
- Possamai V, Hartley B. Voice disorders in children. *Pediatr Clin North Am*. 2013;60(4):879–892.

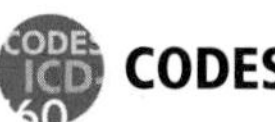

CODES

ICD10

- R47.9 Unspecified speech disturbances
- F80.81 Childhood onset fluency disorder
- R48.2 Apraxia

FAQ

- Q: Does ankyloglossia negatively affect speech production?
- A: The tongue tip is used for speech sounds /t, d, n, l, s, z/. If the child can make one or more of these sounds, then ankyloglossia can go untreated.
- Q: Does "baby sign" help or delay the acquisition of speech and language?
- A: Evidence suggests teaching gestural communication is associated with slightly advanced auditory–verbal language skills before 24 months of age and may decrease toddler–parent frustration. By 30 to 36 months of age, no significant differences are observed between children who used baby sign and those who did not.
- Q: Does chronic otitis media slow the acquisition of speech or language?
- A: Early speech and language may be delayed in the presence of otitis media. If treated, differences in language skills typically resolve by school age.

SPINAL MUSCULAR ATROPHY

Jessica Rose Nance, MS, MD

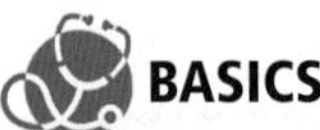

BASICS

DESCRIPTION

- Spinal muscular atrophy (SMA) is a progressive disorder of motor neurons in the spinal cord and brainstem.
- Major symptom is proximal weakness.
- Three forms are described based on clinical features:
  - Type I
    - Also known as Werdnig-Hoffman disease
    - Typically presents by 6 months of age
    - These children never sit.
  - Type II
    - Typically presents between 6 and 18 months of age
    - These children sit independently but never walk.
  - Type III
    - Also known as Kugelberg-Welander disease
    - May be diagnosed later; these children stand and walk at some point.
- There appears to be a spectrum of severity within and between each type.

EPIDEMIOLOGY

- 1 in 6,000 to 10,000 live births
- Carrier frequency 1 in 40 to 50, although some variation between populations seems to exist

RISK FACTORS

Genetics

- Genetic testing is recommended in all cases, even when the diagnosis appears clear.
- Genetic counseling is critical for all families with children affected by SMA, as the chance of recurrence is 25%.
- *SMN2* copy number varies among the general population and is loosely correlated with SMA type (type I likely to have fewer copies); however, all copies of *SMN2* are not equal (some make more SMN protein than others), and an individual patient's *SMN2* copy number should not be used for prognostic purposes.
- Universal newborn screening is strongly recommended by some but is controversial; a pilot study has been approved in limited states.

ETIOLOGY

- All three types of proximal SMA follow an autosomal recessive inheritance and are caused by mutations in the survival motor neuron (*SMN*) gene on 5q11.2 to 13.3.
- Two copies of *SMN* on each chromosome. *SMN1* (SMNt), the telomeric copy, produces stable SMN protein. *SMN2* (SMNc), the centromeric copy, is an inverted duplication of *SMN1* with a single nucleotide change in an exonic splice enhancer, which produces mostly an unstable, truncated protein product and a smaller percentage of stable, full-length SMN protein.
- Individuals with SMA harbor homozygous deletions of exon 7 in the *SMN1* gene, which renders it nonfunctional. The presence of *SMN2* essentially "rescues" individuals with *SMN1* deletions because complete absence of SMN protein appears to be embryonically lethal. The level of SMN protein roughly correlates with the severity of disease, making this a target of therapeutics development.
- The SMN protein plays a role in RNA processing; it is unclear why motor neurons (anterior horn cells) are selectively vulnerable to this defect, although a role in axonal mRNA trafficking and splicing is being explored.
- SMA appears to affect other organ systems, especially in those with the most severe form; cardiovascular, autonomic, and metabolic abnormalities are reported.

COMMONLY ASSOCIATED CONDITIONS

Other anterior horn cell diseases:

- SMA with respiratory distress (SMARD) or diaphragmatic SMA due to mutations in the *IGHMBP2* gene on chromosome 11q
- Distal SMAs, a group of disorders with distal weakness, genetically heterogeneous
- Other variants are associated with arthrogryposis, pontocerebellar hypoplasia, congenital fractures, and congenital heart disease. Few such cases have been shown to have *SMN* mutations.
- Fazio-Londe disease: rare degeneration of anterior horn cells in the brainstem, childhood onset
- Kennedy disease or X-linked spinal and bulbar muscular atrophy: anterior horn cell disease with adult onset; affected men have gynecomastia, bulbar weakness, and reduced fertility.

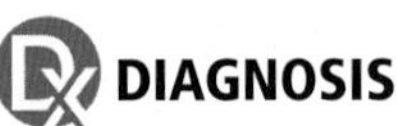

DIAGNOSIS

HISTORY

- Hypotonia and weakness are the primary features. Infants with SMA I will be floppy and less active and have delayed motor milestones, with preserved language/social interaction (a bright, alert demeanor is often remarked on).
- Some babies with type I present with feeding problems and failure to thrive.
- History of reduced vigor of prenatal movements

PHYSICAL EXAM

- Weakness and absent or reduced reflexes suggest a neuromuscular rather than central etiology for hypotonia. A proximal pattern of weakness is consistent with SMA, myopathies, and muscular dystrophies; a distal pattern usually suggests polyneuropathies.
- Weakness is almost universally symmetric, but occasional cases of asymmetric weakness have been reported in SMA III.
- Extraocular movements remain intact in SMA.
- Facial strength diminishes in children with type I over time, and jaw contractures may be present in type II.
- Dysmorphic features, or involvement of other organs, may point to alternative diagnoses. Occasionally, SMA presents with contractures (spectrum of arthrogryposis multiplex congenita).
- Tongue fasciculations strongly suggest SMA, but their absence does not exclude the diagnosis.
- Tremor of a specific type, polyminimyoclonus, is often present in type II and type III.

DIFFERENTIAL DIAGNOSIS

- Other genetic neuromuscular disorders include congenital muscular dystrophy, congenital myopathy, glycogen storage disorders (Pompe disease), myotonic dystrophy, mitochondrial disease, congenital myasthenia gravis, and Prader-Willi syndrome.
- More acute course may suggest infant botulism or Guillain-Barré syndrome, although the latter is rare in this age group.
- Systemic disorders: sepsis, meningitis, acute bowel syndromes
- SMA II differential: congenital muscular dystrophy, congenital myopathy, and congenital myasthenia gravis
- SMA III differential includes Duchenne, Becker, and the limb girdle muscular dystrophies; Lambert-Eaton myasthenic syndrome; and limb girdle congenital myasthenic syndromes.
- Spinal cord mass lesions rarely may resemble SMA.

DIAGNOSTIC TESTS & INTERPRETATION

Initial Tests (screening, lab, imaging)

- Initial screening tests: Serum creatine kinase may be mildly elevated.
- Genetic testing
  - Genetic testing of DNA extracted from blood (*SMN* deletions): now the gold standard in diagnosis, may be done prenatally, >95% sensitive
  - Genetic testing for Prader-Willi syndrome (fluorescence in situ hybridization and methylation) may be indicated if there is no *SMN* gene deletion and electromyography (EMG) is normal in an infant who appears to have SMA.
- Other testing
  - EMG may be helpful if the clinical presentation is atypical for SMA or if genetic testing is negative. EMG shows high-amplitude, long-duration motor units with a reduced recruitment pattern.
  - With the advent of molecular testing, muscle biopsy is rarely performed. Use when genetic testing is unrevealing. The characteristic findings are fiber-type grouping with generalized atrophy of muscle fibers.
  - If the entire evaluation is negative, MRI of the spine may be indicated to evaluate for an anomaly or mass lesion.

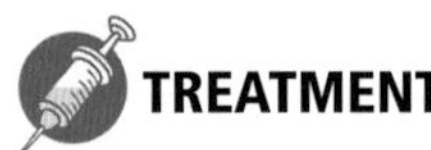

TREATMENT

ALERT

An apparently minor respiratory infection may carry a higher risk of respiratory failure in SMA I and later stages of SMA II and III. Depending on family/patient wishes regarding respiratory support, consider admitting such a patient to the hospital for observation. Infants with SMA may be exquisitely sensitive to postural shifts—watch for hypoventilation, for example, with forward truncal flexion associated with some seating arrangements.

GENERAL MEASURES

- Nusinersen is an antisense oligonucleotide therapy approved by United States Food and Drug Administration (FDA) in late 2016 for all types and ages of SMA patients. The therapy increases the expression of SMN2 protein and significantly improves motor function. Treatment appears to be most effective when given in the neonatal/infantile period, so prompt referral to a neuromuscular center is important.
- A multidisciplinary approach to care is recommended, with early and proactive involvement of orthopedics, nutrition, pulmonary, and physical and occupational therapy as well as social work and psychological support for families and patients.
- Physical therapy is appropriate for all three types; although it may not affect the course in SMA I, it can lessen discomfort and make care easier by improving range of motion and preventing contractures.
- A wheelchair provides mobility in SMA II. Children as young as age 2 years may be considered for a motorized wheelchair, depending on developmental level. Adults with SMA III may require the use of a wheelchair later in their course.
- Bracing of ankles, wrists, and back can help reduce contractures and slow progression of scoliosis.
- Spinal fusion surgery may preserve respiratory function.
- Low threshold for empiric antibiotics for respiratory infection is appropriate.
- Chest physiotherapy and early implementation of cough-assist device can help prevent pneumonia and atelectasis.
- Be wary of symptoms of hypoventilation (disturbed sleep, daytime fatigue, moodiness, morning headaches), which may occur prior to other symptoms of respiratory insufficiency.
- Low threshold to order a sleep study if hypoventilation is suspected
- In acute respiratory illness, supplemental oxygen is appropriate as long as the patient is also evaluated and treated for hypercarbia.
- Noninvasive positive pressure ventilation (bilevel positive airway pressure [BiPAP] and other regimens) may improve quality of life and life expectancy in patients with decreased respiratory function. More aggressive respiratory management is becoming more common and accepted among families and physicians, but the extent of interventions varies widely. Start discussions about family/patient preferences early, as respiratory decompensation can occur very quickly.
- Avoid catabolic state with proactive nutritional support, including tube feeding.
- However, note that type II patients may have increased adiposity, and overweight is also a risk.
- Monitor for osteopenia, which is almost universal in types I and II, and ensure adequate calcium and vitamin D intake.
- Social and psychological support for caregivers and patients

ONGOING CARE

PATIENT EDUCATION

- Cure SMA: http://www.curesma.org
- FightSMA: http://www.fightsma.org
- Muscular Dystrophy Association: http://www.mda.org
- SMA Foundation: http://www.smafoundation.org

PROGNOSIS

- Survival in all three forms has been increasing with improved supportive care and, in type I, ventilatory support. Nusinersen therapy especially in types I and II improves respiratory function and overall survival.
- SMA type I
  - Most children with SMA type I die by 2 years without major pulmonary interventions.
  - With ventilatory support, patients may survive several years longer; survival as long as 2 decades has been observed with tracheostomy and full mechanical ventilation
- SMA type II
  - Children with SMA type II typically survive into late adolescence or early adulthood.
  - This life expectancy is increasing with more aggressive pulmonary management.
- SMA type III
  - Individuals with SMA type III survive well into adulthood and often have a normal life expectancy.
  - In one study of patients with SMA type III with onset $<$3 years, 50% could not walk 20 years later; for those with onset $>$3 years, 30% could not walk 20 years later.
- Intelligence is generally preserved.
- Death typically ensues from respiratory complications.
- Discuss the level of respiratory interventions, including resuscitation, early in SMA I and in the advanced stages of SMA II and III.

COMPLICATIONS

- Recurrent pneumonias, hypoventilation
- Swallowing difficulties may require tube feeding.
- Scoliosis may require surgery.

ADDITIONAL READING

- Arnold WD, Burghes AH. Spinal muscular atrophy: development and implementation of potential treatments. *Ann Neurol*. 2013;74(3):348–362.
- Chung BH, Wong VC, Ip P. Spinal muscular atrophy: survival pattern and functional status. *Pediatrics*. 2004;114(5):e548–e553.
- Hardart MK, Truog RD. Spinal muscular atrophy—type I. *Arch Dis Child*. 2003;88(10):848–850.
- Iannaccone ST, Burghes A. Spinal muscular atrophies. *Adv Neurol*. 2002;88:83–98.
- Khirani S, Colella M, Caldarelli V, et al. Longitudinal course of lung function and respiratory muscle strength in spinal muscular atrophy type 2 and 3. *Eur J Paediatr Neurol*. 2013;17(6):552–560.
- Kolb SJ, Kissel JT. Spinal muscular atrophy: a timely review. *Arch Neurol*. 2011;68(8):979–984.
- Lunn MR, Wang CH. Spinal muscular atrophy. *Lancet*. 2008;371(9630):2120–2133.
- Messina S, Pane M, De Rose P, et al. Feeding problems and malnutrition in spinal muscular atrophy type II. *Neuromuscul Disord*. 2008;18(5):389–393.
- Ogino S, Leonard DG, Rennert H, et al. Genetic risk assessment in carrier testing for spinal muscular atrophy. *Am J Med Genet*. 2002;110(4):301–307.
- Petit F, Cuisset JM, Rouaix-Emery N, et al. Insights into genotype-phenotype correlations in spinal muscular atrophy: a retrospective study of 103 patients. *Muscle Nerve*. 2011;43(1):26–30.
- Prasad AN, Prasad C. The floppy infant: contribution of genetic and metabolic disorders. *Brain Dev*. 2003;25(7):457–476.
- Prior TW, Snyder PJ, Rink BD, et al. Newborn and carrier screening for spinal muscular atrophy. *Am J Med Genet A*. 2010;152A(7):1608–1616.
- Shababi M, Lorson CL, Rudnik-Schöneborn SS. Spinal muscular atrophy: a motor neuron disorder or a multi-organ disease? *J Anat*. 2014;224(1):15–28.
- Wang CH, Finkel RS, Bertini ES, et al; for Participants of the International Conference on SMA Standard of Care. Consensus statement for standard of care in spinal muscular atrophy. *J Child Neurol*. 2007;22(8):1027–1049.
- Zerres K, Rudnik-Schöneborn S. Natural history in proximal spinal muscular atrophy. Clinical analysis of 445 patients and suggestions for a modification of existing classifications. *Arch Neurol*. 1995;52(5):518–523.

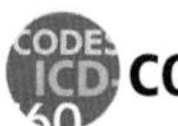

CODES

ICD10

- G12.9 Spinal muscular atrophy, unspecified
- G12.0 Infantile spinal muscular atrophy, type I [Werdnig-Hoffman]
- G12.1 Other inherited spinal muscular atrophy

FAQ

- Q: Can routine vaccinations be given to children with SMA?
- A: Yes. In addition to routine vaccinations, yearly influenza and respiratory syncytial virus (RSV) vaccinations are recommended.
- Q: How much respiratory support should a child with SMA receive?
- A: Standards of care are evolving rapidly, and a consensus remains elusive. Noninvasive respiratory interventions are becoming more widely accepted. Noninvasive respiratory options should be offered to all patients with SMA I and those in the later stages of SMA II. Tracheostomy is more controversial.
- Q: Are more effective therapies for SMA being developed?
- A: There are ongoing studies in animal models and on humans, involving both pharmacologic and gene-based therapies. Patients and families should be informed about clinical trials that may be available to them. Cure SMA, the Muscular Dystrophy Association, and other groups, as well as Clinicaltrials.gov, are sources of information on such research.

SPLENOMEGALY

Tiffany F. Lin, MD

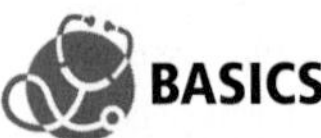

BASICS

DESCRIPTION

- Splenomegaly can be an incidental finding on imaging or examination or it can present with left upper quadrant pain.
- Thorough history often can differentiate the various causes of splenomegaly.
- Normal spleen sizes correlate with height and age. It can range from 5 cm in a newborn to >13 cm for adolescents.
- A palpable spleen is found in most premature infants and in 30% of term infants. A spleen tip is still palpable in 10% of infants at 1 year of age and in 1% of children at 10 years of age.
- The clinical significance of splenomegaly found on a radiologic study but not palpable on physical exam is unclear in the absence of other laboratory or clinical data.

PATHOPHYSIOLOGY

- The spleen is a hematopoietic organ with two main parts:
  - White pulp is the lymphoid tissue.
  - Red pulp is the red cell mass.
- Splenic sinusoids are lined with macrophages that destroy abnormal red cells and other cells or opsonized bacteria that need to be removed from the circulation.
- The lymphoid function of the spleen makes up about 25% of the lymph tissue of the body.
- The spleen also serves as a reservoir for platelets. A normal-sized spleen can hold 1/3 of the circulating platelets; an enlarged spleen can hold up to 90% of the circulating platelet mass.

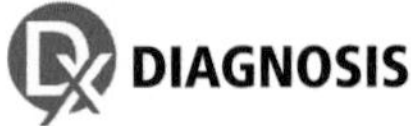

DIAGNOSIS

HISTORY

- Etiologies of pediatric splenomegaly include congenital growths, deposition of lipids or storage disorders, robust hemolytic disease, infiltrative process, inflammatory or infectious causes, or abnormal blood flow (lack of venous drainage in portal hypertension).
- Family history should include history of hemolytic disease or anemia, any need for spleen removal, or history of early childhood death.
- Proceeding illness, symptoms, and travel history can lead to infectious diagnoses.
- Developmental history and growth delay can be related to storage disorders.
- Infiltrative neoplastic processes are associated with other signs or symptoms of neoplasia.

PHYSICAL EXAM

Begin the abdominal examination in the lower left quadrant because an enlarged spleen may be missed in the upper quadrant exam. Stand to the right of the patient; use the right hand to palpate and the left hand to support the patient's left lower rib cage. Flexing the legs at the knees may help to relax the abdominal musculature.

- Normal spleens are generally soft at the midclavicular line, nontender, and often palpable only on deep inspiration.
- Dullness on percussion beyond the 11th intercostal space suggests splenomegaly.
- A spleen edge palpated >2 cm below the costal margin is always an abnormal finding.
- Splenic tenderness is always abnormal.
- Other important exam findings: Check for prominent abdominal veins or hepatomegaly, lymphadenopathy.
- Consider retinal exam if patient has other stigmata of storage disease.

DIFFERENTIAL DIAGNOSIS

- Infectious causes are the most common in an otherwise previously healthy pediatric patient.
  - Viral
    - Epstein-Barr virus (EBV) (mononucleosis)—most common
    - Cytomegalovirus
    - HIV
    - Rubella
    - Herpes
    - Hepatitis A, B, C
  - Bacterial
    - Sepsis
    - Subacute bacterial endocarditis
    - Salmonellosis
    - Tuberculosis
    - Brucellosis
    - Staphylococcal shunt infections
    - Tularemia
    - Syphilis
    - Leptospirosis
  - Rickettsial/protozoan
    - Rocky Mountain spotted fever
    - Malaria
    - Toxoplasmosis
    - Trypanosomiasis
    - Babesiosis
    - Schistosomiasis
    - Visceral larval migrans
    - Kala azar
  - Fungal
    - Histoplasmosis
    - Coccidioidomycosis
- Hematologic disorders can cause mild persistent splenomegaly due to ongoing hemolysis and spleen hyperfunctioning.
  - Hereditary spherocytosis
  - Sickle cell disease in early childhood or during splenic sequestration crisis, later the spleen involutes
  - Hemoglobin C disease
  - Thalassemia major
  - Autoimmune hemolytic anemia
  - Glucose-6-phosphate dehydrogenase deficiency (rare in settings of hemolysis)
  - Infantile pyknocytosis
- Vascular disorders
  - Cavernous transformation of the portal vein
  - Budd-Chiari syndrome
  - Splenic vein thrombosis
  - Congenital portal vein stenosis or atresia
  - Splenic hematoma
  - Splenic hemangioma
- Neoplastic diseases cause splenomegaly by infiltrating the spleen.
  - Leukemia
  - Lymphoma
  - Lymphosarcoma
  - Neuroblastoma
  - Histiocytosis X
  - Familial hemophagocytic lymphohistiocytosis

- Metabolic diseases (storage)
  - Gangliosidoses
  - Mucolipidoses
  - Metachromatic leukodystrophy
  - Wolman disease
  - Gaucher disease
  - Niemann-Pick disease
  - Amyloidosis
- Liver disease/cirrhosis can cause portal hypertension leading to splenic enlargement.
- Miscellaneous
  - Serum sickness
  - Connective tissue disorders
  - Juvenile rheumatoid arthritis
  - Systemic lupus erythematosus
  - Sarcoidosis
  - Splenic hamartoma
  - Splenic cysts: congenital and posttraumatic
  - Trauma: subcapsular hematoma

ALERT

- Life-threatening causes: sepsis, severe hemolytic anemia, trauma, splenic sequestration
- A large-bore IV access route should be rapidly placed when a life-threatening cause is suspected.

DIAGNOSTIC TESTS & INTERPRETATION

- Lab testing should be directed toward the suspected cause of splenomegaly.
- Infectious etiology: cultures, malaria smear, viral testing, and EBV evaluation
- Hemolytic disease: CBC with differential and manual smear review
- Follow platelet counts as they can be decreased in splenic sequestration.
- Imaging can be useful in cases of evaluation of extrasplenic causes of disease.
- If no hemolytic disease, no sign of infection, no sign of congestion:
  - Ultrasound with Doppler
- If no hemolytic disease, no sign of infection but signs of congestion:
  - Ultrasound with Doppler
  - MRI; consider Magnetic Resonance Angiography (MRA)/Magnetic Resonance Venography (MRV).

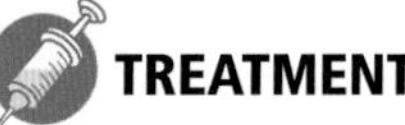

TREATMENT

GENERAL MEASURES

- Treatment depends on underlying etiology.
- Spleen guards can be used to protect from traumatic splenic rupture.

ISSUES FOR REFERRAL

- Increasing size over serial examinations (hepatology, hematology/oncology)
- Unexplained lymphadenopathy (oncology)
- Liver dysfunction and/or ascites (hepatology)
- Signs of storage or metabolic disease (metabolism, GI)
- Howell-Jolly bodies on peripheral smear, suggesting splenic dysfunction (hematology)

SURGERY/OTHER PROCEDURES

Splenectomy indicated in certain situations including symptomatic hematologic disorders, abscess, and neoplasms

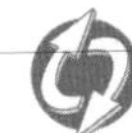

ONGOING CARE

General goal is to determine the etiology of the large spleen.

- Establish the presence of enlarged spleen, not a palpable spleen that is pushed down by inflated lungs.
- Rule out common causes such as a viral infection, bacterial infection, or anemia.
- Rule out malignancy or storage disease or other rare causes of large spleen.
- Ensure proper immunizations or antibiotic prophylaxis (see "FAQ").
- Ongoing care depends on the underlying etiology of the splenomegaly.

ADDITIONAL READING

- Benter T, Klühs L, Teichgräber U. Sonography of the spleen. *J Ultrasound Med*. 2011;30(9):1281–1293.
- Donnelly LF, Foss JN, Frush DP, et al. Heterogeneous splenic enhancement patterns on spiral CT images in children: minimizing misinterpretation. *Radiology*. 1999;210(2):493–497.
- Konuş OL, Ozdemir A, Akkaya A, et al. Normal liver, spleen, and kidney dimensions in neonates, infants, and children: evaluation with sonography. *AJR Am J Roentgenol*. 1998;171(6):1693–1698.
- McCormick PA, Murphy KM. Splenomegaly, hypersplenism and coagulation abnormalities in liver disease. *Baillieres Best Pract Res Clin Gastroenterol*. 2000;14(6):1009–1031.
- Pozo AL, Godfrey EM, Bowles KM. Splenomegaly: investigation, diagnosis and management. *Blood Rev*. 2009;23(3):105–111.

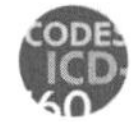

CODES

ICD10

- R16.1 Splenomegaly, not elsewhere classified
- D73.5 Infarction of spleen
- D18.03 Hemangioma of intra-abdominal structures

FAQ

- Q: How long will the enlarged spleen secondary to a viral infection be present?
- A: The enlarged spleen may persist for several months.
- Q: Should patients with decreased splenic function due to splenomegaly be immunized?
- A: Immunization with a pneumococcal conjugate and/or polysaccharide vaccine should be carried out in all patients with compromised splenic function. In those patients who will be undergoing a scheduled splenectomy, the *Streptococcus pneumoniae*, meningococcus, and *Haemophilus influenzae* type B vaccines should be given at least 14 days prior to the operation.
- Q: Should a child with an enlarged spleen refrain from sports?
- A: Contact sports should be avoided for a child with an enlarged spleen. An enlarged spleen is engorged with blood, and a splenic rupture would be a catastrophic event. Children with persistent splenomegaly should be considered for a spleen guard.

SPONDYLOARTHROPATHY

Melissa L. Mannion, MD, MSPH • Randy Q. Cron, MD, PhD

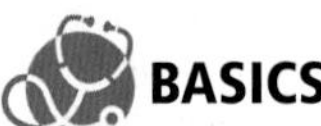

BASICS

DESCRIPTION

A group of rheumatic diseases characterized by axial and/or peripheral arthritis and enthesitis (inflammation at the bony insertion of tendons and ligaments)

- Enthesitis-related arthritis
- Ankylosing spondylitis (AS)
- Psoriatic arthritis
- Inflammatory bowel disease–associated arthropathy
- Reactive arthritis

EPIDEMIOLOGY

- Spondyloarthritis accounts for 15–20% of juvenile arthritis or more.
- Nonradiographic axial spondyloarthritis (male = female)
- AS typically affects adolescent boys (male-to-female ratio is 2 to 3:1).

Prevalence

Prevalence of AS mirrors that of HLA-B27 in a population

- European descent 8% HLA-B27+ and 0.5% AS

RISK FACTORS

Genetics

- HLA-B27 associated
- Risk of developing ERA with HLA-B27 is approximately 1–3%. Usually, there is a family history of a male relative with the disease.
- HLA-B27–positive with a family history of AS have a 10-fold increased risk of AS compared to HLA-B27–positive person with no family history.

PATHOPHYSIOLOGY

- Inflammatory synovitis of joints and inflammation at sites of ligament and tendon attachment to bone (entheses).
- Progression to ankylosis is a result of calcification of the anterior and posterior longitudinal ligaments of the spine.

ETIOLOGY

- Autoimmune or autoinflammatory arthritis of unknown etiology, likely multifactorial
- Microbiome may play a role in disease.

DIAGNOSIS

- Inflammatory back pain (better with exercise, not relieved by rest) of insidious onset that has been present for at least 6 weeks
- Inactivity stiffness resulting in gelling of peripheral joints and back
- Arthritis and/or enthesitis
  - Axial arthritis typically sacroiliitis

HISTORY

- Inflammatory back pain and joint pain/swelling
- Morning stiffness
- Family history

PHYSICAL EXAM

- Sacroiliac (SI) tenderness
  - Indicates site of inflammation
- Pain on direct palpation at insertion of Achilles tendon, metatarsal heads, inferior and superior patellar poles, and plantar fascia at calcaneal insertion (location of entheses)
  - Indicates site of inflammation
- Peripheral arthritis typically asymmetric large joints
- Patrick test (FABER)
  - FABER stands for "Flexion, ABduction and External Rotation"
  - A series of maneuvers to screen for issues with the SI and hip joints
- Psoriasis, nail pitting, or dactylitis

DIFFERENTIAL DIAGNOSIS

- Caution
  - Overdiagnosis in HLA-B27–positive individuals in whom other causes for joint swelling should be considered.
- Infection
  - Reactive arthritis caused by enteric pathogens or *Chlamydia* species
  - Whipple disease
  - Intestinal bypass–associated arthritis
  - Discitis
  - Pott disease (vertebral tuberculosis)
- Tumors
  - Osteoid osteoma
  - Osteoblastoma
- Trauma
  - Traumatic injury causing lower back pain/spasm
  - Herniated disk
  - Spondylolysis/spondylolisthesis
- Metabolic
  - Ochronosis
- Congenital
  - Kyphosis
- Immunologic
  - Oligoarticular juvenile idiopathic arthritis
- Psychological
  - Feigning lower back pain/stiffness
- Miscellaneous
  - Fibromyalgia
  - Muscle stiffness without inflammation

DIAGNOSTIC TESTS & INTERPRETATION

Schober test of lumbar spine flexibility

- Mark 15-cm vertical span at mid-lower back at level of iliac crest while patient is standing.
- Have patient bend forward at the waist as far as possible without bending knees.
- Remeasure span.
- Abnormal if <5 cm increase in span

Initial Tests (screening, lab, imaging)
- CBC, erythrocyte sedimentation rate (ESR), HLA-B27
- ESR is often elevated.
- Rheumatoid factor and antinuclear antibodies are typically negative.
- Imaging
  - SI views
    - Demonstrate evidence of pseudowidening, erosions, and/or sclerosis; fusion is a late finding.
    - Because radiographic findings may take years to develop in the presence of disease, MRI is supplanting radiographs as the initial modality to assess SI involvement in many centers.

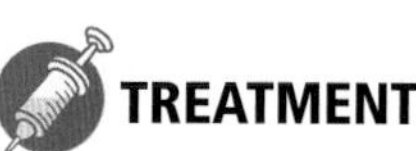

TREATMENT

GENERAL MEASURES
- Therapy may need to be lifelong.
- After initiation of therapy, should see some improvement in stiffness, synovitis, and range of motion over weeks to several months
- Only tumor necrosis factor (TNF) inhibitors are effective for axial involvement.

MEDICATION
- NSAIDs
  - Naproxen
  - Indomethacin
  - Diclofenac
- Disease-modifying drugs
  - Sulfasalazine
  - Methotrexate
  - Leflunomide
  - TNF inhibitors

ADDITIONAL THERAPIES
Physical therapy
- Physical therapy is an essential component of treatment.
- Must encourage range-of-motion exercises and avoid prolonged neck flexion

SURGERY/OTHER PROCEDURES
In advanced cases, total hip replacement, C-spine fusion, and/or spinal wedge osteotomy (the latter if posture is severely affected)

ONGOING CARE

DIET
- Ensure food intake with NSAIDs.
- Ensure folate intake with methotrexate.

PATIENT EDUCATION
Activity
- As tolerated. In cases of severe/advanced disease, modify behaviors accordingly in consideration of reduced spine flexibility and subsequent risk of serious injury.

PROGNOSIS
Poor if disease remains active for 10 years or more

COMPLICATIONS
- Acute anterior uveitis
- Aortic insufficiency
- Worsening stiffness
- Ankylosis with risk of vertebral subluxation, fracture, and nerve damage, including cauda equina syndrome
- Chest pain or shortness of breath

ALERT
A red, painful eye in a patient with HLA-B27–positive spondyloarthropathy should not be assumed to be infectious conjunctivitis. Slit-lamp exam is required to diagnose acute anterior uveitis.

ADDITIONAL READING

- Altaf F, Heran MKS, Wilson LF. Back pain in children and adolescents. *Bone Joint J*. 2014;96-B(6):717–723.
- Colbert RA. Early axial spondyloarthritis. *Curr Opin Rheumatol*. 2010;22(5):603–607.
- Homeff G, Burgos-Vargas R. TNF-alpha antagonists for the treatment of juvenile-onset spondyloarthritides. *Clin Exp Rheumatol*. 2002;20(6 Suppl 28):S137–S142.
- Ramanathan A, Srinivasalu H, Colbert RA. Update on juvenile spondyloarthritis. *Rheum Dis Clin North Am*. 2013;39(4):767–788.
- Sherry DD, Sapp LR. Enthesalgia in childhood: site-specific tenderness in healthy subjects and in patients with seronegative enthesopathic arthropathy. *J Rheumatol*. 2003;30(6):1335–1340.
- Sieper J, Poddubnyy D. Axial spondyloarthritis. *Lancet*. 2017;390(10089):73–84.
- Stoll ML, Cron RQ. The microbiota in pediatric rheumatic disease: epiphenomenon or therapeutic target? *Curr Opin Rheumatol*. 2016;28(5):537–543.
- Stoll ML, Lio P, Sundel RP, et al. Comparison of Vancouver and International League of Associations for rheumatology classification criteria for juvenile psoriatic arthritis. *Arthritis Rheum*. 2008;59(1):51–58.
- Tse SM, Laxer RM. New advances in juvenile spondyloarthritis. *Nat Rev Rheumatol*. 2012;8(5):269–279.
- Tse SM, Laxer RM, Babyn PS, et al. Radiologic improvement of juvenile idiopathic arthritis-enthesitis-related arthritis following anti-tumor necrosis factor-alpha blockade with etanercept. *J Rheumatol*. 2006;33(6):1186–1188.

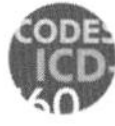

CODES

ICD10
- M12.88 Oth specific arthropathies, NEC, vertebrae
- M46.1 Sacroiliitis, not elsewhere classified
- M45.9 Ankylosing spondylitis of unspecified sites in spine

FAQ
- Q: Should HLA-B27 be checked routinely in boys with back pain?
- A: Inflammatory back, joint, or entheseal pain; family history; and exam findings should increase your suspicion for HLA-B27–positive disease. Detection of HLA-B27 alone should not precipitate an extensive workup because it is so common in the normal healthy population.
- Q: Can affected individuals play contact sports?
- A: This is probably not a good idea in patients with ankylosis because as the spine fuses, the risk for fracture of the spine (especially the cervical spine) increases. However, children with milder forms of disease, such as enthesitis-related arthritis, should not be discouraged from participation in activities.
- Q: What class of medicines has been shown to help prevent spinal ankylosis?
- A: TNF inhibitors

STAPHYLOCOCCAL SCALDED SKIN SYNDROME

Lauren G. Solan, MD, MEd • Craig H. Gosdin, MD, MSHA

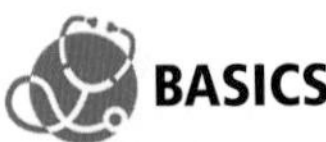

BASICS

DESCRIPTION

- A spectrum of generalized exfoliative skin disease with blistering of the upper layer of skin caused by an epidermolytic toxin produced by certain strains of *Staphylococcus aureus*
- In neonates and young infants, also known as Ritter disease or pemphigus neonatorum
- Classically described as skin tenderness and erythema, with bullae formation and desquamation
- Severity of the disease ranges from
  - Few blisters localized to site of infection
  - Mild illness with desquamation of skinfolds following impetigo
  - Generalized severe exfoliation involving much of the body (typically seen in neonates)
  - Classic staphylococcal scalded skin syndrome (SSSS): tenderness, erythema, desquamation, or bullae formation; may resemble scalding injury

EPIDEMIOLOGY

- Most cases occur in neonates and children <5 years of age, although can occur at any age.
- Rare in adults due to increased circulating antibodies and adult kidney excretion of the toxin

Incidence

- No differences in incidence based on gender in children; however, in adults, the male-to-female ratio is 2:1.
- Increased incidence in children reported during summer and fall months

RISK FACTORS

- Immunocompromised state (in children or adults)
  - Maternal antibodies transferred via breast milk are partially protective, but neonatal cases can still occur.
- Increased *S. aureus* carriage and susceptibility to toxin (usually in adults)
- Renal impairment either due to immature renal clearance of toxin in children or underlying renal disease

GENERAL PREVENTION

- Good hand hygiene practices, including adherence to contact precautions in hospitalized patients, to prevent spread from asymptomatic carriers
- Prevent skin from becoming overly moist or macerated.
- Isolation of hospitalized patient
  - Suspected or documented cases should be placed in contact isolation.

PATHOPHYSIOLOGY

- Results from *S. aureus* infection and subsequent exfoliative toxin production
- Exfoliative toxins circulate throughout the body, causing blisters at sites distant from the infection.
- Destruction of protein desmoglein 1 (attachment protein found only in the superficial epidermis) by exfoliative toxin A (ETA) and exfoliative toxin B (ETB) causes intraepidermal splitting leading to bullae development and skin desquamation.

ETIOLOGY

Exfoliative toxin released by *S. aureus*:

- Two major serotypes of the toxin: ETA and ETB
- Mostly caused by *S. aureus* belonging to phage group II, types 71 and 55

COMMONLY ASSOCIATED CONDITIONS

- Normal skin colonization with *S. aureus* with break in skin leading to systemic infection
- Skin and soft tissue infections or abscesses
- Bullous impetigo

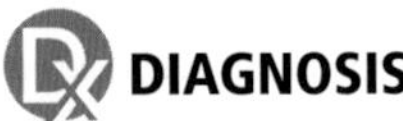

DIAGNOSIS

ALERT

Diagnosis is primarily clinical; cultures and other diagnostic tests are largely confirmatory; late recognition can lead to delayed therapy and shock.

- Differentiation from toxic epidermal necrolysis (TEN) is critical, as therapy is very different.
- Confusion with TEN may lead to use of corticosteroids or discontinuation of antibiotics, resulting in worsening infection from prolonged toxin production.
- Differentiation from streptococcal disease is important, as SSSS requires treatment with penicillinase-resistant antibiotic therapy (e.g., nafcillin).

HISTORY

- Nonspecific virus-like prodrome with irritability, sore throat, conjunctivitis, and upper respiratory infection is typical.
- Usual onset of fever within 48 hours after prodrome
- Rash typically begins periorally, then extends to the trunk and extremities, and finally desquamates.
- Recent localized extracutaneous infection is common.
  - Infections involving the nasopharynx, middle ear, conjunctivae, pharynx, tonsils, umbilicus, or urinary tract are frequently recalled.
- A history of recent drug use suggests other etiology such as TEN.

PHYSICAL EXAM

- Rash initially appears as faint, erythematous, and tender areas.
- Erythroderma: red, painful skin
- Large flaccid bullae that leave behind denuded skin resembling a burn after rupturing appear within 1 to 2 days.
  - Bullae often appear in areas of trauma or in areas that are rubbed or touched, including intertriginous zones.
- Nikolsky sign
  - Gentle friction applied to apparently healthy skin will cause blistering and sloughing.
  - Appears within 1 to 2 days
- Distribution of lesions: most commonly face, neck, axilla, perineum
- Facial edema with perioral and periocular crustiness is typical and may be the primary clinical features.
- Conjunctivitis with or without periorbital edema may also be present.

ALERT

- Nikolsky sign can be seen in both TEN and SSSS, but in SSSS, it is often noted over areas of unaffected skin as well.
- SSSS does NOT involve the mucous membranes, but TEN does.

DIFFERENTIAL DIAGNOSIS

- TEN
- Kawasaki disease
- Bullous impetigo
- Erythema multiforme bullosum
- Erythema multiforme major (Stevens-Johnson syndrome)
- Streptococcal scarlet fever
- Streptococcal or staphylococcal toxic shock syndrome (TSS)
- Bullous varicella
- Burns, including inflicted burns in suspected child abuse
- Primary bullous disorders (e.g., bullous mastocytosis)
- Chronic bullous disease of childhood
- Pemphigus vulgaris or foliaceus
- Epidermolysis bullosa

DIAGNOSTIC TESTS & INTERPRETATION

Initial Tests (screening, lab, imaging)

- Diagnosis is primarily clinical.
- General: CBC may be normal; erythrocyte sedimentation rate (ESR) typically elevated; electrolytes and renal function should be followed closely in severe cases and cases with dehydration.
- Microbiologic diagnosis: Culture of the original infected site, other involved sites/abnormal skin, blood, urine, nasopharynx, and umbilicus should be performed to determine the organism and antibiotic susceptibility.
  - Typically isolate phage group II *S. aureus*
  - Some immunologic methods exist to specifically identify the exfoliative exotoxins.
  - Intact bullae are sterile.
  - Blood cultures are typically negative in children (generally positive in adults).

Diagnostic Procedures/Other
- Skin biopsy can be used for histologic diagnosis to differentiate SSSS from TEN.
- SSSS demonstrates separation of the epidermis at the granular layer, whereas with TEN, there is necrosis of the entire epidermis with a deeper plane of separation at the basement membrane.

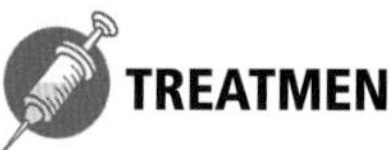

TREATMENT

GENERAL MEASURES
- Hospitalization is necessary for IV antibiotic therapy and supportive care.
- Recommend dermatology consultation.
- Consider consultation with infectious disease.
- Apply principles of good burn care in severe cases, including the following:
  - Consideration of management in a critical care setting, particularly for severe cases and/or high-risk patients
  - Aggressive and early fluid and electrolyte management including daily maintenance requirements in addition to replacement of increased insensible skin losses
  - Petrolatum gauze should cover eroded areas to prevent further skin trauma.
  - Blisters should be left intact.
  - Children should be allowed to rest unclothed on clean linens, and handling of the child should be kept to a minimum.
  - Use of pressure-relieving mattresses
  - Pain control regimen

MEDICATION
- 1st-line agent: parenteral antistaphylococcal antibiotics: nafcillin, oxacillin, or 1st-generation cephalosporin (e.g., cefazolin)
- Some experts add clindamycin to inhibit exotoxin production.
- Clindamycin or vancomycin can be used for penicillin-allergic patients (severe allergies), although clindamycin-resistant strains have been reported.
- 2nd-line agent: vancomycin for severe cases with toxic-appearing patient or concern for methicillin-resistant *S. aureus* (MRSA)
  - MRSA is rare but can occur.
- Antibiotic therapy can be tailored once sensitivities are known.
- Topical antibiotics are of no benefit.
- Oral antibiotics are not effective initially, but once a clear response has been noted with parenteral antibiotics, an oral antibiotic active against *S. aureus* can be used to complete the course of therapy.
- Corticosteroids have been shown to be detrimental both in experimental animal models as well as clinical trials.
- Adequate pain management is essential; consider acetaminophen and opiates.
- Can consider fresh frozen plasma (FFP) in critically ill children to neutralize exotoxin antibodies (success documented only in pediatric case series)
- Can consider IV immunoglobulin (IVIG) in critically ill children to neutralize the exotoxin (benefit shown in pediatric patients but no RCT studies done)

ALERT
- Avoid nonsteroidal anti-inflammatories for pain due to potential for renal impairment.
- Avoid steroids in SSSS.

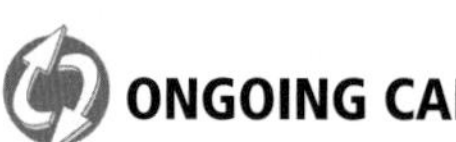

ONGOING CARE

FOLLOW-UP RECOMMENDATIONS
- Close follow-up with primary care provider recommended to ensure patient is recovering as expected
- As dermatology is typically involved in these cases, follow up with dermatology is also recommended.

DIET
No dietary restrictions after discharge

PATIENT EDUCATION
- Oral antibiotics should be continued after discharge for prescribed period of time, typically a total of 14 days.
- Follow-up with primary care provider and dermatology as recommended
- Skin typically heals well without scarring.

PROGNOSIS
- Usually complete recovery within 10 to 14 days *without* scarring if treated
- Prognosis is more guarded in infants and those with underlying illness.
- With early diagnosis and appropriate treatment, childhood mortality typically <5%, whereas adult mortality reported up to >60%
- Does not tend to recur

COMPLICATIONS
- Occasional shedding of hair and nails
- Fungal or bacterial superinfection following desquamation
- Serious fluid and electrolyte disturbances may occur in cases involving large surface areas, which may lead to poor temperature control, sepsis, shock, and death.
- Neonates are particularly susceptible to complications.

ADDITIONAL READING

- Braunstein I, Wanat KA, Abuabara K, et al. Antibiotic sensitivity and resistance patterns in pediatric staphylococcal scalded skin syndrome. *Pediatr Dermatol*. 2014;31(3):305–308.
- Handler MZ, Schwartz RA. Staphylococcal scalded skin syndrome: diagnosis and management in children and adults. *J Eur Acad Dermatol Venereol*. 2014;28(11):1418–1423.
- Patel GK, Finlay AY. Staphylococcal scalded skin syndrome: diagnosis and management. *Am J Clin Dermatol*. 2003;4(3):165–175.
- Schenfeld LA. Images in clinical medicine. Staphylococcal scalded skin syndrome. *N Engl J Med*. 2000;342(16):1178.
- Stanley JR, Amagai M. Pemphigus, bullous impetigo, and the staphylococcal scalded-skin syndrome. *N Engl J Med*. 2006;355(17):1800–1810.

CODES

ICD10
L00 Staphylococcal scalded skin syndrome

FAQ
- Q: Can SSSS recur?
- A: Yes, although it is uncommon.
- Q: Is SSSS contagious?
- A: Yes. The staphylococci are spread primarily from person to person (familial clusters have been reported), even from mother to fetus, most efficiently by someone with lesions, but asymptomatic carriers may also spread infection. Spread of organisms does not necessarily lead to signs of toxin production in those acquiring infection.
- Q: How can one distinguish TEN from SSSS?
- A: TEN is frequently confused with SSSS and may be differentiated by skin biopsy showing cleavage plane at the dermal–epidermal junction. TEN is more common in older children and adults and is usually secondary to drug hypersensitivity (e.g., sulfonamides, barbiturates, pyrazolone derivatives).
- Q: Can *Staphylococcus* be isolated from the bullae?
- A: SSSS bullae are sterile, although organisms may be found in a distant focus, such as the nares or conjunctivae. In bullous impetigo, however, staphylococci may be isolated from the bullae.

STATUS EPILEPTICUS

Rajesh K. Daftary, MD, MPH • Adam L. Numis, MD

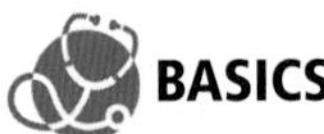

BASICS

DESCRIPTION

- Status epilepticus (SE) is defined as a continuous seizure lasting >30 minutes or recurrent seizures without return to baseline in between. After 30 minutes, ischemic injury to the brain is more likely to occur. Seizures lasting >5 minutes are unlikely to resolve without anticonvulsant therapy and are likely to progress to SE without intervention.
- SE presents in several forms:
  - Generalized SE: continuous or repeated generalized convulsion(s) with persistent loss of consciousness and neurologic function
  - Nonconvulsive SE, myoclonic SE, or absence SE: persistent encephalopathy, often with variable subtle motor signs such as myoclonus or nystagmus
  - Repeated partial seizures with alteration of consciousness (focal SE) or preserved consciousness (epilepsia partialis continua)
- Systemic complications of SE:
  - Hyperthermia, rhabdomyolysis
  - Tachycardia, hypertension early → hypotension late
  - Hypoxia, hypercapnia, aspiration pneumonia
  - Impaired cerebral autoregulation
  - Rare: cardiac arrhythmias, neurogenic pulmonary edema, bone fractures

ALERT

- Neuromuscular blockers used in intubation may obscure ongoing seizures. EEG monitoring is mandatory for all patients who have had any pharmacologic paralysis during SE.
- Continued encephalopathy after convulsions have stopped may indicate ongoing electrographic seizures (nonconvulsive SE), found in up to 30% of children after treated SE.
- Nonepileptic seizures can be mistaken for SE. EEG establishes the diagnosis.

EPIDEMIOLOGY

- Incidence in pediatric patients is 17 to 23/100,000. In children <1 year old, incidence is 135 to 156/100,000.
- ~40–70% of children have no history of seizures.

RISK FACTORS

- Known epilepsy
- Remote or acute central nervous system (CNS) insult
- History of previous SE
- Low anticonvulsant drug levels
- Younger age

GENERAL PREVENTION

- Adherence to the anticonvulsant medication regimen and clinical follow-up in patients with epilepsy
- Avoid rapid changes in anticonvulsants unless urgently needed.
- Prompt treatment of convulsive seizures

PATHOPHYSIOLOGY

SE may be related to acute or chronic factors or frequently of unknown etiology.

- Common acute factors:
  - Fever
  - Infectious meningoencephalitis
  - Metabolic: electrolyte abnormalities, hypoglycemia
  - Intoxications
  - Trauma or hemorrhage
  - Ischemic stroke, hypoxic-ischemic injury
  - Medications: low anticonvulsant drug levels or abrupt withdrawal of anticonvulsants, inappropriate anticonvulsants (e.g., absence SE with phenytoin or carbamazepine use in generalized epilepsy or with tiagabine in focal epilepsy)
- Subacute or chronic factors:
  - Epilepsy of any cause
  - Brain tumors
  - Brain malformations (e.g., lissencephaly, polymicrogyria, hemimegalencephaly, neurocutaneous syndromes)
  - Other structural brain abnormalities such as strokes hypoxic-ischemic encephalopathy (HIE) or periventricular leukomalacia (PVL)
  - Genetic epilepsies: Dravet syndrome (febrile SE), Angelman syndrome (myoclonic SE), progressive myoclonic epilepsy syndromes
  - Inflammatory disorders (e.g., Rasmussen encephalitis, *N*-methyl-D-aspartate [NMDA] receptor antibody syndrome)
  - Acute malfunction of ventriculoperitoneal (VP) shunt

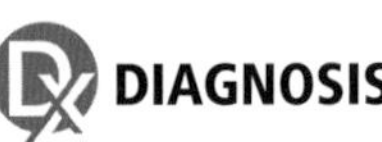

DIAGNOSIS

HISTORY

- Ask about onset of seizure activity, duration, characteristic movements, and similarity to prior episodes. Ask about prior need for anticonvulsants and intubation/coma induction.
- Ask about treatment with antiepileptic drugs (AEDs), adherence to dosing, and other neurologic abnormality, including previous neurologic workup such as MRI brain or EEG.
- Ask specifically about precipitating factors: fever, preceding illness, head trauma, change in antiepileptic medication, and family history of seizures.
- Ask about presence of prior neurosurgical intervention (presence of VP shunt).

PHYSICAL EXAM

- Vital signs: fever, respiratory rate/O_2 saturation (adequacy of air exchange and abnormal breathing patterns), heart rate, BP (Hypertension suggests intracranial hypertension.)
- End-tidal capnography provides earliest sign of hypoventilation.
- Signs of head trauma: retinal hemorrhages, excess bruising, bone fractures, evidence of intracranial hypertension such as bulging fontanelle
- Meningismus signals CNS infection, intracranial hemorrhage, or spine trauma; may be absent in young infants with meningitis
- Signs of systemic infection: fever (also potentiates seizure activity), petechiae, rash, mucosal lesions, lymphadenopathy
- Skin examination: Check for evidence of neurocutaneous disorders (e.g., café au lait spots, ash leaf spots, shagreen patches).
- Signs of electrolyte derangement: dehydration, poor skin turgor, delayed capillary refill, ambiguous genitalia
- Observe clinical presentation, specifically focal features or asymmetry.
- Postictal exam: Transient neurologic abnormalities (e.g., pupillary asymmetries, eye deviation, focal motor weakness [Todd paresis], aphasia) may not correlate with the underlying structural lesion. After seizure has stopped, a neurologic examination should be performed, with attention to mental status, focal weakness, tone, or sensation.

DIFFERENTIAL DIAGNOSIS

- Nonepileptic SE: clinically suspected with eye closure; asynchronous, thrashing limb movements; pelvic thrusting, fluctuating responsiveness, head side-to-side movements, purposeful resistance to passive movement; and normal concurrent EEG. Induction of a seizure by suggestion further supports this diagnosis.
- Movement disorders (including dystonia, chorea, and very frequent tics) can be mistaken for persistent seizure activity.
- Postanoxic myoclonus status after prolonged cardiopulmonary arrest. These movements are usually nonrhythmic and segmental but can appear rhythmic at times. EEG is recommended for diagnosis.
- Gastroesophageal reflux: presents in infants with repetitive back arching and arm flailing while awake and interactive (Sandifer syndrome)

DIAGNOSTIC TESTS & INTERPRETATION

Initial Tests (screening, lab, imaging)

Initial:

- STAT glucose, electrolytes, calcium, magnesium, and blood gas
- Anticonvulsant levels if indicated
- Consider: CBC, liver function tests, toxicology screen, urinalysis

ALERT

Leukocytosis is common after prolonged seizure and may not indicate infection. Hypercapnia and mild to moderate acidosis is expected with prolonged seizure and should not be used in isolation to determine need for intubation.

- Neuroimaging, CT, or MRI: indicated for SE, especially with partial-onset seizures (including aura), focally abnormal EEG, focal neurologic signs, or history of head trauma. MRI is the preferred neuroimaging test, but CT may be more appropriate for urgent imaging or if the patient is medically unstable.

Diagnostic Procedures/Other

- EEG
  - Recommended to determine continued electrographic seizures and to identify focal versus generalized abnormalities
  - Urgent EEG recommended in patients with persistent SE or encephalopathy and in those with concern for nonconvulsive SE and nonepileptic SE
- Lumbar puncture (LP):
  - Indicated to evaluate CNS infection (meningitis or encephalitis)
  - Contraindications include intracranial hypertension known or suspected from exam or CT scan, cerebral mass lesion, and obstructive hydrocephalus.
  - LP may be deferred if suspicion of CNS infection is low (patient is afebrile, and an alternate etiology is present).

- Electrocardiogram (EKG)
  - 1st-time seizure may be acute presentation of underlying arrhythmia and subsequent cerebral hypoperfusion. Additionally, prolonged SE may result in cardiac injury.

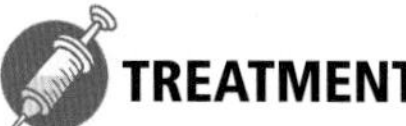

TREATMENT

- ABCs (stabilization of airway, supporting respiration, maintaining BP, and gaining intravascular access)
- Assess for hypoxia, hemodynamics, hyperthermia, hypoglycemia, hyponatremia.
- BP, EKG, and respiratory function should be monitored.
- Airway control may be maintained by head positioning and nasopharyngeal placement; avoid placement of anything in the mouth during active seizure as dental trauma may occur. Provide oxygen supplementation via nonrebreathing mask or bag-valve-mask ventilation if apneic.
- If the need for respiratory assistance persists (poor ventilatory effort, hypoxemia, anticipated coma induction), endotracheal intubation may be required.
- For hypoglycemia: 5 mL/kg of D10
- Rectal acetaminophen for fever

GENERAL MEASURES

- Attempt to establish IV access, but if difficult to establish, immediately consider IM midazolam, IN midazolam, or IO access or rectal diazepam immediately. The most important modifiable treatment parameter is time to initial treatment.
- Consider bedside EEG monitoring in any patient who needs more than the listed 2nd-line treatment.

MEDICATION

Anticonvulsant administration should be initiated when continuous seizure activity persists for >5 minutes.

ALERT

The most important modifiable treatment parameter is timing to treatment, and prompt treatment provides better seizure control.

- First line: benzodiazepines (give up to 2 times)
  - Lorazepam 0.1 mg/kg/dose IV (max 4 mg over 1 minute)
  - If no IV: diazepam 0.2 to 0.5 mg/kg/dose PR (max 20 mg/dose) or midazolam (5 mg/mL concentration, 0.2 mg/kg/dose intranasal or 0.5 mg/kg/dose buccal; max 10 mg)
- Second line
  - Fosphenytoin 20 mg phenytoin sodium equivalents (PE)/kg IV at a rate of 2 mg PE/kg/min not to exceed 150 mg PE/min
  - If fosphenytoin unavailable: phenytoin 20 mg/kg IV at a rate not to exceed 1 mg/kg/min
- Third line: can try one below, or proceed to 4th-line therapies
  - Phenobarbital 20 mg/kg IV; can give additional 10 mg/kg if needed
  - Valproic acid 20 to 40 mg/kg over 5 to 10 minutes
  - Levetiracetam 40 to 60 mg/kg IV over 5 to 10 minutes
- Fourth line: refractory SE
  - Midazolam 0.2 mg/kg IV bolus followed by infusion starting at 0.1 mg/kg/h with increases up to every 5 minutes as needed
  - Pentobarbital continuous infusion to seizure control or burst suppression
  - Alternatives: propofol (beware of propofol infusion syndrome with prolonged use), inhalational anesthetics, ketamine

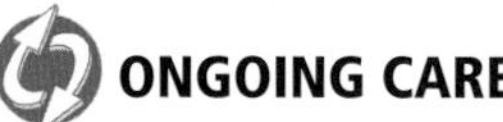

ONGOING CARE

FOLLOW-UP RECOMMENDATIONS

Patient Monitoring

- Cardiorespiratory monitoring, level of care as appropriate for clinical status
- Monitor hydration and creatine kinase (CK) levels in case of convulsive SE.
- Consider need for continued video-EEG monitoring and medication titration.

PATIENT EDUCATION

- Need for long-term anticonvulsant drug therapy after SE depends on the etiology, patient's age, and circumstances in which SE occurred.
  - Chronic anticonvulsant therapy is indicated when SE is caused by structural brain lesions and in other patients with a clear predisposition toward seizures.
  - Chronic anticonvulsant therapy is generally not needed in children who have SE from transient metabolic disturbances (e.g., hyponatremia, intoxication, fever).
- Educate family members regarding first aid for seizures. Discuss potential risks of seizure recurrence even if the child is taking an anticonvulsant drug. Review risks of climbing, swimming, bathing, and head protection for wheeled toys (e.g., bicycles).
- Provide caregivers with rectal diazepam with instructions for its use for seizure ≥5 minutes in duration.
- For patients with known epilepsy, counsel families regarding importance of medication compliance.

PROGNOSIS

The morbidity and mortality of SE reflect etiology and are lower in children than in adults. Recent mortality estimates in children range from 1% to 3%, with risk of new neurologic sequelae estimated at 15% and subsequent epilepsy at 30%. Refractory SE, however, has a morbidity estimated at 32% and a mortality of 17%. Factors associated with outcome include duration of SE, patient age, and underlying cause.

ADDITIONAL READING

- Abend NS, Loddenkemper T. Pediatric status epilepticus management. *Curr Opin Pediatr*. 2014;26(6):668–674.
- Appleton R, Macleod S, Martland T. Drug management for acute tonic-clonic convulsions including convulsive status epilepticus in children. *Cochrane Database Syst Rev*. 2008;(3):CD001905.
- Chin RF, Neville BG, Peckham C, et al. Treatment of community-onset, childhood convulsive status epilepticus: a prospective, population-based study. *Lancet Neurol*. 2008;7(8):696–703.
- El Amrousy D, Abd El-Hafez M, Nashat M, et al. Cardiac injury after convulsive status epilepticus in children. *Eur J Paediatr Neurol*. 2017;21(4):648–653.
- Ostrowsky K, Arzimanoglou A. Outcome and prognosis of status epilepticus in children. *Semin Pediatr Neurol*. 2010;17(3):195–200.
- Riviello JJ Jr, Ashwal S, Hirtz D, et al. Practice parameter: diagnostic assessment of the child with status epilepticus (an evidence-based review): report of the Quality Standards Subcommittee of the American Academy of Neurology and the Practice Committee of the Child Neurology Society. *Neurology*. 2006;67(9):1542–1550.
- Sánchez Fernández I, Abend NS, Arndt DH, et al. Electrographic seizures after convulsive status epilepticus in children and young adults: a retrospective multicenter study. *J Pediatr*. 2014;164(2):339–346.
- Singh RK, Stephens S, Berl MM, et al. Prospective study of new-onset seizures presenting as status epilepticus in childhood. *Neurology*. 2010;74(8):636–642.
- Trinka E, Höfler J, Zerbs A. Causes of status epilepticus. *Epilepsia*. 2012;53(Suppl 4):127–138.

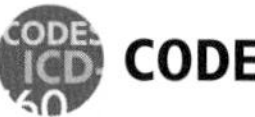

CODES

ICD10

- G40.901 Epilepsy, unsp, not intractable, with status epilepticus
- G40.401 Oth generalized epilepsy, not intractable, w stat epi
- G40.411 Oth generalized epilepsy, intractable, w status epilepticus

FAQ

- Q: Does SE cause brain injury?
- A: Neuronal loss may occur with prolonged SE after 30 minutes. This illness represents a neurologic emergency. Other determinants of outcome are hypoxic brain injury due to hypoventilation or injury due to a primary cause of SE such as encephalitis. Outcome in children with idiopathic SE without hypoxia is usually very good. Outcome of SE due to other brain injury (e.g., hypoxia, encephalitis, trauma) depends on the severity of the inciting process.
- Q: How safe is administration of rectal diazepam for clusters of seizures?
- A: With recommended dosing, this agent is safe and effective and can obviate a trip to the emergency room. Respiratory depression is very rare but can occur.
- Q: How likely is SE to recur?
- A: It is estimated at 17% in the 1st year and predominantly in children with other neurologic conditions.
- Q: When should a patient undergo acute head imaging
- A: If seizure is new in presentation or focality, if the patient does not return to baseline after prolonged observation period, if there is a focal neurologic deficit, or there are signs of neurotrauma
- Q: What should be the disposition of a patient presenting in an ambulatory setting with SE?
- A: Given the usual need for ongoing EEG monitoring and potential need for seizure control, most patients with SE should be admitted for observation. Decisions to manage a patient with known seizure disorder as an outpatient should be made in conjunction with the patient's primary neurologist.

STEVENS-JOHNSON SYNDROME AND TOXIC EPIDERMAL NECROLYSIS

Brianna Castillo, MD • James R. Treat, MD

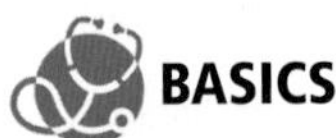

BASICS

DESCRIPTION

- Stevens-Johnson syndrome (SJS) and toxic epidermal necrolysis (TEN) are severe, potentially fatal, mucocutaneous reactions, typically caused by medications. Clinically, they are characterized by epidermal necrosis involving skin and at least two mucous membranes.
- The cutaneous necrosis leads to widespread epidermal detachment and loss of skin barrier function.
- Given the potential risk for infection and fluid and electrolyte imbalances with widespread denudation, SJS and TEN are considered medical emergencies.

EPIDEMIOLOGY

- Overall annual risk of 0.5 to 1.9 per million in the general population
- The precise incidence in children is unknown.
- Patients with HIV have a 1,000-fold increased risk.

RISK FACTORS

- Exposure to inciting medications
- Infection with *Mycoplasma pneumoniae*, HIV
- Genetic background
- Coexistence of cancer
- Concomitant radiotherapy

Genetics

- Strong associations have been made between HLA alleles and SJS/TEN.
- Associations are ethnic population–specific, and therefore universal screening of HLA alleles is rarely recommended.
- The U.S. Food and Drug Administration (FDA) recommends checking for HLA-B*1502 in Asian populations where this HLA subtype is highly prevalent before prescribing carbamazepine.

GENERAL PREVENTION

Once SJS/TEN has occurred, the inciting medication and any cross-reacting medications should be avoided.

PATHOPHYSIOLOGY

- Widespread keratinocyte and mucosal cell death occurs secondary to CD8+ T-cell–mediated apoptosis via Fas and Fas ligand pathways and/or direct granulysin secretion. Fas receptors are located on keratinocytes and, when activated with Fas ligand, induce apoptosis and therefore necrosis of epidermal cells. Granulysin is released from cytotoxic T cells and induces apoptosis by creating holes in target cell membranes.
- The exact mechanism by which the implicated drug or infection triggers activation of cytotoxic T cells and the upregulation of the Fas/FasL pathway is unknown.
- Soluble Fas ligand is increased in patients with SJS/TEN.
- IVIG theoretically acts to block the Fas–FasL connection, thereby interrupting keratinocyte death and epidermal necrosis. Trials that show a benefit of IVIG use demonstrate improvement of disease severity but not complete abolition of symptoms; this incomplete effect may be due to IVIG being started too late in the disease progression or due to a potential alternative pathway to keratinocyte destruction.

ETIOLOGY

- <5% of cases have no known cause.
- Medications
  - >100 medications have been implicated in causing SJS/TEN.
  - High-risk drugs include aromatic amine anticonvulsants such as carbamazepine, phenobarbital and phenytoin, lamotrigine, β-lactam antibiotics, sulfa medications (including trimethoprim-sulfamethoxazole and sulfasalazine), minocycline, cephalosporins, quinolones, NSAIDs (especially piroxicam and meloxicam), allopurinol, and nevirapine.
- Acetaminophen (very rare)
  - The FDA issued a warning about the risk of acetaminophen-related SJS/TEN.
  - Although SJS/TEN is a very rare occurrence in patients taking acetaminophen, the ubiquity of acetaminophen in prescription and over the counter (OTC) products prompted the requirement for new labeling.
- A greater risk of developing SJS/TEN is seen in the first 8 weeks of treatment with these medications, with the highest risk being 1 to 3 weeks after exposure.
- *M. pneumoniae*
  - More commonly implicated in children and adolescents
  - *M. pneumoniae* can cause severe isolated mucositis or mucositis with limited targetoid lesions typically <10% body surface area (BSA).
  - The designation of *M. pneumoniae* mucositis as a distinct entity termed *Mycoplasma-induced recurrent mucosits*, separate from SJS and erythema multiforme (EM) has been recently proposed due to the paucity of skin lesions and less sever clinical course.
- There is scant evidence that vaccines, neoplastic syndromes, and autoimmune disease such as SLE may play a role in etiology.
- Herpes simplex virus (HSV)–associated EM was historically categorized on the spectrum with SJS and TEN, but new classification schemes place it as a separate entity.

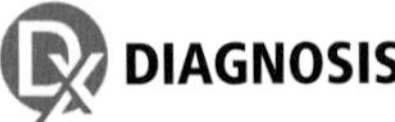

DIAGNOSIS

HISTORY

- Prodromal period for 1 to 7 days of low-grade fever, sore throat or upper respiratory infection or dysphagia, and general malaise; patient may also complain of pain or stinging in the eyes.
- Subsequent development of targetoid red papules and plaques with dusky, blistered, or eroded center as well as mucosal (lip, intraoral, conjunctival, urethral, anal) pain with blistering and erosions
- Recent initiation of high-risk agent (see earlier list) or upper respiratory symptoms such as cough indicative of *Mycoplasma* infection

PHYSICAL EXAM

- Acute phase
  - Early skin lesions are erythematous targetoid macules and patches with a dusky center that then vesiculate.
  - The eruption usually starts on the face, presternal area of chest, and palms and soles. >90% of patients also have ocular and/or genital mucosa involvement consisting of erythema and erosions as well as hemorrhaging, crusting, and blisters.
  - Skin and mucosal lesions are very tender.
- Intraoral lesions may precede the cutaneous findings.
- Ocular involvement at the onset of disease is common. Early ocular disease ranges from acute conjunctivitis, eyelid edema, and ocular discharge to pseudomembrane formation and corneal erosion.
- Secondary phase
  - Over hours to days, necrosis, blistering, and sloughing cause large areas of epidermal detachment.
  - Lesions are characterized by a positive Nikolsky sign (epidermal detachment upon mechanical stress).
- Extensive mucosal involvement may include the esophagus, distal gastrointestinal (GI) tract, and respiratory epithelium.
- Occasionally, *Mycoplasma*-induced SJS can involve only the mucosal surfaces with little or no cutaneous involvement.

ALERT

- The progression of disease to sheets of widespread epidermal necrosis and sloughing may be hours. This is a medical emergency.
- The systemic severity of SJS and TEN is often underestimated based on the severity of skin disease.
- Ocular involvement is often early and severe.

DIFFERENTIAL DIAGNOSIS

- Staphylococcal scalded skin syndrome (SSSS)
- Linear IgA dermatosis
- Primary herpetic gingivostomatitis
- Paraneoplastic pemphigus, pemphigus vulgaris, and bullous pemphigoid
- Acute generalized exanthematous pustulosis
- Disseminated fixed bullous drug eruption
- Drug-induced hypersensitivity syndrome (drug reaction with eosinophilia and systemic symptoms [DRESS])

DIAGNOSTIC TESTS & INTERPRETATION

Initial Tests (screening, lab, imaging)

- CBC with differential, metabolic panel, hepatic function test, coagulation studies, urinalysis, mycoplasma serology, or polymerase chain reaction (PCR), HSV PCR of skin lesions if indicated
- Anemia and lymphocytopenia are common and portend a poor prognosis.
- Symptom-directed imaging may be indicated depending on the extent of mucosal and systemic involvement.
- Clinical diagnosis
  - The diagnosis of SJS and TEN is largely clinical based on history and physical exam.
  - By definition, <10% affected BSA is SJS; 10–30% affected BSA is SJS/TEN overlap; >30% affected BSA is TEN.

Diagnostic Procedures/Other

- Skin biopsy with cryosection can be performed to confirm the clinical diagnosis if in doubt.
- Histologic examination with direct immunofluorescence (DIF) can be performed to rule out other autoimmune blistering diseases such as paraneoplastic pemphigus if in doubt.
- Pathologic and diagnostic findings
  - Skin biopsy shows full-thickness epidermal necrosis and few inflammatory cells; the skin biopsy may additionally show separation at the subepidermal level.
  - DIF shows no immunoglobulin or complement deposition in the epidermis or in the epidermal—dermal zone.

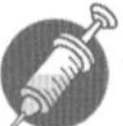

TREATMENT

MEDICATION

First Line

- Stop all potentially offending medications.
- Early admission to burn unit or pediatric intensive care unit for initial stabilization and management of fluid, electrolytes, and nutrition; airway stability; and eye care
- Prompt ophthalmology and dermatology consultation
- Otolaryngology, urology, or gynecology consultation may be needed based on extent of mucosal involvement.
- Meticulous wound care with bland emollients; avoid silver sulfadiazine as it may cause SJS/TEN owing to its sulfa moiety or exacerbate SJS/TEN caused by sulfa medications.
- Topical antibiotics should be used in areas of superinfection. The prophylactic use of topical antibiotics is somewhat controversial. They should be considered in areas with a higher risk of superinfection, such as the perioral, periocular, and intertriginous areas.
- No medication has been tested in large enough randomized controlled trials to be considered a true 1st-line agent. Options are listed below.
  - IVIG: 0.5 to 1 g/kg/dose given in 2 to 4 doses for a total of 2 to 3 g/kg total
  - There have been variable results from a limited number of quality studies looking at the effects of IVIG. Multiple studies have demonstrated a beneficial effect especially if started early in the course.
  - Adverse effects of IVIG include acute renal failure, DIC, osmotic nephrosis, anaphylaxis, serum sickness, aseptic meningitis, and thrombosis, among others.
  - Steroids (prednisolone, dexamethasone, methylprednisolone) were the mainstay of therapy in the 1990s but now are less commonly used because of the increased risk of sepsis, infection, and other complications especially when used in TEN with widespread epidermal loss. Systemic steroid may still play a role in *Mycoplasma*-induced mucositis.
  - Cyclosporine and TNF antagonists, such as etanercept and infliximab, may confer a survival benefit based on small studies.
  - Plasmapheresis and cyclophosphamide have been studied in the treatment of SJS/TEN, with limited data to support their use.
  - Thalidomide was evaluated for the treatment of TEN in a single randomized clinical trial and was found to increase mortality, which resulted in the termination of the trial.
  - Prophylactic systemic antibiotics are not recommended, as they place the patient at an increased risk of candidemia and resistant infections.

ADDITIONAL THERAPIES

- Pain control is key to patient comfort.
- Good oral care using agents such as "magic mouthwash" helps debride dead skin and provide oral anesthesia.

SURGERY/OTHER PROCEDURES

- Surgical debridement. Studies have shown that surgical debridement of wounds prior to wound care yielded no additional benefit.
- Lysis of synechiae and vaginal adhesion
- Ocular amniotic membrane transplantation. Amniotic membranes are sewn into place preventatively early in the course of SJS/TEN. Amniotic membranes have been shown to prevent ocular and lid-related complications, as well as chronic ocular cicatricial sequelae, such as long-term eye pain and permanent visual deficits.

ADMISSION, INPATIENT, AND NURSING CONSIDERATIONS

When afebrile, the loss of skin is clearly done, and reepithelialization has occurred; cleavage of synechiae in the eyes is no longer needed; and the patient can eat and drink appropriately.

ONGOING CARE

FOLLOW-UP RECOMMENDATIONS

- Follow-up with a dermatologist and/or wound care specialist in addition to ophthalmologist
- Reepithelialization often starts within days and may take up to 3 weeks to be completed.

Patient Monitoring

- SCORTEN is a well-validated, widely used scoring system in adults used for its predictive value, which is best at day 3. Variables include age, percentage BSA affected, BUN, serum glucose, HR, serum bicarbonate, and associated malignancy.
- Monitor for skin, urinary tract, and pulmonary infections; synechiae in the eyes; and vaginal and urethral adhesions.

PROGNOSIS

- Mortality is 1–5% in SJS and up to 25–35% in TEN (although most of this data is from the adult literature and likely the mortality is lower in children).
- Prognosis depends on BSA affected, time to cessation of offending medication, and time to initiation of supportive care.

COMPLICATIONS

- Mucosal complications occur in >70% of patients with acute-phase mucosal involvement. Ocular complications occur in 50% of patients with TEN.
- Systemic: sepsis, multiorgan failure, major metabolic dysregulation
- Mucosal: respiratory failure, pneumonia, pulmonary embolus, UTI, GI hemorrhage, obstruction, and perforation
- Cutaneous: skin infections, scarring, hypo- or hyperpigmentation, nail dystrophies
- Ocular: synechiae, dry eyes, bacterial conjunctivitis, suppurative keratitis, endophthalmitis, impaired tear ducts, corneal ulcers, vision loss

ADDITIONAL READING

- Bastuji-Garin S, Rzany B, Stern RS, et al. Clinical classification of cases of toxic epidermal necrolysis, Stevens-Johnson syndrome, and erythema multiforme. *Arch Dermatol*. 1993;129(1):92–96.
- Canavan TN, Mathes EF, Frieden I, et al. *Mycoplasma pneumoniae*-induced rash and mucositis as a syndrome distinct from Stevens-Johnson syndrome and erythema multiforme: a systematic review. *J Am Acad Dermatol*. 2015;72(2):239–245.
- Chong I, Chao A. Stevens-Johnson syndrome/toxic epidermal necrolysis and treatment with a biologic: a case report. *Perm J*. 2017;21. doi:10.7812/TPP/16-060.
- Del Pozzo-Magana BR, Lazo-Langner A, Carleton B, et al. A systematic review of treatment of drug-induced Stevens-Johnson syndrome and toxic epidermal necrolysis in children. *J Popul Ther Clin Pharmacol*. 2011;18:e121–e133.
- Ferrandiz-Pulido C, Garcia-Patos V. A review of causes of Stevens-Johnson syndrome and toxic epidermal necrolysis in children. *Arch Dis Child*. 2013;98(12):998–1003.
- Gregory DG. New grading system and treatment guidelines for the acute ocular manifestations of Stevens-Johnson syndrome. *Ophthalmology*. 2016;123(8):1653–1658.
- Gubinelli E, Canzona F, Tonanzi T, et al. Toxic epidermal necrolysis successfully treated with etanercept. *J Dermatol*. 2009;36(3):150–153.
- Karlin E, Phillips E. Genotyping for severe drug hypersensitivity. *Curr Allergy Asthma Rep*. 2014;14(3):418.
- Levi N, Bastuji-Garin S, Mockenhaupt M, et al. Medications as risk factors of Stevens-Johnson syndrome and toxic epidermal necrolysis in children: a pooled analysis. *Pediatrics*. 2009;123(2):e297–e304.
- Martínez-Pérez M, Imbernón-Moya A, Lobato-Berezo A, et al. *Mycoplasma pneumoniae*-induced mucocutaneous rash: a new syndrome distinct from erythema multiforme? Report of a new case and review of the literature. *Actas Dermosifiliogr*. 2016;107(7):e47–e51.
- Paradisi A, Abeni D, Bergamo F, et al. Etanercept therapy for toxic epidermal necrolysis. *J Am Acad Dermatol*. 2014;71(2):278–283.
- Patmanidis K, Sidiras A, Dolianitis K, et al. Combination of infliximab and high-dose intravenous immunoglobulin for toxic epidermal necrolysis: successful treatment of an elderly patient. *Case Rep Dermatol Med*. 2012;2012:915314.
- Sadighha A. Etanercept in the treatment of a patient with acute generalized exanthematous pustulosis/toxic epidermal necrolysis: definition of a new model based on translational research. *Int J Dermatol*. 2009;48(8):913–914.
- Schneider JA, Cohen PR. Stevens-Johnson syndrome and toxic epidermal necrolysis: a concise review with a comprehensive summary of therapeutic interventions emphasizing supportive measures. *Adv Ther*. 2017;34(6):1235–1244.
- Scott-Lang V, Tidman M, McKay D. Toxic epidermal necrolysis in a child successfully treated with infliximab. *Pediatr Dermatol*. 2014;31(4):532–534.
- Sharma N, Thenarasun SA, Kaur M, et al. Adjuvant role of amniotic membrane transplantation in acute ocular Stevens-Johnson syndrome: a randomized control trial. *Ophthalmology*. 2016;123(3):484–491.
- Treat J. Stevens-Johnson syndrome and toxic epidermal necrolysis. *Pediatr Ann*. 2010;39(10):667–674.
- Wojtkiewicz A, Wysocki M, Fortuna J, et al. Beneficial and rapid effect of infliximab on the course of toxic epidermal necrolysis. *Acta Derm Venereol*. 2008;88(4):420–421.
- Wolkenstein P, Latarjet J, Roujeau JC, et al. Randomised comparison of thalidomide versus placebo in toxic epidermal necrolysis. *Lancet*. 1998;352(9140):1586–1589.
- Zárate-Correa LC, Carrillo-Gómez DC, Ramírez-Escobar AF, et al. Toxic epidermal necrolysis successfully treated with infliximab. *J Investig Allergol Clin Immunol*. 2013;23(1):61–63.
- Zimmermann S, Sekula P, Venhoff M, et al. Systemic immunomodulating therapies for Stevens-Johnson syndrome and toxic epidermal necrolysis: a systematic review and meta-analysis. *JAMA Dermatol*. 2017;153(6):514–522.

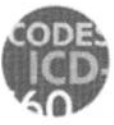

CODES

ICD10

- L51.1 Stevens-Johnson syndrome
- L51.3 Stevens-Johnson synd-tox epdrml necrolysis overlap syndrome
- L51.2 Toxic epidermal necrolysis [Lyell]

S

STOMATITIS

Cara L. Biddle, MD, MPH

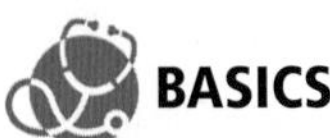

BASICS

DESCRIPTION

- Inflammation of the mucous membranes of the mouth including the cheeks, gingiva, tongue, lips, hard palate, and soft palate
- Also called gingivostomatitis when the gums are specifically involved
- Enteroviruses (causing herpangina and hand-foot-and-mouth disease) and herpes simplex type 1 (HSV-1) are the most common infectious causes of stomatitis.
- Recurrent aphthous stomatitis (or canker sores) is also common in children. The etiology of recurrent aphthous stomatitis is unknown.

EPIDEMIOLOGY

- Enteroviruses (including coxsackie viruses)
  - Infections are more common in the summer and fall months in temperate climates but occur year-round in the tropics.
  - Herpangina and hand-foot-and-mouth disease are most common in infants, toddlers, and young children.
- HSV-1:
  - Infections occur throughout the year.
  - Most primary HSV infections in childhood after the neonatal period are asymptomatic.
  - Primary herpetic gingivostomatitis is most common in infants, toddlers, and young children.
  - Recurrent HSV-1 infections can occur any time after the primary infection.
  - Seroprevalence of HSV-1 in the United States: >25% by age 7 years; >40% by age 21 years
- Recurrent aphthous stomatitis is most common in older children and adolescents.

GENERAL PREVENTION

- Wash hands after contact with the infected individual to help prevent spread of viral stomatitis.
- Disinfect surfaces, toys, and other objects used by an infected child to decrease spread of illness. Enteroviruses can survive on surfaces long enough to allow transmission of infection.
- Use contact precautions for hospitalized patients with viral stomatitis.

PATHOPHYSIOLOGY

- Enteroviral infections:
  - Spread by fecal–oral and respiratory routes; can also be passed from mother to infant prenatally, in the peripartum period, and perhaps via breast milk
  - Result in viremia which spreads virus to target organs
- HSV-1 infections:
  - Spread via contact with mucous membranes or open skin
  - Travel from the skin to the trigeminal sensory ganglion where infection persists for life; reactivates causing recurrent symptoms

ETIOLOGY

- Herpangina—most often coxsackie A viruses; also caused by other enteroviruses
- Hand-foot-and-mouth disease—most often coxsackie A viruses; also coxsackie B, enterovirus 71, and echoviruses
- Primary herpetic gingivostomatitis—typically HSV-1; can also be caused by HSV-2
- Recurrent aphthous stomatitis—possible causative factors: physical and chemical trauma, foods, nutrient deficiencies, immunodeficiency, systemic illness, infections, genetic predisposition, smoking, stress, medications

DIAGNOSIS

HISTORY

- History of present illness:
  - Onset and duration
  - Mouth pain or sores in mouth
  - Drooling
  - Fever
  - Intake of liquids and food
  - Urine output
  - Activity level
  - Close contact with similar symptoms
- Review of systems:
  - Vomiting, diarrhea, abdominal pain
  - Rash on body
  - Headache, mental status changes
  - Respiratory symptoms
  - Previous history of oral lesions
- Chronic health issues and family history: immunodeficiency (including HIV infection), inflammatory bowel disease, gluten enteropathy, anemia, neutropenia, rheumatologic disease. Include recent medication history to assess risk for Stevens-Johnson syndrome.

PHYSICAL EXAM

- Exam of lips and oral cavity:
  - Describe mucous membranes: Moist? Erythematous? Swollen? Friable?
  - Describe oral lesions: Color? Location? Number? Ulceration?
- Additional physical exam
  - General appearance
  - Hydration status
  - Respiratory, cardiovascular, and abdominal exam
  - Skin exam for additional rash
  - Lymphadenopathy
- Typical physical findings
  - Herpangina
    - Vesicles and ulcers surrounded by erythematous ring on tonsillar pillars, soft palate, uvula, tonsils, and/or posterior pharynx
  - Hand-foot-and-mouth
    - Inflamed oropharynx with scattered vesicles and ulcers with an erythematous ring on buccal mucosa, tongue, gingiva, hard and soft palate, and/or posterior pharynx
    - Maculopapular, vesicular, and/or pustular lesions on hands and fingers, feet, and buttocks
    - Hand and foot lesions most commonly on dorsal surface but can also be on palms and soles
  - Primary herpetic gingivostomatitis (herpes labialis)
    - Inflamed gingiva with mucosal hemorrhages
    - Clusters of vesicles throughout the mouth including the lip's mucocutaneous margin and perioral skin
  - Recurrent herpes labialis
    - Cluster of vesicles on lip or mucocutaneous margin
  - Aphthous stomatitis
    - Shallow round or ovoid ulcers with gray base and surrounding erythema
- Also consider:
  - Varicella
    - Grouped vesicles or ulcers on hard palate, buccal mucosa, tongue, or gingiva
    - Diffuse vesicles in various stages of healing on skin of body
  - Stevens-Johnson syndrome
    - Erythema and edema of lips; painful intraoral bullae which rupture leaving erosions
    - Rash on body including urticarial, target lesions, and bullae
  - Behçet syndrome
    - Oral ulcers accompanied by genital ulcers, uveitis, rash, and other systemic symptoms
  - Periodic fever with aphthous stomatitis, pharyngitis, and adenitis (PFAPA syndrome)
    - Prodrome of systemic symptoms, sore throat, and aphthous ulcers on lips or buccal mucosa followed by abrupt onset of fever and chills

DIFFERENTIAL DIAGNOSIS

- Infectious
  - Enteroviruses including coxsackievirus and other enteroviruses
  - HSV
  - Varicella
  - HIV infection
  - Syphilis
  - *Candida*
- Recurrent aphthous stomatitis
- Trauma
- Other:
  - Chemotherapy-associated stomatitis
  - Stevens-Johnson syndrome
  - Behçet syndrome
  - Reiter syndrome
  - PFAPA syndrome

DIAGNOSTIC TESTS & INTERPRETATION

- Diagnosis of stomatitis is typically made by history, location and characteristics of oral lesions, and additional physical findings.
- Confirmatory lab tests are available when needed:
  - Enterovirus can be identified by polymerase chain reaction (PCR) assay or culture of stool, throat swab, blood, urine, tracheal aspirate, conjunctival swab, and tissue biopsy.
  - HSV can be detected by viral culture, PCR, direct fluorescent antibody (DFA) staining, or enzyme immunoassays (EIAs).
  - For HSV culture: Unroof a vesicle with scalpel or sterile needle, and use swab to soak up fluid and scrape the base. Use appropriate viral transport media.

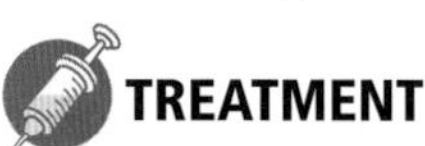

TREATMENT

GENERAL MEASURES

- Maintain hydration. Offer small amounts of cool, nonacidic liquids frequently. Use a syringe to continue giving liquids when children are refusing to drink. Try popsicles as another source of liquids.
- Offer soft, cool foods like ice cream, yogurt, and Jell-O®. Avoid foods that are salty, spicy, hard, or acidic. They are likely to irritate the mouth sores and cause more pain.
- Apply petroleum jelly or other barrier ointment to the lips to limit cracking and prevent adhesions in herpetic gingivostomatitis.

MEDICATION

- Pain control:
  - Acetaminophen or ibuprofen
  - Acetaminophen with an opioid (avoid codeine due to pharmacogenomic risk for toxicity with rapid CYP450 2D6 metabolizers) in severe cases. Use caution due to risk of sedation and constipation. Do not use in combination with regular acetaminophen.
- Antivirals:
  - Oral acyclovir can be used for immunocompetent children with herpetic gingivostomatitis if started within the first 72 to 96 hours of illness. Oral acyclovir may shorten the duration of symptoms and viral shedding.
  - Topical acyclovir is not recommended for primary herpetic gingivostomatitis.
- Topical therapy—"magic mouthwash"
  - 1:1 mixture of diphenhydramine and Maalox® (calcium carbonate) or Kaopectate® (bismuth subsalicylate), and add viscous lidocaine (1:1:1 mixture) in severe cases
  - Use with caution. Many young children cannot "swish and spit" and will swallow the medication. Applying magic mouthwash to ulcers with a swab may cause additional irritation to friable mucosa. Use of viscous lidocaine can result in systemic toxicity (e.g., arrhythmias), anesthesia of the oral mucosa leading to mechanical trauma, and anesthesia of the posterior pharynx leading to choking or aspiration.

ONGOING CARE

FOLLOW-UP RECOMMENDATIONS

Patient Monitoring

- Most children with stomatitis can be cared for at home with pain control and maintenance of hydration.
- Providers should ensure that parents and caregivers are familiar with signs and symptoms of dehydration.
- Children with poor oral intake due to pain may be unable to maintain hydration at home and require admission for IV fluids.

PROGNOSIS

- Primary herpetic gingivostomatitis results in permanent HSV infection. Recurrent infection can be triggered by stress, fever, trauma, sun exposure, immunosuppression, or extremes in termperature. Children may have tingling, pain, itching, or parasthesias before the appearance of recurrent lesions.
- Recurrent aphthous stomatitis causes significant morbidity due to recurrences of painful oral lesions.

COMPLICATIONS

- Enteroviral infection:
  - Respiratory—bronchiolitis, pneumonia, pleurodynia
  - Neurologic—viral meningitis, encephalitis, motor paralysis
  - Gastrointestinal—vomiting, diarrhea, abdominal pain, pancreatitis, hepatitis
  - Genitourinary—orchitis
  - Ophthalmologic—uveitis, acute hemorrhagic conjunctivitis
  - Cardiac—myocarditis, pericarditis
  - Muscular—myositis

ALERT

Enterovirus 71 can cause both hand-foot-and-mouth disease and herpangina. Children with enterovirus 71 can develop severe neurologic disease (including brainstem encephalomyelitis and acute paralysis) followed by secondary pulmonary edema/hemorrhage and cardiopulmonary collapse.

- HSV infection:
  - Herpetic keratitis—herpetic eye infection due to autoinoculation from mouth lesions
  - Herpetic whitlow—development of herpetic lesions on the extremities (typically fingers) due to direct contact with mouth lesions
  - Eczema herpeticum—extensive herpes infection of the skin in children with atopic dermatitis or other chronic skin disease
  - HSV encephalitis
  - Secondary bacteremia

ADDITIONAL READING

- Chattopadhyay A, Shetty K. Recurrent aphthous stomatitis. *Otolaryngol Clin North Am.* 2011;44(1):79–88.
- Faden H. Management of primary herpetic gingivostomatitis in young children. *Pediatr Emerg Care.* 2006;22(4):268–269.
- Gibson AM, Sommerkamp SK. Evaluation and management of oral lesions in the emergency department. *Emerg Med Clin North Am.* 2013;31(2):455–463.
- Le Doare K, Hullah E, Challacombe S, et al. Fifteen-minute consultation: a structured approach to the management of recurrent oral ulceration in a child. *Arch Dis Child Educ Pract Ed.* 2014;99(3):82–86.
- Usatine RP, Tinitigan R. Nongenital herpes simplex virus. *Am Fam Physician.* 2010;82(9):1075–1082.

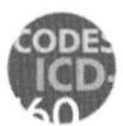

CODES

ICD10

- K12.1 Other forms of stomatitis
- B00.2 Herpesviral gingivostomatitis and pharyngotonsillitis
- B08.4 Enteroviral vesicular stomatitis with exanthem

FAQ

- Q: My child is refusing to drink any liquids. How can I keep her hydrated?
- A: Mouth sores can be very painful. Even if your child is not having fever, give regularly scheduled doses of ibuprofen or acetaminophen around the clock for pain control. Offer cool, nonacidic liquids and foods, which will be less likely to irritate the mouth sores. Use a syringe to put small amounts of liquids in her mouth every few minutes if she refuses to drink anything.
- Q: What should I do at home to prevent spread of the infection?
- A: Frequent hand washing is the most important way to prevent the spread of infection. Avoid sharing contaminated toys, utensils, and other objects until they have been cleaned, and wipe down surfaces to disinfect. For enteroviral infections, it is particularly important to do careful hand washing after diaper changes because the virus is shed in the stool.
- Q: When can my child return to school or daycare?
- A: Viral stomatitis is contagious. Children who drool are the most contagious and should not return to school until the mouth sores heal. Children with aphthous ulcers or recurrent herpes labialis should not be excluded from school.

STRABISMUS

Leah G. Reznick, MD • Allison R. Loh, MD

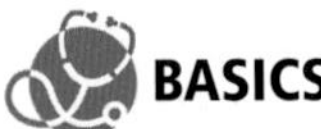

BASICS

DESCRIPTION

- Strabismus is defined as any form of ocular misalignment. It derives from the Greek word *strabismos* (to squint).
- Strabismus can be intermittent or constant.
- There are many types of strabismus, which are defined by the direction of misalignment.
  - Exotropia: out-turning of eyes
  - Esotropia: in-turning of eyes
  - Hypertropia: one eye higher than the other eye
- Strabismus can be comitant (amount of misalignment is the same in all directions of gaze) or incomitant (variable angle of deviation, which is dependent on the direction of gaze).
  - Comitant strabismus is the most common form of strabismus. These children are typically developmentally normal.
  - Incomitant strabismus is less common. It is caused by paralytic strabismus such as cranial nerve palsies or restrictive strabismus such as Brown syndrome.
- Strabismus may cause permanent loss of three-dimensional vision, amblyopia (visual acuity loss), and/or ocular torticollis.
- Strabismus can result in significant psychosocial problems for children, which warrant attention and treatment.
- Patients with intermittent strabismus can also develop lifelong loss of depth perception and visual acuity. These children should be evaluated and potentially treated for their strabismus.

EPIDEMIOLOGY

Prevalence

For children <6 years of age, the prevalence of strabismus is 4–5%.

RISK FACTORS

- Low birth weight
- Maternal cigarette smoking
- Retinopathy of prematurity
- Refractive errors: high hyperopia and anisometropia
- Congenital or acquired vision loss
- Cerebral palsy
- Craniofacial syndromes
- Seizure disorders
- Developmental delays
- Hydrocephalus
- Neurologic problems—stroke, brain tumor
- Family history of strabismus

Genetics

- There is a 4-fold increase in the risk of strabismus for a child with an affected 1st-degree relative.
- There is limited knowledge of the genetic inheritance patterns of common strabismus. There appears to be polygenic pattern, but the *STBMS1* gene has been isolated as a specific locus for a few individuals.

PATHOPHYSIOLOGY

- There is a limited understanding of the pathophysiology of the most common comitant strabismus. There is no specific pathologic abnormality of the cranial nerves, extraocular muscles, or orbits.
- Accommodative esotropia is a common form of strabismus in young children. It is associated with high hyperopia (farsightedness) and anisometropia (see "Refractive Error"). When a child with high hyperopia attempts to focus at any distance, he or she needs to focus his or her intraocular lens (accommodation). This focusing can trigger overconvergence of the eyes (esotropia).
- Paretic strabismus is caused by weakness of cranial nerves and their associated extraocular muscles. Examples of this type of pathology include cranial nerve palsies—III, IV, and VI; Möbius syndrome; or Duane syndrome.
- Neuromuscular diseases such as myasthenia gravis can cause strabismus with decreased extraocular muscle function.
- Restrictive strabismus is a result of muscle tightness causing a limitation in eye movement. Examples include Graves disease, Brown syndrome, or trauma to extraocular muscles.
- Sensory strabismus results from poor visual acuity in one eye.

COMMONLY ASSOCIATED CONDITIONS

- Strabismus can be a sign of a vision- or life-threatening neurologic problem.
  - A physician needs to consider that retinoblastoma, brain tumor, cataract, and other conditions may initially present with ocular misalignment.
- Other ocular problems often coexist with strabismus including amblyopia, nystagmus, and refractive error.

DIAGNOSIS

- It is normal for infants <2 months of age to have intermittent strabismus but not constant strabismus.
- After 4 months of age, any strabismus is abnormal and warrants an ophthalmologic exam.
- Children do not commonly "grow out" of strabismus.
- A delay in diagnosis and treatment can lead to a worse prognosis for normal visual development.
- Signs and symptoms
  - Children are typically asymptomatic. Because the brain suppresses one eye in childhood strabismus, the patient has no diplopia and is not aware of ocular misalignment.
  - Strabismus needs to be screened for and identified by primary care providers and family members.

HISTORY

- Onset of misalignment
- Frequency, duration, and direction of deviation
- Torticollis
- History of eye or head trauma
- Birth and developmental history focusing on prematurity, seizure disorder, or neurologic abnormality
- History of glasses, patching, or other vision therapy
- Family history of strabismus, amblyopia, refractive error, or childhood vision problems

PHYSICAL EXAM

- Patient's visual acuity should be evaluated in an age-appropriate manner individually for each eye (see "Amblyopia" and "Refractive Error").
- The presence of torticollis may indicate strabismus.
- Ocular alignment
  - Corneal light reflex (Hirschberg test): With a patient looking at a light, look for the location of the corneal light reflex. The light reflex should be focused at the center of each pupil symmetrically. If the reflex is located outside of the pupillary center and asymmetric, the child likely has strabismus. If it is positioned laterally, the child has esotropia, and if it is positioned medially, the child has exotropia.
  - Red reflex test (Brückner): With dimmed room lights, an examiner uses a direct ophthalmoscope to look at the red reflex of both eyes simultaneously from 2 to 3 feet. Normally, the pupils should be red and the pupils should symmetrically fill with light. If there is asymmetry to the brightness, a dulled reflex, or a black or white area within the reflex, there is likely an ocular problem, which could be strabismus.
  - Alternate cover test: The examiner should get the patient to focus on a single target. While they are holding fixation, the examiner should occlude each eye for a brief period of time. The examiner should watch for movement of the uncovered eye to pick up fixation. If the eyes remain still while you alternately occlude each eye, then there is no strabismus. If the eyes move from inward to outward, the child has esotropia. If the eyes move from outward to inward, the child has exotropia.

- Ocular rotations
  - Each eye should be evaluated for full movement in horizontal and vertical directions. If the eye has limited movement in a particular direction, then there may be paralytic or restrictive strabismus. If there is limited movement, a patient should be evaluated by an ophthalmologist urgently.
- Complete ophthalmic examination is indicated whenever there is suspicion of strabismus or abnormal vision based on history, screening tests, or examination.

DIFFERENTIAL DIAGNOSIS

- In the initial evaluation, one needs to differentiate between true strabismus and pseudostrabismus.
  - Children with wide epicanthal folds often give the false appearance of esotropia due to minimal amount of conjunctiva showing in the medial canthal region.
  - Rather than looking at the amount of "whites" showing, a practitioner can use the corneal light reflex (Hirschberg test) to see if the light reflex lies in the central pupil and perform a cover test.
  - If there is any doubt about the presence of strabismus, a referral to an ophthalmologist is warranted.
- In children with abnormal eye movements (incomitant strabismus), the differential diagnosis includes the following:
  - Cranial nerve palsies (III, IV, or VI)
  - Craniofacial anomalies
  - Orbital fracture
  - Systemic or localized motor abnormalities such as myasthenia gravis
  - Orbital pseudotumor
  - Thyroid eye disease (Graves)
  - Strabismus syndromes
- Strabismus syndromes include the following:
  - Duane syndrome: congenital aberrant innervation of cranial nerve III
  - Möbius syndrome: congenital absence of cranial nerve VI and VII
  - Brown syndrome: an abnormality of the trochlear-superior oblique tendon causing a monocular elevation deficit
- Sensory strabismus is caused by any form of vision loss. The strabismus can be either esotropia or exotropia. If a child has sensory strabismus, it is crucial to identify the cause of vision loss because it can be life-threatening (such as retinoblastoma or intracranial tumor).

DIAGNOSTIC TESTS & INTERPRETATION

Serologic or radiologic testing is rarely performed to work up the etiology of routine strabismus.

Initial Tests (screening, lab, imaging)

- In select patients, a physician may order antiacetylcholine receptor antibodies testing to test for myasthenia gravis or thyroid function studies to test for thyroid eye disease.
- If orbital or neurologic pathology is suspected, an MRI or CT scan may be performed to evaluate for a restrictive or paralytic strabismus.

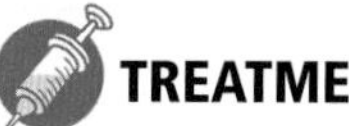

TREATMENT

GENERAL MEASURES

- If a child remains strabismic for a prolonged period, it can result in irreversible loss of depth perception and vision loss (amblyopia). Therefore, it is imperative that a child receives prompt evaluation and treatment.
- Treatment options can include glasses, occlusion therapy, orthoptic exercises, surgery, or a combination of these therapies.
- Glasses are primary treatment for a common form of strabismus—accommodative esotropia.
- Occlusion therapy is typically used for amblyopia rather than strabismus. If occlusion therapy improves vision, occasionally, the strabismus may improve, but more importantly, better vision improves prognosis for strabismus treatment.
- Eye exercises (orthoptic exercises) are useful in patients with convergence insufficiency. There is no evidence that they improve other forms of childhood esotropia and exotropia.

SURGERY/OTHER PROCEDURES

- If patching and glasses do not improve strabismus, then surgery is often recommended to improve binocular vision.
- In strabismus surgery, the eye muscles are either weakened by moving the muscle's insertion or tightened (strengthened) by removing a small piece of muscle tissue.
- For most patients, strabismus surgery is performed in an outpatient setting with minimal risk or morbidity.
- In large-case series, there is ~80% success rate for surgery and a ~20% reoperation risk.

ONGOING CARE

Long-term follow-up is important for children to monitor their vision development until at least 10 years of age. There is a risk for amblyopia and strabismus recurrence even after a successful surgical correction.

ADDITIONAL READING

- American Academy of Ophthalmology Pediatric Ophthalmology/Strabismus Panel. *Preferred Practice Pattern® Guidelines. Esotropia and Exotropia*. San Francisco, CA: American Academy of Ophthalmology; 2012. https://www.aao.org/preferred-practice-pattern/esotropia-exotropia-ppp-2017. Accessed May 8, 2018.
- American Association for Pediatric Ophthalmology and Strabismus. Strabismus surgery. http://www.aapos.org/terms/conditions/102. Accessed May 8, 2018.
- Handler SM, Fierson WM; and Section on Ophthalmology and Council on Children with Disabilities, American Academy of Ophthalmology, American Association for Pediatric Ophthalmology and Strabismus, et al. Learning disabilities, dyslexia, and vision. *Pediatrics*. 2011;127(3):e818–e856.
- Cotter SA, Mohney BG, Chandler DL, et al; for Pediatric Eye Disease Investigator Group. A randomized trial comparing part-time patching with observation for children 3–10 years of age with intermittent exotropia. *Ophthalmology*. 2014;121(12):2299–2310.

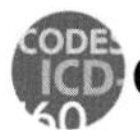

CODES

ICD10

- H50.9 Unspecified strabismus
- H50.10 Unspecified exotropia
- H50.00 Unspecified esotropia

FAQ

- Q: Will a child's strabismus resolve on its own?
- A: In most cases, children do not outgrow strabismus. Diagnosis and treatment should not be delayed.
- Q: Should a child wait to have surgery until he or she is older?
- A: When a child has strabismus, there are anatomic changes to the brain to prevent diplopia. The longer a child spends strabismic, the more adaptation occurs and the harder it is to regain normal depth perception. Therefore, it is important not to delay diagnosis and treatment. There is improved prognosis with prompt treatment.
- Q: Does strabismus cause learning difficulties?
- A: There is no proven association between strabismus and learning disabilities. If a child has learning difficulties and has strabismus, the learning issues should be evaluated outside of the strabismus.
- Q: How does loss of depth perception affect a child?
- A: A child may demonstrate subtle changes in fine motor skills, visual–spatial tasks, and athletic capabilities.
- Q: Will surgery in older children and adults improve their ocular function?
- A: With surgery, older children and adults may expand their visual fields and restore binocularity. The psychosocial effects of strabismus can significantly affect a person's sense of self and social interaction. For this reason, strabismus surgery can dramatically improve quality of life.
- Q: When is vision therapy prescribed for strabismus?
- A: Vision therapy has limited use for patients with strabismus. Eye exercises have been proven effective for one type of exotropia called convergence insufficiency. For most childhood strabismus, there is no evidence that vision therapy successfully treats ocular misalignment.

STREP INFECTION: INVASIVE GROUP A β-HEMOLYTIC *STREPTOCOCCUS*

Maribeth Chitkara, MD

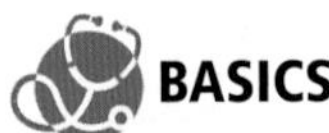

BASICS

DESCRIPTION

Infection associated with isolation of group A β-hemolytic streptococci (GABHS) from a normally sterile body site; includes three clinical syndromes:

- GABHS toxic shock syndrome (STSS)
- GABHS necrotizing fasciitis (NF)
  - Infection characterized by extensive local necrosis of skin and subcutaneous soft tissues
- Isolation of GABHS from normally sterile sites in patients not meeting criteria for STSS or NF (e.g., meningitis, osteomyelitis, septic arthritis, myositis, surgical wound infections) with or without bacteremia
  - Diagnostic criteria for STSS:
    - (I) Isolation of GABHS
      - A: From a normally sterile site (e.g., blood, CSF, tissue, peritoneal fluid)
      - B: From a nonsterile site (e.g., throat, vagina, sputum, open surgical wound)
    - (II) Clinical signs of severity
      - A: Hypotension
      - B: Two or more of the following signs:
        - Renal impairment
        - Coagulopathy
        - Hepatic involvement
        - Acute respiratory distress syndrome
        - A generalized erythematous macular rash that may desquamate
      - C: Soft tissue necrosis, including NF or myositis, or gangrene
  - A *definite* case fulfills criteria IA and II (A and B). A *probable* case fulfills criteria IB and II (A and B) and no other identifiable cause.

EPIDEMIOLOGY

- Overall mortality rates for invasive GABHS infections are lower in children (3.6–8.3%) than in adults (30–80%).
- Most cases occur in winter and early spring.

Incidence

- The average annual incidence in the United States is approximately 3.5 cases per 100,000 persons.
- Incidence is highest in infants and the elderly.
- 85% of cases are sporadic, 10% hospital-acquired, 4% in chronic care facilities, 1% in cases with a close index contact.

RISK FACTORS

- Risk factors for invasive GABHS infections include injuries resulting in bruising or muscle strain, surgical procedures, viral infections such as varicella, and use of NSAIDS.
- High-risk groups include patients with diabetes mellitus, chronic cardiac or pulmonary disease, HIV infection or AIDS, and those with a history of IV drug use.

GENERAL PREVENTION

- Routine immunization against varicella
- Isolation of hospitalized patients
  - In addition to standard precautions, droplet precautions for children with pneumonia
  - Contact precautions should be used for at least 24 hours after the start of antimicrobial therapy in children with extensive or draining cutaneous infections.
- Several GABHS vaccine candidates are in varying stages of development. A 26-valent recombinant M protein vaccine is the only vaccine to have entered into clinical trials.

PATHOPHYSIOLOGY

- The pathogenic mechanism has not been fully defined; however, an association with streptococcal pyrogenic exotoxins (SPE) has been suggested.
- SPE A, B, and C (responsible for rash of scarlet fever) along with streptococcal exotoxins, mitogen factor, and superantigen stimulate activation of T lymphocytes and macrophages to produce large quantities of cytokines resulting in shock and tissue damage.

ETIOLOGY

Streptococcus pyogenes is the only species of β-hemolytic streptococci to be associated with invasive infections.

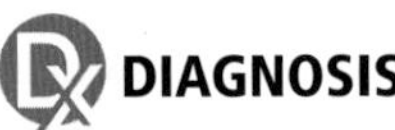

DIAGNOSIS

HISTORY

- Historic features vary depending on the GABHS syndrome.
- Typically presents with fever and the abrupt onset of severe pain
- May have preceding soft tissue infection such as cellulitis
- A preceding clinical pharyngitis is not common.
- Consider GABHS infection in any child with varicella who has any of the following:
  - Localized skin findings of erythema, warmth, swelling, or induration
  - Return of fever after having been afebrile
  - A temperature of $\geq$39°C (102.7°F) beyond the 3rd day of illness
  - Any fever persisting beyond the 4th day of illness
- In children without varicella, presentation can mimic influenza infection (fever, chills, myalgias). Abrupt onset of localized or severe pain and absence of respiratory symptoms or a contact history are clues to help distinguish STSS from influenza.
- Incubation period for STSS is unknown.

PHYSICAL EXAM

- Vital signs
  - Elevated temperature
  - Tachycardia
  - Hypotension (late sign)
- Toxic appearance is common but may not be present, especially early in the disease course.
- There may be no identifiable focus of infection.
- Skin exam varies:
  - Often, there are no cutaneous findings.
  - With varicella infection, vesicular lesions may have underlying erythema, warmth, or induration but can also appear normal.
  - NF should be suspected in child who presents with diffuse swelling of an extremity followed by the development of bullae with fluid that rapidly evolves from clear to violaceous in color.
  - Erythroderma, a generalized macular exfoliative and erythematous rash, is sometimes observed with STSS.
- Deep infections will have exam findings consistent with the specific focus (e.g., joint pain and limitation of mobility in septic arthritis, respiratory symptoms in GABHS pneumonia).
- Pain and/or hyperesthesias out of proportion to clinical findings may be noted.

DIFFERENTIAL DIAGNOSIS

- Bacterial sepsis
- Toxic shock syndrome from *Staphylococcus aureus*
- Other soft tissue infections
  - Cellulitis
  - Erysipelas
  - Clostridial or mixed anaerobic and aerobic fasciitis/gangrene

DIAGNOSTIC TESTS & INTERPRETATION

- CBC (leukocytosis with immature neutrophils may be noted, but WBC can also be normal)
- Electrolytes, BUN, creatinine, and glucose
- Liver function tests
- Screen for disseminated intravascular coagulation.
- Creatine kinase level (may be elevated in NF)
- Blood culture (positive in ~50% of STSS cases)
- Culture of wound and tissue aspirates
- Throat culture
  - If culture negative, a rise in antibody titers to streptolysin O, deoxyribonuclease B, or other streptococcal extracellular products 4 to 6 weeks after infection may help confirm the diagnosis.
  - These antibodies may remain elevated for several months and indicate an infection in the recent past.
- In cases of NF: Consider MRI to confirm diagnosis and extent of infection.

ALERT

- Diagnosis is primarily clinical and requires a high degree of suspicion because of the rapid progression of infection.
- Diagnosis should be considered even in suspect cases with absence of rash, cellulitis, or superinfected varicella lesions.
- In cases of NF, extent of involvement in subcutaneous tissues may be underestimated. Infection may be more widespread than what is apparent on physical exam.
- In STSS cases, care should be taken to search for a localized infection as a possible source of toxin production.

TREATMENT

GENERAL MEASURES

- Volume resuscitation
- Anticipatory management of multisystem organ failure
- Replete electrolytes as indicated
- Inotropes as indicated
- Blood products as indicated for anemia or thrombocytopenia
- Airway support for severe depression of level of consciousness or respiratory insufficiency

MEDICATION

- Parenteral therapy at maximum doses should be instituted promptly to cover both GABHS and *S. aureus* until the results of bacteriologic studies are available, with the capacity to do both of the following:
  - Kills organism with bactericidal cell wall inhibitor
  - Decreases enzyme, toxin, or cytokine production with protein synthesis inhibitor
- Recommended regimens:
  - Oxacillin (200 mg/kg/24 h IV divided q6h) or nafcillin (200 mg/kg/24 h IV divided q4–6h; maximum 12 g/24 h) *plus* clindamycin (25 to 40 mg/kg/24 h IV divided q6h or q8h)
  - In penicillin-allergic patients, consider vancomycin (40 mg/kg/24 h IV divided q6h; monitor serum levels and adjust dose if necessary) *plus* clindamycin.
  - In areas with high prevalence of community-acquired methicillin-resistant *S. aureus*, vancomycin should be used in place of β-lactamase–resistant penicillins.
- Once GABHS has been identified, antibiotic regimen should be changed to high-dose penicillin G (200,000 to 400,000 U/kg/24 h IV in 4 to 6 divided doses) *plus* clindamycin.
  - No penicillin G–resistant isolates of GABHS have been reported.
  - There are strains resistant to clindamycin, so it should not be used alone until shown to be sensitive.
- Antibiotics should be continued for a minimum of 14 days in patients with bacteremia and for 14 days after last positive culture obtained during surgical debridement for patients with deep soft tissue infections.
- The use of IV immune globulin (IVIG) may be considered in cases refractory to aggressive therapy, for infection in an area that precludes drainage, or persistent oliguria with pulmonary edema. Various regimens have been used: 150 to 400 mg/kg/24 h for 5 days or 1 to 2 g/kg as single dose.

SURGERY/OTHER PROCEDURES

Clinical suspicion of NF warrants prompt surgical consultation. Wound drainage, debridement of deep tissues, and Gram stain and culture of surgical specimens are often indicated.

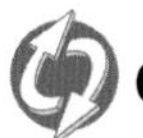

ONGOING CARE

PROGNOSIS

- Fulminant course with rapid deterioration is characteristic of invasive GABHS infections.
- Prognosis is improved with early recognition and aggressive management.
- Case fatality rate for invasive GABHS infections in the United States is 13.7% (36% for STSS and 24% for NF).
- Increased morbidity and mortality reported in cases of coinfection with H1N1 influenza
- Poor prognostic factors:
  - Emm/M strain types 1, 3, or 12
  - Increased age
  - Occurrence in winter/early spring
  - Development of GI symptoms

COMPLICATIONS

- From deep and systemic infections:
  - Sepsis syndrome
  - Hematologic seeding and development of focal infection
  - Infection site–specific complications (e.g., meningitis, neurologic impairment; septic arthritis, joint destruction)
- From NF:
  - Severe tissue necrosis usually requires extensive surgical debridement and may require amputation of involved extremities.
  - Compartment syndrome
  - Functional disabilities
  - Cosmetic sequelae
- From STSS:
  - Multiorgan system failure
  - Acute respiratory distress syndrome
  - Disseminated intravascular coagulation
  - Acute tubular necrosis and renal failure
  - Hepatic failure
  - Cardiac insufficiency
  - Cerebral ischemia and edema
  - Metabolic derangements

ADDITIONAL READING

- American Academy of Pediatrics. Group A streptococcal infections. In: Kimberlin DW, Brady MT, Jackson MA, et al, eds. *Red Book: 2015 Report of the Committee on Infectious Diseases*. 30th ed. Elk Grove Village, IL: American Academy of Pediatrics; 2015:732–744.
- American Academy of Pediatrics Committee on Infectious Diseases. Severe invasive group A streptococcal infections: a subject review. *Pediatrics*. 1998;101(1, Pt 1):136–140.
- Factor SH, Levine OS, Harrison LH, et al. Risk factors for pediatric invasive group A streptococcal disease. *Emerg Infect Dis*. 2005;11(7):1062–1066.
- Lamagni TL, Neal S, Keshishian C, et al. Predictors of death after severe *Streptococcus pyogenes* infection. *Emerg Infect Dis*. 2009;15(8):1304–1307.
- Langlois DM, Andreae M. Group A streptococcal infections. *Pediatr Rev*. 2011;32(10):423–430.
- O'Loughlin RE, Roberson A, Cieslak PR, et al. The epidemiology of invasive group A streptococcal infection and potential vaccine implications: United States, 2000–2004. *Clin Infect Dis*. 2007;45(7):853–862.

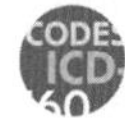

CODES

ICD10

- B95.0 Streptococcus, group A, causing diseases classd elswhr
- B95.1 Streptococcus, group B, causing diseases classd elswhr
- A48.3 Toxic shock syndrome

FAQ

- Q: For whom should the diagnosis of invasive GABHS be entertained?
- A: Consider GABHS in any child with varicella who experiences recrudescence of fever, fever ≥39°C (102.2°F) beyond the 3rd day of illness, or any fever beyond the 4th day of illness. A high index of suspicion should be maintained in patients with septicemia and in febrile patients with pain and hyperesthesia out of proportion to the clinical findings.
- Q: Is NSAID use in patients with varicella associated with GABHS?
- A: There are reports suggesting an association between the use of NSAIDs and the development of invasive GABHS diseases, but a causal relationship has not been established. There is evidence that NSAIDs impair granulocyte function and enhance production of cytokines. Additionally, they may mask signs of disease by suppressing the pain and fever that might encourage a patient with invasive GABHS infection to seek medical attention. No formal recommendations for restricting the use of NSAIDs are being made at this time.
- Q: Should close contacts of patients with invasive GABHS infections receive chemoprophylaxis?
- A: Although the risk of developing disease for household contacts is elevated in comparison to the general population, the risk is not sufficiently high to warrant routine testing or treatment for GABHS colonization. No clearly effective chemoprophylactic regimen has been identified. However, in high-risk populations (people >65 years or those with HIV, varicella, or diabetes mellitus), targeted chemoprophylaxis may be considered. Chemoprophylaxis is not recommended in schools or child-care facilities.

STROKE

Melissa G. Chung, MD • Warren D. Lo, MD

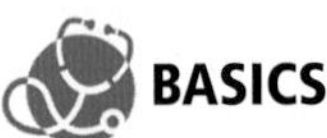

BASICS

DESCRIPTION

- A CNS insult that causes objective evidence (clinical, radiographic, or pathologic) of damage in a vascular territory and clinical symptoms lasting <24 hours
- A stroke can be ischemic due to decreased arterial (arterial ischemic stroke [AIS]) or venous flow (cerebral sinovenous thrombosis [CSVT]) or hemorrhagic. Acute neurologic dysfunction and not causing evidence of brain injury is a transient ischemic attack (TIA) (typically last 1 to 2 hours).
- Acute hemiparesis, sensory loss, aphasia, cranial nerve deficits, ataxia, or altered consciousness (especially if occurring together) should prompt rapid evaluation for possible stroke to prevent delays in diagnosis. Acute neonatal stroke may present with seizures and depressed level of consciousness without focal signs. Silent strokes can occur with sickle cell disease and congenital heart disease.

EPIDEMIOLOGY

- The neonatal period has the highest risk for pediatric stroke. Neonatal stroke occurs in approximately 1 in 4,000 live births.
- Incidence of AIS is 1.2 to 7.9 per 100,000 per year in children over a month of age.
- Hemorrhagic stroke incidence is estimated to be 0.5 to 5.1 per 100,000 children per year.
- CSVT occurs in 0.67 per 100,000 children per year.

RISK FACTORS

Genetics

Pediatric stroke occurs secondary to a plethora of etiologies as noted below. Some risk factors are genetic:

- Sickle cell disease: autosomal recessive (AR)
- Classic homocystinuria: *CBS* gene, AR
- Mitochondrial encephalomyopathy, lactic acidosis, and stroke-like symptoms (MELAS): maternal inheritance
- Cerebral autosomal dominant (AD) arteriopathy with subcortical infarcts and leukoencephalopathy (CADASIL): *NOTCH-3*, AD
- Fabry disease: *GLA* gene, X-linked
- Ehlers-Danlos type IV: *COL3A1* gene, AD
- Marfan syndrome: *FBN1* gene, AD
- Moyamoya syndrome (RNF213, ACTA2)
- *COL4A1* mutation

ETIOLOGY

- Cardiac
  - Complex congenital heart defects with right to left shunt
  - Cardiac rhabdomyoma or myxoma
  - Infectious endocarditis, especially left sided
  - Rheumatic heart disease
  - Prosthetic heart valves
  - Cardiomyopathy/myocarditis
  - Patent foramen ovale (PFO) with atrial septal aneurysm or known deep venous thrombosis (DVT) and large R>L shunt
- Vascular
  - Congenital/genetic vasculopathies associated with Ehlers-Danlos type IV, Marfan syndrome, PHACES, neurofibromatosis type I, Down syndrome
  - Moyamoya disease
  - Fibromuscular dysplasia, postradiation vasculopathy, intracranial aneurysm, arterial agenesis or hypoplasia, dissection, transient cerebral arteriopathy, focal arteriopathy, arteriovenous malformation
- Vasculitis, inflammatory
  - Systemic: systemic infections, varicella, lupus, hemolytic uremic syndrome, AIDS, Takayasu arteritis, drug abuse, Behçet disease
  - Primary angiitis of the CNS
  - Cranial or cervical infections (meningitis, encephalitis, sinusitis mastoiditis)
- Hematologic/coagulation disorders
  - Severe anemia, polycythemia, or thrombocytosis
  - Hemoglobinopathies especially hemoglobin SS (HgbSS) and Hgb S-thal
  - Primary thrombophilia: antithrombin III deficiency, factor V Leiden homozygous mutation, protein S and C deficiencies, prothrombin G20210A homozygous mutation, hemophilia A and B
  - Acquired thrombophilia: leukemia or other neoplasm, L-asparaginase treatment, anticardiolipin/antiphospholipid syndrome, estrogen-containing contraceptives, nephrotic syndrome, pregnancy/postpartum period, inflammatory bowel disease, thrombotic thrombocytopenic purpura
  - Primary or acquired coagulopathies: anticoagulation, disseminated intravascular coagulation
- Trauma
  - Blunt cervical or intraoral trauma (Consider cervical arterial dissection with high-speed MVA or cervical injury.)
  - Carotid ligation (e.g., with extracorporeal membrane oxygenation [ECMO])
  - Fat, air, foreign body, amniotic fluid embolism
  - Catheter angiography
  - Chiropractic manipulation
- Metabolic disorders
  - Hyperhomocysteinemia
  - Mitochondrial and related nuclear disorders
  - Fabry disease
- Miscellaneous
  - Migraine
  - Severe hypotension or hypertension
  - Reversible vasoconstriction syndrome
  - Cervical vessel compression

ALERT

Recent evidence suggests that minor infection may increase the risk of pediatric stroke and that immunizations are protective.

DIAGNOSIS

HISTORY

- Timing and progression of symptoms, including last known time when patient was normal
- Analysis of risk factors/etiology: inquire about
  - History of trauma
  - Recent medication/drug use
  - Cardiac history
  - Infectious history
  - Skin lesions (acute and chronic)
  - Symptoms/signs of inflammatory disorders
  - Personal and family history of excessive bleeding or clotting

ALERT

Acute stroke may present with stuttering symptoms rather than abrupt onset of maximal deficits.

PHYSICAL EXAM

- Note level of alertness, vital signs, presence of cough/gag and respiratory pattern as signs of possible increased intracranial pressure (ICP), and/or need for respiratory support/intubation.
- Age-appropriate neurologic examination including special attention to mental status, funduscopic exam for papilledema, cranial nerve abnormalities, and focal motor deficits. Pediatric National Institutes of Health Stroke Scale (PedNIHSS) use is encouraged.
- General examination: careful cardiac exam for murmurs or dysrhythmias; evaluate for stigmata of neurocutaneous syndromes or connective tissue disorders.

DIFFERENTIAL DIAGNOSIS

Several disorders may mimic an acute stroke:

- Hypoglycemia
- Complicated migraine (hemiplegic, basilar)
- Postepileptic paralysis (Todd paralysis)
- Alternating hemiplegia of childhood
- Posterior reversible encephalopathy syndrome
- Brain tumor
- Conversion disorder
- Metabolic encephalopathies
- Intoxication/toxins
- Syncope
- Acute vestibular disease

DIAGNOSTIC TESTS & INTERPRETATION

- Blood chemistry, particularly glucose
- CBC and platelet count
- Prothrombin time (PT), partial thromboplastin time (PTT), and fibrinogen
- Fasting lipid panel
- Thrombophilia screening (best to consult hematology): antithrombin III, protein C and S levels, factor V Leiden mutation, prothrombin G20210A mutation, and antiphospholipid screen
- Thrombophilia screening in acute neonatal stroke is less important unless other signs of coagulopathy are present.
- Coagulation factors with hemorrhagic stroke
- More extensive testing in unexplained cases should be tailored to the individual patient and may include the following:
  - Homocysteine
  - Mitochondrial disorder: blood +/− CSF lactate, genetic testing including WES when high level suspicion for nuclear disorder, muscle biopsy
  - Connective tissue disorder gene testing
  - Testing for systemic inflammatory disease (best done in consultation with rheumatology) such as erythrocyte sedimentation rate (ESR), C-reactive protein (CRP), antiphospholipid antibodies, antinuclear antibody, etc.
  - Intracranial infection: lumbar puncture (after imaging) with opening pressure, cell counts, glucose and protein, viral studies, and cultures; blood cultures
  - Drug screen when clinically appropriate
- After stabilization, prompt neuroimaging:
  - Non–contrast CT can screen for hemorrhage but may be insensitive to ischemic stroke.
  - Gold standard for diagnosis of ischemic stroke is MRI with diffusion-weighted imaging.
  - Contrast images (CT or MR) should be obtained if there is concern for infection or sinovenous thrombosis.

- Vascular imaging (MR or CT) of the head and neck to evaluate for focal stenosis /thrombosis, dissection, vasculopathy, or congenital malformation
- Perfusion imaging (CT or MR) may be helpful in defining the penumbra to evaluate the possible benefit of endovascular procedures.
- More extensive testing in undiagnosed cases may include the following:
  - ECG to assess for rhythm dysfunction
  - Echocardiography with bubble study
  - Conventional catheter angiography

ALERT

CT scan may be normal in the first 24 hours after nonhemorrhagic stroke.

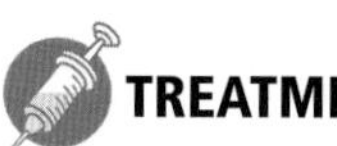

TREATMENT

ALERT

- For children with sickle cell disease and acute AIS, exchange transfusion is the treatment of choice so urgent early hematology consultation is needed.
- Early neurosurgical evaluation is indicated for large hemispheric or posterior fossa ischemic stroke, or intracranial hemorrhage because of potential need for surgical decompression.

GENERAL MEASURES

- Admit patients with acute symptomatic stroke to the hospital for close monitoring for clinical deterioration and for workup for underlying etiology. Chronic stroke discovered incidentally (children with HgbSS or presumed perinatal stroke) can be evaluated as an outpatient.
- Patients with diminished or fluctuating level of alertness, inability to protect airway, large hemispheric strokes, or posterior fossa strokes require monitoring in an intensive care unit (ICU) for respiratory deterioration or signs of increased ICP.
- Bed rest for at least the first 24 hours is recommended for patients with large territory strokes, stuttering symptoms, or increased ICP.
- Consultation with neurology, hematology, and other pediatric subspecialists as clinically indicated (e.g., rheumatology, genetics)
- Immediately attend to airway, breathing, and circulation to avoid hypoxia and hypotension and to reduce secondary brain injury.
- Maintain adequate hydration particularly in patients with CSVT. Avoid hypoglycemia. Aggressively treat fevers to avoid increased cerebral metabolic demand.
- With ischemic stroke, allow a relative degree of normal or elevated blood pressure to maintain cerebral perfusion. Avoid hypotension. Correct anemia if present.
- Strongly consider a swallow study in patients with facial weakness or cranial nerve involvement before allowing oral intake to reduce aspiration risk.
- Start empiric antibiotics if there is clinical concern for acute CNS infection.
- Consider low-molecular-weight heparin or unfractionated heparin for CSVT and with acute AIS to reduce acute recurrence in craniocervical dissection or cardioembolic stroke.
  - Avoid anticoagulation for intracranial dissection due to increased risk of subarachnoid hemorrhage.
  - Avoid anticoagulation in large hemispheric strokes due to risk of hemorrhagic conversion.
- Antiplatelet therapy, such as aspirin 3 to 5 mg/kg/24 h, is reasonable in children whose strokes are not secondary to sickle cell disease, dissection, or cardioembolism.
- Up to 25% of children have seizures with an acute stroke (may be the presenting sign). Acute neonatal stroke may be complicated by status epilepticus (clinical and nonconvulsive). Treat seizures aggressively.
- Isotonic-based fluids, preferably 0.9 NS, should be used to avoid hyponatremia and brain edema.
- Hyperacute (<4.5 hours from symptom onset) IV tissue plasminogen activator (tPA) or mechanical thrombectomy for large vessel occlusion may be considered in highly selected situations with expert consultation and pediatric ICU and neurosurgical support. The time window for thrombectomy in adults is actively being revised.
- Complications
  - Acute complications include increased ICP from cerebral edema, seizures, dysphagia resulting in aspiration. Increased ICP, papilledema, and vision loss can occur with CSVT. Intraventricular hemorrhage and acute hydrocephalus can occur with hemorrhagic stroke.
  - Cerebral edema peaks at 72 to 120 hours after acute ischemia. Edema can cause increased ICP that may require treatment with hypertonic saline. Hyperventilation should be used conservatively because severe hypocarbia can decrease cerebral perfusion and cause secondary ischemic injury.
  - Acute ICP with CSVT or acute hydrocephalus with intraventricular hemorrhage may require emergency CSF drainage.

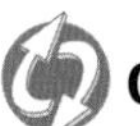

ONGOING CARE

- Initiate rehabilitation (physical, occupational, speech therapies) early.
- For patients with significant acute neurologic deficits, consider discharge to inpatient rehabilitation.
- Consider constraint induced movement therapy (CIMT) for patients with a hemiparesis.
- Therapies for cognitive impairments and aphasia remain limited. Nevertheless, children, particularly those with perinatal stroke, should be monitored for cognitive, speech, and behavioral impairments and provide assistance as needed.
- Neuropsychology consultation should be pursued if there are questions about academic performance or questions about attention span and disorganization.
- Mood disorders can be a complication of stroke.
- Focal arteriopathy has a higher risk of recurrence and requires long-term treatment with antithrombotics.
- Patients with moyamoya disease/syndrome are at high risk for recurrence and should be referred for vascular bypass.

PROGNOSIS

- About half of children with AIS have no to mild motor deficits, whereas the rest have moderate to severe deficits.
- The extent of cognitive impairment is not well known but occurs more often with greater neurologic deficits. Neonates and young children should be followed because deficits may not be evident until they reach school age.
- Predictors of poor outcome after hemorrhagic stroke include Glasgow Coma Scale score ≤7 at admission, infratentorial hemorrhage, age <3 years, or large hemorrhage volume.
- Patients with prolonged or recurrent acute seizures or younger age at the time of stroke are at higher risk for developing epilepsy. Epileptic seizures occur in 10% of children 1 year after AIS.
- Epilepsy tends to occur in patients with greater impairments.
- Mortality from AIS and underlying conditions is 10–12% and from hemorrhagic stroke 7–54%.

ADDITIONAL READING

- Beslow LA, Licht DJ, Smith SE, et al. Predictors of outcome in childhood intracerebral hemorrhage: a prospective consecutive cohort study. *Stroke*. 2010;41(2):313–318.
- Fullerton HJ, Wintermark M, Hills NK, et al. Risk of recurrent arterial ischemic stroke in childhood: a prospective international study. *Stroke*. 2016;47(1):53–59.
- Ichord RN, Benedict SL, Chan AK, et al. Paediatric cerebral sinovenous thrombosis: findings of the International Paediatric Stroke Study. *Arch Dis Child*. 2015;100(2):174–179.
- Jordan LC, Hillis AE. Challenges in the diagnosis and treatment of pediatric stroke. *Nat Rev Neurol*. 2011;7(4):199–208.
- Monagle P, Chan AKC, Goldenberg NA, et al. Antithrombotic therapy in neonates and children: antithrombotic therapy and prevention of thrombosis, 9th ed: American College of Chest Physicians evidence-based clinical practice guidelines. *Chest*. 2012;141(Suppl 2):e737S–e801S.

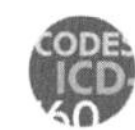

CODES

ICD10

- I63.9 Cerebral infarction, unspecified
- I63.50 Cereb infrc due to unsp occls or stenos of unsp cereb artery
- I61.9 Nontraumatic intracerebral hemorrhage, unspecified

FAQ

- Q: Will my child have another stroke?
- A: Overall risk of recurrent AIS is about 10–12%, depending on the cause of the stroke. Children with focal arterial stenosis, HgbSS, and uncorrectable congenital heart defects have a higher risk for recurrence. Recurrent venous thrombosis is rare, and long-term anticoagulation is typically not needed. Children with neonatal strokes without an identified risk factor are unlikely to have a second stroke. Hemorrhage due to arteriovenous malformation or aneurysm is likely to recur unless the lesion is removed.
- Q: Which therapies will help my child the most?
- A: Small randomized trials have shown CIMT improves motor function in hemiplegic cerebral palsy, but CIMT has not been tested in childhood stroke.
- Q: Will my child get better?
- A: Recovery from a neurologic injury takes time. By 3 months after the stroke, we can get a rough sense if the child will still have some degree of deficit, but the extent of permanent deficit may not be clear until a year or more after the injury, depending on the age of the child.

S

STUTTERING

Gary A. Emmett, MD, FAAP

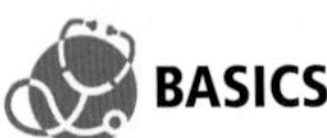

BASICS

DESCRIPTION

Stuttering (also referred to as stammering or dysfluency) is an involuntary disturbance in the normal fluency and timing of speech that is not appropriate for the age of the speaker. Various patterns are seen:

- Prolongation of sounds or syllables
- Repetition of sounds, syllables, or even whole words
- Pauses in the middle of words
- Blocking—either silence or pauses filled with nonsense sounds in the middle of words as if considering what to say next
- Avoidance—word substitutions that are used to skip known problem words; also called circumlocution
- Overemphasis of some syllables or words; also called tension
- Stuttering is significant when it interferes with the patient's life in academic, occupational, or social arenas. Many children with developmental delays have dysfluencies of speech, but it is not considered stuttering unless the dysfluencies are present more frequently than expected for the level of disability.

EPIDEMIOLOGY

- At least 1% of all studied populations affected
- Males stutter 3 times more often than females.
- Stuttering is found in every culture and language. The language spoken in the home does not increase or decrease the amount of stuttering.
- Stuttering begins between 2 and 7 years of age, with 98% of cases presenting by age 10 years.
- Girls start stuttering several months earlier on average than boys; however, they also speak, in general, earlier than boys do.

RISK FACTORS

Genetics

Stuttering does cluster in families:

- Monozygotic twins have a higher concordance for stuttering than dizygotic twins.
- The more closely related one is to a stutterer, the more likely one is to stutter.
- Identical twins have a concordance for stuttering of ≥30%.

GENERAL PREVENTION

There is no known prevention strategy for stuttering.

PATHOPHYSIOLOGY

Stuttering appears to be associated with an excessive amount of dopamine, or closely related vasoactive compounds, in the brain:

- Patients with Parkinson disease often develop adult-onset stuttering.
- PET scans show increased vasoactive substances in the brains of those who stutter.
- Medications that increase brain dopamine (antidepressants) or are dopaminergic (major tranquilizers) can induce stuttering in nonstutterers; medications that lower dopamine (e.g., clomipramine) may stop stuttering.
- Many differences exist between the brains of stutterers and nonstutterers in glucose uptake, dopamine release, and metabolic activity of the basal ganglia, but no single physiologic process has been well defined as the cause of stuttering.

ETIOLOGY

- Specific etiology is not known, but many factors contribute. Stuttering may be more pronounced when a child is fatigued, excited, upset, rushed, or exposed to some other stressor.
- Environmental factors are thought to have a role. Children adopted by a parent who stutters are more likely to stutter than children adopted by a parent who does not stutter.

COMMONLY ASSOCIATED CONDITIONS

- Other language problems: articulation disorders, phonologic disorders
- Learning disabilities
- Dyslexia
- Attention deficit hyperactivity disorder (ADHD)
- Students with developmental delay or intellectual impairment are found to stutter up to 25% of the time.

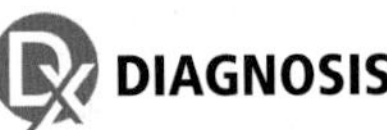

DIAGNOSIS

HISTORY

- Stuttering runs in families by both nature and nurture.
- Age of onset and length of persistence
  - Onset is insidious, with the child often unaware of the problem.
  - If stuttering starts after the 10th birthday, suspect an intracranial mass or brain ischemia.
- Physiologic stuttering is rarely present during oral reading, singing, acting, and reciting in rhythm or while talking to pets or inanimate objects.
- Medications, especially those that increase dopamine, may activate stuttering.
- Increased intracranial pressure from disease or trauma may lead to stuttering.

PHYSICAL EXAM

- There are no specific physical exam findings of stuttering. Observations of children improve the ability to make this diagnosis. Stuttering is 2 or more repetitions of a speech unit.
- Stutterers often improve in one-to-one situations with familiar people, so ask the parents to bring in a video recording of the child in a variety of situations: when talking in public, singing, and talking to a pet or infant.
- Observations that may be made in the office and correlate strongly with the diagnosis of stuttering include the following:
  - Multiple repetitions and/or prolongations
  - Rising pitch with difficult words
  - Grimacing or other physical tension such as taking deep breaths or jerking the head back when speaking
  - Inappropriate emphasis of words not normally emphasized, extremely slow speech, or speech without intonation
- Although unwillingness to speak to the examiner is normal, unwillingness to speak to the parent is not.

DIFFERENTIAL DIAGNOSIS

- Developmental
  - Normal development: dysfluencies associated with rapid onset of full speech capabilities that will usually resolve very quickly
  - Transitory dysfluency is an ill-defined term but generally means stuttering in preschool-aged children that lasts <1 year.
  - Cluttering: Patients with extremely rapid speech will have dysfluencies that resolve with slowing down of speech.
  - Pervasive developmental disorder (autism spectrum disorder): may also have echolalia, tonelessness, and poor eye contact
- Neurologic
  - Tics/Tourette syndrome: similar time of onset, initially somewhat similar symptoms. Stuttering is usually not associated with simultaneous physical movement.
  - Trauma, tumor, or major CNS disease, such as Parkinson disease, may cause late-onset stuttering.
- Medications
  - Any medication that increases the presence of dopamine may worsen (or cause) stuttering. Examples are selective serotonin reuptake inhibitors (SSRI)-type antidepressants or major tranquilizers.

DIAGNOSTIC TESTS & INTERPRETATION

Diagnostic Procedures/Other

- None currently available, but PET scan may be a useful modality in the future.
- If stuttering begins after the age of 10 years, or if the patient has additional neurologic or developmental problems, a workup for brain abnormalities should be considered.

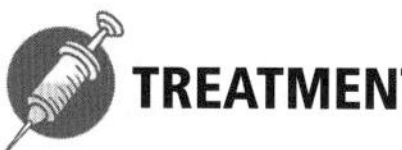

TREATMENT

GENERAL MEASURES

- Therapy must work on improving the child's fluency and increasing acceptance and tolerance of this problem by the patient and his or her family.
- In a multicultural learning atmosphere, sensitivity to the learning styles of each social group is paramount in achieving successful results.
- Current evidence-based analysis suggests that early intervention by a certified speech pathologist is always indicated.

ADDITIONAL THERAPIES

- Speech therapy
  - Stuttering in young children can be resolved with very short courses of therapy, often ≤3 months. Stuttering remains resolved in ≥95% of these early treatment cases. The younger the patient is at the time of referral to speech therapy, the shorter the course of therapy needed and the more likely that the therapy will be successful.
  - Many experts in dysfluency believe that early intervention is more likely to be successful than waiting to start therapy if the stuttering has not spontaneously resolved by the seventh birthday.
  - Among the more successful new programs for young children who stutter is the Lidcombe Program of Early Stuttering Intervention, an intense behavioral therapy program that centers on the belief that stuttering is physical in nature. The program teaches parents and caregivers to praise the child for speaking fluently and to correct them occasionally when they stutter. Parents are supported throughout the process by the clinician. The therapy ultimately enables the child to speak fluently and to monitor his or her own speech.
- Other therapies
  - A successful new therapy for adolescents and adults is a hearing aid–type device (SpeechEasy®, www.speecheasy.com) that feeds the individual's speech directly back into an earpiece.
  - Devices that make hearing monaural or provide a white noise background in the ear also improve stuttering.
  - Information for families is available through organizations such as The Stuttering Foundation, a nonprofit organization (www.stutteringhelp.org).

ALERT

- Because stuttering waxes and wanes with time, temporary improvement does not equal cure.
- Any behavioral therapy must be done under the guidance of a well-trained professional because inappropriate criticism may worsen stuttering.
- Waiting to see if stuttering goes away by age 7 years is not the best strategy for young children, as was often taught in the past.
- The literature does not give a clear time frame for how long stuttering in preschool children should last before requiring evaluation and treatment, but a significant stutter that lasts for >1 year should be referred to a speech therapist.
- No medications are known to reduce stuttering safely. Acupuncture, hypnosis, and yoga have been used with some success but not in controlled studies.

ONGOING CARE

FOLLOW-UP RECOMMENDATIONS

If stuttering is reported by the parents in a preschool-aged child, follow up in 1 to 2 months to see if it was only a transitory dysfluency that has resolved. If not, obtain a speech therapy consult for evaluation.

Patient Monitoring

- Periodic follow-up to ensure that speech therapy is in place and that progress is being made
- Reassessment to ensure that child is adapting to social situations and interacting with others

PATIENT EDUCATION

The following suggestions, although helpful to parents, should be recommended in conjunction with, but not in place of, speech therapy. Parents may be too critical of their own children.

- Take time out of each day to speak with the child one-on-one.
- Model slow speech.
- Wait for the child to speak. Take turns speaking.
- Allow for transition time between activities and tasks.
- Keep a notebook of things that help make speech better and things that elicit stuttering.

PROGNOSIS

- Up to 80% of stuttering cases spontaneously regress by age 16 years.
- Severity of stuttering does not relate to persistence of stuttering.
- The longer stuttering exists, the more likely it will persist.

COMPLICATIONS

- Anxiety and depression, often far out of proportion to the degree of dysfluency
- Blocking and hesitation, giving an impression of delayed intellectual development
- Voluntary withdrawal from social interaction to avoid embarrassment

ADDITIONAL READING

- Craig A, Hancock K, Tran Y, et al. Epidemiology of stuttering in the community across the entire life span. *J Speech Lang Hear Res*. 2002;45(6):1097–1105.
- Frigerio-Domingues C, Drayna D. Genetic contributions to stuttering: the current evidence. *Mol Genet Genomic Med*. 2017;5(2):95–102.
- Jones M, Onslow M, Packman A, et al. Randomised controlled trial of the Lidcombe programme of early stuttering intervention. *BMJ*. 2005;331(7518):659.
- Onslow M, O'Brian S. Management of childhood stuttering. *J Paediatr Child Health*. 2013;49(2):E112–E115.
- Rosenfield DB, Viswanath NS. Neuroscience of stuttering. *Science*. 2002;295(5557):973.
- The Stuttering Foundation. *Videotape No. 70: Stuttering and the Preschool Child. Help for Families*. Memphis, TN: The Stuttering Foundation; 2000. http://www.stutteringhelp.org. Accessed May 8, 2018.
- van Beijsterveldt CE, Felsenfeld S, Boomsma DI. Bivariate genetic analyses of stuttering and nonfluency in a large sample of 5-year-old twins. *J Speech Lang Hear Res*. 2010;53(3):609–619.
- Yairi E, Ambrose N. Epidemiology of stuttering: 21st century advances. *J Fluency Disord*. 2013;38(2):66–87.

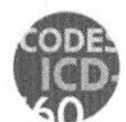

CODES

ICD10

F80.81 Childhood onset fluency disorder

FAQ

- Q: Are some children more prone to stuttering?
- A: Yes. "Sensitive" children (many different definitions in many different studies) are more likely to stutter as are the children of highly critical parents.
- Q: Should family and friends complete the sentences of children who stutter?
- A: No. Children who cannot complete a thought should be gently asked to slow down and try again with no time limit set; others should simply wait until the child has completed his or her sentence. Children with a stuttering problem should also be praised when they do not stutter.

SUBDURAL HEMATOMA

Sabrina E. Smith, MD, PhD

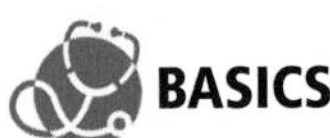

BASICS

DESCRIPTION

A subdural hematoma (SDH) is a collection of blood between the outer pial and inner dural meningeal layers. The bleeding is usually venous in origin, although either cortical arteries or bridging veins may be torn.

EPIDEMIOLOGY

- Heterogeneous causes; occur in all age groups
- Incidence in infants <1 year old estimated at 20 to 25/100,000

RISK FACTORS

- In infants and young children, SDHs are frequently the result of abusive head trauma.
- In older children, SDHs are often the result of motor vehicle collisions.
- Neonatal SDHs occur with spontaneous deliveries but may be more frequent following deliveries with forceps or vacuum extraction. SDHs related to birth usually resolve.
- Abusive head trauma
  - Risk factors for abusive head trauma include disability or prematurity of the child, unstable family situations, parents of young age, and low socioeconomic status.
  - One study found that fathers were the most frequent perpetrators, followed by boyfriends, female babysitters, and mothers, in descending order of frequency.
- Accidental trauma

Genetics

There is no clear genetic predisposition except when hereditary coagulopathy or metabolic disease is implicated.

GENERAL PREVENTION

- Parents should be counseled about appropriate methods to channel frustration and anger toward infants and children. Shaking an infant when the parent is angry is never appropriate.
- Bicycle helmets, car seats, and seat belts are all valuable in preventing head injuries in children.

PATHOPHYSIOLOGY

- SDHs may be acute or chronic:
  - Arterial SDHs grow quickly, whereas venous SDHs may accumulate slowly, remaining undetected for weeks or months.
  - Acute SDHs contain blood, whereas chronic SDHs contain proteinaceous exudate and blood-breakdown products.
  - Rebleeding may be the underlying cause of many chronic SDHs.
- Significant force is usually required for SDH unless there are predisposing circumstances; SDH is only rarely due to trivial or minor trauma. However, SDH can occur with relatively minor trauma in individuals with bleeding disorders, children on chronic dialysis, and those with enlarged extracerebral spaces, arachnoid cysts, or cortical atrophy.
- SDHs in abusive head trauma may be due to the striking of the infant's head against a surface (such as a mattress):
  - The sudden deceleration associated with the impact may tear bridging veins traveling in the subdural space.
- The term shaking-impact syndrome may be more accurate than shaken baby syndrome.

ETIOLOGY

- See "Risk Factors."
- SDHs can also occur after ventricular shunting and extracorporeal membrane oxygenation (ECMO).

COMMONLY ASSOCIATED CONDITIONS

- Some metabolic disorders, such as glutaric aciduria type I and Menkes disease, can be associated with both acute and chronic SDHs.
- Victims of motor vehicle collisions with SDH may have other intracranial injuries such as diffuse axonal injury.
- Traumatic SDHs are often associated with cerebral contusions. Other associated injuries include skull fractures, diffuse axonal injury, and penetrating injuries.

DIAGNOSIS

A careful history and detailed physical exam are essential to explore possible causes of the SDH, assess the child's neurologic status, and look for evidence of other injuries. Prompt neuroimaging is critical.

HISTORY

- Newborns: SDHs due to birth trauma may present with lethargy, pallor, poor feeding, apnea, and seizures. However, many term newborns with small SDHs are asymptomatic.
- Infants and young children: SDHs may also present with a nonspecific history of lethargy, irritability, vomiting, poor feeding, apnea, and seizures.
- Older children: present with a history of trauma and alteration of consciousness
- Caution
  - Be suspicious if the stated history does not fit with the pattern or severity of the injury.
  - Physicians and other health care professionals with experience in child abuse should be consulted early if abuse is suspected.

PHYSICAL EXAM

- Newborns
  - May present with decreased responsiveness, a bulging fontanelle, hypotonia, or hypertonia
  - Retinal hemorrhages are not specific at this age because they are seen in up to 40% of newborns following a vaginal delivery.
- Infants and young children
  - May also present with nonspecific physical signs, but focal neurologic signs may be present
  - Retinal hemorrhages are most often associated with abusive head trauma, but they have been reported after accidental trauma leading to SDH.
  - Bilateral retinal hemorrhages with retinal folds or detachments are particularly associated with abusive head trauma.
- Other signs of child abuse include burns, lacerations, and bruises in various stages of healing and belt marks, choke marks, and multiple fractures of different ages.
- Older children present with signs of external head trauma, decreased responsiveness, and focal neurologic signs.
- SDHs present with nonspecific signs such as vomiting, irritability, lethargy, failure to thrive, anemia, and seizures.

DIFFERENTIAL DIAGNOSIS

- SDHs are usually traumatic, but separating accidental from abusive head trauma may be difficult: Falls in infants may cause linear skull fractures but rarely SDHs. On noncontrast head CT, homogeneous hyperdense SDH is more common following accidental trauma, whereas mixed-density SDH is more common following abusive head trauma.
- Macrocephaly or other signs/symptoms since birth may help to date the origin of the SDH to the perinatal or neonatal period.
- Epidural hematomas, subarachnoid hemorrhages, and acute SDHs cannot be distinguished clinically:
  - The lucid interval sometimes seen with epidural hematomas in adults is not a reliable sign.
  - A head CT should differentiate the different entities.
- Chronic SDHs must be differentiated from benign enlargement of the subarachnoid spaces, a self-limited condition characterized by progressive macrocrania and extra-axial fluid collections with the density of spinal fluid:
  - MRI can differentiate benign enlargement of the subarachnoid spaces from SDH.
  - Rarely, SDH can also occur in children with benign enlargement of the subarachnoid spaces.

DIAGNOSTIC TESTS & INTERPRETATION

- CT scan is the imaging study of choice in acute head trauma with neurologic signs:
  - SDH appears as an extra-axial area of increased density, crescentic in shape, and often associated with cerebral contusion or mass effect.
  - CT also may show evidence of cerebral edema, with loss of gray matter/white matter differentiation and small ventricles.
  - Subacute SDHs may be difficult to distinguish from adjacent gray matter on CT scan.
  - Loss of gray/white matter differentiation may occur.
  - Chronic SDHs appear as areas of low density on CT scan, often bilateral.
- MRI is helpful to clarify subacute and chronic SDHs and to identify small SDHs missed by CT. Early MRI also may reveal shearing injury or hypoxic-ischemic injury and provide information regarding the timing of injury.
- Ultrasound is less helpful because it may be difficult to distinguish the subdural space from the subarachnoid space.

- If child abuse is suspected, a skeletal survey or bone scan is useful to look for fractures of different ages.
- Incidental SDH may be found on neuroimaging studies in newborns; frequently, no intervention is required other than close follow-up.

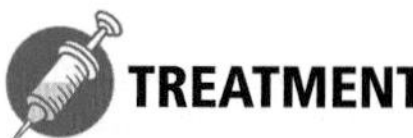

TREATMENT

GENERAL MEASURES

- The treatment of choice for large, acute SDHs is surgical evacuation. Smaller SDHs may be managed conservatively, with careful monitoring for signs of neurologic deterioration.
- While awaiting surgery, attention to airway, breathing, and circulation (ABCs) is critical. Tracheal intubation should be performed if the child's Glasgow Coma Scale score is <8 or if airway protective reflexes are impaired.
- Measures to control intracranial pressure (ICP) include elevating the head of the bed 30 degrees to promote venous drainage and osmotic therapy with mannitol or hypertonic saline:
  - ICP monitoring should be considered.
  - Mild hyperventilation (P_{CO_2} 30 to 35 mm Hg) may be helpful but should not be instituted prophylactically.
  - The efficacy of these measures in improving long-term outcome following large SDHs has not been established. Mild hypothermia and hypertonic saline have been used in some cases of traumatic brain injury in adults, but these are not proven therapies in children.
- Seizures should be treated promptly.
- Treatment of chronic SDHs is more controversial:
  - If there are no signs of elevated ICP, conservative treatment is reasonable, and most collections will resolve.
  - Subdural taps are indicated if ICP rises.
  - If taps are not successful, a subdural peritoneal shunt may be placed.
- Treatment of SDHs that develop after ventricular shunting is particularly challenging.

MEDICATION

Seizures

- Phenytoin/fosphenytoin and levetiracetam are good options if IV medication is needed, with phenobarbital as a reasonable alternative, especially in neonates.
- Prophylactic anticonvulsants given for a few weeks are effective in reducing early posttraumatic seizures but may not affect long-term risk of epilepsy.

ISSUES FOR REFERRAL

Social work services should be consulted in cases of known or suspected child abuse.

SURGERY/OTHER PROCEDURES

The treatment of choice for large, acute SDHs is surgical evacuation.

ADMISSION, INPATIENT, AND NURSING CONSIDERATIONS

- Children with SDHs may be critically ill on presentation.
- The aggressiveness of acute therapy depends on the child's clinical condition.
- Neuroimaging studies and, if necessary, prompt neurosurgical consultation should be performed.
- Isotonic fluids should be given because hypotonic fluids may worsen cerebral edema.

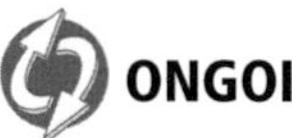

ONGOING CARE

FOLLOW-UP RECOMMENDATIONS

Children with neurologic sequelae from head injury may benefit from admission to a rehabilitation hospital.

PROGNOSIS

- In general, long-term outcome is related to the condition of the child at time of presentation. Prolonged elevation of ICP, concomitant ischemic brain injury, or significant cerebral edema before treatment is worrisome and indicates a poor prognosis.
- Children typically have a better outcome from head injury than do adults, but children <7 years of age often do worse than older children, especially if the SDH is the result of abusive head trauma.

COMPLICATIONS

- SDHs may result in mass effect, focal neurologic signs, and coma.
- Increased ICP and seizures are other serious complications.
- Neurologic sequelae of SDHs are more severe than epidural hematomas because of associated cerebral contusions.
- Long-term problems include headache, seizures, hydrocephalus, cerebral palsy, difficulty concentrating, poor school performance, fixed neurologic deficits, and neurobehavioral problems.
- Epilepsy eventually develops in ~10–15% of patients after severe head injury: This risk generally does not warrant the use of prophylactic anticonvulsants.

ADDITIONAL READING

- Foerster BR, Petrou M, Lin D, et al. Neuroimaging evaluation of non-accidental head trauma with correlation to clinical outcomes: a review of 57 cases. *J Pediatr*. 2009;154(4):573–577.
- Matschke J, Voss J, Obi N, et al. Nonaccidental head injury is the most common cause of subdural bleeding in infants <1 year of age. *Pediatrics*. 2009;124(6):1587–1594.
- Narang S, Clarke J. Abusive head trauma: past, present, and future. *J Child Neurol*. 2014;29(12):1747–1756.
- Piteau SJ, Ward MG, Barrowman NJ, et al. Clinical and radiographic characteristics associated with abusive and nonabusive head trauma: a systematic review. *Pediatrics*. 2012;130(2):315–323.

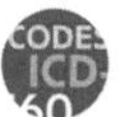

CODES

ICD10

- S06.5X0A Traum subdr hem w/o loss of consciousness, init
- P52.8 Other intracranial (nontraumatic) hemorrhages of newborn
- P10.0 Subdural hemorrhage due to birth injury

FAQ

- Q: When did the bleed occur?
- A: With chronic SDHs, the time and type of injury may be difficult to establish because no trauma may be reported and the trauma may have occurred weeks or months before. Neuroimaging can give some indication of the injury's timing.
- Q: What limitations should be imposed after an acute SDH?
- A: Because SDH may recur with minor trauma, it is prudent to avoid any activities that have significant risk of fall or a blow to the head for weeks to months or until neuroradiologic resolution of the hematoma.
- Q: Why are anticonvulsants not used to prevent seizures following SDHs?
- A: Seizure medications may be given for a few weeks to prevent early seizures following an SDH. After a few weeks, the risks and side effects of the medications outweigh the risk of developing seizures. If seizures begin at a time remote from the injury, then seizure medications can be restarted.
- Q: My baby twisted out of my arms, fell head first onto a tile floor, and suffered a head injury. Will I be reported for child abuse?
- A: Not if the injuries fit with the stated history. In this case, the most likely injury would be a linear skull fracture. If more serious intracranial injuries occur, they will probably not be associated with retinal hemorrhages or other injuries such as older fractures in multiple stages of healing.

S

SUBSTANCE USE DISORDERS

Sara M. Buckelew, MD, MPH

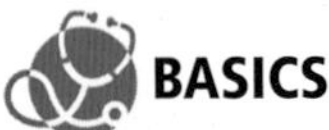

BASICS

DESCRIPTION

- In adolescence, substance use tends to occur along a continuum from abstinence to experimentation to nonproblematic use to problematic use to substance use disorder.
- *DSM-5* defines substance use disorder as a maladaptive pattern of use leading to clinical impairment or distress, which is based on presence of specific criterion including the following:
  - Substance use resulting in failure to fulfill obligations (such as school or work)
  - Substance use in situations that are hazardous (such as driving)
  - Continued use despite interpersonal problems exacerbated by use
  - Development of tolerance
  - Development of withdrawal
  - Craving for the substance
  - Persistent desire or unsuccessful efforts to curb/cut down usage
  - Significant time and energy spent obtaining substances
  - Continued use despite recognition of associated psychological or physical consequences of continued use (with or without physiologic dependence)
- Substance use disorder combines the previous diagnoses of substance abuse and substance dependence from the *DSM-IV*.
- Substance use disorder exists along a continuum from mild to severe depending on the number of criterion met.

EPIDEMIOLOGY

- Substance use estimates vary by substance, age of youth, and geographical location. Up to date, epidemiologic data can be found online at www.monitoringthefuture.org which includes data for cigarette, alcohol, and other illicit drug use among 8th,10th, and 12th graders. Another source of substance abuse data includes the Youth Risk Behavior Survey (YRBS) conducted by the Centers for Disease Control and Prevention.
- Tobacco, alcohol, and marijuana are the most commonly used; however, prescription medication misuse is a significant challenge.
- Adolescent substance use has been associated with increased morbidity and mortality including depression, suicide, motor vehicle accidents, unintentional injuries, teenage pregnancy, high-risk sexual activity, and sexually transmitted infections (STIs).

RISK FACTORS

- Early initiation: Adolescents who begin using alcohol or drugs at an early age have an increased risk of developing an addictive disorder later in life. Later initiation of use may be a protective factor.
- Individual factors such as low self-esteem and impulsivity
- Social factors such as peer use
- Family factors such as a parental tolerance of use, negative parent–child/adolescent relationship, permissive or authoritarian parenting style, parental divorce during adolescence
- Other environmental factors such as school failure and availability of substances within the community
- Individual and family factors may be protective as well such as positive self-esteem and positive, open, and supportive relationships with family.

Genetics

Research demonstrates a genetic predisposition to alcohol dependence. Children of alcoholic parents are 4 to 6 times more prone to developing alcohol dependence.

COMMONLY ASSOCIATED CONDITIONS

- Mood disorders
- Anxiety disorders, including posttraumatic stress disorder
- Eating disorders (specifically bulimia nervosa)
- Attention deficit disorder
- Learning disorders
- Conduct disorders
- Psychotic disorders

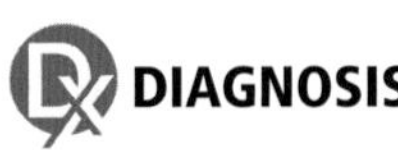

DIAGNOSIS

HISTORY

- Adolescent-appropriate screening using a validated measure should be administered at least annually at every adolescent preventive care visit and appropriate urgent/acute care visits.
- Screening should be performed confidentially and with the adolescent alone (without parents/guardians).
- SBIRT model recommended for adolescents. Includes the following steps: Screening, Brief Intervention, and Referral to Treatment. The Brief Intervention is based in principles of motivational interviewing in addressing behavior change.
- The CRAFFT (an acronym for key components in the questions: Car, Relax, Alone, Forget, Family/Friends, Trouble) screen is one of several tools validated for adolescents.
- All patients who screen positive warrant a more complete assessment including more in-depth substance use history. Questions should include what substances are used, frequency of use, mode of use (nasal, ingestions, smoking, IV), how they are obtaining the substances, and peer group usage.
- The 5 A's was developed to address smoking cessation and includes Asking about use; Advising all smokers to quit; Assessing a patients willingness to quit; Assisting the patient with smoking cessation; and Arranging follow-up.

PHYSICAL EXAM

- Vital signs: increased blood pressure and increased pulse seen in stimulants (such as cocaine, amphetamines), cannabis, phencyclidine (PCP)
- General: odor of alcohol, marijuana, or tobacco; poor personal hygiene; slurred speech; intoxicated appearance
- HEENT: rhinitis and/or nasal mucosa irritation if snorting substances
- Eyes: injected conjunctiva with cannabis; nystagmus with PCP; pupillary constriction with opiates; pupillary dilatation with cocaine, PCP, and opiate withdrawal
- Respiratory depression with opiates, overdose on depressants (such as alcohol and benzodiazepines)
- Respiratory: wheezing/abnormal breath sounds due to smoking substances (tobacco, cannabis, other substances)
- Skin: needle marks in injection users

DIFFERENTIAL DIAGNOSIS

- Mood disorders
- Attention deficit disorder
- Psychotic disorders

DIAGNOSTIC TESTS & INTERPRETATION

Initial Tests (screening, lab, imaging)

- Urine drug screens are most commonly used. Their use in the emergency situation is critical when overdose or acute intoxication is suspected. They can be used effectively as part of a drug treatment program. With limited exceptions, random and routine drug screening is not recommended by the American Academy of Pediatrics and is of limited value.
- Urine drug screens typically include
  - Cannabinoids
  - Cocaine
  - Amphetamines
  - Opiates
  - PCP

Diagnostic Procedures/Other

Screening for STIs including HIV (particularly in IV drug users) and hepatitis B and C is recommended as part of a risk reduction program.

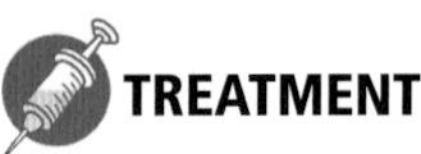

TREATMENT

GENERAL MEASURES

- School-based prevention programs have demonstrated efficacy.
- Treatment can be provided in a number of different settings both outpatient and inpatient with varying intensity, including the following:
  - Outpatient treatment: typically 1 hour weekly, may be individual therapy or family therapy

- Intensive outpatient program or partial hospitalization program: more intensive outpatient program where teen lives at home but may be participating in individual and group therapy multiple hours per day and multiple days per week
- Residential treatment/therapeutic boarding school: where teen is no longer living at home and receiving more intensive services

MEDICATION

- Cigarette/nicotine dependence
  - Nicotine replacement available in number of different forms including nicotine replacement patch, lozenge, inhaler, and gum
  - Bupropion may be recommended in those who have failed with nicotine replacement alone.
  - Varenicline is not approved in those <18 years of age.
- Alcohol dependence
  - Medications available for adults such as naltrexone, disulfiram, and acamprosate are not approved for adolescents.
- Buprenorphine (partial agonist of the mu opioid receptor) for treatment of opioid dependence. Approved in those aged 16 years and older and may be used for maintenance. Methadone has been used for short-term detoxification but not typically used for maintenance due to poor adherence.
- Comorbid and associated psychiatric illnesses such as mood disorders, anxiety disorders, and attention deficit hyperactivity disorder (ADHD) should be medicated appropriately.

ISSUES FOR REFERRAL

- Rates of treatment are low, with only 6–10% of those adolescents with substance use disorders receiving treatment.
- All youth with a concern for substance abuse or comorbid disease should be referred to an experienced mental health professional or addiction specialist.

ADDITIONAL THERAPIES

Strongest body of evidence in the treatment of adolescent substance use disorders is therapy.

- Cognitive behavioral therapy: structured and goal-oriented therapy designed to assist teen in identifying behavioral strategies to address distorted thoughts and subsequent emotions
- Family therapy: Some research demonstrates that family treatments are superior to individual therapy.
- 12-step programs such as Alcoholics Anonymous (AA) and Narcotics Anonymous (NA): typically small group format where participants may provide support for each other
- Brief intervention/brief advice/motivational interviewing: a counseling style that is patient-focused, aimed at exploring benefits and cons of usage in order to direct the patient toward behavior change

ADMISSION, INPATIENT, AND NURSING CONSIDERATIONS

- Detoxification should be considered for youth when there is concern for withdrawal; includes medical management of withdrawal symptoms
- Residential treatment is an intensive, structured program for adolescents who may require this particularly acutely; for those who require 24-hour care and support

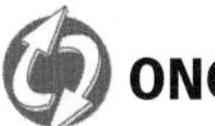

ONGOING CARE

FOLLOW-UP RECOMMENDATIONS

Patient Monitoring

- Patients should be screened annually at all preventive visits.
- When an action plan is created or in those receiving brief advice or brief interventions, patients should be followed closely.
- The pediatrician may play an important role in monitoring for relapse in those who have undergone treatment.

PATIENT EDUCATION

All youth who have not initiated substance use should be given positive reinforcement about their behaviors and encouraged to discuss the topic in the future.

PROGNOSIS

- Youth who receive treatment do better than those who do not.
- Approximately 1/3 to 1/2 of youth who receive treatment will relapse within 12 months following treatment completion.
- Factors associated with relapse include psychiatric comorbidity, poor coping skills, poor familial relationships, and return to prior peer groups.
- Continued involvement in therapy and ongoing support helps to protect against relapse.

COMPLICATIONS

Acute intoxication/overdose can have significant associated morbidity and mortality.

ADDITIONAL READING

- Adger H Jr, Saha S. Alcohol use disorders in adolescents. *Pediatr Rev*. 2013;34(3):103–114.
- Das JK, Salam RA, Arshad A, et al. Interventions for adolescent substance abuse: an overview of systematic reviews. *J Adolesc Health*. 2016;59(Suppl 4):S61–S75.
- Kaplan G, Ivanov I. Pharmacotherapy for substance abuse disorders in adolescence. *Pediatr Clin North Am*. 2011;58(1):243–258.
- Levy SJ, Williams JF; for Committee on Substance Use and Prevention. Substance use screening, brief intervention, and referral to treatment. *Pediatrics*. 2016;138(1):e20161211.
- Ryan SA, Ammerman SD; for Committee on Substance Use and Prevention. Counseling parents and teens about marijuana use in the era of legalization of marijuana. *Pediatrics*. 2017;139(3):e20164069.
- Sanchez-Samper X, Knight J. Drug abuse by adolescents: general considerations. *Pediatr Rev*. 2009;30(3):83–93.

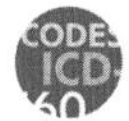

CODES

ICD10

- F19.10 Other psychoactive substance abuse, uncomplicated
- F10.10 Alcohol abuse, uncomplicated
- F12.10 Cannabis abuse, uncomplicated

FAQ

- Q: Should I screen adolescents who use substances for suicide risk?
- A: Yes. All adolescents with a history of substance misuse should be screened for suicide risk and suicidal ideations. Adolescents who use substances have a higher percentage of psychiatric comorbidity and a higher risk of suicide.
- Q: What do I tell parents about their teen's substance use?
- A: The laws about confidentiality pertaining to adolescent substance use and disclosure to parents depend on the state. It is important to know the laws in your state.
- Q: What symptoms would you expect to see based on a patient's blood alcohol level (BAL)?
- A: BAL can be indicative of the severity and may vary due to metabolism and body weight. A BAL of 0.05% is associated with slowing reaction time and altered cognition; 0.1–0.2%: intoxication, drowsiness, and loss of balance; 0.2–0.3% may lead to vomiting and stupor; 0.3–0.4% may lead to hypothermia and coma; and >0.4% may lead to death.

S

SUDDEN INFANT DEATH SYNDROME (SIDS)

Katherine Deye, MD • Rachel Y. Moon, MD

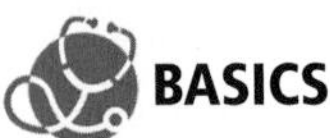

BASICS

DESCRIPTION

- Sudden infant death syndrome (SIDS) is the sudden and unexpected death of an infant <1 year of age, with onset of the lethal episode apparently occurring during sleep, which remains unexplained after a thorough investigation, including the performance of a complete autopsy, review of the circumstances of death, and review of the clinical history.
- SIDS is a subcategory of deaths described as "sudden unexpected deaths in infancy" (SUDI) or "sudden unexpected infant deaths" (SUID). SUID can include both explained deaths, including suffocation, asphyxia, entrapment, trauma (accidental or nonaccidental), cardiac arrhythmia, infection, and metabolic disorders; and unexplained deaths, including SIDS and those with an undetermined/ill-defined cause of death.

EPIDEMIOLOGY

- Most common cause of death in postneonatal (1 month to 1 year old) infants
- Peak age of incidence: 1 to 4 months; uncommon before 2 weeks or after 6 months
- Incidence has been decreasing:
  - 1970s: ∼2.5 SIDS deaths per 1,000 live births: SIDS defined somewhat loosely
  - 1980s: ∼1.4 per 1,000 live births
  - 1990s: ∼1.2 per 1,000 (1992) to 0.7 per 1,000 live births (1999): "Back to Sleep" campaign encouraging supine positioning during sleep in 1994 is associated with steady decline in deaths.
  - 2000s: Since 2001, SIDS rate has declined at a much slower rate. In 2013, the rate was 0.4 per 1,000 live births.
- The rates of accidental suffocation and other undetermined or unspecified causes of death have risen.
  - For example, the death rate from accidental suffocation and strangulation in bed (ASSB) has increased 7-fold between 1994 and 2013.
  - Largely because of improved death scene investigations, many deaths that previously would have been classified as SIDS are now being classified as having resulted from these other causes of death.

RISK FACTORS

- Male gender
- Premature birth or low birth weight
- Inadequate prenatal care
- Poverty
- Lower maternal educational level
- Exposure to prenatal, gestational, and postnatal tobacco smoke
- Alcohol and illicit drug use in utero and after infant's birth
- Maternal substance abuse
- Young maternal age
- Prone and side sleeping position
- Overheating and overbundling
- African American or American Indian/Alaska Native heritage
- Soft sleep surface. Sofas, couches, and cushioned armchairs are particularly hazardous.
- Soft and loose bedding
- Bed sharing, particularly if sharing bed with one or more smokers; if the infant is <4 months of age (even if neither parent is a smoker); if the infant was born preterm or with low birth weight, if sleeping on a surface with soft bedding; if bed sharing adults have consumed alcohol or drugs; if bed sharing with people who are not the infant's parents; and if the sleep surface is very soft (couches, armchairs, waterbeds)
- Potential *protective* factors include the following:
  - Breastfeeding
  - Pacifier use at bedtime and naptime
  - Regular prenatal care
  - Immunizations
  - Room sharing without bed sharing

Genetics

- Most likely represents a heterogeneous group of causes of death
- Genetic factors may play a role in some of these deaths. Candidate genes include those encoding ion channel proteins, serotonin transporters, nicotine-metabolizing enzymes, and those regulating autonomic nervous system development, inflammation, energy production, hypoglycemia, and thermal regulation.
- There appears to be a complex gene and environment interaction.
- Parents should be reassured that the chance of recurrence in future siblings is small and will be examined during the investigation of the SIDS death.

GENERAL PREVENTION

- Place infants on their backs for every sleep until 1 year of life.
  - Preterm infants should be placed supine as soon as possible.
  - The supine sleep position does not increase the risk of aspiration and choking, even in infants with gastroesophageal reflux.
  - Elevating the head of the crib is not recommended as it may result in the infant sliding to the foot of the bed into a position that may comprise respiration.
  - Side positioning has similar risk as prone positioning and should be avoided.
- Use a firm sleep surface.
- Do not use blankets, pillows, bumper pads, sheepskins, or comforters in the infant's sleep area.
- Avoid tobacco smoke exposure during pregnancy and after birth.
- Place the infant for sleep on a separate surface designed for infants in the parental room, close to the parental bed.
- Breastfeed as much and as long as possible.
- Consider offering a pacifier at naptime and bedtime. If breastfeeding, wait until breastfeeding is well established before introducing a pacifier. To decrease the risk of strangulation, do not use pacifiers that attach to infant clothing with sleeping infants.
- Do not use alcohol or illicit drugs during pregnancy or after birth.
- Avoid overheating.
- Do not cover infant's head during sleep.
- Immunize your infant.
- Do not use home cardiorespiratory monitors as a strategy to reduce the risk of SIDS.
- Do not use commercial devices that are inconsistent with safe sleep recommendations.

PATHOPHYSIOLOGY

- The "triple risk" model of SIDS describes the interplay of three factors thought to contribute to these deaths: a vulnerable infant, a critical period of development, and stressful environmental challenges.
  - Individual traits that influence an infant's vulnerability to SIDS are characterized as intrinsic risk factors. Examples include serotonin receptor abnormalities noted in the ventral medulla of up to 70% of SIDS infants at autopsy, suggesting derangements in the neural circuits responsible for arousal and cardiorespiratory functioning. Autopsy studies have also revealed changes in the serotonin transporter gene (*5-HTT*) that ultimately reduce serotonin concentration at these nerve synapses.
  - The period from birth to age 6 months is one of rapid brain growth and maturation, as well as motor skill acquisition, such as the ability to lift and turn the head in the event of life-threatening rebreathing or asphyxia.
  - Exogenous risk factors such as soft bedding, tobacco smoke, side or prone positioning, and overheating place these vulnerable infants at risk for asphyxia or other physiologic disturbances.
- Failure of arousal in the face of asphyxia or other physiologic disturbances likely contributes to the final pathway leading to these infants' deaths. Known risk factors for SIDS have been linked to arousal and cardiorespiratory responses; for example:
  - Prematurely born infants have immature central respiratory responses.
  - When compared with supine-sleeping infants, prone-sleeping infants have increased arousal thresholds.
  - Prenatal and postnatal nicotine exposure blunts arousal responses to hypoxia.

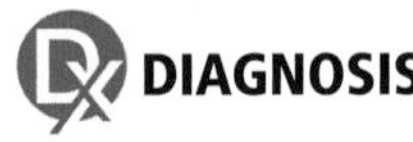

DIAGNOSIS

HISTORY

- SIDS is a diagnosis of exclusion.
  - A thorough postmortem evaluation, including death scene investigation, complete autopsy, and review of the infant's clinical history, should be done.
  - Standardized forms developed by the Centers for Disease Control and Prevention (CDC) for the collection of the circumstances and factors contributing to these deaths and reporting of cases of SUID are available online at https://www.cdc.gov/sids/pdf/suidi-reporting-form.pdf.
- Parents and other caregivers should be interviewed in a sensitive manner so as not to imply that parents or caregivers are blamed for the death. Specifically, the following should be ascertained:
  - Signs and symptoms (such as fever, cough, irritability, easy fatigability, and lethargy) that may be suggestive of an acute or chronic medical condition that may have caused or contributed to the death
  - Family history of sudden death, condition associated with cardiac arrhythmia, epilepsy, metabolic, or genetic disease
  - Known risk factors for SIDS and other SUID, including sleep position when placed and found, sleep environment, bed sharing, prematurity, parental smoking history, and history of maternal substance abuse

- Evidence suggestive of accidental suffocation, strangulation, or entrapment
- Evidence suggestive of nonaccidental traumatic injury and other forms of abuse (including medical child abuse, also known as "Munchausen syndrome by proxy")

PHYSICAL EXAM

- Normal-appearing infant without obvious reason for death
- May have postmortem lividity and/or a pink, frothy discharge from the mouth or nose
- May have signs of terminal motor activity (clenched fists, trismus, or anal dilation)
- Lack of signs of injury or neglect (malnourishment, dehydration, wasting)
- Care must be taken with the deceased body; only medical examiners and coroners have legal authority to establish the cause of death.
- Manipulation or examination of body after the declaration of death may violate applicable laws. All medical paraphernalia used during resuscitation must be left in place.

DIFFERENTIAL DIAGNOSIS

In approximately 10–15% of cases of suspected SIDS, an alternate cause of death is identified. These include the following:

- Environmental: asphyxia (due to such causes as overlaying, wedging, choking, obstruction of nose or mouth, rebreathing, neck compression, immersion in water), hyperthermia, hypothermia, toxic exposures
- Infectious: sepsis (bacterial, viral), pneumonia, bronchiolitis, meningitis, myocarditis, pertussis
- Trauma: accidental and nonaccidental trauma (cranial injuries, abdominal trauma, nonaccidental suffocation, and drowning)
- Metabolic: electrolyte disturbances, inborn errors of metabolism, especially involving energy production or toxic metabolites (e.g., medium chain acyl-CoA dehydrogenase deficiency, defects in glycogenolysis, defects in oxidative phosphorylation, urea cycle defects, aminoacidopathies, glycogen storage disease)
- Congenital/anatomic: congenital heart disease, Arnold-Chiari malformation, malrotation, volvulus
- Miscellaneous: adrenal insufficiency, cardiac arrhythmias (channelopathies)

DIAGNOSTIC TESTS & INTERPRETATION

- A full autopsy, including the cranium and cranial contents, must be performed on all infants who die suddenly and unexpectedly.
- A toxicology screen; microbiologic evaluation for bacterial, viral, and fungal infections; and urine and serum chemistries to evaluate for metabolic disease should be performed—whether these are performed at the hospital or by the medical examiner is dictated by local resources and protocols.
- Skeletal survey
  - Local resources and protocols dictate whether this is performed at the hospital or by the medical examiner.
- Pathologic findings
  - After a review of a thorough death scene investigation, clinical history, and complete autopsy, pathologists can only make the diagnosis of SIDS when no other specific cause of death has been identified.
  - There are no pathologic findings that are pathognomonic. Approximately 80–85% of SIDS infants are noted to have intrathoracic petechiae on examination. Additional common autopsy findings include pulmonary congestion and edema as well as minor airway inflammation.

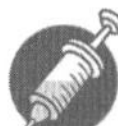

TREATMENT

GENERAL MEASURES

- Prevention rather than treatment is the goal. All caregivers of infants should be educated about SIDS risk reduction strategies, ideally before the infant's birth.
- For families who have experienced a SIDS death, grief counseling may be helpful.
- Families who are contemplating a subsequent pregnancy should be offered genetic and metabolic screening to rule out any hereditary conditions that may mimic SIDS. Avoidance of risk factors should be stressed. However, this discussion should be done with sensitivity, as discussion of risk factors may incur feelings of guilt, particularly if risk factors were associated with the infant's death.
- Health care providers and childcare providers should educate about and model safe sleep practices.
- Media and manufacturers should follow safe sleep guidelines in their messaging and advertising.

ADDITIONAL READING

- Centers for Disease Control and Prevention. What does a safe sleep environment look like? https://www.nichd.nih.gov/publications/pubs/Documents/Safe_Sleep_Environment_English.pdf. Accessed June 3, 2017.
- Hymel KP; and American Academy of Pediatrics, Committee on Child Abuse and Neglect, National Association of Medical Examiners. Distinguishing sudden infant death syndrome from child abuse fatalities. *Pediatrics*. 2006;118(1):421–427.
- Jaafar SH, Jahanfar S, Angolkar M, et al. Effect of restricted pacifier use in breastfeeding term infants for increasing duration of breastfeeding. *Cochrane Database Syst Rev*. 2012;(7):CD007202.
- Kinney HC, Thach BT. The sudden infant death syndrome. *N Engl J Med*. 2009;361(8):795–805.
- Moon RY, Fu L. Sudden infant death syndrome: an update. *Pediatr Rev*. 2012;33(7):314–320.
- Task Force on Sudden Infant Death Syndrome. SIDS and other sleep-related infant deaths: updated 2016 recommendations for a safe infant sleeping environment. *Pediatrics*. 2016;138(5):e20162938.
- Weese-Mayer DE, Ackerman MJ, Marazita ML, et al. Sudden infant death syndrome: review of implicated genetic factors. *Am J Med Genet A*. 2007;143A(8):771–788.
- Willinger M, James LS, Catz C. Defining the sudden infant death syndrome (SIDS): deliberations of an expert panel convened by the National Institute of Child Health and Human Development. *Pediatr Pathol*. 1991;11(5):677–684.

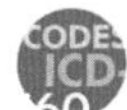

CODES

ICD10

R99 Ill-defined and unknown cause of mortality

FAQ

- Q: What is the difference between SIDS and an undetermined cause of death?
- A: SIDS, which is a subcategory of SUID, is most commonly defined as "the sudden death of an infant <1 year of age, which remains unexplained after a thorough case investigation, including performance of a complete autopsy, examination of the death scene, and a review of the clinical history" (Willinger et al, 1991). When the cause of death cannot be clearly established (e.g., appears to be SIDS, but death occurred in a sleep environment where accidental suffocation cannot be ruled out), cause of death may be "ill-defined" or "undetermined."
- Q: Won't giving a baby a pacifier interfere with breastfeeding?
- A: If a baby is breastfed, there is a theoretical risk of "nipple confusion." A recent Cochrane Collaboration review on the topic (2012) concluded that "for mothers who are motivated to breastfeed their infants, pacifier use before or after breastfeeding was established did not significantly affect the prevalence or duration of exclusive and partial breastfeeding up to 4 months of age." However, long-term data beyond 4 months of age are lacking. If concerned, parents can wait until breastfeeding is well established, usually about 3 to 4 weeks, before introducing a pacifier.
- Q: Is it okay for a baby to take a nap while lying prone on the parent's chest?
- A: No. Parents often fall asleep unintentionally, which can result in a hazardous situation. Falling asleep with the baby while on a couch or sofa is particularly dangerous.
- Q: If an infant rolls into the prone position while he/she sleeps, should the parent place the infant on their back again?
- A: Once an infant possesses the motor skills to roll into the prone position after being placed in the supine position and vice versa, he or she can then be allowed to remain in the sleep position that he or she assumes. All infants should continue to be placed on their back when placed down to sleep until 1 year of age. A predominant risk factor for sleep-related deaths in older infants (4 to 12 months of age) is rolling onto objects in the sleep environment, so caregivers should continue to keep the sleep area free of soft or loose bedding or other objects.
- Q: Is a newborn hearing screen a good screening test for SIDS?
- A: No. Based on current research, the newborn hearing test has not been shown to be a valid screening tool to help determine which infants may be at increased risk to subsequently die of SIDS. Additionally, an increased SIDS risk should not be assumed if an infant has an abnormal newborn hearing screen.
- Q: Can swaddling reduce an infant's risk of SIDS?
- A: There is no evidence that swaddling reduces an infant's risk of SIDS—in fact, an infant who is placed or rolls into the prone position while swaddled has a 12-fold risk of SIDS. If swaddling is used, the infant must always be placed on his or her back, and swaddling must be discontinued once the infant demonstrates attempts to roll. Finally, care must be taken that swaddling is applied in such a manner to minimize the risks of strangulation and head covering.

SUICIDE

Leonard J. Levine, MD • Jonathan R. Pletcher, MD

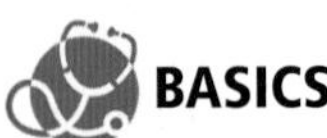

BASICS

DESCRIPTION

- Suicidal behavior is a voluntary self-harming act with the intent of ending one's own life.
- Attempted suicide occurs when the act does not result in death (also, failed or near-suicide).
- Suicidal ideation is any thought, with or without a specific plan, to end one's life.
- Suicidality is the likelihood of an individual completing suicide.
- This chapter will focus on recognizing suicidal ideation and preventing suicide attempt.

EPIDEMIOLOGY

- In 2014, suicide was the 2nd leading cause of death for adolescents and emerging young adults (10 to 24 years) and the 10th overall cause of death in the United States.
- Adolescent mortality from suicide tripled between the 1950s and the 1980s, falling steadily until 1999, then increasing since 1999
- From 1999 to 2014, the age-adjusted suicide rate in the United States has increased 24%, with an increased rate of rise since 2008.
- Females attempt suicide at a rate 2 to 4 times that of males and are most likely to attempt suicide through ingestion.
- Males 15 to 24 years old are 5 times as likely to die by suicide as females and are most likely to use more lethal methods.
- Completed suicide rates are highest in non-Hispanic white (13.9/100,000) and Native American (9.5/100,000) adolescents.
- Gay, lesbian, bisexual, transgender, and questioning youth experience significantly higher rates of suicide thoughts and attempts than their heterosexual peers.
- More than half of all deaths by suicide in the United States involve a firearm.

Incidence

- Annually in the United States, ~2,000 adolescents die from suicide and over a million suicide attempts come to medical attention; there were as many as 11 times the number of attempts as completed suicides.
- Overall, suicide accounted for 11.9 deaths per 100,000 persons aged 15 to 24 years in 2014.
- In 2015, 18% of youth surveyed in grades 9 to 12 reported seriously considering suicide at some point in the preceding year, whereas >8% reported attempting suicide in the previous year.

RISK FACTORS

- Previous suicide attempt(s)
- Mental health disorder
- Social isolation
- Substance/alcohol use disorder
- Family history of suicide
- Family history of severe mental illness or substance abuse
- Past or present sexual or physical abuse
- Family conflict or disruption
- Presence of firearms in the home

GENERAL PREVENTION

- Primary prevention of suicide involves addressing its root causes, including social isolation, childhood trauma, substance use, and depression.
- Predicting which patients will attempt suicide is an emerging science.
- It is possible to identify who may be at risk and to provide resources to address underlying factors.
- Several methods of providing brief, validated screening tools to identify risk factors for suicide are available for primary care and many other medical settings.
- It is recommended to directly ask about suicidal ideation routinely when providing health care to adolescents.
- Talking about or writing about death or suicide, threatening to kill oneself, or looking for ways to kill oneself can all be evidence of suicidal ideation.
- Warning signs, aside from obvious emotional distress, can include the following:
  - Chronic physical symptoms, with or without discrete physiologic etiology (e.g., chronic headache, abdominal pain)
  - Apathy or disengagement with school, work, or home
  - Changes in mood or affect
- If suicidal ideation is suspected, a risk assessment that includes the following components should occur:
  - Frequency and chronicity of suicidal thoughts
  - Evidence of active, detailed planning
  - Access to lethal means such as firearms
  - History of past suicide attempt(s)
  - History of mental health problems, including substance abuse and treatment
  - Acute or anticipated psychosocial stressor
- Referral or consultation with a psychiatrist or mental health professional is indicated with any question or risk for suicide attempt.
- Developing clear referral processes and regular communication with mental health providers is the standard of care for pediatric practitioners.

PATHOPHYSIOLOGY

- Decreased central serotonergic activity may result in aggressive or impulsive behaviors, which may be aimed at oneself.
- An underlying psychiatric or personality disorder acutely worsened by a stressful life event may trigger a suicidal act.
- Feelings of isolation and lack of external support can result in hopelessness and limit opportunities for care.
- Suicide may be an impulsive act to express frustration or rage.
- Suicidal and self-harming behavior may be associated with the onset of other chronic mental health diseases that can occur during adolescence or young adulthood, including schizophrenia.

ETIOLOGY

Suicidal behavior in adolescents results from the interaction of long-standing individual and family factors, social environment, and acute stressors:

- Diagnostic criteria for psychiatric disorders such as major depressive episode and borderline personality disorder include suicidality (*DSM-5*).
- Intense emotional state, in particular shame or humiliation, can be "trigger events" for a suicidal act.
- Personality and social factors, such as antisocial behavior, aggressive or impulsive proclivities, and social isolation, can also contribute.

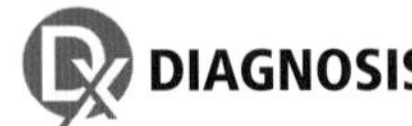

DIAGNOSIS

HISTORY

ALERT

Once suicidal ideation has been disclosed, it is critically important that a prompt suicide risk assessment occur.

- Clinician's confidence and competence in discussing suicidal ideation is a key factor in a successful intervention.
- The provider should establish a quiet environment with clear discussion of confidentiality and limitations before inquiring about suicidal ideation or attempt.
- Brief, to the point, and nonjudgmental questions are key to a successful interview.
- If positive, a comprehensive history should always be obtained or reviewed by a trained mental health worker. Components include the following:
  - Sensitively ascertain any planning, including method and timing.
  - Ask factors that could increase lethality of attempt (e.g., number of pills ingested).
  - Circumstances of attempt (e.g., remote site, public display)
  - History of prior attempts
  - Current psychological status (e.g., feelings and/or level of depression, hopelessness, impulsivity, self-esteem)
  - Family consistency and dynamics
  - Pharmaceuticals available at home; what is missing
  - History of interpersonal conflict or loss
  - Family history of suicide
  - History of substance use
  - History of psychological disorder
  - History of abuse, neglect, or incest
  - Social supports and coping strategies
  - Feelings of regret or continued desire for self-harm

PHYSICAL EXAM

- Regardless of ingestion history, closely observe vital signs, skin, mucous membranes, and pupils for evidence of toxidrome or past drug use.
- Examine skin for signs of physical abuse or self-mutilation, including extremities and torso.
- A complete neurologic examination is essential for the evaluation of intracranial processes, acute mental status changes, and ingestions.

DIAGNOSTIC TESTS & INTERPRETATION

- Different laboratories offer different spectra and sensitivities in their toxicology screens. Testing should be tailored to specific circumstances.
  - Serum and urine toxicology screens
  - Urine pregnancy test: Pregnancy status could be a precipitating factor and, if positive, could affect treatment.

- Acetaminophen level, as it is highly hepatotoxic and is used frequently by teenagers
  - EKG and ongoing cardiac monitoring are indicated for ingestions, including most antidepressants and benzodiazepines.
- Imaging
  - Abdominal plain film: if history of iron or vitamin ingestion or severe trauma

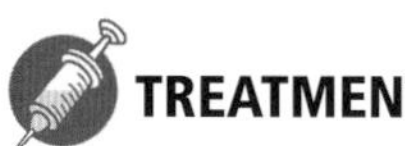

TREATMENT

GENERAL MEASURES

- Medical stabilization is always the first priority, including transfer to the emergency department if there is any question of toxic ingestion or other form of potentially lethal self-injury.
- The objective of any initial intervention for suicidal ideation is to maximize safety until the suicidal ideation diminishes or can be addressed with mental health professionals.
- Parents and professionals should avoid minimizing attempts as "not serious" or as "just seeking attention."
- Engaging the adolescent to develop a safety plan is advisable, while relying on a safety or no-suicide contracts is not recommended.
- When discharge to a caregiver is being considered, the following minimal criteria should be in place at the time of discharge:
  - The patient reliably expresses regret and denies ongoing suicidal thoughts.
  - The patient is medically stable.
  - The patient's adult caregiver reports understanding of the seriousness of the attempt and importance of follow-up.
  - The patient and parents agree to contact a health professional or go to the emergency department if suicidal intent recurs. The patient and family should have 24-hour access to mental health or physical health professionals.
  - The patient must not have impaired mental status (e.g., psychoses, delirium).
  - Lethal methods of self-harm are not immediately available to the patient.
  - Follow-up for underlying mental health disorders have been arranged, including a transfer of key information and clear communication of follow-up locations and times with a behavioral health provider accessible to the patient.
  - Acute precipitants and crises have been addressed.
  - Caregivers and patients are in agreement with the discharge plan.
  - Barriers to obtaining follow-up treatment, in particular insurance and social stigma, have been addressed and will not preclude the next step toward ongoing treatment.

MEDICATION

- Although psychotherapy is an essential component to the care of the suicidal ideation, pharmacotherapy with antidepressants can also play a role.
- Selective serotonin reuptake inhibitors (SSRIs) such as fluoxetine, sertraline, and citalopram, have been shown to be effective in treating depressive disorders in adolescents.
  - Use of SSRIs in patients with the potential for suicidal behavior requires close monitoring.
  - In general, SSRIs may cause a short-term increase from 1% to 2% in the risk of suicidality in depressed teens.
- Tricyclic antidepressants (TCAs) have high lethality potential. TCAs are not indicated in treating depression in children and adolescents.

ISSUES FOR REFERRAL

- Multiple barriers to accessing mental health services can be anticipated, including individual or family resistance due to social stigma, past history of negative experiences, financial and insurance associated restraints, and fear that information may be disclosed.
- If safety is questionable, the disposition should be determined by, or in conjunction with, a mental health professional. Typically occurring in an emergency department setting, assessment for hospital admission takes into account the following criteria:
  - Historical factors indicating high risk for repeated attempt
  - Ongoing suicidal ideation and/or planning
  - Family instability and lack of support
  - Altered mental status
  - Lack of alternative interventions (e.g., intensive psychiatric follow-up, day treatment program)
  - Medication initiation that has risk for increasing suicidal thoughts (e.g., SSRIs)

ADDITIONAL THERAPIES

- Mobile or centralized crisis intervention services may be available to the adolescent and may serve as an effective means to support a safety plan and access to ongoing mental health supports.
- In addition to medication, important psychiatric interventions include acute, short-term, inpatient psychiatric hospitalization; partial hospitalization (with intensive treatment and support); and outpatient therapy.

ADMISSION, INPATIENT, AND NURSING CONSIDERATIONS

- Airway, breathing, circulation (ABCs)
- One-to-one monitoring is typically indicated until formal mental health evaluation is obtained.
- Decontamination of GI tract and circulation is rarely indicated.
- When available, a poison control center or toxicologist will be helpful with evaluation and treatment of most drug ingestions.
- Family engagement and early support with mental health professionals may be key factors in accessing posthospital care.

ONGOING CARE

FOLLOW-UP RECOMMENDATIONS

- Clear plans for outpatient follow-up should be mutually established by the patient, family, and care team at regular intervals, including a plan to identify and coordinate additional supports if follow-up visits are missed.
- In general, continued involvement of the primary health care provider/team is recommended.
- Long-term psychotherapy (individual and family therapy) is often needed for adolescents who attempt suicide.
- Improvement may be slow and punctuated by setbacks.

PROGNOSIS

- 20–50% of those attempting suicide will try again.
- Multiple reports show that a majority of adolescents and young adults who attempt suicide disengage with treatment after a few visits due to a multitude of systemic and societal factors.

COMPLICATIONS

- Long-term organ damage or physical disability, depending on the method used
- Long-lasting emotional sequelae in survivors, resulting from frustration, anger, and guilt
- Repeat suicide attempt or completion

ADDITIONAL READING

- Centers for Disease Control and Prevention. Suicide and self-inflicted injury. https://www.cdc.gov/nchs/fastats/suicide.htm. Accessed May 12, 2017.
- Cooper WO, Callahan ST, Shintani A, et al. Antidepressants and suicide attempts in children. *Pediatrics*. 2014;133(2):204–210.
- National Institute of Mental Health. Statistics. https://www.nimh.nih.gov/health/statistics/suicide/index.shtml#part_153200. Accessed May 12, 2017.
- O'Connor E, Gaynes B, Burda BU, et al. *Screening for Suicide Risk in Primary Care: A Systematic Evidence Review for the U.S. Preventive Services Task Force*. Rockville, MD: Agency for Healthcare Research and Quality; 2013. Evidence Synthesis No. 103. AHRQ Publication No. 13-05188-EF-1.
- Shain B; and Committee on Adolescence. Suicide and suicide attempts in adolescents. *Pediatrics*. 2016;138(1):e20161420.

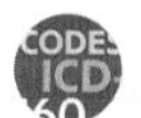

CODES

ICD10

- R45.851 Suicidal ideations
- T14.91 Suicide attempt
- Z91.5 Personal history of self-harm

FAQ

- Q: Should I ever keep suicide attempts or plans confidential?
- A: No. The limits of confidentiality should be clearly outlined to patients and families at the first visit or early in the patient's adolescence. These limits include anything that will directly place the patient's life in danger such as suicidal intent, ongoing or recent abuse, or homicidal intentions.
- Q: If I directly question my patients about suicide, won't that put the idea in their head?
- A: No. In the majority of cases, patients will be relieved by having a professional who wants to talk about suicide. There is only risk in asking if nothing is done with the answer. Appropriate referral to mental health services or counseling will save patients' lives.
- Q: Is a patient who is engaging in self-injurious behavior but denies suicidal ideation actually suicidal?
- A: Any adolescent who is practicing self-mutilation to cope with emotional distress is at risk of developing additional unhealthy coping behaviors. Furthermore, they are likely suffering from a mood disorder that places them at risk for developing suicidality. There is no evidence to support management of self-injurious behavior as if the patient has a secret agenda.

SUPERIOR MESENTERIC ARTERY SYNDROME

Keisha R. Barton, MD • Kristin L. Van Buren, MD, MEd • Eric H. Chiou, MD

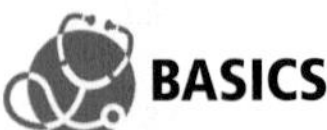

BASICS

DESCRIPTION

- Superior mesenteric artery (SMA) syndrome is the extrinsic compression of the third portion of the duodenum between the SMA and aorta.
- It is also called Wilkie syndrome, Cast syndrome, or aortomesenteric syndrome.
- The diagnosis is somewhat controversial because symptoms do not always correlate with radiologic findings and do not always improve following treatment.

EPIDEMIOLOGY

- Rare
- More common in adolescents
- Also seen following corrective scoliosis surgery with a rate of 0.5–2.4%

ETIOLOGY

- The SMA arises from the abdominal aorta at the L1–L2 vertebral body level and forms an acute downward aortomesenteric angle that is normally between 35 and 65 degrees, due in part to intervening mesenteric fat pad.
- The third portion of the duodenum lies within the aortomesenteric angle, and narrowing of the angle (<25 degrees) can lead to duodenal compression by the SMA anteriorly and the L3 vertebral body posteriorly.
- Any factor that narrows the aortomesenteric angle can cause duodenal compression. Common conditions that predispose to narrowing of this angle are as follows:
  - Conditions associated with significant weight loss leading to loss of the mesenteric fat pad:
    - Anorexia nervosa, malignancy, spinal cord injury, trauma, or burns
  - Rapid linear growth in children
  - Increase in lordosis of the back such as from immobilization by body cast, scoliosis surgery, or prolonged bed rest in a supine position
    - Weight percentile for height of <5% is a risk factor for development of SMA syndrome following scoliosis surgery.
  - Variations of the ligament of Treitz: A short/high-anchoring ligament lifts the third or fourth part of the duodenum into the narrower segment in the aortomesenteric angle.
- If the left renal vein is also compressed, this can lead to microscopic hematuria, also known as nutcracker syndrome.

DIAGNOSIS

HISTORY

- Clinical presentation can be acute or chronic with gradual, progressive symptoms.
- Symptoms are generally consistent with proximal small bowel obstruction, including the following:
  - Nausea
  - Vomiting (bilious and nonbilious, postprandial)
  - Gastroesophageal reflux
  - Epigastric abdominal pain
  - Eructation
  - Weight loss
  - Early satiety
  - Dehydration
  - Bloating
  - Failure to thrive
- Symptoms may be relieved when patient is lying prone, in left lateral decubitus, or in knee-chest positions.

PHYSICAL EXAM

- Nonspecific findings of small bowel obstruction include the following:
  - Abdominal distension
  - Succussion splash
  - High-pitched bowel sounds
- No pathognomonic signs or symptoms, but a history of weight loss, immobilization, or back surgery followed by symptoms of early satiety, bloating, and vomiting after meals would suggest the diagnosis.

DIFFERENTIAL DIAGNOSIS

- Causes of small bowel obstruction
  - Luminal obstruction: foreign body
  - Intramural obstruction: duplication cyst, web, tumor, bezoar, stricture
  - Extramural obstruction: tumor, annular pancreas, bands, adhesions, volvulus, intussusception
- Duodenal dysmotility
  - Intrinsic neuronal disorder
  - Muscular weakness (hollow visceral myopathy, diabetes)
  - Fibrosis (scleroderma, lupus retroperitoneal fibrosis)
  - Collagen vascular diseases
  - Chronic idiopathic intestinal pseudo-obstruction
- Anorexia nervosa/bulimia

DIAGNOSTIC TESTS & INTERPRETATION

Initial Tests (screening, lab, imaging)

- Classic imaging may show duodenal obstruction with dilated stomach and proximal duodenum, active peristalsis, and a narrow angle between the aorta and the SMA.
- Abdominal radiograph is usually the initial diagnostic imaging test.
  - Findings can be nonspecific but may also reveal suggestive findings of obstruction, including a distended stomach or a dilated proximal duodenum with a sharp cutoff of the third portion of the duodenum where the SMA crosses the duodenum.
- Additional evaluation with upper gastrointestinal (UGI) series:
  - Passage of contrast is typically delayed and often stops at the third portion of the duodenum. Contrast passes when the patient is moved to a prone position, where gravity will increase the aortomesenteric angle.
  - Similar findings can be seen with CT.

- Additional imaging may be required if the diagnosis remains unclear.
  - Superior mesenteric arteriography with simultaneous barium contrast radiography to show SMA superimposed on duodenum
  - CT and MR angiography have now replaced superior mesenteric arteriography.
- An aortomesenteric angle <25 degrees is the most useful diagnostic marker, especially if the aortomesenteric distance is <8 mm.
- Determination of the aortomesenteric angle in severe cases may help with decision for surgery.

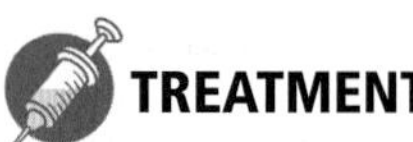

TREATMENT

GENERAL MEASURES

- Correct fluid and electrolyte imbalances.
- Decompress obstruction.
  - Insert nasogastric tube to decompress stomach and proximal duodenum.
- Definitive treatment is aimed at correcting the precipitating factor.
- Feed to improve nutrition and weight gain.
  - Feeding in a prone or left lateral decubitus position can help relieve pain but may require a distal feeding tube (i.e., jejunal tube) to bypass the obstruction.
  - Total parenteral nutrition may be needed if cannot tolerate enteral nutrition.
- If a patient had recent spinal surgery:
  - Frequent repositioning of patients in body casts
  - Reversal of back surgery may be necessary in some patients.

ISSUES FOR REFERRAL

Consider psychiatric evaluation if eating disorder suspected

SURGERY/OTHER PROCEDURES

Surgery is typically unnecessary.

- Surgery is indicated only if supportive care is ineffective.
- Usually performed in patients with a prolonged history of weight loss or pronounced duodenal dilation
- Surgical options include duodenojejunostomy, gastrojejunostomy, or Strong procedure (mobilization of duodenum by dividing the ligament of Treitz).

ONGOING CARE

PROGNOSIS

- Delay in diagnosis of SMA syndrome can result in the following:
  - Electrolyte disturbances
  - Dehydration and malnutrition
  - In severe cases, possible gastric pneumatosis, perforation, formation of a duodenal bezoar, or death
- Most patients do not require surgery and improve with supportive care alone.

ADDITIONAL READING

- Agrawal GA, Johnson PT, Fishman EK. Multidetector row CT of superior mesenteric artery syndrome. *J Clin Gastroenterol*. 2007;41(1):62–65.
- Altiok H, Lubicky JP, DeWald CJ, et al. The superior mesenteric artery syndrome in patients with spinal deformity. *Spine (Phila Pa 1976)*. 2005;30(19):2164–2170.
- Bernotavičius G, Saniukas K, Karmonaitė I, et al. Superior mesenteric artery syndrome. *Acta Med Litu*. 2016;23(3)155–164.
- Jain R. Superior mesenteric artery syndrome. *Curr Treat Options Gastroenterol*. 2007;10(1):24–27.
- Kadji M, Naouri A, Bernard P. Superior mesenteric artery syndrome: a case report [in French]. *Ann Chir*. 2006;131(6–7):389–392.
- Kim IY, Cho NC, Kim DS, et al. Laparoscopic duodenojejunostomy for management of superior mesenteric artery syndrome: two cases report and a review of the literature. *Yonsei Med J*. 2003;44(3):526–529.
- Kurbegov A, Grabb B, Bealer J. Superior mesenteric artery syndrome in a 16-year-old with bilious emesis. *Curr Opin Pediatr*. 2010;22(5):664–667.
- Merrett ND, Wilson RB, Cosman P, et al. Superior mesenteric artery syndrome: diagnosis and treatment strategies. *J Gastrointest Surg*. 2009;13(2):287–292.
- Okugawa Y, Inoue M, Uchida K, et al. Superior mesenteric artery syndrome in an infant: case report and literature review. *J Pediatr Surg*. 2007;42(10):E5–E8.
- Schwartz A. Scoliosis, superior mesenteric artery syndrome, and adolescents. *Orthop Nurs*. 2007;26(1):19–24.
- Vulliamy P, Hariharan V, Gutmann J, et al. Superior mesenteric artery syndrome and the "nutcracker phenomenon." *BMJ Case Rep*. 2013;21:1–2.
- Welsch T, Büchler MW, Kienle P. Recalling superior mesenteric artery syndrome. *Dig Surg*. 2007;24(3):149–156.

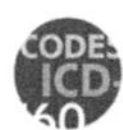

CODES

ICD10

K55.1 Chronic vascular disorders of intestine

FAQ

- Q: When the diagnosis of SMA syndrome is suspected, what are the next steps in management?
- A: The general sequence is to confirm the diagnosis with an imaging study such as an upper GI contrast study and also to initiate supportive care of refeeding and mobilization.
- Q: The following treatment modalities are known to be useful in treatment of SMA syndrome: do nothing, or feed with a jejunal tube, a liquid diet, prone feeding, or total parenteral nutrition. Which program works?
- A: All of the above have been used in SMA syndrome. Weight gain has also been accomplished with total parenteral nutrition.
- Q: Does radiographic testing or a feeding clinical trial help in confirming the diagnosis?
- A: Yes. It may be helpful to confirm the diagnosis and look at the aortomesenteric angle with a CT or MR angiography. In addition, a clinical trial of feeding and weight gain often becomes the criterion for confirmation of the diagnosis.

SUPRAVENTRICULAR TACHYCARDIA

Francesca A. Byrne, MD

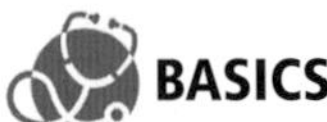

BASICS

DESCRIPTION

- The term supraventricular tachycardia (SVT) is generally used to refer to atrioventricular nodal reentry tachycardia (AVNRT), atrioventricular reciprocating tachycardia (AVRT), and atrial tachycardia (AT) but includes any tachycardia originating at or above the atrioventricular (AV) node.
- The heart rate in SVT in infants generally ranges from 220 to 320 beats per minute (bpm) and in older children from 150 to 250 bpm.

EPIDEMIOLOGY

- SVT is the most common arrhythmia in childhood.
- Incidence of SVT is 35 per 100,000 per year.
- Prevalence of SVT is 1 in 250 to 25,000 children.
- AVRT is the most common type of SVT in children, occurring in ~75% of cases.
- AVNRT rarely occurs before age 2 years.
- 50–60% of pediatric patients with SVT present in the 1st year of life.

RISK FACTORS

- Most children with SVT have structurally normal hearts; however, children with congenital heart disease (CHD) have an increased risk of SVT.
- SVT is commonly observed in patients who have undergone surgery for CHD, for example, after the Mustard/Senning procedure, the Fontan operation, and repair of an atrial septal defect.

Genetics

- Wolff-Parkinson-White syndrome (WPW) syndrome has been noted in several families, and an autosomal dominant (AD) mode of inheritance has been demonstrated:
  - ~15% of cases of WPW have associated CHD, such as Ebstein anomaly, L-looped transposition of the great arteries, and hypertrophic cardiomyopathy.
- ~50% of the cases of junctional ectopic tachycardia (JET) occur in a familial setting with an AD mode of inheritance.

PATHOPHYSIOLOGY

There are two major mechanisms for SVT:

- Reentry tachycardia:
  - This is the most common mechanism for SVT.
  - It involves a circuit rhythm within the atria (atrial flutter), within the AV node (AVNRT), or using an accessory pathway (AVRT); characterized by sudden onset and termination, regular rate, and responsiveness to pacing maneuvers and DC cardioversion
- Automatic tachycardia:
  - Automaticity refers to a group of cells' enhanced ability to spontaneously depolarize, which can overdrive suppress the sinus node.
  - Examples are ectopic atrial tachycardia, multifocal atrial tachycardia, and JET; characterized by warm-up and cool-down phases, an irregular rate that is sensitive to catecholamine states, and lack of responsiveness to pacing and cardioversion

ETIOLOGY

SVT can frequently be precipitated by exercise, infection, fever, or drug exposure.

DIAGNOSIS

HISTORY

- Infants
  - Manifest signs and symptoms of low cardiac output and congestive heart failure (CHF) with prolonged SVT (>48 hours): tachypnea, retractions, irritability, decreased feeding, excessive sweating, hypotension, poor perfusion, and decreased urine output
- A toddler or older child
  - May experience palpitations, shortness of breath, chest pain, anxiety, and dizziness or syncope:
    - It is important to know what the child was doing at the time the arrhythmia started and whether there was an abrupt onset and termination.
    - Older children often report being able to terminate episodes of tachycardia by performing a vagal maneuver.

PHYSICAL EXAM

The following need to be assessed in all patients presenting with SVT:

- Heart rate and regularity
- Respiratory rate
- Blood pressure
- Hydration status
- Peripheral perfusion
- Liver size
- Mental status
- Presence of gallop rhythm

DIFFERENTIAL DIAGNOSIS

- Narrow complex SVT needs to be distinguished from sinus tachycardia.
- Structural heart disease should be excluded in all cases of newly diagnosed SVT.
- Wide-complex tachycardia can be due to SVT with bundle branch block or aberrant conduction, antidromic reciprocating tachycardia with antegrade conduction down an accessory pathway, or preexcited atrial flutter/fibrillation in WPW.
  - This can be difficult to distinguish from ventricular tachycardia.
  - Unless it is known that the patient has SVT, wide-complex tachycardia should always be interpreted as ventricular tachycardia until proven otherwise.
- Differentiating between the types of SVT can be accomplished by evaluating the regularity of the rhythm, modes of onset/termination, and the responsiveness to pacing and cardioversion.

DIAGNOSTIC TESTS & INTERPRETATION

Initial Tests (screening, lab, imaging)

- Electrocardiogram (ECG)
  - 15-lead ECG during SVT if patient is hemodynamically stable and again once sinus rhythm is established
  - Continuous ECG monitoring during therapeutic maneuvers can aid in diagnosis.
- Chest radiograph to assess for pulmonary edema and cardiomegaly
- Echocardiogram to assess underlying cardiac anatomy (with first episode) and ventricular function (if prolonged tachycardia)

Follow-Up Tests & Special Considerations

Repeat imaging may be warranted if there are initial abnormalities.

Diagnostic Procedures/Other

- Outpatient: Diagnosis can be made with ambulatory cardiac monitoring. Patients with WPW pattern have ventricular preexcitation (short PR interval and a delta wave) on the ECG during sinus rhythm.
- An exercise stress test may be indicated in older patients with exercise-induced SVT or those with WPW syndrome to help determine the risk of rapid antegrade conduction through the accessory pathway.
- Electrophysiologic study is often performed to evaluate drug effect, assess risk, or to map in conjunction with catheter ablation.
- Nonpharmacologic maneuvers (ice, vagal) and pharmacologic maneuvers (IV adenosine) may distinguish tachycardias that involve the AV node from other types of SVT.

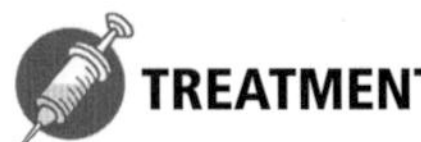

TREATMENT

GENERAL MEASURES

- Short-term treatment goals are to terminate the tachycardia.
  - Nonpharmacologic vagal maneuvers; for example, ice to the face for 15 to 30 seconds, rectal stimulation, Valsalva, gag, and headstand may be helpful. In younger children, Valsalva can be achieved by having the child blow into an obstructed straw or thumb. Pacing maneuvers via an esophageal catheter may also be used. Carotid massage and orbital pressure should not be performed in children.
  - Unstable patients with hemodynamic compromise warrant termination with synchronized DC cardioversion (0.5 to 2.0 J/kg).
- Long-term treatment goals are to reduce the frequency of episodes of SVT. Long-term treatment may not be necessary when the episodes are infrequent, self-terminating, or produce minimal symptoms.

MEDICATION

- In a stable child with acute SVT, adenosine (rapid IV bolus, 0.1 mg/kg and increase by 0.1 mg/kg to a maximum of 0.3 mg/kg or 12 mg) may be used to block the AV node for reentrant SVT that requires the AV node. The half-life of the drug is <10 seconds. Because of the risk of atrial fibrillation, DC cardioversion should be available. Use adenosine with caution in asthmatic patients, as it can cause acute bronchospasm.
- IV verapamil is an effective therapy in older children with SVT but should be avoided in children <12 months of age because of its vasodilatory and negative inotropic effect.
- Long-term preventive pharmacotherapy is an alternative approach in some patients.

- Reentrant SVT
  - β-Blockers (propranolol or atenolol) are 1st-line treatment in individuals with WPW and SVT.
  - Flecainide and amiodarone may be used in cases that are more resistant.
  - Oral digoxin is an option in patients with hemodynamically stable SVT. Digoxin is contraindicated in patients with WPW.
  - Atrial flutter may be treated with digoxin, flecainide, sotalol, or amiodarone as a single agent or in combination.
- Automatic SVT:
  - Automatic tachycardias may be responsive to antiarrhythmics such as β-blockers, flecainide, and amiodarone, either alone or in combination.

ISSUES FOR REFERRAL

Patients suspected of having SVT or those with documented SVT should be referred to a pediatric cardiologist or pediatric electrophysiologist. A copy of the ECG is important.

SURGERY/OTHER PROCEDURES

Catheter ablation using radiofrequency energy or cryoenergy is an alternative to long-term drug therapy and is indicated in the following scenarios:

- SVT refractory to medical therapy
- Side effects from the medical regimen
- Patient choice due to frequency, duration, or poor quality of life
- Life-threatening arrhythmias (syncope)
- Rapid conduction properties of an accessory pathway (e.g., WPW)
- Congenital or acquired heart disease

ADMISSION, INPATIENT, AND NURSING CONSIDERATIONS

- Always assess the child's ABCs (airway, breathing, and circulation).
- Adenosine should be given as a rapid IV push, followed by a normal saline flush due to the short drug half-life <10 seconds.
- Admission for cardiac monitoring is indicated in hemodynamically unstable SVT.
- If the duration of the SVT episode was prolonged, evaluate for tachycardia-induced cardiomyopathy.

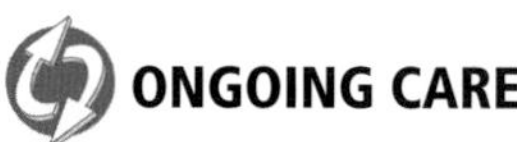

ONGOING CARE

PROGNOSIS

- Of patients who present in infancy, 30–70% will be asymptomatic by 1 year of age. However, ~1/3 of these patients may experience a reappearance of their tachycardia at an average age of 8 years.
- Most older children who present with SVT will have recurrence of SVT.
- 20–30% of those with WPW pattern on the ECG (preexcitation/delta wave) will develop SVT and have WPW *syndrome*. Only 8% of those with intermittent preexcitation on ECG will develop SVT.

FOLLOW-UP RECOMMENDATIONS

- As SVT may recur, neonates and infants have historically received maintenance therapy for the 1st year of life and then been observed off medications if they are not having breakthrough episodes of SVT. This approach has recently been challenged, and studies evaluating the ideal duration for maintenance therapy in the neonate and infant are being conducted.
- In children who present beyond infancy, spontaneous resolution of the tachycardia substrate is less likely, and treatment may need to be continued into adulthood. These patients may be considered for catheter ablation therapy.
- Over-the-counter sympathomimetic cold medications and caffeine should be avoided, as they may increase the likelihood of SVT.

COMPLICATIONS

Complications from SVT can arise from one of three causes:

- Persistent tachycardia can lead to CHF, tachycardia-induced cardiomyopathy, and cardiovascular collapse. This is especially true of the infant whose symptoms go unrecognized for 24 to 48 hours.
- Some patients with WPW syndrome (<5%) can have rapid antegrade conduction through the accessory pathway. A rapid ventricular response to atrial flutter/fibrillation can potentially cause ventricular fibrillation and sudden death. Digoxin and verapamil should not be used in patients with WPW syndrome because they enhance antegrade conduction through the accessory pathway.
- Side effects of pharmacologic agents used to treat SVT include bradycardia, other arrhythmias due to proarrhythmic effects, and noncardiac side effects (gastrointestinal, liver, pulmonary, and thyroid dysfunction).

ADDITIONAL READING

- Cohen MI, Triedman JK, Cannon BC, et al. PACES/HRS expert consensus statement on the management of the asymptomatic young patient with a Wolff-Parkinson-White (WPW, ventricular preexcitation) electrocardiographic pattern: developed in partnership between the Pediatric and Congenital Electrophysiology Society (PACES) and the Heart Rhythm Society (HRS). Endorsed by the governing bodies of PACES, HRS, the American College of Cardiology Foundation (ACCF), the American Heart Association (AHA), the American Academy of Pediatrics (AAP), and the Canadian Heart Rhythm Society (CHRS). *Heart Rhythm*. 2012;9(6):1006–1024.
- Drago F. Paediatric catheter cryoablation: techniques, successes and failures. *Curr Opin Cardiol*. 2008;23(2):81–84.
- Fox DJ, Tischenko A, Krahn AD, et al. Supraventricular tachycardia: diagnosis and management. *Mayo Clin Proc*. 2008;83(12):1400–1411.
- Friedman RA, Walsh EP, Silka MJ, et al. NASPE Expert Consensus Conference: radiofrequency catheter ablation in children with and without congenital heart disease. Report of the writing committee. North American Society of Pacing and Electrophysiology. *Pacing Clin Electrophysiol*. 2002;25(6):1000–1017.
- Manole E, Saladino RA. Emergency department management of the pediatric patient with supraventricular tachycardia. *Pediatr Emerg Care*. 2007;23(3):176–185.
- Paul T, Bertram H, Bökenkamp R, et al. Supraventricular tachycardia in infants, children and adolescents: diagnosis, and pharmacological and interventional therapy. *Paediatr Drugs*. 2000;2(3):171–181.
- Sanatani S, Potts, Reed JH, et al. The study of antiarrhythmic medications in infants (SAMIS): a multicenter, randomized controlled trial comparing the efficacy and safety of digoxin versus propranolol for prophylaxis of supraventricular tachycardia in infants. *Circ Arrhythm Electrophysiol*. 2012;5(5):984–991.

S

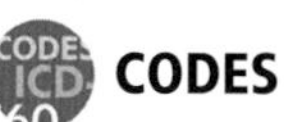

CODES

ICD10

I47.1 Supraventricular tachycardia

FAQ

- Q: How should infants on chronic therapy be monitored?
- A: Parents with infants on chronic therapy for SVT should be educated about counting the heart rate by palpation or auscultation at least 1 or 2 times daily. This method of surveillance is just as effective as apnea/bradycardia monitors. Because alarm monitors are inaccurate and can increase parental anxiety with frequent false alarms, they are generally not recommended. Patients on amiodarone should be monitored with liver function tests and thyroid function tests at baseline and every 3 to 6 months.
- Q: What is the concern with verapamil?
- A: Verapamil is an L-type calcium channel blocker that blocks conduction in the AV node and is very effective in treating SVT in adults. Because myocardial contractility in infants depends mostly on the trans-sarcolemmal L-type calcium channels, hypotension, and cardiovascular collapse have been reported in children <1 year of age.
- Q: What are success rates and risks of catheter ablation?
- A: The success rate of radiofrequency catheter ablation varies from 80% to 97%, depending on the location of the arrhythmia substrate. The incidence of major complications is <2%, with the most common being heart block requiring a pacemaker, cardiac perforation, brachial plexus injury, and embolization. The risk of complete heart block is greater in patients whose accessory pathway is located close to the AV node. In such patients, cryoablation is a safer ablation technique because of its potentially reversible electrical and thermal effect.

SYMPATHOMIMETIC POISONING

Robert J. Hoffman, MD, MS

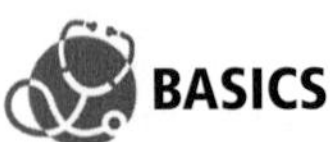

BASICS

DESCRIPTION

- Excess autonomic stimulation by adrenergic agents produces the clinical syndrome typically described as "sympathomimetic."
- The sequelae of sympathomimetic overdose are generally neurologic, cardiovascular, and psychiatric.
- Severe problems may include agitation-induced hyperthermia, cardiac dysrhythmia, hypertension, myocardial ischemia, infarction, cerebrovascular accident (CVA), seizure, and cardiovascular collapse.

EPIDEMIOLOGY

- Cocaine, methamphetamine, and 3,4-methylenedioxymethamphetamine (MDMA; commonly called "Molly" or "ecstasy") are the three most common illicit stimulant drugs causing emergency visits in the United States.
- Prescription stimulants such as methylphenidate and albuterol are often frequent causes of intentional as well as unintentional poisoning.
- Bath salts (mephedrone and methylenedioxypyrovalerone [MDPV] among others) appear to be associated with a much higher incidence of psychotic events than other sympathomimetics.
- A number of potent amphetamine analogs, such as paramethoxymethamphetamine (PMA), which have a high incidence of morbidity and mortality, are increasingly common components of tablets sold as MDMA.

PATHOPHYSIOLOGY

- Relevant pathophysiology is based on the adrenergic receptor type stimulated by the drug in question. The adrenergic receptors of relevance include α_1, β_1, and β_2 receptors.
- Common adverse effects of stimulant toxicity include the following:
  - Tachycardia, palpitations, chest pain, and tremor
  - Hypertension
  - Nausea, vomiting
  - Anxiety, fear, and headache also may occur.
  - More severe symptoms may be associated, if associated with end-organ injury such as stroke or intracranial hemorrhage, myocardial infarction, or other cardiovascular injury.
- Sympathomimetic toxicity is highly variable depending on the half-life. For most amphetamines and cocaine, this typically peaks in 1 to 2 hours and lasts 4 to 8 hours. Sustained-release medications may alter this time course and cause much longer toxicity.
- Ephedrine and pseudoephedrine stimulate both α and β receptors:
  - Excessive cardiovascular stimulation results in symptoms qualitatively similar to those that occur with catecholamines.
  - Ephedrine and pseudoephedrine have weaker penetration of the CNS relative to drugs of abuse.
  - As a result, users may suffer from systemic complications of the relatively larger doses necessary to achieve the CNS "high" of other stimulants.
- Isoproterenol, rarely used, is the prototypical nonselective β-agonist causing the following:
  - Tachycardia, hypotension, tachydysrhythmia, myocardial ischemia, and flushing due to its cardiostimulatory and vasodilatory properties
  - Commonly, CNS effects of anxiety, fear, and headache occur.
- Selective β_2-adrenergic agonists are commonly used, and these include albuterol, levalbuterol, salmeterol, terbutaline, and others. Besides stimulant toxicity, other effects of β_2 agonists include:
  - Hypotension, often with widened pulse pressure
  - Hyperglycemia and hypokalemia
  - Elevation of creatine phosphokinase (CPK) as well as troponin, although myocardial infarction is never expected to occur in otherwise healthy children with selective β_2 agonist exposure
- Selective α_1 agonists include phenylephrine and phenylpropanolamine, although the latter is no longer commercially produced in any meaningful quantity in the United States.
  - Hypertension due to direct vasoconstrictive effects is the most common effect.
  - Reflex bradycardia may occur, particularly with phenylpropanolamine.
  - Headache due to elevated BP and even CVA may occur.

ETIOLOGY

Causative agents:

- Agents with combined α- and β-adrenergic activity: all amphetamines, cocaine, ephedrine, norepinephrine, pseudoephedrine, and dopamine
- α_1-Adrenergic agonists: phenylephrine, phenylpropanolamine
- β-adrenergic agonists: nonselective β-agonist isoproterenol
- Selective β_1 agonists: dobutamine
- Selective β_2 agonists: albuterol, salmeterol, terbutaline
- Overdose from sympathomimetic agents occurs secondary to the use of prescription drugs, nonprescription drugs such as over-the-counter (OTC) cold medicine (e.g., pseudoephedrine), dietary supplements (e.g., ephedra, synephrine), and illicit drugs such as cocaine, amphetamine, and methamphetamine.
- Illicit drugs: cocaine, amphetamine, methamphetamine, MDMA (ecstasy), MDPV (bath salts)
- Recently, many newer amphetamine congeners have come into use. These are available for purchase over the internet, and until specific legislation can be passed against a certain new drug, it can be legal.
  - Examples of new but illegal stimulants are mephedrone and MDPV ("bath salts").
  - 1,3-dimethylamylamine (DMAA) is an example of a stimulant widely sold over the internet. DMAA was briefly banned in the United States but is currently legal again.
- Theophylline and caffeine may cause a clinical syndrome of sympathomimetic poisoning.

COMMONLY ASSOCIATED CONDITIONS

- Many sympathomimetic agents are capable of producing psychiatric symptoms, particularly psychosis.
- This psychosis is similar to or indistinguishable from schizophrenia.
- Two rare results of MDMA use include serotonin syndrome and syndrome of inappropriate antidiuretic hormone (SIADH) with symptomatic hyponatremia.

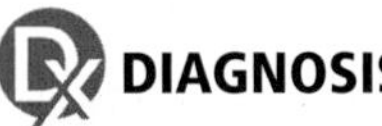

DIAGNOSIS

- The clinical effects of these agents' overdose vary based on their receptor selectivity.
- Most agents have some degree of combined α- and β-adrenergic activity (ephedrine, pseudoephedrine).
- Cardiovascular: palpitations, tremor, headache, chest pain; if intracranial hemorrhage or infarction, signs and symptoms of stroke including visual changes, weakness, paralysis, dysarthria, or coma
- Psychiatric: anxiety, apprehension, psychosis

HISTORY

- History of exposure may be helpful but is often unavailable or deliberately concealed, particularly use of illicit drugs such as cocaine or amphetamines.
- Use of OTC medicines, such as multisymptom cold preparations or dietary supplements
- The onset of symptoms usually occurs within 1 hour.
  - Typically, prescription and OTC sympathomimetic agents are inhaled or orally administered.
  - Inhalation or injection results in immediate symptoms.
  - Cocaine, amphetamine, and methamphetamine or the sympathomimetics are most commonly used in this manner.

PHYSICAL EXAM

Sympathomimetic toxicity is a clinical diagnosis.

- Vital sign derangement is the most common and most reliable indicator of toxicity.
- HEENT: mydriasis, visual changes, epistaxis, poor dentition
- Cardiovascular: Tachycardia and hypertension are typical.
- Skin: diaphoresis, flushing
- CNS: Psychomotor agitation is very common, but delirium or psychosis is also frequent. Focal neurologic findings may occur. Focal cranial nerve abnormalities are particularly concerning for the possibility of CVA.

DIFFERENTIAL DIAGNOSIS

- Anticholinergic syndrome
- Hyperthyroidism/thyroid storm
- Mania/psychosis
- Lithium toxicity
- Neuroleptic malignant syndrome
- Pheochromocytoma
- Serotonin syndrome
- Subarachnoid hemorrhage

- Withdrawal syndromes
- Other situations of increased endogenous catecholamine release

DIAGNOSTIC TESTS & INTERPRETATION

- An EKG should be obtained to assess for ischemia as well as dysrhythmias.
- Sympathomimetic overdose is a clinical diagnosis, and lab assays are only adjunctive.
- Unless there are specific forensic indications, such as malicious poisoning or child abuse, drugs of abuse screening is not recommended and is not useful.
- Serum acetaminophen level should be considered in patients with ingestion with intent of self-harm.
- The measurement of electrolytes, BUN, creatinine, and blood sugar may be useful.
- Cardiac markers (e.g., CPK-MB, troponin) are appropriate to screen for cardiac injury.
- A noncontrast head CT or MRI should be obtained in unresponsive patients or those with focal neurologic deficits.

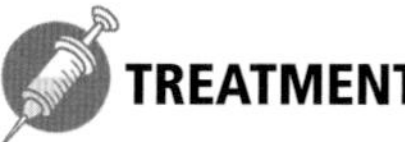

TREATMENT

Managing ABCs should be addressed first, but sympathomimetic toxicity usually does not result in illness requiring any specific airway, breathing, or circulation issues.

GENERAL MEASURES

Maintaining vital signs within acceptable limits and controlling patient agitation are commonly required.

- Managing ABCs is paramount.
- Sedation of agitated patients with a benzodiazepine is often appropriate.
- Benzodiazepines treat both cardiovascular stimulation and psychomotor agitation.
- Use of specific cardiovascular medications to lower blood pressure (BP) and heart rate may be needed.
- Particularly for cocaine toxicity, β blockers are usually avoided to prevent paradoxical hypertension.
- In recent years, a growing body of evidence suggests that ketamine is extremely effective to sedate adolescents or adults with agitated delirium.
- Use of antipsychotics, such as haloperidol or droperidol, is relatively contraindicated both because these medications may lower seizure threshold, impair heat dissipation, and increase risk of cardiac dysrhythmia.
- Special therapy
  - Severe hyperthermia should be treated with active cooling.
  - Patients with core temperature of ≥107°F should be placed in an ice bath or ice packs and have core temperature monitored.
- IV fluids
  - Unless there is a contraindication, at least maintenance IV fluid should be administered.
  - IV fluids may protect against rhabdomyolysis as well as potential dehydration that may occur with stimulant exposure.

MEDICATION

Agitation, vasoconstrictive effects, chronotropic and inotropic effects, are the most common issues requiring mediation therapy for sympathomimetic toxicity.

First Line

- Psychomotor agitation may be managed with benzodiazepines.
- The quantity of benzodiazepine required will directly depend on degree of adrenergic stimulation.
- Large doses may be required for sedation.
  - Lorazepam in doses of 0.1 mg/kg IV q15min until sedation is achieved and then maintenance dosing q4–6h
  - Diazepam 0.1 mg/kg IV q10min until sedation is achieved and then maintenance dosing q2–4h
- Ketamine 1 mg/kg IV or 3 mg/kg IM in a single dose may be used to sedate agitated patients.
- Vasoconstrictive effects may be managed with a variety of medications.
  - Phentolamine 0.1 mg/kg/dose (up to 5 mg/dose) IV repeated q10min PRN
  - A dihydropyridine calcium channel blocker, such as nifedipine or amlodipine, may be used.
  - Sodium nitroprusside 0.3 to 10 mcg/kg/min IV, titrated to effect
- Chronotropic and inotropic effects may be managed with conduction-modulating calcium channel blockers such as diltiazem or verapamil.

Second Line

- A β-blocker may be used only if an α-adrenergic antagonist is concomitantly administered.
- Use of a β-blocker without α-adrenergic blockade may result in paradoxical increase in BP and death.
  - Labetalol has some α-adrenergic blockade and may be used alone as a 2nd-line agent: 0.2 to 0.5 mg/kg/dose IV, maximal dose 20 mg, followed by infusion of 0.25 to 1 mg/kg/h
  - Esmolol 500 mcg/kg IV bolus over 1 minute followed by infusion 50 mcg/kg/min titrated to effect up to 500 mcg/kg/min
- Severe cardiovascular symptoms resulting from β-agonists or methylxanthines such as theophylline or caffeine may be treated with a β-blocker.
  - This treatment may seem counterintuitive in the management of hypotension.
  - Severe β_2 agonist effects resulting in hypotension may be counteracted by using a β-blocker.
  - Such therapy should only be undertaken under the direction of a medical toxicologist, intensivist, or other clinician familiar with and experienced with use of such cardiovascular medications.

ADMISSION, INPATIENT, AND NURSING CONSIDERATIONS

- Any patient with severely deranged vital signs; end-organ manifestations such as chest pain, severe headache, focal neurologic deficit; or other evidence of CVA; and patients with persistent agitation or psychosis should be admitted.
- Any patient with vital signs within safe limits, normal mental status, and no evidence of end-organ damage or manifestations may be discharged from the emergency department or inpatient unit.

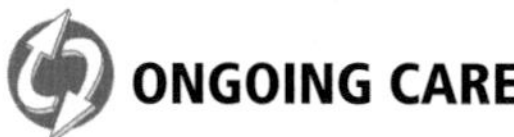

ONGOING CARE

PROGNOSIS

If end-organ damage such as myocardial infarction or CVA is prevented, prognosis for full recovery to premorbid status is excellent.

COMPLICATIONS

The most common catastrophic complications are cardiovascular, including ventricular dysrhythmia, myocardial infarction, and CVA.

ADDITIONAL READING

- Carr BC. Efficacy, abuse, and toxicity of over-the-counter cough and cold medicines in the pediatric population. *Curr Opin Pediatr*. 2006;18(2):184–188.
- Gibbons S. "Legal highs"—novel and emerging psychoactive drugs: a chemical overview for the toxicologist. *Clin Toxicol (Phila)*. 2012;50(1):15–24.
- Isbister GK, Calver LA, Downes MA, et al. Ketamine as rescue treatment for difficult-to-sedate severe acute behavioral disturbance in the emergency department. *Ann Emerg Med*. 2016;67(5):581–587.e1.
- Kuehn BM. Citing serious risks, FDA recommends no cold and cough medicines for infants. *JAMA*. 2008;299(8):887–888.

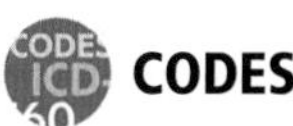

CODES

ICD10

- T44.901A Poisn by unsp drugs aff the autonm nervous sys, acc, init
- T44.991A Poisoning by oth drug aff the autonm nervous sys, acc, init
- T48.5X1A Poisoning by oth anti-cmn-cold drugs, accidental, init

S

SYNCOPE

Nancy A. Drucker, MD

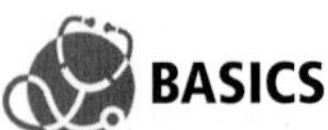

BASICS

DESCRIPTION

Transient loss of consciousness, typically lasting no longer than 1 to 2 minutes, due to a transient drop in cerebral perfusion pressure

GENERAL PREVENTION

- Avoiding circumstances predisposing to the most common form of syncope (vasovagal)
- Sitting or lying down when warning signs occur
- Maintaining adequate hydration, especially during illness/exertion

PATHOPHYSIOLOGY

Most common mechanism is vasovagal or neurocardiogenic, in which a variety of stimuli and conditions—pain, heat, dehydrated state, emotional upset, carotid pressure—trigger increased vagal tone, leading to slowed heart rate, peripheral vasodilation, and decreased cerebral perfusion.

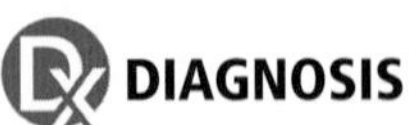

DIAGNOSIS

HISTORY

- **Question:** Did the event occur during exercise or at rest and were there any symptoms prior to the event?
- *Significance*: important information used to distinguish syncope from seizure or head trauma
- **Question:** Does the child or observer recall "presyncopal" signs?
- *Significance*: often present in patients with benign syncope—such as warmth, diaphoresis, lightheadedness, nausea, palpitations, auditory, or visual changes—all lasting only a few seconds before loss of consciousness
- **Question:** Family history?
- *Significance*: Obtaining a careful history is essential. Family history of sudden unexpected death, seizures, syncope, cardiomyopathy, or arrhythmias especially at younger ages or requiring pacemaker/implantable defibrillator should trigger further testing and investigation.
- **Question:** Syncope during exercise or without warning?
- *Significance*: may indicate an underlying arrhythmia, coronary artery anomaly, or myocardial dysfunction
- **Question:** Generalized tonic–clonic movements?
- *Significance*: may occur with syncope due to epilepsy or vasovagal syncope —presyncopal signs point to the nonepileptic nature of the event
- **Question:** Longer duration of unconsciousness or slow recovery?
- *Significance*: greater probability that the event is epileptic rather than syncope
  - Caution: Syncope may be associated with a convulsion in a patient with epilepsy.
  - Epilepsy may rarely mimic a syncopal episode or recurrent presyncopal symptoms; temporal lobe syncope seems to occur principally in adults or adolescents.
- **Question:** Details of body position, eye movements, and respiratory pattern?
- *Significance*: may help determine etiology
- **Question:** Carbon monoxide poisoning?
- *Significance*: may cause syncope-like spells; ask about potential exposure.

PHYSICAL EXAM

Key findings to document include the following:

- Vital signs with orthostatic pulse and BP changes
- Four-extremity BP
- Pulses in arm and leg
- Funduscopy: possible papilledema
- Cranial bruits
- Precordial thrill
- Heart sounds (gallop, click, rub, significant murmur)

DIAGNOSTIC TESTS & INTERPRETATION

Often, only a thorough physical exam, detailed history, and family history are needed if findings are consistent with vasovagal syncope.

- **Test:** EKG and cardiac consultation
- *Significance*: If the event is suggestive of a heart condition or there is a concerning history/family history, an EKG and cardiac consultation may be indicated.
- **Test:** treadmill EKG, Holter monitoring, echocardiogram, EEG, MRI (Chiari malformation)
- *Significance*: Children with unexplained syncope may undergo more extensive testing.
- **Test:** glucose, CBC, blood gases, spinal tap
- *Significance*: Laboratory testing may be appropriate based on clinical suspicion of underlying causes.

ALERT

Pitfall: Recurrent syncope due to prolonged QT interval may be missed on routine EKG; prolongation of QT interval may only be noted on treadmill testing or cardiac monitoring.

DIFFERENTIAL DIAGNOSIS

- Cardiac
  - Congenital heart defect
  - Myocarditis
  - Cardiomyopathy
  - Coronary artery anomaly
  - Heart block (congenital or acquired complete heart block, status postcardiac surgery)
  - Arrhythmia secondary to long QT syndrome
  - Brugada syndrome
  - Arrhythmogenic right ventricular dysplasia
  - Catecholaminergic polymorphic ventricular tachycardia
  - Wolff-Parkinson-White syndrome
  - Syncope due to an arrhythmia may be familial and may occur as unprovoked syncope or as exercise-induced syncope that may resemble an epileptic convulsion.
- Neurologic
  - Migraines (predisposed to orthostatic intolerance)
  - Arteriovenous malformation
  - Intracranial hypertension due to hydrocephalus, mass, pseudotumor
- Pulmonary
  - Pulmonary hypertension
- Other
  - Medications/toxins

- Other causes of syncope by age group include the following:
  - Toddlers
    - Pallid or cyanotic breath-holding spells; these occur in response to pain, fear, excitement, or frustration, begin with a deep inspiration or exhalation, although the precipitating "gasp" may not be apparent (iron deficiency may be associated). A history of pallid breath-holding spells is not uncommon in adolescents with vasovagal syncope.
  - Older children
    - Situational syncope: venipuncture, defecation, hair brushing, stretching
    - Dysautonomia, orthostatic hypotension
    - Dehydration
    - Adrenal insufficiency
- Syncopal spells in children may be accompanied by a convulsion (nonepileptic) that usually lasts <1 minute (EEG shows normal findings or slowing, not epileptiform activity).
- Alternative causes of loss of consciousness not due to syncope include the following:
  - Head trauma
  - Epilepsy ("temporal lobe syncope")
  - Psychogenic
  - Stroke
  - Hypoglycemia (rare except in certain metabolic disorders)
  - Anxiety/hyperventilation

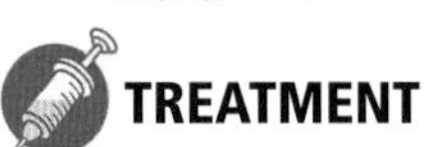

TREATMENT

GENERAL MEASURES

- Clinical intervention is aimed primarily at training the patient in prevention/anticipation:
  - Avoiding circumstances predisposing to the most common form of syncope (vasovagal)
  - Sitting or lying down when warning signs occur
  - Maintaining adequate hydration, especially during illness/exertion
  - Support stockings may be beneficial.
- Therapy is otherwise addressed to underlying causes, in the unusual circumstance that one is found.
- Syncope during exercise always warrants a cardiovascular evaluation, with EKG as initial step.

MEDICATION

Medications are not usually necessary; however, in more extreme clinical presentation, patients may benefit from:

- Midodrine (midodrine hydrochloride): Adult dosing is 10 mg orally, 3 times daily. Dosing should take place during the daytime hours when the patient needs to be upright, pursuing the activities of daily living. A suggested dosing schedule of approximately 4-hour intervals is as follows: shortly before or upon arising in the morning, midday, and late afternoon (not later than 6 p.m.).

ONGOING CARE

- Many children experience a developmental stage in which for unknown reasons they have frequent vasovagal episodes. Most common age group is adolescents; however, syncopal spells may continue through adulthood.
- Persistent and frequent spells may prompt more extensive laboratory testing, as described earlier.

ADDITIONAL READING

- Batra AS, Hohn AR. Consultation with the specialist: palpitations, syncope, and sudden cardiac death in children: who's at risk? *Pediatr Rev*. 2003;24(8):269–275.
- Driscoll DJ, Jacobsen SJ, Porter CJ, et al. Syncope in children and adolescents. *J Am Coll Cardiol*. 1997;29(5):1039–1045.
- Friedman KG, Alexander ME. Chest pain and syncope in children: a practical approach to the diagnosis of cardiac disease. *J Pediatr*. 2013;163(3):896–901.
- Friedman MJ, Mull CC, Sharieff GQ, et al. Prolonged QT syndrome in children: an uncommon but potentially fatal entity. *J Emerg Med*. 2003;24(2):173–179.
- Kapoor WN. Syncope. *N Engl J Med*. 2000;343(25):1856–1862.
- McVicar K. Seizure-like states. *Pediatr Rev*. 2006;27(5):e42–e44.
- Sapin SO. Autonomic syncope in pediatrics: a practice-oriented approach to classification, pathophysiology, diagnosis, and management. *Clin Pediatr (Phila)*. 2004;43(1):17–23.
- Strickberger SA, Benson DW, Biaggioni I, et al. AHA/ACCF scientific statement on the evaluation of syncope. *Circulation*. 2006;113(2):316–327.
- Strieper MJ. Distinguishing benign syncope from life-threatening cardiac causes of syncope. *Semin Pediatr Neurol*. 2005;12(1):32–38.
- Task Force for the Diagnosis and Management of Syncope, European Society of Cardiology, European Heart Rhythm Association, et al. Guidelines for the diagnosis and management of syncope (version 2009). *Eur Heart J*. 2009;30(21):2631–2671.
- Wieling W, Ganzeboom KS, Saul JP. Reflex syncope in children and adolescents. *Heart*. 2004;90(9):1094–1100.
- Willis J. Syncope. *Pediatr Rev*. 2000;21(6):201–204.

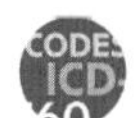

CODES

ICD10

R55 Syncope and collapse

FAQ

- Q: What limitations in activity are appropriate for children with recurrent syncope who have normal heart structure and function?
- A: Precautions should be taken similar to those for children of similar age who have epilepsy—closely monitored water recreation and restrictions on climbing; however, most children with recurrent syncope do not experience spells in the midst of vigorous activity and do not warrant activity restrictions.
- Q: Do breath-holding spells cause brain damage?
- A: Pallid breath-holding spells appear to be uniformly benign; in rare cases, older children with cyanotic breath-holding spells have had neurologic sequelae of recurrent hypoxemia.
- Q: When should I refer a patient with syncope to a cardiologist?
- A: Syncope during exercise or without any preceding symptoms/warning signs, abnormal cardiac exam, or worrisome family history

SYNDROME OF INAPPROPRIATE ANTIDIURETIC HORMONE SECRETION

Todd D. Nebesio, MD, FAAP

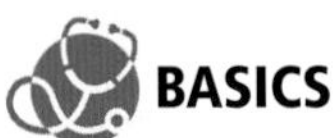

BASICS

DESCRIPTION
Inappropriate secretion of antidiuretic hormone (ADH) or ADH-like peptide in the presence of low serum sodium, low serum osmolality, and high urine osmolality and in the absence of renal, adrenal, or thyroid pathology

EPIDEMIOLOGY
Incidence
The syndrome of inappropriate ADH secretion (SIADH) can occur at any age. Its incidence depends on the various possible etiologies.

RISK FACTORS
Genetics
Genetic causes of SIADH are exceedingly rare. However, rare cases have been described with gain-of-function mutations in the vasopressin-2 receptor contributing to SIADH and undetectable serum ADH levels.

PATHOPHYSIOLOGY
- ADH is synthesized within the neurons of the hypothalamus, transported in conjunction with neurophysin down the supraopticohypophyseal tract, and stored in the posterior pituitary.
- ADH acts on the renal collecting ducts.
- Interaction of ADH with its receptors forms intracellular cyclic AMP (cAMP), which increases water permeability through insertion of aquaporins (water channels) in renal collecting ducts and consequently enhances reabsorption of free water.
- SIADH results when elevated ADH or ADH-like peptide concentrations cause free water retention and hypervolemia, leading to hyponatremia; three possible mechanisms include
  - Increased hypothalamic production of ADH (e.g., CNS disorders such as stroke or meningitis)
  - Independent production of ADH or ADH-like substances from ectopic sources (e.g., oat cell carcinoma of the lung or olfactory neuroblastoma)
  - Decreased venous return that stimulates atrial volume receptors and thereby leads to ADH release (e.g., heart failure, cirrhosis; pulmonary and intrathoracic diseases, such as tuberculosis)

ETIOLOGY
- Idiopathic
- CNS pathology, causing increased secretion of ADH or ADH-like peptides: meningitis, head trauma, neurosurgical procedures, encephalitis, brain tumor, brain abscess, hydrocephalus, hypoxia, subarachnoid hemorrhage, cerebral venous thrombosis
- Ectopic production of ADH or ADH-like peptides: oat cell carcinoma of the lung, bronchogenic carcinoma, olfactory neuroblastoma, and pancreatic carcinoma
- Pulmonary disease (leading to secondary elevation in ADH secretion or ADH-like peptides): tuberculosis, viral or bacterial pneumonia, asthma, cystic fibrosis, pneumothorax, positive pressure ventilation
- Drugs (which mimic ADH or stimulate its release): vincristine, cyclophosphamide, carbamazepine, chlorpropamide, phenothiazines, clofibrate, nicotine, selective serotonin reuptake inhibitors (SSRIs)
- Iatrogenic exogenous ADH administration: vasopressin infusion for treatment of diabetes insipidus, excess desmopressin (DDAVP®) in conjunction with fluid intake
- Severe, prolonged nausea
- Postoperative patient (e.g., as part of triple-phase response after hypothalamic-pituitary surgery, after transsphenoidal pituitary surgery)
- Rocky Mountain spotted fever
- Stem cell transplantation

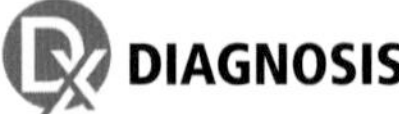

DIAGNOSIS

HISTORY
- Unusual water intake (suspicious for psychogenic polydipsia)
- Review of intake and output for inpatients
- Decreased urine output
- Anorexia, lethargy
- Weight gain or weight loss
- Renal disease
- Vomiting
- Diarrhea
- Diuretic use
- Burns
- Heart disease
- Liver disease
- Brain injury: trauma, surgery, hypoxia, toxin

PHYSICAL EXAM
- A complete neurologic and physical exam must be performed. Classically, patients with SIADH manifest subtle signs of hypervolemia but without increased urine output.
- With or without edema
- No signs of dehydration
- Signs of fluid overload
- Absent hyperpigmentation of skin creases/gums (Presence suggests Addison disease.)
- Hyponatremia; may cause lethargy or irritability and muscle cramps. In severe cases, patients may lose deep tendon reflexes, seize, or be comatose.

ALERT
- Pitfall: Failure to distinguish SIADH from other causes of hyponatremia such as adrenal insufficiency, hypothyroidism, or cerebral salt wasting (CSW) can result in erroneous medical management and lead to worsening hyponatremia.
- Patients with SIADH are still capable of producing urine; basing the diagnosis on urine volume alone can be misleading.

DIAGNOSTIC TESTS & INTERPRETATION
Initial Tests (screening, lab, imaging)
- Specific tests
  - Simultaneous urinary osmolality, serum osmolality, and serum sodium (order a basic metabolic panel)
  - Urine sodium: usually >30 mmol/L (but not usually >100 mmol/L)
  - Serum uric acid: sometimes low in SIADH
  - Presence of hyponatremia (serum sodium <130 mEq/L), decreased serum osmolality (<260 mOsm/kg), with an inappropriately elevated urinary osmolality (>260 mOsm/L)
  - Plasma ADH concentration: diagnostic but not helpful for rapid diagnosis
- Nonspecific tests
  - Fractional renal excretion of sodium: Net sodium loss is normal or elevated and depends on sodium intake.
  - Urinary specific gravity: helpful but not as specific as urine osmolality
  - Blood glucose: Hyperglycemia results in hypertonic hypernatremia (benign).
  - Triglycerides: Hyperlipidemia causes hypertonic hypernatremia (benign).
- Head MRI with special cuts of the pituitary and hypothalamus if concern of CNS etiology

DIFFERENTIAL DIAGNOSIS
- Hypovolemic hyponatremia (e.g., hyponatremic dehydration, seen after running a marathon)
- Euvolemic hyponatremia (e.g., hypothyroidism, adrenal insufficiency)
- Hypervolemic hyponatremia (e.g., CHF, cirrhosis, nephrotic syndrome)
- Diuretics
- Total body sodium loss through vomiting, nasogastric suction, diarrhea, or increased intestinal secretions
- Renal failure
- Severe potassium depletion
- Water intoxication
- CSW: excess production or effects of atrial and/or brain natriuretic peptide hormones
- Reset hypothalamic osmostat.

- Rocky Mountain spotted fever
- Hypertonic hyponatremia (sometimes called "pseudohyponatremia," although blood sodium is low with normal total body sodium stores) with hyperglycemia (diabetic ketoacidosis), severe hyperlipidemia, or after administration of mannitol

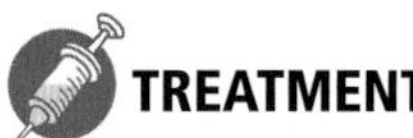

TREATMENT

GENERAL MEASURES

- The most important aspects of therapy for SIADH are diagnosis and treatment of the underlying cause.
- If hyponatremic and sodium >120 mEq/L and no neurologic signs, first step in management is fluid restriction.
- Hyponatremia may result in seizure, which requires immediate treatment with 3% hypertonic saline until the seizure activity stabilizes. Despite the urgent need for correction of hyponatremia to address the severe neurologic symptoms, the rate of sodium correction should not exceed 12 mEq/L in 24 hours.

MEDICATION

- For emergency use only: hypertonic saline (1.5–3% NaCl)
- Diuretics should be avoided because they worsen hyponatremia.
- ADH antagonists, such as tolvaptan and conivaptan, have been shown to be effective for treatment of SIADH in research trials for adults.
- Demeclocycline (for chronic SIADH); avoid using in children <8 years old as it can stain and discolor teeth and inhibit bone growth.
- Oral urea (for chronic SIADH)

ADMISSION, INPATIENT, AND NURSING CONSIDERATIONS

- Patients with severe hyponatremia and/or neurologic manifestations will need to be admitted for correction of hyponatremia under close medical supervision.
- Fluid restriction is essential to treat and prevent worsening hyponatremia. Thus, IV fluids, in general, are not recommended for patients with SIADH. If IV fluids are clinically necessary, a rate comparable to insensible losses (1/3 daily maintenance) is recommended with close attention to serum sodium levels.
- The hyponatremia in SIADH is due to free water retention and not due to decreased total body sodium content. For this reason, changing IV fluids from hypotonic solutions to normal saline without restriction of the IV fluid rate will still result in worsening hyponatremia.
- Discharge criteria
  - Depends on the primary etiology causing SIADH
  - Generally, when the serum sodium is stabilized and the patient is neurologically stable

ONGOING CARE

FOLLOW-UP RECOMMENDATIONS

Patient Monitoring

- When to expect improvement: After about 48 to 72 hours of fluid restriction, the serum sodium level will gradually start to increase.
- Signs to watch for: changes in neurologic status

DIET

Fluid restriction is the most important aspect in the treatment of SIADH. Generally, only fluids for insensible losses (1/3 daily maintenance) are recommended.

PROGNOSIS

Based on the primary cause

COMPLICATIONS

- Severe hyponatremia can cause seizures and, rarely, brain damage. Correcting hyponatremia too quickly can lead to central pontine myelinolysis (CPM), a devastating demyelinating disease that impairs vital functions such as breathing.
- Susceptibility to CPM due to correction of hyponatremia is strongly influenced by the severity and preexisting duration of hyponatremia in the patient.
- Serum sodium should not be increased >12 mEq/L in 24 hours.

ADDITIONAL READING

- Cuesta M, Thompson CJ. The syndrome of inappropriate antidiuresis (SIAD). *Best Pract Res Clin Endocrinol Metab*. 2016;30(2):175–187.
- Ellison DH, Berl T. Clinical practice. The syndrome of inappropriate antidiuresis. *N Engl J Med*. 2007;356(20):2064–2072.
- Feldman BJ, Rosenthal SM, Vargas GA, et al. Nephrogenic syndrome of inappropriate antidiuresis. *N Engl J Med*. 2005;352(18):1884–1890.
- Fenske W, Allolio B. The syndrome of inappropriate secretion of antidiuretic hormone: diagnostic and therapeutic advances. *Horm Metab Res*. 2010;42(10):691–702.
- Palmer BF. Hyponatremia in patients with central nervous system disease: SIADH versus CSW. *Trends Endocrinol Metab*. 2003;14(4):182–187.
- Rivkees SA. Differentiating appropriate antidiuretic hormone secretion, inappropriate antidiuretic hormone secretion and cerebral salt wasting: the common, uncommon, and misnamed. *Curr Opin Pediatr*. 2008;20(4):448–452.

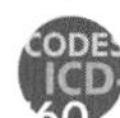

CODES

ICD10

E22.2 Syndrome of inappropriate secretion of antidiuretic hormone

FAQ

- Q: Is diuretic use beneficial in treating SIADH?
- A: No. Although diuretics may relieve the effects of volume overload, they can also worsen hyponatremia. Overall, diuretics usually cause more detriment than benefit in SIADH.
- Q: What distinguishes SIADH from CSW?
- A: CSW occurs because of increased natriuresis from increased plasma and CSF levels of atrial natriuretic peptide (ANP) after neurologic insults (e.g., subarachnoid hemorrhage). Owing to the natriuresis, these patients become dehydrated with notable decreased plasma volume and elevated BUN. In contrast, patients with SIADH have free water overload, causing hyponatremia. CSW is associated with high urine output, in contrast to SIADH, which has low urine output. However, patients with SIADH who are treated with excess solute (3% saline) may exhibit a natural natriuresis and high urine output. Thus, polyuria alone should never be used to distinguish between CSW and SIADH. Net sodium loss is very high in CSW (>100 mmol/L), but SIADH has normal to slightly elevated net sodium loss; thus, urinary sodium levels are often not specific in distinguishing CSW from SIADH. Laboratory features of CSW include suppressed plasma aldosterone and often normal serum uric acid concentration. Note that plasma ADH concentration is high in SIADH and initially in CSW as well. However, in CSW, after the intravascular volume has been restored, ADH will decrease again and patients may not exhibit elevated urine osmolality. In these patients, persistent hyponatremia with elevated urine osmolality is more suggestive of SIADH, which is far more common than CSW.
- Q: Why is it important to distinguish SIADH from CSW?
- A: Therapies differ dramatically for these conditions. Unlike the water and fluid restriction used to treat SIADH, treatment of dehydration in CSW requires replacement of ongoing salt and water losses. However, CSW is much less common than SIADH and appropriate diagnosis of each condition is necessary to avoid worsening of the hyponatremia by the treatment regimen.

SYNOVITIS–TRANSIENT

Jay Mehta, MD, MS

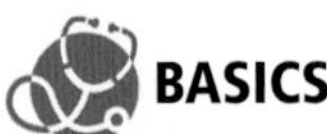

BASICS

DESCRIPTION
Transient inflammatory process resulting in arthralgia and arthritis (especially affecting the hip), often precipitated by an exposure to an infectious agent

EPIDEMIOLOGY
- Any age at risk
- Most common in ages 3 to 8 years
- Males affected ~2 times more frequently

RISK FACTORS
Genetics
No specific associations

PATHOPHYSIOLOGY
Unclear

ETIOLOGY
Usually viral (especially upper respiratory but also enterovirus). Allergic and traumatic causes have been proposed as well.

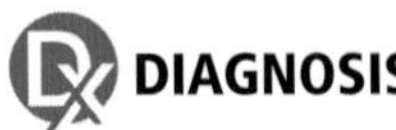

DIAGNOSIS

HISTORY
- Preceding infection (URI, UTI, gastroenteritis) or trauma
- Relatively rapid onset of symptoms, with acute onset of groin or thigh pain or refusal to bear weight
- Non–toxic-appearing child

PHYSICAL EXAM
- General examination usually benign
- Child refuses to bear weight but may tolerate limited ranging of joint.
- Bilateral in 1–4% of cases
- Effusions in peripheral joints are rare and usually small and evanescent.
- Pitfalls
  - Distinctions between transient synovitis and a septic joint may be impossible.
  - Fever, inability to bear weight, extreme pain, and guarding on passive ranging raises suspicion for septic joint.

DIFFERENTIAL DIAGNOSIS
- Infection
  - Lyme disease
  - Septic arthritis
  - Tuberculosis
  - Gonorrhea
- Trauma (fracture or soft tissue injury)
  - Slipped capital femoral epiphysis
  - Avascular necrosis
  - Labral tear
- Tumors
  - Osteoid osteoma
- Immunologic
  - Juvenile idiopathic arthritis
  - Spondyloarthritis
- Psychologic
  - Psychogenic limp
  - Imitative limp
- Miscellaneous
  - Hypothyroidism

DIAGNOSTIC TESTS & INTERPRETATION
Initial Tests (screening, lab, imaging)
- CBC
  - Usually mild leukocytosis
- Erythrocyte sedimentation rate (ESR)
  - Usually mild elevation (20 to 40 mm/h)
  - ESR >40 mm/h raises suspicion for septic joint.
- C-reactive protein (CRP)
  - Mild elevation (1 to 2 mg/dL)
  - CRP >2mg/dL raises suspicion for septic joint.
- Radiography
  - Usually normal findings or joint space widening or small effusion
  - No periosteal changes
- Ultrasound
  - Affected hip joints may have demonstrable effusions.
- MRI
  - Normal bone marrow signal intensity may help differentiate transient synovitis from septic hip.

Diagnostic Procedures/Other
- Joint aspirate culture is usually not needed unless suspicion for septic joint.
- Be wary of contaminated joint aspiration cultures.
- Up to 50% of infected joints are negative on culture.

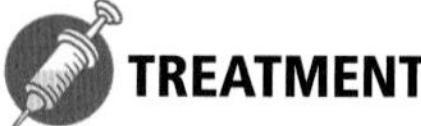

TREATMENT

GENERAL MEASURES

Pitfalls

- Missing a septic hip or, alternatively, overinvestigating transient synovitis with invasive procedures
- Avoid initiation of therapy until septic joint has been ruled out, although rapid resolution of symptoms with one NSAID dose is reassuring against septic hip.

MEDICATION

- Usually responsive to NSAIDs such as oral ibuprofen (up to 10 mg/kg/dose q.i.d.)
  - If not responsive to NSAIDs, consider septic joint.
- Very rarely, a short course of oral steroids is necessary.

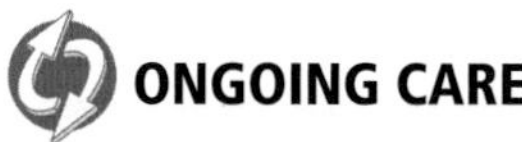

ONGOING CARE

FOLLOW-UP RECOMMENDATIONS

Usually significant improvement in 24 to 48 hours

Patient Monitoring

Ongoing synovitis despite therapeutic levels of NSAIDs or any bony change indicates need to change diagnosis.

PROGNOSIS

Excellent, although on occasion, patients will experience recurrence of symptoms with subsequent viral syndromes or if there is an underlying spondyloarthritis.

COMPLICATIONS

Increased incidence of Legg-Calves-Perthes disease following episode of transient synovitis

ADDITIONAL READING

- Del Baccaro MA, Champoux AN, Bockers T, et al. Septic arthritis versus transient synovitis of the hip: the value of screening laboratory tests. *Ann Emerg Med*. 1992;21(12):1418–1422.
- Do TT. Transient synovitis as a cause of painful limps in children. *Curr Opin Pediatr*. 2000;12(1):48–51.
- Luhmann SJ, Jones A, Schootman M, et al. Differentiation between septic arthritis and transient synovitis of the hip in children with clinical prediction algorithms. *J Bone Joint Surg Am*. 2004;86-A(5):956–962.
- Taekema HC, Landham PR, Maconochie I. Towards evidence based medicine for paediatricians. Distinguishing between transient synovitis and septic arthritis in the limping child: how useful are clinical prediction tools? *Arch Dis Child*. 2009;94(2):167–168.
- Uziel Y, Butbul-Aviel Y, Barash J, et al. Recurrent transient synovitis of the hip in childhood. Long-term outcome among 39 patients. *J Rheumatol*. 2006;33(4):810–811.

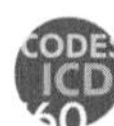

CODES

ICD10

- M67.30 Transient synovitis, unspecified site
- M67.359 Transient synovitis, unspecified hip
- M67.351 Transient synovitis, right hip

FAQ

- Q: Are there any chronic sequelae from transient synovitis?
- A: Not usually. This is generally a benign disease, but there is an increased incidence of Legg-Calve-Perthes disease after transient synovitis.
- Q: Is there an association with chronic arthritis?
- A: No. There is no known increased risk for chronic arthritis in affected children unless this is the first manifestation of a spondyloarthritis.

S

SYPHILIS

Ibukunoluwa C. Akinboyo, MD • Joseph B. Cantey, MD • Pablo J. Sánchez, MD

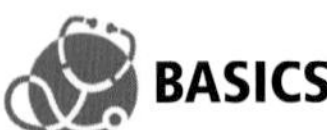

BASICS

DESCRIPTION

- Etiologic agent: *Treponema pallidum*
- Can be congenital or acquired
- Consider sexual abuse when syphilis diagnosed in young children.
- All confirmed cases should be reported to the local public health department.

EPIDEMIOLOGY

- Congenital syphilis
  - Approximately 12.4 cases per 100,000 live births in 2015 (487 cases), mostly among blacks
  - Case fatality rate 6%; 82% of deaths are stillborn.
  - Occurs via vertical transmission and mostly transplacental, but natal transmission possible by contact with infectious lesions at time of delivery
  - Fetal infection can occur at any time of gestation
- Acquired syphilis
  - Sexually transmitted
  - Highest among men who have sex with men (MSM)
  - Often facilitates transmission and acquisition of HIV. All persons with syphilis should be tested for HIV.
  - Open, moist mucocutaneous lesions are highly infectious for up to 24 hours after institution of treatment.

RISK FACTORS

- Congenital syphilis
  - Lack of prenatal care
  - Maternal use of illicit drugs
  - Maternal HIV infection
- Acquired syphilis
  - MSM
  - HIV infection, especially among MSM
  - Illicit drug use (especially crack cocaine)
  - Sexual abuse

DIAGNOSIS

- Congenital syphilis
  - Clinical manifestations range from clinically unapparent to stillbirth (see "Physical Exam").
- Acquired syphilis
  - Primary stage: chancre, single or multiple, at the site of inoculation ~3 weeks after exposure (range, 10 to 90 days); lesions usually resolve without treatment in 3 to 6 weeks.
  - Secondary stage: generalized rash that involves the palms and soles, condyloma lata (see "Physical Exam"); signs appear 3 to 6 weeks after initial chancre and may last 2 to 10 weeks.
  - Latent stage: seroreactive but no clinical manifestations
    - Early latent: syphilis within the past 12 months
    - Late latent: syphilis >1 year duration
    - Unknown duration: timing of infection not known
  - Relapse: symptoms of secondary syphilis that recur during the first 1 to 4 years of latent infection
  - Tertiary stage: Up to 1/3 of untreated secondary syphilis cases progress to tertiary or late disease that occurs 15 to 30 years after the initial infection; gummatous changes of the skin, bone, or viscera; cardiovascular syphilis (aortitis); neurosyphilis (tabes dorsalis, general paresis)
  - Neurosyphilis: CNS involvement in 3–7% of cases; can develop at any stage of disease; signs include headache, altered mood/behavior, meningitis, hyperactive reflexes, impaired memory and/or judgment, dementia, stroke/paralysis, seizures, and cranial nerve dysfunction, Argyll Robertson pupils.
  - Ocular syphilis: posterior uveitis and panuveitis most common but also anterior uveitis, optic neuropathy, retinal vasculitis, and interstitial keratitis; decreased visual acuity including permanent blindness

HISTORY

- Neonates/infants
  - Obtain a detailed prenatal history including possible signs of primary or secondary syphilis.
  - Inquire about past history of syphilis including all syphilis testing and treatment of parents.
    - Pregnant women with penicillin allergy should be desensitized if needed and treated with penicillin.
    - Health departments have information (serologic test results and treatment) on all cases of syphilis.
    - Mothers of infants with congenital syphilis should be tested for HIV, as well as gonorrhea, chlamydia, and hepatitis B virus infection.
- Older children/adolescents and adults
  - Ask about possible sexual abuse.
  - Ask about sexual activity, including experience, MSM, number of partners, age of partners, history of other STDs, and use of barrier contraception.
  - Ask about other high-risk behaviors (e.g., drug use).
  - Ask about risk factors for HIV exposure.

PHYSICAL EXAM

- Majority of infected infants and children are "asymptomatic."
- Early congenital syphilis (<2 years of age)
  - Nonimmune hydrops; prematurity
  - Intrauterine growth restriction, small for gestational age
  - Hepatosplenomegaly with or without jaundice
  - Rhinitis ("snuffles"): clear but may become purulent or blood-tinged
  - Rash: bullous ("pemphigus syphiliticus"), peeling and/or maculopapular (copper-red) with or without desquamation; "blueberry muffin" spots, with symmetric distribution on palms and soles (but can be generalized), petechiae
  - Mucocutaneous lesions with fissures on lips, nares, anus (rhagades); condyloma lata (flat, wart-like, moist lesions) around the anus/vagina; mucous patches
  - Lymphadenopathy
  - Pneumonia alba
  - Pseudoparalysis of an extremity ("of Parrot")
  - Myocarditis
  - Alopecia (scalp and eyebrows)
  - Nephrotic syndrome
  - Chorioretinitis
  - Irritability, bulging fontanel (if neurosyphilis is present)
- Late congenital syphilis (>2 years of age)
  - Musculoskeletal: frontal bossing, saddle nose, protuberant mandible, sternoclavicular joint thickening (Higouménakis sign), saber shins, painless swelling of knees (Clutton joints)
  - Dental: Hutchinson teeth, mulberry molars
  - Skin: Rhagades (perioral fissures)
  - Ophthalmologic: interstitial keratitis
  - Nervous system: intellectual disability, seizures, cranial nerve palsies, 8th cranial nerve deafness
- Acquired syphilis
  - Primary syphilis
    - Painless, indurated ulcer (chancre), most commonly in the genital region but can occur anywhere at point of contact
    - Painless inguinal lymphadenopathy
  - Secondary syphilis
    - Fever, headache, sore throat, generalized arthralgia and myalgia, malaise, generalized painless lymphadenopathy (epitrochlear); hepatosplenomegaly; alopecia
    - Maculopapular rash involving the palms and soles; mucous patches; condyloma lata (moist, papular genital lesions)
    - Signs of meningitis, hepatitis, nephropathy, or ocular involvement

DIFFERENTIAL DIAGNOSIS

- Congenital syphilis
  - Congenital infections due to cytomegalovirus, herpes simplex virus (HSV), *Toxoplasma gondii*, rubella, Zika virus, parvovirus, others
  - Neonatal hepatitis
  - Osteomyelitis
- Acquired syphilis
  - Chancroid (*Haemophilus ducreyi*)
  - Granuloma inguinale
  - Calymmatobacterium granulomatis
  - Lymphogranuloma venereum (*Chlamydia trachomatis*)
  - Scabies
  - Mycotic infections
  - Genital herpes (HSV)
  - Venereal warts (human papillomavirus [HPV])
  - Viral exanthem (e.g., enteroviruses may cause a maculopapular rash involving the palms and soles)

DIAGNOSTIC TESTS & INTERPRETATION

- Nontreponemal tests
  - Rapid plasma reagin (RPR) test, venereal disease research laboratory (VDRL) test
  - Traditional screening test with syphilis infection confirmed by subsequent treponemal test
  - Quantitative serum titers correlate with disease activity, with 4-fold titer change (e.g., from 1:8 to 1:32 or vice versa) necessary to document clinically significant change.
  - RPR titers are generally one to two dilutions higher than VDRL titer; therefore, use the same test (and preferably same lab) when comparing test results.
  - Performed preferably on infant serum rather than umbilical cord blood
  - VDRL (not RPR) is used on CSF to evaluate for neurosyphilis.
  - False-positive nontreponemal test result can occur with autoimmune diseases (e.g., systemic lupus erythematosus [SLE]), tuberculosis, lymphoma, viral infections (e.g., Epstein-Barr, hepatitis, varicella, HIV), malaria, IV drug abuse, and pregnancy.
  - False-negative nontreponemal test (e.g., RPR) result may be seen with prozone phenomenon.
- Treponemal antibody tests
  - *T. pallidum* particle agglutination (TP-PA), fluorescent treponemal antibody-absorption (FTA-ABS), *T. pallidum* chemiluminescence immunoassay (TP-CIA), or *T. pallidum* enzyme immunoassay (TP-EIA); microhemagglutination assay for *T. pallidum* antibodies (MHA-TP) not available

- Used to confirm a reactive nontreponemal test
- Become reactive before nontreponemal tests
- "Reverse sequence syphilis screening": serum first tested by TP-CIA or TP-EIA, and if positive, RPR performed. If RPR is reactive, syphilis confirmed. If RPR nonreactive, then TP-PA is performed: if TP-PA reactive, then syphilis is confirmed, but if negative, then TP-CIA/TP-EIA considered a false-positive result
- False-positive treponemal tests may occur in other spirochetal diseases (i.e., Lyme disease, leptospirosis, yaws) and autoimmune diseases (i.e., SLE) and, rarely, in viral infections.

- Treponemal tests usually remain positive for life so not useful for assessing treatment efficacy or reinfection.
- Dark-field microscopy: performed on clinical lesions for visualization of motile spirochetes
- No commercially available *T. pallidum* IgM test is recommended.
- Placental histopathology
- CSF analysis (neurosyphilis): reactive CSF VDRL test, pleocytosis (mostly mononuclear cells), elevated protein
- Infant evaluation
  - Performed if (i) infant's physical examination is consistent with syphilis; serum nontreponemal titer is 4-fold or greater than maternal titer; dark-field or fluorescent antibody test positive on body fluids; (ii) mother untreated or inadequately treated for syphilis during pregnancy or treated within 4 weeks of delivery
    - CBC: looking for anemia, thrombocytopenia
    - Long bone radiographs: looking for osteochondritis (metaphyseal lucencies) and/or periostitis
    - CSF analysis: VDRL, cell count, and protein
  - Other tests as clinically indicated:
    - Liver function tests
    - Ophthalmologic exam
    - Cranial ultrasound
  - Infants born to mothers coinfected with HIV and syphilis do not require different evaluation, treatment, or follow-up for syphilis.
  - Infants should not be discharged from the nursery until the results of maternal syphilis tests are known at least once during pregnancy. In communities with high prevalence of syphilis, mothers should be screened at the first prenatal visit, 28 to 32 weeks' gestation, and at delivery.

TREATMENT

- Infants with proven or highly probably disease:
  - Infants <28 days of age
    - Aqueous crystalline penicillin G (50,000 U/kg/dose) IV q12h for first 7 days of age and then q8h for a total of 10 days *or* penicillin G procaine (50,000 U/kg/dose) IM daily for 10 days
    - If ≥1 day of treatment is missed, restart 10-day course.
  - Infants >28 days of age
    - Aqueous crystalline penicillin G (50,000 U/kg/dose) IV q4–6h for 10 days
    - If neurosyphilis present, 1 to 3 weekly doses of penicillin G benzathine (50,000 U/kg IM) may be given after the 10-day treatment.
- Infants with a normal physical examination and born to mothers with (i) untreated or inadequately treated syphilis, (ii) treated with nonpenicillin regimen; or (iii) treated <4 weeks before delivery:
  - If complete evaluation (physical examination, CBC and platelets, bone radiographs, CSF analysis) is normal, then a single dose of penicillin G benzathine (50,000 U/kg IM)
- Infants with normal physical exam and born to mothers adequately treated during pregnancy: no evaluation, but treat with a single dose of penicillin G benzathine (50,000 U/kg IM)
- Neonates with a normal physical examination and nonreactive RPR test but born to mother with untreated or inadequately treated syphilis: Infant should receive single IM injection of penicillin G benzathine (50,000 U/kg) but no evaluation needed.
- Primary, secondary, and early latent (<1 year duration) syphilis
  - Children: penicillin G benzathine 50,000 U/kg IM (maximum, 2.4 million units), single dose
  - Adolescent/adult: penicillin G benzathine 2.4 million U IM, single dose
  - Nonpregnant, penicillin-allergic persons: doxycycline 100 mg PO b.i.d. or tetracycline 500 mg PO q.i.d. for 14 days
- Late latent syphilis (>1 year duration) or disease of unknown duration
  - Infant/child: penicillin G benzathine 50,000 U/kg IM (maximum 2.4 million U) weekly for 3 weeks
  - Adolescent/adult: penicillin G benzathine 2.4 million U IM weekly for 3 weeks
  - Nonpregnant, penicillin-allergic persons: doxycycline 100 mg PO b.i.d. or tetracycline 500 mg PO q.i.d. for 28 days
- Tertiary syphilis (normal CSF): penicillin G benzathine 2.4 million U weekly for 3 weeks
- Neurosyphilis: aqueous penicillin G 3 to 4 million U IV q4h or continuous infusion for 10 to 14 days or penicillin G procaine 2.4 million U IM once daily PLUS probenecid 500 mg PO QID for 10 days; may be followed by penicillin G benzathine 2.4 million U weekly for up to 3 weeks
- Pregnant women with penicillin allergy who require therapy for syphilis should be desensitized.
- For penicillin shortage treatment options, see http://www.cdc.gov/std/treatment/drugnotices/penicilling.htm.

ADMISSION, INPATIENT, AND NURSING CONSIDERATIONS

Standard precautions unless rash is present, for which contact precautions should be instituted until 24 hours of penicillin treatment has been completed

ONGOING CARE

FOLLOW-UP RECOMMENDATIONS

Patient Monitoring

- Congenital syphilis
  - Careful follow-up examinations and serologic testing (i.e., a nontreponemal test) of infants and children should be performed every 2 to 3 months until the test becomes nonreactive (preferable) or the titer has decreased 4-fold.
  - If nontreponemal titers increase 4-fold or remain stable after 12 to 18 months, the child should be (re)evaluated (e.g., CSF analysis) and treated with IV penicillin G for 10 days.
  - Infants or children whose initial CSF evaluation was abnormal should undergo a repeat lumbar puncture approximately every 6 months until results are normal. Abnormal results require retreatment.
  - A reactive treponemal test at 18 months of age or older is diagnostic of congenital syphilis.
- Acquired syphilis
  - Quantitative nontreponemal serologic test repeated at 6, 12, and 24 months to document 4-fold decrease in titer after treatment
  - A CSF examination should be performed if
    - A sustained (>2 weeks) 4-fold increase or greater in titer is observed.
    - An initially high titer (≥1:32) fails to decline at least 4-fold within 12 to 24 months of therapy.
    - Signs or symptoms attributable to syphilis develop.
    - If CSF is abnormal, treat for neurosyphilis. If the CSF examination is negative, retreatment for latent syphilis should be administered.
  - Sexual partners require evaluation and treatment.

PROGNOSIS

- Congenital syphilis
  - Infants with congenital syphilis who are treated appropriately in early infancy have excellent neurodevelopmental outcomes.
- Acquired syphilis
  - Appropriate and effective treatment should lead to resolution of skin lesions.
  - Neurologic and ocular damage may not resolve.

COMPLICATIONS

Jarisch-Herxheimer reaction: an acute febrile reaction with headache and myalgia within the first 24 hours after the initiation of any therapy for syphilis; can induce labor or fetal distress in pregnant women

ADDITIONAL READING

- American Academy of Pediatrics. Syphilis. In: Kimberlin DW, Brady MT, Jackson MA, et al, eds. *Red Book: 2015 Report of the Committee on Infectious Diseases*. 30th ed. Elk Grove Village, IL: American Academy of Pediatrics; 2015:755–768.
- Binnicker MJ. Which algorithm should be used to screen for syphilis? *Curr Opin Infect Dis*. 2012;25(1):79–85.
- Mmeje O, Chow JM, Davidson L, et al. Discordant syphilis immunoassays in pregnancy: perinatal outcomes and implications for clinical management. *Clin Infect Dis*. 2015;61(7):1049–1053.
- Workowski KA, Bolan GA; for Centers for Disease Control and Prevention. Sexually transmitted diseases treatment guidelines, 2015. *MMWR Morb Mortal Wkly Rep*. 2015;64(RR-03):1–137.

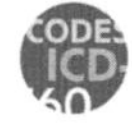

CODES

ICD10

- A53.9 Syphilis, unspecified
- A50.9 Congenital syphilis, unspecified
- A51.5 Early syphilis, latent

FAQ

- Q: What is the prozone phenomenon?
- A: When a nontreponemal test is falsely negative due to high concentrations of nontreponemal IgG antibody; diluting the serum will result in a positive test result.

SYSTEMIC SCLEROSIS (SYSTEMIC SCLERODERMA)

Megan L. Curran, MD • Peter Weiser, MD • Elizabeth R. Volkmann, MD, MS

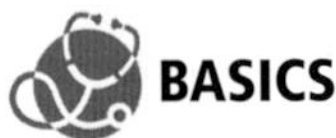

BASICS

DESCRIPTION

- Systemic sclerosis (SSc) is an autoimmune vasculopathic disease causing fibrosis of skin and internal organs.
  - SSc is a type of scleroderma (meaning "hard skin") but should not be confused with localized scleroderma, otherwise known as morphea, which involves only the skin, is more common, and has a much better overall prognosis.
- Characterized by Raynaud phenomenon (RP), skin thickening proximal to the metacarpophalangeal (MCP) joints, and internal organ involvement
- There are two main subtypes of SSc:
  - Diffuse cutaneous SSc (dcSSc):
    - Widespread fibrosis of skin, gastrointestinal (GI), pulmonary, cardiovascular, and renal systems
    - Skin thickening proximal to the elbows or knees, face, chest, abdomen, flanks, legs, feet
    - More rapid progression of skin thickening versus limited cutaneous SSc (lcSSc), associated with joint contractures, myopathy, interstitial lung disease, myocardial and GI involvement, and renal crisis
    - Skin thickening reaches maximal point by 5 years and then softens while internal organ involvement can continue to accrue.
    - Autoantibodies to Scl-70 or other rare autoantibodies
  - lcSSc:
    - Distal skin fibrosis and internal organ involvement
    - Previously known as CREST: **c**alcinosis, **R**aynaud phenomenon, **e**sophageal dysmotility, **s**clerodactyly, **t**elangiectasia
    - Skin thickening restricted to fingers, hands, forearms, lower legs, and feet; can include face
    - Slower progression of skin thickening over years associated with esophageal disease, pulmonary hypertension, and malabsorption
    - Better long-term survival prognosis than dcSSc
    - Can be associated with centromere antibodies

EPIDEMIOLOGY

- SSc—all types
  - Estimated ~3% of all SSc patients have onset in childhood.
  - Mean age of onset 8 to 12.4 years
- dcSSc
  - Adult age of onset generally 30 to 50 years
  - In general population: annual incidence 0.45 to 1.9 cases per 100,000, prevalence 24 in 100,000
  - Sex ratio
    - <8 years, male = female
    - ≥8 years, female > male (3:1)
  - 90% of pediatric patients with SSc have dcSSc.
- lcSSc
  - Earlier age of onset than dcSSc
  - Female > male

RISK FACTORS

Genetics

- Associations with histocompatibility antigens (Choctaw Native Americans in Oklahoma)
- Rare reports of familial and twin occurrences

PATHOPHYSIOLOGY

- Three-part process of dysfunction: endothelial cells, immune system, and extracellular matrix
- Primary insult is endothelial injury and dysfunction causing vasculopathy in skin and organs.
  - Chemical, microbial, autoantibody, and sheer stress injury to endothelial cells
  - Vascular injury activates immune system and contributes to tissue fibrosis.
  - Progressive vascular damage causes obliteration of small vessels in various organs.
- Immune dysfunction
  - Within innate immune system: dendritic cells, toll-like receptors, interferons
  - Within adaptive immune system: autoantibody production, T- and B-cell dysfunction
  - Elevated proinflammatory cytokines in serum, skin
- Extracellular matrix
  - Overactive connective tissue remodeling: fibrotic changes in extracellular matrix
  - Transforming growth factor-β causes fibroblast activation.
  - Collagen accumulation, extracellular matrix deposition, matrix remodeling, and contraction

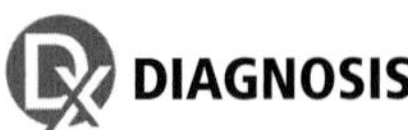

DIAGNOSIS

HISTORY

- Onset is almost always insidious.
- Initial symptoms in SSc
  - Reflection of vasculopathy in microvasculature
    - RP
    - Edematous fingers
    - Nailfold capillary changes and distorted/thickened cuticles
  - RP can precede other manifestations by years, especially in lcSSc.
    - Cold hands > feet
    - Color change of digits: pallor, duskiness, blue or purple discoloration, redness
- Later symptoms in dcSSc and lcSSc
  - Cutaneous complaints
    - Thickening of skin
    - Pruritus
    - Hyper- and hypopigmentation
  - Musculoskeletal complaints
    - Morning stiffness
    - Inability to fully extend fingers: prayer sign
    - Joint swelling and tenderness
    - Loss of range of motion
  - Sicca symptoms: dry mouth and eyes
  - GI complaints
    - Heartburn and reflux
    - Dysphagia, choking
    - Cough with swallowing
- Later symptoms in dcSSc
  - Cardiopulmonary complaints: shortness of breath, dyspnea with exertion, dizziness, syncope
  - GI complaints
    - Poor motility: diarrhea, constipation, loss of continence
    - Malabsorption: bloating, weight loss

PHYSICAL EXAM

- RP: recurrent episodes of vasospasm triggered by cold and strong emotions
  - Affects end-circulatory locations: fingers, toes, nose, ears, tongue
  - Almost always spares thumb
  - Rarely affects viscera
  - Three phases usually demonstrated:
    - Phase 1: Arterial vasoconstriction causes blanching of distal digits with sharp demarcation of normal versus blanched skin.
    - Phase 2: Pooling of venous blood causes cyanosis, often with numbness and pain.
    - Phase 3: Reflex hyperemia from vasodilation causes erythema, tingling.
  - Primary RP
    - More common than secondary
    - Milder symptoms without tissue damage
    - Not associated with underlying autoimmune disease
  - Secondary RP
    - Associated with underlying disease such as SSc, systemic lupus erythematosus (SLE), Sjögren syndrome, mixed connective tissue disease, dermatomyositis
    - Present in 95% of SSc patients
    - Symptoms are more severe than primary RP.
    - Ischemia causing digital ulceration, pulp loss, gangrene
    - Nailfold capillary changes

ALERT

RP is almost always the first presenting sign of SSc. To determine whether RP is more likely to be primary or secondary, perform nailfold capillaroscopy, antinuclear antibody (ANA) by immunofluorescence, and erythrocyte sedimentation rate (ESR). If any are abnormal, secondary RP is likely: Refer to rheumatology.

- Skin: Affected areas in dcSSc and lcSSc are described above.
  - Stage 1: active inflammatory phase
    - First affects fingers then legs
    - Nonpitting edema progressing to warm, sometimes erythematous induration
    - Pruritus, pain
  - Stage 2: dermal fibrosis
    - Diffuse thickening of skin
    - Facial changes: microstomia (small mouth) with thin lips, decreased opening; loss of nasolabial folds
  - Stage 3: atrophy of dermis
    - Shiny appearance, hypo- or hyperpigmentation
  - Sclerodactyly: tight, thickened skin of fingers causing tapering and flexion deformities
  - Telangiectasias of face, lips, other skin
  - Calcinosis over fingertips and extensor joint surfaces
  - Periungual nailfold capillary loop abnormalities visible under magnification or grossly: dilation, tortuosity, hemorrhage, and dropout
- Musculoskeletal
  - Tendon friction rubs felt over joints when performing active or passive range of motion
  - Contractures, especially proximal interphalangeal joints and elbows
  - Arthritis of small and large joints
  - Weakness, myopathy
- GI
  - Sicca syndrome (xerostomia) with parotitis
  - Esophageal disease: esophagitis, occasional ulceration or stricture
  - Gastric antral vascular ectasia (GAVE)
  - Bowel disease: hypomotility, bacterial overgrowth, pneumatosis intestinalis, malabsorption
  - Weight loss secondary to all above problems
- Cardiac in dcSSc: myocarditis, arrhythmia, heart failure
- Pulmonary in dcSSc
  - Combined pulmonary vascular and pulmonary parenchymal disease
  - Primary pulmonary vascular disease with right ventricular failure
  - Signs of interstitial disease: crackles
  - Signs of pulmonary vascular disease: lower extremity edema, accentuated P_2 on cardiac auscultation

- Renal disease
  - Very rare in children, more common in adults
  - Proteinuria, hypertension
  - Scleroderma renal crisis: life-threatening acute onset renal failure and abrupt hypertension
- CNS: cranial nerve involvement, especially sensory branch of trigeminal nerve, carpal tunnel syndrome
- Ocular: keratoconjunctivitis sicca (dry eyes)

DIFFERENTIAL DIAGNOSIS

- Overlapping connective tissue disease and mixed connective tissue disease can have Raynaud, features of SSc and myositis.
  - Can be distinguished by autoantibodies and clinical features
  - PM-Scl (overlap), U1RNP (mixed connective tissue disease)
- SSc sine scleroderma (internal organ involvement without skin fibrosis) is exceedingly rare.
- If patient does not have RP or nailfold capillary abnormalities, consider alternative diagnosis.
- Graft-versus-host disease (GVHD)
- Nephrogenic systemic fibrosis in patients with kidney failure due to gadolinium exposure
- Chemically induced scleroderma-like disease: polyvinyl chloride, bleomycin, toxic oil syndrome
- IgG4-related disease
- Scleromyxedema or scleredema
- Stiff skin syndrome (mucin deposition in the dermis, hardening of the subcutaneous tissue with normal-looking epidermis)
- Eosinophilic fasciitis
- Pansclerotic morphea
- Syndromes of premature aging: progeria, Werner syndrome
- Phenylketonuria
- Porphyria cutanea tarda
- Borrelia infection: acrodermatitis chronica atrophicans

DIAGNOSTIC TESTS & INTERPRETATION

Initial Tests (screening, lab, imaging)

- ANA often positive by immunofluorescence
- Antibodies to specific antinuclear antigens can be tested by enzyme-linked immunosorbent assay (ELISA):
  - Antibodies give risk and prognostic information.
  - Scl-70 (also known as topoisomerase I): present in 34% of children, mainly dcSSc patients
  - Anticentromere antibody: present in 7%, almost exclusively lcSSc
  - Other rare antibodies in dcSSc: RNA polymerase III, U3RNP, Th/To
  - PM-Scl antibodies seen in patients with overlapping connective tissue disease
- Anemia—multifactorial: chronic disease; vitamin B_{12} and folate deficiencies from chronic malabsorption; blood loss from GI ulcer disease, GAVE
- Eosinophilia
- Elevated inflammatory markers in inflammatory stage of disease: ESR, CRP
- Elevated muscle enzymes; muscle biopsy may show signs of myositis.
- Imaging
  - GI
    - Esophagogram or upper GI with small bowel follow through
    - Esophageal manometry and pH probe
  - Chest radiograph: bibasilar pulmonary fibrosis, rib notching, calcifications
  - High-resolution chest CT
    - More sensitive than chest radiograph
    - Ground-glass attenuation
    - Reticulations
    - Honeycombing (rare)
  - Bone radiograph
    - Acroosteolysis: resorption of tufts of distal phalanges, especially with severe RP
    - Periarticular or subcutaneous calcification
    - Bony erosions

Diagnostic Procedures/Other

- Nailfold capillaroscopy can be done with common office equipment: Place surgical lubricant over nailfolds and cuticles, view through otoscope or ophthalmoscope set at 40×.
- For sicca syndrome: Schirmer test for dry eyes, rose bengal staining of cornea, lip biopsy
- ECG
  - 1st-degree block
  - Right and left bundle-branch block
  - Premature atrial contractions and premature ventricular contractions: nonspecific T-wave changes, ventricular hypertrophy
- Pulmonary function tests
  - Restrictive lung disease: present in >30% of patients with SSc
  - Earliest change is decreased diffusion capacity of the lung for carbon monoxide (DLCO).
  - Later declines in forced vital capacity (FVC) and FEV1
- Classification criteria for adult SSc (2013), not yet validated for pediatric disease—diagnosis requires 9 points
  - Finger skin thickening proximal to MCPs (9 points)
  - Finger skin thickening—count either puffy fingers (2 points) or sclerodactyly of fingers proximal to interphalangeal but distal to MCP joints (4 points)
  - Fingertip lesions—count either digital tip ulcers (2 points) or fingertip pitting scars (3 points)
  - Telangiectasia (2 points)
  - Abnormal nailfold capillaries (2 points)
  - Lung disease—count either pulmonary arterial hypertension (2 points) or interstitial lung disease (2 points)
  - RP (3 points)
  - SSc-related autoantibodies centromere, Scl-70, RNA polymerase III (3 points)
- Provisional classification criteria for pediatric SSc (2007)—not yet prospectively validated
  - Requires major criterion: proximal skin sclerosis
  - Requires two or more minor criteria: sclerodactyly, RP, nailfold capillary abnormalities, digital tip ulcers, dysphagia, gastroesophageal reflux, arrhythmia, heart failure, renal crisis, new-onset arterial hypertension, pulmonary fibrosis, decreased DLCO, pulmonary arterial hypertension, neuropathy, carpal tunnel syndrome, tendon friction rubs, arthritis, myositis, ANA, SSc-selective autoantibodies
- The concepts of early SSc and very early diagnosis of systemic sclerosis (VEDOSS) are important in identifying pediatric patients who do not meet classification criteria for SSc but will likely progress to develop complete disease.

TREATMENT

GENERAL MEASURES

- Collaborative care with subspecialists (pulmonary, GI, cardiology), school, social work, physical therapy
- Supportive care: Avoid skin trauma; wound care for digital and other skin ulcers
- Management of RP: Keep extremities warm and dry; avoid excessive cold, smoking, β-blockers, caffeine, and stimulants.

MEDICATION

- Disease modification: Many agents have been tried; however, there are few controlled trials (especially inclusive of children), and no proven treatment exists.
- RP: vasodilators including calcium channel blockers, phosphodiesterase inhibitors, prostacyclins
- Skin disease: methotrexate, mycophenolate mofetil, cyclophosphamide for rapidly progressive skin thickening/inflammation, rituximab
- Pulmonary fibrosis: cyclophosphamide, mycophenolate mofetil
- Pulmonary hypertension: vasodilators
- Other immunosuppressants: steroids, rituximab, tocilizumab
- Stem cell transplant for severe disease shows promise for patients with early, diffuse cutaneous disease with internal organ involvement.

ADDITIONAL THERAPIES

Long-term physical/occupational therapy is required to slow development of contractures and muscle atrophy.

S

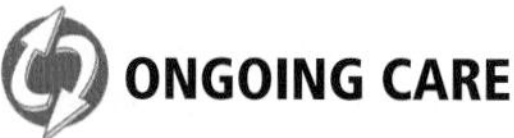

ONGOING CARE

FOLLOW-UP RECOMMENDATIONS

Patient Monitoring

- Physical exam for digital or other skin ulcerations, joint mobility, muscle bulk, weight loss, poor growth
- Pulmonary function tests and echocardiogram to monitor cardiopulmonary decline

PROGNOSIS

- Systemic form is progressive, and ultimate prognosis depends on severity of skin tightness, joint contractures, and visceral involvement.
- Mortality with SSc: males > females, non-whites > whites
- Most common cause of pediatric death is secondary to cardiac and pulmonary complications.

ADDITIONAL READING

- Foeldvari I. Update on juvenile systemic sclerosis. *Curr Opin Rheumatol*. 2015;17(3):18.
- Martini G, Foeldvari I, Russo R, et al; for Juvenile Scleroderma Working Group of the Pediatric Rheumatology European Society. Systemic sclerosis in childhood: clinical and immunologic features of 153 patients in an international database. *Arthritis Rheum*. 2006;54(12):3971–3978.
- McCann LJ, Pain CE. A practical approach to juvenile dermatomyositis and juvenile scleroderma. *Indian J Pediatr*. 2016;83(2):163–171.
- van den Hoogen F, Khanna D, Fransen J, et al. 2013 classification criteria for systemic sclerosis: an American College of Rheumatology/European League against rheumatism collaborative initiative. *Arthritis Rheum*. 2013;65(11):2737–2747.

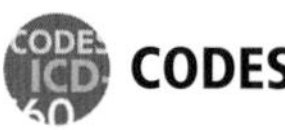

CODES

ICD10

- M34.9 Systemic sclerosis, unspecified
- M34.89 Other systemic sclerosis

TAPEWORM

Brittany B. Hubbell, MD • Samir S. Shah, MD, MSCE

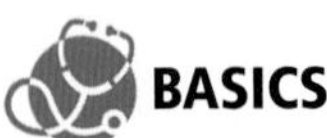

BASICS

DESCRIPTION

- Tapeworms cause two major types of zoonotic disease syndromes, depending on whether humans are the definitive or intermediate host.
- When humans serve as definitive hosts, adult tapeworms infect the GI tract and interfere with nutrition; patients may be asymptomatic.
- When humans serve as intermediate hosts for the larval cestode, serious pathology results.
- Causative organisms include the following:
  - *Taenia saginata* (beef tapeworm)
  - *Taenia solium* (pork tapeworm)
  - *Diphyllobothrium latum* (fish tapeworm)
  - *Dipylidium caninum* (dog tapeworm)
  - *Echinococcus granulosus*

EPIDEMIOLOGY

- Beef tapeworm
  - Estimated 77 million people infested worldwide
  - Widespread in cattle-breeding areas of the world; endemic in Asia, Latin America, Eastern Europe
- Pork tapeworm
  - Estimated >50 million people infested worldwide
  - Taeniasis: typically asymptomatic infection with adult tapeworm (from undercooked pork)
  - Cysticercosis: infection with larval parasite (fecal–oral transmission from carriers)
  - High prevalence in developing areas of Asia, Central and South America
  - Up to 5,000 new cases of neurocysticercosis in United States annually
- Fish tapeworm
  - Infection is most prevalent in temperate climates of Europe (Finland, Estonia, Sweden most common) and Canada.
  - Persons who prepare or eat raw freshwater fish are most at risk.
  - In the United States, infected salmon have been implicated in most cases.
- Dog tapeworm
  - Found in dogs and cats worldwide
- Echinococcosis
  - Associated with the practice of feeding sheep viscera to dogs
  - Hyperendemic in sheep-raising areas of South America, Australia, areas of Africa, China, Central Asia, and the Western United States

GENERAL PREVENTION

- Adult tapeworms
  - Proper cooking prevents transmission of beef, pork, and fish tapeworms.
- Pork tapeworm
  - Storage of pork for 4 days at −5°C (21.2°F) or 1 day at −24°C (−11.2°F) kills most cysticerci.
  - Persons traveling to areas with high endemic rates of cysticercosis should avoid eating uncooked vegetables and fruit that can't be peeled.
- Fish tapeworm
  - Brief cooking (at >56°C [132.8°F] for 5 minutes) or freezing (−18°C [−0.4°F] for 24 to 48 hours) renders the fish safe to consume.
- Dog tapeworm
  - Periodic deworming of pets
- Echinococcosis
  - Careful disposal of sheep viscera and mass chemotherapy of dogs can interrupt the life cycle of *E. granulosus* as the cestode moves between sheep and carnivore hosts.

PATHOPHYSIOLOGY

- Beef tapeworm
  - Cattle (intermediate host) ingests *T. saginata* eggs in contaminated feeds. The eggs hatch, releasing embryos which penetrate intestinal mucosa, enter the bloodstream, and settle in skeletal muscle, where they develop into larvae. Larvae in undercooked meat are consumed by humans and mature into adult tapeworms within the human (definitive host) GI tract.
- Pork tapeworm: Humans are the only definitive host for the adult pork tapeworm. Both humans and pigs are intermediate hosts for its embryonic form, cysticercosis.
  - Pigs ingest *T. solium* eggs. In the intestine, the eggs release embryos that penetrate the mucosa, enter the bloodstream, and settle in various tissues to differentiate into cysticerci (infective larvae). Cysticerci are ingested by humans (definitive host) who consume undercooked pork.
  - Humans ingest food contaminated with human feces containing *T. solium* eggs. The eggs hatch, liberating embryos which penetrate the intestinal mucosa leading to blood-borne distribution to the brain, subcutaneous tissues, muscle, and eye, where they develop into cysticerci.
- Fish tapeworm
  - When sewage containing *D. latum* eggs contaminates freshwater lakes and streams, eggs hatch into the water becoming embryos. Embryos are eaten by crustaceans and then passed on to fresh water fish. Humans are infected when they consume these undercooked fish. The larvae mature into adult tapeworms in the intestines of humans in 3 to 5 weeks' time and can survive up to 10 years. Rarely, the tapeworm migrates thru intestinal wall to other tissues (sparganosis).
- Dog tapeworm
  - Larvae develop in fleas (intermediate host) after ingestion of the eggs; humans are infected through accidental ingestion of infected fleas.
- Echinococcosis (hydatid disease)
  - Humans ingest eggs of *E. granulosus* through contaminated dog feces. After ingestion, the eggs hatch and release embryos (oncospheres) in the small intestine. Penetration through the mucosa leads to blood-borne distribution to the liver, lungs, and other sites, where development of cysts begins. Within the cysts, new larvae (scolices) develop, accumulate fluid, and encroach on surrounding structures.

DIAGNOSIS

HISTORY

- Recent travel or immigration
- Most patients with adult tapeworm infections are asymptomatic.
- Household contacts of persons with adult pork tapeworm infection are at risk of cystercercosis.
- GI tract
  - Nausea, weight loss, diarrhea, change in appetite
  - Beef, pork taperworm: Motile proglottids may cause discomfort as they pass; anal pruritus
  - Dog tapeworm: Proglottids resembling rice or seeds may be observed in stool.
- Respiratory tract
  - Pulmonary hydatid cyst due to *E. granulosus* causes cough, dyspnea, and hemoptysis; rupture of a cyst can cause anaphylaxis.
- Hematologic
  - Anemia from vitamin B_{12} deficiency occurs in 2% of fish tapeworm infections due to competition for absorption in ileum.
- CNS
  - New-onset seizures (partial or generalized) occur with neurocysticercosis and some species of *Echinococcus*.
  - Neurocysticercosis may present with headache, vomiting, visual changes (increased intracranial pressure).
  - Neurocysticercosis and vitamin B_{12} deficiency due to fish tapeworm can mimic psychotic illness with delirium or hallucinations.
  - CNS symptoms in neurocysticercosis typically appear 5 to 7 years after initial infection (range: 6 months to 30 years).
- Note: For echinococcosis, a presymptomatic stage may last for years before the enlarging cysts cause symptoms. The variability of signs and symptoms depends on the target organ.

PHYSICAL EXAM

- GI tract
  - Abdominal tenderness or distention
  - Eggs or proglottids may be visible at anus or in stool.
  - Fish and, rarely, dog tapeworm infections can be complicated by intestinal obstruction.
  - Beef and pork tapeworm proglottids may rarely become lodged in the appendiceal lumen, or pancreatic or bile ducts; biliary tree extension leads to obstructive jaundice and cholangitis.
  - Hepatic cysts from echinococcosis may be palpable in the right upper quadrant.
- Hematologic
  - Fish tapeworm: signs of pernicious anemia, including glossitis, peripheral neuropathy, decreased vibration sense, and ataxia
- CNS
  - Neurocysticercosis: cranial nerve abnormalities, altered mental status, increased intracranial pressure, or meningitis

DIFFERENTIAL DIAGNOSIS

- Enterobiasis (anal pruritus)
- Non-tapeworm gastroenteritis
- Inflammatory bowel disease
- Cholecystitis or biliary obstruction (i.e., gallstones, neoplasms, or liver disease)
- B_{12} deficiency from dietary deficiency or pancreatic insufficiency
- Idiopathic epilepsy
- Echinococcal cysts must be differentiated from benign cysts, cavitary tuberculosis, abscesses, and neoplasms.

DIAGNOSTIC TESTS & INTERPRETATION

Initial Tests (screening, lab, imaging)

- Microscopic identification of eggs and proglottids in feces is diagnostic for taeniasis.
  - Eggs and proglottids are not released into the feces until ~2 to 3 months after initial infection.
  - Examination of 3 stools samples collected on different days increases test sensitivity.
- Beef tapeworm
  - Ziehl–Neelsen stain of stool identifies eggs.
  - Proglottids or eggs in stool with microscopic examination (62% sensitivity)
  - Enzyme-linked immunosorbent assay (ELISA) test detects *Taenia* antigens in stool (85% sensitivity, 95% specificity).

- Pork tapeworm
  - Stool samples for intestinal worms
  - Serum electro immunotransfer blot (most sensitive) and ELISA of serum and/or CSF
- Fish tapeworm
  - Stool samples for eggs and proglottids are diagnostic.
- Dog tapeworm
  - Characteristic egg packets (loose membrane containing up to 20 eggs) or proglottids may be identified in stool or on perianal adhesive tape ("paddle") preparations.
- Echinococcosis
  - Polymerase chain reaction (PCR) of stool
  - IgE levels are elevated. Eosinophilia is present in <25% of infected persons.
  - The Casoni skin test (injection of hydatid fluid into the dermis) yields an erythematous papule in <60 minutes in 50–80% of infected patients; not routinely performed because false-positive rate is 30% in uninfected patients
  - Serologic testing is falsely negative in 10–50% of cases. False-negative results are more likely in patients with pulmonary hydatid cysts and in children. No serologic test excludes the diagnosis of hydatid cysts.
- Pork tapeworm (neurocysticercosis)
  - Contrast-enhanced CT or MRI of the brain may reveal cysticerci; ring-enhancing lesions with surrounding edema represent a dying parasite; calcification represents a resolved infection.
  - Imaging is usually diagnostic.
- Echinococcosis
  - On chest radiograph, pulmonary cysts demonstrate a sharply demarcated, smooth-bordered cyst; there is a crescent-shaped air level after cyst rupture. Liver and spleen lesions may calcify over time.
  - Hydatid cysts: Internal septa or daughter cysts after cyst rupture are detected by CT, MRI, or ultrasound; present in ~50% of patients with unilocular liver cysts

Follow-Up Tests & Special Considerations

- Other blood tests are not routinely necessary but may provide clues to diagnosis and identify complications.
  - Fish tapeworm is associated with low vitamin B_{12} levels (50%) and mild eosinophilia. Megaloblastic anemia is rare.
  - Echinococcosis with hepatic cysts may result in mildly elevated hepatic enzymes.
- Regions and groups at risk for neurocysticercosis are also at risk for tuberculosis and strongyloidiasis; consider testing prior to corticosteroid treatment.

Diagnostic Procedures/Other

Echinococcosis: In seronegative persons, a presumptive diagnosis can be confirmed by demonstrating protoscolices or hydatid membranes in liquid obtained by ultrasound-guided percutaneous cyst aspiration. This procedure is controversial because anaphylaxis may occur with cyst rupture.

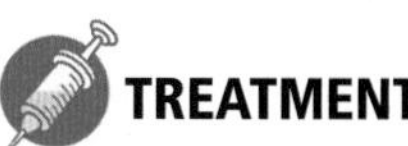

TREATMENT

MEDICATION

- Beef, pork, fish, and dog tapeworm (and most other intestinal cestodes)
  - Praziquantel: 5 to 10 mg/kg as a single oral dose; no safety profile exists for children <4 years of age.
  - Niclosamide (second line for beef tapeworm): 50 mg/kg orally once (max 2 g); not available in the United States
  - Supplement with vitamin B_{12} for fish tapeworm.
- Neurocysticercosis
  - Treatment should be conducted in consultation with a neurologist and/or neurosurgeon and individualized based on number, location, and viability of cysticerci on MRI or CT scan.
  - Treatment may not be indicated for single degenerating cysts, calcifications, or encephalitis. Most experts recommend therapy for patients with nonenhancing or multiple cysticerci.
  - Albendazole: 15 mg/kg/24 h (maximum, 800 mg/24 h) in 2 divided doses for 8 to 30 days or praziquantel 100 mg/kg/24 h in 3 divided doses for 1 day followed by 50 mg/kg/24 h in 3 divided doses for 29 days
  - Steroids (1 mg/kg/24 h of prednisone or 0.5 mg/kg/24 h of dexamethasone), in combination with albendazole, decrease seizure frequency and number of CNS cysts.
  - Antiepileptic drugs are recommended and shunt placement and/or mannitol should be considered for treatment of hydrocephalus.
  - Antiparasitic therapy, which generates an inflammatory response, is contraindicated in patients with diffuse cerebral edema ("cysticercal encephalitis").
  - No definite recommendations exist regarding the use of corticosteroids alone.
- Echinococcosis
  - Albendazole 15 mg/kg/24 h (max 800 mg/24 h) divided b.i.d. for 1 to 6 months
  - May require three courses of therapy with drug-free intervals of 14 days between courses
- Note: The benzimidazoles, including albendazole, are contraindicated in patients with blood dyscrasia, leukopenia, and liver disease. Prolonged courses require monitoring of liver function and hematopoiesis.

SURGERY/OTHER PROCEDURES

- Neurocysticercosis: Intraventricular cysts usually require endoscopic surgical resection due to risk of obstructive hydrocephalus.
- Echinococcosis: surgical resection of intact hydatid cysts, especially if >10 cm, secondarily infected, or causing symptoms
- Subcutaneous sparganosis: surgical resection or ethanol injection

ADMISSION, INPATIENT, AND NURSING CONSIDERATIONS

- Patients with neurocysticercosis should be hospitalized during the 1st week of therapy.
- Isolation: Standard precautions should be observed.

ONGOING CARE

FOLLOW-UP RECOMMENDATIONS

Patient Monitoring

- Beef tapeworm
  - Stool should be checked for eggs and proglottids 1 month after therapy.
- Pork tapeworm
  - Repeat CNS imaging studies at 2-month intervals (with continued therapy) until successful elimination of parenchymal brain cysticerci.
- Fish tapeworm
  - Perform stool examination 12 weeks after therapy to test for cure.
- Dog tapeworm
  - No follow-up stool examination required, but the appearance of proglottids >1 week after therapy indicates treatment failure
- Echinococcosis
  - Requires prolonged follow-up with ultrasound or other imaging procedures

PROGNOSIS

- Taeniasis: Long-term sequelae are uncommon.
- Neurocysticercosis: Seizures recurrence is unlikely with a single parenchymal cyst but likely with multiple cysts.

COMPLICATIONS

- Taeniasis
  - Proglottids may become lodged in the appendiceal lumen, bile, or pancreatic ducts.
- Cysticercosis
  - Cysticerci can develop in the brain, muscle, eye, or other organs. Seizures and obstructive hydrocephalus are the most common life-threatening complications.
  - Ophthalmologic exam is warranted in cases of neurocysticercosis.
- Echinococcosis
  - Cysts grow slowly, causing symptoms only when relatively large.
  - They frequently develop in the liver (50–70%) and lung (20–30%); 5–10% of cysts involve other organs, including the eye, brain, spleen, heart, bone, and kidneys.
  - Rupture of cysts can cause anaphylaxis.
  - Bone involvement can cause pathologic fractures, and renal involvement can cause pain or hematuria.

ADDITIONAL READING

- Garcia HH, Nash TE, Del Brutto OH. Clinical symptoms, diagnosis, and treatment of neurocysticercosis. *Lancet Neurol*. 2014;13(12):1202–1215.
- Ito A, Budke CM. Culinary delights and travel? A review of zoonotic cestodiases and metacestodiases. *Travel Med Infect Dis*. 2014;12(6, Pt A):582–591.
- Zhao BC, Jiang HY, Ma WY, et al. Albendazole and corticosteroids for the treatment of solitary cysticercus granuloma: a network meta-analysis. *PLoS Negl Trop Dis*. 2016;10(2):e0004418.

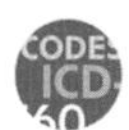

CODES

ICD10

- B71.9 Cestode infection, unspecified
- B68.1 Taenia saginata taeniasis
- B68.0 Taenia solium taeniasis

FAQ

- Q: Can vegetarians develop neurocysticercosis?
- A: Yes. Human cysticercosis results from consuming food/water contaminated by a tapeworm carrier (often a household contact), or when tapeworm carriers autoinfect themselves due to poor hand hygiene. Ingestion of infected pork causes the adult form of *T. solium* infection and results in GI disease alone.
- Q: Is treatment for neurocysticercosis always indicated?
- A: The findings are controversial. In many children, the lesion disappears spontaneously within 2 to 3 months. Guidelines for treatment depend on the number and location of lesions, as well as the viability of the parasites within the nervous system. A growing parasite deserves active management, either with antiparasitic drugs or surgical excision.

T

TEETHING

Karen R. Fratantoni, MD, MPH • Anupama R. Tate, DMD, MHP

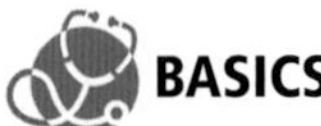

BASICS

DESCRIPTION

Teething is the normal developmental process of primary tooth eruption whereby the tooth moves from its position in the alveolar bone through the mucosa into the mouth. Parents/caregivers, physicians, and dentists often associate many localized and systemic symptoms with the teething process, including mouthing/biting, drooling, changes in appetite, and fever.

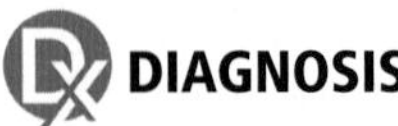

DIAGNOSIS

Consider the following diagnostic approach when evaluating an infant or toddler who presents with chief complaint of teething:

- Careful history and physical exam
- Evaluation of signs/symptoms inconsistent with teething (fever >102°F/38.8°C, irritability, diarrhea) and treatment of possible illness
- If teething is suspected or confirmed and serious illness ruled out, offer education and advice for parents/caregivers around the management of teething symptoms.

HISTORY

Teething is a normal developmental process for which anticipatory guidance should be offered at appropriate well visits. The following questions will be helpful for providers in determining if teething should be considered in the differential diagnosis.

- Is teething likely to be occurring at the child's age?
  - First tooth appears by 6 months of age; however, 1% of children will get their first tooth before 4 months old and 1% after 12 months old.
  - Completion of a set of 20 deciduous/primary teeth by 30 months of age
  - Teeth emerge in pairs, with lower central incisors usually appearing first.
  - Rule of thumb: age (in months) − 6 = average number of teeth (until 24 months old)
- Has the child had fever?
  - General consensus is that temperature >102°F or 38.8°C should not be attributed to teething.
  - One prospective longitudinal study showed an association between mild tympanic temperature elevations (with maximum 36.8°F) and day of tooth eruption.
  - Another study showed mild temperature elevation in the 8-day teething period.
- Does the child have one or more symptoms often attributed to teething?
  - Common symptoms parents often attributed to teething include biting, drooling, gum rubbing, irritability, sucking, wakefulness, ear rubbing, facial rash, and decrease in appetite for solids.
  - One prospective study showed an increase of the above symptoms in the period from 4 days prior to 3 days after tooth eruption, considered to be the 8-day window of teething.
  - There is no consensus in the medical literature about the association of teething and these minor symptoms.
- Is the child irritable?
  - Irritability with an inability to console is concerning and must not be attributed to teething.

ALERT

Fever >38.8°C/102°F, irritability, or diarrhea should NOT be attributed to teething and should prompt a careful history, physical exam, and investigation for possible etiology, including otitis media, meningitis, serious bacterial illness, or viral infection.

- Is the child exhibiting changes in sleep pattern?
  - Teething should not cause significant sleep disturbances.
  - Further history should be obtained regarding the nature of the sleep changes, some of which are common in children between 6 and 12 months old.
- Are there changes in the mouth which make the parent think the child may be teething?
  - Swelling of the gums may be noted prior to tooth eruption.
  - An area of gum swelling with bluish purple discoloration may represent an eruption cyst for which no treatment is required.

PHYSICAL EXAM

- Often, there are no pertinent findings on physical exam.
- Gum swelling and eruption cysts are both normal findings.

DIFFERENTIAL DIAGNOSIS

- Infectious
  - Gingivostomatitis causing pain or drooling
  - Viral or bacterial illnesses causing pain, fever, fussiness, or change in behavior
- Toxic ingestion causing drooling
- Trauma or burn to the mouth
- Normal developmental behaviors: Drooling, gum rubbing, and finger sucking may be consistent with typical development.

DIAGNOSTIC TESTS & INTERPRETATION

No laboratory tests are indicated in the otherwise healthy child with teething.

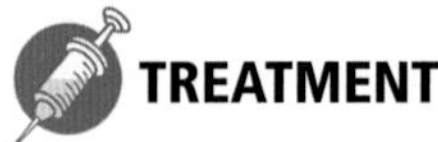

TREATMENT

GENERAL MEASURES

- Nonpharmacologic
  - Application of cold objects onto the gums causes vasoconstriction and reduces inflammation.
  - Biting on teething rings or other objects can offer relief by applying pressure to the gums.
  - Objects used for this purpose include teething rings, pacifiers, or a cold washcloth.
    - Teething rings can be placed in the refrigerator but not the freezer, which could disrupt the integrity of the plastic cover.
    - Discard teething rings made prior to 1998, as they may contain diisononyl phthalate, a plastic softening agent which was later found to be toxic and potentially carcinogenic.
    - Do not attach a teething ring to a tether around the child's neck, as that may cause strangulation.
    - Care should be taken to not give the child an object which could be a potential choking hazard.

- Pharmacologic management
  - Acetaminophen (15 mg/kg PO q4–6h) or ibuprofen (10 mg/kg PO q6–8h) may be used for pain relief as needed.
  - Over-the-counter teething preparations containing benzocaine have been associated with methemoglobinemia and are not recommended for pediatric use. The U.S. Food and Drug Administration (FDA) released a Drug Safety Communication in 2011 to inform the public of this potentially fatal adverse effect.
  - The FDA warns against the use of homeopathic teething gels and tablets sold in retail stores and online.
  - Remedies used in the past that are no longer recommended include alcoholic liquors, honey, emetics, purgatives, and lancing of the gums.

ISSUES FOR REFERRAL

- Children should have a dental home by the age of 12 months.
- Children who have delayed eruption of their first primary tooth beyond 15 months should be evaluated. The following conditions have been associated with delayed eruption:
  - Anodontia
  - Impacted teeth
  - Hypothyroidism
  - Hypopituitarism
  - Calcium/phosphorus metabolism problems
  - Ectodermal dysplasias
  - Gaucher disease
  - Osteopetrosis
  - Apert syndrome
  - Cleidocranial dysplasia
  - Down syndrome
- Referral to a dentist should be considered for children with significant variation in eruption caused by dental infections, additional teeth in the path of eruption, insufficient space in the dental arch, and/or ectopic placement of teeth.
- Presence of or risk for dental caries at an early age should prompt a dental evaluation.
- Natal teeth should be evaluated only if they are loose and pose an aspiration risk or if they interfere with breastfeeding.

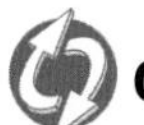

ONGOING CARE

PATIENT EDUCATION

- Information available at http://www.mouthhealthy.org/en/az-topics/t/teething
- Parent handout available at http://patiented.solutions.aap.org/handout.aspx?resultClick=1&gbosid=166311

ADDITIONAL READING

- Kozuch M, Peacock E, D'Auria JP. Infant teething information on the world wide web: taking a byte out of the search. *J Pediatr Health Care*. 2015;29(1):38–45.
- Lehr J, Masters A, Pollack B. Benzocaine-induced methemoglobinemia in the pediatric population. *J Pediatr Nurs*. 2012;27(5):583–588.
- Macknin ML, Piedmonte M, Jacobs J, et al. Symptoms associated with infant teething: a prospective study. *Pediatrics*. 2000;105(4, Pt 1):747–752.
- Markman L. Teething: facts and fiction. *Pediatr Rev*. 2009;30(8):e59–e64.
- Ramos-Jorge J, Pordeus I, Ramos-Jorge M, et al. Prospective longitudinal study of signs and symptoms associated with primary tooth eruption. *Pediatrics*. 2011;128(3):471–476.
- Sood S, Sood M. Teething: myths and facts. *J Clin Pediatr Dent*. 2010;35(1):9–14.
- U.S. Food and Drug Administration. Benzocaine and babies: not a good mix. http://www.fda.gov/ForConsumers/ConsumerUpdates/ucm306062.htm. Accessed January 18, 2017.
- U.S. Food and Drug Administration. FDA warns against the use of homeopathic teething tablets and gels. http://www.fda.gov/NewsEvents/Newsroom/PressAnnouncements/ucm523468.htm. Accessed January 18, 2017.
- Wake M, Hesketh K, Lucas J. Teething and tooth eruption in infants: a cohort study. *Pediatrics*. 2000;106(6):1374–1379.

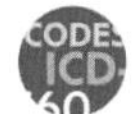

CODES

ICD10

K00.7 Teething syndrome

FAQ

- Q: When does a child need to see the dentist?
- A: Every infant should receive an oral health assessment from the primary care provider by 6 months of age to assess the patient's risk for oral disease or caries. Parents should be provided education on infant oral health and evaluation of fluoride supplementation. The American Academy of Pediatrics (AAP) and the American Academy of Pediatric Dentistry (AAPD) recommend that the patient establish a dental home by 1 year of age or sooner if with concern for dental caries, trauma, teeth staining, or family history of early dental caries.
- Q: What is the proper care of newly erupted teeth?
- A: Brushing with a toothbrush helps reduce bacterial colonization and should be done by a parent twice daily using a soft toothbrush of age-appropriate size with a small smear of toothpaste. Never put the baby to bed with a bottle due to increased risk for early childhood dental caries. Flossing can begin when two teeth touch.
- Q: Will thumb sucking affect my baby's teeth?
- A: Thumb sucking is a normal part of infancy but, if allowed to continue into early childhood, can cause problems with the child's bite. If it continues past the age of 3 years, the primary care or dental provider should counsel parents on strategies to reduce the behavior.
- Q: Is there a cluster of symptoms that can predict when teeth will emerge?
- A: Studies have failed to show a group of symptoms which is predictive of tooth eruption.
- Q: What are natal and neonatal teeth?
- A: Natal teeth are teeth present at birth, most often representing the premature eruption of primary teeth but occasionally can be a third set of teeth. They are usually left in place unless they cause difficulty with nursing or are loose and pose an aspiration risk. Neonatal teeth, however, erupt in the 1st month of life. Occurring in approximately 1 in 2,000 children, natal and neonatal teeth are not usually pathologic but have been associated with various syndromes, including Hallermann-Streiff syndrome, Ellis-van Creveld syndrome, craniofacial dysostosis, pachyonychia congenita, Pierre Robin, adrenogenital syndrome, and Sotos syndrome.

TENDONITIS AND TENDINOSIS

Jay Mehta, MD, MS

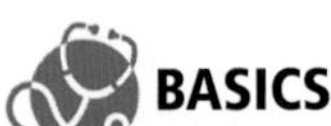

BASICS

DESCRIPTION

- Tendonitis: inflammation of a tendon or along the tendon sheath due to microtears
- Tendinosis: tendon collagen degeneration due to chronic overuse

EPIDEMIOLOGY

- Increases with age and at time of puberty
- May be slightly more common in girls

RISK FACTORS

Genetics

Hypermobile individuals may be prone to tendonitis.

PATHOPHYSIOLOGY

Inflammation and microtearing may be present.

ETIOLOGY

- Tendinosis associated with repetitive motion/overuse activities
- Can also see with inflammatory rheumatic disease
- Tendonitis associated with fluoroquinolone antibiotic use

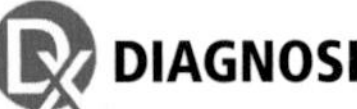

DIAGNOSIS

HISTORY

- Trauma or overuse
  - Verify acute nature of injury.
  - Pop or snap felt at the time of the event
- History of rheumatic disease (juvenile idiopathic arthritis [JIA], spondyloarthritis)
- Fluoroquinolone use
- Signs and symptoms
  - Pain
  - Tenderness

PHYSICAL EXAM

- Evidence of hematoma
  - Palpate around and about affected areas, detecting point tenderness especially at tendon insertions as well as over bony prominences.
- Evidence of bursitis or arthritis
  - Systemic conditions, such as spondyloarthritis, can lead to inflammation of tendons, bursa, and joints.
  - Bursitis can mimic the pain of tendonitis.
- Pop or snap felt on exam
  - Sometimes this is felt when tendons and ligaments are torn or avulsed.
- Caution: false positives
  - Patients may have torn ligaments, fractures, or arthritis, and not just tendonitis on examination.
- Pitfalls
  - Overdiagnosis in young children, in whom overuse is rare and other diagnoses should be considered
  - Underdiagnosis in older children in whom repetitive activities are likely to occur

DIFFERENTIAL DIAGNOSIS

- Infection
  - Gonococcal disease
  - Septic arthritis
  - Osteomyelitis
  - Tuberculosis (rare)
- Environmental
  - Fracture
- Metabolic
  - Homocystinuria
- Congenital
  - Generalized hypermobility
  - Marfan syndrome
  - Ehlers-Danlos

- Immunologic
  - Ankylosing spondylitis or spondyloarthropathy (including inflammatory bowel disease, reactive arthritis)
  - JIA
- Psychological or neuropathic
  - Amplified musculoskeletal pain

DIAGNOSTIC TESTS & INTERPRETATION

- No specific lab abnormalities seen
- If inflammatory markers are elevated, consider spondyloarthritis.
- Plain radiograph of affected area may be indicated to rule out a fracture or avulsion or identify a bone spur.

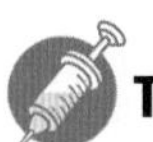

TREATMENT

GENERAL MEASURES

- Rest/reduced use of the affected tendon/muscle group is essential, occasionally requiring splinting.
- Duration of therapy
  - 1 to 4 weeks

MEDICATION

- NSAIDs initially
- Rarely, if ever, do soft tissue steroid injections have a role in children.

ADDITIONAL THERAPIES

- Physical or occupational therapy for eccentric muscle strengthening
- Either self-directed or formal help with resumption of desired activity to improve biomechanics

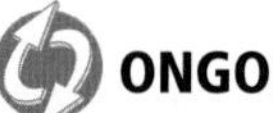

ONGOING CARE

FOLLOW-UP RECOMMENDATIONS

Improvement often takes 2 to 6 weeks or longer, if chronic.

Patient Monitoring

If the provocative activity is resumed too soon, the irritation will recur.

PROGNOSIS

Usually good for children; however, many will suffer recurrences if proper exercises before desired activity are not continued.

COMPLICATIONS

Ongoing pain and predisposition for recurrence

ADDITIONAL READING

- Almekinders LC, Temple JD. Etiology, diagnosis, and treatment of tendonitis: an analysis of the literature. *Med Sci Sports Exerc*. 1998;30(8):1183–1190.
- Jonsson P, Alfredson H. Superior results with eccentric compared to concentric quadriceps training in patients with jumper's knee: a prospective randomised study. *Br J Sports Med*. 2005;39(11):847–850.
- Marsh JS, Daigneault JP. Ankle injuries in the pediatric population. *Curr Opin Pediatr*. 2000;12(1):52–60.
- Millar NL, Murrell GA, McInnes IB. Inflammatory mechanisms in tendinopathy—towards translation. *Nat Rev Rheumatol*. 2017;13(2):110–122.
- Pommering TL, Kluchurosky L. Overuse injuries in adolescents. *Adolesc Med State Art Rev*. 2007;18(1):95–120.

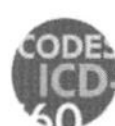

CODES

ICD10

M77.9 Enthesopathy, unspecified

FAQ

- Q: Which activities can result in overuse syndromes and tendonitis?
- A: Virtually, any repetitive activity in which children engage can cause tendonitis. For example, pain in the tendons of the thumb has occurred in children overusing video games.

TESTICULAR TORSION

Christopher E. Bayne, MD • Michael H. Hsieh, MD, PhD

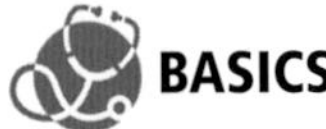

BASICS

DESCRIPTION

- Although the term "testicular torsion" (TT) is most commonly used, it is a pathologic misnomer. "Torsion of the spermatic cord" is the anatomically correct description of the urologic emergency in which the testis twists on its spermatic cord axis, occluding blood flow to the testis.
- TT is classified as extravaginal torsion (predominant in the neonatal period) or intravaginal torsion (most common during the pubertal period).
- Rapid diagnosis and correction is necessary to save testicular tissue. Duration of ischemia and degree of spermatic cord twisting are the primary determinants of testis viability.

EPIDEMIOLOGY

Incidence

- Reported to be as high as 1 per 4,000 and as low as 4.5 per 100,000 males ≤25 years
- Peak incidence is bimodal: the 1st year of life (likely the 1st month) and the pubertal period

RISK FACTORS

- The only known risk factor is the anatomic "bell-clapper" deformity (see "Pathophysiology").
- There have been reports of increased incidence of extravaginal TT in colder climates. Large database studies have refuted this observation.
- Family history
- There are associated conditions that do not increase risk of TT itself but may alter the entity's presentation, thus increasing the risk of delayed presentation and initial misdiagnosis.
  - Onset of symptoms with physical activity or genital trauma
  - Undescended (cryptorchid) testis

Genetics

- Clear predispositions have not been identified.
- A meta-analysis found up to 10% of unilateral torsion patients have an affected 1st-degree relative. Incidence among family members may be higher in bilateral cases.

GENERAL PREVENTION

- Paramount are awareness of genital pathology unique to pubertal boys and promptly seeking medical attention at onset of symptoms.
- Caretakers of patients with developmental, cognitive, or social disorders should be educated about scrotal pathology unique to the adolescent period (including TT and testis tumors) as these patients are less likely to report symptoms.

PATHOPHYSIOLOGY

- Testicular compartment anatomy
  - The spermatic cord suspends the testis in a compartment between parietal and visceral layers of tunica vaginalis (TV; derived from peritoneum).
  - The parietal and visceral TV are fused at the posterolateral border (forming a mesentery).
  - The gubernaculum fuses the testis to the TV at the inferior pole.
  - These points of fusion fix the testis in the scrotum. If either the tunical mesentery or gubernacular fixation is deficient, the testis is free to rotate within the TV compartment (commonly called the "bell-clapper deformity").
  - The incidence of bell-clapper deformity in autopsy series has been reported to be ~12%, much higher than the incidence of TT.
- Blood supply to the testis
  - The primary arterial supply is the testicular (gonadal) arteries (branches off the aorta).
  - The deferential artery (branch off the inferior vesical artery) and cremasteric artery (branch off the inferior epigastric artery) provide supplemental arterial support.
  - The testicular, deferential, and cremasteric arteries have collateral connections at the tail of the epididymis; thus, torsion of the spermatic cord effectively occludes all blood flow to the testis.
- Extravaginal torsion
  - Primarily occurs in the neonatal period (only 11% of torsion after 1 month of age has been reported as extravaginal)
  - 10% of all TT
  - In the neonatal period, the TV may not be fused within the scrotum, allowing the spermatic cord and TV to twist as a unit.
  - This mechanism of neonatal torsion is distinct from that of a pubertal/postpubertal male.
  - The incidence of contralateral bell-clapper deformity noted during surgical exploration of neonatal torsion has been reported.
  - There is controversy on whether or not to surgically explore cases of neonatal torsion without acute changes given the unknown duration of ischemia (e.g., potentially as long as labor), decreased likelihood of contralateral bell-clapper deformity, and risks of general anesthesia in the newborn period.
  - Cases of occult contralateral testis ischemia have been reported at time of preventative fixation.
  - Extravaginal torsion may occur prior to birth (e.g., a "vanishing testis"). These children may only have a palpable testis remnant.
- Intravaginal torsion
  - Commonly the result of bell-clapper anatomy
  - The spermatic cord twists medially/inward approximately 2/3 of the time.
  - A clear explanation for the increased incidence of TT in the pubertal period is lacking. Most theorize a connection with increased testicular growth and hormonal changes.
  - Given the high incidence of a contralateral bell-clapper deformity, preventative fixation of the contralateral side is standard practice.

COMMONLY ASSOCIATED CONDITIONS

Intermittent TT (extravaginal)

- Patients will report history of recurrent episodes characteristic of TT (see "History" and "Physical Exam").

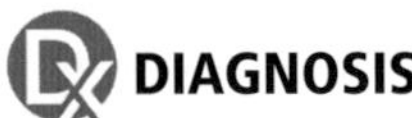

DIAGNOSIS

ALERT

TT has a diverse spectrum of presentation, from the "classic presentation" to complete absence of ipsilateral scrotal pain. The "classic" history, exam, and imaging findings are helpful in suggesting a diagnosis, but the absence of these features does not exclude TT.

HISTORY

- Acute-onset scrotal pain
  - The classic chief complaint, although pain can develop more gradually or after abdominal pain
  - Pain may have occurred at rest, awoken the boy from sleep, or been initiated by activity or trauma.
- Acute-onset abdominal pain
  - Usually lower quadrant (ipsilateral to affected testicle) in isolation or combination with scrotal pain
  - Isolated abdominal pain may be the only initial complaint (explained by testicular innervation originating from retroperitoneum as opposed to cutaneous innervation of the scrotum).
- Nausea and/or vomiting
- Patients may unintentionally or intentionally downplay or withhold symptoms due to embarrassment or perceived association with masturbation or other sexual activity.

PHYSICAL EXAM

- Low-grade fever may be present.
- Tender, edematous hemiscrotum, which may be firm to palpation
- Testis is often "high riding" in the scrotum compared to the contralateral side (as the spermatic cord twists, the testis is pulled into the inguinal canal).
- Scrotal skin may be normal at first but erythematous or darker in the delayed setting.
- Absence of a cremasteric reflex is a classic finding in TT. There are nuances to this finding:
  - Scratching the inner thigh normally causes elevation of the testis within the scrotum.
  - Absence is based on comparison to the contralateral, unaffected hemiscrotum.
  - The genitofemoral nerve reflex arc may be underdeveloped in children <2 years.
  - An intact reflex has been reported in cases of TT throughout the literature, and the reflex may be absent in normal boys.
  - The exam finding may be hard to discern in the setting of significant edema, a reactive hydrocele, and/or an already high-riding testis.
- TT of an undescended testis will alter the typical exam findings.
- In neonates, an erythematous, swollen hemiscrotum may be the only finding. This may appear similar to the scrotal changes typical of child birth (e.g., traumatic scrotal ecchymoses).
  - Caretakers and providers may be unsure of the exact timing or duration of changes.
  - It is important to establish whether a normal exam was ever documented.
- A dark, hardened hemiscrotum in a neonate is suggestive of prolonged TT.

DIFFERENTIAL DIAGNOSIS

- Torsion of the appendix testis (TAT)
  - The appendix testis is a small remnant of the paramesonephric duct (müllerian duct) structure at the upper pole of the testis.
  - The presentation of TAT can mimic TT.
  - Exam may reveal classic "blue dot" discoloration of the scrotal skin. This is essentially diagnostic but not always present and has been reported in the setting of concurrent TT.
- Epididymitis, orchitis, or epididymoorchitis
  - Caused by nonspecific inflammation, bacterial or viral infection, or reflux of urine through ejaculatory ducts and vas deferens ("reflux" epididymoorchitis caused by neuropathic or nonneuropathic dysfunctional voiding against a contracted external urethral sphincter)
  - Exam may be similar to TT but with preserved cremasteric reflex (see "Physical Exam") and positive "Prehn sign" (pain relief with manual elevation of testis suggestive of epididymitis or epididymoorchitis over TT).
  - Color Doppler ultrasonography (CDUS) will likely show signs of inflammation, including hyperemia, reactive hydrocele.
  - See "Epididymitis" chapter.
- Hydrocele (see "Hydrocele" chapter)
- Inguinal hernia (see "Inguinal Hernia" chapter)
- Testicular rupture
  - Traumatic rupture of testis capsule
  - Exam is variable and may be inconclusive.
  - CDUS may show tunica defect, scrotal hematoma, testicular hyperemia (or ischemia from distorting hematoma), irregular testis contour, or echotexture.

ALERT

TT should be included in the differential diagnosis of any male with acute abdominal pain or history of recent genital trauma.

DIAGNOSTIC TESTS & INTERPRETATION

Initial Tests (screening, lab, imaging)

- Urinalysis (UA) with pyuria and/or bacteriuria may help distinguish TT from epididymitis, but UA from a young patient epididymitis may be sterile, and UA from a patient with TT may have pyuria.
- CDUS
  - Nearly 100% specific but only 60–90% sensitive
  - Used to evaluate spermatic cord architecture, testicular blood flow, and intratesticular echotexture
  - Absence of testicular arterial Doppler waveforms is the most specific finding for TT with near 100% specificity.
  - Heterogeneous intratesticular echotexture suggests prolonged ischemia and necrosis.
  - CDUS is operator- and reader-dependent.
  - CDUS has ability to differentiate between TT and other conditions of the scrotum.
- Scrotal nuclear scintigraphy
  - Not commonly used due to poor sensitivity and specificity compared to high-resolution CDUS
  - The test has poor ability to differentiate other conditions of the scrotum.

ALERT

In atypical cases, surgical exploration may be the only definitive way to exclude the diagnosis of TT.

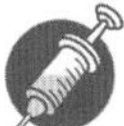

TREATMENT

GENERAL MEASURES

- Acute TT requires emergent detorsion.
- In most circumstances, time of symptom onset equals ischemia time.
- Rates of orchiectomy sharply increase 6 to 8 hours after symptom onset.

MEDICATION

Treat pain and emesis appropriately.

ISSUES FOR REFERRAL

- If the clinical history, exam, or imaging are inconclusive, consult a pediatric urologist.
- In the case of neonates at a general hospital, it may be useful to discuss the circumstances with a pediatric urologist prior to initiating transfer to a dedicated pediatric facility.
- In the case of pubertal and teenage boys, retrospective reviews have consistently shown routine transfer to a dedicated pediatric facility does not improve orchiectomy rate and may result in worse outcomes.

SURGERY/OTHER PROCEDURES

- Once a diagnosis of TT has been made or is strongly suspicious, some advocate providers attempt manual detorsion.
  - Involves manually attempting to rotate the testis within the hemiscrotal sac
  - Because approximately 2/3 of cases of TT involve internal rotation, an attempt at 360 degrees external rotation (the "open the book" technique) is often described.
  - The advantage of this maneuver: It can be performed prior to the operating room, thus possibly restoring blood flow faster.
  - The disadvantages of this maneuver: It may be extremely painful; it is impossible to know if 360 degrees is enough rotation (or too much); in approximately 1/3 of cases, the testis turns internally (thus, attempting detorsion may worsen blood flow).
  - It is critical to monitor symptomatic response to manual detorsion.
  - Postmanual detorsion CDUS may clarify if blood flow has been restored.
  - Successful manual detorsion does not obviate the need for testis fixation within the scrotum as the risk of recurrence is extremely high.
- Emergent surgical exploration and detorsion is the only definitive treatment for TT.
  - Surgeons expose the testis and detorse the spermatic cord.
  - Orchiectomy is performed if the testis is deemed nonviable.
  - The affected (if viable) and contralateral testis are usually secured in the scrotum with suture to prevent recurrence.

ONGOING CARE

PROGNOSIS

- How TT may affect fertility, regardless of whether a testis was saved or removed, is unclear.
- Some testicular atrophy, even after short-duration TT, is common.
- Previous TT is a rare complaint among patients undergoing fertility workup.
- After TT sperm quality is usually within normal range but may correlate with duration of ischemia

ADDITIONAL READING

- Bayne CE, Villanueva J, Davis TD, et al. Factors associated with delayed presentation and misdiagnosis of testicular torsion: a case-control study. *J Pediatr*. 2017;186:200–204.
- DaJusta DG, Granberg CF, Villanueva C, et al. Contemporary review of testicular torsion: new concepts, emerging technologies and potential therapeutics. *J Pediatr Urol*. 2013;9(6 Pt A):723–730.
- Mellick LB. Torsion of the testicle: it is time to stop tossing the dice. *Pediatr Emerg Care*. 2012;28(1): 80–86.

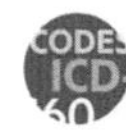

CODES

ICD10

- N44.00 Torsion of testis, unspecified
- N44.0 Torsion of testis
- N44.02 Intravaginal torsion of spermatic cord

FAQ

- Q: Does decreased or increased flow on CDUS rule out TT?
- A: No. In fact, TT in this setting is reported throughout the literature.
- Q: Can a testis be salvaged despite symptoms of >6 hours duration?
- A: Yes, albeit at a decreased rate.
- Q: Should TT of long duration (>24 hours) be treated emergently?
- A: This is dependent on the surgeon's assessment of probability of testis viability. Intermittently torsed testes may be more likely to be viable in this setting.

TETANUS

Eimear Kitt, MB, BCh, BAO (NUI) • Hamid Bassiri, MD, PhD

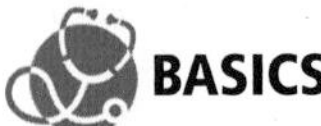

BASICS

DESCRIPTION

- Tetanus is characterized by muscle rigidity and spasms due to production of a neurotoxin in infected wounds by *Clostridium tetani*, an anaerobic spore-forming gram-positive bacillus.
- There are four clinical forms of tetanus: generalized, neonatal, localized, and cephalic.

EPIDEMIOLOGY

- Tetanus is rare in the United States, with an average of 29 reported cases per year. Nearly all cases are in unvaccinated individuals.
  - Rare cases have been reported in patients with protective levels of antitetanus antibodies.
- Tetanus continues to occur in countries in which mothers are not immunized and nonsterile care of the umbilical cord is practiced. Worldwide, it is estimated that >250,000 deaths from neonatal tetanus occurred between 2000 and 2003.
- Generalized tetanus is the most common form of disease.

RISK FACTORS

- Inadequate immunization
- Neonate born to unimmunized mother
- Elderly with declining immune status
- Injection drug use
- Chronic wounds
- Acute traumatic injury
- Foreign bodies
- Nonsterile delivery conditions and practice of applying mud or feces to umbilical cord

GENERAL PREVENTION

- All wounds should be cleaned with soap and water and foreign bodies should be removed.
- Universal immunization with tetanus toxoid (For details and information on catch-up schedules, refer to Centers for Disease Control and Prevention (CDC) Web site.)
- Tetanus postexposure prophylaxis should be initiated at the time of injury:
  - For clean minor wounds:
    - If patient has had ≥3 prior doses of tetanus toxoid (DTaP, Tdap, or Td) and it has been <10 years since the last dose, no prophylaxis is indicated; if it has been ≥10 years since last dose, give tetanus toxoid.
    - If patient has had <3 prior doses of tetanus toxoids, give tetanus toxoid.
  - For all other wounds:
    - If patient has had ≥3 prior doses of tetanus toxoid and it has been <5 years since the last dose, no prophylaxis is indicated; if it has been ≥5 years since the last dose, give tetanus toxoid.
    - Patients with <3 prior doses of tetanus toxoid should receive tetanus immune globulin (TIG) and tetanus toxoid at separate sites.
    - Patients with HIV or severe immunodeficiency should receive TIG regardless of prior immunization history.
  - In neonates or infants <6 months of age who have not received 3 doses of DTaP, the decision to use TIG should be based on mother's tetanus immunization status; if unknown or inadequate, should give TIG
  - Type of tetanus toxoid to use for prophylaxis:
    - For children <7 years old, use DTaP; if pertussis vaccine is contraindicated, use DT.
    - For a child 7 to 10 years old, use Tdap.
    - For an adolescent 11 to 18 years old who has not received Tdap, use Tdap; for those who have received Tdap or for those whom pertussis is contraindicated, use Td.
  - TIG dose is 250 U IM for wound prophylaxis (regardless of age or weight); if TIG is unavailable, use IV immunoglobulin (IVIG) or tetanus antitoxin (TAT).
    - Because TAT is equine in origin, test patient for sensitivity prior to use.
    - TAT is no longer available in the United States.

PATHOPHYSIOLOGY

- *C. tetani* produces tetanospasmin, a powerful metalloprotease neurotoxin.
- Tetanospasmin can be absorbed directly into skeletal muscles adjacent to the injury.
- Tetanospasmin can travel to the CNS via retrograde axonal transport through peripheral nerves or via lymphocytes.
  - In the CNS, tetanospasmin prevents the release of γ-aminobutyric acid (GABA) and glycine in inhibitory nerve terminals, resulting in sustained excitatory discharges (motor spasms and increased muscle tone) and autonomic instability; tetanospasmin does not directly affect cognitive processes.
  - In the peripheral nervous system, tetanospasmin may block inhibitory impulses to motor neurons.
  - Loss of regulation of adrenal catecholamine release precipitates tachycardia, hypertension, and sweating.
- Infection does not confer immunity; all patients need to be immunized during recovery.

ETIOLOGY

- Tetanus is caused by *C. tetani*, a spore-forming, anaerobic gram-positive bacillus.
- *C. tetani* is found in soil, animal and human feces, house dust, and salt and fresh water.
- Under anaerobic conditions, spores become vegetative and produce tetanospasmin; anaerobic conditions in wounds are promoted by extensive necrosis, foreign bodies, or other suppurative infections.

DIAGNOSIS

HISTORY

- Incubation period is 3 to 21 days (usually 10 days) but varies as inoculations distal to CNS are associated with longer incubation periods.
- Generalized tetanus
  - "Lockjaw" or trismus is initial symptom in 50–75% of cases.
  - Other early complaints include dysphagia, neck pain and stiffness, stiffness and pain in other muscle groups, urinary retention, restlessness, irritability, and headache.
  - More muscle groups involved as disease progresses
  - Noise, light, touch, and other stimuli can trigger painful spasms.
- Neonatal tetanus (generalized tetanus during neonatal period)
  - Occurs following vaginal delivery to unimmunized mothers
  - Usually due to umbilical stump infections
  - Typically presents at around 1 week of life with irritability and poor feeding but progresses rapidly to generalized tetanic spasms
- Local tetanus
  - Painful muscle contractions and stiffness limited to the area near the wound
  - Can persist for several weeks
  - Can progress to generalized tetanus
- Cephalic tetanus (local tetanus of head/neck affecting cranial nerves [CNs])
  - Caused by *C. tetani* infections of head/neck including chronic infections of the head/neck (e.g., chronic otitis media)
  - Unlike generalized tetanus, flaccid CN palsies (especially CN VII) predominate; trismus may develop; however, if trismus is absent, could be confused with Bell palsy due to other etiologies.

PHYSICAL EXAM

- Vital sign abnormalities
  - Severe, labile episodes of hypertension and tachycardia; hypotension is a late feature.
  - Initially, patients are afebrile but may develop hyperthermia with sustained contractions or from superinfections.
- Trismus is often initial presenting sign.
- Persistent trismus causes *risus sardonicus*, wrinkling of the forehead, and distortion of the eyebrows and the corners of the mouth.
- With disease progression, other muscle groups develop tetanic contractions and spasms:
  - Can lead to a severe opisthotonic posture
  - Can mimic seizures
  - Can be extremely painful
  - Can be associated with laryngospasm and tetany of respiratory musculature
  - The anxiety and pain associated with these spasms may precipitate additional spasms.
- Sweating can occur from autonomic instability.
- Normal mental status is the norm.
- In cephalic tetanus, CN palsies can be seen.
  - Look for underlying wounds or chronic infections of the face, scalp, neck, or ear.

DIFFERENTIAL DIAGNOSIS

- Infections
  - Dental infections, retropharyngeal and peritonsillar abscesses, poliomyelitis, viral encephalitis, and meningoencephalitis may present with trismus and/or CN findings.
- Toxins and medications
  - Dystonic reactions to phenothiazine medications may resemble tetanus.
  - Strychnine poisoning may mimic generalized tetanus.
  - Malignant neuroleptic syndrome causes increased muscular rigidity resembling tetanic spasms.

- Metabolic
  - Hypocalcemic tetany is usually not as severe as that seen in tetanus.
- Stiff man syndrome can result in fluctuating tonic contractions resembling tetanic spasms.
- Bell palsy may resemble cephalic tetanus.

DIAGNOSTIC TESTS & INTERPRETATION

- Lab tests often yield little information; WBC is usually normal or mildly elevated and CSF studies are unremarkable, but serum calcium levels may help exclude hypocalcemic tetany.
- Gram stain and anaerobic wound cultures yield *C. tetani* in <1/3 of cases.
- Presence of protective tetanus antibody titer does not exclude possibility of disease.
- EEG and EMG findings are nonspecific.

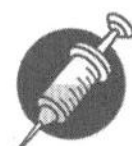

TREATMENT

GENERAL MEASURES

- Tetanus is not a transmissible disease.
- Keep patient in a quiet, darkened room with minimum stimulus.
- Monitor cardiac and respiratory status closely.
- Be prepared to perform a tracheotomy to prevent fatal laryngospasm.
- Monitor for and treat urinary retention and constipation.
- Parenteral nutrition is usually required to maintain adequate nutrition and hydration.
- Monitor for and correct electrolyte abnormalities, especially hyperkalemia.

ALERT

Tetanus infections may not result in immunity, as even a small amount of toxin can result in significant disease. Because of this, active immunization against tetanus should always be undertaken once the patient has recovered from the acute illness.

MEDICATION

First Line

- Neutralization of unbound neurotoxin:
  - Human TIG 3,000 to 6,000 U IM as a single dose; part of the dose may be infiltrated around the wound.
  - Administer prior to antibiotics and wound manipulation.
- Tetanus toxoid should be administered IM at a site contralateral to where TIG is given.
- Antibiotics can decrease burden of vegetative *C. tetani* that produce tetanospasmin:
  - First line: metronidazole 30 mg/kg/24 h PO or IV in 4 divided doses; maximum 4 g/24 h
  - Alternative: parenteral penicillin G 100,000 to 200,000 U/kg/24 h IV in 4 to 6 divided doses; maximum 12,000,000 U/24 h
  - Treat for 10 to 14 day.
  - Cephalosporins are not effective.
- Sedation and muscle relaxation
  - Diazepam 0.1 to 0.2 mg/kg IV q4–6h
  - Phenothiazines, especially chlorpromazine, may be helpful.
  - Titrate sedation to desired effect and monitor for respiratory depression.
- Nondepolarizing neuromuscular blockade and mechanical ventilation:
  - Use if spasms cannot be adequately controlled or if spasm of airway and respiratory musculature compromises ventilation:
    - Vecuronium 0.08 to 0.1 mg/kg IV followed by continuous infusion or hourly dosing
    - Avoid succinylcholine due to increased risk of hyperkalemia and arrhythmia.
- Management of autonomic dysfunction
  - β-Blockers (e.g., labetalol 0.4 to 1 mg/kg/h) can control hypertension or arrhythmias.
  - Magnesium sulfate can significantly reduce cardiovascular instability and act as an adjunctive agent to control muscle spasms.

Second Line

If TIG is not available:

- IVIG 200 to 400 mg/kg may be used (not FDA approved for this use).
- TAT can be given in doses of 1,500 to 3,000 U IM or IV (to achieve a serum concentration of 0.1 IU/mL) but only after a negative skin test or desensitization:
  - TAT is not available in the United States.
  - Anaphylactic reactions can occur with varying severity in up to 20% of patients.

SURGERY/OTHER PROCEDURES

Aggressive surgical debridement of wounds and removal of foreign bodies is critical.

ADMISSION, INPATIENT, AND NURSING CONSIDERATIONS

- Prompt recognition of clinical signs of tetanus and initiation of emergency care are crucial.
- All suspected cases of tetanus should be rapidly transferred to a tertiary care center capable of providing ventilatory and cardiovascular support in an intensive care setting.
- In the emergency department, treatment with TIG should be initiated to neutralize unbound neurotoxin; however, supportive care including aggressive airway management, ventilatory support, and pharmacologic interventions (sedation, muscle relaxation) are also critical to ameliorate the effects of bound neurotoxin.

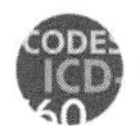

ONGOING CARE

PROGNOSIS

- Signs and symptoms usually progress for ~1 week, then plateau for ~1 week, and gradually improve over the next 2 to 6 weeks.
- Overall mortality rates have decreased with advances in the ability to provide respiratory support in an intensive care setting.
- Mortality rates vary from 1% to 18% for localized tetanus, 15–30% for cephalic tetanus, to 45–55% for generalized tetanus. Neonatal tetanus has the highest mortality rates of between 50% and 100%, with low birth weight and age of onset between 5 and 7 days of life associated with increased risk of death.
- Children and young adults have a better prognosis than older individuals or neonates.
- A more rapid onset and progression of disease from trismus to generalized spasms is associated with a more severe course.
- In the absence of complications, survivors usually recover fully without sequelae.

COMPLICATIONS

- Most complications are related to the severe tetanic muscle contractions:
  - Rhabdomyolysis and hyperkalemia
  - Vertebral body and other fractures
  - Muscle hemorrhages
- Respiratory failure from spasms of the upper airway or diaphragm is the most common cause of death in acute phase, whereas arrhythmia and myocardial infarction are most common cause of death later in disease.
- Cerebrovascular hemorrhages may be seen in rare cases, especially in neonatal tetanus.
- Pneumonia, including aspiration, can occur.

ADDITIONAL READING

- Brook I. Tetanus in children. *Pediatr Emerg Care*. 2004;20(1):48–51.
- Hassel B. Tetanus: pathophysiology, treatment, and the possibility of using botulinum toxin against tetanus-induced rigidity and spasms. *Toxins (Basel)*. 2013;5(1):73–83.
- Lambo JA, Anokye EA. Prognostic factors for mortality in neonatal tetanus: a systematic review and meta-analysis. *Int J Infect Dis*. 2013;17(12):e1100–e1110.
- Rhee P, Nunley MK, Demetriades D, et al. Tetanus and trauma: a review and recommendations. *J Trauma*. 2005;58(5):1082–1088.
- Thwaites CL, Farrar JJ. Preventing and treating tetanus. *BMJ*. 2003;326(7381):117–118.

CODES

ICD10

- A35 Other tetanus
- A33 Tetanus neonatorum

FAQ

- Q: What types of wounds are tetanus-prone?
- A: Punctures, avulsion wounds, crush injuries, burns, wounds from frostbite or missiles, and wounds contaminated with saliva, soil, or feces.
- Q: How is tetanus diagnosed?
- A: Tetanus is a clinical diagnosis. Laboratory testing is typically not helpful as *C. tetani* usually cannot be recovered from the wound of the patient.
- Q: Where can I find a schedule of the recommended childhood vaccine series for tetanus?
- A: The CDC Web site contains all current official recommended immunization series (www.cdc.gov/vaccines/schedules/downloads/child/0-18yrs-child-combined-schedule.pdf).

T

TETRALOGY OF FALLOT

Lauren Andrade, MD • Arvind Hoskoppal, MD, MHS

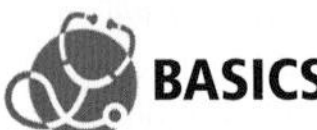

BASICS

DESCRIPTION

Anatomic hallmark is anterior malalignment of infundibular (outlet) septum, which results in

- A large and unrestrictive ventricular septal defect (VSD)
- Various degrees of right ventricular outflow tract obstruction (RVOTO)
- Overriding aorta
- Right ventricular hypertrophy (RVH) secondary to exposure to systemic pressure

EPIDEMIOLOGY

- The most common cyanotic congenital heart disease
- 3.5–10% of all congenital heart disease

RISK FACTORS

Genetics

About 20% of cases of tetralogy of Fallot are associated with a chromosome 22q11 microdeletion or duplication.

PATHOPHYSIOLOGY

- Severity of clinical signs and symptoms depends on the degree of RVOTO and related right-to-left shunt at the VSD.
- Physiology is a spectrum ranging from too little pulmonary blood flow and right-to-left shunt at the VSD due to severe RVOT obstruction ("blue tet") to moderate pulmonary overcirculation and left-to-right shunt at the VSD with minimal RVOTO ("pink tet").

COMMONLY ASSOCIATED CONDITIONS

- May be associated with other syndromes including trisomy 21, Alagille syndrome, fetal alcohol syndrome, and those involving a variety of limb abnormalities
- Tetralogy of Fallot may also be associated with midline abdominal defects (e.g., omphalocele) as in the pentalogy of Cantrell.

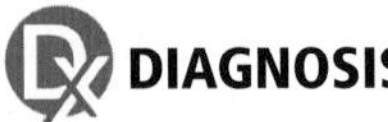

DIAGNOSIS

Signs and symptoms

- Varying degree of cyanosis, especially when crying or during and after physical activity
- "Blue tets"
  - Present with cyanosis at or shortly after birth
- "Pink tets"
  - May not present until 4 to 6 weeks of age (once pulmonary vascular resistance drops)
  - Present with signs of pulmonary overcirculation and heart failure (failure to thrive, diaphoresis with feeds, increased work of breathing)

PHYSICAL EXAM

- Cyanosis may be present at birth or may appear later during infancy or childhood as a result of progressive RVOTO.
- Normal S1 and single loud S_2 secondary to a more anteriorly located aorta
- Systolic ejection murmur at the left sternal border secondary to RVOTO

DIFFERENTIAL DIAGNOSIS

- Tetralogy of Fallot should be considered in all infants with a heart murmur and/or various degrees of cyanosis as well as acyanotic infants or children with a history of hypercyanotic episodes.
- Other forms of cyanotic congenital heart disease should be considered, including the following:
  - Double outlet right ventricle (DORV)
  - Transposition of the great arteries (TGA)
  - Pulmonary atresia with a VSD (PA-VSD)

DIAGNOSTIC TESTS & INTERPRETATION

- Electrocardiography
  - Right axis deviation (+90 to 180 degrees)
  - RVH
- Chest radiograph
  - Right aortic arch (30%)
  - Decreased pulmonary vascular markings in "blue tets" (may be increased markings in "pink tets")
  - Boot-shaped heart (*coeur en sabot*) with concave main pulmonary artery segment
- Echocardiogram
  - Anterior malalignment VSD
  - Presence of additional VSDs
  - Degree of RVOTO
  - Appearance of pulmonary valve and presence of valvar pulmonary stenosis, pulmonary valve size, and/or branch pulmonary artery stenosis
  - Overriding aorta, arch sidedness
  - Coronary artery anatomy (Most common anomaly is left anterior descending coronary artery originating from the right coronary artery in 4% of patients.)
- Cardiac catheterization
  - Generally not indicated unless there is concern regarding the branch pulmonary artery anatomy, coronary anatomy, or additional VSDs that need to be defined before surgery

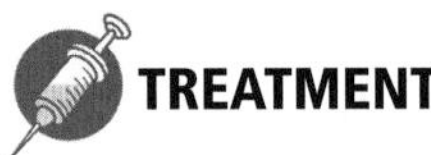

TREATMENT

MEDICATION

- Preoperatively all patients should receive subacute bacterial endocarditis (SBE) prophylaxis prior to dental procedures; postoperatively, patients should receive SBE prophylaxis for 6 months.
- Hypercyanotic episodes ("tet spells")
  - The goal is to increase preload and promote pulmonary blood flow, decreasing right-to-left shunt at the VSD.
  - Knee-chest position increases systemic vascular resistance.
  - IV fluid bolus increases preload.
  - $NaHCO_3$ to treat acidosis
  - Oxygen decreases pulmonary vascular resistance.
  - Morphine sulfate (0.1 mg/kg IV or IM) to decrease pain resulting in lower heart rate and improved ventricular filling time (i.e., increase preload)
  - β-Blocker (esmolol infusion for immediate therapy, propranolol for long-term prophylaxis) to lower heart rate and improve ventricular filling time (i.e., increase preload)
  - Phenylephrine (0.02 mg/kg IV) to increase systemic vascular resistance and oppose the right-to-left shunt

- Postoperatively, patients with prosthetic valves or residual defects adjacent to prosthetic material should receive SBE prophylaxis prior to dental procedures indefinitely.
- Postoperatively, patients with prosthetic valves should take aspirin daily indefinitely.

SURGERY/OTHER PROCEDURES

- Palliative surgery:
  - Blalock-Taussig systemic-to-pulmonary artery shunt (also known as the Blalock-Taussig-Thomas shunt)
  - No longer commonly performed
- Corrective surgery:
  - VSD patch closure and right ventricular outflow tract reconstruction
  - Sometimes requiring a right ventricle to pulmonary artery conduit depending on the degree of RVOTO

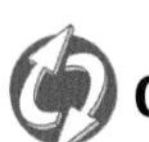

ONGOING CARE

PROGNOSIS

- 35-year survival is approximately 85%.
- >90% of children with tetralogy of Fallot are expected to survive to adulthood.
- Higher risk of adverse outcomes in patients with repair at age >3 years.
- There is a higher risk of developmental delay in children with tetralogy of Fallot (as with all congenital heart disease).
- Residual hemodynamic abnormalities are common:
  - Pulmonary insufficiency (with transannular patch repair disrupting the pulmonary valve)
  - Residual RVOTO
  - Right ventricular dysfunction in adulthood due to chronic volume overload
  - Left pulmonary artery stenosis is particularly common in tetralogy of Fallot.
  - Residual VSD
  - Commonly, adults develop aortic root dilation and subsequent aortic valve insufficiency.
- Conduction abnormalities (e.g., complete heart block, atrial, and ventricular tachyarrhythmias)
  - Incidence of sudden death is 2.5% per decade of follow-up and is generally attributed to ventricular arrhythmias.
  - Almost all patients have right bundle branch block following surgical repair.
- The need for reintervention (pulmonary valve replacement) increases after the 2nd decade of life, most frequently for severe pulmonary insufficiency.
  - Right ventricular end-diastolic volume >150 mL/m^2, QRS > 180 ms, history of tachyarrhythmias, RVOTO, exercise intolerance, and syncope are indications for intervention
  - Options are surgical versus transcatheter intervention (Melody valve) for pulmonary valve replacement.

COMPLICATIONS

- Preoperatively
  - Paroxysmal hypoxic episodes (i.e., hypercyanotic episodes, also called "tet spell")
  - Bacterial endocarditis
  - Cerebrovascular accident secondary to cyanosis, polycythemia, and microcytic anemia
- Postoperatively
  - Right ventricular dysfunction
  - Progressive pulmonary insufficiency
  - Ventricular arrhythmias
  - Sudden death (ventricular arrhythmias and/or complete heart block)

ADDITIONAL READING

- Apitz C, Webb G, Redington A. Tetralogy of Fallot. *Lancet*. 2009;374(9699):1462–1471.
- Cobanoglu A, Schultz JM. Total correction of tetralogy of Fallot in the first year of life: late results. *Ann Thorac Surg*. 2005;74(1):133–138.
- Geva T. Indications for pulmonary valve replacement in repaired tetralogy of Fallot: the quest continues. *Circulation*. 2013;128(17):1855–1857.
- Hirsch JC, Bove EL. Tetralogy of Fallot. In: Mavroudis C, Backer CL, eds. *Pediatric Cardiac Surgery*. 3rd ed. Philadelphia, PA: Mosby; 2003:383–397.
- Martinez RM, Ringewald J, Fontanet HL, et al. Management of adults with tetralogy of Fallot. *Cardiol Young*. 2013;23(6):921–932.
- Murphy AM, Cameron DE. The Blalock-Taussig-Thomas collaboration. A model for medical progress. *JAMA*. 2008;300(3):328–330.
- Siwik ES. *Moss and Adams Heart Diseases in Infants, Children and Adolescents*. 5th ed. Baltimore, MD: Williams & Wilkins; 2001:880–902.
- Walker WT, Temple IK, Gnanapragasam JP, et al. Quality of life after repair of tetralogy of Fallot. *Cardiol Young*. 2002;12(6):549–553.
- Warnes CA, Williams RG, Bashore TM, et al. ACC/AHA 2008 guidelines for the management of adults with congenital heart disease: a report of the American College of Cardiology/American Heart Association Task Force on Practice Guidelines (writing committee to develop guidelines on the management of adults with congenital heart disease). *Circulation*. 2008;118(23):e714–e833.

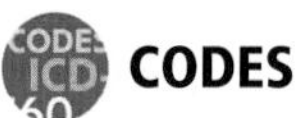

CODES

ICD10

Q21.3 Tetralogy of Fallot

FAQ

- Q: What is the etiology of the "tet spell"?
- A: There is an increase in resistance to flow through the right ventricular outflow tract and/or pulmonary vascular bed that leads to a dramatic decrease in pulmonary blood flow and increased right-to-left shunt at the level of the VSD. Therefore, treatment should be aimed at increasing pulmonary blood flow either by decreasing pulmonary vascular resistance (e.g., oxygen, morphine), increasing systemic vascular resistance (e.g., knee-chest position, phenylephrine), or decreasing dynamic obstruction by decreasing heart rate and thus increasing right ventricular preload (e.g., β-blockers).
- Q: When is an optimal time for surgical repair of tetralogy of Fallot?
- A: Surgical correction should be guided by symptoms. Progressive hypoxemia or recurrent tet spells indicate a need for emergent surgical intervention. A "pink tet" can be referred for elective repair in early infancy (3 to 6 months) and before the end of the 1st year of life.

THALASSEMIA

Irina B. Pateva, MD

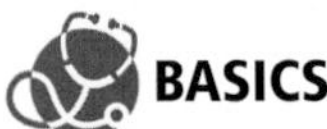

BASICS

DESCRIPTION

- Thalassemia syndromes are hereditary microcytic anemias that result from mutations that quantitatively reduce globin synthesis.
- Normal hemoglobin (Hb) is a tetramer of 2 α and 2 β chains:
  - α-Thalassemia: reduced or absent α-globin production
  - β-Thalassemia: reduced or absent β-globin production

EPIDEMIOLOGY

- α-Thalassemia:
  - Predominantly in Chinese subcontinent, Malaysia, Indochina, and Africa
  - African Americans
- β-Thalassemia:
  - Mediterranean countries, Africa, India, Pakistan, Middle East, and China

RISK FACTORS

Genetics

- α-Thalassemia
  - Normally, there are four α-globin genes, two on each chromosome 16.
  - Most mutations in α-thalassemia are large deletions.
  - Deletions may be in *trans* conformation (one deletion on each chromosome, common in African Americans) or *cis* conformation (two genes deleted on same chromosome, common in Asians).
  - Hb Constant Spring is an α-globin gene mutation caused by a point mutation that reduces or eliminates production of α-globin, leading to a more severe phenotype.
  - The four α-thalassemia syndromes reflect the inheritance of molecular defects affecting the output of 1, 2, 3, or 4 α genes.
- β-Thalassemia
  - Normally, there are two β-globin genes, one on each chromosome 11.
  - Most mutations in β-thalassemia are point mutations.
  - Many mutations abolish the expression completely (β^0), whereas others variably decrease quantitative expression (β^+).
  - Heterozygous state for β-globin mutation produces β-thalassemia trait.
  - Homozygous state produces β-thalassemia major or β-thalassemia intermedia.
  - Note: Rare dominant β-thalassemia mutations exist, causing ineffective erythropoiesis with a single mutation (due to creation of unstable β-globin variants).

Genotype	Name	Degree of Anemia
α-Thalassemia		
$\alpha\alpha/\alpha-$	Silent carrier	Asymptomatic
$\alpha-/\alpha-$ or $\alpha\alpha/-{>}-$	α-Thalassemia trait	Asymptomatic
$\alpha-/--$	α-Thalassemia intermedia, HbH disease	Moderate to severe
$--/--$	α-Thalassemia major	Hydrops fetalis
β-Thalassemia		
β/β^+ or β/β^0	β-Thalassemia trait	Asymptomatic
β/β^0 or β^+/β^+	β-Thalassemia intermedia	Variable, intermittent, or chronic transfusions
β^0/β^+ or β^0/β^0	β-Thalassemia major	Severe, chronic transfusions

PATHOPHYSIOLOGY

- Decrease in either α- or β-globin synthesis leads to fewer completed α_2–β_2 tetramers produced per RBC, which results in a decrease in intracellular Hb and microcytosis.
- Unpaired globin chains precipitate, resulting in apoptosis of red cell precursors (ineffective erythropoiesis) and damage to the RBC membrane leading to hemolysis.
- Ineffective erythropoiesis causes hepatosplenomegaly and osseous changes.
- The erythrocyte's lifespan is shortened by hemolysis and splenic trapping.
- Degree of anemia varies depending on the specific gene defect.
- Chronic transfusion therapy and, to a lesser degree, increased absorption of dietary iron in thalassemia major lead to iron accumulation.
- Increased absorption of dietary iron and intermittent transfusions in thalassemia intermedia lead to iron accumulation.
- Iron overload leads to cardiac arrhythmias and congestive heart failure (CHF) that can be fatal, liver inflammation and fibrosis, and endocrinopathies (e.g., diabetes mellitus, hypothyroidism, gonadal failure, osteoporosis).

DIAGNOSIS

HISTORY

- Severe α-thalassemia (4 gene deletion) presents prenatally by ultrasound or at birth with hydrops fetalis and severe anemia.
- Severe β-thalassemia usually presents between 3 and 12 months old, as production of the normal fetal Hb decreases.
- α-Thalassemia syndromes will present with microcytosis in infancy. Hemoglobin H (HbH) disease may present later, with mild to moderate anemia on screening or after worsening hemolysis related to intercurrent infection.
- Mediterranean, African, or Asian ethnic backgrounds are common in patients with thalassemia.
- Familial history of anemia, long-term transfusions, recurrent iron therapy for presumed iron deficiency anemia, or splenectomy
- Newborn screening varies by state but can contribute to a presumptive diagnosis of α-thalassemia or β-thalassemia major. Abnormal patterns include presence of Hb Barts (consistent with α-thalassemia) or isolated HbF (consistent with β-thalassemia major). Extreme prematurity and previous blood transfusions can obscure results, and confirmatory testing is required.

PHYSICAL EXAM

- Pallor indicates anemia.
- Heart murmur: Flow murmurs are often heard in significant anemia. Patients with severe anemia may present with CHF.
- Variable degrees of icterus: Hemolysis leads to increased bilirubin production.
- Abnormal facies (frontal bossing and maxillary hyperplasia): facial bone expansion by hypertrophic marrow in poorly transfused patients with β-thalassemia
- Failure to thrive: related to anemia and energy expended in ineffective erythropoiesis
- Variable degrees of hepatosplenomegaly (or CHF) due to extramedullary hematopoiesis

DIFFERENTIAL DIAGNOSIS

- Iron deficiency anemia can be distinguished with iron studies.
- Anemia of chronic inflammation (can be distinguished with soluble transferrin receptor assay)
- Lead poisoning

DIAGNOSTIC TESTS & INTERPRETATION

Initial Tests (screening, lab, imaging)

- CBC with RBC indices
  - Mean cell volume (MCV), mean cell hemoglobin (MCH), and mean cell hemoglobin concentration (MCHC) are all decreased in α- and β-thalassemia.
  - RBC volume distribution width (RDW) is usually normal.
  - Peripheral smear may reveal microcytosis, hypochromia, anisocytosis, poikilocytosis, target cells, nucleated RBCs, and/or polychromasia.
  - Hb 9 to 12 g/dL in α- or β-thalassemia trait
  - Hb usually 7 to 10 g/dL in HbH disease
  - Hb usually 7 to 10 g/dL in β-thalassemia intermedia
  - Hb $<$7 g/dL in thalassemia major (without transfusions)
- Reticulocyte count: usually mildly elevated in HbH and β-thalassemia intermedia and major
- Indirect bilirubin: may be elevated in severe thalassemia where there is significant red cell destruction

- Hb electrophoresis
  - α-Thalassemia trait (two defective genes) will have 5–10% Hb Barts (a tetramer of four γ chains) at birth, which should be detected on the newborn's screen. This disappears in 1 to 2 months, after which time the electrophoresis will be normal in α-thalassemia trait.
  - β-Thalassemia trait: HbF 1–5%, HbA2 3.5–8%, remainder HbA. The elevated HbA2 will distinguish α- from β-thalassemia trait.
  - HbH disease (three defective α genes): 5–30% HbH (β_4), remainder HbA
  - Hydrops fetalis (four defective α genes): mainly Hb Barts (γ_4)
  - β-Thalassemia major (two defective β genes): HbF 20–100%, HbA2 2–7%. In most cases, little or no HbA is detected unless recently transfused.
- Iron studies, serum ferritin: useful to help distinguish thalassemia from iron deficiency
- Mentzer index: MCV/RBC <13 is more likely thalassemia, >13 more likely iron deficiency

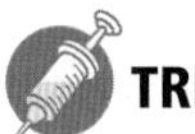

TREATMENT

- Silent carriers (single α gene deletion) and α- and β-thalassemia trait
  - Genetic counseling only
  - Distinguish from iron deficiency microcytosis to avoid excess iron supplementation
- For HbH disease:
  - Folic acid daily
  - Transfusions whenever necessary (aplastic episode, infection)
  - Splenectomy if with evidence of hypersplenism
  - Cholecystectomy if necessary
- For β-thalassemia intermedia:
  - Folic acid daily
  - No iron supplements
  - Transfusions whenever necessary (aplastic episode, infection, acute complication)
  - Splenectomy is less commonly performed due to increased risk of thrombosis and pulmonary hypertension.
  - Cholecystectomy if necessary
  - HbF-inducing agents such as hydroxyurea may be beneficial.
  - Monitoring and treatment of iron overload
- β-Thalassemia major
  - Stem cell transplantation (umbilical cord blood or bone marrow) using histocompatible sibling donor can cure the disease and is being used more frequently.
  - Regular transfusions of RBCs every 3 to 4 weeks to maintain Hb at 9 to 10 g/dL
  - Chelation therapy: It is important to balance the treatment of iron overload with the dangers of overchelation (toxicity to ears, eyes, bone).
  - Chelation options include the following:
    - Deferoxamine (SC or IV infusion over 8 to 24 hours)
    - Deferasirox (q.d. PO chelator). Side effects include GI discomfort, rash, renal failure +/− proteinuria, hepatic failure.
    - Deferiprone (t.i.d. PO chelator), United States Food and Drug Administration (FDA)-approved for iron overload in thalassemia syndromes. Especially useful for cardiac iron removal. Side effects include arthropathy, GI upset, and agranulocytosis.
  - Folic acid daily
  - Penicillin V potassium oral prophylaxis (125 to 250 mg b.i.d.) for splenectomized patients
  - *Pneumococcus*, *Meningococcus*, and *Haemophilus influenzae* vaccines before splenectomy and annual influenza A vaccination
  - Cholecystectomy if indicated
  - No iron supplements
  - Genetic counseling for those with any thalassemia syndrome
  - There are multiple completed and ongoing early phase clinical trials in adult patients of novel therapeutics in β-thalassemia.
    - Janus kinase 2 (JAK2) and transforming growth factor (TGF)-β inhibitors are studied in phase II trials.
    - Gene therapies (most commonly with lentiviral vectors) are currently in phase I trials in Europe and in the United States.

ALERT

Thalassemia trait is often treated incorrectly as presumptive iron deficiency anemia. Iron studies should be performed to confirm the diagnosis if there is no improvement in Hb level after a few weeks of iron therapy.

ISSUES FOR REFERRAL

Parents who can have children with thalassemia can be referred for genetic counseling. Diagnosis can be made in early pregnancy by chorionic villus sampling.

ONGOING CARE

For patients with thalassemia major and intermedia:

- Serum ferritin and liver function tests should be monitored.
- Close monitoring of kidney function is necessary as some chelating agents are associated with impaired renal tubular function, particularly in pediatric patients.
- Annual monitoring for cardiac complications (echocardiogram, EKG) and endocrine function is recommended.
- Liver iron quantitation by biopsy, MRI, or other techniques are necessary intermittently to quantitate the status of iron overload accurately.
- Newer cardiac T_2* MRI techniques to assess the degree of cardiac iron loading, which correlates with risk of cardiac complications
- Annual audiologic and ophthalmologic screening is recommended for persons receiving chelation therapy (to monitor for chelator toxicity).
- Dual-energy x-ray absorptiometry (DEXA) scan or bone peripheral quantitative computed tomography (PQCT) annually

PROGNOSIS

- Life expectancy for patients with β-thalassemia major has improved over the years because of regular transfusions and chelation therapy.
- Bone marrow transplant from a histocompatible sibling donor may be curative.

COMPLICATIONS

Most complications occur in patients with β-thalassemia intermedia or major and can be divided into two categories:

- Complications related to anemia/ineffective erythropoiesis and hemolysis (seen mostly in thalassemia intermedia):
  - Skeletal abnormalities secondary to hyperplastic marrow
  - Osteopenia, osteoporosis, and fractures
  - Growth retardation
  - Extramedullary hematopoiesis
  - Leg ulcers
  - CHF owing to severe anemia
  - Thrombophilia, particularly in thalassemia intermedia after splenectomy
  - Hypercoagulability: deep vein thrombosis, pulmonary embolus
  - Gallstones from hemolysis
  - Pulmonary hypertension
  - Allo- or autoimmunization with RBC antibodies
- Complications of iron overload:
  - Cardiac abnormalities: pericarditis, arrhythmias, CHF
  - Hepatic abnormalities: cirrhosis and liver failure (onset usually after 2nd decade)
  - Endocrine disturbances: delayed puberty, growth retardation, diabetes mellitus, hypothyroidism, hypoparathyroidism
  - Infection: particularly *Yersinia* species

T

ADDITIONAL READING

- de Dreuzy E, Bhukhai K, Leboulch P, et al. Current and future alternative therapies for beta-thalassemia major. *Biomed J*. 2016;39(1):24–38.
- Higgs DR, Engel JD, Stamatoyannopoulos G. Thalassaemia. *Lancet*. 2012;379(9813):373–383.
- Makis A, Hatzimichael E, Papassotiriou I, et al. 2017 Clinical trials update in new treatments of β-thalassemia. *Am J Hematol*. 2016;91(11):1135–1145.
- Olivieri NF, Brittenham GM. Management of the thalassemias. *Cold Spring Harb Perspect Med*. 2013;3(6):a011767.
- Peters M, Heijboer H, Smiers F, et al. Diagnosis and management of thalassaemia. *BMJ*. 2012;344:e228.
- Rachmilewitz EA, Giardina PJ. How I treat thalassemia. *Blood*. 2011;118(13):3479–3488.

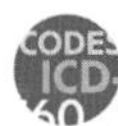

CODES

ICD10

- D56.9 Thalassemia, unspecified
- D56.0 Alpha thalassemia
- D56.1 Beta thalassemia

FAQ

- Q: Is prenatal testing available?
- A: Yes.
- Q: In a transfused patient, when does iron overload become a problem and when is chelation started?
- A: Usually after the age of 3 to 4 years
- Q: At what age should monitoring for cardiac iron overload begin in β-thalassemia major?
- A: 6 to 10 years of age

THORACIC INSUFFICIENCY SYNDROME

Stamatia Alexiou, MD • Robert M. Campbell Jr., MD • Oscar Henry Mayer, MD

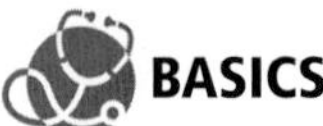

BASICS

DESCRIPTION

- Thoracic insufficiency syndrome (TIS) is the inability of the thorax to support normal respiration or lung growth.
- Patients are skeletally immature with varied anatomic deformities that often include the following:
  - Flail chest syndrome: rib absence due to a congenital malformation or chest wall tumor resection, rib instability in cerebrocostomandibular syndrome, and others
  - Constrictive chest wall syndrome, including rib fusion and scoliosis: VACTERL association, chest wall scarring from radiation treatment, windswept deformity of the chest from progressive scoliosis, and others
  - Hypoplastic thorax syndrome including Jeune syndrome, Ellis–van Creveld syndrome, Jarcho-Levin syndrome, or spondylothoracic dysplasia (STD)
  - Scoliosis (without rib anomaly) or neuromuscular scoliosis
- The recognizable anatomic abnormalities often occur before respiratory insufficiency, with patients compensating for low lung volumes and poor respiratory mechanics by increasing their respiratory rate.
- Subsequently decreased activity and chronic respiratory insufficiency

PATHOPHYSIOLOGY

- The thorax is the respiratory pump, requiring adequate diaphragm (abdominal) and chest wall movement. Limitation in resting lung volume (functional residual capacity [FRC]) and/or the ability of the rib cage to expand during respiration can significantly alter respiratory function and cause TIS.
- The window of rapid lung growth and alveolar development is during the first 3 years of life.
  - Although alveolar development is felt to continue up until 5 or 8 years of age, recent evidence suggests that it can occur through childhood and adolescence.
  - Without concurrent thoracic growth, however, the lung cannot grow normally.
- Growth of the thoracic pump is also necessary so that the respiratory system can continue to meet a patient's metabolic demands.
  - Thoracic spinal height (TSH) directly contributes to thoracic volume and lung volume.
  - At birth, the TSH is 13 cm normally, then during the first 5 years of life, thoracic spinal growth is 1.4 cm/year, 0.6 cm/year from 5 to 10 years, and 1.2 cm/year from 10 to 18 years of age.
  - A thoracic length of 22 cm at skeletal maturity, the normal TSH of a 10-year-old, appears to be the minimum height necessary for normal respiration.
- Complex scoliosis with spinal rotation and lordosis into the convex hemithorax, the "windswept" deformity of the thorax, can further restrict lung volume.
- In neuromuscular disorders, unilateral caudal rotation of the ribs, the "collapsing parasol deformity," typically occurs on the convex side of the scoliosis and may also severely narrow the thorax, worsen thoracic mechanics, and further increase work of breathing.

ETIOLOGY

- The etiologies of TIS can be grouped into unilateral or bilateral volume depletion deformities (VDDs) of the thorax that reduce the volume available for the lungs in certain subsets of patients with rare syndromes. This causes primary TIS or deformity of the chest from scoliosis.
  - Type I: absent ribs and scoliosis
  - Type II: fused ribs and scoliosis
  - Type III: hypoplastic thorax
  - Type IIIa: foreshortening (Jarcho-Levin)
  - Type IIIb: narrowed (Jeune)
- In addition, progressive congenital scoliosis without rib anomalies can result in TIS from a variant of type II VDD of the thorax.
- Type IIIb VDD of the thorax can also develop in neurogenic scoliosis, as in spinal muscular atrophy with marked intercostal muscle weakness.
- Spinal deformity, such as lumbar kyphosis in spina bifida, collapses the torso into the pelvis, raising abdominal pressure blocking diaphragm excursion, and causing secondary TIS.

COMMONLY ASSOCIATED CONDITIONS

- Congenital renal abnormalities can occur in 25–30% of congenital scoliosis.
- Cervical spine abnormalities, causing stenosis and proximal instability
- Spinal cord abnormalities, including spinal cord syrinx and tethered cord, which are especially prevalent in meningomyelocele
- Jeune syndrome
  - Congenital renal abnormalities
  - Hepatic fibrosis
  - Cervical spinal stenosis in 60% of cases
  - Retinal dystrophy
- Ellis–van Creveld syndrome: tracheomalacia
- STD: congenital diaphragmatic hernia
- Cerebrocostomandibular syndrome, Pierre Robin sequence: micrognathia
- Severe tracheal compression and narrowing can occur in advanced scoliosis or severe anteroposterior narrowing.

DIAGNOSIS

HISTORY

- Prenatal ultrasound showing a hypoplastic thorax
- Onset of clinical scoliosis
- Onset of respiratory symptoms:
  - Relative exertional intolerance
  - Ineffective cough resulting in recurrent respiratory infections
  - Need for supplemental oxygen or noninvasive ventilatory support (bilevel positive airway pressure [BLPAP] or continuous positive airway pressure [CPAP])
- Progression of the spinal or chest wall deformity
- Signs and symptoms:
  - Exertional limitation relative to age and gross motor capability
  - Recurrent respiratory illnesses
  - Balance problems
  - Back pain

PHYSICAL EXAM

- Comprehensive respiratory examination:
  - Assessment of work of breathing including accessory muscle use and thoracoabdominal asynchrony
  - Abnormalities in vitals such as respiratory rate, heart rate, Spo_2, and weight can be a result of ventilatory insufficiency and increased work of breathing.
  - Qualitative assessment of chest wall compliance and motion
  - Symmetry of aeration during auscultation
- Thoracic circumference is usually found to be <75% of head circumference at birth.
- Thumb excursion test: The palms of each hand are loosely positioned posteriorly over each side of the chest with the thumbs aligned on either side of the spinal column, and relative excursion is assessed by the amount of lateral thumb movement.
- Assessment for rib hump by having the patient bend forward while standing upright.
- Measure of liver size to evaluate for hepatomegaly and possible cor pulmonale

DIAGNOSTIC TESTS & INTERPRETATION

Initial Tests (screening, lab, imaging)

- Serum bicarbonate as an indirect assessment for chronic hypoventilation
- Arterial blood gas if there is a concern for acute respiratory failure
- Liver function testing to assess for coincident liver failure
- Brain-type natriuretic peptide to help assess for progressive heart strain or failure
- Genetic testing as indicated based on suspected underlying condition
- Standing anteroposterior and lateral radiographs to establish severity of scoliosis in the sagittal and coronal planes; bending films to establish the flexibility of the curve
- Chest CT scan with 5-mm cuts noncontrast with optimal pediatric settings to minimize radiation, with spinal and chest wall reconstruction to assess three-dimensional anatomy
- MRI of spine and spinal cord to look for spinal cord abnormality
- Dynamic MRI to assess motion of chest wall, diaphragm, and abdomen

- Additional radiologic testing may be employed in certain cases (e.g., ventilation–perfusion scan of the lungs to quantify right vs. left functional perfusion asymmetry).
- Echocardiogram to evaluate for cor pulmonale and pulmonary hypertension

Diagnostic Procedures/Other

- Pulmonary assessment: baseline and subsequent pulmonary function testing at each clinic visit
  - Dynamic lung volumes and flows
    - Forced vital capacity (FVC)
    - Timed expiratory volume (forced expiratory volume in 0.5 or 1 second) and the ratio to FVC
    - Forced expiratory flow (FEF) between 25% and 75% of vital capacity (FEF 25–75%)
  - Static lung volume measurements
    - Total lung capacity (TLC), FRC, residual volume (RV), and RV/TLC
    - Maximal inspiratory pressure (MIP) and maximal expiratory pressure (MEP) measurements
- Specialized measurements of respiratory system compliance (stiffness) and partitioned measurements of chest wall and lung compliance
- Pulse oximetry and end-tidal carbon dioxide measurement
- Overnight polysomnography to assess the degree of underlying respiratory insufficiency and need for supplemental oxygen or noninvasive ventilation
- Exercise testing adapted for the capabilities of the patient (6-minute walk test) can be used to assess for exertional limitation.
- If there is significant thoracospinal abnormality and certainly if there is other dysmorphology, a genetics assessment is very helpful to comprehensively assess for other comorbidities and help anticipate future problems.

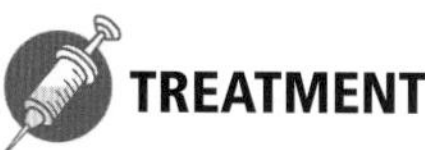

TREATMENT

GENERAL MEASURES

- Bracing and halo-gravity traction can be used as a temporizing procedure and at best has been shown to control some forms of scoliosis or partially improve, but not correct, scoliosis.
- Physical and occupational therapy

SURGERY/OTHER PROCEDURES

- The goal of surgical treatment is to stabilize the chest and spine in order to support normal growth until skeletal maturity is attained, at which point procedures such as a spinal fusion can be considered.
- Vertical expandable prosthetic titanium rib (VEPTR) expansion thoracoplasty techniques enable five types of acute thoracic reconstructions to handle each of the subtypes of TIS.
  - The procedure can be performed as early as 4 to 6 months of age to exploit the growth potential of the developing lungs and provide additional thoracic volume and compensatory lung growth.
  - After implantation to stabilize the initial thoracospinal reconstruction, it can then be expanded about every 6 months commensurate with patient growth until skeletal maturity.
- Magnetic expansion control (MAGEC) rods have been used more recently as an alternative to VEPTR with the advantage of nonsurgical expansion. Long-term efficacy studies have not been reported yet.

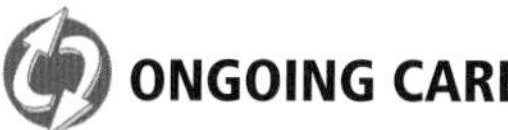

ONGOING CARE

FOLLOW-UP RECOMMENDATIONS

- After TIS surgery, patients are followed with radiographs at regular intervals.
- Pulmonary follow-up should include careful assessment for respiratory insufficiency.
- Longitudinal measure of lung function and growth to demonstrate an improvement in respiratory status or lung function, or at the very least a decrease in the rate of decline, in the most severely affected patients

PROGNOSIS

- Prognosis will vary depending on the underlying cause of TIS, severity of respiratory insufficiency, and the age of the patient at surgery.
  - In infants and toddlers, however, there may be preservation of lung growth, but there has not been evidence to support regaining lung function that has been lost.
  - The expectation in infancy would be for growth preservation and an increase in lung volume above the preoperative value as a percent of predicted. There does appear to be an inverse relationship between the age of the patient at the time of surgery and the level of positive impact of VEPTR insertion on lung function.
  - In school-aged and older children, lung volume remains stable.
  - For older patients near skeletal maturity, the focus is chest wall reconstruction, spinal stabilization, and stabilization in pulmonary function.
- Jeune syndrome is one of the more severe forms of TIS, with 60–70% mortality in early infancy from respiratory failure. However, after VEPTR insertion, there has been a 50% decrease in mortality.
- Of those patients with TIS due to an STD, 47% die in infancy from respiratory complications and pulmonary hypertension. VEPTR treatment of STD remains controversial.
- Improved quality of life following VEPTR insertion

COMPLICATIONS

- In the immediate postoperative period—wound infection, skin slough, and bleeding
- Implant-related complication such as device breakage or dislodgement is uncommon.
- Decreased chest wall compliance
- Neurologic complications are rare.

ADDITIONAL READING

- Campbell RM Jr. VEPTR: past experience and the future of VEPTR principles. *Eur Spine J*. 2013;22(Suppl 2):S106–S117.
- Gadepalli SK, Hirschl RB, Tsai WC, et al. Vertical expandable prosthetic titanium rib device insertion: does it improve pulmonary function? *J Pediatr Surg*. 2011;46(1):77–80.
- Mayer OH. Management of thoracic insufficiency syndrome. *Curr Opin Pediatr*. 2009;21(3):333–343.
- Mayer O, Campbell R, Cahill P, et al. Thoracic insufficiency syndrome. *Curr Probl Pediatr Adolesc Health Care*. 2016;46(3):72–97.
- Watts SL. Use of a vertical expandable prosthetic titanium rib in children with thoracic insufficiency syndrome and scoliosis. *Crit Care Nurse*. 2016; 36(2):52–61.

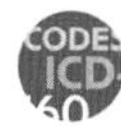

CODES

ICD10

- Q76.8 Other congenital malformations of bony thorax
- Q76.6 Other congenital malformations of ribs
- Q77.2 Short rib syndrome

FAQ

- Q: What criteria need to be met before a patient can undergo VEPTR insertion?
- A: The patient can be as young as 6 months and should not have reached skeletal maturity.
- Q: What is the average length of stay?
- A: In a 2004 study by Campbell et al., the mean total hospital length of stay for an initial VEPTR insertions was 14 days. About half of those days were spent in the intensive care unit (ICU). This time can be longer in patients with more complex medical issues or more involved surgery, such as the procedure for chest all hypoplasia. Patients undergoing VEPTR expansion procedures remain hospitalized for an average of about 3 days. Some patients are able to be discharged the same day.
- Q: Are patients able to be weaned from respiratory support following VEPTR procedure?
- A: Due to a VEPTR ability to increase the longitudinal chest wall diameter and spinal length, some patients have been shown to benefit with a >50% increase in lung volume by chest CT. Outcomes are variable, but studies have reported that over the course of several years, patients have had ventilator support decreased or discontinued.

THROMBOSIS

Char M. Witmer, MD, MSCE

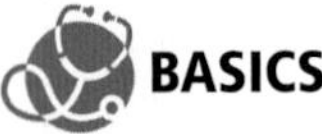

BASICS

DESCRIPTION

Pathologic arterial or venous intravascular occlusion secondary to abnormal thrombus formation. The following are common thrombotic events:

- Deep venous thrombosis (DVT): involves large systemic veins outside the central nervous system (CNS)
- Cerebral sinovenous thrombosis (CSVT): involves intracranial venous sinuses
- Ischemic stroke: CNS arterial occlusion with infarction of brain tissue
- Intracardiac thrombosis: mural, valvular, or foreign body associated
- Femoral artery thrombosis: can be associated with vessel catheterization
- Renal vein thrombosis: commonly in the neonatal period; may be unilateral or bilateral
- Myocardial infarction: Kawasaki disease, antiphospholipid antibody syndrome, or with severe familial hypercholesterolemia
- Budd-Chiari syndrome: thrombosis of the hepatic vein
- Portal vein thrombosis: most commonly seen in neonates with umbilical catheters

EPIDEMIOLOGY

- Incidence of venous thrombosis in children is estimated at 4.9 per 100,000 per year.
- Age distribution is bimodal; peak rates are found in the neonatal and adolescent age groups.
- Idiopathic thrombosis is rare in children.
- >90% of pediatric venous thrombosis is associated with additional risk factors.
- Central venous lines are the most common risk factor for venous thrombosis in children.

RISK FACTORS

- Neonatal
  - Prematurity
  - Maternal diabetes
  - Umbilical catheters or other central lines
  - Sepsis
  - Polycythemia
  - Perinatal asphyxia
- Malignancy/bone marrow disorders
  - Leukemia (hyperleukocytosis, acute promyelocytic leukemia)
  - Myeloproliferative disorders
  - Paroxysmal nocturnal hemoglobinuria
- Medications
  - L-Asparaginase
  - Oral contraceptives (with estrogen)
  - Heparin-induced thrombocytopenia
  - Steroids
- Anatomic
  - Indwelling catheters
  - Congenital heart disease
  - Prosthetic heart valves
  - Intracardiac baffles
  - Tumor compression
  - Atresia of the inferior vena cava
  - Thoracic outlet obstruction (Paget-Schroetter syndrome)
  - May-Thurner syndrome (compression of the left iliac vein by the right iliac artery)
- Miscellaneous
  - Infection
  - Trauma
  - Surgery
  - Obesity
  - Prolonged immobilization or paralysis
  - Dehydration
  - Antiphospholipid syndrome
  - Inherited prothrombotic state
- Risk factors/conditions specific for arterial disease
  - Kawasaki disease
  - Takayasu arteritis
  - Hyperlipidemia
  - Antiphospholipid syndrome

COMMONLY ASSOCIATED CONDITIONS

- Nephrotic syndrome
- Inflammatory disorders
- Liver disease
- Sickle cell disease
- Diabetes mellitus
- Congenital heart disease (hypoplastic left heart syndrome)

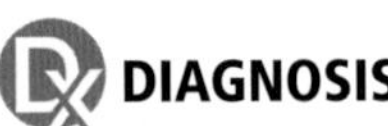

DIAGNOSIS

Approach to patient

- Phase 1
  - Perform complete history and physical exam.
  - Establish diagnosis using the appropriate radiographic study.
- Phase 2
  - Send initial laboratory studies (CBC, PT/aPTT, D-dimer, β-hCG testing in postmenarchal females).
  - If deemed safe, begin anticoagulation therapy with unfractionated heparin or low-molecular-weight heparin (i.e., enoxaparin).
  - *Patients with life- or limb-threatening thrombosis may require thrombolysis.*
- Phase 3
  - If appropriate, consider sending a complete lab workup for a hypercoagulable state; outpatient anticoagulation; follow thrombosis radiologically; *not indicated for an isolated central line–associated clot*

HISTORY

- Presence of risk factors previously listed
- Family history of thrombosis
- Personal history of thrombosis
- Neonatal seizure: common and often the only presenting sign for CSVT or arterial ischemic stroke in neonates

PHYSICAL EXAM

- Extremity DVT: unilateral swelling/edema of a limb
- Thrombosis of the inferior vena cava: bilateral lower extremity edema of a limb, visible superficial veins on the abdomen
- Superior vena cava syndrome: plethoric, swollen head and neck
- Arterial thrombosis: pale extremity with decreased perfusion/pulses
- Renal vein thrombosis: abdominal mass in neonate with hematuria
- Pulmonary embolism: tachypnea, shallow respirations
- Peripheral venous collateral formation: superficial dilated cutaneous veins
- Postthrombotic syndrome: chronic discoloration (darkening) of the skin, ulcerations, pain, intermittent swelling

DIFFERENTIAL DIAGNOSIS

- Other disorders that cause extremity swelling:
  - Low albumin
  - Obstruction of venous flow by a catheter without thrombus formation
  - Hemihypertrophy
- A high hematocrit in neonates can make the cerebral veins appear "dense" on a head CT and be misinterpreted as thrombosis.
- Arterial stroke mimics: complex migraine, demyelinating disease, metabolic disease, tumor

ALERT

- Normal ranges for coagulation tests are age dependent: Diagnosing an inherited deficiency in any of the anticoagulant proteins can be difficult in the neonatal period. Repeat testing at 6 to 12 months of age is necessary.
- Consumption can occur during acute thrombosis; therefore, low levels of the anticoagulant proteins must be repeated.
- Warfarin will decrease the levels of protein C, protein S, and clotting factors II, VII, IX, and X.

DIAGNOSTIC TESTS & INTERPRETATION

- The following tests can be used to investigate for a prothrombotic state:
  - Factor V Leiden mutation analysis
  - Prothrombin 20210A mutation analysis
  - Lupus anticoagulant screen (dilute Russell viper venom time, aPTT)
  - Anticardiolipin antibodies (IgG, IgM)
  - Anti-β2-glycoprotein antibodies (IgG, IgM)

- Protein C activity
- Protein S activity
- Antithrombin activity
- Homocysteine
- Lipoprotein(a)
- Factor VIII activity

- Radiologists should be consulted for choosing the best imaging study for diagnosis and follow-up.
  - Contrast angiography: gold standard but invasive and sometimes technically difficult to perform in small children
  - Ultrasound: most commonly used imaging study because of noninvasiveness, absence of radiation, and ability to be performed at the bedside
  - In the diagnosis of upper extremity–related DVT, often a combination of ultrasound and venography is necessary:
    - Compression ultrasound of the upper central veins may be impeded by the distal end of the clavicle.
    - Venography has poor sensitivity for diagnosing thrombosis of the internal jugular veins.
    - Recommended approach for diagnosis of an upper extremity thrombosis is to start with ultrasound and proceed to venography if the ultrasound is normal and there is a high clinical suspicion for thrombosis.
  - Echocardiogram may be useful in evaluating atrial thrombi, which may result from central venous catheters.
  - Pulmonary angiography, ventilation–perfusion scans, and spiral CT scans are the imaging studies used for the diagnosis of pulmonary embolism, although none of these have been studied in children.
  - In patients with a pulmonary embolism, it is important to look for a source of thrombosis in the upper and lower extremities.
  - Other diagnostic imaging options include CT or Magnetic Resonance Venography (MRV):
    - Noninvasive
    - Sensitivity and specificity not known
    - May be helpful in evaluating proximal thrombosis
  - For diagnosis of CSVT, the most sensitive imaging study is a brain MRI with venography.

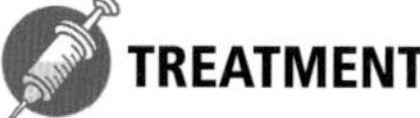

TREATMENT

GENERAL MEASURES

- Therapy for acute thrombosis and long-term management is individualized.
- Consult a pediatric hematologist or someone with expertise in pediatric anticoagulant therapy.

MEDICATION

- Unfractionated heparin:
  - Given as a bolus followed by an infusion, adjusted to maintain the aPTT at 1.5 to 2.5 times baseline
  - Younger children require higher doses of heparin to achieve a therapeutic level secondary to physiologically decreased antithrombin levels.
- Low-molecular-weight heparin (i.e., enoxaparin)
  - More predictable dose response
  - Given subcutaneously twice a day
  - Equivalent in efficacy to unfractionated heparin in the acute management of uncomplicated DVT
  - Renal clearance
- Thrombolytic therapy
  - Recombinant tissue plasminogen activator
  - May be given systemically or locally
  - High risk of bleeding
- Warfarin
  - Oral anticoagulant
  - Initially started when a patient is already receiving a form of heparin. The heparin is discontinued when the warfarin is in the therapeutic range.
  - Warfarin is adjusted to maintain an international normalized ratio (INR) of 2 to 3 for treatment of DVT.
  - Used for outpatient management
- Aspirin
  - Beneficial in stroke and other arterial events
  - Irreversibly inhibits platelet function
- Direct oral anticoagulants (i.e., rivaroxaban, apixaban, edoxaban, or dabigatran)
  - Currently are not approved for in children
  - Clinical trials are ongoing.

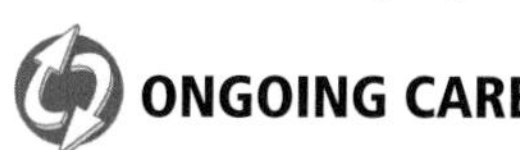

ONGOING CARE

COMPLICATIONS

- Inferior vena cava filters are used to prevent pulmonary embolism. There are limited pediatric studies. They should only be considered in the setting of a lower extremity DVT with a contraindication to anticoagulation (i.e., recent extensive surgery or active bleeding) or if a patient experiences a pulmonary embolism while on therapeutic anticoagulation. Temporary filters should be placed and removed as soon as possible, as they are a nidus for further thrombosis formation. The risk/benefit ratio needs to be considered individually.
- Vary depending on the location and severity of the thrombosis
- In acute DVT, pulmonary embolism is the most significant complication.
- Recurrent thrombosis and postthrombotic syndrome are common chronic complications.
- In arterial thromboembolic disease, the ischemic injury to the involved organ determines the acute and long-term complications.

ALERT

- Central venous catheter–related thrombosis may be subtle despite extensive damage to the venous system. Recurrent line infection, line occlusion, and prominent venous collaterals on the chest suggest upper extremity DVT. The long-term consequences of this are not known.
- Warfarin can cause purpura fulminans if started in a nonheparinized patient.

ADDITIONAL READING

- Goldenberg N, Bernard T. Venous thromboembolism in children. *Pediatr Clin North Am*. 2008;55(2):305–322.
- Monagle P, Chan AK, Goldenberg NA, et al. Antithrombotic therapy in neonates and children: antithrombotic therapy and prevention of thrombosis, 9th ed: American College of Chest Physicians evidence-based clinical practice guidelines. *Chest*. 2012;141(Suppl 2):e737S–e801S.
- Raffini L. Thrombolysis for intravascular thrombosis in neonates and children. *Curr Opin Pediatr*. 2009;21(1):9–14.
- Witmer CM, Ichord R. Crossing the blood-brain barrier: clinical interactions between neurologists and hematologists in pediatrics—advances in childhood arterial ischemic stroke and cerebral venous thrombosis. *Curr Opin Pediatr*. 2010;22(1):20–27.

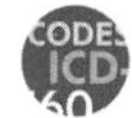

CODES

ICD10

- I82.90 Acute embolism and thrombosis of unspecified vein
- I82.409 Acute embolism and thrombosis of unspecified deep veins of unspecified lower extremity
- G08 Intracranial and intraspinal phlebitis and thrombophlebitis

FAQ

- Q: When is it appropriate to use low-molecular-weight heparin (i.e., enoxaparin) rather than unfractionated heparin?
- A: There are several advantages to low-molecular-weight heparin. The pharmacokinetics is predictable, and frequent monitoring is not necessary. It is administered subcutaneously, not intravenously. Alternatively, low-molecular-weight heparin cannot be completely reversed with protamine and it is renally cleared.
- Q: When is it appropriate to use thrombolytic therapy?
- A: If a thrombus is high risk (i.e., limb-threatening), thrombolytic therapy can be used. Intracranial bleeding, other active bleeding, and surgery within 7 days are contraindications to thrombolytic therapy. For arterial thrombotic events, thrombolytic therapy is often the treatment of choice because of the rapid resolution of the clot and restoration of blood flow.
- Q: What precautions should be taken for invasive procedures and for athletics when a patient is on anticoagulant therapy?
- A: Lumbar punctures, arterial punctures, and surgical procedures should be avoided. If they are necessary, then the anticoagulant should be reversed or held prior to the procedure. While on anticoagulation, participation in contact sports such as football, karate, or boxing is discouraged.

TICK FEVER

Amaran Moodley, MD

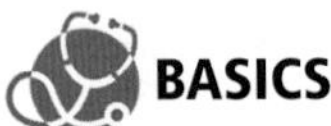

BASICS

DESCRIPTION

- Tick-borne relapsing fever (TBRF) and Colorado tick fever (CTF) is discussed in this chapter.
- TBRF is a vector-borne infection characterized by recurrent fevers caused by several species of spirochetes of the genus *Borrelia*. In the United States, the vector for TBRF is the soft-bodied tick of the genus *Ornithodoros*.
- CTF is an acute, febrile, usually benign systemic illness caused by a coltivirus in the family Reoviridae and transmitted by a tick bite. Although the primary reservoir for infection is the *Dermacentor andersoni* tick (wood tick), the causative organism has been isolated from many other ticks.

EPIDEMIOLOGY

- TBRF
  - Reported in almost all western states up to and including Texas with the highest incidence reported in the states of California, Washington, and Colorado
  - *Ornithodoros* ticks inhabit the burrows and nests of rodents living in caves and coniferous forests at elevations between 1,500 and 8,000 feet.
  - The most important risk factor for human infection is sleeping in a rodent-infested cabin or house in endemic, forested areas.
  - Most cases present during June through September.
  - Approximately 20 cases were reported annually in the United States between 1990 and 2011.
  - Age distribution is bimodal, with peaks among persons aged 10 to 14 years and 40 to 44 years, with a male preponderance.
- CTF
  - Human infections typically occur in areas where *D. andersoni* is found: western United States and southwestern Canada at elevations of 4,000 to 10,000 feet.
  - The U.S. states with the highest incidence include Wyoming, Montana, and Utah.
  - <15 cases are reported annually in the United States, typically between May and July when adult ticks are most active.
  - Infection is more common in males and people aged ≥40 years, but 15% of cases occur in those <20 years.
- Transfusion-related and laboratory-associated infection are rare but have been reported.

GENERAL PREVENTION

- Both of these infections can be prevented by avoidance or protection from ticks.
- Light-colored, long-sleeved shirts and pants should be worn when tick-infested areas cannot be avoided.
- Permethrin should be applied to clothing and N,N-Diethyl-meta-toluamide (DEET) and picaridin applied to exposed skin to help repel ticks.
- Persons who enter endemic areas should inspect themselves and each other frequently for adherent ticks.
- Avoid rodent-infested homes in endemic areas. If necessary, rodent-nesting materials should be removed with protective gloves.
- Other measures include the application of acaricides to nesting sites in human habitations in endemic areas and eliminating rodent access to unnatural food sources.
- Confirmed cases should be reported to health authorities so that control measures can be instituted.

PATHOPHYSIOLOGY

- TBRF
  - When an *Ornithodoros* tick feeds on a natural host (e.g., squirrels, chipmunks, and rodents), *Borrelia* subsequently invade all tissues of the tick including the salivary glands. Ticks in the larval stage are unlikely to be infectious.
  - *Borrelia* is often transmitted to humans through a painless and brief (<30 minutes) nocturnal tick bite. Transmission may occur within minutes of the start of a blood meal. After transmission, spirochetemia develops, resulting in systemic symptoms.
  - Between episodes of spirochetemia, organisms likely persist in the CNS, bone marrow, liver, and spleen.
  - The relapsing fever pattern is attributed to antigenic variation which allows the spirochete to temporarily evade host immunity and rebound.
  - Pathologic findings in humans include petechial hemorrhages on visceral surfaces, hepatosplenomegaly, and a histiocytic myocarditis.
- CTF
  - Ticks are infected during their larval stage when they feed on viremic, intermediate hosts such as chipmunks, ground squirrels, and porcupines.
  - Once infected, ticks remain infected for life (as long as 3 years).
  - Human infection typically occurs during outdoor recreational (camping, hiking) or occupational activities when the adult *D. andersoni* wood tick attaches and ingests a blood meal from an incidental human host.
  - CTF virus is thought to infect hematopoietic cells, causing leukopenia and prolonged viremia for up to 3 to 4 months.

ETIOLOGY

- TBRF is caused by several species of spirochetes in the genus *Borrelia*. *Borrelia hermsii*, *Borrelia turicatae*, and *Borrelia parkeri* are the most common species found in the United States.
- CTF is caused by CTF virus, a double-stranded RNA coltivirus in the family Reoviridae.

DIAGNOSIS

HISTORY

- Both TBRF and CTF most commonly present with high fever, headache, myalgia, and chills. A thorough history documenting recent travel and a description of the fever curve are necessary to help direct the clinician to either diagnosis.
- TBRF
  - Fevers present after a mean incubation period of 5 to 7 days (range 4 to 18 days). Symptoms resolve after 3 to 6 days but then recur within 7 days. Relapses may be less severe than the initial episode with prolonged asymptomatic intervals. Average number of relapses is 3 to 5 in untreated patients.
  - Patients commonly complain of headache, myalgia, nausea, vomiting, arthralgias, and abdominal pain.
  - Confusion, dry cough, diarrhea, photophobia, rash, and dysuria are less common.
  - Patients rarely report a recent tick bite.
- CTF
  - CTF has an usual incubation period of 3 to 4 days (range 1 to 14 days).
  - In ~50% of patients, fever will present in a "saddleback" pattern. The fever persists for 2 to 3 days with resolution for 2 to 3 days. Fever then recurs and lasts for another 2 to 3 days. Some patients will have a third febrile period.
  - Patients may complain of lethargy, myalgia, headache, photophobia, retro-orbital pain, and conjunctival injection.
  - Less commonly, patients will have gastrointestinal symptoms, pharyngitis, nuchal rigidity, and a maculopapular or petechial rash.
  - Unlike TBRF, 90% of patients presenting with CTF have a history of tick exposure.

PHYSICAL EXAM

The presentation for TBRF and CTF are varied. High fevers (39–41°C) are common to both. Additional findings for each may include:

- TBRF
  - Elevated pulse and BP are common.
  - Tender hepatosplenomegaly with jaundice
  - Nuchal rigidity suggesting meningitis
  - Gallop on cardiac auscultation suggesting underlying myocarditis
  - A macular rash starting on the trunk that becomes generalized and or petechial in nature
  - Neurologic deficits are less common but can include delirium, cranial nerve deficits (7th or 8th nerve palsy), and visual impairment from iridocyclitis.
- CTF
  - A small, red painless papule may be seen.
  - A maculopapular rash with petechial lesions has been reported in ~10% of cases.
  - Pharyngitis is reported in 20% of cases.
  - Hepatosplenomegaly has been found in some patients.
  - Nuchal rigidity and delirium are rare but, if present, suggest meningitis or encephalitis.

DIFFERENTIAL DIAGNOSIS

- TBRF and CTF are similar clinically. The presence of biphasic or relapsing fever along with a history of travel to an area where appropriate vectors are found are helpful clues in diagnosing either disease. Leukopenia and a history of a tick bite may differentiate CTF from TBRF. TBRF and CTF may be misdiagnosed as influenza or enteroviral infections, especially with the first febrile episode.

- Other infectious illnesses that may present with recurrent fevers include:
  - Louse-borne relapsing fever
  - Yellow fever
  - Dengue fever
  - Brucellosis
  - Malaria
  - Leptospirosis
  - Rat bite fever
  - Chronic meningococcemia
  - Other tick-borne infections
- The patient's travel history and animal exposure should help differentiate some of these diagnoses.

DIAGNOSTIC TESTS & INTERPRETATION

- TBRF
  - The diagnosis can be readily made by identification of loosely coiled spirochetes on thick and thin smears of Wright or Giemsa-stained peripheral blood. Blood samples taken at the time of fever have the highest yield.
  - Increased sensitivity can be obtained by examining acridine orange–stained preparations of dehemoglobinized thick smears or buffy coat preparations.
  - The organism can only be cultured on special culture medium. Intraperitoneal inoculation of mice with the patient's blood can lead to spirochetemia in the mice.
  - Multiple serologic antibody studies exist, including direct and indirect immunofluorescence, enzyme-linked immunosorbent assay (ELISA), and immunoblot analysis:
    - A 4-fold rise in titers between acute and convalescent studies is considered confirmatory.
    - Antibody tests may not be helpful in the acute setting, and false-positive reactions may occur in patients with prior spirochete infections such as Lyme disease and syphilis.
  - Polymerase chain reaction (PCR) analysis can be useful in identifying the causative organism but is not readily available.
  - Other nonspecific laboratory findings may include leukocytosis, anemia, thrombocytopenia, unconjugated hyperbilirubinemia, elevated hepatic transaminases, and proteinuria.
  - If myocarditis is present, an electrocardiogram can reveal abnormalities such as a prolonged corrected QT interval.
  - In cases complicated by meningitis, the CSF will typically have moderately elevated protein and a mononuclear pleocytosis.
- CTF
  - Leukopenia (2,000 to 4,000/mm^3) with relative lymphocytosis is a hallmark of this illness.
  - Thrombocytopenia may also occur.
  - Direct immunofluorescent examination of blood smears for intraerythrocytic viral antigen is a rapid approach to the diagnosis.
  - PCR testing and viral cultures are available in certain laboratories. PCR testing is the most sensitive and timely approach for diagnosing acute infection.
  - Various techniques (e.g., complement fixation, indirect immunofluorescence, enzyme immunoassay (EIA), and Western blot) have been used to establish a serologic diagnosis:
    - Serologic testing may not be diagnostic in the acute phase of the illness as antibodies only become detectable after 2 weeks. Presence of a 4-fold rise in neutralizing antibody titers at >2 weeks after onset can be confirmatory.
  - In patients with meningitis or encephalitis, CSF studies may reveal elevated protein and a lymphocytic pleocytosis.

TREATMENT

MEDICATION

- TBRF
  - The treatment of choice is oral tetracycline/doxycycline for 7 to 10 days. Children <8 years of age and pregnant women should receive erythromycin or penicillin.
  - Newer macrolides may be effective but are not routinely recommended.
  - In >50% of cases, treatment results in a Jarisch-Herxheimer reaction (severe fevers, rigors, diaphoresis, and hypotension) related to rapid clearing of the spirochetemia. Close observation, IV fluids, and good supportive care are important in treating possible reactions.
  - Some experts support the use of an initial single dose of oral penicillin V potassium (7.5 mg/kg) or IV penicillin G (100,000 U/kg given >30 minutes) in patients presenting with systemic symptoms. It is thought that this initial dose of penicillin leads to gradual clearance of spirochetes, decreasing the risk of the Jarisch-Herxheimer reaction. These patients should then receive a 10-day course of tetracycline or erythromycin because penicillin has been associated with an increased rate of relapse.
  - Single-dose tetracycline or erythromycin has been successful for the treatment of louse-borne epidemic relapsing fever in Ethiopia.
- CTF
  - There is no specific therapy for patients with CTF, as the treatment is primarily supportive.
  - Avoidance of aspirin may help reduce the risk of bleeding in patients with thrombocytopenia

ONGOING CARE

PATIENT EDUCATION

CTF

- Patients should avoid donating blood for 6 months after onset of illness.

PROGNOSIS

- TBRF
  - Generally responds rapidly to appropriate antibiotic therapy without sequelae
  - Mortality in patients treated appropriately is thought to be ~1%.
- CTF
  - Usually a self-limiting illness without sequelae
  - Death is rare but has been reported in children with generalized bleeding likely secondary to thrombocytopenia; thus, thrombocytopenia should be monitored closely.
  - Prolonged weakness may persist for ≥3 weeks and is more likely in those patients >30 years old.

COMPLICATIONS

- TBRF
  - May be associated with splenic rupture, diffuse histiocytic interstitial myocarditis, hepatitis, pneumonia, ARDS, and iridocyclitis
  - CNS complications include meningitis, meningoencephalitis, and focal deficits such as cranial nerve palsy.
  - Pregnant women often experience severe disease and in-utero infection may result in fetal loss, preterm delivery, or severe neonatal infection.
- CTF
  - Complications are rare but most commonly occur in children.
  - May lead to aseptic meningitis, encephalitis, myocarditis, pneumonitis, hepatitis, hemorrhage, and epididymo-orchitis

T

ADDITIONAL READING

- Brackney MM, Marfin AA, Staples JE, et al. Epidemiology of Colorado tick fever in Montana, Utah, and Wyoming, 1995–2003. *Vector Borne Zoonotic Dis*. 2010;10(4):381–385.
- Cutler SJ. Relapsing fever—a forgotten disease revealed. *J Appl Microbiol*. 2010;108(4):1115–1122.
- Dworkin MS, Schwan TG, Anderson DE Jr, et al. Tick-borne relapsing fever. *Infect Dis Clin North Am*. 2008;22(3):449–468.
- Forrester JD, Kjemtrup AM, Fritz CL, et al. Tickborne relapsing fever—United States, 1990–2011. *MMWR Morb Mortal Wkly Rep*. 2015;64(3):58–60.
- Romero JR, Simonsen KA. Powassan encephalitis and Colorado tick fever. *Infect Dis Clin North Am*. 2008;22(3):545–559.
- Yendell SJ, Fischer M, Staples JE. Colorado tick fever in the United States, 2002–2012. *Vector Borne Zoonotic Dis*. 2015;15(5):311–316.

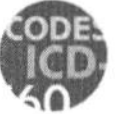

CODES

ICD10

- A68.1 Tick-borne relapsing fever
- A93.2 Colorado tick fever

FAQ

- Q: When should a clinician suspect tick fever?
- A: A history of recurring or relapsing fever in the appropriate epidemiologic setting (such as travel history to the western parts of the United States, summertime illness, history of tick exposure) should raise the possibility of a tick fever.

TICS

Jordan F. Garris, MD • Donald L. Gilbert, MD, MS, FAAN, FAAP

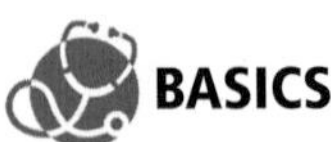

BASICS

DESCRIPTION

- Tics are sudden, repetitive, patterned movements (e.g., blinking, grimacing, gesturing) or vocalizations (e.g., throat clearing, grunting, shouting words). Tics may occur sporadically for short periods on one or more occasions during childhood or they may persist for months to years. When they persist, tics characteristically change in anatomic location, frequency, type, complexity, and severity. Multiple concurrent tics may occur. Most older children are able to suppress their tics for brief periods of time and endorse having premonitory sensory urges that precede at least some of their tics. Tics tend not to interrupt continuous purposeful movements in the same muscle group. Tics may increase during stress or relaxation. Tics typically diminish or stop during engagement in performance of skilled activities and during sleep.
- *DSM-5* classification of tic disorders:
  - Tourette disorder also known as Tourette syndrome (TS):
    - Both ≥2 motor and ≥1 vocal tics have been present at some time, although not necessarily concurrently.
    - Tics have been present for >1 year since first tic onset (regardless of the duration of tic-free periods).
    - Onset <18 years
  - Persistent (chronic) motor or vocal tic disorder:
    - Designates ≥1 year of either motor or vocal tics but not both (Note subtle vocal tics such as throat clearing are easily overlooked; thus, most cases are actually TS.)
    - Onset <18 years
  - Provisional tic disorder:
    - ≥1 motor and/or vocal tics; tics have been present for <1 year since first tic onset.
    - Onset <18 years
  - Note: When tics occur secondary to other brain processes (via induction by medications, after brain injury, as part of autoimmune Sydenham chorea, or as part of Wilson or other degenerative diseases), the diagnosis of TS should not be used.
- Pediatric autoimmune neuropsychiatric disorders associated with streptococcal infections (PANDAS)/pediatric acute-onset neuropsychiatric syndrome (PANS):
  - PANDAS has recently been subsumed under the broader (in etiology as well as symptoms) and less specific umbrella of PANS. As tics are now a minor criterion, this discussion lies outside the scope of this section.

EPIDEMIOLOGY

- Described in almost all ethnic groups
- Affects males > females
- Typical onset is between ages 3 and 10 years.

Prevalence

- The prevalence of tics in school-age children is 6–12%, with transient tics occurring in 20–25% at some time during childhood.
- The prevalence of TS is 0.5–1% in school-age children.

RISK FACTORS

Genetics

A positive family history of tics and/or obsessive-compulsive disorder (OCD), with a pattern often consistent with autosomal dominant transmission is very common. Incomplete penetrance frequently occurs, with greater penetrance in males. However, genetics are complex, with large cohort genetic studies demonstrating that a large number of genes exert small effects.

GENERAL PREVENTION

Tics cannot be prevented.

PATHOPHYSIOLOGY

The pathophysiology underlying tics and TS is thought to involve genetically influenced abnormalities in dopamine neurotransmission within the basal ganglia and/or cortex. Evidence also implicates differences in signaling involving gamma-aminobutyric acid (GABA), serotonin, and possibly norepinephrine in prefrontal brain regions. Environmental processes and unknown age- and sex-dependent factors may play a role in symptom induction and expression.

ETIOLOGY

Unknown. Is highly heritable but not contagious. Increased tic severity can occur acutely with psychosocial stresses.

COMMONLY ASSOCIATED CONDITIONS

- The majority of children with TS have associated comorbid conditions, with attention-deficit/hyperactivity disorder (ADHD) and OCD most frequently present.
- Anxiety, learning disabilities (LD), oppositional defiant disorder, conduct disorder, and rage episodes are also common in TS.

DIAGNOSIS

The diagnosis of tics is based on history and observation. Physical examination is typically otherwise normal.

HISTORY

- Document a description of the patient's past and current tics, including age of onset, type, anatomic location(s), duration, number, frequency, complexity, severity, exacerbating or alleviating factor(s), presence of premonitory urges/sensations, and suppressibility.
- Determine the degree to which the tics are causing interference and/or impairment in social, home, and school environments.
- Assess for commonly associated conditions.

PHYSICAL EXAM

Physical examination is usually normal. Tics may not be seen. Having the child intentionally reproduce the sound(s) and/or movement(s) of concern and/or having the parents provide video can aid in differentiating tics from other movement disorders.

DIFFERENTIAL DIAGNOSIS

- Certain simple tics (eye blinking, sniffing, throat clearing) may be mistaken for allergy symptoms, whereas more complex tics may be mistaken for purposeful, voluntary movements.
- Stereotypies are patterned, episodic, repetitive, purposeless, continuous, sometimes rhythmic movements, usually bilateral and with onset prior to age 3 years. The movements are more constant in pattern and location, with limited variation over time. Examples include rocking and arm flapping.
- Chorea designates rapid, random-appearing, purposeless movements, and movement fragments that often have a "dance-like" quality. Unlike tics, choreic movements do not have premonitory urges and usually interfere with purposeful movement.
- Dystonia is characterized by repetitive, sustained muscle contractions that cause abnormal postures, often with a twisting quality. Dystonic tics result in sustained postures and can be difficult to distinguish from dystonia; however, the presence of a premonitory urge suggests tics.
- Myoclonus is a sudden, brief, shock-like movement. It is not suppressible, can occur during actions, and is not associated with a premonitory sensation.
- Automatisms, seen in some focal or absence epilepsies, may look like tics but are neither associated with premonitory sensations nor suppressible.
- Hemifacial spasm (HFS) is a rare condition that results in frequent, involuntary muscle contractions involving one side of the face. Early cases of HFS may be difficult to distinguish from motor tics, but HFS is limited to one side of the face, does not involve premonitory urges, and the spasms last longer than tics.

DIAGNOSTIC TESTS & INTERPRETATION

Initial Tests (screening, lab, imaging)

Blood tests are not indicated in most cases.

Diagnostic Procedures/Other

Other tests such as brain imaging or EEG are not needed in most cases. Standard clinical rating scales for common conditions such as ADHD are often helpful. In more complex cases, psychological or educational testing may clarify whether OCD, anxiety, depression, autism spectrum disorder, or LD are present.

TREATMENT

GENERAL MEASURES

- Educating the child and family about tics is essential. Providing educational resources for the family to access after the clinic visit and for school personnel may also be useful.
- The decision to treat tics or associated symptoms should be based on functional impairment for the child in school, social, or home settings. Severe tics that cause pain and injury also warrant treatment. The waxing and waning nature of tics and the slow onset of medication and behavioral treatment effects make treatment assessment difficult (improvement may be from treatment or from natural symptom waning).
- Specific behavioral interventions (see "Additional Therapies") are considered first line by many practitioners and can therefore be considered prior to prescribing medications.

MEDICATION

- Mild/occasional tics: Medication is not needed.
- Moderate or severe tics causing impairment: α-2 Agonist or dopamine antagonist may reduce severity/frequency.
- Often, treatment of comorbidities is a primary goal, and typical OCD and ADHD treatment guidelines can be followed.

First Line

- Clonidine and guanfacine are used off-label as 1st-line treatments for tics based on safety, despite overall limited efficacy. Both may reduce tics and ADHD symptoms. Both are available in immediate- and extended-release forms.
  - Clonidine: Start 0.05 mg at bedtime. Increase by 0.05 mg every 3 to 7 days until benefit, side effects, or a maximum of 0.4 mg/24 h, divided 3 or 4 times per day; available as a tablet and transdermal patch
  - Guanfacine: Start 0.5 mg at bedtime. Increase by 0.5 to 1 mg every 3 to 7 days until benefit, side effects, or a maximum of 4 mg/24 h, divided 2 or 3 times per day.
- Sedation and orthostatic hypotension are common initial adverse effects, more so with clonidine than guanfacine. Encourage hydration.
- Avoid abrupt discontinuation, which can cause rebound hypertension.

Second Line

- Consider referral to child neurologist/child psychiatrist/specialist before initiating any 2nd-line medications.
- Dopamine D2 receptor–blocking agents (antipsychotic medications) are considered 2nd-line treatments by many because of much greater potential side effects. Therefore, some clinicians prescribe other medications, for example, topiramate or baclofen, as second line.
- Weight gain is common with antipsychotic medications.
- Atypical antipsychotics can be better tolerated overall and are less likely to cause extrapyramidal side effects. Commonly used atypical agents include aripiprazole, risperidone, ziprasidone, and olanzapine.
- Typical antipsychotics (haloperidol, pimozide, fluphenazine) are potent, but due to higher risks, should only be used for those with refractory, disabling tics. Common side effects: sedation, weight gain, metabolic syndrome, and galactorrhea; serious side effects: extrapyramidal reactions, neuroleptic malignant syndrome, and tardive dyskinesia

ALERT

Poor metabolizers of pimozide may be at increased risk for QT prolongation and cardiac arrhythmias; therefore, the U.S. Food and Drug Administration (FDA) has stated that CYP2D6 genotyping should be performed before exceeding 4 mg of pimozide in adults or 0.05 mg/kg/24 h in children, and that the dose of pimozide should not be increased earlier than 14 days in patients who are known CYP2D6 poor metabolizers.

ADDITIONAL THERAPIES

- Comprehensive behavioral intervention for tics (CBIT), consisting of awareness training, competing response training, relaxation training, and social support has been shown effective for tic suppression.
- Randomized controlled trials of CBIT in both children and adults with TS and chronic tic disorder resulted in greater improvement in tic severity than supportive therapy and education alone. The effect size of the intervention was on par with that of medication but was greater when patients were not taking medications.
- Focal motor (or vocal) tics, especially those that are dystonic, may be treated with botulinum toxin injections to the affected muscles.

SURGERY/OTHER PROCEDURES

Recent experimental data have shown deep brain stimulation (DBS) as a potential treatment for adults with severe and refractory tics.

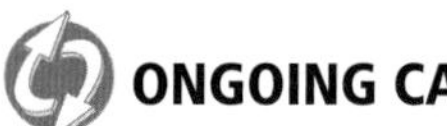

ONGOING CARE

DIET

There is no evidence that dietary modifications alter the course of tic disorders.

PATIENT EDUCATION

The Tourette Association of America (tourette.org) is a valuable resource for information. There are also local chapters.

PROGNOSIS

Although common, tics cause impairment in a minority of children. Peak severity occurs in preadolescence to mid-adolescence. Most patients have partial or complete resolution of tics as adults. Long-term outcome depends on associated comorbidities.

COMPLICATIONS

Tics can be emotionally distressing and can result in social disability. Injuries—due to complex tics, compulsions, impulsivity, inattention, and other factors—may be more common in patients with TS than in the general population. More rarely, chronic, repetitive, and forceful tics can cause musculoskeletal problems (e.g., cervical spine arthritis, disc herniation) or other neurologic problems (e.g., cervical myelopathy, stroke secondary to vertebral artery dissection).

ADDITIONAL READING

- Barfell KSF, Snyder RR, Isaacs-Cloes KM, et al. Parent and patient perceptions of functional impairment due to Tourette syndrome: development of a shortened version of the Child Tourette Syndrome Impairment Scale. *J Child Neurol*. 2017;32(8):725–730.
- Cavanna AE, Luoni C, Selvini C, et al. Parent and self-report health-related quality of life measures in young patients with Tourette syndrome. *J Child Neurol*. 2013;28(10):1305–1308.
- Gilbert DL, Jankovic J. Pharmacological treatment of Tourette syndrome. *J Obsessive-Compulsive Relat Disord*. 2014;3(4):407–414.
- Sukhodolsky DG, Woods DW, Piacentini J, et al. Moderators and predictors of response to behavior therapy for tics in Tourette syndrome. *Neurology*. 2017;88(11):1029–1036.

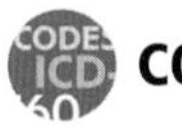

CODES

ICD10

- F95.9 Tic disorder, unspecified
- F95.2 Tourette's disorder
- F95.0 Transient tic disorder

FAQ

- Q: Can a child with tics and ADHD be treated with stimulant medication?
- A: Although there have been concerns of stimulants making tics worse, there is no evidence that stimulants cause chronic tics. Furthermore, several recent studies have shown that treatment of ADHD with stimulants does not worsen tics and may lead to improvement.
- Q: Should mild tics be treated if they lead to teasing?
- A: The best approach is to educate the child, parents, and teacher about tics. The child can be armed with a response to questions, such as "Those are tics. It's a neurologic symptom."

TOXIC ALCOHOLS

Amin Salem, MD, MRCPCH, DCH, DPP • Robert J. Hoffman, MD, MS

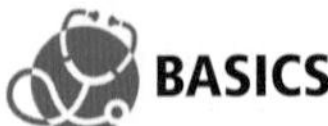

BASICS

DESCRIPTION

- Toxic alcohols discussed here include ethylene glycol, isopropyl alcohol, and methanol.
- Ethylene glycol is a sweet, odorless, colorless liquid, commonly used as automobile antifreeze solution as well as for other uses.
- Isopropyl alcohol is used as rubbing alcohol as well as in liquid soaps and for other uses.
- Methanol is wood alcohol used in windshield wiper fluid, Sterno®, and other products.

GENERAL PREVENTION

Poison proofing homes and giving parents poison prevention advice is the most effective way to prevent toxic alcohol exposures in children.

RISK FACTORS

Toxicity via dermal absorption can occur in infants or young children with permeable skin.

PATHOPHYSIOLOGY

All toxic alcohols have direct effects as intoxicants. Ethylene glycol and methanol are metabolized to toxic by-products that result in severe morbidity or mortality.

- All toxic alcohols may result in CNS depression or coma. This coma may result in respiratory depression requiring ventilatory support.
- Ethylene glycol is metabolized to oxalic acid and glycolic acid, ultimately forming calcium oxalate crystals, which may precipitate in the renal tubules and cause renal failure.
- Methanol is metabolized to formaldehyde and then formic acid, which may damage the retina and cause visual impairment or blindness.
- The metabolism of ethylene glycol and methanol to their toxic metabolites may be prevented by competitively inhibiting alcohol dehydrogenase with either fomepizole or ethanol.
- Therapy to inhibit alcohol dehydrogenase is used for ethylene glycol and methanol exposure.
- Isopropyl alcohol is metabolized to acetone. Isopropyl alcohol may cause severe gastrointestinal irritation or hemorrhage.

DIAGNOSIS

HISTORY

- Typically, a history of exposure is available. In absence of this history, an osmolal gap or anion gap with metabolic acidemia is suggestive of toxic alcohol exposure.
- Visual complaints may include blurred vision, diplopia, hazy vision, or nystagmus.
- Neurologic abnormalities may include ataxia, CNS depression, coma, dysarthria, seizure, and visual impairment or loss.
- Gastrointestinal effects may include pain, emesis, or hematemesis, most typically with isopropyl alcohol.

PHYSICAL EXAM

- Patients commonly have depressed mental status or coma.
- Tachycardia and hypotension are the most frequent vital sign abnormalities that occur.
- Hyperpnea or tachypnea often accompanies metabolic acidemia. Neurologic findings may include ataxia, CNS depression, coma, dysarthria, focal neurologic changes, hyporeflexia, hypotonia, and nystagmus,
- Ophthalmologic findings may include constricted visual fields, decreased visual acuity, hyperemic optic disc with retinal edema, specifically associated with methanol.

DIFFERENTIAL DIAGNOSIS

Drugs and disorders that may alter lab values include acetone, diethylene glycol, ethanol, iron, isoniazid, lactic acidemia, mannitol, methanol, propylene glycol, renal failure, salicylates, toluene, and various forms of ketoacidosis.

DIAGNOSTIC TESTS & INTERPRETATION

- Check serum electrolytes, BUN, creatinine, and glucose.
  - Elevated anion gap metabolic acidemia supports the diagnosis of ethylene glycol or methanol exposure.
  - Absence of this gap early after ingestion is expected and does not rule out ingestion.
  - Acidemia is an indication for use of fomepizole as well as a potential indication for hemodialysis.
  - Fomepizole treatment should not be delayed waiting to determine if acidemia will develop.
  - Anion gap metabolic acidemia does not result from isopropyl alcohol poisoning.
  - Fluid and electrolyte abnormalities from ethylene glycol or methanol may include hypoglycemia, hypokalemia, hypocalcemia, hypomagnesemia, and elevated anion gap metabolic acidosis.
  - A spurious rise in creatinine may occur.
  - Serum ionized calcium is useful in managing ethylene glycol toxicity.
  - Hematuria, renal insufficiency, or renal failure may occur, particularly from ethylene glycol.
  - Acetonemia and ketonemia may result from isopropyl alcohol ingestion.
- Blood gas analysis can assess for degree of metabolic acidemia in any patient with low serum bicarbonate.
  - Initial use of capillary or venous blood gas to screen for abnormality is preferable.
  - Repeated blood gas analysis should occur every 1 to 2 hours if acidemia results.
- Serum osmolality or osmolarity is used to predict the level of ethylene glycol, isopropyl alcohol, or methanol before laboratory quantification is performed.
- Serum ethanol level should simultaneously be performed to determine quantity of ethanol contribution to osmolal gap.
  - An elevated osmolal gap can be used to rule in, but not exclude, toxic alcohol exposure.
  - An elevated osmolal gap indicates the presence of unmeasured solute such as ethanol, ethylene glycol, isopropyl alcohol, or methanol.
  - Absence of an osmolal gap does not exclude the possibility of toxic alcohol exposure.
  - Osmolal gap is calculated as follows: osmolal gap = (calculated serum osmolality − measured osmolality).
  - The measured osmolality is determined by the laboratory.
  - The calculated osmolality is determined as follows: 2 × [Na (mEq/L)] + [BUN (mg/dL)/2.8] + [glucose (mg/dL)/18].
  - Normal osmolal gap is <15 mEq/L.
  - Any patient with increased osmolal gap should be presumed to have toxic alcohol exposure.
  - Initially before the toxic alcohol is metabolized, an elevated osmol gap without anion gap will be present.
  - As metabolism occurs, the osmol gap will decrease; an increased anion gap metabolic acidemia results with ethylene glycol or methanol toxicity.
  - Isopropyl alcohol causes elevation of osmol gap without metabolic acidemia, unlike ethylene glycol and methanol, which cause anion gap metabolic acidemia after they are metabolized.
- Serum concentration of ethylene glycol, isopropyl alcohol, or methanol should be obtained if possible.
  - An ethylene glycol or methanol level >20 mg/dL is an indication for fomepizole or ethanol infusion.
  - An ethylene glycol or methanol level >50 mg/dL is an indication for hemodialysis.
- Urinalysis with microscopic examination may be used adjunctively with ethylene glycol exposure.
  - Presence of oxalate crystals corroborates poisoning.
  - Absence of crystals does not exclude the possibility of ethylene glycol toxicity.
  - Fluorescence of urine is unreliable and is neither sensitive nor specific for exposure.
  - Proteinuria and hematuria may be present with ethylene glycol or isopropyl alcohol exposure.
- Additional tests may include ECG to detect cardiac conduction disturbance or serum acetaminophen and salicylate levels in patients with intentional ingestion or with presumed intent of self-harm.
- Cardiovascular effects may include hypocalcemic QT prolongation and myocarditis.
- Tests necessary to rule out differential diagnoses should be obtained when appropriate.
- Neuroimaging to rule out intracranial pathology may rarely be indicated.

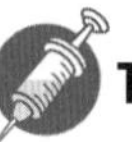

TREATMENT

- Prompt evaluation of airway, breathing, circulation, serum glucose, and ECG ("A,B,C,D,E") is critical.
- Consultation with a medical toxicologist or poison center is recommended.

GENERAL MEASURES

Supportive care is the most important general principle. The illness is managed with intent of close monitoring and addressing issues as they arise.

- For ingestion <1 hour previously, an attempt to aspirate gastric contents with a nasogastric tube is reasonable.
- Treatment for ethylene glycol or methanol exposure should focus on acid–base correction and preventing organ damage.

- Hemodialysis should be considered for the following:
  - Any patient with severe metabolic acidemia from ethylene glycol or methanol
  - Any patient with evidence of end-organ damage, particularly if metabolic acidemia is present
  - Any patient with profound hypotension or life-threatening symptoms resulting from isopropyl alcohol toxicity

MEDICATION

- For ethylene glycol or methanol poisoning (but NOT isopropyl alcohol), either fomepizole or ethanol are used to competitively inhibit alcohol dehydrogenase.
- Fomepizole is highly preferable to ethanol for this purpose, as ethanol has many severe, adverse side effects and fomepizole does not.
- Indications for fomepizole or ethanol include the following:
  - Serum level of ethylene glycol or methanol >20 mg/dL
  - Metabolic acidemia with any quantity of detectable ethylene glycol or methanol
- Use of fomepizole or ethanol will prolong the half-life of ethylene glycol and methanol.
  - Without therapy, the ethylene glycol half-life is 3 to 4 hours and methanol 14 to 20 hours.
  - With fomepizole or ethanol, the ethylene glycol half-life is 12 hours and methanol 30 to 50 hours.
- Some clinicians consider a necessary duration of therapy longer than several days to be an indication for hemodialysis. Successful use of prolonged therapy with fomepizole to avoid hemodialysis has been reported.
- Fomepizole is contraindicated in patients with documented allergic reaction to the drug. The loading dose of fomepizole is dose of 15 mg/kg IV.
  - Initial maintenance dosing is 10 mg/kg q12h for 4 doses. Because fomepizole induces its own metabolism, the subsequent maintenance dose is increased to 15 mg/kg q12h thereafter. Hemodialysis should be considered in patients with renal failure, significant/worsening metabolic acidosis, or ethylene glycol or methanol concentrations ≥50 mg/dL.
  - Each dose is diluted into normal saline or D_5W (<25 mg/mL) and infused over 30 minutes.
  - Each time after hemodialysis is performed, a loading dose must be readministered.
- Ethanol is administered as a 10% solution in D_5W. This dilution requirement often results in a very large quantity of free water administration.
  - Ethanol should be used with extreme caution in Asians, as aldehyde dehydrogenase deficiency may result in severe illness and hypotension.
  - The ethanol loading dose is 6 to 7 mL/kg (max 200 mL) of a 10% solution infused IV over 1 hour.
  - A maintenance dose of 0.8 mL/kg/h of 10% ethanol is then given IV. Consider 1.6 mL/kg/h for patients who are chronic drinkers.
  - Target blood ethanol level is 100 to 125 mg/dL.
  - Patients receiving ethanol should have the ethanol level and serum glucose checked hourly.
  - Oral ethanol may be used when IV is not available or if the patient is willing and capable of drinking. This is possibly feasible in adolescents.
  - Oral dosing is similar to IV dosing, with the advantage being lower chance for free water intoxication.
- Adjunctive treatment with folate or leucovorin for methanol, and thiamine and pyridoxine for ethylene glycol may be given:
  - This continues until methanol or ethylene glycol levels are undetectable.
  - Leucovorin 1 to 2 mg/kg or 100 mg IV q6h
  - Tetrahydrofolate (leucovorin) may hasten the elimination of formic acid resulting from methanol exposure.
  - Pyridoxine 1 mg/kg or 50 mg IV q6h. Pyridoxine and thiamine hasten elimination of ethylene glycol metabolites.

ADMISSION, INPATIENT, AND NURSING CONSIDERATIONS

- Admission criteria
  - Any patient requiring therapy with fomepizole, ethanol, or hemodialysis
  - Any patient with renal impairment, visual impairment, or other organ effect
  - Any patient for whom consequential ingestion is suspected and ethylene glycol or methanol levels are unavailable
- Protect inebriated patients from falls.
- For the duration of inebriation or therapy with ethanol, vigilance for detection of hypoglycemia should be maintained.
- IV fluid to maintain adequate blood pressure may be necessary.
- Maintenance IV fluid may be required in patients who are unable to take PO.
- IV fluid may be necessary to aid in prevention of calcium oxalate crystals in the urine.
- IV fluid may be helpful to prevent renal injury if rhabdomyolysis occurs.
- 8.4% sodium bicarbonate may be used in resistant acidosis and should be given via a central line if available.
- Discharge criteria
  - Asymptomatic patients with undetectable ethylene glycol or methanol levels and no metabolic acidemia may be safely discharged.
  - Inpatients who have received therapy with fomepizole, ethanol, or hemodialysis must be medically and metabolically stable for at least 12 to 24 hours prior to discharge.
  - From the hospital, patients with ethylene glycol or methanol level <20 mg/dL, no anion gap, no metabolic acidemia, and stable renal function and vision may be discharged.
  - Patients with isopropyl alcohol exposure who develop no symptoms or have only mild symptoms may be discharged within 4 to 6 hours.

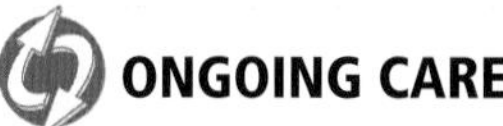

ONGOING CARE

FOLLOW-UP RECOMMENDATIONS

- Most exposures for which ethylene glycol or methanol levels cannot be obtained should be followed for 12 to 24 hours to detect development of metabolic acidemia or other symptoms.
- From the hospital, patients with ethylene glycol or methanol level <20 mg/dL, no anion gap, no metabolic acidemia, and stable renal function and vision may be discharged.
  - Patients with isopropyl alcohol exposure who develop no symptoms or have only mild symptoms may be discharged within 4 to 6 hours.

Patient Monitoring

Symptomatic exposure to ethylene glycol or methanol may warrant intensive care monitoring.

PROGNOSIS

- For ethylene glycol and methanol exposure, prognosis depends on the degree of toxin metabolism as well as adequacy of care.
- Speed and adequacy of therapy with fomepizole or ethanol as well as prompt hemodialysis when indicated is critical.
- For isopropyl alcohol, prognosis depends on severity of intoxication and adequacy of supportive care.

COMPLICATIONS

Blindness, coma, hepatic injury, hypertension or hypotension, myocarditis, temporary or permanent neurologic injury, pancreatitis, renal failure, respiratory depression, rhabdomyolysis, seizure may occur as a result of toxic alcohol exposure.

ADDITIONAL READING

- Barceloux DG, Bond GR, Krenzelok EP, et al; for American Academy of Clinical Toxicology Ad Hoc Committee on the Treatment Guidelines for Methanol Poisoning. American Academy of Clinical Toxicology practice guidelines on the treatment of methanol poisoning. *J Toxicol Clin Toxicol*. 2002;40(4):415–446.
- Barceloux DG, Krenzelok EP, Olson K, et al. American Academy of Clinical Toxicology practice guidelines on the treatment of ethylene glycol poisoning. Ad hoc committee. *J Toxicol Clin Toxicol*. 1999;37(5):537–560.
- Brent J. Fomepizole for the treatment of pediatric ethylene and diethylene glycol, butoxyethanol, and methanol poisonings. *Clin Toxicol (Phila)*. 2010;48(5):401–406.

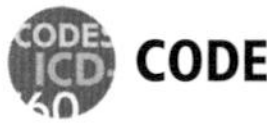

CODES

ICD10

- T52.8X1A Toxic effect of organic solvents, accidental, init
- T51.2X1A Toxic effect of 2-Propanol, accidental (unintentional), initial encounter
- T51.1X1A Toxic effect of methanol, accidental (unintentional), initial encounter

TOXIC SHOCK SYNDROME

Amanda C. Schondelmeyer, MD, MSc • Erin E. Shaughnessy, MD, MSHCM

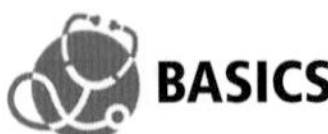

BASICS

DESCRIPTION

Toxic shock syndrome (TSS) is an acute febrile illness characterized by hypotension and gastrointestinal and respiratory distress progressing to multisystem organ failure. The clinical syndrome is caused by bacterial exotoxins produced most commonly by the following:

- TSS toxin-1 (TSST-1)–producing strains of *Staphylococcus aureus*—referred to as TSS in this section
- Group A β-hemolytic streptococci (GAS or *Streptococcus pyogenes*), referred to as streptococcal toxic shock–like syndrome (STSS) in this section
- Cases have also been reported in association with groups B, C, and G1 streptococci and *Streptococcus mitis*.

EPIDEMIOLOGY

- In the 1980s, most cases were associated with superabsorbent tampon use.
  - Subsequent decline in menstrual-related staphylococcal TSS after removal of these products from the market
  - Currently, ~50% of cases are non–menstrual related.
- Higher burden for STSS in developing countries

Incidence

- TSS: 3.4 cases per 100,000 in 2003
- Current incidence of menses-related TSS: 1 to 5 per 100,000 women of menstrual age per year
- STSS: 2 to 4 cases per 100,000 in developed countries with $>$10 per 100,000 per year in developing countries
- STSS incidence is highest among young children and associated with focal infections, pneumonia, or bacteremia.

RISK FACTORS

- Use of superabsorbent tampon, diaphragm, or contraceptive sponge; local or invasive staphylococcal or streptococcal infection
- Recent gynecologic procedure
- Focal infections including surgical and postpartum wounds, sinus, soft tissue, and musculoskeletal infections and respiratory infections
- STSS most often occurs with skin and soft tissue infections.
  - Preceding varicella infection increases risk.

GENERAL PREVENTION

- Scrupulous wound care
- Limitation of intravaginal foreign body use (e.g., tampon, sponge) and strict adherence to manufacturer's directions
- Early recognition and appropriate treatment of infections

PATHOPHYSIOLOGY

- Both *S. aureus* and *S. pyogenes* can produce exotoxins.
- Some exotoxins function as superantigens, interacting with immune cells to induce massive cytokine production leading to the predominant symptoms.
- Cytokines result in fever, capillary leak, hypotension, and end-organ dysfunction.

DIAGNOSIS

HISTORY

- Patients may report use of tampons, contraceptive sponge, or diaphragm.
  - TSS may occur at any time during menses.
- Inquire about recent wounds or surgical procedures including catheters (e.g., IV, peritoneal dialysis).
  - Incubation period for postoperative TSS may be as short as 12 hours.
- Patient may report recent childbirth or abortion.
- Patients may report abrupt onset of high fever, chills, malaise, headache, pharyngitis, erythroderma, fatigue, and dizziness or syncope.
- Gastrointestinal symptoms including profuse watery diarrhea, vomiting, abdominal pain may occur.

PHYSICAL EXAM

- Initial exam should include an assessment of hemodynamic status including vital signs, perfusion, and mental status.
  - Patients are typically ill-appearing.
  - Mental status may be altered, somnolent, agitated, disoriented, or obtunded.
  - Vitals sign assessment may reveal fever, tachycardia, tachypnea, orthostasis, or frank hypotension, although tachycardia and normotension may occur early in disease.
- Exam should include evaluation for soft tissue or musculoskeletal focus of infection or retained foreign body.
- Skin findings include erythroderma, peripheral cyanosis, and edema.
  - Erythroderma may be less prominent with severe hypotension.
  - There may be vesicle or bullae formation or presence of violaceous hue.
- Mucosal exam may show bulbar conjunctival injection and oral mucosal hyperemia.
- Caveats for physical exam
  - Patients may not have all symptoms upon presentation.

DIFFERENTIAL DIAGNOSIS

- Septic shock from other bacterial or viral
- Streptococcal scarlatiniform eruption
- Leptospirosis
- Rickettsial diseases, if travel to or living in endemic areas
- Kawasaki disease:
  - TSS may present simultaneously with Kawasaki disease.
  - Coronary artery dilatation has been reported in cases presenting as TSS.
- Toxic epidermal necrolysis (TEN)
- Drug-induced hypersensitivity reaction

DIAGNOSTIC TESTS & INTERPRETATION

- U.S. Centers for Disease Control and Prevention (CDC) criteria for diagnosis of staphylococcal TSS requires six criteria for confirmed cases and five for probable:
  - Fever 38.9°C (102.0°F) or higher
  - Diffuse macular erythroderma
  - Desquamation 1 to 2 weeks after onset, particularly affecting palms and soles
  - Hypotension defined as systolic blood pressure $<$5th percentile for children, orthostatic changes $>$15 mm Hg, or orthostatic syncope or dizziness
  - Involvement of three or more organ systems: gastrointestinal, muscular, mucous membrane, renal, hepatic, hematologic, or neurologic
  - Negative blood (may be positive for *S. aureus*), throat, or CSF cultures and/or negative titers for Rocky Mountain spotted fever (RMSF), leptospirosis, or measles
- For CDC criteria for diagnosis of STSS; confirmed cases meet clinical definition in addition to isolation of GAS from normally sterile site; probable cases meet clinical definition with isolation of GAS from nonsterile site:
  - Hypotension as defined above
  - Any two of the following: renal impairment, coagulopathy, hepatic impairment, acute respiratory distress syndrome (ARDS), erythematous macular rash that may desquamate, or soft tissue necrosis

Initial Tests (screening, lab, imaging)

Initial laboratory evaluation should be aimed at diagnosing organ dysfunction to guide supportive therapy and identifying potential source and pathogen to guide antimicrobial therapy.

- Cultures
  - Blood cultures: ideally obtained prior to antimicrobial therapy but still helpful if patient has been on outpatient therapy prior to presentation
    - Positive in 60% of STSS but $<$5% of staphylococcal TSS
  - Other cultures
    - Culture of other fluids (abscess, pleural, cerebrospinal) should be guided by clinical presentation.
    - *S. aureus* may be isolated from vagina or cervix in menstrual TSS, although asymptomatic carriage can occur.
    - Culture of GAS from the throat or other nonsterile site may be helpful although does not confirm STSS.
- Antibodies (Ab)
  - TSST-1 Ab are available for informational purposes/research only.
  - Antistreptolysin O (ASO), antideoxyribonuclease B, or other streptococcal extracellular products
    - May increase 4 to 6 weeks after infection in streptococcal-mediated disease, although not helpful in acute phases of disease
- Arterial blood gas
  - Helpful in cases of respiratory distress and poor perfusion to help guide ventilation strategies
- Complete blood count
  - Leukocytosis with left shift (Neutropenia is an ominous sign.)
  - Thrombocytopenia may indicate ongoing disseminated intravascular coagulation (DIC).
- Renal profile: may reflect acute kidney injury with elevated creatinine
- Hepatic profile: may have elevations in liver enzymes

- Coagulation studies
  - May reveal prolonged prothrombin and partial thromboplastin times (PT/PTT) with or without evidence of DIC; low fibrinogen, elevated fibrin degradation products
- Urinalysis
  - May reveal sterile pyuria
- Lumbar puncture
  - May reveal CSF pleocytosis
  - Gram stain positive for organisms or overt abnormalities indicating meningitis argue against STSS or TSS.
- Creatine phosphokinase (CPK)
  - May be elevated, reflecting skeletal muscle involvement
- Chest radiograph should be obtained if there is evidence of respiratory distress or oxygen requirement.
  - May show diffuse bilateral infiltrates in ARDS

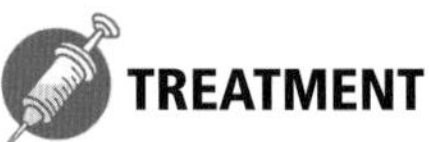

TREATMENT

MEDICATION

1st-line therapy should be broad initially and guided by local rates of methicillin-resistant *S. aureus* (MRSA).

- Vancomycin IV (15 mg/kg every 6 hours, max daily dose 4,000 mg) should be administered as first line if MRSA is a consideration.
  - Renal toxicity is a known adverse effect.
  - Dose should be adjusted for renal impairment and serum creatinine followed.
  - Trough levels (before fourth dose) should be used to adjust dose under the guidance of an experienced pharmacist.
- Clindamycin IV (40 mg/kg/24 h divided every 6 to 8 hours, max daily dose 2,700 mg) should be administered in addition to 1st-line therapy to end production of toxins.
- Ceftriaxone (100 mg/kg/24 h divided every 12 to 24 hours, max daily dose 2,000 mg) should be added empirically for gram-negative coverage until organism or diagnosis is confirmed.
- Antistaphylococcal penicillins (i.e., nafcillin, oxacillin, dicloxacillin) may be considered in place of vancomycin if local MRSA rates are low and can be substituted for vancomycin if the organisms are susceptible.
- IVIG is commonly used as adjunct therapy to antibiotics, but its efficacy is unclear.
  - Proposed mechanism is by providing neutralizing antibodies to exotoxins and inhibiting T-cell activation.
- Continue antibiotic therapy for at least 10 to 14 days; total treatment length should be guided by initial focus of infection if present.
- Consultation with infectious disease specialist is recommended in cases where the diagnosis is unclear.
- Therapy can be changed to oral when there is resolution of hemodynamic instability, clear clinical improvement, and patient is tolerating oral nutrition.

SURGERY/OTHER PROCEDURES

- Remove all foreign bodies.
- Incision and drainage and or surgical debridement for abscess, myositis, and necrotizing fasciitis

ADMISSION, INPATIENT, AND NURSING CONSIDERATIONS

Treatment of suspected TSS or STSS should occur ideally at a tertiary care center with close access to a pediatric intensive care unit.

- Initial resuscitation should proceed rapidly to support adequate tissue perfusion and oxygenation.
  - IV isotonic fluid bolus should be given initially with further fluid boluses and pressor therapy guided by perfusion and vital signs.
    - Be mindful of potential cardiac dysfunction when providing fluid resuscitation.
  - Stabilize airway if respiratory distress is present.
- Antibiotic therapy should be administered as soon as possible.

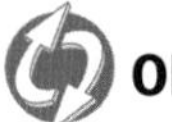

ONGOING CARE

Aside from antimicrobial therapy, the mainstays of treatment are supportive care for organ dysfunction.

FOLLOW-UP RECOMMENDATIONS

Patient Monitoring

- Temperature usually returns to normal within 2 days if on effective therapy.
- Gastrointestinal, hepatic, and musculoskeletal changes resolve rapidly with rare permanent sequelae except for muscle weakness.
- Full-thickness desquamation of fingers, toes, palms, and soles begins 10 to 12 days after onset.
  - Hair and nail loss may occur 4 to 16 weeks after illness onset; should resolve within 5 to 6 months
- Encephalopathy is common but rarely causes seizures; usually resolves within 4 to 5 days
- Poor prognosis is often heralded by development of pulmonary edema and worsening cardiac function.
  - Cardiac and pulmonary failure are the most common causes of death.
  - Toxin-mediated cardiomyopathy should resolve with effective treatment.

PROGNOSIS

- Nonmenstrual TSS has a case fatality rate of 5%; menstrual TSS case fatality rate was approximately 1.8% between 1987 and 1996.
- STSS case fatality rate exceeds 50%.
- Recurrences are associated with inadequate treatment or persistent focus.
- Death usually occurs within the first few days but may occur as late as 2 weeks following onset.

COMPLICATIONS

Multisystem organ failure secondary to distributive shock/hypotension, including the following:

- Pulmonary edema
- DIC
- Acute renal failure (oliguric and nonoliguric)
- Hepatic failure
- Myocardial dysfunction; may have arrhythmias
- Cerebral edema with toxic or ischemic encephalopathy
- Metabolic disturbances
- Tissue death and potentially limb amputation
- Neuropsychological disturbances including memory loss; abnormal electroencephalograms (EEGs) are rare.

ADDITIONAL READING

- Adalat S, Dawson T, Hackett S, et al. Toxic shock syndrome surveillance in UK children. *Arch Dis Child*. 2014;99(12):1078–1082.
- Bisno AL, Stevens DL. Streptococcal infections of skin and soft tissues. *N Engl J Med*. 1996;334(4):240–245.
- Byer RL, Bachur RG. Clinical deterioration among patients with fever and erythroderma. *Pediatrics*. 2006;118(6):2450–2460.
- Low DE. Toxic shock syndrome: major advances in pathogenesis, but not treatment. *Crit Care Clin*. 2013;29(3):651–675.
- O'Loughlin RE, Roberson A, Cieslak PR, et al; for Active Bacterial Core Surveillance Team. The epidemiology of invasive group A streptococcal infection and potential vaccine implications: United States, 2000–2004. *Clin Infect Dis*. 2007;45(7):853–862.
- Shah SS, Hall M, Srivastava R, et al. Intravenous immunoglobulin in children with streptococcal toxic shock syndrome. *Clin Infect Dis*. 2009;49(9):1369–1376.

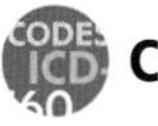

CODES

ICD10

- A48.3 Toxic shock syndrome
- B95.61 Methicillin suscep staph infct causing dis classd elswhr
- B95.0 Streptococcus, group A, causing diseases classd elswhr

FAQ

- Q: Can TSS recur?
- A: Yes. Inadequate eradication of the nidus of infection or inadequate treatment may result in recurrence. Poor immune function may also contribute to recurrence.
- Q: Can TSS be diagnosed in patients who have no risk factors?
- A: Yes. There have been reports meeting the case definition where none of the known associated factors was present.
- Q: Should I wait for confirmation of the diagnosis prior to treating with antibiotics?
- A: No. Empiric antibiotic therapy should be initiated immediately in any patient suspected of having TSS.
- Q: Are special isolation precautions required?
- A: Although medical personnel may use standard precautions when treating patients with TSS, the diagnosis may not be confirmed on initial presentation. Therefore, it is important to consider other potential diagnoses and isolate accordingly during initial treatment phase.

TOXOPLASMOSIS

Rimsha Iqbal, MD • Rebecca Schein, MD

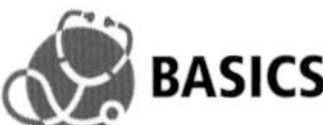

BASICS

DESCRIPTION

Toxoplasmosis is caused by *Toxoplasma gondii*, an obligate intracellular protozoan parasite with a complex life cycle, which can cause a wide range of clinical symptoms depending on individual strain virulence and the host immune system.

- Primary infection is often asymptomatic and may result in fever, lymphadenopathy, and eye disease.
- Congenital infection classically presents with triad of chorioretinitis, hydrocephalus, and brain calcifications.
- Reactivation of disease may develop after either primary or congenital infection and most commonly presents as chorioretinitis.
- Patients with immune deficiency can develop brain abscesses, encephalitis, fever of unknown origin, or pneumonia.

EPIDEMIOLOGY

- Toxoplasmosis infects about a third of the world's population.
- Toxoplasmosis is the leading cause of death due to foodborne illness in the United States.
- *T. gondii* is found worldwide and can infect most warm-blooded animals.
- Cats are the definitive hosts, and the parasite replicates sexually in the feline small intestine.
- Vertical transmission is more common with primary infection during pregnancy or within 3 months prior to conception. Treatment of primary maternal infection can decrease fetal transmission rate by half from 50–60% to 25–30%.

Incidence

Congenital infection in the United States occurs in an estimated 1 in 1,000 to 1 in 10,000 live births annually.

Prevalence

- Worldwide, the rate of infection varies greatly and ranges from 7% to 80%.
- In the United States, overall seroprevalence is 11% but may be as high as 40% in areas with lower socioeconomic status.

RISK FACTORS

- Main risk factors for *T. gondii* infection are eating raw or rare meat, consuming local cured or smoked meat, working with meat, drinking unpasteurized goat milk, or having more than three kittens.
- Untreated or contaminated water is also a risk factor and has been responsible for outbreaks of toxoplasmosis.
- Immunocompromised individuals are at increased risk for toxoplasmosis, including reactivation of chronic disease.

GENERAL PREVENTION

Pregnant women should be counseled to avoid cat feces exposure including gardening, landscaping, and changing litter boxes and to avoid consuming undercooked meat.

PATHOPHYSIOLOGY

- Cats shed oocysts in feces, which then sporulate and become infectious.
- Humans are infected by eating raw or undercooked meat infested with oocytes; accidental ingestion of contaminated soil, food, or water; contaminated blood transfusion or organ donation; or via transplacental transmission from mother to fetus.
- In the human host, tissue cysts are formed in skeletal muscle, myocardium, brain, and eyes.
- Tissue cysts persist for the life of the host.
- Reactivation can occur when the immune system is compromised particularly due to T-cell deficiency.

COMMONLY ASSOCIATED CONDITIONS

- Reactivation of disease may develop after either primary or congenital infection and most commonly presents as chorioretinitis.
- Patients with immune deficiency can develop brain abscesses, encephalitis, fever of unknown origin, or pneumonia.

DIAGNOSIS

HISTORY

- Exposure to raw meat, unfiltered water, cats or kittens
- Immune deficiency disease
- Maternal illness during pregnancy
- Primary infection may be asymptomatic.
- Symptoms are nonspecific and include lymphadenopathy, fever, headache, sore throat, malaise, myalgia, or arthralgia. A mononucleosis-like syndrome with rash and hepatosplenomegaly is seen occasionally.

PHYSICAL EXAM

- Congenital infection is asymptomatic at birth in 70–90% of patients. Visual impairment, learning disabilities, or mental retardation commonly develop over time.
- Signs of symptomatic congenital infection include rash, generalized lymphadenopathy, hepatosplenomegaly, jaundice, pericarditis, thrombocytopenia, meningoencephalitis, hydrocephalus, microcephaly, and brain calcifications.
- The classic triad of toxoplasmosis in neonates is chorioretinitis, hydrocephalus, and brain calcifications.
- Ocular toxoplasmosis commonly is due to reactivation of chronic infection.
- In persons with secondary immunodeficiency, reactivation disease can result encephalitis, pneumonia, or systemic toxoplasmosis.

DIFFERENTIAL DIAGNOSIS

- Primary infection
  - Epstein-Barr virus (EBV)
  - Cytomegalovirus (CMV)
  - HIV
  - Lymphoma
- Congenital infection
  - CMV (Calcifications are periventricular.)
  - Herpes simplex virus (HSV)
  - Rubella
  - Syphilis
  - Zika virus
  - Lymphocytic choriomeningitis virus syndrome

DIAGNOSTIC TESTS & INTERPRETATION

Initial Tests (screening, lab, imaging)

- Serology testing for *T. gondii*–specific antibodies is the primary means of diagnosis.
- The presence of immunoglobulin G (IgG) determines if a person has ever been infected, whereas immunoglobulin M (IgM) or IgG avidity test detects primary infection.
- Pregnant women in high-prevalence area should be screened with both IgM to detect acute infection and IgG for latency. If IgG is present, an avidity test will determine if infection occurred within the last 3 to 4 months.

- Infants suspected of congenital toxoplasmosis should be tested for the presence of *T. gondii* immunoglobulin A (IgA) in addition to IgG and IgM due to higher sensitivity in this age group.
- Amniotic fluid may be tested for *T. gondii* DNA.
- Diagnosis can be made by direct observation of the parasite in tissue specimens, cerebral spinal fluid, or biopsy material.
- As serology testing can vary, any positive tests should be confirmed by a reference laboratory such as Palo Alto Medical Foundation Toxoplasma Serology Laboratory (PAMF-TSL).
- Immunocompromised patients including those with HIV should be tested for *T. gondii*–specific IgG, prior to starting therapy.
- Prenatal ultrasound is useful to detect signs of congenital infection including hydrocephalus, brain calcifications, or pericarditis.
- Head CT or MRI will detect calcifications and hydrocephalus.

Diagnostic Procedures/Other

- Ophthalmologic examinations for characteristic retinal lesions
- Hearing exams, as hearing loss may be absent in infancy and develop over time

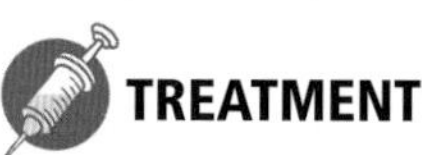

TREATMENT

GENERAL MEASURES

- Most cases of acute infection do not require treatment.
- Persons with eye disease, severe organ damage, pregnant women, congenital infection (symptomatic or asymptomatic), and immunocompromised hosts should be treated.
- Treatment is prolonged, and congenital infection is treated for 1 year.

MEDICATION

First Line

- Therapy is a combination of pyrimethamine and sulfadiazine.
- Folinic acid is also given to protect against the hematologic side effects of pyrimethamine.
- Trimethoprim/sulfamethoxazole should be used for prophylaxis to prevent disease in those with HIV infection and CD4 count $<100/\mu L$ or severe immunosuppression with known IgG antibody to toxoplasma.

Second Line

- Spiramycin treatment of pregnant women may reduce congenital transmission.
- Spiramycin is currently only available as an investigational drug in the United States.

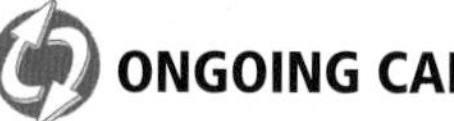

ONGOING CARE

FOLLOW-UP RECOMMENDATIONS

Patient Monitoring

- Children with congenital infection should be monitored for neurologic manifestations, including hearing loss and chorioretinitis that may develop over time.
- Ophthalmologic exams and audiometry should be performed periodically for at least the first 10 years of life after congenital infection.
- Head circumference should be monitored due to development of hydrocephalus in congenital infections.

PATIENT EDUCATION

Immunocompetent women infected while pregnant should be educated that they are not at risk for transmitting disease in the future.

PROGNOSIS

- Congenital infections are also mostly asymptomatic at birth; however, hearing loss, vision loss, and seizures may present months to years later.
- Bad neurologic outcomes are associated with early maternal infection, lack of prenatal treatment, presence of chorioretinitis, and clinical signs noted at birth.
- Treatment improves clinical outcomes, including cognitive function.
- Immunocompromised patients require chronic suppressive therapy until demonstrated immune recovery.

COMPLICATIONS

- Congenital infection
  - Chorioretinitis
  - Hydrocephalus
  - Seizures
  - Intellectual delay
  - Sensorineural hearing loss
  - Microcephaly
- Primary infection: Rare complications are myocarditis, pericarditis, pneumonia, meningitis, or encephalitis.

ADDITIONAL READING

- Berrébi A, Assouline C, Bessières MH, et al. Long-term outcome of children with congenital toxoplasmosis. *Am J Obstet Gynecol*. 2010;203(6):552.e1–e6.
- Del Pizzo J. Focus on diagnosis: congenital infections (TORCH). *Pediatr Rev*. 2011;32(12):537–542.
- McLeod R, Boyer K, Karrison T, et al; for Toxoplasmosis Study Group. Outcome of treatment for congenital toxoplasmosis, 1981–2004: the National Collaborative Chicago-Based, Congenital Toxoplasmosis Study. *Clin Infect Dis*. 2006;42(10):1383–1394.
- Robert-Gangneux F, Dardé M. Epidemiology of and diagnostic strategies for toxoplasmosis. *Clin Microbiol Rev*. 2012;25(2):264–296.

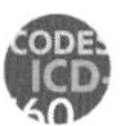

CODES

ICD10

- B58.9 Toxoplasmosis, unspecified
- P37.1 Congenital toxoplasmosis
- B58.3 Pulmonary toxoplasmosis

FAQ

- Q: What newborns require evaluation for congenital toxoplasmosis?
- A: Newborns with known maternal disease or concerning exposure and those with hydrocephalus, intracranial calcifications, strabismus, intrauterine growth restriction, or other concern for congenital infection should have serologic testing for *T. gondii*–specific IgG, IgM, and IgA.
- Q: How do people get toxoplasmosis?
- A: By ingesting oocytes from undercooked meat, drinking unpasteurized milk, or by exposure to cat feces in litter or soil
- Q: Who is at risk developing severe toxoplasmosis?
- A: Infants born to mother infected with *T. gondii* during pregnancy and persons with immune suppression due to AIDS, chemotherapy, or organ transplantation
- Q: How can I prevent toxoplasmosis?
- A: Thoroughly cook meat, wash all fruits and vegetables well, eat only pasteurized dairy products, and wash hands well after contact with sand or soil.

TRACHEITIS

Charles A. Pohl, MD

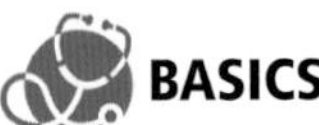

BASICS

DESCRIPTION

Infection of the trachea associated with airway inflammation and obstruction

- Acute tracheitis: sudden onset; higher morbidity and mortality
- Subacute tracheitis: indolent presentation and course; more common among children with prolonged intubation, tracheostomy, and/or underlying respiratory or neurologic conditions

EPIDEMIOLOGY

- Viral prodrome common
- Increased incidence during viral respiratory season (fall and winter): up to 75% coinfected with influenza A
- Gender predisposition unclear (1.3:1 male-to-female ratio has been reported.)
- 2–3% mortality rate

RISK FACTORS

- Antecedent viral infection, especially croup
- Tracheal trauma

GENERAL PREVENTION

- Routine childhood immunization with *Haemophilus influenzae* type b, influenza, measles, and pneumococcal vaccines
- Avoid overaggressive suctioning of children with artificial airways.

PATHOPHYSIOLOGY

- Epithelial damage from a viral infection or mechanical trauma (e.g., endotracheal intubation, surgical procedure) occurs in the trachea at the level of the cricoid cartilage. As a result, the damaged tissue is more susceptible to bacterial superinfection.
- Mucosal damage characterized by marked subglottic edema, copious purulent secretions, and a pseudomembrane (mucosal lining, inflammatory products, and bacteria). These changes lead to marked airway obstruction.
- Toxic shock syndrome may be a consequence if the infection is associated with toxin-producing strains of *Staphylococcus aureus* or *Streptococcus pyogenes*.

ETIOLOGY

- Bacteria
  - *S. aureus* (most common), group A β-hemolytic *Streptococcus, Moraxella catarrhalis*, nontypeable *H. influenzae*, *Streptococcus pneumoniae*
  - *Pseudomonas aeruginosa* and other gram-negative enteric bacteria have been associated with health care–associated infections.
  - *Mycobacterium tuberculosis, Mycoplasma pneumoniae, Corynebacterium diphtheriae*, *H. influenzae* type b, and respiratory anaerobic bacteria are uncommon pathogens.
- Viruses: Influenza, parainfluenza, respiratory syncytial, herpes simplex, and measles viruses have been found with bacterial pathogen(s).
- Fungi: seen with underlying immunodeficiency disorders or chronic steroid use

DIAGNOSIS

HISTORY

- Hyperpyrexia; nonpainful, brassy cough; noisy respirations; lethargy; dyspnea; rapid progression of airway occlusion (hours to a few days)
- Hoarseness, dysphagia, neck pain, drooling, and croupy cough are less common with bacterial tracheitis.
- Presence of upper airway infection and/or croup
- Lack of clinical improvement with racemic epinephrine should raise the suspicion for tracheitis.
- An indolent progression of symptoms, including increase of supplemental oxygen requirement and tracheal secretions (thicker and color changes), may be seen in subacute tracheitis.
- Affects any age (peak age 1 to 6 years)

PHYSICAL EXAM

- Toxic appearance; anxious, agitated, or lethargic
- Labored breathing with signs of severe respiratory distress (e.g., air hunger posture, retractions)
- Pallor or cyanosis
- Severe stridor
- Concomitant signs of pneumonia
- Deviated uvula suggests a peritonsillar abscess.
- Asymmetric lung sounds are often found in patients with foreign bodies in the airway.
- Generalized lymphadenopathy and splenomegaly are clues for infectious mononucleosis.

DIFFERENTIAL DIAGNOSIS

- Infectious
  - Epiglottitis/supraglottitis (presence of supraglottic inflammation)
  - Laryngotracheitis (croup)
  - Peritonsillar and parapharyngeal abscesses
  - Retropharyngeal abscess
  - Infectious mononucleosis (Epstein-Barr virus)
  - Diphtheria (rare)
- Environmental
  - Aspiration or inhalation of a caustic substance, including alkali products (e.g., oven cleaner) or smoke
  - Foreign body aspiration
  - Generalized allergic reaction or anaphylaxis leading to angioedema
- Tumors (rare)
  - Papillomas secondary to human papillomavirus
  - Hamartoma and inflammatory pseudotumor
  - Laryngeal tumors
- Trauma
  - Posttraumatic tracheal stenosis
  - Blunt trauma to neck
- Congenital
  - Tracheal stenosis
  - Vascular ring and slings
  - Laryngotracheal web and clefts
  - Laryngotracheomalacia
  - Vocal cord paralysis
  - Arnold-Chiari malformation

DIAGNOSTIC TESTS & INTERPRETATION

Initial Tests (screening, lab, imaging)

- Radiographs must be completed in controlled settings by personnel who are trained in airway management.
- Lateral and anteroposterior neck films: Findings include distention of the hypopharynx, subglottic narrowing, and irregularity of the tracheal wall owing to mucosal sloughing or the presence of a pseudomembrane.
- Chest radiograph: Obtain if pneumonia, which may be concurrent, is suspected.

Diagnostic Procedures/Other

- Laryngoscopy or bronchoscopy
  - Direct visualization and suctioning of obstructed airway is both diagnostic and therapeutic.
  - Findings include a red, edematous, and/or eroded trachea and bronchi with purulent secretions and pseudomembrane.
  - Consider in an ill-appearing child with an unclear diagnosis or when the child's condition does not respond to current management.
- Tracheal bacterial culture (for aerobic and anaerobic bacteria): the gold standard for microbiologic diagnosis
- Tracheal Gram stain for pathogens and white blood cells (especially polymorphonuclear leukocytes): helps differentiate bacterial infection from colonization
- Blood culture: rarely helpful in diagnosis (<50% positive)
- CBC: little diagnostic value but may show leukocytosis with a left shift
- ESR and/or C-reactive protein: may be elevated

ALERT

- Watch for sudden deterioration from tracheal inflammation and secretions. Continuous monitoring is necessary.
- Bacterial tracheitis must be considered in all children with sudden upper respiratory distress and hyperpyrexia.

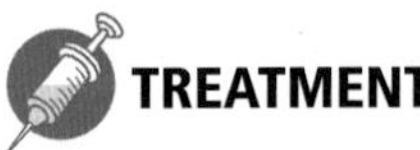

TREATMENT

GENERAL MEASURES

- Support by stabilizing circulation, airway, breathing (ABCs).
- Maintain airway.
- Initiate IV, oxygen, and monitor.
- Rapid assessment of ABCs is essential with emphasis on airway control.
- Supplemental oxygen is usually needed.
- Pediatric intensive care unit (ICU) care is initially recommended.

- Anticipate and prepare for emergent endotracheal intubation and tracheostomy.
- Endoscopy with suctioning and debridement is often necessary for diagnosis and therapy.
- Subsequent airway suctioning and monitoring prevents adverse outcomes.
- Increased ventilatory support is often required for children with preexisting artificial airways.

MEDICATION

Select antibiotic therapy based on Gram stain and culture results of tracheal secretions and the most likely pathogens. Also consider known prior colonization and institutional pathogens in children with preexisting artificial airway and hospital-acquired infections:

- Mild illness
  - Empiric therapy with amoxicillin-clavulanic acid or a 2nd-generation cephalosporin for 10 to 14 days
  - Consider a semisynthetic penicillin such as dicloxacillin (40 mg/kg/24 h PO divided q6h) if *H. influenzae* type b vaccine completed and clindamycin (10 to 30 mg/kg/24 h PO divided q6–8h) if presence of a penicillin allergy or MRSA suspected.
  - These oral agents should be reserved for children with subacute tracheitis who are not toxic and do not have respiratory distress.
- Moderate to severe illness
  - Empiric therapy with an antistaphylococcal agent such as clindamycin plus a 3rd-generation cephalosporin or with ampicillin-sulbactam
  - Consider vancomycin IV if a hospital-acquired infection (MRSA) is present or in severe illness or cases of toxic shock syndrome pending culture results.
- Anaerobic, *Pseudomonas*, and other gram-negative coverage should be considered in children not responding to initial therapy or having preexisting artificial airways.
- In contrast to croup, nebulized racemic epinephrine, bronchodilators, and steroids do not provide significant relief.
- Duration: based on clinical response; usually 7 to 10 days
- Consider antiviral therapy if ill child with documented influenza illness.

ADMISSION, INPATIENT, AND NURSING CONSIDERATIONS

- Majority of bacterial tracheitis cases require hospitalization with ICU monitoring for 1 to 15 weeks.
- Up to 75% patients are intubated for 2 to 7 days.
- Consider extubation with clinical improvement, decrease in secretions and/or air leaks.
- Clinical improvement usually seen within 2 to 3 days

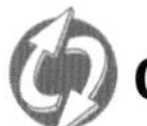

ONGOING CARE

FOLLOW-UP RECOMMENDATIONS

Patient Monitoring

- Routine surveillance cultures in children with artificial airways are not recommended. They usually represent colonization in an asymptomatic patient.
- Signs to watch for:
  - Toxic appearance, excessive secretions, persistent fever, or worsening respiratory distress after introducing antibiotics suggests a resistant organism, an unusual pathogen, or a different diagnosis.
  - Recurrent respiratory distress, especially stridor, with subsequent respiratory tract infections suggests underlying tracheal stenosis.
  - Sudden deterioration on a ventilator may indicate endotracheal tube obstruction, pneumothorax, or mechanical problems.

DIET

NPO until the airway is stabilized and the patient is able to tolerate oral foods

PROGNOSIS

- Most children recover without any sequelae.
- Younger patients are more likely to require intubations and longer hospital stays.
- Children at risk for subacute tracheitis are more likely to have recurrent episodes.

COMPLICATIONS

- Atelectasis
- Pulmonary edema and pneumonia
- Hypotension
- Septicemia
- Toxic shock syndrome (staphylococcal or streptococcal)
- Prolonged mechanical ventilation with associated complications (including air leak, infection, pneumothorax, and tracheal stenosis)
- Subglottic stenosis
- Respiratory failure and arrest
- Death (2–3%)

ADDITIONAL READING

- Dawood FS, Chaves SS, Pérez A, et al; for Emerging Infections Program Network. Complications and associated bacterial coinfections among children hospitalized with seasonal or pandemic influenza, United States, 2003–2010. *J Infect Dis*. 2014;209(5):686–694.
- Hopkins A, Lahiri T, Salerno R, et al. Changing epidemiology of life-threatening upper airway infections: the reemergence of bacterial tracheitis. *Pediatrics*. 2006;118(4):1418–1421.
- Salamone FN, Bobbitt DB, Myer CM, et al. Bacterial tracheitis reexamined: is there a less severe manifestation? *Otolaryngol Head Neck Surg*. 2004;131(6):871–876.
- Tebruegge M, Pantazidou A, Thorburn K, et al. Bacterial tracheitis: a multi-centre perspective. *Scand J Infect Dis*. 2009;41(8):548–557.
- Tebruegge M, Pantazidou A, Yau C. Bacterial tracheitis—tremendously rare, but truly important: a systemic review. *J Pediatr Infect Dis*. 2009;4: 199–209.

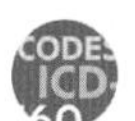

CODES

ICD10

- J04.10 Acute tracheitis without obstruction
- J04.11 Acute tracheitis with obstruction
- J05.10 Acute epiglottitis without obstruction

FAQ

- Q: How can you differentiate a child with severe croup from one with tracheitis?
- A: Infectious croup and tracheitis can present with similar features of fever, toxic appearance, respiratory distress, and stridor. Direct endoscopic visualization and culture of the upper airway is the test of choice to distinguish these medical conditions. Croup is commonly associated with parainfluenza virus and a "steeple sign" of the upper trachea on an anteroposterior neck radiograph. A "worsening" of an uncomplicated case of croup, manifested by high fever, toxicity, and respiratory distress, should make one suspicious for bacterial tracheitis.
- Q: Is influenza A virus a common pathogen of tracheitis?
- A: This subject is controversial. Influenza A virus is frequently recovered from tracheal cultures in children who present with tracheitis. It remains unclear, though, whether this virus is a pathogen or predisposing factor in tracheitis.
- Q: Is the supraglottic area usually involved in tracheitis?
- A: No. Unlike with epiglottitis, the supraglottic region is usually spared in tracheitis. Lack of supraglottic involvement suggests bacterial tracheitis rather than epiglottitis.
- Q: How does the presentation of bacterial tracheitis differ from epiglottitis?
- A: Children with bacterial tracheitis may appear toxic but typically are not drooling and are able to speak, whereas children with epiglottitis are drooling, apprehensive, and not able to speak. A prodrome of upper respiratory tract symptoms is common with bacterial tracheitis but very uncommon with epiglottitis.

TRACHEOESOPHAGEAL FISTULA AND ESOPHAGEAL ATRESIA

Daniel E. Levin, MD • F. Dylan Stewart, MD, FACS

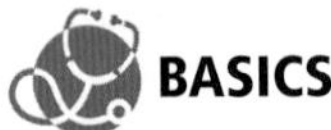

BASICS

DESCRIPTION

- Esophageal atresia with tracheoesophageal fistula (EA-TEF) is a congenital condition of incomplete formation of the esophagus. In most cases, the atretic (blind-ending) esophagus has an aberrant fistula to the trachea (TEF).
- Five types are described:
  - EA with distal TEF is the most common (Gross type C, 85%).
  - Pure EA without TEF occurs in 10% (Gross type A).
  - EA with proximal TEF and EA with both distal and proximal TEFs are quite rare (1% each, gross types B and D).
  - Pure TEF without EA occurs in 3–4% ("H type fistula", Gross type E).

EPIDEMIOLOGY

- The prevalence of EA-TEF is 1 in 2,500 to 4,000 live births. This frequency appears to be consistent worldwide.
- Slight male predominance (1.2:1)

RISK FACTORS

- Many maternal exposures have been postulated to contribute, but none are well established.
- Maternal diabetes (nongestational) during first trimester, older age, maternal diethylstilbestrol (DES) exposure, horticultural work, alcohol, and smoking have all been implicated.

Genetics

- No specific genetic cause of EA-TEF has been established.
- Twin concordance is only 2.5%.

ETIOLOGY

- The foregut diverticulum separates into the trachea and esophagus by 5th week of gestation, thus, factors leading to EA-TEF are present prior to week 5.
- In EA-TEF, it is postulated that the lateral folds that fuse to separate the trachea and esophagus fail to form.
- Disruption of signalling in the *Wnt* and *Bmp* pathways has been implicated in this chain of development. This theory remains controversial, and the exact nature of the defect is unresolved.

COMMONLY ASSOCIATED CONDITIONS

- Up to 50% are associated with another anomaly.
- Congenital heart disease is most common (found in 27% of EA-TEF babies).
- VACTERL (vertebral defects, anal atresia, cardiac defects, TEF, radial or renal anomalies, and limb anomalies)
  - EA-TEF is associated with the VACTERL sequence of congenital anomalies.
  - 10–25% of EA-TEF infants
- Trisomy 13
- Trisomy 18
- Trisomy 21
- CHARGE (coloboma, heart disease, choanal atresia, retarded growth, genital hypoplasia, and ear anomalies with deafness) syndrome
- Feingold syndrome
- DiGeorge syndrome

DIAGNOSIS

HISTORY

- Prenatal ultrasound may demonstrate features suggestive of EA-TEF such as absence of a stomach bubble, a dilated proximal pouch, or polyhydramnios.
  - Only a minority of patients are prenatally identified (9–24%), and the positive predictive value is low (50% of suspected prenatal scans prove to have EA-TEF).
  - Prenatal diagnosis most common in cases of pure EA without TEF
- In patients without a prenatal suspicion of EA-TEF, the diagnosis is usually first entertained when a newborn has excessive secretions and repeated bouts of choking and spitting up during attempts at feeding.
- In patients with an H-type fistula, diagnosis may be delayed. These patients often present with recurrent respiratory infections or aspiration events later in childhood.

PHYSICAL EXAM

- Infants with EA-TEF are frequently normal in physical appearance.
- Failure of passage of a stiff 10F or 12F nasogastric tube at 10 to 12 cm is the major diagnostic test.
- Exam should focus on evidence of VACTERL anomalies.
- Careful cardiac auscultation
- Respiratory auscultation may reveal crackles or other signs of aspiration.
- Documentation of patent anus
- Examination of limbs for skeletal abnormalities (absent radii or thumbs)
- Observation of other congenital anomalies consistent with genetic syndromes

DIFFERENTIAL DIAGNOSIS

- Congenital esophageal stricture
- Severe gastroesophageal reflux disease (GERD)
- Vascular ring
- Tracheal bronchus (H-type fistula)
- Laryngotracheoesophageal cleft (H-type fistula)
- Iatrogenic esophageal perforation, particularly in VLBW infants (Appearance of Replogle tip in mediastinum on chest radiograph may look similar to esophageal pouch.)

DIAGNOSTIC TESTS & INTERPRETATION

- There are no specific laboratory findings associated with EA-TEF.
- Underlying pathology may lead to expected laboratory findings (e.g., electrolyte derangement with severe renal anomalies).
- Chest/abdominal radiograph: first recommended test
  - Nasogatric tube coiled in the proximal pouch in the upper chest or neck
  - Bowel gas present distally (type C)
  - No bowel gas with pure atresia (type A)
  - Possible vertebral and rib anomalies
  - Rule out "double bubble" of coincident duodenal atresia.
- Additional required imaging studies include a renal ultrasound, echocardiogram, and spinal ultrasound to rule out other VACTERL anomalies.
- Limb radiographs are indicated if abnormalities are seen on physical exam.
- Echocardiogram is crucial for operative planning as well as to assess for cardiac defects.
  - Ask the cardiologist to comment specifically on the sidedness of the aortic arch.
  - An anomalous right-sided arch may prompt the surgeon to explore the chest through a left thoracotomy rather than the usual right thoracotomy or thoracoscopy.
- Esophagram
  - For a suspected H-type fistula: Prone pressure esophagram may demonstrate the communication between the trachea and esophagus; however, the finding can be subtle and repeated studies may be necessary.
  - Esophagram is otherwise contraindicated in patients with EA-TEF because of high risk of aspiration.

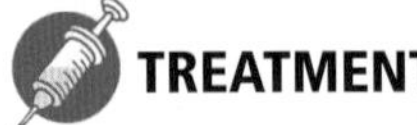

TREATMENT

GENERAL MEASURES

Preoperative management

- Strict NPO until surgical correction is undertaken
- Maintain a Replogle suction tube in the proximal pouch to decrease aspiration from pooled secretions.
- Initiate acid suppression therapy.
- Maintain head of bed (HOB) elevated to 45 degrees.

ADDITIONAL THERAPIES

Complete workup for VACTERL anomalies as described above

SURGERY/OTHER PROCEDURES

- Surgical repair is required for all forms of EA-TEF.
- Repair is performed as early as feasible in the newborn period to avoid ongoing lung damage from repeated aspiration events.
- Extremely premature or ill infants can undergo fistula ligation and gastrostomy tube placement without esophageal repair. The esophagus can be reconstructed at a later date when the infant is more stable.
- Bronchoscopy at time of repair is controversial. It may identify the rare case of dual TEF or laryngotracheoesophageal cleft.
- Repair via thoracotomy or thoracoscopy at the surgeon's discretion
- The fistula is ligated by sutures or clips; the proximal esophageal pouch is mobilized and the esophagus brought together with a sutured anastomosis.
- In a long-gap atresia (esophageal ends separated by more than three vertebral bodies) where the esophageal ends do not meet, a gastric pull-up or esophageal growth induction (Foker) process may be used. Alternately, a gastrostomy tube can be placed for nutrition and esophageal anastomosis performed in delayed fashion.

- Most surgeons place a nasogastric feeding tube across the esophageal anastomosis to act as a stent and allow early enteral feeding.
- Chest tube placement is at the discretion of the surgeon and is often maintained on water seal until the anastomosis has healed.
- Postoperative paralysis and prolonged intubation are sometimes employed to reduce tension on the repair, but there is no strong evidence in favor of this practice.
- Pure H-type TEF can often be repaired by a cervical incision, avoiding entry into the chest.

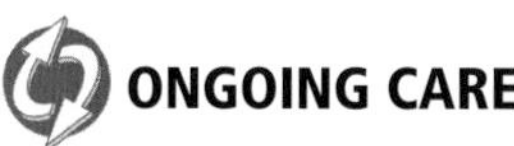

ONGOING CARE

FOLLOW-UP RECOMMENDATIONS

- EA-TEF patients require long-term follow-up for GERD, dysphagia, and esophageal motility issues.
- Surveillance endoscopy may be considered in young adulthood for risk of esophageal cancer, but this strategy is not yet established.

DIET

No change in diet. As infants and toddlers transition to solid food, dysphagia may become apparent and be related to esophageal stricture and/or GERD.

PATIENT EDUCATION

- Parents of EA-TEF patients may be informed that asthma, bronchitis, and pneumonia are common and may continue into adolescence.
- Esophageal dysmotility and GERD may persist throughout life.
- Adults with history of EA-TEF repair report very good quality of life, although some deficits neurocognitive outcomes have been noted in those patients with severe associated anomalies.

PROGNOSIS

- Survival depends predominantly on the presence or absence of cardiac anomalies.
- Overall survival is approximately 95%.
- Survival of babies >1.5 kg without cardiac anomalies is 98%.

COMPLICATIONS

- Esophageal leak
  - Early complication of EA-TEF repair
  - Seen on contrast esophagram
  - Will usually resolve with conservative management (NPO, TPN, and chest tube drainage of any collection)
  - Predisposes to the subsequent development of esophageal stricture and recurrent TEF
- Esophageal stricture
  - Common complication of EA-TEF repair
  - Symptoms include coughing and choking during feeds.
  - An esophagram is diagnostic.
  - Serial esophageal dilations may relieve symptoms.
  - Acid suppression can improve response to dilation and fundoplication may be required in refractory cases.
- Tracheomalacia
  - Symptomatic tracheomalacia occurs in 20% of patients with EA-TEF.
  - Diagnose by rigid or flexible bronchoscopy
  - Presents at 2 to 3 months of age with barking cough or stridor; may improve with positive airway pressure
  - Although children will outgrow tracheomalacia, the occurrence of "death spells" may mandate a surgical aortopexy to reduce severity of symptoms.
- GERD
  - Very common in EA-TEF patients due to disordered esophageal motility and anatomic alteration of the lower esophageal sphincter (LES) by esophageal traction
  - Unlike typical pediatric patients, reflux does not improve with age.
  - 15–70% of TEF patients eventually require fundoplication.
  - Predisposes the patient to Barrett esophagus, and recent data suggest that the lifetime risk of esophageal carcinoma may be 50 times higher than average
- Recurrent TEF is a difficult problem requiring endoscopic or operative correction.
- As most complications of EA-TEF present with choking, coughing, and cyanosis, it can be hard to distinguish between potential etiologies. A rational strategy of esophagram and bronchoscopy is needed to determine the appropriate treatment plan.

ALERT

- Positive pressure ventilation (PPV) preoperatively may lead to preferential ventilation of the fistula. Avoidance of PPV is preferred when feasible.
- If intubation is required, placement of the endotracheal tube past the fistula is the textbook recommendation. However, the fistula is frequently at the carina, which can render this process impossible.
- In case of dislodgement, the postoperative nasogastric feeding tube should not be replaced without consultation with the surgeon to avoid disruption of the esophageal repair.
- If a postoperative EA-TEF infant requires urgent reintubation, mask-ventilate as gently as possible during induction to avoid disruption of the esophageal anastomosis. Maximize visualization of the vocal cords, as inadvertent esophageal intubation can be catastrophic.

ADDITIONAL READING

- Burge DM, Shah K, Spark P, et al; for British Association of Paediatric Surgeons Congenital Anomalies Surveillance System. Contemporary management and outcomes for infants born with oesophageal atresia. *Br J Surg*. 2013;100(4):515–521.
- Gibreel W, Zendejas B, Antiel RM, et al. Swallowing dysfunction and quality of life in adults with surgically corrected esophageal atresia/tracheoesophageal fistula as infants: forty years of follow-up. *Ann Surg*. 2017;266(2):305–310.
- Kunisaki SM, Foker JE. Surgical advances in the fetus and neonate: esophageal atresia. *Clin Perinatol*. 2012;39(2):349–361.
- Lal DR, Gadepalli SK, Downard CD, et al; for Midwest Pediatric Surgery Consortium. Perioperative management and outcomes of esophageal atresia and tracheoesophageal fistula. *J Pediatr Surg*. 2017;52(8):1245–1251.
- Sfeir RS, Bonnard BA, Rousseaux RV, et al. P-25: risk factors for morbidity and mortality in esophageal atresia type III: data from a population based register. *Dis Esophagus*. 2016;29(3):295–296.
- Solomon BD, Baker LA, Bear KA, et al. An approach to the identification of anomalies and etiologies in neonates with identified or suspected VACTERL (vertebral defects, anal atresia, tracheoesophageal fistula with esophageal atresia, cardiac anomalies, renal anomalies, and limb anomalies) association. *J Pediatr*. 2014;164(3):451–457.e1.

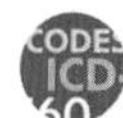

CODES

ICD10

- Q39.1 Atresia of esophagus with tracheoesophageal fistula
- Q39.2 Congenital tracheo-esophageal fistula without atresia
- Q39.0 Atresia of esophagus without fistula

FAQ

- Q: What is the diagnostic workup for suspected TEF?
- A: A chest radiograph with gentle forward pressure held on the nasogastric tube is the preferred diagnostic study. Without pressure, the film may imply a falsely high level of the cervical pouch. Once TEF is confirmed, the recommended evaluation includes echocardiogram, spinal and renal ultrasounds, and a surveillance radiograph of the spine.
- Q: How is this defect fixed surgically?
- A: Surgery is always required. Surgeon preference, patient's size and hemodynamic stability will determine an open (thoracotomy) or minimally invasive (thoracoscopy) repair. The fistula will be divided through the right chest and the proximal and distal ends of the esophagus anastomosed. If the two ends do not reach, the surgeon may initiate one of several techniques to either elongate or replace the esophagus and may provide interim feeding access via gastrostomy tube.
- Q: What is the prognosis for babies with TEF?
- A: Overall survival is approximately 95%, with most mortalities occurring in very preterm babies and those with congenital cardiac defects. Reflux is common and may require fundoplication in some cases. Esophageal dysmotility is nearly universal, but the long-term implications of this problem are unclear.

TRACHEOMALACIA/LARYNGOMALACIA

Thomas G. Saba, MD • Amy G. Filbrun, MD, MS

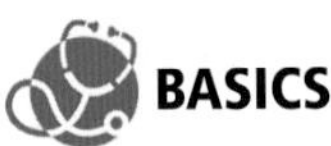

BASICS

DESCRIPTION

- Malacia refers to "softness" of airway structures.
- Laryngomalacia
  - Dynamic collapse of the supraglottic structures of the larynx resulting in airway obstruction
  - Most common congenital anomaly of the larynx
  - Most common noninfectious cause of stridor in children
- Tracheomalacia
  - Dynamic collapse of the trachea resulting in airway obstruction during forceful respiratory maneuvers
  - Common cause of chronic wheezing in infants and children
  - Clinical manifestations depend on if lesion is part of the intrathoracic or extrathoracic portions of the trachea.
    - Intrathoracic tracheomalacia: Airway collapse occurs during exhalation because pleural pressure exceeds luminal pressure.
    - Extrathoracic tracheomalacia: Airway collapse occurs during inhalation because atmospheric pressure exceeds luminal pressure.

ETIOLOGY

- Laryngomalacia
  - Anatomic abnormalities:
    - Short aryepiglottic folds
    - Elongated, flaccid, omega-shaped epiglottis prolapses posteriorly.
    - Redundant arytenoid mucosa
  - Neurologic abnormalities:
    - Immaturity of neuromuscular control results in hypotonia of pharyngeal muscles.
- Tracheomalacia
  - Weakness of the tracheal wall secondary to softening of the anterior cartilaginous rings and/or decreased tone of the posterior membranous wall
  - Classified as primary or secondary
    - Primary: congenital; most common congenital tracheal abnormality occurring in 1:2,100 children; results from immature development of the tracheal structures; may occur with other congenital anomalies such as tracheoesophageal fistula, laryngomalacia, and facial anomalies
    - Secondary: acquired in a normally developed trachea after some insult such as prolonged positive pressure ventilation, recurrent infection or aspiration, or external compression
  - With increasing age, the length, area, thickness, and amount of cartilage increases in the anterior rings as well as the size and contractility of the membranous wall.

DIAGNOSIS

HISTORY

- Laryngomalacia
  - Symptoms may be present at birth or delayed until 1 to 2 months of age.
  - Inspiratory stridor
  - May be asymptomatic during sleep or quiet breathing
  - Worsens with crying, agitation, feeding, upper respiratory infections, supine positioning
  - Often associated with feeding difficulties
- Tracheomalacia
  - Primary: Symptoms may be delayed until 2 to 3 months of age.
  - Secondary: Symptoms delayed until after causative insult occurs
  - Expiratory wheeze, if intrathoracic portion of trachea involved
  - Inspiratory stridor, if extrathoracic portion of trachea involved
  - Harsh barking cough
  - Symptoms worsen with crying, agitation, feeding, and infections.
  - Impaired mucus clearance, frequent infections
  - Rarely, cyanosis, hyperextension of neck, breath-holding spells, feeding difficulties

PHYSICAL EXAM

- Laryngomalacia
  - High-pitched or vibratory, inspiratory stridor
  - Suprasternal retractions
  - Positional changes noted: usually worsens with flexion of neck, supine position
  - Stridor transmitted throughout the chest on auscultation
- Tracheomalacia
  - Homophonous expiratory wheeze (intrathoracic malacia)
  - High-pitched inspiratory stridor (extrathoracic malacia)
  - Intercostal retractions, worse during activity, and acute respiratory infections

DIFFERENTIAL DIAGNOSIS

- Laryngomalacia: differential diagnosis of chronic stridor
  - Vocal cord abnormalities: vocal cord paralysis/paresis
  - Laryngeal abnormalities: laryngeal cleft, laryngeal web, subglottic hemangioma, papilloma
  - Subglottic stenosis (biphasic stridor)
- Tracheomalacia: differential diagnosis of chronic homophonous wheeze
  - Structural abnormalities: vascular compression/ring, tracheal stenosis/web, cystic lesion, mass/tumor
  - Nonstructural abnormalities: gastroesophageal reflux disease (GERD), retained foreign body, persistent bacterial bronchitis

ALERT

- The differential diagnosis for stridor in children includes life-threatening causes.
- If history or clinical course deviates from expected pattern, consider comorbidities (asthma, GERD) or investigating for alternative diagnosis.
- Investigate lower airways in more severe cases of laryngomalacia for other airway anomalies.
- The use of β_2 agonists may increase the tracheal wall collapsibility by decreasing muscular tone, thereby making the symptoms worse.
- Bronchoscopy should ideally be done under conscious sedation during spontaneous breathing to avoid altering vocal cord movement and airway dynamics.
- The use of rigid bronchoscopy may stent open the trachea, making tracheomalacia more difficult to identify; flexible bronchoscopy is a more appropriate test.

DIAGNOSTIC TESTS & INTERPRETATION

Diagnostic Procedures/Other

- Flexible fiberoptic laryngo/bronchoscopy
  - Usually the only study needed to diagnose laryngomalacia; additional tests exist for tracheomalacia.
  - Gold standard for diagnosis of dynamic airway collapse
  - Visualize the degree, extent, and location of laryngomalacia and/or tracheomalacia.
  - Evaluate for other airway lesions in the differential diagnosis.
  - Laryngomalacia
    - Redundant arytenoid mucosa or cuneiform cartilage, shortened aryepiglottic folds, or retroflexed epiglottis
  - Tracheomalacia
    - At least 50% tracheal lumen narrowing during spontaneous breathing
    - Severity based on extent of lumen collapse but not well defined

- Computed tomography
  - Paired end-inspiratory and end-expiratory studies, dynamic end-expiratory studies and cine cough studies
  - Requires patient participation, exposure to radiation
- Airway fluoroscopy
  - Insensitive except in severe cases; unable to visualize antero-posterior and lateral caliber simultaneously
- Barium esophagography
  - Used to evaluate for external vascular compression of the esophagus
  - Might help to identify gastroesophageal reflux
- Chest radiograph
  - Usually normal in both laryngomalacia and tracheomalacia
  - Important to rule out other causes of chronic cough or abnormalities that may cause external airway compression
- Magnetic resonance imaging
  - Useful to evaluate for extrinsic vascular airway compression
- Pulmonary function tests
  - Might show flow limitation, typical notching in expiratory portion of flow-volume loop

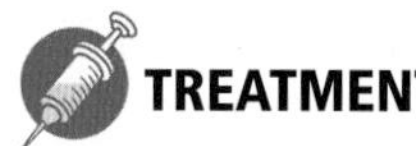

TREATMENT

GENERAL MEASURES

- Laryngomalacia
  - Most cases resolve spontaneously by 15 to 18 months of age.
  - Observation and reassurance
  - Consider feeding modifications (pacing, positioning, texture change).
  - Strong association with GERD. Treat if symptomatic; empiric treatment is controversial.
  - Consider swallow evaluation with video fluoroscopic swallow study (VFSS) and/or fiberoptic endoscopic evaluation of swallowing (FEES) when choking, cough, feeding difficulty, poor weight gain.
- Tracheomalacia
  - Usually resolves spontaneously by 18 to 24 months of age
  - Observation and reassurance, chest physiotherapy for mucus clearance
  - Treatment of exacerbating factors, such as upper respiratory infections, asthma, or GERD

SURGERY/OTHER PROCEDURES

- Laryngomalacia
  - 10% of cases of laryngomalacia are severe (apnea, cyanosis, severe retractions, failure to thrive, feeding difficulty, obstructive apnea) and require further investigation and treatment.
    - Supraglottoplasty: excision of redundant arytenoid mucosa, trimming of epiglottis, division of tight aryepiglottic folds
    - Tracheostomy
  - Postoperative complications: scarring, dysphagia
- Tracheomalacia
  - For severe cases, little evidence supporting noninvasive and surgical therapies
  - Tracheostomy may be needed in severe cases to bypass lesion or to provide continuous positive airway pressure.
  - Consider aortopexy (suspending the anterior trachea to widen the airway), in severe cases, refractory to more conservative management.
  - Airway stents are associated with significant complications; reserved for children with otherwise poor prognosis
  - External airway splints currently under investigation

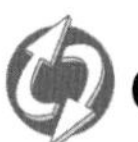

ONGOING CARE

FOLLOW-UP RECOMMENDATIONS

Monitor for recurrent respiratory symptoms, poor growth, and other exacerbating conditions (asthma, GERD).

PROGNOSIS

- In cases of isolated laryngomalacia and/or tracheomalacia, prognosis is usually excellent.
- In patients with history of tracheoesophageal fistula, vascular ring, or other airway anomalies, tracheal dysfunction may persist after corrective surgery.

ADDITIONAL READING

- Ambrosio A, Brigger MT. Pediatric supraglottoplasty. *Adv Otorhinolaryngol*. 2012;73:101–104.
- Carter J, Rahbar R, Brigger M, et al. International Pediatric ORL Group (OPIG) laryngomalacia consensus recommendations. *Int J Pediatr Otorhinolaryngol*. 2016;86:256–261.
- Hysinger EB, Panitch HB. Paediatric tracheomalacia. *Paediatr Respir Rev*. 2016;17:9–15.
- Snijders D, Barbato A. An update on diagnosis of tracheomalacia in children. *Eur J Pediatr Surg*. 2015;25(4):333–335.
- Thorne MC, Garetz SL. Laryngomalacia: review and summary of current clinical practice in 2015. *Paediatr Respir Rev*. 2016;17:3–8.

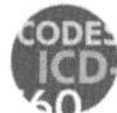

CODES

ICD10

- Q32.0 Congenital tracheomalacia
- Q31.5 Congenital laryngomalacia

FAQ

- Q: When will the symptoms improve?
- A: As anatomic structures mature with age, laryngomalacia symptoms may improve by 6 months of age, with usual resolution by 18 months of age. Primary tracheomalacia may last longer, but in both entities, symptoms usually resolve completely by age 2 years. Natural history of secondary tracheomalacia is dependent on cause.
- Q: Should all patients have an endoscopic evaluation?
- A: No. Diagnosis is usually made based on the history and physical examination. Infants with mild to moderate typical presentation need only careful monitoring for recurrence or worsening of symptoms and for poor growth. However, airway evaluation should be performed in all cases where a different pathology is considered or when symptoms worsen or persist past the expected age of resolution.

T

TRANSFUSION REACTION

Kristin A. Shimano, MD

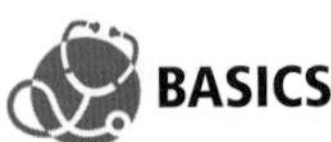

BASICS

DESCRIPTION

- Any acute or subacute adverse reaction that develops as a consequence of the administration of blood components
- Types include the following:
  - Acute reactions: hemolytic, febrile, allergic, anaphylactic, septic, transfusion-related acute lung injury (TRALI), transfusion-associated circulatory overload (TACO)
  - Delayed reactions: delayed hemolytic, transfusion-associated graft-versus-host disease (TA-GVHD)
  - Late complications of transfusion: infection, alloimmunization, iron overload

EPIDEMIOLOGY

- 1% of pediatric blood product recipients develop some type of transfusion reaction.
- Transfusion associated with death in 1 in 200,000 to 420,000 transfused units

PATHOPHYSIOLOGY

- Acute hemolytic transfusion reaction
  - Antigen–antibody interaction leads to complement activation on the surface of the transfused RBCs, resulting in acute intravascular hemolysis and vasomotor instability.
  - Usually ABO blood group incompatibility
  - Most commonly due to medical error
- Febrile nonhemolytic transfusion reaction (FNHTR)
  - Cytokines released by leukocytes in the product
  - 40% of patients with one febrile reaction will have a subsequent one.
- Urticarial (allergic)
  - IgE-mediated
  - Recipient allergic response to donor plasma proteins or other constituents of plasma
  - Sporadic and donor dependent
- Anaphylactic
  - Overwhelming acute allergic reaction; can be mediated by anti-IgA formed by a recipient who is IgA deficient and receives blood products containing IgA
- Bacterial sepsis
  - Intravascular infusion of viable bacteria and endotoxins leads to fever, chills, and/or acute septic shock.
  - Contaminated blood product; most commonly a platelet product near the end of shelf life
- Delayed hemolytic transfusion reaction (DHTR)
  - Previously transfused patients who are sensitized to a minor blood group antigen, especially Jk^a or Jk^b (Kidd antigen), develop an anamnestic response on reexposure.
  - Antibody is below detectable levels in antibody screen and crossmatch; after transfusion, titers rise (usually within 2 to 10 days) and extravascular hemolysis occurs.
- TRALI
  - Antileukocyte antibodies or neutrophil-activating factors in transfused product interact with recipient neutrophils, causing leukocyte aggregates that deposit in the lung.
  - Multiparous female donors with HLA sensitization often are implicated.
- TACO
  - Circulatory overload leading to heart failure
  - Administration of an excessive volume of a blood product or infusion at an excessive rate
- TA-GVHD
  - Patients with inherited or acquired T-cell immunodeficiency can develop TA-GVHD from transfused immunocompetent T cells.
  - Can also occur if the donor and recipient are related and share HLA types

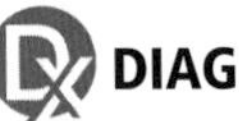

DIAGNOSIS

HISTORY

- Acute hemolytic
  - Fever/chills
  - Abdominal or flank pain
  - Pink or tea-colored urine
  - Tachycardia
  - Hypotension
  - Oliguria
- FNHTR
  - Fever, chills 1 to 6 hours after transfusion
- Urticarial
  - Urticaria
  - Flushing
  - Pruritus
- Anaphylactic
  - Urticaria
  - Bronchospasm
  - Hypotension
- Bacterial sepsis
  - Fever
  - Chills
  - Hypotension
- DHTR
  - Fever
  - Malaise
  - Dark urine
  - Jaundice
  - Shock (rarely)
  - Renal failure 2 to 10 days after transfusion
- TRALI
  - Acute dyspnea, tachypnea, rales, decreased oxygenation within 6 hours of transfusion
- TACO
  - Hypertension
  - Dyspnea
  - Rales
  - Cardiac arrhythmia
- TA-GVHD
  - Fever
  - Rash
  - Diarrhea
  - Cough 4 to 30 days after transfusion

DIAGNOSTIC TESTS & INTERPRETATION

Initial Tests (screening, lab, imaging)

- Acute hemolytic
  - Direct Coombs test: positive
  - CBC: anemia
  - Urinalysis: hemoglobinuria
  - Prothrombin time (PT), partial thromboplastin time (PTT), fibrinogen, fibrin split products: disseminated intravascular coagulation (DIC)
- FNHTR
  - Direct Coombs test: negative or no change from pretransfusion
  - Immediate Gram stain of the product
  - Blood culture of the patient and product
  - All results should be negative; a diagnosis of exclusion
- Urticarial
  - No specific testing
- Anaphylactic
  - IgA level in recipient. If undetectable, test for anti-IgA antibody (of the IgE class).
- Bacterial sepsis
  - Immediate Gram stain and blood culture of the transfused product: result positive for bacteria
- DHTR
  - CBC: anemia
  - Bilirubin: elevated
  - Indirect Coombs test (antibody screen): positive
  - Direct Coombs test: positive (mixed field) if done early
- TRALI
  - Leukocyte antibody testing in the implicated donor(s)
- Chest radiograph: increased pulmonary vascular markings or infiltrates for hypervolemia (TACO) and TRALI

TREATMENT

GENERAL MEASURES

- Acute hemolytic
  - Stop transfusion immediately.
  - Supportive care with hydration, pressors, and diuretics to maintain circulation and urine output
- FNHTR
  - Stop transfusion.
  - Antipyretics (acetaminophen)
  - Demerol for severe chills and rigors
  - May resume transfusion if patient is stable and acute hemolytic transfusion reaction and bacterial sepsis are ruled out
- Urticarial
  - Stop transfusion.
  - Antihistamine (diphenhydramine)
  - Steroids or epinephrine in severe reactions
  - Transfusion may be resumed if mild reaction.
- Anaphylactic
  - Epinephrine
  - IV fluids, pressors
  - Respiratory support
- Bacterial sepsis
  - Stop transfusion.
  - Fluids if hypotensive
  - Antibiotics to eradicate *Staphylococcus* and Gram negatives including *Yersinia* species
- DHTR
  - Depends on degree of hemolysis; if profound, management as acute hemolytic reaction. If mild, no therapy may be needed.
- TRALI
  - Supportive care; usually resolves in 12 to 24 hours
- TACO: diuretics (furosemide)
- TA-GVHD: no treatment; almost always fatal
- General prevention
  - Acute hemolytic
    - Proper labeling of blood specimens and products and adherence to procedures for correct identification of product and recipient will eliminate most acute hemolytic transfusion reactions.
  - FNHTR
    - Administration of leukodepleted blood products, especially for long-term transfused patients who have a high incidence of febrile transfusion reactions
    - No evidence to support premedication with acetaminophen or diphenhydramine to prevent FNHTR
  - Urticarial
    - Administration of washed erythrocyte products (in patients with repeated or severe allergic reactions)
    - No conclusive evidence to support premedication with antihistamines
  - Anaphylactic
    - If due to anti-IgA in an IgA-deficient recipient, provision of IgA-deficient products may be possible.
  - Bacterial sepsis
    - Sterile technique in blood collection, storage, and administration; inspection of product before transfusion
    - Bacterial screening of platelet products before they are transfused
  - DHTR
    - Appropriately performed antibody screen and crossmatch as pretransfusion testing
    - Check blood bank records for previous antibodies.
  - TRALI
    - Deferral of donors is implicated in proven TRALI cases.
  - TACO
    - Administer appropriate volumes (typically 10 to 15 mL/kg) at appropriate rate, usually over 3 to 4 hours unless hypovolemic or actively bleeding.
    - Patients with chronic anemia are euvolemic and should be transfused with smaller volumes over longer time periods.
  - TA-GVHD
    - Patients at risk (immunocompromised, neonates) must receive irradiated blood products.

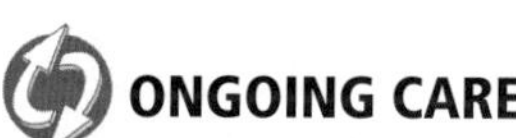

ONGOING CARE

COMPLICATIONS

- Posttransfusion hepatitis: caused by hepatitis B or C viruses, others
- AIDS: caused by HIV
- Cytomegalovirus (CMV)
  - Symptomatic infection in patients with inherited or acquired immunodeficiency states, premature neonates
  - These individuals should receive CMV-safe products.
- Other transfusion-transmissible infections
  - Epstein-Barr virus, syphilis, malaria, toxoplasmosis, human T-cell lymphotropic virus I (HTLV-I), Chagas disease, babesiosis, filariasis, West Nile virus, parvovirus B19
- Alloimmunization
  - Formation of antibodies to erythrocyte, platelet, and HLA antigens can develop in some multiply transfused patients; may cause delays in pretransfusion testing, febrile transfusion reactions, DHTR, and platelet transfusion refractoriness
  - HLA alloimmunization may also affect eligibility and organ procurement for solid organ transplantation.
- Iron overload
  - Long-term transfusion recipients will accumulate iron as a by-product of erythrocyte breakdown.
  - An iron-chelating drug will enhance its excretion.

ADDITIONAL READING

- Delaney M, Wendel S, Bercovitz RS, et al. Transfusion reactions: prevention, diagnosis, and treatment. *Lancet*. 2016;388(10061):2825–2836.
- Lindholm PF, Annen K, Ramsey G. Approaches to minimize infection risk in blood banking and transfusion practice. *Infect Disord Drug Targets*. 2011;11(1):45–56.
- Slonim AD, Joseph JG, Turenne WM, et al. Blood transfusions in children: a multi-institutional analysis of practices and complications. *Transfusion*. 2008;48(1):73–80.
- Tobian AA, King KE, Ness PM. Transfusion premedications: a growing practice not based on evidence. *Transfusion*. 2007;47(6):1089–1096.
- Vamvakas EC, Blajchman MA. Transfusion-related mortality: the ongoing risks of allogeneic blood transfusion and the available strategies for their prevention. *Blood*. 2009;113(15):3406–3417.

CODES

ICD10

- T80.92XA Unspecified transfusion reaction, initial encounter
- T80.919A Hemolytic transfusion reaction, unspecified incompatibility, unspecified as acute or delayed, initial encounter
- R50.84 Febrile nonhemolytic transfusion reaction

FAQ

- Q: What is the risk of acquiring certain viral infections?
- A: Hepatitis B: 1:300,000 transfused units; hepatitis C: 1:1,800,000 transfused units; HIV: 1:2,300,000 transfused units
- Q: What is the risk of developing bacterial sepsis?
- A: 1:1,000,000 red cell units; 1:13,000 to 100,000 platelet units
- Q: Is directed donor blood safer?
- A: No. There is no evidence that the infection risk is lower, and some studies suggest that the infection risk may be higher.
- Q: Is it safe to give a transfusion to a patient with fever?
- A: Yes. However, if the temperature rises during the transfusion or if symptoms such as chills or hypotension develop, the transfusion should be stopped and the patient evaluated for a transfusion reaction.

TRANSGENDER YOUTH

Stanley R. Vance Jr., MD • Stephen M. Rosenthal, MD

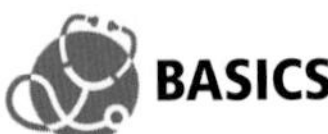

BASICS

DESCRIPTION

Transgender describes youth with incongruent gender identity and birth-assigned sex. These youth may have gender identities that are opposite from the birth-assigned sex, neither female nor male, a combo of female and male, or fluid.

- They may experience gender dysphoria, which is distress stemming from gender identity/birth-assigned sex incongruence.
- Gender dysphoria is also a psychiatric diagnosis in the *Diagnostic and Statistical Manual of Mental Disorders,* 5th edition (*DSM-5*), with primary criteria of long-standing distress and decreased psychosocial function.
- Some youth desire to socially and/or medically transition to their affirmed gender.

EPIDEMIOLOGY

- Recent data from state-level population-based surveys and Centers for Disease Control and Prevention (CDC) surveys indicate the prevalence of transgender adolescents (13 to 17 years) in the United States is 0.7%, equivalent to 150,000 youth.
- There has been an increase in the number of transgender youth presenting to specialty clinics.

ETIOLOGY

Not well understood. Gender identity development and gender nonconformity are thought to be due to interplay between biologic (genetic, endocrine, neurologic), cultural, and environmental factors.

COMMONLY ASSOCIATED CONDITIONS

Transgender youth are at risk for following psychosocial morbidities:

- Depression
- Anxiety
- Suicidality and nonsuicidal self-injury
- Physical and verbal victimization/bullying
- Poor school performance
- Drug and alcohol abuse
- Homelessness
- Eating disorders
- Obesity

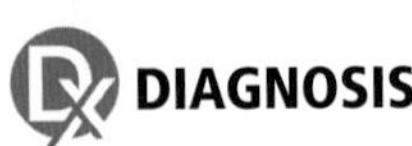

DIAGNOSIS

HISTORY

During well visits, ask children and their parents if there are concerns about the child's gender development. During the confidential portion of adolescent visit, ask adolescents if they have concerns about their gender identity. Early identification of transgender youth facilitates early referrals for psychosocial support and medical interventions.

- If there are concerns about gender identity:
  - Determine the youth's chosen name and preferred pronouns. Documentation is crucial for other staff to refer to the youth appropriately.
  - Take a gender history:
    - Gender preferences for clothing, haircuts, toys, types of play, playmates/friends and the duration of those preferences
    - Distress with body parts
    - Duration of current gender identity
    - Who knows about youth's gender identity? Whether the youth has "come out" as transgender and to whom
    - Whether youth has socially transitioned (outward gender expression consistent with gender identity) and in what environments
  - Pubertal history:
    - Onset of breast development, menarche for birth-assigned females
    - Male-pattern hair growth, voice changes for birth-assigned males
    - Screen for distress around development of or anticipation of these changes.
  - Psychosocial history:
    - Can use HEADSS assessment as framework
    - Home (family acceptance/rejection). Education (do teachers use chosen name/pronoun if youth is "out" at school; ability to use preferred bathroom; school functioning; bullying). Activity (social networks; ability to participate in activities as affirmed gender). Drugs (drug/alcohol use; use of nonphysician-prescribed hormones). Sexuality (assess sexual identity, behavior, and attraction; assess for high-risk sexual behaviors). Suicide/depression (Screen for depression, anxiety, suicidality, self-harm.)
- Diagnosis of gender dysphoria is made using *DSM-5* criteria. This diagnosis may not be applicable to all transgender youth as some do not experience distress.
  - *DSM-5* criteria for gender dysphoria in children require a marked incongruence between experienced/expressed gender and assigned gender for at least 6 months with impairment and at least six of the following:
    - Strong desire to be or insistence that one is the other or alternative gender from birth-assigned sex
    - In birth-assigned boys, strong preference for simulating traditional female attire; in birth-assigned girls, strong preference for wearing typical masculine clothing and strong resistance to wearing of typical feminine clothing
    - Strong preference for cross-gender roles in fantasy play or make-believe
    - Strong preference for toys, games, or activities stereotypically associated with other gender
    - Strong preference for playmates of the other gender
    - In birth-assigned boys, a strong rejection of typically masculine toys and activities and strong avoidance of rough and tumble play, or in birth-assigned girls, strong rejection of typically feminine toys and activities
    - Strong dislike of one's sexual anatomy
    - Strong desire for primary and/or secondary sex characteristics that match one's gender identity
  - *DSM-5* criteria for gender dysphoria in adolescents and adults require a marked incongruence between experienced/expressed gender and assigned gender for at least 6 months with impairment and at least two of the following:
    - Marked incongruence between one's gender identity and 1° and/or 2° sex characteristics (in young adolescents, the anticipated 2° sex characteristics)
    - Strong desire to be rid of one's 1° and/or 2° sex characteristics (or in young adolescents, a desire to prevent development of anticipated 2° sex characteristics)
    - Strong desire to have 1° and/or 2° sex characteristics of other gender
    - Strong desire to be the other or alternative gender
    - Strong desire to be treated as the other or alternative gender
    - Strong conviction that one has typical feelings of the other or alternative gender

PHYSICAL EXAM

- Vital signs
  - Underweight or obesity may be noted as some youth try to minimize 2° sex characteristics (e.g., lose weight to stop menses in transgender males; pseudogynecomastia from obesity may be desired in transgender females)
  - Height should be measured to determine height potential with sexual maturity.
- Pubertal development: Endocrine Society and World Professional Association for Transgender Health guidelines recommend consideration of medical treatment only if patient has at least sexual maturity rating (SMR) $\geq$2.
  - Perform sensitive pubertal assessment (e.g., referring to body parts according to patient's preference; appropriately draping breasts and genitalia).
    - Onset of puberty in birth-assigned females is heralded by development of breast buds.
    - Onset of puberty in birth-assigned males is heralded by testicular volume $>$4 mL.
- Youth may use methods to minimize appearance of unwanted 2° sex characteristics.
  - Tucking: practice by which some transgender females move testicles into the inguinal canal and penis into the perineal area. Prolonged tucking can potentially result in genital discomfort/irritation, and urinary tract infections.
  - Binding: practice by which some transgender males flatten the breast contour by use of tightly fitted sports bra, shirts, or specially made garment called a chest binder. Prolonged chest binding can cause chest pain, breast pain, skin irritation, and fungal infections.
- Skin: Assess for evidence of self-injurious behavior (e.g., scars from self-cutting). For birth-assigned females who wear chest binders to minimize appearance of breasts, check for skin breakdown from prolonged use or fungal infections.

DIAGNOSTIC TESTS & INTERPRETATION

Initial Tests (screening, lab, imaging)

There are no laboratory tests to determine one's gender identity. This is optimally determined through careful evaluation by a skilled mental health provider or medical provider who has expertise with working with transgender youth.

- Youth in early puberty
  - Laboratory tests may be a useful aide in the determination of pubertal status. This includes ultrasensitive gonadotropins (luteinizing hormone [LH]; follicle-stimulating hormone [FSH]) and sex steroid levels (estrogen and total testosterone).
  - Baseline evaluation of bone mineral density using a dual-energy x-ray absorptiometry (DEXA) scan and 25-hydroxy vitamin D (25(OH)D) status are helpful as pubertal suppression with gonadotropin-releasing hormone (GnRH) agonist may adversely impact bone mineral density therapy.
- Youth in late puberty
  - Laboratory tests may be useful in confirming pubertal status and as a baseline for subsequent surveillance for potential adverse effects of testosterone or estrogen treatment or spironolactone treatment (see below).

Follow-Up Tests & Special Considerations

Laboratory surveillance is used to demonstrate adequacy of hormonal interventions, whether pubertal suppression or pubertal induction and to screen for potential adverse effects (e.g., abnormal hemoglobin or lipid profile with testosterone use, abnormal potassium with use of spironolactone, abnormal prolactin with use of estrogen).

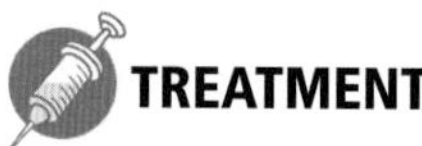

TREATMENT

GENERAL MEASURES

Published studies indicate that pubertal suppression in early pubertal transgender youth with gender dysphoria and pubertal induction with gender-affirming hormones (estrogen or testosterone) in older transgender youth with gender dysphoria significantly improve psychological functioning and sense of well-being. Of note, GnRH agonists, spironolactone, testosterone, estrogen are off-label medications for gender dysphoria in youth

MEDICATION

- Youth in early puberty
  - Pubertal suppression in early pubertal transgender youth is optimally achieved with GnRH agonists. GnRH agonists can be given via intramuscular or subcutaneous injections every 1 to 4 months or via subcutaneous implant that can last 1 to 2 years.
- Youth in late puberty
  - In transgender males, masculinization is achieved with subcutaneous or intramuscular testosterone every 1 to 2 weeks.
  - In transgender females, feminization is optimally achieved with 17-beta estradiol (transdermally, orally, sublingually, or parenterally) and concurrent administration of a GnRH agonist or spironolactone (a potassium-sparring diuretic which inhibits testosterone's production and action).
- In both transgender males and transgender females who were on a GnRH agonist at early pubertal stages, pubertal induction with gender-affirming hormones is carried out over 2 to 3 years. Bone mineral density should also be monitored in those youth who were blocked at early puberty and subsequently treated with cross-sex hormones. For those who are in late puberty at presentation, gender-affirming hormones for puberty transition are titrated to goal doses over 2 to 3 months.

ISSUES FOR REFERRAL

- Transgender youth who require psychosocial support regarding their gender should be referred to a mental health provider with experience with gender expansive youth.
- Transgender youth who would potentially benefit from gender-affirming medications are typically referred to pediatric endocrinologists, adolescent medicine specialists, or primary care providers knowledgeable in this treatment.

SURGERY/OTHER PROCEDURES

For transgender persons desiring gender-affirming surgeries, procedures involving the gonads and genitalia are typically not carried out before the age of 18 years. Breast reduction procedures in transgender males are occasionally done before age 18 years.

- For transgender males, gender-affirming surgeries may include mastectomy, hysterectomy and oophorectomy, and metoidioplasty or phalloplasty (creation of a penis from skin flap).
- For transgender females, gender-affirming surgeries may include vaginoplasty (creation of a vagina—penile inversion procedure and orchiectomy).

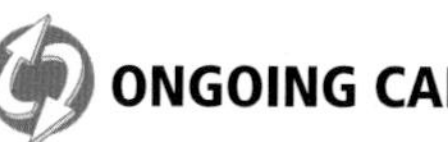

ONGOING CARE

FOLLOW-UP RECOMMENDATIONS

- Youth in pubertal suppression
  - Follow-up with medical visit every 3 months to monitor height, weight, and sexual maturity rating to ensure pubertal suppression.
  - Yearly DEXA scans and monitoring of vitamin D status, dietary calcium intake, and encouragement of weight-bearing exercise
- Youth on gender-affirming hormones
  - Follow-up with medical visit every 3 months in the 1st year monitoring height, weight, and desired secondary sexual characteristics.
  - Medical follow-up visits may occur less frequently after the 1st year of treatment.

COMPLICATIONS

- Potential side effects of GnRH agonists include:
  - Decreased bone mineral density
  - Mood changes
  - Potential effects on cognitive development
  - Impaired fertility
- Potential side effects of estradiol (less common with physiological doses of 17-beta estradiol) include:
  - Thromboembolic disease
  - Gallstones
  - Elevated prolactin
  - Headache
  - Mood changes
  - Unclear impact on fertility
- Potential side effects of testosterone include:
  - Polycythemia
  - Dyslipidemia
  - Acne
  - Hypertension
  - Mood changes
  - Unclear impact on fertility

ADDITIONAL READING

- American Psychiatric Association. *Diagnostic and Statistical Manual of Mental Disorders*. 5th ed. Arlington, VA: American Psychiatric Association; 2013.
- de Vries AL, McGuire JK, Steensma TD, et al. Young adult psychological outcome after puberty suppression and gender reassignment. *Pediatrics*. 2014;134(4):696–704.
- Hembree WC, Cohen-Kettenis P, Delemarre-van de Waal HA, et al; for Endocrine Society. Endocrine treatment of transsexual persons: an Endocrine Society clinical practice guideline. *J Clin Endocrinol Metab*. 2009;94(9):3132–3154.
- Herman JL, Flores AR, Brown TNT, et al. *Age of Individuals Who Identify as Transgender in the United States*. Los Angeles, CA: The Williams Institute; 2017.
- Rosenthal SM. Approach to the patient: transgender youth: endocrine considerations. *J Clin Endocrinol Metab*. 2014;99(12):4379–4389.
- Vance SR Jr, Ehrensaft D, Rosenthal SM. Psychological and medical care of gender nonconforming youth. *Pediatrics*. 2014;134(6):1184–1192.

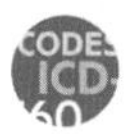

CODES

ICD10

- F64.9 Gender identity disorder, unspecified
- F64.8 Other gender identity disorders
- F64.2 Gender identity disorder of childhood

FAQ

- Q: Does being transgender in childhood predict being transgender in adulthood?
- A: The majority of gender nonconforming children do not go on to be transgender in adolescence or adulthood. It is not possible to predict with certainty a child's gender trajectory, but a gender-nonconforming child being persistent, consistent, and insistent in his or her gender identification may be more likely to persist as transgender during adulthood.
- Q: What is the role a primary care provider can play in providing care to transgender youth?
- A: For primary care providers not comfortable with providing gender-affirming medications, providing a gender-affirming environment (signage, communication) and providing referral to a gender specialist can be crucial.
- Q: When is the optimal time to start cross-sex hormones in a transgender adolescent?
- A: Although some guidelines recommend initiation of such treatment at "about" 16 years of age, there may be compelling reasons to begin treatment earlier. Such decisions are complex and should be made on a case-by-case basis in consultation with a multidisciplinary team including medical providers and mental health providers/gender specialists.

TRANSIENT ERYTHROBLASTOPENIA OF CHILDHOOD

Julie W. Stern, MD

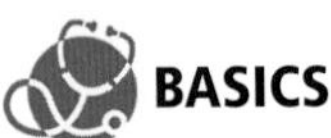

BASICS

DESCRIPTION

An acquired, self-limited suppression of red cell production in an otherwise healthy child

EPIDEMIOLOGY

- Mean age at diagnosis is 26 months.
- <10% are >3 years of age at diagnosis.
- Slight male predominance (male/female 5.1:3.1)
- No seasonal predominance

Incidence

The incidence of transient erythroblastopenia of childhood is unknown due to limited data about unreported asymptomatic cases.

RISK FACTORS

Genetics

- There is no simple genetic pattern.
- Familial transient erythroblastopenia of childhood has been reported (rarely), suggesting a combination of environmental factors and genetic propensity.

GENERAL PREVENTION

There is no known way to prevent transient erythroblastopenia of childhood.

PATHOPHYSIOLOGY

Transient erythroblastopenia of childhood is due to the absence of red cell precursors in bone marrow.

ETIOLOGY

- Unknown
- Possible viral causes include parvovirus B19 and human herpesvirus 6 (HHV-6), but this remains hypothetical.
- A serum inhibitor, such as an IgG directed at the committed erythroid stem cell progenitor, has also been proposed but not yet proven.

DIAGNOSIS

HISTORY

- Pallor
  - Typically slow in onset and therefore often missed by parents
  - Often noted by an adult who sees the child less frequently
- Activity level
  - Often preserved because of slow onset of anemia
  - An extremely anemic child may be irritable, sleepy, and/or lethargic.
- History of fever, easy bruisability, or frequent/severe infections (especially bacterial): should alert the clinician to consider other diagnoses such as leukemia and bone marrow failure syndromes

PHYSICAL EXAM

- Child is generally well appearing and not chronically ill.
- Pallor
- Tachycardia secondary to anemia
- Usually no organomegaly, ecchymosis, petechiae, or jaundice

DIFFERENTIAL DIAGNOSIS

- Environmental: iron deficiency anemia
- Metabolic: hypothyroidism
- Diamond-Blackfan anemia (this diagnosis usually made within 1st year of life)
- Neoplasm
  - Leukemia
  - Myelodysplastic syndromes
- Miscellaneous
  - Renal disease
  - Anemia of chronic disease
  - Blood loss (usually GI)

DIAGNOSTIC TESTS & INTERPRETATION

Initial Tests (screening, lab, imaging)

- CBC
  - Low hemoglobin, normal mean corpuscular volume, normal RBC morphology
  - Total WBC count/morphology and platelet count should be normal; if not, consider leukemias.
  - Absolute neutrophil count may be decreased (rarely <500/μL), but morphology must be normal.
  - Red cell distribution width may be elevated during recovery.
- Reticulocyte count
  - Low to zero during anemic phase
  - Should be high during recovery
- Chemistry/blood bank
  - Bilirubin, lactate dehydrogenase, ferritin, iron levels, and direct and indirect Coombs testing should be normal to rule out iron deficiency anemia and immune hemolysis.
- Parvovirus titers, parvovirus polymerase chain reaction (PCR) testing
- Immunoglobulin (Ig) levels in some cases
- Hemoglobin electrophoresis with quantitative fetal hemoglobin
  - Should be normal in transient erythroblastopenia of childhood
  - Fetal Hgb elevated in Diamond-Blackfan anemia
- Chest radiograph: to determine degree of cardiomegaly

Follow-Up Tests & Special Considerations

Follow CBC and reticulocyte count 2 to 3 times a week to monitor for recovery and need for transfusions.

Diagnostic Procedures/Other

Bone marrow aspiration

- Not mandatory to make diagnosis
- May be necessary to rule in transient erythroblastopenia of childhood and rule out other diagnoses such as Diamond-Blackfan and the leukemias

Test Interpretation

- Presence or absence of early RBC precursors may help predict time to recovery.
- Maturation of megakaryocytes and the myeloid cell line must be normal, especially if neutropenia is present.
- Transient erythroblastopenia of childhood must be an isolated normocytic, normochromic anemia. If the other cell lines are affected (except for mild neutropenia) or if the anemia is macrocytic, consider bone marrow failure syndromes.

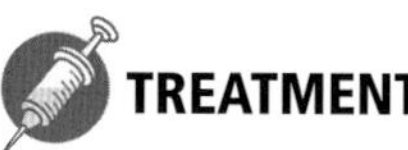

TREATMENT

GENERAL MEASURES

- Normal activity and diet for age, as tolerated
- Instruct family on signs and symptoms of severe anemia.

MEDICATION

- No role for prednisone, iron supplements, anabolic steroids, or other immunosuppressive agents
- Short-term folic acid may be indicated during reticulocytosis.
- Iron therapy has no place in the treatment of transient erythroblastopenia of childhood. Be sure to check RBC indices and reticulocyte count prior to instituting iron therapy for anemia.

ADMISSION, INPATIENT, AND NURSING CONSIDERATIONS

- Initial inpatient observation for complications of severe anemia; daily CBC at least initially to gauge rate of fall of hemoglobin/rise of reticulocyte count and to estimate time to recovery
- Packed RBC transfusion
  - Indicated for evidence of cardiovascular compromise
  - Transfuse slowly to prevent fluid overload. A good rule of thumb is to transfuse the same number of mL/kg as the patient's hemoglobin over 3 to 4 hours. Should a second transfusion be needed, attempt to use a second aliquot of the same unit to decrease donor exposure.
- Nursing issues include monitoring vital signs to assess cardiac status, administering blood, family education.
- Isolation is necessary because of possible teratogenicity of parvovirus B19 and contagion within the hospital.

ISSUES FOR REFERRAL

Follow-up with a hematologist 1 week postdischarge and then as needed until counts fully recovered.

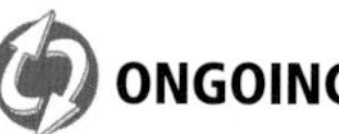

ONGOING CARE

FOLLOW-UP RECOMMENDATIONS

Patient Monitoring

- Clinic visits weekly to monitor hemoglobin and reticulocytes. These visits may need to be more frequent in the beginning of the illness and less frequent as recovery becomes evident.
- Elevation of reticulocyte count is the first sign of recovery.

DIET

No special diet is recommended.

PATIENT EDUCATION

- Parents should understand the signs and symptoms of anemia.
- Patients may resume regular activities as tolerated.

PROGNOSIS

- All children recover usually within 1 to 2 months from diagnosis (may take up to 8 to 12 months for full recovery).
- Prognosis is excellent.
- Recurrence is rare.

COMPLICATIONS

- Cardiovascular compromise secondary to severe anemia is often less than expected given the level of anemia. High-output congestive heart failure (CHF) is unusual.
- Neurologic symptoms including confusion and transient hemiparesis have been reported but are rare.
- A significant number of patients also have neutropenia (absolute neutrophil count $\leq$1,500/μL) during either the acute or recovery phase of the illness.

ADDITIONAL READING

- Bhambhani K, Inoue S, Sarnaik SA. Seasonal clustering of transient erythroblastopenia of childhood. *Am J Dis Child*. 1988;142(2):175–177.
- Huang L, Portwine C, Miller C. Transient erythroblastopenia of childhood. https://emedicine.medscape.com/article/959644-overview. Updated May 10, 2017. Accessed May 11, 2018.
- Shaw J, Meeder R. Transient erythroblastopenia of childhood in siblings: case report and review of the literature. *J Pediatr Hematol Oncol*. 2007;29(9):659–660.
- Skeppner G, Kreuger A, Elinder G. Transient erythroblastopenia of childhood: prospective study of 10 patients with special reference to viral infections. *J Pediatr Hematol Oncol*. 2002;24(4):294–298.

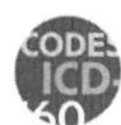

CODES

ICD10

D60.1 Transient acquired pure red cell aplasia

FAQ

- Q: Can other children in a family get this illness?
- A: The cause(s) of this illness in otherwise normal children is unknown. It is very rare for other family members to be affected. It is appropriate to reassure parents regarding this issue.
- Q: Are transfusions always necessary?
- A: No. Only in cases of heart failure is a transfusion necessary. Most often, children can be managed with watchful waiting.
- Q: How can transient erythroblastopenia of childhood be distinguished from Diamond-Blackfan syndrome?
- A: Children with Diamond-Blackfan syndrome are usually <1 year old and can have elevated hemoglobin F levels. If a bone marrow aspirate is obtained during the recovery phase of transient erythroblastopenia of childhood, the diagnosis will be clear. Often, however, only time will tell. Children with transient erythroblastopenia of childhood always recover; those with Diamond-Blackfan syndrome do not.
- Q: Is transient erythroblastopenia of childhood a precursor to leukemia?
- A: No. However, if recovery does not occur in a timely manner, or if neutropenia worsens, a bone marrow aspirate may be indicated if not previously completed.

TRANSIENT TACHYPNEA OF THE NEWBORN

Colleen A. Hughes Driscoll, MD • Bernadette A. Hillman, MD

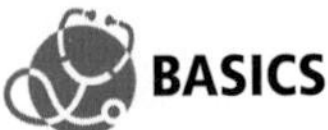

BASICS

DESCRIPTION
- Early onset of tachypnea (respiratory rate >60 breaths/minute) in the newborn following an uneventful delivery
- Symptoms of respiratory distress including mild retractions, expiratory grunting, and nasal flaring may occur. Cyanosis is rarely involved.

EPIDEMIOLOGY
- Estimated 4 to 6 per 1,000 live births
- Incidence is likely underestimated.
- Most common cause of respiratory distress in newborns
- Higher in males

RISK FACTORS
- Early gestation
- Cesarean section delivery (with or without preceding labor)
- Male gender
- Maternal diabetes
- Macrosomia
- Low birth weight
- Maternal history of asthma
- Unexplained transient tachypnea of the newborn (TTN) in individuals belonging to the same family suggests a genetic predisposition.

GENERAL PREVENTION
- Vaginal delivery should be recommended in the absence of maternal or fetal indications for cesarean section.
- Elective cesarean section before 39 weeks' gestation should be avoided.

PATHOPHYSIOLOGY
Transient pulmonary edema due to delayed clearance of fetal lung fluid

ETIOLOGY
- During fetal life, pulmonary epithelial cells are secretory, delivering chloride into the alveolar space.
- Sodium and water follow chloride into the alveoli, establishing and maintaining fetal lung fluid.
- During labor and delivery, fetal lung fluid is absorbed through a variety of proposed mechanisms:
  - Epithelial cells transition from secretory cells to absorptive cells in response to circulating epinephrine levels, which trigger opening of epithelial sodium channels (ENaC).
  - Compression of the fetal thorax from uterine contractions and passage through the vaginal canal contributes to removal of fluid from the lungs through the pulmonary circulation.
  - Prostaglandin-mediated dilation of lymphatic vessels occurs with resultant absorption of interstitial lung fluid into the lymphatic system.
- TTN occurs when there is inadequate fluid clearance from the lungs.
- It is believed that this excess interstitial lung fluid contributes to decreased lung compliance.

DIAGNOSIS

HISTORY
- Tachypnea presenting within the first few hours of life
- Presence of familial risk factors
  - Maternal diabetes
  - Maternal asthma
  - Family history of unexplained TTN
- Birth-related risk factors
  - Perinatal depression
  - Absence of labor
  - Precipitous delivery
- Absence of risk factors that suggest an infectious, metabolic, or anatomic disease process such as the following:
  - Maternal chorioamnionitis or other untreated maternal infections
  - Meconium or blood-stained amniotic fluid
  - Prolonged rupture of membranes
  - Long-standing oligohydramnios or anhydramnios
  - Advanced resuscitation at delivery
- Presence of risk factors for other conditions should prompt additional investigations.

PHYSICAL EXAM
- Sustained respiratory rate >60 breaths/minute
- Grunting, nasal flaring, mild to moderate retractions; rarely, cyanosis
- Symmetric breath sounds on auscultation
- Symmetry of thoracic cavity, possibly with barrel-shaped chest appearance due to lung hyperinflation
- Lungs are generally clear on auscultation, but crackles may be present.
- Absence of stridor
- Absence of signs, symptoms, or other abnormalities in one or more additional organ systems (i.e., fever, acidosis)

DIFFERENTIAL DIAGNOSIS
- Respiratory
  - Delayed adaption of the newborn
  - Meconium/blood/amniotic fluid aspiration
  - Respiratory distress syndrome
  - Pulmonary hypoplasia
  - Persistent pulmonary hypertension of the newborn
  - Pneumothorax
  - Pneumomediastinum
- Infection
  - Pneumonia
  - Sepsis
- Neurologic
  - Hypoxic brain injury
  - Conditions that present with central hypotonia
- Cardiac
  - Congenital cyanotic heart disease
  - Cardiovascular anatomy that contributes to pulmonary overcirculation
- Metabolic
  - Conditions that present with metabolic acidosis or hyperammonemia
- Miscellaneous
  - Disorders related to abnormal embryonic pulmonary development (e.g., congenital diaphragmatic hernia, congenital pulmonary airway malformation, formerly congenital cystic adenomatoid malformation [CCAM], congenital emphysema)
  - Congenital airway abnormalities (e.g., Pierre Robin sequence, choanal atresia)

ALERT
TTN is a diagnosis of exclusion. A thorough review of the maternal history, birth history, and physical examination is essential in determining the degree of workup needed to exclude more severe etiologies.

DIAGNOSTIC TESTS & INTERPRETATION
- TTN is a diagnosis of exclusion.
- Degree of diagnostic workup will vary and will depend on risk factors and clinical manifestations of the mother and baby.
- Risk factors or physical findings consistent with other disease processes should prompt diagnostic testing as clinically indicated.
- CBC
  - Leukopenia or leukocytosis with increased immature to total neutrophil count suggests infection.
- C-reactive protein
  - May be elevated within the first 24 hours with infectious etiology

- If abnormalities exist on these laboratory evaluations, a workup for infection is warranted and should minimally include a blood culture and chest radiograph.
- Arterial blood gas
  - Respiratory acidosis (particularly for P_{CO_2} >60 mm Hg), metabolic acidosis, or metabolic alkalosis suggest alternative etiologies for respiratory distress.
  - A significantly elevated A–a gradient may suggest an extrapulmonary or intrapulmonary right-to-left shunt.
- Pulse oximetry
  - Typically, preductal saturations will be >95% on room air.
  - Supplemental oxygen is rarely required; oxygen supplementation of more >40% FiO_2 suggests an alternative etiology.
- Echocardiogram
  - Respiratory distress and cyanosis may be a manifestation of congenital heart disease.
- Chest radiograph
  - Findings are variable but generally include pronounced perihilar vascular marking and fluid opacity in the interlobar spaces.
  - Slight flattening of the diaphragms and increase in the intercostal spaces can be present if air trapping occurs.
- Of note, there may be poor concordance between the clinical diagnosis of TTN and the presence of radiographic findings of TTN, as radiographic interpretation in cases of TTN is relatively variable.

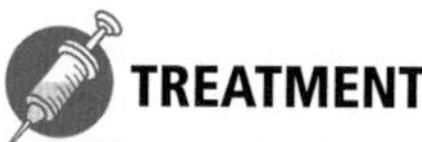

TREATMENT

GENERAL MEASURES

- Resolution of symptoms will occur in time, most often within the first 2 days of life.
- Initial management
  - Direct observation under radiant heat (maintaining thermoregulation) for signs of worsening tachypnea/distress or other abnormal vital signs
  - NPO for initial observation period
  - Monitoring for hypoglycemia
  - Continuous cardiorespiratory monitoring and pulse oximeter monitoring—preductal saturation goal of >95% as the infant transitions to extrauterine circulation
  - Administration of antibiotics and appropriate diagnostic workup if infection or metabolic condition is suspected

ONGOING CARE

FOLLOW-UP RECOMMENDATIONS

Patient Monitoring

Admission to a special care nursery or neonatal intensive care unit and chest radiography are indicated for the following:

- Symptoms persisting beyond 2 hours from onset
- Worsening of symptoms or onset of additional symptoms
- Infection is suspected.
- Persistent need for oxygen
- Chest radiograph is abnormal.
- IV fluids are required to maintain nutrition/hydration/glycemic control.

DIET

- NPO for RR deemed not safe to feed
- D10W +/− electrolytes with total fluid volume appropriate for gestational age and weight

PATIENT EDUCATION

Infant can transition to routine care when

- There has been steady improvement in symptoms during the observation period
- The respiratory rate permits adequate oral nutrition
- Oxygen is no longer required to maintain normal oxygen saturations

PROGNOSIS

- TTN is typically self-resolved, and few, if any, long-term sequelae exist.
- Limited studies have shown an association between TTN and developing wheezing symptoms at school age.

COMPLICATIONS

- Hypoxia requiring oxygen administration
- Occasionally, mechanical ventilation is necessary, and rarely, extracorporeal membrane oxygenation is needed if persistent pulmonary hypertension develops.

ADDITIONAL READING

- Abughalwa M, Taha S, Sharaf N, et al. Antibiotics therapy in classic transient tachypnea of the newborn: a necessary treatment or not? A prospective study. *Neonatology Today*. 2010;7(6):3–8.
- American College of Obstetricians and Gynecologists. ACOG Committee Opinion No. 559: cesarean delivery on maternal request. *Obstet Gynecol*. 2013;121(4):904–907.
- Costa S, Rocha G, Leitão A, et al. Transient tachypnea of the newborn and congenital pneumonia: a comparative study. *J Matern Fetal Neonatal Med*. 2012;25(7):992–994.
- Guglani LG, Lakshminrusimha S, Ryan R. Transient tachypnea of the newborn. *Pediatr Rev*. 2008;29(11):e59–e65.
- Hermansen CL, Lorah KN. Respiratory distress in the newborn. *Am Fam Physician*. 2007;76(7):987–994.
- Hibbard JU, Wilkins I, Sun L, et al; and Consortium on Safe Labor. Respiratory morbidity in late preterm births. *JAMA*. 2010;304(4):419–425.
- Liem JJ, Hug SI, Ekuma O, et al. Transient tachypnea of the newborn may be an early clinical manifestation of wheezing symptoms. *J Pediatr*. 2001;151(1):29–33.
- Mendola P, Männiatö TI, Leishear K, et al. Neonatal health of infants born to mothers with asthma. *J Allergy Clin Immunol*. 2014;133(1):85–90.e4.
- Silasi M, Coonrod DV, Kim M, et al. Transient tachypnea of the newborn: is labor prior to cesarean delivery protective? *Am J Perinatol*. 2010;27(10):797–802.
- Yurdakök M. Transient tachypnea of the newborn: what is new? *J Matern Fetal Neonatal Med*. 2010;23(Suppl 3):24–26.

CODES

ICD10

P22.1 Transient tachypnea of newborn

FAQ

- Q: When does the tachypnea in neonates with TTN begin?
- A: Tachypnea usually starts within 6 hours of birth.
- Q: How long does the tachypnea generally last?
- A: Most babies' respiratory rates improve within 72 hours of onset; in some cases, it may last longer.
- Q: What respiratory rate is safe for trial of oral feeds?
- A: A respiratory <70 breaths/minute without significant increased work of breathing will allow for attempts at oral feeds, although gavage feeds may be considered in the presence of tachypnea if no other clinical issues are present.
- Q: What respiratory rate is safe for hospital discharge?
- A: <60 breaths/minute for >12 hours to ensure resolution of symptoms and confirm the diagnosis of TTN

TRANSPOSITION OF THE GREAT ARTERIES

Kim Haberer, MD, FRCPC

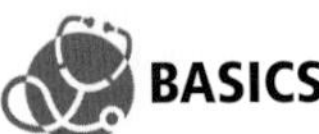

BASICS

DESCRIPTION

Abnormal anatomic relationship between the great arteries and the ventricles in which the aorta arises from the anatomic right ventricle and the pulmonary artery arises from the anatomic left ventricle

EPIDEMIOLOGY

Incidence

Incidence is 20 to 30 per 100,000 live births, with a 60–70% male predilection.

Prevalence

Transposition of the great arteries (TGA) represents up to 7% of all cases of congenital heart disease.

PATHOPHYSIOLOGY

- Systemic and pulmonary circulations are separated and function in parallel.
- Desaturated systemic venous blood is ejected from the right heart to the aorta, whereas the oxygenated pulmonary venous blood is ejected from the left ventricle into the lungs.
- Degree of hypoxemia depends on amount of intercirculatory mixing (patent ductus arteriosus [PDA], patent foramen ovale [PFO], ventricular septal defect [VSD]).
  - Degree of left-to-right shunting is the effective systemic blood flow, whereas right-to-left shunting determines effective pulmonary flow.

COMMONLY ASSOCIATED CONDITIONS

- PDA and PFO with intact ventricular septum (50%)
- VSD (40%)
- Posterior malalignment VSD with left ventricular outflow tract obstruction (e.g., subpulmonic stenosis, pulmonary stenosis, pulmonary atresia) (10%)
- Anterior malalignment VSD with right ventricular outflow tract obstruction (e.g., subaortic stenosis, aortic stenosis, coarctation of the aorta, or interruption of the aortic arch) (10%)
- Leftward juxtaposition of the atrial appendages (5%)
- Straddling of the atrioventricular valve

DIAGNOSIS

HISTORY

- Infants are of normal birth weight or sometimes large for gestational age.
- Association with maternal diabetes
- Cyanosis
- Tachypnea often without retractions
- Poor feeding

PHYSICAL EXAM

- General
  - Moderate to severe cyanosis
- Cardiovascular
  - Single loud S_2
  - In infants with intact ventricular septum, there may be only a ductal murmur or no murmur at all.
  - A soft systolic murmur can be heard in those infants with a VSD, and a systolic ejection murmur of valvar or subvalvar aortic or pulmonic stenosis may be present.
- Respiratory
  - Generally, "quiet" tachypnea present without retractions in the neonate
  - With a large VSD and congestive heart failure (CHF), retractions may develop.
- Abdomen
  - Hepatomegaly may occur with a large VSD and CHF.

DIFFERENTIAL DIAGNOSIS

The differential diagnosis for the neonate with TGA is that for the cyanotic neonate.

- Cardiac
  - Lesions with ductal-dependent pulmonary blood flow
    - Tricuspid atresia with normally related great arteries
    - Tetralogy of Fallot
    - Tetralogy of Fallot with pulmonic atresia
    - Critical pulmonic stenosis
    - Pulmonary atresia with intact ventricular septum
    - Ebstein anomaly
    - Heterotaxy (most forms)
  - Ductal-independent mixing lesions
    - Total anomalous pulmonary venous connection
    - Truncus arteriosus
  - Lesions with ductal-dependent systemic blood flow
    - Hypoplastic left heart syndrome
    - Interrupted aortic arch
    - Critical coarctation of the aorta
    - Critical aortic stenosis
- Persistent pulmonary hypertension of the newborn
- Pulmonary
  - Primary lung disease
  - Airway obstruction
  - Extrinsic compression of the lungs
- Neurologic
  - Central nervous system dysfunction
  - Respiratory neuromuscular dysfunction
- Hematologic
  - Methemoglobinemia
  - Polycythemia

DIAGNOSTIC TESTS & INTERPRETATION

- Arterial blood gas
  - Hypoxemia (Po_2 often in low 30s) unchanged in 100% FiO_2. Infants with inadequate mixing have Po_2 <25 torr with metabolic acidosis.
  - Glucose; may be hypoglycemic in the newborn period
- Chest radiograph
  - Mild cardiomegaly with an "egg-shaped" heart with narrow superior mediastinum (so-called egg on a string) and increased pulmonary vascular markings
- ECG
  - Initially normal, progressing to right ventricular hypertrophy and right axis deviation
- Echocardiogram (ECHO)
  - 2D ECHO and color-flow Doppler studies usually provide all anatomic and functional information required for management of infants with D-TGA.
  - The study should focus on the alignment of the great arteries and other associated anomalies, specifically defects that promote intercirculatory mixing (ASD, PDA, VSD), the presence of left or right ventricular outflow tract obstruction, coarctation, and the coronary anatomy.
  - The most important mixing in D-TGA is at the atrial level. Without an adequate atrial communication, the baby will remain cyanotic.
- Pathologic findings
  - In the normal heart, the aorta arises posteriorly from the left ventricle and carries oxygenated blood to the body; there is fibrous continuity between the aortic and mitral valves, and subpulmonary conus is present.
  - In D-TGA, the aorta is oriented anteriorly and rightward from the pulmonary artery and originates from the right ventricle, carrying desaturated blood to the body. The pulmonary artery originates posteriorly from the left ventricle and carries oxygenated blood to the lungs. There is fibrous continuity between the pulmonary and mitral valves; subaortic conus (infundibulum) is present.
  - TGA types
    - The most common type of TGA, known as D-TGA, has transposed great arteries with cardiac segments S, D, and D: situs solitus of the atria and viscera (S), dextroventricular segment situs (D), aortic valve annulus to the right of the pulmonary artery (D). There is atrioventricular concordance and ventriculoarterial discordance.
    - L-TGA, or "corrected transposition," has transposed great arteries with cardiac segments S, L, and L: situs solitus of the atria and viscera (S), levoventricular segment situs (L), and the aortic valve annulus is to the left of the pulmonary artery (L). There is atrioventricular discordance and ventriculoarterial discordance.
  - Abnormal coronary artery (CA) branching occurs in 33%.
    - Circumflex artery off the right CA (16%), single right CA (4%), single left CA (2%)

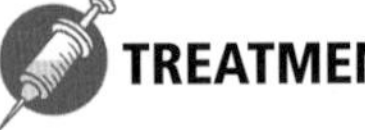

TREATMENT

MEDICATION

- Correction of metabolic acidosis, hypoglycemia, and hypocalcemia improves myocardial function. The neonate may require fluid resuscitation.
- Prostaglandin E_1 (PGE_1) is used for severe cyanosis to promote left (aorta) to right (pulmonary artery) shunting at the ductus arteriosus, thereby increasing pulmonary blood flow, return of blood to the left atrium, and improved mixing at the atrial level. Side effects of PGE_1 include apnea, fever, and hypotension.

SURGERY/OTHER PROCEDURES

- Interventional catheterization
  - Balloon atrial septostomy (Rashkind procedure) is used in the severely hypoxemic infant with an intact or restrictive atrial septum to promote intercirculatory mixing at the atrial level and stabilize the neonate before definitive or palliative surgery.
- Definitive surgery for D-TGA includes procedures that redirect the pulmonary and systemic venous return at the atrial, ventricular, and great artery levels.
  - Atrial inversion: Atrial inversion procedures involve baffling the pulmonary venous blood flow to the tricuspid valve (systemic circulation) and the systemic venous blood flow to the mitral valve (pulmonary circulation). The two atrial inversion operations include the Mustard procedure, in which prosthetic or pericardial baffles are used to redirect the blood, and the Senning procedure, in which the baffles are composed of an atrial septal flap and the right atrial free wall. The Senning or Mustard procedures were the original surgeries performed for D-TGA. Now, they are sometimes used in the following infants:
    - Infants with D-TGA with intact ventricular septum who have not had surgical repair within the 1st month of life
    - Neonates with D-TGA with intact ventricular septum and severe pulmonic stenosis. Most centers would perform a Rastelli procedure for this anatomic variant (see subsequent list items).
    - Neonates with D-TGA with "unswitchable coronaries" (<1% of cases)
  - Ventricular inversion
    - D-TGA with a VSD and severe pulmonic stenosis: The Rastelli operation may be used to redirect blood flow at the ventricular level. In this operation, the proximal main pulmonary artery is divided and oversewn, and the left ventricular blood flow is baffled to the aorta by creating an intraventricular tunnel between the VSD and the aortic valve. A conduit is placed from the right ventricle to the pulmonary artery to redirect the right ventricular blood flow.
    - Nikaidoh and REV procedures are modifications developed primarily for D-TGA with a VSD.
  - Arterial switch
    - D-TGA with intact ventricular septum and "switchable" coronaries: The arterial switch operation (ASO) is performed in which the great arteries are transected above their respective semilunar valves and switched with reimplantation of the CAs into the neoaortic root (native pulmonary valve root). In the Lecompte maneuver, the pulmonary arteries are brought anterior to the ascending aorta.
    - D-TGA with anterior malalignment VSD with severe aortic stenosis: ASO with VSD patch closure and transannular patch of the right ventricular outflow tract; if coarctation is present, may require coarctation repair

ONGOING CARE

PROGNOSIS

- Without treatment, mortality is 30% within the 1st week of life, 50% within the 1st month, 70% within the first 6 months, and 95% within the 1st year.
- In most centers, the mortality rate after ASO for D-TGA with intact ventricular septum or D-TGA with a VSD is <3%. Factors that have been shown to increase the mortality risk include an intramural course of the left CA, retropulmonary course of the left CA, complex arch abnormalities, right ventricular hypoplasia, multiple VSDs, and straddling atrioventricular valves.

COMPLICATIONS

- Complications of intra-atrial surgeries include absence of sinus rhythm (>50% of cases), supraventricular arrhythmias (50%), moderately to severely depressed systemic right ventricular function (20%), intra-atrial baffle leak (20% of cases), tricuspid regurgitation (5–10% of cases), obstruction of systemic venous return (5% of cases), and obstruction of pulmonary venous return (<2% of cases). Follow-up observation is recommended every 12 months to detect arrhythmias, tricuspid regurgitation, or depressed right ventricular function that generally occurs years after surgery. Arrhythmias include sinus node dysfunction and supraventricular tachycardia, especially atrial flutter. Many require pacemaker insertion in later life.
- Complications after the Rastelli operation include left ventricular outflow tract obstruction, conduit obstruction, and complete heart block. Follow-up observation is recommended every 12 months to monitor for conduit obstruction, left ventricular outflow tract obstruction, and heart block.
- The most common complication after the ASO is neoaortic root dilation with or without neoaortic insufficiency. Other rarer complications include supravalvar pulmonary stenosis at the anastomotic site (5% of cases), supravalvar aortic stenosis at the anastomotic site (5% of cases), branch pulmonary artery stenosis, and coronary stenosis or obstruction, which may lead to ischemia and infarction. These complications are uncommon and usually hemodynamically insignificant. Mortality varies depending on the period of time being assessed:
  - Early mortality is usually related to kinking or obstruction of the CAs during transfer to the neoaorta, an "unprepared" left ventricle, or hemorrhage from the multiple suture lines.
  - Late mortality (i.e., 1–2%) usually results from myocardial ischemia, pulmonary vascular obstructive disease, or during reoperation for supravalvar stenosis.
- Follow-up observation is recommended every 12 months to monitor for neoaortic root dilation, neoaortic valve insufficiency, supravalvar aortic or pulmonic stenosis, and CA ischemia.

ADDITIONAL READING

- Bellinger DC, Wypij D, duPlessis AJ, et al. Neurodevelopmental status at eight years in children with dextro-transposition of the great arteries: the Boston Circulatory Arrest Trial. *J Thorac Cardiovasc Surg*. 2003;126(5):1385–1396.
- Culbert EL, Ashburn DA, Cullen-Dean G, et al; and Congenital Heart Surgeons Society. Quality of life of children after repair of transposition of the great arteries. *Circulation*. 2003;108(7):857–862.
- Formigari R, Toscano A, Giardini A, et al. Prevalence and predictors of neoaortic regurgitation after arterial switch operation for transposition of the great arteries. *J Thorac Cardiovasc Surg*. 2003;126(6): 1753–1759.
- Langley SM, Winlaw DS, Stumper O, et al. Midterm results after restoration of the morphologically left ventricle to the systemic circulation in patients with congenitally corrected transposition of the great arteries. *J Thorac Cardiovasc Surg*. 2003;125(6): 1229–1241.
- Marino BS, Wernovsky G, McElhinney D, et al. Neo-aortic valvar function after the arterial switch. *Cardiol Young*. 2006;16(5):481–489.
- Mavroudis C, Backer CL. Physiologic versus anatomic repair of congenitally corrected transposition of the great arteries. *Semin Thorac Cardiovasc Surg Pediatr Card Surg Annu*. 2003;6:16–26.
- Pasquali SK, Hasselblad V, Li JS, et al. Coronary artery pattern and outcome of arterial switch operation for transposition of the great arteries: a meta-analysis. *Circulation*. 2002;106(20): 2575–2580.
- Warnes CA. Transposition of the great arteries. *Circulation*. 2006;114(24):2699–2709.
- Williams WG, McCrindle BW, Ashburn DA, et al; for Congenital Heart Surgeon's Society. Outcomes of 829 neonates with complete transposition of the great arteries 12–17 years after repair. *Eur J Cardiothorac Surg*. 2003;24(1):1–9.

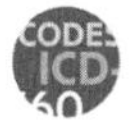

CODES

ICD10

- Q20.3 Discordant ventriculoarterial connection
- Q20.5 Discordant atrioventricular connection

T

TRANSVERSE MYELITIS

Benjamin M. Greenberg, MD, MHS • Cynthia X. Wang, MD

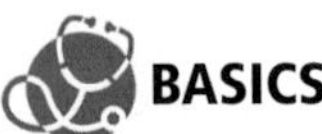

BASICS

DESCRIPTION

An acquired, immune-mediated inflammatory process in the spinal cord presenting as rapid onset (acute to subacute) weakness, sensory change, and/or autonomic dysfunction. Classically described with a sensory level (hence, "transverse") although not required and less often described in children. Transverse myelitis (TM) is typically associated with MRI and CSF abnormalities consistent with acute inflammation. TM can be idiopathic (usually monophasic) or be a manifestation of a chronic relapsing inflammatory disorder such as multiple sclerosis (MS) or neuromyelitis optica spectrum disorder (NMOSD).

EPIDEMIOLOGY

- Incidence: estimated 1 to 8 per million cases per year, or 1,400 new cases, in the United States
- 20% are children (approximately 300 children affected per year).
- Bimodal age distribution is observed with peaks between ages 0 and 5 years and 10 and 17 years in children.
- Prevalence: estimated 34,000 people with chronic morbidity from TM in the United States
- No difference in ethnicity prevalence
- Female-to-male ratio is approximately 1:1 for children with idiopathic TM; female predominance can be observed if TM is a part of a relapsing syndrome such as MS or NMOSD.

RISK FACTORS

- Prodromal infections in up to 66% and vaccination in up to 28% in 30 days preceding onset of TM symptoms in children (although most data suggest that there is not a link between TM and vaccination)
- >1/3 may be disease associated (secondary TM).

GENERAL PREVENTION

Avoid unnecessary exposure to communicable diseases and obtain routine immunizations to protect against preventable diseases. Because some autoimmune disorders are linked to vitamin D deficiency, supplementation of vitamin D_3 may help prevent CNS inflammatory conditions.

PATHOPHYSIOLOGY

Multiple mechanisms have been implicated due to the diverse spectrum of disease from idiopathic to disease-associated myelitis. Histopathology may reveal perivascular infiltration by monocytes and lymphocytes, demyelination, and axonal loss.

ETIOLOGY

Unknown, although molecular mimicry has been implicated, leading to immune response against infectious antigens with cross-reactivity to CNS proteins. Other theories include direct microbial infection of the spinal cord and superantigen-mediated disease.

COMMONLY ASSOCIATED CONDITIONS

- Predominately idiopathic, occurring as a postinfectious autoimmune process
- Infectious etiologies include but are not limited to West Nile Virus, human T-lymphotropic virus (HTLV)-1, HIV, Zika, influenza, enteroviruses, and herpes family viruses, mycoplasma, syphilis, Lyme disease.
- Can be a manifestation of a multifocal CNS disease (MS, NMOSD, acute disseminated encephalomyelitis [ADEM]) or paraneoplastic syndrome
- TM can be associated with systemic inflammatory diseases such as sarcoidosis, Sjögren disease, systemic lupus erythematosus, Behçet disease, antiphospholipid syndrome, scleroderma, ankylosing spondylitis, juvenile idiopathic arthritis, mixed connective tissue disease.

DIAGNOSIS

HISTORY

- Children may present with:
  - Sensory changes (positive and/or negative) (91%)
  - Extremity weakness (89%)
  - Urinary and bowel dysfunction (85%)
  - Pain (75%)
  - Gait disturbance
- A sensory level may not be evident in up to 40% of children.
- Symptoms typically evolve over 2 to 4 days and peak at 5 to 6 days.
- A hyperacute time course (minutes to hours) should prompt consideration of vascular and traumatic etiologies.
- Recent history may reveal fever or acute illness.
- If past history includes episodes of transient neurologic dysfunction such as sensory disturbance, weakness, or vision change, a relapsing disease should be considered.

PHYSICAL EXAM

- A complete neurologic examination should be performed at presentation and followed closely for progression of weakness, sensory level, respiratory difficulty, bladder and/or bowel dysfunction.
- Children may have a sensory level with decreased sensation and weakness of extremities below level.
- Reflexes may be initially decreased due to spinal shock but over time often become increased and accompanied by spasticity.
- Babinski sign is often present when corticospinal tracts are affected.
- Persistent flaccid weakness or asymmetric limb involvement should prompt consideration of variants of TM including acute flaccid myelitis (AFM).
- Meningismus, fever, and altered mental status should prompt consideration of meningitis and encephalitis.

DIFFERENTIAL DIAGNOSIS

- Compressive myelopathy
  - Traumatic
  - Arteriovenous malformation
  - Disk herniation
  - Epidural abscess
  - Vertebral osteomyelitis
  - Neoplasm
- Vascular myelopathies
  - Anterior spinal cord infarction
  - Spinal-dural arteriovenous fistula
  - Angiitis/vasculitis
  - Fibrocartilaginous embolism
- Metabolic and nutritional myelopathies: deficiency in vitamin B_{12}, D, E, or copper; nitrous oxide toxicity
- Autoimmune
  - Acquired demyelination syndromes
  - Systemic autoimmune disease
- Infectious myelitis
- Postradiation myelopathy
- Paraneoplastic syndrome
- Non-myelopathic:
  - Guillain-Barre syndrome (although a sensory level should always argue against this diagnosis)

DIAGNOSTIC TESTS & INTERPRETATION

Initial Tests (screening, lab, imaging)

- Serum: complete blood cell count and differential, neuromyelitis optica (NMO)/aquaporin-4 IgG
- LP and CSF analysis: cell count, differential, protein, glucose, Gram stain, culture, IgG index, oligoclonal bands, NMO IgG
- Infectious: enterovirus, human herpesvirus (HHV), varicella zoster virus (VZV), Epstein-Barr virus (EBV), HIV, rapid plasma reagin (RPR), *Mycoplasma*, *Bartonella*, *Borrelia*, HTLV
- Nutritional/metabolic: serum vitamin B_{12}, copper, methylmalonic acid, TSH
- Inflammatory/rheumatologic: antinuclear antibody (ANA), anti-Sjögren syndrome A (SSA)/anti-Sjögren syndrome B (SSB), ESR, C-reactive protein (CRP), extractable nuclear antigen (ENA), antiphospholipid antibody (APA), antineutrophil cytoplasmic antibodies (ANCA)
- Prothrombotic evaluation
- Paraneoplastic panel
- Acute myelopathic symptoms constitute a neurologic emergency and mandates emergent spinal imaging.
- An MRI complete spine with and without gadolinium contrast is preferred, although consider partial study if time-critical concern or child cannot tolerate full study.
- Imaging entire neuraxis may reveal clinically silent lesions or serve as baseline imaging.
- MRI spine lesions are often centrally located with high T2-signal intensity involving gray and neighboring white matter.
- Predominantly gray matter involvement is seen in AFM, although this can also affect white matter tracts.
- Spinal nerve root or cauda equina enhancement may be observed in setting of some patterns of TM.
- Asymptomatic lesions on brain MRI are seen in >1/3 and predict MS or NMOSD.

Follow-Up Tests & Special Considerations

- Consultation of physical therapy, occupational therapy, physical medicine, and rehabilitation
- Consider use of electrical stimulation with therapy to prevent muscle atrophy.

Diagnostic Procedures/Other

Electrodiagnostic studies: An electromyogram and nerve conduction studies can be used in clinically ambiguous cases to differentiate GBS from TM. Visual-evoked potentials can evaluate for prior optic neuritis.

Test Interpretation

- Inflammation of the spinal cord identified by imaging or CSF findings is required for a diagnosis of TM.
- CSF is abnormal in approximately 50–80% of patients.

- Moderate pleocytosis (<100/mm^3) and elevated protein (100 to 120 mg/dL) are most common abnormalities.
- Children may have higher values, as reported in one case series; mean WBC was 136/mm^3 and mean protein was 173 mg/dL.
- Glucose is usually normal (low glucose suggestive of infection).
- Oligoclonal bands usually not present in idiopathic TM, may be seen in 90% of MS or 30% NMOSD
- Serum and CSF NMO-IgG (aquaporin-4) antibodies should be investigated; longitudinally extensive TM (≥3 vertebral segments) is not as specific for NMOSD in children.
- Myelin oligodendrocyte glycoprotein (MOG) antibody syndromes can also cause NMOSD-like picture, although testing not universally available.
- Longitudinally extensive TM (T2 hyperintense lesion spanning ≥3 segments) is typical of idiopathic TM or NMO, not MS.
- Selective enhancement of the nerve roots without cord involvement suggests GBS.

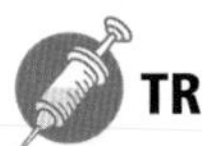

TREATMENT

GENERAL MEASURES

- Most patients will have urinary and bowel dysfunction so this should be assessed proactively and an appropriate regimen (i.e., intermittent catheterization, bowel regimen) be implemented.
- Short-term and long-term pain management plans may be indicated.

MEDICATION

There are no rigorous controlled studies in children with TM or U.S. Food and Drug Administration (FDA) approved treatments of acute TM; most data come from experience and retrospective studies.

First Line

- Methylprednisolone IV (dose: 30 mg/kg/24 h or a maximum dose of 1 g/24 h) or an oral equivalent is recommended initial treatment for noninfectious TM.
- Typical treatment length is 3 to 5 days followed by oral corticosteroid taper starting at dose of 1 mg/kg/24 h (maximum 60 mg/24 h prednisone equivalent) over 3 to 4 weeks.

Second Line

- If steroids are not effective or contraindicated, plasma exchange (PLEX) is an alternative. Evidence exists for efficacy of PLEX treatment in children (especially in TM associated with NMOSD). Typically, five to seven exchanges (1.1 to 1.5 plasma volumes) are performed. In severe cases (significant visual or motor impairment), consider concurrent use of PLEX and IV steroids.
- IV immunoglobulin G (IVIG; dose: 2 g/kg divided over 2 to 5 days) is an alternative or adjunctive treatment.
- Cyclophosphamide (dose: 500 to 750 mg/m^2) administered once is reportedly effective in refractory TM cases and particularly effective for SLE-associated TM.
- Immunomodulatory therapies for MS can begin after acute treatment. Immunosuppression (e.g., rituximab or mycophenolate mofetil) is an option for TM due to NMOSD.

ISSUES FOR REFERRAL

- Follow-up with neurologist or PM&R physician for management of residual symptoms of TM including weakness, pain, and bowel and bladder dysfunction
- Neurologist can provide evaluation and counseling for risk of disease recurrence.
- If urinary symptoms are severe, consider referral to urologist/neuro-urologist.

ADDITIONAL THERAPIES

Physical, occupational, or speech/language therapists should be engaged as soon as possible to maintain function during hospitalization and assess indication for inpatient rehabilitation or provide recommendations for outpatient follow-up.

SURGERY/OTHER PROCEDURES

Spasticity not sufficiently treated with medication may improve with botulinum toxin injections; botulinum toxin may also been very effective in treating neurogenic bladder. Intrathecal baclofen pump could be considered in patients unable to tolerate sufficient doses of oral antispasmotic medications due to sedation.

COMPLEMENTARY & ALTERNATIVE THERAPIES

- Yoga, stretching exercises may improve spasticity.
- Acupuncture and biofeedback may be beneficial for pain management.

ADMISSION, INPATIENT, AND NURSING CONSIDERATIONS

- Acute onset of myelopathic symptoms warrants emergent testing and inpatient monitoring.
- Monitor heart rate, blood pressure, respiratory status closely with lesions affecting brainstem to upper thoracic cord given potential for autonomic dysreflexia and compromise of respiratory muscles.

ONGOING CARE

FOLLOW-UP RECOMMENDATIONS

Patient Monitoring

- Respiratory and autonomic dysfunction may require ICU level monitoring.
- Outpatient neurology follow frequency typically ranges from 6 to 12 months.
- If serum aquaporin-4 IgG is negative, consider repeating after 6 months.

DIET

Insufficient evidence to support any specific dietary regimen or restrictions. Optimizing vitamin D level (50 to 100 nmol/L) may be protective against future inflammatory events.

PATIENT EDUCATION

- Patient with TM should be counseled on possibility of exacerbation of prior symptoms with physiologic stress (acute illness, fever, dehydration, sleep deprivation).
- Any new symptoms warrant evaluation for new inflammatory event.

PROGNOSIS

- Children generally have a better outcome than adults with idiopathic TM with one half making a full recovery within 2 years.
- Pain and motor deficits often improve before bladder function and sensory deficits.
- 40% have some form of persistent disability; 20% may have significant residual disabilities (nonambulatory, require urinary catheterization).
- Recovery can occur even after many years with continued rehabilitation therapy.
- Factors associated with poor prognosis include onset in infancy, short time to maximal deficits, long time of peak neurologic deficits, need for ventilation, and secondary infection.
- Mortality due to acute TM is <5% and associated with respiratory failure and high cervical lesion.

COMPLICATIONS

- Recurrent urinary tract infections related to neurogenic lower urinary tract dysfunction may lead to vesiculoureteral reflex and renal failure.
- Lack of mobility may increase risk for deep venous thrombosis, pulmonary embolism, and pressure ulcers.

ADDITIONAL READING

- Absoud M, Greenberg BM, Lim M, et al. Pediatric transverse myelitis. *Neurology*. 2016;87(9 Suppl 2): S46–S52.
- Deiva K, Absoud M, Hemingway C, et al; for United Kingdom Childhood Inflammatory Demyelination Study and French Kidbiosep Study. Acute idiopathic transverse myelitis in children: early predictors of relapse and disability. *Neurology*. 2015;84(4): 341–349.
- Krupp LB, Tardieu M, Amato MP, et al. International Pediatric Multiple Sclerosis Study Group criteria for pediatric multiple sclerosis and immune-mediated central nervous system demyelinating disorders: revisions to the 2007 definitions. *Mult Scler*. 2013;19(10):1261–1267.
- Scott TF, Frohman EM, De Seze J, et al. Evidence-based guideline: clinical evaluation and treatment of transverse myelitis: report of the Therapeutics and Technology Assessment Subcommittee of the American Academy of Neurology. *Neurology*. 2011;77(24):2128–2134.
- Thomas T, Branson HM, Verhey LH, et al. The demographic, clinical, and magnetic resonance imaging (MRI) features of transverse myelitis in children. *J Child Neurol*. 2012;27(1):11–21.
- Wolf VL, Lupo PJ, Lotze TE. Pediatric acute transverse myelitis overview and differential diagnosis. *J Child Neurol*. 2012;27(11):1426–1436.

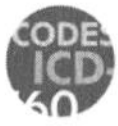

CODES

ICD10

- G37.3 Acute transverse myelitis in demyelinating disease of central nervous system
- A89 Unspecified viral infection of central nervous system

FAQ

- Q: What is the typical clinical timeline of TM?
- A: TM symptoms typically begin over 2 to 3 days. Functional nadir can occur within hours to 1 month of onset. This nadir averages 7 days before recovery. Patient recovery can be rapid (within weeks) or span years.
- Q: What is the likelihood of recurrence?
- A: 60–80% of pediatric TM is monophasic. Approximately 15% of patients with TM will be diagnosed with MS or NMO and therefore would be at risk for a relapse.

TRICHINOSIS

Carolyn A. Paris, MD, MPH • George A. (Tony) Woodward, MD, MBA

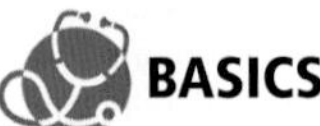

BASICS

DESCRIPTION

- Infection caused by ingestion of undercooked meat containing nematode (roundworm) larval cysts of the *Trichinella* genus
- Clinical disease in humans characterized by an intestinal phase followed by a muscular phase
- Extremely wide host range and geographic distribution

EPIDEMIOLOGY

- Historically, most U.S. infections are due to *Trichinella spiralis* in commercial pork.
- Currently, more U.S. infections are associated with wild game meat (especially bear) or through spillover to domestic animals.
- *Trichinella* parasites found in animals from all continents except Antartica
- Occasional grouped outbreaks (e.g., families and communities with common exposure)
- Reservoir hosts include rodents, domesticated animals (e.g., dogs, cats), raccoons, opossums, and skunks.

Incidence

- Estimated 10,000 cases per year worldwide, with a mortality rate of 0.2% in main 55 countries reporting
- Incidence worldwide highly variable due to variations in reporting and cultural and religious practices
- Between 2002 and 2007 in the United States, average of 11 cases annually
- Decreasing reported case numbers attributed to decline in prevalence of *Trichinella* in commercial swine (1.41% in 1900, 0.125% in 1966, and 0.013% in 1995), federal regulation preventing uncooked meat consumption by commercial swine, and increased public awareness regarding proper meat handling and preparation
- Likely underreported, particularly in developing countries with modest health controls

Prevalence

~4% of cadavers in 1970 study with evidence of previous infection (additional estimates range from 10% to 20% prevalence)

RISK FACTORS

- Consumption of inadequately cooked meat, even in small quantities
- Consumption of foreign meat (e.g., horse in France, dog in China) or wild game (e.g., bear, cougar, hyena, lion, panther, fox, horse, seal, walrus)
- Exposure to adulterated food (e.g., pork mixed in beef product)
- Traveling to underdeveloped countries
- Compromised immune status of host

GENERAL PREVENTION

- Consume only fully cooked meat, pork, and wild game; meat should reach >145°F internally, no pink color.
- Freezing kills *T. spiralis* in pork (<6 inches thick) at −20°F for 6 days, −10°F for 10 days, and −5°F for 20 days.
- Freezing may not kill other *Trichinella* species, particularly in wild game.
- Curing, smoking, salting, and drying meat (including jerky) are not reliable sterilization methods.
- Routinely clean meat processing equipment.
- Irradiation may not kill *Trichinella* but should prevent replication.
- Avoid feeding swine uncooked meat scraps.
- Actively control reservoir hosts (e.g., rodents).

PATHOPHYSIOLOGY

- *Trichinella* are obligate intracellular parasites capable of infecting warm-blooded animals.
- Currently 11 *Trichinella* species identified: *T. spiralis* (most common), *Trichinella nelsoni*, *Trichinella patagoniensis*, *Trichinella britovi*, *Trichinella* murrelli, *Trichinella* T6, *Trichinella* T8, *Trichinella* T9, (encapsulated species), *Trichinella pseudospiralis*, *Trichinella papuae*, and *Trichinella zimbabwensis* (nonencapsulated)
- Life cycle of all species comprises two generations in the same host (broad range of >100 species—mammal, birds, and reptiles), but only humans become clinically affected.
- Disease not transmissible person to person
- Larvae in undercooked meat eaten by the patient are released after cyst wall digestion by gastric enzymes, pass to the small intestine, invade mucosa, and then develop into adult worms.
- Incubation period is 1 to 2 weeks.
- Fertilized females release larvae (~500) over 2 to 3 weeks; adult worms do not multiply in human host and are expelled in feces.
- Newborn larvae travel the bloodstream to seed skeletal muscles, where they grow 10-fold, coil, encyst, and cause muscle fibers to enlarge and become edematous. Nonskeletal muscle may have granulomatous reactions, but larvae are found only in skeletal muscle.
- Cysts (hyaline capsules) may calcify over several months to years.
- Growing body of research on the ability of parasites to modulate the immune system and implications of this for immune-mediated diseases

ETIOLOGY

T. spiralis is the most common organism that causes trichinosis and is acquired by the consumption of raw or undercooked, infected meat.

COMMONLY ASSOCIATED CONDITIONS

- Rheumatic syndromes: polyarteritis nodosa–like systemic necrotizing vasculitis, symmetric polyarteritis, glomerulonephritis
- Immunocompromised hosts are at risk for more serious or prolonged infection.

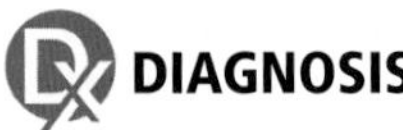

DIAGNOSIS

HISTORY

- Ingestion of inadequately cooked meat (commercial and noncommercial pork, game animals, foreign meat)
- Others with similar symptoms and same dietary exposure
- Signs and symptoms
  - Clinical severity varies, from asymptomatic (most common) to fatal (rare); depends on *Trichinella* species and inoculum size
  - Children often have fewer and milder symptoms than adults.
  - Many signs and symptoms (i.e., periorbital and muscle edema, eosinophilia) due to allergic reaction to parasite antigens
  - Nonspecific signs and symptoms may mimic other illnesses.
  - Enteral phase (24 hours to 7 days after infection): symptoms due to intestinal ulceration from mucosal invasion by adult worms
    - Diarrhea, abdominal pain, nausea, vomiting, anorexia
    - May persist for weeks
  - Parenteral phase (1 to 8 weeks after infection): symptoms due to systemic invasion
    - General: fever (begins at 2 weeks, peaks after 4 weeks, night spikes to 40–41°C), weakness, malaise, myalgias
    - Ocular: periorbital edema, subconjunctival hemorrhage, conjunctivitis, disturbed vision, ocular pain, chemosis
    - Muscular: myalgias, myositis (usually in extraocular muscles, then masseters, tongue, neck, limb flexors, lumbar muscles, intercostals, and diaphragm) with dyspnea, cough, hoarseness
    - Neurologic: headache, focal paralysis, delirium, psychosis
    - Skin: urticarial rash, subungual hemorrhages
    - Parenteral phase symptoms typically peak 2 to 3 weeks after infection.
    - Malaise and weakness may persist for weeks.
    - Cardiac: myocarditis, arrhythmias secondary to myocarditis
  - Convalescent phase is somewhat controversial (begins 2nd month, may last months to years): myalgias, muscle weakness

PHYSICAL EXAM
Fever, periorbital and generalized edema, muscular tenderness, urticaria, plus findings related to neurologic or cardiac involvement mentioned in "History" section

DIFFERENTIAL DIAGNOSIS
- Infection: viral syndromes, parasitic, spirochete, gastroenteritis, influenza, sinusitis, typhoid fever, measles, scarlet fever, meningitis, rheumatic fever, encephalitis, encephalomyelitis, poliomyelitis, tetanus, schistosomiasis, hookworm, strongyloides, or helminthic infection
- Miscellaneous: fever of unknown origin, dermatomyositis, myocarditis, inflammatory bowel disease, angioneurotic edema, rheumatoid arthritis, glomerulonephritis, polyneuritis, eosinophilic leukemia, polyarteritis nodosa, nonabsorption syndromes

DIAGNOSTIC TESTS & INTERPRETATION
Initial Tests (lab, imaging)
- Stool ova and parasite examination
- CBC and differential: leukocytosis (moderate) with eosinophilia (up to 70%, peaks 10 to 21 days postinoculation but prior to clinical symptoms)
- Elevation of muscle enzymes (lactate dehydrogenase [LDH], creatinine phosphokinase [CPK], aldolase)
- Specific anti-*Trichinella* antibody detection
- Serologic tests are available through the U.S. Centers for Disease Control and Prevention or state and some private labs.
- Detection of *Trichinella*-specific DNA by polymerase chain reaction (availability limited)
- *Trichinella* serology
  - Two tests required to ensure accurate diagnosis: first to detect antigen (enzyme-linked immunosorbent assay [ELISA]) and the second to detect antibodies to parasite surface antigens (FA)
  - Bentonite flocculation (1:5- or 4-fold increase), latex flocculation test, ELISA, or immunofluorescence
- Radiograph: may show calcified cysts in muscle (6 to 24 months postinfection) or enlarged heart
- EKG: Myocarditis may cause premature contractions, prolonged PR interval, small QRS with intraventricular block, and/or T-wave flattening or inversion.
- CT: small CNS lesions, IV enhancing ring calcifications
- Electromyography: Results resemble those of polymyositis and inflammatory myopathies.

Diagnostic Procedures/Other
- Skeletal muscle biopsy (especially deltoid or gastrocnemius muscle from the patient at least 17 days after infection)
  - Inflammatory cells surround encysted larvae in necrotic muscle fibers.
  - Granulomatous reaction present in nonskeletal muscle but not encysted larvae.
  - Usually unnecessary, negative result possible in infected patient due to sampling error
- Can test suspected meat if available

TREATMENT

GENERAL MEASURES
- Most patients recover without specific therapy.
- Symptomatic treatment: acetaminophen or NSAIDs, bed rest

MEDICATION
First Line
- Systemic corticosteroids for severe symptoms (not recommended as monotherapy, may prolong adult worm survival in intestines) *plus*
- Albendazole (Albenza®)
  - 10 mg/kg/24 h PO divided b.i.d. for 15 days
  - Max dose 800 mg/24 h
  - Teratogenic/embryotoxic in rats
  - Approved <2 years
- Mebendazole and albendazole are predominantly efficacious during the enteral phase (active against intestinal worms, little effect on muscle-embedded larvae).

Second Line
Pyrantel pamoate (Antiminth®)
- Used during pregnancy; not approved <2 years
- Effective only against adult worms, not encysted larvae

ISSUES FOR REFERRAL
Cardiac, neurologic, pulmonary complications

ADMISSION, INPATIENT, AND NURSING CONSIDERATIONS
- Admission criteria: cardiac, neurologic, or pulmonary complications indicate more severe disease
- Discharge criteria: resolution of cardiac symptoms

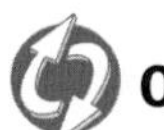

ONGOING CARE

FOLLOW-UP RECOMMENDATIONS
- Expect improvement over several weeks.
- At 3 to 4 weeks, retreatment may be indicated if symptoms persist or there are ova in the feces.

Patient Monitoring
Cardiopulmonary monitoring

DIET
Avoid further exposures.
- Breastfeeding may continue; the single case report of cessation of milk production was associated with parenteral mebendazole.

PATIENT EDUCATION
If concern for trichinosis exposure or symptoms, seek medical care early. Treatment is most efficacious the 1st week after exposure.

PROGNOSIS
- Mild to moderate illness usually resolves spontaneously with minimal sequelae. Muscle swelling and weakness may persist.
- Poorer prognosis (can be fulminant and fatal) with cardiac, CNS, or pulmonary involvement
- Children usually are less symptomatic, have fewer complications, and recover more quickly.

COMPLICATIONS
- Cardiac: myocarditis (may result in death 4 to 8 weeks after infection), secondary arrhythmias, hypotension, pericardial effusion
- Neurologic: meningoencephalitis, CNS granulomas, headaches
- Pulmonary: pneumonia, pneumonitis, pleural effusion, pulmonary embolism or infarct
- Renal: glomerulonephritis
- Hepatic: fatty change
- Muscular: prolonged myalgias
- Ocular: retinal hemorrhages
- Complications rarely are permanent.

ADDITIONAL READING

- American Academy of Pediatrics. Trichinellosis. In: Kimberlin DW, Brady MT, Jackson MA, et al, eds. *Red Book: 2015 Report of the Committee on Infectious Diseases*. 30th ed. Elk Grove, Village, IL: American Academy of Pediatrics; 2015:796–797.
- Bruschi F. Trichinellosis in developing countries: is it neglected? *J Infect Dev Ctries*. 2012;6(3):216–222.
- Gottstein B, Pozio E, Nöckler K. Epidemiology, diagnosis, treatment, and control of trichinellosis. *Clin Microbiol Rev*. 2009;22(1):127–145.
- Ilic N, Gruden-Movsesijan A, Sofronic-Milosavljevic L. *Trichinella spiralis*: shaping the immune response. *Immunol Res*. 2012;52(1–2):111–119.
- Murrell KD, Pozio E. Worldwide occurrence and impact of human trichinellosis, 1986–2009. *Emerg Infect Dis*. 2011;17(12):2194–2202.
- Ozdemir D, Ozkan H, Akkoc N, et al. Acute trichinellosis in children compared with adults. *Pediatr Infect Dis J*. 2005;24(10):897–900.
- Roy SL, Lopez AS, Schantz PM. Trichinellosis surveillance—United States, 1997–2001. *MMWR Surveill Summ*. 2003;52(6):1–8.
- Shimoni Z, Froom P. Uncertainties in diagnosis, treatment and prevention of trichinellosis. *Expert Rev Anti Infect Ther*. 2015;13(10):1279–1288.

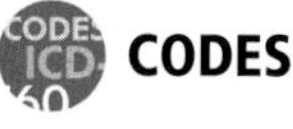

CODES

ICD10
- B75 Trichinellosis
- M63.80 Disorders of muscle in diseases classd elswhr, unsp site

FAQ
- Q: Is trichinosis contagious from person to person?
- A: No, except through infected breast milk
- Q: Do special precautions need to be taken when treating a patient with presumed trichinosis?
- A: Only thorough hand washing; no isolation required
- Q: What should we recommend for a patient who has eaten contaminated meat?
- A: Treatment with albendazole should be considered.
- Q: What are the classic hallmark signs of trichinosis?
- A: Diarrhea, abdominal pain, periorbital edema, myositis, fever, and eosinophilia, especially when combined with history of ingestion of potentially poorly cooked meat.

T

TRICHOTILLOMANIA

Carol A. Mathews, MD

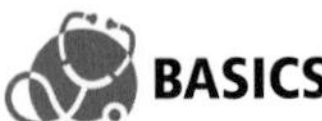

BASICS

DESCRIPTION

Trichotillomania (TTM) is the recurrent pulling out of one's hair resulting in hair loss. Pulling causes clinically significant distress or functional impairment, is accompanied by repeated efforts to stop, and is not due to another mental disorder or a general medical condition.

- Hair pulling can occur in any region of the body, but the most common sites are the scalp, eyelashes, and eyebrows. Other relatively common sites include the axilla, face, and pubic area. Sites may vary over time.
- Pulling can occur in brief episodes throughout the day or in sustained bouts.
- Automatic pulling is outside the patient's awareness.
- Focused pulling is in response to identifiable affective triggers.
- Some patients experience tension immediately before pulling or when attempting to resist the behavior, whereas others experience pleasure or relief when pulling.
- Patients may search for and pull hairs with specific qualities (e.g., thick hairs or short hairs).
- More than half of patients engage in a "ritual" with the hair before discarding it.
- TTM does not include habitual hair twirling.

EPIDEMIOLOGY

- Typical onset in childhood or adolescence: often coincides with the onset of puberty
- In childhood, girls and boys are equally affected.
- In adulthood, the ratio of affected females to males is 10:1.

Prevalence

1–3% lifetime prevalence

RISK FACTORS

TTM is more common in individuals with obsessive-compulsive disorder (OCD) and in their 1st-degree relatives.

Genetics

- A study of >5,400 female twins suggests that the heritability of TTM is ~30%, and that it has substantial genetic overlap with excoriation disorder (ExD), also known as skin picking disorder. Approximately 1/3 of genetic risk for TTM is shared with other obsessive-compulsive and related disorders.
- No specific genes implicated, although animal models of TTM exist

COMMONLY ASSOCIATED CONDITIONS

- Trichophagia (ingesting hair), which can lead to trichobezoar. It is estimated that between 5% and 18% of patients with TTM ingest their hair.
- Psychiatric comorbidity is common (seen in 1/3 to 2/3 of children with TTM) and includes autism, pervasive developmental disorder (PDD), anxiety, attention deficit, substance use, and eating disorders.
- Patients may also engage in nail-biting, skin-picking, or other pathologic grooming behaviors.

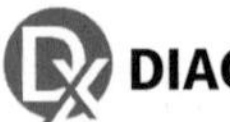

DIAGNOSIS

HISTORY

Patients may present with a complaint of hair loss or with concern regarding pulling behavior.

PHYSICAL EXAM

- Areas of hair loss do not show complete alopecia; instead, they contain hairs of different lengths, hairs with blunt ends, and remnants of hair bulbs. Hair density is normal in other areas.
- In some cases, pulling is widely distributed and hair loss may not be readily apparent.
- In children, patches of loss may be more prevalent on the side of the patient's dominant hand.

DIFFERENTIAL DIAGNOSIS

- Alopecia areata
- Tinea capitis
- Dermatologic conditions causing pruritus; normative hair removal (e.g., for cosmetic reasons)
- Other obsessive-compulsive or related disorders where pulling is part of a symmetry or other ritual
- Body dysmorphic disorder

DIAGNOSTIC TESTS & INTERPRETATION

Diagnostic Procedures/Other

Several instruments are available for clinical use; the Massachusetts General Hospital Hair Pulling Scale is one tool commonly used to monitor symptom severity and response to treatment.

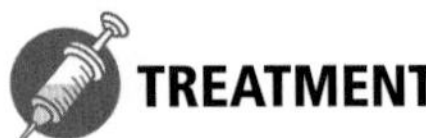

TREATMENT

GENERAL MEASURES

- Triggers should be identified and minimized with a focus on stress management strategies.
- Parent and family education about TTM and associated conditions is essential.
- The Trichotillomania Learning Center (www.trich.org) has valuable educational materials for patients, parents, and clinicians as well as a list of mental health providers with experience treating TTM and online programs focused on TTM treatment.

MEDICATION

- Few placebo-controlled randomized trials have included children or adolescents.
- *N*-acetylcysteine
  - A randomized controlled trial (RCT) of 50 adults demonstrated efficacy of *N*-acetylcysteine (56% of patients responded to treatment compared to 16% of patients on placebo).
  - A similarly designed study of 34 children showed no effect, with clinically modest but statistically significant improvements in symptoms in both treatment and control groups.
- Olanzapine
  - Has been shown to be efficacious in a study of 25 adults (85% of treatment group responded as compared to 17% of placebo group)
  - However, 84% of treatment group reported undesirable side effects.
- Selective serotonin reuptake inhibitors (SSRIs) do not reduce hair pulling but are efficacious for treating comorbid conditions and are used in some adults with TTM.

ADDITIONAL THERAPIES

- For mild cases in young children, reward systems or "home remedies" like a hat or adhesive bandages on fingers may help.
- Behavior modification programs, habit reversal training (HRT) methods, and cognitive behavioral therapy (BT) are the most effective forms of treatment.
- An RCT of 24 children showed sustained effect of BT (75% in BT group were responders as compared with 0% in minimal attention control group at 8 weeks; effect sustained over 8-week maintenance period).
- An RCT of HRT compared to treatment as usual (TAU) in 40 children resulted in a 76% response rate in the HRT group compared with 21% in the TAU group. Gains were maintained at 1 and 3 months' posttreatment in over half of the responders.

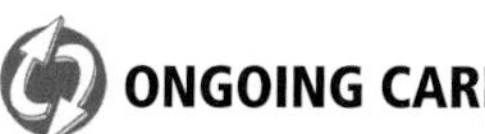

ONGOING CARE

FOLLOW-UP RECOMMENDATIONS

- Patients with TTM should be referred to a mental health professional with training in BT and, ideally, with experience treating patients with TTM.
- Online treatments can help in cases where mental health professionals with specific experience are not available.

PROGNOSIS

TTM often waxes and wanes, with symptoms reemerging at times of stress or transition.

COMPLICATIONS

- TTM can lead to significant academic, social, and developmental impairment.
  - 55% of children reported that TTM made it more difficult to study, and 35% reported academic impairment as a direct result of pulling.
  - 55% of parents of children with TTM reported that their child avoided social events as a direct result of pulling.
  - 80% of parents of children with TTM felt that their child's pulling contributed to another psychiatric problem.
- Trichobezoar resulting from trichophagia can cause serious gastrointestinal complications including obstruction and perforation.

ADDITIONAL READING

- American Psychiatric Association. *Diagnostic and Statistical Manual of Mental Disorders*. 5th ed. Arlington, VA: American Psychiatric Association; 2013.
- Bloch MH, Landeros-Weisenberger A, Dombrowski P, et al. Systematic review: pharmacological and behavioral treatment for trichotillomania. *Biol Psychiatry*. 2007;62(8):839–846.
- Bloch MH, Panza KE, Grant JE, et al. *N*-Acetylcysteine in the treatment of pediatric trichotillomania: a randomized, double-blind, placebo-controlled add-on trial. *J Am Acad Child Adolesc Psychiatry*. 2013;52(3):231–240.
- Duke DC, Keeley ML, Geffken GR, et al. Trichotillomania: a current review. *Clin Psychol Rev*. 2010;30(2):181–193.
- Franklin ME, Flessner CA, Woods DW, et al. The child and adolescent trichotillomania impact project: descriptive psychopathology, comorbidity, functional impairment, and treatment utilization. *J Dev Behav Pediatr*. 2008;29(6):493–500.
- Franklin ME, Zagrabbe K, Benavides KL. Trichotillomania and its treatment: a review and recommendations. *Expert Rev Neurother*. 2011;11(8):1165–1174.
- Grant JE, Odlaug BL, Kim SW. *N*-acetylcysteine, a glutamate modulator, in the treatment of trichotillomania: a double-blind, placebo-controlled study. *Arch Gen Psychiatry*. 2009;66(7):756–763.
- Monzani B, Rijsdijk F, Harris J, et al. The structure of genetic and environmental risk factors for dimensional representations of DSM-5 obsessive-compulsive spectrum disorders. *JAMA Psychiatry*. 2014;71(2):182–189.
- Novak CE, Keuthen NJ, Stewart SE, et al. A twin concordance study of trichotillomania. *Am J Med Genet B Neuropsychiatr Genet*. 2009;150B(7):944–949.
- Rahman O, McGuire J, Storch EA, et al. Preliminary randomized controlled trial of habit reversal training for treatment of hair pulling in youth. *J Child Adolesc Psychopharmacol*. 2017;27(2):132–139.
- Van Ameringen M, Mancini C, Patterson B, et al. A randomized, double-blind, placebo-controlled trial of olanzapine in the treatment of trichotillomania. *J Clin Psychiatry*. 2010;71(10):1336–1343.

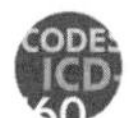

CODES

ICD10

- F63.3 Trichotillomania
- F50.8 Other eating disorders

FAQ

- Q: What are signs and symptoms of trichobezoar?
- A: Patients can present with abdominal pain, nausea, vomiting, weight loss, or gastrointestinal bleeding. Abdominal radiograph shows a characteristic abdominal mass, and hair may be present in the patient's stool.
- Q: Which patients with hair pulling behaviors should be referred for evaluation and treatment?
- A: Patients with patches of alopecia, distress related to their alopecia or pulling behavior, and those with deliberate pulling should be referred.
- Q: To whom should I refer patients with suspected or diagnosed TTM?
- A: Ideally, a psychologist or other mental health professional with training in BT, cognitive BT, or exposure-response management therapy.

TUBERCULOSIS

Andrew P. Steenhoff, MBBCh, DCH

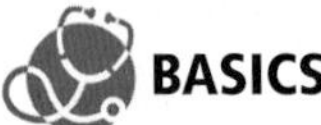

BASICS

DESCRIPTION

- Pediatric tuberculosis (TB) is the disease state caused by *Mycobacterium tuberculosis*, an acid-fast bacillus (AFB). Pediatric TB should be regarded as a spectrum of exposure through infection to disease because progression from an infected person (exposure) to infection and disease can occur much faster (within 1 to 6 months) in children <2 years of age (occurring within the incubation of the disease stated below).
- Progression through this spectrum depends on age; such disease progression being 40–50% for children up to 2 years old, ~20% for those 2 to 4 years old, and 10–15% for those ≥5 years old. 5- to 10-year-old children are the most protected age group. Adolescence is another vulnerable age group.

EPIDEMIOLOGY

- Most common route of infection is via the respiratory tract. TB is spread from a person with disease by droplet nuclei that are inhaled by other people. Infection occurs after close and prolonged contact with an adult or adolescent who has active untreated infectious disease, usually pulmonary TB, in a poorly ventilated space. However, there are people who develop TB without knowledge of an infectious contact.
- Congenital infection occurs, although rarely, in the setting of an untreated mother in the last trimester of pregnancy.
- Infection with the tubercle bacillus needs to be differentiated from disease (i.e., TB infection vs. TB disease).
- The interval between onset of TB infection (previously called "latent TB") and TB disease is usually 10 to 12 weeks. This interval is occasionally faster than 10 weeks and, not infrequently, may be significantly longer than 12 weeks.
- Following TB exposure, the greatest chance of infection occurring (i.e., of a positive result in tests using purified protein derivative [PPD], now renamed tuberculin skin test [TST]) is within the first 2 years after infection.
- The speed of progression through the spectrum of pediatric TB (exposure–infection–disease) is age dependent for infants and children <5 years of age (see "Description").
- Postpubertal adolescents and immunosuppressed people including people with diabetes, HIV, chronic renal failure, the malnourished, and those taking steroids for any reason have higher risks for progression of infection to disease.

GENERAL PREVENTION

- There are now several treatment regimens available for the treatment of TB infection in the absence of TB disease. The reader is referred to the Centers for Disease Control and Prevention (CDC) Web site in the "Additional Reading" section.
- Preferred regimen is isoniazid (isonicotinic acid hydrazide [INH]), 10 to 20 mg/kg/24 h PO for 9 months or, if compliance is not anticipated, 2 times a week as direct observed therapy at 20 to 30 mg/kg, with a maximum dose of 900 mg usually administered by a school nurse, child care worker, or the local TB control program, ideally without breaks in treatment, although the patient has 12 months to complete the course. If a break occurs near the end of treatment, it need not be restarted because such treatment is ~90% effective against development of active TB for 20 years in nonimmunosuppressed children. This recommendation prevents disease in the treated patient and, as a public health measure, interrupts transmission to contacts of that infected person with 90% efficacy.
- Other drugs for latent TB when INH cannot be tolerated or case patient has INH-resistant but rifampicin-susceptible TB include 6 months of rifampin 10 to 20 mg/kg by direct observed therapy (for a total of 180 doses).
- For adults and children 12 years and older, a once-weekly 3-month course of INH and rifapentine can be considered via direct observed therapy (12 doses total).
- Bacillus Calmette-Guérin (BCG) vaccine is recommended in the United States only for infants and children who test negative to PPD and who are continually exposed to and cannot be separated from either (i) contagious adults or (ii) adults with TB that is resistant to both INH and rifampin.

COMMONLY ASSOCIATED CONDITIONS

- HIV infection
- Lymphoma
- Diabetes
- Chronic renal failure
- Malnutrition
- Immunosuppression, including chronic daily steroid use, high-dose steroid use or tumor necrosis factor-α (TNF-α) agonists, cancer chemotherapy
- Social issues: incarcerated adolescents, infants, and children in homeless shelters

DIAGNOSIS

HISTORY

- Exposure: family member with TB or positive skin test
- Migrant farm workers
- Immigration from a TB-endemic geographic area (e.g., Haiti, Southeast Asia, Africa, South and Central America, Russia, and elsewhere in Eastern Europe, where greater concern about drug-resistant strains ought to be exercised); visit by individuals from those countries; or visited the above countries
- Higher incidence in Native Americans
- Contact with adults who have active TB
- HIV-positive people
- Immunosuppressed state
- Incarcerated adolescents and their relatives who visit
- Homeless people
- Poor people in urban areas
- Exposure to milk from untested herds
- Malnutrition
- Long-term steroid usage

PHYSICAL EXAM

- Cervical and/or axillary adenopathy
- May reflect underlying disease or state (e.g., HIV, malnutrition, long-term steroid use)
- Pulmonary rales or clear chest
- Enlarged liver or spleen
- Site-specific findings (e.g., gibbus [vertebral TB]) or focal neurologic signs (TB meningitis)
- Signs and symptoms:
  - Failure to thrive
  - Cervical or axillary lymphadenopathy without any other cause or that is prolonged
  - Cough >2 weeks
  - Weight loss
  - Change in sensorium
  - Fever in infants and adolescents, rarely in children 5 to 10 years of age
  - Decreased energy level/playfulness >2 weeks

DIFFERENTIAL DIAGNOSIS

- Malignancy
- Cervical or axillary adenopathy: nontuberculous mycobacteria, malignancy
- Pulmonary infiltrate: other chronic organisms, disorders, and conditions (e.g., *Nocardia*, histoplasmosis). Infiltrates owing to bacterial or viral pathogens resolve faster than TB; thus, reevaluation of a suspect in 8 to 12 weeks clarifies this differential.
- Hilar adenopathy: in TB, is usually unilateral, but Epstein-Barr virus, adenovirus, pertussis, and malignancy may possibly mimic symptoms
- GI disease: Most common differential diagnosis is Crohn disease.
- Meningitis: fungal meningitis, partially treated bacterial meningitis (rarely)

DIAGNOSTIC TESTS & INTERPRETATION

Initial Tests (screening, lab, imaging)

- Smear for AFB
- Culture for TB: sputum, three gastric washings (early morning) or induced sputum, pleural fluid, CSF, urine
- Culture may take 2 to 3 weeks by the radiometric method.
- Positive cultures are found in <50% of children. If MTB is cultured, the isolate should be sent for drug susceptibility testing to detect any drug resistance.
- Pathology of TB-infected tissue may show caseating granulomas and/or Langhans giant cells.
- Chest radiographs may show hilar adenopathy with or without atelectasis. However, any infiltrate or pleural effusion in a child with a positive TST result and a risk factor for TB should be considered a TB suspect until proven otherwise. Infiltrates from bacterial or viral pathogens generally clear within 6 to 8 weeks; TB infiltrates generally, do not clear so rapidly.

Diagnostic Procedures/Other

- Skin testing: TST
  - The Mantoux test comprises 5 tuberculin units with PPD administered intradermally. Details may be found at http://www.cdc.gov/tb.
  - The CDC does not recommend routine skin testing in low-risk groups in communities with low prevalence of TB.
  - Children at high risk should be tested annually:
    - Those in contact with adults from regions with high TB prevalence
    - Children who spend time in homeless shelters
  - Those in contact with adults with TB, HIV, and other disease-producing immunosuppressed states: A skin test result may become positive 3 to 6 weeks after exposure; however, most commonly, it does not turn positive for 2 to 3 months—hence the rationale for treating an exposed child with INH and retesting with a PPD in 3 months.
  - A positive TST is a Sentinel public health event indicating TB transmission in a community even if all other tests and examinations are negative.

- Interferon-γ release assays (IGRA) are being used with more frequency to diagnose TB exposure in children. These tests can be used as an alternative to TST in screening high-risk children; they are most helpful in children who have received BCG vaccine in the past, as these tests are more specific for TB. There are limited data on the use of these tests in children <4 years of age.
- A promising new molecular diagnostic test, Xpert® multidrug resistant tuberculosis/resistant to isoniazid and rifampin (MTB/RIF), is both simple and accurate but performs less well in children compared to adults. Selected laboratories do TB polymerase chain reaction (PCR), but this is not yet widely available.

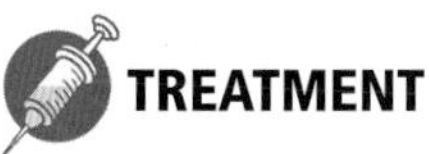

TREATMENT

GENERAL MEASURES

- Hospitalization (if the patient has disease)
  - In cases of extensive disease (e.g., miliary TB or meningitis), and when an adult source case is not known, aggressive attempts should be made to obtain an organism from gastric aspirates, induced sputum, lymph node biopsy, bronchoalveolar lavage, CSF, pleural or joint aspirate, bone aspirate, liver or tissue biopsy, and, in some cases, blood cultures (generally low yield).
- Isolation policies
  - Unless the clinician can verify that the parent or any adult visitors are not themselves contagious, many infection control units require isolation of the child because the family members' state of contagion remains unknown at admission.
  - Nonpulmonary TB (e.g., GI TB, meningitis, bone TB, and TB with joint involvement) does not require isolation.
- Of those with pulmonary TB, children >8 years of age and adolescents should be isolated until they are both smear negative and until they have completed at least 10 days of therapy. Occasionally, immunocompromised children <8 years old also have cavitary disease; and hence, they, too, should be isolated.

MEDICATION

- Initial treatment in areas with multidrug-resistant TB >4%: Until sensitivities are known, a 4-drug oral regimen should be started: INH, 10 to 15 mg/kg/24 h; rifampin, 10 to 20 mg/kg/24 h; pyrazinamide (PZA), 30 to 40 mg/kg/24 h; and ethambutol, 15 to 25 mg/kg/24 h.
- If the organism is sensitive to therapy, treatment with the initial four primary drugs should continue for the first 2 months; by then, all sputum specimens should have a negative result on culture, followed by 4 months of INH and rifampin. When this regimen is adhered to, favorable prognosis and a complete cure are achieved in 97–98% of patients.
- If sputum specimens continue to test positive, the initiation phase is longer. For meningeal TB, the duration of treatment is always longer (12 months). For bone TB, treatment is longer still (12 to 18 months).

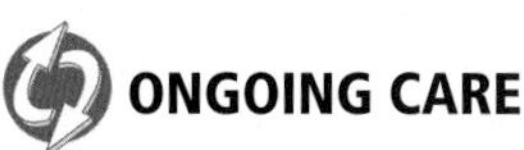

ONGOING CARE

FOLLOW-UP RECOMMENDATIONS

Patient Monitoring

Both follow-up and contact tracing are key to diagnosing, managing, and preventing TB.

PROGNOSIS

- Mortality for untreated TB is 40% over 4 years.
- For miliary TB and meningeal TB, prognosis depends on the stage of presentation.
- For outbreaks of multidrug-resistant TB, death rates range from 70% to 90% within 4 months of diagnosis.

COMPLICATIONS

- Missed diagnosis: failure to consider TB in a child who is failing to thrive and whose TST is negative
- TB meningitis: Outcome depends on the stage at which anti-TB medication starts:
  - If pharmacotherapy is started at stage I, complete recovery occurs in 94%, with neurologic sequelae in 6%.
  - If delayed until stage II, complete recovery occurs in 51%, with neurologic sequelae in 40% and death in 7%.
  - If delayed until stage III, complete recovery occurs in 18%, with neurologic sequelae in 61% and death in 20%.
- Miliary TB: at least two organ systems involved
- Bone TB: most commonly spinal manifestation
- Renal TB: presents as a fever of undetermined origin (FUO), with or without urinary symptoms, may have "sterile pyuria"
- Congenital TB manifests with hepatosplenomegaly; may have CSF abnormalities and abnormalities on CSF testing and chest radiograph. Patients are too young for TST to be useful.
- Drug toxicity: Pediatric patients are much more tolerant of anti-TB medications than adults; thus, regular monitoring of liver function test results is not routinely required, although clinical monitoring for symptoms such as abdominal pain and loss of appetite on a monthly basis remains the cornerstone for identifying any toxicity.
- Hepatitis with INH, rifampin, and pyrazinamide; neurologic and hematologic complications with INH; skin rashes predominantly with rifampin and INH, but reports have occurred with all anti-TB medications; ototoxicity with streptomycin; but ocular toxicity with ethambutol in the pediatric age group has not been documented, and therefore it is a safe drug to use. Management of common side effects and drug interactions may be found in the 2006 American Thoracic Society/CDC/Infectious Diseases Society of America statements (see "Additional Reading").

ADDITIONAL READING

- Boehme CC, Nabeta P, Hillemann D, et al. Rapid molecular detection of tuberculosis and rifampin resistance. *N Engl J Med*. 2010;363(11):1005–1015.
- Centers for Disease Control and Prevention. Drug-resistant TB. https://www.cdc.gov/tb/topic/drtb/default.htm. Accessed June 7, 2018.
- Centers for Disease Control and Prevention. Latent tuberculosis infection: a guide for primary health care providers. https://www.cdc.gov/tb/publications/ltbi/default.htm. Accessed June 7, 2018.
- Cruz AT, Starke JR, Lobato MN. Old and new approaches to diagnosing and treating latent tuberculosis in children in low-incidence countries. *Curr Opin Pediatr*. 2014;26(1):106–113.
- Lewinsonh DM, Leonard MK, LoBue PA, et al. Official American Thoracic Society/Infectious Diseases Society of America/Centers for Disease Control and Prevention clinical practice guidelines: diagnosis of tuberculosis in adults and children. *Clin Infect Dis*. 2017;64(2):111–115.
- Nahid P, Dorman SE, Alipanah N, et al. Official American Thoracic Society/Centers for Disease Control and Prevention/Infectious Diseases Society of America clinical practice guidelines: treatment of drug-susceptible tuberculosis. *Clin Infect Dis*. 2016;63(7):e147–e195.
- Perez-Velez CM, Marais BJ. Tuberculosis in children. *N Engl J Med*. 2012;367(4):348–361.
- World Health Organization. Global tuberculosis report 2016. http://apps.who.int/medicinedocs/en/d/Js23098en/. Accessed June 7, 2018.
- World Health Organization. Use of high burden country lists for TB by WHO in the post-2015 era. http://www.tbfacts.org/wp-content/uploads/2016/06/high_tb_burdencountrylists2016-2020-1.pdf. Accessed June 7, 2018.

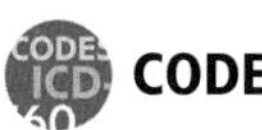

CODES

ICD10

- A15.9 Respiratory tuberculosis unspecified
- P37.0 Congenital tuberculosis
- A15.0 Tuberculosis of lung

FAQ

- Q: Should all children in close proximity to inner city areas with a prevalence of TB be screened annually with PPD?
- A: The American Academy of Pediatrics (AAP) and CDC encourage targeted screening based on risk factors indicated earlier. The targeted screening questionnaire should be administered at every visit until age 2 years then annually thereafter. See tools at http://www.cdc.gov/tb.
- Q: Can the whole blood assay, IGRA (e.g., "QuantiFERON-TB Gold"), be used instead of the TST to differentiate children who were born in other countries and had BCG?
- A: Yes. The IGRA tests can be used as an alternative to TST, although additional larger studies are needed to evaluate the test characteristics of IGRAs in children. See www.cdc.gov/mmwr/pdf/rr/rr5905.pdf and Cruz et al. in the section "Additional Reading."
- Q: What is the difference between "TB infection" and "TB disease"?
- A: TB infection (previously termed "latent TB") denotes TB infection which has been controlled by the body, is without end-organ damage, and can usually be treated with a single agent. TB disease encompasses TB infection with ongoing replication of organisms resulting in end-organ damage and usually requires four medications to treat with duration depending on the site of disease.

T

TUBEROUS SCLEROSIS COMPLEX

Francis J. DiMario Jr., MD

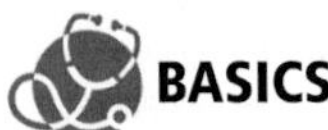

BASICS

DESCRIPTION

- Tuberous sclerosis complex (TSC) is an autosomal dominant, neurocutaneous, multisystem disorder characterized by clinical signs and symptoms that are highly variable and individual.
- Désiré-Magloire Bourneville has been credited with the first detailed description of the neurologic symptoms and neuropathology of TSC and coined the term "tuberous sclerosis of the cerebral convolutions" in 1880. Numerous other clinicians highlighted the clinical features now recognized as diagnostic of TSC.

EPIDEMIOLOGY

- Population studies have consistently approximated the prevalence of TSC to be 1 in 6,000 to 9,000 people.
- Noninherited sporadic mutation rates approach 65–75% of those affected with TSC.

RISK FACTORS

Genetics

- TSC is caused by mutations in two different genes.
  - *TSC1* identified on 9q34 and *TSC2* on 16p13
  - Genetic mutations in TSC to account for as many as 80–90% of those affected with identified genetic mutations; however, there remain up to 15% of affected individuals with no identifiable mutation.
  - The coating region of *TSC2* is 1.5 times larger than that of *TSC1*. This accounts for several differences in the types of mutations found within these genes. Missense mutations and large deletions and duplications are rare in *TSC1*, whereas these are relatively common in *TSC2*. Although there are no specific mutation "hot spots," individuals with *TSC2* have a higher prevalence of cognitive impairment, renal and cardiac lesions compared to *TSC1*.
- Because TSC is an autosomal dominant disorder, there is full penetrance but variable expressivity. Affected individuals carry a 50% risk of passing the disease on to each prospective progeny.
  - Gonadal mosaicism, where only the gonads and their affected gametes is the only affected organ with the TSC mutation, allows for multiple affected offspring from a parent who is otherwise "clinically unaffected."
  - The recurrence risk for all clinically unaffected parents with an affected child is estimated to be <2% due to this mechanism.

PATHOPHYSIOLOGY

- The protein products of *TSC1* and *TSC2* are hamartin and tuberin respectively. These proteins combine with a third intracellular protein, TBC1D7, to form the TSC protein complex.
- This protein complex in turn serves to regulate multiple cellular processes that includes suppression of the mechanistic target of rapamycin (mTOR) complex 1 (mTORC1). This latter complex is central to cell growth, proliferation, differentiation, metabolism, and cellular organization.
- Consequently, loss of function mutations in either TSC1 or TSC2 results in enhanced mTORC1 activation and increased cellular protein synthesis, anabolic pathways, and the cellular machinery for energy production.

DIAGNOSIS

- TSC should be considered in patients who are identified with any of the following:
  - Prenatally identified cardiac rhabdomyoma, infantile spasms
  - Autism
  - Cognitive impairment/developmental delay
  - Multiple hypomelanotic macules (often best identified using a Wood lamp)
  - "Acne" in a preteenaged child
- A definite diagnosis of TSC is made after the identification of two major or one major and two minor clinical features (see "Physical Exam" section).

HISTORY

- The earliest manifestation of TSC can be identified prenatally in the fetus as cardiac rhabdomyoma.
- Skin lesions are often the first clinically identifiable sign of TSC postnatally. Hypomelanotic macules (three or more) should prompt consideration of a TSC diagnosis.
- Cognitive impairment and behavioral problems are identified in 70–80% of patients with TSC.
- Autism spectrum disorders can be identified in 40–50% of those individuals. Patients who are affected with autism spectrum disorders or cognitive impairment have an additional prevalence of concurrent epilepsy approaching 90–100%.
- A family history that includes any of the clinical hallmarks of TSC can be significant for assessing an individual's risk of inheritance.
- Women of young adult age with TSC may present with a spontaneous pneumothorax or progressive dyspnea from pulmonary lymphangioleiomyomatosis.

PHYSICAL EXAM

- Major diagnostic criteria
  - Hypomelanotic macules (three or more at least 5 mm in diameter)
    - May be evident shortly after birth and gradually become more apparent in the 1st year to 2 years of life
    - When hair is contained within the macule, it also appears hypomelanotic and referred to as poliosis. Large macules with a pointed and rounded base are referred to as an ash leaf.
  - Cephalic plaques
    - Typically noted along the scalp line and forehead
    - They evolve into firm, raised, and waxy textured lesions that eventually harden and calcify by adulthood.
  - Facial angiofibromas (>3)
    - Often develop in early school-aged children
    - The initial erythematous macules later evolve into fleshy nodules around the nasolabial folds, nares, and cheek region.
    - These are present in 85% of patients >4 years.
  - Shagreen patches
    - May become evident in late childhood and early adolescence as elongated nummular patches with a puckered appearance that eventually resembles an orange peel surface
    - Most often seen along the lumbar flanks
  - Ungual fibromas (>2)
    - Generally adjacent to the nail or underneath it
    - May produce a longitudinal groove along the nail
    - Noted in 15–20% of people with TSC
  - Multiple retinal hamartomas (>1)
    - Present in about 20–25% of TSC-affected individuals
    - On direct ophthalmoscopy examination, a smooth translucent whitish-yellow patch along the retina near the optic nerve head. Alternatively, these can be raised, nodular calcified lesions.
  - Cortical dysplasia
    - Incorporates lesions identified as tubers and cerebral white matter migration lines on neuroimaging. They may be localized to several millimeters of cortex or encompass an entire cerebral lobe.
    - Identifiable in 80–90% of patients affected with TSC
  - Subependymal nodules
    - Located along the ventricular walls and evident on neuroimaging
    - Frequently exhibit calcification and most remain static in size
  - Subependymal giant cell astrocytomas (SEGAs)
    - Located within the frontal ventricular system in and around the foramen of Monro
    - Noted in approximately 10–15% of patients with TSC and have a higher likelihood of enlarging during childhood
    - By virtue of their location, obstructive hydrocephalus can be a consequence.
  - Cardiac rhabdomyoma
    - Primary benign tumors of the heart noted in 50–60% of patients with TSC
    - Infants born with an isolated cardiac rhabdomyoma have an estimated 80% risk of having TSC.
    - Wolff-Parkinson-White syndrome can be a complication.
  - Lymphangioleiomyomatosis
    - Most common pulmonary manifestation of TSC and is typically identified in women of childbearing age
    - Patients suffer from progressive exertional dyspnea, pneumothorax, hemoptysis, and respiratory insufficiency.
  - Angiomyolipomas (>2)
    - Benign tumors comprised of smooth muscle, vascular, and adipose tissues
    - Identified in 50% of young children with an increasing prevalence to 80% by adolescence and young adulthood
    - Most commonly identified in the kidney but may be seen in pancreas, spleen, and liver
- Minor diagnostic criteria
  - "Confetti" skin lesions
    - Identifiable as hypomelanotic macules smaller than 5 mm in diameter
    - Often clustered along the lower legs
  - Dental enamel pits (>3)
    - Almost all patients with TSC develop these in their permanent teeth.
  - Intraoral fibromas (>2)
    - Identifiable as fleshy protrusions of the gum between the teeth
    - They may disrupt tooth alignment but are more often a source of bleeding and are identifiable in 40–50% of patients with TSC.
  - Retinal achromic patch are small patches on the retina or along retinal vessels without pigment.

- Multiple renal cysts
  - Recognizable in 40–50% of patients with TSC
  - Identified as five or fewer in number with a mean diameter of 2 cm or smaller
- Nonrenal hamartomas are infrequently encountered and generally are without clinical consequence. Individual organ identification is considered as single criteria. These can be identified within the thyroid, pituitary, pancreas, gonads, and rectal polyps.

DIFFERENTIAL DIAGNOSIS

Neurocutaneous syndromes in which skin lesions, intellectual disability, and seizures are characteristic features should be considered:

- Neurofibromatosis
- Sturge-Weber syndrome
- Neurocutaneous melanosis
- Incontinentia pigmenti
- Linear sebaceous nevus

DIAGNOSTIC TESTS & INTERPRETATION

Initial Tests (screening, lab, imaging)

- All individuals suspected of having TSC on the basis of clinical suspicion should undergo further evaluation to confirm diagnosis.
- Genetic counseling with a three-generation family history is a first step and consideration for targeted genetic testing as confirmation.
- In infancy and early childhood, specific assessment of behavioral difficulties, autism spectrum disorders, and cognitive impairments should be assessed.
- Brain MRI
  - All individuals suspected of having TSC should undergo brain MRI with and without gadolinium to identify tubers, subependymal nodules, migration lines, and SEGA.
  - CT scanning or head ultrasound in neonates may be used when necessary but are considered suboptimal.
- EEG
  - All pediatric patients should have a baseline EEG when undergoing evaluation for TSC even when clinical seizures are not recognized.
  - Infantile spasms are associated with hypsarrhythmia; a pattern of extremely disorganized, bursts of high-amplitude asynchronous spike, and sharp waves
- Abdominal MRI
  - All pediatric patients should undergo baseline abdominal MRI to assess for the presence of renal angiomyolipoma and cysts.
  - Blood pressure measurements to screen for hypertension and renal function tests are also recommended.
- EKG
  - All pediatric patient should undergo baseline EKG to assess for conduction defects.
  - WPW arrhythmia can be identified among other disturbances. An echocardiogram is recommended for children age <3 years.
- Ophthalmologic exam
  - All pediatric patients should undergo ophthalmologic examination including dilated funduscopy to assess for retinal lesions and visual field defects.
- Pathologic findings
  - Findings reflect the primary tissue in which lesions are:
    - In tubers, the cerebral cortical architecture is disrupted, and these regions may undergo calcification, which can be visible on skull radiographs or brain CT.
    - Subependymal glial nodules (SENs) consist of large abnormal astrocytes emanating from the lateral ventricular surface.
    - SEGAs are low-grade benign astrocytic neoplasms.
    - Skin
      - Facial angiofibromas may be mistaken for acne and are highly suggestive of tuberous sclerosis; they appear as pinkish-yellow plaques on the malar regions and nasolabial folds.
    - Ash leaf spots are hypopigmented hypomelanotic macules occurring anywhere on the body.
    - Ungual fibromas are fleshy growths along the lateral borders of the nail bed.
    - Shagreen patches are areas of shaggy leathery skin typically in the lumbosacral area.
  - Retina
    - Whitish-yellow hamartomas occur near the optic nerve head or the retinal periphery and may calcify.
  - Heart
    - Rhabdomyomas in the ventricular walls and septum occur in infancy and contain abundant nodules of large eosinophilic cells. The majority regress by age 6 years; 4% of the time will occur in the absence of TSC.
  - Kidney
    - Renal cysts, polycystic kidneys, angiomyolipomas, and, more rarely, renal carcinomas

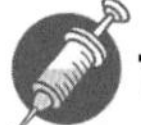

TREATMENT

MEDICATION

- Organ and symptom specific treatments are indicated (e.g., anticonvulsants for seizures).
- Clinical evidence supports the use of mTOR inhibitors in many TSC-associated disease manifestations, including SEGAs, renal angiomyolipoma, skin manifestations, and epilepsy. Everolimus is approved for use with SEGAs and angiomyolipomas.
- Vigabatrin is 1st-line treatment for infantile spams.

ONGOING CARE

FOLLOW-UP RECOMMENDATIONS

- Once a diagnosis of TSC is established and baseline evaluations completed, surveillance for progression of known problems or the development of new lesions is needed.
- Brain MRI with and without gadolinium is suggested every 1 to 3 years and asymptomatic TSC patients age <25 years. Patients with symptoms or growing SEGAs may need more frequent imaging to assess for obstructive hydrocephalus.
- Continued assessment for TSC-associated neuropsychiatric disorders should be obtained periodically throughout early adulthood.
- Abdominal MRI with and without gadolinium is suggested every 1 to 3 years throughout life to assess for the presence and potential progression of angiomyolipoma. Yearly blood pressure measurements and renal function testing is also suggested.
- Clinical screening and high-resolution CT scanning should be obtained by late adolescence and every 5 to 10 years in asymptomatic individuals at risk for lymphangioleiomyomatosis.
- Repeat echocardiogram every 1 to 3 years and asymptomatic pediatric patients with cardiac rhabdomyoma until regression is documented. Obtaining an EKG every 3 to 5 years in asymptomatic individuals of all ages is suggested.
- Annual ophthalmologic examination in patients with previously identified retinal lesions or visual problems at baseline is suggested.
- Routine EEG and prolonged video EEG should be determined by clinical need. Children with intractable epilepsy, especially after infantile spasms, may develop Lennox-Gastaut syndrome, an epilepsy syndrome that consists of cognitive impairment, prominent sleep-related tonic seizures, and an EEG pattern characterized by generalized slow spike wave (<2.5 Hz).

PROGNOSIS

Aggressive control of seizures can improve cognitive outcomes. mTOR inhibitors are under study for cognitive and epilepsy control.

ADDITIONAL READING

- Curatolo P, Bjørnvold M, Dill PE, et al. The role of mTOR inhibitors in the treatment of patients with tuberous sclerosis complex: evidence-based and expert opinions. *Drugs*. 2016;76(5):551–565.
- Curatolo P, Jóźwiak S, Nabbout R; for TSC Consensus Meeting for SEGA and Epilepsy Management. Management of epilepsy associated with tuberous sclerosis complex (TSC): clinical recommendations. *Eur J Paediatr Neurol*. 2012;16(6):582–586.
- De Vries P, Humphrey A, McCartney D, et al; for TSC Behaviour Consensus Panel. Consensus clinical guidelines for the assessment of cognitive and behavioural problems in tuberous sclerosis. *Eur Child Adolesc Psychiatry*. 2005;14(4):183–190.
- Franz DN, Bissler JJ, McCormack FX. Tuberous sclerosis complex: neurological, renal and pulmonary manifestations. *Neuropediatrics*. 2010;41(5):199–208.
- Krueger DA, Care MM, Holland K, et al. Everolimus for subependymal giant-cell astrocytomas in tuberous sclerosis. *N Engl J Med*. 2010;363(19):1801–1811.
- Krueger DA, Northrup H; for International Tuberous Sclerosis Complex Consensus Group. Tuberous sclerosis complex surveillance and management: recommendations of the 2012 International Tuberous Sclerosis Complex Consensus Conference. *Pediatr Neurol*. 2013;49(4):255–265.
- Northrup H, Kruger DA, on behalf of the International Tuberous Sclerosis Complex Consensus Group. Tuberous sclerosis complex diagnostic criteria update: recommendations of the 2012 International Tuberous Sclerosis Complex Consensus Conference. *Pediatr Neurol*. 2013;49(4):243–254.

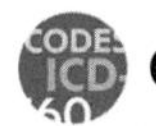

CODES

ICD10

Q85.1 Tuberous sclerosis

FAQ

- Q: Can tuberous sclerosis be transmitted in subsequent pregnancies?
- A: An affected patient with the tuberous sclerosis gene mutation has a 50% chance of transmitting the mutation to his or her children.
- Q: Is genetic testing available?
- A: Molecular genetic testing for mutations at the *TSC1* and *TSC2* loci are available but are not required for diagnosis because not all clinical cases of TSC have identifiable mutations.
- Q: Will my child need brain surgery?
- A: In the event of refractory seizures, removal of cortical tubers may help seizure control. Surgery may also be indicated in cases of obstructive hydrocephalus. If a brain tumor is detected by MRI, neurosurgical evaluation is indicated.

T

TULAREMIA

Amaran Moodley, MD

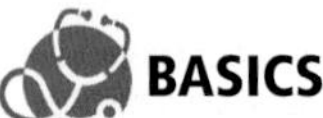

BASICS

DESCRIPTION

- Tularemia is an infection caused by *Francisella tularensis*, often presenting with fever, myalgia, and headache 3 to 6 days after initial exposure. The extent of the illness depends on infecting dose, subspecies, and route of entry.
- Six clinical forms are typically described:
  - Ulceroglandular tularemia
    - Constitutes 75% of all cases
    - A papule, which ruptures and ulcerates, occurs at the site of entry.
  - Glandular tularemia
    - Identical to the ulceroglandular form however does not have an identified primary skin lesion
  - Oculoglandular tularemia
    - Occurs when the organism gains access via the conjunctival sac
    - Usually from the patient rubbing the eyes with contaminated fingers
    - Yellow nodules and ulcers may appear on the palpebral conjunctiva associated with enlarged preauricular nodes.
  - Oropharyngeal tularemia
    - Occurs after the ingestion of contaminated food or water
    - An ulcerative or membranous tonsillitis accompanies a painful sore throat.
    - Lower GI tract involvement with vomiting, diarrhea, and abdominal pain may be associated.
  - Typhoidal tularemia
    - Presents with fever of unknown origin, without localizing lymphadenopathy or skin findings
    - Shock, pleuropulmonary findings, odynophagia, diarrhea, and bowel necrosis are often associated.
  - Pneumonic tularemia
    - Occurs after inhalation of the organism
    - It can also be present in association with ulceroglandular and typhoidal tularemia.
    - Pulmonary tularemia is the most fulminant and lethal form.
    - Symptoms include fever, dry cough, and pleuritic chest pain.
    - Tularemia in this form is a feared potential biologic weapon because an exposure to only 1 to 10 colony-forming units can result in infection. Although not transmitted person to person, laboratory workers working with organism on an agar plate are at risk for this form of disease.

ALERT

- *F. tularensis* is currently listed as a class A bioterrorism agent because of its potential ease for dissemination and infection as well as potential for high case fatality rates.
- In the past, resistant forms of *F. tularensis* have been engineered, but the actual use of this organism as a bioterrorism agent has not been documented.
- The diagnosis of inhalation tularemia should raise the suspicion of bioterrorism.

EPIDEMIOLOGY

- *F. tularensis* is found primarily in the Northern hemisphere from the 30- to 70-degree latitudes. Wild and domestic mammals (e.g., cats, rabbits, hares, squirrels, boars, beavers, deer, and rodents) may be infected as well as invertebrates (e.g., ticks, deerflies, horseflies, and mosquitoes).
- Humans acquire tularemia after a bite by an infected arthropod or through contact with tissues or body fluids of an infected animal. The subspecies *holarctica* has been shown to persist in various water sources, and waterborne transmission to humans has been reported.
- Inhalational exposure can happen in the laboratory setting or after the organism is aerosolized during meat preparation or certain outdoor activities.
- Most commonly reported during the summer months in children between 5 and 9 years of age and adults >55 years old with a male preponderance
- Annual incidence is 0.041 cases per 100,000 persons.
- U.S. states with an increased incidence in recent years include Wyoming, Nebraska, Kansas, South Dakota, Colorado, Missouri, and Arkansas.

RISK FACTORS

- Most frequently infected groups include hunters, trappers, farmers, and veterinarians.
- Activities involving wild animals or exposure to various arthropod vectors
- Tick exposure is a common mode of transmission in children in the United States.
- Infection has been linked to landscapers using lawn mowers and brush cutters.
- Laboratory personnel working with samples known to be or potentially infected with *Francisella*

GENERAL PREVENTION

- Isolation of the hospitalized patient
  - Standard precautions are recommended for protection against secretions. Human-to-human transmission has not been reported.
- Control measures
  - Protective clothing and insect repellent should be used to minimize insect bites.
  - Inspection for ticks and their immediate removal should be routine after outdoor activity in endemic areas.
  - Rubber gloves should be worn while handling or cooking wild animals (e.g., rabbits, lemmings) possibly contaminated with *Francisella*.
  - Game meat should be cooked thoroughly.
  - Laboratory workers should wear rubber gloves and masks in a biosafety level 3 environment when working with specimens potentially containing *Francisella*.
- Vaccine
  - Significant research into various vaccine techniques continues to evolve given concerns of *F. tularensis* as an agent of bioterrorism.

PATHOPHYSIOLOGY

- Human infection can result from various modes of entry:
  - Skin contact with infected animals
  - Vector-borne infection described after the bite of a tick (dog tick, wood tick, lone star tick), mosquito, horsefly, or deerfly
  - Inhalation of aerosolized organism seen in laboratory workers, crop harvesting, disturbance of contaminated hay, and grass cutting
  - Ingestion of contaminated food products or water
- A primary lesion develops at the site of exposure.
- Local tender lymph node swelling ensues.
- After skin inoculation or inhalation, the organism can spread via the bloodstream to various organs.

ETIOLOGY

Tularemia is caused by a small, fastidious, nonmotile, gram-negative coccobacillus; four distinct subspecies have been described:

- *Tularensis* (type A): found primarily in North America; causes the most severe cases of tularemia in humans
- *Holarctica* (type B): subspecies found primarily in Europe and Asia; less virulent than *tularensis*
- *Novicida*: rarely isolated but can be found worldwide
- *Mediasiatica*: recovered from ticks and animals in Central Asia; not associated with disease in immunocompetent humans
- An additional species, *Francisella philomiragia* (formerly *Yersinia philomiragia*), has also been reported. This is a rare cause of human disease and is possibly associated with salt water exposure.

DIAGNOSIS

HISTORY

- In the right clinical setting, a history of occupational exposure or recreational activity previously noted as risk factors should raise suspicion for tularemia.
- History of a recent tick or fly bite may be recalled among affected patients.
- A history of a papule that became ulcerated is classic for the ulceroglandular form.
- Fever >101°F for 2 to 3 weeks is common with associated weight loss, myalgia, headache, and fatigue.

PHYSICAL EXAM

- A papule or ulcer with raised edges may be seen at the inoculation site.
- Skin lesions should be sought, especially when lymphadenopathy is present.
- Lymph node swelling is typically tender with overlying erythema.
- Hepatosplenomegaly, purulent conjunctivitis, and tonsillitis are other localized findings.

DIFFERENTIAL DIAGNOSIS

- Depending on the form of tularemia, the infection can mimic other illnesses such as streptococcal or staphylococcal infection, cat-scratch disease, mononucleosis, cutaneous anthrax, pasteurellosis, Q fever, legionellosis, typhoid fever, or mycobacterial disease.
- In general, tularemia should be considered in the following differential diagnoses:
  - Fever of unknown origin
  - Fever with purulent conjunctivitis
  - Fever with hepatosplenomegaly
  - Fever with skin ulcer
  - Fever with painful lymphadenopathy, especially in the cervical or occipital region in children

DIAGNOSTIC TESTS & INTERPRETATION

- Serum tube agglutination titers of 1:160 or greater are generally considered positive. Patients do not develop antibodies until the 2nd week of illness.
- A 4-fold rise in titers over a 2-week period is necessary to define a current infection.
- Nonspecific cross reactions can occur in the presence of heterophile antibodies or specimens containing antibodies to *Brucella* species, *Legionella* species, or other gram-negative bacteria.
- Cultures of blood, skin, ulcers, lymph nodes, gastric washings, and respiratory secretions require special media containing cysteine.
- Laboratory personnel should be made aware of the infection risk from specimens. Growth of the organism requires a biosafety level 3 laboratory.
- Polymerase chain reaction (PCR) tests are more sensitive than culture; however, they are not widely available.
- Fluorescent in situ hybridization techniques have been used in the research setting to differentiate subspecies.

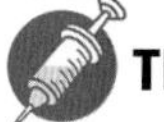

TREATMENT

MEDICATION

- IV/IM gentamicin for 7 to 10 days is considered 1st-line therapy in children.
- 2nd-line therapeutic options include streptomycin, ciprofloxacin, or doxycycline. Relapses have been associated with the latter two, and they are generally only used in adults or in specific situations. In severe disease, some experts recommend combination therapy such as gentamicin with ciprofloxacin or doxycycline.
- *F. tularensis* is resistant to β-lactam drugs and carbapenems.

ADMISSION, INPATIENT, AND NURSING CONSIDERATIONS

- If respiratory compromise is present, oxygen supplementation and/or assisted ventilation may be required.
- Recognition and prompt aggressive treatment of shock should be a major priority.

ONGOING CARE

PROGNOSIS

- When recognized and treated with appropriate antibiotics, the course is generally <1 month.
- Mortality is low, except in cases of fulminant disease or in immunocompromised patients.
- The subspecies *tularensis* is thought to be more virulent than the others.
- Both typhoidal and pneumonic forms of tularemia are associated with the highest risk for mortality.

COMPLICATIONS

- Lymph node suppuration, meningitis, endocarditis, hepatitis, and renal failure have all been associated with tularemia. Lymph node suppuration despite adequate therapy may occur in up to 25% of patients with ulceroglandular or glandular disease.
- Infection with *F. tularensis* may be complicated by necrotic and granulomatous lesions in the liver and spleen as well as parenchymal degeneration.
- A sepsis syndrome with shock, fever, myalgia, and severe headache can be seen.
- Skin manifestations, including vesiculopapular rash, erythema nodosum, and erythema multiforme have been associated with tularemia.

ADDITIONAL READING

- Cross JT Jr, Schutze GE, Jacobs RF. Treatment of tularemia with gentamicin in pediatric patients. *Pediatr Infect Dis J*. 1995;14(2):151–152.
- Eliasson H, Broman T, Forsman M, et al. Tularemia: current epidemiology and disease management. *Infect Dis Clin North Am*. 2006;20(2):289–311.
- Nelson C, Kugeler K, Petersen J, et al. Tularemia—United States, 2001–2010. *MMWR Morb Mortal Wkly Rep*. 2013;62(47):963–966.
- Nigrovic LE, Wingerter SL. Tularemia. *Infect Dis Clin North Am*. 2008;22(3):489–504.
- Oyston PC. Francisella tularensis: unravelling the secrets of an intracellular pathogen. *J Med Microbiol*. 2008;57(Pt 8):921–930.
- Pedati C, House J, Hancock-Allen J, et al. Notes from the field: increase in human cases of tularemia—Colorado, Nebraska, South Dakota, and Wyoming, January-September 2015. *MMWR Morb Mortal Wkly Rep*. 2015;64(47):1317–1318.
- Snowden J, Stovall S. Tularemia: retrospective review of 10 years' experience in Arkansas. *Clin Pediatr (Phila)*. 2011;50(1):64–68.
- Weber IB, Turabelidze G, Patrick S, et al. Clinical recognition and management of tularemia in Missouri: a retrospective records review of 121 cases. *Clin Infect Dis*. 2012;55(10):1283–1290.

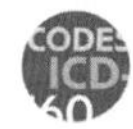

CODES

ICD10

- A21.9 Tularemia, unspecified
- A21.0 Ulceroglandular tularemia
- A21.1 Oculoglandular tularemia

FAQ

- Q: If a tick is removed from my child, should antibiotics be started?
- A: No. Empiric antimicrobial therapy will not prevent tularemia.
- Q: Can my child get tularemia again?
- A: No. It appears once infection has occurred, the patient is protected from future infections.
- Q: Where did tularemia get its name?
- A: Tularemia was identified in 1911 from squirrels who died of a plague-like disease. When attempts to culture the organism for plague failed, more selective media were used that identified the novel bacteria. The bacteria was named for Tulare County, California, the location where the bacteria was first isolated.

TURNER SYNDROME

John S. Fuqua, MD

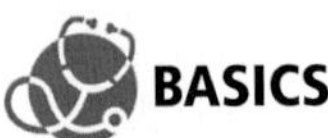

BASICS

DESCRIPTION

Presence of typical findings in a phenotypic female with complete or partial absence of the second sex chromosome

EPIDEMIOLOGY

Prevalence: 1:2,000 to 5,000 liveborn females

RISK FACTORS

Genetics

- Genotype frequencies
  - 45,X 55%
  - 46,Xi(Xq) 17%
  - 45,X/46,XX 13%
  - 46,Xr(X) 5%
  - 45,X/46,XY 5%
  - Other 5%
- Recurrence risk is low in subsequent pregnancies in the absence of familial X chromosome defects.

PATHOPHYSIOLOGY

- Deletion of the *SHOX* gene at Xp22.33 is responsible for the majority of the height deficit in affected patients.
- Fetuses with Turner syndrome have accelerated loss of germ cells from the second half of gestation through the first few years of life, with eventual gonadal failure.

COMMONLY ASSOCIATED CONDITIONS

- Short stature (~100%)
- Hypogonadism (90%)
- Sensorineural hearing loss in adults (60%)
- Hypertension (50%)
- Glucose intolerance in adults (40–50%)
- Autoimmune thyroiditis (27%)
- ADHD (24%)
- Conductive hearing loss (21%)
- Renal collecting system abnormalities (20%)
- Strabismus/hyperopia (17%)
- Bicuspid aortic valve (16%)
- Coarctation of the aorta (11%)
- Horseshoe kidney (10%)
- Celiac disease (6%)
- Aortic dissection (1–2%)

DIAGNOSIS

HISTORY

- Intrauterine growth retardation
- Slow postnatal growth, beginning in infancy
  - Eventual short stature
- Lymphedema, especially in infancy
- Frequent otitis media and middle ear effusions
- Normal overall intelligence, with performance IQ less than verbal IQ
  - Focused difficulties in math, visuospatial skills, executive functioning
- Decreased social cognition, with problems reading facial expressions, body language, and other nonverbal cues
- Lack of pubertal maturation for age, especially breast development

PHYSICAL EXAM

- HEENT
  - Down slanting palpebral fissures, ptosis, epicanthal folds
  - Low set, posteriorly rotated ears
  - Arched palate
  - Micrognathia
  - Neck webbing (pterygium colli)
  - Low set posterior hairline
- Musculoskeletal
  - Short stature
  - Wide carrying angle (cubitus valgus)
  - Short 4th metacarpals
  - Broad chest relative to height
  - Scoliosis
  - Genu valgum
  - Madelung deformity of wrist (bowed radial shaft secondary to deformity at the distal epiphysis of the radius)
- Other:
  - Increased number of pigmented nevi
  - Absent breast development, normal pubic hair for age
  - Edema of feet and/or hands
  - Hyperconvex fingernails, dystrophic toenails

DIAGNOSTIC TESTS & INTERPRETATION

Laboratory diagnosis of Turner syndrome is based on karyotype. Once the diagnosis is established, additional tests should be performed to identify associated conditions or complications.

Initial Tests (screening, lab, imaging)

- If >4 years old: TSH, free T_4, screening for celiac disease
- If >10 years old: TSH, free T_4, celiac disease screening, LFTs, fasting lipids, CBC, renal function, LH, FSH
- In all patients, regardless of age: renal ultrasonography and 2D echocardiography with color Doppler or cardiac MRI

Diagnostic Procedures/Other

- EKG
- Audiologic evaluation
- Orthodontic assessment
- Educational/psychosocial evaluation
- Scoliosis screening

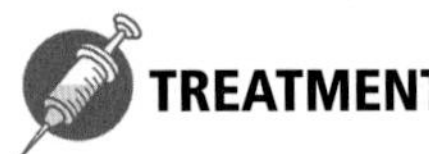

TREATMENT

GENERAL MEASURES

- Treatment of girls with Turner syndrome focuses on promoting linear growth and pubertal maturation as well as screening for and managing other associated conditions.
- Spontaneous puberty, manifested as breast development, occurs in 14% of girls with a 45,X karyotype and 32% of girls with other Turner syndrome karyotypes. Up to 50% of those with spontaneous puberty may go on to have menses that persist into late adolescence or early adulthood.
- Nearly all girls with Turner syndrome eventually have ovarian failure.

MEDICATION

- Growth hormone administration is part of standard care for girls with Turner syndrome.
  - Treatment should start when growth failure is recognized.
  - Recommended dose for girls with Turner syndrome is 54 mcg/kg/24 h or 0.375 mg/kg/week.
- Addition of oxandrolone, a nonaromatizable androgen, may be considered in girls >9 years to help promote growth.
  - This treatment may accelerate pubic and axillary hair growth, so oxandrolone is generally reserved for peripubertal patients.
  - The recommended dose is 0.05 mg/kg/24 h or less.

- Estrogen is required for pubertal-aged girls without spontaneous breast development who have elevated FSH levels.
  - Induction of puberty should ideally occur at a physiologic age but may be delayed to accrue additional linear growth. Early diagnosis and treatment with growth hormone should normalize height and make such a delay unnecessary, allowing for estrogen treatment at a normal age.
  - There are many estrogen treatment regimens available, including oral and transdermal routes. Treatment is usually initiated at doses that are 1/8 to 1/10 of the adult doses.
  - Doses are gradually increased to adult values over 2 to 4 years. After 2 to 4 years, intermittent progestin treatment is given to induce menstrual bleeding.

ADDITIONAL THERAPIES

Associated conditions may require treatment, including antihypertensives, subacute bacterial endocarditis (SBE) prophylaxis, levothyroxine, gluten-free diet, myringotomy tubes, and strabismus care.

ONGOING CARE

FOLLOW-UP RECOMMENDATIONS

- Age 4 to 5 years
  - Assessment of social skills, psychoeducational evaluation prior to school entry
- Age 5 to 12 years
  - Every year: blood pressure (BP), TSH, LFTs, educational and social progress
  - Every 1 to 5 years: audiology and ENT
  - Every 2 to 5 years: celiac disease screening
  - As needed: dental and orthodontic evaluations
- Age 12 years to adult
  - Every year: BP, TSH, LFTs, fasting lipids, blood glucose
  - Every 1 to 5 years: audiology and ENT
  - Assessment of pubertal development and psychosexual adjustment
  - Every 5 to 10 years: cardiac MRI
  - As needed: celiac disease screening

PROGNOSIS

- Height percentile at diagnosis is highly predictive of adult height if not treated with growth hormone or estrogen, with a correlation coefficient of 0.95.
- Height loss in untreated girls with Turner syndrome is approximately 20 cm compared to the midparental target height.
- Mean adult height in untreated girls is 144 cm.
- The presence of webbed neck (pterygium colli) on physical exam is predictive of both aortic coarctation and ovarian failure.
- Low antimüllerian hormone (AMH) concentrations may predict ovarian failure in prepubertal girls.
- 90% of women with Turner syndrome have ovarian failure.
- 40–50% of adults with Turner syndrome have insulin resistance or abnormal glucose tolerance.
- Girls and women with Turner syndrome have an increased risk for depression, anxiety, and social withdrawal.

ALERT

Girls and women with Turner syndrome are at increased risk for aortic dissection, manifested as chest or back pain. Those with a bicuspid aortic valve or with an ascending aortic size index >2.5 cm/m^2 are at highest risk.

ADDITIONAL READING

- Bondy CA; and Turner Syndrome Study Group. Care of girls and women with Turner syndrome: a guideline of the Turner Syndrome Study Group. *J Clin Endocrinol Metab*. 2007;92(1):10–25.
- Carlson M, Airhart N, Lopez L, et al. Moderate aortic enlargement and bicuspid aortic valve are associated with aortic dissection in Turner syndrome: report of the international Turner syndrome aortic dissection registry. *Circulation*. 2012;126(18):2220–2226.
- Cintron D, Rodriguez-Gutierrez R, Serrano V, et al. Effect of estrogen replacement therapy on bone and cardiovascular outcomes in women with Turner syndrome: a systematic review and meta-analysis. *Endocrine*. 2017;55(2):366–375.
- Davenport ML, Crowe BJ, Travers SH, et al. Growth hormone treatment of early growth failure in toddlers with Turner syndrome: a randomized, controlled, multicenter trial. *J Clin Endocrinol Metab*. 2007;92(9):3406–3416.
- Gault EJ, Perry RJ, Cole TJ, et al; for British Society for Paediatric Endocrinology and Diabetes. Effect of oxandrolone and timing of pubertal induction on final height in Turner's syndrome: randomised, double blind, placebo controlled trial. *BMJ*. 2011;342:d1980.
- Gonzalez L, Witchel SF. The patient with Turner syndrome: puberty and medical management concerns. *Fertil Steril*. 2012;98(4):780–786.
- Lunding SA, Aksglaede L, Anderson RA, et al. AMH as predictor of premature ovarian insufficiency: a longitudinal study of 120 Turner syndrome patients. *J Clin Endocrinol Metab*. 2015;100(7):E1030–E1038.
- Mårild K, Størdal K, Hagman A, et al. Turner syndrome and celiac disease: a case-control study. *Pediatrics*. 2016;137(2):e20152232.
- Pinsker JE. Clinical review: Turner syndrome: updating the paradigm of clinical care. *J Clin Endocrinol Metab*. 2012;97(6):E994–E1003.
- Ross JL, Quigley CA, Cao D, et al. Growth hormone plus childhood low-dose estrogen in Turner's syndrome. *N Engl J Med*. 2011;364(13):1230–1242.
- Schoemaker MJ, Swerdlow AJ, Higgins CD, et al; for United Kingdom Clinical Cytogenetics Group. Mortality in women with Turner syndrome in Great Britain: a national cohort study. *J Clin Endocrinol Metab*. 2008;93(12):4735–4742.

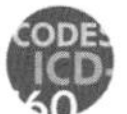

CODES

ICD10

- Q96.9 Turner's syndrome, unspecified
- Q96.0 Karyotype 45, X
- Q96.1 Karyotype 46, X iso (Xq)

FAQ

- Q: Are older parents at increased risk to have a child with Turner syndrome?
- A: No. Turner syndrome is not associated with either advanced maternal or paternal age.
- Q: Are there special precautions for girls with bicuspid aortic valve?
- A: Affected patients with bicuspid aortic valves should receive SBE prophylaxis.
- Q: Can assisted reproductive technology allow women with Turner syndrome to carry a pregnancy?
- A: In vitro fertilization of donor oocytes has been performed in women with Turner syndrome. However, pregnant women with Turner syndrome have a significantly increased risk for hypertension and gestational diabetes. Importantly, they also are at high risk for aortic dissection. Thus, pregnancy is controversial and usually discouraged at this time.

ULCERATIVE COLITIS

Naamah Levy Zitomersky, MD

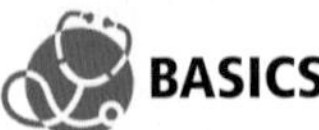

BASICS

DESCRIPTION

Ulcerative colitis (UC) is a chronic, relapsing, inflammatory disease of the colon, which extends continuously from the rectum proximally to a varying extent. UC is categorized as an inflammatory bowel disease (IBD), along with Crohn disease (CD). Unlike CD, UC does not affect the small bowel.

EPIDEMIOLOGY

- The incidence of pediatric-onset UC is between 1 and 4 per 100,000 children per year in most North American and European regions.
- Roughly 15–20% of patients with UC develop the disease before the age of 18 years.
- Incidence peaks between 15 and 30 years of age.

ETIOLOGY

The precise cause of UC, as with IBD in general, is unknown but is thought to involve both genetic predisposition and environmental triggers.

RISK FACTORS

Genetics

- Family history of IBD in ~15–20% of patients with UC
- Higher concordance in monozygotic than in dizygotic twins
- Genome-wide association studies (GWAS) have identified multiple loci associated with UC. Mutations in genes involving intestinal barrier functions are seen in UC more often than healthy controls.

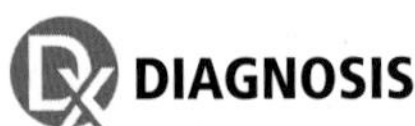

DIAGNOSIS

Patients with UC typically present with bloody diarrhea, tenesmus, and lower quadrant abdominal pain. When symptoms become severe, weight loss, fatigue, and vomiting can be seen. Colonoscopy with histopathologic review of biopsies is the gold standard in diagnosis of UC.

HISTORY

A detailed history is important in making the diagnosis:

- Rectal bleeding (90%)
- Abdominal pain (90%)
- Diarrhea (50%)
- Weight loss (10%)
- Growth failure
- Recent travel (enteric infections)
- Antibiotic use (*Clostridium difficile*)
- Family history of IBD

PHYSICAL EXAM

- Fever, tachycardia
- Evidence of weight loss or poor growth
- Signs of anemia
- Uveitis
- Mouth sores
- Arthritis
- Abdominal tenderness typically in lower quadrants or abdominal distention
- Perianal/rectal examination
  - UC is not typically associated with perianal disease, but hemorrhoids or rash from diarrhea can be seen.
  - Perianal disease (skin tags or fistula) are more common with CD, which can have a similar presentation.

DIFFERENTIAL DIAGNOSIS

- Infectious colitis: *C. difficile*, *Salmonella*, *Shigella*, *Campylobacter*, *Yersinia*, *Escherichia coli* (enterohemorrhagic), *Aeromonas*, cytomegalovirus
- CD
- Congenital Hirschsprung enterocolitis
- Bleeding juvenile polyps
- Milk protein allergy especially in infants
- Immunodeficiency states (rare), characterized by onset of colitis within the first 2 years of life, often with perianal involvement; skin folliculitis or eczema; other fungal or bacterial infections
- Solitary rectal ulcer syndrome
- Eosinophilic colitis
- Autoimmune enteropathy
- Hemolytic-uremic syndrome
- Henoch-Schönlein purpura
- Trauma due to anal sex or sexual abuse

DIAGNOSTIC TESTS & INTERPRETATION

Initial Tests (screening, lab, imaging)

- CBC
  - Iron deficiency anemia and anemia of chronic disease can be seen.
  - Thrombocytosis is another frequent finding.
- Iron studies (iron deficiency)
- ESR, CRP; disease activity (can be normal)
- Electrolytes (hydration)
- Serum albumin may be low; hypoalbuminemia may be present in fulminant colitis.
- Liver panel (hepatobiliary disease—primary sclerosing cholangitis [PSC])
- Perinuclear antineutrophil cytoplasmic antibody (pANCA)
  - Positive in 80% of UC patients, 20% of CD patients
  - This test is not typically needed to make the diagnosis.
- Stool for blood, white cells (colitis)
- Fecal calprotectin and fecal lactoferrin (leukocyte byproducts not typically present in stool): may be elevated during times of active inflammation
- Stool cultures:
  - *C. difficile*, *Salmonella*, *Shigella*, *Campylobacter*, *Yersinia*, *E. coli* (enterohemorrhagic), *Aeromonas*, amebiasis
- Plain abdominal radiograph
  - Important in diagnosing perforation, ileus, obstruction, and toxic megacolon
- Magnetic resonance enterography (MRE)
  - Can help identify small bowel inflammation not seen with endoscopy and colonoscopy
  - MRI may have a role in differentiating transmural and mucosal inflammation and is useful for demonstrating perianal fistulas more consistent with CD than UC.
- MRE is a preferred modality for imaging suspected or known UC in pediatric patients as it has the advantage of avoiding radiation exposure.
- CT enterography with low-dose radiation protocol is also used to look for small bowel inflammation to suggest CD.
- Previously upper GI with small bowel follow-through (UGI/SBFT) was used more often to exclude small intestinal inflammation indicative of CD. It is now used less often because it involves more radiation exposure.
- Right upper quadrant ultrasound may be useful for evaluating associated hepatobiliary disease if it is suspected (PSC).
- Endoscopic retrograde cholangiopancreatography (ERCP) or MRCP are also useful in diagnosing PSC (3% of UC patients).

Diagnostic Procedures/Other

- Colonoscopy (with biopsies) is the gold standard and is necessary to confirm the diagnosis of UC. It is critical to visualize and biopsy the entire colon, including terminal ileum, to differentiate CD from UC.
- Upper endoscopy may increase chances of detecting CD and may detect chronic gastritis sometimes seen with UC.
- Video capsule endoscopy (VCE) is more sensitive than UGI/SBFT for diagnosing small bowel disease indicative of CD rather than UC.
- Pitfalls:
  - Infectious colitis (especially *C. difficile*) can mimic the findings of UC so this should first be ruled out with stool culture. Recurrent *C. difficile* occurs frequently in UC.
  - Differentiating Crohn colitis from UC: Small intestinal inflammation and perianal disease (fistula, abscess) are more indicative of CD.
  - Serum inflammatory markers and CBC may be normal in children with active colitis especially with mild disease.
  - The combination of positive pANCA and negative anti-*Saccharomyces cerevisiae* antibody (ASCA) has a reported sensitivity of 60–70% and a specificity of 95–97% for UC in adults. The sensitivity and specificity are lower for pediatric patients.
- Pathologic findings
  - Chronic or chronic active colitis, with continuous inflammation limited to the mucosa
  - Crypt architectural distortion (branching), cryptitis (aggregation of inflammatory cells in the crypt epithelium), crypt abscesses
  - Site of colon affected:
    - Rectum (virtually 100%)
    - Left side (50–60%)
    - Pancolitis (10%)
  - Small intestine is technically not involved, but occasionally the terminal ileum of patients with UC can be found to have mild inflammation on radiologic or histologic examination. This finding is thought to be from refluxed colonic contents (backwash ileitis).
  - Skip lesions are not typically seen in UC. Some patients can have rectal sparing or a gap of inflammation in the transverse colon and a cecal patch of inflammation.
  - Chronic gastritis may be present in patients with UC.

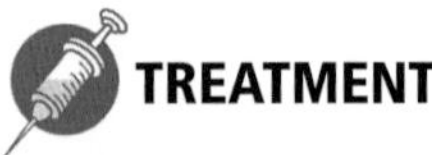

TREATMENT

MEDICATION

- Mild disease can be treated with oral mesalamine, topical corticosteroid enema or foam, or mesalamine enema/suppositories.
- For mild to moderate disease, Budesonide MMX® is a once-daily, extended-release budesonide, which has been shown to induce remission in adults with mild to moderate UC and has fewer side effects than systemic corticosteroids.

- For moderate disease, mesalamine, a short course of oral corticosteroid and the addition of an immunomodulators such as azathioprine or 6-mercaptopurine may help to maintain disease remission and minimize the need for recurrent steroid use.
- Antibodies against tumor necrosis factor (TNF)-α include infliximab and adalimumab; both are used in the treatment of moderate to severe UC or steroid-resistant UC.
- If treatment of acute symptoms with IV steroids fails (after 3 to 5 days), therapy with tacrolimus, cyclosporine, or infliximab can be started.
- Pediatric Ulcerative Colitis Activity Index (PUCAI): obtained on day 3 to 5; may identify patients with severe UC who will require escalation of therapy; prevents unnecessary prolonged exposure to corticosteroids
- Short-term medications for severe colitis should be used as a bridge to surgery or to transition to another steroid-sparing agent, such as an immunomodulator or biologic.
- Tacrolimus (PO) 0.1 mg/kg/dose every 12 hours with goal trough levels of 10 to 15 ng/mL after 2 days
- Cyclosporine (IV): 4 mg/kg/24 h for 2 weeks (Therapeutic levels vary depending on the technique used in the laboratory.)
- Cyclosporine (PO): 6 to 8 mg/kg/24 h for 6 to 8 months
- Tacrolimus and cyclosporine are both nephrotoxic; should only be used by experienced clinicians who follow serial blood pressures and electrolytes
- Trimethoprim/sulfamethoxazole should be given for *Pneumocystis jiroveci* (formerly known as *Pneumocystis carinii*) prophylaxis.
- 5-aminosalicylates:
  - Mesalamine (PO): 40 to 60 mg/kg/24 h (maximum 4.8 g/24 h)
  - Mesalamine (enema): 4 g at bedtime (for proctitis or isolated left-sided disease)
  - Mesalamine (suppository): 500 mg b.i.d.
- Corticosteroids:
  - Methylprednisolone (IV): 1 to 2 mg/kg/24 h (equivalent to prednisone 60 mg maximum)
  - Prednisone (PO): 1 to 2 mg/kg/24 h oral (up to maximum 60 mg/day)
  - For proctitis and isolated left-sided disease
  - Hydrocortisone enema: 100 mg once to twice daily
  - Hydrocortisone foam: 80 mg once to twice daily
  - Budesonide multimatrix system 9 mg/24 h orally
- Immunomodulators:
  - Mercaptopurine (6-MP) (PO): 1 to 1.5 mg/kg/24 h or azathioprine (PO): 2 mg/kg/24 h
  - Check thiopurine methyltransferase genetics or activity prior to initiation to avoid pancytopenia in those who lack this enzyme. Also monitor CBC and lipase every 2 weeks on initiation and with dosing changes to look for cytopenias or pancreatitis.
- Biologics:
  - Infliximab (IV): 5 mg/kg weeks 0, 2, 6 and then every 8 weeks; dose and frequency can be increased to capture symptoms.
  - Adalimumab (IM): for patients weighing 40 kg and greater, 160 mg on week 0, 80 mg on week 2, followed by 20 or 40 mg every 2 weeks starting on week 4. Reduce dosage by 50% for patients <40 kg.
- Anti-integrin
  - Vedolizumab (adult dosage) 300 mg IV weeks 0, 2, 6, and then every 8 weeks and can be increased to every 4 weeks to capture symptoms

ADMISSION, INPATIENT, AND NURSING CONSIDERATIONS

Hospitalization for fulminant disease:

- If concern for toxic megacolon—complete bowel rest with total parenteral nutrition
- Broad-spectrum antibiotics
- Discontinuation of anticholinergics and narcotics
- Avoidance of endoscopy
- IV corticosteroids
- Monitoring
  - Serial abdominal radiographs
  - Frequent examinations
  - Stool (frequency, amount of blood, and volume of stool output)
- Early surgical consult

SURGERY/OTHER PROCEDURES

- Patients with fulminant disease who fail medical therapy should be referred for colectomy.
- Patients with chronically active disease unresponsive to medication, growth failure, or with corticosteroid dependence should also consider colectomy.
- Because UC is limited to the colon, colectomy is considered a curative procedure. It also eliminates the elevated colon cancer risk.
- Sometimes surgery is urgently required for perforation, significant and persistent bleeding, toxic megacolon, and failure of medical treatment.
- Can be electively performed for chronic incapacitating disease, growth failure, corticosteroid dependence, dysplastic changes in the colon, or long-standing disease (usually after 10 years)
- Ileoanal anastomosis and pouch construction is surgery of choice for most pediatric patients.
  - Usually is performed in three stages over 6 months
  - 10% of cases are subsequently found to have CD after colectomy.

ONGOING CARE

FOLLOW-UP RECOMMENDATIONS

- Pediatric gastroenterology outpatient follow-up
- Important parameters to follow routinely include abdominal symptoms, rectal bleeding, stool frequency/consistency, height/weight, hemoglobin, WBC count (for patients on immunosuppressives), ESR, albumin, bilirubin, and liver enzymes.
- There is ongoing debate about monitoring for mucosal healing in UC. Adult studies have shown better outcomes, reduction in disease progression, and fewer complications in individuals who achieve mucosal healing.
- Colon cancer screening with colonoscopy should be performed within 10 years of diagnosis.

COMPLICATIONS

- Bleeding
- Anemia
- Toxic megacolon
  - A life-threatening complication of UC characterized by total or segmental nonobstructive intestinal dilation
  - The dilated colon is at risk of loss of barrier function and release of bacterial toxins into systemic circulation.
  - Plain abdominal radiograph shows a segment or total colonic dilatation. Risk factors include new diagnosis of UC, pancolitis, concurrent use of opiates and/or anticholinergics, and recent colonoscopy.
  - Diagnostic criteria include:
    - Radiographic evidence of colonic distension plus at least three of the following:
      - Fever >38°C
      - Heart rate >120 bpm
      - Neutrophilic leukocytosis >10,500/μL
      - Anemia
    - Plus at least one of the following:
      - Dehydration
      - Altered sensorium
      - Electrolyte disturbances
      - Hypotension
- Extraintestinal manifestations include hepatobiliary disease (3–5%), uveitis (up to 4%), arthritis affecting large joints (10%), spondylitis (6%), erythema nodosum (>5%), pyoderma gangrenosum (>1%), renal calculi (5%).
- Malignancy risk is 8%, 10 to 25 years after colitis is diagnosed and it increases ~10% for every subsequent decade.
- Colonic stricture
- Thrombosis:
  - Patients with IBD have a 3-fold higher risk of thrombosis compared to individuals without IBD. This risk rises further to 15-fold with disease flares.
  - Presentation with calf pain or shortness of breath should prompt evaluation for deep vein thrombosis or pulmonary embolism.
  - Anticoagulation with subcutaneous low-molecular-weight heparin should be strongly considered in hospitalized individuals with UC and those within 1 month of surgery.

ADDITIONAL READING

- Bousvaros A, Antonioli DA, Colletti RB, et al. Differentiating ulcerative colitis from Crohn disease in children and young adults: report of a working group of the North American Society for Pediatric Gastroenterology, Hepatology, and Nutrition and the Crohn's and Colitis Foundation of America. *J Pediatr Gastroenterol Nutr*. 2007;44(5):653–674.
- Hyams JS, Lerer T, Griffiths A, et al; for Pediatric Inflammatory Bowel Disease Collaborative Research Group. Outcome following infliximab therapy in children with ulcerative colitis. *Am J Gastroenterol*. 2010;105(6):1430–1436.
- Loftus EV Jr. Epidemiology and risk factors for colorectal dysplasia and cancer in ulcerative colitis. *Gastroenterol Clin North Am*. 2006;35(3):517–531.
- Turner D, Levine A, Escher JC, et al. Management of pediatric ulcerative colitis: joint ECCO and ESPGHAN evidence-based consensus guidelines. *J Pediatr Gastroenterol Nutr*. 2012;55(3):340–361.

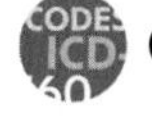

CODES

ICD10

- K51.90 Ulcerative colitis, unspecified, without complications
- K51.80 Other ulcerative colitis without complications
- K51.311 Ulcerative (chronic) rectosigmoiditis with rectal bleeding

UPPER GASTROINTESTINAL BLEEDING

Michael A. Manfredi, MD

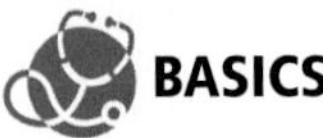

BASICS

DESCRIPTION

Upper gastrointestinal bleeding (UGIB) is classified based on its origin of bleeding being proximal to the ligament of Treitz. The classic clinical symptom is hematemesis which is emesis of bright red blood or coffee grounds. Other symptoms include melena, occult blood loss, and in the case of severe UGIB, hematochezia.

EPIDEMIOLOGY

- The incidence of GI bleeding in children is not well established in the general population.
- Large, prospective studies have assessed the prevalence of upper GI bleeding in pediatric critical care settings to range from 6.4% to 25% of admissions.
- 80% of UGIB stop bleeding spontaneously.

ETIOLOGY

- Neonatal period (birth to 1 month)
  - Swallowed maternal blood
  - Necrotizing enterocolitis
  - Duodenal web, antral web
  - Hemorrhagic disease of the newborn
  - Esophagitis
  - Gastritis
  - Stress ulcer
  - Foreign body irritation
  - Vascular malformation
  - GI malformation
- Infancy (1 month to 2 years)
  - Esophagitis/gastritis
  - Stress ulcer
  - Mallory-Weiss tear
  - Pyloric stenosis
  - Vascular malformation
  - Duplication cysts
  - Metabolic disease
- Preschool age (2 to 5 years)
  - Esophageal varices
  - Esophagitis/gastritis/ulcer
  - Foreign body/bezoar
  - Mallory-Weiss tear
  - Vascular malformation
  - Meckel diverticulum
- School age (>5 years)
  - Esophageal varices
  - Infection
  - Esophagitis/gastritis/ulcer
  - Mallory-Weiss tear
  - Inflammatory bowel disease
  - Drugs: NSAIDS, α-adrenergic antagonists
  - *Helicobacter pylori*
- All ages: liver failure—coagulopathy

GENERAL PREVENTION

- Avoid or minimize the use of drugs that can lead to peptic ulcers, for example, NSAIDs and aspirin.
- Correct coagulopathy.
- In patients with chronic GI conditions, optimize therapy and monitoring.
- Use prophylactic medical or endoscopic therapy in patients with a history of variceal bleeding.

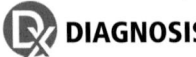

DIAGNOSIS

The initial evaluation of patients presenting with GI bleeding focuses on assessment of vital signs, history of present illness, focused medical history, physical examination, and lab testing. It is important for the clinician to differentiate upper GI bleeding from non-GI causes such as hemoptysis (coughing up blood), nosebleeds, and bleeding from the mouth and pharynx. Interpreting all of the above factors allows for early diagnosis, aggressive resuscitation, and timely management.

- General goals: Determine location of the bleeding and etiology, begin stabilization, and start treatment.
- **Phase 1:** Determine whether the emesis contains blood; red food coloring, fruit-flavored drinks and juices, vegetables, and some medicines may resemble blood. A pH-buffered Gastroccult test identifies blood in the vomitus.
- **Phase 2:** Assess severity of bleeding. Is there a change in vital signs, hematocrit, blood pressure (BP), capillary filling, pulse?
- **Phase 3:** Stabilize patient; decide if emergency treatment or referral is needed.

HISTORY

The key aspects in the medical history of patients who present with UGIB:

- GI symptoms:
  - May provide a clue to the etiology of the bleeding
  - Emesis prior to hematemesis may suggest Mallory-Weiss tear.
  - Odynophagia and GERD may suggest esophageal ulcer.
  - Epigastric pain may suggest peptic ulcer.
- Color of blood:
  - Emesis: bright red blood versus coffee ground
  - Stool: melena versus maroon-colored versus hematochezia
- Amount of blood
  - Drops versus 1 teaspoon versus 1 tablespoon?
  - May indicate severity of bleeding
- Duration of symptoms: may help determine if UGIB is an acute or chronic issue
- Medication history
  - The patient's current or recently used medications can help determine the cause.
  - Inquire about known gastrotoxic and/or antithrombotic medications (i.e., NSAIDs, aspirin, anticoagulants, etc.).
  - In addition, a history of medications in the house should also be obtained due to possible ingestion in younger children.
- Prior history of UGIB
  - May help determine the location of current bleed
  - If the prior bleed was recent, this may expedite proper specialty consultation with gastroenterology, surgery, and/or interventional radiology.
- Prior GI history
  - Gastroesophageal reflux, peptic ulcer disease, or previous GI surgery may suggest symptoms are due to recurrence of disease.
- Medical comorbidities
  - Liver disease may suggest portal hypertension and or coagulopathy.
  - Renal disease may suggest gastritis or angiodysplasia.
  - Renal failure or cirrhosis may suggest gastric antral vascular ectasia.
  - Recent stress (e.g., burns, head trauma, surgery) may suggest an stress ulcer or gastritis.
- History of alcohol abuse could suggest gastritis or Mallory-Weiss tear.

PHYSICAL EXAM

ALERT

- Assess for hemodynamic stability immediately.
  - Heart rate: Tachycardia may be an early sign of intravascular volume depletion.
  - BP: Hypotension is a late sign and may not be present even with significant blood loss, because vasoconstriction maintains BP until decompensation occurs.
  - In the setting of normal BP, obtain orthostatic BP.
  - Capillary refill: Delayed capillary refill suggests intravascular volume depletion.
  - Oxygen saturation: may be decreased due to decreased oxygen-carrying capacity
  - Evaluate for signs of shock:
    - Vitals signs
    - Cool clammy extremities
    - Poor mentation
- Abdominal examination:
  - Evaluate bowel sounds for evidence of possible bowel obstruction.
  - Abdominal tenderness which may suggest peptic disease
  - Ascites which may suggest liver disease

- Evaluate for signs of chronic liver disease of portal hypertension:
  - Hepatomegaly
  - Splenomegaly
  - Spider angioma
  - Caput medusa
  - Palmar erythema
- Rectal examination:
  - Heme-positive stool may or may not be present.
  - If positive, this may confirm the presence of upper GI bleeding.
- Skin examination:
  - Skin petechiae, ecchymosis, or hemangiomas may suggest a coagulopathy or a vascular anomaly.
- HEENT
  - Evaluate for nasopharyngeal source of bleeding.
  - Evaluate the buccal mucosa for syndromic findings: freckles (Peutz-Jeghers syndrome) and telangiectasias (Osler-Weber-Rendu syndrome).

DIAGNOSTIC TESTS & INTERPRETATION

- NG tube lavage
  - No longer required in patients with suspected upper GI bleeding for diagnosis, prognosis, visualization, or therapeutic effect
- Gastric occult blood testing (Gastrocult®)
  - If possible, confirm that visualized red substances are blood.
  - In neonates, may need to check for fetal hemoglobin with the Apt test—a test to identify fetal hemoglobin
- CBC
  - Initial hemoglobin values may be unreliable because a delay in hemodilution may falsely elevate values. Therefore, hemoglobin should be measured serially.
  - If leukopenia or thrombocytopenia is present, consider chronic liver disease and portal hypertension.
  - If anemia is present with normal erythrocyte indices, there is truly an acute cause for bleeding.
  - If erythrocyte indices indicate iron-deficiency anemia, consider varices or a mucosal lesion (i.e., chronic blood loss).
- Coagulation profile
  - If PT/PTT/INR are abnormal, consider liver disease or disseminated intravascular coagulation (DIC) with sepsis.
  - If DIC screen is negative, consider liver disease. Make sure, however, that blood sample was not contaminated with heparin.
- Liver function test results
  - Abnormal in chronic liver disease
- Barium tests:
  - Not useful in the acute setting and can actually obscure view if esophagogastroduodenoscopy (EGD) is performed for diagnosis and/or hemostasis
- Abdominal radiograph
  - Useful if suspicious for small bowel obstruction or foreign body
- Ultrasound: useful if portal hypertension is suspected
- Bleeding scan:
  - Useful in the patient with significant bleeding that precludes endoscopy or in whom endoscopy is undiagnostic
  - Technetium-99m tagged erythrocyte scan detects rapid bleeding at a rate of 0.1 to 0.5 mL/min; can be performed at 30-minute intervals for up to 24 hours
- Meckel scan: Technetium-99m pertechnetate tagged can detect a Meckel diverticulum that contains gastric mucosa.
- Angiography:
  - Useful in detecting vascular causes of upper GI bleeding; can also be therapeutic (i.e., injection of coils into a vascular malformation may occlude it)
  - Requires bleeding rate of 0.5 to 1 mL/min
- Upper endoscopy
  - Upper endoscopy has become the prime diagnostic and therapeutic tool for UGIB.
  - 90–95% sensitive at locating bleeding site

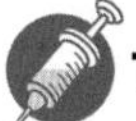

TREATMENT

GENERAL MEASURES

- Initial management:
  - Patients should be made NPO.
  - Have stable IV access.
  - Obtain blood type, and cross-match RBCs.
  - Stabilize the patient with IV fluids and blood products if necessary (target hemoglobin ≥7 g/dL).
  - Target INR <2.5
- Disease-specific therapy:
  - Peptic ulcer disease (medical therapy):
    - Proton pump inhibitors
    - H_2 blockers
    - Sucralfate
    - Prokinetic agents
    - *H. pylori* eradication
  - Peptic ulcer disease (endoscopic therapy)
    - Hemoclip
    - Thermal therapy
      - Bipolar
      - Argon plasma coagulation
    - Injection therapy with 1:10,000 epinephrine
  - Esophageal varices:
    - Octreotide infusion
    - Esophageal band ligation
    - Sclerotherapy
    - Sengstaken-Blakemore tube
    - Portosystemic shunts

ISSUES FOR REFERRAL

Immediate referral if bleeding is profuse, if patient is hemodynamically unstable, or if bleeding will not stop. Refer any patient with evidence of chronic iron-deficiency anemia and heme-positive stools.

SURGERY/OTHER PROCEDURES

- Patients with significant UGIB should generally undergo endoscopy within 24 hours of admission, following resuscitative efforts to optimize hemodynamic parameters.
- If rebleeding occurs after endoscopy or if endoscopy is unable to achieve initial hemostasis, then surgery or angiography should be considered.

ONGOING CARE

- Monitor hemoglobin in the hospital until patient's condition is stable.
- If bleeding has stopped, endoscopy should still be strongly considered to diagnose source of bleeding.
- Once patient is discharged, monitor patient's hemoglobin weekly as well as hemoccult cards until stable.
- More specific follow-up depends on the underlying condition.

ADDITIONAL READING

- Chawla S, Seth D, Mahajan P, et al. Upper gastrointestinal bleeding in children. *Clin Pediatr (Phila)*. 2007;46(1):16–21.
- Kato S, Sherman PM. What is new related to *Helicobacter pylori* infection in children and teenagers? *Arch Pediatr Adolesc Med*. 2005;159(5):415–421.
- Kim SJ, Kim KM. Recent trends in the endoscopic management of variceal bleeding in children. *Pediatr Gastroenterol Hepatol Nutr*. 2013;16(1):1–9.
- Pai N, Manfredi MA. Endoscopic Management of gastrointestinal bleeding in pediatrics. *Tech Gastrointest Endosc*. 2013;15(1):18–24.
- Uppal K, Tubbs RS, Matusz P, et al. Meckel's diverticulum: a review. *Clin Anat*. 2011;24(4):416–422.

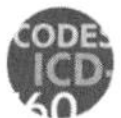

CODES

ICD10

- K92.2 Gastrointestinal hemorrhage, unspecified
- K92.0 Hematemesis
- K92.1 Melena

FAQ

- Q: When do you refer a patient with suspected active upper GI bleeding?
- A: Immediately, especially if the patient is hemodynamically unstable; urgently, in patients with evidence of chronic iron-deficiency anemia and heme-positive stools
- Q: What makes upper GI bleeding an emergency?
- A: Any persistent bleed with a change in vital signs and a significant drop in hemoglobin

URETEROPELVIC JUNCTION OBSTRUCTION

J. Christopher Austin, MD • Michael C. Carr, MD, PhD

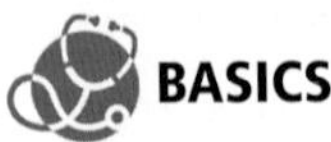

BASICS

DESCRIPTION

Ureteropelvic junction (UPJ) obstruction is a partial blockage of the kidney at the point where the renal pelvis transitions into the proximal ureter.

EPIDEMIOLOGY

- 45% of all cases of significant prenatal hydronephrosis are due to UPJ obstruction.
- Occurs more commonly in males (M/F 2:1)
- Left-sided lesion more common (66%)
- Bilateral in 10–40%

PATHOPHYSIOLOGY

- The obstruction can cause varying degrees of hydronephrosis.
- Mild forms of UPJ obstruction result in dilation of the renal pelvis without loss of function.
- More severe forms result in dilation of the renal pelvis and calyces with loss of renal parenchyma and decreased function.
- In the most severe cases, the kidney may have cystic dysplasia and very poor function.
- Congenital hydronephrosis owing to an intrinsic narrowing is nearly always asymptomatic.
- When the obstruction is intermittent owing to a crossing vessel, the renal pelvis becomes distended (most commonly owing to a transient increase in urine output), which drapes it over the vessel and kinks the ureter, resulting in an acute obstruction. The acute distention of the renal pelvis results in severe pain (renal colic).

ETIOLOGY

- Intrinsic: a congenital narrowing of the UPJ, which is most commonly due to abnormal musculature and fibrosis of this area, resulting in an adynamic segment
- Extrinsic: kinking at the UPJ, which is most commonly due to the renal pelvis draping over a lower pole crossing vessel. This type of obstruction can be intermittent.

COMMONLY ASSOCIATED CONDITIONS

- Patients with UPJ may have an additional genitourinary malformation, most commonly
  - Vesicoureteral reflux
  - Contralateral UPJ obstruction
  - Multicystic dysplastic kidney
  - Renal agenesis
- Of patients with VATER association, 21% have UPJ obstruction and thus should be screened with renal ultrasound. (VATER stands for vertebral defects, anal atresia, tracheoesophageal fistula with esophageal atresia, and radial and renal anomalies.)

DIAGNOSIS

HISTORY

- Antenatal
  - If unilateral, timing and severity of hydronephrosis and status of the contralateral kidney are factors.
  - When bilateral or affecting a solitary kidney, renal insufficiency is a concern.
  - The presence of oligohydramnios, increased renal echogenicity, and cystic changes are indicators of poor renal function and dysplasia.
- Postnatal
  - Feeding intolerance/respiratory distress (very rarely caused by UPJ obstruction)
- Older children
  - History of episodic abdominal (may not lateralize well), flank, or back pain
  - Length of episodes (usually 30 minutes to several hours); associated nausea and vomiting
  - Relation of episodes to fluid intake; history of urinary tract infections (UTIs) or gross hematuria

PHYSICAL EXAM

- Newborn
  - Palpate kidneys.
  - Affected kidney may feel enlarged but should not be tense.
  - A tense mass can indicate a severe obstruction and should be imaged promptly.
- Older child
  - Careful abdominal exam for enlarged kidney and tenderness
  - Costovertebral angle tenderness

DIFFERENTIAL DIAGNOSIS

- Vesicoureteral reflux: Higher grades of reflux will result in the dilation of the upper urinary tract.
- Megaureter: obstruction at the level of the bladder owing to ureterovesical junction obstruction, ureterocele, or an ectopic ureter
- Bladder outlet obstruction: dilation of the upper urinary tract secondary to obstruction of the lower urinary tract owing to posterior urethral valves, urethral atresia, or stricture
- Megacalycosis: congenital dilation and increased numbers of calyces without significant renal pelvis dilation or obstruction
- Multicystic dysplastic kidney: can be difficult to differentiate severe hydronephrosis from cysts by ultrasound. Renal scan will demonstrate no function in multicystic dysplastic kidneys.
- Triad syndrome: a triad of hypoplastic abdominal wall musculature, bilateral undescended testes, and dilation of the urinary tract (also known as prune belly syndrome or Eagle-Barrett syndrome)

DIAGNOSTIC TESTS & INTERPRETATION

- Newborn
  - If bilateral or a solitary kidney, serial assessments of renal function are necessary (serum electrolytes and creatinine), starting at 24 to 48 hours of age.
  - With a normal contralateral kidney, no immediate laboratory testing is necessary.
- Older children
  - Urinalysis to detect hematuria or pyuria; culture if infection is suspected
- Antenatally detected hydronephrosis: Infants with moderate to severe unilateral or bilateral antenatally detected hydronephrosis typically are evaluated with three imaging studies—renal/bladder ultrasound, voiding cystourethrogram (VCUG), and renal scan:
  - Renal/bladder ultrasound: In most cases, immediate imaging is not necessary. Because of a period of relative oliguria of a newborn in the first 24 to 48 hours of life, an ultrasound may underestimate the degree of hydronephrosis. This should not preclude evaluating an infant during this time as long as any normal study is followed up with a repeat study after 48 hours of life and <1 month of age. Evaluation should reveal the severity of dilation of the renal pelvis and calyces, changes in the amount and echogenicity of the parenchyma, and the presence of cortical cysts:
    - The evaluation of the full bladder is important for excluding dilated distal ureters, thickening of the bladder wall owing to outlet obstruction, and ureteroceles.
    - In cases of bilateral hydronephrosis, a solitary hydronephrotic kidney, or a tense kidney on physical examination, imaging should be promptly performed.
    - In older children with intermittent symptoms, it is now often used in place of an intravenous pyelogram (IVP) to evaluate for worsening hydronephrosis.
  - VCUG: This study will detect the presence of vesicoureteral reflux as well as exclude the presence of posterior urethral valves and other abnormalities of the bladder:
    - The test can be delayed until after discharge from the nursery unless there is concern about posterior urethral valves, in which case it should be performed early.
    - The presence of ureteral dilation on ultrasound strengthens the argument to perform a VCUG. The detection of vesicoureteral reflux, particularly in a circumcised male patient, may not confer benefit in their clinical management.
    - In cases of mild, unilateral hydronephrosis, the necessity of a VCUG is controversial and may be delayed until other imaging is completed.

- Renal scan: This study quantifies the differential renal function or the amount each kidney contributes to overall renal function (the normal differential is 50% ± 5% for each kidney) and gives information about how well the kidney is draining.
  - The two most commonly used radionuclides are mercaptoacetyltriglycine (MAG-3) and diethylenetriamine pentaacetic acid (DTPA). In addition to the ability to detect diminished function, if there is poor drainage of the affected kidney, furosemide is given to wash out the radiotracer.
  - The time for washing out half of the accumulated radiotracer (T1/2) is often given in the report.
  - A prompt T1/2 (<10 minutes) is indicative of a nonobstructed kidney.
  - A slower T1/2 may be indicative of obstruction when it is >20 minutes. An intermediate T1/2 (10 to 20 minutes) is indeterminate for obstruction. Owing to effects of hydration, the amount of hydronephrosis, and variables in the timing of the diuretic administration, the T1/2 may be unreliable.
- IVP: This study is being done less frequently due to the need for IV contrast and exposure to ionizing radiation. It is used to evaluate the anatomy of the kidney and the ureters:
  - It can also be used for evaluating an older child with intermittent symptoms if it can be done during a symptomatic episode.
- Magnetic resonance urography (MRU): A less commonly performed study that provides both anatomic and functional detail. Dynamic contrast-enhanced MRI requires sedation and placement of a bladder catheter. The images are obtained following infusion of gadolinium-diethylene-triamine pentacetate (DTPA). Furosemide is given at the start of the study. This study is being used instead of renal scans as a more precise study for deciding whether or not the child requires surgical repair.

TREATMENT

GENERAL MEASURES

- The decision to observe or surgically correct a UPJ obstruction depends on several factors. One must consider the age and overall health of the neonate, the amount of functional impairment of the kidney, whether it is a unilateral or bilateral process, the drainage pattern on renal scan, and whether or not it is symptomatic. There is no strict rule for who should be observed and who should undergo surgery. This decision should be made on an individual basis.
- Antibiotic prophylaxis
  - Newborns with severe hydronephrosis may be started on a once-a-day daily dose of amoxicillin (10 to 15 mg/kg daily) or cephalexin (10 to 15 mg/kg daily).
  - The antibiotic can be switched to trimethoprim (2 mg/kg daily), trimethoprim/sulfamethoxazole (2 mg/kg of trimethoprim daily), or nitrofurantoin (1 to 2 mg/kg daily) when patients are >2 months old.
  - The duration and indications that infants should be left on antibiotics is controversial, but infants with a UPJ obstruction and severe hydronephrosis are at increased risk of UTI.
- Observation
  - Infants with the hydronephrosis thought to be owing to a narrowing at the UPJ are typically observed when there is preserved function (>40%) in the affected kidney, and the contralateral kidney is normal.
  - The pattern of drainage is taken into account, and if there is prompt drainage and normal differential function (50% ± 5%), these patients are followed with less frequent follow-up studies than those with less function or poor drainage.
  - Most patients have follow-up imaging studies done at 3- to 6-month intervals during their 1st year of life, and they are gradually spaced out as time goes by if the hydronephrosis remains stable or improves.
- Older children with hydronephrosis owing to a UPJ obstruction are often detected during a symptomatic episode. If the UPJ obstruction is noted as an incidental finding and the child is asymptomatic with the function of the kidney preserved, the child can be observed clinically.

SURGERY/OTHER PROCEDURES

- The gold standard for the repair of the UPJ obstruction has been a pyeloplasty:
  - During the procedure, the narrowed UPJ is most commonly excised, and the ureter is reanastomosed to the renal pelvis.
  - This procedure is successful 95% of the time.
- Robotic or laparoscopic pyeloplasty is being performed in children and adolescents commonly now. Robotically assisted procedures are laparoscopic but involve using a surgical robot such as the DaVinci, which allows the surgeon greater dexterity and movement of the laparoscopic instruments and facilitates suturing. Both offer a similar rate of success to a traditional pyeloplasty with smaller incisions. The benefits are most significant for older children, but it has been safely done in infants.
- Less invasive approaches include endoscopically incising the narrowing (endopyelotomy) or balloon dilation:
  - These approaches have been used in adults with rates of success in the 50–70% range but are considerably less invasive.
  - Endoscopic procedures have not been routinely offered as a 1st-line therapy for the treatment of UPJ obstructions because of their limited experience in children and the lower rates of success.

ADDITIONAL READING

- Carr MC, Casale P. Anomalies in surgery of the ureter in children. In: Wein AJ, Kavoussi LR, Novick AC, et al, eds. *Campbell-Walsh Urology*. 10th ed. Philadelphia, PA: W.B. Saunders; 2012:590–593.
- Darge K, Higgins M, Hwang TJ, et al. Magnetic resonance and computed tomography in pediatric urology: an imaging overview for current and future daily practice. *Radiol Clin North Am*. 2013;51(4):583–598.

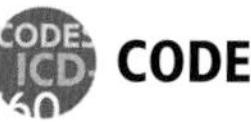

CODES

ICD10

- Q62.39 Other obstructive defects of renal pelvis and ureter
- Q62.11 Congenital occlusion of ureteropelvic junction
- N13.8 Other obstructive and reflux uropathy

FAQ

- Q: My unborn baby has hydronephrosis. My obstetrician told me that it is most likely a UPJ obstruction. Is my baby going to need surgery to correct this?
- A: Not necessarily; only ~1/3 of babies with significant hydronephrosis ultimately require surgical correction.
- Q: Will my child's kidney look normal after the surgery to fix it?
- A: Often the kidney has less dilation and an improved appearance but not completely normal. Of greater importance is that there is no longer obstruction, and the kidney function is preserved or improved.

URINARY TRACT INFECTION

Mercedes M. Blackstone, MD

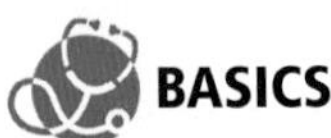

BASICS

DESCRIPTION

- Urinary tract infection (UTI) is defined by having pyuria and ≥50,000 CFUs/mL of a single urinary tract pathogen from an appropriately collected specimen.
- Upper tract infection or pyelonephritis: infection of the renal parenchyma; most febrile babies with a positive culture have upper tract infection.
- Lower tract infection or cystitis: infection limited to the bladder, not involving the kidneys; occurs more in older children and adolescents; usually no fever
- Cystitis and pyelonephritis can be clinically indistinguishable.

EPIDEMIOLOGY

- Bimodal age distribution with peak incidence in infants <1 year of age (40 per 1,000)
- Second peak in adolescent females
- Overall prevalence of about 7% in febrile infants and young children; varies according to risk factors below
- Higher prevalence in Caucasian girls

RISK FACTORS

- Sex/age: Boys are most at risk for UTI during 1st year of life; girls until school age and again in adolescence
- Circumcision status: Uncircumcised males <1 year of age have increased risk of UTI; prevalence is 10 times higher for uncircumcised males versus circumcised males <3 months of age.
- Race/ethnicity: Caucasian children are 2 to 4 times more likely than African American children to have UTI:
  - May be due in part to genetic differences in blood group antigens on the surfaces of uroepithelial cells, which affect bacterial adherence
- Abnormal urinary tract: Children with vesicoureteral reflux (VUR) are at higher risk for UTI.
- Poor bladder emptying (neurogenic bladder, obstructive uropathies) increase risk of bacterial growth in stagnant urine.
- Bowel and bladder dysfunction is a major risk factor in toilet-trained children.
- Requiring frequent catheterization
- Sexual activity
- Conditions that alter vaginal flora such as use of spermicidal birth control methods or recent antibiotics
- Clinical decision rule in febrile girls 2 to 24 months of age. Consider testing if ≥3 of following are present:
  - Temperature ≥39°C, fever for ≥2 days, non-African American race, age <1 year, absence of another potential source of fever

GENERAL PREVENTION

- Teach correct wiping—front to back—to young children.
- Consider prophylactic antibiotics for select children with recurrent infection, high-grade VUR, bowel/bladder dysfunction, and urologic anomalies.
  - There is controversy in the literature about the effectiveness of antimicrobial prophylaxis. It has not been shown to reduce renal scarring.
- Attention to good voiding and stooling habits; treat constipation.
- Consider single-dose postcoital antibiotics for adolescents with recurrent UTI.
- Cranberry juice has not been shown to help.

PATHOPHYSIOLOGY

- Flora from skin or gut ascend the urethra and adhere to the uroepithelium, triggering local inflammation.
- Various virulence factors make certain bacteria more likely to ascend and adhere.
- Shorter urethra in females may put them at increased risk; in young infants, can be from hematogenous spread

ETIOLOGY

Urinary tract pathogens

- *Escherichia coli* is responsible for >80% of UTIs in children.
- Other fairly common microbes include *Klebsiella* species, *Enterococcus*, and *Proteus mirabilis*.
- Less common: *Enterobacter cloacae*, group B hemolytic streptococci, *Citrobacter*, *Pseudomonas* species, *Staphylococcus aureus*, *Serratia* species, and *Staphylococcus saprophyticus* (teenage girls)
  - Viral or fungal causes of UTI also possible

COMMONLY ASSOCIATED CONDITIONS

- ~5–10% of babies with febrile UTIs (pyelonephritis) are bacteremic, but the clinical course is likely unchanged.
- Unless they are ill-appearing on presentation or have significant underlying medical problems, infants with UTI have a very low risk of meningitis or other adverse events.
- VUR, urinary abnormalities, bowel and bladder dysfunction

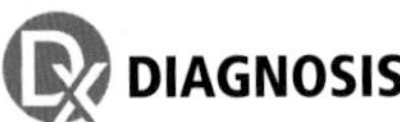

DIAGNOSIS

HISTORY

- Babies
  - Nonspecific symptoms, often fever alone
  - Can have vomiting, irritability, poor feeding, and lethargy
  - Rarely, failure to thrive or jaundice
- Older children
  - Classic symptoms of the lower tract include urgency, frequency, dysuria, hesitancy, suprapubic discomfort, hematuria, and malodorous urine. Classic symptoms of the upper tract include fever, chills, nausea, and flank pain.
  - May have history of constipation, poor voiding and stooling habits, incontinence
  - Can also present with secondary enuresis
  - Ask older children about sexual activity and contraceptive methods.
- Special question
  - Has the young child had a history of UTI, unexplained fevers, or urinary tract anomaly?

PHYSICAL EXAM

- Temperature and blood pressure should be documented.
- Babies and toddlers: often no physical findings or high fever alone
  - Less common: suprapubic tenderness, abdominal distention, poor growth or weight gain
  - Associated findings: may see evidence of foreign body, phimosis, labial adhesions, or midline abnormality of the lower back, which could indicate a neurogenic bladder
- Older children
  - Lower tract: suprapubic tenderness; may see evidence of constipation
  - Upper tract: fever; costovertebral angle tenderness

DIFFERENTIAL DIAGNOSIS

- True UTI can easily be confused with asymptomatic bacteriuria.
- The differential diagnosis of isolated or prolonged fever is very broad.
- Infants: gastroenteritis, occult bacteremia, occult pneumonia, meningitis, viral syndrome
- Older children and adolescents
  - Common: vaginal foreign body, vulvovaginitis/urethritis, epididymitis, gastroenteritis, sexually transmitted infection, pelvic inflammatory disease
  - Less common: excessive drinking, urinary calculi, diabetes mellitus or insipidus, appendicitis, Kawasaki disease, tuboovarian abscess, ovarian torsion, group A streptococcal infection
  - Rare: mass adjacent to bladder, spinal cord process (tumor, abscess), hypercalcemia

DIAGNOSTIC TESTS & INTERPRETATION

Initial Tests (screening, lab, imaging)

- Urine culture collected sterilely is the gold standard for diagnosis:
  - Bladder catheterization in young children (or less commonly, suprapubic aspirate)
  - Midstream clean-catch method for older cooperative children
  - A specimen for culture should not be obtained by applying a bag to the perineum; contamination rates are too high.
- False positives
  - Contaminated urine by perineum or stool organisms
- Cultures take 24 to 48 hours, so several rapid screening tests are available:
  - A two-step approach with a bag used to obtain a screening urinalysis is an appropriate option.
  - Conventional urinalysis: ≥5 WBC/HPF (uses centrifuged urine) and bacteria suggest UTI.
  - Enhanced urinalysis (combines microscopy on uncentrifuged urine with Gram stain): ≥10 WBC/mm^3 and positive Gram stain consistent with infection
    - High sensitivity and specificity; helpful in neonates
  - Urine dipstick alone equivalent to conventional microscopy
    - Leukocyte esterase (LE) indicates presence of urinary leukocytes.
    - Remember that conditions other than UTI may also present with pyuria.
    - Nitrites are formed by nitrate-splitting bacteria (high rate of false negatives because urine has to sit in the bladder for ≥4 hours for nitrites to be detected).
    - LE or nitrites alone suggest UTI; together they are more specific.
- Serum testing is not routinely indicated in the patient with suspected UTI.
  - Blood culture: not indicated in the well-appearing patient ≥2 months because bacteremia does not alter management
  - Inflammatory markers: WBC count, C-reactive protein (CRP), erythrocyte sedimentation rate (ESR), and procalcitonin (PCT) may all be elevated in UTIs but are not particularly helpful in predicting diagnosis or distinguishing between upper and lower tract disease.
  - Serum creatinine: not necessary for routine UTI but should be obtained in patients with recurrent disease or renal anomalies

ALERT

Pitfalls

- 10–15% of infants will have a negative urinalysis despite culture- or nuclear scan–documented UTI, so a culture should always be obtained in this population.
- Conversely, there are very high rates of asymptomatic bacteriuria in the pediatric population, so a mildly positive urinalysis should be weighed in the context of the pretest probability for UTI.
- Failure to culture by sterile means: leads to a contaminated culture that is difficult to interpret
- Failure to send urine promptly to the lab: can confound results in either direction
- Failure to screen a young child with another possible source of fever; children with otitis media, upper respiratory infections, and gastroenteritis can have a concurrent UTI.

Follow-Up Tests & Special Considerations

- There is controversy surrounding indications for imaging in routine febrile UTIs. UTI without fever does not require radiologic evaluation.
- Renal bladder ultrasound (RBUS): identifies hydronephrosis, congenital anomalies, and abscesses; not good at detecting scars or VUR
  - Recommended by the American Academy of Pediatrics (AAP) clinical practice guideline for febrile children 2 to 24 months of age with first UTI
  - Normal prenatal US beyond 32 weeks' gestation substantially reduces the likelihood of an abnormal US.
  - Also recommended for recurrent febrile UTIs or children not improving as expected on appropriate antibiotics
  - If following predicted clinical course, optimal timing is as an outpatient, after acute UTI (to avoid a false positive result)
- Voiding cystourethrogram (VCUG): test of choice to detect and characterize VUR
  - No longer routinely recommended by the AAP after first febrile UTI
  - Indicated for young children with recurrent febrile UTIs or an abnormal renal US
  - Consider for children w/ high fever and non-*E. coli* UTI because these risk factors have been associated with high grade VUR.
- In addition to the children covered by the AAP parameter, consider imaging for UTIs in boys, children with recurrent infections, and children with persistent voiding dysfunction, urinary abnormalities, poor growth, hypertension, or concerning family history.
- Renal cortical scan: detects acute pyelonephritis and renal scarring. Unclear use in clinical setting; consider in febrile children if diagnosis is unclear.

TREATMENT

MEDICATION

First Line

- Empiric antibiotic therapy should be initiated in febrile children with suspected UTI in order to prevent scarring.
- *E. coli* is the most common pathogen associated with first UTI; it is typically sensitive to multiple antimicrobials.
- Gram staining, when available, can help guide empiric therapy as can local patterns of susceptibility.
- Empiric inpatient therapy: IV therapy with a 3rd-generation cephalosporin such as cefotaxime (120 mg/kg/24 h divided t.i.d.) or ceftriaxone (75 mg/kg/24 h) or the combination of ampicillin (100 mg/kg/24 h divided q.i.d.) and gentamicin (7.5 mg/kg/24 h divided t.i.d.)
  - High-risk patients who are immunocompromised, have indwelling catheters, or have recurrent UTIs should initially receive broad-spectrum antibiotics that cover the causative organisms from prior infections.
- Empiric outpatient therapy: Options include cefixime (8 mg/kg/24 h once daily), cefdinir (14 mg/kg once daily), amoxicillin-clavulanate (45 mg/kg of amoxicillin component per 24 h divided b.i.d.), co-trimoxazole (6 to 12 mg TMP/kg/24 h divided b.i.d.), or cephalexin (50 to 100 mg/kg/24 h divided q6–8h).
  - Many communities have high rates of resistance to amoxicillin and co-trimoxazole; resistance to amoxicillin-clavulanate and cephalexin is also on the rise.
- Antibiotic duration (IV/oral)
  - Children ≤2 years of age with a febrile UTI, UTI, or urinary tract abnormalities should receive a total of 7 to 14 days of antibiotic therapy.
  - Older children without fever or significant history likely have an uncomplicated cystitis are eligible for a short course of antibiotics (5 to 7 days).
- Antibiotic prophylaxis after UTI
  - Benefit somewhat unclear; AAP no longer recommends prophylactic antibiotics after first febrile UTI.
  - Consider prophylaxis for patients with high-grade VUR in consultation with an urologist.

ADMISSION, INPATIENT, AND NURSING CONSIDERATIONS

- The majority of patients with UTI can receive outpatient therapy with close follow-up.
- Consider hospitalization for young infants (consider hospitalization <6 months, hospitalize <2 months).
- The following patient groups may benefit from hospitalization:
  - Ill patients with concern for development of urosepsis
  - Complex or immunocompromised host
  - Concern for dehydration or inability to tolerate medications
  - Social concerns, lack of follow-up
  - Failed outpatient management

ONGOING CARE

FOLLOW-UP RECOMMENDATIONS

Patient Monitoring

- Consider a repeat urine culture after 2 days of therapy if the patient is not improving on an appropriate antibiotic regimen.
- Such patients should also receive imaging.
- Urinalysis and urine culture for subsequent febrile illnesses in young children

PROGNOSIS

- Prompt treatment of febrile UTIs reduces the risk for scarring and its sequelae. These children generally have a very good prognosis.
- High grade VUR, signs of significant inflammation, non-*E. coli* UTIs, and delays in treatment are associated with risk of scarring.

COMPLICATIONS

- Repeated febrile UTIs in young children may lead to renal scarring.
- Renal scarring in childhood carries a risk of hypertension, preeclampsia, and end-stage renal disease as an adult.

ADDITIONAL READING

- Gorelick MH, Shaw KN. Clinical decision rule to identify young febrile young girls at risk for urinary tract infection. *Arch Pediatr Adolesc Med*. 2000;154(4):386–390.
- Hoberman A, Greenfield SP, Mattoo TK, et al; and RIVUR Trial Investigators. Antimicrobial prophylaxis for children with vesicoureteral reflux. *N Engl J Med*. 2014;370(25):2367–2376.
- Lavelle JM, Blackstone MM, Funari MK, et al. Two-step process for ED UTI screening in febrile young children: reducing catheterization rates. *Pediatrics*. 2016;138(1):e20153023.
- Montini G, Rigon L, Zucchetta P, et al; for IRIS Group. Prophylaxis after first febrile urinary tract infection in children? A multicenter, randomized, controlled non-inferiority trial. *Pediatrics*. 2008;122(5):1064–1071.
- Montini G, Tullus K, Hewitt I. Febrile urinary tract infections in children. *N Engl J Med*. 2011;365(3):239–250.
- Roberts KB; and Subcommittee on Urinary Tract Infection, Steering Committee on Quality Improvement and Management. Urinary tract infection: clinical practice guideline for the diagnosis and management of the initial UTI in febrile infants and children 2 to 24 months. *Pediatrics*. 2011;128(3):595–610.
- Schnadower D, Kuppermann N, Macias CG, et al; for American Academy of Pediatrics Pediatric Emergency Medicine Collaborative Research Committee. Febrile infants with urinary tract infections at very low risk for adverse events and bacteremia. *Pediatrics*. 2010;126(6):1074–1083.
- Shaikh N, Craig JC, Rovers MM, et al. Identification of children and adolescents at risk for renal scarring after a first urinary tract infection: a meta-analysis with individual patient data. *JAMA Pediatr*. 2014;168(10):893–900.
- Shaikh N, Morone NE, Bost JE, et al. Prevalence of urinary tract infection in childhood: a meta-analysis. *Pediatr Infect Dis J*. 2008;27(4):302–308.
- Shaikh N, Morone NE, Lopez J, et al. Does this child have a urinary tract infection? *JAMA*. 2007;298(24):2895–2904.
- Subcommittee on Urinary Tract Infection. Reaffirmation of AAP clinical practice guideline: the diagnosis and management of the initial urinary tract infection in febrile infants and young children 2–24 months of age. *Pediatrics*. 2016;138(6):e20163026.

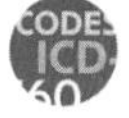

CODES

ICD10

- N39.0 Urinary tract infection, site not specified
- N12 Tubulo-interstitial nephritis, not spcf as acute or chronic
- N30.90 Cystitis, unspecified without hematuria

FAQ

- Q: Which children should have a radiologic evaluation after a UTI?
- A: Boys; febrile children <2 years, and anyone with recurrent febrile UTIs, hypertension, or family history of urinary tract abnormalities
- Q: Does a urine culture need to be done if the catheterized dipstick or urinalysis is negative?
- A: >10% of febrile young infants with pyelonephritis will have a false-negative screening test (dipstick, urinalysis). A sterile urine culture should be done in these young patients.

U

UROLITHIASIS

Kara N. Saperston, MD • Michael DiSandro, MD

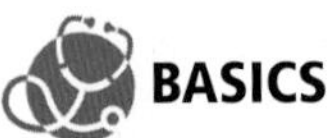

BASICS

DESCRIPTION

- Urolithiasis is the occurrence of calculi (stones) within the urinary tract, including the kidney, ureter, or bladder.
- Stones may be composed of calcium oxalate, calcium phosphate, uric acid, cystine, magnesium ammonium phosphate, xanthine, indinavir, or triamterene.

EPIDEMIOLOGY

The incidence of stones in children of both sexes has increased over the last 25 years. In the adolescent population, the prevalence is about 50 per 100,000.

RISK FACTORS

- Poor fluid intake
- Immobility
- Urinary tract obstruction
- Urinary tract infection (UTI) (*Proteus mirabilis or Escherichia coli*)
- Bladder augmentation
- Dumping syndrome
- In children, 50% have a metabolic syndrome associated with urolithiasis.
- 75% have a metabolic predisposition to forming stones.

PATHOPHYSIOLOGY

- The urine contains multiple solutes; some help prevent crystallization and some contribute to crystal formation.
- The likelihood of a solute crystalizing varies with the pH of the urine (e.g., uric acid crystal formation is more likely at lower pH).
- When enough crystals form in the urine and urine flow out of the kidney is slow or obstructed
- Crystals then coalesce into a small nidus upon which more crystals will form. This process then leads to stone formation.

COMMONLY ASSOCIATED CONDITIONS

Children who present with urolithiasis age <6 years are more likely to develop hypertension (HTN) and diabetes mellitus (DM) later in life.

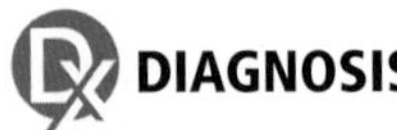

DIAGNOSIS

HISTORY

- Sudden or gradual onset of flank pain
- Location of stone is guided by the pain.
  - Midabdominal or suprapubic pain may indicate ureteral location of stone.
  - Testicular or labial pain indicates the stone is near the ureteral orifice.
  - Younger children are more likely to have nonspecific and/or nonlocalized pain.
- Nausea and/or vomiting
- Vague midabdominal pain
- Gross or microscopic hematuria is seen in only 50% of patients.
- UTI or fever
- Recent furosemide exposure
- Immobilization (postsurgical, wheelchair use)

PHYSICAL EXAM

- +/− Costovertebral angle (CVA) tenderness
- Abdominal tenderness, without rebound tenderness. Patient will have peritonitis only if a stone is accompanied by severe pyelonephritis.
- +/− Restless and unable to find a comfortable position
- +/− Blood in the urine

DIFFERENTIAL DIAGNOSIS

- UTI, upper or lower tract
- Appendicitis
- Gastroenteritis
- Congenital ureteropelvic junction (UPJ) obstruction
- Henoch-Schönlein purpura
- Tumor
- Papillary necrosis
- Trauma
- Renal artery/vein thrombosis
- Nutcracker phenomenon

ALERT

A stone causing urinary obstruction with an associated UTI is high risk and a surgical emergency.

DIAGNOSTIC TESTS & INTERPRETATION

- Urinalysis and urine culture
- 24-hour urine collection for calcium, citrate, creatinine, magnesium, oxalate, pH, phosphate, and uric acid
- Basic metabolic panel including calcium, phosphorus, and uric acid
- If hypercalciuria, then obtain vitamin D and PTH levels.
- CBC: if infection suspected
- Renal ultrasound: limited ability to visualize ureteral stones
- Plain abdominal radiograph
- CT scan of abdomen and pelvis, only if absolutely necessary
  - Consider radiation ALARA (as low as reasonably achievable) goal.

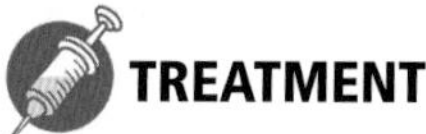

TREATMENT

GENERAL MEASURES

- After diagnosis, referral to pediatric urology for surgical management and to pediatric urology or pediatric nephrology for complete metabolic evaluation and treatment
- Stones <3 mm may pass without surgical intervention.
- Regardless of the size, further metabolic evaluation by a specialist should occur.

MEDICATION

- Increase fluid intake to achieve greater urine volume.
- Analgesia (with admission as needed for IV analgesis administration)
- Watchful waiting
- Consider expulsion therapy
  - α-Blockers: Flomax®
    - May cause headache and hypotension
    - Not approved by U.S. Food and Drug Administration (FDA)

ADDITIONAL THERAPIES

- Approximately 20% of pediatric patients will require surgical removal.
- Surgical removal
  - Ureteroscopy
  - Extracorporeal shock wave lithotripsy (ESWL)
  - Percutaneous nephrolithotomy (PCNL)
  - Open pyelolithotomy (large stones)

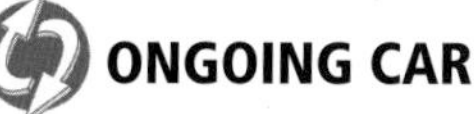

ONGOING CARE

FOLLOW-UP RECOMMENDATIONS

- All stones passed should be sent for chemical analysis.
- Increase fluid intake: Urine should be clear.
- Avoid vitamin D and C supplementation until metabolic workup is complete.
- Calcium in the diet should not be restricted even for patients with calcium stones. Patient should receive the age-appropriate recommended daily intake for calcium.
- Minimize sodium intake and reduce animal protein intake.
- Targeted reduction of specific foods such as oxalate-containing foods if hyperoxaluria present

PROGNOSIS

- 1/2 to 1/3 of children with metabolic abnormality will form another stone.
- Approximately, 25% of pediatric patients requiring surgical or ESWL therapy will require one or more additional procedures.
- Severe hyperoxaluria is associated with primary hyperoxaluria that can cause early renal failure and may require kidney transplant to correct renal failure and simultaneous liver transplant to correct the hereditary metabolic defect.
- Cystinuria: Treatment with Thiola® and D-penicillamine can be associated with myelosuppression.

ADDITIONAL READING

- Dwyer ME, Krambeck AE, Bergstralh EJ, et al. Temporal trends in incidence of kidney stones among children: a 25-year population based study. *J Urol*. 2012;188(1):247–252.
- Erturhan S, Bayrak O, Sarica K, et al. Efficacy of medical expulsive treatment with doxazosin in pediatric patients. *Urology*. 2013;81(3):640–643.
- Hernandez JD, Ellison JS, Lendvay TS. Current trends, evaluation, and management of pediatric nephrolithiasis. *JAMA Pediatr*. 2015;169(10):964–970.

CODES

ICD10

- N20.9 Urinary calculus unspecified
- N20.0 Calculus of kidney
- N20.1 Calculus of ureter

FAQ

- Q: When should a child with a stone be admitted for management?
- A: If the stone has obstructed a solitary kidney, if the child has an elevated white blood cell count or UTI in the setting of obstruction, and if the child is immunocompromised and shows signs of a UTI. In addition, some pediatric patients may require admission for pain control while a stone is passing.
- Q: What is the most common type of kidney stone?
- A: Like adults, for children, kidney stones are most commonly composed of calcium oxalate (60–90%) of cases.

U

URTICARIA (HIVES)

Christopher P. Raab, MD

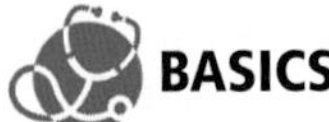

BASICS

DESCRIPTION

- Urticarial lesions are best described as raised, pruritic, circumscribed erythematous papules.
  - Single lesions may coalesce as they enlarge, forming generalized, raised, erythematous areas.
  - Transient, typically lasting several hours
  - Also known as "hives" or "nettle rash"
  - Acute: <6 weeks' duration
  - Chronic: >6 weeks' duration
- Other similar but non-urticarial entities:
  - Angioedema
    - Urticarial-like lesions
    - Form in the deep dermal, subcutaneous, and submucosal layers
  - Anaphylaxis
    - Hypersensitivity reaction after exposure to an antigen
    - Producing respiratory compromise secondary to airway edema, urticarial rash, pruritus, and hypotension; can lead to shock

EPIDEMIOLOGY

- Female-to-male ratio of 3:2
- No variation in race

Incidence

Lifetime incidence of 15–25%

GENERAL PREVENTION

When a trigger is identified, avoidance is the main preventive measure.

PATHOPHYSIOLOGY

- Immune mediated
  - Antigen is cross-linked to IgE on a mast cell.
  - This event causes mast cell activation, leading to the release of vasoactive mediators, such as histamine, leukotrienes, prostaglandin D2, platelet-activating factor, and other vasoactive mediators.
  - These vasoactive mediators cause pruritus, vasodilatation, and capillary leak, which lead to the characteristic findings.
  - Common triggers include some medications such as penicillins, foods such as milk or eggs, and envenomations.
- Non–immune mediated
  - Degranulation of mast cells secondary to other non-IgE reactions such as physical changes, chemicals, some medications such as β-lactams and sulfa-containing drugs, and some foods
- Autoimmune mediated
  - Degranulation of mast cells caused by cross-linking of IgE by IgG or IgG binding to the high-affinity IgE (FcεRI) receptor on mast cells

ETIOLOGY

- Acute urticaria
  - Viral infections are thought to make up approximately 80% of all cases of acute urticaria in children. Most commonly isolated causes include the following viruses:
    - Picornavirus
    - Coronavirus
    - Epstein-Barr
    - Hepatitis A, B, and C
  - Parasitic infections
  - Bacterial infections (especially group A strep)
  - Medications: most frequently reported include the following:
    - NSAIDs
    - Opiates
    - β-lactams
    - Vancomycin
  - Radiocontrast
  - Foods
  - Transfusion of blood products
  - Food additives and dyes
  - Natural remedies including cranberry, feverfew, glucosamine, and ginger
  - Insect venom including bees, wasps, hornets
- Chronic urticaria
  - Idiopathic: Most have an unknown cause, but many feel that an association with an autoimmune mechanism is likely.
  - Physical (~20–30%)
    - Dermatographism (9%): Stroking of skin using mild-to-moderate pressure with fingernail or hard object causes linear urticaria at site of contact.
    - Cholinergic (5%): diffuse erythema and elevated but pale urticarial lesions; intense pruritus; associated with sweating reflex, so often associated with overheating or exertion; may be worsened in combination with other triggers in specific combinations
    - Cold (3%): urticarial lesions present at areas of skin exposed to low temperatures; familial and nonhereditary forms
    - Aquagenic: Urticarial lesions arise when the patient is exposed to water (e.g., bathtub, swimming pool).
    - Delayed pressure/vibratory: Deep or prolonged pressure on skin produces significant urticaria and often angioedema. Vibratory urticaria is a form of delayed pressure urticaria caused by repetitive vibration (e.g., use of a jackhammer).
  - Mast cell disease
    - Urticaria pigmentosa: excessive number of mast cells in skin, bone marrow, lymph nodes, and other tissues; flares characterized by pruritus, flushing, tachycardia, nausea, and vomiting
    - Systemic mastocytosis
  - Systemic disease
    - Rheumatologic
      - Urticarial vasculitis: erythematous wheals that resemble urticaria but histologically appear as leukocytoclastic vasculitis; often presents with systemic symptoms and lasts >24 hours
      - Cryopyrin-associated periodic syndromes can present with urticaria, such as Muckle-Wells syndrome: chronic recurrent urticaria, deafness, amyloidosis, and arthritis.
    - Neoplasms
    - Infections: parasites especially noted to cause chronic urticaria
    - Autoimmune: antibodies to IgE or IgE receptor (FcεRI)
    - Hashimoto disease, hypothyroidism

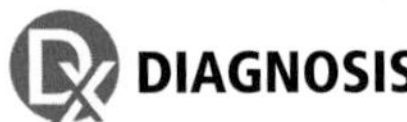

DIAGNOSIS

HISTORY

- Description of rash:
  - Lesions may not be present at time of exam due to transient nature.
  - Digital photos are often useful.
- Duration of symptoms, acute versus chronic:
  - If acute (<6 weeks), ask about
    - Viral symptoms including rhinorrhea, cough, fever, congestion, malaise
    - Any medications (prescription or over the counter) or any herbal remedies
    - Any new foods or beverages
    - Any new exposures to perfumes, chemicals, or other skin products
  - If chronic (>6 weeks)
    - History of previous episodes including timing, exposures, any past history of urticaria or angioedema
    - Other symptoms or variations in presentation
    - Symptoms of systemic diseases, such as hyperthyroidism, systemic lupus erythematosus (SLE), juvenile idiopathic arthritis, myositis, amyloidosis, infections, and lymphoma
    - Duration of lesions

PHYSICAL EXAM

- Appearance of rash: classic wheal and flare appearance
- Respiratory: Look for evidence of stridor, wheezing, or dyspnea. If present, be concerned for airway compromise or lower airway edema from an anaphylactic reaction.
- Facial or neck swelling: concern for possible airway compromise
- A full physical exam should be performed to look for signs of systemic disease or malignancy, such as
  - Upper respiratory tract infections
  - Thyromegaly
  - Lymphadenopathy or splenomegaly to suggest lymphoma
  - Joint examination for any evidence of connective tissue disease, arthritis, or SLE

DIFFERENTIAL DIAGNOSIS

- Viral exanthema
- Atopic dermatitis
- Contact dermatitis
- Insect bites
- Maculopapular drug rash
- Erythema multiforme
- Plant-induced eruptions
- Henoch-Schönlein purpura
- SLE
- Autoinflammatory disease
  - Systemic onset juvenile idiopathic arthritis
  - Cryopyrin-associated periodic syndromes: familial cold autoinflammatory syndrome, Muckle-Wells syndrome, neonatal onset multisystem inflammatory disease (NOMID)
  - Mevalonate kinase deficiency
  - Tumor necrosis factor-receptor–associated periodic syndrome (TRAPS)

DIAGNOSTIC TESTS & INTERPRETATION
- Testing is often fruitless unless indicated by history and physical examination.
- Skin testing may be performed if the causative agent is thought to be one of several food items.
- If symptoms are difficult to handle or persist >3 months, consider
  - CBC with differential
  - ESR
  - Thyroid studies (thyroid-stimulating hormone [TSH], free T_4, antithyroglobulin, and antithyroid peroxidase antibody)
- If symptoms are atypical, last >1 year, or are suggestive of urticarial vasculitis
  - Complement studies
  - ANA titer
  - Liver function tests
  - Skin punch biopsy

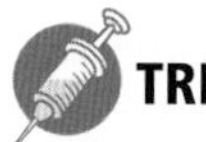

TREATMENT

Emergent treatment: If with any difficulty breathing, stridor or wheezing, or other signs of anaphylaxis, give epinephrine 0.01 mL/kg of the 1:1,000 solution SC/IM.

MEDICATION
- Acute urticaria
  - Usually self-resolving but can treat with 2nd-generation nonsedating antihistamines
  - 1st-generation antihistamines: diphenhydramine 1 mg/kg/dose or total 5 mg/kg/24 h divided PO q6h or hydroxyzine 2 mg/kg/24 h PO divided q6h for pruritus
- Chronic urticaria: See below.

First Line
- Antihistamines/H_1 antagonists:
  - Less sedating, longer acting, and should be mainstay of therapy
    - Cetirizine (Zyrtec®): Dosing varies by age from 2.5 to 10 mg daily.
    - Loratadine (Claritin®): Dosing varies by age from 5 to 10 mg daily.
- Fexofenadine (Allegra®): 6 months to <2 years of age, 15 mg twice daily; 2 to 11 years of age, 30 mg twice daily; and >12 years of age, 60 mg twice daily. 1st-generation antihistamines are effective but more sedating:
  - Diphenhydramine (Benadryl®): 5 mg/kg/24 h divided q6h
  - Hydroxyzine (Atarax®): 0.5 mg/kg/dose q6h
  - Cyproheptadine (Periactin®): 2 mg up to 3 times a day: primary treatment for cold urticaria

Second Line
Increase 2nd-generation H_1 antagonist dose to maximum for age. In adult guidelines, increasing the dose up to 4-fold is more effective.

Third Line
- Addition of a second nonsedating 2nd-generation H_1 antihistamine
- Leukotriene inhibitors: minimal additive response noted in clinical studies
  - Montelukast (Singulair®): 5 mg daily
- Combined H_1 and H_2 antagonists
  - H_2 antagonists: added as second agent because skin cells have both H_1 and H_2 receptors and a synergistic effect can be achieved by addition of an H_2 blocker
  - Ranitidine (Zantac®): 2 to 4 mg/kg/24 h divided twice daily
- Doxepin (Sinequan®): a tricyclic antidepressant. >12 years of age, 10 to 50 mg/24 h and can slowly titer up to 100 mg/24 h; potent antihistamine but poorly tolerated due to sedation, hypotension, anticholinergic side effects, and massive weight gain
- Other immune-modifying agents used in chronic urticaria:
  - Other nonstandard therapies have been tried in small case studies: cyclosporine, colchicine, dapsone, IV immunoglobulin (IVIG), plasmapheresis, methotrexate, cyclophosphamide, calcium channel blockers, ephedrine.
  - Corticosteroids: Titer to lowest effective dose. Start with standard dose of 0.5 to 1 mg/kg/24 h of prednisone; often poorly tolerated secondary to substantial side effects including hypertension, immunosuppression, hyperglycemia, physical changes
  - Omalizumab: Anti-IgE antibody has been shown to reduce signs and symptoms of chronic urticaria in those at maximum standard therapies.

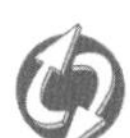

ONGOING CARE

FOLLOW-UP RECOMMENDATIONS

Patient Monitoring
- Watch for signs and symptoms of anaphylaxis; this is the major complication.
- Patients with chronic urticaria should follow up with their physician on a regular basis to monitor symptoms and response to therapies.

PROGNOSIS
- Chronic urticaria
- Resolution in 50% by 12 months
- Another 20% resolve by 5 years.
- 10–20% >20 years; many of those who continue to have symptoms are felt to have an autoimmune etiology.
- May have recurrences; physical urticaria subtypes are more likely to recur.

COMPLICATIONS
Anaphylaxis with resulting edema of the upper airway is the major life-threatening complication. The patient should seek immediate medical attention.

ADDITIONAL READING

- Bailey E, Shaker M. An update on childhood urticaria and angioedema. *Curr Opin Pediatr*. 2008;20(4):425–430.
- Bernstein J, Lang D, Khan D, et al. The diagnosis and management of acute and chronic urticaria: 2014 update. *J Allergy Clin Immunol*. 2014;133(5):1270–1277.
- Dibbern DA Jr. Urticaria: selected highlights and recent advances. *Med Clin North Am*. 2006;90(1):187–209.
- Kaplan A, Ledford D, Ashby M, et al. Omalizumab in patients with symptomatic chronic idiopathic/spontaneous urticaria despite standard combination therapy. *J Allergy Clin Immunol*. 2013;132(1):101–109.
- Krause K, Grattan CE, Bindslev-Jensen C, et al. How not to miss autoinflammatory disease masquerading as urticaria. *Allergy*. 2012;67(12):1465–1474.
- Powell RJ, Du Toit GL, Siddique N, et al; for British Society for Allergy and Clinical Immunology. BSACI guidelines for the management of chronic urticaria and angio-oedema. *Clin Exp Allergy*. 2007;37(5):631–650.
- Zuberbier T, Asero R, Bindslev-Jensen C, et al. EAACI/GA(2)LEN/EDF/WAO guideline: management of urticaria. *Allergy*. 2009;64(10):1427–1443.

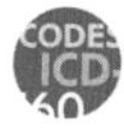

CODES

ICD10
- L50.9 Urticaria, unspecified
- L50.0 Allergic urticaria
- L50.6 Contact urticaria

FAQ
- Q: When should I refer patients to a specialist, and to what specialty should I send them?
- A: Often, referral is made when a trigger cannot be identified, if it is felt to be a food or medication trigger, and/or the symptoms persist for >6 weeks. Refer to a dermatologist or allergist–immunologist experienced in the evaluation and workup of urticaria.
- Q: When should treatment with corticosteroids or other nonstandard therapies be used to treat chronic urticaria?
- A: Typically, these medications carry significant side effects and should be reserved for those patients in whom the urticaria is causing significant alterations in activities of daily living.
- Q: When does a patient need to be hospitalized or observed during an episode of urticaria?
- A: Concerning signs include extensive angioedema, respiratory symptoms such as stridor or wheezing, or nausea/vomiting. Symptoms of anaphylaxis should be treated with epinephrine and the patient observed for several hours to ensure that symptoms do not recur.

U

VACCINE ADVERSE EVENTS

Kristen A. Feemster, MD, MPH, MSHP

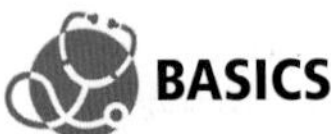

BASICS

ALERT
Adverse events after immunization may be a true vaccine-associated event or may be a coincidental event that would happen without immunization. Epidemiologic studies are important to establish causation.

DESCRIPTION

- A clinically significant event that occurs after administration of a vaccine and has been causally related to the vaccine
- All suspected adverse events should be reported; however, reporting does not imply causation.
- Contraindication to immunization = condition that increases risk of a serious adverse reaction
- Precaution for immunization = condition that might increase risk of an adverse event or may decrease effectiveness of vaccine to generate an immune response
  - Usually a temporary condition
  - Immunization indicated with a precaution if benefits outweigh risk

EPIDEMIOLOGY

Adverse events monitored prelicensure to establish safety and postlicensure to identify rare adverse events that would not be detected in prelicensure studies. Reporting is guided by:

- National Vaccine Injury Compensation Program:
  - Established by National Childhood Vaccine Injury Act of 1986 to establish a no-fault mechanism to manage claims of vaccine injury outside of the civil law system and provide compensation
  - Petitioners can file claims based on the Vaccine Injury Table (see "Patient Education") created by the program or can attempt to prove causation for an injury that is not listed.
  - Covers vaccines recommended for routine administration to children
  - Program also mandates reporting of adverse events by health care professionals and creation of vaccine information materials.
- Vaccine Adverse Event Reporting System (VAERS)
  - Passive surveillance system to monitor all vaccines licensed in the United States
  - All reports reviewed by U.S. Food and Drug Administration (FDA) and Centers for Disease Control and Prevention (CDC) medical officers
  - Can detect possible unrecognized adverse events but unable to determine true causal relationships
  - Health care providers, vaccine recipients, or vaccine manufacturers can submit a report to VAERS.
- Vaccine Safety Datalink
  - Active surveillance system formed by CDC in partnership with managed care organizations covering 9 million people
  - Can perform better observational studies to help determine causation
- Clinical Immunization Safety Assessment Network
  - Network of six academic centers established by CDC in 2001 to develop research protocols to diagnose, evaluate, and manage adverse events
  - Develops evidence-based guidelines for immunizing people at risk for serious adverse events after vaccination
- Post-licensure Rapid Immunization Safety Monitoring (PRISM) program
  - Established in 2009 by the FDA to monitor safety of pandemic influenza vaccine
  - Links electronic health record data to data from nine state immunization registries

Incidence

- Difficult to measure incidence owing to current reporting systems for adverse events
- There are ~30,000 reports each year to VAERS.
  - 13% are considered serious adverse events.
- Between 2006 to 2014, 3,451 petitions were reviewed by the National Vaccine Injury Compensation Program and 2,199 were compensated.

DIAGNOSIS

- Common mild adverse events after vaccination include:
  - Fever
  - Local erythema, swelling, and/or tenderness
  - Sleepiness and decreased appetite
  - Increased fussiness
  - Mild rash: occurs in 1 of 25 people up to 1 month after varicella vaccination
- Moderate to serious adverse events to currently recommended vaccines are rare but include:
  - Syncope, particularly among adolescents
  - Febrile seizures (measles, mumps, rubella [MMR], varicella, and diphtheria-tetanus-acellular pertussis [DtaP] vaccines)
  - Temporary joint pain or stiffness (MMR)
  - Temporary thrombocytopenia (MMR)
  - High fever
  - Shoulder injury related to vaccination
- To minimize the possibility of vaccine adverse events and to maximize the effectiveness of vaccination, the following contraindications and precautions, listed below, should be followed.

DIFFERENTIAL DIAGNOSIS

- Allergic reaction to an unrelated exposure
- Intercurrent illness

ONGOING CARE

- Approach
  - Before vaccination:
    - Discuss benefits and potential known adverse events so that families know what to expect.
    - Actively review vaccine information sheets.
    - Solicit concerns that they can be addressed.
    - Review medical history for conditions that are contraindications or precautions for vaccination.
- Contraindications
  - General *contraindications* for vaccination include:
    - History of an *anaphylactic* reaction to a vaccine component:
      - History of egg allergy no longer contraindication to influenza vaccination unless documented history of anaphylactic reaction
    - Pregnancy for *live-virus vaccines* unless mother is at high risk for the vaccine-preventable condition
    - Primary T-cell immunodeficiencies (i.e., severe combined immunodeficiency [SCID]):
      - No live vaccines
      - Inactivated vaccines can be safely administered but may not generate an adequate immune response.
    - Primary B-cell immunodeficiencies:
      - If severe (i.e., X-linked agammaglobulinemia), no live bacterial vaccines, live-attenuated influenza vaccine (LAIV), or yellow fever vaccine
      - Less severe antibody deficiencies can receive live vaccines except for OPV.
    - Phagocyte dysfunction:
      - No live bacterial vaccines
      - All live-virus and inactivated vaccines probably safe and effective
    - Secondary immunosuppression (transplant, malignancy, autoimmune disease):
      - No live vaccines depending on degree of immunosuppression
      - Can achieve adequate response to vaccination within 3 months to 2 years after stopping immunosuppressive therapy
    - HIV/AIDS:
      - Can give MMR and varicella vaccine unless severely immunocompromised
      - No OPV or LAIV
    - High-dose corticosteroids >14 days:
      - No live-virus vaccines until therapy discontinued for at least 1 month
    - Vaccine-specific contraindications
      - DTaP/Tdap
        - Encephalopathy within 7 days of previous DTP, DTaP, or Tdap dose not attributable to another cause
      - Rotavirus
        - SCID
        - Previous history intussusception
      - Hib conjugate vaccine should not be given to infants <6 weeks of age.
      - LAIV: Advisory Committee on Immunization Practices recommends against use in multiple groups (please see "Influenza" chapter).
- Precautions
  - General *precautions* for receiving a vaccine include moderate to severe acute illness with or without fever. Vaccine-specific *precautions* include:
    - DTaP/DTP
      - Fever ≥104°F or shock-like state within 48 hours of previous DTaP/DTP dose
      - Persistent, inconsolable crying >3 hours within 48 hours of previous DTaP/DTP dose
      - Seizure within 3 days of previous DTaP/DTP dose

- Any tetanus toxoid–containing vaccine:
  - Guillain-Barré within 6 weeks of a previous tetanus toxoid–containing vaccine dose
  - Progressive neurologic disorder (infantile spasms, poorly controlled epilepsy)
  - History of Arthus hypersensitivity reaction after previous tetanus toxoid–containing dose
    - Wait 10 years between doses of tetanus toxoid–containing vaccines.
- Inactivated influenza vaccines (IIVs)
  - History of Guillain-Barré within 6 weeks of a previous dose of influenza vaccine
  - Egg allergy other than hives (angioedema, respiratory distress, emesis)
    - May receive IIV in an outpatient or inpatient medical setting under supervision of a health care provider who can manage severe allergic reactions
- Human papillomavirus (HPV) vaccines:
  - Pregnancy
- Varicella:
  - Receipt of antibody-containing blood product within past 11 months
  - Immunocompromised household contacts are not a contraindication or precaution, but if rash develops 7 to 25 days after vaccination, should avoid direct contact with immunocompromised individual.
  - Receipt of certain antiviral drugs within 24 hours before vaccination
- MMR:
  - Receipt of antibody-containing blood product within past 11 months
  - History of thrombocytopenic purpura
  - Need for tuberculin skin test or interferon-γ release assay (IGRA) testing
- Rotavirus:
  - Immunosuppression (other than SCID)
  - Chronic gastrointestinal disease
  - Spina bifida or bladder exstrophy
- The following are NOT precautions or contraindications to the receipt of any vaccine:
  - Mild or recent illness
  - History of a mild to moderate local reaction to vaccine in the past
  - Concurrent antimicrobial therapy
  - Breastfeeding
  - History of other nonvaccine allergies
  - Stable neurologic conditions (e.g., cerebral palsy, developmental delay)
- For all precautions, decision to give vaccine based on assessment of benefits versus risks of vaccination

- Management
  - If a patient presents with a potential adverse event:
    - Take thorough history and perform exam to characterize symptoms and determine timing of symptom onset.
    - Evaluate for other potential causes of symptoms.
    - Determine likelihood of causality.
    - Report all adverse events to VAERS.
    - If the family would like to file a claim, refer to National Vaccine Injury Compensation Program.
  - Addressing safety concerns:
    - Nearly 20% of parents from a national telephone survey refused or delayed at least one recommended vaccine.
    - Growing prevalence of misinformation about vaccines challenges provider–parent communication.
    - Despite increasing vaccine safety concerns, health care professionals are one of the most trusted sources of information regarding vaccines.
    - Provide tailored information emphasizing benefits of vaccination and potential consequences of not accepting vaccination.
    - Actively solicit concerns before vaccination.
    - If parents have specific concerns, refer to additional information sources for reliable and accurate information (see references in "Patient Education").
    - Document vaccine discussions.
  - Reporting adverse events:
    - VAERS is the primary reporting site for suspected adverse events. Health care providers, vaccine recipients, or parents of vaccine recipients and vaccine manufacturers can all report.
    - Health care providers are required to report:
      - Any adverse event listed by vaccine manufacturer as a contraindication for the receipt of additional doses of the vaccine
      - Any adverse event included on the VAERS table of reportable events that occurred within the specified time period
  - Vaccine Injury Compensation Program:
    - Covers all vaccines recommended for routine administration by the Advisory Committee on Immunization Practices
    - To qualify for compensation, must prove there was an injury listed in the Vaccine Injury Table that occurred within prescribed time period, prove that a vaccine caused an injury not listed on the table, or prove that a vaccine aggravated a preexisting condition
    - Burden of proof is based on "presumption of causation."
    - Effects of injury must last >6 months after vaccination and have resulted in hospitalization, surgery, or death.

PATIENT EDUCATION

- Vaccine Adverse Event Reporting System: http://vaers.hhs.gov
- Vaccine Safety Datalink Project: www.cdc.gov/od/science/iso/vsd
- Clinical Immunization Safety Assessment Network: http://www.cdc.gov/vaccinesafety/cisa/
- National Vaccine Injury Compensation Program: http://www.hrsa.gov/vaccinecompensation/
- Vaccine Injury Table: http://www.hrsa.gov/vaccinecompensation/table.html
- Vaccine Education Center at the Children's Hospital of Philadelphia: http://www.chop.edu/service/vaccine-education-center/home.html
  - Vaccine education information for health care providers, educators, and parents
- Immunization Action Coalition: www.immunize.org
- World Health Organization Vaccine Safety Net: www.vaccinesafetynet.org
- American Academy of Pediatrics (AAP) Immunization Initiatives Web site: https://www2.aap.org/immunization/
  - Refusal to vaccinate waivers

ADDITIONAL READING

- American Academy of Pediatrics. Active immunization. In: Kimberlin DW, ed. *Red Book: Report of the Committee on Infectious Diseases*. 30th ed. Washington, DC: American Academy of Pediatrics; 2015:43–56.
- American Academy of Pediatrics. Immunization in special clinical circumstances. In: Kimberlin DW, ed. *Red Book: Report of the Committee on Infectious Diseases*. 30th ed. Washington, DC: American Academy of Pediatrics; 2015:68–101.
- Cook KM, Evans G. The National Vaccine Injury Compensation Program. *Pediatrics*. 2011;127(Suppl 1):S74–S77.
- Edwards KM, Hackell JM; for Committee on Infectious Diseases, The Committee on Practice and Ambulatory Medicine. Countering Vaccine Hesitancy. *Pediatrics*. 2016;138(3):e20162146.
- Stratton K, Ford A, Rusch E, et al, eds. *Adverse Effects of Vaccines: Evidence and Causality*. Washington, DC: The National Academies Press; 2012.
- Rubin LG, Levin MJ, Ljungman P, et al; for Infectious Diseases Society of America. 2013 IDSA clinical practice guideline for vaccination of the immunocompromised host. *Clin Infect Dis*. 2014;58(3):309–318.

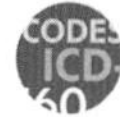

CODES

ICD10

- T88.1XXA Oth complications following immunization, NEC, init
- T80.62XA Other serum reaction due to vaccination, initial encounter
- T80.52XA Anaphylactic reaction due to vaccination, initial encounter

FAQ

- Q: Many parents request spacing vaccines. Is there evidence that giving multiple vaccines at a time is too much for a child's immune system?
- A: Recommended vaccines have a very small amount of antigen compared to natural infection and they activate a small proportion of immune system memory. Additionally, all vaccines given together have been tested when given at the same time to make sure they remain safe and effective.
- Q: What is the bottom line regarding autism and vaccines?
- A: Multiple studies including a recent Institute of Medicine report have not shown any causal relationship between thimerosal-containing vaccines and autism or MMR and autism. Additionally, the U.S. court system through the Omnibus Autism Proceedings has recently ruled that there is insufficient evidence to show any causal relationship between thimerosal-containing vaccines or MMR and autism.

VACCINE REFUSAL

Kristen A. Feemster, MD, MPH, MSHP • Renee D. Boss, MD, MHS

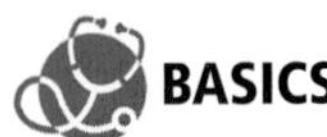

BASICS

DESCRIPTION

- A decision by a patient or parent to delay or refuse a vaccine recommended by a health care provider
- Comprises a range of behaviors from unquestioning acceptance of vaccines to cautious or selective acceptance to refusal of all vaccines
- Influenced by the interaction of several factors related to: confidence, complacency, and convenience
  - Confidence: lack of trust in vaccines, health care providers, and/or health care system
  - Complacency: low prioritization of vaccination related to low perceived risk of vaccine preventable diseases
  - Convenience: barriers to accessing immunization services (e.g., vaccine cost or difficulty getting to immunization provider)

EPIDEMIOLOGY

- Majority of adults in the United States believe vaccination is extremely or very important, but increasing proportion believe vaccines are more dangerous than diseases they prevent.
- Majority of pediatricians report >1 vaccine refusal/month.
- >1/3 of pediatricians will accept requests to delay certain vaccines, but fewer than 10% agree with such requests.
- Among a cohort of undervaccinated young children, 13% were undervaccinated due to parental choice.
- Rate of infants who receive first vaccine dose at age 4 to 5 months increased from ~50/10,000 to 100/10,000 across five successive birth cohorts (2004 to 2008).
- In the 2015 to 2016 school year, exemption rates for kindergarten school entry requirements rose from 0.4% to 6.2% across U.S. states.

RISK FACTORS

Because of the heterogeneity of vaccine hesitancy, there is no one singular set of risk factors. However, contributors to refusal include:

- Less experience with vaccine preventable diseases due to decreased disease incidence. This leads to underappreciation of disease risk and severity and parents may question need for vaccines.
- Vaccine safety concerns—especially as concerns about risk of vaccine—preventable diseases decreases, parents may worry more about potential risks of vaccination.
- Rapid dissemination of information increases likelihood of access to misinformation about vaccines, which may reinforce vaccine safety concerns,
- Anti-vaccine advocacy by prominent public figures that call attention to anti-vaccine beliefs.
- Increase in scientific denialism, which is rejection of facts for which there is well-established scientific consensus.

GENERAL PREVENTION

- Early communication about vaccines with parents can help identify and address concerns to prevent vaccine refusal or delay.
- Opportunities may include prenatal visits, in the nursery prior to discharge from the hospital after or at the newborn visit.

COMMONLY ASSOCIATED CONDITIONS

- For some parents, vaccine refusal may be associated with refusal of other health care interventions.
- Some parents may accept all recommended vaccines but request an alternative schedule. Alternative vaccine schedules spread out the recommended vaccine doses, resulting in immunization delay for some vaccines.
- Reasons for request of alternative vaccine schedules:
  - Belief that receiving multiple injections at same time overwhelms the immune system
  - Belief that recommended schedule exposes infants to too much aluminum

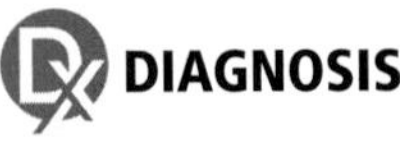

DIAGNOSIS

HISTORY

- Likelihood of vaccine refusal or hesitancy may not be evident until the time that a vaccine recommendation is made.
- Evidence of delayed/missing vaccines when reviewing a child's immunization schedule
- Diagnosis of a vaccine preventable disease

DIAGNOSTIC TESTS & INTERPRETATION

- Emerging screening tools to identify parents who are more likely to refuse or delay vaccines including the Parent Attitudes about Childhood Vaccines (PACV)
  - 15-item self-administered survey covering three domains: safety and efficacy, general attitudes, and behavior
  - Reliably predicts likelihood of delaying or refusing vaccines → as score increases, percent days underimmunized increases
- The Vaccine Confidence Index is an additional tool developed by the World Health Organization Strategic Advisory Group of Experts (SAGE) Vaccine Confidence Project and Gallup International
  - 18-item survey covering: safety and effectiveness, attitudes toward immunization requirements and trust

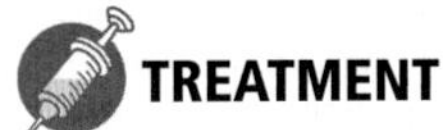

TREATMENT

GENERAL MEASURES

- Provider recommendation is the *most* important predictor of vaccine acceptance.
  - Evidence suggests that a presumptive recommendation is more effective than a participatory recommendation. Use clear, declarative statement such as "These are the vaccines your child needs today" or "There are the vaccines I recommend for your child today."
  - Targeted messages can be used to address specific concerns that are most salient to the parent. For example, parents who question the need for vaccines may respond to information about outbreaks.
  - Motivational interviewing in which questions about vaccine are actively elicited and acknowledged, then addressed using the OARS technique (open questions, affirmations, reflections, summary ask, acknowledge, advise).
  - OARS: Begin discussion about vaccines before time of recommendation to give time to address concerns.
- Vaccine policy can also address vaccine hesitancy by imposing a cost to the decision not to vaccinate (or an incentive to the decision to vaccinate). Vaccine policies also address access to immunization services.
  - Immunization requirements for school entry increase immunization rates, promote equity, and make immunization for school-aged children the default from which parents must actively opt out
  - Immunization requirements are upheld by constitutional law (*Jacobson v. Massachusetts* [1905] and others) which holds that there may be restraints placed on individual liberty in the interest of common good.
  - States also have medical, religious, or philosophical exemptions from school entry requirements. All states have medical exemptions, 47 allow religious exemptions, 17 also allow philosophical exemptions.
  - Steps required to obtain an exemption vary—the ease of obtaining an exemption has been associated with exemption rates (easy exemptions associated with higher exemption rates) as well as risk of vaccine preventable disease outbreaks.
- Policies to increase access to vaccines, such as the Vaccines for Children program or policies that allow for vaccine delivery in alternative locations like pharmacies or schools, can help increase rates by addressing convenience.

ADDITIONAL THERAPIES

- Media campaigns to raise public awareness about vaccines and vaccine preventable diseases and promote positive vaccine messages.
  - Important to leverage social media and Internet-based communication as a growing proportion of parents seek health information from these sources
- Practice-based policies such as the use of signed declination forms to document refusal or dismissal of families who refuse vaccines may also influence decision making by parents.
  - If family continues to refuse vaccines after working to address concerns, may consider referring family to another practice, especially if vaccine refusal affects overall trust. Family dismissal endorsed in a recent American Academy of Pediatrics policy statement as a potential approach when other strategies have been unsuccessful.

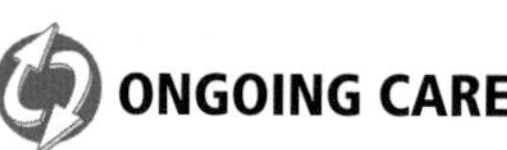

ONGOING CARE

FOLLOW-UP RECOMMENDATIONS

Families who express hesitancy about vaccines or who have delayed or refused a vaccine should be followed closely with ongoing counseling and education toward goal of scheduled vaccination.

- If family unwilling to consent to vaccination, clinician may dismiss family from the medical practice if no compromise available.

Patient Monitoring

Children with inadequate vaccination should be monitored closely for the development of vaccine preventable diseases such as pertussis.

- Susceptible family members and other close contacts should also be aware of risk.
- Underimmunized children may need to be restricted from certain activities, including school attendance, during an outbreak.

PATIENT EDUCATION

It is important to provide families with reliable sources of vaccine information when addressing hesitancy. Health care providers should also be able to comfortably address questions and concerns. Sources of reliable information include:

- Vaccine Education Center (www.vaccine.chop.edu)
- Immunization Action Coalition (www.immunize.org)
- Parents of Kids with Infections Diseases (www.pkids.org)
- Every Child By Two (www.ecbt.org)
- Voices for Vaccines (www.voicesforvaccines.org)

PROGNOSIS

- Ability to increase vaccine acceptance among parents with firmly held beliefs who refuse all vaccines is particularly challenging, but interventions to address concerns may increase acceptance among most vaccine hesitant parents.
- Ongoing studies are evaluating the effectiveness of communication strategies—both the content of a message and the way in which it is delivered are important.

COMPLICATIONS

Vaccine refusal and subsequent undervaccination has been associated with disease outbreaks.

- In a review of measles outbreaks, the majority (72.1%) of cases were unvaccinated or had unknown vaccination status. Among unvaccinated individuals, 70.6% were unvaccinated due to nonmedical exemption.
- Children with vaccine exemptions have 35 times higher risk of acquiring measles compared to fully vaccinated children.
- Counties with higher rates of vaccine exemptions are more likely to have outbreaks.

ADDITIONAL READING

- Edwards KM, Hackell JM; for Committee on Infectious Diseases, Committee on Practice and Ambulatory. Countering vaccine hesitancy. *Pediatrics*. 2016;138(3):e20162146.
- Glanz JM, Newcomer SR, Narwaney KJ, et al. A population-based cohort study of undervaccination in 8 managed care organizations across the United States. *JAMA Pediatr*. 2013;167(3):274–281.
- National Vaccine Advisory Committee. Assessing the state of vaccine confidence in the United States: recommendations from the National Vaccine Advisory Committee. *Public Health Rep*. 2015;130(6):573–595.
- Phadke VK, Bednarczyk RA, Salmon DA, et al. Association between vaccine refusal and vaccine-preventable diseases in the United States: a review of measles and pertussis. *JAMA*. 2016;315(11):1149–1158.
- Schwartz JL, Caplan AL. Vaccination refusal: ethics, individual rights, and the common good. *Prim Care*. 2011;38(4):717–728, ix.
- World Health Organization. Immunization, vaccines and biologicals: addressing vaccine hesitancy. http://www.who.int/immunization/programmes_systems/vaccine_hesitancy/en/. Accessed May 10, 2018.

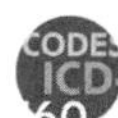

CODES

ICD10

- Z28.82 Immunization not carried out because of caregiver refusal
- Z28.8 Immunization not carried out for other reason
- Z28.89 Immunization not carried out for other reason

FAQ

- Q: Are alternative vaccine schedules safer?
- A: The routine recommended schedule was evaluated by the Institute of Medicine (now National Academy of Medicine) who found no increased risk for several outcomes, including neurodevelopmental conditions such as autism. In fact, alternative schedules are less safe, as they increase the amount of time a child is susceptible to vaccine preventable diseases. Spreading out doses also does not reduce stress; studies have shown that children have a similar cortisol response to the receipt of one or more than one shot at the same time.
- Q: What is the legal justification for mandatory immunization policies?
- A: Requirements for immunization at school entry are based on state-level public health laws aimed at reducing vaccine preventable diseases. All states have school entry requirements and while there is no federal law dictating such requirements, they have been upheld by constitutional law (see *Jacobson v. Massachusetts* [1905], *Zucht v. King* [1922], and *Prince v. Massachusetts* [1944]). However, states differ in their approach to providing exemptions to school entry requirements.
- Q: What should I do if a family refuses vaccination despite repeated counseling?
- A: Ongoing support and education of the family is the best way to address vaccine hesitancy. If these efforts are exhausted, and the clinician has concerns about the impact on other patients in the medical practice, the clinician can refuse to continue to provide care for the child and family.

VAGINITIS

Sara M. Buckelew, MD, MPH

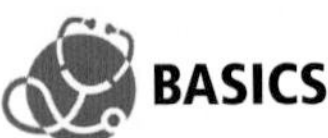

BASICS

DESCRIPTION

- Vaginitis is inflammation or irritation of the vagina causing typical symptoms of vaginal discharge, burning, and itching.
  - May be due to infection such as trichomoniasis, candidiasis, or bacterial vaginosis (BV); see Appendix, Table 7.
  - Noninfectious causes include foreign body or exposure to an irritant or allergen.
- Vulvovaginitis is irritation or inflammation of both the vulva and the vagina; most often due to *Candida albicans*
- In postpubertal females, BV is the most prevalent cause of vaginal discharge and typically causes a fishy odor.
- Physiologic leukorrhea (i.e., "physiologic discharge") is usually associated with pubertal onset and frequently precedes menarche. It is typically thin, white, and mucoid.

EPIDEMIOLOGY

- Vaginitis affects females of all ages.
- In prepubescent girls, 25–75% of vaginitis is nonspecific in etiology.
- Approximately 75% of women have had at least one episode of vulvovaginitis due to candida in their lifetime.
- The most common causes of postpubertal vaginitis are as follows:
  - BV (22–50%)
  - Vulvovaginal candidiasis (17–39%)
  - *Trichomonas vaginalis* (4–35%)

RISK FACTORS

- For prepubertal females, poor hygiene is a common risk factor.
- Irritant risk factors often include soaps, tampons, topical products and medications, extreme cleansing, clothing, and douching.
- For BV:
  - Vaginal douching
  - Smoking
  - Intrauterine device usage
  - Non-white race
  - Prior pregnancy
  - Unprotected sexual intercourse
  - Use of spermicide
  - Homosexual relationships
- For trichomoniasis:
  - Multiple sexual partners
  - Other sexually transmitted infections
  - Lack of condom use
  - Smoking
- For vulvovaginal candidiasis:
  - Use of systemic antibiotics
  - Uncontrolled diabetes mellitus
  - Diet high in refined sugars

PATHOPHYSIOLOGY

- In prepubescent females, with prepubertal hormones, the vagina has a neutral pH, atrophic mucosa, and a warm environment that easily allow for bacterial overgrowth.
- Physiologic leukorrhea
  - Estrogen levels; the volume of discharge varies with the menstrual cycle and is especially heavy at the time of ovulation.
- Candida vulvovaginitis
  - Use of antibiotics increases the occurrence of candidiasis by eliminating competitive organisms.
- BV
  - Caused by shift in vaginal flora
  - Normal *Lactobacillus* species decrease and overgrowth of bacteria, including *Gardnerella vaginalis*, *Mycoplasma hominis*, and anaerobes such as *Prevotella* and *Mobiluncus* species

ETIOLOGY

- All ages:
  - Chemical, irritant, allergy
  - Nonspecific vaginitis (may be associated with hygiene)
  - Foreign body or material such as rolled up toilet paper
  - Candidiasis associated with antibiotic use
  - Trauma, mechanical irritation
  - Sexual abuse
- More common in prepubertal females:
  - Group A β-hemolytic *Streptococcus*
  - *Haemophilus influenzae*
  - *Shigella*
  - Pinworms or scabies
  - Congenital abnormalities
- More common in postpubertal females:
  - Physiologic leukorrhea (may cause discharge but not irritation)
  - BV
  - Trichomoniasis
  - Sexually transmitted infections (STIs) such as gonorrhea and chlamydia
  - Pubic lice

DIAGNOSIS

HISTORY

- For many preadolescent and adolescent girls, vaginal symptoms may be uncomfortable to talk about. Important to meet alone with an adolescent.
- Symptoms alone cannot distinguish between the different causes of vaginitis but can assist the clinician.
- Describe the discharge including color (white, green-yellow, gray?), consistency (frothy? thick?), amount, odor, and duration of symptoms.
- Is there pain? Pain with intercourse? Burning?
- Bladder/urinary symptoms: Is there dysuria? Frequency? Urgency?
- Is there itching? Is it worse at night? Is it present in other family members?
- Exposure to any new possible irritants (e.g., new soap, spermicides, douching)
- Anything that makes symptoms better or worse?
- Prior history of similar symptoms? Prior treatment for past vaginitis?
- Sexual history including number of partners, use of barrier methods, history of STI
- Any medications, such as systemic antibiotics
- STI risk factors
- Any chronic diseases such as diabetes or other immunocompromised conditions

PHYSICAL EXAM

- Vital signs, including height, weight, BMI, and temperature
- Inspect pubic hair for sexual maturity rating (tanner staging) and evidence of infection or irritation.
- External genital or vaginal evidence of erythema, excoriation, and discharge. In younger children, this can be done in the "frog-leg" position.
- Discharge should be sampled.
- Examination of other evidence for irritation or inflammation such as warts, injury, and ulceration
- Consistency, color of discharge
- If patient is sexually active, speculum exam may need to be performed to evaluate the cervix. "Strawberry cervix" can be a sign of inflammation seen in trichomoniasis.
- Bimanual exam also should be considered if symptoms suggest risk for pelvic inflammatory disease.

DIFFERENTIAL DIAGNOSIS

Can be age dependent, similar to etiology

- Skin conditions including psoriasis, eczema
- Lichen sclerosis (hypotrophic dystrophy of the vulva)
- Congenital abnormalities, such as ectopic ureter
- Sexual abuse
- Mechanical irritation from lack of lubrication, trauma
- Pinworm infection
- Physiologic leukorrhea
- Candidiasis
- BV
- Trichomonas
- Other STIs including chlamydia, gonorrhea, herpes simplex virus infection, human papillomavirus (HPV)

DIAGNOSTIC TESTS & INTERPRETATION

In order to best evaluate etiology, a sample of discharge should be collected. The sample can be obtained by the clinician or by the patient typically using a cotton-tipped applicator.

- Odor/"whiff" or "amine" test:
  - Slide prepared with drop of 10% KOH
  - The examiner should whiff the slide for presence of a fishy odor suggestive of BV, also seen in trichomoniasis, negative in candida.

- Wet mount of the vaginal discharge mixed with saline for microscopy
  - This slide is examined for evidence of trichomonads, clue cells, and yeast.
  - Clue cells are vaginal epithelial cells with adherent coccobacilli seen on wet mount and when >20% of epithelial cells suggestive of BV.
- Wet mount with 10% KO
  - May demonstrate budding yeast ("spaghetti with meatballs" appearance) suggestive of candida
- Nitrazine paper
  - Measures pH of sample
  - Vaginal pH >5 seen in BV, >5.4 seen in trichomoniasis, <4.9 candidiasis
- Urinalysis may be helpful if patient complains of dysuria.
- STI testing as warranted based on risk factors. Chlamydia polymerase chain reaction (PCR) can be obtained by cervical or vaginal swab or urine; gonorrhea PCR or culture (cervical or vaginal swab)
- Consider a pregnancy test as indicated.

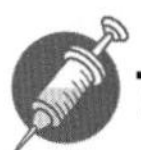

TREATMENT

GENERAL MEASURES

- Good hygiene and avoidance/removal of irritants includes hand washing following toileting, encourage wiping from front to back, clean with a mild nonscented soaps or lotions, wear cotton underwear, and avoid bubble baths and douching.
- Warm bath/Sitz baths followed by air-drying
- Use of topical emollients, zinc creams, or topical low-potency steroids to assist with itching and/or inflammation especially in patients with nonspecific vaginitis

MEDICATION

- Medication management depends on the etiology. Sensitivity culture results should drive treatment management.
- Vulvovaginal candidiasis
  - Topical antifungals such as clotrimazole, butoconazole, miconazole, or terconazole are available over the counter.
  - Oral fluconazole 6 mg/kg up to a maximum of 150 mg as a single dose can be given.
  - Longer treatments may be necessary for recurrent or severe infections.
- BV
  - Antibiotics are treatment of choice.
  - Oral metronidazole 500 mg twice daily for 7 days or intravaginal metronidazole gel for 5 days or clindamycin cream (7 days) or suppository (100 mg ovules for 3 days)
  - Higher rates of recurrence are seen with single-dose therapy for BV. Relapse may require longer courses of treatment.
- Trichomonas
  - Metronidazole 2 g orally in a single dose
  - Sexual partners should be treated simultaneously if possible to avoid reinfection.
- Chlamydia cervicitis
  - Azithromycin 1 g orally for 1 dose or doxycycline 100 mg orally twice daily for 7 days
- Gonorrhea cervicitis
  - Ceftriaxone 125 mg IM for 1 dose
  - PLUS azithromycin 1 g orally for 1 dose or doxycycline 100 mg orally twice daily for 7 days
- HSV
  - For initial outbreak: acyclovir 400 mg orally 3 times daily for 7 to 10 days or 200 mg 5 times daily for 7 to 10 days; can use valacyclovir or famciclovir alternatively
  - Suppressive therapy for recurrent infections can use acyclovir, valacyclovir, or famciclovir.
- Lichen sclerosus
  - Mild pruritus, consider emollient.
  - For itching, consider an antihistamine.
  - More severe symptoms, consider topical steroids.
- Group A β-hemolytic *Streptococcus* and *H. influenzae*
  - Amoxicillin 40 mg/kg/24 h to max 500 mg divided twice daily for 7 days
- *Shigella*
  - Trimethoprim/sulfamethoxazole
- Pinworm infestations
  - Mebendazole 100 mg orally, consider repeat dosage 2 weeks later.
  - Launder all clothing and bedding and consider treatment of entire family.

COMPLEMENTARY & ALTERNATIVE THERAPIES

Specific probiotic strains may be helpful in preventing recurrence in BV and candida vulvovaginitis; however most studies have been conducted in adult populations.

ONGOING CARE

FOLLOW-UP RECOMMENDATIONS

Patient Monitoring

- If symptoms persist following over the counter or other treatment, patients need to be reevaluated by a clinician as may be another etiology.
- Patients with an STI such as trichomonas, gonorrhea, or chlamydia should make certain that all sexual partners receive treatment in order to prevent reinfection.

ALERT

Patients taking metronidazole for trichomonas or BV should be told explicitly to avoid alcohol.

PATIENT EDUCATION

- In prepubescent females: Encourage good hygiene to prevent recurrence.
- In sexually active adolescents: Encourage regular condom usage and consider discussion of contraceptive options.

PROGNOSIS

With treatment, vaginitis typically resolves quickly with no complications.

COMPLICATIONS

- BV is associated with premature labor and preterm birth, premature rupture of membranes, and increased risk of acquiring STIs.
- Gonorrhea and chlamydial infections that are not treated can lead to pelvic inflammatory disease.

ADDITIONAL READING

- Freeto JP, Jay MS. "What's really going on down there?" A practical approach to the adolescent who has gynecologic complaints. *Pediatr Clin North Am*. 2006;53(3):529–545.
- Hainer BL, Gibson MV. Vaginitis. *Am Fam Physician*. 2011;83(7):807–815.
- Loveless M, Myint O. Vulvovaginitis—presentation of more common problems in pediatric and adolescent gynecology. *Best Pract Res Clin Obstet Gynaecol*. 2018;48:14–27.
- Zuckerman A, Romano M. Clinical recommendation: vulvovaginitis. *J Pediatr Adolesc Gynecol*. 2016;29(6):673–679.

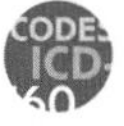

CODES

ICD10

- N76.0 Acute Vaginitis
- N89.8 Other specified noninflammatory disorders of vagina
- B37.3 Candidiasis of vulva and vagina

FAQ

- Q: How do you diagnose BV?
- A: BV is a clinical diagnosis based on having three out of four Amsel criteria:
  - Thin, homogenous discharge
  - Vaginal pH >4.5
  - Positive "whiff" test
  - >20% clue cells on wet mount or Gram stain
- Q: Should sex partners of patients with vaginitis be treated?
- A: It depends on the etiology of the vaginitis. For BV and candida, there are no treatment recommendations for sex partners. For patients with trichomonas, partners should be treated, and to reduce recurrence, partners should avoid sexual intercourse until both have been treated and are asymptomatic.
- Q: In prepubescent females, is a positive culture definitive for infection?
- A: One common issue in prepubertal females is how to distinguish between normal vaginal flora and potential pathogens. Growth of normal pathogens even in girls who are symptomatic is not diagnostic.

VARICOCELE

Adam B. Hittelman, MD, PhD, FACS

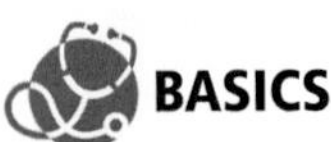

BASICS

DESCRIPTION

A varicocele is an abnormal tortuosity and dilation of the testicular veins and the pampiniform venous plexus of the spermatic cord.

EPIDEMIOLOGY

- Rare in prepubertal boys, increases with age to approximately 15% in late adolescence and healthy adult population
  - 2 to 10 years old, <1%
  - 11 to 14 years old, 7.8%
  - 15 to 19 years old, 14.1%
- Based on World Health Organization observational study (1992), 15–20% of adult varicocele patients have fertility problems.
  - Varicocele presents in 25% of men with abnormal semen analysis and 12% of men with normal semen parameters.
  - Present in 35–40% of males with primary infertility
- Left-sided predominance, 90%
- No racial predilection

RISK FACTORS

- Exact mechanisms have not been fully elucidated.
- May be related to physiologic changes in puberty, such as rapid testicular growth and increased testicular blood flow
- Associated with increased height and low body mass index
- Increased risk in 1st-degree relatives of patients with a varicocele

PATHOPHYSIOLOGY

- Association between varicocele and testicular dysfunction/fertility compromise
  - Impaired spermatogenesis: decreased motility, decreased density, and increased number of pathologic sperm forms; decreased total sperm count
- Ipsilateral testicular hypotrophy
  - Recent data demonstrates correlation between varicocele grade and testicular hypotrophy although not observed in prior studies.
  - Testicular "catch-up growth" can be seen after varicocelectomy.
  - Catch-up growth can all be seen in 30–50% of patients managed conservatively.
- Potentially caused by an embryonic field defect, affecting growth of bilateral testicles
- Exact mechanisms not clearly elucidated—multiple theories:
  - Hyperthermia: Varicocele increases intratesticular temperature, likely by interfering with the pampiniform plexus' ability to provide countercurrent cooling system.
  - Potential reflux of renal and adrenal metabolites, potentially causing testicular damage
  - Increased production of nitric oxide and reactive oxygen species correlate with severity of varicocele.
  - Endocrine abnormalities are found in subset of patients with varicocele, including low testosterone, abnormal response to gonadotropin-releasing hormone (GnRH), and impaired Leydig cell function.

ETIOLOGY

Associated with anatomy of left testicular vein

- Inserts into renal vein at right angle (right testicular vein drains into vena cava)
- Incompetent or absent valves
- Left testicular vein 8 to 10 cm longer than right, with increased pressure
- Increased venous pressure from "nutcracker phenomenon": compression of left renal vein as it passes between aorta and superior mesenteric artery

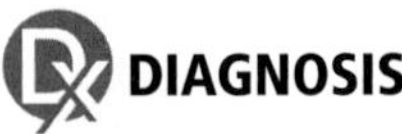

DIAGNOSIS

HISTORY

- Often asymptomatic and incidentally noted on routine physical exam
  - Infertility uncommon issue in adolescent population
  - Associated pain/heaviness/dull ache in 2–11% of cases
- Laterality
- Age of onset
- When and how testicular abnormality first detected
- Change in size of varicocele with positioning or Valsalva
- Prior surgery or trauma
- Prior imaging

PHYSICAL EXAM

- Examine in warm room with patient supine and standing.
- Palpate at rest and with Valsalva.
- Para- and supratesticular mass; feels like a "bag of worms"
- Assess testicular size and consistency.
- Estimate testicular volume with orchidometer, calipers, or color Doppler ultrasound.
  - Right testicle serves as control for left.
  - >2 mL or >20% size discrepancy, right > left, is significant.
- Varicocele grade
  - Grade 1 (small): palpable only with Valsalva
  - Grade 2 (medium): easily palpable but not visible
  - Grade 3 (large): visible through scrotal skin
- Varicocele should decompress in supine position.

ALERT

Solitary right varicocele or failure of vessels to decompress in supine position raises concern for potential retroperitoneal or abdominal mass.

DIFFERENTIAL DIAGNOSIS

- Inguinal hernia
- Hydrocele
- Epididymal cyst/spermatocele
- Testicular mass
- Epididymal mass
- Paratesticular mass
- Cord lipoma

DIAGNOSTIC TESTS & INTERPRETATION

Initial Testing (screening, lab, imaging)

- Color Doppler scrotal ultrasound to diagnose varicocele and quantitate testicular volume
  - Size discrepancy used as surrogate to predict future fertility compromise
- Semen analysis in age-appropriate patients (Tanner V)
  - Total sperm count
  - Sperm motility

Follow-Up Tests & Special Considerations

- Serial trans-scrotal US to follow testicular growth/volume (left vs. right)
- Prior surgery/injury to right testicle can complicate comparison between left and right testicular growth.

ALERT

Secondary varicocele, especially right-sided, can be a clinical indicator of retroperitoneal mass or venous obstruction. Left-sided varicocele that does not decompress in supine position also a concern for venous obstruction/retroperitoneal mass. It is important to do physical exam standing and in supine position to assess for decompression of varicocele in supine position.

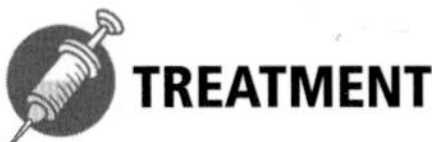

TREATMENT

GENERAL MEASURES

- Treatment is not indicated in all children/adolescents with varicocele.
- Annual ultrasound assessment of testicular volume recommended
  - Potential for interobserver variability for imaging
  - Spontaneous catch-up growth in some patients with hypotrophy followed conservatively (30–50%).
- 80–85% of men with varicocele do not exhibit effect on fertility.
- Semen analysis on Tanner V adolescents can guide care.

SURGERY/OTHER PROCEDURES

- Definitive treatment is recommended for the following:
  - Size discrepancy between right and left testicle of >2 mL or 20%
  - Adolescents with abnormal semen analysis and high-grade varicocele
  - Adolescents with symptoms: pain, heaviness
  - Adolescents with bilateral varicocele
- Treatment options
  - Surgical ligation/division of testicular veins (laparoscopic vs. subinguinal approach)
    - Testicular artery- and lymphatic-sparing reduces risk of secondary hydrocele.
  - Endovascular/IV embolization of testicular veins

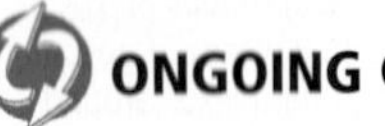

ONGOING CARE

FOLLOW-UP RECOMMENDATIONS

- Persistence should be assessed by surveillance ultrasound 6 months after repair.
- Trans-scrotal US to assess for testicular catch-up growth
- Semen analysis to see if improvement in semen parameters

PROGNOSIS

After repair, recurs in 1–16% of patients (depending on surgical technique)

COMPLICATIONS

- Recurrent/persistent varicocele
- Secondary hydrocele
  - May require surgery if symptomatic
  - More common in laparoscopic approach
- Testicular hypotrophy/atrophy
  - 1% in subinguinal surgical approach
- Persistent fertility compromise

ADDITIONAL READING

- de Los Reyes T, Locke J, Afshar K. Varicoceles in the pediatric population: diagnosis, treatment, and outcomes. *Can Urol Assoc J*. 2017;11(1–2 Suppl 1):S34–S39.
- Evers JH, Collins J, Clarke J. Surgery or embolisation for varicoceles in subfertile men. *Cochrane Database Syst Rev*. 2008;(3):CD000479.
- Preston MA, Carnat T, Flood T, et al. Conservative management of adolescent varicoceles: a retrospective review. *Urology*. 2008;72(1):77–80.
- Robinson SP, Hampton LJ, Koo HP. Treatment strategy for the adolescent varicocele. *Urol Clin North Am*. 2010;37(2):269–278.
- Sack BS, Schäfer M, Kurtz MP. The dilemma of adolescent varicoceles: do they really have to be repaired? *Curr Urol Rep*. 2017;18(5):38.
- Serefoglu EC, Saitz TR, La Nasa JA Jr, et al. Adolescent varicocoele management controversies. *Andrology*. 2013;1(1):109–115.

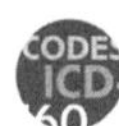

CODES

ICD10

I86.1 Scrotal varices

FAQ

- Q: What are long-term benefits of surgical repair of varicoceles?
- A: If varicocele is corrected, testicular catch-up growth can occur when performed in adolescents. The risk for infertility is also decreased. In adult population, 2/3 of patients will have improvement in semen analysis, and 40% of their partners will become pregnant.
- Q: Is there benefit of surgical repair of varicocele after puberty? Will this improve fertility?
- A: Testicular hypotrophy does not improve after adult varicocelectomy. Although it appears to be a progressive process, studies have not clearly demonstrated clear benefit in fertility improvement if corrected in adolescence versus when fertility compromise is diagnosed.
- Q: What happens if a varicocele is left untreated?
- A: There is good evidence to show that when left untreated, a varicocele will continue to affect testicular growth with loss of volume and progressive deterioration in semen analysis.
- Q: What is the risk of recurrence after repair?
- A: Recurrence can occur in 1–16% of adolescents, depending on surgical technique.

VASCULAR BRAIN LESIONS (CONGENITAL)

Sabrina E. Smith, MD, PhD

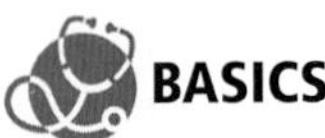

BASICS

DESCRIPTION

- Developmental venous anomalies (DVAs) are the most common vascular malformation of the brain, representing 60% of all central nervous system (CNS) vascular malformations. Also known as venous angiomas, DVAs are made up of a cluster of venous radicles that drain into a collecting vein. They occur in 2.5–3% of the general population.
- Cavernous malformations (CMs), also known as cavernous hemangiomas or cavernomas, are multilobulated, low-pressure, and slow-flow vascular structures filled with blood, thrombus, or both. They do not contain elastin or smooth muscle. There is no intervening brain tissue except at the periphery of the lesion.
- Arteriovenous malformations (AVMs) are abnormal clusters of vessels that connect arteries and veins without a true capillary bed and have intervening gliotic brain tissue.
- Vein of Galen malformations (VOGMs) are a specific type of congenital AVM that involves the vein of Galen, which flows into the straight sinus after draining the internal cerebral veins and basal veins.
- Sturge-Weber syndrome (SWS), also known as encephalotrigeminal angiomatosis, is characterized by leptomeningeal angiomatosis, facial port-wine stain (capillary malformation), and glaucoma. Some patients have all three findings, whereas others have just one or two features.

PATHOPHYSIOLOGY

- DVAs are an extreme variation of normal venous development. Typically, venous drainage in the brain occurs through a superficial system and a deep system. DVAs result when a deep venous territory drains toward the surface or when a superficial territory drains to the deep venous system instead of draining in the expected direction. Intervening brain tissue is normal. The mechanism responsible for DVA formation is unknown.
- The pathogenesis of CMs is unknown, although the report of cases of new cavernoma development adjacent to a DVA suggests that DVAs may lead to CM formation. Most CMs occur sporadically, although familial syndromes exist. Several genes have been associated with familial CMs.
- The cause of AVM formation is unknown. A failure of normal capillary development with dysplastic vessels forming between primordial arteriovenous connections has been suggested.
- VOGMs are embryonic AVMs consisting of choroidal arteries draining into the precursor of the vein of Galen. They develop between weeks 6 and 11 of fetal life.
- SWS occurs sporadically in 1/40,000 to 50,000 births and is associated with a somatic mosaic mutation in guanine nucleotide–binding protein G(q) subunit alpha. The pathophysiology is thought to be venous dysplasia, in which the primordial venous plexus that is normally present at 5 to 8 weeks of gestation fails to regress. The location of this plexus around the cephalic end of the neural tube and under the ectoderm destined to form the facial skin accounts for the clinical features. Venous stasis occurs due to the absence of normal cortical venous structures, and hypoperfusion of brain tissue occurs. These findings are unilateral in the majority but can be bilateral in up to 20% of cases.

COMMONLY ASSOCIATED CONDITIONS

- DVAs are associated with CMs in 8–40% of cases, and 20% of patients with mucocutaneous venous malformations of the head and neck have DVAs.
- DVAs are also associated with sinus pericranii, a communication between intracranial and extracranial venous drainage pathways in which blood may circulate bidirectionally.

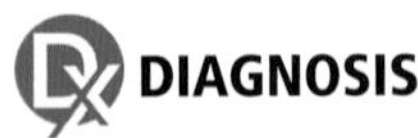

DIAGNOSIS

HISTORY

- DVAs are usually benign and asymptomatic, coming to clinical attention as an incidental finding on a neuroimaging study.
- Headache, seizure, and intracerebral hemorrhage are common in patients with CMs and AVMs. Focal neurologic deficits may result from intracerebral hemorrhage or compression of underlying brain structures by the vascular malformation.
- 95% of newborns with VOGMs present with congestive heart failure (CHF). Others present with hydrocephalus, subarachnoid hemorrhage, intraventricular hemorrhage, or failure to thrive.
- Infants and older children usually present with hydrocephalus, headache, seizures, exercise-induced syncope, or subarachnoid hemorrhage.
- Facial port-wine stain, seizures, and glaucoma are common in SWS. Other neurologic symptoms include hemiparesis, developmental delay, intellectual disability, and stroke-like episodes presenting with hemiparesis and visual field defects.

PHYSICAL EXAM

- Physical exam is normal in children with DVAs and children with CMs or AVMs that have not ruptured. Focal neurologic deficits may persist following intracerebral hemorrhage associated with CMs or AVMs.
- In newborns with VOGMs, signs of CHF such as tachycardia, respiratory distress, and hepatomegaly may occur. A continuous cranial bruit may be heard over the posterior skull, and bounding carotid pulses and peripheral pulses may be present. Scalp veins may be dilated.
- Older infants and children with VOGMs also may present with CHF but more often demonstrate increased head circumference, focal neurologic signs, and failure to thrive. Proptosis may be noted.
- Children with SWS often have a facial port-wine stain, most often in the V_1 distribution. Glaucoma is also common. Hemiparesis or seizures may develop.

DIFFERENTIAL DIAGNOSIS

- The differential diagnosis for headaches and seizures, common presenting symptoms of brain vascular malformations, is broad. CNS infection, intracerebral hemorrhage, hydrocephalus, and mass lesion can result in both. Other causes of seizure include dysplasia, remote brain injury, and genetic conditions. Other causes of headache include benign conditions such as migraine and tension headaches and structural abnormalities such as Chiari I malformations.
- VOGMs must be considered in any newborn with unexplained CHF (especially high-output failure), hydrocephalus, or intracranial hemorrhage. Other causes of high-output CHF in the newborn include anemia, hyperthyroidism, and other AVMs.
- Intracerebral hemorrhage may result from AVMs, CMs, aneurysms, bleeding diatheses, hypertension, or trauma in neonates and children. In older children, sickle cell disease, vasculopathies including moyamoya syndrome, and vasculitis also can lead to hemorrhage.

DIAGNOSTIC TESTS & INTERPRETATION

Routine blood studies are usually normal. Chest x-ray studies and electrocardiogram may reveal typical changes of high-output CHF in patients with VOGMs.

Initial Tests (screening, lab, imaging)

- Neuroimaging studies are required for definitive diagnosis.
- DVAs can be visualized on contrast-enhanced CT or MRI. Diagnosis is made by visualization of the typical "caput medusa" appearance of the radially arranged veins draining into a collecting vein, seen as a linear or curvilinear focus of enhancement. They can also be visualized with conventional angiography, although this is not required unless a patient presents with an acute hemorrhage.
- MRI is better than CT at demonstrating CMs, which have a mulberry appearance. On MRI, they are well-circumscribed lesions of mixed signal intensity on T1- and T2-weighted sequences. Contrast enhancement is variable. They are best seen on gradient-echo T2-weighted images or susceptibility-weighted images, which are sensitive to hemosiderin or deoxyhemoglobin.
- AVMs can be seen with CT/CTA, MR/MRA, and conventional angiography. Dynamic sequences are required to characterize the anatomy of feeding and draining vessels. Conventional angiography is the gold standard.

- VOGMs can be diagnosed on fetal ultrasound or MRI. In newborns, cranial ultrasound shows a large, hypoechoic structure in the region of the vein of Galen. CT shows a high-density mass that enhances with contrast. MRI shows an area of decreased signal intensity or signal void because of high flow within the malformation. CT and MRI also show areas of cerebral ischemia or hemorrhage. Conventional angiography is required before intervention.
- In SWS, CT may show calcifications or atrophy. Gadolinium-enhanced MRI is the most sensitive study, showing leptomeningeal enhancement due to pial angiomatosis. Initial CT and MRI are often normal in the newborn period, so follow-up imaging is required.

TREATMENT

GENERAL MEASURES

- DVAs do not typically require treatment.
- Anticonvulsants should be used to treat seizures.
- Surgical resection is the only treatment option for CMs, although conservative management may be indicated if the risk of surgery outweighs the potential benefit.
- Treatment options for AVMs include resection via microsurgery, embolization, stereotactic radiosurgery, and conservative management. Risk of hemorrhage ranges 0.9–34% per year, so decisions about treatment should be guided by symptoms at presentation and structural features of the AVM.
- Treatment of choice for VOGMs in all ages is endovascular embolization. Direct surgical intervention has unacceptable risks and is no longer recommended. Radiosurgery has been used in a small number of clinically stable older patients. Refractory CHF prompts intervention in neonates. Treatment in older infants and children is indicated to prevent cerebral ischemia (from arterial steal or from venous infarction) and to prevent hydrocephalus. Embolization can be completed in stages over a few months after CHF is controlled.
- Ventriculoperitoneal shunts may be required in patients who develop hydrocephalus following intracerebral hemorrhage related to CM or AVM or in patients with VOGMs.
- Treatment in SWS is targeted to symptoms, using anticonvulsants for seizures and eye drops or ocular shunts for glaucoma. Low-dose aspirin is recommended at the time of diagnosis to prevent further brain injury due to impaired cerebral blood flow. Seizures can lead to ongoing brain injury by increasing metabolic demand in brain tissue that has abnormal perfusion at baseline, so aggressive seizure management is recommended. Some children with intractable epilepsy may be good candidates for epilepsy surgery.

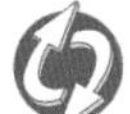

ONGOING CARE

- Generally, no specific follow-up is required for patients with DVAs.
- Follow-up with a neurologist is indicated for patients with CMs, AVMs, VOGMs, and SWS.
- Neurosurgical consultation is indicated for patients with CMs, AVMs, and VOGMs.
- A follow-up CT or MRI is indicated to evaluate patients with new neurologic signs or symptoms.
- Ophthalmologic follow-up is indicated for patients with SWS and most patients with VOGMs, especially prior to treatment when hydrocephalus may develop.

PROGNOSIS

- Prognosis is excellent for patients with isolated DVAs.
- Prognosis for patients with CMs and AVMs depends on the size, location, presenting symptoms, and specific characteristics of the lesion. Patients who have experienced an intracerebral hemorrhage have worse prognosis than those who have not.
- For patients with VOGMs, earlier age of symptoms is associated with worse prognosis. Mortality in neonates with symptomatic lesions is 36%. In a recent meta-analysis of endovascular embolization, 84% had a good or fair clinical outcome, and mortality was 16%.
- Prognosis in patients with SWS depends on the extent and location of involvement. Seizures occur in the majority (~85%), with low normal intelligence or intellectual disability in ~35%.

COMPLICATIONS

- Death can occur in patients with intracerebral hemorrhage due to CMs or AVMs.
- Mortality approaches 100% in untreated patients with VOGMs.
- In severe cases of VOGMs, 80% of cardiac output may be delivered to the head because of the low vascular resistance within the malformation. Cardiac ischemia may occur because of decreased coronary artery blood flow.
- Intracerebral hemorrhage may occur as a result of CMs, AVMs, and VOGMs or as a complication of treatment.
- Longer term complications from CMs, AVMs, and VOGMs include intellectual disability, seizures, hydrocephalus, and chronic motor impairment.
- In patients with SWS, visual impairment can result if glaucoma is difficult to control. Persistent hemiparesis can develop.

PATIENT MONITORING

- Serial neuroimaging should be performed in patients with CMs, AVMs, and VOGMs to guide the timing of treatment and to assess for recurrence.
- Head circumference should be monitored in patients with VOGMs as a marker of hydrocephalus.

ADDITIONAL READING

- Comi A. Current therapeutic options in Sturge-Weber syndrome. *Semin Pediatr Neurol*. 2015;22(4):295–301.
- Niazi TN, Klimo P Jr, Anderson RC, et al. Diagnosis and management of arteriovenous malformations in children. *Neurosurg Clin N Am*. 2010;21(3):443–456.
- Recinos PF, Rahmathulla G, Pearl M, et al. Vein of Galen malformations: epidemiology, clinical presentations, management. *Neurosurg Clin N Am*. 2012;23(1):165–177.
- San Millán Ruíz D, Gailloud P. Cerebral developmental venous anomalies. *Childs Nerv Syst*. 2010;26(10):1395–1406.
- Smith ER, Scott RM. Cavernous malformations. *Neurosurg Clin N Am*. 2010;21(3):483–490.

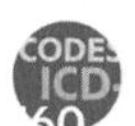

CODES

ICD10

- Q28.3 Other malformations of cerebral vessels
- Q85.8 Other phakomatoses, not elsewhere classified
- D18.02 Hemangioma of intracranial structures

FAQ

- Q: Can the AVM recur after treatment?
- A: AVMs have a propensity to recur. Imaging studies give a good indication of the likelihood of recurrence.
- Q: How does a vascular malformation cause seizures?
- A: Seizures can result from ischemia, hemorrhage, or acute hydrocephalus associated with the malformation.

V

VENTRICULAR SEPTAL DEFECT

Shabnam Peyvandi, MD

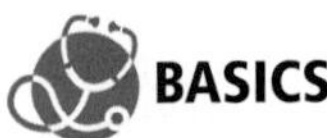

BASICS

DESCRIPTION

- A ventricular septal defect (VSD) is an opening in the ventricular septum, resulting in a communication between the left ventricle (LV) and the right ventricle (RV). The ventricular septum can be divided into four major areas:
  - Inlet/canal septum
  - Membranous/conoventricular septum
  - Muscular septum (largest)
  - Conal/infundibular/outlet septum (includes conal septal hypoplasia and malalignment types)
- There are several corresponding types of VSDs that have different natural histories and associated problems:
  - Inlet/canal VSDs: usually part of an atrioventricular (AV) canal defect, 5–7% of all VSDs
  - Membranous/conoventricular VSDs: 80% of all VSDs by classic teaching; fewer than muscular VSDs by echocardiographic data
  - Muscular VSDs: usually single and small but can be multiple and of variable size; 5–20% of all VSDs by classic teaching, but a large percentage are inaudible
  - Conal septal hypoplasia/outlet VSDs: usually large and unrestrictive; associated with aortic valve (AoV) cusp prolapse and aortic insufficiency
  - Anterior malalignment VSDs: usually associated with RV outflow tract obstruction; paradigms: tetralogy of Fallot, double outlet RV
  - Posterior malalignment VSDs: usually associated with LV outflow tract obstruction; paradigms: subaortic stenosis with coarctation or interrupted aortic arch
- There may also be multiple VSDs of different types in a single patient. Many complex forms of congenital heart disease include a VSD.

EPIDEMIOLOGY

- VSDs are the most common form of congenital heart disease, occurring in ~1.5 to 5.7 per 1,000 term births and ~4.5 to 7 per 1,000 preterm births, by classic teaching.
- Echocardiographic data show a higher incidence of ~50 per 1,000 live births, mostly asymptomatic muscular VSDs.

RISK FACTORS

Genetics

- Sibling and offspring recurrence risk for VSDs is estimated to be ~3–4%.
- VSD is the most common lesion in trisomy 21, 13, and 18, but >95% of children with VSDs have normal chromosomes.
- Congenital heart disease that includes a conal septal malalignment VSD (e.g., tetralogy of Fallot) or VSD with a conotruncal malformation (e.g., truncus arteriosus or interrupted aortic arch type B) has a 13–50% incidence of microdeletion of chromosome 22 (22q11.2 deletion syndrome). In a recent series, 7% of patients with an isolated membranous/conoventricular VSD had a 22q11.2 deletion.

PATHOPHYSIOLOGY

- Both the size of the VSD and the ratio of pulmonary (PVR) to systemic vascular resistance (SVR) determine the direction and amount of shunting.
  - Small VSD: The VSD imposes high resistance to flow with a large LV-to-RV pressure gradient, usually resulting in normal RV pressures. The restrictive size results in a small left-to-right shunt. The VSD size is usually ≤1/4 the size of the AoV annulus. The workload of the ventricles is normal.
  - Moderate VSD: The VSD imposes modest resistance to flow, usually resulting in mildly elevated RV pressures. The amount of shunting can still be large and is determined by the PVR/SVR ratio. The VSD size is usually 1/3 to 2/3 the size of the AoV annulus. The workload of the ventricles is increased.
  - Large VSD: The VSD imposes no resistance to flow and is unrestrictive, resulting in systemic RV pressures and RV hypertension. The workload of the ventricles is markedly increased.
- The lower the PVR/SVR ratio, the greater the degree of left-to-right shunting. A large left-to-right shunt leads to pulmonary vascular congestion, tachypnea, tachycardia, and hepatomegaly, all signs of congestive heart failure (CHF). The amount of CHF correlates directly with shunt size and usually peaks at 6 to 8 weeks of age, timed with the nadir of PVR and physiologic anemia. Lack of significant CHF in patients with a large VSD signifies elevated PVR and requires careful evaluation. Cardiac catheterization may be required in these patients to provide additional data.
- If a large VSD is left untreated, pulmonary vascular obstructive disease will eventually develop, leading to reversal of the shunt, cyanosis, and RV failure (Eisenmenger syndrome).

DIAGNOSIS

HISTORY

- Small VSD: The child is usually asymptomatic, with normal growth and development. Most commonly, a murmur is detected at 1 to 6 weeks of age.
- Moderate VSD: The child is usually symptomatic with slow weight gain and sparing of longitudinal growth. There is often an increased incidence of respiratory infections. Sweating and fatigue with feeding may be present.
- Large VSD: The child is usually quite symptomatic, especially with a larger shunt, showing signs of CHF, and marked failure to thrive.
- Children with Eisenmenger syndrome have cyanosis, fatigue, and symptoms of right heart failure.

PHYSICAL EXAM

- Small VSD
  - The child usually appears healthy with normal growth.
  - The heart action is quiet, but there is often an associated systolic thrill along the left sternal border with a membranous VSD, in contrast to a small muscular VSD.
  - Heart sounds are normal. A high-frequency, pansystolic murmur is present in membranous VSDs, whereas in muscular VSDs the murmur is not pansystolic.
  - The murmur is loudest over the region of the VSD.
- Moderate VSD
  - The child usually appears in mild distress with tachycardia and tachypnea.
  - The heart action is increased, and there is often still an associated thrill.
  - The P_2 component of S_2 may be normal or accentuated.
  - A medium frequency, pansystolic murmur is present over the location of the VSD.
  - A mid-diastolic rumble is present over the mitral listening area (apex), as a result of a significant shunt and indicates ≥2:1 pulmonary to systemic flow ratio. Hepatomegaly may be present.
- Large VSD
  - The child usually appears ill with marked distress and marked tachycardia and tachypnea, proportional to the size of the left-to-right shunt.
  - The heart action is markedly increased without a thrill. The P_2 component of S_2 is loud and narrowly split as a result of pulmonary hypertension.
  - A soft, low-frequency pansystolic murmur is present over the VSD.
  - The loudness of the mid-diastolic rumble is proportional to the size of the left-to-right shunt.
  - CHF physical exam signs are proportional to the size of the left-to-right shunt but are usually present to a significant degree.
- If significant aortic insufficiency develops, a high-frequency, early diastolic murmur is heard along the left sternal border.
- In newborns whose PVR has not yet fallen, the increased heart action remains the key to diagnosis as auscultation may be unimpressive.
- Likewise, in children with elevated PVR, the increased heart action remains the key to diagnosis. Auscultation shows a narrowly split S_2 with a loud P_2. The murmur loudness is dependent on VSD size and shunt but often is soft or absent and unimpressive.

- Once Eisenmenger syndrome develops (secondary to pulmonary vascular obstructive changes), patients manifest cyanosis, clubbing, an increased RV impulse, a narrowly split S_2 with a loud P_2 component, and a soft or absent VSD murmur. There may be a systolic murmur of tricuspid insufficiency at the left lower sternal border (LLSB), a high-frequency early diastolic murmur of pulmonary insufficiency, or an S_3 at the LLSB. There is usually associated jugular venous distention and hepatomegaly, indicating high right-sided filling pressures.

DIAGNOSTIC TESTS & INTERPRETATION

Initial Tests (screening, lab, imaging)

- Electrocardiogram:
  - Small VSD: normal
  - Moderate VSD: left ventricular hypertrophy (LVH)
  - Large VSD: biventricular hypertrophy (BVH) and left atrial enlargement (LAE)
  - Eisenmenger syndrome: right ventricular hypertrophy (RVH) and right atrial enlargement (RAE)
- Cardiac catheterization:
  - Generally reserved for patients with difficult VSD anatomy, associated lesions, or for the assessment of the ratio of pulmonary to systemic flow and pulmonary vascular reactivity
- Chest radiograph:
  - Small VSD: normal
  - Moderate VSD: hyperinflation, cardiomegaly, increased pulmonary vascular markings
  - Large VSD: cardiomegaly, markedly increased pulmonary vascular markings, Kerley B lines
  - Eisenmenger syndrome: normal heart size, prominent central pulmonary arteries, and decreased peripheral vascular markings
- Echocardiogram:
  - All children with a murmur consistent with a VSD should undergo an echocardiogram to define the location, size, and number of VSDs and any associated defects. Color/spectral Doppler allows visualization of the shunt direction and the amount of restriction to the VSD, if any.

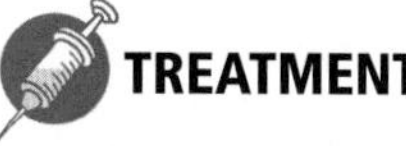

TREATMENT

GENERAL MEASURES

- Small VSD: no intervention; continued observation
- Moderate VSD: If signs of CHF develop, digoxin, diuretics, afterload reduction, and increased caloric intake are indicated.
- Large VSD: CHF often develops and requires aggressive therapy as noted above.
- Membranous and muscular VSDs often become smaller or close spontaneously. Generally, observation and/or medical therapy is indicated for a few months.
- Conoseptal hypoplasia and malalignment VSDs do not close spontaneously and therefore require surgical closure.
- After 1 year of life, a significant left-to-right shunt (Qp:Qs $\geq$2:1) or elevated pulmonary artery pressures are an indication for surgery.
- Children with elevated pulmonary artery pressures ($\geq$1/2 systemic) should undergo repair before 2 years of age, even if CHF symptoms are controlled.
- Development of complications, including aortic insufficiency, subaortic membrane, and double-chamber RV, is usually an indication for surgical repair.
- Surgical correction may be contraindicated if the PVR is >8 Wood units/m^2.
- Recent series of surgical VSD closure report a mortality of <2%.
- Complete heart block occurs in <2% of patients postoperatively but requires pacemaker therapy when it occurs.
- A small percentage of patients with muscular or membranous VSDs may have successful transcatheter device closure.

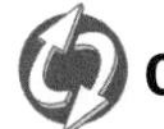

ONGOING CARE

PROGNOSIS

- Spontaneous closure: usually by age 2 years; 90% of small muscular VSDs and 8–35% of small conoventricular/membranous VSDs
- Prognosis with surgical closure is excellent.
- The risk of Eisenmenger syndrome is considered minimal if large VSDs are surgically closed by 2 years of age.
- Caveat: Despite timely VSD surgical closure, a tiny percentage of patients still go on to develop Eisenmenger syndrome.

COMPLICATIONS

- All VSDs: endocarditis—overall rate of 15 cases per 10,000 person-years of follow-up
- Moderate-to-large VSDs: LV volume overload, left atrial hypertension, CHF, poor growth, Eisenmenger syndrome
- Specific types:
  - Inlet/canal VSDs: often associated with cleft mitral valve with possible AV valve insufficiency
  - Membranous/conoventricular VSDs: risk for development of aortic insufficiency typically due to prolapse of the right aortic cusp, subaortic membrane, or double-chamber RV
  - Muscular VSDs: isolated—near-zero risk for the development of subsequent lesions
  - Conal septal hypoplasia VSDs: risk for development of aortic insufficiency
  - Malalignment VSDs: usually associated with outflow tract obstruction and distal great artery hypoplasia/obstruction

FOLLOW-UP RECOMMENDATIONS

Patient Monitoring

Subacute bacterial endocarditis (SBE) prophylaxis is recommended for 6 months after complete closure (surgical or catheter based) of a VSD.

ADDITIONAL READING

- Aguilar NE, Eugenio Lopez J. Ventricular septal defects. *Bol Asoc Med P R*. 2009;101(4):23–29.
- Hoffman JI, Kaplan S. The incidence of congenital heart disease. *J Am Coll Cardiol*. 2002;39(12):1890–1900.
- McDaniel NL. Ventricular and atrial septal defects. *Pediatr Rev*. 2001;22(8):265–270.
- Penny DJ, Vick GW III. Ventricular septal defect. *Lancet*. 2011;377(9771):1103–1112.
- Schipper M, Slieker MG, Schoof PH, et al. Surgical repair of ventricular septal defect; Contemporary results and risk factors for a complicated course. *Pediatr Cardiol*. 2017;38(2):264–270.

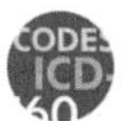

CODES

ICD10

- Q21.0 Ventricular septal defect
- Q24.8 Other specified congenital malformations of heart

FAQ

- Q: Should children with a murmur consistent with a VSD undergo echocardiogram?
- A: Yes, to define the location, size, and number of VSDs and any associated lesions
- Q: Should children with VSD have SBE prophylaxis?
- A: Based on the revised 2007 American Heart Association guidelines, isolated VSD does not warrant SBE prophylaxis. However, SBE prophylaxis is recommended for 6 months following complete surgical or interventional catheterization closure (no residual defect) of a VSD.
- Q: Should asymptomatic children with a small VSD have activity restrictions?
- A: No, if there are no other problems

VENTRICULAR TACHYCARDIA

Walter L. Li, MD

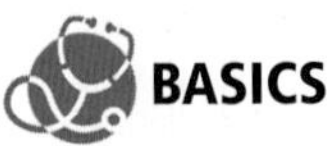

BASICS

DESCRIPTION

- Ventricular tachycardia (VT) is a series of three or more repetitive beats originating from the ventricle at a rate faster than the upper limit of normal for age. The QRS complex is always different from sinus rhythm and is usually wide but can appear narrow in infants. VT may, but not always, have atrioventricular (AV) dissociation; nonsustained VT: >3 beats and <30 seconds
- Sustained VT: lasts >30 seconds
- VT may be monomorphic or polymorphic.
- Torsades de pointes: a polymorphic variant
  - The QRS complexes gradually change shape and axis throughout the tachycardia.
  - Associated with congenital long QT syndrome (LQTS), acquired long QT, and Brugada syndrome

RISK FACTORS

- Metabolic disturbances (hypoxia, acidosis, hypo/hyperkalemia, hypomagnesemia, hypothermia)
- Drug toxicity (e.g., digitalis toxicity, antiarrhythmic agents)
- Substance abuse (cocaine, methamphetamine)
- Myocardial ischemia (e.g., Kawasaki disease, congenital coronary anomalies)
- Trauma
- Invasive lines or catheters
- Pericardial effusion

Genetics

- LQTS may be inherited in an autosomal recessive or autosomal dominant pattern. It is mostly commonly associated with potassium cardiac ion channel defects and may be associated with hearing loss and/or a family history of sudden death.
- Brugada syndrome may be inherited in an autosomal dominant pattern. It is most commonly associated with a defect in the cardiac sodium channel (SCN5A) and appears to be inherited in an autosomal dominant pattern.

PATHOPHYSIOLOGY

VT may result from a reentrant, triggered, or abnormal automaticity mechanism.

ETIOLOGY

- Diverse and often overlapping
- LQTS
- Brugada syndrome
- Catecholaminergic polymorphic VT
- Myocarditis
- Dilated cardiomyopathy
- Hypertrophic cardiomyopathy
- Arrhythmogenic right ventricular cardiomyopathy
- Before and after surgery for congenital heart disease (CHD) (e.g., tetralogy of Fallot, transposition of the great arteries, aortic stenosis, Ebstein anomaly, and pulmonary vascular occlusive disease)
- Myocardial tumors
- Heart failure
- Idiopathic

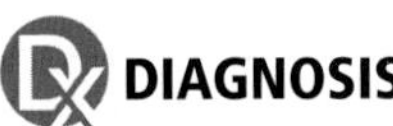

DIAGNOSIS

Based on electrocardiogram (ECG), rhythm strip, Holter, or event monitor

HISTORY

- Varies widely, ranging from asymptomatic to sudden cardiac arrest/death
- Other symptoms include palpitations, presyncope or syncope, exercise intolerance, and dizziness.

PHYSICAL EXAM

- Can be normal; occasional heart rhythm irregularity secondary to premature ventricular complexes (PVCs) may be auscultated.
- Acute, sustained VT may have signs of hemodynamic compromise, including lack of palpable pulse.
- Signs of underlying heart disease may be present.

DIFFERENTIAL DIAGNOSIS

Wide complex tachyarrhythmia

- Suspect VT until proven otherwise.
- Supraventricular tachycardia (SVT) with aberrancy
- Antidromic tachycardia (antegrade conduction down an accessory pathway during an AV reciprocating tachycardia [e.g., Wolff-Parkinson-White syndrome]).
- Atrial flutter or atrial fibrillation with rapid antegrade conduction over an accessory pathway
- Sinus tachycardia or SVT with underlying bundle branch block

DIAGNOSTIC TESTS & INTERPRETATION

Initial Tests (screening, lab, imaging)

- Serum electrolytes, including magnesium and potassium levels, blood gas, and serum drug levels as appropriate
- Urine toxicology screen
- ECG
  - AV dissociation during tachycardia is diagnostic but not always present or easily seen.
  - Bundle branch morphology (right or left) and QRS axis during tachycardia may help localize the site of origin.
  - Typically, repolarization (T wave) abnormalities are present.
  - A prolonged QTc interval during sinus rhythm may help establish a LQTS diagnosis.
  - Brugada pattern: right bundle branch block with coved-type ST elevation and T-wave inversion in leads V1 and V2 during sinus rhythm. Brugada pattern may be more obvious when the patient is febrile and/or with leads V1 and V2 placed one intercostal space higher than standard.
- Echocardiogram
  - Rule out CHD, pericardial effusion, tumors, hypertrophic and dilated cardiomyopathy, myocarditis.
- Ambulatory Holter monitor
  - Quantitative assessment of ventricular ectopy, and frequency, rate, and duration of VT
  - Less frequent episodes may need longer term monitoring with an event monitor or implantable loop recorder.
- Exercise stress test (>5 years old)
  - Benign PVCs are characteristically suppressed with exercise and return in the immediate recovery period.
  - Exacerbation or worsening of ventricular arrhythmias is concerning.
- Cardiac magnetic resonance imaging: assessment for arrhythmogenic right ventricular cardiomyopathy and abnormalities that are beyond the resolution of echocardiography

Diagnostic Procedures/Other

- Cardiac catheterization: hemodynamic assessment, endomyocardial biopsy, and coronary artery angiography
- Electrophysiologic study indications
  - Confirm diagnosis and mechanism of a wide complex rhythm.
  - Determine appropriate medical therapy in a patient with inducible VT.
  - Evaluate for suspected VT in the setting of structural or functional heart disease, syncope, or cardiac arrest.
  - Risk assessment of VT. Evaluate syncope in the setting of palpitations.
  - Characterize VT with consideration for catheter ablation.

TREATMENT

GENERAL MEASURES

- If the patient is hemodynamically compromised, prompt synchronized direct-current (pediatric, 1 to 2 joules/kg; adult, 100 to 400 joules/kg) cardioversion is indicated.
- Asynchronous defibrillation is needed for ventricular fibrillation or pulseless VT.
- Cardiopulmonary resuscitation is needed for persistent hemodynamic compromise.

MEDICATION

- Acute
  - Some forms of VT in structurally normal hearts may respond to adenosine (pediatric, 0.1 to 0.3 mg/kg rapid push; adult 6 to 12 mg).
  - Esmolol IV (bolus, 0.5 mg/kg; infusion, 50 to 300 mcg/kg/min).
  - Procainamide IV (bolus, 5 to 15 mg/kg over 20 to 60 minutes; infusion, 20 to 100 mcg/kg/min).
  - Amiodarone IV (bolus, 2 to 5 mg/kg over 30 minutes; infusion, 5 to 10 mcg/kg/min).
  - Lidocaine IV (bolus,1 mg/kg over 1 minute; infusion, 20 to 50 mcg/kg/min).
  - $MgSO_4$ is indicated for torsades de pointes.
  - Overdrive ventricular pacing may terminate the tachycardia but should be used cautiously as it may accelerate the VT or induce ventricular fibrillation.
- Chronic
  - Class IB (mexiletine and phenytoin)
  - β-Blockers (propranolol, nadolol, metoprolol) are used in LQTS and may be effective in exercise-induced VT and postoperative CHD.
  - Class III agents (amiodarone and sotalol) should be avoided in patients with LQTS.
  - Class IC agents (flecainide) may be proarrhythmic and sudden death has been reported in patients with structural heart disease.
  - Verapamil is often effective for right ventricular outflow tract VT and left ventricular fascicular VT.

ISSUES FOR REFERRAL

Cardiology consultation and close follow-up is needed.

SURGERY/OTHER PROCEDURES

- An implantable cardioverter defibrillator is indicated for survivors of sudden cardiac arrest without a reversible cause and those at risk for sudden cardiac arrest.
- Pacing may help suppress ectopy that causes VT.
- Catheter ablation using radiofrequency energy or cryothermal energy

ADMISSION, INPATIENT, AND NURSING CONSIDERATIONS

Patient with hemodynamically unstable forms of VT should be stabilized and admitted.

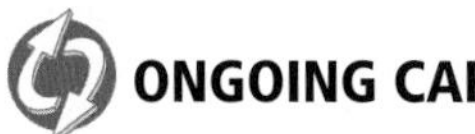

ONGOING CARE

FOLLOW-UP RECOMMENDATIONS

Patient Monitoring

- Monitoring in an intensive care unit is needed for transition to a stable chronic suppressive medical regimen.
- Frequency of outpatient follow-up is dependent on the underlying cause and clinical severity.
- ECG, Holter monitor, and exercise stress test are helpful in titrating and assessing efficacy of medical therapy.

PATIENT EDUCATION

Patients should be counseled about potential triggers of VT, which is dependent on the underlying etiology. Exercise-related VT should prompt exercise restrictions. LQTS patients should avoid QT prolonging medications. Brugada syndrome patients should receive antipyretics promptly during times of fever.

PROGNOSIS

- Generally, very good in patients with idiopathic VT and a structurally normal heart
- Suppression of ventricular ectopy with exercise has a favorable prognosis.
- In patients with heart disease (congenital or acquired) or LQTS and other channelopathies, VT may increase the risk of presyncope, syncope, and possibly sudden death.

COMPLICATIONS

- Sudden cardiac arrest/sudden cardiac death
- Acquired cardiomyopathy (from chronic, persistent VT and a lack of AV synchrony)

ADDITIONAL READING

- Ceresnak SR, Liberman L, Avasarala K, et al. Are wide complex tachycardia algorithms applicable in children and patients with congenital heart disease? *J Electrocardiol*. 2010;43(6):694–700.
- Escudero C, Carr R, Sanatani S. The medical management of pediatric arrhythmias. *Current Treat Options Cardiovasc Med*. 2012;14(5):455–472.
- Kleinman ME, Chameides L, Schexnayder SM, et al. Part 14: pediatric advanced life support: 2010 American Heart Association Guidelines for Cardiopulmonary Resuscitation and Emergency Cardiovascular Care. *Circulation*. 2010;122(18 Suppl 3):S876–S908.
- McBride ME, Marino BS, Webster G, et al. Amiodarone versus lidocaine for pediatric cardiac arrest due to ventricular arrhythmias: a systematic review. *Pediatr Crit Care Med*. 2017;18(2):183–189.
- Wang S, Zhu W, Hamilton RM, et al. Diagnosis-specific characteristics of ventricular tachycardia in children with structurally normal hearts. *Heart Rhythm*. 2010;7(12):1725–1731.

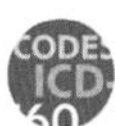

CODES

ICD10

- I47.2 Ventricular tachycardia
- I45.81 Long QT syndrome
- Q24.8 Other specified congenital malformations of heart

FAQ

- Q: Should siblings of patients with LQTS be evaluated?
- A: Yes. Siblings and parents (even if asymptomatic) should have an ECG, Holter monitor, and exercise stress test for evaluation of the QT interval. Commercial genetic testing is currently available to detect mutations in the most common genes that cause the LQTS. The test will positively identify ~75% of patients with the LQTS. Genetic testing may be considered in patients in whom there is a high suspicion of LQTS.
- Q: Can patients with underlying substrates for VT be identified before onset of symptoms?
- A: Family history suspicious for sudden cardiac death may prompt evaluation for inheritable forms of LQTS, cardiomyopathy, and CHD. Early identification of patients with underlying substrates for VT may lead to preventative therapy.
- Q: Who should be screened for VT?
- A: Children with syncope and palpitations should be screened for CHD and underlying substrates for VT. Families with a history of unexplained sudden death, frequent miscarriages, and sudden infant death syndrome may have an inheritable substrate for VT.

V

VESICOURETERAL REFLUX

Christopher E. Bayne, MD • Michael H. Hsieh, MD, PhD

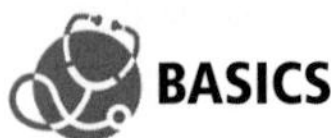

BASICS

DESCRIPTION

- Vesicoureteral reflux (VUR) occurs when urine passes from the bladder to the ureters or kidneys. VUR is either a primary (congenital) or acquired process secondary to bladder dysfunction (congenital, acquired, or behavioral) or outlet obstruction (e.g., posterior urethral valves [PUVs]).
- VUR can be subgrouped according to presentation type. It is usually detected in two scenarios: the postnatal evaluation of an infant with prenatal hydronephrosis (HN) or during imaging evaluation after urinary tract infection (UTI).
- Children in the latter category are at higher risk for recurrent UTI (rUTI) and renal scarring (RS). RS is primarily a risk after febrile UTI (fUTI). Breakthrough UTI (btUTI) is a UTI that occurs while on continuous antibiotic prophylaxis (CAP).

EPIDEMIOLOGY

Prevalence

- VUR occurs in ~1% of children.
- In those detected in the postnatal evaluation of an infant with prenatal HN:
  - ~20–30% of patients with prenatal HN have VUR. Screening this population for VUR is controversial (see "Diagnostic Tests & Interpretation" section).
  - Ratio of males to females in this group is 3:1, which is believed to reflect a period of high-pressure voiding in boys that resolves by 18 months.
- In those detected during imaging evaluation of a UTI:
  - Up to 30–50% of children with fUTI will have VUR.

RISK FACTORS

It is important to distinguish between associations that increase risk for VUR and conditions in which VUR is more commonly found.

- VUR is more likely to be detected in those with prenatal HN and/or r/fUTI. fUTIs are not thought to cause VUR, although some data suggest high-grade VUR may be a risk for fUTI.
- It is unknown whether some pathologies of the urinary tract associated with VUR (e.g., ureteropelvic junction obstruction [UPJO]) reflect a single event (e.g., ureteral bud defect) or represent separate abnormalities.
- Primary VUR (see "Pathophysiology")
  - Young age (There is debate whether normal infant voiding patterns may predispose to VUR.)
  - UPJO (ipsilateral VUR in 10–20%)
  - Ureteral duplication (see "Pathophysiology")
  - Dysplastic kidney (contralateral VUR in 30–40%)
  - Bladder diverticula, especially periureteral location
  - Prune belly (Eagle-Barrett) syndrome
  - Severe congenital anomalies, including bladder exstrophy and cloacal anomalies, VACTERL and CHARGE, and imperforate anus
- Secondary VUR (see "Pathophysiology")
  - Bladder neck and/or urethral obstruction (e.g., prolapsing ureterocele, PUV, urethral atresia)
  - Neurologic conditions predisposing to neuropathic bladder (e.g., spina bifida, tethered cord)
  - Bladder and bowel dysfunction (BBD)

Genetics

- 30% of siblings will have VUR (usually low grade). The majority will be asymptomatic with only rare RS.
- Parents with VUR have a 60% chance of having a child with VUR.
  - Screening siblings is controversial. Low-grade VUR usually resolves without sequelae.
  - Consider screening siblings with history of febrile illnesses, even in absence of definitive UTIs.
  - Siblings of children with VUR are more likely to show renal cortical abnormalities if diagnosed after a previous UTI than after screening.

PATHOPHYSIOLOGY

- The ureterovesical junction (UVJ) is a flap valve. During storage and voiding, pressure within the bladder compresses the intramural ureter against detrusor backing to prevent flow of urine up the ureter.
- VUR can result from either abnormal anatomy, abnormal storage, abnormal voiding pressure, or a combination of the three.
- Primary VUR results from either a short ureteral tunnel through the bladder wall or transient high-pressure voiding, which occurs normally in the first 18 months of life (particularly in boys).
  - Patients with primary VUR generally improve and even resolve with time as the ureteral tunnel grows or bladder pressures decrease.
- In complete ureteral duplication, an early forming ureteric (refluxing in 30–40%) bud drains the lower pole renal moiety, and a late forming ureteric bud drains the upper pole renal moiety.
- Any circumstance that increases pressure storage of urine and/or impairs or obstructs urine outflow can overwhelm the UVJ and create secondary VUR.
  - The distinction between primary and secondary reflux is important because large prospective trials have been conducted on patients with primary reflux and it is not appropriate to extend those findings to patients with secondary reflux.
- VUR is classified as five grades by the International Reflux Study based on the voiding cystourethrogram (VCUG):
  - Grade I: reflux into ureter
  - Grade II: reflux to renal pelvis without calyceal dilation
  - Grade III: calyceal blunting, mild dilatation of ureter
  - Grade IV: gross ureteral dilatation, moderate calyceal dilation, papillary impressions maintained
  - Grade V: gross urinary tract dilatation, loss of papillary impressions
- General consensus is that VUR alone does not damage kidneys, but renal damage results from reflux of infected urine.
  - As VUR grade increases, risk of spontaneous resolution decreases and risk of rUTI, RS increases.
  - To this end, in the literature, VUR is often classified as either (i) low (I to II), moderate (III), or high grade (IV to V) *or* (ii) nondilating (I to II) versus dilating (≥III).
  - From the perspective of preventing r/btUTI and RS, dilating and high-grade VUR are more concerning than low-grade and nondilating VUR (ndVUR).

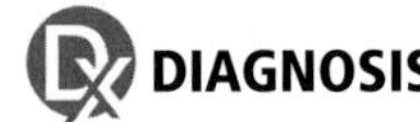

DIAGNOSIS

HISTORY

- Prenatal evaluations, including prenatal ultrasound findings of HN
- Family history of renal disease, VUR, or UTI (may suggest inheritance of UTI-susceptible uroepithelium)
- Voiding history: age at toilet training, daytime or nighttime incontinence, frequency of urination
- Sensation of emptying the bladder completely
- Signs of BBD:
  - Frequency and/or urgency
  - Damp underwear
  - Associated constipation, infrequent bowel movements (may suggest pelvic floor immaturity)
  - "Vincent curtsy": holding urine during bladder contraction by squatting, crossing legs so heel compresses urethra

PHYSICAL EXAM

- Blood pressure
- Abdominal palpation (primarily to check for hard stool)
- In girls, inspect the urethral meatus and vaginal introitus. Look for pooling of urine in the vaginal vault (e.g., ectopic ureteral insertion, suggesting possible ureteral duplication), discharge, or skin irritation.
- In boys, inspect foreskin for phimosis, location and caliber of urethral meatus, and complete scrotal exam.
- Examine spine, sacrum for occult spinal dysraphism.

DIFFERENTIAL DIAGNOSIS

Prenatal HN and UN can also be due to UPJO or UVJO. The important task is differentiating primary from secondary VUR so patients can be appropriately managed and parents appropriately counseled.

DIAGNOSTIC TESTS & INTERPRETATION

Initial Tests (screening, lab, imaging)

- Serum creatinine and urinalysis for proteinuria may be obtained if imaging shows solitary kidney, decreased function, RS, or severe bilateral VUR.
  - Serum creatinine <24 hours of life reflects maternal renal function.
- Serum procalcitonin (sPCT) at initial presentation for fUTI may screen for VUR.
  - In children ≤2 years, sPCT ≥1 ng/mL is 94.3% sensitive and 53.5% specific for dilating VUR (dVUR) and predicts dVUR on multivariate analysis.
- Non-*Escherichia coli* fUTI is a predictor for dVUR compared to *E. coli* fUTI.
- Renal and bladder ultrasound (RBUS)
  - Usually obtained between 2nd day and 1st week of life if the child had prenatal HN or UN. RBUS <48 hours after birth may underestimate HN or UN.
  - After fUTI, RBUS has been recommended as a screen for VUR. HN, UN, renal parenchymal defects, or other abnormalities constitute an abnormal test and prompt VCUG to assess for VUR (see "Pyelonephritis" chapter).
    - After UTI in children ≤19 years, pooled sensitivity and specificity for RBUS in predicting dVUR (on VCUG) are 59% (45–72%) and 79% (65–88%). Post-test probability of dVUR given an abnormal RBUS is 30%. Post-test probability of dVUR given negative RBUS is 8%.

    - Accuracy of predicting dVUR may be improved by looking for specific RBUS findings, including renal pelvis uroepithelial thickening and kidney length.
    - Others have found highly sophisticated modeling techniques improve RBUS specificity to detect dVUR to 98% but decrease sensitivity to 18%.
  - After fUTI in children ≤18 years, normal RBUS may miss renal function loss and/or cortical defects on delayed phase dimercaptosuccinic acid (DMSA) in up to 19%.
  - An unremarkable RBUS does not exclude significant GU pathology, dVUR.
  - RBUS is a useful tool for following renal growth.
  - In children with prenatal HN, the presence of ureteral dilatation, renal dysplasia, or ureteral duplication significantly increases the chance of findings VUR on postnatal VCUG.
- VCUG
  - Performed with radiopaque contrast instilled in bladder via urethral catheter (contrast VCUG) or IV radionucleotide (nuclear VCUG)
  - Contrast study is necessary for first VCUG to accurately grade the reflux in both sexes and evaluate urethral anatomy in boys.
    - Age-appropriate volume should be instilled in bladder and repeated for second cycle.
    - The voiding portion of the study is important because ~20% of VUR can be missed if voiding not observed.
  - American Academy of Pediatrics (AAP) does not recommend a VCUG after a first fUTI in children age 2 to 24 months. National Institute for Health and Clinical Excellence (NICE) guidelines do not routinely recommend VCUG to detect VUR. There are some shortcomings to these guidelines (also see "Pyelonephritis" chapter).
- ^{99m}Tc-DMSA renography
  - Gold standard for diagnosing acute pyelonephritis (APN) and RS
    - Used acutely (≤7 days after UTI) to detect APN or in delayed setting (≥5 months after APN) to identify RS
    - Without a baseline DMSA, congenital (dysplasia) and acquired (RS) lesions appear similar.
  - If differentiating upper tract infection versus cystitis in setting of fUTI is important; acute DMSA is useful.
  - Some advocate using DMSA to identify high-risk patients requiring VCUG ("top-down approach")

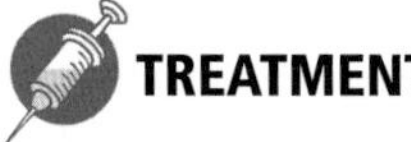

TREATMENT

GENERAL MEASURES

There are four management arms for children with VUR:

- Surveillance
- CAP with the goal of preventing UTI and RS until VUR spontaneously downgrades or resolves
  - CAP does not treat VUR or RS.
  - CAP does not involve treatment-dose therapy. Antibiotics are chosen based on higher urine concentration at low daily dosages.
  - Common agents: amoxicillin at 10 to 15 mg/kg/24 h used for first 2 months of life and then trimethoprim/sulfamethoxazole (40 mg/200 mg/5 mL) at 0.25 mL/kg/24 h (equivalent to 2 to 3 mg/kg daily of trimethoprim), and nitrofurantoin at 1 to 2 mg/kg/24 h
- Endoscopic subureteric injection of a bulking agent (dextranomer/hyaluronic acid copolymer [Deflux] is the only FDA-approved agent for this use in United States)
- Surgical ureteral reimplant (ureteroneocystostomy)
- Historically, randomized controlled trials have suggested CAP and surgery have equitable outcomes. These studies have been criticized for heterogeneous populations, methodology, and reporting.
- More recently, the Swedish Reflux Trial compared CAP to endoscopic injection or surveillance in children 1 to 2 years with VUR grade III to IV. The RIVUR trial compared CAP to placebo in children 2 to 72 months with VUR grade I to IV.
- Swedish Reflux Trial showed CAP and endoscopic management significantly reduced fUTI and new RS compared to surveillance in girls. There was no difference between treatment groups in boys.
- RIVUR showed CAP reduced rUTI by 50% compared to placebo and was particularly effective in those whose first UTI was febrile and had BBD. There was no difference in RS between groups.
- Two meta-analyses have evaluated the efficacy of CAP versus placebo/no treatment in preventing fUTI in children ≤18 years with VUR since completion of RIVUR:
  - Wang (2015) reported pooled OR 0.63 (0.42 to 0.96) in favor of CAP (no difference in RS).
  - De Bessa (2015) reported pooled RR 0.72 (0.56 to 0.92) and 0.51 (0.32 to 0.79) in favor of CAP for dVUR and ndVUR.
- The primary criticism against CAP is the risk of creating antibiotic resistance. Both RIVUR and Wang reported btUTIs while on CAP were more likely to be caused by resistant bacteria.
- Injectable bulking agents have a 80–85% success rate (no postoperative VUR) 1 year after one treatment of low-grade VUR. Success rates progressively decrease and need to repeat, injection increases as VUR grade increases. Injection is less effective in setting of BBD.
- Open ureteral reimplantation has a high success rate (≥95%) and low complication rate (≤5%) in most circumstances. Laparoscopic and robotic techniques have lower success and higher complication rates, which has been attributed to a steep learning curve.
- Indications for crossing from CAP to surgery:
  - Patient or parental preference
  - Nonadherence with medical therapy
  - btUTI while on CAP and/or new RS, especially in setting of reduced renal function and when careful review identifies optimal management of BBD
  - Persistence of high-grade VUR after a lengthy period of CAP
- In toilet-trained children, BBD is an independent risk factor for r/btUTI. Risk is especially prominent in setting of dVUR. Risk of BBD on RS has not yet been clearly delineated, although consensus in BBD generally increases RS risk.
  - American Urological Association (2010) recommends CAP for children with BBD and VUR and treating BBD before surgery.
- Maintenance of a regular voiding and bowel habits decreases the risk of fUTI and increases the chance of VUR resolution.

ONGOING CARE

FOLLOW-UP RECOMMENDATIONS

Patient Monitoring

Patients with RS should have annual blood pressure and urinalysis for proteinuria through adolescence.

PROGNOSIS

The majority of patients with VUR can be managed nonoperatively.

- Traditionally, spontaneous resolution of VUR was the outcome of interest.
  - In primary VUR, 80–90% of grades I and II, 70% of grade III, 40% of grade IV, and 25% of grade V resolve over a 5-year period.
  - The annual rate of spontaneous resolution is between 15% and 20% for grades I to III.
  - Bilateral VUR is less likely to resolve than unilateral VUR.
  - VUR in patients ≥5 years at presentation are less likely to resolve than those who present <5 years.
  - VUR that appears in the filling phase of VCUG ("passive reflux") may be less likely to resolve than reflux that only appears during voiding phase.
  - Distal ureteral diameter on VCUG may be a better predictor of spontaneous resolution than VUR grade.
  - The vesicoureteral reflux index (VURx) is a retrospectively, multi-institutionally validated tool for predicting resolution of VUR in children <2 years.
- Ultimately, the outcome of interest is prevention of UTI and RS rather than resolution of VUR.
- In children with APN on DMSA, there is a higher rate of RS in the setting of VUR versus no VUR.
- It is clinically useful to stratify VUR prognosis in terms of improvement ≥2 grades (rather than complete resolution) and risk of btUTI (which can lead to RS).
  - Risk of btUTI is significantly higher in girls, VUR grade ≥IV, presentation after UTI (versus prenatal HN or UN), and in presence of BBD.
  - iReflux is a calculator for stratifying children with primary VUR into 2-year risk groups for btUTI (http://choc.org/programs-services/urology/ireflux-risk-calculator/).
- Data on resolution rates when VUR is associated with duplication anomalies and periureteral diverticula relative to isolated VUR is mixed.

ADDITIONAL READING

- Hoberman A, Greenfield SP, Mattoo TK, et al; and RIVUR Trial Investigators. Antimicrobial prophylaxis for children with vesicoureteral reflux. *N Engl J Med*. 2014;370(25):2367–2376.
- Nelson CP, Johnson EK, Logvinenko T, et al. Ultrasound as a screening test for genitourinary anomalies in children with UTI. *Pediatrics*. 2014;133(3):e394–e403.
- Peters CA, Skoog SJ, Arant BS Jr, et al. Summary of the AUA guideline on management of primary vesicoureteral reflux in children. *J Urol*. 2010;184(3):1134–1144.
- Shaikh N, Spingarn RB, Hum SW. Dimercaptosuccinic acid scan or ultrasound in screening for vesicoureteral reflux among children with urinary tract infections. *Cochrane Database Syst Rev*. 2016;(7):CD010657.

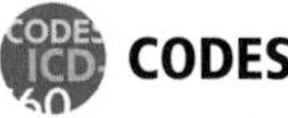

CODES

ICD10

- N13.70 Vesicoureteral-reflux, unspecified
- Q62.7 Congenital vesico-uretero-renal reflux
- N13.71 Vesicoureteral-reflux without reflux nephropathy

V

VIRAL HEPATITIS

Scott A. Elisofon, MD

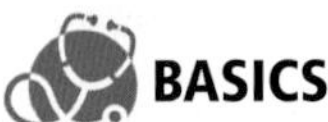

BASICS

DESCRIPTION

- Viral hepatitis is defined as a systemic viral infection, in which the predominant manifestation is that of hepatic injury and dysfunction.
- It is primarily caused by hepatotropic viruses, which include hepatitis A to E.
- 10% of cases are caused by other viruses, such as Epstein-Barr virus (EBV), cytomegalovirus (CMV), herpes simplex virus (HSV), varicella-zoster virus (VZV), rubella, parvovirus, adenovirus, enteroviruses, and others.

EPIDEMIOLOGY

Incidence

- Hepatitis A: ~2,500 cases per year in the United States
- Hepatitis B: 140,000 to 320,000 infections per year worldwide; ~20,000 U.S. cases per year
- Hepatitis C: 30,000 infections per year in the United States
- Hepatitis E: common in poorly developed countries but rare in the United States

Prevalence

- Hepatitis B: United States has a low prevalence with <1% of the population infected; higher rates in certain subgroups such as immigrants from endemic areas, men who have sex with men, and parenteral drug users
- Hepatitis C: United States has prevalence of 1.8%, representing ~3.9 million people (85% chronically infected).

RISK FACTORS

- Hepatitis A (transmission: fecal–oral)
  - Day care attendance, household exposure, travel to endemic areas, men who have sex with men
  - Maximum infectivity 2 weeks before jaundice
- Hepatitis B and C (transmission: blood, body fluids, and sexual contact)
  - Recipients of blood or blood products
  - IV drug users
  - Multiple sexual partners
  - Men who have sex with men
  - Body piercing and tattoos
  - HIV-positive status
  - Infants born to a mother with hepatitis B or C
  - Household contacts with hepatitis B or C

GENERAL PREVENTION

- Good sanitation, hygiene, vaccination, screening blood products, condom use, safe disposal of needles
- Hepatitis A
  - Vaccination of all children between the ages of 1 and 18 years, especially those travelling to endemic regions or those with liver disease
  - Vaccine (Havrix, Vaqta): 0.5-mL dose IM and second dose 6 to 12 months later
  - Prior to travel to an endemic region, immune globulin 0.02 mL/kg should be given to children <1 year of age and considered for children who are immunocompromised or have liver disease.
  - Infected patients should avoid return to day care center for 2 weeks after illness subsides.
  - Postexposure prophylaxis for healthy children >1 year of age: hepatitis A vaccine
  - Postexposure prophylaxis for <1 year of age, immunocompromised individuals or patients with chronic liver disease: immune globulin 0.02 mL/kg IM
- Hepatitis B
  - Screen all pregnant women.
  - Hepatitis B vaccine to all infants at birth; complete 3-vaccine series 0.5-mL dose IM during infancy.
  - Vaccine and hepatitis B immunoglobulin (HBIG) to high-risk infants
  - Mother's with high viral loads or previous vertical transmission should consult a high-risk obstetrician and hepatitis B expert at least 3 to 6 months prior to delivery of another infant.
- Hepatitis C
  - Elective C-section has not been shown to reduce vertical transmission.
  - During vaginal delivery, avoid fetal scalp monitoring and prolonged rupture of membranes >8 hours.
  - Avoid sharing of toothbrushes, nail clippers, and razors.
  - Breastfeeding is contraindicated only if mother has active bleeding from nipples.

PATHOPHYSIOLOGY

- Acute viral hepatitis tends to affect the liver parenchyma, whereas chronic viral hepatitis affects portal and periportal areas.
- Chronic viral hepatitis (B or C) is defined by continuing viral replication and inflammation of the liver for >6 months.
- Worsening injury leads to extensive fibrosis that occurs between portal tracts (portal bridging), nodular changes, and finally, cirrhosis.

DIAGNOSIS

HISTORY

- History should focus on risk factors for viral exposure, sick contacts, travel history, and high-risk behaviors.
- Family history of liver or autoimmune disease, medications, or drug and alcohol use should also be explored.

PHYSICAL EXAM

- Jaundice, hepatomegaly, or tenderness over the liver may or may not be present during acute infection.
- Signs and symptoms during acute infection:
  - Fever
  - Malaise and fatique
  - Nausea and vomiting, anorexia
  - Jaundice: in hepatitis A, seen in 88% of adults but only 65% of children
  - Hepatomegaly
  - Right upper quadrant (RUQ) abdominal pain
  - Dark urine and pale stools
  - Arthralgias/arthritis
  - The vast majority of affected patients are minimally symptomatic or asymptomatic, especially with chronic infection.

DIFFERENTIAL DIAGNOSIS

- Many disorders give rise to elevated transaminases, and clues to a viral origin are based on the history, serology, and histologic findings.
- The diagnosis of "non A to E hepatitis" is often used when the cause is almost certainly viral, but no virus is isolated.
- Other possibilities include drug-induced, ischemic, alcoholic, autoimmune hepatitis, as well as Wilson disease or α_1-antitrypsin deficiency.

DIAGNOSTIC TESTS & INTERPRETATION

Initial Tests (screening, lab, imaging)

- Liver tests
  - Marked elevation of aspartate aminotransferase/alanine aminotransferase (AST/ALT) during acute infection
  - May be normal to mildly elevated in chronically infected individuals
  - Bilirubin from mild to marked elevation
  - In severe hepatitis, monitor PT/INR, albumin, electrolytes, glucose, and CBC.
- Biochemical markers for each virus for diagnosis, management, and monitoring
  - Hepatitis A
    - Virus (HAV) IgM: recent infection
    - Anti-HAV IgG: past exposure or immunization-acquired
  - Hepatitis B
    - Surface antigen (HBsAg): current infection, acute or chronic
    - Surface antibody (HBsAb): immunized or resolved infection
    - "e" antigen (HBeAg): active viral replication; "infectious"
    - "e" antibody (HBeAb): end of severe infectivity (except in precore mutants); end point for many hepatitis B therapies and studies
    - Core antigen (HBcore) IgM: early phase of acute infection, not present in chronic HBV
    - Core total Ab: exposed to HBV
    - HBV DNA: quantification useful to assess viral load
    - HBV mutations: useful to assess resistance to treatment
    - HBV genotyping can sometimes be helpful in determining if interferon therapy would be beneficial (genotype D unfavorable for interferon use).
  - Hepatitis C
    - HCV Ab: exposure to HCV
    - HCV RNA: Quantitative, assess viral load; qualitative, assess presence/absence of virus.
    - HCV genotype: useful to determine duration of treatment and likelihood of response
  - Hepatitis D
    - HDV Ab: exposure to hepatitis D

Diagnostic Procedures/Other

- Liver biopsy is often needed to determine type and extent of liver damage. It is usually indicated prior to initiation of antiviral therapy in children with hepatitis B or C.
- Transient elastography, a noninvasive tool for liver fibrosis, may be used to assess the extent of liver damage.

- Pathologic findings
  - A wide array of histologic features is possible on liver biopsy, including inflammation, necrosis, and fibrosis, based on the severity and chronicity of disease.

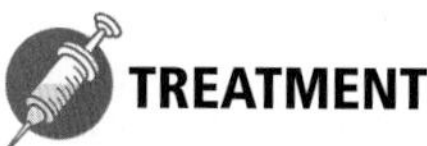

TREATMENT

GENERAL MEASURES

- Most cases of acute hepatitis do not require hospitalization.
- Dehydration, coagulopathy, or severe cases need inpatient care; monitor and correct coagulation defects and fluid, electrolyte, and acid–base imbalances.
- Report acute cases to public health department.
- Patients with acute liver failure should be transferred to a pediatric transplant center.

MEDICATION

- Hepatitis A
  - No specific therapy is necessary for previously immunized or infected patients.
  - Postexposure prophylaxis is recommended for nonimmunized patients household contacts, intimate exposure contacts, and children and staff in nursery or day care centers with outbreaks.
  - Hepatitis A vaccine for children >1 year of age. Children <1 year of age or immunocompromised individuals should receive immune globulin 0.02 mL/kg IM × 1.
- Hepatitis B
  - Postexposure prophylaxis with hepatitis B vaccine and HBIG is indicated for neonates born to mothers who are hepatitis B carriers and for unvaccinated individuals after sexual contact with carriers or accidental exposure to infected blood products.
  - Persons previously vaccinated with known titer >10 mIU/mL do not require any intervention, and children vaccinated with low titer need only a booster HBV vaccine.
  - There is no treatment for acute hepatitis B, although lamivudine is reported to be effective in fulminant HBV hepatitis.
  - Treatment is not usually considered when patients are immune tolerant (normal ALT, HBeAg positive, with high HBV DNA).
  - Children should be monitored every 6 to 12 months with ALT, HBeAg, and HBeAb. When ALT is elevated, treatment is considered by hepatitis B experts.
  - Some pediatric studies suggest that antiviral therapy hastens but does not increase the rate of HBeAg seroconversion.
  - Medications that have been used for chronic hepatitis B include the following: interferon, peginterferon, lamivudine, adefovir, tenofovir, or entecavir.
  - Lamivudine is no longer routinely recommended in chronic HBV due to a high rate of resistance with prolonged treatment.
  - Adefovir dipivoxil and tenofovir are approved for children >12 years of age and entecavir for children >2 years of age.
  - The factor most predictive of treatment response in children with chronic hepatitis B is an elevated pretreatment ALT.
  - Each year, approximately 5% of children spontaneously clear HBeAg, at which point the disease usually becomes inactive, although a few will later reactivate.
- Hepatitis C
  - For acute hepatitis C, treatment with interferon in first 3 months after acquiring infection has been quite successful in adults and should be considered in children.
  - Antiviral therapy for chronic infection can be initiated at any time after 3 years of age and is indicated for children with progressive or advanced disease.
  - Pegylated interferon and ribavirin is currently the only FDA-approved treatment for chronic hepatitis C in children >3 years of age.
  - Despite Pegylated interferon and ribavirin being approved for children, there are many new oral therapies approved for adults that have much more success with much fewer side effects. These direct-acting antiviral medications are currently being studied in pediatric drug trials.

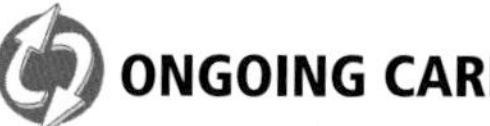

ONGOING CARE

FOLLOW-UP RECOMMENDATIONS

- For hepatitis B and C, serial measurement of serum AST/ALT, viral markers, α-fetoprotein, and ultrasound of the liver
- Liver biopsy pretreatment and for evaluation of disease progression

PROGNOSIS

- Hepatitis A
  - Mild disease usual
  - Rarely results in relapsing, fulminant, or cholestatic disease
  - No chronic liver disease
  - Mortality <1%
  - Protective antibodies develop in response to infection and persist for life.
- Hepatitis B
  - Fulminant hepatitis 1–2%
  - Mortality 0.8%
  - Chronic sequelae:
    - Rate of chronicity is inversely proportional to age of acquisition: 90% in infants, 25% in ages 1 to 5 years, and 6–10% in older children
    - Cirrhosis <5%
    - Hepatocellular carcinoma
- Hepatitis C
  - Fulminant hepatitis 1%
  - Chronic sequelae:
    - Infants infected via vertical transmission have 60–80% chance of chronic infection.
    - Cirrhosis is uncommon.
    - Hepatocellular carcinoma is rare in children and adolescents.
    - If untreated, HCV can lead to advanced liver disease in adults.
  - HCV is the most common indication for liver transplantation in adults.

COMPLICATIONS

- Patients with advanced liver disease due to chronic hepatitis B or C are at risk of complications associated with cirrhosis and portal hypertension.
- Patients with chronic hepatitis B or with cirrhosis due to hepatitis C are at increased risk of hepatocellular carcinoma.
- Hepatitis B
  - Hepatitis D coinfection: Acute hepatitis B and D virus infection occur simultaneously.
  - Hepatitis D superinfection: Acute hepatitis D occurs in a chronic carrier of hepatitis B.

Pregnancy Considerations

Hepatitis E: mortality of 20% caused by acute liver failure in pregnant women

ADDITIONAL READING

- Daniels D, Grytdal S, Wasley A; for Centers for Disease Control and Prevention. Surveillance for acute viral hepatitis—United States, 2007. *MMWR Surveill Summ*. 2009;58(3):1–27.
- Haber BA, Block JM, Jonas MM, et al; for Hepatitis B Foundation. Recommendations for screening, monitoring, and referral of pediatric chronic hepatitis B. *Pediatrics*. 2009;124(5):e1007–e1013.
- Mack CL, Gonzalez-Peralta RP, Gupta N, et al. NASPGHAN practice guidelines: diagnosis and management of hepatitis C infection in infants, children, and adolescents. *J Pediatr Gastroenterol Nutr*. 2012;54(6):838–855.
- Mohan N, González-Peralta RP, Fujisawa T, et al. Chronic hepatitis C virus infection in children. *J Pediatr Gastroenterol Nutr*. 2010;50(2):123–131.
- Murray KF, Shah U, Mohan N, et al. Chronic hepatitis. *J Pediatr Gastroenterol Nutr*. 2008;47(2): 225–233.

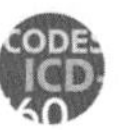

CODES

ICD10

- B19.9 Unspecified viral hepatitis without hepatic coma
- B19.10 Unspecified viral hepatitis B without hepatic coma
- B19.20 Unspecified viral hepatitis C without hepatic coma

FAQ

- Q: Why do infants who acquire HBV at birth have a higher incidence of chronicity?
- A: The immaturity of the neonatal immune system contributes to the higher incidence of chronicity in this population.
- Q: Should a mother with HCV positivity breastfeed?
- A: Transmission of HCV via breast milk is unlikely.

VOLVULUS

Mitchell R. Ladd, MD, PhD • Jeffrey R. Lukish, MD, FACS

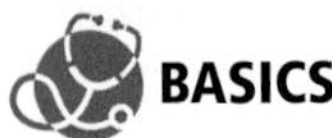

BASICS

DESCRIPTION

Volvulus represents an abnormal rotation (torsion) of the viscera that results in ischemia. Gastric, cecal, and midgut volvulus can occur. Midgut volvulus is the most common form in infants and children and is an acute complication of malrotation in which the viscera twist around the superior mesenteric artery (SMA).

EPIDEMIOLOGY

- Malrotation with midgut volvulus occurs in 1 in 6,000 live births.
- Because malrotation can be asymptomatic, the true incidence and prevalence are not known.
- Malrotation with volvulus is slightly more common in boys.
- Most children with midgut volvulus present in the 1st month of life.
- Malrotation can present at older ages, even in adulthood.

RISK FACTORS

- Children with malrotation have a narrow mesenteric vascular pedicle and are predisposed to volvulus around the SMA.
- Familial associations of malrotation can occur.
- The risk of volvulus in patients with malrotation does not decrease with age.

ETIOLOGY

- Malrotation occurs due to failure of the fetal gut to undergo normal in utero rotation and fixation resulting in a narrow mesenteric vascular pedicle.
- Volvulus occurs when the viscera twist around the narrow vascular pedicle (i.e., the SMA) resulting in intestinal ischemia.

COMMONLY ASSOCIATED CONDITIONS

- Nearly 100% of infants with congenital diaphragmatic hernia have some form of malrotation.
- Congenital heart disease is associated with malrotation in about 40–90% of cases, especially in the setting of heterotaxy.
- 31–45% of infants with omphalocele have malrotation.

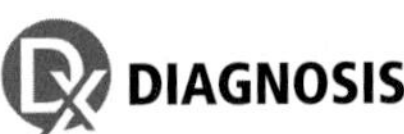

DIAGNOSIS

HISTORY

- The primary presenting sign of malrotation in infants is the sudden onset of bilious emesis, especially in the setting of volvulus.
- In older children, symptoms of malrotation are variable and range from vague abdominal pain to malabsorption to failure to thrive to an acute abdomen if volvulus occurs.
- Consideration should be given to screening patients with heterotaxy for malrotation.

ALERT

Infants and children with bilious emesis require evaluation to rule out malrotation and volvulus. Other presenting symptoms can include:

- Recurrent colicky abdominal pain
- Feeding intolerance
- Chylous ascites and/or protein-losing enteropathy due to lymphatic congestion and bacterial overgrowth
- In older children, recurrent abdominal pain with or without emesis or constipation
- Bloody stools or blood-tinged mucus per rectum can occur and can be late manifestations of ischemic bowel.

PHYSICAL EXAM

- Infants with volvulus may manifest complaints of severe pain without significant physical exam findings (out of proportion to physical exam).
- Abdominal tenderness (mild to severe)
- Irritability, lethargy
- Palpable abdominal mass
- Edema of abdominal wall (late finding)
- Flexion of legs
- Tachypnea and tachycardia
- Hypotension (late finding)

ALERT

Pitfalls in management include the following:

- Delay in diagnosis
- Failure to recognize the key sign of bilious emesis
- Failure to recognize colicky pain (in infants) or cyclic bilious emesis (in older children) as possible manifestations of malrotation
- Failure to order the diagnostic study (a limited upper gastrointestinal series ["upper GI"]) to evaluate the duodenal sweep

DIFFERENTIAL DIAGNOSIS

- Ileus
- Intestinal atresia
- Perforated viscus
- Necrotizing enterocolitis
- Meconium ileus or meconium plug syndrome
- Hirschsprung enterocolitis
- Appendicitis
- Intussusception
- Pyelonephritis

DIAGNOSTIC TESTS & INTERPRETATION

Initial Tests (screening, lab, imaging)

- Associated lab abnormalities may include elevated acute phase reactants, leukocytosis, metabolic acidosis, and thrombocytopenia but may not always be present.
- No imaging modality is 100% sensitive.
  - The goal is to delineate whether the duodenum follows a normal sweep to the left of the vertebral bodies before transition to the jejunum.
  - The 3rd portion of the duodenum crosses behind the SMA to the left of the vertebral body at L1 and rises to the level of the pyloric bulb before transition into the jejunum.
- Plain radiographs
  - Can be normal or show a paucity of bowel gas
  - A dilated stomach and duodenum (double bubble) can be present.
  - Used as first imaging test in unstable patient to rule out pneumoperitoneum and perforation (Applegate)
- Abdominal ultrasound
  - May show inversion of normal position of SMA and superior mesenteric vein (SMV)
  - If SMA is to the right of the SMV, malrotation may be present.
  - The ultrasound has a sensitivity of 80%.
- Upper GI tract (contrast) radiography
  - May show abnormal position of the ligament of Treitz and, if volvulus is present, a corkscrew appearance of the midgut
  - The upper GI is approximately 95% sensitive for identifying malrotation and is the gold standard test.
  - False positives may occur in children with a distended stomach or ileus; in these cases, the ligament of Treitz is then pushed into an abnormal position.
- Barium enema (BE)
  - Can be useful in evaluating the position of the colon and cecum
  - The sensitivity of BE for diagnosing malrotation and volvulus is 80%.
  - In cases of cecal, sigmoid, or transverse colonic volvulus, contrast enema shows a beak deformity at site of volvulus.

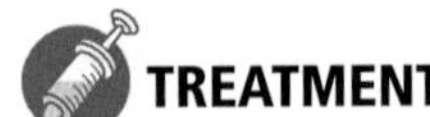

TREATMENT

GENERAL MEASURES

- Any child who presents with bilious emesis and an acute abdomen may require emergent surgical exploration; the concern for midgut volvulus is paramount, and delays for further workup may not be warranted.
- IV fluid resuscitation is indicated, until normal urine output is established.
- Nasogastric decompression and IV antibiotics are indicated.

SURGERY/OTHER PROCEDURES

- In malrotation with volvulus, laparotomy with reduction of the torsion and inspection of the bowel for necrosis or ischemia is indicated.
- Detorsion is the first part of the Ladd procedure, whose goal is to widen the mesenteric base and fix the viscera in place to prevent recurrent volvulus.
- The Ladd procedure does not put the intestines into normal anatomic position.
- The Ladd procedure consists of four components:
  - Reduction and untwisting of the volvulus (if present) by a 360-degree counterclockwise rotation of the midgut
  - Division of abnormal adhesions extending over the duodenum (Ladd bands) that are transfixing the cecum in the right upper quadrant
  - Division and opening of the mesenteric attachments to provide a wider vascular base to the midgut
  - Removal of the appendix: The appendix is removed because it is in an unusual anatomic position and would result in a diagnostic dilemma should the child develop appendicitis in the future.
- The Ladd procedure is also performed for malrotation without volvulus.
- Many surgeons can perform the Ladd procedure laparoscopically when malrotation is present without volvulus.
- In acute volvulus, laparoscopy can be attempted safely, but many surgeons will do an open operation.
- Second-look operations may be indicated if a large portion of the midgut is ischemic; the volvulus may be reduced with reexploration in 12 to 24 hours.
- On rare occasions, bowel resection and ostomy may be necessary.

ONGOING CARE

FOLLOW-UP RECOMMENDATIONS

Patient Monitoring

- Prognosis depends on extent of involvement and degree of bowel ischemia.
- Most of these children develop a profound ileus and require total parenteral nutrition (TPN) for days to weeks postoperatively.
- Third-space volume loss is common postoperatively; monitoring of intake/output is critical to maintain euvolemia.
- Postoperative small bowel obstruction and even recurrent volvulus can occur.

COMPLICATIONS

- Recurrent volvulus occurs in <1% of patients after open surgery, but it is more common if Ladd procedure is done laparoscopically (5.6–19%).
- Short bowel syndrome
- Adhesive bowel obstruction; more common when open Ladd procedure is performed
- Wound infection
- Intra-abdominal abscess
- Mortality is 4–9%.

ADDITIONAL READING

- Aboagye J, Goldstein SD, Salazar JH, et al. Age at presentation of common pediatric surgical conditions: reexamining dogma. *J Pediatr Surg*. 2014;49(6):995–999.
- Andrassy RJ, Mahour H. Malrotation of the midgut in infants and children: a 25-year review. *Arch Surg*. 1981;116(2):158–160.
- Applegate KE. Evidence-based diagnosis of malrotation and volvulus. *Pediatr Radiol*. 2009;39(Suppl 2): S161–S163.
- Draus JM Jr, Foley DS, Bond SJ. Laparoscopic Ladd procedure: a minimally invasive approach to malrotation without midgut volvulus. *Am Surg*. 2007;73(7):693–696.
- El-Gohary Y, Alagtal M, Gillick J. Long-term complications following operative intervention for intestinal malrotation: a 10-year review. *Pediatr Surg Int*. 2010;26(2):203–206.
- Ferrero L, Ahmed YB, Philippe P, et al. Intestinal malrotation and volvulus in neonates: laparoscopy versus open laparotomy. *J Laparoendosc Adv Surg Tech A*. 2017;27(3):318–321.
- Filston HC, Kirks DR. Malrotation—the ubiquitous anomaly. *J Pediatr Surg*. 1981;16(4 Suppl 1): 614–620.
- Graziano K, Islam S, Dasgupta R, et al. Asymptomatic malrotation: diagnosis and surgical management: an American Pediatric Surgical Association outcomes and evidence based practice committee systematic review. *J Pediatr Surg*. 2015;50(10):1783–1790.
- Hagendoorn J, Vieira-Travassos D, van der Zee D. Laparoscopic treatment of intestinal malrotation in neonates and infants: retrospective study. *Surg Endosc*. 2011;25(1):217–220.
- Lodwick DL, Minneci PC, Deans KJ. Current surgical management of intestinal rotational abnormalities. *Curr Opin Pediatr*. 2015;27(3):383–388.
- Malek MM, Burd RS. Surgical treatment of malrotation after infancy: a population-based study. *J Pediatr Surg*. 2005;40(1):285–289.
- Messineo A, MacMillan JH, Palder SB, et al. Clinical factors affecting mortality in children with malrotation of the intestine. *J Pediatr Surg*. 1992;27(10):1343–1345.
- Nagdeve NG, Qureshi AM, Bhingare PD, et al. Malrotation beyond infancy. *J Pediatr Surg*. 2012;47(11):2026–2032.
- Stanfill AB, Pearl RH, Kalvakuri K, et al. Laparoscopic Ladd's procedure: treatment of choice for midgut malrotation in infants and children. *J Laparoendosc Adv Surg Tech A*. 2010;20(4):369–372.
- Stephens LR, Donoghue V, Gillick J. Radiological versus clinical evidence of malrotation, a tortuous tale—10-year review. *Eur J Pediatr Surg*. 2012;22(3):238–242.

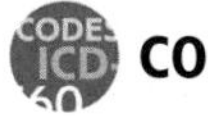

CODES

ICD10

- K56.2 Volvulus
- K31.89 Other diseases of stomach and duodenum
- Q43.8 Other specified congenital malformations of intestine

FAQ

- Q: When should workup for volvulus be initiated?
- A: In any child with bilious emesis
- Q: What is the best diagnostic study to confirm the diagnosis?
- A: Limited upper GI to evaluate the duodenal sweep and position of the ligament of Treitz
- Q: What is the most common age of presentation of volvulus?
- A: In the 1st month of life; however, it can occur in any age.
- Q: What are the other types of volvulus that have been reported in children?
- A: Gastric, small bowel, and colonic volvulus can occur in children. Gastric volvulus presents with abdominal pain and retching. Two types occur: meso-axial (rotation about the lesser and greater curvature) and organo-axial (rotation around the longitudinal axis of the stomach). A majority of these children have structural abnormality of the stomach such as asplenia or abnormal fixation to the esophagus. Both small bowel and colonic volvulus present similarly to midgut volvulus, with high-grade bowel obstruction, abdominal pain, and bilious emesis.
- Q: Can volvulus occur in teenagers and young adults?
- A: Yes. Age is not a determinant of presentation of volvulus and may occur in older children and adults.
- Q: Can volvulus recur after surgery?
- A: Yes, but recurrence is not common.
- Q: Who developed the Ladd procedure?
- A: William Edwards Ladd, MD (1880 to 1967) first described the procedure in 1936. He was a pioneer in the field of pediatric surgery. He was the first surgeon-in-chief at Boston Children's Hospital and coauthored the first pediatric surgical textbook.

VOMITING

T. Matthew Shields, MD

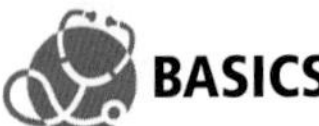

BASICS

DESCRIPTION

- Vomiting is the forceful expulsion of gastric contents through the mouth.
  - A prominent feature of many disorders of infancy and childhood
  - Often the only presenting symptom
- Regurgitation is defined as small, effortless mouthfuls of food or stomach contents.
- Retching is contraction of the abdominal musculature against a closed glottis, restricting expulsion of stomach contents (also referred to as "dry heaves").

PATHOPHYSIOLOGY

Vomiting may be indicative of a number of different physiologic pathways, including as:

- A defense mechanism to expel ingested toxins
- An abnormality of, or damage to, the postrema area of the brain (a.k.a. the chemoreceptor trigger zone or vomiting center), which is located at the base of the 4th ventricle
- A result of intestinal obstruction leading to bowel dilation
- A reaction to chronic gastrointestinal mucosal disease
- A result of a generalized metabolic disease
- A sequela of increased intracranial pressure

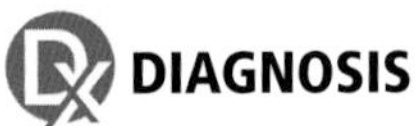

DIAGNOSIS

HISTORY

- Special attention should be directed to the timing of the emesis, relationship to meals, position and time of day, as well as to the chronicity of symptoms.
- Ask about medication, alcohol and drug use trauma, travel history, personal and/or family history of acute and chronic gastrointestinal diseases, and personal and/or family history of migraine.
- Fever: may suggest an infectious etiology
- Abdominal pain and frequent, forceful, or bilious emesis
  - Often associated with anatomic or obstructive intestinal disorder
  - For example, obstruction of a lumen (i.e., small bowel obstruction, common bile duct stone or ureteropelvic junction [UPJ] obstruction) can each present as vomiting.
- Age of patient
  - Some etiologies of vomiting may be aged-based.
  - In infants, pyloric stenosis or inborn errors of metabolism should be considered especially with vomiting, dehydration, and biochemical abnormalities.
  - In adolescents, disordered eating patterns (bulimia) and the possibility of pregnancy should be considered.
- Pica and patchy baldness can be the result of a foreign body or hair ingestion and the development of a gastric bezoar.
- Nausea and epigastric pain related to meals support delayed gastric emptying or gallbladder disease.
- Symptoms alleviated by meals may signify gastroesophageal reflux or a gastric ulcer.
- Alternating vomiting and lethargy with periods of well appearance support intussusception.
- Chronic headaches, fatigue, weakness, weight loss, early morning vomiting, or focal neurologic deficits may suggest vomiting secondary to increased intracranial pressure.
- Right- or left-sided abdominal pain may suggest renal disease.
- Periumbilical abdominal pain may be consistent with increased fecal load and/or constipation.
- Recurrent, intermittent episodes of vomiting interspersed with long-standing periods of wellness may suggest cyclic vomiting syndrome (CVS).
- Recurrent vomiting and other gastrointestinal symptoms are commonly seen with mucosal diseases such as celiac disease, eosinophilic esophagitis, and inflammatory bowel disease.

PHYSICAL EXAM

A careful and complete physical examination can often contribute to determining the cause of vomiting in children:

- Abdominal distention with tympanitic bowel sounds may suggest a bowel obstruction.
- Rectal examination is important to evaluate for hard, impacted stool within the rectum suggestive of constipation.
- Jaundice and/or icteric sclera suggests a hepatic etiology.
- Unusual odors support a diagnosis of a metabolic disease, diabetic ketoacidosis.
- Evidence of neurologic dysfunction, including nystagmus, papilledema, abnormal reflexes, and weakness is seen with increased intracranial pressure.
- Enlarged parotid glands are seen in bulimia and other feeding disorders.
- A palpable "olive-shaped" mass and peristaltic wave can be seen in infants with pyloric stenosis.

DIFFERENTIAL DIAGNOSIS

- Gastrointestinal tract:
  - Anatomic
    - Esophageal: stricture, web, ring, atresia
    - Stomach: pyloric stenosis, antral web, hiatal hernia
    - Intestine: malrotation with or without volvulus
    - Colon: Hirschsprung disease, imperforate anus
  - Motility
    - Achalasia
    - Gastroesophageal reflux
    - Intestinal pseudoobstruction
    - Gastroparesis
    - Ileus
  - Obstruction
    - Foreign body/bezoar
    - Intussusception
    - Intestinal-stricturing Crohn disease
    - Duodenal hematoma
    - Superior mesenteric artery syndrome
  - Other
    - Hepatobiliary disease
    - Appendicitis
    - Eosinophilic esophagitis
    - Necrotizing enterocolitis
    - Peritonitis
    - Celiac disease
    - Peptic ulcer disease
    - Pancreatitis
- Neurologic
  - Intracranial mass lesions:
    - Tumor
    - Cyst
    - Subdural hematoma
  - Cerebral edema
  - Hydrocephalus
  - Pseudotumor cerebri
  - Arnold-Chiari malformation
  - Migraine (head, abdominal)
  - Cyclical vomiting syndrome
  - Seizures
  - Postconcussion syndrome
- Renal
  - Obstructive uropathy
    - UPJ obstruction
    - Hydronephrosis
    - Nephrolithiasis
    - Renal insufficiency
    - Glomerulonephritis
    - Renal tubular acidosis
- Metabolic
  - Inborn errors of metabolism:
    - Galactosemia
    - Fructose intolerance
    - Hereditary fructose intolerance
    - Amino acid or organic acid metabolism
    - Urea cycle defects
    - Fatty acid oxidation disorders
    - Lactic acidosis
- Infection
  - Sepsis
  - Meningitis
  - UTI
  - *Helicobacter pylori*
  - Parasites
  - *Giardia*
  - Viral/bacterial gastroenteritis
  - Viral hepatitis (A, B, C)
  - Pneumonia
  - *Bordetella pertussis*
  - Streptococcal pharyngitis

- Endocrine
  - Diabetes
    - Diabetic ketoacidosis
    - Diabetic gastroparesis
    - Adrenal insufficiency
- Respiratory
  - Sinusitis
  - Laryngitis
- Immunologic
  - Food allergy (IgE vs. non-IgE)
  - Food protein-induced enterocolitis syndrome
  - Anaphylaxis
  - Graft-versus-host disease
  - Chronic granulomatous disease
- Other:
  - Pregnancy
  - Rumination
  - Bulimia
  - Overfeeding
  - Pain
  - ETOH intoxication
  - Cannabinoid hyperemesis syndrome
  - Medications:
    - Drugs (chemotherapy)
    - Vitamin toxicity
  - Porphyria
  - Familial dysautonomia

ALERT

Vomiting accompanied by hematemesis, intestinal obstruction (bilious vomiting), dehydration, neurologic dysfunction, or an acute abdomen should be treated as a medical emergency, and hospitalization should be considered.

DIAGNOSTIC TESTS & INTERPRETATION

Initial Tests (screening, lab, imaging)

- CBC
  - Anemia and iron deficiency can occur with gastritis/esophagitis, inflammatory bowel disease, celiac disease, and ulcer disease.
- Blood chemistry
  - Electrolyte abnormalities (hypokalemic, hypochloremic metabolic alkalosis) are found in pyloric stenosis.
  - An elevated alanine aminotransferase, conjugated bilirubin, and γ-glutamyl transferase (GGT) can indicate liver, gallbladder, or metabolic disease.
- Urine toxicology screening for drugs of abuse
- Urinalysis: UTI, pyelonephritis, nephrolithiasis
- Amylase/lipase: pancreatitis
- BUN/creatinine: Elevated levels can occur with renal disease.
- Stool for occult blood, *H. pylori* antigen
- Celiac serology
  - Tissue transglutaminase IgA, endomysial antibody, or deamidated gliadin IgA and serum IgA
- Plain abdominal radiographic study
  - Can detect ileus and/or obstruction
  - May also need upright or left lateral decubitus films
- Abdominal ultrasound
  - Liver, gallbladder, renal, pancreatic, ovarian, or uterine disease
  - In infants, abdominal ultrasound is the test of choice for pyloric stenosis.
  - Useful when considering abdominal abscess and appendicitis
  - Can detect intussusception but best performed when the patient is symptomatic
- Contrast radiography
  - Intestinal anatomic abnormalities (e.g., malrotation, intussusception, volvulus, hiatal hernia), gastric bezoar, achalasia
- Gastric scintigraphy (gastric emptying study)
  - Evaluate rate of gastric emptying; assess for gastroparesis.
- Abdominal CT
  - Not generally indicated for evaluation of vomiting, although it is an effective tool when more anatomic abdominal detail is required (abscess, tumor)
- Head CT
  - Can be helpful in evaluation of acute neurologic causes of vomiting (i.e., intracranial bleeding, hydrocephalus)
- Brain MRI
  - Provides superior imaging of the brain stem, without radiation exposure
  - Test of choice if considering intracranial mass

Diagnostic Procedures/Other

- Upper endoscopy
  - Can identify esophageal, gastric, and duodenal inflammation (reflux esophagitis, eosinophilic esophagitis, gastritis, ulcer disease, celiac disease)
  - Provides means to obtain biopsies or cultures for infections (*H. pylori*, duodenal *Giardia*, cytomegalovirus gastritis)
- Gastroesophageal and antroduodenal manometry: can be used to evaluate for primary or secondary motility disorders, evaluation of suspected rumination syndrome

TREATMENT

- Potential therapeutic interventions are broad, and therapy should be directed toward the underlying etiology.
- Historically, empiric antiemetic medications were contraindicated in cases of acute vomiting, although more recent studies suggest ondansetron may reduce frequency of admission.
- Oral rehydration therapy is typically the first line of treatment. IV fluids are appropriate if oral rehydration therapy fails or are contraindicated.
- Neurotransmitters involved in vomiting include dopamine, acetylcholine, histamine, endorphins, serotonin, and neurokinins. The mechanism of many antiemetic medications is blockade of these neurotransmitters.

ISSUES FOR REFERRAL

- Chronic vomiting (2 to 3 weeks)
- Weight loss
- Severe abdominal pain or irritability
- Gastrointestinal bleeding
- Bilious emesis
- Evidence of intestinal obstruction
- Serum electrolyte abnormalities
- Abnormal neurologic examination
- Papilledema
- Dehydration
- Signs of acute abdomen
- Lethargy

ADDITIONAL READING

- Fedorowicz Z, Jagannath VA, Carter B. Antiemetics for reducing vomiting related to acute gastroenteritis in children and adolescents. *Cochrane Database Syst Rev*. 2011;(9):CD005506.
- Freedman SB, Adler M, Seshadri R, et al. Oral ondansetron for gastroenteritis in a pediatric emergency department. *N Engl J Med*. 2006;354(16):1698–1705.
- Li B, Misiewicz L. Cyclic vomiting syndrome: a brain-gut disorder. *Gastroenterol Clin North Am*. 2003;32(3):997–1019.
- Li HK, Sunku BK. Vomiting and nausea. In: Wyllie R, Hyams JS, eds. *Pediatric Gastrointestinal and Liver Disease*. 4th ed. Philadelphia, PA: Saunders; 2011:88–105.

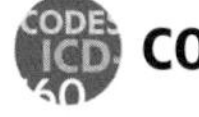

CODES

ICD10

- R11.10 Vomiting, unspecified
- P92.1 Regurgitation and rumination of newborn

FAQ

- Q: What are the most common causes of nonbilious vomiting in an infant?
- A: Gastroesophageal reflux and milk protein allergy, although hypertrophic pyloric stenosis, sepsis, and malrotation must be considered
- Q: What is appropriate management of a 6-month-old presenting with an episode of bilious emesis and lethargy?
- A: Referral for emergent abdominal ultrasound and surgical consult for possible intussusception
- Q: Is bilious emesis always associated with small bowel obstruction?
- A: Repeated episodes of vomiting can cause duodenal contents to reflux into the stomach resulting in bile-stained emesis without small bowel obstruction. Nevertheless, evaluation should include high suspicion and workup for possible obstruction.

VON WILLEBRAND DISEASE

Char M. Witmer, MD, MSCE

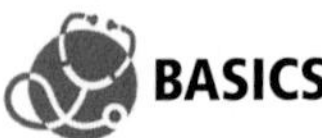

BASICS

DESCRIPTION

- An inherited bleeding disorder caused by either a quantitative or qualitative defect of the von Willebrand protein
- Characterized by mucocutaneous bleeding or bleeding after surgical procedures

EPIDEMIOLOGY

Prevalence

The prevalence of von Willebrand disease in the general pediatric population is estimated to be ~1%.

RISK FACTORS

Genetics

- The gene for von Willebrand factor is found on chromosome 12.
- Type 1 (see "Pathophysiology") follows an autosomal dominant inheritance pattern with variable penetrance.
- Type 2 can be autosomal dominant or recessive.
- Type 3 follows an autosomal recessive inheritance pattern.

GENERAL PREVENTION

- Avoid contact sports.
- For patients with recurrent epistaxis, measures should be taken to avoid drying of the mucosa by applying petroleum jelly, humidifying the air, and reducing trauma to the nasal mucosa by keeping the fingernails short and discouraging nose picking.
- It may be advisable for patients to wear an emergency ID bracelet indicating that they have von Willebrand disease in the event they are involved in an accident that renders them unconscious.
- Avoid medications that negatively affect platelet function (i.e., ibuprofen, aspirin).
- Combination oral contraceptive pills are very effective for some patients with menorrhagia.
- Appropriate hemostatic therapy is needed prior to dental or surgical procedures to prevent bleeding.

PATHOPHYSIOLOGY

- von Willebrand factor is a large multimeric protein that allows platelets to adhere to sites of endothelial injury, initiating the primary step in hemostasis—formation of the platelet plug.
- von Willebrand factor also serves as a carrier for factor VIII in the peripheral circulation, protecting it from degradation. Deficiency of von Willebrand factor results in a shorter factor VIII half-life, causing a lower level of circulating factor VIII.
- When von Willebrand factor is either deficient or defective, primary hemostasis is compromised, resulting in a bleeding diathesis characterized by easy bruising, frequent epistaxis, menorrhagia, and prolonged bleeding following surgical or dental procedures.
- Acquired forms of von Willebrand disease have been described in association with hypothyroidism, Wilms tumor, other neoplasms, cardiovascular disorders with increased shear stress (aortic stenosis), myeloproliferative disorders, uremia, and medications, including ciprofloxacin, griseofulvin, and valproate therapy.
- Classification: There are three major categories of von Willebrand disease:
  - Type 1
    - Mild to moderate quantitative deficiency
    - The most common type, accounting for 70–80% of patients
    - Generally a mild bleeding disorder
  - Type 2
    - Qualitative deficiency of von Willebrand factor
    - Diagnosed in 15–20% of patients
    - Tend to have more significant bleeding symptoms than in type 1
    - Type 2 von Willebrand disease is further classified into four subtypes.
      - Type 2A: loss of the intermediate- and high-molecular-weight multimers. The loss is secondary to either abnormal assembly or secretion of multimers or increased proteolytic degradation. The multimer deficiency results in decreased platelet binding.
      - Type 2B: an abnormal von Willebrand factor that spontaneously binds to normal platelets, resulting in accelerated clearance of these platelets and loss of high-molecular-weight multimers. This can result in mild thrombocytopenia.
      - Type 2N: The abnormal von Willebrand factor does not bind factor VIII optimally. This decrease in binding results in a shorter plasma half-life of factor VIII, resulting in reduced plasma factor VIII levels. Type 2N can be confused with mild hemophilia.
      - Type 2M: The abnormal von Willebrand factor fails to bind normally to platelets; normal multimers
  - Type 3
    - Near-complete quantitative deficiency of von Willebrand factor, which also results in a secondary deficiency of factor VIII
    - Accounts for <5% of patients and results in a severe bleeding disorder

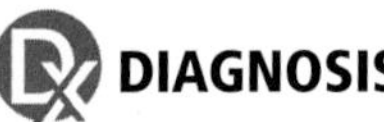

DIAGNOSIS

HISTORY

- A family history of von Willebrand disease or bleeding tendency is an important question in the evaluation for von Willebrand disease. However, be aware that variation in frequency and severity of bleeding symptoms can occur from person to person, even within an affected family.
- Bruising is common, with increased quantity, increased size (>5 cm), raised bruises, and often in unusual locations with minimal trauma.
- Recurrent and/or prolonged epistaxis
- Menorrhagia occurs in 70–90% of women with von Willebrand disease.
- Excessive posttraumatic or postsurgical bleeding

PHYSICAL EXAM

- Bruises: increased number, size, raised, and/or unusual location
- May be entirely normal

DIFFERENTIAL DIAGNOSIS

- Primary hemostatic disorders
  - Platelet function abnormalities, congenital thrombocytopenia
  - Mild inherited coagulation factor deficiencies
  - Hemophilia A
- Acquired and secondary hemostatic disorders
  - Liver disease
  - Uremia
  - Acquired thrombocytopenia
  - Drugs that affect platelet function
  - Acquired factor inhibitors (extremely rare in children)
- Connective tissue disorders
  - Ehlers-Danlos syndrome
  - Scurvy
- Prolonged activated partial thromboplastin time (aPTT) but no bleeding symptoms
  - Inhibitor
  - Factor XII deficiency

DIAGNOSTIC TESTS & INTERPRETATION

- Screening tests for a bleeding disorder:
  - Prothrombin time (PT) is normal in von Willebrand disease.
  - aPTT may be prolonged if there is a decrease in factor VIII levels but can be normal.
  - Platelet count is normal except in type 2B patients, who may have mild thrombocytopenia.
  - Bleeding time is usually prolonged but may be normal in patients with mild type 1 von Willebrand disease (not recommended as a screening test).

- Platelet function assay (PFA)-100 is usually prolonged but may be normal in mild type 1 von Willebrand disease (not recommended as a screening test).
- Specific tests for von Willebrand disease include the following:
  - von Willebrand factor antigen: quantitation of von Willebrand factor by immunoassay
  - von Willebrand factor activity (ristocetin cofactor): assesses the function of von Willebrand factor using the antibiotic ristocetin, which induces platelet aggregation in the presence of von Willebrand factor
  - Factor VIII: factor VIII clotting activity
  - von Willebrand factor multimers: multiple molecular forms of von Willebrand factor evaluated on agarose gel
    - Multimer analysis is important in delineating the type of von Willebrand disease. Do not send as part of the initial screening for von Willebrand disease.

ALERT
- The diagnosis of von Willebrand disease is not always straightforward.
- Because of normal physiologic variation in plasma levels of von Willebrand factor, repeated measurements over time may be necessary to establish the diagnosis.
- Conditions that may increase von Willebrand factor levels:
  - The newborn period
  - Surgery
  - Liver disease
  - Hyperthyroidism
  - High-stress states
  - Pregnancy
  - Inflammatory or infectious disease
  - Steroids
  - Oral contraceptives (high-dose estrogen)
  - Other estrogens

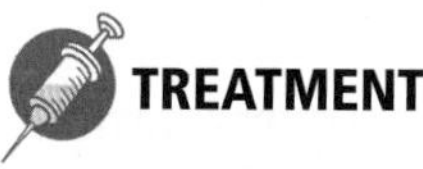

TREATMENT

GENERAL MEASURES
- There are several options for the management of bleeding in patients with von Willebrand disease. Superficial bleeding can usually be stopped by applying local pressure, ice, or topical thrombin, particularly in type 1.
- There are two main approaches to systemic therapy in von Willebrand disease: increasing the release of endogenous von Willebrand factor or exogenous replacement of von Willebrand factor. The appropriate therapy depends on the type of von Willebrand disease and the clinical scenario.

MEDICATION
- Desmopressin (DDAVP®) is a synthetic analog of vasopressin that stimulates endothelial cell release of von Willebrand factor. It is effective in patients who have a functional von Willebrand factor, as in type 1 von Willebrand disease. It may be used for some patients with type 2 von Willebrand disease but is ineffective in type 3 and contraindicated in type 2B:
  - Available in IV and intranasal formulations
  - An infusion of 0.3 mcg/kg results in a 3- to 5-fold increase in von Willebrand factor and factor VIII; nasal administration is slightly less effective.
  - Side effects include facial flushing, lightheadedness, hypotension, or nausea.
  - Prior to use in a surgical setting, patients should have a trial to demonstrate an appropriate response (10% of patients do not respond).
  - May worsen thrombocytopenia in type 2B; it is not recommended.
  - DDAVP® may not be useful when prolonged hemostasis is required. After 24 to 48 hours, there is depletion of stored von Willebrand factor, causing it to be ineffective (tachyphylaxis).
  - It is important to remember that DDAVP® will also cause fluid retention and, in some cases, hyponatremia. This can be avoided with fluid restriction for 24 hours following treatment.
- Factor concentrates
  - Humate-P® or Alphanate®:
    - Plasma-derived, intermediate-purity factor VIII concentrate products with adequate levels (especially large multimers) of von Willebrand factor
    - Therapy of choice for some patients with type 2 von Willebrand disease and all patients with type 3 von Willebrand disease
    - Useful in type 1 von Willebrand disease when prolonged hemostasis is necessary
  - Recombinant von Willebrand factor:
    - Approved for use only in severe von Willebrand disease
    - Factor VIII replacement is initially needed if the patient's baseline factor VIII is low.
- Antifibrinolytics: aminocaproic acid or tranexamic acid
  - Stabilize the fibrin clot by inhibiting the physiologic process of clot lysis.
  - Best for oral mucosal bleeding

ONGOING CARE

PROGNOSIS
- von Willebrand disease type 1 is often a very mild bleeding disorder and may go undetected.
- Most patients with von Willebrand disease have a normal life expectancy and, with proper education and treatment, minimal risk for permanent disability.
- Type 3 von Willebrand disease is a severe bleeding disorder, and life-threatening hemorrhage can occur.

COMPLICATIONS
- Significant perioperative bleeding can occur, especially with tonsillectomy, but the most common complications are recurrent epistaxis, prolonged bleeding with cuts and abrasions, and menorrhagia.
- Patients with type 3 von Willebrand disease have a more severe bleeding disorder and can have bleeding complications similar to those seen in hemophilia such as hemarthroses and intracranial hemorrhage.

ADDITIONAL READING

- Cox Gill J. Diagnosis and treatment of von Willebrand disease. *Hematol Oncol Clin North Am*. 2004;18(6):1277–1299.
- Mannucci PM. Treatment of von Willebrand's disease. *N Engl J Med*. 2004;351(7):683–694.
- Mohri H. Acquired von Willebrand syndrome: features and management. *Am J Hematol*. 2006;81(8): 616–623.
- Pruthi RK. A practical approach to genetic testing for von Willebrand disease. *Mayo Clin Proc*. 2006;81(5):679–691.
- Robertson J, Lillicrap D, James PD. Von Willebrand disease. *Pediatr Clin North Am*. 2008;55(2): 377–392.

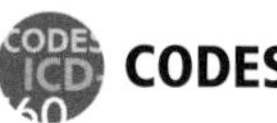

CODES

ICD10
D68.0 Von Willebrand's disease

FAQ
- Q: What sports activities can a person with von Willebrand disease participate in safely?
- A: People with type 1 von Willebrand disease can participate in most activities, although it is usually advised to avoid situations in which significant trauma takes place, like contact sports such as football or boxing. Patients with type 3 von Willebrand disease should avoid activities with moderate trauma. For type 2 patients, the risk of bleeding varies.
- Q: Is life expectancy lower in people with von Willebrand disease?
- A: For most patients with von Willebrand disease, their life expectancy and quality of life will be normal.
- Q: Are there any medications contraindicated in a patient with von Willebrand disease?
- A: Aspirin should not be given, as it interferes with platelet function. Nonsteroidal anti-inflammatory agents cause a milder effect on platelets and should also be avoided when possible. Patients should use acetaminophen for fever or pain.

V

WARTS

Prina P. Amin, MD • [illegible] Abramson, MD, MS

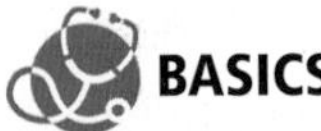

BASICS

DESCRIPTION

- Warts (verrucae) are common, benign, and frequently self-limited epithelial growths caused by human papillomavirus (HPV) infection of keratinocytes.
- Types of warts
  - Cutaneous
    - Common warts (verruca vulgaris)
    - Flat warts (verruca plana)
    - Plantar warts (weight-bearing)
  - Anogenital
  - Laryngeal (laryngeal papillomatosis)

EPIDEMIOLOGY

Prevalence

- Cutaneous warts
  - Mostly affect children and young adults
  - Affect girls more than boys
  - 5.3% prevalence from age 6 to 15 years of age
  - Up to 1/3 of school-aged children have had warts.
- Anogenital warts
  - Exact prevalence in children and adolescents is unknown.
  - Approximately 1% of sexually active adults have external genital warts.
- Laryngeal warts
  - Rare with no known cure; transmission occurs in utero or through birth canal.

RISK FACTORS

- Direct or indirect contact
- Autoinoculation can cause persistent infection and spread.
- Use of communal pool surfaces, bathrooms, and shower rooms increases risk.
- Areas of skin trauma and breakdown have increased susceptibility to HPV infection.
- Regularly walking barefoot outside also increases risk.
- Excessive foot perspiration
- Immunosuppressed patients, particularly transplant patients, are highly vulnerable.
- Individual susceptibility factors related to developing warts after exposure to HPV are less clear.

GENERAL PREVENTION

- Cutaneous warts
  - Use protective footwear in warm, moist environments and communal areas.
  - Wear cotton socks and change twice a day, especially if significant perspiration.
  - Avoid sharing nail files.
  - Avoid scratching and nail-biting to prevent autoinoculation.
- Anogenital warts
  - Avoid sexual contact with multiple partners.
  - Condoms may be protective.
  - Quadrivalent HPV vaccine protects against HPV subtypes 6, 11, 16, and 18.
    - Recommended universally for males and females, ages 9 to 26 years

PATHOPHYSIOLOGY

- Warts are caused by HPV infection of the epithelium.
- HPV replication leads to cell proliferation and formation of characteristic lesions.

ETIOLOGY

- >150 subtypes of HPV exist.
- Certain subtypes have a predilection for particular body sites and produce characteristic lesions:
  - Plantar and common palmar warts often caused by HPV 1 and 2
  - Anogenital warts commonly caused by HPV 6, 11, 16, 18, 31, and 45
  - Laryngeal papillomatosis is associated with HPV 6 and 11.

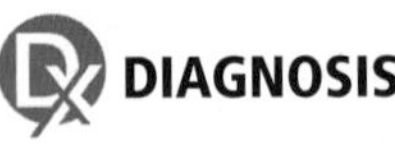

DIAGNOSIS

HISTORY

- Ask about risk factors for warts.
- Assess history of warts in close contacts (caregiver).
- Assess for immunosuppression.
- For anogenital warts: Take detailed sexual history and assess risk for sexual abuse.
- Assess symptoms: Warts are usually asymptomatic with the exception of plantar warts or warts near nails, which may be painful.
- Assess duration: Warts may be present for months to years without intervention.

PHYSICAL EXAM

- Common warts (verruca vulgaris)
  - Rough keratotic papules and nodules that can be single or grouped
  - Often dome-shaped
  - Appear anywhere but most often affect fingers, hands, knees, and elbows
- Flat warts (verruca plana)
  - Generally 2 to 4 mm, slightly elevated, flat-topped lesions with minimal scale
- Plantar warts (weight-bearing warts)
  - Thick, hyperkeratotic lesions that may be tender to palpation
  - Tend to occur at pressure points on soles of feet
  - May have punctate black dots representing thrombosed capillaries
  - Disrupt normal skin markings
- Anogenital warts
  - Usually multiple, clustered soft lesions that are pink or gray
  - Four morphologic types: condyloma acuminata (cauliflower-shaped), smooth papules (dome-shaped, flesh-colored), keratotic papules (resemble common warts), flat warts
- Laryngeal warts (laryngeal papillomatosis)
  - Visible only under direct airway examination
  - Children may present with stridor, hoarseness, and signs of airway obstruction.
  - In children, laryngeal warts are diagnosed most often between 2 and 3 years, with most children presenting before age 5 years.

DIFFERENTIAL DIAGNOSIS

- Common warts
  - Molluscum contagiosum
  - Moles
  - Skin tag
  - Squamous cell carcinoma or melanoma
- Flat warts
  - Lichen planus
  - Lichenoid keratosis
- Plantar warts
  - Callus
  - Corns
  - Squamous cell carcinoma or melanoma
  - Foreign body
- Anogenital warts
  - Pearly penile papules
  - Molluscum contagiosum
  - Condylomata lata (secondary syphilis lesions)
  - Vulvar carcinoma
  - Lichen planus
  - Squamous cell carcinoma

ALERT

- Any child or adolescent with anogenital warts should prompt consideration for sexual abuse and consultation with a child abuse specialist as necessary.
- Testing for other sexually transmitted infections should occur in any pediatric patient with anogenital warts.
- In any patient with extensive HPV infection, consideration must be given to underlying immunodeficiencies including HIV.

DIAGNOSTIC TESTS & INTERPRETATION

- Diagnosis is based on visual identification.
- Biopsy may be indicated when the diagnosis is uncertain or warts are resistant to treatment.
- In anogenital warts, testing for other sexually transmitted infections is recommended.

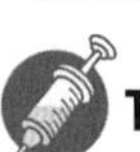

TREATMENT

- General
  - Warts are often self-limited and resolve without treatment.
  - 2/3 of warts will resolve within 2 years with no treatment.
  - Earlier treatment may be warranted for warts that are painful or cause significant social stigma.
  - Goal of treatment is to destroy or damage the infected epithelium by either chemical or physical means.

- Cutaneous warts
  - Salicylic acid
    - 1st-line therapy for cutaneous warts
    - Over-the-counter (OTC) formulations contain 5–27% salicylic acid and are applied topically 1 to 2 times daily for up to 12 weeks.
    - Prescription strength 40% adhesive plaster is available to be applied for 24 to 48 hours and is particularly useful for plantar warts.
    - Repetitive filing of the wart with either an emery board, pumice stone, or metal file and soaking the wart for 10 to 20 minutes prior to treatment may improve response to topical salicylic acid.
    - Applying a thin layer of petrolatum around the wart to protect the surrounding healthy tissue may prevent pain during treatment.
    - Adverse reactions include local irritation and chemical burn.
  - Duct tape or moleskin
    - Used as 1st-line therapy
    - May be helpful, although studies on effectiveness are mixed
    - To use, cut tape or moleskin approximately 1/4 inch larger than wart and cover for 6 days.
    - After 6 days, remove, soak wart, and file with an emery board, pumice stone, or metal file; leave uncovered overnight.
    - Reapply duct tape in 6-day cycles until resolution.
  - Cryotherapy
    - 2nd-line therapy
    - Involves freezing the wart using one of several methods, the most commonly used being liquid nitrogen
    - Can be painful and is more expensive than 1st-line agents
    - Newer data support its efficacy as comparable to salicylic acid.
    - Most commonly used in the office, although newer OTC cryotherapy products are available
  - Other therapies (if needed) are generally performed in conjunction with a pediatric dermatologist.
    - Phototherapy
    - Immunotherapies
    - Intralesional therapies
    - Antimitotic therapies
    - Curettage
    - Laser ablation
- Anogenital warts
  - Treatment issues
    - Main goal of treatment is to remove symptomatic warts.
    - Most warts will clear within 3 months after initiation of therapy.
    - Treatment does not eradicate HPV, prevent recurrence, or reduce cancer risk.
  - Podofilox (0.5% gel) or imiquimod (3.75% or 5% cream) are 1st-line therapy (avoid in pregnancy).
    - Podofilox gel is applied topically q12h for 3 days; no treatment for 4 days; then repeat cycles until warts disappear; avoid unprotected sexual activity during treatment due to possible irritant effect.
    - Imiquimod: for patients aged 12 years and older
      - 3.75%: once daily at bedtime; wash off ~8 hours later for up to a maximum of 8 weeks.
      - 5%: Apply 3 times per week at bedtime; wash off 6 to 10 hours later for up to a maximum of 16 weeks.
  - Cryotherapy for anogenital warts is an option for experienced providers.
  - 2nd-line options include podophyllin resin, intralesion treatments, trichloroacetic acid, surgical removal, laser therapy, and photodynamic therapy.

ISSUES FOR REFERRAL

- Consider referral to pediatric dermatology if
  - Lesions are atypical or extensive.
  - Lesions progress during therapy.
  - Multiple failed treatments
  - Lesions are located on the face.
  - Frequent or prompt recurrence occurs.
  - Warts are pigmented, indurated, ulcerated, or fixed to underlying structures.
  - Individual warts are >1 cm.
  - Patients are immunocompromised.
- Consider referral to a child abuse specialist if anogenital warts are present AND
  - Caregivers suspect sexual abuse.
  - A sexual predator has access to the child.
  - Child discloses abuse.
  - Child is >48 months of age.
  - Any other sexually transmitted infection is detected.
  - Physical exam suggests any type of abuse.
  - Provider is uncomfortable with evaluating for sexual abuse.

COMPLEMENTARY & ALTERNATIVE THERAPIES

Psychological (hypnosis), homeopathic, and herbal treatments have all been studied and have not been found to be efficacious.

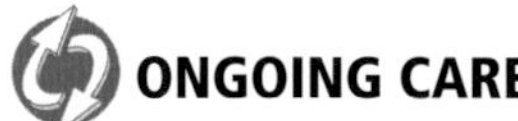

ONGOING CARE

FOLLOW-UP RECOMMENDATIONS

Patient Monitoring

Patients should be seen at regular intervals to assess clearance of the lesions and monitor for side effects.

PROGNOSIS

- 2/3 of warts clear without treatment within 2 years.
- However, early treatment is recommended while warts are small and few in number to prevent enlargement and spread.

COMPLICATIONS

- Bacterial infection such as cellulitis or abscess can occur if patients pick at warts.
- Other complications are generally related to treatment and can include pain and scarring.
- Malignant transformation to squamous cell carcinoma can rarely occur for both cutaneous and anogenital warts; this is most problematic in immunosuppressed patients.

ADDITIONAL READING

- Kwok CS, Gibbs S, Bennett C, et al. Topical treatments for cutaneous warts. *Cochrane Database Syst Rev*. 2012;(9):CD001781.
- Kwok CS, Holland R, Gibbs S. Efficacy of topical treatments for cutaneous warts: a meta-analysis and pooled analysis of randomized controlled trials. *Br J Dermatol*. 2011;165(2):233–246.
- Mulhem E, Pinelis S. Treatment of nongenital cutaneous warts. *Am Fam Physician*. 2011;84(3): 288–293.
- Sinclair K, Woods C, Sinal S. Venereal warts in children. *Pediatr Rev*. 2011;32(3):115–121.
- Sterling JC, Gibbs S, Haque Hussain SS, et al. British Association of Dermatologists' guidelines for the management of cutaneous warts 2014. *Br J Dermatol*. 2014;171(4):696–712.

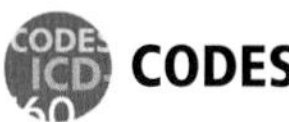

CODES

ICD10

- B07.9 Viral wart, unspecified
- B07.0 Plantar wart
- A63.0 Anogenital (venereal) warts

FAQ

- Q: Do condoms protect against HPV?
- A: Condoms lower the risk of HPV; however, HPV can infect areas not covered by the condom and so condoms are not fully protective.
- Q: Does a patient with cutaneous warts need to be excluded from school or sports?
- A: No. Exclusion is not fully effective because asymptomatic transmission can occur. In addition, risk of transmission is low.
- Q: How can a callus and wart be differentiated?
- A: Careful paring with a #15 scalpel of a callus shows preserved skin markings and no bleeding. Paring of a wart often reveals black dots, which are thrombosed blood vessels.

WEIGHT LOSS

Kendall Purcell, MD, MPH

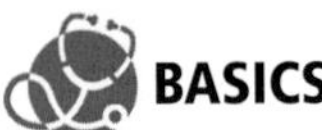

BASICS

DESCRIPTION

Documented decrease in weight from a previous measurement. Can be acute or chronic, intentional or unintentional. Unintentional weight loss is an unusual and worrisome symptom, regardless of the percentage decline.

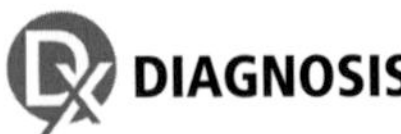

DIAGNOSIS

HISTORY

Determine that weight loss is real and not due to scale error, different scales, different technique (e.g., clothed vs. unclothed, diaper vs. no diaper).

- **Question:** Child's diet?
- *Significance*: A 3-day dietary record can be useful for demonstrating insufficient caloric intake or intake of empty calories (e.g., juice).
- **Question:** Age?
- *Significance*: The patient's age can help direct questions in the history to the most likely causes of weight loss.
  - Age <2 weeks old: physiologic weight loss, underfeeding, inappropriate feeding, breastfeeding difficulties, postpartum depression, short frenulum, congenital heart disease, inborn error of metabolism
  - Age <4 months old: malnutrition, improper formula preparation, low breast milk supply, cystic fibrosis, pyloric stenosis, congenital heart disease, gastroesophageal reflux, congenital adrenal hyperplasia, inborn error of metabolism
  - Age 4 months to 8 years old: chronic infection, cystic fibrosis, malabsorption, renal disease, liver disease, constipation, diabetes, neglect/abuse
  - Age >8 years old: eating disorder, chronic infection, neoplasm, renal disease, substance abuse, depression, diabetes, thyroid disorder, inflammatory bowel disease
- **Question:** Emesis, especially projectile vomiting?
- *Significance*: suggests intestinal obstruction, gastroesophageal reflux, inborn error of metabolism
- **Question:** Cramping, bloating, or abnormally greasy, voluminous stools?
- *Significance*: possible malabsorption
- **Question:** Tiring during feeding or difficulty feeding due to cough and dyspnea?
- *Significance*: suggests congestive heart failure in newborn/infant
- **Question:** Seizures, unusual body/fluid odors?
- *Significance*: possible inborn error of metabolism
- **Question:** Foreign travel?
- *Significance*: possible chronic infection (e.g., tuberculosis, parasitic disease)
- **Question:** History of severe infections, persistent candidal infections?
- *Significance*: possible immunodeficiency
- **Question:** Increased appetite with weight loss?
- *Significance*: suggests hyperthyroidism, cystic fibrosis, pheochromocytoma
- **Question:** Polyuria, polydipsia, and polyphagia?
- *Significance*: possible new-onset diabetes
- **Question:** Concomitant delayed puberty?
- *Significance*: suggests chronic severe weight loss, pituitary abnormalities, anorexia nervosa
- **Question:** Fear of fatness, preoccupation with food, distorted body image, and/or amenorrhea?
- *Significance*: possible eating disorder
- **Question:** Chronic sadness or irritability, insomnia, or hypersomnia?
- *Significance*: possible depression/affective disorder
- **Question:** Trouble affording food or running out of money to buy food?
- *Significance*: suggests food insecurity

PHYSICAL EXAM

- **Finding:** Hypothermia, bradycardia?
- *Significance*: suggests anorexia nervosa
- **Finding:** Tachycardia, resting?
- *Significance*: suggests hyperthyroidism, anemia, acute weight loss, pheochromocytoma
- **Finding:** Orthostatic changes?
- *Significance*: Hemodynamically significant weight loss suggests anorexia, acute dehydration.
- **Finding:** Oral lesions, perianal skin tags, or fissures?
- *Significance*: suggests inflammatory bowel disease
- **Finding:** Goiter?
- *Significance*: suggests hyperthyroidism
- **Finding:** Heart murmur?
- *Significance*: suggests congenital heart disease
- **Finding:** Clubbing?
- *Significance*: suggests chronic cardiac or pulmonary disease
- **Finding:** Significant abdominal distension?
- *Significance*: suggests celiac disease, constipation, obstruction
- **Finding:** Enlarged liver and/or spleen?
- *Significance*: suggests heart failure, malignancy, chronic infection, storage disease, inborn error of metabolism
- **Finding:** Muscle weakness?
- *Significance*: suggests electrolyte abnormality, muscular dystrophy
- **Finding:** Swollen joint(s)?
- *Significance*: suggests juvenile idiopathic arthritis, inflammatory bowel disease
- **Finding:** Thinning hair, brittle nails, lanugo?
- *Significance*: suggests anorexia
- **Finding:** Erosion of teeth enamel, calluses on knuckles?
- *Significance*: suggests bulimia
- **Finding:** Eczema?
- *Significance*: suggests immunodeficiency, eosinophilic esophagitis
- **Finding:** Lymphadenopathy?
- *Significance*: suggests malignancy, immunodeficiency, infection, autoimmune disease

ALERT

- Confirm the weight loss is real. In some studies, up to 25% of weight loss is artifactual, resulting from measurement errors.
- Newborns with weight loss, especially at the 2-week visit, may manifest paradoxical lack of interest in feeding due to low energy stores.
- Observation of the feeding technique by a practitioner with expertise or a lactation consultant for breastfed babies is vital.

DIFFERENTIAL DIAGNOSIS

- Nutritional
  - Malnutrition
  - Dieting
  - Iron deficiency/zinc deficiency
  - Postoperative recovery
  - Inability to eat (new orthodontic appliances, loss of teeth, chronic mouth ulcerations)
- Congenital/anatomic
  - Congenital heart disease
  - Pyloric stenosis
  - GI malformation (duodenal atresia, annular pancreas, and volvulus)
  - Short-bowel syndrome
  - Lymphangiectasia
  - Superior mesenteric artery syndrome
  - Gastroesophageal reflux
  - Immunodeficiency disorders
  - Hirschsprung disease
- Infectious
  - Urinary tract infection (UTI)
  - Tuberculosis
  - Stomatitis
  - Osteomyelitis
  - HIV
  - Hepatitis
  - Parasitic disease
  - Gastroenteritis
  - Postinfectious malabsorption
  - Disseminated histoplasmosis
  - Acute severe febrile illness (pyelonephritis, pneumonia, septic arthritis)
- Malignancy
  - Diencephalic syndrome
  - Leukemia
  - Lymphoma
  - Pheochromocytoma
  - Other neoplasms
- Endocrine
  - Type 1 and type 2 diabetes
  - Diabetes insipidus
  - Hyperthyroidism
  - Adrenal insufficiency
  - Congenital adrenal hyperplasia
  - Hypopituitarism
  - Hypercalcemia
- Genetic/metabolic
  - Cystic fibrosis
  - Shwachman-Diamond syndrome
  - Renal tubular acidosis
  - Chronic renal failure
  - Inborn errors of metabolism
  - Storage diseases
  - Muscular dystrophy
  - Lipodystrophy

- Allergic/inflammatory
  - Inflammatory bowel disease
  - Juvenile idiopathic arthritis
  - Systemic lupus erythematosus
  - Sarcoidosis
  - Pancreatitis
  - Hepatitis
  - Celiac disease (gluten enteropathy)
  - Eosinophilic esophagitis
- Psychiatric
  - Rumination syndrome
  - Depression including postpartum depression
  - Anorexia nervosa/bulimia nervosa
- Toxic, environmental, drugs
  - Lead poisoning
  - Mercury poisoning
  - Vitamin A poisoning
  - Chronic methylphenidate, dextroamphetamine, or valproic acid use
  - Substance abuse, especially amphetamines and crack cocaine
- Miscellaneous
  - Child abuse, neglect
  - Food insecurity
  - Chronic illness (e.g., pulmonary disease, renal disease)
  - Cerebral palsy
  - Factitious (e.g., scale error)

ALERT

Emergency care is indicated for the following:

- Significant dehydration
  - Abnormal vital signs with orthostasis, decreased urine output, decreased skin turgor, delayed capillary refill (>3 seconds)
  - Mandates cardiovascular support (IV hydration) and a more urgent diagnosis (e.g., inborn error of metabolism, obstructive GI disease, congenital adrenal hyperplasia, diabetic ketoacidosis)
- Abnormal mental status or significant lethargy which may be seen in the following:
  - Severe dehydration
  - Adrenal insufficiency
  - Hypoxic states
  - Toxic ingestions
  - Renal or respiratory failure
  - Increased intracranial pressure
  - Severe electrolyte abnormalities
- Increasing vomiting in the setting of known weight loss in infants
  - High risk for dehydration, hypoglycemia, and electrolyte abnormalities
  - Need to evaluate for treatable conditions (e.g., obstructive GI disease, inborn errors of metabolism, congenital adrenal hyperplasia, congenital heart disease) in which a delay is life-threatening
- Severe malnutrition (weight loss >20% of ideal body weight)
  - High risk for metabolic derangements, including dysrhythmias secondary to electrolyte abnormalities
- Aggressive evaluation is warranted.

DIAGNOSTIC TESTS & INTERPRETATION

- **Test:** CBC for evidence of the following:
- *Significance*:
  - Anemia—macrocytic associated with folate/vitamin B_{12} deficiency, microcytic with iron deficiency, normocytic with chronic infection
  - Polycythemia—suggestive of chronic pulmonary or cardiac disease
  - Neutropenia—suggestive of hematologic malignancy, Shwachman-Diamond syndrome, immunodeficiency
  - Lymphopenia—suggestive of immunodeficiency
  - Eosinophilia—suggestive of parasitic disease, eosinophilic esophagitis
  - Leukocytosis—suggestive of infection
  - Lymphoblasts—suggestive of leukemia
  - Thrombocytosis—suggestive of chronic infection, malignancy
- **Test:** serum electrolytes
- *Significance*: abnormalities in dehydration, adrenal insufficiency (low sodium, high potassium), renal disease, anorexia nervosa, pyloric stenosis
- **Test:** BUN, creatinine
- *Significance*: abnormal in renal disease, dehydration
- **Test:** erythrocyte sedimentation rate
- *Significance*: may be elevated in inflammatory bowel disease, chronic infections, rheumatoid diseases
- **Test:** stool for occult blood and pH, reducing substances (Clinitest®)
- *Significance*:
  - Occult blood suggests inflammatory bowel disease.
  - Low pH and positive reducing substances suggest malabsorption.
- **Test:** urinalysis
- *Significance*:
  - Hematuria and/or proteinuria suggest renal disease.
  - Glycosuria suggests diabetes mellitus.
  - Very low specific gravity suggests diabetes insipidus, chronic renal failure, hypercalcemia.
  - Pyuria suggests UTI.
  - pH >6 suggests renal tubular acidosis (type I).
- **Test:** urine culture
- *Significance*: evaluation for UTI
- **Test:** serum protein levels
- *Significance*: Very low levels imply impaired liver function, severe chronic weight loss, or protein malabsorption.
- **Test:** tuberculosis skin test
- *Significance*: possible chronic infection
- **Test:** liver function tests
- *Significance*: evaluation for hepatitis, chronic liver disease
- **Other tests:** Depending on age and clinical findings, other tests to consider include the following: serum calcium, thyroid function tests (TSH, T_4), sweat test, tests for malabsorption (e.g., lactose breath test, stool fat, stool for trypsin), tests for metabolic disease (e.g., plasma ammonia, lactate, serum/urine amino acids, urine organic acids), imaging studies (e.g., CT, MRI, bone scan), immunologic studies.

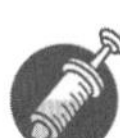

TREATMENT

- Establish if the weight loss is voluntary or involuntary.
- Determine the acuity or chronicity and severity of weight loss, and the need for hospitalization versus close, serial outpatient follow-up.
- Attempt to narrow the diagnostic possibilities by history and physical exam, particularly by assessing if the loss might be attributable to diminished intake, diminished absorption, or increased metabolic requirements.
- Treatment is then based on the most likely diagnosis following evaluation.

ADDITIONAL READING

- Flaherman VJ, Schaefer EW, Kuzniewicz MW, et al. Early weight loss nomograms for exclusively breastfed newborns. *Pediatrics*. 2015;135(1):e16–e23.
- Kyle UG, Shekerdemian LS, Coss-Bu JA. Growth failure and nutrition considerations in chronic childhood wasting diseases. *Nutr Clin Pract*. 2015;30(2):227–238.
- Schechter M. Weight loss/failure to thrive. *Pediatr Rev*. 2000;21(7):238–239.
- Seligman HK. Food insecurity and "unexplained" weight loss. *JAMA Intern Med*. 2017;177(3):421–422. doi:10.1001/jamainternmed.2016.8697.

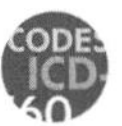

CODES

ICD10

- R63.4 Abnormal weight loss
- K21.9 Gastro-esophageal reflux disease without esophagitis
- E46 Unspecified protein-calorie malnutrition

FAQ

- Q: How common is weight loss in the first 2 weeks of life?
- A: Formula-fed babies may lose up to 7% of birth weight and breastfed newborns up to 10% before regaining their birth weight by 2 weeks of age. An infant who has not regained his or her birth weight by 2 weeks requires evaluation and intervention.
- Q: How important a finding is weight loss?
- A: Involuntary weight loss requires prompt evaluation—a cause must be found or the loss self-resolved. If a diagnosis is not uncovered in the setting of continued weight loss, referral to a pediatric diagnostic center is indicated.
- Q: What is standard laboratory evaluation for weight loss in a pediatric patient?
- A: There is no established laboratory evaluation for weight loss. The workup should be guided by history and physical exam findings, both of which can elucidate cause of weight loss and prevent extraneous testing and imaging.
- Q: When is it appropriate to refer a patient with weight loss to a subspecialty provider?
- A: Subspecialty referral is indicated when workup is inconclusive and further subspecialty diagnostic testing is required (e.g., endoscopy) or when workup suggests disease process requiring subspecialty care.

WEST NILE VIRUS (AND OTHER ARBOVIRUS ENCEPHALITIS)

Jessica R. Newman, DO

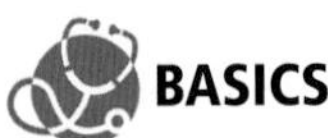

BASICS

DESCRIPTION

- Viruses transmitted by an arthropod vector that can cause CNS infections, undifferentiated febrile illness, acute polyarthropathy, and hemorrhagic fevers
- Most arboviral infections are asymptomatic.
- West Nile virus (WNV) is an arbovirus in the flavivirus family.
- WNV was first recognized in the United States in 1999 during an outbreak of encephalitis in New York City and is now the most common epidemic viral encephalitis in the United States.
- >150 arboviruses are known to cause human disease.
- Other arboviruses can produce similar syndromes or acute hemorrhagic fevers.

EPIDEMIOLOGY

- Arboviruses are spread by mosquitoes, ticks, and sand flies. The major vector for WNV in the United States is the Culex mosquito. WNV has been spread through blood transfusions, transplanted organs, and, rarely, intrauterine.
- Arboviruses are maintained in nature through cycles of transmission among birds, horses, and small animals. Humans and domestic animals are infected incidentally as "dead-end" hosts.
- Disease among birds has been a hallmark of WNV in the United States and has served as a sensitive surveillance indicator of WNV activity.
- Each North American arbovirus has specific geographic distributions and is associated with a different ratio of asymptomatic to clinical infections. These agents cause disease of variable severity and have distinct age-dependent effects. WNV has now been identified throughout the United States and is also found in Europe, Africa, and Asia.

Incidence

- The peak incidence of arboviral encephalitis occurs during the late summer and early fall. Seasonality depends on the breeding and feeding seasons of the arthropod host.
- WNV is the leading cause of arboviral CNS disease. Encephalitis is most commonly seen in older adults, generally aged >60 years, and severe WNV disease is more common in immunocompromised individuals. Symptomatic cases of WNV in children are unusual.
- Fewer than 10 cases each of Eastern equine encephalitis and Western equine encephalitis are reported nationally each year. Eastern equine encephalitis tends to produce a more fulminant illness than LaCrosse or Western equine encephalitis.

GENERAL PREVENTION

- Public health department efforts focus on surveillance of viral activity to predict and prevent outbreaks:
  - Active bird surveillance to detect the presence of WNV activity
  - Active mosquito surveillance to detect viral activity in mosquito populations
  - Passive surveillance by veterinarians and human health care professionals to detect neurologic illnesses consistent with encephalitis
  - Screening of blood and organ donors
- Personal precautions to avoid mosquito bites including use of repellents, protective clothing, and screens; avoiding peak feeding times (dawn and dusk); and installation of air conditioners
- Coordination of mosquito control programs in endemic infection areas
- Vaccines for prevention of most arbovirus infections are not available. A vaccine is available for Japanese encephalitis, yellow fever (YF), and tick-borne encephalitis for travelers to endemic areas who are planning prolonged stays.
- Infection control measures
  - Standard precautions are recommended for the hospitalized patient.
  - Respiratory precautions are recommended when vector mosquitoes are present.
  - Patients with dengue and YF can be viremic and should be protected against vector mosquitoes to avoid potential transmission.

PATHOPHYSIOLOGY

- The incubation period for WNV and other arboviral encephalitis agents is 2 to 14 days (up to 21 days in immunocompromised hosts).
- The incubation period reflects the time necessary for viral replication, viremia, and subsequent invasion of the CNS.
- Virus replication begins locally at the site of the insect bite; transient viremia leads to spread of virus to liver, spleen, and lymph nodes. With continued viral replication and viremia, seeding of other organs including the CNS occurs.
- Virus can rarely be recovered from blood within the 1st week of onset of illness but not after neurologic symptoms have developed.

ETIOLOGY

- Arboviruses can be divided into two groups based on the predominant clinical syndrome.
  - In the United States, seven arboviruses are important causes of encephalitis: WNV, California encephalitis virus (LaCrosse strain), Eastern equine encephalitis, Western equine encephalitis, St. Louis encephalitis, Powassan encephalitis virus, and Venezuelan equine encephalitis virus.
  - Arboviruses such as YF, dengue fever, chikungunya, and Colorado tick fever typically cause acute febrile diseases and hemorrhagic fevers and are not characterized by encephalitis.
- Clinical manifestations of WNV
  - Asymptomatic: most common
  - Self-limited febrile illness: 67% of symptomatic cases
  - Neuroinvasive disease: aseptic meningitis, encephalitis, or flaccid paralysis—1% cases

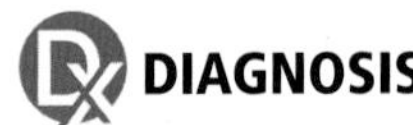

DIAGNOSIS

HISTORY

- The diagnosis of arboviral infections of the CNS is difficult.
- Characteristic epidemiology that suggests a specific etiology is an important part of the history.
- The season of disease, prevalent diseases within the community, and animal exposures may provide clues to the diagnosis:
  - Enteroviral infections are seen in the warmer months (summer and early fall) in temperate climates.
  - Mosquito propagation in damp climates or standing water during the summer months may increase the likelihood of arthropod-borne viruses.
  - History of an animal bite or bat exposure may suggest the possibility of rabies.
- Approximately 20% of infected individuals develop clinical disease. WNV (symptomatic infection) is characterized by sudden onset of fever, headache, myalgias, muscle weakness, and GI symptoms (nausea, vomiting, or diarrhea).
- Neuroinvasive WNV affects around 1% of infected individuals and can be characterized by neck stiffness and headache, mental status changes, movement disorders, or flaccid paralysis.
- Encephalitis caused by arboviruses is characterized by acute onset of fever and headache in almost all patients. Associated symptoms may include seizures, altered consciousness, disorientation, and behavioral disturbances.

PHYSICAL EXAM

- Neurologic signs are more commonly diffuse but may be focal. These clinical findings can help to distinguish patients with meningitis, which is characterized by nuchal rigidity and fever usually without an altered sensorium.
- Other signs possibly observed in WNV infection:
  - A rash is seen in 25–50% of patients and is described as nonpruritic, roseolar, or maculopapular on the chest, back, and arms, which lasts 1 week.
  - Diffuse lymphadenopathy is also common.
- Neurologic examination in WNV infection may reveal motor weakness or flaccid paralysis, increased deep tendon reflexes and extensor plantar responses, and tremor or abnormal movement of extremities.

DIFFERENTIAL DIAGNOSIS

- Infectious
  - Viral
    - Herpes simplex virus
    - Enterovirus
    - HIV
    - HHV-6
    - Epstein-Barr virus
    - Cytomegalovirus
    - Lymphocytic choriomeningitis virus
    - Rabies
    - Mumps
    - Influenza
    - Adenovirus

- Nonviral
  - Cat-scratch disease (*Bartonella henselae*)
  - *Mycoplasma pneumoniae*
  - Postinfectious encephalomyelitis: generally follows a vague viral syndrome, usually upper respiratory tract, by days to weeks
  - Abscess/subdural empyema
  - Meningitis
    - Tuberculous
    - Cryptococcal or other fungal (histoplasmosis, coccidioidomycoses, blastomycoses)
    - Bacterial
    - *Listeria*
  - Toxoplasmosis
  - *Plasmodium falciparum* infection (malaria)
  - Parasites (cysticercosis, echinococcus, amebiasis, trypanosomiasis)
- Noninfectious: tumor, carcinomatous meningitis, systemic lupus erythematosus, sarcoidosis, vasculitis, hemorrhage, toxic encephalopathy, metabolic disorders

DIAGNOSTIC TESTS & INTERPRETATION

The diagnosis of arboviral encephalitis depends on the recognition of epidemiologic risk factors and typical signs and symptoms with the aid of laboratory and radiographic studies.

Initial Tests (screening, lab, imaging)

- Routine laboratory tests
  - CBC typically reveals a mild leukocytosis.
  - Mild increase in erythrocyte sedimentation rate (ESR)
  - Mild to moderate CSF pleocytosis, predominately mononuclear cells
  - Elevated CSF protein
  - Normal CSF glucose
- Serology
  - IgM and IgG enzyme-linked immunosorbent assay (ELISA) or indirect fluorescent antibody (IFA) for WNV and other arboviruses
  - The diagnosis of arbovirus encephalitis is made by one of the following:
    - Detection of virus-specific IgM antibodies in the CSF is confirmatory.
    - A 4-fold rise in serum antibody titers is confirmatory. Acute-phase titers should be collected 0 to 8 days after onset of symptoms. Convalescent phase titers should be collected 14 to 21 days after acute specimen. A single negative acute-phase specimen is inadequate for diagnosis, but a positive test can provide evidence of recent infection.
  - Isolation of the virus from tissue, blood, or CSF
  - Polymerase chain reaction (PCR) to detect viral RNA
- Imaging studies such as MRI or CT can assist in ruling out other potential causes of encephalopathy or encephalitis.
- MRI has proved useful in differentiating postinfectious encephalomyelitis from acute viral encephalitis. The former is characterized by enhancement of multifocal white matter lesions.

Diagnostic Procedures/Other

- In WNV poliomyelitis-like acute flaccid paralysis, EMG studies may show increased insertional activity and fasciculations. In contrast to Guillain-Barré, no evidence of significant demyelination is seen.
- EEG
  - Diffuse generalized slowing of brain waves
  - Periodic high-voltage spike waves originating in the temporal lobe region and slow-wave complexes at 2- to 3-second intervals are suggestive of herpes simplex virus infection.

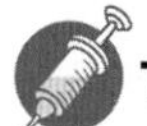

TREATMENT

GENERAL MEASURES

- No specific antiviral therapy is available.
- Supportive therapy including cardiorespiratory function, fluid and electrolyte balance, seizure control, and reduction of intracranial pressure is important.

MEDICATION

Consider IV immunoglobulin (IVIG)/plasmapheresis for associated Guillain-Barré syndrome; IVIG has been used in cases of flaccid paralysis with some response.

ONGOING CARE

FOLLOW-UP RECOMMENDATIONS

Patient Monitoring

- Neurobehavioral follow-up should be considered in children with severe or complicated disease.
- If WNV is diagnosed during pregnancy, detailed fetal ultrasound (US) should be considered 2 to 4 weeks after illness onset with evaluation for congenital anomalies and neurologic deficits.
- Infant serum should be tested for WNV IgM at birth and 6 months with IgG at 6 months.

PROGNOSIS

- Prognosis for recovery depends on the specific infecting agent and host factors such as age and underlying illness.
- Eastern equine and Japanese encephalitis have the worst prognoses, with mortality occurring in 30% of cases.
- Recovery can be seen after prolonged periods of coma.

COMPLICATIONS

- Optic neuritis
- Seizures
- Coma
- Death
- Guillain-Barré syndrome
- Severe neurologic sequelae
- Myocarditis
- Pancreatitis
- Hepatitis

ADDITIONAL READING

- Beckham JD, Tyler KL. Arbovirus infections. *Continuum (Minneap Minn)*. 2015;21(6, Neuroinfectious Disease):1599–1611.
- Hayes EB. West Nile virus disease in children. *Pediatr Infect Dis J*. 2006;25(11):1065–1066.
- Lindsey NP, Hayes EB, Staples JE, et al. West Nile virus disease in children, United States, 1999–2007. *Pediatrics*. 2009;123(6):e1084–e1089.
- Rizzo C, Esposito S, Azzari C, et al; for Italian Society of Pediatric Allergy, Immunology. West Nile virus infections in children: a disease pediatricians should think about. *Pediatr Infect Dis J*. 2011;30(1):65–66.
- Romero JR, Newland JG. Viral meningitis and encephalitis: traditional and emerging viral agents. *Semin Pediatr Infect Dis*. 2003;14(2):72–82.

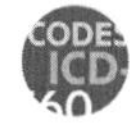

CODES

ICD10

- A92.30 West Nile virus infection, unspecified
- A92.31 West Nile virus infection with encephalitis
- A85.2 Arthropod-borne viral encephalitis, unspecified

FAQ

- Q: Should testing for arboviruses, including WNV, be performed on all patients with encephalitis?
- A: Diagnostic testing for arboviruses is not recommended for all patients with encephalitis. The prevalence of these diseases is low, and the diagnosis of more common causes of childhood encephalitis (e.g., herpes simplex virus) should be pursued initially. Patients with no other identifiable cause of encephalitis who have epidemiologic risk factors such as geographic location, season, and exposure history suggestive of arbovirus encephalitis should be evaluated. Testing of patients with aseptic meningitis or Guillain-Barré syndrome is low yield.
- Q: Which is the most severe of the arbovirus encephalitides?
- A: Arbovirus encephalitis is generally rare; Eastern equine encephalitis virus, occurring in North, Central, and South America and the Caribbean has a mortality of >30%.
- Q: Are vaccines available for at-risk travelers?
- A: Vaccinations are commercially available for Japanese encephalitis, YF, and tick-borne encephalitis for those traveling to endemic areas.

WHEEZING

Samuel B. Goldfarb, MD • Lee J. Brooks, MD

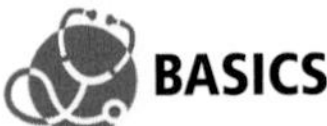

BASICS

DESCRIPTION

Wheezing is a continuous sound that is caused by turbulent airflow through an obstructed airway.

- Often described as musical in nature and with a variable pitch
- Wheezing is an expiratory sound; stridor is an inspiratory sound.
- Wheezing occurs from obstruction in the intrathoracic airway, whereas stridor is caused by an obstruction in the extrathoracic airway.
- If heard in both inspiration and expiration, there may be a fixed obstruction or separate lesions in both the intrathoracic and extrathoracic airways.

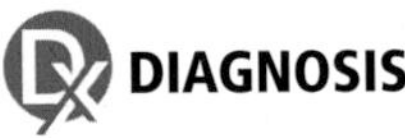

DIAGNOSIS

Approach to the patient

- Phase 1: Determine the severity of the patient's general status and degree of respiratory distress and triage accordingly.
- Phase 2: Construct a differential diagnosis.
- Phase 3: Initiate appropriate therapies.

HISTORY

- **Question:** Pattern of the wheezing?
- *Significance*:
  - A rapid onset suggests a foreign body or a post-exposure exacerbation of asthma.
  - Unilateral versus bilateral wheezing suggests foreign body or other focal process.
  - A slow onset suggests an infection.
  - Periods of recurrent wheezing suggest asthma.
  - Nocturnal and early morning wheezing or coughing are consistent with gastroesophageal reflux, sinusitis, and/or sensitivity to common bedroom allergens.
  - Wheezing in association with or soon after a meal can be seen in swallowing dysfunction, gastroesophageal reflux, or, less commonly, tracheoesophageal fistula (TEF).
  - Wheezing that worsens with crying is suggestive of tracheomalacia and/or bronchomalacia or a fixed intraluminal or extraluminal obstruction.
- **Question:** Wheezing correlated with exertion?
- *Significance*: suggests asthma triggered by exercise
- **Question:** Multiple exacerbations with recurrent or chronic symptoms?
- *Significance*:
  - Recurrent cycles of exacerbations, with clearing in between, suggest a process such as asthma, cystic fibrosis, ciliary dyskinesia, and bronchopulmonary dysplasia.
  - Chronic or persistent wheezing is more common with fixed anatomic abnormalities.
- **Question:** Common triggers?
- *Significance*: could be
  - Smoke
  - Dust
  - Animal dander
  - Change in humidity or temperature
  - Change in seasons (pollens, grasses, molds)
  - Exercise
  - Infections (usually viral)
  - Inflammation of any sort
  - Meals (aspiration, gastroesophageal reflux disease [GERD], TEF)
- **Question:** Family history?
- *Significance*: A family history of wheezing, asthma, allergic rhinitis, or atopy suggests a diagnosis of asthma.
- **Question:** An episode of choking preceding the first onset of wheezing?
- *Significance*: suggests foreign body aspiration
- **Question:** History of recurrence, reactivity, and reversibility (3 *R*'s)?
- *Significance*: The 3 *R*'s suggest asthma.
  - Recurrence: symptoms that recur multiple times with full resolution in between episodes
  - Reactivity: symptoms that can be triggered during exposures (temperature extremes, smoke, dust, humid or dry air, aromas, etc.)
  - Reversibility: symptoms that resolve with bronchodilator therapy

PHYSICAL EXAM

- **Finding:** Patient's degree of respiratory difficulty?
- *Significance*:
  - Tachypnea
  - Accessory muscle usage: Use of intercostal and sternocleidomastoid muscles and abdominal musculature indicates increased expiratory effort to overcome airway obstruction.
  - Nasal flaring: With increasing respiratory difficulty, the nares will be dilated to decrease the resistance to air flow.
- **Finding:** Auscultate: Assess airflow, adventitious sounds, and the inspiratory-to-expiratory ratio. Is the wheezing diffuse or localized?
- *Significance*:
  - Aeration: Decreased aeration is much worse prognostically than wheezing because it is directly related to the amount of aeration and ventilation. With decreased aeration, wheezing may not be audible.
  - Ratio of inspiration to exhalation: With increased intrathoracic airway obstruction, the time needed to exhale will become greater because of a greater decrease in airway caliber during exhalation. Normal ratio is 1:3.
  - Localized wheezing may suggest a foreign body.
- **Finding:** Presence of nasal crease, the "allergic salute" (i.e., rubbing the nose with the palm of the hand), atopic dermatitis, boggy nasal turbinates, clear postnasal drainage, allergic shiners, or Dennie lines?
- *Significance*: suggestive of allergic rhinitis or atopic disease including asthma
- **Finding:** Patients with first-time, persistent, or atypical episodes of wheezing?
- *Significance*: "All that wheezes is not asthma": Although most episodes of wheezing will represent viral infections or asthma, clinicians need to be mindful of alternative diagnoses.

DIFFERENTIAL DIAGNOSIS

- Extrathoracic (usually results in stridor or stertor rather than wheezing)
  - Nasal/nasopharynx
    - Acute: nasal turbinate edema or secretions, foreign body
    - Chronic: adenoidal enlargement, nasal polyps, choanal stenosis, midface hypoplasia
  - Oropharynx
    - Acute: peritonsillar abscess, retropharyngeal abscess, palatine tonsillitis
    - Chronic: adenotonsillar hypertrophy, macroglossia, micrognathia
  - Hypopharynx
    - Acute: acute nasal, nasopharyngeal, or oropharyngeal obstruction
    - Chronic: hypopharyngeal hypotonia, glossoptosis, obesity, neoplasia
  - Larynx
    - Acute: laryngospasm, laryngotracheobronchitis (croup), epiglottitis, foreign body (large and irregular)
    - Chronic: laryngomalacia, papillomatosis, hemangioma, granuloma, congenital cyst or web, laryngocele
  - Glottis
    - Acute: vocal cord paralysis or paresis, vocal cord inflammation or polyp, psychogenic wheezing
    - Chronic: paradoxical vocal cord motion (vocal cord dysfunction); psychogenic wheezing; brainstem compression; injury to the vagus, glossopharyngeal, or recurrent laryngeal nerves; papillomatosis
  - Subglottis/extrathoracic trachea
    - Acute: laryngotracheobronchitis (croup), bacterial tracheitis, recent endotracheal extubation
    - Chronic: subglottic stenosis (congenital or after prolonged intubation), papillomatosis
- Intrathoracic
  - Trachea (extrinsic compression)
    - Acute: uncommon
    - Chronic
      - Vascular: vascular ring/sling, compression by an aberrant pulmonary artery
      - Cardiac: left main bronchus compression, recurrent laryngeal nerve compression "cardiovocal syndrome"
      - Anterior mediastinum: lymphoma, thymoma, teratoma
      - Middle mediastinum: lymphoma, lymphadenopathy (tuberculosis, mycotic infection, sarcoidosis)
      - Posterior mediastinum: neurogenic tumors, esophageal duplication or cyst, bronchogenic cyst

- Trachea (intramural lesions)
  - Acute: uncommon
  - Chronic: tracheomalacia
    - Congenital: cartilaginous defect (Campbell-Williams syndrome), muscular defect (Mounier-Kuhn syndrome), status post TEF repair, external compression/distortion, complete tracheal rings
    - Acquired: chronic inflammation (recurrent infection, gastroesophageal reflux, recurrent aspiration), prolonged positive pressure ventilation, external compression
- Trachea (intraluminal lesions)
  - Acute: foreign body (irregularly shaped and elongated), bacterial tracheitis (with chronic tracheostomy tube usage)
  - Chronic: tracheal granulomas, hemangioma, papillomatosis, tracheal web
- Bronchi/bronchioles
  - Acute: viral bronchiolitis, bronchopneumonia, foreign body (small, smooth shape), immune defect (transient hypogammaglobulinemia of the newborn is most common), granuloma, neoplasia
  - Chronic: asthma, bronchopulmonary dysplasia, bronchomalacia, carcinoid, adenoma

DIAGNOSTIC TESTS & INTERPRETATION

- **Test:** bronchodilator responsiveness
- *Significance*:
  - A postbronchodilator improvement in wheezing indicates a reversible process such as asthma.
  - A bronchodilator may worsen wheezing in disorders of airway wall rigidity such as bronchomalacia or tracheomalacia.
  - There may be no change following a bronchodilator in situations with foreign bodies, fixed airway obstruction due to significant inflammation (i.e., status asthmaticus), or airway remodeling.
- **Test:** pulmonary function testing (spirometry)
- *Significance*:
  - Spirometry remains the standard and most helpful measure of pulmonary function.
  - Normative data have been described in children >5 years of age.
  - Normal spirometry does not rule out asthma.
  - Methacholine challenge test is a provocative test to evaluate for asthma.
  - Exercise test with spirometry to evaluate for exercise-induced asthma
- **Test:** pulse oximetry measurement of oxygen saturation (Spo_2)
- *Significance*: Pulse oximetry is an insensitive measure of mild to moderate respiratory difficulty during wheezing, but oxyhemoglobin saturation <92% may be seen in severe compromise.
- **Test:** arterial blood gas
- *Significance*:
  - Arterial blood gases provide a direct measure of oxygenation (Pao_2) and ventilation ($Paco_2$) and can also help to determine severity.
  - A normal or high normal $Paco_2$ in a tachypneic patient (when it should be low) may be a sign of impending respiratory failure.

Initial Tests (screening, lab, imaging)

- **Test:** microbiologic studies
- *Significance*:
  - Positive bacterial culture of sputum is helpful in directing or focusing antibiotic therapy. A Gram stain showing sheets of polymorphonuclear leukocytes and a predominant organism is helpful to differentiate a potentially causative organism from the multitude of normal flora.
  - Positive respiratory virus screen (often within 12 hours) can prevent needless antibiotic therapy and may be helpful in predicting future disease.
- **Test:** tuberculosis skin test
- *Significance*: Mantoux purified protein derivative—tuberculosis. May be falsely positive in a patient who received BCG vaccine; may be falsely negative in a patient who is anergic
- **Test:** CBC including eosinophil count, quantitative immunoglobulins, IgE, complement, allergy skin testing, blood test for specific allergens
- *Significance*: screening for immune defects, atopy
- Chest radiography (posteroanterior and lateral views)
  - Should be strongly considered in all patients with new-onset wheezing or an asymmetric lung exam
  - Can show findings suggestive of airway obstruction (hyperinflation, hyperlucency, flattening of the diaphragms)
  - Asymmetry in aeration on right and left lateral decubitus films suggests foreign body or other obstructing lesions on the side having the greatest air trapping.

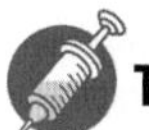

TREATMENT

GENERAL MEASURES

- A trial of bronchodilator therapy (e.g., albuterol) may be both therapeutic and diagnostic of the reversible airway obstruction characteristic of asthma.
- For acute asthma exacerbation: corticosteroids PO or IV
- Ipratropium bromide may be helpful in reducing airway secretions and reducing airway obstruction; may be helpful in tracheomalacia as might bethanechol
- Inhaled corticosteroids, antileukotriene agents, and less frequently, methylxanthines (aminophylline and theophylline) are used as maintenance medications.
- Antibiotics should be used in patients with suspected pneumonia.
- In emergency setting, epinephrine, terbutaline, and magnesium sulfate can be used along with supportive care such as supplemental oxygen.

ALERT

Factors that may indicate a respiratory emergency:

- Signs of mild to moderate respiratory difficulty: tachypnea, intercostal and suprasternal retractions, nasal flaring, head bobbing and exaggerated shoulder movement during breathing, abdominal breathing and subcostal retractions (may be normal in infants, especially during active [REM] sleep), relative difficulty speaking in complete sentences, significant wheezing, prolonged exhalation, and low $Paco_2$ in the face of tachypnea
- Signs of impending respiratory failure: cyanosis, fatigue, inability to speak in >1- or 2-word phrases, altered mental status (e.g., confusion, agitation), decreased respiratory drive, inadequate ventilation (poor air flow), no audible wheezing, high normal or rising $Paco_2$ in the face of tachypnea or respiratory distress
- Determine which patients require assisted ventilation (e.g., bag-mask ventilation, noninvasive [nasal] ventilation, or endotracheal intubation).
- Lack of response to aggressive bronchodilator therapy, without a history of asthma or recurrent wheeze, or biphasic adventitious sounds should immediately raise the suspicion of a fixed lesion.

ADDITIONAL READING

- Castro-Rodriguez JA, Rodrigo GJ. Efficacy of inhaled corticosteroids in infants and preschoolers with recurrent wheezing and asthma: a systemic review with meta-analysis. *Pediatrics*. 2009;123(3):e519–e525.
- Cowan K, Guilbert TW. Pediatric asthma phenotypes. *Curr Opin Pediatr*. 2012;24(3):344–351.
- Jurca M, Pescatore AM, Goutaki M, et al. Age-related changes in childhood wheezing characteristics: a whole population study. *Pediatr Pulmonol*. 2017;52(10):1250–1259.
- Nelson KA, Zorc JJ. Asthma update. *Pediatr Clin North Am*. 2013;60(5):1035–1048.
- Piippo-Savolainen E, Korppi M. Long-term outcomes of early childhood wheezing. *Curr Opin Allergy Clin Immunol*. 2009;9(3):190–196.

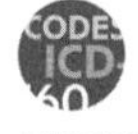

CODES

ICD10

R06.2 Wheezing

FAQ

- Q: What percentage of recurrent wheezing resolves by school age?
- A: Roughly 40% of children with ≥1 episode of wheezing before 3 years clear by 6 years of age.
- Q: Should chest radiographs be routinely obtained in children experiencing their first episodes of wheezing?
- A: For a child with new-onset asymmetric wheezing, a chest radiograph should be obtained. For a child with symmetric wheezing, chest radiography may not be helpful and should be ordered judiciously.

WILMS TUMOR

Nicholas F. Evageliou, MD

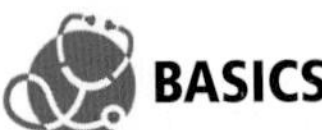

BASICS

DESCRIPTION

Wilms tumor is a malignant tumor of the kidney occurring in the pediatric age group. It is also referred to as nephroblastoma.

EPIDEMIOLOGY

Slightly more common in girls than boys; 90% of patients present by age 6 years

Incidence

1 in 10,000 live births

Prevalence

- Most common primary malignant renal tumor of childhood
- 5–6% of all childhood cancers

RISK FACTORS

Genetics

- 5–10% present in the context of a predisposing syndrome
- Familial cases represent 1–2% of cases and are more often bilateral and occur at an earlier age.
- A tumor suppressor gene related to Wilms tumor (*WT1*) has been localized to chromosome 11p13. Mutations in this gene occur in 10–20% of Wilms tumors.
- Another tumor suppressor gene, *WT2*, has been localized on 11p15.

ETIOLOGY

- 10–20% of Wilms tumors have a mutation in the *WT1* tumor suppressor gene.
- Causes in the remaining 80% of patients are complex and involve the WNT signaling pathway and *IGF2* overexpression.

COMMONLY ASSOCIATED CONDITIONS

- 12–15% of patients have other congenital anomalies.
- May be associated with aniridia, hemihypertrophy, and cryptorchidism
- Associated syndromes
  - WAGR (Wilms tumor, aniridia, genitourinary [GU] abnormalities, mental retardation)
  - Beckwith-Wiedemann syndrome (macroglossia, omphalocele, visceromegaly, hemihypertrophy)
  - Denys-Drash syndrome (ambiguous genitalia, progressive renal failure, and increased risk of Wilms tumor)
- Nephroblastomatosis is a condition where islands of embryonic renal tissue develop. This is a generally benign condition which carries a risk of developing into Wilms tumor.

DIAGNOSIS

HISTORY

- Abdominal distention, most often painless
- Abdominal pain (20–30% of cases)
- Hematuria (20–30% of cases)
- Fever, anorexia, vomiting
- Family history of Wilms tumor
- Rapid increase in abdominal size (suggestive of hemorrhage in the tumor)

PHYSICAL EXAM

- Asymptomatic abdominal mass extending from flank toward midline (most common presentation)
- Anemia (secondary to hemorrhage in the tumor)
- Fever
- Hypertension (owing to increased renin production in 25% of cases)
- Check for signs of Beckwith-Wiedemann or other syndromes (aniridia, hemihypertrophy, cryptorchidism, hypospadias, other GU abnormalities).

DIFFERENTIAL DIAGNOSIS

- Polycystic kidney
- Renal hematoma
- Renal abscess
- Neuroblastoma
- Other neoplasms of kidney: clear cell carcinoma, rhabdoid tumor, renal cell carcinoma

DIAGNOSTIC TESTS & INTERPRETATION

Initial Tests (screening, lab, imaging)

- CBC
- Electrolytes
- Urine analysis: for microscopic hematuria
- Liver and kidney function tests
- Coagulation factors
- Ultrasound of abdomen
  - Diagnostic of mass of renal origin
  - Evaluate for extension of tumor into inferior vena cava and possibly into right atrium.
- CT or MRI scan of abdomen and chest CT: to evaluate for metastatic disease
- Bone scan: only if clear cell sarcoma, renal cell carcinoma, or rhabdoid tumor on pathology
- MRI of head: only for clear cell sarcoma and rhabdoid tumors
- EKG and echocardiogram in patients who will receive anthracycline chemotherapy
- Pathologic findings
  - Gross pathology
    - Often cystic with hemorrhages and necrosis
    - Usually no calcification (useful in differentiating from neuroblastoma, which is calcified on plain radiograph)
    - May extend into the inferior vena cava
  - Histology
    - Triphasic pattern blastemal, epithelial, and stromal cell
    - Blastemal cells aggregate into nodules like primitive glomeruli; the presence of diffuse anaplasia indicates a poor prognosis.

- Lymph node positivity confers somewhat poorer EFS.
- Loss of heterozygosity (LOH) of 1p and 16q useful in treatment decision
- Clinicopathologic staging
  - Stage I: Tumor is restricted to one kidney and completely resected. The renal capsule is intact.
  - Stage II: Tumor extends beyond the kidney but is completely excised.
  - Stage III: Residual nonhematogenous tumor is confined to the abdomen.
  - Stage IV: There is hematogenous spread to lungs, liver, bone, or brain.
  - Stage V: bilateral disease

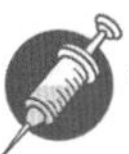

TREATMENT

Radiotherapy

- Not required for stage I and II patients unless anaplastic, clear cell, or rhabdoid
- Radiotherapy to tumor bed with 1,080 cGy for stages III and IV; if gross tumor spillage or peritoneal seeding, whole abdomen radiation indicated
- Whole-lung radiation (1,200 cGy) for pulmonary metastasis which do not resolve with upfront chemotherapy

MEDICATION

- Chemotherapy
  - For stages I and II favorable histology: vincristine and actinomycin D every for 5 months
  - For stages III and IV favorable histology, stage I to III focal anaplasia, and stage I diffuse anaplasia: vincristine, actinomycin D, and doxorubicin for 6 to 15 months
  - Add cyclophosphamide, etoposide, and/or carboplatin for higher stage anaplastic tumors (stage IV focal or II to IV diffuse).
- Side effects of therapy
  - Temporary loss of hair
  - Peripheral neuropathy
  - Hepatotoxicity
  - Neutropenia/infection depending on regimen

SURGERY/OTHER PROCEDURES

Nephrectomy

- In general, upfront nephrectomy preferred
- Preoperative chemotherapy in case of very large tumors with inferior vena cava extension
- For bilateral disease, partial nephrectomy following 6 to 12 weeks of chemotherapy

ONGOING CARE

FOLLOW-UP RECOMMENDATIONS

Patient Monitoring

- Every 3 months for 18 months, every 6 months for 1 year, and then yearly
- Chest radiograph, urinalysis, and abdominal ultrasound at regular intervals

PROGNOSIS

- Stages I and II: >90% cured
- Stage III: 85–90% cured
- Stage IV: 80–90% cured
- Favorable prognostic factors
  - Tumor weight <550 g
  - Age at presentation <24 months
  - Stage I disease
  - Favorable histology
- Poor prognostic factors
  - Diffuse anaplastic pathology
  - Clear cell sarcoma variant
  - Rhabdoid tumor variant
  - Lymph node involvement
  - Distant metastasis
  - Tumors with LOH of chromosomes 1p and/or 16q

COMPLICATIONS

- Extension into inferior vena cava
- Metastasis to lungs and liver
- Cardiac toxicity secondary to doxorubicin
- Pulmonary fibrosis if lung radiation received
- Second malignancies due to XRT/chemotherapy agents
- Impaired fertility if cyclophosphamide or radiation

ADDITIONAL READING

- Davidoff AM. Wilms tumor. *Adv Pediatr*. 2012;59(1):247–267.
- Dome JS, Graf N, Geller JI, et al. Advances in Wilms tumor treatment and biology: progress through international collaboration. *J Clin Oncol*. 2015;33(27):2999–3007.
- Hohenstein P, Hastie ND. The many facets of the Wilms' tumour gene, WT1. *Hum Mol Genet*. 2006;15(2):R196–R201.
- Irtan S, Ehrlich PF, Pritchard-Jones K. Wilms tumor: "State-of-the-art" update, 2016. *Semin Pediatr Surg*. 2016;25(5):250–256.
- Malkan AD, Loh A, Bahrami A, et al. An approach to renal masses in pediatrics. *Pediatrics*. 2015;135(1):142–158.
- Martinez CH, Dave S, Izawa J. Wilms' tumor. *Adv Exp Med Biol*. 2010;685:196–209.

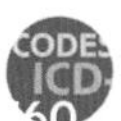

CODES

ICD10

- C64.9 Malignant neoplasm of unsp kidney, except renal pelvis
- C64.1 Malignant neoplasm of right kidney, except renal pelvis
- C64.2 Malignant neoplasm of left kidney, except renal pelvis

FAQ

- Q: Can a child grow and live normally with one kidney?
- A: Yes. Studies of children with unilateral nephrectomy show a rate of chronic renal failure at 25 years of <1%.
- Q: What is my child's risk of late effects of therapy?
- A: This depends on the specific regimen received, but late effects are minimal for lower stage tumors.

WILSON DISEASE

Anthony F. Porto, MD, MPH

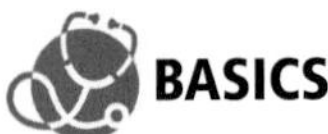

BASICS

DESCRIPTION

Wilson disease (WD), also known as hepatolenticular degeneration, is an autosomal recessive disorder of copper transport affecting several organs, most notably the liver, brain, and cornea.

EPIDEMIOLOGY

Children usually present with hepatic manifestations; adolescents and young adults may present with neurologic symptoms.

- Worldwide carrier rate is 1:100.
- Prevalence is 1:30,000 to 40,000.
- Most cases present between ages 5 and 35 years.
- No gender predilection
- Worldwide distribution with higher risk in Sardinia (1:7,000 to 10,000) and Costa Rica (1:20,400)

RISK FACTORS

Genetics

- Autosomal recessive inheritance with 1 of >500 known defects of the WD gene (*ATP7B*) on chromosome 13q14.3 membrane (ATPase)
- The affected protein facilitates biliary excretion of excess copper; incorporates copper into apoceruloplasmin for transport
- Heterozygotes are generally asymptomatic.
- Siblings have 25% risk of disease, 50% chance of being an asymptomatic carrier, and a 25% chance of being unaffected and not a carrier.
- Clinical phenotype of WD is modified by mutations in other genes, including *MTHFR*, *COMMD1*, *ATOX1*, and *XIAP*.
- Use of direct mutational analysis to phenotype WD is limited by the high number of mutations.

PATHOPHYSIOLOGY

- Loss of ATP7B function causes; (i) impaired biliary copper excretion (the only route for elimination of copper) and (ii) failure to incorporate copper to apoceruloplasmin during ceruloplasmin biosynthesis, leading to ceruloplasmin deficiency
- Copper accumulates preferentially in the liver, leading to cirrhosis.
- After liver is saturated, copper overflows and settles in the brain (primarily in the basal ganglia leading to impaired motor control), as well as other tissues including kidneys, heart, blood, and cornea.
- Excess copper damages mitochondria, causing oxidative damage to cells. In addition, toxic intracellular copper deposition promotes apoptotic cell death by the inhibition of inhibitor of apoptosis proteins (IAPs).

DIAGNOSIS

HISTORY

- Issues with presentation of disease:
  - WD has a variable presentation that requires a high level of suspicion.
  - 45% of all patients present with liver disease, 35% with neurologic symptoms, and 10% psychiatric.
  - Remaining 10%: Coombs negative hemolytic anemia, jaundice, cardiomyopathy, other
  - Consider WD in all cases of liver abnormality in which viral and autoimmune causes have been excluded.
  - Also consider WD in every young patient with unexplained neuropsychiatric symptoms including with a movement disorder
  - Up to 10% of patients may be asymptomatic with diagnosis made after elevated ALT/AST, noted on routine testing.
- Hepatic
  - In children, symptoms of hepatic disease predominate, ranging from asymptomatic hepatomegaly and elevated transaminases to chronic hepatitis, cirrhosis, and fulminant hepatic failure.
  - Mean age for onset of hepatic symptoms ~10 years
  - Fulminant liver failure is associated with hemolysis and coagulopathy unresponsive to vitamin K.
- Neurologic
  - Neurologic symptoms are rare before age 10 years and may develop 1 decade later than hepatic symptoms.
  - Neurologic signs in children: Early signs include poor concentration, change in penmanship, behavior change, decline in school performance, poor hand–eye coordination, motor abnormalities—dystonia, tremors, dysphagia, dysarthria with drooling, chorea, ataxia, and parkinsonism (slowness of movements with rigidity and bradykinesia typically symmetric in WD and may be asymmetric in Parkinson disease)
  - Other manifestations include seizures, myoclonus, and dysautonomia.
- Psychiatric: development of depression, anxiety, psychosis, and/or obsessive-compulsive disorder
- Other: Nonspecific complaints are common—abdominal pain, nausea, anorexia, and fatigue.

PHYSICAL EXAM

- Ophthalmologic
  - Kayser-Fleischer (KF) rings: copper deposits on Descemet membrane of cornea (at limbus)
    - Not pathognomonic for WD; may be seen in cholestatic liver disease
    - Golden-brown pigment noted with naked eye
    - May require slit-lamp examination to detect
  - 95% with neurologic signs have KF rings.
  - 50–65% with hepatic presentation has KF rings.
- Cardiovascular: signs of cardiomyopathy, dysrhythmia, congestive heart failure
- Abdominal
  - Hepatomegaly, ascites
  - Splenomegaly from portal hypertension
- Skin
  - Jaundice due to hemolysis
  - Bleeding diathesis from liver disease
  - Edema
- Neurologic
  - Movement disorders
  - Neurologic deficits

DIFFERENTIAL DIAGNOSIS

- Liver disease
  - Viral hepatitis
  - Autoimmune hepatitis (AIH)/primary biliary cirrhosis
  - Menkes disease (low ceruloplasmin)
  - Cholestatic disease from parenteral nutrition (KF rings)
- Neurologic disease
  - Essential tremor
  - Sydenham or Huntington chorea
  - Hereditary dystonia
  - Other neurodegenerative diseases
- Psychiatric disease: depression, psychoses
- Protein loss from GI or renal abnormalities

DIAGNOSTIC TESTS & INTERPRETATION

Initial Tests (screening, lab, imaging)

- Serum ceruloplasmin
  - An acute-phase reactant; increased with inflammation, infection, or trauma; also high with use of estrogen-based oral contraceptives; level may increase to reference range.
  - Made mostly in the liver; it is the major carrier of copper (<90% of total copper) in blood.
  - Low serum ceruloplasmin can be helpful in diagnosing WD.
    - Very low (<20 mg/L): strong evidence for WD
    - Low (<200 mg/L) plus symptoms and KF rings: diagnostic of WD
  - Ceruloplasmin levels also low in renal or GI protein loss, Menkes disease, and end-stage liver disease
- Serum copper
  - Low total serum copper (<80 mcg/dL) in WD
  - Level is decreased in proportion to decreased ceruloplasmin in circulation.
  - In acute fulminant liver failure, serum copper is increased owing to sudden release of stores (most is not bound to ceruloplasmin).
- Free copper estimation
  - Measure of nonceruloplasmin toxic copper in the blood; normal values 1.3 to 1.9 μmol/L (8 to 12 mcg/dL), in WD >3.9 μmol/L (25 mcg/dL)
  - Useful in cases where false elevation of ceruloplasmin is suspected; when a measurement of urinary copper is difficult to obtain, as well to monitor chelators efficacy during maintenance phase of therapy (goal <25 mcg/dL)
  - Calculated by the formula: total serum copper in mcg/mL × 100 − (ceruloplasmin in mg/dL × 3) = free copper
- Urinary copper excretion
  - Reflects unbound copper in blood
  - Normal: <40 to 50 mcg/24 h
  - Level is high in WD: >100 mcg/24 h in symptomatic (neurologic and psychiatric phenotype) patient is diagnostic; may also be high in AIH and chronic cholestasis so additional tests may be needed to differentiate
  - In equivocal cases, marked increase in urinary copper output (>1,600 mcg/24 h) after initiation of chelation therapy may help in diagnosis.
- Other:
  - Mutational analysis if familial mutation is known especially if urinary copper is equivocal, such as in children <10 years of age
- Abdominal ultrasound for liver size and pathology
- MRI of the brain/basal ganglia should be obtained prior to initiation of therapy.
- "Face of the giant panda" sign that is characteristic of WD (hyperintense signal in the midbrain around the red nuclei and substantia nigra)

Diagnostic Procedures/Other

- Liver biopsy to assess copper content is the definitive procedure for tissue diagnosis and hepatic disease staging.
- Biopsy should be obtained when diagnosis is not straightforward and in younger patients.
- Hepatic parenchymal copper concentration >250 mcg/g dry weight; also increased in cholestasis but not as high as seen in WD
- Hepatic copper level <50 mcg/g dry weight excludes WD.

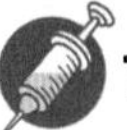

TREATMENT

- Lifetime therapy aimed at treating copper overload
- Consists of two phases
  - (1) Removing or detoxifying the tissue copper (achieved by chelators)
  - (2) Preventing reaccumulation without leading to copper deficiency (low-dose chelators, dosages reduced by about 33% from original induction dose and/or by use of zinc salts)
- Outcomes are best with therapy started within 1 month of the onset of symptoms.
- Successful therapy is measured in terms of a restoration of normal levels of free serum copper and its excretion in the urine.

GENERAL MEASURES

- Immunize for hepatitis A, B.
- Avoid excess alcohol.
- Well water or water via copper pipes needs to be tested: If >0.1 ppm Cu, find alternative source.

MEDICATION

- Penicillamine
  - Mode of action (MOA)
    - Chelates copper and promotes renal excretion
    - Also induces metallothionein (which forms a nontoxic combination with copper)
    - Efficacy: improvement in clinical features noted after 2 to 3 months, continuing over a period of 1 to 2 years
  - Dosages and monitoring:
    - Initial dose: 1 to 1.5 g/24 h in 2 to 4 divided doses PO, maximum total daily dose 20 mg/kg, taken 1 or 2 hours after food (absorption decreased by approximately 50% when taken with food)
    - May start at a lower dose (250 to 500 mg/24 h) with gradual escalation over a few weeks
    - Monitoring: clinical assessment + hematologic, biochemical (transaminases), and urinary parameters every week for 1 month and then every month for 6 months, and subsequently every 6 months
    - While on therapy, 24-hour urine copper exceeds ≥2,000 mcg/24 h, with gradual decline over 6 to 12 months to values below ≤200 to 500 mcg/24 h.
    - Once this level achieved and free serum copper <15 mcg/dL, the maintenance dose can be lowered to 0.5 to 1 g/24 h in divided doses (usually after 4 to 6 months).
    - At this point, a zinc salt could be added to the treatment regimen, preferably before meals to avoid any interaction with penicillamine.
    - The goal of treatment is a 24-hour urine copper excretion of 50 to 100 mcg.
  - Side effects in 20–30%
    - Acute neurologic deterioration caused by rapid mobilization of hepatic copper stores leading to increased brain copper deposition or from the development of intracellular copper complexes
    - Reduce dose to 250 mg/24 h or switch to trientine or zinc.
    - Pyridoxine deficiency, risk factors include intercurrent infection or a growth spurt; vitamin B_6 supplementation 25 to 50 mg/24 h
    - Skin diseases such as elastosis perforans serpiginosa (skin degeneration due to interference with collagen and elastin formation)
    - Hypersensitivity reactions (rash, fever, lymphadenopathy), bone marrow suppression, myasthenia gravis, optic neuritis, nephritis, lupuslike syndrome
    - Discontinue if the total white blood cell count <3,000 cells per mm^3, neutrophils <2,000 cells per mm^3, platelets <120,000 per mm^3, or if a steady decline over three successive tests even if the values are above the earlier mentioned parameters for discontinuation.
    - Discontinue also if >2+ proteinuria on a dipstick, red cell or white casts or >10 red cells seen per high-power field on urine microscopy.
- Trientine
  - MOA: chelates copper/promotes renal excretion
  - Dosages and monitoring:
    - Has become initial drug of choice
    - Used in combination with zinc
  - Dosages: pediatric dose 20 mg/kg/24 h PO divided 2 to 3 times per day up to a maximum of 1,500 mg/24 h. Round dose to the nearest 250 mg.
  - Maintenance therapy: 750 to 1,000 mg/24 h 2 to 3 times per day; avoid taking with food.
  - Monitoring: same as penicillamine
  - Side effects: fewer than penicillamine
    - Risk of sideroblastic anemia (drug's effects on mitochondrial iron metabolism), hemorrhagic gastritis, nephritis, arthritis, worsened neurologic signs
    - Serum copper increases during treatment.
    - Also chelates iron, creating toxic complex; do not give supplemental iron (if iron supplementation required, administer iron in short courses, separated by trientine by at least 2 hours).
- Zinc
  - Routinely combined with trientine
  - Also used alone as maintenance therapy
  - Used successfully in asymptomatic or presymptomatic affected family members of individuals with WD
  - MOA
    - Interferes with absorption from GI tract by inducing metallothionein in enterocytes, which chelates metals. Copper is bound within the enterocyte and not absorbed into the portal circulation. It is shed in stool along with normal shedding of enterocytes.
    - Also induces copper-binding metallothionein in the liver
    - May create a negative copper balance, removing all extra copper stores, resulting in improvement of hepatic and brain function, and loss of KF rings
  - Dosage: 50 mg t.i.d. PO, empty stomach
  - Side effects:
    - Few side effects: gastric irritation, nausea
    - Overtreatment may result in anemia, decreased wound healing, or neuromyelopathy from copper deficiency.
  - No altered dose needed for surgery
  - Compliance with overall therapy monitored by urine zinc levels, which should be >2 mg
  - After chelation for 4 to 6 months, with normal labs, usually OK to change to zinc for maintenance
- Ammonium tetrathiomolybdate
  - Not United States Food and Drug Administration (FDA)-approved, available in Europe, although bis-choline tetrathiomolybdate is in phase II trials in the United States
  - If taken with food, complex with copper in the intestinal tract, preventing absorption
  - When taken without food, absorbed drug forms a complex with copper and albumin in blood, which is metabolized by liver and excreted in bile.
  - Particularly suited for treatment of neurologic manifestation in WD, as it is not associated with exacerbation on initiation of treatment
  - Side effects: bone marrow suppression, elevated aminotransferases
- Antioxidants and experimental therapies
  - Antioxidants (vitamin E/*N*-acetylcysteine) may protect against oxidative damage.
  - Organ-specific chelators
  - Human hepatocyte transplantation (as done for metabolic diseases), using mesenchymal stem cells that differentiate into hepatocytes, is being currently under investigation.

SURGERY/OTHER PROCEDURES

- Orthotopic liver transplant required for fulminant liver failure or end-stage liver cirrhosis, which is resistant to chelation therapy
- Uncertain indication for therapy-resistant neurologic symptoms. Several case reports suggest improved neurologic symptoms after transplantation.
- 5% with WD need liver transplants.

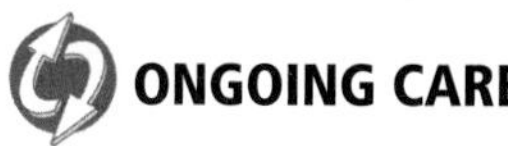

ONGOING CARE

FOLLOW-UP RECOMMENDATIONS

Patient Monitoring

- Patients require lifelong dietary copper restriction and chelation therapy. Dosing of chelation therapy, although not zinc, needs to be adjusted during pregnancy.
- Continual monitoring for compliance and side effects of medications is crucial.
- Sudden discontinuation of therapy may precipitate fulminant hepatic failure.
- 1st-degree relatives age >3 years should be screened with history, physical exam, LFTs, CBC, serum ceruloplasmin, 24-hour urine copper, and ophthalmologic examination for KF rings.
- Reproductive and genetic counseling for carriers should be offered; prenatal testing

DIET

Low-copper diet for life: Avoid liver and other organ meats, shellfish, nuts, mushrooms, and chocolate.

COMPLICATIONS

- Renal: Copper accumulation leads to Fanconi syndrome (tubular dysfunction, glycosuria, hypophosphatemia, and low uric acid).
- Hematologic: Coombs-negative hemolytic anemia, coagulopathy from liver failure
- Cardiac: cardiomyopathy/dysrhythmias
- Rare associations include renal stones, gallstones, osteomalacia, osteoporosis, arthralgias, pancreatitis, hypoparathyroidism, skin pigmentation, and a bluish discoloration at the base of the fingernails (azure lunulae).

PROGNOSIS

- If WD is recognized early and treated, most patients experience complete recovery.
- Progression to hepatocellular carcinoma is rare, unlike hemochromatosis.

ADDITIONAL READING

- Ala A, Walker AP, Ashkan K, et al. Wilson's disease. *Lancet*. 2007;369(9559):397–408.
- Brewer GJ, Askari F, Dick RB, et al. Treatment of Wilson's disease with tetrathiomolybdate: V. Control of free copper by tetrathiomolybdate and a comparison with trientine. *Transl Res*. 2009;154(2):70–77.
- European Association for Study of Liver. EASL clinical practice guidelines: Wilson's disease. *J Hepatol*. 2012;56(3):671–685.
- Hedera P. Update on the clinical management of Wilson's disease. *Appl Clin Genet*. 2017;10:9–19.

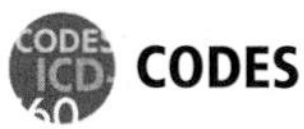

CODES

ICD10

E83.01 Wilson's disease

W

WISKOTT-ALDRICH SYNDROME

Elena E. Perez, MD, PhD

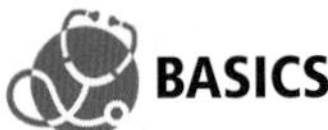

BASICS

DESCRIPTION

- An X-linked primary immunodeficiency caused by a mutation in the Wiskott-Aldrich syndrome (*WAS*) gene
- Originally described as clinical triad of thrombocytopenia with small platelets, eczema, and recurrent infections with opportunistic and pyogenic organisms
- Increased bleeding tendency secondary to thrombocytopenia likely results from impaired platelet production, increased turnover, and defective function.
- Disease variants also resulting from *WAS* gene mutations include X-linked thrombocytopenia (XLT) and X-linked neutropenia (XLN).
- Classic WAS is characterized by broad immunodeficiency, decreased number and function of T cells, disturbed marginal B-cell homeostasis, and skewed immunoglobulin isotypes, with defective antibody responses to vaccinations, impaired NK-cell cytotoxicity, and abnormal regulatory T-cell function as well as reduced phagocyte chemotaxis.

EPIDEMIOLOGY

- Presents in infancy with serious bleeding episodes secondary to thrombocytopenia (such as circumcision with increased bleeding, bloody diarrhea, ecchymoses)
- Recurrent infections usually start after 6 months of age:
  - Bacterial: otitis media, sinusitis, meningitis, sepsis and pneumonia
  - Viral infections: herpes simplex virus, varicella with systemic complications
- Milder phenotypes may lack history of recurrent infections.
- Decline in T- and B-cell numbers with time
- Eczema is usually present by 1 year of age (may be resistant to therapy, sometimes requiring systemic antibiotics).

Incidence

- For WAS/XLT, estimate is 10 in 1 million live births.
- Prevalence of XLT equal to WAS

RISK FACTORS

Genetics

- X-linked recessive disease
- Defective WAS protein gene located on X p11.22p–11.23
- ~60% of cases will have a positive family history for WAS.
- XLT without the other findings is caused by mutations of the same gene.
- Genotype/phenotype correlation
  - Lack of WAS protein (WASP) expression correlates with classic WAS phenotype: increased infections, severe eczema, intestinal hemorrhage, death from intracranial bleeding, and malignancies
  - Survival rate significantly lower in WASP-negative patients
  - WASP-positive patients have expression of mutated protein and often have XLT phenotype.

ETIOLOGY

- Mutations in the gene for the WASP
- WASP is involved in the reorganization of the actin cytoskeleton in hematopoietic cells:
  - Following activation of WASP, reorganization of actin cytoskeleton results in polarization of cells (e.g., polarized actin mesh in platelets for clotting and in macrophages for phagocytosis and polarization of T or B cells to form immunologic synapses).
- WASP is a cytoplasmic protein involved in cell mobility, immune regulation, cell signaling, cell-to-cell interactions, signaling, and cytotoxicity.
- Defects in WASP can lead to dysfunction in adaptive and innate immunity, immune surveillance, and platelet homeostasis and function as well as neutropenia.
- "Classic" WAS and XLT result from loss-of-function mutations.
- XLT can be misdiagnosed as idiopathic thrombocytopenic purpura (ITP) that does not carry increased risk of malignancy, so testing for WASP expression and *WAS* gene mutation is important in any male with thrombocytopenia and small platelets.
- XLN results from "activating" mutations in WAS that lead to increased actin polymerization; profound neutropenia, with or without associated lymphopenia; decreased T-cell proliferation in vitro; and increased risk of myelodysplastic changes in bone marrow.
- WASP is also important for regulatory T-cell function.

COMMONLY ASSOCIATED CONDITIONS

- IgA nephropathy
- Autoimmune disorders
- Increased incidence of B-cell lymphomas

DIAGNOSIS

- Diagnosis should be considered in any boy who has congenital or early-onset thrombocytopenia with small platelets.
- Definitive diagnosis
  - Male patient
  - Congenital thrombocytopenia ($<$70,000/mm^3)
  - Small platelets (mean platelet volume $<$0.5 fL)
  - Mutation in the *WASP* gene or absent WASP mRNA

HISTORY

- Persistent or severe bleeding in infancy due to thrombocytopenia
- Recurrent infections, especially by bacteria with capsular polysaccharides (e.g., *pneumococcus*)
- Eczema can be of variable severity:
  - "Acute or chronic"
  - 80% of cases associated with eczema
  - May result from imbalance of cytokines skewed toward Th_2
- Older patients may report recurrent viral infections.
- Most common autoimmune features include autoimmune hemolytic anemia, cutaneous vasculitis, arthritis, and nephropathy.
- Less common autoimmune features include inflammatory bowel disease, ITP, and neutropenia.
- Autoimmune features are poor prognostic indicators and can occur simultaneously.
- Maternal family history of WAS or XLT

PHYSICAL EXAM

- Evaluation should focus on presence of infection.
- Dermatologic examination is significant for the extent of eczema and the presence of petechiae or ecchymoses.
- Splenomegaly

DIFFERENTIAL DIAGNOSIS

- Other causes of thrombocytopenia such as ITP
  - In one cohort, approximately 7% of patients diagnosed as having ITP actually had WAS as an underlying cause of thrombocytopenia.
- Severe atopic disease with dermatitis and secondary skin infections
- HIV infection
- Hyper-IgE syndrome

DIAGNOSTIC TESTS & INTERPRETATION

Initial Tests (screening, lab, imaging)

- CBC with differential
- Small platelets, decreased mean platelet volume, decreased platelet count
- Normal IgG, decreased IgM, increased IgA and IgE (reflecting immune dysregulation)
- Reduced or absent responses to polysaccharide antigens and isohemagglutinins to ABO antigens
- T- and B-lymphocyte enumeration and mitogen stimulation studies may progressively deteriorate with increasing age.

Diagnostic Procedures/Other

- WAS disease scoring system useful for defining clinical phenotypes associated with WAS mutations (XLN, XLT vs. classic WAS)
- Sequencing of *WAS* gene
- Lymph node biopsy in suspected malignancy
- Bone marrow aspirate to evaluate thrombocytopenia

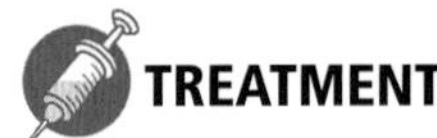

TREATMENT

GENERAL MEASURES

- Antibiotics for acute infections and prophylactically in postsplenectomy patients
- Splenectomy
  - May be helpful for persistent severe thrombocytopenia in select patients. However, this may greatly increase the risk of overwhelming infections with encapsulated organisms.
  - Splenectomy should be reserved for emergencies in classic WAS patients who are candidates for hematopoietic stem cell transplantation (HSCT) because splenectomy is a risk factor for death.
  - Splenectomy in XLT with severe bleeding may increase platelet counts, but risk of severe infection requires lifelong antibiotic prophylaxis.
- Thrombocytopenia precautions
  - No aspirin
  - Avoidance of situations in which trauma (especially head trauma) is likely to occur, such as contact sports
- Platelet transfusions
  - May be necessary for severe bleeding
  - Use irradiated blood products to avoid graft-versus-host disease and cytomegalovirus-negative products in case of bone marrow transplantation.

- Immunoglobulin replacement therapy is helpful in managing recurrent infections in some patients:
  - HSCT is the treatment of choice for the classic WAS phenotype.
  - Allogeneic stem cell transplant from human leukocyte antigen (HLA) genotypically identical sibling or 9/10 or 10/10 allele matched unrelated donor for any WAS patient with disease score 3 to 5 (see "Additional Reading") or with absent WASP expression
  - Outcomes are improving with 5-year survival rates >80% for matched sibling donors and similar for matched unrelated donor grafts <5 years of age.
  - Transplant outcomes for patients >5 years of age with matched sibling or matched unrelated are improving over time.
- Consider food allergy as exacerbating factor for eczema.
- First retroviral-based gene therapy trial in WAS recently completed in Germany with good immune reconstitution and increase in platelet counts in 9 of 10 patients.
- Lentiviral-based gene therapy trials have started in Italy, United States, France, and England and are showing promising results.
- A safe dose of IL-2 has been identified as an immunostimulant therapy; further study of efficacy is needed.
- XLT patients have excellent long-term survival with supportive treatment, but HLA-matched sibling transplant can be considered owing to morbidity.
- Umbilical cord blood transplantation may be an option for young children with WAS lacking an HLA identical stem cell donor.

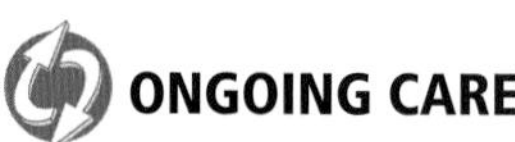

ONGOING CARE

FOLLOW-UP RECOMMENDATIONS

Patient Monitoring

- Signs and symptoms of malignancy should be evaluated expeditiously.
- As patients age, a progressive increase in infectious and autoimmune complications may occur.
- Signs of skin infection, worsening eczema
- Signs of bruising, bleeding
- IgG level and frequency of infections if on gammaglobulin replacement

PATIENT EDUCATION

Sources available to patients and families:

- Immune Deficiency Foundation: http://primaryimmune.org
- International Patient Organisation for Primary Immunodeficiencies: www.ipopi.org
- The Jeffrey Modell Foundation: www.jmfworld.org
- National Institute of Allergy and Infectious Diseases: www.niaid.nih.gov

COMPLICATIONS

- Progressive decline in immunologic function with an increase in infections. Humoral and cellular immune systems are affected.
- Increased frequency of autoimmune phenomena such as arthritis and vasculitis. The most common is hemolytic anemia. Vasculitis, Henoch-Schönlein purpura, inflammatory polyarthritis, and inflammatory bowel disease are also observed.
- Approximately 100-fold increased risk of malignancy compared with the general pediatric population
  - Malignancy is more common in adolescents.
  - Associated with Epstein-Barr virus
- Bleeding episodes can be life-threatening.
- Immune reconstitution via stem cell transplant or gene therapy needed to prevent autoimmune disorders, lymphoma, and other malignancy
- Success of bone marrow transplant in last 10 years significantly improved.
- Splenectomy not recommended for classic WAS but may have role in XLT

ADDITIONAL READING

- Aiuti A, Biasco L, Scaramuzza S, et al. Lentiviral hematopoietic stem cell gene therapy in patients with Wiskott-Aldrich syndrome. *Science*. 2013;341(6148):1233151.
- Albert MH, Notarangelo LD, Ochs HD. Clinical spectrum, pathophysiology and treatment of the Wiskott-Aldrich syndrome. *Curr Opin Hematol*. 2011;18(1):42–48.
- Aldrich RA, Steinberg AG, Campbell DC. Pedigree demonstrating a sex-linked recessive condition characterized by draining ears, eczematoid dermatitis and bloody diarrhea. *Pediatrics*. 1954;13(2):133–139.
- Binder V, Albert M, Kabus M, et al. The genotype of the original Wiskott phenotype. *N Engl J Med*. 2006;355(17):1790–1793.
- Bosticardo M, Marangoni F, Aiuti A, et al. Recent advances in understanding the pathophysiology of Wiskott-Aldrich syndrome. *Blood*. 2009;113(25):6288–6295.
- Bryant N, Watts R. Thrombocytopenic syndromes masquerading as childhood immune thrombocytopenic purpura. *Clin Pediatr (Phila)*. 2011;50(3):225–230.
- Candotti F. Advances of gene therapy for primary immunodeficiencies. *F1000Res*. 2016;5. doi:10.12688/f1000research.7512.1.
- Charrier S, Dupré L, Scaramuzza S, et al. Lentiviral vectors targeting WASp expression to hematopoietic cells, efficiently transduce and correct cells from WAS patients. *Gene Ther*. 2007;14(5):415–428.
- Jyonouchi S, Gwafila B, Gwalani LA, et al. Phase I trial of low-dose interleukin 2 therapy in patients with Wiskott-Aldrich syndrome. *Clin Immunol*. 2017;179:47–53.
- Kohn DB, Kuo CY. New frontiers in the therapy of primary immunodeficiency: from gene addition to gene editing. *J Allergy Clin Immunol*. 2017;139(3):726–732.
- Massaad MJ, Ramesh N, Geha RS. Wiskott-Aldrich syndrome: a comprehensive review. *Ann N Y Acad Sci*. 2013;1285:26–43.
- Schurman SH, Candotti F. Autoimmunity in Wiskott-Aldrich syndrome. *Curr Opin Rheumatol*. 2003;15(4):446–453.
- Shcherbina A, Candotti F, Rosen F, et al. High incidence of lymphomas in a subgroup of Wiskott-Aldrich syndrome patients. *Br J Haematol*. 2003;121(3):529–530.
- Shekhovtsova Z, Bonfim C, Ruggeri A, et al. A risk factor analysis of outcomes after unrelated cord blood transplantation for children with Wiskott-Aldrich syndrome. *Haematologica*. 2017;102(6):1112–1119.
- Wiskott A. Familiärer, angeborener Morbus Werlhofii? [Familial congenital Werlhof's disease?]. *Montsschr Kinderheilkd*. 1937;68:212–216.
- Xu X, Tailor CS, Grunebaum E. Gene therapy for primary immune deficiencies: a Canadian perspective. *Allergy Asthma Clin Immunol*. 2017;13:14.

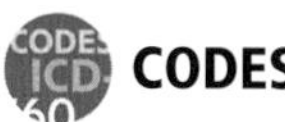

CODES

ICD10

D82.0 Wiskott-Aldrich syndrome

FAQ

- Q: What is the life expectancy for patients with WAS?
- A: Before currently available therapies, most affected patients died in childhood. Currently, many patients live into their 3rd and 4th decades, even without bone marrow transplantation. Major causes of mortality are infections (44%), bleeding (23%), and malignancies (26%). Incidence of malignancy increases in 3rd decade of life. Successfully transplanted patients have a prolonged life expectancy. Patients with no gene expression have a poorer outcome.
- Q: Should patients with WAS receive live viral vaccines?
- A: These vaccines should be avoided because of the variable cellular immune defects associated with WAS. In general, patients receiving IV immunoglobulin do not require vaccinations.
- Q: What is the chance of a sibling having WAS?
- A: As with any X-linked disease, there is a 50% chance of another affected male child or asymptomatic carrier female. Genetic counseling should be offered to carrier females.
- Q: Can WAS be diagnosed prenatally?
- A: In families with affected males, fetal blood sampling can be performed in male fetuses to assess the size of the platelets. Small platelet size and family history of WAS suggest an affected infant.
- Q: Who was Wiskott?
- A: Alfred Wilhelm Wiskott, MD (1898 to 1978) received his medical degree at Ludwig Maximilian University in Munich, Germany. He trained in pediatrics at the von Haunersches Kinderspital in Munich. In 1937, he published a report of three brothers who had thrombocytopenia, eczema, and recurrent ear infections. The boys eventually died due to bleeding and infectious complications; however, Wiskott noted the sisters in the family were completely unaffected. He initially described the condition as "familial congenital ITP." In 1939, Dr. Wiskott served as Chair of the Department of Pediatrics at Ludwig Maximilian University.
- Q: Who was Aldrich?
- A: Robert A. Aldrich, MD (1917 to 1998) received his MD at Northwestern University and completed his pediatrics residency at the University of Minnesota and the Mayo Clinic. In 1954, while working at the University of Oregon, he described a "pedigree demonstrating a sex-linked recessive condition characterized by draining ears, eczematoid dermatitis, and bloody diarrhea." In 1956, he served as Chair of the Department of Pediatrics at the University of Washington. In 1962, he served as the first director of the National Institute of Child Health & Human Development.

YERSINIA ENTEROCOLITICA

Camille Sabella, MD

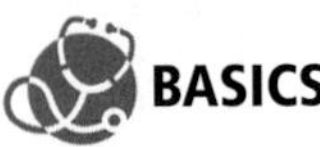

BASICS

DESCRIPTION

Yersinia enterocolitica is a gram-negative bacillus that produces an enteric infection characterized by fever, diarrhea, and abdominal pain that may mimic acute appendicitis.

EPIDEMIOLOGY

- According to surveillance by the Foodborne Diseases Active Surveillance Network (FoodNet) from 2015, the annual incidence of *Y. enterocolitica* infections was 0.28 per 100,000 persons.
- 16% of infections occurred in children <5 years, and almost 30% occurred in children <19 years.
- Transmission of *Y. enterocolitica*
  - Occurs through ingestion of contaminated food or water (particularly raw or undercooked pork or unpasteurized milk products) or contact with infected animals (swine are the principal reservoir)
  - Fecal–oral and person-to-person transmission are also possible.
  - In the United States, most epidemics have been related to the improper handling of raw pork intestine (chitterlings), most often during winter holiday festivities among African American households in the South.
  - Transmission to young children occurs through contact with adult caregivers preparing the chitterlings.
- Transmission through transfusion of contaminated blood products is also possible. The U.S. Food and Drug Administration (FDA) has reported that contamination of the U.S. blood supply by bacteria, although rare, is most frequently due to *Y. enterocolitica*.
- The incubation period is ~1 to 14 days (average 4 to 6). The mean duration of organism excretion is 42 days; however, asymptomatic carriage can persist even longer.
- Systemic disease or bacteremia occurs more commonly in young infants or those with predisposing conditions, including:
  - A clinical state of iron overload or deferoxamine therapy
  - Immunosuppression
  - Diabetes mellitus
  - Malnutrition
  - Cirrhosis or other liver diseases

GENERAL PREVENTION

- Infection control
  - Contact precautions are indicated for patients with enterocolitis until diarrhea resolves.
- General measures
  - Attempts to eliminate reservoirs and reduce frequency of ingesting contaminated foods and beverages are necessary.
  - Ingestion of undercooked meats, especially pork and unpasteurized milk, should be avoided.
  - Meticulous hand hygiene before and after handling uncooked meat products and avoidance of preparation of meats near or during preparation of infant bottles for feeding are essential.

PATHOPHYSIOLOGY

- The portal of entry for *Y. enterocolitica* is the gastrointestinal tract.
- *Y. enterocolitica* adheres to epithelial cells and mucus, producing heat-stable enterotoxins, which play a role in the development of watery diarrhea.
  - Another cytotoxin then directly injures the distal small and large bowel, producing stools characterized by blood and mucus.
  - Release of these toxins leads to the development of an enterocolitis, most commonly in younger age groups.
- Mesenteric adenitis and/or terminal ileitis may lead to a pseudoappendicitis syndrome, typically in the older child or young adult.
- Bacteremia may lead to focal abscesses in a variety of organs, including the lung, liver, spleen, and kidney.

ETIOLOGY

- The genus *Yersinia* consists of 11 species, of which *Y. enterocolitica*, *Yersinia pseudotuberculosis*, and *Yersinia pestis* are the three most commonly encountered pathogens.
- *Y. enterocolitica* is a facultative, non–lactose-fermenting, urease-positive, gram-negative bacillus.
- >60 serotypes and six biotypes of *Y. enterocolitica* have been identified. Serotypes O:3, O:5.27, O:8, and O:9 and biotypes 2, 3, and 4 are most commonly isolated from patients. Serotype O:3 is the most common type in the United States.

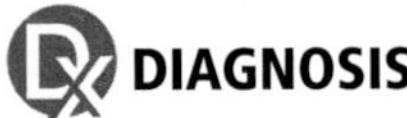

DIAGNOSIS

Diagnosis depends on elucidation of the pertinent exposure history as well as recognition of typical symptoms and laboratory testing.

HISTORY

- Enterocolitis is the most common manifestation of *Y. enterocolitica* infection in young children and is characterized by fever, abdominal pain, and diarrhea with blood or mucus.
  - 25% of patients have hematochezia.
  - Typical duration of illness is 1 to 3 weeks but may be longer (up to several months).
  - The history taking should include questions regarding exposure to unpasteurized milk products and raw pork or poultry, especially the preparation of pork chitterlings.
- Pseudoappendicitis syndrome
  - Due to mesenteric adenitis and/or terminal ileitis predominates in older children and adults
  - It is associated with fever, right lower quadrant abdominal pain, and leukocytosis.
- *Yersinia* bacteremia is found most commonly in infants <1 year of age or those with predisposing conditions, particularly states of iron overload (e.g., sickle cell disease, thalassemia).
- Extraintestinal manifestations of *Y. enterocolitica* infection are uncommon and include pharyngitis, suppurative lymphadenitis, pyomyositis, osteomyelitis, abscess, UTI, pneumonia, endocarditis, meningitis, peritonitis, panophthalmitis, conjunctivitis, and septic arthritis.

PHYSICAL EXAM

Because of the wide range of clinical symptoms, including extraintestinal manifestations, the physical exam is nonspecific for this infection.

DIFFERENTIAL DIAGNOSIS

- *Y. enterocolitica* should be considered in all patients with fever, abdominal pain, and stools with blood or mucus as well as in patients with the extraintestinal manifestations described earlier.
- Pitfalls
  - Not all bacterial colitis presents with bloody or mucus-appearing diarrhea. Therefore, suspicion should exist if the diarrhea is prolonged or environmental exposures pose a risk for developing infection.
  - The possibility of *Y. enterocolitica* bacteremia should be considered in blood transfusion–related illnesses, thalassemia, or prior history of liver disease.

DIAGNOSTIC TESTS & INTERPRETATION

- *Y. enterocolitica* can be isolated from blood, sputum, CSF, urine, and bile; these specimens do not require selective culture media techniques.
  - Stool samples should be plated on selective media such as cefsulodin-triclosan-novobiocin agar.
  - If routine enteric media (MacConkey) are used, a cold enrichment technique will increase recovery of the organism.
  - The laboratory should be notified that *Yersinia* is suspected if not routinely sought.
- Serologic methods (tube agglutination assay, enzyme-linked immunosorbent assay [ELISA]) are available with a rise in titers noted 1 week after onset of symptoms and peak titers observed by the 2nd week of illness. These tests identify IgM, IgG, and IgA antibodies against *Y. enterocolitica*.
- Cross-reactivity between *Y. enterocolitica* and *Brucella abortus*, *Rickettsia* species, *Morganella morganii*, *Salmonella* species, and thyroid tissue antigen makes serodiagnosis of limited usefulness.
- Imaging
  - Abdominal ultrasound can be used to distinguish pseudoappendicitis from acute appendicitis through demonstration of bowel wall edema in the terminal ileum and cecum.

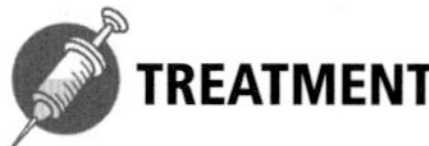

TREATMENT

GENERAL MEASURES

The benefit of treatment of uncomplicated enterocolitis, mesenteric adenitis, or pseudoappendicitis has not been established in immunocompetent hosts.

MEDICATION

- Antimicrobial therapy is indicated for neonates, immunocompromised patients, and those with systemic and focal extraintestinal infections. For most isolates, trimethoprim/sulfamethoxazole, chloramphenicol, aminoglycosides, tetracycline or doxycycline, fluoroquinolones, and 3rd-generation cephalosporins are effective treatment options.
- *Y. enterocolitica* is usually resistant to most penicillins and 1st-generation cephalosporins.

ONGOING CARE

FOLLOW-UP RECOMMENDATIONS

- Symptoms of enterocolitis usually abate within 2 weeks of the onset of illness.
- Shedding of the organism in stool can last >6 weeks after diagnosis.
- For extraintestinal manifestations, the expected course depends on the specific organ system involved.

PROGNOSIS

- The prognosis is usually quite good, as most infections are gastrointestinal.
- Systemic disease (i.e., septicemia with subsequent secondary spread) has higher morbidity and mortality. Mortality related to septicemia can be as high as 50%.

COMPLICATIONS

- Postinfectious sequelae may occur 1 to 2 weeks after gastrointestinal symptoms and include erythema nodosum as well as reactive arthritis involving weight-bearing joints. These complications are seen most often in adults, particularly those with HLA-B27 antigen.
- Reactive arthritis syndrome, myocarditis, glomerulonephritis, erysipelas, chronic diarrhea persisting for months, and hemolytic anemia have also been reported.
- Intestinal perforation and ileocolic intussusception are possible.

ADDITIONAL READING

- Abdel-Haq NM, Asmar BI, Abuhammour WM, et al. *Yersinia enterocolitica* infection in children. *Pediatr Infect Dis J*. 2000;19(10):954–958.
- American Academy of Pediatrics. *Yersinia enterocolitica* and *Yersinia pseudotuberculosis* infections. In: Kimberlin DW, Brady MT, Jackson MA, et al, eds. *Red Book: 2015 Report of the Committee on Infectious Diseases*. 30th ed. Elk Grove Village, IL: American Academy of Pediatrics; 2015:868–870.
- Committee on Infectious Diseases, Committee on Nutrition, American Academy of Pediatrics. Consumption of raw or unpasteurized milk and milk products by pregnant women and children. *Pediatrics*. 2014;133(1):175–179.
- Guinet F, Carniel E, Leclercq A, et al. Transfusion-transmitted *Yersinia enterocolitica* sepsis. *Clin Infect Dis*. 2011;53(6):583–591.
- Ong KL, Gould LH, Chen DL, et al. Changing epidemiology of *Yersinia enterocolitica* infections: markedly decreased rates in young black children, Foodborne Diseases Active Surveillance Network (FoodNet), 1996–2009. *Clin Infect Dis*. 2012;54(Suppl 5):S385–S390.
- Scallan E, Hoekstra RM, Angulo FJ, et al. Foodborne illness acquired in the United States—major pathogens. *Emerg Infect Dis*. 2011;17(1):7–15. doi:10.3201/eid1701.091101p1.

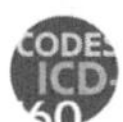

CODES

ICD10

- A04.6 Enteritis due to Yersinia enterocolitica
- A05.8 Other specified bacterial foodborne intoxications

FAQ

- Q: How long is a child considered infectious with *Y. enterocolitica*?
- A: Although the typical course of enterocolitis is ~14 days, shedding of the organism in the stool can last 6 weeks or longer. Strict adherence to hand hygiene should be discussed with the child's parent or caregiver, particularly for those with incontinent or diapered children, to ensure infection control.
- Q: If there is no history of stools with blood or mucus, can you exclude *Y. enterocolitica* as the likely infectious agent in a child with diarrhea?
- A: No. In fact, early in the course of illness, the diarrhea is more likely to be watery owing to the enterotoxins produced (see "Pathophysiology").

ZIKA VIRUS INFECTIONS IN CHILDREN

Anna Sick-Samuels, MD, MPH • Jeanne S. Sheffield, MD • W. Christopher Golden, MD

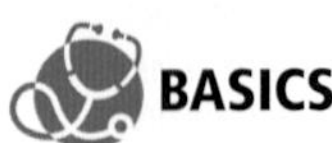

BASICS

DESCRIPTION

- Zika virus is a single-stranded RNA flavivirus discovered in 1947 in the Zika forest in Uganda.
- It is transmitted via mosquitoes (including *Aedes aegypti* and *Aedes albopictus*), sexual intercourse with an infected person (symptomatic or asymptomatic), vertical exposure (mother-to-child transmission), and blood transfusions.
- The incubation period is 3 to 10 days.
- In adults and in most children outside the neonatal period, Zika virus infection causes an acute, self-limited viral syndrome (acute Zika infection).

ALERT

Zika virus is a relatively new medical concern in the United States. Recommendations are constantly evolving. Health care providers can monitor resources via the Centers for Disease Control and Prevention (CDC) website (www.cdc.gov) for up to date information. Zika virus infection is a reportable condition.

EPIDEMIOLOGY

- An epidemic of Zika virus infections and an associated congenital Zika syndrome (CZS), with central nervous system, musculoskeletal, and eye anomalies was noted in the Americas beginning in Brazil in 2015, with >50 countries affected by early 2017.
- As of December 6, 2017, the CDC reported:
  - A total of 226 locally acquired Zika virus cases (in Florida and Texas), 5,324 travel-associated cases in the United States, and 37,087 cases in U.S. territories
  - A total of 2,311 pregnant women in the United States and 4,621 pregnant women within U.S. territories with laboratory evidence of Zika virus infection
  - A total of 98 liveborn infants with birth defects and nine pregnancy losses with birth defects within the United States
- The incidence of birth defects of pregnant women in the U.S. Zika Pregnancy Registry (January to September, 2016) was 58.8 per 1,000 live births, compared to 2.86 per 1,000 live births in a "pre-Zika" cohort (2013 to 2014).

RISK FACTORS

- Travel to a Zika-endemic region
- Sexual intercourse with a person who has travelled to a Zika-endemic region
- In utero exposure via a mother infected with the Zika virus

GENERAL PREVENTION

- Prevention of primary acquisition via mosquito bites (i.e., use of insect repellent containing N,N-diethyl-meta-toluamide [DEET] in adults and in children >2 months of age, air conditioning in warm weather climates, mosquito nets in endemic areas)
- Barrier contraceptive methods or abstinence to prevent sexual transmission to pregnant women or women wishing to conceive
- Avoidance of travel to Zika-endemic regions by pregnant women, women wishing to conceive, and their male sexual partners
- No current vaccine for Zika is available.

PATHOPHYSIOLOGY

- Mosquitoes ingest the virus after feeding on a human or animal host and transmit the virus to humans.
- In humans, Zika virus has been shown to disrupt the placental barrier and target neural progenitor cells and immature neurons, leading to abnormal fetal brain development.
- Fetal demise and congenital anomalies occur as a result of intrauterine Zika virus infection.

COMMONLY ASSOCIATED CONDITIONS

Zika virus infection has been associated with Guillain-Barré syndrome during epidemics in French Polynesia and Brazil.

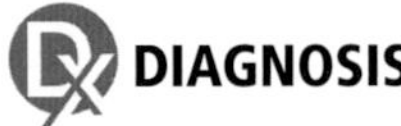

DIAGNOSIS

HISTORY

- Travel history, including travel to or residence within a Zika-endemic region
- Sexual relations with a person who has traveled to or resides within a Zika-endemic region
- Abnormal fetal sonography or MRI findings (microcephaly with skull abnormalities, ventriculomegaly, intracranial calcifications [usually subcortical], intrauterine growth restriction [IUGR])

PHYSICAL EXAM

- Acute Zika infection:
  - About 20% of patients are symptomatic.
  - The most common findings include fever (65%), macular or papular rash (90%), arthralgia (65%), conjunctivitis (55%), myalgia (48%), and headache (45%).
- CZS:
  - IUGR
  - Fetal brain disruption sequence (FBDS) characterized by microcephaly, skull collapse with overriding sutures, prominent occipital bone, and redundant scalp skin
  - Neurologic/neuromuscular abnormalities: hypo- or hypertonia, spasticity, hyperreflexia, irritability, seizures, hearing loss, dysphagia, diaphragmatic paralysis, club feet, and congenital joint contractures
  - Ocular anomalies: microphthalmia, coloboma, cataracts, intraocular calcifications, chorioretinal atrophy, focal pigmentary retinal mottling, optic nerve atrophy
  - Endocrine abnormalities due to hypothalamic-pituitary axis disturbance in the setting of abnormal brain development
  - Delayed onset of microcephaly, postnatal hydrocephalus, and developmental delays

DIFFERENTIAL DIAGNOSIS

- Acute Zika infection:
  - Infection with other arboviruses such as chikungunya and dengue viruses
  - Other infections such as adenovirus, influenza virus, coxsackievirus, Epstein-Barr virus, parvovirus, leptospirosis, Lyme disease
  - Autoimmune diseases such as systemic lupus erythematosus, systemic juvenile idiopathic arthritis, and dermatomyositis
- CZS:
  - Congenital infections such as toxoplasmosis, congenital rubella syndrome, congenital cytomegalovirus (CMV) infection, and intrauterine herpes simplex virus (HSV) infection
  - Note: CZS is *not* known to cause hepatic or renal abnormalities seen in other congenital infections.
  - Neuronal migration defects (i.e., lissencephaly, polymicrogyria)
  - Genetic, chromosomal, or metabolic disorders (i.e., trisomy 18, peroxisomal disorders)
  - Intrauterine insults (i.e., maternal drug exposure, intracranial hemorrhage)

DIAGNOSTIC TESTS & INTERPRETATION

Initial Tests (screening, lab, imaging)

- Acute Zika infection: Serum and urine nucleic acid testing (NAT) for Zika virus and serum testing for Zika IgM must be approved by the local health department.
  - Positive PCR results confirm active viral infection.
  - Positive IgM serology supports recent or previous exposure to Zika virus. There is high cross reactivity of the serologic tests with Zika and other flaviviruses, particularly dengue virus.
  - Positive IgM serology should be confirmed with a plaque reduction neutralization test (PRNT), which measures virus-specific neutralizing antibodies.
- CZS: The following evaluation should be performed within the first few days of age (2 days of age, optimally) for neonates with clinical findings consistent with CZS and a maternal history of possible Zika virus exposure during pregnancy OR for asymptomatic neonates with maternal laboratory evidence of possible Zika virus infection during pregnancy.
  - Comprehensive physical exam (including weight, length and occipitofrontal circumference [OFC], age-appropriate vision, hearing [auditory brainstem response preferred], and developmental surveillance and screening)
  - Serum and urine Zika NAT and serum Zika IgM testing
  - Cerebrospinal fluid (CSF) NAT and IgM testing, if CSF is obtained for evaluation of another condition (such as meningitis) OR if the infant has abnormalities consistent with CZS, urine and serum Zika testing is negative, and other etiologies for the clinical presentation are ruled out.
  - Placental pathology
  - Cord blood testing *is not* recommended because of false-positive and false-negative rate.
- Interpretation of test results for CZS in neonates/infants:
  - A positive NAT result with any IgM result represents *confirmed* congenital Zika virus infection.
  - A negative NAT result with nonnegative IgM result in a neonate is interpreted as *probable* congenital Zika virus infection.
  - Negative NAT and negative IgM results suggest congenital Zika virus infection is *unlikely*.
  - False-positive and false-negative results are possible, and results must be interpreted within the context of maternal history and the patient's evaluation.
- Other laboratory tests, including a complete blood count, metabolic panel, and transaminases/liver function tests should be sent in children with high suspicion of CZS and may aid in diagnosis of or exclusion of other conditions.

- For infants with concern for CZS, coordination of care between health care facilities, local and regional health departments, and the CDC is important to ensure appropriate procurement and processing of samples and neonatal/infant follow-up.
- By 1 month of age, a head ultrasound should be performed on an infant with abnormalities consistent with CZS born to a mother with possible Zika virus infection during pregnancy OR a newborn without CZS findings born to a mother with laboratory confirmed Zika virus infection during pregnancy.
- If abnormalities are present or the infant has a fontanelle limiting visualization of the intracranial anatomy, a head MRI or CT should be considered.
- Abnormalities may include intracranial calcifications (usually subcortical); ventriculomegaly; abnormal gyral patterns (polymicrogyria, hypogyria, pachygyria); hemimegalencephaly; grey matter heterotopias; decreased brain volume; cortical atrophy or malformation; cerebellar, vermian, or brainstem hypoplasia; or delayed myelination.
- Ventral spinal cord hypoplasia also may be seen on spinal imaging.

Follow-Up Tests & Special Considerations

- Babies with abnormalities consistent with CZS born to a mother with laboratory evidence of Zika virus infection during pregnancy OR asymptomatic infants born to a mother with laboratory confirmed Zika virus infection during pregnancy should undergo the following additional evaluations by 1 month of age:
  - Comprehensive ophthalmologic exam
  - Automated auditory brainstem response hearing evaluation
- Clinically asymptomatic infants with negative laboratory testing should receive standard pediatric care.
- Clinically asymptomatic infants born to mothers with possible Zika virus exposure in pregnancy but without maternal testing or with negative maternal laboratory results should receive standard pediatric care, with no additional Zika-specific testing or evaluation.
  - However, health care providers should remain alert to the possibility of CZS and development of its sequelae. Should a child demonstrate abnormalities consistent with CZS, he or she should undergo a complete evaluation.

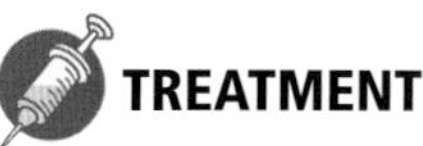

TREATMENT

GENERAL MEASURES

- Acute Zika infection
  - Supportive care fluids, rest, symptomatic treatment (acetaminophen for fever, antihistamines for pruritus)
  - Avoid salicylates (Reye syndrome risk).
  - Use nonsteroidal anti-inflammatory drugs (NSAIDs) with caution in the setting of dehydration (nephrotoxicity in infants) or possible dengue infection (worsening hemorrhagic complications).
  - Although more commonly seen in adults, children with acute Zika infection should be monitored for signs and symptoms of Guillain-Barré syndrome.
- CZS
  - Treatment of underlying complications (i.e., antiepileptic drugs for seizures)
  - Consultation with subspecialists in neurology, developmental pediatrics, infectious diseases, ophthalmology, and genetics to confirm the diagnosis and rule out other etiologies
  - Consultation with orthopedics, physical/occupational therapy to assist with joint contractures, hypertonia, club foot abnormalities
  - Consultation with gastroenterology/pediatric surgery and speech language pathology for feeding support/swallowing difficulties
  - Consultation with social work and/or psychology to provide psychosocial support to the family

ISSUES FOR REFERRAL

- For acute Zika infection, no follow-up needed, unless issues with vision or neurologic function occur
- For CZS, routine newborn care with neurologic exams, consultant follow-up as necessary, referral to developmental specialists, and early intervention service programs for infants and toddlers

ALERT

Infants with laboratory evidence of Zika infection but without evidence of CZS may develop evidence of CZS in later infancy. These babies should undergo head imaging, auditory brainstem response hearing testing, ophthalmologic evaluation, and full evaluation for any detected abnormalities.

SURGERY/OTHER PROCEDURES

- Orthopedic interventions may be needed for joint contractures.
- Pediatric gastroenterology or pediatric surgery may be needed for assistive feeding device placement.

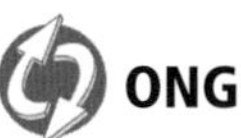

ONGOING CARE

PROGNOSIS

Acute Zika infection: Expect full recovery without sequelae within days up to 1 week. Severe disease requiring hospitalization is uncommon.

COMPLICATIONS

- A proportion of women with acute Zika virus during pregnancy may have infants born with gross brain abnormalities or microcephaly at birth.
- Clinicians and families may wish to pursue palliative care in severely affected children.
- Some infants may have no obvious manifestations at birth but are at risk to develop complications of developmental delay or vision abnormalities that are detected later.
- Delayed hearing abnormalities have not been noted in CZS (different than congenital CMV infection).
- All infants with confirmed or suspected CZS require close follow-up through their 1st year.
- Other long-term complications may include decreases in weight, length and OFC as they grow, irritability, seizures, pyramidal and extrapyramidal abnormalities, contractures, and endocrine dysfunction from hypothalamic or pituitary insufficiency.

ADDITIONAL READING

- Adebanjo T, Godfred-Cato S, Viens L, et al. Update: Interim guidance for the diagnosis, evaluation, and management of infants with possible congenital Zika virus infection—United States, October 2017. *MMWR Morb Mortal Wkly Rep.* 2017;66(41):1089–1099.
- Cragan JD, Mai CT, Petersen EE, et al. Baseline prevalence of birth defects associated with congenital Zika virus infection—Massachusetts, North Carolina, and Atlanta, Georgia, 2013–2014. *MMWR Morb Mortal Wkly Rep.* 2017;66(8):219–222.
- Goodman AB, Dziuban EJ, Powell K, et al. Characteristics of children aged <18 years with Zika virus disease acquired postnatally—U.S. states, January 2015–July 2016. *MMWR Morb Mortal Wkly Rep.* 2016;65(39):1082–1085.
- Honein MA, Dawson AL, Petersen EE, et al; and U.S. Zika Pregnancy Registry Collaboration. Birth defects among fetuses and infants of US women with evidence of possible Zika virus infection during pregnancy. *JAMA.* 2017;317(1):59–68.
- Karwowski MP, Nelson JM, Staples JE, et al. Zika virus disease: a CDC update for pediatric health care providers. *Pediatrics.* 2016;137(5):e20160621.
- Moore CA, Staples JE, Dobyns WB, et al. Characterizing the pattern of anomalies in congenital Zika syndrome for pediatric clinicians. *JAMA Pediatr.* 2017;171(3):288–295.
- Noronha Ld, Zanluca C, Azevedo ML, et al. Zika virus damages the human placental barrier and presents marked fetal neurotropism. *Mem Inst Oswaldo Cruz.* 2016;111(5):287–293.
- Petersen LR, Jamieson DJ, Powers AM, et al. Zika virus. *N Engl J Med.* 2016;374(16):1552–1563.
- Poretti A, Huisman TAGM. Neuroimaging findings in congenital Zika syndrome. *AJNR Am J Neuroradiol.* 2016;37(10):1764–1765.
- Russell K, Oliver SE, Lewis L, et al. Update: interim guidance for the evaluation and management of infants with possible congenital Zika virus infection—United States, August 2016. *MMWR Morb Mortal Wkly Rep.* 2016;65(33):870–878.

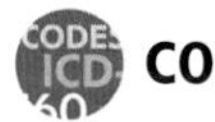

CODES

ICD10

A92.5 Zika virus disease

FAQ

- Q: Can infants of women with suspected or confirmed Zika virus breastfeed?
- A: Yes. At this time, although there has been evidence of viral RNA in breast milk, there have been no documented cases of infants acquired Zika virus via breastfeeding. Suspected benefits outweigh risks.
- Q: When should CZS be considered as an explanation of neonatal abnormalities?
- A: When mother has had confirmed or suspected Zika infection or signs/symptoms of Zika virus infection during pregnancy AND risk factors for Zika virus exposure (travel to or resides in area with active Zika virus transmission or unprotected sex with a partner who travels or resides to such an area) OR if an infant has findings consistent with CZS and a epidemiologic history suggesting possible transmission regardless of maternal testing
- Q: Should pregnant women with risk factors and symptoms of Zika virus be tested?
- A: Yes. The CDC has guideline for health care providers caring for pregnant women (http://www.cdc.gov/zika/hc-providers/pregnant-woman.html).
- Q: How long should couples wait to conceive if the male partner has a possible exposure to Zika virus?
- A: 6 months, but optimal duration is not yet known

Appendix I

The 5-Minute Educator

Part 1: Precepting
Part 2: Direct Observation
Part 3: Feedback
Part 4: Clinical Reasoning

PART 1: PRECEPTING

Cara Lichtenstein, MD, MPH

DESCRIPTION

Precepting is the education and teaching of learners in a clinical care setting.

TECHNIQUES USED BEFORE THE VISIT

Orient the learner at the start of the rotation:

- Gather information on background, strengths, and weaknesses of the learner.
- Communicate goals and set expectations for the rotation.
- Discuss your style of feedback and how frequently it will be given.
- Introduce trainee to office staff they will work with.
- Familiarize trainee with recordkeeping including electronic health record (EHR), what they will be permitted to enter in the EHR, and whether use of templates is encouraged, allowed, or restricted.

Maximize the Schedule

- Use wave scheduling to build in preceptor teaching time without reducing overall number of patients.
- Book several urgent care visits for yourself while your learner sees a complex visit.
- Double book your first appointment so you can block your last appointment for teaching.
- Review schedule at the start of the day to determine which patients are appropriate for learners so they can preview charts.

Prime learners before they enter room:

- Prompt learner to retrieve stored information and prepare for immediate use.
- Orient the learner to the patient or possible medical problem.
  - For example: cc ear tugging: What will help you determine what the origin of the ear tugging is?
  - For example: cc speech delay: What is the typical speech of a 2-year-old like?
  - For example: cc 2-week well-child visit: What do you think the purpose(s) of this visit is?
- Give the learner a task and goal.
  - For example: cc "1st-time wheeze": The task may be to gather a focused history, and the goal may be to formulate a broad differential diagnosis of causes of wheezing.
- Make a plan for when to meet to discuss the case.

TECHNIQUES USED DURING THE VISIT

Reflective Modeling

- Allows learners to observe the preceptor interacting with and examining the patient
- Preceptor talks aloud during the visit explaining to patient AND to learner what's going on, what they think the diagnosis or next steps are, and why they don't think something else is going on.

Activated Demonstration

- Goal is for trainee to learn by observing preceptor's interaction with a patient.
- Briefly prime them in advance for what to look for.
- Set up the observation.
  - Determine student's relevant knowledge.
  - Identify what student should learn from observation.
    - Watch technique the preceptor uses for examining the ear, exposing the oropharynx, etc.
    - Watch how the preceptor enlists the help of the parent.
    - Watch how the preceptor navigates excusing parent from the room so preceptor can talk with the teen (patient) privately.
  - Provide clear guidelines for what student should do while observing.
    - For example: Quietly observe; jot notes with what you are observing.

Student Clinical Observation of Preceptor (SCOOP)

- Allows learner to observe preceptor's interaction with patient and family
- Learner uses a tool or writes three things they observed.
- Items discussed together afterwards

Structured Clinical Observation (SCO)

- Allows assessment of learners skill level through direct observation
- Preceptor spends short period of time (5 minutes) observing part of visit (can be history, physical, or information giving).
- Uses a tool to give immediate feedback to learner on directly observed performance

Presenting in the Room

- After confirming there are no sensitive issues, learner presents in front of family.
- Saves time, as preceptor can examine patient while learner is presenting
- Family can correct any misinformation or clarify questions on the spot.
- Patients perceive increased time spent with doctor, better care, and better explanation of problems.

TECHNIQUES USED AFTER THE VISIT

One-Minute Preceptor

- A structure allowing preceptors to assess learners effectively, teach key points of a case, and provide feedback efficiently, using five "microskills"
  - **Get a commitment** about diagnosis or treatment.
  - **Probe for supporting evidence** for that diagnosis or treatment.
  - **Teach general rules** about the case or diagnosis.
  - **Reinforce what was correct** (+ feedback).
  - **Correct mistakes** with suggestions for future improvements.

SNAPPS

- Presentation method focusing on clinical reasoning and self-directed learning that is learner driven
- Preceptor sets expectation that learner will present using SNAPPS:
  - **Summarize** the history and findings.
  - **Narrow** the differential.
  - **Analyze** the differential diagnosis by comparing/contrasting possibilities.
  - **Probe** (student probes preceptor) for further understanding about areas of uncertainty.
  - **Plan** for patient management.
  - **Self**-directed learning: **Select** an issue to learn more about.

GENERAL TEACHING TIPS

- Wait 3 seconds after asking a question.
- Focus only on 1 to 2 teaching points per encounter.
- If you don't know, say you don't know.
- Examples speak louder than words.

PITFALLS TO AVOID

- "Taking over" the case by providing answers instead of questions
- Inappropriately long, esoteric, or noninteractive lectures
- Not waiting long enough to get an answer
- Preprogrammed answers
- Not appreciating the level of the learners and teaching beyond their ability

ADDITIONAL READING

- Allevi AM, Lane JL. Microskills in office teaching. *Pediatr Ann*. 2010;39(2):72–77.
- Biagioli FE, Chappelle K. How to be an efficient and effective preceptor. *Fam Pract Manag*. 2010;17(3):18–21.
- Ferenchick G, Simpson D, Blackman J, et al. Strategies for efficient and effective teaching in the ambulatory care setting. *Acad Med*. 1997;72(4):277–280.
- Hammoud MM, Dalymple JL, Christner JG, et al. Medical student documentation in electronic health records: a collaborative statement from the Alliance for Clinical Education. *Teach Learn Med*. 2012;24(3):257–266.
- Neher JO, Stevens NG. The one-minute preceptor: shaping the teaching conversation. *Fam Med*. 2003;35(6):391–393.

FAQS

- Q: What preceptor qualities do students most appreciate?
- A: Learners value preceptors who are enthusiastic, organized, willing to answer questions and explore clinical reasoning, and who provide timely feedback.
- Q: Are there other ways to teach in the office setting besides direct patient care?
- A: Yes, learners can be asked to work with ancillary staff, look up answers to patient questions, and review lab or imaging results. Also remember that there may be other providers in your office who can help precept.
- Q: What are pros/cons of the EHR in precepting?
- A: Some pros: increased learning via clinical decision support systems, efficiency in accessing patient history, tracking of clinical activity, and facilitating "just in time" learning. Some cons: the need to learn a new system at each site, learning how to communicate with patient while using EHR, and restrictions on student documentation in EHR for billing purposes by Centers for Medicare & Medicaid Services (CMS)

PART 2: DIRECT OBSERVATION

Sandra Cuzzi, MD

BASICS

- **Definition:** the process of observing a learner (e.g., student, resident) during an actual patient encounter for the purpose of assessing clinical skills
- **Aim:** to help preceptors gather accurate information about a learner's performance in real-life clinical scenarios
- **Assessment:** communication skills, history taking, physical exam techniques, information giving, procedural skills, professionalism, entrustable professional activities (EPAs), and evaluation of competence

GETTING STARTED

Primary Purpose

Defining the primary purpose of direct observation is important in choosing the tool, setting, scope, and skills to be observed.

- **Formative:** timely feedback given to initiate discussion and promote reflection, with the goal of improving clinical skills and modifying behavior
- **Summative:** scheduled summary evaluation to "grade" or rank, with the goal of assessing global performance
- **Assessment of EPAs:** Observation of a clinical interaction can help the preceptor decide whether a learner can be entrusted to perform a particular professional activity including how much supervision is needed.
- **Documentation of competency:** Direct observation is required by the accrediting bodies for both medical student and resident education.

Using an Observation Tool

- Advantages of using a tool are that it:
  - Clarifies expectations for all involved
  - Standardizes what preceptors watch for
  - Guides feedback to make it more specific
  - Fulfills documentation requirements
- Formative assessment: Primary focus of tool is to facilitate feedback so proven reliability and validity is not as important.
- Summative assessment: critical for the tool to be well-studied, valid, and reliable
- Use an existing tool for direct observation that fits the primary purpose.
- Mini-clinical evaluation exercise (mini-CEX)
  - Best studied tool with excellent validity used for formative or summative assessment
  - Requires observation over 10 to 20 minutes, which can make it difficult to incorporate into a busy clinical setting
- Structured clinical observation (SCO)
  - Most commonly used tool in pediatrics for formative assessment
  - Divided into three to four specific sections, one for each part of the clinical encounter, with a behavioral checklist to guide feedback
  - Used for 3- to 5-minute observations; complete only the section observed.

Determine Setting, Scope, and Skills

- Look for opportunities where an observer is already present during a clinical encounter.
- For example, a physician working in the newborn nursery may be present to observe learner's newborn physical exam skills or a social worker present at family meetings where learners are leading the discussion can engage in direct observation.
- Opportunities can lend themselves to shorter observation (e.g., inpatient or outpatient visit) or longer ones (e.g., counseling session).
- Shorter observations tend to work best as formative feedback; longer ones can be used for summative evaluations.

IMPLEMENTATION

Potential Barriers to Direct Observation

- Lack of time
- Inadequate training, discomfort, or difficulty in observation and/or feedback
- Hawthorne effect: Presence of observer changes behavior of those observed.
- Family perception regarding observation
- Logistical barriers (scheduling, patient flow, space configuration)

Orienting the Preceptor and Learner

- Clearly state expectations once setting, scope, and skills are defined.
- Understand preceptor and learner attitudes, experience, and knowledge regarding direct observation.
- If setting up a direct observation program institution-wide, then determine what content areas need to be covered and provide preceptor faculty development.
- Orient all to the process and logistics.

Number of Observations

- When paired with feedback, every observation has value to the learner as formative assessment.
- 4 to 5 observations will probably identify an "outlier" in terms of minimal competency.
- Ideally, 10 to 12 observations are needed over time to reliably assess competency for summative assessment.

Practical Tips

- Multiple short observations allow for less time commitment, observation in a variety of clinical scenarios, and can monitor improvement over time.
- A preceptor may want to routinely set up direct observation with the first patient in a clinical session (e.g., first afternoon patient).
- Set up the specific observation beforehand with the learner and family.
- Brief 3- to 5-minute observations
- Take notes while observing: Set up two columns, one for "things done well," the other for "things to improve," or consider filling out the tool's checklist as you observe.
- Be a "fly on the wall": Sit away from line of sight of the patient, avoid the temptation to interrupt.
- At times, the preceptor can get involved at a certain predetermined stage of the process (e.g., after physical exam, preceptor confirms findings and advises on technique).
- Provide timely focused feedback right after observing.

Creating a Culture of Observation

- Goal: Create a culture in which observation is understood, expected, nonthreatening, and routine for everyone including patients, parents, learners, and preceptors.
- Orient the participants and set expectations.
- Make it a joint responsibility between learner and preceptor to arrange.
- Observe at regular intervals so it becomes routine.
- Consistently give feedback after observing.
- Identify "champions" of direct observation as role models and mentors.
- Encourage opportunities for preceptors to be observed by learners too.

ADDITIONAL READING

- Hanson JL, Bannister SL. To trust or not to trust? An introduction to entrustable professional activities. *Pediatrics*. 2016;138(5):e20162373.
- Hanson JL, Bannister SL, Clark A, et al. Oh, what you can see: the role of observation in medical student education. *Pediatrics*. 2010;126(5):843–845.
- Hamburger EK, Cuzzi S, Coddington DA, et al. Observation of resident clinical skills: outcomes of a program of direct observation in the continuity clinic setting. *Acad Pediatr*. 2011;11(5):394–402.
- Hauer KE, Holmboe ES, Kogan JR. Twelve tips for implementing tools for direct observation of medical trainees' clinical skills during patient encounters. *Med Teach*. 2011;33(1):27–33.
- Holmboe ES. Faculty and the observation of trainees' clinical skills: problems and opportunities. *Acad Med*. 2004;79(1):16–22.
- Lane JL, Gottlieb RP. Structured clinical observations a method to teach clinical skills with limited time and financial resources. *Pediatrics*. 2000;105(4, Pt 2):973–977.

PART 3: FEEDBACK

Terry Kind, MD, MPH • Dewesh Agrawal, MD

BASICS

Description

Feedback

- Formative, nonevaluative, objective appraisal of performance aimed at modifying and improving clinical skills, correcting deficits, and improving future performance
- Targeted to specific (observed) behaviors the trainee already does well and those in need of improvement
- Immediate and *formative*, not summative
- Formative feedback sometimes called "low stakes"
- Presents information, not judgment
- Can be positive (reinforcing) or negative (constructive or corrective) or both
- Feedback involves a specific event or occurrence versus compliment/criticism, which are more vague and general.
- Like evaluation, should ideally be based on objective observations

Evaluation

- Summative judgment
- Equivalent to grading and/or assigning a final grade for the rotation
- Intent is to tell learners how they performed.
- Like feedback, should ideally be based on objective observations

Compliment and Criticism

- COMPLIMENT: a polite expression of praise or admiration
- CRITICISM: an expression of disapproval based on perceived faults or mistakes
- These are typically general, judgmental, and are not goal based or not based on specific observations.

BARRIERS

- Potential barriers to providing effective feedback:
  - Insufficient time; competing demands
  - Insufficient observation; gathering essential information is difficult.
  - Don't have the necessary skills; didn't have good role models
  - Difficult to give negative feedback; want to be "popular"
  - Fears of student reprisals or failure to recruit into specialty
  - Not my responsibility; unimportant
  - Don't know where to start
  - Lack of sufficient structure
  - Defensive learner or one who lacks insight into his or her deficiencies
  - Lack of well-defined, mutually agreed upon goals established
- Conditions that promote appropriate feedback
  - Feedback is part of the institutional culture and is given frequently.
  - Adequate time and timing (promptly)
  - Private setting
  - Learner knows when/where it will happen.
  - Based on specific, observed, and potentially modifiable behaviors
  - Based on objective observations, not on interpretations of the learner's motives
  - Matches with well-defined learning goals
  - Nonjudgmental language

ALERT
Remember that the GOAL of feedback is to improve performance.

MODELS

Fast

- **F** = frequently given and in digestible chunks
- **A** = accurate, based on observation
- **S** = specific, focused on modifiable behaviors
- **T** = timely

Insight

- **I** = INQUIRY: How does the resident/student/learner think it went?
- **N** = NEEDS: What learning needs does the resident/student/learner identify?
- **S** = SPECIFIC: Was your feedback specific?
- **I** = INTERCHANGE: Was there a discussion?
- **G** = GOALS: What are the next steps?
- **H** = HELP: Are there ways you can help?
- **T** = TIMING: When will follow-up occur?

Feedback Grid (Walsh, 2006)

- **Continue:** Comment on aspects of performance that were effective and should be done in the future.
- **Start or do more:** Comment on behaviors that the student knows how to do and should start doing or do so more often.
- **Consider:** Comment on "doable challenges" for the future growth of the student.
- **Stop, or do less:** Comment on observed actions that were not helpful and/or could be harmful.

Pearls (Milan et al., 2006)

- **P** = partnership for joint problem solving
- **E** = empathic understanding
- **A** = apology for barriers to the learner's success
- **R** = respect for learner's values and choices
- **L** = legitimation of feelings and intentions
- **S** = support for efforts at correction

Adapt (Johnston, Pauwels, Patton, Fainstad; University of Washington)

Prepare for and perform the observation, then ADAPT

- **A** = Ask for feedback about the observation.
- **D** = Discuss modifiable, specific behaviors.
- **A** = Ask for clarification.
- **P** = Plan next steps between coach and learner . . .
- **T** = Together

Sandwich

- Provide a compliment or some reinforcing feedback, then provide some constructive feedback, then close with another compliment or additional reinforcing feedback.
- The negative feedback is sandwiched between two positive statements.

SOAP Feedback

- **S** = subjective self-assessment by learner; ask learner how he or she thinks it went.
- **O** = objective balanced; descriptive feedback is provided.
- **A** = assess and summarize; ask learner to summarize two "take-home" points.
- **P** = plan for next steps incorporating new strategies.

ADDITIONAL READING

- Bing-You R, Hayes V, Varaklis K, et al. Feedback for learners in medical education: what is known? a scoping review. *Acad Med*. 2017;92(9):1346–1354.
- Branch WT Jr, Paranjape A. Feedback and reflection: teaching methods for clinical settings. *Acad Med*. 2002;77(12, Pt 1):1185–1188.
- Ende J. Feedback in clinical medical education. *JAMA*. 1983;250(6):777–781.
- Hewson MG, Little ML. Giving feedback in medical education: verification of recommended techniques. *J Gen Intern Med*. 1998;13(2):111–116.
- Milan FB, Parish SJ, Reichgott MJ. A model for educational feedback based on clinical communication skills strategies: beyond the "feedback sandwich." *Teach Learn Med*. 2006;18(1):42–47.
- Ramani S, Krackov SK. Twelve tips for giving feedback effectively in the clinical environment. *Med Teach*. 2012;34(10):787–791.
- Reddy ST, Zegarek MH, Fromme HB, et al. Barriers and facilitators to effective feedback: a qualitative analysis of data from multispecialty resident focus groups. *J Grad Med Educ*. 2015;7(2):214–219.
- Richardson BK. Feedback. *Acad Emerg Med*. 2004;11(12):e1–e5.
- Walsh A. Working with IMGs: delivering effective feedback. In: Walsh A, ed. *A Faculty Development Program for Teachers of International Medical Graduates*. Ottawa, Ontario, Canada: Association Of Faculties of Medicine of Canada; 2006. https://afmc.ca/timg/modules_en.htm. Accessed February 15, 2017.

FAQ

- Q: Is there anything wrong with just using the "feedback sandwich"?
- A: It can either confuse or dilute the real message. It may be perceived as insulting or condescending by the learner. Sometimes the learner only focuses on positives or negatives and fails to understand the big picture.
- Q: Is it ever okay to say "good job"?
- A: Compliments are best used when paired with reinforcing feedback that is more specific and based on observed behavior.

PART 4: CLINICAL REASONING

Mary C. Ottolini, MD, MPH, MEd • Terry Kind, MD, MPH

BASICS

Description

- The process of acquiring and interpreting clinical data to determine the etiology of a patient's presenting complaint
- Involves having a framework for storing and organizing medical knowledge effectively, which is critical for avoiding diagnostic error
- The experienced clinician uses problem representation, searches through "illness scripts" to make a diagnosis, and employs strategies to avoid cognitive biases.

DEVELOPMENTAL PROGRESSION

Clinical educators simultaneously diagnose the patient and diagnose the learner's developmental level of clinical reasoning.

- **Analytic reasoning:** Through basic pathophysiology, differential diagnoses are considered in "silos" or "disembodied" unrelated to patient's specific findings.
- **Development of illness scripts:** linking signs and symptoms of current patient to patterns of signs and symptoms seen in previous patients, filtering and grouping the data gathered into illness scripts
- **Problem representation:** creating a nuanced illness script for a current patient by synthesizing information into "semantic qualifiers," reflecting cognitive processing based on prior experience

THE CLINICAL REASONING PROCESS

PATIENT STORY

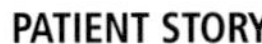

DATA ACQUISITION

PROBLEM REPRESENTATION

HYPOTHESIS GENERATION

SEARCH FOR ILLNESS SCRIPT

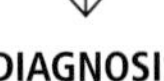

DIAGNOSIS

Problem Representation

SUMMARY statement of mental model of patient

- Key features of HPI/PE+
- Semantic qualifiers (adjectives)

Illness Scripts

- Prototypical disease presentations based on the following:
  - Epidemiology: Who gets the illness? (age, exposure, travel, etc.)
  - Timing: onset and progression
  - Classic/exclusionary findings
  - Pathophysiology/anatomic explanation
- Problem representation and illness scripts promote the "CHUNKING" of data or compiling information into a clinical syndrome, based on patterns and experience.

"Vertical versus Horizontal Reading"

Deliberately compare/contrast illness scripts for two to three diagnoses for a clinical syndrome (vertically), rather than one diagnosis at a time (horizontally).

Type 1 versus Type 2 Reasoning

Experts move back and forth between types (i.e., dual-processing) depending on prior experience with illness presentation:

- **Type 1:** heuristics or "rules of thumb" as mental shortcuts if a pattern of signs and symptoms or illness script is recognized
- **Type 2:** analytical/deductive reasoning used when the presentation is unusual; slow and deliberate process

FACTORS LEADING TO DIAGNOSTIC ERRORS

Cognitive Biases

- Predictable errors in reasoning occurring particularly with type 1 (heuristic) processing; can make gathering essential information and clinical reasoning difficult
- Common biases:
  - Premature closure: relying on initial diagnostic impression despite subsequent information to the contrary
  - Anchoring bias: relying too heavily on one piece of information
  - Confirmation bias: searching for, interpreting, and remembering information in a way that confirms one's preconceptions
  - Diagnostic momentum: sticking with one diagnostic label due to frequent repetition
  - Availability bias: overreliance on what easily comes to mind
  - Base-rate neglect: ignoring the true prevalence of a disease

ALERT
Diagnostic error is currently a leading cause of serious medical errors. Improved clinical reasoning can be taught as a strategy to decrease diagnostic errors.

Strategies to Overcome Biases

- Guided reflection:
  - Prompt the learner to identify findings that support and that oppose their initial hypothesis, list findings were expected but not present, and list alternative hypotheses.
- Metacognition: deliberately reflecting "in-action" and thinking about thinking
  - Did the diagnosis come too easily?
  - Is there any data that doesn't fit?
  - Am I investing too much in one finding?
  - Do I dislike the patient/parent?
- Take a "diagnostic time-out"
  - Recognize when time pressure may lead to premature closure on the wrong diagnosis.

Oral Presentation Framework

Encourage students to include clinical reasoning in their presentations:

P: PROBLEM REPRESENTATION: assessment-driven presentation

BE: BACKGROUND EVIDENCE: Focus on pertinent positives and negatives.

A: ANALYSIS: Compare and contrast two likely illness scripts.

R: RECOMMENDATION: Plan based on a problem rather than system.

ADDITIONAL READING

- Bowen J. Educational strategies to promote clinical diagnostic reasoning. *N Engl J Med*. 2006;355(21):2217–2225.
- Croskerry P. Achieving quality in clinical decision making: cognitive strategies and detection of bias. *Acad Emerg Med*. 2002;9(11):1184–1204.
- Lambe KA, O'Reilly G, Kelly BD, et al. Dual-process cognitive interventions to enhance diagnostic reasoning: a systematic review. *BMJ Qual Saf*. 2016;25(10):808–820.
- Newman-Toker DE, Pronovost PJ. Diagnostic errors—the next frontier for patient safety. *JAMA*. 2009;301(10):1060–1062.
- Schmidt HG, Norman GR, Boshuizen HP. A cognitive perspective on medical expertise: theory and implication. *Acad Med*. 1990;65(10):611–621.
- Schmidt HG, Rikers RM. How expertise develops in medicine: knowledge encapsulation and illness script formation. *Med Educ*. 2007;41(12):1133–1139.
- Thammasitboon S, Cutrer WB. Diagnostic decision-making and strategies to improve diagnosis. *Curr Probl Pediatr Adolesc Health Care*. 2013;43(9):232–241.

FAQ

- Q: Can the clinical reasoning process be taught?
- A: Yes, promoting "problem representation" and comparing and contrasting the differentiating features using illness scripts helps trainees to organize and store their patient experiences so that they can recall them in future similar situations.
- Q: Can one overcome cognitive errors?
- A: Yes. Using metacognition, or "thinking about your thinking," a form of situational awareness, one can develop a habit of taking a "diagnostic time-out."

Appendix II
Cardiology Laboratory

Kieran Leong, DO • Gurumurthy Hiremath, MD, FACC, FSCAI

BLOOD PRESSURE MEASUREMENT

- **All children >3 years old should have blood pressure (BP) measured as part of their physical exam.**
- If <3 years old, measure BP if there are comorbidities present that predispose them to hypertension (congenital heart disease, NICU stay, recurrent UTI, proteinuria, renal disease).
- **Measure BP in right upper arm** for purposes of consistency, comparability to standard tables, and to avoid a spurious value in cases of coarctation.
- BP by auscultation is the preferred method.
- Abnormal BPs obtained by oscillometry should be confirmed by auscultation.
- **Optimal BP cuff size (Table 1):**
  - Bladder length covers 80–100% of the circumference of the arm.
  - Bladder width covers 40% of the upper arm circumference.
- **Refer to BP standards based on gender, age, and height** that now include 50th, 90th, 95th, and 99th percentiles **(Tables 2 and 3)**.
- **Hypertension** is defined as average systolic BP (SBP) and/or diastolic BP (DBP) that are ≥95th percentile for gender, age, and height on three occasions.
- **Prehypertension**: If the SBP or DBP is ≥90th percentile and <95th percentile, it is called "Prehypertension."
- **Aortic coarctation**: If suspected, check BP in all four extremities. A difference >10 mm Hg between upper and lower extremity BPs is pathologic and suggests the presence of aortic coarctation, aortic arch hypoplasia, or interrupted aortic arch.

PULSE OXIMETRY

- **Systemic arterial blood oxygen content** is a combination of oxygen bound to hemoglobin (Hgb) and dissolved oxygen and is represented by the following formula:
  - **Oxygen content** = (**Hgb** in gm/dL × **1.36** in mL O_2/gm of Hgb × **O_2 saturation in percent**) + (Pao_2 × 0.003 O_2/dL per mm Hg)
  - Decreased arterial oxygen content is called **"hypoxemia"** and could result in **"hypoxia"** which is failure to oxygenate at tissue level (manifesting as metabolic acidosis). **"Cyanosis"** is the clinical manifestation of bluish discoloration of skin or mucosa resulting from hypoxemia.
  - **Systemic arterial desaturation causes:**
    - Pulmonary venous desaturation (lung disease)
    - Right-to-left shunting (cardiac disease)
    - Hgb disorders
- **Clinical manifestation of cyanosis depends on many factors including Hgb level. Clinically apparent central cyanosis occurs when the absolute concentration of deoxygenated Hgb is >3 gm/dL.**

Contrasting Examples

- **Polycythemic neonate** (Hgb = 20 g/dL) with an arterial saturation of 80% will have *4 g/dL* of deoxygenated Hgb *and will appear cyanotic.*
- **Anemic neonate** (Hgb = 10 g/dL) with an arterial saturation of 80% will have *only 2 g/dL* of deoxygenated Hgb *and will not appear cyanotic.*
- **Pulse oximetry is now an established screening tool to detect critical congenital heart disease in newborns.** See **Figure 1** for most recent recommendations endorsed by American Heart Association and American Academy of Pediatrics.

How to Measure Saturations Properly

- **Preductal**: Measure saturation in the right ear lobe or right arm.
  - *Right ear lobe saturation is always preductal unlike the right arm (such as in the presence of an aberrant right subclavian artery).*
- **Postductal:** Measure saturation in either leg.

Differential Saturation Interpretation

- Lower postductal saturation might suggest coarctation of aorta, pulmonary hypertension, critical left-sided obstructive lesions, or infradiaphragmatic total anomalous pulmonary venous return.
- Higher postductal saturation in the legs suggests transposition or supracardiac total anomalous pulmonary venous return.

Table 1. Recommended Dimensions for BP Cuff Bladders

Age Range	Width, cm	Length, cm	Maximum Arm Circumference, cm[a]
Newborn	4	8	10
Infant	6	12	15
Child	9	18	22
Small adult	10	24	26
Adult	13	30	34
Large adult	16	38	44
Thigh	20	42	52

[a]Calculated so that the largest arm would still allow the bladder to encircle arm by at least 80%.
BP, blood pressure.
Source: National Heart, Lung, and Blood Institute; National Institutes of Health; U.S. Department of Health and Human Services.

Table 2. BP Levels for Boys by Age and Height Percentile

		SBP, mm Hg							DBP, mm Hg						
		Percentile of Height							Percentile of Height						
Age, y	BP Percentile	5th	10th	25th	50th	75th	90th	95th	5th	10th	25th	50th	75th	90th	95th
1	50th	80	81	83	85	87	88	89	34	35	36	37	38	39	39
	90th	94	95	97	99	100	102	103	49	50	51	52	53	53	54
	95th	98	99	101	103	104	106	106	54	54	55	56	57	58	58
	99th	105	106	108	110	112	113	114	61	62	63	64	65	66	66
2	50th	84	85	87	88	90	92	92	39	40	41	42	43	44	44
	90th	97	99	100	102	104	105	106	54	55	56	57	58	58	59
	95th	101	102	104	106	108	109	110	59	59	60	61	62	63	63
	99th	109	110	111	113	115	117	117	66	67	68	69	70	71	71
3	50th	86	87	89	91	93	94	95	44	44	45	46	47	48	48
	90th	100	101	103	105	107	108	109	59	59	60	61	62	63	63
	95th	104	105	107	109	110	112	113	63	63	64	65	66	67	67
	99th	111	112	114	116	118	119	120	71	71	72	73	74	75	75
4	50th	88	89	91	93	95	96	97	47	48	49	50	51	51	52
	90th	102	103	105	107	109	110	111	62	63	64	65	66	66	67
	95th	106	107	109	111	112	114	115	66	67	68	69	70	71	71
	99th	113	114	116	118	120	121	122	74	75	76	77	78	78	79
5	50th	90	91	93	95	96	98	98	50	51	52	53	54	55	55
	90th	104	105	106	108	110	111	112	65	66	67	68	69	69	70
	95th	108	109	110	112	114	115	116	69	70	71	72	73	74	74
	99th	115	116	118	120	121	123	123	77	78	79	80	81	81	82
6	50th	91	92	94	96	98	99	100	53	53	54	55	56	57	57
	90th	105	106	108	110	111	113	113	68	68	69	70	71	72	72
	95th	109	110	112	114	115	117	117	72	72	73	74	75	76	76
	99th	116	117	119	121	123	124	125	80	80	81	82	83	84	84
7	50th	92	94	95	97	99	100	101	55	55	56	57	58	59	59
	90th	106	107	109	111	113	114	115	70	70	71	72	73	74	74
	95th	110	111	113	115	117	118	119	74	74	75	76	77	78	78
	99th	117	118	120	122	124	125	126	82	82	83	84	85	86	86
8	50th	94	95	97	99	100	102	102	56	57	58	59	60	60	61
	90th	107	109	110	112	114	115	116	71	72	72	73	74	75	76
	95th	111	112	114	116	118	119	120	75	76	77	78	79	79	80
	99th	119	120	122	123	125	127	127	83	84	85	86	87	87	88
9	50th	95	96	98	100	102	103	104	57	58	59	60	61	61	62
	90th	109	110	112	114	115	117	118	72	73	74	75	76	76	77
	95th	113	114	116	118	119	121	121	76	77	78	79	80	81	81
	99th	120	121	123	125	127	128	129	84	85	86	87	88	88	89
10	50th	97	98	100	102	103	105	106	58	59	60	61	61	62	63
	90th	111	112	114	115	117	119	119	73	73	74	75	76	77	78
	95th	115	116	117	119	121	122	123	77	78	79	80	81	81	82
	99th	122	123	125	127	128	130	130	85	86	86	88	88	89	90
11	50th	99	100	102	104	105	107	107	59	59	60	61	62	63	63
	90th	113	114	115	117	119	120	121	74	74	75	76	77	78	78
	95th	117	118	119	121	123	124	125	78	78	79	80	81	82	82
	99th	124	125	127	129	130	132	132	86	86	87	88	89	90	90

Table 2. BP Levels for Boys by Age and Height Percentile *(continued)*

Age, y	BP Percentile	SBP, mm Hg							DBP, mm Hg						
		Percentile of Height							Percentile of Height						
		5th	10th	25th	50th	75th	90th	95th	5th	10th	25th	50th	75th	90th	95th
12	50th	101	102	104	106	108	109	110	59	60	61	62	63	63	64
	90th	115	116	118	120	121	123	123	74	75	75	76	77	78	79
	95th	119	120	122	123	125	127	127	78	79	80	81	82	82	83
	99th	126	127	129	131	133	134	135	86	87	88	89	90	90	91
13	50th	104	105	106	108	110	111	112	60	60	61	62	63	64	64
	90th	117	118	120	122	124	125	126	75	75	76	77	78	79	79
	95th	121	122	124	126	128	129	130	79	79	80	81	82	83	83
	99th	128	130	131	133	135	136	137	87	87	88	89	90	91	91
14	50th	106	107	109	111	113	114	115	60	61	62	63	64	65	65
	90th	120	121	123	125	126	128	128	75	76	77	78	79	79	80
	95th	124	125	127	128	130	132	132	80	80	81	82	83	84	84
	99th	131	132	134	136	138	139	140	87	88	89	90	91	92	92
15	50th	109	110	112	113	115	117	117	61	62	63	64	65	66	66
	90th	122	124	125	127	129	130	131	76	77	78	79	80	80	81
	95th	126	127	129	131	133	134	135	81	81	82	83	84	85	85
	99th	134	135	136	138	140	142	142	88	89	90	91	92	93	93
16	50th	111	112	114	116	118	119	120	63	63	64	65	66	67	67
	90th	125	126	128	130	131	133	134	78	78	79	80	81	82	82
	95th	129	130	132	134	135	137	137	82	83	83	84	85	86	87
	99th	136	137	139	141	143	144	145	90	90	91	92	93	94	94
17	50th	114	115	116	118	120	121	122	65	66	66	67	68	69	70
	90th	127	128	130	132	134	135	136	80	80	81	82	83	84	84
	95th	131	132	134	136	138	139	140	84	85	86	87	87	88	89
	99th	139	140	141	143	145	146	147	92	93	93	94	95	96	97

BP, blood pressure; SBP, systolic blood pressure; DBP, diastolic blood pressure.
Source: National Heart, Lung, and Blood Institute; National Institutes of Health; U.S. Department of Health and Human Services.

Table 3. BP Levels for Girls by Age and Height Percentile

		SBP, mm Hg							DBP, mm Hg						
		Percentile of Height							Percentile of Height						
Age, y	BP Percentile	5th	10th	25th	50th	75th	90th	95th	5th	10th	25th	50th	75th	90th	95th
1	50th	83	84	85	86	88	89	90	38	39	39	40	41	41	42
	90th	97	97	98	100	101	102	103	52	53	53	54	55	55	56
	95th	100	101	102	104	105	106	107	56	57	57	58	59	59	60
	99th	108	108	109	111	112	113	114	64	64	65	65	66	67	67
2	50th	85	85	87	88	89	91	91	43	44	44	45	46	46	47
	90th	98	99	100	101	103	104	105	57	58	58	59	60	61	61
	95th	102	103	104	105	107	108	109	61	62	62	63	64	65	65
	99th	109	110	111	112	114	115	116	69	69	70	70	71	72	72
3	50th	86	87	88	89	91	92	93	47	48	48	49	50	50	51
	90th	100	100	102	103	104	106	106	61	62	62	63	64	64	65
	95th	104	104	105	107	108	109	110	65	66	66	67	68	68	69
	99th	111	111	113	114	115	116	117	73	73	74	74	75	76	76
4	50th	88	88	90	91	92	94	94	50	50	51	52	52	53	54
	90th	101	102	103	104	106	107	108	64	64	65	66	67	67	68
	95th	105	106	107	108	110	111	112	68	68	69	70	71	71	72
	99th	112	113	114	115	117	118	119	76	76	76	77	78	79	79
5	50th	89	90	91	93	94	95	96	52	53	53	54	55	55	56
	90th	103	103	105	106	107	109	109	66	67	67	68	69	69	70
	95th	107	107	108	110	111	112	113	70	71	71	72	73	73	74
	99th	114	114	116	117	118	120	120	78	78	79	79	80	81	81
6	50th	91	92	93	94	96	97	98	54	54	55	56	56	57	58
	90th	104	105	106	108	109	110	111	68	68	69	70	70	71	72
	95th	108	109	110	111	113	114	115	72	72	73	74	74	75	76
	99th	115	116	117	119	120	121	122	80	80	80	81	82	83	83
7	50th	93	93	95	96	97	99	99	55	56	56	57	58	58	59
	90th	106	107	108	109	111	112	113	69	70	70	71	72	72	73
	95th	110	111	112	113	115	116	116	73	74	74	75	76	76	77
	99th	117	118	119	120	122	123	124	81	81	82	82	83	84	84
8	50th	95	95	96	98	99	100	101	57	57	57	58	59	60	60
	90th	108	109	110	111	113	114	114	71	71	71	72	73	74	74
	95th	112	112	114	115	116	118	118	75	75	75	76	77	78	78
	99th	119	120	121	122	123	125	125	82	82	83	83	84	85	86
9	50th	96	97	98	100	101	102	103	58	58	58	59	60	61	61
	90th	110	110	112	113	114	116	116	72	72	72	73	74	75	75
	95th	114	114	115	117	118	119	120	76	76	76	77	78	79	79
	99th	121	121	123	124	125	127	127	83	83	84	84	85	86	87
10	50th	98	99	100	102	103	104	105	59	59	59	60	61	62	62
	90th	112	112	114	115	116	118	118	73	73	73	74	75	76	76
	95th	116	116	117	119	120	121	122	77	77	77	78	79	80	80
	99th	123	123	125	126	127	129	129	84	84	85	86	86	87	88
11	50th	100	101	102	103	105	106	107	60	60	60	61	62	63	63
	90th	114	114	116	117	118	119	120	74	74	74	75	76	77	77
	95th	118	118	119	121	122	123	124	78	78	78	79	80	81	81
	99th	125	125	126	128	129	130	131	85	85	86	87	87	88	89

Table 3. BP Levels for Girls by Age and Height Percentile *(continued)*

		SBP, mm Hg							DBP, mm Hg						
		Percentile of Height							Percentile of Height						
Age, y	BP Percentile	5th	10th	25th	50th	75th	90th	95th	5th	10th	25th	50th	75th	90th	95th
12	50th	102	103	104	105	107	108	109	61	61	61	62	63	64	64
	90th	116	116	117	119	120	121	122	75	75	75	76	77	78	78
	95th	119	120	121	123	124	125	126	79	79	79	80	81	82	82
	99th	127	127	128	130	131	132	133	86	86	87	88	88	89	90
13	50th	104	105	106	107	109	110	110	62	62	62	63	64	65	65
	90th	117	118	119	121	122	123	124	76	76	76	77	78	79	79
	95th	121	122	123	124	126	127	128	80	80	80	81	82	83	83
	99th	128	129	130	132	133	134	135	87	87	88	89	89	90	91
14	50th	106	106	107	109	110	111	112	63	63	63	64	65	66	66
	90th	119	120	121	122	124	125	125	77	77	77	78	79	80	80
	95th	123	123	125	126	127	129	129	81	81	81	82	83	84	84
	99th	130	131	132	133	135	136	136	88	88	89	90	90	91	92
15	50th	107	108	109	110	111	113	113	64	64	64	65	66	67	67
	90th	120	121	122	123	125	126	127	78	78	78	79	80	81	81
	95th	124	125	126	127	129	130	131	82	82	82	83	84	85	85
	99th	131	132	133	134	136	137	138	89	89	90	91	91	92	93
16	50th	108	108	110	111	112	114	114	64	64	65	66	66	67	68
	90th	121	122	123	124	126	127	128	78	78	79	80	81	81	82
	95th	125	126	127	128	130	131	132	82	82	83	84	85	85	86
	99th	132	133	134	135	137	138	139	90	90	90	91	92	93	93
17	50th	108	109	110	111	113	114	115	64	65	65	66	67	67	68
	90th	122	122	123	125	126	127	128	78	79	79	80	81	81	82
	95th	125	126	127	129	130	131	132	82	83	83	84	85	85	86
	99th	133	133	134	136	137	138	139	90	90	91	91	92	93	93

BP, blood pressure; SBP, systolic blood pressure; DBP, diastolic blood pressure.
Source: National Heart, Lung, and Blood Institute; National Institutes of Health; U.S. Department of Health and Human Services.

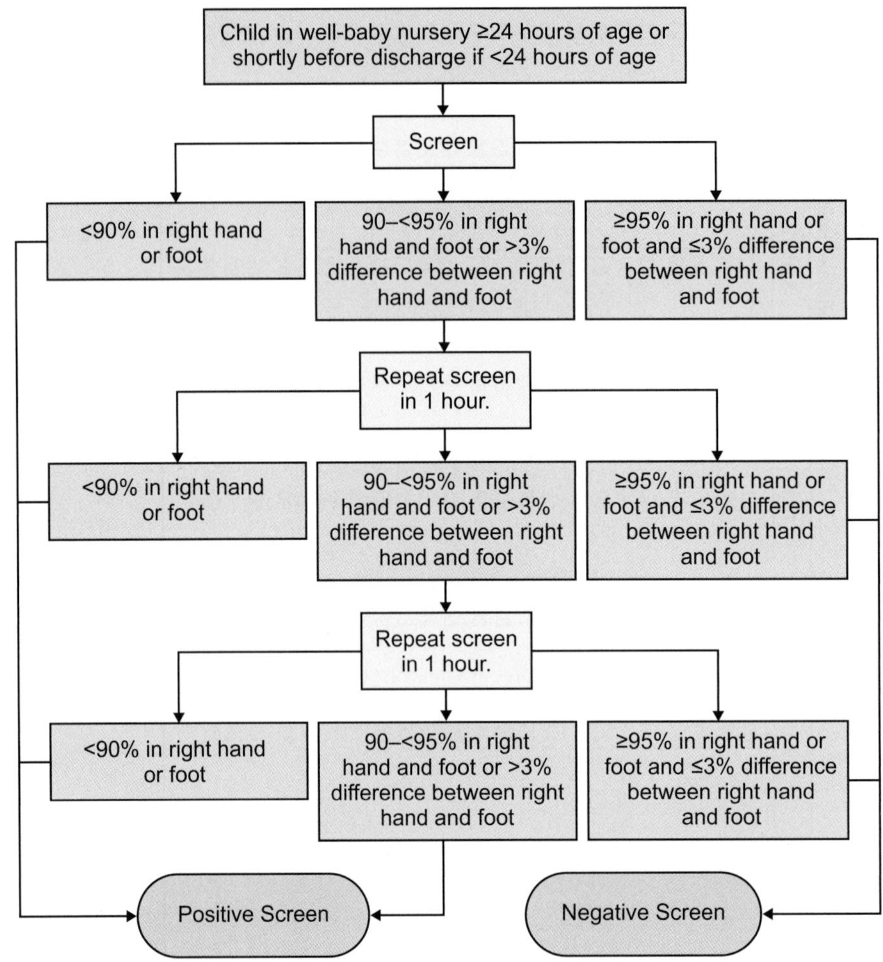

FIGURE 1. Pulse-oximetry screening protocol based on results from the right hand and either foot. (Reproduced with permission from Kemper AR, Mahle WT, Martin GR, et al. Strategies for implementing screening for critical congenital heart disease. *Pediatrics*. 2011;128[5]:e1259–e1267, Copyright 2011 American Academy of Pediatrics.)

Hyperoxia Test

In infants with cyanosis, a hyperoxia test using arterial blood gas is performed to differentiate cyanotic congenital heart disease from other etiologies of hypoxia. If a right radial arterial Pao_2 on 100% FiO_2 is <150 mm Hg, cyanotic congenital heart disease is likely **(Table 4)**.

ELECTROCARDIOGRAPHY

- The standard ECG consists of 12 leads that include 3 limb leads (I, II, III), 3 augmented limb leads (aVR, aVL, aVF), and 6 precordial leads (V1 to V6). In children, additional precordial leads are often used making it a 15-lead ECG (V3R, V4R, and V7).
- The standard ECG paper speed is 25 mm/sec with amplitude of 1 mV/mm (Figure 2). Each small box is 40 ms, and each large box is 200 ms.
- **Pediatric ECG parameters are age dependent**. Please see **Table 5** for comprehensive standards of normal ECG in children.

Rate and Rhythm

Heart rate is calculated by dividing 60,000 ms/min by the measured cycle length. The rhythm is considered sinus if each QRS is preceded by a P wave and the P wave is upright in I, II, and aVF.

Axes

- Axes can be calculated in a hexaxial reference plane for all three waves of the ECG. P-wave axis helps in determining if the rhythm is originating from the sinus node or an alternative pacemaker.
- **The normal QRS axis changes with age.** In the newborn period, the mean vector of depolarization is rightward, reflecting the dominance of the right ventricle in early infancy. As the left ventricular mass increases relative to the right side, the QRS axis shifts more leftward.
- **When the QRS axis is superior (northwest axis), an endocardial cushion defect or tricuspid atresia is possible.**
- The T wave represents ventricular repolarization. Within the first 72 hours of life, the T wave should invert in lead V1. Persistence of upright T wave beyond 7 days of age till adolescence is a sensitive indicator of increased right ventricular pressure. As the left ventricle becomes progressively more dominant, the T-wave axis parallels the QRS axis. Thus, during adolescence, the T wave becomes upright in lead V1, and the T-wave axis becomes leftward.
- The QRS-T angle should be ≤90 degrees. Abnormally wide QRS-T angle may be a result of ventricular hypertrophy with strain pattern or ventricular conduction disturbance.

Atrioventricular Conduction and Intervals

- The PR interval is measured from the onset of the P wave to the beginning of the QRS complex and reflects the time for atrial depolarization and delay through the AV node. In general, with age, the heart rate is slower, and the PR interval is longer.
- A **short PR interval** occurs when there is Wolff-Parkinson-White syndrome, Lown-Ganong-Levine syndrome, glycogen storage disease, or low atrial pacemaker.

Table 4. Diagnostic Testing in Cyanosis

Test	Pulmonary Parenchymal Disease	Intra- or Extrapulmonary Right-to-Left Shunt	Central Hypoventilation	Transposition Physiology	Hemoglobin Disorders
Respiratory distress?	Present; may have fever	No	No; apnea/hypoventilation+	Mild distress, usually tachypnea due to increased PBF	No
Cardiac exam	Normal	May have single S2, RV heave, thrill, and murmurs	Normal	Single S2, flow murmur, RV heave	Normal
Chest radiograph	Pulmonary pathology	Variable cardiac silhouette; usually clear lung fields	Normal	Egg on end appearance, pulmonary venous congestion +/−	Normal
Differential saturation (preductal vs. postductal)	Absent	Present if right-to-left shunt at ductus; postductal < preductal	Absent	Postductal > preductal	Absent
CBC	Elevated white count	Polycythemia if chronic	Normal	Polycythemia if chronic	Normal
Arterial blood gas on 100% FiO_2	$Pao_2 > 150$ Pco_2 variable	$Pao_2 < 150$ Normal Pco_2	$Pao_2 > 150$, usually much higher; elevated Pco_2	$Pao_2 < 150$, usually < 50 Normal Pco_2	Normal Pao_2 and Pco_2

PBF, pulmonary blood flow; RV, right ventricle; CBC, complete blood count.
From Hiremath G, Kamat D. Diagnostic considerations in infants and children with cyanosis. *Pediatr Ann*. 2015;44(2):76–80, with permission.

Abnormal AV conduction

- **1st-degree AV block** is PR prolongation for age and heart rate.
- **2nd-degree AV block** can be Mobitz Type I (Wenckebach), where there is progressive PR prolongation before a dropped beat, or Mobitz Type II, where there is abrupt failure of AV conduction without previous PR prolongation.
- **3rd-degree AV block** involves no conduction of atrial impulses to the ventricle.
- **QRS widening** is seen with a bundle branch block, preexcitation (e.g., Wolff-Parkinson-White syndrome), intraventricular block, ventricular arrhythmias, and ventricular paced rhythms.
- **Left bundle branch block** is diagnosed when there is slurred R wave in left precordial leads (V6) and slurred S wave in right precordial leads (V1).
- **Right bundle branch block** is diagnosed when there is a wide and slurred S wave in leads I and V6, slurred R (RSR′ pattern or M-shaped) QRS complex in lead V1. Left anterior hemiblock can be diagnosed in the setting of left axis deviation associated with right bundle branch block.
- **QT interval** represents the time it takes for ventricular depolarization and repolarization and is measured from the onset of the Q wave to the termination of the T wave. Given that the QT interval should shorten with increasing heart rates, the QT measurement should be adjusted for heart rate using **Bazett formula**:

$$\text{QTc} = \frac{\textbf{measured QT}}{\textbf{square root of the R-R interval}}$$

- **The QTc interval is <0.45 seconds for infants/younger children and <0.46 for adolescent females.**
- The QTc is prolonged in **long QT syndrome** wherein there are genetic abnormalities of either the cardiac potassium or sodium channels. Other conditions that prolong the QTc interval include head injury, myocarditis, medications (such as procainamide, amiodarone, quinidine), and electrolyte abnormalities (e.g., hypocalcemia, hypomagnesemia, hypokalemia).

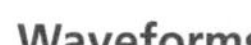

Waveforms

- When the P-wave amplitude is >3 mm in lead II or lead V1, **right atrial enlargement** is present. If the P wave has duration >0.1 seconds in lead II or is biphasic with a prominent negative component in lead V1, **left atrial enlargement** is present.
- Abnormally tall R waves in lead V1 or deep S-waves in V5 and V6 represent **right ventricular hypertrophy**. Similarly, tall R-waves in leads V5 and V6 or deep S waves in lead V1 **represent left ventricular hypertrophy**.
- Low-voltage QRS complexes suggest myocarditis, pericarditis, pericardial effusion, or hypothyroidism.
- Tall, peaked T waves can be seen with ventricular hypertrophy associated with strain, myocardial infarction, or hyperkalemia.
- Low-voltage, flat T-waves are associated with electrolyte abnormalities (hypokalemia, hypoglycemia), hypothyroidism, myocarditis, pericarditis, ischemia, or medications (i.e., digitalis).

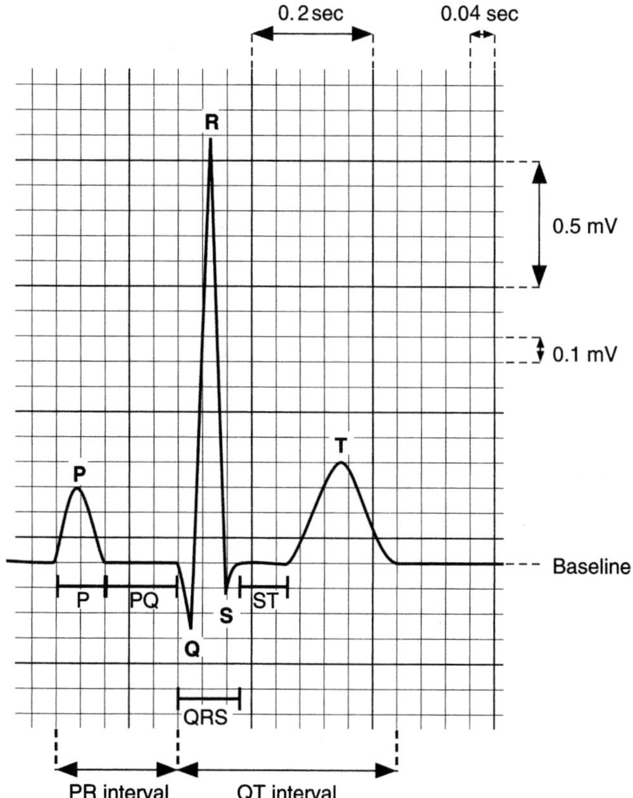

FIGURE 2. A normal electrocardiogram showing waveforms and intervals. The standard paper speed is 25 mm/sec; therefore, a single 1-mm box equals 0.04 second and a large (5-mm) box equals 0.20 second.

Table 5. Normal ECG Standards for Children by Age

	0–1 d	1–3 d	3–7 d	7–30 d	1–3 mo	3–6 mo	6–12 mo	1–3 y	3–5 y	5–8 y	8–12 y	12–16 y
Heart rate per minute	94–155 (122)	91–158 (122)	90–166 (128)	06–182 1 (149)	120–179 (149)	105–185 (141)	108–169 (131)	89–152 (119)	73–137 (109)	65–133 (100)	62–130 (91)	60–120 (80)
Frontal plane QRS axis (degrees)	59–189 (135)	64–197 (134)	76–191 (133)	0–160 7 (109)	30–115 (75)	7–105 (60)	6–98 (55)	7–102 (55)	6–104 (56)	10–139 (65)	6–116 (60)	9–128 (59)
PR lead II (s)	0.08–0.16 (0.107)	0.08–0.14 (0.138)	0.07–0.15 (0.102)	0.07–0.14 (0.100)	0.07–0.13 (0.098)	0.07–0.15 (0.105)	0.07–0.16 (0.106)	0.08–0.15 (0.113)	0.08–0.16 (0.119)	0.09–0.16 (0.123)	0.09–0.17 (0.128)	0.09–0.18 (0.135)
QRS duration, V5 (s)	0.02–0.07 (0.05)	0.02–0.07 (0.05)	0.02–0.07 (0.05)	0.02–0.08 (0.05)	0.02–0.08 (0.05)	0.02–0.08 (0.05)	0.03–0.08 (0.05)	0.03–0.08 (0.06)	0.03–0.07 (0.06)	0.03–0.08 (0.06)	0.04–0.09 (0.06)	0.04–0.09 (0.07)
P-wave amplitude lead II	0.5–2.8 (1.6)	0.3–2.8 (1.5)	0.7–2.9 (1.7)	0.7–3.0 (1.9)	0.7–2.6 (1.5)	0.4–2.7 (1.6)	0.6–2.5 (1.6)	0.7–2.5 (1.5)	0.3–2.5 (1.4)	0.4–2.5 (1.4)	0.3–2.5 (1.4)	0.3–2.5 (1.4)
Q-wave amplitude, aVF	0.1–3.4 (1.0)	0.1–3.3 (1.0)	0.1–3.5 (1.1)	0.1–3.5 (1.2)	0.1–3.4 (0.9)	0–3.2 (0.9)	0–3.3 (1.0)	0–3.2 (0.9)	0–2.9 (0.6)	0–2.5 (00.6)	0–2.7 (0.5)	0–2.4 (0.4)
Q-wave amplitude, V6	0–1.7 (0.1)	0–2.2 (0.1)	0–2.8 (0.1)	0–2.8 (0.4)	0–2.6 (0.3)	0–2.6 (0.3)	0–3.0 (0.4)	0–2.8 (0.6)	0.1–3.3 (0.8)	0.1–4.6 (0.8)	0.1–2.8 (0.6)	0–2.9 (0.4)
R amplitude, V1	5–26 (13)	5–27 (15)	3–25 (12)	3–12 (10)	3–19 (10)	3–20 (10)	2–20 (9)	2–18 (8)	1–18 (8)	1–14 (7)	1–12 (5)	1-10 (4)
S amplitude, V1	1–23 (8)	1–20 (9)	1–17 (7)	0–11 (4)	0–13 (5)	0–17 (6)	1–18 (7)	1–21 (8)	2–22 (10)	3–23 (12)	3–25 (12)	3–22 (11)
R amplitude, V6	0–12 (4)	0–12 (5)	1–12 (5)	3–16 (8)	5–21 (12)	6–22 (13)	6–23 (13)	6–23 (13)	8–25 (15)	8–26 (16)	9–25 (16)	7–23 (14)
S amplitude, V6	0–10 (4)	0–9 (3)	0–10 (4)	0–10 (3)	0–7 (3)	0–10 (3)	0–8 (2)	0–7 (2)	0–6 (2)	0–4 (1)	0–4 (1)	0–4 (1)
R/S ratio, V1	0.1–9.9 (2.2)	0–11.6 (2.0)	0.1–9.8 (2.8)	1.0–7.0 (2.9)	0.3–7.4 (2.2)	0.1–6.0 (2.3)	0.1–4.0 (1.8)	0.1–4.3 (1.4)	0.03–2.7 (0.9)	0.02–2.0 (0.8)	0.02–1.9 (0.6)	0.02–1.8 (.5)
R/S ratio, V6	0.1–9 (2)	0.1–12 (3)	0.1–10 (2)	0.1–12 (4)	0.2–14 (5)	0.2–18 (7)	0.2–22 (8)	0.3–27 (10)	0.6–30 (11)	0.9–30 (12)	1.5–33 (14)	1.4–39 (15)

ECG, electrocardiogram.
From Hugh DA. The normal electrocardiogram. In: Hugh DA, ed. *Moss & Adams' Heart Disease in Infants, Children, and Adolescents, Including the Fetus and Young Adult*. 9th ed. Philadelphia, PA: Lippincott Williams & Wilkins; 2016:372, with permission.

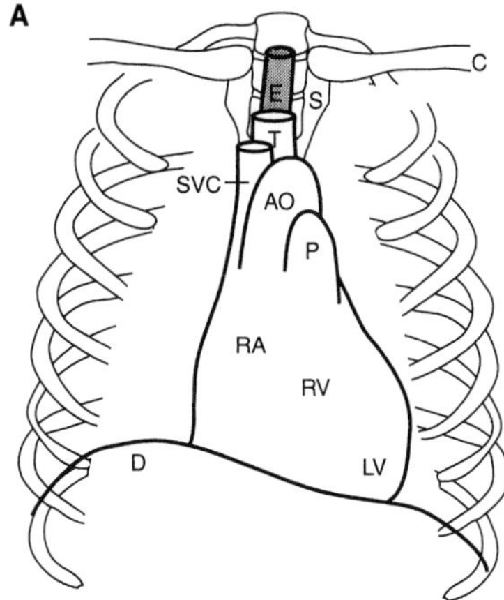

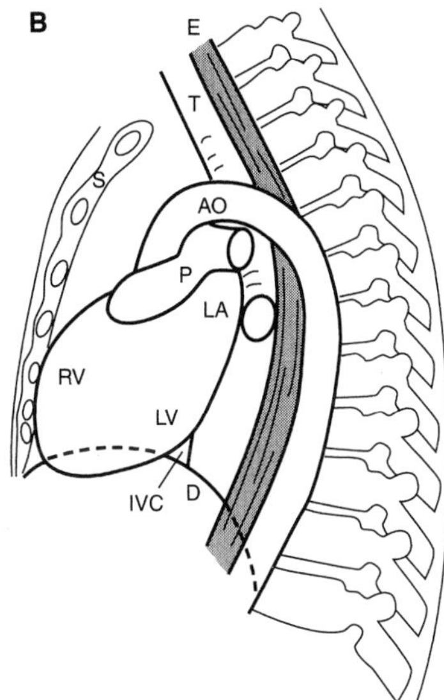

FIGURE 3. Normal cardiac silhouette. A: Anterior-posterior view. B: Lateral view. AO, aorta; C, clavicle; D, diaphragm; E, esophagus; IVC, inferior vena cava; LA, left atrium; LV, left ventricle; P, pulmonary outflow tract; RA, right atrium, RV, right ventricle; S, sternum; T, trachea; SVC, superior vena cava. (Modified from Sapire DW. *Understanding and Diagnosing Pediatric Heart Disease*. East Norwalk, CT: Appleton & Lange, 1991:64.)

CHEST ROENTGENOGRAM

The plain chest roentgenogram is inexpensive, expedient, readily available, and continues to provide important information to the clinician when cardiac disease is suspected. The normal cardiac silhouette in the anteroposterior and lateral views are shown in **Figure 3**.

Heart Size

- **Cardiomegaly** can be due to dilated cardiac chambers or pericardial effusion. A quantitative assessment of cardiac size should be made on the inspiratory film, when 9 to 10 ribs are visualized above the level of the diaphragm.
- **The cardiothoracic ratio** is then determined by comparing the transverse dimension of the heart relative to the width of the thoracic cavity. **The heart is considered enlarged if the cardiothoracic ratio exceeds 60%.**

Pulmonary Vascularity

- When there is a suspicion of congenital heart disease, the appearance of the pulmonary vascular markings plays an important role in understanding the pathophysiology.
- **Increased vascularity** is seen when a large left-to-right shunt is present (as in atrial septal defect, ventricular septal defect, patent ductus arteriosus). Increased pulmonary arterial flow makes the vessels appear sharp and prominent.
- **Decreased vascularity** is seen in right-sided obstructive lesion that results in decreased pulmonary blood flow or in Eisenmenger syndrome.
- **Pulmonary venous congestion** indicated by bronchial cuffing and Kerley B lines (horizontal lines seen at periphery of lung fields suggesting fluid-filled interlobar septa) suggest pulmonary venous obstructive disease or congestive heart failure.

Specific Cardiac Lesions

Distinctive radiographic configurations of the cardiac silhouette have been associated with specific cardiac lesions as listed below:

- **Tetralogy of Fallot:** "boot-shaped" heart
- **Total anomalous pulmonary venous return (supracardiac type):** "snowman" or "figure of eight"
- **Coarctation of aorta:** "figure of three"
- **D-transposition of great arteries:** "egg on a string"
- **L-transposition of great arteries:** "box-shaped heart"
- **Ebstein anomaly:** "wall-to-wall" heart

ECHOCARDIOGRAPHY

- Echocardiography involves the use of ultrasound technology to image the heart. It is an invaluable tool that gives immense details of the cardiac anatomy, function, and physiology and is the pillar of cardiac diagnostic laboratory. Echocardiography can be done bedside and is very valuable in emergently ruling out pericardial effusions and checking ventricular function.
- Transesophageal echo is done when more detailed information is needed or to guide cardiac surgery or catheterization procedures, using a probe inserted through the esophagus.
- Normal values for cardiac valves and dimensions vary with age and are available in literature for comparison.
- **Ejection fraction (EF)** is calculated by using left ventricular end-diastolic and end-systolic volumes in two planes; **normal value range for EF: 56–75%**
- **Shortening fraction (SF)** is also a measure of left ventricular function and is measured in M-mode; **normal value range for the SF: 28–38%, independent of age**

CARDIAC CATHETERIZATION

- Cardiac catheterization helps us obtain direct oximetric, hemodynamic information and, in conjunction with angiography, provides complete anatomic and physiologic data.
- **The normal pressures and oxygen saturations for children are shown in Figure 4.**

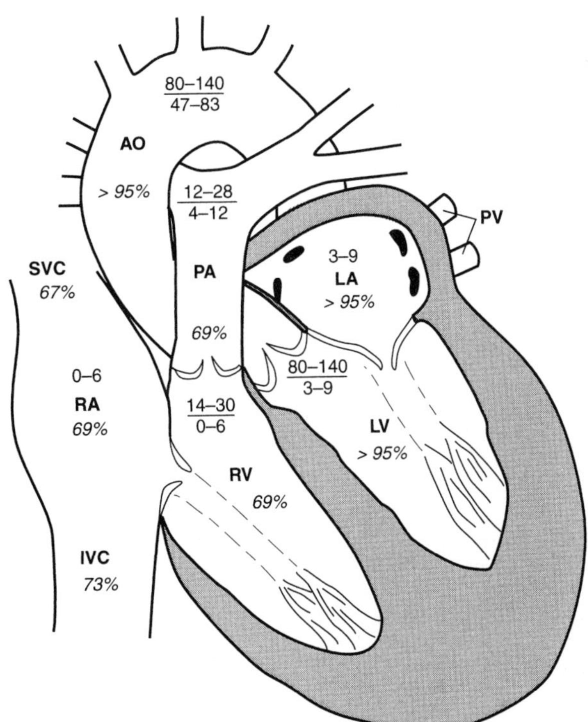

FIGURE 4. Normal pressures (systolic over diastolic, in mm Hg), mean pressures, and oxygen saturations for children during cardiac catheterization. The data are based on information compiled from healthy patients between the ages of 2 months and 20 years. AO, aorta; IVC, inferior vena cava; LA, left atrium; LV, left ventricle; PA, pulmonary artery; PV, pulmonary vein; RA, right atrium; RV, right ventricle; SVC, superior vena cava.

- The technique also has therapeutic applications, including device closure of atrial septal defects, ventricular septal defects, and patent ductus arteriosus; performance of pulmonary artery angioplasty and stent placement; balloon valvuloplasty of valvar aortic/pulmonary stenosis; angioplasty or stent repair of coarctation; and transcatheter replacement of pulmonary valves.

Calculation of Flows, Shunts, and Resistances

- Cardiac output can be calculated using thermodilution or Fick principle. When using Fick principle, oxygen is used as an indicator, and blood flow can be calculated using oxygen consumption (measured or assumed) divided by the arteriovenous oxygen content difference.

$$\text{Qs (cardiac output)} = \frac{\text{(oxygen consumption)}}{\text{(systemic arterial oxygen content} - \text{systemic venous oxygen content)}}$$

- In most instances, the fraction of dissolved oxygen as a percentage of total oxygen content is negligible and can be ignored. That makes the equation for cardiac output simpler as shown below:

$$\text{Qs (systemic blood flow in L/min)} = \frac{O_2 \text{ consumption (L/min)}}{(1.36) \times (10) \times \text{(Hgb gm/dL)} \times \text{(aorta sat} - \text{superior vena cava sat)}}$$

Similarly,

$$\text{Qp (pulmonary blood flow in L/min)} = \frac{O_2 \text{ consumption (L/min)}}{(1.36) \times (10) \times \text{(Hgb in gm/dL)} \times \text{(pulmonary vein sat} - \text{pulmonary artery sat)}}$$

- **Normal cardiac output is 3 to 4.5 L/min/m^2.**
- Mathematically, the ratio of pulmonary blood flow to systemic blood flow is easier to calculate and is expressed as:

$$\text{Qp/Qs} = \frac{\text{aortic sat} - \text{SVC sat}}{\text{pulmonary venous sat} - \text{pulmonary arterial sat}}$$

- **Using the mixed venous saturation, systemic saturation, and Hgb, one can use the same principle to calculate cardiac output in any patient who has a central venous line.**

Resistance

- Systemic and pulmonary vascular resistance (SVR and PVR) can also be calculated using the catheterization data. This calculation is based on Ohm law (resistance equals the pressure change across the vascular bed divided by flow):

SVR = (AO − RA)/Qs
PVR = (PA − LA)/Qp

in which
AO = mean systemic (aorta) pressure
RA = mean right atrial pressure
PA = mean pulmonary artery pressure
LA = mean left atrial pressure

- **A PVR (Rp) of 1 to 3 Wood units/m^2 is considered to be within the normal range.**

Appendix III
Syndromes Glossary

Angela E. Scheuerle, MD

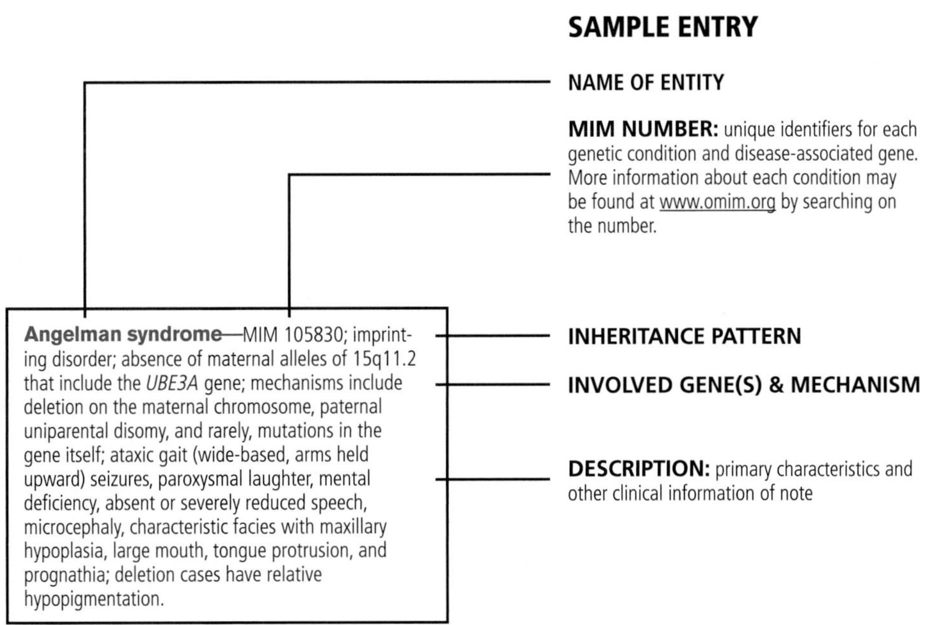

SAMPLE ENTRY
NAME OF ENTITY
MIM NUMBER: unique identifiers for each genetic condition and disease-associated gene. More information about each condition may be found at www.omim.org by searching on the number.
Angelman syndrome—MIM 105830; imprinting disorder; absence of maternal alleles of 15q11.2 that include the UBE3A gene; mechanisms include deletion on the maternal chromosome, paternal uniparental disomy, and rarely, mutations in the gene itself; ataxic gait (wide-based, arms held upward) seizures, paroxysmal laughter, mental deficiency, absent or severely reduced speech, microcephaly, characteristic facies with maxillary hypoplasia, large mouth, tongue protrusion, and prognathia; deletion cases have relative hypopigmentation.
INHERITANCE PATTERN
INVOLVED GENE(S) & MECHANISM
DESCRIPTION: primary characteristics and other clinical information of note

4p syndrome (Wolf-Hirschhorn syndrome; deletion 4p; monosomy 4p)—MIM 194190; characterized by growth failure of prenatal onset, microcephaly, "Greek helmet" facies (high forehead, prominent glabella, arched eyebrows, straight nose), hypertelorism, hypotonia, neurocognitive impairment, seizures, scoliosis

5α-reductase deficiency—MIM 264600; autosomal recessive; mutations in *SRD5A2*; results in defective dihydrotestosterone formation and decreased plasma levels; 46,XY males show ambiguous external genitalia at birth but develop masculinization at puberty.

22q11.2 deletion syndrome—see "22q11.2 Deletion Syndrome."

22 tetrasomy syndrome—see Glossary entry "cat eye syndrome."

Aarskog syndrome—MIM 305400; X-linked recessive; mutations in *FGD1*; characterized by short stature, characteristic facies, "shawl" scrotum (penoscrotal transposition), syndactyly, various ocular findings, and prominent umbilicus; delayed bone age; mild to moderate intellectual disability in 1/3; female carriers may show mild features.

Achondrogenesis type I—MIM 200600 and 600972; autosomal recessive; mutations in *TRIP11* or *SLC26A2*; short-limbed dwarfism; most severe form of chondrodysplasia; characterized by deficient ossification of lumbar vertebrae and absent ossification of pelvic bones; stillbirth or early death

Achondroplasia—MIM 100800; autosomal dominant; mutations in *FGFR3*; characterized by disproportionate short stature with rhizomelia, macrocephaly, small foramen magnum (risk of cord compression), caudal narrowing of spinal canal, mild hypotonia, and relative glucose intolerance; cognitive development is normal; 90% result from new mutations, usually paternal in origin; American Academy of Pediatrics (AAP) Health Maintenance Guidelines published

Acidotic newborns, metabolic diseases in—see "Metabolic Diseases in Acidotic Newborns."

Acrodermatitis enteropathica—MIM 201100; autosomal recessive; mutations in *SLC39A4*; characterized by abnormal intestinal absorption of zinc, resulting in zinc deficiency; secondary effects include vesiculobullous and eczematous skin lesions in the perioral and perineal areas, cheeks, knees, and elbows; photophobia, conjunctivitis, corneal dystrophy; chronic diarrhea; nail dystrophy; growth retardation; superinfections and candidal infections; treatment requires lifelong zinc supplementation.

Acute intermittent porphyria—MIM 176000; autosomal dominant; mutations in *HMBS*; characterized by recurrent attacks of severe abdominal pain, GI dysfunction, and neurologic disturbances; attacks may be precipitated by medications, alcohol, endocrine factors, stress, infections, or caloric restriction; attacks are rare before puberty and are more likely in women than in men.

Adrenoleukodystrophy—MIM 300100; X-linked recessive; mutations in *ABCD1*; defect in peroxisomal β-oxidation and accumulation of very long chain fatty acids (VLCFA); onset ranges from childhood to adulthood; progressive neurodegeneration; carrier females may have symptoms; currently included in many state; newborn screening programs in the United States

Agenesis of corpus callosum—multifactorial; complete or partial absence of the major tracts connecting the right and left hemispheres; can be associated with hydrocephalus, seizures, developmental delay, spasticity, and hypertelorism; can be isolated or found with other brain malformations and in many multiple anomaly and chromosomal syndromes

Aicardi syndrome—MIM 304050; apparently X-linked dominant; gene remains unknown; characterized by microcephaly, various brain malformations including cysts and heterotopias, infantile spasms, chorioretinal lacunae, and costovertebral skeletal abnormalities; lethal in males

Alagille syndrome (arteriohepatic dysplasia)—MIM 118450 and 610205; autosomal dominant; mutations in *JAG1* or *NOTCH2*; characterized by paucity or absence of intrahepatic bile ducts with progressive destruction of bile ducts and five clinical abnormalities: cholestasis, cardiac disease characteristic facies (broad forehead, deep-set eyes that are widely spaced and underdeveloped, a small, pointed mandible), skeletal defects, and eye abnormalities; 39% also have renal involvement.

Albright syndrome—see Glossary entry "McCune-Albright syndrome."

Alexander disease—MIM 203450; autosomal dominant; mutations in *GFAP*; three subtypes: infantile, juvenile, adult; characterized by macrocephaly in infants, neurocognitive delay, spasticity and seizures; older patients show bulbar or pseudobulbar symptoms and spasticity; progressive neurodegenerative with death within 10 years of onset; see also Glossary entry "Canavan disease."

Alopecia areata—MIM 104000; multifactorial and heterogeneous; genetically determined, immune-mediated; one of the most common human autoimmune conditions; spectrum of severity; includes nail abnormalities

α_1-antitrypsin deficiency—MIM 613490; autosomal recessive; mutations in *SERPINA1*; liver disease in children and adults, emphysema in adults; testing most commonly done by protein phenotype; M allele is normal; the most common pathogenic allele is Z.

Alport syndrome—MIM 301050; X-linked dominant; mutations in *COL4A5*; characterized by renal failure due to glomerulonephropathy, sensorineural hearing loss, and variable eye anomalies. Usually presents in infancy with hematuria; proteinuria and hearing loss are later findings; carrier mothers may show microscopic hematuria; less common autosomal recessive and dominant forms

Andersen disease—see Glossary entry "glycogen storage disease IV (GSD4)."

Androgen insensitivity—MIM 300068; X-linked recessive; mutations in *AR*; affected 46,XY males have female external genitalia with blind-ending vagina, absent uterus, and otherwise female features; testes are present; androgen levels are normal to high with inability of physiologic response.

Angelman syndrome—MIM 105830; imprinting disorder; absence of maternal alleles of 15q11.2 that include the *UBE3A* gene; mechanisms include deletion on the maternal chromosome, paternal uniparental disomy, and rarely, mutations in the gene itself; ataxic gait (wide-based, arms held upward) seizures, paroxysmal laughter, mental deficiency, absent or severely reduced speech, microcephaly, characteristic facies with maxillary hypoplasia, large mouth, tongue protrusion, and prognathia; deletion cases have relative hypopigmentation.

Apert syndrome—MIM 101200; autosomal dominant; mutations in *FGFR2*; characterized by craniosynostosis (typically coronal), turribrachycephaly, underdevelopment of the middle third of the face, hypertelorism and proptosis, variable but pronounced syndactyly. Other anomalies include characteristic facies, malrotation and gastrointestinal atresias, and congenital heart defects; neurocognitive delays are present, but intelligence can be normal.

Aplasia cutis congenita (nonsyndromic)—MIM 107600; mutations in *BMS1*; congenitally localized absence of skin on the scalp vertex, may be associated with underlying skull defects; may also be found in numerous syndromes including trisomy 13

Arthrogryposis multiplex congenita—a category of conditions rather than a single entity; congenital contracture(s) of many if not all major joints; some syndromes with identified genes and defined heritability; pathogenically variable with origin anywhere along the axis from motor cortex to muscle cell

Ataxia telangiectasia syndrome (Louis-Bar)—MIM 208900; autosomal recessive; mutations in *ATM*; characterized by progressive ataxia within the 1st year, telangiectasias by age 8 years, neurodegeneration, lymphopenia, immune deficit (low to absent IgA and IgE), and growth deficiency; increased risk of lymphomas and leukemias in patients and carrier parents

Axenfeld-Rieger syndrome—MIM 180500; autosomal dominant; mutations in *PITX2*; characterized by Rieger anomaly of the eye (anterior segment dysgenesis), glaucoma, hypodontia, maxillary hypoplasia, and umbilical abnormalities

Bardet-Biedl syndrome—MIM 209900; autosomal recessive; mutations in various genes; caused by abnormalities in nonmotile cilia; characterized by mental retardation, retinitis pigmentosa, obesity, polydactyly, renal anomalies, hypogonadism, and neurocognitive impairments (looks superficially like Prader-Willi syndrome with polydactyly)

Bart syndrome—see Glossary entry "epidermolysis bullosa dystrophica, autosomal dominant."

Barth syndrome—MIM 302060; X-linked recessive; mutations in *TAZ*; affected males have skeletal myopathy and cardiomyopathy, neutropenia, growth delay, and characteristic facies; carrier females usually unaffected

Bartter syndrome—see "Bartter Syndrome."

Basal cell nevus syndrome—MIM 109400; autosomal dominant; mutations in *PTCH1*, *PTCH2*, or *SUFU*; characterized by basal cell carcinomas, macrocephaly, odontogenic keratocysts of jaws, bifid ribs, pits in the palms and soles, and calcification of the falx cerebri

Becker muscular dystrophy—see "Muscular Dystrophies."

Beckwith-Wiedemann syndrome—MIM 130650; imprinting disorder of chromosome 11 or autosomal dominant due to mutations in *CDKN1C*; characterized by overgrowth of prenatal onset, omphalocele, macroglossia, hemihyperplasia, and characteristic facies; significant risk of Wilms tumor and hepatoblastoma especially in patients with hemihyperplasia; neurocognitive impairment if neonatal hypoglycemia is unrecognized or uncontrolled

Behçet syndrome—MIM 109650; presumed autosomal dominant; gene unidentified; disease mechanism unknown; recurrent inflammatory lesions, oral and genital ulcers, various skin and eye lesions

Bloch-Sulzberger syndrome—see Glossary entry "incontinentia pigmenti."

Bloom syndrome—MIM 210900; autosomal recessive chromosome instability syndrome; mutations in *BLM*; characterized by growth deficiency of prenatal onset, microcephaly, facial telangiectatic erythema in a butterfly pattern, skin pigmentation changes, mild neurocognitive impairment, and characteristic facies; high risk of malignancy; increased prevalence in Ashkenazi Jews

Blue diaper syndrome—MIM 211000; probably autosomal recessive; gene unidentified; defect in intestinal transport of tryptophan; bacterial degradation of the intraluminal tryptophan forms water-soluble metabolites that turn blue on exposure to oxygen; may be a nongenetic *Pseudomonas aeruginosa* metabolite; only two brothers have been documented with the transport defect.

Bourneville disease, Bourneville–Pringle disease—see "Tuberous Sclerosis Complex."

Branchio-Oto-Renal syndrome—MIM 113650; autosomal dominant; mutations in gene *EYA1*; characterized by ear malformations, hearing impairment, branchial fistulae and cysts, and renal malformations

Byler disease—see Glossary entry "progressive familial intrahepatic cholestasis."

Caffey disease—see Glossary entry "infantile cortical hyperostosis."

Campomelic dysplasia—MIM 114290; autosomal dominant; mutations in *SOX9*; skeletal dysplasia with bowing of long bones, laryngotracheomalacia, and ambiguous genitalia or sex reversal in 46,XY patients

Canavan disease—MIM 271900; autosomal recessive; mutations in *ASPA*; progressive, degenerative demyelination and leukodystrophy; usually begins in infancy with macrocephaly, hypotonia, and developmental regression; increased prevalence in Ashkenazi Jews; features similar to Alexander disease—see Glossary entry "Alexander Disease."

Caroli disease—MIM 600643; inheritance pattern unclear; gene unidentified; overlaps significantly with the polycystic kidney syndromes and may not represent a separate entity; characterized by cystic dilatation of the intrahepatic bile ducts; recurrent bouts of cholangitis and biliary abscesses secondary to bile stasis and gallstones

Cat eye syndrome (22 Tetrasomy syndrome)—MIM 115470; presence of an extra chromosome comprising two identical segments of chromosome 22 (i.e., the patient has four total copies of chromosome 22); characterized by coloboma of iris, down-slanting palpebral fissures, anal atresia, cardiac defects, renal agenesis; mild neurocognitive impairment; growth is usually normal.

Charcot-Marie-Tooth disease (hereditary motor and sensory neuropathy [HMSN] or peroneal muscular atrophy)—MIM 118200; various inheritance patterns; mutations in various genes; group of sensorineural peripheral polyneuropathies that are most common cause of chronic peripheral neuropathy; characterized by insidious onset of slowly progressive weakness and atrophy of distal limb muscles, impaired sensation

CHARGE syndrome—MIM 214800; autosomal dominant; mutations in *CHD7*; characterized by Coloboma, Heart disease, choanal Atresia, Retarded growth and development and/or CNS anomalies, Genital anomalies and/or hypogonadism, and Ear anomalies and/or deafness. The ear malformation is characteristic: Mondini defect and hypoplastic semicircular canals of the inner ear in the presence of other typical malformations are diagnostic for CHARGE.

Chédiak-Higashi syndrome—MIM 214500; autosomal recessive; mutations in *LYST*; characterized by oculocutaneous albinism, lack of natural killer cells, decreased neutrophil and monocyte migration, anemia, neurodegeneration, hepatomegaly, and splenomegaly

Chondrodysplasia punctata 2, X-linked dominant—MIM 302960; X-linked dominant; mutations in *EBP*; characterized by short stature, skeletal changes including stippling of epiphyses and rhizomelic limb shortening, linear or blotchy ichthyosis, and eye findings including cataracts and microphthalmia. Most affected patients are female; germline inheritance considered lethal to males

Ciliary dyskinesia—see Glossary entry "primary ciliary dyskinesia."

Cockayne syndrome—MIM 216400; autosomal recessive; mutations in *ERCC6* and *ERCC8*; characterized by postnatal growth deficiency, microcephaly, neurocognitive impairment, ataxia, hearing loss, seizures, characteristic facies, hypertension, renal dysfunction, and photosensitivity

Coffin-Lowry syndrome—MIM 303600; X-linked dominant; mutations in *RSK2*; characterized by severe intellectual disability in affected males, microcephaly, characteristic facies, short stature, fleshy hands; stimulus-induced drop attacks in 20%; carrier females can have intellectual disability.

Cohen—MIM 216550; autosomal recessive; mutations in *VSP13B*; characterized by intellectual disability, microcephaly, progressive retinopathy, characteristic facies, obesity, and intermittent congenital neutropenia

Cole-Carpenter syndrome—MIM 112240; autosomal dominant; mutations in *P4HB* or *SEC24D*; characterized by bone fragility, craniosynostosis, proptosis, hydrocephalus, and characteristic facies

Congenital adrenal hyperplasia—see "Congenital Adrenal Hyperplasia."

Congenital amegakaryocytic thrombocytopenia—MIM 604498; autosomal recessive; mutations in *MPL*; characterized by thrombocytopenia and megakaryocytopenia

Congenital disorders of glycosylation—any different types, most are autosomal recessive; enzymatic defects in synthesis of glycoproteins; two main groups: type I and type II. Type I defects are abnormalities in glycoprotein assembly. Type II defects involved abnormal processing of protein-bound glycans; more likely a disease mechanism than a set of discrete conditions

Congenital hypothyroidism—see "Hypothyroidism, Congenital."

Congenital insensitivity to pain—MIM 243000; autosomal recessive; mutations in *SCN9A*; MIM 147430; autosomal dominant; gene unidentified; characterized by absence of pain perception and hyposmia/anosmia

Congenital rubella syndrome—see Glossary entry "fetal rubella syndrome."

Conradi-Hünermann syndrome—see Glossary entry "chondrodysplasia punctata 2, X-linked dominant."

Cornelia de Lange syndrome (Brachmann-De Lange syndrome, de Lange syndrome)—MIM 122470; autosomal dominant; mutations in various genes, most commonly *NIPBL*; characterized by growth failure of prenatal onset microcephaly, hirsutism, limb reduction defects (particularly ulnar ray defects) gastroesophageal reflux, congenital heart defects, neurocognitive impairment, and characteristic facies

Costello syndrome—MIM 218040; autosomal dominant; mutations in *HRAS*; characterized by coarse facial features, short stature, postnatal feeding problems, curly or sparse fine hair, loose soft skin, hypertrophic cardiomyopathy, arrhythmias especially chaotic atrial rhythm/multifocal atrial tachycardia; 15% lifetime risk for malignant tumors

Crigler-Najjar syndrome, types I and II—MIM 218800 and 606785; autosomal recessive; mutations in *UGT1A1*; absence of hepatic uridine 5′-diphospho-glucuronosyltransferase activity leading to unconjugated hyperbilirubinemia on 1st day of life without evidence of hemolysis; type I treatment requires phototherapy to prevent kernicterus; type II treatable with phenobarbital treatment

Crouzon syndrome (craniofacial dysostosis)—MIM 123500; autosomal dominant; mutations in *FGFR2*; characterized by craniosynostosis (most often coronal), exophthalmos due to shallow orbits, hypertelorism, high palate, and hypoplasia of maxilla; obstructive sleep apnea is common; hands and feet are not involved.

Cyclic neutropenia—MIM 162800; autosomal dominant; mutations in *ELANE*; lack of granulocyte macrophage colony-stimulating factor (GM-CSF); characterized by fever, mouth lesions, cervical adenitis, and gastroenteritis; underlying regular 21-day cyclic fluctuation in number of blood leukocytes

Cystic fibrosis—see "Cystic Fibrosis."

Cystinosis—MIM 219800; autosomal recessive; mutations in *CTNS*; lysosomal storage of cysteine; patients normal at birth with development of rickets, nephrolithiasis, corneal crystal accumulation, peripheral retinopathy, hepatosplenomegaly and pancreatic insufficiency. Multiple organs affected; normal intelligence with deterioration over time

Cystinuria—MIM 220100; both autosomal dominant and autosomal recessive forms; mutations in *SLC3A1* or *SLC7A9*; characterized by nephrolithiasis

Dent syndrome—MIM 300009; X-linked recessive; mutations in *CLCN5* or *OCRL*; proximal renal tubular dysfunction; proteinuria, hypercalcuria, nephrocalcinosis, nephrolithiasis, and chronic kidney disease; end-stage renal disease by 30 to 50 years of age in affected males. Carrier females rarely develop chronic kidney disease.

De Sanctis-Cacchione syndrome—MIM 278800; autosomal recessive; mutations in *ERCC6*; characterized by xeroderma pigmentosum, dwarfism, gonadal hypoplasia, and neurocognitive impairment with degeneration; see also Glossary entry "xeroderma pigmentosum."

Diamond-Blackfan syndrome—MIM 105650; autosomal dominant; mutations in *RPS19*; congenital pure red cell aplasia due to failure of erythropoiesis; characterized by normochromic macrocytic anemia, postnatal growth retardation, craniofacial, limb, heart, and urinary system malformations in 30–50%

DiGeorge syndrome—see Glossary entry "22q11.2 deletion syndrome."

Down syndrome—see "Down Syndrome (Trisomy 21)."

Dubin-Johnson Syndrome—MIM 237500; autosomal recessive; mutations in *ABCC2*; characterized by elevated conjugated bilirubin, large amounts of coproporphyrin I in urine, and deposits of melanin-like pigment in hepatocellular lysosomes; otherwise normal liver function

Dubowitz syndrome—MIM 223370; autosomal recessive; gene unidentified; characterized by growth failure of prenatal onset, microcephaly, eczema-like skin disorder, brachydactyly, various ocular abnormalities, neurocognitive impairment, characteristic facies that resemble fetal alcohol syndrome

Duchenne muscular dystrophy—see "Muscular Dystrophies."

Dyskeratosis congenita—many types; various inheritance patterns; mutations in various genes; abnormality in telomere stability; characterized by triad of reticulated skin hyperpigmentation, nail dystrophy, and leukoplakia; bone marrow failure and dysplasia that can include leukemia; higher risk of other cancers and other conditions usually associated with aging

Eagle-Barrett syndrome—see Glossary entry "prune belly syndrome."

Ectodermal dysplasia—many types; various inheritance patterns; mutations in various genes; most common type is X-linked recessive; characterized by poor development, or absence, of teeth, nails, hair, and sweat glands

Ectrodactyly-ectodermal dysplasia-clefting syndrome—MIM 129900; autosomal dominant; mutations in *TP63* cause about half; characterized by split-hand/split-foot, ectodermal dysplasia with keratitis, and cleft lip and/or cleft palate

Edwards syndrome—see Glossary entry "trisomy 18."

Ehlers-Danlos syndrome—MIM 130000 (classic type); autosomal dominant and autosomal recessive group of conditions classified by type; mutations in some of the collagen genes; hypermobile joints and hyperextensible or fragile skin are characteristic features across the types, but the specific phenotypes vary; classic type (type I) is caused my mutations in *COL5A1* or *COL5A2*. Abnormalities of the vasculature and hollow organs are characteristic of vascular type (type IV), caused by mutations in *COL3A1*.

Epidermolysis bullosa—four major types: simplex, junctional, dystrophic, and Kindler syndrome; fragility of the skin that manifests as blisters and erosions with minimal trauma; severity varies with type.

Epidermolysis bullosa dystrophica, autosomal dominant—MIM 131750; autosomal dominant; mutations in *COL7A1*; characterized by congenital aplasia of the skin on the lower legs and feet; nail defects and recurrent blistering of the skin and mucous membranes

Fabry disease—MIM 301500; X-linked; mutations in *GLA*; deficiency α-galactosidase A leading to lysosomal storage of glycosphingolipids; characterized by angiofibromas (buttocks, inguinal area, fingernails, and lips) and vascular involvement; secondary effects of vascular involvement include renal failure, cardiovascular disease, stroke, GI complaints, anhidrosis, and tingling/burning sensation in the periphery; carrier females frequently manifest symptom; enzyme replacement therapy is available.

Familial adenomatous polyposis—MIM 171500; autosomal dominant; mutations in *APC*; characterized by multiple GI polyps with malignant transformation, skin cysts, supernumerary teeth, and multiple osteoma; Gardner syndrome is a variant in which desmoid tumors and other neoplasms occur along with the colon and rectum adenomas.

Familial dysautonomia (hereditary sensory and autonomic neuropathy)—MIM 223900; autosomal recessive; mutations in *IKBKAP*; characterized by aberrant sensory and autonomic functions; progressive course of poor growth, alacrima, decreased taste sense, postural hypotension, episodic hyperhidrosis, hypotonia, and decreased pain sensation; increased prevalence in Ashkenazi Jews

Familial Mediterranean fever—MIM 249100; usually autosomal recessive; mutations in *MEFV*; characterized by recurrent fever with painful inflammation of the peritoneum, synovium, and/or pleura, and amyloidosis with renal failure

Fanconi anemia—MIM 227650; most are autosomal recessive; mutations in various genes; characterized by bone marrow failure, increased risk of malignancy, and physical abnormalities including short stature, abnormal skin pigmentation, skeletal malformations, microcephaly, and eye and genitourinary tract anomalies; radial ray defect that usually includes absent or hypoplastic thumbs, which can distinguish it clinically from thrombocytopenia absent radius (TAR) syndrome, in which the thumbs are spared

Farber lipogranulomatosis—MIM 228000; autosomal recessive; mutations in *ASAH1*; lysosomal storage disease caused by deficiency of acid ceramidase; characterized by subcutaneous nodules, painful and progressively deformed joints, and laryngeal involvement with hoarseness

Fetal alcohol spectrum disorder (FASD)—see "Fetal Alcohol Syndrome" chapter.

Fetal alcohol syndrome—see "Fetal Alcohol Syndrome" chapter.

Fetal brain disruption sequence—brain destruction resulting in collapse of the fetal skull, microcephaly, scalp rugae, and neurologic impairment; has come to recent attention because it can be a result of in utero Zika virus infection

Fetal hydantoin syndrome—hydantoin (phenytoin) exposure during pregnancy; 5–10% of exposed fetuses; characterized by growth deficiency of prenatal onset, characteristic facies, neurocognitive impairment, and nail hypoplasia/aplasia; may have cleft lip and palate, and cardiac defects

Fetal rubella syndrome—rubella virus infection, especially in the first trimester; characterized by mental deficiency, microcephaly, deafness, cataract, glaucoma, patent ductus arteriosus, cardiac septal defects, hepatosplenomegaly, anemia, and thrombocytopenia; hearing impairment is the most common defect; vaccine-preventable disease

Fetal valproate syndrome—valproate exposure in the first trimester; characterized by neurocognitive impairments, neural tube defects, cardiovascular anomalies, and characteristic facies

Fetal warfarin syndrome—warfarin exposure during pregnancy; features vary with exposure window: 6- to 9-week exposure characterized by defects associated with aberrant cartilage: nasal hypoplasia, stippled epiphyses, hypoplastic distal phalanges; 14- to 20-week exposure characterized by central nervous system defects, eye anomalies, and intrauterine growth retardation. Exposure in the third trimester is less concerning.

Fibrodysplasia ossificans progressiva (FOP)—MIM 135100; autosomal dominant; mutations in *ACVR1*; characterized by short hallux, progressive ossification of muscles and subcutaneous tissues, and hearing loss; any trauma (including iatrogenic such as needle sticks) can cause ectopic ossification.

Five-alpha reductase deficiency—see Glossary entry "5α- reductase deficiency."

Focal dermal hypoplasia—MIM 305600; X-linked dominant; mutations in *PORCN*; characterized by linear atrophy of the skin with fat herniation through the dermis, linear pigmentation abnormalities, and papillomata; may have eye, oral, or limb abnormalities; 90% of affected patients are female; germline inheritance considered lethal to males

Fragile X syndrome—MIM 600624; X-linked; triplet repeat mutation in *FMR1* with expansion risk increased when inherited from mother; full expansion (>200 repeats) characterized by mental deficiency, autism spectrum disorders, macrocephaly, prognathism, large ears, mild connective tissue dysplasia, and macroorchidism after puberty; female full mutation carriers can manifest the phenotype; female carriers of premutations (55 to 200 repeats) have increased risk of premature ovarian insufficiency; male and female premutation carriers have increased risk of fragile X–associated tremor ataxia syndrome as adults.

Fragile XE syndrome—MIM 309548; X-linked recessive; triplet repeat mutations in *AFF2*; characterized by mild to moderate intellectual disability and other neurocognitive problems

Friedreich ataxia—MIM 229300; autosomal recessive; triplet repeat mutations in *FXN*; progressive loss of large myelinated axons in peripheral nerves; characterized by progressive cerebellar and spinal cord dysfunction; symptoms usually appearing in late childhood or adolescence; patients have high-arched foot, hammer toes, and cardiac failure.

Fukuyama muscular dystrophy—see Glossary entry "muscular dystrophy-dystroglycanopathy with brain and eye anomalies."

Galactosemia—MIM 230400; autosomal recessive; mutations most commonly in *GALT*; inability to metabolize lactose; characterized by jaundice, hepatosplenomegaly, liver failure, renal tubular dysfunction, hypotonia, cataracts, and risk of infection; usually symptomatic in the neonatal period; may present with sepsis, particularly from *Escherichia coli*; treated by restricting lactose; currently included in most state newborn screening programs in the United States

Gardner syndrome—see Glossary entry "familial adenomatous polyposis."

Gaucher disease—MIM 230800; autosomal recessive; mutations in *GBA*; deficiency of glucocerebrosidase, leading to accumulation and storage of glucocerebroside in the reticuloendothelial system; three types: type I includes adult-onset hepatosplenomegaly, cytopenia, and pulmonary disease; type II presents in infancy with the features of type I and bulbar and pyramidal signs as well as cognitive impairment; type III includes the features of type I with juvenile onset as well as oculomotor apraxia, seizure, and progressive myoclonic epilepsy. There are also perinatal-lethal and cardiovascular forms. Enzyme replacement therapy is available.

Gilbert syndrome—MIM 143500; autosomal recessive; mutations in *UGT1A1*; reduced activity of glucuronyltransferase activity leading to mild unconjugated hyperbilirubinemia that worsens with stresses on the body, such as fasting; carriers can manifest symptoms.

Gilles de la Tourette syndrome—see "Tics."

Glanzmann thrombasthenia—MIM 273800; autosomal recessive; mutations in *ITGA2B* and *ITGB3*; involves defective primary platelet aggregation (size and survival of platelets is normal); presents as bleeding dyscrasia

Glucose-6-phosphate dehydrogenase deficiency or G6PD deficiency—see "Glucose-6-Phosphate Dehydrogenase."

Glutauric aciduria I—MIM 231670; autosomal recessive; mutations in *GCDH*; inability to metabolize lysine, hydroxylysine, and tryptophan; characterized by basal ganglia atrophy and scarring with progressive movement disorder, macrocephaly, hepatomegaly; currently included in many state newborn screening programs in the United States

Glycine encephalopathy—MIM 605899; autosomal recessive; mutations in genes of the glycine cleavage system *AMT*, *GLDC*, or *GCSH*; most patients present in the neonatal period with lethargy, hypotonia, and myoclonus progressing to apnea; survivors have intractable seizures and profound intellectual disability; currently included in many state newborn screening programs in the United States

Glycogen storage disease 1A (GSD1A; von Gierke)—MIM 232200; autosomal recessive; mutations in *G6PC*; accumulation of glycogen and defective gluconeogenesis; characterized by fasting hypoglycemia, growth retardation, hepatomegaly, lactic acidosis, hyperlipidemia, and hyperuricemia

Glycogen storage disease IV (GSD4; Andersen disease)—MIM 232500; autosomal recessive; mutations in *GBE1*; defect of glycogen-branching enzyme; classic form characterized by hepatomegaly and failure to thrive in the 1st few months of life, progressing to liver cirrhosis and splenomegaly; neuromuscular forms can present at any age.

GM1 gangliosidosis—MIM 230500; autosomal recessive; mutations in *GLB1*; lysosomal storage disease with accumulation of ganglioside substrates. Three types: Type I presents in infancy with CNS dysfunction and life expectancy of 2 to 3 years; type II has onset between 1 and 10 years with developmental delays and regression and may include skeletal dysplasia; type III begins in 2nd or 3rd decade with parkinsonian features and cardiomyopathy.

Goldenhar syndrome— see Glossary entry "oculo-auriculo-vertebral."

Goltz syndrome—see Glossary entry "focal dermal hypoplasia."

Gorlin syndrome—see Glossary entry "basal cell nevus syndrome."

Hallerman-Streif syndrome—MIM 234100; inheritance undefined; gene unidentified; characterized by hypotrichosis, microphthalmia, cataracts, beaked nose, micrognathia, dental anomalies, and proportionate short stature; typically normal intelligence

Hartnup disorder—MIM 234500; autosomal recessive; mutations in *SLC6A19*; defect in transport of monoamine monocarboxylic amino acids by intestinal mucosa and renal tubules; characterized by photosensitivity and a pellagra-like skin rash, cerebellar ataxia, emotional instability, and amino aciduria

Hemochromatosis—MIM 235200; autosomal recessive; mutations in *HFE* or *BMP2*; excessive iron storage in multiple organs leading to compromise or failure of those organs, especially the liver and pancreas; can have increased apparent skin pigmentation from iron deposition; early symptoms include abdominal pain, weakness/lethargy, and weight loss; treatment is phlebotomy; men have earlier and more severe problems than women, who many not manifest until after menopause.

Hemophilia—see "Hemophilia."

Hereditary angioedema—see "Hereditary Angioedema (C1 Esterase Deficiency)."

Hereditary fructose intolerance—MIM 229600; autosomal recessive; mutations in *ALDOB*; deficiency of fructose-1-phosphate aldolase or fructose 1,6-diphosphatase; characterized by vomiting, diarrhea, hypoglycemic seizures, and jaundice upon exposure to fructose or sucrose

Hereditary spherocytosis—see "Hereditary Spherocytosis."

Hermanski-Pudlak syndrome—MIM 203300; autosomal recessive; mutations in *HPS1*; characterized by oculocutaneous albinism, bleeding, and lysosomal ceroid storage; electron micrography shows absence of platelet dense granules and can be diagnostic; increased incidence in Puerto Rico

Holt-Oram syndrome—MIM 142900; autosomal dominant; mutations in *TBX5*; characterized by upper limb defects, typically radial ray defects, and cardiac anomalies; most common combination is a missing or hypoplastic thumb and atrial septal defect.

Homocystinuria—MIM 236200; autosomal recessive; mutations in *CBS*; deficient cystathionine synthetase activity leading to marfanoid habitus and neurocognitive impairment, also thrombotic events, generalized hypopigmentation, and, with progression, seizures; currently included in many state newborn screening programs in the United States

Hunter syndrome—see Glossary entry "mucopolysaccharidosis II."

Huntington disease—MIM 143100; autosomal dominant; triplet repeat mutations in *HHT* with expansion risk increased when inherited from father; characterized in adults by progressive neurodegeneration including chorea, dystonia, incoordination, and cognitive decline; childhood Huntington manifests as developmental delay and seizures which worsen with time. Youngest documented patient is 2 years of age.

Hurler syndrome—see Glossary entry "mucopolysaccharidosis I."

Hutchinson-Gilford progeria syndrome—MIM 176670; autosomal dominant; mutations in *LMNA*; all cases to date have been de novo mutations; characterized by the appearance of premature aging, severe growth failure, atherosclerosis, lipodystrophy, alopecia, and decreased joint mobility; cognitive development is normal.

Hyperammonemic newborns, metabolic diseases in—see "Metabolic Diseases in Hyperammonemic Newborns."

Hyperekplexia—MIM 149400; autosomal dominant and autosomal recessive types; mutations in *GLRA1*; characterized by exaggerated startle response with intense generalized hypertonia that may be prolonged; prolonged episodes put an infant at risk for apnea or aspiration; residual effects in adulthood include nocturnal myoclonus and startle-induced falls.

Hyperimmunoglobulinemia E syndrome—see "Hyperimmunoglobulinemia E Syndrome."

Hyperinsulinism—see "Hyperinsulinism."

Hypoglycemic newborns, metabolic diseases in—see "Metabolic Diseases in Hypoglycemic Newborns."

Hypogonadotropic hypogonadism with or without anosmia—MIM 308700; X-linked or autosomal dominant; some digenic inheritance; multiple genes involved; characterized by some degree of hypogonadism and altered or absent sense of smell due to olfactory lobe agenesis; bimanual synkinesia; not all affected persons are infertile.

Hypophosphatasia—see "Hypophosphatemic Disorders."

Hypothyroidism, congenital—see "Hypothyroidism, Congenital."

Ichthyosis—a group of conditions that result from abnormal hyperkeratosis; the most common and least severe type is ichthyosis vulgaris, an autosomal dominant condition caused by mutations in *FLG*. The X-linked type of Ichthyosis is caused by steroid sulfatase deficiency and mutations in *STS*. Most of the remainder are autosomal recessive, caused by mutations in a variety of genes. They can be severe, especially at birth when they can present with a collodion membrane.

Immune deficiency—see "Immune Deficiency."

Immune dysregulation, polyendocrinopathy, enteropathy X-linked syndrome (IPEX)—MIM 304790; X-linked recessive; mutations in *FOXP3*; characterized by enteropathy and severe diarrhea in infancy, type I diabetes mellitus, and dermatitis

Incontinentia pigmenti (IP)—MIM 308300; X-linked dominant; mutations in *IKBKG* (*NEMO*); characterized by four-stage evolving skin lesions and abnormalities of skin appendages, eosinophilia, high risk of neonatal stroke; neurocognitive problems in patients with stroke or CNS anomalies, but majority of patients are neurocognitively normal; malformations of internal organs and the skeleton are not characteristic of IP.

Infantile cortical hyperostosis—MIM 114000; autosomal dominant; mutations in *COL1A1*; inflammation of bone with cortical changes that appears before 5 months of age and usually resolves by 2 years

Jansen metaphyseal chondrodysplasia—MIM 156400; autosomal dominant; mutations in *PTHR1*; metaphyseal chondrodysplasia; characterized by severe short stature, short bowed limbs, small jaw, and hypercalcemia/hypophosphatemia despite normal parathyroid function

Job syndrome—see "Hyperimmunoglobulinemia E Syndrome."

Johanson-Blizzard syndrome—MIM 243800; autosomal recessive; mutations in *UBR1*; characterized by growth failure, hypoplastic alae nasae, abnormal hair patterns, oligodontia, hypothyroidism, sensorineural hearing loss, imperforate anus, and exocrine pancreatic insufficiency

Kabuki syndrome—MIM 147920; autosomal dominant; mutations in *KMT2D* or *KDM6A*; characterized by growth deficiency of postnatal onset, intellectual disability, hypotonia, characteristic facies resembling Kabuki dance makeup (long palpebral fissures with lateral ectropion, ptosis, arching eyebrows), skeletal anomalies, cardiac defects, and neurocognitive impairment

Kallmann syndrome—see Glossary entry "hypogonadotropic hypogonadism with or without anosmia."

Kartagener syndrome—see Glossary entry "primary ciliary dyskinesia."

Kleine-Levin hibernation syndrome—MIM 148840; inheritance undefined; gene unidentified; characterized by episodes of compulsive megaphagia, somnolence, and abnormal behavior predominantly in males

Klinefelter syndrome—47 XXY karyotype; paternal meiosis error; characterized by hypogonadism, tall stature with long limbs, mild neurocognitive impairments, although many are cognitively normal. Infertility is not universal.

Klippel-Feil anomaly—multifactorial; cervical spine fusion of varying degrees; characterized by a short neck, limited neck motion, and low occipital hairline; isolated defect or can appear as part of a multisystem syndrome

Krabbe leukodystrophy—MIM 245200; autosomal recessive; mutations in *GALC*; deficiency in galactosylceramidase; lysosomal storage disorder primarily affecting white matter of the central and peripheral nervous systems; characterized classically by early, severe neurodegeneration leading, in the infantile form, to death by 2 years of age. There are later onset forms.

***L1CAM*/X-linked hydrocephalus**—MIM 307000; X-linked recessive; mutations in *L1CAM*; hydrocephalus due to aqueductal stenosis, adducted thumbs, spasticity, and severe intellectual disability; one manifestations of *L1CAM* mutations, of which there is a spectrum

Larsen syndrome—MIM 150250; autosomal recessive; mutations in *B3GAT3*; characterized by osteochondrodysplasia, hyperlaxity, multiple congenital dislocations, short stature, heart defects, and characteristic facies

Laurence-Moon-Biedl syndrome—see Glossary entry "Bardet-Biedl syndrome."

Leber hereditary optic neuropathy—MIM 535000; mitochondrial inheritance; mutations in any of a number of genes active in mitochondria; characterized by central vision loss leading to blindness; most commonly presents in adults

LEOPARD syndrome (Noonan syndrome with multiple lentigines)—MIM 151100; autosomal dominant; mutations in *PTPN11*, *RAF1*, or *BRAF*; characterized by Lentigines, EKG abnormalities, Ocular hypertelorism, Pulmonic stenosis, Abnormalities of genitalia, Retardation of growth, and sensorineural Deafness

Lesch-Nyhan syndrome—MIM 300322; X-linked recessive; mutations in *HPRT1*; diminished or absent hypoxanthine guanine phosphoribosyl transferase (HPRT) activity leading to abnormal purine metabolism; characterized by hyperuricemia, spastic cerebral palsy, choreoathetosis, uric acid urinary stones; compulsive self-mutilation, and neurocognitive impairment

Letterer-Siwe disease—see "Histiocytosis" chapter.

Li-Fraumeni syndrome—MIM 151623; autosomal dominant; various genes, the most common being *TP53*; this is a cancer predisposition syndrome that increases the risk of many different cancers, classically but not limited to soft tissue sarcoma, osteosarcoma, premenopausal breast cancer, brain tumors, adrenocortical carcinoma, and leukemias; there is some genotype-phenotype correlation with the type of mutation; there are currently two genetic modifiers which lead to earlier or more severe tumor growth.

Loeys-Dietz syndrome—MIM 609192; autosomal dominant; mutations in *TGFBR1* or *TGFBR2*; characterized by skeletal findings similar to Marfan syndrome and vascular abnormalities including aneurysms and tortuous blood vessels as well as craniofacial malformations; vascular abnormalities include aggressive arterial aneurysms anywhere in the body; high incidence of pregnancy-related complications including uterine rupture

Long QT interval—see "Long QT Syndrome."

Louis-Bar syndrome—see Glossary entry "ataxia telangiectasia syndrome."

Lowe oculocerebrorenal syndrome—MIM 309000; X-linked recessive; mutations in *OCRL*; characterized by congenital cataracts, microphthalmia, vitamin D-resistant rickets, amino aciduria, hyporeflexia, hypotonia, renal Fanconi syndrome, and neurocognitive impairment; carrier females have characteristic lens findings on slit-lamp examination.

Lymphedema-distichiasis syndrome—MIM 153400; autosomal dominant; mutations in *FOXC2*; characterized by lymphedema of the lower limbs and double rows of eyelashes; complications include corneal irritation and ulceration, cardiac defects, varicose veins, cleft palate, extradural spinal cysts, and photophobia; lymphedema usually appears in late childhood or at puberty and is more severe in males.

Lysosomal acid lipase deficiency (Wolman disease)—MIM 278000; autosomal recessive; mutations in *LIPA*; lysosomal storage disease leading to cholesteryl ester and triglyceride deposition in visceral organs; characterized by intractable vomiting, failure to thrive, abdominal distention, steatorrhea, hepatosplenomegaly, and adrenal calcification; lethal in infancy

Maffucci syndrome—see Glossary entry "multiple enchondromatosis, Maffucci type."

Malignant hyperthermia, susceptibility to—MIM 145600; autosomal dominant; mutations in *RYR1*; pharmacogenetic disorder of skeletal muscle calcium metabolism precipitated by some volatile anesthetics (e.g., halothane) alone or used with succinylcholine; characterized by muscle contracture and increased cellular metabolism leading to hyperthermia, compartment syndrome, and rhabdomyolysis, the latter of which can precipitate renal failure via myoglobinuria or cardiac arrhythmia via hyperkalemia

Mandibulofacial syndrome—see Glossary entry "Treacher Collins syndrome."

Marfan syndrome—MIM 154700; autosomal dominant; mutations in *FBN1*; characterized by ectopia lentis, dilatation of the aorta, scoliosis, pneumothorax, pectus deformities, and long, thin extremities. Diagnostic criteria have been published.

Maternal phenylketonuria (PKU) effects—in children born to women with poorly controlled phenylketonuria, high maternal plasma phenylalanine is a teratogen; characterized by microcephaly, intellectual disability, behavior abnormalities, congenital heart defects, and other malformations; PKU is a recessive condition, so the infants usually are not affected and do not need dietary management; dietary control during pregnancy is necessarily stricter than baseline because phenylalanine concentrates in the fetus.

McCune-Albright syndrome—MIM 174800; autosomal dominant; mutations in *GNAS*; surviving cases are somatic mosaics as the nonmosaic state is presumed to be an embryonic lethal; characterized by polyostotic fibrous dysplasia, café-au-lait skin pigmentation, and peripheral precocious puberty; diagnosis most appropriately made via biopsy of affected tissue

Meckel-Gruber syndrome—MIM 249000; autosomal recessive; there are 12 types differentiated by mutations in various genes, most commonly *MKS1*; caused by abnormalities in nonmotile cilia; characterized by cystic renal disease, CNS malformation, and hepatic abnormalities, +/− postaxial polydactyly

Medium-chain acyl-CoA dehydrogenase (MCAD) deficiency—MIM 201450; autosomal recessive; mutations in *ACADM*; abnormal mitochondrial fatty acid oxidation and intolerance of fasting; can present as hypoketotic hypoglycemia, vomiting, lethargy, seizures, and sudden death; prognosis is excellent with dietary and medical management; currently included in many state newborn screening programs in the United States

Meige disease—MIM 153200; inheritance and gene unidentified; characterized by edema, primarily below the waist, which develops at puberty; may be associated with facial swelling, cleft palate, and/or yellow nails

MELAS syndrome—MIM 540000; mitochondrial or autosomal recessive; mutations in any of a number of genes active in mitochondria most commonly *MTTL1*; characterized by Mitochondrial myopathy, Encephalopathy, Lactic Acidosis, and Strokelike episodes; causes seizures, hemiparesis, hemianopsia, or cortical blindness, and episodic vomiting

Menkes disease (kinky hair disease)—MIM 309400; X-linked recessive; mutations in *ATP7A*; impaired GI transport of copper results in copper deficiency; characterized by low serum copper and ceruloplasmin, short, friable, colorless scalp hair, growth failure of postnatal onset, microcephaly, progressive neurocognitive impairment; death usually by 3 years of age

Metabolic diseases in acidotic newborns—see "Metabolic Diseases in Acidotic Newborns."

Metabolic diseases in hyperammonemic newborns—see "Metabolic Diseases in Hyperammonemic Newborns."

Metabolic diseases in hypoglycemic newborns—see "Metabolic Diseases in Hypoglycemic Newborns."

Metachromatic leukodystrophy—MIM 250100; autosomal recessive; mutations in *ARSA*; characterized by progressive neurologic dysfunction and MRI evidence of leukodystrophy; three types: late infantile, juvenile, and adult. Types run within families; infantile type presents with physical neurologic features, others start with neurocognitive and behavioral changes.

Miller-Dieker syndrome—MIM 247200; autosomal dominant; contiguous gene deletion syndrome of 17p13.3; characterized by lissencephaly, microcephaly, characteristic facies, heart malformations, male hypogonadism, growth deficiency, and neurologic abnormalities including seizures; often fatal in infancy

Milroy disease—see "Lymphedema."

Mismatch repair cancer syndrome—MIM 276300; autosomal dominant inheritance, autosomal recessive in manifestation; dominant inheritance of one mutated allele, with somatic mutation ("second hit") of the other; mutations in any of four separate genes; characterized by adenomatous colonic polyposis associated with malignant brain tumors, especially medulloblastoma and glioblastoma; there may be skin findings similar to those in neurofibromatosis type I.

Möbius (or Moebius) syndrome—MIM 157900; mostly isolated cases, may be autosomal dominant; gene unidentified; classically characterized by cranial nerve dysfunction causing bilateral facial weakness, feeding difficulties, and impairment of ocular abduction; the term has come to include any condition that includes congenital cranial nerve VII palsy and is, therefore, less useful than previously.

Monilethrix—MIM 158000; autosomal dominant; mutations in *KRT86*, *KRT81*, or *KRT83*; characterized by normal hair at birth that transitions in a few months to brittle, easily broken hair and dystrophic alopecia; spectrum of involvement from just the occipital scalp to facial and axillary/pubertal hair; follicular hyperkeratosis often present; may improve with puberty and pregnancy

Morquio syndrome—see Glossary entry "mucopolysaccharidosis IV."

Mucopolysaccharidosis I (Hurler, Scheie)—MIM 607014; autosomal recessive; mutations in *IDUA*; lysosomal storage disease; deficiency of α-L-iduronidase causing accumulation of heparan sulfate and dermatan sulfate; characterized by coarse facial features, growth arrest, dysostosis multiplex, glaucoma, arthritis, cardiac valvular disease, and neurocognitive impairment. There is a spectrum of involvement from severe (Hurler phenotype) to mild (Scheie phenotype), and both may be found in the same family. Enzyme replacement therapy is available.

Mucopolysaccharidosis II (Hunter syndrome)—MIM 309900; X-linked recessive; mutations in *IDS*; lysosomal storage disease; deficiency of l-iduronate sulfatase causing accumulation of heparan sulfate and dermatan sulfate; characterized by macrocephaly, coarse facial features, hypertrophy of internal organs, dysostosis multiplex, and neurocognitive impairment; female carriers are unaffected; this is the only mucopolysaccharidosis that is not autosomal recessive; enzyme replacement therapy is available.

Mucopolysaccharidosis III (Sanfilippo syndrome)—MIM 252900; autosomal recessive; deficiency in one of four enzymes with clinically similar manifestations; lysosomal storage disease; characterized by accumulation of heparan sulfate and progressive neurocognitive impairment with mild somatic features. Type A—mutations in *SGSH* and deficiency of heparin *N*-sulfatase; type B—mutations in *NAGLU* and deficiency of *N*-α-acetylglucosaminidase; type C—mutations in *HGSNAT* and deficiency of acetyl CoA:alpha-glucosaminide *N*-acetyltransferase; type D—mutations in *GNS* and deficiency of *N*-acetylglucosamine-6-sulfatase

Mucopolysaccharidosis IV (Morquio syndrome)—MIM 253000; autosomal recessive; mutations in *GALNS*; lysosomal storage disease; deficiency of galactosamine-6-sulfate sulfatase causing accumulation of keratin sulfate and chondroitin-6-sulfate; characterized by skeletal dysplasia with short-trunk dwarfism, corneal clouding, small joint hyperlaxity, and cardiac valve disease; patients have laxity of the odontoid processes and are at risk for life-threatening atlantoaxial subluxation. Enzyme replacement therapy is available.

Multiple enchondromatosis, Maffucci type—MIM 614569; all cases to date have been sporadic; presumed to be somatic mosaicism for mutations in currently unidentified gene; characterized by multiple enchondromas of the bone and soft tissue hemangiomas; patients have short stature, skeletal deformities, scoliosis, and high risk of malignant transformation.

Multiple endocrine neoplasia type I—MIM 131100; autosomal dominant; mutations in *MEN1*; characterized by varying combinations of endocrine and non-endocrine tumors, primarily parathyroid tumors, prolactinomas of the pituitary, endocrine tumors of the GI tract and pancreas, carcinoid, and adrenocortical tumors

Multiple endocrine neoplasia types 2A, 2B—MIM 171400 and 162300; autosomal dominant; mutations in *RET*; characterized by medullary thyroid carcinoma; type 2A has pheochromocytoma and parathyroid adenomas; type 2B has variable pheochromocytoma and ganglioneuromas of lips, tongue, and colon, without hyperparathyroidism.

Multiple epiphyseal dysplasia—MIM 132400; autosomal dominant; mutations in various genes, most commonly *COMP*; short-limbed skeletal dysplasia clinically affecting the lower extremities more; presents in childhood with hip and/or knee pain with intolerance of long-distance walking; waddling gait; early onset osteoarthritis; adult height is around the lower range of normal.

Multiple exostoses, type I—MIM 133700; autosomal dominant; mutations in *EXT1*; characterized by multiple osteochondromas (exostoses) occurring most commonly on the long bone metaphyses, but any bone can be involved except the skull. Secondary deformity of legs, forearms, and hands typically occur.

Multiple hereditary exostosis—see Glossary entry "multiple exostoses, type I."

Muscle-eye-brain disease—see Glossary entry "muscular dystrophy-dystroglycanopathy with brain and eye anomalies."

Muscular dystrophies—see "Muscular Dystrophies."

Muscular dystrophy-dystroglycanopathy with brain and eye anomalies—MIM 235800; autosomal recessive; mutations in *FKTN*; characterized by cobblestone lissencephaly, cerebellar and retinal malformations, muscular dystrophy, profound intellectual disability, and early death. The most severe dystroglycanopathy is Walker-Warburg syndrome.

Myelofibrosis—MIM 254450; somatic (acquired) activating mutations in various genes; kinase activation leads to uncontrolled cells expansion; characterized by bone marrow fibrosis and reduced hematopoiesis; myelofibrosis associated with mutations in *MPL* includes myeloid metaplasia.

Myotonic dystrophy—MIM 160900; autosomal dominant; triplet repeat mutations in *DMPK* with expansion risk increased when inherited from mother; characterized by myotonia, muscular dystrophy, cataracts, hypogonadism, frontal balding, and cardiomyopathy. Mild type (50 to 150 repeats) includes cataracts and mild myotonia with adult onset. Classic type (100 to 1,000 repeats) includes weakness, myotonia, cataracts, balding, cardiac arrhythmia, and other features. Congenital (>1,000 repeats) includes infantile hypotonia, respiratory distress, intellectual disability, and classic signs presenting if there is survival to adulthood.

Nail-patella syndrome—MIM 161200; autosomal dominant; mutations in *LMX1B*; characterized by dystrophic and hypoplastic nails, hypoplastic patellae, iliac horns, malformed radial heads, and nephrotic syndrome

Nephronophthisis—MIM 256100; autosomal recessive; mutations in *NPHP1*; caused by abnormalities in nonmotile cilia; characterized by progressive renal disease starting from reduced concentrating ability progressing through tubulointerstitial nephritis and cystic renal disease to end-stage renal disease before age 30 years. Infantile type can present prenatally with oligohydramnios and related malformations; can also manifest in teenage years; 80–90% of patients have isolated renal problems.

Neurofibromatosis I—see "Neurofibromatosis-1" chapter.

Neurofibromatosis II—MIM 101000; autosomal dominant; mutations in *NF2*; characterized by tumors of cranial nerve VIII, brain meningiomas, and dorsal root schwannomas; can have subcapsular lens opacities; no characteristic skin findings

Netherton syndrome—MIM 256500; autosomal recessive; mutations in *SPINK5*; characterized by trichorrhexis nodosa ("bamboo hair"), congenital ichthyosiform erythroderma, and atopic diathesis including hypereosinophilia, elevated IgE, urticaria, angioedema, and enteropathy; all reported patients to date are female.

Niemann-Pick types A and B—MIM 257200 and 607616; autosomal recessive; mutations in *SMPD1*; lipid storage disorder; deficiency of acid sphingomyelinase causes accumulation of sphingomyelin in reticuloendothelial and other cells; characterized by failure to thrive, organomegaly, macular cherry red spot, and rapidly progressive neurodegeneration; in its most severe form, patients are normal at birth but by 6 months experience delayed development and loss of developmental milestones with death by 3 years; increased prevalence in Ashkenazi Jews

Niemann-Pick type C—MIM 257220; autosomal recessive; mutations in *NPC1*; lipid storage disorder; can present as neonatal liver disease with respiratory failure; otherwise characterized by neurologic abnormalities in infants—hypotonia and delays—or children—ataxia, vertical supranuclear gaze palsy, and dementia; dystonia seizures, dysarthria, and dysphagia are major problems; death in 2nd or 3rd decade; adult onset presents with psychiatric symptoms.

Nonketotic hyperglycinemia—see Glossary entry "glycine encephalopathy."

Noonan syndrome—MIM 163950; autosomal dominant; mutations in various genes, most commonly *PTPN11*; characterized by short stature, heart defects (most commonly pulmonic stenosis and hypertrophic cardiomyopathy), bleeding diathesis, and characteristic facies; neurocognitive function varies and is often average.

Norrie disease—MIM 310600; X-linked recessive; mutations in *NDP*; characterized by retinal vasculopathy leading to detachment and pseudogliomas causing congenital blindness; about half of patients have progressive mental disorders including psychosis, and about a third develop sensorineural hearing loss.

Oculo-auriculo-vertebral spectrum (OAV, hemifacial microsomia, Goldenhar)—multifactorial; characterized by craniofacial malformations—typically unilateral—starting with microtia and involving ipsilateral skull and face bones, globe, and facial soft tissue structures. Severe cases may also involve vertebrae. Cognitive function tends to be normal.

Oculomandibulofacial syndrome—see Glossary entry "Hallerman-Streif syndrome."

Omenn syndrome—MIM 603554; autosomal recessive; mutations in *RAG1*, *RAG2*, or *DCLRE1C*; severe combined immunodeficiency (SCID) syndrome with reticuloendotheliosis and eosinophilia; characterized otherwise by generalized erythroderma, alopecia, hepatosplenomegaly, and short stature; documented in the Irish Traveller population

Omphalocele-exstrophy-imperforate anus-spina bifida (OEIS)—see "Exstrophy–Epispadias Complex."

Opitz syndrome—There are seven syndromes that in some fashion are or have been referred to as Opitz syndrome. In this text, it is mentioned in the differential of fetal alcohol syndrome neurocognitive problems. This may be true of all conditions referred to as Opitz. Other sources indicate a similarity with some physical features. It is best remembered that there are single gene syndromes in the differential diagnosis of fetal alcohol syndrome, and in the absence of a clear history and classic presentation, further evaluation is warranted.

Orofacialdigital syndrome type I—MIM 311200; X-linked dominant, mutations in *OFD1*; characterized by malformations of the face, mouth, and digits but also has polycystic kidney disease; 15 types differing by gene and inheritance pattern

Osler-Weber-Rendu syndrome (hereditary hemorrhagic telangiectasia)—MIM 187300; autosomal dominant; mutations in *ENG*; vascular dysplasia; characterized by telangiectasias and arteriovenous malformation of the skin, mucosa, and viscera (lung, liver, brain)

Osteogenesis imperfecta—see "Osteogenesis Imperfecta."

Osteopetrosis—MIM 259700 and 166600; various inheritance patterns; mutations in various genes; widely varying phenotypes; characterized by dense bones that are prone to fracture, mild anemia, and craniofacial disproportion; radiologic changes include increased cortical bone density, longitudinal and transverse dense striations at the ends of the long bones, lucent and dense bands in the vertebrae, and thickening at the base of the skull; bone marrow insufficiency limits survival.

Paroxysmal nocturnal hemoglobinuria—MIM 300818; acquired; somatic mutations in *PIGA*; characterized by complement-mediated hemolysis and anemia manifesting as hemoglobinuria, abdominal pain, smooth muscle dystonia, fatigue, and thrombosis

Patau syndrome—see Glossary entry "trisomy 13."

Pearson syndrome—MIM 557000; mitochondrial inheritance; contiguous gene deletion syndrome of mitochondrial DNA; characterized by sideroblastic anemia and exocrine pancreas dysfunction; typically lethal in infancy

Pelizaeus-Merzbacher disease—MIM 312080; X-linked recessive; mutations in *PLP1*; characterized by failure of normal CNS myelination, nystagmus, spastic quadriplegia, ataxia, and neurocognitive impairment; patients may also have optic atrophy and seizures; infantile and adult onset subtypes

Pendred syndrome—MIM 274600; autosomal recessive; mutations in *SLC26A4*; characterized by prelingual (congenital) severe-to-profound bilateral sensorineural hearing loss, vestibular dysfunction, enlarged vestibular aqueducts, and euthyroid goiter

Peutz-Jeghers syndrome—MIM 175200; autosomal dominant; mutations in *STK11*; characterized by melanotic macules on the lips, mucous membranes, and digits, intestinal polyposis, and increased risk of malignancy

Pfeiffer syndrome—MIM 101600; autosomal dominant; mutations in *FGFR1* or *FGFR2*; characterized by craniosynostosis and limb anomalies; presentation ranges from limited craniosynostosis with broad thumbs and toes to a severe form with cloverleaf skull, ankylosis of knees and elbows, and high risk of early mortality.

PFIC—see Glossary entry "progressive familial intrahepatic cholestasis."

PHACES association—MIM 606519; sporadic; no identified gene; characterized by Posterior fossa brain malformations, large or complex Hemangiomas of the face, Arterial anomalies, Cardiac anomalies, Eye abnormalities, +/− Sternal clefting; definite diagnosis requires presence of characteristic facial/scalp hemangioma plus one major and two minor additional criteria involving other body systems.

Phenylketonuria—MIM 261600; autosomal recessive; mutations in *PAH*; inability to catalyze phenylalanine into tyrosine causes accumulation of phenylalanine, which is toxic; characterized by impaired cognitive development, relative hypopigmentation, "mousy" odor; treatable with phenylalanine-restricted diet; currently included in most state newborn screening programs in the United States

PHP1A—see Glossary entry "pseudohypoparathyroidism IA."

Pierre Robin sequence—multifactorial; characterized by micrognathia, glossoptosis, and cleft soft palate; may be found as an isolated entity or a component of multisystem syndromes, most commonly 22q11.2 deletion syndrome and Stickler syndrome.

Poland anomaly—multifactorial; characterized by a unilateral absence or hypoplasia of the pectoralis major muscle with ipsilateral breast hypoplasia and sometimes associated upper limb abnormalities; may be found as an isolated entity or a component of multisystem syndromes

Polycystic kidney disease—see "Polycystic Kidney Disease."

Pompe disease—MIM 232300; autosomal recessive; mutations in *GAA*; lysosomal storage disease involving glycogen, so also a glycogen storage disease; deficiency of acid maltase causes accumulation of glycogen; infantile type characterized by profound hypotonia and cardiomegaly with a characteristic high-voltage EKG; hepatomegaly, hypoglycemia, and acidosis do not occur; usually lethal in the 1st year of life; later onset types involve skeletal muscle more than cardiac; enzyme replacement therapy is available.

Porphyrias—inherited defects of heme biosynthesis. See also Glossary entry "acute intermittent porphyria."

Prader-Willi syndrome—MIM 176270; imprinting disorder; absence of paternal alleles of 15q11.2 that include *SNRPN*; mechanisms include deletion on the paternal chromosome, maternal uniparental disomy or, rarely, mutations in the gene itself; characterized by hypotonia and initial failure to thrive due to poor feeding, followed by marked obesity due to an insatiable appetite; other features include mental retardation, hypogonadism, small hands and feet, and short stature; appropriate treatment with growth hormone and diet control ameliorates the obesity, increased lean muscle mass, and raises height.

Primary ciliary dyskinesia—MIM 244400; autosomal recessive except for type 36, which is X-linked recessive; mutations in various genes; results from loss of function of the primary ciliary apparatus, most often the dynein arms; characterized by heterotaxy, mucociliary dysfunction in the respiratory tract, immotile sperm, and hydrocephalus

Progeria syndrome—see Glossary entry "Hutchinson-Gilford progeria syndrome."

Progressive familial intrahepatic cholestasis (PFIC) (Byler disease)—MIM 211600; autosomal recessive; mutations in *ATP8B1*, *PFIC2*, or *PFIC3*; characterized by intrahepatic cholestasis leading to cirrhosis and end-stage liver disease before adulthood and anticipated secondary effects of liver failure; short stature, failure to thrive, splenomegaly

Proximal focal femoral deficiency—multifactorial; high association with maternal pregestational diabetes; partial or complete absence of the femur, with pelvis and sometimes sacral abnormalities

Prune belly sequence—multifactorial; characterized by deficiency of the abdominal musculature; may be primary malformation of the abdominal wall or secondary to fetal abdominal distention; abdominal distention most commonly due to a grossly distended urinary system with bladder outlet obstruction; the primary defect is variable, even within the urinary system; obstruction and dilation of other viscera or presence of a mass can lead to prune belly as a secondary feature.

Pseudohypoparathyroidism IA—MIM 103580; autosomal dominant with imprinting; mutations in *GNAS* inherited from the mother; characterized by parathyroid hormone resistance as well as resistance to other hormones including thyroid-stimulating hormone and gonadotropins; additionally, there are physical features of Albright hereditary osteodystrophy such as short stature, obesity, round face, subcutaneous ossifications, and skeletal anomalies.

***PTEN* macrocephaly/autism**—MIM 605309; autosomal dominant; mutations in *PTEN*; characterized by large head circumference, abnormal facies, and neuropsychiatric abnormalities including autism; mutations in *PTEN* are also associated with some genetic cancer syndromes.

***RASA1* syndromes**—MIM 608354; autosomal dominant; capillary malformation–arteriovenous malformation syndrome and Parkes Weber syndrome; characterized by multiple small capillary malformations and arteriovenous malformations and/or fistulas which can be life-threatening due to bleeding, congestive heart failure, and/or neurologic impairment; Parkes Weber includes hemihyperplasia; somatic mutations can cause basal cell carcinoma.

Retinitis pigmentosa—MIM 268000; various inheritance patterns; mutations in various genes; can be found as an isolated problem or part of a syndrome; characterized by progressive retinal degeneration including night blindness, tunnel vision, and progressive decreased macular vision; there are characteristic findings on retinal exam.

Rett syndrome—MIM 312750; X-linked dominant; mutations in *MECP2*; characterized by a period of normal growth and development over weeks to months with onset of developmental regression, lack of head growth leading to microcephaly, lack of purposeful hand use, autistic features, seizures, and fits of screaming; "classic" features include hand wringing, bruxism, and stereotypic breathing patterns; vast majority of affected patients are female; germline inheritance considered lethal to males

Rieger syndrome—see Glossary entry "Axenfeld-Rieger syndrome."

Riley-Day syndrome—see Glossary entry "familial dysautonomia."

Rotor syndrome—MIM 237450; autosomal recessive; digenic inheritance of homozygous mutations in *SLCO1B1* and *SLCO1B3*; characterized by mild conjugated bilirubinemia and jaundice that may be exacerbated by infection, surgery, pregnancy, or drugs; usually asymptomatic with normal life expectancy; clinically, similar to Dubin-Johnson syndrome, but patients with Rotor have normal-appearing hepatocytes

Rubinstein-Taybi syndrome—MIM 180840; autosomal dominant; mutations in *CREBBP*: characterized by growth deficiency of postnatal onset, microcephaly, broad thumbs and halluces, neurocognitive impairment, and characteristic facies; increased risk of neoplasia

Russell-Silver syndrome—MIM 180860; multifactorial; 20–60% caused by imprinting abnormalities of chromosome 11, 10% by maternal uniparental disomy of chromosome 7; characterized by growth failure and short stature of prenatal onset with head sparing (relative but not absolute macrocephaly) and characteristic facies; can have 5th finger clinodactyly, body asymmetry due to hemihypoplasia, and hyperpigmented macules

Sandhoff Disease (GM2-gangliosidosis type II)—MIM 268800; autosomal recessive; mutations in *HEXB*; deficiency of hexosaminidase B leading to accumulation of GM2 gangliosides, particularly in neurons; progressive neurodegenerative disorder; hypotonia in the first 6 months of life, startle reaction, macular cherry-red spots, macrocephaly, organomegaly, and progressive neurocognitive impairment; manifestations similar to Tay-Sachs disease; no ethnic predilection

Sanfilippo syndrome, types A, B, C, and D—see Glossary entry "mucopolysaccharidosis III."

Scheie syndrome—see Glossary entry "mucopolysaccharidosis I."

Seckel syndrome—MIM 210600; autosomal recessive; multiple subtypes differentiated by gene involved; characterized by growth failure of prenatal onset, extreme short stature, microcephaly, neurocognitive impairment, and characteristic facies

Short-rib thoracic dysplasia (with or without polydactyly)—MIM 208500; autosomal recessive; mutations in various genes; a set of conditions caused by abnormalities in nonmotile cilia; characterized by skeletal dysplasia, short ribs, polydactyly, orofacial clefts, and abnormalities of the brain, eye, heart, kidneys, liver, pancreas, intestines, and genitalia; includes Jeune, Ellis-van Creveld syndrome, hydrolethalus, and others

Shwachman-Diamond syndrome—MIM 260400; autosomal recessive; mutations in *SBDS*; characterized by exocrine pancreatic dysfunction, bone marrow dysfunction with risk of malignant transformation, and skeletal abnormalities with disproportionate short stature

Sickle cell—see "Sickle Cell Disease."

Smith-Lemli-Opitz syndrome—MIM 270400; autosomal recessive; mutations in *DHCR7*; disorder of cholesterol synthesis; characterized by growth retardation, microcephaly, hypospadias with cryptorchidism, characteristic 2 to 3 toe Y-shaped syndactyly, photosensitivity, neurocognitive impairment, and characteristic facies; dietary cholesterol supplementation may result in clinical improvement of behavior.

Sotos syndrome (cerebral gigantism)—MIM 117550; autosomal dominant; mutations in *NSD1*; characterized by macrocephaly, rapid somatic growth (final height usually average for the family), large hands and feet, neurocognitive impairment that may be mild, and characteristic facies

Spinal cerebellar ataxia—MIM 164400; autosomal dominant; mutations in various genes; characterized by cerebellar degeneration with progressive ataxia, dysarthria, and deterioration of bulbar functions; onset typically in 20s and 30s

Spinal muscular atrophy—see "Spinal Muscular Atrophy."

Spondyloepiphyseal dysplasia—MIM 183900; autosomal dominant; mutations in *COL2A1*; chondrodysplasia characterized by short-trunk dwarfism, abnormal epiphyses, and platyspondyly; may include myopia and/or retinal detachment and cleft palate

Stargardt disease—MIM 248200; autosomal recessive; mutations in *ABCA4* or *CNGB3*; characterized by macular degeneration and central retinitis pigmentosa; onset usually by age 20 years

Stickler syndrome—MIM 108300; autosomal dominant; mutation in *COL2A1*, *COL11A1* or *COL11A2*; characterized by Pierre Robin anomaly at birth and mild skeletal features with more obvious problems later, vitreous and retinal abnormalities, high-frequency hearing loss, and osteoarthritis before age 40 years; cognition usually normal

Stiff man syndrome—see Glossary entry "hyperekplexia."

Stiff skin syndrome—MIM 184900; autosomal dominant; mutations in *FBN1*; characterized by hard, thick skin throughout, limited joint mobility, and flexion contractures; can include hypotonia and lipodystrophy

Sturge-Weber syndrome—MIM 185300; multifactorial, can be caused by autosomal dominant somatic mutation of *GNAQ*; characterized by facial port-wine stain at the 1st branch of the trigeminal nerve, ipsilateral leptomeningeal angiomatosis with intracranial calcifications leading to seizures and intellectual disability; possible ocular complications such as glaucoma

Tay-Sachs disease (GM2-gangliosidosis type I)—MIM 272800; autosomal recessive; mutations in *HEXA*; deficiency of hexosaminidase A activity leading to accumulation of GM2 gangliosides in the CNS; characterized by motor development regression, seizures, macular cherry-red spot, and progressive neurodegeneration leading to blindness, paralysis, and death within the 2nd or 3rd year of life; highest prevalence in Ashkenazi Jews and Cajuns

Testicular regression syndrome—see Glossary entry "vanishing testes syndrome."

Tetrasomy 22—see Glossary entry "cat eye syndrome."

Thalassemia (includes β-thalassemia)—see "Thalassemia."

Thanatophoric dysplasia—MIM 187600; autosomal dominant; mutations in *FGFR3*; characterized by severe short-limb dwarfism, cloverleaf skull; usually neonatal lethal due to respiratory insufficiency

Thrombocytopenia-absent radius (TAR)—MIM 274000; autosomal recessive; mutations in *RBM8A*; characterized by bilateral absence of the radius with thumbs present and waxing/waning thrombocytopenia; cow milk allergy is common and can exacerbate thrombocytopenia; can be clinically differentiated from Fanconi anemia in which the radial ray defect usually includes absent or hypoplastic thumbs

Tourette syndrome—see Glossary entry "Gilles de la Tourette syndrome."

Townes-Brock syndrome—MIM 107480; autosomal dominant; mutations in *SALL1*; characterized by imperforate anus, thumb polydactyly, and dysplastic ears; high incidence of structural and functional renal involvement, congenital heart malformations, and other skeletal involvement

Treacher Collins syndrome—MIM 154500; autosomal dominant; mutations in *TCOF1*; characterized by mandibulofacial dysostosis with characteristic finding of hypoplastic zygomatic arches and mandibles, micrognathia, downward slanting palpebral fissures, coloboma of the lower eyelid, microtia with associated conductive hearing deficits, and a cleft palate with or without cleft lip; cognitive function is usually normal.

Trichorhinophalangeal—MIM 190350; autosomal dominant; mutations in *TRPS1*; characterized by distinctive facies (particularly the nose), abnormalities of hair and other skin appendages, short stature with other skeletal anomalies; cognitive development is usually normal; when *TRPS1* is included in a contiguous gene deletion, the manifestations include exostoses and a higher incidence of intellectual disability.

Triploidy—sporadic; the presence of an entire extra set of chromosomes resulting in 69 total chromosomes: 69,XXX, 69,XXY, or 69,XYY; most often the result of two sperm fertilizing a single ovum; the vast majority will spontaneously abort.

Trisomy 13 (Patau syndrome)—characterized by holoprosencephaly, aplasia cutis congenita, cleft lip and/or cleft palate, microphthalmia, postaxial polydactyly; cardiovascular anomalies in 80%; majority abort spontaneously; median survival is 7 days.

Trisomy 18 (Edwards syndrome)—characterized by severe neurocognitive impairment, growth failure of prenatal onset, and characteristic facies, prominent occiput, and micrognathia; other common features are clenched hands with overriding fingers, a short sternum, and rocker bottom feet; cardiac and renal anomalies in up to 50% of cases; the majority abort spontaneously.

Trisomy 21 (Down Syndrome)—see "Down Syndrome (Trisomy 21)."

Tuberous sclerosis (Bourneville disease, Bourneville-Pringle disease)—see "Tuberous Sclerosis Complex."

Turcot syndrome—see Glossary entry "mismatch repair cancer syndrome."

Turner syndrome (monosomy X)—see "Turner Syndrome."

Tyrosinemia—MIM 276700; autosomal recessive; mutations in *FAH*; characterized by progressive liver disease and secondary renal tubulopathy leading to hypophosphatemic rickets; may present with acute liver failure after birth; currently included in many state newborn screening programs in the United States

Usher syndrome—MIM 276900; autosomal recessive; mutations in various genes; characterized by early retinitis pigmentosa, vestibular dysfunction, and sensorineural hearing loss

VACTERL association—statistical association of common malformations; characterized by Vertebral defects, Anal atresia, Congenital heart defects, Tracheoesophageal fistula with Esophageal atresia, Renal and Limb anomalies; at least two noncardiac components must be present for the diagnosis; overlaps with diagnosable genetic conditions which must be considered; VACTERL is a diagnosis of exclusion rather than a primary diagnosis.

van der Woude syndrome—MIM 119300; autosomal dominant; mutations in *IRF6*; characterized by cleft lip and/or cleft palate and pits or sinuses of the lower lip

Vanishing testes syndrome—MIM 273250; gene remains unknown; characterized by bilateral gonadal absence in a person with 46 XY karyotype; phenotype depends on the amount of early testicular tissue present and active and ranges from unambiguous female to anorchic but unambiguous male.

von Gierke disease—see Glossary entry "glycogen storage disease IA (GSD1A)."

von Hippel–Lindau disease—MIM 193300; autosomal dominant; mutations in *VHL* or *CCND1*; familial cancer syndrome; benign and malignant tumors, most frequently retinal, cerebellar, and spinal hemangioblastoma, renal cell carcinoma, pheochromocytoma, and pancreatic tumors

von Willebrand—see "von Willebrand Disease."

Waardenburg syndrome—MIM 193500; autosomal dominant; mutations most commonly in *PAX3*; multiple types and subtypes; pigmentary abnormalities of the hair, skin, and eyes, (white forelock, heterochromia iridis, premature graying of hair), congenital sensorineural hearing loss, and characteristic facies

WAGR (Wilms tumor, Aniridia, Genitourinary anomalies, and mental Retardation)—MIM 194072; autosomal dominant; contiguous gene deletion syndrome of 11p13 involving the *WT1* and *PAX6* genes; characterized by aniridia, genitourinary anomalies (hypospadias or uterine malformations), and high risk of Wilms tumor

Walker-Warburg syndrome—MIM 236670; autosomal recessive; mutations in *POMT1*; most severe of the dystroglycanopathies; characterized by congenital muscular dystrophy, cobblestone lissencephaly, cerebellar and retinal malformations; death often before a year of age

Wegener granulomatosis—MIM 608710; complex genetics; necrotizing granulomatous vasculitis involving (i) the airways, leading to rhinorrhea, chronic sinusitis, nasal ulceration; (ii) the lungs, causing hemoptysis, dyspnea, and cough; (iii) the kidneys, manifested as hematuria and/or proteinuria due to glomerulonephritis; other symptoms include fever, malaise, weight loss, myalgias, arthralgias, ophthalmic involvement, neuropathies, and cutaneous nodules or ulcers.

Werner syndrome—MIM 277700; autosomal recessive; mutations in *RECQL2*; characterized by scleroderma-like skin changes, premature arteriosclerosis, diabetes mellitus, an appearance of premature aging, short stature, slender limbs, and a stocky trunk.

Williams syndrome—MIM 194050; autosomal dominant; hemizygous deletion of 7q11.23; characterized by hypercalcemia in infants; supravalvular aortic stenosis; peripheral pulmonary artery stenosis; short stature; neurocognitive impairment, particularly in math; hypersocial with affinity for music; hyperacusis; characteristic facies

Wilson disease—see "Wilson Disease."

Wiskott-Aldrich syndrome—see "Wiskott-Aldrich Syndrome."

Wolff-Parkinson-White syndrome—MIM 194200; can be autosomal dominant or acquired; when inherited, caused by mutations in *PRKAG2*; Accessory conduction pathway found in 25% of patients with supraventricular tachycardia; typical electrocardiographic findings include a short PR interval and slow upstroke of the QRS (delta wave); may be an isolated finding, or related to structural cardiac defects

Wolman disease—see Glossary entry "Lysosomal Acid Lipase Deficiency."

Xeroderma pigmentosum—MIM 278700; autosomal recessive; mutations in *XPA*; defective DNA repair after exposure to ultraviolet light; characterized by extreme sunlight sensitivity, slowly progressive neurocognitive impairment, photophobia, and cutaneous and ocular malignancies; patients may have freckling, progressive skin atrophy, erythema, scaling bullae, and crusting telangiectasia.

Zellweger syndrome (cerebrohepatorenal syndrome; peroxisome biogenesis disorder 1A)—MIM 214100; autosomal recessive; mutations in *PEX1*; disorder of peroxisome biogenesis (absence of peroxisomes); characterized by severe neurologic dysfunction, hepatic cirrhosis, and characteristic facies; the vast majority of patients die within the 1st year of life.

Appendix IV
Tables and Figures

Michael D. Cabana, MD, MPH

Table 1. Developmental Milestones from Birth to 5 Years

Age (mo)	Adaptive/Fine Motor	Language	Gross Motor	Personal–Social
1	Grasp reflex (hands fisted)	Facial response to sounds	Lifts head in prone position	Stares at face
2	Follows object with eyes past midline	Coos (vowel sounds)	Lifts head in prone position to 45 degrees	Smiles in response to others
4	Hands open Brings objects to mouth	Laughs and squeals Turns toward voice	Sits: head steady Rolls to supine	Smiles spontaneously
6	Palmar grasp of objects	Babbles (consonant sounds)	Sits independently Stands, hands held	Reaches for toys Recognizes strangers
9	Pincer grasp	Says "mama," "dada" nonspecifically, comprehends "no"	Pulls to stand	Feeds self Waves bye-bye
12	Helps turn pages of book	2–4 words Follows command with gesture	Stands independently Walks, one hand held	Points to indicate wants
15	Scribbles	4–6 words Follows command no gesture	Walks independently	Drinks from cup Imitates activities
18	Turns pages of book	10–20 words Points to 4 body parts	Walks up steps	Feeds self with spoon
24	Solves single-piece puzzles	Combines 2–3 words Uses "I" and "you"	Jumps Kicks ball	Removes coat Verbalizes wants
30	Imitates horizontal and vertical lines	Names all body parts	Rides tricycle using pedals	Pulls up pants Washes, dries hands
36	Copies circle Draws person with 3 parts	Gives full name, age, and sex Names 2 colors	Throws ball overhand Walks up stairs (alternating feet)	Toilet-trained Puts on shirt, knows front from back
42	Copies cross	Understands "cold," "tired," "hungry"	Stands on 1 foot for 2–3 s	Engages in associative play
48	Counts 4 objects Identifies some numbers and letters	Understands prepositions (under, on, behind, in front of) Asks "how" and "why"	Hops on 1 foot	Dresses with little assistance Shoes on correct feet
54	Copies square Draws person with 6 parts	Understands opposites	Broad-jumps 24 inches	Bosses and criticizes Shows off
60	Prints first name Counts 10 objects	Asks meaning of words	Skips (alternating feet)	Ties shoes

REFRACTIVE ERROR

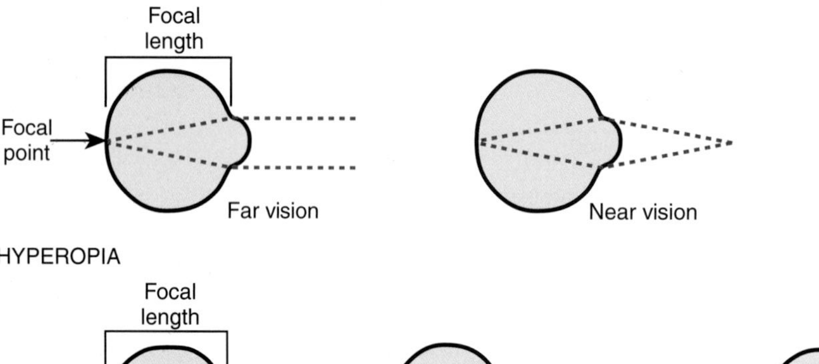

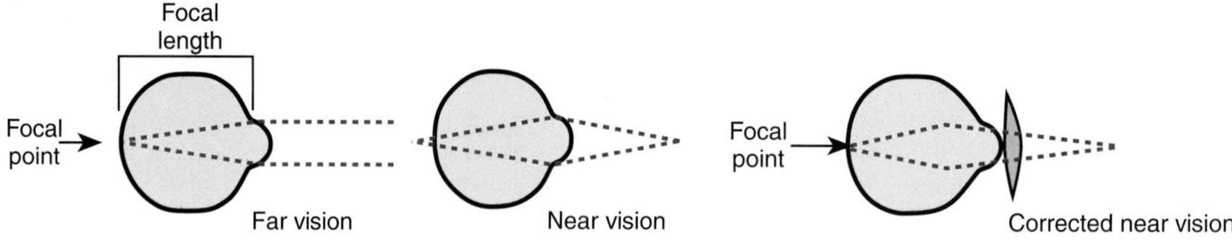

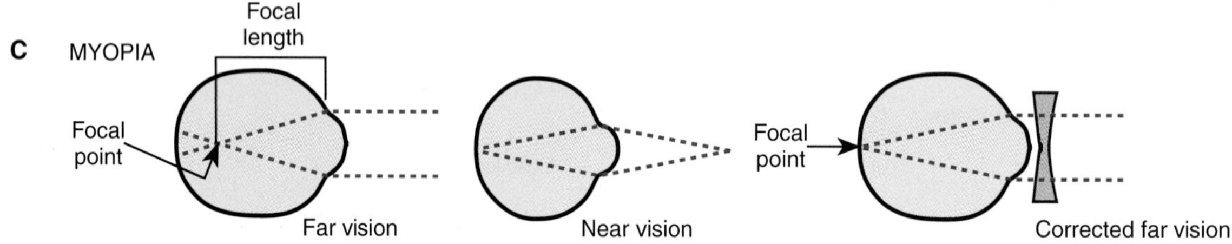

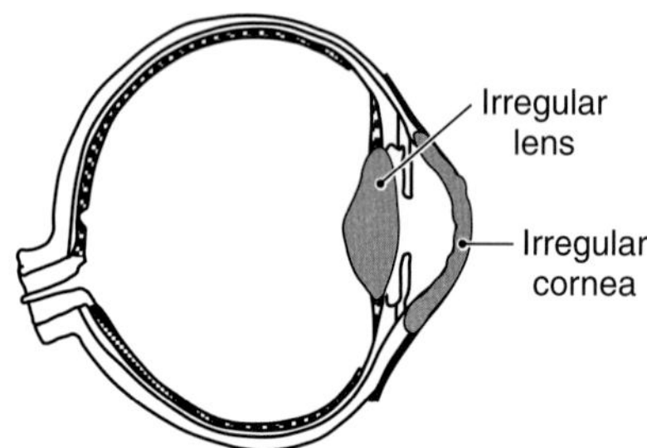

FIGURE 1. The normally refractive eye, common refractive errors, and their corrections. **A:** In a normal (emmetropic) eye, light rays from a near or far object are adequately refracted so that the rays converge directly on the retina, enabling formation of a clear image. **B:** In a farsighted (hypermetropic, hyperopic) eye, an image from a near point is focused behind the retina. The resulting condition can be corrected with convex lenses. **C:** In a nearsighted (myopic) eye, an image from a far point is focused in front of the retina. This refractive condition can be corrected with concave lenses. **D:** Refractive errors of astigmatism result from irregular curvatures of the cornea, lens, or both. Consequently, horizontal and vertical points from various visual fields are focused at two different focal points on the retina, resulting in distorted vision. (From Bhatnagar SC. *Neuroscience for the Study of Communicative Disorders*. 4th ed. Philadelphia, PA: Lippincott Williams & Wilkins; 2012.)

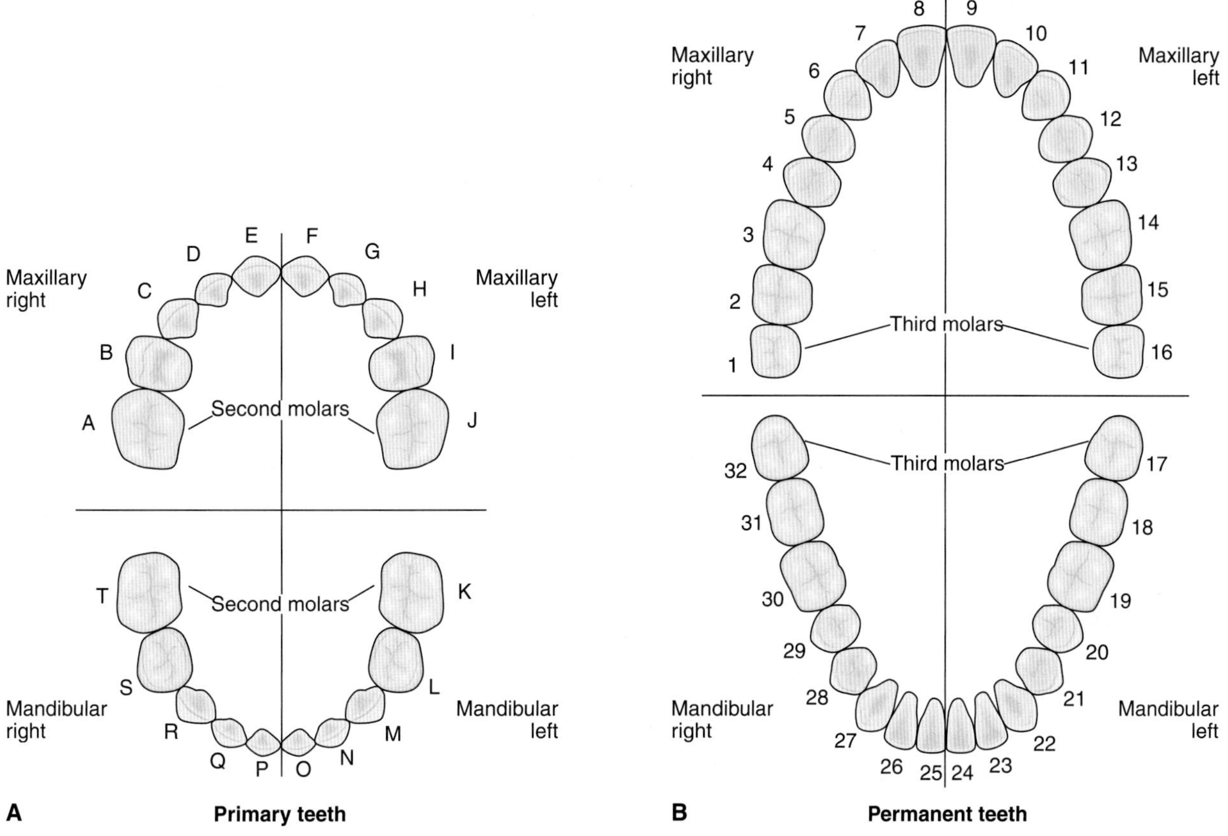

FIGURE 2. The Universal Numbering System. **A:** Primary teeth. **B:** Permanent teeth. (From Lippincott Williams & Wilkins. *Lippincott Williams & Wilkins' Comprehensive Dental Assisting.* Philadelphia, PA: Lippincott Williams & Wilkins; 2011.)

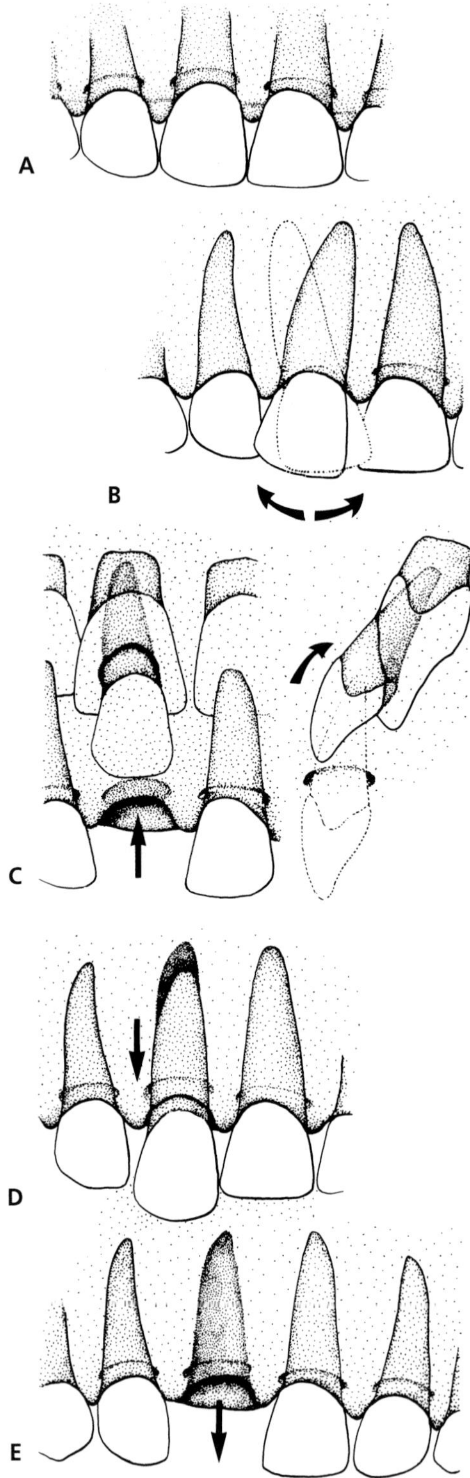

FIGURE 3. The various types of trauma to the periodontal structures: concussion/subluxation **(A)**, lateral luxation **(B)**, intrusion (if primary tooth is intruded, note location of developing permanent tooth bud) **(C)**, extrusion **(D)**, and avulsion **(E)**. Refer emergencies B through E to the dental staff as soon as possible. (From Fleisher GR, Ludwig S, Henretig FM, et al, eds. *Textbook of Pediatric Emergency Medicine*. 5th ed. Philadelphia, PA: Lippincott Williams & Wilkins; 2005.)

Table 2. Clinical Signs of Dehydration in Children

Parameter	Mild	Moderate	Severe
Activity	Normal	Lethargic	Lethargic to comatose
Color	Pale	Gray	Mottled
Urine output	Decreased (<2–3 mL/kg/h)	Oliguric (<1 mL/kg/h)	Anuric
Fontanelle	Flat	Depressed	Sunken
Mucous membranes	Dry	Very dry	Cracked
Skin turgor	Slightly decreased	Markedly decreased	Tenting
Pulse	Normal to increased	Increased	Grossly tachycardic
Blood pressure	Normal	Normal	Decreased
Weight loss	5%	10%	15%

Hypernatremic dehydration may be accompanied by moderate clinical signs.
Reprinted with permission from Rogers MC. Shock. In: Rogers MC, Helfaer MA, eds. *Handbook of Pediatric Intensive Care*. 2nd ed. Baltimore: Williams Wilkins; 1994:140.

Table 3. Characteristics of the Three Stages of Parapneumonic Pleural Effusions

	Exudative Stage	Fibrinolytic Stage	Organizing Stage (Empyema)
Appearance	Nonpurulent, not turbid	Nonpurulent, not turbid	Purulent, turbid
Fluid consistency	Free-flowing	Loculated	Organized
Gram stain and culture results	Negative	Transitional	Positive (before antibiotic treatment)
Glucose	>100 mg/dL	<50 mg/dL	<50 mg/dL
Protein	<3 g/dL	>3 g/dL	>3 g/dL
pH	>7.30	<7.30	<7.30
WBCs	Few	PMNs	PMNs

PMNs, polymorphonuclear neutrophils; WBCs, white blood cells.

Table 4. Pleural Fluid Diagnostic Studies

Study	Transudate	Exudate
Biochemical		
Pleural LDH	<200 IU	≥200 IU
Pleural fluid/serum LDH ratio[a]	<0.6	≥0.6
Pleural fluid/serum protein ratio[a]	<0.5	≥0.5
Specific gravity	<1.016	≥1.016
Protein level	<3.0 g/dL	≥3.0 g/dL
Other studies		
Glucose	Usually >40 mg/dL	Typically <40 mg/dL
Amylase	May be elevated in some neoplasms, GI trauma, or surgery	
Rheumatoid factor, LE prep, ANA	Are occasionally helpful if collagen vascular disorders are within the differential	
Hematologic		
WBC count	Although high counts (>100/mm3) are suggestive of an exudate, the results are quite variable.	
WBC differential	May actually provide more useful information	
Lymphocyte count	May be elevated in neoplasms, tuberculosis, and some fungal infections	
Segmented neutrophils	May be elevated in bacterial infections, connective tissue disease, pancreatitis, or pulmonary infarction	
Eosinophil count	May be elevated in bacterial infections, neoplasms, and connective tissue diseases	
RBC count	If >100,000/mm^3, is suggestive of trauma, neoplasms, or pulmonary infarction	
Cytology and chromosomal studies	May show evidence of malignant cells or chromosomal abnormalities	
Microbiology		
Gram stain		
Fluid culture for aerobes and anaerobes		
Acid-fast stain (if tuberculosis is in the differential)		
Fungal culture		
Viral culture		
Counterimmune electrophoresis may aid in the detection of a bacterial infection.		

[a]These tests are more reliable in differentiating transudate from exudate than specific gravity or protein level.
LDH, lactate dehydrogenase; LE prep, lupus erythematosus cell preparation; ANA, antinuclear antibody; WBC, white blood cell; RBC, red blood cells.

Table 5. Glasgow Coma Scale

Eyes open		Best motor response	
Spontaneously	4	Obey commands	6
To speech	3	Localize pain	5
To pain	2	Withdrawal	4
None	1	Flexion to pain	3
Best verbal response		Extension to pain	2
Oriented	5	None	1
Confused	4		
Inappropriate	3		
Incomprehensible	2		
None	1		

Adapted from Fleisher G, Ludwig S, eds. *Textbook of Pediatric Emergency Medicine*. 3rd ed. Baltimore, MD: Lippincott Williams & Wilkins; 1993:272.

Table 6. Glasgow Coma Scale for Adults and Children and Modified Score for Infants

	Glasgow Coma Score (Adults/Older Children)		Modified Glasgow Coma Score (Infants)
Eye opening	Spontaneous	4	Spontaneous
	To verbal stimuli	3	To speech
	To pain	2	To pain
	None	1	None
Best verbal response	Oriented	5	Coos and babbles
	Confused speech	4	Irritable, cries
	Inappropriate words	3	Cries to pain
	Nonspecific sounds	2	Moans to pain
	None	1	None
Best motor response	Follows commands	6	Normal spontaneous movements
	Localizes pain	5	Withdraws to touch
	Withdraws to pain	4	Withdraws to pain
	Flexes to pain	3	Abnormal flexion
	Extends to pain	2	Abnormal extension
	None	1	None

VAGINITIS: PHYSICAL EXAM

Table 7. Key Characteristics of Vaginal Discharges

	Presenting Symptoms	Discharge	Nonmenstrual pH	Amine/ Whiff Test	Vaginal Smear	Treatment
Nonspecific vaginitis	Foul-smelling discharge Itching	Scant to copious Brown to green in color	Variable	Negative	Leukocytes Bacteria and other debris	Improve perineal hygiene.
Physiologic leukorrhea	None	Variable Scant to moderate Clear to white	<4.5	Negative	Normal epithelial cells Lactobacilli predominate	None
Bacterial vaginosis	Foul-smelling discharge	Gray-white	>4.7	Positive	Epithelial cells with bacteria ("clue cells") Gram-negative rods	Metronidazole Clindamycin
Candidiasis	Severe itching Vulvar inflammation	White, "curd-like"	<4.5	Negative	Fungal hyphae and buds	Topical or intra-vaginal imidazoles, triazoles Oral ketoconazole
Trichomonal vaginitis	Copious discharge Itching	Profuse Yellow to green	5.0–6.0	Occasionally present	Motile flagellated organisms	Metronidazole
Foreign body	Foul-smelling discharge	Foul-smelling Purulent Dark brown	Variable (usually >4.7)	Occasionally present	Leukocytes Epithelial cells with bacteria and debris	Remove foreign body. Irrigate vagina.
Contact vulvovaginitis	Vulvar inflammation Itching Edema	Scant White to yellow	Variable (usually <4.5)	Negative	Leukocytes Epithelial cells	Remove irritant. Topical steroids

FOOD POISONING OR FOODBORNE ILLNESS

Table 8. Epidemiologic Aspects of Food Poisoning

Organism	Pathogenesis	Source	Prevention
Salmonella	Infection	Meats, poultry, eggs, dairy products	Proper cooking and food handling, pasteurization
Staphylococcus	Preformed enterotoxin	Meats, poultry, potato salad, cream-filled pastry, cheese, sausage	Careful food handling, rapid refrigeration
Clostridium perfringens	Enterotoxin	Meats, poultry	Avoid delay in serving foods; avoid cooling and rewarming foods.
Clostridium botulinum	Preformed neurotoxin	Honey, home-canned foods, uncooked foods	Proper refrigeration (see text)
Vibrio parahaemolyticus	Infection enterotoxin	Sea fish, seawater, shellfish	Proper refrigeration
Bacillus cereus			
Diarrheal type	Sporulation enterotoxin	Many prepared foods	Proper refrigeration
Vomiting type	Preformed toxin	Cooked or fried rice, vegetables, meats, cereal, puddings	Proper refrigeration of cooked rice and other foods
Enterohemorrhagic including STEC 0157-H7	Cytotoxins	Milk, beef	Thorough cooking of beef, consumption of pasteurized milk products
Enterotoxigenic *Escherichia coli* (traveler's diarrhea)	Enterotoxin	Food or water	Travelers should drink only bottled or canned beverages and water, and avoid ice, raw produce including salads, and peeled fruit. Cooked foods should be eaten hot.

STEC, Shiga toxin–producing *Escherichia coli*.

Table 9. Clinical Aspects of Food Poisoning

Organism	Incubation	Symptoms	Duration
Bacillus cereus	Vomiting toxin 1–6 h Diarrhea toxin 6–24 h	Vomiting ± diarrhea; fever uncommon	8–24 h
Brucella	Several days to months; usually >30 d	Weakness, fever, headache chills, arthralgia, weight loss; splenomegaly	
Campylobacter	2–10 d; usually 2–5 d	Diarrhea (often bloody), abdominal pain, fever	
Clostridium botulinum	2 h to 8 d; usually 12–48 h	Poor feeding, weak cry, constipation, diplopia, blurred vision, respiratory weakness; symmetric descending paralysis	
Clostridium perfringens	6–24 h	Diarrhea, abdominal cramps, vomiting and fever uncommon	<24 h
Escherichia coli	→	→	
E. coli 0157:H7	1–10 d; usually 3–4 d	Diarrhea (often bloody), abdominal cramps, little or no fever can cause HUS	5–10 d
ETEC	6–48 h	Diarrhea, abdominal cramps, nausea, fever, and vomiting; uncommon	5–10 d
Listeria monocytogenes	2–6 wk	Meningitis, neonatal sepsis, fever	Variable
Nontyphoidal *Salmonella*	6–72 h	Diarrhea often with fever and abdominal cramps	<7 d
Salmonella typhi	3–60 d; usually 7–14 d	Fever, anorexia, malaise, headache, myalgias ± diarrhea or constipation	3–4 wk
Shigella	12 h to 6 d; usually 2–4 d	Diarrhea (often bloody), frequently fever, abdominal cramps	1 d to 1 mo
Staphylococcus aureus	30 min to 8 h; usually 2–4 h	Vomiting, diarrhea	<24 h
Vibrio	4–30 h	Diarrhea, cramps, nausea, vomiting	Self-limited
Yersinia enterocolitica	1–10 d; usually 4–6 d	Diarrhea, abdominal pain (often severe), mesenteric adenitis, pseudoappendicular syndrome	1–3 wk

ETEC, enterotoxigenic *Escherichia coli*; HUS, hemolytic uremic syndrome.

Table 10. U.S. Food and Drug Administration Pharmaceutical Pregnancy Categories

Pregnancy Category A	Adequate and well-controlled human studies have failed to demonstrate a risk to the fetus in the first trimester of pregnancy (and there is no evidence of risk in later trimesters).
Pregnancy Category B	Animal reproduction studies have failed to demonstrate a risk to the fetus, and there are no adequate and well-controlled studies in pregnant women OR animal studies have shown an adverse effect, but adequate and well-controlled studies in pregnant women have failed to demonstrate a risk to the fetus in any trimester.
Pregnancy Category C	Animal reproduction studies have shown an adverse effect on the fetus, and there are no adequate and well-controlled studies in humans, but potential benefits may warrant use of the drug in pregnant women despite potential risks.
Pregnancy Category D	There is positive evidence of human fetal risk based on adverse reaction data from investigational or marketing experience or studies in humans, but potential benefits may warrant use of the drug in pregnant women despite potential risks.
Pregnancy Category X	Studies in animals or humans have demonstrated fetal abnormalities and/or there is positive evidence of human fetal risk based on adverse reaction data from investigational or marketing experience, and the risks involved in use of the drug in pregnant women clearly outweigh potential benefits.

Table 11. Assessment of Etiology of Rickets Based on Laboratory Results

	Ca	Phos	Alk phos	iPTH	25-(OH)D	1,25-$(OH)_2$D	Urine Ca/Cr	TRP
Nutritional/insufficient sunlight	N or ↓	↓	↑	↑	↓	↑	↓	↑
Malabsorption	N or ↓	↓	↑	↑	↓	↑	↓	↑
Renal tubular defects	N or ↓	↓	↑	↑	N	↑	↑	N or ↓
Altered vitamin D metabolism	N or ↓	↓	↑	↑	↓	↑	↓	↑
Genetic forms of rickets								
X-linked, AD, and AR hypophosphatemic rickets	N	↓	↑	N or ↑	N	N or ↑	N or ↓	↓
1α-hydroxylase deficiency	↓	↓	↑	↑	N	↓	↓	↑
Vitamin D receptor mutations (vitamin D resistance)	↓	↓	↑	↑	N	↑	↓	↑
Hereditary hypophosphatemic rickets with hypercalciuria	N or ↓	↓	↑	↑	N	↑	↑	↓
Hypophosphatasia	N or ↑	N or ↑	↓	N or ↓	N	N or ↓	N or ↑	N

Ca, calcium; phos, phosphorus; alk phos, alkaline phosphatase; iPTH, intact parathyroid hormone; 25-(OH)-D, 25-hydroxy vitamin D; 1,25-(OH)2-D, 1,25-dihydroxy vitamin D; Ca/Cr, calcium/creatinine ratio; TRP, tubular reabsorption of phosphorus ([1 − (U phos × P Cr/U Cr × S Phos)] × 100, normal 85–95%); AD, autosomal dominant; AR, autosomal recessive; N, normal.

Table 12. Dietary Reference Intake for Calcium and Vitamin D

	Calcium			Vitamin D		
Age	Estimated Average Requirement (mg/d)	Recommended Dietary Allowance (mg/d)	Upper Level Intake (mg/d)	Estimated Average Requirement (IU/d)	Recommended Dietary Allowance (IU/d)	Upper Level Intake (IU/d)
0–6 mo	200	200	1,000	400	400	1,000
6–12 mo	260	260	1,500	400	400	1,500
1–3 y	500	700	2,500	400	600	2,500
4–8 y	800	1,000	2,500	400	600	3,000
9–18 y	1,100	1,300	3,000	400	600	4,000
19–30 y	800	1,000	2,500	400	600	4,000

Adapted from Ross AC, Abrams SA, Aloia JF, et al. Dietary reference intakes for calcium and vitamin D. http://www.iom.edu/~/media/Files/Report%20Files/2010/Dietary-Reference-Intakes-for-Calcium-and-Vitamin-D/Vitamin%20D%20and%20Calcium%202010%20Report%20Brief.pdf. Accessed March 1, 2015.

Table 13. Clinical and Biochemical Features of Congenital Adrenal Hyperplasia

Enzyme Defect	Sexual Ambiguity: Female	Sexual Ambiguity: Male	Additional Clinical Manifestations	Predominant Steroids
Desmolase	−	+	Salt wasting	—
3β-hydroxysteroid dehydrogenase	+	+	Salt wasting	17-OH-pregnenolone, DHEA
21-hydroxylase	+	−	Salt wasting	17-OH-progestone, androstenedione
11-hydroxylase	+	−	Hypertension	11-deoxycortisol
17-hydroxylase	−	+	Hypertension	DOC, corticosterone

DHEA, dehydroepiandrosterone; DOC, deoxycorticosterone.

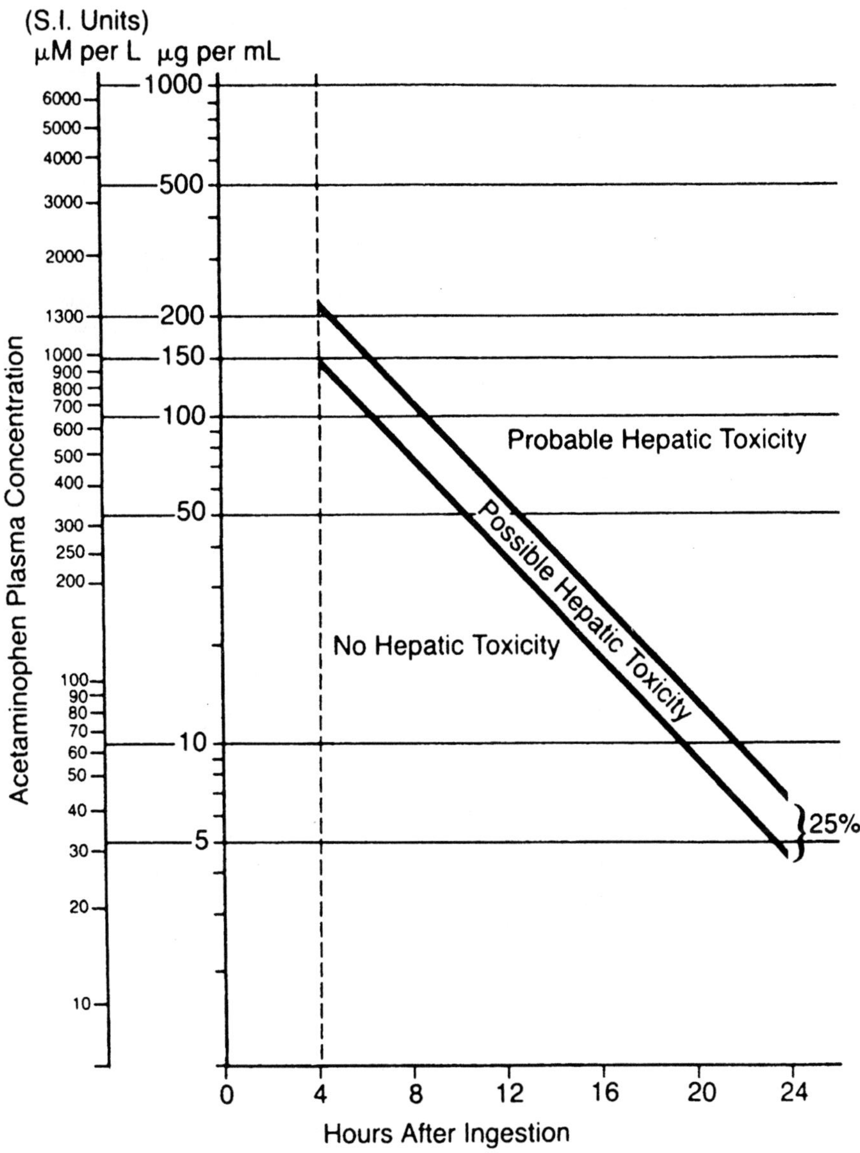

FIGURE 4. Nomogram for estimating severity of acute poisoning. (Reprinted with permission from Rumack BH, Matthew H. Acetaminophen poisoning and toxicity. *Pediatrics*. 1975;55(6):871–876.)

STEPWISE APPROACH FOR MANAGING ASTHMA LONG TERM

The stepwise approach tailors the selection of medication to the level of asthma severity (see page 5) or asthma control (see page 6). The stepwise approach is meant to help, not replace, the clinical decisionmaking needed to meet individual patient needs.

ASSESS CONTROL:

STEP UP IF NEEDED (first, check medication adherence, inhaler technique, environmental control, and comorbidities)

STEP DOWN IF POSSIBLE (and asthma is well controlled for at least 3 months)

At each step: Patient education, environmental control, and management of comorbidities

0–4 years of age

	STEP 1	STEP 2	STEP 3	STEP 4	STEP 5	STEP 6
	Intermittent Asthma	**Persistent Asthma: Daily Medication** Consult with asthma specialist if step 3 care or higher is required. Consider consultation at step 2.				
Preferred Treatment†	SABA* as needed	low-dose ICS*	medium-dose ICS*	medium-dose ICS* + either LABA* or montelukast	high-dose ICS* + either LABA* or montelukast	high-dose ICS* + either LABA* or montelukast + oral corticosteroids
Alternative Treatment†,‡		cromolyn or montelukast				
	If clear benefit is not observed in 4–6 weeks, and medication technique and adherence are satisfactory, consider adjusting therapy or alternate diagnoses.					
Quick-Relief Medication	▪ SABA* as needed for symptoms; intensity of treatment depends on severity of symptoms. ▪ With viral respiratory symptoms: SABA every 4–6 hours up to 24 hours (longer with physician consult). Consider short course of oral systemic corticosteroids if asthma exacerbation is severe or patient has history of severe exacerbations. ▪ Caution: Frequent use of SABA may indicate the need to step up treatment.					

5–11 years of age

	STEP 1	STEP 2	STEP 3	STEP 4	STEP 5	STEP 6
	Intermittent Asthma	**Persistent Asthma: Daily Medication** Consult with asthma specialist if step 4 care or higher is required. Consider consultation at step 3.				
Preferred Treatment†	SABA* as needed	low-dose ICS*	low-dose ICS* + either LABA,* LTRA,* or theophylline(b) **OR** medium-dose ICS	medium-dose ICS* + LABA*	high-dose ICS* + LABA*	high-dose ICS* + LABA* + oral corticosteroids
Alternative Treatment†,‡		cromolyn, LTRA,* or theophylline§		medium-dose ICS* + either LTRA* or theophylline§	high-dose ICS* + either LTRA* or theophylline§	high-dose ICS* + either LTRA* or theophylline§ + oral corticosteroids
		Consider subcutaneous allergen immunotherapy for patients who have persistent, allergic asthma.**				
Quick-Relief Medication	▪ SABA* as needed for symptoms. The intensity of treatment depends on severity of symptoms: up to 3 treatments every 20 minutes as needed. Short course of oral systemic corticosteroids may be needed. ▪ Caution: Increasing use of SABA or use >2 days/week for symptom relief (not to prevent EIB*) generally indicates inadequate control and the need to step up treatment.					

≥12 years of age

	STEP 1	STEP 2	STEP 3	STEP 4	STEP 5	STEP 6
	Intermittent Asthma	**Persistent Asthma: Daily Medication** Consult with asthma specialist if step 4 care or higher is required. Consider consultation at step 3.				
Preferred Treatment†	SABA* as needed	low-dose ICS*	low-dose ICS* + LABA* **OR** medium-dose ICS*	medium-dose ICS* + LABA*	high-dose ICS* + LABA* **AND** consider omalizumab for patients who have allergies††	high-dose ICS* + LABA* + oral corticosteroid§§ **AND** consider omalizumab for patients who have allergies††
Alternative Treatment†,‡		cromolyn, LTRA,* or theophylline§	low-dose ICS* + either LTRA,* theophylline,§ or zileuton‡‡	medium-dose ICS* + either LTRA,* theophylline,§ or zileuton‡‡		
		Consider subcutaneous allergen immunotherapy for patients who have persistent, allergic asthma.**				
Quick-Relief Medication	▪ SABA* as needed for symptoms. The intensity of treatment depends on severity of symptoms: up to 3 treatments every 20 minutes as needed. Short course of oral systemic corticosteroids may be needed. ▪ Caution: Use of SABA >2 days/week for symptom relief (not to prevent EIB*) generally indicates inadequate control and the need to step up treatment.					

* **Abbreviations:** EIB, exercise-induced bronchospasm; ICS, inhaled corticosteroid; LABA, inhaled long-acting $beta_2$-agonist; LTRA, leukotriene receptor antagonist; SABA, inhaled short-acting $beta_2$-agonist.

† Treatment options are listed in alphabetical order, if more than one.

‡ If alternative treatment is used and response is inadequate, discontinue and use preferred treatment before stepping up.

§ Theophylline is a less desirable alternative because of the need to monitor serum concentration levels.

** Based on evidence for dust mites, animal dander, and pollen; evidence is weak or lacking for molds and cockroaches. Evidence is strongest for immunotherapy with single allergens. The role of allergy in asthma is greater in children than in adults.

†† Clinicians who administer immunotherapy or omalizumab should be prepared to treat anaphylaxis that may occur.

‡‡ Zileuton is less desirable because of limited studies as adjunctive therapy and the need to monitor liver function.

§§ Before oral corticosteroids are introduced, a trial of high-dose ICS + LABA + either LTRA, theophylline, or zileuton, may be considered, although this approach has not been studied in clinical trials.

FIGURE 5. National Heart, Lung, and Blood Institute, National Institutes of Health. Asthma care quick reference: http://www.nhlbi.nih.gov/files/docs/guidelines/asthma_qrg.pdf. Accessed March 1, 2015.

Table 14. Estimated Comparative Daily Dosages: Inhaled Corticosteroids for Long-Term Asthma Control

	0–4 years of age			5–11 years of age			≥12 years of age		
Daily Dose	**Low**	**Meduim***	**High***	**Low**	**Meduim***	**High***	**Low**	**Meduim***	**High***
MEDICATION									
Beclomethasone MDI†	N/A	N/A	N/A	80–160 mcg	>160–320 mcg	>320 mcg	80–240 mcg	>240–480 mcg	>480 mcg
40 mcg/puff				1–2 puffs 2×/day	3–4 puffs 2×/day		1–3 puffs 2×/day	4–6 puffs 2×/day	
80 mcg/puff				1 puff 2×/day	2 puffs 2×/day	≥3 puffs 2×/day	1 puff am, 2 puffs pm	2–3 puffs 2×/day	≥4 puffs 2×/day
Budesonide DPI†	N/A	N/A	N/A	180–360 mcg	>360–720 mcg	>720 mcg	180–540 mcg	>540–1,080 mcg	>1,080 mcg
90 mcg/inhalation				1–2 inhs† 2×/day	3–4 inhs† 2×/day		1–3 inhs† 2×/day		
180 mcg/inhalation					2 inhs† 2×/day	≥3 inhs† 2×/day	1 inh† am, 2 inhs† pm	2–3 inhs† 2×/day	≥4 inhs† 2×/day
Budesonide Nebules	0.25–0.5 mg	>0.5–1.0 mg	>1.0 mg	0.5 mg	1.0 mg	2.0 mg	N/A	N/A	N/A
0.25 mg	1–2 nebs†/day			1 neb† 2×/day					
0.25 mg	1 neb†/day	2 nebs†/day	3 nebs†/day	1 neb†/day	1 neb† 2×/day				
1.0 mg		1 neb†/day	2 nebs†/day		1 neb†/day	1 neb†2×/day			
Ciclesonide MDI†	N/A	N/A	N/A	80–160 mcg	>160–320 mcg	>320 mcg	160–320 mcg	>320–640 mcg	>640 mcg
80 mcg/puff				1–2 puffs/day	1 puff am, 2 puffs pm– 2 puffs 2×/day	≥3 puffs 23/day	1–2 puffs 2×/day	3–4 puffs 2×/day	
160 mcg/puff				1 puff/day	1 puff 2×/day	≥2 puffs 2×/day		2 puffs 2×/day	≥3 puffs 2×/day
Flunisolide MDI†	N/A	N/A	N/A	160 mcg	320–480 mcg	≥480 mcg	320 mcg	>320–640 mcg	>640 mcg
80 mcg/puff				1 puff 2×/day	2–3 puffs 2×/day	≥4 puffs 2×/day	2 puffs 2×/day	3–4 puffs 2×/day	≥5 puffs 2×/day
Fluticasone MDI†	176 mcg	>176–352 mcg	>352 mcg	88–176 mcg	>176–352 mcg	>352 mcg	88–264 mcg	>264–440 mcg	>440 mcg
44 mcg/puff	2 puffs 2×/day	3–4 puffs 2×/day		1–2 puffs 2×/day	3–4 puffs 2×/day		1–3 puffs 2×/day		
110 mcg/puff		1 puff 2×/day	≥2 puffs 2×/day		1 puff 2×/day	≥2 puffs 2×/day		2 puffs 2×/day	3 puffs 2×/day
220 mcg/puff								1 puff 2×/day	≥2 puffs 2×/day
Fluticasone DPI†	N/A	N/A	N/A	100–200 mcg	>200–400 mcg	>400 mcg	100–300 mcg	>300–500 mcg	>500 mcg
50 mcg/inhalation				1–2 inhs† 2×/day	3–4 inhs† 2×/day		1–3 inhs† 2×/day		
100 mcg/inhalation				1 inh† 2×/day	2 inhs† 2×/day	>2 inhs† 2×/day		2 inhs† 2×/day	≥3 inhs† 2×/day
250 mcg/inhalation						1 inh† 2×/day		1 inh† 2×/day	≥2 inhs† 2×/day
Mometasone DPI†	N/A	N/A	N/A	110 mcg	220–440 mcg	>440 mcg	110–220 mcg	>220–440 mcg	>440 mcg
110 mcg/inhalation				1 inh†/day	1–2 inhs† 2×/day	≥3 inhs† 2×/day	1–2 inhs† pm	3–4 inhs† pm or 2 inhs† 2×/day	≥3 inhs† 2×/day
220 mcg/inhalation					1–2 inhs†/day	≥3 inhs† divided in 2 doses	1 inh† pm	1 inh† 2×/day or 2 inhs† pm	≥3 inhs† divided in 2 doses

*It is preferable to use a higher mcg/puff or mcg/inhalation formulation to achive as low a number of puffs or inhalations as possible.
†**Abbreviations:** DPI, dry power inhaler (requires deep, fast inhalation); inh, inhalation; MDI, metered dose inhaler (releases a puff of medication); neb, nebule.
National Heart, Lung, and Blood Institute, National Institutes of Health. Asthma care quick reference: http://www.nhlbi.nih.gov/files/docs/guidelines/asthma_qrg.pdf. Accessed March 1, 2015.

Table 15. Relative Potencies of Topical Corticosteroids

Class	Drug	Dosage form(s)	Strength (%)
I. Very high potency	Augmented betamethasone dipropionate	Ointment	0.05
	Clobetasol propionate	Cream, foam, ointment	0.05
	Diflorasone diacetate	Ointment	0.05
	Halobetasol propionate	Cream, ointment	0.05
II. High potency	Amcinonide	Cream, lotion, ointment	0.1
	Augmented betamethasone dipropionate	Cream	0.05
	Betamethasone dipropionate	Cream, foam, ointment, solution	0.05
	Desoximetasone	Cream, ointment	0.25
	Desoximetasone	Gel	0.05
	Diflorasone diacetate	Cream	0.05
	Fluocinonide	Cream, gel, ointment, solution	0.05
	Halcinonide	Cream, ointment	0.1
	Mometasone furoate	Ointment	0.1
	Triamcinolone acetonide	Cream, ointment	0.5
III–IV. Medium potency	Betamethasone valerate	Cream, foam, lotion, ointment	0.1
	Clocortolone pivalate	Cream	0.1
	Desoximetasone	Cream	0.05
	Fluocinolone acetonide	Cream, ointment	0.025
	Flurandrenolide	Cream, ointment	0.05
	Fluticasone propionate	Cream	0.05
	Fluticasone propionate	Ointment	0.005
	Mometasone furoate	Cream	0.1
	Triamcinolone acetonide	Cream, ointment	0.1
V. Lower-medium potency	Hydrocortisone butyrate	Cream, ointment, solution	0.1
	Hydrocortisone probutate	Cream	0.1
	Hydrocortisone valerate	Cream, ointment	0.2
	Prednicarbate	Cream	0.1
VI. Low potency	Alclometasone dipropionate	Cream, ointment	0.05
	Desonide	Cream, gel, foam, ointment	0.05
	Fluocinolone acetonide	Cream, solution	0.01
VII. Lowest potency	Dexamethasone	Cream	0.1
	Hydrocortisone	Cream, lotion, ointment, solution	0.25, 0.5, 1
	Hydrocortisone acetate	Cream, ointment	0.5–1

From Paller AS, Mancini AJ. Eczematous eruptions in childhood. In: Paller AS, Mancini AJ, eds. *Hurwitz Clinical Pediatric Dermatology: A Textbook of Skin Disorders of Childhood and Adolescence*. 4th ed. St. Louis, MO: Elsevier; 2011: 49, with permission from Elsevier.

INDEX

C

H

M